Davidson's
Principles and Practice of
Medicine

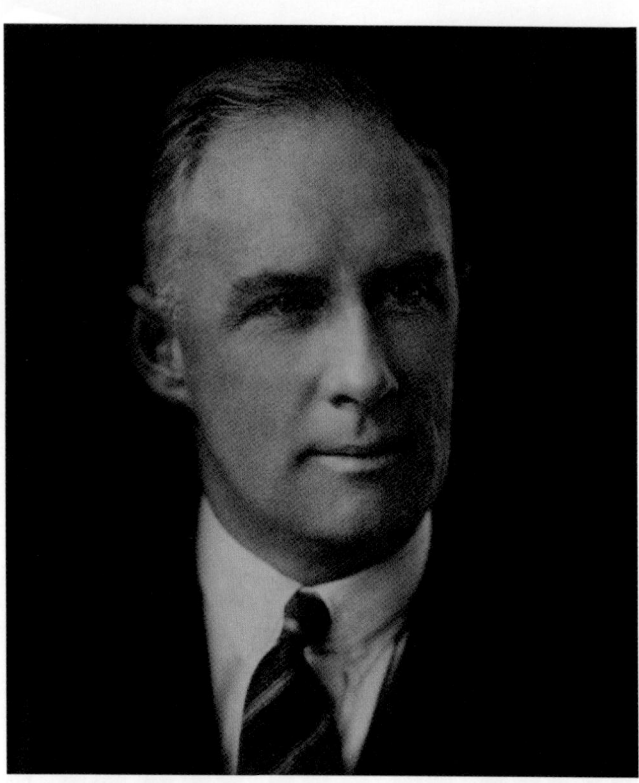

Sir Stanley Davidson (1894–1981)

This famous textbook was the brainchild of one of the great Professors of Medicine of the 20th century. Stanley Davidson was born in Sri Lanka and began his medical undergraduate training at Trinity College, Cambridge; this was interrupted by World War I and later resumed in Edinburgh. He was seriously wounded in battle, and the carnage and shocking waste of young life that he encountered at that time had a profound effect on his subsequent attitudes and values.

In 1930 Stanley Davidson was appointed Professor of Medicine at the University of Aberdeen, one of the first full-time Chairs of Medicine anywhere and the first in Scotland. In 1938 he took up the Chair of Medicine at Edinburgh and was to remain in this post until retirement in 1959. He was a renowned educator and a particularly gifted teacher at the bedside, where he taught that everything had to be questioned and explained. He personally gave most of the systematic lectures in Medicine, which were made available as typewritten notes that emphasised the essentials and far surpassed any textbook available at the time.

Principles and Practice of Medicine was conceived in the late 1940s with its origins in those lecture notes. The first edition, published in 1952, was a masterpiece of clarity and uniformity of style. It was of modest size and price, but sufficiently comprehensive and up to date to provide students with the main elements of sound medical practice. Although the format and presentation have seen many changes in 23 subsequent editions, Sir Stanley's original vision and objectives remain. More than half a century after its first publication, his book continues to inform and educate students, doctors and health professionals all over the world.

Davidson's
Principles and Practice of
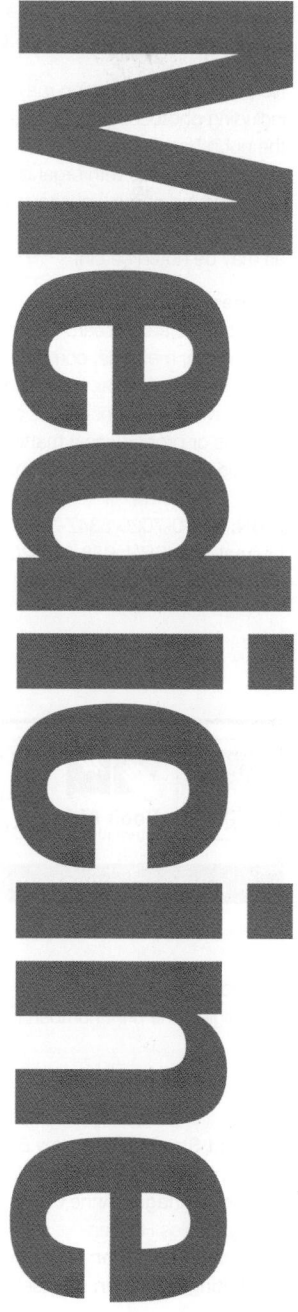

24th Edition

Edited by

Ian D Penman

BSc(Hons), MBChB, MD, FRCPE

Consultant Gastroenterologist, Royal Infirmary of Edinburgh;
Honorary Senior Lecturer, University of Edinburgh, UK

Stuart H Ralston

MBChB, MD, FRCP, FMedSci, FRSE, FFPM(Hon)

Professor of Rheumatology, Centre for Genomic and Experimental Medicine,
Institute of Genetics and Cancer University of Edinburgh;
Honorary Consultant Rheumatologist, Western General Hospital,
Edinburgh, UK

Mark WJ Strachan

BSc(Hons), MBChB(Hons), MD, FRCPE

Consultant Endocrinologist, Metabolic Unit, Western General Hospital,
Edinburgh; Honorary Professor, University of Edinburgh, UK

Richard P Hobson

MBBS, LLM, PhD, MRCP(UK), FRCPath

Consultant Microbiologist, Harrogate and District NHS Foundation Trust;
Honorary Senior Lecturer, University of Leeds, UK

Illustrations by Robert Britton

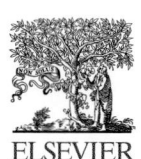

ELSEVIER

London New York Oxford Philadelphia St Louis Sydney 2023

First edition 1952
Second edition 1954
Third edition 1956
Fourth edition 1958
Fifth edition 1960
Sixth edition 1962
Seventh edition 1964
Eighth edition 1966

Ninth edition 1968
Tenth edition 1971
Eleventh edition 1974
Twelfth edition 1977
Thirteenth edition 1981
Fourteenth edition 1984
Fifteenth edition 1987
Sixteenth edition 1991

Seventeenth edition 1995
Eighteenth edition 1999
Nineteenth edition 2002
Twentieth edition 2006
Twenty-first edition 2010
Twenty-second edition 2014
Twenty-third edition 2018
Twenty-fourth edition 2022

Notices

Practitioners and researchers must always rely on their own experience and knowledge in evaluating and using any information, methods, compounds or experiments described herein. Because of rapid advances in the medical sciences, in particular, independent verification of diagnoses and drug dosages should be made. To the fullest extent of the law, no responsibility is assumed by Elsevier, authors, editors or contributors for any injury and/or damage to persons or property as a matter of products liability, negligence or otherwise, or from any use or operation of any methods, products, instructions, or ideas contained in the material herein.

ISBN: 978-0-7020-8347-1
International ISBN: 978-0-7020-8348-8

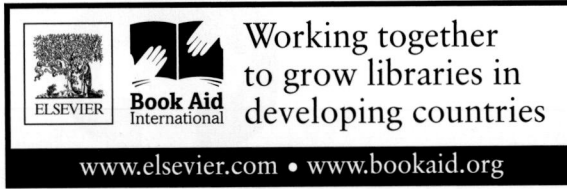

Printed in India
Last digit is the print number: 9 8 7 6 5 4 3 2

Content Strategist: Jeremy Bowes
Content Development Specialist: Siân Jarman
Project Manager: Anne Collett
Design: Miles Hitchen
Illustration Manager: Narayanan Ramakrishnan
Marketing Manager: Kathleen Patton

Contents

Get the most out of your Davidson's!

Redeem your unique e-content PIN code today (see inside front cover) to access:

- **The complete, downloadable eBook** – for quick reference, anytime access
- **BONUS NEW self-assessment material** – 166 interactive questions and answers supplement each chapter, to help test your understanding of key points and aid exam preparation

Preface

Well over 2.5 million copies of *Davidson's Principles and Practice of Medicine* have been sold since it was first published in 1952. Now in its 24th Edition, *Davidson's* is regarded as a 'must-have' textbook for thousands of medical students, doctors and health professionals across the world, describing the pathophysiology and clinical features of the most important conditions encountered in the major specialties of adult medicine and explaining how to investigate, diagnose and manage them. The book is the winner of numerous prizes and awards and has been translated into many languages. Taking its origins from Sir Stanley Davidson's much-admired lecture notes, the book has endured because it continues to keep pace with how modern medicine is taught and to provide a wealth of information in an easy-to-read, concise and beautifully illustrated format.

Davidson's strives to ensure that readers can not only recognise the clinical features of a disease, but also understand the underlying causes. To achieve this, each chapter begins with a summary of the relevant pre-clinical science, linking pathophysiology with clinical presentation and treatment so that students can use the book from the start of their medical studies right through to their final examinations and beyond.

The regular introduction of new authors and editors is important for maintaining freshness. On this occasion, 21 new authors have joined our existing contributors to make up an outstanding team of authorities in their respective fields. As well as recruiting authors from around the globe, particularly for topics such as infectious diseases, HIV and envenomation, we welcome members from 10 countries on to our International Advisory Board. These leading experts provide detailed comments that are crucial to our revision of each new edition. A particularly important aspect in planning the revision is for the editors to meet students and faculty in medical schools in those countries where the book is most widely read, so that we can respond to the feedback of our global readership and their tutors. We use this feedback, along with the information we gather via detailed student reviews and surveys, to craft each edition. The authors, editors and publishing team aim to ensure that readers all over the world are best served by a book that integrates medical science with clinical medicine to convey key knowledge and practical advice in an accessible and readable format. The amount of detail is tailored to the needs of medical students working towards their final examinations, as well as candidates preparing for Membership of the Royal Colleges of Physicians (MRCP) or its equivalent.

With this new edition we have introduced several changes in both structure and content. The opening eight chapters provide an account of the principles of genetics, immunology, infectious diseases, population health, oncology and pain management, along with a discussion of the core principles behind clinical decision-making and good prescribing.

Subsequent chapters discuss medical emergencies in poisoning, envenomation and medicine in austere environments, while common presentations in acute medicine, including recognition and management of the critically ill patient, are also addressed. The disease-specific chapters that follow cover the major medical specialties, each one thoroughly revised and updated to ensure that readers have access to the 'cutting edge' of medical knowledge and practice. As we publish the 24th edition, the world is in the grip of the COVID-19 pandemic and while our knowledge of virology, epidemiology, clinical impact and management of SARS-CoV-2 is still evolving, we have dedicated a new section on core aspects of this hugely important topic in Chapter 13, but also in Chapter 6 and, as appropriate, elsewhere throughout the book.

The innovations introduced in recent editions have been maintained and, in many cases, developed. The highly popular 'Clinical Examination' overviews have been extended and updated. The 'Presenting Problems' sections continue to provide an invaluable overview of the most common presentations in each disease area. The 'Emergency' and 'Practice Point' boxes have been retained along with the 'In Old Age', 'In Pregnancy' and 'In Adolescence' boxes, which emphasise key practical points in the presentation and management of the older adult, women with medical disorders who are pregnant or planning pregnancy, and adolescents transitioning between paediatric and adult services.

Education is achieved by assimilating information from many sources and readers of this book can enhance their learning experience by using several complementary resources. We developed a self-testing companion book entitled *Davidson's Assessment in Medicine*, containing over 1250 multiple choice questions specifically tailored to the contents of *Davidson's* for the 23rd edition and have added more new online MCQs to accompany this edition. The long-standing association of *Davidson's* with its sister books, *Macleod's Clinical Examination* and *Principles and Practice of Surgery*, still holds good. Our 'family' has also expanded with the publication of *Davidson's Essentials of Medicine*, a pocket-sized version of the main text, now in its 3rd edition; and *Macleod's Clinical Diagnosis*, which describes a systematic approach to the differential diagnosis of symptoms and signs. We congratulate the editors and authors of these books for continuing the tradition of easily digested and expertly illustrated texts.

We all take immense pride in continuing the great tradition first established by Sir Stanley Davidson and in producing an outstanding book for the next generation of doctors.

IDP, SHR, MWJS, RPH
Edinburgh 2022

Contributors

Brian J Angus MD, FRCP, DTM&H
Associate Professor, Nuffield Department of Medicine,
Oxford University, Oxford, UK

Adam C Baker BM, BMedSci(Hons), MSc ExMed
Pre-Hospital Emergency Medicine Fellow, Honorary Senior Clinical
Research Fellow, Department of Emergency Medicine,
University Hospitals Plymouth NHS Trust, Devon Air Ambulance,
University of Exeter, Devon, UK

James G Boyle MBChB, MD, MSc, FRCP
Consultant Diabetologist, Department of Diabetes, Endocrinology and
Clinical Pharmacology, Glasgow Royal Infirmary; Honorary Associate
Clinical Professor, School of Medicine, Dentistry and Nursing,
University of Glasgow, Glasgow, UK

Harry Campbell MBChB, MD, FRCPE, FFPH, FRSE, FMedSci
Professor of Genetic Epidemiology and Public Health,
Centre for Global Health, Usher Institute, University of Edinburgh,
Edinburgh, UK

Thean Soon Chew MBChB, MRCP, PhD
Consultant Gastroenterologist and Honorary Senior Lecturer in
Gastroenterology, Academic Unit of Gastroenterology,
University of Sheffield, Sheffield, UK

Ian J Clifton MD, FRCP
Consultant Respiratory Physician and Honorary Senior Lecturer,
Department of Respiratory Medicine, St James's University Hospital,
Leeds, UK

Sally Clive BMedSci(Hons), MBChB, MD, FRCPE
Consultant Medical Oncologist, Edinburgh Cancer Centre, Western
General Hospital, Edinburgh, UK

Gavin PR Clunie MD, FRCP
Consultant Rheumatologist and Metabolic Bone Physician,
Department of Rheumatology, Cambridge University Hospital NHS
Foundation Trust, Addenbrooke's Hospital, Cambridge, UK

Daniel J Clutterbuck BSc(Hons), FRCP
Consultant in Genitourinary and HIV Medicine, NHS Lothian;
Chalmers Sexual Health Centre, Edinburgh, UK

Lesley A Colvin MBChB, PhD, FRCA, FFPMRCA, FRCPE
Professor of Pain Medicine, Division of Population Health
and Genomics, University of Dundee School of Medicine,
Dundee, UK

Myles D Connor MBBCh, FCP(SA), FCNeurol(SA), PhD, FRCPE
Consultant Neurologist, Department of Neurology, NHS Borders,
Melrose, UK; Honorary Senior Lecturer, Centre for Clinical Brain
Sciences, University of Edinburgh, Edinburgh, UK; Honorary Senior
Researcher, School of Public Health,
University of the Witwatersrand, Johannesburg, South Africa

Bryan Conway MB, MRCP, PhD
Senior Lecturer and Honorary Consultant Nephrologist, Department of
Renal Medicine, University of Edinburgh and Edinburgh Royal Infirmary,
Edinburgh, UK

Nicola Cooper MBChB, MMedSci, FRCPE, FRACP, FAcadMEd,
SFHEA
Consultant Physician and Clinical Associate Professor in Medical
Education, Department for Acute Internal Medicine, University Hospitals
of Derby & Burton NHS Foundation Trust, Derby, UK

Alison L Cracknell MBChB, FRCP
Consultant in Medicine for Older People, Department of Medicine for
Older People, Leeds Teaching Hospitals NHS Trust; Honorary Clinical
Associate Professor, University of Leeds, Leeds, UK

Dominic J Culligan BSc, MD, FRCP, FRCPath
Consultant Haematologist and Honorary Senior Lecturer,
Department of Haematology, Aberdeen Royal Infirmary,
Aberdeen, UK

David H Dockrell MD, FRCPI, FRCPG, FACP
Chair of Infection Medicine, Centre for Inflammation Research,
University of Edinburgh; Professor of Infection Medicine,
UoE Centre for Inflammation Research, University of Edinburgh,
Edinburgh, UK

Deborah AB Ellames BSc(Hons), MBChB
Consultant Physician in Respiratory Medicine, Department of
Respiratory Medicine, Leeds Teaching Hospitals NHS Trust, Leeds, UK

Marie Fallon MBChB, MD, FRCPG, FRCPE, DCH, DRCOG,
MRCGP
St Columba's Hospice Chair of Palliative Medicine, Edinburgh Cancer
Research Centre, Institute for Genetics and Cancer, University of
Edinburgh, Edinburgh, UK

Fraser W Gibb MBChB, BSc(Hons), FRCP, PhD
Consultant Physician/Honorary Clinical Reader, Edinburgh Centre for
Endocrinology and Diabetes, Royal Infirmary of Edinburgh/
University of Edinburgh, Edinburgh, UK

Timothy T Gordon-Walker MBChB, PhD, MRCP
Consultant Hepatologist, Department of Gastroenterology and
Scottish Liver Transplant Unit, The Royal Infirmary of Edinburgh,
Edinburgh, UK

Neil R Grubb MD, FRCP
Consultant in Cardiology and Cardiac Electrophysiology,
Department of Cardiology, Royal Infirmary of Edinburgh, Edinburgh, UK

David PJ Hunt MB BChir, PhD, FRCP
Wellcome Senior Clinical Fellow, Department of Clinical Brain Sciences,
University of Edinburgh, Edinburgh, UK

Sally H Ibbotson BSc(Hons), MD, FRCPE
Professor of Photodermatology, University of Dundee; Honorary
Consultant Dermatologist and Head of Photobiology Unit,
Ninewells Hospital and Medical School, Dundee, UK

Sara J Jenks MBChB, MRCP, FRCPath
Consultant in Metabolic Medicine, Department of Clinical Biochemistry,
Royal Infirmary of Edinburgh, Edinburgh, UK

Sarah L Johnston FRCP, FRCPath
Consultant Immunologist, Department of Immunology and
Immunogenetics, North Bristol NHS Trust, Bristol, UK

Stephen M Lawrie MD(Hons), FRCPsych, Hon FRCPE, FRSE
Professor of Psychiatry and Neuroimaging, Division of Psychiatry,
Centre for Clinical Brain Sciences, University of Edinburgh,
Edinburgh, UK

Michael EJ Lean MA, MB, BChir, MD, FRCP, FRSE
Professor of Human Nutrition, Human Nutrition, University of Glasgow,
Glasgow, UK

Gary Maartens MBChB, MMed, FCP(SA)
Chair of Clinical Pharmacology, Department of Medicine,
University of Cape Town, Cape Town, South Africa

Lucy H Mackillop BM BCh, MA(Oxon), FRCP
Consultant Obstetric Physician, Oxford University Hospitals,
NHS Foundation Trust; Honorary Senior Clinical Lecturer,
Nuffield Department of Women's and Reproductive Health,
University of Oxford, Oxford, UK

Michael J MacMahon FRCA, EDIC
Consultant Intensivist, Department of Anaesthesia and Intensive Care,
Victoria Hospital, Kirkcaldy, UK

Rebecca J Mann BMedSci, BMBS, MRCP, FRCPCh
Consultant Paediatrician, Department of Paediatrics, Taunton and
Somerset NHS Foundation Trust, Taunton, UK

Lynn M Manson MBChB, MD
Consultant Haematologist, Department of Transfusion Medicine,
Royal Infirmary of Edinburgh, Edinburgh, UK

Amanda Mather MBBS, FRACP, PhD
Renal Staff Specialist, Department of Renal Medicine, Royal North
Shore Hospital; Conjoint Senior Lecturer, Faculty of Medicine,
University of Sydney, Sydney, NSW, Australia

Simon RJ Maxwell MD, PhD, FRCP, FRCPE, FBPhS
Professor of Student Learning (Clinical Pharmacology and Prescribing),
Clinical Pharmacology Unit, University of Edinburgh, Edinburgh, UK

David A McAllister MBChB, MPH, MD, MRCP, MFPH
Wellcome Trust Intermediate Clinical Fellow and Beit Fellow and
Honorary Consultant in Public Health Medicine, Institute of Health and
Wellbeing, University of Glasgow, Glasgow, UK

Eve Miller-Hodges MBChB, PhD
Senior Clinical Lecturer and Honorary Consultant in Inherited Metabolic
Disorders and Renal Medicine, Centre for Cardiovascular Science &
Scottish IMD Service, University of Edinburgh, Edinburgh, UK

Francesca EM Neuberger MBChB, FRCP
Consultant Physician in Acute and Obstetric Medicine, Medical Division,
North Bristol NHS Trust, Bristol, UK

David E Newby BA BSc(Hons), PhD, BM DM DSc, FRSE, FESC, FACC, FMedSci
British Heart Foundation Duke of Edinburgh Chair of Cardiology, Centre
for Cardiovascular Science, University of Edinburgh, Edinburgh, UK

John DC Newell-Price MA, PhD, FRCP
Professor of Endocrinology, Department of Oncology and Metabolism,
University of Sheffield, Sheffield, UK

John A Olson MD, FRCPE, FRCOphth
Consultant Ophthalmic Physician, Aberdeen Royal Infirmary; Honorary
Reader, University of Aberdeen, Aberdeen, UK

John R Petrie BSc, MBChB, PhD, FRCPE, FRCPG
Professor of Diabetic Medicine, Institute of Cardiovascular and Medical
Sciences, University of Glasgow, Glasgow, UK

Paul J Phelan MD, FRCPE
Consultant Nephrologist and Renal Transplant Physician,
Department of Nephrology, Royal Infirmary of Edinburgh, Edinburgh, UK

Terence J Quinn FRCP, MD, MBChB, BSc
Senior Clinical Lecturer and Honorary Consultant in Geriatric Medicine,
Institute of Cardiovascular and Medical Sciences, University of
Glasgow, Glasgow, UK

Stuart H Ralston MBChB, MD, FRCP, FFPM(Hon), FMedSci, FRSE
Professor of Rheumatology, Centre for Genomic and Experimental
Medicine, Institute of Genetics and Cancer, University of Edinburgh,
Western General Hospital, Edinburgh, UK

Anupam Rej MBChB, BMedSci(Hons), MRCP(UK)
Clinical Research Fellow, Academic Unit of Gastroenterology,
Royal Hallamshire Hospital, Sheffield, UK

David S Sanders MBChB, MD, FACG
Professor of Gastroenterology, Academic Unit of Gastroenterology,
Royal Hallamshire Hospital and University of Sheffield, Sheffield, UK

Jonathan AT Sandoe FRCPath, PhD
Associate Clinical Professor, Consultant Microbiologist,
Department of Microbiology, University of Leeds and
Leeds Teaching Hospitals NHS Trust, Leeds, UK

Alan G Shand MD, FRCPE
Consultant Gastroenterologist, Gastrointestinal Unit,
Western General Hospital, Edinburgh, UK

Mark Stares MBBS, MD(Res), MRes, BSc, MRCP
Medical Oncologist, Edinburgh Cancer Centre, Western General
Hospital, NHS Lothian, Edinburgh, UK

Robby M Steel MA, MD, FRCPsych
Consultant Liaison Psychiatrist and Honorary (Clinical) Senior Lecturer in Psychiatry, Department of Psychological Medicine, Royal Infirmary of Edinburgh, Edinburgh, UK

Grant D Stewart BSc, MBChB, PhD Edin, MA Cantab, FRCSE (Urol)
Professor of Surgical Oncology, Department of Surgery, University of Cambridge, Cambridge, and Honorary Consultant Urological Surgeon, Addenbrooke's Hospital, Cambridge, UK

David R Sullivan MBBS, FRACP, FRCPA, FCSANZ
Head of Department, Department of Chemical Pathology, NSW Health Pathology, Sydney, NSW, Australia

Shyam Sundar MD, FRCP, FAMS, FASc, FNA
Distinguished Professor, Department of Medicine, Institute of Medical Sciences, Banaras Hindu University, Varanasi, India

Victoria R Tallentire MBChB, MD, FRCP
Consultant Acute Physician and Associate Postgraduate Dean, Medical Directorate, NHS Education for Scotland, Edinburgh, UK

Katrina Tatton-Brown BM BCh, BA, MD
Professor of Clinical Genetics and Genomic Education and Consultant in Clinical Genetics, South West Thames Regional Genetics Service, St George's University Hospitals NHS Foundation Trust, London, UK

Simon HL Thomas BSc, MD, FRCP, FRCPE, FEAPCCT, FACCT
Professor of Clinical Pharmacology and Therapeutics, Translational and Clinical Research Institute, Newcastle University, Newcastle-upon-Tyne, UK

Henry G Watson MD, FRCP, FRCPath
Consultant Haematologist and Honorary Professor of Medicine, Department of Haematology, Aberdeen Royal Infirmary, Aberdeen, UK

Julian White MD, FACTM
Clinical Toxinologist and Head of Toxinology, Toxinology Department and University of Adelaide Department of Paediatrics, Women's & Children's Hospital, North Adelaide, SA, Australia

William Whiteley BA, BM BCh, MSc, PhD, FRCP
Reader in Neurology, Centre for Clinical Brain Sciences, University of Edinburgh, Edinburgh, UK; Senior Research Fellow, Nuffield Department of Population Health, University of Oxford, Oxford, UK

Michael J Williams BM BCh, PhD
Consultant Hepatologist, Scottish Liver Transplant Unit, Royal Infirmary of Edinburgh, Edinburgh, UK

Rebecca Woodfield MA, MB BChir, MRCP, PhD
Consultant Geriatrician and Stroke Physician, Department of Medicine for the Elderly, Western General Hospital, Edinburgh, UK

International Advisory Board

Acknowledgements

The editors would like to acknowledge and offer grateful thanks for the input of all previous editions' contributors, without whom this new edition would not have been possible.

In particular we are indebted to those former authors who step down with the arrival of this new edition. They include Quentin M Anstee, Leslie Burnett, Mark Byers, Graham G Dark, Richard J Davenport, Emad El-Omar, David R FitzPatrick, J Alastair Innes, David EJ Jones, Peter Langhorne, John Paul Leach, Sara E Marshall, Rory J McCrimmon, Mairi H McLean, Ewan R Pearson, Peter T Reid, Gordon R Scott, Peter Stewart, John PH Wilding and Miles D Witham.

We are grateful to members of the International Advisory Board, all of whom provided detailed suggestions that have improved the book. Several members have now retired from the Board and we are grateful for their support during the preparation of previous editions. They include Ragavendra Bhat, Khalid I Bzeizi, Piotr Kuna, Pravin Manga, Moffat Nyirenda, Tommy Olsson, KR Sethuraman, Ibrahim Sherif, Ian J Simpson, SG Siva Chidambaram and Josanne Vassallo. We are equally grateful to new members of our International Advisory Board, who have given us valuable advice as we prepared this new edition, including ABM Abdullah, Quazi T Islam, Viswanathan Neelakantan and Jacek Rozanski.

We would like to extend special thanks to Professor Dilip Karnad, Jupiter Hospital, Thane, India, who thoroughly reviewed all chapters of this 24th edition in draft form, to help ensure the coverage of this edition is more relevant than ever to our large readership in India, Pakistan and Bangladesh. He provided invaluable advice to the editorial team during preparation of the 24th edition and exhaustive feedback on how the content aligns with competencies in the current Indian National Medical Commission undergraduate curriculum. Readers of the International Edition of this book can now access a comprehensive Competency Mapping Guide with full page references for the first time as a result of this thorough review.

Detailed chapter reviews were commissioned to help plan this new edition and we are grateful to all those who assisted, including Professor Rustam Al-Shahi, Dr Daniel Beckett, Dr Helen Cohen, Dr Ian Edmond, Dr David Enoch, Professor Tonks Fawcett, Dr Colin Forfar, Professor Richard Gilson, Dr Helena Gleeson, Dr Peter Hall, Dr Greg Heath, Dr Richard Herriot, Dr Robert Lindsay, Dr Catherine Nelson-Piercy and Dr Alex Rowe.

The Editors and Publisher would like to thank all those who have provided valuable feedback on this textbook and whose comments have helped shape this new edition. We would particularly like to extend our thanks to the many readers who contact us with suggestions for improvements. This input has been invaluable and is much appreciated; we regret the names are too numerous to mention individually.

The authors of Chapter 20 would like to thank Dr Drew Henderson, who reviewed the 'Diabetic nephropathy' section, and we are indebted to Dr Ruth Darbyshire for assistance with the Ophthalmology multiple choice questions to accompany Chapter 30.

Two short sections in Chapter 3 on array comparative genomic hybridisation and single-molecule sequencing are adapted from Dr K Tatton-Brown's Massive Open Online Course for FutureLearn. We would like to thank the Open University and St George's, University of London, for permission to use this material.

We are especially grateful to Laurence Hunter and Wendy Lee from Elsevier for their endless support and expertise in the shaping, collation and publication of Davidson's over many years and who have now retired. We have thoroughly enjoyed working with a new team including Jeremy Bowes, Siân Jarman and Anne Collett who have seamlessly taken over the reins. We are delighted that Robert Britton continues to work on the book and illustrate it beautifully. We are proud of this new edition and are confident it will remain an essential and invaluable resource for readers the world over.

Introduction

The opening chapters of the book, making up Part 1 on 'Fundamentals of Medicine', provide an account of the principles of genetics, immunology, infectious diseases and population health, oncology and pain management, along with a discussion of the core principles behind clinical decision-making and good prescribing. Subsequent chapters in Part 2, 'Emergency and Critical Care Medicine', discuss medical emergencies in poisoning, envenomation and medicine in austere environments, while Chapter 9 explores common presentations in acute medicine, as well as the recognition and management of the critically ill. The third part, 'Clinical Medicine', is devoted to the major medical specialties. Each chapter has been written by experts in the field to provide the level of detail expected of trainees in their discipline. To maintain the book's virtue of being concise, care has been taken to avoid unnecessary duplication between chapters.

The system-based chapters in Part 3 follow a standard format, beginning with an overview of the relevant aspects of clinical examination, followed by an account of functional anatomy, physiology and investigations, then the common presentations of disease, and details of the individual diseases and treatments relevant to that system. In chapters that describe the immunological, cellular and molecular basis of disease, this problem-based approach brings the close links between modern medical science and clinical practice into sharp focus.

The methods used to present information are described below.

Clinical examination overviews

The value of good clinical skills is highlighted by a two-page overview of the important elements of the clinical examination at the beginning of most chapters. The left-hand page includes a mannikin to illustrate key steps in examination of the relevant system, beginning with simple observations and progressing in a logical sequence around the body. The right-hand page expands on selected themes and includes tips on examination technique and interpretation of physical signs. These overviews are intended to act as an aide-mémoire and not as a replacement for a detailed text on clinical examination, as provided in our sister title, *Macleod's Clinical Examination*.

Presenting problems

Medical students and junior doctors must not only assimilate a great many facts about various disorders, but also develop an analytical approach to formulating a differential diagnosis and a plan of investigation for patients who present with particular symptoms or signs. In *Davidson's* this is addressed by incorporating a 'Presenting Problems' section into all relevant chapters. Nearly 250 presentations are included, which represent the most common reasons for referral to each medical specialty.

Boxes

Boxes are a popular way of presenting information and are particularly useful for revision. They are classified by the type of information they contain, using specific symbols.

General Information

These include causes, clinical features, investigations, treatments and other useful information.

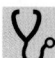
Practice Point

There are many practical skills that students and doctors must master. These vary from inserting a nasogastric tube to reading an ECG or X-ray, or interpreting investigations such as arterial blood gases or thyroid function tests. 'Practice Point' boxes provide straightforward guidance on how these and many other skills can be acquired and applied.

Emergency

These boxes describe the management of many of the most common emergencies in medicine.

In Old Age

Life expectancy is increasing in many countries and older people are the chief users of health care. While they contract the same diseases as those who are younger, there are often important differences in the way they present and how they are best managed. Chapter 34, 'Ageing and disease', concentrates on the principles of managing the frailest group, who suffer from multiple comorbidity and disability, and who tend to present with non-specific problems such as falls or delirium. Many older people, though, also suffer from specific single-organ pathology. 'In Old Age' boxes are thus included in each chapter and describe common presentations, implications of physiological changes of ageing, effects of age on investigations, problems of treatment in old age, and the benefits and risks of intervention in older people.

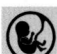
In Pregnancy

Many conditions are different in the context of pregnancy, while some arise only during or shortly after pregnancy. Particular care must be taken with investigations (for example, to avoid radiation exposure to the fetus) and treatment (to avoid the use of drugs that harm the fetus). These issues are highlighted by 'In Pregnancy' boxes distributed throughout the book, which complement Chapter 32, 'Maternal medicine'.

In Adolescence

Although paediatric medicine is not covered in *Davidson's*, many chronic disorders begin in childhood, and physicians who look after adults often contribute to multidisciplinary teams that manage young patients 'in transition' between paediatric and adult health-care services. This group of patients often presents a particular challenge, due to the physiological and psychological changes that occur in adolescence, and which can have a major impact on the disease and its management. Adolescents can be encouraged to take over responsibility from their parents/carers in managing their disease, but are naturally rebellious and often struggle to adhere to the impositions of chronic treatment. Chapter 33, 'Adolescent and transition medicine', highlights these issues, alongside the 'In Adolescence' boxes that appear in relevant chapters.

Terminology

The recommended International Non-proprietary Names (INNs) are used for all drugs, with the exception of adrenaline and noradrenaline. British spellings have been retained for drug classes and groups (e.g. amphetamines not amfetamines).

Units of measurement

The International System of Units (SI units) is the recommended means of presentation for laboratory data and has been used throughout *Davidson's*. We recognise, however, that many laboratories around the world continue to provide data in non-SI units, so these have been included in the text for the commonly measured analytes. Both SI and non-SI units are also given in Chapter 35, which describes the reference ranges used in laboratories in Edinburgh. It is important to appreciate that these reference ranges may vary from those used in other laboratories.

Finding what you are looking for

A contents list is given on the opening page of each chapter. In addition, the book contains cross-references to help readers find their way around, along with an extensive index. A list of up-to-date reviews and useful websites with links to management guidelines appears at the end of each chapter.

Giving us your feedback

The Editors and Publisher hope that you will find this edition of *Davidson's* informative and easy to use. We would be delighted to hear from you if you have any comments or suggestions to make for future editions of the book. Please contact us by e-mail at: davidson.feedback@elsevier.com. All comments received will be much appreciated and will be considered by the editorial team.

N Cooper
AL Cracknell

1

Clinical decision-making

Introduction

A great deal of knowledge and skill is required to practise as a doctor. Physicians in the 21st century need to have a comprehensive knowledge of basic and clinical sciences, have good communication skills, be able to perform procedures, work effectively in a team and demonstrate professional and ethical behaviour. But how doctors think, reason and make decisions is arguably their most critical skill. Knowledge is necessary, but not sufficient on its own for good performance and safe care. This chapter describes the principles of clinical decision-making, also known as 'clinical reasoning'.

The problem of diagnostic error

It is estimated that diagnosis is wrong 10%–15% of the time in specialties such as emergency medicine, internal medicine and general practice. Diagnostic error is associated with greater morbidity than other types of medical error, and the majority is considered to be preventable. For every diagnostic error there are usually several root causes. Studies identify three main categories, shown in Box 1.1. However, 'human cognitive error' appears to play a significant role in the majority of diagnostic errors.

Human cognitive error occurs when the clinician has all the information necessary to make the diagnosis, but then makes the wrong diagnosis. Why does this happen? Three main reasons have been identified:

- knowledge gaps
- misinterpretation of diagnostic tests
- cognitive biases.

Examples of errors in these three categories are shown in Box 1.2. Clearly, clinical knowledge is required for sound clinical reasoning, and an incomplete knowledge base or inadequate experience can lead to diagnostic error. However, this chapter will focus on some other aspects of knowledge that are important for effective clinical reasoning, including use and interpretation of diagnostic tests, cognitive biases and human factors.

Clinical reasoning: definitions

'Clinical reasoning' describes the thinking and decision-making processes associated with clinical practice. Our understanding of clinical reasoning derives from the fields of education, cognitive psychology, studies of expertise and the diagnostic error and health systems literature.

Clinical reasoning can be conceptualised as a process with different components, each requiring specific knowledge, skills and behaviours.

1.1 Root causes of diagnostic error in studies

Error category	Examples
No fault	Unusual presentation of a disease Missing information
System error	Inadequate diagnostic support Results not available Error-prone processes Poor supervision of inexperienced staff Poor team communication
Human cognitive error	Inadequate data-gathering Errors in reasoning

Adapted from Graber M, Gordon R, Franklin N. Reducing diagnostic errors in medicine: what is the goal? Acad Med 2002; 77:981–992.

1.2 Reasons for errors in clinical reasoning

Source of error	Examples
Knowledge gaps	Telling a patient she cannot have biliary colic because she has had her gallbladder removed – gallstones can form in the bile ducts in patients who have had a cholecystectomy
Misinterpretation of diagnostic tests	Deciding a patient has not had a stroke because his brain scan is normal – computed tomography and even magnetic resonance imaging, especially when performed early, may not identify an infarct
Cognitive biases	Accepting a diagnosis handed over to you without question (the 'framing effect') instead of asking yourself 'What is the evidence that supports this diagnosis?'

The UK Clinical Reasoning in Medical Education group (see 'Further information') broadly lists these components as:

- history and physical examination
- use and interpretation of diagnostic tests
- problem identification and management
- shared decision-making.

Not all of these components are necessary for effective clinical reasoning and they do not necessarily happen in this order. They also occur in contexts that impact on decision-making, which will be explored later. Underpinning all of this is formal and experiential knowledge of basic sciences and clinical medicine. The knowledge required for effective clinical reasoning includes factual knowledge, but also conceptual knowledge (how things fit together) as well as procedural knowledge (how to do something, what techniques to use) plus an awareness of and an ability to think about one's own thinking (also known as metacognitive knowledge). This is where an understanding of cognitive biases and human factors is important.

Fig. 1.1 shows the key components involved in clinical reasoning that will be explored further in this chapter.

History and physical examination

Even with major advances in medical technology, the history remains the most important part of the clinical decision-making process. Studies show that physicians make a diagnosis in 70%–90% of cases from the history alone. It is important to remember that the history is explored not only with the patient, but also (and with consent if required) from all available sources if necessary: for example, paramedic and emergency department notes, eye-witnesses, relatives and/or carers.

However, clinicians need to be aware of the diagnostic usefulness of clinical features in the history and physical examination. For example, students are often taught that meningitis classically presents with the following features:

- headache
- fever
- meningism (photophobia, neck stiffness and other signs of meningeal irritation, such as Kernig's and Brudzinski's signs).

However, knowing the frequency with which patients present with certain features and the diagnostic weight of each feature are important in clinical decision-making. Many patients with meningitis do not

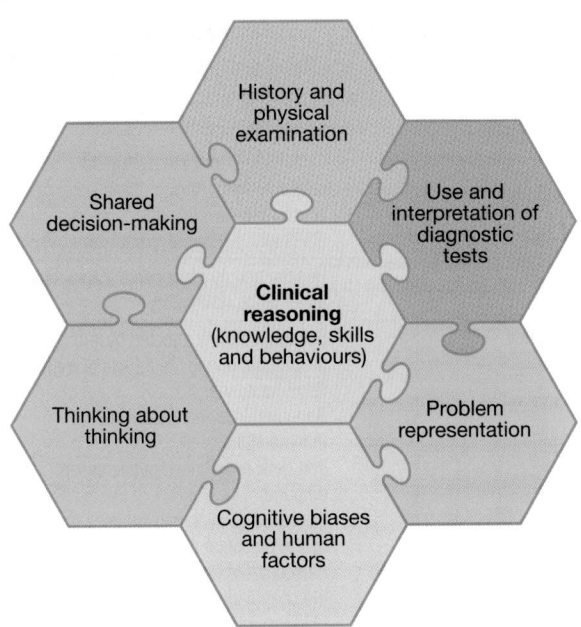

Fig. 1.1 Elements of clinical reasoning.

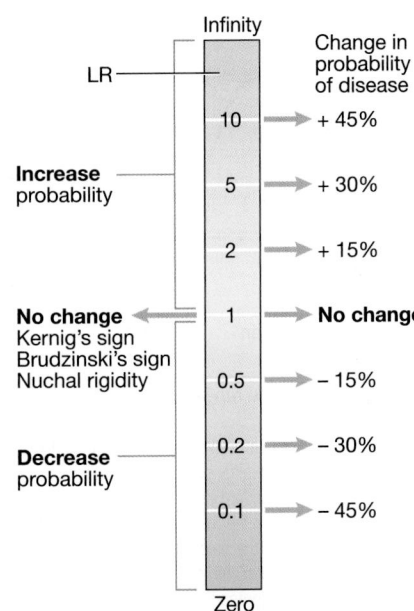

Fig. 1.2 Likelihood ratio (LR) of Kernig's sign, Brudzinski's sign and nuchal rigidity in the clinical diagnosis of meningitis.

$$LR = \frac{\text{probability of finding in patients with disease}}{\text{probability of finding in patients without disease}}$$

LRs are also used for diagnostic tests; here a physical examination finding can be considered a diagnostic test. *Data from Thomas KE, Hasbun R, Jekel J, et al. The diagnostic accuracy of Kernig's sign, Brudzinski's sign, and nuchal rigidity in adults with suspected meningitis. Clin Infect Dis 2002; 35:46–52.*

have classical signs of meningism and the clinical presentation varies among different patient populations and in different parts of the world. In one prospective study conducted in the United States, nearly all adult patients with meningitis had headache and a fever, but less than half had neck stiffness on examination and only 5% of patients had Kernig's and Brudzinski's signs. All three signs had a likelihood ratio of around 1, meaning their presence or absence was of little use in deciding whether a patient had meningitis or not (Fig. 1.2).

Likelihood ratios (LR) are clinical diagnostic weights. An LR of greater than 1 increases the probability of disease (the higher the value, the greater the probability). Similarly, an LR of less than 1 decreases the probability of disease. LRs are developed against a diagnostic standard (in the case of meningitis, lumbar puncture results), so do not exist for all clinical findings. LRs illustrate how an individual clinical finding changes the probability of a disease. For example, in a person presenting with headache and fever, the clinical finding of neck stiffness may carry little weight in deciding whether to perform a lumbar puncture because LRs do not determine the prior probability of disease; they reflect only how a single clinical finding changes it. Clinicians have to take all the available information from the history and physical examination into account. If the overall clinical probability is high to begin with, a clinical finding with an LR of around 1 does not change this.

'Evidence-based history and examination' is a term used to describe how clinicians incorporate knowledge about the prevalence and diagnostic weight of clinical findings into their decision-making. In studies, students who are taught the probabilities of features being present in specific diseases rather than lists of features have better diagnostic accuracy. This is improved further by understanding the basic science explanation for symptoms and signs: bedside signs of meningism identify patients with severe meningeal inflammation but do not pick up those with early or mild inflammation.

Evidence-based history and examination is important because estimating the clinical (pre-test) probability is vital not only for diagnostic accuracy, but also in the use and interpretation of diagnostic tests.

Use and interpretation of diagnostic tests

There is no such thing as a perfect diagnostic test. Test results give us test probabilities, not real probabilities. Test results have to be interpreted because they are affected by the following:

- how 'normal' is defined
- factors other than disease
- operating characteristics
- sensitivity and specificity
- prevalence of disease in the population.

Normal values

Most tests provide quantitative results (i.e. a value on a continuous numerical scale). In order to classify quantitative results as normal or abnormal, it is necessary to define a cut-off point. Many quantitative measurements in populations have a Gaussian or 'normal' distribution. By convention, the normal range is defined as those values that encompass 95% of the population, or 2 standard deviations above and below the mean. This means that 2.5% of the normal population will have values above, and 2.5% will have values below the normal range. For this reason, it is more appropriate to talk about the 'reference range' rather than the 'normal range' (Fig. 1.3).

Test results in abnormal populations also have a Gaussian distribution, with a different mean and standard deviation. In some diseases there is no overlap between results from the abnormal and normal population. However, in many diseases there is overlap; in these circumstances, the greater the difference between the test result and the limits of the reference range, the higher the chance that the person has the disease.

However, there are also situations in medicine when 'normal' is abnormal and 'abnormal' is normal. For example, in the context of a severe asthma attack a 'normal' $PaCO_2$ is abnormal and means the patient has life-threatening asthma. Conversely, a low ferritin in a young menstruating woman is not considered to be abnormal at all.

Laboratory results (e.g. cholesterol, thyroid-stimulating hormone) also vary from day to day in the same person in the absence of a real change because of biological variation and laboratory variation. The extent to which a blood test is allowed to vary before it has truly changed is called

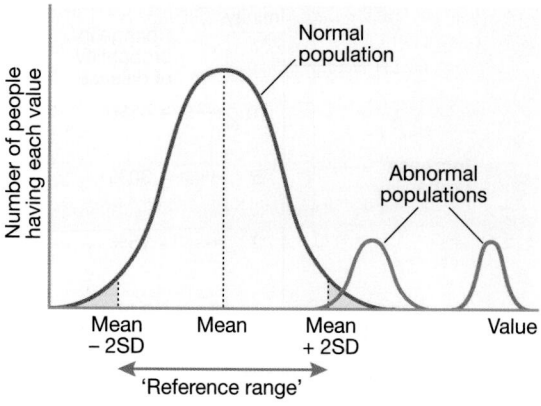

Fig. 1.3 Normal distribution and reference range. For many tests, the frequency distribution of results in the normal healthy population (red line) is a symmetrical bell-shaped curve. The mean ±2 standard deviations (SD) encompasses 95% of the normal population and usually defines the 'reference range'; 2.5% of the normal population have values above, and 2.5% below, this range (shaded areas). For some diseases (blue line), test results overlap with the normal population or even with the reference range. For other diseases (green line), tests may be more reliable because there is no overlap between the normal and abnormal population.

the 'critical difference'. The critical difference is different for each test, and can be high – 17% in the case of cholesterol and higher for some other tests.

Factors other than disease that influence test results

A number of factors other than disease influence test results:

- age
- ethnicity
- pregnancy
- sex
- spurious (in vitro) results.

Box 1.3 gives some examples.

Operating characteristics

Tests are also subject to operating characteristics. This refers to the way the test is performed. Patients need to be able to comply fully with some tests, such as spirometry (p. 501), and if they cannot, the test result will be affected. Some tests are very dependent on the skill of the operator and are also affected by the patient's body habitus and clinical state; ultrasound of the heart and abdomen are examples. A common mistake is when doctors refer to a test result as 'no abnormality detected' when, in fact, the report describes a technically difficult and incomplete scan that should more accurately be described as 'non-diagnostic'.

Some conditions are paroxysmal. For example, around half of patients with epilepsy have a normal standard electroencephalogram (EEG). A normal EEG therefore does not exclude epilepsy. On the other hand, around 10% of patients who do *not* have epilepsy have epileptiform discharges on their EEG. This is referred to as an 'incidental finding'. Incidental findings are common in medicine, and are increasing in incidence with the greater availability of more sensitive tests. Test results should always be interpreted in the light of the patient's history and physical examination.

Sensitivity and specificity

Diagnostic tests have characteristics termed 'sensitivity' and 'specificity'. Sensitivity is the ability to detect true positives; specificity is the ability to

1.3 Examples of factors other than disease that influence test results

Factor	Examples
Age	Creatinine is lower in old age (due to relatively lower muscle mass) – an older person can have a significantly reduced eGFR with a 'normal' creatinine
Ethnicity	Healthy people of African ancestry have lower white cell counts
Pregnancy	Several tests are affected by late pregnancy, due to the effects of a growing fetus, including: Reduced urea and creatinine (haemodilution) Iron deficiency anaemia (increased demand) Increased alkaline phosphatase (produced by the placenta) Raised D-dimer (physiological changes in the coagulation system) Mild respiratory alkalosis (physiological maternal hyperventilation) ECG changes (tachycardia, left axis deviation)
Sex	Males and females have different reference ranges for many tests, e.g. haemoglobin
Spurious (in vitro) results	A spurious high potassium is seen in haemolysis and in thrombocytosis ('pseudohyperkalaemia')

(ECG = electrocardiogram; eGFR = estimated glomerular filtration rate, a better estimate of renal function than creatinine)

detect true negatives. Even a very good test, with 95% sensitivity, will miss 1 in 20 people with the disease. Every test therefore generates 'false positives' and 'false negatives' (Box 1.4).

A very sensitive test will detect most disease but may generate abnormal findings in healthy people. A negative result will therefore reliably exclude disease but a positive result does not mean the disease is present – it means further evaluation is required. On the other hand, a very specific test may miss significant pathology but is likely to establish the diagnosis beyond doubt when the result is positive. All tests differ in their sensitivity and specificity, and clinicians require a working knowledge of the tests they use in order to accurately interpret them.

In choosing how a test is used to guide decision-making there is a trade-off between sensitivity versus specificity. For example, defining an exercise electrocardiogram (p. 393) as abnormal if there is at least 0.5 mm of ST depression would ensure that very few cases of coronary artery disease are missed but would generate many false-positive results (high sensitivity, low specificity). On the other hand, a cut-off point of 2.0 mm of ST depression would detect most cases of important coronary artery disease with far fewer false positives. This trade-off is calculated using the receiver operating characteristic curve of the test (Fig. 1.4).

An extremely important concept in clinical decision-making is this: the probability that a person has a disease depends on the pre-test probability, and the sensitivity and specificity of the test. For example, imagine an older woman has fallen and hurt her left hip. On examination, the hip is extremely painful to move and she cannot stand. However, her hip X-rays are normal. Does she have a fracture?

The sensitivity of plain X-rays of the hip performed in the emergency department for suspected hip fracture is around 95%. A small percentage of fractures are therefore missed. If our patient has (or is at risk of) osteoporosis, has severe pain on hip movement and cannot bear weight on the affected side, then the clinical probability of hip fracture is high. If, on the other hand, she is unlikely to have osteoporosis, has no pain on

i 1.4 Sensitivity and specificity

	Disease	No disease
Positive test	A (True positive)	B (False positive)
Negative test	C (False negative)	D (True negative)

Sensitivity = A/(A+C) × 100
Specificity = D/(D+B) × 100

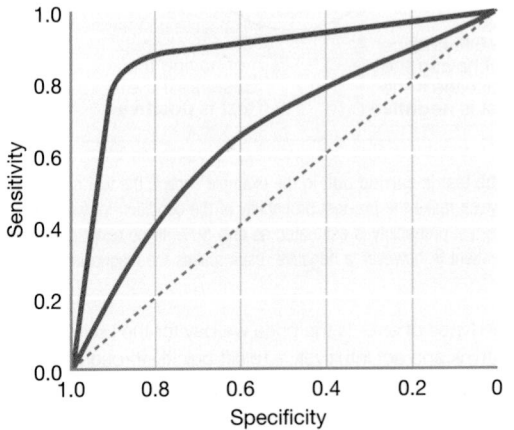

Fig. 1.4 Receiver operating characteristic graph illustrating the trade-off between sensitivity and specificity for a given test. The curve is generated by 'adjusting' the cut-off values defining normal and abnormal results, calculating the effect on sensitivity and specificity and then plotting these against each other. The closer the curve lies to the top left-hand corner, the more useful the test. The red line illustrates a test with useful discriminant value and the green line illustrates a less useful, poorly discriminant test.

hip movement and is able to bear weight, then the clinical probability of hip fracture is low.

Doctors are continually making judgements about whether something is true, given that something else is true. This is known as 'conditional probability'. Bayes' Theorem (named after English clergyman Thomas Bayes, 1702–1761) is a mathematical way to describe the post-test probability of a disease by combining pre-test probability, sensitivity and specificity. In clinical practice, doctors are not able to make complex mathematical calculations for every decision they make. In practical terms, the answer to the question of whether there is a fracture is that in a high-probability patient a normal test result does not exclude it, but in a low-probability patient it (virtually) does. This principle is illustrated in Fig. 1.5.

Sox and colleagues (see 'Further information') state a fundamental assertion, which they describe as a profound and subtle principle of clinical medicine: the interpretation of new information depends on what you believed beforehand. In other words, the interpretation of a test result depends on the probability of disease before the test.

Prevalence of disease

Consider this problem that was posed to a group of Harvard doctors. The problem originates from a 1978 article in the *New England Journal of Medicine* (Casscells et al, see 'Further information'): if a test to detect a disease whose prevalence is 1:1000 has a false-positive rate of 5%, what is the chance that a person found to have a positive result actually has the disease, assuming you know nothing about the person's symptoms and signs? Assume the test generates no false negatives and take a moment to work this out. In this problem, we have removed clinical probability and are only considering prevalence. The answer is at the end of the chapter (p. 11).

Predictive values combine sensitivity, specificity and prevalence. Sensitivity and specificity are characteristics of the test; the population

does not change this. However, as doctors, we are interested in the question, 'What is the probability that a person with a positive test actually has the disease?' This is illustrated in Box 1.5.

Post-test probability and predictive values are different. Post-test probability is the probability of a disease after taking into account new information from a test result. Bayes' Theorem can be used to calculate post-test probability for a patient in any population. The pre-test probability of disease is decided by the doctor; it is a judgement based on information gathered prior to ordering the test. Predictive value is the proportion of patients with a test result who have the disease (or no disease) and is calculated from a table of results in a specific population (see Box 1.5). It is not possible to transfer this value to a different population. This is important to realise because published information about the performance of diagnostic tests may not apply to different populations.

In deciding the pre-test probability of disease, clinicians often neglect to take prevalence into account and this distorts their estimate of probability. To estimate the probability of disease in a patient more accurately, clinicians should anchor on the prevalence of disease in the subgroup to which the patient belongs and then adjust to take the individual factors into account.

Dealing with uncertainty

Clinical findings are imperfect and diagnostic tests are imperfect. It is important to recognise that clinicians frequently deal with uncertainty. By expressing uncertainty as probability, new information from diagnostic tests can be incorporated more accurately. However, subjective estimates of probability can sometimes be unreliable. As the section on cognitive biases will demonstrate (see below), intuition can be a source of error.

Knowing the patient's true state is often unnecessary in clinical decision-making. Sox and colleagues (see 'Further information') argue that there is a difference between knowing that a disease is present and acting as if it were present. The requirement for diagnostic certainty depends on the penalty for being wrong. Different situations require different levels of certainty before starting treatment. How we communicate uncertainty to patients will be discussed later in this chapter (see Fig. 1.9).

The 'treatment threshold' combines factors such as the risks of the test, and the risks versus benefits of treatment. The point at which the factors are all evenly weighed is the threshold. If a test or treatment for a disease is effective and low risk (e.g. giving antibiotics for a suspected urinary tract infection), then there is a lower threshold for going ahead. On the other hand, if a test or treatment is less effective or high risk (e.g. starting chemotherapy for a malignant brain tumour), then greater confidence is required in the clinical diagnosis and potential benefits of treatment first. In principle, if a diagnostic test will not change the management of the patient, then careful consideration should be given to whether it is necessary to do the test at all.

In summary, test results shift our thinking, but rarely give a 'yes' or a 'no' answer in terms of a diagnosis. Sometimes tests shift the probability of disease by less than we realise. Pre-test probability is key, and this is derived from the history and physical examination, combined with a sound knowledge of medicine and an understanding of the prevalence of disease in the particular care setting or the population to which the patient belongs.

Problem representation

Many students are taught to formulate a differential diagnosis after the history, physical examination and initial test results, but the ability to accurately articulate a 'problem representation' (or problem list) first and *then* construct a prioritised differential diagnosis based on this, including relevant 'must-not-miss' diagnoses, is a key step in the clinical reasoning process. A problem representation refers to how information about a problem is mentally organised. Studies show that expert clinicians spend far more time on defining a problem before trying to solve it compared with novices, and novices are more likely to be unsuccessful in solving

Percentage probability of having the disease

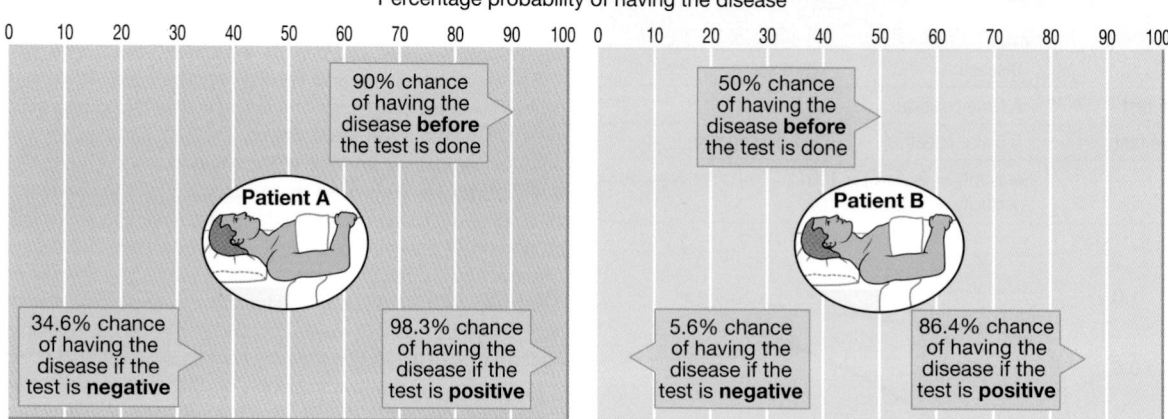

Fig. 1.5 The interpretation of a test result depends on the probability of the disease before the test is carried out. In the example shown, the test being carried out has a sensitivity of 95% and a specificity of 85%. Patient A has very characteristic clinical findings, which make the pre-test probability of the condition for which the test is being used very high – estimated as 90%. Patient B has more equivocal findings, such that the pre-test probability is estimated as only 50%. If the result in Patient A is negative, there is still a significant chance that he has the condition for which he is being tested; in Patient B, however, a negative result makes the diagnosis very unlikely.

i **1.5 Predictive values: 'What is the probability that a person with a positive test actually has the disease?'**

	Disease	No disease
Positive test	A (True positive)	B (False positive)
Negative test	C (False negative)	D (True negative)

Positive predictive value = A/(A+B) × 100
Negative predictive value = D/(D+C) × 100

a problem because they have not accurately represented the problem in the first place. The ability to synthesise all the available information and encapsulate it into a problem representation using precise medical language is an important skill that helps to organise and retrieve knowledge from long-term memory relevant to the case and is associated with significantly higher diagnostic accuracy, particularly in complex cases (Bordage, 1994; see 'Further information').

Formulating a problem representation (e.g. a 30-year-old pregnant woman with acute left-sided pleuritic chest pain and breathlessness) or a problem list (e.g. persistent vomiting, hypokalaemia, acute kidney injury), not only helps to organise and retrieve knowledge relevant to the case which helps in diagnosis, it also helps to formulate an action plan while further information is being gathered when a diagnosis is not yet possible.

Cognitive biases

Advances in cognitive psychology in recent decades have demonstrated that human thinking and decision-making are prone to error. Cognitive biases are subconscious errors that lead to inaccurate judgement and illogical interpretation of information. They are prevalent in everyday life; as the famous saying goes, 'to err is human'.

Take a few moments to look at this simple puzzle. Do not try to solve it mathematically but listen to your intuition:

A bat and ball cost £1.10.
The bat costs £1 more than the ball.
How much does the ball cost?

The answer is at the end of the chapter. Most people get the answer to this puzzle wrong – even though they have all the knowledge and experience they need to solve this problem. Why? British psychologist and patient safety pioneer James Reason said that, 'Our propensity

for certain types of error is the price we pay for the brain's remarkable ability to think and act intuitively – to sift quickly through the sensory information that constantly bombards us without wasting time trying to work through every situation anew.' This property of human thinking is highly relevant to clinical decision-making.

Type 1 and type 2 thinking

Decades of studies in cognitive psychology and, more recently, functional magnetic resonance imaging demonstrate two distinct types of processes when it comes to decision-making: humans have a fast, intuitive, pattern-recognising way of thinking which uses little cognitive effort (known as type 1 thinking) and a more deliberate, analytical one which engages our working memory (known as type 2 thinking). This is known as 'dual process theory' and Box 1.6 explains this in more detail.

Psychologists estimate that we spend 95% of our daily lives engaged in type 1 thinking – the intuitive, fast, subconscious mode of decision-making. Imagine driving a car, for example: it would be impossible to function efficiently if every decision and movement were as deliberate, conscious, slow and effortful as in our first driving lesson. With experience, complex procedures become automatic, fast and effortless. The same applies to medical practice. There is evidence that expert decision-making is well served by intuitive thinking. The problem is that although intuitive processing is highly efficient in many circumstances, in others it is prone to error.

Clinicians use both type 1 and type 2 thinking, and both types are important in clinical decision-making. When encountering a problem that is familiar, clinicians employ pattern recognition and reach a working diagnosis or differential diagnosis quickly (type 1 thinking). When encountering a problem that is more complicated, they use a slower, systematic approach (type 2 thinking). Both types of thinking interplay – they are not mutually exclusive in the diagnostic process. Fig. 1.6 illustrates the interplay between type 1 and type 2 thinking in clinical practice.

Errors can occur in both type 1 and type 2 thinking. For example, people can apply the wrong rules or make errors in their application while using type 2 thinking. However, it has been argued that the common cognitive biases encountered in medicine tend to occur when clinicians are engaged in type 1 thinking.

For example, imagine being asked to see a young woman who is drowsy. She is handed over to you as a 'probable overdose' because she has a history of depression and a packet of painkillers was found beside her at home. Her observations show she has a Glasgow Coma Scale score of 10/15, heart rate 100 beats/min, blood pressure 100/60 mmHg, respiratory rate 14 breaths/min, oxygen saturations 98% on air and temperature 37.5°C. Already your mind has reached a working diagnosis. It fits a pattern (type 1 thinking). You think she has taken an overdose. At

i	1.6 Type 1 and type 2 thinking	
Type 1	**Type 2**	
Intuitive, heuristic (pattern recognition)	Analytical, systematic	
Automatic, subconscious	Deliberate, conscious	
Fast, effortless	Slow, effortful	
Low/variable reliability	High/consistent reliability	
Vulnerable to error	Less prone to error	
Highly affected by context	Less affected by context	
High emotional involvement	Low emotional involvement	
Low scientific rigour	High scientific rigour	

this point you can stop to think about your thinking (rational override in Fig. 1.6): 'What is the evidence for this diagnosis? What else could it be?'

On the other hand, imagine being asked to assess a patient who has been admitted with syncope. There are several different causes of syncope and a systematic approach is required to reach a diagnosis (type 2 thinking). However, you recently heard about a case of syncope due to a painless leaking abdominal aortic aneurysm. At the end of your assessment, following evidence-based guidelines, it is clear the patient can be discharged. Despite this, you decide to observe the patient overnight *just in case* (irrational override in Fig. 1.6). In this example, your intuition is actually 'availability bias' (when things are at the forefront of your mind) which has significantly distorted your estimate of probability.

Common cognitive biases in medicine

Figure 1.7 illustrates the common cognitive biases prevalent in medical practice. Biases often work together; for example, in overconfidence bias (the tendency to believe we know more than we actually do), too much faith is placed in opinion instead of gathered evidence. This bias can be augmented by the availability bias and finally by commission bias (the tendency towards action rather than inaction) – sometimes with disastrous results.

The mark of a well-calibrated thinker is the ability to recognise what mode of thinking is being employed and to anticipate and recognise situations in which cognitive biases and errors are more likely to occur.

Thinking about thinking

Research has highlighted the importance of being aware of and being able to think about one's own thinking (also known as metacognition). Several studies have demonstrated that engaging in reflection during diagnostic decision-making improves performance (Prakash et al, see 'Further information'). This can be as simple as asking, 'What is the evidence for this diagnosis? What else could it be?' Reflection is most effective when the case is more complex (relative to the clinician).

Some people have a natural tendency to look for evidence, weigh things up, be aware of context, not take things at face value, and think about their own thinking. Others can learn to do so. Psychologists consider this 'reflective mind' a subset of analytical type 2 thinking. The tendency to engage in reflection during decision-making is independent of knowledge and cognitive ability, and accounts for the greatest variation in individual performance on many reasoning tasks.

With increasing knowledge and experience, intuitive type 1 thinking is used more; it is fast and highly accurate and commonly used by experts. Novices cannot do this because they have not yet built a database of patterns in their long-term memory, known as illness scripts. Reflection interrupts type 1 processing, even briefly, to simulate alternatives. So as you can see, good decision-making relies on knowledge and experience, but also the ability to 'stop and think' when needed. However, this requires cognitive effort (type 2 thinking), which may be impaired by things like fatigue, interruptions and cognitive overload.

Human factors

'Human factors' is the science of the limitations of human performance, and how technology, the work environment and team communication can adapt for this to reduce diagnostic and other types of error. Analysis of serious adverse events in clinical practice shows that human factors and poor team communication play a significant role when things go wrong.

Research shows that many errors are beyond an individual's conscious control and are precipitated by many factors. The discipline of human factors seeks to understand interactions between:

- people and tasks or technology
- people and their work environment
- people in a team.

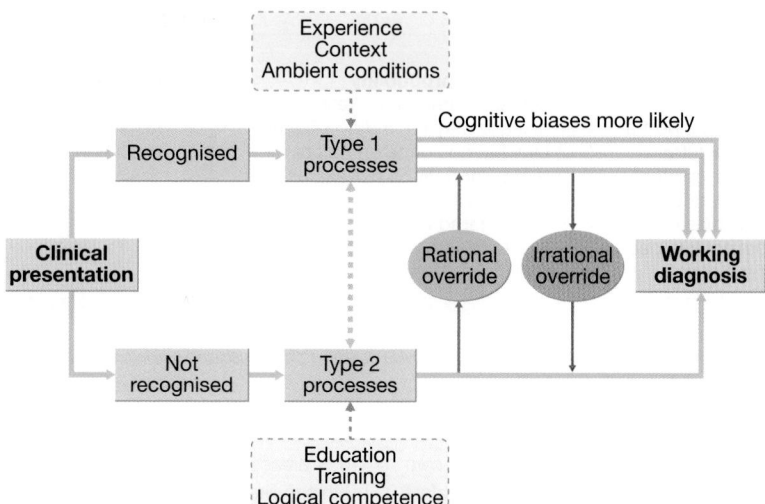

Fig. 1.6 The interplay between type 1 and type 2 thinking in the diagnostic process. *Adapted from Croskerry P. A universal model of diagnostic reasoning. Acad Med 2009; 84:1022–1028.*

Anchoring
The common human tendency to rely too heavily on the first piece of information offered (the 'anchor') when making decisions

Diagnostic momentum
Once a diagnostic label has been attached to a patient (by the patient or other health-care professionals), it can gather momentum with each review, leading others to exclude other possibilities in their thinking

Premature closure
The tendency to close the decision-making process prematurely and accept a diagnosis before it, and other possibilities, have been fully explored

Ascertainment bias
We sometimes see what we expect to see ('self-fulfilling prophecy'). For example, a frequent self-harmer attends the emergency department with drowsiness; everyone assumes he has taken another overdose and misses a brain injury

Framing effect
How a case is presented – for example, in handover – can generate bias in the listener. This can be mitigated by always having 'healthy scepticism' about other people's diagnoses

Psych-out error
Psychiatric patients who present with medical problems are under-assessed, under-examined and under-investigated because problems are presumed to be due to, or exacerbated by, their psychiatric condition

Availability bias
Things may be at the forefront of your mind because you have seen several cases recently or have been studying that condition in particular. For example, when one of the authors worked in an epilepsy clinic, all blackouts were possible seizures

Hindsight bias
Knowing the outcome may profoundly influence the perception of past events and decision-making, preventing a realistic appraisal of what actually occurred – a major problem in learning from diagnostic error

Search satisficing
We may stop searching because we have found something that fits or is convenient, instead of systematically looking for the best alternative, which involves more effort

Base rate neglect
The tendency to ignore the prevalence of a disease, which then distorts Bayesian reasoning. In some cases, clinicians do this deliberately in order to rule out an unlikely but worst-case scenario

Omission bias
The tendency towards inaction, rooted in the principle of 'first, do no harm.' Events that occur through natural progression of disease are more acceptable than those that may be attributed directly to the action of the health-care team

Triage-cueing
Triage ensures patients are sent to the right department. However, this leads to 'geography is destiny'. For example, a diabetic ketoacidosis patient with abdominal pain and vomiting is sent to surgery. The wrong location (surgical ward) stops people thinking about medical causes of abdominal pain and vomiting

Commission bias
The tendency towards action rather than inaction, on the assumption that good can come only from doing something (rather than 'watching and waiting')

Overconfidence bias
The tendency to believe we know more than we actually do, placing too much faith in opinion instead of gathered evidence

Unpacking principle
Failure to 'unpack' all the available information may mean things are missed. For example, if a thorough history is not obtained from either the patient or carers (a common problem in geriatric medicine), diagnostic possibilities may be discounted

Confirmation bias
The tendency to look for confirming evidence to support a theory rather than looking for disconfirming evidence to refute it, even if the latter is clearly present. Confirmation bias is common when a patient has been seen first by another doctor

Posterior probability
Our estimate of the likelihood of disease may be unduly influenced by what has gone on before for a particular patient. For example, a patient who has been extensively investigated for headaches presents with a severe headache, and serious causes are discounted

Visceral bias
The influence of either negative or positive feelings towards patients, which can affect our decision-making

Fig. 1.7 **Common cognitive biases in medicine.** *Adapted from Croskerry P. Achieving quality in clinical decision-making: cognitive strategies and detection of bias. Acad Emerg Med 2002; 9:1184–1204.*

An understanding of these interactions makes it easier for health-care professionals, who are committed to 'first, do no harm', to work in the safest way possible. For example, performance is adversely affected by factors such as poorly designed processes and equipment, fatigue and poor communication. So simple, clear processes, good design of equipment and shift patterns, and clear team communication all help to minimise errors.

The areas of the brain required for type 2 processing are most affected by things like fatigue and cognitive overload, and the brain reverts to type 1 processing to conserve cognitive energy. Figure 1.8 illustrates some of the internal and external factors that affect human judgement and decision-making. An awareness of the factors that impact on decision-making can allow clinicians to take steps to mitigate these.

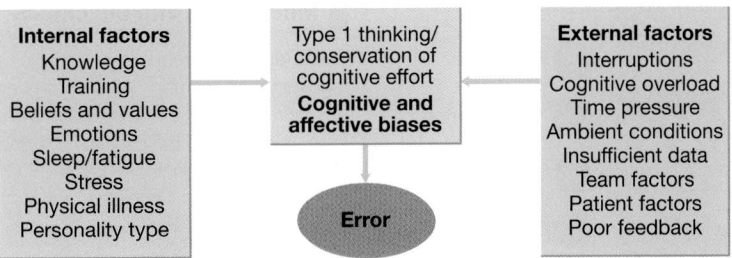

Fig. 1.8 Factors that affect our judgement and decision-making. (Type 1 thinking = fast, intuitive, subconscious, low effort)

Several studies demonstrate that we focus our attention to filter out distractions. This is advantageous in many situations (for example, when performing a procedure), but in focusing on what we are trying to see we may not notice the unexpected. In a team context, what is obvious to one person may be completely missed by someone else. Safe and effective team communication therefore requires us never to assume, and to verbalise things, even though they may seem 'obvious'.

Shared decision-making

Shared decision-making refers to the fact that clinical reasoning does not necessarily take place solely within a clinician's head. Good decision-making is often shared with patients, relatives and carers, within teams, and by using guidelines, clinical prediction rules and other decision aids. Integral to all of this is the ability to engage in optimal decision-making behaviours: involving the patient and/or carers in the diagnostic and management process, listening to others, following evidence-based guidelines, asking for help when needed, and using clear communication, especially when handing over care.

Patient-centred evidence-based medicine

'Patient-centred evidence-based medicine' refers to the application of best available research evidence while taking individual patient factors into account; these include both clinical and non-clinical factors (e.g. the patient's social circumstances, values and wishes). For example, a 95-year-old man with dementia and a recent gastrointestinal bleed is admitted with an inferior myocardial infarction. He is clinically well. Should he be treated with dual antiplatelet therapy and low-molecular-weight heparin as recommended in clinical guidelines?

As this chapter has described, clinicians frequently deal with uncertainty/probability. Clinicians need to be able to explain risks and benefits of treatment in an accurate and understandable way. Providing the relevant statistics is seldom sufficient to guide decision-making because a patient's perception of risk may be influenced by irrational factors as well as individual values.

Research evidence provides statistics but these can be confusing. Terms such as 'common' and 'rare' are nebulous. Whenever possible, clinicians should quote numerical information using consistent denominators (e.g. '90 out of 100 patients who have this operation feel much better, 1 will die during the operation and 2 will suffer a stroke'). Visual aids can be used to present complex statistical information (Fig. 1.9).

How uncertainty is conveyed to patients is important. Many studies demonstrate a correlation between effective clinician–patient communication and improved health outcomes. If patients feel they have been listened to and understand the problem and proposed treatment plan, they are more likely to follow the plan and less likely to re-attend.

Effective team communication

In increasingly complex health-care systems, patients are looked after by a wide variety of professionals, each of whom has access to important information required to make clinical decisions. Strict hierarchies are hazardous to patient safety if certain members of the team do not feel able to speak up.

The SBAR system of communication has been recommended by the UK's Patient Safety First campaign. It is a structured way to communicate about a patient with another health-care professional (e.g. during handover or when making a referral) and increases the amount of relevant information being communicated in a shorter time. It is illustrated in Box 1.7.

Using clinical prediction rules and other decision aids

A clinical prediction rule is a statistical model of the diagnostic process. When clinical prediction rules are matched against the opinion of experts, the model usually outperforms the experts, because it is applied consistently in each case. However, it is important that clinical prediction rules are used correctly – that is, applied to the patient population that was used to create the rule. Clinical prediction rules force a scientific assessment of the patient's symptoms, signs and other data to develop a numerical probability of a disease or an outcome. They help clinicians to estimate probability more accurately.

A good example of a clinical prediction rule to estimate pre-test probability is the Wells score in suspected deep vein thrombosis (see Box 9.18). Other commonly used clinical prediction rules predict outcomes and therefore guide the management plan. These include the GRACE score in acute coronary syndromes (see Fig. 16.61) and the CURB-65 score in community-acquired pneumonia (see Fig. 17.32).

Reducing errors in clinical decision-making

Deliberate practice

Studies of expertise reveal that extensive experience is necessary to achieve high levels of performance, but extensive experience does not by itself lead to expert levels of achievement. Something else is required, encapsulated in the term 'deliberate practice'. This involves *effortful* practice, coaching and feedback, and the ability of an individual to plan, assess, reflect and adjust so their performance improves.

Cognitive debiasing strategies

Knowledge and experience alone, however, do not eliminate errors. There are some simple and established techniques that can be used to avoid cognitive biases and errors in clinical decision-making.

History and physical examination

Taking a history and performing a physical examination may seem obvious, but these are sometimes carried out inadequately. This is the 'unpacking principle': failure to unpack all the available information means things can be missed and lead to error.

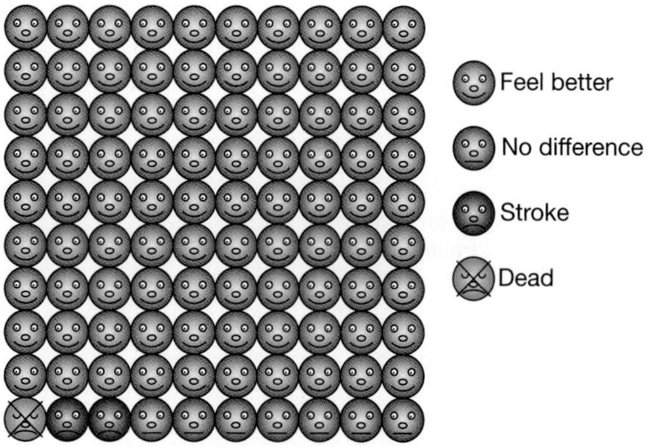

Fig. 1.9 Visual portrayal of benefits and risks. The image refers to an operation that is expected to relieve symptoms in 90% of patients, but cause stroke in 2% and death in 1%. *From Edwards A, Elwyn G, Mulley A. Explaining risks: turning numerical data into meaningful pictures. BMJ 2002; 324:827–830, reproduced with permission from the BMJ Publishing Group.*

i	**1.7 The SBAR system of communicating**	
SBAR		**Example (a telephone call to the Intensive Care team)**
Situation		I am [name] calling from [place] about a patient with a NEWS* of 10.
Background		[Patient's name], 30-year-old woman, no past medical history, was admitted last night with community-acquired pneumonia. Since then her oxygen requirements have been steadily increasing.
Assessment		Her vital signs are: blood pressure 115/60 mmHg, heart rate 120 beats/min, temperature 38°C, respiratory rate 32 breaths/min, oxygen saturations 89% on 15 L via reservoir bag mask. An arterial blood gas shows H^+ 50 nmol/L (pH 7.3), $PaCO_2$ 4.0 kPa (30 mmHg), PaO_2 7 kPa (52.5 mmHg), standard bicarbonate 14 mmol/L. Chest X-ray shows extensive right lower zone consolidation.
Recommendation		Please can you come and see her as soon as possible? I think she needs admission to Intensive Care.

*NEWS = National Early Warning Score; a patient with normal vital signs scores 0. See Royal College of Physicians. National Early Warning Score (NEWS) 2: Standardising the assessment of acute-illness severity in the NHS. Updated report of a working party. London: RCP; December 2017.

Problem representation/list and differential diagnosis

Once all the available data from history, physical examination and (sometimes) initial test results are available, these need to be synthesised into a problem representation or problem list. The process of generating a problem list ensures nothing is missed. The process of generating a differential diagnosis works against anchoring on a particular diagnosis too early, thereby avoiding search satisficing and premature closure (see Fig. 1.6).

Mnemonics and checklists

These are used frequently in medicine in order to reduce reliance on fallible human memory. ABCDE (airway, breathing, circulation, disability, exposure/examination) is probably the most successful checklist in medicine, used during the assessment and treatment of critically ill patients (ABCDE is sometimes prefixed with 'C' for 'control of any obvious problem'; see p. 191). Checklists ensure that important issues have been considered and completed, especially under conditions of complexity, stress or fatigue.

Red flags and ROWS ('rule out worst-case scenario')

These are strategies that force doctors to consider serious diseases that can present with common symptoms. Red flags in back pain are listed in Box 26.19. Considering and investigating for possible pulmonary embolism in patients who present with pleuritic chest pain and breathlessness is a common example of ruling out a worst-case scenario, as pulmonary embolism can be fatal if missed. Red flags and ROWS help to avoid cognitive biases such as the 'framing effect' and 'premature closure'.

Newer strategies to avoid cognitive biases and errors in decision-making are emerging. These involve explicit training in clinical reasoning and human factors. In theory, if doctors are aware of the science of human thinking and decision-making, then they are more able to think about their thinking, understand situations in which their decision-making may be affected, and take steps to mitigate this.

Clinical decision-making: putting it all together

The following is a practical example that brings together many of the concepts outlined in this chapter:

A 25-year-old woman presents with right-sided pleuritic chest pain and breathlessness. She reports that she had an upper respiratory tract infection a week ago and was almost back to normal when the symptoms started. The patient has no past medical history and no family history, and her only medication is the combined oral contraceptive pill. On examination, her vital signs are normal (respiratory rate 19 breaths/min, oxygen saturations 98% on air, blood pressure 115/60 mmHg, heart rate 90 beats/min, temperature 37.5°C) and the physical examination is also normal. You have been asked to assess her for the possibility of a pulmonary embolism.

(More information on pulmonary embolism can be found in Chapter 17.)

Evidence-based history and examination

Information from the history and physical examination is vital in deciding whether this could be a pulmonary embolism. Pleurisy and breathlessness are common presenting features of this disease but are also common presenting features in other diseases. There is nothing in the history to suggest an alternative diagnosis (e.g. high fever, productive cough, recent chest trauma). The patient's vital signs are normal, as is the physical examination. However, very few individual findings help to distinguish patients with pulmonary embolism from those without it. The presence of wheeze and a high fever modestly decrease the probability of pulmonary embolism. The presence of hypoxaemia is unhelpful (likelihood ratio not significant).

Deciding pre-test probability

The prevalence of pulmonary embolism (PE) in 25-year-old women is low. We anchor on this prevalence and then adjust for individual patient factors. This patient has no major risk factors for pulmonary embolism. To assist our estimate of pre-test probability, we could use a clinical prediction rule: in this case, the modified Wells score for pulmonary embolism, which would give a score of 3 (low probability – answering yes only to the criterion 'PE is the number one diagnosis, an alternative is less likely').

Interpreting test results

Imagine the patient went on to have a normal chest X-ray and blood results, apart from a raised D-dimer of 900 (normal <500 ng/mL). A normal chest X-ray is a common finding in pulmonary embolism. Several studies have shown that the D-dimer assay has at least 95% sensitivity in acute pulmonary embolism but it has a low specificity. A very sensitive test will detect most disease but generate abnormal findings in healthy people. On the other hand, a negative result virtually, but not completely, excludes the disease. It is important at this point to realise that a raised D-dimer result does not mean this patient has a pulmonary embolism; it just means that we have not been able to exclude it. Since pulmonary embolism is a potentially fatal condition we need to rule out the worst-case scenario (ROWS), and the next step is therefore to arrange further imaging. What kind of imaging depends on individual patient characteristics and what is available.

Treatment threshold

The treatment threshold combines factors such as the risks of the test, and the risks versus benefits of treatment. A CT pulmonary angiogram (CTPA) could be requested for this patient, although in some circumstances ventilation–perfusion single-photon emission computed tomography (V̇/Q̇SPECT, p. 547) may be a more suitable alternative. However, what if the scan cannot be performed until the next day? Because pulmonary embolism is potentially fatal and the risks of treatment in this case are low, the patient should be started on treatment while awaiting the scan.

Post-test probability

The patient's scan result is subsequently reported as 'no pulmonary embolism'. Combined with the low pre-test probability, this scan result reliably excludes pulmonary embolism.

Cognitive biases

Imagine during this case that the patient had been handed over to you as 'nothing wrong – probably a pulled muscle'. Cognitive biases (subconscious tendencies to respond in a certain way) would come into play, such as the 'framing effect', 'confirmation bias' and 'search satisficing'. The normal clinical examination might confirm the diagnosis of musculoskeletal pain in your mind, despite the examination being entirely consistent with pulmonary embolism and despite the lack of history and examination findings (e.g. chest wall tenderness) to support the diagnosis of musculoskeletal chest pain.

Human factors

Imagine that, after you have seen the patient, a colleague hands you some blood forms and asks you what tests you would like to request on 'this lady'. You request blood tests including a D-dimer on the wrong patient. Luckily, this error is intercepted.

Shared decision-making

The diagnosis of pulmonary embolism can be difficult. Clinical prediction rules (e.g. modified Wells score), guidelines (e.g. from the UK's National Institute for Health and Care Excellence, or NICE) and decision aids (e.g. simplified pulmonary embolism severity index, or PESI) are frequently used in combination with the doctor's opinion, derived from information gathered in the history and physical examination.

The patient is treated according to evidence-based guidelines that apply to her particular situation. Tests alone do not make a diagnosis and at the end of this process the patient is told that the combination of history, examination and test results mean she is extremely unlikely to have a pulmonary embolism. Viral pleurisy is offered as an alternative diagnosis and she is reassured that her symptoms are expected to settle over the coming days with analgesia. She is advised to re-present to hospital if her symptoms get worse.

Answers to problems

Harvard problem (p. 5)

Almost half of doctors surveyed said 95%, but they neglected to take prevalence into account. If 1000 people are tested, there will be 51 positive results: 50 false positives and 1 true positive (assuming 100% sensitivity). The chance that a person found to have a positive result actually has the disease is therefore only 1/51 or ~2%.

Bat and ball problem (p. 6)

This puzzle is from the book *Thinking, Fast and Slow*, by Nobel laureate Daniel Kahneman (see 'Further information'). He writes, 'A number came to your mind. The number, of course, is 10p. The distinctive mark of this easy puzzle is that it evokes an answer that is intuitive, appealing – and wrong. Do the math, and you will see.' The correct answer is 5p.

Further information

Books and journal articles

Bordage G. Elaborated knowledge: a key to successful diagnostic thinking. Acad Med 1994;69:883–885.
Casscells W, Schoenberger A, Graboys TB. Interpretation by physicians of clinical laboratory results. N Engl J Med 1978;299:999–1001.
Cooper N, Frain J, eds. ABC of clinical reasoning. Oxford: Wiley–Blackwell; 2016.
Croskerry P. A universal model of diagnostic reasoning. Acad Med 2009;84:1022–1028.
Kahneman D. Thinking, fast and slow. London: Penguin; 2012.
McGee S. Evidence-based physical diagnosis, 4th edn. Philadelphia: Elsevier; 2018.
Prakash S, Sladek RM, Schuwirth L. Interventions to improve diagnostic decision making: a systematic review and meta-analysis on reflective strategies. Med Teacher 2019;41:517–524.
Sox H, Higgins MC, Owens DK. Medical decision making, 2nd edn. Chichester: Wiley–Blackwell; 2013.

Websites

creme.org.uk *UK Clinical Reasoning in Medical Education Group.*
improvediagnosis.org *Society to Improve Diagnosis in Medicine (USA).*
chfg.org *UK Clinical Human Factors Group.*
clinical-reasoning.org *Clinical reasoning resources.*
vassarstats.net/index.html *Suite of calculators for statistical computation (Calculator 2 is a calculator for predictive values and likelihood ratios).*

SRJ Maxwell

2

Clinical therapeutics and good prescribing

Prescribing medicines is the major tool used by doctors to restore or preserve the health of patients. Medicines contain drugs (the specific chemical substances with pharmacological effects), either alone or in combination with additional drugs, in a formulation mixed with other ingredients. The beneficial effects of medicines must be weighed against their cost and potential adverse drug reactions and interactions. The latter two factors are sometimes caused by injudicious prescribing decisions and by prescribing errors. The modern prescriber must meet the challenges posed by the increasing number of drugs and formulations available, of indications for prescribing them and the greater complexity of treatment regimens followed by individual patients ('polypharmacy', a particular challenge in the ageing population). The purpose of this chapter is to elaborate on the principles and practice that underpin good prescribing (Box 2.1).

2.1 Steps in good prescribing

- Make a diagnosis
- Consider factors that might influence the patient's response to therapy (age, concomitant drug therapy, renal and liver function etc.)
- Establish the therapeutic goal*
- Choose the therapeutic approach*
- Choose the drug and its formulation (the 'medicine')
- Choose the dose, route and frequency
- Choose the duration of therapy
- Write an unambiguous prescription (or 'medication order')
- Inform the patient about the treatment and its likely effects
- Monitor treatment effects, both beneficial and harmful
- Review/alter the prescription

*These steps in particular take the patient's views into consideration to establish a therapeutic partnership that aims to achieve 'concordance' based on shared decision-making.

Principles of clinical pharmacology

Prescribers need to understand what the drug does to the body (pharmacodynamics) and what the body does to the drug (pharmacokinetics) (Fig. 2.1). Although this chapter is focused on the most common drugs, which are synthetic small molecules, the same principles apply to the increasingly numerous 'biologic' therapies (sometimes abbreviated to 'biologics') now in use, which include peptides, proteins, enzymes and monoclonal antibodies.

Pharmacodynamics

Drug targets and mechanisms of action

Modern drugs are usually discovered by screening compounds for activity either to stimulate or to block the function of a specific molecular target, which is predicted to have a beneficial effect in a particular disease (Box 2.2). Other drugs have useful but less selective chemical properties, such as chelators (e.g. for treatment of iron or copper overload), osmotic agents (used as diuretics in cerebral oedema) or general anaesthetics (that alter the biophysical properties of lipid membranes). The following characteristics of the interaction of drugs with receptors illustrate some of the important determinants of the effects of drugs:

- *Affinity* describes the propensity for a drug to bind to a receptor and is related to the 'molecular fit' and the strength of the chemical bond. Some drug–receptor interactions are *irreversible*, either because the affinity is so strong or because the drug modifies the structure of its molecular target.
- *Selectivity* describes the propensity for a drug to bind to one target rather than another. Selectivity is a relative term, not to be confused with absolute specificity. It is common for drugs targeted

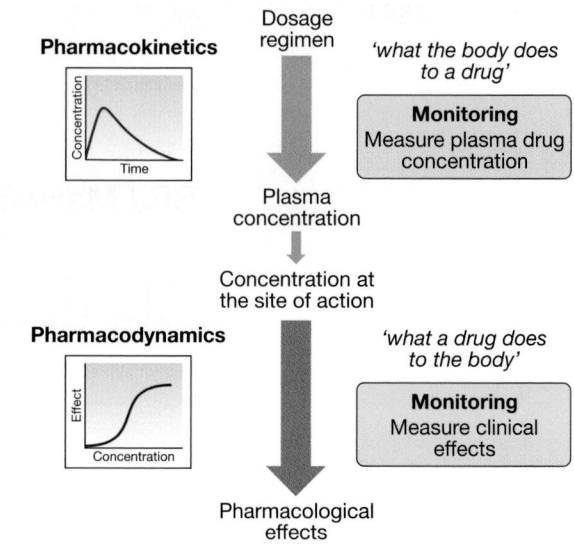

Fig. 2.1 Pharmacokinetics and pharmacodynamics.

at a particular subtype of receptor to exhibit some effect at other subtypes. For example, β-adrenoceptors can be subtyped on the basis of their responsiveness to the endogenous agonist noradrenaline (norepinephrine): the concentration of noradrenaline required to cause bronchodilatation (via β_2-adrenoceptors) is 10 times higher than that required to cause tachycardia (via β_1-adrenoceptors). 'Cardioselective' β-adrenoceptor antagonists (β-blockers) have anti-anginal effects on the heart (β_1), but may still cause bronchospasm in the lung (β_2) and are contraindicated for asthmatic patients.
- *Agonists* bind to a receptor to produce a conformational change that is coupled to a biological response. As agonist concentration increases, so does the proportion of receptors occupied, and hence the biological effect. *Partial agonists* activate the receptor, but cannot produce a maximal signalling effect equivalent to that of a full agonist even when all available receptors are occupied.
- *Antagonists* bind to a receptor, but do not produce the conformational change that initiates an intracellular signal. A *competitive antagonist* competes with endogenous agonist ligands to occupy receptor-binding sites, with the resulting antagonism depending on the relative affinities and concentrations of the antagonist drug and endogenous agonist. *Non-competitive antagonists* inhibit the effect of an agonist by mechanisms other than direct competition for receptor binding with the agonist (e.g. by affecting post-receptor signalling).

Dose–response relationships

Plotting the logarithm of drug dose against drug response typically produces a sigmoidal dose–response curve (Fig. 2.2). Progressive increases in drug dose (which, for most drugs, is proportional to the plasma drug concentration) produce increasing response, but only within a relatively narrow range of dose; further increases in dose beyond this range produce little extra effect. The following characteristics of the drug response are useful in comparing different drugs:

- *Efficacy* describes the extent to which a drug can produce a target-specific response when all available receptors or binding sites are occupied (i.e. E_{max} on the dose–response curve). A full agonist can produce the maximum response of which the receptor is capable, while a partial agonist at the same receptor will have lower efficacy. *Therapeutic efficacy* describes the effect of the drug on a desired biological endpoint and can be used to compare drugs that act via different pharmacological mechanisms (e.g. loop diuretics

i 2.2 Examples of target molecules for drugs

Drug target	Description	Examples
Receptors		
Channel-linked receptors	Ligand binding controls a linked ion channel, known as 'ligand-gated' (in contrast to 'voltage-gated' channels that respond to changes in membrane potential)	Nicotinic acetylcholine receptor GABA receptor Sulphonylurea receptor
G-protein-coupled receptors (GPCRs)	Ligand binding affects one of a family of 'G-proteins' that mediate signal transduction either by activating intracellular enzymes (such as adenylate or guanylate cyclase, producing cyclic AMP or GMP, respectively) or by controlling ion channels	Muscarinic acetylcholine receptor β-adrenoceptors Dopamine receptors 5-Hydroxytryptamine (5-HT, serotonin) receptors Opioid receptors
Kinase-linked receptors	Ligand binding activates an intracellular protein kinase that triggers a cascade of phosphorylation reactions	Insulin receptor Cytokine receptors
Transcription factor receptors	Intracellular and also known as 'nuclear receptors'; ligand binding promotes or inhibits gene transcription and hence synthesis of new proteins	Steroid receptors Thyroid hormone receptors Vitamin D receptors Retinoid receptors PPARγ and α receptors
Other targets		
Voltage-gated ion channels	Mediate electrical signalling in excitable tissues (muscle and nervous system)	Na^+ channels Ca^{2+} channels
Enzymes	Catalyse biochemical reactions. Drugs interfere with binding of substrate to the active site or of co-factors	Cyclo-oxygenase ACE Xanthine oxidase
Transporter proteins	Carry ions or molecules across cell membranes	5-HT re-uptake transporter Na^+/K^+ ATPase
Cytokines and other signalling molecules	Small proteins that are important in cell signalling (autocrine, paracrine and endocrine), especially affecting the immune response	Tumour necrosis factors Interleukins
Cell surface antigens	Block the recognition of cell surface molecules that modulate cellular responses	Cluster of differentiation molecules (e.g. CD20, CD80)

(ACE = angiotensin-converting enzyme; AMP = adenosine monophosphate; ATPase = adenosine triphosphatase; GABA = γ-aminobutyric acid; GMP = guanosine monophosphate; PPAR = peroxisome proliferator-activated receptor)

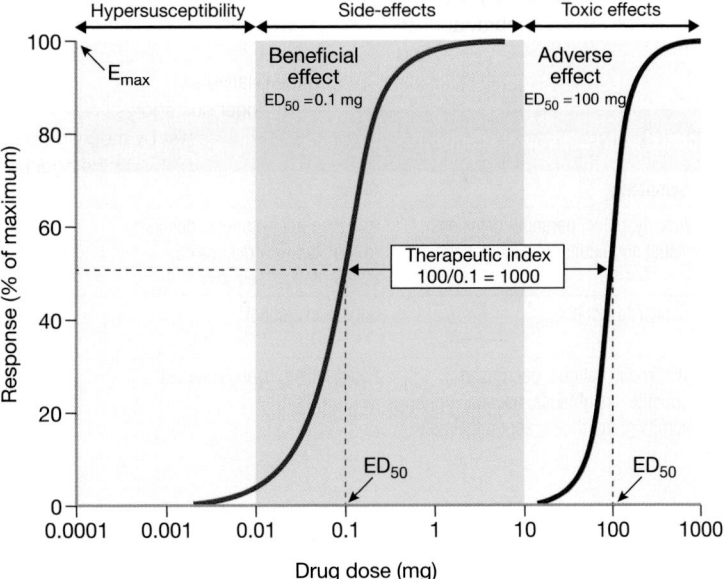

Fig. 2.2 Dose–response curve. The green curve represents the beneficial effect of the drug. The maximum response on the curve is the E_{max} and the dose (or concentration) producing half this value ($E_{max}/2$) is the ED_{50} (or EC_{50}). The red curve illustrates the dose–response relationship for the most important adverse effect of this drug. This occurs at much higher doses; the ratio between the ED_{50} for the adverse effect and that for the beneficial effect is the 'therapeutic index', which indicates how much margin there is for prescribers when choosing a dose that will provide beneficial effects without also causing this adverse effect. Adverse effects that occur at doses above the therapeutic range are normally called 'toxic effects', while those occurring within the therapeutic range are 'side-effects' and those below it are 'hyper-susceptibility effects'.

induce a greater diuresis than thiazide diuretics and so have greater therapeutic efficacy).

- *Potency* describes the amount of drug required for a given response. More potent drugs produce biological effects at lower doses, so they have a lower ED_{50}. A less potent drug can still have an equivalent or greater efficacy if it is given in higher doses.

The dose–response relationship for a specific drug varies between patients because of variations in the many determinants of pharmacokinetics and pharmacodynamics. In clinical practice, the prescriber is unable to construct a dose–response curve for each individual patient. Therefore, most drugs are licensed for use within a recommended range of doses that is expected to reach close to the top of the dose–response curve for most patients. However, it is sometimes possible to achieve the desired therapeutic efficacy at doses towards the lower end of, or even below, the recommended range.

Therapeutic index

The adverse effects of drugs are often dose-related in a similar way to the beneficial effects, although the dose–response curve for these adverse effects is normally shifted to the right (see Fig. 2.2). The ratio of the ED_{50} for therapeutic efficacy and for a major adverse effect is known as the 'therapeutic index'. In reality, drugs have multiple potential adverse effects, but the concept of therapeutic index is usually based on adverse effects that might require dose reduction or discontinuation. For most drugs, the therapeutic index is greater than 100, but there are some notable exceptions with therapeutic indices of less than 10 (e.g. digoxin, warfarin, insulin, phenytoin, opioids). The doses of such drugs have to be titrated carefully for individual patients to maximise benefits, but avoid adverse effects.

Desensitisation and withdrawal effects

Desensitisation refers to the common situation in which the biological response to a drug diminishes when it is given continuously or repeatedly. It may be possible to restore the response by increasing the dose of the drug but, in some cases, the tissues may become completely refractory to its effect.

- *Tachyphylaxis* describes desensitisation that occurs very rapidly, sometimes with the initial dose. This rapid loss of response implies depletion of chemicals that may be necessary for the pharmacological actions of the drug (e.g. a stored neurotransmitter released from a nerve terminal) or receptor phosphorylation.
- *Tolerance* describes a more gradual loss of response to a drug that occurs over days or weeks. This slower change implies changes in receptor numbers or the development of counter-regulatory physiological changes that offset the actions of the drug (e.g. accumulation of salt and water in response to vasodilator therapy).
- *Drug resistance* is a term normally reserved for describing the loss of effectiveness of an antimicrobial (p. 113) or cancer chemotherapy drug.
- In addition to these pharmacodynamic causes of desensitisation, reduced response may be the consequence of lower plasma and tissue drug concentrations as a result of altered *pharmacokinetics* (see below).

When drugs induce chemical, hormonal and physiological changes that offset their actions, discontinuation may allow these changes to cause 'rebound' withdrawal effects (Box 2.3).

Pharmacokinetics

Understanding 'what the body does to the drug' (Fig. 2.3) is extremely important for prescribers because this forms the basis on which the optimal route of administration and dose regimen are chosen and explains the majority of inter-individual variation in the response to drug therapy.

Drug absorption and routes of administration

Absorption is the process by which drug molecules gain access to the blood stream. The rate and extent of drug absorption depend on the route of administration (see Fig. 2.3).

Enteral administration

These routes involve administration via the gastrointestinal tract:

- *Oral.* This is the most common route of administration because it is simple, convenient and readily used by patients to self-administer their medicines. Absorption after an oral dose is a complex process that depends on the drug being swallowed, surviving exposure to gastric acid, avoiding unacceptable food binding, being absorbed across the small bowel mucosa into the portal venous system, and surviving metabolism by gut wall or liver enzymes

i	2.3 Examples of drugs associated with withdrawal effects			
Drug	**Symptoms**	**Signs**	**Treatment**
Alcohol	Anxiety, panic, paranoid delusions, visual and auditory hallucinations	Agitation, restlessness, delirium, tremor, tachycardia, ataxia, disorientation, seizures	Treat immediate withdrawal syndrome with benzodiazepines
Barbiturates, benzodiazepines	Similar to alcohol	Similar to alcohol	Transfer to long-acting benzodiazepine then gradually reduce dosage
Glucocorticoids	Weakness, fatigue, decreased appetite, weight loss, nausea, vomiting, diarrhoea, abdominal pain	Hypotension, hypoglycaemia	Prolonged therapy suppresses the hypothalamic–pituitary–adrenal axis and causes adrenal insufficiency requiring glucocorticoid replacement. Withdrawal should be gradual after prolonged therapy (p. 684)
Opioids	Rhinorrhoea, sneezing, yawning, lacrimation, abdominal and leg cramping, nausea, vomiting, diarrhoea	Dilated pupils	Transfer addicts to long-acting agonist methadone
Selective serotonin re-uptake inhibitors (SSRIs)	Dizziness, sweating, nausea, insomnia, tremor, delirium, nightmares	Tremor	Reduce SSRIs slowly to avoid withdrawal effects

('first-pass metabolism'). As a consequence, absorption is frequently incomplete following oral administration. The term 'bioavailability' describes the proportion of the dose that reaches the systemic circulation intact.

- *Buccal and sublingual (SL)*. These routes have the advantage of enabling rapid absorption into the systemic circulation without the uncertainties associated with oral administration (e.g. organic nitrates for angina pectoris, triptans for migraine, opioid analgesics).
- *Rectal (PR)*. The rectal mucosa is occasionally used as a site of drug administration when the oral route is compromised because of nausea and vomiting or unconsciousness (e.g. diazepam in status epilepticus).

Parenteral administration

These routes avoid absorption via the gastrointestinal tract and first-pass metabolism in the liver:

- *Intravenous (IV)*. The IV route enables all of a dose to enter the systemic circulation reliably, without any concerns about absorption or first-pass metabolism (i.e. the dose is 100% bioavailable), and rapidly achieve a high plasma concentration. It is ideal for very ill patients when a rapid, certain effect is critical to outcome (e.g. benzylpenicillin for meningococcal meningitis).
- *Intramuscular (IM)*. IM administration is easier to achieve than the IV route (e.g. adrenaline (epinephrine) for acute anaphylaxis), but absorption is less predictable and depends on muscle blood flow.
- *Subcutaneous (SC)*. The SC route is ideal for drugs that have to be administered parenterally because of low oral bioavailability, are absorbed well from subcutaneous fat and can ideally be injected by patients themselves (e.g. insulin, heparin).
- *Transdermal*. A transdermal patch can enable a drug to be absorbed through the skin and into the circulation (e.g. oestrogens, nicotine, nitrates).
- *Nasal*. The nasal mucosa provides another potential route for absorption of some drugs with systemic action (e.g. sumatriptan, calcitonin, naloxone, testosterone, desmopressin).

Other routes of administration

- *Topical* application of a drug involves direct administration to the site of action (e.g. skin, eye, ear). This has the advantage of achieving sufficient concentration at this site while minimising systemic exposure and the risk of adverse effects elsewhere.
- *Inhaled (INH)* administration allows drugs to be delivered directly to a target in the respiratory tree, usually the small airways (e.g. salbutamol, beclometasone). However, a significant proportion of the inhaled dose may be absorbed from the lung or is swallowed and can reach the systemic circulation. The most common mode of delivery is the metered-dose inhaler, but its success depends

on some degree of manual dexterity and timing (see Fig. 17.23). Patients who find these difficult may use a 'spacer' device to improve drug delivery. A special mode of inhaled delivery is via a nebulised solution created by using pressurised oxygen or air to break up solutions and suspensions into small aerosol droplets that can be directly inhaled from the mouthpiece of the device.

Drug distribution

Distribution is the process by which drug molecules transfer between the circulating blood, interstitial space and intracellular fluid. This is influenced by the drug's molecular size and lipid solubility, the extent to which it binds to proteins in plasma, its susceptibility to drug transporters expressed on cell surfaces and its binding to its molecular target and to other cellular proteins (which can be irreversible). Most drugs diffuse passively across capillary walls down a concentration gradient into the interstitial fluid until the concentration of free drug molecules in the interstitial fluid is equal to that in the plasma. As drug molecules in the blood are removed by metabolism or excretion, the plasma concentration falls and drug molecules diffuse back from the tissue compartment into the blood until eventually all are eliminated. Note that this reverse movement of drug away from the tissues will be prevented if further drug doses are administered and absorbed into the plasma.

Volume of distribution

The apparent volume of distribution (V_d) is the volume into which a drug appears to have distributed following intravenous injection. It is calculated from the equation

$$V_d = D.C_0$$

where D is the amount of drug given and C_0 is the initial plasma concentration (Fig. 2.4A). Drugs that are highly bound to plasma proteins may have a V_d below 10 L (e.g. warfarin, aspirin), while those that diffuse into the interstitial fluid but do not enter cells because they have low lipid solubility may have a V_d between 10 and 30 L (e.g. gentamicin, amoxicillin). It is an 'apparent' volume because those drugs that are lipid-soluble and highly tissue-bound may have a V_d of greater than 100 L (e.g. digoxin, amitriptyline). Drugs with a larger V_d have longer half-lives (see below), take longer to reach steady state on repeated administration and are eliminated more slowly from the body following discontinuation.

Drug elimination

Drug metabolism

Metabolism is the process by which drugs are chemically altered from a lipid-soluble form suitable for absorption and distribution to a more water-soluble form that is necessary for excretion. Some drugs, known as 'prodrugs', are inactive in the form in which they are administered, but are converted to an active metabolite in vivo.

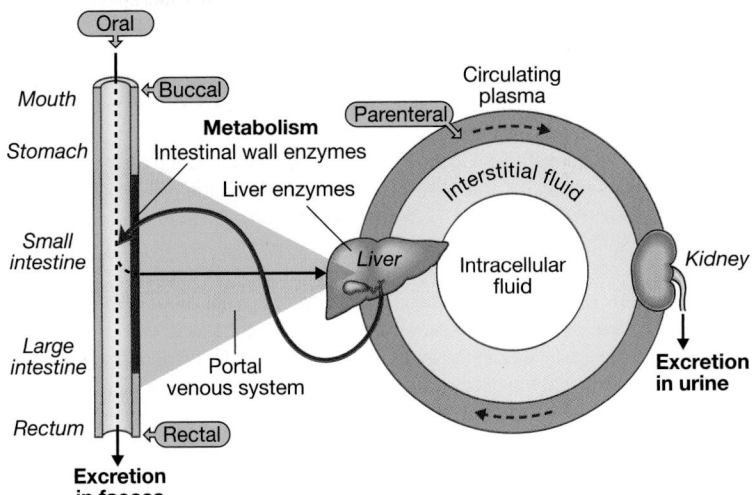

Fig. 2.3 Pharmacokinetics summary. Most drugs are taken orally, are absorbed from the intestinal lumen and enter the portal venous system to be conveyed to the liver, where they may be subject to first-pass metabolism and/or excretion in bile. Active drugs then enter the systemic circulation, from which they may diffuse (or sometimes be actively transported) in and out of the interstitial and intracellular fluid compartments. Drug that remains in circulating plasma is subject to liver metabolism and renal excretion. Drugs excreted in bile may be reabsorbed, creating an enterohepatic circulation. First-pass metabolism in the liver is avoided if drugs are administered via the buccal or rectal mucosa, or parenterally (e.g. by intravenous injection).

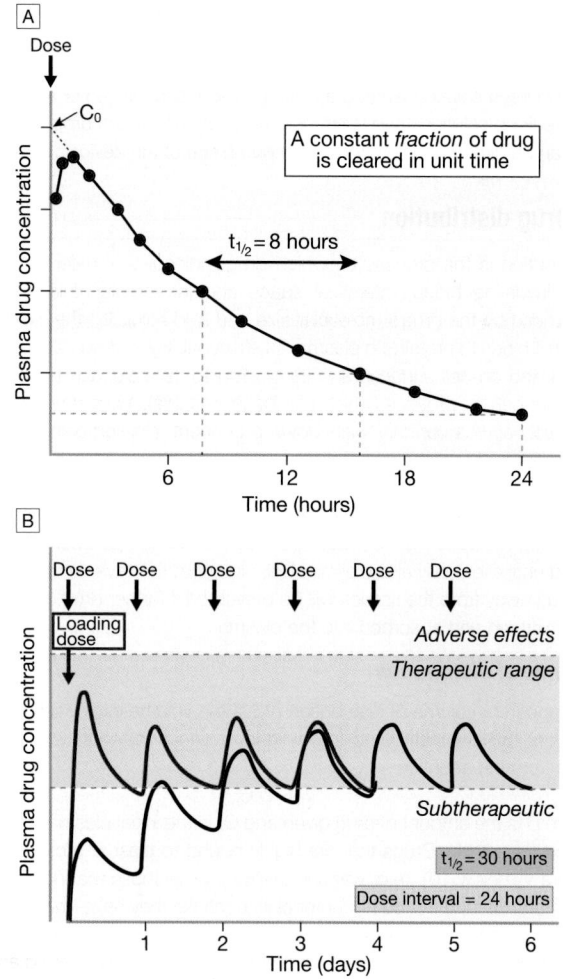

Fig. 2.4 Drug concentrations in plasma following single and multiple drug dosing. **A** In this example of first-order kinetics following a single intravenous dose, the time period required for the plasma drug concentration to halve (half-life, $t_{1/2}$) remains constant throughout the elimination process. **B** After multiple dosing, the plasma drug concentration rises if each dose is administered before the previous dose has been entirely cleared. In this example, the drug's half-life is 30 hours, so that with daily dosing the peak, average and trough concentrations steadily increase as drug accumulates in the body (black line). Steady state is reached after approximately 5 half-lives, when the rate of elimination (the product of concentration and clearance) is equal to the rate of drug absorption (the product of rate of administration and bioavailability). The long half-life in this example means that it takes 6 days for steady state to be achieved and, for most of the first 3 days of treatment, plasma drug concentrations are below the therapeutic range. This problem can be overcome if a larger loading dose (red line) is used to achieve steady-state drug concentrations more rapidly.

Phase I metabolism involves oxidation, reduction or hydrolysis to make drug molecules suitable for phase II reactions or for excretion. Oxidation is by far the most common form of phase I reaction and chiefly involves members of the cytochrome P450 family of membrane-bound enzymes in the endoplasmic reticulum of hepatocytes.

Phase II metabolism involves combining phase I metabolites with an endogenous substrate to form an inactive conjugate that is much more water-soluble. Reactions include glucuronidation, sulphation, acetylation, methylation and conjugation with glutathione. This is necessary to enable renal excretion, because lipid-soluble metabolites will simply diffuse back into the body after glomerular filtration (p. 617).

Drug excretion

Excretion is the process by which drugs and their metabolites are removed from the body.

Renal excretion is the usual route of elimination for drugs or their metabolites that are of low molecular weight and sufficiently water-soluble to avoid reabsorption from the renal tubule. Drugs bound to plasma proteins are not filtered by the glomeruli. The pH of the urine is more acidic than that of plasma, so that weakly acidic drugs (e.g. salicylates) become un-ionised and tend to be reabsorbed. Alkalination of the urine can hasten excretion (e.g. after a salicylate overdose; p. 225). For some drugs, active secretion into the proximal tubule lumen, rather than glomerular filtration, is the predominant mechanism of excretion (e.g. methotrexate, penicillins).

Faecal excretion is the predominant route of elimination for drugs with high molecular weight, including those that are excreted in the bile after conjugation with glucuronide in the liver and any drugs that are not absorbed after enteral administration. Molecules of drug or metabolite that are excreted in the bile enter the small intestine where they may, if they are sufficiently lipid-soluble, be reabsorbed through the gut wall and return to the liver via the portal vein (see Fig. 2.3). This recycling between the liver, bile, gut and portal vein is known as 'enterohepatic circulation' and can significantly prolong the residence of drugs in the body (e.g. digoxin, morphine, levothyroxine).

Elimination kinetics

The net removal of drug from the circulation results from a combination of drug metabolism and excretion and is usually described as 'clearance', i.e. the volume of plasma that is completely cleared of drug per unit time.

For most drugs, elimination is a high-capacity process that does not become saturated, even at high dosage. The rate of elimination is, therefore, directly proportional to the drug concentration because of the 'law of mass action', whereby higher drug concentrations will drive faster metabolic reactions and support higher renal filtration rates. This results in 'first-order' kinetics, when a constant fraction of the drug remaining in the circulation is eliminated in a given time and the decline in concentration over time is exponential (see Fig. 2.4A). This elimination can be described by the drug's half-life ($t_{1/2}$), i.e. the time taken for the plasma drug concentration to halve, which remains constant throughout the period of drug elimination. The significance of this phenomenon for prescribers is that the effect of increasing doses on plasma concentration is predictable – a doubled dose leads to a doubled concentration at all time points.

For a few drugs in common use (e.g. phenytoin, alcohol), elimination capacity is exceeded (saturated) within the usual dose range. This is called 'zero-order' kinetics. Its significance for prescribers is that, if the rate of administration exceeds the maximum rate of elimination, the drug will accumulate progressively, leading to serious toxicity.

Repeated dose regimens

The goal of therapy is usually to maintain drug concentrations within the therapeutic range (see Fig. 2.2) over several days (e.g. antibiotics) or even for months or years (e.g. antihypertensives, lipid-lowering drugs, thyroid hormone replacement therapy). This goal is rarely achieved with single doses, so prescribers have to plan a regimen of repeated doses. This involves choosing the size of each individual dose and the frequency of dose administration.

As illustrated in Figure 2.4B, the time taken to reach drug concentrations within the therapeutic range depends on the half-life of the drug. Typically, with doses administered regularly, it takes approximately 5 half-lives to reach a 'steady state' in which the rate of drug elimination is equal to the rate of drug administration. This applies when starting new drugs and when adjusting doses of current drugs. With appropriate dose selection, steady-state drug concentrations will be maintained within the therapeutic range. This is important for prescribers because it means that the effects of a new prescription, or dose titration, for a drug with a long half-life (e.g. digoxin – 36 hours) may not be known for a few days. In contrast, drugs with a very short half-life (e.g. dobutamine – 2 minutes) have to be given continuously by infusion, but reach a new steady state within minutes.

For drugs with a long half-life, if it is unacceptable to wait for 5 half-lives until concentrations within the therapeutic range are achieved, then an initial 'loading dose' can be given that is much larger than the maintenance dose and equivalent to the amount of drug required in the body at steady state. This achieves a peak plasma concentration close to the plateau concentration, which can then be maintained by successive maintenance doses.

'Steady state' actually involves fluctuations in drug concentrations, with peaks just after administration followed by troughs just prior to the next administration. The manufacturers of medicines recommend dosing regimens that predict that, for most patients, these oscillations result in troughs within the therapeutic range and peaks that are not high enough to cause adverse effects. The optimal dose interval is a compromise between convenience for the patient and a constant level of drug exposure. More frequent administration (e.g. 25 mg 4 times daily) achieves a smoother plasma concentration profile than 100 mg once daily, but is much more difficult for patients to sustain. A solution to this need for compromise in dosing frequency for drugs with half-lives of less than 24 hours is the use of 'modified-release' (m/r) formulations. These allow drugs to be absorbed more slowly from the gastrointestinal tract and reduce the oscillation in plasma drug concentration profile, which is especially important for drugs with a low therapeutic index (e.g. levodopa).

Inter-individual variation in drug responses

Prescribers have numerous sources of guidance about how to use drugs appropriately (e.g. dose, route, frequency, duration) for many conditions. However, this advice is based on average dose–response data derived from observations in many individuals. When applying this information to an individual patient, prescribers must take account of inter-individual variability in response. Some of this variability is predictable and good prescribers are able to anticipate it and adjust their prescriptions accordingly to maximise the chances of benefit and minimise harm. Inter-individual variation in responses also mandates that effects of treatment should be monitored (p. 35).

Some inter-individual variation in drug response is accounted for by differences in pharmacodynamics. For example, the beneficial natriuresis produced by the loop diuretic furosemide is often significantly reduced at a given dose in patients with renal impairment, while delirium caused by opioid analgesics is more likely in the elderly. However, it is differences in pharmacokinetics that more commonly account for different drug responses. Examples of factors influencing the absorption, metabolism and excretion of drugs are shown in Box 2.4.

It is hoped that a significant proportion of the inter-individual variation in drug responses can be explained by studying genetic differences in single genes ('pharmacogenetics'; Box 2.5) or the effects of multiple gene variants ('pharmacogenomics'). The aim is to identify those patients most likely to benefit from specific treatments and those most susceptible to adverse effects. In this way, it may be possible to select drugs and dose regimens for individual patients to maximise the benefit-to-hazard ratio ('personalised medicine').

Adverse outcomes of drug therapy

The decision to prescribe a drug always involves a judgement of the balance between therapeutic benefits and risk of an adverse outcome. Both prescribers and patients tend to be more focused on the former, but a truly informed decision requires consideration of both.

Adverse drug reactions

Some important definitions for the adverse effects of drugs are:

- *Adverse event*. A harmful event that occurs while a patient is taking a drug, irrespective of whether the drug is suspected of being the cause.
- *Adverse drug reaction (ADR)*. An unwanted or harmful reaction that is experienced following the administration of a drug or combination of drugs under normal conditions of use and is suspected to be related to the drug. An ADR will usually require the drug to be discontinued or the dose reduced.
- *Side-effect*. Any effect caused by a drug other than the intended therapeutic effect, whether beneficial, neutral or harmful. The term 'side-effect' is often used interchangeably with 'ADR', although the former usually implies an ADR that occurs during exposure to normal therapeutic drug concentrations (e.g. vasodilator-induced ankle oedema).
- *Hypersensitivity reaction*. An ADR that occurs as a result of an immunological reaction and often after exposure to subtherapeutic drug concentrations. These include: (1) acute anaphylaxis (p. 183) – the result of an interaction between drug antigens and immunoglobulin E (IgE) on mast cells and basophils, resulting in a release of vasoactive biomolecules (e.g. penicillin, suxamethonium); this is also known as a type I hypersensitivity reaction. (2) 'Anaphylactoid'

---

i 2.4 Patient-specific factors that influence pharmacokinetics

Age
- Drug metabolism is low in the fetus and newborn, may be enhanced in young children, and becomes less effective with age
- Drug excretion falls with the age-related decline in renal function

Sex
- Women have a greater proportion of body fat than men, increasing the volume of distribution and half-life of lipid-soluble drugs

Body weight
- Obesity increases volume of distribution and half-life of lipid-soluble drugs
- Patients with higher lean body mass have larger body compartments into which drugs are distributed and may require higher doses

Liver function
- Metabolism of most drugs depends on several cytochrome P450 enzymes that are impaired in patients with advanced liver disease
- Hypoalbuminaemia influences the distribution of drugs that are highly protein-bound

Kidney function
- Renal disease and the decline in renal function with ageing may lead to drug accumulation

Gastrointestinal function
- Small intestinal absorption of oral drugs may be delayed by reduced gastric motility
- Absorptive capacity of the intestinal mucosa may be reduced in disease (e.g. Crohn's or coeliac disease) or after surgical resection

Food
- Food in the stomach delays gastric emptying and reduces the rate (but not usually the extent) of drug absorption
- Some food constituents bind to certain drugs and prevent their absorption

Smoking
- Tar in tobacco smoke stimulates the oxidation of certain drugs

Alcohol
- Regular alcohol consumption stimulates liver enzyme synthesis, while binge drinking may temporarily inhibit drug metabolism

Drugs
- Drug–drug interactions cause marked variation in pharmacokinetics (see Box 2.12)

i	2.5 Examples of pharmacogenetic variations that influence drug response	
Genetic variant	**Drug affected**	**Clinical outcome**
Pharmacokinetic		
Aldehyde dehydrogenase-2 deficiency	Ethanol	Elevated blood acetaldehyde causes facial flushing and increased heart rate in ~50% of Japanese, Chinese and other Asian populations
Acetylation	Isoniazid, hydralazine, procainamide	Increased responses in slow acetylators, up to 50% of some populations
Oxidation (CYP2D6)	Nortriptyline Codeine	Increased risk of toxicity in poor metabolisers Reduced responses with slower conversion of codeine to more active morphine in poor metabolisers, 10% of European populations Increased risk of toxicity in ultra-fast metabolisers, 3% of Europeans but 25% of North Africans
Oxidation (CYP2C9)	Warfarin	Polymorphisms known to influence dosages
Oxidation (CYP2C19)	Clopidogrel Proguanil	Reduced enzymatic activation results in reduced antiplatelet effect Reduced efficacy with slower conversion to active cycloguanil in poor metabolisers
Sulphoxidation	Penicillamine	Increased risk of toxicity in poor metabolisers
Pseudocholinesterase deficiency	Suxamethonium (succinylcholine)	Decreased drug inactivation leads to prolonged paralysis and sometimes persistent apnoea requiring mechanical ventilation until the drug can be eliminated by alternate pathways; occurs in 1 in 1500 people
Pharmacodynamic		
Glucose-6-phosphate dehydrogenase (G6PD) deficiency	Oxidant drugs, including antimalarials (e.g. chloroquine, primaquine)	Risk of haemolysis in G6PD deficiency
Acute intermittent porphyria	Enzyme-inducing drugs	Increased risk of an acute attack
SLC01B1 polymorphism	Statins	Increased risk of rhabdomyolysis
HLA-B*5701 polymorphism	Abacavir	Increased risk of skin hypersensitivity reaction
HLA-B*5801 polymorphism	Allopurinol	Increased risk of rashes in Han Chinese
HLA-B*1502 polymorphism	Carbamazepine	Increased risk of serious dermatological reactions (e.g. Stevens–Johnson syndrome)
Hepatic nuclear factor 1 alpha (HNF1A) polymorphism	Sulphonylureas	Increased sensitivity to the blood glucose-lowering effects
Human epidermal growth factor receptor 2 (HER2)-positive breast cancer cells	Trastuzumab	Increased sensitivity to the inhibitory effects on growth and division of the target cancer cells

reactions – these present in a similar manner to acute anaphylaxis, but are a consequence of non-IgE-mediated degranulation of mast cells and basophils or direct complement activation (e.g. aspirin, non-steroidal anti-inflammatory drugs, opiates). (3) Types II–IV hypersensitivity reactions – these occur via other mechanisms, such as antibody-dependent (IgM or IgG), immune complex-mediated or cell-mediated pathways (p. 78); examples of such reactions are listed in Box 2.6.

- *Drug toxicity.* Adverse effects of a drug that occur because the dose or plasma concentration has risen above the therapeutic range, either unintentionally or intentionally (drug overdose; see Fig. 2.2 and p. 224).
- *Drug misuse.* The misuse of recreational or therapeutic drugs that may lead to addiction or dependence, serious physiological injury (such as liver damage), psychological harm (abnormal behaviour patterns, hallucinations, memory loss) or death (p. 1240).

Prevalence of ADRs

ADRs are a common cause of illness, accounting in the UK for approximately 3% of consultations in primary care, 7% of emergency admissions to hospital and affecting around 15% of hospital inpatients. Many 'disease' presentations are eventually attributed to ADRs, emphasising the importance of always taking a careful drug history (Box 2.7). Factors

accounting for the rising prevalence of ADRs are the increasing age of patients, polypharmacy (higher risk of drug interactions), increasing availability of over-the-counter medicines, increasing use of herbal or traditional medicines and the increase in medicines available via the Internet that can be purchased without a prescription from a health-care professional. Risk factors for ADRs are shown in Box 2.8.

ADRs are important because they reduce quality of life for patients, reduce adherence to and therefore efficacy of beneficial treatments, cause diagnostic confusion, undermine the confidence of patients in their health-care professional(s) and consume health-care resources.

Retrospective analysis of ADRs has shown that more than half could have been avoided if the prescriber had taken more care in anticipating the potential hazards of drug therapy. For example, non-steroidal anti-inflammatory drug (NSAID) use accounts for many thousands of emergency admissions, gastrointestinal bleeding episodes and a significant number of deaths. In many cases, the patients are at increased risk due to their age, interacting drugs (e.g. aspirin, warfarin) or a past history of peptic ulcer disease. Drugs that commonly cause ADRs are listed in Box 2.9.

Prescribers and their patients ideally want to know the frequency with which ADRs occur for a specific drug. Although this may be well characterised for more common ADRs observed in clinical trials, it is less clear for rarely reported ADRs when the total numbers of reactions and patients exposed are not known. The words used to describe frequency

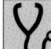

2.6 Examples of drug-mediated types I–IV hypersensitivity reactions[1]

Type I (mediated by IgE antibodies and mast cell degranulation)

Acute anaphylaxis

- Penicillins
- Chemotherapy
- Monoclonal antibodies
- Neuromuscular blocking drugs

Type II (mediated by IgM and IgG antibodies)

Haemolytic anaemia (latency less than 7 days)

- Methyldopa
- Penicillins
- Cephalosporins
- NSAIDs
- Quinidine/quinine

Neutropenia/agranulocytosis (latency days to weeks)

- Antiarrhythmics
- Antibiotics
- NSAIDs
- Antimalarials
- Antithyroid drugs
- Clozapine
- Ticlopidine

Thrombocytopenia (latency 1–2 weeks)

- Carbamazepine
- Heparin
- Penicillins
- Cephalosporins
- NSAIDs
- Quinidine/quinine
- Thiazide diuretics

Type III (mediated by immune complex deposition)

Glomerulonephritis, serum sickness, vasculitis

- Penicillins
- Cephalosporins
- Sulphonamides

Type IV (mediated by T cells)

Skin eruptions, including maculopapular rash, lichenoid or pemphigoid-like reaction, drug rash with eosinophilia and systemic symptoms (DRESS), Stevens–Johnson syndrome (SJS), toxic epidermal necrolysis (TEN)[2]

- Carbamazepine
- Abacavir
- Trimethoprim
- Dapsone

Drug-induced lupus

- Allopurinol
- Thiazide diuretics
- Hydralazine

[1]Type I is often known as 'immediate' hypersensitivity while types II–IV are known as 'delayed' hypersensitivity. [2]See also Boxes 27.34 and 27.35.

2.7 How to take a drug history

Information from the patient (or carer)

Use language that patients will understand (e.g. 'medicines' rather than 'drugs', which may be mistaken for drugs of abuse) while gathering the following information:
- Current prescribed drugs, including formulations (e.g. modified-release tablets), doses, routes of administration, frequency and timing, duration of treatment
- Other medications that are often forgotten (e.g. contraceptives, over-the-counter drugs, herbal remedies, vitamins)
- Drugs that have been taken in the recent past and reasons for stopping them
- Previous drug hypersensitivity reactions, their nature and time course (e.g. rash, anaphylaxis)
- Previous ADRs, their nature and time course (e.g. ankle oedema with amlodipine)
- Adherence to therapy (e.g. 'Are you taking your medication regularly?')

Information from GP medical records and/or pharmacist

- Up-to-date list of medications
- Previous ADRs
- Last order dates for each medication

Inspection of medicines

- Drugs and their containers (e.g. blister packs, bottles, vials) should be inspected for name, dosage and the number of dosage forms taken since dispensed

(ADR = adverse drug reaction)

2.8 Risk factors for adverse drug reactions

Patient factors

- Advanced age (e.g. low physiological reserve)
- Gender (e.g. ACE inhibitor-induced cough in women)
- Polypharmacy (e.g. drug interactions)
- Genetic predisposition (see Box 2.5)
- Hypersensitivity/allergy (e.g. β-lactam antibiotics)
- Diseases altering pharmacokinetics (e.g. hepatic or renal impairment) or pharmacodynamic responses (e.g. bladder instability)
- Adherence problems (e.g. cognitive impairment)

Drug factors

- Steep dose–response curve (e.g. insulin)
- Low therapeutic index (e.g. digoxin, cytotoxic drugs)

Prescriber factors

- Inadequate understanding of the principles of clinical pharmacology
- Inadequate knowledge of the patient
- Inadequate knowledge of the prescribed drug
- Inadequate instructions and warnings provided to patients
- Inadequate monitoring arrangements planned

(ACE = angiotensin-converting enzyme)

can be misinterpreted by patients, but widely accepted meanings include: very common (10% or more), common (1%–10%), uncommon (0.1%–1%), rare (0.01%–0.1%) and very rare (0.01% or less).

Classification of ADRs

ADRs have traditionally been classified into two major groups:

- *Type A ('augmented') ADRs.* These are predictable from the known pharmacodynamic effects of the drug and are dose-dependent, common (detected early in drug development) and usually mild. Examples include constipation caused by opioids, hypotension caused by antihypertensives and dehydration caused by diuretics.
- *Type B ('bizarre') ADRs.* These are not predictable, are not obviously dose-dependent in the therapeutic range, are rare (remaining undiscovered until the drug is marketed) and often severe. Patients

who experience type B reactions are generally 'hyper-susceptible' because of unpredictable immunological or genetic factors (e.g. anaphylaxis caused by penicillin, peripheral neuropathy caused by isoniazid in poor acetylators).

This simple classification has shortcomings, and a more detailed classification based on dose (see Fig. 2.2), timing and susceptibility (DoTS) is now used by those analysing ADRs in greater depth (Box 2.10). The AB classification can be extended as a reminder of some other types of ADR:

- *Type C ('chronic/continuous') ADRs.* These occur only after prolonged continuous exposure to a drug. Examples include osteoporosis caused by glucocorticoids, retinopathy caused by (hydroxy)chloroquine and tardive dyskinesia caused by phenothiazines.
- *Type D ('delayed') ADRs.* These are delayed until long after drug exposure, making diagnosis difficult. Examples include malignancies that may emerge after immunosuppressive treatment post-transplantation (e.g. azathioprine, tacrolimus) and vaginal cancer occurring many years after exposure to diethylstilboestrol.
- *Type E ('end-of-treatment') ADRs.* These occur after abrupt drug withdrawal (see Box 2.3).

i 2.9 Drugs that are common causes of adverse drug reactions

Drug or drug class	Common adverse drug reactions
ACE inhibitors (e.g. lisinopril)	Renal impairment Hyperkalaemia
Antibiotics (e.g. amoxicillin)	Nausea Diarrhoea
Anticoagulants (e.g. warfarin, heparin)	Bleeding
Antipsychotics (e.g. haloperidol)	Falls Sedation Delirium
Aspirin	Gastrotoxicity (dyspepsia, gastrointestinal bleeding)
Benzodiazepines (e.g. diazepam)	Drowsiness Falls
β-blockers (e.g. atenolol)	Cold peripheries Bradycardia
Calcium channel blockers (e.g. amlodipine)	Ankle oedema
Digoxin	Nausea and anorexia Bradycardia
Diuretics (e.g. furosemide, bendroflumethiazide)	Dehydration Electrolyte disturbance (hypokalaemia, hyponatraemia) Hypotension Renal impairment
Insulin	Hypoglycaemia
NSAIDs (e.g. ibuprofen)	Gastrotoxicity (dyspepsia, gastrointestinal bleeding) Renal impairment
Opioid analgesics (e.g. morphine)	Nausea and vomiting Delirium Constipation

(ACE = angiotensin-converting enzyme; NSAID = non-steroidal anti-inflammatory drug)

i 2.10 DoTS classification of adverse drug reactions

Category	Example
Dose	
Below therapeutic dose	Anaphylaxis with penicillin
In the therapeutic dose range	Nausea with morphine
At high doses	Hepatotoxicity with paracetamol
Timing	
With the first dose	Anaphylaxis with penicillin
Early stages of treatment	Hyponatraemia with diuretics
On stopping treatment	Benzodiazepine withdrawal syndrome
Significantly delayed	Clear-cell cancer with diethylstilboestrol
Susceptibility	See patient factors in Box 2.8

i 2.11 TREND analysis of suspected adverse drug reactions

Factor	Key question	Comment
*T*emporal relationship	What is the time interval between the start of drug therapy and the reaction?	Most ADRs occur soon after starting treatment and within hours in the case of anaphylactic reactions
*R*e-challenge	What happens when the patient is re-challenged with the drug?	Re-challenge is rarely possible because of the need to avoid exposing patients to unnecessary risk
*E*xclusion	Have concomitant drugs and other non-drug causes been excluded?	ADR is a diagnosis of exclusion following clinical assessment and relevant investigations for non-drug causes
*N*ovelty	Has the reaction been reported before?	The suspected ADR may already be recognised and mentioned in the SPC approved by the regulatory authorities
*D*e-challenge	Does the reaction improve when the drug is withdrawn or the dose is reduced?	Most, but not all, ADRs improve on drug withdrawal, although recovery may be slow

(ADR = adverse drug reaction; SPC = summary of product characteristics)

A teratogen is a drug with the potential to affect the development of the fetus in the first 10 weeks of intrauterine life (e.g. phenytoin, warfarin). The thalidomide disaster in the early 1960s highlighted the risk of teratogenicity and led to mandatory testing of all new drugs. Congenital defects in a live infant or aborted fetus should provoke suspicion of an ADR and a careful exploration of maternal drug exposures (including self-medication and herbal remedies).

Detecting ADRs – pharmacovigilance

Type A ADRs become apparent early in the development of a new drug. By the time a new drug is licensed and launched on to a possible worldwide market, however, a relatively small number of patients (just several hundred) may have been exposed to it, meaning that rarer but potentially serious type B ADRs may remain undiscovered. Pharmacovigilance is the process of detecting ('signal generation') and evaluating ADRs in order to help prescribers and patients to be better informed about the risks of drug therapy. Drug regulatory agencies may respond to this information by placing restrictions on the licensed indications, reducing the recommended dose range, adding special warnings and precautions for prescribers in the product literature, writing to all health-care professionals or withdrawing the product from the market.

Voluntary reporting systems allow health-care professionals and patients to report suspected ADRs to the regulatory authorities. A good example is the 'Yellow Card' scheme that was set up in the UK in response to the thalidomide tragedy. Reports are analysed to assess the likelihood that they represent a true ADR (Box 2.11). Although voluntary reporting is a continuously operating and effective early-warning system for previously unrecognised rare ADRs, its weaknesses include low reporting rates (only 3% of all ADRs and 10% of serious ADRs are ever reported), an inability to quantify risk (because the ratio of ADRs to prescriptions is unknown) and the influence of prescriber awareness on likelihood of reporting (reporting rates rise rapidly following publicity about potential ADRs).

More systematic approaches to collecting information on ADRs include 'prescription event monitoring', in which a sample of prescribers of a particular drug are issued with questionnaires concerning the clinical outcome for their patients and the collection of population statistics. Many health-care systems routinely collect patient-identifiable data on prescriptions (a surrogate marker of exposure to a drug), health-care events (e.g. hospitalisation, operations, new clinical diagnoses) and other clinical data (e.g. haematology, biochemistry). If these records can be linked, with appropriate safeguards for confidentiality and data protection, they may provide a much more powerful mechanism for assessing both the harms and benefits of drugs.

All prescribers will inevitably see patients experiencing ADRs caused by prescriptions written by themselves or their colleagues. It is important that these are recognised early. In addition to the features in Box 2.11, features that should raise suspicion of an ADR and the need to respond (by drug withdrawal, dosage reduction or reporting to the regulatory authorities) include:

- concern expressed by a patient that a drug has harmed them
- abnormal clinical measurements (e.g. blood pressure, temperature, pulse, blood glucose and weight) or laboratory results (e.g. abnormal liver or renal function, low haemoglobin or white cell count) while on drug therapy
- new therapy started that could be in response to an ADR (e.g. omeprazole, allopurinol, naloxone)
- the presence of risk factors for ADRs (see Box 2.8).

Drug interactions

A drug interaction has occurred when the administration of one drug increases or decreases the beneficial or adverse responses to another drug. Although the number of potential interacting drug combinations is very large, only a small number are common in clinical practice. Important drug interactions are most likely to occur when the affected drug has a low therapeutic index, steep dose–response curve, high first-pass or saturable metabolism, or a single mechanism of elimination.

Mechanisms of drug interactions

Pharmacodynamic interactions occur when two drugs produce additive, synergistic or antagonistic effects at the same drug target (e.g. receptor, enzyme) or physiological system (e.g. electrolyte excretion, heart rate). These are the most common interactions in clinical practice and some important examples are given in Box 2.12.

i | 2.12 Common drug interactions

Mechanism	Object drug	Precipitant drug	Result
Pharmaceutical*			
Chemical reaction	Sodium bicarbonate	Calcium gluconate	Precipitation of insoluble calcium carbonate
Pharmacokinetic			
Reduced absorption	Tetracyclines	Calcium, aluminium and magnesium salts	Reduced tetracycline absorption
Reduced protein binding	Phenytoin	Aspirin	Increased unbound and reduced total phenytoin plasma concentration
Reduced metabolism:			
CYP3A4	Amiodarone	Grapefruit juice	Cardiac arrhythmias because of prolonged QT interval (p. 418)
	Warfarin	Clarithromycin	Enhanced anticoagulation
CYP2C19	Phenytoin	Miconazole	Phenytoin toxicity
CYP2D6	Haloperidol	Fluoxetine	Haloperidol toxicity
Xanthine oxidase	Azathioprine	Allopurinol	Azathioprine toxicity
Monoamine oxidase	Catecholamines	Monoamine oxidase inhibitors	Hypertensive crisis due to monoamine toxicity
Increased metabolism (enzyme induction)	Ciclosporin	St John's wort	Loss of immunosuppression
Reduced renal elimination	Lithium	Diuretics	Lithium toxicity
	Methotrexate	NSAIDs	Methotrexate toxicity
Pharmacodynamic			
Direct antagonism at same receptor	Opioids	Naloxone	Reversal of opioid effects used therapeutically
	Salbutamol	Atenolol	Inhibits bronchodilator effect
Direct potentiation in same organ system	Benzodiazepines	Alcohol	Increased sedation
	ACE inhibitors	NSAIDs	Increased risk of renal impairment
Indirect potentiation by actions in different organ systems	Digoxin	Diuretics	Digoxin toxicity enhanced because of hypokalaemia
	Warfarin	Aspirin, NSAIDs	Increased risk of bleeding because of gastrotoxicity and antiplatelet effects
	Diuretics	ACE inhibitors	Blood pressure reduction (may be therapeutically advantageous) because of the increased activity of the renin–angiotensin system in response to diuresis

*Pharmaceutical interactions are related to the formulation of the drugs and occur before drug absorption.
(ACE = angiotensin-converting enzyme; NSAID = non-steroidal anti-inflammatory drug)

Pharmacokinetic interactions occur when the administration of a second drug alters the concentration of the first at its site of action. There are numerous potential mechanisms:

- *Absorption interactions*. Drugs that either delay (e.g. anticholinergic drugs) or enhance (e.g. prokinetic drugs) gastric emptying influence the rate of rise in plasma concentration of other drugs, but not the total amount of drug absorbed. Drugs that bind to form insoluble complexes or chelates (e.g. aluminium-containing antacids binding with ciprofloxacin) can reduce drug absorption.
- *Distribution interactions*. Co-administration of drugs that compete for protein binding in plasma (e.g. phenytoin and diazepam) can increase the unbound drug concentration, but the effect is usually short-lived due to increased elimination and hence restoration of the pre-interaction equilibrium.
- *Metabolism interactions*. Many drugs rely on metabolism by different isoenzymes of cytochrome P450 (CYP) in the liver. CYP enzyme inducers (e.g. phenytoin, rifampicin) generally reduce plasma concentrations of other drugs, although they may enhance activation of prodrugs. CYP enzyme inhibitors (e.g. clarithromycin, cimetidine, grapefruit juice) have the opposite effect. Enzyme induction effects usually take a few days to manifest because of the need to synthesise new CYP enzyme, in contrast to the rapid effects of enzyme inhibition.
- *Excretion interactions*. These primarily affect renal excretion. For example, drug-induced reduction in glomerular filtration rate (e.g. diuretic-induced dehydration, angiotensin-converting enzyme (ACE) inhibitors, NSAIDs) can reduce the clearance and increase the plasma concentration of many drugs, including some with a low therapeutic index (e.g. digoxin, lithium, aminoglycoside antibiotics). Less commonly, interactions may be due to competition for a common tubular organic anion transporter (e.g. methotrexate excretion may be inhibited by competition with NSAIDs).

Avoiding drug interactions

Drug interactions are increasing as patients are prescribed more medicines (polypharmacy). Prescribers can avoid the adverse consequences of drug–drug interactions by taking a careful drug history (see Box 2.7) before prescribing additional drugs, only prescribing for clear indications and taking special care when prescribing drugs with a narrow therapeutic index (e.g. warfarin). When prescribing an interacting drug is unavoidable, good prescribers will seek further information and anticipate the potential risk. This will allow them to provide special warnings for the patient and arrange for monitoring, either of the clinical effects (e.g. coagulation tests for warfarin) or of plasma concentration (e.g. digoxin).

Medication errors

A medication error is any *preventable* event that may lead to inappropriate medication use or patient harm while the medication is in the control of the health-care professional or patient. Errors may occur in prescribing, dispensing, preparing solutions, administration or monitoring. Many ADRs are considered in retrospect to have been 'avoidable' with more care or forethought; in other words, an adverse event considered by one prescriber to be an unfortunate ADR might be considered by another to be a prescribing error.

Medication errors are very common. Several thousand medication orders are dispensed and administered each day in a medium-sized hospital. Recent UK studies suggest that 7%–9% of hospital prescriptions contain an error, and most are written by junior doctors. Common prescribing errors in hospitals include omission of medicines (especially failure to prescribe regular medicines at the point of admission or discharge, i.e. 'medicines reconciliation'), dosing errors, unintentional prescribing and poor use of documentation (Box 2.13).

Most prescription errors result from a combination of failures by the individual prescriber and the health-service systems in which they work

i	2.13 Hospital prescribing errors	
Error type		**Approximate % of total**
Omission on admission		30
Underdose		11
Overdose		8
Strength/dose missing		7
Omission on discharge		6
Administration times incorrect/missing		6
Duplication		6
Product or formulation not specified		4
Incorrect formulation		4
No maximum dose		4
Unintentional prescribing		3
No signature		2
Clinical contraindication		1
Incorrect route		1
No indication		1
Intravenous instructions incorrect/missing		1
Drug not prescribed but indicated		1
Drug continued for longer than needed		1
Route of administration missing		1
Start date incorrect/missing		1
Risk of drug interaction		< 0.5
Controlled drug requirements incorrect/missing		< 0.5
Daily dose divided incorrectly		< 0.5
Significant allergy		< 0.5
Drug continued in spite of adverse effects		< 0.5
Premature discontinuation		< 0.5
Failure to respond to out-of-range drug level		< 0.5

(Box 2.14). Health-care organisations increasingly encourage reporting of errors within a 'no-blame culture' so that they can be subject to 'root cause analysis' using human error theory (Fig. 2.5). Prevention is targeted at the factors in Box 2.14 and can be supported by prescribers communicating and cross-checking with colleagues (e.g. when calculating doses adjusted for body weight, or planning appropriate monitoring after drug administration). Prescription errors may also be reduced by clinical pharmacist support (e.g. to check the patient's previous medications and current prescriptions) and electronic prescribing (which avoids errors due to illegibility or serious dosing mistakes and may be combined with a clinical decision support system to take account of patient characteristics and drug history, and provide warnings of potential contraindications and drug interactions).

Responding when an error is discovered

All prescribers will make errors. When they do, their first duty is to protect the patient's safety. This will involve a clinical review and the taking of any steps that will reduce harm (e.g. remedial treatment, monitoring, recording the event in the notes, informing colleagues). Patients should be informed if they have been exposed to potential harm. For errors that do not reach the patient, it is the prescriber's duty to report them, so that others can learn from the experience and take the opportunity to reflect on how a similar incident might be avoided in the future.

2

Systems factors

- Working hours of prescribers (and others)
- Patient throughput
- Professional support and supervision by colleagues
- Availability of information (medical records)
- Design of prescription forms
- Distractions
- Availability of decision support
- Checking routines (e.g. clinical pharmacy)
- Reporting and reviewing of incidents

Prescriber factors

Knowledge

- Clinical pharmacology principles
- Drugs in common use
- Therapeutic problems commonly encountered
- Knowledge of workplace systems

Skills

- Taking a good drug history
- Obtaining information to support prescribing
- Communicating with patients
- Numeracy and calculations
- Prescription writing

Attitudes

- Coping with risk and uncertainty
- Monitoring of prescribing
- Checking routines

Phase I

- Healthy volunteers (20–80)
- These involve initial single-dose, 'first-into-man' studies, followed by repeated-dose studies. They aim to establish the basic pharmacokinetic and pharmacodynamic properties, and short-term safety
- Duration: 6–12 months

Phase II

- Patients (100–200)
- These investigate clinical effectiveness ('proof of concept'), safety and dose–response relationship, often with a surrogate clinical endpoint, in the target patient group to determine the optimal dosing regimen for larger confirmatory studies
- Duration: 1–2 years

Phase III

- Patients (100s–1000s)
- These are large, expensive clinical trials that confirm safety and efficacy in the target patient population, using relevant clinical endpoints. They may be placebo-controlled studies or comparisons with other active compounds
- Duration: 1–2 years

Phase IV

- Patients (100s–1000s)
- These are undertaken after the medicine has been marketed for its first indication to evaluate new indications, new doses or formulations, long-term safety or cost-effectiveness

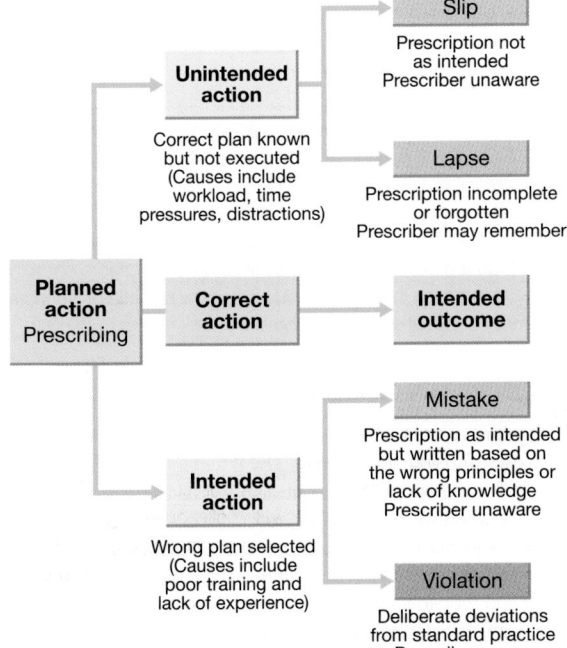

Fig. 2.5 Human error theory. Unintended errors may occur because the prescriber fails to complete the prescription correctly (a slip; e.g. writes the dose in 'mg' not 'micrograms') or forgets part of the action that is important for success (a lapse; e.g. forgets to co-prescribe folic acid with methotrexate); prevention requires the system to provide appropriate checking routines. Intended errors occur when the prescriber acts incorrectly due to lack of knowledge (a mistake; e.g. prescribes atenolol for a patient with known severe asthma because of ignorance about the contraindication); prevention must focus on training the prescriber.

Drug regulation and management

Given the powerful beneficial and potentially adverse effects of drugs, the production and use of medicines are strictly regulated (e.g. by the Food and Drug Administration in the United States, Medicines and Healthcare Products Regulatory Agency in the UK, and Central Drugs Standard Control Organisation in India). Regulators are responsible for licensing medicines, monitoring their safety (pharmacovigilance), approving clinical trials, and inspecting and maintaining standards of drug development and manufacture.

In addition, because of the high costs of drugs and their adverse effects, health-care services must prioritise their use in light of the evidence of their benefit and harm, a process referred to as 'medicines management'.

Drug development and marketing

Naturally occurring products have been used to treat illnesses for thousands of years and some remain in common use today. Examples include morphine from the opium poppy (*Papaver somniferum*), digitalis from the foxglove (*Digitalis purpurea*), curare from the bark of a variety of species of South American trees, and quinine from the bark of the *Cinchona* species. Although plants and animals remain a source of discovery, the majority of new drugs come from drug discovery programmes that aim to identify small-molecule compounds with specific interactions with a molecular target that will induce a predicted biological effect.

The usual pathway for development of these small molecules includes: identifying a plausible molecular target by investigating pathways in disease; screening a large library of compounds for those that interact with the molecular target in vitro; conducting extensive medicinal chemistry to optimise the properties of lead compounds; testing efficacy and toxicity of these compounds in vitro and in animals; and undertaking a clinical development programme (Box 2.15). This process typically takes longer than 10 years and may cost up to US$2 billion. Manufacturers have a defined period of exclusive marketing of the drug while it remains protected by an original patent, typically 10–15 years, during which time they must recoup the costs of developing the drug. Meanwhile, competitor companies will often produce similar 'me too' drugs of the same class. Once the drug's patent has expired, 'generic' manufacturers may step in to produce cheaper formulations of the drug. Paradoxically, if a generic drug is produced by only one manufacturer, the price may actually rise, sometimes substantially.

i 2.16 Novel therapeutic alternatives to conventional small-molecule drugs		
Approaches	**Therapeutic indications**	**Challenges**
Monoclonal antibodies Targeting of receptors or other molecules with relatively specific antibodies	Cancer Chronic inflammatory diseases (e.g. rheumatoid arthritis, inflammatory bowel disease)	Selectivity of action Complex manufacturing process
Small interfering RNA (siRNA) Inhibition of gene expression	Macular degeneration	Delivery to target
Gene therapy Delivery of modified genes that supplement or alter host DNA	Cystic fibrosis Cancer Cardiovascular disease	Delivery to target Adverse effects of delivery vector (e.g. virus)
Stem cell therapy Stem cells differentiate and replace damaged host cells	Parkinson's disease Spinal cord injury Ischaemic heart disease	Delivery to target Immunological compatibility Long-term effects unknown

New therapeutic agents

The traditional approach of targeting membrane-bound receptors and enzymes with small molecules (see Box 2.2) is now giving way to drug development that focuses on new targets, such as complex second-messenger systems, cytokines, nucleic acids and cellular networks (Box 2.16). These require the development of novel therapeutic agents, which are typically large molecules (e.g. human recombinant antibodies) manufactured by biological processes ('biologics') (Fig. 2.6). These present new challenges for 'translational medicine', the discipline of converting scientific discoveries into a useful medicine with a well-defined benefit–risk profile, and also for health-care providers and prescribers.

Manufacturers

There are multiple challenges at every stage of the development and quality assurance of high-quality biological products. These include the initial molecular cloning process, development of clone expression by stable cell lines, purification and characterisation procedures, performing post-translation modifications, ensuring chemical stability, deploying novel sensitive bio-analytical methods and meeting stringent regulatory expectations. There are also new hurdles to overcome in the clinical development phase, including definition of the clinical indication with linked inclusion and exclusion criteria, study design and appropriate comparator product, selecting the appropriate therapeutic dose based on interpretation of pharmacokinetic/pharmacodynamic (PK/PD) data, and addressing specific safety concerns (notably immunogenicity) that arise after exposure to large biological molecules.

Health services

Biological drugs are often much more expensive than conventional synthetic molecules because of the complex manufacturing process outlined above, but also because they often have much narrower indications for use based on specific molecular profiling of the recipients. This means that the development costs have to be recouped from a relatively smaller patient group. After the patent for the originator product expires, other manufacturers may develop similar products ('biosimilars') that have the same pharmacological actions, but are not completely identical because of inevitable differences that arise during a complex manufacturing process (e.g. glycosylation). For that reason, 'biosimilars' are not considered to be 'generic' medications, although they are usually considerably cheaper than the originator product. Nevertheless, the use of expensive biological agents is subject to particular scrutiny with regard to cost-effectiveness and health services may put additional requirements in place prior to access (e.g. failure of conventional treatments).

Prescribers

For prescribers there are some important considerations when assessing the balance of beneficial and adverse effects of biologics, for example, the use of recombinant antibodies for autoimmune inflammatory conditions. Drugs such as infliximab or adalimumab carry a significantly increased risk of infection when compared to classical disease-modifying anti-rheumatic drugs (cDMARDs) and this risk is increased by age, co-morbidities and concomitant use of other immunosuppressant drugs (e.g. glucocorticoids). Patients should be protected with appropriate vaccinations (e.g. influenza, pneumococcus) and treatment is contra-indicated in the presence of active infection (e.g. hepatitis B, tuberculosis). The increased immunogenicity of large biological molecules has two important consequences. First, there is an increased chance of immediate and delayed hypersensitivity reactions (see Box 2.6). Second, the development of anti-drug antibodies can precipitate loss of effect. A recent Cochrane review of exposure to nine commonly used biologics for up to 5 years concluded that there was a 5% absolute increase in all adverse effects combined, a 1% absolute increase in risk of serious infection, but little or no increased risk of cancer or other serious outcomes.

Licensing new medicines

New drugs are given a 'market authorisation', based on the evidence of quality, safety and efficacy presented by the manufacturer. The regulator not only will approve the drug, but also will take great care to ensure that the accompanying information reflects the evidence that has been presented. The summary of product characteristics (SPC), or 'label', provides detailed information about indications, dosage, adverse effects, warnings and monitoring requirements. If approved, drugs can be made available with different levels of restriction:

- *Controlled drug (CD)*. These drugs are subject to strict legal controls on supply and possession, usually due to their abuse potential (e.g. opioid analgesics).
- *Prescription-only medicine (PoM)*. These are available only from a pharmacist and can be supplied only if prescribed by an appropriate practitioner.
- *Pharmacy (P)*. These are available only from a pharmacist, but can be supplied without a prescription.
- *General sales list (GSL)*. These medicines may be bought 'over the counter' (OTC) from any shop and without a prescription.

Although the regulators take great care to agree the exact indications for prescribing a medicine, based on the evidence provided by the manufacturer, there are some circumstances in which prescribers may

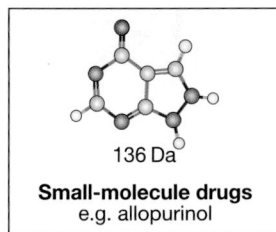

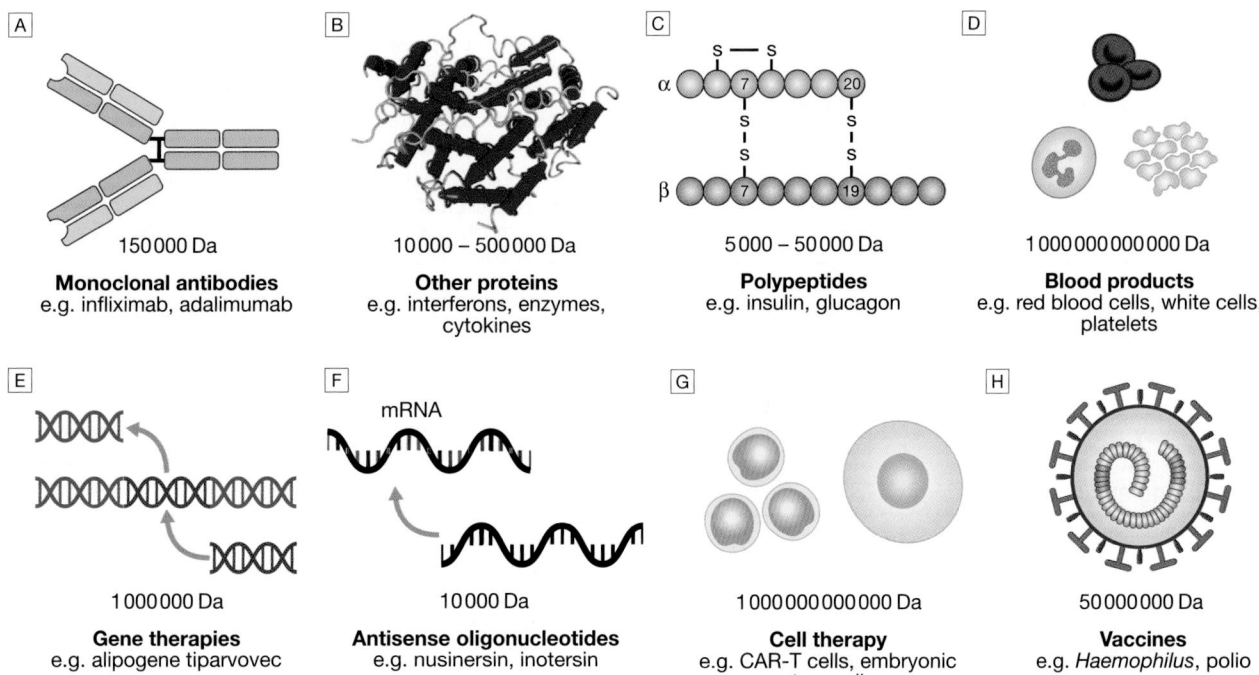

Fig. 2.6 **The mechanism of action and molecular weight of various types of biologic therapies.** [A] Monoclonal antibodies are synthesised proteins that act like human antibodies in the immune system to sequester specific molecules involved in cell signalling (e.g. TNF-alpha) or enhance the response to exogenous antigens. [B] Other proteins include analogues of cytokines involved in cell signalling and enzymes that increase the activity of metabolic pathways. [C] Polypeptides are typically analogues of endogenous peptide hormones. [D] Blood products are given as replacement for natural blood constituents. [E] Gene therapies are used to regulate, repair, replace, add to, or remove a nucleic acid sequence in native DNA. [F] Antisense oligonucleotides are short, synthetic, single-stranded oligodeoxynucleotides that can alter RNA and reduce, restore, or modify protein expression. [G] Cell therapies include injection of cells that replace damaged cells (e.g. embryonic stem cells) or manipulated immune cells that are targeted against cancer cells (e.g. CAR-T cells). [H] Vaccines are used to stimulate the immune system to respond to and remember specific antigens associated with viral or bacterial infections. (CAR-T cells = chimeric antigen recipient T cells; Da = Daltons; mRNA = messenger ribonucleic acid; TNF = tumour necrosis factor)

direct its use outside the terms stated in the SPC ('off-label' prescribing). Common situations where this might occur include prescribing outside the approved age group (e.g. prescribing for children) or using an alternative formulation (e.g. administering a medicine provided in a solid form as an oral solution). Other important examples might include prescribing for an indication for which there are no approved medicines or where all of the approved medicines have caused unacceptable adverse effects. Occasionally, medicines may be prescribed when there is no marketing authorisation in the country of use. Examples include when a medicine licensed in another country is imported for use for an individual patient ('unlicensed import') or when a patient requires a specific preparation of a medicine to be manufactured ('unlicensed special'). When prescribing is 'off-label' or 'unlicensed', there is an increased requirement for prescribers to be able to justify their actions and to inform and agree the decision with the patient.

Drug marketing

The marketing activities of the pharmaceutical industry are well resourced and are important in the process of recouping the massive costs of drug development. In some countries, such as the United States, it is possible to promote a new drug by direct-to-consumer advertising, although this is illegal in the UK and countries of the European Union. A major focus is on promotion to prescribers via educational events, sponsorship of meetings, advertisements in journals, involvement with opinion leaders and direct contact by company representatives. Such largesse has the potential to cause significant conflicts of interest and might tempt prescribers to favour one drug over another, even in the face of evidence on effectiveness or cost-effectiveness.

Managing the use of medicines

Many medicines meet the three key regulatory requirements of quality, safety and efficacy. Although prescribers are legally entitled to prescribe any of them, it is desirable to limit the choice so that treatments for specific diseases can be focused on the most effective and cost-effective options, prescribers (and patients) gain familiarity with a smaller number of medicines, and pharmacies can concentrate stocks on them.

The process of ensuring optimal use of available medicines is known as 'medicines management' or 'quality use of medicines'. It involves careful evaluation of the evidence of benefit and harm from using the medicine, an assessment of cost-effectiveness and support for processes to implement the resulting recommendations. These activities usually involve both national (e.g. National Institute for Health and Care Excellence (NICE) in the UK) and local organisations (e.g. drug and therapeutics committees).

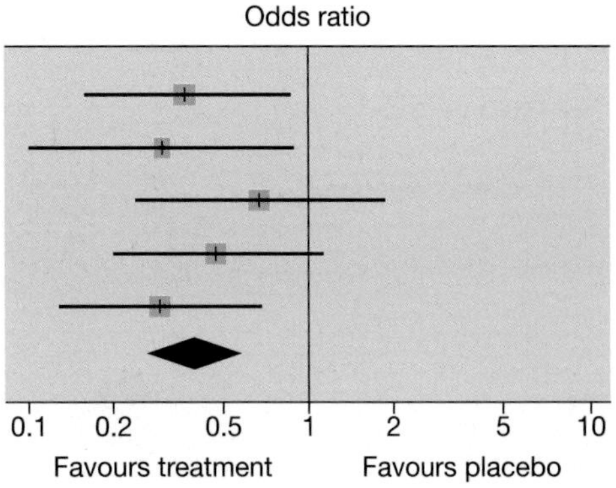

Odds ratio

Favours treatment   Favours placebo

Fig. 2.7 Systematic review of the evidence from randomised controlled clinical trials. This forest plot shows the effect of warfarin compared with placebo on the likelihood of stroke in patients with atrial fibrillation in five randomised controlled trials that passed the quality criteria required for inclusion in a meta-analysis. For each trial, the purple box is proportionate to the number of participants. The tick marks show the mean odds ratio and the black lines indicate its 95% confidence intervals. Note that not all the trials showed statistically significant effects (i.e. the confidence intervals cross 1.0). However, the meta-analysis, represented by the black diamond, confirms a highly significant statistical benefit. The overall odds ratio is approximately 0.4, indicating a mean 60% risk reduction with warfarin treatment in patients with the characteristics of the participants in these trials.

Evaluating evidence

Drugs are often evaluated in high-quality randomised controlled trials, the results of which can be considered in systematic reviews (Fig. 2.7). Ideally, data are available not only for comparison with placebo, but also for 'head-to-head' comparison with alternative therapies. Trials are conducted in selected patient populations and so may not be representative of every clinical scenario; therefore, extrapolation to individual patients is not always straightforward. Other subtle bias may be introduced because of the sources of funding (e.g. pharmaceutical industry) and the interests of the investigators in being involved in research that has a 'positive' impact. These biases may be manifest in the way the trials are conducted or in how they are interpreted or reported. A common example of the latter is the difference between relative and absolute risk of clinical events reported in prevention trials. If a clinical event is encountered in the placebo arm at a rate of 1 in 50 patients (2%), but only 1 in 100 patients (1%) in the active treatment arm, then the impact of treatment can be described as either a 50% relative risk reduction or 1% absolute risk reduction. Although the former sounds more impressive, it is the latter that is of more importance to the individual patient. It means that the number of patients that needed to be treated (NNT) for 1 to benefit (compared to placebo) was 100. This illustrates how large clinical trials of new medicines can produce highly statistically significant and impressive relative risk reductions and still predict a very modest clinical impact.

Evaluating cost-effectiveness

New drugs often represent an incremental improvement over the current standard of care, but are usually more expensive. Health-care budgets are limited in every country and so it is impossible to fund all new medicines. This means that very difficult financial decisions have to be taken with due regard to the principles of ethical justice. The main approach taken is cost-effectiveness analysis (CEA), where a comparison is made between the relative costs and outcomes of different courses of action. CEA is usually expressed as a ratio where the denominator is a gain in health and the numerator is the cost associated with the health gain. A major challenge is to compare the value of interventions for different clinical outcomes. One method is to calculate the quality-adjusted life years (QALYs) gained if the new drug is used rather than standard treatment. This analysis involves estimating the 'utility' of various health states between 1 (perfect health) and 0 (dead). If the additional costs and any savings are known, then it is

---

i   2.17 Cost-effectiveness analysis

A clinical trial lasting 2 years compares two interventions for the treatment of colon cancer:
- Treatment A: standard treatment, cost £1000/year, oral therapy
- Treatment B: new treatment, cost £6000/year, monthly intravenous infusions, often followed by a week of nausea.

The new treatment (B) significantly increases the average time to progression (18 months versus 12 months) and reduces overall mortality (40% versus 60%). The health economist models the survival curves from the trial in order to undertake a cost–utility analysis and concludes that:
- Intervention A: allows an average patient to live for 2 extra years at a utility 0.7 = 1.4 QALYs (cost £2000)
- Intervention B: allows an average patient to live for 3 extra years at a utility 0.6 = 1.8 QALYs (cost £18 000).

The health economists conclude that treatment B provides an extra 0.4 QALYs at an extra cost of £16 000, meaning that the ICER = £40 000/QALY. They recommend that the new treatment should not be funded on the basis that their threshold for cost acceptability is £30 000/QALY.

(ICER = incremental cost-effectiveness ratio; QALY = quality-adjusted life year)

---

possible to derive the incremental cost-effectiveness ratio (ICER) in terms of cost/QALY. These principles are exemplified in Box 2.17. There are, however, inherent weaknesses in this kind of analysis: it usually depends on modelling future outcomes well beyond the duration of the clinical trial data; it assumes that QALYs gained at all ages are of equivalent value; and the appropriate standard care against which the new drug should be compared is often uncertain.

These pharmacoeconomic assessments are challenging and resource-intensive, and are undertaken at national level in most countries, e.g. in the UK by NICE.

Implementing recommendations

Many recommendations about drug therapy are included in clinical guidelines written by an expert group after systematic review of the evidence. Guidelines provide recommendations rather than obligations for prescribers and are helpful in promoting more consistent and higher-quality prescribing. They are often written without concern for cost-effectiveness, however, and may be limited by the quality of available evidence. Guidelines cannot anticipate the extent of the variation between individual patients who may, for example, have unexpected contraindications to recommended drugs or choose different priorities for treatment. When deviating from respected national guidance, prescribers should be able to justify their practice.

Additional recommendations for prescribing are often implemented locally or imposed by bodies responsible for paying for health care. Most health-care units have a drug and therapeutics committee (or equivalent) comprised of medical staff, pharmacists and nurses, as well as managers (because of the implications of the committee's work for governance and resources). This group typically develops local prescribing policy and guidelines, maintains a local drug formulary and evaluates requests to use new drugs. The local formulary contains a more limited list than any national formulary (e.g. *British National Formulary*) because the latter lists all licensed medicines that can be prescribed legally, while the former contains only those that the health-care organisation has approved for local use. The local committee may also be involved, with local specialists, in providing explicit protocols for management of clinical scenarios.

Prescribing in practice

Decision-making in prescribing

Prescribing should be based on a rational approach to a series of challenges (see Box 2.1).

Making a diagnosis

Ideally, prescribing should be based on a confirmed diagnosis but, in reality, many prescriptions are based on the balance of probability, taking into account the differential diagnosis (e.g. proton pump inhibitors for post-prandial retrosternal discomfort).

Establishing the therapeutic goal

The goals of treatment are usually clear, particularly when relieving symptoms (e.g. pain, nausea, constipation). Sometimes the goal is less obvious to the patient, especially when aiming to prevent future events (e.g. ACE inhibitors to prevent hospitalisation and extend life in chronic heart failure). Prescribers should be clear about the therapeutic goal against which they will judge success or failure of treatment. It is also important to establish that the value placed on this goal by the prescriber is shared by the patient (concordance).

Choosing the therapeutic approach

For many clinical problems, drug therapy is not absolutely mandated. Having taken the potential benefits and harms into account, prescribers must consider whether drug therapy is in the patient's interest and is preferred to no treatment or one of a range of alternatives (e.g. physiotherapy, psychotherapy, surgery). Assessing the balance of benefit and harm is often complicated and depends on various features associated with the patient, disease and drug (Box 2.18).

Choosing a drug

For most common clinical indications (e.g. type 2 diabetes, depression), more than one drug is available, often from more than one drug class. Although prescribers often have guidance about which represents the rational choice for the average patient, they still need to consider whether this is the optimal choice for the individual patient. Certain factors may influence the choice of drug:

Absorption

Patients may find some formulations easier to swallow than others or may be vomiting and require a drug available for parenteral administration.

Distribution

Distribution of a drug to a particular tissue sometimes dictates choice (e.g. tetracyclines and rifampicin are concentrated in the bile, and lincomycin and clindamycin in bones).

Metabolism

Drugs that are extensively metabolised should be avoided in severe liver disease (e.g. opioid analgesics).

Excretion

Drugs that depend on renal excretion for elimination (e.g. digoxin, aminoglycoside antibiotics) should be avoided in patients with impaired renal function if suitable alternatives exist.

Efficacy

Prescribers normally choose drugs with the greatest efficacy in achieving the goals of therapy (e.g. proton pump inhibitors rather than H_2-receptor

---

i	**2.18 Factors to consider when balancing benefits and harms of drug therapy**

- Seriousness of the disease or symptom
- Efficacy of the drug
- Seriousness of potential adverse effects
- Likelihood of adverse effects
- Efficacy of alternative drugs or non-drug therapies
- Safety of alternative drugs or non-drug therapies

---

antagonists). It may be appropriate, however, to compromise on efficacy if other drugs are more convenient, safer to use or less expensive.

Avoiding adverse effects

Prescribers should be wary of choosing drugs that are more likely to cause adverse effects (e.g. cephalosporins rather than alternatives for patients allergic to penicillin) or worsen coexisting conditions (e.g. β-blockers as treatment for angina in patients with asthma).

Features of the disease

This is most obvious when choosing antibiotic therapy, which should be based on the known or suspected sensitivity of the infective organism.

Severity of disease

The choice of drug should be appropriate to disease severity (e.g. paracetamol for mild pain, morphine for severe pain).

Coexisting disease

This may be either an indication or a contraindication to therapy. Hypertensive patients might be prescribed a β-blocker if they also have left ventricular impairment, but not if they have asthma.

Avoiding adverse drug interactions

Prescribers should avoid giving combinations of drugs that might interact, either directly or indirectly (see Box 2.12).

Patient adherence to therapy

Prescribers should choose drugs with a simple dosing schedule or easier administration (e.g. the ACE inhibitor lisinopril once daily rather than captopril 3 times daily for hypertension).

Cost

Prescribers should choose the cheaper drug (e.g. a generic or biosimilar) if two drugs are of equal efficacy and safety. Even if cost is not a concern for the individual patient, it is important to remember that unnecessary expenditure will ultimately limit choices for other prescribers and patients. Sometimes a more costly drug may be appropriate (e.g. if it yields improved adherence).

Genetic factors

There are already a small number of examples where genotype influences the choice of drug therapy (see Box 2.5).

Choosing a dosage regimen

Prescribers have to choose a dose, route and frequency of administration (dosage regimen) to achieve a steady-state drug concentration that provides sufficient exposure of the target tissue without producing toxic effects. Manufacturers draw up dosage recommendations based on average observations in many patients, but the optimal regimen that will maximise the benefit to harm ratio for an individual patient is never certain. Rational prescribing involves treating each prescription as an experiment and gathering sufficient information to amend it if necessary. There are some general principles that should be followed, as described below.

Dose titration

Prescribers should generally start with a low dose and titrate this slowly upwards as necessary. This cautious approach is particularly important if the patient is likely to be more sensitive to adverse pharmacodynamic effects (e.g. delirium or postural hypotension in the elderly), if there may be altered pharmacokinetic handling (e.g. renal or hepatic impairment) and when using drugs with a low therapeutic index (e.g. benzodiazepines, lithium, digoxin). However, there are some exceptions. Some drugs must achieve therapeutic concentration quickly because of the clinical circumstance (e.g. antibiotics, glucocorticoids, carbimazole). When early effect is important, but there may be a delay in achieving steady state because of a drug's long half-life (e.g. digoxin, warfarin, amiodarone), an initial loading dose is given prior to establishing the appropriate maintenance dose (see Fig. 2.4).

i	**2.19 Factors influencing the route of drug administration**

Reason	Example
Only one route possible	Dobutamine (IV) Gliclazide (oral)
Patient adherence	Phenothiazines and thioxanthenes (2 weekly IM depot injections rather than daily tablets, in schizophrenia)
Poor absorption	Furosemide (IV rather than oral, in severe heart failure)
Rapid action	Haloperidol (IM rather than oral, in acute behavioural disturbance)
Vomiting	Phenothiazines (PR or buccal rather than oral, in nausea)
Avoidance of first-pass metabolism	Glyceryl trinitrate (SL, in angina pectoris)
Certainty of effect	Amoxicillin (IV rather than oral, in acute chest infection)
Direct access to the site of action (avoiding unnecessary systemic exposure)	Bronchodilators (INH rather than oral, in asthma) Local application of drugs to skin, eyes etc.
Ease of access	Diazepam (PR, if IV access is difficult in status epilepticus) Adrenaline (epinephrine) (IM, if IV access is difficult in acute anaphylaxis)
Comfort	Morphine (SC rather than IV in terminal care)

(IM = intramuscular; INH = by inhalation; IV = intravenous; PR = per rectum; SC = subcutaneous; SL = sublingual)

If adverse effects occur, the dose should be reduced or an alternative drug prescribed; in some cases, a lower dose may suffice if it can be combined with another synergistic drug (e.g. the immunosuppressant azathioprine reduces glucocorticoid requirements in patients with inflammatory disease). It is important to remember that the shape of the dose–response curve (see Fig. 2.2) means that higher doses may produce little added therapeutic effect and might increase the chances of toxicity.

Route

There are many reasons for choosing a particular route of administration (Box 2.19).

Frequency

Frequency of doses is usually dictated by a manufacturer's recommendation. Less frequent doses are more convenient for patients, but result in greater fluctuation between peaks and troughs in drug concentration (see Fig. 2.4). This is relevant if the peaks are associated with adverse effects (e.g. dizziness with antihypertensives) or the troughs are associated with troublesome loss of effect (e.g. anti-Parkinsonian drugs). These problems can be tackled either by splitting the dose or by employing a modified-release formulation, if available.

Timing

For many drugs the time of administration is unimportant. There are occasionally pharmacokinetic or therapeutic reasons, however, for giving drugs at particular times (Box 2.20).

Formulation

For some drugs there is a choice of formulation, some for use by different routes. Some are easier to ingest, particularly by children (e.g. elixirs). The formulation is important when writing repeat prescriptions for drugs with

a low therapeutic index that come in different formulations (e.g. lithium, phenytoin, theophylline). Even if the prescribed dose remains constant, an alternative formulation may differ in its absorption and bioavailability, and hence plasma drug concentration. These are examples of the small number of drugs that should be prescribed by specific brand name rather than 'generic' international non-proprietary name (INN).

Duration

Some drugs require a single dose (e.g. thrombolysis post-myocardial infarction), while for others the duration of the course of treatment is certain at the outset (e.g. antibiotics). For most, the duration will be largely at the prescriber's discretion and will depend on response and disease progression (e.g. analgesics, antidepressants). For many, the treatment will be long-term (e.g. insulin, antihypertensives, levothyroxine).

Involving the patient

Patients should, whenever possible, be engaged in making choices about drug therapy. Their beliefs and expectations affect the goals of therapy and help in judging the acceptable benefit/harm balance when selecting treatments. Very often, patients may wish to defer to the professional expertise of the prescriber. Nevertheless, they play key roles in adherence to therapy and in monitoring treatment, not least by providing early warning of adverse events. It is important for them to be provided with the necessary information to understand the choice that has been made, what to expect from the treatment, and any measurements that must be undertaken (Box 2.21).

A major drive to include patients has been the recognition that up to half of the drug doses for chronic preventative therapy are not taken. This is often termed 'non-compliance', but is more appropriately called 'non-adherence', to reflect a less paternalistic view of the doctor–patient relationship; it may or may not be intentional. Non-adherence to the dose regimen reduces the likelihood of benefits to the patient and can be costly in terms of wasted medicines and unnecessary health-care episodes. An important reason may be lack of concordance with the prescriber about the goals of treatment. A more open and shared decision-making process might resolve any misunderstandings at the outset and foster improved adherence, as well as improved satisfaction with health-care services and confidence in prescribers. Considerable efforts are now made to help patients to access the reliable information they require to engage more fully with clinicians. Patient-focused websites and leaflets provided by national services, local health-care providers and charities are increasingly supplementing the Patient Information Leaflet (PIL) approved by the regulatory authorities and supplied with all medicines. Fully engaging patients in shared decision-making is sometimes constrained by various factors, such as limited consultation time, language barriers and challenges in communicating complex numerical data.

Writing the prescription

The culmination of the planning described above is writing an accurate and legible prescription so that the drug will be dispensed and administered as planned (see 'Writing prescriptions' below).

Monitoring treatment effects

Rational prescribing involves monitoring for the beneficial and adverse effects of treatment so that the balance remains in favour of a positive outcome (see 'Monitoring drug therapy' below).

Stopping drug therapy

It is also important to review long-term treatment at regular intervals to assess whether continued treatment is required. Elderly patients are keen to reduce their medication burden and are often prepared to compromise on the original goals of long-term preventative therapy to achieve this.

i	**2.20 Factors influencing the timing of drug therapy**	
Drug	**Recommended timing**	**Reasons**
Diuretics (e.g. furosemide)	Once in the morning	Night-time diuresis undesirable
Statins (e.g. simvastatin)	Once at night	HMG CoA reductase activity is greater at night
Antidepressants (e.g. amitriptyline)	Once at night	Allows adverse effects to occur during sleep
Salbutamol	Before exercise	Reduces symptoms in exercise-induced asthma
Glyceryl trinitrate	When required	Relief of acute symptoms only
Paracetamol		
Regular nitrate therapy (e.g. isosorbide mononitrate)	Eccentric dosing regimen (e.g. twice daily at 8 a.m. and 2 p.m.)	Reduces development of nitrate tolerance by allowing drug-free period each night
Aspirin	With food	Minimises gastrotoxic effects
Alendronate	Once in the morning before breakfast, sitting upright	Minimises risk of oesophageal irritation
Tetracyclines	2 hours before or after food or antacids	Divalent and trivalent cations chelate tetracyclines, preventing absorption
Hypnotics (e.g. temazepam)	Once at night	Maximises therapeutic effect and minimises daytime sedation
Antihypertensive drugs (e.g. amlodipine)	Once in the morning	Blood pressure is higher during the daytime

(HMG CoA = 3-hydroxy-3-methylglutaryl-coenzyme A)

i	**2.21 What patients need to know about their medicines***	
Knowledge	**Comment**	
The reason for taking the medicine	Reinforces the goals of therapy	
How the medicine works		
How to take the medicine	May be important for the effectiveness (e.g. inhaled salbutamol in asthma) and safety (e.g. alendronate for osteoporosis) of treatment	
What benefits to expect	May help to support adherence or prompt review because of treatment failure	
What adverse effects might occur	Discuss common and mild effects that may be transient and might not require discontinuation. Mention rare but serious effects that might influence the patient's consent	
Precautions that improve safety	Explain symptoms to report that might allow serious adverse effects to be averted, monitoring that will be required and potentially important drug–drug interactions	
When to return for review	This will be important to enable monitoring	

*Many medicines are provided with patient information leaflets, which the patient should be encouraged to read.

Prescribing in special circumstances

Prescribing for patients with renal disease

Patients with renal impairment are identified by a low estimated glomerular filtration rate (eGFR < 60 mL/min/1.73 m²), based on their serum creatinine, age, sex and ethnic group (see Box 18.1). This group includes a large proportion of elderly patients. If a drug (or its active metabolites) is eliminated predominantly by the kidneys, it will tend to accumulate and so the maintenance dose must be reduced. For some drugs, renal impairment makes patients more sensitive to their adverse pharmacodynamic effects. Examples of drugs that require extra caution in patients with renal disease are listed in Box 2.22.

Prescribing for patients with hepatic disease

The liver has a large capacity for drug metabolism and hepatic insufficiency has to be advanced before drug dosages need to be modified. Patients who may have impaired metabolism include those with jaundice, ascites, hypoalbuminaemia, malnutrition or encephalopathy. Hepatic drug clearance may also be reduced in acute hepatitis, in hepatic congestion due to cardiac failure and in the presence of intra-hepatic arteriovenous shunting (e.g. in hepatic cirrhosis). There are no good tests of hepatic drug-metabolising capacity or of biliary excretion, so dosage should be guided by the therapeutic response and careful monitoring for adverse effects. The presence of liver disease also increases the susceptibility to adverse pharmacological effects of drugs. Some drugs that require extra caution in patients with hepatic disease are listed in Box 2.22.

Prescribing for older patients

The issues around prescribing in old age are discussed in Box 2.23.

Prescribing for women who are pregnant or breastfeeding

Prescribing in pregnancy should be avoided if possible to minimise the risk of adverse effects in the fetus. Drug therapy in pregnancy may, however, be required either for a pre-existing problem (e.g. epilepsy, asthma, hypothyroidism) or for problems that arise during pregnancy (e.g. morning sickness, anaemia, prevention of neural tube defects, gestational diabetes, hypertension). About 35% of women take drug

2.22 Some drugs that require extra caution in patients with renal or hepatic disease

Kidney disease	Liver disease
Pharmacodynamic effects enhanced	
ACE inhibitors and ARBs (renal impairment, hyperkalaemia) Metformin (lactic acidosis) Spironolactone (hyperkalaemia) NSAIDs (impaired renal function) Sulphonylureas (hypoglycaemia) Insulin (hypoglycaemia)	Warfarin (increased anticoagulation because of reduced clotting factor synthesis) Metformin (lactic acidosis) Chloramphenicol (bone marrow suppression) NSAIDs (gastrointestinal bleeding, fluid retention) Sulphonylureas (hypoglycaemia) Benzodiazepines (coma)
Pharmacokinetic handling altered (reduced clearance)	
Aminoglycosides (e.g. gentamicin) Vancomycin Other antibiotics (e.g. ciprofloxacin) Digoxin Lithium Atenolol Allopurinol Cephalosporins Methotrexate Opioids (e.g. morphine)	Phenytoin Rifampicin Propranolol Warfarin Diazepam Lidocaine Opioids (e.g. morphine)

(ACE = angiotensin-converting enzyme; ARB = angiotensin receptor blocker; NSAID = non-steroidal anti-inflammatory drug)

therapy at least once during pregnancy and 6% take drug therapy during the first trimester (excluding iron, folic acid and vitamins). The most commonly used drugs are simple analgesics, antibacterial drugs and antacids. Some considerations when prescribing in pregnancy are listed in Box 2.24.

Drugs that are excreted in breast milk may cause adverse effects in the baby. Prescribers should always consult the SPC for each drug or a reliable formulary when treating a pregnant woman or breastfeeding mother.

Writing prescriptions

A prescription is a means by which a prescriber communicates the intended plan of treatment to the pharmacist who dispenses a medicine and to a nurse or patient who administers it. It should be precise, accurate, clear and legible. The two main kinds of prescription are those written, dispensed and administered in hospital and those written in primary care (in the UK by a GP), dispensed at a community pharmacy and self-administered by the patient. The information supplied must include:

- the date
- the identification details of the patient
- the name of the drug
- the formulation
- the dose
- the frequency of administration
- the route and method of administration
- the amount to be supplied (primary care only)
- instructions for labelling (primary care only)
- the prescriber's signature.

Prescribing in hospital

Although primary care prescribing is increasingly electronic, many hospital prescriptions continue to be based around the prescription and administration record (the 'drug chart') (Fig. 2.8). A variety of charts are

2.23 Prescribing in old age

- **Reduced drug elimination**: partly due to impaired renal function.
- **Increased sensitivity to drug effects**: notably in the brain (leading to sedation or delirium) and as a result of comorbidities.
- **More drug interactions**: largely as a result of polypharmacy.
- **Lower starting doses and slower dose titration**: often required, with careful monitoring of drug effects.
- **Drug adherence**: may be poor because of cognitive impairment, difficulty swallowing (dry mouth) and complex polypharmacy regimens. Supplying medicines in pill organisers (e.g. dosette boxes or calendar blister packs), providing automatic reminders, and regularly reviewing and simplifying the drug regimen can help.
- **Some drugs that require extra caution, and their mechanisms**:
  Digoxin: increased sensitivity of Na^+/K^+ pump; hypokalaemia due to diuretics; renal impairment favours accumulation→increased risk of toxicity.
  Antihypertensive drugs: reduced baroreceptor function→increased risk of postural hypotension.
  Antidepressants, hypnotics, sedatives, tranquillisers: increased sensitivity of the brain; reduced metabolism→increased risk of toxicity.
  Warfarin: increased tendency to falls and injury and to bleeding from intra- and extracranial sites; increased sensitivity to inhibition of clotting factor synthesis→increased risk of bleeding.
  Amitriptyline, diltiazem, lidocaine, metoprolol, morphine, propranolol, theophylline: metabolism reduced→increased risk of toxicity.
  Non-steroidal anti-inflammatory drugs: poor renal function→increased risk of renal impairment; susceptibility to gastrotoxicity→increased risk of upper gastrointestinal bleeding.

2.24 Prescribing in pregnancy

- **Teratogenesis**: a potential risk, especially when drugs are taken between 2 and 8 weeks of gestation (4–10 weeks from last menstrual period). Common teratogens include retinoids (e.g. isotretinoin), cytotoxic drugs, angiotensin-converting enzyme inhibitors, antiepileptics (e.g. sodium valproate) and warfarin. If there is inadvertent exposure, then the timing of conception should be established, counselling given and investigations undertaken for fetal abnormalities.
- **Adverse fetal effects in late gestation**: e.g. tetracyclines may stain growing teeth and bones; sulphonamides displace fetal bilirubin from plasma proteins, potentially causing kernicterus; opioids given during delivery may be associated with respiratory depression in the neonate.
- **Altered maternal pharmacokinetics**: extracellular fluid volume and V_d increase. Plasma albumin falls but other binding globulins (e.g. for thyroid and steroid hormones) increase. Glomerular filtration increases by approximately 70%, enhancing renal clearance. Placental metabolism contributes to increased clearance, e.g. of levothyroxine and glucocorticoids. The overall effect is a fall in plasma concentration of many drugs.
- **In practice**:
  Avoid any drugs unless the risk:benefit analysis is in favour of treating (usually the mother).
  Use drugs for which there is some record of safety in humans.
  Use the lowest dose for the shortest time possible.
  Choose the least harmful drug if alternatives are available.

in use and prescribers must familiarise themselves with the local version. Most contain the following sections:

- *Basic patient information*: will usually include name, age, date of birth, hospital number and address. These details are often 'filled in' using a sticky addressograph label, but this increases the risk of serious error.
- *Previous adverse reactions/allergies*: communicates important patient safety information based on a careful drug history and/or the medical record.
- *Other medicines charts*: notes any other hospital prescription documents that contain current prescriptions being received by the patient (e.g. anticoagulants, insulin, oxygen, fluids).
- *Once-only medications*: for prescribing medicines to be used infrequently, such as single-dose prophylactic antibiotics and other pre-operative medications.

Monitoring drug therapy

Prescribers should measure the effects of the drug, both beneficial and harmful, to inform decisions about dose titration (up or down), discontinuation or substitution of treatment. Monitoring can be achieved subjectively by asking the patient about symptoms or, more objectively, by measuring a clinical effect, which may be possible to assess by clinical examination (e.g. eczematous rash), physiological measurement (e.g. blood pressure, pulse oximetry), imaging (e.g. chest X-ray, CT scan) or laboratory tests (e.g. haemoglobin, INR (International Normalised Ratio)). Alternatively, if the pharmacodynamic effects of the drug are difficult to assess, the plasma drug concentration may be measured, if this is closely related to the effect of the drug (see Fig. 2.2). Rational prescribing ultimately rests on continuous monitoring of the balance between the risks and benefits of drug therapy. Common examples are ACE inhibitors (negative impact on renal function versus blood pressure-lowering), cancer chemotherapy (bone marrow suppression versus radiological tumour regression) and disease-modifying anti-rheumatic drugs (liver toxicity versus anti-inflammatory effect). Advances in therapeutics have also led to increasing complexity of ongoing monitoring

requirements. The recognition that hospital specialist clinics cannot take on the responsibility for monitoring of all chronic disease therapy has led to the development of 'shared care protocols' that aim to share monitoring activities between specialists and primary care physicians with the aim of maximising efficient use of health-care resources and convenience for patients.

Clinical and surrogate endpoints

Ideally, clinical endpoints are measured directly and the drug dosage titrated to achieve the therapeutic goal and avoid toxicity (e.g. control of ventricular rate in a patient with atrial fibrillation, monitoring anticoagulation using INR). Sometimes this is impractical because the clinical endpoint is a future event (e.g. prevention of myocardial infarction by statins or resolution of a chest infection with antibiotics); in these circumstances, it may be possible to select a 'surrogate' endpoint that will predict success or failure. This may be an intermediate step in the pathophysiological process (e.g. serum cholesterol as a surrogate for risk of myocardial infarction) or a measurement that follows the pathophysiology, even if it is not a key factor in its progression (e.g. serum C-reactive protein as a surrogate for resolution of inflammation in chest infection, TSH as a surrogate for adequate replacement of levothyroxine). Such surrogates are sometimes termed 'biomarkers'.

Plasma drug concentration

The following criteria must be met to justify routine monitoring by plasma drug concentration:

- Clinical endpoints and other pharmacodynamic (surrogate) effects are difficult to monitor.
- The relationship between plasma concentration and clinical effects is predictable.
- The therapeutic index is low. For drugs with a high therapeutic index, any variability in plasma concentrations is likely to be irrelevant clinically.

Some examples of drugs that fulfil these criteria are listed in Box 2.26.

Measurement of plasma concentration may be useful in planning adjustments of drug dose and frequency of administration; to explain an inadequate therapeutic response (by identifying subtherapeutic concentration or incomplete adherence); to establish whether a suspected ADR is likely to be caused by the drug; and to assess and avoid potential drug interactions.

Timing of samples in relation to doses

The concentration of drug rises and falls during the dosage interval (see Fig. 2.4B). Measurements made during the initial absorption and

---

> **i** | **2.25 High-risk prescribing moments**
>
> - Trying to amend an active prescription (e.g. altering the dose/timing) – *always avoid and start again*
> - Writing up drugs in the immediate presence of more than one prescription chart or set of notes – *avoid*
> - Allowing one's attention to be diverted in the middle of completing a prescription – *avoid*
> - Prescribing 'high-risk' drugs (e.g. anticoagulants, opioids, insulin, sedatives) – *ask for help if necessary*
> - Prescribing parenteral drugs – *take care*
> - Rushing prescribing (e.g. in the midst of a busy ward round) – *avoid*
> - Prescribing unfamiliar drugs – *consult the formulary and ask for help if necessary*
> - Transcribing multiple prescriptions from an expired chart to a new one – *take care to review the rationale for each medicine*
> - Writing prescriptions based on information from another source such as a referral letter (the list may contain errors and some of the medicines may be the cause of the patient's illness) – *review the justification for each as if it is a new prescription*
> - Writing up 'to take out' drugs (because these will become the patient's regular medication for the immediate future) – *take care and seek advice if necessary*
> - Calculating drug doses – *ask a colleague to perform an independent calculation or use approved electronic dose calculators*
> - Prescribing sound-alike or look-alike drugs (e.g. chlorphenamine and chlorpromazine) – *take care*

> **i** | **2.26 Drugs commonly monitored by plasma drug concentration**
>
> | Drug | Half-life (hrs)* | Comment |
> | --- | --- | --- |
> | Digoxin | 36 | Steady state takes several days to achieve. Samples should be taken 6 hrs post dose. Measurement is useful to confirm the clinical impression of toxicity or non-adherence but clinical effectiveness is better assessed by ventricular heart rate. Risk of toxicity increases progressively at concentrations > 1.5 μg/L, and is likely at concentrations > 3.0 μg/L (toxicity is more likely in the presence of hypokalaemia) |
> | Gentamicin | 2 | Measure pre-dose trough concentration (should be < 1 mg/L) to ensure that accumulation (and the risk of nephrotoxicity and ototoxicity) is avoided; see Fig. 6.18 |
> | Lithium | 24 | Steady state takes several days to achieve. Samples should be taken 12 hrs post dose. Target range 0.4–1 mmol/L |
> | Phenytoin | 24 | Measure pre-dose trough concentration (should be 10–20 mg/L) to ensure that accumulation is avoided. Good correlation between concentration and toxicity. Concentration may be misleading in the presence of hypoalbuminaemia |
> | Theophylline (oral) | 6 | Steady state takes 2–3 days to achieve. Samples should be taken 6 hrs post dose. Target concentration is 10–20 mg/L but its relationship with bronchodilator effect and adverse effects is variable |
> | Vancomycin | 6 | Measure pre-dose trough concentration (should be 10–15 mg/L) to ensure clinical efficacy and that accumulation and the risk of nephrotoxicity are avoided |
>
> *Half-lives vary considerably with different formulations and between patients.

distribution phases are unpredictable because of the rapidly changing concentration, so samples are usually taken at the end of the dosage interval (a 'trough' or 'pre-dose' concentration). This measurement is normally made in steady state, which usually takes 5 half-lives to achieve after the drug is introduced or the dose changed (unless a loading dose has been given).

Interpreting the result

A target range is provided for many drugs, based on average thresholds for therapeutic benefit and toxicity. Inter-individual variability means that these can be used only as a guide. For instance, in a patient who describes symptoms that could be consistent with toxicity, but has a drug concentration in the top half of the target range, toxic effects should still be suspected. Another important consideration is that some drugs are heavily protein-bound (e.g. phenytoin), but only the unbound drug is pharmacologically active. Patients with hypoalbuminaemia may, therefore, have a therapeutic or even toxic concentration of unbound drug, despite a low 'total' concentration.

Further information

Websites

bnf.org *The British National Formulary (BNF) is a key reference resource for UK NHS prescribers, with a list of licensed drugs, chapters on prescribing in renal failure, liver disease, pregnancy and during breastfeeding, and appendices on drug interactions.*

cochrane.org *The Cochrane Collaboration is a leading international body that provides evidence-based reviews (around 7000 so far).*

evidence.nhs.uk *NHS Evidence provides a wide range of health information relevant to delivering quality patient care.*

icp.org.nz *The Interactive Clinical Pharmacology site is designed to increase understanding of principles in clinical pharmacology.*

medicines.org.uk/emc/ *The electronic medicines compendium (emc) contains up-to-date, easily accessible information about medicines licensed by the UK Medicines and Healthcare Products Regulatory Agency (MHRA) and the European Medicines Agency (EMA).*

nice.org.uk *The UK National Institute for Health and Care Excellence makes recommendations to the UK NHS on new and existing medicines, treatments and procedures.*

who.int/health-topics/medicines *The World Health Organization Essential Medicines and Pharmaceutical Policies.*

K Tatton-Brown

3

Clinical genetics

We have entered a genomic era. Powerful new technologies are driving forward transformational change in health care. Genetic sequencing has evolved from the targeted sequencing of a single gene to the parallel sequencing of multiple genes. In addition to improving the chances of identifying a genetic cause of rare diseases, these technologies are increasingly directing therapies and, in the future, are likely to be used in the diagnosis and prevention of common diseases such as diabetes. In this chapter we explore the fundamentals of genomics, the basic principles underlying these new genomic technologies and how the data generated can be applied safely for patient benefit. We will review the use of genomic technology across a breadth of medical specialties, including obstetrics, paediatrics, oncology and infectious disease, and consider how health care is being transformed by these new genomic technologies. Finally, we will consider the ethical impact that these technologies are likely to have, both for the individual and for their wider family.

The fundamental principles of genomics

The packaging of genes: DNA, chromatin and chromosomes

Genes are functional units encoded in double-stranded deoxyribonucleic acid (DNA), packaged as chromosomes and located in the nucleus of the cell: a membrane-bound compartment found in all cells except erythrocytes and platelets (Fig. 3.1). DNA consists of a linear sequence of just four

bases: adenine (A,) cytosine (C), thymine (T) and guanine (G.) It forms a 'double helix', a twisted ladder-like structure formed from two complementary strands of DNA joined by hydrogen bonds between bases on the opposite strand that can form only between a C and a G base and an A and a T base. It is this feature of DNA that enables faithful DNA replication and is the basis for many of the technologies designed to interrogate the genome: when the DNA double helix 'unzips', one strand can act as a template for the creation of an identical strand.

A single copy of the human genome comprises approximately 3.1 billion base pairs of DNA, wound around proteins called histones. The unit consisting of 147 base pairs wrapped around four different histone proteins is called the nucleosome. Sequences of nucleosomes (resembling a string of beads) are wound and packaged to form chromatin: tightly wound, densely packed chromatin is called heterochromatin and open, less tightly wound chromatin is called euchromatin.

The chromatin is finally packaged into the chromosomes. Humans are diploid organisms: the nucleus contains two copies of the genome, visible microscopically as 23 chromosome pairs (known as the karyotype). Chromosomes 1 through to 22 are known as the autosomes and consist of identical chromosome pairs. The 23rd 'pair' of chromosomes are the two sex chromosomes: females have two X chromosomes and males an X and Y chromosome. A normal female karyotype is therefore written as 46,XX and a normal male is 46,XY.

From DNA to protein

Genes are functional elements on the chromosome that are capable of transmitting information from the DNA template via the production of messenger ribonucleic acid (mRNA) to the production of proteins. The human genome contains over 20000 genes, although many of these are inactive or silenced in different cell types, reflecting the variable gene expression responsible for cell-specific characteristics. The central dogma is the pathway describing the basic steps of protein production: transcription, splicing, translation and protein modification (Fig. 3.2). Although this is now recognised as an over-simplification (contrary to this linear relationship, a single gene will often encode many different proteins), it remains a useful starting point to explore protein production.

Transcription: DNA to messenger RNA

Transcription describes the production of ribonucleic acid (RNA) from the DNA template. For transcription to commence, an enzyme called RNA polymerase binds to a segment of DNA at the start of the gene: the promoter. Once bound, RNA polymerase moves along one strand of DNA, producing an RNA molecule complementary to the DNA template. In protein-coding genes this is known as messenger RNA (mRNA). A DNA sequence close to the end of the gene, called the polyadenylation signal, acts as a signal for termination of the RNA transcript (Fig. 3.3).

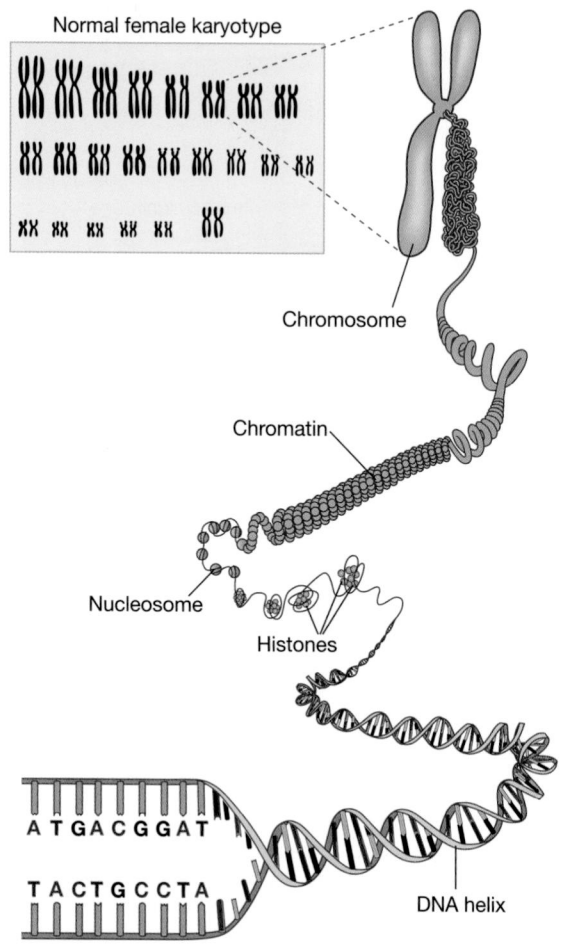

Fig. 3.1 **The packaging of DNA, genes and chromosomes.** From bottom to top: the double helix and the complementary DNA bases; chromatin; and a normal female chromosome pattern – the karyotype.

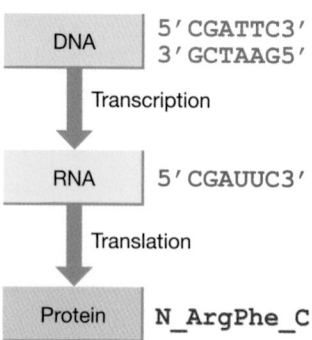

Fig. 3.2 **The central dogma of protein production.** Double-stranded DNA as a template for single-stranded RNA, which codes for the production of a peptide chain of amino acids. Each of these chains has an orientation. For DNA and RNA, this is 5′ to 3′. For peptides, this is N-terminus to C-terminus.

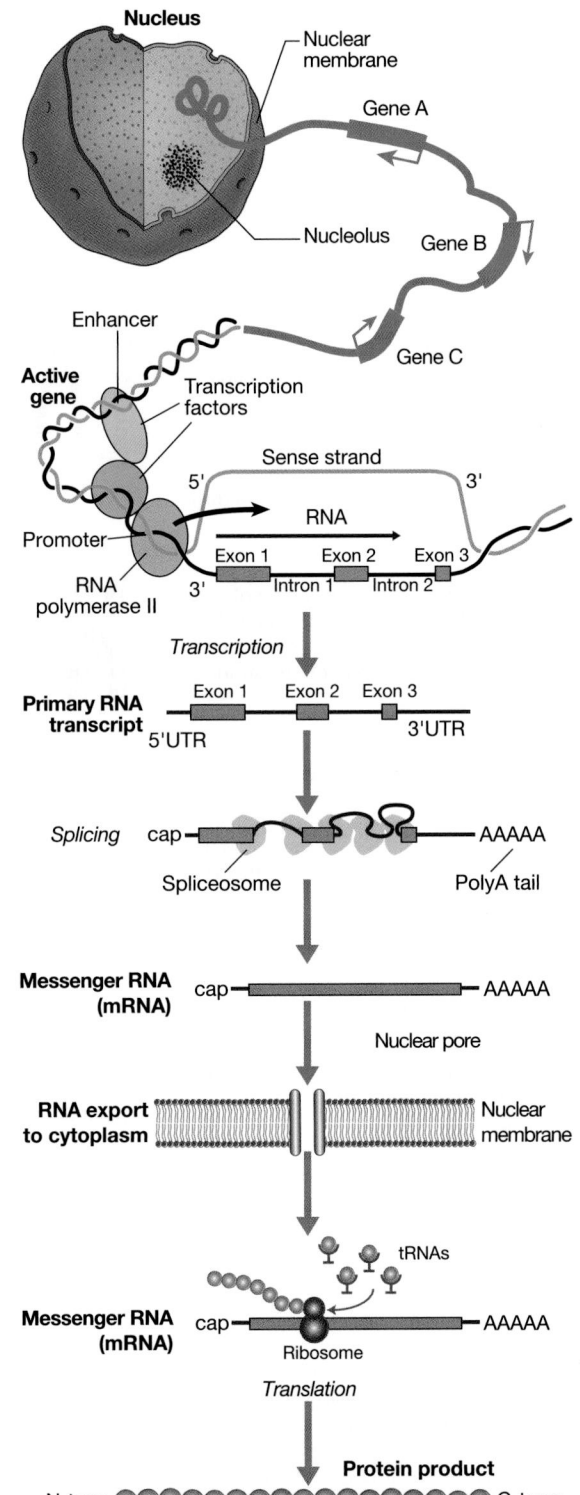

Fig. 3.3 RNA synthesis and its translation into protein. Gene transcription involves binding of RNA polymerase II to the promoter of genes being transcribed with other proteins (transcription factors) that regulate the transcription rate. The primary RNA transcript is a copy of the whole gene and includes both introns and exons, but the introns are removed within the nucleus by splicing and the exons are joined to form the messenger RNA (mRNA). Prior to export from the nucleus, a methylated guanosine nucleotide is added to the 5′ end of the RNA ('cap') and a string of adenine nucleotides is added to the 3′ ('polyA tail'). This protects the RNA from degradation and facilitates transport into the cytoplasm. In the cytoplasm, the mRNA binds to ribosomes and forms a template for protein production. (tRNA = transfer RNA; UTR = untranslated region)

RNA differs from DNA in three main ways:

- RNA is single-stranded.
- The sugar residue within the nucleotide is ribose, rather than deoxyribose.
- It contains uracil (U) in place of thymine (T).

The activity of RNA polymerase is regulated by transcription factors. These proteins bind to specific DNA sequences at the promoter or to enhancer elements that may be many thousands of base pairs away from the promoter; a loop in the chromosomal DNA brings the enhancer close to the promoter, enabling the bound proteins to interact. The human genome encodes more than 1200 different transcription factors. Mutations (now more frequently referred to as gene variants) within transcription factors, promoters and enhancers can cause disease. For example, the blood disorder alpha-thalassaemia is usually caused by gene deletions (see Box 3.4). However, it can also result from a variant in an enhancer located more than 100 000 base pairs (bp) from the α-globin gene promoter, leading to greatly reduced transcription.

Gene activity, or expression, is influenced by a number of complex interacting factors, including the accessibility of the gene promoter to transcription factors. DNA can be modified by the addition of a methyl group to cytosine molecules (methylation). If DNA methylation occurs in promoter regions, transcription is silenced, as methyl cytosines are usually not available for transcription factor binding. A second mechanism determining promoter accessibility is the structural configuration of chromatin. In open chromatin, called euchromatin, gene promoters are accessible to RNA polymerase and transcription factors; therefore it is transcriptionally active. This contrasts with heterochromatin, which is densely packed and transcriptionally silent. The chromatin configuration is determined by modifications (such as methylation or acetylation) of specific amino acid residues of histone protein tails.

Modifications of DNA and histone protein tails are termed epigenetic ('epi-' meaning 'above' the genome), as they do not alter the primary sequence of the DNA code but have biological significance in chromosomal function. Abnormal epigenetic changes are increasingly recognised as important events in the progression of cancer, allowing expression of normally silenced genes that result in cancer cell de-differentiation and proliferation. They also afford therapeutic targets. For instance, the histone deacetylase inhibitor vorinostat has been successfully used to treat cutaneous T-cell lymphoma, due to the re-expression of genes that had previously been silenced in the tumour. These genes encode transcription factors that promote T-cell differentiation as opposed to proliferation, thereby causing tumour regression.

RNA splicing, editing and degradation

Transcription produces an RNA molecule that is a copy of the whole gene, termed the primary or nascent transcript. This nascent transcript then undergoes splicing, whereby regions not required to make protein (the intronic regions) are removed while those segments that are necessary for protein production (the exonic regions) are retained and rejoined.

Splicing is a highly regulated process that is carried out by a multimeric protein complex called the spliceosome. Following splicing, the mRNA molecule is exported from the nucleus and used as a template for protein synthesis. Many genes produce more than one form of mRNA (and thus protein) by a process termed alternative splicing, in which different combinations of exons are joined together. Different proteins from the same gene can have entirely distinct functions. For example, in thyroid C cells the calcitonin gene produces mRNA encoding the osteoclast inhibitor calcitonin, but in neurons the same gene produces an mRNA with a different complement of exons via alternative splicing that encodes a neurotransmitter, calcitonin-gene-related peptide.

Translation and protein production

Following splicing, the segment of mRNA containing the code that directs synthesis of a protein product is called the open reading frame (ORF). The inclusion of a particular amino acid in the protein is specified by a codon composed of three contiguous bases. There are 64 different codons with some redundancy in the system: 61 codons encode one of the 20 amino acids, and the remaining three codons – UAA, UAG and UGA (known as stop codons) – cause termination of the growing polypeptide chain. ORFs in humans most commonly start with the amino acid methionine. All mRNA molecules have domains before and after the ORF called the 5′ untranslated region (UTR) and 3′UTR, respectively. The start of the 5′UTR contains a cap structure that protects mRNA from enzymatic degradation, and other elements within the 5′UTR are required for efficient translation. The 3′UTR also contains elements that regulate efficiency of translation and mRNA stability, including a stretch of adenine bases known as a polyA tail (see Fig. 3.3).

The mRNAs then leave the nucleus via nuclear pores and associate with ribosomes, the sites of protein production (see Fig. 3.3). Each ribosome consists of two subunits (40S and 60S), which comprise non-coding rRNA molecules (see Fig. 3.9) complexed with proteins. During translation, a different RNA molecule known as transfer RNA (tRNA) binds to the ribosome. The tRNAs deliver amino acids to the ribosome so that the newly synthesised protein can be assembled in a stepwise fashion. Individual tRNA molecules bind a specific amino acid and 'read' the mRNA ORF via an 'anticodon' of three nucleotides that is complementary to the codon in mRNA (see Fig. 3.3). A proportion of ribosomes is bound to the membrane of the endoplasmic reticulum (ER), a complex tubular structure that surrounds the nucleus.

Proteins synthesised on these ribosomes are translocated into the lumen of the ER, where they undergo folding and processing. From here, the protein may be transferred to the Golgi apparatus, where it undergoes post-translational modifications, such as glycosylation (covalent attachment of sugar moieties), to form the mature protein that can be exported into the cytoplasm or packaged into vesicles for secretion. The clinical importance of post-translational modification of proteins is shown by the severe developmental, neurological, haemostatic and soft tissue abnormalities that are associated with the many different congenital disorders of glycosylation. Post-translational modifications can also be disrupted by the synthesis of proteins with abnormal amino acid sequences. For example, the most common *CFTR* gene variant that causes cystic fibrosis (ΔF508) results in an abnormal protein that cannot be exported from the ER and Golgi (see Box 3.4).

Non-coding RNA

Approximately 4500 genes in humans encode non-coding RNAs (ncRNA) rather than proteins. There are various categories of ncRNA, including transfer RNA (tRNA), ribosomal RNA (rRNA), ribozymes and microRNA (miRNA). The miRNAs, which number over 1000, have a role in post-translational gene expression: they bind to mRNAs, typically in the 3′UTR, promoting target mRNA degradation and gene silencing. Together, miRNAs affect over half of all human genes and have important roles in normal development, cancer and common degenerative disorders. This is the subject of considerable research interest at present.

Cell division, differentiation and migration

In normal tissues, molecules such as hormones, growth factors and cytokines provide the signal to activate the cell cycle: a controlled programme of biochemical events that culminates in cell division. In all cells of the body, except the gametes (the sperm and egg cells, also known as the germ line), mitosis completes cell division, resulting in two diploid daughter cells. In contrast, the sperm and eggs cells complete cell division with meiosis, resulting in four haploid daughter cells (Fig. 3.4).

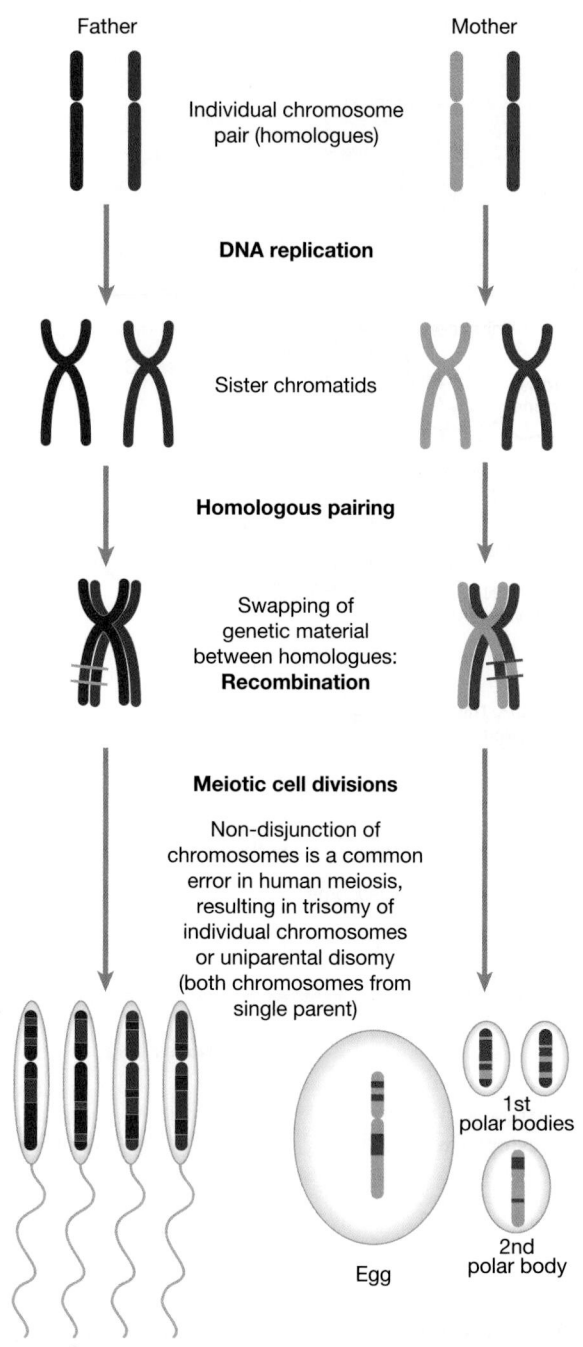

Fig. 3.4 Meiosis and gametogenesis: the main chromosomal stages of meiosis in both males and females. A single homologous pair of chromosomes is represented in different colours. The final step is the production of haploid germ cells. Each round of meiosis in the male results in four sperm cells; in the female, however, only one egg cell is produced, as the other divisions are sequestered on the periphery of the mature egg as peripheral polar bodies.

The stages of cell division in the non-germ-line, somatic cells are shown below:

- Cells not committed to mitosis are said to be in G_0.
- Cells committed to mitosis must go through the preparatory phase of interphase consisting of G_1, S and G_2:
  - G_1 (first gap): synthesis of the cellular components necessary to complete cell division
  - S (synthesis): DNA replication producing identical copies of each chromosome called the sister chromatids

- G$_2$ (second gap): repair of any errors in the replicated DNA before proceeding to mitosis.
- *Mitosis* (M) consists of four phases:
  - Prophase: the chromosomes condense and become visible, the centrioles move to opposite ends of the cell and the nuclear membrane disappears.
  - Metaphase: the centrioles complete their migration to opposite ends of the cell and the chromosomes – consisting of two identical sister chromatids – line up at the equator of the cell.
  - Anaphase: spindle fibres attach to the chromosome and pull the sister chromatids apart.
  - Telophase: the chromosomes decondense, the nuclear membrane reforms and two daughter cells – each with 46 chromosomes – are formed.

The progression from one phase to the next is tightly controlled by cell-cycle checkpoints. For example, the checkpoint between G$_2$ and mitosis ensures that all damaged DNA is repaired prior to segregation of the chromosomes. Failure of these control processes is a crucial driver in the pathogenesis of cancer, as discussed on page 130.

- *Meiosis* is a special, gamete-specific, form of cell division (see Fig. 3.4). Like mitosis, meiosis consists of four phases (prophase, metaphase, anaphase and telophase) but differs from mitosis in the following ways:
  - It consists of two separate cell divisions known as meiosis I and meiosis II.
  - It reduces the chromosome number from the diploid to the haploid number via a tetraploid stage, i.e. from 46 to 92 (MI S) to 46 (MI M) to 23 (MII M) chromosomes, so that when a sperm cell fertilises the egg, the resulting zygote will return to a diploid, 46, chromosome complement. This reduction to the haploid number occurs at the end of meiosis II.
  - The 92 chromosome stage consists of 23 homologous pairs of sister chromatids, which then swap genetic material, a process known as recombination. This occurs at the end of MI prophase and ensures that the chromosome that a parent passes to his or her offspring is a mix of the chromosomes that the parent inherited from his or her own mother and father.

The individual steps in meiotic cell division are similar in males and females. However, the timing of the cell divisions is very different. In females, meiosis begins in fetal life but does not complete until after ovulation. A single meiotic cell division can thus take more than 40 years to complete. As women become older, the separation of chromosomes at meiosis II becomes less efficient. That is why the risk of trisomies (p. 42) due to non-disjunction grows greater with increasing maternal age. In males, meiotic division does not begin until puberty and continues throughout life. In the testes, both meiotic divisions are completed in a matter of days.

Cell death, apoptosis and senescence

With the exception of stem cells, human cells have only a limited capacity for cell division. The Hayflick limit is the number of divisions a cell population can go through in culture before division stops and enters a state known as senescence. This 'biological clock' is of great interest in the study of the normal ageing process. Rare human diseases associated with premature ageing, called progeric syndromes, have been very helpful in identifying the importance of DNA repair mechanisms in senescence. For example, in Werner syndrome, a DNA helicase (an enzyme that separates the two DNA strands) is mutated, leading to failure of DNA repair and premature ageing. A distinct mechanism of cell death is seen in apoptosis, or programmed cell death.

Apoptosis is an active process that occurs in normal tissues and plays an important role in development, tissue remodelling and the immune response. The signal that triggers apoptosis is specific to each tissue or cell type. This signal activates enzymes, called caspases, which actively destroy cellular components, including chromosomal DNA. This degradation results in cell death, but the cellular corpse contains characteristic vesicles called apoptotic bodies. The corpse is then recognised and removed by phagocytic cells of the immune system, such as macrophages, in a manner that does not provoke an inflammatory response.

A third mechanism of cell death is necrosis. This is a pathological process in which the cellular environment loses one or more of the components necessary for cell viability. Hypoxia is probably the most common cause of necrosis.

Genomics, health and disease

Classes of genetic variant

There are many different classes of variation in the human genome, categorised by the size of the DNA segment involved and/or by the mechanism giving rise to the variation.

Nucleotide substitutions

The substitution of one nucleotide for another is the most common type of genomic variation. This is caused by misincorporation of a nucleotide during DNA synthesis or by chemical modification of the base. When these substitutions occur within ORFs of a protein-coding gene, they are further classified into:

- *synonymous* – resulting in a change in the codon without altering the amino acid
- *non-synonymous* (also known as a missense variant) – resulting in a change in the codon and the encoded amino acid
- *stop gain* (or *nonsense variant*) – introducing a premature stop codon and resulting in truncation of the protein
- *splicing* – disruption of normal splicing and therefore most frequently occurring at the junctions between an intron and an exon.

These different types of gene variants are illustrated in Box 3.1 and examples are shown in Figs. 3.5 and 3.6.

Insertions and deletions

One or more nucleotides may be inserted or lost in a DNA sequence, resulting in an insertion/deletion (indel) variant (see Box 3.1 and Fig. 3.5). If a multiple of three nucleotides is involved, this is in-frame. If an indel change affects one or two nucleotides within the ORF of a protein-coding gene, this can have serious consequences because the triple nucleotide sequence of the codons is disrupted, resulting in a frameshift variant. The effect on the gene is typically severe because the amino acid sequence is totally disrupted.

Simple tandem repeat variants

Variations in the length of simple tandem repeats of DNA are thought to arise as the result of slippage of DNA during meiosis and are termed microsatellite (small) or minisatellite (larger) repeats. These repeats are unstable and can expand or contract in different generations. This instability is proportional to the size of the original repeat, in that longer repeats tend to be more unstable. Many microsatellites and minisatellites occur in introns or in chromosomal regions between genes and have no obvious adverse effects. However, some genetic diseases are caused by microsatellite repeats that result in duplication of amino acids within the affected gene product or affect gene expression (Box 3.2).

3.1 Classes of genetic variant

The classes of genetic variant can be illustrated using the sentence
'THE FAT FOX WAS ILL COS SHE ATE THE OLD CAT'

Synonymous

Silent polymorphism with no amino acid change	THE FAT FOX WAS ILL COS SHE ATE THE OLD KAT where the C is replaced with a K but the meaning remains the same

Non-synonymous

Causing an amino acid change	THE FAT BOX WAS ILL COS SHE ATE THE OLD CAT where the F of FOX is replaced by B and the original meaning of the sentence is lost

Stop-gain (also called a nonsense variant)

Causing the generation of a premature stop codon	THE CAT where the F of FAT is replaced by a C, generating a premature stop codon

Indel

Where the bases are either inserted or deleted; disruption of the reading frame is dependent on the number of bases inserted or deleted	THE FAT FOX WAS ILL ILL COS SHE ATE THE OLD CAT where the insertion of three bases results in maintenance of the reading frame THE FAT FOX WAW ASI LLC OSS HEA TET HEO LDC AT where the insertion of two bases results in disruption of the reading frame

Copy number variations

Variation in the number of copies of an individual segment of the genome from the usual diploid (two copies) content can be categorised by the size of the segment involved. Rarely, individuals may gain (trisomy) or lose (monosomy) a whole chromosome. Such numerical chromosome anomalies most commonly occur by a process known as non-disjunction, where pairs of homologous chromosomes do not separate at meiosis II (p. 40). Common trisomies include Down syndrome (trisomy 21), Edwards syndrome (trisomy 18) and Patau syndrome (trisomy 13). Monosomy of the autosomes (present in all the cells, as opposed to in a

mosaic distribution) does not occur, but Turner syndrome, in which there is monosomy for the X chromosome, affects approximately 1 in 2500 live births (Box 3.3).

Large insertions or deletions of chromosomal DNA also occur and are usually associated with a learning disability and/or congenital malformations. Such structural chromosomal anomalies usually arise as the result of one of two different processes:

- non-homologous end-joining
- non-allelic homologous recombination.

Random double-stranded breaks in DNA are a necessary process in meiotic recombination and also occur during mitosis at a predictable rate. The rate of these breaks is dramatically increased by exposure to ionising radiation. When such breaks take place, they are usually repaired accurately by DNA repair mechanisms within the cell. However, in a proportion of breaks, segments of DNA that are not normally contiguous will be joined ('non-homologous end-joining'). If the joined fragments are from different chromosomes, this results in a translocation. If they are from the same chromosome, this will result in either inversion, duplication or deletion of a chromosomal fragment (Fig. 3.7). Large insertions and deletions may be cytogenetically visible as chromosomal deletions or duplications. If the anomalies are too small to be detected by microscopy, they are termed microdeletions and microduplications. Many microdeletion syndromes have been described and most result from non-allelic homologous recombination between repeats of highly similar DNA sequences, which leads to recurrent chromosome anomalies – and clinical syndromes – occurring in unrelated individuals (see Fig. 3.7 and Box 3.3).

Consequences of genomic variation

The consequence of an individual genomic variant depends on many factors, including the variant type, the nature of the gene product and the position of the variant in the protein. Variants can have profound or subtle effects on gene and cell function. Variations that have profound effects are responsible for 'classical' genetic diseases, whereas those with subtle effects may contribute to the pathogenesis of common disease where there is a genetic component, such as diabetes.

- *Neutral variants* have no effect on quality or type of protein produced.

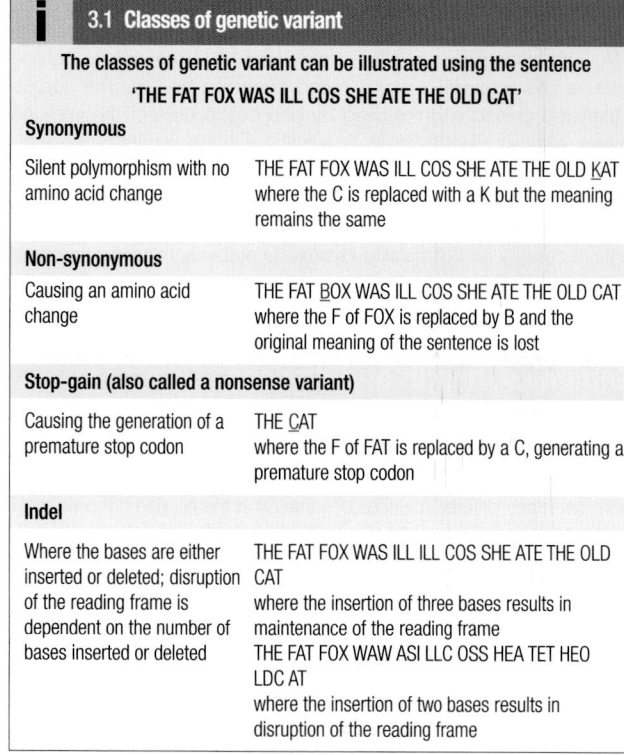

Fig. 3.5 Different types of mutation affecting coding exons. A Normal sequence. B A synonymous nucleotide substitution changing the third base of a codon; the resulting amino acid sequence is unchanged. C A missense variant in which the nucleotide substitution results in a change in a single amino acid from the normal sequence (AAG) encoding lysine to glutamine (CAG). D Insertion of a G residue (boxed) causes a frameshift variant, completely altering the amino acid sequence downstream. This usually results in a loss-of-function variant. E A nonsense variant resulting in a single nucleotide change from a lysine codon (AAG) to a premature stop codon (TAG).

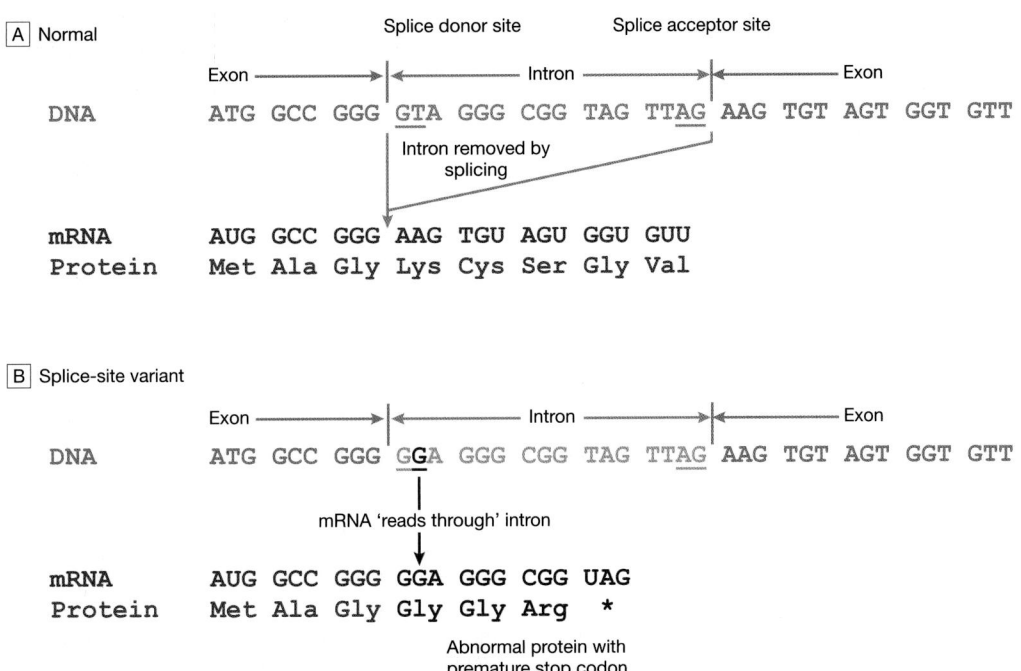

Fig. 3.6 Splice-site variants. [A] The normal sequence is shown, illustrating two exons, and intervening intron (blue) with splice donor (AG) and splice acceptor sites (GT) underlined. Normally, the intron is removed by splicing to give the mature messenger RNA that encodes the protein. [B] In a splice-site variant the donor site is mutated. As a result, splicing no longer occurs, leading to read-through of the mRNA into the intron, which contains a premature termination codon downstream of the variant.

i	**3.2 Diseases associated with triplet and other repeat expansions***					
	Repeat	**No. of repeats**		**Gene**	**Gene location**	**Inheritance**
		Normal	**Mutant**			
Coding repeat expansion						
Huntington's disease	[CAG]	6–34	>35	*Huntingtin*	4p16	AD
Spinocerebellar ataxia (type 1)	[CAG]	6–39	>40	*Ataxin*	6p22–23	AD
Spinocerebellar ataxia (types 2, 3, 6, 7)	[CAG]	Various	Various	Various	Various	AD
Dentatorubral-pallidoluysian atrophy	[CAG]	7–25	>49	*Atrophin*	12p12–13	AD
Machado–Joseph disease	[CAG]	12–40	>67	*MJD*	14q32	AD
Spinobulbar muscular atrophy	[CAG]	11–34	>40	Androgen receptor	Xq11–12	XL recessive
Non-coding repeat expansion						
Myotonic dystrophy	[CTG]	5–37	>50	*DMPK-3′ UTR*	19q13	AD
Friedreich's ataxia	[GAA]	7–22	>200	*Frataxin-intronic*	9q13	AR
Progressive myoclonic epilepsy	[CCCCGCCCCGCG]₄₋₈	2–3	>25	*Cystatin B-5′ UTR*	21q	AR
Fragile X mental retardation	[CGG]	5–52	>200	*FMR1–5′ UTR*	Xq27	XL dominant
Fragile site mental retardation 2 (FRAXE)	[GCC]	6–35	>200	*FMR2*	Xq28	XL, probably recessive

*The triplet repeat diseases fall into two major groups: those with disease stemming from expansion of [CAG]n repeats in coding DNA, resulting in multiple adjacent glutamine residues (polyglutamine tracts), and those with non-coding repeats. The latter tend to be longer. Unaffected parents usually display 'pre-mutation' allele lengths that are just above the normal range.
(AD/AR = autosomal dominant/recessive; UTR = untranslated region; XL = X-linked)

- *Loss-of-function variants* result in loss or reduction in the normal protein function. Whole-gene deletions are the archetypal loss-of-function variants but stop-gain or indel variants (early in the ORF), missense variants affecting a critical domain and splice-site variants can also result in loss of protein function.
- *Gain-of-function variants* result in a gain of protein function. They are typically non-synonymous variants that alter the protein structure, leading to activation/alteration of its normal function through causing

either an interaction with a novel substrate or a change in its normal function.
- *Dominant negative variants* are the result of non-synonymous substitutions or in-frame deletions/duplications but may also, less frequently, be caused by triplet repeat expansions. Dominant negative variants are heterozygous changes that result in the production of an abnormal protein that interferes with the normal functioning of the wild-type protein.

i **3.3 Chromosome and contiguous gene disorders**

Disease	Locus	Incidence	Clinical features
Numerical chromosomal abnormalities			
Down syndrome (trisomy 21)	47,XY,+21 or 47,XX,+21	1 in 800	Characteristic facies, IQ usually < 50, congenital heart disease, reduced life expectancy
Edwards syndrome (trisomy 18)	47,XY,+18 or 47,XX,+18	1 in 6000	Early lethality, characteristic skull and facies, frequent malformations of heart, kidney and other organs
Patau syndrome (trisomy 13)	47,XY,+13 or 47, XX,+13	1 in 15000	Early lethality, cleft lip and palate, polydactyly, small head, frequent congenital heart disease
Klinefelter syndrome	47,XXY	1 in 1000	Phenotypic male, infertility, gynaecomastia, small testes
XYY	47,XYY	1 in 1000	Usually asymptomatic, some impulse control problems
Triple X syndrome	47,XXX	1 in 1000	Usually asymptomatic, may have reduced IQ
Turner syndrome	45,X	1 in 5000	Phenotypic female, short stature, webbed neck, coarctation of the aorta, primary amenorrhoea
Recurrent deletions, microdeletions and contiguous gene defects			
Di George/velocardiofacial syndrome	22q11.2	1 in 4000	Cardiac outflow tract defects, distinctive facial appearance, thymic hypoplasia, cleft palate and hypocalcaemia. Major gene seems to be *TBX1* (cardiac defects and cleft palate)
Prader–Willi syndrome	15q11–q13	1 in 15000	Distinctive facial appearance, hyperphagia, small hands and feet, distinct behavioural phenotype. Imprinted region, deletions on paternal allele in 70% of cases
Angelman syndrome	15q11–q13	1 in 15000	Distinctive facial appearance, absent speech, electroencephalogram (EEG) abnormality, characteristic gait. Imprinted region, deletions on maternal allele encompassing *UBE3A*
Williams syndrome	7q11.23	1 in 10000	Distinctive facial appearance, supravalvular aortic stenosis, learning disability and infantile hypercalcaemia. Major gene for supravalvular aortic stenosis is *elastin*
Smith–Magenis syndrome	17p11.2	1 in 25000	Distinctive facial appearance and behavioural phenotype, self-injury and rapid eye movement (REM) sleep abnormalities. Major gene seems to be *RAI1*

A How structural chromosomal anomalies are described

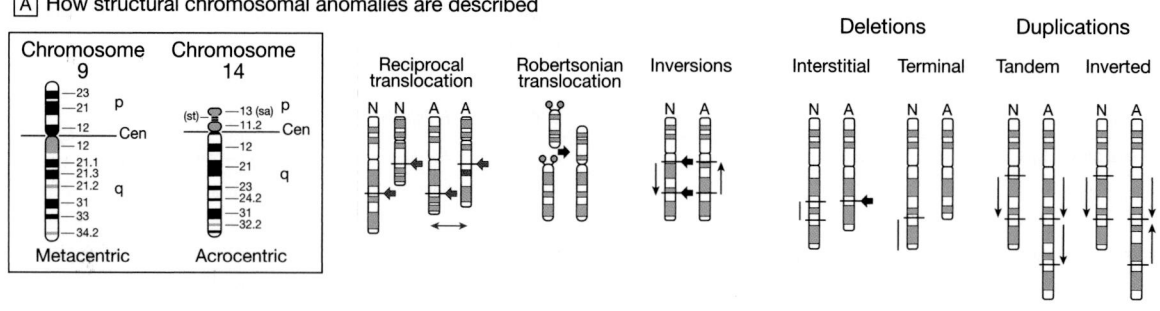

B Mechanism underlying recurrent deletions and duplication: non-allelic homologous recombination

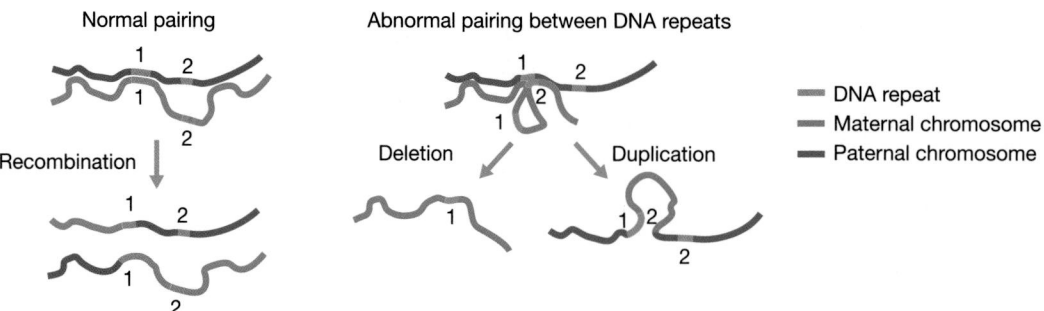

Fig. 3.7 Chromosomal analysis and structural chromosomal disorders. A Human chromosomes can be classed as metacentric if the centromere is near the middle, or acrocentric if the centromere is at the end. The bands of each chromosome are given a number, starting at the centromere and working out along the short (p) arm and long (q) arm. Translocations and inversions are balanced structural chromosome anomalies where no genetic material is missing but it is in the wrong order. Translocations can be divided into reciprocal (direct swap of chromosomal material between non-homologous chromosomes) and Robertsonian (fusion of acrocentric chromosomes). Deletions and duplications can also occur due to non-allelic homologous recombination (illustrated in part B). Deletions are classified as interstitial if they lie within a chromosome, and terminal if the terminal region of the chromosome is affected. Duplications can be either in tandem (where the duplicated fragment is inserted next to the region that is duplicated and orientated in the correct direction) or inverted (where the duplicated fragment is in the wrong direction). (N = normal; A = abnormal) B A common error of meiotic recombination, known as non-allelic homologous recombination, can occur (right panel), resulting in a deletion on one chromosome and a duplication in the homologous chromosome. The error is induced by tandem repeats in the DNA sequences (green), which can misalign and bind to each other, thereby 'fooling' the DNA into thinking the pairing prior to recombination is correct.

Normal genomic variation

We each have 3–5 million variants in our genome, occurring approximately every 300 bases. These variants are mostly polymorphisms, arising in more than 1% of the population; they have no or subtle effects on gene and cell function, and are not associated with a high risk of disease. Polymorphisms can occur within exons, introns or the intergenic regions that comprise 98%–99% of the human genome. Each of the classes of genetic variant discussed in this chapter (Box 3.1) is present in the genome as a common polymorphism. However, the most frequent is the single nucleotide polymorphism, or SNP (pronounced 'snip'), describing the substitution of a single base.

Polymorphisms and common disease

The protective and detrimental polymorphisms associated with common disease have been identified primarily through genome-wide association studies (GWAS, p. 52) and are the basis for many direct-to-consumer tests that purport to determine individual risk profiles for common diseases or traits such as cardiovascular disease, diabetes and even male-pattern baldness! An example is the polymorphism in the gene *SLC2A9* that not only explains a significant proportion of the normal population variation in serum urate concentration but also predisposes 'high-risk' allele carriers to the development of gout. However, the current reality is that, until we have a more comprehensive understanding of the full genomic landscape and knowledge of the complete set of detrimental and protective polymorphisms, we cannot accurately assess risk.

Evolutionary selection

Genetic variants play an important role in evolutionary selection, with advantageous variants resulting in positive selection via improved reproductive fitness, and variations that decrease reproductive fitness becoming excluded through evolution. Given this simple paradigm, it would be tempting to assume that common variants are all advantageous and all rare variants are pathogenic. Unfortunately, it is often difficult to classify any common variant as either advantageous or deleterious – or, indeed, neutral. Variants that are advantageous in early life and thus enhance reproductive fitness may be deleterious in later life. There may be variants that are advantageous for survival in particular conditions (e.g. famine or pandemic) that may be disadvantageous in more benign circumstances by causing a predisposition to obesity or autoimmune disorders.

Constitutional genetic disease

Familial genetic disease is caused by constitutional variants, which are inherited through the germ line. However, different variants in the same gene can have different consequences, depending on the genetic mechanism underlying that disease. About 1% of the human population carries constitutional pathogenic variants that cause disease.

Constructing a family tree

The family tree – or pedigree – is a fundamental tool of the clinical geneticist, who will routinely take a three-generation family history, on both sides of the family, enquiring about details of all medical conditions in family members, consanguinity, dates of birth and death, and any history of pregnancy loss or infant death. The basic symbols and nomenclature used in drawing a pedigree are shown in Fig. 3.8.

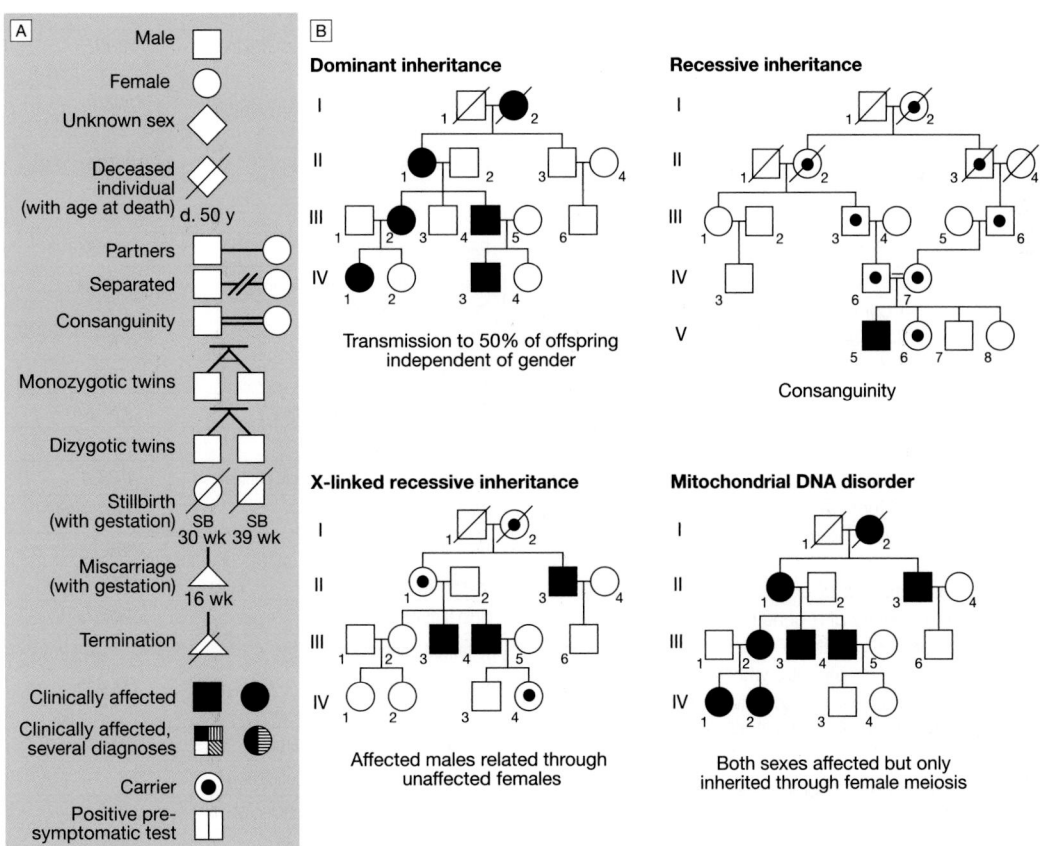

Fig. 3.8 Drawing a pedigree and patterns of inheritance. A The main symbols used to represent pedigrees in diagrammatic form. B The main modes of disease inheritance (see text for details).

Patterns of disease inheritance

Autosomal dominant inheritance

Take some time to draw out the following pedigree:

Anne is referred to Clinical Genetics to discuss her personal history of colon cancer (she was diagnosed at the age of 46 years) and family history of colon/endometrial cancer: her mother was diagnosed with endometrial cancer at the age of 60 years and her cousin through her healthy maternal aunt was diagnosed with colon cancer in her fifties. Both her maternal grandmother and grandfather died of 'old age'. There is no family history of note on her father's side of the family. He has one brother and both his parents died of old age, in their eighties. Anne has two healthy daughters, aged 12 and 14 years, and a healthy full sister.

This family history is typical of an autosomal dominant condition (see Fig. 3.8): in this case, a colon/endometrial cancer susceptibility syndrome known as Lynch syndrome, associated with disruption of one of the mismatch repair genes: *MSH2*, *MSH6*, *MLH1* and *PMS2* (see Ch. 23 and Box 3.11).

Features of an autosomal dominant pedigree include:

- There are affected individuals in each generation (unless the pathogenic variant has arisen de novo, i.e. for the first time in an affected individual). However, variable penetrance and expressivity can influence the number of affected individuals and the severity of disease in each generation. Penetrance is defined as the proportion of individuals bearing a mutated allele who develop the disease phenotype. The variant is said to be fully penetrant if all individuals who inherit a variant develop the disease. Expressivity describes the level of severity of each aspect of the disease phenotype.
- Males and females are usually affected in roughly equal numbers (unless the clinical presentation of the condition is gender-specific, such as an inherited susceptibility to breast and/or ovarian cancer).

The offspring risk for an individual affected with an autosomal dominant condition is 1 in 2 (or 50%). This offspring risk is true for each pregnancy, since half the affected individual gametes (sperm or egg cells) will contain the affected chromosome/gene and half will contain the normal chromosome/gene.

There is a long list of autosomal dominant conditions, some of which are shown in Box 3.4.

Autosomal recessive inheritance

As above, take some time to draw a pedigree representing the following:

Mr and Mrs Kent, a non-consanguineous couple, are referred because their son, Jamie, had severe neonatal liver disease. Included among the many investigations that the paediatric hepatologist undertook was testing for α_1-antitrypsin deficiency (Box 3.5). Jamie was shown to have the PiZZ phenotype. Testing confirmed both parents as carriers with PiMZ phenotypes. In the family, Jamie has an older sister who has no medical problems. Mr Kent is one of four children with two brothers and a sister and Mrs Kent has a younger brother. Both sets of grandparents are alive and well. There is no family history of α_1-antitrypsin deficiency.

This family history is characteristic of an autosomal recessive disorder (see Fig. 3.8), where both alleles of a gene must be mutated before the disease is manifest in an individual; an affected individual inherits one mutant allele from each of their parents, who are therefore healthy carriers for the condition. An autosomal recessive condition might be suspected in a family where:

- Males and females are affected in roughly equal proportions.
- Parents are blood-related; this is known as consanguinity. Where there is consanguinity, the variant are usually homozygous, i.e. the same mutant allele is inherited from both parents.
- Individuals within one sibship in one generation are affected and so the condition can appear to have arisen 'out of the blue'.

i | **3.4 Genetic conditions dealt with by clinicians in other specialties**

Name of condition	Gene	Reference
Autosomal dominant conditions		
Autosomal dominant polycystic kidney disease (ADPKD)	PKD1 (85%), PKD2 (15%)	p. 579 Box 18.28
Tuberous sclerosis	TSC1 TSC2	p. 1114
Marfan syndrome	FBN1	p. 445
Long QT syndrome	KCNQ1	p. 418
Brugada syndrome	SCN5A	p. 418
Neurofibromatosis type 1	NF1	p. 1185 Box 28.76
Neurofibromatosis type 2	NF2	p. 1185 Box 28.76
Hereditary spherocytosis	ANK1	p. 956
Vascular Ehlers–Danlos syndrome (EDS type 4)	COL3A1	p. 980
Hereditary haemorrhagic telangiectasia	ENG, ALK1, GDF2	p. 980
Osteogenesis imperfecta	COL1A1, COL1A2	p. 1058
Charcot–Marie–Tooth disease	PMP22, MPZ, GJB1	p. 1193
Hereditary neuropathy with liability to pressure palsies	PMP22	
Autosomal recessive conditions		
Familial Mediterranean fever	MEFV	p. 76
Mevalonic aciduria (mevalonate kinase deficiency)	MVK	p. 76
Autosomal recessive polycystic kidney disease (ARPKD)	PKHD1	Box 18.28
Kartagener syndrome (primary ciliary dyskinesia)	DNAI1	Box 17.30
Cystic fibrosis	CFTR1	p. 510 Box 17.30 p. 854
Pendred syndrome	SLC26A4	p. 667
Congenital adrenal hyperplasia-21 hydroxylase deficiency	CYP21A	p. 689 Box 20.27
Haemochromatosis	HFE	p. 906
Wilson's disease	ATP7B	p. 907
Alpha-1-antitrypsin deficiency	SERPINA1	p. 908
Gilbert syndrome	UGT1A1	p. 908
Benign recurrent intrahepatic cholestasis	ATP8B1	p. 912
Alpha-thalassaemia	HBA1, HBA2	p. 962
Beta-thalassaemia	HBB	p. 962
Sickle cell disease	HBB	p. 960
Spinal muscular atrophy	SMN1	p. 1171
X-linked conditions		
Alport syndrome	COL4A5	Box 18.28 p. 577
Primary agammaglobulinaemia	BTK	p. 74
Haemophilia A (factor VIII deficiency)	F8	p. 981
Haemophilia B (factor IX deficiency)	F9	p. 984
Duchenne muscular dystrophy	DMD	p. 1196 Box 28.90

3.5 Alpha-1-antitrypsin deficiency

Inheritance pattern

- Autosomal recessive

Genetic cause

- Two common variants in the *SERPINA1* gene: p.Glu342Lys and p.Glu264Val

Prevalence

- 1 in 1500–3000 of European ancestry

Clinical presentation

- Variable presentation from neonatal period through to adulthood
- Neonatal period: prolonged jaundice with conjugated hyperbilirubinaemia or (rarely) liver disease
- Adulthood: pulmonary emphysema and/or cirrhosis. Rarely, the skin disease, panniculitis, develops

Disease mechanism

- *SERPINA1* encodes α_1-antitrypsin, which protects the body from the effects of neutrophil elastase. The symptoms of α_1-antitrypsin deficiency result from the effects of this enzyme attacking normal tissue

Disease variants

- M variant: if an individual has normal *SERPINA1* genes and produces normal levels of α_1-antitrypsin, they are said to have an M variant
- S variant: p.Glu264Val variant results in α_1-antitrypsin levels reduced to about 40% of normal
- Z variant: p.Glu342Lys variant results in very little α_1-antitrypsin
- PiZZ: individuals who are homozygous for the p.Glu342Lys variant are likely to have α_1-antitrypsin deficiency and the associated symptoms
- PiZS: individuals who are compound heterozygous for p.Glu342Lys and p.Glu264Val are likely to be affected, especially if they smoke, but usually to a milder degree

3.6 Duchenne muscular dystrophy

Inheritance pattern

- X-linked recessive

Genetic cause

- Deletions/variants encompassing/within the *DMD* (dystrophin) gene located at Xp21

Prevalence

- 1 in 3000–4000 live male births

Clinical presentation

- Delayed motor milestones
- Speech delay
- Grossly elevated creatine kinase levels (in the thousands)
- Ambulation is usually lost between the ages of 7 and 13 years
- Lifespan is reduced, with a mean age of death, usually from respiratory failure, in the mid-twenties
- Cardiomyopathy affects almost all boys with Duchenne muscular dystrophy and some female carriers

Disease mechanism

- *DMD* encodes dystrophin, a major structural component of muscle
- Dystrophin links the internal cytoskeleton to the extracellular matrix

Disease variants

- Becker muscular dystrophy, although a separate disease, is also caused by variants in the dystrophin gene
- In Duchenne muscular dystrophy, there is no dystrophin protein, whereas in Becker muscular dystrophy there is a reduction in the amount or alteration in the size of the dystrophin protein

Approximately 1 in 4 children born to carriers of an autosomal recessive condition will be affected. The offspring risk for carrier parents is therefore 25% and the chances of an unaffected child, with an affected sibling, being a carrier is 2/3.

Examples of some autosomal recessive conditions, discussed elsewhere in this book, are shown in Box 3.4.

X-linked inheritance

The following is an exemplar of an X-linked recessive pedigree (see Fig. 3.8):

Edward has a diagnosis of Duchenne muscular dystrophy (DMD, Box 3.6). His parents had suspected the diagnosis when he was 3 years old because he was not yet walking and there was a family history of DMD: Edward's maternal uncle had been affected and died at the age of 24 years. Edward's mother has no additional siblings. After Edward demonstrated a very high creatinine kinase level, the paediatrician also requested genetic testing, which identified a deletion of exons 2–8 of the dystrophin gene. Edward has a younger, healthy sister and grandparents on both sides of the family are well, although the maternal grandmother has recently developed a cardiomyopathy. Edward's father has an older sister and an older brother who are both well.

Genetic diseases caused by variants on the X chromosome have specific characteristics:

- X-linked diseases are mostly recessive and predominantly affect males who carry the mutant allele. This is because males have only one X chromosome, whereas females have two (see Fig. 3.1). Occasionally, female carriers may exhibit signs of an X-linked disease due to a phenomenon called skewed X-inactivation. All female embryos, at about 100 cells in size, stably inactivate one of their two X chromosomes in each cell. Where this inactivation is random, approximately 50% of the cells will express the genes from one X chromosome and 50% of cells will express genes from the other. Where there is a mutant gene, there is often skewing away from the associated X chromosome, resulting in an unaffected female carrier. However, if, by chance, there is a disproportionate inactivation of the normal X chromosome with skewing towards the mutant allele, then an affected female carrier may be affected (albeit more mildly than males).
- The gene can be transmitted from female carriers to their sons: in families with an X-linked recessive condition, there are often a number of affected males related through unaffected females.
- Affected males cannot transmit the condition to their sons (but all their daughters would be carriers).

The risk of a female carrier having an affected child is 25% or half of her male offspring.

Mitochondrial inheritance

The mitochondrion is the main site of energy production within the cell. Mitochondria arose during evolution via the symbiotic association with an intracellular bacterium. They have a distinctive structure with functionally distinct inner and outer membranes. Mitochondria produce energy in the form of adenosine triphosphate (ATP). ATP is mostly derived from the metabolism of glucose and fat (Fig. 3.9). Glucose cannot enter mitochondria directly but is first metabolised to pyruvate via glycolysis. Pyruvate is then imported into the mitochondrion and metabolised to acetyl-co-enzyme A (acetyl-CoA). Fatty acids are transported into the mitochondria following conjugation with carnitine and are sequentially catabolised by a process called β-oxidation to produce acetyl-CoA. The acetyl-CoA from both pyruvate and fatty acid oxidation is used in the citric acid (Krebs) cycle – a series of enzymatic reactions that produces CO_2, the reduced form of nicotinamide adenine dinucleotide (NADH) and the reduced form of flavine adenine dinucleotide ($FADH_2$). Both NADH and $FADH_2$ then donate electrons to the respiratory chain. Here these elections are transferred via a complex series of reactions, resulting in the formation of a proton gradient across the inner mitochondrial membrane. The gradient is used by an inner mitochondrial membrane protein, ATP synthase, to produce ATP, which is then transported to other parts of the cell. Dephosphorylation of ATP is used to produce the energy required for many cellular processes.

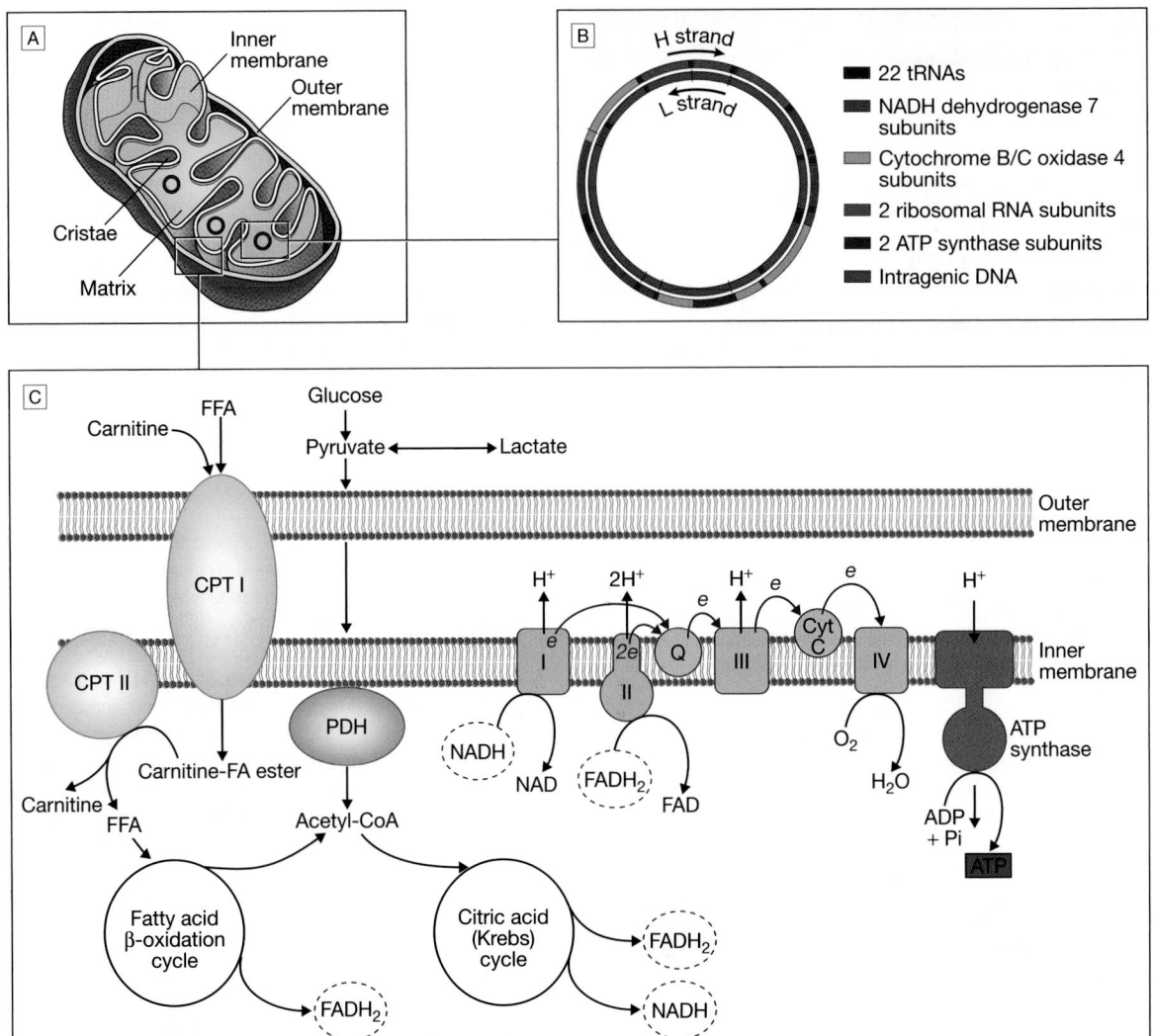

Fig. 3.9 Mitochondria. [A] Mitochondrial structure. There is a smooth outer membrane surrounding a convoluted inner membrane, which has inward projections called cristae. The membranes create two compartments: the inter-membrane compartment, which plays a crucial role in the electron transport chain, and the inner compartment (or matrix), which contains mitochondrial DNA and the enzymes responsible for the citric acid (Krebs) cycle and the fatty acid β-oxidation cycle. [B] Mitochondrial DNA. The mitochondrion contains several copies of a circular double-stranded DNA molecule, which has a non-coding region, and a coding region that encodes the genes responsible for energy production, mitochondrial transfer RNA (tRNA) molecules and mitochondrial ribosomal RNA (rRNA) molecules. [C] Mitochondrial energy production. Fatty acids enter the mitochondrion conjugated to carnitine by carnitine-palmityl transferase type 1 (CPT I) and, once inside the matrix, are unconjugated by CPT II to release free fatty acids (FFA). These are broken down by the β-oxidation cycle to produce acetyl-co-enzyme A (acetyl-CoA). Pyruvate can enter the mitochondrion directly and is metabolised by pyruvate dehydrogenase (PDH) to produce acetyl-CoA. The acetyl-CoA enters the Krebs cycle, leading to the production of NADH and flavine adenine dinucleotide (reduced form) (FADH$_2$), which are used by proteins in the electron transport chain to generate a hydrogen ion gradient across the inter-membrane compartment. Reduction of NADH and FADH$_2$ by proteins I and II, respectively, releases electrons (e), and the energy released is used to pump protons into the inter-membrane compartment. Coenzyme Q$_{10}$/ubiquinone (Q) is an intensely hydrophobic electron carrier that is mobile within the inner membrane. As electrons are exchanged between proteins in the chain, more protons are pumped across the membrane, until the electrons reach complex IV (cytochrome oxidase), which uses the energy to reduce oxygen to water. The hydrogen ion gradient is used to produce ATP by the enzyme ATP synthase, which consists of a proton channel and catalytic sites for the synthesis of ATP from ADP. When the channel opens, hydrogen ions enter the matrix down the concentration gradient, and energy is released that is used to make ATP. (ATP = adenosine triphosphate; NADH = the reduced form of nicotinamide adenine dinucleotide)

Each mitochondrion contains 2–10 copies of a 16-kilobase (kB) double-stranded circular DNA molecule (mtDNA). This mtDNA contains 13 protein-coding genes, all involved in the respiratory chain, and the ncRNA genes required for protein synthesis within the mitochondria (see Fig. 3.9). The mutational rate of mtDNA is relatively high due to the lack of protection by chromatin. Several mtDNA diseases characterised by defects in ATP production have been described. Mitochondria are most numerous in cells with high metabolic demands, such as muscle, retina and the basal ganglia, and these tissues tend to be the ones most severely affected in mitochondrial diseases (Box 3.7). There are many other mitochondrial diseases that are caused by pathogenic variants in nuclear genes, which encode proteins that are then imported into the mitochondrion and are critical for energy production, e.g. most forms of Leigh syndrome (although Leigh syndrome may also be caused by a mitochondrial gene variant).

The inheritance of mtDNA disorders is characterised by transmission from females, but males and females generally are equally affected (see Fig. 3.8). Unlike the other inheritance patterns mentioned above, mitochondrial inheritance has nothing to do with meiosis but reflects the fact that mitochondrial DNA is transmitted by oöcytes: sperm do not contribute mitochondria to the zygote. Mitochondrial disorders tend to be variable in penetrance and expressivity within families, and this is mostly accounted for by the fact that only a proportion of multiple mtDNA molecules within mitochondria contain the causal variant (the degree of mtDNA heteroplasmy).

Imprinting

Several chromosomal regions (loci) have been identified where gene expression is inherited in a parent-of-origin-specific manner; these are called imprinted loci. Within these loci the paternally inherited gene may be active while the maternally inherited may be silenced, or vice versa. Variants within imprinted loci lead to an unusual pattern of inheritance where the phenotype is manifest only if inherited from the parent who contributes the transcriptionally active allele. Examples of imprinting disorders are given in Box 3.8.

Somatic genetic disease

Somatic variants are not inherited but instead occur during post-zygotic mitotic cell divisions at any point from embryonic development to late adult life. An example of this phenomenon is polyostotic fibrous dysplasia (McCune–Albright syndrome), in which a somatic variant in the G_s alpha gene causes constitutive activation of downstream signalling, resulting in focal lesions in the skeleton and endocrine dysfunction.

The most important example of human disease caused by somatic variants is cancer (see Ch. 7). Here, 'driver mutations' occur within genes that are involved in regulating cell division or apoptosis, resulting in abnormal cell growth and tumour formation. The two general categories of cancer-causing variant are gain-of-function variants in growth-promoting genes (oncogenes) and loss-of-function variants in growth-suppressing genes (tumour suppressor genes). Whichever mechanism is acting, most tumours require an initiating variant in a single cell that can then escape from normal growth controls. This cell replicates more frequently or fails to undergo programmed death, resulting in clonal expansion. As the size of the clone increases, one or more cells may acquire additional variants that confer a further growth advantage, leading to proliferation of these subclones, which may ultimately result in aggressive metastatic cancer. The cell's complex self-regulating machinery means that more than one variant is usually required to produce a malignant tumour (see Fig. 7.3). For example, if a variant results in activation of a growth factor gene or receptor, then that cell will replicate more frequently as a result of autocrine stimulation. However, this mutant cell will still be subject to normal cell-cycle checkpoints to promote DNA integrity in its progeny. If additional variants in the same cell result in defective cell-cycle checkpoints, however, it will rapidly accumulate further genomic variants, which may allow completely unregulated growth and/or separation from its matrix and cellular attachments and/or resistance to apoptosis. As cell growth becomes increasingly dysregulated, cells de-differentiate, lose their response to normal tissue environment and cease to ensure appropriate mitotic chromosomal segregation. These processes combine to generate the classical malignant characteristics of disorganised growth, variable levels of differentiation and numerical and structural chromosome abnormalities. An increase in somatic variant rate can occur on exposure to external mutagens, such as ultraviolet light or cigarette smoke, or if the cell has defects in DNA repair systems. Cancer is thus a disease that affects the fundamental processes of molecular and cell biology.

i | 3.7 The structure of the respiratory chain complexes and the diseases associated with their dysfunction

Complex	Enzyme	nDNA subunits[1]	mtDNA subunits[2]	Diseases
I	NADH dehydrogenase	38	7	MELAS, MERRF bilateral striatal necrosis, LHON, myopathy and exercise intolerance, parkinsonism, Leigh syndrome, exercise myoglobinuria, leucodystrophy/myoclonic epilepsy
II	Succinate dehydrogenase	4	0	Phaeochromocytoma, Leigh syndrome
III	Cytochrome bc₁ complex	10	1	Parkinsonism/MELAS, cardiomyopathy, myopathy, exercise myoglobinuria, Leigh syndrome
IV	Cytochrome c oxidase	10	3	Sideroblastic anaemia, myoclonic ataxia, deafness, myopathy, MELAS, MERRF mitochondrial encephalomyopathy, motor neuron disease-like, exercise myoglobinuria, Leigh syndrome
V	ATP synthase	14	2	Leigh syndrome, NARP, bilateral striatal necrosis

[1]nDNA subunits. [2]mtDNA subunits = number of different protein subunits in each complex that are encoded in the nDNA and mtDNA, respectively.
(ATP = adenosine triphosphate; LHON = Leber hereditary optic neuropathy; MELAS = myopathy, encephalopathy, lactic acidosis and stroke-like episodes; MERRF = myoclonic epilepsy and ragged red fibres; mtDNA = mitochondrial DNA; NADH = the reduced form of nicotinamide adenine dinucleotide; NARP = neuropathy, ataxia and retinitis pigmentosa; nDNA = nuclear DNA)

i | 3.8 Imprinting disorders

Disorder	Locus	Genes	Notes
Beckwith–Wiedemann syndrome	11p15	CDKN1C, IGF2, H19	Increased growth, macroglossia, hemihypertrophy, abdominal wall defects, ear lobe pits/creases and increased susceptibility to developing childhood tumours
Prader–Willi syndrome	15q11–q13	SNRPN, Necdin and others	Obesity, hypogonadism and learning disability. Lack of paternal contribution (due to deletion of paternal 15q11–q13, or inheritance of both chromosome 15q11–q13 regions from the mother)
Angelman syndrome (AS)	15q11–q13	UBE3A	Severe mental retardation, ataxia, epilepsy and inappropriate laughing bouts. Due to loss-of-function variants in the maternal UBE3A gene. The neurological phenotype results because most tissues express both maternal and paternal alleles of UBE3A, whereas the brain expresses predominantly the maternal allele
Pseudohypoparathyroidism	20q13	GNAS1	Inheritance of the variant from the mother results in hypocalcaemia, hyperphosphataemia, raised parathyroid hormone (PTH) levels, ectopic calcification, obesity, delayed puberty and shortened 4th and 5th metacarpals (the syndrome known as Albright hereditary osteodystrophy, AHO). When the gene variant is inherited from the father, PTH, calcium and phosphate levels are normal but the other features are present. These differences are due to the fact that, in the kidney (the main target organ through which PTH regulates serum calcium and phosphate), the paternal allele is silenced and the maternal allele is expressed, whereas both alleles are expressed in other tissues

Interrogating the genome: the changing landscape of genomic technologies

Looking at chromosomes

The analysis of metaphase chromosomes by light microscopy was the mainstay of clinical cytogenetic analysis for decades, the aim being to detect gain or loss of whole chromosomes (aneuploidy) or large chromosomal segments (>4 million bp). More recently, genome-wide microarrays (array comparative genomic hybridisation or array CGH) have replaced chromosome analysis, allowing rapid and precise detection of segmental gain or loss of DNA throughout the genome (see Box 3.3). Microarrays consist of grids of multiple wells containing short DNA sequences (reference DNA) that are complementary to known sequences in the genome. Patient and reference DNA are each labelled with a coloured fluorescent dye (generally, patient DNA is labelled with a green fluorescent dye and reference DNA with a red fluorescent dye) and added to the microarray grid. Where there is an equal quantity of patient and reference DNA bound to the spot, this results in yellow fluorescence. Where there is too much patient DNA (representing a duplication of a chromosome region), the spot will be greener; it will be more red (appears orange) where there is 2:1 ratio of the control:patient DNA (representing heterozygous deletion of a chromosome region; Fig. 3.10).

Array CGH and other array-based approaches can detect small chromosomal deletions and duplications. They are also generally more sensitive than conventional karyotyping at detecting mosaicism (where there are two or more populations of cells, derived from a single fertilised egg, with different genotypes). However, array-based approaches will not detect balanced chromosome rearrangements where there is no loss or gain of genes/chromosome material, such as balanced reciprocal translocations, or a global increase in copy number, such as triploidy.

The widespread use of array-based approaches has brought a number of challenges for clinical interpretation, including the identification of copy number variants (CNVs) of uncertain clinical significance, CNVs of variable penetrance and incidental findings. A CNV of uncertain clinical significance describes a loss or gain of chromosome material where there are insufficient data to conclude whether or not it is associated with a learning disability and/or medical problems. While this uncertainty can be difficult to prepare families for and can be associated with considerable anxiety, it is likely that there will be greater clarity in the future as we generate larger CNV datasets.

A CNV of variable penetrance, also known as a neurosusceptibility locus, describes a chromosome deletion or duplication associated with a lower threshold for manifesting a learning disability or autistic spectrum disorder. CNVs of variable penetrance are therefore identified at greater frequencies among individuals with a learning disability and/or autistic spectrum disorder than in the general population. The current understanding is that additional modifying factors (genetic, environmental or stochastic) must influence the phenotypic expression of these neurosusceptibility loci.

Finally, an incidental CNV finding describes a deletion or duplication encompassing a gene or genes that are causative of a phenotype or risk unrelated to the presenting complaint. For instance, if, through the array CGH investigation for an intellectual disability, a deletion encompassing the *BRCA1* gene were identified, this would be considered an incidental finding.

Looking at genes

Gene amplification: polymerase chain reaction

The polymerase chain reaction (PCR) is a fundamental laboratory technique that amplifies targeted sections of the human genome for further analyses – most commonly, DNA sequencing. The method utilises thermal cycling: repeated cycles of heating and cooling allow the initial separation of double-stranded DNA into two single strands (known as denaturation), each of which serves as a template during the subsequent replication step, guided by primers designed to anneal to a specific genomic region. This cycle of heating/cooling and denaturation/replication is repeated many times, resulting in the exponential amplification of DNA between primer sites (Fig. 3.11).

Gene sequencing

In the mid-1970s, a scientist called Fred Sanger pioneered a DNA sequencing technique ('Sanger sequencing') that determined the precise order and nucleotide type (thymine, cytosine, adenine and guanine) in a molecule of DNA. Modern Sanger sequencing uses fluorescently labelled, chain-terminating nucleotides that are sequentially incorporated into the newly synthesised DNA, generating multiple DNA chains of differing lengths. These DNA chains are subject to capillary electrophoresis, which separates them by size, allowing the fragments to be 'read' by a laser and producing a sequence chromatogram that corresponds to the target sequence (Fig. 3.12). Although transformative, Sanger sequencing was difficult and costly to scale, as exemplified by the Human Genome Project, which took 12 years to sequence the entire human genome at a cost approaching 3 billion US$. Recently, DNA sequencing has been transformed again by a group of technologies collectively known as 'next-generation sequencing' (NGS; Fig. 3.13). This refers to a family of post-Sanger sequencing technologies that utilise the same five basic principles:

- *Library preparation*: DNA samples are fragmented (by enzyme cleavage or ultrasound) and then modified with a custom adapter sequence.
- *Amplification*: the library fragment is amplified to produce DNA clusters, each originating from a single DNA fragment. Each cluster will act as a single sequencing reaction.
- *Capture*: if an entire genome is being sequenced, this step will not be included. The capture step is required if targeted resequencing is necessary, such as for a panel gene test or an exome (Box 3.9).

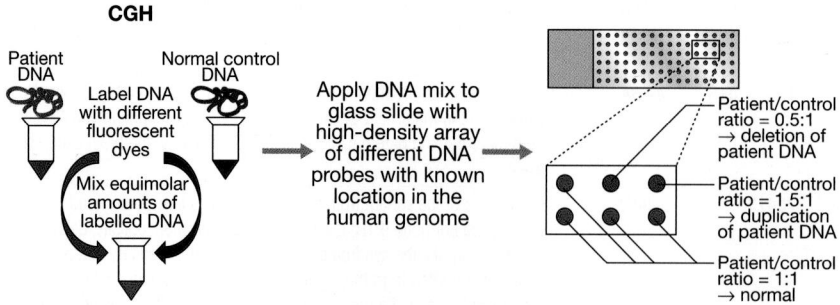

CGH

Patient DNA | Normal control DNA

Label DNA with different fluorescent dyes

Mix equimolar amounts of labelled DNA

Apply DNA mix to glass slide with high-density array of different DNA probes with known location in the human genome

Patient/control ratio = 0.5:1 → deletion of patient DNA

Patient/control ratio = 1.5:1 → duplication of patient DNA

Patient/control ratio = 1:1 → normal

Fig. 3.10 Detection of chromosome abnormalities by comparative genomic hybridisation (CGH). Deletions and duplications are detected by looking for deviation from the 1:1 ratio of patient and control DNA in a microarray. Ratios in excess of 1 indicate duplications, whereas ratios below 1 indicate deletions.

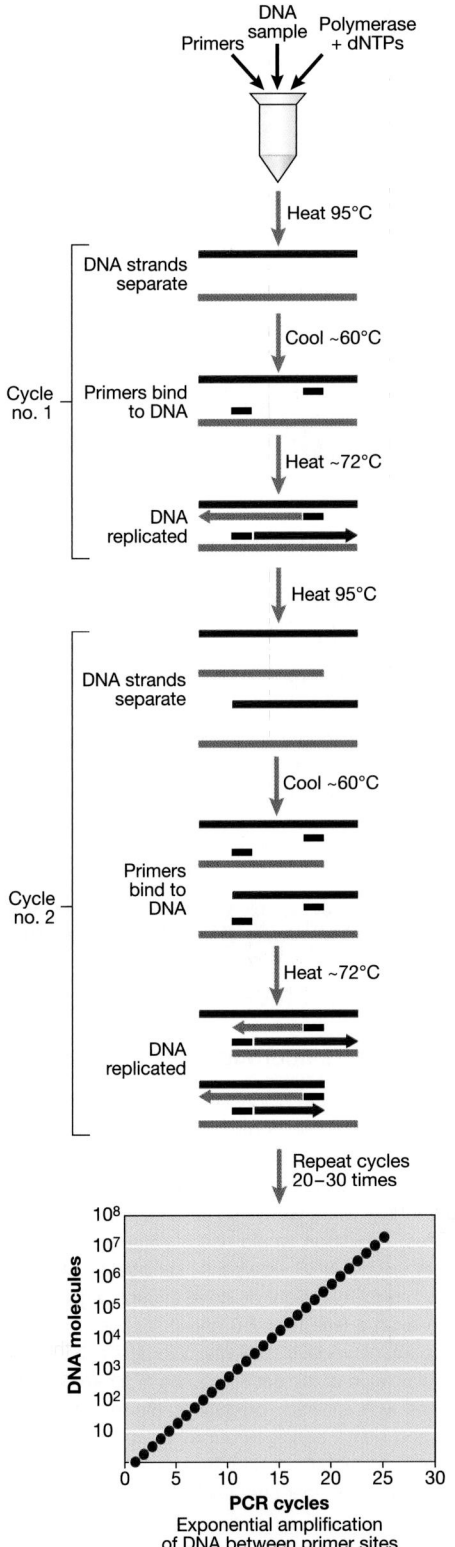

Fig. 3.11 The polymerase chain reaction (PCR). PCR involves adding a tiny amount of the patient's DNA to a reaction containing primers (short oligonucleotides 18–21 bp in length, which bind to the DNA flanking the region of interest) and deoxynucleotide phosphates (dATP, dCTP, dGTP, dTTP), which are used to synthesise new DNA and a heat-stable polymerase. The reaction mix is first heated to 95°C, which causes the double-stranded DNA molecules to separate. The reaction is then cooled to 50–60°C, which allows the primers to bind to the target DNA. The reaction is then heated to 72°C, at which point the polymerase starts making new DNA strands. These cycles are repeated 20–30 times, resulting in exponential amplification of the DNA fragment between the primer sites. The resulting PCR products can then be used for further analysis – most commonly, DNA sequencing (see Fig. 3.12).

- *Sequencing*: each DNA cluster is simultaneously sequenced and the data from each captured; this is known as a 'read' and is usually between 50 and 300 bases long (see Box 3.10 for a detailed description of the three most commonly used sequencing methods: synthesis, ligation and ion semiconductor sequencing).
- *Alignment and variant identification*: specialised software analyses read sequences and compare the data to a reference template. This is known as 'alignment' or 'mapping' and, although there are approximately 3 billion bases in the human genome, allows the remarkably accurate determination of the genomic origin where a read consists of 25 nucleotides or more. Variants are identified as differences between the read and the reference genome. For instance, if there is a different nucleotide in half the reads at a given position compared to the reference genome, this is likely to represent a heterozygous base substitution. The number of reads that align at a given point is called the 'depth' or 'coverage'. The higher the read depth, the more accurate the variant call. However, in general, a depth of 30 or more reads is generally accepted as producing diagnostic-grade results.

Rather than sequencing only one small section of DNA at a time, NGS allows the analysis of many hundreds of thousands of DNA strands in a single experiment and so is also commonly referred to as multiple parallel sequencing technology. Today's NGS machines can sequence the entire human genome in a single day at a cost of less than 1000 US$.

NGS capture

Although we now have the capability to sequence the entire genome in a single experiment, whole-genome sequencing is not always the optimal use of NGS. NGS capture refers to the 'pull-down' of a targeted region of the genome and may constitute several to several hundred genes associated with a given phenotype (a gene panel), the exons of all known coding genes (an exome), or the exons of all coding genes known to be associated with disease (a clinical exome). Each of these targeted resequencing approaches is associated with a number of advantages and disadvantages (see Box 3.9). In order for NGS to be used for optimal patient benefit, it is essential for the clinician to have a good understanding of which test is the best one to request in any given clinical presentation.

Challenges of NGS technologies

Genomic technologies are transforming the way that we practise medicine, and ever faster and cheaper DNA sequencing offers increasing opportunities to prevent, diagnose and treat disease. However, genomic technologies are not without their challenges: for instance, storing the enormous quantities of data generated by NGS. While the A, C, T and G of our genomic code could be stored on the memory of a smartphone, huge computers, able to store several petabytes of data (where 1 petabyte is 1 million gigabytes of data), are required to store the information needed to generate each individual's genome.

Even if we can store and handle these huge datasets successfully, we then need to be able to sift through the millions of normal variants to identify the single (or, rarely, several) pathogenic, disease-causing variant. While this can, to an extent, be achieved through the application of complex algorithms, these take time and considerable expertise to develop and are not infallible.

Furthermore, even after these data have been sifted by bioinformaticians, it is highly likely that clinicians will be left with some variants for which there are insufficient data to enable their definitive categorisation as either pathogenic or non-pathogenic. This may be because we simply do not know enough about the gene, because the particular variant has not previously been reported and/or it is identified in an unaffected parent. These variants must be interpreted with caution and, more usually, their interpretation will require input from a genetics expert in the context of the clinical presentation, where an 'innocent until proven guilty' approach is often adopted.

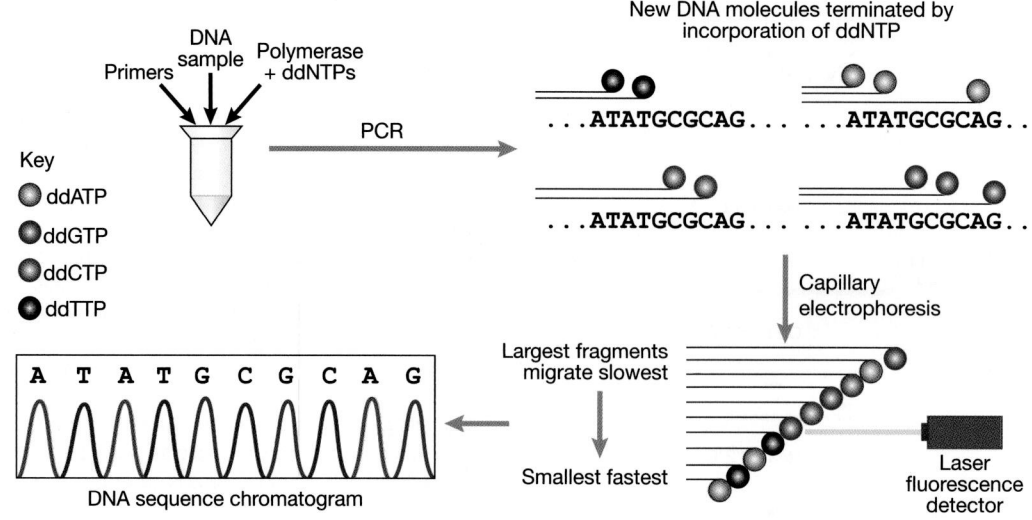

Fig. 3.12 Sanger sequencing of DNA, which is very widely used in DNA diagnostics. This is performed using polymerase chain reaction (PCR)-amplified fragments of DNA corresponding to the gene of interest. The sequencing reaction is carried out with a combination dNTP and fluorescently labelled di-deoxy-dNTP (ddATP, ddTTP, ddCTP and ddGTP), which become incorporated into the newly synthesised DNA, causing termination of the chain at that point. The reaction products are then subject to capillary electrophoresis and the different-sized fragments are detected by a laser, producing a sequence chromatogram that corresponds to the target DNA sequence.

Finally, if we are to interrogate the entire genome or even the exome, it is foreseeable that we will routinely identify 'incidental' or secondary findings – in other words, findings not related to the initial diagnostic question. Whether or not to report these incidental findings is a topic of much debate in the UK, although there is growing support to feedback incidental findings where there is an intervention that could slow or halt development/progress of the associated disease.

Uses of NGS

NGS is now frequently used, within diagnostic laboratories, to identify base substitutions and indels (although the latter were initially problematic). The current NGS challenge is to detect large deletions or duplications spanning several hundreds or thousands of bases and therefore exceeding any single read copy number variants and triplet repeat disorders such as those that cause Huntington's disease, myotonic dystrophy and fragile X syndrome, although techniques to detect both are improving (see Box 3.2). Increasingly, however, disorders caused by both copy number variants and triplet repeat expansions are being diagnosed using sophisticated computational methods. Additional potential uses of NGS include detection of balanced and unbalanced translocations and mosaicism: NGS has proved remarkably sensitive at detecting the latter when there is high read coverage for a given region. Of note, however, NGS is still not able to interrogate the epigenome and so will not identify conditions caused by a disruption of imprinting, such as Beckwith–Wiedemann, Silver–Russell, Angelman and Prader–Willi syndromes (see Boxes 3.8 and 3.2).

Third-generation sequencing

Increasingly, third-generation or single-molecule sequencing is entering the diagnostic arena. As with next- or second-generation sequencing, a number of different platforms are commercially available. One of the most successful is SMRT technology (single-molecule sequencing in real time), developed by Pacific Biosciences. This system utilises a single-stranded DNA molecule (as compared to the amplified clusters used in NGS), which acts as a template for the sequential incorporation, using a polymerase, of fluorescently labelled nucleotides. As each complementary nucleotide is added, the fluorescence (and therefore the identity of the nucleotide) is recorded before it is removed and another nucleotide is added.

A key advantage of third-generation sequencing is the long length of the read it generates: in the region of 10–15 kilobases. It is also cheaper than NGS, as fewer reagents are required. Given these inherent advantages, third-generation sequencing is likely to supersede NGS in the near future. Given the confusion surrounding the terminology of NGS and third-generation sequencing, these technologies are increasingly referred to as 'massively parallel sequencing'.

Genomics and clinical practice

Genomics and health care

Genomics in rare neurodevelopmental disorders

Although, by definition, the diagnosis of a rare disorder is made infrequently, rare diseases, when considered together, affect about 3 million people in the UK, the majority of whom are children. NGS has transformed the ability to diagnose individuals affected by a rare disease. Whereas previously, when we were restricted to the sequential analysis of single genes, a clinician would need to make a clinical diagnosis in order to target testing, NGS allows the interrogation of multiple genes in a single experiment. This might be done through a gene panel, a clinical exome or an exome (see Box 3.9 and p. 51), and has increased the diagnostic yield in neurodevelopmental disorders to 35%–50%. Not only does the identification of the genetic cause of a rare disorder potentially provide families with answers, prognostic information and the opportunity to meet and derive support from other affected families but also it can provide valuable information for those couples planning further children and wishing to consider prenatal testing in the future.

Genomics and common disease

Most common disorders are determined by interactions between a number of genes and the environment. In this situation, the genetic contribution to disease is termed polygenic. Until recently, very little progress had been made in identifying the genetic variants that predispose to common disorders, but this has been changed by the advent of genome-wide association studies. A GWAS typically involves genotyping many (> 500 000) genetic markers (SNPs) spread across the genome in a large group of individuals with the disease and in controls. By comparing the SNP genotypes in cases and controls, it is possible to identify regions of the genome, and therefore genes, more strongly associated with a given

1 Library preparation

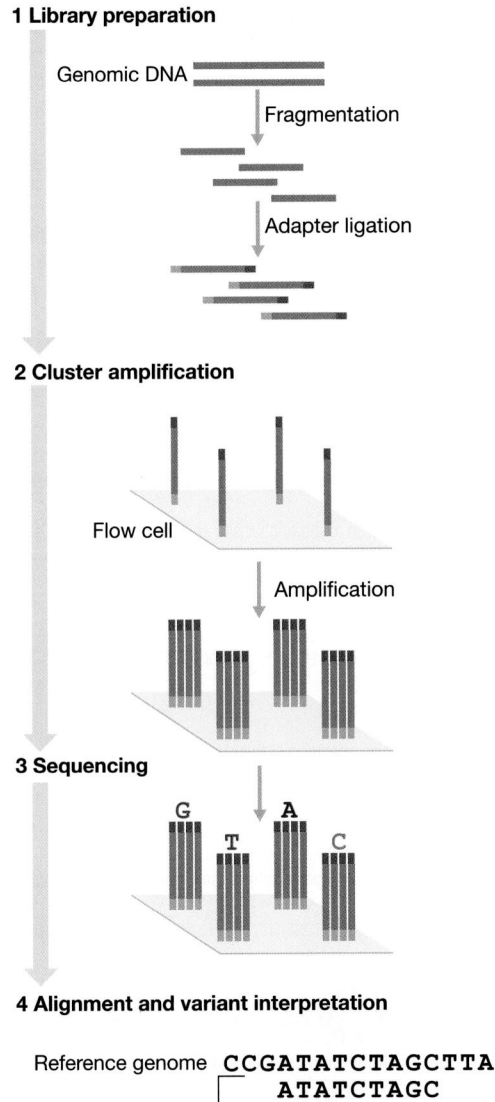

Genomic DNA

Fragmentation

Adapter ligation

2 Cluster amplification

Flow cell

Amplification

3 Sequencing

G   A
T   C

4 Alignment and variant interpretation

Reference genome CCGATATCTAGCTTA
                  ATATCTAGC
Reads   CGATAGC
              TATCTAGC
           CCGATAGCTAGCTTA

Fig. 3.13 Sequencing by synthesis as used in the Illumina system. (1) Library preparation: DNA is fragmented and specialist adapters are ligated to the fragmented ends. (2) Cluster amplification: the library is loaded to a flow cell and the adapters hybridise to the flow-cell surface. Each bound fragment is hybridised. (3) Sequencing. (4) Alignment and variant interpretation: reads are aligned to a reference sequence using complex software and differences between reference and case genomes are identified.

i | **3.9 The advantages and disadvantages of whole-genome sequencing, whole-exome sequencing and gene panels**

Test	Advantages	Disadvantages
Whole-genome sequencing (WGS)	The most comprehensive analysis of the genome available. More even coverage of genes, allowing better identification of dosage abnormalities. Will potentially detect all gene variants, including intronic variants	More expensive to generate and store. Will detect millions of variants in non-coding DNA, which can be very difficult to interpret. Associated with a greater risk of identifying incidental findings. Shallow sequencing (few reads per gene) and so less sensitive and less able to detect mosaicism
Whole-exome sequencing (WES)	Cheaper than whole-genome sequencing. Analysis is not restricted to only those genes known to cause a given condition. Fewer variants detected than in WGS and so easier interpretation. Deeper sequencing than WGS increases sensitivity and detection of mosaicism	Less even coverage of the genome and so dosage abnormalities are more difficult to detect. Less comprehensive analysis (1%–2% of the genome) than WGS. Increased risk of identifying incidental findings over targeted gene sequencing
Gene panels	Cost-effective. Very deep sequencing, increasing the chances of mosaicism being detected. Fewer variants detected and so data easier to interpret. As analysis is restricted to known genes, the likelihood of a variant being pathogenic is greatly increased	Will only detect variation in genes known to cause a given condition. Difficult to add new genes to the panel as they are discovered

SNP profile and therefore more likely to contribute to the disease under study. Increasingly there is a move to develop disease-specific polygenic risk scores (PRS) in order to stratify individual risk and determine personalised management strategies. Whilst not yet in mainstream practice, it is likely that PRS will be integrated into clinical management in the next few years.

Genomics and obstetrics

Prenatal genetic testing may be performed where a pregnancy is considered at increased risk of being affected with a genetic condition, either because of the ultrasound/biochemical screening results or because of the family history. While invasive tests, such as amniocentesis and chorionic villus sampling, have been the mainstay of prenatal diagnosis for many years, they are increasingly being superseded by non-invasive testing of cell-free fetal DNA (cffDNA), originating from placental trophoblasts and detectable in the maternal circulation from 4–5 weeks' gestation; it is present in sufficient quantities for testing by 9 weeks.

- *Non-invasive prenatal testing (NIPT)*: the sequencing and quantification, using NGS, of cffDNA chromosome-specific DNA sequences to identify trisomy 13, 18 or 21. The accuracy of NIPT in detecting pregnancy-specific aneuploidy approaches 98%. A false-negative result can occur when there is too little cffDNA (possibly due to early gestation or high maternal body mass index) or when aneuploidy has arisen later in development and is confined to the embryo and not represented in the placenta. False positives can occur with confined placental mosaicism (describing aneuploidy in the placenta, not the fetus) or with an alternative cause of aneuploidy in the maternal circulation, such as cell-free tumour DNA.

i 3.10 Next-generation sequencing methods

Sequencing by synthesis (Fig. 3.13)

- The most frequently used NGS method
- Used in Illumina systems (commonly used in diagnostic laboratories)
- Uses fluorescently labelled, terminator nucleotides that are sequentially incorporated into a growing DNA chain
- Library DNA samples (fragmented DNA flanked by DNA adapter sequences) are anchored to a flow cell by hybridisation of the DNA adapter sequence to probes on the flow-cell surface
- Amplification occurs by washing the flow cell in a mixture containing all four fluorescently labelled terminator nucleotides: A, C, T and G
- Once the nucleotide, complementary to the first base of the DNA template, is incorporated, no further nucleotides can be added until the mixture is washed away
- The nucleotide terminator is shed and the newly incorporated nucleotide reverts to a regular, non-fluorescent nucleotide that can be extended
- The process is then repeated with the incorporation of a second base etc.
- Sequencing by synthesis is therefore space- and time-dependent: a sensor will detect the order of fluorescent emissions for each spot on the plate (representing the cluster) and determine the sequence for that read

Sequencing by ligation

- Used in SOLiD systems
- Uses DNA ligase rather than DNA polymerase (as is used in sequencing by synthesis) and short oligonucleotides (as opposed to single nucleotides)
- Library DNA samples are washed in a mixture containing oligonucleotide probes representing 4–16 dinucleotide sequences. Only one nucleotide in the probe is fluorescently labelled
- The complementary oligo probes will hybridise, using DNA ligase, to the target sequence, initially at a primer annealed to the anchor site and then progressively along the DNA strand
- After incorporation of each probe, fluorescence is measured and the dye is cleaved off
- Eventually, a new strand is synthesised (composed of a series of the oligo probes)
- A new strand is then synthesised but is offset by one nucleotide
- The process is repeated a number of times (5 rounds in the SOLiD system), providing overlapping templates that are analysed and a composite of the target sequence determined

Ion semiconductor sequencing

- When a nucleotide is incorporated into a growing DNA strand, a hydrogen ion is released that can be detected by an alteration in the pH of the solution. This hydrogen ion release forms the basis of ion semiconductor sequencing
- Each amplified DNA cluster is located above a semiconductor transistor, capable of detecting differences in the pH of the solution
- The DNA cluster is washed in a mixture containing only one type of nucleotide
- If the correct nucleotide, complementary to the next base on the DNA template, is in the mixture and incorporated, a hydrogen ion is released and detected
- If a homopolymer (sequence of two or more identical nucleotides) is present, this will be detected as a decrease in pH proportionate to the number of identical nucleotides in the sequence

i 3.11 Inherited cancer predisposition syndromes

Syndrome name	Gene	Associated cancers	Additional clinical features
Birt–Hogg–Dubé syndrome	FLCN	Renal tumour (oncocytoma, chromophobe (and mixed), renal cell carcinoma)	Fibrofolliculoma Trichodiscoma Pulmonary cysts
Breast/ovarian hereditary susceptibility	BRCA1 BRCA2	Breast carcinoma Ovarian carcinoma Pancreatic carcinoma Prostate carcinoma	
Cowden syndrome	PTEN	Breast carcinoma Thyroid carcinoma Endometrial carcinoma	Macrocephaly Intellectual disability/autistic spectrum disorder Trichilemmoma Acral keratosis Papillomatous papule Thyroid cyst Lipoma Haemangioma Intestinal hamartoma
Gorlin syndrome/basal cell naevus syndrome	PTCH1	Basal cell carcinoma Medulloblastoma	Odontogenic keratocyst Palmar or plantar pits Falx calcification Rib abnormalities (e.g. bifid, fused or missing ribs) Macrocephaly Cleft lip/palate
Li–Fraumeni syndrome	TP53	Sarcoma (e.g. osteosarcoma, chondrosarcoma, rhabdomyosarcoma) Breast carcinoma Brain cancer (esp. glioblastoma) Adrenocortical carcinoma Brain	

i | 3.11 Inherited cancer predisposition syndromes

Syndrome name	Gene	Associated cancers	Additional clinical features
Lynch syndrome/hereditary non-polyposis colon cancer	MLH1 MSH2 MSH6 PMS2	Colorectal carcinoma (majority right-sided) Endometrial carcinoma Gastric carcinoma Cholangiocarcinoma Ovarian carcinoma (esp. mucinous)	
Multiple endocrine neoplasia 1	MEN1	Parathyroid tumour Endocrine pancreatic tumour Anterior pituitary tumour	Lipoma Facial angiofibroma
Multiple endocrine neoplasia 2a and 2b (formerly known as type 2 and 3, respectively)	RET	Medullary thyroid tumour Phaeochromocytoma Parathyroid tumour	
Polyposis, familial adenomatous (FAP)	APC	Colorectal adenocarcinoma (FAP is characterised by thousands of polyps from the second decade; without colectomy, malignant transformation of at least one of these polyps is inevitable) Duodenal carcinoma Hepatoblastoma	Desmoid tumour Congenital hypertrophy of the retinal pigment epithelium (CHRPE)
Polyposis, MYH-associated	MYH (MUTYH)	Colorectal adenocarcinoma Duodenal adenocarcinoma	
Retinoblastoma, familial	RB1	Retinoblastoma Osteosarcoma	

- *Non-invasive prenatal diagnosis (NIPD)*: the identification of a fetal single-gene defect that either has been paternally inherited or has arisen de novo and so is not identifiable in the maternal genome. Examples of conditions that are currently amenable to NIPD include achondroplasia and the craniosynostoses. Increasingly, however, NIPD is being used for autosomal recessive conditions such as cystic fibrosis, where parents are carriers for different gene variants and research is under way to perform more agnostic fetal gene sequencing through whole-exome or whole-genome sequencing.

Where a genetic diagnosis is known in a family, a couple may opt to undertake pre-implantation genetic diagnosis (PGD). PGD is used as an adjunct to in vitro fertilisation and involves the genetic testing of a single cell from a developing embryo, prior to implantation.

Genomics and oncology

Until recently, individuals were stratified to genetic testing if they presented with a personal and/or family history suggestive of an inherited cancer predisposition syndrome (Box 3.11). Relevant clinical information included the age of cancer diagnosis and number/type of tumours. For example, the diagnosis of bilateral breast cancer in a woman in her thirties with a mother who had ovarian cancer in her forties is suggestive of BRCA1/2-associated familial breast/ovarian cancer. In many familial cancer syndromes, somatic gene variants act together with an inherited variant to cause specific cancers (p. 49). Familial cancer syndromes may be due to germ-line loss-of-function variants in tumour suppressor genes encoding DNA repair enzymes or proto-oncogenes. At the cellular level, loss of one copy of a tumour suppressor gene does not have any functional consequences, as the cell is protected by the remaining normal copy. However, a somatic variant affecting the normal allele is likely to occur in one cell at some point during life, resulting in complete loss of tumour suppressor activity and a tumour developing by clonal expansion of that cell. This two-hit mechanism (one inherited, one somatic) for cancer development is known as the Knudson hypothesis. It explains why tumours may not develop for many years (or ever) in some members of these cancer-prone families. In DNA repair diseases, the inherited variants increase the somatic mutation rate. Autosomal dominant variants

in genes encoding components of specific DNA repair systems are relatively common causes of familial colon cancer and breast cancer (e.g. BRCA1).

Increasingly, genetics is moving into the mainstream, becoming integrated into routine oncological care as new gene-specific treatments are introduced. Testing for a genetic predisposition to cancer is therefore moving from the domain of clinical genetics, where it has informed diagnosis, cascade treatment and screening/prophylactic management, to oncology, where it is informing the immediate management of the patient following cancer diagnosis. This is exemplified by BRCA1 and BRCA2 (BRCA1/2)-related breast cancer. Previously, women with a pathogenic variant in either the BRCA1 or BRCA2 gene would have received similar first-line chemotherapy to women with a sporadic breast cancer without a known genetic association. More recently, it has been shown that BRCA1/2 mutation-positive tumours are sensitive to poly ADP ribose polymerase (PARP) inhibitors. PARP inhibitors block the single-strand break-repair pathway. In a BRCA1/2 mutation-positive tumour – with compromised double-strand break repair – the additional loss of the single-strand break-repair pathway will drive the cell towards apoptosis. Indeed, PARP inhibitors have been shown to be so effective at destroying BRCA1/2 mutation-positive tumour cells, and with such minimal side-effects, that BRCA1/2 gene testing is increasingly determining patient management. It is likely, with a growing understanding of the genomic architecture of tumours, increasing accessibility of NGS and an expanding portfolio of gene-directed therapies, that testing for many of the other inherited cancer susceptibility genes will, in time, move into the mainstream.

Genomics in infectious disease

NGS technologies are also transforming infectious disease. Given that a microbial genome can be sequenced within a single day at a current cost of less than 100 US$, microbiologists are able to identify a causative microorganism and target effective treatment rapidly and accurately. Moreover, microbial genome sequencing enables the effective surveillance of infections to reduce and prevent transmission. Finally, an understanding of the microbial genome will drive the development of vaccines and antibiotics, essential in an era characterised by increasing microbial resistance to established antibiotic agents.

Treatment of genetic disease

Pharmacogenomics

Pharmacogenomics is the science of dissecting the genetic determinants of drug kinetics and effects using information from the human genome. For more than 50 years it has been appreciated that polymorphic variants within genes can affect individual responses to some drugs, such as loss-of-function variants in *CYP2D6* that cause hypersensitivity to debrisoquine, an adrenergic-blocking medication formerly used for the treatment of hypertension, in 3% of the population. This gene is part of a large family of highly polymorphic genes encoding cytochrome P450 proteins, mostly expressed in the liver, which determine the metabolism of a host of specific drugs. Polymorphisms in the *CYP2D6* gene also determine codeine activation, while those in the *CYP2C9* gene affect warfarin inactivation. Polymorphisms in these and other drug metabolic genes determine the persistence of drugs and, therefore, should provide information about dosages and toxicity. With the increasing use of NGS, genetic testing for assessment of drug response is seldom employed routinely, but in the near future it may be possible to predict the best specific drugs and dosages for individual patients based on genetic profiling: so-called 'personalised medicine'. An example is the enzyme thiopurine methyltransferase (TPMT), which catabolises azathioprine, a drug that is used in the treatment of autoimmune diseases and in cancer chemotherapy. Genetic screening for polymorphic variants of TPMT can be useful in identifying patients who have increased sensitivity to the effects of azathioprine and who can be treated with lower doses than normal.

Gene therapy and genome editing

Replacing or repairing mutated genes (gene therapy) is challenging in humans. Retroviral-mediated ex vivo replacement of the defective gene in bone marrow cells for the treatment of severe combined immune deficiency syndrome has been successful. The major problems with clinical use of virally delivered gene therapy have been oncogenic integration of the exogenous DNA into the genome and severe immune response to the virus.

Other therapies for genetic disease include PTC124, a compound that can 'force' cells to read through a nonsense variant that results in a premature termination codon in an ORF with the aim of producing a near-normal protein product. This therapeutic approach could be applied to any genetic disease caused by nonsense variants.

The most exciting development in genetics for a generation has been the discovery of accurate, efficient and specific techniques to enable editing of the genome in cells and organisms. This technology is known as CRISPR/Cas9 (clustered regularly interspaced short palindromic repeats and CRISPR-associated) genome editing. It is likely that ex vivo correction of genetic disease will become commonplace over the next few years. In vivo correction is not yet possible and will take much longer to become part of clinical practice.

Induced pluripotent stem cells and regenerative medicine

Adult stem-cell therapy has been in wide use for decades in the form of bone marrow transplantation. The identification of adult stem cells for other tissues, coupled with the ability to purify and maintain such cells in vitro, now offers exciting therapeutic potential for other diseases. It was recently discovered that many different adult cell types can be trans-differentiated to form cells (induced pluripotent stem cells or iPS cells) with almost all the characteristics of embryonal stem cells derived from the early blastocyst. In mammalian model species, such cells can be taken and used to regenerate differentiated tissue cells, such as in heart and brain. They have great potential both for the development of tissue models of human disease and for regenerative medicine.

Pathway medicine

The ability to manipulate pathways that have been altered in genetic disease has tremendous therapeutic potential for Mendelian disease, but a firm understanding of both disease pathogenesis and drug action at a biochemical level is required. An exciting example has been the discovery that the vascular pathology associated with Marfan syndrome is due to the defective fibrillin molecules causing up-regulation of transforming growth factor (TGF)-β signalling in the vessel wall. Losartan is an antihypertensive drug that is marketed as an angiotensin II receptor antagonist. However, it also acts as a partial antagonist of TGF-β signalling and is effective in preventing aortic dilatation in a mouse model of Marfan syndrome, showing promising effects in early human clinical trials.

Ethics in a genomic age

As genomic technology is increasingly moving into mainstream clinical practice, it is essential for clinicians from all specialties to appreciate the complexities of genetic testing and consider whether genetic testing is the right thing to do in a given clinical scenario. To exemplify the ethical considerations associated with genetic testing, it may be helpful to think about them in the context of a clinical scenario. As you read the scenario, try to think what counselling/ethical issues might arise:

A 32-year-old woman is referred to discuss *BRCA2* testing; she is currently pregnant with her second child (she already has a 2-year-old daughter) and has an identical twin sister. Her mother, a healthy 65-year-old with Ashkenazi Jewish ancestry, participated in direct-to-consumer testing (DCT) for 'a bit of fun' and a *BRCA2* gene variant – common in the Ashkenazi Jewish population – was identified. There is no significant cancer family history of note.

Consider the following issues:

- *Pre-symptomatic/predictive testing*: this describes testing for a known familial gene variant in an unaffected individual (compared with diagnostic testing, where genetic testing is undertaken in an affected individual). Although this could be considered for the unaffected patient, in the current scenario any testing would also have implications for her identical twin sister. This needs to be fully explored with the patient and her sister prior to testing. There is also the potential issue of predictive testing in the patient's first child. A fundamental tenet in clinical genetics is that predictive genetic testing should be avoided in childhood for adult-onset conditions. This is because, if no benefit to the patient is accrued through childhood testing, it is better to retain the child's right to decide for herself, when she is old enough, whether she wishes to participate in genetic testing or not.
- *Prenatal testing*: the principles behind predictive genetic testing in childhood can be extended to prenatal testing, i.e. if a pregnancy is being continued, a baby should not be tested for an adult-onset condition that cannot be prevented or treated in childhood. However, prenatal testing itself is hugely controversial and there is much debate as to how severe a condition should be to justify prenatal diagnosis, which would determine ongoing pregnancy decisions.
- *DCT*: while DCT can be interesting and empowering for individuals wishing to find out more about their genetic backgrounds, it also has several drawbacks. Perhaps the main one is that, unlike face-to-face genetic counselling (which usually precedes any genetic testing, certainly where there are serious health implications for the individual and their family, such as is associated with *BRCA1/2* variants), DCT is undertaken in isolation with no direct access to professional support. Furthermore, in addition to some (common) single-gene variants, such as the founder *BRCA1/2* variants frequently identified in the Ashkenazi Jewish population and discussed in this example, current DCT packages utilise a series of SNPs to determine an overall risk profile; they evaluate the number of detrimental and

protective SNPs for a given disease. However, given that only a minority of the risk SNPs have so far been characterised, this is often inaccurate. Individuals may be falsely reassured that they are not at increased risk of a genetic condition despite a family history suggesting otherwise, resulting in inadequate surveillance and/or management.

The ethical considerations listed in this clinical scenario give just a flavour of some of the issues frequently encountered in clinical genetics. They are not meant to be an exhaustive summary and whole textbooks and meetings are devoted to the discussion of hugely complex ethical issues in genetics. However, a guiding principle is that, although each counselling situation will be unique with specific communication and ethical challenges, a genetic result is permanent and has implications for the whole family, not just the individual. Where possible, therefore, an informed decision regarding genetic testing should be taken by a competent adult following counselling by an experienced and appropriately trained clinician.

Further information

Books and journal articles

Alberts B, Bray D, Hopkin K, et al. Essential cell biology, 4th edn. New York: Garland Science; 2013.

Firth H, Hurst JA. Oxford desk reference: clinical genetics. Oxford: Oxford University Press; 2005.

Read A, Donnai D. New clinical genetics, 2nd edn. Banbury: Scion; 2010.

Strachan T, Read A. Human molecular genetics, 4th edn. New York: Garland Science; 2010.

Websites

bsgm.org.uk *British Society for Genetic Medicine; has a report on genetic testing of children.*

decipher.sanger.ac.uk *Excellent, comprehensive genomic database.*

ensembl.org *Annotated genome databases from multiple organisms.*

futurelearn.com/courses/the-genomics-era *Has a Massive Open Online Course on genomics, for which the author of the current chapter is the lead educator.*

genome.ucsc.edu *Excellent source of genomic information.*

ncbi.nlm.nih.gov *Online Mendelian Inheritance in Man (OMIM).*

ncbi.nlm.nih.gov/books/NBK1116/ *Gene Reviews: excellent US-based source of information about many rare genetic diseases.*

orpha.net/consor/cgi-bin/index.php *Orphanet: European-based database on rare disease.*

3

4

Clinical immunology

The immune system has evolved to identify and destroy pathogens while minimising damage to host tissue. Despite the ancient observation that recovery from an infectious disease frequently results in protection against that condition, the existence of the immune system as a functional entity was not recognised until the end of the 19th century. More recently, it has become clear that the immune system not only protects against infection but also regulates tissue repair following injury, and when dysregulated, governs the responses that can lead to autoimmune and auto-inflammatory diseases. Dysfunction or deficiency of the immune response can lead to a wide variety of diseases that may potentially involve every organ system in the body.

The aim of this chapter is to provide a general understanding of the immune system, how it contributes to human disease and how manipulation of the immune system can be put to therapeutic use. A review of the key components of the immune response is followed by sections that illustrate the clinical presentation of the most common forms of immune dysfunction: immune deficiency, inflammation, autoimmunity and allergy. More detailed discussion of individual conditions can be found in the relevant organ-specific, emergency and critical care medicine chapters

Functional anatomy and physiology

The immune system consists of an intricately linked network of lymphoid organs, cells and proteins that are strategically placed to protect against infection (Fig. 4.1). Immune defences are normally categorised into the innate immune response, which provides immediate protection against an invading pathogen, and the adaptive or acquired immune response, which takes more time to develop but confers exquisite specificity and long-lasting protection. Innate and adaptive immunity do not work in isolation, but rather in concert, largely driven by cytokines produced by the specific immune cell populations.

The innate immune system

Innate defences against infection include anatomical barriers, phagocytic cells, soluble molecules such as complement and acute phase proteins, and natural killer cells. The innate immune system recognises generic microbial structures present on non-mammalian tissue and can be mobilised within minutes. A specific stimulus will elicit essentially identical responses in different individuals, in contrast with adaptive antibody and T-cell responses, which vary greatly between individuals.

Physical barriers

The tightly packed keratinised cells of the skin physically limit colonisation by microorganisms. The hydrophobic oils that are secreted by sebaceous glands further repel water and microorganisms, and microbial growth is inhibited by the skin's low pH and low oxygen tension. Sweat also contains lysozyme, an enzyme that destroys the structural integrity of bacterial cell walls; ammonia, which has antibacterial properties; and several antimicrobial peptides such as defensins. Similarly, the mucous membranes of the respiratory, gastrointestinal and genitourinary tracts provide a physical barrier to infection. Secreted mucus traps invading pathogens, and immunoglobulin A (IgA), generated by the adaptive immune system, prevents bacteria and viruses attaching to and penetrating epithelial cells. As in the skin, lysozyme and antimicrobial peptides within mucosal membranes directly kill invading pathogens, and lactoferrin acts to starve invading bacteria of iron. Within the respiratory tract, cilia directly trap pathogens and contribute to removal of mucus, assisted by physical manœuvres such as sneezing and coughing. In the gastrointestinal tract, hydrochloric acid and salivary amylase chemically destroy bacteria, while normal peristalsis and induced vomiting or diarrhoea assist clearance of invading organisms.

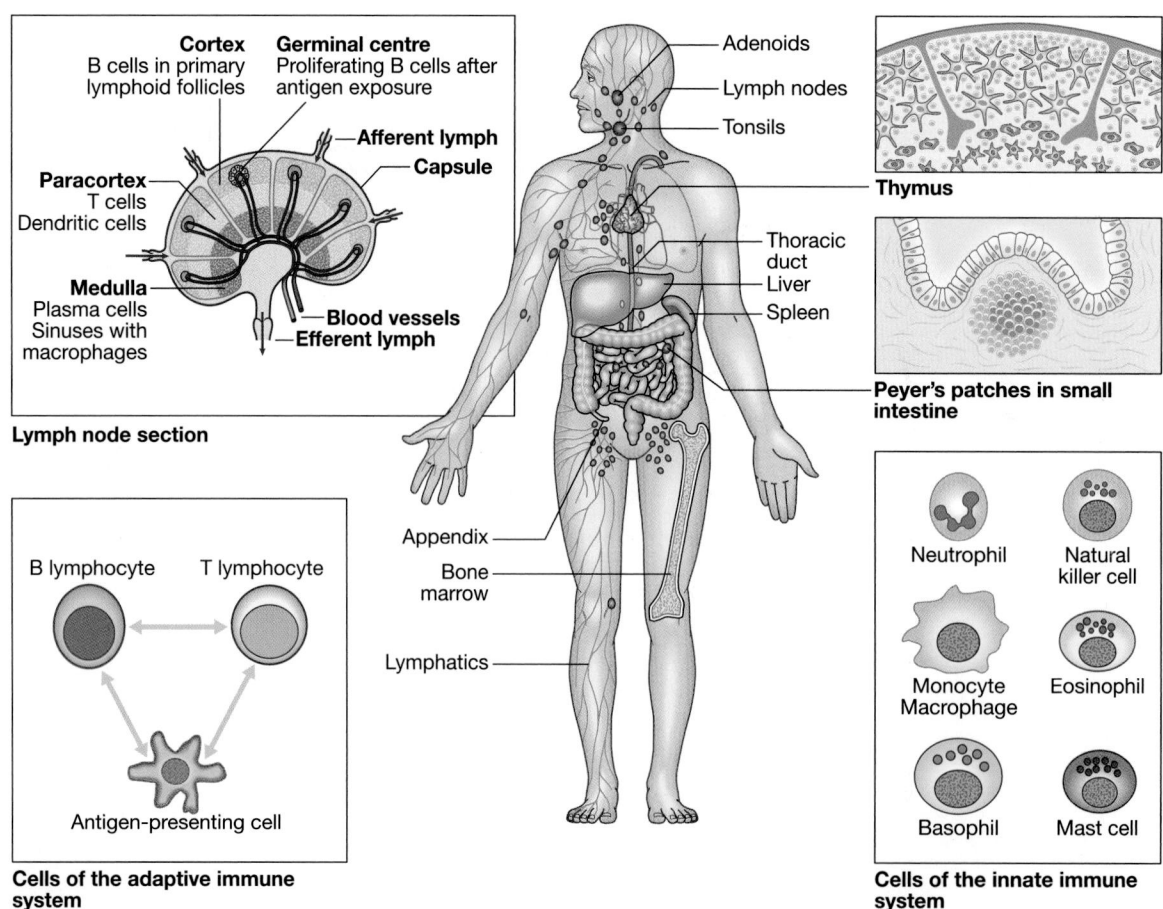

Fig. 4.1 Anatomy of the immune system.

The microbiome, which is made up of endogenous commensal bacteria, provides an additional constitutive defence against infection. Approximately 10^{14} bacteria normally reside at epithelial surfaces in symbiosis with the human host. They compete with pathogenic microorganisms for scarce resources, including space and nutrients, and produce fatty acids and bactericidins that inhibit the growth of many pathogens. In addition, recent research has demonstrated that commensal bacteria help to shape the immune response by inducing specific regulatory T cells within the intestine. Eradication of the normal flora with broad-spectrum antibiotics commonly results in opportunistic infection by organisms such as *Clostridioides difficile*, which rapidly colonise an undefended ecological niche.

These constitutive barriers are highly effective, but if external defences are breached by a wound or pathogenic organism, the specific soluble proteins and cells of the innate immune system are activated.

Phagocytes

Phagocytes ('eating cells') are specialised cells that ingest and kill microorganisms, scavenge cellular and infectious debris, and produce inflammatory molecules that regulate other components of the immune system. They include neutrophils, monocytes and macrophages, and are particularly important for defence against bacterial and fungal infections. Phagocytes express a wide range of surface receptors, including pattern recognition receptors (PRRs), which recognise pathogen-associated molecular patterns (PAMPs) on invading microorganisms, allowing their identification. The PRRs include Toll-like receptors, nucleotide oligomerisation domain (NOD) protein-like receptors and mannose receptors, whereas the PAMPs they recognise are molecular motifs not present on mammalian cells, including bacterial cell wall components, bacterial DNA and viral double-stranded RNA. Interaction between the PRRs and their PAMPs leads to activation of nuclear factor kappa B (NFκB), which stimulates expression of pro-inflammatory genes, and of nucleotide-binding

oligomerisation domain (NOD)-like receptor proteins (NLRP), which form complexes with other intracellular proteins to form the inflammasome (Fig. 4.2). The inflammasome results in activation of interleukin-1 beta (IL-1β), which is excreted extracellularly and plays a key pathogenic role in familial fever syndromes (p. 76) and acute gout (Ch. 26). While phagocytes can recognise microorganisms through PRRs alone, engulfment of microorganisms is greatly enhanced by opsonisation. Opsonins include acute phase proteins produced by the liver, such as C-reactive protein and complement component C3b. Antibodies generated by the adaptive immune system also act as opsonins. They bind both to the pathogen and to phagocyte receptors, acting as a bridge between the two to facilitate phagocytosis (see Fig. 4.2). This is followed by intracellular pathogen destruction and downstream activation of pro-inflammatory genes, resulting in the generation of pro-inflammatory cytokines as discussed below.

Neutrophils

Neutrophils, also known as polymorphonuclear leucocytes, are derived from the bone marrow and circulate freely in the blood. They are short-lived cells with a half-life of 6 hours, and are produced at the rate of 10^{11} cells daily. Their functions are to kill microorganisms, to facilitate rapid transit of cells through tissues and to amplify the immune response non-specifically. These functions are mediated by enzymes contained in granules, which also provide an intracellular milieu for the killing and degradation of microorganisms.

Two main types of granule are recognised: primary or azurophil granules, and the more numerous secondary or specific granules. Primary granules contain myeloperoxidase and other enzymes important for intracellular killing and digestion of ingested microbes. Secondary granules are smaller and contain lysozyme, collagenase and lactoferrin, which can be released into the extracellular space. Enzyme production is increased in response to infection, which is reflected by more intense granule staining on microscopy, known as 'toxic granulation'.

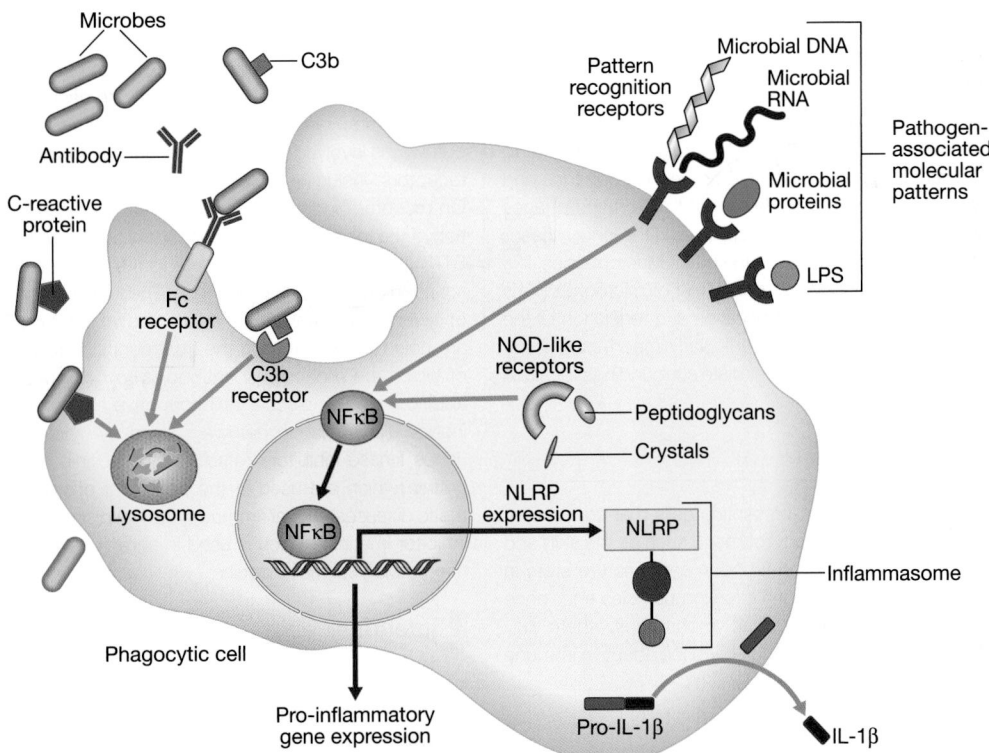

Fig. 4.2 Phagocytosis and opsonisation. Phagocytosis of microbes can be augmented by several opsonins, such as C-reactive protein, antibodies and complement fragments like C3b, which enhance the ability of phagocytic cells to engulf microorganisms and destroy them. Phagocytes also recognise components of microbes, such as lipopolysaccharide, peptidoglycans, DNA and RNA, collectively known as pathogen-associated molecular patterns (PAMPs). These activate pattern recognition receptors (PRRs), such as Toll-like receptors and nucleotide oligomerisation domain (NOD)-like receptors, which promote inflammatory gene expression through the nuclear factor kappa B (NFκB) pathway. Uric acid and other crystals can also promote inflammation through the NOD pathway. (IL = interleukin; LPS = lipopolysaccharide; NLRP = nucleotide-binding oligomerisation domain (NOD)-like receptor proteins)

Changes in damaged or infected cells trigger local production of inflammatory molecules and cytokines. These cytokines stimulate the production and maturation of neutrophils in the bone marrow, and their release into the circulation. Neutrophils are recruited to specific sites of infection by chemotactic agents, such as interleukin 8 (IL-8), and by activation of local endothelium. Up-regulation of cellular adhesion molecules on neutrophils and the endothelium also facilitates neutrophil migration. The transit of neutrophils through the blood stream is responsible for the rise in neutrophil count that occurs in early infection. Once present within infected tissue, activated neutrophils seek out and engulf invading microorganisms. These are initially enclosed within membrane-bound vesicles, which fuse with cytoplasmic granules to form the phagolysosome. Within this protected compartment, killing of the organism occurs through a combination of oxidative and non-oxidative killing. Oxidative killing, also known as the respiratory burst, is mediated by the nicotinamide adenine dinucleotide phosphate (NADPH)–oxidase enzyme complex, which converts oxygen into reactive oxygen species such as hydrogen peroxide and superoxide that are lethal to microorganisms. The myeloperoxidase enzyme within neutrophils produces hypochlorous acid, which is a powerful oxidant and antimicrobial agent. Non-oxidative (oxygen-independent) killing occurs through the release of bactericidal enzymes into the phagolysosome. Each enzyme has a distinct antimicrobial spectrum, providing broad coverage against bacteria and fungi.

An additional, recently identified form of neutrophil-mediated killing is neutrophil extracellular trap (NET) formation. Activated neutrophils can release chromatin with granule proteins such as elastase to form an extracellular matrix that binds to microbial proteins. This can immobilise or kill microorganisms without requiring phagocytosis. The process of phagocytosis and NET formation (NETosis) depletes neutrophil glycogen reserves and is followed by neutrophil death. As the cells die, their contents are released and lysosomal enzymes degrade collagen and other components of the interstitium, causing liquefaction of closely adjacent tissue. The accumulation of dead and dying neutrophils results in the formation of pus, which, if extensive, may lead to abscess formation.

Monocytes and macrophages

Monocytes are the precursors of tissue macrophages. They are produced in the bone marrow and enter the circulation, where they constitute about 5% of leucocytes. From the blood stream they migrate to peripheral tissues, where they differentiate into tissue macrophages and reside for long periods. Specialised populations of tissue macrophages include Kupffer cells in the liver, alveolar macrophages in the lung, mesangial cells in the kidney, and microglial cells in the brain. Macrophages, like neutrophils, are capable of phagocytosis and killing of microorganisms but also play an important role in the amplification and regulation of the inflammatory response (Box 4.1). They are particularly important in tissue surveillance and constantly survey their immediate surroundings for signs of tissue damage or invading organisms.

Dendritic cells

Dendritic cells are specialised antigen-presenting cells that are present in tissues in contact with the external environment, such as the skin and mucosal membranes. They can also be found in an immature state in the blood. They sample the environment for foreign particles and, once activated, carry microbial antigens to regional lymph nodes, where they interact with T cells and B cells to initiate and shape the adaptive immune response.

Cytokines

Cytokines are signalling proteins produced by cells of the immune system and a variety of other cell types. More than 100 have been identified. Cytokines have complex and overlapping roles in cellular communication and regulation of the immune response. Subtle differences in cytokine production, particularly at the initiation of an immune response, can have a major impact on outcome. Cytokines bind to specific receptors on

i 4.1 Functions of macrophages

Amplification of the inflammatory response
- Stimulate the acute phase response (through production of IL-1 and IL-6)
- Activate vascular endothelium (IL-1, TNF-α)
- Stimulate neutrophil maturation and chemotaxis (IL-1, IL-8)
- Stimulate monocyte chemotaxis

Killing of microorganisms
- Phagocytosis
- Microbial killing through oxidative and non-oxidative mechanisms

Clearance, resolution and repair
- Scavenging of necrotic and apoptotic cells
- Clearance of toxins and other inorganic debris
- Tissue remodelling (elastase, collagenase, matrix proteins)
- Down-regulation of inflammatory cytokines
- Wound healing and scar formation (IL-1, platelet-derived growth factor, fibroblast growth factor)

Link between innate and adaptive immune systems
- Activate T cells by presenting antigen in a recognisable form
- T cell-derived cytokines increase phagocytosis and microbicidal activity of macrophages in a positive feedback loop

(IL = interleukin; TNF = tumour necrosis factor)

target cells and activate downstream intracellular signalling pathways, ultimately leading to changes in gene transcription and cellular function. Two important signalling pathways are illustrated in Figure 4.3. The nuclear factor kappa B (NFκB) pathway is activated by tumour necrosis factor (TNF), by other members of the TNF superfamily such as receptor activator of nuclear kappa B ligand (RANKL), and by the Toll-like receptors and NOD-like receptors (see Fig. 4.2). In the case of TNF superfamily members, receptor binding causes the inhibitor of kappa B kinase (IKK) complex of three proteins to be recruited to the receptor by binding TNF receptor-associated proteins (TRAF). This activates IKK, which in turn leads to phosphorylation of the inhibitor of nuclear factor kappa B protein (IκB), causing it to be degraded by the proteasome, allowing NFκB to translocate to the nucleus and activate gene transcription. The Janus kinase/signal transducers and activators of transcription (JAK-STAT) pathway is involved in transducing signals downstream of many cytokine receptors, including those for IL-2, IL-6 and interferon-gamma (IFN-γ). On receptor binding, JAK proteins are recruited to the intracellular portion of the receptor and are phosphorylated. These in turn phosphorylate STAT proteins, which translocate to the nucleus and activate gene transcription, altering cellular function. The function and disease associations of several important cytokines are shown in Box 4.2. Cytokine inhibitors are now routinely used in the treatment of autoimmune diseases, most of which are monoclonal antibodies to cytokines or their receptors. In addition, small-molecule inhibitors have been developed that inhibit the intracellular signalling pathways used by cytokines. These include the Janus kinase inhibitors tofacitinib, baracitinib and upadacitinib and filgotinib which are used in the treatment of various inflammatory rheumatic diseases and inflammatory bowel disease, and the tyrosine kinase inhibitor imatinib, which is used in chronic myeloid leukaemia and other haematological malignancies.

Integrins

Integrins are transmembrane proteins that play important roles in cell–cell and cell–matrix interactions. They are expressed on lymphocytes as well as a variety of other cell types and mediate attachment of cells to the endothelium and the extracellular matrix, affecting cell migration and signal transduction. Their role in autoimmune disease has been extensively studied and therapeutic agents are now being developed which modify binding of integrins to their targets. For example, natalizumab is a monoclonal antibody which targets the α4 integrin which is expressed on lymphocytes. Natalizumab prevents α4β1 integrin binding to VCAM-1 and the α4β7 integrin binding to MAdCAM-1 resulting in an anti-inflammatory

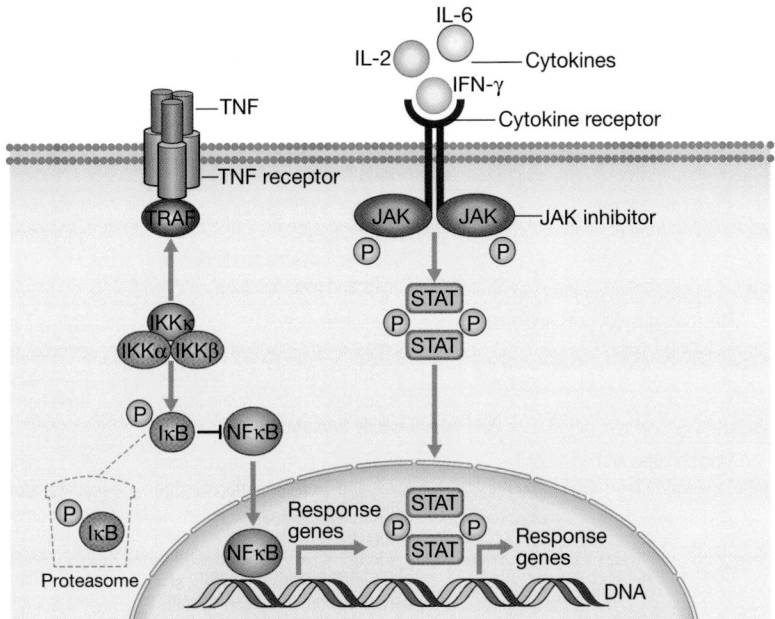

Fig. 4.3 Cytokines signalling pathways and the immune response. Cytokines regulate the immune response through binding to specific receptors that activate a variety of intracellular signalling pathways, two of which are shown. Members of the tumour necrosis factor (TNF) superfamily and the Toll-like receptors and NOD-like receptors (see Fig. 4.2) signal through the nuclear factor kappa B (NFκB) pathway. Several other cytokines, including IL-2, IL-6 and interferons, employ the Janus kinase/signal transducer and activator of transcription (JAK-STAT) pathway to regulate cellular function (see text for more details). (IFN, interferon; IκB = inhibitor of kappa B; IKK = I kappa B kinase; IL = interleukin; P = phosphorylation of the signalling protein; TRAF = tumour necrosis factor receptor-associated factor)

effect. It is an effective treatment for multiple sclerosis, which works by preventing immune cells from entering the central nervous system by interfering with lymphocyte binding the α4β1 integrin. This treatment is not without risk, however, since there are reports of progressive multifocal leucoencephalopathy (PML) in MS treated patients, as a result of JC virus infection of the central nervous system. Similarly, vedolizumab, a monoclonal antibody directed against the α4/β7 integrin, is an effective treatment for Crohn's disease and ulcerative colitis which works selectively by preventing lymphocytes entering gut endothelium by inhibiting the interaction with MAdCAM-1.

Complement

The complement system comprises a group of more than 20 tightly regulated, functionally linked proteins that act to promote inflammation and eliminate invading pathogens. Complement proteins are produced in the liver and are present in inactive form in the circulation. When the complement system is activated, it sets in motion a rapidly amplified biological cascade analogous to the coagulation cascade.

There are three mechanisms by which the complement cascade can be activated (Fig. 4.4):

- *The alternate pathway* is triggered directly by binding of C3 to bacterial cell-wall components, such as lipopolysaccharide of Gram-negative bacteria and teichoic acid of Gram-positive bacteria.
- *The classical pathway* is initiated when two or more IgM or IgG antibody molecules bind to antigen. The associated conformational change exposes binding sites on the antibodies for the first protein in the classical pathway, C1, which is a multiheaded molecule that can bind up to six antibody molecules. Once two or more 'heads' of a C1 molecule are bound to antibody, the classical cascade is triggered. An important inhibitor of the classical pathway is C1 inhibitor (C1inh), as illustrated in Figure 4.4.
- *The lectin pathway* is activated when mannose-binding lectin interacts with microbial cell surface carbohydrates. This directly stimulates the classical pathway at the level of C4, bypassing the need for immune complex formation.

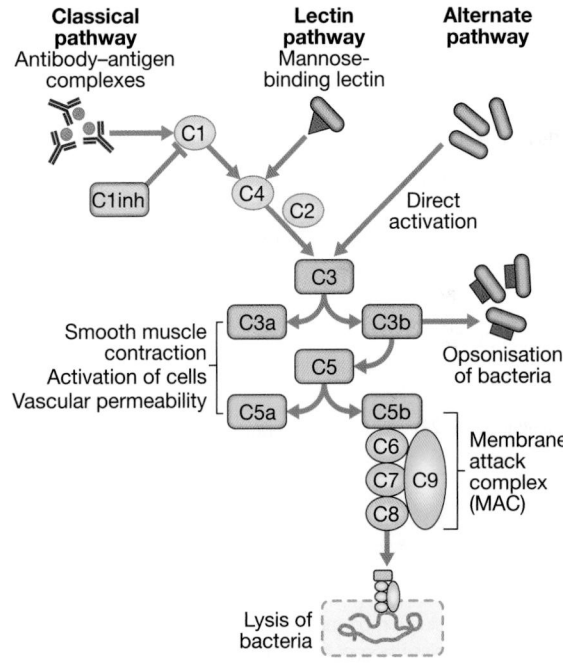

Fig. 4.4 The complement pathway. The classical pathway is activated by binding of antigen–antibody complexes to C1 but is blocked by C1 inhibitor (C1inh), whereas mannose-binding lectins, which are macromolecules that bind to carbohydrates on the surface of various microorganisms, activate the pathway by binding C4. Bacteria can directly activate the pathway through C3, which plays a pivotal role in complement activation through all three pathways.

Activation of complement by any of these pathways results in activation of C3. This in turn activates the final common pathway, in which the complement proteins C5–C9 assemble to form the membrane attack complex (MAC). This can puncture the cell wall, leading to osmotic lysis of target cells.

| i | 4.2 | Important cytokines in the regulation of the immune response |

Cytokine	Source	Actions	Biologic therapies
Interferon-alpha (IFN-α)	T cells and macrophages	Antiviral activity Activates NK cells, CD8+ T cells and macrophages	Recombinant IFN-α used in hepatitis C and some malignancies
Interferon-gamma (IFN-γ)	T cells and NK cells	Increases antimicrobial activity of macrophages Regulates cytokine production by T cells and macrophages	Interferon-γ used in chronic granulomatous disease
Tumour necrosis factor alpha (TNF-α)	Macrophages, NK cells and others, including T cells	Pro-inflammatory Increases expression of other cytokines and adhesion molecules Causes apoptosis of some target cells Directly cytotoxic	TNF-α inhibitors used in rheumatoid arthritis, inflammatory bowel disease, psoriasis and many other inflammatory conditions
Interleukin-1 (IL-1)	Macrophages and neutrophils	Stimulates neutrophil recruitment, fever, and T-cell and macrophage activation as part of the inflammatory response	IL-1 inhibitors used in systemic juvenile rheumatoid arthritis, periodic fever syndromes and acute gout
Interleukin-2 (IL-2)	CD4+ T cells	Stimulates proliferation and differentiation of antigen-specific T lymphocytes	IL-2 inhibitors used in the treatment of transplant rejection
Interleukin-4 (IL-4)	CD4+ T cells	Stimulates maturation of B and T cells, and production of IgE antibody	Antibodies to IL-4 receptor used in severe atopic dermatitis
Interleukin-5 (IL-5)	CD4+ T cells, mast cells, eosinophils and basophils	Growth and differentiation factor for B cells and eosinophils	Antibodies to IL-5 or the IL-5 receptor used in treatment refractory eosinophilic asthma and more recently anti-IL-5 antibodies used in eosinophilic vasculitis
Interleukin-6 (IL-6)	Monocytes and macrophages	Stimulates neutrophil recruitment, fever, and T-cell and macrophage activation as part of the inflammatory response, stimulates maturation of B cells into plasma cells	Antibodies to IL-6 receptor used in rheumatoid arthritis and giant cell arteritis
Interleukin-12 (IL-12)	Monocytes and macrophages	Stimulates IFN-γ and TNF-α release by T cells Activates NK cells	Antibody to p40 subunit of IL-12 used in psoriasis and psoriatic arthritis
Interleukin-17 (IL-17)	Th17 cells (T helper), NK cells, NK-T cells	Pro-inflammatory cytokine Involved in mucosal immunity and control of extracellular pathogens, synergy with IL-1 and TNF	Antibody to IL-17 used in psoriasis, psoriatic arthritis and ankylosing spondylitis
Interleukin-22 (IL-22)	Th17 cells	Induction of epithelial cell proliferation and antimicrobial proteins in keratinocytes	
Interleukin-23 (IL-23)	Activated macrophages and dendritic cells in peripheral tissues	Pro-inflammatory cytokine, proliferation of Th17 T cells with induction of IL-17	Antibody to IL-23 used in psoriasis, psoriatic arthritis and inflammatory bowel disease

(IgE = immunoglobulin E; NK = natural killer)

This step is particularly important in the defence against encapsulated bacteria such as *Neisseria* spp. and *Haemophilus influenzae*.

Complement fragments generated by activation of the cascade can also act as opsonins, rendering microorganisms more susceptible to phagocytosis by macrophages and neutrophils (see Fig. 4.2). In addition, they are chemotactic agents, promoting leucocyte trafficking to sites of inflammation. Some fragments act as anaphylotoxins, binding to complement receptors on mast cells and triggering release of histamine, which increases vascular permeability. The products of complement activation also help to target immune complexes to antigen-presenting cells, providing a link between the innate and the adaptive immune systems. Finally, activated complement products dissolve the immune complexes that triggered the cascade, minimising bystander damage to surrounding tissues.

There are a number of control proteins within the complement system that prevent activation on host cells, thereby preventing host cell damage, some of which are membrane bound, others soluble, such as C1 inhibitor. Factor H is an important example in control of the alternate pathway, CD59 and decay accelerating factor (DAF) are important in the terminal complement pathway. Deficiencies in factor H can lead to atypical haemolytic uraemic syndrome and failure of binding of CD59 and DAF due to deficiency in the anchoring glycosylphosphatidylinositol on red blood cells can lead to paroxysmal nocturnal haemoglobulinuria as a result of complement-mediated haemolysis. A monoclonal antibody directed against the central complement molecule C5, eculizumab, has been developed for therapeutic use in these conditions. Invasive infection, including meningococcal sepsis, has been reported with eculizumab therapy, highlighting the importance of the complement system in preventing such infections.

Mast cells and basophils

Mast cells and basophils are bone marrow-derived cells that play a central role in allergic disorders. Mast cells reside predominantly in tissues exposed to the external environment, such as the skin and gut, while basophils circulate in peripheral blood and are recruited into tissues in response to inflammation. Both contain large cytoplasmic granules that enclose vasoactive substances such as histamine (see Fig. 4.14). Mast cells and basophils express IgE receptors on their cell surface, which bind IgE antibody. On encounter with specific antigen, the cell is triggered to release histamine and other mediators present within the granules and to synthesise additional mediators, including leukotrienes, prostaglandins and cytokines. An inflammatory cascade is initiated that increases local blood flow and vascular permeability, stimulates smooth muscle contraction and increases secretion at mucosal surfaces.

Natural killer cells

Natural killer (NK) cells are large granular lymphocytes that play a major role in defence against tumours and viruses. They exhibit features of both the adaptive and the innate immune systems in that they are morphologically similar to lymphocytes and recognise similar ligands, but they are not antigen-specific and cannot generate immunological memory. NK cells express a variety of cell surface receptors, some of which are stimulatory and others inhibitory. The effects of inhibitory receptors normally predominate. These recognise human leucocyte antigen (HLA) molecules that are expressed on normal nucleated cells, preventing NK cell-mediated attack, whereas the stimulatory receptors recognise molecules that are expressed primarily when cells are damaged. This allows NK cells to remain tolerant to healthy cells but not to damaged ones. When cells become infected by viruses or undergo malignant change, expression of HLA class I molecules on the cell surface can be down-regulated. This is an important mechanism by which these cells then evade adaptive T-lymphocyte responses. In this circumstance, however, NK cell defences becomes important, as down-regulation of HLA class I abrogates the inhibitory signals that normally prevent NK activation. The net result is NK attack on the abnormal target cell. NK cells can also be activated by binding of antigen–antibody complexes to surface receptors. This physically links the NK cell to its target in a manner analogous to opsonisation and is known as antibody-dependent cellular cytotoxicity (ADCC).

Activated NK cells can kill their targets in various ways. They secrete pore-forming proteins such as perforin into the membrane of the target cell, and proteolytic enzymes called granzymes into the target cell, which cause apoptosis. In addition, NK cells produce a variety of cytokines such as TNF-α and IFN-γ, which have direct antiviral and anti-tumour effects.

The adaptive immune system

If the innate immune system fails to provide effective protection against an invading pathogen, the adaptive immune system is mobilised (see Fig. 4.1). This has three key characteristics:

- It has exquisite specificity and can discriminate between very small differences in molecular structure.
- It is highly adaptive and can respond to an almost unlimited number of molecules.
- It possesses immunological memory, and changes consequent to initial activation by an antigen allow a more effective immune response on subsequent encounters.

There are two major arms of the adaptive immune response. Humoral immunity involves the production of antibodies by B lymphocytes, and cellular immunity involves the activation of T lymphocytes, which synthesise and release cytokines that affect other cells, as well as directly killing target cells. These interact closely with each other and with the components of the innate immune system to maximise effectiveness of the immune response.

Lymphoid organs

The primary lymphoid organs are involved in lymphocyte development. They include the bone marrow, where T and B lymphocytes differentiate from haematopoietic stem cells and where B lymphocytes also mature, and the thymus, the site of T-cell maturation (see Fig. 4.1). After maturation, lymphocytes migrate to the secondary lymphoid organs. These include the spleen, lymph nodes and mucosa-associated lymphoid tissue. These trap and concentrate foreign substances and are the major sites of interaction between naïve lymphocytes and microorganisms.

The thymus

The thymus is a bi-lobed structure in the anterior mediastinum, and is organised into cortical and medullary areas. The cortex is densely populated with immature T cells, which migrate to the medulla to undergo selection and maturation. The thymus is most active in the fetal and neonatal period, and involutes after puberty. Failure of thymic development is associated with profound T-cell immune deficiency but surgical removal of the thymus in childhood (usually during major cardiac surgery) is not associated with significant immune dysfunction.

The spleen

The spleen is the largest of the secondary lymphoid organs. It is highly effective at filtering blood and is an important site of phagocytosis of senescent erythrocytes, bacteria, immune complexes and other debris, and of antibody synthesis. It is important for defence against encapsulated bacteria, and asplenic individuals are at risk of overwhelming *Streptococcus pneumoniae* and *H. influenzae* infection (see Box 4.5).

Lymph nodes

These are positioned to maximise exposure to lymph draining from sites of external contact, and are highly organised (see Fig. 4.1).

- The *cortex* contains primary lymphoid follicles, which are the site of B-lymphocyte interactions. When B cells encounter antigen, they undergo intense proliferation, forming germinal centres.
- The *paracortex* is rich in T lymphocytes and dendritic cells.
- The *medulla* is the major site of antibody-secreting plasma cells.
- Within the medulla there are many *sinuses*, which contain large numbers of macrophages.

Mucosa-associated lymphoid tissue

Mucosa-associated lymphoid tissue (MALT) consists of diffusely distributed lymphoid cells and follicles present along mucosal surfaces. It has a similar function to the more organised, encapsulated lymph nodes. They include the tonsils, adenoids and Peyer's patches in the small intestine.

Lymphatics

Lymphoid tissue is connected by a network of lymphatics, with three major functions: lymphatics provide access to lymph nodes, return interstitial fluid to the venous system and transport fat from the small intestine to the blood stream (see Fig. 19.12). The lymphatics begin as blind-ending capillaries, which come together to form lymphatic ducts, entering and leaving regional lymph nodes as afferent and efferent ducts, respectively. They eventually coalesce and drain into the thoracic duct and left subclavian vein. Lymphatics may be either deep or superficial, and follow the distribution of major blood vessels.

Humoral immunity

Humoral immunity is mediated by B lymphocytes, which differentiate from haematopoietic stem cells in the bone marrow. Their major functions are to produce antibody and interact with T cells, but they are also involved in antigen presentation. Mature B lymphocytes can be found in the bone marrow, lymphoid tissue, spleen and, to a lesser extent, the blood stream. They express a unique immunoglobulin receptor on their cell surface, the B-cell receptor, which binds to soluble antigen targets (Fig. 4.5).

Encounters with antigen usually occur within lymph nodes. If provided with appropriate cytokines and other signals from nearby T lymphocytes, antigen-specific B cells respond by rapidly proliferating in a process known as clonal expansion (see Fig. 4.5). This is accompanied by a highly complex series of genetic rearrangements known as somatic hypermutation, which generates B-cell populations that express receptors with greater affinity for antigen than the original. These cells differentiate into either long-lived memory cells, which reside in the lymph nodes, or plasma cells, which produce antibody. Memory cells allow production of a more rapid and more effective response on subsequent exposure to that pathogen.

Immunoglobulins

Immunoglobulins (Ig) play a central role in humoral immunity. They are soluble proteins produced by plasma cells and are made up of two heavy and two light chains (Fig. 4.6). The heavy chain determines the antibody class or isotype, such as IgG, IgA, IgM, IgE or IgD. Subclasses of IgG and IgA also occur. The antigen is recognised by the antigen-binding regions (F_{ab}) of both heavy and light chains, while the consequences of antibody binding are determined by the constant region of the heavy chain (F_c) (Box 4.3). Antibodies have several functions. They facilitate phagocytosis by acting as opsonins (see Fig. 4.2) and facilitate cell killing by cytotoxic cells, particularly NK cells by antibody-dependent cellular cytotoxicity. Binding of antibodies to antigen can trigger activation of the classical complement pathway (see Fig. 4.4). In addition, antibodies can directly neutralise the biological activity of their antigen target. This is a particularly important feature of IgA antibodies, which act predominantly at mucosal surfaces.

The humoral immune response is characterised by immunological memory, in which the antibody response to successive exposures to an antigen is qualitatively and quantitatively improved from the first exposure. When a previously unstimulated or 'naïve' B lymphocyte is activated by antigen, the first antibody to be produced is IgM, which appears in the serum after 5–10 days. Depending on additional stimuli provided by T lymphocytes, other antibody classes (IgG, IgA and IgE) are produced 1–2 weeks later. If the memory B cell is subsequently re-exposed to the same antigen, the lag time between exposure and production of antibody is decreased to 2–3 days, the amount of antibody produced is increased, and the response is dominated by IgG antibodies of high affinity. Furthermore, in contrast to the initial antibody response, secondary antibody responses do not require additional input from T lymphocytes. This allows the rapid generation of highly specific responses on re-exposure to a pathogen and is an important mechanism in vaccine efficacy.

Cellular immunity

Cellular immunity is mediated by T lymphocytes, which play important roles in defence against viruses, fungi and intracellular bacteria. They also play an important immunoregulatory role, by orchestrating and regulating the responses of other components of the immune system. T-lymphocyte precursors differentiate from haematopoietic stem cells in the bone marrow and are exported to the thymus when they are still immature (see Fig. 4.1). Individual T cells express a unique receptor that is highly specific for a single antigen. Within the thymus T cells undergo a process of stringent selection to ensure that autoreactive cells are destroyed. Mature T lymphocytes leave the thymus and expand to populate other organs of the immune system. It has been estimated that an individual possesses 10^7–10^9 T-cell clones, each with a unique T-cell receptor, ensuring at least partial coverage for any antigen encountered.

Unlike B cells, T cells cannot recognise intact protein antigens in their native form. Instead, the protein must be broken down into component peptides by antigen-presenting cells for presentation to T lymphocytes in association with HLA molecules on the antigen-presenting cell surface (Fig. 4.7). This process is known as antigen processing and presentation, and it is the complex of peptide and HLA together that is recognised by individual T cells. The structure of HLA molecules varies widely between individuals. Since each HLA molecule has the capacity to present a subtly different peptide repertoire to T lymphocytes, this ensures enormous diversity in recognition of antigens by the T-cell population. All nucleated cells have the capacity to process and present antigens, but cells with specialised antigen-presenting functions include dendritic cells, macrophages and B lymphocytes. These cells carry additional co-stimulatory molecules, such as CD80 and CD86, providing the necessary 'second signal' for full T-cell activation (Fig. 4.8). Mechanisms also exist to inhibit activation of T-cells. One of the most important is the programmed cell death 1 (PD-1) pathway. The PD1 receptor is expressed on lymphocytes and inhibits lymphocyte activation when bound by its ligand (PDL-1) which is a molecule expressed on antigen-presenting cells, endothelial; cells and come tumour cells (Fig. 4.8). Monoclonal antibodies which inhibit this interaction are important treatments for certain types of cancer (see tumour immunology later in this chapter).

T lymphocytes can be divided into two subgroups on the basis of function and recognition of HLA molecules. These are designated CD4+ and CD8+ T cells, according to the 'cluster of differentiation' (CD) antigen number of key proteins expressed on their cell surface.

CD8+ T lymphocytes

These cells recognise antigenic peptides in association with HLA class I molecules (HLA-A, HLA-B, HLA-C). They kill infected cells directly

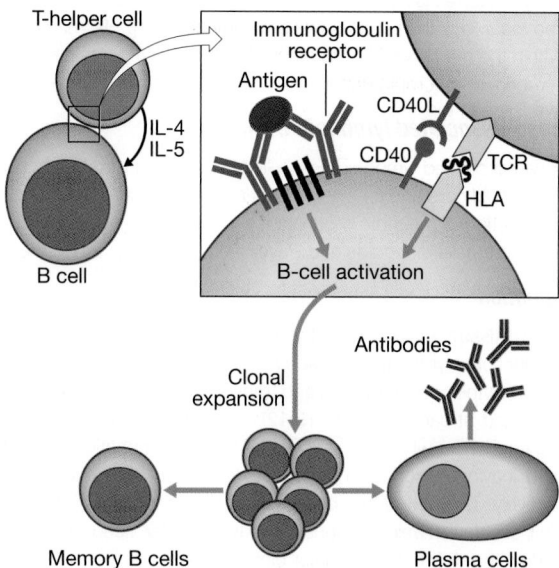

Fig. 4.5 B-cell activation. Activation of B cells is initiated through binding of an antigen with the immunoglobulin receptor on the cell surface. For activation to proceed, an interaction with T-helper cells is also required, providing additional signals through binding of CD40 ligand (CD40L) to CD40; an interaction between the T-cell receptor (TCR) and processed antigenic peptides presented by human leucocyte antigen (HLA) molecules on the B-cell surface; and cytokines released by the T-helper cells. Fully activated B cells undergo clonal expansion with differentiation towards plasma cells that produce antibody. Following activation, memory cells are generated that allow rapid antibody responses when the same antigen is encountered on a second occasion. (IL = interleukin)

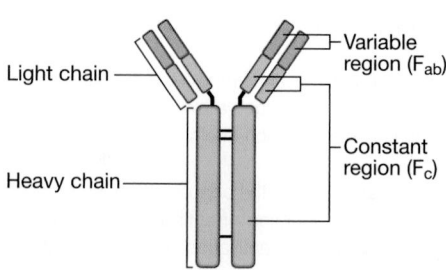

Fig. 4.6 The structure of an immunoglobulin (antibody) molecule. The variable region is responsible for antigen binding, whereas the constant region can interact with immunoglobulin receptors expressed on immune cells.

i	**4.3 Classes and properties of antibody**					
Antibody	Concentration in adult serum	Complement activation*	Opsonisation	Presence in external secretions	Other properties	
IgG	6.0–16.0 g/L	IgG1 +++ IgG2 + IgG3 +++	IgG1 ++ IgG3 ++	++	Four subclasses: IgG1, IgG2, IgG3, IgG4 Distributed equally between blood and extracellular fluid, and transported across placenta IgG2 is particularly important in defence against polysaccharides antigens	
IgA	1.5–4.0 g/L	–	–	++++	Two subclasses: IgA1, IgA2 Highly effective at neutralising toxins Particularly important at mucosal surfaces	
IgM	0.5–2.0 g/L	++++	–	+	Highly effective at agglutinating pathogens	
IgE	0.003–0.04 g/L	–	–	–	Majority of IgE is bound to mast cells, basophils and eosinophils Important in allergic disease and defence against parasite infection	
IgD	Not detected	–	–	–	Function in B-cell development	

*Activation of the classical pathway, also called 'complement fixation'.
(IgG = immunoglobulin)

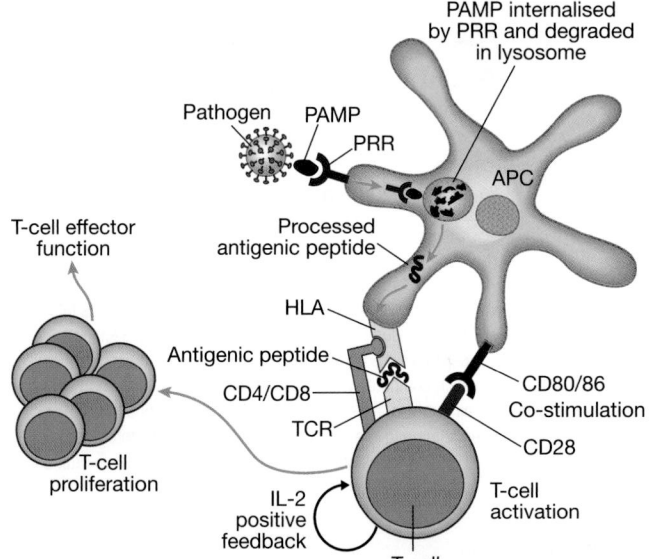

Fig. 4.7 Antigen presentation. For T-cell activation, antigen has to be processed via antigen-presenting cells (APC). Pathogens, bearing pathogen-associated molecular patterns (PAMPs) on their surface, are recognised by pattern recognition receptors (PRRs) on the APC. Following endocytosis, the pathogen is broken down intracellularly. Antigenic peptides are then loaded onto human leucocyte antigens (HLA), also known as major histocompatibility complexes (MHC), and presented at the APC surface. The combination of peptide and HLA is then recognised by the T-cell receptor (TCR). For T-cell activation, a second, co-stimulatory signal is required through binding of CD80 or CD86 on the APC to CD28 on the T cell (see also Fig. 4.8). (CD28 and CD80/86 = co-stimulatory molecules; IL = interleukin)

through the production of pore-forming molecules such as perforin and release of digesting enzymes triggering apoptosis of the target cell, and are particularly important in defence against viral infection.

CD4+ T lymphocytes

These cells recognise peptides presented on HLA class II molecules (HLA-DR, HLA-DP and HLA-DQ) and have mainly immunoregulatory functions. They produce cytokines and provide co-stimulatory signals that support the activation of CD8+ T lymphocytes and assist the production of mature antibody by B cells. In addition, their close interaction

with phagocytes determines cytokine production by both cell types. CD4+ lymphocytes can be further subdivided into subsets on the basis of the cytokines they produce:

- Th1 (T-helper) cells typically produce IL-2, IFN-γ and TNF-α, and support the development of delayed-type hypersensitivity responses.
- Th2 cells typically produce IL-4, IL-5, IL-10 and IL-13, and promote allergic responses.
- T-regulatory cells (T-regs) are a further subset of specialised CD4+ lymphocytes that are important in actively suppressing activation of other cells and preventing autoimmune disease. They produce cytokines such as TGF-β and IL-10.
- Th17 cells are pro-inflammatory cells defined by their production of IL-17. They are related to regulatory T cells. Th17 cells have a key role in defence against extracellular bacteria and fungi. They also have a role in the development of autoimmune disease.

T-cell activation is regulated by a balance between co-stimulatory molecules, the second signal required for activation, and inhibitory molecules that down-regulate T-cell activity. One such inhibitory molecule, CTLA4, has been harnessed therapeutically in the form of abatacept, which is a fusion protein comprised of the Fc fragment of immunoglobulin linked to CTLA4. This is used to inhibit T-cell activation in rheumatoid arthritis and solid organ transplantation.

The inflammatory response

Inflammation is the response of tissues to injury or infection, and is necessary for normal repair and healing. This section focuses on the general principles of the inflammatory response and its multisystem manifestations. The role of inflammation in specific diseases is discussed in many other chapters of this book.

Acute inflammation

Acute inflammation is the result of rapid and complex interplay between the cells and soluble molecules of the innate immune system. The classical external signs include heat, redness, pain and swelling (Fig. 4.9). The inflammatory process is initiated by local tissue injury or infection. Damaged epithelial cells produce cytokines and antimicrobial peptides, causing early infiltration of phagocytic cells. Production of leukotrienes,

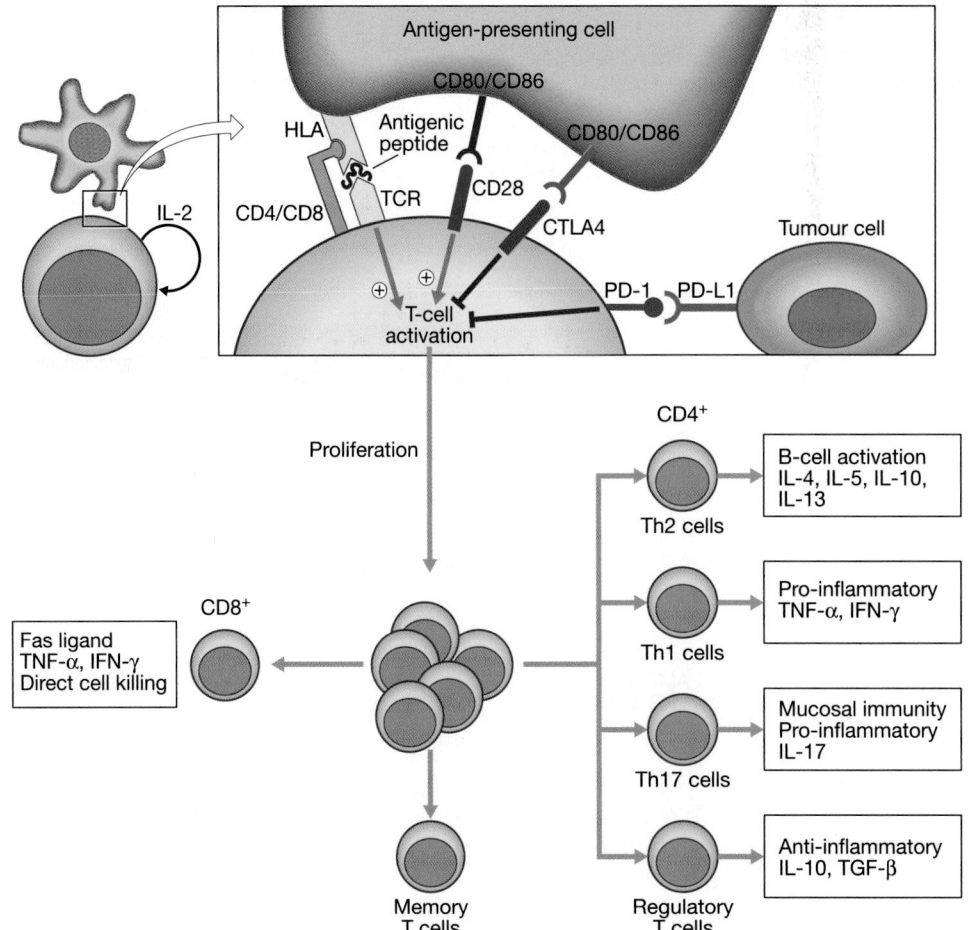

Fig. 4.8 T-cell activation. Activation of T cells is initiated when an antigenic peptide bound to a human leucocyte antigen (HLA) molecule on antigen-presenting cells interacts with the T-cell receptor expressed by T lymphocytes. Additional signals are required for T-cell activation, however. These include binding of the co-stimulatory molecules CD80 and CD86 with CD28 on the T cell, and interleukin 2 (IL-2), which is produced in an autocrine manner by T cells that are undergoing activation. Other molecules are present that can inhibit T-cell activation, however, including cytotoxic T-lymphocyte-associated protein 4 (CTLA4), which competes with CD28 for binding to CD80 and CD86; and PD-1, which, by binding PD-L1, is also inhibitory. Following activation, T cells proliferate and, depending on their subtype, have various functions with distinct patterns of cytokine production, as indicated. Memory cells are also generated that can mount a rapid immune response on encountering the same antigen. (IFN-γ = interferon-gamma; IL = interleukin; PD-1 = programmed cell death 1; PD-L1 = programmed death ligand 1; TCR = T-cell receptor; TGF-β = transforming growth factor beta; TNF-α = tumour necrosis factor alpha)

prostaglandins, histamine, kinins, anaphylotoxins and inducible nitric oxide synthase also occurs within inflamed tissue. These mediators cause vasodilatation and increased vascular permeability, causing trafficking of fluid and cells into the affected tissue. In addition, pro-inflammatory cytokines, such as IL-1, TNF-α and IL-6 produced at the site of injury, are released systemically and act on the hypothalamus to cause fever, and on the liver to stimulate production of acute phase proteins.

The acute phase response

The acute phase response refers to the production of a variety of proteins by the liver in response to inflammatory stimuli. These proteins have a wide range of activities. Circulating levels of C-reactive protein (CRP) and serum amyloid A may be increased 100- to 1000-fold, contributing to host defence and stimulating repair and regeneration. Fibrinogen plays an essential role in wound healing, and α$_1$-antitrypsin and α$_1$-antichymotrypsin control the pro-inflammatory cascade by neutralising the enzymes produced by activated neutrophils, preventing widespread tissue destruction. In addition, antioxidants such as haptoglobin and manganese superoxide dismutase scavenge for oxygen free radicals, while increased levels of iron-binding proteins such as ferritin and lactoferrin decrease the iron available for uptake by bacteria. Immunoglobulins are not acute phase proteins but are often increased in chronic inflammation.

Septic shock

Septic shock is the clinical manifestation of overwhelming inflammation. It is characterised by excessive production of pro-inflammatory cytokines by macrophages, causing hypotension, hypovolaemia and tissue oedema. In addition, uncontrolled neutrophil activation causes release of proteases and oxygen free radicals within blood vessels, damaging the vascular endothelium and further increasing capillary permeability. Direct activation of the coagulation pathway combines with endothelial cell disruption to form clots within the damaged vessels. The clinical consequences include cardiovascular collapse, acute respiratory distress syndrome, disseminated intravascular coagulation, multi-organ failure and often death. Septic shock most frequently results from infection with Gram-negative bacteria, because lipopolysaccharide produced by these organisms is particularly effective at activating the inflammatory cascade. Early recognition and appropriate early intervention can improve patient outcome. More details on the diagnosis and management of septic shock are provided in Chapter 9.

Resolution of inflammation

Resolution of an inflammatory response is crucial for normal healing. This involves active down-modulation of inflammatory stimuli and repair

4

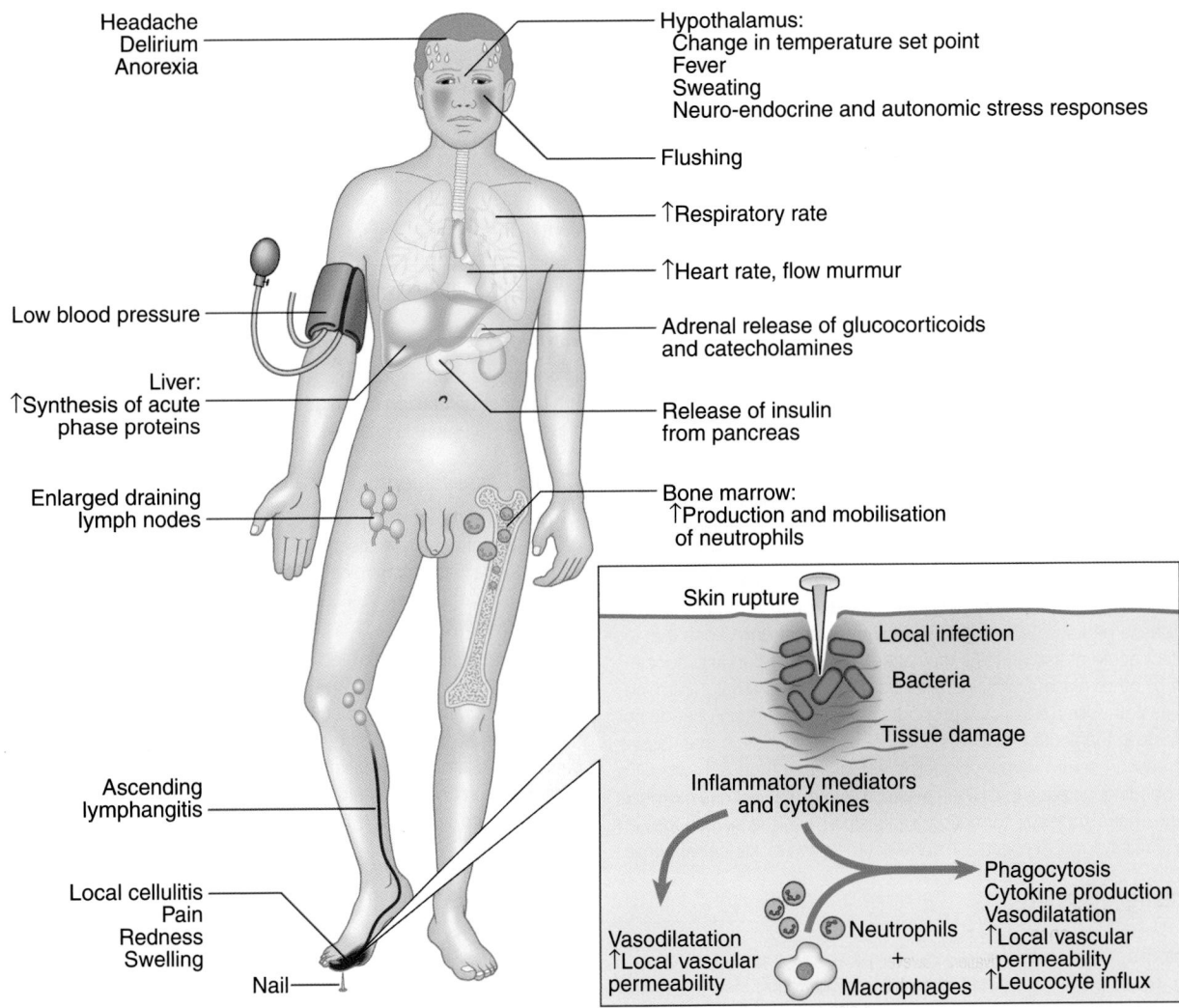

Headache
Delirium
Anorexia

Hypothalamus:
Change in temperature set point
Fever
Sweating
Neuro-endocrine and autonomic stress responses

Flushing

↑Respiratory rate

↑Heart rate, flow murmur

Low blood pressure

Adrenal release of glucocorticoids
and catecholamines

Liver:
↑Synthesis of acute
phase proteins

Release of insulin
from pancreas

Enlarged draining
lymph nodes

Bone marrow:
↑Production and mobilisation
of neutrophils

Skin rupture

Local infection

Bacteria

Tissue damage

Inflammatory mediators
and cytokines

Ascending
lymphangitis

Phagocytosis
Cytokine production
Vasodilatation
↑Local vascular
permeability
↑Leucocyte influx

Neutrophils

Local cellulitis
Pain
Redness
Swelling

Vasodilatation
↑Local vascular
permeability

+

Nail

Macrophages

Fig. 4.9 Clinical features of acute inflammation. In this example, the response is to a penetrating injury and infection of the foot.

of bystander damage to local tissues. Extravasated neutrophils undergo apoptosis and are phagocytosed by macrophages, along with the remains of microorganisms. Macrophages also synthesise collagenase and elastase, which break down local connective tissue and aid in the removal of debris. Normal tissue homeostasis is also associated with reversion of parenchymal cells to a non-inflammatory phenotype. Macrophage-derived cytokines, including transforming growth factor-beta (TGF-β) and platelet-derived growth factor, stimulate fibroblasts and promote the synthesis of new collagen, while angiogenic factors stimulate new vessel formation.

Chronic inflammation

In most instances, the development of an active immune response results in clearance and control of the inflammatory stimulus and resolution of tissue damage. Failure of this process may result in chronic inflammation, with significant associated bystander damage, known as hypersensitivity responses. Persistence of microorganisms can result in ongoing accumulation of neutrophils, macrophages and activated T lymphocytes within the lesion. If this is associated with local deposition of fibrous tissue, a granuloma may form. Granulomas are characteristic of tuberculosis and leprosy (Hansen's disease), in which the microorganism is protected by a robust cell wall that shields it from killing, despite phagocytosis.

Laboratory features of inflammation

Inflammation is associated with changes in many laboratory investigations. Leucocytosis is common, and reflects the transit of activated neutrophils and monocytes to the site of infection. The platelet count may also be increased. The most widely used laboratory measure of acute inflammation is CRP. Circulating levels of many other acute phase reactants, including fibrinogen, ferritin and complement components, are also increased in response to acute inflammation, while albumin levels are reduced. Chronic inflammation is frequently associated with a normocytic normochromic anaemia.

C-reactive protein

C-reactive protein (CRP) is an acute phase reactant synthesised by the liver, which opsonises invading pathogens. Circulating concentrations of CRP increase within 6 hours of the start of an inflammatory stimulus. Serum concentrations of CRP provide a direct biomarker of acute inflammation and, because the serum half-life of CRP is 18 hours, levels fall promptly once the inflammatory stimulus is removed. Sequential measurements are useful in monitoring disease activity (Box 4.4). For reasons that remain unclear, some diseases are associated with only minor elevations of CRP despite unequivocal evidence of active inflammation. These include systemic lupus erythematosus (SLE), systemic sclerosis, ulcerative colitis and leukaemia. An important practical point is that if the CRP is raised in these conditions, it suggests intercurrent infection rather than disease activity. Since the CRP is a more sensitive early indicator of the acute phase response, it is generally used in preference to the erythrocyte sedimentation rate (ESR). If both ESR and CRP are used, any discrepancy should be resolved by assessing the individual determinants of the ESR, which are discussed below.

Erythrocyte sedimentation rate

The ESR is an indirect measure of inflammation. It measures how fast erythrocytes fall through plasma, which is determined by the composition of plasma proteins and the morphology of circulating erythrocytes. These factors govern the propensity of red cells to aggregate, the major determinant of the ESR. Erythrocytes are inherently negatively charged, which prevents them from clumping together in the blood stream. Since plasma proteins such as fibrinogen and immunoglobulins are positively charged, increased concentrations of these proteins neutralise an increase in plasma protein concentrations neutralises the negative charge of erythrocytes, overcoming their inherent repulsive forces and causing them aggregate, resulting in rouleaux formation. Rouleaux have a higher mass-to-surface area ratio than single red cells, and therefore sediment faster. The most common reason for an increased ESR is an acute phase response, which causes an increase in the concentration of acute phase proteins, including CRP. However, other conditions that do not affect acute phase proteins may alter the composition and concentration of other plasma proteins (see Box 4.4). For example, immunoglobulins comprise a significant proportion of plasma proteins but do not participate in the acute phase response. Thus any condition that causes an increase in serum immunoglobulins will increase the ESR without a corresponding increase in CRP. In addition, abnormal red cell morphology can make rouleaux formation impossible. For these reasons, an inappropriately low ESR occurs in spherocytosis and sickle-cell anaemia.

Plasma viscosity

Plasma viscosity is another surrogate measure of plasma protein concentration. Like the ESR, it is affected by the concentration of large plasma proteins, including fibrinogen and immunoglobulins. It is not affected by

properties of erythrocytes and is generally considered to be more reliable than the ESR as a marker of inflammation.

Presenting problems in immune disorders

Recurrent infections

Infections can occur in otherwise healthy individuals but recurrent infection raises suspicion of an immune deficiency. Depending on the component of the immune system affected, the infections may involve bacteria, viruses, fungi or protozoa, as summarised in Box 4.5. T-cell deficiencies can involve pathogens from all groups.

Aetiology

Infections secondary to immune deficiency occur because of defects in the number or function of phagocytes, B cells, T cells or complement, as described later in this chapter.

Clinical assessment

Clinical features that may indicate immune deficiency are listed in Box 4.6. Frequent or severe infections, or ones caused by unusual organisms or at unusual sites, are typical of immune deficiency.

Investigations

Initial investigations should include full blood count and white cell differential, CRP, renal and liver function tests, urine dipstick, serum immunoglobulins with protein electrophoresis, and HIV testing. Additional microbiological tests, virology and imaging are required to identify the causal organism and localise the site of infection, as outlined in Box 4.7. If primary immune deficiency is suspected on the basis of initial investigations, more specialised tests should be considered, as summarised in Box 4.8.

Management

If an immune deficiency is suspected but has not yet been formally characterised, patients should not receive live vaccines because of the risk of vaccine-induced disease. Further management depends on the underlying cause and details are provided later.

i	4.4 Conditions commonly associated with abnormal C-reactive protein (CRP) and/or erythrocyte sedimentation rate (ESR)			
Condition	Consequence	Effect on CRP[1]	Effect on ESR[2]
Acute bacterial, fungal or viral infection	Stimulates acute phase response	Increased (range 50–150 mg/L; in severe infections may be > 300 mg/L)	Increased
Necrotising bacterial infection	Stimulates profound acute inflammatory response	Greatly increased (may be > 300 mg/L)	Increased
Chronic bacterial or fungal infection Localised abscess, bacterial endocarditis or tuberculosis	Stimulates acute and chronic inflammatory response with polyclonal increase in immunoglobulins, as well as increased acute phase proteins	Increased (range 50–150 mg/L)	Increased disproportionately to CRP
Acute inflammatory diseases Crohn's disease, polymyalgia rheumatica, inflammatory arthritis	Stimulates acute phase response	Increased (range 50–150 mg/L)	Increased
Systemic lupus erythematosus, Sjögren syndrome, ulcerative colitis	Chronic inflammatory response	Normal	Increased
Multiple myeloma	Monoclonal increase in serum immunoglobulin without acute inflammation	Normal	Increased
Pregnancy, old age, end-stage renal disease	Increased fibrinogen	Normal	Moderately increased

[1]Reference range <5 mg/L. [2]Reference range: adult males <10 mm/hr, adult females <3–15 mm/hr.

i 4.5 Immune deficiencies and common patterns of infection

Phagocyte deficiency	Complement deficiency	Antibody deficiency	T-lymphocyte deficiency
Bacteria			
Staphylococcus aureus Pseudomonas aeruginosa Serratia marcescens Burkholderia cenocepacia Nocardia Mycobacterium tuberculosis Atypical mycobacteria	Neisseria meningitidis Neisseria gonorrhoeae Haemophilus influenzae Streptococcus pneumoniae	Haemophilus influenzae Streptococcus pneumoniae Staphylococcus aureus	Mycobacterium tuberculosis Atypical mycobacteria
Fungi			
Candida spp. Aspergillus spp.	–	–	Candida spp. Aspergillus spp. Pneumocystis jirovecii
Viruses	–	–	Cytomegalovirus (CMV) Enteroviruses Epstein–Barr virus (EBV) Herpes zoster virus Human papillomavirus Human herpesvirus 8
Protozoa	–	Giardia lamblia	Toxoplasma gondii Cryptosporidia

i 4.6 Warning signs of primary immune deficiency*

In children	In adults
≥ 4 new ear infections within 1 year	≥ 2 new ear infections within 1 year
≥ 2 serious sinus infections within 1 year	≥ 2 new sinus infections within 1 year, in the absence of allergy
≥ 2 months on antibiotics with little effect	Recurrent viral infections
≥ 2 pneumonias within 1 year	≥ 1 pneumonia per year for more than 1 year
Failure of an infant to gain weight or grow normally	Chronic diarrhoea with weight loss
Recurrent deep skin or organ abscesses	Recurrent deep skin or organ abscesses
Persistent thrush in mouth or elsewhere on skin after infancy	Persistent thrush or fungal infection on skin or elsewhere
Need for intravenous antibiotics to clear infections	Recurrent need for intravenous antibiotics to clear infections
≥ 2 deep-seated infections such as sepsis, meningitis or cellulitis	Infection with atypical mycobacteria
A family history of primary immune deficiency	A family history of primary immune deficiency

*The presence of two or more of the listed features may indicate the presence of an underlying primary immunodeficiency.
©Jeffrey Modell Foundation.

i 4.7 Initial investigations in suspected immune deficiency

Test	Value	Comment
Full blood count	Full white cell differential	May define pathway for further investigation
Acute phase reactants	Help determine presence of active infection	
Serum immunoglobulins	Detection of antibody deficiency	
Serum protein electrophoresis	Detection of paraprotein	May be the cause of immune paresis; paraprotein should be excluded prior to diagnosis of primary antibody deficiency
Serum free light chains/Bence Jones proteins	Detection of paraprotein	
Human immunodeficiency virus (HIV) test	To exclude HIV as cause of secondary immune deficiency	
Imaging according to history and examination findings	Detection of active infection/end-organ damage	To support treatment decisions

Intermittent fever

Intermittent fever has a wide differential diagnosis, including recurrent infection, malignancy and certain rheumatic disorders, such as Still's disease, vasculitis and SLE but a familial fever syndrome is a potential cause.

Aetiology

Familial fever syndromes are genetic disorders caused by mutations in genes responsible for regulating the inflammatory response. The symptoms are caused by activation of intracellular signalling pathways involved in the regulation of inflammation, with over-production of pro-inflammatory cytokines such as IL-1.

Clinical assessment

A full clinical history and physical examination should be performed, paying attention to the patient's ethnic background and any family history of a similar disorder. If this assessment shows no evidence of underlying infection, malignancy or a rheumatic disorder and there is a positive

4.8 Specialist investigations in suspected immune deficiency		
Test	**Value**	**Comment**
Complement (C3/C4/CH50/AP50)	Investigation of recurrent pyogenic bacterial infection	Inherited complement deficiency likely to give low/absent results on functional assays
Test vaccination	Determination of functional humoral immune response	Helpful in patients with borderline low or normal immunoglobulins but confirmed recurrent infection
Neutrophil function	Investigation of recurrent invasive bacterial and fungal infection, especially with catalase-positive organisms	Respiratory burst low/absent in chronic granulomatous disease
	Investigation of leucocyte adhesion deficiency	Leucocytosis with absent CD11a, b, c expression
Lymphocyte immunophenotyping (by flow cytometry)	Determination of specific lymphocyte subsets, T cell, B cell, NK cell	May define specific primary immune deficiency, e.g. absent B cells in X-linked agammaglobulinaemia
Lymphocyte proliferation	Determination of lymphocyte proliferation in response to mitogenic stimulation	Poor responses seen in certain T-cell immune deficiencies
Cytokine production	To determine T-cell immune function in response to antigen stimulation; limited availability, not routine	Can be helpful, for example, in investigation of atypical mycobacterial infection
Genetic testing	Under specialist supervision when specific primary immune deficiency suspected	May confirm genetic cause, with implications for family members and future antenatal testing
(NK = natural killer)		

family history and early age at onset, then the likelihood of a familial fever syndrome is increased.

Investigations

Blood should be taken for a full blood count, measurement of ESR and CRP, and assessment of renal and liver function. Serum ferritin should be checked, as very high levels support the diagnosis of Still's disease. Blood and urine cultures should also be performed, along with an autoimmune screen that includes measurement of antinuclear antibodies and consideration of antineutrophil cytoplasmic antibodies to check for evidence of SLE or vasculitis, respectively. Imaging may be required to exclude occult infection. If these investigations provide no evidence of infection or another cause, then genetic analysis should be considered to confirm the diagnosis of a familial fever syndrome. Negative genetic testing does not, however, entirely exclude a periodic fever syndrome.

Management

Symptomatic management with non-steroidal anti-inflammatory drugs (NSAIDs) should be initiated, pending the results of investigations. If the response to NSAIDs is inadequate, glucocorticoids can be tried, provided that infection has been excluded. If a familial fever syndrome is confirmed, then definitive therapy should be initiated, depending on the underlying diagnosis, as discussed later in this chapter (p. 76).

Anaphylaxis

Anaphylaxis is a potentially life-threatening, systemic allergic reaction characterised by circulatory collapse, bronchospasm, laryngeal stridor, often associated with angioedema, and urticaria. The risk of death is increased in patients with pre-existing asthma, particularly if this is poorly controlled, and in situations where treatment with adrenaline (epinephrine) is delayed. Further details are provided in the 'Presenting problems in acute medicine' section in Chapter 9.

Immune deficiency

The consequences of immune deficiency include recurrent infection, autoimmunity as a result of immune dysregulation, and increased susceptibility to malignancy, especially malignancy driven by viral infections such as Epstein–Barr virus. Immune deficiency may arise through intrinsic defects in immune function but is much more commonly due to secondary causes, including infection, drug therapy, malignancy and ageing. This section gives an overview of primary immune deficiencies. More than a hundred such deficiencies have been described, most of which are genetically determined and present in childhood or adolescence. The presentation of immune deficiency depends on the component of the immune system that is defective (see Box 4.5). There is considerable overlap and redundancy in the immune network, however, and some diseases do not fall easily into this classification.

Primary phagocyte deficiencies

Primary phagocyte deficiencies typically present with recurrent bacterial and fungal infections, which may involve unusual sites. Affected patients require aggressive management of infections, including intravenous antibiotics and surgical drainage of abscesses, and long-term prophylaxis with antibacterial and antifungal agents. The most important examples are illustrated in Figure 4.10 and discussed below.

Chronic granulomatous disease

This is caused by mutations in genes that encode NADPH oxidase enzymes, which results in failure of oxidative killing. The defect leads to susceptibility to catalase-positive organisms such as *Staphylococcus aureus*, *Burkholderia cenocepacia* and *Aspergillus*. Intracellular killing of mycobacteria in macrophages is also impaired. Infections most commonly involve the lungs, lymph nodes, soft tissues, bone, skin and urinary tract, and are characterised histologically by granuloma formation. Most cases are X-linked

Leucocyte adhesion deficiencies

These very rare disorders of phagocyte migration occur because of failure to express adhesion molecules on the surface of leucocytes, resulting in their inability to exit the blood stream. The most common cause is loss-of-function mutations affecting the *ITGB2* gene, which encodes the integrin β-2 chain, a component of the adhesion molecule LFA1. They are characterised by recurrent bacterial infections but sites of infection lack evidence of neutrophil infiltration, such as pus formation. Peripheral blood neutrophil counts may be very high during acute infection because of the failure of mobilised neutrophils to exit blood vessels. Specialised tests show reduced or absent expression of adhesion molecules on neutrophils.

Normal

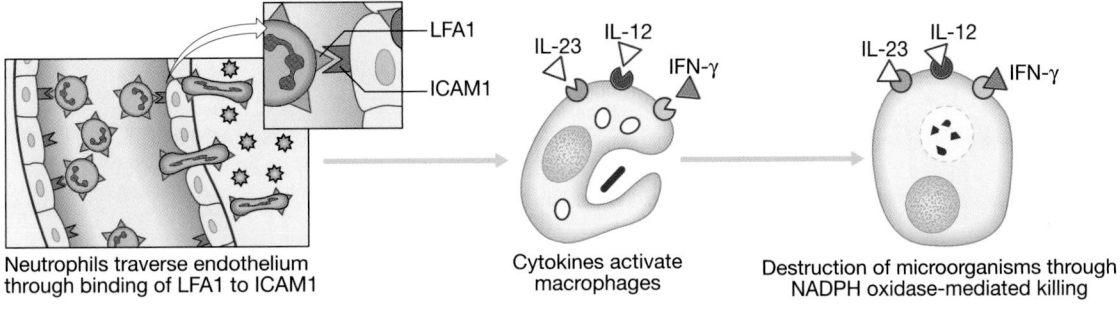

Neutrophils traverse endothelium through binding of LFA1 to ICAM1

Cytokines activate macrophages

Destruction of microorganisms through NADPH oxidase-mediated killing

Primary phagocyte deficiency

Leucocyte adhesion deficiency

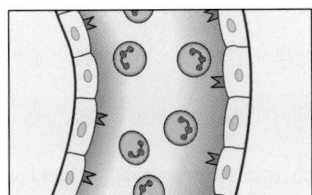

Neutrophils cannot traverse endothelium due to defects in *ITGB2*, a component of LFA1

Cytokine defects

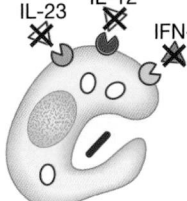

Phagocytes cannot be activated due to defects in cytokines or their receptors

Chronic granulomatous disease

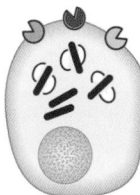

Microorganisms cannot be destroyed in lysosomes due to NADPH oxidase deficiency

Fig. 4.10 Normal phagocyte function and mechanisms of primary phagocyte deficiency. Under normal circumstances, neutrophils traverse the endothelium to enter tissues by the cell surface molecule lymphocyte function-associated antigen 1 (LFA1), which binds to intercellular adhesion molecule 1 (ICAM1) on endothelium. In order for macrophages to engulf and kill microorganisms, they need to be activated by cytokines and also require nicotinamide adenine dinucleotide phosphate (NADPH) oxidase to generate free radicals. Primary phagocyte deficiencies can occur as the result of leucocytes being unable to traverse endothelium due to defects in LFA1, because of mutations in cytokines or their receptors, or because of defects in NADPH oxidase. (IFN-γ = interferon-gamma; IL = interleukin)

Defects in cytokines and cytokine receptors

Mutations of the genes encoding cytokines such as IFN-γ, IL-12, IL-23 or their receptors result in failure of intracellular killing by macrophages, and affected individuals are particularly susceptible to mycobacterial infections.

Complement pathway deficiencies

Loss-of-function mutations have been identified in almost all the complement pathway proteins (see Fig. 4.4). While most complement deficiencies are rare, mannose-binding lectin deficiency is common and affects about 5% of the northern European population, many of whom are asymptomatic (see below).

Clinical features

Patients with deficiency in complement proteins can present in different ways. In some cases, the presenting feature is recurrent infection with encapsulated bacteria, particularly *Neisseria* spp., reflecting the importance of the membrane attack complex in defence against these organisms. However, genetic deficiencies of the classical complement pathway (C1, C2 and C4) also present with an increased risk of autoimmune disease, particularly SLE. Individuals with mannose-binding lectin deficiency have an increased incidence of bacterial infections if subjected to an additional cause of immune compromise, such as premature birth or chemotherapy. The significance of this condition has been debated, however, since population studies have shown no overall increase in infectious disease or mortality in patients with this disorder. Deficiency of the regulatory protein Cl inhibitor is not associated with recurrent infection but causes recurrent angioedema.

Investigations

Screening for complement deficiencies usually involves specialised functional tests of complement-mediated haemolysis. These are known as the CH50 (classical haemolytic pathway 50) and AP50 (alternative pathway 50) tests. If abnormal, haemolytic tests are followed by measurement of individual complement components.

Management

Patients with complement deficiencies should be vaccinated with meningococcal, pneumococcal and *H. influenzae* B vaccines to boost their adaptive immune responses. Lifelong prophylactic penicillin to prevent meningococcal infection is recommended, as is early access to acute medical assessment in the event of infection. Patients should also carry a MedicAlert or similar. At-risk family members should be screened for complement deficiencies with functional complement assays. The management of C1 esterase deficiency is discussed elsewhere.

Primary antibody deficiencies

Primary antibody deficiencies occur as the result of abnormalities in B-cell function, as summarised in Figure 4.11. They are characterised by recurrent bacterial infections, particularly of the respiratory and gastrointestinal tract. The most common causative organisms are encapsulated bacteria such as *Streptococcus pneumoniae* and *H. influenzae*. These disorders usually present in infancy, when the protective benefit of placental transfer of maternal immunoglobulin has waned. The most important causes are discussed in more detail below.

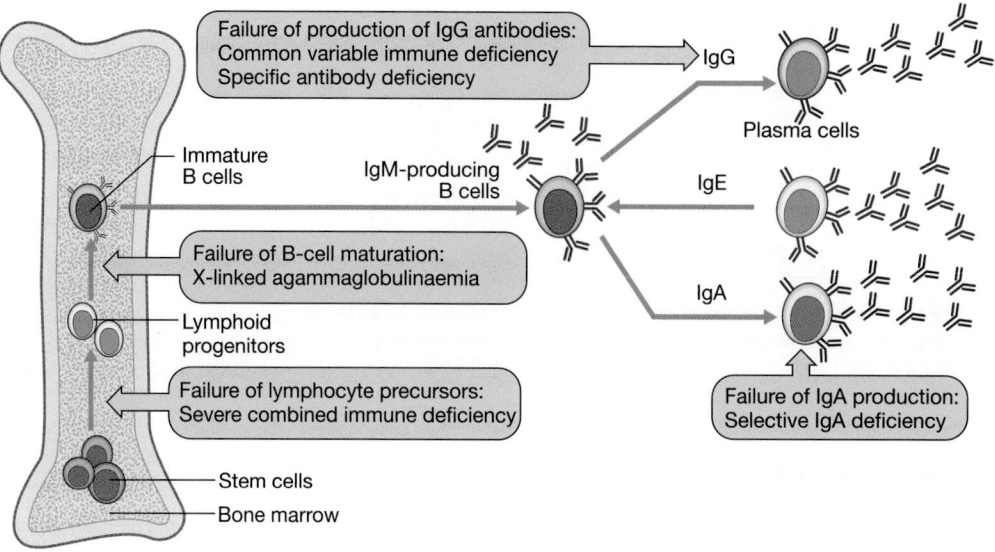

Fig. 4.11 B lymphocytes and primary antibody deficiencies (green boxes). (Ig = immunoglobulin)

i 4.9 Investigation of primary antibody deficiencies

	Serum immunoglobulin (Ig) concentrations				Circulating lymphocyte numbers		Test immunisation
	IgM	IgG	IgA	IgE	B cells	T cells	
Selective IgA deficiency	Normal	Often elevated	Absent	Normal	Normal	Normal	Not applicable*
Common variable immune deficiency	Normal or low	Low	Low or absent	Low or absent	Variable	Variable	No antibody response
Specific antibody deficiency	Normal	Normal	Normal	Normal	Normal	Normal	No antibody response to polysaccharide antigens

*Test immunisation is not usually performed in IgA deficiency but some patients may have impaired responses.

X-linked agammaglobulinaemia

This rare X-linked disorder is caused by mutations in the *BTK* gene, which encodes Bruton tyrosine kinase, a signalling protein that is required for B-cell development. Affected males present with severe bacterial infections during infancy. There is a marked reduction in B-cell numbers and immunoglobulin levels are low or undetectable. Management is with immunoglobulin replacement therapy and antibiotics to treat infections.

Selective IgA deficiency

This is the most common primary antibody deficiency, affecting 1:600 northern Europeans. Although IgA deficiency is usually asymptomatic with no clinical sequelae, about 30% of individuals experience recurrent mild respiratory and gastrointestinal infections. The diagnosis can be confirmed by measurement of IgA levels, which are low or undetectable (< 0.05 g/L). In some patients, there is a compensatory increase in serum IgG levels. Specific treatment is generally not required.

Common variable immune deficiency

Common variable immune deficiency (CVID) is characterised by low serum IgG levels and failure to make antibody responses to exogenous pathogens. It is a heterogeneous adult-onset primary immune deficiency, the underlying cause is unknown in most cases, although genetic mutations have been identified in a minority of patients. The presentation is with recurrent infections, and bronchiectasis is a recognised complication. Paradoxically, antibody-mediated autoimmune diseases, such as idiopathic thrombocytopenic purpura and autoimmune haemolytic anaemia, are common in CVID. It is also associated with an increased risk of malignancy, particularly lymphoproliferative disease.

Specific antibody deficiency

This is a poorly characterised condition resulting in defective antibody responses to polysaccharide antigens. Some patients are also deficient in the antibody subclasses IgG2 and IgG4, and this condition was previously called IgG subclass deficiency. There is overlap between specific antibody deficiency, IgA deficiency and CVID, and some patients may progress to a more global antibody deficiency over time.

Investigations

Serum immunoglobulins (Box 4.9) should be measured in conjunction with protein and urine electrophoresis to exclude secondary causes of hypogammaglobulinaemia, and B- and T-lymphocyte subsets should be measured. Specific antibody responses to known pathogens should be assessed by measuring IgG antibodies against tetanus, *H. influenzae* and *Strep. pneumoniae* (most patients will have been exposed to these antigens through infection or immunisation). If specific antibody levels are low, immunisation with the appropriate killed vaccine should be followed by repeat antibody measurement 6–8 weeks later; failure to mount a response indicates a significant defect in antibody production. These functional tests have generally superseded IgG subclass quantitation.

Management

The mainstay of treatment in most patients with antibody deficiency is immunoglobulin replacement therapy. Human normal immunoglobulin (Box 4.10) is derived from plasma from hundreds of donors and contains IgG antibodies to a wide variety of common organisms. Replacement immunoglobulin may be administered either intravenously or subcutaneously, with the aim of maintaining trough IgG levels (the IgG level just prior to an infusion) within the normal range. This has been shown to minimise progression of end-organ damage and improve clinical outcome. Patients with antibody deficiencies also require aggressive treatment of infections when they occur; prophylactic antibiotics may be indicated. Treatment may be self-administered and is life-long. Benefits of immunisation are limited because of the defect in IgG antibody production, but patients may derive some T cell benefit from vaccination. As with all primary immune deficiencies, live vaccines should be avoided.

Primary T-lymphocyte deficiencies

These are a group of diseases characterised by recurrent viral, protozoal and fungal infections (see Box 4.5). Many T-cell deficiencies are also associated with defective antibody production because of the importance of T cells in providing help for B cells. These disorders generally present in childhood. Several causes of T-cell deficiency are recognised. These are summarised in Figure 4.12 and discussed in more detail below.

DiGeorge syndrome

This results from failure of development of the third and fourth pharyngeal pouches, and is usually caused by a deletion of chromosome 22q11. The immune deficiency is accounted for by failure of thymic development; however, the immune deficiency can be very heterogeneous. Affected patients can have very low numbers of circulating T cells despite normal development in the bone marrow. It is associated with multiple developmental anomalies, including congenital heart disease, hypoparathyroidism, tracheo-oesophageal fistulae, cleft lip and palate.

 4.10 Types of immunoglobulin preparations for therapeutic use

Normal human Immunoglobulin

Derived from multiple plasma donors and provides passive immunity to those unable to produce immunoglobulin, be that as a result of primary or secondary antibody deficiency. Immunoglobulin replacement therapy provides short-term protection, lasting for the duration of the passively transferred antibodies, IgG having a half-life of approximately 21 days. Treatment is therefore required on an ongoing basis

Hyperimmune globulin

Concentrated antibody products, initially derived from animal sources (diphtheria and tetanus anti-toxins), but more recently of human origin, developed for the prevention of a number of infectious diseases, including rabies as post-exposure treatment, hepatitis B and varicella zoster virus as post-exposure prophylaxis and cytomegalovirus as prophylaxis in patients on immune suppressive therapy, particularly transplant recipients

Convalescent plasma

Convalescent plasma derived from individual donors with high antibody levels against certain pathogens following recovery from natural infection, recently under investigation for the treatment of epidemic/pandemic infection, such as Ebola virus infection and more recently COVID-19, where clinical trials of ABO-compatible convalescent plasma for severe COVID-19 pneumonia have to date proved disappointing, possibly as a result of such intervention being given too late in the course of infection.

Bare lymphocyte syndromes

These very rare disorders are caused by mutations in a variety of genes that regulate expression of HLA molecules or their transport to the cell surface. If HLA class I molecules are affected, CD8+ lymphocytes fail to develop normally, while absent expression of HLA class II molecules affects CD4+ lymphocyte maturation. In addition to recurrent infections, failure to express HLA class I is associated with systemic vasculitis caused by uncontrolled activation of NK cells.

Severe combined immune deficiency

Severe combined immune deficiency (SCID) results from mutations in a number of genes that regulate lymphocyte development, with failure of T-cell maturation, with or without accompanying B- and NK-cell maturation. The most common cause is X-linked SCID, resulting from loss-of-function mutations in the interleukin-2 receptor gamma (*IL2RG*) gene. The gene product is a component of several interleukin receptors, including those for IL-2, IL-7 and IL-15, which are absolutely required for T-cell and NK development. This results in T-cell-negative, NK-cell-negative, B-cell-positive SCID. Another cause is deficiency of the enzyme adenosine deaminase (ADA), which causes lymphocyte death due to accumulation of toxic purine metabolites intracellularly, resulting in T-cell-negative, B-cell-negative and NK-cell-negative SCID.

The absence of an effective adaptive immune response causes recurrent bacterial, fungal and viral infections soon after birth. Stem cell transplantation (SCT) is the treatment option of first choice. Gene therapy has been approved for treatment of ADA deficiency when there is no suitable donor for SCT, has been used successfully in X-linked SCID and is under investigation for a number of other causes of SCID.

Investigations

The principal tests for T-lymphocyte deficiencies are a total lymphocyte count and quantitation of individual lymphocyte subpopulations. Serum immunoglobulins should also be measured. Second-line, functional tests of T-cell activation and proliferation may be indicated. Patients in whom T-lymphocyte deficiencies are suspected should be tested for HIV infection. Genetic testing to identify the underlying cause is usually undertaken following specialist referral.

Management

Patients with T-cell deficiencies should be considered for anti-*Pneumocystis* and antifungal prophylaxis, and require aggressive management of infections when they occur. Immunoglobulin replacement is indicated for associated defective antibody production. Stem cell transplantation or gene therapy may be appropriate in some disorders. Where a family history is known and antenatal testing confirms a specific defect, stem cell therapy prior to recurrent invasive infection can improve outcome.

Autoimmune lymphoproliferative syndrome

This rare disorder is caused by failure of normal lymphocyte apoptosis, most commonly due to mutations in the *FAS* gene, which encodes Fas, a signalling protein that regulates programmed cell death in lymphocytes. This results in massive accumulation of autoreactive T cells, which cause autoimmune-mediated anaemia, thrombocytopenia and neutropenia. Other features include lymphadenopathy, splenomegaly and a variety of other autoimmune diseases. Susceptibility to infection is increased because of the neutropenia.

Secondary immune deficiencies

Secondary immune deficiencies are much more common than primary immune deficiencies and occur when the immune system is compromised by external factors (Box 4.11). Common causes include infections, such as HIV and measles, and cytotoxic and immunosuppressive drugs, particularly those used in the management of transplantation, autoimmunity and cancer. Physiological immune deficiency occurs at the extremes of

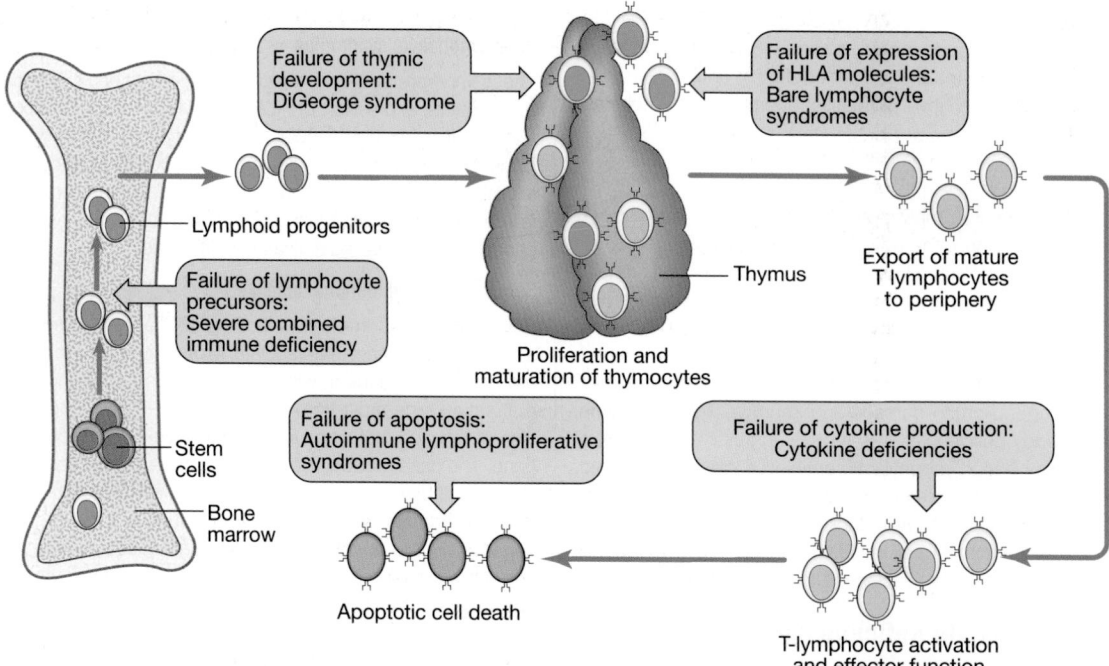

Fig. 4.12 T-lymphocyte function and dysfunction (green boxes). (HLA = human leucocyte antigen)

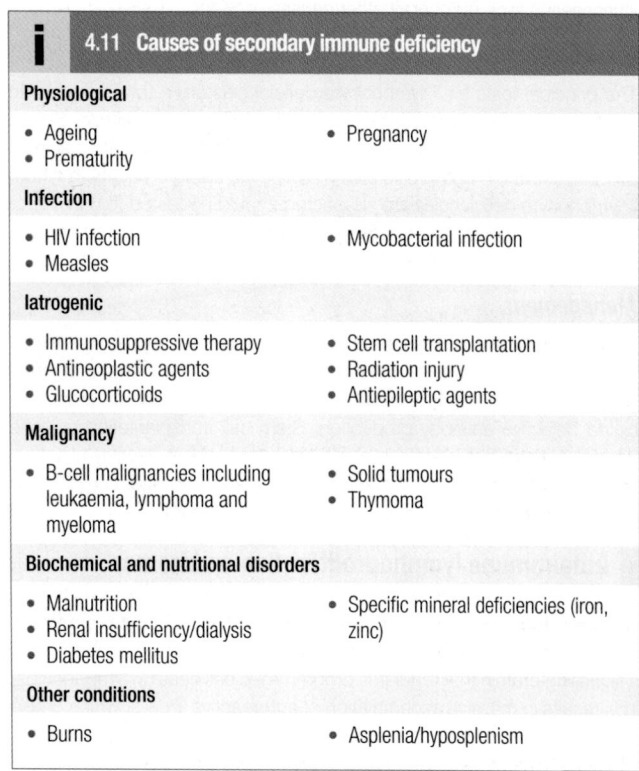

i	4.11 Causes of secondary immune deficiency

Physiological

- Ageing
- Prematurity
- Pregnancy

Infection

- HIV infection
- Measles
- Mycobacterial infection

Iatrogenic

- Immunosuppressive therapy
- Antineoplastic agents
- Glucocorticoids
- Stem cell transplantation
- Radiation injury
- Antiepileptic agents

Malignancy

- B-cell malignancies including leukaemia, lymphoma and myeloma
- Solid tumours
- Thymoma

Biochemical and nutritional disorders

- Malnutrition
- Renal insufficiency/dialysis
- Diabetes mellitus
- Specific mineral deficiencies (iron, zinc)

Other conditions

- Burns
- Asplenia/hyposplenism

life; the decline of the immune response in the elderly is known as immune senescence (Box 4.12). Management of secondary immune deficiency is described in the relevant chapters on infectious diseases (Ch. 13), HIV (Ch. 14), haematological disorders (Ch. 25) and oncology (Ch. 7).

Periodic fever syndromes

These rare disorders are characterised by recurrent episodes of fever and organ inflammation, associated with an elevated acute phase response.

Familial Mediterranean fever

Familial Mediterranean fever (FMF) is the most common of the familial periodic fevers, predominantly affecting Mediterranean people, including Arabs, Turks, Sephardic Jews and Armenians. It results from mutations of the *MEFV* gene, which encodes a protein called pyrin that regulates neutrophil-mediated inflammation by indirectly suppressing the production of IL-1. FMF is characterised by recurrent painful attacks of fever associated with peritonitis, pleuritis and arthritis, which last for a few hours to 4 days and are associated with markedly increased CRP levels. Symptoms resolve completely between episodes. Most individuals have their first attack before the age of 20. The major complication of FMF is AA amyloidosis (see below). Colchicine significantly reduces the number of febrile episodes in 90% of patients but is ineffective during acute attacks. Anti-cytokine therapy blocking IL-1, for example anakinra or the monoclonal antibody canakinumab, can be effective for patients with colchicine refractory symptoms.

Mevalonate kinase deficiency

Mevalonate kinase deficiency, previously known as hyper-IgD syndrome, is an autosomal recessive disorder that causes recurrent attacks of fever, abdominal pain, diarrhoea, lymphadenopathy, arthralgia, skin lesions and aphthous ulceration. Most patients are from Western Europe, particularly the Netherlands and northern France. It is caused by loss-of-function mutations in the gene encoding mevalonate kinase, which is involved in the metabolism of cholesterol. It remains unclear why this causes an inflammatory periodic fever. Serum IgD and IgA levels may be persistently elevated, and CRP levels are increased during acute attacks. Standard anti-inflammatory drugs, including colchicine and glucocorticoids, are ineffective in suppressing the attacks but IL-1 inhibitors, such as anakinra, and TNF inhibitors, such as etanercept, may improve symptoms and can induce complete remission in some patients.

TNF receptor-associated periodic syndrome

TNF receptor-associated periodic syndrome (TRAPS) also known as Hibernian fever, is an autosomal dominant syndrome caused by mutations in the *TNFRSF1A* gene. The presentation is with recurrent attacks of

4

4.12 Immune senescence

- **T-cell responses**: decline, with reduced delayed-type hypersensitivity responses.
- **Antibody production**: decreased for many exogenous antigens. Although autoantibodies are frequently detected, autoimmune disease is less common.
- **Response to vaccination**: reduced; 30% of healthy older people may not develop protective immunity after influenza vaccination.
- **Allergic disorders and transplant rejection**: less common.
- **Susceptibility to infection**: increased; community-acquired pneumonia by threefold and urinary tract infection by 20-fold. Latent infections, including tuberculosis and herpes zoster, may be reactivated.
- **Manifestations of inflammation**: may be absent, with lack of pyrexia or leucocytosis.
- **Secondary immune deficiency**: common.

fever, arthralgia, myalgia, serositis and rashes. Attacks may be prolonged for 1 week or more. During a typical attack, laboratory findings include neutrophilia, increased CRP and elevated IgA levels. The diagnosis can be confirmed by low serum levels of the soluble type 1 TNF receptor and by mutation screening of the *TNFRSF1A* gene. As in FMF, the major complication is amyloidosis, and regular screening for proteinuria is advised. Acute episodes respond to systemic glucocorticoids. Therapy with IL-1 inhibitors, such as anakinra, can be effective in preventing attacks.

Cryopyrin-associated periodic syndrome (CAPS)

This disorder includes three phenotypes: familial cold auto-inflammatory syndrome, Muckle–Wells syndrome and neonatal-onset multisystem inflammatory disease. CAPS results from gain of function mutation of the *NLRP3* gene coding cryopyrin, which forms part of the inflammasome. Defects lead to overproduction of IL-1, resulting in the inflammatory manifestations. Treatments are now targeted at the IL-1 pathway.

Amyloidosis

Amyloidosis is the name given to a group of acquired and hereditary disorders characterised by the extracellular deposition of insoluble proteins.

Pathophysiology

Amyloidosis is caused by deposits consisting of fibrils of the specific protein involved, linked to glycosaminoglycans, proteoglycans and serum amyloid P. Protein accumulation may be localised or systemic, and the clinical manifestations depend on the organ(s) affected. Amyloid diseases are classified by the aetiology and type of protein deposited (Box 4.13).

Clinical features

The clinical presentation may be with nephrotic syndrome, cardiomyopathy or peripheral neuropathy. Amyloidosis should always be considered as a potential diagnosis in patients with these disorders when the cause is unclear.

Investigations

The diagnosis is established by biopsy, which may be of an affected organ, rectum or subcutaneous fat. The pathognomonic histological feature is apple-green birefringence of amyloid deposits when stained with Congo red dye and viewed under polarised light. Immunohistochemical staining can identify the type of amyloid fibril present. Quantitative scintigraphy with radiolabelled serum amyloid P is a valuable tool in determining the overall load and distribution of amyloid deposits.

Management

The aims of treatment are to support the function of affected organs and, in acquired amyloidosis, to prevent further amyloid deposition through treatment of the primary cause. When the latter is possible, regression of existing amyloid deposits may occur.

4.13 Causes of amyloidosis

Disorder	Pathological basis	Predisposing conditions	Other features
Acquired systemic amyloidosis			
Reactive (AA) amyloidosis	Increased production of serum amyloid A as part of prolonged or recurrent acute inflammatory response	Chronic infection (tuberculosis, bronchiectasis, chronic abscess, osteomyelitis) Chronic inflammatory diseases (untreated rheumatoid arthritis, familial Mediterranean fever)	90% of patients present with non-selective proteinuria or nephrotic syndrome
Light chain amyloidosis (AL)	Increased production of monoclonal light chain	Monoclonal gammopathies, including myeloma, benign gammopathies and plasmacytoma	Restrictive cardiomyopathy, peripheral and autonomic neuropathy, carpal tunnel syndrome, proteinuria, spontaneous purpura, amyloid nodules and plaques Macroglossia occurs rarely but is pathognomonic Prognosis is poor
Dialysis-associated (Aβ_2M) amyloidosis	Accumulation of circulating β_2-microglobulin due to failure of renal catabolism in kidney failure	Renal dialysis	Carpal tunnel syndrome, chronic arthropathy and pathological fractures secondary to amyloid bone cyst formation Manifestations occur 5–10 years after the start of dialysis
Senile systemic amyloidosis	Normal transthyretin protein deposited in tissues	Age > 70 years	Feature of normal ageing (affects > 90% of 90-year-olds) Usually asymptomatic
Hereditary systemic amyloidosis			
> 20 forms of hereditary systemic amyloidosis	Production of protein with an abnormal structure that predisposes to amyloid fibril formation. Most commonly due to mutations in *transthyretin* gene	Autosomal dominant inheritance	Peripheral and autonomic neuropathy, cardiomyopathy Renal involvement unusual 10% of gene carriers are asymptomatic throughout life

Autoimmune disease

Autoimmunity can be defined as the presence of immune responses against self-tissue. This may be a harmless phenomenon, identified only by the presence of low-titre autoantibodies or autoreactive T cells. However, if these responses cause significant organ damage, autoimmune diseases occur. These are a major cause of chronic morbidity and disability, affecting up to 1 in 30 adults at some point during life.

Pathophysiology

Autoimmune diseases result from the failure of immune tolerance, the process by which the immune system recognises and accepts self-tissue. Central immune tolerance occurs during lymphocyte development, when T and B lymphocytes that recognise self-antigens are eliminated before they develop into fully immunocompetent cells. This process is most active in fetal life but continues throughout life as immature lymphocytes are generated. Some autoreactive cells inevitably evade deletion and escape into the circulation, however, and are controlled through peripheral tolerance mechanisms. Peripheral immune tolerance mechanisms include the suppression of autoreactive cells by regulatory T cells; the generation of functional hyporesponsiveness (anergy) in lymphocytes that encounter antigen in the absence of the co-stimulatory signals that accompany inflammation; and cell death by apoptosis. Autoimmune diseases develop when self-reactive lymphocytes escape from these tolerance mechanisms.

Multiple genetic and environmental factors contribute to the development of autoimmune disease. Autoimmune diseases are much more common in women than in men, for reasons that remain unclear. Many are associated with genetic variations in the HLA loci, reflecting the importance of HLA genes in shaping lymphocyte responses. Other important susceptibility genes include those determining cytokine activity, co-stimulation (the expression of second signals required for full T-cell activation; see Figs. 4.7 and 4.8) and cell death. Many of the same gene variants underlie multiple autoimmune disorders, reflecting their common pathogenesis (Box 4.14). Even though some of these associations are the strongest that have been identified in complex genetic diseases, they have very limited predictive value and are generally not useful in determining management of individual patients. Several environmental factors may be associated with autoimmunity in genetically predisposed individuals, including infection, cigarette smoking and hormone levels. The most widely studied of these is infection, as occurs in acute rheumatic fever following streptococcal infection or reactive arthritis following bacterial infection. Several mechanisms

have been invoked to explain the autoimmunity that occurs after an infectious trigger. These include cross-reactivity between proteins expressed by the pathogen and the host (molecular mimicry), such as Guillain–Barré syndrome and *Campylobacter* infection; release of sequestered antigens from tissues that are damaged during infections that are not usually visible to the immune system; and production of inflammatory cytokines that overwhelm the normal control mechanisms that prevent bystander damage. Occasionally, autoimmune disease may be an adverse effect of drug treatment. For example, metabolic products of the anaesthetic agent halothane can bind to liver enzymes, resulting in a structurally novel protein that is recognised as a foreign antigen by the immune system. This can provoke the development of autoantibodies and activated T cells, which can cause hepatic necrosis.

Clinical features

The clinical presentation of autoimmune disease is highly variable. Autoimmune diseases can be classified by organ involvement or by the predominant mechanism responsible for tissue damage. The Gell and Coombs classification of hypersensitivity is the most widely used, and distinguishes four types of immune response that result in tissue damage (Box 4.15).

- *Type I hypersensitivity* is relevant in allergy but is not associated with autoimmune disease.
- *Type II hypersensitivity* causes injury to a single tissue or organ and is mediated by specific autoantibodies.
- *Type III hypersensitivity* results from deposition of immune complexes, which initiates activation of the classical complement cascade, as well as recruitment and activation of phagocytes and CD4+ lymphocytes. The site of immune complex deposition is determined by the relative amount of antibody, size of the immune complexes, nature of the

---

i 4.14 Association of specific gene polymorphisms with autoimmune diseases

Gene	Function	Diseases
HLA complex	Key determinants of antigen presentation to T cells	Most autoimmune diseases
PTPN22	Regulation of T- and B-cell receptor signalling	Rheumatoid arthritis, type 1 diabetes, systemic lupus erythematosus
CTLA4	Important co-stimulatory molecule that transmits inhibitory signals to T cells	Rheumatoid arthritis, type 1 diabetes
IL23R	Cytokine-mediated control of T cells	Inflammatory bowel disease, psoriasis, ankylosing spondylitis
TNFRSF1A	Control of tumour necrosis factor network	Multiple sclerosis
ATG5	Autophagy	Systemic lupus erythematosus

---

i 4.15 Gell and Coombs classification of hypersensitivity diseases

Type	Mechanism	Example of disease in response to exogenous agent	Example of autoimmune disease
Type I Immediate hypersensitivity	IgE-mediated mast cell degranulation	Allergic disease	None described
Type II Antibody-mediated	Binding of cytotoxic IgG or IgM antibodies to antigens on cell surface causes cell killing	ABO blood transfusion reaction Hyperacute transplant rejection	Autoimmune haemolytic anaemia Idiopathic thrombocytopenic purpura Goodpasture's disease
Type III Immune complex-mediated	IgG or IgM antibodies bind soluble antigen to form immune complexes that trigger classical complement pathway activation	Serum sickness Farmer's lung	Systemic lupus erythematosus Cryoglobulinaemia
Type IV Delayed type	Activated T cells, and phagocytes	Acute cellular transplant rejection Nickel hypersensitivity	Type 1 diabetes Hashimoto's thyroiditis

antigen and local haemodynamics. Generalised deposition of immune complexes gives rise to systemic diseases such as SLE.

- *Type IV hypersensitivity* is mediated by activated T cells and macrophages, which together cause tissue damage.

Investigations

Autoantibodies

Many autoantibodies have been identified and are used in the diagnosis and monitoring of autoimmune diseases, as discussed elsewhere in this book. Antibodies can be quantified either by titre (the maximum dilution of the serum at which the antibody can be detected) or by concentration in standardised units using an enzyme-linked immunosorbent assay (ELISA) in which the antigen is used to coat microtitre plates to which the patient's serum is added (Fig. 4.13A). Immunoblotting (Fig. 4.13B) can also be employed for autoantibody detection as well as qualitative tests in which the pattern of immunofluorescence staining is recorded

(Fig. 4.13C). Antibody testing can also be performed using Luminex technology. In this case multiple test antigens are individually bound to red and infra-red fluorescently labelled polystyrene or paramagnetic beads. Each antigen-coated bead is coated with a unique proportion of red and infrared dyes. The patient sample is incubated with these beads and if antibodies are present in the sample these will bind to the test antigens coating the beads. After washing to remove unbound antibodies, a third fluorescent dye is added and the sample is processed through a dual laser Luminex analyser, which can detect the unique spectral signatures arising from beads coated with different test antigens allowing detection of multiple antibodies present in a single patient sample.

Complement

Measurement of complement components can be useful in the evaluation of immune complex-mediated diseases. Classical complement pathway activation leads to a decrease in circulating C4 levels and is

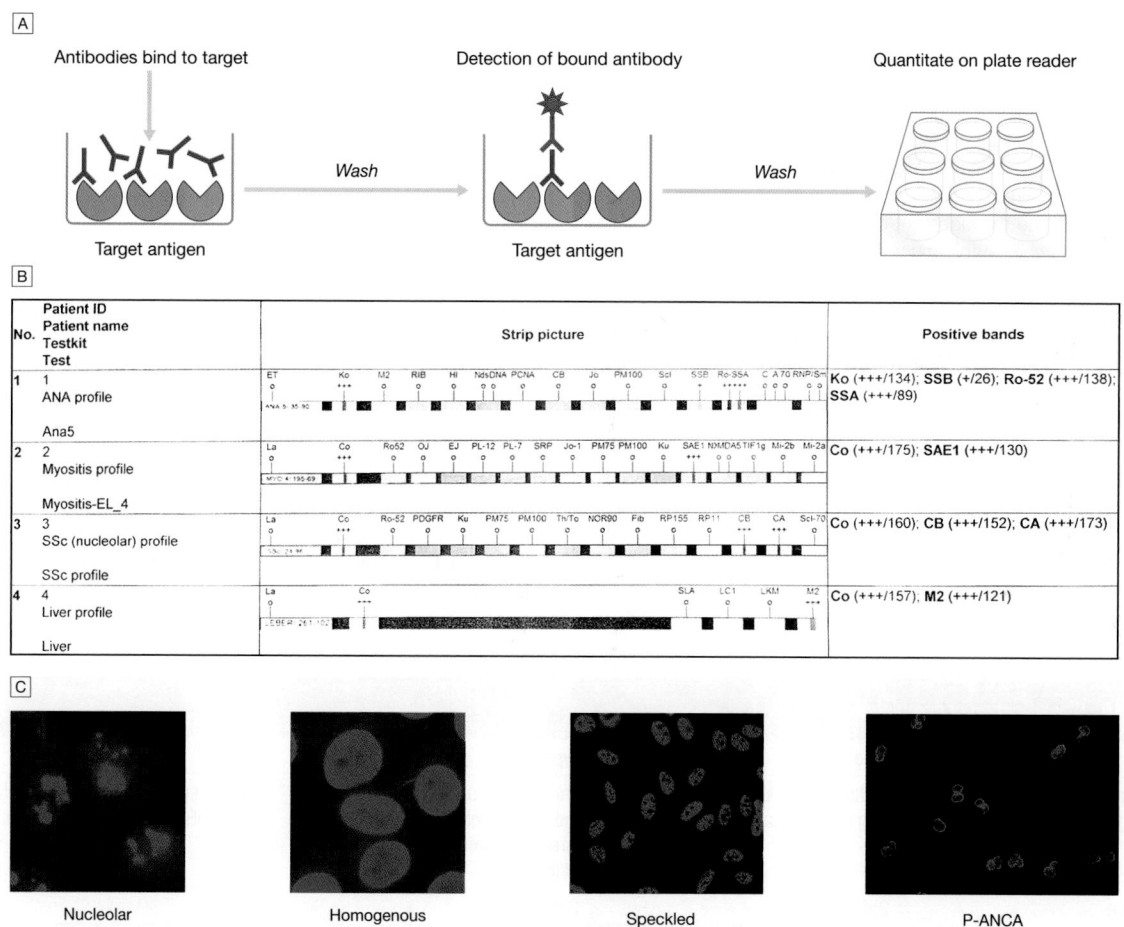

Fig. 4.13 Autoantibody testing. **A** Measurement of autoantibody levels by enzyme-linked immunosorbent assay (ELISA). The antigen of interest is used to coat microtitre plates to which patient serum is added. If autoantibodies are present, these bind to the target antigen on the microtitre plate. The amount of bound antibody is quantitated by adding a secondary antibody linked to an enzyme that converts a colourless substrate to a coloured one, which can be detected by a plate reader. **B** Detection of autoantibodies by immunoblotting. Test strips are coated with purified antigens in parallel lines. The strips are incubated with patient serum or plasma and controls. After washing to remove unbound antibody, strips are incubated with enzyme-conjugated alkaline phosphatase-labelled anti-human IgG. After washing and addition of a chromogenic substrate, an enzyme-mediated colour reaction develops. After a final wash, the strips are dried and any observed banding pattern is scanned for band intensity against an electronic template. The black bars on the strip separate the antigens being tested. Positive results are seen as vertical grey lines below the test antigen and the intensity of staining corresponds to the concentration of antibody in the patient's serum. The strength of staining is expressed both as a number and as a grade from + (weak) to +++ (strong). Note that all strips contain an internal quality control (marked as Ko or Co) to ensure the assay has worked. In the example shown, the patient sample was positive for multiple auto-antibodies in the ANA profile, the Myositis profile, the Systemic sclerosis (SSc) profile and the Liver profile. **C** Qualitative analysis of autoantibodies by patterns of indirect immunofluorescence staining. In this assay, patient serum is added to cell substrate and a secondary antibody is added with a fluorescent label to detect any bound antibody. If antibodies are present, they are detected as bright green staining using a fluorescence microscope. Different antinuclear antibody patterns may be seen in different types of connective tissue disease using a HEp2 or HEp2000 (human epithelial cell line) as substrate (see Ch. 26). Immunofluorescence can be undertaken using different substrates, according to the autoantibody under investigation. An antinucleolar ANA can be seen in systemic sclerosis, a homogenous ANA can be seen in SLE and a speckled ANA can be seen in SLE or Sjögren syndrome. In the context of small vessel vasculitis, the tissue substrate is ethanol-fixed neutrophils. Two main staining patterns of anti-neutrophil cytoplasmic antibodies (ANCA) are clinically relevant, cytoplasmic and perinuclear, seen in granulomatosis with polyangiitis and microsopcopic polyangiitis (see Ch. 26), the autoantibodies recognising proteinase 3 and myeloperoxidase respectively. *(B and C, Nucleolar and Homogenous) Courtesy of Juliet Dunphy, Biomedical Scientist, Royal United Hospital Bath, UK; (C, Speckled and P-ANCA) Courtesy of Mr Richard Brown, Clinical Scientist in Immunology, Southwest Pathology Services, UK.*

often also associated with decreased C3 levels. Serial measurement of C3 and C4 can be helpful as a surrogate measure of disease activity in conditions such as SLE.

Cryoglobulins

Cryoglobulins are antibodies that can be directed against other immunoglobulins, which form immune complexes that precipitate in the cold. They can lead to type III hypersensitivity reactions, with typical clinical manifestations including purpuric rash, often of the lower extremities, arthralgia and peripheral neuropathy. Cryoglobulins are classified into three types, depending on the properties of the immunoglobulin involved (Box 4.16). Testing for cryoglobulins requires the transport of a serum specimen to the laboratory at 37°C. Cryoglobulins should not be confused with cold agglutinins; the latter are autoantibodies specifically directed against the I/i antigen on the surface of red cells, which can cause intravascular haemolysis in the cold (p. 958).

Management

The management of autoimmune disease depends on the organ system involved and further details are provided elsewhere in this book. In general, treatment of autoimmune diseases involves the use of glucocorticoids and immunosuppressive agents, which are increasingly used in combination with biologic agents targeting disease-specific cytokines and their receptors. Not all conditions require immune suppression, however. For example, the management of coeliac disease involves dietary gluten withdrawal, while autoimmune hypothyroidism requires appropriate thyroxine supplementation.

Allergy

Allergic diseases are a common and increasing cause of illness, affecting between 15% and 20% of the population at some time. They comprise a range of disorders from mild to life-threatening and affect many organs. Atopy is the tendency to produce an exaggerated IgE immune response to otherwise harmless environmental substances, while an allergic disease can be defined as the clinical manifestation of this inappropriate IgE immune response.

Pathophysiology

The immune system does not normally respond to the many environmental substances to which it is exposed on a daily basis. In allergic individuals, however, an initial exposure to a normally harmless exogenous substance (known as an allergen) triggers the production of specific IgE antibodies by activated B cells. These bind to high-affinity IgE receptors on the surface of mast cells, a step that is not itself associated with clinical sequelae. However, re-exposure to the allergen binds to and cross-links membrane-bound IgE, which activates the mast cells, releasing a variety of vasoactive mediators (the early phase response; Fig. 4.14 and see Chapter 9). This type I hypersensitivity reaction forms the basis of an allergic reaction, which can range from sneezing and rhinorrhea to anaphylaxis (Box 4.17). In some individuals, the early phase response is followed by persistent activation of mast cells, manifest by ongoing swelling and local inflammation. This is known as the late phase reaction and is mediated by mast cell metabolites, basophils, eosinophils and macrophages. Long-standing or recurrent allergic inflammation may give rise to a chronic inflammatory response characterised by a complex infiltrate of macrophages, eosinophils and T lymphocytes, in addition to mast cells and basophils. Once this has been established, inhibition of mast cell mediators with antihistamines is clinically ineffective in isolation. Mast cell activation may also be non-specifically triggered through other signals, such as neuropeptides, anaphylotoxins and bacterial peptides.

The increasing incidence of allergic diseases is largely unexplained but one widely held theory is the 'hygiene hypothesis'. This proposes that infections in early life are critically important in maturation of the immune response and bias the immune system against the development of allergies; the high prevalence of allergic disease is the penalty for the decreased exposure to infection that has resulted from improvements in sanitation and health care. Genetic factors also contribute strongly to the development of allergic diseases. A positive family history is common in patients with allergy, and genetic association studies have identified a wide variety of predisposing variants in genes controlling innate immune responses, cytokine production, IgE levels and the ability of the epithelial barrier to protect against environmental agents. The expression of a genetic predisposition is complex; it is governed by environmental factors, such as pollutants and cigarette smoke, and the incidence of bacterial and viral infection.

i 4.16 Classification of cryoglobulins

	Type I	Type II	Type III
Immunoglobulin (Ig) isotype and specificity	Isolated monoclonal IgM paraprotein with no particular specificity	Immune complexes formed by monoclonal IgM paraprotein directed towards constant region of IgG	Immune complexes formed by polyclonal IgM or IgG directed towards constant region of IgG
Prevalence	25%	25%	50%
Disease association	Lymphoproliferative disease, especially Waldenström macroglobulinaemia	Infection, particularly hepatitis C; lymphoproliferative disease	Infection, particularly hepatitis C; autoimmune disease, including rheumatoid arthritis and systemic lupus erythematosus
Symptoms	*Hyperviscosity:* Raynaud's phenomenon Acrocyanosis Retinal vessel occlusion Arterial and venous thrombosis	*Small-vessel vasculitis:* Purpuric rash Arthralgia Neuropathy Cutaneous ulceration, hepatosplenomegaly, glomerulonephritis, Raynaud's phenomenon	*Small-vessel vasculitis:* Purpuric rash, arthralgia Cutaneous ulceration hepatosplenomegaly, glomerulonephritis Raynaud's phenomenon
Protein electrophoresis	Monoclonal IgM paraprotein	Monoclonal IgM paraprotein	No monoclonal paraprotein
Rheumatoid factor	Negative	Strongly positive	Strongly positive
Complement	Usually normal	Decreased C4	Decreased C4
Serum viscosity	Raised	Normal	Normal

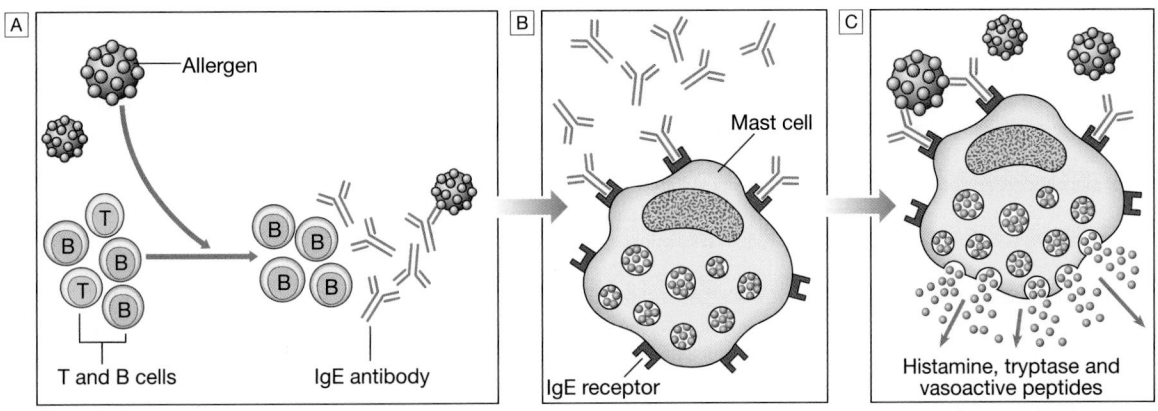

Fig. 4.14 Type I (immediate) hypersensitivity response. [A] After an encounter with allergen, B cells produce immunoglobulin E (IgE) antibody against the allergen. [B] Specific IgE antibodies bind to circulating mast cells via high-affinity IgE cell surface receptors. [C] On re-encounter with allergen, the allergen binds to the IgE antibody-coated mast cells. This cross-linking of the IgE triggers mast cell activation with release of vasoactive mediators.

---

i 4.17 Clinical manifestations of allergy

Dermatological
- Urticaria
- Atopic eczema if chronic
- Allergic contact eczema
- Angioedema

Respiratory
- Asthma
- Atopic rhinitis

Ophthalmological
- Allergic conjunctivitis

Gastrointestinal
- Food allergy

Other
- Anaphylaxis
- Drug allergy
- Allergy to insect venom

Clinical features

Common presentations of allergic disease are shown in Box 4.17. Those that affect the respiratory system and skin are discussed in more detail in Chapters 17 and 27, respectively. Here we focus on general principles of the approach to the allergic patient and some specific allergies. The management of acute anaphylaxis is discussed in Chapter 9.

Insect venom allergy

Local non-IgE-mediated reactions to insect stings are common and may cause extensive swelling around the site lasting up to 7 days. These usually do not require specific treatment. Toxic reactions to venom after multiple (50–100) simultaneous stings may mimic anaphylaxis. In addition, exposure to large amounts of insect venom frequently stimulates the production of IgE antibodies, and thus may be followed by allergic reactions to single stings. Allergic IgE-mediated reactions vary from mild to life-threatening. Antigen-specific immunotherapy (desensitisation; see below) with bee or wasp venom can reduce the incidence of recurrent anaphylaxis from 50% to 60% to approximately 10%, but requires 3–5 years of treatment or more.

Peanut allergy

Peanut allergy is the most common food-related allergy. More than 50% of patients present before the age of 3 years and some individuals react to their first known exposure to peanuts, thought to result from sensitisation to arachis oil in topical creams. Peanuts are ubiquitous in the Western diet, and every year up to 25% of peanut-allergic individuals experience a reaction as a result of inadvertent exposure.

Birch oral allergy syndrome

This syndrome is characterised by the combination of birch pollen hay fever and local oral symptoms, including itch and angioedema, after contact with certain raw fruits, raw vegetables and nuts. Cooked fruits and vegetables are tolerated without difficulty. It is due to shared or cross-reactive allergens that are destroyed by cooking or digestion, and can be confirmed by skin-prick testing using fresh fruit. Severe allergic reactions are unusual.

Diagnosis

When assessing a patient with a complaint of allergy, it is important to identify what the patient means by the term, as up to 20% of the UK population describe themselves as having a food allergy; in fact, less than 1% have true allergy, as defined by an IgE-mediated hypersensitivity reaction confirmed on double-blind challenge. The nature of the symptoms should be established and specific triggers identified, along with the predictability of a reaction, and the time lag between exposure to a potential allergen and onset of symptoms. An allergic reaction usually occurs within minutes of exposure and provokes predictable, reproducible symptoms such as angioedema, urticaria and wheezing. Specific enquiry should be made about other allergic symptoms, past and present, and about a family history of allergic disease. Potential allergens in the home and workplace should be identified. A detailed drug history should always be taken, including details of adherence to medication, possible adverse effects and the use of over-the-counter or complementary therapies.

Investigations

Skin-prick tests

Skin-prick testing is a key investigation in the assessment of patients suspected of having allergy. A droplet of diluted standardised allergen is placed on the forearm and the skin is superficially punctured through the droplet with a sterile lancet. Positive and negative control material must be included in the assessment. After 15 minutes, a positive response is indicated by a local weal and flare response 2 mm or more larger than the negative control. A major advantage of skin-prick testing is that the patient can clearly see the results, which may be useful in gaining adherence to avoidance measures. Disadvantages include the remote risk of a severe allergic reaction, so resuscitation facilities should be available. Results are unreliable in patients with extensive skin disease. Antihistamines inhibit the magnitude of the response and should be discontinued for at least 3 days before testing; low-dose glucocorticoids do not influence test results. A number of other prescribed medicines can also lead to false-negative results, including amitriptyline and risperidone.

Specific IgE tests

An alternative to skin-prick testing is the quantitation of IgE directed against the suspected allergen. The sensitivity and specificity of specific IgE tests (previously known as radioallergosorbent tests, RAST) are lower than those of skin-prick tests. However, IgE tests may be very useful if skin testing is inappropriate, such as in patients taking antihistamines or those with severe skin disease or dermatographism. They can also be used to test for cross-reactivity – for example, with multiple insect venoms, where component-resolved diagnostics, using recombinant allergens, is now increasingly used rather than crude allergen extract. Component resolved diagnostics (CRD) is a more recent development in allergic investigation. CRD uses purified native or recombinant allergens to detect specific IgE directed against individual allergenic molecules. CRD can discriminate genuine sensitisation from sensitisation due to cross reactivity and in some cases can be used in risk stratification. For example, in patients with hazelnut allergy, the clinical features can be mild and most consistent with the oral allergy syndrome rather than primary nut allergy, in which case CRD may confirm specific IgE to Cor a1, a birch pollen homologue, hence the association with the oral allergy syndrome, whereas patients with primary hazelnut allergy positive for Cor a9 or Cor a14 tend to have more severe allergy. Severity of reaction in peanut allergy can also be associated with specific Ara h allergens, which are present in peanuts. Such risk stratification can impact on patient management, for example, identifying patients who may require an adrenaline auto-injector.

Supervised exposure to allergen

Tests involving supervised exposure to an allergen (allergen challenge) are usually performed in specialist centres on carefully selected patients, and include bronchial provocation testing, nasal challenge, and food or drug challenge. These may be particularly useful in the investigation of occupational asthma or food allergy. Patients can be considered for challenge testing when skin tests and/or IgE tests are negative, as they can be helpful in ruling out allergic disease.

Mast cell tryptase

Measurement of serum mast cell tryptase is extremely useful in investigating a possible anaphylactic event. Ideally, measurements should be made at the time of the reaction following appropriate resuscitation, and 3 hours and 24 hours later. The basis of the test is the fact that circulating levels of mast cell degranulation products rise dramatically to peak 1–2 hours after a systemic allergic reaction. Tryptase is the most stable of these and is easily measured in serum.

Serum total IgE

Serum total IgE measurements are not routinely indicated in the investigation of allergic disease, other than to aid in the interpretation of specific IgE results, as false-positive specific IgEs are common in patients with atopy, who often have a high total IgE level. Although atopy is the most common cause of an elevated total IgE in developed countries, there are many other causes, including parasitic and helminth infections, lymphoma, drug reactions and eosinophilic granulomatosis with polyangiitis (previously known as Churg–Strauss vasculitis). Normal total IgE levels do not exclude allergic disease.

Eosinophilia

Peripheral blood eosinophilia is common in atopic individuals but lacks specificity. Eosinophilia of more than 20% or an absolute eosinophil count over 1.5×10^9/L should initiate a search for a non-atopic cause, such as eosinophilic granulomatosis with polyangiitis or parasitic infection.

Management

Several approaches can be deployed in the management of allergic individuals, as discussed below.

Avoidance of the allergen

This is indicated in all cases and should be rigorously attempted, with the advice of specialist dietitians and occupational physicians as necessary.

Antihistamines

Antihistamines are useful in the management of allergy as they inhibit the effects of histamine on tissue H_1 receptors. Long-acting, non-sedating preparations are particularly useful for prophylaxis.

Glucocorticoids

These are highly effective in allergic disease, and if used topically, adverse effects can be minimised.

Sodium cromoglicate

Sodium cromoglicate stabilises the mast cell membrane, inhibiting release of vasoactive mediators. It is effective as a prophylactic agent in asthma and allergic rhinitis but has no role in management of acute attacks. It is poorly absorbed and therefore generally ineffective in the management of food allergies.

Antigen-specific immunotherapy

This involves the sequential administration of increasing doses of allergen extract over a prolonged period of time. The mechanism of action is not fully understood but it is highly effective in the prevention of insect venom anaphylaxis and of allergic rhinitis secondary to grass pollen allergy. The traditional route of administration is by subcutaneous injection, which carries a risk of anaphylaxis and should be performed only in specialised centres. Sublingual immunotherapy is also increasingly used. Clinical studies to date do not support the use of allergen immunotherapy for food hypersensitivity, although this is an area of active investigation.

Omalizumab

Omalizumab is a monoclonal antibody directed against IgE; it inhibits the binding of IgE to mast cells and basophils. It is licensed for treatment of refractory chronic spontaneous urticaria and also for severe persistent allergic asthma that has failed to respond to standard therapy. The dose and frequency are determined by baseline IgE (measured before the start of treatment) and body weight. It is under investigation for allergic rhinitis but not yet approved for this indication.

Adrenaline (epinephrine)

Adrenaline given by injection in the form of a pre-loaded self-injectable device can be life-saving in the acute management of anaphylaxis (see Ch. 9).

Angioedema

Angioedema is an episodic, localised, non-pitting swelling of submucous or subcutaneous tissues.

Pathophysiology

The causes of angioedema are summarised in Box 4.18. It may be a manifestation of allergy or non-allergic degranulation of mast cells in response to drugs and toxins. In these conditions the main cause is mast cell degranulation with release of histamine and other vasoactive mediators. In hereditary angioedema, the cause is C1 inhibitor deficiency, which leads to increased local release of bradykinin. Angiotensin-converting enzyme (ACE) inhibitor-induced angioedema also occurs as the result of increased bradykinin levels due to inhibition of its breakdown.

Clinical features

Angioedema is characterised by soft-tissue swelling that most frequently affects the face (Fig. 4.15) but can also affect the extremities and genitalia. Involvement of the larynx or tongue may cause life-threatening respiratory tract obstruction, and oedema of the intestinal mucosa may cause abdominal pain and distension.

Investigations

Differentiating the mechanism of angioedema is important in determining the most appropriate treatment. A clinical history of allergy or drug

i 4.18 Types of angioedema				
	Allergic reaction to specific trigger	**Idiopathic angioedema**	**Hereditary angioedema**	**ACE-inhibitor associated angioedema**
Pathogenesis	IgE-mediated degradation of mast cells	Non-IgE-mediated degranulation of mast cells	C1 inhibitor deficiency, with resulting increased local bradykinin concentration	Inhibition of breakdown of bradykinin
Key mediator	Histamine	Histamine	Bradykinin	Bradykinin
Prevalence	Common	Common	Rare autosomal dominant disorder	0.1%–0.2% of patients treated with ACE inhibitors
Clinical features	Usually associated with urticaria\nHistory of other allergies common\nFollows exposure to specific allergen, in food, animal dander or insect venom	Usually associated with urticaria\nMay be triggered by physical stimuli such as heat, pressure or exercise\nDermatographism common\nOccasionally associated with underlying infection or thyroid disease	Not associated with urticaria or other features of allergy\nDoes not cause anaphylaxis\nMay cause life-threatening respiratory tract obstruction\nCan cause severe abdominal pain	Not associated with urticaria\nDoes not cause anaphylaxis\nUsually affects the head and neck, and may cause life-threatening respiratory tract obstruction\nCan occur years after the start of treatment
Investigations	Specific IgE tests or skin-prick tests	Specific IgE tests and skin-prick tests often negative\nHypothyroidism should be excluded	Complement C4 (invariably low in acute attacks)\nC1 inhibitor levels	No specific investigations
Treatment	Allergen avoidance\nAntihistamines	Antihistamines are mainstay of treatment and prophylaxis	Unresponsive to antihistamines\nAnabolic steroids\nC1 inhibitor concentrate or icatibant for acute attacks	ACE inhibitor should be discontinued\nARBs should be avoided if possible unless there is a strong indication
Associated drug reactions	Specific drug allergies	NSAIDs\nOpioids, radiocontrast media		ACE inhibitors, ARBs

(ACE = angiotensin-converting enzyme; ARBs = angiotensin II receptor blockers; IgE = immunoglobulin E; NSAIDs = non-steroidal anti-inflammatory drugs)

exposure can give clues to the underlying diagnosis. If no obvious trigger can be identified, measurement of complement C4 is useful in differentiating hereditary and acquired angioedema from other causes. If C4 levels are low, further investigations should be initiated to look for evidence of C1 inhibitor deficiency.

Management

Management depends on the underlying cause. Angioedema associated with allergen exposure generally responds to antihistamines and glucocorticoids. Following acute management of angioedema secondary to drug therapy, drug withdrawal should prevent further attacks, although ACE inhibitor-induced angioedema can continue for a limited period post drug withdrawal. Management of angioedema associated with C1 inhibitor deficiency is discussed below.

Hereditary angioedema

Hereditary angioedema (HAE), also known as inherited C1 inhibitor deficiency, is an autosomal dominant disorder caused by decreased production or activity of C1 inhibitor protein. This complement regulatory protein inhibits spontaneous activation of the classical complement pathway (see Fig. 4.4). It also acts as an inhibitor of the kinin cascade, activation of which increases local bradykinin levels, giving rise to local pain and swelling.

Clinical features

The angioedema in HAE may be spontaneous or triggered by local trauma or infection. Multiple parts of the body may be involved, especially the face, extremities, upper airway and gastrointestinal tract. Oedema of the intestinal wall causes severe abdominal pain and many patients with undiagnosed HAE undergo exploratory laparotomy. The most important complication is laryngeal obstruction, often associated with minor dental procedures, which can be fatal. Episodes of angioedema are self-limiting

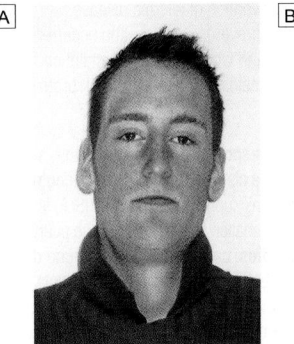 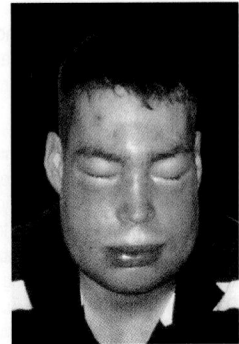

Fig. 4.15 Angioedema. This young man has hereditary angioedema. **A** Normal appearance. **B** During an acute attack. *From Helbert M. Flesh and bones of immunology. Edinburgh: Churchill Livingstone, Elsevier Ltd; 2006.*

and usually resolve within 48 hours. Patients with HAE generally present in adolescence but may go undiagnosed for many years. A family history can be identified in 80% of cases. HAE is not associated with allergic diseases and is specifically not associated with urticaria.

Investigations

Acute episodes are accompanied by low C4 levels; a low C4 during an episode of angioedema should therefore trigger further investigation. The diagnosis can be confirmed by measurement of C1 inhibitor levels and function.

Management

Severe acute attacks should be treated with plasma-derived or recombinant C1 inhibitor or the bradykinin receptor antagonist icatibant. Anabolic steroids, such as danazol, can be used to prevent attacks and act by increasing endogenous production of complement proteins, but is limited by treatment toxicity. Tranexamic acid can be helpful as prophylaxis in some patients. C1 inhibitor concentrate can also be used as prophylaxis, for example for surgical or dental intervention. Patients can be taught to self-administer therapy and should be advised to carry a MedicAlert or similar. More recently, a humanised monoclonal antibody which inhibits plasma kallikrein activity, limiting the production of bradykinin, has been developed for the prevention of recurrent attacks in patients with C1 inhibitor deficiency. This is not licensed for acute attacks.

Acquired C1 inhibitor deficiency

This rare disorder is clinically indistinguishable from HAE but presents in late adulthood. It is associated with autoimmune and lymphoproliferative diseases. Most cases are due to the development of autoantibodies to C1 inhibitor, but the condition can also be caused by autoantibodies that activate C1. Treatment of the underlying disorder may induce remission of angioedema. As with HAE, a low C4 is seen during acute episodes.

Pregnancy and the immune system

Major adaptations occur in the immune system during pregnancy so that the mother does not mount an immune response to the developing fetus. These adaptations can influence the risk and severity of certain infectious diseases such as varicella pneumonia (see p. 1271) as well as the activity of some autoimmune diseases. Some considerations for the development and management of immunological diseases during pregnancy and breastfeeding are summarised in Box 4.19.

Transplantation and graft rejection

Transplantation provides the opportunity for definitive treatment of end-stage organ disease. The major complications are graft rejection, drug toxicity and infection consequent to immunosuppression. Transplant survival continues to improve, as a result of the introduction of less toxic immunosuppressive agents and increased understanding of the processes of transplant rejection. Stem cell transplantation and its complications are discussed in more detail in Chapter 25.

Transplant rejection

Solid organ transplantation inevitably stimulates an aggressive immune response by the recipient, unless the transplant is between monozygotic twins. The type and severity of the rejection response is determined by the genetic disparity between the donor and recipient, the immune status of the host and the nature of the tissue transplanted (Box 4.20). The most important genetic determinant is the difference between donor and recipient HLA proteins. The extensive polymorphism of these proteins means that donor HLA antigens are almost invariably recognised as foreign by the recipient immune system, unless an active attempt has been made to minimise incompatibility.

- *Hyperacute rejection* results in rapid and irreversible destruction of the graft (see Box 4.20). It is mediated by pre-existing recipient antibodies against donor HLA antigens, which arise as a result of previous exposure through transplantation, blood transfusion or pregnancy. It is very rarely seen in clinical practice, as the use of screening for anti-HLA antibodies and pre-transplant cross-matching ensures the prior identification of such recipient–donor incompatibility.
- *Acute cellular rejection* is the most common form of graft rejection. It is mediated by activated T lymphocytes and results in deterioration in graft function. If allowed to progress, it may cause fever, pain and tenderness over the graft. It is usually amenable to increased immunosuppressive therapy.
- *Acute vascular rejection* is mediated by antibody formed de novo after transplantation. It is more curtailed than the hyperacute response because of the use of intercurrent immunosuppression but it is also associated with reduced graft survival. Aggressive immunosuppressive therapy is indicated and physical removal of antibody through plasmapheresis may be indicated in severe causes. Not all post-transplant anti-donor antibodies cause graft damage; their consequences are determined by specificity and ability to trigger other immune components, such as the complement cascade.

4.19 Immunological diseases in pregnancy

Allergic disease

- **Maternal dietary restrictions during pregnancy or lactation**: current evidence does not support these for prevention of allergic disease.
- **Breastfeeding for at least 4 months**: prevents or delays the occurrence of atopic dermatitis, cow's milk allergy and wheezing in early childhood, as compared with feeding formula milk containing intact cow's milk protein.

Autoimmune disease

- **Suppressed T-cell-mediated immune responses in pregnancy**: may suddenly reactivate post-partum. Some autoimmune diseases may improve during pregnancy but flare immediately after delivery. Systemic lupus erythematosus (SLE) is an exception, however, as it is prone to exacerbation in pregnancy or the puerperium.
- **Passive transfer of maternal antibodies**: can mediate autoimmune disease in the fetus and newborn, including SLE, Graves' disease and myasthenia gravis.
- **Antiphospholipid syndrome** (p. 987): an important cause of fetal loss, intrauterine growth restriction and pre-eclampsia.
- **HIV in pregnancy**: see p. 367.

4.20 Classification of transplant rejection

Type	Time	Pathological findings	Mechanism	Treatment
Hyperacute rejection	Minutes to hours	Thrombosis, necrosis	Pre-formed antibody to donor antigens results in complement activation (type II hypersensitivity)	None – irreversible graft loss
Acute cellular rejection	5–30 days	Cellular infiltration	CD4+ and CD8+ T cells (type IV hypersensitivity)	Increase immunosuppression
Acute vascular rejection	5–30 days	Vasculitis	Antibody and complement activation	Increase immunosuppression
Chronic allograft failure	> 30 days	Fibrosis, scarring	Immune and non-immune mechanisms	Minimise drug toxicity, control hypertension and hyperlipidaemia

i 4.21 Immunosuppressive drugs used in transplantation

Drug	Mechanism of action	Major adverse effects
Anti-proliferative agents Azathioprine, mycophenolate mofetil	Inhibit lymphocyte proliferation by blocking DNA synthesis May be directly cytotoxic at high doses	Increased susceptibility to infection Leucopenia Hepatotoxicity
Calcineurin inhibitors Ciclosporin, tacrolimus	Inhibit T-cell signalling; prevent lymphocyte activation; block cytokine transcription	Increased susceptibility to infection Hypertension Nephrotoxicity Diabetogenic (especially tacrolimus) Gingival hypertrophy, hirsutism (ciclosporin)
Glucocorticoids	Decrease phagocytosis and release of proteolytic enzymes; decrease lymphocyte activation and proliferation; decrease cytokine production; decrease antibody production	Increased susceptibility to infection Multiple other complications
Anti-thymocyte globulin (ATG)	Antibodies to cell surface proteins deplete or block T cells	Profound non-specific immunosuppression Increased susceptibility to infection
Basiliximab	Monoclonal antibody directed against CD25 (IL-2Rα chain), expressed on activated T cells	Increased susceptibility to infection Gastrointestinal side-effects
Belatacept	Selectively inhibits T-cell activation through blockade of CD80/CD86	Increased susceptibility to infection and malignancy Gastrointestinal side-effects Hypertension Anaemia/leucopenia

- *Chronic allograft failure*, also known as chronic rejection, is a major cause of graft loss. It is associated with proliferation of transplant vascular smooth muscle, interstitial fibrosis and scarring. The pathogenesis is poorly understood but contributing factors include immunological damage caused by subacute rejection, hypertension, hyperlipidaemia and chronic drug toxicity.

Investigations

Pre-transplantation testing

HLA typing determines an individual's HLA polymorphisms and facilitates donor–recipient matching. Potential transplant recipients are also screened for the presence of anti-HLA antibodies. The recipient is excluded from receiving a transplant that carries these alleles.

Donor–recipient cross-matching is a functional assay that directly tests whether serum from a recipient (which potentially contains anti-donor antibodies) is able to bind and/or kill donor lymphocytes. It is specific to a prospective donor–recipient pair and is done immediately prior to transplantation. A positive cross-match is a contraindication to transplantation because of the risk of hyperacute rejection.

Post-transplant biopsy: C4d staining

C4d is a fragment of the complement protein C4 (see Fig. 4.4). Deposition of C4d in graft capillaries indicates local activation of the

classical complement pathway and provides evidence of antibody-mediated damage. This is useful in the early diagnosis of vascular rejection.

Complications of transplant immunosuppression

Transplant recipients require indefinite treatment with immunosuppressive agents. In general, two or more immunosuppressive drugs are used in synergistic combination in order to minimise adverse effects (Box 4.21). The major complications of long-term immunosuppression are infection and malignancy. The risk of some opportunistic infections may be minimised through the use of prophylactic medication, such as ganciclovir for cytomegalovirus prophylaxis and trimethoprim–sulfamethoxazole for *Pneumocystis* prophylaxis. Immunisation with killed vaccines is appropriate, although the immune response may be curtailed. Live vaccines should not be given.

The increased risk of malignancy arises because T-cell suppression results in failure to control viral infections associated with malignant transformation. Virus-associated tumours include lymphoma (associated with Epstein–Barr virus), Kaposi's sarcoma (associated with human herpesvirus 8) and skin tumours (associated with human papillomavirus). Immunosuppression is also linked with a small increase in the incidence of common cancers not associated with viral infection (such as lung, breast and colon cancer), reflecting the importance of T cells in anti-cancer surveillance.

Organ donation

The major problem in transplantation is the shortage of organ donors. Cadaveric organ donors are usually previously healthy individuals who experience brainstem death, frequently as a result of road traffic accidents or cerebrovascular events. Even if organs were obtained from all potential cadaveric donors, though, their numbers would be insufficient to meet current demands. An alternative is the use of living donors. Altruistic living donation, usually from close relatives, is widely used in renal transplantation. Living organ donation is inevitably associated with some risk to the donor and it is highly regulated to ensure appropriate appreciation of the risks involved. Because of concerns about coercion and exploitation, non-altruistic organ donation (the sale of organs) is illegal in most countries.

Tumour immunology

Surveillance by the immune system is critically important in monitoring and removing damaged and mutated cells as they arise. The ability of the immune system to kill cancer cells effectively is influenced by tumour immunogenicity and specificity. Many cancer antigens are poorly expressed and specific antigens can mutate, either spontaneously or in response to treatment, which can result in evasion of immune responses. In addition, the inhibitory pathways that are used to maintain self-tolerance and limit collateral tissue damage during antimicrobial immune responses can be co-opted by cancerous cells to evade immune destruction. Recognition and understanding of these immune checkpoint pathways has led to the development of a number of new treatments for cancers that are otherwise refractory to treatment. Immune checkpoint blockade enhances anti-tumour immunity by blocking down-regulators of immune activation. Immune checkpoint inhibitors targeting CTLA-4, PD1 and PD-L1, such as ipilimimab, nivolumab, and pembrolizumab, have shown benefit in a number of tumour types, including melanoma, non-small cell lung cancer, urothelial cancers, colorectal malignancy and classic Hodgkin's lymphoma. These agents can, however, have serious inflammatory side effects, with immune-related adverse events most commonly involving the skin, liver, endocrine and gastrointestinal tracts, which may be treatment limiting. The effects of the different agents vary, with lung and thyroid involvement being more common with anti-PD1 therapy, colitis and hypophysitis being more common with anti-CTLA-4 therapy, with anti-CTLA-4 therapy-related events often being more severe. However, patients who have had a favourable response to immune checkpoint blockade but discontinue as a result of immune-related adverse events may maintain their anti-tumour response. Glucocorticoids are considered first line therapy for these side effects, with additional immune suppression if required. The development of autoimmunity reflects the importance of these pathways in the control of self-tolerance.

Another recent advance is CAR-T cell therapy, in which genetically engineered, chimaeric antigen receptor T cells are specifically developed for an individual patient, with effective reprogramming of the patient's immune cells, which are then used to target their cancer. This has been applied to certain otherwise treatment-refractory haematological malignancies (Ch. 25). Not only is it a very expensive treatment, but cytokine storm and subsequent antibody deficiency are predictable side effects of the CAR T-cell therapies directed at B-cell antigens, requiring management in their own right.

Further information

Websites

allergy.org.au *An Australasian site providing information on allergy, asthma and immune diseases.*

allergyuk.org *UK site for patients and health-care professionals.*

anaphylaxis.org.uk *Provides information and support for patients with severe allergies.*

info4pi.org *A US site managed by the non-profit Jeffrey Modell Foundation, which provides extensive information about primary immune deficiencies.*

niaid.nih.gov *National Institute of Allergy and Infectious Diseases: provides useful information on a variety of allergic diseases, immune deficiency syndromes and autoimmune diseases.*

H Campbell
DA McAllister

5

Population health and epidemiology

The UK Faculty of Public Heath defines public health as 'The science and art of promoting and protecting health and well-being, preventing ill-health and prolonging life through the organised efforts of society'. This recognises that there is a collective responsibility for the health of the population which requires partnerships between government, health services and other partners to promote and protect health and prevent disease. Population health has been defined as 'the health outcomes of a group of individuals, including the distribution of such outcomes within the group'. Medical doctors can play a role in all these efforts to improve health both as part of their clinical work but also through supporting broader actions to improve public health.

Global burden of disease and underlying risk factors

The Global Burden of Disease (GBD) exercise was initiated by the World Bank in 1992, with first estimates appearing in the World Development Report in 1993. Regular updated estimates have been published since that time together with projections of future disease burden. The aim of the exercise was to produce reliable and internally consistent estimates of disease burden for all diseases and injuries and to assess their physiological, behavioural and social risk factors so that this information could be made available to health workers, researchers and policy-makers.

The GBD exercise adopted the metric 'disability life year' or DALY to describe population health. This combines information about premature mortality in a population (measured as Years of Life Lost from an 'expected' life expectancy) and years of life lived with disability (Years of Life lived with Disability (YLD), which is weighted by a severity factor). The International Classification of Disease (ICD) rules, which assign one cause to each death, are followed. All estimates are presented by age and sex groups and by regions of the world. Many countries now also report their own national burden of disease data.

Life expectancy

Global life expectancy at birth increased from 61.7 years in 1980 to 73.0 years in 2017, an increase of about 0.3 years per calendar year. This change is due to a substantial fall in child mortality (mainly due to common infections) partly offset by rises in mortality from adult conditions such as diabetes and chronic kidney disease. Some areas have not shown these increases in life expectancy in men, often due to war and interpersonal violence.

Global causes of death and disability

Box 5.1 shows a ranked list of the major causes of global deaths in 2019. Communicable, maternal, neonatal and nutritional causes accounted for about one-quarter of deaths worldwide – down from about one-third in 1990. In contrast, deaths from non-communicable diseases are increasing in importance and now account for about two-thirds of all deaths globally,: including about 18.5 million from cardiovascular disease (ischaemic heart disease and stroke), 10 million from cancer and about 4 million from chronic respiratory diseases. The age standardised death rates for most diseases globally are falling. However, despite this, the numbers of deaths from many diseases are rising due to global population growth and the change in age structure of the population to older ages and this is placing an increasing burden on health systems. For a few conditions (e.g. HIV/AIDS, diabetes mellitus and chronic kidney disease) age-standardised death rates continue to rise. Within this overall pattern, significant regional variations exist – for example, communicable, maternal, neonatal and nutritional causes still account for about two-thirds of premature mortality in sub-Saharan Africa.

GBD also provides estimates of disability from disease (Box 5.2). This has raised awareness of the importance of conditions like depression and other common mental health conditions, low back and neck pain

---

i | **5.1 Global causes of death – top 15 ranked causes 2019 [rank in 1990]**

1. Cardiovascular disease   [1]
2. Neoplasms   [2]
3. Chronic respiratory   [6]
4. Respiratory infections and TB   [3]
5. Diabetes and CKD   [10]
6. Digestive diseases   [8]
7. Neurological disorders   [15]
8. Maternal and neonatal   [15]
9. Unintentional injuries   [9]
10. Enteric infections   [5]
11. Transport injuries   [13]
12. Self harm and violence   [12]
13. Other non-communicable diseases   [11]
14. HIV/AIDS and STIs   [17]
15. NTDs and malaria   [14]

(CKD = chronic kidney disease; TB = tuberculosis; STIs = sexually transmitted infections; NTDs = neglected tropical diseases)
From GBD 2019. https://vizhub.healthdata.org/gbd-compare/.

---

i | **5.2 Global disability – top 15 ranked causes 2019 [rank in 1990]***

1. Musculoskeletal disorders   [1]
2. Mental disorders   [2]
3. Other non-communicable diseases   [3]
4. Sense organ diseases   [5]
5. Neurological disorders   [4]
6. Diabetes and CKD   [12]
7. Skin diseases   [7]
8. Unintentional injuries   [8]
9. Nutritional deficiencies   [6]
10. Cardiovascular diseases   [11]
11. Chronic respiratory diseases   [9]
12. Substance use   [13]
13. Maternal and neonatal conditions   [17]
14. Transport injuries   [16]
15. Digestive diseases   [15]

*By years of life lived with disability (YLD).
(CKD = chronic kidney disease)
From GBD 2019. https://vizhub.healthdata.org/gbd-compare/.

---

and other musculo-skeletal conditions, and asthma, which account for a relatively large disease burden but relatively few deaths. This in turn has resulted in greater health policy priority given to these conditions. Since the policy focus in national health systems is increasingly on keeping people healthy rather than only on reducing premature deaths it is important to have measures of these health outcomes.

It is important to recognise that although these estimates represent the best overall picture of burden of disease globally, they are based on limited and imperfect data. Nevertheless, the quality of data underlying the estimates and the modelling processes are improving steadily over time and provide an increasingly robust basis for evidence-based health planning and priority setting.

Risk factors underlying disease

Box 5.3 shows a ranked list of the main risk factors underlying GBD in 2019 and how this ranking has changed over the past 29 years. A number of key insights have been identified in this, the most recent, GBD exercise:

- Socio-demographic development has been progressing steadily since 1990 but it has increased faster in countries with the highest socio-demographic development index and thus gaps have been widening.

i **5.3 Global risk factors – top 10 ranked causes 2019 [rank in 1990]***

1. High blood pressure   [7]
2. Smoking/second hand smoke exposure   [5]
3. High fasting blood glucose   [11]
4. Low birth weight   [2]
5. High BMI   [16]
6. Short gestation   [3]
7. Ambient particulate matter pollution   [13]
8. High LDL cholesterol   [14]
9. Alcohol use   [15]
10. Household air pollution   [4]

*Risk factors ranked by % of burden of disease they cause.
(BMI = body mass index; LDL = low density lipoprotein)
From GBD 2019 Diseases and Injuries Collaborators. Global burden of 369 diseases and injuries in 204 countries and territories, 1990–2019: a systematic analysis for the Global Burden of Disease Study 2019. Lancet 2020; 396:1204–1222.

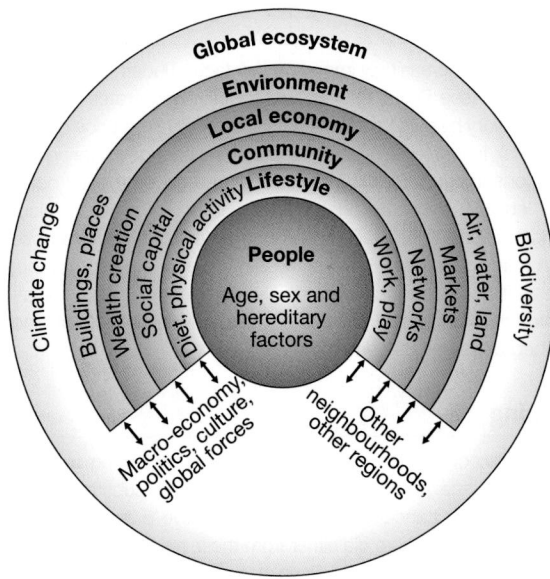

Fig. 5.1 Hierarchy of systems that influence population health. *Adapted from an original model by Whitehead M, Dahlgren G. What can be done about inequalities in health? Lancet 1991; 338:1059–1063.*

- Health systems need to transform to be better able to respond to the changing pattern of NCDs and disabilities.
- The Millennium Development Goal (MDG) programme from 2000 to 2015 has led to faster progress in reducing deaths from maternal, child and neonatal conditions/TB/HIV/malaria but this level of attention now needs to be directed at NCDs.
- Public health is not giving sufficient priority to important global risk factors which are increasing over time, such as high blood pressure, high fasting glucose, high BMI, ambient particulate matter pollution and drug and alcohol use.
- There are many challenges resulting from the change in global population pyramid structures, which have become inverted over recent decades and now pose many health, financial and political challenges.

Social determinants of health

Health emerges from a highly complex interaction between a person's genetic background and environmental factors (aspects of the physical, biological (microbes), built and social environments and also distant influences such as the global ecosystem) (Fig. 5.1).

The hierarchy of systems – from molecules to ecologies

Influences on health exist at many levels and extend beyond the individual to include the family, community, population and ecology. Box 5.4 shows an example of this for determinants of coronary heart disease and demonstrates the importance of considering not only the disease process in a patient but also its context. Health care is not the only determinant – and is usually not the major determinant – of health status in the population. The concept of 'global health' recognises the global dimension of health problems, whether these be, for example, emerging or pandemic infections or global economic influences on health internationally.

The life course

The determinants of health operate over the whole lifespan. Values and behaviours acquired during childhood and adolescence have a profound influence on educational outcomes, job prospects and risk of disease. These can have a strong influence, for example, on whether a young person takes up a damaging behaviour like smoking, risky sexual activity and drug misuse. Influences on health can even operate before birth. Low birth weight can lead to higher risk hypertension and

i **5.4 'Hierarchy of systems' applied to ischaemic heart disease**

Level in the hierarchy	Example of effect
Molecular	ApoB mutation causing hypercholesterolaemia
Cellular	Foam cells accumulate in vessel wall
Tissue	Atheroma and thrombosis of coronary artery
Organ	Ischaemia and infarction of myocardium
System	Cardiac failure
Person	Limited exercise capacity, impact on employment
Family	Passive smoking, diet
Community	Shops and leisure opportunities
Population	Prevalence of obesity
Society	Policies on smoking, screening for risk factors
Ecology	Agriculture influencing fat content in diet

type 2 diabetes in young adults and of cardiovascular disease in middle age. It has been suggested that under-nutrition during middle to late gestation permanently 'programmes' cardiovascular and metabolic responses.

This 'life course' perspective highlights the cumulative effect (through each stage of life) on health of exposures to illness, adverse environmental conditions and behaviours that damage health.

Preventive medicine

The complexity of the interactions between physical, social and economic determinants of health means that successful prevention is often difficult. Moreover, the life course perspective illustrates that it may be necessary to intervene early in life or even before birth, to prevent important disease in later life. Successful prevention is likely to require many interventions across the life course and at several levels in the hierarchy of systems. The examples below illustrate this principle.

Alcohol

Alcohol use is an increasingly important risk factor underlying global burden of disease (see Box 5.3). Reasons for increasing rates of alcohol-related harm vary by place and time but include the falling price of alcohol (in real terms), increased availability and cultural change fostering higher levels of consumption. Public, professional and governmental concern has now led to a minimum price being charged for a unit of alcohol, tightening of licensing regulations and curtailment of some promotional activity in many countries. However, even more aggressive public health measures will be needed to reverse the levels of harm in the population. The approach for individual patients suffering adverse effects of alcohol is described on pages 892 and 1240.

Smoking

Smoking is also one of the top three risk factors underlying global burden of disease (see Box 5.3). It is responsible for a substantial majority of cases of lung cancer and chronic obstructive pulmonary disease (COPD), and most smokers die either from these respiratory diseases or from ischaemic heart disease. Smoking also causes cancers of the upper respiratory and gastrointestinal tracts, pancreas, bladder and kidney, and increases risks of peripheral vascular disease, stroke and peptic ulceration. Maternal smoking is an important cause of fetal growth retardation. Moreover, there is increasing evidence that passive ('second hand') smoking has adverse effects on cardiovascular and respiratory health.

The decline in smoking rates in many high-income countries has been achieved not only by warning people of the health risks but also increased taxation of tobacco, banning of advertising, banning of smoking in public places and support for smoking cessation to maintain a decline in smoking rates. However, smoking rates remain high in many poorer areas and are increasing amongst young women. In many low-income countries, tobacco companies have found new markets and rates are rising.

There is a complex hierarchy of systems that interact to cause smokers to initiate and maintain their habit. At the molecular and cellular levels, nicotine acts on the nervous system to create dependence and acts to maintain the smoking habit. There are also strong influences at the personal and social level, such as young female smokers being motivated to 'stay thin' or 'look cool' and peer pressure. Other important influences in the wider environment include cigarette advertising, with the advertising budget of the tobacco industry being much greater than that of health services. Strategies to help individuals quit smoking (such as nicotine replacement therapy, anti-smoking advice and behavioural support) are cost-effective and form an important part of the overall anti-tobacco strategy.

Obesity

Obesity is an increasingly important risk factor underlying global burden of disease (see Box 5.3). The weight distribution of almost the whole population is shifting upwards – the slim are becoming less slim while the overweight and obese are becoming more so. In the UK, this translates into a 1-kilogram increase in weight per adult per year (on average over the adult population). The current obesity epidemic cannot be explained simply by individual behaviour and poor choice but also requires an understanding of the obesogenic environment that encourages people to eat more and exercise less. This includes the availability of cheap and heavily marketed energy-rich foods, the increase in labour-saving devices (e.g. elevators and remote controls) and the increase in passive transport (cars as opposed to walking, cycling, or walking to public transport hubs). To combat the health impact of obesity, therefore, we need to help those who are already obese but also develop strategies that impact on the whole population and reverse the obesogenic environment.

Poverty and affluence

The adverse health and social consequences of poverty are well documented: high birth rates, high death rates and short life expectancy.

Typically, with industrialisation, the pattern changes: low birth rates, low death rates and longer life expectancy. Instead of infections, chronic conditions such as heart disease dominate in an older population. Adverse health consequences of excessive affluence are also becoming apparent. Despite experiencing sustained economic growth for the last 50 years, people in many high-income countries are not growing any happier and the litany of socioeconomic problems – crime, congestion, inequality, mental health problems – persists.

Many countries are now experiencing a 'double burden'. They have large populations still living in poverty who are suffering from problems such as diarrhoea and malnutrition, alongside affluent populations (often in cities) who suffer from chronic illness such as diabetes and heart disease.

Atmospheric pollution

Emissions from industry, power plants and motor vehicles of sulphur oxides, nitrogen oxides, respirable particles and metals are severely polluting cities and towns in Asia, Africa, Latin America and Eastern Europe. Increased death rates from respiratory and cardiovascular disease occur in vulnerable adults, such as those with established respiratory disease and older people, while children experience an increase in bronchitic symptoms. Low-income countries also suffer high rates of respiratory disease as a result of indoor pollution caused mainly by heating and cooking combustion.

Carbon dioxide and global warming

Climate change is arguably the world's most important environmental health issue. A combination of increased production of carbon dioxide and habitat destruction, both caused primarily by human activity, seems to be the main cause. The temperature of the globe is rising, climate is being affected, and if the trend continues, sea levels will rise and rainfall patterns will be altered so that both droughts and floods will become more common. These have already claimed millions of lives during the past 20 years and have adversely affected the lives of many more. The economic costs of property damage and the impact on agriculture, food supplies and prosperity have also been substantial. The health impacts of global warming will also include changes in the geographical range of some vector-borne infectious diseases. Currently, politicians cannot agree on an effective framework of actions to tackle the problem. Meanwhile, the industrialised world continues with lifestyles and levels of waste that are beyond the planet's ability to sustain.

Principles of screening and immunisation

Screening

Screening is the application of a screening test to a large number of asymptomatic people with the aim of reducing morbidity or mortality from a disease. WHO have identified a set of (Wilson and Jungner) criteria to guide health systems in deciding when it is appropriate to implement screening programmes. The essential criteria are:

- Is the disease an important public health problem?
- Is there a suitable screening test available?
- Is there a recognisable latent or early stage?
- Is there effective treatment for the disease at this stage which improves prognosis?

A suitable screening test is one that is cheap, acceptable, easy to perform, safe and gives a valid result in terms of sensitivity and specificity. Screening programmes should always be evaluated in trials so that robust evidence is provided in favour of their adoption. These evaluations are prone to several biases – self-selection bias, lead-time bias and length bias – and these need to be accounted for in the analysis. Examples of large-scale screening programmes in the UK include breast, colorectal and cervical cancer national screening programmes (https://www.gov.uk/topic/population-screening-programmes) and a number of screening tests carried out in pregnancy and in the newborn, such as the:

- diabetic eye screening programme
- fetal anomaly screening programme
- infectious diseases in pregnancy screening programme
- newborn and infant physical examination screening programme
- newborn blood spot screening programme
- newborn hearing screening programme
- sickle-cell anaemia and thalassaemia screening programme.

These are illustrated in Figure 5.2.
Problems with screening include:

- over-diagnosis (of a disease that would not have come to clinical attention on its own or would not have led to death)
- false reassurance
- diversion of resources from investments that could control the disease more cost-effectively.

Immunisation

Immunisation can confer immunity to specific infectious diseases and be either passive (through injected antibodies, such as the monoclonal palivizumab against respiratory syncytial virus (RSV) infection given to premature infants) or active (through administration of a vaccine). Immunisation invokes antibody and/or cell-mediated immunity and can lead to both short- and longer-term protection in the person who is vaccinated. Immunisation has also been used to eradicate a disease such as occurred in the smallpox eradication programme and is currently being targeted in the polio eradication programme. As well as direct effects of vaccination a number of indirect effects can occur – such as protection of individuals who are vaccinated through altering disease transmission leading to 'herd immunity'; or reduction of antibiotic resistance through selective reduction of pneumococcal serogroups that are associated with antibiotic resistance. The UK immunisation schedule is described in detail and regularly updated in the UK government publication 'Immunisation against infectious disease' (Green Book).

Epidemiology

Epidemiologists study disease in free-living humans, seeking to describe patterns of health and disease and to understand how different exposures cause or prevent disease (Box 5.5). Chronic diseases and risk factors (e.g. smoking, obesity etc.) are often described in terms of their prevalence. A prevalence is simply a proportion, for example the prevalence of diabetes among people aged 80 and older in developed countries is around 10%.

Events such as deaths, hospitalisations and first occurrences of a disease are described using incidence rates, so, for example, if there are 100 new cases of a disease in a single year in a population of 1000, the incidence rate is 105 per 1000 person-years. The rate is 105 rather than 100 because the denominator is person-time, the sum of the total 'exposed' time for the population, which in this example is 950 person-years. Person-time is the sum of the total 'exposed' time for the population and in this example is 950 person-years. The reason the person-time is less than 1000 is that 100 people experienced the event. These 100 people are assumed to have had an event, on average, half-way through the time-period, removing 100 ×0.5 person-years from the exposure-time (as it is not possible to have a first occurrence of a disease twice).

A similar measure to the incidence rate is the cumulative incidence or risk, which is the number of new cases as a proportion of the total people at risk at the beginning of the exposure time. If in the example above the same 1000 people were observed for a year (i.e. with no one joining or leaving the group) then the one-year risk is 10% (100/1000). The time-period should always be specified for risks.

These rates and proportions are used to describe how diseases (and risk factors) vary according to time, person and place. Temporal variation may occur seasonally; for example, malaria occurs in the wet season but not the dry, or as longer-term 'secular' trends, e.g. malaria may re-emerge due to drug resistance. Person comparisons include age, sex, socio-economic status, employment, and lifestyle characteristics. Place comparisons include the local environment (e.g. urban versus rural) and international comparisons.

Understanding causes and effect

Epidemiological research complements that based on animal, cell and tissue models, the findings of which do not always translate to humans. For example, only a minority of drug discoveries from laboratory research are found to be effective when tested in people.

However, differentiating causes from mere non-causal associations is a considerable challenge for epidemiology. This is because while laboratory researchers can directly manipulate conditions to isolate and understand causes, such approaches are impossible in free-living populations. Epidemiologists have developed a different approach, based around a number of study designs (Box 5.6). Of these, the clinical trial is closest to the laboratory experiment. An early example of a clinical trial is shown in Figure 5.3, along with 'effect measures' which are used to quantify the difference in rates and risks.

In clinical trials, patients are usually randomly allocated to treatments so that, on average, groups are similar apart from the intervention of interest. Nevertheless, for any particular trial, especially a small trial, the laws of probability mean that differences can and do occur by chance. Poorly designed or executed trials can also limit comparability between groups. Allocation may not truly be random (e.g. because of inadequate concealment of the randomisation sequence), and there may be systematic differences (biases) in the way people allocated to different groups are treated or studied.

Such biases also occur in observational epidemiological study designs, such as cohort, case–control and cross-sectional studies (see Box 5.6). These designs are also much more subject to the problem of confounding than are randomised trials.

Confounding is where the relationship between an exposure and outcome of interest is confused by the presence of some other causal factor. For example, coffee consumption may be associated with lung cancer because smoking is commoner among coffee-drinkers. Here, smoking is said to confound the association between coffee and lung cancer.

Despite these limitations, for most causes of diseases, randomised controlled trials are not feasible because of ethical, or more often practical, considerations. Epidemiologists therefore seek to minimise bias and confounding by good study design and analysis. Epidemiologists subsequently make causal inferences by balancing the probability that an observed association has been caused by chance, bias and/or confounding against the alternative probability that the relationship is causal. This weighing-up requires an understanding of the frequency and importance of different sources of bias and confounding as well as the scientific rationale of the putative causal relationship. It was this approach, collectively and over a number of years, that settled the fact that smoking causes lung cancer, and, subsequently, heart disease.

Mendelian randomisation

Mendelian randomisation (MR) is a method to study whether the relationship between a (modifiable) risk factor and a disease may be causal. It uses genetic variation in a gene that influences the level of the risk factor under consideration and studies the impact of this variation on

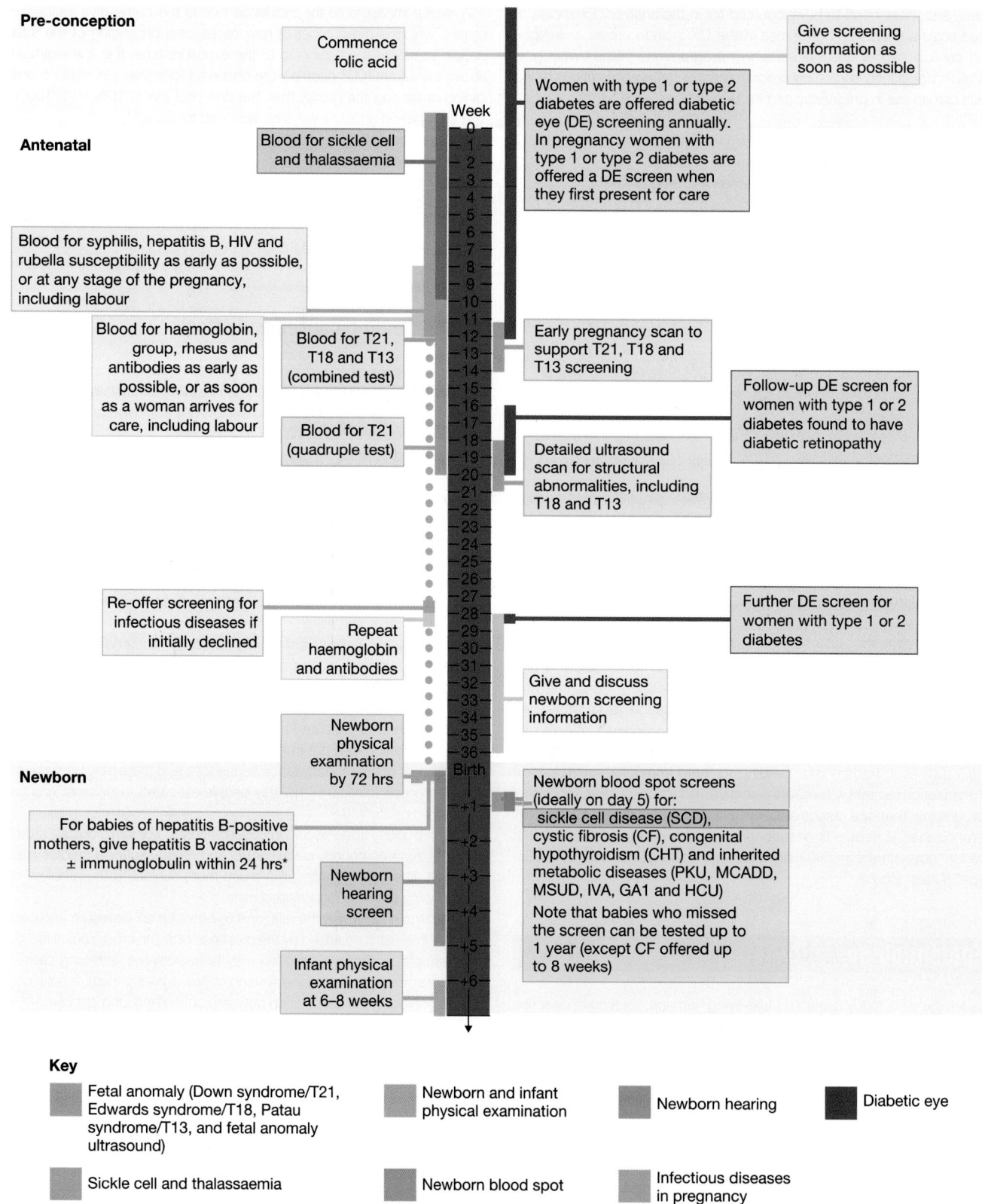

Pre-conception

Commence folic acid

Give screening information as soon as possible

Antenatal

Blood for sickle cell and thalassaemia

Week

Women with type 1 or type 2 diabetes are offered diabetic eye (DE) screening annually. In pregnancy women with type 1 or type 2 diabetes are offered a DE screen when they first present for care

Blood for syphilis, hepatitis B, HIV and rubella susceptibility as early as possible, or at any stage of the pregnancy, including labour

Blood for haemoglobin, group, rhesus and antibodies as early as possible, or as soon as a woman arrives for care, including labour

Blood for T21, T18 and T13 (combined test)

Early pregnancy scan to support T21, T18 and T13 screening

Follow-up DE screen for women with type 1 or 2 diabetes found to have diabetic retinopathy

Blood for T21 (quadruple test)

Detailed ultrasound scan for structural abnormalities, including T18 and T13

Re-offer screening for infectious diseases if initially declined

Repeat haemoglobin and antibodies

Further DE screen for women with type 1 or 2 diabetes

Give and discuss newborn screening information

Newborn physical examination by 72 hrs

Newborn

Newborn blood spot screens (ideally on day 5) for: sickle cell disease (SCD), cystic fibrosis (CF), congenital hypothyroidism (CHT) and inherited metabolic diseases (PKU, MCADD, MSUD, IVA, GA1 and HCU)

Note that babies who missed the screen can be tested up to 1 year (except CF offered up to 8 weeks)

For babies of hepatitis B-positive mothers, give hepatitis B vaccination ± immunoglobulin within 24 hrs*

Newborn hearing screen

Infant physical examination at 6–8 weeks

Key

Fetal anomaly (Down syndrome/T21, Edwards syndrome/T18, Patau syndrome/T13, and fetal anomaly ultrasound)

Newborn and infant physical examination

Newborn hearing

Diabetic eye

Sickle cell and thalassaemia

Newborn blood spot

Infectious diseases in pregnancy

Fig. 5.2 UK NHS pregnancy and newborn screening programmes. Antenatal and newborn screening timeline. *To stop mother-to-baby transmission of infection follow up all infection screens in pregnancy that are positive: carry out paediatric assessment and follow-up of mothers who are found to be HIV-positive or had syphilis treatment in pregnancy; and if mothers are found to be susceptible to rubella then offer the mother MMR vaccination postnatally and refer to GP for second dose. (GA1 = glutaric aciduria type 1; HCU = homocystinuria; IVA = isovaleric acidaemia; MCADD = medium-chain acyl-CoA dehydrogenase deficiency; MSUD = maple syrup urine deficiency; PKU = phenylketonuria) *Based on Version 8.4, January 2019. Gateway Ref: 20144696. www.gov.uk/phe/screening.*

5.5 Calculation of risk using descriptive epidemiology

Prevalence

- The ratio of the number of people with a longer-term disease or condition at a specified time, to the number of people in the population who are at risk

Incidence

- The number of events (new cases or episodes) occurring in the population at risk during a defined period of time

Attributable risk

- The difference between the risk (or incidence) of disease in exposed and non-exposed populations

Attributable fraction

- The ratio of the attributable risk to the incidence

Relative risk

- The ratio of the risk (or incidence) in the exposed population to the risk (or incidence) in the non-exposed population

5.6 Epidemiological study designs

Design	Description	Example
Clinical trial	Enrols a sample from a population and compares outcomes after randomly allocating patients to an intervention	The Medical Research Council (MRC) streptomycin trial – demonstrated effectiveness of streptomycin in tuberculosis
Cohort	Enrols a sample from a population and compares outcomes according to exposures	The Framingham Study – identified risk factors for cardiovascular disease
Case–control	Enrols cases with an outcome of interest and controls without that outcome, and compares exposures between the groups	Doll and Hill's study on smoking and carcinoma of the lung (BMJ 1950, 2) demonstrated that smoking caused lung cancer
Cross-sectional	Enrols a cross-section (sample) of people from the population of interest. Obtains data on exposures and outcomes	World Health Organization Demographic and Health Survey. Captures risk factor data in a uniform way across many countries

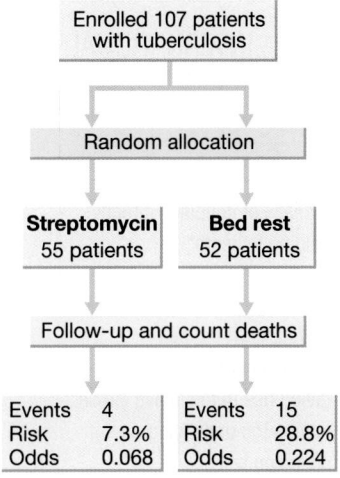

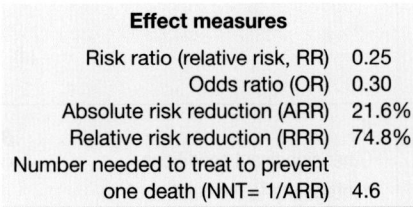

Fig. 5.3 **An example of a clinical trial: streptomycin versus bed rest in tuberculosis.** Both prevalences and risks are, in fact, proportions and are therefore frequently expressed as odds. The reasons for doing so are beyond the scope of this text.

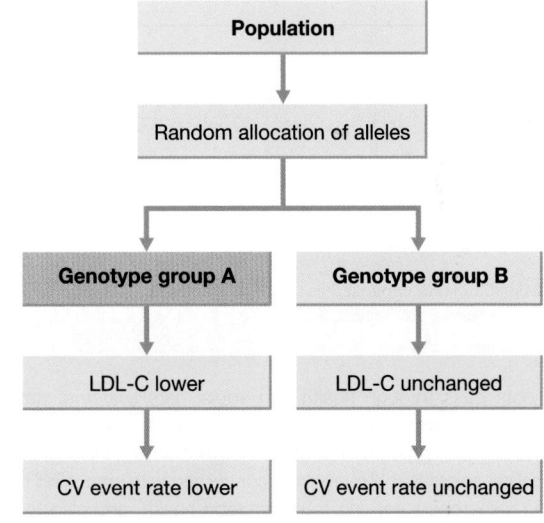

Fig. 5.4 **Mendelian randomisation.** An example showing comparison of a conventional trial with a Mendelian randomisation study. (CV = cardiovascular; LDL-C = low-density lipoprotein cholesterol) *Adapted with permission from Bennett DA, Holmes MV. Heart 2017; 103:1400–1407.*

disease risk (see Fig. 5.4 for an example). The genetic variant (or multiple variants or genetic risk score) is used as an instrumental variable under certain assumptions. MR investigates the effect of differences in the risk factor level through the life course which have been determined by the genetic variants. This approach uses observational data to test a proposed causal relationship and to estimate the size of effect. Guidelines such as STROBE-MR have been published for the proper conduct of these studies and analytic software packages are now available which contain a range of methods and tools. The selection of the most appropriate method depends on the research question and the data structure.

The MR approach requires very large sample sizes to have sufficient power and very large databases of genetic and health data such as UK Biobank are often used. MR can be conducted using either individual level data or summary data from genome-wide association studies (GWAS); and data from one study (one sample) or two studies with the variant–risk factor association measure from one and the risk factor–outcome association from the other (two sample).

Correct interpretation of MR results is challenging and multiple analytic methods are often employed. This includes methods to detect and adjust for pleiotropy (having more than one effect) which is a common problem in data interpretation. The strength of the conclusions depends on the degree to which instrumental variable assumptions are met and the level of consistency of findings across different methods. MR has proven useful in both identifying new causal relationships or confirming trial results but also in redirecting research interest away from relationships that have been shown not to be causal. MR can be considered

INTERNATIONAL FORM OF MEDICAL CERTIFICATE OF CAUSE OF DEATH

	Cause of death		Approximate interval between onset and death
I Disease or condition directly leading to death*	(a)	*Acute myocardial infarction*　　I21.9	*2 days*
	due to (or as a consequence of)		
Antecedent causes Morbid conditions, if any, giving rise to the above cause, stating the underlying condition last	(b)	*Familial hypercholesterolaemia*　E78.0	*30 years*
	due to (or as a consequence of)		
	(c)		
	due to (or as a consequence of)		
	(d)		
II Other significant conditions contributing to the death, but not related to the disease or condition causing it		*Bronchiectasis*　　J47	*10 years*

*This does not mean the mode of dying, e.g. heart failure, respiratory failure. It means the disease, injury, or complication that caused death.

Fig. 5.5 Completed death certificate. International Classification of Diseases 10 (ICD-10) codes are appended in red. *Based on World Health Organization, ICD-10, vol. 2. Geneva: WHO; 1990. Form retrieved from* https://commons.m.wikimedia.org/wiki/File:International_form_of_medical_certificate_of_cause_of_death.png.

to provide further evidence for or against a causal relationship but care should be taken in interpretation of the size of the expected impact from an intervention.

Health data/informatics

As patients pass through health and social care systems, data are recorded concerning their family background, lifestyle and disease states, which is of potential interest to health-care organisations seeking to deliver services, policy-makers concerned with improving health, scientific researchers seeking to understand health, and also to pharmaceutical and other commercial organisations seeking to identify markets.

There is a long tradition of maintaining health information systems. In most countries, the registration of births and deaths is required by law, and in the majority, the cause of death is also recorded (Fig. 5.5). There are numerous challenges in ensuring such data are useful, especially for making comparisons across time and place. First, a system of standard terminologies is needed, such as the World Health Organization International Classification of diseases, which provides a list of diagnostic codes attempting to cover every diagnostic entity. Secondly, these terms must be understood to refer to the same, or at least similar diseases in different places. Thirdly, access to diagnostic skill and facilities is required, fourthly standard protocols for assigning clinical diagnoses to ICD-10 codes are needed and fifthly, robust quality control processes are needed to maintain some level of data completeness and accuracy.

Many countries employ similar systems for hospitalisations, either to allow recovery of healthcare utilisation costs, or to manage and plan services. Similar data are, however, rarely collected for community-based healthcare. Nor are detailed data on health-care process generally included in national data systems.

Consequently, there has been considerable interest in using data from information technology systems used to deliver care – such as electronic patient records, drug-dispensing databases, radiological software, and clinical laboratory information systems.

Data from such systems are, of course, much less structured than those obtained from vital registrations. Moreover, the completeness of such data depends greatly on local patterns of healthcare utilisation as well as how clinicians and others use IT systems within different settings. As such, deriving useful unbiased information from such data is a considerable challenge.

Much of the discipline of health informatics is concerned with addressing this challenge. One approach has been to develop comprehensive standard classification systems such as SNOMED-CT 'a standardised, multilingual vocabulary of terms relating to the care of the individual' which has been designed for electronic health-care records. An alternative has been to use statistical methods such as natural language processing to automatically derive information from free text (such as culling diagnoses from radiological reports), or to employ 'machine learning', in which software algorithms are applied to data in order to derive useful insights. Such approaches are suited to large, messy data where the costs of systematisation would be prohibitive. It is likely that such innovations will over the coming years provide useful information to complement that obtained from more traditional health information systems.

Management of epidemics

An epidemic, as defined by the World Health Organization, occurs when 'in a community or region [the] cases of an illness, specific health-related behaviour, or other health-related events [are] clearly in excess of normal expectancy'. Epidemics that are small-scale or confined to a small geographic area are informally referred to as 'outbreaks'.

Epidemics are regularly caused where preventative measures break down; examples include breaches of food safety procedures in restaurants resulting in outbreaks of enteropathogenic *E. coli* infection, failure to adequately maintain cooling towers causing *Legionella* infections and falls in vaccination coverage resulting in measles epidemics.

Epidemics can also arise from novel infectious agents such as the SARS-CoV-1, MERS, SARS-CoV-2 and H1N1 viruses, for which new preventative measures require to be developed. Where epidemics from novel agents are not controlled locally, but instead spread beyond international borders, these are termed pandemics, of which SARS-CoV-2 and H1N1 are examples.

To detect epidemics early, public health agencies undertake surveillance. Surveillance involves the collection and review of cases that have been identified via statutory notifications, or health information systems (such as microbiology reporting systems). For some infections such as *E. coli* and *Legionella*, one challenge for public health agencies is to distinguish epidemics from 'sporadic' cases at an early stage. This is done using human judgement, for example, if a large number of cases of *E. coli* occur in individuals who ate a specific food, although this task is sometimes supported using computer algorithms.

Epidemics require an incident management team, some of whose members have legal powers to impose measures to control infection. The team establish a formal case definition for confirmed, probable and possible cases (based on epidemiological features as well as clinical and/or microbiological findings), interview individuals with whom cases have had significant contact (termed contact tracing), test potential sources of infections (e.g. foodstuffs or industrial cooling towers), and implement control measures. The latter might include requiring infected individuals to isolate for a time period (e.g. until they are asymptomatic or until they test negative depending on the infectious agent), and/or ordering temporary closure of businesses thought to be sources of infection (e.g. a restaurant with poor food hygiene practices).

Epidemic curves are crucial to the monitoring and management of epidemics. Figure 5.6 shows a notional epidemic curve for an epidemic caused by a single source, which is eliminated after 31 days. However, they are also used in more complex epidemics where there is person-to-person spread. In the latter, epidemic curves are used to estimate key statistics such as the basic reproduction number (R0) in the population, as well as to make projections about future infections. Where the source of an epidemic is not apparent, comparative epidemiological methods can be used to identify the likely source, for example, a case–control design may identify a higher than expected consumption of a given food – for example uncooked legumes – among cases compared to controls prompting testing of foods, an education campaign and/or product recalls.

The principles for managing pandemics are similar to those for managing epidemics but operate on a national or international scale. The universality of pandemics, however, means that they pose special problems. First, they pose risks to the society-wide infrastructure needed to deal with diseases, including, but not limited to health-care facilities. Secondly, pandemics, unlike local and regional epidemics are rare, so

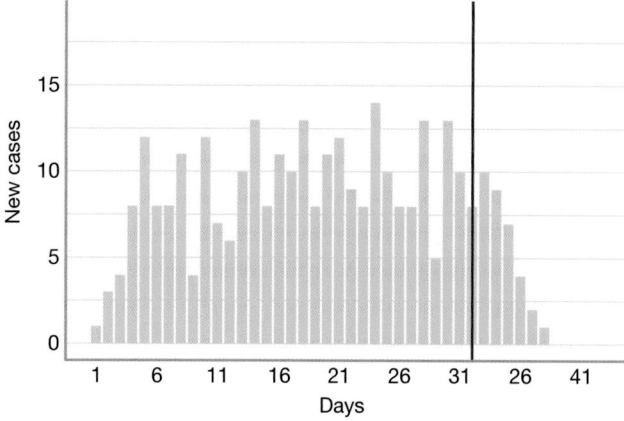

Fig. 5.6 Epidemic curve for a notional outbreak within a single ongoing source. Red line indicates time point where source of infection was removed (e.g. closure of a restaurant).

agencies have little direct experience with their management. For this reason, most settings develop pandemic plans and undertake regular table-top simulations to test and improve their preparedness. The COVID-19 pandemic, caused by SARS-CoV-2, is a key example and is discussed in detail in Chapter 13.

Further information

Kindig D, Stoddart G. What is population health? Am J Publ Health 2003;93: 380–383.
UK Faculty of Public Health. What is public health? http://www.fph.org.uk/what_is_public_health.

Burden of disease

GBD Diseases and Injuries Collaborators. Global burden of 369 diseases and injuries in 204 countries and territories, 1990–2019: a systematic analysis for the Global Burden of Disease Study 2019. Lancet 2019; 2020(396): 1204–1222.
GBD Risk Factors Collaborators. Global burden of 87 risk factors in 204 countries and territories, 1990–2019: a systematic analysis for the Global Burden of Disease Study 2019. Lancet 2019; 2020(396):1223–1249.
GBD Viewpoint Collaborators. Five insights from the Global Burden of Disease Study 2019. Lancet 2019; 2020(396):1135–1159.

Screening

Gov.UK. Population screening programmes. https://www.gov.uk/topic/population-screening-programmes. *Detailed information on 11 NHS population screening programmes.*

Immunisation

Gov.UK. Immunisation against infectious disease. https://www.gov.uk/government/collections/immunisation-against-infectious-disease-the-green-book. *The Green Book has the latest information on vaccines and vaccination procedures, for vaccine-preventable infectious diseases in the UK.*

Epidemiology

Burgess S, Davey Smith G, Davies NM, et al. Guidelines for performing Mendelian randomization investigations. Wellcome Open Res 2020;4:186.
STROBE-MR Steering Group: STROBE-MR: Guidelines for strengthening the reporting of Mendelian randomization studies. PeerJ https://peerj.com/preprints/27857/.

JAT Sandoe
DH Dockrell

6

Principles of infectious disease

'Infection' in its strict sense describes the situation where microorganisms or other infectious agents become established in the host organism's cells or tissues, replicate, induce a host response, and result in pathologic changes in tissues. If a microorganism survives and replicates on an epithelial surface without causing pathological change the host is said to be 'colonised' by that organism. If a microorganism survives and lies dormant after invading host cells or tissues, infection is said to be 'latent'. When a microorganism, or the host response to it, is sufficient to cause illness or harm, then the process is said to have caused infection, which may manifest by symptoms or signs. In milder cases there can be asymptomatic infection that may be identified by detection of a pathogen or the host response to the pathogen. Most pathogens (agents that can cause infection) are microorganisms but some are multicellular organisms. The manifestations of disease may aid pathogen dissemination (e.g. diarrhoea or coughing).

The term 'infection' is often used interchangeably with 'infectious disease' but not all infections are 'infectious', i.e. transmissible from person to person, and not all infections result in symptomatic disease. Infectious diseases caused by pathogens that are transmitted between hosts can also be called 'communicable diseases', whereas infection caused by organisms that are already colonising the host are described as 'endogenous'. The distinction is blurred in some situations, including health care-associated infections such as meticillin-resistant *Staphylococcus aureus* (MRSA) or *Clostridioides* (formerly *Clostridium*) *difficile* infection (CDI), in which colonisation precedes infection but the colonising bacteria may have been recently transmitted between patients. The chain of infection (Fig. 6.1) describes elements for communicable disease transmission.

Despite dramatic advances in hygiene, immunisation and antimicrobial therapy, infections still cause a massive burden of disease worldwide.

Key challenges remain in tackling infection in resource-poor countries. Microorganisms are continually mutating and evolving; the emergence of new infectious agents (e.g. SARS-CoV-2, see Ch. 13) and antimicrobial-resistant microorganisms is therefore inevitable. This chapter describes the biological and epidemiological principles of infectious diseases and the general approach to their prevention, diagnosis and treatment. Specific infectious diseases are described in Chapters 13–15 and many of the organ-based chapters.

Agents causing infection

The concept of an infectious agent was established by Robert Koch in the 19th century (Box 6.1). Although fulfilment of 'Koch's postulates' became the standard for confirming the cause of an infection, many infectious agents do not fulfil Koch's postulates (e.g. uncultivable organisms and the causes of endogenous infections), and the postulates are now of mainly historical interest. The groups of infectious agents that are now recognised are described in the following sections.

---

i   **6.1 Definition of an infectious agent – Koch's postulates**

1. The same organism must be present in every case of the disease.
2. The organism must be isolated from the diseased host and grown in pure culture.
3. The isolate must cause the disease, when inoculated into a healthy, susceptible animal.
4. The organism must be re-isolated from the inoculated, diseased animal.

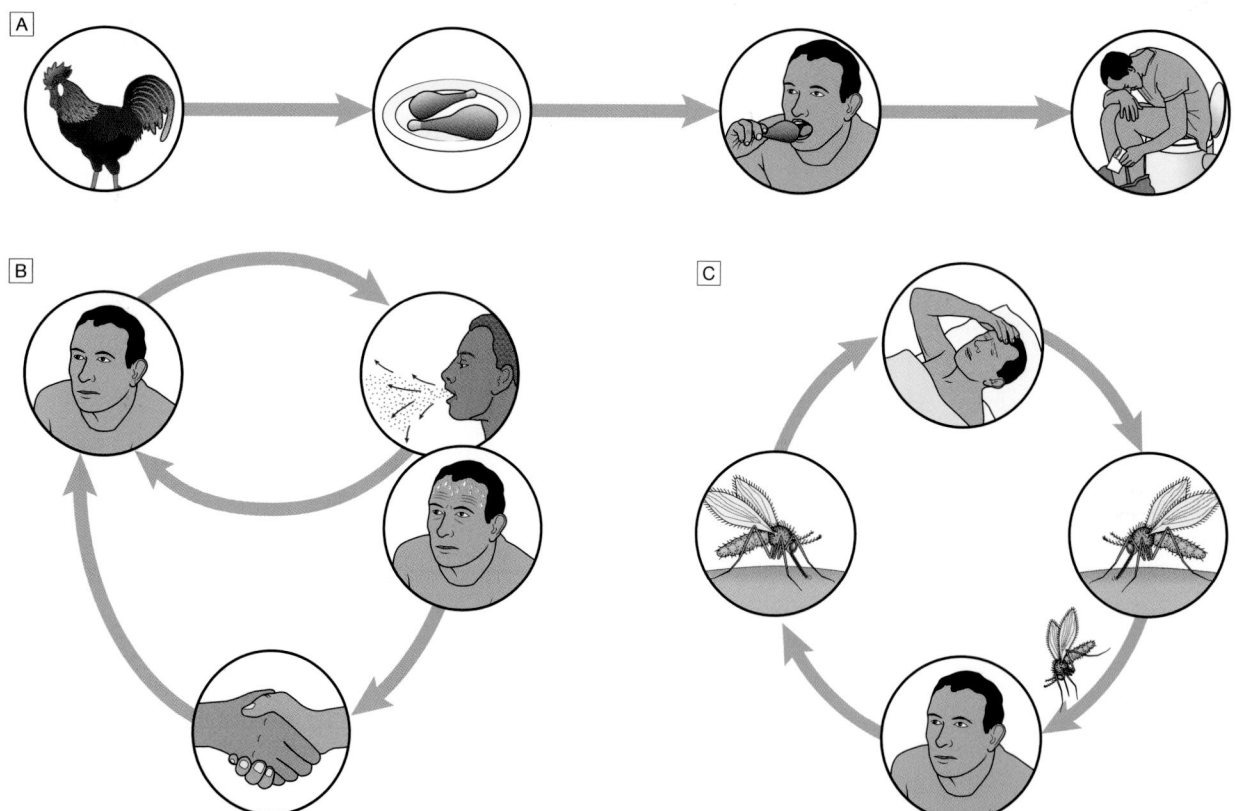

Fig. 6.1 The chain of infection can be linear (A) and cyclical (B and C). [A] Infections with an animal reservoir (e.g. *Campylobacter* enteritis) require a portal of exit from the reservoir and a vehicle for transmission to a susceptible human host (often water or a contaminated item of food). [B] Infections with person-to-person transmission (e.g. respiratory virus infection) require a mode of exit from the infected person, a mode of transmission (e.g. contaminated respiratory droplets or transmission via the surface of an intermediate fomite) and a portal of entry to a susceptible host. [C] Infections with an insect vector (e.g. malaria) require a mode of transmission from the insect reservoir to a susceptible human host and a mode of transmission back to the insect vector. Many infections involve a combination of these modes of transmission (e.g. Lyme disease, which has both an animal host and an insect vector) or several different modes of transmission.

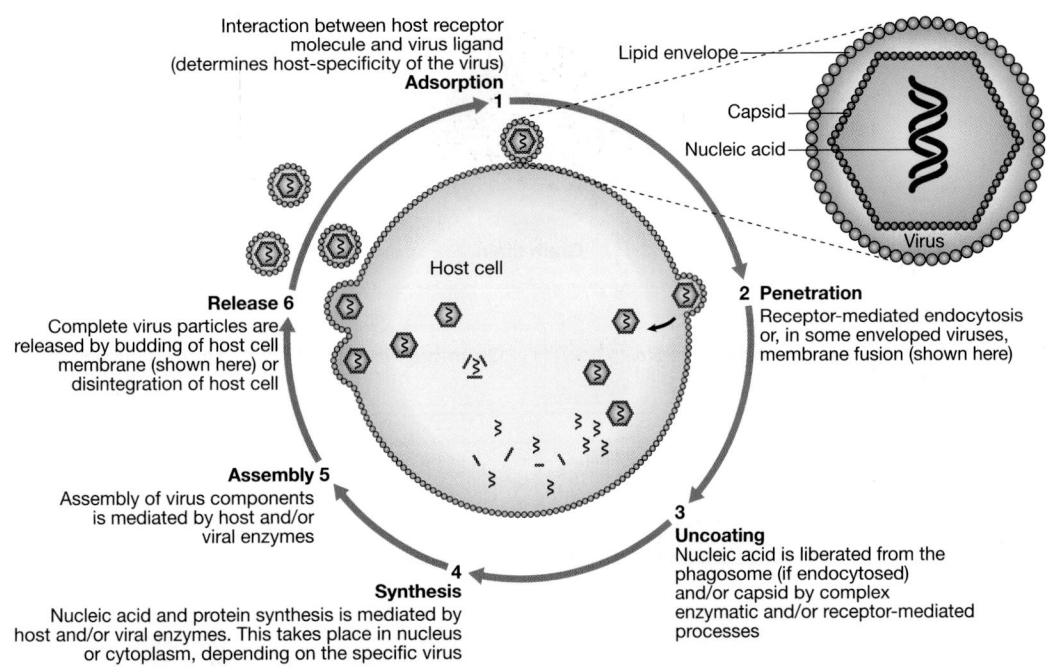

Fig. 6.2 A generic virus life cycle. Life cycle components common to most viruses are host cell attachment and penetration, virus uncoating, nucleic acid and protein synthesis, virus assembly and release. Virus release is achieved either by budding, as illustrated, or by lysis of the cell membrane. Life cycles vary between viruses.

Viruses

Viruses are incapable of independent replication. Instead, they subvert host cellular processes to ensure synthesis of their nucleic acids and proteins. Viruses' genetic material (the genome) consists of single- or double-stranded DNA or RNA. Retroviruses transcribe their RNA into DNA in the host cell by reverse transcription. An antigenically unique protein coat (capsid) encloses the genome, and together these form the nucleocapsid. In many viruses, the nucleocapsid is packaged within a lipid envelope. Enveloped viruses are less able to survive in the environment and are spread by respiratory, sexual or blood-borne routes, including arthropod-based transmission. Non-enveloped viruses survive better in the environment and are predominantly transmitted by faecal–oral or, less often, respiratory routes. A generic virus life cycle is shown in Figure 6.2. A virus that infects a bacterium is a bacteriophage (phage).

Prokaryotes: bacteria (including mycobacteria and actinomycetes)

Prokaryotic cells can synthesise their own proteins and nucleic acids, and are able to reproduce autonomously, although they lack a nucleus. The bacterial cell membrane is bounded by a peptidoglycan cell wall, which is thick (20–80 nm) in Gram-positive organisms and thin (5–10 nm) in Gram-negative ones. The Gram-negative cell wall is surrounded by an outer membrane containing lipopolysaccharide. Genetic information is contained within a chromosome but bacteria may also contain rings of extra-chromosomal DNA, known as plasmids, which can be transferred between organisms, without cells having to divide. Bacteria may be embedded in a polysaccharide capsule, and motile bacteria are equipped with flagella. Although many prokaryotes are capable of independent existence, some (e.g. *Chlamydia trachomatis*, *Coxiella burnetii*) are obligate intracellular organisms. Bacteria that can grow in artificial culture media are classified and identified using a range of characteristics (Box 6.2); examples are shown in Figures 6.3 and 6.4.

Eukaryotes: fungi, protozoa and helminths

Eukaryotic cells contain membrane-bound organelles, including nuclei, mitochondria and Golgi apparatus. Pathogenic eukaryotes are unicellular (e.g. yeasts, protozoa) or complex multicellular organisms (e.g. nematodes, trematodes and cestodes).

6.2 How bacteria are identified

Gram stain reaction (see Fig. 6.3)

• Gram-positive (thick peptidoglycan layer), Gram-negative (thin peptidoglycan) or unstainable

Microscopic morphology

• Cocci (round cells) or bacilli (elongated cells)
• Presence or absence of capsule

Cell association

• Association in clusters, chains or pairs

Colonial characteristics

• Colony size, shape or colour
• Effect on culture media (e.g. β-haemolysis of blood agar in haemolytic streptococci; see Fig. 6.4)

Atmospheric requirements

• Strictly aerobic (requires O_2), strictly anaerobic (requires absence of O_2), facultatively aerobic (grows with or without O_2) or micro-aerophilic (requires reduced O_2)

Biochemical reactions

• Expression of enzymes (oxidase, catalase, coagulase)
• Ability to ferment or hydrolyse various biochemical substrates

Motility

• Motile or non-motile

Antibiotic susceptibility

• Identifies organisms with invariable susceptibility (e.g. to optochin in *Streptococcus pneumoniae* or metronidazole in obligate anaerobes)

Matrix-assisted laser desorption/ionisation time-of-flight mass spectrometry (MALDI-TOF-MS)

• A rapid technique that identifies bacteria and some fungi from their specific molecular composition

Sequencing bacterial 16S ribosomal RNA gene

• A highly specific test for identification of organisms in pure culture and in samples from normally sterile sites

Whole-genome sequencing

• Although not yet in routine use, whole-genome sequencing (WGS) offers the potential to provide rapid and simultaneous identification, sensitivity testing and typing of organisms from pure culture and/or directly from clinical samples. As such, WGS is likely to replace many of the technologies described above over the next few years

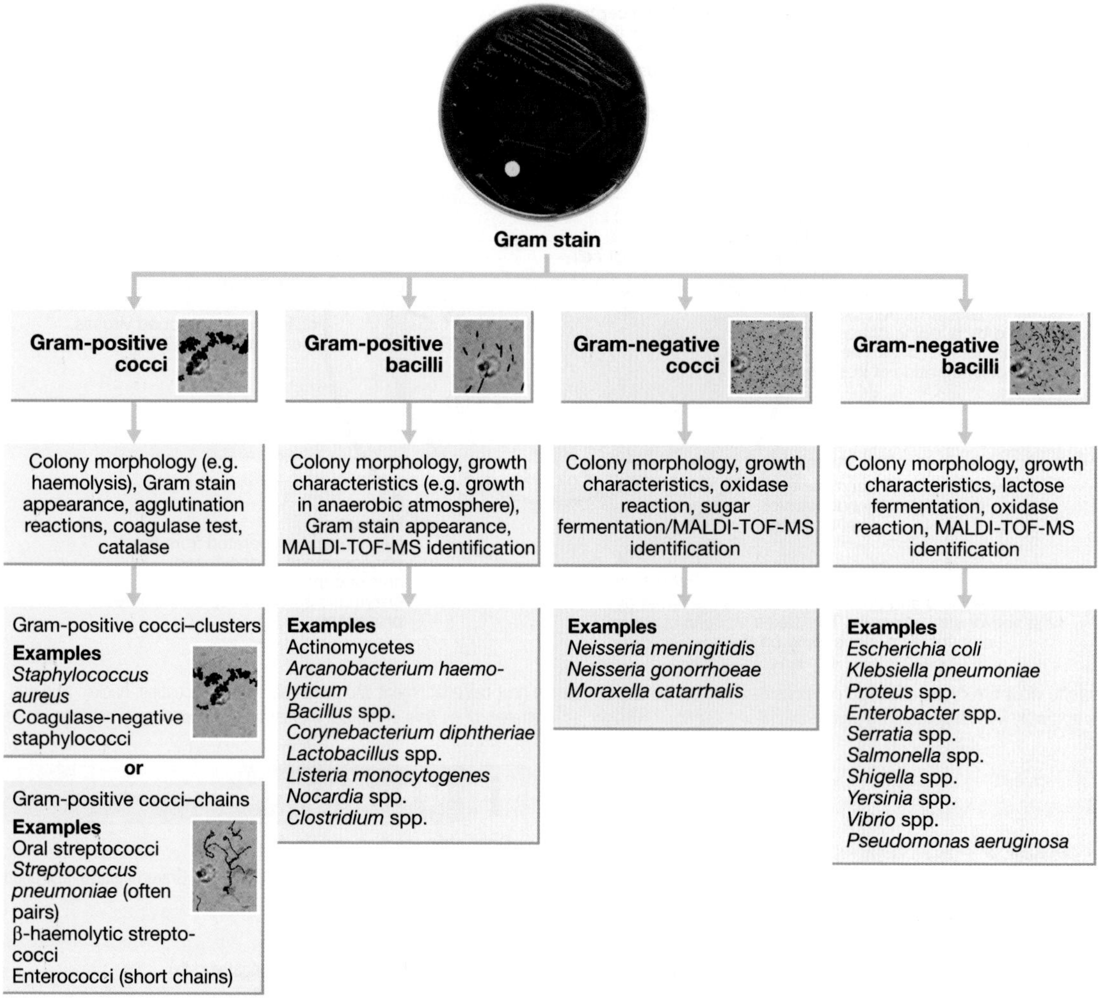

Gram stain

Gram-positive cocci	Gram-positive bacilli	Gram-negative cocci	Gram-negative bacilli
Colony morphology (e.g. haemolysis), Gram stain appearance, agglutination reactions, coagulase test, catalase	Colony morphology, growth characteristics (e.g. growth in anaerobic atmosphere), Gram stain appearance, MALDI-TOF-MS identification	Colony morphology, growth characteristics, oxidase reaction, sugar fermentation/MALDI-TOF-MS identification	Colony morphology, growth characteristics, lactose fermentation, oxidase reaction, MALDI-TOF-MS identification

Gram-positive cocci–clusters

Examples
Staphylococcus aureus
Coagulase-negative staphylococci

or

Gram-positive cocci–chains

Examples
Oral streptococci
Streptococcus pneumoniae (often pairs)
β-haemolytic streptococci
Enterococci (short chains)

Examples
Actinomycetes
Arcanobacterium haemolyticum
Bacillus spp.
Corynebacterium diphtheriae
Lactobacillus spp.
Listeria monocytogenes
Nocardia spp.
Clostridium spp.

Examples
Neisseria meningitidis
Neisseria gonorrhoeae
Moraxella catarrhalis

Examples
Escherichia coli
Klebsiella pneumoniae
Proteus spp.
Enterobacter spp.
Serratia spp.
Salmonella spp.
Shigella spp.
Yersinia spp.
Vibrio spp.
Pseudomonas aeruginosa

Fig. 6.3 Flow chart for bacterial identification, including Gram film appearances on light microscopy (×100). (MALDI-TOF-MS = matrix-assisted laser desorption/ionisation time-of-flight mass spectroscopy).

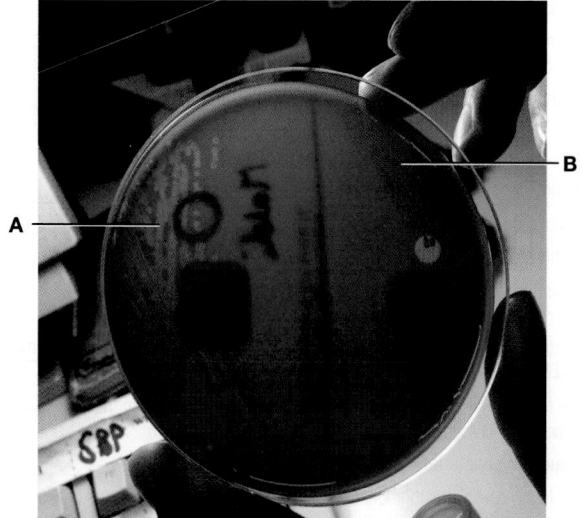

Fig. 6.4 β-haemolytic streptococci (A) and α-haemolytic streptococci (B) spread on each half of a blood agar plate (backlit). This image is half life-size. × 0.5. ß-haemolysis renders the agar transparent around the colonies (A) and α-haemolysis imparts a green tinge to the agar (B).

Fungi exist as either moulds (filamentous fungi) or yeasts. Dimorphic fungi exist in either form, depending on environmental conditions (see Fig. 13.62). The fungal plasma membrane differs from the human cell membrane in that it contains the sterol, ergosterol. Fungi have a cell wall made up of polysaccharides, chitin and mannoproteins. In most fungi, the main structural component of the cell wall is β-1,3-D-glucan, a polysaccharide. These differences from mammalian cells are important because they offer useful therapeutic targets.

Protozoa and helminths are often referred to as parasites. Many parasites have complex multistage life cycles, which involve animal and/or plant hosts in addition to humans.

Prions

Although prions are transmissible and have some of the characteristics of infectious agents, they are not microorganisms, and are discussed on page 1181.

Normal microbial flora

The human body is colonised by large numbers of microorganisms (collectively termed the human microbiota). Colonising bacteria, also referred to as the 'normal bacterial flora', are able to survive and replicate on epithelial

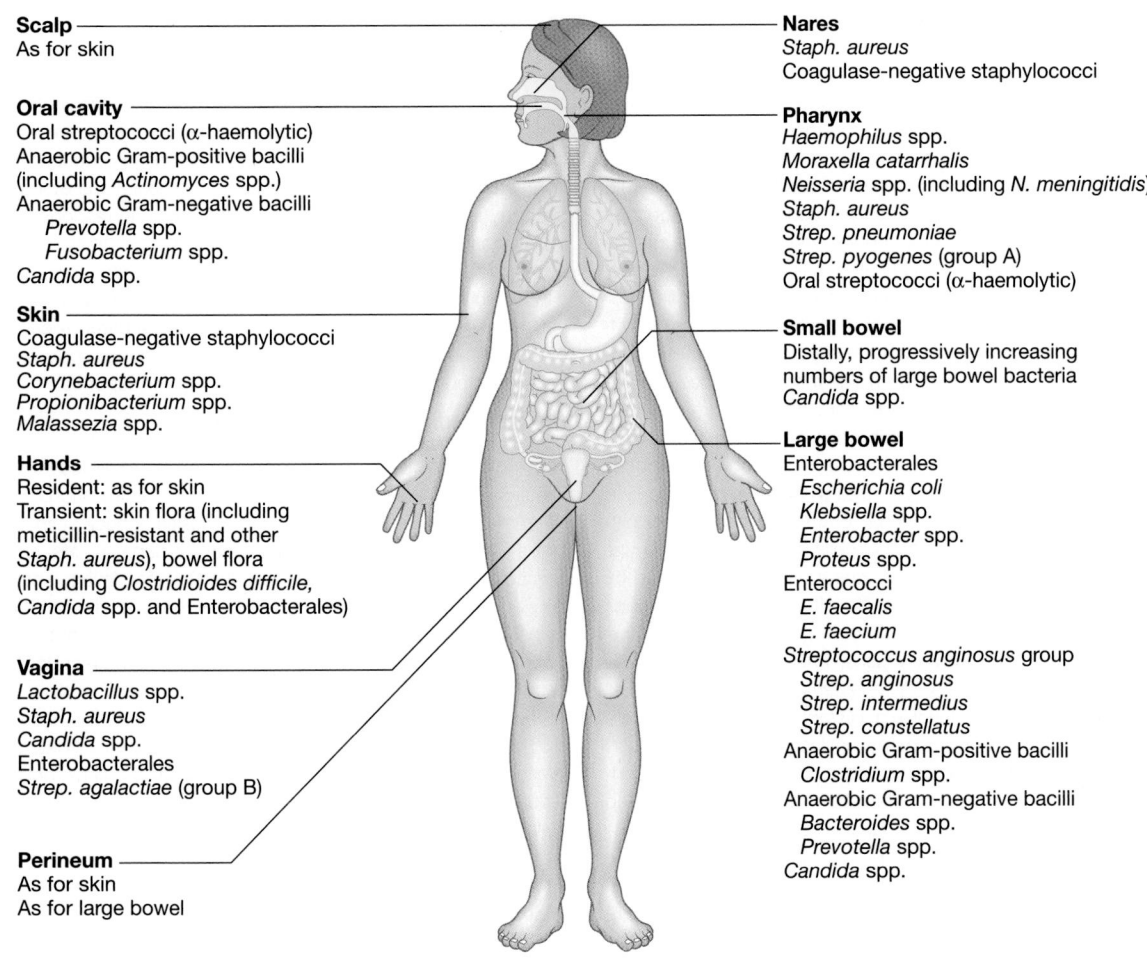

Scalp
As for skin

Oral cavity
Oral streptococci (α-haemolytic)
Anaerobic Gram-positive bacilli
(including *Actinomyces* spp.)
Anaerobic Gram-negative bacilli
    Prevotella spp.
    Fusobacterium spp.
Candida spp.

Skin
Coagulase-negative staphylococci
Staph. aureus
Corynebacterium spp.
Propionibacterium spp.
Malassezia spp.

Hands
Resident: as for skin
Transient: skin flora (including
meticillin-resistant and other
Staph. aureus), bowel flora
(including *Clostridioides difficile*,
Candida spp. and Enterobacterales)

Vagina
Lactobacillus spp.
Staph. aureus
Candida spp.
Enterobacterales
Strep. agalactiae (group B)

Perineum
As for skin
As for large bowel

Nares
Staph. aureus
Coagulase-negative staphylococci

Pharynx
Haemophilus spp.
Moraxella catarrhalis
Neisseria spp. (including *N. meningitidis*)
Staph. aureus
Strep. pneumoniae
Strep. pyogenes (group A)
Oral streptococci (α-haemolytic)

Small bowel
Distally, progressively increasing
numbers of large bowel bacteria
Candida spp.

Large bowel
Enterobacterales
    Escherichia coli
    Klebsiella spp.
    Enterobacter spp.
    Proteus spp.
Enterococci
    E. faecalis
    E. faecium
Streptococcus anginosus group
    Strep. anginosus
    Strep. intermedius
    Strep. constellatus
Anaerobic Gram-positive bacilli
    Clostridium spp.
Anaerobic Gram-negative bacilli
    Bacteroides spp.
    Prevotella spp.
Candida spp.

Fig. 6.5 Human non-sterile sites and normal flora in health.

surfaces, e.g. skin and mucosal surfaces. The gastrointestinal tract and the mouth are the two most heavily colonised sites in the body and they have distinct microbiota, in both composition and function. Knowledge of non-sterile body sites and their normal bacterial flora is required to inform microbiological sampling strategies and interpret culture results (Fig. 6.5).

The microbiota is the total burden of microorganisms, their genes and their environmental interactions, and is now recognised to have a profound influence on human health and disease. Maintenance of the normal flora is beneficial to normal immune function. Other functions include: lower gastrointestinal tract bacteria synthesise and excrete vitamins (e.g. vitamins K and B$_{12}$); colonisation with normal flora confers 'colonisation resistance' to infection with pathogenic organisms by altering the local environment (e.g. lowering pH), producing antibacterial agents (e.g. bacteriocins (small antimicrobial peptides/proteins), fatty acids and metabolic waste products), and inducing host antibodies that cross-react with pathogenic organisms.

Conversely, some body sites are either sterile or contain very low numbers of colonising bacteria. For example, the submucosal tissues, blood stream, peritoneal and pleural cavities are maintained as sterile by physical separation from the external environment; and the lower airways and bladder, sites that were formerly believed to be sterile but are now known to support limited microbiota, are protected from excessive contamination by the mucociliary escalator and urethral sphincter respectively, as well as local immune responses.

Members of the normal flora can cause (endogenous) infection by 'translocation' from their normal habitat to other body sites or by excessive growth at the 'normal' site (overgrowth). Overgrowth is exemplified by dental caries and 'blind loop' syndrome (p. 821). Translocation results from spread along a surface or penetration through a colonised surface, e.g. urinary tract infection caused by perineal/enteric flora, and surgical

site infections, particularly of prosthetic materials, caused by skin flora such as staphylococci. Normal flora also contribute to disease by cross-infection; organisms colonising one individual can cause disease when transferred to another, more susceptible, individual.

The importance of limiting antimicrobial-induced perturbations of microbiota is increasingly recognised. 'Probiotics' are proprietary microbes or mixtures of microbes administered with the aim of restoring a beneficial profile of gastrointestinal normal flora. Faecal microflora transplantation (FMT) has the same aim, by giving gastrointestinal microbiota from healthy people (filtered extract of faeces) to a patient. Although the clinical effectiveness of probiotics remains a subject of debate, FMT has proven benefit in recurrent *C. difficile* infection.

Host–pathogen interactions

A 'pathogen' is a microorganism that can cause infection. The manifestations of infection, including a pathogen's ability to cause severe disease in a previously healthy host, are affected by its 'virulence'. Virulence is determined by the number and type of disease-causing proteins and other factors that it can produce ('virulence factors').

- *Primary pathogens* cause disease in a proportion of individuals to whom they are exposed, regardless of the host's immunological status.
- *Opportunistic pathogens* cause disease only in individuals whose host defences are compromised, e.g. by an intravascular catheter, or when the immune system is compromised, by genetic susceptibility or immunosuppressive therapy.

Determinants of virulence

For a primary pathogen to cause infection in a healthy host it must compete with colonising flora to reach target host cells. It can do this in various ways, including sequestration of nutrients, adapting metabolism to exploit metabolites not used by commensal flora, production of bacteriocins, and using motility to 'swim' to the site of infection. Many microorganisms, including viruses, use 'adhesins' to initiate their attachment to host cells. Some pathogens can invade through tissues. Many bacteria and fungi multiply after initial adhesion to a host surface to form 'biofilms'. These are complex three-dimensional structures surrounded by a matrix of host and bacterial products, which afford protection to the colony and limit the effectiveness of antimicrobials. Biofilm-related infections on man-made medical devices such as vascular catheters or grafts can be particularly difficult to treat.

Pathogens may produce toxins, microbial molecules that cause adverse effects on host cells, either at the site of infection, or remotely following carriage through the blood stream. Endotoxin is the lipid component of Gram-negative bacterial outer membrane lipopolysaccharide. It is released when bacterial cells are damaged and has generalised inflammatory effects. Exotoxins are proteins released by living bacteria, which often have specific effects on target organs (Box 6.3).

Intracellular pathogens, including viruses, bacteria (e.g. *Salmonella* spp., *Listeria monocytogenes* and *Mycobacterium tuberculosis*), parasites (e.g. *Leishmania* spp.) and fungi (e.g. *Histoplasma capsulatum*), are able to survive in intracellular environments, including after phagocytosis by macrophages. Pathogenic bacteria express different genes, depending on environmental stress (pH, iron starvation, O_2 starvation etc.) and anatomical location.

Genetic diversity enhances the pathogenic capacity of bacteria. Some virulence factor genes are found on plasmids or in phages and are exchanged between different strains or species. The ability to acquire genes from the gene pool of all strains of the species increases diversity and the potential for pathogenicity. Viruses exploit their rapid reproduction and potential to exchange nucleic acid with other strains of the virus to enhance diversity. Once a new strain acquires sufficient virulence genes, including those enhancing infectivity, it may become an epidemic or pandemic strain, resulting in regional or global transmission, respectively. This phenomenon accounts for influenza and COVID-19 pandemics (see Box 6.10 and Ch. 13).

The host response

Innate and adaptive immune and inflammatory responses, which humans use to control the normal flora and respond to pathogens, are reviewed in Chapter 4.

i	6.3 Exotoxin-mediated bacterial diseases	
Disease	**Organism**
Antibiotic-associated diarrhoea/pseudomembranous colitis	*Clostridioides difficile*
Botulism	*Clostridium botulinum*
Cholera	*Vibrio cholerae*
Diphtheria	*Corynebacterium diphtheriae*
Haemolytic uraemic syndrome	Enterohaemorrhagic *Escherichia coli* (*E. coli* 0157 and other strains)
Necrotising pneumonia	*Staphylococcus aureus*
Tetanus	*Clostridium tetani*
Toxic shock syndrome	*Staph. aureus* *Streptococcus pyogenes*

Pathogenesis of infectious disease

The severity of an infection is determined by the virulence of the pathogen and the host response. Whilst an intact host response protects against infection or reduces its severity, an excessive response can be damaging. Both the host immune response and pathogen-produced factors can contribute to tissue injury and systemic manifestations of infection (see 'Sepsis', p. 198). The contribution of the immune response to disease manifestations is exemplified by the immune reconstitution inflammatory syndrome (IRIS), which can be seen in human immunodeficiency virus (HIV) infection, post-transplantation neutropenia or tuberculosis (which causes suppression of T-cell function): there is a paradoxical worsening of the clinical condition as the immune dysfunction is corrected, caused by an exuberant but dysregulated inflammatory response.

Clinical manifestations of infection

The clinical manifestations of infection can be localised to the site of infection or generalised. Examples of local manifestations include the inflammation of cellulitis, facial pain of sinusitis or neck stiffness of meningitis (Ch. 13). Generalised manifestations include sweats, chills (feeling very cold, even with extra clothes/blankets), rigors, fevers, anorexia, lethargy and generalised aches, and many of these result from the immune response to infection. While the presence of infection may be clinically clear in some settings, often it is not. Identifying the responsible pathogen in patients with infection is usually not possible on clinical grounds, neither is prediction of pathogen susceptibility and resistance to antimicrobial agents. Hence there is a need to carefully investigate suspected infections to optimise, or avoid unnecessary, antimicrobial therapy. Rigors are a clinical symptom (or sign if they are witnessed) characterised by feeling very cold ('chills') and uncontrollable shivering, usually followed by fever and sweating. Rigors occur when the thermoregulatory centre attempts to correct a core temperature to a higher level by stimulating skeletal muscle activity and shaking.

Thermoregulation can be altered during infection, causing both hyperthermia (fever) and hypothermia. Fever is mediated mainly by 'pyrogenic cytokines' (e.g. interleukins IL-1 and IL-6, and tumour necrosis factor (TNF)), which are released in response to various stimuli. including activation of pattern recognition receptors (PRRs) by microbial products (e.g. lipopolysaccharide) and factors released by injured cells (Ch. 4). This induces prostaglandin E_2 production, which binds to specific receptors in the preoptic nucleus of the hypothalamus (thermoregulatory centre), causing the core temperature to rise.

Investigation of infection

The aims of investigating a patient with suspected infection are: to confirm the presence of infection; identify the specific pathogen(s); and, where appropriate, identify its susceptibility to specific antimicrobial agents in order to optimise therapy. Pathogens may be detected directly (e.g. by culturing a normally sterile body site) or their presence may be inferred by identifying the host response to the organism ('indirect detection', Box 6.4), e.g. C-reactive protein or procalcitonin as part of the acute phase response (p. 68), although these are activated to varying extents by other inflammatory stimuli. Careful sampling increases the likelihood of diagnosis (Box 6.5). Culture results must be interpreted in the context of the normal flora at the sampled site (see Fig. 6.5). The extent to which a microbiological test result supports or excludes a particular diagnosis depends on its statistical performance (e.g. sensitivity, specificity, positive and negative predictive value). Sensitivity and specificity vary according to the type of test, sampling and processing techniques, and time between infection and testing. Positive and negative predictive values depend on the prevalence of the condition in the test population. The complexity of test interpretation is illustrated in Figure 6.8 below, which shows the 'windows of opportunity' afforded by various testing methods. Given this complexity, coordinated thought and action ensures appropriate test application and timing; effective communication between clinicians and the microbiologists facilitates optimal results and interpretation.

6.4 Tests used to diagnose infection

Non-specific markers of inflammation/infection

- e.g. White cell count in blood sample (WCC), plasma C-reactive protein (CRP), procalcitonin (PCT)*, serum lactate, cell counts in urine or cerebrospinal fluid (CSF), CSF protein and glucose

Direct detection of organisms or organism components

- Microscopy
- Detection of organism components (e.g. antigen, toxin)
- Nucleic acid amplification tests (e.g. polymerase chain reaction)

Culture of organisms

- ± Antimicrobial susceptibility testing

Tests of the host's specific immune response

- Antibody detection
- Interferon-gamma release assays (IGRA)

*Although PCT is used increasingly in clinical practice, further evidence is required to establish its precise role in distinguishing bacterial infections from other causes of inflammation.

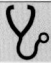

6.5 How to provide samples for microbiological sampling

Communicate with the laboratory

- Discuss samples that require processing urgently or that may contain hazardous or unusual pathogens with laboratory staff *before* collection
- Communication is key to optimising microbiological diagnosis. If there is doubt about any aspect of sampling, it is far better to discuss it with laboratory staff beforehand than to risk diagnostic delay by inappropriate sampling or sample handling

Take samples based on a clinical diagnosis

- Sampling in the absence of clinical evidence of infection is rarely appropriate (e.g. collecting urine, or sputum for culture)

Use the correct container

- Certain tests (e.g. nucleic acid and antigen detection tests) require proprietary sample collection equipment

Follow sample collection procedures

- Failure to follow sample collection instructions precisely can result in false-positive (e.g. contamination of blood culture samples) or false-negative (e.g. collection of insufficient blood for culture) results

Label sample and request form correctly

- Label sample containers and request forms according to local policies, with demographic identifiers, specimen type and time/date collected
- Include clinical details on request forms
- Identify samples carrying a high risk of infection (e.g. blood liable to contain a blood-borne virus) with a hazard label

Use appropriate packaging

- Close sample containers tightly and package securely (usually in sealed plastic bags)
- Attach request forms to samples but not in the same compartment (to avoid contamination, should leakage occur)

Manage storage and transport

- Transport samples to the microbiology laboratory quickly
- Consider pre-transport storage, conditions (e.g. refrigeration, incubation, storage at room temperature) vary with sample type
- Notify the receiving laboratory prior to arrival of unusual or urgent samples, to ensure timely processing

Direct detection of pathogens

Some direct detection methods provide rapid results and enable detection of organisms that cannot be grown easily on artificial culture media, such as *Chlamydia* spp.; they can also provide information on antimicrobial susceptibility, e.g. *M. tuberculosis*.

Detection of whole organisms

Whole organisms are detected by examination of biological fluids or tissue using a microscope.

- *Bright field microscopy* (in which the test sample is interposed between the light source and the objective lens) uses stains to enhance visual contrast between the organism and its background. Examples include Gram staining of bacteria and Ziehl–Neelsen or auramine staining of acid- and alcohol-fast bacilli (AAFB) in tuberculosis (the latter requires an ultraviolet light source). In histopathological examination of tissue samples, stains are used to demonstrate not only the presence of microorganisms but also features of disease pathology.
- *Dark field microscopy* (in which light is scattered to make organisms appear bright on a dark background) is used, for example, to examine genital chancre fluid in suspected syphilis.
- *Electron microscopy* may be used to examine stool and vesicle fluid to detect enteric and herpesviruses, respectively, but its use has largely been supplanted by nucleic acid detection (see below).
- *Flow cytometry* can be used to analyse liquid samples (e.g. urine) for the presence of particles based on properties such as size, impedance and light scatter. This technique can detect bacteria but may misidentify other particles as bacteria too.

Detection of components of organisms

Components of microorganisms detected for diagnostic purposes include nucleic acids, cell wall molecules, toxins and other antigens. Commonly used examples include SARS-CoV-2 antigen in respiratory secretions, *Legionella pneumophila* serogroup 1 antigen in urine and cryptococcal polysaccharide antigen in cerebrospinal fluid (CSF). Most antigen detection methods are based on in vitro binding of specific antigen/antibody and are therefore described with serological tests below. Other methods may be used, such as tissue culture cytotoxicity assay for *C. difficile* toxin. In toxin-mediated disease, detection of toxin may be of greater relevance than identification of the organism itself (e.g. stool *C. difficile* toxin).

Nucleic acid amplification tests

In a nucleic acid amplification test (NAAT), specific sequences of microbial DNA or RNA are identified using a nucleic acid primer that is amplified exponentially by enzymes to generate multiple copies of a target nucleotide sequence. The most commonly used NAAT is the polymerase chain reaction (PCR; see Fig. 3.11). Reverse transcription PCR (RT-PCR) is used to detect RNA from RNA viruses. The use of fluorescent labels in the reaction enables 'real-time' detection of amplified DNA; quantification is based on the principle that the time taken to reach the detection threshold is proportional to the initial number of copies of the target nucleic acid sequence. In 'broad range' (bacterial) PCR the primers are targeted to parts of the gene that encode 16S ribosomal RNA (rRNA) that have shared DNA sequences across most bacteria. Between these shared DNA sequences, the 16S rRNA gene varies between species; so, using PCR, nucleotide sequencing of the product and comparison of the DNA sequence information with large databases, bacterial detection and species identification can be achieved. In multiplex PCR, multiple primer pairs are used to enable detection of several different organisms in a single reaction.

Determination of nucleotide sequences in a target gene(s) can be used to assign microorganisms to specific strains, which may be relevant to treatment and/or prognosis (e.g. in hepatitis C infection). Genes that are relevant to virulence (such as toxin genes) or antimicrobial resistance can also be detected; for example, the *mecA* gene can be used to screen for MRSA.

NAATs are the most sensitive direct detection methods and are also relatively rapid. They are used widely in virology, where the possibility of false-positive results from colonising or contaminating organisms is remote, and are applied to blood, respiratory samples, stool and urine. In bacteriology, PCR is used to examine CSF, blood, tissue and genital samples, and multiplex PCR is being developed for use in faeces. PCR is particularly helpful for microorganisms that cannot be readily cultured, e.g. *Tropheryma whipplei*, and is being used increasingly in mycology and parasitology.

Culture

Microorganisms may be both detected and further characterised by culture from clinical samples (e.g. tissue, swabs and body fluids).

- *Ex vivo culture* (tissue or cell culture) was widely used in the isolation of viruses but has been largely supplanted by NAATs.
- *In vitro culture* (in artificial culture media) of bacteria and fungi is used to confirm the presence of pathogens, allow identification, test antimicrobial susceptibility and subtype the organism for epidemiological purposes.

Culture has its limitations: results are not immediate, even for organisms that are easy to grow, and negative cultures rarely exclude infection. Organisms such as *M. tuberculosis* are slow-growing, typically taking at least 2 weeks, even in rapid-culture systems. Certain organisms, such as *Mycobacterium leprae* and *Tropheryma whipplei*, cannot be cultivated on artificial media, and others (e.g. *Chlamydia* spp. and viruses) grow only in culture systems, which are slow and labour-intensive.

Blood culture

The terms 'bacteraemia' and 'fungaemia' describe the presence of bacteria and fungi in the blood without implication of clinical significance, while the term 'blood stream infection' means bacteraemia or fungaemia are present together with symptoms or signs infection; this is discussed on p. 270. Bacteraemia/fungaemia is identified by inoculating a liquid culture medium with freshly drawn blood, which is then incubated in a system that monitors it constantly for growth of microorganisms (e.g. by detecting products of microbial respiration using fluorescence; Fig. 6.6). If growth is detected, organisms are identified and sensitivity testing is performed. Traditionally, identification has been achieved by Gram stain appearance and biochemical reactions. However, matrix-assisted laser desorption/ionisation time-of-flight mass spectroscopy (MALDI-TOF-MS; see Box 6.2) is being used increasingly to identify organisms. MALDI-TOF-MS produces a profile of proteins of different sizes from the target microorganism and uses databases of such

---

1 Patient sampling
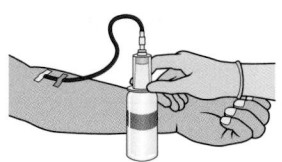
Contamination minimised by aseptic technique. Maximise sensitivity by sampling correct volume

2 Sample handling
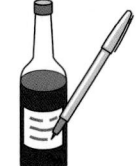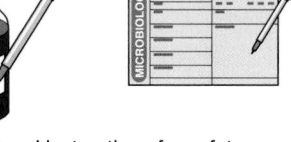
Follow local instructions for safety, labelling, and numbers of samples and bottles required

3 Specimen transport
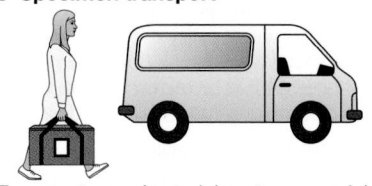
Transport samples to laboratory as quickly as possible. Follow manufacturer's instructions for the blood culture system used if temporary storage is required

4 Incubation
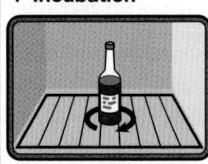
Incubate at 35–37°C for 5–7 days. Microbial growth is usually detected by constant automatic monitoring of CO_2. **If no growth, specimen is negative and discarded**

5 Growth detection
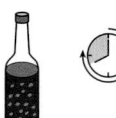
Time to positivity (TTP) is usually 12–24 hrs in significant bacteraemia, but may be shorter in overwhelming sepsis or longer with fastidious organisms (e.g. *Brucella* spp.)

6 Preliminary results*
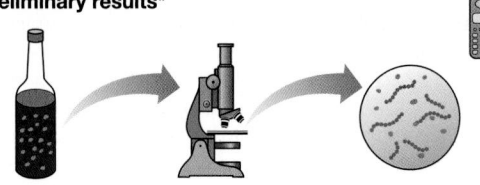
A Gram film of the blood culture medium is examined and **results are communicated immediately to the clinician** to guide antibiotic therapy

7 Incubation
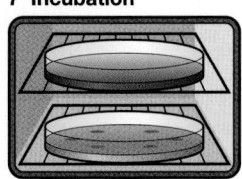
A small amount of the medium is incubated on a range of culture media. Preliminary susceptibility testing may be carried out

8 Culture results*
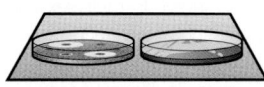
Preliminary susceptibility results are communicated to the clinician

9 Definitive results
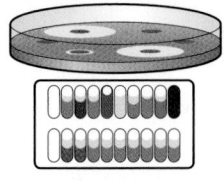
Further overnight incubation is often required for definitive identification of organisms (by biochemical testing) and additional susceptibility testing; identification by MALDI-TOF-MS (Fig. 6.7) is more rapid

10 Reporting
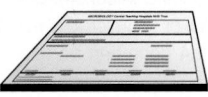
A final summary is released when all testing is complete. For clinical care, communication of interim results (Gram film, preliminary identification and susceptibility) is usually more important than the final report. **Effective clinical–laboratory communication is vital**

 Overnight incubation required

 Urgent communication required

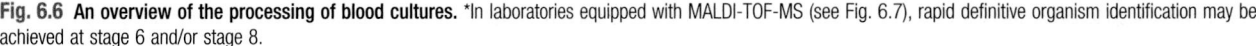

Fig. 6.6 An overview of the processing of blood cultures. *In laboratories equipped with MALDI-TOF-MS (see Fig. 6.7), rapid definitive organism identification may be achieved at stage 6 and/or stage 8.

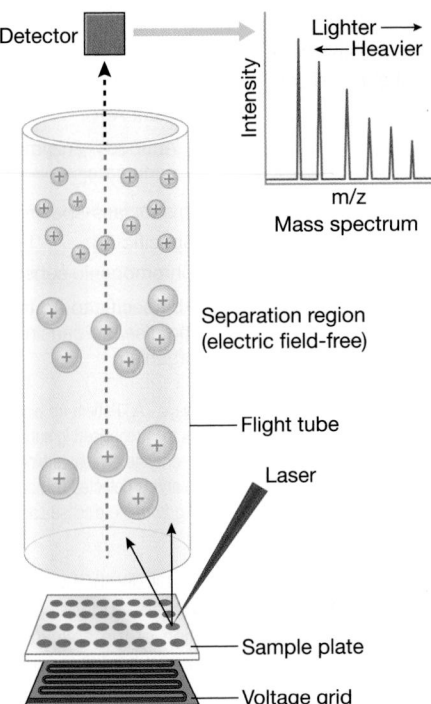

Fig. 6.7 The workings of matrix-assisted laser desorption/ionisation time-of-flight mass spectrometry (MALDI-TOF MS). *Adapted from Sobin K, Hameer D, Ruparel T. Digital genotyping using molecular affinity and mass spectrometry. Nature Rev Genet 2003; 4:1001–1008.*

profiles to identify the organism (Fig. 6.7). It is rapid and accurate. Taking multiple blood samples for culture at different times allows differentiation of transient (one positive sample) and persistent (majority are positive) bacteraemia. This can be clinically important in identifying the source of infection.

Indirect detection of pathogens

Tests may be used to detect the host's immune (antibody) response to a specific microorganism, and can enable the diagnosis of infection with organisms that are difficult to detect by other methods or are no longer present in the host. The term 'serology' describes tests carried out on serum and includes both antigen (direct) and antibody (indirect) detection. Antigen detection tests used on other fluids (e.g. CSF and respiratory secretions) are also described in this section, as they largely share the same methodology as serological tests.

Antibody detection

Organism-specific antibody detection is applied mainly to blood (Fig. 6.8). Results are typically expressed as titres: that is, the reciprocal of the highest dilution of the serum at which antibody is detectable (e.g. detection at serum dilution of 1:64 gives a titre of 64). 'Seroconversion' is defined as either a change from negative to positive detection or a fourfold rise in titre between acute and convalescent serum samples. An acute sample is usually taken during the first week of disease and the convalescent sample 2–4 weeks later. Earlier diagnosis can be achieved by detection of immunoglobulin M (IgM) antibodies, which are produced early in infection. A limitation of these tests is that antibody production requires a fully functional host immune system, so there may be false-negative results in immunocompromised patients. Also, other than in chronic infections and with IgM detection, antibody tests usually provide a retrospective diagnosis. False-positive results can occur when there is cross-reactivity of the test reagents with other molecules or when patients have been given blood products containing other people's antibodies. Serological testing methods are described below.

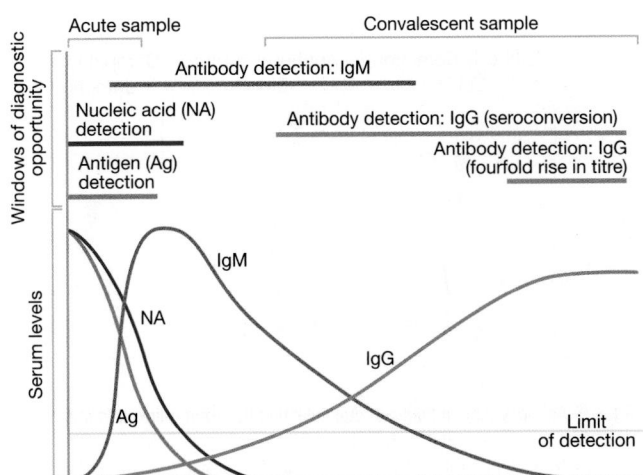

Fig. 6.8 Detection of antigen, nucleic acid and antibody in infectious disease. The acute sample is usually taken during the first week of illness, and the convalescent sample 2–4 weeks later. Detection limits and duration of detectability vary between tests and diseases, although in most diseases immunoglobulin M (IgM) is detectable within the first 1–2 weeks.

Enzyme-linked immunosorbent assay

The principles of the enzyme-linked immunosorbent assay (ELISA, EIA) are illustrated in Figure 6.9. These assays rely on linking an antibody with an enzyme that generates a colour change on exposure to a chromogenic substrate. Various configurations allow detection of antigens or specific subclasses of immunoglobulin (e.g. IgG, IgM, IgA). ELISA may also be adapted to detect PCR products, using immobilised oligonucleotide hybridisation probes and various detection systems.

Immunoblot (Western blot)

Microbial proteins are separated according to molecular weight by polyacrylamide gel electrophoresis (PAGE) and transferred (blotted) on to a nitrocellulose membrane, which is incubated with patient serum. Binding of specific antibody is detected with an enzyme–anti-immunoglobulin conjugate similar to that used in ELISA, and specificity is confirmed by its location on the membrane. Immunoblotting is a highly specific test, which may be used to confirm the results of less specific tests such as ELISA (e.g. in Lyme disease).

Immunofluorescence assays

Indirect immunofluorescence assays (IFAs) detect antibodies by incubating a serum sample with immobilised antigen (e.g. virus-infected cells on a glass slide); any virus-specific antibody present in the serum binds to antigen and is then detected by fluorescence microscopy using a fluorescent-labelled anti-human immunoglobulin ('secondary' antibody). This method can also detect organisms in clinical samples (usually tissue or centrifuged cells) using a specific antibody in place of immobilised antigen to achieve capture.

Complement fixation test (CFT)

In a CFT, patient serum is heat-treated to inactivate complement and mixed with test antigen. Any specific antibody in the serum will complex with the antigen. Complement is then added to the reaction. If antigen–antibody complexes are present, the complement will be 'fixed' (consumed). Sheep erythrocytes, coated with an anti-erythrocyte antibody, are added. The degree of erythrocyte lysis reflects the remaining complement and is inversely proportional to the quantity of the specific antigen–antibody complex present.

Agglutination tests

When antigens are present on the surface of particles (e.g. cells, latex particles or microorganisms) and cross-linked with antibodies, visible clumping (or 'agglutination') occurs.

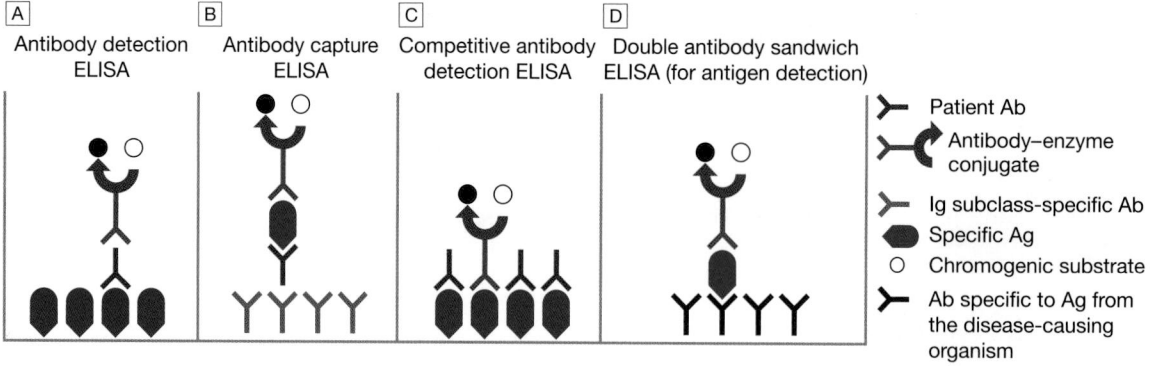

Fig. 6.9 Antibody (Ab) and antigen (Ag) detection by enzyme-linked immunosorbent assay (ELISA). This can be configured in various ways. [A] Patient Ab binds to immobilised specific Ag and is detected by addition of anti-immunoglobulin–enzyme conjugate and chromogenic substrate. [B] Patient Ab binds to immobilised Ig subclass-specific Ab and is detected by addition of specific Ag, followed by antibody–enzyme conjugate and chromogenic substrate. [C] Patient Ab and antibody–enzyme conjugate bind to immobilised specific Ag. Magnitude of colour change reaction is inversely proportional to concentration of patient Ab. [D] Patient Ag binds to immobilised Ab and is detected by addition of antibody–enzyme conjugate and chromogenic substrate. In A, the conjugate Ab is specific for human immunoglobulin. In B–D, it is specific for Ag from the disease-causing organism.

- In *direct agglutination*, patient serum is added to a suspension of organisms that express the test antigen. The Widal agglutination test uses a suspension of *Salmonella typhi* and *S. paratyphi* 'A' and 'B', treated to retain only 'O' and 'H' antigens. These antigens are kept to detect corresponding antibodies in serum from a patient suspected of having typhoid fever.
- In *indirect (passive) agglutination*, specific antigen is attached to the surface of carrier particles, which agglutinate when incubated with patient samples that contain specific antibodies.
- In *reverse passive agglutination* (an antigen detection test), the carrier particle is coated with antibody rather than antigen.

Immunodiffusion

Immunodiffusion involves antibodies and antigen migrating through gels and forming insoluble complexes where they meet. The complexes are seen on staining as 'precipitin bands'. Immunodiffusion is used in the diagnosis of dimorphic fungi and some forms of aspergillosis.

Lateral flow immunochromatography

Lateral flow (LF) immunochromatography is mainly used to detect antigens, and often in fluids other then blood (e.g. respiratory secretions, urine). The system consists of a porous test strip (e.g. a nitrocellulose membrane), at one end of which there is target-specific antibody, complexed with coloured microparticles. Further specific antibody is immobilised in a transverse narrow line some distance along the strip. Test material is added to the antibody–particle complexes, which then migrate along the strip by capillary action. If these are complexed with antigen, they will be immobilised by the specific antibody and visualised as a transverse line across the strip. If the test is negative, the antibody–particle complexes will bind to a line of immobilised anti-immunoglobulin antibody placed further along the strip, which acts as a negative control. Immunochromatographic tests are rapid and relatively cheap to perform, and are appropriate for point-of-care testing, e.g. in HIV-1, COVID-19 and malaria.

Antibody-independent specific immunological tests

Interferon-gamma release assays (IGRA) are used to diagnose latent tuberculosis infection. The principle behind IGRA is illustrated in Fig. 17.42. IGRA cannot distinguish between latent and active tuberculosis infection and is therefore appropriate for use only in regions where the background incidence of tuberculosis is low.

Antimicrobial susceptibility testing

If growth of microorganisms in culture is inhibited by the addition of an antimicrobial agent, the organism is considered to be susceptible to that antimicrobial. Bacteriostatic agents cause reversible inhibition of

replication and bactericidal agents cause cell death; the terms fungistatic/fungicidal are equivalent for antifungal agents, and virustatic/virucidal for antiviral agents. The lowest concentration of the antimicrobial agent at which growth is inhibited is the minimum inhibitory concentration (MIC), and the lowest concentration that causes cell death is the minimum bactericidal concentration (MBC). If the MIC is less than or equal to a predetermined breakpoint threshold, the organism is considered susceptible, and if the MIC is greater than the breakpoint, it is resistant. Breakpoints are determined for antimicrobial agents using a combination of pharmacokinetic and clinical data. The relationship between in vitro antimicrobial susceptibility and clinical response is complex, as response also depends on severity of illness, site of infection, pharmacokinetics, immune status, comorbidities and antibiotic dosing. Thus, although treating a patient according to the results of susceptibility testing increases the likelihood of recovery, it does not guarantee therapeutic success.

Susceptibility testing is often carried out by disc diffusion (Fig. 6.10). Antibiotic-impregnated filter paper discs are placed on agar plates containing bacteria; antibiotic diffuses into the agar, resulting in a concentration gradient centred on the disc. Bacteria are unable to grow where the antibiotic concentration exceeds the MIC, which may therefore be inferred from the size of the zone of inhibition. The MIC is commonly measured in diagnostic laboratories using 'diffusion strips'.

Epidemiology of infection

The communicability of many infections means that, once a clinician has diagnosed an infectious disease, potential exposure of other patients must also be considered. Measures to control spread may be required at a patient level (e.g. separation from other patients ('isolation')), at an organisation or institutional levels (e.g. in a nursing home (Ch. 5) or hospital) at a national level, or, in the case of a pandemic, at an international level. The approach will be specific to the microorganism involved (Chs. 11–13) but the principles are outlined below.

Geographical and temporal patterns of infection

Endemic disease

Endemic disease has a constant presence within a given geographical area or population. The infectious agent may have a reservoir, vector or intermediate host that is geographically restricted, or may itself have restrictive environmental requirements (e.g. temperature range, humidity). The population affected may be geographically isolated or the disease may be limited to unvaccinated populations. Factors that alter geographical restriction include:

- expansion of an animal reservoir (e.g. Lyme disease from reforestation)
- vector escape (e.g. airport malaria)

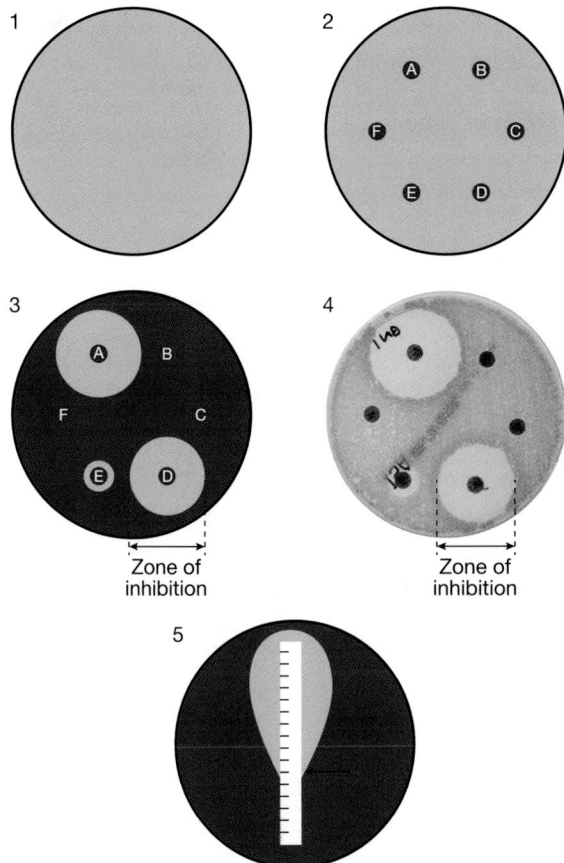

Fig. 6.10 Antimicrobial susceptibility testing by disc diffusion (panels 1–4) and minimum inhibitory concentration (MIC, panel 5). 1 The test organism is spread over the surface of an agar plate. **2** Antimicrobial-impregnated discs (A–F) are placed on the surface and the plate is incubated (e.g. overnight). **3–4** After incubation, zones of growth inhibition may be seen. The organism is considered susceptible if the diameter of the zone of inhibition exceeds a predetermined threshold. **5** In a 'diffusion strip' test, the strip is impregnated with antimicrobial at a concentration gradient that decreases steadily from top to bottom. The system is designed so that the MIC value is the point at which the ellipse cuts a scale on the strip (arrow). *(4) Kindly supplied by Charlotte Symes.*

- extension of host range (e.g. schistosomiasis from dam construction)
- importation of foods
- human migration (e.g. carbapenemase-producing *Klebsiella pneumoniae*)
- public health service breakdown (e.g. diphtheria in unvaccinated areas)
- climate change (e.g. dengue virus and Rift Valley fever).

Emerging and re-emerging disease

An emerging infectious disease is one that has newly appeared in a population, or has been known for some time but is increasing in incidence or geographical range. If the disease was previously known and thought to have been controlled or eradicated, it is considered to be re-emerging. Many emerging diseases are caused by organisms that infect animals and have undergone adaptations that enable them to infect humans. This is exemplified by HIV-1, which originated in higher primates in Africa, and SARS-CoV-2, from bats potentially via intermediate hosts. The geographical pattern of some recent emerging and re-emerging infections is shown in Figure 6.11.

Reservoirs of infection

The US Centers for Disease Control (CDC) define a reservoir of infection as any person, other living organism, environment or combination of these in which the infectious agent lives and replicates and on which the infectious agent is dependent for its survival. The infectious agent is transmitted from this reservoir to a susceptible host.

Human reservoirs

Both colonised and infected individuals can act as human reservoirs, and infected human reservoirs may be asymptomatic. The organism must be long-lasting in at least a proportion of those affected, to facilitate onward transmission. Infections in which humans act as reservoirs include tuberculosis, MRSA, HIV and COVID-19. For some infections (e.g. measles) humans are the only known reservoir.

Animal reservoirs

The World Health Organization (WHO) defines a zoonosis as 'a disease or infection that is naturally transmissible from vertebrate animals to

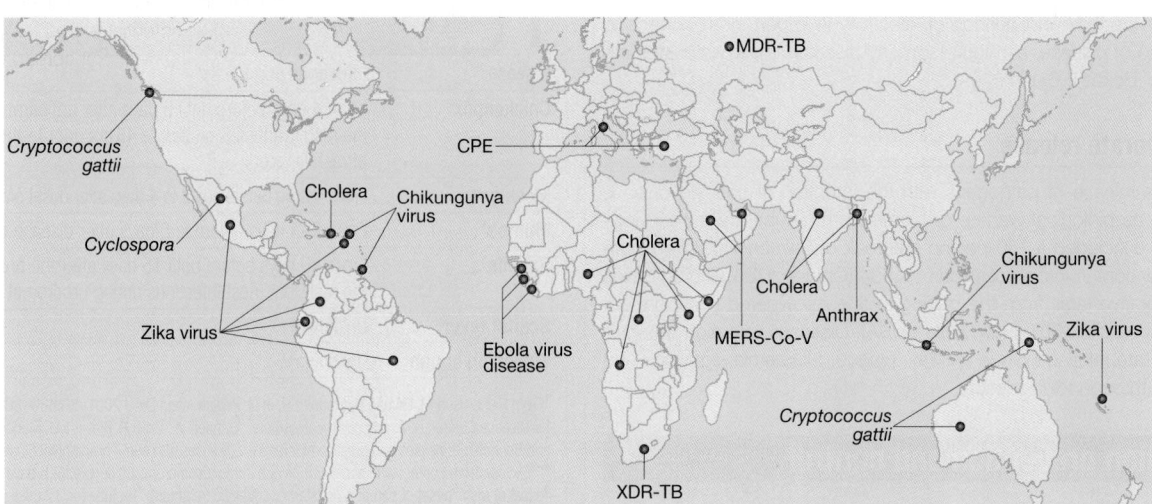

Fig. 6.11 Geographical locations of some infectious disease outbreaks, with examples of emerging and re-emerging diseases. (CPE = carbapenemase-producing *Enterobacterales*; MDR-TB = multidrug-resistant tuberculosis; MERS-Co-V = Middle East respiratory syndrome coronavirus; XDR-TB = extensively drug-resistant tuberculosis)

humans'. Infected animals may be asymptomatic. Zoonotic agents may be transmitted via any of the routes described below. Primary infection with zoonoses may be transmitted onward between humans, causing secondary disease (e.g. Q fever, brucellosis, Ebola virus disease).

Environmental reservoirs

Some pathogens are acquired from an environmental source (e.g. *Pseudomonas aeruginosa* from hospital water supplies). However, some of these are maintained in human or animal reservoirs, with the environment acting only as a conduit for infection.

Transmission of infection

Communicable diseases may be transmitted by one or more of the following routes:

- Respiratory route: airborne/droplet spread (see p. 293).
- Faecal–oral route: ingestion of material originating from faeces.
- Sexually transmitted infections: direct contact between mucous membranes.
- Blood-borne infections: direct inoculation of blood.
- Direct contact: very few organisms are capable of causing infection by direct contact with intact skin. Most infection by this route requires contact with damaged skin (e.g. surgical wound).
- Via a vector or fomite: the vector/fomite bridges the gap between the infected host or reservoir and the uninfected host. Vectors are animate, and include mosquitoes in malaria and dengue virus infection and humans in MRSA. Fomites are inanimate objects such as door handles, water taps and ultrasound probes, which are particularly associated with health care-associated infection (HCAI).

The basic reproduction number (R_0) is a measure of the propensity for a communicable disease to spread between people; it is the average number of people one person with an infection is likely to pass on infection to. R_0 is calculated by mathematical models that take into account infection rates, the period of infectivity (known or estimated), opportunities for transmission and susceptibility to infection. R_0 assumes everyone is susceptible, whereas 'effective R' (R_e) takes into account the development of herd immunity within the population (e.g. from infection or vaccination) and therefore varies with time. R_0 and R_e are calculated for whole populations, so will hide local variations in transmission.

The likelihood of infection following transmission of a pathogen depends on the virulence of the organism and the susceptibility of the host. The incubation period is the time between exposure and development of symptoms, and the period of infectivity is the period after exposure during which the patient is infectious to others. Knowledge of incubation periods and periods of infectivity is important in controlling the spread of disease, although for many diseases these estimates are imprecise (Boxes 6.6 and 6.7).

Deliberate release

Deliberate release of pathogens with the intention of causing disease is known as biological warfare or bioterrorism. Deliberate release incidents have included a 750-person outbreak of *Salmonella typhimurium* caused by contamination of salads in 1984 (Oregon, USA) and 22 cases of anthrax (five fatal) from the mailing of finely powdered (weaponised) anthrax spores in 2001 (New Jersey, USA). Diseases with high potential for deliberate release include anthrax, plague, tularaemia, smallpox and botulism (through toxin release).

Infection prevention and control

Infection prevention and control (IPC) describes the measures applied to populations with the aim of breaking the chain of infection (see Fig. 6.1).

---

i 6.6 Incubation periods of important infections[1]

Infection	Incubation period
Short incubation periods	
Anthrax, cutaneous[2]	9 hrs to 2 weeks
Anthrax, inhalational[2]	2 days[3]
Bacillary dysentery[4]	1–6 days
Cholera[2]	2 hrs to 5 days
Dengue haemorrhagic fever[5]	3–14 days
Diphtheria[5]	1–10 days
Gonorrhoea[6]	2–10 days
Influenza[4]	1–3 days
Meningococcaemia[2]	2–10 days
Norovirus	1–3 days
SARS[2]	2–7 days[3]
Scarlet fever[4]	2–4 days
Intermediate incubation periods	
Amoebiasis[5]	1–4 weeks
Brucellosis[6]	5–30 days
Chickenpox[4]	11–20 days
COVID-19 (SARS-CoV-2)	5–6 days[2]
Lassa fever[2]	3–21 days
Malaria[2]	10–15 days
Measles[4]	6–19 days
Mumps[4]	15–24 days
Poliomyelitis[5]	3–35 days
Psittacosis[6]	1–4 weeks
Rubella[4]	15–20 days
Typhoid[4]	5–31 days
Whooping cough[4]	5–21 days
Long incubation periods	
Hepatitis A[4]	3–7 weeks
Hepatitis B[6]	6 weeks to 6 months
Leishmaniasis, cutaneous[5]	Weeks to months
Leishmaniasis, visceral[5]	Months to years
Leprosy (Hansen's disease)[2]	5–20 years
Rabies[6]	3–12 weeks[3]
Trypanosoma brucei gambiense infection[5]	Months to years
Tuberculosis[4]	1–12 months

[1]Incubation periods are approximate and may differ from local or national guidance. [2]World Health Organization. [3]Longer incubation periods have been reported. [4]Richardson M, et al. Paediatr Infect Dis J 2001; 20:380–88. [5]Centers for Disease Control, USA. [6]Public Health England. (SARS = severe acute respiratory syndrome)

---

i 6.7 Periods of infectivity in common childhood infectious diseases

Disease	Infectious period
Chickenpox[1]	From 4 days before until 5 days after appearance of the rash (transmission before 48 hrs prior to the onset of rash is rare)[4]
Measles[2]	From 4 days before onset to 4 days after onset of the rash
Mumps[3]	From 2–3 days before to 5 days after disease onset[5]
Rubella[3]	From 10 days before until 15 days after the onset of the rash, but most infectious during prodromal illness[4]
Scarlet fever[1]	Unknown[6]
Whooping cough[1]	Unknown[6,7]

[1]From Richardson M, Elliman D, Maguire H, et al. Pediatr Infect Dis J 2001; 20:380–388. [2]Centers for Disease Control, USA; cdc.gov/measles/hcp/. [3]Bennett JE, Dolin R, Blaser MJ. Mandell, Douglas and Bennett's Principles and practice of infectious diseases, 8th edn. Philadelphia: Elsevier; 2015. [4–6]Exclude from contact with non-immune and immunocompromised people for 5 days from [4]onset of rash [5]onset of parotitis, or [6]start of antibiotic treatment. [7]Exclude for 3 weeks if untreated. Durations are approximate and vary between information sources, and these recommendations may differ from local or national guidance.

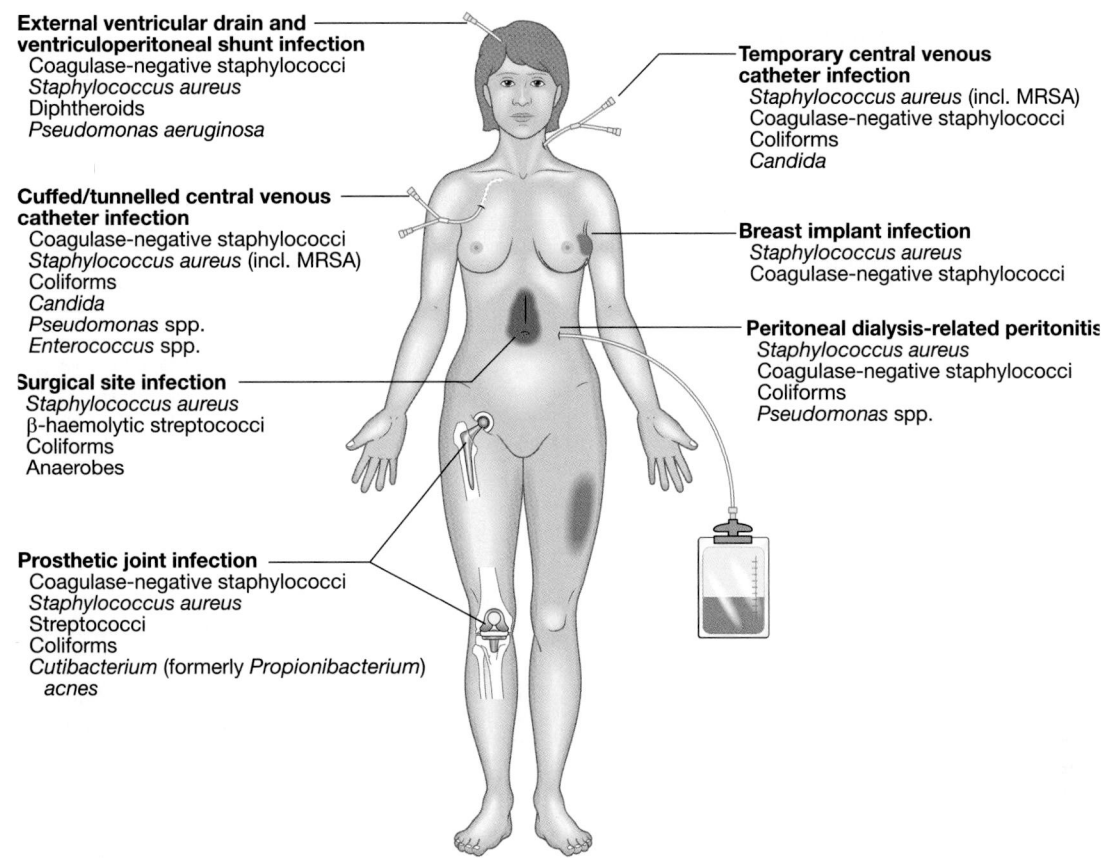

Fig. 6.12 Commonly encountered health care-associated infections (HCAIs) and the factors that predispose to them.

Health care-associated infection

The risk of developing infection following admission to a health-care facility (health care-associated infection, HCAI) in the developed world is about 10%. Many nosocomial bacterial infections are caused by organisms that are resistant to numerous antibiotics (multi-resistant bacteria), including MRSA, extended-spectrum β-lactamases (ESBLs) and carbapenemase-producing *Enterobacterales* (CPE), and glycopeptide-resistant enterococci (GRE). Other infections of particular concern in hospitals include *C. difficile* and norovirus. Some examples are shown in Figure 6.12.

IPC measures are described in Box 6.8. The most important is maintenance of good hand hygiene (Fig. 6.13). Hand decontamination (e.g. using alcohol gel or washing) is mandatory before and after every patient contact. Decontamination with alcohol gel is usually adequate but hand-washing (with hot water, liquid soap and complete drying) is required after any procedure that involves more than casual physical contact, or if hands are visibly soiled. In situations where the prevalence of *C. difficile* is high (e.g. a local outbreak), alcohol gel decontamination between patient contacts is inadequate as it does not kill *C. difficile* spores, and hands must be washed.

Some infections necessitate additional measures to prevent cross-infection (Box 6.9) and sometimes these are combined, e.g. both droplet and contact precautions in the case of SARS-CoV-2. To minimise risk of infection, invasive procedures must be performed using strict aseptic technique.

Outbreaks of infection

Descriptive terms for infectious disease outbreaks are defined in Box 6.10. Confirmation of an infectious disease outbreak usually requires evidence from 'typing' that the causal organisms have identical

6.8 Measures used in infection prevention and control (IPC)

Organisational measures
- Handling, storage and disposal of clinical waste
- Containment and safe removal of spilled blood and body fluids
- Cleanliness of environment and medical equipment
- Specialised ventilation (e.g. laminar flow, air filtration, controlled pressure gradients)
- Sterilisation and disinfection of instruments and equipment
- Food hygiene
- Laundry management

Health-care staff interventions
- Education
- Hand hygiene, including hand-washing (see Fig. 6.13)
- Sharps management and disposal
- Use of personal protective equipment (PPE, e.g. masks, sterile and non-sterile gloves, gowns and aprons)
- Screening health workers for disease (e.g. tuberculosis, hepatitis B virus, MRSA)
- Immunisation and post-exposure prophylaxis

Clinical practice
- Antibiotic stewardship
- Aseptic technique
- Perioperative antimicrobial prophylaxis
- Screening patients for colonisation or infection (e.g. MRSA, GRE, CPE)

Response to infections
- Surveillance to detect alert organism (see text) outbreaks and antimicrobial resistance
- Antibiotic chemoprophylaxis in infectious disease contacts, if indicated (see Box 6.19)
- Isolation (see Box 6.9)
- Reservoir control
- Vector control

Population measures
- See Box 6.12 and p. 293

(CPE = carbapenemase-producing *Enterobacterales*; GRE = glycopeptide-resistant enterococci; MRSA = meticillin-resistant *Staphylococcus aureus*)

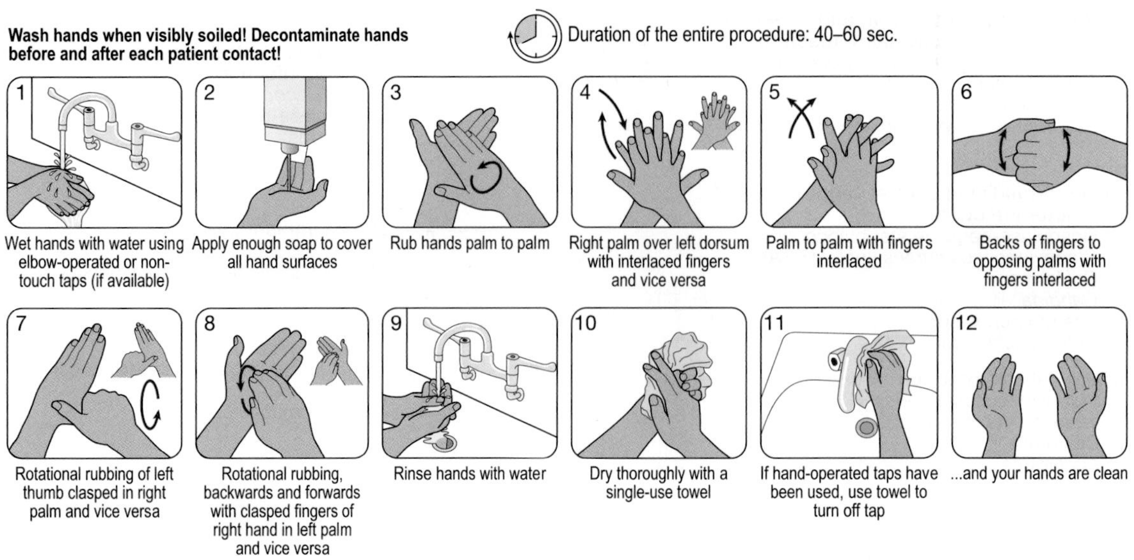

Wash hands when visibly soiled! Decontaminate hands before and after each patient contact!

Duration of the entire procedure: 40–60 sec.

1	2	3	4	5	6
Wet hands with water using elbow-operated or non-touch taps (if available)	Apply enough soap to cover all hand surfaces	Rub hands palm to palm	Right palm over left dorsum with interlaced fingers and vice versa	Palm to palm with fingers interlaced	Backs of fingers to opposing palms with fingers interlaced

7	8	9	10	11	12
Rotational rubbing of left thumb clasped in right palm and vice versa	Rotational rubbing, backwards and forwards with clasped fingers of right hand in left palm and vice versa	Rinse hands with water	Dry thoroughly with a single-use towel	If hand-operated taps have been used, use towel to turn off tap	...and your hands are clean

Fig. 6.13 Hand-washing. Good hand hygiene, whether with soap/water or alcohol handrub, includes areas that are often missed, such as fingertips, web spaces, palmar creases and the backs of hands. *Adapted from the 'How to Handwash' URL: who.int/gpsc/5may/How_To_Handwash_Poster.pdf © World Health Organization 2009. All rights reserved.*

i 6.9 Types of isolation precaution[1]

Airborne transmission	Contact transmission	Droplet transmission
Precautions		
Negative pressure room with air exhausted externally or filtered N95 masks or personal respirators for staff Avoid using non-immune staff	Private room preferred (otherwise, inter-patient spacing ≥1 m) Gloves and gown for staff in contact with patient or contaminated areas	Private room preferred (otherwise, inter-patient spacing ≥1 m) Surgical masks for staff in close contact with patient
Examples of infections managed with these precautions		
Measles Tuberculosis, pulmonary or laryngeal, suspected	Enteroviral infections in young children (diapered or incontinent) Norovirus *Clostridioides difficile* infection Multidrug-resistant organisms (e.g. MRSA, ESBL, GRE, VRSA, penicillin-resistant *Streptococcus pneumoniae*)[2] Parainfluenza in infants and young children Rotavirus RSV in infants, children and immunocompromised Viral conjunctivitis, acute	Diphtheria, pharyngeal *Haemophilus influenzae* type b infection Herpes simplex infection, disseminated or severe Influenza Meningococcal infection Mumps *Mycoplasma pneumoniae* Parvovirus (erythrovirus) B19 (erythema infectiosum, fifth disease) Pertussis Plague, pneumonic Rubella *Streptococcus pyogenes* (group A), pharyngeal
Infections managed with multiple precautions		
← Smallpox, monkeypox, VZV (chickenpox or disseminated disease)[3] →		
← SARS-CoV-2,[4] adenovirus pneumonia →		
← SARS, viral haemorrhagic fever →		

[1]Recommendations based on 2007 CDC guideline for isolation precautions, revised in July 2019. May differ from local or national recommendations. [2]Subject to local risk assessment. [3]Or in any immunocompromised patient until possibility of disseminated infection excluded. [4]SARS-CoV-2 and other respiratory viruses are managed with airborne precautions in certain circumstances (see p. 293). (ESBL = extended-spectrum β-lactamase; GRE = glycopeptide-resistant enterococci; MRSA = meticillin-resistant *Staphylococcus aureus*; RSV = respiratory syncytial virus; SARS = severe acute respiratory syndrome; VRSA = vancomycin-resistant *Staphylococcus aureus*; VZV = varicella zoster virus)

phenotypic and/or genotypic characteristics. When an outbreak of infection is suspected, a case definition is agreed. The number of cases that meet the case definition is then assessed by case-finding, using methods ranging from administration of questionnaires to national reporting systems. Case-finding usually includes microbiological testing, at least in the early stages of an outbreak. Temporal changes in cases are noted in order to plot an outbreak curve, and demographic details are collected to identify possible sources of infection. A case–control study, in which recent activities (potential exposures) of affected 'cases' are compared to those of unaffected 'controls', may be undertaken to establish the outbreak source, and measures are taken to manage the outbreak and control its spread. Good communication between relevant personnel during and after the outbreak is important to inform practice in future outbreaks.

Surveillance ensures that disease outbreaks are either prevented or identified early. In hospitals, staff are made aware of the isolation of 'alert organisms', which have the propensity to cause outbreaks, and 'alert conditions', which are likely to be caused by such organisms. Analogous

6.10 Terminology in outbreaks of infection

Term	Definition
Classification of related cases of infectious disease*	
Cluster	An aggregation of cases of a disease that are closely grouped in time and place, and may or may not exceed the expected number
Epidemic	The occurrence of more cases of disease than expected in a given area or among a specific group of people over a particular period of time
Outbreak	Synonymous with epidemic. Alternatively, a localised, as opposed to generalised, epidemic
Pandemic	An epidemic occurring over a very wide area (several countries or continents) and usually affecting a large proportion of the population
Classification of affected patients (cases)	
Index case	The first case identified in an outbreak
Primary cases	Cases acquired from a specific source of infection
Secondary cases	Cases acquired from primary cases
Types of outbreak	
Common source outbreak	Exposure to a common source of infection (e.g. water-cooling tower, medical staff member shedding MRSA). New primary cases will arise until the source is no longer present
Point source outbreak	Exposure to a single source of infection at a specific point in time (e.g. contaminated food at a party). Primary cases will develop disease synchronously
Person-to-person spread	Outbreak with both primary and secondary cases. May complicate point source or common source outbreak

*Adapted from cdc.gov. (MRSA = meticillin-resistant *Staphylococcus aureus*)

6.11 Reasons for including an infectious disease on a regional/national list of reportable diseases*

Reason for inclusion	Examples
Endemic/local disease with the potential to spread and/or cause outbreaks	Influenza, *Salmonella*, tuberculosis
Imported disease with the propensity to spread and/or cause outbreaks	Typhoid, cholera (depending on local epidemiology)
Evidence of a possible breakdown in health protection/public health functions	*Legionella*, *Cryptosporidium*
Evidence of a possible breakdown in food safety practices	Botulism, verotoxigenic *Escherichia coli*
Evidence of a possible failure of a vaccination programme	Measles, poliomyelitis, pertussis
Disease with the potential to be a novel or increasing threat to human health	COVID-19, MERS-CoV, multi-resistant bacteria
Evidence of expansion of the range of a reservoir/vector	Lyme disease, rabies, West Nile encephalitis
Evidence of possible deliberate release	Anthrax, tularaemia, plague, smallpox, botulism

*Given the different geographical ranges of individual diseases and wide national variations in public health services, vaccination programmes and availability of resources, reporting regulations vary between regions, states and countries. Many diseases are reportable for more than one reason.
(MERS-CoV = Middle East respiratory syndrome)

6.12 Pandemic response*

- International travel restrictions
- National entry screening (e.g. testing for fever or pathogen) and quarantining new arrivals from areas with high infection rates
- Isolation of disease contacts
- Social isolation
- Shielding (strict separation of the vulnerable)
- Social distancing (maintaining physical separation between people and restricting public gatherings)
- Encouraging home working
- Restricting commuting and work-related travel to 'key workers' (workers required to maintain a functioning society)
- Home education
- Curfews
- Closure or reduction in public transport
- Requirement for PPE use in public areas (e.g. face coverings, eye protection)
- Litigation and imposition of legal sanctions to enforce the above responses

*Pandemic control measures vary widely by jurisdiction and depend on the stage and extent of the outbreak and political considerations such as the acceptability of restriction of personal freedoms and the economic consequences of the interventions. See also p. 293.

systems are used nationally; many countries publish lists of organisms and diseases, which, if detected (or suspected), must be reported to public health authorities. Reasons why a disease might be reportable are shown in Box 6.11.

A pandemic is the most extensive form of outbreak, in which the disease spreads over a wide area and may affect a large proportion of the population. The most recent pandemic was the COVID-19 pandemic of 2019 onwards. The measures that may be put in place in an attempt to control a pandemic are shown in Box 6.12.

Immunisation

Immunisation may be passive or active. Passive immunisation is achieved by administering antibodies targeting a specific pathogen. Antibodies are obtained from blood, so confer some of the infection risks associated with blood products. The protection afforded by passive immunisation is immediate but of short duration (a few weeks or months); it is used to prevent or attenuate infection before or after exposure (Box 6.13).

Vaccination

Active immunisation is achieved by vaccination with whole organisms, organism components or nucleic acids (DNA/RNA) (Box 6.14).

Types of vaccine

Whole-cell vaccines consist of live or inactivated (killed) microorganisms. Component vaccines contain only extracted or synthesised components of microorganisms (e.g. polysaccharides or proteins). Live vaccines contain organisms with attenuated (reduced) virulence, which cause only

mild symptoms but induce T-lymphocyte and humoral responses and are therefore more immunogenic than inactivated whole-cell vaccines. The use of live vaccines in immunocompromised individuals is not generally recommended, but they may be used by specialists following a risk/benefit assessment.

Component vaccines consisting only of polysaccharides, such as the pneumococcal polysaccharide vaccine (PPV), are poor activators of T lymphocytes and produce a short-lived antibody response without long-lasting memory. Conjugation of polysaccharide to a protein, as in the *Haemophilus influenzae* type B (Hib) vaccine and the protein conjugate pneumococcal vaccine (PCV), activates T lymphocytes, which results in a sustained response and immunological memory. Toxoids are bacterial toxins that have been modified to reduce toxicity but maintain antigenicity. Vaccine response can be improved by co-administration with mildly pro-inflammatory adjuvants, such as aluminium hydroxide.

6.13 Indications for post-exposure prophylaxis with immunoglobulins

Human normal immunoglobulin (pooled immunoglobulin)

- Hepatitis A (unvaccinated contacts*)
- Measles (exposed child with heart or lung disease)

Human specific immunoglobulin

- Hepatitis B (sexual partners, inoculation injuries, infants born to infected mothers)
- Tetanus (high-risk wounds or incomplete or unknown immunisation status)
- Rabies
- Chickenpox (immunosuppressed children and adults, pregnant women)

*Active immunisation is preferred if contact is with a patient who is within 1 week of onset of jaundice.

6.14 Vaccines in current clinical use

Live attenuated vaccines

- Measles, mumps, rubella (MMR)
- Oral poliomyelitis (OPV, not used in UK)
- Rotavirus
- Tuberculosis (bacille Calmette–Guérin, BCG)
- Typhoid (oral typhoid vaccine)
- Varicella zoster virus

Inactivated (killed) whole-cell vaccines

- Cholera
- Hepatitis A
- Influenza
- Poliomyelitis (inactivated polio virus, IPV)
- Rabies

Component vaccines

- Anthrax (adsorbed extracted antigens)
- COVID-19
- Diphtheria (adsorbed toxoid)
- Hepatitis B (adsorbed recombinant hepatitis B surface antigen, HBsAg)
- *Haemophilus influenzae* type B (conjugated capsular polysaccharide)
- Human papillomavirus (recombinant capsid proteins)
- Meningococcal, quadrivalent A, C, Y, W135 (conjugated capsular polysaccharide)
- Meningococcal, serogroup C (conjugated capsular polysaccharide)
- Pertussis (adsorbed extracted antigens)
- Pneumococcal conjugate (PCV; conjugated capsular polysaccharide, 13 serotypes)
- Pneumococcal polysaccharide (PPV; purified capsular polysaccharide, 23 serotypes)
- Tetanus (adsorbed toxoid)
- Typhoid (purified Vi capsular polysaccharide)

Viral vector vaccines

- Dengue virus (containing Yellow fever 17D vaccine strain with dengue virus genes)
- Ebola virus (vesicular stomatitis virus expressing Ebola virus glycoproteins)
- COVID-19

Nucleic acid vaccines

- COVID-19 (RNA vaccines)
- Ebola virus (DNA in clinical trials)

Recent and emerging vaccine approaches include nucleic acid (DNA or RNA)-based vaccines, in which the vaccine nucleic acid encodes the microbial component of interest; when the vaccine enters the vaccinee's cells they are induced to express viral antigens. They have several advantages over component vaccines: antigen is expressed for a period of time and with the modifications that the host cell would normally produce; antigen is presented by both major histocompatibility class I and II and induces broad B- and T-lymphocyte responses; vaccines are stable and cost-effective; production can be at large scale. DNA and RNA vaccines can be administered directly or may be added with other components to aid cell entry, e.g. liposomses for DNA vaccines or lipid nanoparticles for RNA vaccines. Long-term persistence and chromosomal integration with the potential for mutagenesis remain theoretical concerns for DNA vaccines.

Another approach is to use viral vectors in which an unrelated and modified virus expresses the antigen of interest. These vectors include pox viruses (e.g. modified vaccinia virus Ankara or canary pox virus), adenovirus or adeno-associated viruses. The vector may replicate or be non-replicating. These vaccines work on the same basis as DNA vaccines and are safe and stable. Pre-existing immunity can influence efficacy but use of rare human or related animal strains or a strategy of priming with a non-viral DNA vaccine can help overcome this ('prime-boost' strategy). Nucleic acid vaccines are administered intramuscularly or intradermally while viral vector vaccines can be given by these routes but also intranasally or orally. The first viral vector vaccine to receive clinical approval was for dengue virus, while to date DNA vaccines have only been used in veterinary settings. However, both strategies are employed in studies investigating a range of approaches against Ebola virus and pandemic infections. For COVID-19, vaccines in use or development include viral vectored, RNA, DNA, live attenuated, inactivated (killed) virus, subunit and virus-like particle (lacking genetic material) vaccines. The first types to be used widely were mRNA and adenovirus vector RNA vaccines (see Box 13.38).

Use of vaccines

Vaccination may be applied to entire populations or to subpopulations at specific risk through travel, occupation or other activities. In ring vaccination, the population immediately surrounding a case or outbreak of infectious disease is vaccinated to curtail further spread. This strategy has been used for Ebola in West Africa. Vaccination is aimed mainly at preventing infectious disease. However, vaccination against human papillomavirus (HPV) was introduced to prevent cervical and other cancers that complicate HPV infection. Vaccination guidelines for individuals are shown in Box 6.15.

Vaccination becomes successful for a population once the number of susceptible hosts falls below the level required to sustain continued transmission of the target organism, i.e. when R_e is less than 1 ('herd immunity'). Naturally acquired smallpox was declared to have been eradicated worldwide in 1980 through mass vaccination. In 1988, the WHO resolved to eradicate poliomyelitis by vaccination; the number of cases of wild polio virus infection worldwide has since fallen from approximately 350 000 per annum to 176 in 2019. Recommended vaccination schedules, including catch-up schedules for people who join vaccination programmes late, vary between countries.

Antimicrobial stewardship

Antimicrobial stewardship (AMS) refers to the systems and processes applied to a population to optimise the use of antimicrobial agents. The populations referred to here may be a nation, region, hospital, or a unit within a health-care organisation (e.g. ward or clinic). AMS aims to improve patient outcomes and reduce antimicrobial resistance (AMR). IPC and AMS complement each other (Fig. 6.14). Elements of AMS include treatment guidelines, antimicrobial formularies and ward rounds by infection specialists.

6.15 Guidelines for vaccination against infectious disease

- The principal contraindication to inactivated vaccines is an anaphylactic reaction to a previous dose or a vaccine component
- Live vaccines should not be given during an acute infection, to pregnant women or to the immunosuppressed, unless the immunosuppression is mild and the benefits outweigh the risks
- If two live vaccines are required, they should be given either simultaneously in opposite arms or 4 weeks apart
- Live vaccines should not be given for 3 months after an injection of human normal immunoglobulin (HNI)
- HNI should not be given for 2 weeks after a live vaccine
- Hay fever, asthma, eczema, sickle-cell disease, topical glucocorticoid therapy, antibiotic therapy, prematurity and chronic heart and lung diseases, including tuberculosis, are not contraindications to vaccination

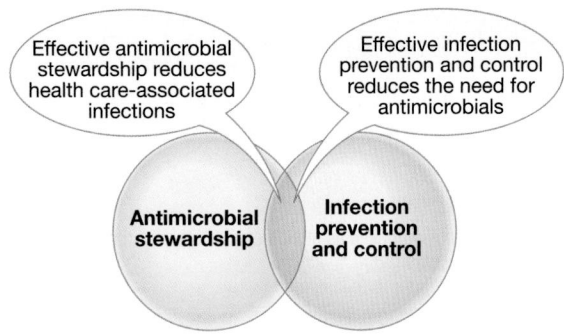

Fig. 6.14 The relationship between infection prevention and control (IPC) and antimicrobial stewardship (AMS).

Treatment of infectious diseases

Key components of treating infection are:

- prompt initiation of antimicrobial therapy in severe infections, e.g. sepsis, meningitis
- optimising antimicrobial therapy while minimising selection for antimicrobial resistance and the impact on the normal microbial flora
- addressing predisposing factors, e.g. glycaemic control in diabetes mellitus; viral load control in HIV-1 infection
- achieving source control, e.g. removal of an infected medical device, pus or necrotic tissue
- managing complications, e.g. sepsis and acute kidney injury.

For communicable disease, treatment must also take into account contacts of the infected patient, and may include IPC interventions such as isolation, antimicrobial prophylaxis, vaccination and contact tracing.

Principles of antimicrobial therapy

In some situations (e.g. pneumonia, meningitis, sepsis) it is important to start appropriate antimicrobial therapy promptly, whereas in others prior confirmation of the diagnosis and pathogen is preferred. The principles underlying the choice of antimicrobial agent(s) are discussed below. The WHO 'World Antibiotic Awareness Week' campaign is a yearly event aimed at highlighting the importance of prudent antimicrobial prescribing (see 'Further information').

Antimicrobial action and spectrum

Antimicrobial agents may kill or inhibit microorganisms by targeting essential and non-essential cellular processes, respectively. The range, or spectrum, of microorganisms that is killed or inhibited by a particular antimicrobial agent needs consideration when selecting therapy. Mechanisms of action of the major classes of antibacterial agent are listed in Box 6.16 and appropriate agents for some common infecting organisms are shown in Box 6.17. In severe infections and/or immunocompromised patients, it is customary to use bactericidal agents in preference to bacteriostatic agents.

Empiric versus targeted therapy

Empiric antimicrobial therapy is selected to treat a suspected infection (e.g. meningitis) before the microbiological cause is known. Targeted or 'directed' therapy can be prescribed when the pathogen(s) is known. Empirical antimicrobial regimens need to have activity against the range of pathogens potentially causing the infection; because broad-spectrum agents affect a wide range of bacteria they select for antimicrobial resistance. 'Start Smart – Then Focus' (Fig. 6.15) describes the principle of converting from empiric therapy to narrow-spectrum targeted therapy. Optimum empiric therapy depends on the site of infection,

> **i 6.16 Target and mechanism of action of common antibacterial agents**
>
> **Aminoglycosides, chloramphenicol, macrolides, lincosamides, oxazolidinones**
> - Inhibition of bacterial protein synthesis by binding to subunits of bacterial ribosomes
>
> **Tetracyclines**
> - Inhibition of protein synthesis by preventing transfer RNA binding to ribosomes
>
> **ß-lactams**
> - Inhibition of cell wall peptidoglycan synthesis by competitive inhibition of transpeptidases ('penicillin-binding proteins')
>
> **Cyclic lipopeptide (daptomycin)**
> - Insertion of lipophilic tail into plasma membrane causing depolarisation and cell death
>
> **Fluoroquinolones**
> - Inhibition of DNA replication by binding to DNA topoisomerases (DNA gyrase and topoisomerase IV), preventing supercoiling and uncoiling of DNA
>
> **Glycopeptides**
> - Inhibition of cell wall peptidoglycan synthesis by forming complexes with D-alanine residues on peptidoglycan precursors
>
> **Nitroimidazoles**
> - The reduced form of the drug causes strand breaks in DNA
>
> **Rifamycins**
> - Inhibition of RNA synthesis by inhibiting DNA-dependent RNA polymerase
>
> **Sulphonamides and trimethoprim**
> - Inhibition of folate synthesis by dihydropteroate synthase (sulphonamides) and dihydrofolate reductase (trimethoprim) inhibition

patient characteristics and local antimicrobial resistance patterns. National or local guidelines should inform antimicrobial prescribing decisions.

Combination therapy

It is sometimes appropriate to combine antimicrobial agents:

- when there is a need to increase clinical effectiveness (e.g. biofilm infections)
- when no single agent's spectrum covers all potential pathogens (e.g. polymicrobial infection)
- when there is a need to reduce development of antimicrobial resistance in the target pathogen, as the organism would need to develop resistance to multiple agents simultaneously (e.g. antituberculous chemotherapy and antiretroviral therapy (ART) for HIV.

Antimicrobial resistance

Microorganisms have evolved in the presence of naturally occurring antibiotics and have therefore developed resistance mechanisms to all classes of antimicrobial agent (antibiotics and their derivatives) (Fig. 6.16). Intrinsic resistance is an innate property of a microorganism, whereas acquired resistance arises by spontaneous mutation or horizontal transfer of genetic material from another organism, usually via a plasmid. Plasmids can be easily transferred between bacteria (especially *Enterobacterales*) and often encode resistance to multiple antibiotics.

Penicillin-binding proteins (PBP) are enzymes involved in bacterial cell wall synthesis. The *mecA* gene encodes a PBP, which has a low affinity for penicillins and therefore confers resistance to β-lactam antibiotics in staphylococci. Extended-spectrum β-lactamases (ESBLs) are bacterial-produced enzymes that break down β-lactam antibiotics, and are frequently encoded on plasmids in *Enterobacterales*. Plasmid-encoded carbapenemases have been detected in strains of *Klebsiella pneumoniae* (e.g. New Delhi metallo-β-lactamase 1, NDM-1). Strains of MRSA have been described that also have reduced susceptibility to glycopeptides through the development of a relatively impermeable cell wall.

6.17 Antimicrobial options for common infecting bacteria

Organism	Antimicrobial options*
Gram-positive organisms	
Enterococcus faecalis	Ampicillin, vancomycin/teicoplanin
Enterococcus faecium	Vancomycin/teicoplanin, linezolid
Glycopeptide-resistant enterococci	Linezolid, tigecycline, daptomycin
MRSA	Clindamycin, vancomycin, rifampicin (never used as monotherapy), linezolid, daptomycin, tetracyclines, tigecycline, co-trimoxazole
Staphylococcus aureus	Flucloxacillin, clindamycin
Streptococcus pyogenes	Penicillin, clindamycin, vancomycin
Streptococcus pneumoniae	Penicillin, cephalosporins, levofloxacin, vancomycin
Gram-negative organisms	
E. coli, 'coliforms' (enteric Gram-negative bacilli)	Amoxicillin, trimethoprim, cefuroxime, ciprofloxacin, co-amoxiclav
Enterobacter spp., *Citrobacter* spp.	Ciprofloxacin, meropenem, ertapenem, aminoglycosides
ESBL-producing *Enterobacterales*	Ciprofloxacin, meropenem, ertapenem (if sensitive), temocillin, aminoglycosides
Carbapenemase-producing *Enterobacterales*	Ciprofloxacin, aminoglycosides, tigecycline, colistin
Haemophilus influenzae	Amoxicillin, co-amoxiclav, macrolides, cefuroxime, cefotaxime, ciprofloxacin
Legionella pneumophila	Azithromycin, levofloxacin, doxycycline
Neisseria gonorrhoeae	Ceftriaxone/cefixime, spectinomycin
Neisseria meningitidis	Penicillin, cefotaxime/ceftriaxone, chloramphenicol
Pseudomonas aeruginosa	Ciprofloxacin, piperacillin–tazobactam, aztreonam, meropenem, aminoglycosides, ceftazidime/cefepime
Salmonella typhi	Ceftriaxone, azithromycin (uncomplicated typhoid), chloramphenicol (resistance common)
Strict anaerobes	
Bacteroides spp.	Metronidazole, clindamycin, co-amoxiclav, piperacillin–tazobactam, meropenem
Clostridioides difficile	Metronidazole, vancomycin (oral), fidaxomicin
Clostridium spp.	Penicillin, metronidazole, clindamycin
Fusobacterium spp.	Penicillin, metronidazole, clindamycin
Other organisms	
Chlamydia trachomatis	Azithromycin, doxycycline
Treponema pallidum	Penicillin, doxycycline

*Antibiotic selection depends on multiple factors, including local susceptibility patterns, which vary enormously between geographical areas. There are many appropriate alternatives to those listed. (ESBL= extended-spectrum β-lactamase; MRSA = meticillin-resistant *Staphylococcus aureus*)

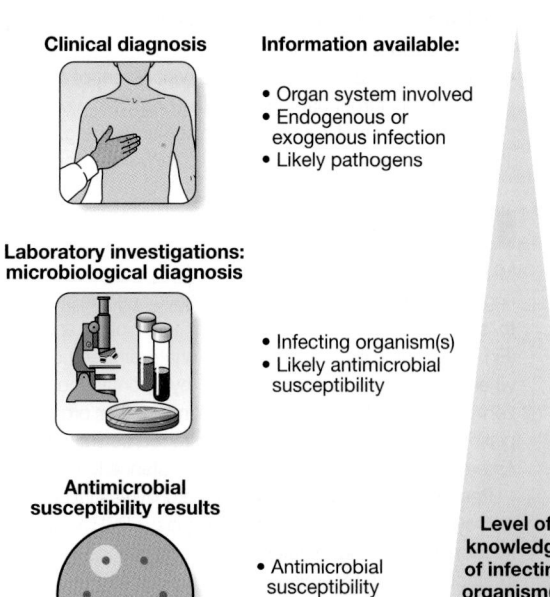

Fig. 6.15 Stages in the selection and refinement of antimicrobial therapy: 'Start Smart – Then Focus'.

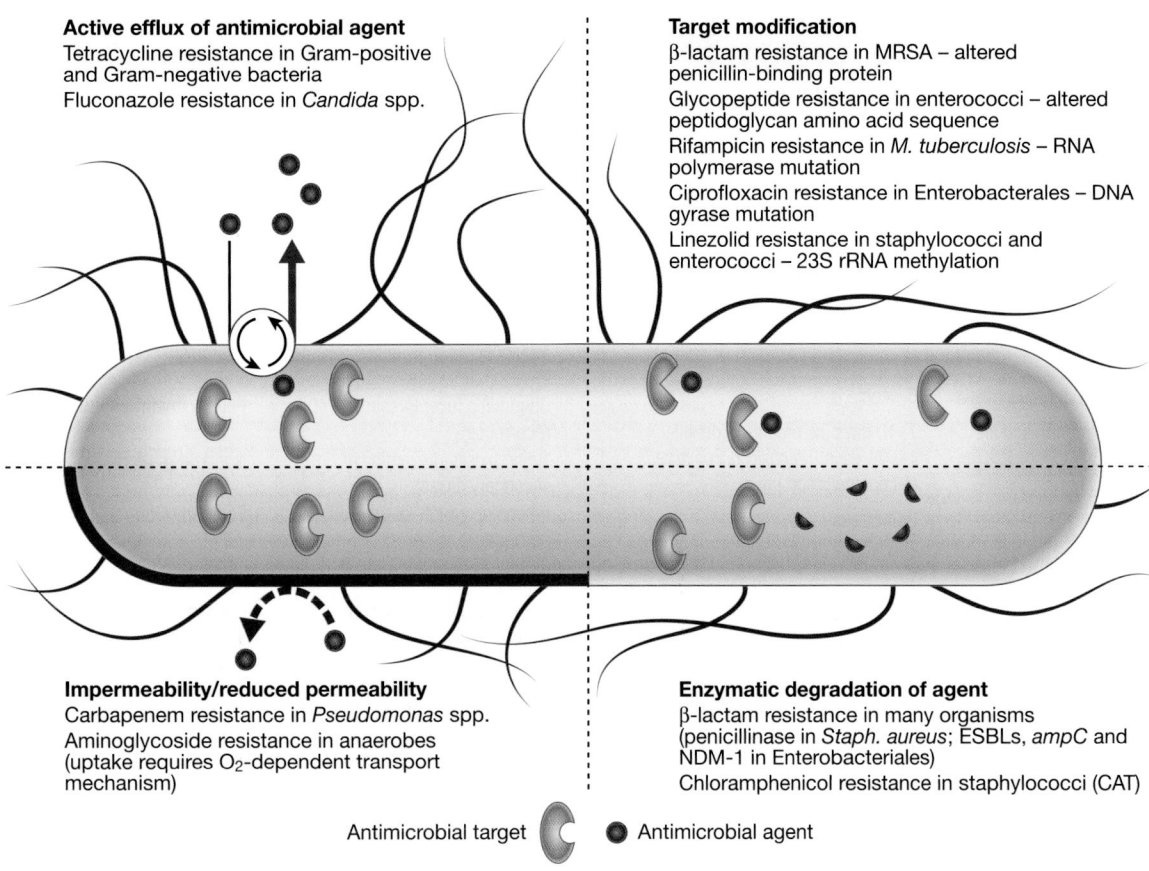

Active efflux of antimicrobial agent
Tetracycline resistance in Gram-positive and Gram-negative bacteria
Fluconazole resistance in *Candida* spp.

Target modification
β-lactam resistance in MRSA – altered penicillin-binding protein
Glycopeptide resistance in enterococci – altered peptidoglycan amino acid sequence
Rifampicin resistance in *M. tuberculosis* – RNA polymerase mutation
Ciprofloxacin resistance in Enterobacterales – DNA gyrase mutation
Linezolid resistance in staphylococci and enterococci – 23S rRNA methylation

Impermeability/reduced permeability
Carbapenem resistance in *Pseudomonas* spp.
Aminoglycoside resistance in anaerobes (uptake requires O_2-dependent transport mechanism)

Enzymatic degradation of agent
β-lactam resistance in many organisms (penicillinase in *Staph. aureus*; ESBLs, *ampC* and NDM-1 in Enterobacterales)
Chloramphenicol resistance in staphylococci (CAT)

Antimicrobial target   ● Antimicrobial agent

Fig. 6.16 Examples of mechanisms of antimicrobial resistance. (CAT = chloramphenicol acetyltransferase; ESBLs = extended-spectrum β-lactamases; MRSA = meticillin-resistant *Staph. aureus*; NDM-1 = New Delhi metallo-β-lactamase 1).

Factors promoting antimicrobial resistance include the inappropriate use of antibiotics (e.g. to treat viral infections), inadequate dosage or unnecessarily prolonged treatment, and use of antimicrobials as growth promoters in agriculture. However, *any* antimicrobial use exerts a selection pressure that favours the development of resistance. Combination antimicrobial therapy may reduce the emergence of resistance in the target pathogen but not in the normal flora that it also affects. Despite use of combination therapy for *M. tuberculosis*, multi-resistant tuberculosis (MDR-TB) and extremely drug-resistant tuberculosis (XDR-TB) have been reported worldwide and are increasing in incidence (see p. 524).

The term 'post-antibiotic era' was coined to describe a future in which widespread antimicrobial resistance will render antimicrobials useless. At present there is a gradual but inexorable progression of resistance globally, necessitating the use of more expensive antimicrobials or older antimicrobials with significant toxicity.

Duration of therapy

Treatment duration reflects the severity of infection and accessibility of the infected site to antimicrobial agents. For most infections, there is limited evidence available to support a specific duration of treatment (Box 6.18). Depending on the indication, initial intravenous therapy can often be switched to oral as soon as the patient is apyrexial and improving. In the absence of specific guidance, antimicrobial therapy should be stopped when there is no longer any clinical evidence of infection.

Pharmacokinetics and pharmacodynamics

Pharmacokinetics of antimicrobial agents is the study of how antibiotics are absorbed, distributed and excreted from the body. Septic patients often have poor gastrointestinal absorption, so the preferred initial route of therapy is intravenous. Knowledge of anticipated antimicrobial drug concentrations at sites of infection is critical. For example, achieving a 'therapeutic' blood level of gentamicin is of little practical use in treating meningitis, as CSF penetration of the drug is poor. Knowledge of routes of antimicrobial elimination is also critical; for instance, urinary tract infection is ideally treated with a drug that is excreted unchanged in the urine.

Pharmacodynamics describes the complex relationship between antimicrobial concentrations and microbial killing in the body. For many agents, antimicrobial effect can be categorised as 'concentration-dependent' or 'time-dependent'. The concentration of antimicrobial achieved after a single dose is illustrated in Figure 6.17. The maximum concentration achieved is C_{max} and the measure of overall exposure is the area under the curve (AUC). The efficacy of antimicrobial agents whose killing is concentration-dependent (e.g. aminoglycosides) increases with the amount by which C_{max} exceeds the minimum inhibitory concentration (C_{max}:MIC ratio). For this reason, it has become customary to administer aminoglycosides (e.g. gentamicin) infrequently at high doses (e.g. 7 mg/kg) rather than frequently at low doses. This has the added advantage of minimising toxicity by reducing the likelihood of drug accumulation. Conversely, the β-lactam antibiotics and vancomycin exhibit time-dependent killing, and their efficacy depends on C_{max} exceeding the MIC for a certain time (which is different for each class of agent). This is reflected in the dosing interval of benzylpenicillin, which is usually given every 4 hours in severe infection (e.g. meningococcal meningitis), and may be administered by continuous infusion. For other antimicrobial agents, the pharmacodynamic relationships are more complex and often less well understood. With some agents, bacterial inhibition persists after antimicrobial exposure (post-antibiotic and post-antibiotic sub-MIC effects).

Therapeutic drug monitoring

Therapeutic drug monitoring is used to confirm that levels of antimicrobial agents with a low therapeutic index (e.g. aminoglycosides) are not

6.18 Duration of antimicrobial therapy for some common infections*

Infection	Duration of therapy
Viral infections	
Herpes simplex encephalitis	2–3 weeks
Bacterial infections	
Gonorrhoea	Single dose
Infective endocarditis (streptococcal, native valve)	4 weeks ± gentamicin for first 2 weeks
Infective endocarditis (prosthetic valve)	6 weeks
Osteomyelitis	6 weeks
Pneumonia (community-acquired, severe)	7–10 days (no organism identified), 14–21 days (*Staphylococcus aureus* or *Legionella* spp.)
Septic arthritis	2–4 weeks
Urinary tract infection (male)	1–2 weeks depending on severity
Urinary tract infection, upper tract, uncomplicated (female)	7 days
Urinary tract infection, lower (female)	3 days
Mycobacterial infections	
Tuberculosis (meningeal)	12 months
Tuberculosis (pulmonary)	6 months
Fungal infections	
Invasive pulmonary aspergillosis	Until clinical/radiological resolution and reversal of predisposition
Candidaemia (acute disseminated)	2 weeks after last positive blood culture and resolution of signs and symptoms

*All recommendations are indicative. Actual duration takes into account predisposing factors, specific organisms and antimicrobial susceptibility, source control, current guidelines and clinical response.

6.19 Recommendations for antimicrobial prophylaxis in adults*

Infection risk	Recommended antimicrobial
Bacterial	
Diphtheria (prevention of secondary cases)	Erythromycin
Gas gangrene (after high amputation or major trauma)	Penicillin or metronidazole
Lower gastrointestinal tract surgery	Cefuroxime + metronidazole, gentamicin + metronidazole, or co-amoxiclav (single dose only)
Meningococcal disease (prevention of secondary cases)	Rifampicin or ciprofloxacin
Rheumatic fever (prevention of recurrence)	Phenoxymethylpenicillin or sulfadiazine
Tuberculosis (prevention of secondary cases)	Isoniazid ± rifampicin
Whooping cough (prevention of secondary cases)	Erythromycin
Viral	
HIV, occupational exposure (sharps injury)	Combination tenofovir/emtricitabine and raltegravir. Modified if index case's virus known to be resistant
Influenza A (prevention of secondary cases in adults with chronic respiratory, cardiovascular or renal disease, immunosuppression or diabetes mellitus)	Oseltamivir
Fungal	
Aspergillosis (in high-risk haematology patients)	Posaconazole (voriconazole or itraconazole alternatives if intolerant)
Pneumocystis pneumonia (prevention in HIV and other immunosuppressed states)	Co-trimoxazole, pentamidine or dapsone
Protozoal	
Malaria (prevention of travel-associated disease)	Specific antimalarials depend on travel itinerary. Specialist guidance should be consulted

*These are based on current UK practice. Recommendations may vary locally or nationally. Antimicrobial prophylaxis for infective endocarditis during dental procedures is not currently recommended in the UK.

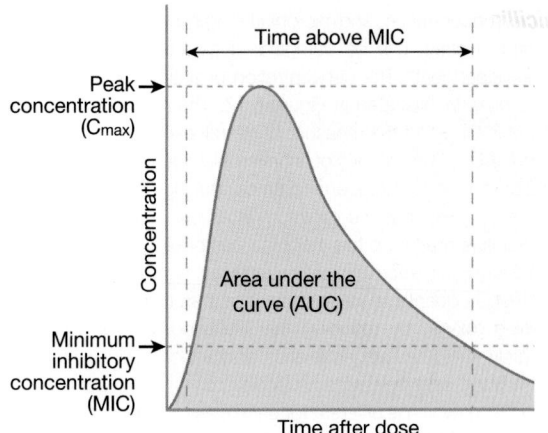

Fig. 6.17 Antimicrobial pharmacodynamics. The curve represents drug concentrations after a single dose of an antimicrobial agent. Factors that determine microbial killing are C_{max}:MIC ratio (concentration-dependent killing), time above MIC (time-dependent killing) and AUC:MIC ratio.

excessive, and that levels of agents with marked pharmacokinetic variability (e.g. vancomycin) are adequate. Specific recommendations for monitoring depend on individual clinical circumstances; for instance, different pre- and post-dose levels of gentamicin are recommended, depending on whether it is being used in traditional divided doses, once daily or for synergy in infective endocarditis (p. 462).

Antimicrobial prophylaxis

Antimicrobial prophylaxis is the use of antimicrobial agents to prevent infection. Primary prophylaxis is used to reduce the risk of infection following certain medical procedures (e.g. colonic resection or prosthetic hip insertion), following exposure to a specific pathogen (e.g. *Bordetella pertussis*) or in specific situations such as post-splenectomy (Box 6.19). Antimicrobial prophylaxis should be chosen to have minimal adverse effects and based on robust evidence. In the case of exposure, it may be combined with passive immunisation (see Box 6.13). Secondary prophylaxis is used in patients who have been treated successfully for an infection but remain predisposed to it. It is used in haemato-oncology patients in the context of fungal infection and in HIV-positive individuals with an opportunistic infection until a defined level of immune reconstitution is achieved.

Antibacterial agents

For details of antibacterial usage in pregnancy and old age, see Boxes 6.20 and 6.21.

6.20 Antimicrobial agents in pregnancy[1]

Contraindicated

- Chloramphenicol: neonatal 'grey baby' syndrome – collapse, hypotension and cyanosis
- Fluconazole: teratogenic in high doses
- Quinolones: arthropathy in animal studies
- Sulphonamides: neonatal haemolysis and methaemoglobinaemia
- Tetracyclines, glycylcyclines: skeletal abnormalities in animals in first trimester; fetal dental discoloration and maternal hepatotoxicity with large parenteral doses in second or third trimesters
- Trimethoprim: teratogenic in first trimester
- Macrolides[2]: major malformations in first trimester and genital malformations any trimester

Relatively contraindicated

- Aminoglycosides: potential damage to fetal auditory and vestibular nerves in second and third trimesters
- Metronidazole: avoidance of high dosages is recommended[3]

Not known to be harmful; use only when necessary

- Aciclovir
- Penicillins and cephalosporins
- Clindamycin
- Glycopeptides
- Linezolid
- Meropenem

[1]Data extracted from Joint Formulary Committee. British National Formulary (online). London: BMJ Group and Pharmaceutical Press; (medicinescomplete.com) [accessed 16 March 2013]. [2]Fan H, Gilbert R, O'Callaghan F, Li L. Associations between macrolide antibiotics prescribing during pregnancy and adverse child outcomes in the UK: population based cohort study. BMJ 2020; 368:m331. [3]Theoretical risk of teratogenicity, not supported by available clinical evidence.

6.21 Problems with antimicrobial therapy in old age

- ***Clostridioides difficile* infection**: all antibiotics predispose to some extent, but second- and third-generation cephalosporins, co-amoxiclav and clindamycin especially so.
- **Hypersensitivity reactions**: rise in incidence due to increased previous exposure.
- **Renal impairment**: may be significant in old age, despite creatinine levels being within the reference range.
- **Nephrotoxicity**: more likely, e.g. aminoglycosides.
- **Accumulation of β-lactam antibiotics**: may result in myoclonus, seizures or coma.
- **Reduced gastric acid production**: gastric pH is higher, which causes increased penicillin absorption.
- **Reduced hepatic metabolism**: results in a higher risk of isoniazid-related hepatotoxicity.
- **Quinolones**: associated with delirium and may increase the risk of seizures.

β-lactam antibiotics

These antibiotics have a β-lactam ring structure and exert a bactericidal action by inhibiting PBPs and cell wall synthesis. They are classified in Box 6.22.

Pharmacokinetics

- Good drug levels are achieved in lung, kidney, bone, muscle and liver, and in pleural, synovial, pericardial and peritoneal fluids.
- CSF levels are low, except when meninges are inflamed.
- 'Inoculum effect': the activity of β-lactams is reduced in the presence of a high organism burden, although the clinical relevance of this effect is a subject of debate.
- Generally safe in pregnancy (except imipenem/cilastatin).

Adverse effects

Immediate (IgE-mediated) allergic reactions are rare but life-threatening. Approximately 90% of patients who report a penicillin allergy do not have a true IgE-mediated allergy, highlighting the importance of careful allergy histories and documentation of reactions. Other reactions, such as rashes, fever and haematological effects (e.g. low white cell count), usually follow more prolonged therapy (more than 2 weeks). Patients with

6.22 β-lactam antibiotics

Penicillins

- Natural penicillins: benzylpenicillin, phenoxymethylpenicillin
- Penicillinase-resistant penicillins: methicillin*, flucloxacillin, nafcillin, oxacillin
- Aminopenicillins: ampicillin, amoxicillin
- Carboxy- and ureido-penicillins: ticarcillin, piperacillin, temocillin

Cephalosporins

- See Box 6.23

Monobactams

- Aztreonam

Carbapenems

- Imipenem, meropenem, ertapenem, doripenem

*Not used for treatment.

infectious mononucleosis may develop a rash if given aminopenicillins; this does not imply lasting allergy. The relationship between allergy to penicillin and allergy to cephalosporins depends on the specific cephalosporin used. Avoidance of cephalosporins, however, is recommended in patients who have IgE-mediated penicillin allergy (p. 80). Cross-reactivity between penicillin and carbapenems is rare (approximately 1% by skin testing) and carbapenems may be administered if there are no suitable alternatives and appropriate resuscitation facilities are available.

Gastrointestinal upset and diarrhoea are common, and a mild reversible hepatitis is recognised with many β-lactams. More severe forms of hepatitis can be observed with flucloxacillin and co-amoxiclav. Leucopenia, thrombocytopenia, coagulation deficiencies, interstitial nephritis and potentiation of aminoglycoside-mediated kidney damage are also recognised. Seizures and encephalopathy have been reported, particularly with high doses in the presence of renal insufficiency. Thrombophlebitis occurs in up to 5% of patients receiving parenteral β-lactams.

Drug interactions

Synergism occurs in combination with aminoglycosides in vitro. Ampicillin decreases the biological effect of oral contraceptives and the whole class is significantly affected by concurrent administration of probenecid, producing a 2–4-fold increase in the peak serum concentration.

Penicillins

Natural penicillins are primarily effective against Gram-positive organisms (except staphylococci, most of which produce a penicillinase) and anaerobic organisms. *Streptococcus pyogenes* has remained sensitive to natural penicillins worldwide. According to the European Antimicrobial Resistance Surveillance Network (EARS-Net), the prevalence of non-susceptibility to penicillin in *Streptococcus pneumoniae* in Europe in 2018 varied widely from 0.1% (Belgium) to 40% (Romania).

Penicillinase-resistant penicillins are the mainstay of treatment for infections with *Staph. aureus*, other than MRSA. However, EARS-Net data from 2018 indicate that MRSA rates in Europe vary widely from 0% (Iceland) to 43% (Romania).

Aminopenicillins have the same spectrum of activity as the natural penicillins, with additional Gram-negative cover against *Enterobacterales*. Amoxicillin has better oral absorption than ampicillin. Unfortunately, resistance to these agents is widespread (*Escherichia coli* Europe-wide in 2018, range 35.3%–67.6%), so they are no longer appropriate for empiric use in Gram-negative infections. In many organisms, resistance is due to β-lactamase production, which can be overcome by the addition of β-lactamase inhibitors (clavulanic acid or sulbactam).

Carboxypenicillins (e.g. ticarcillin) and ureidopenicillins (e.g. piperacillin) are particularly active against Gram-negative organisms, especially *Pseudomonas* spp., which are resistant to the aminopenicillins. β-lactamase inhibitors may be added to extend their spectrum of activity (e.g. piperacillin–tazobactam). Temocillin is derived from ticarcillin; it has good activity against *Enterobacterales*, including those that produce ESBL enzymes, but poor activity against *P. aeruginosa* and Gram-positive bacteria.

Cephalosporins and cephamycins

Cephalosporins are broad-spectrum agents. Unfortunately, their use is associated with *C. difficile* infection. With the exception of ceftobiprole, the group has no activity against enterococci. Only the cephamycins have anti-anaerobic activity. All cephalosporins are inactivated by ESBL. Cephalosporins are arranged in 'generations' (Box 6.23).

- *First-generation compounds* have excellent activity against Gram-positive organisms and some activity against Gram-negatives.
- *Second-generation drugs* retain Gram-positive activity but have extended Gram-negative activity. Cephamycins (e.g. cefoxitin), included in this group, are active against anaerobic Gram-negative bacilli.
- *Third-generation agents* have improved anti-Gram-negative coverage. For some (e.g. ceftazidime), this is extended to include *Pseudomonas* spp. Cefotaxime and ceftriaxone have excellent Gram-negative activity and retain good activity against *Strep. pneumoniae* and β-haemolytic streptococci. Ceftriaxone is administered once daily and is therefore a suitable agent for outpatient intravenous (parenteral) antimicrobial therapy (OPAT).
- *Fourth-generation agents*, e.g. cefepime, have a broad spectrum of activity, including streptococci and some Gram-negatives, including *P. aeruginosa*.
- *Fifth-generation agents*, such as ceftobiprole and ceftaroline, have an enhanced spectrum of Gram-positive activity that includes MRSA, and also have activity against Gram-negative bacteria; some, such as ceftobiprole, are active against *P. aeruginosa*.
- Cefiderocol is a novel siderophore cephalosporin, which is also active in the presence of ESBLs and carbapenamases.

The spectrum of cephalosporins has also been enhanced by adding β-lactamase inhibitors, e.g. ceftazidime/avibactam and ceftolazone/tazobactam.

Monobactams

Aztreonam is the only available monobactam. It is active against Gram-negative bacteria, except ESBL-producing organisms, but inactive against Gram-positive organisms or anaerobes. It is a parenteral-only agent and may be used safely in most penicillin-allergic patients other than those with an allergy to ceftazidime, which shares a common side chain.

Carbapenems

These intravenous agents have the broadest antibiotic activity of the β-lactam antibiotics, covering most clinically significant bacteria, including anaerobes (e.g. imipenem, meropenem, ertapenem). Carbapenems are also being combined with β-lactamase inhibitors in response to emergence of carbapenemase enzymes that inactivate this class (e.g. meropenem-vaborbactam).

Macrolide and lincosamide antibiotics

Macrolides (e.g. erythromycin, clarithromycin and azithromycin) and lincosamides (e.g. clindamycin) are bacteriostatic agents. Both classes bind to the same component of the ribosome, so they are not administered together. Macrolides are used for *Legionella*, *Mycoplasma*, *Chlamydia* and *Bordetella* infections. Azithromycin is employed for single-dose/short-course therapy for genitourinary *Chlamydia/Mycoplasma* spp. infections. Clindamycin is used primarily for skin, soft tissue, bone and joint infections.

Pharmacokinetics

Macrolides

- Variable bioavailability (intravenous and oral preparations available).
- Frequency of administration: erythromycin is administered 4 times daily, clarithromycin twice daily, azithromycin once daily.
- High protein binding.
- Excellent intracellular accumulation.

Lincosamides (e.g. clindamycin)

- Good oral bioavailability.
- Food has no effect on absorption.
- Good bone/joint penetration; limited CSF penetration.

Adverse effects

- Gastrointestinal upset, especially in young adults (erythromycin 30%).
- Cholestatic jaundice with erythromycin estolate.
- Prolongation of QT interval can cause torsades de pointes (p. 418).
- Clindamycin predisposes to CDI.

Aminoglycosides and spectinomycin

Aminoglycosides are effective mainly in Gram-negative infections and are therefore commonly used in regimens for intra-abdominal infection. Some aminoglycosides, e.g. amikacin, are important components of therapy for MDR-TB. Because they act synergistically with β-lactam antibiotics they are used in combinations to treat biofilm infections, including infective endocarditis and orthopaedic implant infections. They cause very little local irritation at injection sites and negligible allergic responses. Oto- and nephrotoxicity must be avoided by monitoring of renal function and drug levels and by use of short treatment regimens. Aminoglycosides are not subject to an inoculum effect and they all exhibit a post-antibiotic effect. Resistance is mediated mainly through inactivation by aminoglycoside-modifying enzymes (AMEs). Plazomicin is a novel aminoglycoside that is not yet inactivated by AMEs.

Pharmacokinetics

- Negligible oral absorption.
- Hydrophilic, so excellent penetration to extracellular fluid in body cavities and serosal fluids, but poor penetration into adipose tissue.
- Very poor intracellular penetration (except hair cells in cochlea and renal cortical cells).
- Negligible CSF and corneal penetration.
- Peak plasma levels 30 minutes after infusion.
- Exhibit a post-antibiotic effect.
- Monitoring of therapeutic levels required.

Gentamicin dosing

- Gentamicin should be dosed according to actual body weight or ideal body weight if obese.
- Except in certain forms of endocarditis, pregnancy, severe burns, end-stage renal disease and paediatric patients, gentamicin can be administered at 7 mg/kg body weight. The appropriate dose interval

---

i 6.23 **Cephalosporins**

First generation
- Cefalexin, cefradine (oral)
- Cefazolin (IV)

Second generation
- Cefuroxime (oral/IV)
- Cefaclor (oral)
- Cefoxitin (IV)

Third generation
- Cefixime (oral)
- Cefotaxime (IV)
- Ceftriaxone (IV)
- Ceftazidime (IV)

Fourth generation
- Cefepime (IV)

Fifth generation (also referred to as 'next generation')
- Ceftobiprole (IV)
- Ceftaroline (IV)

(IV = intravenous)

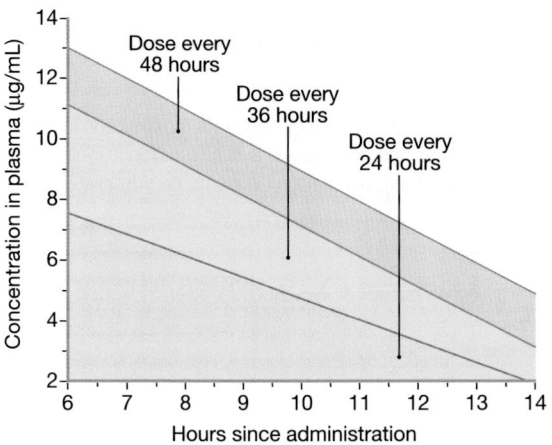

Fig. 6.18 Dosing of aminoglycosides using the Hartford nomogram. The nomogram is used to determine the dose interval for 7 mg/kg doses of gentamicin or tobramycin, using measurements of drug levels in plasma 6–14 hours after a single dose.

depends on drug clearance and is determined by reference to the Hartford nomogram (Fig. 6.18).

- In most other situations, gentamicin is usually administered twice or 3 times daily at 3–5 mg/kg/day with target pre- and post-dose levels of <1 mg/L and 5–10 mg/L.
- In streptococcal and enterococcal endocarditis, gentamicin is used with a cell wall active agent (usually a β-lactam), to provide synergy. Lower doses and target levels are used in this situation.
- For all aminoglycoside dosing local guidance should be consulted.

Adverse effects

- Renal toxicity (usually reversible) accentuated by other nephrotoxic agents.
- Cochlear toxicity (permanent) more likely in older people and those with a predisposing mitochondrial gene mutation.
- Neuromuscular blockade after rapid intravenous infusion (potentiated by calcium channel blockers, myasthenia gravis and hypomagnesaemia).

Spectinomycin

Chemically similar to the aminoglycosides and given intramuscularly, spectinomycin was developed to treat strains of *Neisseria gonorrhoeae* resistant to β-lactam antibiotics. Unfortunately, resistance to spectinomycin is very common. Its only indication is the treatment of gonococcal urethritis in pregnancy or in patients allergic to β-lactam antibiotics.

Quinolones and fluoroquinolones

These are effective and generally well-tolerated bactericidal agents. The quinolones have purely anti-Gram-negative activity, whereas the fluoroquinolones are broad-spectrum agents (Box 6.24). Ciprofloxacin has anti-pseudomonal activity but resistance emerges rapidly. In 2018, European surveillance showed that resistance to fluoroquinolones in *E. coli* ranged between 8.4% (Finland) and 42.4% (Cyprus). Quinolones and fluoroquinolones are used for a variety of infections, including pyelonephritis, osteomyelitis and less common problems like MDR-TB.

Pharmacokinetics

- Well absorbed after oral administration but delayed by food, antacids, ferrous sulphate and multivitamins.
- Wide volume of distribution; tissue concentrations twice those in serum.
- Good intracellular penetration, concentrating in phagocytes.

i | 6.24 Quinolones and fluoroquinolones

Agent	Route of administration	Typical antimicrobial spectrum
Quinolones		
Nalidixic acid	Oral	Enteric Gram-negative bacilli (not *Pseudomonas aeruginosa*)
Fluoroquinolones		
Ciprofloxacin	IV/oral	Enteric Gram-negative bacilli,
Norfloxacin	Oral	*P. aeruginosa, Haemophilus*
Ofloxacin	IV/oral/topical	spp., 'atypical' respiratory pathogens*
Levofloxacin (L-isomer of ofloxacin)	IV/oral	*Haemophilus* spp., *Streptococcus pneumoniae*, 'atypical' respiratory pathogens*
Moxifloxacin	Oral	*Strep. pneumoniae. Staphylococcus aureus*, 'atypical' respiratory pathogens,* mycobacteria and anaerobes

*'Atypical' pathogens include *Mycoplasma pneumoniae* and *Legionella* spp. Fluoroquinolones have variable activity against *Mycobacterium tuberculosis* and other mycobacteria.

Adverse effects

- Gastrointestinal side-effects in 1%–5%.
- Rare skin reactions (phototoxicity).
- Tendinitis and Achilles tendon rupture, especially in older people.
- Central nervous system effects (delirium, tremor, dizziness and occasional seizures in 5%–12%), especially in older people.
- Reduces clearance of xanthines and theophyllines, potentially inducing insomnia and increased seizure potential.
- Prolongation of QT interval on ECG, cardiac arrhythmias.
- Ciprofloxacin use is associated with acquisition of MRSA and strains of *C. difficile*.

Glycopeptides

Glycopeptides (vancomycin and teicoplanin) are effective against Gram-positive organisms only, and are used mainly against staphylococci (including MRSA) and enterococci. Some staphylococci and enterococci are resistant, and glycopeptide use should be restricted to limit the emergence of resistance. Glycopeptides are not absorbed after oral administration but vancomycin is used orally to treat CDI.

Dalbavancin and telavancin are semisynthetic derivatives of glycopeptide (lipoglycopeptides). Dalbavancin is used primarily for skin and skin structure infections. Telavancin has a dual mechanism of action, inhibiting both cell wall synthesis and membrane polarisation; it is reserved for hospital-acquired pneumonia when other agents cannot be used.

Pharmacokinetics

- Vancomycin is administered by slow intravenous infusion. It has good tissue distribution and a short half-life, and enters the CSF only in the presence of inflammation. Therapeutic drug monitoring is recommended, to maintain pre-dose levels of >10 mg/L (15–20 mg/L in serious staphylococcal infections).
- Teicoplanin is administered intravenously or intramuscularly. Its long half-life allows once-daily dosing
- Telavancin and dalbavancin are administered intravenously. Telavancin has a long half-life that allows once-daily dosing; dalbavancin has a very long half-life, allowing once-weekly dosing.

Adverse effects

- Rapid infusion of vancomycin can cause histamine release ('red man' syndrome), although this is rare with modern preparations.
- Vancomycin and teicoplanin are associated with nephrotoxicity and ototoxicity.
- Vancomycin and teicoplanin can cause DRESS (drug reaction with eosinophilia and systemic symptoms, see Box 27.35).

Lipopeptides

Daptomycin is a cyclic lipopeptide with bactericidal activity against Gram-positive organisms only, including MRSA and glycopeptide-resistant enterococci. It is not absorbed orally, and is used intravenously to treat Gram-positive infections, such as soft tissue infections and *Staph. aureus* infective endocarditis. Daptomycin is inactivated by pulmonary surfactant and is not effective for pneumonia. Treatment can be associated with increased levels of creatine kinase and eosinophilic pneumonitis.

Polymyxins

Colistin is a polymyxin antibiotic that binds and disrupts the outer cell membrane of Gram-negative bacteria, including *P. aeruginosa* and *Acinetobacter baumannii*. Its use has increased with the emergence and spread of multi-resistant Gram-negative bacteria, including CPEs. It can be administered by oral, intravenous and nebulised routes. Significant adverse effects include neurotoxicity, including encephalopathy, and nephrotoxicity.

Folate antagonists

These are bacteriostatic antibacterials. A combination of a sulphonamide and either trimethoprim or pyrimethamine is most commonly used, which interferes with two consecutive steps in the folate metabolic pathway. Available combinations include trimethoprim/sulfamethoxazole (co-trimoxazole) and pyrimethamine with either sulfadoxine (used to treat malaria) or sulfadiazine (used in toxoplasmosis). Co-trimoxazole is the first-line drug for *Pneumocystis jirovecii* infection, the second-line drug for treatment and prevention of *B. pertussis* infection, and is also used for a variety of other infections, including *Staph. aureus*. Dapsone is used to treat leprosy (Hansen's disease) and to prevent toxoplasmosis and pneumocystis when patients are intolerant of other medications. Folinic acid should be given to prevent myelosuppression if these drugs are used long-term or unavoidably in early pregnancy.

Pharmacokinetics

- Well absorbed orally.
- Sulphonamides are hydrophilic, distributing well to the extracellular fluid.
- Trimethoprim is lipophilic with high tissue concentrations.

Adverse effects

- Trimethoprim is generally well tolerated, with few adverse effects.
- Sulphonamides and dapsone may cause haemolysis in glucose-6-phosphate dehydrogenase deficiency.
- Sulphonamides and dapsone cause skin and mucocutaneous reactions, including Stevens–Johnson syndrome and 'dapsone syndrome' (rash, fever and lymphadenopathy).
- Dapsone causes methaemoglobinaemia and peripheral neuropathy.

Tetracyclines and glycylcyclines

Tetracyclines

Of this mainly bacteriostatic class, the newer drugs doxycycline and minocycline show better absorption and distribution than older ones. Resistance is common in streptococci and Gram-negative bacteria. Tetracyclines are indicated for infections caused by *Mycoplasma* spp., *Chlamydia* spp., *Rickettsia* spp., *Coxiella* spp., *Bartonella* spp., *Borrelia* spp., *Helicobacter pylori*, *Treponema pallidum* and atypical mycobacteria. Tetracyclines can also be used for malaria prevention.

Pharmacokinetics

- Best oral absorption is in the fasting state (doxycycline is 100% absorbed unless gastric pH rises) and absorption is inhibited by cations, e.g. calcium or iron, which should not be administered at the same time.

Adverse effects

- All tetracyclines except doxycycline are contraindicated in renal failure.
- Dizziness with minocycline.
- Binding to metallic ions in bones and teeth causes discoloration (avoid in children and pregnancy) and enamel hypoplasia.
- Oesophagitis/oesophageal ulcers with doxycycline.
- Phototoxic skin reactions.

Glycylcyclines (tigecycline)

Chemical modification of tetracycline has produced tigecycline, a broad-spectrum, parenteral-only antibiotic with activity against resistant Gram-positive and Gram-negative pathogens, such as MRSA and ESBL (but excluding *Pseudomonas* spp.). Re-analysis of trial data has shown that there was excess mortality following tigecycline treatment as opposed to comparator antibiotics, so tigecycline should be used only when there has been adequate assessment of risk versus benefit.

Nitroimidazoles

Nitroimidazoles (e.g. metronidazole) are highly active against strictly anaerobic bacteria, especially *Bacteroides fragilis*, *C. difficile* and *Clostridium* spp. Both metronidazole and tinidazole have significant anti-protozoal activity against amoebae and *Giardia lamblia*. Nitroimidazoles are almost completely absorbed after oral administration (60% after rectal administration) and well distributed, especially to brain and CSF. They can be used in pregnancy after a risk assessment.

Adverse effects include: metallic taste (dose-dependent), severe vomiting if taken with alcohol ('Antabuse effect') and peripheral neuropathy with prolonged use.

Phenicols (chloramphenicol)

Chloramphenicol use is best reserved for severe and life-threatening infections when other antibiotics are either unavailable or impractical, due to toxicity. It is bacteriostatic to most organisms and has a very broad spectrum of activity against aerobic and anaerobic organisms. It competes with macrolides and lincosamides for ribosomal binding sites, so should not be used in combination with these agents. Significant adverse effects are 'grey baby' syndrome in infants (cyanosis and circulatory collapse due to inability to conjugate drug and excrete the active form in urine); reversible dose-dependent bone marrow depression in adults receiving high cumulative doses; and severe aplastic anaemia in 1 in 25000–40000 exposures (unrelated to dose, duration of therapy or route of administration).

Oxazolidinones

Linezolid and tedizolid are examples and have good activity against Gram-positive organisms. They are primarily used in infection caused by resistant Gram-positive bacteria, including MRSA and GRE, but also for resistant *Mycobacterium tuberculosis*. Administration can be intravenous or oral. Common linezolid adverse effects include mild gastrointestinal upset and tongue discoloration. Myelodysplasia and peripheral and optic neuropathy can occur with prolonged use. Linezolid has monoamine oxidase inhibitor (MAOI) activity, and co-administration with other MAOIs or serotonin re-uptake inhibitors should be avoided, as this may precipitate a 'serotonin syndrome'.

Other antibacterial agents

Fusidic acid

This antibiotic, active against Gram-positive bacteria, is available in intravenous, oral or topical formulations. It is lipid-soluble and distributes well to tissues. Its antibacterial activity is, however, unpredictable. Fusidic acid is used in combination, typically with antistaphylococcal penicillins, or for MRSA with clindamycin or rifampicin. It interacts with coumarin derivatives and oral contraceptives.

Nitrofurantoin

This drug has very rapid renal elimination and is active against aerobic Gram-negative and Gram-positive bacteria, including enterococci. It is used only for treatment of lower urinary tract infection, being generally safe in pregnancy and childhood. With prolonged treatment, however, it can cause eosinophilic lung infiltrates, fever, pulmonary fibrosis, peripheral neuropathy, hepatitis and haemolytic anaemia so its use must be carefully balanced against risks.

Fidaxomicin

Fidaxomicin is an RNA synthesis inhibitor, and was introduced for the treatment of CDI in 2012. The registration trial found fidaxomicin was non-inferior to oral vancomycin in non-severe CDI and was associated with a lower recurrence rate. Its effectiveness for severe CDI has not been assessed in trials.

Fosfomycin

Fosfomycin acts by inhibiting cell wall synthesis. It has activity against Gram-negative and Gram-positive bacteria and can demonstrate in vitro synergy against MRSA when combined with other antimicrobials. It is used for treatment of urinary tract infections but can be employed in other situations against multi-resistant bacteria.

Lefamulin

Lefamulin is a pleuromutilin antibiotic that inhibits the 50S ribosome and inhibits protein synthesis. It has recently been licensed for use in community-acquired pneumonia and is available orally and intravenously. It should not be used in pregnancy and prolongs the QT interval.

Antimycobacterial agents

Isoniazid

Isoniazid is bactericidal for replicating bacteria and bacteriostatic for non-replicating bacteria. It is activated by mycobacterial catalase-peroxidase (KatG) and inhibits the InhA gene product, a reductase involved in mycolic acid synthesis. Mutations in KatG or InhA result in isoniazid resistance, which was reported in 15% of cases of M. tuberculosis infection globally in 2013. Isoniazid is well absorbed orally and metabolised by acetylation in the liver. The major side-effects are hepatitis, neuropathy (ameliorated by co-administration of pyridoxine) and hypersensitivity reactions.

Rifampicin

Rifampicin inhibits DNA-dependent RNA polymerase and is bactericidal against replicating bacteria. It is also active in necrotic foci, where mycobacteria have low levels of replication, and is therefore important in sterilisation and sputum conversion. Resistance most often involves the β-subunit of RNA polymerase and most often occurs with isoniazid-resistant MDR-TB. Rifampicin is well absorbed orally. It is metabolised by the liver via the microsomal cytochrome P450 system and is one of the most potent inducers of multiple P450 isoenzymes, so is subject to extensive drug–drug interactions. Common side-effects include hepatitis, influenza-like symptoms and hypersensitivity reactions. Orange discoloration of urine and body secretions is expected.

Pyrazinamide

The mechanism of action of pyrazinamide is incompletely defined but includes inhibition of fatty acid synthase and ribosomal trans-translation, a quality control system for mRNA and protein synthesis. Pyrazinamide is often bacteriostatic but can be bactericidal and is active against semi-dormant bacteria in a low-pH environment. Primary resistance is rare but MDR-TB strains are frequently pyrazinamide-resistant and intrinsic resistance is a feature of Mycobacterium bovis strains. Pyrazinamide is well absorbed orally and metabolised by the liver. Side-effects include nausea, hepatitis, asymptomatic elevation of uric acid and myalgia.

Ethambutol

Ethambutol is a bacteriostatic agent. It inhibits arabinosyl transferase, which is involved in the synthesis of arabinogalactan, a component of the mycobacterial cell wall. Resistance is usually seen when resistance to other antimycobacterial agents is also present, e.g. in MDR-TB strains. It is orally absorbed but, in contrast to the first-line agents described above, it achieves poor CSF penetration and is renally excreted. The major side-effect is optic neuritis with loss of red–green colour discrimination and impaired visual acuity.

Streptomycin

Streptomycin is an aminoglycoside whose mechanism of action and side-effects are similar to those of other aminoglycosides. It is administered intramuscularly.

Other antituberculous agents

Second-line agents used in MDR or XDR strains (p. 524) include aminoglycosides (amikacin, capreomycin or kanamycin) and fluoroquinolones (moxifloxacin or levofloxacin), discussed above. Other established second-line agents administered orally are cycloserine (which causes neurological side-effects); ethionamide or prothionamide (which are not active with InhA-gene-mediated resistance but have reasonable CSF penetration; their side-effect profile includes gastrointestinal disturbance, hepatotoxicity and neurotoxicity); and paraminosalicylic acid (which causes rashes and gastrointestinal upset). Linezolid may also be used and has good CSF penetration, while meropenem with co-amoxiclav is occasionally chosen. New drugs developed for XDR-TB include delamanid and bedaquiline (which targets the ATP synthase); their adverse effects include QT prolongation and cardiac arrhythmias. Their co-administration with other agents with a similar side-effect profile (e.g. fluoroquinolones) therefore requires careful risk assessment. Pretomanid is used in combinations with bedaquiline for drug-resistant strains and improves the bactericidal activity of combination therapy which may enable shorter durations. Its side-effects include nerve damage, headaches, gastrointestinal upset, abnormal liver function tests, low glucose and skin rash.

Clofazimine

Clofazimine is used against M. leprae and resistant strains of M. tuberculosis. Its mode of action may involve induction of oxidative stress and it is weakly bactericidal. Oral absorption is variable and it is excreted in the bile. Side-effects include gastrointestinal upset, dry eyes and skin, and skin pigmentation, especially in those with pigmented skin.

Antifungal agents

See Box 6.25.

Azole antifungals

The azoles (imidazoles and triazoles) inhibit synthesis of ergosterol, a constituent of the fungal cell membrane. Side-effects vary but include gastrointestinal upset, hepatitis and rash. Azoles are inhibitors of cytochrome P450 enzymes, so tend to increase exposure to cytochrome P450-metabolised drugs.

Imidazoles

Miconazole, econazole, clotrimazole and ketoconazole are relatively toxic and therefore administered topically. Clotrimazole is used extensively to treat superficial fungal infections. Triazoles are used for systemic treatment because they are less toxic.

i 6.25 Antifungal agents

Agent	Usual route(s) of administration	Clinically relevant antifungal spectrum
Imidazoles		
Miconazole Econazole Clotrimazole	Topical	*Candida* spp., dermatophytes
Ketoconazole	Topical, oral	*Malassezia* spp., dermatophytes, agents of eumycetoma
Triazoles		
Fluconazole	Oral, IV	Yeasts (*Candida* and *Cryptococcus* spp.)
Itraconazole	Oral, IV	Yeasts, dermatophytes, dimorphic fungi (p. 342), *Aspergillus* spp.
Voriconazole	Oral, IV	Yeasts and most filamentous fungi (excluding mucoraceous moulds)
Posaconazole	Oral, IV	Yeasts and many filamentous fungi (including most mucoraceous moulds)
Isavuconazole	Oral, IV	Yeasts and many filamentous fungi (variable activity against mucoraceous moulds)
Echinocandins		
Anidulafungin Caspofungin Micafungin	IV only	*Candida* spp., *Aspergillus* spp. (no activity against *Cryptococcus* spp. or mucoraceous moulds)
Polyenes		
Amphotericin B	IV	Yeasts and most dimorphic and filamentous fungi (including mucoraceous moulds)
Nystatin	Topical	
Others		
5-fluorocytosine	Oral, IV	Yeasts
Griseofulvin	Oral	Dermatophytes
Terbinafine	Topical, oral	Dermatophytes

(IV = intravenous)

Triazoles

Fluconazole is effective against yeasts (*Candida* and *Cryptococcus* spp.) and has a long half-life (approximately 30 hours) and an excellent safety profile. The drug is highly water-soluble and distributes widely to all body sites and tissues, including CSF. Itraconazole is lipophilic and distributes extensively, including to toenails and fingernails. Its CSF penetration is poor. Because oral absorption of itraconazole is erratic, therapeutic drug monitoring is required. Voriconazole is well absorbed orally but variability in levels requires therapeutic drug monitoring. It is used mainly in aspergillosis. Side-effects include photosensitivity, hepatitis and transient retinal toxicity. Posaconazole and isavuconazole are broad-spectrum azoles, with activity against *Candida* spp., *Aspergillus* spp. and some mucoraceous moulds. Isavuconazole is non-inferior to voriconazole in the management of invasive aspergillosis and may be considered as an alternative when voriconazole cannot be used.

Echinocandins

The echinocandins inhibit β-1,3-glucan synthesis in the fungal cell wall. They have few significant adverse effects. Caspofungin, anidulafungin and micafungin are used to treat systemic candidosis, and caspofungin is also used in aspergillosis.

Polyenes

Amphotericin B (AmB) deoxycholate causes cell death by binding to ergosterol and damaging the fungal cytoplasmic membrane. Its use in resource-rich countries has been largely supplanted by less toxic agents. Its long half-life enables once-daily administration. CSF penetration is poor.

Adverse effects include immediate anaphylaxis, other infusion-related reactions and nephrotoxicity. Nephrotoxicity may be sufficient to require dialysis and occurs in most patients who are adequately dosed. It may be ameliorated by concomitant infusion of normal saline. Irreversible nephrotoxicity occurs with large cumulative doses of AmB.

Nystatin has a similar spectrum of antifungal activity to AmB. Its toxicity limits it to topical use, e.g. in oral and vaginal candidiasis.

Lipid formulations of amphotericin B

Lipid formulations of AmB have been developed to reduce AmB toxicity and have replaced AmB deoxycholate in many regions. They consist of AmB encapsulated in liposomes (liposomal AmB, L-AmB) or complexed with phospholipids (AmB lipid complex, ABLC). The drug becomes active on dissociating from its lipid component. Adverse effects are similar to, but considerably less frequent than, those with AmB deoxycholate, and efficacy is similar. Lipid formulations of AmB are used in invasive fungal disease, as empirical therapy in patients with neutropenic fever and also in visceral leishmaniasis.

Other antifungal agents

Flucytosine

Flucytosine (5-fluorocytosine) has particular activity against yeasts. When it is used as monotherapy, acquired resistance develops rapidly, so it should be given in combination with another antifungal agent. Adverse effects include myelosuppression, gastrointestinal upset and hepatitis.

Griseofulvin

Griseofulvin has been largely superseded by terbinafine and itraconazole for treatment of dermatophyte infections, except in children, for whom these agents remain largely unlicensed. It is deposited in keratin precursor cells, which become resistant to fungal invasion.

Terbinafine

Terbinafine distributes with high concentration to sebum and skin, with a half-life of more than 1 week. It is used topically for dermatophyte skin infections and orally for onychomycosis. The major adverse reaction is hepatic toxicity (approximately 1:50000 cases). Terbinafine is not recommended for breastfeeding mothers.

Antiviral agents

Most viral infections in immunocompetent individuals resolve without intervention. Antiviral therapy is available for a limited number of infections only (Box 6.26).

Antiretroviral agents

These agents, used predominantly against HIV, are discussed on page 366.

Anti-herpesvirus agents

Aciclovir, valaciclovir, penciclovir and famciclovir

These antivirals are acyclic analogues of guanosine, which inhibit viral DNA polymerase after being phosphorylated by virus-derived thymidine kinase (TK). Aciclovir is poorly absorbed after oral dosing; better levels are achieved intravenously or by use of the prodrug valaciclovir. Famciclovir is the prodrug of penciclovir. Resistance is mediated by viral TK or polymerase mutations.

i 6.26 Antiviral agents

Drug	Route(s) of administration	Indications	Significant side-effects
Antiretroviral therapy			
(ART, p. 366)	Oral	HIV infection (including AIDS)	CNS symptoms, anaemia, lipodystrophy
Anti-herpesvirus agents			
Aciclovir	Topical/oral/IV	Herpes zoster; Chickenpox (esp. in immunosuppressed); Herpes simplex infections: encephalitis (IV only), genital tract, oral, ophthalmic	Significant side-effects rare. Hepatitis, renal impairment and neurotoxicity reported rarely
Valaciclovir	Oral	Herpes zoster, herpes simplex	As for aciclovir
Famciclovir	Oral	Herpes zoster, herpes simplex (genital)	As for aciclovir
Penciclovir	Topical	Labial herpes simplex	Local irritation
Ganciclovir	IV	Treatment and prevention of CMV infection in immunosuppressed	Gastrointestinal symptoms, liver dysfunction, neurotoxicity, myelosuppression, renal impairment, fever, rash, phlebitis at infusion sites. Potential teratogenicity
Valganciclovir	Oral	Treatment and prevention of CMV infection in immunosuppressed	As for ganciclovir but neutropenia is predominant
Cidofovir	IV/topical	HIV-associated CMV infections and occasionally other viruses (see text)	Renal impairment, neutropenia
Foscarnet	IV	CMV and aciclovir-resistant HSV and VZV infections in immunosuppressed	Gastrointestinal symptoms, renal impairment, electrolyte disturbances, genital ulceration, neurotoxicity
Anti-influenza agents			
Zanamivir	Inhalation	Influenza A and B	Allergic reactions (very rare)
Oseltamivir	Oral	Influenza A and B	Gastrointestinal side-effects, rash, hepatitis (very rare)
Peramivir	IV, IM		
Amantadine, rimantadine	Oral	Influenza A (but see text)	CNS symptoms, nausea
Agents used in other virus infections*			
Ribavirin	Oral/IV/inhalation	Lassa fever (IV); RSV infection in infants (inhalation)	Haemolytic anaemia, cough, dyspnoea, bronchospasm and ocular irritation (when given by inhalation)
Remdesivir	IV	COVID-19 (experimental, not recommended for clinical use at the time of writing)	Significant side-effects rare

*Antiviral agents used in viral hepatitis are discussed on pages 884–890.
(AIDS = acquired immunodeficiency syndrome; CMV = cytomegalovirus; CNS = central nervous system; HIV = human immunodeficiency virus; HSV = herpes simplex virus; IM = intramuscular; IV = intravenous; RSV = respiratory syncytial virus; VZV = varicella zoster virus)

Ganciclovir

Chemical modification of the aciclovir molecule allows preferential phosphorylation by protein kinases of cytomegalovirus (CMV) and other β-herpesviruses (e.g. human herpesvirus (HHV) 6/7) and hence greater inhibition of the DNA polymerase, but at the expense of increased toxicity. Ganciclovir is administered intravenously or as a prodrug (valganciclovir) orally.

Cidofovir

Cidofovir inhibits viral DNA polymerases with potent activity against CMV, including most ganciclovir-resistant CMV. It also has activity against aciclovir-resistant herpes simplex virus (HSV) and varicella zoster virus (VZV), HHV6 and occasionally adenovirus, poxvirus, papillomavirus or polyoma virus, and may be used to treat these infections in immunocompromised hosts.

Foscarnet

This analogue of inorganic pyrophosphate acts as a non-competitive inhibitor of HSV, VZV, HHV6/7 or CMV DNA polymerase. It does not require significant intracellular phosphorylation and so may be effective when HSV or CMV resistance is due to altered drug phosphorylation. It has variable CSF penetration.

Letermovir

Letermovir is a CMV DNA terminase inhibitor that plays a role in cleavage of viral DNA for packaging into mature virions. It is available in oral and intravenous formulations. It is well tolerated and is approved for prophylaxis of CMV in allogeneic haematopoeitic stem cell transplant recipients. Gastrointestinal disturbance and drug–drug interactions occur and resistance may develop.

Anti-influenza agents

Zanamivir and oseltamivir

These agents inhibit influenza A and B neuraminidase, which is required for release of virus from infected cells (see Fig. 6.2). They are used in the treatment and prophylaxis of influenza. Administration within 48 hours of disease onset reduces the duration of symptoms by approximately 1–1½ days. In the UK, their use is limited mainly to adults with chronic respiratory or renal disease, significant cardiovascular disease, immunosuppression or diabetes mellitus, during known outbreaks. Peramivir has been developed as a distinct chemical structure, which means that it retains activity against some oseltamivir- and zanamivir-resistant strains. It has poor oral bioavailability and has been developed as an intravenous or intramuscular formulation for treatment of severe cases of influenza, e.g. in intensive care units. It is now approved for use in adults in a number of countries. An intravenous formulation of zanamivir is also in development for critically ill patients. Laninamivir is approved as an intranasal formulation in Japan.

Other anti-influenza agents

Amantidine and rimantadine inhibit viral M2 protein ion channel function, which is required for uncoating (see Fig. 6.2). Resistance is widespread, and these are only used to treat oseltamivir-resistant influenza A in patients unable to take zanamivir (e.g. ventilated patients) and when the strain is susceptible to these agents. Baloxavir marboxil inhibits a component of viral RNA synthesis. It is licensed for uncomplicated influenza but is likely to be reserved for neuraminidase-resistant strains. Faviparvir is an oral or intravenous RNA-dependent RNA polymerase that may also play a role against resistant strains of influenza but also other RNA viruses and has been studied against SARS-CoV-2.

Other agents used to treat viruses

Antiviral agents used to treat hepatitis B and C virus are discussed on pages 886 and 889, and those used against HIV-1 are described on page 366.

Remdesivir

Remdesivir is an intravenous RNA-dependent RNA polymerase inhibitor that has a broad antiviral spectrum in vitro and has decreased the time to recovery following SARS-Cov-2 infection. So far it has not demonstrated efficacy against other viruses clinically. Initial studies have not shown significant effects on SARS-CoV-2 viral replication, suggesting it may need to be used early in the course of infection before peak viral replication. The main side-effects include abnormal liver function tests and infusion reactions.

Ribavirin

Ribavirin is a guanosine analogue that inhibits nucleic acid synthesis in a variety of viruses. It is used in particular in the treatment of hepatitis C virus but also against certain viral haemorrhagic fevers, e.g. Lassa fever, although it has not been useful against Ebola virus.

Antiparasitic agents

Antimalarial agents

Artemisinin (qinghaosu) derivatives

Artemisinin originates from a herb (sweet wormwood, *Artemisia annua*), which was used in Chinese medicine to treat fever. Its derivatives, artemether and artesunate, were developed for use in malaria in the 1970s. Their mechanism of action is unknown. They are used in the treatment, but not prophylaxis, of malaria, usually in combination with other antimalarials, and are effective against strains of *Plasmodium* spp. that are resistant to other antimalarials. Artemether is lipid-soluble and may be administered via the intramuscular and oral routes. Artesunate is water-soluble and is administered intravenously or orally. Serious adverse effects are uncommon. Current advice for malaria in pregnancy is that the artemisinin derivatives should be used to treat uncomplicated *falciparum* malaria in the second and third trimesters, but should not be prescribed in the first trimester until more information becomes available.

Atovaquone

Atovaquone inhibits mitochondrial function. It is an oral agent, used for treatment and prophylaxis of malaria, in combination with proguanil (see below), without which it is ineffective. It is also employed in the treatment of mild cases of *Pneumocystis jirovecii* pneumonia, or as prophylaxis, where there is intolerance to co-trimoxazole. Significant adverse effects are uncommon.

Folate synthesis inhibitors (proguanil, pyrimethamine–sulfadoxine)

Proguanil inhibits dihydrofolate reductase and is used for malaria prophylaxis. Pyrimethamine–sulfadoxine may be used in the treatment of malaria.

Quinoline-containing compounds

Chloroquine and quinine are believed to act by intraparasitic inhibition of haem polymerisation, resulting in toxic build-up of intracellular haem.

The mechanisms of action of other agents in this group (quinidine, amodiaquine, mefloquine, primaquine, etc.) may differ. They are employed in the treatment and prophylaxis of malaria. Primaquine is used for radical cure of malaria due to *Plasmodium vivax* and *P. ovale* (destruction of liver hypnozoites). Chloroquine may also be given for extraintestinal amoebiasis.

Chloroquine can cause significant pruritus. If used in long-term, high-dose regimens, it causes an irreversible retinopathy. Overdosage leads to life-threatening cardiotoxicity. The side-effect profile of mefloquine includes neuropsychiatric effects ranging from mood change, nightmares and agitation to hallucinations and psychosis. Quinine may cause hypoglycaemia and cardiotoxicity, especially when administered parenterally. Primaquine causes haemolysis in people with glucose-6-phosphate dehydrogenase deficiency, which should be excluded before therapy. Chloroquine is considered safe in pregnancy but mefloquine should be avoided in the first trimester.

Chloroquine (and its metabolite hydroxychloroquine) exhibits in vitro activity against the virus SARS-CoV-2 but has not demonstrated clinical efficacy.

Lumefantrine

Lumefantrine is used in combination with artemether to treat uncomplicated *falciparum* malaria, including chloroquine-resistant strains. Its mechanism of action is unknown. Significant adverse effects are uncommon.

Drugs used in trypanosomiasis

The antiparasitic agents used to treat human African trypanosomiasis (HAT) and American trypanosomiasis (Chagas' disease) (benznidazole, eflornithine, fexinidazole, melarsoprol, nifurtimox, pentamidine and suramin) are discussed in detail on pages 324 and 325.

In addition to its use in HAT, pentamidine is used in leishmaniasis (p. 327) and in severe *Pneumocystis jirovecii* pneumonia, if co-trimoxazole cannot be tolerated or is ineffective. It is administered via intravenous or intramuscular routes. It is a relatively toxic drug, commonly causing rash, renal impairment, profound hypotension (especially on rapid infusion), electrolyte disturbances, blood dyscrasias and hypoglycaemia.

Other antiprotozoal agents

Pentavalent antimonials

Sodium stibogluconate and meglumine antimoniate inhibit protozoal glycolysis by phosphofructokinase inhibition. They are used parenterally (intravenous or intramuscular) to treat leishmaniasis. Adverse effects include arthralgia, myalgias, raised hepatic transaminases, pancreatitis and electrocardiogram changes. Severe cardiotoxicity leading to death is not uncommon.

Diloxanide furoate

This oral agent is used to eliminate luminal cysts following treatment of intestinal amoebiasis, or in asymptomatic cyst excreters. The drug is absorbed slowly (enabling luminal persistence) and has no effect in hepatic amoebiasis. It is a relatively non-toxic drug, the most significant adverse effect being flatulence.

Iodoquinol (di-iodohydroxyquinoline)

Iodoquinol is a quinoline derivative with activity against *Entamoeba histolytica* cysts and trophozoites. It is used orally to treat asymptomatic cyst excreters or, in association with another amoebicide (e.g. metronidazole), to treat extraintestinal amoebiasis. Long-term use of this drug is not recommended, as neurological adverse effects include optic neuritis and peripheral neuropathy.

Nitazoxanide

Nitazoxanide is an inhibitor of pyruvate–ferredoxin oxidoreductase-dependent anaerobic energy metabolism in protozoa. It is a broad-spectrum agent, active against various nematodes, tapeworms, flukes and intestinal protozoa. Nitazoxanide also has activity against some anaerobic bacteria and viruses. It is administered orally in giardiasis and cryptosporidiosis. Adverse effects are usually mild and involve the gastrointestinal tract (e.g. nausea, diarrhoea and abdominal pain).

Paromomycin

Paromomycin is an aminoglycoside that is used to treat visceral leishmaniasis and intestinal amoebiasis. It is not significantly absorbed when administered orally, and is therefore given orally for intestinal amoebiasis and by intramuscular injection for leishmaniasis. It showed early promise in the treatment of HIV-associated cryptosporidiosis but subsequent trials have demonstrated that this effect is marginal at best.

Drugs used against helminths

Benzimidazoles (albendazole, mebendazole)

These agents act by inhibiting both helminth glucose uptake, causing depletion of glycogen stores, and fumarate reductase. Albendazole is used for hookworm, ascariasis, threadworm, *Strongyloides* infection, trichinellosis, *Taenia solium* (cysticercosis) and hydatid disease. Mebendazole is used for hookworm, ascariasis, threadworm and whipworm. The drugs are administered orally. Absorption is relatively poor but is increased by a fatty meal. Significant adverse effects are uncommon.

Bithionol

Bithionol is used to treat fluke infections with *Fasciola hepatica*. It is well absorbed orally. Adverse effects are mild (e.g. nausea, vomiting, diarrhoea, rashes) but relatively common (approximately 30%).

Diethylcarbamazine

Diethylcarbamazine (DEC) is an oral agent used to treat filariasis and loiasis. Treatment of filariasis is often followed by fever, headache, nausea, vomiting, arthralgia and prostration. This is caused by the host response to dying microfilariae, rather than the drug, and may be reduced by pre-treatment with glucocorticoids.

Ivermectin

Ivermectin binds to helminth nerve and muscle cell ion channels, causing increased membrane permeability. It is an oral agent, used in *Strongyloides* infection, filariasis and onchocerciasis. Significant side-effects are uncommon.

Niclosamide

Niclosamide inhibits oxidative phosphorylation, causing paralysis of helminths. It is an oral agent, used in *Taenia saginata* and intestinal *T. solium* infection. Systemic absorption is minimal and it has few significant side-effects.

Piperazine

Piperazine inhibits neurotransmitter function, causing helminth muscle paralysis. It is an oral agent, used in ascariasis and threadworm (*Enterobius vermicularis*) infection. Significant adverse effects are uncommon but include neuropsychological reactions such as vertigo, delirium and convulsions.

Praziquantel

Praziquantel increases membrane permeability to Ca^{2+}, causing violent contraction of worm muscle. It is the drug of choice for schistosomiasis and is also used in *T. saginata*, *T. solium* (cysticercosis) and fluke infections (*Clonorchis*, *Paragonimus*) and in echinococcosis. It is administered orally and is well absorbed. Adverse effects are usually mild and transient, and include nausea and abdominal pain.

Pyrantel pamoate

This agent causes spastic paralysis of helminth muscle through a suxamethonium-like action. It is used orally in ascariasis and threadworm infection. Systemic absorption is poor and adverse effects are uncommon.

Thiabendazole

Thiabendazole inhibits fumarate reductase, which is required for energy production in helminths. It is used orally in *Strongyloides* infection and topically to treat cutaneous larva migrans. Significant adverse effects are uncommon.

Further information

Websites

cdc.gov. *Centers for Disease Control and Prevention, Atlanta, USA. Provides information on all aspects of communicable disease, including prophylaxis against malaria.*

gov.uk/government/collections/immunisation-against-infectious-disease-the-green-book. *UK Department of Health recommendations for immunisation.*

ecdc.europa.eu. *European Centre for Disease Prevention and Control. Includes data on prevalence of antibiotic resistance in Europe.*

gov.uk/government/organisations/public-health-england. *Public Health England. Provides information on infectious diseases relating mainly to England, including community infection control.*

idsociety.org. *Infectious Diseases Society of America. Publishes up-to-date, evidence-based guidelines.*

who.int. *World Health Organization. Provides up-to-date information on global aspects of infectious disease, including outbreak updates. Also has information on the 'World Antibiotic Awareness Week' campaign.*

6

S Clive
M Stares

7

Oncology

Clinical examination of the cancer patient

6 Face

Conjunctival pallor
Icterus
Horner syndrome
Cushingoid features

5 Lymph nodes (see p. 923)

Cervical
Supraclavicular
Axillary
Inguinal

4 Respiratory

Stridor
Consolidation
Pleural effusion (see p. 481)

3 Breast asymmetry, lump

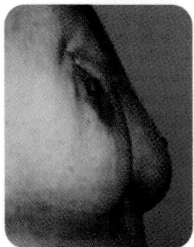

▲ Skin tethering above the nipple

2 Hands

Clubbing
Signs of smoking
Pallor

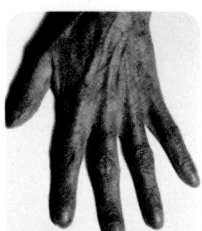

▲ Finger clubbing in lung cancer

1 Periphery

Calf tenderness, venous thrombosis
Rash, skin changes (see also p. 1065)

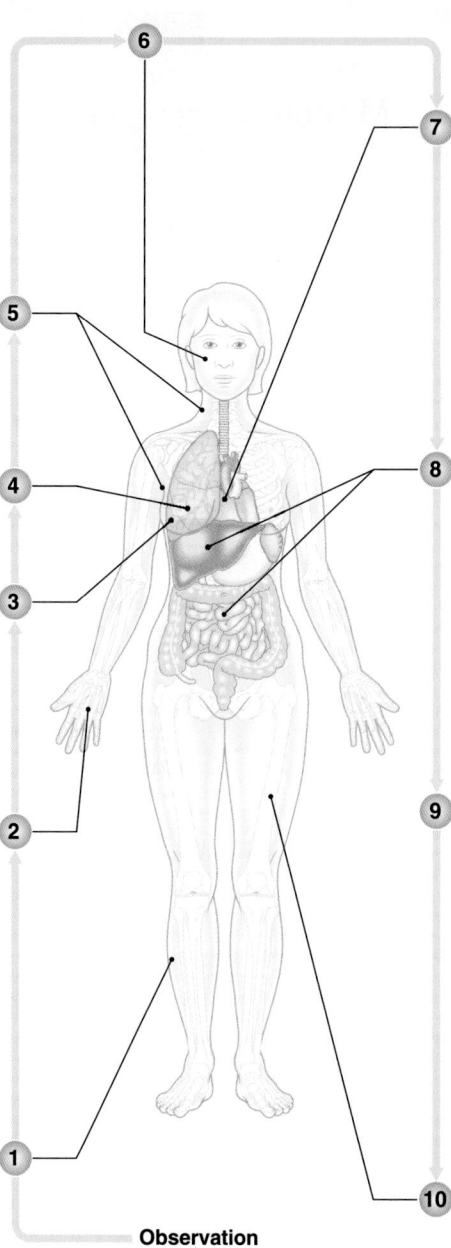

Observation
• Cachexia
• Dehydration
• Asymmetry/lumps

7 Cardiovascular

Superior vena cava obstruction (SVCO) (see Box 7.15)
Atrial fibrillation
Pericardial effusion (see Ch. 16)
Hypo-/hypertension

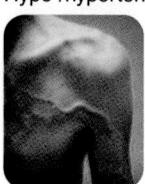

▲ SVCO in a patient with a mediastinal mass

8 Abdomen (see p. 783)

Surgical scars
Umbilical nodule
Mass in epigastrium
Visible peristalsis
Abdominal distension
Ascites
Hepatomegaly
Splenomegaly
Renal mass
Pelvic or adnexal mass

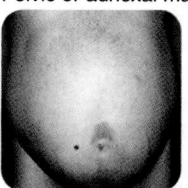

▲ Ascites (ovarian carcinoma)

9 Neurological

Focal neurological signs
Sensory deficit
Spinal cord compression
Memory deficit
Personality change

10 Skeletal survey

Focal bone tenderness (pelvis, spine, long bones)
Wrist tenderness (hypertrophic pulmonary osteoarthropathy)

Clinical examination of the patient on cancer treatment

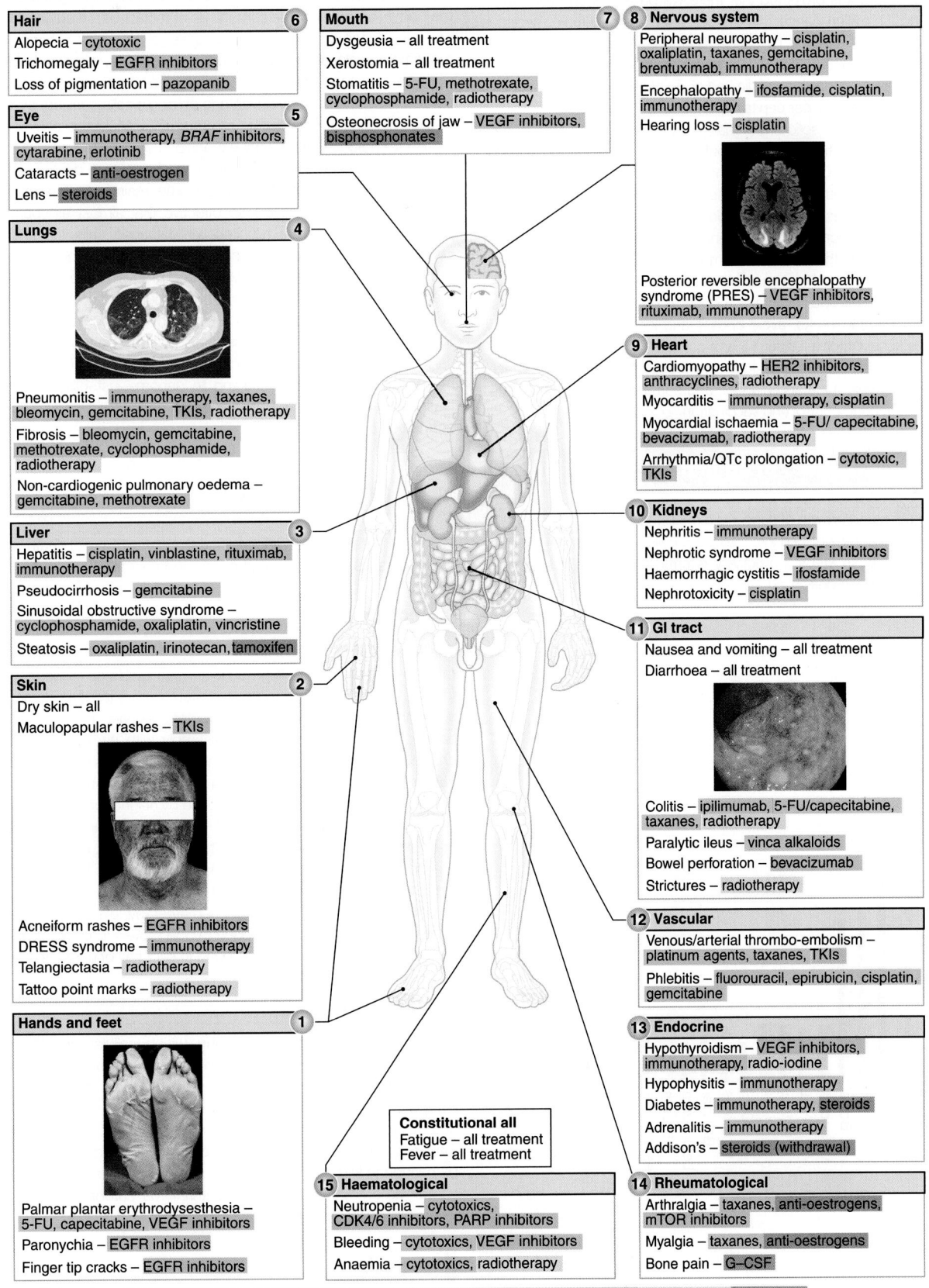

Hair 6
Alopecia – cytotoxic
Trichomegaly – EGFR inhibitors
Loss of pigmentation – pazopanib

Eye 5
Uveitis – immunotherapy, *BRAF* inhibitors, cytarabine, erlotinib
Cataracts – anti-oestrogen
Lens – steroids

Lungs 4
Pneumonitis – immunotherapy, taxanes, bleomycin, gemcitabine, TKIs, radiotherapy
Fibrosis – bleomycin, gemcitabine, methotrexate, cyclophosphamide, radiotherapy
Non-cardiogenic pulmonary oedema – gemcitabine, methotrexate

Liver 3
Hepatitis – cisplatin, vinblastine, rituximab, immunotherapy
Pseudocirrhosis – gemcitabine
Sinusoidal obstructive syndrome – cyclophosphamide, oxaliplatin, vincristine
Steatosis – oxaliplatin, irinotecan, tamoxifen

Skin 2
Dry skin – all
Maculopapular rashes – TKIs

Acneiform rashes – EGFR inhibitors
DRESS syndrome – immunotherapy
Telangiectasia – radiotherapy
Tattoo point marks – radiotherapy

Hands and feet 1

Palmar plantar erythrodysesthesia – 5-FU, capecitabine, VEGF inhibitors
Paronychia – EGFR inhibitors
Finger tip cracks – EGFR inhibitors

Mouth 7
Dysgeusia – all treatment
Xerostomia – all treatment
Stomatitis – 5-FU, methotrexate, cyclophosphamide, radiotherapy
Osteonecrosis of jaw – VEGF inhibitors, bisphosphonates

Constitutional all
Fatigue – all treatment
Fever – all treatment

Haematological 15
Neutropenia – cytotoxics, CDK4/6 inhibitors, PARP inhibitors
Bleeding – cytotoxics, VEGF inhibitors
Anaemia – cytotoxics, radiotherapy

Nervous system 8
Peripheral neuropathy – cisplatin, oxaliplatin, taxanes, gemcitabine, brentuximab, immunotherapy
Encephalopathy – ifosfamide, cisplatin, immunotherapy
Hearing loss – cisplatin

Posterior reversible encephalopathy syndrome (PRES) – VEGF inhibitors, rituximab, immunotherapy

Heart 9
Cardiomyopathy – HER2 inhibitors, anthracyclines, radiotherapy
Myocarditis – immunotherapy, cisplatin
Myocardial ischaemia – 5-FU/ capecitabine, bevacizumab, radiotherapy
Arrhythmia/QTc prolongation – cytotoxic, TKIs

Kidneys 10
Nephritis – immunotherapy
Nephrotic syndrome – VEGF inhibitors
Haemorrhagic cystitis – ifosfamide
Nephrotoxicity – cisplatin

GI tract 11
Nausea and vomiting – all treatment
Diarrhoea – all treatment

Colitis – ipilimumab, 5-FU/capecitabine, taxanes, radiotherapy
Paralytic ileus – vinca alkaloids
Bowel perforation – bevacizumab
Strictures – radiotherapy

Vascular 12
Venous/arterial thrombo-embolism – platinum agents, taxanes, TKIs
Phlebitis – fluorouracil, epirubicin, cisplatin, gemcitabine

Endocrine 13
Hypothyroidism – VEGF inhibitors, immunotherapy, radio-iodine
Hypophysitis – immunotherapy
Diabetes – immunotherapy, steroids
Adrenalitis – immunotherapy
Addison's – steroids (withdrawal)

Rheumatological 14
Arthralgia – taxanes, anti-oestrogens, mTOR inhibitors
Myalgia – taxanes, anti-oestrogens
Bone pain – G–CSF

Colour key Cytotoxic chemotherapy Hormone therapy Targeted therapy Immunotherapy Radiotherapy Supportive

(CDK = cyclin-dependent kinase; EGFR = epidermal growth factor receptor; G–CSF = granulocyte–colony stimulating factor; PARP = poly-ADP ribose polymerase; TKI = tyrosine kinase inhibitor; VEGF = vascular endothelial growth factor) *(Acneiform rashes) From Potthoff K, Hofheinz R, Hassel JC, et al. Interdisciplinary management of EGFR-inhibitor-induced skin reactions: a German expert opinion. Ann Oncol 2011; 22(3):524–535. (Colitis) From Som A, Mandaliya R, Alsaadi D, et al. Immune checkpoint inhibitor-induced colitis: A comprehensive review. World J Clin Cases 2019; 7(4):405–418.*

7

Cancer represents a significant global health, social and economic burden. In 2018 there were 17 million new cases of cancer worldwide and 9.6 million cancer deaths, making it the second leading cause of death. By 2030, it is projected that there will be 26 million new cancer cases and 17 million cancer deaths per year. The developing world is disproportionately affected by cancer and in 2018 approximately 70% of cancer deaths occurred in low- and middle-income countries. These deaths happen in countries with limited or no access to investigations or treatment and with low per capita expenditure on health care.

The most common solid organ malignancies arise in the lung, breast and gastrointestinal tract (Fig. 7.1), but the most common form worldwide is skin cancer. Cigarette smoking accounts for more than 20% of all global cancer deaths, 80% of lung cancer cases in men and 50% of lung cancer cases in women worldwide, which could be prevented by smoking cessation. Diet and alcohol contribute to a further 30% of cancers, including those of the stomach, colon, oesophagus, breast and liver. Lifestyle modification could reduce these if steps were taken to avoid animal fat and red meat, reduce alcohol, increase fibre, fresh fruit and vegetable intake, avoid obesity and increase physical activity. Infections account for a further 15% of cancers (25% of cancers in low- and middle-income countries), including those of the cervix, stomach, liver, nasopharynx, anus and bladder, and some of these could be prevented by infection control and vaccination.

The 10 hallmarks of cancer

The formation and growth of cancer is a multistep process, during which normal cells are transformed into malignant cells. Ten key characteristics that underlie these steps, collectively referred to as the *'Hallmarks of Cancer'*, have been described.

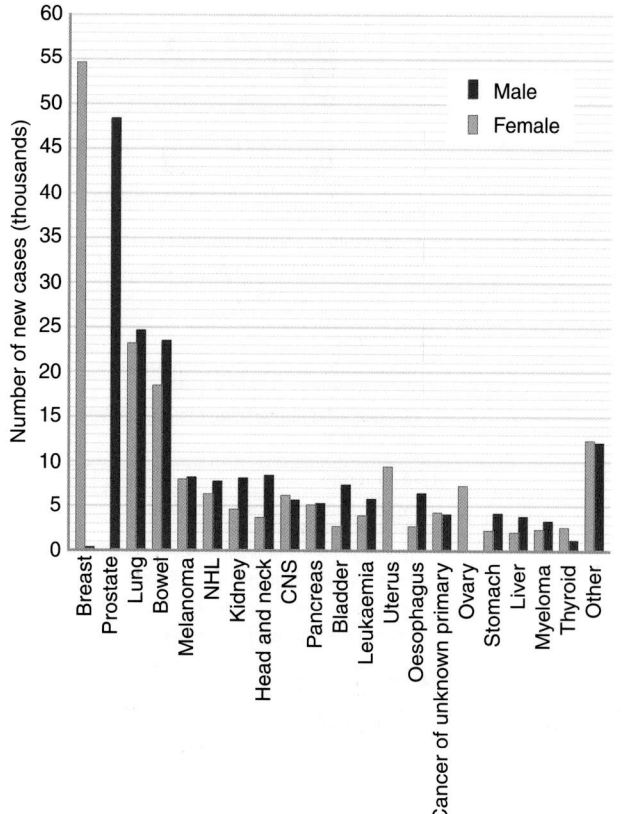

Fig. 7.1 The most commonly diagnosed cancers in the UK.
(CNS = central nervous system; NHL = non-Hodgkin lymphoma) *Statistics from Cancer Research UK website* (http://info.cancerresearchuk.org).

1. Genome instability and mutation

Random genomic aberrations occur continuously throughout all cells of the body. This may include somatic point mutations, insertions, deletions and chromosome structural changes (i.e. copy number changes, chromosomal translocations). Epigenomic aberrations, such as DNA methylation and histone modification, may also occur. Rarely, aberrations will confer a selective survival advantage on single cells, 'driving' overgrowth and dominance in local tissue environments. Multistep carcinogenesis results from successive clonal expansions of pre-malignant cells, each expansion being triggered by acquisition of a random driver aberration.

Under normal circumstances, genome maintenance systems and DNA repair mechanisms are so effective that almost all spontaneous genomic aberrations are repaired, or damaged cells are forced into senescence or apoptosis. In cancer cells, though, the accumulation of mutations can be accelerated by compromising these maintenance mechanisms. In turn, this leads to the accumulation of driver genomic aberrations which lead to cancer growth and progression. Genomic sequencing technology demonstrates that the pattern of aberrations vary dramatically between cancer types. However, defects in genome maintenance mechanisms leading to genome instability are common findings across all cancers. This enabling characteristic may lead to the acquisition of other hallmarks.

2. Resisting cell death

There are three principal mechanisms through which cell death occurs in healthy tissues: apoptosis, autophagy and necrosis.

Apoptosis

This is programmed cell death. It is frequently found at markedly reduced rates in cancers, particularly those of high grade or those resistant to treatment. The cellular apoptotic system has regulatory elements that sense intrinsic and extrinsic pro-apoptotic signals. This initiates a cascade of proteolysis and cell disassembly with nuclear fragmentation, chromosomal condensation and shrinking of the cell with loss of intercellular contact, followed by cellular fragmentation and the formation of apoptotic bodies that are phagocytosed by neighbouring cells. The most important regulator of apoptosis is the *TP53* tumour suppressor gene, often described as the 'guardian of the genome' as it is able to induce apoptosis in response to sufficient levels of genomic damage. The largest initiator of apoptosis via *TP53* is cellular injury, particularly that due to DNA damage from cytotoxic chemotherapy, oxidative damage and ultraviolet (UV) radiation. Disruption of p53 protein function as a result of mutations in the *TP53* gene are found in over half of cancers.

Autophagy

This is a catabolic process during which cellular constituents are degraded by lysosomal machinery within the cell. It is an important physiological mechanism; it usually occurs at low levels in cells but can be induced in response to environmental stresses, particularly radiotherapy and cytotoxic chemotherapy, which induce elevated levels of autophagy that are cytoprotective for malignant cells, thus impeding rather than perpetuating the killing actions of these stress situations. Severely stressed cancer cells have been shown to shrink via autophagy to a state of reversible dormancy.

Necrosis

This is the premature death of cells and is characterised by the release of cellular contents into the local tissue microenvironment, in marked contrast to apoptosis, where cells are disassembled in a step-by-step fashion and the resulting cellular fragments are phagocytosed. Necrotic cell death results in the recruitment of inflammatory immune cells, promotion of angiogenesis and release of stimulatory factors that increase cellular proliferation and tissue invasion, thereby enhancing rather than inhibiting carcinogenesis.

3. Sustaining proliferative signalling

The 'cell cycle' is tightly controlled at different stages. Normal cells grow and divide in response to external signals, typically growth factors. These are able to bind to cell surface-bound receptors that activate an intracellular tyrosine kinase-mediated signalling cascade, ultimately leading to changes in gene expression that promote cellular proliferation and growth.

The cell cycle

The cell cycle is composed of four ordered, strictly regulated phases referred to as G_1 (gap 1), S (DNA synthesis), G_2 (gap 2) and M (mitosis) (Fig. 7.2). Normal cells grown in culture will stop proliferating and enter a quiescent state called G_0 once they become confluent or are deprived of serum or growth factors. The first gap phase (G_1) prior to the initiation of DNA synthesis represents the period of commitment that separates M and S phases as cells prepare for DNA duplication. Cells in G_0 and G_1 are receptive to growth signals, but once they have passed a restriction point, they are committed to enter DNA synthesis (S phase). Cells demonstrate arrest at different points in G_1 in response to different inhibitory growth signals. Mitogenic signals promote progression through G_1 to S phase, utilising phosphorylation of the retinoblastoma gene product (pRB, p. 40). Following DNA synthesis, there is a second gap phase (G_2) prior to mitosis (M), allowing cells to repair errors that have occurred during DNA replication and thus preventing propagation of these errors to daughter cells. Although the duration of individual phases may vary, depending on cell and tissue type, most adult cells are in a G_0 state at any one time.

Stimulation of the cell cycle

Many cancer cells produce growth factors, which drive their own proliferation by a positive feedback mechanism known as autocrine stimulation.

Examples include transforming growth factor-alpha (TGF-α) and platelet-derived growth factor (PDGF). Other cancer cells express growth factor receptors at increased levels due to gene amplification or express abnormal receptors that are permanently activated. This results in abnormal cell growth in response to physiological growth factor stimulation or even in the absence of growth factor stimulation (ligand-independent signalling). The epidermal growth factor receptor (EGFR) is often over-expressed in lung and gastrointestinal tumours and the human epidermal growth factor receptor 2 (HER2)/neu receptor is frequently over-expressed in breast cancer. Both receptors activate the Ras–Raf–mitogen activated protein (MAP) kinase pathway, causing cell proliferation.

4. Evading growth suppressors

The cell cycle is orchestrated by a number of molecular mechanisms, most importantly by cyclins and cyclin-dependent kinases (CDKs). Cyclins bind to CDKs and are regulated by both activating and inactivating phosphorylation, with two main checkpoints at G_1/S and G_2/M transition. The genes that inhibit progression play an important part in tumour prevention and are referred to as tumour suppressor genes (e.g. *TP53*, *TP21*, *TP16* genes). The products of these genes deactivate the cyclin–CDK complexes and are thus able to halt the cell cycle. The complexity of cell cycle control is susceptible to dysregulation, and mutations within inhibitory proteins are common in cancer.

5. Enabling replicative immortality

Normal cells have a limited number of divisions before they are unable to divide further (senescence) or before they die (crisis). These limits are controlled by telomeric DNA sequences, which protect and stabilise chromosomal ends. During replication, telomeres shorten progressively as small fragments of telomeric DNA are lost with successive cycles of replication. This shortening process represents a mitotic clock and eventually prevents the cell from dividing further. Telomerase, a specialised polymerase enzyme, adds nucleotides to telomeres, allowing continued cell division and thus preventing premature arrest of cellular replication. The telomerase enzyme is almost absent in normal cells but is expressed at significant levels in the majority of human cancers.

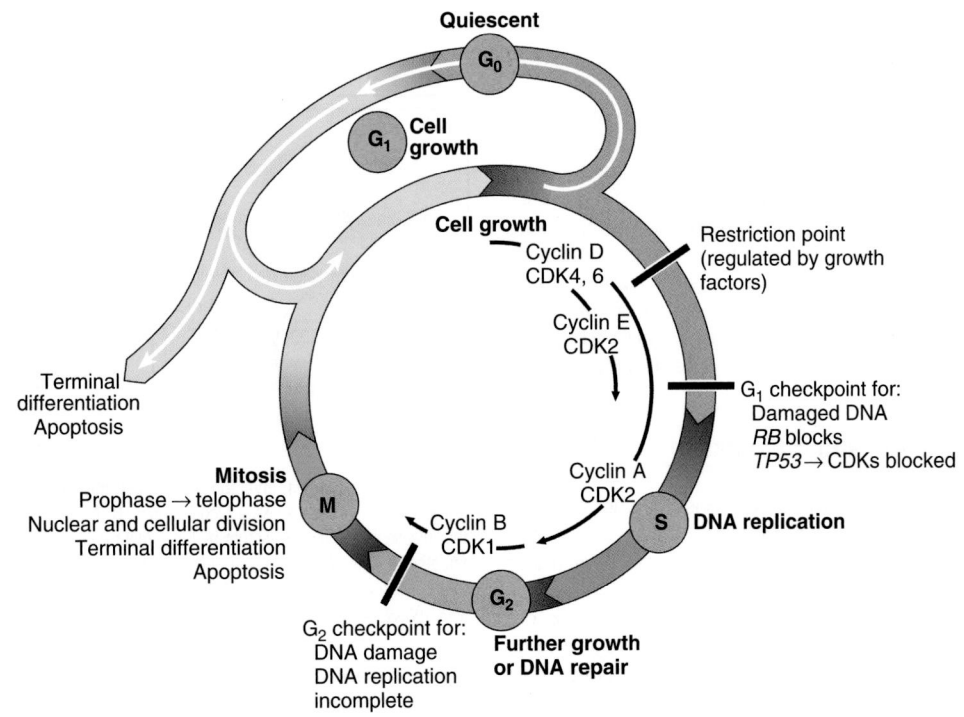

Fig. 7.2 The cell cycle and sites of action of chemotherapeutic agents. (CDK = cyclin-dependent kinase; *RB* = retinoblastoma gene)

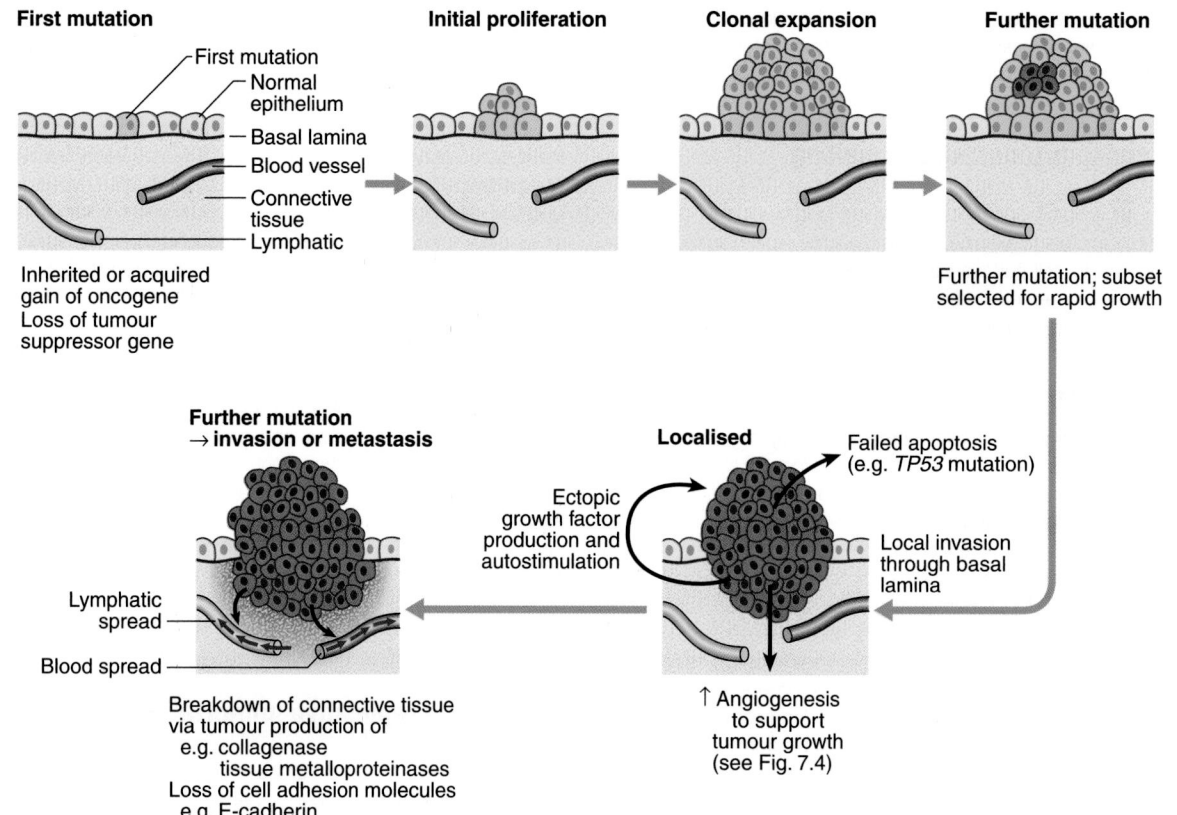

Fig. 7.3 Oncogenesis. The multistep origin of cancer, showing events implicated in cancer initiation, progression, invasion and metastasis.

6. Inducing angiogenesis

All cells and body tissues require sustenance in the form of nutrients and oxygen, as well as an ability to evacuate metabolic waste products and carbon dioxide. Tumours require a functional vascular network to ensure continued growth and are unable to grow beyond $1\,mm^3$ without stimulating the development of a vascular supply through angiogenesis (Figs. 7.3 and 7.4).

Angiogenesis is dependent on the production of angiogenic growth factors, of which vascular endothelial growth factor (VEGF) and platelet-derived growth factor (PDGF) are the best characterised. During tumour progression, an angiogenic switch is activated and remains on, causing normally quiescent vasculature to develop new vessels continually to help sustain expanding tumour growth. Angiogenesis is governed by a balance of pro-angiogenic stimuli and angiogenesis inhibitors, such as thrombospondin (TSP)-1, which binds to transmembrane receptors on endothelial cells and evokes suppressive signals. A number of cells can contribute to the maintenance of a functional tumour vasculature and therefore sustain angiogenesis. These include pericytes and a variety of bone marrow-derived cells such as macrophages, neutrophils, mast cells and myeloid progenitors.

7. Activating invasion and metastasis

The ability to invade neighbouring tissue determines whether a tumour is benign or malignant. Clinically, the presence of metastases often determines whether a cancer can be cured. The invasion-metastatic cascade is a complex multistep process. The initiation of this process is enabled by epithelial-mesenchymal transition (EMT). Cancer cells in a tumour lose normal cell–cell adhesion through the down-regulation or, occasionally, mutational inactivation of E-cadherin, a calcium-dependent cell–cell adhesion glycoprotein. After breaking through the basement membrane, cancer cells enter the blood stream (intravasation). These circulating tumour cells (CTCs) then exit the blood stream into distant tissues (extravasation) to form small nodules of cancer cells (micrometastases).

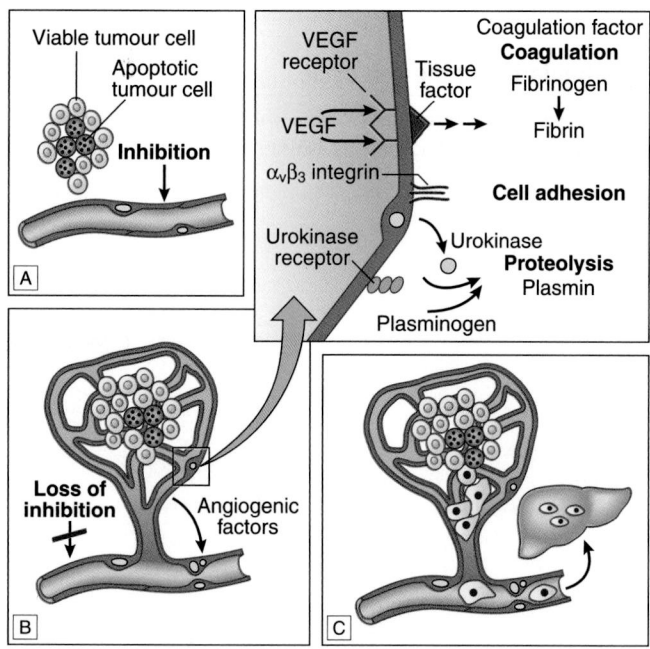

Fig. 7.4 Angiogenesis, invasion and metastasis. [A] For any cancer to grow beyond $1\,mm^3$, it must evoke a blood supply. [B] New vessel formation results from the release of angiogenic factors by the tumour cells and loss of inhibition of the endothelial cells. [C] The loss of cellular adhesion and disruption of the extracellular matrix allow cells to extravasate into the blood stream and metastasise to distant sites. (VEGF = vascular endothelial growth factor)

Following mesenchymal–epithelial transition these micrometastatic lesions develop into macroscopic tumours (colonisation) (see Fig. 7.3).

Cross-talk between cancer cells and cells of the surrounding stromal tissue is involved in the acquired capability for invasive growth and metastasis. Mesenchymal stem cells in tumour stroma have been found to secrete CCL5, a protein chemokine that helps recruit leucocytes into inflammatory sites. With the help of particular T-cell-derived cytokines (interleukin (IL)-2 and interferon-gamma (IFN-γ)), CCL5 induces proliferation and activation of natural killer cells and then acts reciprocally on cancer cells to stimulate invasive behaviour. Macrophages at the tumour periphery can foster local invasion by supplying matrix-degrading enzymes such as metalloproteinases and cysteine cathepsin proteases.

8. Deregulating cellular energetics

Under aerobic conditions, oxidative phosphorylation functions as the main metabolic pathway for energy production; cells process glucose, first to pyruvate via glycolysis and thereafter to carbon dioxide in the mitochondria. While under anaerobic conditions, glycolysis is favoured to produce adenosine triphosphate (ATP). Cancer cells can reprogram their glucose metabolism to limit energy production to glycolysis, even in the presence of oxygen. This has been termed 'aerobic glycolysis'. Up-regulation of glucose transporters, such as GLUT1, is the main mechanism through which aerobic glycolysis is achieved.

This reprogramming of energy metabolism appears paradoxical, as overall energy production from glycolysis is significantly lower (18-fold) than that from oxidative phosphorylation. One explanation may be that the increased production of glycolytic intermediates can be fed into various biosynthetic pathways, including those that generate the nucleosides and amino acids, necessary for the production of new cells.

9. Tumour-promoting inflammation

Almost all tumours show infiltration with immune cells on pathological investigation and historically this finding was thought to represent an attempt of the immune system to eradicate the cancer. It is now clear that tumour-associated inflammatory responses contribute to several hallmark capabilities and promote tumour formation and cancer progression. Immune cells may promote invasive behaviour, and bioactive molecules such as cytokines, growth factors and pro-angiogenic factors may be released into the tumour microenvironment. In particular, the release of reactive oxygen species, which are actively mutagenic, will accelerate the genetic evolution of surrounding cancer cells, enhancing growth and contributing to cancer progression.

10. Evading immune destruction

Cancer cells continuously shed antigens into the circulatory system, prompting an immune response that includes cytotoxic T-cell, natural killer cell and macrophage production. The immune system is thought to provide continuous surveillance, with resultant elimination of cells that undergo malignant transformation. However, if not all cancer cells are eliminated there may be a period of equilibrium where tumour growth is controlled by the immune system and cancer cells may enter a dormant state, sometimes for many years. Alternatively, cancer cells may escape immune control and grow into clinically apparent tumours. Several factors may contribute to immune escape, including reduced immune recognition, increased resistance or survival and the development of an immunosuppressive tumour microenvironment.

Immune checkpoints are increasingly recognised as key factors in the immune escape of tumours. These pathways are crucial for regulating the immune response to normal cells by down-regulating the immune system and promoting self-tolerance by suppressing T-cell immune activity. However, some cancers co-opt these protective mechanisms by stimulating immune checkpoint molecular targets such as the programmed cell death ligand (PD-L1), a protein that helps stop immune cells from attacking other cells in the body (see Fig. 7.12).

Environmental and genetic determinants of cancer

The majority of cancers do not have a single cause but rather are the result of a complex interaction between genetic factors and exposure to environmental carcinogens. These are often tumour type-specific but some general principles do apply.

Environmental factors

Environmental triggers for cancer have mainly been identified through epidemiological studies that examine patterns of distribution of cancers in patients in whom parameters such as age, sex, presence of other illnesses, social class, geography and diet differ. Sometimes, these give strong pointers to the molecular or cellular causes of the disease, such as the association between aflatoxin production within contaminated food supplies and hepatocellular carcinomas. For most solid cancers, however, there is evidence of a multifactorial pathogenesis, even when there is a principal environmental cause (Box 7.1).

Smoking is now established beyond all doubt as a major cause of lung cancer, but there are additional predisposing factors since not all smokers develop cancer. Similarly, most carcinomas of the cervix are related to infection with human papillomavirus (HPV subtypes 16 and 18). For carcinomas of the bowel and breast, there is strong evidence of an environmental component. For example, the risk of breast cancer in women of Far Eastern origin remains relatively low when they first migrate to a country with a Western lifestyle, but rises in subsequent generations to approach that of the resident population of the host country. The precise environmental factors that cause this change are unclear but may include diet (higher intake of saturated fat and/or dairy products), reproductive patterns (later onset of first pregnancy) and lifestyle (increased use of artificial light and shift in diurnal rhythm).

Genetic factors

A number of inherited cancer syndromes are recognised and account for 5%–10% of all cancers (Box 7.2). Their molecular basis is discussed in Chapter 3, but in general they result from inherited mutations in driver genes that regulate cell growth, cell death and apoptosis. Although carriers of these gene mutations have a greatly elevated risk of cancer, none has 100% penetrance and additional modulating factors, both genetic and environmental, are likely to be operative. Exploration of a possible genetic contribution is a key part of cancer management. It may inform anti-cancer therapy decisions in people with cancer. Patients and their family members may also benefit from screening investigations to detect cancer early, or preventative treatments such as prophylactic mastectomy in women who carry a BRCA1 or BRCA2 mutation.

Investigations

When a patient is suspected of having cancer, a full history should be taken. Attention should be paid to potential risk factors such as smoking and occupational exposures, any family history of cancer and elucidating potential complications of the disease. A thorough clinical examination is essential to identify both the primary cancer site and possible sites of metastases, and to discover any other conditions that may have a bearing on the management plan.

In order to plan the most appropriate investigations and management, information is needed on:

- the extent of disease
- the type of cancer
- the patient's fitness.

Determining the extent of disease (staging)

The extent of disease, such as how large a tumour is and if it has spread, is determined by the process of staging. It entails clinical examination, imaging (e.g. CT, MRI, PET), specialised investigations (e.g. colonoscopy, endoscopy, laparoscopy, mediastinoscopy) and, in some cases, surgery. The outcome is recorded using a standard staging classification that

i	7.1 Environmental factors that predispose to cancer

Environmental aetiology	Processes	Diseases
Occupational exposure (see 'Radiation' below)	Dye and rubber manufacturing (aromatic amines)	Bladder cancer
	Asbestos mining, construction work, shipbuilding (asbestos)	Lung cancer and mesothelioma
	Vinyl chloride (PVC) manufacturing	Liver angiosarcoma
	Petroleum industry (benzene)	Acute leukaemia
Chemicals	Cytotoxic chemotherapy (e.g. melphalan, cyclophosphamide)	Acute myeloid leukaemia
Cigarette smoking	Exposure to carcinogens from inhaled smoke	Lung, throat, oesophagus and bladder cancer
Viral infection	Epstein–Barr virus	Burkitt lymphoma and nasopharyngeal cancer
	Human papillomavirus	Cervical cancer, anal cancer, oropharyngeal cancer
	Hepatitis B and C viruses	Hepatocellular carcinoma
Bacterial infection	*Helicobacter pylori*	Gastric MALT lymphomas, gastric cancer
Parasitic infection	Liver fluke (*Opisthorchis sinensis*)	Cholangiocarcinoma
	Schistosoma haematobium	Squamous cell bladder cancer
Dietary factors	Low-roughage/high-fat content diet	Colonic cancer
	High nitrosamine intake	Gastric cancer
	Aflatoxin from contamination of *Aspergillus flavus*	Hepatocellular cancer
Obesity	Reduced physical activity, increased insulin	Colon cancer
	Increased oestrogen	Breast and endometrial cancer
Radiation	UV exposure	Basal cell carcinoma
		Melanoma
		Non-melanocytic skin cancer
	Nuclear fallout following explosion (e.g. Hiroshima, Chernobyl)	Leukaemia
		Solid tumours, e.g. thyroid
	Diagnostic exposure (e.g. CT)	Cholangiocarcinoma following Thorotrast usage
	Occupational exposure (e.g. beryllium and strontium mining)	Lung cancer
	Therapeutic radiotherapy	Medullary thyroid cancer
		Sarcoma
Inflammatory diseases	Ulcerative colitis	Colon cancer
Hormonal	Use of diethylstilbestrol	Vaginal cancer
	Oestrogens	Endometrial cancer
		Breast cancer

(CT = computed tomography; MALT = mucosa-associated lymphoid tissue; UV = ultraviolet)

allows comparisons to be made between different groups of patients. One of the most commonly used systems is the T (tumour), N (regional lymph nodes), M (metastatic sites) approach of the International Union against Cancer (UICC, see Box 7.3). For most cancers staging will define patients into having:

- *early, localised disease*, which can be cured with surgery or other localised therapy (e.g. radiotherapy or ablative therapies)
- *locally advanced disease*, which can often be cured with a combination of surgery and/or systemic anti-cancer therapy and radiotherapy
- *metastatic disease*, where the cancer has spread to distant sites, which can only rarely be cured with systemic anti-cancer therapy, radiotherapy and/or surgery.

Imaging plays a critical role in the diagnosis and staging of cancer. It is also used to determine the response to treatment. The imaging modality employed depends primarily on the site of the disease and likely patterns of spread.

Computed tomography

Computed tomography (CT) is a key investigation in cancer patients and is particularly useful in imaging the thorax and abdomen (Fig. 7.5). With modern scanners it is possible to visualise the large bowel if it is prepared (CT colonography), allowing accurate detection of colorectal cancers and adenomas ≥10 mm.

Ultrasound

Ultrasound is useful in characterising lesions within the liver, kidney, pancreas and reproductive organs. It may be used for guiding biopsies of tumours in the breast and liver. Endoscopic ultrasound is helpful in staging upper gastrointestinal and pancreatic cancers, involving a special endoscope with an ultrasound and biopsy probe attached.

Magnetic resonance imaging

Magnetic resonance imaging (MRI) has a high resolution and is the preferred technique for brain, bone and pelvic imaging. It is widely employed for the staging of rectal, cervical and prostate cancers.

Positron emission tomography

Positron emission tomography (PET) visualises metabolic activity of tumour cells and is often used in combination with CT (PET–CT) to evaluate the extent of the disease, particularly in the assessment of potential distant metastases when a radical treatment approach is being considered. Not all tumour types are 'PET-avid' and the metabolic activity of

i 7.2 Inherited cancer predisposition syndromes

Syndrome	Malignancies	Inheritance	Gene
Ataxia telangiectasia	Leukaemia, lymphoma, ovarian, gastric, brain, colon	AR	*AT*
Bloom syndrome	Leukaemia, tongue, oesophageal, colonic, Wilms' tumour	AR	*BLM*
Breast/ovarian	Breast, ovarian, colonic, prostatic, pancreatic	AD	*BRCA1, BRCA2*
Cowden syndrome	Breast, thyroid, gastrointestinal tract, pancreatic	AD	*PTEN*
Familial adenomatous polyposis	Colonic, upper gastrointestinal tract	AD	*APC, MUTYH*
Familial atypical multiple mole melanoma (FAMMM)	Melanoma, pancreas	AD	*CDKN2A (TP16)*
Fanconi anaemia	Leukaemia, oesophageal, skin, hepatoma	AR	*FACA, FACC, FACD*
Gorlin syndrome	Basal cell skin, brain	AD	*PTCH*
Hereditary diffuse gastric cancer	Diffuse gastric cancer	AD	*E-cadherin*
Hereditary non-polyposis colon cancer (HNPCC)	Colonic, endometrial, ovarian, pancreatic, gastric	AD	*MSH2, MLH1, MSH6, PMS1, PMS2*
Li–Fraumeni syndrome	Sarcoma, breast, osteosarcoma, leukaemia, glioma, adrenocortical	AD	*TP53*
Multiple endocrine neoplasia (MEN) 1	Pancreatic islet cell, pituitary adenoma, parathyroid adenoma and hyperplasia	AD	*MEN1*
MEN 2	Medullary thyroid, phaeochromocytoma, parathyroid hyperplasia	AD	*RET*
Neurofibromatosis 1	Neurofibrosarcoma, phaeochromocytoma, optic glioma	AD	*NF1*
Neurofibromatosis 2	Vestibular schwannoma	AD	*NF2*
Papillary renal cell cancer syndrome	Renal cell cancer	AD	*MET*
Peutz–Jegher syndrome	Colonic, ileal, breast, ovarian	AD	*STK11*
Prostate cancer	Prostate	AD	*HPC1*
Retinoblastoma	Retinoblastoma, osteosarcoma	AD	*RB1*
von Hippel–Lindau syndrome	Haemangioblastoma of retina and CNS, renal cell, phaeochromocytoma	AD	*VHL*
Wilms' tumour	Nephroblastoma, neuroblastoma, hepatoblastoma, rhabdomyosarcoma	AD	*WT1*
Xeroderma pigmentosum	Skin, leukaemia, melanoma	AR	*XPA, XPC, XPD (ERCC2), XPF*

(AD = autosomal dominant; AR = autosomal recessive; CNS = central nervous system)

small but malignant lymph nodes may not be detected, limiting the sensitivity of PET-CT.

Biochemical markers

Many cancers produce substances called tumour markers, some of which may assist in diagnosis, response evaluation and detection of relapse. Unfortunately, most tumour markers are neither sufficiently sensitive nor sufficiently specific to be used in isolation for diagnosis and need to be interpreted in the context of other clinical features. Some can be used for antibody-directed therapy or imaging, where they have a greater role in diagnosis. Tumour markers in routine use are outlined in Box 7.4.

Establishing the type of cancer

In most cases a biopsy is required in order to establish the tumour type. Biopsies can be taken at endoscopy, laparoscopy, surgery or by ultrasound- or CT- guided biopsy with the help of interventional radiology. At times a diagnosis can be obtained by examination of cells (cytology) from fluid (e.g. pleural or peritoneal), from a smear (e.g. cervical) or by doing fine needle aspiration of a palpable or visible lump (Box 7.5).

i 7.3 TNM classification

Extent of primary tumour*

TX	Not assessed
T0	No tumour
T1	
T2	Increase in primary tumour size or
T3	depth of invasion
T4	

Increased involvement of nodes*

NX	Not assessed
N0	No nodal involvement
N1	
N2/3	Increases in involvement

Presence of metastases

MX	Not assessed
M0	Not present
M1	Present

*Exact criteria for size and region of nodal involvement have been defined for each anatomical site.

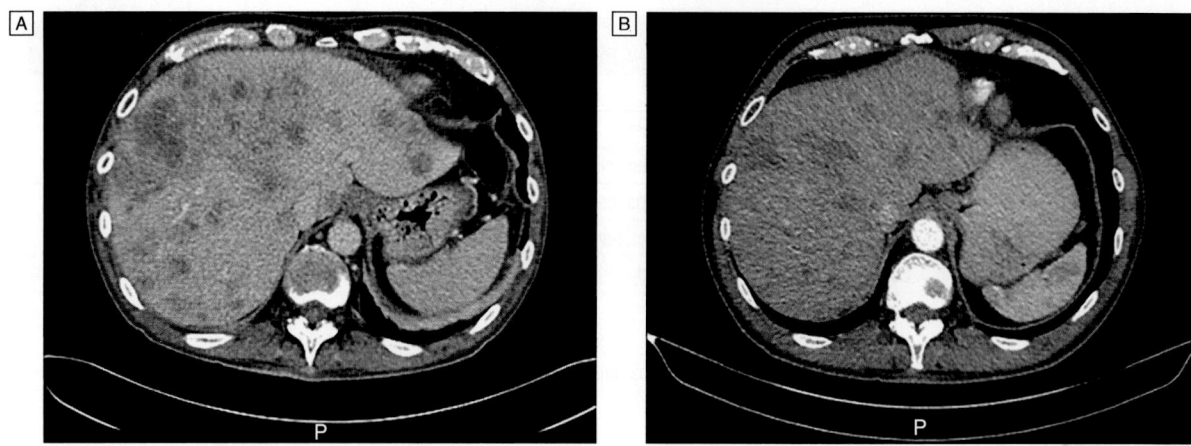

Fig. 7.5 Computed tomography (CT) images. A Extensive liver metastases in a patient with a high-grade neuro-endocrine cancer of unknown primary. B Repeat imaging after cytotoxic chemotherapy showing a partial radiological response to treatment. These remain stable 9 years later.

7.4 Commonly used serum tumour markers

Name	Natural occurrence	Tumours
Alpha-fetoprotein (AFP)	Glycoprotein found in yolk sac and fetal liver tissue. Transient elevation in liver diseases. Has a role in screening during pregnancy for the detection of neural tube defects and Down syndrome	Ovarian non-seminomatous germ cell tumours (80%), testicular teratoma (80%), hepatocellular cancer (50%)
Beta-2-microglobulin	A human leucocyte antigen (HLA) common fragment present on surface of lymphocytes, macrophages and some epithelial cells. Can be elevated in autoimmune disease and renal glomerular disease	Non-Hodgkin lymphoma, myeloma
Calcitonin	32-amino-acid peptide from C cells of thyroid. Used to screen for MEN 2	Medullary cell carcinoma of thyroid
Cancer antigen 125 (CA-125)	Differentiation antigen of coelomic epithelium (Müller's duct). Raised in any cause of ascites, pleural effusion or heart failure. Can be raised in inflammatory conditions	Ovarian epithelial cancer (75%), gastrointestinal cancer (10%), lung cancer (5%) and breast cancer (5%)
CA-19.9	A mucin found in epithelium of fetal stomach, intestine and pancreas. It is eliminated exclusively via bile and so any degree of cholestasis can cause levels to rise	Pancreatic cancer (80%), mucinous tumour of the ovary (65%), gastric cancer (30%), colon cancer (30%)
Carcinoembryonic antigen (CEA)	Glycoprotein found in intestinal mucosa during embryonic and fetal life. Elevated in smokers, cirrhosis, chronic hepatitis, ulcerative colitis, pneumonia	Colorectal cancer, particularly with liver metastasis, gastric cancer, breast cancer, lung cancer, mucinous cancer of the ovary
Human chorionic gonadotrophin (hCG)	Glycoprotein hormone, 14 kD α subunit and 24 kD β subunit from placental syncytiotrophoblasts. Used for disease monitoring in hydatidiform mole and as the basis of a pregnancy test	Choriocarcinoma (100%), hydatidiform moles (97%), ovarian non-seminomatous germ cell tumours (50%–80%), seminoma (15%)
Placental alkaline phosphatase (PLAP)	Isoenzyme of alkaline phosphatase	Seminoma (40%), ovarian dysgerminoma (50%)
Prostate-specific antigen (PSA)	Glycoprotein member of human kallikrein gene family. PSA is a serine protease that liquefies semen in excretory ducts of prostate. Can be elevated in benign prostatic hypertrophy and prostatitis	Prostate cancer (95%)
Thyroglobulin	Matrix protein for thyroid hormone synthesis in normal thyroid follicles	Papillary and follicular thyroid cancer
(MEN = multiple endocrine neoplasia)		

Histopathology

Histopathological analysis of tumour tissue is pivotal in identifying the type of cancer and provides information that may direct subsequent management. The results of histopathological analysis are most informative when combined with knowledge of the clinical picture; biopsy results should therefore be reviewed and discussed within the context of a multidisciplinary team meeting.

Light microscopy

Examination of tumour samples by light microscopy remains the core method of cancer diagnosis and, in cases where the primary site is unclear, may give clues to the origin of the tumour:

- Signet-ring cells favour a gastric primary.
- Presence of melanin favours melanoma.

- Ensure the patient is in a comfortable position with the lesion accessible to the operator.
- Identify the tumour, confirm that it is easily palpable and make sure there are no nearby critical structures.
- If tumour is not palpable or concern about nearby critical structures then perform FNA under ultrasound guidance.
- Clean the skin over the lesion.
- Inject local anaesthetic (if required) into the skin over the lesion.
- Label glass slide(s) and have ready near to the patient.
- Immobilise the lesion between thumb and forefinger of one hand.
- Introduce needle (usually with syringe attached) into lesion with the other hand.
- When the needle tip is at the edge of the lesion, apply negative pressure by pulling on the syringe and continue to enter the lesion.
- Make multiple rapid passes through the lesion, varying the angles if necessary.
- Stop sampling if blood is seen in the syringe hub as blood reduces the quality of the sample.
- Release the negative pressure while the needle is still in the lesion.
- Withdraw the needle and expel the cellular material from the needle onto the labelled glass slide(s) for pathological evaluation.

i 7.6 Eastern Cooperative Oncology Group (ECOG) performance status scale

0	Fully active, able to carry on all usual activities without restriction and without the aid of analgesics
1	Restricted in strenuous activity but ambulatory and able to carry out light work or pursue a sedentary occupation. This group also contains patients who are fully active, as in grade 0, but only with the aid of analgesics
2	Ambulatory and capable of all self-care but unable to work. Up and about more than 50% of waking hours
3	Capable of only limited self-care, confined to bed or chair more than 50% of waking hours
4	Completely disabled, unable to carry out any self-care and confined totally to bed or chair

 7.7 Cancer in old age

- **Incidence**: around 50% of cancers occur in the 15% of the population aged over 65 years.
- **Screening**: women over 65 in the UK are not invited to breast cancer screening but can request it. Uptake is low despite increasing incidence with age.
- **Presentation**: may be later for some cancers. When symptoms are non-specific, patients (and their doctors) may initially attribute them to age alone.
- **Life expectancy**: an 80-year-old woman can expect to live 8 years, so cancer may still shorten life and an active approach remains appropriate.
- **Prognosis**: histology, stage at presentation and observation for a brief period are better guides to outcome than age.
- **Rate of progression**: malignancy may have a more indolent course. This is poorly understood but may be due to reduced effectiveness of angiogenesis with age, inhibiting the development of metastases.
- **Response to treatment**: equivalent to that in younger people – well documented for a range of cancers and for surgery, radiotherapy, cytotoxic chemotherapy and hormonal therapy.
- **Toxicity of treatment**: may be greater due to subclinically reduced baseline hepatic, renal and bone marrow function and reduced baseline energy.
- **Treatment selection**: chronological age is of minor importance compared to comorbid illness and patient choice. Although older patients can be treated effectively and safely, aggressive intervention is not appropriate for all. Symptom control may be all that is possible or desired by the patient.

- Mucin is common in gut/lung/breast/endometrial and ovarian cancers.
- Psammoma bodies are a feature of ovarian cancer (mucin +) and thyroid cancer (mucin –).

Immunohistochemistry

Immunohistochemical (IHC) staining for tumour markers can provide useful diagnostic information and may help with treatment decisions. Commonly used examples of IHC in clinical practice include:

- Oestrogen (ER) and progesterone (PR) receptor positivity indicate that the cancer may be sensitive to hormonal manipulation.
- Alpha-fetoprotein (AFP) and human chorionic gonadotrophin (hCG) favour germ-cell tumours.
- Prostate-specific antigen (PSA) favours prostate cancer.
- Cytokeratins and epithelial membrane antigen (EMA) favour epithelial carcinomas.
- HER2 receptor positivity in breast or gastric cancers indicate that the tumour may respond to HER2 inhibitor targeted therapy.
- T-cell receptor and cluster designation (CD) antigen expression aid in the diagnosis and classification of lymphomas.

Molecular pathology

Molecular profiling of individual tumours is used to better understand their clinical behaviour and to stratify treatment options. Treatment selection is increasingly tailored to specific 'druggable' molecular pathways which include:

- *EGFR* mutations – predict response to EGFR inhibitor targeted therapy in lung cancer
- *RAS* mutations – predict resistance to EGFR inhibitor targeted therapy in colon cancer
- *ALK* fusion oncogene rearrangement – predict response to ALK inhibitor targeted therapy in lung cancer
- microsatellite instability – predict response to checkpoint inhibitor immunotherapy in several cancer types

Cytogenetic analysis

Some tumours demonstrate typical chromosomal changes that help in diagnosis. The utilisation of fluorescent in situ hybridisation (FISH) techniques can be useful in Ewing's sarcoma and peripheral neuro-ectodermal tumours where there is a translocation between chromosome 11 and 22: t(11;22)(q24;q12). In some cases, gene amplification can be detected via FISH (e.g. determining over-expression of HER2/neu).

Assessing fitness

When making decisions about investigations and management in patients with cancer it is important to consider an individual's general condition and comorbidities. The Eastern Cooperative Oncology Group (ECOG) performance status (PS) scale is used to formally assess a patient's fitness (Box 7.6). Outcomes for patients with PS 3–4 are worse in almost all malignancies than for those with PS 0–2, and this has a strong influence on the approach to treatment in the individual patient. Additionally, outcomes are typically worse for patients with a low albumin and raised inflammatory markers (i.e. white blood cell count, C-reactive protein). Comorbidities also frequently influence treatment options. For example, hepatic or renal dysfunction means some systemic therapies cannot be used or can only be given in lower doses. In some patients poor fitness or comorbidities may preclude any anti-cancer therapy options, in which case comprehensive diagnostic and staging investigations add little clinical value and may not be in the best interests of the patient.

Although the incidence of cancer increases with patient age, the approach to investigation and management is similar at all ages (Box 7.7). However, assessing fitness in this group of patients can be difficult, with increasing comorbidity and declining physiological reserve in particular placing patients at increased risk of treatment toxicity. Geriatric assessment tools to assess patient fitness and toxicity risks have been developed.

Multidisciplinary teams

The multidisciplinary team (MDT) is well established in oncology and meets on a regular basis to discuss patient progress and provide a forum for patient-centred, interdisciplinary communication to coordinate care and decision-making. It is a platform on which individual clinicians can discuss complex cases or situations and draw on the collective experience of the team membership to decide on the best approach for an individual patient. This can be particularly important when discussing patients with a rare condition or in an unusual situation. As a minimum, most MDTs include a radiologist, pathologist, specialist physician, specialist surgeon, radiation oncologist, medical oncologist, nurse specialist, auditor and scheduler. Additional staff may be relevant to different MDTs, e.g. dermatologists in skin cancer MDTs, dieticians in upper gastrointestinal cancer MDTs, stoma nurses in colorectal cancer MDTs, palliative care doctors in pancreatic cancer or cancer of unknown primary (CUP) MDTs. Specific roles of the MDT are outlined in Box 7.8.

Acute oncology

Cancer centres are usually based in cities and have busy radiotherapy and systemic anti-cancer therapy units containing specialist equipment and teams of highly trained physicians, surgeons, nurses, pharmacists, radiographers, physicists and support workers amongst others. Most patients with cancer undergo investigations, assessments and treatment as outpatients. However, patients may present acutely to any specialty in any hospital with a new cancer, cancer-related symptoms, emergency complications of cancer or with treatment-related toxicities.

Acute presentation of new cancer

Despite cancer screening initiatives, most patients still present with symptomatic disease. They may have symptoms related to the local effect of a primary tumour or metastatic deposit, such as finding a lump, dysphagia or persistent pain. These are sometimes called 'red flag' symptoms of cancer (Box 7.9). Patients may present with constitutional symptoms such as unexplained weight loss, fatigue or fevers. Paraneoplastic syndromes due to the production of biologically active hormones by the tumour, or as the result of an immune response to the tumour, may also be the presenting symptom of new cancer (Box 7.10). The pattern of

i 7.9 Red flag symptoms of malignancy

Symptom	Typical site or possible tumour
Lump	Breast, lymph node (any site), testicle
Skin abnormality	Melanoma, basal cell carcinoma
Bleeding	Stomach, colon, lung, endometrium, bladder, kidney
Dysphagia, odynophagia	Oesophagus, bronchus, gastric, head and neck
Change in bowel habit	Colon, rectum, ovary
Cough, hoarseness, stridor	Lung, head and neck, thyroid
Bone pain or fracture	Bone (primary sarcoma, secondary metastasis from breast, prostate, bronchus, thyroid, kidney)
Abdominal swelling (ascites)	Ovary, stomach, pancreas
Unexplained weight loss, anorexia	Lung, gastrointestinal tract, CUP
Unexplained fatigue	Any

(CUP = cancer of unknown primary)

i 7.10 Paraneoplastic syndromes

Feature	Common cancer site associations
Lambert–Eaton myasthenic syndrome	Small cell lung cancer
Subacute cerebellar degeneration	Small cell lung cancer, ovarian cancer
Encephalomyelitis	Small cell lung cancer
Retinopathy	Non-small cell lung cancer
Dermatomyositis/polymyositis	Gastric, lung cancer
Acanthosis nigricans	Gastric, oesophageal cancer
Vitiligo	Melanoma
Pruritus	Lymphoma, leukaemia, central nervous system tumours
Pemphigus	Lymphoma, Kaposi's sarcoma, thymic
Dermatitis herpetiformis	Enteropathy-associated T-cell lymphoma (EATL)

symptoms, detailed clinical history and examination will most often direct the initial investigations and early referral to the appropriate specialist multidisciplinary team.

Cancer of unknown primary (CUP)

When a patient is found to have advanced or metastatic cancer but history, examination and imaging is unable to define a primary cancer site, an assessment of patient fitness, disease extent, comorbidities and patient wishes should be made. Selected investigations should be carried out (Box 7.11). However, a primary cancer site does not need to be 'hunted down' in all patients and investigations should be limited to those that will help management. Specialist investigations (e.g. endoscopies) are only indicated when there is radiological suspicion or if there are localising symptoms.

In some cases, such as those with clinical suspicion of germ cell tumours, high-grade lymphoma or small cell cancer, or those presenting with oncological emergencies, urgent referral directly to oncology or haematology is essential to allow rapid initiation of anti-cancer therapy, sometimes before investigations are completed (Fig. 7.6).

If patients are fit to undergo investigations and fit enough to be considered for treatment then a core biopsy of the most accessible metastatic

7.11 Initial diagnostic tests in patients presenting with carcinoma of unknown primary

- Detailed medical history and examination, including breast, nodal areas, skin, genital, rectal and pelvic regions
- Full blood count, urea and electrolytes, renal function, liver function tests, albumin, calcium, urinalysis, lactate dehydrogenase, CRP
- Myeloma screen (if lytic bone lesions)
- CT scan of chest, abdomen and pelvis
- CT neck if thyroid lump or neck nodes
- Histological examination by biopsy, with immunohistochemistry and/or molecular pathology if required
- Upper or lower gastrointestinal endoscopy if gastrointestinal symptoms
- Mammography and/or breast MRI for women with axillary nodes or adenocarcinoma
- Breast MRI for women with adenocarcinoma limited to axillary nodes
- Testicular ultrasound (if midline disease in young man or clinical features suggest germ cell tumour)
- Naso-endoscopy for squamous neck nodes
- PET scan for single-site disease or squamous neck nodes with no primary on endoscopic evaluation
- Tumour markers: prostate-specific antigen (PSA) in men with bone lesions, cancer antigen 125 (CA-125) in women with peritoneal malignancy or ascites, α-fetoprotein (AFP) in liver-limited disease, α-fetoprotein (AFP) and human chorionic gonadotrophin (hCG) in midline disease in young men

(CRP = C-reactive protein; CT = computed tomography; MRI = magnetic resonance imaging; PET = positron emission tomography)

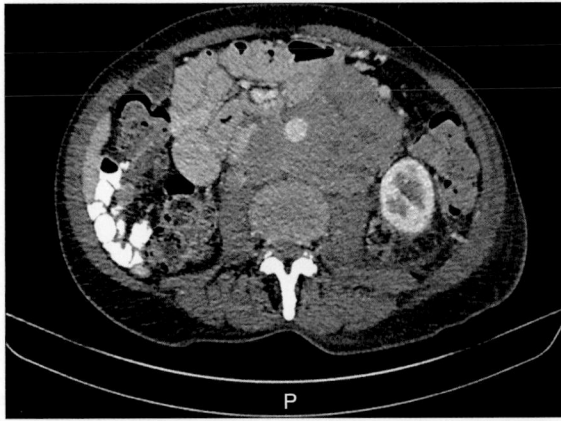

Fig. 7.6 Young male patient presenting with a bulky midline tumour and elevated hCG and AFP suggestive of a non-seminomatous testicular cancer.

lesion is usually the quickest way of obtaining tissue for pathological evaluation of cancer type. Review of tumour morphology, immunohistochemistry and molecular pathology will usually be sufficient to plan appropriate treatment. Patients with clinico-pathological features suggestive of a particular cancer should be identified early and referred promptly to the appropriate multidisciplinary/oncology team for consideration of further investigations and treatment. Where the primary site remains unclear following comprehensive investigations, a patient is said to have a cancer of unknown primary (CUP).

Whilst it is crucial to identify patients with highly treatable CUPs (Box 7.12), some of whom can live for years (see Fig. 7.5), or even be cured by treatment, most CUPs are poorly differentiated cancers or adenocarcinomas with liver and/or multi-site metastases. These cancers often behave aggressively so early discussion with oncology, within the context of a specialist MDT, is essential to streamline investigations and assess fitness for anti-cancer treatment. Whilst responses to generic systemic anti-cancer treatment are modest, gene expression tests or molecular tumour profiling are increasingly providing greater information about likely tissue of origin or possible treatment targets which may ultimately lead to improved understanding of CUP and better outcomes.

7.12 Cancer of unknown primary – favourable clinicopathological features

Clinicopathological features	Management
Women with serous papillary adenocarcinoma of the peritoneal cavity	Treat like ovarian cancer
Women with isolated adenocarcinoma of axillary lymph nodes	Treat like breast cancer
Men with poorly differentiated carcinoma with midline distribution	Treat like germ cell cancer
Poorly differentiated neuro-endocrine carcinoma of unknown origin	Treat like small cell cancer
Well-differentiated neuro-endocrine tumour (NET)	Treat with somatostatin analogues or as per NETs of known primary sites
Squamous cell carcinoma of non-supraclavicular cervical lymph nodes	Treat like head and neck squamous cell cancer
Adenocarcinoma with a colorectal-IHC profile (CK20+, CK7−, CDX2+)	Treat like colon cancer
Men with blastic bone metastases or elevated prostate-specific antigen (adenocarcinoma)	Treat like prostate cancer
Isolated inguinal adenopathy squamous carcinoma	Treat like anogenital squamous cancer
Patients with one small, potentially resectable tumour	Assess for surgical resection

Metastatic malignant disease of undefined primary origin (MUO)

Patients who present as emergencies to hospital with symptomatic new metastatic cancer often have a short prognosis. Features associated with poor prognosis, irrespective of subsequent diagnosis, include: poor performance status (PS 3–4), requirement for hospital admission, bulky or multi-organ metastatic disease, significant comorbidity, raised LDH, raised inflammatory markers and low albumin. Further investigations, including biopsy, may not be warranted and honest conversations about palliative care and end-of-life planning are often preferable. Appropriate analgesia, palliative radiotherapy (for bleeding or pain) and interventional/surgical palliation can all help improve symptoms.

Oncological emergencies

Oncological emergencies are a group of potentially life-threatening conditions that occur as a direct result of cancer or its treatment. Positive outcomes depend upon prompt recognition and implementation of appropriate management.

Malignant spinal cord compression

Malignant spinal cord compression complicates 5% of cancers and is most common in myeloma, prostate, breast and lung cancers that most frequently involve bone. Malignant spinal cord compression often results from posterior extension of a vertebral body mass but intrathecal spinal cord metastases can cause similar signs and symptoms. The thoracic region is most commonly affected (Fig. 7.7).

Clinical features

The earliest sign is back pain, often rapidly worsening or in a 'band', most marked on coughing and lying flat. Subsequently, sensory changes develop in dermatomes below the level of compression, and motor weakness distal to the block occurs. Finally, sphincter disturbance, causing urinary retention and bowel incontinence, is observed.

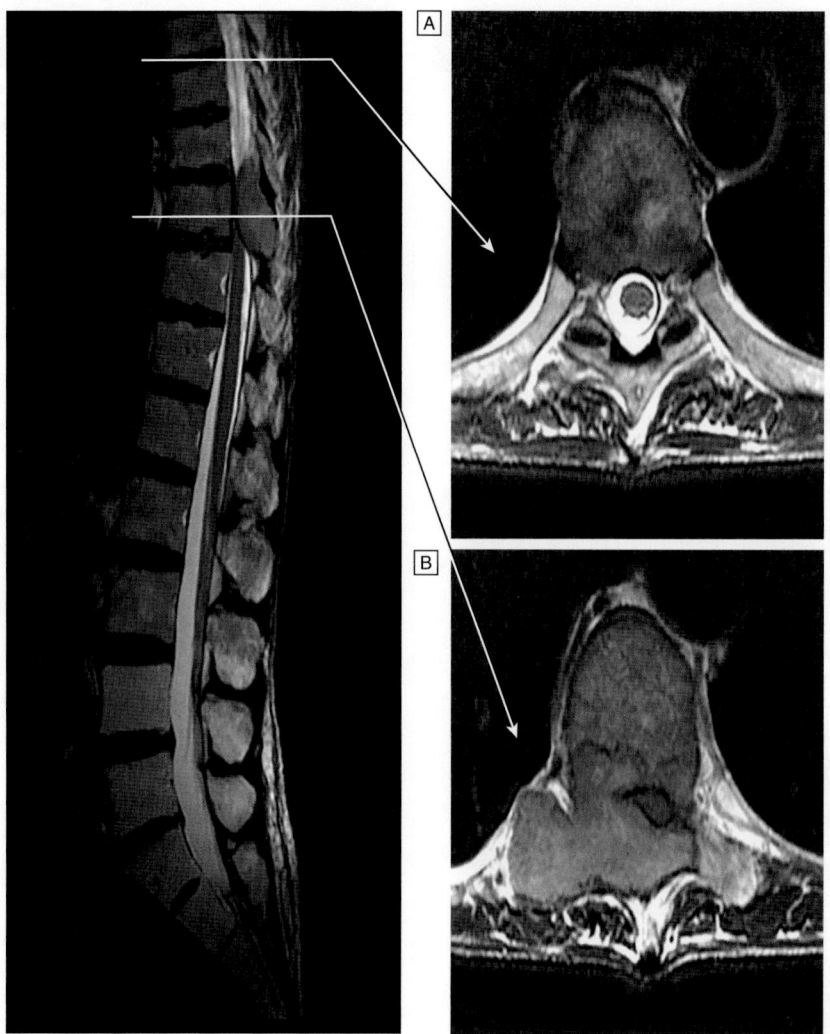

Fig. 7.7 MRI images of patient presenting with back pain and lower limb neurological disturbance. **A** Normal appearances of spinal cord. **B** Metastatic disease arising from thoracic vertebra compressing spinal cord.

i 7.13 Comparison of features of neurological deficit

Clinical feature	Spinal cord	Conus medullaris	Cauda equina
Weakness	Symmetrical and profound	Symmetrical and variable	Asymmetrical, may be mild
Reflexes	Increased (or absent) knee and ankle reflexes with extensor plantar reflex	Increased knee reflex, decreased ankle reflex, extensor plantar reflex	Decreased knee and ankle reflexes with flexor plantar reflex
Sensory loss	Symmetrical, sensory level	Symmetrical, saddle distribution	Asymmetrical, radicular pattern
Sphincters	Late loss	Early loss	Often spared
Progression	Rapid	Variable	Variable

Involvement of the lumbar spine may cause conus medullaris or cauda equina compression (Box 7.13). Physical examination findings consistent with an upper motor neuron lesion, but lower motor neuron findings, may predominate early on or in cases of nerve root or cauda equina compression.

Management

Malignant spinal cord compression is a medical emergency and should be treated with analgesia and high-dose glucocorticoid therapy (Box 7.14). Neurosurgical intervention produces superior outcomes and survival compared to radiotherapy alone, and should be considered first for all patients. It is the preferred treatment if there is a single site of disease, low volume metastatic disease, if a biopsy is required to make a diagnosis or if it is a treatable cancer (e.g. lymphoma, breast cancer). Radiotherapy is used for the remaining patients and selected tumour

✚ 7.14 Management of suspected spinal cord compression

- Confirm diagnosis with urgent MRI scan of whole spine
- Administer high-dose glucocorticoids:
    Dexamethasone 16 mg IV or oral stat
    Dexamethasone 8 mg twice daily orally
- Ensure adequate analgesia
- Refer for surgical decompression or urgent radiotherapy

(IV = intravenous; MRI – magnetic resonance imaging)

types when the cancer is likely to be radiosensitive. The prognosis varies considerably, depending on tumour type, but the degree of neurological dysfunction at presentation is the strongest predictor of outcome, irrespective of the underlying diagnosis. Mobility can be preserved in more than 80% of patients who are ambulatory at presentation, but neurological function is seldom regained in patients with established deficits such as paraplegia.

Superior vena cava obstruction

Superior vena cava obstruction (SVCO) is a common complication of cancer that can occur through extrinsic compression or intravascular blockage. The most common causes of extrinsic compression are lung cancer, lymphoma and metastatic tumours (Fig. 7.8). Patients with cancer can also develop SVCO due to intravascular blockage in association with a central catheter or thromboembolism secondary to the tumour.

Clinical features

The classical presentation is with breathlessness, oedema of the arms and face, distended neck and arm veins and dusky skin coloration over the chest, arms and face. Collateral vessels may develop over a period of weeks and the flow of blood in the collaterals helps to confirm the diagnosis. Headache secondary to cerebral oedema arising from the back-flow pressure may also occur and tends to be aggravated by bending forwards, stooping or lying down. The severity of symptoms is related to the rate of obstruction and the development of a venous collateral circulation. Accordingly, symptoms may develop rapidly or gradually. Clinical features are summarised in Box 7.15.

Investigations and management

The investigation of choice is a CT scan of the thorax to confirm the diagnosis and distinguish between extra- and intravascular causes.

A biopsy should be obtained when the tumour type is unknown because tumour type has a major influence on treatment. CT of the

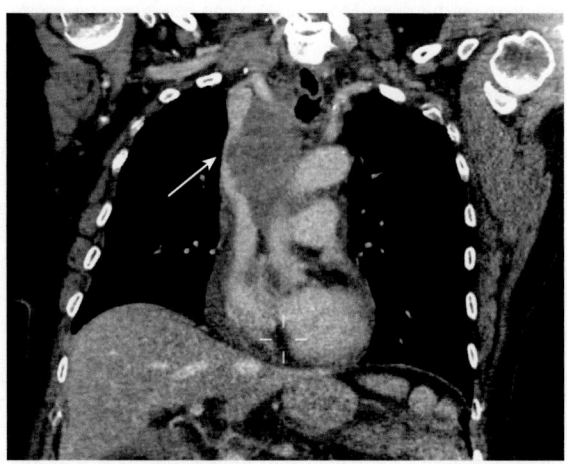

Fig. 7.8 Computed tomography (CT) image of extrinsic compression of the superior vena cava by a small cell lung cancer (arrow) performed as part of investigations for an acute presentation of cancer.

7.15 Common symptoms and physical findings in superior vena cava obstruction*

Symptoms

- Dyspnoea (63%)
- Facial swelling and head fullness (50%)
- Cough (24%)
- Arm swelling (18%)
- Chest pain (15%)
- Dysphagia (9%)

Physical findings

- Venous distension of neck (66%)
- Venous distension of chest wall (54%)
- Elevated, non-pulsatile jugular venous pulse (66%)
- Facial oedema (46%)
- Cyanosis (20%)
- Plethora of face (19%)
- Oedema of arms (14%)

*Percentage of patients affected.

head may be indicated if cerebral oedema is suspected. Tumours that are exquisitely sensitive to cytotoxic chemotherapy, such as germ cell tumours and lymphoma, can be treated with cytotoxic chemotherapy alone. For most other patients with symptomatic SVCO, SVC stenting provides the best outcomes although mediastinal radiotherapy may also be considered. Where possible, these measures should be followed by treatment of the primary tumour, as long-term outcome is strongly dependent on the prognosis of the underlying cancer.

Neutropenic fever

Neutropenia is a common complication of malignancy. It is usually secondary to cytotoxic chemotherapy but may occur with radiotherapy, if large amounts of bone marrow are irradiated, and some targeted therapy agents; it may also be a component of pancytopenia due to malignant infiltration of the bone marrow. After cytotoxic chemotherapy neutropenic fever is most commonly defined as a single oral temperature of $\geq 38.3°C$ or a temperature of $\geq 38°C$ sustained for over 1 hour in a patient with a neutrophil count of $<0.5 \times 10^9/L$ (or $<1.0 \times 10^9/L$ if the nadir is anticipated to drop to $<0.5 \times 10^9/L$ in the next 48 hours). The risk of sepsis is greater with profound neutropenia (neutrophil count $<0.1 \times 10^9/L$), prolonged neutropenia (<0.5 neutrophils for ≥ 7 days) or a rapid rate of decline in neutrophils as well as the presence of other risk factors, such as intravenous cannulae or urinary catheters. Neutropenic fever is an emergency in cancer patients as, if left untreated, it can result in sepsis with a high mortality rate.

Clinical features

The typical presentation is with high fever, and affected patients may feel non-specifically unwell. If patients have been taking paracetamol or steroids then fever or symptoms may be masked. Examination is usually unhelpful in defining a primary source of the infection. Hypotension is an adverse prognostic feature and may progress to systemic circulatory shutdown and organ failure.

Investigations and management

An infection screen should be performed, including blood cultures (both peripheral and from central lines), urine culture, chest X-ray and swabs for culture (throat, central line, wound). High-dose intravenous antibiotics should be commenced (ideally within 1 hour of admission) for all febrile patients on systemic anti-cancer therapy, without awaiting test results. The standard approach is to commence empirical broad-spectrum antibiotics according to local hospital policies agreed with microbiologists and based on local antibiotic resistance patterns. Depending on the patient's MASCC risk index score (Box 7.16) and likely organisms this

7.16 MASCC* risk index score for neutropenic fever

Characteristic	Score
Burden of current illness	
No or mild symptoms (normal function)	5
Moderate symptoms (uncomfortable or influences daily activities)	3
Severe symptoms (significant discomfort or limits daily activities)	0
No hypotension (systolic BP > 90 mmHg)	5
No chronic obstructive pulmonary disease	4
Solid tumour or lymphoma with no previous fungal infection	4
No dehydration requiring parenteral fluids	3
Outpatient at onset of fever	3
Age <60 years	2
Score ≥21 = low risk febrile neutropenia Score <21 = high risk febrile neutropenia	

*Multinational Association of Supportive Care in Cancer.

may be either monotherapy (e.g. piperacillin–tazobactam or meropenem) or combination therapy (e.g. with the addition of gentamicin if high risk on MASCC score, metronidazole if anaerobic infection is suspected, or vancomycin/teicoplanin where Gram-positive infection is suspected). Antibiotics should be adjusted according to culture results, although these are often negative. If there is no clinical improvement after 36–48 hours antibiotics should be reviewed with microbiological advice, and antifungal cover should be considered (e.g. fluconazole or liposomal amphotericin B). Granulocyte–colony-stimulating factor (G–CSF) can be used to hasten neutrophil recovery in some patients with febrile neutropenia, in line with local guidelines. Other supportive therapy, including intravenous fluids, oxygen, inotrope therapy, ventilation or haemofiltration, may be required.

Hypercalcaemia of malignancy

Hypercalcaemia is the most common metabolic disorder in patients with cancer and has a prevalence of up to 20% in cancer patients. The incidence is highest in myeloma and breast cancer (approximately 40%), intermediate in non-small cell lung cancer, and uncommon in colon, prostate and small cell lung carcinomas. It is most commonly due to over-production of PTHrP (80%), which binds to the PTH receptor and elevates serum calcium by stimulating osteoclastic bone resorption and increasing renal tubular reabsorption of calcium. Direct invasion of bone by metastases accounts for around 20% of cases while other mechanisms, such as ectopic PTH secretion, are rare.

Clinical features

The symptoms of hypercalcaemia are often non-specific and may mimic those of the underlying malignancy. They include drowsiness, delirium, nausea and vomiting, constipation, polyuria, polydipsia and dehydration.

Investigations and management

The diagnosis is made by measuring serum total calcium and adjusting for albumin. It is especially important to correct for albumin in cancer because hypoalbuminaemia is common and total calcium values under-estimate the level of ionised calcium. The principles of management are outlined in Box 7.17.

Patients should initially be treated with intravenous 0.9% saline to improve renal function and increase urinary calcium excretion. This alone often results in clinical improvement. Concurrently, intravenous bisphosphonates should be given to inhibit bone resorption. Calcitonin acts rapidly to increase calcium excretion and to reduce bone resorption, and can be combined with fluid and bisphosphonate therapy for the first 24–48 hours in patients with life-threatening hypercalcaemia. Bisphosphonates will usually reduce the serum calcium levels to normal within 5 days, but, if not, treatment can be repeated. The duration of action is up to 4 weeks and repeated therapy can be given at 3–4-weekly intervals in the outpatient department. Hypercalcaemia is frequently a sign of tumour progression and the patient requires further investigation to establish disease status and review the anti-cancer treatment strategy.

Immune-related adverse events

Immunotherapy has revolutionised the treatment of many cancers (see 'Immunotherapy' below). Checkpoint inhibitor immunotherapy, in particular, is now widely used in the treatment of many different cancers. Side-effects of checkpoint inhibitor immunotherapy agents occur when the immune system is stimulated to attack healthy cells and tissues in the body. These immune-related adverse events (IRAEs) are increasingly being recognized as oncological emergencies.

Clinical features

Almost any body system may be affected, but inflammation of the colon, endocrine organs (thyroid, adrenal and pituitary glands) lungs, liver, skin and nervous system are most frequently seen (see p. 129). IRAEs may occur at any point in a patient's treatment, or even after they have stopped receiving the checkpoint inhibitor immunotherapy agent.

Investigations and management

Investigation and management of IRAEs requires a multidisciplinary approach including oncologists and relevant system specialists. Specialist investigations may be required depending on the body system affected. The focus of treatment is on dampening the immune response, often using high-dose steroids. Additional immunosuppressant therapies are sometimes required. In the case of endocrine organ inflammation, replacement of deficient hormones is also important. In patients who experience severe IRAEs, checkpoint inhibitor immunotherapy treatment will usually be permanently discontinued. In other cases, and in patients with endocrine IRAEs who commence replacement hormone therapy, it may be possible to reintroduce checkpoint inhibitor immunotherapy treatment.

Tumour lysis syndrome

The acute destruction of a large number of cells can be associated with metabolic sequelae and is called tumour lysis syndrome. It is usually related to bulky, chemosensitive disease, including lymphoma, leukaemia and germ cell tumours. More rarely, it can occur spontaneously.

Clinical features

Cellular destruction results in the release of potassium, phosphate, nucleic acids and purines that can cause transient hypocalcaemia, hyperphosphataemia, hyperuricaemia and hyperkalaemia. This can lead to acute impairment of renal function and the precipitation of uric acid crystals in the renal tubular system. These can manifest with symptoms associated with multiple underlying electrolyte abnormalities, including fatigue, nausea, vomiting, cardiac arrhythmia, heart failure, syncope, tetany, seizures and sudden death.

Investigations and management

Serum biochemistry should be monitored regularly for 48–72 hours after treatment in patients at risk. Elevated serum potassium may be the earliest biochemical marker but pre-treatment serum lactate dehydrogenase (LDH) correlates with tumour bulk and may indicate increased risk. Good hydration and urine output should be maintained throughout treatment administration. Prophylaxis with allopurinol should be considered and recombinant urate oxidase (rasburicase) can be used to reduce uric acid levels when other treatments fail. Adequate hydration is vital, as it has a dilution effect on the extracellular fluid, improving electrolyte imbalance, and increases circulating volume, improving filtration in the kidneys. In high-risk patients, hydration and rasburicase should be commenced 24 hours before the start of treatment. If normal treatment methods fail to correct the problems, haemodialysis should be considered at an early stage to prevent progression to irreversibility.

Other acute presentations in oncology

Venous thromboembolism

Venous thromboembolism (VTE) is the second leading cause of death amongst patients with cancer. Malignancy is a strong risk factor for

---

7.17 Medical management of severe hypercalcaemia

- IV 0.9% saline 2–4 L/day
- Zoledronic acid 4 mg IV *or* pamidronate 60–90 mg IV
- For patients with severe, symptomatic hypercalcaemia that is refractory to zoledronic acid, denosumab (initial dose 60 mg SC, with repeat dosing based on response) is an alternative option

(IV = intravenous; SC = subcutaneous)

VTE and may be the first presenting feature of an underlying cancer. Several mechanisms lead to a prothrombotic state in cancer. This includes the ability of cancer cells to produce procoagulant/fibrinolytic substances and inflammatory cytokines and the physical interaction between tumour cells and blood (monocytes, neutrophils, platelets) or endothelial cells. Anti-cancer therapy (i.e. surgery, cytotoxic chemotherapy, hormone therapy and radiotherapy) and any in-dwelling access devices (i.e. central venous catheters) further increase the risk. As in patients without cancer, the management of cancer-associated VTE primarily involves anticoagulation therapy. However, the choice of therapy must take into account bleeding risk and possible interactions with anti-cancer therapies and their side-effects, such as thrombocytopenia. In patients with metastatic cancer, anticoagulation therapy will often be lifelong.

Ectopic hormone production

Some cancers are associated with metabolic abnormalities due to ectopic production of hormones by tumour cells, including insulin, ACTH, vasopressin (antidiuretic hormone, ADH), fibroblast growth factor (FGF)-23, erythropoietin and parathyroid hormone-related protein (PTHrP). This can result in a wide variety of presentations, as summarised in Box 7.18.

Neurological paraneoplastic syndromes

These form a group of conditions associated with cancer that are thought to be due to an immunological response to the tumour that results in damage to the nervous system or muscle (see Box 7.10). The cancers most commonly implicated are those of the lung, pancreas, breast, prostate, ovary and lymphoma. Many are associated with specific detectable immune biomarkers such as antibodies to pre-synaptic calcium channels (Lambert–Eaton syndrome), anti-Hu antibodies (encephalomyelitis) and anti-Yo or anti-Tr antibodies (cerebellar degeneration). However, these are not always specific and negative results do not exclude the diagnosis. The management of these syndromes is multidisciplinary and includes treatment of the underlying cancer itself and treatment of the syndrome primarily with immunosuppressive agents.

Cutaneous manifestations of cancer

Cancers can present with skin manifestations that are not due to metastases (see Box 7.10). The clinical features and management of these skin conditions are discussed in Chapter 27.

i	7.18 Ectopic hormone production by tumours	
Hormone	**Consequence**	**Tumours**
ACTH	Cushing's syndrome	SCLC
Erythropoietin	Polycythaemia	Kidney, HCC, cerebellar haemangioblastoma, uterine fibroids
FGF-23	Hypophosphataemic osteomalacia	Mesenchymal tumours
PTHrP	Hypercalcaemia	NSCLC (squamous cell), breast, kidney
Vasopressin (ADH)	Hyponatraemia	SCLC

(ACTH = adrenocorticotrophic hormone; ADH = antidiuretic hormone; FGF = fibroblast growth factor; HCC = hepatocellular carcinoma; NSCLC = non-small cell lung cancer; PTHrP = parathyroid hormone-related protein; SCLC = small cell lung cancer)

Symptoms from locally advanced cancer or metastatic sites

Metastatic disease is the major cause of death in cancer patients and the principal cause of morbidity. For the majority of patients with metastatic disease the goal of treatment is to control cancer, maintain quality of life, treat symptoms and prolong life (i.e. 'palliative treatment'). Patients of PS 3–4 (Box 7.6) or with low albumin plus high inflammatory markers often have a limited prognosis irrespective of anti-cancer treatments. Systemic anti-cancer therapies have resulted in improved survival for many cancers so that some patients live a good quality life for many years with metastatic cancer. Treatment of a solitary metastasis or highly treatable cancers (e.g. germ cell) can be curative.

Brain metastases

Brain metastases occur in 10%–30% of adults and 6%–10% of children with cancer and are an increasingly important cause of morbidity. Cancers of lung, breast, melanoma and gastrointestinal tract most commonly metastasise to the brain. Most involve the brain parenchyma but can also affect the meninges, cranial nerves, the blood vessels and other intracranial structures. In cases of solitary metastasis to the brain, the use of surgery followed by adjuvant radiotherapy, or alternatively stereotactic radiotherapy, has been shown to increase survival in patients whose disease is otherwise controlled. Outcomes for patients with more advanced brain metastases depends on the primary cancer, extent of extracranial disease and what systemic treatment options are available. For patients with advanced untreatable cancer and multiple brain metastases, prognosis is often short. Glucocorticoids can improve symptoms, particularly where there is evidence of peri-lesional oedema. In treatable cancers whole brain radiotherapy can allow steroid dose to be reduced whilst systemic therapy is used to treat the remaining cancer. With improved systemic therapies, including targeted therapies and immunotherapy, some patients are now living for several years with brain metastases.

Clinical features

Presentation is with headaches and nausea (40%–50%), focal neurological dysfunction (20%–40%), cognitive dysfunction (35%), seizures (10%–20%) and papilloedema (<10%).

Investigations and management

The diagnosis can be confirmed by CT or contrast-enhanced MRI. Treatment options include high-dose glucocorticoids for tumour-associated oedema (dexamethasone 4–12 mg daily depending on amount of oedema), anticonvulsants for seizures, whole-brain radiotherapy and systemic anti-cancer therapy. Surgery may be considered for single sites of disease and can be curative; stereotactic radiotherapy may also be considered for solitary site involvement or where surgery is more difficult or not possible.

Lung metastases

Lung metastases are common in breast cancer, colon cancer, renal cancer, sarcoma and tumours of the head and neck. The presentation is usually with a lesion on chest X-ray or CT. Solitary lesions require investigation, as single metastases can be difficult to distinguish from a primary lung tumour. Patients with two or more pulmonary nodules can be assumed to have metastases. The approach to treatment depends on the extent of disease in the lung and elsewhere. For solitary lesions, surgery should be considered, with a generous wedge resection, or radiofrequency ablation if available. Radiotherapy and systemic anti-cancer therapies can be used, dependent on the underlying primary cancer diagnosis (Fig. 7.9).

Liver metastases

Metastatic cancer in the liver can represent the sole or life-limiting component of disease for many with colorectal cancer, ocular melanoma,

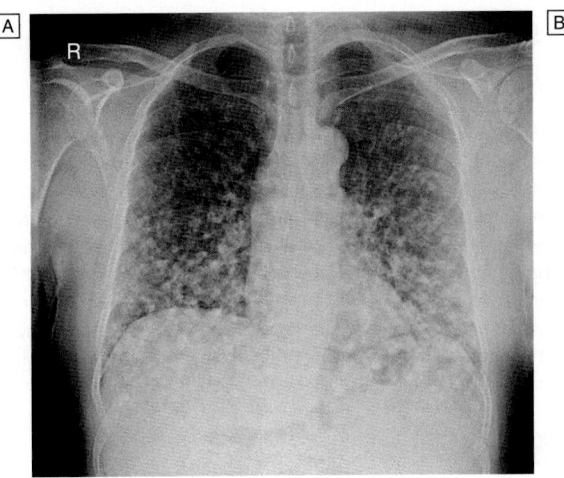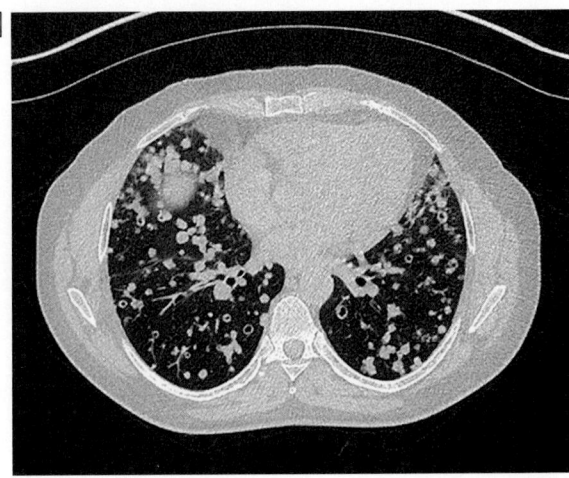

Fig. 7.9 [A] Chest X-ray and [B] computed tomography (CT) images of diffuse metastatic lung lesions in a symptomatic patient.

neuro-endocrine tumours (NETs) and, less commonly, other tumour types. The most common clinical presentations are with right upper quadrant pain due to stretching of the liver capsule, jaundice, deranged liver function tests or an abnormality detected on imaging. In selected cases, resection of the metastasis can be contemplated. In colorectal cancer, successful resection of metastases improves 5-year survival from 3% to 30%–40%. Other techniques, such as chemoembolisation, radiofrequency ablation or microwave ablation, can also be used, provided the number and size of metastases remain small. If these are not feasible, symptoms may respond to systemic anti-cancer therapy (Fig. 7.5).

Bone metastases

Bone is the third most common organ involved by metastasis, after lung and liver. Bone metastases are a major clinical problem in patients with myeloma and breast or prostate cancers, but other tumours that commonly metastasise to bone include those of the kidney and thyroid. Bone metastases are increasingly seen in other tumour types that do not classically target bone, due to effective anti-cancer treatments prolonging survival of patients with many cancers. Accordingly, effective management of bony metastases has become a focus in the treatment of patients with many incurable cancers.

Clinical features

The main presentations are with pain, pathological fractures, spinal cord compression (see above) and hypercalcaemia. Pain tends to be progressive and worst at night, and may be partially relieved by activity, but subsequently becomes more constant in nature and is exacerbated by movement. Most pathological fractures occur in metastatic breast cancer (53%); other tumour types associated with fracture include the kidney (11%), lung (8%), thyroid (5%), lymphoma (5%) and prostate (3%).

Investigations and management

The most sensitive way of detecting bone metastases is by isotope bone scan. This can have false-positive results in healing bone, particularly as a flare response following treatment and false-negative results occur in multiple myeloma due to suppression of osteoblast activity. Plain X-ray films or MRI scans are therefore preferred for any sites of bone pain, as lytic lesions may not be detected by a bone scan. In patients with a single lesion, it is especially important to perform a biopsy to obtain a tissue diagnosis, since primary bone tumours may look very similar to metastases on X-ray. The main goals of management are:

- pain relief
- preservation and restoration of function

- skeletal stabilisation
- local tumour control (e.g. relief of tumour impingement on normal structure).

Surgical intervention may be warranted where there is evidence of skeletal instability (e.g. anterior or posterior spinal column fracture) or an impending fracture (e.g. a large lytic lesion on a weight-bearing bone with more than 50% cortical involvement). Intravenous bisphosphonates (pamidronate, zoledronic acid or denosumab) are widely used for bone metastases and are effective at improving pain and in reducing further skeletal related events, such as fractures and hypercalcaemia. In certain types of cancer, such as breast and prostate, hormonal therapy may be effective. Radiotherapy, in the form of external beam therapy or systemic radionuclides (strontium treatment), can also help pain. In some settings (e.g. breast carcinoma), systemic anti-cancer therapy may be used in the management of bony metastases.

Malignant pleural effusion

This is a common complication of cancer and 40% of all pleural effusions are due to malignancy. The most common causes are lung and breast cancers, and the presence of an effusion indicates incurable disease. The presentation may be with dyspnoea, cough or chest discomfort, which can be dull or pleuritic in nature. Diagnosis and management of pleural effusion is discussed on page 494.

Investigations and management

Pleural aspirate is the key investigation and may show the presence of malignant cells. Malignant effusions are commonly blood-stained and are exudates with a raised fluid to serum LDH ratio (> 0.6) and a raised fluid to serum protein ratio (>0.5). Treatment should focus on palliation of symptoms and be tailored to the patient's physical condition, treatment options and prognosis. Aspiration alone may be an appropriate treatment in frail patients with a limited life expectancy. Those who present with malignant pleural effusion as the initial manifestation of breast cancer, small cell lung cancer, germ cell tumours or lymphoma should have the fluid aspirated and should be given systemic anti-cancer therapy to try to treat disease in the pleural space. Treatment options for patients with recurrent pleural effusions include pleurodesis, implanted drainage catheters, pleurectomy and pleuroperitoneal shunt.

Other common symptoms

Other symptoms that commonly arise from metastatic cancer are: gastrointestinal obstruction, malignant abdominal ascites, hydronephrosis and cancer cachexia.

Treatment-related toxicities

Whilst most anti-cancer therapies cause some side-effects, most of these can be managed with supportive medicines at home. Some patients will develop severe toxicities and an acute assessment will be needed. Examination of the patient on anti-cancer treatment (p. 128) should consider the type of anti-cancer treatment, duration since the last treatment and other concurrent toxicities. Patients on anti-cancer therapy can deteriorate quickly and prompt assessment and management is required. There may be specific management protocols to help manage treatment-related toxicities and advice should be sought from the patient's cancer centre or acute oncology team.

Therapeutics in oncology

Anti-cancer therapy may be used with either curative or palliative intent, and this distinction influences the approach to management of individual patients. The goal of treatment should be recorded in the medical notes.

- *Curative therapy* is given with the aim of achieving complete remission. Surgery to remove all macroscopic disease is most frequently the primary curative intervention. However, in some circumstances radiotherapy, systemic anti-cancer therapy or a combination of these may be used with curative, or radical, intent.
- *Adjuvant therapy* is additional therapy given after the primary curative intervention to lower the risk of disease recurrence. Radiotherapy and/or systemic anti-cancer therapy may be given after surgery with the intention of eradicating any micrometastatic disease that remains.
- *Neoadjuvant therapy* is additional therapy given prior to the primary curative intervention. Systemic anti-cancer therapy may be administered prior to planned surgery. The principal aim is to lower the risk of disease recurrence. Any reduction in the volume of disease, or 'downstaging', may also allow less extensive surgery, increase the likelihood of successful debulking and improve subsequent surgical morbidity. Direct evaluation of the surgical specimen allows assessment of the effectiveness of neoadjuvant therapies, guiding subsequent management and lending this approach to translational research.
- *Palliative therapy* is primarily used to treat patients with metastatic disease, or where curative treatment is not possible. The goal is to control cancer, with the aim of improving or maintaining quality of life, treating and preventing symptoms and improving survival. The choice of therapy depends on the clinical situation and a careful evaluation of the risks and benefits of the intervention.

Surgical treatment

Surgery has a pivotal role in the management of cancer. It is the main curative management of most solid cancers. In early localised cases of colorectal, breast and lung cancer, cure rates are high with surgery. There is evidence that outcome is related to surgical expertise, and most multi-disciplinary teams include surgeons experienced in the management of a particular cancer. There are some cancers for which surgery is one of two or more options for primary management, and the role of the MDT is to recommend appropriate treatment for an individual patient. Examples include prostate and transitional cell carcinoma of the bladder, in which radiotherapy and surgery may be equally effective. Specialised surgical, or interventional radiology techniques may also be employed with curative intent. Radiofrequency ablation, microwave ablation or cryotherapy may be used to treat small renal cell carcinomas or hepatocellular carcinomas. Surgery has less of a role in lymphoma, high-grade neuro-endocrine tumours or small cell cancer, where systemic anti-cancer therapy is the main treatment used.

Surgical procedures are often the quickest and most effective way of palliating symptoms in patients with metastatic disease. Examples include the treatment of faecal incontinence with a defunctioning colostomy; fixation of pathological fractures; decompression of spinal cord compression; and the treatment of fungating skin lesions by 'toilet' surgery. Debulking cytoreductive surgery may improve survival in some cancers, including renal cell carcinoma and ovarian cancer. In very selected cases, such as patients with oligometastatic disease, resection of metastases may improve survival and reduce the need for other therapies.

Radiotherapy

Radiotherapy (radiation therapy) involves treating the cancer with ionising radiation such as X-rays, gamma rays, electrons or charged atoms. Ionising radiation kills cancer cells by two mechanisms; directly damaging cancer DNA or indirectly by triggering the formation of very reactive molecules (free radicals) that also damage cancer DNA.

Two main types of radiation therapy exist: external beam radiotherapy, and brachytherapy (internal radiotherapy). External beam radiotherapy is most commonly delivered by a linear accelerator, which produces electron or photon beams. As normal tissues can also be damaged by radiotherapy, treatments are planned to ensure maximum exposure of the tumour and minimal exposure of surrounding normal tissues. Improved localisation of the target volume, or tumour, can be achieved by the use of surgical clips at the site of resection and fusion of radiotherapy-planning CT scans with diagnostic MRI or PET-CT scans. Treatment-planning software controls the size and shape of the beam. Intensity modulated radiotherapy (which allows for more homogeneous dose distribution), and volumetric radiotherapy (in which the shape of the radiation beam is designed to closely fit the tumour), have largely replaced conventional methods that use a limited number of square or rectangular beams. Stereotactic radiotherapy is a highly targeted method to deliver focused radiation beams from many different angles which converge on the tumour to deliver high doses precisely. Proton therapy uses a cyclotron to produce beams of high-energy protons, which deposit their radiation dose by a means that allows further sparing of normal tissues.

Brachytherapy, or internal radiation therapy, involves the direct application of a radioactive source onto or into a tumour. This allows the delivery of a high, localised dose of radiation. Brachytherapy is a common treatment for cancers of the prostate, uterus and cervix. Most commonly, an applicator device is used to deliver a radioactive source to the tumour for a set time, typically 10–20 minutes. In other cases, such as in prostate cancer, small radioactive seeds may be permanently placed, releasing radiation slowly over several months. Radioactive liquid treatments, such as ^{223}radium for bone metastases from prostate cancer or ^{131}iodine for thyroid cancers are other examples of internal radiation therapy.

Biological differences between normal and tumour tissues are exploited to obtain therapeutic benefit. Fundamental to this is fractionation, which entails delivering the radiation as a number of small doses on a daily basis. This allows normal cells to recover from radiation damage but recovery occurs to a lesser degree in malignant cells. Fractionation regimens vary depending on the tumour being treated, the total radiation dose to be delivered and the intent of treatment. Curative, or radical treatments typically deliver a higher overall dose in 20–35 fractions over 4–7 weeks. For palliative treatments a smaller dose given over 1–10 fractions is usually adequate. Malignant tissues vary widely in their sensitivity to radiotherapy. Germ cell tumours and lymphomas are extremely radiosensitive, and relatively low doses are adequate for cure. However, most other cancers require higher doses. Normal tissue also varies in its radiosensitivity, with the central nervous system, small bowel and lung being among the most sensitive.

The side-effects of radiotherapy depend on the site being treated, the tissue's radiosensitivity and the dose delivered. For example, skin reactions are common with high-dose radical head and neck cancer treatments, or proctitis and cystitis with treatment to the bladder or prostate. These acute reactions typically settle within a few weeks after treatment. Late effects of radiotherapy develop more than 6 weeks after treatment and occur in 5%–10% of patients. Examples include brachial nerve damage and subcutaneous fibrosis after breast cancer treatment. There is also a risk of inducing new cancer after radiotherapy, which varies depending on the site treated and on whether the patient has had other treatment such as cytotoxic chemotherapy.

Systemic anti-cancer therapy

Systemic anti-cancer therapy (SACT) is a collective term to describe the growing number of differing drug therapies used to treat cancer. These drugs reach throughout the body to treat cancer cells wherever they may be. Increasingly, treatment is tailored to a patient's particular cancer and its molecular profile, allowing more personalised therapy.

Cytotoxic chemotherapy

Cytotoxic chemotherapy drugs work by interfering with the processes involved in cell division. They are sub-classified by their mode of action (Fig. 7.10). Cytotoxic chemotherapies have their greatest activity in proliferating cells and this provides the rationale for their use in the treatment

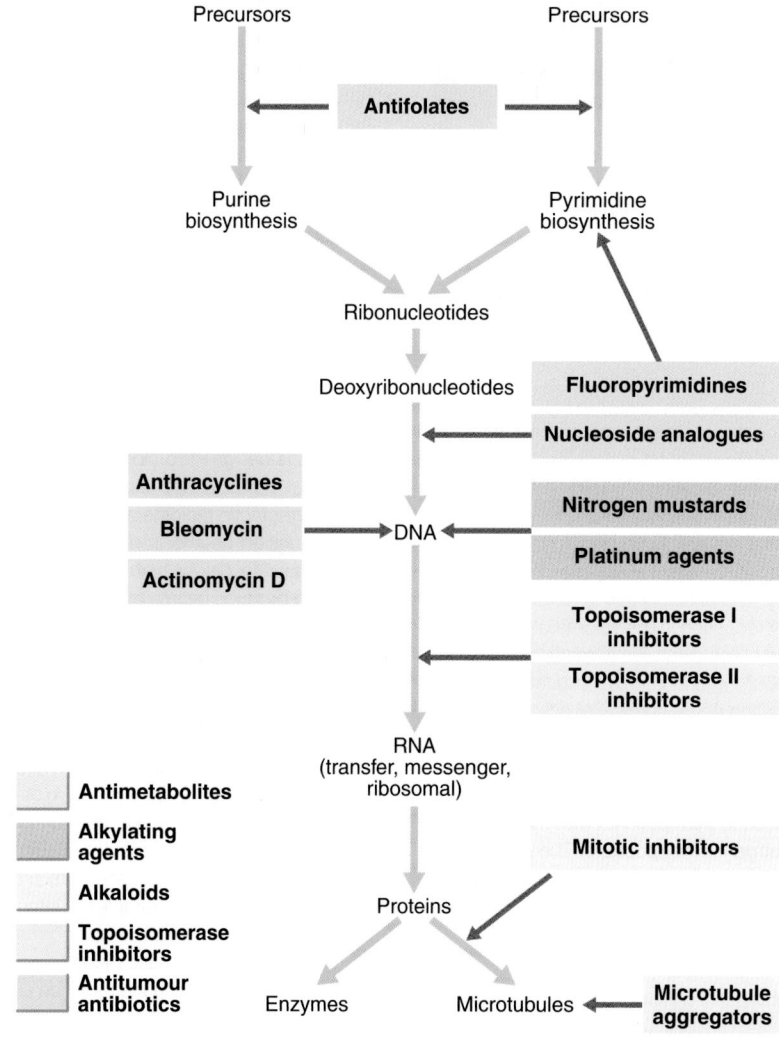

	Antifolates	Fluoropyrimidines	Nucleoside analogues	Nitrogen mustards	Platinum agents	Topoisomerase I/II inhibitors	Mitotic inhibitors	Microtubule aggregators	Others – acting on DNA
Mechanism of action	Inhibit dihydrofolate reductase and so purine and pyrimidine synthesis	Inhibit thymidylate synthase and so pyrimidine synthesis	Incorporated into DNA during synthesis, leading to irreparable errors	Form covalent cross-links between DNA molecules by adding an alkyl group to DNA	Form inter-/intra-strand cross-links between DNA molecules, not by adding an alkyl group, so considered alkylating-like agents	Prevent re-ligation of DNA strands by topoisomerase I/II	Bind tubulin, blocking microtubule formation	Stabilise the microtubule polymer preventing its disassembly	1. Intercalate with DNA and inhibit the progression of topoisomerase I 2. Induce DNA strand breaks by oxidative damage 3. Bind to DNA to prevent transcription
Examples	Methotrexate	5-Fluorouracil, capecitabine	Gemcitabine, fludarabine	Cyclophosphamide, ifosfamide	Cisplatin, carboplatin, oxaliplatin	Etoposide (II); topotecan, irinotecan (I)	Vinca alkaloids: vincristine, vinblastine, vinorelbine	Taxanes: paclitaxel, docetaxel	1. Anthracyclines: epirubicin, doxorubicin 2. Bleomycin 3. Actinomycin D

Fig. 7.10 Commonly used cytotoxic chemotherapy agents and their mechanisms of action.

of cancer. However, they are not specific for cancer cells and the side-effects of treatment are largely a result of their antiproliferative actions in normal tissues such as the bone marrow, skin and gut (p. 129). Other organs, such as the heart, kidney and peripheral nervous system, may also be affected by some cytotoxic drugs.

The choice of cytotoxic chemotherapy agent, or combination of treatments, is determined by the cancer type. The dosing schedule is determined by the choice of treatments and recovery of normal tissues, usually the bone marrow. For most common cytotoxic chemotherapy regimens the treatment is administered in cycles. A course of treatment may constitute a pre-defined number of cycles, or may continue indefinitely until evidence of disease progression or until limiting side-effects. Supportive therapy is used to enable patients to tolerate therapy and achieve benefit. Nausea and vomiting are common, but with modern antiemetics, regimens such as the combination of dexamethasone and highly selective 5-hydroxytryptamine (5-HT$_3$, serotonin) receptor antagonists such as ondansetron, most patients now receive cytotoxic chemotherapy without any significant problems. Myelosuppression is common to almost all cytotoxics and this not only limits the dose of drug but also can cause life-threatening complications. The risk of neutropenia can be reduced with the use of specific growth factors that accelerate the repopulation of myeloid precursor cells. The most commonly employed is G–CSF, which is widely used in conjunction with cytotoxic chemotherapy regimens that induce a high rate of neutropenia.

Hormone therapy

Hormones are important cell-signalling molecules and, in some cancers, may be key drivers of tumour growth. Blocking hormonal signalling pathways in these cancers may be a very effective treatment strategy.

Approximately 80% of breast tumours are positive for expression of the oestrogen receptor (ER). Assessment of ER status is now standard in the diagnostic workup of breast cancer. Drugs that reduce oestrogen levels or block the effects of oestrogen on the receptor are widely used in the management of ER-positive breast cancer. Adjuvant hormone therapy may reduce the risk of relapse and death at least as much as cytotoxic chemotherapy and in advanced cases can induce stable disease and remissions that may last months to years, with acceptable toxicity.

Hormonal manipulation may be effective in other cancers. In prostate cancer, hormonal therapy (e.g. luteinising hormone releasing hormone (LHRH) analogues such as goserelin and/or anti-androgens such as bicalutamide) aimed at reducing androgen levels can provide good long-term control of advanced disease. The side-effects of hormone therapies are linked to their hormonal targets.

Targeted therapies

Advances in knowledge about the molecular basis of cancer have resulted in the development of treatments to target specific genes and proteins that are involved in the growth and survival of cancer cells (Fig. 7.11). These signalling pathways may have broad importance to a range of cancer types or be specific to certain cancers. They may not be important in all tumours of the same cancer type, requiring specific molecular testing to predict whether the patient may benefit.

Targeted therapies are broadly divided into two groups: monoclonal antibodies (-mab) and small molecule inhibitors (-ib). The -mab family are typically utilised for targets that are overexpressed on the outside of the cancer cell. The -ib family typically target processes within the cell, such as the cytoplasmic tyrosine kinase, and are designed to be small enough to enter the cell.

A wide range of targeted therapies are now used routinely in oncological practice. Some of these are described below. The side effects of targeted therapies are determined by the molecular pathway being targeted (p. 129).

Epidermal growth factor receptor (EGFR) is an important transmembrane signalling protein. Mutations in the *EGFR* gene lead to overexpression of the EGFR protein or constitutive activation of the cell-signalling

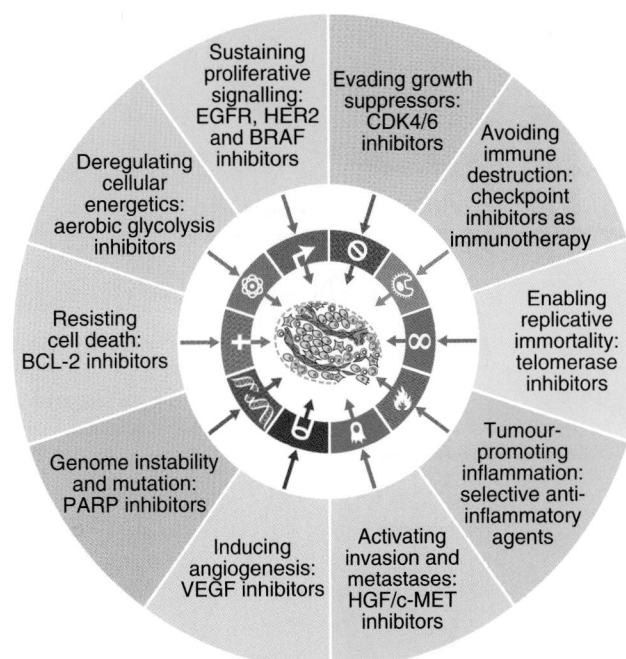

Fig. 7.11 Examples of targeted anti-cancer therapies and their actions in relation to the Hallmarks of Cancer. (For abbreviations see text.)

pathway, leading to uncontrolled cell division, in several cancer types. Approximately 15% of lung adenocarcinomas have activating mutations of *EGFR*, which may be targeted with drugs such as gefitinib, erlotinib or osimertinib. The latter of these agents has been designed to overcome a particular mutation (i.e. T790M) responsible for 50% of resistance to older EGFR inhibitors. In colorectal cancer drugs such as cetuximab and panitumumab are active in patients where molecular testing does not detect resistance inferred by mutations in the *RAS/RAF* family of genes.

Vascular endothelial growth factor receptor (VEGFR) inhibitors such as sunitinib, pazopanib and cabozantinib have been a pillar of renal cell carcinoma treatment for over a decade. Activation of members of the VEGFR family play an important role in tumour angiogenesis. VEGFR small molecule inhibitors are commonly used in the management of hepatocellular carcinoma and thyroid cancer. Bevacizumab, a monoclonal antibody therapy targeted at VEGF-A, is active in a number of cancers, including ovarian, colorectal and breast.

HER2 is a member of the epidermal growth factor receptor family. Amplification or over-expression of HER2 is found in breast, gastric, pancreatic, lung and some uterine cancers. Approximately 20% of breast cancers are HER2-positive, where it is associated with increased risk of recurrence and poor prognosis. Several agents have been developed to target HER2, including trastuzumab and pertuzumab. The agent trastuzumab emtansine is an antibody-drug conjugate consisting of trastuzumab covalently linked to the cytotoxic chemotherapy agent emtansine which is delivered specifically to the HER2-positive breast cancer cell.

Immunotherapy

The term immunotherapy encompasses a range of anti-cancer therapies that work by harnessing the immune system to attack cancer cells. Cytokines, such as interferon alpha and interleukin-2, have been used with some success in melanoma and renal cell carcinoma. However, in recent years the development of other immunotherapy treatments has revolutionized the management of several cancer types.

Immune checkpoints are key regulators of the immune system which work to prevent the immune response from attacking normal healthy cells. Cancers may co-opt this mechanism to evade immune destruction. Targeted therapies that inhibit these checkpoint molecules (CTLA4, PD-1) or their ligands (PD-L1) (Fig. 7.12) are now licensed in

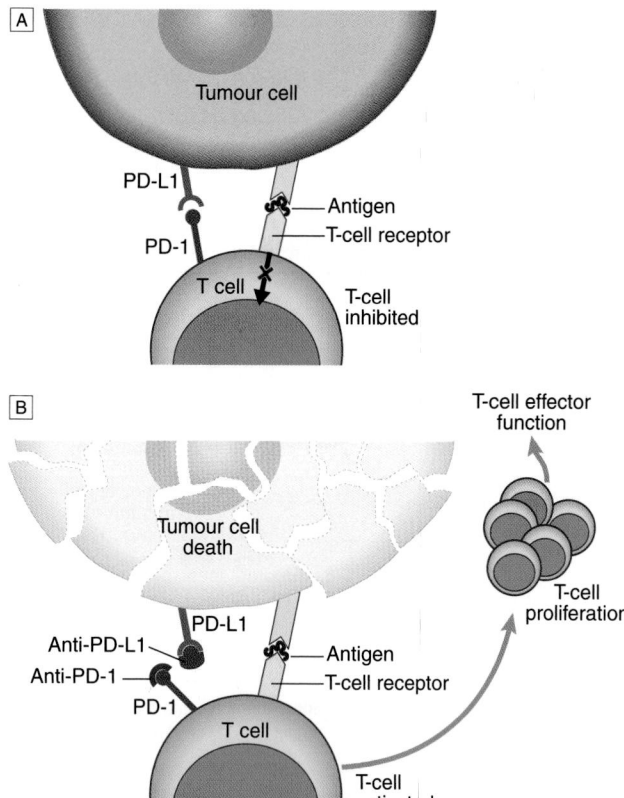

Fig. 7.12 **A** PD-L1 expressed on tumour cells inhibits T-cell activation by binding PD-1. **B** Checkpoint inhibitors block this PD-1–PD-L1 interaction, leading to T-cell activation and tumour cell death. (PD-1 = programmed cell death protein 1; PD-L1 = programmed cell death ligand 1)

7.19 Response evaluation criteria in solid tumours (RECIST)

Response	Criteria
Complete response (CR)	Disappearance of all target lesions
Partial response (PR)	At least a 30% decrease in the sum of the longest diameter (LD) of target lesions, taking as reference the baseline sum LD
Progressive disease (PD)	At least a 20% increase in the sum of the LD of target lesions, taking as reference the smallest sum LD recorded since the treatment started and at least 5 mm increase or the appearance of one or more new lesions
Stable disease (SD)	Neither sufficient shrinkage to qualify for PR nor sufficient increase to qualify for PD, taking as reference the smallest sum LD since the treatment started

the management of many cancers, including melanoma, renal cell carcinoma, lung, bladder, head and neck, and, more broadly, any cancers demonstrating microsatellite instability. Checkpoint inhibitor immunotherapies may be used alone, or in combination with other checkpoint inhibitor immunotherapies, targeted therapies or cytotoxic chemotherapy.

Adoptive cell therapy, also known as cellular immunotherapy, is increasingly being used, particularly in haematological malignancies. Immune cells isolated from either the patient's tumour or bloodstream may be activated and expanded, before being infused back into the patient to attack cancer cells (i.e. tumour infiltrating lymphocyte (TIL) therapy). The immune cells may also be genetically modified to improve the likelihood that they identify the cancer cells (i.e. engineered T-cell (TCR) therapy, chimeric antigen receptor T-cell (CAR-T) therapy). Cancer treatment vaccines are also in development. These aim to boost the immune system's ability to recognise and destroy antigens using a number of different techniques.

Immunotherapy treatment is likely to become more prevalent in the future for many types of cancers and indications. In patients with advanced or metastatic disease a key observation has been the potential for durable treatment responses. For example, average survival for patients with metastatic melanoma has improved from 6–8 months in the pre-immunotherapy era to over 5 years with the use of combination anti-CTLA4 and anti-PD-1 checkpoint inhibitors in clinical trials. However, many patients do not respond and others are affected by potentially life-threatening immune-related adverse events (see above).

Evaluation of treatment

In advanced or metastatic cancer the evaluation of treatment is an ongoing process and includes assessments of treatment response, toxicity and quality of life. Clinical evaluation alongside radiological imaging or biochemical monitoring are commonly used to determine whether a treatment is being effective. Uniform criteria have been established to measure these, including the response evaluation criteria in solid tumours (RECIST, Box 7.19) and common toxicity criteria (e.g. common terminology criteria for adverse events (CTCAE)). This allows clinicians to inform patients accurately about the prognosis, effectiveness and toxicity of systemic anti-cancer therapy and empowers patients to take an active role in treatment decisions.

Late toxicity of therapy

The late toxicities of treatment for cancer are particularly important for patients where multimodality therapy is given with curative intent, where the patient is young and as more patients are living longer. This can cause considerable morbidity: for example, radiotherapy can retard bone and cartilage growth, impair intellect and cognitive function, and cause dysfunction of the hypothalamus, pituitary and thyroid glands. Late consequences of cytotoxic chemotherapy include heart failure due to cardiotoxicity, pulmonary fibrosis, nephrotoxicity and neurotoxicity.

Premature gonadal failure can result from cytotoxic chemotherapy or radiotherapy and leave a patient subfertile. Patients should be made aware of this before treatment is initiated, as it may be possible to store sperm for male patients before treatment starts; this should always be offered, if practical. Egg storage or embryo banking after in vitro fertilisation may be an option for young women. Sterility develops at higher radiotherapy doses but erectile dysfunction is seen in patients receiving high radiotherapy doses to the pelvis, as in prostate cancer. Additional social or psychological support may be required to address these issues. Infertility and pubertal delay are potential late effects of therapy in children, especially boys.

Second malignancies may be induced by cancer treatment and occur at greatest frequency following chemoradiation. Secondary acute leukaemia (mostly AML) can occur 1–2 years after treatment with topoisomerase II inhibitors, or 2–5 years after treatment with alkylating agents. The most common second malignancy within a radiation field is osteosarcoma but others include soft tissue sarcoma and leukaemia.

Cancer clinical trials

Cancer clinical trials are embedded within routine practice in oncology. Close collaboration with laboratory scientists, active recruitment of cancer patients into clinical trials and robust translational research have led to many new cancer treatments, personalised therapies and a transformation of cancer management over the last 20 years. As many anti-cancer drugs are expected to have toxicities, which may ultimately limit the deliverable dose, clinical trials in cancer differ from trials of other medicines.

- Phase I cancer clinical trials take treatments of interest from laboratory studies and test them in patients with advanced cancer for whom no other standard anti-cancer treatment exists. Phase I trials assess the safety of a treatment and identify an optimal dose and dosing schedule. Initial doses are very low and each sequential cohort of patients receives a higher dose. Doses are escalated in controlled cohorts of 1–6 patients, according to toxicities, pharmacokinetics and pharmacodynamics, until the maximum tolerated dose is reached.
- Phase II cancer clinical trials treat patients with specific cancers of interest with the trial drug, using the dose established in phase I trials. Phase II trials may be randomised or non-randomised but will recruit enough patients to further assess the safety of the treatment and whether it results in enough anti-cancer activity in a specific cancer to develop the drug further by way of phase III trials.
- Phase III cancer trials are large, multi-centre randomised controlled trials to compare the new treatment of interest with the current established therapy for this indication. Cancer response, toxicity, quality of life and survival data will usually be assessed. Phase III trials may also compare current standard treatment with a different treatment, either looking for improved outcome or improved quality of life with non-inferior outcome. If a treatment is deemed to be safe and effective it will be licensed for clinical use.
- Phase IV trials involve the continuing safety surveillance of a treatment after it receives a licence for clinical use. This can be particularly useful to detect any rare or long-term adverse effects in a much larger population and longer time period than was possible during Phase I–III trials.

Specific cancers

As cancer management becomes more complex and personalised, and incorporates multi-modality treatment approaches, oncology teams are increasingly subspecialised and work as part of tumour-specific multidisciplinary teams. The diagnosis and management of specific cancers are discussed in more detail elsewhere in the book (Box 7.20). Here we discuss the pathogenesis, clinical features, investigation and management of some common tumours that are not covered elsewhere.

Breast cancer

Globally, the incidence of breast cancer is second only to that of lung cancer, and the disease represents the leading cause of cancer-related deaths among women. Invasive ductal carcinoma with or without ductal carcinoma in situ (DCIS) is the most common histology, accounting for 70%, whilst invasive lobular carcinoma accounts for most of the remaining cases. DCIS constitutes 20% of breast cancers detected by mammography screening. It is multifocal in one-third of women and has a high risk of becoming invasive (10% at 5 years following excision only). Pure DCIS does not cause lymph node metastases, although these are found in 2% of cases where nodes are examined, owing to undetected invasive cancer. Lobular carcinoma in situ (LCIS) is a predisposing risk factor for developing cancer in either breast (7% at 10 years). The survival for breast cancer by stage is outlined in Box 7.21.

Pathogenesis

Both genetic and hormonal factors play a role: about 5%–10% of breast cancers are hereditary and occur in patients with mutations of *BRCA1*, *BRCA2*, *AT* or *TP53* genes. Prolonged oestrogen exposure associated with early menarche, late menopause and use of hormone replacement therapy (HRT) has been associated with an increased risk. Other risk

i	7.20 Specific cancers covered in other chapters	
Bladder cancer		p. 607
Colorectal cancer		p. 826
Familial cancer syndromes		p. 55
Gastric cancer		p. 817
Hepatocellular carcinoma		p. 901
Leukaemia		p. 963
Lung cancer		p. 528
Lymphoma		p. 971
Mesothelioma		p. 546
Myeloma		p. 976
Oesophageal cancer		p. 809
Pancreatic cancer		p. 855
Prostate cancer		p. 610
Renal cancer		p. 606
Seminoma		p. 611
Skin cancer		p. 1082
Teratoma		p. 611
Thyroid cancer		p. 665

i	7.21 Five-year survival rates for breast cancer by stage		
Tumour stage	**Stage definition**	**5-year survival (%)**	
I	Tumour <2 cm, no lymph nodes	98	
II	Tumour 2–5 cm and/or mobile axillary lymph nodes	90	
III	Chest wall or skin fixation and/or fixed axillary lymph nodes	72	
IV	Metastasis	26	

factors include obesity, alcohol intake, nulliparity and late first pregnancy. There is no definite evidence linking use of the contraceptive pill to breast cancer.

Clinical features

Breast cancer usually presents as a result of mammographic screening or as a palpable mass with nipple discharge in 10% and pain in 7% of patients. Less common presentations include inflammatory carcinoma with diffuse induration of the skin of the breast, and this confers an adverse prognosis. Around 40% of patients will have axillary nodal disease, with likelihood correlating with increasing size of the primary tumour. Distant metastases are infrequently present at diagnosis and the most common sites of spread are bone (70%), lung (60%), liver (55%), pleura (40%), adrenals (35%), skin (30%) and brain (10%–20%).

Investigations

Following clinical examination, patients should undergo imaging with mammography or ultrasound evaluation, and a biopsy using fine needle aspiration for cytology or core biopsy for histology. Histological assessment should be carried out to assess tumour type and to determine oestrogen and progesterone receptor (ER/PR) status and HER2 status. If distant spread is suspected, CT of the thorax and abdomen and an isotope bone scan are required. Molecular subtyping is being used to classify tumours into four major subtypes: luminal A, luminal B, HER2 type and basal-like (often called 'triple negative', as these tumours are ER-, PR- and HER2-negative). This may allow more targeted selection of therapies in future.

Management

Surgery is the mainstay of curative treatment. This can range from a lumpectomy, where only the tumour is removed, to mastectomy, where the whole breast is removed. Breast-conserving surgery is as effective as mastectomy if complete excision with negative margins can be achieved. Lymph node sampling is performed at the time of surgery.

There is significant evidence to support the use of additional therapies to reduce the risk of breast cancer recurrence. Adjuvant radiotherapy is given to reduce the risk of local recurrence. In those patients considered at high risk of recurrence (i.e. tumour of >1 cm, ER-negative disease or the presence of involved axillary lymph nodes) cytotoxic chemotherapy may be offered. In patients with HER2-positive breast cancer adjuvant trastuzumab, a humanised monoclonal antibody to HER2, may be used alongside standard cytotoxic chemotherapy. These treatments are increasingly being used in the neoadjuvant setting, with the aim of achieving a complete pathological response when the cancer is resected, often with a more organ-preserving surgical procedure. In patients with ER-positive tumours adjuvant hormonal therapy may gain additional disease-free and overall survival benefits. Patients at low risk of recurrence (i.e. small, ER-positive disease) may require only adjuvant hormonal therapy. In post-menopausal women adjuvant bisphosphonate therapy may also be used.

The treatment of metastatic breast cancer is complex. Radiotherapy may be used to palliate painful bone metastases. SACT decisions are made with consideration of ER status, HER2 status, the distribution of metastatic disease and previous neo/adjuvant treatment, alongside assessments of performance status (PS) and comorbidities. For example, in a post-menopausal patient with ER-positive, HER2-negative bone-only metastatic disease who is PS 0, hormonal therapy (i.e. an aromatase inhibitor) in combination with a CDK4/6 targeted therapy (i.e. palbociclib, abemaciclib or ribociclib) may be used as first-line treatment. In a similar patient with additional symptomatic liver metastases, cytotoxic chemotherapy may be more appropriate.

Ovarian cancer

Ovarian cancer is the most common gynaecological tumour in Western countries. Most ovarian cancers are epithelial in origin (90%), and up to 7% of women with ovarian cancer have a positive family history. Patients often present late in ovarian cancer with vague abdominal discomfort, low back pain, bloating, altered bowel habit and weight loss. Occasionally, peritoneal deposits are palpable as an omental 'cake' and nodules in the umbilicus (Sister Mary Joseph nodules).

Pathogenesis

Genetic and environmental factors play a role. The risk of ovarian cancer is increased in patients with *BRCA1* or *BRCA2* mutations, and Lynch type II families (a subtype of hereditary non-polyposis colon cancer, HNPCC) can have ovarian, endometrial, colorectal and gastric tumours due to mutations of mismatch repair enzymes. Advanced age, nulliparity, ovarian stimulation and European descent all increase the risk of ovarian cancer, while suppressed ovulation appears to protect, so pregnancy, prolonged breastfeeding and the contraceptive pill have all been shown to reduce the risk of ovarian cancer.

Investigations

Initial workup for patients with suspected ovarian cancer includes imaging in the form of ultrasound and CT. Serum levels of the tumour marker CA-125 are often measured. Surgery plays a key role in the diagnosis, staging and treatment of ovarian cancer, and in early cases, palpation of viscera, peritoneal washings and biopsies are generally performed to define disease extent.

Management

In early disease, surgery followed by adjuvant cytotoxic chemotherapy with carboplatin, or carboplatin plus paclitaxel, is the treatment of choice.

Surgery should include removal of the tumour along with total abdominal hysterectomy, bilateral salpingo-oophorectomy, and omentectomy. Even in advanced disease, surgery is undertaken to maximally debulk the tumour and is followed by cytotoxic chemotherapy, typically using carboplatin and paclitaxel. Bevacizumab, a targeted therapy against VEGFR, is indicated for patients with high-grade tumours that are suboptimally debulked or those with a more aggressive biological pattern. Subsequent treatment decisions are made with consideration of response to first-line cytotoxic chemotherapy and germline BRCA mutation status. Options include further platinum/paclitaxel combination, liposomal doxorubicin or targeted therapy against poly-ADP ribose polymerase (PARP, e.g. olaparib, niraparib or rucaparib).

The serum tumour marker CA-125 and clinical examination may be used to monitor treatment response in ovarian cancer, with CT imaging for those with suspected progressive disease.

Endometrial cancer

Endometrial cancer accounts for 4% of all female malignancies, producing a 1 in 73 lifetime risk. The majority of patients are post-menopausal, with a peak incidence at 50–60 years of age. Mortality from endometrial cancer is currently falling. The most common presentation is with post-menopausal bleeding, which often results in detection of the disease before distant spread has occurred.

Pathogenesis

Oestrogen plays an important role in the pathogenesis of endometrial cancer, and factors that increase the duration of oestrogen exposure, such as nulliparity, early menarche, late menopause and unopposed HRT, increase the risk. Endometrial cancer is 10 times more common in obese women and this is thought to be due to elevated levels of oestrogens.

Investigations

The diagnosis is confirmed by endometrial biopsy.

Management

Surgery is the treatment of choice and is used for staging. A hysterectomy and bilateral salpingo-oophorectomy are performed with peritoneal cytology and, in some cases, lymph node dissection. Where the tumour extends beyond the inner 50% of the myometrium or involves the cervix and local lymph nodes, or there is lymphovascular space invasion, adjuvant pelvic radiotherapy is recommended. Cytotoxic chemotherapy is used as adjuvant therapy, and hormonal therapy and cytotoxic chemotherapy are used to palliate symptoms in recurrent disease.

Cervical cancer

Cervical cancer is the fourth most common cancer in women and the leading cause of death from gynaecological cancer worldwide. The incidence is decreasing in high-income industrialised countries but continues to rise in low- and middle-income nations. The most common presentation in the UK is with an abnormal smear test, but with locally advanced disease the presentation is with vaginal bleeding, discomfort, discharge or symptoms attributable to involvement of adjacent structures, such as bladder, or rectal or pelvic wall. Occasionally, patients present with distant metastases to bone and lung.

Pathogenesis

Almost all cases of cervical cancer are linked to high-risk human papillomaviruses (HPV), transmitted through sexual contact. This has underpinned the introduction of programmes to immunise adolescents against HPV in an effort to prevent up to 90% of cervical cancer.

Investigations

Diagnosis is made by smear or cone biopsy. Further examination may require cystoscopy and flexible sigmoidoscopy if there are symptoms referable to the bladder, colon or rectum. In contrast to other gynaecological malignancies, cervical cancer is a clinically staged disease, although MRI is often used to characterise the primary tumour. CT of the chest, abdomen and pelvis is performed to look for metastases in the lungs, liver and lymph nodes, and to exclude hydronephrosis and hydroureter.

Management

This depends on the stage of disease. Pre-malignant disease can be treated with laser ablation or diathermy, whereas in microinvasive disease a large loop excision of the transformation zone (LLETZ) or a simple hysterectomy is employed. Invasive but localised disease requires radical surgery, while cytotoxic chemotherapy and radiotherapy, including brachytherapy, may be given as primary treatment, especially in patients with adverse prognostic features such as bulky or locally advanced disease, or lymph node or parametrium invasion. In metastatic disease, platinum-based cytotoxic chemotherapy may be beneficial in improving symptoms but does not increase survival significantly.

Head and neck tumours

Head and neck cancers are typically squamous tumours that arise in the nasopharynx, hypopharynx and larynx. They are most common in older adult males but oropharyngeal cancers now occur with increasing frequency in a younger cohort of patients, including in women. The rising incidence of oropharyngeal cancers, especially in high-income countries, is thought to be secondary to HPV infection. Presentation depends on the location of the primary tumour and the extent of disease. For example, early laryngeal cancers may present with hoarseness, while more extensive local disease may present with pain due to invasion of local structures or with a lump in the neck. Patients who present late often have pulmonary symptoms, as this is the most common site of distant metastases (Box 7.22).

Pathogenesis

The tumours are strongly associated with a history of smoking and excess alcohol intake, but other recognised risk factors include Epstein–Barr virus for nasopharyngeal cancer and HPV infection for oropharyngeal tumours.

Investigations

Careful inspection of the primary site is required as part of the staging process, and most patients will require endoscopic evaluation and examination under anaesthesia. Tissue biopsies should be taken from the most accessible site. CT of the primary site and the thorax is the investigation of choice for visualising the tumour, while MRI may be useful in certain cases.

i	7.22 Common presenting features by location in head and neck cancer
Hypopharynx	
• Dysphagia	• Referred otalgia
• Odynophagia	• Enlarged lymph nodes
Mouth and tongue	
• Non-healing ulcers	• Ipsilateral otalgia
Nasal cavity and sinuses	
• Discharge (bloody) or obstruction	
Nasopharynx	
• Nasal discharge or obstruction	• Diplopia
• Conduction deafness	• Hoarse voice
• Atypical facial pain	• Horner syndrome
Oropharynx	
• Dysphagia	• Otalgia
• Pain	
Salivary gland	
• Painless swelling	• Facial nerve palsy

Management

In general, the majority of patients with early or locally advanced disease are treated with curative intent. In localised disease where there is no involvement of the lymph nodes, long-term remission can be achieved in up to 90% of patients with surgery or radiotherapy. The choice of surgery versus radiotherapy often depends on patient preference, as surgical treatment can be mutilating with an adverse cosmetic outcome. Patients with lymph node involvement are treated with a combination of surgery and radiotherapy (often with a radiosensitising agent such as cisplatin or cetuximab), and this produces long-term remission in approximately 60%–70% of patients. Recurrent or metastatic tumours may be palliated with further surgery or radiotherapy to aid local control, or systemic cytotoxic chemotherapy or immunotherapy may be used. Second malignancies are common (3% per year) following successful treatment for primary disease, and all patients should be encouraged to give up smoking and drinking alcohol to lower their risk.

Survivorship

Advances in cancer prevention, diagnosis and treatment mean that more people are surviving cancer. Cancer survival has doubled in the last 40 years in the UK. There are an estimated 2 million people living with, or beyond, cancer in the UK today and 50% of those diagnosed with cancer will survive their disease for 10 years or more. Cancer survivorship has at least two common meanings:

- completing treatment for cancer and having no signs of cancer after finishing treatment
- living with, through and beyond cancer, thus including people who receive curative treatment and people who receive intermittent anti-cancer treatment to control their cancer over a longer time.

Many people feel that life is never the same after a cancer diagnosis. There are often long-lasting physical, social and emotional consequences of both cancer and its treatment. These start at diagnosis and last through first treatment (acute survivorship), continue through and beyond cancer treatments (extended survivorship) and can be long-lasting, even when risk of cancer recurrence is low (permanent survivorship). An increasing awareness of survivorship, the impact of a cancer diagnosis and its wide-ranging effects on patients has highlighted the need for holistic and patient-centred care, support and services throughout and after cancer treatment.

Further information

Books and journal articles

Cassidy J, Bissett D, Spence RAJ, et al. Oxford handbook of oncology, 4th edn. Oxford: Oxford University Press; 2015.
Hanahan D, Weinberg RA. The hallmarks of cancer: perspectives for cancer medicine. In: Kerr DJ, Haller DG, van de Velde CJH, Baumann M, eds. Oxford textbook of oncology, 3rd edn. Oxford: Oxford University Press; 2016. Oxford Medicine Online DOI: 10.1093/med/9780199656103.003.0001.
Tobias J, Hochhauser D. Cancer and its management, 7th edn. Chichester: Wiley–Blackwell; 2014.

Websites

cancer.org *American Cancer Society: clinical practice guidelines.*
ctep.cancer.gov/reporting/ctc.html *Common toxicity criteria.*
info.cancerresearchuk.org/cancerstats/ *Cancer statistics that can be sorted by type or geographical location.*

LA Colvin
M Fallon

8

Pain and palliative care

Clinical examination in pain and palliative care

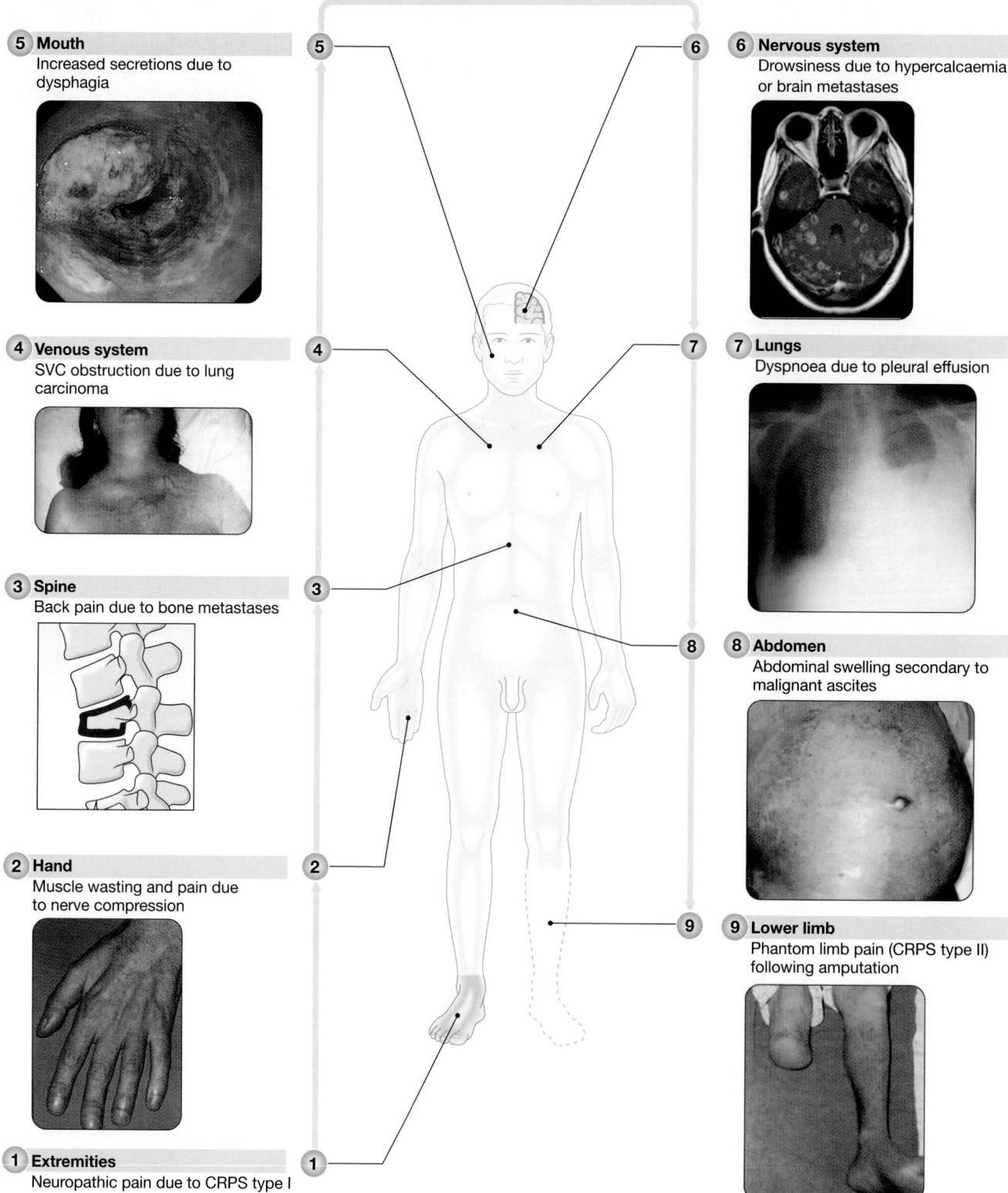

5 Mouth
Increased secretions due to dysphagia

4 Venous system
SVC obstruction due to lung carcinoma

3 Spine
Back pain due to bone metastases

2 Hand
Muscle wasting and pain due to nerve compression

1 Extremities
Neuropathic pain due to CRPS type I

6 Nervous system
Drowsiness due to hypercalcaemia or brain metastases

7 Lungs
Dyspnoea due to pleural effusion

8 Abdomen
Abdominal swelling secondary to malignant ascites

9 Lower limb
Phantom limb pain (CRPS type II) following amputation

Insets (SVC obstruction, wasting in the hand, pleural effusion, ascites, amputation) From Forbes CD, Jackson WF. Color atlas and text of clinical medicine, 3rd edn. Edinburgh: Mosby; 2002. (CRPS = chronic regional pain syndrome; SVC = superior vena cava)

Clinical evaluation and management in a patient with chronic pain or in the palliative care setting

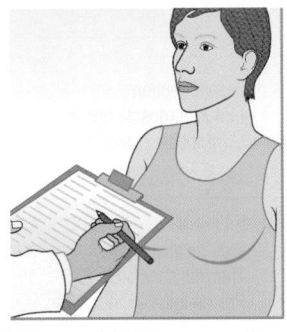

Take careful history, recording character and radiation of pain

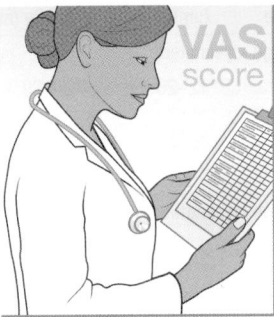

Record severity of pain

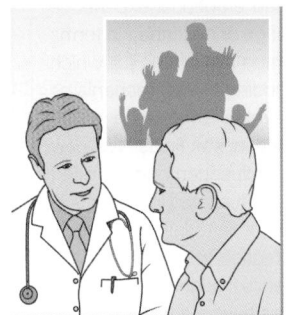

Conduct biopsychosocial assessment

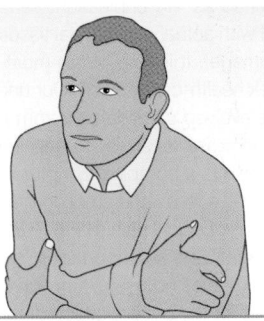

Assess mood and screen for depression

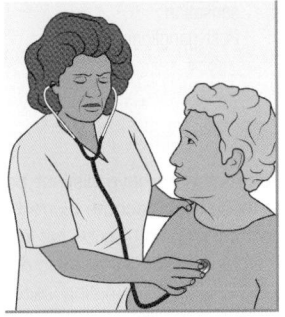

Conduct general examination

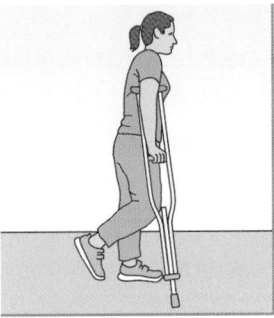

Check gait and whether using a walking aid

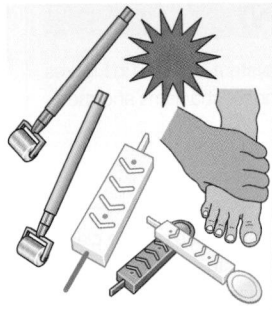

Assess pinprick, fine touch and heat/cold sensation

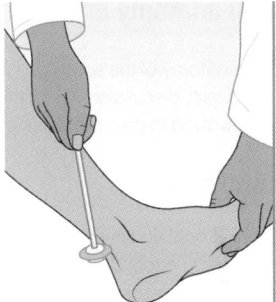

Conduct neurological examination

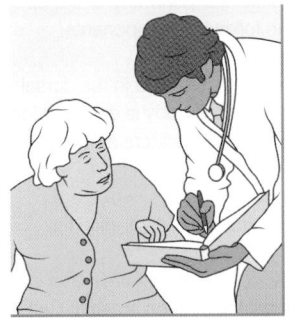

Educate patient on nature of pain and promote self-management

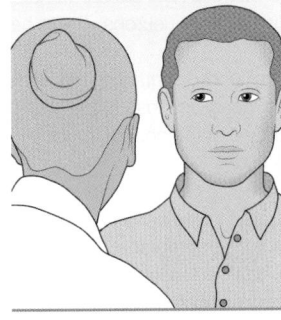

Formulate management plan with patient and set goals

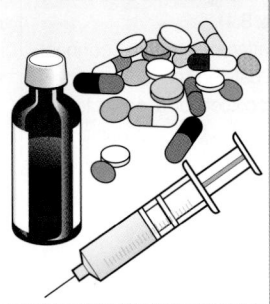

Optimise medication

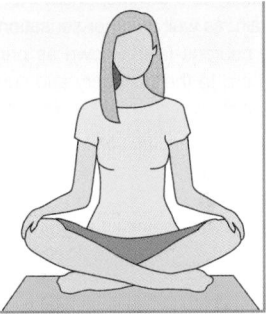

Consider psychological therapies and mindfulness

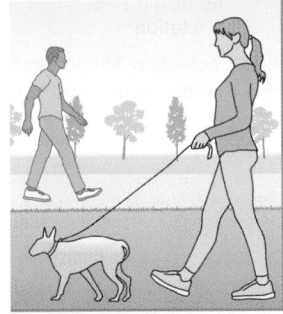

Increase physical activity

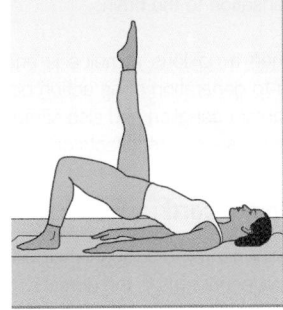

Consider yoga, pilates or tai chi

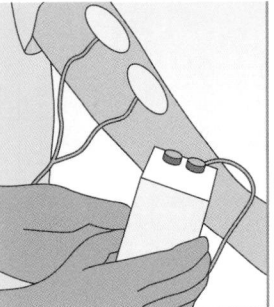

Consider TENS and acupuncture

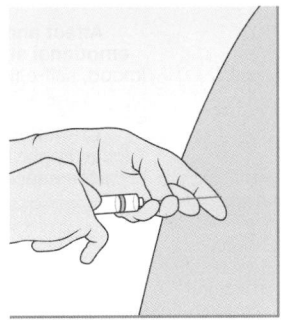

Consider nerve block or ablation

(TENS = transcutaneous electrical nerve stimulation)

Pain

Pain is defined as 'an unpleasant sensory and emotional experience associated with actual or potential tissue damage or described in terms of such damage'. It is one of the most common symptoms for which people seek health-care advice. Our understanding of the mechanisms of pain has evolved considerably from Hippocrates' suggestion in 450 BC that pain arose as a result of an imbalance in vital fluids. We now know that pain is a complex symptom that is influenced and modified by many social, cultural and emotional factors, as illustrated in Figure 8.1. The sensation of acute pain that occurs in response to inflammation or tissue damage plays an important role in protection from further injury. Chronic pain serves no useful function but results in significant distress and suffering for the patient affected, as well as having a wider societal impact.

Functional anatomy and physiology

The functional anatomy of the somatosensory system is shown in Figures 28.3 and 28.6. Here, discussion will focus on the mechanisms and mediators that are involved in pain processing.

Peripheral nerves

Peripheral nerves contain several types of neuron. These can be classified into two groups, depending on whether or not they are surrounded by a myelin sheath. Myelinated neurons have a fast conduction velocity and are responsible for transmission of various sensory signals, such as proprioception, light touch, heat and cold, and the detection of localised pains, such as pin-prick. Unmyelinated fibres have a much slower conduction velocity and are responsible for transmitting diffuse and poorly localised pain, as well as other sensations (Box 8.1).

Sensory neurons (also known as primary afferent neurons) connect the spinal cord to the periphery and supply a defined territory or a dermatome, which can be used to identify the position of a nerve lesion

8.1 Types of nerve fibre			
Fibre type	Diameter (µm)	Conduction velocity (ms⁻¹)	Function
Large myelinated			
Aα	12–20	70–120	Proprioception Motor to muscle fibres
Aβ	5–12	30–70	Light touch, pressure
A–	3–6	15–30	Motor to muscle spindles
Small myelinated			
A	2–5	12–30	Well-localised pain Thermal sensation
B	<3	3–15	Pre-ganglionic autonomic
Unmyelinated			
C	0.4–1.3	0.5–3	Diffuse pain Poorly localised thermal sensation Post-ganglionic autonomic

(see Fig. 28.10). In healthy individuals, dermatomes have distinct borders, but in pathological pain syndromes these may become blurred as the result of neuronal plasticity, which means that pain may be felt in an area adjacent to that supplied by a specific nerve root. Autonomic neurons also contain pain fibres and are responsible for transmitting visceral sensations, such as colic. In general, visceral pain is diffuse and less well localised than pain transmitted by sensory neurons.

Anatomical features of the afferent pain pathway are illustrated in Figure 8.2. Pain signals are transmitted from the periphery to the spinal cord by sensory neurons. These have the following components:

- *A cell body*, containing the nucleus, which is situated in the dorsal root ganglion close to the spinal cord. The cell body is essential for survival of the neuron, production of neurotransmitters and neuronal function.
- *The nerve fibre (axon) and peripheral nerve endings*, which are located in the periphery and contain a range of receptors in the neuronal membrane.
- *Specialised receptors* in the periphery, consisting of bare nerve endings known as nociceptors or pain receptors, which are activated by various mediators. They are situated mainly in the epidermis.
- *The central termination*, which travels to the dorsal horn of the spinal cord to form the first central synapse with neurons that transmit pain sensation to the brain.

When a noxious stimulus is encountered, activation of nociceptors leads to generation of an action potential, which travels upwards to the dorsal root ganglion and also stimulates the release of neurotransmitters that have secondary effects on surrounding neurons.

Spinal cord

Sensory neurons, through their central termination, synapse with second-order neurons in the dorsal horn of the spinal cord. There is considerable modulation of pain messages at this site, both from local neurons within the spinal cord and from neurons that descend from the brain, as depicted in Figure 28.11. Several neurotransmitters are involved in pain processing at this level and these are summarised in Box 8.2. They include amino acids, such as glycine and γ-aminobutyric acid (GABA), which are inhibitory, and glutamate, which is excitatory; neuropeptides, such as substance P and calcitonin gene-related peptide (CGRP); and endorphins. Whether or not they increase or decrease pain perception depends on the connectivity of the neurons on which they act.

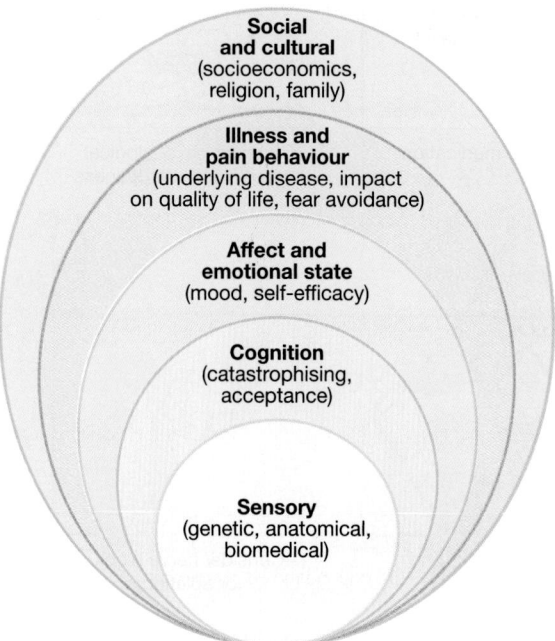

Fig. 8.1 The biopsychosocial model of pain. The perception of pain as a symptom is dependent not only on sensory inputs but also on the individual's cognitive reaction to the pain, their emotional state, their underlying disease and their social and cultural background.

Social and cultural (socioeconomics, religion, family)

Illness and pain behaviour (underlying disease, impact on quality of life, fear avoidance)

Affect and emotional state (mood, self-efficacy)

Cognition (catastrophising, acceptance)

Sensory (genetic, anatomical, biomedical)

8

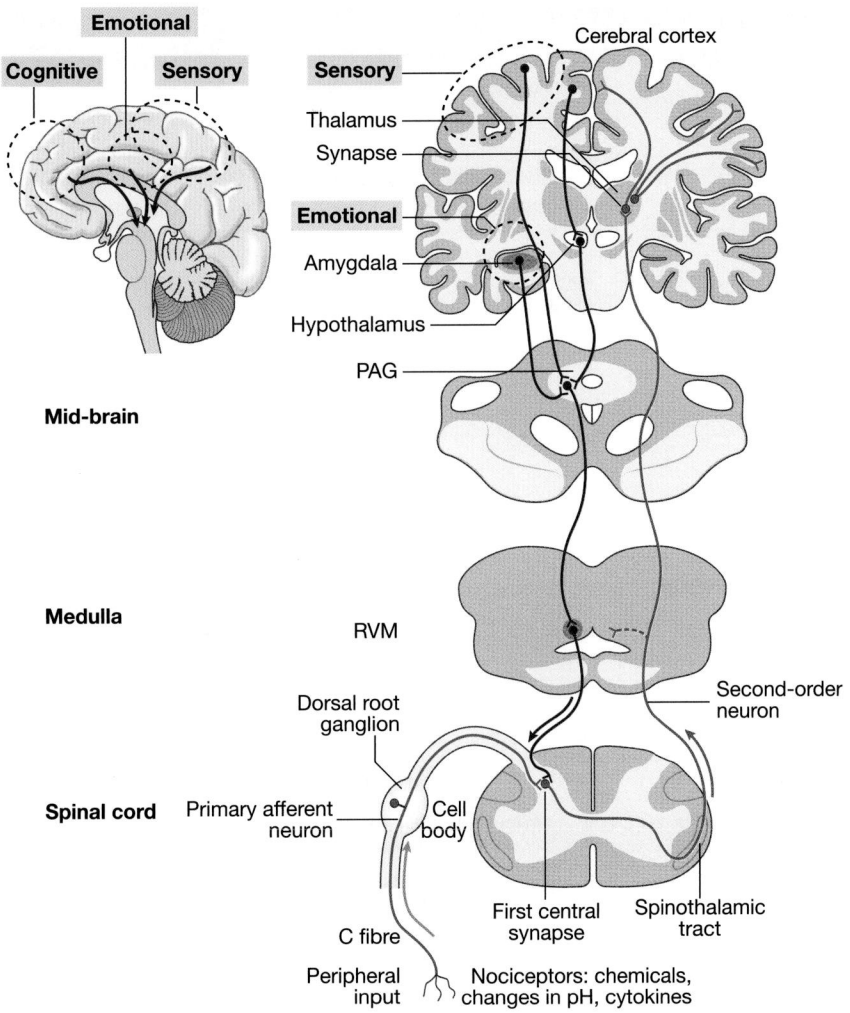

Fig. 8.2 Ascending and descending pain pathways. Ascending pathways are shown in blue and descending in red. Pain signals are detected in the periphery by nociceptors, which are activated by chemicals, changes in pH and cytokines. The signal is transmitted by the primary afferent neuron to the spinal cord, where there is a synapse with a second-order neuron, which transmits the signal onwards to the thalamus. Thereafter, the pain signal is transmitted to the cerebral cortex. The intensity of pain signals is subject to extensive modulation at several levels within the nervous system. Cognitive influences derived from the frontal lobe, coupled with sensory influences from cortex and emotional influences from the amygdyla, affect pain perception in the mid-brain around the periaqueductal grey matter (PAG) and the rostroventrolateral medulla (RVM) in the medulla. These structures form part of the descending modulatory systems, which, under normal circumstances, inhibit pain perception. In some chronic pain states, however, dysfunction of the descending pathways can occur, increasing pain.

Central processing of pain

The signals transmitted by second-order neurons in the spinal cord are relayed to the sensory cortex by third-order neurons, which synapse with second-order neurons in the thalamus. At this site, perception of pain is influenced by interactions between a range of structures in the brain, where sensory, cognitive and emotional aspects are integrated. This is termed the pain neuromatrix (see Fig. 8.2). Signals within the neuromatrix are multidirectional in nature, involving modulation of incoming messages by the cerebral cortex (top-down regulation), as well as a complex network of connections between other subcortical structures. Under normal conditions, there is a degree of descending inhibition from the brainstem that reduces input from peripheral stimuli.

It is thought that chronic widespread pain (CWP) and opioid-induced hyperalgesia may result, at least in part, from abnormalities in central processing of pain signals. It has also been suggested that variations in the levels of descending inhibition between individuals may make some people more vulnerable than others to developing chronic pain. Over recent years, there has been increasing interest in the role that glial cells (see Fig. 28.1) play in pain processing. Both astrocytes and microglial cells can become activated in chronic pain states and release pro-inflammatory cytokines, as well as altering re-uptake of excitatory neurotransmitters

such as glutamate, which can influence pain perception considerably. As our understanding of these processes improves, there is increasing potential to develop novel therapies targeted at these mediators, with some early clinical studies in neuropathic pain (pain related to nerve injury or disease, with characteristic neurobiological changes).

Sensitisation

Sensitisation is one of the key features of pain processing. It refers to the fact that both peripheral and central nervous systems adapt rapidly to the presence of pain, especially in response to tissue damage. This adaptive process is called neuronal plasticity. In some situations, neuronal plasticity can lead to prolonged changes in the pathways that are involved in detecting and processing nociceptive stimuli, resulting in chronic pain syndromes. The specific changes in key neurotransmitters and receptors differ between chronic pain states, with implications for the efficacy of treatments. For example, mu opioid receptors are down-regulated in neuropathic pain, potentially leading to limited opioid responsiveness.

Peripheral sensitisation

Peripheral sensitisation can occur in association with a variety of clinical conditions, including sepsis, cancer, inflammatory disease, injury,

| i | 8.2 Neurotransmitters and receptors involved in pain processing in the spinal cord |

Neurotransmitter	Receptor(s)	Receptor type	Comments*
Amino acids			
Glutamate	AMPA	Ion channel	Excitatory; permeable to cations: can be Ca^{2+}, Na^+ or K^+, depending on subunit structure
	NMDA	Ion channel	Excitatory; blocked by Mg^{2+} in the resting state; block can be altered if membrane potential changes; permeable to Ca^{2+}, Na^+ and K^+
	Kainate	Ion channel	Post synaptic – excitatory
	Gp I	GPCR	Pre-synaptic – inhibitory through GABA release; permeable to Na^+ and K^+
	Gp II	GPCR	Activates a range of signalling pathways; long-term effects on synaptic excitability
	Gp III	GPCR	Probably inhibitory; can decrease cAMP production; pre-synaptic; decreases glutamate release
Glycine	GlyR	Ion channel	Mainly inhibitory; permeable to Cl^-; blocked by caffeine
GABA	GABA$_A$	Ion channel	Mainly inhibitory in spinal cord; permeable to Cl^-; indirectly modulated by benzodiazepines (increased ion channel opening); not specifically involved in nociception, generally depressant effect on spinal cord activity
	GABA$_B$	GPCR	Predominantly inhibitory; activated by baclofen
Neuropeptides			
Substance P	Neurokinin receptors	GPCR	Mainly excitatory; increased in inflammation, decreased in neuropathic pain
Cholecystokinin	CCKRs1–8	GPCR	Excitatory; clinical trials of antagonists in progress
Calcitonin gene-related peptide	CALCRL	GPCR	Excitatory; slows degradation of substance P; implicated in migraine
Opioids			
Dynorphin	DOP	GPCR	Excitatory?; may be pro-nociceptive
β-endorphin	MOP	GPCR	Inhibitory
Nociceptin	NOP	GPCR	Inhibitory; also expressed by immune cells

(AMPA = α-amino 3-hydroxy, 5-methyl, 4-isoxazole propionic acid; CALCRL = calcitonin receptor-like receptor; cAMP = cyclic adenosine monophosphate; CCKR = cholecystokinin receptor; DOP = delta opioid receptor; GABA = γ-aminobutyric acid; Gp = group; GPCR=G-protein-coupled receptor; MOP = mu opioid receptor; NMDA = N-methyl-D-aspartate; NOP = nociceptin/orphan receptor)
*Excitatory = increased pain; inhibitory = reduced pain.

surgery and obesity. The final common pathway by which sensitisation takes place in all of these conditions is inflammation. Inflammation is accompanied by increased capillary permeability and tissue oedema with the release of a diverse range of mediators, including bradykinin, hydrogen ions, prostaglandins and adenosine, which bind to receptors and ion channels on nociceptors of primary afferent neurons (Fig. 8.3). The signalling pathways activated by these mediators generate action potentials, which are transmitted by sensory neurons to the spinal cord. If these pain-provoking stimuli persist, the activation threshold of sensory neurons is reduced, resulting in an increased transmission of pain signals to the spinal cord.

Central sensitisation

Sensitisation may also take place at the level of the spinal cord in response to a sustained painful stimulus. It can occur acutely and rapidly, such as immediately after surgery, or may progress to chronic changes, such as chronic infection, cancer, repeated surgery or multiple traumatic episodes. Glutamate, acting via the N-methyl-D-aspartate (NMDA) receptor complex, plays a key role in central sensitisation (Fig. 8.4). In response to a sustained peripheral painful stimulus, increased amounts of glutamate are released in the spinal cord, overcoming the inhibitory action of magnesium ions and resulting in activation of the NMDA receptor. This initiates a cascade of intracellular signalling events that lead to prolonged modifications of somatosensory processing, with amplification of pain responses within the spinal cord and continued neuronal firing, even after the noxious stimulus has stopped. This phenomenon is termed 'after-discharge'. In neuropathic pain, prolonged activation of the NMDA pathway results in a decrease in the number of inhibitory interneurons, which further potentiates pain.

Genetic determinants of pain perception

There are marked ethnic and individual variations in how people respond to painful stimuli and studies in twins have estimated that the heritability of CWP ranges between 30% and 50%. In the general population, the individual variants in response to pain and perception of pain are most likely due to a complex interaction between genetic and environmental influences. Few variants have been identified with robust evidence of association with CWP. Several rare syndromes have been described, however, in which insensitivity to pain or heightened pain responses occur as the result of a single gene disorder, as summarised in Box 8.3. Most are due to mutations affecting ion channels that play a key role in neurotransmission (see Fig. 8.3), but other causes include mutations in the *NTKR1* gene, which encodes the receptor for nerve growth factor, and mutations in the *PDRM12* transcription factor, which is involved in neuron development.

Investigations

Pain can be a presenting feature of a wide range of disorders and the first step in evaluation of a patient with pain should be to perform whatever investigations are required to define the underlying cause of the pain, unless this is already known. However, with most chronic pain syndromes, such as fibromyalgia, complex regional pain syndrome and CWP, investigations are negative and the diagnosis is made on the basis of clinical history and exclusion of other causes. Specific investigations that are useful in the assessment of selected patients with chronic pain are discussed below.

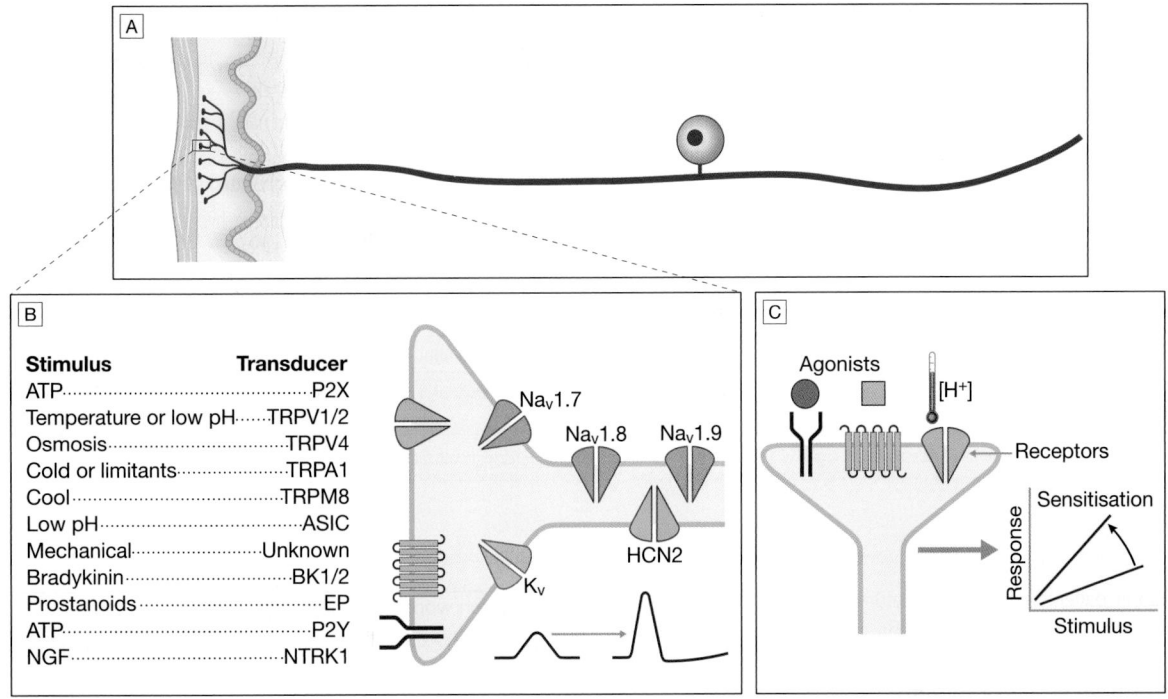

Fig. 8.3 Mechanisms of peripheral sensitisation. [A] Sensory nerve terminating with nociceptor in skin. [B] Peripheral nociceptors express various receptors and ion channels that act as mediators of pain. They include sodium channels implicated in congenital pain syndromes; the purinergic 2X (P2X) and purinergic 2Y (P2Y) receptor for adenosine triphosphate (ATP); members of the transient receptor potential (TRP) superfamily of ion channel receptors, which detect changes in osmolality and temperature; acid-sensing ion channel (ASIC) receptors, which detect hydrogen ions; G-protein-coupled receptors, which detect bradykinin (BK), prostaglandins and ATP; sodium-potassium hyperpolarization-activated cyclic nucleotide-gated channels (HCN2), and voltage gated potassium channels (Kv) and the neurotrophic tyrosine kinase 1 (NTRK1) receptor, which detects nerve growth factor (NGF). [C] Activation of these receptors by ligands, hydrogen ion [H+] and high temperature (> 42°C) amplifies action potentials, which increase pain signals and cause peripheral sensitisation. (EP = E-prostanoid receptor) *Adapted from Bennett DL, Woods CG. Painful and painless channelopathies. The Lancet Neurol 2014; 13:587–599; reproduced with permission from Elsevier.*

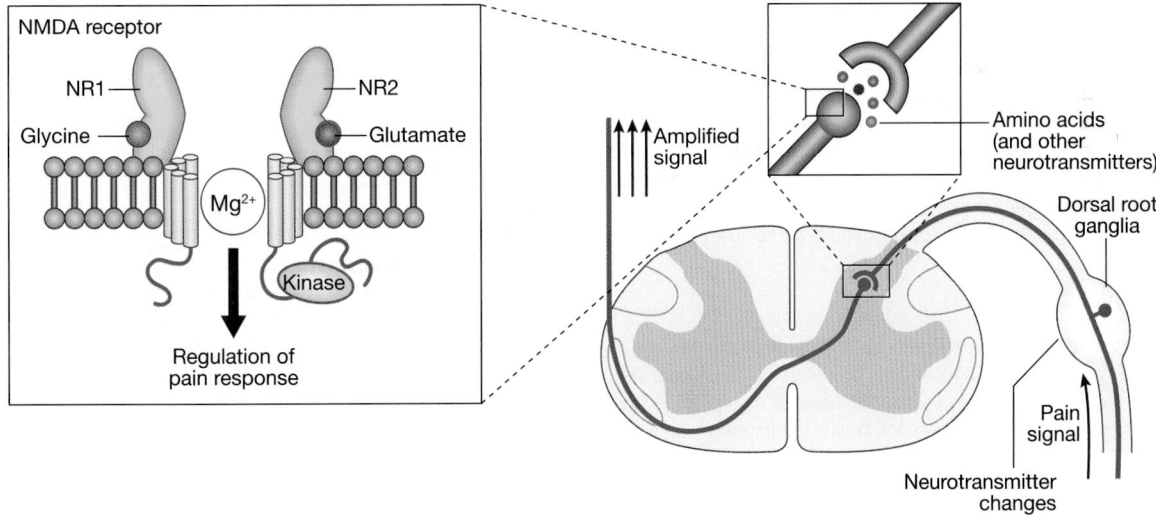

Fig. 8.4 Mechanisms of central sensitisation. Post-synaptic activation of the *N*-methyl-D-aspartate (NMDA) receptor requires the amino acids glycine and glutamate, which bind to the NR1 and NR2 subunits, respectively; these amplify pain signals at the level of the spinal cord. In contrast, magnesium ions block receptor activation.

Magnetic resonance imaging

Magnetic resonance imaging (MRI) can be helpful in the assessment of an underlying cause in patients with focal pain that follows a nerve root or peripheral nerve distribution. Imaging is seldom helpful in individuals with CWP.

Blood tests

Blood tests are not generally helpful in the diagnosis of chronic pain, except in patients with peripheral neuropathy; in this case, a number of blood tests may be required to investigate the underlying causes of the neuropathy. Full details are provided in Box 28.85. Genetic testing may

8.3 Genetic regulators of pain perception			
Gene (protein)	Mutation (inheritance)	Protein function	Phenotypes
SCN9A (Na,1.7)	LoF (AR)	Ion channel	Absent pain, hypohydrosis, anosmia
SCN9A (Na,1.7)	GoF (AD)	Ion channel	Erythromelalgia, paroxysmal pain, burning pain, autonomic dysfunction
SCN11A (Na,1.9)	GoF (AD)	Ion channel	Absent pain, hyperhydrosis, muscular weakness, gut dysmotility
SCN10A (Na,1.8)	GoF (AD)	Ion channel	Burning pain, autonomic dysfunction
TRPA1 (TRPA1)	GoF (AD)	Ion channel	Absent pain
PDRM12 (PDRM12)	LoF (AR)	Transcription factor; neuron development	Absent pain
NTRK1 (high-affinity NGF receptor)	LoF (AR)	Tyrosine kinase; promotes neuron development	Absent pain; anhydrosis, mental retardation, increased cancer risk

(AD = autosomal dominant; AR = autosomal recessive; GoF = gain of function; LoF = loss of function; NGF = nerve growth factor)

be of value in patients with clinical features that point to an inherited disorder of pain processing (see Box 8.3).

Quantitative sensory testing

Quantitative sensory testing can be helpful in the detailed assessment of patients with chronic pain. A simple set of tools can be used in the clinical setting (Fig. 8.5). Lightly touching the skin with a brush, swab or cotton-wool ball can be used to test for abnormalities of fine touch. This may include allodynia, where a normally non-painful stimulus is perceived as painful. Assessing the patient's response to a pin-prick can be used to test for abnormalities in mechanical hyperalgesia. Finally, touching the patient's skin with warm and cool thermal rollers can be used to test for abnormalities of thermal sensation. An unaffected area of skin should be tested first, to establish normal sensation, before testing the affected area.

Nerve conduction studies

Nerve conduction studies can be helpful in demonstrating and quantifying a definitive nerve lesion, either peripherally or centrally. They can be used to help differentiate between central and peripheral neuropathic pain. They do not, however, effectively examine small nerve fibre function.

Nerve blocks

Performing a nerve block with infiltration of a local anaesthetic such as 1% lidocaine can be used diagnostically, in assessing whether a pain syndrome is due to involvement of a specific nerve or nerve root. Where inflammation and or swelling may be contributing to the underlying pain – for example, if there is compression of a nerve root – then a mixture of local anaesthetic and depot glucocorticoid may be helpful in alleviating pain. Nerve blockade can also be used to determine whether more radical therapies, such as nerve ablation, might be helpful in controlling pain, particularly that related to cancer.

Pain scoring systems

Various questionnaires and other instruments have been devised to localise pain, rate its severity and assess its impact on quality of life. Some of the most widely used are listed in Box 8.4. The distribution of pain can be documented on a diagram of the body, on which the patient can mark the sites that are painful. Similarly, other methods have been developed with which to assess the severity of pain using verbal, numerical and behavioural rating scales. Visual scoring systems employing different facial expressions may be of value in paediatric patients and those

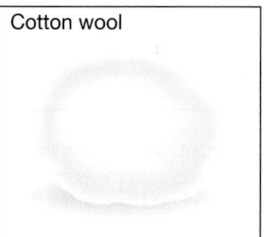

Cotton wool

Allodynia

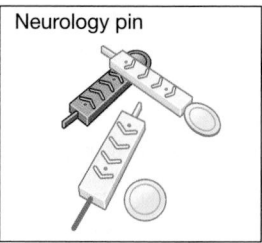

Neurology pin

Hyperalgesia

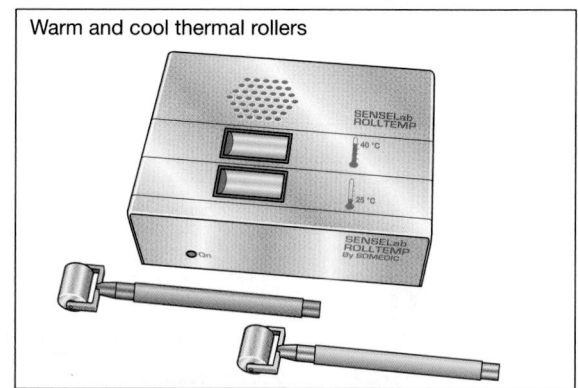

Warm and cool thermal rollers

Increased or decreased thermal sensation

Fig. 8.5 Equipment for bedside sensory testing.

with cognitive impairment. Documenting changes in pain scores using questionnaires can be helpful in indicating to what extent drug treatments have been successful and can reduce the time taken to achieve pain control.

Principles of management

Effective management of chronic pain depends in part on the underlying cause but some general principles can be applied. In general terms, the treatment goals are to:

- educate the patient
- promote self-management
- optimise function
- enhance quality of life
- control pain.

Clinical history

Biopsychosocial assessment

A full biopsychosocial assessment should be performed in all patients with chronic pain. Although this is time-consuming, the time invested is likely to pay dividends in improving the long-term outcome for patients. A biopsychosocial assessment takes account of the underlying neurobiology of the condition in the context of wider influences, including cognition and beliefs, emotions, and social and cultural factors. For example, an individual with abdominal pain might respond differently if a close relative had recently died of gastric cancer than if a colleague had been off work with gastric upset.

An accurate clinical history is important, taking note of the duration of pain, any precipitating and relieving factors, its location and, if the pain is located at more than one site, which site is the one that impacts most on the patient's quality of life. The characteristics of the pain should be documented, by assessing whether it is described as dull, sharp, aching or burning. Associated features, such as hypersensitivity to fine touch or temperature, numbness, paraesthesia, tingling and formication (the feeling of insects crawling over the skin), should be noted. It is important to determine to what extent the pain is interfering with normal daily activities, such as work, leisure pursuits and sleep. The patient's social circumstances and cultural background should be documented, including any caring responsibilities, employment status and social and family support. The intensity of pain should also be recorded, preferably using a validated questionnaire (see Box 8.4). The patient's mood should be assessed and, if evidence of low mood is detected, a suicide risk assessment should be considered (see Box 31.14). The past medical and medication history should be recorded and specific enquiry made about substance misuse and any previous history of physical or mental abuse. This should be approached sympathetically, with information about how to access appropriate support if required. It is also useful to enquire specifically about the patient's beliefs as to what is causing their pain, as well as what their expectation of treatment is; unless these are addressed, management may be less effective. There are some patient populations in whom particular challenges arise, often related to differences in communication ability. Strategies that can be used to overcome these difficulties are summarised in Box 8.5.

Examination

The patient's general appearance should be noted, including ability to walk and use of a walking aid. In those with focal pain, neurological examination should be performed, focusing particularly on any areas of abnormal sensation, reflexes and evidence of muscle wasting. A general examination should be carried out to determine whether there is any evidence of an underlying physical disorder that can account for the pain. In addition to the use of investigations to find the underlying cause of pain, patients with persistent or chronic pain may benefit from sensory testing or diagnostic nerve blocks to explore the underlying mechanisms and direct treatment. For example, a combined femoral and sciatic nerve block may be used in a patient with lower limb amputation to assess whether the pain is predominantly peripherally or centrally generated. If the pain is not improved by an effective nerve block, then peripherally directed therapies are unlikely to be effective.

i 8.4 Instruments used in the assessment of pain and its impact

Instrument	Comments
Brief Pain Inventory	Developed for use in cancer pain, validated and widely employed for chronic pain; based on 0–10 ratings of pain intensity and the impact of pain on a range of domains, including sleep, work and enjoyment of life
Pain Detect, s-LANSS, DN-4	A number of screening questionnaires to aid diagnosis of neuropathic pain
Pain Catastrophising Scale	Developed to assess individual levels of catastrophising, encompassing three different domains: helplessness, rumination and magnification
Tampa Scale of Kinesiophobia	Measures how much an individual is fearful of movement
Pain Self-efficacy Questionnaire	Assesses individual beliefs about self-efficacy in the context of chronic pain, and how this impacts on function
Visual analogue scale (VAS)	Patient marks pain intensity on a horizontal line
Localisation of pain	Body chart, allowing the patient to indicate where pain is situated
Beck Depression Inventory	Assesses emotional function
SF-36/EQ-5D	Assesses health-related quality of life

(DN-4 = Douleur Neuropathique questionnaire; EQ-5D = EuroQol 5-Domain questionnaire; SF-36 = Short Form 36; s-LANSS = self-completed Leeds Assessment of Neuropathic Signs and Symptoms)

i 8.5 Challenges in pain assessment in particular patient populations

Patient population	Challenges	Solutions
Paediatric	Assessment needs to be appropriate to developmental stage	Consider visual tools to aid pain assessment
Older adults	May have impaired cognitive function Cultural factors may reduce self-reporting of pain Risk of adverse effects of medication increased	Consider formal assessment of cognitive function Consider non-verbal assessment Consider visual tools to assess pain Employ a number of tools assessing pain behaviours
Cognitive impairment	Reporting and expression of pain may change Increased sensitivity to central nervous system effects of analgesics	Perform formal assessment of cognitive function Use non-verbal assessment: facial expressions, vocalisations, body movements, changes in social interactions
Substance misuse	Response to analgesics altered Increased tolerance Increased risk of addiction Substance misuse may affect reporting of pain	Seek specialist support early Ensure prescribing is safe

Interventions

Probably the most effective mode of treatment for pain is to identify the underlying cause. Examples include the use of immunosuppressive medication in inflammatory disease, chemotherapy, radiotherapy or hormone therapy in cancer, and antimicrobial therapy in patients with infection. There are many circumstances, however, in which the underlying cause of pain cannot be treated or the treatments available are incompletely effective. Under these circumstances, several management options are available. In all cases, a multidisciplinary approach is necessary that combines pharmacological management with supported self-management, and other specific interventions when appropriate.

Supported self-management

Self-management strategies are useful in the treatment of chronic pain. Self-management works best if the patient has some understanding of their chronic pain, and acceptance that it is unlikely to resolve completely. The aim is for patients to maximise their quality of life and function *despite* ongoing pain. Support for self-management can be delivered by healthcare professionals, patients who suffer from the same condition or lay people, either on an individual basis, in a group setting or, increasingly, through web-based resources. There is a strong educational component to supported self-management, which seeks to generate an interaction between patient and tutor. The key aspects include:

- increasing activity levels, while understanding and practising pacing techniques (not overdoing things and cycling between over- and under-activity)
- using relaxation and mindfulness techniques as part of daily management
- using medication when appropriate
- having a plan to manage pain flares.

All these are covered in formal pain management programmes (see 'Psychological therapies'), where a structured approach is used, in a group-based setting, to address all these aspects with expert multidisciplinary input, that may include psychologists, occupational therapists, nurses, pharmacists and pain medicine specialists.

For less complex cases, or to provide ongoing support, there are a number of useful online self-help resources (see 'Further information').

Physical therapies

There is strong evidence that exercise can help in the management of chronic pain. Several types of exercise have been successfully delivered in various ways, through physiotherapists, exercise classes or individual tuition. In choosing a form of exercise therapy, it is important to tailor the approach most likely to be acceptable to the individual patient. A successful exercise programme can help overcome 'fear avoidance', a well-recognised problem in chronic pain, where patients associate activity with an increase in pain and therefore do progressively less activity, with resultant deconditioning. Because of this it is important to pace physical activity to ensure that patients do not cycle from over-activity,

i	8.6 Physical therapies for chronic pain

Land-based

- Walking
- Gym work
- Exercise classes
- Yoga
- Pilates
- Tai-chi

Water-based

- Hydrotherapy
- Swimming
- Exercise classes

with a flare in pain, to fatigue and deconditioning. This can be done by working with patients to establish their baseline level of activity and using an individually tailored, graded exercise programme (Box 8.6). This may include normal household activities, as well as targeted exercises and stretches. Manual therapy covers a variety of hands-on treatments, including manipulation, mobilisation and massage. Manual therapy can be provided by a range of therapists, including physiotherapists, osteopaths and chiropractors. There is some evidence of short-term benefit for manual therapy but limited evidence of long-term efficacy.

Pharmacological therapies

A range of analgesics can be used in the management of chronic pain but, for most of these, the evidence of long-term benefit is limited, and there may be considerable risks associated with long-term use for some agents. If using analgesics as part of a holistic treatment plan (e.g. to manage short-term flare-ups, or target neuropathic pain), in general, it is advisable to use a multimodal approach, choosing different drugs to target pain processing at multiple points (Box 8.7). By employing different classes of analgesic, it is possible to use lower doses of each, thereby improving the side-effect profile and reducing risk. There is considerable inter-individual variability in response to analgesics, even within the same class. There are many reasons for this, including genetic variations in the enzymes that metabolise drugs. For example, the *CYP2D6* gene encodes for a liver enzyme, cytochrome P450 2D6, which metabolises a number of commonly used analgesics. Genetic variation in *CYP2D6* can influence circulating levels of many drugs, depending on whether someone is a rapid or poor metaboliser. This is particularly important if metabolites are active, as is the case with codeine and dihydrocodeine, which are metabolised to morphine. Genetic variations have also been described in the opioid receptors and downstream pathways that they affect, with good pre-clinical evidence that variations in mu opioid receptors alter analgesic response to different opioids. Because of this there is a good rationale to try different drugs, even ones from the same class, if there is an inadequate response or there are unacceptable side-effects with one agent.

Whatever drug or combination of drugs is chosen, the key to successful pharmacological management is careful assessment and review, aiming for an acceptable balance between the benefits of treatment in providing pain relief, maximising function, and improving quality of life and adverse effects. Specific drug treatments are described below.

Non-opioid analgesics

Paracetamol

Paracetamol is widely used in the treatment of mild to moderate pain. Its mechanism of action is incompletely understood but it is known to be a weak inhibitor of the cyclo-oxygenase type 1 (COX-1) and cyclo-oxygenase type 2 (COX-2) enzymes, providing weak anti-inflammatory properties. There is also some evidence that it activates inhibitory descending spinal pathways, via a serotonergic mechanism. Other postulated mechanisms include endocannabinoid re-uptake inhibition, and inhibition of nitric oxide and tumour necrosis factor alpha. For migraine and tension-type headache it has moderate efficacy at a dose of 1000 mg. It is used widely for musculoskeletal disorders and osteoarthritis, with very little high-quality evidence that it is much better than placebo, even at doses of up to 4000 mg per day. Acute liver failure is a well-recognised complication of paracetamol overdose but this risk may also be increased with long-term use, even within the recommended dose range. In view of this, it should be employed with caution in older patients and those weighing less than 50 kg.

Non-steroidal anti-inflammatory drugs

Non-steroidal anti-inflammatory drugs (NSAIDs) are widely used in the treatment of inflammatory pain and osteoarthritis. These drugs can be given systemically or locally and are discussed in more detail in Chapter 26. They are also useful in the management of pain in cancer patients, as discussed later in this chapter. Although widely prescribed, there is

	8.7 Pharmacological management of chronic pain	

Drug or class of drug	Mechanism of action
Paracetamol	Central inhibition of COX-1 and COX-2 enzymes Mechanisms of action incompletely understood
Non-steroidal anti-inflammatory drugs	Inhibition of prostaglandin production
Opioids	Agonists at opioid receptors at multiple levels in the central nervous system Blockade of ascending pain pathways
Ketamine	Antagonist of NMDA receptors Reduction of central sensitisation
Gabapentin and pregabalin	Inhibition of glutamate release by primary afferent neurons at first central synapse Decrease of excitatory neuronal activity
Tricyclic antidepressants	Inhibition of serotonin and noradrenaline (norepinephrine) re-uptake at synapses in the spinal cord, and also potential effects in the limbic system Inhibition of Na^+ channels in neurons
Serotonin (5-hydroxytryptamine, 5-HT) and noradrenaline (norepinephrine) re-uptake inhibitors	Inhibition of serotonin and noradrenaline re-uptake at synapses in the spinal cord, and also potential effects in the limbic system
Lidocaine patches	Inhibition of Na^+ in sensory neurons
Capsaicin patch	Activation of TRPV1 channels on subset of C fibres, causing selective pharmacological denervation, with a decrease in intra-epidermal nerve fibre density
Nerve blocks with lidocaine and glucocorticoids	Temporary denervation due to blockade of Na^+ channels in sensory neurons Local anti-inflammatory effect

(COX = cyclo-oxygenase; NMDA = *N*-methyl-D-aspartate; OP = opioid; TRPV1 = transient receptor potential vanilloid 1)

limited high-quality evidence of long-term efficacy in chronic pain, and concerns about risks of long-term use particularly around cardiovascular and renal effects. There is a clear need for further studies in this area.

Topical analgesics

Topical capsaicin cream (0.025 or 0.075%) has some efficacy for osteoarthritis and may be used for neuropathic pain, although evidence of benefit is limited. A single application (done by a trained health-care professional) of a high-dose 8% capsaicin patch can give around 12 weeks of pain relief for neuropathic pain and can be repeated thereafter. Capsaicin is an agonist at the transient receptor potential vanilloid 1 (TRPV1) ion channel, found on some C fibres. Capsaicin activates the channel, causing an initial sensation of heat, but an analgesic effect subsequently results due to desensitisation of the channel, with a reduction in intra-epidermal nerve fibre density.

Lidocaine 5% patches can also be helpful in focal neuropathic pain and should be applied for 12 hours out of 24 hours, with up to 4–6 weeks before maximum benefit is seen. The mode of action is blockade of sodium channels in primary afferent neurons and nociceptors, which reduces peripheral input to the spinal cord.

Anti-neuropathic agents

Anti-neuropathic agents are also termed 'adjuvant analgesics'. This term is used to cover a range of medicines that are employed in the treatment of neuropathic pain, and in certain patients with CWP. It should be noted that these medicines should only be used as part of a holistic management plan, including physical and psychological therapies, sometimes in combination with classical analgesics. Typically, these agents do not produce an immediate reduction in pain, but rather exert an analgesic effect over a longer timeframe through their effects on central processing of pain. They are of particular value when used in combination in the management of pain with a neuropathic component but require careful dose titration over a number of weeks, to reach a dose that balances efficacy with side-effects. While the response to individual agents is variable, it is often possible to find an agent or combination of agents that works for most patients.

In the majority of current recommendations, including those from the International Association for the Study of Pain, first-line treatments include antidepressants such as serotonin noradrenaline reuptake inhibitors (mainly duloxetine) or tri-cyclic anti-depressants such as amitriptyline and nortriptyline. Anti-epileptic agents such as gabapentin or pregabalin are also recommended for use as second-line treatments, although there is increasing concern around their abuse potential and association with an increase in drug deaths.

Opioid analgesics

Opioids have been used for centuries to reduce pain, and were originally obtained from the resin of the opium poppy (*Papaver somniferum*). Over recent years, new synthetic opioids such as fentanyl, oxycodon and tramadol have been introduced. The pharmacological effects of opioids are mediated by binding to a number of opioid receptors which are G-protein-coupled receptors, as summarised in Box 8.8. When opioids bind to their receptors, several intracellular signalling pathways are activated, increasing cyclic adenosine monophosphate (cAMP) levels and altering calcium and potassium permeability of neurons. Opioids are traditionally divided into subclasses of weak opioids, such as codeine and dihydrocodeine, and strong opioids, such as morphine and oxycodone. While tramadol is a weak agonist at the mu opioid receptor, it is classified as a strong opioid in some countries. Codeine and dihydrocodeine are metabolised in the liver to morphine by *CYP2D6* at a rate that is genetically determined. Similarly, tramadol is metabolised by *CYP2D6* to yield o-desmethyltramadol, which has greater affinity than tramadol for opioid receptors. Up to 10% of people are rapid metabolisers and this may be associated with differences in efficacy and adverse effects of these drugs between individuals (see Box 2.5). The dosages and characteristics of commonly prescribed opioids are shown in Box 8.9. There has been a large increase in the use of strong opioids for chronic pain over the last few decades, to the extent that it has been referred to as an 'opioid epidemic'. A number of factors contribute to this, including a rising incidence of chronic pain with an ageing population, reluctance to use NSAIDs because of cardiovascular and gastrointestinal adverse effects, changes in patient expectation, societal attitudes and availability of new formulations of opioids. There is very limited evidence of short- to medium-term benefit for strong opioids in low back pain and osteoarthritis with more recent longer-term evidence finding no improvement in function, worse pain and increased side-effects in people on opioids compared to non-opioid analgesia. More good-quality studies of

i 8.8 Endogenous opioids and opioid receptors

Endogenous ligand	Receptor (IUPHAR)	Alternative classification	Potential sites	Pharmacological effects
Endomorphin 1 and 2 Met-enkephalin Dynorphin A Dynorphin B	MOP	Mu	Brain, spinal cord, peripheral nerves, immune cells	Analgesia, reduced gastrointestinal motility, respiratory depression, pruritus
Leu-enkephalin Met-enkephalin β-endorphin	DOP	Delta	Brain, spinal cord, peripheral nerves	Analgesia, cardioprotection, thermoregulation
Dynorphin A Dynorphin B β-endorphin	KOP	Kappa	Brain (nucleus accumbens, neocortex, brainstem, cerebellum)	Analgesia, neuroendocrine (hypothalamic–pituitary axis), diuresis, dysphoria
Orphanin FQ (nociceptin)	NOP	Orphan	Nucleus raphe magnus, spinal cord, afferent neurons	Opioid tolerance, anxiety, depression, increased appetite

It is thought that opioids used clinically act through the MOP.
(IUPHAR = International Union of Basic and Clinical Pharmacology)

i 8.9 Commonly used opioids

Opioid	Typical starting dose	Route	Oral morphine equivalent	Comments
Morphine	10 mg	Oral	10 mg	Most widely used
Codeine	30–60 mg; max 240 mg/24 hr	Oral	3–6 mg	Metabolised to morphine by *CYP2D6* enzyme
Dihydrocodeine	60 mg; max 240 mg/24 hr	Oral	6 mg	Metabolised to morphine by *CYP2D6* enzyme
Tramadol	100 mg; max 400 mg/24 hr	Oral	10 mg	Metabolised to o-desmethyl tramadol by *CYP2D6* enzyme
Oxycodone	6.6 mg	Oral	10 mg	More predictable bioavailability than morphine
Buprenorphine	5 µg/hr	Transdermal	12 mg/day	Patch change usually every 7 days (frequency of change dependent on manufacturer and dose); advantages in impaired renal function
Fentanyl	12 µg/hr	Transdermal	30 mg/day	Use with care in opioid-naïve patients; patch change usually every 72 hrs
Tapentadol	50 mg; max 600 mg/24 hr	Oral	20 mg	Use with care in opioid-naïve patients
Hydromorphone	2 mg	Oral	10 mg	Semi-synthetic; hepatic metabolism
Morphine	3 mg	Subcutaneous, intramuscular, intravenous	10 mg	Mainly used for acute pain or palliative care

long-term use are needed. Additionally, there is increasing concern about potential harm from long-term use. This includes addiction, dependence, opioid-induced hyperalgesia, endocrine dysfunction, fracture risk (especially in older people), overdose and cardiovascular events, with many of these adverse effects being dose-related. Doses of more than 50 mg morphine equivalents per day may be detrimental, with an increased in harm at doses of >90 mg morphine equivalents per day. National and international guidelines have changed to reflect this, with most only recommending short- to medium-term use of opioids in carefully selected patients, as part of a holistic management plan. Regular review is essential to assess ongoing benefit, and any opioid trial should have clear goals, and a plan for cessation if these are not reached. A suggested strategy for using strong opioids in chronic pain is shown in Box 8.10.

Psychological therapies

The aims of psychological therapy are to increase coping skills and improve quality of life when facing the challenges of living with chronic pain. There are a range of ways in which psychological therapies can be delivered, including individual one-to-one sessions, group sessions, multidisciplinary pain management programmes, or web-based or telephone-based programmes.

There is good evidence for the use of a cognitive behavioural therapy (CBT)-based approach for chronic pain, delivered either individually or in a group. The overall aim is to reduce negative thoughts and beliefs, and develop positive coping strategies. The interaction between thoughts, behaviours and emotions is explored, and a problem-focused approach is used in therapy delivery.

Relaxation techniques, such as biofeedback and mindfulness meditation, require a degree of stillness and withdrawal, with regular practice required for sustained benefit (see 'Further information'). Acceptance and commitment therapy (ACT) is based on CBT principles but also uses components of mindfulness to improve psychological flexibility in the context of living with chronic pain.

Stimulation therapies

These range from minimally invasive procedures like acupuncture and transcutaneous electrical nerve stimulation (TENS) to more invasive techniques such as spinal cord stimulation.

i 8.10 Use of opioids in chronic pain: Always use as part of a holistic management plan

Step	Factors to take into account	Comment
1. Assess suitability for opioids	Type of pain Likelihood of dependence Co-morbidity	Neuropathic pain and chronic widespread pain less likely to respond Increased risk in those with history of alcohol and substance misuse Avoid use in conditions where adverse effects more likely: 　Chronic obstructive pulmonary disease 　Chronic liver disease 　Chronic kidney disease
2. Discuss with patient	Discuss potential benefits Discuss adverse effects Establish treatment goal	Improvement in pain Improvement in function Nausea Constipation Drowsiness Improvement in function
3. Plan treatment trial	Set timescale Agree on dose Agree on stopping rules	Define duration of treatment Agree frequency of review Aim for lowest effective dose Set upper dose limit Consider stopping if: 　Treatment goal is not met 　There is no dose response 　Tolerance develops rapidly

Acupuncture (Fig. 8.6) has been used successfully in Eastern medicine for centuries. The mechanisms are incompletely understood, although endorphin release may explain, in part, the analgesic effect. Acupuncture is particularly effective in pain related to muscle spasm, with some evidence of short-term benefit for patients with low back pain. Similar mechanisms probably apply to TENS, which is worth considering in many types of chronic pain. Neuromodulation, using implanted electrodes in the epidural space (or, more recently, adjacent to peripheral nerves), has been shown to be an effective option for neuropathic pain, including failed back surgery syndrome and chronic regional pain syndrome (see below). Specialist assessment and ongoing support is necessary, as there are many potential complications, including infection, malfunction and battery failure. The likelihood of success is increased when this technique is used within the context of multidisciplinary assessment and management.

Complementary and alternative therapies

Complementary techniques, such as herbal medicines, vitamins, homeopathy and reflexology, have been used for the treatment of chronic pain but with little evidence of efficacy. It should be noted that herbal medications may interact with conventional drugs, causing adverse effects as the result of drug–drug interactions. St John's wort (*Hypericum perforatum*) interacts with many drugs, including many antidepressants used in chronic pain, with increased serotonergic effects. Grapefruit may also increase the risk of serotonergic effects with some antidepressants. *Ginkgo biloba* may interact with paracetamol to increase bleeding time.

Nerve blocks and nerve ablation

The use of specialist nerve blocks and nerve ablation therapy can be considered for pain that is unresponsive to less invasive approaches. If these are being considered, they should form part of a multidisciplinary management plan, with the aim of restoring function and reducing pain. Local anaesthetic with or without depot glucocorticoid (non-particulate for neuraxial administration) can be effective in some circumstances. Examples include occipital nerve blocks for migraine or cervicogenic headache and trigger point injections for myofascial pain. If there is limited compression of a spinal nerve root, the nerve root injections into the epidural space may help settle symptoms and

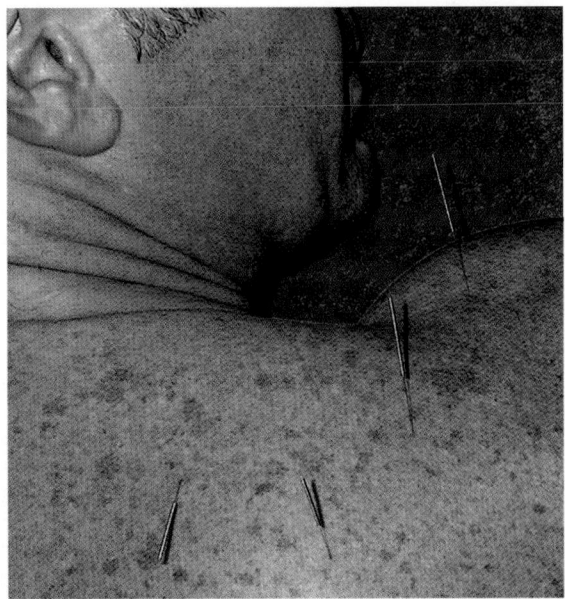

Fig. 8.6 Acupuncture.

avoid the need for surgical intervention. Neurodestructive procedures can also be employed for intractable pain but are rarely used outside the palliative care setting.

Chronic pain syndromes

Chronic pain is a feature of several recognised syndromes, which are discussed in more detail below.

Neuropathic pain

Neuropathic pain is defined as 'pain associated with a lesion or disease of the somatosensory nervous system'. Neuropathic pain may be acute, such as in sciatica, which occurs as the result of a prolapsed disc, but is most problematic when it becomes chronic. Neuropathic pain causes major morbidity; in a recent study, 17% of those affected rated their

i	**8.11 Clinical features of neuropathic pain**	
Characteristic	Symptom or clinical feature*	Descriptive term
Spontaneous pain	No stimulus required to evoke pain	
Positive sensory disturbance	Light touch painful Pressure painful Increased pain on pin-prick Cool and warm temperatures painful	Dynamic allodynia Punctate allodynia Hyperalgesia Thermal allodynia
Negative sensory disturbance	Numbness Tingling Loss of temperature sensitivity	Loss of sensation Paraesthesia
Other features	Feeling of insects crawling over skin Affected area feels abnormal	Formication Dysaesthesia

*Symptoms may cluster, with a predominance of either positive or negative symptoms, or a mixture of both, reflecting differences in underlying mechanisms.

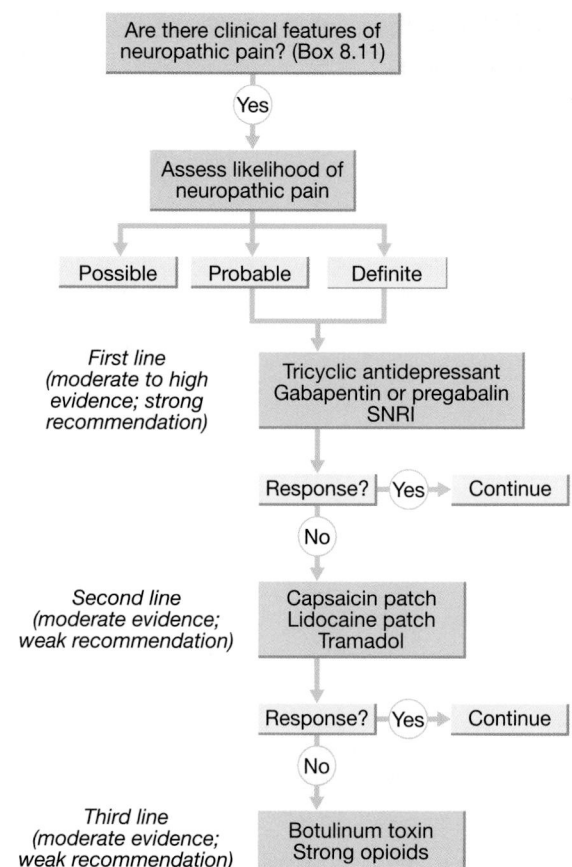

Fig. 8.7 Algorithm for pharmacological management of neuropathic pain. (SNRI = serotonin noradrenaline (norepinephrine) re-uptake inhibitor) *Adapted from SIGN 136 and NeuPSIG recommendations; reproduced from Finnerup NB, Attal N, Haroutounian S, et al. Pharmacotherapy for neuropathic pain in adults: a systematic review and meta-analysis. The Lancet Neurol 2015; 14:162–173, with permission from Elsevier.*

quality of life as 'worse than death'. The clinical features of neuropathic pain are summarised in Box 8.11. The diagnosis is easily missed and so careful assessment is vital, in order to make the diagnosis in the first place and then to direct management appropriately. An algorithm for the management of neuropathic pain is provided in Figure 8.7. It is important to recognise the negative impact of neuropathic pain on quality of life, which has been shown to be greater than with other types of chronic pain. As a result, appropriate support and multidisciplinary management should always be considered in addition to pharmacological therapies.

Complex regional pain syndrome

Complex regional pain syndrome (CRPS) is a type of neuropathic pain that affects one or more limbs. It was previously termed reflex sympathetic dystrophy (RSD), reflecting the fact the disease is thought to be caused in part by an abnormality in the autonomic nervous system. It is a rare syndrome, occurring in about 20 per 100 000 individuals, and is more common in females, typically presenting between the ages of 35 and 50. It is classified into type 1 CRPS, which may be precipitated by a traumatic event such as a fracture but is not associated with peripheral nerve damage, and type 2 CRPS, which is associated with a peripheral nerve lesion. The diagnosis is primarily clinical, with the current standard being based on the Budapest criteria, as outlined in Box 8.12. Other diagnostic tools, none of which provide a definitive diagnosis, include thermography (temperature difference of >1°C), and electromyography (if myoclonus is a feature). Increased tracer uptake on radionuclide bone scan and bone marrow oedema on MRI scan may be observed in CRPS but the diagnosis is primarily clinical, as outlined in Box 8.12.

Prompt diagnosis and early treatment with physiotherapy, and additional approaches such as desensitisation, and graded motor imagery, may prevent progression of symptoms. Pharmacological management is similar to that for neuropathic pain. Specific approaches (with variable quality evidence) that may be considered include bisphosphonates or calcitonin. Intravenous regional block with guanethidine is not recommended, as there is limited evidence of benefit, and an increased risk of adverse effects. If medical management is incompletely effective, consideration should be given to the appropriateness of a spinal cord stimulator, with reasonable evidence of efficacy.

Phantom limb pain

Phantom limb is a common complication of amputation, occurring in up to 70% of patients. It is a form of neuropathic pain but can

be particularly distressing, as the pain is felt in the area where the absent limb was previously. Although usually presenting after limb amputation, reports of phantom pain in other body parts have been reported, such as phantom breast pain following mastectomy. It is very often associated with phantom sensations, which are described as non-painful sensations in the absent body part and pain in the stump.

Diagnostic nerve blocks may be helpful in directing therapy, with use of anti-neuropathic medications as outlined in Box 8.7. If there is a definite neuroma at the stump site that is interfering with prosthesis use, surgical review may be necessary. Management should use rehabilitation approaches with physical therapy. Additional approaches such as mirror visual feedback and desensitisation may also be considered.

Chronic widespread pain

Chronic widespread pain (CWP) is often associated with other features, such as fatigue and irritable bowel syndrome. Fibromyalgia is a subtype of CWP in which there are myofascial trigger points, and is often associated with sleep disturbance. Clinical features and management of fibromyalgia are discussed in more detail in Chapter 26.

Joint hypermobility syndrome

Hypermobility can be associated with chronic musculoskeletal pain that often targets the joints and periarticular tissues. It is thought to be caused by abnormal stresses being placed on the joints and surrounding

8.12 The Budapest criteria for diagnosis of complex regional pain syndrome (CRPS)	
Category	**Symptom or sign**

Sensory	Allodynia to:
	    Temperature
	    Light touch
	    Deep somatic pressure
	    Movement
	Hyperalgesia to pin-prick

Vasomotor	Temperature asymmetry Skin colour change and/or asymmetry
Sudomotor	Oedema Sweating change and/or asymmetry

Motor/trophic	Reduced range of motion
	Motor dysfunction:
	    Weakness
	    Tremor
	    Dystonia
	Trophic changes:
	    Hair
	    Nails
	    Skin

Type 1 CRPS: without evidence of major nerve damage; type 2 CRPS: evidence of major nerve damage. For a positive diagnosis, the patient should report at least one symptom in at least three out of the four categories, and at least one sign should be detected in two out of the four categories. Other causes that might explain the signs and symptoms should be excluded.

soft tissues due to ligament laxity, although the mechanisms are poorly understood since many people with hypermobile joints do not suffer pain. It is described in more detail in Chapter 26.

Palliative care

Palliative care is the term used to describe the active total care of patients with incurable disease. It can be distinguished from end-of-life care, which refers to the care of patients with far advanced, rapidly progressive disease that will soon prove fatal. The focus of palliative care is on symptom control alongside supportive care. While palliative care can and should be delivered at any stage of an incurable illness alongside optimal disease control, the focus of end-of-life care is on quality of life rather than prolongation of life or cure. Palliative care encompasses a distinct body of knowledge and skills that all good physicians must possess to allow them to care effectively for patients. Palliative care is seen traditionally as a means of managing distress and symptoms in patients with cancer, when metastatic disease has been diagnosed and death is seen as inevitable. However, prognosis in metastatic cancers has evolved significantly with the emergence of improved anti-cancer treatments, hence the principle of delivering palliative and supportive care whenever a patient needs it, as opposed to a specific stage of disease, is now even more important. There is also a growing recognition that the principles of palliative care and some of the interventions it uses are equally applicable in other conditions. Palliative care may be applied to any chronic disease state. Which elements are used will depend on the individual patient's need.

For conditions other than cancer, the challenge is recognising when patients have entered the terminal phase of their illness, as there are fewer clear markers and the course of the illness is much more variable. Different chronic disease states progress at different rates, allowing some general trajectories of illness or dying to be defined (Fig. 8.8). These trajectories are useful in decision-making for individual patients but also in the planning of services.

The 'rapid decline' trajectory following a gradual decline, as occurs in cancer, is the best-recognised pattern of the need for palliative care,

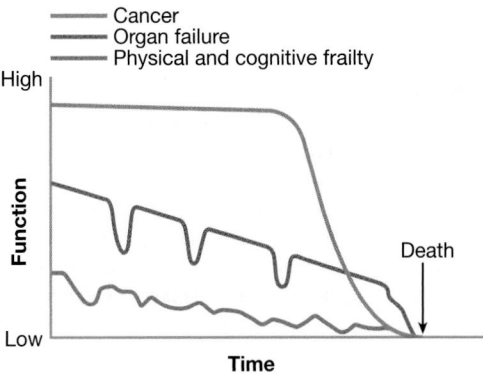

Fig. 8.8 Archetypal trajectories of dying. *From Murray SA, Kendall M, Boyd K, et al. Illness trajectories and palliative care. BMJ 2005; 330:7498; reproduced with permission from the BMJ Publishing Group.*

although a similar trajectory may be observed in other conditions, such as motor neuron disease. Many traditional hospice services are designed to meet the needs of people on this trajectory. Over recent years, improvements in management of malignant disease mean that some types of cancer may follow an erratic or intermittent decline trajectory.

Many chronic diseases, such as advanced chronic obstructive pulmonary disease (COPD) and intractable congestive heart failure, carry as high a burden of symptoms as cancer, as well as psychological and family distress. The 'palliative phase' of these illnesses may be more difficult to identify because of periods of relative stability interspersed with acute episodes of severe illness. However, it is still possible to recognise those patients who may benefit from a palliative approach to their care. The challenge is that symptom management needs to be delivered at the same time as treatment for acute exacerbations. This leads to difficult decisions as to the balance between symptom relief and aggressive management of the underlying disease. The starting point of need for palliative care in these conditions is the point at which consideration of comfort and individual values becomes important in decision-making, often alongside management of the underlying disease.

The third major trajectory is categorised by years of poor function and frailty before a relatively short terminal period; it is exemplified by dementia but is also increasingly true for patients with many different chronic illnesses. As medical advances extend survival, this mode of dying is being experienced by increasing numbers of people. The main challenge lies in providing nursing care and ensuring that plans are agreed for the time when medical intervention is no longer beneficial.

In a situation where death is inevitable and foreseeable, palliative care aims to strike a balance between addressing the wishes, expectations and values of the patient with a realistic assessment of the benefits of medical interventions. This often results in a greater focus on comfort, symptom control and support for patient and family, and may enable withdrawal of both futile and burdensome interventions. In cases of prognostic uncertainty, open, honest and gentle communication with the patient and family is important. The most common symptoms in palliative care are discussed in the next section. The central networks we have heard about above in relation to chronic pain also exist for all other symptoms. In addition there is an extra complexity in cancer as a result of the additional layer of biological complexity resulting from the factors released by the tumour such as pro-inflammatory cytokines and the body's response to these factors.

Presenting problems in palliative care

Pain

Pain is a common problem in palliative care. It has been estimated that about two-thirds of patients with cancer experience moderate or severe pain, and a quarter have three or more different sites of pain. Many of these are of a mixed aetiology and about half of patients with cancer-associated pain have a neuropathic element.

Clinical assessment

The commonest barrier to assessment of pain is the development of idiosyncratic shortcuts in the belief that these are also easier for the patient. A common example is, 'How is your pain?' The patient will often give a reflex response such as, 'OK', which might be documented by the clinician as 0, 1 or 2 out of 10. If the same patient were asked, 'Have you had any pain in the last 24 hours, on a scale of 0–10, where 0 is none at all and 10 is the worst imaginable?' the same patient might record a score as high as 8 or 9 out of 10. This emphasises the importance of using a validated question that screens for pain effectively.

Improved control of cancer-associated pain has been demonstrated with use of the Edinburgh Pain Assessment and management Tool (EPAT). This involves administration of a simple screening question about worst pain on a scale of 0–10 in the last 24 hours, followed by questions to identify specific pain/s such as neuropathic or bone, in addition to distress. The identified pains are linked to management algorithms. Review of pain and opioid side-effects completes the loop (see 'Further information').

Clinical features and suggested management strategies for common types of pain in cancer are shown in Box 8.13. The majority of patients with cancer-associated pain can be managed effectively using a step-wise approach, as outlined below.

Management: pharmacological treatments

Pharmacological treatments are the mainstay of management in cancer-associated pain, however, they have to be underpinned by an appropriate assessment of pain and associated symptoms. In addition, non-pharmacological treatments and disease-modifying treatments run through each step of pain control. A stepwise approach is adopted, following the principles of the World Health Organization (WHO) analgesic ladder (Fig. 8.9), in which analgesia that is appropriate for the degree of pain is prescribed first. Patients with mild pain should be started on a non-opioid analgesic drug, such as paracetamol (maximum: 1 g 4 times daily) or an NSAID (step 1). If the patient fails to respond adequately or has moderate pain, a weak opioid, such as codeine (60 mg 4 times daily), should be added (step 2). This can be prescribed separately or in the form of the compound analgesic co-codamol. If pain relief is still not achieved or if the patient has severe pain, a strong opioid should be substituted for the weak opioid (step 3). If the pain is severe at the outset, strong opioids should be prescribed and increased or titrated according to the patient's response. It is important not to move 'sideways' (change from one drug to another of equal potency), which is a common problem during step 2 of the analgesic ladder.

In recent years there has been a tendency to use a low dose of a step 3 opioid rather than a traditional step 2 opioid such as codeine. It has now been demonstrated that it is safe, effective and has cost savings to miss out step 2 of the analgesic ladder. This is of great importance in low- and middle-income countries where step 2 drugs are usually much more expensive than morphine.

Opioids

Opioid analgesia plays a key role in patients with moderate to severe pain. Its successful use depends on appropriate assessment and a detailed explanation to the patient and carer about the benefits and potential side-effects of therapy. Morphine is the most commonly prescribed strong opioid, although there are several alternatives, as outlined in Box 8.9.

Oral morphine takes about 20 minutes to exert an effect and usually provides pain relief for 4 hours. Most patients with continuous pain should be prescribed oral morphine every 4 hours initially, as this will provide continuous pain relief over the whole 24-hour period. Controlled-release morphine lasts for 12 or 24 hours, depending on the formulation, and if clinical circumstances dictate, a controlled-release formulation can be used to initiate and titrate morphine. The median effective morphine equivalent dose for cancer pain is about 200 mg per 24 hours.

i	8.13 Common types of pain in cancer		
Type of pain	**Features**		**Management options**
Bone pain	Tender area over bone Possible pain on movement		NSAIDs Bisphosphonates Radiotherapy
Increased intracranial pressure	Headache, worse in the morning, associated with vomiting and occasionally delirium		Glucocorticoids Radiotherapy Opioid
Abdominal colic	Intermittent, severe, spasmodic, associated with nausea or vomiting		Antispasmodics Hyoscine butylbromide Antiemetic and opioid may be required for intestinal obstruction
Liver capsule pain	Right upper quadrant abdominal pain, often associated with tender enlarged liver Responds poorly to opioids		Glucocorticoids
Neuropathic pain	Spontaneous pain Light touch, pressure and temperature changes are painful; increased pain on pin-prick Numbness, tingling or loss of temperature sensation Skin feels abnormal		Anticonvulsants: Gabapentin Pregabalin Antidepressants: Amitriptyline Duloxetine Ketamine
Ischaemic pain	Diffuse, severe, aching pain associated with evidence of poor perfusion Responds poorly to opioids		NSAIDs Ketamine
Incident pain	Episodic pain usually related to movement		Intermittent short-acting opioids Nerve block

(NSAIDs = non-steroidal anti-inflammatory drugs)

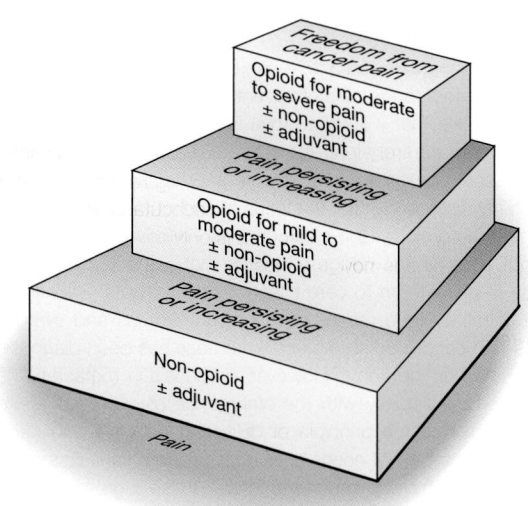

Fig. 8.9 The WHO analgesic ladder. *From WHO. Cancer pain relief, 2nd edn. Geneva: WHO; 1996.*

In addition to the regular dose of morphine, an extra dose of immediate-release (IR) morphine should be prescribed 'as required' for the treatment of breakthrough pain that has not been controlled by the regular prescription. As a rule of thumb, this additional dose should be one-sixth of the total 24-hour dose of opioid. The frequency of breakthrough doses should be dictated by their efficacy and any side-effects, rather than by a fixed time interval. A patient may require breakthrough analgesia as frequently as hourly if pain is severe, but this should lead to early review of the regular prescription. The patient or carer should note the timing of any breakthrough doses and the reason for them. These should be reviewed daily and the regular 4-hourly dose increased for the next 24 hours on the basis of:

- the frequency of and reasons for breakthrough analgesia
- the degree and acceptability of side-effects.

The regular dose should be increased by adding the total of the breakthrough doses over the previous 24 hours, unless there are significant problems with unacceptable side-effects. When the correct dose has been established, a continuous release (CR) preparation can be prescribed, usually twice daily. Breakthrough analgesia used for movement-related pain is generally not included in background opioid dose titration. Attempts to control movement-related pain with background opioid dose will usually lead to over-dosing and opioid-related side-effects. This can be a risk in metastatic bone pain.

Some patients may have concerns about using opioids and it is vital for these to be explored. Patients should be reassured that psychological dependence is rare when opioids are used for cancer pain, unless a pre-existing dependence problem exists. Recent survey data from the United States have suggested that opioid abuse may occur in up to 20% of cancer patients, but to-date, these data have not been replicated in other countries. In fact, the majority of the world's population do not have any access to opioids for cancer pain relief. Good prescribing practice, clear communication and reassessment of benefits and side-effects are all critical in achieving good cancer pain relief. Pharmacological tolerance is not usually a clinically relevant problem; however, physical dependence, which is physiological, as manifest by a physical withdrawal syndrome, can occur if opioids are suddenly discontinued.

Nearly all types of cancer pain respond to morphine to some degree but there is a spectrum of response, such that in some patients the dose of opioid required to control neuropathic pain and all elements of metastatic bone pain may be high and associated with unacceptable side-effects. In these situations, other methods of analgesia, both pharmacological and non-pharmacological, should be explored and considered at an early stage.

The most effective and appropriate route of morphine administration is oral but transdermal preparations of strong opioids (usually fentanyl) are useful in certain situations, such as in patients with dysphagia or those who are reluctant to take tablets on a regular basis. Diamorphine is a highly soluble strong opioid used for subcutaneous infusions, particularly in the last few days of life, but is only available in certain countries and morphine is now the most commonly prescribed parenteral opioid.

Opioid-related adverse effects

Adverse effects are a common problem with opioids, especially on initiating treatment and on increasing the dose. The most common side-effects are nausea, drowsiness, constipation and dry mouth, as summarised in Box 8.14. Nausea and vomiting can occur initially but usually settle after a few days. Drowsiness is usually transient at opioid initiation and dose increase. If it is persistent, an alternative opioid and/or a non-opioid should be considered. In acute dosing, respiratory depression can occur but this is rare in patients on regular opioids or in those starting on small, regular doses with appropriate titration.

Tolerance usually develops to nausea, vomiting and drowsiness but not to constipation or dry mouth. All patients should therefore be prescribed a laxative, unless suffering from diarrhoea, and have access to an antiemetic and good mouth care, along with rationalisation of any concomitant medication that might exacerbate drowsiness. Newer developments include the use of preparations in which opioids are combined with opioid antagonists, such as naloxone. The naloxone is poorly absorbed and does not antagonise the systemic analgesic effect but

Side-effect	Management
Constipation	Regular laxative Opioid/naloxone oral combination, in resistant constipation
Dry mouth	Frequent sips of iced water, soft white paraffin to lips, chlorhexidine mouthwashes twice daily, sugar-free gum, water or saliva sprays
Nausea/vomiting	Oral haloperidol 0.5–1 mg at night, oral metoclopramide 10 mg 3 times daily or oral domperidone 10 mg 3 times daily If constant, haloperidol or levomepromazine may be given parenterally to break the nausea cycle
Sedation	Explanation is very important Symptoms usually settle in a few days Avoid other sedating medication where possible Ensure appropriate use of adjuvant analgesics that can have an opioid-sparing effect May require an alternative opioid

8.14 Opioid side-effects

rather acts locally to block opioid receptors in the gut, thereby reducing opioid-related constipation. Vivid dreams, visual hallucinations (often consisting of a sense of movement at the periphery of vision), delirium and myoclonus are typical of opioid-related toxicity and, if present, require urgent reassessment of the opioid dose. Biochemistry should also be checked to exclude renal impairment, dehydration, electrolyte disturbance or hypercalcaemia.

Since opioid toxicity can occur at any dose, side-effects should be assessed regularly, but particularly after a dose increase. Pain should be reassessed to ensure that appropriate adjuvants are being used. Parenteral rehydration is often helpful to speed up excretion of active metabolites of morphine. The dose of opioid may need to be reduced or the opioid changed to a strong alternative.

Different opioids have different side-effect profiles in different people. If a patient develops side-effects, switching to an alternative strong opioid may be helpful. Options include oxycodone, transdermal fentanyl, hydromorphone and occasionally methadone, any of which may produce a better balance of benefit against side-effects. Fentanyl has no renally excreted active metabolites and may be particularly useful in patients with renal failure. Buprenorphine is also particularly useful in significant renal impairment. It is possible to switch between opioids but great care must be taken when doing so to make sure the dose is correct and to avoid prescribing too much or too little opioid.

Adjuvant analgesics

An adjuvant analgesic is a drug that has a primary indication other than pain but which provides analgesia in some painful conditions and may enhance the effect of the primary analgesic. Commonly used adjuvant analgesics in the palliative care setting are shown in Box 8.15. Some adjuvant analgesics may enhance the side-effect profile of the primary analgesic, and dose reductions of opioids may be required when an adjuvant analgesic is added. At each step of the WHO analgesic ladder, an adjuvant analgesic should be considered, the choice depending on the type of pain.

Management: non-pharmacological treatments
Neurodestructive interventions

Neurodestructive techniques have an important role in the management of cancer pain, where life expectancy is limited. They should be used as part of an overall management plan and considered when the response to drug treatment has been inadequate. Intrathecal analgesia, delivered via either an external pump or a fully implanted device, is a good option,

i | **8.15 Adjuvant analgesics in cancer pain**

Drug	Example	Indications	Side-effects*
NSAIDs	Diclofenac	Bone metastases, soft tissue infiltration, liver pain, inflammatory pain	Gastric irritation and bleeding, fluid retention, headache Caution in renal impairment
Glucocorticoids	Dexamethasone 8–16 mg per day, titrated to lowest dose that controls pain	Raised intracranial pressure, nerve compression, soft tissue infiltration, liver pain	Gastric irritation if used together with NSAID, fluid retention, proximal muscle myopathy, delirium, Cushingoid appearance, candidiasis, hyperglycaemia
Anticonvulsants	Evidence strongest for: Duloxetine Gabapentin Pregabalin	Neuropathic pain of any aetiology	Mild sedation, tremor, delirium Exacerbation of opioid-related side-effects
Tricyclic antidepressants	Amitriptyline Nortriptyline (less sedative)	Neuropathic pain of any aetiology	Sedation, dizziness, delirium, dry mouth, constipation, urinary retention Avoid in cardiac disease Exacerbation of opioid-related side-effects
NMDA receptor blockers	Ketamine	Severe neuropathic pain (only under specialist supervision)	Delirium, anxiety, agitation, hypertension

*In old age, all drugs can cause delirium.
(NMDA = N-methyl-D-aspartate; NSAIDs = non-steroidal anti-inflammatory drugs)

particularly where life expectancy is more than 3 months. Coeliac plexus blocks can be helpful for visceral pain, such as in pancreatic cancer. Lateral cordotomy to disrupt the spinothalamic tracts (either open or percutaneous) may be considered for unilateral chest wall pain, such as may occur in mesothelioma, where life expectancy is limited.

Radiotherapy

Radiotherapy is the treatment of choice for pain from bone metastases (see Box 8.13) and can also be considered for metastatic involvement at other sites. All patients with pain secondary to bone metastases should be considered for palliative radiotherapy, which can usually be given in a single dose. Some patients experience a transient flare of pain after radiotherapy and this can be managed by 24–48 hours of dexamethasone (4–8 mg once in the morning).

Physiotherapy

Physiotherapy has a key role in the multidisciplinary approach to a wide spectrum of cancer-related symptoms, including the prevention and management of pain, muscle spasm, reduced mobility, muscle wasting and lymphoedema. Rehabilitation in palliative care has expanded and now includes pre-habilitation, which involves the use of proactive focused exercise to maintain muscle mass during cancer chemotherapy and in other chronic conditions such as COPD.

Psychological techniques

As with chronic pain, there is increasing use of psychological techniques in cancer pain management, which train the patient to use coping strategies and behavioural techniques. Other issues related to the specific experience of a cancer diagnosis and cancer treatment may be complex, and individual therapy in addition to group-based approaches can be helpful.

Stimulation therapies

Acupuncture and TENS are low-risk stimulation therapies that may be useful in palliative care for management of pain and nausea. Both are particularly useful for secondary muscle spasm and TENS is increasingly used for bone pain.

Complementary and alternative therapies

Palliative care patients often seek symptom relief from both complementary and alternative therapies. While the evidence base is poorly developed, individual patients can gain significant benefits from the complementary therapies as outlined earlier in this chapter. It is critically important that patients are encouraged to discuss any alternative medicines they are considering, given the potential interactions with other therapies.

Breathlessness

Breathlessness is one of the most common symptoms in palliative care and is distressing for both patients and carers. Patients with breathlessness should be fully assessed to determine whether there is a reversible cause, such as a pleural effusion, heart failure or bronchospasm; if so, this should be managed in the normal way. If symptoms persist, additional measures may be necessary. There are many potential causes of dyspnoea in cancer patients and in other chronic diseases; apart from direct involvement of the lungs, muscle loss secondary to cachexia, anxiety and fear can all contribute. A cycle of panic and breathlessness, often associated with fear of dying, can be dominant. Exploration of precipitating factors is important and patient education about breathlessness and effective breathing has been shown to be effective. Non-pharmacological approaches that include using a hand-held fan, pacing and following a tailored exercise programme can help. There is no evidence to suggest that oxygen therapy reduces the sensation of breathlessness in advanced cancer any better than cool airflow, and oxygen is indicated only if there is significant hypoxia. Opioids, through both their central and their peripheral action, can palliate breathlessness. Both oral and parenteral opioids are effective and are now licensed for this indication in Australia. A low dose should be used initially and titrated against symptoms, unless opioids are already being prescribed for pain, in which case the existing dose can be increased further. If anxiety is considered to be playing a significant role, a quick-acting benzodiazepine, such as lorazepam (used sublingually for rapid absorption), may also be useful.

Cough

Persistent unproductive cough can be helped by opioids, which have an antitussive effect. Troublesome respiratory secretions can be treated with hyoscine hydrobromide (400–600 µg every 4–8 hours), although dry mouth is a common adverse effect. As an alternative, glycopyrronium can be useful and is given by subcutaneous infusion (0.6–1.2 mg in 24 hours).

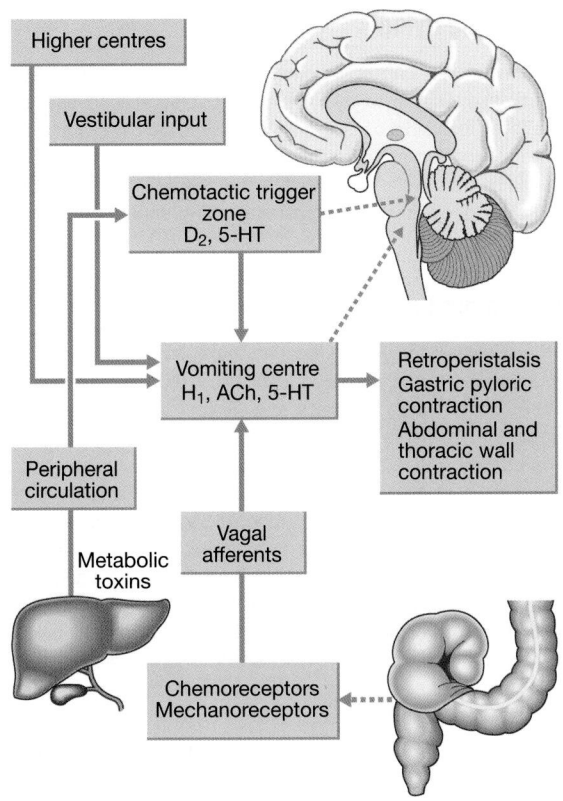

Fig. 8.10 Mechanisms of nausea. (ACh = acetylcholine; D_2 = dopamine; 5-HT = 5-hydroxytryptamine, serotonin; H_1 = histamine)

8.16 Receptor site activity of antiemetic drugs		
Area	**Receptors**	**Drugs**
Chemotactic trigger zone	Dopamine$_2$ 5-HT	Haloperidol Metoclopramide
Vomiting centre	Histamine$_1$ Acetylcholine	Cyclizine Levomepromazine Hyoscine
Gut (gastric stasis)		Metoclopramide
Gut distension (vagal stimulation)	Histamine$_1$	Cyclizine
Gut (chemoreceptors)	5-HT	Levomepromazine

(5-HT = 5-hydroxytryptamine, serotonin)

Nausea and vomiting

The presentation of nausea and vomiting differs depending on the underlying cause, of which there are many. Large-volume vomiting with little nausea is common in intestinal obstruction, whereas constant nausea with little or no vomiting is often due to metabolic abnormalities or adverse effects of drugs. Vomiting related to raised intracranial pressure is worse in the morning. Different receptors are activated, depending on the cause or causes of the nausea (Fig. 8.10). For example, dopamine receptors in the chemotactic trigger zone in the fourth ventricle are stimulated by metabolic and drug causes of nausea, whereas gastric irritation stimulates histamine receptors in the vomiting centre via the vagus nerve. Reversible causes, such as hypercalcaemia and constipation, should be treated appropriately. Drug-induced causes should be considered and the offending drugs stopped if possible. As different classes of antiemetic drug act at different receptors, antiemetic therapy should be based on a careful assessment of the probable causes and a rational decision to use a particular class of drug (Box 8.16). The subcutaneous route is often required initially to overcome gastric stasis and poor absorption of oral medicines.

Gastrointestinal obstruction

Gastrointestinal obstruction is a frequent complication of intra-abdominal cancer. Patients may have multiple levels of obstruction and symptoms may vary greatly in nature and severity. Surgical mortality is high in patients with advanced disease and obstruction should normally be managed without surgery. The key to effective management is to address the presenting symptoms – colic, abdominal pain, nausea, vomiting, intestinal secretions – individually or in combination, using parenteral drugs that do not cause or worsen other symptoms. This can be problematic when a specific treatment worsens another symptom. Cyclizine improves nausea and colic responds well to anticholinergic agents, such

as hyoscine butylbromide, but both slow gut motility. Nausea will improve with metoclopramide, although this is usually contraindicated in the presence of colic because of its prokinetic effect. There is some low-quality evidence that glucocorticoids (dexamethasone 8 mg) can shorten the length of obstructive episodes. Somatostatin analogues, such as octreotide, will reduce intestinal secretions and therefore large-volume vomits. Occasionally, a nasogastric tube is required to reduce gaseous or fluid distension.

Weight loss

Patients with cancer lose weight for a variety of reasons, including reduced appetite or the effects of drug treatment, or as a consequence of low mood and anxiety. There is, however, a particularly challenging syndrome associated with weight loss, which is known as cancer cachexia. This results from an alteration of metabolism caused by a complex interaction of tumour-related factors and the body's response to these factors, resulting in muscle loss, along with anorexia. Treatment involves prescribing exercise to maintain muscle mass and strengthen muscles, ensuring that there is an adequate calorie intake and providing nutritional supplements. Anti-inflammatory medication to attenuate systemic inflammation is the subject of research and many patients self-medicate with fish oil. Glucocorticoids can temporarily boost appetite and general well-being but may cause false weight gain by promoting fluid retention. Their benefits need to be weighed against the risk of side-effects, and glucocorticoids should generally be used on a short-term basis only.

Anxiety and depression

Anxiety and depression are common in palliative care but the diagnosis may be difficult, since the physical symptoms of depression are similar to those of advanced cancer. It is therefore important to acknowledge that these symptoms are not inevitable in advanced cancer. Patients should still expect to look forward to things and to enjoy them, within the context of the situation. Simply asking the question 'Do you think you are depressed?' can be very useful in deciding with the patient whether antidepressants or psychological interventions may be of benefit. In this regard, psycho-oncology has been evolving rapidly and there is now good evidence for the role of 'talk therapy' in palliative care, along with other appropriate management of anxiety and depression. If antidepressants are required, citalopram and mirtazapine are good choices since they are generally well tolerated in patients with advanced disease.

Delirium and agitation

Many patients become confused or agitated in the last days of life. It is important to identify and treat potentially reversible causes unless the patient is too close to death for this to be feasible. Early diagnosis and effective management of delirium are extremely important. As in other palliative situations, it may not be possible to identify and treat the underlying cause, and the focus of management should be to ensure that the patient is comfortable. It is important to distinguish between behavioural change due to pain and that due to delirium, as opioids will improve one and worsen the other. The management of delirium is detailed in Chapter 34. It is important, even in the care of the actively dying patient, to treat delirium with antipsychotic medicines, such as haloperidol, or olanzapine if under 70 years, rather than to regard it as distress or anxiety and use benzodiazepines only.

Dehydration

Deciding whether to give intravenous fluids can be difficult when a patient is very unwell and the prognosis is uncertain. A patient with a major stroke, who is unable to swallow but is expected to survive the event, will develop renal impairment and thirst if not given fluids and should be hydrated. On the other hand, when a patient has been deteriorating and is clearly dying, parenteral hydration needs very careful consideration and it is very important to manage this on an individual basis. Patient comfort and avoidance of distress in the family are the primary aims. Where a patient and family are happy with meticulous oral hygiene and care to reduce the sensation of dryness in the mouth, this is usually more appropriate and effective at the end of life than parenteral hydration, which by itself will not necessarily improve the sensation of dryness. In some patients, parenteral hydration will simply exacerbate pooling of secretions, causing noisy and distressing breathing. Each decision should be individual and discussed with the patient's family.

Death and dying

Planning for dying

There have been dramatic improvements in the medical treatment and care of patients with cancer and other illnesses over recent years but the inescapable fact remains that everyone will die at some time. Planning for death should be actively considered in patients with chronic diseases when the death is considered to be foreseeable or inevitable. Doctors rarely know exactly when a patient will die but are usually aware that an individual is about to die and that medical interventions are unlikely to extend life or improve its quality significantly. Most people wish their doctors to be honest about this situation to allow them time to think ahead, make plans and address practical issues. A few do not wish to discuss future deterioration or death; if this is felt to be the case, avoidance of discussion should be respected. For doctors, it is helpful to understand an individual's wishes and values about medical interventions at this time, as this can help guide decisions about interventions. It is important to distinguish between interventions that will not provide clinical benefit (a medical decision) and those that do not confer sufficient benefit to be worthwhile (a decision that can only be reached with a patient's involvement and consent). A common example of this would be decisions about not attempting cardiopulmonary resuscitation.

In general, people wish for a dignified and peaceful death and most, but not all, prefer to die at home. Families also are grateful for the chance to prepare themselves for the death of a relative, by timely and gentle discussion with the doctor or other health professionals. Early discussion and effective planning improve the chances that an individual's wishes will be achieved. There are two important caveats: firstly, wishes can and do change as the terminal situation evolves, and secondly, planning in general can only be done over time as patients form a relationship with professionals and evolve an understanding of the situation in which they find themselves. Attempts to carry out and finalise advanced care planning at a single consultation, especially if a first meeting, are usually unsatisfactory.

Structures for assessment and planning around end-of-life care are for guidance only and the focus should evolve with the individual patient.

Diagnosing dying

When patients with cancer or other conditions become bed-bound, semi-comatose, unable to take tablets and only able to take sips of water, with no reversible cause, they are likely to be dying and many will have died within 2 days. Doctors are sometimes poor at recognising this and should be alert to the views of other members of the multidisciplinary team. A clear decision that the patient is dying should be agreed and recorded.

Management of dying

Once the conclusion has been reached that a patient is going to die in days to a few weeks, there is a significant shift in management (Box 8.17). Symptom control, relief of distress and care for the family become the most important elements of care. Medication and investigation are justifiable only if they contribute to these ends. When patients can no longer drink because they are dying, intravenous fluids are usually not necessary and may cause worsening of bronchial secretions; however, this is a decision that can be made only on an individual basis. Management should not be changed without discussion with the patient and/or family. Medicines should always be prescribed for the relief of symptoms. For example, morphine or diamorphine may be used to control pain, levomepromazine to control nausea, haloperidol to treat delirium, diazepam or midazolam to treat distress, and hyoscine hydrobromide to reduce respiratory secretions. Side-effects, such as drowsiness, may be acceptable if the principal aim of relieving distress is achieved. It is important to discuss and agree the aims of care with the patient's family. Poor communication with families at this time is one of the most common reasons for family distress afterwards and for formal complaints.

Ethical considerations

The overwhelming force in caring for any patient must be to listen to that patient and family and take their wishes on board. Patients know

---

8.17 How to manage a patient who is dying

Patient and family awareness
- Assess patient's and family's awareness of the situation
- Ensure patient, if able, and family understand plan of care

Medical interventions
- Stop non-essential medications that do not contribute to symptom control
- Stop inappropriate investigations and interventions, including routine observations

Resuscitation
- Complete Do Not Attempt Cardiopulmonary Resuscitation (DNACPR) form
- Deactivate implantable defibrillator

Symptom control
- Ensure availability of parenteral medication for symptom relief

Support for family
- Make sure you have contact details for family, that you know when they want to be contacted and that they are aware of facilities available to them

Religious and spiritual needs
- Make sure any particular wishes are identified and followed

Ongoing assessment
- Family's awareness of condition
- Management of symptoms
- Need for parenteral hydration

Care after death
- Make sure family know what they have to do
- Notify other appropriate health professionals

when health-care professionals are just receiving the information, as opposed to receiving and understanding the information in the context of the patient, their illness and needs, their carers and the socioeconomic context. It is impossible to provide holistic care for a patient without this comprehension. Every patient is unique and it is important to avoid slipping into a tick-box mentality in addressing items that should be covered in patients with advanced, incurable disease. While the key to successful palliative care is effective interdisciplinary working, every patient needs to know who has overall responsibility for their care. Trust in the whole team will come through a solid lead working with a team who are appropriately informed and in sympathy with the patient's situation, each having a clear role.

Families and other carers are often unprepared for the challenge of caring for a dying person. It can be an exhausting experience, both emotionally and physically, and without a critical number of carers battle fatigue can ensue, resulting in urgent admissions. With much discussion about advance directives, we should not lose sight of the reality of changing circumstances and wishes. Good anticipatory care means not just providing for new physical symptoms, but also planning for any time when care at home becomes no longer possible.

Capacity and advance directives

The wishes of the patient are paramount in Western societies, whereas in other cultures the views of the family are equally important. If a patient is unable to express their view because of communication or cognitive impairment, that person is said to lack 'capacity'. In order to decide what the patient would have wished, as much information as possible should be gained about any previously expressed wishes, along with the views of relatives and other health professionals. An advance directive is a previously recorded, written document of a patient's wishes. It should carry the same weight in decision-making as a patient's expressed wishes at that time, but may not be sufficiently specific to be used in a particular clinical situation. The legal framework for decision-making varies in different countries.

Euthanasia

In the UK and Europe, between 3% and 6% of dying patients will ask a doctor to end their life. Many of these requests are transient; some are associated with poor control of physical symptoms or a depressive illness. All expressions of a wish to die are an opportunity to help the patient discuss and address unresolved issues and problems. Reversible causes, such as pain or depression, should be treated. Sometimes, patients may choose to discontinue life-prolonging treatments, such as diuretics or anticoagulation, following discussion and the provision of adequate alternative symptom control. However, there remain a small number of patients who have a sustained, competent wish to end their lives, despite good control of physical symptoms. Euthanasia is now permitted or legal under certain circumstances in some countries but remains illegal in many others; public, ethical and legal debate over this issue continues and is often influenced by many complex non-palliative care issues. The European Association for Palliative Care does not see euthanasia or physician-assisted suicide as part of the role of palliative care physicians. The British Medical Association (BMA) has published results from its recent poll on assisted dying in the *BMJ* (8 October 2020). Respect for others' freedom is reflected in this poll as, even though 50% supported a change in the law to permit assisted dying, only 36% of those polled would be personally willing to prescribe lethal drugs. The results were similar for euthanasia, with 37% supporting a change in the law, but only 26% willing to participate in any way in the process of administering drugs with the intention of ending an eligible patient's life. It can be inferred from the poll, that although some BMA members would support a legal framework, thereby respecting freedom of opinion and demonstrating a toleration of others' views, the majority would not be prepared to be involved in assisted dying or in euthanasia themselves, even if legal (see 'Further information').

Further information

Journal articles

Fallon M, Walker J, Colvin L, Rodriguez A, Murray G, Sharpe M, on behalf of the EPAT© Study Group. Does the institutionalisation of pain assessment using the EPAT package reduce pain in cancer unit inpatients more than usual care; a cluster randomised trial. J Clin Oncol 2018; 36(13):1284–1290.

Finnerup NB, Attal N, Haroutounian S, et al. Pharmacotherapy for neuropathic pain in adults: a systematic review and meta-analysis. Lancet Neurol 2015;14:162–173. *A comprehensive, high-quality review of the current evidence for the pharmacological management of neuropathic pain.*

McDonald J, Lambert DG. Opioid receptors. Cont Edu Anaesth Crit Care Pain. 2005;5(1):22–25. https://bjaed.org/article/S1743-1816(17)30577-2/pdf. *A concise review of opioid receptors.*

Websites

bma.org.uk/advice-and-support/ethics/end-of-life/physician-assisted-dying-survey *Survey on UK doctors' views on assisted dying.*

breathworks-mindfulness.org.uk *An online resource to support learning the use of mindfulness to deal with pain, illness or stress.*

cuh.org.uk/breathlessness *Information and resources from Cambridge University Hospital on managing breathlessness.*

ed.ac.uk/cancer-centre/research/fallon-group/epat *Edinburgh Pain Assessment Tool (EPAT)*

hospiceuk.org *A resource from UK hospices.*

mdanderson.org *Brief Pain Inventory (Short Form) questionnaire.*

nhmrc.gov.au *Australia and New Zealand College of Anaesthetists and Faculty of Pain Medicine. Acute pain management: scientific evidence, 3rd edn; 2010.*

npcrc.org *Short-form McGill Pain questionnaire.*

paintoolkit.org *Pain toolkit self-help resource for managing pain.*

palliativecareguidelines.scot.nhs.uk *Regularly reviewed, evidence-based clinical guidelines.*

palliativedrugs.com *Practical information about drugs used in palliative care.*

rcplondon.ac.uk/guidelines-policy/complex-regional-pain-syndrome-adults *Guidelines on CRPS, providing recommendations for diagnosis, treatment and referral in a variety of clinical settings (updated 2018).*

sign.ac.uk/assets/sign136.pdf *SIGN guideline 136 – Management of chronic pain (updated Aug 2019). A comprehensive review of the evidence for assessment and management of chronic pain.*

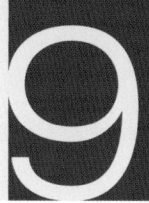

VR Tallentire
MJ MacMahon

9

Acute medicine and critical illness

Clinical examination in critical care

A Airway
Is the airway patent?
Is the end-tidal CO_2 trace normal?
Are there any signs of airway obstruction?

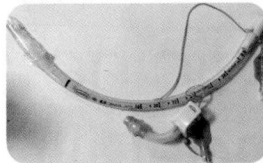

I Infection
What is the temperature?
Review recent infective markers and trend
What antibiotics are being given and what is the duration of treatment?

H Haematology
What are the haemoglobin/platelet levels?
Are there any signs of bleeding?

G Glucose
What is the glucose level?
Is insulin being administered?

F Fluids, electrolytes and renal system
What is the fluid balance?
Urine volume and colour?
Is there any oedema?
Review the renal biochemistry and electrolyte levels

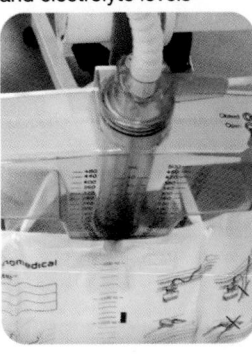

B Breathing
Is the physiology normal (SpO_2, respiratory rate, tidal volume)?
What is the level of support?
Are there any abnormal signs on chest examination?
Review the ventilator settings, arterial blood gases and recent chest X-ray

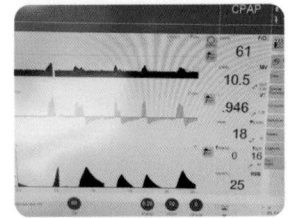

C Circulation
Is the physiology normal (heart rate, blood pressure, peripheral temperature, lactate, urine output)?
How much support is required (inotrope, vasopressor)?

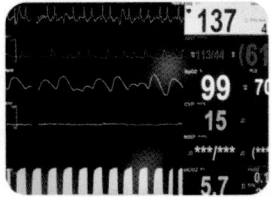

E Enteral/exposure
Feeding regimen
Stool frequency
Abdominal tenderness/bowel sounds present?

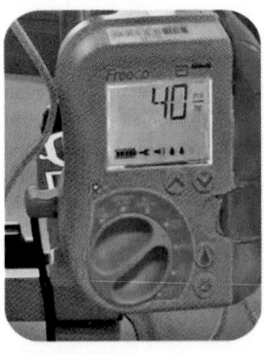

D Disability
Level of responsiveness
Delirium screen
Pupillary responses
Doses of sedative drugs

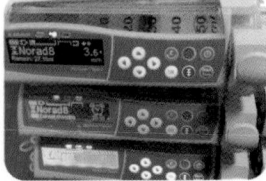

Monitoring

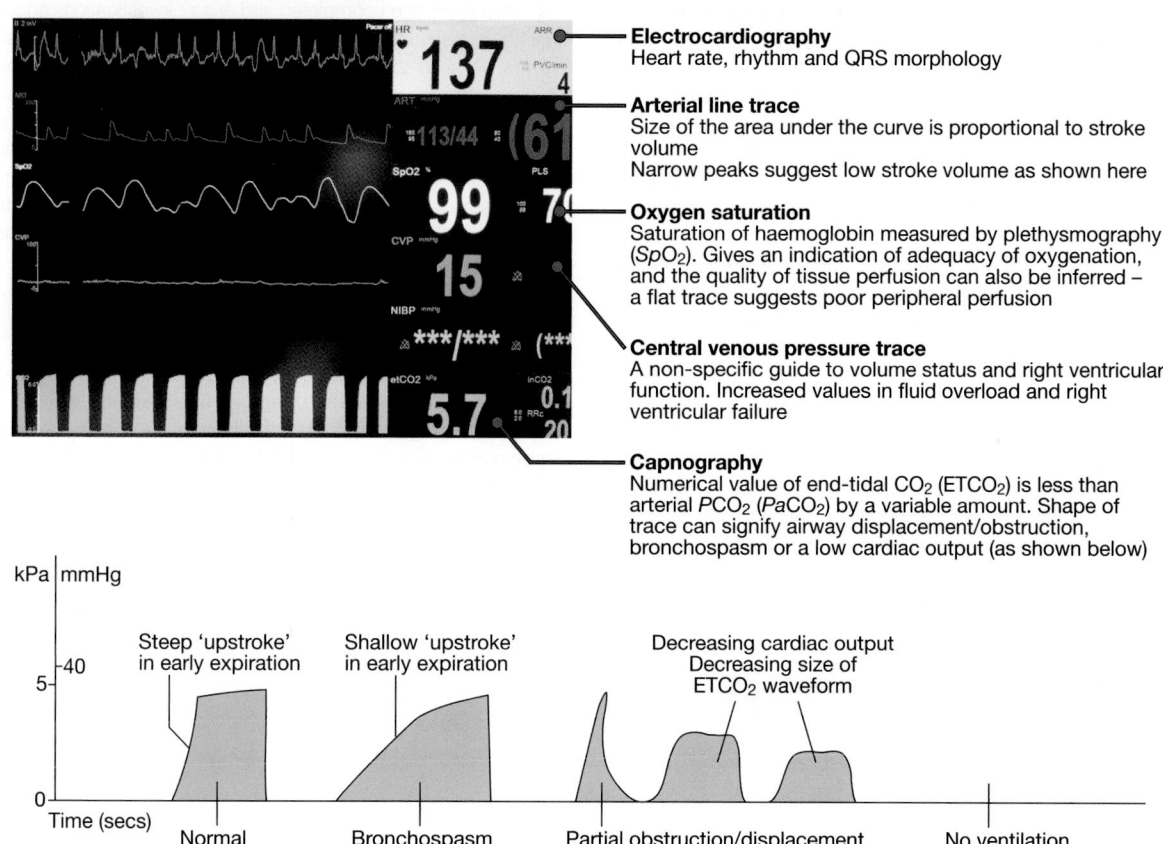

Electrocardiography
Heart rate, rhythm and QRS morphology

Arterial line trace
Size of the area under the curve is proportional to stroke volume
Narrow peaks suggest low stroke volume as shown here

Oxygen saturation
Saturation of haemoglobin measured by plethysmography (SpO_2). Gives an indication of adequacy of oxygenation, and the quality of tissue perfusion can also be inferred – a flat trace suggests poor peripheral perfusion

Central venous pressure trace
A non-specific guide to volume status and right ventricular function. Increased values in fluid overload and right ventricular failure

Capnography
Numerical value of end-tidal CO_2 ($ETCO_2$) is less than arterial PCO_2 ($PaCO_2$) by a variable amount. Shape of trace can signify airway displacement/obstruction, bronchospasm or a low cardiac output (as shown below)

Bedside physiological data commonly monitored in an intensive care unit setting.

Pulse oximetry (SpO_2)

Basic principles

- Uses the different red and infrared absorption profiles of oxyhaemoglobin and deoxyhaemoglobin to estimate arterial oxyhaemoglobin saturation (SaO_2)
- Only pulsatile absorption is measured
- A poor trace correlates with poor perfusion

Sources of error

- Carboxyhaemoglobin – absorption profile is the same as oxyhaemoglobin: falsely elevated SpO_2
- Methaemoglobinaemia – SpO_2 will tend towards 85%
- Ambient light/poor application of probe/severe tricuspid regurgitation (pulsatile venous flow): falsely depressed SpO_2
- Reduced accuracy below 80% saturation
- Hyperbilirubinaemia does not affect SpO_2

Hospital medicine is becoming ever-more specialised and people are living longer while accruing increasing numbers of chronic disease diagnoses. Rather than diminishing the role of the generalist, these factors paradoxically create a need for experts in the undifferentiated presentation. In the UK such physicians are known as 'general physicians', while in the United States they are referred to as 'hospitalists'.

Acute illness can present in a large variety of ways, depending on the nature of the illness, the underlying health of the individual, and their cultural and religious background. The skills of prompt diagnosis formation and provision of appropriate treatment rely on the integration of information from all the available sources, along with careful consideration of underlying chronic health problems.

Patients who deteriorate while in hospital make up a small but important cohort. If they are well managed, in-hospital cardiac arrest rates will be low. This can be achieved through the combined effects of prompt resuscitation and appropriate end-of-life decision-making. Early recognition of deterioration by ward teams and initial management by healthcare professionals operating within a functioning rapid response system are the central tenets of any system designed to improve the outcomes of deteriorating ward patients.

Intensive care medicine has developed into a prominent specialty, central to the safe functioning of a modern acute hospital. Scientific endeavour has resulted in a much better understanding of the molecular pathophysiology of processes such as sepsis and acute respiratory distress syndrome, which account for much premature death worldwide.

Acute medicine

Acute medicine is the part of general medicine that is concerned with the immediate and early management of medical patients who require urgent care. As a specialty, it is closely aligned with emergency medicine and intensive care medicine, but is firmly rooted within general medicine. Acute physicians manage the adult medical take and lead the development of acute care pathways that aim to reduce variability, improve care and cut down hospital admissions. In order to achieve these aims, acute physicians must use their knowledge, combined with high-level clinical reasoning and decision-making skills, to minimise both diagnostic error and the risks of over-investigation. These concepts are explained more fully in Chapter 1.

The decision to admit to hospital

Every patient presenting to hospital should be assessed by a clinician who is able to determine whether or not admission is required. The requirement for admission is determined by many factors, including the severity of illness, the patient's physiological reserve, the need for urgent investigations, the nature of proposed treatments and the patient's social circumstances. In many cases, it is clear early in the assessment process

that a patient requires admission. In such cases, a move into a medical receiving unit – often termed a medical admissions unit (MAU) or acute medical unit (AMU) – should be facilitated as soon as the initial assessment has been completed and urgent investigations and/or treatments have been instigated. In hospitals where such units do not exist, patients will need to be moved to a downstream ward once treatment has been commenced and they have been deemed sufficiently stable. In suspected cases of airborne-transmissible infectious diseases, patients should be isolated initially and may require cohorting in specific areas of the hospital once diagnoses have been confirmed. Following the initial assessment, it may be possible to discharge stable patients home with a plan for early follow-up (such as a rapid-access specialist clinic appointment).

Ambulatory care

In some hospitals, it is increasingly possible for patient care to be coordinated in an ambulatory setting, negating the need for a patient to remain in hospital overnight. In the context of acute medicine, ambulatory care can be employed for conditions that are perceived by either the patient or the referring practitioner as requiring prompt clinical assessment by a competent decision-maker with access to appropriate diagnostic resources. The patient may return on several occasions for investigation, observation, consultation or treatment. Some presentations, such as a unilateral swollen leg (p. 188), lend themselves to this type of management (Box 9.1). If indicated, a Doppler ultrasound can be arranged, and patients with confirmed deep vein thrombosis can be anticoagulated on an outpatient basis. Successful ambulatory care requires careful patient selection; while many patients may cherish the opportunity to sleep at home, others may find frequent trips to hospital or clinic too difficult due to frailty, poor mobility or transport difficulties.

Presenting problems in acute medicine

This section details some of the most common presentations to acute medicine. However, many people present to hospital with physical complaints that do not appear to be the symptoms of a medical condition, referred to as 'medically unexplained' or 'functional' symptoms (see Chs 23, 28 and 31). It is thought that such symptoms may account for up to half of all new visits to hospital in the UK. Rather than providing reassurance, a lack of understanding of the cause of the symptoms can result in more distress for patients. When the unexplained symptoms relate to the nervous system (such as limb weakness, numbness, shaking or blackouts), the term 'functional neurological disorder' is used (see p. 1152). Medically unexplained symptoms are more common in women, younger people, those who have previously suffered from depression or anxiety, recently bereaved people and those recovering from a recent physical

i	9.1 Groups of patients who are potentially suitable for ambulatory care		
Group	**Example(s)**	**Quality and safety issues**
Diagnostic exclusion group	Chest pain – possible myocardial infarction; breathlessness – possible pulmonary embolism	Even when a specific condition has been excluded, there is still a need to explain the patient's symptoms through the diagnostic process
Low-risk stratification group	Non-variceal upper gastrointestinal bleed with low Blatchford score (Box 23.16); community-acquired pneumonia with low CURB-65 score (see Fig. 17.32)	Appropriate treatment plans should be in place
Specific procedure group	Replacement of percutaneous endoscopic gastrostomy (PEG) tube; drainage of pleural effusion/ascites	The key to implementation is how ambulatory care for this group of patients can be delivered when they present out of hours
Outpatient group with supporting infrastructure	Deep vein thrombosis (DVT); cellulitis	These are distinct from the conditions listed above because the infrastructure required to manage them is quite different

illness. For every acute medical presentation, there will be a cohort of patients for whom the diagnosis remains elusive. In such circumstances, consideration should be given to the potential harm of over-investigation and the alternative approaches required to manage medically unexplained symptoms. Further detail can be found on p. 1256.

Chest pain

Chest pain is a common symptom in patients presenting to hospital. The differential diagnosis is wide (Box 9.2), and a detailed history and thorough clinical examination are paramount to ensure that the subsequent investigative pathway is appropriate.

Presentation

Chest 'pain' is clearly a subjective phenomenon and may be described by patients in a variety of different ways. Whether the patient describes 'pain', 'discomfort' or 'pressure' in the chest, there are some key features that must be elicited from the history.

Site and radiation

Pain secondary to myocardial ischaemia is typically located in the centre of the chest. It may radiate to the neck, jaw and upper or even lower arms. Occasionally, it may be experienced only at the sites of radiation or in the back. The pain of myocarditis or pericarditis is characteristically felt retrosternally, to the left of the sternum, or in the left or right shoulder. The severe pain of aortic dissection is typically central with radiation through to the back. Central chest pain may also occur with tumours affecting the mediastinum, oesophageal disease (p. 806) or disease of the thoracic aorta (p. 342). Pain situated over the left anterior chest and radiating

laterally is unlikely to be due to cardiac ischaemia and may have many causes, including pleural or lung disorders, musculoskeletal problems or anxiety. Rarely, sharp, left-sided chest pain that is suggestive of a musculoskeletal problem may be a feature of mitral valve prolapse (p. 455).

Characteristics

Pleurisy, a sharp or 'catching' chest pain aggravated by deep breathing or coughing, is indicative of respiratory pathology, particularly pulmonary infection or infarction. However, the pain associated with myocarditis or pericarditis is often also described as 'sharp' and may 'catch' during inspiration, coughing or lying flat. It typically varies in intensity with movement and the phase of respiration. A malignant tumour invading the chest wall or ribs can cause gnawing, continuous local pain. The pain of myocardial ischaemia is typically dull, constricting, choking or 'heavy', and is usually described as squeezing, crushing, burning or aching. Patients often emphasise that it is a discomfort rather than a pain. Angina occurs during (not after) exertion and is promptly relieved (in less than 5 minutes) by rest. It may also be precipitated or exacerbated by emotion but tends to occur more readily during exertion, after a large meal or in a cold wind. In crescendo or unstable angina, similar pain may be precipitated by minimal exertion or at rest. The increase in venous return or preload induced by lying down may also be sufficient to provoke pain in vulnerable patients (decubitus angina). Patients with reversible airways obstruction, such as asthma, may also describe exertional chest tightness that is relieved by rest. This may be difficult to distinguish from myocardial ischaemia. Bronchospasm may be associated with wheeze, atopy and cough (p. 489). Musculoskeletal chest pain is variable in site and intensity but does not usually fall into any of the patterns described above. The pain may vary with posture or movement of the upper body, or be associated with a specific movement (bending, stretching, turning). Many minor soft tissue injuries are related to everyday activities, such as driving, manual work and sport.

Onset

The pain associated with myocardial infarction (MI) typically takes several minutes or even longer to develop to its maximal intensity; similarly, angina builds up gradually in proportion to the intensity of exertion. Pain that occurs after, rather than during, exertion is usually musculoskeletal or psychological in origin. The pain of aortic dissection (severe and 'tearing'), massive pulmonary embolism (PE) or pneumothorax is usually very sudden in onset. Other causes of chest pain tend to develop more gradually, over hours or even days.

Associated features

The pain of MI, massive PE or aortic dissection is often accompanied by autonomic disturbance, including sweating, nausea and vomiting. Some patients describe a feeling of impending death, referred to as 'angor animi'. Breathlessness, due to pulmonary congestion arising from transient ischaemic left ventricular dysfunction, is often a prominent feature of myocardial ischaemia. Breathlessness may also accompany any of the respiratory causes of chest pain and can be associated with cough, wheeze or other respiratory symptoms. Patients with myocarditis or pericarditis may describe a prodromal viral illness. Gastrointestinal disorders, such as gastro-oesophageal reflux or peptic ulceration, may present with chest pain that is hard to distinguish from myocardial ischaemia; it may even be precipitated by exercise and be relieved by nitrates. However, it is usually possible to elicit a history relating chest pain to supine posture or eating, drinking or oesophageal reflux. The pain of gastro-oesophageal reflux often radiates to the interscapular region and dysphagia may be present. Severe chest pain arising after retching or vomiting, or following oesophageal instrumentation, should raise the possibility of oesophageal perforation.

Anxiety-induced chest pain may be associated with breathlessness (without hypoxaemia), throat tightness, perioral tingling and other evidence of emotional distress. It is important to remember, however, that chest pain itself can be an extremely frightening experience, and so psychological and organic features often coexist. Anxiety may amplify the effects of organic disease and a confusing clinical picture may result.

---

i | **9.2 Differential diagnosis of chest pain**

Central

Cardiac

- Myocardial ischaemia (angina)
- Myocardial infarction
- Myocarditis
- Pericarditis
- Mitral valve prolapse syndrome

Aortic

- Aortic dissection
- Aortic aneurysm

Oesophageal

- Oesophagitis
- Oesophageal spasm
- Mallory–Weiss syndrome
- Oesophageal perforation (Boerhaave syndrome)

Pulmonary embolus

Mediastinal

- Malignancy

Anxiety/emotion[1]

Peripheral

Lungs/pleura

- Pulmonary infarct
- Pneumonia
- Pneumothorax
- Malignancy
- Tuberculosis
- Connective tissue disorders

Musculoskeletal[2]

- Osteoarthritis
- Rib fracture/injury
- Acute vertebral fracture
- Costochondritis (Tietze syndrome)
- Intercostal muscle injury
- Epidemic myalgia (Bornholm disease)

Neurological

- Prolapsed intervertebral disc
- Herpes zoster

[1]May also cause peripheral chest pain. [2]Can sometimes cause central chest pain.

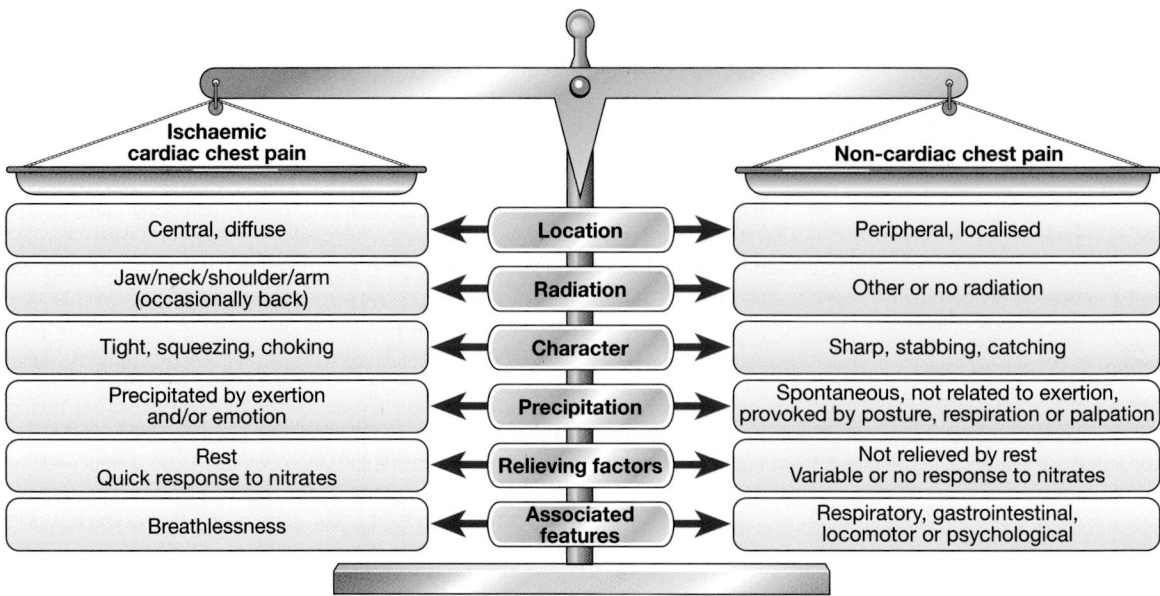

Fig. 9.1 Identifying ischaemic cardiac pain: the 'balance' of evidence.

A detailed and clear history is key to narrowing the differential diagnosis of chest pain. Figure 9.1 shows how certain features of the history, particularly when combined, can tip the balance of evidence towards or away from ischaemic cardiac chest pain.

Clinical assessment

Cardiorespiratory examination may detect clinical signs that help guide ongoing investigation. Patients with a history compatible with myocardial ischaemia should have a 12-lead electrocardiogram (ECG) performed while clinical examination proceeds. Ongoing chest pain with clinical features of shock or pulmonary oedema, or ECG evidence of ventricular arrhythmia or complete heart block, should prompt urgent cardiology review and referral to a higher level of care.

Chest pain that is accompanied by clinical evidence of increased intracardiac pressure (especially a raised jugular venous pressure) increases the likelihood of myocardial ischaemia or massive PE. The legs should be examined for clinical evidence of deep vein thrombosis.

A large pneumothorax should be evident on clinical examination, with absent breath sounds and a hyper-resonant percussion note on the affected side. Other unilateral chest signs, such as bronchial breathing or crackles, are most likely to indicate a respiratory tract infection, and a chest X-ray should be expedited.

Pericarditis may be accompanied by a pericardial friction rub. In aortic dissection, syncope or neurological deficit may occur. Examination may reveal asymmetrical pulses, features of undiagnosed Marfan syndrome (p. 445) or a new early diastolic murmur representing aortic regurgitation.

Any disease process involving the pleura may restrict rib movement and a pleural rub may be audible on the affected side. Local tenderness of the chest wall is likely to indicate musculoskeletal pain but can also be found in pulmonary infarction.

Subdiaphragmatic inflammatory pathology, such as a liver abscess, cholecystitis or ascending cholangitis, can mimic pneumonia by causing fever, pleuritic chest pain and a small sympathetic pleural effusion, usually on the right. Likewise, acute pancreatitis can present with thoracic symptoms, and an amylase or lipase level should be requested where appropriate. It is imperative that the abdomen is examined routinely in all patients presenting with pleuritic chest pain.

Initial investigations

Chest X-ray, ECG and biomarkers (e.g. troponin, D-dimer) play a pivotal role in the evaluation of chest pain. However, indiscriminate ordering of such investigations may result in diagnostic confusion and over-investigation. The choice of investigation(s) is intimately linked to the history and examination findings. A chest X-ray and 12-lead ECG should be performed in the vast majority of patients presenting to hospital with chest pain. Pregnancy is not a contraindication to chest X-ray, but particular consideration should be given to whether the additional diagnostic information justifies breast irradiation.

The chest X-ray may confirm the suspected diagnosis, particularly in the case of pneumonia. Small pneumothoraces are easily missed, as are rib fractures or small metastatic deposits, and all should be considered individually during chest X-ray review. A widened mediastinum suggests acute aortic dissection but a normal chest X-ray does not exclude the diagnosis. Provided it has been more than 1 hour since the onset of pain, chest X-ray in oesophageal rupture may reveal subcutaneous emphysema, pneumomediastinum or a pleural effusion.

Patients with a history compatible with myocardial ischaemia require an urgent 12-lead ECG. Acute chest pain with ECG changes indicating a ST segment elevation myocardial infarction (STEMI) suggests that the patient is likely to benefit from immediate reperfusion therapy. Specific information relating to cocaine or amphetamine use should be sought, particularly in younger patients. In the context of a compatible history, an ECG showing ischaemic changes that do not meet STEMI criteria should prompt regular repeat ECGs and treatment for non-ST segment elevation myocardial infarction (NSTEMI)/unstable angina. Measurement of serum troponin concentration on admission is often helpful in cases where there is diagnostic doubt, but a negative result should always prompt a repeat sample 6–12 hours after maximal pain. Acute coronary syndrome may be diagnosed with confidence in patients with a convincing history of ischaemic pain (see Fig. 9.1) and either ECG evidence of ischaemia or an elevated serum troponin. If an elevated serum troponin is found in a patient who has an atypical history or is at low risk of ischaemic heart disease, then alternative causes of raised troponin should be considered (Box 9.3). Further management of acute coronary syndromes is discussed on page 432.

In the absence of convincing ECG evidence of myocardial ischaemia, other life-threatening causes of chest pain, such as aortic dissection, massive PE and oesophageal rupture, should be considered. Suspicion of aortic dissection (background of hypertension, trauma, pregnancy or previous aortic surgery) should prompt urgent thoracic computed tomography (CT) or transoesophageal echocardiography. An ECG in the context of massive PE most commonly reveals only a sinus tachycardia, but may show new right axis deviation, right bundle branch block or a dominant R wave in V_1. The classical finding of $S_1Q_3T_3$ (a deep S wave in

i **9.3 Causes of elevated serum troponin other than acute coronary syndrome**

Cardiorespiratory causes

- Pulmonary embolism
- Acute pulmonary oedema
- Tachyarrhythmias
- Myocarditis/myopericarditis
- Aortic dissection
- Cardiac trauma
- Cardiac surgery/ablation

Non-cardiorespiratory causes

- Prolonged hypotension
- Severe sepsis
- Severe burns
- Stroke
- Subarachnoid haemorrhage
- End-stage renal failure

lead I, with a Q wave and T wave inversion in lead III) is rare. If massive PE is suspected and the patient is haemodynamically unstable, a transthoracic echocardiogram, to seek evidence of right heart strain and exclude alternative diagnoses such as tamponade, is extremely useful.

If the patient is deemed to be at low risk of PE, a D-dimer test can be informative, as a negative result effectively excludes the diagnosis. The D-dimer test should be performed only if there is clinical suspicion of PE, as false-positive results can lead to unnecessary investigations. If the D-dimer is positive, there is high clinical suspicion, or there is other convincing evidence of PE (such as features of right heart strain on the ECG), prompt imaging should be arranged (p. 546 and Fig. 17.67).

Acute breathlessness

In acute breathlessness, the history, along with a rapid but careful examination, will usually suggest a diagnosis that can be confirmed by routine investigations including chest X-ray, 12-lead ECG and arterial blood gas (ABG) sampling.

Presentation

A key feature of the history is the speed of onset of breathlessness. Acute severe breathlessness (over minutes or hours) has a distinct differential diagnosis list to chronic exertional breathlessness. The presence of associated cardiovascular (chest pain, palpitations, sweating and nausea) or respiratory (cough, wheeze, haemoptysis, stridor) symptoms can narrow the differential diagnosis yet further. A previous history of left ventricular dysfunction, asthma or exacerbations of chronic obstructive pulmonary disease (COPD) is important. A high temperature, cough (productive or non-productive) and/or viral prodrome may indicate respiratory infection and, if so, relevant infection control precautions should be taken from initial assessment. In the severely ill patient, it may be necessary to obtain the history from accompanying witnesses. In children, the possibility of inhalation of a foreign body (Fig. 9.2) or acute epiglottitis should always be considered. There is often more than one underlying diagnosis; a thorough assessment should continue, even after a possible diagnosis has been reached, particularly if the severity of symptoms does not seem to be adequately explained. The causes of acute severe breathlessness are covered here; chronic exertional dyspnoea is discussed further on page 489).

Clinical assessment

Airway obstruction, anaphylaxis and tension pneumothorax require immediate identification and treatment. If any of these is suspected, treatment should not be delayed while additional investigations are performed, and anaesthetic support is likely to be required. In the absence of an immediately life-threatening cause, the following should be assessed and documented:

- level of consciousness
- degree of central cyanosis
- work of breathing (rate, depth, pattern, use of accessory muscles)
- adequacy of oxygenation (SpO_2)

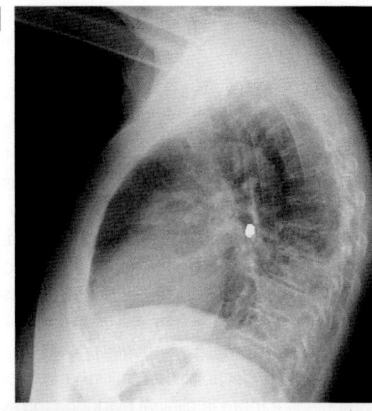

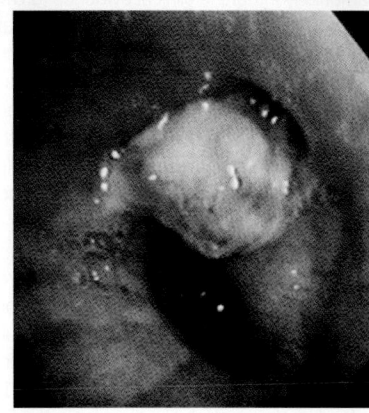

Fig. 9.2 Inhaled foreign body. **A** Chest X-ray showing a tooth lodged in a main bronchus. **B** Bronchoscopic appearance of inhaled foreign body (tooth) with a covering mucous film.

- ability to speak (in single words or sentences)
- cardiovascular status (heart rate and rhythm, blood pressure (BP) and peripheral perfusion).

Pulmonary oedema is suggested by a raised jugular venous pressure and bi-basal crackles or diffuse wheeze, while asthma or COPD is characterised by wheeze and prolonged expiration. A hyper-resonant hemithorax with absent breath sounds raises the possibility of pneumothorax, while severe breathlessness with normal breath sounds may indicate PE. Leg swelling may suggest cardiac failure or, if asymmetrical, venous thrombosis.

The presence of wheeze is not always indicative of bronchospasm. In acute left heart failure, an increase in the left ventricular diastolic pressure causes the pressure in the left atrium, pulmonary veins and pulmonary capillaries to rise. When the hydrostatic pressure of the pulmonary capillaries exceeds the oncotic pressure of plasma (about 25–30 mmHg), fluid moves from the capillaries into the interstitium. This stimulates respiration through a series of autonomic reflexes, producing rapid, shallow respiration, and congestion of the bronchial mucosa may cause wheeze (sometimes known as cardiac asthma). Sitting upright or standing may provide some relief by helping to reduce congestion at the apices of the lungs. The patient may be unable to speak and is typically distressed, agitated, sweaty and pale. Respiration is rapid, with recruitment of accessory muscles, coughing and wheezing. Sputum may be profuse, frothy and blood-streaked or pink. Extensive crepitations and rhonchi are usually audible in the chest and there may also be signs of right heart failure.

Any arrhythmia may cause breathlessness, but usually does so only if the heart is structurally abnormal, such as with the onset of atrial fibrillation in a patient with mitral stenosis. In such cases, the classic mid-diastolic rumbling murmur may be heard. Patients sometimes describe chest tightness as 'breathlessness'. However, myocardial ischaemia may also induce true breathlessness by provoking transient left ventricular dysfunction. When breathlessness is the dominant or sole feature of myocardial ischaemia, it is known as 'angina equivalent'. A history of chest tightness or close correlation with exercise should be sought.

Initial investigations

As shown in Box 9.4, amalgamation of a clear history and thorough clinical examination with chest X-ray, ECG and ABG findings will usually indicate the primary cause of breathlessness. In cases of suspected infection, a viral throat swab should be obtained early in the course of the assessment; increasingly point-of-care testing of viral throat swabs is available, providing important and rapid diagnostic information. If available, sputum should be sent for culture. If bronchospasm is suspected, measurement of peak expiratory flow will assist in the assessment of severity and should be performed whenever possible.

An ABG will often provide additional information to SpO_2 measurement alone, particularly if there is clinical evidence (drowsiness, delirium, asterixis) or a strong likelihood of hypercapnia. An acute rise in $PaCO_2$ will increase the HCO_3^- by only a small amount, resulting in inadequate buffering and acidaemia. Renal compensation and a large rise in HCO_3^- will take at least 12 hours. In acute type II respiratory failure (p. 496), the rate of rise of $PaCO_2$ is a better indicator of severity than the absolute value. An ABG can also give a carboxyhaemoglobin level after smoke inhalation (although this can also be measured on a venous sample), and is central to the identification of metabolic acidosis or the diagnosis of psychogenic hyperventilation (see Box 9.4).

If pulmonary embolism is suspected, calculating pre-test probability (Ch. 1) is key. In a patient with a pre-test probability of less than 15%, the pulmonary embolism rule-out criteria (PERC) can rule out pulmonary embolism clinically, negating the need for further imaging, if none of the criteria listed in Box 9.5 is met. Further detail on the investigation and management of pulmonary embolus is given on page 546.

Procalcitonin (PCT) and N-terminal pro-hormone brain natriuretic protein (NT-proBNP) can be measured in venous blood. While these biomarkers can give an indication of aetiology in shortness of breath, they are probably of more value in tracking clinical progression and response to treatment. Elevated PCT is a biomarker for bacterial infection and may be useful, in addition to clinical assessment, in helping decide the need for and duration of antibiotic therapy in patients with confirmed viral respiratory disease (such as COVID-19) who may have additional bacterial super-infection. Elevated NT-proBNP is suggestive of underlying left ventricular failure (p. 393), although it can be elevated in other conditions such as renal failure, COPD, pulmonary hypertension and pulmonary embolism. Measurement of NT-proBNP may be considered if there is no clear-cut evidence of pulmonary oedema on a chest X-ray and can be particularly useful as a 'rule-out' test, as a normal NT-proBNP has high negative predictive value for heart failure. Individuals with suspected heart failure should undergo early echocardiography (p. 402).

CT imaging (with or without pulmonary angiography) is a useful investigation in many respiratory conditions as interstitial changes, tumours or consolidation may not be evident on chest X-ray. If breathlessness is suspected to be an 'angina equivalent', objective evidence

---

| **i** | **9.5 PERC rule for pulmonary embolism** |

Rules out PE if none of the eight criteria is present and pre-test probability is less than or equal to 15% (1.8% was chosen as the point of equipoise between the benefits and risks of further investigations for PE, and the benefits and risks of *not* investigating further).

- Age ≥ 50
- Heart rate ≥ 100
- Oxygen saturation on room air < 95%
- Unilateral leg swelling
- Haemoptysis
- Recent surgery or trauma (≤ 4 weeks ago requiring hospitalisation)
- Prior venous thromboembolism (VTE)
- Hormone use (oral contraceptives), hormone replacement or oestrogenic hormone use in male or female patients

---

| **i** | **9.4 Clinical features in acute breathlessness** |

Condition	History	Signs	Chest X-ray	ABG	ECG
Pulmonary oedema	Chest pain, palpitations, orthopnoea, cardiac history*	Central cyanosis, ↑JVP, sweating, cool extremities, basal crackles*	Cardiomegaly, oedema/pleural effusions*	↓PaO_2 ↓$PaCO_2$	Sinus tachycardia, ischaemia*, arrhythmia
Massive pulmonary embolus	Risk factors, chest pain, pleurisy, syncope*, dizziness*	Central cyanosis, ↑JVP*, absence of signs in the lung*, shock (tachycardia, hypotension)	Often normal Prominent hilar vessels, oligaemic lung fields*	↓PaO_2 ↓$PaCO_2$	Sinus tachycardia, RBBB, $S_1Q_3T_3$ pattern ↑T(V_1–V_4)
Acute severe asthma	History of asthma, asthma medications, wheeze*	Tachycardia, pulsus paradoxus, cyanosis (late), →JVP*, ↓peak flow, wheeze*	Hyperinflation only (unless complicated by pneumothorax)*	↓PaO_2 Normal $PaCO_2$ (↑$PaCO_2$ in extremis)	Sinus tachycardia (bradycardia in extremis)
Acute exacerbation of COPD	Previous episodes*, smoker. If in type II respiratory failure, may be drowsy	Cyanosis, hyperinflation*, signs of CO_2 retention (flapping tremor, bounding pulses)*	Hyperinflation*, bullae, complicating pneumothorax	↓ or ↓↓PaO_2 ↑$PaCO_2$ in type II failure ± ↑H^+, ↑HCO_3^- in chronic type II failure	Normal, or signs of right ventricular strain
Pneumonia/ lower respiratory tract infection	Prodromal illness*, fever*, rigors*, pleurisy*	Fever, delirium, pleural rub*, consolidation*, cyanosis (if severe)	Pneumonic consolidation*	↓PaO_2 ↓$PaCO_2$ (↑ in extremis)	Tachycardia
Metabolic acidosis	Evidence of diabetes mellitus or renal disease, aspirin or ethylene glycol overdose	Fetor (ketones), hyperventilation without heart or lung signs*, dehydration*, air hunger	Normal	PaO_2 normal ↓↓$PaCO_2$, ↑H^+ ↓HCO_3^-	
Psychogenic	Previous episodes, digital or perioral dysaesthesia	No cyanosis, no heart or lung signs, carpopedal spasm	Normal	PaO_2 normal* ↓↓$PaCO_2$, ↓H^{+*}	

*Valuable discriminatory feature.
(ABG = arterial blood gas; COPD = chronic obstructive pulmonary disease; JVP = jugular venous pressure; RBBB = right bundle branch block)

of myocardial ischaemia from stress testing may help to establish the diagnosis, although coronary artery angiography (either by CT or cardiac catheterisation) is often performed early in the investigation pathway (p. 432).

Anaphylaxis

Anaphylaxis is a potentially life-threatening, systemic allergic reaction characterised by a variable combination of circulatory collapse, bronchospasm, laryngeal stridor, angioedema and urticaria. The risk of death is increased in patients with pre-existing asthma, particularly if this is poorly controlled, and in situations where treatment with adrenaline (epinephrine) is delayed.

Presentation

Anaphylaxis occurs when an allergen binds to and cross-links membrane-bound IgE on mast cells in a susceptible individual, causing release of histamine, tryptase and other vasoactive mediators from mast cells. These mediators have a variety of effects, including vasodilatation, increased capillary permeability leading to hypotension, and bronchoconstriction. It can be difficult to distinguish IgE-mediated anaphylaxis clinically from non-specific degranulation of mast cells on exposure to drugs, chemicals or other triggers where IgE is not involved, previously known as anaphylactoid reactions.

Clinical assessment

The clinical features of anaphylaxis are summarised in Figure 9.3. Several other conditions can mimic anaphylaxis and these are listed in Box 9.6.

It is important to assess the severity of the reaction, and the time between allergen exposure and onset of symptoms provides a guide. Enquiry should be made about potential triggers. If a trigger is immediately obvious, a detailed history of the previous 24 hours may be helpful. The most common triggers of anaphylaxis are foods, latex, insect venom and drugs. A history of previous local allergic responses to the offending agent is common. The route of allergen exposure may influence the principal clinical features of a reaction; for example, if an allergen is inhaled, the major symptom is frequently wheezing. Features of anaphylaxis may overlap with the direct toxic effects of drugs and venoms (Chs 7 and 8). Potentiating factors, such as exercise alcohol or fatigue, can lower the threshold for an anaphylactic event. It is important to identify precipitating factors so that appropriate avoidance measures may be taken in the longer term.

Investigations and management

Measurement of serum mast cell tryptase concentrations is useful to confirm the diagnosis. It is important to measure tryptase in serial tests to demonstrate the temporal relationship to the triggering event. Specific IgE tests may be useful in confirming hypersensitivity and may be preferable to skin-prick tests when investigating patients with a history of anaphylaxis. The cornerstone of management of a severe case is the early administration of adrenaline (epinephrine), which supports the cardiovascular system, reduces bronchospasm and has some disease-modifying effects. Secondary management depends upon which organs are most affected. The emergency management of anaphylaxis is summarised in Box 9.7. If present, angioedema of the orofacial area requires careful observation and timely intervention, possibly with endotracheal intubation. The investigation and management of angioedema is discussed further on page 82.

Individuals who have recovered from an anaphylactic event should be referred for specialist assessment. The aims are to identify the trigger, educate the patient regarding avoidance and management of subsequent episodes, and to establish whether specific treatment, such as immunotherapy, is indicated. If the trigger factor cannot be identified or avoided, recurrence is common. Patients who have previously

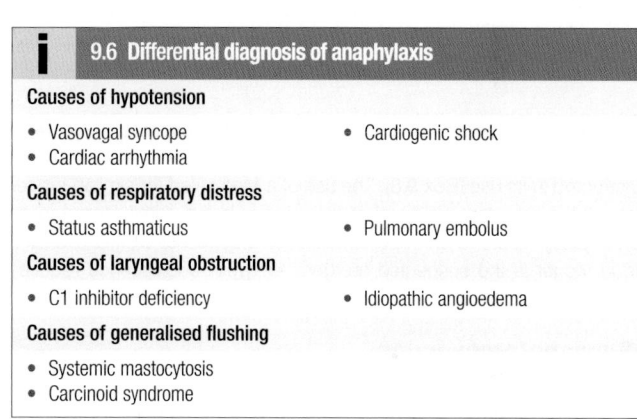

i | **9.6 Differential diagnosis of anaphylaxis**

Causes of hypotension
- Vasovagal syncope
- Cardiac arrhythmia
- Cardiogenic shock

Causes of respiratory distress
- Status asthmaticus
- Pulmonary embolus

Causes of laryngeal obstruction
- C1 inhibitor deficiency
- Idiopathic angioedema

Causes of generalised flushing
- Systemic mastocytosis
- Carcinoid syndrome

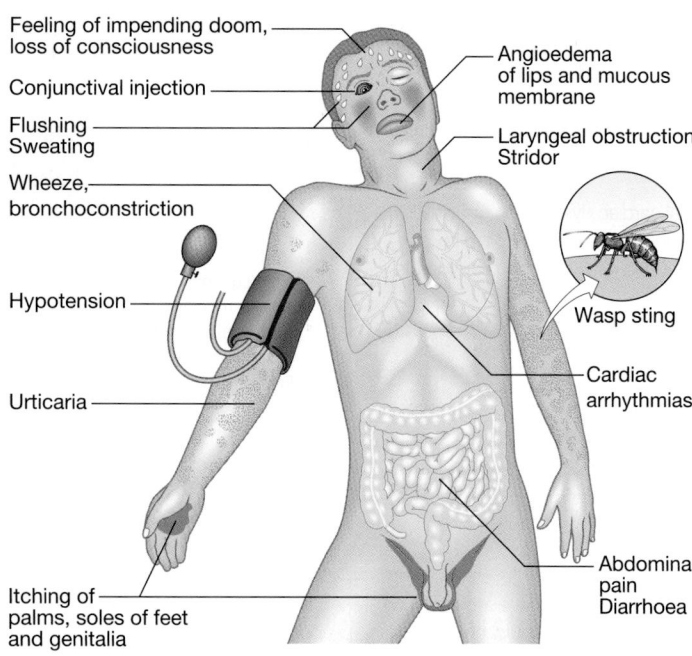

Fig. 9.3 Clinical manifestations of anaphylaxis. In this example, the response is to an insect sting containing venom to which the patient is allergic. This causes release of histamine and other vasoactive mediators, which lead to the characteristic features of anaphylaxis that are illustrated.

9.7 Emergency management of anaphylaxis

Treatment	Comment
Prevent further contact with allergen	Prevents ongoing mast cell activation
Ensure airway patency	Prevents hypoxia
Administer adrenaline (epinephrine) promptly: 0.3–0.5 mL 1:1000 solution IM in adults (0.3–0.5 mg) Repeat at 5–10 min intervals if initial response is inadequate	Intramuscular route important because of peripheral vasoconstriction Acts within minutes Increases blood pressure Reverses bronchospasm
Administer antihistamines: Chlorphenamine 10 mg IM or slow IV injection	Blocks effect of histamine on target cells
Administer glucocorticoids: Hydrocortisone 200 mg IV	Reduces cytokine release Prevents rebound symptoms in severe cases
Provide supportive treatment: Nebulised adrenaline (epinephrine) (e.g. 3 mg) Nebulised β₂-agonists (e.g. salbutamol 5 mg) IV fluids Oxygen	Reduces airway oedema Reverses bronchospasm Restores plasma volume Reverses hypoxia

(IM = intramuscular; IV = intravenous)

9.8 How to prescribe self-injectable adrenaline (epinephrine)

Prescription (normally initiated by an immunologist or allergist)

- Specify the brand of autoinjector, as they have different triggering mechanisms
- Prescribe two devices

Indications

- Anaphylaxis to allergens that are difficult to avoid:
  - Insect venom
  - Foods
- Idiopathic anaphylactic reactions
- History of severe localised reactions with high risk of future anaphylaxis:
  - Reaction to trace allergen
  - Likely repeated exposure to allergen
- History of severe localised reactions with high risk of adverse outcome:
  - Poorly controlled asthma
  - Lack of access to emergency care

Patient and family education

- Know when and how to use the device
- Carry the device at all times
- Seek medical assistance immediately after use
- Wear an alert bracelet or necklace
- Include the school in education for young patients

Other considerations

- Caution with β-adrenoceptor antagonists (β-blockers) in anaphylactic patients as they may increase the severity of an anaphylactic reaction and reduce the response to adrenaline (epinephrine)

experienced an anaphylactic event should be prescribed self-injectable adrenaline (epinephrine) and they and their families or carers should be instructed in its use (Box 9.8). The use of a MedicAlert (or similar) bracelet will increase the likelihood of the injector being administered in an emergency. There is an important role for a specialist dietitian when a food trigger is the suspected allergen. Allergy in adolescence requires additional consideration and management, as set out in Box 9.9.

Syncope/presyncope

The term 'syncope' refers to sudden loss of consciousness due to reduced cerebral perfusion. 'Presyncope' refers to lightheadedness, in which the individual thinks he or she may 'black out'. Dizziness and presyncope are particularly common in old age (Box 9.10). Symptoms are disabling, undermine confidence and independence, and can affect a person's ability to work or to drive.

There are three principal mechanisms that underlie recurrent presyncope or syncope:

- *cardiac syncope* due to mechanical cardiac dysfunction or arrhythmia
- *neurocardiogenic syncope (also known as vasovagal or reflex syncope)*, in which an abnormal autonomic reflex causes bradycardia and/or hypotension
- *postural hypotension*, in which physiological peripheral vasoconstriction on standing is impaired, leading to hypotension.

There are, however, other causes of loss of consciousness, and differentiating syncope from seizure is a particular challenge. Psychogenic blackouts (also known as non-epileptic seizures or pseudoseizures) also need to be considered in the differential diagnosis.

Presentation

The history from the patient *and* a witness is the key to establishing a diagnosis. The terms used for describing the symptoms associated with syncope vary so much among patients that they should not be taken for granted. Some patients use the term 'blackout' to describe a purely visual symptom, rather than loss of consciousness. Some may understand 'dizziness' to mean an abnormal perception of movement (vertigo),

9.9 Allergy in adolescence

- **Resolution of childhood allergy**: most children affected by allergy to milk, egg, soybean or wheat will grow out of their food allergies by adolescence, but allergies to peanuts, tree nuts, fish and shellfish are frequently life-long.
- **Risk-taking behaviour and fatal anaphylaxis**: serious allergy is increasingly common in adolescents and this is the highest risk group for fatal, food-induced anaphylaxis. This is associated with increased risk-taking behaviour, and food-allergic adolescents are more likely than adults to eat unsafe foods, deny reaction symptoms and delay emergency treatment.
- **Emotional impact of food allergies**: some adolescents may neglect to carry a prescribed adrenaline (epinephrine) autoinjector because of the associated nuisance and/or stigma. Surveys of food-allergic teenagers reveal that many take risks because they feel socially isolated by their allergy.

9.10 Dizziness in old age

- **Prevalence**: common, affecting up to 30% of people aged > 65 years.
- **Symptoms**: most frequently described as a combination of unsteadiness and lightheadedness.
- **Most common causes**: postural hypotension and cardiovascular disease. Many patients have more than one underlying cause.
- **Arrhythmia**: can present with lightheadedness either at rest or on activity.
- **Anxiety**: frequently associated with dizziness but rarely the only cause.
- **Falls**: multidisciplinary workup is required if dizziness is associated with falls.

some will consider this a feeling of faintness, and others will regard it as unsteadiness. The clinician thus needs to elucidate the exact nature of the symptoms that the patient experiences. The potential differential diagnosis of syncope and presyncope, on the basis of the symptoms described, is shown in Figure 9.4.

The history should always be supplemented by *a direct eye-witness account* if available. Careful history with corroboration will usually establish whether there has been full consciousness, altered consciousness, vertigo, transient amnesia or something else. Attention should be paid to potential triggers (e.g. medication, micturition, exertion, prolonged standing), the

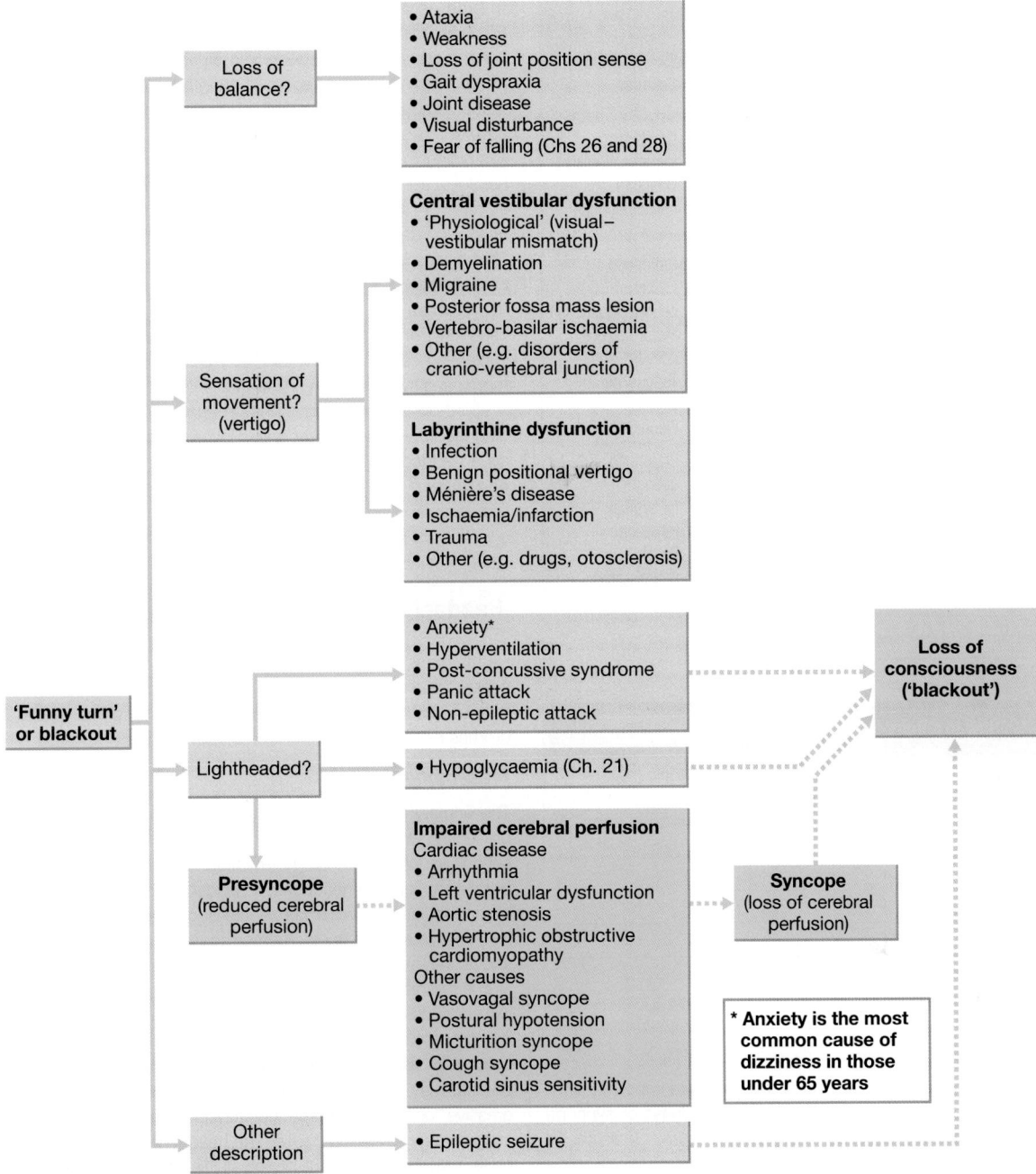

Fig. 9.4 The differential diagnosis of syncope and presyncope.

patient's appearance (e.g. colour, seizure activity), the duration of the episode, and the speed of recovery (Box 9.11). Cardiac syncope is usually sudden, but can be associated with premonitory lightheadedness, palpitation or chest discomfort. The blackout is usually brief and recovery rapid. Exercise-induced syncope can be the presenting feature of a number of serious pathologies (such as hypertrophic obstructive cardiomyopathy or exercise-induced arrhythmia) and always requires further investigation. Neurocardiogenic syncope will often be associated with a situational trigger (such as pain or emotion), and the patient may experience flushing, nausea, malaise and clamminess for several minutes afterwards. Recovery is usually quick and without subsequent delirium, provided the patient has assumed a supine position. There is often some brief stiffening and limb-twitching, which requires differentiation from seizure-like movements. It is rare for syncope to cause injury or to cause amnesia after regaining awareness. Patients with seizures do not exhibit pallor, may have abnormal movements, usually take more than 5 minutes to recover and are often

confused. Aspects of the history that can help to differentiate seizure from syncope are shown in Box 9.12.

A diagnosis of psychogenic blackout (also known as non-epileptic seizure, pseudoseizure or psychogenic seizure) may be suggested by specific emotional triggers, dramatic movements or vocalisation, or by very prolonged duration (hours). A history of rotational vertigo is suggestive of a labyrinthine or vestibular disorder (p. 1143). Postural hypotension is normally obvious from the history, with presyncope or, less commonly, syncope occurring within a few seconds of standing. The history should include enquiry about predisposing medications (diuretics, vasodilators, antidepressants) and conditions (such as diabetes mellitus and Parkinson's disease).

Clinical assessment

Examination of the patient may be entirely normal, but may reveal clinical signs that favour one form of syncope. The systolic murmurs of aortic

i **9.11 Typical features of cardiac syncope, neurocardiogenic syncope and seizures**

	Cardiac syncope	Neurocardiogenic syncope	Seizures
Premonitory symptoms	Often none Lightheadedness Palpitation Chest pain Breathlessness	Nausea Lightheadedness Sweating	Delirium Hyperexcitability Olfactory hallucinations 'Aura'
Unconscious period	Extreme 'death-like' pallor	Pallor	Prolonged (> 1 min) unconsciousness Motor seizure activity* Tongue-biting Urinary incontinence
Recovery	Rapid (< 1 min) Flushing	Rapid Nausea Lightheadedness	Prolonged delirium (> 5 mins) Headache Focal neurological signs

*N.B. Cardiac syncope can also cause convulsions by inducing cerebral anoxia.

9.12 How to differentiate seizures from syncope

	Seizure	Syncope
Aura (e.g. olfactory)	+	−
Cyanosis	+	−
Lateral tongue-biting	+	−/+
Post-ictal delirium	+	−
Post-ictal amnesia	+	−
Post-ictal headache	+	−
Rapid recovery	−	+

stenosis or hypertrophic obstructive cardiomyopathy are important findings, particularly if paired with a history of lightheadedness or syncope on exertion. BP taken when supine and then after 1 and 3 minutes of standing may, when combined with symptoms, provide robust evidence of symptomatic postural hypotension.

Clinical suspicion of hypersensitive carotid sinus syndrome (sensitivity of carotid baroreceptors to external pressure such as a tight collar) should prompt monitoring of the ECG and BP during carotid sinus pressure, provided there is no carotid bruit or history of cerebrovascular disease. A positive cardio-inhibitory response is defined as a sinus pause of 3 seconds or more; a positive vasodepressor response is defined as a fall in systolic BP of more than 50 mmHg. Carotid sinus pressure will produce positive findings in about 10% of older adults, but fewer than 25% of these experience spontaneous syncope. Symptoms should not, therefore, be attributed to hypersensitive carotid sinus syndrome unless they are reproduced by carotid sinus pressure.

Initial investigations

A 12-lead ECG is essential in all patients presenting with syncope or presyncope. Lightheadedness may occur with many arrhythmias, but blackouts (Stokes–Adams attacks) are usually due to profound bradycardia or malignant ventricular tachyarrhythmias. The ECG may show evidence of conducting system disease (e.g. sinus bradycardia, atrioventricular block, bundle branch block), which would predispose a patient

to bradycardia, but the key to establishing a diagnosis is to obtain an ECG recording *while symptoms are present*. Since minor rhythm disturbances are common, especially in older adults, symptoms must occur at the same time as a recorded arrhythmia before a diagnosis can be made. Ambulatory ECG recordings are helpful only if symptoms occur several times per week. Patient-activated ECG recorders are useful for examining the rhythm in patients with recurrent dizziness, but are not helpful in assessing sudden blackouts. When these investigations fail to establish a cause in patients with presyncope or syncope, an implantable ECG recorder can be sited subcutaneously over the upper left chest. This device continuously records the cardiac rhythm and will activate automatically if extreme bradycardia or tachycardia occurs. The ECG memory can also be tagged by the patient, using a hand-held activator as a form of 'symptom diary'. Stored ECGs can be accessed by the implanting centre, using a telemetry device in a clinic, or using a home monitoring system via an online link.

Head-up tilt-table testing is a provocation test used to establish the diagnosis of vasovagal syncope. It involves positioning the patient supine on a padded table that is then tilted to an angle of 60–70° for up to 45 minutes, while the ECG and BP responses are monitored. A positive test is characterised by bradycardia (cardio-inhibitory response) and/or hypotension (vasodepressor response), associated with typical symptoms.

Headache

Headache is common and causes considerable worry amongst both patients and clinicians, but rarely represents sinister disease. The causes may be divided into primary or secondary, with primary headache syndromes being vastly more common (Box 9.13).

Presentation

The primary purpose of the history and clinical examination in patients presenting with headache is to identify the small minority of patients with serious underlying pathology. Key features of the history include the temporal evolution of a headache; a headache that reached maximal intensity immediately or within 5 minutes of onset requires rapid assessment for possible subarachnoid haemorrhage. Other 'red flag' symptoms are shown in Box 9.14.

It is important to establish whether the headache comes and goes, with periods of no headache in between (usually migraine), or whether it is present all or almost all of the time. Associated features, such as preceding visual symptoms, nausea/vomiting or photophobia/phonophobia, may support a diagnosis of migraine but others, such as progressive focal symptoms or constitutional upset like weight loss, may suggest a more sinister cause. The headache of cerebral venous thrombosis may be 'throbbing' or 'band-like' and associated with nausea, vomiting or hemiparesis. Raised intracranial pressure (ICP) headache

i **9.13 Primary and secondary headache syndromes**

Primary headache syndromes

- Migraine (with or without aura)
- Tension-type headache
- Trigeminal autonomic cephalalgia (including cluster headache)
- Primary stabbing/coughing/exertional/sex-related headache
- Thunderclap headache
- New daily persistent headache syndrome

Secondary causes of headache

- Medication overuse headache (chronic daily headache)
- Intracranial bleeding (subdural haematoma, subarachnoid or intracerebral haemorrhage)
- Raised intracranial pressure (brain tumour, idiopathic intracranial hypertension)
- Infection (meningitis, encephalitis, brain abscess)
- Inflammatory disease (temporal arteritis, other vasculitis, arthritis)
- Referred pain from other structures (orbit, temporomandibular joint, neck)

9.14 'Red flag' symptoms in headache

Symptom	Possible explanation
Sudden onset (maximal immediately or within 5 min)	Subarachnoid haemorrhage Cerebral venous sinus thrombosis Pituitary apoplexy Meningitis
Focal neurological symptoms (other than for typically migrainous)	Intracranial mass lesion: Vascular Neoplastic Infection
Constitutional symptoms: Weight loss General malaise Pyrexia Meningism Rash	Meningitis Encephalitis Neoplasm (lymphoma or metastases) Inflammation (vasculitis)
Raised intracranial pressure (worse on waking/lying down, associated vomiting)	Intracranial mass lesion
New-onset aged > 60 years	Temporal arteritis

9.15 Identification of bacterial meningitis

In patients presenting with headache, identification of those with bacterial meningitis is a top priority to facilitate rapid antibiotic treatment. In almost all cases there will be one of the following features:

- meningism (neck stiffness, photophobia, positive Kernig's sign)
- fever > 38°C
- signs of shock (tachycardia, hypotension, elevated serum lactate)
- rash (not always petechial).

tends to be worse in the morning and when lying flat or coughing, and associated with nausea and/or vomiting.

A description of neck stiffness along with headache and photophobia should raise the suspicion of meningitis (Box 9.15), although this may present in atypical ways in immunosuppressed, alcoholic or pregnant patients. The behaviour of the patient during headache is often instructive; migraine patients typically retire to bed to sleep in a dark room, whereas cluster headache often induces agitated and restless behaviour. The pain of a subarachnoid haemorrhage frequently causes significant distress.

Headache duration is also important to elicit; headaches that have been present for months or years are almost never sinister, whereas new-onset headache, especially in older adults, is more of a concern. In a patient over 60 years with head pain localised to one or both temples, scalp tenderness or jaw claudication, temporal arteritis (Ch. 26) should be considered.

Clinical assessment

An assessment of conscious level (using the Glasgow Coma Scale (GCS); Fig. 9.5) should be performed early and constantly reassessed. A decreased conscious level suggests raised ICP and urgent CT scanning (with airway protection if necessary) is indicated. A full neurological examination may provide clues as to the pathology involved; for example, brainstem signs in the context of acute-onset occipital headache may indicate vertebrobasilar dissection. Neurological signs may, however, be 'falsely localising', as in large subarachnoid haemorrhage or bacterial meningitis. Care should be taken to examine for other evidence of meningitis such as a rash (not always petechial), fever or signs of shock.

Unilateral headache with agitation, ipsilateral lacrimation, facial sweating and conjunctival injection is typical of cluster headache. Conjunctival injection may also be seen in acute glaucoma, accompanied by peri- or

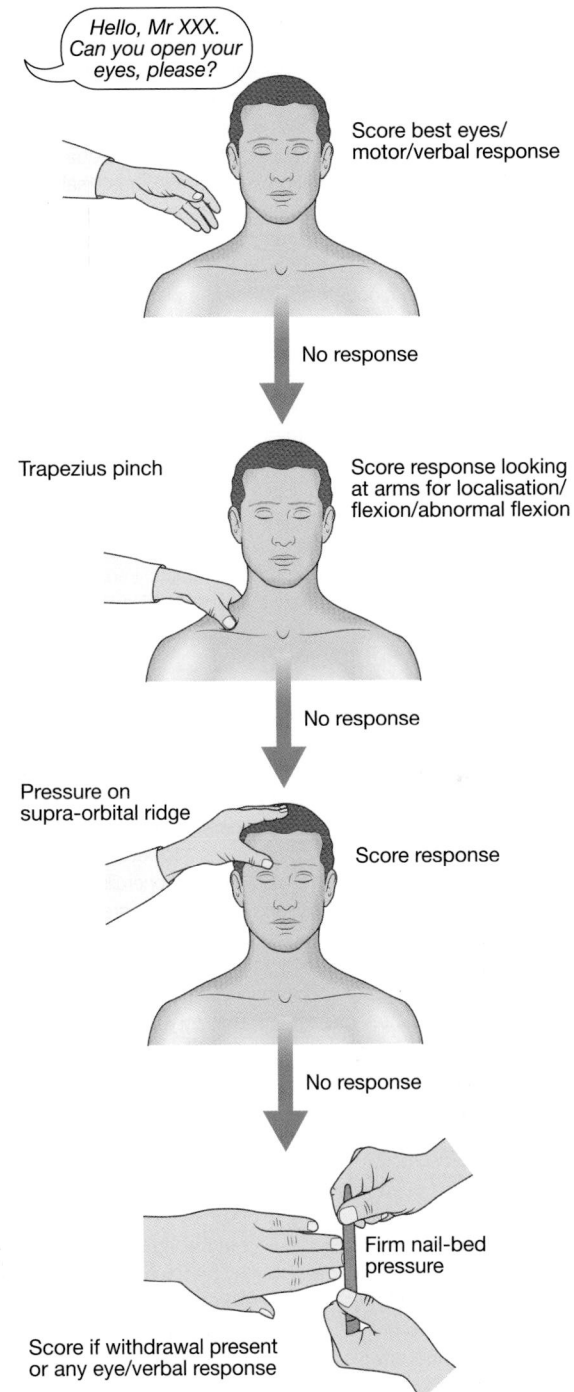

Fig. 9.5 Assessment of the Glasgow Coma Scale (GCS) score in an obtunded patient. Avoid using a sternal rub, as it causes bruising.

retro-orbital pain, clouding of the cornea, decreased visual acuity and, often, systemic upset. Temporal headaches in patients over 60 should prompt examination for enlarged or tender temporal arteries and palpation of temporal pulses (often absent in temporal arteritis). Visual acuity should be assessed promptly, as visual loss is an important complication of temporal arteritis.

Initial investigations

If there is any alteration of conscious level, focal neurological signs, new-onset seizures or a history of head injury, then CT scanning of the head is indicated. The urgency of scanning will depend on the clinical picture and trajectory but in many circumstances will be immediately required. Intracranial haemorrhage or a space-occupying lesion with mass effect should prompt urgent neurosurgical referral. If bacterial meningitis is suspected (see Box 9.15), cerebrospinal fluid (CSF) analysis is required to make a definite diagnosis. Antibiotics should not be delayed for lumbar puncture (LP), which needs to be preceded by CT scanning only if raised ICP is suspected. In cases of thunderclap headache (peak intensity within 5 minutes and lasting over an hour), a normal CT scan should be followed by an LP performed more than 12 hours after headache onset, to look for evidence of xanthochromia. A negative CT scan within 6 hours of headache onset has a high degree of sensitivity for detecting subarachnoid blood. In such cases, a discussion of risks and benefits with the patient may conclude that an LP is not necessary to exclude subarachnoid haemorrhage, although a CT angiogram may be considered to exclude other pathology, such as arterial dissection. Many headaches require prompt involvement of specialists. Features of acute glaucoma, for example, require immediate ophthalmological review for measurement of intraocular pressures. Suspected temporal arteritis with an erythrocyte sedimentation rate (ESR) of >50 mm/hr should prompt immediate glucocorticoid therapy and rheumatological referral (see Ch. 26 for management). Features of raised ICP in the absence of a mass lesion on neuroimaging may indicate idiopathic intracranial hypertension; CSF opening pressure is likely to be informative.

Unilateral leg swelling

Most leg swelling is caused by oedema, the accumulation of fluid within the interstitial space. There are three explanatory mechanisms for development of oedema, which are described in Box 9.16. Unilateral swelling usually indicates a localised pathology in either the venous or the lymphatic system, while bilateral oedema often represents generalised fluid overload combined with the effects of gravity. However, all causes of unilateral leg swelling may present bilaterally, and generalised fluid overload may present with asymmetrical (and therefore apparently unilateral) oedema. Fluid overload may be the result of cardiac failure, pulmonary hypertension (even in the absence of right ventricular failure), renal failure, hypoalbuminaemia or drugs (calcium channel blockers, glucocorticoids, mineralocorticoids, non-steroidal anti-inflammatory drugs (NSAIDs) and others); see Box 16.14 for other causes. The remainder of this section focuses on the causes of 'unilateral' oedema.

Presentation

Any patient who presents with unilateral leg swelling should be assessed with the possibility of deep vein thrombosis (DVT) in mind. The pain and swelling of a DVT is often fairly gradual in onset, over hours or even days. Sudden-onset pain in the posterior aspect of the leg is more consistent with gastrocnemius muscle tear (which may be traumatic or spontaneous) or a ruptured Baker's cyst. Leg swelling and pain associated with paraesthesia or paresis, or in the context of lower limb injury or reduced conscious level, should always prompt concern regarding the possibility of compartment syndrome (Box 9.17).

Clinical assessment

Lower limb DVT characteristically starts in the distal veins, causing an increase in temperature of the limb and dilatation of the superficial veins. Often, however, symptoms and signs are minimal.

Cellulitis is usually characterised by erythema and skin warmth localised to a well-demarcated area of the leg and may be associated with an obvious source of entry of infection (e.g. leg ulcer or insect bite). The patient may be febrile and systemically unwell. Superficial thrombophlebitis is more localised; erythema and tenderness occur along the course of a firm, palpable vein.

Examination of any patient presenting with leg swelling should include assessment for malignancy (evidence of weight loss, a palpable mass or lymphadenopathy). Malignancy is a risk factor for DVT, but pelvic or lower abdominal masses can also produce leg swelling by compressing the pelvic veins or lymphatics. Early lymphoedema is indistinguishable from other causes of oedema. More chronic lymphoedema is firm

9.16 Mechanisms of oedema

There are three explanatory mechanisms for the development of oedema that may occur in isolation or combination:

- increased hydrostatic pressure in the venous system due to increased intravascular volume or venous obstruction
- decreased oncotic pressure secondary to a decrease in the plasma proteins that retain fluid within the circulation
- obstruction to lymphatic drainage ('lymphoedema').

✚ 9.17 Identification of compartment syndrome

- Compartment syndrome classically occurs following extrinsic compression of a limb due to trauma or reduced conscious level (especially when caused by drugs or alcohol).
- It usually presents with a tense, firm and exquisitely painful limb.
- The pain is characteristically exacerbated by passive muscle stretching or squeezing the compartment.
- Altered sensation may be evident distally.
- Absent peripheral pulses are a late sign and their presence does not exclude the diagnosis.
- Clinical suspicion of compartment syndrome should prompt measurement of creatine kinase and urgent surgical review.

and non-pitting, often with thickening of the overlying skin, which may develop a 'cobblestone' appearance.

Chronic venous insufficiency is a cause of long-standing oedema that, particularly when combined with another cause of leg swelling, may acutely worsen. Characteristic skin changes (haemosiderin deposition, hair loss, varicose eczema, ulceration) and prominent varicosities are common, and sometimes cause diagnostic confusion with cellulitis. See Box 9.17 for the examination findings associated with compartment syndrome.

Initial investigations

Factors predisposing to venous thromboembolism are covered in detail in Chapter 25. Clinical criteria can be used to rank patients according to their likelihood of DVT, by using scoring systems that determine pre-test probability (see Ch. 1), such as the Wells score (Box 9.18). Figure 9.6 gives an algorithm for investigation of suspected DVT based on initial Wells score. In patients with a low ('unlikely') pre-test probability of DVT, D-dimer levels can be measured; if these are normal, further investigation for DVT is unnecessary. Further information on the interpretation of D-dimer is given in Box 9.19. In those with a moderate or high ('likely') probability of DVT or with elevated D-dimer levels, objective diagnosis of DVT should be obtained using appropriate imaging, usually a Doppler ultrasound scan. Therefore, in the same way as for pulmonary embolus, the investigative pathway for DVT differs according to the pre-test probability of DVT. For low-probability DVT, the negative predictive value of the D-dimer test (the most important parameter in this context) is over 99%; if the test is negative, the clinician can discharge the patient with confidence. In patients with a high probability of DVT, the negative predictive value of a D-dimer test falls to somewhere in the region of 97%–98%. While this may initially appear to be a high figure, to discharge 2 or 3 patients in every 100 incorrectly would generally be considered an unacceptable error rate. Hence, with the exception of pregnancy (Box 9.20), a combination of clinical probability and blood test results should be used in the diagnosis of DVT.

If cellulitis is suspected, serum inflammatory markers, skin swabs and blood cultures should be sent, ideally before antibiotics are given. Ruptured Baker's cyst and calf muscle tear can both be readily diagnosed on ultrasound. If pelvic or lower abdominal malignancy is suspected, a prostate-specific antigen (PSA) level should be measured in males and appropriate imaging with ultrasound (transabdominal or transvaginal) or CT should be undertaken.

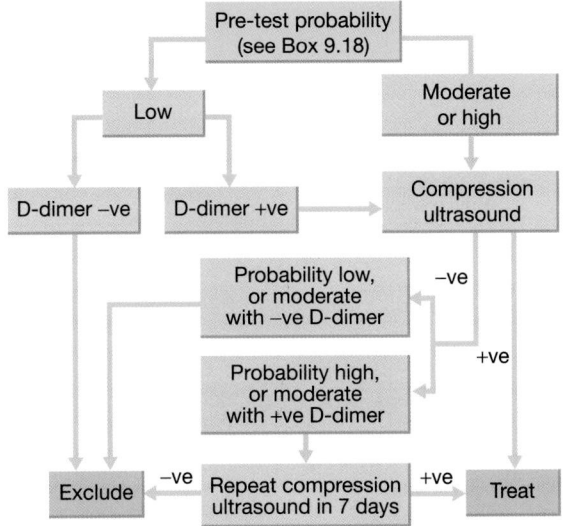

Fig. 9.6 Investigation of suspected deep vein thrombosis. Pre-test probability is calculated in Box 9.18. See also page 10.

---

i 9.18 Predicting the pre-test probability of deep vein thrombosis (DVT) using the Wells score*

Clinical characteristic	Score
Previous documented DVT	1
Active cancer (patient receiving treatment for cancer within previous 6 months or currently receiving palliative treatment)	1
Paralysis, paresis or recent plaster immobilisation of lower extremities	1
Recently bedridden for ≥ 3 days, or major surgery within previous 12 weeks	1
Localised tenderness along distribution of deep venous system	1
Entire leg swollen	1
Calf swelling at least 3 cm larger than that on asymptomatic side (measured 10 cm below tibial tuberosity)	1
Pitting oedema confined to symptomatic leg	1
Collateral superficial veins (non-varicose)	1
Alternative diagnosis at least as likely as DVT	−2

Clinical probability	Total score
DVT low probability	<1
DVT moderate probability	1–2
DVT high probability	>2

*A dichotomised revised Wells score, which classifies patients as 'unlikely' or 'likely', may also be used.
From Wells PS. Evaluation of D-dimer in the diagnosis of suspected deep vein thrombosis. N Engl J Med 2003; 349:1227; copyright © 2003 Massachusetts Medical Society.

Acute abdomen

The acute abdomen accounts for approximately 50% of all urgent admissions to general surgical units, but a significant proportion of patients present via acute medicine.

Presentation

The acute abdomen is a consequence of one or more of the following pathological processes (Box 9.21):

- *Inflammation*. Pain develops gradually, usually over several hours. It is initially rather diffuse until the parietal peritoneum is involved, when

---

i 9.19 D-dimer

- D-dimers are specific cross-linked fibrin degradation products which are small protein fragments present in blood after a blood clot is degraded by fibrinolysis.
- D-dimers are present in human blood when the coagulation system has been activated, usually because of the presence of thrombosis, disseminated intravascular coagulation or venom-induced consumptive coagulopathy.
- As the sensitivity of D-dimer decreases with time, it should not be used in the assessment of patients who present with symptoms for 7 days or more.
- D-dimer increases with age; for patients aged over 50 years with suspected venous thromboembolism (VTE), a cut-off equal to the patient's age in years × 10 µg/L (or × 0.056 nmol/L) has therefore been proposed.
- Although their safety is still being evaluated, age-adjusted D-dimers appear to decrease the false-positive rate without substantially increasing the false-negative rate

---

9.20 Swollen legs in pregnancy

- **Benign swollen legs**: common in pregnancy; this is usually benign.
- **DVT**: pregnancy is a significant risk factor; however
- **D-dimer**: should not be measured in pregnancy; it has not been validated in this group.
- **Imaging**: should be arranged on the basis of clinical suspicion alone, and the threshold for undertaking a definite diagnostic test should be low.

---

i 9.21 Causes of acute abdominal pain

Inflammation

- Appendicitis
- Diverticulitis
- Cholecystitis
- Pelvic inflammatory disease
- Pancreatitis
- Pyelonephritis
- Intra-abdominal abscess

Perforation/rupture

- Peptic ulcer
- Diverticular disease
- Ovarian cyst
- Aortic aneurysm

Obstruction

- Intestinal obstruction
- Biliary colic
- Ureteric colic

Other (rare)

- See Box 23.22

---

it becomes localised. Movement exacerbates the pain; abdominal rigidity and guarding occur.
- *Perforation*. When a viscus perforates, pain starts abruptly; it is severe and leads to generalised peritonitis.
- *Obstruction*. Pain is colicky, with spasms that cause the patient to writhe around and double up. Colicky pain that does not disappear between spasms suggests complicating inflammation.
- *Ischaemia*. Signs are variable; pain may come on acutely or more gradually and the abdomen can be soft or rigid. A raised venous lactate is usually only a late sign once hepatic lactate clearance is overwhelmed (see Fig. 9.14).

Clinical assessment

If there are signs of peritonitis (guarding and rebound tenderness with rigidity), the patient should be resuscitated with titrated oxygen, intravenous fluids and antibiotics; urgent surgical input is required. In other circumstances, further investigations may be necessary, as detailed below (Fig. 9.7).

Initial investigations

Patients should have a full blood count, urea and electrolytes, glucose and amylase taken to look for evidence of dehydration, leucocytosis and

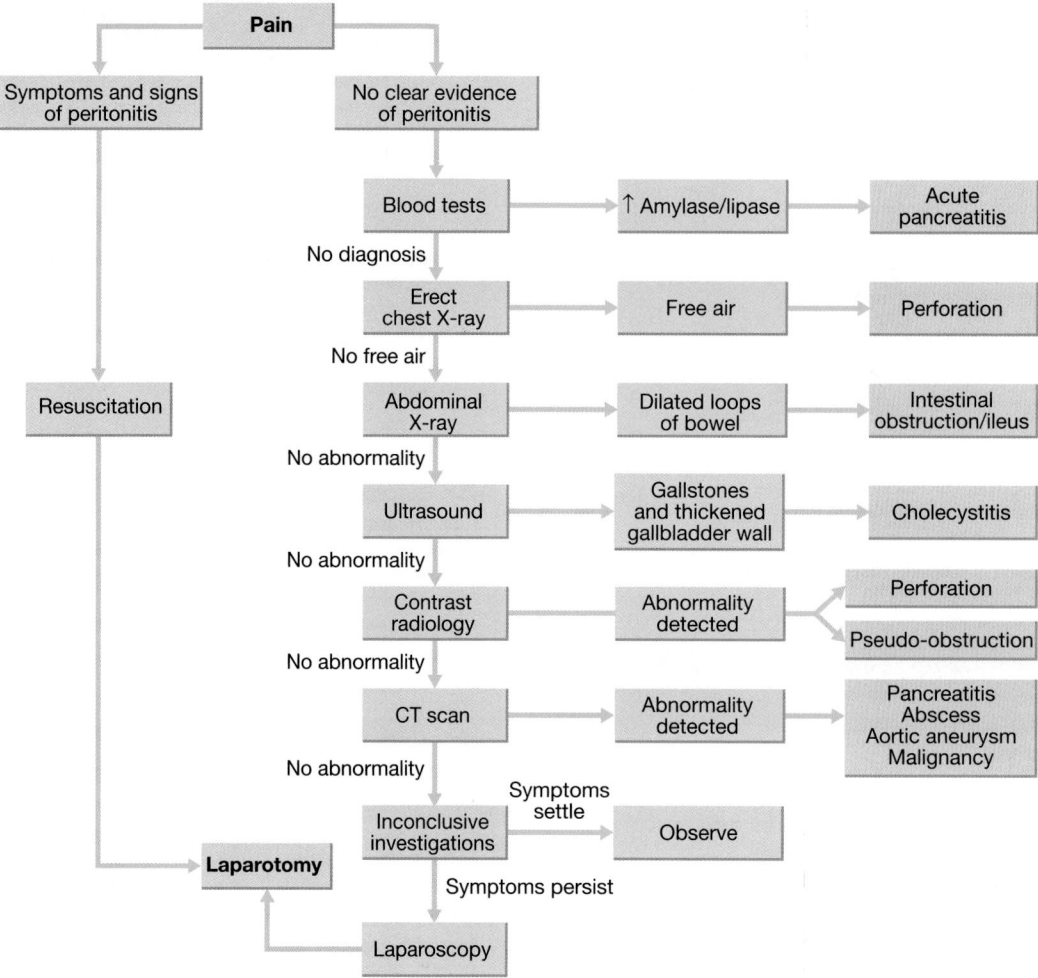

Fig. 9.7 Management of acute abdominal pain: an algorithm.

pancreatitis. Urinalysis is useful in suspected renal colic and pyelone-phritis. An erect chest X-ray may show air under the diaphragm, sug-gestive of perforation, and a plain abdominal film may show evidence of obstruction or ileus (see Fig. 23.11). An abdominal ultrasound may help in identifying gallstones, renal stones, free fluid or an intra-abdominal abscess. Abdominal CT scanning is the most useful investigation, and is essential in differentiating pseudo-obstruction and mechanical large bowel obstruction. Concerns regarding contrast-induced nephropathy should be secondary to the imperative to reach an early diagnosis. CT may also be useful to seek evidence of pancreatitis, retroperitoneal col-lections or masses, including aortic aneurysm.

Diagnostic laparotomy should be considered when the diagnosis has not been revealed by other investigations. All patients must be carefully and regularly reassessed (every 2–4 hours) so that any change in condi-tion that might alter both the suspected diagnosis and clinical decision can be observed and acted on early.

Management

The general approach is to close perforations, treat inflammatory condi-tions with antibiotics or resection, and relieve obstructions. Aspiration of gastric contents is a major risk in all acute abdominal conditions, espe-cially intestinal obstruction. This occurs once the laryngeal reflexes are overwhelmed by the volume of regurgitated material, and is particularly common in frailer individuals or where there is a coexisting reduction in conscious level. The placement of a large-bore nasogastric tube should therefore be considered whenever bowel obstruction is suspected. The speed of intervention and the necessity for surgery depend upon vari-ous factors, of which the presence of peritonitis is the most pertinent.

A treatment summary of some of the more common surgical conditions follows:

- *Acute appendicitis:* This should be treated by early surgery, since there is a risk of perforation and recurrent attacks with non-operative treatment. The appendix can be removed through a conventional right iliac fossa skin crease incision or by laparoscopic techniques.
- *Acute cholecystitis*: This can be successfully treated non-operatively but the high risk of recurrent attacks and the low morbidity of sur-gery have made early laparoscopic cholecystectomy the treatment of choice unless there are other considerations (such as pregnancy).
- *Acute diverticulitis:* Conservative therapy is standard, but if perfora-tion has occurred, resection is advisable. Depending on peritoneal contamination and the degree of shock (risk of anastomotic leak correlates with severity of shock), primary anastomosis is pref-erable to a Hartmann's procedure (oversew of rectal stump and end-colostomy).
- *Small bowel obstruction*: If the cause is obvious and surgery inevita-ble (such as with a strangulated hernia), an early operation is appro-priate. If the suspected cause is adhesions from previous surgery, only those patients who do not resolve within the first 48 hours or who develop signs of strangulation (colicky pain becoming constant, peritonitis, tachycardia, fever, leucocytosis) should have surgery.
- *Large bowel obstruction:* Pseudo-obstruction should be treated non-operatively. Some patients benefit from colonoscopic decom-pression, but mechanical obstruction merits resection, usually with a primary anastomosis. Differentiation between the two can be made by water-soluble contrast enema.

- *Mesenteric ischaemia*: This can be due to an arterial or venous thrombosis, or a structural abnormality of the gut such as a volvulus. Early surgery can be successful in revascularisation of the gut or removing ischaemic tissue, although acute mesenteric arterial thrombosis has a poor prognosis, especially when the diagnosis is delayed.
- *Acute pancreatitis*: CT scanning can be useful to rule out other pathologies that may be amenable to operative management (e.g. retroperitoneal perforation), but is not essential in the early management of the disease. Management is usually conservative, and the majority of patients will improve. A minority will develop pancreatic necrosis that will require prolonged supportive care and organ support. Antibiotics are not usually indicated in the early phase of the disease.
- *Perforated peptic ulcer*: Surgical closure of the perforation is standard practice, but some patients without generalised peritonitis can be treated non-operatively once a water-soluble contrast meal has confirmed spontaneous sealing of the perforation. Adequate and aggressive resuscitation with intravenous fluids, antibiotics and analgesia is mandatory before surgery.

For a more detailed discussion of acute abdominal pain, the reader is referred to the companion volume of this text, *Principles and Practice of Surgery*.

Identification and assessment of deterioration

Early warning scores and the role of the medical emergency team

There are many systems that have been developed with the aim of rapidly identifying and managing physiological deterioration. These are referred to as 'rapid response systems'. One popular example of a rapid response system is a medical emergency team (MET). A MET system operates on the basis that when a patient meets certain physiological criteria, the team is alerted. The team is expected to make a rapid assessment and institute immediate management. This may include escalation to critical care or, following liaison with the parent clinical team, ongoing ward-based care.

The trigger for a 'MET' call may be a single parameter – such as a low BP or tachycardia – or may consist of a composite early warning score. Early warning score systems function by the observer allocating a value between 0 and 3 for abnormalities in respiratory rate, SpO_2, temperature, BP, heart rate and neurological response (Fig. 9.8). The values are summed and the composite score gives an indication of the severity of physiological derangement. Early warning systems can be automated into an electronic format that calculates the score and even alerts the responsible clinician(s) by email or text message.

There are advantages and disadvantages to having a separate MET system, compared with allowing the responsible clinical team to manage deterioration, and to having a composite score or a single parameter detection system. These are outlined in Box 9.22.

Immediate assessment of the deteriorating patient

An approach to assessment of the deteriorating patient can be summarised by the mnemonic 'C-A-B-C-D-E'.

C – Control of obvious problem

For example, if the patient has ventricular tachycardia on the monitor or significant blood loss is apparent, immediate action is required.

A and B – Airway and breathing

If the patient is talking in full sentences, then the airway is clear and breathing is adequate. A rapid history should be obtained while the initial assessment is undertaken. Breathing should be assessed with a focused respiratory examination. Oxygen saturations and ABGs should be checked early (p. 194).

C – Circulation

A focused cardiovascular examination should include heart rate and rhythm, blood pressure, jugular venous pressure, evidence of bleeding, signs of shock and abnormal heart sounds. The carotid pulse should be palpated in the collapsed or unconscious patient, but peripheral pulses also should be checked in conscious patients. The radial, brachial, foot and femoral pulses may disappear as shock progresses, and this indicates the severity of circulatory compromise.

D – Disability

Conscious level should be assessed using the GCS (see Fig. 9.5 and Box 9.29). A brief neurological examination looking for focal signs should be performed. Capillary blood glucose should always be measured to exclude hypoglycaemia or severe hyperglycaemia.

E – Exposure and evidence

'Exposure' indicates the need for targeted clinical examination of the remaining body systems, particularly the abdomen and lower limbs. 'Evidence' may be gathered via a collateral history from other health-care professionals or family members, recent investigations, prescriptions or monitoring charts.

Selecting the appropriate location for ongoing management and anticipatory care planning

Two groups of patients frequently gain benefit from admission to critical care: those with organ dysfunction severe enough to require organ support and those in whom the disease process is clearly setting them on a downward trajectory and in whom early, aggressive management may alter the outcome. Whether an individual patient should be admitted to the intensive care or high-dependency unit (ICU/HDU) will depend on local arrangements. A useful tool to assist with the decision regarding location is the 'level of care' required (Box 9.23). Many intensive care units are a mix of level 2 and level 3 beds, which streamlines the admission process. When a patient requires admission with a suspected transmissible disease that poses a risk to other patients and staff, the patient should be admitted to an isolated room located within an appropriate area of the hospital that can provide an appropriate level of care.

Anticipatory care planning (ACP) refers to the process of decision-making relating to treatments or support that would be appropriate if a patient's condition was to deteriorate. Admission can be a valuable opportunity for discussion with the patient and family members/carers about the appropriate 'ceiling of care'; for example, would resuscitation in the event of a cardiac arrest and/or admission to a critical care area be appropriate. Such discussions may result in the placement of a 'do not resuscitate order' and a decision that 'ward-level' care may be the 'ceiling' for that individual. It is important that discussions and decisions are clearly documented in the patient record. Further details of ACP decision-making are found on page 206.

Common presentations of deterioration

As patients become critically unwell, they usually manifest physiological derangement. The principle underpinning critical care is the simultaneous assessment of illness severity and the stabilisation of life-threatening physiological abnormalities. The goal is to prevent deterioration and

A

NEWS key 0 1 2 3	Full Name		Date of Admission
	Date of Birth		

			Date																Date
			Time																Time

A+B (Respiration rate)

	Score	
≥25	3	≥25
21–24	2	21–24
18–20		18–20
15–17		15–17
12–14		12–14
9–11	1	9–11
≤8	3	≤8

A+B (SpO₂ Scale 1)

	Score	
≥96		≥96
94–95	1	94–95
92–93	2	92–93
≤91	3	≤91

SpO₂ Scale 2†
Oxygen saturation (%)
Use Scale 2 if target range is 88–92%, e.g. in hypercapnic respiratory failure

†ONLY use Scale 2 under the direction of a qualified clinician

	Score	
≥97 on O₂	3	≥97 on O₂
95–96 on O₂	2	95–96 on O₂
93–94 on O₂	1	93–94 on O₂
≥93 on air		≥93 on air
88–92		88–92
86–87	1	86–87
84–85	2	84–85
≤83%	3	≤83%

A=Air		A=Air
O₂ L/min	2	O₂ L/min
Device		Device

C (Blood pressure, systolic)

	Score	
≥220	3	≥220
201–219		201–219
181–200		181–200
161–180		161–180
141–160		141–160
121–140		121–140
111–120		111–120
101–110	1	101–110
91–100	2	91–100
81–90		81–90
71–80		71–80
61–70	3	61–70
51–60		51–60
≤50		≤50

C (Pulse)

	Score	
≥131	3	≥131
121–130	2	121–130
111–120		111–120
101–110		101–110
91–100	1	91–100
81–90		81–90
71–80		71–80
61–70		61–70
51–60		51–60
41–50	1	41–50
31–40	3	31–40
≤30		≤30

D (Consciousness)

	Score	
Alert		Alert
Confusion		Confusion
V	3	V
P		P
U		U

E (Temperature)

	Score	
≥39.1	2	≥39.1
38.1–39.0	1	38.1–39.0
37.1–38.0		37.1–38.0
36.1–37.0		36.1–37.0
35.1–36.0	1	35.1–36.0
≤35.0	3	≤35.0

Monitoring frequency		Monitoring
Escalation of care Y/N		Escalation
Initials		Initials

Fig. 9.8 Identifying and responding to physiological deterioration. A An example of an early warning score chart. (NEWS = National Early Warning Score; V/P/U = Verbal/Pain/Unresponsive). B (opposite) Responses to physiological deterioration. (ICU = intensive care unit; NEWS = National Early Warning Score) *(A and B) From Royal College of Physicians. National Early Warning Score (NEWS) 2: Standardising the assessment of acute-illness severity in the NHS. Updated report of a working party. London: RCP; December 2017.*

B

NEW score	Frequency of monitoring	Clinical response
0	Minimum 12 hourly	• Continue routine NEWS monitoring
Total 1–4	Minimum 4–6 hourly	• Inform registered nurse, who must assess the patient • Registered nurse decides whether increased frequency of monitoring and/or escalation of care is required
3 in single parameter	Minimum 1 hourly	• Registered nurse to inform medical team caring for the patient, who will review and decide whether escalation of care is necessary
Total 5 or more Urgent response threshold	Minimum 1 hourly	• Registered nurse to immediately inform the medical team caring for the patient • Registered nurse to request urgent assessment by a clinician or team with core competencies in the care of acutely ill patients • Provide clinical care in an environment with monitoring facilities
Total 7 or more Emergency response threshold	Continuous monitoring of vital signs	• Registered nurse to immediately inform the medical team caring for the patient – this should be at least at specialist registrar level • Emergency assessment by a team with critical care competencies, including practitioner(s) with advanced airway management skills • Consider transfer to a level 2 or 3 clinical care facility, i.e. higher-dependency unit or ICU • Clinical care in an environment with monitoring facilities

Fig. 9.8, cont'd

i **9.22 Advantages and disadvantages of different rapid response systems**

System	Advantages	Disadvantages
Single parameter trigger	High sensitivity. Will probably pick up subclinical deterioration and allow optimisation	Low specificity. Much time will be spent with patients who are not deteriorating
Composite early warning scoring system, e.g. NEWS2	Combines good sensitivity with improved specificity	May miss single parameter deterioration that is still significant, e.g. a drop of 2 GCS points may not trigger an alert
MET system	Brings expertise in deteriorating patients immediately to the bedside	Expensive to have well-trained individuals who are free from other clinical duties. May de-skill the ward-based teams in acute care. May not have expertise in highly specific areas of medicine
Clinical team review	Patient is seen by clinicians familiar with the patient and condition	Clinical team may be busy with other urgent duties. There may not be expertise in acute care within the ward-based team

(GCS = Glasgow Coma Scale; MET = Medical Emergency Team; NEWS2 = National Early Warning Score 2)

effect improvements, as the diagnosis is established and treatment of the underlying disease process is initiated.

It can be useful to consider the physiological changes as a starting point to help delineate urgent investigations and supportive treatment, which should proceed alongside the search for a definitive diagnosis.

Tachypnoea

Pathophysiology

A raised respiratory rate (tachypnoea) is the earliest and most sensitive sign of clinical deterioration. Tachypnoea may be primary (i.e. a problem within the respiratory system) or secondary to pathology elsewhere in the body. Cardiopulmonary causes of tachypnoea have been covered on page 179. Secondary tachypnoea is usually due to a metabolic acidosis, most commonly observed in the context of sepsis, haemorrhage, ketoacidosis or visceral ischaemia. More detailed information on metabolic acidosis can be found on page 630.

Assessment and management

A simple assessment of a patient's clinical status and basic physiology will usually indicate whether urgent intervention is required. In the examination, attention should be paid to the adequacy of chest expansion, air entry and the presence of added sounds such as wheeze.

Analysis of an arterial blood sample is especially helpful in narrowing the differential diagnosis and confirming clinical suspicion of severity. The 'base excess' provides rapid quantification of the component of disease that is metabolic in origin. A base excess lower than −2 mEq/L (or, put another way, a 'base deficit' of more than 2 mEq/L) is likely to represent a metabolic acidosis. A simple rule of thumb is that a lactate of more than 4 mmol/L (36 mg/dL) or a base deficit of more than 10 mEq/L should cause concern and trigger escalation to a higher level of care. In addition to clinical examination, chest radiography and bedside ultrasound can help to distinguish the cause of poor air entry; consolidation and effusion can be readily identified and a significant pneumothorax can be excluded (as shown in Fig. 9.9).

Level of care	Criteria	Appropriate location
i	**9.23 Levels of care and the corresponding admission criteria for intensive care unit (ICU) and high-dependency unit (HDU)**	
3	Patients requiring/likely to require endotracheal intubation and invasive mechanical ventilatory support Patients requiring support of two or more organ systems (e.g. inotropes and haemofiltration) Patients with chronic impairment of one or more organ systems (e.g. COPD or severe ischaemic heart disease) who require support for acute reversible failure of another organ	ICU
2	Patients requiring detailed observation or monitoring that cannot be provided at ward level: Direct arterial BP monitoring CVP monitoring Fluid balance Neurological observations, regular GCS recording Patients requiring support for a single failing organ system, excluding invasive ventilatory support (IPPV): Non-invasive respiratory support (p. 207) Moderate inotropic or vasopressor support Renal replacement therapy in an otherwise stable patient Step-down from intensive care requiring additional monitoring or single organ support	HDU
1	Patients in whom frequent but intermittent observations and medical review are sufficient	General ward setting

(BP = blood pressure; COPD = chronic obstructive pulmonary disease; CVP =central venous pressure; GCS = Glasgow Coma Scale; IPPV = intermittent positive pressure ventilation)

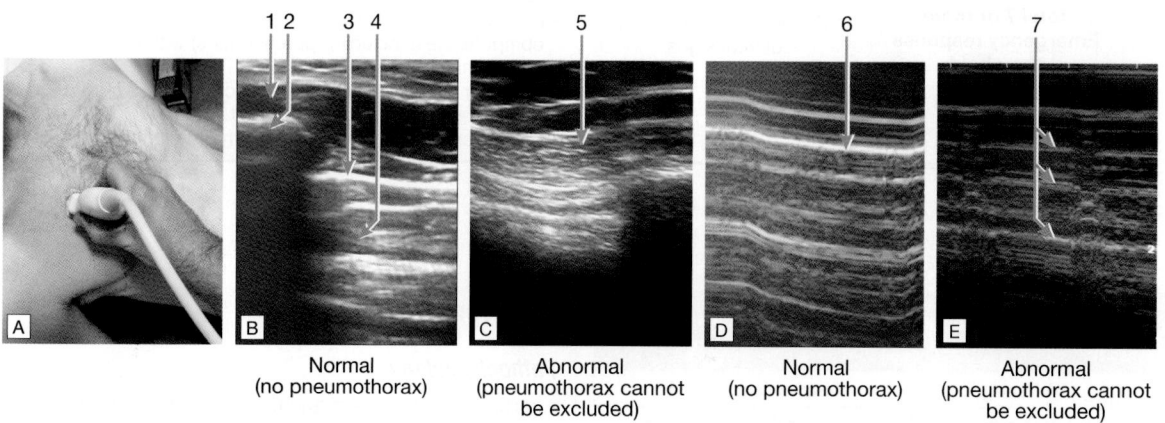

Fig. 9.9 Using ultrasound to rule out an anterior pneumothorax. [A] Probe position and orientation. [B] and [C] Two-dimensional (2D) ultrasound images. [D] and [E] M-mode ultrasound images. Key: (1) Intercostal muscle. (2) Rib. (3) Normal bright pleural line –'shimmering appearance' of sliding pleura. (4) Lung. (5) Absent 'shimmering' in pneumothorax and lung not visible. (6) Normal – 'sea shore' sign excludes pneumothorax at that location. The 'sea shore' is represented by the bright granular line with lung (sea) deeper to the bright line. (7) Absent granular pleural line and a repeating linear pattern or 'barcode' sign suggest the presence of pneumothorax.

Hypoxaemia

Pathophysiology

Low arterial partial pressure of oxygen (PaO_2) is termed hypoxaemia. It is a common presenting feature of deterioration. Hypoxia is defined as an inadequate amount of oxygen in tissues (or the inability of cells to use the available oxygen for cellular respiration). Hypoxia may be due to hypoxaemia, or may be secondary to impaired cardiac output, the presence of inadequate or dysfunctional haemoglobin, or intracellular dysfunction (such as in cyanide poisoning, where oxygen utilisation at the cellular level is impaired).

Over 97% of oxygen carried in the blood is bound to haemoglobin. The haemoglobin–oxygen dissociation curve delineates the relationship between the percentage saturation of haemoglobin with oxygen (SO_2) and the partial pressure (PO_2) of oxygen in the blood. A shift in the curve will influence the uptake and release of oxygen by the haemoglobin molecule. As capillary PCO_2 rises, the curve moves to the right, increasing the offloading of oxygen in the tissues (the Bohr effect). This increases capillary PO_2 and hence cellular oxygen supply. Shifts of the oxyhaemoglobin dissociation curve can have significant implications in certain disease processes (Fig. 9.10).

Due to the shape of the curve, a small drop in arterial PO_2 (PaO_2) below 8 kPa (60 mmHg) will cause a marked fall in SaO_2.

Relative hypoxaemia refers to the comparison between the observed PaO_2 and that which might be expected for a given fraction of inspired oxygen (FiO_2). With the patient breathing air, PaO_2 of 12–14 kPa (90–105 mmHg) would be expected; with the patient breathing 100% oxygen, a PaO_2 of > 60 kPa (450 mmHg) would be normal.

Assessment and management

Oxygen therapy should be titrated to avoid hyperoxia (too high a PaO_2; Box 9.24). Hyperoxia is theoretically harmful via a number of mechanisms. This has a clinically significant effect in patients with acute stroke, those with MI and those who chronically retain CO_2. Adverse effects of hyperoxia include:

- free radical-induced tissue damage
- less efficient buffering of carbon dioxide by oxyhaemoglobin (compared to deoxyhaemoglobin)
- less efficient ventilation–perfusion matching in lung units (due to loss of hypoxic vasoconstriction of under-ventilated lung units)
- decreased hypoxic respiratory drive in individuals with chronic hypercapnia.

When attempting to determine the cause of hypoxaemia, it is useful to consider whether the primary physiological mechanism is a type of

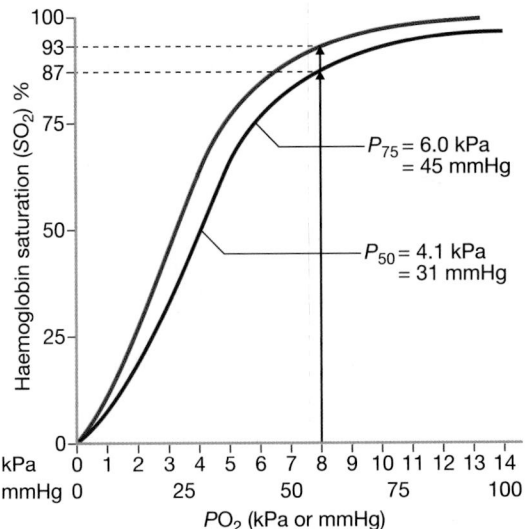

Fig. 9.10 The haemoglobin–oxygen dissociation curve and the effect of CO_2 on oxygen saturations. In pulmonary embolism, compensatory hyperventilation often occurs. $PaCO_2$ decreases, shifting the oxyhaemoglobin saturation curve to the left (green line). Therefore, despite a low PaO_2 (8 kPa/60 mmHg), the oxygen saturation reading is 93%.

9.24 Prescribing oxygen in critical illness

- Oxygen should be prescribed to achieve a target saturation of 94%–98% for most critically unwell patients.
- 88%–92% is a more appropriate target range for those at risk of hypercapnic respiratory failure.
- In patients with acute myocardial infarction or stroke, do not start oxygen unless SpO_2 is below 92%, as hyperoxia may be harmful.

shunt, or one of the many causes of ventilation–perfusion mismatch, such as alveolar or central hypoventilation (Fig. 9.11). A classification of common causes of hypoxaemia in hospitalised patients is shown in Box 9.25. In reality, the observed physiological abnormality may represent a combination of inter-related processes, such as severe pulmonary oedema leading to exhaustion, which in turn causes hypoventilation.

Evaluation of risk factors, history and examination will help to differentiate the likely aetiology and guide specific management. Further management of respiratory failure is discussed on page 207.

Tachycardia

Pathophysiology

A heart rate of >110 beats/min in an adult should always be considered abnormal and not attributed to anxiety until other causes have been excluded. Intrinsic cardiac causes (atrial fibrillation (AF), atrial flutter, supraventricular tachycardia and ventricular dysrhythmias) are less common in the general inpatient population than secondary causes of tachycardia.

A cardiac monitor or 12-lead ECG early in the examination will help both determine severity (heart rate >160 beats/min should prompt urgent escalation to a higher level of care) and narrow the differential diagnosis. AF with a rapid ventricular response should usually be regarded as secondary to another insult (most commonly, infection) until other diagnoses have been excluded. Hypovolaemia should not be missed. Concealed bleeding (e.g. into the pleura, gastrointestinal tract or retroperitoneum) may not be apparent initially and assessment of haemoglobin in an acute haemorrhage, when <30 mL/kg of fluid has been administered, can be misleadingly high. Sepsis and other hyper-metabolic

conditions may present with a tachycardia that is accompanied by tachypnoea, peripheral vasodilatation and a raised temperature. Other organ dysfunction should be noted from a brief general examination and salient points from the history.

Assessment and management

The management of a tachycardic patient should focus on treating the cause. Treating the rate alone with beta-blockade in an unwell or deteriorating patient should be done only under specialist guidance, in controlled conditions and when a clear evaluation of the risk–benefit ratio has been undertaken.

The recognition and management of primary cardiac dysrhythmias are discussed on page 408. The most appropriate method of rate control in AF depends primarily on the degree of haemodynamic compromise. An intravenous loading dose of amiodarone is well tolerated and efficacious in the majority of critically ill patients with AF and a very rapid ventricular rate. There are thromboembolic concerns regarding chemical cardioversion of AF of unknown duration. However, in deteriorating patients, the low incidence of embolic events makes this concern of secondary importance to achieving haemodynamic stability.

Digoxin continues to have a role in the treatment of AF in critically unwell but haemodynamically stable patients, when its inotropic properties can be helpful. Electrical cardioversion is reserved for dysrhythmias with extremely high heart rates, following failure of pharmacological management, and/or for those of ventricular origin. It is rarely successful in dysrhythmias secondary to systemic illness.

Hypotension

Pathophysiology

Low BP (hypotension) should always be defined in relation to a patient's usual BP. The calculation of mean arterial pressure (MAP) is shown in Box 9.26; it unifies the systolic and diastolic BPs into a single reference value. A MAP of >65 mmHg will maintain renal perfusion in the majority of patients, although a MAP of up to 80 mmHg may be required in patients with chronic hypertension.

Assessment and management

The first stage of assessment is to decide if the hypotension is physiological or pathological. The MAP is useful as, despite low systolic pressures, it is rare to see a physiological MAP of <65 mmHg. Urine output is particularly useful in the determination of the desirable MAP for an individual patient; oliguria suggests that measures to increase the MAP should be sought (p. 210). If the hypotension is pathological, an assessment of severity should look at whether it is causing physiological harm to the patient (i.e. the patient is shocked).

Shock

Shock means 'circulatory failure'. It can be defined as a level of oxygen delivery (DO) that fails to meet the metabolic requirements of the tissues (Box 9.27). Hypotension is a common presentation of shock but the terms are not synonymous. Patients can be hypotensive but not shocked, and oxygen delivery can be critically low in the context of a 'normal' BP. Along with the signs of low cardiac output (Box 9.28), objective markers of inadequate tissue oxygen delivery, such as increasing base deficit, elevated blood lactate and reduced urine output, can aid early identification. If shock is suspected, resuscitation should be commenced (p. 210).

Hypotensive patients who do not have any evidence of shock are still at significant risk of organ dysfunction. Hypotension should serve as a 'red flag' that there may be serious underlying pathology. Organ failure occurs despite normal or elevated oxygen delivery, so a full assessment of the patient is indicated. A review of the drug chart is essential, as many inpatients will be on antihypertensive medications that are contributing to hypotension. Non-cardiac medications may also have a negative influence on BP; for example, some drugs used for urine outflow tract obstruction, such as tamsulosin, have an α-adrenoceptor-blocking effect.

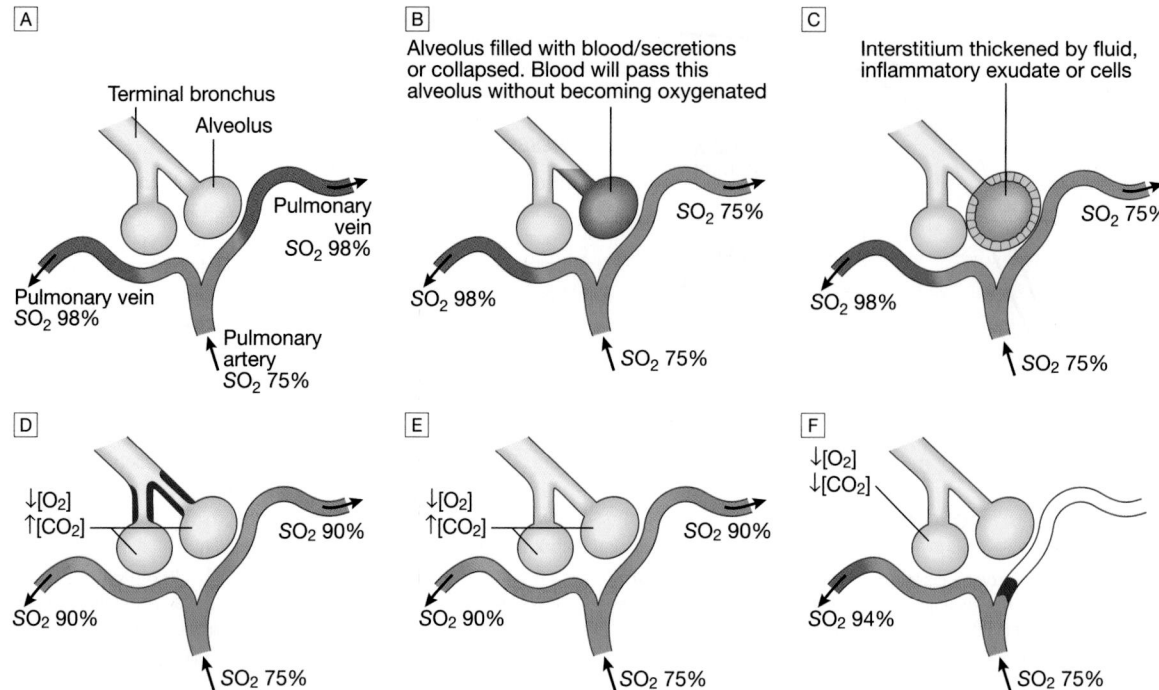

Fig. 9.11 Theoretical mechanisms of hypoxaemia. [A] Normal physiology. [B] Shunt caused by alveolar filling, e.g. in pneumonia or alveolar haemorrhage. The mixture of oxygenated and deoxygenated blood causes arterial desaturation. [C] Shunt caused by interstitial pathology, e.g. pulmonary oedema or fibrosis. Interstitial thickening causes inadequate transfer of oxygen from the alveolus to the blood, leading to shunting and arterial desaturation. Because minute volume is usually maintained, this causes type I respiratory failure. [D] Ventilation–perfusion (V/Q) mismatch caused by alveolar hypoventilation, e.g. in chronic obstructive pulmonary disease (COPD)/asthma. Alveoli are under-ventilated relative to perfusion. Alveolar PO_2 falls and PCO_2 rises, causing type II respiratory failure. [E] (V/Q) mismatch caused by central hypoventilation, e.g. in neuromuscular disease or narcotic use. The alveoli are relatively over-perfused, causing type II respiratory failure. [F] (V/Q) mismatch caused by a perfusion defect, e.g. a small pulmonary embolism. Pulmonary blood flow is diverted to other alveoli, causing them to be relatively over-perfused and thus reducing alveolar PO_2. Minute volume is increased, so PCO_2 is not elevated.

---

i 9.25 Common causes of hypoxaemia in hospitalised patients

Hypoxaemia due to shunt

- Lung collapse
- Consolidation/alveolar haemorrhage
- Interstitial oedema or interstitial infiltration (e.g. fibrosis)
- Silent aspiration of gastric contents

Hypoxaemia due to ventilation–perfusion mismatch

- Pulmonary embolism
- Acute exacerbation of asthma
- COPD (with high minute volume)

Hypoxaemia from hypoventilation

- Effects of opiates
- Severe COPD (with low minute volume)
- Neuromuscular disease/general weakness from other illness

(COPD = chronic obstructive pulmonary disease)

---

i 9.26 Calculation of mean arterial pressure (MAP)

$$MAP = \text{Diastolic blood pressure} + \frac{(\text{systolic} - \text{diastolic})}{3}$$

At normal heart rates, the heart, on average, spends two-thirds of the cycle in diastole. The MAP reflects this by weighting the value towards the diastolic blood pressure.

---

i 9.27 Oxygen content and delivery

- Oxygen content of blood = Haemoglobin concentration* × oxygen saturation × constant
- Cardiac output = Heart rate × stroke volume
- Stroke volume is dependent on cardiac filling (preload) and contractility.
- In shock, the most productive measures to improve oxygen delivery are optimising the haemoglobin level and the cardiac output.

*Oxygen is almost exclusively bound to haemoglobin; only tiny amounts are dissolved in blood at atmospheric pressure.

---

i 9.28 Hypotension in relation to cardiac output: clinical signs and possible causes

	High cardiac output	Low cardiac output
Signs	Warm hands	Cold/clammy peripheries
	Pulsatile head movement	Peripheral cyanosis
	High-volume/strong pulse	Raised venous pressure
	Low venous pressure	(except in haemorrhage)
Causes	Sepsis	Bleeding
	Allergy	Aortic stenosis and failed
	Drug overdose (e.g.	compensation
	antihypertensive)	Dysrhythmia
	Acidosis (e.g. diabetic	Obstructive (pulmonary embolism/
	ketoacidosis)	tamponade/dynamic hyperinflation
	Thyrotoxicosis	as in severe asthma)
	Beri-beri	Chronic heart failure

Hypertension

Pathophysiology

High BP (hypertension) is common and is usually benign in a critical care context. However, it can be the presenting feature of a number of serious disease processes. Furthermore, acute hypertension can result in an acute rise in vascular tone that increases left ventricular end-systolic pressure (afterload). The left ventricle may be unable to eject blood against the increased aortic pressure, and acute pulmonary oedema can result (referred to as 'flash' pulmonary oedema.)

Assessment and management

Before treating an acute rise in BP, it is worth considering a few important diagnoses that may impact on the immediate management:

- *Intracranial event*. Ischaemia of the brainstem (commonly via a pressure effect) will cause acute increases in BP. A neurological examination and CT scan of the head should be considered.
- *Fluid overload*. Once the capacity of the venous blood reservoir becomes saturated, increases in fluid volume will lead to increases in BP. This can occur in younger patients without the onset of peripheral oedema and originate from myocardial dysfunction or impaired renal clearance.
- *Underlying medical problems*. A brief search for a history of renal disease, spinal injury and less common metabolic causes such as phaeochromocytoma can be worthwhile. In women of child-bearing age, pregnancy-induced hypertension and pre-eclampsia must always be considered.
- *Primary cardiac problems*. Myocardial ischaemia, acute heart failure and aortic dissection can all present with hypertension.
- *Drug-related problems*. Most commonly, these involve a missed antihypertensive medication, but sympathomimetic drugs such as cocaine and amphetamines can be implicated.

The management of hypertension is discussed further on page 447.

Decreased conscious level

Assessment

A reduction in conscious level should prompt an urgent assessment of the patient, a search for the likely cause and an evaluation of the risk of airway loss. The GCS was developed to risk-stratify head injury, but it has become the most widely recognised assessment tool for conscious level (see Box 9.29 for a breakdown of GCS assessment, Box 9.30 for how to communicate the findings and Fig. 9.5 for how to assess GCS). While disorders that affect language or limb function (e.g. left hemisphere stroke, locked-in syndrome) may reduce its usefulness, evaluation of the GCS usually provides helpful prognostic information, and serial recordings can plot improvement or deterioration. It is not possible to define a total score below which a patient is unlikely to be able to protect the airway (from aspiration or obstruction), but a motor score of less than 5 would suggest significant risk.

Coma is defined as a persisting state of deep unconsciousness. In practice, this means a sustained GCS of 8 or less. There are many causes of coma (Box 9.31), including neurological (structural or non-structural brain disease) and non-neurological (e.g. type II respiratory failure) ones. The mode of onset of coma and any precipitating event is crucial to establishing the cause, and should be obtained from witnesses. Failure to obtain an adequate history for patients in coma is a common cause of diagnostic delay.

Once the patient is stable from a cardiorespiratory perspective, examination should include accurate assessment of conscious level and a thorough general medical examination, looking for clues such as needle tracks indicating drug abuse, rashes, fever and focal signs of infection, including neck stiffness or evidence of head injury. Focal neurological

---

i 9.29 Glasgow Coma Scale (GCS)*

Eye opening (E)

• Spontaneous	4
• To speech	3
• To pain	2
• Nil	1

Best motor response (M)

• Obeys commands	6
• Localises to painful stimulus	5
• Flexion to painful stimulus or withdraws hand from pain	4
• Abnormal flexion (internal rotation of shoulder, flexion of wrist)	3
• Extensor response (external rotation of shoulder, extension of wrist)	2
• Nil	1

Verbal response (V)

• Orientated	5
• Confused conversation	4
• Inappropriate words	3
• Incomprehensible sounds	2
• Nil	1

Coma score = E + M + V

Always present GCS as breakdown, not a sum score (unless 3 or 15)

• Minimum sum	3
• Maximum sum	15

*Record the best score observed. When the patient is intubated, there can be no verbal response. The suffix 'T' should replace the verbal component of the score, and the remainder of the score is therefore a maximum of 10.

 9.30 How to communicate conscious level to other health-care professionals

- It is best to state the physical response along with the numerical score.
- For example, 'a patient who doesn't open his eyes, withdraws to pain and makes groaning noises, having a GCS of E1, M4, V2, making a total of 7' is preferable to 'a male with a GCS of 7'.

---

i 9.31 Causes of coma

Metabolic disturbance

- Drug overdose
- Diabetes mellitus
  - Hypoglycaemia
  - Ketoacidosis
  - Hyperosmolar coma
- Hyponatraemia
- Uraemia
- Hepatic failure (hyperammonaemia)
- Inborn errors of metabolism causing hyperammonaemia
- Hyperammonaemia on refeeding following profound anorexia
- Respiratory failure
- Hypothermia
- Hypothyroidism

Trauma

- Cerebral contusion
- Extradural haematoma
- Subdural haematoma
- Diffuse axonal injury

Vascular disease

- Subarachnoid haemorrhage
- Brainstem infarction/haemorrhage
- Intracerebral haemorrhage
- Cerebral venous sinus thrombosis

Infections

- Meningitis
- Encephalitis
- Cerebral abscess
- Systemic sepsis

Others

- Epilepsy
- Brain tumour
- Functional ('pseudo-coma')

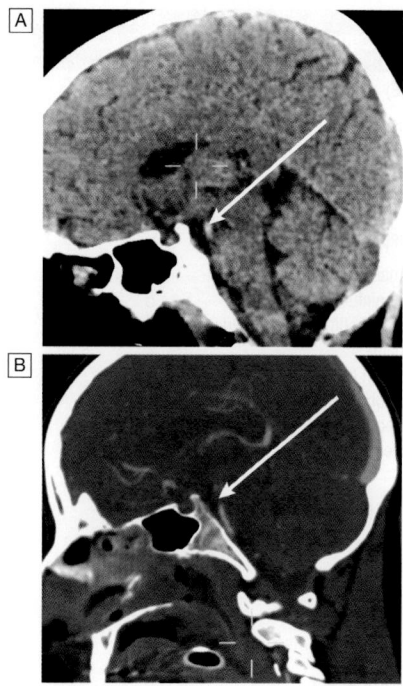

Fig. 9.12 Hyperacute changes in conscious state are commonly of vascular origin. CT of the brain is unlikely to identify many vascular causes but a CT angiogram of the circle of Willis is a high-yield investigation in this context. A Non-contrast CT of the head showing hyperdense thrombus in the basilar artery (arrow). This is a specific, but not sensitive, sign. B CT angiogram of the circle of Willis demonstrating thrombosis in the basilar artery (arrow). This has better sensitivity for acute vascular occlusion.

signs may suggest a structural explanation (stroke or tumour) or may be falsely localising (for example, 6th nerve palsy can occur as a consequence of raised intracerebral pressure). It is vital to exclude non-neurological causes of coma. Sodium and glucose should be measured urgently as part of the initial assessment, as acute hyponatraemia (Ch. 19) and hypoglycaemia (see Box 21.17) are easily corrected and can cause irreversible brain injury if missed.

Further investigations should be guided by the clinical presentation and examination findings; a sudden onset suggests a vascular cause. An early CT scan of the brain may demonstrate any gross pathology but if a brainstem stroke is suspected (Fig. 9.12), a CT angiogram of the circle of Willis will provide more useful information, as a non-contrast CT is frequently negative in this context. If there are features suggestive of cerebral venous thrombosis, such as thrombophilia or sinus infection, a CT venogram should be performed. Meningitis or encephalitis may be suggested by the history, signs of infection or subtle radiological findings. If these diagnoses are considered, it is best to commence treatment with broad-spectrum antibiotics and antivirals while awaiting more definitive diagnostic information.

Other drug, metabolic and hepatic causes of reduced conscious level are dealt with in the relevant chapters. An ammonia level (sent on ice) can narrow the differential diagnosis to a metabolic or hepatic cause if there is diagnostic doubt; levels > 140 μg/dL (100 μmol/L) are significantly abnormal. Psychiatric conditions such as catatonic depression or neurological conditions such as the autoimmune encephalitides can cause a reduced level of consciousness, but they are diagnoses of exclusion and will require specialist input.

Management

Moving an unconscious patient into the recovery position is best for airway protection while preparations are made for escalation to a higher level of care. The decision regarding intubation for airway protection is always difficult. Length of stay in intensive care is significantly reduced

if there is no secondary organ dysfunction. Therefore, early intubation and the prevention of lung injury constitute the safer option if there is any doubt about a patient's ability to protect the airway from obstruction or aspiration.

Decreased urine output/deteriorating renal function

Assessment

A urine output of 0.5 mL/kg/hr is a commonly quoted, though arbitrary target. Although some patients can produce urine volumes below this level with no change in their renal biochemistry, such low volumes should alert the clinician to the possibility of suboptimal renal perfusion.

Oliguria in association with hypotension or an increase in serum creatinine level (even if small) should prompt examination for the underlying cause. Pre-renal causes predominate in the general inpatient population, so optimising the MAP by administration of intravenous fluids (and possibly vasopressors) is the first priority. In the majority of inpatients there is no role for high volumes (i.e. > 30 mL/kg) of intravenous fluid if the MAP is normal. Exceptions to this rule include patients with clinical dehydration or high fluid losses such as in burns, diabetes emergencies (see Ch. 21) and diabetes insipidus (Ch. 20), where fluid management should be guided by local protocols.

Diagnosis and management

Further assessment and management of oliguria are explained on page 566. Two other important causes of renal failure in the inpatient population are abdominal compartment syndrome and rhabdomyolysis.

Abdominal compartment syndrome

Abdominal compartment syndrome occurs when raised pressure within the abdomen reduces perfusion to the abdominal organs. It is most commonly seen in surgical patients, but can occur in medical conditions with extreme fluid retention such as liver cirrhosis. When it is suspected, intra-abdominal pressure can be monitored via a pressure transducer connected to a urinary catheter (following instillation of 25 mL of 0.9% saline into the bladder). Values over 20 mmHg suggest abdominal compartment syndrome is present. Urgent measures should be taken to reduce the pressure, such as decompression of the stomach, bladder and peritoneum if ascites is present. If conservative measures fail, a laparostomy can be considered.

Rhabdomyolysis

Rhabdomyolysis occurs when there is an injury to a large volume of skeletal muscle, usually because a single limb or muscle compartment has been ischaemic for a prolonged period. It can also occur following trauma and crush injury or after over-exertion of muscles. Over-exertion can occur after intense physical exercise or as part of a medical condition that causes widespread muscular activity, such as malignant hyperpyrexia or neuroleptic malignant syndrome. A creatine kinase (CK) level of > 1000 U/L is highly suggestive, although it can rise to tens of thousands in severe cases. Management should focus on identification and correction of the underlying cause and support for multi-organ dysfunction. Forced alkaline diuresis (using intravenous bicarbonate infusion and furosemide) can be used to maintain a good flow of less acidic fluid within the renal tubules and reduce myoglobin precipitation.

Disorders causing critical illness

Sepsis and the systemic inflammatory response

Sepsis is one of the most common causes of multi-organ failure. Sepsis requires the presence of infection with a resultant systemic inflammatory state; organ dysfunction occurs from a combination of the two processes. The definition of sepsis has undergone various iterations and

i **9.32 Definitions of sepsis and septic shock***

Sepsis

Patients with suspected infection who have two or more of:
- *Hypotension* – systolic blood pressure < 100 mmHg
- *Altered mental status* – Glasgow Coma Scale score ≤ 14
- *Tachypnoea* – respiratory rate ≥ 22 breaths/min

Sepsis can also be diagnosed by suspected infection and an increase of ≥ 2 points on the Sequential Organ Failure Assessment (SOFA) score (Box 9.55).

Septic shock

A subset of sepsis with underlying circulatory or cellular/metabolic abnormalities associated with a substantially increased mortality:
- Sepsis and both of (after fluid resuscitation):
  1. Persistent hypotension requiring vasopressors to maintain a MAP > 65 mmHg
  2. Serum lactate > 2 mmol/L (18 mg/dL)

(MAP = mean arterial pressure)
*From the Third International Consensus Definitions for Sepsis and Septic Shock (Sepsis-3).

there is still a lack of consensus as to the exact wording that best reflects this complex, multisystem process (Box 9.32).

Aetiology and pathogenesis

To understand how an infection can lead to progressive multi-organ failure, it is essential to have a grasp of the pathophysiology.

Initiation of the inflammatory response

The process begins with infection in one part of the body that triggers a localised inflammatory response. Appropriate source control and a competent immune system will, in most cases, contain the infection at this stage. However, if certain factors are present, the infection may become systemic. The causative factors are not fully elucidated but probably include:

- a genetic predisposition to sepsis
- a large microbiological load
- high virulence of the organism
- delay in source control (either surgical or antimicrobial)
- resistance of the organism to treatment
- patient factors (immune status, nutrition, frailty).

Mediators are released from damaged cells (called 'alarmins') and these, coupled with direct stimulation of immune cells by the molecular patterns of the microorganism, trigger the inflammatory response. An example of such direct stimulation is that of lipopolysaccharide, which is found on the surface of Gram-negative bacteria. It strongly stimulates an immune response and is commonly used in research settings to initiate a septic cascade.

Viral and fungal infections can cause a syndrome that is clinically indistinguishable from bacterial sepsis. Likewise, numerous non-infective processes, such as pancreatitis, burns, trauma, major surgery and drug reactions, can cause alarmins to be released and initiate the process of systemic inflammation.

Propagation of the inflammatory response

Once activated, immune cells such as macrophages release the inflammatory cytokines interleukin-2 (IL-2), IL-6 and tumour necrosis factor alpha, which, in turn, activate neutrophils. Activated neutrophils express adhesion factors and release various other inflammatory and toxic substances; the net effects are vasodilatation (via activation of inducible nitric oxide synthase enzymes) and damage to the endothelium. Neutrophils migrate into the interstitial space; fluid and plasma proteins will also leak through the damaged endothelium, leading to oedema and intravascular fluid depletion.

Activation of the coagulation system

Damaged endothelium triggers the coagulation cascade (via tissue factor, factor VII, and reduced activity of proteins C and S) and thrombus forms within the microvasculature. A vicious circle of endothelial injury,

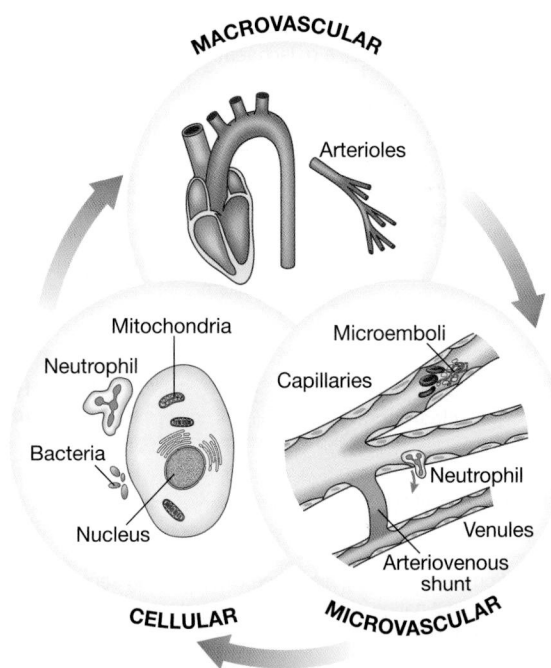

Fig. 9.13 Pathophysiology of organ damage in sepsis. *Macrovascular.* Severe hypovolaemia, vasodilatation or septic cardiomyopathy can reduce oxygen delivery, causing tissue hypoxia. Paradoxically, most patients with sepsis have an increased cardiac output and oxygen delivery. *Microvascular.* Tissue injury can occur from hypoxia secondary to microvascular injury and thrombosis. Damaged epithelium permits neutrophils, proteins and fluid to leak out. *Shunting.* Organs fail in sepsis despite supranormal blood flow. It is likely that arteriovenous shunt pathways exist within vascular beds; these shunts open up in septic shock. *Cellular.* Cells are damaged by a number of mechanisms in sepsis: (1) direct injury by microorganisms; (2) injury from toxins produced by immune cells, e.g. oxygen free radicals; (3) mitochondrial injury causing cytopathic hypoxia – cells are unable to metabolise oxygen; (4) apoptosis – if the cell injury is sufficient, caspase enzymes are activated within the nucleus and programmed cell death occurs; (5) hypoxia from micro- and macrovascular pathology.

intravascular coagulation and microvascular occlusion develops, causing more tissue damage and further release of inflammatory mediators. In severe sepsis, intravascular coagulation can become widespread. This is referred to as disseminated intravascular coagulation (DIC) and usually heralds the onset of multi-organ failure. Specific aspects of the diagnosis and management of DIC are discussed on page 988.

Organ damage from sepsis

Any and all organs may be injured by severe sepsis. The pathological mechanisms are shown in Figure 9.13.

Lactate physiology

Lactate is an excellent biomarker for the severity of sepsis. Hyperlactataemia (serum lactate > 2.4 mmol/L or 22 mg/dL) is used as a marker of severity. Figure 9.14 explains the physiology of hyperlactataemia; it is caused by all types of shock and therefore is not specific to sepsis. A lactate level of > 8 mmol/L (72 mg/dL) is associated with an extremely high mortality and should trigger immediate escalation. Measures to optimise oxygen delivery should be sought, and the adequacy of resuscitation measured by lactate clearance.

The anti-inflammatory cascade

As the inflammatory state develops, a compensatory anti-inflammatory system is activated involving the release of anti-inflammatory cytokines such as IL-4 and IL-10 from immune cells. While such mechanisms are necessary to keep the inflammatory response in check, they may lead to a period of immunosuppression after the initial septic episode. Patients

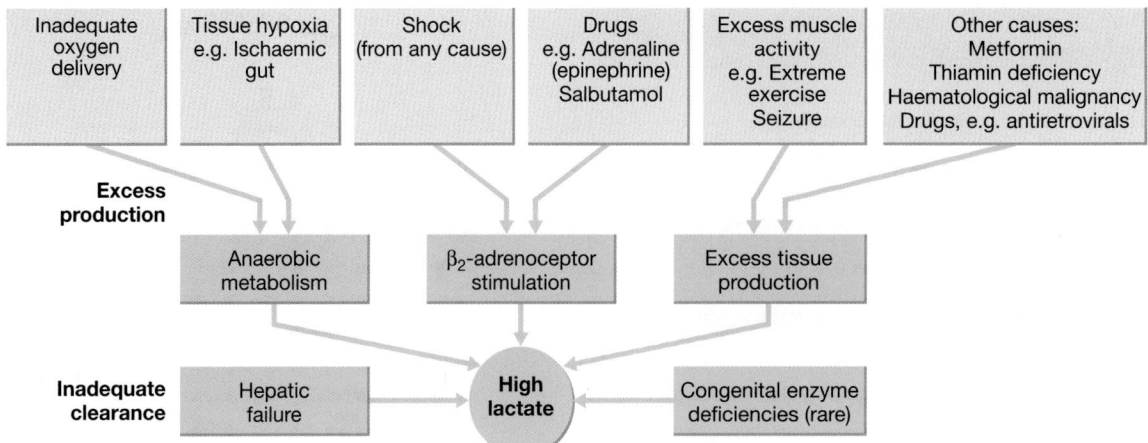

Fig. 9.14 Physiology of hyperlactataemia.

recovering from severe sepsis are prone to developing secondary infections due to a combination of this immunosuppression and the presence of indwelling devices.

Management

The most important action is to consider sepsis as the cause of a patient's deterioration. Aligned to this is the requirement to consider other diagnoses that could be causing the presentation, such as haemorrhage, PE, anaphylaxis or a low cardiac output state.

Resuscitation in sepsis

General resuscitative measures are discussed on page 208. Early resuscitation can be aided by following the requirements of the 'Sepsis Six' (Box 9.33). Red cell transfusion should be used to target a haemoglobin concentration of 70–90 g/L. Albumin 4% can be used as colloid solution and has the theoretical benefit of remaining in the intravascular space for longer than crystalloid. Early intubation is recommended in severe cases to facilitate further management and reduce oxygen demand.

Appropriate antibiotics should be administered as early as possible (Box 9.34). Specific points in the history should be reviewed, such as underlying immune system status, risk factors for human immunodeficiency virus (HIV) and contacts with highly transmissible infections such as tuberculosis, pertussis or COVID-19. Immunocompromised patients will be susceptible to a far broader spectrum of infectious microorganisms (p. 268). The antibiotic choice will depend on local patterns of resistance, patient risk factors and the likely source of infection. Information on likely organisms and appropriate antibiotics can be found on pages 113 and 271. Microbiological samples (such as blood cultures, urine or CSF) should be taken, but this should not delay antibiotic administration, if obtaining samples is difficult.

Early source control

Source control requires an accurate diagnosis; urgent investigations should be performed as soon as physiological stability has been established. A CT scan of the chest and abdomen with contrast is a high-yield test in this context. Specific actions may be required to control infection, such as drainage of an abscess or surgical débridement/resection of infected and/or necrotic tissue. Removal of potentially infected urine catheters or venous/arterial catheters should be promptly undertaken. Infected prosthetic devices, e.g. joint replacements, can be particularly challenging and require early specialist input.

Noradrenaline (norepinephrine) for refractory hypotension

Central venous access should be established early in the resuscitation process and a noradrenaline infusion commenced. If there is severe hypotension, it is not necessary to wait until 30 mL/kg of fluid has been administered before commencing noradrenaline; early vasopressor use

9.33 The 'Sepsis Six'*

- Deliver high-flow oxygen
- Take blood cultures
- Administer intravenous antibiotics
- Measure serum lactate and send full blood count
- Start intravenous fluid replacement
- Commence accurate measurement of urine output

*International recommendations for the immediate management of suspected sepsis from the Surviving Sepsis Campaign (all to be delivered within 1 hr of the initial diagnosis of sepsis).

9.34 Early administration of antibiotics in suspected sepsis

- Broad-spectrum antibiotics should be administered as soon as possible after sepsis is suspected.
- Every hour of delayed treatment is associated with a 5%–10% increase in mortality.

9.35 Central and mixed venous oxygen saturations

- Saturation of venous blood is sampled from the right atrium or superior vena cava (central) or pulmonary artery (mixed venous).
- Both values reflect the balance of supply and demand of oxygen to the tissues.
- Mixed venous oxygen saturation is a measure of whole-body supply and demand of oxygen; central venous oxygen saturation measures the supply and demand of oxygen from the upper body. Normal mixed venous oxygen saturation is 70%. Lower values than this suggest inadequate oxygen delivery.
- Central venous oxygen saturation is more variable, depending on whether the patient is awake or anaesthetised, but a value of 70% is considered normal.
- Where cytopathic hypoxia occurs, oxygen extraction is impaired and the central and mixed venous oxygen saturations may be > 80%. This is often a poor prognostic sign.

may improve the outcome from acute kidney injury. Measurement of central and mixed venous oxygen saturations may provide additional prognostic information (Box 9.35).

Other therapies for refractory hypotension

Refractory hypotension is due to either inadequate cardiac output or inadequate systemic vascular resistance (vasoplegia). When vasoplegia is suspected, it may be necessary to add vasopressin (antidiuretic hormone, ADH). This is a potent vasoconstrictor that may be used to augment noradrenaline (norepinephrine) in achieving an acceptable MAP.

i | **9.36 Sepsis mimics**

- Pancreatitis
- Drug reactions – e.g. reactions to immunotherapy
- Widespread vasculitis – catastrophic antiphospholipid syndrome, Goodpasture's disease
- Autoimmune diseases – inflammatory bowel disease, rheumatoid arthritis, systemic lupus erythematosus
- Malignancy – carcinoid syndrome
- Haematological conditions – haemophagocytic syndrome, diffuse lymphoma, thrombotic thrombocytopenic purpura

Intravenous glucocorticoids are also commonly used in refractory hypotension. There is little evidence that they improve the overall outcome, but they do lead to a more rapid reversal of the shocked state. There is a small increased risk of secondary infection following glucocorticoid use.

Septic cardiomyopathy

The myocardium can be affected by the septic process, presenting as either acute left or right ventricular dysfunction. A bedside echocardiogram is particularly useful to confirm the diagnosis, as ECG changes are usually non-specific. Dobutamine or adrenaline (epinephrine) can be used to augment cardiac output, and intravenous calcium should be replaced if ionised calcium is low.

Other interventions such as intravenous bicarbonate in profound metabolic acidosis, high-volume haemofiltration/haemodialysis and extracorporeal support are sometimes used, but currently lack evidence of benefit.

Review of the underlying pathology

While sepsis is the most common cause of acute systemic inflammation, up to 20% of patients initially treated for sepsis will have a non-infectious cause: that is, a sepsis mimic (Box 9.36). These conditions should be considered where the clinical picture is not typical, no source of sepsis can be found, or the inflammatory response seems excessive in the context of local infection. Early reconsideration of the diagnosis of sepsis is crucial, as many of the 'sepsis mimics' offer a finite time window for specific intervention, after which irreversible organ damage will have occurred.

Acute respiratory distress syndrome

Aetiology and pathogenesis

Acute respiratory distress syndrome (ARDS) is a diffuse neutrophilic alveolitis caused by a range of conditions and characterised by bilateral radiographic infiltrates and hypoxaemia (Box 9.37). Activated neutrophils are sequestered into the lungs and capillary permeability is increased, with damage to cells within the alveoli. The pathophysiology is part of the inflammatory spectrum described in 'Sepsis' above, and the triggers are similar: infective and non-infective inflammatory processes. These processes result in exudation and accumulation of protein-rich cellular fluid within alveoli and the formation of characteristic 'hyaline membranes'. Local release of cytokines and chemokines by activated macrophages and neutrophils results in progressive recruitment of inflammatory cells. Secondary effects include loss of surfactant and impaired surfactant production. The net effect is alveolar collapse and reduced lung compliance, most marked in dependent regions of the lung (mainly dorsal in supine patients). The affected airspaces become fluid-filled and can no longer contribute to ventilation, resulting in hypoxaemia (due to increased pulmonary shunt) and hypercapnia (due to inadequate ventilation in some areas of the lung): that is, ventilation–perfusion mismatch.

Diagnosis and management

ARDS can be difficult to distinguish from fluid overload or cardiac failure. Classic chest X-ray and CT appearances are shown in Figures 9.15 and 9.16, respectively. Occasionally, conditions may

i | **9.37 Berlin definition of ARDS**

- Onset within 1 week of a known clinical insult, or new or worsening respiratory symptoms
- Bilateral opacities on chest X-ray, not fully explained by effusions, lobar/lung collapse or nodules
- Respiratory failure not fully explained by cardiac failure or fluid overload. Objective assessment (e.g. by echocardiography) must exclude hydrostatic oedema if no risk factor is present
- Impaired oxygenation (see Box 9.38)

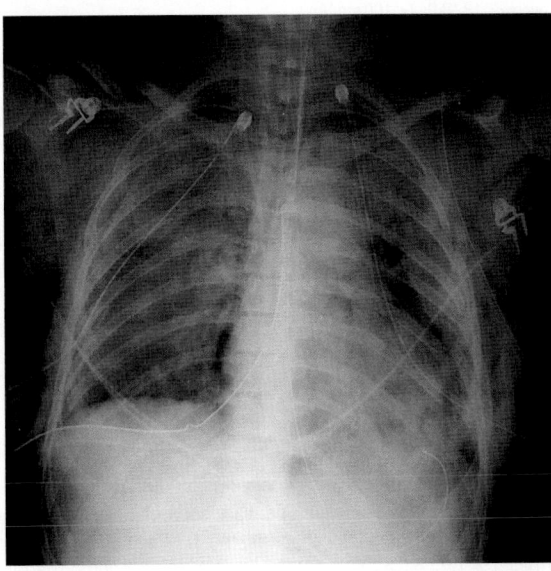

Fig. 9.15 Chest X-ray in acute respiratory distress syndrome (ARDS). Note bilateral lung infiltrates, pneumomediastinum, pneumothoraces with bilateral chest drains, surgical emphysema and fractures of the ribs, right clavicle and left scapula.

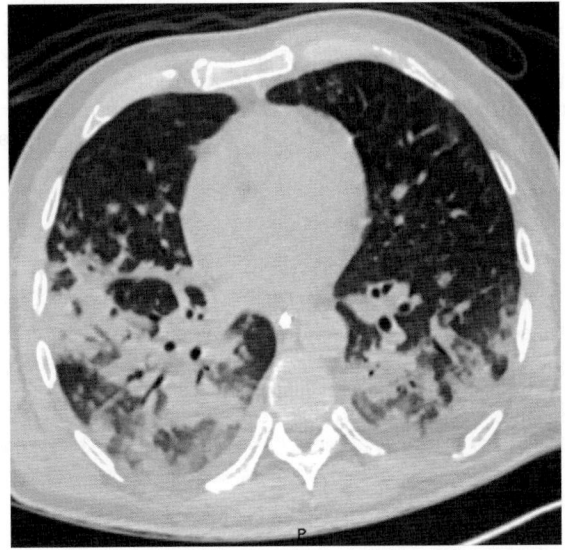

Fig. 9.16 CT scan of the thorax in a patient with severe ARDS. Note the pathology is mainly in the dorsal (dependent) parts of the lung.

present in a similar way to ARDS but respond to alternative treatments; an example of this might be a glucocorticoid-responsive interstitial pneumonia (p. 533). There is debate within the intensive care community as to whether severe COVID-19 pneumonitis causes ARDS. Clinically and pathologically COVID-19 does appear to be a separate entity in which glucocorticoids may be useful. However, glucocorticoids

9.38 Determining the severity of ARDS

Severity of hypoxaemia is calculated using a Pa/FiO_2 ratio. This is a number calculated by using the PaO_2 from an arterial blood gas measurement divided by the fraction of inspired oxygen (FiO_2, expressed as a fraction).

For example, a patient with a PaO_2 of 10 kPa (75 mmHg) on 50% oxygen, i.e. FiO_2 of 0.5, would have a Pa/FiO_2 ratio of 20 kPa (150 mmHg). This would be defined as moderately severe ARDS, if the other Berlin criteria were met (see Box 9.37). All measurements should be taken on a minimum of 5 cmH₂O of PEEP or CPAP.

- Mild: 40–26.6 kPa (300–200 mmHg)
- Moderate: 26.6–13.3 kPa (200–100 mmHg)
- Severe: ≤ 13.3 kPa (≤ 100 mmHg)

(CPAP = continuous positive airway pressure; PEEP = positive end-expiratory pressure)

remain of unproven benefit in ARDS from other causes. Safely reaching an accurate pathological diagnosis of respiratory failure is one of the key research areas within intensive care.

Management of ARDS is supportive, including use of lung-protective mechanical ventilation, inducing a negative fluid balance and treating the underlying cause. Establishing the severity of ARDS (Box 9.38) is useful, as severe disease will require more proactive management such as prone positioning or extracorporeal membrane oxygenation (ECMO; Fig. 9.24).

Acute circulatory failure (cardiogenic shock)

Definition and aetiology

Cardiogenic shock is defined as hypoperfusion due to inadequate cardiac output or, more technically, a cardiac index of < 2.2 L/min/m² (see Box 9.47). While cardiogenic shock is the final common pathway of many disease processes (e.g. sepsis, anaphylaxis, haemorrhage), the important primary causes of acute heart failure or cardiogenic shock (Fig. 9.17) are described here.

Myocardial infarction

In the majority of cases, cardiogenic shock following acute MI is due to left ventricular dysfunction. However, it may also be due to infarction of the right ventricle, or a variety of mechanical complications, including tamponade (due to infarction and rupture of the free wall), an acquired ventricular septal defect (due to infarction and rupture of the septum) and acute mitral regurgitation (due to infarction or rupture of the papillary muscles).

Severe myocardial systolic dysfunction causes a fall in cardiac output, BP and coronary perfusion pressure. Diastolic dysfunction causes a rise in left ventricular end-diastolic pressure, pulmonary congestion and oedema, leading to hypoxaemia that worsens myocardial ischaemia. This is further exacerbated by peripheral vasoconstriction. These factors combine to create the 'downward spiral' of cardiogenic shock (Fig. 9.18). Hypotension, oliguria, delirium and cold, clammy peripheries are the manifestations of a low cardiac output, whereas breathlessness, hypoxaemia, cyanosis and inspiratory crackles at the lung bases are typical features of pulmonary oedema. If necessary, a Swan–Ganz catheter can be used to measure the pulmonary artery pressures and cardiac output (Fig. 9.25). These findings can be used to categorise patients with acute MI into four haemodynamic subsets (Box 9.39) and titrate therapy accordingly.

In cardiogenic shock associated with acute MI, immediate percutaneous coronary intervention should be performed. The viable myocardium surrounding a fresh infarct may contract poorly for a few days and then recover. This phenomenon is known as myocardial stunning and means that acute heart failure should be treated intensively because overall cardiac function may subsequently improve.

Acute massive pulmonary embolism

Massive PE may complicate leg or pelvic vein thrombosis and usually presents with sudden collapse. The clinical features and treatment are discussed on page 546. Bedside echocardiography may demonstrate a small, under-filled, vigorous left ventricle with a dilated right ventricle; it is sometimes possible to see thrombus in the right ventricular outflow tract or main pulmonary artery. In practice, it can be difficult to distinguish massive PE from a right ventricular infarct on transthoracic echocardiogram. CT pulmonary angiography usually provides a definitive diagnosis.

Acute valvular pathology, aortic dissection and cardiac tamponade

These conditions should be considered in an undifferentiated presentation of shock. The diagnosis and management of these conditions is discussed in Chapter 16.

Cardiac arrest

Cardiac arrest is the cessation of functional cardiac contraction and is the final common pathway in death from any pathology. In the clinical context, cardiac arrest refers to the sudden loss of cardiac output that prompts an emergency response. Pathogenesis, prognosis and management of in-hospital and out-of-hospital cardiac arrest are subtly different; however, the basic principles of cardiopulmonary resuscitation (CPR) are to maintain forward flow of oxygenated blood, correct the causative factor and restore spontaneous circulation.

Out-of-hospital cardiac arrest (OHCA)

This is the sudden and complete loss of cardiac output occurring in the community. The clinical diagnosis is based on the victim being unconscious and pulseless; breathing may take some time to stop completely after cardiac arrest. Death is virtually inevitable, unless effective treatment is given promptly.

Pathogenesis

Cardiac arrest may be caused by ventricular fibrillation (Fig. 9.19), pulseless ventricular tachycardia (see Ch. 16), asystole or pulseless electrical activity. Myocardial ischaemia is the most common trigger of OHCA. This can be due to an acute infarct, acute on chronic coronary insufficiency, post-infarct ventricular scarring or structural cardiac disease (cardiomyopathy, aortic stenosis). Ventricular fibrillation can occur in the absence of recognised structural abnormalities, e.g. congenital syndromes such as Brugada syndrome. Occasionally, sudden cardiac death can occur from an acute mechanical catastrophe such as cardiac rupture or aortic dissection. The causes are listed in Chapter 16, Box 16.7.

Survivors of OHCA

The 'Chain of Survival' (Fig. 9.20) refers to the sequence of events that is necessary to maximise the chances of a cardiac arrest victim surviving. Survival is most likely if all links in the chain are strong: that is, if the arrest is witnessed, help is called immediately, basic life support is administered by a trained individual, the emergency medical services respond promptly, and defibrillation is achieved within a few minutes. CPR from bystanders, often assisted by ambulance service telephone dispatchers, is crucial. Good training in both basic and advanced life support is essential and should be maintained by regular refresher courses. Automated external defibrillators (AEDs) are increasingly available in public places, particularly where traffic congestion may impede the response of emergency services, and should be used as soon as possible. Designated individuals can respond to a cardiac arrest using basic life support and an automated external defibrillator.

For OHCA, survival rates of approximately 10% have been reported internationally. When type I myocardial infarction Box 16.47 is the suspected pathology, early coronary revascularisation should be considered. Those with reversible causes, such as exercise-induced ischaemia or aortic stenosis, should have the underlying cause treated if possible. Survivors of a ventricular tachycardia or ventricular fibrillation arrest, in whom no reversible cause can be identified, may be at risk of another episode and should be considered for an implantable cardiac defibrillator (p. 418) and anti-arrhythmic drug therapy.

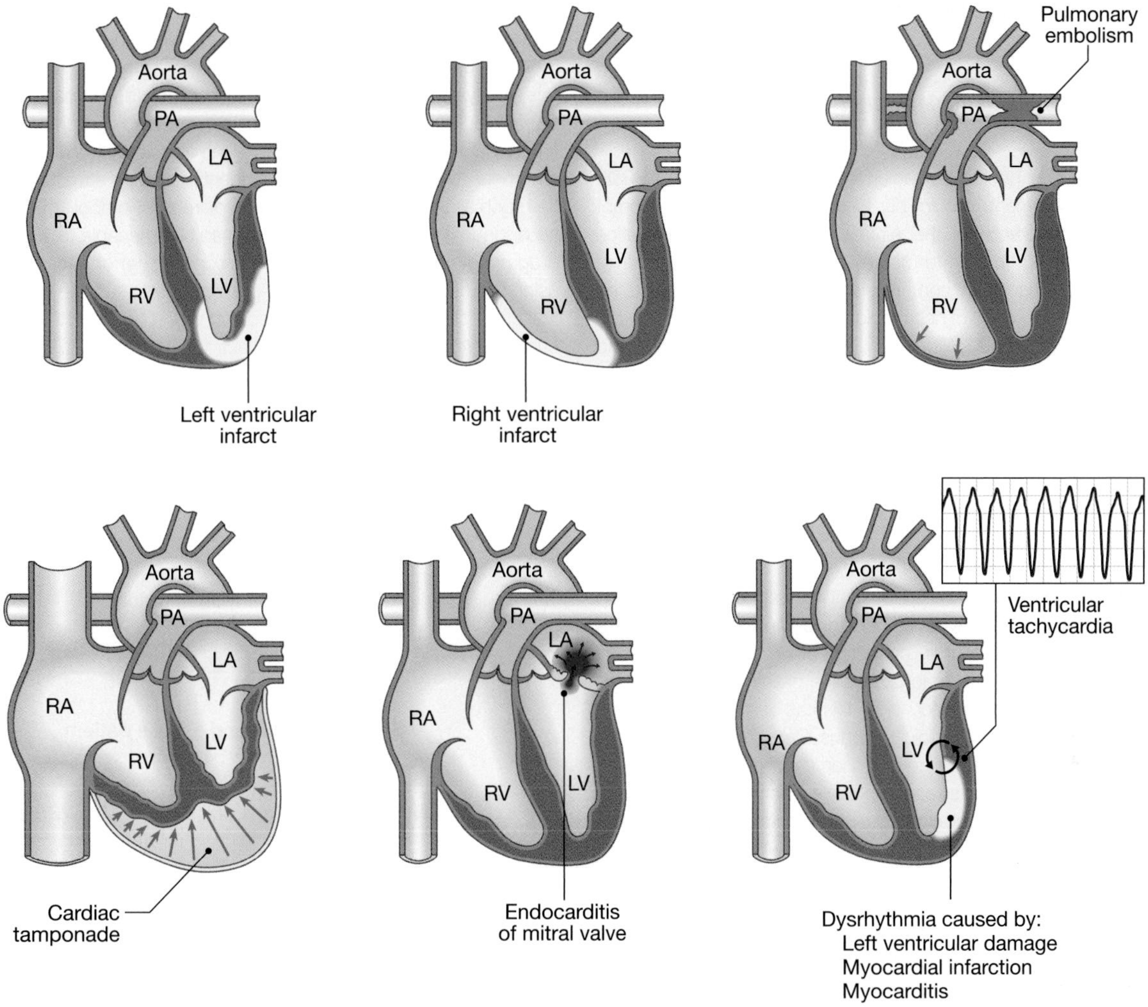

Left ventricular
infarct

Right ventricular
infarct

Pulmonary
embolism

Ventricular
tachycardia

Cardiac
tamponade

Endocarditis
of mitral valve

Dysrhythmia caused by:
Left ventricular damage
Myocardial infarction
Myocarditis

Fig. 9.17 Some common causes of cardiogenic shock. (LA = left atrium; LV = left ventricle; PA = pulmonary artery; RA = right atrium; RV = right ventricle)

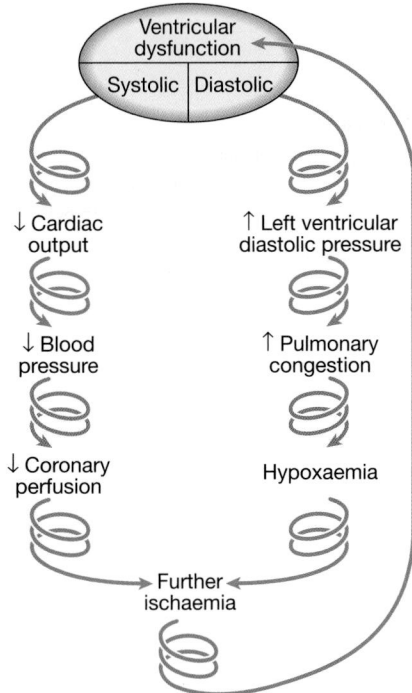

Fig. 9.18 The downward spiral of cardiogenic shock.

9.39 Acute myocardial infarction: haemodynamic subsets		
Cardiac output	**Pulmonary oedema**	
	No	**Yes**
Normal	Good prognosis and requires no treatment for heart failure	Due to moderate left ventricular dysfunction. Treat with vasodilators and diuretics
Low	Due to right ventricular dysfunction or concomitant hypovolaemia. Give fluid challenge and consider pulmonary artery catheter to guide therapy	Extensive myocardial infarction and poor prognosis. Consider intra-aortic balloon pump, vasodilators, diuretics and inotropes

In-hospital cardiac arrest (IHCA)

Historically, outcomes from IHCA were extremely poor. However, with appropriate anticipatory care planning and prompt intervention of hospital resuscitation teams, outcomes can be significantly better than for OHCA.

Pathogenesis

Although primary cardiac causes are the most common cause of IHCA, additional factors such as organ failure, sepsis or respiratory decompensation are often more pertinent. Correction of hypoxaemia with early tracheal intubation and ventilation is therefore of higher importance in this group than in OHCA, provided it can be achieved without interruption of chest compressions.

Clinical assessment and management

Basic life support

When a patient with suspected cardiac arrest is encountered, the ABCDE approach to management should be followed; this involves prompt assessment and restoration of the **A**irway, maintenance of ventilation using rescue **B**reathing ('mouth-to-mouth' breathing), and maintenance of the **C**irculation using chest compressions; **D**isability, in resuscitated patients, refers to assessment of neurological status, and **E**xposure entails removal of clothes to enable defibrillation, auscultation of the chest and assessment for a rash caused by anaphylaxis, for injuries and so on (Fig. 9.21). The term basic life support (BLS) encompasses manoeuvres that aim to maintain a low level of circulation until more definitive treatment with advanced life support can be given. Chest compression-only ('hands-only') CPR is easier for members of the public to learn and administer, and is now advocated in public education campaigns.

Advanced life support

Advanced life support (ALS) (Fig. 9.22) aims to restore normal cardiac rhythm by defibrillation when the cause of cardiac arrest is a tachyarrhythmia, or to restore cardiac output by correcting other reversible causes of cardiac arrest. The initial priority is to assess the patient's cardiac rhythm by attaching a defibrillator or monitor. Once this has been done, treatment should be instituted based on the clinical findings. Only a minority of patients will have a shockable rhythm at the commencement of resuscitation.

Ventricular fibrillation or pulseless ventricular tachycardia should be treated with immediate defibrillation. Defibrillation is more likely to be effective if a biphasic shock defibrillator is used, where the polarity of the shock is reversed midway through its delivery. Defibrillation is usually administered using a 150 Joule biphasic shock, and CPR resumed immediately for 2 minutes without attempting to confirm restoration of a pulse, because restoration of mechanical cardiac output rarely occurs immediately after successful defibrillation. If, after 2 minutes, a pulse is not restored, a further biphasic shock of 150–200 J should be given. Thereafter, additional biphasic shocks of 150–200 J are given every 2 minutes after each cycle of CPR. During resuscitation, adrenaline (epinephrine, 1 mg IV) should be given every 3–5 minutes and consideration

given to the use of intravenous amiodarone, especially if ventricular fibrillation or ventricular tachycardia re-initiates after successful defibrillation.

Ventricular fibrillation of low amplitude, or 'fine VF', may mimic asystole. If asystole cannot be confidently diagnosed, the patient should be treated for VF and defibrillated. Bedside echocardiography can be a useful clinical aid. The subcostal views can frequently be obtained without detriment to CPR quality, and can identify cardiac structural abnormalities such as an enlarged right heart in pulmonary embolism, aortic stenosis or ongoing fine VF. Refractory VF can be amenable to supplementary drugs (e.g. lidocaine, magnesium, procainamide) or alternative ways of using the defibrillator, e.g. antero-posterior pad placement.

If an electrical rhythm is observed that would be expected to produce a cardiac output, 'pulseless electrical activity' is present. Pulseless electrical activity should be treated by continuing CPR and adrenaline (epinephrine) administration while seeking causes. Asystole should be treated similarly although prolonged asystole has an extremely poor prognosis.

There are many potentially reversible causes of cardiac arrest; the main ones can be remembered as a list of four Hs and four Ts (see Fig. 9.22). In specialist centres and in appropriate candidates, the use of extracorporeal life support (has been used in cardiac arrest with good

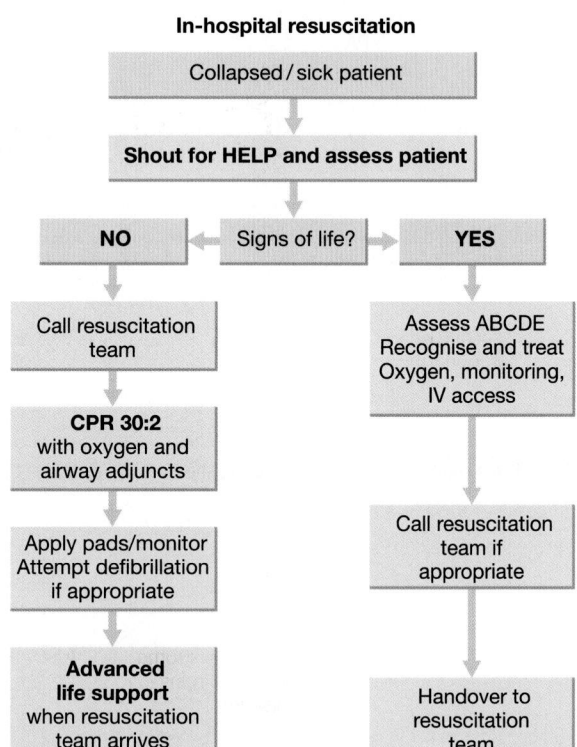

In-hospital resuscitation

Collapsed / sick patient

↓

Shout for HELP and assess patient

↓

NO ← Signs of life? → YES

NO →
Call resuscitation team
↓
CPR 30:2 with oxygen and airway adjuncts
↓
Apply pads/monitor Attempt defibrillation if appropriate
↓
Advanced life support when resuscitation team arrives

YES →
Assess ABCDE Recognise and treat Oxygen, monitoring, IV access
↓
Call resuscitation team if appropriate
↓
Handover to resuscitation team

Fig. 9.21 Algorithm for adult basic life support. For further information, see www.resus.org.uk. (CPR = cardiopulmonary resuscitation) *From Resuscitation Council (UK) guidelines:* https://www.resus.org.uk/resuscitation-guidelines/in-hospital-resuscitation/.

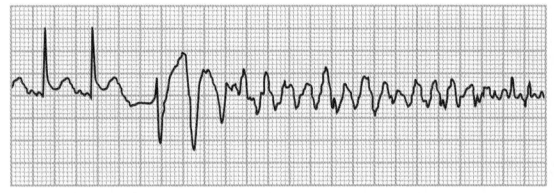

Fig. 9.19 Ventricular fibrillation. A bizarre chaotic rhythm, initiated in this case by two ventricular ectopic beats in rapid succession.

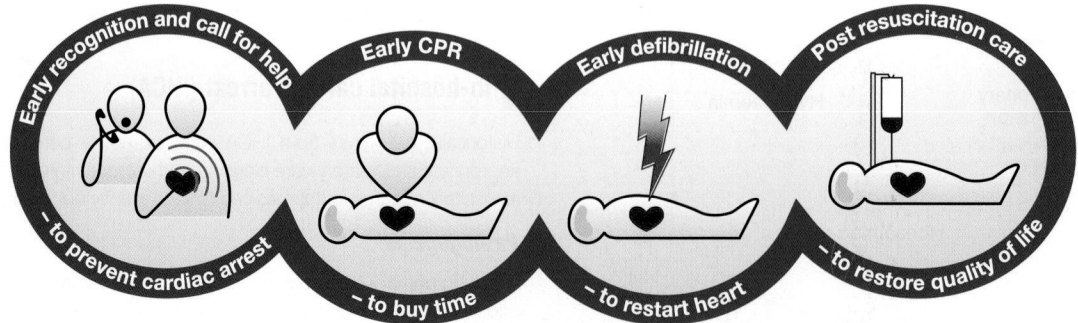

Early recognition and call for help – to prevent cardiac arrest

Early CPR – to buy time

Early defibrillation – to restart heart

Post resuscitation care – to restore quality of life

Fig. 9.20 The Chain of Survival in cardiac arrest. (ALS = advanced life support; CPR = cardiopulmonary resuscitation)

effect. However, this is not generally available outside of large urban centres. The use of automated chest compression devices is becoming more common and their use should be considered in patients in whom a prolonged resuscitation is expected (e.g. when thrombolytic has been administered or in profound hypothermia). Injuries from CPR are common; their management is summarised in the section on 'Complications and outcomes of critical illness'.

Post cardiac arrest

The majority of cardiac arrest survivors will need a period of time in intensive care to achieve physiological stability, identify and manage the underlying cause of the arrest, and optimise neurological recovery.

Acute management

A MAP of >70 mmHg should be maintained to optimise cerebral perfusion. Shock is common following return of spontaneous circulation (ROSC) and is caused by a combination of the underlying condition leading to the arrest, myocardial stunning and a post-arrest vasodilated state. Support

with inotropes, vasopressors and occasionally mechanical support from an intra-aortic balloon pump or venous–arterial ECMO (Fig. 9.24) may be required. Specific cardiac interventions and their indications are described in Chapter 16. Other physiological targets are listed in Box 9.40.

Prognosis

Predicting which patients will not recover from the brain injury sustained at the time of cardiac arrest is very difficult. Certain features suggest that the outcome will be poor: for example, the absence of pupillary and corneal reflexes, absence of a motor response and persistent myoclonic jerking.

Tools to assist prognostication following cardiac arrest are shown in Box 9.41. The clinician should, where feasible, delay prognostication until a period of 72 hours of targeted temperature management has been completed. The bilateral absence of the 'N20' spike on the somatosensory evoked potential is the most specific test to predict irrecoverable brain injury. This test is performed by administering an electrical impulse over a peripheral nerve and recording the electrical impulses measured by the scalp electrodes overlying the part of the brain expected to receive the

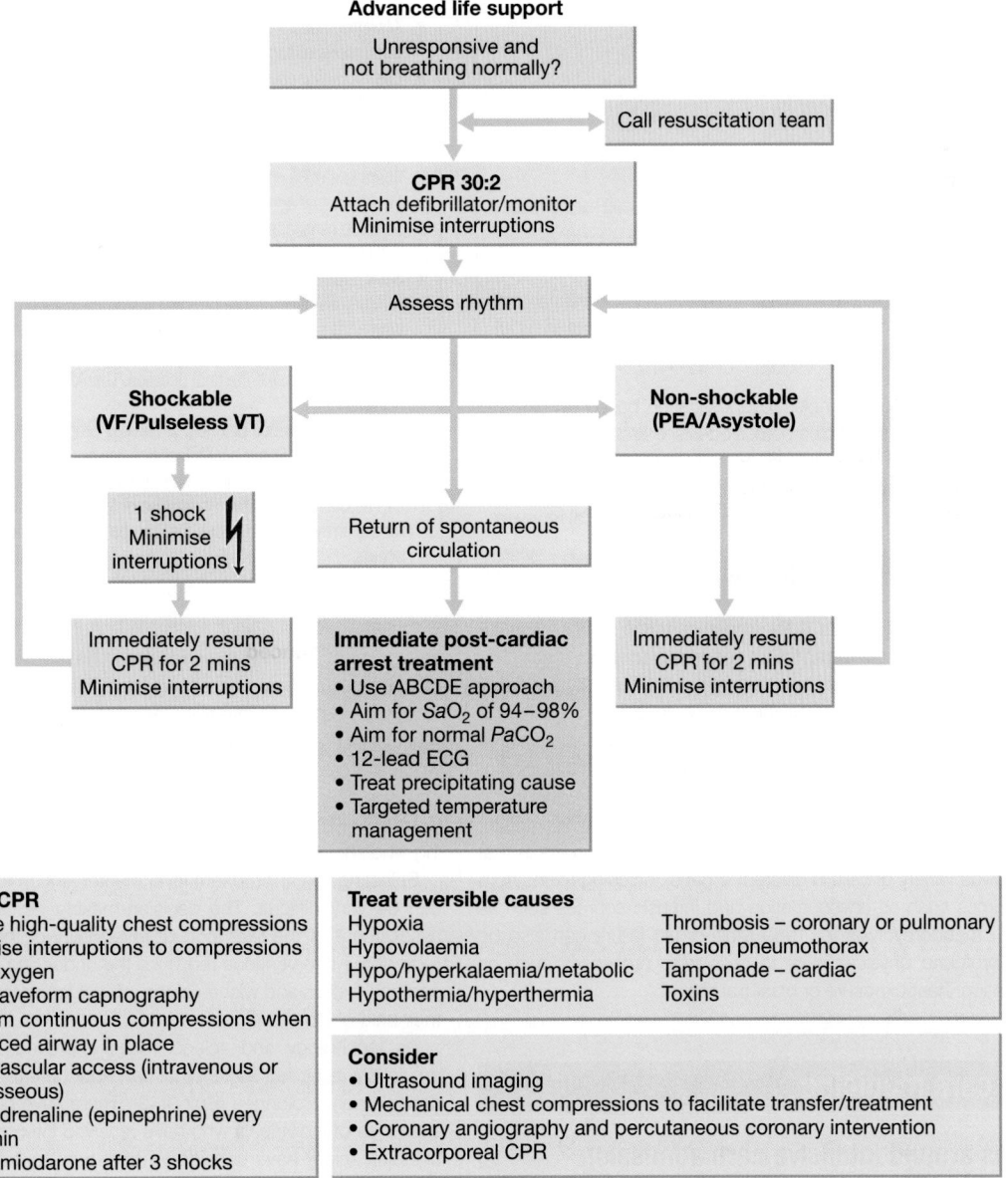

Fig. 9.22 Algorithm for adult advanced life support. For further information, see www.resus.org.uk. (CPR = cardiopulmonary resuscitation: PEA = pulseless electrical activity; VF = ventricular fibrillation; VT = ventricular tachycardia) *From Resuscitation Council (UK) guidelines:* https://www.resus.org.uk/resuscitation-guidelines/adult-advanced-life-support/.

9.40 Physiological targets following a return of spontaneous circulation (ROSC)

- *Temperature management.* Facilitate maintenance of temperature at 36°C and avoidance of pyrexia using a cooling blanket. This should be continued for 72 hrs. Muscle relaxants may be required to prevent shivering.
- *Blood pressure management.* Aim for a MAP of at least 70 mmHg and a systolic blood pressure of > 120 mmHg.
- *Glucose control.* Control the glucose to 6–10 mmol/L (108–180 mg/dL).
- *Normal CO_2* (4.5–6 kPa, 33–45 mmHg) *and oxygen saturation* (94%–98%). Avoid both hypoxaemia and hyperoxia.

 9.41 Prognostication after cardiac arrest: predictors of poor neurological recovery

Coexisting problems

- Multi-organ failure
- Significant comorbidities

Clinical

- Persisting and generalised myoclonus
- Absence of pupillary or corneal reflexes
- Poor motor response (absent or extensor response)

Biochemical

- Neuron-specific enolase > 33 µg/L

Imaging

- CT showing loss of grey–white differentiation
- Focal cause or consequence of cardiac arrest, e.g. subarachnoid haemorrhage

Electrophysiology

- EEG patterns may suggest brain injury, e.g. burst suppression
- Somatosensory evoked potentials – bilateral absence of the N20 spike (recorded from scalp electrodes from cutaneous electrical impulse over the median nerve)

impulse. Where this is not available, prognostication based on all other available information, along with the perceived wishes relating to the level of disability the individual would be prepared to accept, should allow a decision regarding ongoing treatment to be made. Where there is doubt, more time should be given to allow assessment of neurological recovery.

Other causes of multi-organ failure

As previously discussed, sepsis is the most common cause of multi-organ failure. However, multi-organ failure secondary to single organ dysfunction, such as cardiac failure, liver failure, renal failure or respiratory failure, is also common. The multisystem insult in these disease processes goes beyond the direct biochemical damage and tissue hypoxia caused by the primary organ dysfunction. It probably reflects cellular signalling pathways and the release of other systemic toxins by the failing organ, referred to as organ 'crosstalk'.

Multi-organ failure can also be caused by a physiological insult that damages a wide variety of cells in different organs, including toxins from extrinsic sources such as envenomation and intrinsic sources such as myoglobin in rhabdomyolysis (p. 198). Multi-organ failure can also be caused by profound physical injury to cells from processes such as nuclear radiation, heat exposure or blast trauma.

Critical care medicine

Decisions around intensive care admission

Being a patient in intensive care is seldom a pleasant experience. The interventions are usually painful and the loss of liberties that are normally taken for granted can be devastating. While much of the unpleasant

 9.42 Critical illness in the context of congenital conditions

- **Longer survival**: there are many congenital conditions that would, in the past, have been fatal in childhood, but now patients survive into adulthood. Decision-making can be difficult when the adolescent has impaired decision-making capacity.
- **Parental views**: in such circumstances, the views of the parent or legal guardian become paramount.
- **Goals of care**: often a detailed explanation of what is, and is not, achievable in intensive care allows the direction of care to be switched to palliative when life expectancy is poor and quality of life is severely impaired.
- **Decision-making**: such conversations may require input from experts in the patient's congenital condition(s), and advanced decision-making regarding ICU admission should be encouraged whenever patients and families feel able to discuss such issues.

 9.43 Techniques to improve admission decision-making

- *Always act in the best interests of the patient*: external influences are commonly present but these should be of only secondary importance.
- *Maximise patient capacity*: wherever possible, the patient should be involved in discussions of escalation and resuscitation status.
- *Communicate openly and honestly with the next of kin*: when communicating potential outcomes, it is best to use natural frequencies rather than percentages. For example, 'If we had 100 patients with the same illness as your mother, only 10 would survive' is easier for most people to understand than 'there is a 90% chance of death'.
- *Reach mutual agreement with the next of kin*: it is rare for there to be discord between clinicians and family, and in most cases the most appropriate course of action is clear.
- *Seek additional opinions*: other clinicians involved in the care of the patient will provide useful input. The premise should be to err on the side of escalation where the most appropriate course of action is unclear. Where there is an unresolvable difference in opinion, a mediation process or court ruling may be required to make the final decision. Thankfully, this is a very infrequent occurrence.
- *Plan ahead*: advance planning in chronic, progressive disease can make the decision easier. Some health facilities use an escalation form, which specifies the interventions that should be offered or are acceptable to the patient. This can be useful as the binary decision of for/not for resuscitation fails to account for the array of interventions that can be performed before cardiac arrest occurs.

sensory and emotional experience can be modified with high-quality care and analgesia, there is a strong case that it can only be morally 'right' to admit a patient to intensive care if 'the ends justify the means'. There must be a realistic hope that the patient will regain a quality of life that would be worth the pain and suffering that he or she will experience in intensive care. Few patients are able to comprehend fully what it means to be critically ill, so the physician should guide the process of determining who should be admitted to intensive care.

Selecting the appropriate level of intervention for an individual patient can be very difficult. The decision-making process should involve an assessment of the likelihood of reversibility of the disease, the magnitude of the interventions required, the underlying level of frailty, and the personal beliefs and wishes of the patient (commonly expressed through their next of kin).

As technology and science have improved, conditions that were previously regarded as terminal can now be supported and life can be considerably prolonged (Box 9.42). There have been several prominent examples of individuals who have received intensive care, but where an onlooker might have considered treatment to be futile owing to frailty, comorbidity or profound neurological injury. Such cases will, in part, shape the views and expectations of society, and it is unlikely that making decisions in this area will become any easier. Some suggested techniques to aid decision-making are listed in Box 9.43.

Stabilisation and institution of organ support

In order to stabilise a critically unwell patient, the primary problem should be corrected as quickly as possible: for example, source control in sepsis and control of the bleeding point in haemorrhage. Immediate resuscitation and prioritisation of the safety of the patient are clearly important, but there is only a limited role for 'optimising' the patient if such measures may significantly delay a definitive treatment, such as laparotomy for a perforated viscus. In some cases, the definitive treatment is not readily apparent or treatments take time to have their full effect. In these cases, adequate organ support to stabilise the patient while the treatment is given becomes the main goal of care.

Respiratory support

Non-invasive respiratory support

Non-invasive respiratory support provides a bridge between simple oxygen delivery devices and invasive ventilation. It can be used in patients who are in respiratory distress but do not have an indication for invasive ventilation, or in those who are not suitable for intubation and ventilation for chronic health reasons. Patients must be cooperative, able to protect their airway, and have the strength to breathe spontaneously and cough effectively. Clinicians should avoid using non-invasive respiratory support to prolong the dying process in irreversible conditions such as end-stage lung disease. Likewise, a failure to respond to treatment or further deterioration should trigger a decision regarding intubation, as delayed invasive ventilation in this context is associated with worse outcome.

High-flow nasal cannulae

High-flow nasal cannulae (HFNCs) are devices that provide very high gas flows of fully humidified oxygen and air. They offer distinct advantages over non-invasive ventilation (NIV) in selected patients, mainly those with type I respiratory failure (particularly pneumonia) who have not reached an indication for invasive ventilation. They allow patient comfort and increased expectoration while providing some degree of positive end-expiratory pressure (PEEP) and a high oxygen concentration that can be titrated to the SO_2.

Continuous positive pressure ventilation

Continuous positive pressure ventilation therapy involves the application of a continuous positive airway pressure (CPAP) throughout the patient's breathing cycle, typically 5–10 cmH$_2$O. It helps to recruit collapsed alveoli and can enhance clearance of alveolar fluid. It is particularly effective at treating pulmonary atelectasis (which may be post-operative) and pulmonary oedema. It can be delivered using a simpler device than NIV, may be better tolerated and avoids compounding the hypocapnia that sometimes occurs in type I respiratory failure.

Non-invasive ventilation or bi-level ventilation

NIV provides ventilatory support via a tight-fitting nasal or facial mask. It can be delivered by using a simple bi-level ventilation (BiPAP) turbine ventilator, or an intensive care ventilator. These machines can deliver pressure at a higher level (approximately 15–25 cmH$_2$O) for inspiration and a lower pressure (usually 4–10 cmH$_2$O) to allow expiration. Ventilation can be spontaneous (triggered by a patient's breaths) or timed (occurring at a set frequency). Systems that synchronise with a patient's efforts are better tolerated and tend to be more effective in respiratory failure. Timed breaths are used for patients with central apnoea. NIV is the first-line therapy in patients with type II respiratory failure secondary to an acute exacerbation of COPD because it reduces the work of breathing and offloads the diaphragm, allowing it to recover strength. It is also useful in pulmonary oedema, obesity hypoventilation syndromes and some neuromuscular disorders. It should be initiated early, especially when severe respiratory acidosis secondary to hypercapnia is present. NIV can also be used to support selected patients with hypercapnia secondary to

pneumonia, or during weaning from invasive ventilation, but its effectiveness in these contexts is less certain; early intubation or re-intubation is probably more beneficial.

Intubation and intermittent positive pressure ventilation

Taking control of the respiratory system in a critically ill patient is one of the most significant and risky periods in a patient's journey. Critical incidents are common because the patient is often deteriorating rapidly and is exhausted. The potential for cardiovascular collapse is further exacerbated by the negatively inotropic and vasodilating drugs used to induce anaesthesia, and the period of apnoea invoked to facilitate intubation (Box 9.44).

The main aims of intermittent positive pressure ventilation (IPPV) are to avoid critical hypoxaemia and hypercapnia while minimising damage to the alveoli and encouraging the patient to breathe spontaneously once it is safe to do so. The determination of what constitutes *critical* will depend on the status of each patient. For example, a patient with raised ICP will have a strong indication for normocapnia (because hypercapnia increases ICP). Unfortunately, achieving the minute volumes required to maintain normocapnia can be harmful to the lungs.

Ventilator modes

Following intubation, most patients have a period of paralysis from the muscle relaxation. Mandatory ventilation is, therefore, required for a variable period, depending on the severity of the lung injury, the underlying disease process and the general condition of the patient. Mandatory ventilation means that the ventilator will deliver set parameters (either a set tidal volume or a set inspiratory pressure), regardless of patient effort. A physician can choose to support additional patient effort in between mandatory breaths with pressure support. This requires sufficient patient effort to 'trigger' the ventilator to deliver a synchronised breath, in time with the patient's own ventilation. Other parameters that should be considered when using mechanical ventilation are shown in Figure 9.23.

As a patient's illness resolves, or if the lung injury necessitating intubation is not severe, periods of spontaneous breathing with pressure support are commenced. While spontaneous breathing is preferable to mandatory ventilation modes, the shearing forces of patient effort can exacerbate lung injury in patients with severely damaged lungs. It is, therefore, important that a patient is permitted to breathe in a planned and controlled way.

Ventilator-induced lung injury

Every positive pressure breath causes cyclical inflation of alveoli followed by deflation. The resultant damage to alveoli occurs via several possible mechanisms:

- distending forces from the tidal volume, termed 'volutrauma'
- the pressure used to inflate the lung, referred to as 'barotrauma'

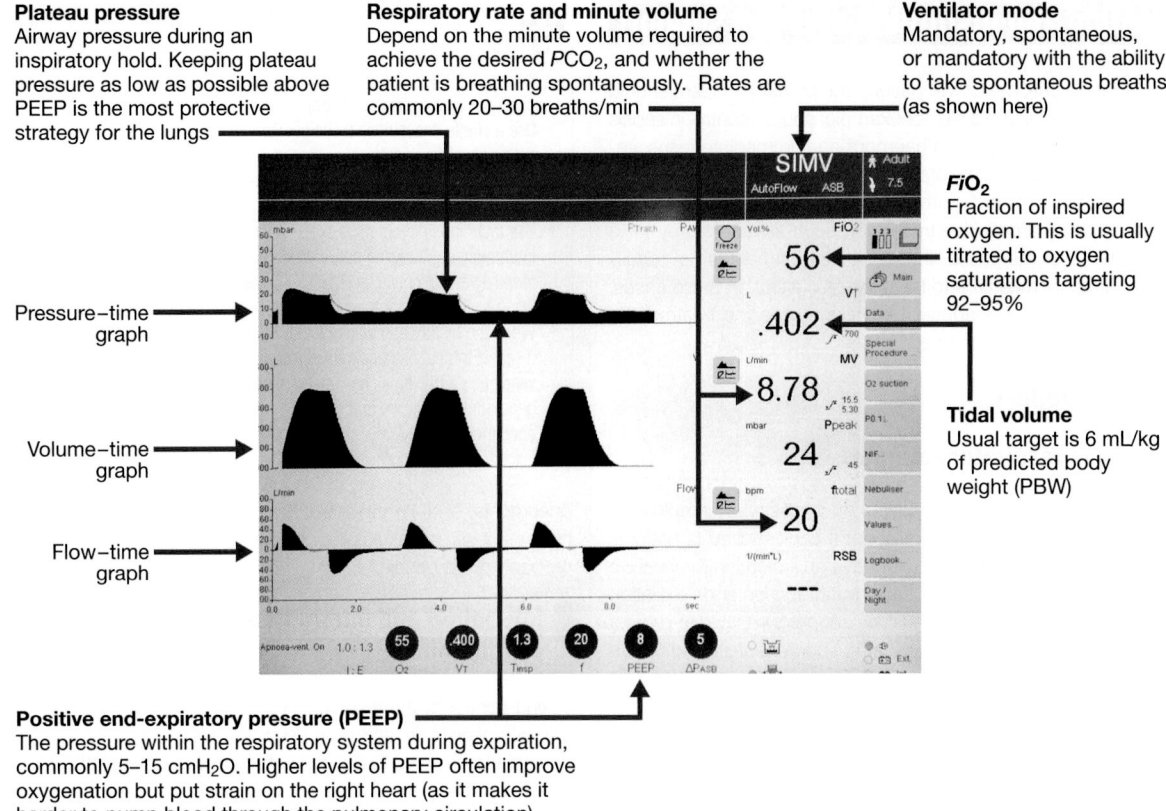

Plateau pressure
Airway pressure during an inspiratory hold. Keeping plateau pressure as low as possible above PEEP is the most protective strategy for the lungs

Respiratory rate and minute volume
Depend on the minute volume required to achieve the desired PCO_2, and whether the patient is breathing spontaneously. Rates are commonly 20–30 breaths/min

Ventilator mode
Mandatory, spontaneous, or mandatory with the ability to take spontaneous breaths (as shown here)

FiO_2
Fraction of inspired oxygen. This is usually titrated to oxygen saturations targeting 92–95%

Tidal volume
Usual target is 6 mL/kg of predicted body weight (PBW)

Pressure–time graph

Volume–time graph

Flow–time graph

Positive end-expiratory pressure (PEEP)
The pressure within the respiratory system during expiration, commonly 5–15 cmH$_2$O. Higher levels of PEEP often improve oxygenation but put strain on the right heart (as it makes it harder to pump blood through the pulmonary circulation)

Fig. 9.23 Settings to be considered when commencing mechanical ventilation.

- alveoli collapsing at the end of expiration, called 'atelectotrauma'
- the release of inflammatory cytokines in response to cyclical distension, called 'biotrauma'.

The threshold of injurious ventilation is unique to each patient. Moderate ventilator pressures and volumes used to ventilate healthy lungs may not cause ventilator-induced lung injury (VILI), but the same settings may cause significant VILI if delivered to a patient with lungs that are already damaged from another disease process.

Strategies that may reduce the incidence and severity of VILI include:

- *Permissive hypercapnia.* In the majority of patients who are ventilated for respiratory failure, it is preferable to tolerate moderate degrees of hypercapnia rather than strive for normal blood gases at the expense of VILI. For example, in a patient with isolated respiratory failure, a physician may choose to tolerate a $PaCO_2$ of up to 10 kPa (75 mmHg), provided the H+ is < 63 nmol/L (pH > 7.2).
- *'Open lung' ventilation.* Maintaining a positive pressure within the airways at the end of expiration prevents atelectotrauma. This can be facilitated by the use of low tidal volumes and higher levels of PEEP (see Fig. 9.23). Recruitment manoeuvres (occasional short periods of sustained high airway pressures to open up alveoli that have collapsed) can reduce the incidence of VILI in patients who do not have ARDS.
- *Paralysis.* When respiratory failure is severe, patient effort may worsen VILI. An infusion of muscle relaxant can be used to moderate dyssynchrony with the ventilator.

Advanced respiratory support

Airway pressure release ventilation

Airway pressure release ventilation (APRV) is a mode of ventilation that lengthens the inspiratory time to the extreme, with a very short period of

time for expiration. It relies on spontaneous movement of the diaphragm from patient effort to facilitate the mixing of gas within the respiratory system during the long period in full inspiration, followed by a very short period of low pressure to allow passive expiration. It has not, however, been demonstrated to be superior to conventional modes of ventilation, but may have a role in some patients with moderate to severe ARDS.

Prone positioning

In ARDS, the posterior parts of the lung lose airspaces due to atelectasis and inflammatory exudate. By placing patients on their front, the pattern of fluid distribution within the lung changes, and ventilation–perfusion matching is improved. This is used to enhance oxygenation in moderate to severe ARDS, and may have some disease-modifying effects as the dependent areas of the lung are changed periodically. Although there are risks associated with nursing a patient in the prone position, it is a widely used therapy. Patients are usually placed in the prone position for 12–24 hours and then rotated back to the supine position for a similar period. This cycle continues until there is evidence of resolving lung injury. Using prone positioning in the awake and cooperative patient on high-flow oxygen or CPAP may be a useful technique in some patients.

Extracorporeal respiratory support

Sometimes, despite optimal invasive ventilation, it is not possible to maintain adequate oxygenation or prevent a profound respiratory acidosis. When a patient has a reversible cause of respiratory failure (or is a potential lung transplant recipient) and facilities are available, extracorporeal respiratory support should be considered.

Venous–venous extracorporeal membrane oxygenation

In venous–venous extracorporeal membrane oxygenation (VV ECMO), large-bore central venous cannulae are inserted into the superior vena cava (SVC) and/or the inferior vena cava (IVC) via the femoral or jugular veins, and advanced under ultrasound or fluoroscopic guidance (Fig. 9.24). Venous blood is then pumped through a membrane oxygenator. This device has thousands of tiny silicone tubes with air/oxygen gas on the other side of the tubes (the membrane). This facilitates the passage of oxygen into the blood and diffusion of carbon dioxide across the membrane, where it is removed by a constant flow of gas (sweep gas). The oxygenated blood is then returned to the right atrium, from where it flows through the lungs as it would in the physiological state. This means that even if the lungs are contributing no oxygenation or carbon dioxide removal, a patient can remain well oxygenated and normocapnic.

9

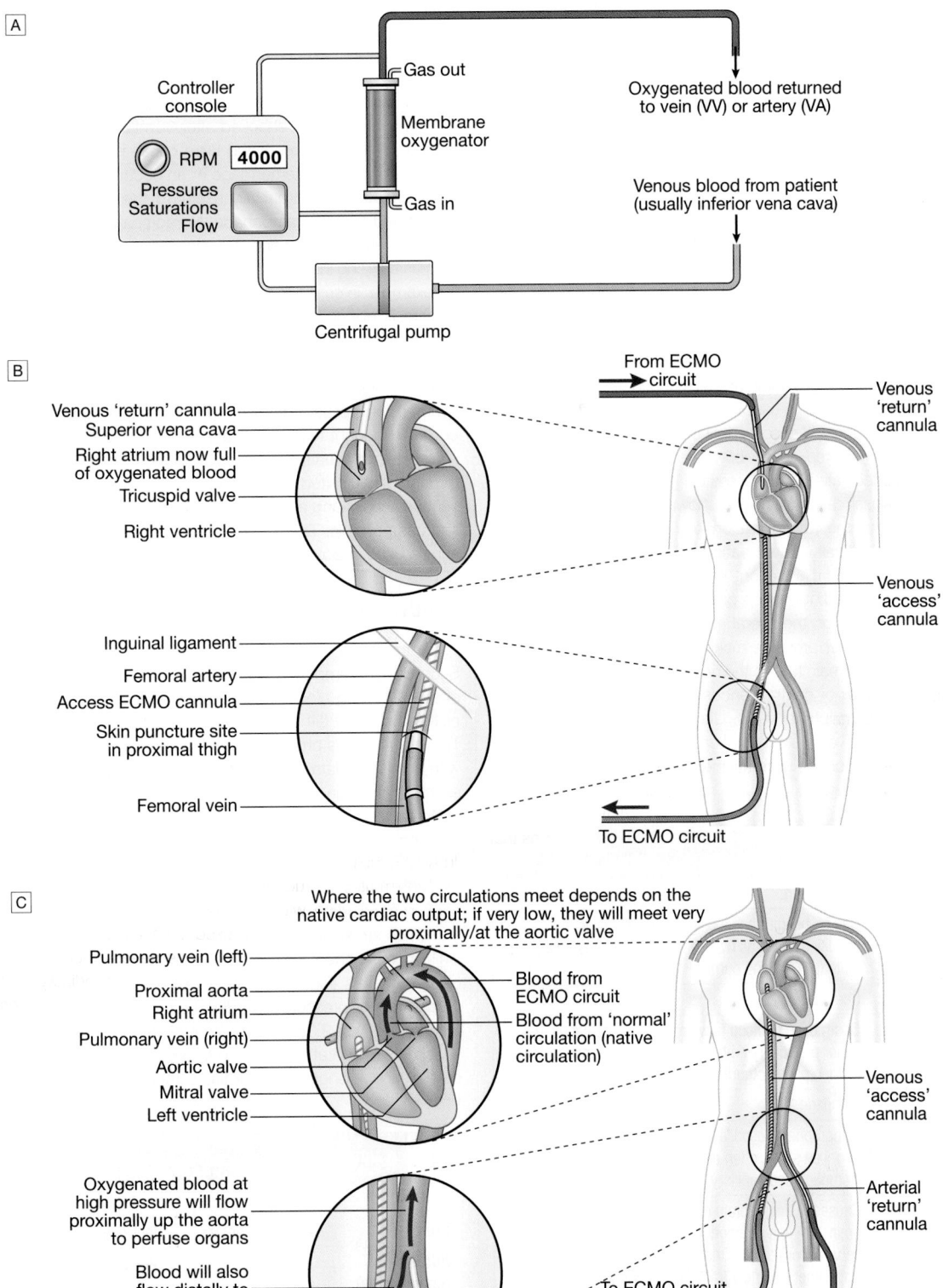

Fig. 9.24 Principles of extracorporeal membrane oxygenation (ECMO). A Basic ECMO circuit: venous–arterial (VA) and venous–venous (VV). B Example of a VV ECMO circuit. C Example of a VA ECMO circuit.

Extracorporeal carbon dioxide removal

In some patients it is possible to maintain oxygenation but there is refractory hypercapnia. There are devices available that can remove carbon dioxide using a much lower blood flow rate than VV ECMO. Consequently, smaller venous cannulae, similar to those used in renal dialysis, can be sufficient to have a 'CO_2 dialysis' effect. This can be useful in patients in whom normocapnia is essential (such as those with a raised ICP), or those with refractory hypercapnia and adequate oxygenation. In addition, extracorporeal carbon dioxide removal can be used to reduce the required minute volume, which is a beneficial strategy for protecting the lungs against VILI or facilitating early extubation.

Cardiovascular support

Initial resuscitation

A brief assessment can usually yield enough information to determine whether a patient is at significant risk of an imminent cardiac arrest. If the patient is obtunded and there is no palpable radial or brachial pulse, then treatment should proceed as described on page 204.

In a peri-arrest situation, a single dose of intramuscular adrenaline (epinephrine) 0.5 mg (0.5 mL of 1:1000) can be life-saving. If expertise is available, a small dose of intravenous adrenaline (epinephrine) can delay cardiac arrest long enough to identify the cause of shock and institute other supportive measures; a suggested dose would be 50 μg (0.5 mL of 1:10000). If haemorrhage is considered a possibility, a 'major haemorrhage' alert should be activated, facilitating rapid access to large volumes of blood and blood products. A classification of shock is shown in Box 9.45.

Venous access for the administration of drugs and fluids is vital but often difficult in critically unwell patients. Wide-bore cannulae are required for rapid fluid administration. In extremis, the external jugular vein can be cannulated; it is often prominent in low cardiac output states and readily visible on the lateral aspect of the neck. Occluding the vein distally with finger pressure makes it easier to cannulate, but care must be taken to remain high in the neck to avoid causing a pneumothorax. Intra-osseous or central venous access can be established if there are no visible peripheral veins. Ultrasound can provide assistance for rapid and safe venous cannulation. Rapid infusion devices are widely available and should be used for the delivery of warmed, air-free fluid and blood products.

i	9.45 Categories of shock	
Category	**Description**	
Hypovolaemic	Can be haemorrhagic or non-haemorrhagic in conditions such as hyperglycaemic hyperosmolar state (p. 723) and burns	
Cardiogenic	See page 202	
Obstructive	Obstruction to blood flow around the circulation, e.g. major pulmonary embolism, cardiac tamponade, tension pneumothorax	
Septic	See page 198	
Anaphylactic	Inappropriate vasodilatation triggered by an allergen (e.g. bee sting), often associated with endothelial disruption and capillary leak (p. 183)	
Neurogenic	Caused by major brain or spinal injury, which disrupts brainstem and neurogenic vasomotor control. High cervical cord trauma may result in disruption of the sympathetic outflow tracts, leading to inappropriate bradycardia and hypotension. Guillain–Barré syndrome (p. 1192) can involve the autonomic nervous system, resulting in periods of severe hypo- or hypertension	
Others	e.g. Drug-related such as calcium channel blocker overdose; Addisonian crisis	

Fluid and vasopressor use

Resuscitation of the shocked patient should usually include a 10 mL/kg fluid challenge. Using colloid or crystalloid is acceptable; starch solutions are associated with additional renal dysfunction and should be avoided. The fluid challenge can be repeated if shock persists, to a maximum total of 30 mL/kg of fluid. However, commencing vasopressor therapy early in resuscitation is better than delaying until a large volume of fluid has been given. Amongst other beneficial effects, vasopressors induce venoconstriction, reducing the capacitance of the circulation and effectively mobilising more fluid into the circulation.

If a patient remains shocked after 30 mL/kg of fluid has been administered, a re-evaluation of the likely cause is required, looking particularly for concealed haemorrhage or an obstructive pathology. A bedside echocardiogram is especially useful at this stage to evaluate cardiac output and exclude tamponade. Noradrenaline (norepinephrine) should be commenced as the first-line vasoactive agent in most cases, unless there is a strong indication to use a pure inotropic or chronotropic agent: for example, in cardiogenic shock or shock associated with bradycardia. If there is evidence of low cardiac output, adrenaline (epinephrine) or dobutamine should be commenced. Both agents are equally effective, but dobutamine causes more vasodilatation and additional noradrenaline may be required to maintain an adequate MAP. Vasopressin is added if hypotension persists despite high doses of noradrenaline and cardiac output is thought to be adequate.

In extreme situations it is acceptable to start infusions of inotropes through a well-sited, large-bore peripheral cannula, although central venous access and an arterial line (for monitoring) should be inserted as soon as possible. The actions of commonly used vasoactive drugs are summarised in Box 9.46.

Advanced haemodynamic monitoring

There are many different devices available to estimate cardiac output. Such devices employ a variety of mechanisms, including the Doppler effect of moving blood, changes in electrical impedance of the thorax, or the dilution of either an indicator substance or heat (thermodilution). The information is processed within the equipment, and often integrated with additional data, such as the arterial pressure waveform, to give an estimate of cardiac output and stroke volume.

When the aetiology of shock is straightforward and the patient is responding as predicted to treatment, the value of devices that estimate cardiac output is limited. Portable echocardiography has the advantage of giving qualitative information – for example, demonstrating aortic stenosis or a regional wall motion abnormality – as well as quantitative information on stroke volume, but it requires technical expertise.

Pulmonary artery (PA) catheters, sometimes referred to as Swan–Ganz catheters (Fig. 9.25), are invasive but provide useful information on pulmonary pressures, cardiac output, mixed venous oxygen saturations (see Box 9.35) and, by extrapolation, whether the cause of the shock is vasodilatation or pump failure. They can be helpful in complex cases, such as shock after cardiac surgery, or in patients with suspected

i	9.46 Actions of commonly used vasoactive agents		
	Action		
Drug	**Vasoconstrictor**	**Inotrope**	**Chronotrope**
Adrenaline (epinephrine)	++	+++	++
Noradrenaline (norepinephrine)	++++	+	+
Dobutamine	–	++++	+++
Vasopressin	+++++	No action	– (reflex bradycardia)

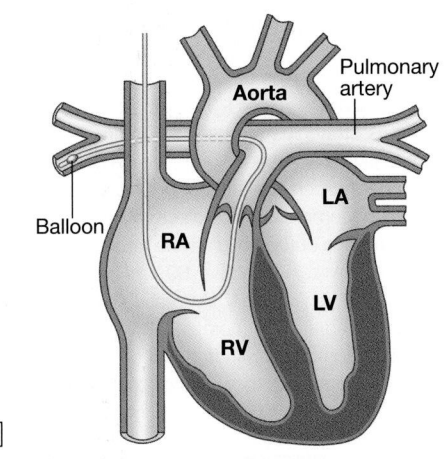

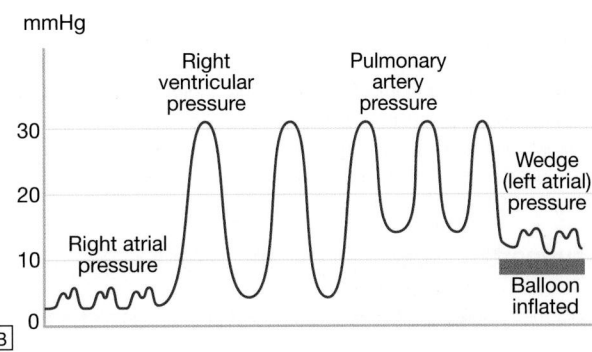

Fig. 9.25 A pulmonary artery (Swan–Ganz) catheter. **A** There is a small balloon at the tip of the catheter and pressure can be measured through the central lumen. The catheter is inserted via an internal jugular, subclavian or femoral vein and advanced through the right heart until the tip lies in the pulmonary artery. When the balloon is deflated, the pulmonary artery pressure can be recorded. **B** Advancing the catheter with the balloon inflated will 'wedge' the catheter in the pulmonary artery. Blood cannot then flow past the balloon, so the tip of the catheter will now record the pressure transmitted from the pulmonary veins and left atrium (known as the pulmonary artery capillary wedge pressure), which provides an indirect measure of the left atrial pressure. (LA = left atrium; LV = left ventricle; RA = right atrium; RV = right ventricle)

9.47 Interpreting haemodynamic data			
Variable	**Units**	**Reference range**	**Interpretation**
Cardiac output (CO)	L/min	4–8 L/min	Low cardiac output suggests pump failure
Cardiac index (CI) Cardiac output referenced to the size of the patient	L/min/m²	2.5–4 L/min/m²	More useful than raw cardiac output alone, especially in smaller patients
Central venous pressure (CVP)	mmHg	0–6 mmHg	Reflects right atrial pressure – a non-specific measurement of right ventricular (RV) function and volume status Low levels suggest good RV function or hypovolaemia
Pulmonary artery systolic pressure (PA systolic)	mmHg	15–30 mmHg	Difficult to interpret in isolation Low levels suggest vasodilatation, hypovolaemia or right heart failure High levels are seen in many pathologies, e.g. left heart failure, primary pulmonary arterial hypertension (PAH), fluid overload
Pulmonary artery diastolic pressure (PA diastolic)	mmHg	5–15 mmHg	As with PA systolic pressure, difficult to interpret in isolation
Pulmonary artery capillary wedge pressure (PACWP)	mmHg	2–10 mmHg (should be within a few mmHg of PA diastolic)	Reasonable indication of left atrial pressure – raised in left heart failure and fluid overload Measurement is associated with injury to PA so should only be taken occasionally
Transpulmonary gradient (PA diastolic – PACWP)	mmHg	1–5 mmHg	A high gradient suggests the pathology is in the pulmonary arteries, e.g. primary PAH

pulmonary hypertension (Box 9.47). However, PA catheters are associated with some rare but serious complications, including lung infarction, PA rupture and thrombosis of the catheter itself. Such complications occur infrequently in centres that use PA catheters regularly; it should be stressed that a lack of familiarity within the wider clinical team is a relative contraindication to their use.

Mechanical cardiovascular support

When shock is so severe that it is not possible to maintain sufficient organ perfusion with fluids and inotropic support, it is sometimes necessary to use an internal device to augment or replace the inadequate native cardiac output.

Intra-aortic balloon pump

An intra-aortic balloon counter-pulsation device is a long tube that is usually inserted into the femoral artery and fed proximally into the thoracic aorta. The basic principle is that a helium-filled balloon is able to inflate and deflate rapidly in time with the cardiac cycle. It is inflated in diastole,

thus augmenting forward flow of blood to the abdominal organs and improving diastolic pressure proximal to the balloon, thereby optimising coronary perfusion. While the principle is appealing, and an intra-aortic balloon pump (IABP) is often effective in achieving predetermined physiological goals, this does not translate into improved survival in cardiogenic shock. There are risks associated with thrombosis formation on the balloon, mesenteric ischaemia and femoral artery pseudo-aneurysm following removal of the device.

Venous–arterial extracorporeal membrane oxygenation

Venous–arterial extracorporeal membrane oxygenation (VA ECMO) can be life-saving in profound cardiogenic shock and has even been used effectively in refractory cardiac arrest. The circuit and principles are very similar to those described in 'VV ECMO' above (see Fig. 9.24) with one important difference: oxygenated blood is returned to the arterial system (rather than into the right atrium). This means that the pump needs to generate sufficient pressure to allow blood to flow through the systemic circulation. The sites of venous and arterial access can be either central (via a thoracotomy or sternotomy) or peripheral via cannulae in the IVC/SVC and the femoral/subclavian artery. If the return cannula is peripherally sited (e.g. in the femoral artery), blood will flow back up the aorta from distal to proximal and perfuse the organs.

The outcome depends on the avoidance of complications (primarily, bleeding at the cannula site, intracranial haematoma, air embolism, infection and thrombosis) and improvement of the underlying condition. Most causes of profound cardiogenic shock are unlikely to resolve, and the potential availability of a longer-term solution, such as cardiac transplantation or insertion of a ventricular assist device, is a prerequisite for commencing VA ECMO in most centres.

Renal support

Renal replacement therapy (RRT) is explained in detail on page 593. The key points relating to RRT in an intensive care context are:

- Haemodynamic instability is common. Continuous therapies are widely believed to cause less haemodynamic instability than intermittent dialysis. However, many units use intermittent dialysis without significant problems.
- Haemodialysis and haemofiltration are equally good. Although there are theoretical benefits to removing inflammatory cytokines with haemofiltration, this does not translate into improved survival.
- Anticoagulation is usually achieved using citrate or heparin. Citrate has a better profile for anticoagulating the extracorporeal circuit without inducing an increased bleeding risk, but may accumulate in patients with profound multi-organ failure.
- Most patients who survive intensive care will regain adequate renal function to live without long-term renal support.
- A thorough investigation for reversible causes of renal dysfunction should always be undertaken in conjunction with instigation of renal support (see Fig. 18.18).
- Shock appears to reverse more rapidly when renal support is instituted. Commencing renal support soon after a patient develops renal 'injury' (when serum creatinine is more than two times higher than baseline) is probably beneficial in the context of septic shock.

Neurological support

A diverse range of neurological conditions require management in intensive care. These include the various causes of coma, spinal cord injury, peripheral neuromuscular disease and prolonged seizures.

The goals of care in such cases are to:

- Protect the airway, if necessary by endotracheal intubation.
- Provide respiratory support to correct hypoxaemia and hypercapnia.
- Treat circulatory problems, e.g. neurogenic pulmonary oedema in subarachnoid haemorrhage, autonomic disturbances in Guillain–Barré syndrome, and spinal shock following high spinal cord injuries.
- Manage acute brain injury with control of ICP.
- Manage status epilepticus using antiepileptic agents such as levetiracetam, phenytoin and benzodiazepines. In refractory cases an infusion of sodium thiopental or ketamine may be required.

The aim of management in acute brain injury is to optimise cerebral oxygen delivery by maintaining normal arterial oxygen content and a cerebral perfusion pressure (CPP) of > 60 mmHg. Secondary insults to the brain, such as hypoxaemia, hyper/hypoglycaemia and prolonged seizures, must be avoided. ICP rises in acute brain injury as a result of haematoma, contusions, oedema or ischaemic swelling. Raised ICP causes damage to the brain in two ways: direct damage to the brainstem and motor tracts as a result of downward pressure and herniation through the tentorium cerebelli and foramen magnum, and indirect damage by reducing CPP. Cerebral blood flow is dependent on an adequate CPP. The CPP is determined by the formula:

$$CPP = MAP - ICP$$

ICP can be measured by pressure transducers that are inserted directly into the brain tissue. The normal upper limit for ICP is 15 mmHg and an upper acceptable limit of 20 mmHg is usually adopted in intensive care. Sustained pressures of > 30 mmHg are associated with a poor prognosis. Various strategies are used to control ICP: maintaining normocapnia, preventing any impedance to venous drainage from the head, giving osmotic agents such as mannitol and hypertonic saline, and using hypothermia and decompressive craniectomy. No single technique has been shown to improve outcome in severe intracranial hypertension.

CPP should be maintained above 60 mmHg by ensuring adequate fluid replacement and, if necessary, by treating hypotension with a vasopressor such as noradrenaline (norepinephrine). Complex neurological monitoring must be combined with frequent clinical assessment of GCS, pupillary response to light and focal neurological signs.

Daily clinical management in intensive care

Clinical review

In intensive care, detailed clinical examination should be performed daily to identify changes to a patient's condition and review the latest diagnostic information. Further focused clinical reviews are usually incorporated into twice-daily ward rounds. Each ward round offers an ideal opportunity to monitor and document adherence with relevant care bundles. A care bundle is a group of interventions that, when implemented concurrently, have provided evidence of clinical benefit. The mnemonic 'FAST HUG' provides a useful checklist of interventions that reduce intensive care complications: feeding/fluids, analgesia, sedation, thromboprophylaxis, head of bed elevation (to reduce the incidence of passive aspiration), ulcer prophylaxis and glucose control.

Other key aspects of the daily review are outlined on page 176. The over-arching aim of the review is to identify the issues that are impeding recovery from critical illness, and make alterations to address them. In addition, specific and realistic goals for each relevant organ system should be defined, facilitating the autonomous titration of therapy by the bedside critical care nurse. An example of daily goals may be: 'Titrate the noradrenaline (norepinephrine) to achieve a MAP of 65 mmHg, aim for a negative fluid balance, titrate FiO_2 to achieve oxygen saturations of 92%–95% and titrate sedation to a RASS score of 0 to −1' (see Box 9.49).

Infection surveillance

Infection surveillance is an important part of the daily review as nosocomial infection is common in critically ill patients. Trends in temperature, heart/respiratory rate and secretion load can all be early indicators of ventilator-associated pneumonia (VAP). Likewise leucocytosis and a raised C-reactive protein are measured frequently, but are not specific enough to guide therapy alone. Procalcitonin (PCT) is increasingly used to give more specific information on bacterial infection. A rapidly reducing trend can allow for a shortening of antibiotic courses (reducing the likelihood of generating resistant organisms) and a persistently low PCT in a shocked patient can alert the clinician to the possibility of an aetiology other than sepsis. Severe viral and fungal infections, e.g. COVID-19, can cause an elevated PCT and occasionally sepsis can develop before the PCT has risen, so as with all investigations the result should be used as adjunct to clinical assessment.

Sedation and analgesia

Most patients require some degree of sedation and analgesia to ensure comfort, relieve anxiety and tolerate mechanical ventilation. Some conditions, such as critically high ICP or critical hypoxaemia, require deep sedation to reduce tissue oxygen requirements and protect the brain from the peaks in ICP associated with coughing or gagging. For the

i	9.48 Properties of sedative and analgesic agents used in ICU			
Drug	**Mode of action**	**Advantages**	**Disadvantages**	
Propofol	Intravenous anaesthetic	Rapid onset and offset	Large cumulative doses can cause multi-organ failure, especially in children – the 'propofol infusion syndrome'	
Alfentanil	Potent opiate analgesic	Rapid onset and offset	High doses may be required Agitation may persist	
Morphine	Opioid	Analgesia	Active metabolites and accumulation cause slow offset	
Midazolam	Benzodiazepine sedative	Can be used in children	Active metabolites and accumulation cause slow offset	
Remifentanil	Very potent opiate	Analgesia and tube tolerance	Respiratory depression – extreme caution in non-intubated patients	
Dexmedetomidine	α_2-adrenergic agonist	Excellent tube tolerance Less delirium Can be used in awake patients	Cost and availability	

9

majority of patients, however, optimal sedation is an awake and lucid patient who is comfortable and able to tolerate an endotracheal tube (termed 'tube tolerance').

Over-sedation is associated with longer ICU stays, a higher prevalence of delirium, prolonged requirement for mechanical ventilation, and an increased incidence of ICU-acquired infection. Box 9.48 compares the various agents used for sedation in intensive care. The key principles are that the patient should primarily receive analgesia, rather than anaesthesia, and caution should be used with drugs that accumulate in hepatic and renal dysfunction. Often a combination of drugs is used to achieve the optimal balance of sedation and analgesia.

Sedation is monitored via clinical sedation scales that record responses to voice and physical stimulation. The Richmond Agitation–Sedation Scale (RASS) is the best-recognised tool (see Box 9.49 for details). Regular use of a scoring system to adjust sedation is associated with a shorter ICU stay. Many ICUs also have a daily 'sedation break', when all sedation is stopped in appropriate cases for a short period. This is commonly combined with a trial of spontaneous breathing aiming to shorten the duration of mechanical ventilation.

Delirium in intensive care

Delirium is discussed in Chapter 34. It is extremely common in critically ill patients and often becomes apparent as sedation is reduced. Hypoactive delirium is far more common than hyperactive delirium, but is easily missed unless routine screening is undertaken. A widely used bedside assessment is the CAM-ICU score. The patient is requested to squeeze the examiner's hand in response to instruction and questions, aiming to ascertain whether disordered thought or sensory inattention are present.

Delirium of any type is associated with poorer outcome. Management is focused on non-pharmacological interventions such as early mobilisation, reinstatement of day–night routine, noise reduction, cessation of drugs known to precipitate delirium, and treatment of potential underlying causes such as thiamine replacement in patients at risk of Wernicke's encephalopathy. Patients with agitated delirium that is refractory to verbal de-escalation should initially be managed with small doses of parenteral antipsychotics, changed to the enteral route once control is established. Atypical antipsychotics such as olanzapine and quetiapine can be more efficacious than traditional drugs such as haloperidol. Pharmacological interventions are not useful as prophylaxis or in hypoactive delirium. Additional information on diagnosis and management of delirium can be found on page 1304.

Weaning from respiratory support

As the condition that necessitated ventilation resolves, respiratory support is gradually reduced: the process of 'weaning' from ventilation. Some approaches to weaning are described below.

i	9.49 Richmond Agitation–Sedation Scale (RASS)		
Score	**Term**	**Description**	
+4	Combative	Overtly combative, violent or immediate danger to staff	
+3	Very agitated	Pulls on/removes tubes or catheters, or aggressive to staff	
+2	Agitated	Frequent non-purposeful movement or patient–ventilator dyssynchrony	
+1	Restless	Anxious or apprehensive but no aggressive or vigorous movements	
0	Alert and calm		
−1	Drowsy	Not fully alert but sustained awakening (> 10 secs) with eye opening/contact to voice	
−2	Light sedation	Brief awakening (< 10 secs) with eye contact to voice	
−3	Moderate sedation	Movement but no eye contact to voice	
−4	Deep sedation	Movement to physical stimulation but no response to voice	
−5	Unrousable	No response to voice or physical stimulation	

Spontaneous breathing trials

A spontaneous breathing trial involves the removal of all respiratory support followed by close observation of how long the patient is able to breathe unassisted. The technique is particularly effective when linked to a reduction in sedation. PEEP and pressure support are reduced to low levels, or patients are disconnected from the ventilator and breathe oxygen or humidified air through the endotracheal tube. Signs of failure include rapid shallow breathing, hypoxaemia, rising $PaCO_2$, sweating and agitation. Patients who pass a spontaneous breathing trial are assessed for suitability of extubation (endotracheal tube removal).

Progressive reduction in pressure support ventilation

Progressive reduction in pressure support ventilation (PSV) is applied to each breath over a period of hours or days, according to patient response. Some ICU ventilators have software that allows the facility to wean the support provided automatically.

A useful tool to guide the weaning process is the rapid shallow breathing index (RSBI). This composite score of a patient's spontaneous respiratory rate and tidal volume (respiratory rate divided by tidal volume in litres) gives a numerical indication of how difficult the patient is finding breathing at that particular level of support. A RSBI value of > 100 suggests that a patient is working at a level that would be unsustainable for longer periods.

Extubation

It is not possible to predict whether a patient is ready to be extubated accurately; the timing relies heavily on clinical judgement. There are, however, some principles that can aid decision-making. Patients must have stable ABGs with resolution of hypoxaemia and hypercapnia despite minimal ventilator pressure support and a low FiO_2. Conscious level must be adequate to protect the airway, comply with physiotherapy and cough. Furthermore, an assessment must be made as to whether the patient can sustain the required minute volume without ventilator support. This depends on the condition of patients' lungs, their strength and other factors affecting the $PaCO_2$, such as temperature and metabolic rate. Frequently it is not possible to meet all of these criteria and the decision to extubate relies on a balance of risks and benefits. The need for re-intubation following extubation is associated with poorer outcome, but patients who are not given the opportunity to breathe without a ventilator will also be at increased risk of ventilator-associated complications such as pneumonia and myopathy.

Tracheostomy

A tracheostomy is a percutaneous tube passed into the trachea (usually between the first and second, or second and third tracheal rings) to facilitate longer-term ventilation. The advantages and disadvantages of tracheostomy insertion are listed in Box 9.50. When ventilation weaning has been unsuccessful, a tracheostomy provides a bridge between intubation and extubation; the patient can have increasing periods free of ventilator support but easily have support reinstated. A tracheostomy can be inserted percutaneously, using a bronchoscope in the trachea for guidance, or surgically under direct vision. Occasionally, a patient will have a tracheostomy in situ following a laryngectomy. Such patients are important to identify, as emergency management in the event of a tracheostomy problem (blockage or displacement) must be through the tracheostomy site; access will not be possible via the upper airway.

Nutrition

It is crucial that critically ill patients receive adequate calories, protein and essential vitamins and minerals. Calculation of exact requirements is complex and requires the expertise of a dietitian. It is, however, useful to make a rough estimation of requirements (see Ch. 22). Under-feeding leads to muscle wasting and delayed recovery, while over-feeding can lead to

biliary stasis, jaundice and steatosis. Enteral feeding is preferred where possible because it avoids the infective complications of total parenteral nutrition (TPN) and helps to maintain gut integrity. However, TPN is recommended for patients who are likely to have a sustained period without effective enteral feeding, or who are already malnourished. Caution must be taken to avoid the consequences of refeeding syndrome (p. 768).

Other essential components of intensive care

Survival after critical illness depends, to a large extent, on the prevention of medical complications during recovery from the primary insult.

Thromboprophylaxis

DVT, venous catheter-related thrombosis and PE are common in critically ill patients. Low-molecular-weight heparin (LMWH) should be administered to all patients, unless there is a contraindication. Often patients at highest risk of thrombosis, such as those with hepatic dysfunction or those who have suffered major trauma, have a relative contraindication to heparin. Such cases mandate daily evaluation of the risk–benefit ratio, and LMWH should be administered as soon as it is deemed safe to do so. Mechanical thromboprophylaxis, such as intermittent calf compression devices, are useful adjuvants in high-risk patients.

Glucose control

Hyperglycaemia is harmful in critical illness and may occur in people with pre-existing diabetes or undiagnosed diabetes, following administration of high-dose glucocorticoids, or as a consequence of 'stress hyperglycaemia'. Hyperglycaemia is commonly managed by infusion of intravenous insulin titrated against a 'sliding scale'. Intensive management of hyperglycaemia with insulin can result in hypoglycaemia, which may also be harmful in critical illness. Therefore, a compromise is to titrate insulin to a blood glucose level of 6–10 mmol/L (108–180 mg/dL).

Blood transfusion

Many critically ill patients become anaemic due to reduced red cell production and red cell loss through bleeding and blood sampling. However, red cell transfusion carries inherent risks of immunosuppression, fluid overload, organ dysfunction from microemboli and transfusion reactions. In stable patients, a haemoglobin level of 70 g/L is a safe compromise between optimisation of oxygen delivery and the risks of transfusion. This transfusion threshold should be adjusted upwards for situations where oxygen delivery is critical, such as in patients with active myocardial ischaemia.

Peptic ulcer prophylaxis

Stress ulceration during critical illness is a serious complication. Proton pump inhibitors or histamine-2 receptor antagonists are effective at reducing the incidence of ulceration. There is, however, a suggestion that the use of these agents, particularly in conjunction with antibiotics, may increase the incidence of nosocomial infection, especially with Clostridoides difficile (p. 311). It is therefore common practice to stop ulcer prophylaxis once consistent absorption of enteral feed is established.

Complications and outcomes of critical illness

The majority of patients will survive their episode of critical illness. While some will return to full, active lives, there are many who have ongoing physical, emotional and psychological problems.

---

i	**9.50 Advantages and disadvantages of tracheostomy**

Advantages

- Patient comfort
- Improved oral hygiene
- Access for tracheal toilet
- Ability to speak with cuff deflated and a speaking valve attached
- Reduced equipment 'dead space' (the volume of tubing)
- Earlier weaning and ICU discharge
- Reduced sedation requirement
- Reduced vocal cord damage

Disadvantages

- Immediate complications: hypoxaemia, haemorrhage
- Tracheostomy site infection
- Tracheal damage; late stenosis

Adverse neurological outcomes

Brain injury

Head injury, hypoxic–ischaemic injury and infective, inflammatory and vascular pathologies can all irreversibly injure the brain. If treatment is unsuccessful, patients will either die or be left with a degree of disability. In the latter situation, the provision of ongoing organ support will depend on the severity of the injury, the prognosis, and the wishes of the patient (usually expressed via relatives). Brain death is a state in which cortical and brainstem function is irreversibly lost. Diagnostic criteria for brain death vary between countries (Box 9.51); if satisfied, these criteria allow physicians to withdraw active treatment and discuss the potential for organ donation. Diagnosing brain death is complex and should be done only by physicians with appropriate expertise, as clinical differentiation from reduced consciousness can be challenging (Box 9.52). Where there is doubt – for example, in patients with coexisting spinal injury or localised brainstem pathology – additional investigations should be performed, such as a brain perfusion scan.

The 'locked-in' syndrome occurs when a patient is paralysed but has preserved hemispheric function. This is usually caused by a lesion in the pons and is frequently of vascular origin. Communication can usually be maintained via vertical eye movements or blinking if these functions are preserved. The term 'vegetative state' implies some retention of brainstem function and minimal cortical function, with loss of awareness of the environment. In contrast, 'minimally conscious state' implies that there is some degree of awareness and intact brainstem function. Confident distinction between these states is important and requires careful assessment, often over a period of time. Brain death is, by definition, irreversible but other states may offer hope for improvement.

ICU-acquired weakness

Weakness is common among survivors of critical illness. It is usually symmetrical, proximal and most marked in the lower limbs. Critical illness polyneuropathy and myopathy can occur simultaneously and, within the constraints of an altered sensorium, it can be impossible to distinguish the two conditions clinically. Risk factors for both processes include the severity of multi-organ failure, poor glycaemic control and the use of muscle relaxants and glucocorticoids.

Critical illness polyneuropathy

This is due to peripheral nerve axonal loss and characteristically presents as proximal muscle weakness with preserved sensation. It may also manifest as failure to wean from the ventilator secondary to respiratory muscle weakness. Electrophysiological studies of the affected nerves can be helpful, especially to rule out other potential causes such as Guillain–Barré syndrome. Conduction studies typically show reduced amplitude of transmitted voltage action potential with preserved velocity (compare with findings in Guillain–Barré syndrome; pp. 1133 and 1192). There are no specific treatments aside from resolution of the underlying cause and rehabilitation. Weakness may persist long into the convalescence stage of illness. In some cases, the clinical picture may be more in keeping with individual nerve involvement. This may be due to local pressure effects or part of a generalised picture. Great care must be taken to avoid pressure on high-risk areas such as the neck of the fibula where the common peroneal nerve navigates a superficial course. Nerve palsies such as foot drop can be permanent.

Critical illness myopathy

Although loss of muscle bulk is related to immobility and the catabolic state of critical illness, it is likely that microvascular and intracellular pathophysiological processes are also involved in critical illness myopathy. These processes result in loss of actin myofibrils and muscle weakness. Typically, the CK is normal or only mildly elevated. Like critical illness polyneuropathy, critical illness myopathy is usually a clinical diagnosis.

9.51 UK criteria for the diagnosis of brain death

Preconditions for considering a diagnosis of brain death

- The patient is deeply comatose:
  a. There must be no suspicion that coma is due to depressant drugs, such as narcotics, hypnotics, tranquillisers
  b. Hypothermia has been excluded – rectal temperature must exceed 35°C
  c. There is no profound abnormality of serum electrolytes, acid–base balance or blood glucose concentrations, and any metabolic or endocrine cause of coma has been excluded
- The patient is maintained on a ventilator because spontaneous respiration has been inadequate or has ceased. Drugs, including neuromuscular blocking agents, must have been excluded as a cause of the respiratory failure
- The diagnosis of the disorder leading to brain death has been firmly established. There must be no doubt that the patient is suffering from irremediable structural brain damage

Tests for confirming brain death

- All brainstem reflexes are absent:
  a. The pupils are fixed and unreactive to light
  b. The corneal reflexes are absent
  c. The vestibulo-ocular reflexes are absent – there is no eye movement following the injection of 20 mL of ice-cold water into each external auditory meatus in turn
  d. There are no motor responses to adequate stimulation within the cranial nerve distribution
  e. There is no gag reflex and no reflex response to a suction catheter in the trachea
- No respiratory movement occurs when the patient is disconnected from the ventilator for long enough to allow the carbon dioxide tension to rise above the threshold for stimulating respiration ($PaCO_2$ must reach 6.7 kPa/50 mmHg)

The diagnosis of brain death should be made by two doctors of a specified status and experience. The tests are usually repeated after a short interval to allow blood gases to normalise before brain death is finally confirmed.

Nerve conduction studies and electromyography may be suggestive of critical illness myopathy, and helpful in ruling out other pathology. A muscle biopsy is required to confirm the diagnosis (p. 1133), although it is seldom used in clinical practice as there are no specific treatment options. Biopsies typically show selective loss of the thick myofibrils and muscle necrosis. Management is conservative and the prognosis is good in ICU survivors.

Airway complications

Prolonged instrumentation of the airway is occasionally associated with injuries that may have long-term consequences. Vocal cord oedema is common after intubation, especially in female patients. This may require urgent re-intubation, a short course of systemic steroids or the insertion of a tracheostomy to allow oedema to settle. Long-term vocal cord problems occur in a small number of ICU survivors. This may include vocal cord palsies or chronically increased vocal cord tone causing either a weak voice or stridor.

Both tracheal intubation and tracheostomy can cause damage to the trachea (either at the insertion point or from ischaemia at the level of the cuff). This may be associated with tracheal stenosis or a tracheoesophageal fistula. If any of these complications is suspected, referral to a throat specialist is recommended.

Micro- and macrovascular complications

Areas of tissue ischaemia can occur during an episode of critical illness. Causative mechanisms may include: micro-emboli; reduced tissue perfusion from vasoconstriction or poor cardiac output; pressure from positioning or medical devices such as those securing a tracheostomy; invasive arterial lines causing arterial thrombosis. Vascular surgical opinion may be helpful in recommending specific treatments or management of necrotic tissue. Wherever possible, steps should be taken to reduce

i | **9.52 Classification of brain death and reduced conscious states**

Diagnosis	Features	Investigation	Prognosis
Brain death	See Box 9.51	Often not required if cranial imaging shows compatible cause and patient meets clinical criteria In diagnostic doubt: four-vessel angiogram (fluoroscopic or CT) of cerebral vessels or isotope scan of brain to demonstrate absence of cerebral blood flow	Time of confirmed brain death is recorded as time of death Potential to donate organs – donation after brain death (DBD) donor
Vegetative state (VS) 'Persistent VS' >1 month 'Permanent VS' >1 year	No reaction to verbal stimuli Some reaction to noxious stimuli Sleep–wake cycles (periods of eye opening) Maintained respiratory drive Intact brainstem reflexes Occasional automatic movements (yawning, swallowing)	Cranial imaging for primary cause Maintained cortical blood flow	Poor. May be better with traumatic aetiology
Minimally conscious state	Some reaction to verbal stimuli Some reaction to noxious stimuli Spontaneous movements Intact brainstem reflexes	EEG demonstrates reactivity	Variable. Recovery of function more likely than in VS
Locked-in syndrome	Cortex is intact but bilateral motor tracts are damaged Can be partial or complete, i.e. some response to verbal stimuli (e.g. vertical eye movements to communicate) Variable brainstem reflexes No limb movement to noxious stimuli	Imaging for primary cause – commonly MRI or CT will show brainstem or pontine infarction	Variable and depends on cause – progress can continue over months to years

the incidence of these complications, e.g. active pressure management. However, in critically unwell patients, peripheral ischaemia can occur despite optimal management.

Other complications

Cardiopulmonary resuscitation can frequently lead to damage to the integrity of the chest wall. This appears to be more common with the use of automated compression devices although it is possible this reflects increased survivorship in this cohort. Anterior rib fractures and sternocostal dislocation are seen most commonly and this pattern of injury can lead to a flail segment of the chest wall, or a flail sternum. The segment moves independently from the rest of the chest; this is a problem when ventilation is spontaneous as the negative pressure draws the flail segment inwards. Simple rib fractures can usually be managed with analgesia but flail segments frequently benefit from surgical fixation (Fig. 9.26). The experience of critical illness and the necessary invasive management can leave patients with profound psychological sequelae akin to the post-traumatic stress syndrome seen in many survivors of conflict. Specialist psychological help is required in managing these issues. Sometimes recovering patients benefit from returning to the ICU to see the environment in a different way and gain a better understanding of the processes and procedures that haunt them.

Long-term physical consequences are also common. Many diseases are not completely cured, but follow a relapsing–remitting course; patients who have been critically ill with sepsis are far more likely than others in the general population to suffer from it again. Intensive care follow-up clinics provide an excellent forum for addressing such issues, and for coordinating care involving a variety of medical specialties.

The older patient

Critically ill older patients present additional challenges following intensive care discharge (Box 9.53). As the ability to make a full recovery depends on frailty rather than chronological age, it can be helpful to use a validated frailty scoring system (p. 1300) to inform admission decision-making.

Rehabilitation medicine has much to offer survivors of critical illness, and an early referral is beneficial when it is clear that a patient is likely to survive with significant morbidity.

Withdrawal of active treatment and death in intensive care

Futility

The idea of futility is not new: Hippocrates stated that physicians should 'refuse to treat those who are overmastered by their disease, realising that in such cases medicine is powerless'. In intensive care, where the concept of futility is often used as a criterion to limit or withdraw life-sustaining treatment, it is helpful to have a working definition on which families and physicians can agree. It is, therefore, reasonable to define futility in such circumstances as the point at which recovery to a quality of life that the patient would find acceptable has passed. The primary insult may be neurological (irreversible brain injury not meeting criteria for brain death), or multi-organ failure that is refractory to treatment.

Death

While most patients prefer to die at home, many spend their final days in hospital. Chapter 8 details the medical, legal and ethical priorities that should guide patient management once the decision to withdraw active treatment has been made. The decision to shift the focus of care to palliation should not change its intensity; it is the over-arching objective that changes. Only interventions that will improve the quality of a patient's remaining life should be offered. In the ICU, it is often appropriate to continue infusions of sedatives and analgesics, as reducing or stopping them may cause unnecessary pain and agitation. Measures that were instituted to prolong life should be withdrawn (usually including cessation of inotropes and extubation) to allow the patient to die peacefully with their family and friends present.

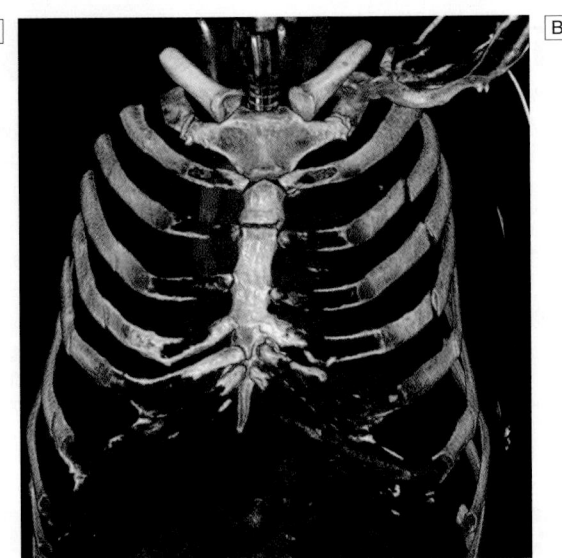 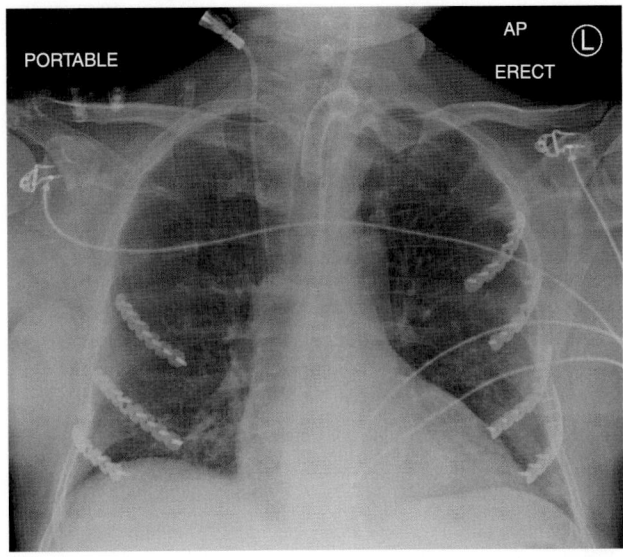

Fig. 9.26 Anterior chest wall injuries are common after CPR. A Here is shown a flail sternum with multiple bilateral chest wall fractures. The patient underwent rib fixation following unsuccessful attempts at weaning. B The post-fixation chest radiograph is shown and weaning was successful shortly afterwards. *Images courtesy of Dr Jonathan Serhan.*

9

9.53 The critically ill older patient

- **ICU demography**: increasing numbers of critically ill older patients are admitted to the ICU; more than 50% of patients in many general ICUs are over 65 years old.
- **Outcome**: affected to some extent by age, as reflected in APACHE II (see Box 9.55), but age should not be used as the sole criterion for withholding or withdrawing ICU support.
- **Cardiopulmonary resuscitation (CPR)**: successful hospital discharge following in-hospital CPR is rare in patients over 70 years old in the presence of significant chronic disease.
- **Functional independence**: tends to be lost during an ICU stay and prolonged rehabilitation may subsequently be necessary.
- **Specific problems**:
  Skin fragility and ulceration
  Poor muscle strength: difficulty weaning from ventilator and mobilising
  Delirium: compounded by sedatives and analgesics
  High prevalence of underlying nutritional deficiency

Organ donation

Donation after brain death

The diagnosis of brain death is discussed on page 215. Once brain death has been confirmed, consideration should be given to organ donation, termed 'donation after brain death' (DBD). Time of death is recorded as the time when the first series of brain death tests are undertaken, although the deceased patient continues to be ventilated. The practice of organ donation varies throughout the world but the principles remain the same.

Organ donation specialists are contacted and they begin the process of establishing the suitability of any organs for transplantation and matching potential recipients. Many patients will have expressed their wishes through an organ donor registration scheme but agreement of family and next of kin is a moral (and sometimes legal) prerequisite. Once the organ retrieval theatre team have been assembled and all preliminary tests have been completed, the deceased patient is transferred to the operating theatre and the organs are sequentially removed.

Donation after cardiac death

If a patient does not meet brain death criteria but withdrawal of treatment has been agreed, donation of organs with residual function may be appropriate. This is termed 'donation after cardiac death' (DCD). If the patient dies within a short period following the commencement of 'warm ischaemic time' (the time to asystole following the onset of physiological derangement after the withdrawal of active treatment), then DCD can proceed. The deceased patient is transferred to an operating theatre and the agreed organs (lungs, liver, kidney and pancreas and occasionally heart) are retrieved. As heart valves and corneas can be retrieved later (within a longer time frame), tissue retrieval may occur in the mortuary.

Post-mortem examination or autopsy

There are several indications to request a post-mortem examination. A coroner (or legal equivalent) may initiate the process if a death is unexpected or violent, or has occurred under suspicious circumstances. The treating physician(s) may request one if they are unable to establish a cause of death or there is agreement that it may yield information of interest to the family or clinical team. The post-mortem diagnosis is occasionally at odds with the ante-mortem diagnosis and it is a very useful learning exercise to review the results with all those involved in the patient's care.

Discharge from intensive care

Discharge is appropriate when the original indication for admission has resolved and the patient has sufficient physiological reserve to continue to recover without the facilities of intensive care. Many ICUs and HDUs function as combined units, allowing 'step-down' of patients to HDU care without changing the clinical team involved. Discharge from ICU is stressful for patients and families, and clear communication with the clinical team accepting responsibility is vital. Nursing ratios change from 1:1 (one nurse per patient) or 1:2 to much lower staffing levels. Discharges from ICU or HDU to standard wards should take place within normal working hours to ensure adequate medical and nursing support and detailed handover. Discharge outside normal working hours is associated with higher ICU re-admission rates and increased mortality. The receiving team should be provided with a written summary, including the information listed in Box 9.54. The ICU team should remain available for advice; many ICU teams provide an outreach service to supply advice and facilitate continuity of care.

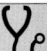

9.54 How to write an ICU discharge summary: information to be included

- Summary of diagnosis and progress in intensive care
- Current medications and changes to regular medications with justifications
- Antibiotic regimen and suggested review dates
- Results of positive microbiological tests
- Positions of invasive devices and insertion dates
- Escalation plan in the event of deterioration
- Pending investigations and specialty consultations
- If the physiology remains abnormal due to chronic disease, rapid response triggers should be adjusted accordingly

Critical care scoring systems

Admission and discharge criteria vary between ICUs, so it is important to define the characteristics of the patients admitted in order to assess the effects of the care provided on the outcomes achieved. Two systems are widely used to measure severity of illness (see Box 9.55 for further details):

- *APACHE II*: Acute Physiology Assessment and Chronic Health Evaluation
- *SOFA score*: Sequential Organ Failure Assessment tool.

When combined with the admission diagnosis, scoring systems have been shown to correlate well with the risk of death in hospital. Such outcome predictions are useful at a population level but lack the specificity to be of use in decision-making for individual patients.

i 9.55 Comparison of APACHE II and SOFA scores

APACHE II score

- An assessment of admission characteristics (e.g. age and pre-existing organ dysfunction) and the maximum/minimum values of 12 routine physiological measurements during the first 24 hours of admission (e.g. temperature, blood pressure, GCS) that reflect the physiological impact of the illness
- Composite score out of 71
- Higher scores are given to patients with more serious underlying diagnoses, medical history or physiological instability; higher mortality correlates with higher scores

SOFA score

- A score of 1–4 is allocated to six organ systems (respiratory, cardiovascular, liver, renal, coagulation and neurological) to represent the degree of organ dysfunction, e.g. platelet count $> 150 \times 10^9$/L scores 1 point, $< 25 \times 10^9$/L scores 4 points
- Composite score out of 24
- Higher scores are associated with increased mortality

Further information

Websites

criticalcarereviews.com *Reviews and appraisal of ICU topics*.
emcrit.org *Online podcasts and general information on emergency medicine and critical care*.
emcrit.org *European Society of Intensive Care Medicine: guidelines, recommendations, consensus conference reports*.
lifeinthefastlane.com *Information on a range of intensive care and emergency medicine topics*.
survivingsepsis.org *Surviving Sepsis website*.

SHL Thomas

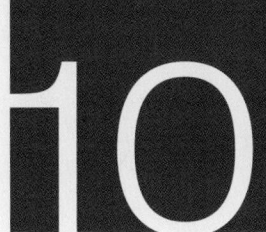

Poisoning

Comprehensive evaluation of the poisoned patient

1 Airway, breathing, circulation
Respiration rate,
oxygen saturation,
pulse, BP,
dysrhythmias

2 Level of consciousness
Presence of seizures,
delirium, agitation
or psychosis

3 Chest
Evidence of aspiration,
bronchoconstriction

4 Movement and muscles
Tone, fasciculations,
myoclonus, tremor,
paralysis, ataxia

5 Reflexes
Tendon reflexes, plantar
responses, inducible clonus

6 Eyes
Miosis or mydriasis,
diplopia or strabismus,
lacrimation

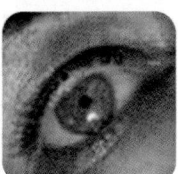

▲ Pinpoint pupil

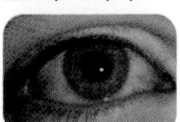

▲ Injected conjunctiva

7 Abdomen
Hepatic or epigastric
tenderness, ileus,
palpable bladder

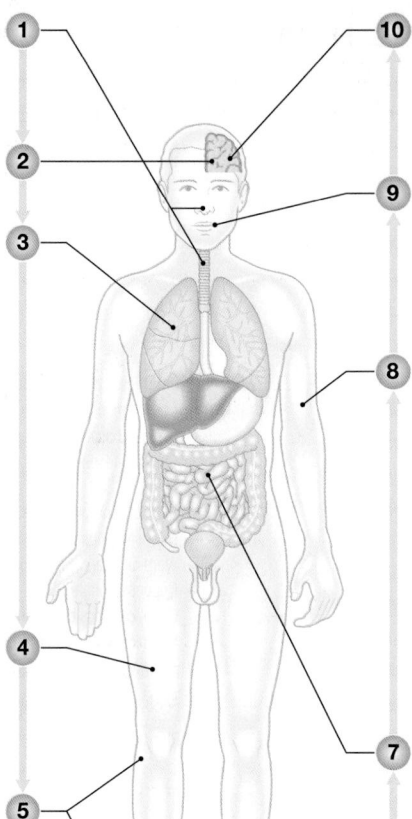

10 Psychiatric evaluation
Features of psychiatric illness,
mental capacity

9 Mouth
Dry mouth, excessive salivation

8 Skin
Temperature, cyanosis,
flushing, sweating,
blisters, pressure areas,
piloerection,
evidence of self-harm

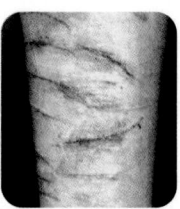

▲ Self-cutting

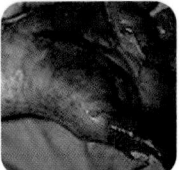

▲ Chemical burn

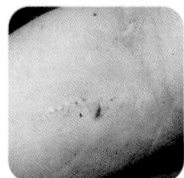

▲ Needle tracks

Insets (Self-cutting) From Douglas G, Nicol F, Robertson C (eds). Macleod's Clinical examination, 11th edn. Churchill Livingstone, Elsevier Ltd; 2005. (Chemical burn) www.firewiki.net. (Needle tracks) www.deep6inc.com. (Pinpoint pupil) http://drugrecognition. com/images. (Injected conjunctiva) http://knol.google.com.

---

i Taking a history in poisoning

- What toxin(s) have been taken and how much?
- What time were they taken and by what route?
- Have alcohol or other substances (including drugs of misuse) also been taken?
- Obtain details from witnesses (e.g. family, friends, ambulance personnel) of the circumstances of the overdose
- Assess immediate suicide risk in those with apparent self-harm (full psychiatric evaluation when patient has recovered physically)

- Assess capacity to make decisions about accepting or refusing treatment
- Establish past medical history, drug history and allergies, social and family history
- Record all information carefully

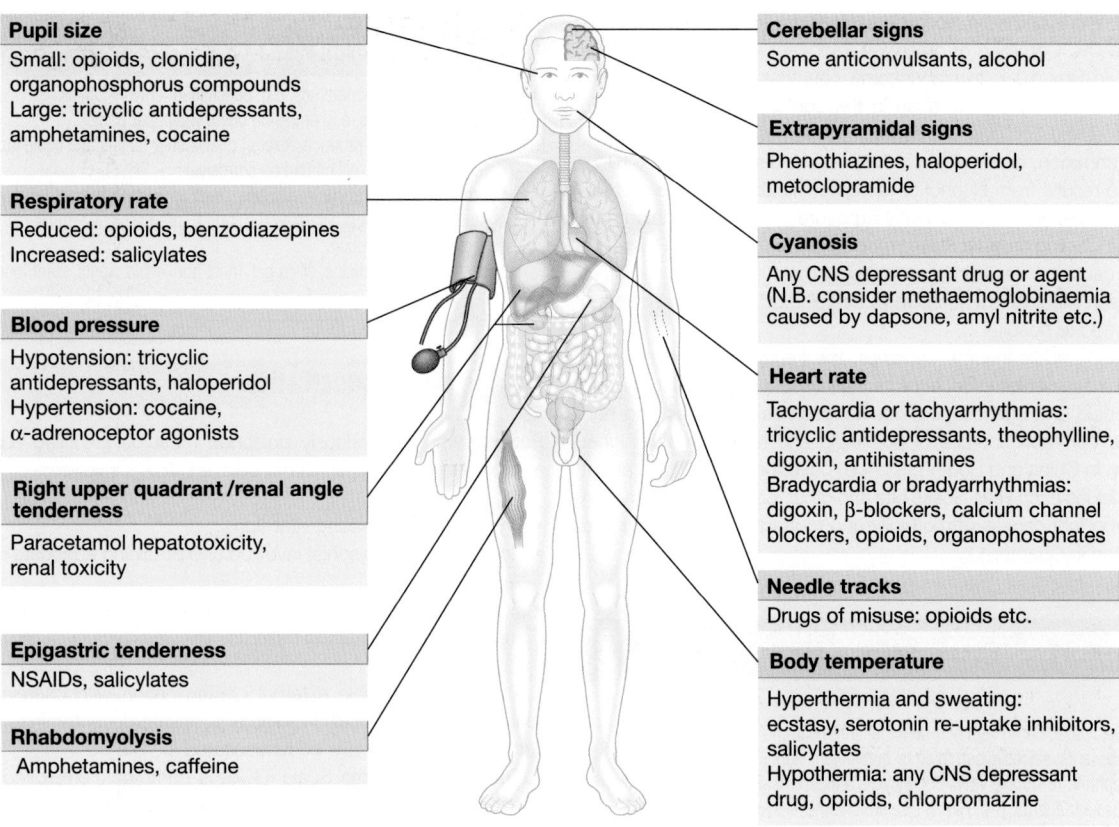

Pupil size
Small: opioids, clonidine, organophosphorus compounds
Large: tricyclic antidepressants, amphetamines, cocaine

Respiratory rate
Reduced: opioids, benzodiazepines
Increased: salicylates

Blood pressure
Hypotension: tricyclic antidepressants, haloperidol
Hypertension: cocaine, α-adrenoceptor agonists

Right upper quadrant /renal angle tenderness
Paracetamol hepatotoxicity, renal toxicity

Epigastric tenderness
NSAIDs, salicylates

Rhabdomyolysis
Amphetamines, caffeine

Cerebellar signs
Some anticonvulsants, alcohol

Extrapyramidal signs
Phenothiazines, haloperidol, metoclopramide

Cyanosis
Any CNS depressant drug or agent (N.B. consider methaemoglobinaemia caused by dapsone, amyl nitrite etc.)

Heart rate
Tachycardia or tachyarrhythmias: tricyclic antidepressants, theophylline, digoxin, antihistamines
Bradycardia or bradyarrhythmias: digoxin, β-blockers, calcium channel blockers, opioids, organophosphates

Needle tracks
Drugs of misuse: opioids etc.

Body temperature
Hyperthermia and sweating: ecstasy, serotonin re-uptake inhibitors, salicylates
Hypothermia: any CNS depressant drug, opioids, chlorpromazine

Clinical signs of poisoning by pharmaceutical agents and drugs of misuse.

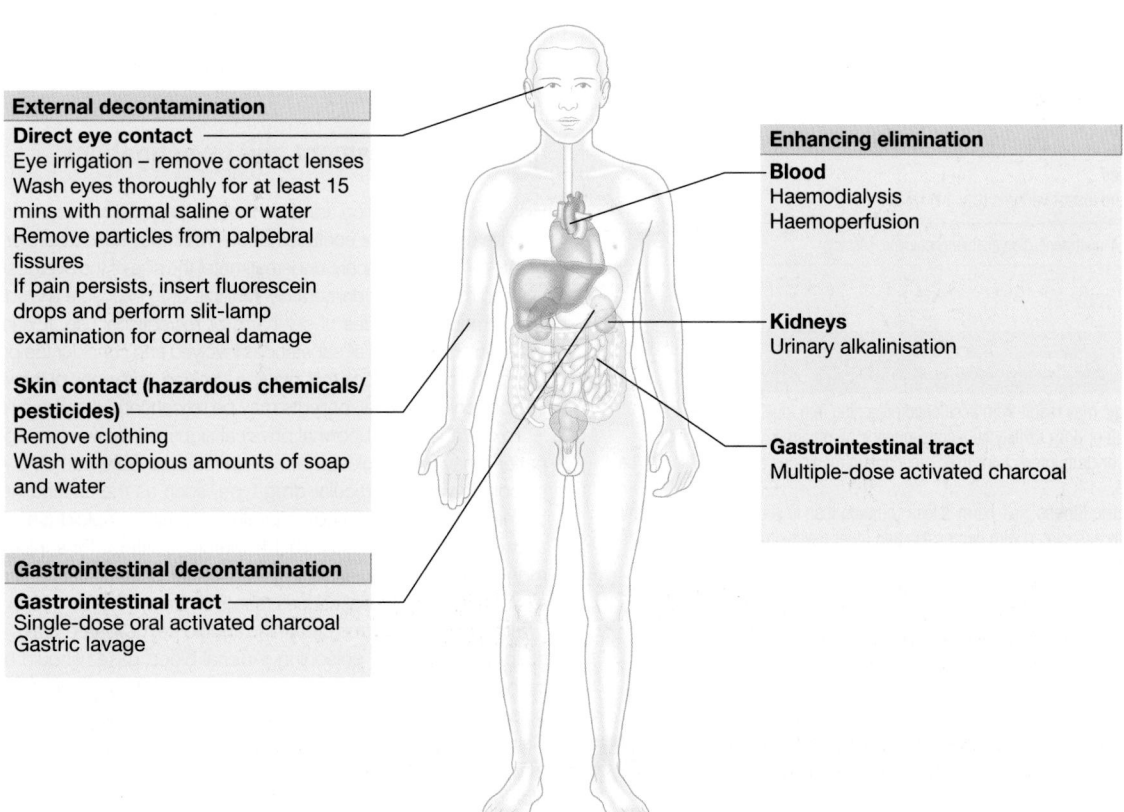

External decontamination
Direct eye contact
Eye irrigation – remove contact lenses
Wash eyes thoroughly for at least 15 mins with normal saline or water
Remove particles from palpebral fissures
If pain persists, insert fluorescein drops and perform slit-lamp examination for corneal damage

Skin contact (hazardous chemicals/ pesticides)
Remove clothing
Wash with copious amounts of soap and water

Gastrointestinal decontamination
Gastrointestinal tract
Single-dose oral activated charcoal
Gastric lavage

Enhancing elimination
Blood
Haemodialysis
Haemoperfusion

Kidneys
Urinary alkalinisation

Gastrointestinal tract
Multiple-dose activated charcoal

Decontamination and enhanced elimination. One of the key aspects in the evaluation of a poisoned patient is deciding if decontamination and/or enhanced elimination is required.

Acute poisoning is common, accounting for about 1% of hospital admissions in the UK. Common or otherwise important substances involved are shown in Box 10.1. In high-income countries, the most frequent cause is intentional drug overdose in the context of self-harm, often involving prescribed or 'over-the-counter' medicines. Accidental poisoning is also common, especially in children and older people (Box 10.2). Toxicity also results from alcohol or recreational substance use and following occupational or environmental exposure. Criminal poisoning may also occur, including drug-facilitated robbery or sexual assault. Poisoning is a major cause of death in young adults; most deaths occur before patients reach medical attention, while overall mortality is low (< 1%) in those admitted to hospital.

In low- and middle-income countries, the frequency of self-harm is more difficult to estimate. Because of their widespread availability and use, household and agricultural products, such as pesticides and herbicides, are common sources of poisoning and have a much higher case fatality. In China and South-east Asia, pesticides account for about 300 000 suicides each year. Snake bite and other forms of envenomation are also important causes of morbidity and mortality internationally and are discussed in Chapter 11.

10.1 Important substances involved in poisoning

In the UK

- Analgesics: paracetamol and non-steroidal anti-inflammatory drugs (NSAIDs)
- Antidepressants: selective serotonin re-uptake inhibitors (SSRIs), serotonin-norepinephrine re-uptake inhibitors (SNRIs), tricyclic antidepressants (TCAs) and lithium
- Cardiovascular agents: β-blockers, calcium channel blockers and cardiac glycosides
- Drugs of misuse: depressants (e.g. opiates, benzodiazepines), stimulants and entactogens (e.g. amphetamines, MDMA, mephedrone, cocaine), hallucinogens (e.g. cannabis, synthetic cannabinoid receptor agonists)
- Carbon monoxide
- Alcohol

In South and South-east Asia

- Organophosphorus and carbamate insecticides
- Aluminium and zinc phosphide
- Paraquat
- Oleander
- Corrosives
- Snake and insect venoms (Ch. 11)

(MDMA = 3,4-methylene-dioxymethamphetamine, ecstasy)

10.2 Poisoning in old age

- **Aetiology**: may result from accidental poisoning (e.g. due to delirium or dementia) or drug toxicity as a consequence of impaired renal or hepatic function or drug interaction. Toxic prescription medicines are more likely to be available.
- **Psychiatric illness**: self-harm is less common than in younger adults, but more frequently associated with depression and other psychiatric illness, as well as chronic illness and pain. There is a higher risk of subsequent suicide.
- **Severity of poisoning**: increased morbidity and mortality result from reduced renal and hepatic function, lower functional reserve, increased sensitivity to sedative agents and frequent comorbidity.

General approach to the poisoned patient

A general approach is shown on pages 220–221. In many countries, poisons centres are available to provide advice on management of suspected poisoning with specific substances and the use of antidotes. Information is also available online see 'Further information'.

10.3 Substances of very low toxicity

- Writing/educational materials, e.g. pencil lead, crayons, chalk
- Decorating products, e.g. emulsion paint, wallpaper paste
- Cleaning/bathroom products (except dishwasher tablets and liquid laundry detergent capsules, which can be corrosive)
- Pharmaceuticals: oral contraceptives, most antibiotics (but not tetracyclines or antituberculous drugs), vitamins B, C and E, prednisolone, emollients and other skin creams, baby lotion
- Miscellaneous: Plasticine, silica gel, most household plants, plant food, pet food, soil

Triage and resuscitation

Patients who are seriously poisoned must be identified early so that appropriate management is not delayed. Triage involves:

- immediately assessing vital signs
- identifying the poison(s) involved and obtaining adequate information about them
- identifying patients at risk of further attempts at self-harm and removing any remaining hazards.

Those with possible external contamination with chemical or environmental toxins should undergo appropriate decontamination (p. 221). Critically ill patients must be resuscitated (p. 176).

The Glasgow Coma Scale (GCS) is commonly employed to assess conscious level, although not specifically validated in poisoning. The AVPU (alert/verbal/painful/unresponsive) scale is also a rapid and simple method. An electrocardiogram (ECG) should be performed and cardiac monitoring instituted in all patients with cardiovascular features or where exposure to potentially cardiotoxic substances is suspected. Patients who may need antidotes should be weighed if possible, so that appropriate weight-related doses can be prescribed.

Substances involved that are unlikely to be toxic in humans should be identified so that inappropriate admission and intervention are avoided (Box 10.3).

Clinical assessment and investigations

History and examination are described on page 220. Occasionally, patients may be unaware of or confused about what they have taken, or may exaggerate (or, less commonly, underestimate) the size of the overdose, but rarely mislead medical staff deliberately. Multiple drug exposure (including alcohol) is common in episodes of self-harm or recreational use. It is important to obtain information on all substances involved and consider the potential toxicity of the combinations that may be involved. In regions of the world where self-poisoning is illegal, patients may be reticent about giving a history.

Toxic causes of abnormal physical signs are shown on page 221. The patient may have a cluster of clinical features ('toxidrome') suggestive of poisoning with a particular drug type, such as the anticholinergic, serotoninergic (see Box 10.10), stimulant, sedative, opioid (see Box 10.12) and cholinergic (see Box 10.14) feature clusters. Poisoning is a common cause of coma, especially in younger people, but it is important to exclude other potential causes (see Box 9.31).

Urea, electrolytes and creatinine should be measured in all patients with suspected systemic poisoning. Arterial blood gases should be checked in those with significant respiratory or circulatory compromise, or after poisoning with substances likely to affect acid–base status (Box 10.4). Calculation of anion and osmolar gaps may help to inform diagnosis and management (Box 10.5). Potent oxidising agents may cause methaemoglobinaemia, with consequent blue discoloration of skin and blood, and reduced tissue oxygen delivery (Fig. 10.1).

For some substances, management may be facilitated by measurement of the amount of toxin in the blood. Qualitative urine screens for potential toxins, including near-patient testing kits, have a limited clinical role.

Psychiatric assessment

Patients presenting with drug overdose in the context of self-harm should undergo psychiatric evaluation prior to discharge by a health professional with appropriate training (see p. 1243). This should occur after they have recovered from poisoning, unless there is an urgent issue, such as uncertainty about their capacity to decline medical treatment.

10.4 Causes of acidosis in the poisoned patient

Cause	Normal lactate*	High lactate
Toxic	Salicylates Methanol Ethylene glycol Paraldehyde	Metformin Iron Cyanide Sodium valproate Carbon monoxide
Other	Renal failure Ketoacidosis Severe diarrhoea	Shock

*Unless circulatory shock is present, when it will be high in any case.

10.5 Anion and osmolar gaps in poisoning

	Anion gap	Osmolar gap
Calculation	$[Na^+ + K^+] - [Cl^- + HCO_3^-]$	[Measured osmolality] − [(2 × Na) + Urea + Glucose][1]
Reference range	12–16 mmol/L	<10
Common toxic causes of elevation[2]	Ethanol Ethylene glycol Methanol Salicylates Iron Cyanide	Ethanol Ethylene glycol Methanol

[1]All units should be in mmol/L, except osmolality, which should be in mOsmol/kg. For non-SI units, the corresponding formula is [Measured osmolality (mOsmol/kg)] − [(2 × Na (mEq/L)) + Urea/2.8 (mg/dL) + Glucose/18 (mg/dL)]. [2]Box 19.19 gives non-toxic causes.

General management

Patients presenting with eye/skin contamination should undergo local decontamination measures. These are described on page 221.

Gastrointestinal decontamination

Patients who have ingested toxins in potentially harmful amounts may be considered for gastrointestinal decontamination if poisoning has been recent.

Activated charcoal

Given orally as a slurry, activated charcoal absorbs toxins in the bowel as a result of its large surface area. It can prevent absorption of an important proportion of the ingested dose of toxin, but efficacy decreases with time. Activated charcoal is most effective if given within 1 hour of overdose, but may have useful efficacy later than this, for example if a sustained-release preparation has been taken or when gastric emptying is delayed. Use is ineffective for some toxins that do not bind to activated charcoal (Box 10.6). In patients with impaired swallowing or a reduced level of consciousness, activated charcoal given via a nasogastric tube carries a risk of aspiration pneumonitis, but this can be reduced (though not eliminated) by protecting the airway using a cuffed endotracheal tube.

Multiple doses of oral activated charcoal (50 g 6 times daily in an adult) may enhance the elimination of some substances at any time after poisoning (Box 10.7). This interrupts enterohepatic circulation or reduces the concentration of free drug in the gut lumen, to the extent that drug diffuses from the blood back into the bowel to be absorbed on to the charcoal ('gastrointestinal dialysis'). A laxative is generally given with the charcoal to reduce the risk of constipation or intestinal obstruction by charcoal 'briquette' formation in the gut lumen.

Evidence suggests that single or multiple doses of activated charcoal do not improve clinical outcomes after poisoning with pesticides or oleander.

Gastric aspiration and lavage

Gastric aspiration and/or lavage is very infrequently indicated in acute poisoning, as it is no more effective than activated charcoal for most substances and complications are common, especially pulmonary aspiration.

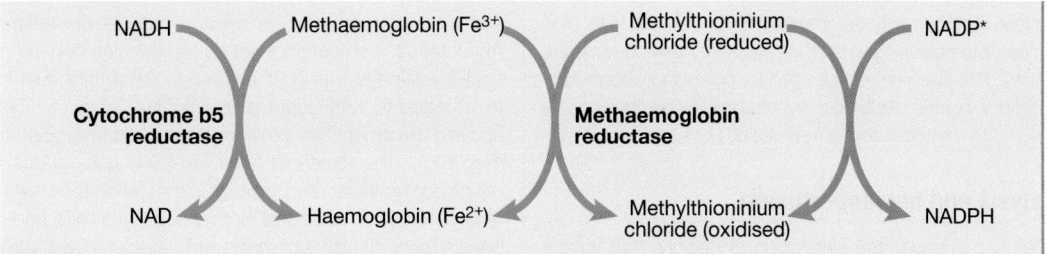

Causes
Non-toxic
• Congenital methaemoglobinaemias
Toxic (Oxidising agents)
• Organic nitrites
• Nitrates
• Benzocaine
• Dapsone
• Chloroquine
• Aniline dyes
• Chlorobenzene
• Naphthalene
• Copper sulphate

Consequences
• Haemoglobin–oxygen dissociation curve is shifted to the left (see Fig. 25.5)
• Oxygen delivery to tissues is reduced
• There is apparent 'cyanosis'
• Breathlessness, fatigue, headache and chest pain occur
• Delirium, impaired consciousness and seizures may occur in severe cases

Treatment
• Methylthioninium chloride ('methylene blue') 1–2 mg/kg (intravenous) is given
• Reduces methaemoglobin (see below)
• Used for symptomatic patients with severe methaemoglobinaemia (e.g. >30%)
• Patients with anaemia or other comorbidities may need treatment at lower concentrations

Fig. 10.1 Methaemoglobinaemia. (NAD = nicotinamide adenine dinucleotide, H = hydrogen, P = phosphate)

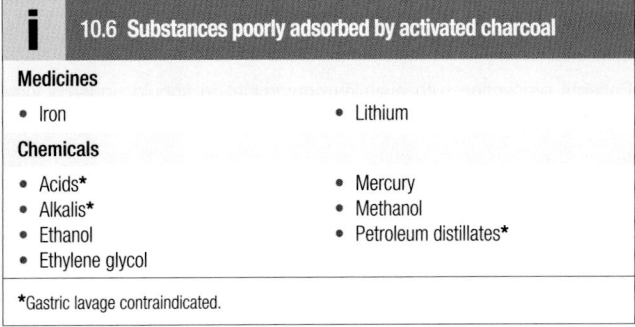

i | **10.6 Substances poorly adsorbed by activated charcoal**

Medicines

- Iron
- Lithium

Chemicals

- Acids*
- Mercury
- Alkalis*
- Methanol
- Ethanol
- Petroleum distillates*
- Ethylene glycol

*Gastric lavage contraindicated.

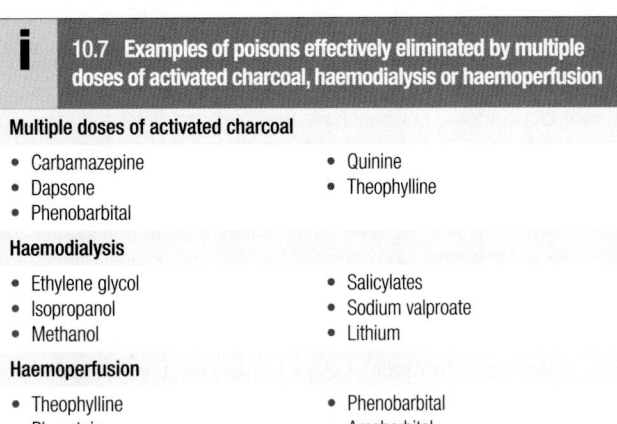

i | **10.7 Examples of poisons effectively eliminated by multiple doses of activated charcoal, haemodialysis or haemoperfusion**

Multiple doses of activated charcoal

- Carbamazepine
- Quinine
- Dapsone
- Theophylline
- Phenobarbital

Haemodialysis

- Ethylene glycol
- Salicylates
- Isopropanol
- Sodium valproate
- Methanol
- Lithium

Haemoperfusion

- Theophylline
- Phenobarbital
- Phenytoin
- Amobarbital
- Carbamazepine

It is contraindicated if strong acids, alkalis or petroleum distillates have been ingested. Use may be justified for life-threatening overdoses of those substances that are not absorbed by activated charcoal (see Box 10.6).

Whole bowel irrigation

This involves the administration of large quantities of osmotically balanced polyethylene glycol and electrolyte solution (1–2 L/hr for an adult), usually by a nasogastric tube, until the rectal effluent is clear. It is occasionally indicated to enhance the elimination of ingested packets of illicit drugs or slow-release tablets such as iron and lithium that are not absorbed by activated charcoal. Contraindications include inadequate airway protection, haemodynamic instability, gastrointestinal haemorrhage, obstruction or ileus. Whole bowel irrigation may precipitate nausea and vomiting, abdominal pain and electrolyte disturbances.

Urinary alkalinisation

Urinary excretion of weak acids and bases is affected by urinary pH, which changes the extent to which they are ionised. Highly ionised molecules pass poorly through lipid membranes and therefore little tubular reabsorption occurs and urinary excretion is increased. If the urine is alkalinised (pH > 7.5) by the administration of sodium bicarbonate (e.g. 1.5 L of 1.26% sodium bicarbonate over 2 hrs), weak acids (e.g. salicylates, methotrexate) are highly ionised, resulting in enhanced urinary excretion.

Urinary alkalinisation is currently recommended for patients with clinically significant salicylate poisoning when the criteria for haemodialysis are not met (see below). It is also sometimes used for poisoning with methotrexate. Complications include alkalaemia, hypokalaemia and occasionally alkalotic tetany (Ch. 19). Hypocalcaemia may occur, but is rare.

Haemodialysis and haemoperfusion

These techniques can enhance the elimination of poisons that have a small volume of distribution and a long half-life after overdose; use is appropriate when poisoning is sufficiently severe. The toxin must be small enough to cross the dialysis membrane (haemodialysis) or must bind to activated charcoal (haemoperfusion) (see Box 10.7). Haemodialysis can also correct acid–base and metabolic disturbances associated with poisoning.

Lipid emulsion therapy

Lipid emulsion therapy is increasingly used for poisoning with lipid-soluble agents. Evidence for efficacy is most compelling for local anaesthetics, especially bupivacaine. The treatment has also been used with anecdotal reports of success for poisoning with tricyclic antidepressants, calcium channel blockers and lipid-soluble β-adrenoceptor antagonists (β-blockers) such as propranolol. It involves intravenous administration of 20% lipid emulsion (e.g. Intralipid, suggested initial dose 1.5 mL/kg, followed by a continued infusion of 0.25 mL/kg/min until there is clinical improvement). It is thought that lipid-soluble toxins partition into the intravenous lipid, reducing target tissue concentrations. The elevated myocardial free fatty acid concentrations may also have beneficial effects on myocardial metabolism and performance by counteracting the inhibition of myocardial fatty acid oxidation produced by some cardiotoxins, enabling increased adenosine triphosphate (ATP) synthesis and energy production. Some animal studies have suggested efficacy and case reports of use in human poisoning have also been encouraging, with recovery of circulatory collapse reported in cases where other treatment modalities have been unsuccessful. No controlled trials of this technique have been performed, however, and efficacy remains uncertain, especially for substances other than local anaesthetics.

Supportive care

For most poisons, antidotes and methods to accelerate elimination are inappropriate, unavailable or incompletely effective. Outcome is dependent on appropriate nursing and supportive care, and treatment of complications (Box 10.8).

Antidotes

Antidotes are available for some poisons and work by a variety of mechanisms (Box 10.9). The use of some of these in the management of specific poisons is described below.

Poisoning by specific pharmaceutical agents

Analgesics

Paracetamol

Paracetamol (acetaminophen) is the drug most commonly used in overdose in the UK. Toxicity is caused by an intermediate reactive metabolite that binds covalently to cellular proteins, causing cell death. This results in hepatic and occasionally renal failure. In therapeutic doses, the toxic metabolite is detoxified in reactions requiring glutathione, but in overdose, glutathione reserves become exhausted.

Management

Activated charcoal may be used in patients presenting within 1 hour. Antidotes for paracetamol act by replenishing hepatic glutathione, and acetylcysteine is the most commonly used. It should be administered to all patients with acute poisoning and paracetamol concentrations above a 'treatment line' provided on paracetamol poisoning nomograms (Fig. 10.2). The threshold used for these nomograms varies between countries, however, and local guidance should be followed. Liver and renal function, International Normalised Ratio (INR) and a venous bicarbonate should also be measured. Arterial blood gases and lactate should be assessed in patients with reduced bicarbonate or severe liver function abnormalities; metabolic acidosis indicates severe poisoning.

10.8 Complications of poisoning and their management

Complication	Examples of causative agents	Management
Coma	Sedative agents	Appropriate airway protection and ventilatory support Oxygen saturation and blood gas monitoring Pressure area and bladder care Identification and treatment of aspiration pneumonia
Seizures	NSAIDs Anticonvulsants TCAs Theophylline	Appropriate airway and ventilatory support IV benzodiazepine (e.g. diazepam 10–20 mg or lorazepam 2–4 mg) Correction of hypoxia, acid–base and metabolic abnormalities
Acute dystonias	Typical antipsychotics Metoclopramide	Procyclidine, benzatropine or diazepam
Hypotension		
Due to vasodilatation	Vasodilator antihypertensives Anticholinergic agents TCAs	IV fluids Vasopressors (rarely indicated; p. 210)
Due to myocardial suppression	β-blockers Calcium channel blockers TCAs	Optimisation of volume status Inotropic agents (p. 210)
Ventricular tachycardia		
Monomorphic, associated with QRS prolongation	Sodium channel blockers	Correction of electrolyte and acid–base abnormalities and hypoxia Sodium bicarbonate (e.g. 50 mL 8.4% solution, repeated if necessary)
Torsades de pointes, associated with QT$_c$ prolongation	Anti-arrhythmic drugs (quinidine, amiodarone, sotalol) Antimalarials Organophosphate insecticides Antipsychotic agents Antidepressants Antibiotics (erythromycin)	Correction of electrolyte and acid–base abnormalities and hypoxia Magnesium sulphate, 2 g IV (adults) over 1–2 mins, repeated if necessary

(IV = intravenous; NSAID = non-steroidal anti-inflammatory drug; TCA = tricyclic antidepressant)

10.9 Specific antidotes used to treat poisoning

Mechanism of action	Examples of antidote	Poisoning treated
Receptor antagonists (block actions of toxin)	Naloxone	Opioids
	Flumazenil	Benzodiazepines
	Atropine	Organophosphorus compounds Carbamates
Effects on enzymes Correct functional deficiencies		
Glutathione	Acetylcysteine Methionine	Paracetamol
Pyridoxine	Pyridoxine	Isoniazid
Vitamin K	Vitamin K	Warfarin
Alcohol dehydrogenase inhibitors (prevent formation of toxic metabolites)	Fomepizole Ethanol	Ethylene glycol Methanol
Cholinesterase reactivators (restore cholinesterase function)	Pralidoxime Obidoxime	Organophosphorus compounds
Hydrolysing enzymes (metabolise toxin)	Glucarpidase	Methotrexate
Rhodanase enhancers (enhance enzyme-related detoxification by donating sulphur)	Sodium thiosulphate	Cyanide
Binding agents (prevent toxicity by binding to toxin)		
Chelating agents	Desferrioxamine	Iron
	Hydroxocobalamin Dicobalt edetate	Cyanide
	DMSA Sodium calcium edetate	Lead
	Protamine	Heparins
Decoy receptor	Andexanet alfa,	Apixaban, rivaroxaban
Antibody fragments	Digoxin Fab fragments	Digoxin
	Idarucizumab	Dabigatran etexilate
Reducing agents (convert methaemoglobin to haemoglobin)	Methylthioninium chloride	Aniline dyes, organic nitrites, phenacetin, sulphonamides
Oxidising agents (convert haemoglobin to methaemoglobin, which has high affinity for binding cyanide)	Sodium nitrite	Cyanide

(DMSA = dimercaptosuccinic acid)

If multiple ingestions of paracetamol have taken place over several hours ('staggered overdose') or days (e.g. chronic therapeutic excess), acetylcysteine may be indicated, but paracetamol treatment nomograms are not useful for assessing this; specific treatment recommendations are based on the reported dose ingested and vary between countries.

When indicated, acetylcysteine given intravenously (or orally in some countries) is highly efficacious if administered within 8 hours of overdose. However, efficacy declines thereafter, so administration should not be delayed to await a paracetamol blood concentration result in patients presenting after 8 hours. The antidote can be stopped if the paracetamol concentration is subsequently shown to be below the nomogram treatment line. High-dose acetylcysteine regimens are increasingly used in patients with very large paracetamol overdoses.

Non-allergic anaphylactic ('anaphylactoid') reactions are the most important adverse effects of acetylcysteine and are caused by dose-related histamine release. Common features are itching and urticaria, and in severe cases, bronchospasm and hypotension. Most cases can be managed by temporary discontinuation of acetylcysteine and administration of an antihistamine.

An alternative antidote is methionine 2.5 g orally (adult dose) every 4 hours to a total of four doses, but this may be less effective, especially after delayed presentation. Liver transplantation should be considered for paracetamol poisoning with life-threatening liver failure (p. 872).

Salicylates (aspirin)

Clinical features

Salicylate overdose commonly causes nausea, vomiting, sweating, tinnitus and deafness. Direct stimulation of the respiratory centre produces

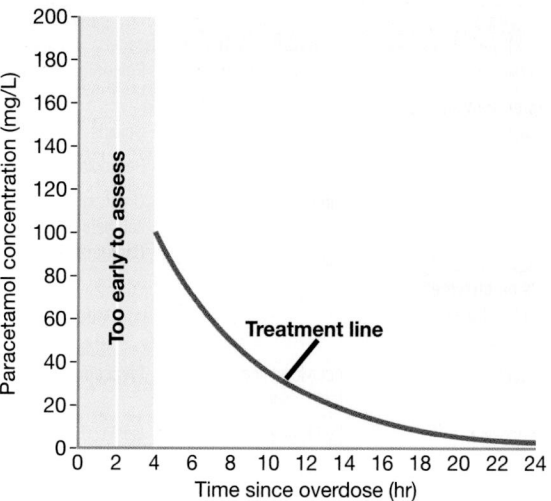

Fig. 10.2 Paracetamol treatment nomogram (UK). Above the treatment line, benefits of treatment outweigh risk. Below it, risks of treatment outweigh benefits.

hyperventilation and respiratory alkalosis. Peripheral vasodilatation with bounding pulses and profuse sweating occurs in moderately severe cases. Serious poisoning is associated with metabolic acidosis, hypoprothrombinaemia, hyperglycaemia, hyperpyrexia, renal failure, pulmonary oedema, shock and cerebral oedema. Agitation, delirium, coma and fits may occur, especially in children. Toxicity is enhanced by acidosis, which increases salicylate transfer across the blood–brain barrier.

Management

Activated charcoal should be administered if the patient presents sufficiently early. Multiple doses may enhance salicylate elimination, but are not routinely recommended.

The plasma salicylate concentration should be measured at least 2 (symptomatic patients) or 4 hours (asymptomatic patients) after overdose and repeated in suspected serious poisoning, as concentrations may continue to rise for several hours. Clinical status, however, is more important than the salicylate concentration when assessing severity.

Dehydration should be corrected carefully because of the risk of pulmonary oedema. Metabolic acidosis should be treated with intravenous sodium bicarbonate (8.4%), after plasma potassium has been corrected. Urinary alkalinisation is indicated for adults with salicylate concentrations above 500 mg/L.

Haemodialysis is very effective for removing salicylate and correcting associated acid–base and fluid balance abnormalities. It should be considered when serum concentrations are above 700 mg/L in adults with severe toxic features, or in renal failure, pulmonary oedema, coma, convulsions or refractory acidosis.

Non-steroidal anti-inflammatory drugs

Clinical features

Overdose of most non-steroidal anti-inflammatory drugs (NSAIDs) usually causes only minor abdominal discomfort, vomiting and/or diarrhoea, but convulsions can occur occasionally, especially with mefenamic acid. Coma, prolonged seizures, apnoea, liver dysfunction and renal failure may follow substantial overdose but are rare. Features of toxicity are unlikely to develop in patients who are asymptomatic more than 6 hours after overdose.

Management

Electrolytes, liver function tests and a full blood count should be checked in all but the most trivial cases. Activated charcoal may be given if the patient presents within 1 hour. Symptomatic treatment for nausea and gastrointestinal irritation may be needed.

Antidepressants

Tricyclic antidepressants

Overdose with tricyclic antidepressants (TCAs) carries a high morbidity and mortality because of their sodium channel-blocking, anticholinergic and α-adrenoceptor-blocking effects.

Clinical features

Anticholinergic effects are common (Box 10.10). Severe complications include convulsions, coma and arrhythmias (ventricular tachycardia, ventricular fibrillation and, less commonly, heart block). Hypotension results from inappropriate vasodilatation or impaired myocardial contractility. Serious complications appear more common with dosulepin and amitriptyline.

Management

Activated charcoal should be administered if the patient presents within 1 hour. A 12-lead ECG should be taken and continuous cardiac monitoring maintained for at least 6 hours. Prolongation of the QRS interval (especially if >0.16 secs) indicates severe sodium channel blockade and a high risk of arrhythmia (Fig. 10.3). QT interval prolongation may also occur. Arterial blood gases should be measured in suspected severe poisoning.

In patients with arrhythmias, significant QRS or QT prolongation or acidosis, intravenous sodium bicarbonate (50 mL of 8.4% solution) should be administered and repeated to correct pH. The correction of the acidosis and the increased extracellular sodium loading that improve sodium channel function and may bring about rapid improvement in ECG features and arrhythmias. Hypoxia and electrolyte abnormalities should also be corrected. Anti-arrhythmic drugs should be given only on specialist

	10.10 Anticholinergic and serotonergic feature clusters	
	Anticholinergic	**Serotonin syndrome**
Common causes	Benzodiazepines Antipsychotics TCAs Antihistamines Scopolamine Benzatropine Belladonna Some plants and mushrooms (see Box 10.18)	SSRIs MAOIs TCAs Amphetamines Tryptamines Buspirone Bupropion (especially in combination)
Clinical features		
Cardiovascular	Tachycardia, hypertension	Tachycardia, hyper- or hypotension
Central nervous system	Delirium, hallucinations, sedation	Delirium, hallucinations, sedation, coma
Muscle	Myoclonus	Shivering, tremor, myoclonus, raised creatine kinase
Temperature	Fever	Fever
Eyes	Diplopia, mydriasis	Normal pupil size
Abdomen	Ileus, palpable bladder	Diarrhoea, vomiting
Mouth	Dry	
Skin	Flushing, hot, dry	Flushing, sweating
Complications	Seizures	Seizures Rhabdomyolysis Renal failure Metabolic acidosis Coagulopathies

(MAOI = monoamine oxidase inhibitor; SSRI = selective serotonin re-uptake inhibitor; TCA = tricyclic antidepressant)

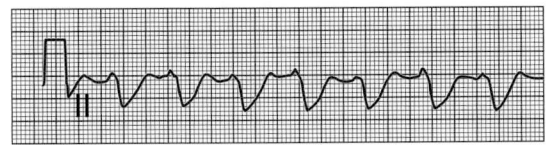

Fig. 10.3 ECG in severe tricyclic antidepressant poisoning. This rhythm strip shows a broad QRS complex due to impaired conduction.

advice. Prolonged seizures should be treated initially with intravenous benzodiazepines (see Box 10.8).

Selective serotonin and noradrenaline re-uptake inhibitors

Selective serotonin re-uptake inhibitor (SSRI) antidepressants (e.g. fluoxetine, paroxetine, fluvoxamine, sertraline, citalopram, escitalopram) are commonly used to treat depression and are less toxic in overdose than TCAs. The related serotonin–noradrenaline re-uptake inhibitors (SNRIs), such as venlafaxine and duloxetine, are also commonly used and are more toxic than SSRIs in overdose. The pre-synaptic alpha$_2$-antagonist mirtazapine, which increases central noradrenergic and serotinergic neurotransmission, is also increasingly encountered in overdose.

Clinical features and management

Overdose of SSRIs may produce nausea and vomiting, tremor, insomnia and sinus tachycardia. Agitation, drowsiness and convulsions occur infrequently and may be delayed for several hours. Serotonin syndrome may occur (see Box 10.10), especially if SSRIs are taken in combination or with other serotonergic agents. Cardiac arrhythmias occur infrequently and most patients require supportive care only. The toxic effects of SNRIs are similar but tachycardia, hypertension or hypotension and ECG changes (QRS and QT prolongation) may be more prominent and hypoglycaemia can also arise. Mirtazapine has lower toxicity, but high doses may cause sedation, tachycardia and serotonin syndrome.

Lithium

Severe lithium toxicity is uncommon after intentional acute overdose, but is more often encountered in patients taking therapeutic doses as a result of interactions with drugs such as diuretics or NSAIDs or because of worsening renal function. Severe toxicity is more common after acute overdose in patients already taking chronic therapy ('acute on chronic' poisoning).

Clinical features

Nausea, diarrhoea, polyuria, dizziness and tremor may progress to muscular weakness, drowsiness, delirium, myoclonus, fasciculations, choreoathetosis and renal failure. Coma, seizures, ataxia, cardiac dysrhythmias such as heart block, blood pressure disturbances and renal failure may occur in severe poisoning.

Management

Activated charcoal is ineffective. Early gastric lavage is of theoretical benefit, but lithium tablets are likely to remain intact in the stomach and may be too large for aspiration via a lavage tube. Whole bowel irrigation is often used after substantial overdose, but efficacy is unproven.

Lithium concentrations should be measured immediately (symptomatic patients) or after at least 6 hours (asymptomatic patients) following acute overdose. The usual therapeutic range is 0.4–1.0 mmol/L. Adequate hydration should be maintained with intravenous fluids. Seizures should be treated as in Box 10.8.

Haemodialysis should be considered for severe toxicity associated with high lithium concentrations (e.g. >4.0 mmol/L after chronic or 'acute on chronic' poisoning, or >7.5 mmol/L after acute poisoning). Lithium

concentrations are reduced substantially during dialysis, but rebound increases occur after discontinuation and multiple sessions are usually required.

Cardiovascular medications

Although not common, cardiovascular drug overdose is important because features of toxicity are often severe.

Beta-blockers

Major features of toxicity are bradycardia and hypotension; heart block, pulmonary oedema and cardiogenic shock occur in severe poisoning. Those with additional sodium channel-blocking effects (e.g. propranolol, acebutolol, carvedilol) may cause seizures, delirium and coma, while sotalol, which also blocks potassium channels, may cause QT$_c$ prolongation and torsades de pointes (see Box 10.8 and p. 418).

Management

Intravenous fluids may reverse hypotension, but care is required to avoid pulmonary oedema. Bradycardia and hypotension may respond to high doses of atropine (up to 3 mg in an adult) or an infusion of isoproterenol. Glucagon (5–10 mg IV over 10 mins, then 50–150 microgram/kg/hr by infusion) counteracts β-blockade by stimulating intracellular cyclic adenosine monophosphate (cAMP) production and is now more commonly used. In severe cases, 'hyperinsulinaemia euglycaemic therapy' has been used, as described under calcium channel blockers below. The efficacy of lipid emulsion therapy in severe poisoning with lipid-soluble β-blockers, such as propranolol, carvedilol and oxprenolol, is uncertain.

Calcium channel blockers

In therapeutic doses, dihydropyridine calcium channel blockers (e.g. nifedipine, amlodipine) cause vasodilatation, whereas diltiazem and verapamil have predominantly cardiac effects, including bradycardia and reduced myocardial contractility. All L-type calcium channel blockers, however, are highly toxic in overdose.

Clinical features

Hypotension due to vasodilatation or myocardial depression is common and bradycardias and heart block may also occur, especially with verapamil and diltiazem. Gastrointestinal disturbances, delirium, metabolic acidosis, hyperglycaemia and hyperkalaemia may also be present.

Management

Hypotension should be corrected with intravenous fluids, taking care to avoid pulmonary oedema. Persistent hypotension may respond to intravenous calcium gluconate (10 mg IV over 5 mins, repeated as required). Isoproterenol and glucagon may also be useful. Successful use of high-dose intravenous insulin with glucose (10%–20% dextrose with insulin initially at 0.5–2.0 U/kg/hr, increasing to 5–10 U/kg/hr according to clinical response), so-called 'hyperinsulinaemia euglycaemic therapy', has been reported in patients unresponsive to other strategies. The mechanism of action remains to be fully elucidated, but in states of shock myocardial metabolism switches from use of free fatty acids to glucose. Calcium channel blocker poisoning is also associated with hypoinsulinaemia and insulin resistance, impeding glucose uptake by myocytes. High doses of insulin inhibit lipolysis and increase glucose uptake and the efficiency of glucose utilisation. Cardiac pacing may be needed for severe unresponsive bradycardias or heart block. Lipid emulsion therapy has also been used in severe poisoning with apparent benefit, although evidence is largely anecdotal.

Digoxin and oleander

Poisoning with digoxin (a cardiac glycoside; p. XXX) is usually accidental, arising from prescription of an excessive dose, impairment of renal function or drug interactions. In South Asia, deliberate self-poisoning with

10

the plant yellow oleander (*Thevetia peruviana*), which contains cardiac glycosides, is common.

Clinical features

Cardiac effects include tachyarrhythmias (either atrial or ventricular) and bradycardias, with or without atrioventricular block. Ventricular bigeminy is common and atrial tachycardia with evidence of atrioventricular block is highly suggestive of the diagnosis. Severe poisoning is often associated with hyperkalaemia. Non-cardiac features include delirium, headache, nausea, vomiting, diarrhoea and (rarely) altered colour vision. Digoxin poisoning can be confirmed by elevated plasma concentration (usual therapeutic range 1.3–2.5 mmol/L). After chronic exposure, concentrations >5 mmol/L suggest serious poisoning, although this may sometimes also occur with lower concentrations.

Management

Activated charcoal is commonly administered to patients presenting soon after acute ingestion, although evidence of benefit is lacking. Urea, electrolytes and creatinine should be measured, a 12-lead ECG performed and cardiac monitoring instituted. Hypoxia, hypokalaemia (sometimes caused by concurrent diuretic use), hypomagnesaemia and acidosis increase the risk of arrhythmias and should be corrected. Significant bradycardias may respond to atropine, although temporary pacing is sometimes needed. Ventricular arrhythmias may respond to intravenous magnesium (see Box 10.8). If available, digoxin-specific antibody fragments should be administered when there are severe refractory ventricular arrhythmias or bradycardias. These are effective for both digoxin and yellow oleander poisoning.

Iron

Overdose with iron can cause severe and sometimes fatal poisoning, with toxicity of individual iron preparations related to their elemental iron content.

Clinical features

Early features include gastrointestinal disturbance with the passage of grey or black stools, progressing to hyperglycaemia, leucocytosis, haematemesis, rectal bleeding, drowsiness, convulsions, coma, metabolic acidosis and cardiovascular collapse in severe cases. Early symptoms may improve or resolve within 6–12 hours, but hepatocellular necrosis can develop 12–24 hours after overdose and occasionally progresses to hepatic failure. Gastrointestinal strictures are late complications.

Management

Activated charcoal is ineffective, but gastric lavage or whole bowel elimination may be considered in patients presenting soon after substantial overdose, although efficacy is unknown. Serum iron concentration should be measured at least 4 hours after overdose or earlier if there are features of toxicity. Desferrioxamine chelates iron and should be administered immediately in patients with severe features (e.g. coma, shock, metabolic acidosis, haemolysis), without waiting for serum iron concentrations, as well as symptomatic patients with high serum iron concentrations (e.g. >5 mg/L). Desferrioxamine may cause hypotension, allergic reactions and occasionally pulmonary oedema. Otherwise, treatment is supportive and directed at complications.

Antipsychotic drugs

Antipsychotic drugs (see Box 31.26) are often prescribed for patients at high risk of self-harm or suicide and are often taken in overdose.

Clinical features

Anticholinergic features (see Box 10.10) including drowsiness, tachycardia and hypotension are common and convulsions may occur. Acute dystonias, including oculogyric crisis, torticollis and trismus, may occur after overdose with typical antipsychotics like haloperidol or

chlorpromazine (Box 10.8). QT interval prolongation and torsades de pointes can occur with some typical (e.g. haloperidol) and atypical (e.g. quetiapine, amisulpride, ziprasidone) agents.

Management

Activated charcoal may be of benefit if given early. Cardiac monitoring should be undertaken for at least 6 hours. Management is largely supportive, with treatment directed at complications (see Box 10.8).

Antidiabetic agents

Overdose is uncommon, but toxic effects can be severe.

Clinical features

Sulphonylureas, meglitinides (e.g. nateglinide, repaglinide) and parenteral insulin cause hypoglycaemia when taken in overdose, although insulin is non-toxic if ingested by mouth. The duration of hypoglycaemia depends on the half-life or release characteristics of the preparation and may be prolonged over several days with long-acting agents such as glibenclamide, insulin degludec or insulin glargine.

Features of hypoglycaemia include nausea, agitation, sweating, aggression, delirium, tachycardia, hypothermia, drowsiness, convulsions and coma (p. 719). Permanent neurological damage can occur if hypoglycaemia is prolonged. Hypoglycaemia can be diagnosed using bedside glucose strips, but venous blood should also be sent for laboratory confirmation.

Metformin is uncommonly associated with hypoglycaemia. Its major toxic effect is lactic acidosis, which can have a high mortality, and is particularly common in older patients and those with renal or hepatic impairment, or when ethanol has been co-ingested. Other features of metformin overdose are nausea, vomiting, diarrhoea, abdominal pain, drowsiness, coma, hypotension and cardiovascular collapse.

There is limited experience of overdose involving thiazolidinediones (e.g. pioglitazone) and dipeptidyl peptidase 4 (DPP-4) inhibitors (e.g. sitagliptin), but significant hypoglycaemia is unlikely.

Management

Activated charcoal should be considered for recent substantial overdose. Venous blood glucose and urea and electrolytes should be measured and measurement repeated regularly. Hypoglycaemia should be corrected using oral or intravenous glucose (50 mL of 50% dextrose); an infusion of 10%–20% dextrose may be required to prevent recurrence. Intramuscular glucagon can be used as an alternative, especially if intravenous access is unavailable. If the patient remains hypoglycaemic in spite of these measures, subcutaneous or intravenous octreotide may be used. Failure to regain consciousness within a few minutes of normalisation of the blood glucose can indicate that a central nervous system (CNS) depressant has also been ingested, the hypoglycaemia has been prolonged, or there is another cause of coma (e.g. cerebral haemorrhage or oedema).

Arterial blood gases and plasma lactate should be taken after metformin overdose; acidosis should be corrected with intravenous sodium bicarbonate (250 mL 1.26% solution or 50 mL 8.4% solution, repeated as necessary). In severe cases, haemodialysis or haemodiafiltration is used.

Pharmaceutical agents less commonly taken in poisoning

An overview of the clinical features and management for drugs less commonly involved in poisoning is provided in Box 10.11.

Drugs of misuse

Drugs of misuse are common causes of toxicity causing presentation to hospitals. Management has recently become more complex because of the emergence of 'new psychoactive substances' (NPS). These are often chemically related to traditional drugs of misuse, but with structural modifications made to evade legal control. The constituents of branded NPS products are often unknown and knowledge about the clinical features and management of NPS toxicity is limited.

Depressants

These produce CNS depression, including drowsiness, ataxia, delirium and coma, sometimes with respiratory depression, airway compromise, aspiration pneumonia and respiratory arrest (Box 10.12). Other complications of coma include pressure blisters or sores and rhabdomyolysis. Effects are potentiated by other CNS depressants, including alcohol.

Essential supportive care is detailed in Box 10.8. Antidotes are available for some depressants.

Benzodiazepines

Benzodiazepines (e.g. diazepam, lorazepam, midazolam) and related substances (e.g. zopiclone) are of low toxicity when taken alone in overdose, but can enhance CNS and respiratory depression when taken with other sedative agents, including alcohol or heroin. They are more hazardous in older people and those with chronic lung or neuromuscular disease (see Box 10.12). Dependency develops after chronic use over a few weeks and features of withdrawal commonly occur after rapid discontinuation of use. Highly potent novel benzodiazepines, such as etizolam, flualprazolam and flubromazolam, have recently been encountered, especially in counterfeit tablets purchased from dealers or via the internet; these can cause toxic effects after very low doses.

The specific benzodiazepine antagonist flumazenil (0.5 mg IV, repeated if needed) increases conscious level in patients with benzodiazepine overdose, but carries a risk of seizures and is contraindicated in patients co-ingesting pro-convulsants (e.g. TCAs, cocaine) and in those with a history of epilepsy.

Opioids

Toxicity may result from misuse of illicit drugs such as heroin or from intentional or accidental overdose of medicinal opiates. In recent years, fentanyl and its analogues have increasingly been used to fortify heroin preparations in North America. These synthetic compounds are highly potent, their presence increases the risk of overdose and there has been a sharp increase in deaths related to opioid overdose in the United States and Canada.

---

i | **10.11 Clinical features and specific management of drugs less commonly involved in poisoning**

Substance	Clinical features	Management
Anticonvulsants		
Carbamazepine, phenytoin	Cerebellar signs Convulsions Cardiac arrhythmias Coma	Multiple-dose activated charcoal (carbamazepine)
Sodium valproate	Coma Metabolic acidosis Hepatotoxicity	Haemodialysis for severe poisoning L-carnitine may be useful for severe cases with hyperammonaemia or hepatotoxicity
Isoniazid	Peripheral neuropathy Convulsions	Activated charcoal IV pyridoxine
Theophylline	Cardiac arrhythmias Convulsions Coma	Multiple-dose activated charcoal
Antimalarial drugs		
Chloroquine	Acidosis and hypokalaemia Visual loss Convulsions, coma ECG changes and arrhythmias	Correction of pH (but not potassium) Monitoring and treatment of cardiac rhythm High-dose diazepam with mechanical ventilation
Quinine	Tremor, tinnitus, deafness, ataxia, convulsions, coma Haemolysis ECG changes and arrhythmias Retinal toxicity	Correction of pH (but not potassium) Monitoring and treatment of cardiac rhythm Multiple-dose activated charcoal No effective treatment for visual loss

---

i | **10.12 Stimulant, sedative and opioid feature clusters**

	Stimulant	Sedative hypnotic	Opioid
Common causes	Amphetamines MDMA ('ecstasy') Ephedrine Pseudoephedrine Cocaine Cannabis Phencyclidine Cathinones (e.g. mephedrone) Benzylpiperazine	Benzodiazepines Barbiturates Ethanol GHB	Heroin Morphine Methadone Fentanyl and derivatives Oxycodone Dihydrocodeine Codeine Pethidine Buprenorphine Dextropropoxyphene Tramadol
Clinical features			
Respiratory	Tachypnoea	Reduced respiratory rate and ventilation[1]	Reduced respiratory rate and ventilation
Cardiovascular	Tachycardia, hypertension	Hypotension[1]	Hypotension, relative bradycardia
Central nervous system	Restlessness, anxiety, anorexia, insomnia	Delirium, hallucinations, slurred speech	Delirium, hallucinations, slurred speech
	Hallucinations	Sedation, coma[1]	Sedation, coma[2]
Muscle	Tremor	Ataxia, reduced muscle tone	Ataxia, reduced muscle tone
Temperature	Fever	Hypothermia	Hypothermia
Eyes	Mydriasis	Diplopia, strabismus, nystagmus Normal pupil size	Miosis
Abdomen	Abdominal pain, diarrhoea	–	Ileus
Mouth	Dry	–	–
Skin	Piloerection	Blisters, pressure sores	Needle tracks[2]
Complications	Seizures Myocardial infarction Dysrhythmias Rhabdomyolysis Renal failure Intracerebral haemorrhage or infarction	Respiratory failure[1] Aspiration	Respiratory failure[2] Non-cardiogenic pulmonary oedema Aspiration

[1]Especially barbiturates. [2]Intravenous use.
(GHB = gamma hydroxybutyrate; MDMA = 3,4-methylene-dioxymethamphetamine)

10

Intravenous or smoked heroin gives a rapid, intensely pleasurable experience, often accompanied by heightened sexual arousal. Physical dependence occurs within a few weeks of regular high-dose use. Withdrawal can start within 12 hours, causing intense craving, rhinorrhoea, lacrimation, yawning, perspiration, shivering, piloerection, vomiting, diarrhoea and abdominal cramps. Examination reveals tachycardia, hypertension, mydriasis and facial flushing.

Commonly encountered opioids and clinical features of poisoning are shown in Box 10.12. Needle tracks may be visible in intravenous users and there may be drug-related paraphernalia. Methadone may also cause QT_c prolongation and torsades de pointes. Features of opioid poisoning can be prolonged for up to 48 hours after use of long-acting agents such as methadone or oxycodone.

Use of the specific opioid antagonist naloxone (0.4–2 mg IV in an adult, repeated if necessary) may obviate the need for intubation, although excessive doses may precipitate acute withdrawal in chronic opiate users and breakthrough pain in those receiving opioids for pain management. Repeated doses or an infusion are often required because the half-life of the antidote is short compared to that of most opiates, especially those with prolonged elimination. Patients should be monitored for at least 6 hours after the last naloxone dose. Rare complications of naloxone therapy include fits, ventricular arrhythmias and pulmonary oedema.

Gamma hydroxybutyrate

Gamma hydroxybutyrate (GHB), and the related compounds gamma butyrolactone (GBL), 1,4 butanediol, gamma-hydroxyvaleric acid (GHV) and gamma-valerolactone (GVL), are sedative substances with psychedelic and body-building effects. They are usually supplied as clear fluids and have been administered surreptitiously to enable drug-facilitated sexual assaults or other crimes.

As well as sedative hypnotic features (see Box 10.12), toxicity may cause nausea, diarrhoea, vertigo, tremor, myoclonus, extrapyramidal signs, euphoria, bradycardia, convulsions, metabolic acidosis, hypokalaemia and hyperglycaemia. Coma usually resolves abruptly within a few hours, but occasionally persists for several days. Dependence may develop in regular users, who experience severe, prolonged withdrawal effects if use is discontinued suddenly.

Management is largely supportive. All patients should be observed for a minimum of 2 hours and until symptoms resolve, with monitoring of blood pressure, heart rate, respiratory rate and oxygenation. Withdrawal symptoms may require treatment with very high doses of benzodiazepine.

Stimulants and entactogens

These are sympathomimetic and serotonergic amines that have overlapping clinical features, depending on the balance of their stimulant (see Box 10.12) and serotonergic (see Box 10.10) effects. As well as traditional drugs such as cocaine, amphetamines and ecstasy, the group includes many more recently emerging new psychoactive substances, including cathinones (e.g. mephedrone), piperazines (e.g. benzylpiperazine), piperadines (e.g. ethylphenidate), benzofurans (e.g. 5-aminopropylbenzofuran) and NBOMe compounds (e.g. 25I-NBOMe).

Cocaine

Cocaine is available as a water-soluble hydrochloride salt powder suitable for nasal inhalation ('snorting'), or as insoluble free-base ('crack' cocaine) 'rocks' that, unlike the hydrochloride salt, vaporise at high temperature and can be smoked, giving a more rapid and intense effect.

Effects appear rapidly after inhalation and especially after smoking. Sympathomimetic stimulant effects predominate (see Box 10.12). Serious complications usually occur within 3 hours of use and include coronary artery spasm, leading to myocardial ischaemia or infarction, hypotension and ventricular arrhythmias. Cocaine toxicity should be considered in younger adults presenting with ischaemic chest pain.

Hyperpyrexia, rhabdomyolysis, acute renal failure and disseminated intravascular coagulation may occur.

A 12-lead ECG and ECG monitoring should be undertaken. ST segment elevation may occur in the absence of myocardial infarction and troponin T estimations are the most sensitive and specific markers of myocardial damage. Benzodiazepines and intravenous nitrates are useful for managing patients with chest pain or hypertension. Acidosis should be corrected and physical cooling measures used for hyperpyrexia. Beta-blockers may be contraindicated because of the risk of unopposed α-adrenoceptor stimulation, but this is debated. Coronary angiography should be considered in patients with myocardial infarction or acute coronary syndromes.

Amphetamines and cathinones

Amphetamine-related compounds include amphetamine sulphate ('speed'), methylamphetamine ('crystal meth') and 3,4-methylenedioxymethamphetamine (MDMA, 'ecstasy'). Synthetic cathinones include mephedrone, methylenedioxypyrovalerone (MDPV) and n-ethyl pentylone. Tolerance is common, leading regular users to seek ever-higher doses.

Toxic features usually appear within a few minutes of use and last 4–6 hours, or substantially longer after a large overdose. Sympathomimetic stimulant and serotonergic effects are common (see Boxes 10.10 and 10.12). Some users develop hyponatraemia as a result of excessive water-drinking or inappropriate vasopressin (antidiuretic hormone, ADH) secretion. Muscle rigidity, pain and bruxism (clenching of the jaw), hyperpyrexia, rhabdomyolysis, metabolic acidosis, acute renal failure, disseminated intravascular coagulation, hepatocellular necrosis, acute respiratory distress syndrome (ARDS) and cardiovascular collapse have all been described following MDMA use. Cerebral infarction and haemorrhage have been reported, especially after intravenous amphetamine use.

Management is supportive and directed at complications (see Box 10.8).

Hallucinogens

Cannabis

Derived from the dried leaves and flowers of *Cannabis sativa*, cannabis produces euphoria, perceptual alterations and conjunctival injection, followed by enhanced appetite, relaxation and occasionally hypertension, tachycardia, slurred speech and ataxia. Effects occur 10–30 minutes after smoking or 1–3 hours after ingestion, and last 4–8 hours. Solutions are also available for 'vaping' using electronic cigarettes. High doses of cannabis may produce anxiety, delirium, hallucinations and psychosis, but serious acute toxicity is uncommon and supportive treatment is all that is required. Psychological dependence is common, but tolerance and withdrawal symptoms are unusual. Long-term use is thought to increase the lifetime risk of psychosis and a cannabis hyperemesis syndrome is also recognised, involving episodes if vomiting that respond poorly to antiemetics, but improve on discontinuation of cannabis use.

Synthetic cannabinoid receptor agonists

Synthetic cannabinoid receptor agonists (SCRAs), sometimes referred to collectively as 'spice', have recently been in common use as legal alternatives to cannabis. More than 150 different SCRAs have been encountered, with recently prevalent examples including MDMB-CHMICA, 5F-MDMB-PINACA and AMB-FUBINACA. They are usually sprayed on to a herbal smoking mix and packaged as smoking products with appealing brand names. These may contain more than one SCRA and content may change with time. 'Vaping' of SCRA solutions has also been reported.

The toxic effects of SCRAs differ from those of cannabis, being generally more marked and including agitation, panic, delirium, hallucinations, tachycardia, ECG changes, hypertonia, dyspnoea and vomiting. Coma, respiratory acidosis, seizures, hypokalaemia and renal dysfunction may also occur. There is increasing evidence of pharmacological tolerance and dependence with SCRA use and features of withdrawal may occur after discontinuation. Treatment of intoxication is supportive.

Tryptamines

These are predominantly 5-hydroxytryptamine (5-HT, serotonin; especially 5-HT2A) agonists with associated stimulant effects. Typical clinical features include hallucinations, agitation, delirium, hypertension, tachycardia, sweating, anxiety and headache. Serotonin syndrome may occur (see Box 10.10), especially if tryptamines are used in combination with other serotonergic agents. Naturally occurring examples are psilocin and psilocybin, found in 'magic mushrooms', and dimethyltryptamine (DMT) in traditional ayahuasca brews. Synthetic tryptamines, such as alpha-methyltryptamine (AMT), have also been encountered.

D-Lysergic acid diethylamide

D-Lysergic acid diethylamide (LSD) is a synthetic ergoline usually ingested as small squares of impregnated absorbent paper (often printed with a distinctive design) or as 'microdots'. The drug causes perceptual effects, such as heightened visual awareness of colours or distortion of images. Hallucinations may be pleasurable or terrifying ('bad trip'). Other features are delirium, agitation, aggression, dilated pupils, hypertension, pyrexia and metabolic acidosis. Psychosis may sometimes last several days.

Patients with psychotic reactions or CNS depression should be observed in hospital, preferably in a quiet, dimly lit room to minimise external stimulation. A benzodiazepine can be used for sedation if required, avoiding antipsychotics if possible because these may precipitate cardiovascular collapse or convulsions.

Dissociative drugs

Ketamine, its *N*-ethyl derivative methoxetamine and phencyclidine (now rarely encountered) produce a sense of dissociation from reality, often associated with visual and auditory distortions. Memory loss, impaired consciousness, agitation, hallucinations, tremors and numbness may also occur. Long-term ketamine or methoxetamine use can cause severe chronic cystitis with dysuria, frequency, urgency, haematuria and incontinence. These features are often severe, debilitating and difficult to treat. Management of acute intoxication is supportive.

Volatile substances

Inhalation of volatile nitrites (e.g. amyl nitrite, isobutyl nitrite), often sold in bottles or vials as 'poppers', is reported to produce a feeling of pleasure and warmth, relax the anal sphincter and prolong orgasm. These potent vasodilators commonly provoke headache, dizziness, hypotension and tachycardia. They also oxidise haemoglobin to produce methaemoglobinaemia, with resulting breathlessness and delirium. Severe methaemoglobinaemia is treated with methylthioninium chloride ('methylene blue', see Fig. 10.1) Regular use may also precipitate maculopathy with visual loss.

Several volatile solvents found in household products, such as propane, butane, toluene and trichloroethylene, have a mild euphoriant effect if inhaled. Serious toxic effects can occur, including reduced level of consciousness, seizures and cardiac arrhythmias; there is also a risk of asphyxia from some methods of inhalation.

Nitrous oxide is an anaesthetic gas, but small canisters of it are sold for the domestic production of whipped cream and the contents of these can be transferred to balloons for inhalation. The gas has euphoriant effects ('laughing gas'), but hazards include asphyxia from inhalation without oxygen, or vitamin B_{12} inactivation from chronic use leading to megaloblastic anaemia, psychosis and other neurological sequelae.

Body packers and body stuffers

Body packers ('mules') attempt to smuggle illicit drugs (usually cocaine, heroin or amphetamines) by ingesting multiple small packages wrapped in several layers of clingfilm or in condoms. Body stuffers are those who have ingested unpackaged or poorly wrapped substances, often to avoid

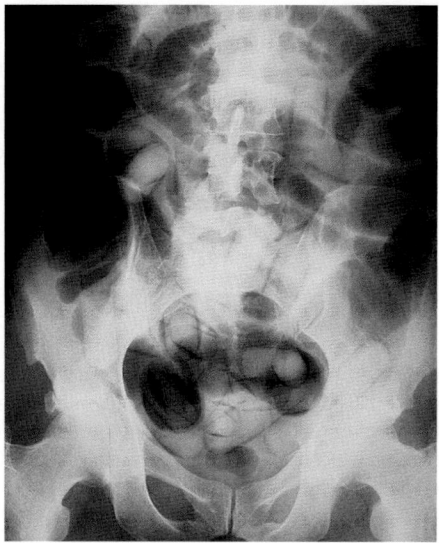

Fig. 10.4 Abdominal X-ray of a body packer showing multiple drug-filled condoms.

arrest. Both groups are at risk of severe toxicity if the packages rupture. This is more likely for body stuffers, who may develop symptoms of poisoning within 8 hours of ingestion. The risk of poisoning depends on the quality of the wrapping, and the amount and type of drug ingested. Cocaine, for example, presents a much higher risk than heroin because of its high toxicity and lack of a specific antidote.

Patients suspected of body packing or stuffing should be admitted for observation. A careful history taken in private is important, but for obvious reasons patients may withhold details of the drugs involved. Examination of the mouth, rectum and vagina as possible sites for concealed drugs should be arranged with patient consent, consistent with local laws. A urine toxicology screen performed at intervals may provide evidence of leakage, although positive results may reflect earlier drug use. Packages may be visible on plain abdominal films (Fig. 10.4), but ultrasound and computed tomography (CT) are more sensitive. One of these (preferably CT) should be performed in all suspected body packers.

Antimotility agents are often used by body packers to prevent premature passage of packages; it can take several days for packages to pass spontaneously, during which the carrier is at risk from package rupture. Whole bowel irrigation is commonly used to accelerate passage and is continued until all packages have passed. Surgery may be required when there is mechanical bowel obstruction or when evolving clinical features suggest package rupture, especially with cocaine.

Chemicals and pesticides

Carbon monoxide

Carbon monoxide (CO) is a colourless, odourless gas produced by faulty appliances burning organic fuels. It is also present in vehicle exhaust fumes and sometimes in smoke from house fires or barbeques. It binds with haemoglobin (to form carboxyhaemoglobin) and cytochrome oxidase, reducing tissue oxygen delivery and inhibiting cellular respiration. CO is a common cause of death by poisoning and most patients die before reaching hospital.

Clinical features

Early features include headache, nausea, irritability, weakness and tachypnoea. The cause of these non-specific features may not be obvious if the exposure is occult, such as from a faulty domestic appliance. Subsequently, ataxia, nystagmus, drowsiness and hyper-reflexia may develop, progressing to coma, convulsions, hypotension, respiratory

10

depression, cardiovascular collapse and death. Myocardial ischaemia may result in arrhythmias or myocardial infarction. Cerebral oedema is common and rhabdomyolysis may cause myoglobinuria and renal failure. In those who recover from acute toxicity, longer-term neuropsychiatric effects are common, such as personality change, memory loss and concentration impairment. Extrapyramidal effects, urinary or faecal incontinence, and gait disturbance may also occur. Poisoning during pregnancy may cause fetal hypoxia and intrauterine death.

Management

Patients should be removed from exposure as soon as possible and resuscitated as necessary. A high concentration of oxygen should be administered via a tightly fitting facemask; this reduces the half-life of carboxyhaemoglobin from 4–6 hours to about 40 minutes. Measurement of carboxyhaemoglobin is useful for confirming exposure; levels > 20% suggest significant exposure, but do not correlate well with the severity of poisoning, partly because concentrations fall rapidly after removal of the patient from exposure, especially if supplemental oxygen has been given.

An ECG should be performed in all patients with acute CO poisoning, especially those with pre-existing heart disease. Arterial blood gas analysis should be checked in those with serious poisoning. Pulse oximetry may provide misleading oxygen saturation levels because the devices do not distinguish between carboxyhaemoglobin and oxyhaemoglobin. Excessive intravenous fluid administration should be avoided, particularly in the older patients, because of the risk of pulmonary and cerebral oedema. Convulsions should be controlled with diazepam.

Hyperbaric oxygen therapy is controversial. At 2.5 atmospheres, the half-life of carboxyhaemoglobin is reduced to about 20 minutes and the amount of oxygen dissolved in plasma is increased 10-fold, but systematic reviews have not consistently shown improved clinical outcomes. The logistical difficulties of transporting sick patients to hyperbaric chambers and managing them therein are substantial.

Organophosphorus insecticides and nerve agents

Organophosphorus (OP) compounds (Box 10.13) have been widely used as pesticides, especially in low- and middle-income countries. Case fatality following deliberate ingestion is high (5%–20%). Legal controls banning the most toxic examples have substantially reduced local rates of suicide, for example in Sri Lanka.

Nerve agents, developed for chemical warfare, are derived from OP insecticides and are much more toxic. They are commonly classified as G (originally synthesised in Germany) or V ('venomous') agents. The 'G' agents, such as tabun, sarin and soman, are volatile, absorbed by inhalation or via the skin, and dissipate rapidly after use. 'V' agents, such as

VX, are contact poisons unless aerosolised and contaminate ground for weeks or months. Novichok agents, originally developed in the former Soviet Union, have also recently been encountered.

The toxicology and management of nerve agent and pesticide poisoning are similar.

Mechanism of toxicity

OP compounds inactivate acetylcholinesterase (AChE), resulting in the accumulation of acetylcholine (ACh) in cholinergic synapses (Fig. 10.5). Initially, spontaneous hydrolysis of the OP–enzyme complex allows reactivation of the enzyme but, subsequently, loss of a chemical group from the OP–enzyme complex prevents further enzyme reactivation. After this process (termed 'ageing') has taken place, new enzyme needs to be synthesised before function can be restored. The rate of 'ageing' is an important determinant of toxicity and is more rapid with dimethyl (3.7 hours) than diethyl (31 hours) compounds (see Box 10.13) and especially rapid after exposure to nerve agents (soman in particular), which cause 'ageing' within minutes.

Clinical features and management

OP poisoning causes an acute cholinergic phase, which may occasionally be followed by the 'intermediate syndrome' and organophosphate-induced delayed polyneuropathy (OPIDN). The onset, severity and duration depend on the route of exposure and agent involved.

Acute cholinergic syndrome

This usually starts within a few minutes of exposure and nicotinic or muscarinic features may be present (Box 10.14). Vomiting and profuse diarrhoea are typical following ingestion. Bronchoconstriction, bronchorrhoea and salivation may cause severe respiratory compromise. Excess sweating and miosis are characteristic and the presence of muscular fasciculations strongly suggests the diagnosis, although this feature is often absent, even in serious poisoning. Subsequently, generalised flaccid paralysis may develop and affect respiratory and ocular muscles,

| i | 10.13 Organophosphorus compounds |

Nerve agents

- G agents: sarin, tabun, soman
- V agents: VX, VE
- Novichok agents

Insecticides

Dimethyl compounds

- Dichlorvos
- Fenthion
- Malathion
- Methamidophos

Diethyl compounds

- Chlorpyrifos
- Diazinon
- Parathion-ethyl
- Quinalphos

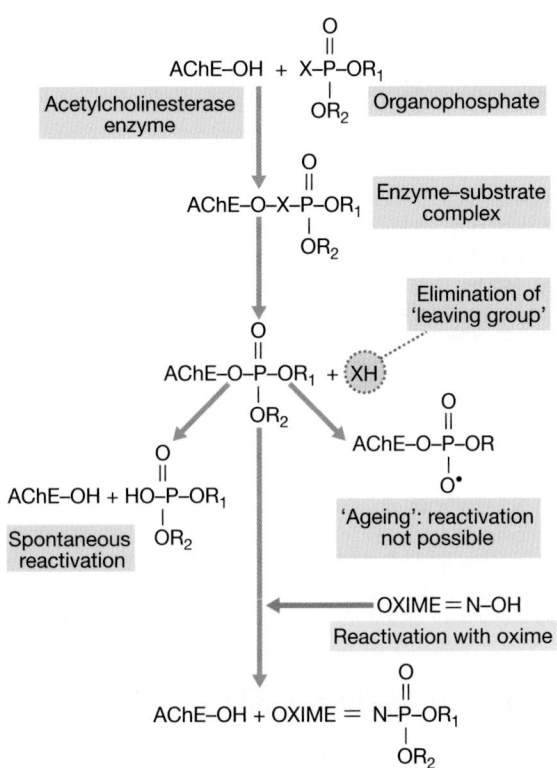

Fig. 10.5 Mechanism of toxicity of organophosphorus compounds and treatment with oxime.

i	**10.14 Cholinergic features in poisoning***	
	Muscarinic	**Nicotinic**
Respiratory	Bronchorrhoea, bronchoconstriction	Reduced ventilation
Circulation	Bradycardia, hypotension	Tachycardia, hypertension
Higher mental function	Anxiety, delirium, psychosis	
Muscle	–	Fasciculation, paralysis
Temperature	Fever	–
Eyes	Diplopia, miosis, lacrimation	Mydriasis
Abdomen	Vomiting, profuse diarrhoea	–
Mouth	Salivation	–
Skin	Sweating	–
Complications	Coma, seizures, respiratory depression	

*Both muscarinic and nicotinic features occur in OP poisoning. Nicotinic features occur in nicotine poisoning and Black Widow spider bites. Cholinergic features are sometimes seen with some mushrooms.

resulting in respiratory failure. Ataxia, coma, convulsions, cardiac repolarisation abnormalities and torsades de pointes may occur.

Management

The airway should be cleared of excessive secretions, breathing and circulation assessed, high-flow oxygen administered and intravenous access obtained. Appropriate external decontamination is needed (p. 221). Gastric lavage or activated charcoal may be considered if the patient presents sufficiently early. Seizures should be treated as described in Box 10.8. The ECG, oxygen saturation, blood gases, temperature, urea and electrolytes, amylase and glucose should be monitored closely.

Early use of sufficient doses of atropine is potentially life-saving in patients with severe toxicity. Atropine reverses ACh-induced bronchospasm, bronchorrhoea, bradycardia and hypotension. When the diagnosis is uncertain, a marked increase in heart rate associated with skin flushing after a 1 mg intravenous dose makes OP poisoning unlikely. In OP poisoning, atropine (2 mg IV) should be administered and this dose should be doubled every 5–10 minutes until clinical improvement occurs. Further bolus doses should be given until secretions are controlled, the skin is dry, blood pressure is adequate and heart rate is >80 bpm. Large doses may be needed, but excessive doses may cause anticholinergic effects (see Box 10.10).

In severe poisoning requiring atropine, an oxime (such as pralidoxime chloride or obidoxime) is generally recommended if available, although efficacy is debated. This may reverse or prevent muscle weakness, convulsions or coma, especially if given rapidly after exposure. Oximes reactivate AChE that has not undergone 'ageing' and are therefore less effective with dimethyl compounds and nerve agents, especially soman. Oximes may provoke hypotension, especially if administered rapidly.

Intravenous magnesium sulphate has been reported to increase survival in animals and in small human studies of OP poisoning; however, further clinical trial evidence is needed before this can be recommended routinely.

Ventilatory support should be instituted before the patient develops respiratory failure. Benzodiazepines may be used to treat agitation, fasciculations and seizures and for sedation during mechanical ventilation.

Exposure is confirmed by measurement of plasma or red blood cell cholinesterase activity, but antidote use should not be delayed pending results. Plasma cholinesterase is reduced more rapidly, but is less specific than red cell cholinesterase. Values correlate poorly with the severity of clinical features, but are usually < 10% in severe poisoning, 20%–50% in moderate poisoning and > 50% in subclinical poisoning.

The acute cholinergic phase usually lasts 48–72 hours, with most patients requiring intensive cardiorespiratory support and monitoring. Cholinergic features may be prolonged over several weeks with some lipid-soluble agents.

Intermediate syndrome

About 20% of patients with OP poisoning develop weakness that spreads rapidly from the ocular muscles to those of the head and neck, proximal limbs and the muscles of respiration, resulting in ventilatory failure. This 'intermediate syndrome' generally develops 1–4 days after exposure, often after resolution of the acute cholinergic syndrome and may last 2–3 weeks. There is no specific treatment and supportive care is needed, including maintenance of airway and ventilation.

Organophosphate-induced delayed polyneuropathy

Organophosphate-induced delayed polyneuropathy (OPIDN) is a rare complication that usually occurs 2–3 weeks after acute exposure. It is a mixed sensory/motor polyneuropathy, affecting long myelinated neurons especially, and appears to result from inhibition of enzymes other than AChE. It is a feature of poisoning with some OPs such as triorthocresyl phosphate, but is less common with nerve agents. Early clinical features are muscle cramps followed by numbness and paraesthesiae, proceeding to flaccid paralysis of the lower and subsequently the upper limbs, with foot and wrist drop and a high-stepping gait, progressing to paraplegia. Sensory loss may also be present but is variable. Initially, tendon reflexes are reduced or lost but mild spasticity may develop later.

There is no specific therapy for OPIDN. Regular physiotherapy may limit deformity caused by muscle wasting. Recovery is often incomplete and may be limited to the hands and feet, although substantial functional recovery after 1–2 years may occur, especially in younger patients.

Carbamate insecticides

Carbamate insecticides such as bendiocarb, carbofuran, carbaryl and methomyl inhibit a number of tissue esterases, including AChE. The mechanism, clinical features and management of toxicity are similar to those of OP compounds. However, clinical features are usually less severe and of shorter duration, because the carbamate–AChE complex dissociates quickly, with a half-life of 30–40 minutes, and does not undergo ageing. Also, carbamates penetrate the CNS poorly. Intermediate syndrome and OPIDN are not common features of carbamate poisoning. In spite of this, case fatality can be high for some carbamates, depending on their formulation.

Atropine may be given intravenously as for OP poisoning (see above, this section) is unnecessary.

Paraquat

Paraquat is a herbicide that has been widely used across the world, although it has been banned in the European Union and some other countries for many years. It is highly toxic if ingested, with clinical features including oral burns, vomiting and diarrhoea, progressing to pneumonitis, pulmonary fibrosis and multi-organ failure.

Exposure can be confirmed by a urinary dithionite test, while the plasma paraquat concentration gives an indication of prognosis. There is no specific antidote, but activated charcoal is commonly administered. Immunosuppression with glucocorticoids and cyclophosphamide is sometimes used, but evidence for benefit is weak. Irrespective of treatment, death is common and may occur within 24 hours with substantial poisoning or after 1–2 weeks with lower doses.

Alcohols and glycols

Ethanol (alcohol, ethyl alcohol) is commonly consumed in alcoholic beverages but is also found in some cosmetics, perfumes and antiseptic hand gels. It may also be used as an industrial solvent or produced illicitly. It can also be used as an antidote in ethylene glycol or methanol poisoning (see below). The health effects of chronic alcohol use are described in Chapter 31.

Acute alcohol consumption causes concentration-related toxicity, although it is unusual for ethanol toxicity alone to precipitate hospital admission. Severe and fatal toxicity, however, is more likely in children or when alcohol has been used with other sedative substances such as opioids or benzodiazepines. High concentrations of alcohol produce incoordination and slurred speech, and this may progress to unconsciousness with respiratory depression, loss of airway reflexes, hypotension, metabolic acidosis and occasionally hypothermia, hypoglycaemia and convulsions. Investigations should include measurement of blood alcohol concentration, arterial blood gases as well as full blood count, glucose, renal and hepatic function. Management involves protection of the airway, maintenance of ventilation and oxygenation, fluid resuscitation, correction of hypoglycaemia with glucose and treatment of convulsions. Thiamine should be administered if chronic excess alcohol use is suspected. Haemodialysis is effective for increasing alcohol clearance and should be considered in severe cases associated with very high ethanol concentrations.

Ethylene glycol (1,2-ethanediol) is found in antifreeze, brake fluids and, in lower concentrations, windscreen washes. Methanol is present in some antifreeze products and commercially available industrial solvents, and in low concentrations in some screen washes and methylated spirits. It may also be an adulterant of illicitly produced alcohol. Both are rapidly absorbed after ingestion. Methanol and ethylene glycol are not of high intrinsic toxicity, but are converted via alcohol dehydrogenase to toxic metabolites that are largely responsible for their clinical effects (Fig. 10.6).

Early features of poisoning with either methanol or ethylene glycol include vomiting, ataxia, drowsiness, dysarthria and nystagmus. As toxic metabolites are formed, metabolic acidosis, tachypnoea, coma and seizures may develop.

Toxic effects of ethylene glycol include ophthalmoplegia, cranial nerve palsies, hyporeflexia and myoclonus. Renal pain and acute tubular necrosis occur because of renal calcium oxalate precipitation. Hypocalcaemia, hypomagnesaemia and hyperkalaemia are common.

Methanol poisoning causes headache, delirium and vertigo. Visual impairment and photophobia develop, associated with optic disc and retinal oedema and impaired pupil reflexes. Blindness may be permanent, although some recovery may occur over several months. Pancreatitis and abnormal liver function have also been reported.

Urea and electrolytes, chloride, bicarbonate, glucose, calcium, magnesium, albumin, plasma osmolarity and arterial blood gases should be measured in all patients with suspected methanol or ethylene glycol toxicity. The osmolar and anion gaps should be calculated (see Box 10.5).

Initially, poisoning is associated with an increased osmolar gap, but as toxic metabolites are produced an increased anion gap develops associated with metabolic acidosis. The diagnosis can be confirmed by measurement of ethylene glycol or methanol concentrations, but assays are not widely available.

An antidote, ideally fomepizole or otherwise ethanol, should be administered to all patients with suspected significant exposure while awaiting the results of laboratory investigations. These block alcohol dehydrogenase and delay the formation of toxic metabolites until the parent drug is eliminated in the urine or by dialysis. The antidote should be continued until ethylene glycol or methanol concentrations are undetectable. Metabolic acidosis should be corrected with sodium bicarbonate (e.g. 250 mL of 1.26% solution, repeated as necessary). Convulsions should be treated with an intravenous benzodiazepine. In ethylene glycol poisoning, hypocalcaemia should be corrected only if there are severe ECG features or if seizures occur, as this may increase calcium oxalate crystal formation. In methanol poisoning, folinic acid should be administered to enhance the metabolism of the toxic metabolite, formic acid.

Haemodialysis or haemodiafiltration should be used in severe poisoning, especially if renal failure is present or there is visual loss in the context of methanol poisoning. It should be continued until acute toxic features are no longer present and ethylene glycol/methanol concentrations are undetectable.

Corrosive substances

Products containing acids (e.g. hydrochloric or sulphuric acid) or alkalis (e.g. sodium hydroxide, calcium carbonate) may be ingested accidentally or intentionally, causing gastrointestinal pain, ulceration and necrosis, with risk of perforation. Severity depends on the volume and pH of the substance ingested.

External decontamination (p. 221), if needed, should be performed after initial resuscitation. Gastric lavage should not be attempted and neutralising chemicals should not be administered after large ingestions because of the risk of tissue damage from heat release. Cardiorespiratory monitoring is necessary and full blood count, renal function, coagulation and acid–base status should be assessed. An erect chest X-ray should be performed if perforation is suspected and may show features of mediastinitis or gas under the diaphragm. Strong analgesics should be administered for pain.

Severe abdominal or chest pain, abdominal distension, shock or acidosis may indicate perforation and should prompt an urgent CT scan of chest and abdomen and surgical review. In the absence of perforation, drooling, dysphagia, stridor or oropharyngeal burns suggest possible severe oesophageal damage and early endoscopy by an experienced operator should be considered. Delayed endoscopy (e.g. after several days) may carry a higher risk of perforation.

Aluminium and zinc phosphide

These rodenticides and fumigants are a common means of self-poisoning in northern India. The mortality rate for aluminium phosphide ingestion has been estimated at 60%; zinc phosphide ingestion appears less toxic (mortality about 2%). When ingested, both compounds react with gastric acid to form phosphine, a potent pulmonary and gastrointestinal toxicant. Clinical features include severe gastrointestinal disturbances, chest tightness, cough and breathlessness progressing to ARDS and respiratory failure, tremor, paraesthesiae, convulsions, coma, tachycardia, metabolic acidosis, electrolyte disturbances, hypoglycaemia, myocarditis, liver and renal failure, and leucopenia. Ingestion of a few tablets can be fatal.

Treatment is supportive and directed at correcting electrolyte abnormalities and treating complications; there is no specific antidote. Early gastric lavage is sometimes used, often with vegetable oil to reduce the release of toxic phosphine, but the benefit is uncertain.

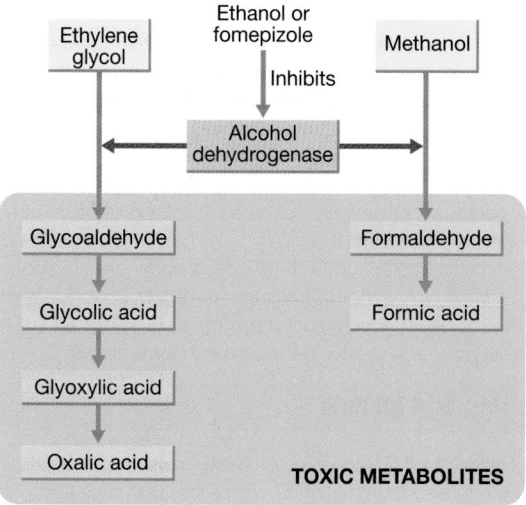

Fig. 10.6 Metabolism of methanol and ethylene glycol.

Copper sulphate

This is used as a fungicide. If ingested, clinical features of toxicity include nausea, vomiting, abdominal pain, diarrhoea, discoloured (blue/green) secretions, corrosive effects on the gastrointestinal tract, renal or liver failure, methaemoglobinaemia, haemolysis, rhabdomyolysis, convulsions and coma. Treatment is as for other corrosive substances (see above) and should address complications, including use of methylthioninium chloride for methaemoglobinaemia (see Fig. 10.1). Chelation therapy is unlikely to be beneficial after acute exposure.

Chemicals less commonly taken in poisoning

An overview of the clinical features and management for chemicals less commonly involved in poisoning is provided in Box 10.15.

Chemical warfare agents

Some toxins have been developed for use as chemical warfare agents. These are summarised in Box 10.16.

10.15 Clinical features and specific management of chemicals less commonly involved in poisoning

Substance	Clinical features	Management
Lead e.g. chronic occupational exposure, leaded paint, water contaminated by lead pipes, use of kohl cosmetics	Abdominal pain Microcytic anaemia with basophilic stippling Headache and encephalopathy Motor neuropathy Nephrotoxicity Hypertension Hypocalcaemia	Prevention of further exposure Measurement of blood lead concentration, full blood count and blood film, urea and electrolytes, liver function tests and calcium Abdominal X-ray in children to detect pica Bone X-ray for 'lead lines' Chelation therapy with DMSA or sodium calcium edetate
Barium salts	GI upset, haematemesis, hypersalivation, perioral paraesthesia, Cyanosis, bradycardia, chest pain, breathlessness. Profound hypokalaemia	Abdominal X-ray to confirm ingestion of radio-opaque material. Aggressive correction of hypokalaemia Haemodialysis in severe cases (removes barium and may correct hypokalaemia)
Strychnine	Rapid onset of gastrointestinal symptoms Agitation, sweating, tachycardia, chest pain, Muscular stiffness and twitching, convulsions and respiratory arrest.	Supportive care including treatment of agitation and convulsions
Thallium	Gastrointestinal disturbances including bleeding Subsequently pancreatitis, parotid swelling, confusion, peripheral neuropathy, alopecia, renal, liver, cardiac or bone marrow failure Coma and death developing over 7–21 days.	Oral Prussian blue or repeated doses of activated charcoal (adsorb thallium in the gut). Supportive care including treatment of convulsions and cardiac complications
Petroleum distillates e.g. white spirit, kerosene	Vomiting Aspiration pneumonitis	Gastric lavage contraindicated Activated charcoal ineffective Oxygen and nebulised bronchodilators Chest X-ray to assess pulmonary effects
Organochlorines e.g. DDT, lindane, dieldrin, endosulfan	Nausea, vomiting Agitation Fasciculation Paraesthesiae (face, extremities) Convulsions Coma Respiratory depression Cardiac arrhythmias Hyperthermia Rhabdomyolysis Pulmonary oedema Disseminated intravascular coagulation	Activated charcoal (with nasogastric aspiration for liquid preparations) within 1 hr of ingestion Cardiac monitoring
Pyrethroid insecticides e.g. cypermethrin, permethrin, imiprothrin	Skin contact: dermatitis, skin paraesthesiae. Systemic features may occur after substantial exposure Eye contact: lacrimation, photophobia and oedema of the eyelids Inhalation: dyspnoea, nausea, headaches Ingestion: epigastric pain, nausea, vomiting, hypersalivation, headache, coma, convulsions, pulmonary oedema	Symptomatic and supportive care Washing contaminated skin makes irritation worse Hyoscine (20 mg subcutaneously every 4 hrs) may be useful for severe hypersalivation
Anticoagulant rodenticides e.g. brodifacoum, bromadialone and warfarin	Abnormal bleeding (prolonged)	Monitor INR/prothrombin time Vitamin K_1 by slow IV injection if there is coagulopathy Fresh frozen plasma or specific clotting factors for bleeding

(DMSA = dimercaptosuccinic acid; INR = International Normalised Ratio; IV = intravenous)

10.16 Chemical warfare agents

Examples	Clinical effects	Antidotes*
Nerve agents		
Tabun Sarin Soman VX Novichok agents	Eyes: miosis (sometimes painful) GI tract: diarrhoea, vomiting, salivation Respiratory: bronchoconstriction, respiratory paralysis/failure Neurological: fasciculations, tremor, ataxia, convulsions, flaccid muscular paralysis See also p. 232 and Box 10.13	Atropine Oximes (e.g. pralidoxime, obidoxime) (see Fig. 10.5)
Blistering agents		
Nitrogen/sulphur Mustard Lewisite	Eyes: watering, blepharospasm, corneal ulceration Skin: erythema, blistering Respiratory: cough, hoarseness, dyspnoea, pneumonitis	None
Choking agents		
Chlorine Phosgene	Eyes: watering, blepharospasm, corneal ulceration Respiratory: cough, hoarseness, dyspnoea, pneumonitis	None
Blood agents		
Cyanide	Cardiovascular: dizziness, shock Respiratory: dyspnoea, cyanosis CNS: anxiety, headache, delirium, convulsions, coma, fixed dilated pupils Other: vomiting, lactic acidosis	Dicobalt edetate Hydroxocobalamin Sodium nitrite Sodium thiosulphate

*Appropriate resuscitation, decontamination and supportive care are essential after exposure to all chemical warfare agents. Use appropriate personal protective equipment.

Environmental poisoning

Arsenism

Chronic arsenic exposure from drinking water has been reported in many countries, especially India, Bangladesh, Nepal, Thailand, Taiwan, China, Mexico and South America, where a large proportion of the drinking water (ground water) has a high arsenic content, placing large populations at risk. The World Health Organization (WHO) guideline value for arsenic content in tube well water is 10 μg/L.

Health effects associated with chronic exposure to arsenic in drinking water are shown in Box 10.17. In exposed individuals, high concentrations of arsenic are present in bone, hair and nails. Specific treatments are of no benefit in chronic arsenic toxicity and recovery from the peripheral neuropathy may never be complete, so the emphasis should be on prevention.

Fluorosis

Fluoride poisoning can result from exposure to excessive quantities of fluoride (>10 ppm) in drinking water, industrial exposure to fluoride dust or consumption of brick teas. Clinical features include yellow staining

10.17 Clinical features of chronic arsenic poisoning

Gastrointestinal tract
- Anorexia, vomiting, weight loss, diarrhoea, increased salivation, metallic taste

Neurological
- Peripheral neuropathy (sensory and motor) with muscle wasting and fasciculation, ataxia

Skin
- Hyperpigmentation, palmar and plantar keratosis, alopecia, multiple epitheliomas, Mee's lines (transverse white lines on fingernails)

Eyes
- Conjunctivitis, corneal necrosis and ulceration

Bone marrow
- Aplastic anaemia

Other
- Low-grade fever, vasospasm and gangrene, jaundice, hepatomegaly, splenomegaly

Increased risk of malignancy
- Lung, liver, bladder, kidney, larynx and lymphoid system

and pitting of permanent teeth, osteosclerosis, soft tissue calcification, deformities (e.g. kyphosis) and joint ankylosis. Changes in the bones of the thoracic cage may lead to rigidity that causes dyspnoea on exertion. Very high doses of fluoride may cause abdominal pain, nausea, vomiting, seizures and muscle spasm. In calcium-deficient children, the toxic effects of fluoride manifest even at marginally high exposures to fluoride.

In endemic areas, such as Jordan, Turkey, Chile, India, Bangladesh, China and Tibet, fluorosis is a major public health problem, especially in communities engaged in physically strenuous agricultural or industrial activities. Dental fluorosis is endemic in East Africa and some West African countries.

Food-related poisoning

Paralytic shellfish poisoning

Paralytic shellfish poisoning is caused by consumption of bivalve molluscs (e.g. mussels, clams, oysters, cockles and scallops) contaminated with saxitoxins, which are concentrated in the shellfish as a result of constant filtration of toxic algae during algal blooms (e.g. 'red tide'). Symptoms develop within 10–120 minutes of eating the contaminated shellfish and include gastrointestinal disturbances, paraesthesia around the mouth or in the extremities, ataxia, mental state changes and dysphagia. In severe cases, paralysis and respiratory failure can develop. There is no specific antidote and treatment is supportive. Most cases resolve over a few days.

Ciguatera poisoning

Ciguatera toxin and related toxins are produced by dinoflagellate plankton that adhere to algae and seaweed. These accumulate in the tropical herbivorous fish that feed on these and in their larger predators (e.g. snapper, barracuda), especially in the Pacific and Caribbean. Human exposure occurs through eating contaminated fish, even if well cooked. Nausea, vomiting, diarrhoea and abdominal pain develop within a few hours, followed by paraesthesia, ataxia, blurred vision, ataxia and tremor. Convulsions and coma can occur, although death is uncommon. Fatigue and peripheral neuropathy can be long-term effects. There is no specific treatment. In the South Pacific and Caribbean, there are approximately 50000 cases per year, with a case fatality of 0.1%.

| **i** | **10.18 Some poisonous plants and fungi, with their clinical effects** |

Species (common name)	Toxins	Important features of toxicity
Plants		
Abrus precatorius (jequirity bean)	Abrin	Gastrointestinal effects, drowsiness, delirium, convulsions, multi-organ failure
Ricinus communis (castor oil plant)	Ricin	
Aconitum napellus (aconite, wolf's bane, monkshood)	Aconite	Gastrointestinal effects, paraesthesiae, convulsions, ventricular tachycardia
Aconitum ferox (Indian aconite, bikh)		
Atropa belladonna (deadly nightshade)	Atropine, scopolamine, hyocyamine	Anticholinergic toxidrome (see Box 10.10)
Datura stramonium (Jimson weed, thorn apple)		
Brugmansia spp. (angel's trumpet)		
Colchicum autumnale (autumn crocus)	Colchicine	Gastrointestinal effects, hypotension, cardiogenic shock
Conium maculatum (hemlock)	Toxic nicotinic alkaloids	Hypersalivation, gastrointestinal effects, followed by muscular paralysis
Digitalis purpurea (foxglove)	Cardiac glycosides	Nausea, vomiting, bradycardia and heart block, supraventricular and ventricular tachyarrhythmias, visual disturbances, confusion (p. 224)
Nerium oleander (pink oleander)		
Thevetia peruviana (yellow oleander)		
Laburnum anagyroides (laburnum)	Cytosine	Gastrointestinal effects; convulsions in severe cases
Taxus baccata (yew)	Taxane alkaloids	Hypotension, bradycardia, respiratory depression, convulsions, coma, arrhythmias
Fungi		
Amanita phalloides (death cap mushroom)	Amatoxins	Gastrointestinal effects, progressing to liver failure
Cortinarius spp.	Orellanine	Gastrointestinal effects, fever, progressing to renal failure
Psilocybe semilanceata ('magic mushrooms')	Psilocybin, psilocin	Hallucinations

10

Scombrotoxic fish poisoning

Under poor storage conditions, histidine in scombroid fish (e.g. tuna, mackerel, bonito, skipjack and the dark meat of canned sardines) may be converted by bacteria to histamine and other chemicals. Within minutes of consumption, flushing, burning, sweating, urticaria, pruritus, headache, colic, nausea and vomiting, diarrhoea, bronchospasm and hypotension may occur. Management is with nebulised salbutamol, intravenous antihistamines and, occasionally, intravenous fluid replacement.

Tetrodotoxin poisoning

The highly toxic tetrodotoxin is found in the skin and viscera of Puffer fish. Tetrodotoxin blocks voltage-gated sodium channels, inhibiting action potential generation and propagation. Clinical features include paraesthesiae, salivation, gastrointestinal disturbances, sweating, headache, tachycardia, hypokalaemia, twitching or tremor, vertigo, dysphonia and dysphagia. In severe cases ataxia, paralysis and fixed dilated pupils occur, mimicking brain death. Without appropriate ventilator support, respiratory paralysis can be fatal. Otherwise there is no specific treatment and management is supportive.

Plant poisoning

A substantial number of plants and fungi are potentially toxic if consumed, with patterns of poisoning depending on their geographical distribution. Some toxic examples and the clinical features of toxicity are shown in Box 10.18.

Further information

Books and journal articles

Bateman DN, Jefferson R, Thomas SHL, eds. Oxford desk reference: toxicology. Oxford: Oxford University Press; 2014.

Benson BE, Hoppu K, Troutman WG, et al. Position paper update: gastric lavage for gastrointestinal decontamination. Clin Toxicol 2013;51:140–146.

Gosselin S, Hoegberg LCG, Hoffman RS, et al. Evidence-based recommendations on the use of intravenous lipid emulsion therapy in poisoning. Clin Toxicol 2016;54(10):899–923.

Thanacoody R. Position paper update: Whole bowel irrigation for gastrointestinal decontamination of overdose patients. Clin Toxicol 2015;53:5–12.

Thompson JP, Watson ID, Thanacoody HK, et al. Guidelines for laboratory analyses for poisoned patients in the United Kingdom. Ann Clin Biochem 2014;51:312–325.

Websites

toxbase.org *Toxbase, the clinical toxicology database of the UK National Poisons Information Service. Free for UK health professionals but registration is required. Access for overseas users by special arrangement. Low-cost smartphone app available.*

wikitox.org/doku.php?id=wikitox:wikitox_home *WikiTox, an open access curriculum project to improve the treatment of people who are poisoned.*

apps.who.int/poisoncentres *World directory of poisons centres, as of 28 February 2019 (interactive map).*

J White

11

Envenomation

Comprehensive evaluation of the envenomed patient

1 Airway, breathing, circulation
Blood pressure
Pulse
Respiration rate
Oxygen saturation
Dysrhythmias

2 Level of consciousness
Confusion
Agitation
Seizures

3 Mouth, gums
Evidence of bleeding
Increased salivation
Drooling

4 Cranial nerves
Drooling
Dysarthria
Dysphagia
Upper airway compromise

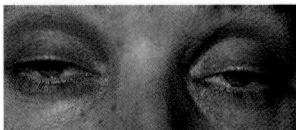

▲ Bilateral mild ptosis

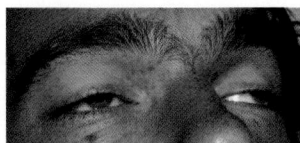

▲ Ptosis and lateral ophthalmoplegia

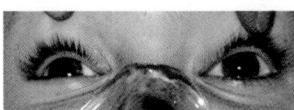

▲ Fixed dilated pupils

5 Chest
Pulmonary oedema
Diminished respiration

Copyright © Julian White.

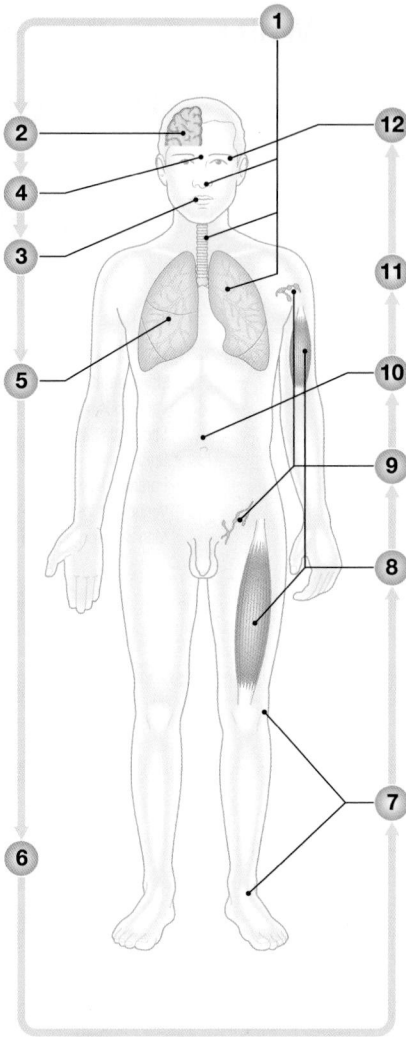

6 Bite/sting site
Pain
Swelling
Bruising
Discoloration
Necrosis

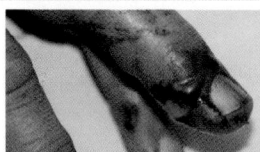

▲ Local bleeding, blistering

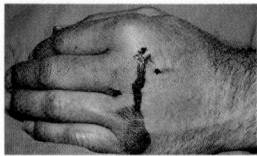

▲ Local bleeding

12 Eyes
Miosis or mydriasis
Increased lacrimation
Corneal injury (venom spit injury)

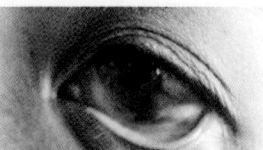

▲ Chemosis – can indicate capillary leak syndrome

11 Skin
In addition to (6):
Piloerection
Erythema
Blistering
Infection

▲ Local increased sweating

10 Abdomen
Intra-abdominal, retroperitoneal or renal pathology

9 Lymph nodes
Tender or enlarged nodes draining bite/sting area

8 Muscles
Weakness
Tenderness
Pain

7 Reflexes
Decreased or absent reflexes

Geographical distribution of venomous snakes

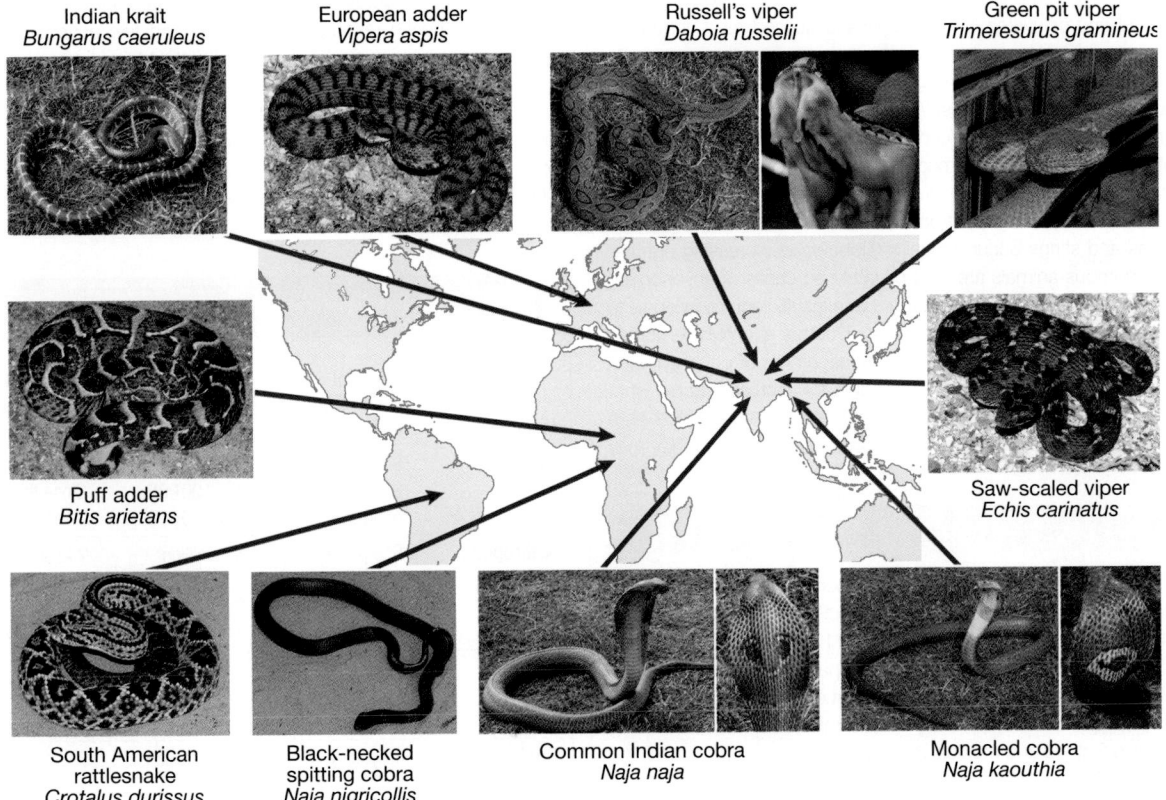

Indian krait
Bungarus caeruleus

European adder
Vipera aspis

Russell's viper
Daboia russelii

Green pit viper
Trimeresurus gramineus

Puff adder
Bitis arietans

Saw-scaled viper
Echis carinatus

South American rattlesnake
Crotalus durissus

Black-necked spitting cobra
Naja nigricollis

Common Indian cobra
Naja naja

Monacled cobra
Naja kaouthia

The geographical location of a snakebite determines the likely animal(s) involved and the nature and risks of the envenomation. *Copyright © Julian White.*

Bedside tests in the envenomed patient

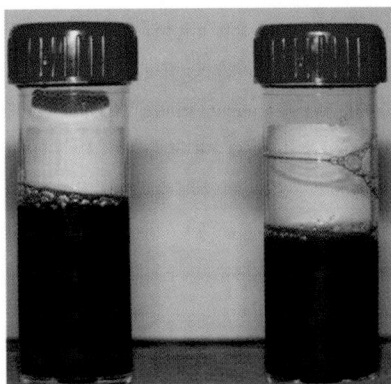

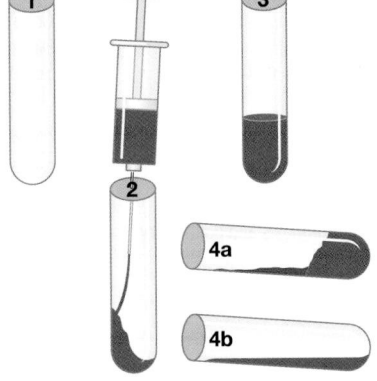

1 Obtain a clean **glass** container (test tube or bottle) that is either new, or has only been washed with water (not detergent/soap)

2 Place 2–3 mL venous blood in the **glass** container

3 Allow to stand undisturbed for 20 mins

4 Gently invert/tip the glass container checking for presence of a blood clot

4a Clot present = negative test (no coagulopathy present)

4b Clot absent = positive test (coagulopathy present)

Examination of urine. Haematuria may indicate a coagulopathy. Dark urine is suggestive of myoglobinuria, which is a sign of extensive rhabdomyolysis. *Copyright © Julian White.*

Twenty-minute whole-blood clotting test (20WBCT). The presence of coagulopathy is a key indicator of major envenoming for some species. While full laboratory coagulation studies may be the ideal, the 20WBCT has emerged as a simple standardised bedside test of coagulopathy, applicable even in areas with limited health facilities. *Copyright © Julian White.*

Overview of envenomation

Envenomation occurs when a venomous animal injects sufficient venom by a bite or a sting into a prey item or perceived predator to cause deleterious local and/or systemic effects. This is defined as a venom-induced disease (VID). Venomous animals generally use their venom to acquire and, in some cases, pre-digest prey, with defensive use a secondary function for many species. Where defensive use of venom is an important evolutionary driver, immediate and severe local pain is a common feature, though the toxin mechanisms causing pain are diverse. Accidental encounters between venomous animals and humans are frequent, particularly in the rural tropics, where millions of cases of venomous bites and stings occur annually. Globally, an increasing number of exotic venomous animals are kept privately, so cases of envenoming may present to hospitals where doctors have insufficient knowledge to manage potentially complex presentations. Doctors everywhere should thus be aware of the basic principles of management of envenomation and how to seek expert support. It is important for doctors to know what types of venomous animal are likely to occur in their geographical area (hospital hinterland; see p. 241) and the types of envenoming they may cause.

Venom

Venom is a complex mixture of diverse components, often with several separate toxins that can cause adverse effects in humans, with each potentially capable of multiple effects (Box 11.1). Venom is produced at considerable metabolic cost, so is used sparingly; only some bites/stings by venomous animals result in significant envenoming, the remainder are 'dry bites'. The concept of dry bites is important in understanding approaches to first aid and medical management.

Venomous animals

There are many animal groups that contain venomous species (Box 11.2). The epidemiological estimates of envenomation episodes reflect the importance of snakes and scorpions as causes of severe or lethal envenomation, but also the fragmentary nature of the data. For snakebites, recent studies have proposed widely varying estimates, but even the higher estimates may be too low. In India, studies indicate there are at least 45000 snakebite-related deaths annually, far above both government figures and previous estimates. In many areas of the rural tropics, health resources are limited and few envenoming cases are either seen or recorded within the official hospital system, compared to the actual community burden of disease. While fatal cases may gain most attention, long-term disability from envenomation affects significantly more people and has a major social and economic cost. The World Health Organization (WHO) has recently recognised snakebite as a 'Neglected Tropical Disease' and this may improve access to funding.

---

i 11.2 Venomous animals and human envenoming

Phyla	Principal venomous animal groups	Estimated number of human cases/year	Estimated number of human deaths/year
Chordata	Snakes	> 2.5 million	> 100 000
	Spiny fish	? > 100 000	Close to zero
	Stingrays	? > 100 000	? < 10
Arthropoda	Scorpions	> 1 million	? < 5000
	Spiders	? > 100 000	? < 100
	Paralysis ticks	? > 1000	? < 10
	Insects	? > 1 million	? > 1000*
Mollusca	Cone snails	? < 1000	? < 10
	Blue-ringed octopus	? < 100	? < 10
Coelenterata	Jellyfish	? > 1 million	? < 10

*Social insect stings cause death by anaphylaxis rather than primary venom toxicity, except for massive multiple sting attacks.
Copyright © Julian White.

---

i 11.1 Key venom effects*

Venom component	Clinical effects	Type of venomous animal
Neurotoxin		
Paralytic	Flaccid paralysis (may develop in a *descending* pattern, commencing first in cranial nerves, or in an *ascending* pattern, with early ataxia)	Some snakes (descending) Paralysis ticks (ascending) Cone snails (descending) Blue-ringed octopus (descending)
Excitatory	Neuroexcitation: autonomic storm, cardiotoxicity, pulmonary oedema	Some scorpions, spiders, jellyfish (irukandji)
Myotoxins	Systemic or local myolysis	Some snakes
Cardiotoxins	Direct or indirect cardiotoxicity; cardiac collapse, shock	Some snakes, scorpions, spiders and jellyfish (box jellyfish)
Haemostasis system toxins	Variation from rapid coagulopathy and bleeding to thrombosis, deep venous thrombosis and pulmonary emboli	Many snakes and a few scorpions (*Hemiscorpius*) Brazilian caterpillars (*Lonomia*)
Haemorrhagic toxins	Local vessel damage, fluid extravasation, blistering, ecchymosis, shock	Mainly some snakes
Nephrotoxins (direct or indirect)	Renal damage	Some snakes, massed bee and wasp stings
Necrotoxins	Local tissue injury/necrosis, shock	Some snakes, a few scorpions (*Hemiscorpius*), spiders (recluse spiders), jellyfish and stingrays
Allergic toxins	Induction of acute allergic response (direct and indirect)	Almost all venoms but particularly those of social insects (i.e. bees, wasps, ants)

*All venom components have lethal potential.
Copyright © Julian White.

Snakebite occurs frequently in low resource areas of the rural tropics and so is an important poverty trap; it is also a predominantly occupational disease, with farmers and other agricultural workers at particularly high risk. Although snakebite is undoubtedly the most impactful form of envenoming globally, there are some areas where scorpion stings have a higher impact on health systems than snakebite.

Stings by social insects such as bees and wasps may also cause lethal anaphylaxis and mass stings may cause severe, even, lethal, envenomation. Other venomous animals may commonly envenom humans, but cause mostly non-lethal effects. A few animals only rarely envenom humans, but have a high potential for severe or lethal envenoming. These include box jellyfish, cone snails, blue-ringed octopus, paralysis ticks and Australian funnel web spiders. Within any given group, particularly snakes, there may be a wide range of clinical presentations. Some are described here, but for a more detailed discussion of the types of venomous animal, their venoms and their effects on humans, see toxinology.com.

Clinical effects

With the exception of dry bites, where no significant toxin effects occur, venomous bites/stings can result in three broad classes of effect.

Local effects

These vary from trivial to severe (Box 11.3). There may be minimal or no local effects with some snakebites (not even pain), yet lethal systemic envenoming may still be present (e.g. kraits in Asia). For other species, local effects predominate over systemic, and for some, (e.g. certain snakes) both are important (p. 240). Some species commonly cause local necrosis, notably some snakes, brown recluse spiders, an Iranian scorpion (*Hemiscorpius lepturus*) and some stingrays. Globally, amputations secondary to snakebite are an important cause of long-term morbidity and social disadvantage.

General systemic effects

By definition, these are non-specific (see Box 11.3). Shock is an important complication of major local envenoming by some snake species and if inadequately treated can prove lethal, especially in children.

11.3 Local and systemic effects of envenomation

Local effects

- Pain
- Sweating
- Erythema
- Major direct tissue trauma (e.g. stingray injuries)
- Blistering
- Necrosis
- Swelling
- Bleeding and bruising

Non-specific systemic effects

- Headache
- Nausea
- Vomiting and diarrhoea
- Abdominal pain
- Tachycardia or bradycardia
- Hypertension or hypotension
- Pulmonary oedema
- Dizziness
- Collapse
- Convulsions
- Shock
- Cardiac arrest

Specific systemic effects

- Neurotoxic flaccid paralysis (descending or ascending)
- Excitatory neurotoxicity (catecholamine storm-like and similar)
- Rhabdomyolysis (systemic or local)
- Coagulopathy (procoagulants, anticoagulants, fibrinolytics and platelet-active toxins)
- Cardiotoxicity (decreased/abnormal cardiac function or arrhythmia or arrest)
- Acute kidney injury (polyuria or oliguria or anuria or isolated elevated creatinine/urea)

Copyright © Julian White.

Specific systemic effects

These are important in both diagnosis and treatment.

- *Neurotoxic flaccid paralysis* can develop very rapidly, progressing from mild weakness to full respiratory paralysis in less than 30 minutes (blue-ringed octopus bite, cone snail sting), or may develop far more slowly, over hours (e.g. kraits, some cobras) to days (paralysis tick). For neurotoxic snakes, the cranial nerves are usually involved first, with bilateral ptosis a common initial sign, often progressing to partial and later complete ophthalmoplegia, fixed dilated pupils, drooling and loss of upper airway protection (p. 240). From this, paralysis may extend to the limbs, with weakness and loss of deep tendon reflexes, the neck ('broken neck' sign), then finally respiratory paralysis affecting the diaphragm.
- *Excitatory neurotoxins* cause an 'autonomic storm', often with profuse sweating (p. 240), variable cardiac effects and cardiac failure, sometimes with pulmonary oedema (notably, Australian funnel web spider bite, some scorpions such as Indian red scorpion). This type of envenomation can be rapidly fatal (many scorpions, funnel web spiders), or may cause distressing symptoms with a lesser risk of death (widow spiders, banana spiders).
- *Myotoxicity* can be localised in the bitten limb, or systemic, affecting mostly skeletal muscles. It can initially be silent, then present with generalised muscle pain, tenderness, myoglobinuria (p. 241) and substantial rises in serum creatine kinase (CK). Secondary renal failure can precipitate potentially lethal hyperkalaemic cardiotoxicity.
- *Cardiotoxicity* is often secondary, but symptoms and signs are non-specific in most cases. For some scorpions, envenomation can cause direct cardiac effects, including decreased cardiac output, arrhythmias and pulmonary oedema.
- *Haemostasis system toxins* cause a variety of effects, depending on the type of toxin (Fig. 11.1). Coagulopathy may present as bruising and bleeding from the bite site (p. 240), gums and intravenous sites. Surgical interventions are high risk in such cases. Other venoms cause thrombosis, usually presenting as deep venous thrombosis (DVT), pulmonary embolus or stroke (particularly Caribbean/ Martinique vipers).
- *Haemorrhagic toxins* (associated with some snakebites) cause vascular damage, especially in the bitten limb, with extravasation of fluid and sometimes hypotensive shock. They may also cause internal bleeding such as retroperitoneal haemorrhage. The role of these toxins in causing late-developing capillary leak syndrome (p. 240) is uncertain (seen notably with Russell's viper),
- *Renal damage* in envenoming is mostly secondary, although some species (such as Russell's vipers) can cause primary renal damage. The presentation is similar in both scenarios, with changes in urine output (polyuria, oliguria or anuria), proteinuria, or rises in creatinine and urea. In cases with intravascular haemolysis, secondary renal damage is likely. The clinical effects of specific animals in different regions of the world are shown in Boxes 11.4–11.6.

General approach to the envenomed patient

First aid

First aid can be crucial in determining the outcome for envenomed patients, yet throughout much of the world inappropriate and dangerous first aid is often administered.

A significant proportion of venom is transported from the bite/sting site via the lymphatic system, particularly for venoms with larger molecular weight toxins, such as many snake venoms. It is recommended that for most forms of envenoming, the patient should be kept still, the bitten limb immobilised with a splint and vital systems supported, where required. A patent upper airway should be ensured and respiratory

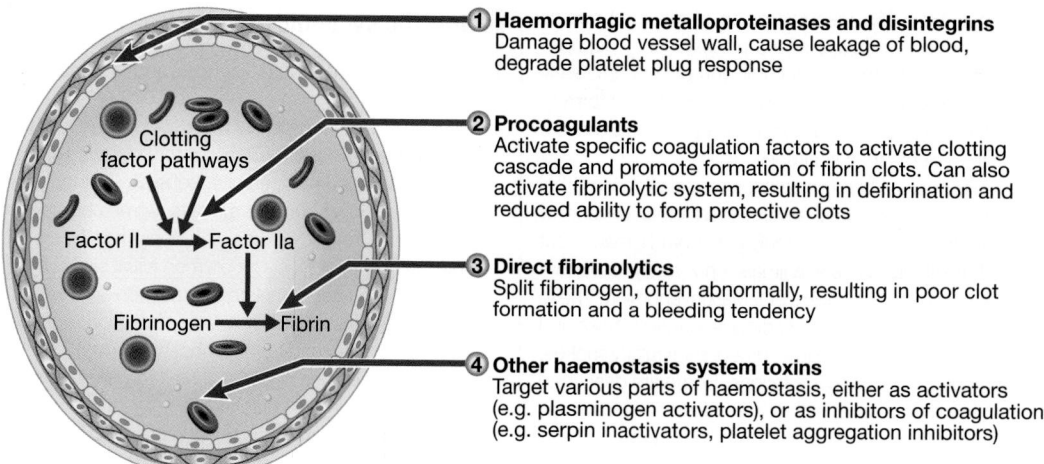

1 **Haemorrhagic metalloproteinases and disintegrins**
Damage blood vessel wall, cause leakage of blood, degrade platelet plug response

2 **Procoagulants**
Activate specific coagulation factors to activate clotting cascade and promote formation of fibrin clots. Can also activate fibrinolytic system, resulting in defibrination and reduced ability to form protective clots

3 **Direct fibrinolytics**
Split fibrinogen, often abnormally, resulting in poor clot formation and a bleeding tendency

4 **Other haemostasis system toxins**
Target various parts of haemostasis, either as activators (e.g. plasminogen activators), or as inhibitors of coagulation (e.g. serpin inactivators, platelet aggregation inhibitors)

Fig. 11.1 Sites of action of venoms on the haemostasis system. *Copyright © Julian White.*

i 11.4 Selected important venomous animals in Asia

Scientific name[1]	Common name	Clinical effects	Antivenom/antidote/treatment
South Asia			
Bungarus spp. (E)	Kraits	Flaccid paralysis[2,3], myolysis[4], hyponatraemia[5]	Indian PV or specific
Naja spp. (E)	Cobras	Flaccid paralysis[3], local necrosis/blistering, shock	Indian PV or specific
Ophiophagus hannah (E)	King cobra	Flaccid paralysis[3], local necrosis, shock	Indian PV or specific
Echis spp. (Vv)	Saw-scaled vipers	Procoagulant coagulopathy, local necrosis/blistering, renal failure	Indian PV or specific
Daboia russelii (Vv)	Russell's viper	Procoagulant coagulopathy, local necrosis/blistering, myolysis, renal failure, shock, flaccid paralysis[2]	Indian PV or specific
Hypnale spp. (Vc)	Hump-nosed vipers	Procoagulant coagulopathy, shock, renal failure	No available AV; Indian PV unlikely to be effective
Trimeresurus[6] spp. (Vc)	Green pit vipers	Procoagulant coagulopathy, local necrosis, shock	Indian PV unlikely to be effective; consider specific AV from Thailand
Hottentotta spp. (Sc)	Indian scorpions	Neuroexcitation, cardiotoxicity	Indian specific AV Prazosin
East Asia			
Bungarus spp. (E)	Kraits	Flaccid paralysis[2,3]	Specific AV from country
Naja spp. (E)	Cobras (some spitters)	Flaccid paralysis[3], local necrosis/blistering, shock	Specific AV from country
Ophiophagus hannah (E)	King cobra	Flaccid paralysis[3], local necrosis, shock	King cobra AV
Calloselasma rhodostoma (Vc)	Malayan pit viper	Procoagulant coagulopathy, local necrosis/blistering, renal failure, shock	Specific AV from country
Daboia siamensis (Vv)	Russell's viper	Procoagulant coagulopathy, local necrosis/blistering, renal failure, capillary leak syndrome, shock, anterior pituitary haemorrhage and failure	Specific AV from country
Gloydius spp. (Vc)	Mamushis, pit vipers	Procoagulant coagulopathy, local necrosis/blistering, shock, renal failure, flaccid paralysis[2]	Specific AV from country
Trimeresurus[6] spp. (Vc)	Green pit vipers, habus	Procoagulant coagulopathy, local necrosis/blistering, shock	Specific AV from country
Hydrophis schistosus + other species	Sea snakes (all species globally)	Flaccid paralysis and/or myolysis	Seqirus sea snake AV

[1]Family names: C = 'Colubridae' (mostly 'non-venomous'; family subject to major taxonomic revisions); E = Elapidae (all venomous); Sc = Scorpionoidea; Vc = Viperidae Crotalinae (New World and Asian vipers); Vv = Viperidae viperinae (Old World vipers). [2]Pre-synaptic. [3]Post-synaptic. [4]Only reported so far for *B. candidus*, *B. niger* and *B. caeruleus*. [5]Only reported so far for *B. multicinctus* and *B. candidus*. [6]Genus is subject to major taxonomic change (split into at least eight genera).
(AV = antivenom; PV = polyvalent)
More information is available from the World Health Organization, Regional Office for South-East Asia and from toxinology.com. See 'Further Information'.
Copyright © Julian White.

| i | 11.5 | Selected important venomous animals in the Americas and Australia |

Scientific name[1]	Common name	Clinical effects	Antivenom/antidote/treatment
North America			
Crotalus spp. (Vc)	Rattlesnakes	Procoagulant coagulopathy, local necrosis/blistering (flaccid paralysis[2] rare), shock	CroFab (Fab') AV or Anavip (F(ab')$_2$) AV
Sistrurus spp. (Vc)	Massasaugas	Procoagulant coagulopathy, local necrosis/blistering, shock	CroFab (Fab') AV or Anavip (F(ab')$_2$) AV
Agkistrodon spp. (Vc)	Copperheads and moccasins	Procoagulant coagulopathy, local necrosis/blistering, shock	CroFab (Fab') AV or Anavip (F(ab')$_2$) AV
Micrurus spp. (E)	Coral snakes	Flaccid paralysis[3]	Bioclon Coralmyn AV
Latrodectus mactans	Widow spider	Neuroexcitation	MSD Widow spider AV
Centruroides sculpturatus	Arizona bark scorpion	Neuroexcitation	Bioclon Anascorp AV
Central and South America			
Crotalus spp. (Vc)	Rattlesnakes	Flaccid paralysis[2], myolysis, procoagulant coagulopathy, shock, renal failure	Specific AV from country
Bothrops spp. (Vc)	Lancehead vipers	Procoagulant coagulopathy, local necrosis/blistering, shock, renal failure	Specific AV from country
Bothriechis spp. (Vc)	Eyelash pit vipers	Shock, pain and swelling	Specific AV from country
Lachesis spp. (Vc)	Bushmasters	Procoagulant coagulopathy, shock, renal failure, local necrosis/blistering	Specific AV from country
Micrurus spp. (E)	Coral snakes	Flaccid paralysis[2,3], myolysis, renal failure	Specific AV from country
Tityus serrulatus	Brazilian scorpion	Neuroexcitation, shock	Instituto Butantan scorpion AV
Loxosceles spp.	Recluse spiders	Local necrosis	Instituto Butantan spider AV
Phoneutria nigriventer	Banana spider	Neuroexcitation, shock	Instituto Butantan spider AV
Potamotrygon, Dasyatis spp.	Freshwater stingrays	Necrosis of bite area, shock, severe pain and oedema	No available AV; good wound care
Australia			
Pseudonaja spp. (E)	Brown snakes	Procoagulant coagulopathy, renal failure, flaccid paralysis[2] (rare)	Seqirus brown snake AV or PVAV
Notechis spp. (E)	Tiger snakes	Procoagulant coagulopathy, myolysis, flaccid paralysis[2,3], renal failure	Seqirus tiger snake AV or PVAV
Oxyuranus spp. (E)	Taipans	Procoagulant coagulopathy, flaccid paralysis[2,3], myolysis, renal failure	Seqirus taipan or PVAV
Acanthophis spp. (E)	Death adders	Flaccid paralysis[3]	Seqirus death adder or PVAV
Pseudechis spp.	Black and mulga snakes	Anticoagulant coagulopathy, myolysis, renal failure	Seqirus black snake AV or PVAV
Hydrophis schistosus + other species	Sea snakes (all species globally)	Flaccid paralysis and/or myolysis	Seqirus sea snake AV
Atrax, Hadronyche spp.	Funnel web spiders	Neuroexcitation, shock	Seqirus funnel web spider AV
Latrodectus hasseltii	Red back spider	Neuroexcitation, pain and sweating	Seqirus red back spider AV
Chironex fleckeri	Box jellyfish	Neuroexcitation, cardiotoxicity, local necrosis	Seqirus box jellyfish AV
Synanceia spp.	Stonefish	Severe local pain	Seqirus stonefish AV

[1]For family name, see Box 11.4. [2]Pre-synaptic. [3]Post-synaptic.
(AV = antivenom; MSD = Merck, Sharpe & Dohme; PV = polyvalent)
Copyright © Julian White.

11

support provided, if required. For some animals, notably snakes in certain regions, the use of a local pressure pad bandage over the bite site (Myanmar) or a pressure immobilisation bandage (Australia, New Guinea) is recommended.

Ineffective or dangerous first aid, such as suction devices, 'cut and suck', local chemicals, snake stones (stones of some sort placed over the snakebite), electric shock devices and tourniquets, should not be used. Tourniquets, in particular, have the potential to cause catastrophic ischaemic distal limb injuries in snakebite when applied too narrowly or too tightly, or left on too long. Caution is required when removing tourniquets or other constricting first aid, as there may be a sudden rush of venom into the circulation causing rapid effects and cardiorespiratory collapse.

Transporting patients

Where possible, transport should be brought to the patient. It is vital to obtain medical assessment and intervention at the earliest opportunity, so any delay in transporting the patient to a medical facility should be avoided. Severely envenomed patients may develop life-threatening problems during transport, such as shock or respiratory failure, so ideally the transport method should allow for management of these problems en route.

In resource-poor environments, simple solutions for rapid transport have been successfully employed, such as motorbikes or similar with the patient supported between the driver in front and another person behind the patient. However, this method cannot cope with a patient developing airway compromise or respiratory failure, such as from developing neurotoxicity.

| i | 11.6 Selected important venomous animals in Africa and Europe |

Scientific name[1]	Common name	Clinical effects	Antivenom/antidote/treatment
Africa			
Naja spp. (E)	Cobras		
	Non-spitters	Flaccid paralysis[3] ± local necrosis/blistering	South African PV or other appropriate African-specific AV
	Spitters	Local necrosis/blistering (flaccid paralysis[3] uncommon)	South African PV or other appropriate African-specific AV
Dendroaspis spp. (E)	Mambas	Mamba neurotoxic flaccid paralysis and muscle fasciculation, shock, necrosis (uncommon)	South African PV or other appropriate African-specific AV
Hemachatus haemachatus (E)	Rinkhals	Flaccid paralysis[3], local necrosis, shock	South African PV
Atheris spp. (Vv)	Bush vipers	Procoagulant coagulopathy, shock, pain and swelling	No available AV (can try South African AV)
Bitis spp. (Vv)	Puff adders etc.	Procoagulant coagulopathy, shock, cardiotoxicity, local necrosis/blistering	South African PV or other appropriate African-specific AV
Causus spp. (Vv)	Night adders	Pain and swelling	No available AV
Echis spp. (Vv)	Carpet vipers	Procoagulant coagulopathy, shock, renal failure, local necrosis/blistering	Specific anti-*Echis* AV for species/geographical region or other appropriate African-specific AV
Cerastes spp. (Vv)	Horned desert vipers	Procoagulant coagulopathy, local necrosis, shock	Specific or polyspecific AV covering *Cerastes* from country of origin
Dispholidus typus (C)	Boomslang	Procoagulant coagulopathy, shock	Boomslang AV
Androctonus spp.	North African scorpions	Neuroexcitation	Specific scorpion AV (Algeria, Tunisia, Sanofi Pasteur Scorpifav)
Leiurus quinquestriatus	Yellow scorpion	Neuroexcitation, shock	Specific scorpion AV (Algeria, Tunisia, Sanofi Pasteur Scorpifav)
Europe			
Vipera spp. (Vv)	Vipers and adders	Shock, local necrosis/blistering, procoagulant coagulopathy (flaccid paralysis[2] rare)	ViperaTab AV or Zagreb AV or Sanofi Pasteur Viperfav AV

[1]For family name, see Box 11.4. [2]Pre-synaptic. [3]Post-synaptic.
(AV = antivenom; PV = polyvalent)
More information is available from the World Health Organization, Regional Office for Africa and from toxinology.com. See 'Further Information'.
Copyright © Julian White.

Assessment and management in hospital

On arrival at a health station or hospital, there are two immediate priorities:

- identifying and treating any life-threatening problems (e.g. circulatory shock, respiratory failure; see Ch. 16)
- determining whether envenomation has occurred and if that requires urgent treatment.

Assessment and management of life-threatening problems

Patients who are seriously envenomed must be identified early so that appropriate management is not delayed. Critically ill patients must be resuscitated (Ch. 9) and this takes precedence over administration of any antivenom. Clinicians should look for signs of:

- shock/hypotension
- airway and/or respiratory compromise (likely to be secondary to flaccid paralysis)
- major bleeding, including internal bleeding (especially intracranial, intra- or retro-peritoneal)
- impending limb compromise from inappropriate first aid (e.g. a tourniquet).

In a patient with severe neurotoxic flaccid paralysis, who is still able to maintain sufficient respiratory function for survival, clinical assessment may erroneously suggest irretrievable brain injury (fixed dilated pupils, absent reflexes, no withdrawal response to painful stimuli, no movement of limbs, fixed forward gaze with gross ptosis; p. 240) when, in fact, the patient is conscious and terrified.

Assessment for evidence of envenoming

As in other areas of medicine, comprehensive assessment of a patient bitten/stung by a venomous animal requires a good history, a careful targeted examination and, where appropriate, 'laboratory' testing (though the latter may just consist of simple bedside tests performed by the doctor; p. 241). Animals that are unlikely to cause serious envenomation in humans should be identified so that inappropriate admission and intervention are avoided. Occasionally, patients may be unaware they have been bitten/stung and thus provide a misleading history. In regions of the world where keeping or handling venomous animals is illegal, patients may be reticent in giving a truthful history. Multiple bites or stings are more likely to cause major envenoming.

The following key questions should be asked:

- When was the patient exposed to the venomous bite/sting?
- Was the organism causing it seen and what did it look like (size, colour)?
- What were the circumstances (on land, in water etc.)?
- Was there more than one bite/sting? (multiple bites/stings are more likely to be severe)

- What first aid was used, how quickly was it applied and how long has it been in place?
- What symptoms has the patient had (local and systemic)?
- Are there symptoms suggesting systemic envenomation (paralysis, rhabdomyolysis, coagulopathy etc.)?
- Is there any significant past medical history and medication use?
- Is there a past exposure to antivenom/venom and allergies?

If patients state that they have been bitten by a particular species, ensure this information is accurate. Private keepers of venomous animals may not have accurate knowledge of what they are keeping and misidentification of a snake, scorpion or spider can have dire consequences if the wrong antivenom is used.

An outline of some principal findings on examination of the envenomed patient is shown on page 240. The patient may have a cluster of clinical features suggestive of a particular type of envenoming (see Box 11.1). There are documented envenoming syndromes for some groups of snakes that, in some regions, can guide diagnosis and treatment (see Box 11.7). Detail of this syndromic approach is available in free WHO guides on snakebite in Asia and in Africa.

Even with dangerously venomous animals, some bites/stings will be dry bites and will not require antivenom. The time to onset of first symptoms and signs of envenomation is variable, depending on both animal and patient factors. It may range from a matter of minutes post-bite/sting to 24 hours later in some cases. Therefore, if the initial assessment is normal, it must be repeated multiple times during the first 24 hours. Some types of envenomation will not cause symptoms or signs at all, or may appear very late, long after the optimum time for treatment has passed. Evidence of envenomation may become apparent only through laboratory testing.

Laboratory investigations

Specific tests for venom are currently commercially available only for Australian snakebites, but may be developed for snakebites in other regions. They are not available for other types of envenomation, where venom concentrations are low. For snakebite, a screen for envenomation includes full blood count, coagulation screen, urea and electrolytes, creatinine, CK and electrocardiogram (ECG). Lung function tests, peripheral oximetry or arterial blood gases may be indicated in cases with potential or established respiratory failure. In areas without access to routine laboratory tests, the 20-minute whole-blood clotting test (20WBCT) is useful (p. 241).

Treatment

Once a diagnosis of likely envenoming has been made, the next and urgent decision is whether to give antivenom. However, antivenom may not be the only crucial treatment required. For a snakebite by a potentially lethal species such as Russell's viper, the patient may have local effects with oedema, blistering, necrosis and resultant fluid shifts causing shock, and at the same time have systemic effects such as intractable vomiting, coagulopathy, paralysis and secondary renal failure. Specific treatment with antivenom will be required to reverse the coagulopathy and may prevent worsening of the paralysis and reduce the vomiting, but will not greatly affect the local tissue damage or the renal failure or shock. The latter will require intravenous fluid therapy, possibly respiratory support, renal dialysis and local wound care, perhaps including antibiotics. In Myanmar at least, each hour of delay in giving antivenom after Russell's viper bite markedly increases the likelihood of developing renal failure.

Each venomous animal will cause a particular pattern of envenomation, requiring a tailored response (envenoming syndrome). Listing all of these is beyond the scope of this chapter (see 'Further information').

11.7 Snakebite envenomation syndromes for South-East Asia

Clinical definition/characteristics of syndrome	Likely snakes causing the syndrome
Syndrome 1	
Local envenoming (swelling etc.) + bleeding, clotting disturbances	Viper bite (many possible species)
Syndrome 2	
Local envenoming (swelling etc.) + bleeding, clotting disturbances + shock or AKI	Russell's viper
2a – ± conjunctival oedema and acute pituitary insufficiency	2a – Russell's viper in Myanmar and South India
2b – ± bilateral ptosis, external ophthalmoplegia, flaccid paralysis, dark urine (myoglobinuria)	2b – Russell's viper in Sri Lanka and South India
Syndrome 3	
Local envenoming (swelling etc.) + flaccid paralysis (bilateral ptosis, ophthalmoplegia, etc.)	Cobra or king cobra
Syndrome 4	
Minimal or no local envenoming + flaccid paralysis (bilateral ptosis, ophthalmoplegia, etc.)	
4a – If bitten on land (patient sleeping on ground at night) ± abdominal pain	4a – krait
4b – If bitten in water (sea, some lakes) ± dark urine (myoglobinuria)	4b – sea snake
4c – If bitten on land in New Guinea ± coagulopathy	4c – Australasian Elapid (taipan, small-eyed snake, etc.)
Syndrome 5	
Variable local effects + flaccid paralysis + dark urine (myoglobinuria) and AKI	
5a – If bitten on land (sleeping on ground)	5a – krait
5b – If bitten in water (sea, some lakes) + no coagulopathy	5b – sea snake
5c – If bitten on land + coagulopathy/bleeding	5c – Russell's viper (Sri Lanka and South India)

(AKI = acute kidney injury).
After World Health Organization, Regional Office for South-East Asia. Guidelines for the management of snake-bites, 2nd edn; 2016.

Antivenom

Antivenom, sometimes inappropriately labelled as 'anti-snake venom' (ASV), is the most important tool in treating envenomation. It is made by hyperimmunising an animal, usually horses, to produce antibodies against venom. Once refined, these bind to venom toxins and render them inactive or allow their rapid clearance. Antivenom is available only for certain venomous animals and cannot reverse all types of envenomation. With a few exceptions, it should be given intravenously, with adrenaline (epinephrine) ready in case of anaphylaxis. It should be used only when clearly indicated and indications will vary between venomous animals (Box 11.8). It is critical that the correct antivenom is used at the appropriate dose. Doses vary widely between antivenoms. In some situations (such as South Asia), pre-treatment with subcutaneous adrenaline may reduce the chance of anaphylaxis to antivenom.

Antivenom can sometimes reverse post-synaptic neurotoxic paralysis (α-bungarotoxin-like neurotoxins), but will not usually reverse established pre-synaptic paralysis (β-bungarotoxin-like neurotoxins), so should be given before major paralysis has occurred (Fig. 11.2). Coagulopathy is best reversed by antivenom, but even after all venom is neutralised, there

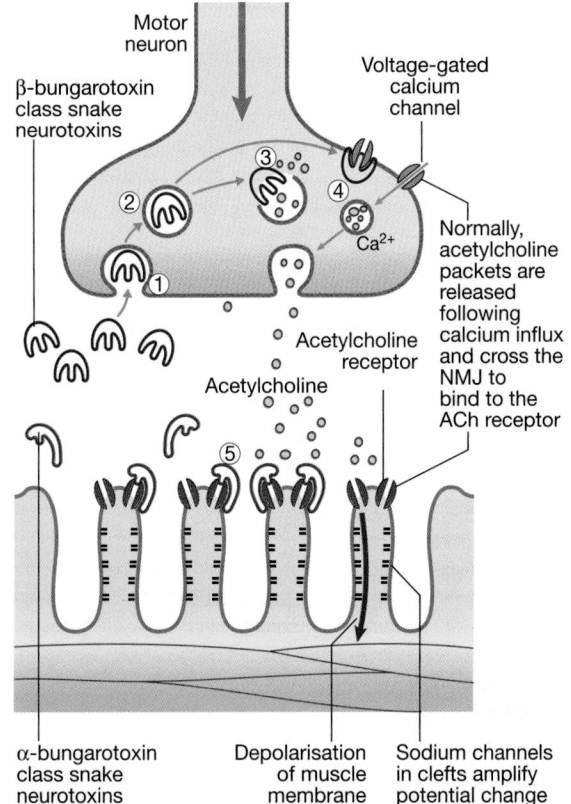

Fig. 11.2 Principal snake venom neurotoxins acting at the neuromuscular junction (NMJ). The pre-synaptic neurotoxins (β-bungarotoxin-like) bind to the cell membrane of the terminal axon (1), form a synaptosome (2) and enter the cell, where they disrupt acetylcholine (ACh) production (3) and damage intracellular structures, including ion channels (4). On initial entry, they cause release of excess ACh, followed by cessation of all ACh release, causing irreversible paralysis until the cell is repaired (days to weeks later). The post-synaptic neurotoxins (α-bungarotoxin-like) bind adjacent to the ACh receptor on the external surface of the muscle end plate and block ACh binding (5), thereby ceasing neurotransmission. Because this action is external to the cell and does not cause cell damage, it is potentially a reversible paralysis. *Copyright © Julian White.*

may be a delay of hours before normal coagulation is restored. More antivenom should not be given because coagulopathy has failed to normalise fully in the first 1–3 hours (except in very particular circumstances). Thrombocytopenia may persist for days despite antivenom. The role of antivenom in reversing established rhabdomyolysis and renal failure is uncertain. Antivenom may help limit local tissue effects or injury in the bitten limb, but this is quite variable and time-dependent. Neuroexcitatory envenoming can respond very well to antivenom (Australian funnel web

spider bites and Mexican, South American and Indian scorpion stings), but there is controversy about the effectiveness of antivenom for some species (some North African and Middle Eastern scorpions). The role of antivenom in limiting local venom effects, including necrosis, is also controversial; it is most likely to be effective when given early.

All patients receiving antivenom are at risk of both early and late adverse reactions, including anaphylaxis (early; not always related to immunoglobulin E (IgE)) and serum sickness (late).

Non-antivenom treatments

Anticholinesterases are used as an adjunctive treatment for post-synaptic paralysis.

Prazosin, an α-adrenoceptor antagonist (α-blocker) has been used in the management of hypertension or pulmonary oedema in scorpion sting cardiotoxicity, particularly for Indian red scorpion stings, though antivenom is now the preferred treatment.

Antibiotics are not routinely required for most bites/stings, though a few animals, such as some South American pit vipers and stingrays, regularly cause significant wound infection or abscess. Tetanus is a risk in some types of bite or sting, such as snakebite, but intramuscular toxoid should not be given until any coagulopathy is reversed.

Mechanical ventilation (p. 207) is vital for established respiratory paralysis that will not reverse with antivenom and may be required for prolonged periods (up to several months in some cases).

Fasciotomy as a treatment for potential compartment syndrome or severe limb swelling is an overused and often disastrous surgical intervention in snakebite and is associated with poor functional outcomes. It should be reserved as a treatment of last resort and used only in cases where compartment syndrome is confirmed by intra-compartment pressure measurement and after first trying limb elevation, antivenom and ensuring that any coagulopathy has resolved.

Follow-up

Cases with significant envenomation and those receiving antivenom should be followed up to ensure any complications have resolved and to identify any delayed envenoming.

Prevention

Community education promoting prevention should be an important part of health delivery, particularly in low resource nations where access to health care may be suboptimal. For snakebite, avoiding sleeping on the ground, walking barefoot or without illumination at night should be emphasised. Use of mosquito netting over raised beds may prevent both mosquito-borne diseases and nocturnal snakebite (kraits in Asia). Use of boots in paddy fields may reduce the risk of snakebite. Installation of glossy tiles around the base of buildings may discourage scorpion entry in endemic areas.

Envenomation by specific animals

Venomous snakes

Venomous snakes represent the single most important cause of envenomation globally, affecting millions of humans annually and resulting in large numbers of deaths and patients left with long-term disability. Of the 3000-plus snake species, more than 1000 either are venomous or produce oral toxins. The most important venomous snake families are the Viperidae (vipers; includes typical vipers (subfamily Viperinae) and pit vipers, with heat-sensing pit organs (subfamily Crotalinae)) and the Elapidae (cobras, kraits, mambas, coral snakes, sea snakes, Australian snakes). However, there are also dangerous species among the Atractaspidinae (side-fanged burrowing vipers of Africa and the Middle East) and the non-front-fanged colubroids (NFFC snakes; several families, including the 'back-fanged' boomslang and vine snakes of Africa and the keelbacks of Asia).

A selection of important species is included in Boxes 11.4–11.6.

Clinical features and management

As with other forms of envenomation, the management of snakebite follows the standard assessment guidelines described previously (p. 240). The nature of the risks posed will depend on the specific snake fauna in a given region (p. 241). For example, in South Asia, the major snakebite risks are claimed to come from the 'big four': cobras, kraits, Russell's viper and saw-scaled vipers. This list is misleading, though, as it omits other important snakes, including the hump-nosed vipers, king cobra and green pit vipers, all of which can cause severe or lethal envenoming and may not be covered by current Indian antivenoms. Even for those snakes recognised as causing envenoming, there may be major geographical variation in venom and features of envenoming. For Russell's viper (*Daboia* spp.), Sri Lankan specimens can cause rhabdomyolysis and flaccid paralysis, in addition to classic severe coagulopathy, haemorrhage, local bite site injury and acute kidney injury (AKI). Most Indian populations of the same snake are not associated with either rhabdomyolysis or paralysis, but in parts of Southern India may cause anterior pituitary haemorrhage and/or capillary leak syndrome (hypotensive shock plus vascular leakage resulting in pulmonary oedema). Capillary leak syndrome is also encountered with populations of Burmese Russell's viper (Myanmar), where AKI is especially common and severe.

Antivenom raised against venom from one population of snakes may be poorly effective against bites from snakes from other regions; this is particularly true for Russell's vipers. Similarly, each of the several species of saw-scaled vipers (*Echis* spp.) spread from West Africa across the Middle East to South Asia (including Sri Lanka) has specific venoms that may not be neutralised by antivenoms raised against other species in the genus; Indian antivenoms are ineffective against African species. It follows that, in managing snakebite envenomation, it is critically important to choose the appropriate antivenom and to understand that this may not include every antivenom claimed to cover a given species.

It is unwise to assume that everything is known about envenoming by snakes because new clinical information and syndromes are emerging as more detailed studies are carried out. For instance, krait bites (*Bungarus* spp.), long associated with 'painless' bites, later development of devastating flaccid paralysis and a high mortality rate, are now known to have some venom diversity. At least some species can cause rhabdomyolysis (black krait, Bangladesh) and/or severe hyponatraemia, and while bites may be painless, systemic envenomation can cause severe abdominal pain in at least some patients. Among cobra bites, the previous division into 'non-spitting', neurotoxic species and 'spitting', less neurotoxic species that cause local necrosis is less clear. Non-spitters are now known to spit in parts of their range (e.g. *Naja kaouthia* in West Bengal) and may cause local necrosis in addition to paralysis. Previously clear diagnostic indicators for envenomation by particular types of snakes, such as Russell's vipers and saw-scaled vipers causing coagulopathy, have also become less sure, as other snakes, such as hump-nosed vipers (*Hypnale* spp.) and green pit vipers (*Trimeresurus* spp.), found in similar regions, can also cause marked coagulopathy and yet are often not covered by available antivenoms. The ability to cause life-threatening coagulopathy, associated with snakes previously considered harmless, such as the keelbacks in Asia (*Rhabdophis* spp.), can further complicate the diagnostic and management process, as antivenom against these snakes is currently available only in Japan.

Scorpions

Scorpions are second only to snakes in their venomous impact on humankind. Most medically important scorpions are in the family Buthidae and have complex neuroexcitatory venoms with highly specific ion-channel toxins. Classically, stings by these scorpions (some key genera listed in Boxes 11.4–11.6) cause moderate to severe local pain and

rapid-onset systemic envenoming with development of a catecholamine storm-like syndrome as the toxins target the nervous system. There may be tachycardia or bradycardia, hyper- or hypotension, profuse sweating, salivation, cardiac dysfunction and pulmonary oedema. Cardiac collapse can occur, especially in children. Other clinical features may vary, depending on the scorpion species.

The Iranian scorpion, *Hemiscorpius lepturus* (principally south-west Iran), causes a quite different presentation, with an initial minor sting, followed by progressive development of bite site or limb necrosis and a potentially lethal systemic envenoming, characterised by intravascular haemolysis, disseminated intravascular coagulation (DIC), secondary renal failure and shock.

Clinical features and management

The approach to management varies with species and region. In South America, specific antivenoms are routinely used and associated with improved outcomes and reduced mortality. In India, the past reliance on prazosin has been replaced with use of specific antivenom, again with improved outcomes. In contrast, in parts of North Africa, past reliance on antivenom has been replaced with use of cardiac support and arguably poorer outcomes.

In Iran, *H. lepturus* stings are treated with antivenom, though as presentation is often delayed because the sting initially appears to be minor, the role of late antivenom is unclear.

Spiders

There are vast numbers and great species diversity of spiders, with two broad taxonomic groupings: the more 'primitive' Mygalomorphs (several medically important species, especially Australian funnel web spiders (*Atrax, Hadronyche* and *Illawarra*)) and the far more diverse Araneomorphs (main clinically important species in the genera *Latrodectus* (widow spiders), *Loxosceles* (brown recluse spiders) and *Phoneutria* (banana or wandering spiders)).

Clinical features and management

While spiders and spider bites are common, only those genera noted above commonly cause medically significant effects. In most cases this is a neuroexcitatory envenoming, sometimes similar to severe scorpion envenoming (notable from Australian funnel web spiders), but the recluse spiders cause an often painless bite that develops into local skin necrosis and sometimes a systemic illness similar to that caused by the Iranian scorpion, *H. lepturus*, and with similar lethal potential. Widow spiders cause 'latrodectism', with initial local pain and sweating. In some, the pain becomes severe, sometimes spreading regionally followed by generalised pain, with associated hypertension, nausea and malaise.

For most of these spiders, antivenom remains the key treatment and is life-saving in some cases. Studies suggesting that anti-*Latrodectus* antivenom is ineffective have not been confirmed by independent studies and are in contrast to decades of positive clinical experience.

Paralysis ticks

Most ticks are vectors for disease but a few species in Australia, North America and parts of Africa can cause flaccid paralysis. Toxins in the saliva act as potent pre-synaptic neurotoxins that can cause gradual-onset *ascending* flaccid paralysis.

There are no antivenoms for tick paralysis. Treatment is based on removal of all ticks and supportive care, including intubation/ventilation where required. The paralysis usually resolves by about 48 hours following removal of all ticks, although embedded ticks may be hard to find, hiding in the scalp, ears and skin folds.

Venomous insects

A number of insects are venomous, but very few cause significant envenoming in humans.

Venomous lepidopterans

The *Lonomia* caterpillars of South America, especially Brazil, have numerous protective venomous spines that, on contact with the skin, can discharge a potent procoagulant venom that can cause a progressive and sometimes fatal consumptive coagulopathy, with terminal haemorrhagic and/or organ failure events. Treatment includes use of a Brazilian specific antivenom and supportive care.

Venomous hymenopterans

Many bees, wasps, hornets and some ants have modified ovipositors in the abdomen that act as stings, attached to venom glands. The quantity of venom injected in a single sting is insufficient to cause significant envenomation, but as many of these venoms are potently allergenic, it can cause severe and sometimes fatal anaphylaxis in sensitised persons (p. 183). Massed stings by hundreds of these insects in a swarm, however, can cause life-threatening systemic envenoming, often with intravascular haemolysis, DIC, shock and multi-organ failure. 'Africanised' bees are a particular risk for such attacks in South America and now in parts of North America. The giant wasps and hornets of Asia can similarly cause systemic envenoming with multiple attacks, even from a few individual insects. Invasive ants, such as *Solenopsis* spp., are colonising new regions and can cause both allergic reactions and unpleasant local reactions.

Marine venomous and poisonous animals

The marine environment is dominated by animal life, and many species utilise toxins, either self-produced or taken up from the environment, to arm themselves for either defence or predation. Many of these animals can cause adverse effects in humans, either as a direct venom effect on bites/stings (venomous spiny fish, sea snakes, stingrays, jellyfish, sea urchins, some starfish, cone snails, selected octopuses etc.), or through poisoning if eaten (fugu, ciguatera, scombroid, several types of shellfish poisoning; p. 236).

For venomous marine animals, there is antivenom available only for sea snakes, which can cause rhabdomyolysis and/or paralytic neurotoxicity; box jellyfish, which can cause very rapid cardiac collapse; and stonefish, which cause intense sting-site pain and sometimes local necrosis. In general, marine venoms respond to heat; thus a hot water immersion or shower (about 45°C) is effective at reducing local pain, particularly for jellyfish, stinging fish and stingray stings. For stingray stings, the venom may cause local tissue damage both through sting trauma and a venom effect. Wounds penetrating the abdomen or chest are potentially lethal and should be adequately explored, cleaned and allowed to heal by secondary intention, with antibiotic treatment of secondary infection if indicated. For bites by the blue-ringed octopus and stings by cone snails, rapid-acting venom can cause early cardiovascular collapse and flaccid paralysis. Supportive care is crucial in ensuring survival from these potentially lethal and seemingly trivial local wounds. Sea urchin and venomous starfish wounds can result in multiple penetrating spines, which cause pain and act as a nidus for secondary infection, but surgical removal of spines can be difficult and unrewarding. Contact with venomous sessile animals (coral, anemones, some sponges etc.) can result in painful local envenoming.

Further information

Books and journal articles

Brent J, Burkhart K, Dargan P, Hatten B, Megarbane B, Palmer R, White J, eds. Critical care toxicology, 2nd edn. Cham: Springer; 2017.

Meier J, White J. Handbook of clinical toxicology of animal venoms and poisons. Boca Raton: CRC Press; 1995.

World Health Organization, Regional Office for Africa. Guidelines for the prevention and clinical management of snakebite in Africa; 2010. https://www.who.int/snakebites/resources/9789290231684/en/

World Health Organization, Regional Office for South-East Asia. Guidelines for the management of snake-bites, 2nd edn; 2016. https://www.who.int/snakebites/resources/9789290225300/en/.

Websites

toxinology.com *Clinical toxinology guide from the University of Adelaide.*

who.int *Information from the World Health Organization on snakes, snakebite and antivenoms.*

AC Baker

12

Medicine in austere environments

'Wilderness medicine' can be defined as medical care delivered in environments greater than one hour away from definitive care, however in practice it often represents the care of patients that are multiple hours, if not days, away from the nearest hospital. This covers a broad range of scenarios from expeditions to commercial work and research projects, often in austere conditions. Adventure tourism is also becoming increasingly popular, and projected to grow further in the future.

Delivery of exemplary care in this context is summarised in Box 12.1. It involves a core understanding of the interaction between the environment and human health, alongside strong situational awareness and consideration of human factors. As the environment continually alters, whether through population growth, economic development or climate change, it plays an important role in disease causation – one that may increase over time. This chapter deals principally with the acute effects of environmental hazards on individuals and should be read in conjunction with the chapters on Acute Medicine and Critical Illness (Ch. 9) and Poisoning (Ch. 10).

Extremes of temperature

Thermoregulation

Body heat is generated by basal metabolic activity and muscle movement, and lost by four main mechanisms: conduction, convection, evaporation and radiation (Fig. 12.1). Body temperature is controlled in the hypothalamus, which is directly sensitive to changes in core temperature and indirectly responds to temperature-sensitive neurons in the skin. The normal 'set-point' of core temperature is tightly regulated within the range $37 \pm 0.5°C$, which is necessary to preserve the normal function of many enzymes and metabolic processes. Aspects of thermoregulation specific to old age are detailed in Box 12.2.

The cold environment

Protective mechanisms in a cold environment include activation of the sympathetic nervous system with cutaneous vasoconstriction, shivering and increases in both heart rate and cardiac contractility. Shivering, an involuntary contraction and relaxation of muscles, is an early adaptive cold response that results in a two- to fivefold increase in heat generation. As core temperature drops these protective mechanisms fail; shivering stops between 29°C and 31°C.

Physiological effects

The cold environment has six main effects on physiological systems:

Metabolism

Regional organ blood flow is reduced in the cold environment with marked variation; the kidneys demonstrate the most significant change, similar in response to that seen with haemorrhage or sepsis. The stress response results in glycogenolysis and gluconeogenesis with a relatively defective insulin efficacy resulting in hyperglycaemia.

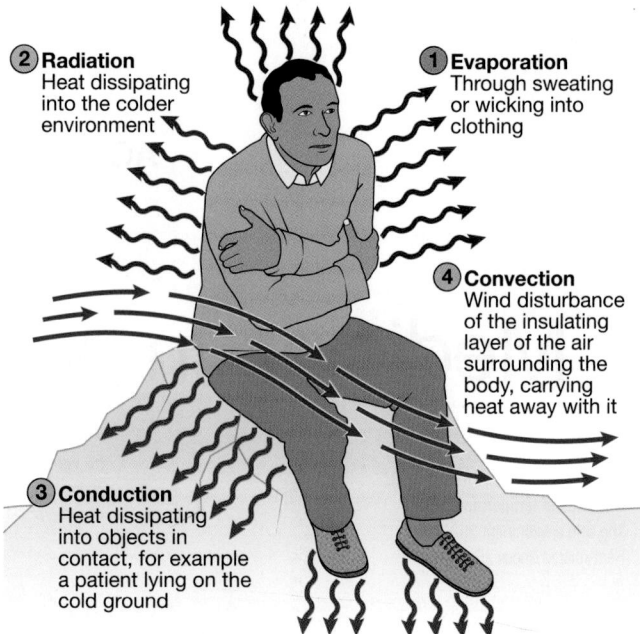

2 Radiation Heat dissipating into the colder environment

1 Evaporation Through sweating or wicking into clothing

4 Convection Wind disturbance of the insulating layer of the air surrounding the body, carrying heat away with it

3 Conduction Heat dissipating into objects in contact, for example a patient lying on the cold ground

Fig. 12.1 Mechanisms of heat loss.

12.2 Thermoregulation in old age

- **Age-associated changes**: impairments in vasomotor function, skeletal muscle response and sweating mean that older people react more slowly to changes in temperature.
- **Increased comorbidity**: thermoregulatory problems are more likely in the presence of pathology such as atherosclerosis and hypothyroidism, and medication such as sedatives and hypnotics.
- **Hypothermia**: this may arise as a primary event, but more commonly complicates other acute illness, e.g. pneumonia, stroke or fracture.
- **Ambient temperature**: financial pressures and older equipment may result in inadequate heating during cold weather.

Fluid and electrolytes

As the body cools there is a relative decrease in plasma volume as fluid moves intracellularly with subsequent inadequate tissue perfusion. There is a decrease in intracellular potassium below a core temperature of 25°C, which is linked to the risk of arrhythmias.

Respiratory

For every 1°C reduction in core temperature there is a 6% drop in oxygen consumption. The initial increased respiratory rate declines with ongoing cooling, with animal studies suggesting a cessation of breathing at a core temperature of 24°C. There is direct respiratory centre depression from a reduction in both oxygen expenditure and production of carbon dioxide.

Cardiovascular

As the core temperature falls there is a reduction in cardiac output with initial maintenance of stroke volume. At around 28°C the heart rate is reduced by 50% with a subsequent increased risk of arrythmias. Initial conduction abnormalities include a sinus bradycardia, progressing to slow atrial fibrillation (AF) and then to ventricular fibrillation (VF). VF may be induced below 30°C with excessive stimulation/movement, which is why handling of a hypothermic patient needs to be performed with great care.

Haematological

There is an increased plasma viscosity, with a 150% rise in haematocrit documented at a core temperature of 25°C. Enzymatic reactions within the coagulation cascade are prolonged, alongside platelet trapping within the liver and spleen, resulting in an increased bleeding risk.

---

i 12.1 Key factors in the delivery of exemplary wilderness medicine

- Optimise participant fitness (e.g. pre-departure health screening)
- Understand the patterns of injury and anticipate issues
- Appropriate technical equipment, medical kit and drugs
- Effective logistical support
- Multiple communication options (awareness of limitations of each)
- Understand environmental factors that affect ingress and egress
- Proactive rather than reactive approach (e.g. daily skin checks/blister care)
- Established standard operating procedures (SOPs)

Neurological

There is a decline in cognitive function in the cold environment with unconsciousness occurring at a core temperature around 28–30°C. Slurred speech, ataxia and paradoxical undressing are all described with lowering core temperatures. Absence of brain electrical activity is seen below 20°C; this is generally considered to be neuroprotective. It is believed that the cold stabilises the blood–brain barrier and cerebral cell membranes that would otherwise be disrupted by hypoxia.

Hypothermia

Hypothermia is defined as a core temperature below 35°C and can be sub-categorised into primary hypothermia due to environmental exposure and secondary hypothermia due to abnormal thermoregulatory mechanisms as a result of an underlying altered physiological state. Measurement of core temperature can be challenging, with tympanic measurements often considered inaccurate; monitors are often not calibrated below 35.5°C. Alternatives such as oesophageal temperature can be difficult to achieve in practice, and rectal measurements (considered the gold standard measurement) can lag behind the true core temperature.

Traditionally, hypothermia is categorised as mild (32–35°C), moderate (28–32°C) and severe (< 28°C), however, newer staging systems, such as the Swiss Staging System, adopted by some ambulance services, define the level of hypothermia based on symptoms (Fig. 12.2). This has been shown to overestimate the degree of hypothermia in around 20% of cases but remains a helpful classification when an accurate core temperature cannot be obtained.

Management

Following resuscitation, the objectives of management are to rewarm the patient in a controlled manner whilst treating associated hypoxia (by oxygenation and ventilation if necessary), fluid and electrolyte disturbance, and cardiovascular abnormalities. Careful handling is essential to avoid precipitating arrhythmias. The Swiss Staging System can be used to guide treatment at various levels of hypothermia (see Fig. 12.2).

Mild hypothermia

Continued heat loss can be prevented by sheltering the patient from the cold, replacing wet clothing, covering the head and insulating the patient from the ground. Hibler's method is the best available technique for packaging a patient, which involves wrapping the patient in an insulating layer, followed by an outer vapour-tight layer. Warm drinks and active movement can raise the core temperature by 2°C per hour. Forced-air re-warming blankets and heat packs can increase core temperature by 0.1–3.4°C per hour. Warmed intravenous fluids have been shown to provide no active warming but they do prevent further cooling.

Severe hypothermia

For severe hypothermia a number of invasive warming methods can be instigated in hospital. This includes bladder lavage, which involves flushing the bladder with 300 mL of warm saline resulting in a 1–2°C rise in core temperature per hour. Thoracic lavage through two unilateral chest drains (anterior and lateral) can result in a 2–3°C rise per hour. A single chest drain approach can be used by clamping a 32–36 French tube for 2–3 minutes after flushing in 300 mL of warm saline, then allowing it to drain.

Extracorporeal membrane oxygenation (ECMO) and cardiopulmonary bypass (CPB) are performed in specialist hospitals and represent the best warming strategies, with increases in core temperature of 6–10°C per hour.

Cardiac arrest

There are a number of adaptations to resuscitation algorithms for hypothermic patients in cardiac arrest (Box 12.3). There is an old adage that 'you're not dead until you're warm and dead' with documented cases of full recovery following extended periods of ECMO and CPB (Box 12.4). There are, however, some markers of futility. These include: obvious

Stage/core temperature	Symptoms	Treatment
01: 32–35°	Alert and shivering	Pragmatic support. Warm environment and clean warm clothes. Hot sugary drinks. Active movement – can increase temperature generation by 20 times the basal metabolic rate
02: 28–<32°	Drowsy and not shivering	Insulate whole body, wind and vapour barrier and external rewarming (warming blanket or chemical packs around axilla and groin). Warm fluids (this prevents further cooling but doesn't actively warm). Try to reduce movement to avoid arrhythmias. Keep horizontal.
03: 24–<28°	Unconscious with vital signs, no shivering	Same as stage 2 but added airway support as needed. May require more invasive warming methods including extracorporeal membrane oxygenation (ECMO) or cardiopulmonary bypass (CPB)
04: <24°	Unconscious with no vital signs	Same as stage 3 but manage as cardiac arrest

Fig. 12.2 Swiss Staging System and the treatment of hypothermia.

12.3 Management of cardiac arrest in hypothermic patients

- Assessment for signs of life should be extended to 1 minute
- Ventricular fibrillation and ventricular tachycardia can be defibrillated, however if after three shocks there is no response, additional shocks should be delayed until core temperature is > 30°C (3-shock 'stacked' sequences are not recommended)
- Withhold adjunctive medications (adrenaline, amiodarone etc.) if the temperature is below 30°C; or double the interval between doses when temperature is 30–35°C

12.4 Cases of full recovery following extended periods of ECMO and CPB

- In 1999 a 29-year-old Norwegian radiology registrar fell whilst skiing into an ice waterfall gully. She was cut out after 1 hour and 20 minutes with a core temperature of 13.7°C. Following 9 hours of CPR and CPB she survived with no neurological impairment.
- In 2011 a 7-year-old Swedish girl fell from a cliff into the sea and was found in the water after 3–4 hours with a core temperature of 13.2°C. Following CPR and warming she survived with no neurological impairment.

(CPB = cardiopulmonary bypass; CPR = cardiopulmonary resuscitation; ECMO = extracorporeal membrane oxygenation)

lethal injury, prolonged asphyxia (mouthful of snow etc.), incompressible thorax (distinct from a stiff chest which is common), frozen abdomen, or potassium > 12 mmol/L.

Cold injury

Freezing cold injury ('frostbite')

Hypothermia-induced vasoconstriction results in tissue cooling and frostbite refers to ice formation and freezing within the tissue, most commonly affecting the hands and feet (around 90% of cases). Risk factors include alcohol consumption (which impairs decision-making and results in peripheral vasodilatation), previous frostbite, drug use, inappropriate clothing, fatigue and dehydration. There are two distinct phases to cold injury: a 'cooling–supercooling–freezing' stage during exposure; and a vascular stage during re-warming. When skin tissues cool to below 0°C ice crystal formation causes microvascular and cell damage. During warming, this results in a degree of circulatory failure and fluid loss. The release of inflammatory mediators causes ischaemia and clot production. Re-freezing following warming is particularly destructive, resulting in massive cell inflammatory changes, therefore re-warming should only be initiated if there is no risk of further re-freezing.

Patients often describe an initial numbness and woody sensation followed by a severe pain during warming with a persistent throbbing sensation. Pain can endure for months alongside potentially permanent sensory changes. The skin can look waxy, discoloured or blistered (Fig. 12.3), however prognostication using initial skin changes can be very challenging.

Management

If concerned about the possibility of cold injury, immediate pre-hospital treatment is to try to shelter from the environment, consume warm drinks, remove shoes, wet clothing and jewellery and re-dress in warm, dry clothing. If there is absolutely no risk of re-freezing then warming the area can be achieved by placing the area into a companion's armpit or groin. Aspirin 75–300 mg and ibuprofen 800 mg are recommended. Do not rub the area and do not place heat sources directly onto the area. Evacuation for formal medical review should be obtained. Warmed areas need to be made non-load-bearing and therefore prior thought about extraction needs to be considered. Aloe vera gel has anti-prostaglandin effects and can be applied before application of a non-adherent dressing, splinting and elevation of the affected region.

Definitive warming involves placing the affected area into circulating water between 37°C and 42°C with small amounts of antiseptic for around an hour, avoiding contact with the sides of the container. Additional treatment involves fluid replacement with warmed fluids (due to cold diuresis), strong analgesia and blister care. Blisters may present as clear, cloudy or haemorrhagic. Blister management remains controversial, with current evidence recommending débridement of all blisters in hospital (likely under a general anaesthetic) to improve wound healing. There is no evidence for prophylactic antibiotics and tetanus prophylaxis should be given according to local protocols; frostbite wounds are not considered tetanus-prone.

In-hospital management includes specialist imaging (e.g. angiography and technetium bone scanning) to inform prognosis. A combination of thrombolysis and vasodilators (such as nitroglycerin), given within 24 hours, has evidence of good outcomes. Iloprost, a prostacyclin analogue that causes vasodilation and reduces the requirement for amputation, can be given intravenously after 24 hours of injury. Early

amputations have a higher morbidity and surgery should be delayed unless there is evidence of sepsis. There is also a potential role for hyperbaric oxygen treatment and this is an area of current research.

Non-freezing cold injury

This results from prolonged exposure to cold, damp conditions and is often seen in individuals who become wet but are unable to dry out. The important distinction from frostbite is that the tissues do not freeze. It is almost exclusively seen in the lower limb and feet, however concomitant injury to the hands is sometimes seen. It is often described as a patch of numbness, which when rewarmed, changes in colour from pale to red, with associated swelling and pain. These symptoms can last for months or indefinitely; often far longer than an equivalent freezing injury. The pathology remains uncertain but probably involves endothelial injury. Gradual re-warming is associated with less pain than rapid re-warming. The pain and associated paraesthesia are difficult to control with conventional analgesia and may benefit from early use of amitriptyline. The patient is at risk of further damage on subsequent exposure to the cold.

Heat-related illness

Heat-related illness defines a spectrum of pathology from benign heat oedema to lethal heat stroke, the definitions of which are found in Box 12.5. There is a growing risk of heat-related illness with global temperatures predicted to rise by between 1.7°C and 5.6°C within this century alone; the World Health Organization predicts over 250 000 additional deaths a year from 2050 as a result of heat exposure.

Heat-related illness is often categorised as either environmental or exertional heat illness depending on the primary underlying mechanism. Environmental heat illness results from elevated ambient temperatures,

i	**12.5 Definitions of heat-related illness**
Heat-related illness	**Definition**
Heat oedema	Mild swelling to the limbs during the first few days of heat exposure due to increased plasma volume, peripheral vasodilation and interstitial pooling of blood
Heat cramps	Muscle spasms related to sodium loss. Generally occur after exercise in non-acclimatised individuals who sweat freely and replace losses with water or other hypotonic solutions, so they become salt depleted. Salt supplementation reduces the incidence
Heat syncope	Heat syncope refers to a multi-factorial syndrome involving transient loss of consciousness in the context of heat exposure with a relatively rapid return to normal function and baseline. Contributing factors may include peripheral vasodilation, orthostatic pooling of blood, prolonged standing, advanced age and dehydration, as well as coexisting medical conditions such as ischaemic heart disease that reduce cardiac output
Heat exhaustion	Characterised by volume and salt depletion. It is an inability to continue an activity due to heat stress. It presents with thirst, lethargy, headache, nausea but importantly a normal mental status. Some literature describes it as benign as it may be protective in the development of heat stroke, causing an individual to stop an activity and thus the generation of heat
Heat stroke	Neurological impairment with core body temperature ≥ 40°C (rectal temperature is gold standard in a pre-hospital environment). Symptoms can involve a coarse muscle tremor, confusion, aggression and loss of consciousness. Sweating may be absent due to dehydration and failure of thermoregulatory mechanisms

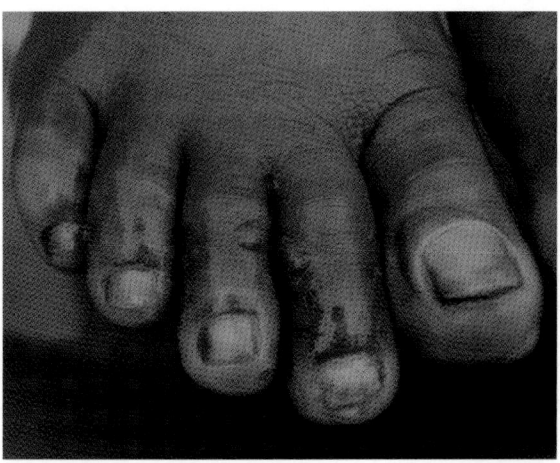

Fig. 12.3 Frostbite in a female Everest sherpa.

with increased incidence seen at the extremes of age, due to sub-optimal homeostatic thermoregulation. Peaks of incidence are common during heatwaves, exemplified by the 70 000 heat-related deaths reported during the 2003 European heatwave. Conversely, exertional heat illness predominantly affects young, physically fit individuals (such as soldiers and athletes), reflecting a failure to dissipate intrinsic heat production from physical activity.

Risk factors for the development of heat illness are well established (Box 12.6).

Pathophysiology of heat stroke

The pathophysiology of heat stroke can be summarised as organ dysfunction from the high temperature itself, and end-organ ischaemia from diminished blood flow. Increased sweating results in dehydration and blood pools in vasodilated peripheral vasculature resulting in a decreased effective blood volume. The blood viscosity increases resulting in heart strain. Enzymes denature at 40°C and at 41°C mitochondrial activity stops; the subsequent loss of oxidative phosphorylation results in organ ischaemia. The muscles and gastrointestinal tract are affected first, followed by the central nervous system, circulatory and clotting systems. The pathophysiology is similar to sepsis, severe trauma and extensive burns (Box 12.7).

Management

Mortality of heat illness is around 30% and is directly proportional to the duration and magnitude of hyperthermia, therefore immediate cooling should begin at the scene, before transfer to hospital. The aim should be to reduce core temperature to approximately 39°C.

A patient should be removed from the heat source and put into shade to reduce radiant heat gain. Resting in an air-conditioned room has cooling rates of 0.03–0.06°C/min. Clothes should be removed, high-flow oxygen administered, intravenous access established and a rectal temperature taken. If temperature measurement is unavailable but the history and clinical findings are consistent with heat illness, initiation of treatment with cooling techniques should not be delayed.

A number of cooling strategies exist (Box 12.8), and their implementation will depend on what is feasible within each particular environment. Two meta-analyses have concluded that ice water immersion is the most effective treatment strategy with cooling rates of 0.20–0.35°C/min for iced water and 0.11°C/min for wet towels. Immersion is unlikely to be feasible in the wilderness environment and many hospitals, with further consideration of the potential dangers of immersing a patient with a reduced conscious level. Immersing the hands and forearms in cold water results in reduction of heat stress in normal subjects, but has not been evaluated in the treatment of heat stroke patients.

The placement of ice/cold packs in the axillae, groin and neck has been recommended as an easy method to use in the field, but when compared with evaporative cooling in healthy subjects, cooling times were longest when the ice packs were used alone and shortest when both methods were used simultaneously. Evaporative cooling involves the removal of clothing, spraying tepid or cool water over the patient, and facilitating evaporation and convection with the use of a fan.

The role of invasive cooling methods such as gastric, bladder or peritoneal lavage has not been fully established. Neither hyperhydration nor dantrolene (used in the treatment of malignant hyperthermia) have

12.6 Risk factors for the development of heat-related illness	
Risk factor	**Mechanism**
High ambient temperatures	Increased radiant heat gain
High humidity	Ineffective evaporative heat loss at humidities > 75%
Little shade	Increased radiant heat gain
Intercurrent illness	Raised core temperature
Extremes of age	Suboptimal homeostatic thermoregulation
Overweight/unfit	The main identifiable risk factor for heat illness during military training was a body mass index (BMI) $\geq$ 30 kg/m^2
Effects of alcohol and medication (diuretics, ACE inhibitors, β-adrenoceptor antagonists, vasodilators, antidepressants, anticholinergics, antihistamines and stimulants)	Either through dehydration, decreased cardiovascular and peripheral response to dissipate heat, reduced sweating or increased metabolic rate
Inappropriate clothing	Reduced heat loss through combination of radiation, convection and evaporation
Dehydration	Regardless of body habitus or fitness level, fluid losses that result in a 2%–3% decrease in body weight correlate with decreased aerobic performance, increased perception of fatigue, and greater core temperatures at a given workload
Previous heat-related illness	Impaired homeostatic thermoregulation
No acclimatisation	Body fluid deficits are reduced by around 30% in acclimatised individuals, despite increased sweat rates of up to 18%, as a result of a more accurate thirst response
Intense work/duration	Increased heat generation

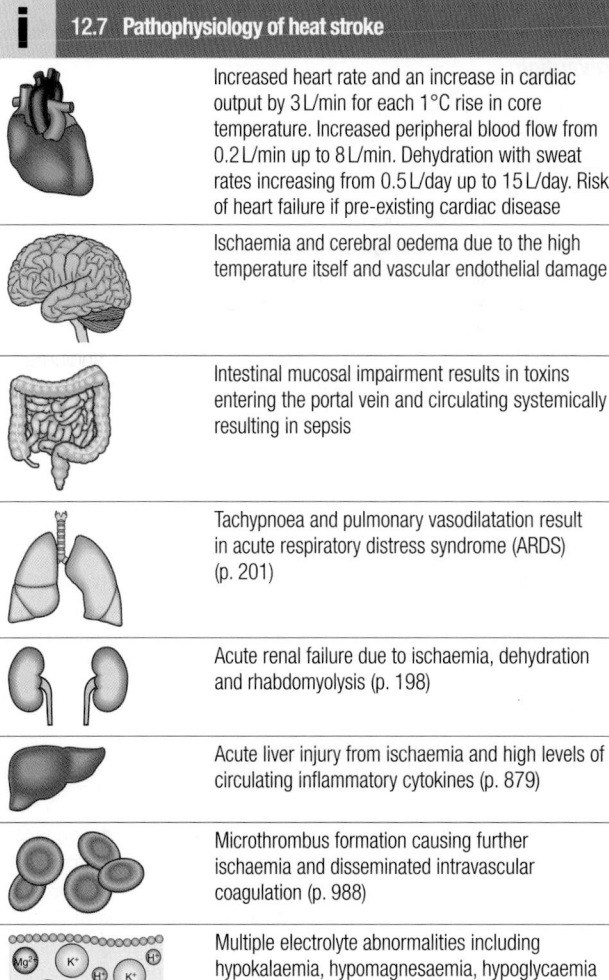

12.7 Pathophysiology of heat stroke	
	Increased heart rate and an increase in cardiac output by 3 L/min for each 1°C rise in core temperature. Increased peripheral blood flow from 0.2 L/min up to 8 L/min. Dehydration with sweat rates increasing from 0.5 L/day up to 15 L/day. Risk of heart failure if pre-existing cardiac disease
	Ischaemia and cerebral oedema due to the high temperature itself and vascular endothelial damage
	Intestinal mucosal impairment results in toxins entering the portal vein and circulating systemically resulting in sepsis
	Tachypnoea and pulmonary vasodilatation result in acute respiratory distress syndrome (ARDS) (p. 201)
	Acute renal failure due to ischaemia, dehydration and rhabdomyolysis (p. 198)
	Acute liver injury from ischaemia and high levels of circulating inflammatory cytokines (p. 879)
	Microthrombus formation causing further ischaemia and disseminated intravascular coagulation (p. 988)
	Multiple electrolyte abnormalities including hypokalaemia, hypomagnesaemia, hypoglycaemia and metabolic acidosis

12

ℹ 12.8 Summary of cooling rates

Cooling technique (target < 39°C)	Cooling rate
Ice water immersion	0.20–0.35°C/min
Wet towels	0.11°C/min
Evaporative and convective combined	0.034–0.31°C/min
Air-conditioned room	0.03–0.06°C/min
Intravenous cold saline	0.03°C/min
Intravenous room-temperature saline	0.015°C/min

ℹ 12.9 Wet Bulb Globe Temperature (WBGT)

Meteorological conditions affect environmental temperatures and a widely used index to calculate this is the WBGT, originally developed by the US Marines. WBGT is an apparent temperature measurement taking into account temperature, humidity, wind speed and solar radiation. This gives a much more accurate representation of the degree of heat stress experienced. WBGT is used to formulate a set of guidelines that guide activity levels, hydration and rest periods. For example, a 'do not start' WBGT of 21°C has been suggested for American marathons based on an unsuccessful attempt of 160 per 1000 finishers above this level, although the incidence of heat-related illness is not well described.

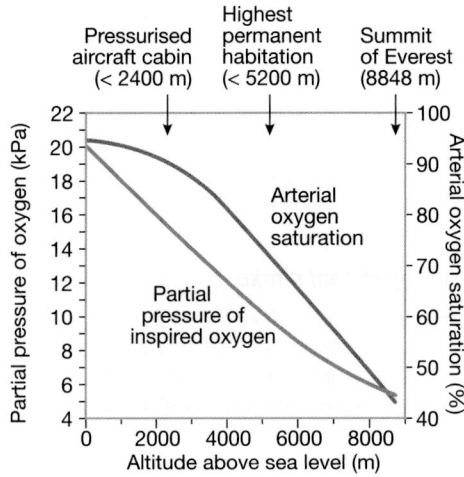

Fig. 12.4 Change in inspired oxygen tension and blood oxygen saturation at altitude. The blue curve shows changes in oxygen availability at altitude and the red curve shows the typical resultant changes in arterial oxygen saturation in a healthy person. Oxygen saturation varies between individuals according to the shape of the oxygen–haemoglobin dissociation curve and the ventilatory response to hypoxaemia. (To convert kPa to mmHg, multiply by 7.5.)

evidence of benefit. Cold intravenous fluids may supplement cooling. In a study of healthy volunteers, infusion of 4°C saline over 30 minutes cooled the body by 1°C, compared to 0.5°C with room-temperature saline.

Prevention

Cooling in a wilderness setting may be incredibly challenging, with likely no access to ice or cold fluids. Prevention of heat illness is therefore paramount. Strategies include:

1. Ensuring adequate hydration. The 2019 Wilderness Medical Society heat illness guidelines identify hydration as the 'most readily modifiable physiologic risk factor'. Fluid ingestion is also identified as the most effective approach to mitigate the rise in core temperature amongst athletes. Military guidelines recommend a 0.25–1.25 L/hr hydration strategy that varies for work rates (low/medium/high/very high) at a given Wet Bulb Globe Temperature (WBGT) (Box 12.9).
2. Consider accepted WBGT cut-offs for activities (Box 12.9).
3. Expedition participants should receive high-level education pre-departure on the dangers of heat-related illness with evidence-based advice on risk reduction. Increased hydration and cooling strategies have been documented following educational material targeting older people prior to heatwaves.
4. If possible, implementing a period of acclimatisation with at least 1–2 hours of mild exertion in a hot environment for at least 8 days. Body fluid deficits are reduced by around 30% in acclimatised individuals as a result of a more accurate thirst response.

Acute high altitude illness

Illness due to high altitudes represents over a quarter of all serious medical incidents from reviews of expeditions in a range of environments. High altitude is generally considered to be over 2500 m and extreme altitude over 5500 m. The summit of Mount Everest stands at 8848 m, where the barometric pressure and atmospheric partial pressure of oxygen (PO_2) is around one-third of that at sea level; the percentage of oxygen remains the same at 20.9%.

Unconsciousness secondary to hypoxia normally occurs within 3 minutes if the body is exposed to an altitude over 8000 m. However, with a

period of acclimatisation, the body is able to adapt and overcome even profound hypoxaemia with arterial partial pressures of oxygen (PaO_2) of 2.55 kPa recorded at 8400 m in a healthy climber (normally > 10.6 kPa at sea level).

Physiological effects of high altitude

There are a number of physiological systems affected by altitude.

Respiratory

Reduction in oxygen tension results in a fall in arterial oxygen saturation (Fig. 12.4). This varies widely between individuals, depending on the shape of the sigmoid oxygen–haemoglobin dissociation curve (see Fig. 25.5) and the ventilatory response. Alveolar ventilation increases with altitude, lowering carbon dioxide and resulting in a respiratory alkalosis, with metabolic compensation via renal bicarbonate loss. At high altitude, individuals are at the steep section of the oxygen dissociation curve whereby a small fall in PaO_2 can result in a substantial decrease in oxygen saturation. The initial respiratory alkalosis shifts the curve to the left but with a period of acclimatisation, increased production of 2,3-diphosphoglycerate moves the curve rightwards towards a sea-level position.

Haematological

Measured haemoglobin concentration increases with acclimatisation – a 20% fall in plasma volume causes haemoconcentration and erythropoietin release (stimulated by hypoxia) leads to increased production of haemoglobin.

Cardiovascular

There is an initial increase in cardiac output due to increased sympathetic activity and heart rate. The reduction in plasma volume causes a fall in preload and stroke volume. Cardiac output returns to baseline over several weeks but the stroke volume remains lowered.

Illness at high altitude

Neurological and respiratory complications from high altitude occur in individuals who ascend rapidly and are not acclimatised. Acute mountain sickness (AMS) is seen in over a third of people who ascend to 3000 m. Serious illness includes high altitude pulmonary oedema (HAPE) and high altitude cerebral oedema (HACE), occurring in 0.1–4% of people climbing over 4000 m. Prevention is essential and achievable through controlled ascents.

Acute mountain sickness

AMS is a syndrome comprised principally of non-specific symptoms including headache, fatigue, anorexia, nausea and vomiting, insomnia and dizziness. The pathophysiology of AMS is not fully understood but it is thought that hypoxia results in vasodilation and increased capillary hydrostatic pressure causing a fluid leak and a raised intracranial venous volume with risk of raised intracranial pressure. There is believed to be an increase in CSF production with a reduced buffering capacity. Non-acclimatised individuals show impaired gas exchange and a lower degree of hyperventilation, alongside fluid retention and a heightened sympathetic activation. Symptoms can occur within 4 hours, with the diagnostic definition specifying an ascent to >2500 m within the prior 4 days. The symptoms can vary in severity, from trivial to completely incapacitating.

Management

Treatment of mild cases consists of rest and symptomatic control with simple analgesia; symptoms usually resolve after 1–3 days at a stable altitude, but may recur with further ascent. Occasionally there is progression to cerebral oedema (HACE). Persistent symptoms indicate the need to descend, which is considered the definitive treatment.

Medication options include acetazolamide and dexamethasone. Acetazolamide is used in both the prophylaxis of AMS and as a treatment option. It works as a carbonic anhydrase inhibitor in the kidneys, increasing bicarbonate excretion and inducing a metabolic acidosis, thereby offsetting the hyperventilation-induced alkalosis seen at altitude. It also decreases CSF production, reducing intracranial pressure and risk of progression to HACE. Ideal dosing strategies are debated, however 125 mg twice daily may be used as prophylaxis and 250 mg three times daily for treatment. Higher doses (750 mg) have greater efficacy but also increased side-effects. Dexamethasone (8 mg) moderates capillary leak and reduces the inflammatory response, improving symptoms to allow for a safe descent.

High altitude cerebral oedema

HACE is considered a severe sequela of AMS, presenting as ataxia or cognitive impairment in addition to the symptoms described above. It very rarely occurs without being preceded by milder AMS symptoms, making early recognition and treatment of AMS essential. Untreated HACE can progress to coma within 24 hours.

Management

Management is directed at improving oxygenation. Descent is essential and dexamethasone (8 mg immediately, followed by 4 mg four times daily) should be given. If descent is impossible, descent can be simulated with the use of portable hyperbaric chambers, such as a Gamow bag. Use of these devices, however, can be difficult in patients with vomiting or a reduced level of consciousness.

High altitude pulmonary oedema

HAPE is a life-threatening condition that usually occurs in the first 4 days after ascent above 2500 m and is the leading cause of mortality from high altitude illness. It is defined as an imbalance of hydrostatic pressure within the alveoli with no evidence of inflammatory changes. Hypoxic pulmonary vasoconstriction causes alveolar capillary stress failure and subsequent pulmonary hypertension. This results in capillary fluid leak which is exacerbated by exercise and compounded by impaired epithelial sodium transport, normally essential for fluid reabsorption. Initial symptoms include a dry cough, exertional dyspnoea and extreme fatigue. Later, the cough becomes wet with haemoptysis and orthopnoea. Tachycardia

and tachypnoea occur at rest and crepitations may often be heard in both lung fields. Fever may also be present. There may be profound hypoxaemia and radiological evidence of diffuse alveolar oedema. HAPE may occur without the preceding signs of AMS, although around 50% of patients with HAPE have concurrent AMS and 14% have HACE.

Management

Treatment is directed at reversal of hypoxia, with immediate descent (by a minimum of 1000 m) and oxygen administration targeting saturations >90%. A portable hyperbaric chamber should be used if descent is delayed. Nifedipine (60 mg modified release divided into 2–3 doses) is recommended prophylactically, starting 1 day before attempting ascent above 2500 m and continued for a further 5 days at altitude or until descent below 2500 m. For treatment of HAPE there is no evidence of benefit for any pharmacological therapy compared to descent and oxygen.

Subaquatic medicine

Drowning

Drowning remains a leading cause of death globally and is defined as 'the process of experiencing respiratory impairment from submersion/immersion in liquid'. Immersion refers to the upper airway being above the water surface and submersion below it. The drowning process involves initial breath holding, followed by a period of laryngospasm. Gas exchange is prevented resulting in hypoxia, hypercarbia and acidosis. Respiratory movements are stimulated by the respiratory centre due to hypercarbia, however the laryngospasm results in obstruction of the airway. The laryngospasm eventually falters with continued hypoxia resulting in the aspiration of liquid of a variable amount, usually < 4 mL/kg.

Aspiration of either saltwater or freshwater results in changes to the alveolar surfactant and the alveolar capillary barrier causing atelectasis, ventilation–perfusion mismatch and hypoxia. Saltwater is hypertonic resulting in bronchoconstriction, inflammation and pulmonary oedema; aspiration of 2.5 mL/kg of seawater results in a 75% increase in right-to-left shunting of deoxygenated blood. Fresh water is hypotonic and is generally absorbed through the pulmonary circulation, entering the systemic circulation and damaging the alveolar capillary membrane. This can also generate foam which further decreases ventilation efficiency. The clinical significance of swallowing water into the stomach during the drowning process remains unclear. Clinically significant electrolyte abnormalities from aspiration and swallowing of both hypotonic and hypertonic fluids are uncommon requiring >22 mL/kg of fluid, although both hyper- and hyponatraemia have been described.

The majority of drownings occur in cold water that results in body cooling, water being considered thermoneutral at around 35°C. Skin cooling (cold shock) and tissue cooling (hypothermia) are important factors in drowning. The historical term 'dry-drowning' refers to the 10% of drowning cases that are documented to have 'macroscopically dry lungs' on examination, attributed to laryngospasm from water irritation on contact. This remains controversial but is no longer felt to be true, with newer evidence demonstrating the presence of microscopic liquid in the lungs of all drowned patients. 'Secondary drowning', referring to patients who develop acute respiratory distress syndrome (ARDS), is now also considered a misnomer as there is no second submersion and ARDS is a recognised complication of the drowning process.

Cold shock

The cold shock response is believed to be responsible for the majority of drowning deaths. Sudden cold-water immersion results in an uncontrolled reflex inspiratory gasping, hyperventilation with profound hypocapnia and tachycardia from activation of peripheral sub-epidermal cold receptors. There is a 75% reduction in breath hold time, which can therefore result in the aspiration of water. The response is maximal at water temperatures of 10–15 °C and peaks within the first 30 seconds of immersion, waning over 2–3 minutes. Continued immersion then results in physical incapacitation from neuromuscular cooling, with peripheral paralysis occurring at regional limb temperatures of 5–15 °C. Hypothermia develops after around 30 minutes in cold water.

Autonomic conflict

Simultaneous positive and negative chronotropic triggers are considered arrhythmogenic. Bradycardia from vagal stimulation (initiated when face down in water – dive reflex) coupled with a tachycardia from sympathetic activation (cold, stress or exercise) can generate arrhythmias in previously healthy individuals and can be fatal in those with structural cardiac abnormalities.

Pre-hospital management

In-water CPR and rescue breaths are no longer recommended. In-water rescue is not recommended for untrained individuals – remember 'Reach, Throw, Row, Don't Go'. If extracting someone from the water following prolonged immersion, the patient should be kept horizontal to prevent post-immersion hypotension; the loss of hydrostatic pressure that the water was applying can result in venous pooling and a sudden circulatory collapse. The patient should be kept warm, with life support commenced at the earliest opportunity. Cervical spine precautions should be considered as there may be a traumatic precursor to the drowning incident (e.g. tombstoning), although these injuries are uncommon (0.5% of cases). Postural drainage techniques to try to clear fluid from the lungs have no proven benefit.

In-hospital management

Treatment is often focused on re-warming and organ support including non-invasive ventilation (CPAP) and protective lung ventilation strategies for acute lung injury/ARDS. Prolonged immersion can result in hypovolaemia due to the hydrostatic pressure effect of water and the patient may require IV fluid. Prophylactic antibiotics are not recommended unless submersion was in grossly contaminated water. Asymptomatic patients, with no respiratory compromise, a normal chest X-ray and normal arterial blood gas can be discharged home after 6–8 hours' observation.

CPR modifications

Five initial rescue ventilations are recommended given the hypoxic nature of a cardiac arrest in drowning. The patient's chest should be dried before application of defibrillation pads; however less than 5% of drowned patients are in a shockable rhythm. The common progression of cardiac rhythm is from bradycardia, to pulseless electrical activity, to asystole. Submersion in ice-cold water (less than 6°C) may confer improved survival due to neuroprotection from rapid brain cooling before the onset of severe hypoxia; children in particular appear to have greater protection, believed in part to be due to a greater surface area to mass ratio allowing quicker cooling. For submersion times greater than 30 minutes in water warmer than 6°C, resuscitation is likely to be futile. If water temperature is below 6°C resuscitation is likely to be futile following a submersion over 90 minutes long. Submersion within a vehicle may prolong these times due to the potential presence of an air bubble. International guidelines do vary on the futility associated with submersion duration. The overall mortality of drowned patients who present in cardiac arrest is 93%.

Decompression illness

Changes in environmental pressure (as seen in diving) can result in decompression illness due to intravascular or extravascular bubbles, the clinical manifestations of which include both arterial gas embolism and decompression sickness. Diagnosis of decompression illness is based on the history and clinical features in patients following a dive; 90% of cases are symptomatic within 6 hours, however, delays up to 72 hours are described.

A brief review of the physics and physiology of diving is essential in understanding the medical issues encountered. The two most important gas laws are Boyle's law and Henry's law (Fig. 12.5).

Decompression sickness

Nitrogen bubble formation on ascent can cause direct mechanical damage to the vascular endothelium and an inflammatory response. The bubbles occur almost anywhere in the body; therefore, the clinical presentation is broad ranging from malaise and headache to paraesthesiae, lymphoedema, rash, joint pain and neurological manifestations including ataxia, paralysis and altered mentation. The overall incidence is low (0.03%) for recreational divers. Decompression sickness is very uncommon for diving depths less than 10 m and is normally seen following multiple dives.

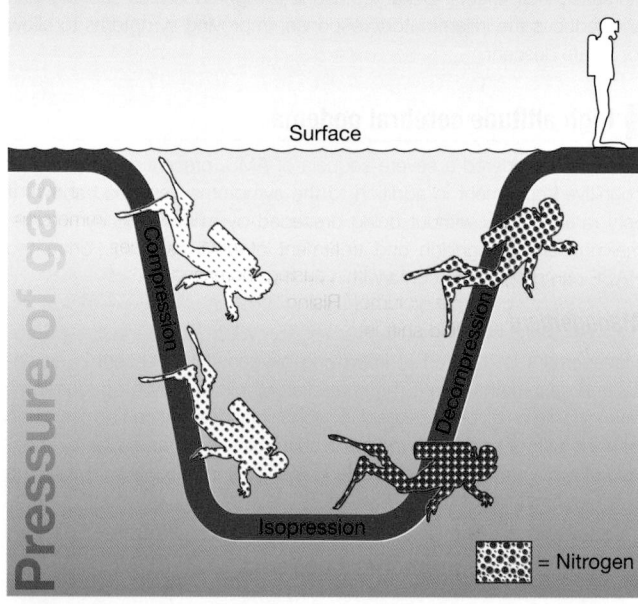

A Boyle's law

Depth in metres	Pressure in atmospheres	Volume of a sealed container	Lung volume
0	1	1	6 L
10	2	1/2	3 L
20	3	1/3	2 L
30	4	1/4	1.5 L
40	5	1/5	1.2 L

B Henry's law

Fig. 12.5 Boyle's law and Henry's law. **A** Boyle's law: The volume of a gas is inversely proportional to the pressure. Atmospheric pressure increases with depth, increasing by 1 atmosphere for each 10 m of depth in water. During diving this increasing pressure compresses the gas within the human body, including the lungs, ears, sinuses and bowels. During ascent this gas expands and can cause barotrauma if the ascent is too rapid. **B** Henry's law: The amount of gas that dissolves in a liquid is proportional to the partial pressure of the gas. Nitrogen is not metabolised by the body and increasingly dissolves into the blood on descent. The reverse occurs on ascent, which if ascending too quickly can cause bubbles to form, resulting in decompression sickness.

Arterial gas embolism

Expanding gases during ascent from diving, from depths as little as 1 metre, can rupture the alveolar capillary membrane (barotrauma), introducing alveolar gas into the arterial circulation. The brain is the most commonly affected organ. Small venous gas emboli are common with diving and usually are of no clinical consequence due to pulmonary capillary filtering. A patent foramen ovale is seen in around a quarter of the population which can result in these emboli transferring to the arterial circulation, causing neurological sequelae. Overall, the risk of arterial gas embolism is rare, representing only around 4% of documented decompression illnesses. Risks include rapid ascents, breath holding and pre-existing pulmonary disease. If there is rapid onset of neurological signs, including seizures or a reduced consciousness following ascent, arterial gas embolism should be suspected.

Management

Any obtunded patient should have appropriate first aid. Definitive treatment for decompression illness is providing 100% oxygen to wash out gas from the tissues to the lungs and remove bubbles. This should be instigated for all patients regardless of their oxygen saturations.

Chamber recompression is the gold standard therapy and should be performed as soon as possible causing a theoretical crushing of bubbles (as per Boyle's law) and providing improved oxygenation to damaged tissues. Extraction to a recompression chamber may require aeromedical retrieval and helicopters at low altitude (less than 300 m) or those with cabins pressurised to 1 atmosphere are recommended. In-water recompression is controversial and is recommended only for divers, including the patient, with specific training in decompression procedures underwater. Previous recommendations of a head-down position to stop cranial spread of bubbles is no longer recommended due to the increased risk of cerebral oedema; patients should be kept horizontal. One litre of intravenous fluid should be given to correct the intravascular fluid loss from endothelial bubble injury and dehydration associated with immersion. Analgesia should be avoided; non-steroidal anti-inflammatory drugs can result in haemorrhage whilst opiates raise the risk of oxygen toxicity. The Divers Alert Network can be contacted for international advice and support.

Immersion pulmonary oedema

Immersion pulmonary oedema can affect surface swimmers as well as divers and is believed to be a leading cause of death during the swim stage of triathlons, previously felt to be due to drowning. Immersion results in exposure to hydrostatic pressure which collapses veins and redistributes blood to the thorax, causing increased preload, cardiac contractility and stroke volume. Rising pulmonary alveolar capillary pressure results in a fluid shift into the lung interstitium initially, followed by the alveoli. This is normally balanced by the release of natriuretic peptides (ANP and BNP) causing a natriuresis and diuresis, however in immersion pulmonary oedema this compensation is overwhelmed. Risk factors include overhydration, overexertion, heart disease, hypertension and cold water, all resulting in raised ventricular filling pressures. Breathing into a snorkel or scuba equipment can result in higher negative pressures in the alveoli with a subsequent greater fluid transudation into them (the opposite of positive pressure ventilation used to treat pulmonary oedema). Symptoms range from shortness of breath to haemoptysis and frothy sputum, generally occurring within 10 minutes of starting swimming, and of variable onset with diving. Treatment involves extraction from the water to remove the hydrostatic pressure, which in turn decreases ventricular filling pressures. Patients should be kept warm to prevent vasocontriction, sat upright and given 100% oxygen. In-hospital management involves a combination of vasodilators (nitrates), diuretics and positive-pressure ventilation (CPAP). Recurrence rates are around 30%.

Shallow-water blackout

This condition refers to the loss of consciousness underwater when hyperventilation is followed by breath holding. It generally occurs in water less than 5 m in depth and can affect even experienced swimmers. Hyperventilation (as rapid shallow breaths before diving) preceding a breath hold lowers the arterial CO_2 and delays the hypercarbic stimulus to breathe, which may not occur before hypoxaemia and unconsciousness develop. Unconsciousness usually occurs on ascent as the hydrostatic pressure decreases, reducing the thoracic shunting of blood and gas exchange, coupled with a decreasing partial pressure of oxygen (Boyle's law) and resulting in a significant hypoxaemia.

Further information

Books

Edmonds C, Bennett M, Lippmann J, Mitchell S. Diving and subaquatic medicine, 5th edn. Boca Raton: CRC Press; 2016. *An excellent review of subaquatic medicine.*

Websites

rgs.org *Royal Geographical Society. Multiple downloadable expedition guidance documents for a range of environments.*

christopherimray.co.uk/highaltitudemedicine *Extensive publications on high altitude medicine and cold injury by Professor Chris Imray.*

altitude.org *A website written by doctors with expertise and experience of expedition and altitude medicine.*

scholar.google.co.uk/citations?user=ZJRI2HEAAAAJ&hl=en *Lists publications by Professor Mike Tipton of the Extreme Environments Laboratory, University of Portsmouth, on cold water immersion, thermoregulation and environmental physiology.*

12

DH Dockrell
S Sundar
BJ Angus

13

Infectious disease

Clinical examination of patients with infectious disease

5 Eyes
Conjunctival petechiae
Painful red eye in uveitis
Loss of red reflex in endophthalmitis
Roth spots in infective endocarditis
Haemorrhages and exudates
of cytomegalovirus retinitis
Choroidal lesions of tuberculosis

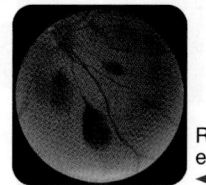

▲ Roth spots in
endocarditis

4 Head and neck
Lymphadenopathy
Parotidomegaly
Abnormal tympanic membranes

3 Oropharynx
Dental caries
Tonsillar enlargement or exudate
Candidiasis

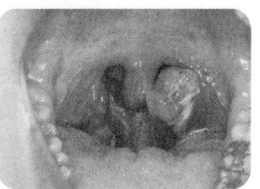

▲ Streptococcal tonsillitis

2 Hands and nails
Finger clubbing
Splinter haemorrhages
Janeway lesions
Signs of chronic liver disease
Vasculitis lesions

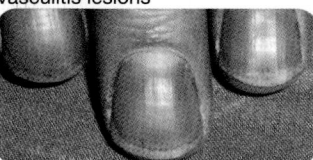

▲ Splinter haemorrhages
in endocarditis

1 Skin
Generalised erythema
Rash (see opposite)
IV injection track marks
Surgical scars
Prosthetic devices, e.g. central
venous catheters
Tattoos

6 Neurological
Neck stiffness
Photophobia
Delirium
Focal neurological signs

7 Heart and lungs
Tachycardia, hypotension
Murmurs or prosthetic heart
sounds
Pericardial rub
Signs of consolidation
Pleural or pericardial effusion

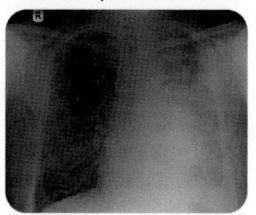

▲ Chest X-ray consolidation
in pneumonia

8 Abdomen
Hepatosplenomegaly
Ascites
Renal angle tenderness
Localised tenderness or
guarding with decreased bowel
sounds, e.g. in left iliac fossa
with diverticulitis
Mass lesions
Surgical drains

9 Musculoskeletal
Joint swelling, erythema or
tenderness
Localised tender spine suggestive
of epidural abscesses or discitis
Draining sinus of
chronic osteomyelitis

10 Genitalia and rectum
Ulceration or discharge
Testicular swelling or nodules
Inguinal lymphadenopathy
Prostatic tenderness
Rectal fluctuance

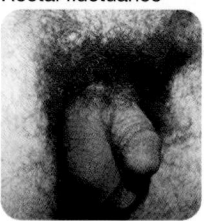

▲ Testicular swelling
in adult mumps

Observation
- Temperature
- Sweating
- Weight loss
- Respiratory distress
- Altered consciousness
- Pallor
- Jaundice

Insets: (splinter haemorrhages) Courtesy of Dr Nick Beeching, Royal Liverpool University Hospital; (Roth spots) Courtesy of Prof. Ian Rennie, Royal Hallamshire Hospital, Sheffield.

(A–C opposite) Courtesy of Dr Ravi Gowda, Royal Hallamshire Hospital, Sheffield.

ℹ️ Fever

Documentation of fever

- 'Feeling hot' or sweaty does not necessarily signify fever – diagnosed only when a body temperature of over 38.0°C is recorded
- Axillary and aural measurement is less accurate than oral or rectal
- Outpatients may be trained to keep a temperature chart

Rigors

- Shivering (followed by excessive sweating) occurs with a rapid rise in body temperature from any cause

Night sweats

- Associated with particular infections (e.g. TB, infective endocarditis); sweating from any cause is worse at night

Excessive sweating

- Alcohol, anxiety, thyrotoxicosis, diabetes mellitus, acromegaly, lymphoma and excessive environmental heat all cause sweating without temperature elevation

Recurrent fever

- There are various causes, e.g. *Borrelia recurrentis*, bacterial abscess

Accompanying features

- Severe headache and photophobia, although characteristic of meningitis, may accompany other infections, including parameningeal infections such as sinusitis or mastoiditis
- Delirium during fever is more common in young children and older people
- Myalgia may occur with viral infections, such as influenza, and with sepsis including meningococcal sepsis
- Shock may accompany severe infections and sepsis

ℹ️ History-taking in suspected infectious disease*

Presenting complaint

- Diverse manifestations of infectious disease make accurate assessment of features and duration critical; e.g. fever and cough lasting 2 days imply an acute respiratory tract infection but raise suspicion of TB if they last 2 months

Review of systems

- Must be comprehensive

Past medical history

- Define the 'host', comorbidities and likelihood of infection(s)
- Include surgical and dental procedures involving prosthetic materials
- Document previous infections and antimicrobial-resistant infections

Medication history

- Include non-prescription drugs, use of antimicrobials and immunosuppressants
- Identify medicines that interact with antimicrobials or that may cause fever

Allergy history

- Esp. to antimicrobials, noting allergic manifestation (e.g. rash versus anaphylaxis)

Family and contact history

- Note infections and their duration
- Sensitively explore exposure to key infections, e.g. TB and HIV

Travel history

- Include countries visited and where previously resident (relevant to exposure and likely vaccination history, e.g. likelihood of BCG vaccination in childhood)

Occupation

- e.g. Anthrax in leather tannery workers

Recreational pursuits

- e.g. Leptospirosis in canoeists and windsurfers

Animal exposures

- Include pets, e.g. dogs/hydatid disease

Dietary history

- Consider under-cooked meats, shellfish, unpasteurised dairy products or well water
- Establish who else was exposed, e.g. to food-borne pathogens

History of intravenous drug injection or receipt of blood products

- Risks for blood-borne viruses, e.g. HIV-1, HBV and HCV

Sexual history

- Explore in a confidential manner (Ch. 15); remember HIV-1 transmission is most frequently heterosexual (Ch. 14)

Vaccination history and use of prophylactic medicines

- Consider occupation- or age-related vaccines
- In a traveller or infection-predisposed patient, establish adherence to prophylaxis

*Always consider non-infectious aetiologies in the differential diagnosis. (HBV/HCV = hepatitis B/C virus; HIV-1 = human immunodeficiency virus-1; TB = tuberculosis)

13

① Skin lesions in infectious diseases

- Diffuse erythema, e.g. A
- Migrating erythema, e.g. enlarging rash of erythema migrans in Lyme disease (see Fig. 13.24)
- Purpuric or petechial rashes, e.g. B
- Macular or papular rashes, e.g. primary infection with HIV (see Box 14.9)
- Vesicular or blistering rash, e.g. C
- Erythema multiforme (see Fig. 27.54 and Box 27.33)
- Nodules or plaques, e.g. Kaposi's sarcoma
- Erythema nodosum (D and Box 27.34)

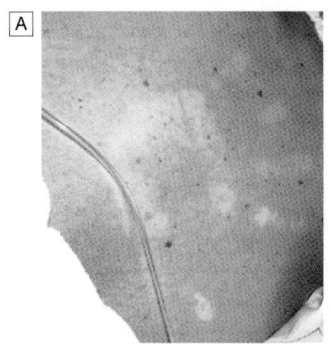
Streptococcal toxic shock syndrome.

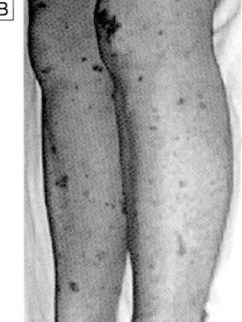
Meningococcal sepsis.

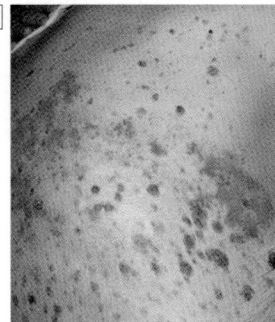
Shingles.

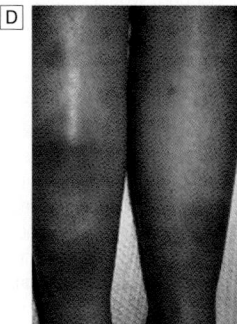
Erythema nodosum.

(HIV = human immunodeficiency virus)

The principles of infection and its investigation and therapy are described in Chapter 6. This chapter and the following ones on human immunodeficiency virus/acquired immunodeficiency syndrome (HIV/AIDS) and sexually transmitted infection (STI) describe the approach to patients with potential infectious disease, the individual infections and the resulting syndromes.

Presenting problems in infectious diseases

Infectious diseases present with myriad clinical manifestations. Many of these are described in other chapters.

Fever

'Fever' implies an elevated core body temperature of more than 38.0°C. Fever is a response to cytokines and acute phase proteins (pp. 62 and 67), and occurs both in infections and non-infectious conditions.

Clinical assessment

The differential diagnosis is broad so clinical features are used to guide the most appropriate investigations. The systematic approach described in this chapter should be followed. Box 13.1 describes the assessment of older patients.

Investigations

If the clinical features do not suggest a specific infection, then initial investigations should include:

- a full blood count (FBC) with differential, including eosinophil count
- urea and electrolytes, liver function tests (LFTs), blood glucose and muscle enzymes
- inflammatory markers: erythrocyte sedimentation rate (ESR), C-reactive protein (CRP) and/or procalcitonin (PCT) (depending on local use and availability)
- an HIV-1 antigen/antibody test
- autoantibodies, including antinuclear antibodies (ANA)
- chest X-ray and electrocardiogram (ECG)
- urinalysis and urine culture
- blood culture
- throat swab for culture or respiratory pathogen nucleic acid detection (usually by polymerase chain reaction (PCR))
- other specimens, as indicated by history and examination, e.g. wound swab; sputum culture; stool culture, microscopy for ova and parasites, and *Clostridioides difficile* toxin assay
- specific tests and their priority, indicated by geographical location: malaria films on three consecutive days or a malaria rapid diagnostic test (RDT), a test for non-structural protein 1 (NS1) in dengue (antigen detection) and blood cultures for *Salmonella* Typhi, as well as abdominal ultrasound, would be standard initial tests in many areas where these infections are prevalent.

13.1 Fever in old age

- **Temperature measurement**: fever may be missed because oral temperatures are unreliable. Rectal measurement may be needed but core temperature is increasingly measured using eardrum reflectance.
- **Delirium**: common with fever, especially in those with underlying cerebrovascular disease or dementia.
- **Prominent causes of pyrexia of unknown origin**: include tuberculosis and intra-abdominal abscesses, complicated urinary tract infection and infective endocarditis. Non-infective causes include polymyalgia rheumatica/temporal arteritis and tumours. A smaller fraction of cases remain undiagnosed than in young people.
- **Diagnostic pitfalls**: conditions such as stroke or thromboembolic disease can cause fever but every effort must be made to exclude concomitant infection.
- **Common infectious diseases in the very frail** (e.g. nursing home residents): pneumonia, urinary tract infection, soft tissue infection and gastroenteritis.

Subsequent investigations in patients with HIV-related, nosocomial or travel-related pyrexia, immunocompromised patients and patients with clinical features suggesting infection in the respiratory, gastrointestinal or neurological systems are described elsewhere.

Management

Fever and its associated systemic symptoms can be treated with paracetamol, and tepid sponging to cool the skin. Replacement of salt and water is important in patients with drenching sweats. Further management is focused on the underlying cause.

Fever with localising symptoms or signs

In most patients, the site of infection is apparent after clinical evaluation, and the likelihood of infection is reinforced by investigation results (e.g. neutrophilia with raised CRP in bacterial infections). Not all apparently localising symptoms are reliable, however; headache, breathlessness and diarrhoea can occur in systemic infection, such as sepsis or malaria, without localised infection in the central nervous system (CNS), respiratory tract or gastrointestinal tract. Abdominal pain may be a feature of basal pneumonia. Careful interpretation of the clinical features is vital (e.g. severe headache associated with photophobia, rash and neck stiffness suggests meningitis, whereas moderate headache with cough and rhinorrhoea is consistent with a viral upper respiratory tract infection).

Common infections that present with fever are shown in Figure 13.1. Further investigation and management are specific to the cause, but may include empirical antimicrobial therapy (Fig. 6.15) pending confirmation of the microbiological diagnosis.

Pyrexia of unknown origin

Pyrexia of unknown origin (PUO) was classically defined as a temperature above 38.0°C on multiple occasions for more than 3 weeks, without diagnosis, despite initial investigation in hospital for 1 week. The definition has been relaxed to allow for investigation over 3 days of inpatient care, three outpatient visits or 1 week of intensive ambulatory investigation. Subsets of PUO are described as HIV-1 related, immune-deficient or nosocomial.

Clinical assessment

Major causes of PUO are outlined in Box 13.2. Periodic fever syndromes are rare causes that should be considered in those with a family history. Children and younger adults are more likely to have infectious causes. Older adults are more likely to have certain infectious and non-infectious causes (see Box 13.1). Detailed history and examination should be repeated at regular intervals to detect emerging features (e.g. rashes, signs of infective endocarditis or features of vasculitis). In men, the prostate should be considered as a potential source of infection.

Clinicians should be alert to the possibility of factitious fever, in which high temperature recordings are engineered by the patient (Box 13.3).

Investigations

If initial investigations are negative, further microbiological and non-microbiological investigations should be considered (Boxes 13.4 and 13.5). As with initial investigation of fever described above, the prioritisation of tests will be influenced by the geographical location of potential exposure to pathogens (see Box 13.4). These will usually include:

- induced sputum or other specimens for mycobacterial stains and culture
- serological tests, including an HIV test and ferritin estimation
- imaging of the abdomen by ultrasonography or computerised tomography (CT)
- echocardiography.

Lesions identified on imaging should usually be biopsied in order to seek evidence of relevant pathogens by culture, histopathology or

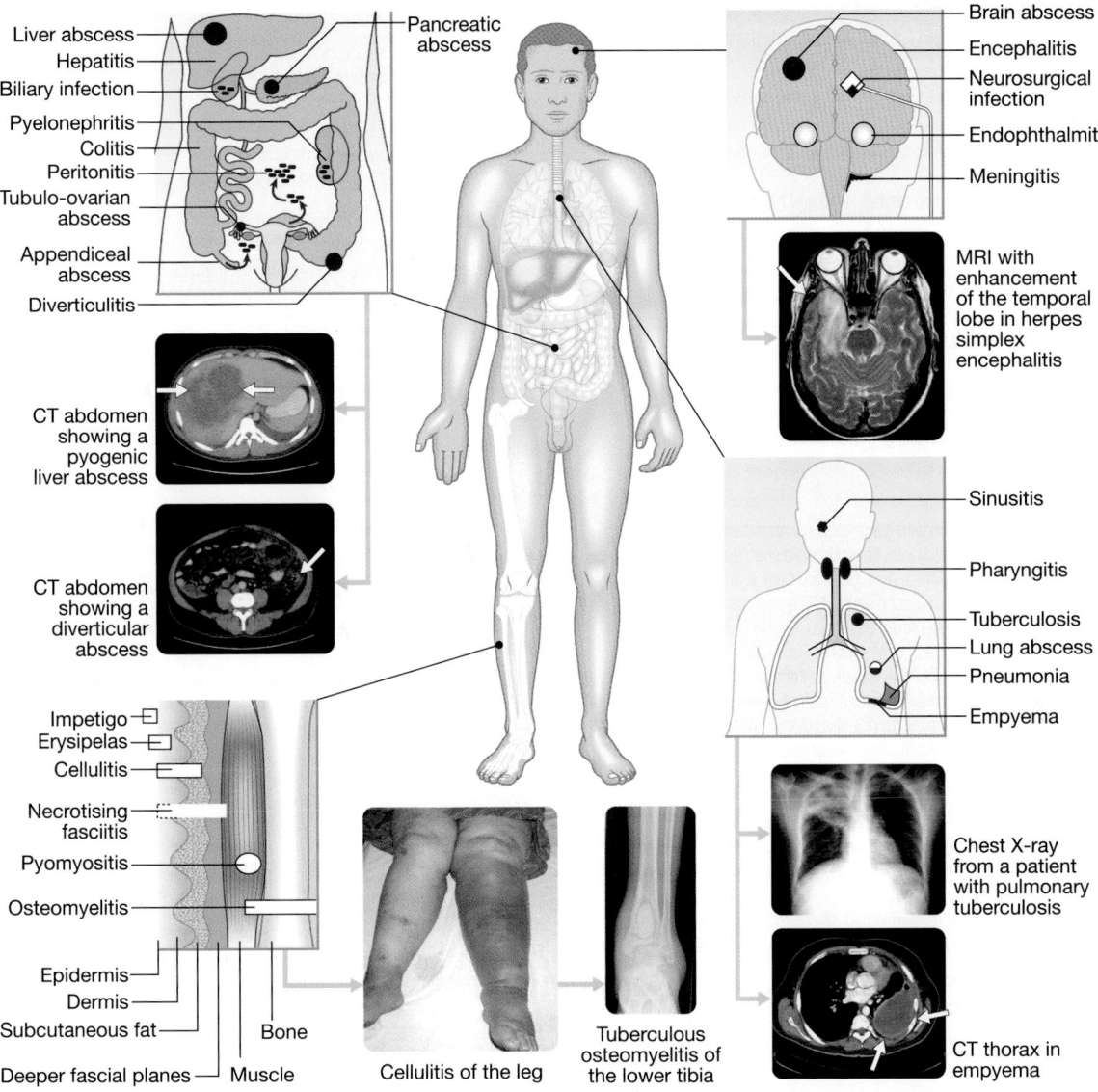

Fig. 13.1 **Common infectious syndromes presenting with fever and localised features.** Major causes are grouped by approximate anatomical location and include central nervous system infection; respiratory tract infections; abdominal, pelvic or urinary tract infections; and skin and soft tissue infections (SSTIs) or osteomyelitis. For each site of infection, particular syndromes and their common causes are described elsewhere in the book. The causative organisms vary, depending on host factors, which include whether the patient has lived in or visited a tropical country or particular geographical location, has acquired the infection in a health-care environment or is immunocompromised. *Insets (cellulitis of the leg) Courtesy of Dr Ravi Gowda, Royal Hallamshire Hospital, Sheffield; (pulmonary tuberculosis) Courtesy of Dr Ann Chapman, Royal Hallamshire Hospital, Sheffield; (empyema, pyogenic liver abscess, diverticular abscess, tuberculous osteomyelitis) Courtesy of Dr Robert Peck, Royal Hallamshire Hospital, Sheffield.*

13

nucleic acid detection. Particularly in patients who have received prior antimicrobials, 16S rRNA analysis (Box 6.2) may aid diagnosis if a microorganism is not cultured. The chance of a successful diagnosis is greatest if procedures for obtaining and transporting the correct samples in the appropriate media are carefully planned between the clinical team, the radiologist or surgeon performing the procedure, and the local microbiologist and histopathologist. Fluorodeoxyglucose (FDG)-positron emission tomography (PET) scans may aid diagnosis of vasculitis or help selection of biopsy sites. Liver biopsy may be justified – for example, to identify idiopathic granulomatous hepatitis – if there are biochemical or radiological abnormalities. Bone marrow biopsies have a diagnostic yield of up to 15%, most often revealing haematological malignancy, myelodysplasia or tuberculosis, and also identifying brucellosis, typhoid fever or visceral leishmaniasis. Bone marrow should be sent for culture, as well as microscopy. Laparoscopy is occasionally undertaken with biopsy of abnormal tissues. Splenic aspiration in specialist centres is the diagnostic test of choice for suspected visceral leishmaniasis. Diagnostic tests for giant cell arteritis should be considered in patients over the age of 50 years, even in the absence of physical signs or a raised ESR.

'Blind' biopsy of other structures in the absence of localising signs or laboratory or radiology results is unhelpful.

Prognosis

No cause is found in up to one-half of PUO cases, but as long as there is no significant weight loss or signs of another disease, the long-term mortality is low.

Fever in the injection drug-user

Intravenous injection of recreational drugs is a global problem. Infective organisms are introduced by non-sterile (often shared) injection equipment (see Fig. 13.2). Approximately 50% of people who inject drugs (PWID) report a recent bacterial infection, with *Streptococcus pyogenes* (group A ß-haemolytic streptococci) and *Staphylococcus aureus* infections increasing in particular. Risk factors for these infections include increasing age, homelessness and injection in prison. The risks increase with prolonged drug use and injection into large veins of the groin and neck necessitated by progressive thrombosis of superficial peripheral veins. The most common causes of fever are soft tissue or respiratory infections.

13.2 Aetiology of pyrexia of unknown origin (PUO)

Infections (~30%)

Specific locations

- Abscesses: hepatobiliary, diverticular, urinary tract (including prostate), pulmonary, CNS
- Infections of oral cavity (including dental), head and neck (including sinuses)
- Bone and joint infections
- Infective endocarditis

Specific organisms

- TB (particularly extrapulmonary)*
- HIV-1 infection
- Other viral infections: cytomegalovirus (CMV), Epstein–Barr virus (EBV)
- Fungal infections (e.g. *Aspergillus* spp., *Candida* spp. or dimorphic fungi)
- Infections with fastidious organisms (e.g. *Bartonella* spp., *Tropheryma whipplei*)

Specific patient groups

- Recently spent time in a region with geographically restricted infection:
  - Malaria*, dengue, rickettsial infections, *Brucella* spp., amoebic liver abscess, enteric fevers (Africa, Asia, Oceania, Central and South America), *Leishmania* spp. (southern Europe, India, Africa and Latin America), *Burkholderia pseudomallei* (South-east Asia), Middle East respiratory syndrome coronavirus (MERS-CoV; Arabian Peninsula)
- Residence in or travel to a region with endemic infection:
  - TB* (Africa, Asia, Central and South America), extensively drug-resistant TB (XDR-TB; South Africa), *Brucella* spp. (Africa, Asia, Central and South America), HIV-1 (Africa, Asia), *Trypanosoma cruzi* (Central and South America)
- Nosocomial infections:
  - Pneumonia*, infections related to prosthetic materials and surgical procedures, urinary tract infections, central venous catheter infections
- HIV-positive individuals:
  - Acute retroviral syndrome
  - AIDS-defining infections (disseminated *Mycobacterium avium* complex (DMAC), *Pneumocystis jirovecii* pneumonia, CMV and others)

Malignancy (~20%)

Haematological malignancy

- Lymphoma*, leukaemia and myeloma

Solid tumours

- Renal, liver, colon, stomach, pancreas

Connective tissue disorders (~15%)

Older adults

- Temporal arteritis/polymyalgia rheumatica*

Younger adults

- Still's disease (juvenile rheumatoid arthritis)*
- Systemic lupus erythematosus (SLE)
- Vasculitic disorders, including polyarteritis nodosa, rheumatoid disease with vasculitis and granulomatosis with polyangiitis (formerly known as Wegener's granulomatosis)
- Polymyositis
- Behçet's disease
- Rheumatic fever (in regions where still endemic, e.g. Asia, Oceania and parts of Africa)

Miscellaneous (~20%)

Cardiovascular

- Atrial myxoma, aortitis, aortic dissection

Respiratory

- Sarcoidosis, pulmonary embolism and other thromboembolic disease, extrinsic allergic alveolitis

Gastrointestinal

- Inflammatory bowel disease, granulomatous hepatitis, alcoholic liver disease, pancreatitis

Endocrine/metabolic

- Thyrotoxicosis, thyroiditis, hypothalamic lesions, phaeochromocytoma, adrenal insufficiency, hypertriglyceridaemia

Haematological

- Haemolytic anaemia, paroxysmal nocturnal haemoglobinuria, thrombotic thrombocytopenic purpura, myeloproliferative disorders, Castleman's disease, graft-versus-host disease (after allogeneic haematopoietic stem cell transplantation)

Inherited

- Familial Mediterranean fever and periodic fever syndromes

Drug reactions*

- e.g. Antibiotic fever, drug hypersensitivity reactions etc.

Factitious fever

Idiopathic (~15%)

*Most common causes within each group. (AIDS = acquired immunodeficiency syndrome; CNS = central nervous system; HIV-1 = human immunodeficiency virus-1; TB = tuberculosis; XDR = extensively drug-resistant)

 13.3 Clues to the diagnosis of factitious fever

- A patient who looks well
- Bizarre temperature chart with absence of diurnal variation and/or temperature-related changes in pulse rate
- Temperature > 41°C
- Absence of sweating during defervescence
- Normal erythrocyte sedimentation rate and C-reactive protein despite high fever
- Evidence of self-injection or self-harm
- Normal temperature during supervised (observed) measurement
- Infection with multiple commensal organisms (e.g. enteric or mouth flora)

Clinical assessment

The history should address the following risk factors:

- *Site of injection*. Femoral vein injection is associated with vascular complications such as deep venous thrombosis (DVT; 50% of which are septic) and accidental arterial injection with false aneurysm formation or a compartment syndrome due to swelling within the fascial sheath. Local complications include ilio-psoas abscess, and septic arthritis of the hip joint or sacroiliac joint. Injection of the jugular vein can be associated with cerebrovascular complications.

Subcutaneous and intramuscular injection has been related to infection by clostridial species, the spores of which contaminate heroin. *Clostridium novyi* causes a local lesion with significant toxin production, leading to shock and multi-organ failure. Tetanus, wound botulism, anthrax and gas gangrene also occur.

- *Technical details of injection*. Sharing of needles and other injecting paraphernalia (including spoons and filters) increases the risk of blood-borne virus infection (e.g. HIV-1, hepatitis B or C virus). Some users lubricate their needles by licking them prior to injection, thus introducing mouth organisms (e.g. anaerobic streptococci, *Fusobacterium* spp. and *Prevotella* spp.). Contamination of commercially available lemon juice, used to dissolve heroin before injection, has been associated with blood-stream infection with *Candida* spp. Excessive use of citric acid to dissolve heroin is associated with DVT and skin and soft tissue infection.
- *Substances injected*. Injection of cocaine is associated with a variety of vascular complications. Psychoactive drugs increase risk taking and bacterial infections. Certain formulations of heroin have been linked with particular infections, e.g. wound botulism with black tar heroin. Drugs are often mixed with other substances, e.g. talc.

13.4 Microbiological investigation of pyrexia of unknown origin[1]

Location-independent investigations

Microscopy

- Blood for atypical lymphocytes (EBV, CMV, HIV-1, hepatitis viruses or *Toxoplasma gondii*)
- Respiratory samples for mycobacteria and fungi
- Stool for ova, cysts and parasites
- Biopsy for light microscopy (bacteria, mycobacteria, fungi) and/or electron microscopy (viruses, protozoa (e.g. microsporidia) and other fastidious organisms (e.g. *Tropheryma whipplei*))
- Urine for white or red blood cells and mycobacteria (early morning urine ×3)

Culture

- Aspirates and biopsies (e.g. joint, deep abscess, débrided tissues)
- Blood, including prolonged culture and special media conditions
- Sputum for mycobacteria
- CSF
- Gastric aspirate for mycobacteria
- Stool
- Swabs
- Urine ± prostatic massage in older men

Antigen detection

- Blood, e.g. HIV p24 antigen (usually combined with an antibody test), cryptococcal antigen, *Aspergillus* galactomannan ELISA and (1,3)-β-D-glucan (for fungi other than mucoraceous moulds and *Cryptococcus*)
- CSF for cryptococcal antigen
- Bronchoalveolar lavage fluid for *Aspergillus* galactomannan
- Nasopharyngeal aspirate/throat swab for respiratory viruses, e.g. IAV or RSV
- Urine, e.g. for *Legionella* antigen

Nucleic acid detection

- Blood for *Bartonella* spp. and viruses
- CSF for viruses and key bacteria (meningococcus, pneumococcus, *Listeria monocytogenes*)

- Nasopharyngeal aspirate/throat swab for respiratory viruses
- Sputum for *Mycobacterium tuberculosis* (MTB) and rifampicin (RIF) resistance with geneXpert MTB/RIF cartridge-based nucleic acid amplification test (NAAT)
- Bronchoalveolar lavage fluid, e.g. for respiratory viruses
- Tissue specimens, e.g. for *T. whipplei*
- Urine, e.g. for *Chlamydia trachomatis*, *Neisseria gonorrhoeae*
- Stool, e.g. for norovirus, rotavirus

Immunological tests

- Serology (antibody detection) for viruses, including HIV-1, and some bacteria
- Interferon-gamma release assay for diagnosis of exposure to tuberculosis (but note this will not distinguish latent from active disease and can only be used to trigger further investigations of active disease)

Geographically restricted tests[2]

Microscopy

- Blood for trypanosomiasis, malaria and *Borrelia* spp.
- Stool for geographically restricted ova, cysts and parasites
- Biopsy for light microscopy (dimorphic fungi, *Leishmania* spp. and other parasites)
- Urine for red blood cells and schistosome ova

Antigen detection

- Blood, e.g. dengue virus NS1 antigen, *Histoplasma* antigen (restricted availability) and malaria antigen (e.g. HRP-2 for *Plasmodium falciparum* or parasite-specific LDH for *P. falciparum* and *P. vivax*)

Nucleic acid detection

- Blood for causes of viral haemorrhagic fever
- CSF for geographically restricted viruses, e.g. Japanese encephalitis virus
- Nasopharyngeal aspirate/throat swab or bronchoalveolar lavage fluid for geographically restricted respiratory viruses, e.g. MERS-CoV

Immunological tests

- Serology (antibody detection) for viruses, dimorphic fungi and protozoa

[1]This list does not apply to every patient with a pyrexia of unknown origin. Appropriate tests should be selected in a stepwise manner, according to specific predisposing factors, epidemiological exposures and local availability, and should be discussed with a microbiologist. [2]Addition of these tests should be guided by the location of presentation or travel history.
(CMV = cytomegalovirus; CSF = cerebrospinal fluid; EBV = Epstein–Barr virus; ELISA = enzyme-linked immunosorbent assay; HIV-1 = human immunodeficiency virus-1; HRP-2 = histidine-rich protein 2; IAV = influenza A virus; LDH = lactate dehydrogenase; MERS-CoV = Middle East respiratory syndrome coronavirus; NS1 = non-structural 1; RSV = respiratory syncytial virus)

13

---

i 13.5 Additional investigations to be considered in pyrexia of unknown origin (PUO)

- Serological tests for connective tissue disorders:
  - Autoantibody screen
  - Complement levels
  - Immunoglobulins
  - Cryoglobulins
- Ferritin
- Echocardiography
- Ultrasound of abdomen
- CT/MRI of thorax, abdomen and/or brain
- Imaging of the skeletal system:
  - Plain X-rays
  - CT/MRI spine
  - Isotope bone scan

- Labelled white cell scan
- Fluorodeoxyglucose-positron emission tomography (FDG-PET)/single-photon emission computed tomography (SPECT)
- Biopsy:
  - Bronchoscopy and lavage ± transbronchial biopsy
  - Lymph node aspirate or biopsy
  - Biopsy of radiological lesion
  - Biopsy of liver
  - Bone marrow aspirate and biopsy
  - Lumbar puncture
  - Laparoscopy and biopsy
  - Temporal artery biopsy

- *Blood-borne virus status.* Results of previous HIV-1 and hepatitis virus tests or vaccinations for hepatitis viruses should be recorded.
- *Surreptitious use of antimicrobials.* Addicts may use antimicrobials to self-treat infections, masking initial blood culture results.

Key findings on clinical examination are shown in Figure 13.2. It can be difficult to distinguish the effects of infection from the effects of drugs or drug withdrawal (excitement, tachycardia, sweating, marked myalgia, delirium). Stupor and delirium may result from drug administration but may also indicate meningitis or encephalitis. Non-infected venous thromboembolism is also common in this group.

Investigations

The initial investigations are as for any fever (see above), including a chest X-ray and blood cultures. Since blood sampling may be difficult, contamination is often a problem. Echocardiography (transthoracic or transoesophageal) to detect infective endocarditis should be performed in all injection drug-users with bacteraemia due to *Staph. aureus* or other organisms associated with endocarditis (Fig. 13.3A); thrombo-embolic phenomena; or a new or previously undocumented murmur. Endovascular infection should also be suspected if lung abscesses or pneumatoceles are detected radiologically. Infected thrombus at injection sites, such as the groin, is common and may lead to abscess

6 Cardiovascular system
Systolic 'V' waves in JVP of tricuspid regurgitation (Ch. 16)
Regurgitant murmurs in endocarditis

5 Nervous system
Signs of drug intoxication
Encephalopathy
Signs of meningitis
Focal neurological features or seizures in septic embolism/ mycotic aneurysm/abscess
Cranial nerve palsies of botulism
Trismus, muscle rigidity or spasms in tetanus
Localised pain over vertebrae with epidural abscess

4 Optic fundi
Roth spots
Candidal cotton wool spots

3 Oropharynx
Dental infections
Oropharyngeal candidiasis or other signs of HIV-1 infection

2 Hands and nails
Splinter haemorrhages
Signs of chronic liver disease

1 Skin and soft tissues (any site)
Cellulitis
Purulent drainage
Abscesses
Ulcers
Bullae or extreme pain suggestive of necrotising fasciitis

7 Respiratory system
Consolidation in pneumonia
Upper lobe signs in tuberculosis
Pleural rub with septic pulmonary emboli

8 Abdomen
Jaundice ± tender liver edge with hepatitis
Pain in left upper quadrant with splenic abscess

9 Bone and joints
Osteomyelitis
Septic arthritis

10 Injection sites
Abscesses
Fistula
Haematoma
Pseudoaneurysm

11 Femoral stretch test
Passive extension of the hip joint causes pain and reflex muscle spasm in ilio-psoas abscess

12 Legs
Signs of DVT
Vasculitis or ischaemic signs of septic emboli, endocarditis or vasospasm
Compartment syndrome

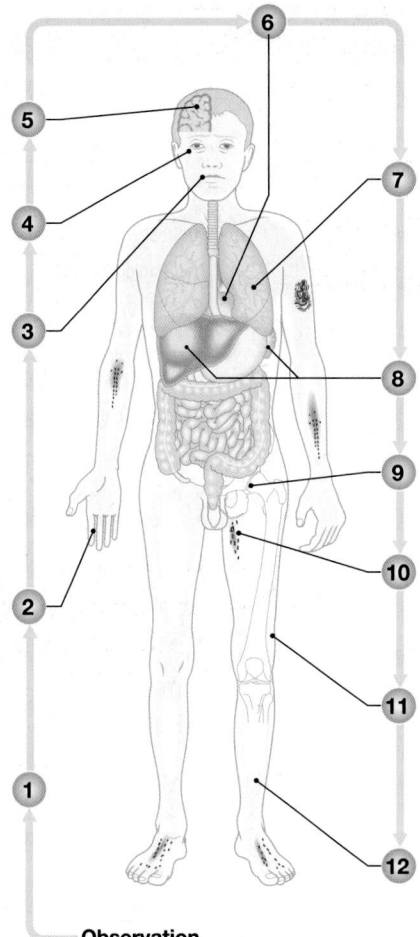

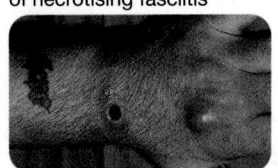

▲ Skin abscesses in an injection drug-user

Observation

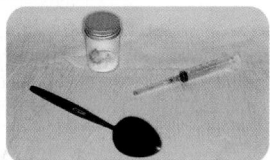

▲ Sharing injecting equipment may transmit blood-borne viruses

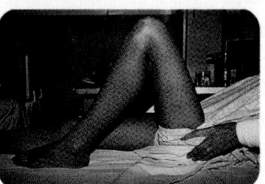

▲ Hip flexor spasm in an injection drug-user with ilio-psoas abscess

Fig. 13.2 Fever in the injection drug-user: key features of clinical examination. Full examination is required but features most common amongst injection drug-users are shown here. (DVT = deep venous thrombosis; HIV = human immunodeficiency virus; JVP = jugular venous pulse)

formation. Additional imaging should be focused on sites of injection or of localising symptoms (Fig. 13.3B). Any pathological fluid collections should be sampled.

Urinary toxicology tests may suggest a non-infectious cause of the presenting complaint. While being investigated, all injection drug-users should be tested for infection with hepatitis B and C virus and HIV-1.

Injection drug-users may have more than one infection. Skin and soft tissue infections are most often due to *Staph. aureus* or streptococci, and sometimes to *Clostridium* spp. or anaerobes. Pulmonary infections are most often due to the common pathogens causing community-acquired pneumonia, tuberculosis or septic emboli (Fig. 13.3C). Endocarditis with septic emboli commonly involves *Staph. aureus* and viridans streptococci, but *Pseudomonas aeruginosa* and *Candida* spp. are also encountered.

Management

Empirical therapy of fever in the injection drug-user includes an anti-staphylococcal penicillin (e.g. flucloxacillin) or, where meticillin-resistant *Staph. aureus* (MRSA) is prevalent, a glycopeptide (e.g. vancomycin) or lipopeptide (e.g. daptomycin). Once microbiological results are available,

therapy can be narrowed to focus on the microorganism identified. In injection drug-users, meticillin-sensitive *Staph. aureus* is customarily treated with high-dose intravenous (IV) flucloxacillin, with a 2-week duration for uncomplicated right-sided endocarditis. Right-sided endocarditis caused by MRSA is usually treated with 4 weeks of vancomycin. Specialist advice should be sought.

For localised infections of the skin and soft tissues, oral therapy with agents active against staphylococci, streptococci and anaerobes is appropriate (e.g. flucloxacillin or clindamycin). Non-adherence to prescribed antimicrobial regimens leads to a high rate of complications.

Fever in the immunocompromised host

Immunocompromised hosts include those with congenital immunodeficiency, HIV infection and iatrogenic immunosuppression induced by chemotherapy, or immunosuppressant medicines, including high-dose glucocorticoids. Metabolic abnormalities, such as under-nutrition or hyperglycaemia, may also contribute. Multiple elements of the immune system are potentially compromised. A patient may have impaired

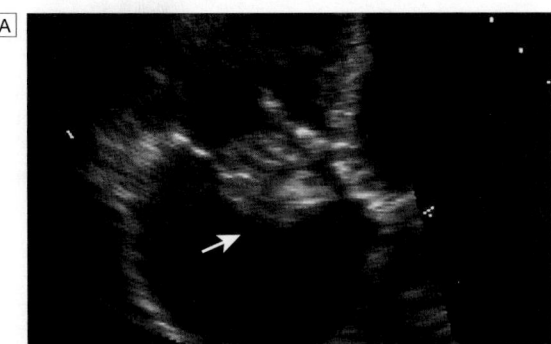

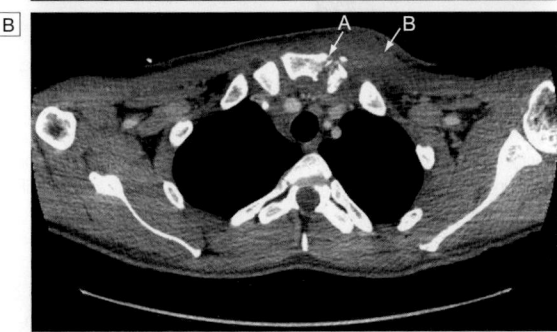

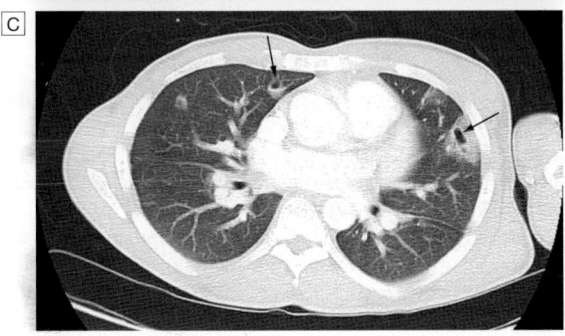

Fig. 13.3 Causes of fever in injection drug-users. [A] Endocarditis: large vegetation on the tricuspid valve (arrow). [B] Septic arthritis of the left sternoclavicular joint (arrow A) (note the erosion of the bony surfaces at the sternoclavicular joint) with overlying soft tissue collection (arrow B). [C] Tricuspid valve endocarditis caused by *Staph. aureus.* Thoracic CT scan shows multiple embolic lesions with cavitation (arrows). The patient presented with haemoptysis. *(C) Courtesy of Dr Julia Greig, Royal Hallamshire Hospital, Sheffield.*

neutrophil function from chemotherapy, impaired T-cell and/or B-cell responses due to underlying malignancy, T-cell and phagocytosis defects due to glucocorticoids, mucositis from chemotherapy and an impaired skin barrier due to insertion of a central venous catheter.

Fever may result from infectious or non-infectious causes, including drugs, vasculitis, neoplasm, lymphoproliferative disease, graft-versus-host disease (in recipients of haematopoietic stem cell transplants (HSCT)), organising pneumonitis or Sweet syndrome (reddish nodules or plaques with fever and leucocytosis, in association with haematological malignancy).

Although many infections in immunocompromised patients are caused by common organisms they may also be infected with organisms that cause infection in the non-immunocompromised host rarely, or not at all (opportunistic pathogens/opportunistic infections).

Clinical assessment

The following should be addressed in the history:

- identification of the immunosuppressant factors and nature of the immune defect
- any past infections and their treatment, including antimicrobial-resistant or recurrent infections

- epidemiological risk factors increasing exposure to infections, including opportunistic infections that would not cause disease in an immunocompetent host
- prophylactic medicines and vaccinations administered.

Examination should include inspection of the skin, any central venous catheters, the mouth, sinuses, ears and perianal area (digital rectal examination should be avoided). Disseminated infections can manifest as cutaneous lesions. The areas around fingernails and toenails should also be inspected closely.

Investigations

Initial screening tests are as described above. Immunocompromised hosts often have decreased inflammatory responses leading to attenuation of physical signs, such as neck stiffness with meningitis, radiological features and laboratory findings, such as leucocytosis. Chest CT scan should be considered in addition to chest X-ray when respiratory symptoms occur. Abdominal imaging may also be warranted, particularly if there is right lower quadrant pain, which may indicate typhlitis (inflammation of the caecum) in neutropenic patients. Blood cultures from a central venous catheter, urine cultures and stool cultures if diarrhoea is present are also recommended.

Nasopharyngeal aspirates are sometimes diagnostic, as immunocompromised hosts may shed respiratory viruses for prolonged periods. Skin lesions should be biopsied if nodules are present, and investigation should include fungal stains. Useful molecular techniques include PCR for cytomegalovirus (CMV) and *Aspergillus* spp. DNA. Antigen assays that may be used include blood tests for cryptococcal antigen (CrAg), *Aspergillus* galactomannan, (1,3)-β-D-glucan (for *Pneumocystis jirovecii* and fungi other than *Cryptococcus* spp. and mucoraceous moulds) and a urine test for *Legionella pneumophila* type 1. Antibody detection is rarely useful in immunocompromised patients. Patients with respiratory signs or symptoms should be considered for bronchoalveolar lavage to detect *Pneumocystis jirovecii*, other fungi, bacteria and viruses.

Neutropenic fever

Patients with neutropenia are highly susceptible to bacterial and fungal infection, the risk of which increases progressively as the neutrophil count drops below 1.0×10^9/L. Gram-positive organisms are the most common pathogens, particularly in association with in-dwelling catheters. There is no universal definition of neutropenic fever, but most authorities define neutropenia as a neutrophil count of $<0.5 \times 10^9$/L (p. 935) and fever as a single measurement >38.5°C or sustained temperature >38°C.

Empirical broad-spectrum antimicrobial therapy is commenced when cultures have been obtained. The most common regimens for neutropenic fever are broad-spectrum penicillins, e.g. piperacillin–tazobactam. The routine addition of aminoglycosides to these agents is not supported by trial data. If fever has not resolved after 3–5 days, empirical antifungal therapy (e.g. caspofungin) is added (p. 122). An alternative antifungal strategy is to use azole prophylaxis in high-risk patients and markers of early fungal infection, such as galactomannan, (1,3)-β-D-glucan and/or fungal PCR, to guide initiation of antifungal treatment (a 'pre-emptive approach').

Post-transplantation fever

Fever in transplant recipients may be due to infection, episodes of graft rejection in solid organ transplant recipients, or graft-versus-host disease following haematopoietic stem cell transplantation.

Infections in solid organ transplant recipients are grouped according to the time of onset (Box 13.6). Those in the first month are mostly related to the underlying condition or surgical complications. Those occurring 1–6 months after transplantation are characteristic of impaired T-cell function. Risk factors for CMV infection have been identified; patients commonly receive either prophylaxis or intensive monitoring involving regular testing for CMV DNA by PCR and early initiation of anti-CMV therapy using

13

i 13.6 Infections in transplant recipients

Time post-transplantation	Infections
Solid organ transplant recipients	
0–1 month	Bacterial or fungal infections related to the underlying condition or surgical complications
1–6 months	CMV, other opportunistic infections (e.g. *Pneumocystis jirovecii* pneumonia)
>6 months	Bacterial pneumonia, other bacterial community-acquired infections, shingles, cryptococcal infection, PTLD
Myeloablative haematopoietic stem cell transplant recipients	
Pre-engraftment (typically 0–4 weeks)	Bacterial and fungal infections, respiratory viruses or HSV reactivation
Post-engraftment:	
Early (<100 days)	CMV, *Pneumocystis jirovecii* pneumonia, moulds or other opportunistic infections
Late (>100 days)	Community-acquired bacterial infections, shingles, CMV, PTLD

(CMV = cytomegalovirus; HSV = herpes simplex virus; PTLD = post-transplant lymphoproliferative disorder)

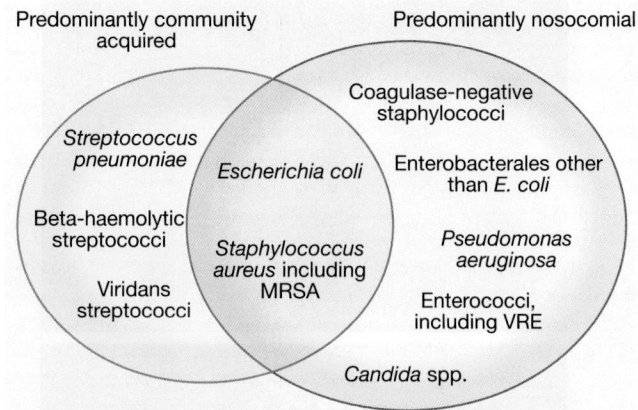

Fig. 13.4 Common causes of blood-stream infection. Causes of community- and hospital-acquired blood-stream infection are subject to significant regional and geographic location. (MRSA = meticillin-resistant *Staphylococcus aureus*; VRE = vancomycin-resistant *Enterococcus* spp.)

intravenous ganciclovir or oral valganciclovir if tests become positive. Greater use of prophylactic regimens, despite reducing infections overall, is extending the period of risk so that some opportunistic infections, e.g. CMV, may be seen after this initial 6-month period.

Following HSCT, infections in the first 4 weeks are more common in patients receiving a myeloablative-conditioning regimen (see Box 13.6). Later infections are more common if an allogeneic, as opposed to autologous, procedure is performed.

Post-transplant lymphoproliferative disorder (PTLD) is an Epstein–Barr virus (EBV)-associated lymphoma that can complicate transplantation, particularly when primary EBV infection occurs after transplantation.

Positive blood culture

Blood-stream infection (BSI) is a frequent presentation of infection. This can be community-acquired or hospital-acquired ('nosocomial'). Common causes are shown in Fig. 13.4. In immunocompromised hosts, a wider range of microorganisms may be isolated, e.g. fungi.

Primary BSI refers to cases in which an extravascular source of infection (e.g. pneumonia or urinary tract infection) is not identified, and is commonly caused by *Staph. aureus*. In community-acquired *Staph. aureus* bacteraemia, 20%–30% of cases are associated with infectious endocarditis and up to 10% are due to osteomyelitis. Peripheral and central venous catheters are an important source of nosocomial BSI.

BSI has an associated mortality of 15%–40%, depending on the setting, host and microbial factors.

Clinical assessment

The history should determine the setting in which BSI has occurred. Host factors predisposing to infection include skin disease, diabetes mellitus, injection drug use, the presence of a central venous, urinary or haemodialysis catheter, and surgical procedures, especially those involving the implantation of prosthetic materials (in particular, endovascular prostheses).

Physical examination should focus on signs of infective endocarditis (p. 462), evidence of bone (especially spinal) or joint infection (tenderness or restriction of movement), and abdominal or flank tenderness. Central venous catheters should be examined for erythema or purulence

at the exit site. Particularly in cases with *Candida* spp. infection or suspected infectious endocarditis, fundoscopy after pupil dilatation should be performed.

Investigations

Positive blood cultures may be caused by contaminants. When isolated from only one bottle, or from all bottles from one venesection, coagulase-negative staphylococci often represent contamination. Repeated isolation of coagulase-negative staphyloccoci, however, should raise suspicion of infective endocarditis or, in a patient with any form of prosthetic material, prosthesis infection. Viridans streptococci occasionally cause transient non-significant bacteraemia or blood culture contamination but, in view of their association with infective endocarditis, significant infection must always be excluded. *Bacillus* spp. ('aerobic spore bearers') and *Clostridium* spp. often represent incidental transient bacteraemia or contamination, but certain species (e.g. *C. septicum*) are more likely to be genuine pathogens.

Further investigations are influenced by the causative organism and setting. Initial screening tests are similar to those for fever and should include chest X-ray, urine culture and, in many cases, ultrasound or other imaging of the abdomen. Imaging should also include any areas of bone or joint pain and any prosthetic material, e.g. a prosthetic joint or an aortic graft.

Echocardiography should be considered for those patients with BSI who have valvular heart disease or clinical features of endocarditis, those whose cultures reveal an organism that is a common cause of endocarditis (e.g. *Staph. aureus*, viridans streptococci or enterococci), those in whom multiple blood cultures are positive for the same organism, and those with a rapid positive result on culture. The sensitivities of transthoracic echocardiography (TTE) and transoesophageal echocardiography (TOE) for the detection of vegetations are 50%–90% and over 95%, respectively. Therefore, if TTE is negative, TOE should be considered.

Certain rare causes of BSI have specific associations that warrant further investigation. Endocarditis caused by *Streptococcus gallolyticus* subsp. *gallolyticus* (formerly *Strep. bovis* biotype I) and BSI with *C. septicum* are both associated with colonic carcinoma and should lead to appropriate investigation.

Management

BSI is treated with antimicrobial therapy and, where possible, source control (surgical drainage, joint washout etc.). Two weeks of therapy may be sufficient for *Staph. aureus* BSI from central and peripheral venous catheter infections when the source is identified and removed, for uncomplicated skin and soft tissue infections, and for uncomplicated right-sided infective endocarditis. Other *Staph. aureus* BSIs are usually treated for 4–6 weeks.

Central venous catheter infections

Infections of central venous catheters typically involve the catheter lumen and are associated with fever, positive blood cultures and, in some cases, signs of purulence or exudate at the site of insertion. Infection is more common in temporary catheters inserted into the groin or jugular vein than in those in the subclavian vein. Tunnelled catheters, e.g. Hickman catheters, may also develop tunnel site infections.

Staphylococci account for 70%–90% of catheter infections, with coagulase-negative staphylococci more common than *Staph. aureus*. Other causes include enterococci and Gram-negative bacilli. Unusual Gram-negative organisms, such as *Citrobacter freundii* and *Pseudomonas fluorescens*, raise the possibility of non-sterile infusion equipment or infusate. *Candida* spp. are a common cause of line infections, particularly in association with total parenteral nutrition. Non-tuberculous mycobacteria may cause tunnel infections.

Investigations and management

In bacteraemic patients with fever and no other obvious source of infection, a catheter infection is likely. Local evidence of erythema, purulence or thrombophlebitis supports the diagnosis but microbiological confirmation is essential. If the line is removed a semi-quantitative culture of the tip may confirm the presence of 15 or more colony-forming units, but this technique is retrospective and does not detect luminal infection. If the catheter remains in place, paired blood cultures (with approximately equal volumes) should be taken through the catheter and from a peripheral vein. A differential time to positive culture of 2 hours or more, with the catheter sample coming up positive first, suggests a luminal catheter infection.

For coagulase-negative staphylococcal line infections, the options are to remove the line and provide 5–7 days' therapy or, particularly in the case of tunnelled catheters, to treat empirically with a glycopeptide antibiotic, e.g. vancomycin, with or without the use of antibiotic-containing lock therapy to the catheter for approximately 14 days. For *Staph. aureus* infection, the chance of curing an infection with the catheter in situ is low and the risks from infection are high. Therefore, unless the risks of catheter removal outweigh the benefits, treatment involves catheter removal, followed by 14 days of antimicrobial therapy; the same applies to infections with *Pseudomonas aeruginosa*, *Candida* spp., atypical mycobacteria or *Bacillus* spp. Infections complicated by endocarditis, thrombophlebitis, metastatic infection or tunnel infection also require catheter removal.

Infection prevention is a key component of the management of vascular catheters. Measures include strict attention to hand hygiene, optimal siting, full aseptic technique on insertion and subsequent interventions, skin antisepsis with chlorhexidine and isopropyl alcohol, daily assessment of catheter sites (e.g. with visual infusion phlebitis (VIP) score; see Box 13.39), and daily consideration of the continuing requirement for catheterisation. The use of catheters impregnated with antimicrobials, such as chlorhexidine or silver, is advocated in some settings.

Sepsis

Sepsis is discussed on page 198 and there are many causes (Box 13.7). The results of blood cultures and pre-existing host factors guide initial investigations. Patients who are immunocompromised may have a broader range of causal pathogens that may be harder to culture, including mycobacteria and fungi. In many regions, malaria and dengue must also be excluded.

Severe skin and soft tissue infections

Skin and soft tissue infections (SSTIs) are an important cause of sepsis. Cases can be classified as in Box 13.8, according to the clinical features and microbiological findings. In some cases, severe systemic features may be out of keeping with mild local features.

i 13.7 Causes of sepsis	
Infection	**Setting**
Bacterial	
Staph. aureus, coagulase-negative staphylococci	Bacteraemia may be associated with endocarditis, intravascular cannula infection, or skin or bone foci
Streptococcus pneumoniae	Invasive pneumococcal disease, usually with pneumonia or meningitis; asplenia
Other streptococci	Invasive streptococcal disease, especially necrotising fasciitis Viridans streptococci in neutropenic host with severe mucositis
Staphylococcal or streptococcal toxic shock syndrome	Toxin-mediated, blood cultures negative; clues include erythrodermic rash and epidemiological setting
Enterococci	Most often with abdominal focus
Neisseria meningitidis	Sepsis in children or young adults with petechial rash and/or meningitis
Escherichia coli, other Gram-negative bacteria	Urinary or biliary tract infection, or other abdominal infections
Pseudomonas aeruginosa, multidrug-resistant Gram-negative bacteraemia	Nosocomial infection
Salmonella Typhi or Paratyphi	In countries with a high incidence of enteric fever
Yersinia pestis	In plague
Burkholderia pseudomallei	Endemic in areas of Thailand; more likely to involve patients with diabetes mellitus or immunocompromised
Capnocytophaga canimorsus	Associated with dog bites and asplenic individuals
Clostridioides difficile	Severe colitis, particularly in older adults
Polymicrobial infection with Gram-negatives and anaerobes	Bowel perforation, bowel ischaemia
Mycobacterium tuberculosis, *M. avium* complex (MAC)	HIV-positive or immunocompromised with miliary tuberculosis or disseminated MAC
Fungal	
Candida spp.	Line infection or post-operative complication, nosocomial or immunocompromised host
Histoplasma capsulatum, other dimorphic fungi	Immunocompromised host
Parasitic	
Falciparum malaria	Malaria with high-level parasitaemia and multi-organ failure or as a complication of bacterial superinfection
Babesia microti	Asplenic individual
Strongyloides stercoralis hyperinfection syndrome	Gram-negative infection complicating *Strongyloides* infection in immunocompromised host

(HIV = human immunodeficiency virus)

Necrotising fasciitis

In necrotising fasciitis, cutaneous erythema and oedema progress to bullae or areas of necrosis. Unlike in cellulitis, pain may be disproportionate to the visible cutaneous features or may spread beyond the zone of erythema. The infection spreads quickly along the fascial plane. Type 1 necrotising fasciitis is a mixed infection with Gram-negative bacteria and anaerobes, often seen post-operatively in diabetic or immunocompromised hosts. Subcutaneous gas may be present. Type 2 necrotising fasciitis is caused by group A or other streptococci. Approximately

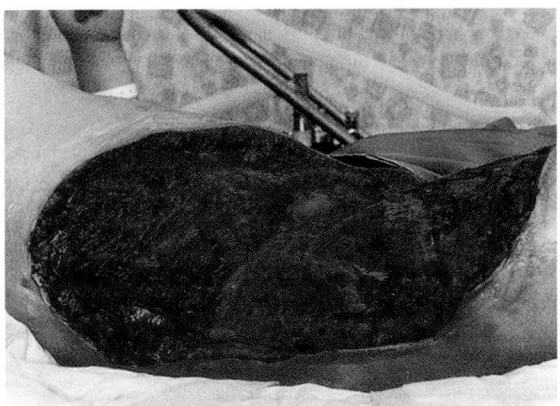

Fig. 13.5 Excision following necrotising fasciitis in an injection drug-user.

60% of cases are associated with streptococcal toxic shock syndrome (p. 302). Type 3 infection involves organisms such as *Aeromonas hydrophila* and *Vibrio vulnificus*, which is found in tropical to subtropical regions and is associated with marine exposure. Type 4 is caused by fungi such as mucoraceous moulds and may also vary geographically in incidence, with recent reports of increased cases in India and other regions.

Necrotising fasciitis is a medical emergency, requiring immediate surgical débridement with inspection of the involved muscle groups, in addition to antimicrobial therapy (Fig. 13.5). Empirical treatment is with broad-spectrum agents (e.g. piperacillin–tazobactam plus clindamycin; meropenem with clindamycin). Ceftazidime or ciprofloxacin with doxycycline may be used where marine exposure is a factor, and antifungals for suspected fungal necrotising fasciitis, but it is important to combine these with effective coverage against streptococcal infection. MRSA-associated necrotising fasciitis has emerged in some regions, where glycopeptides or linezolid should be added to the empirical regimen to cover MRSA until microbiological results allow focused therapy. Hyperbaric oxygen therapy may be considered for polymicrobial infection. Group A streptococcal infection is treated with benzylpenicillin plus clindamycin, and often immunoglobulin, though to date clinical trials have not provided clear evidence of the benefit of immunoglobulin.

Gas gangrene

Although *Clostridium* spp. may colonise or contaminate wounds, no action is required unless there is evidence of spreading infection.

Anaerobic cellulitis occurs when *C. perfringens*, or other clostridia, infect devitalised tissue, usually following a wound. Gas forms locally and extends along tissue planes but bacteraemia does not occur. Prompt surgical débridement of devitalised tissue and therapy with penicillin or clindamycin is usually effective.

Gas gangrene (clostridial myonecrosis) is defined as acute invasion of healthy living muscle undamaged by previous trauma, and is most commonly caused by *C. perfringens*. In at least 70% of cases it follows deep penetrating injury sufficient to create an anaerobic (ischaemic)

environment, allowing clostridial proliferation. Severe pain at the site of the injury progresses rapidly over 18–24 hours. Skin colour changes from pallor to bronze/purple discoloration and the skin is tense, swollen, oedematous and exquisitely tender. Gas in tissues may be obvious, with crepitus on clinical examination, or visible on X-ray, CT or ultrasound. Signs of systemic toxicity develop rapidly, with high leucocytosis, multi-organ dysfunction, raised creatine kinase and evidence of disseminated intravascular coagulation and haemolysis. Antibiotic therapy with high-dose intravenous penicillin and clindamycin is recommended, coupled with aggressive surgical débridement of the affected tissues. Alternative agents include cephalosporins and metronidazole. Hyperbaric oxygen has a putative but controversial role.

Other SSTIs

'Synergistic gangrene' is a polymicrobial infection with anaerobes and other bacteria (*Staph. aureus* or Gram-negatives). When this affects the genital/perineal area, it is known as 'Fournier's gangrene'. Severe gangrenous cellulitis in immunocompromised hosts may involve Gram-negative bacteria or fungi. *Entamoeba histolytica* can cause soft tissue necrosis following abdominal surgery in areas of the world where infection is common. Contact with sea water or shellfish consumption in tropical to subtropical regions worldwide, such as the Gulf of Mexico, can lead to infection with *Vibrio vulnificus*. This infection causes soft tissue necrosis and bullae, and may lead to necrotising fasciitis. Patients with chronic liver disease are particularly susceptible to this infection and can develop sepsis.

Acute diarrhoea and vomiting

Acute diarrhoea, sometimes with vomiting, is the predominant symptom in infective gastroenteritis (Box 13.9). Acute diarrhoea may also be a symptom of other infectious and non-infectious diseases (Box 13.10). Stress, whether psychological or physical, can also produce loose stools.

Global Burden of Disease 2016 estimates suggest acute diarrhoea causes 1.7 million deaths annually, a quarter in children under 5. In high-income countries older people are most susceptible (Box 13.11). The majority of episodes are due to infections spread by the faecal–oral route and transmitted either on fomites, on contaminated hands or in food or water. Provision of clean drinking water, appropriate disposal of human and animal sewage, and the application of simple principles of food hygiene all limit gastroenteritis (water, sanitation and hygiene – *WASH*).

Some organisms (*Bacillus cereus*, *Staph. aureus* and *Vibrio cholerae*) elute exotoxins that cause vomiting and/or so-called 'secretory' diarrhoea (watery diarrhoea without blood or faecal leucocytes, reflecting

13

---

i | **13.10 Differential diagnosis of acute diarrhoea and vomiting**

Infectious causes

- Gastroenteritis
- *Clostridioides difficile* infection
- Acute diverticulitis (p. 832)
- Sepsis (p. 198)
- Pelvic inflammatory disease (p. 375)

- Meningococcaemia
- Pneumonia (especially 'atypical disease', p. 512)
- Malaria

Non-infectious causes

Gastrointestinal

- Inflammatory bowel disease (p. 835)
- Bowel malignancy (p. 826)

- Overflow from constipation (p. 833)
- Enteral tube feeding

Metabolic

- Diabetic ketoacidosis (p. 721)
- Thyrotoxicosis (p. 652)
- Uraemia (p. 588)

- Neuro-endocrine tumours releasing (e.g.) VIP or 5-HT

Drugs and toxins

- NSAIDs
- Cytotoxic agents
- Antibiotics
- Proton pump inhibitors
- Dinoflagellates (p. 236)
- Plant toxins (p. 237)

- Heavy metals
- Ciguatera fish poisoning (p. 236)
- Scombrotoxic fish poisoning (p. 237)

(5-HT = 5-hydroxytryptamine, serotonin; NSAIDs = non-steroidal anti-inflammatory drugs; VIP = vasoactive intestinal peptide)

---

i | **13.12 Foods associated with infectious illness, including gastroenteritis**

Raw seafood

- Norovirus
- *Vibrio* spp.

- Hepatitis A

Raw eggs

- *Salmonella* serovars

Under-cooked meat or poultry

- *Salmonella* serovars
- *Campylobacter* spp.
- EHEC

- Hepatitis E (pork products)
- *Clostridium perfringens*

Unpasteurised milk or juice

- *Salmonella* serovars
- *Campylobacter* spp.

- EHEC
- *Yersinia enterocolitica*

Unpasteurised soft cheeses

- *Salmonella* serovars
- *Campylobacter* spp.
- ETEC

- *Yersinia enterocolitica*
- *Listeria monocytogenes*

Home-made canned goods

- *Clostridium botulinum*

Raw hot dogs, pâté

- *Listeria monocytogenes*

(EHEC = enterohaemorrhagic *Escherichia coli*; ETEC = enterotoxigenic *E. coli*)

 | **13.11 Infectious diarrhoea in old age**

- **Incidence**: not increased but the impact is greater.
- **Mortality**: most deaths due to gastroenteritis in high-income countries are in adults aged over 70. Most are presumed to be caused by dehydration leading to organ failure.
- ***Clostridioides difficile* infection (CDI)**: more common, especially in hospital and nursing home settings, usually following antibiotic exposure.

---

small bowel dysfunction). In general, the time from ingestion to the onset of symptoms is short and, other than dehydration, little systemic upset occurs. Other organisms, such as *Shigella* spp., *Campylobacter* spp. and enterohaemorrhagic *Escherichia coli* (EHEC), may directly invade the mucosa of the small bowel or produce cytotoxins that cause mucosal ulceration, typically affecting the terminal small bowel and colon. The incubation period is longer and more systemic upset occurs, with prolonged bloody diarrhoea. *Salmonella* spp. are capable of invading enterocytes and of causing both a secretory response and invasive disease with systemic features. This is seen with *Salmonella* Typhi and *Salmonella* Paratyphi (enteric fever without diarrhoea), but may occasionally be seen with other non-typhoidal *Salmonella* spp., particularly in the immunocompromised host and older people.

Clinical assessment

The history should address foods ingested (Box 13.12), duration and frequency of diarrhoea, presence of blood or steatorrhoea, abdominal pain and tenesmus, and whether other people have been affected. Fever and bloody diarrhoea suggest an invasive, colitic, dysenteric process. An incubation period of less than 18 hours suggests toxin-mediated food poisoning, and longer than 5 days suggests diarrhoea caused by protozoa or helminths. Person-to-person spread suggests infections, such as shigellosis or cholera.

Examination including assessment of the degree of dehydration such as thirst, headache, altered skin turgor, dry mucous membranes and postural hypotension, is important, particularly in tropical regions, where dehydration progresses rapidly. Signs of more marked dehydration include supine hypotension and tachycardia, decreased urinary output,

delirium and sunken eyes. The blood pressure, pulse rate, urine output and ongoing stool losses should be monitored closely.

The severity of diarrhoea may be assessed by reference to the Bristol stool form scale (Bristol stool chart), which allows an objective assessment of stool consistency by providing a verbal and visual reference scale (Fig. 13.6). The Bristol stool form scale guides (at least in UK hospitals) decisions on stool sampling and infection prevention precautions in hospital inpatients, especially in relation to *C. difficile*.

Investigations

These include stool inspection for blood and microscopy for leucocytes, and also an examination for ova, cysts and parasites if the history indicates residence or travel to areas where these infections are prevalent. Stool culture should be performed and *C. difficile* toxin sought. FBC and serum electrolytes indicate the degree of inflammation and dehydration. Where cholera is prevalent, examination of a wet film with dark-field microscopy for darting motility aids diagnosis. In a malarious area, a blood film for malaria parasites should be obtained. Blood and urine cultures and a chest X-ray may identify alternative sites of infection, particularly if the clinical features suggest a syndrome other than gastroenteritis.

Management

All patients with acute, potentially infective diarrhoea should be appropriately isolated to minimise person-to-person spread of infection. If the history suggests a food-borne source, public health measures must be implemented to identify the source and to establish whether other linked cases exist.

Fluid replacement

Replacement of fluid losses in diarrhoeal illness is crucial and may be life-saving.

Normal daily fluid intake in an adult is only 1–2 L, but there is considerable additional fluid movement in and out of the gut in secretions (see Fig. 23.7). Altered gut resorption with diarrhoea causes substantial isotonic fluid loss; up to 10–20 L per day in cholera. Water and electrolytes need to be replaced, but electrolyte absorption from the gut is an active

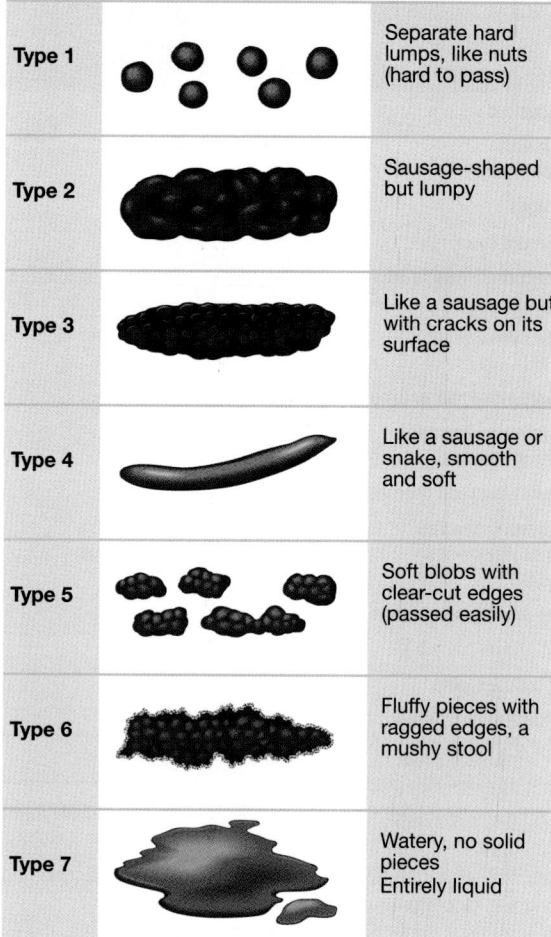

Type 1		Separate hard lumps, like nuts (hard to pass)
Type 2		Sausage-shaped but lumpy
Type 3		Like a sausage but with cracks on its surface
Type 4		Like a sausage or snake, smooth and soft
Type 5		Soft blobs with clear-cut edges (passed easily)
Type 6		Fluffy pieces with ragged edges, a mushy stool
Type 7		Watery, no solid pieces Entirely liquid

Fig. 13.6 Bristol stool chart. The stool is given a 'score' of 1–7 by reference to the verbal and visual description. This is recorded on a chart (usually known as a 'Bristol stool chart') or in a patient monitoring database. *Adapted from Lewis SJ, Heaton KW. Stool form scale as a useful guide to intestinal transit time. Scand J Gastroenterol 1997; 32:920–924.*

energy-requiring process. Infected mucosa is capable of very rapid fluid and electrolyte transport if carbohydrate is available as an energy source. Oral rehydration solutions (ORS) therefore contain sugars, as well as water and electrolytes (Box 13.13). ORS are as effective as intravenous replacement fluid, even for cholera. In mild to moderate gastroenteritis, adults should be encouraged to drink fluids and continue normal dietary food intake. If this is impossible – due to vomiting, for example – intravenous fluid administration is required. In very sick patients or those with cardiac or renal disease, monitoring of urine output and central venous pressure may be necessary.

The volume of fluid replacement required should be estimated based on the following considerations:

- *Replacement of established deficit.* The average adult's diarrhoeal stool accounts for a loss of 200 mL of isotonic fluid. After 48 hours of moderate diarrhoea (6–10 stools per 24 hours), the average adult will be 2–4 L depleted. This requires rapid replacement of 1–1.5 L, either orally (ORS) or by intravenous infusion (normal saline), within the first 2–4 hours of presentation. Longer symptomatology, additional vomiting or more persistent/severe diarrhoea rapidly produces fluid losses comparable to diabetic ketoacidosis and is a metabolic emergency requiring active intervention.
- *Replacement of ongoing losses.* Stool losses should be accurately recorded and an estimate of ongoing losses calculated. Commercially available rehydration sachets provide 200 mL of ORS; one sachet per diarrhoea stool replaces losses.

i	**13.13 Composition of oral rehydration solution and other replacement fluids***			
Fluid	Na	K	Cl	Energy
WHO	90	20	80	54
Dioralyte	60	20	60	71
Pepsi	6.5	0.8	–	400
7UP	7.5	0.2	–	320
Apple juice	0.4	26	–	480
Orange juice	0.2	49	–	400
Breast milk	22	36	28	670

*Values given in mmol/L for electrolyte and kcal/L for energy components. (WHO = World Health Organization)

- *Replacement of normal daily requirement.* The average adult has a daily requirement of 1–1.5 L of fluid in addition to the calculations above. This will be increased substantially in fever or a hot environment.

Antimicrobial agents

In non-specific gastroenteritis, routine use of antimicrobials does not improve outcome and may lead to antimicrobial resistance or side-effects. They are usually used where there is systemic involvement, immunocompromise or significant comorbidity.

Evidence suggests that, in EHEC infections, antibiotics should not be used since they can enhance haemolytic uraemic syndrome (HUS; p. 582) due to increased toxin release.

Conversely, antibiotics are indicated in *Shigella dysenteriae* infection and in invasive salmonellosis – in particular, typhoid fever. Antibiotics may also be advantageous in cholera epidemics, reducing infectivity and controlling infection spread.

Antidiarrhoeal, antimotility and antisecretory agents

These agents are not recommended in acute infective diarrhoea. Loperamide, diphenoxylate and opiates are potentially dangerous in dysentery in childhood, causing intussusception. Antisecretory agents, such as bismuth and chlorpromazine, may make the stools appear bulkier but do not reduce stool fluid losses and may cause significant sedation. Adsorbents, such as kaolin or charcoal, have little effect.

Non-infectious causes of food poisoning

Although less common non-infectious causes must also be considered in the differential diagnosis of gastroenteritis. These are discussed on page 236.

Antimicrobial-associated diarrhoea

Antimicrobial-associated diarrhoea (AAD) is a common complication of antimicrobial therapy, especially with broad-spectrum agents. It is most common in older people but can occur at all ages. Although the specific mechanism is unknown in most cases of AAD, *C. difficile* is implicated in 20%–25% of cases and is the most common cause among patients with evidence of colitis. *Clostridium perfringens* is a rarer cause that usually remains undiagnosed, and *Klebsiella oxytoca* may also cause antibiotic-associated haemorrhagic colitis.

Infections acquired in the tropics

Recent decades have seen unprecedented increases in long-distance travel, as well as extensive migration. Some infections maintain a fixed geographical distribution, being dependent on specific vectors or weather conditions, while others move with their human hosts and some

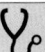

13.14 How to assess health needs in travellers before departure*

- Destination
- Personal details, including previous travel experience
- Dates of trip
- Itinerary and purpose of trip
- Personal medical history, including pregnancy, medication and allergies (e.g. to eggs, vaccines, antibiotics)
- Past vaccinations:
    Childhood schedule followed? Diphtheria, tetanus, pertussis, polio, *Neisseria meningitidis* types B/C, *Haemophilus influenzae* B (HiB)
    Travel-related? Typhoid, yellow fever, hepatitis A, hepatitis B, meningococcal ACW135Y, rabies, Japanese B encephalitis, tick-borne encephalitis
- Malaria prophylaxis: questions influencing the choice of antimalarial drugs are destination, past experience with antimalarials, history of epilepsy or psychiatric illness

Further information is available at fitfortravel.nhs.uk.

13.15 How to obtain a history from travellers to the tropics with fever	
Questions	**Factors to ascertain**
Countries visited and dates of travel	Relate travel to known outbreaks of infection or antimicrobial resistance
Determine the environment visited	Travel to rural environments, forests, rivers or lakes
Clarify where the person slept	Sleeping in huts, use of bed nets, sleeping on the ground
Establish what he/she was doing	Exposure to people with medical illness, animals, soil, lakes and rivers
History of insect bites	Type of insect responsible, circumstances (location, time of day etc.), preventative measures
Dietary history	Ingestion of uncooked foods, salads and vegetables, meats (especially if under-cooked), shellfish, molluscs, unpasteurised dairy products, unbottled water and sites at which food prepared
Sexual history	History of sexual intercourse with commercial sex workers, local population or travellers from other countries
Malaria prophylaxis	Type of prophylaxis
Vaccination history	Receipt of pre-travel vaccines and appropriateness to area visited
History of any treatments received while abroad	Receipt of medicines, local remedies, blood transfusions or surgical procedures

13

may then be transmitted to other people. This means that the pattern of infectious diseases seen in each country changes constantly, and travel history and information on countries previously lived in, particularly during childhood, are crucial.

In general, the diversity of infectious diseases is greater in tropical than in temperate countries, and people in temperate countries have immunity to a narrower range of infections, reflecting less exposure in childhood and less ongoing boosting of immunity later in life, so that the most common travel-associated infections are those that are acquired by residents of temperate countries during visits to the tropics. In addition, those who have lived in tropical areas may lose immunity when they move to temperate countries and become susceptible when visiting their homeland.

Most travel-associated infections are preventable. Pre-travel advice is tailored to the destination and the traveller (Box 13.14). It includes avoidance of insect bites (using at least 20% diethyltoluamide (DEET)), sun protection (sunscreen with a sun protection factor (SPF) of at least 15), food and water hygiene ('Boil it, cook it, peel it or forget it!'), how to respond to travellers' diarrhoea (seek medical advice if bloody or if it lasts more than 48 hours) and, if relevant, safe sex (condom use).

Fever acquired in tropical regions

Presentation with unexplained fever is common in travellers who are visiting or have recently travelled to tropical areas. Fever may also occur in those living in tropical regions if they lack immunity to endemic pathogens or if immunity is compromised by factors such as pregnancy. Common causes are malaria, enteric fever, viral hepatitis and dengue fever. Travellers to affected areas may have viral haemorrhagic fevers (VHFs) such as Ebola, Lassa, Crimean–Congo and Marburg (see Box 13.35), avian influenza (H5N1) or Middle East respiratory syndrome (MERS), which require special isolation precautions (High Consequence Infectious Diseases; HCID).

Clinical assessment

The approach to unexplained fever is as described above and key questions relating to infections acquired in tropical regions are listed in Box 13.15. Medicines purchased in some countries may have reduced efficacy, e.g. for malaria prophylaxis. Consult reliable up-to-date sources about resistance to antimalarial drugs in the country visited. Vaccinations against yellow fever and hepatitis A and B are sufficiently effective to virtually exclude these infections. Oral and injectable typhoid vaccinations are 70%–90% effective.

The differential diagnosis is guided by the clinical scenario, presence of specific exposures (Box 13.16) and incubation period (Box 13.17). *Falciparum* malaria typically presents 7–28 days after exposure. VHF, dengue and rickettsial infection can usually be excluded if more than 21 days have passed between leaving the area and onset of illness.

Clinical examination is summarised on page 262. Particular attention should be paid to the skin, throat, eyes, nail beds, lymph nodes, abdomen and heart. Patients may be unaware of tick bites or eschars. Body temperature should be measured at least twice daily.

Investigations and management

Initial investigations include blood films and a rapid diagnostic test (RDT; antigen detection) for malaria parasites, FBC, urinalysis and chest X-ray if indicated. Box 13.18 lists diagnoses and investigations to consider in unexplained acute fever.

Management is directed at the underlying cause. In patients with suspected HCID, such as VHF, strict infection control measures with isolation and barrier nursing are implemented to prevent contact with the patient's body fluids. The risk of VHF should be determined using epidemiological risk factors and clinical signs (Fig. 13.7), and further management undertaken as described in this chapter.

Diarrhoea acquired in the tropics

Gastrointestinal illness is the most common infection amongst visitors to the tropics, with *Salmonella* spp., *Campylobacter* spp. and *Cryptosporidium* spp. infections prevalent worldwide (Box 13.19). *Shigella* spp. and *Entamoeba histolytica* (amoebiasis) are usually acquired in South Asia or sub-Saharan and southern Africa.

The approach to patients with acute diarrhoea is described on page 272. The benefits of treating travellers' diarrhoea with antimicrobials are marginal, with slight reductions in stool frequency and likelihood of cure at 72 hours offset by increased side-effects. The differential diagnosis of diarrhoea persisting for more than 14 days is wide (see Box 23.19). The differential of chronic diarrhoea includes parasitic and bacterial causes, tropical malabsorption, inflammatory bowel disease and neoplasia. Causes particularly associated with the tropics include giardiasis, strongyloidiasis, chronic intestinal schistosomiasis, intestinal flukes, enteropathogenic *E. coli*, HIV enteropathy, hypolactasia (lactase

i 13.16 Specific exposures and causes of fever in the tropics	
Exposure	**Infection or disease**
Mosquito bite	Malaria, dengue fever, chikungunya, filariasis, tularaemia
Tsetse fly bite	African trypanosomiasis
Tick bite	Rickettsial infections including typhus, Lyme disease, tularaemia, Crimean–Congo haemorrhagic fever, Kyasanur forest disease, babesiosis, tick-borne encephalitis
Louse bite	Typhus
Flea bite	Plague
Sandfly bite	Leishmaniasis, arbovirus infection
Reduviid bug	Chagas' disease
Animal contact	Q fever, brucellosis, anthrax, plague, tularaemia, viral haemorrhagic fevers, rabies
Freshwater swimming	Schistosomiasis, leptospirosis, *Naegleria fowleri*
Exposure to soil	Inhalation: dimorphic fungi Inhalation or inoculation: *Burkholderia pseudomallei* Inoculation (most often when barefoot): hookworms, *Strongyloides stercoralis*
Raw or under-cooked fruit and vegetables	Enteric bacterial infections, hepatitis A or E virus, *Fasciola hepatica*, *Toxocara* spp., *Echinococcus granulosus* (hydatid disease), *Entamoeba histolytica*
Under-cooked pork	*Taenia solium* (cysticercosis)
Crustaceans or molluscs	Paragonimiasis, gnathostomiasis, *Angiostrongylus cantonensis* infection, hepatitis A virus, cholera
Unpasteurised dairy products	Brucellosis, salmonellosis, abdominal tuberculosis, listeriosis
Untreated water	Enteric bacterial infections, giardiasis, *Cryptosporidium* spp. (chronic in immunocompromised), hepatitis A or E virus

i 13.17 Incubation times and illnesses in travellers

<2 weeks

Non-specific fever
- Malaria
- Chikungunya
- Dengue
- Scrub typhus
- Spotted group rickettsiae
- Acute HIV
- Acute hepatitis C virus
- *Campylobacter*
- Salmonellosis
- Shigellosis
- East African trypanosomiasis
- Leptospirosis
- Relapsing fever
- Influenza
- Yellow fever

Fever and coagulopathy (usually thrombocytopenia)
- Malaria
- VHF
- Meningococcaemia
- Enteroviruses
- Leptospirosis and other bacterial pathogens associated with coagulopathy

Fever and central nervous system involvement
- Malaria
- Typhoid fever
- Rickettsial typhus (epidemic caused by *Rickettsia prowazekii*)
- Meningococcal meningitis
- Arboviral encephalitis
- East African trypanosomiasis
- Tick-borne encephalitis
- Other causes of encephalitis or meningitis
- Angiostrongyliasis
- Rabies

Fever and pulmonary involvement
- Influenza
- Pneumonia, including *Legionella* pneumonia
- Acute histoplasmosis
- Acute coccidioidomycosis
- Q fever
- COVID-19 (SARS-CoV-2)
- SARS

Fever and rash
- Viral exanthems (rubella, measles, varicella, mumps, HHV-6, enteroviruses)
- Chikungunya
- Dengue
- Spotted or typhus group rickettsiosis
- Typhoid fever
- Parvovirus B19
- HIV-1

2–6 weeks
- Malaria
- Tuberculosis
- Hepatitis A, B, C and E viruses
- Visceral leishmaniasis
- Acute schistosomiasis
- Amoebic liver abscess
- Leptospirosis
- African trypanosomiasis
- VHF
- Q fever
- Acute American trypanosomiasis
- Viral causes of mononucleosis syndromes

>6 weeks
- Non-*falciparum* malaria
- Tuberculosis
- Hepatitis B and E viruses
- HIV-1
- Visceral leishmaniasis
- Filariasis
- Onchocerciasis
- Schistosomiasis
- Amoebic liver abscess
- Chronic mycoses
- African trypanosomiasis
- Rabies
- Typhoid fever

(HHV-6 = human herpesvirus-6; HIV-1 = human immunodeficiency virus-1; SARS = severe acute respiratory syndrome; VHF = viral haemorrhagic fever)
Adapted from Traveller's Health Yellow Book, CDC Health Information for International Travel, 2008.

deficiency) and chronic calcific pancreatitis. The workup should include tests for parasitic causes of chronic diarrhoea, such as examination of stool and duodenal aspirates for ova and parasites, and serological investigation.

Giardia lamblia infection (giardiasis) may progress to a malabsorption syndrome. If no cause is found, empirical treatment for giardiasis with metronidazole is often helpful.

HIV-1 may cause chronic diarrhoea due to medications or infection. Causes such as HIV enteropathy or infection with agents such as *Cryptosporidium* spp., *Cystoisospora belli* or microsporidia are uncommon once antiretroviral therapy is commenced, and AIDS-associated diarrhoea due to CMV or disseminated *Mycobacterium avium* complex infection is uncommon in tropical regions.

Eosinophilia acquired in the tropics

Eosinophilia occurs in a variety of haematological, allergic and inflammatory conditions discussed on page 935. It may also arise in HIV-1 and human T-cell lymphotropic virus (HTLV)-1 infection. However, eosinophils are important in the immune response to parasitic infections, especially those with a tissue migration phase. In the context of travel to or residence in the tropics, a patient with an eosinophil count of more than

0.4×10^9/L should be investigated for both non-parasitic (see Box 25.9) and parasitic causes (Box 13.20).

The response to parasite infections is often different when travellers to and residents of endemic areas are compared. Travellers often have recent and light infections associated with eosinophilia. Residents who have been infected for a long time often have chronic pathology without eosinophilia.

Clinical assessment

A history of travel to known endemic areas for schistosomiasis, onchocerciasis and the filariases will indicate possible causes. Assessment

i	**13.18 Investigation of tropically acquired acute fever without localising signs**

Features on full blood count	Further investigations
Neutrophil leucocytosis	
Bacterial sepsis	Blood culture
Leptospirosis	Culture of blood and urine, serology
Borreliosis (tick- or louse-borne relapsing fever)	Blood film
Amoebic liver abscess	Ultrasound
Normal white cell count and differential	
Malaria (may have low platelets or anaemia)	Blood film, antigen test
Typhoid fever	Blood and stool culture
Typhus	Serology
Lymphocytosis	
Viral fevers, including VHF	Serology, PCR
Infectious mononucleosis	Monospot test, serology
Malaria	Blood film, antigen test
Rickettsial fevers	Serology
Atypical lymphocytes	
Dengue and other VHF	Serology, antigen, PCR
Infectious mononucleosis-like syndromes	Serology, PCR
HIV (acute retroviral syndrome)	Serology, antigen
Hepatitis viruses	Serology, antigen, PCR
Parasitic, malaria, trypanosomiasis	Blood film, antigen test, PCR

(HIV = human immunodeficiency virus; PCR = polymerase chain reaction; VHF = viral haemorrhagic fever)

i	**13.19 Most common causes of travellers' diarrhoea**

- Enterotoxigenic *E. coli* (ETEC)
- *Shigella* spp.
- *Campylobacter jejuni*
- *Salmonella* serovars
- *Plesiomonas shigelloides*
- Non-cholera *Vibrio* spp.
- *Aeromonas* spp.

Ascaris lumbricoides and *Strongyloides stercoralis*, can cause abdominal symptoms, including intestinal obstruction and diarrhoea. In the case of heavy infestation with *Ascaris*, this may be due to fat malabsorption and there may be associated nutritional deficits. *Schistosoma haematobium* can cause haematuria or haematospermia. *Toxocara* spp. can give rise to choroidal lesions with visual field defects. *Angiostrongylus cantonensis* and gnathostomiasis induce eosinophilic meningitis, and the hyperinfection syndrome caused by *S. stercoralis* in immunocompromised hosts induces meningitis due to Gram-negative bacteria. Myositis is a feature of trichinosis (trichinellosis) and cysticercosis. Periorbital oedema can occur with trichinosis.

Investigations

The diagnosis of a parasitic infestation requires direct visualisation of adult worms, larvae or ova. Serum antibody detection may not distinguish between active and past infection and is often unhelpful in those born in endemic areas. Radiological investigations may provide circumstantial evidence of parasite infestation. Box 13.21 describes initial investigations for eosinophilia.

Management

A specific diagnosis guides therapy. In the absence of a specific diagnosis, many clinicians will give an empirical course of praziquantel if the individual has potentially been exposed to schistosomiasis, or with albendazole/ivermectin if strongyloidiasis or intestinal nematodes are likely causes.

Skin conditions acquired in the tropics

Community-based studies in the tropics consistently show that skin infections (bacterial and fungal), scabies and eczema are the most common skin problems (Box 13.22). Scabies and eczema are discussed on pages 1093 and 1096. Cutaneous leishmaniasis and onchocerciasis have defined geographical distributions. In travellers, secondarily infected insect bites, pyoderma, cutaneous larva migrans and non-specific dermatitis are common.

should establish duration of exposure and the history should address all the elements in Box 13.15.

Physical signs or symptoms that suggest a parasitic cause for eosinophilia include transient rashes (schistosomiasis or strongyloidiasis), fever (Katayama syndrome), pruritus (onchocerciasis) or migrating subcutaneous swellings (loiasis, gnathostomiasis) (see Box 13.21). Paragonimiasis can give rise to haemoptysis, and the migratory phase of intestinal nematodes or lymphatic filariasis may cause cough, wheezing and transient pulmonary infiltrates. Schistosomiasis, strongyloidiasis and gnathostomiasis induce transient respiratory symptoms with infiltrates in the acute stages and, when eggs reach the pulmonary vasculature in chronic schistosomiasis infection, can result in shortness of breath with features of right heart failure due to pulmonary hypertension. Fever and hepatosplenomegaly are seen in schistosomiasis, *Fasciola hepatica* infection and toxocariasis (visceral larva migrans). Intestinal worms, such as

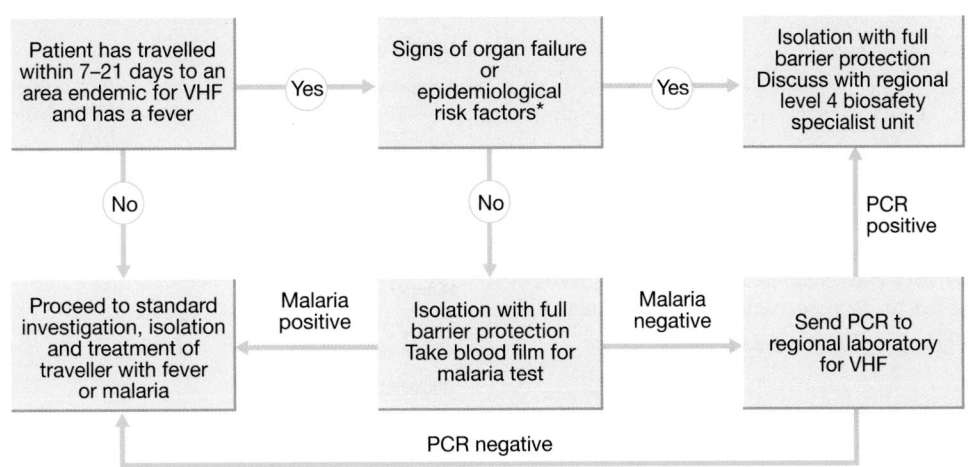

Fig. 13.7 Approach to the patient with suspected viral haemorrhagic fever (VHF). See Box 13.35. *Epidemiological risk factors: staying with a febrile individual, caring for a sick individual, or contact with body fluids from a suspected human or animal case of VHF. (PCR = polymerase chain reaction)

13.20 Parasite infections that cause eosinophilia

Infestation	Pathogen	Clinical syndrome with eosinophilia
Strongyloidiasis	Strongyloides stercoralis	Larva currens
Soil-transmitted helminthiases		
Hookworm	Necator americanus	Anaemia
	Ancylostoma duodenale	Anaemia
Ascariasis	Ascaris lumbricoides	Löffler syndrome
Toxocariasis	Toxocara canis	Visceral larva migrans
Schistosomiasis	Schistosoma haematobium	Katayama fever
	S. mansoni, S. japonicum	Chronic infection
Filariases		
Loiasis	Loa loa	Skin nodules
Wuchereria bancrofti	W. bancrofti	Lymphangitis, lymphadenopathy, orchitis, intermittent bouts of cellulitis, lymphoedema and elephantiasis
Brugia malayi	B. malayi	Brugian elephantiasis similar but typically less severe than that caused by W. bancrofti
Mansonella perstans	M. perstans	Asymptomatic infection, occasionally subconjunctival nodules
Onchocerciasis	Onchocerca volvulus	Visual disturbance, dermatitis
Other nematode infections	Trichinella spiralis	Myositis
	Gnathostoma spinigerum	Pruritus, migratory nodules, eosinophilic meningitis
Cestode infections	Taenia saginata, T. solium	Usually asymptomatic; eosinophilia associated with migratory phase
	Echinococcus granulosus	Lesions in liver or other organ; eosinophilia associated with leakage from cyst
Liver flukes	Fasciola hepatica	Hepatic symptoms; eosinophilia associated with migratory phase
	Clonorchis sinensis	As for fascioliasis
	Opisthorchis felineus	As for fascioliasis
Lung fluke	Paragonimus westermani	Lung lesions

13.21 Initial investigation of eosinophilia

Investigation	Pathogens sought
Stool microscopy	Ova, cysts and parasites
Terminal urine	Ova of Schistosoma haematobium
Duodenal aspirate	Filariform larvae of Strongyloides, liver fluke ova
Day bloods	Microfilariae Brugia malayi, Loa loa
Night bloods	Microfilariae Wuchereria bancrofti
Skin snips	Onchocerca volvulus
Slit-lamp examination	Onchocerca volvulus
Serology	Schistosomiasis, filariasis, strongyloidiasis, hydatid, trichinosis, gnathostomiasis etc.

13.22 Rash in tropical travellers/residents

Maculopapular rash
- Dengue
- HIV-1
- Typhoid
- *Spirillum minus*
- Rickettsial infections
- Measles

Petechial or purpuric rash
- Viral haemorrhagic fevers
- Yellow fever
- Meningococcal sepsis
- Leptospirosis
- Rickettsial spotted fevers
- Malaria

Vesicular rash
- Monkeypox
- Insect bites
- Rickettsial pox

Urticarial rash
- Katayama fever (schistosomiasis)
- *Toxocara* spp.
- *Strongyloides stercoralis*
- Fascioliasis

Ulcers
- Leishmaniasis
- *Mycobacterium ulcerans* (Buruli ulcer)
- Dracunculosis
- Anthrax
- Rickettsial eschar
- Tropical ulcer (*Fusobacterium ulcerans* and *Treponema vincenti*)
- Ecthyma (staphylococci, streptococci)

Papules
- Scabies
- Insect bites
- Prickly heat
- Ringworm
- Onchocerciasis

Nodules or plaques
- Leprosy
- Chromoblastomycosis
- Dimorphic fungi
- Trypanosomiasis
- Onchocerciasis
- Myiasis (larvae of tumbu fly or botfly)
- Tungiasis (*Tunga penetrans*)

Migratory linear rash
- Cutaneous larva migrans (CLM; dog hookworms)
- *Strongyloides stercoralis* (larva currens, more rapid than CLM)

Migratory papules/nodules
- Loa loa
- Gnathostomiasis
- Schistosomiasis

Thickened skin
- Mycetoma (actinomycetoma/ eumycetoma)
- Elephantiasis (filariasis)

(CLM = cutaneous larva migrans; HIV-1 = human immunodeficiency virus-1)

During the investigation of skin lesions, enquiry should be made about habitation, activities undertaken and regions visited (see Box 13.15). Examples of skin lesions in tropical disease are shown in Figure 13.8.

Skin biopsies are helpful in diagnosing aetiology. Culture of biopsy material may be needed to diagnose bacterial, fungal, parasitic and mycobacterial infections.

Infections in adolescence

Particular issues of relevance in adolescent patients are shown in Box 13.23.

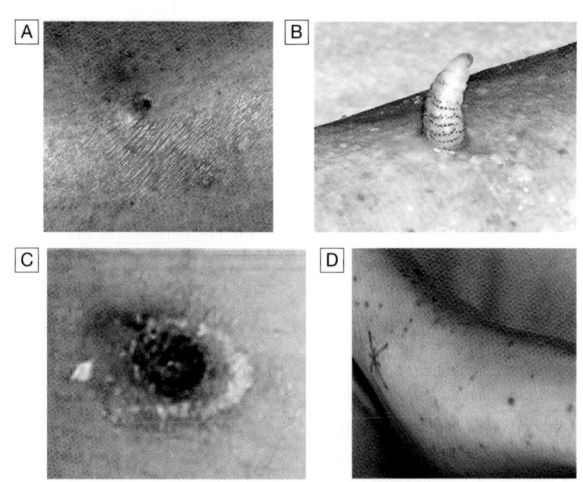

Fig. 13.8 Examples of skin lesions in patients with fever in the tropics. A Subcutaneous nodule due to botfly infection. B Emerging larva after treatment with petroleum jelly. C Eschar of scrub typhus. D Rat bite fever. *(A, B and D) Courtesy of Dr Ravi Gowda, Royal Hallamshire Hospital, Sheffield. (C) Courtesy of Dr Rattanaphone Phetsouvanh, Mahosot Hospital, Vientiane, PDR Laos.*

 13.23 Key issues in infectious diseases in adolescence

- **Common infectious syndromes**: infectious mononucleosis, bacterial pharyngitis, whooping cough, pneumonia, staphylococcal skin/soft tissue infections, urinary tract infections, acute gastroenteritis.
- **Life-threatening infections**: meningococcal infection (sepsis and/or meningitis).
- **Sexually transmitted infections**: human papillomavirus (HPV), human immunodeficiency virus-1 (HIV-1), hepatitis B virus and chlamydia. These may reflect either voluntary sexual activity or sexual coercion/abuse.
- **Travel-related infections**: diarrhoea, malaria etc. are relatively common.
- **Infections in susceptible groups**: patients with cystic fibrosis, congenital immunodeficiency, acute leukaemia and other adolescent malignancies are vulnerable to specific groups of infections.
- **Infections requiring prolonged antimicrobial use**: adherence to chronic therapy is challenging, for both oral (antituberculous or antiretroviral) and systemic (osteomyelitis, septic arthritis or post-operative infections) treatments. Outpatient antimicrobial therapy is preferred to minimise hospitalisation.
- **Vaccination**: engagement with age-specific vaccine programmes should be ensured, e.g. HPV, childhood booster vaccines and meningococcal vaccine.
- **Risk reduction**: education relating to sexual health and alcohol and recreational drug usage is important.

Infections in pregnancy

Box 13.24 shows some of the infections encountered in pregnancy.

Viral infections

Systemic viral infections with exanthem

Childhood exanthems are characterised by fever and widespread rash. Maternal antibody usually gives protection for the first 6–12 months of life. Comprehensive immunisation programmes have dramatically reduced the number of paediatric infections but incomplete uptake results in infections in later life.

Measles

The World Health Organization (WHO) has set the objective of eradicating measles globally using the live attenuated vaccine. However, vaccination of more than 95% of the population is required to prevent outbreaks due to the high basic reproduction number (R_0 value; see p. 108). Clusters of infection in young adults are associated with mass gatherings, e.g. music festivals and sub-populations with lower vaccination coverage. Natural illness produces life-long immunity.

Clinical features

Infection is by respiratory droplets with an incubation period of 6–19 days. A prodromal illness occurs, 1–3 days before the rash, with upper respiratory symptoms, conjunctivitis and the presence of the pathognomonic Koplik's spots: small white spots surrounded by erythema on the buccal mucosa (Fig. 13.9A). As natural antibody develops, the maculopapular rash appears, spreading from the face to the extremities (Fig. 13.9B). Generalised lymphadenopathy and diarrhoea are common. Complications are more common in older children and adults, and include otitis media, bacterial pneumonia, transient hepatitis, pancreatitis and clinical encephalitis (approximately 0.1% of cases). A rare late complication is subacute sclerosing panencephalitis (SSPE), which occurs up to 7 years after infection (see Ch. 28).

Measles is a serious disease in the malnourished, vitamin-deficient or immunocompromised. Persistent infection with a giant cell pneumonitis or encephalitis may occur but rash may be absent. In tuberculosis infection, measles suppresses cell-mediated immunity and may exacerbate disease; for this reason, measles vaccination should be deferred until after commencing antituberculous treatment. Measles does not cause congenital malformation but may be more severe in pregnant women.

Mortality clusters at the extremes of age and is highly dependent on health economic status. In 2018 there were approximately 15 deaths per 1000 cases globally, ranging from 0.2 : 1000 in Europe to 30 : 1000 in the Africa region (WHO data). Death usually results from a bacterial superinfection, occurring as a complication of measles: most often pneumonia, diarrhoeal disease or noma/cancrum oris, a gangrenous stomatitis. Death may also result from complications of measles encephalitis.

Diagnosis

Clinical diagnosis is challenging but supported by detection of antibodies (immunoglobulin (Ig) M and IgG) and/or measles RNA in oral fluid. It is a notifiable disease in the UK.

Management and prevention

Immunoglobulin therapy attenuates the disease in the immunocompromised (regardless of vaccination status) and in non-immune pregnant women, but must be given within 6 days of exposure. Vaccination can be used in outbreaks and vitamin A may improve the outcome in uncomplicated disease. Antibiotic therapy is reserved for bacterial complications. In the UK children are offered vaccination with a combined measles, mumps and rubella vaccine (MMR; a live attenuated vaccine) at 1 year of age, with a pre-school booster at 3 years 4 months.

Rubella (German measles)

Rubella causes exanthem in the non-immunised.

Clinical features

Rubella is spread by respiratory droplet, with infectivity from up to 10 days before to 2 weeks after the onset of the rash. The incubation period is 15–20 days. In childhood, most cases are subclinical, although clinical features may include fever, maculopapular rash spreading from the face, and lymphadenopathy. Complications are rare but include thrombocytopenia and hepatitis. Encephalitis and haemorrhage are occasionally reported. In adults, arthritis involving hands or knees is relatively common, especially in women.

If transplacental infection takes place in the first trimester or later, persistence of the virus is likely and severe congenital disease may result (Box 13.25). Even if normal at birth, there is an increased incidence of other diseases, e.g. diabetes mellitus, later in life.

Diagnosis

Laboratory confirmation of rubella is required if there has been contact with a pregnant woman. This is achieved either by detection of rubella

13

13.24 Infections of specific importance in pregnancy

Infection	Consequence	Prevention and management
Rubella	Congenital malformation	Childhood vaccination and vaccination of non-immune mothers post-delivery
Cytomegalovirus	Neonatal infection, congenital malformation	Limited prevention strategies
Zika virus	Congenital malformation	Avoidance of travel, delay in pregnancy if infected
Varicella zoster (VZ) virus	Neonatal infection, congenital malformation, severe infection in mother	VZ immunoglobulin, antiviral prophylaxis (see Box 13.29)
Herpes simplex virus (HSV)	Congenital or neonatal infection	Aciclovir and consideration of caesarean section for mothers who shed HSV from genital tract at time of delivery. Aciclovir for infected neonates
Hepatitis B virus	Chronic infection of neonate	Hepatitis B immunoglobulin and active vaccination of newborn
Hepatitis E virus	Fulminant hepatitis, pre-term delivery, fetal loss	Maintenance of standard food hygiene practices
Human immunodeficiency virus-1 (HIV-1)	Chronic infection of neonate	Antiretroviral drugs for mother and infant and consideration of caesarean section if HIV-1 viral load detectable. Avoidance of breastfeeding
Parvovirus B19	Congenital infection	Avoidance of individuals with acute infection if pregnant
Measles	More severe infection in mother and neonate, fetal loss	Childhood vaccination, human normal immunoglobulin in non-immune pregnant contacts and vaccination post-delivery
Dengue	Neonatal dengue if mother has infection <5 weeks prior to delivery	Vector (mosquito) control
Syphilis	Congenital malformation	Serological testing in pregnancy with prompt treatment of infected mothers
Neisseria gonorrhoeae and *Chlamydia trachomatis*	Neonatal conjunctivitis (ophthalmia neonatorum, see Ch. 15)	Treatment of infection in mother and neonate
Listeriosis	Neonatal meningitis or bacteraemia, bacteraemia or pyrexia of unknown origin in mother	Avoidance of unpasteurised cheeses and other dietary sources
Brucellosis	Possibly increased incidence of fetal loss	Avoidance of unpasteurised dairy products
Group B streptococcal infection	Neonatal meningitis and sepsis. Sepsis in mother after delivery	Risk- or screening-based antimicrobial prophylaxis in labour (recommendations vary between countries)
Toxoplasmosis	Congenital malformation	Diagnosis and prompt treatment of cases, avoidance of under-cooked meat while pregnant
Malaria	Fetal loss, intrauterine growth retardation, severe malaria in mother	Avoidance of insect bites. Intermittent preventative treatment during pregnancy to decrease incidence in high-risk countries

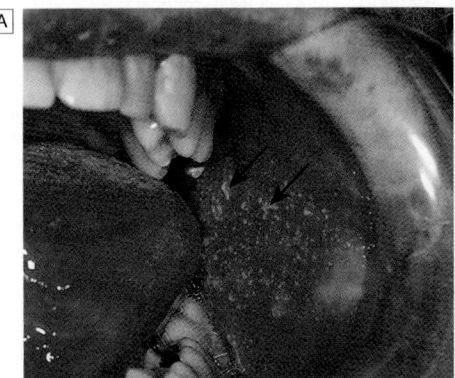
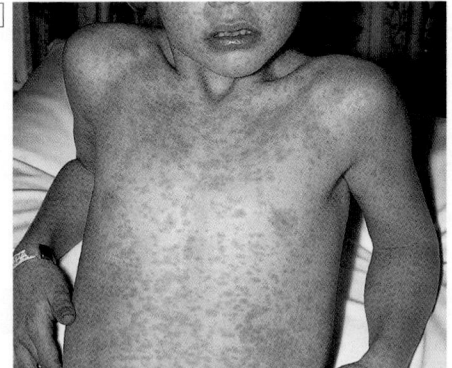

Fig. 13.9 **Measles.** [A] Koplik's spots (arrows) seen on buccal mucosa in the early stages of clinical measles. [B] Typical measles rash.

IgM in serum or by IgG seroconversion. In the exposed pregnant woman, absence of rubella-specific IgG confirms the potential for congenital infection.

Prevention

All children should be immunised with MMR vaccine. Congenital rubella syndrome may be controlled by testing women of child-bearing age for rubella antibodies and offering vaccination if seronegative. Antenatal rubella screening for pregnant mothers in the UK ceased in 2016 because of the rarity of rubella in the target population.

Parvovirus B19

Parvovirus B19 causes exanthem and other clinical syndromes. Some 50% of children and 60%–90% of adults are seropositive. Most infections are spread by the respiratory route, although spread via contaminated blood is also possible. The virus has particular tropism for red cell precursors.

Clinical features

Many infections are subclinical. Clinical manifestations result after an incubation period of 14–21 days (Box 13.26). The classic exanthem

13.25 Rubella infection: risk of congenital malformation

Stage of gestation	Likelihood of malformations
1–2 months	65%–85% chance of illness, multiple defects/spontaneous abortion
3 months	30%–35% chance of illness, usually a single congenital defect (most frequently deafness, cataract, glaucoma, mental retardation or congenital heart disease, especially pulmonary stenosis or patent ductus arteriosus)
4 months	10% risk of congenital defects, most commonly deafness
> 20 weeks	Occasional deafness

13.26 Clinical features of parvovirus B19 infection

Affected age group	Clinical manifestations
Fifth disease (erythema infectiosum) Small children	Three clinical stages: a 'slapped cheek' appearance, followed by a maculopapular rash progressing to a reticulate eruption on the body and limbs, then a final stage of resolution. Often the child is quite well throughout
Gloves and socks syndrome Young adults	Fever and an acral purpuric eruption with a clear margin at the wrists and ankles. Mucosal involvement also occurs
Arthropathies Adults and occasionally children	Symmetrical small-joint polyarthropathy. In children it tends to involve the larger joints in an asymmetrical distribution
Impaired erythropoiesis Adults, those with haematological disease, the immunosuppressed	Mild anaemia; in an individual with an underlying haematological abnormality it can precipitate transient aplastic crisis, or in the immunocompromised a more sustained but often milder pure red cell aplasia
Hydrops fetalis Transplacental fetal infection	Asymptomatic or symptomatic maternal infection that can cause fetal anaemia with an aplastic crisis, leading to non-immune hydrops fetalis and spontaneous abortion

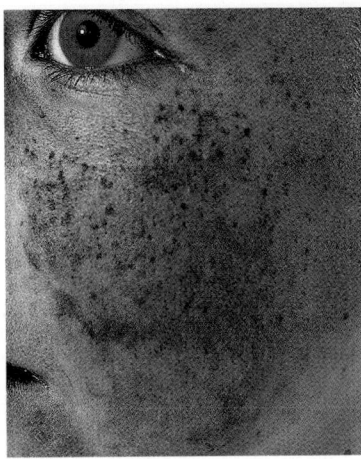

Fig. 13.10 Slapped cheek syndrome. The typical facial rash of parvovirus B19 infection.

Detection of parvovirus B19 DNA in blood is particularly useful in immunocompromised patients. Giant pronormoblasts or haemophagocytosis may be demonstrable in the bone marrow.

Management

Infection is usually self-limiting. Symptomatic relief for arthritic symptoms may be required. Severe anaemia requires transfusion. Persistent viraemia in immunocompromised hosts may require immunoglobulin therapy to clear the virus.

Pregnant women should avoid contact with parvovirus B19 infection; if they are exposed, serology should be performed to establish whether they are immune (IgG-positive).

Passive prophylaxis with immunoglobulin therapy has been suggested for non-immune pregnant women exposed to infection but there are limited data to support this recommendation. Pregnancy should be closely monitored by ultrasound scanning, so that hydrops fetalis can be treated by fetal transfusion.

Human herpesvirus 6 and 7

Human herpesvirus 6 (HHV-6) is a lymphotropic virus that causes a childhood viral exanthem (exanthem subitum), rare cases of an infectious mononucleosis-like syndrome and infection in the immunocompromised host. Infection is almost universal, with approximately 95% of children acquiring this virus by 2 years of age. Transmission is via saliva.

HHV-7 is very closely related to HHV-6 and is believed to be responsible for a proportion of cases of exanthem subitum. Like HHV-6, HHV-7 causes an almost universal infection in childhood, with subsequent latent infection and occasional infection in the immunocompromised host.

Clinical features

Exanthem subitum is also known as roseola infantum or sixth disease (Box 13.27). A high fever is followed by a maculopapular rash as the fever resolves. Fever and/or febrile convulsions may also occur without a rash. Rarely, older children or adults may develop an infectious mononucleosis-like illness, hepatitis or rash. In the immunocompromised, infection is rare but can cause fever, rash, hepatitis, pneumonitis, cytopenia or encephalitis.

Diagnosis and management

Exanthem subitum is usually a clinical diagnosis but can be confirmed by antibody and/or DNA detection. The disease is self-limiting. Treatment with ganciclovir or foscarnet is used in immunocompromised hosts infected with HHV-6.

(erythema infectiosum) is preceded by a prodromal fever and coryzal symptoms. A 'slapped cheek' rash is characteristic (Fig. 13.10) but the rash is very variable, including 'glove and stocking'. In adults, polyarthropathy is common. Infected individuals have a transient block in erythropoiesis for a few days. This is of no clinical consequence except in individuals with increased red cell turnover due to haemoglobinopathy or haemolytic anaemia, who develop an acute anaemia that may be severe (transient aplastic crisis). Erythropoiesis usually recovers spontaneously after 10–14 days. Immunocompromised individuals can develop a more sustained block in erythropoiesis in response to the chronic viraemia that results from their inability to clear the infection. Infection during the first two trimesters of pregnancy can result in intrauterine infection and impact on fetal bone marrow; it causes 10%–15% of non-immune (non-Rhesus-related) hydrops fetalis, a rare complication of pregnancy.

Diagnosis

IgM to parvovirus B19 suggests recent infection but may persist for months and false positives occur. Seroconversion to IgG positivity confirms infection but in isolation a positive IgG is of little diagnostic utility.

13

13.27 Herpesvirus infections

Virus	Infection
Herpes simplex virus (HSV)	
HSV-1	Herpes labialis ('cold sores') Stomatitis, pharyngitis Corneal ulceration Finger infections ('whitlows') Eczema herpeticum Encephalitis
HSV-2	Genital ulceration and neonatal infection (acquired during vaginal delivery) Acute meningitis or transverse myelitis; rarely, encephalitis
Varicella zoster virus (VZV)	Chickenpox (varicella) Shingles (herpes zoster)
Cytomegalovirus (CMV)	Congenital infection Infectious mononucleosis (heterophile antibody-negative) Hepatitis Disease in immunocompromised patients: retinitis, encephalitis, pneumonitis, hepatitis, enteritis Fever with abnormalities in haematological parameters
Epstein–Barr virus (EBV)	Infectious mononucleosis Burkitt and other lymphomas Nasopharyngeal carcinoma Oral hairy leucoplakia (AIDS patients) Other lymphomas, post-transplant lymphoproliferative disorder
Human herpesvirus 6 and 7 (HHV-6, HHV-7)	Exanthem subitem Disease in immunocompromised patients
Human herpesvirus 8 (HHV-8)	Kaposi's sarcoma, primary effusion lymphoma, multicentric Castleman's disease

Chickenpox (varicella)

Varicella zoster virus (VZV) is a dermotropic and neurotropic virus that produces primary infection, usually in childhood, which may reactivate in later life. VZV is spread by aerosol and direct contact. It is highly infectious to non-immune individuals. Disease in children is usually well tolerated. Manifestations are more severe in adults, pregnant women and the immunocompromised.

Clinical features

The incubation period is 11–20 days, after which a vesicular eruption begins (Fig. 13.11), often on mucosal surfaces first, followed by rapid dissemination in a centripetal distribution (most dense on trunk and sparse on limbs). New lesions occur every 2–4 days and each crop is associated with fever. The rash progresses from small pink macules to vesicles and pustules within 24 hours. Infectivity lasts from up to 4 days (but usually 48 hours) before the lesions appear until the last vesicles crust over. Due to intense itching, secondary bacterial infection from scratching is the most common complication of primary chickenpox. Self-limiting cerebellar ataxia and encephalitis are rare complications.

Adults, pregnant women and the immunocompromised are at increased risk of visceral involvement, which presents as pneumonitis, hepatitis or encephalitis. Pneumonitis can be fatal and is more likely to occur in smokers. Maternal infection in early pregnancy carries up to 2% risk of neonatal damage with developmental abnormalities of eyes, CNS and limbs. Chickenpox within 5 days of delivery leads to severe neonatal varicella with visceral involvement and haemorrhage.

Diagnosis

Diagnosis is primarily by recognition of the rash. If necessary, this can be confirmed by detection of antigen (direct immunofluorescence) or DNA in aspirated vesicular fluid. Serology is used to identify seronegative individuals at risk of infection.

Management and prevention

The benefit of antivirals for uncomplicated primary VZV infection in children is marginal, shortening the duration of rash by only 1 day, and is not normally required. Antivirals are, however, used for uncomplicated chickenpox in adults when the patient presents within 24–48 hours of onset of vesicles, in all patients with complications, and in those who are immunocompromised, including pregnant women, regardless of duration of vesicles (Box 13.28). More severe disease, particularly in immunocompromised hosts, requires initial parenteral therapy. Immunocompromised patients may have prolonged viral shedding and may require prolonged treatment until all lesions crust over.

Post-exposure prophylaxis is used to attenuate infection in people who have had significant contact with VZV, are susceptible to infection (i.e. have no history of chickenpox or shingles and are seronegative for VZV IgG) and are at risk of severe disease (e.g. immunocompromised or pregnant) (Box 13.29). Shortages of human VZ immunoglobulin (VZIG) have resulted in greater use of antiviral prophylaxis. Ideally, where indicated, VZIG should be given within 7 days of exposure, but it may attenuate disease even if given up to 10 days afterwards. Susceptible contacts who develop severe chickenpox after receiving VZIG should be treated with antiviral therapy.

A live, attenuated VZV vaccine is available and in routine use in the USA and other countries, but in the UK its use is restricted to non-immune health-care workers and household contacts of immunocompromised individuals. Children receive one dose after 1 year of age and a second dose at 4–6 years of age; seronegative adults receive two doses at least 1 month apart. The vaccine may also be used prior to planned iatrogenic immunosuppression, e.g. before transplant and for people aged over 70 to prevent shingles.

Shingles (herpes zoster)

After initial infection, VZV persists in latent form in the dorsal root ganglion of sensory nerves and can reactivate in later life.

Clinical features

Burning discomfort occurs in the affected dermatome following reactivation and discrete vesicles appear 3–4 days later. Brief viraemia can produce distant satellite 'chickenpox' lesions. Occasionally, paraesthesia occurs without rash ('zoster sine herpete'). Severe disease, a prolonged duration of rash, multiple dermatomal involvement or recurrence suggests underlying immune deficiency. Chickenpox may be contracted from a case of shingles but not vice versa.

Although thoracic dermatomes are most commonly involved (see Fig. 13.11B), the ophthalmic division of the trigeminal nerve is also frequently affected; vesicles may appear on the cornea and lead to ulceration. This condition can lead to blindness and urgent ophthalmology review is required. Geniculate ganglion involvement causes the Ramsay Hunt syndrome of facial palsy, ipsilateral loss of taste and buccal ulceration, plus a rash in the external auditory canal. This may be mistaken for Bell's palsy, which is discussed on page 1140. Bowel and bladder dysfunction occur with sacral nerve root involvement. The virus occasionally causes cranial nerve palsy, myelitis or encephalitis. Granulomatous cerebral angiitis is a cerebrovascular complication that leads to a stroke-like syndrome in association with shingles, especially in an ophthalmic distribution.

In post-herpetic neuralgia, pain from shingles persists for 3 months or longer following healing of the rash. It is more common with advanced age.

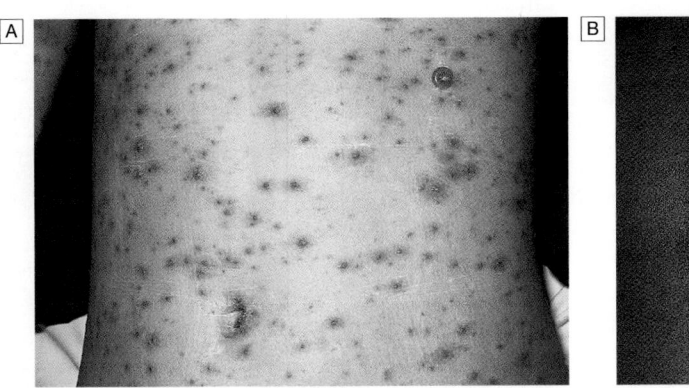 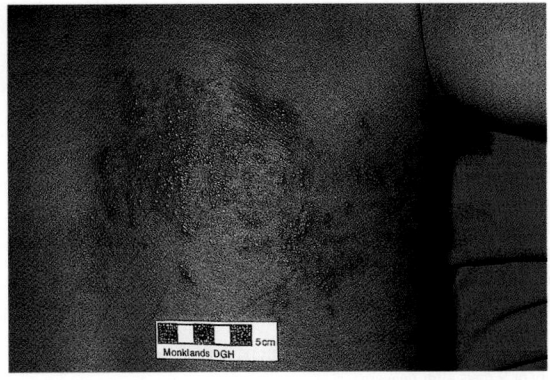

Fig. 13.11 Varicella zoster virus infection. [A] Chickenpox. [B] Shingles in a thoracic dermatome.

	13.28 Therapy for herpes simplex and varicella zoster virus infection
Disease state	**Treatment options**
Primary genital HSV	Famciclovir 250 mg 3 times daily for 7–10 days Valaciclovir 1 g twice daily for 7–10 days Oral aciclovir 200 mg 5 times daily or 400 mg 3 times daily for 7–10 days
Severe and preventing oral intake	Aciclovir 5 mg/kg 3 times daily IV until patient can tolerate oral therapy
Recurrent genital HSV-1 or 2	Oral aciclovir 200 mg 5 times daily or 400 mg 3 times daily for 5 days Famciclovir 125 mg twice daily for 5 days Valaciclovir 500 mg twice daily for 3–5 days or 2 g twice daily for 1 day. Shorter durations increasingly favoured
Primary or recurrent oral HSV	Usually no treatment If required, usually short duration, e.g. valaciclovir 2 g twice daily for 1 day
Mucocutaneous HSV infection in immunocompromised host	Aciclovir 5 mg/kg 3 times daily IV for 7–10 days Oral aciclovir 400 mg 4 times daily for 7–10 days Famciclovir 500 mg 3 times daily for 7–10 days Valaciclovir 1 g twice daily for 7–10 days
Chickenpox in adult or child	Oral aciclovir 800 mg 5 times daily for 5 days Famciclovir 500 mg 3 times daily for 5 days Valaciclovir 1 g 3 times daily for 5 days
Immunocompromised host/pregnant woman	Aciclovir 5 mg/kg 3 times daily IV until patient is improving, then complete therapy with oral therapy until all lesions are crusting over
Shingles	Treatment and doses as for chickenpox but duration typically 7–10 days
Visceral involvement (non-CNS) in HSV	Aciclovir IV 5 mg/kg 3 times daily for 14 days
Visceral involvement (non-CNS) in VZV	Aciclovir IV 5 mg/kg 3 times daily for 7 days
Severe complications (encephalitis, disseminated infection)	Aciclovir IV 10 mg/kg 3 times daily (up to 20 mg/kg in neonates) for 14–21 days
HSV disease suppression	Aciclovir 400 mg twice daily Famciclovir 250 mg twice daily Valaciclovir 500 mg daily
(CNS = central nervous system; HSV = herpes simplex virus; IV = intravenous; VZV = varicella zoster virus)	

13

Management

Early therapy with aciclovir or related antivirals has been shown to reduce both early- and late-onset pain, especially in patients over 65 years. Post-herpetic neuralgia requires aggressive analgesia, along with agents such as amitriptyline 25–100 mg daily, gabapentin (commencing at 300 mg daily and building slowly to 300 mg twice daily or more) or pregabalin (commencing at 75 mg twice daily and building up to 100 mg or 200 mg 3 times daily if tolerated). Capsaicin cream (0.075%) may be helpful. Glucocorticoids have not been demonstrated to reduce post-herpetic neuralgia.

The zoster vaccine is a live attenuated vaccine with a higher dose of VZV than the chickenpox vaccine. It reduces the incidence of shingles and of post-herpetic neuralgia. It is recommended in the UK for people aged over 70 years. A recombinant vaccine is available in the USA.

Enteroviral exanthems

Coxsackievirus or echovirus infections can lead to a maculopapular eruption or roseola-like rash that occurs after fever falls. Enteroviral infections are discussed further under viral infections of the skin (see below).

Systemic viral infections without exanthem

Other systemic viral infections present with features other than a rash suggestive of exanthem. Rashes may occur in these conditions but differ from those seen in exanthems or are not the primary presenting feature.

13.29 Indications for varicella zoster post-exposure prophylaxis (UK guidance)

An adult should satisfy all three of the following conditions:

1. Significant contact

Contact with chickenpox (any time from 48 hrs before the rash until crusting of lesions) or zoster (exposed, disseminated or, with immunocompromised contacts, localised zoster; between development of the rash until crusting) defined as:

- Prolonged household contact, sharing a room for ≥15 mins or face-to-face contact (includes direct contact with zoster lesions)
- Hospital contact with chickenpox in another patient, health-care worker or visitor
- Intimate contact (e.g. touching) with person with shingles lesions
- Newborn whose mother develops chickenpox no more than 5 days before delivery or 2 days after delivery

2. Susceptible contact

- Individual with no history of chickenpox, ideally confirmed by negative test for VZV IgG

3. Predisposition to severe chickenpox

- Immunocompromised due to disease (e.g. acute leukaemia, human immunodeficiency virus, other primary or secondary immunodeficiency)
- Medically immunosuppressed (e.g. following solid organ transplant; current or recent (<6 months) cytotoxic chemotherapy or radiotherapy; current or recent (<3 months) high-dose glucocorticoids; haematopoietic stem cell transplant)
- Pregnant (any stage)
- Infants: newborn whose mother has had chickenpox as above; premature infants <28 weeks

Choice of prophylaxis*

- Immunocompromised adults: acyclovir 800 mg four times a day orally or valaciclovir 1 g three times daily orally, started 7 days after exposure or 7 days after first day of rash in person exposed to. Consider varicella zoster immune globulin (VZIG) only if renal impairment or malabsorption.
- Pregnant women (first 20 weeks): VZIG 1 g by slow intramuscular injection
- Pregnant women (after 20 weeks): VZIG (same dose as first 20 weeks) or aciclovir. Valaciclovir as alternative, all antiviral doses as above.
- Neonate VZIG, dose adjusted

*Based on revised UK 2019 Public Health England Guidelines. https://assets.publishing. service.gov.uk/government/uploads/system/uploads/attachment_data/file/811544/VZIG_ issuing_guidance.pdf.

Mumps

Mumps is a systemic viral infection characterised by swelling of the parotid glands. Infection is endemic worldwide and peaks at 5–9 years of age. Vaccination has reduced the incidence in children but incomplete coverage and waning immunity with time have led to outbreaks in young adults. Infection is spread by respiratory droplets.

Clinical features

The median incubation period is 19 days, with a range of 15–24 days. Classical tender parotid enlargement, which is bilateral in 75%, follows a prodrome of pyrexia and headache (Fig. 13.12). Meningitis complicates up to 10% of cases. The cerebrospinal fluid (CSF) reveals a lymphocytic pleocytosis or, less commonly, neutrophils. Rare complications include encephalitis, transient hearing loss, labyrinthitis, electrocardiographic abnormalities, pancreatitis and arthritis.

Approximately 25% of post-pubertal males with mumps develop epididymo-orchitis but, although testicular atrophy occurs, sterility is unlikely. Oophoritis is less common. Abortion may occur if infection takes place in the first trimester of pregnancy. Complications may occur in the absence of parotitis.

Diagnosis

The diagnosis is usually clinical. In atypical presentations without parotitis, serology for mumps-specific IgM or IgG seroconversion (fourfold rise in IgG convalescent titre) confirms the diagnosis. Virus can also be cultured from urine in the first week of infection or detected by PCR in urine, saliva or CSF.

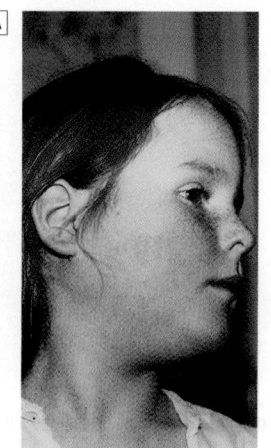
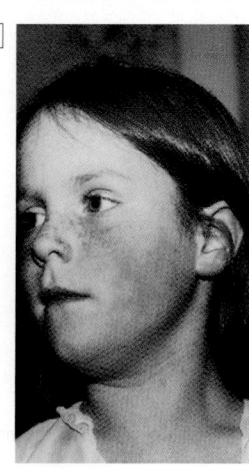

Fig. 13.12 Typical unilateral mumps. [A] Note the loss of angle of the jaw on the affected (right) side. [B] Comparison showing normal (left) side.

Management and prevention

Treatment is with analgesia. There is no evidence that glucocorticoids are of value for orchitis. Mumps vaccine is one of the components of the combined MMR vaccine.

Influenza

Influenza is an acute systemic viral infection that primarily affects the respiratory tract and carries a significant mortality. It is caused by influenza A virus or, in milder form, influenza B virus. Infection is seasonal, and variation in the haemagglutinin (H) and neuraminidase (N) glycoproteins on the surface of the virus leads to disease of variable intensity each year. Minor changes in haemagglutinin are known as 'genetic drift', whereas a switch in the haemagglutinin or neuraminidase antigen is termed 'genetic shift'. Nomenclature of influenza strains is based on these glycoproteins, e.g. H1N1, H3N2 etc. Genetic shift results in the circulation of a new influenza strain within a community to which few people are immune, potentially initiating an influenza epidemic or pandemic in which there is a high attack rate and there may be increased disease severity. Re-assortment of swine, avian and human influenza strains can occur in pigs and lead to outbreaks of swine 'flu' in humans, as occurred in 2009, with the outbreak of H1N1pdm2009 influenza.

Clinical features

After an incubation period of 1–3 days, uncomplicated disease leads to fever, malaise and cough. Viral pneumonia may occur, although pulmonary complications are most often due to superinfection with *Strep. pneumoniae*, *Staph. aureus* or other bacteria. Rare extrapulmonary manifestations include myositis, myocarditis, pericarditis and neurological complications (Reye syndrome in children, encephalitis or transverse myelitis). Mortality is greatest in older people, those with medical comorbidities and pregnant women. Polymorphisms in the gene encoding an antiviral protein, interferon-induced transmembrane protein 3 (IFITM3), are associated with more severe influenza.

Diagnosis

Acute infection is diagnosed by viral antigen or RNA detection in a nasopharyngeal sample. The disease may also be diagnosed retrospectively by serology.

Management and prevention

Management involves early microbiological identification of cases and good infection control, with an emphasis on hand hygiene and preventing dissemination of infection by coughing and sneezing. Administration of a neuraminidase inhibitor, e.g. oral oseltamivir, inhaled zanamivir, intravenous peramivir or the oral cap-dependent endonuclease inhibitor baloxavir, can reduce the severity of symptoms if started within 48 hours of symptom onset (or possibly later in immunocompromised individuals). Antiviral drugs can also be used as prophylaxis in high-risk individuals during the 'flu' season. Resistance can emerge to neuraminidase inhibitors and so updated local advice should be followed with regard to the sensitivity to antivirals of the circulating strain.

Prevention relies on seasonal vaccination of older age groups, children 2–7 years of age and individuals with chronic medical illnesses that place them at increased risk of the complications of influenza, such as chronic cardiopulmonary diseases or immune compromise, as well as their health-care workers. The vaccine composition changes each year to cover the 'predicted' seasonal strains but vaccination may fail when a new pandemic strain emerges.

Avian influenza

Avian influenza is caused by transmission of avian influenza A viruses to humans. Avian viruses, such as H5N1, possess alternative haemagglutinin antigens to seasonal influenza strains. Most cases have had contact with sick poultry, predominantly in South-east Asia, and person-to-person spread has been limited to date. Infections with H5N1 viruses have been severe, with enteric features and respiratory failure. Treatment depends on the resistance pattern but often involves oseltamivir. Vaccination against seasonal 'flu' does not adequately protect against avian influenza. There is a concern that adaptation of an avian strain to allow effective person-to-person transmission is likely to lead to a global pandemic of life-threatening influenza.

Infectious mononucleosis and Epstein–Barr virus

Infectious mononucleosis (IM) is a clinical syndrome characterised by pharyngitis, cervical lymphadenopathy, fever and lymphocytosis (known colloquially as glandular fever). It is most often caused by Epstein–Barr virus (EBV) but other infections can produce a similar clinical syndrome (Box 13.30).

EBV is a gamma herpesvirus. In lower- or middle-income countries (LMIC), subclinical infection in childhood is virtually universal. In high income countries, primary infection may be delayed until adolescence or early adult life. Under these circumstances, about 50% of infections result in typical IM. The virus is usually acquired from asymptomatic excreters via saliva, either by droplet infection or environmental contamination in childhood, or by kissing among adolescents and adults. EBV is not highly contagious and isolation of cases is unnecessary.

Clinical features

EBV infection has a prolonged but undetermined incubation period, followed in some cases by a prodrome of fever, headache and malaise. This is followed by IM with severe pharyngitis, which may include tonsillar exudates and non-tender anterior and posterior cervical lymphadenopathy. Palatal petechiae, periorbital oedema, splenomegaly, inguinal or axillary lymphadenopathy and macular, petechial or erythema multiforme rashes may occur. In most cases, fever resolves over 2 weeks, and fatigue and other abnormalities settle over a further few weeks. Complications are listed in Box 13.31. Death is rare but can occur due to respiratory obstruction, haemorrhage from splenic rupture, thrombocytopenia or encephalitis.

The diagnosis of EBV infection outside the usual age in adolescence and young adulthood is more challenging. In children under 10 years the illness is mild and short-lived, but in adults over 30 years of age it can be severe and prolonged. In both groups, pharyngeal symptoms are often absent. EBV may present with jaundice, as a PUO or with a complication.

Long-term complications of EBV infection

Lymphoma complicates EBV infection in immunocompromised hosts (e.g. post-transplant lymphoproliferative disorder), and some forms of Hodgkin lymphoma are EBV-associated. The endemic form of Burkitt lymphoma complicates EBV infection in areas of sub-Saharan Africa

---

i 13.30 Causes of infectious mononucleosis syndrome

- Epstein–Barr virus infection
- Cytomegalovirus
- HHV-6 or 7
- HIV-1 primary infection
- Toxoplasmosis

(HHV = human herpes virus; HIV = human immunodeficiency virus)

---

i 13.31 Complications of Epstein–Barr virus infection

Common

- Severe pharyngeal oedema
- Antibiotic-induced rash (80%–90% with ampicillin)
- Hepatitis (80%)
- Prolonged post-viral fatigue (10%)
- Jaundice (<10%)

Uncommon

Neurological
- Cranial nerve palsies
- Polyneuritis
- Transverse myelitis
- Meningoencephalitis

Haematological
- Haemolytic anaemia
- Thrombocytopenia

Renal
- Abnormalities on urinalysis
- Interstitial nephritis

Cardiac
- Myocarditis
- ECG abnormalities
- Pericarditis

Rare

- Ruptured spleen
- Respiratory obstruction
- Agranulocytosis
- X-linked lymphoproliferative syndrome

EBV-associated malignancy

- Nasopharyngeal carcinoma
- Burkitt lymphoma
- Hodgkin lymphoma (certain subtypes only)
- Primary CNS lymphoma
- Lymphoproliferative disease in immunocompromised

---

where *falciparum* malaria is endemic. Nasopharyngeal carcinoma is a geographically restricted tumour seen in China and Alaska that is associated with EBV infection. X-linked lymphoproliferative (Duncan) syndrome is a familial lymphoproliferative disorder that follows primary EBV infection in boys without any other history of immunodeficiency; it is due to mutation of the *SAP* gene, causing failure of T-cell and NK-cell activation and inability to contain EBV infection.

Investigations

Atypical lymphocytes are common in EBV infection but also occur in other causes of IM, acute retroviral syndrome with HIV infection, viral hepatitis, mumps and rubella (Fig. 13.13A). They are also a feature of dengue, malaria and other geographically restricted infections (see Box 13.18). A 'heterophile' antibody is present during the acute illness and convalescence, which is detected by the Paul–Bunnell or 'Monospot' test. A heterophile antibody is an antibody that has affinity for antigens other than the specific one, in this case animal immunoglobulins; the Paul–Bunnell and Monospot tests exploit this feature by detecting the ability of test serum to agglutinate sheep and horse red blood cells, respectively. Sometimes antibody production is delayed, so an initially negative test should be repeated. However, many children and 10% of adolescents with IM do not produce heterophile antibody at any stage.

Specific EBV serology confirms the diagnosis. Acute infection is characterised by IgM antibodies against the viral capsid, antibodies to EBV early antigen and the initial absence of antibodies to EBV nuclear antigen (anti-EBNA). Seroconversion of anti-EBNA at approximately 1 month after the initial illness may confirm the diagnosis in retrospect. CNS infections may be diagnosed by detection of viral DNA in CSF.

13

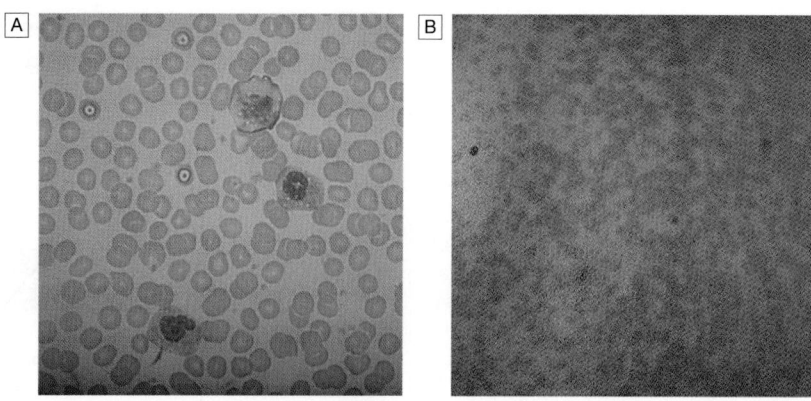

Fig. 13.13 Features of infectious mononucleosis. A Atypical lymphocytes in peripheral blood. B Skin reaction to ampicillin.

Management

Treatment is symptomatic. If a throat culture yields a β-haemolytic streptococcus, penicillin should be given. Administration of ampicillin or amoxicillin in this condition commonly causes an itchy macular rash and should be avoided (Fig. 13.13B). When pharyngeal oedema is severe, a short course of glucocorticoids, e.g. prednisolone 30 mg daily for 5 days, may help. Current antiviral drugs are not active against EBV.

Return to work or school is governed by physical fitness rather than laboratory tests; contact sports should be avoided until splenomegaly has resolved because of the danger of splenic rupture. Unfortunately, about 10% of patients with IM suffer a chronic relapsing syndrome.

Cytomegalovirus

Cytomegalovirus (CMV), like EBV, circulates readily among children. A second period of virus acquisition occurs among adolescents and young adults, peaking between the ages of 25 and 35 years, rather later than with EBV infection. CMV infection is persistent, and is characterised by subclinical cycles of active virus replication and by persistent low-level virus shedding. Most post-childhood infections are therefore acquired from asymptomatic excreters who shed virus in saliva, urine, semen and genital secretions. Sexual transmission and oral spread are common among adults but infection may also be acquired through caring for children with asymptomatic infections.

Clinical features

Most post-childhood CMV infections are subclinical, although some young adults develop an IM-like syndrome and some have a prolonged influenza-like illness lasting 2 weeks or more. Physical signs resemble IM but in CMV infections hepatomegaly is more common, while lymphadenopathy, splenomegaly, pharyngitis and tonsillitis occur less often. Jaundice is uncommon and usually mild. Complications include meningoencephalitis, Guillain–Barré syndrome, autoimmune haemolytic anaemia, thrombocytopenia, myocarditis and skin eruptions, such as ampicillin-induced rash. Immunocompromised patients can develop hepatitis, oesophagitis, colitis, pneumonitis, retinitis, encephalitis and polyradiculitis.

Women who develop a primary CMV infection during pregnancy have about a 40% chance of passing CMV to the fetus, causing congenital infection and disease at any stage of gestation. Features include petechial rashes, hepatosplenomegaly and jaundice; 10% of infected infants will have long-term CNS sequelae, such as microcephaly, cerebral calcifications, chorioretinitis and deafness. Infections in the newborn usually are asymptomatic or have features of an IM-like illness, although subtle sequelae affecting hearing or mental development may occur.

Investigations

Atypical lymphocytosis is not as prominent as in EBV infection and heterophile antibody tests are usually negative. LFTs are often abnormal, with an alkaline phosphatase level raised out of proportion to transaminases. Serological diagnosis depends on the detection of CMV-specific IgM antibody plus a fourfold rise or seroconversion of IgG. In the immuno-compromised, antibody detection is unreliable and detection of CMV in an involved organ by PCR, antigen detection, culture or histopathology establishes the diagnosis. Detection of CMV in the blood may be useful in transplant populations but not in HIV-positive individuals, since in HIV infection CMV reactivates at regular intervals, but these episodes do not correlate well with episodes of clinical disease. Detection of CMV in urine is not helpful in diagnosing infection, except in neonates, since CMV is intermittently shed in the urine throughout life following infection.

Management

Only symptomatic treatment is required in the immunocompetent patient. Immunocompromised individuals are treated with intravenous ganciclovir 5 mg/kg twice daily or with oral valganciclovir 900 mg twice daily for at least 14 days. Foscarnet or cidofovir is also used in CMV treatment of immunocompromised patients who are resistant to or intolerant of ganciclovir-based therapy. They can be given intravitreally if required. Maribavir is an investigational agent also being studied for resistant strains of CMV. Letermovir is a newer antiviral used in the prevention of CMV in high-risk transplant patients, e.g. some haematopoietic stem cell transplant recipients.

Dengue

Dengue is a febrile illness caused by a flavivirus transmitted by mosquitoes. It is endemic in Asia, the Pacific, Africa and the Americas (Fig. 13.14). Approximately 400 million infections and 100 million clinically apparent infections occur annually, and dengue is the most rapidly spreading mosquito-borne viral illness. The principal vector is the mosquito *Aedes aegypti*, which breeds in standing water; collections of water in containers, water-based air coolers and tyre dumps are a good environment for the vector in large cities. *Aedes albopictus* is a vector in some South-east Asian countries. There are four serotypes of dengue virus, all producing a similar clinical syndrome; type-specific immunity is life-long but immunity against the other serotypes lasts only a few months. Dengue haemorrhagic fever (DHF) and dengue shock syndrome (DSS) occur in individuals immune to one dengue virus serotype who are subsequently infected with a different serotype. Prior immunity results in increased uptake of virus by cells expressing the antibody Fc receptor and increased T-cell activation with resultant cytokine release, causing capillary leak and disseminated intravascular coagulation (DIC; Ch. 25). Previously, dengue was seen in small children and DHF/DSS in children 2–15 years old, but these conditions are now being seen in children less than 2 years old, and most frequently in those 16–45 years of age or older, in whom severe organ dysfunction is more common. Other epidemiological changes include the spread of dengue into rural communities and greater case fatality in women.

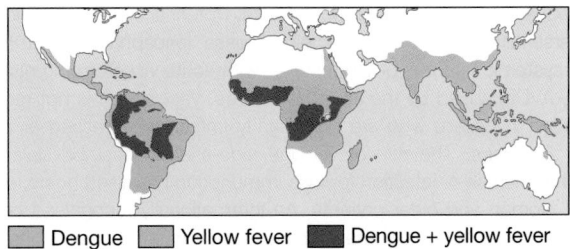

Dengue   Yellow fever   Dengue + yellow fever

Fig. 13.14 Endemic zones of yellow fever and dengue.

13.32 Clinical features of dengue fever

Incubation period
- 2–7 days

Prodrome
- 2 days of malaise and headache

Acute onset
- Fever, backache, arthralgias, headache, generalised pains ('break-bone fever'), pain on eye movement, lacrimation, scleral injection, anorexia, nausea, vomiting, pharyngitis, upper respiratory tract symptoms, relative bradycardia, prostration, depression, hyperaesthesia, dysgeusia, lymphadenopathy

Fever
- Continuous or 'saddle-back', with break on 4th or 5th day and then recrudescence; usually lasts 7–8 days

Rash
- Initial flushing faint macular rash in first 1–2 days. Maculopapular, scarlet morbilliform blanching rash from days 3–5 on trunk, spreading centrifugally and sparing palms and soles; onset often with fever defervescence. May desquamate on resolution or give rise to petechiae on extensor surfaces

Convalescence
- Slow and may be associated with prolonged fatigue syndrome, arthralgia or depression

Complications
- Dengue haemorrhagic fever and disseminated intravascular coagulation
- Dengue shock syndrome
- Severe organ involvement
- Vertical transmission if infection within 5 weeks of delivery

13.33 Differential diagnosis of thrombocytopenia with fever in dengue endemic areas

Common	Less frequent
• Malaria	• Rickettsial infection
• Sepsis	• Leptospirosis
• Typhoid	• Other viruses, e.g. chikungunya, viral haemorrhagic fevers, yellow fever

13.34 WHO case definitions of dengue, 2015

Probable dengue fever
- Exposure in an endemic area
- Fever
- Two of:
  Nausea/vomiting
  Rash
  Aches/pains
  Positive tourniquet test
  Leucopenia
  Any warning sign

Laboratory confirmation important
Needs regular medical observation and instruction in observing for the 'warning signs'
If there are no 'warning signs', need for hospitalisation is influenced by age, comorbidities, pregnancy and social factors

Dengue with warning signs
- Probable dengue plus one of:
  Abdominal pain or tenderness
  Persistent vomiting
  Signs of fluid accumulation, e.g. pleural effusion or ascites
  Mucosal bleed
  Hepatomegaly >2 cm
  Rapid increase in haematocrit with fall in platelet count

Needs medical intervention, e.g. intravenous fluid

Severe dengue
- Severe plasma leakage leading to:
  Shock (dengue shock syndrome)
  Fluid accumulation with respiratory distress
- Severe haemorrhagic manifestations, e.g. gastrointestinal haemorrhage
- Severe organ involvement (atypical features):
  Liver AST or ALT ≥1000 U/L
  CNS: impaired consciousness, meningoencephalitis, seizures
  Cardiomyopathy, conduction defects, arrhythmias
  Other organs, e.g. acute kidney injury, pancreatitis, acute lung injury, disseminated intravascular coagulopathy, rhabdomyolysis

Needs emergency medical treatment and specialist care with intensive care input

(ALT = alanine aminotransferase; AST = aspartate aminotransferase; CNS = central nervous system; WHO = World Health Organization)
Adapted from https://wwwn.cdc.gov/nndss/conditions/dengue-virus-infections/case-definition/2015/.

Clinical features

Many cases of dengue infection are asymptomatic in children. Clinical disease presents with undifferentiated fever termed 'dengue-like illness'. When dengue infection occurs with characteristic symptoms or signs it is termed 'dengue' (Box 13.32). A rash frequently follows the initial febrile phase as the fever settles. Laboratory features include leucopenia, neutropenia, thrombocytopenia and elevated alanine aminotransferase (ALT) or aspartate aminotransferase (AST). The differential diagnosis of thrombocytopenia with fever in dengue endemic areas is shown in Box 13.33. Many symptomatic infections run an uncomplicated course but complications or a protracted convalescence may ensue. Warning signs justify intense medical management and monitoring for progression to severe dengue. Atypical clinical features of dengue are increasingly common, especially in infants or older patients, and in rural locations (Box 13.34). These, along with DHF or DSS, are recognised as features of severe dengue in the 2015 case definition and contribute to mortality, mandating urgent medical management.

The period 3–7 days after onset of fever is termed the 'critical' phase, during which signs of DHF or DSS may develop. In mild forms, petechiae occur in the arm when a blood pressure cuff is inflated to a point between systolic and diastolic blood pressure and left for 5 minutes (the positive 'tourniquet test') – a non-specific test of capillary fragility and thrombocytopenia. As the extent of capillary leak increases, DSS develops, with a raised haematocrit, tachycardia and hypotension, pleural effusions and ascites. This may progress to metabolic acidosis and multi-organ failure, including acute respiratory distress syndrome (ARDS). Minor (petechiae, ecchymoses, epistaxis) or major (gastrointestinal or vaginal) haemorrhage, a feature of DHF, may occur. Cerebrovascular bleeding may be a complication of severe dengue.

Diagnosis

In endemic areas, mild dengue must be distinguished from other viral infections. The diagnosis can be confirmed by seroconversion of IgM or a fourfold rise in IgG antibody titres. Serological tests may detect cross-reacting antibodies from infection or vaccination against other flaviviruses, including yellow fever virus, Japanese encephalitis virus and West Nile virus. Isolation of dengue virus or detection of dengue virus RNA by PCR in blood or CSF is available in specialist laboratories. Commercial enzyme-linked immunosorbent assay (ELISA) kits to detect the NS1 viral antigen, although less sensitive than PCR, are available in many endemic areas.

Management and prevention

Treatment is supportive, emphasising fluid replacement and appropriate management of shock and organ dysfunction, which is a major determinant of morbidity and mortality. With intensive care support, mortality rates are 1% or less. Aspirin should be avoided due to bleeding risk. Glucocorticoids have not been shown to help. No existing antivirals are effective.

Breeding places of *Aedes* mosquitoes should be eliminated and the adults destroyed by insecticides. A live attenuated tetravalent chimeric vaccine was licensed in 2019 for children. It is recommended only for children who have already had a first infection and live in a dengue endemic area. Other vaccines are also in development.

Yellow fever

Yellow fever is a haemorrhagic fever of the tropics, caused by a flavivirus. It is a zoonosis of monkeys in West and Central African, and South and Central American tropical rainforests, and may cause epidemics (see Fig. 13.14). Transmission is by tree-top mosquitoes, *Aedes africanus* (Africa) and *Haemagogus* spp. (America). The infection is introduced to humans either by infected mosquitoes when trees are felled, or by monkeys raiding human settlements. In towns, yellow fever may be transmitted between humans by *Aedes aegypti*, which breeds efficiently in small collections of water. The distribution of this mosquito is far wider than that of yellow fever, threatening geographical spread.

Yellow fever causes up to 170000 infections each year, mainly in sub-Saharan Africa. Mortality varies but is approximately 15%. Humans are infectious during the viraemic phase, which starts 3–6 days after the bite of the infected mosquito and lasts for 4–5 days.

Clinical features

After an incubation period of 3–6 days, yellow fever is often a mild febrile illness lasting less than 1 week, with headache, myalgia, conjunctival erythema and bradycardia. This is followed by fever resolution (defervescence) but, in some cases, fever recurs after a few hours to days. In more severe disease, fever recrudescence is associated with lower back pain, abdominal pain and somnolence, prominent nausea and vomiting, bradycardia and jaundice. Liver damage and DIC lead to bleeding with petechiae, mucosal haemorrhages and gastrointestinal bleeding. Shock, hepatic failure, renal failure, seizures and coma may ensue.

Diagnosis

The differential diagnosis includes malaria, typhoid, viral hepatitis, leptospirosis, haemorrhagic fevers and aflatoxin poisoning. Diagnosis of yellow fever can be confirmed by detection of virus in the blood in the first 3–4 days of illness by culture or reverse transcription polymerase chain reaction (RT-PCR), by the presence of IgM or by a fourfold rise in IgG antibody titre. Leucopenia is characteristic. Liver biopsy should be avoided due to the risk of fatal bleeding. Postmortem features, such as acute mid-zonal necrosis and Councilman bodies with minimal inflammation in the liver, are suggestive but not specific. Immunohistochemistry for viral antigens improves specificity.

Management and prevention

Treatment is supportive, with meticulous attention to fluid and electrolyte balance, urine output and blood pressure. Blood transfusions, plasma expanders and peritoneal dialysis may be necessary. Patients should be isolated, as their blood and body products may contain virus particles.

A single vaccination with a live attenuated vaccine gives full protection and travellers do not require a booster unless specified by individual countries' travel requirements. Potential side-effects include hypersensitivity, acute neurotropic disease (encephalitis) (YEL-NVD) and systemic features of yellow fever with acute viscerotropic disease (YEL-AVD) caused by the attenuated virus. Vaccination is not recommended in people who are significantly immunosuppressed or aged over 60 years. The risk of vaccine side-effects must be balanced against the risk of infection for less immunocompromised hosts, pregnant women and older patients. An internationally recognised certificate of vaccination is sometimes necessary when crossing borders. The Eliminate Yellow Fever Epidemics strategy was launched in 2017 and aims to protect a billion people living in at-risk countries in Africa and the Americas by 2026.

Viral haemorrhagic fevers

Viral haemorrhagic fevers (VHFs) are zoonoses caused by several different viruses (Box 13.35). They are geographically restricted and previously occurred in rural settings or in health-care facilities. The largest outbreak of VHF to date started in 2014, with Ebola circulating in Guinea, Liberia and Sierra Leone. The outbreak resulted in more than 28000 cases by 2016. Since 2018–19 there has been an ongoing Ebola outbreak in the eastern part of the Democratic Republic of Congo (DRC).

Serological surveys have shown that Lassa fever is widespread in West Africa and may lead to up to 500000 infections annually. Mortality overall may be low, as 80% of cases are asymptomatic, but in hospitalised cases mortality averages 15%. Marburg has been documented less frequently, with outbreaks in the DRC and Uganda, but the largest outbreak to date involved 163 cases in Angola in 2005. Mortality rates of Ebola and Marburg vary but are high.

VHFs have extended into Europe, with an outbreak of Congo–Crimean haemorrhagic fever (CCHF) in Turkey in 2006, and cases of haemorrhagic fever with renal syndrome in the Balkans and Russia. An outbreak of CCHF in 2011 in Gujarat, India, involved several health-care workers and emphasised the importance of maintaining a high index of suspicion for VHF and implementing appropriate infection control measures at the first opportunity. Kyasanur forest disease is a tick-borne VHF currently confined to a small focus in Karnataka, India; there are about 500 cases annually. Monkeys are the principal hosts but, with forest felling, there are fears that this disease will increase. Severe fever with thrombocytopenia syndrome (SFTS) is a tick-borne VHF that has emerged in rural China, South Korea and Japan since 2009.

New outbreaks and new agents are identified sporadically. Details on recent disease outbreaks can be found at the WHO website (see 'Further information').

Clinical features

VHFs present with non-specific fever, malaise, body pains, sore throat and headache. On examination, conjunctivitis, throat injection, an erythematous or petechial rash, haemorrhage, lymphadenopathy and bradycardia may be noted. Endothelial dysfunction causes capillary leak. Bleeding is due to endothelial damage and platelet dysfunction. Hypovolaemic shock and ARDS may develop

Haemorrhage is a late feature of most VHFs and many patients present with earlier features. In Lassa fever, joint and abdominal pain is prominent. A macular blanching rash may be present but bleeding is unusual, occurring in only 20% of hospitalised patients. Encephalopathy may develop and deafness affects 30% of survivors. In CCHF, bleeding, manifest by haematemesis or bleeding per rectum, may be an early feature, accompanied by derangement of LFTs.

The clue to the viral aetiology comes from the travel and exposure history. Travel to an outbreak area, activity in a rural environment and contact with sick individuals or animals within 21 days all increase the risk of VHF. Enquiry should be made about insect bites, hospital visits and attendance at ritual funerals (Ebola virus infection). For Lassa fever, retrosternal pain, pharyngitis and proteinuria have a positive predictive value of 80% in West Africa.

i	13.35 Viral haemorrhagic fevers

Disease	Reservoir	Transmission	Incubation period	Geography	Mortality rate	Clinical features of severe disease[1]
Lassa fever	Multimammate rats (*Mastomys natalensis*)	Urine from rat Body fluids from patients	6–21 days	West Africa	15%	Haemorrhage, shock, encephalopathy, ARDS (responds to ribavirin), deafness in survivors
Ebola fever	Fruit bats (Pteropodidae family) and bush meat	Body fluids from patients Handling infected primates	2–21 days	Central Africa Outbreaks as far north as Sudan	25%–90%	Haemorrhage and/or diarrhoea, hepatic failure and acute kidney injury
Marburg fever	Undefined	Body fluids from patients Handling infected primates	3–9 days	Central Africa Outbreak in Angola	25%–90%	Haemorrhage, diarrhoea, encephalopathy, orchitis
Yellow fever	Monkeys	Mosquitoes	3–6 days	See Fig. 13.14	~15%	Hepatic failure, acute kidney injury, haemorrhage
Dengue	Humans	*Aedes aegypti*	2–7 days	See Fig. 13.14	<10%[2]	Haemorrhage, shock
Crimean–Congo haemorrhagic fever	Small vertebrates	*Ixodes* tick	1–3 days up to 9 days	Africa, Asia, Eastern Europe	30%	Encephalopathy, early haemorrhage, hepatic failure, acute kidney injury, ARDS
	Domestic and wild animals	Body fluids	3–6 days up to 13 days			
Rift Valley fever	Domestic livestock	Contact with animals, mosquito or other insect bites	2–6 days	Africa, Arabian peninsula	1%	Haemorrhage, blindness, meningoencephalitis (complications only in a minority)
Kyasanur fever	Monkeys	Ticks	3–8 days	Karnataka State, India	5%–10%	Haemorrhage, pulmonary oedema, neurological features, iridokeratitis in survivors
Bolivian and Argentinian haemorrhagic fever (Junin and Machupo viruses)	Rodents (*Calomys* spp.)	Urine, aerosols Body fluids from case (rare)	5–19 days (3–6 days for parenteral)	South America	15%–30%	Haemorrhage, shock, cerebellar signs (may respond to ribavirin)
Haemorrhagic fever with renal syndrome (Hantaan fever)	Rodents	Aerosols from faeces	5–42 days (typically 14 days)	Northern Asia, northern Europe, Balkans	5%	Acute kidney injury, cerebrovascular accidents, pulmonary oedema, shock (hepatic failure and haemorrhagic features only in some variants)
Severe fever with thrombocytopenia syndrome (SFTS)	Domestic and wild animals	*Ixodes* ticks	5–14 days, average 9 days	China, South Korea, Japan	7%	Organ failure (liver, heart, kidney, lungs), haemorrhage and disseminated intravascular coagulopathy, neuropsychiatric, prominent thrombocytopenia

[1]All potentially have circulatory failure. [2]Mortality of uncomplicated and haemorrhagic dengue fever, respectively.
(ARDS = acute respiratory distress syndrome)

13

Investigations and management

Non-specific findings include leucopenia, thrombocytopenia and proteinuria. In Lassa fever, an AST of >150U/L is associated with a 50% mortality. It is important to exclude other causes of fever, especially malaria, typhoid and respiratory tract infections. In the UK, most patients suspected of having a VHF turn out to have malaria.

A febrile patient from an endemic area within the 21-day incubation period, who has specific epidemiological risk factors (see Fig. 13.7) or signs of organ failure or haemorrhage, should be treated as being at high risk of VHF; appropriate infection control measures must be implemented and the patient transferred to a centre with biosafety level (BSL) 4 facilities if they test positive. Individuals with a history of travel within 21 days and fever, but without the relevant high-risk epidemiological

features or signs of VHF, are classified as medium-risk and should have an initial blood sample tested to exclude malaria. If this is negative, relevant specimens (blood, throat swab, urine and pleural fluid, if available) are collected and sent to an appropriate reference laboratory for nucleic acid detection (PCR), virus isolation and serology. If patients are still felt to be at significant risk of VHF or if infection is confirmed, they should be transferred to a specialised HCID unit. All further laboratory tests should be performed at BSL 4. Transport requires an ambulance with BSL 3 facilities.

In addition to general supportive measures, ribavirin is given intravenously (100mg/kg, then 25mg/kg daily for 3 days and 12.5mg/kg daily for 4 days) when Lassa fever or South American haemorrhagic fevers are suspected.

Prevention

Ribavirin has been used as prophylaxis in close contacts in Lassa fever but there are no formal trials of its efficacy.

Ebola virus disease (EVD)

Ebola virus disease (EVD) is thought to spread to human populations from fruit bats, sometimes indirectly via contact with infected primates or other animals. Person-to-person spread, via contact with blood, secretions or body parts, establishes EVD in populations. Family members, health-care workers and people performing traditional burials are at particular risk. The 2014 outbreak involved the Zaire strain of Ebola virus.

Clinical features

The incubation period is 2–21 days but typically 8–10 days. Fever and non-specific signs are accompanied by abdominal pain, diarrhoea, vomiting and hiccups. A maculopapular rash occurs after 5–7 days in some. Although bleeding from the gums or venepuncture sites or in the stool occurs, haemorrhage may be less prominent than in other VHFs and is often a terminal event. In contrast, fluid losses from diarrhoea are more marked and reach 10 L per day. Complications include meningoencephalitis, uveitis and miscarriages in pregnant women.

Investigations

Lymphopenia occurs, followed by neutrophilia, atypical lymphocytosis, thrombocytopenia and coagulation abnormalities. Elevations of AST/ALT, features of acute kidney injury, electrolyte disturbances and proteinuria are also observed. The virus is detected by a PCR in blood or body fluids, but may need retesting if the duration of symptoms is less than 3 days. Antigen detection has also been used in rural settings. Serology provides a retrospective diagnosis.

Management

Treatment is supportive and aimed at fluid replacement. Bacterial super-infections should be promptly treated. Mortality varies but is approximately 50% (range 25%–90%). Survivors recover from the second week of illness but experience late sequelae, including arthritis (76%), uveitis (60%) and deafness (24%), while skin sloughing is common. Relapse with meningitis is reported months after recovery. Monoclonal antibodies are a promising therapeutic approach.

Prevention

Ebola virus may be detected in the semen months after recovery. Male survivors are therefore encouraged to practise safe sex for 12 months after symptom onset or until two negative semen tests, but recommendations vary. Public health measures are essential for outbreak control and involve contact surveillance and monitoring through the incubation period, separating healthy from sick individuals, practising safe burial methods and ensuring appropriate infection control measures to protect health-care and laboratory workers, including provision of personal protective equipment such as gloves, gowns and full-face protection (face shield or masks combined with goggles). An Ebola glycoprotein vaccine, rVZV-ZEBOV, was shown to be effective in 2016 after a trial in West Africa and has been used in DRC as well as another viral vector vaccine, Ad26.ZEBOV/MVA-BN-Filo.

Zika virus

Zika virus is a flavivirus spread from primate hosts by *Aedes aegypti* and *Aedes albopictus*, which bite during the day. Described in Africa and Asia since 2015, it has been epidemic in the Americas, where a mosquito–man–mosquito transmission cycle is established. It also can be transmitted in semen.

Clinical features

The incubation period is 3–12 days. Infection is asymptomatic or mild, resembling dengue with fever, arthralgia, conjunctivitis and maculopapular rash. Complications include increased reports of Guillain–Barré syndrome. Zika-related complications occur in 5%–15% of pregnant women with infection. The major concern has been a marked increase in microcephaly in pregnant women infected with Zika virus, as well as increased rates of cerebral calcification, deafness, visual problems such as chorioretinal scarring, joint contractures (arthrogryposis), hydrops fetalis and growth retardation.

Investigations

Routine blood tests are usually normal but may show leucopenia, thrombocytopenia or increased transaminases. PCR detects virus in the first week of illness or in urine up to 14 days. Serology provides a retrospective diagnosis but cross-reacts with other flaviviruses. Plaque-reduction neutralisation testing can be used to detect virus-specific neutralising antibodies and distinguish between cross-reacting antibodies in primary flavivirus infections.

Prevention

Prevention focuses on avoiding mosquito bites. Since Zika virus may be found in the semen or genital secretions for prolonged periods, infected individuals should practise safe sex for at least 6 months and planned pregnancy should be postponed for at least 6 months. WHO guidance recommends individuals who have travelled to an endemic area but are asymptomatic should practise safe sex for 6 months in men and 2 months in women, but updated guidance should be sought. There is currently no vaccine.

Viral infections of the skin

Herpes simplex virus 1 and 2

Herpes simplex viruses (HSVs) cause recurrent mucocutaneous infection; HSV-1 typically involves the mucocutaneous surfaces of the head and neck (Fig. 13.15), while HSV-2 predominantly involves the genital mucosa (see p. 380), although there is overlap (see Box 13.27). The seroprevalence of HSV-1 is 30%–100%, varying by socioeconomic status, while that of HSV-2 is 20%–60%. Infection is acquired by inoculation of viruses shed by an infected individual on to a mucosal surface in a susceptible person. The virus infects sensory and autonomic neurons and establishes latent infection in the nerve ganglia. Primary infection is followed by life-long episodes of reactivation.

Clinical features

Primary HSV-1 or 2 infection is more likely to be symptomatic later in life, causing gingivostomatitis, pharyngitis or painful genital tract lesions. The primary attack may be associated with fever and regional lymphadenopathy.

Recurrence

Recurrent attacks occur, most often in association with concomitant medical illness, menstruation, mechanical trauma, immunosuppression, psychological stress or, for oral lesions, ultraviolet light exposure. HSV reactivation in the oral mucosa produces the classical 'cold sore' or 'herpes labialis'. Prodromal hyperaesthesia is followed by rapid vesiculation, pustulation and crusting. Recurrent HSV genital disease is a common cause of recurrent painful ulceration. An inoculation lesion on the finger may cause a paronychia, termed a 'whitlow', in contacts of patients with herpetic lesions (Fig. 13.15B).

Complications

Disseminated cutaneous lesions can occur in individuals with underlying dermatological diseases, such as eczema (eczema herpeticum) (Fig. 13.15C). Herpes keratitis presents with pain and blurring of vision; characteristic dendritic ulcers are visible on slit-lamp examination and may produce corneal scarring and permanent visual impairment.

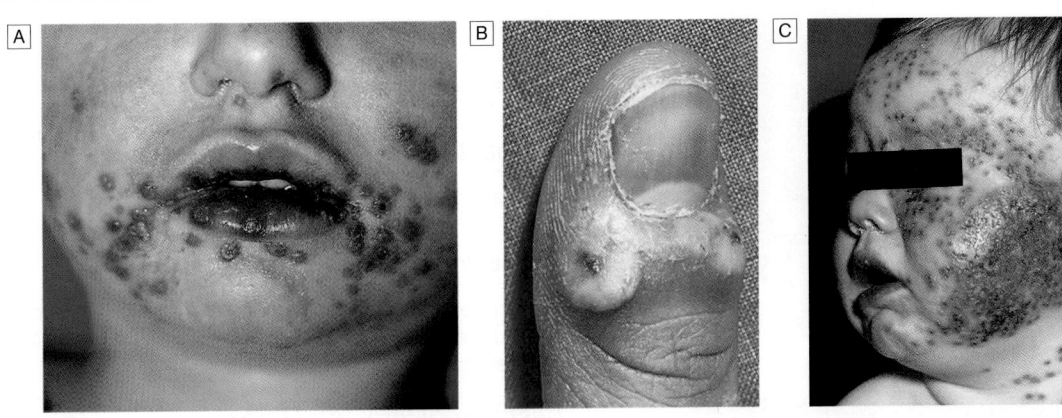

Fig. 13.15 Cutaneous manifestations of herpes simplex virus 1 (HSV-1). A Acute HSV-1. There were also vesicles in the mouth – herpetic stomatitis. B Herpetic whitlow. C Eczema herpeticum. HSV-1 infection spreads rapidly in eczematous skin.

Primary HSV-2 can cause meningitis or transverse myelitis. HSV is the leading cause of sporadic viral encephalitis; this follows either primary or secondary disease, usually with HSV-1. A haemorrhagic necrotising temporal lobe cerebritis produces temporal lobe epilepsy and altered consciousness/coma. Without treatment, mortality is 80%. HSV is also implicated in the pathogenesis of Bell's palsy with a lower motor neuron 7th nerve palsy, although antivirals have not been demonstrated to improve outcome.

Neonatal HSV disease is usually associated with primary infection of the mother at term (see Box 13.24). In excess of two-thirds of cases develop disseminated disease with cutaneous lesions, hepatitis, pneumonitis and, frequently, encephalitis.

Immunocompromised hosts can develop visceral disease with oesophagitis, hepatitis, pneumonitis, encephalitis or retinitis.

Diagnosis

Differentiation from other vesicular eruptions is achieved by demonstration of virus in vesicular fluid, usually by direct immunofluorescence or PCR. HSV encephalitis is diagnosed by a positive PCR for HSV in CSF. Serology is of limited value.

Management

Therapy of localised disease must commence in the first 48 hours of clinical disease (primary or recurrent); thereafter it is unlikely to influence clinical outcome. Oral lesions in an immunocompetent individual may be treated with topical aciclovir. All severe manifestations should be treated, regardless of the time of presentation (see Box 13.28). Suspicion of HSV encephalopathy requires immediate antiviral therapy. Aciclovir resistance is encountered occasionally in immunocompromised hosts, in which case foscarnet is recommended.

Human herpesvirus 8

Human herpesvirus 8 (HHV-8) (see Box 13.27) causes Kaposi's sarcoma in both AIDS-related and endemic non-AIDS-related forms. HHV-8 is spread via saliva, and men who have sex with men have an increased incidence of infection. Seroprevalence varies widely, being highest in sub-Saharan Africa. HHV-8 also causes two rare haematological malignancies: primary effusion lymphoma and multicentric Castleman's disease. Kaposi's sarcoma inflammatory cytokine syndrome is an HHV-8-associated syndrome that mimics sepsis. Current antivirals are not effective and treatment is with rituximab plus chemotherapy.

Enterovirus infections

Hand, foot and mouth disease

This systemic infection is caused by enteroviruses (mainly coxsackievirus A16 and enterovirus 71) and echoviruses. It affects children and occasionally adults, resulting in local or household outbreaks, particularly in the summer months, with recent epidemics in South-east Asia. A relatively mild illness with fever and lymphadenopathy develops after an incubation period of approximately 10 days; 2–3 days later, a painful papular or vesicular rash appears on palmoplantar surfaces of the hands and feet, with associated oral lesions on the buccal mucosa and tongue that ulcerate rapidly. A papular erythematous rash may appear on the buttocks and thighs. Enterovirus A71 and coxsackie A6 have been associated with more severe illness, including acute flaccid paralysis. Antiviral treatment is not available, and management consists of symptom relief with analgesics.

Herpangina

This infection, mainly caused by coxsackieviruses, primarily affects children and adolescents in the summer months. It is characterised by a small number of vesicles at the soft/hard palate junction, often associated with high fever, an extremely sore throat and headache. The lesions are short-lived, rupturing after 2–3 days and rarely persisting for more than 1 week. Treatment is with analgesics if required. Culture of the virus from vesicles or DNA detection by PCR differentiates herpangina from HSV.

Poxviruses

These DNA viruses are rare but potentially important pathogens.

Smallpox (variola)

Smallpox, which has high mortality, was eradicated worldwide by a global vaccination programme but remains a potential bioweapon. The virus is spread by the respiratory route or contact with lesions, and is highly infectious.

The incubation period is 7–17 days. A prodrome with fever, headache and prostration leads, in 1–2 days, to the rash, which develops through macules and papules to vesicles and pustules, worst on the face and distal extremities. Lesions in one area are all at the same stage of development with no cropping (unlike chickenpox). Vaccination can lead to a modified course of disease with milder rash and lower mortality.

If a case of smallpox is suspected, national public health authorities must be contacted. Electron micrography (like Fig. 13.16) and DNA detection tests (PCR) are used to confirm diagnosis.

Monkeypox

Despite the name, the animal reservoirs for this virus are small squirrels and rodents. It causes a rare zoonotic infection in communities in the rainforest belt of Central Africa, producing a vesicular rash that is indistinguishable from smallpox, but differentiated by the presence of lymphadenopathy. Little person-to-person transmission occurs. Outbreaks outside Africa have been linked to importation of African animals as exotic pets. Diagnosis is by electron micrography or DNA detection (PCR).

13

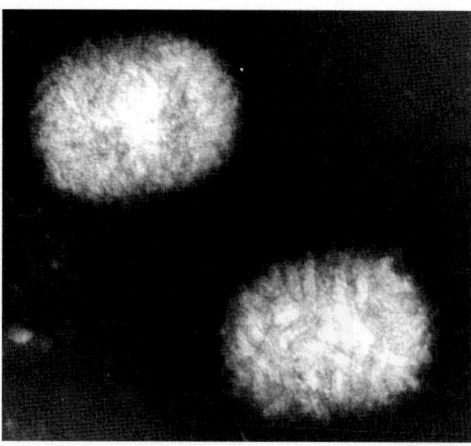

Fig. 13.16 Electron micrograph of molluscum contagiosum, a poxvirus. *Courtesy of Prof. Goura Kudesia, Northern General Hospital, Sheffield.*

Cowpox

Humans in contact with infected cows develop large vesicles, usually on the hands or arms and associated with fever and regional lymphadenitis. The reservoir is thought to be wild rodents.

Vaccinia virus

This laboratory strain is used as the smallpox vaccine. Widespread vaccination is no longer recommended due to the likelihood of local spread from the vaccination site (potentially life-threatening in those with eczema (eczema vaccinatum) or immune deficiency) and of encephalitis. However, vaccination may still be recommended for key medical staff.

Other poxviruses: orf and molluscum contagiosum

See page 1091 and Figure 13.16.

Gastrointestinal viral infections

Norovirus

Norovirus is the most common UK cause of infectious gastroenteritis and causes outbreaks in hospital wards, cruise ships and military camps. Food handlers may transmit this virus, which is relatively resistant to decontamination procedures. The incubation period is 24–48 hours. High attack rates and prominent vomiting are characteristic. Diagnosis may be achieved by antigen or DNA detection (PCR) in stool samples, although the characteristic clinical and epidemiological features mean that microbiological confirmation is not always necessary. The virus is highly infectious and cases should be isolated and environmental surfaces cleaned with detergents and disinfected with bleach.

Astrovirus

Astroviruses cause diarrhoea in small children and occasionally in immunocompromised adults.

Rotavirus

Rotaviruses infect enterocytes and are a major cause of diarrhoeal illness in young children worldwide. Winter epidemics are common in high-income countries, particularly in nurseries. Adults in close contact with cases may develop disease. The incubation period is 48 hours and patients present with watery diarrhoea, vomiting, fever and abdominal pain. Dehydration is prominent. Diagnosis is aided by commercially available enzyme immunoassay kits, which require fresh or refrigerated stool samples. Immunity develops to natural infection. Monovalent and multivalent vaccines have been licensed in many countries and have now demonstrated efficacy in large trials in Africa and the Americas.

Hepatitis viruses (A–E)

See Chapter 24.

Other viruses

Adenoviruses are frequently identified from stool culture and implicated as a cause of diarrhoea in children. They have also been linked to cases of intussusception.

Respiratory viral infections

These infections are described further on page 512.

Adenoviruses, rhinoviruses and enteroviruses (coxsackieviruses and echoviruses) often produce non-specific upper respiratory tract symptoms but may cause viral pneumonia. Parainfluenza and respiratory syncytial viruses cause upper respiratory tract disease, croup and bronchiolitis in small children and pneumonia in the immunocompromised. Respiratory syncytial virus also causes pneumonia in nursing home residents and may be associated with nosocomial pneumonia. Metapneumovirus and bocavirus cause upper and occasionally lower respiratory tract infection, especially in immunosuppressed individuals.

Coronaviruses

Coronaviruses are single-strand positive-sense RNA viruses that cause widespread infection in animals and humans.

Coronaviruses HCoV-229E, HCoV-NL63, HCoVH-KU1 and HCoV-OC43 have a worldwide distribution. They usually cause mild upper respiratory tract infection, but occasionally more serious respiratory infection at extremes of age or in immunocompromised hosts.

Three coronaviruses have emerged in recent years that cause more serious infections. These are SARS-CoV (severe acute respiratory syndrome coronavirus), MERS-CoV (Middle East respiratory syndrome coronavirus) and SARS-CoV-2 (the cause of coronavirus disease 2019; COVID-19). These coronaviruses have emerged as zoonoses from bats and potentially intermediate hosts. The intermediate hosts for SARS-CoV and MERS-CoV include palm civets and camels respectively, but the identity of the intermediate host(s) for SARS-CoV-2 remains elusive.

It has been suggested that both SARS-CoV and SARS-CoV-2 may have been spread to humans through contact with wild animals in wild food markets.

Pathogenesis

The coronaviruses contain non-structural proteins including RNA-polymerases and proteases and structural proteins including the envelope, spike (S) glycoprotein and nucleocapsid protein. RNA replication occurs in double membrane vesicles originating from the endoplasmic reticulum and is incorporated into virions which are released from infected cells. The coronaviruses infect a range of cells, including respiratory and gastrointestinal epithelial cells. Initial interactions involve the S glycoprotein, which binds to the surface receptor. For SARS, SARS-CoV-2 and HCoV-NL63 the receptor is the human angiotensin-converting enzyme 2 (hACE2). Infection with SARS-CoV-2 results in reduced expression of hACE2, a protein that normally plays important anti-inflammatory roles in the lung, and it is thought that reduced expression may contribute to pathogenesis. In SARS-CoV-2 infection the S glycoprotein requires priming by the human serine protease TMPRSS2 to allow optimal engagement with its receptor, hACE2. For MERS-CoV the receptor is the dipeptidyl peptidase 4 (DPP4). The receptor-binding domain of the S glycoprotein undergoes mutation to allow adaptation during cross-species transmission from bats to other species, including man.

Coronaviruses induce suboptimal early interferon responses, in part thought to be because the RNA is shielded from pattern recognition receptors, since it is contained in the double membrane vesicles. Furthermore, several coronaviruses contain a nucleocapsid protein that suppresses interferon production. However, despite suppression of interferon in some cells, other cells such as macrophages and dendritic cells do produce interferon, and excessive production of interferon and other pro-inflammatory cytokines by these cells is associated with failure to clear virus and poor outcomes. Antiviral immunity requires production of neutralising antibody and effective CD4+ and CD8+ T-cell responses. These same antiviral responses, however, also appear to cause tissue injury. In SARS-CoV and SARS-CoV-2 infection pulmonary complications typically emerge after 1–2 weeks and are thought to result from dysregulation of innate and adaptive immune responses. For SARS-CoV-2 it is suggested that suboptimal innate immune responses and recruitment of pro-inflammatory CCR2+ monocytes contribute to inflammation, while apoptotic cell death of CD8+ T-cells is prominent. Disease is more severe in older individuals and it is thought this may correlate with suboptimal T-cell responses and enhanced pro-inflammatory responses with ageing. Skewing of immune responses away from early protective interferon responses and suboptimal antiviral immunity may lead to dysregulated immune responses and prolonged inflammatory responses that lead to tissue injury in multiple organs. For SARS-CoV-2, activation of the clotting cascade in association with marked inflammation appears to be a distinct feature. Microthrombi occur around the body and both venous thromboembolism and arterial clots in the heart and brain may be prominent features.

SARS coronavirus (SARS-CoV)

SARS-CoV emerged as a major respiratory pathogen during an outbreak of SARS in 2002–2003, in which there were approximately 8000 cases. The virus originated in Guangdong, China, and spread to several other countries, with secondary transmission reported in Canada (Toronto), Hong Kong, Taiwan, Singapore and Vietnam during the outbreak. SARS presented as a flu-like illness with non-specific symptoms, including fever, malaise, myalgia, headache, diarrhoea and shivering. In severe cases these progressed to pneumonia, requiring intensive care admission. The case fatality rate was approximately 11%.

According to the World Health Organization, SARS infection has been recorded only four times since the global epidemic, three times from laboratory accidents and once in southern China from an unknown source.

Middle East respiratory syndrome coronavirus (MERS-CoV)

In 2012, a novel coronavirus, distantly related to SARS-CoV, caused several deaths connected with pneumonia in patients originating from the Middle East. The Middle East respiratory syndrome coronavirus (MERS-CoV) appears to be a zoonosis, involving transmission from bats to camels and then to humans. Over 20 countries have reported cases, although most cases have a history of travel to Saudi Arabia or other countries in the Arabian Peninsula. By 2020 there had been over 2500 reported cases. MERS-CoV remains an important but still geographically restricted coronavirus.

Clinical features

The incubation period in person-to-person transmission is 2–14 (average 5) days. Any age may be infected but the patients over 50 with medical comorbidities are particularly susceptible to severe disease. Initial symptoms are fever, chills, headache, myalgia, dry cough and dyspnoea. Abdominal pain and diarrhoea may be prominent. The mean period from symptom onset to hospitalisation is 4 days, and 5 days to intensive care unit admission. Illness is complicated by rapid development of respiratory failure and features of ARDS and multi-organ failure. Mortality is 35%.

Diagnosis and management

Laboratory features include lymphopenia, thrombocytopenia and raised lactate dehydrogenase (LDH). Diagnosis is confirmed by detection of virus RNA (PCR) in serum, nasopharyngeal or other respiratory samples. Antibody detection may also be useful. Treatment is supportive.

Strict infection control measures should be implemented for anyone with fever, severe respiratory illness and epidemiological risk factors. Patients should be managed in an airborne infection isolation room with contact and airborne infection control measures, including personal protective equipment for health-care workers.

SARS-CoV-2

SARS-CoV-2 was first identified in December 2019 in Wuhan, China, where it caused an outbreak that spread rapidly to other parts of China and then the rest of the world. The virus is believed to have been transmitted to humans via horseshoe bats (*Rhinolophus sinicus*) and potentially other intermediate hosts, to whom individuals may have been exposed at wild food markets.

SARS-CoV-2 appears to be more easily transmissible than SARS-CoV and MERS-CoV. Consequently, early efforts to contain the virus were unsuccessful and it spread rapidly. The earliest secondary outbreaks were identified in Iran, Italy and Spain, but most of the world was affected within a few weeks (Fig. 13.17). The World Health Organization declared COVID-19 to be a global pandemic in March 2020, just 3 months after it was first identified in China. By late 2020 new variants had emerged carrying several amino acid substitutions. As the virus mutates variants of interest and variants of concern have been identified to aid public health measures to monitor transmission and research. The nomenclature of new variants developed alongside the pandemic. The variants were initially assigned 'Pango' lineage codes (letters and numbers) or identified with designations associated with clade (GISAID or Nexstrain), although as these were difficult for the public to use the variants tended to be referred to according to the geographic location where they were first identified, e.g. B1.1.7 ('Kent', United Kingdom), B1.351 (South Africa) and P.1 (Brazil). In May 2021, to both simplify the nomenclature and avoid the pejorative connotations of geographic associations, the WHO started to assign Greek characters to the variants, and these strains were named Alpha (e.g. B1.1.7), Beta (e.g. B1.351), Gamma (e.g. P.1) and Delta (e.g. B1.617.2). The Greek letter names are designed to facilitate discussion in non-scientific audiences and do not replace the scientific names. The variants have higher R numbers than the native virus and are more transmissible due to mutations in the receptor-binding domain of the S protein, such as the replacement of asparagine with tyrosine at amino acid position 501 (N501Y). B1.1.7 (Alpha) was found to cause increased mortality compared to previous SARS-CoV-2 strains in several studies. Mutation may also modify interactions with antibody, as suggested for the E484K mutation (where a glutamic acid residue is replaced by lysine) found in the Beta and Gamma variants. The highly transmissible B1.617.2 (Delta) variant emerged in December 2020 causing a '2nd wave' in India before spreading across the world. The pattern was repeated in November 2021 with the B.1.1.529 (Omicron) variant, first reported in South Africa. However, Omicron tended to cause disease of less severity than earlier variants, presumably because of a combination of altered virulence factors and herd immunity from vaccination and natural infection.

As well as exhibiting differences in transmissibility, symptomatology and case-fatality, infection by the variants is prevented to different extents by the separate COVID-19 vaccines available. For example, the Delta variant was found to have a greater propensity to infect individuals who had received only single doses of vaccines, most of which are designed to be given as a two-dose 'course'; and the Omicron variant had a propensity to infect people who were fully vaccinated but had not had 'booster' doses. SARS-CoV-2 is therefore very much a 'moving target' with respect to disease prevention strategies.

Responses to control the pandemic

The rapid emergence and exponential increase in COVID-19 case numbers as the pandemic developed raised significant challenges to the control of its transmission in both health-care settings and the wider community. Particular infection prevention and control (IPC) challenges raised by the pandemic included the rapid depletion of personal protective equipment (PPE), the lag between the spread of

13

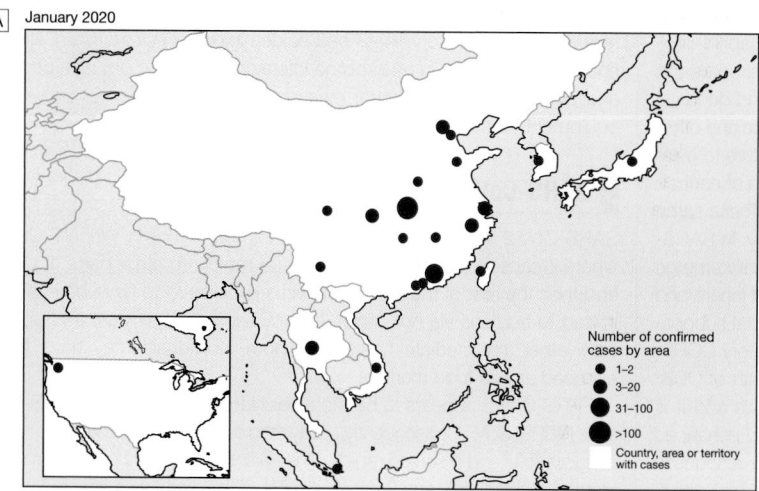

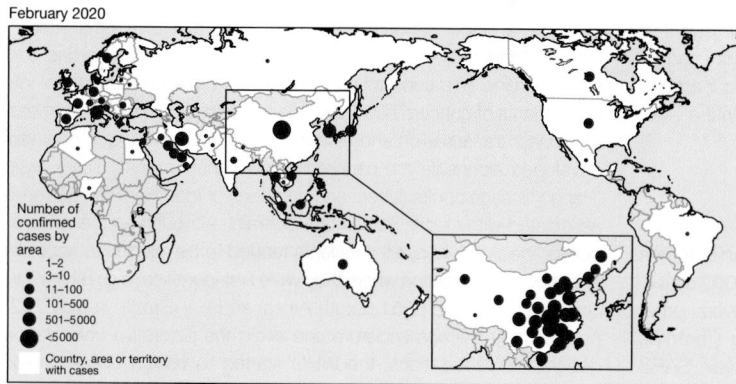

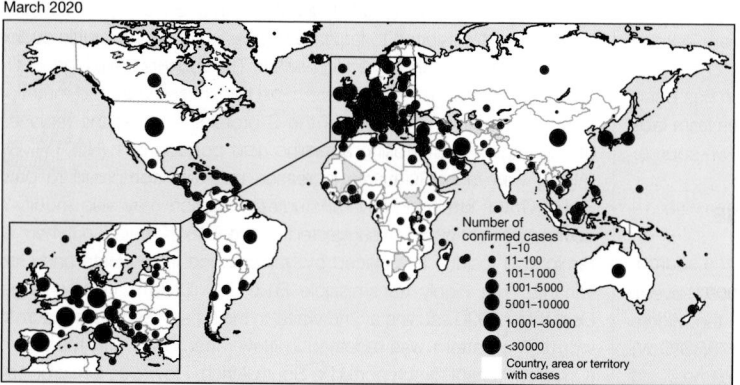

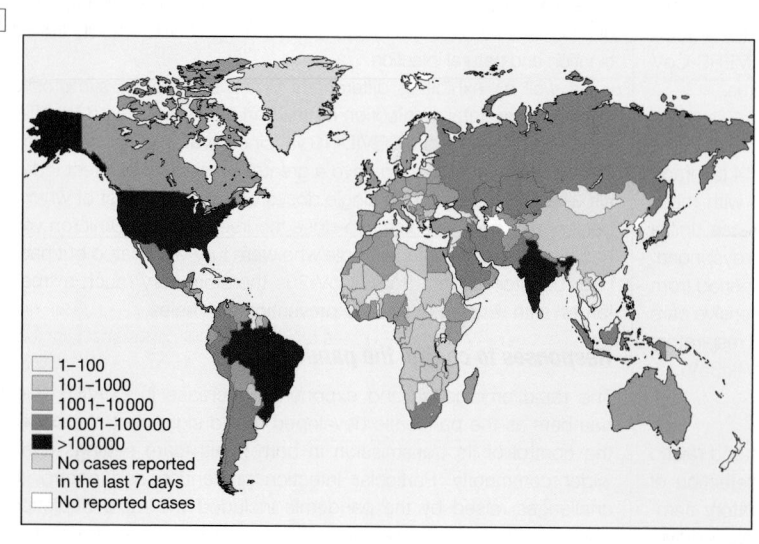

Fig. 13.17 Global spread of COVID-19 in 2020. A The spread of COVID-19 from late January with an epicentre in China to foci in Asia and Europe in late February, with more widespread cases in late March is shown, while in B the established pandemic is shown in July 2020. *Redrawn with permission from WHO.*

i 13.36 Infection prevention and control strategies used for COVID-19 in the health-care setting*	
'Standard' precautions	• Hand hygiene • Use of personal protective equipment (PPE), e.g. masks, gloves, aprons, gowns and eye protection, according to the clinical circumstances • Spillage, sharps, laundry and clinical waste management • Environmental cleaning and disinfection
Transmission-based precautions	• A combination of airborne, contact and droplet precautions (see Box 6.9) with airborne precautions often reserved for situations in which aerosol-generating procedures (AGPs) are carried out • Different precautions may be applied depending on the level of patient risk (e.g. confirmed vs. suspected COVID-19)
Isolation, cohorting and quarantining	• Isolation or cohorting to minimise the risk of onward transmission (cohorting should be reserved for confirmed cases, or it carries the risk of uninfected patients being exposed to infected patients) • Quarantining patients prior to elective procedures • Quarantining staff who test positive for SARS-CoV-2
Screening	• Admission screening to identify asymptomatic infected patients • Interval screening of inpatients to identify and prevent health care-acquired COVID-19 • Pre-procedure screening for patients having elective procedures • Staff screening to identify asymptomatic infected staff
Visitor restriction	• To minimise the possibility of uninfected patients being infected by visitors, and vice versa
Contact tracing	• Detection (and subsequent isolation) of uninfected patients who have been exposed to infected patients (e.g. in a bay/hospital ward) and staff

*Infection prevention and control measures vary with time, in different countries and according to resource availability.

13

infection and the acquisition of evidence required to inform IPC precautions to control its spread, the requirement by health-care providers to implement frequent changes in IPC guidance in response to the availability of PPE, and huge fluctuations in case numbers as the periodic introduction and relaxation of population-based control measures brought about 'waves' of infection, which had the potential to repeatedly overwhelm the ability of health services to function effectively.

Infection prevention and control in health-care settings

SARS-CoV-2 is acquired predominantly from the oropharyngeal and respiratory secretions of infected patients. Respiratory transmission has traditionally been categorized into 'airborne' (or 'aerosol') and 'droplet' spread, which are distinguished by the size of respiratory particles in which viable organisms are carried, with a cut-off size of 5 μm. The theoretical basis for the distinction is that particles of 5–10 μm diameter ('respiratory droplets') tend to fall out of the air soon after being produced. They are therefore unlikely to travel more than 1 m or so from the source patient and are transmitted mainly by settling on mucous membranes (direct transmission) or by being transported to mucous membranes via fomites (indirect transmission). Conversely, particles of <5 μm ('droplet nuclei') can remain suspended in the air for prolonged periods of time and can therefore travel longer distances and be taken into air passages by inhalation. In reality, both the size of respiratory particles produced by an infected person and the distance they can travel is likely to fall on a spectrum. The range of particle sizes will be affected by factors such as the speed of the passage of air across the infected person's respiratory tract mucous membranes, the volume and character of secretions being produced and the extent to which droplets are converted to droplet nuclei by evaporation; and the duration of airborne suspension and distance travelled will be influenced by environmental factors such as temperature, humidity and prevailing air currents. Therefore, the distinction between airborne/aerosol and droplet transmission is not absolute, and different precautions may be required for the same infection in different circumstances.

SARS-CoV-2 is believed to be predominantly transmitted by droplet spread in most circumstances (e.g. when an infected patient is breathing rapidly or coughing) but can be transmitted by the airborne route when the patient is subjected to an 'aerosol-generating procedure' (AGP). AGPs include (but are not limited to) tracheal intubation, manual ventilation, non-invasive ventilation and the use of certain high flow oxygenation treatments. For this reason, in the UK (at the time of writing) 'droplet'

precautions are considered adequate for the management of patients with COVID-19 (and other infections transmitted in a similar manner, such as influenza) in most circumstances, but 'airborne' precautions are used when an infected (or suspected) patient is subjected to an AGP. Unfortunately, the evidence-base for the distinction between airborne and droplet transmission in any given circumstance is weak and subject to repeated interpretation, so precautions used for COVID-19 tend to vary with time and geographical location.

The control of COVID-19 in health-care settings therefore requires a combination of measures, as shown in Box 13.36.

Public health measures

A major strategy for limiting spread of SARS-CoV-2 has been the introduction of physical distancing measures, the most extreme of which have been termed 'lockdowns'. The components and restrictiveness of lockdowns vary between countries, but they have typically included: the closure of schools, workplaces, non-essential shops, sporting and entertainment venues; a move to remote (i.e. computer- based) working where possible; banning mass gatherings; curfews; stay-at-home orders; and other local, national and international travel restrictions. Not all countries have employed lockdowns. Physical distancing measures are designed to slow the spread of the virus and limit the burden of serious illness on overstretched health services, rather than to eradicate the virus. However, in some countries where they were employed early (e.g. New Zealand), they resulted in complete, although temporary, eradication of virus in the community.

Other important measures in limiting virus spread are ensuring high levels of case identification, ramping up testing to identify cases, ensuring public health follow-up of potential cases and enforcing quarantine measures for cases, contacts and travellers from high-incidence countries. The combination of such strategies has been termed 'test, trace and isolate' (TTI). Countries have tended to increase TTI measures as they have eased lockdowns, in an attempt to prevent rebound increases in cases and the need for subsequent lockdowns, which are economically damaging. Novel approaches to TTI have been developed, including the use of mobile phone apps, CCTV footage and tracking of a contact's digital signature, depending on jurisdiction and legal constraints. Surveillance sampling of all adults combined with advice to stay at home have been implemented as measures against emerging variant viruses.

Social distancing strategies employed when lockdown is not considered necessary have included keeping people physically separate (a target of ≥2 metres has been used in the UK), promoting frequent hand hygiene and enforcing the use of face coverings in places where close contact is likely.

Vulnerable adults, including older and immunocompromised people, have been advised to limit social interactions, a strategy termed 'shielding' in the UK.

Clinical features

The incubation period for COVID-19 is 5-6 days on average but can range from 2-14 days. Many infections, probably between 80% and 90%, are asymptomatic. Where patients do experience symptoms, these are very variable and depend on the vaccination status of the patient and the SARS-CoV-2 variant with which they are infected.

In unvaccinated patients and with variants predominating in the first year of the pandemic, typical symptoms include high fever, persistent cough, shortness of breath and loss of taste or smell. Myalgia, fatigue, dizziness or headache are also frequent, as are chest pain, vomiting and diarrhoea. Vomiting and diarrhoea may be prominent features and may precede fever, and gastrointestinal symptoms are often also prominent in children. Confusion or delirium occur, particularly in older people. Variant strains seen in the UK are associated with a greater range of symptoms, for example cough, sore throat, fatigue, myalgia and headaches appear more common, whereas loss of smell or taste are less common, than with the original virus. Variant B1.617.2 (Delta) became the dominant variant in many countries by summer 2021, and commonly presented with coryzal symptoms, myalgia and headache, with cough and loss of taste or smell being a less common presentation.

Before the introduction of vaccination, approximately 15% of symptomatic patients would develop severe symptoms and 5% critical illness. Physical examination of such patients may reveal tachycardia, hypotension, cyanosis, hypoxia or bilateral crackles in the lung fields. Bronchial breath sounds and focal consolidation may suggest bacterial superinfection. Skin lesions are common and include maculopapular lesions, vesicles, pustules and urticarial lesions. Chilblain-like lesions with oedema or haemorrhage under the skin are also described. The differential diagnosis with a predominant respiratory presentation will include community-acquired pneumonia, influenza and other severe respiratory virus infections, including MERS-CoV.

If complications occur they usually develop in the second week. These are most commonly due to acute respiratory distress syndrome (ARDS). Bacterial pneumonia complicates a minority of infections and sepsis may occur. Superinfections occur, in particular in those with critical illness, including fungal infection due to *Aspergillus*, for which prolonged intubation is a risk factor. In India especially, mucormycosis (p. 345) emerged as a specific complication, especially in patients with pre-existing diabetes mellitus who were treated with steroids. Disseminated intravascular coagulation is seen in the majority of those who do not survive and is associated with severe disease and multi-organ failure. Venous thromboembolism occurs in 20%–30% of critically ill patients but may occur in any patients.

Microthrombi can form in the lung and some have proposed the term 'microvascular COVID-19 lung vessels obstructive thrombo-inflammatory syndrome' (MicroCLOTS) to distinguish this syndrome from conventional pulmonary embolism. Acute myocardial injury is reported in 5%–31% and acute coronary syndromes, myocarditis or arrhythmia occur. Acute kidney injury is common in hospitalised patients and up to a third of those requiring mechanical ventilation may require renal dialysis. Neurological complications are diverse and include cerebrovascular disease, cerebral venous thrombosis, meningitis, encephalitis, seizures, impaired consciousness, ataxia, neuropathies and Guillain-Barré syndrome. Rhabdomyolysis and secondary bacterial infections can occur. Hypothyroidism can be a long-term complication.

A striking characteristic of SARS-CoV-2 is its varying severity in different age groups. In broad terms the severity of infection ranges from mild or asymptomatic in children (in whom a fatal outcome is exceedingly rare) to severe and life-threatening in older adults. A specific but

13.37 Features of COVID-19 in older age and frailty

- **Pathogenesis:** reduced expression of hACE2 may predispose to more severe respiratory presentation
- **Immunity:** increased inflammatory responses in general and reduced antiviral responses may reduce viral clearance and increase complications
- **Clinical features:** atypical presentations with confusion, delirium and falls
- **Complications:** increased complication rates
- **Mortality:** case fatality rate doubled in those > 65 years and increases with age
- **Investigations:** lack of data on PCR sensitivity in older age
- **Treatment:** may be less likely to be admitted to intensive care
- **Preventative strategies:** more likely to be asked to 'shield' (minimise social interaction), with consequences for general well-being. Older adults are associated with lower vaccine responses in other diseases

rare manifestation in children is the 'paediatric inflammatory multisystem syndrome: temporally associated with SARS-CoV-2' (PIMS-TS), also referred to as multisystem inflammatory syndrome in children (MIS-C). This severe complication consists of fever, abdominal symptoms, rash, conjunctivitis and markers of a high inflammatory response. Myocardial dysfunction, shock and respiratory failure are common complications, and some children meet a clinical definition of Kawasaki disease with features such as coronary artery dilatation or vascular aneurysms. This syndrome appears distinct from Kawasaki disease, however, since it involves an older age group with more marked elevation of inflammatory biomarkers, and is associated with COVID-19. There is also a variant of MIS in adults.

The true case fatality rate for SARS-CoV-2 infection is not known because the apparent incidence of disease is influenced by many different factors. These factors include sampling strategies (i.e. testing a larger number of asymptomatic individuals will reduce the apparent mortality); the definition of a COVID-19-associated death (which varies with both time and jurisdiction); the period of follow-up or extent to which late deaths are attributed to COVID-19; the stage of the pandemic at which sampling was carried out (as mortality has fallen with the introduction of specific treatments); and the proportion of vaccinated vs. unvaccinated cases (as mortality is much lower in patients infected post-vaccination). However, at the time of writing there have been 4.6 million deaths and 222 million confirmed cases (2.1% overall mortality). The case fatality rate is therefore lower than for SARS-CoV and MERS-CoV, which have 11% and 34% mortality, respectively. Where death occurs, it is most often in the third week due to respiratory failure.

Virus is shed in respiratory secretions for approximately 17–24 days. Infection rates appear higher in urban or socially deprived areas. Mortality is higher with male gender, age and frailty (Box 13.37) and medical comorbidity (e.g. diabetes, heart disease, hypertension, chronic lung disease). In the UK mortality is higher in people with African Caribbean and South Asian origin, compared to individuals who have primarily European ancestry. A genome-wide association study linked severity to blood group A as opposed to blood group O, as well as a gene cluster in chromosome 3 that includes several chemokine receptors. The role of immunocompromise on COVID-19 is still being established. Immunocompomised patients may have atypical presentations and prolonged viral shedding, but may be less susceptible to severe COVID-19 if they are on anti-inflammatory treatments that modify COVID-19 pathogenesis. Early data suggested that patients immunosuppressed due to cancer or organ transplant recipients may present with more severe disease, while those receiving biologics do not. Increased age and medical comorbidity are associated with severe disease and mortality, and care homes have experienced outbreaks with high mortality.

'Long COVID' is a term that has been used to describe both prolonged COVID-19 and a post-COVID-19 syndrome that may involve almost any body system. In the UK, the National Institute for Health and Care Excellence (NICE) has defined acute COVID-19 as 'signs and symptoms of COVID-19 for up to 4 weeks', ongoing symptomatic COVID-19 as 'signs and symptoms of COVID-19 from 4 to 12 weeks' and the post-COVID-19 syndrome as 'signs and symptoms that develop during or after an infection consistent with COVID-19, continue for more than 12 weeks and are not explained by an alternative diagnosis'. 'Long COVID' would encompass the latter two scenarios. The World Health Organization has developed a definition for 'post COVID-19 condition' that specifies a symptom duration of at least two months, with symptoms being either a continuation of the initial infection or new symptoms after initial recovery. This too would accord with the popular understanding of 'long COVID'. Whatever definition is used, the most common unifying feature of long COVID/the post-COVID syndrome is fatigue, which can be prolonged and extreme. Other common presentations have included multisystem inflammatory symptoms, persistent fevers and evidence of organ dysfunction affecting almost any organ, but particularly the heart and lungs. Persistent headache, memory problems, insomnia and mental health symptoms such as depression are frequently reported, as are loss of taste and smell, deafness and tinnitus, arthralgia, skin rashes and paraesthaesias. In reality, the post-COVID syndrome is likely to be a conflation of different conditions, not all of which are specific to COVID-19 (e.g. COVID-19 itself, the sequelae of complications of COVID-19 and the various causes of ICU acquired weakness, p. 215). Optimal management strategies for long COVID have not yet been established.

Investigations

Laboratory abnormalities can include an increased neutrophil to lymphocyte ratio; elevated ALT, D-dimer and inflammatory markers, including C-reactive protein (CRP) and ferritin; hypoalbuminaemia and lymphopenia. However, these findings are non-specific and of very little help in distinguishing COVID-19 from other infections. Procalcitonin (PCT) may be elevated and may raise suspicion of secondary bacterial infection, though there is currently insufficient evidence to recommend its routine use or on which to base decisions on whom to give antimicrobials on this test. Acute kidney injury is common in severe disease. Hypokalaemia and hypocalcaemia are common. Hyperglycaemia is also reported and may be observed in patients not known to be diabetic. Hypoxia may be accompanied by hypocapnia so that it appears inappropriately well tolerated ('happy hypoxia').

Chest radiology shows bilateral predominantly basal and peripheral infiltrates, or in a minority, unilateral infiltrates. CT scan of the chest shows 'ground glass' abnormalities, consolidation, septal thickening or crazy-pavement patterning (Fig. 13.18). Lesions are most often basal, peripheral and bilateral. Pulmonary vascular enlargement, pleural or pericardial effusions may be observed in a minority. CT changes may occur in those with negative chest radiography and negative PCR and can be used in patients in whom COVID-19 is strongly suspected but not confirmed. In general CT is reserved for severe cases or those with other indications for performing a CT.

Microbiological diagnosis is by nasopharyngeal or oropharyngeal swab and reverse-transcription PCR (RT-PCR) to detect viral RNA. Sensitivity is approximately 60%–70% and specificity is high (approximately 98%). Nasotracheal aspirates or deep sputum samples may have greater sensitivity. Antibody detection can confirm prior exposure but may cross-react with antibodies from other coronaviruses. Lateral flow immunochromatography (p. 106) is also used to detect SARS-CoV-2 antigens. It is rapid (around 30 minutes) and can be used at home but is less sensitive and specific than PCR.

Management

Treatment is supportive, with high flow oxygen and proning. Non-invasive ventilation or mechanical ventilation are required for those with more severe respiratory failure. Fluid resuscitation is frequently required for hospitalised patients and antimicrobials are added if there are signs or symptoms suggestive of secondary infection. Inotropic support may be required for shock. Renal replacement therapy may be required for acute kidney injury, and anticoagulation if there is evidence of venous thromboembolism. Dexamethasone improves survival and is recommended for hospitalised patients requiring supplemental oxygen or mechanical ventilation. Anti-interleukin (IL)-6 monoclonal antibodies (e.g. tocilizumab) reduce mortality and reduce time to recovery in critically ill patients if administered within 24 hours of admission to an intensive care unit. In the UK tocilizumab is also used in patients with oxygen saturations <92% on repeated measurement on room air with a CRP ≥75 mg/L. An initial randomised clinical trial of the nucleotide analogue remdesivir (Chapter 6) found that it decreased the time to recovery when used within 10 days of symptom onset in patients requiring supplemental oxygen but not mechanical ventilation. However, it has not been found to significantly improve survival and is not currently recommended by the WHO. Antiviral agents are being developed with the goal of administering these early after symptom onset to prevent the later inflammatory complications. Preliminary trial results indicate that the oral antiviral agents molnupiravir and Paxlovid reduce hospitalisation and death if given within the first 3-5 days of symptoms. Molnupiravir is a prodrug, which is metabolised into a form that causes viral RNA-dependent RNA polymerase to introduce fatal mutations into nascent RNA strands. Paxlovid is a combination of two protease inhibitors, the investigational compound PF-07321332, and ritonavir; PF-07321332 is targeted against SARS-CoV-2 3CL protease and ritonavir inhibits the breakdown of PF-07321332. However, both drugs remain experimental at the time of writing, and there are many other potential SARS-CoV-2 antiviral agents at various stages of development. An alternative antiviral strategy is to use antibodies against the virus. The use of single monoclonal antibodies to variable regions of the S protein is limited by rapid emergence of viral resistance and they have not demonstrated efficacy. In contrast, combinations of two monoclonal antibodies (e.g. casirivimab and imdevimab (REGEN-COV)

13

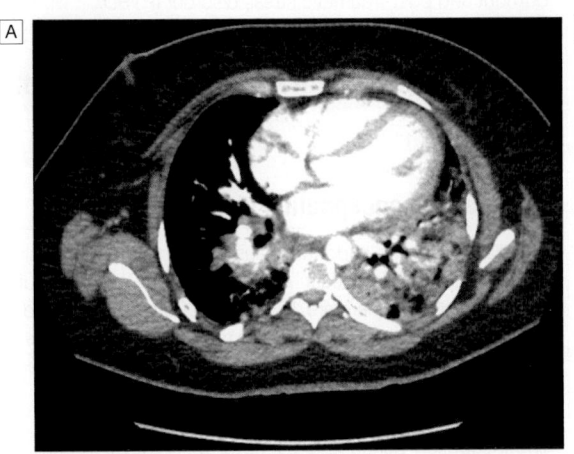
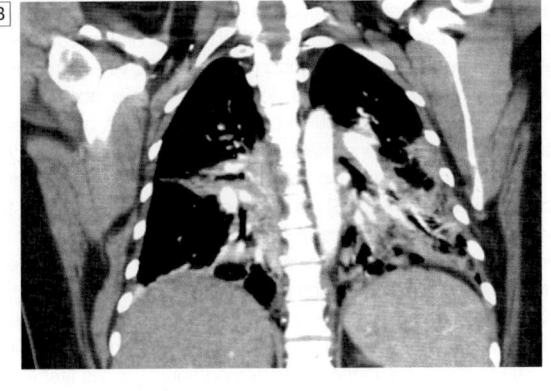

Fig. 13.18 Chest computerised tomography (CT) scan of a patient with COVID-19. The images show widespread areas of consolidation in both lungs.

i	**13.38 SARS-CoV-2 vaccines licensed or at a late stage of development***				
Manufacturer	**Vaccine type**	**Number of doses administered**	**Reported efficacy**	**Storage requirements**	
Oxford/AstraZeneca	Viral vector, ChAdOx (chimpanze adenovirus)	2	62%–90%	4°C	
Moderna	mRNA	2	95%	−20°C	
Pfizer–BioNTech	mRNA	2	95%	−70°C	
Gamaleya (Sputnik V)	Viral vector, Ad5 and Ad26 (human adenoviruses)	2	92%	4°C	
Janssen (Johnson & Johnson)	Viral vector, Ad26 (human adenovirus)	1	66%	4°C	
Novovax	Protein subunit	2	95%	4°C	
Sinopharm	Inactivated virus	2	80%	4°C	
Sinovac	Inactivated virus	2	50%	4°C	
Sinopharm–Wuhan	Inactivated virus	2	70%	4°C	
Bharat Biotech	Inactivated virus	2	80%	4°C	

*This list was accurate at the time of writing (mid-2021). However, because of the rapid speed of vaccine development this is not a complete list of available SARS-CoV-2 vaccines.

or bamlanivimab and etesevimab) are anticipated to represent a greater barrier to escape mutants and preserve efficacy. Initial studies demonstrate these reduce viral load and medical visits in outpatients and reduce hospital stay length and mortality in patients who have not mounted a natural antibody response following vaccination. The efficacy of monoclonal antibodies against the S protein may be challenged by the emergence of variants with mutations such as E484K, and approaches being developed in response include the use of 'broadly neutralizing' antibodies that target more conserved regions of the S protein. Trials using convalescent serum have not shown efficacy.

Vaccination

Because of the global impact of the SARS-CoV-2 pandemic vaccine development started very soon after the virus was identified and sequenced. Vaccines approved or in development include inactivated vaccines, RNA and DNA vaccines, protein subunit vaccines and recombinant RNA vaccines delivered in virus vectors (Box 13.38). The SARS-CoV-2 vaccines induce T-cell immunity in addition to neutralizing antibody but the extent and longevity as well as the ability to block transmission are still being assessed. In general, vaccines have been shown to be efficacious and some have reported efficacy against variant strains after single doses, although the efficacy of single dose vaccination is markedly reduced for the B1.617.2 (Delta) variant. Vaccines have a more dramatic effect on reduction of hospitalised cases than they do on reduction of overall infection but they still play a major role in reducing community transmission. Vaccines are being developed to combat variant strains, including potentially addition of booster doses with modified RNA vaccines. Vaccines have demonstrated safety after billions of administered doses. Side-effects have been minimal and dwarfed by the ongoing mortality of COVID-19 in those without vaccination. Reported severe complications have occurred at incidences approximating 1 per million or less. At least two of the adenoviral vector COVID-19 vaccines have been linked to very rare cases of thrombosis with thrombocytopenia ('vaccine-induced thrombosis with thrombocytopenia syndrome (TTS)'), a condition with some similarities to heparin-induced thrombocytopenia (p. 948). Guillain-Barré syndrome is also reported after the adenoviral vaccines. The RNA vaccines have been linked to rare cases of myocarditis and pericarditis.

Vaccination programmes were rolled out at different rates in different countries. The strategy of rollout used in the UK and some other countries was to target the highest-risk demographic groups first (e.g. older people and those with underlying health conditions). As infection is less severe in patients who have been vaccinated, this strategy gradually converted COVID-19 from a severe disease with high mortality affecting the older population to a predominantly non-severe disease with low mortality affecting younger people. Other strategies may have been used in different countries. The duration of immunity conferred by vaccines and natural infection is not yet known, and booster doses are likely to be required depending on the evidence that emerges.

The need to maintain the 'cold chain' from manufacture to administration is vital for any vaccine. However, it is a particular challenge the pure RNA SARS-CoV-2 vaccines, as they need to be stored at either −20°C or −70°C at all times. This is likely to reduce their use in low- and middle-income countries, where the logistical infrastructure required to maintain the cold chain is less likely to be available.

'Vaccine hesitancy' refers to a heterogenous process in which individuals may refuse or delay vaccination. Vaccine hesitancy has been encountered in many countries and may be more prominent in populations with demographics that vary in different regions. This can represent a major challenge to ensuring high levels of vaccine uptake in a population.

Other considerations

The COVID-19 pandemic has necessitated changes in the law, e.g. to enable governments to mandate the use of masks in public, enforce lockdowns and streamline the processes of death certification to deal with surges in deaths. It has caused health services to become overwhelmed with acutely ill patients, with a knock-on effect of delaying the treatment of less urgent cases. An as yet unquantified problem is the burden of psychological illness in staff who work in patient-facing roles with COVID-19 patients and face issues such as physical exhaustion, burnout and post-traumatic stress disorder (PTSD).

Viral infections with neurological involvement

See also page 1175.

Japanese encephalitis virus (JEV)

This flavivirus is an important cause of endemic encephalitis in Japan, China, Russia, South-east Asia, India and Pakistan; outbreaks also occur elsewhere. There are 10 000–20 000 cases reported to the WHO annually. Pigs and aquatic birds are the reservoirs and transmission is by *Culex* mosquitoes. Exposure to rice paddies is a recognised risk factor.

Clinical features

The incubation period is 4–21 days. Most infections are subclinical in childhood and 1% or less of infections lead to encephalitis. Initial systemic illness with fever, malaise and anorexia is followed by headache, photophobia, vomiting and changes in brainstem function. Other neurological features include meningism, seizures, cranial nerve palsies, flaccid or spastic paralysis and extrapyramidal syndromes. Mortality with neurological disease is 25%. Some 50% of survivors have neurological sequelae.

Investigations, management and prevention

Other infectious causes of encephalitis should be excluded. There is neutrophilia and often hyponatraemia. CSF analysis reveals lymphocytosis and elevated protein. Serological testing of serum and CSF aids diagnosis but may cross-react with dengue and other flaviviruses.

Treatment is supportive. Vaccination is recommended for travellers to endemic areas during the monsoon. Some endemic countries include vaccination in their childhood schedules.

Tick-borne encephalitis virus

This flavivirus is endemic in an area from northern Europe (including the UK) that extends across Siberia to China and Japan. Its incidence is increasing, and it is transmitted from domestic or wild animals by *Ixodes* ticks or sometimes by unpasteurised dairy products. The incubation period is up to 28 days but averages 7 days. A third of cases cause symptoms, with fever, myalgia and headache followed by an interval of up to a month before meningitis, encephalitis or radiculitis occur. The Far Eastern sub-type tends to be more severe. Diagnosis is by IgM ELISA or detection of viral RNA by RT-PCR of blood or CSF. IgG serology cross-reacts with other flaviviruses. Treatment is supportive. Prevention is by avoidance of tick bites. A vaccine is also available.

West Nile virus

This flavivirus is an important cause of neurological disease throughout Australia, India and Russia through Africa and Southern Europe and across to North America. The disease has an avian reservoir and a *Culex* mosquito vector. Older people are at increased risk of neurological disease.

Clinical features

Most infections are asymptomatic. After 2–6 days' incubation, a mild febrile illness and arthralgia may occur. A prolonged incubation may be seen in immunocompromised individuals. Children may develop a maculopapular rash. Neurological disease is seen in 1% and is characterised by encephalitis, meningitis or asymmetric flaccid paralysis with 10% mortality.

Diagnosis and management

Diagnosis is by serology or detection of viral RNA in blood or CSF. Serological tests may show cross-reactivity with other flaviviruses, including vaccine strains. Treatment is supportive.

Nipah virus encephalitis

Nipah virus is a paramyxovirus in the Henipavirus genus, which caused an epidemic of encephalitis in Malaysia and subsequently outbreaks in Bangladesh and India. Mortality is around 30%. Diagnosis is by PCR or serology.

Human T-cell lymphotropic virus type I

Human T-cell lymphotropic virus type I (HTLV-1) is a retrovirus that causes chronic infection with development of adult T-cell leukaemia/lymphoma (ATL) or HTLV-1-associated myelopathy (HAM) in a subset of those infected (see Box 25.57). It is found mainly in Japan, the Caribbean, Central and South America, and the Seychelles. The lifetime risk of ATL in those with chronic HTLV-1 infection is estimated at 2.5%–4%. HAM or tropical spastic paraparesis occurs in less than 5% of those with chronic infection, and presents with gait disturbance, spasticity of the lower extremities, urinary incontinence, impotence and sensory disturbance. Myositis and uveitis may also occur with HTLV-1

infection. Serology, sometimes confirmed with PCR, establishes the diagnosis. Treatment is supportive.

Viral infections with rheumatological involvement

Rheumatological syndromes characterise a variety of viral infections ranging from exanthems, such as rubella and parvovirus B19, to blood-borne viruses, such as HBV and HIV-1 and the sequelae of EVD.

Chikungunya virus

Chikungunya is an alphavirus that causes fever, rash and arthropathy. The disease occurs mainly in Africa and throughout Asia, but is becoming commoner in other areas, including South America and the Carribbean. Cases occur sporadically or in epidemics, with notable epidemics occurring in Réunion and Mauritius (>272 000 cases in 2005–06) and India (1 400 000 cases in 2006). Humans and non-human primates are the main reservoir. The vectors are *Aedes* mosquitoes including *Ae. aegyptii* and *Ae. albopictus*.

The incubation period is 2–12 days. A period of fever may be followed by an afebrile phase and then recrudescence of fever. Children may develop a maculopapular rash. Adults are susceptible to arthritis, which causes early morning pain and swelling, most often in the small joints. Arthritis can persist for months and may become chronic in individuals who are positive for human leucocyte antigen (HLA)-B27. Related alphaviruses causing similar syndromes include Sindbis virus (Scandinavia and Africa), O'nyong-nyong virus (Central Africa), Ross River virus (Australia) and Mayaro virus (Caribbean and South America).

Diagnosis is by serology but cross-reactivity between alphaviruses occurs. Treatment is symptomatic. The disease may be debilitating but is rarely fatal.

Prion diseases

Prions cause transmissible spongiform encephalopathies and are discussed in Chapter 28.

Bacterial infections

Bacterial infections of the skin, soft tissues and bones

Most infections of the skin, soft tissues and bone are caused by either *Staph. aureus* or streptococci (mainly *Strep. pyogenes*) (see pp. 1025 and 1090).

Staphylococcal infections

Staphylococci are usually found colonising the anterior nares and skin. Some staphylococci produce coagulase, an enzyme that converts fibrinogen to fibrin in rabbit plasma, causing it to clot. *Staph. aureus* is coagulase-positive, and most other species are coagulase-negative.

Staph. aureus is the main cause of staphylococcal infections. *Staphylococcus intermedius* is another coagulase-positive staphylococcus, which causes infection following dog bites. Among coagulase-negative organisms, *Staphylococcus epidermidis* is the predominant commensal organism of the skin, and can cause severe infections in those with central venous catheters or implanted prosthetic materials. *Staphylococcus saprophyticus* is part of the normal vaginal flora and causes urinary tract infections in sexually active young women. *Staphylococcus lugdunensis*, *Staphylococcus schleiferi*, *Staphylococcus haemolyticus* and *Staphylococcus caprae* are also human pathogens.

Staphylococcal blood-stream infections can disseminate widely (Fig. 13.19). In any patient with staphylococcal bacteraemia, especially

13

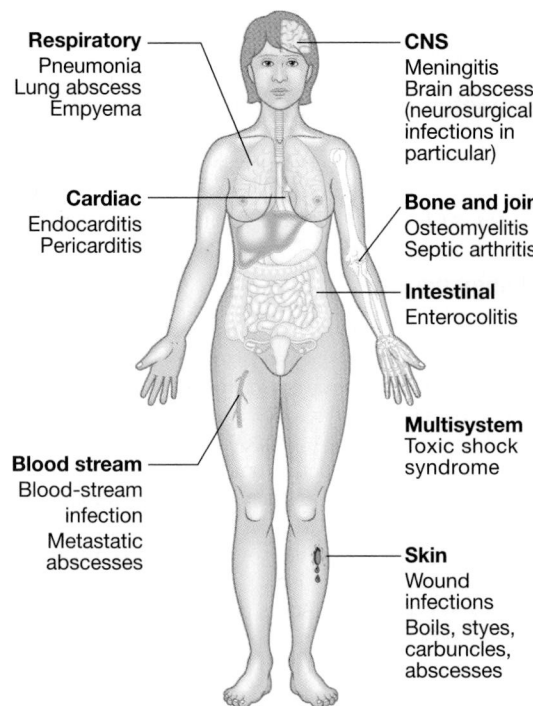

Respiratory
Pneumonia
Lung abscess
Empyema

CNS
Meningitis
Brain abscess
(neurosurgical
infections in
particular)

Cardiac
Endocarditis
Pericarditis

Bone and joint
Osteomyelitis
Septic arthritis

Intestinal
Enterocolitis

Multisystem
Toxic shock
syndrome

Blood stream
Blood-stream
infection
Metastatic
abscesses

Skin
Wound
infections
Boils, styes,
carbuncles,
abscesses

Fig. 13.19 Infections caused by *Staphylococcus aureus*. (CNS = central nervous system)

injection drug-users, the possibility of endocarditis must be considered (see p. 462). Growth of *Staph. aureus* in blood cultures should not be dismissed as a 'contaminant'. Spreading cellulitis mandates the urgent need for an antistaphylococcal antibiotic, such as flucloxacillin, cefazolin or a glycopeptide if MRSA is suspected. This is particularly true for mid-facial cellulitis, which can result in cavernous sinus thrombophlebitis.

In addition, *Staph. aureus* can cause severe systemic disease due to the effects of toxin produced at superficial sites in the absence of tissue invasion by bacteria.

Skin infections

Staphylococci cause ecthyma, folliculitis, furuncles, carbuncles, bullous impetigo and the scalded skin syndrome, which are discussed in Chapter 27. They may also be involved in necrotising infections of the skin and subcutaneous tissues.

Wound infections

Many wound infections, which prolong post-operative care, are caused by staphylococci (Fig. 13.20A). Prevention involves careful attention to hand hygiene, skin preparation and aseptic technique, and the use of topical and systemic antibiotic prophylaxis.

Treatment is by early drainage of any abscesses, removal of prosthetic materials if possible, plus adequate dosage of antistaphylococcal antibiotics.

Cannula-related infection

Staphylococcal infection associated with cannula sepsis (Fig. 13.20B) and thrombophlebitis is an important and common reason for morbidity following hospital admission. The visual infusion phlebitis (VIP) score aids cannula evaluation (Box 13.39). Staphylococci have a predilection for plastic, rapidly forming a biofilm on cannulae, which is a source of bacteraemia. Local poultice application may relieve symptoms but cannula removal and antibiotic treatment with flucloxacillin (or a glycopeptide) are necessary if there is spreading infection.

Meticillin-resistant Staphylococcus aureus

Resistance to meticillin is due to a penicillin-binding protein mutation in *Staph. aureus*, which confers resistance to almost all ß-lactam antibiotics.

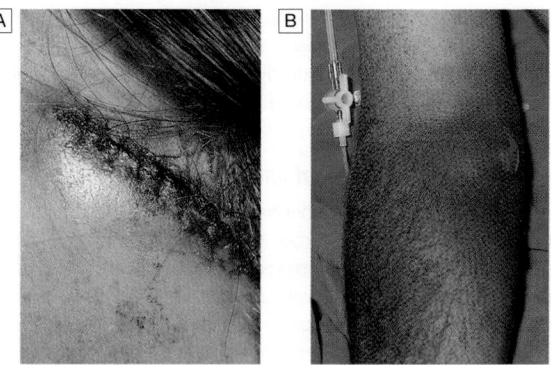

Fig. 13.20 Manifestations of skin infection with *Staphylococcus aureus*. [A] Wound infection. [B] Cannula-related infection.

13.39 How to assess an intravenous (IV) cannula using the visual infusion phlebitis (VIP) score		
Clinical features	**Score**	**Assessment and management**
IV site appears healthy	0	**No signs of phlebitis** Observe cannula
One of the following is evident: Slight pain near IV site Slight redness near IV site	1	**Possible first signs of phlebitis** Observe cannula
Two of the following are evident: Pain near IV site Erythema Swelling	2	**Early stage of phlebitis** Resite cannula
ALL of the following are evident and extensive: Pain along path of cannula Erythema Induration	3	**Medium stage of phlebitis** Resite cannula Consider treatment
ALL of the following are evident and extensive: Pain along path of cannula Erythema Induration Palpable venous cord	4	**Advanced stage of phlebitis or start of thrombophlebitis** Resite cannula Consider treatment
ALL of the following are evident: Pain along path of cannula Erythema Induration Palpable venous cord Pyrexia	5	**Advanced stage of thrombophlebitis** Initiate treatment Resite cannula

Adapted from Jackson A. Infection control: a battle in vein infusion phlebitis. Nursing Times 1997; 94:68–71.

Resistance to vancomycin/teicoplanin (glycopeptides) in either glycopeptide intermediate *Staph. aureus* (GISA) or, rarely, vancomycin-resistant (VRSA) strains threatens management of serious staphylococcal infections. Meticillin-resistant *Staph. aureus* (MRSA) is now a major worldwide health care-acquired pathogen, accounting for up to 40% of staphylococcal bacteraemia in high-income countries. Community-acquired MRSA (c-MRSA) currently accounts for 50% of all MRSA infections in the USA. These organisms have also acquired other toxins, such as Panton–Valentine leukocidin (PVL), and can cause rapidly fatal infection in young people. Clinicians must be aware of the potential danger of these infections and implement appropriate locally approved infection control measures.

Treatment options for MRSA are shown in Box 6.16. Treatment should always be based on the results of antimicrobial susceptibility testing, since resistance to all these agents occurs. Milder MRSA infections may be treated with clindamycin, tetracyclines or co-trimoxazole. Glycopeptides, linezolid and daptomycin are reserved for treatment of more severe infections. Toxin-producing MRSA infections should be treated with the addition of protein-inhibiting antibiotics (clindamycin, linezolid).

Staphylococcal toxic shock syndrome

Staphylococcal toxic shock syndrome (TSS) is a life-threatening disease associated with infection by *Staph. aureus* producing a specific toxin (toxic shock syndrome toxin 1, TSST1). Formerly seen in young women in association with the use of highly absorbent intravaginal tampons, it can occur with any infection involving a TSST1-producing *Staph. aureus* strain. The toxin acts as a 'super-antigen', triggering significant T-cell activation and massive cytokine release.

TSS has an abrupt onset with high fever, generalised systemic upset (myalgia, headache, sore throat and vomiting), a widespread erythematous blanching rash resembling scarlet fever, and hypotension. It rapidly progresses over a few hours to multi-organ failure, leading to death in 10%–20%. Recovery is accompanied at 7–10 days by desquamation (Fig. 13.21).

The diagnosis is clinical and may be confirmed in menstrual cases by finding a retained tampon with staphylococci on Gram stain. Subsequent culture and demonstration of toxin production are confirmatory.

Management

Treatment is with immediate and aggressive fluid resuscitation and an intravenous antistaphylococcal antimicrobial, usually with the addition of a protein synthesis inhibitor (e.g. clindamycin) to inhibit toxin production. Intravenous immunoglobulin is occasionally added in the most severe cases. Women who recover from tampon-associated TSS should avoid tampons for at least 1 year and they should be advised that the condition can recur.

Streptococcal infections

Streptococci are oropharyngeal and gut commensals, which appear as Gram-positive cocci in chains (see Fig. 6.3). They were classified by the pattern of haemolysis they produce on blood agar (see Fig. 6.4), by their 'Lancefield serogroups' (Box 13.40) but are now usually identified and classified by matrix-assisted laser desorption/ionisation time-of-flight (MALDI-TOF) mass spectrometry. Some streptococci (e.g. *Strep. milleri* group) defy simple classification.

Strep. pyogenes (group A streptococcus, GAS) is the leading cause of bacterial pharyngitis. Although the presence of fever, tender anterior lymphadenopathy and purulent tonsillar exudate and the absence of cough make streptococcal pharyngitis more likely than viral infection, clinical features alone are unreliable for diagnosing streptococcal pharyngitis. GAS are the major cause of cellulitis, erysipelas and impetigo. They also cause the post-streptococcal syndromes of glomerulonephrits and rheumatic fever, which are described in Chapters 14 and 16, respectively. The closely related *Streptococcus dysgalactiae* subsp. *equisimilis* (SDSE) (formerly groups C and G) cause cellulitis, particularly in older people, diabetic or immunocompromised patients. *Streptococcus agalactiae* (group B streptococci (GBS)) colonise the gut and vagina. They cause post-partum and neonatal sepsis, as well as other deep infections (infective endocarditis, septic arthritis, osteomyelitis etc.), especially in older people.

Streptococcal scarlet fever

Strep. pyogenes (or occasionally SDSE) causing pharyngitis, tonsillitis or other infection may lead to scarlet fever, if the infecting strain produces a streptococcal pyrogenic exotoxin. Scarlet fever is most common in school-age children, but can also occur in young adults who have contact with young children. A diffuse erythematous rash occurs, which blanches on pressure (Fig. 13.22A), classically with circumoral pallor. The tongue, initially coated, becomes red and swollen ('strawberry tongue', Fig. 13.22B). The disease lasts about 7 days, the rash disappearing in 7–10 days, followed by a fine desquamation. Residual petechial lesions in the antecubital fossa, 'Pastia's sign', can occur (Fig. 13.22C).

Treatment involves intravenous benzylpenicillin or an oral penicillin plus symptomatic measures.

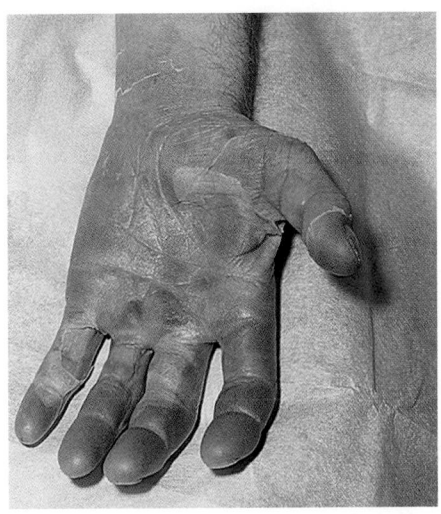

Fig. 13.21 Full-thickness desquamation after staphylococcal toxic shock syndrome.

13

> **i 13.40 Streptococcal and related infections**
>
> **β-haemolytic group A (*Streptococcus pyogenes*)**
>
> - Skin and soft tissue infection (including erysipelas, impetigo, necrotising fasciitis)
> - Streptococcal toxic shock syndrome
> - Puerperal sepsis
> - Scarlet fever
> - Glomerulonephritis
> - Rheumatic fever
> - Bone and joint infection
> - Tonsillitis
>
> **β-haemolytic streptococci group B (*Strep. agalactiae*)**
>
> - Neonatal infections, including meningitis
> - Female pelvic infections
> - Cellulitis
>
> **β-haemolytic streptococci groups C and G**
>
> - Cellulitis
> - Endocarditis
> - Pharyngitis
> - Septic arthritis
>
> **α-, β- or non-haemolytic group D (*Enterococcus faecalis, E. faecium*)**
>
> - Endocarditis
> - Intra-abdominal infections
> - Urinary tract infection
>
> **α- or non-haemolytic group D (*Strep. gallolyticus* subsp. *gallolyticus/S. bovis* biotype I)**
>
> - Bacteraemia/endocarditis associated with large bowel malignancy
>
> **α-haemolytic optochin-resistant (viridans streptococci – *Strep. mitis, Strep. sanguis, Strep. mutans, Strep. salivarius*)**
>
> - Sepsis in immunosuppressed
> - Endocarditis
>
> **α-haemolytic optochin-sensitive (*Strep. pneumoniae*)**
>
> - Pneumonia
> - Meningitis
> - Endocarditis
> - Otitis media
> - Sepsis
> - Spontaneous bacterial peritonitis
> - Sinusitis
>
> **Variable haemolysis (*Strep. milleri* group – *Strep. anginosus, Strep. intermedius, Strep. constellatus*)**
>
> - Endocarditis
> - Intra-abdominal infections
> - Urinary tract infection
>
> **Anaerobic streptococci (*Peptostreptococcus* spp.)**
>
> - Sepsis in immunosuppressed
> - Endocarditis
>
> **N.B.** All streptococci can cause sepsis.

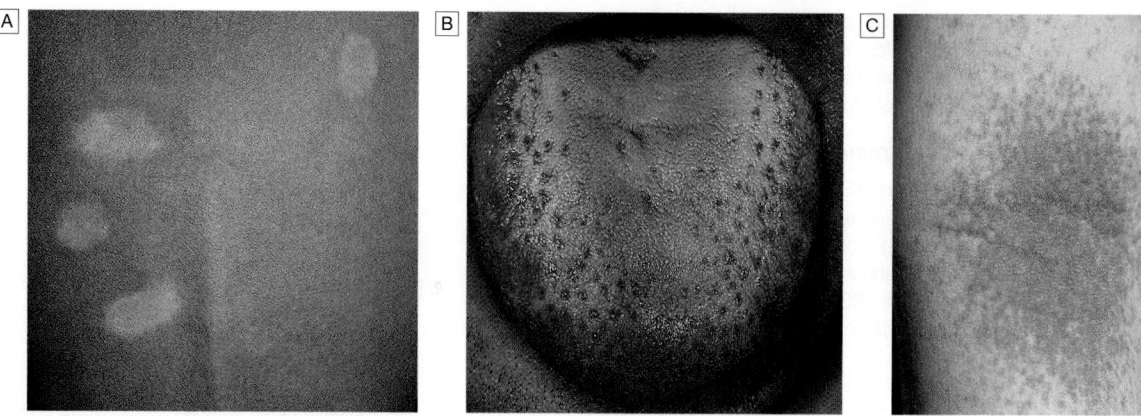

Fig. 13.22 Clinical features of scarlet fever. [A] Characteristic rash with blanching on pressure. [B] 'Strawberry tongue'. [C] Pastia's sign: a petechial rash in the cubital fossa.

Streptococcal toxic shock syndrome

Strep. pyogenes and SDSE can produce one of a variety of toxins, such as streptococcal pyogenic exotoxin A. Like staphylococcal TSST1 (see above), these act as super-antigens. Initially, an influenza-like illness occurs, with signs of localised infection in 50% of cases, most often involving the skin and soft tissues. A faint erythematous rash, mainly on the chest, rapidly progresses to circulatory shock. Without aggressive management, multi-organ failure will develop.

Judicious fluid resuscitation is combined with parenteral antistreptococcal antibiotic therapy, usually with benzylpenicillin and clindamycin, to inhibit toxin production. Intravenous immunoglobulin is often administered. If necrotising fasciitis is present, it should be treated as described on page 272 with urgent débridement.

Treponematoses

Syphilis

This disease is described in Chapter 15.

Endemic treponematoses

Yaws

Yaws is a granulomatous disease, mainly involving the skin and bones, caused by *Treponema pertenue*. It is morphologically and serologically indistinguishable from the microorganisms causing syphilis and pinta. The geographical origin and sexual history of patients helps exclude false-positive syphilis serology due to endemic treponemal infections. Between 1950 and 1960, WHO campaigns treated over 60 million people and eradicated yaws from many areas, but the disease has persisted throughout the tropics. A resurgence occurred in the 1980s and 1990s in West and Central Africa and the South Pacific.

Organisms are transmitted by bodily contact from a patient with infectious yaws through minor skin abrasions of the recipient, usually a child. After 3–4 weeks' incubation, a proliferative granuloma containing numerous treponemes develops at the inoculation site. This primary lesion is followed by secondary eruptions. In addition, there may be hypertrophic periosteal bone lesions, with underlying cortical rarefaction. Lesions of late yaws are characterised by destructive changes that closely resemble the osteitis and gummas of tertiary syphilis. These heal with scarring and deformity. Investigations and management are outlined in Box 13.41. Improved housing and hygiene, combined with mass chemotherapy programmes, have achieved dramatic success in the control of yaws.

Pinta and bejel

These two treponemal infections occur in poor rural populations with low standards of domestic hygiene but are found in separate parts of the world. They have features in common, notably that they are transmitted

---

> **i** | **13.41 Diagnosis and treatment of yaws, pinta and bejel**
>
> **Diagnosis of early stages**
> - Detection of spirochaetes in exudate of lesions by dark ground microscopy
>
> **Diagnosis of latent and early stages**
> - Positive serological tests, as for syphilis (see Box 15.8)
>
> **Treatment of all stages**
> - Single intramuscular injection of 1.2 g long-acting penicillin, e.g. benzathine benzylpenicillin

by contact, usually within the family and not sexually, and in the case of bejel, through common eating and drinking utensils. Their diagnosis and management are as for yaws (see Box 13.41).

- *Pinta.* Pinta is found only in South and Central America, where its incidence is declining. The infection is confined to the skin. The early lesions are scaly papules or dyschromic patches on the skin. The late lesions are often depigmented and disfiguring.
- *Bejel.* Bejel is the Middle Eastern name for non-venereal syphilis, which has a patchy distribution across sub-Saharan Africa, the Middle East, Central Asia and Australia. It has been eradicated from Eastern Europe. Transmission is most commonly from the mouth of the mother or child and the primary mucosal lesion is seldom seen. The early and late lesions resemble those of secondary and tertiary syphilis but cardiovascular and neurological disease is rare.

Tropical ulcer

Tropical ulcer is due to a synergistic bacterial infection caused by a fusobacterium (*Fusobacterium ulcerans*, an anaerobe) and *Treponema vincentii*. It is common in hot, humid regions. The ulcer commonly involves the lower legs, developing as a papule that rapidly breaks down to form a sharply defined, painful ulcer. The ulcer base has a foul slough. Penicillin and metronidazole are useful in the early stages but rest, elevation and dressings are the mainstays of treatment.

Buruli ulcer

Mycobacterium ulcerans causes Buruli ulcer in tropical rainforests. Cases were declining until 2016 but have risen since, with 2713 cases reported in 2018. Outside West and Central Africa occasional cases have been reported in Australia.

The initial lesion is a small subcutaneous nodule on the arm or leg. This breaks down to form a shallow, necrotic ulcer with deeply undermined edges, which extends rapidly. Healing may occur after 6 months but granuloma formation and the accompanying fibrosis cause contractures and deformity. Clumps of acid-fast bacilli are detected in the ulcer floor.

A combination of rifampicin and clarithromycin can cure the infection. Infected tissue should be removed surgically. Wound and lymphoedema management, surgery, including skin grafting, and physiotherapy all play a role in management and prevention of disability.

Systemic bacterial infections

Brucellosis

Brucellosis is an enzootic infection (i.e. endemic in animals) caused by Gram-negative coccobacilli. The four species causing human disease and their animal hosts are: *Brucella melitensis* (goats, sheep and camels in Europe, especially the Mediterranean basin, the Middle East, Africa, India, Central Asia and South America), *B. abortus* (cattle, mainly in Africa, Asia and South America), *B. suis* (pigs in South Asia) and *B. canis* (dogs). *B. melitensis* causes the most severe disease; *B. suis* is often associated with abscess formation.

Infected animals may excrete *Brucella* spp. in their milk for prolonged periods and human infection is acquired by ingesting contaminated dairy products (especially unpasteurised milk), uncooked meat or offal. Animal urine, faeces, vaginal discharge and uterine products may transmit infection through abraded skin or via splashes and aerosols to the respiratory tract and conjunctiva.

Clinical features

Brucella spp. are intracellular organisms that survive for long periods within the reticulo-endothelial system. This favours chronicity and relapse, even after antimicrobial therapy.

Acute illness is characterised by a high swinging temperature, rigors, lethargy, headache, arthralgia, myalgia and scrotal pain. Occasionally, there is delirium, abdominal pain and constipation. Physical signs are non-specific, e.g. enlarged lymph nodes. Splenomegaly may cause thrombocytopenia.

Localised infection (Fig. 13.23) occurs in approximately 30% of patients, particularly if treatment is delayed.

Diagnosis

Definitive diagnosis depends on culture of the organism. Blood cultures are positive in 75%–80% of *B. melitensis* and 50% of *B. abortus* infections. Bone marrow culture is not routine but may increase the diagnostic yield if antibiotics have been used prior to culture. CSF culture in neurobrucellosis is positive in about 30% of cases. The laboratory should be informed of suspected brucellosis, to allow appropriate laboratory steps to prevent laboratory worker infection.

Serology may aid diagnosis. In endemic areas, a single high antibody titre of more than 1/320 or a fourfold rise in titre supports a diagnosis of acute infection. The test usually takes several weeks to become positive but should eventually detect 95% of acute infections.

Management

Aminoglycosides show synergistic activity with tetracyclines and treatment regimens for different forms of brucellosis are outlined in Box 13.42.

Borrelia infections

Borrelia are flagellated spirochaetal bacteria that infect humans after bites from ticks or lice. They cause a variety of human infections worldwide (Box 13.43).

Lyme disease

Lyme disease is caused by *B. burgdorferi*, which occurs in the USA, Europe, Russia, China, Japan and Australia. In Europe, two additional genospecies are also encountered, *B. afzelii* and *B. garinii*. The reservoir of infection is ixodid (hard) ticks that feed on a variety of large mammals, particularly deer. Birds spread ticks over a wide area. The organism is transmitted to humans via the bite of larval, nymphal or adult ticks.

Ehrlichiosis is a common co-infection with Lyme disease. Two forms occur: *Anaplasma phagocytophilum*, human granulocytic anaplasmosis (HGA); and *Ehrlichia chaffeensis*, human monocytic ehrlichiosis (HME).

Clinical features

There are three stages of disease. Progression may be arrested at any stage.

- *Early localised disease.* The characteristic feature is a skin reaction around the site of the tick bite, known as erythema migrans (Fig. 13.24). Initially, a red 'bull's eye' macule or papule appears 2–30 days after the bite. It then enlarges peripherally with central

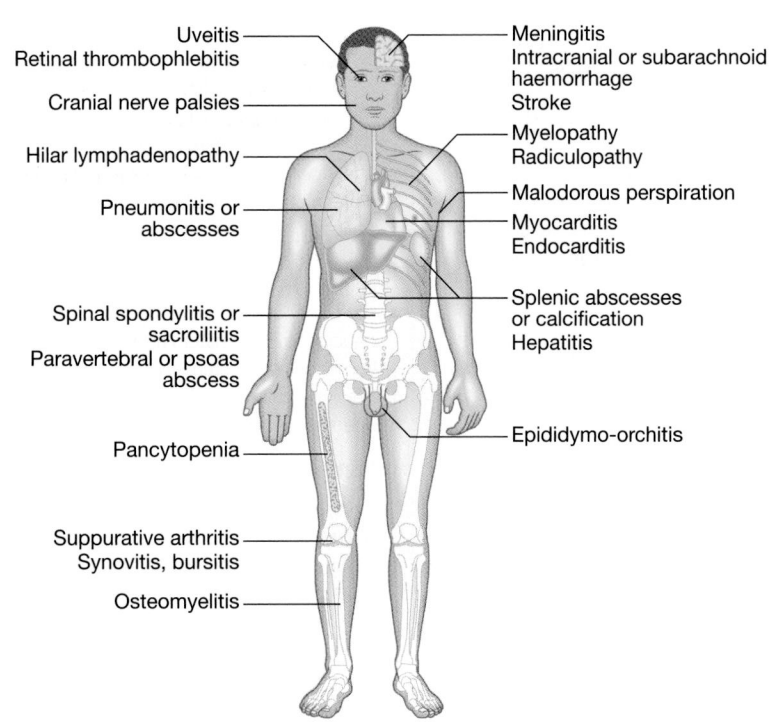

Fig. 13.23 Clinical features of brucellosis.

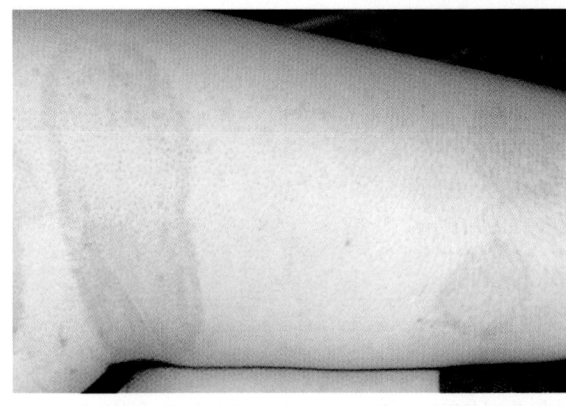

Fig. 13.24 Rash of erythema migrans in Lyme disease with metastatic secondary lesions. *Courtesy of Dr Ravi Gowda, Royal Hallamshire Hospital, Sheffield.*

clearing and may persist for months. Atypical forms are common. The lesion is not pathognomonic of Lyme disease since similar lesions can occur after tick bites. Acute manifestations, such as fever, headache and regional lymphadenopathy, may develop with or without the rash.

- *Early disseminated disease.* Dissemination occurs via the blood stream and lymphatics. There may be a systemic reaction with malaise, arthralgia and, occasionally, metastatic areas of erythema migrans (see Fig. 13.24). Neurological involvement may follow weeks or months after infection. Common features include lympho-cytic meningitis, cranial nerve palsies (especially unilateral or bilateral facial nerve palsy) and peripheral neuropathy. Radiculopathy, often painful, may present a year or more after initial infection. Carditis, sometimes accompanied by atrioventricular conduction defects, occurs in the USA but is rare in Europe.
- *Late disease.* Late manifestations include arthritis, polyneuritis and encephalopathy. Prolonged arthritis, particularly affecting large joints, and brain parenchymal involvement, causing neuropsychiatric abnormalities, may occur but are rare in the UK. Acrodermatitis chronica atrophicans is an uncommon late complication seen more frequently in Europe than North America. Doughy, patchy discoloration occurs on the peripheries, eventually leading to shiny atrophic skin. The lesions are mistaken for those of peripheral vascular disease. In patients with facial nerve palsy coming from an endemic area or having risk factors, Lyme disease should be excluded.

Diagnosis

The diagnosis of early Lyme borreliosis is clinical. Culture from biopsy material is rarely available, has a low yield and may take over 6 weeks. Antibody detection is frequently negative early in the course of the disease but sensitivity increases to 90%–100% in disseminated or late disease. Immunofluorescence or ELISA can give false-positive reactions in a number of conditions, including other spirochaetal infections, infectious mononucleosis, rheumatoid arthritis and systemic lupus erythematosus (SLE). Immunoblot (Western blot) techniques are more specific and should be used to confirm the diagnosis. Microorganism DNA detection by PCR has been applied to blood, urine, CSF and biopsies of skin and synovium.

Management

Asymptomatic patients with positive antibody tests do not require treatment. However, erythema migrans always requires therapy because organisms may persist and cause progressive disease, even if the skin lesions resolve. Standard therapy consists of a 14-day course of doxycycline (200 mg daily) or amoxicillin (500 mg 3 times daily). Some 15% of patients with early disease will develop a mild febrile reaction (Jarisch–Herxheimer JHR) during the first 24 hours of therapy. In pregnant women and small children with penicillin allergy, or in those allergic to amoxicillin and doxycycline, 14-day treatment with cefuroxime axetil (500 mg twice daily) or azithromycin (500 mg once daily) may be used.

Disseminated disease and arthritis require therapy for a minimum of 28 days. Arthritis may respond poorly and prolonged or repeated courses may be necessary. Neuroborreliosis is treated with parenteral β-lactam antibiotics for 3–4 weeks; third-generation cephalosporins such as ceftriaxone are preferred.

Prevention

Protective clothing and insect repellents should be used in tick-infested areas. Since the risk of borrelial transmission is lower in the first few hours of a blood feed, prompt removal of ticks is advisable. Unfortunately, larval and nymphal ticks are tiny and may not be noticed. Where risk of transmission is high, a single 200 mg dose of doxycycline, given within 72 hours of exposure, has been shown to prevent erythema migrans.

Louse-borne relapsing fever

The human body louse, *Pediculus humanus*, causes itching. Borreliae (*B. recurrentis*) are released from infected lice when they are crushed during scratching, inoculating borreliae into the skin. The disease occurs worldwide, with epidemic relapsing fever most often seen in Central/East Africa and South America.

The borreliae multiply in the blood, where they are abundant in the febrile phases, and invade most tissues, especially the liver, spleen and meninges.

Clinical features

Onset is sudden with fever. The temperature rises to 39.5–40.5°C, accompanied by a tachycardia, headache, generalised aching, injected conjunctivae (Fig. 13.25) and herpes labialis. Thrombocytopenia is associated with a petechial rash and epistaxis. As the disease progresses tender hepatosplenomegaly, jaundice and elevated transaminases are common. There may be severe serosal and intestinal haemorrhage, delirium and meningism. The fever ends in crisis between the fourth and tenth days, often associated with profuse sweating, hypotension and circulatory and cardiac failure. Fever may resolve but, in a proportion of patients, after an afebrile period of about 7 days, there are one or more febrile relapses, which are usually milder and less prolonged. Without specific treatment, the mortality rate is up to 40%, especially among older and malnourished patients.

Investigations and management

Dark ground microscopy of a wet film or Wright–Giemsa-stained thick and thin films demonstrate the organism in blood from a febrile patient.

Treatment aims to eradicate the organism and prevent relapses, while minimising the severe JHR that inevitably follows successful chemotherapy. The safest treatment is procaine penicillin 300 mg intramuscularly, followed the next day by 0.5 g tetracycline. Tetracycline alone is effective and prevents relapse, but may give rise to a worse reaction. Doxycycline 200 mg once orally in place of tetracycline has the advantage of also being curative for typhus, which often accompanies epidemics of relapsing fever. JHR is best managed in a high-dependency unit with expert nursing and medical care.

The patient, clothing and all contacts must be freed from lice, as in epidemic typhus.

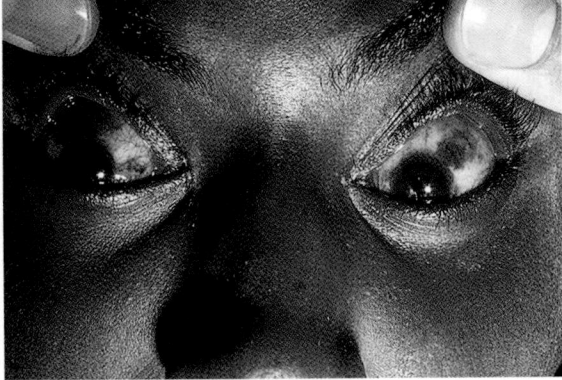

Fig. 13.25 Louse-borne relapsing fever. Injected conjunctivae.

Tick-borne relapsing fever

Soft ticks (*Ornithodoros* spp.) transmit *B. duttonii* (and other *Borrelia* species) through saliva while feeding on their host. People sleeping in mud houses are at risk, as the tick hides in crevices during the day and feeds on humans during the night. Rodents are the reservoir except in East Africa, where humans are the reservoir. Clinical manifestations are similar to those seen with the louse-borne disease but microorganisms are detected in fewer patients on dark-field microscopy. A 7-day course (due to a higher relapse rate than in louse-borne relapsing fever) of treatment with either tetracycline (500 mg 4 times daily) or erythromycin (500 mg 4 times daily) is needed.

Leptospirosis

Microbiology and epidemiology

Leptospirosis is one of the most common zoonotic diseases, favoured by a tropical climate and flooding during the monsoon but occurring worldwide. Leptospires are tightly coiled, thread-like organisms about 5–7 μm in length, which are actively motile; each end is bent into a hook. *Leptospira interrogans* is pathogenic for humans. The genus can be separated into more than 200 serovars (subtypes) belonging to 23 serogroups.

Leptospirosis is ubiquitous in wildlife and in many domestic animals. The organisms persist indefinitely in the convoluted tubules of the kidney and are shed into the urine in massive numbers, but infection is asymptomatic in the host. The most frequent hosts are rodents, especially the common rat (*Rattus norvegicus*). Particular leptospiral serogroups are associated with characteristic animal hosts; for example, *L. icterohaemorrhagiae* is the classical parasite of rats and *L. canicola* of dogs. There is nevertheless considerable overlap in host–serogroup associations.

Leptospires can penetrate intact skin or mucous membranes but human infection is facilitated by cuts and abrasions. Prolonged immersion in contaminated water facilitates invasion, as the spirochaete survives in water for months. Leptospirosis is common in the tropics and also in freshwater sports enthusiasts.

Clinical features

After a relatively brief bacteraemia, invading organisms are distributed throughout the body, mainly in kidneys, liver, meninges and brain. The incubation period averages 1–2 weeks. Four main clinical syndromes can be discerned and clinical features can involve multiple different organ systems (Fig. 13.26).

Bacteraemic leptospirosis

Bacteraemia with any serogroup can produce a non-specific illness with high fever, weakness, muscle pain and tenderness (especially of the calf and back), intense headache and photophobia, and sometimes diarrhoea and vomiting. Conjunctival congestion is the only notable physical sign. The illness comes to an end after about 1 week, or else merges into one of the other forms of infection.

Aseptic meningitis

Classically associated with *L. canicola* infection, this illness is very difficult to distinguish from viral meningitis. The conjunctivae may be congested but there are no other differentiating signs. Laboratory clues include a neutrophil leucocytosis, abnormal LFTs and the occasional presence of albumin and casts in the urine.

Icteric leptospirosis (Weil's disease)

Fewer than 10% of symptomatic infections result in severe icteric illness. Weil's disease is a dramatic life-threatening event, characterised by fever, haemorrhages, jaundice and acute kidney injury. Conjunctival hyperaemia is a frequent feature. The patient may have a transient macular erythematous rash but the characteristic skin changes are purpura and large areas of bruising. In severe cases there may be epistaxis, haematemesis and melaena, or bleeding into the pleural, pericardial or

13

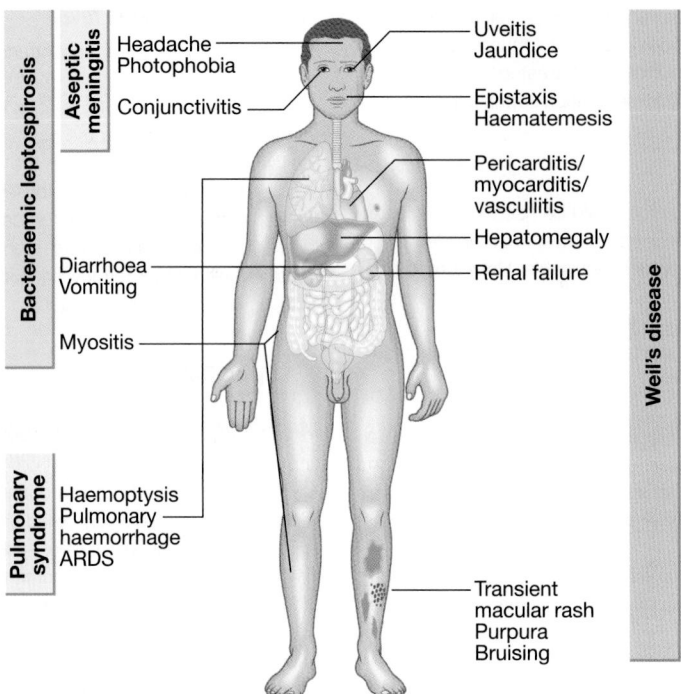

Fig. 13.26 Clinical syndromes of leptospirosis. (ARDS = acute respiratory distress syndrome)

subarachnoid spaces. Thrombocytopenia, probably related to activation of endothelial cells with platelet adhesion and aggregation, is present in 50% of cases. Jaundice and hepatomegaly usually occur without hepatic failure or encephalopathy. Acute kidney injury, primarily caused by impaired renal perfusion and acute tubular necrosis, causes oliguria or anuria, with albumin, blood and casts in the urine.

Weil's disease may also be associated with myocarditis, encephalitis and aseptic meningitis. Uveitis and iritis may appear months after apparent clinical recovery.

Pulmonary syndrome

This syndrome has long been recognised in the Far East and has been described during an outbreak of leptospirosis in Nicaragua. It is characterised by haemoptysis, patchy lung infiltrates on chest X-ray, and respiratory failure. Total bilateral lung consolidation and ARDS with multi-organ dysfunction may develop, with a high mortality (over 50%).

Diagnosis

A polymorphonuclear leucocytosis is accompanied in severe infection by thrombocytopenia and elevated blood levels of creatine kinase. In jaundiced patients, there is hepatitis and the prothrombin time may be prolonged. The CSF in leptospiral meningitis shows a variable cellular response, a moderately elevated protein level and normal glucose content. Acute kidney injury due to interstitial nephritis is common.

In the tropics, dengue, malaria, typhoid fever, scrub typhus and hantavirus infection are important differential diagnoses.

Definitive diagnosis of leptospirosis depends on isolation of the organism, serological tests or detection of specific DNA. In general, however, it is probably under-diagnosed.

- Blood cultures are most likely to be positive if taken before day 10 of illness. Special media are required and cultures may have to be incubated for several weeks.
- Leptospires appear in the urine during the second week of illness, and in untreated patients may be recovered on culture for several months.
- Serological tests are diagnostic if seroconversion or a fourfold increase in titre is demonstrated. The microscopic agglutination test

(MAT) is the investigation of choice and can become positive by the end of the first week. IgM ELISA and immunofluorescent techniques are easier to perform, however, while rapid immunochromatographic tests are specific they are of only moderate sensitivity in the first week of illness.

- Detection of leptospiral DNA by PCR is possible in blood in early symptomatic disease, and in urine from day 8 of illness and for many months thereafter.

Management and prevention

The general care of the patient is critically important. Blood transfusion for haemorrhage and careful attention to renal function, the usual cause of death, are especially important. Acute kidney injury is potentially reversible with adequate support, such as dialysis. Most infections are self-limiting. Therapy with either oral doxycycline (100 mg twice daily for 1 week) or intravenous penicillin (900 mg 4 times daily for 1 week) is effective but may not prevent the development of renal failure. Parenteral ceftriaxone (1 g daily) is as effective as penicillin. JHR may occur but is usually mild. Uveitis is treated with a combination of systemic antibiotics and local glucocorticoids. There is no role for the routine use of glucocorticoids in the management of leptospirosis.

Trials in military personnel have shown that infection with *L. interrogans* can be prevented by taking prophylactic doxycycline 200 mg weekly.

Plague

Plague is caused by *Yersinia pestis*, a small Gram-negative bacillus that is spread between rodents by their fleas. If domestic rats become infected, infected fleas may bite humans. Hunters and trappers can contract plague from handling rodents. In the late stages of human plague, *Y. pestis* may be expectorated and spread between humans by droplets, causing 'pneumonic plague'.

Epidemics of plague, such as the 'Black Death', have occurred since ancient times. It is often said that the first sign of plague is the appearance of dead rats. Plague foci are widely distributed throughout the world, including the USA; human cases are reported from about 10 countries per year (Fig. 13.27).

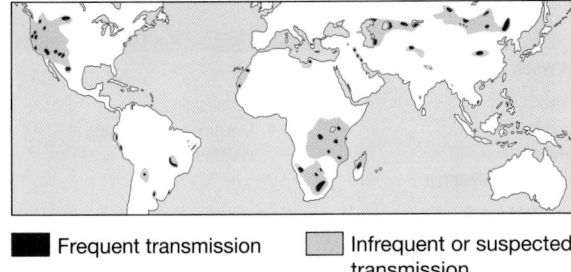

Frequent transmission   Infrequent or suspected
                         transmission

Fig. 13.27 Foci of the transmission of plague. *Reproduced by permission of the World Health Organization.*

Y. pestis is a potential bioweapon because of the possibility of person-to-person spread and the high fatality rate associated with pneumonic plague.

Clinical features

Organisms inoculated through the skin are transported rapidly to the draining lymph nodes, where they elicit a severe inflammatory response that may be haemorrhagic. If the infection is not contained, sepsis ensues and necrotic, purulent or haemorrhagic lesions develop in many organs. Oliguria and shock follow, and disseminated intravascular coagulation may result in widespread haemorrhage. Inhalation of *Y. pestis* causes alveolitis. The incubation period is 3–6 days but shorter in pneumonic plague.

Bubonic plague

In this, the most common form of the disease, onset is usually sudden, with a rigor, high fever, dry skin and severe headache. Soon, aching and swelling at the site of the affected lymph nodes begin. The groin is the most common site of the 'bubo', a collection of swollen lymph nodes and surrounding tissue. Some infections are relatively mild but, in the majority, toxaemia quickly increases, with a rapid pulse, hypotension and delirium. The spleen is usually palpable.

Septicaemic plague

Those without a bubo usually deteriorate rapidly, with high associated mortality. Older people are more prone to septicaemic plague. The patient is toxic and may have gastrointestinal symptoms, such as nausea, vomiting, abdominal pain and diarrhoea. DIC may occur, manifested by bleeding from various orifices or puncture sites, along with ecchymoses. Hypotension, shock, renal failure and ARDS may develop. Meningitis, pneumonia and expectoration of blood-stained sputum containing *Y. pestis* may complicate septicaemic, or occasionally bubonic, plague.

Pneumonic plague

Following primary infection in the lung, the onset of disease is very sudden, with cough and dyspnoea. The patient expectorates copious blood-stained, frothy, highly infective sputum, becomes cyanosed and dies. Chest radiology reveals bilateral infiltrates, which may be nodular and progress to an ARDS-like picture.

Investigations

The organism may be cultured from blood, sputum and bubo aspirates. For rapid diagnosis, Gram, Giemsa and Wayson's stains (the latter containing methylene blue) are applied to smears from these sites. *Y. pestis* is seen as bipolar staining coccobacilli, sometimes referred to as having a 'safety pin' appearance. Smears are also subjected to antigen detection by immunofluorescence, using *Y. pestis* F1 antigen-specific antibodies. The diagnosis may be confirmed by seroconversion or a single high titre (>128) of anti-F1 antibodies in serum. DNA detection by PCR is under evaluation.

Plague is a notifiable disease under international health regulations.

Management

If the diagnosis is suspected on clinical and epidemiological grounds, treatment must be started as soon as, or even before, samples have been collected for laboratory diagnosis. Streptomycin (1 g twice daily) or gentamicin (1 mg/kg 3 times daily) is the drug of choice. Tetracycline (500 mg 4 times daily) and chloramphenicol (12.5 mg/kg 4 times daily) are alternatives. Fluoroquinolones (ciprofloxacin and levofloxacin) may be as effective but there is less clinical experience. Treatment may also be needed for acute circulatory failure, DIC and hypoxia.

Prevention and infection control

Rats and fleas should be controlled. In endemic areas, people should avoid handling and skinning wild animals. The patient should be isolated for the first 48 hours or until clinical improvement begins. Attendants must wear gowns, masks and gloves. Symptomatic or asymptomatic close contacts of cases of pneumonic plague should receive post-exposure antibiotic prophylaxis (doxycycline 100 mg or ciprofloxacin 500 mg twice daily) for 7 days.

A recombinant subunit vaccine (protein antigens F1 + V) is in development.

Listeriosis

Listeria monocytogenes is an environmental Gram-positive bacillus that can contaminate food. Outbreaks have been associated with raw vegetables, soft cheeses, under-cooked chicken, fish, meat and pâtés. The bacterium demonstrates 'cold enrichment', outgrowing other contaminating bacteria during refrigeration. Although food-borne outbreaks of gastroenteritis have been reported in immuno-competent individuals, *Listeria* causes more significant invasive infection, especially in pregnant women, older adults (over 55 years) and the immunocompromised.

In pregnancy, in addition to systemic symptoms of fever and myalgia, listeriosis causes chorioamnionitis, fetal deaths, abortions and neonatal infection. In other susceptible individuals, it causes systemic illness due to bacteraemia without focal symptoms. Meningitis, similar to other bacterial meningitis but with normal CSF glucose, is the next most common presentation; CSF usually shows increased neutrophils but occasionally only the mononuclear cells are increased (see Box 28.6).

Investigations and management

Diagnosis is made by blood and CSF culture. The organism grows readily in culture media.

The most effective regimen consists of a combination of intravenous amoxicillin or ampicillin plus an aminoglycoside. A sulfamethoxazole/trimethoprim combination can be used in those with penicillin allergy. Cephalosporins are of no use in this infection, as the organism is inherently resistant, an important consideration when treating meningitis empirically.

Proper treatment of foods before eating is the key to preventing listeriosis. Pregnant women are advised to avoid high-risk products, including soft cheeses.

Enteric fevers (typhoid and paratyphoid)

Typhoid and paratyphoid fevers, which are transmitted by the faecal–oral route, are important causes of fever in South Asia, sub-Saharan Africa and Latin America. Elsewhere, they are relatively rare. Enteric fevers are caused by infection with *Salmonella enterica* serotypes Typhi and Paratyphi A, B and C, but invasive disease is occasionally observed with non-typhoidal *Salmonella* spp. After a few days of bacteraemia, the bacilli localise, mainly in the lymphoid tissue of the small intestine, resulting in typical lesions in the Peyer's patches and follicles. These swell at first, then ulcerate and usually heal. After clinical recovery, about 5% of patients become chronic carriers (i.e. continue to excrete the bacteria after 1 year); the bacilli may live in the gallbladder for months or years and pass intermittently in the stool and, less commonly, in the urine.

13

Clinical features

Typhoid fever

Clinical features are outlined in Box 13.44. The incubation period is typically about 10–14 days but can be longer, and the onset may be insidious. The temperature rises in a stepladder fashion for 4 or 5 days with malaise, increasing headache, drowsiness and aching in the limbs. Constipation may be caused by swelling of lymphoid tissue around the ileocaecal junction, although in children diarrhoea and vomiting may be prominent early in the illness. The pulse is often slower than would be expected from the height of the temperature, i.e. a relative bradycardia.

At the end of the first week, a rash may appear on the upper abdomen and on the back as sparse, slightly raised, rose-red spots, which fade on pressure. Cough and epistaxis occur. Around the 7th–10th day, the spleen becomes palpable. Constipation is followed by diarrhoea and abdominal distension with tenderness. Bronchitis and delirium may develop. If untreated, by the end of the second week the patient may be profoundly ill.

Paratyphoid fever

The course tends to be shorter than that of typhoid fever and the onset is often more abrupt, with acute enteritis. The rash may be more abundant and the intestinal complications less frequent.

Complications

These are given in Box 13.45. Haemorrhage from, or a perforation of, the ulcerated Peyer's patches may occur at the end of the second week or during the third week of the illness. A drop in temperature to normal or subnormal levels may be falsely reassuring in patients with intestinal haemorrhage. Additional complications may involve almost any viscus or system because of the bacteraemia present during the first week. Bone and joint infection is common in children with sickle-cell disease.

Investigations

In the first week, diagnosis may be difficult because, in this invasive stage with bacteraemia, the symptoms are those of a generalised infection without localising features. Typically, there is a leucopenia. Blood culture establishes the diagnosis and multiple cultures increase the yield. Stool cultures are often positive in the second and third weeks. The Widal test detects antibodies to the O and H antigens but is not specific.

Management

Antibiotic therapy must be guided by in vitro sensitivity testing. Chloramphenicol (500 mg 4 times daily), ampicillin (750 mg 4 times daily) and co-trimoxazole (960 mg PO or IV twice daily) are losing their effect due to resistance in many areas of the world, especially in South and South-east Asia. Fluoroquinolones are the drugs of choice (e.g. ciprofloxacin 500 mg twice daily), if nalidixic acid screening predicts susceptibility, but resistance is common, especially in South Asia and also in the UK. Extended-spectrum cephalosporins (ceftriaxone and cefotaxime) are useful alternatives but have a slightly increased treatment failure rate. Azithromycin (500 mg once daily) is an alternative when fluoroquinolone resistance is present but has not been validated in severe disease. Treatment should be continued for 14 days. Extensively drug-resistant ('XDR') typhoid has been causing an ongoing outbreak in Pakistan since 2016 and azithromycin is the only currently reliable oral therapy. Pyrexia may persist for up to 5 days after the start of specific therapy. Even with effective chemotherapy, there is still a danger of complications, recrudescence of the disease and the development of a carrier state.

Chronic carriers were formerly treated for 4 weeks with ciprofloxacin but may require an alternative agent and duration, as guided by antimicrobial sensitivity testing. Cholecystectomy may be necessary.

Prevention

Improved sanitation and living conditions reduce the incidence of typhoid. Travellers to countries where enteric infections are endemic

should receive typhoid vaccination. In young children a tetanus conjugate vaccine containing Vi polysaccharide conjugated to tetanus toxoid has over 80% efficacy and is superior to older inactivated injectable or oral live attenuated vaccines.

Tularaemia

Tularaemia is primarily a zoonotic disease of the northern hemisphere. It is caused by a highly infectious Gram-negative bacillus, *Francisella tularensis*. *F. tularensis* is passed transovarially (ensuring transmission from parent to progeny) in ticks, which allows persistence in nature without the absolute requirement for an infected animal reservoir. It is a potential bioweapon. Wild rabbits, rodents and domestic dogs or cats are potential reservoirs, and ticks, mosquitoes or other biting flies are the vectors.

Infection is introduced either through an arthropod or animal bite or via contact with infected animals, soil or water through skin abrasions. The most common 'ulceroglandular' variety of the disease (70%–80%) is characterised by skin ulceration with regional lymphadenopathy. There is also a purely 'glandular' form. Alternatively, inhalation of the infected aerosols may result in pulmonary tularaemia, presenting as pneumonia. Rarely, the portal of entry of infection may be the conjunctiva, leading to a nodular, ulcerated conjunctivitis with regional lymphadenopathy (an 'oculoglandular' form). Typhoidal tularaemia is a rare and serious form of tularaemia with vomiting, diarrhoea and hepatosplenomegaly, which may be complicated by pneumonia and meningitis.

Investigations and management

Demonstration of a single high titre (≥1:160) or a fourfold rise in 2–3 weeks in the tularaemia tube agglutination test confirms the diagnosis. Bacterial yield from the lesions is extremely poor. DNA detection methods to enable rapid diagnosis are in development.

Treatment consists of a 10–21-day course of parenteral aminoglycosides, streptomycin (7.5–10 mg/kg twice daily) or gentamicin (1.7 mg/kg 3 times daily), with doxycycline or ciprofloxacin offered as alternatives.

Melioidosis

Melioidosis is caused by *Burkholderia pseudomallei*, a saprophyte found in soil and water (rice paddy fields). Infection is by inoculation or inhalation, leading to bacteraemia, which is followed by the formation of abscesses in the lungs, liver and spleen. Patients with diabetes, renal stones, thalassaemia or severe burns are particularly susceptible. The disease is most common in South-east Asia and northern Australia, and carries a significant mortality. Disease may present years or decades after the initial exposure.

Clinical features

Pneumonia is the most common feature but localised skin nodules and abscesses, or sepsis, especially in diabetics, may occur. Diarrhoea and hepatosplenomegaly may be observed. The chest X-ray can resemble cavitary tuberculosis. In chronic forms, multiple abscesses occur in subcutaneous tissue, liver, spleen and bone, accompanied by profound weight loss.

Investigations and management

Culture of blood, sputum or pus on selective media, e.g. Ashdown agar, may yield *B. pseudomallei*. Latex agglutination has been developed as a rapid diagnostic test in Thailand and PCR-based tests are also available. Indirect haemagglutination testing can be helpful in travellers; however, most people in endemic areas are seropositive.

In the acute illness, prompt initiation of empirical therapy is life-saving. Ceftazidime 100 mg/kg (2 g 3 times daily) or meropenem (0.5–1 g 3 times daily) is given for 2–3 weeks, followed by maintenance therapy of co-trimoxazole (sulfamethoxazole 1600 mg plus trimethoprim 320 mg twice daily) or doxycycline 200 mg daily for 3–6 months. Abscesses should be drained surgically.

Actinomycete infections

Nocardiosis

Nocardiosis is caused by aerobic Actinomycetes of the genus *Nocardia*, found in the soil. Infection occurs follows direct traumatic inoculation or occasionally inhalation or ingestion. Nocardiosis can result in localised cutaneous ulcers or nodules, most often in the lower limbs. Chronic destructive infection in tropical countries can result in actinomycetoma, involving soft tissues with occasional penetration to the bone. Actinomycetoma may also be caused by other aerobic Actinomycetes, and a similar clinical syndrome, eumycetoma, is caused by filamentous fungi. Both conditions are discussed on page 344. Systemic *Nocardia* infection, most commonly in immunocompromised individuals, results in suppurative disease with lung and brain abscesses.

On microscopy, *Nocardia* spp. appear as long, filamentous, branching Gram-positive rods, which are also weakly acid-fast. They are easily grown in culture but require prolonged incubation.

Treatment of systemic infection is guided by sensitivity testing and typically requires combinations of imipenem with ceftriaxone, amikacin or co-trimoxazole, often for 6–12 months or longer. Meropenem, tigecycline, linezolid and minocycline may also be used with severe disease or with allergy, or when intolerance prevents use of the preferred agents. Abscesses are drained surgically when this is feasible. Localised cutaneous infection is usually treated with a single agent for 1–3 months. Treatment of actinomycetoma is discussed on page 344.

Actinomyces spp.

Actinomyces are anaerobic Actinomycetes, which are predominantly commensals of the oral cavity. They are capable of causing deep, suppurating infection in the head and neck (cervicofacial actinomycosis) and the lungs (thoracic actinomycosis). They also cause suppurating disease in the pelvis, associated with intrauterine contraceptive devices (IUCDs). Modern diagnostic techniques demonstrate that actinomycosis is caused by many different *Actinomyces* species, the most common of which is *Actinomyces israelii*. Treatment of established disease requires approximately 6–12 months of penicillin or doxycycline. Early disease may respond to shorter antibiotic courses.

Gastrointestinal bacterial infections

The approach to patients presenting with acute gastroenteritis is described on page 272.

Staphylococcal food poisoning

Staph. aureus is transmitted via the hands of food handlers to foodstuffs such as dairy products, including cheese, and cooked meats. Inappropriate storage of these foods allows growth of the organism and production of one or more heat-stable enterotoxins.

Nausea and profuse vomiting develop within 1–6 hours. Diarrhoea may not be marked. The toxins that cause the syndrome act as 'superantigens' and induce a significant neutrophil leucocytosis that may be clinically misleading. Most cases settle rapidly but severe dehydration can occasionally be life-threatening.

Antiemetics and appropriate fluid replacement are the mainstays of treatment. Suspect food should be cultured for staphylococci and demonstration of toxin production. Public health authorities should be notified if food vending is involved.

Bacillus cereus food poisoning

Ingestion of pre-formed heat-stable exotoxins of *B. cereus* causes rapid onset of vomiting and some diarrhoea within hours of food consumption, which resolves within 24 hours. Fried rice and freshly made sauces are frequent sources; the organism grows and produces enterotoxin during storage (Fig. 13.28). If viable bacteria are ingested and toxin formation takes place within the gut lumen, then the incubation period is longer (12–24 hours) and watery diarrhoea and cramps are the predominant symptoms. The disease is self-limiting but can be severe.

Appropriate fluid replacement and notification of the public health authorities are indicated.

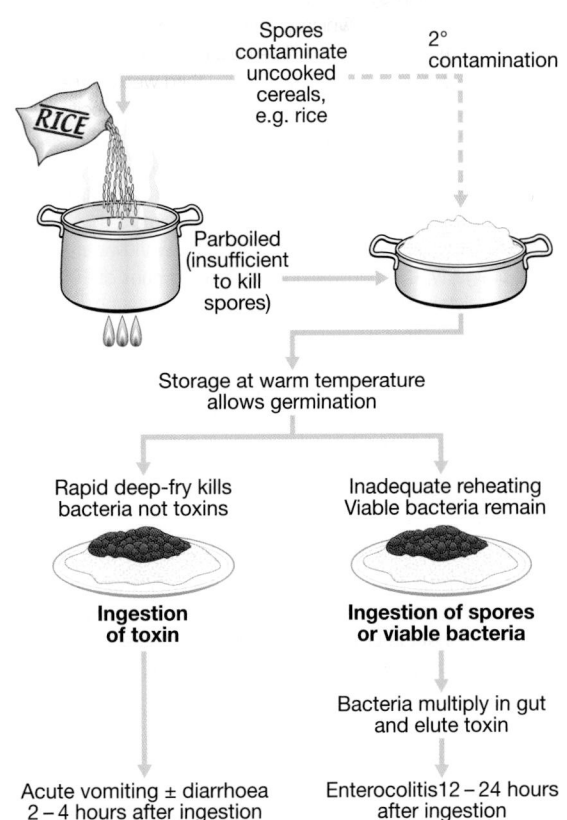

Fig. 13.28 *Bacillus cereus* food poisoning.

Clostridium perfringens food poisoning

Spores of *C. perfringens* are widespread in the guts of large animals and in soil. If contaminated meat products are incompletely cooked and stored in anaerobic conditions, *C. perfringens* spores germinate and viable organisms multiply. Subsequent reheating of the food causes release of enterotoxin. Symptoms (diarrhoea and cramps) occur 6–12 hours following ingestion. The illness is usually self-limiting.

Clostridial enterotoxins are potent and most people who ingest them will be symptomatic. 'Point source' outbreaks, in which a number of cases all become symptomatic following ingestion, classically occur after school or canteen lunches where meat stews are served.

Clostridial necrotising enteritis (CNE) or pigbel is an often-fatal type of food poisoning caused by a β-toxin of *C. perfringens*, type C. The toxin is normally inactivated by certain proteases or by normal cooking. Pigbel is more likely in protein malnutrition or in the presence of trypsin inhibitors, either in foods such as sweet potatoes or during infection with *Ascaris* sp. roundworms.

Campylobacter infection

This infection (caused by *Campylobacter jejuni* or *C. coli*) is essentially a zoonosis, although contaminated water may be implicated, as the organism can survive for many weeks in fresh water. The most common sources of the infection are chicken, beef and contaminated milk products. Pet puppies have also been sources. *Campylobacter* infection is now the most common cause of bacterial gastroenteritis in the UK, accounting for some 100 000 cases per annum, most of which are sporadic.

The incubation period is 2–5 days. Colicky abdominal pain may be severe and mimic acute appendicitis or other surgical pathology. Nausea, vomiting and significant diarrhoea, frequently containing blood, are common features. The majority of *Campylobacter* infections affect fit young adults and are self-limiting after 5–7 days. About 10%–20% will be prolonged, occasionally meriting treatment with a macrolide, most often azithromycin, as many organisms are resistant to ciprofloxacin.

Approximately 1 in 1000–2000 cases will develop bacteraemia and possible distant foci of infection. *Campylobacter* spp. have been linked to Guillain–Barré syndrome and post-infectious reactive arthritis (see Chs 26 and 28).

Salmonella spp. infection

Salmonella enterica serovars other than Typhi and Paratyphi, of which there are more than 2000, are widespread in animals and can cause gastroenteritis. Two serovars are most important worldwide: *Salmonella* Enteritidis phage type 4 and *Salmonella* Typhimurium dt.104. The latter may be resistant to commonly used antibiotics such as ciprofloxacin. Some strains have a clear relationship to particular animals, e.g. *Salmonella* Arizonae and pet reptiles. Transmission is by contaminated water or food, particularly poultry, egg products and minced beef, direct person-to-person spread or the handling of exotic pets such as salamanders, lizards or turtles. The incidence of *Salmonella* enteritis is falling in the UK due to an aggressive culling policy in broiler chicken stocks, coupled with vaccination.

The incubation period of *Salmonella* gastroenteritis is 12–72 hours and the predominant feature is diarrhoea, sometimes with passage of blood. Vomiting may be present at the outset. Approximately 5% of cases are bacteraemic and invasive non-typhoidal salmonellosis is a leading cause of bacteraemia in sub-Saharan Africa especially in people living with HIV. Reactive (post-infective) arthritis occurs in approximately 2%.

Antibiotics are not indicated for uncomplicated *Salmonella* gastroenteritis but are prescribed for bacteraemia. Salmonellae can cause persistent infection and can seed endothelial surfaces such as an atherosclerotic aorta. Mortality, as with other forms of gastroenteritis, is higher in older people (see Box 13.11).

Escherichia coli infection

Many serotypes of *E. coli* constitute part of the human gut microbiome. Clinical disease requires either colonisation with a new or previously unrecognised strain, or the acquisition by current colonising bacteria of a particular pathogenicity factor for mucosal attachment or toxin production. Travel to unfamiliar areas of the world allows contact with different strains of endemic *E. coli* and the development of travellers' diarrhoea. Enteropathogenic strains may be found in the gut of healthy individuals and, if these people move to a new environment, close contacts may develop symptoms.

At least five different clinico-pathological patterns of diarrhoea are associated with specific strains of *E. coli* with characteristic virulence factors.

Enterotoxigenic *E. coli*

Enterotoxigenic *E. coli* (ETEC) is the most common cause of travellers' diarrhoea (see Box 13.19). The organisms produce either a heat-labile or a heat-stable enterotoxin, causing marked secretory diarrhoea and vomiting after 1–2 days' incubation. The illness is usually mild and self-limiting after 3–4 days. Antibiotics are of questionable value.

Entero-invasive *E. coli*

Illness caused by entero-invasive *E. coli* (EIEC) is very similar to *Shigella* dysentery and is caused by invasion and destruction of colonic mucosal cells. No enterotoxin is produced. Acute watery diarrhoea, abdominal cramps and some scanty blood-staining of the stool are common. The symptoms are rarely severe and are usually self-limiting.

Enteropathogenic *E. coli*

Enteropathogenic *E. coli* (EPEC) organisms are very important in infant diarrhoea. They are able to attach to the gut mucosa, inducing a specific 'attachment and effacement' lesion and causing destruction of microvilli and disruption of normal absorptive capacity. The symptoms vary from mild non-bloody diarrhoea to quite severe illness without bacteraemia.

Entero-aggregative *E. coli*

Entero-aggregative *E. coli* (EAEC) strains adhere to the mucosa and produce a locally active enterotoxin. These demonstrate a particular 'stacked brick' aggregation to tissue culture cells when viewed by microscopy. EAEC have been associated with prolonged diarrhoea in children in South America, South-east Asia and India.

Enterohaemorrhagic *E. coli*

A number of distinct 'O' serotypes of *E. coli* possess both the genes necessary for adherence (see 'EPEC' above) and plasmids encoding two distinct enterotoxins (verotoxins), which are identical to the toxins produced by *Shigella* ('shiga toxins 1 and 2'). *E. coli* O157:H7 is perhaps the best known of these verotoxin-producing *E. coli* (VTEC) but others, including types O126 and O11, are also implicated. In 2011, an outbreak of food-borne illness linked to fenugreek seeds occurred in Germany and was due to *E. coli* O104:H4, an EAEC strain that had acquired genes encoding shiga toxin 2a. Although the incidence of enterohaemorrhagic *E. coli* (EHEC) is considerably lower than that of *Campylobacter* and *Salmonella* infection, it is increasing in lower-income countries.

The reservoir of infection is in the gut of herbivores. The organism has an extremely low infecting dose (10–100 organisms). Runoff water from pasture lands where cattle have grazed, which is used to irrigate vegetable crops, as well as contaminated milk, meat products (especially hamburgers that have been incompletely cooked), lettuce, radish shoots and apple juice have all been implicated as sources (Fig. 13.29).

The incubation period is 1–7 days. Initial watery diarrhoea becomes uniformly blood-stained in 70% of cases and is associated with severe abdominal pain. There is little systemic upset, vomiting or fever.

Enterotoxins have both a local effect on the bowel and a distant effect on particular body tissues, such as renal glomeruli, heart and brain. The potentially life-threatening haemolytic uraemic syndrome (HUS) occurs in

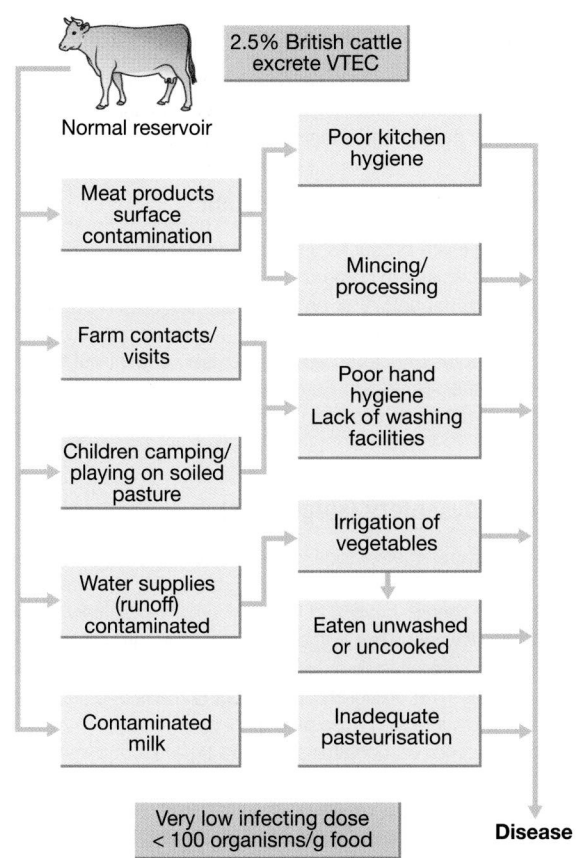

Fig. 13.29 Verocytotoxigenic *Escherichia coli* (VTEC) infections.

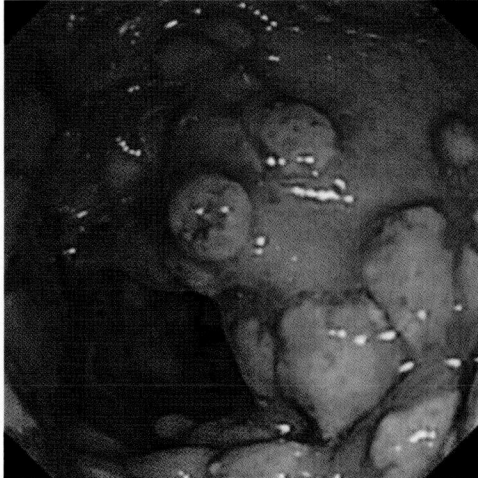

Fig. 13.30 *Clostridioides difficile* infection. Colonoscopic view showing numerous adherent 'pseudomembranes' on the mucosa.

10%–15% of sufferers from this infection, arising 5–7 days after symptom onset. It is most frequent at the extremes of age, is heralded by a high peripheral leucocyte count, and may be induced, particularly in children, by antibiotic therapy.

HUS is treated by dialysis if necessary and may be averted by plasma exchange. Antibiotics should be avoided since they can stimulate toxin release.

Clostridioides difficile infection

Clostridioides (formerly *Clostridium*) *difficile* is the most common cause of antibiotic-associated diarrhoea, and is an occasional constituent of the gut microbiome. *C. difficile* can produce two toxins (A and B). *C. difficile* infection (CDI) usually follows antimicrobial therapy, which alters the composition of the gastrointestinal flora and may facilitate colonisation with toxigenic *C. difficile*, if the patient is exposed to *C. difficile* spores. The combination of toxin production and the ability to produce environmentally stable spores accounts for the clinical features and transmissibility of CDI. A hypervirulent strain of *C. difficile*, ribotype 027, has emerged, which produces more toxin and more severe disease than other *C. difficile* strains.

Clinical features

Disease manifestations range from diarrhoea to life-threatening pseudomembranous colitis. Around 80% of cases occur in people over 65 years of age, many of whom are frail with comorbid diseases. Symptoms usually begin in the first week of antibiotic therapy but can occur up to 6 weeks after treatment has finished. The onset is often insidious, with lower abdominal pain and diarrhoea that may become profuse and watery. The presentation may resemble acute ulcerative colitis with bloody diarrhoea, fever and even toxic dilatation and perforation. Ileus is also seen in pseudomembranous colitis.

Investigations

C. difficile can be isolated from stool culture in 30% of patients with antibiotic-associated diarrhoea and over 90% of those with pseudomembranous colitis, but also from 5% of healthy adults and up to 20% of older adults in residential care. The diagnosis of CDI therefore rests on detection of toxins A or B in the stool. Current practice in the UK is to screen stool from patients with a compatible clinical syndrome by detection either of glutamate dehydrogenase (GDH), an enzyme produced by *C. difficile*, or of *C. difficile* nucleic acid (e.g. by PCR); if screening is positive, *C. difficile* toxin is sought, usually with a sensitive ELISA assay.

The rectal appearances at sigmoidoscopy may be characteristic, with erythema, white plaques or an adherent pseudomembrane (Fig. 13.30), or may resemble ulcerative colitis. In some cases, the rectum is spared and abnormalities are observed in the proximal colon. Patients who are ill require abdominal and erect chest X-rays to exclude perforation or toxic dilatation. CT may be useful when the diagnosis is in doubt.

Management

The precipitating antibiotic should be stopped and the patient should be isolated. Supportive therapy includes intravenous fluids and bowel rest. First-line antimicrobial therapy is usually vancomycin (125 mg orally 4 times daily for 7–10 days), which has replaced the use of metronidazole. Fidaxomicin is associated with a lower relapse rate than vancomycin but is more expensive. Intravenous immunoglobulin and/or glucocorticoids are sometimes given in the most severe or refractory cases, and faecal transplantation from a healthy donor is increasingly used to manage relapses by restoring a more advantageous gut microbiome profile. Bezlotoxumab is a monoclonal antibody against toxin B designed to prevent recurrence but its current role is uncertain. Surgical intervention needs to be considered early in severe cases.

Yersiniosis

Yersinia enterocolitica and *pseudotuberculosis*, commonly found in pork, cause mild to moderate gastroenteritis and can produce significant mesenteric adenitis after an incubation period of 3–7 days. They predominantly cause disease in children but adults may also be affected. The illness resolves slowly and may be mistaken for appendicitis (pseudoappendicitis). Complications include reactive arthritis (10%–13% of cases), which may be persistent, and anterior uveitis.

13

Cholera

Cholera, caused by *Vibrio cholerae* serotype O1, is the archetypal tox-in-mediated bacterial cause of acute watery diarrhoea. The enterotoxin activates adenylate cyclase in the intestinal epithelium, inducing net secretion of chloride and water. *V. cholerae* O1 has two biotypes, classical and El Tor, and each of these has two distinct serotypes, Inaba and Ogawa. Following its origin in the Ganges valley, devastating epidemics have occurred, often in association with large religious festivals, and pandemics have spread worldwide. The seventh pandemic, due to the El Tor biotype, began in 1961 and spread via the Middle East to become endemic in Africa, subsequently spreading throughout South and Central America. Numbers of cases of cholera have been increasing, with ongoing outbreaks in Yemen and Somalia. El Tor is more resistant to commonly used antimicrobials than classical *Vibrio*, and causes prolonged carriage in 5% of infections. An atypical serotype, O139, has been responsible for localised outbreaks in Bangladesh.

Infection spreads via the stools or vomit of symptomatic patients or of the much larger number of subclinical cases. Organisms survive for up to 2 weeks in fresh water and 8 weeks in saltwater. Transmission is normally through infected drinking water, shellfish and food contaminated by flies, or on the hands of carriers.

Clinical features

Severe diarrhoea without pain or colic begins suddenly and is followed by vomiting. Following the evacuation of normal gut faecal contents, typical 'rice water' material is passed, consisting of clear fluid with flecks of mucus. Classical cholera produces enormous loss of fluid and electrolytes, leading to intense dehydration with muscular cramps. Shock and oliguria develop. Death from acute circulatory failure may occur rapidly unless fluid and electrolytes are replaced. Improvement is rapid with proper treatment.

The majority of infections, however, cause mild illness with slight diarrhoea. Occasionally, a very intense illness, 'cholera sicca', occurs, with loss of fluid into dilated bowel, killing the patient before typical gastrointestinal symptoms appear. The disease is more dangerous in children.

Diagnosis and management

Clinical diagnosis is easy during an epidemic. Otherwise, the diagnosis should be confirmed bacteriologically. Stool dark-field microscopy shows the typical 'shooting star' motility of *V. cholerae*. Rectal swab or stool cultures allow identification. Cholera is notifiable under international health regulations.

Maintenance of circulation by replacement of water and electrolytes is paramount. Ringer's lactate is recommended for intravenous replacement. Vomiting usually stops once the patient is rehydrated, and fluid should then be given orally up to 500 mL hourly. Early intervention with oral rehydration solutions that include resistant starch, based on either rice or cereal, shortens the duration of diarrhoea and improves prognosis. Severe dehydration, as indicated by altered consciousness, skin tenting, very dry tongue, decreased pulses, low blood pressure or minimal urine output, mandates intravenous replacement. Total fluid requirements may exceed 50 L over a period of 2–5 days. Accurate records are greatly facilitated by the use of a 'cholera cot', which has a reinforced hole under the patient's buttocks, beneath which a graded bucket is placed.

Three days' treatment with tetracycline 250 mg 4 times daily, a single dose of doxycycline 300 mg or ciprofloxacin 1 g in adults reduces the duration of excretion of *V. cholerae* and the total volume of fluid needed for replacement.

Prevention

Strict personal hygiene is vital and drinking water should come from a clean piped supply or be boiled. Flies must be denied access to food. Oral vaccines containing killed *V. cholerae* with or without the B subunit of cholera toxin are used in outbreaks and in long-term control strategies.

In epidemics, improvements in sanitation and access to clean water, public education and control of population movement are vital. Mass single-dose vaccination and tetracycline treatment are valuable control measures. Disinfection of discharges and soiled clothing, and scrupulous handwashing by medical attendants reduce spread.

Vibrio parahaemolyticus infection

This marine organism produces a disease similar to enterotoxigenic *E. coli* (see above). It is very common where ingestion of raw seafood is widespread (e.g. Japan). After an incubation period of approximately 20 hours, explosive diarrhoea, abdominal cramps and vomiting occur. Systemic symptoms of headache and fever are frequent but the illness is self-limiting after 4–7 days. Rarely, a severe septic illness arises; in this case, *V. parahaemolyticus* can be isolated using specific halophilic culture.

Bacillary dysentery (shigellosis)

Shigellae are Gram-negative rods, closely related to *E. coli*, that invade the colonic mucosa. There are four main groups: *Sh. dysenteriae*, *flexneri*, *boydii* and *sonnei*. In tropical regions bacillary dysentery is usually caused by *Sh. flexneri*, while in the UK most cases are caused by *Sh. sonnei*. Shigellae are often resistant to multiple antibiotics, especially in tropical countries. The organism only infects humans and its spread is facilitated by a low infecting dose of around 10 organisms.

Spread may occur via contaminated food or flies, but person-to-person transmission by unwashed hands after defaecation is the most important factor. Outbreaks occur in psychiatric hospitals, residential schools and other closed institutions, and dysentery is a constant accompaniment of wars and natural catastrophes, due to overcrowding and poor sanitation. *Shigella* infection may spread rapidly among men who have sex with men.

Clinical features

Disease severity varies from mild *Sh. sonnei* infections that escape detection to more severe *Sh. flexneri* infections, while those due to *Sh. dysenteriae* may be fulminating and cause death within 48 hours.

In a moderately severe illness, the patient complains of diarrhoea, colicky abdominal pain and tenesmus. Stools are small, and after a few evacuations contain blood and purulent exudate with little faecal material. Fever, dehydration and weakness occur, with tenderness over the colon. Reactive arthritis or iritis occasionally complicate bacillary dysentery (p. 1035).

Management and prevention

Oral rehydration therapy or, if diarrhoea is severe, intravenous fluid replacement is necessary. Antibiotic therapy is with ciprofloxacin (500 mg twice daily for 3 days). Azithromycin and ceftriaxone are alternatives but resistance occurs to all agents, especially in Asia. The use of antidiarrhoeal medication should be avoided.

The prevention of faecal contamination of food and milk and the isolation of cases may be difficult, except in limited outbreaks. Handwashing is essential.

Respiratory bacterial infections

Most of these infections are described in Chapter 17.

Diphtheria

Infection with *Corynebacterium diphtheriae* occurs most commonly in the upper respiratory tract and is usually spread by droplet infection. Infection may also complicate skin lesions, especially in alcoholics. The organisms remain localised at the site of infection but release of a soluble exotoxin damages the heart muscle and the nervous system.

Diphtheria has been eradicated from many parts of the world by mass vaccination using a modified exotoxin but remains important in areas where vaccination is incomplete, e.g. in Russia and South-east Asia. The disease is notifiable in all countries of Europe and North America, and international guidelines have been issued by the WHO for the management of infection.

Clinical features

The incubation period averages 2–4 days. The disease begins insidiously with a sore throat (Box 13.46). Despite modest fever, there is usually marked tachycardia. The diagnostic feature is the 'wash-leather' elevated, greyish-green membrane on the tonsils. It has a well-defined edge, is firm and adherent, and is surrounded by a zone of inflammation. There may be swelling of the neck ('bull neck') and tender enlargement of the lymph nodes. In the mildest infections, especially where there is a high degree of immunity, a membrane may not appear and inflammation is minimal.

With anterior nasal infection there is nasal discharge, frequently blood-stained. In laryngeal diphtheria, a husky voice and high-pitched cough signal potential respiratory obstruction requiring urgent tracheostomy. If infection spreads to the uvula, fauces and nasopharynx, the patient is gravely ill.

Death from acute circulatory failure may occur within the first 10 days. Late complications arise as a result of toxin action on the heart or nervous system. About 25% of survivors of the early toxaemia may later develop myocarditis with arrhythmias or cardiac failure. These are usually reversible, with no permanent damage other than heart block in survivors.

Neurological involvement occurs in 75% of cases. After tonsillar or pharyngeal diphtheria, it usually starts after 10 days with palatal palsy. Paralysis of accommodation often follows, manifest by difficulty in reading small print. Generalised polyneuritis with weakness and paraesthesia may follow in the next 10–14 days. Recovery from such neuritis is always ultimately complete.

Management

A clinical diagnosis of diphtheria must be notified to the public health authorities and the patient sent urgently to a specialist infectious diseases unit. Empirical treatment should commence after collection of appropriate swabs.

Diphtheria antitoxin is produced from hyperimmune horse serum. It neutralises circulating toxin but not toxin already fixed to tissues, so it must be injected intramuscularly without awaiting the result of a throat swab. However, reactions to this foreign protein include a potentially lethal immediate anaphylactic reaction and a 'serum sickness' with fever, urticaria and joint pains, which occurs 7–12 days after injection. A careful history of previous horse serum injections or allergic reactions should be taken and a small test injection of serum should be given half an hour before the full dose in every patient. Epinephrine (adrenaline) solution must be available to treat any immediate type of reaction (0.5–1.0 mL of 1/1000 solution intramuscularly). An antihistamine is also given. In a severely ill patient, the risk of anaphylactic shock is outweighed by the mortal danger of diphtheritic toxaemia. A dose of up to 100 000 IU of antitoxin is injected intravenously if the test dose is tolerated. For disease of moderate severity, 16 000–40 000 IU intramuscularly will suffice, and for mild cases 4000–8000 IU.

13.46 Clinical features of diphtheria

Acute infection

- Membranous tonsillitis
- *or* Nasal infection
- *or* Laryngeal infection
- *or* Skin/wound/conjunctival infection (rare)

Complications

- Laryngeal obstruction or paralysis
- Myocarditis
- Peripheral neuropathy

Penicillin (1200 mg 4 times daily IV) or amoxicillin (500 mg 3 times daily) should be administered for 2 weeks to eliminate *C. diphtheriae*. Patients allergic to penicillin can be given erythromycin. Due to poor immunogenicity of primary infection, all sufferers should be immunised with diphtheria toxoid following recovery.

Patients must be managed in strict isolation and attended by staff with a clearly documented immunisation history until three swabs 24 hours apart are culture-negative.

Prevention

Active immunisation is recommended for all children. If diphtheria occurs in a closed community, contacts should be given erythromycin, which is more effective than penicillin in eradicating carriage.

All contacts should also be immunised or given a booster dose of toxoid. Booster doses are required every 10 years to maintain immunity.

Pneumococcal infection

Streptococcus pneumoniae (the pneumococcus) is the leading cause of community-acquired pneumonia globally and one of the leading causes of infection-related mortality. Otitis media, meningitis and sinusitis are also frequently caused by *Strep. pneumoniae*. Occasional patients present with bacteraemia without obvious focus. Asplenic individuals are at risk of fulminant pneumococcal disease with purpuric rash.

Increasing rates of penicillin resistance have been reported around the world for *Strep. pneumoniae*, although they remain low in the UK. Strains with cephalosporin resistance causing meningitis require treatment with a combination of cephalosporins, glycopeptides and rifampicin. Macrolide resistance is also increasing. Newer quinolones are also used (e.g. levofloxacin and moxifloxacin) but rates of resistance are rising.

Vaccination of infants with the protein conjugate pneumococcal vaccine decreases *Strep. pneumoniae* infection in infants and in their relatives. The polysaccharide pneumococcal vaccine is used in individuals predisposed to *Strep. pneumoniae* infection and older people, but only modestly reduces pneumococcal bacteraemia and does not prevent pneumonia. All asplenic individuals should receive vaccination against *Strep. pneumoniae*.

Anthrax

Anthrax is an endemic zoonosis in many countries; it causes human disease following inoculation of the spores of *Bacillus anthracis*. *B. anthracis* was the first bacterial pathogen described by Koch and the model pathogen for 'Koch's postulates' (see Box 6.1). It is a Gram-positive organism with a central spore. The spores can survive for years in soil. Infection is commonly acquired from contact with animals, particularly herbivores. The ease of production of *B. anthracis* spores makes this infection a candidate for biological warfare or bioterrorism. *B. anthracis* produces a number of toxins that mediate the clinical features of disease.

Clinical features

These depend on the route of entry of the anthrax spores.

Cutaneous anthrax

This skin lesion is associated with occupational exposure to anthrax spores during processing of hides and bone products. It accounts for the majority of clinical cases. Animal infection is a serious problem in Africa, India, Pakistan and the Middle East.

Spores are inoculated into exposed skin. A single lesion develops as an irritable papule on an oedematous haemorrhagic base. This progresses to a depressed black eschar. Despite extensive oedema, pain is infrequent.

Gastrointestinal anthrax

This is associated with the ingestion of contaminated meat. The caecum becomes infected, which produces nausea, vomiting, anorexia and fever, followed in 2–3 days by severe abdominal pain and bloody diarrhoea. Toxaemia and death can develop rapidly thereafter.

13

Inhalational anthrax

Inhalational anthrax is extremely rare but has been associated with bio-terrorism. Without rapid and aggressive therapy at the onset of symptoms, the mortality is 50%–90%. Fever, dyspnoea, cough, headache and sepsis develop 3–14 days following exposure. Typically, the chest X-ray shows only widening of the mediastinum and pleural effusions, which are haemorrhagic. Meningitis may occur.

Management

B. anthracis can be cultured from skin swabs from lesions. Skin lesions are readily curable with early antibiotic therapy. Treatment is with cipro-floxacin (500 mg twice daily) until penicillin susceptibility is confirmed; the regimen can then be changed to benzylpenicillin with doses up to 2.4 g IV given 6 times daily or phenoxymethylpenicillin orally 500–1000 mg 4 times daily administered for 10 days. The addition of an aminoglycoside may improve the outlook in severe disease. In view of concerns about concomitant inhalational exposure, particularly in the era of bioterrorism, a further 2-month course of ciprofloxacin 500 mg twice daily or doxy-cycline 100 mg twice daily orally is added to eradicate inhaled spores. Inhalational anthrax is treated with ciprofloxacin and clindamycin for at least 14 days, followed by therapy to eradicate spores. Monoclonal anti-bodies against *B. anthracis* protective antigen can be added for systemic infection. Prophylaxis with ciprofloxacin (500 mg twice daily for 2 months) is recommended for anyone at high risk of inhalational exposure to anthrax spores and is combined with three doses of anthrax vaccine adsorbed (AVA).

Bacterial infections with neurological involvement

Infections affecting the CNS, including bacterial meningitis, botulism and tetanus, are described on page 1171.

Mycobacterial infections

Tuberculosis

Tuberculosis is predominantly, although by no means exclusively, a respiratory disease and is described in Chapter 17.

Leprosy

Leprosy (Hansen's disease) is a chronic granulomatous disease affecting skin and nerves and caused by *Mycobacterium leprae*, a slow-growing mycobacterium that cannot be cultured in vitro. The clinical manifestations are determined by the degree of the patient's cell-mediated immunity (CMI) towards *M. leprae* (Fig. 13.31). High levels of CMI with elimination of leprosy bacilli produces tuberculoid leprosy, whereas absent CMI results in lepromatous leprosy. Complications arise due to nerve damage, immunological reactions and bacillary infiltration. People with leprosy are frequently stigmatised and using the word 'leper' is inappropriate.

Epidemiology and transmission

The WHO estimates there are around 200 000 new cases detected annually. About 70% of the world's leprosy patients live in India, with the disease endemic in Brazil, Indonesia, Mozambique, Madagascar, Tanzania and Nepal.

Untreated lepromatous patients discharge bacilli from the nose. Infection occurs through the nose, followed by haematogenous spread to skin and nerve. The incubation period is 2–5 years for tuberculoid cases and 8–12 years for lepromatous cases. Leprosy incidence peaks at 10–14 years, and is more common in males and in household contacts of leprosy cases.

Pathogenesis

M. leprae has tropism for Schwann cells and skin macrophages. In tuberculoid leprosy, effective CMI controls bacillary multiplication

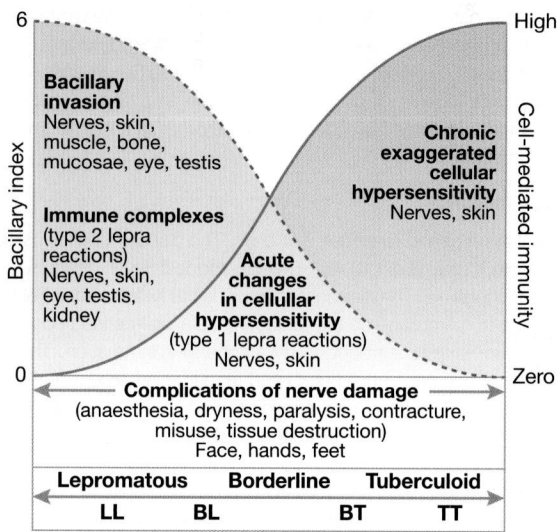

Fig. 13.31 Leprosy: mechanisms of damage and tissue affected. Mechanisms under the broken line are characteristic of disease near the lepromatous end of the spectrum, and those under the solid line are characteristic of the tuberculoid end. They overlap in the centre where, in addition, instability predisposes to type 1 lepra reactions. At the peak in the centre, neither bacillary growth nor cell-mediated immunity has the upper hand. (BL = borderline lepromatous; BT = borderline tuberculoid; LL = lepromatous leprosy; TT = tuberculoid leprosy) *Adapted from Bryceson ADM, Pfaltzgraff RE. Leprosy, 3rd edn. Churchill Livingstone, Elsevier Ltd; 1990.*

('paucibacillary') and organised epithelioid granulomata form. In lepromatous leprosy, there is abundant bacillary multiplication ('multibacillary'), e.g. in Schwann cells and perineurium. Between these two extremes is a continuum, varying from patients with moderate CMI (borderline tuberculoid) to patients with little cellular response (borderline lepromatous).

Immunological reactions evolve as the immune response develops and the bacillary antigenic stimulus varies, particularly in borderline patients. Delayed hypersensitivity reactions produce type 1 (reversal) reactions, while immune complexes contribute to type 2 (erythema nodosum leprosum) reactions.

HIV/leprosy co-infected patients have typical lepromatous and tuberculoid leprosy skin lesions and typical leprosy histology and granuloma formation. Surprisingly, even with low circulating CD4 counts, tuberculoid leprosy may be observed and there is not an obvious shift to lepromatous leprosy.

Clinical features

Box 13.47 gives the cardinal features of leprosy. Types of leprosy are compared in Box 13.48.

- *Skin*. The most common skin lesions are macules or plaques. Tuberculoid patients have few, hypopigmented lesions (Fig. 13.32A). In lepromatous leprosy, papules, nodules or diffuse infiltration of the skin occur. The earliest lesions are ill defined; gradually, the skin becomes infiltrated and thickened. Facial skin thickening leads to the characteristic leonine facies (Fig. 13.32B).
- *Anaesthesia*. In skin lesions, the small dermal sensory and autonomic nerve fibres are damaged, causing localised sensory loss and loss of sweating. Anaesthesia can occur in the distribution of a damaged large peripheral nerve. A 'glove and stocking' sensory neuropathy is also common in lepromatous leprosy.
- *Nerve damage*. Peripheral nerve trunks are affected at 'sites of predilection'. These are the ulnar (elbow), median (wrist), radial (humerus), radial cutaneous (wrist), common peroneal (knee), posterior tibial and sural nerves (ankle), facial nerve (zygomatic arch) and great auricular nerve (posterior triangle of the neck). Damage to peripheral nerve trunks produces characteristic signs with regional

i 13.47 Cardinal features of leprosy

- Skin lesions, typically anaesthetic at tuberculoid end of spectrum
- Thickened peripheral nerves
- Acid-fast bacilli on skin smears or biopsy

i 13.48 Clinical characteristics of the polar forms of leprosy

Clinical and tissue-specific features	Lepromatous	Tuberculoid
Skin and nerves		
Number and distribution	Widely disseminated	One or a few sites, asymmetrical
Skin lesions		
Definition:		
Clarity of margin	Poor	Good
Elevation of margin	Never	Common
Colour:		
Dark skin	Slight hypopigmentation	Marked hypopigmentation
Light skin	Slight erythema	Coppery or red
Surface	Smooth, shiny	Dry, scaly
Central healing	None	Common
Sweat and hair growth	Impaired late	Impaired early
Loss of sensation	Late	Early and marked
Nerve enlargement and damage	Late	Early and marked
Bacilli (bacterial index)	Many (5 or 6+)	Absent (0)
Natural history	Progressive	Self-healing
Other tissues	Upper respiratory mucosa, eye, testes, bones, muscle	None
Reactions	Immune complexes (type 2)	Cell-mediated (type 1)

sensory loss and muscle dysfunction (Fig. 13.32C). All these nerves should be examined for enlargement and tenderness, and tested for motor and sensory function. The CNS is not affected.

- *Eye involvement*. Blindness is a devastating complication for a patient with anaesthetic hands and feet. Eyelid closure is impaired when the facial nerve is affected. Damage to the trigeminal nerve causes anaesthesia of the cornea and conjunctiva. The cornea is then susceptible to trauma and ulceration.
- *Other features*. Many organs can be affected. Nasal collapse occurs secondary to bacillary destruction of the nasal cartilage and bone. Diffuse infiltration of the testes causes testicular atrophy and the acute orchitis that occurs with type 2 reactions. This results in azoospermia and hypogonadism.

Leprosy reactions

Leprosy reactions (Box 13.49) are events superimposed on the cardinal features shown in Box 13.47.

- *Type 1 (reversal) reactions*. These occur in 30% of borderline patients (BT, BB or BL – see below) and are delayed hypersensitivity reactions. Skin lesions become erythematous (Fig. 13.32D). Peripheral nerves become tender and painful, with sudden loss of nerve function. These reactions may occur spontaneously, after starting treatment and also after completion of multidrug therapy (MDT).
- *Type 2 (erythema nodosum leprosum, ENL) reactions*. These are partly due to immune complex deposition and occur in BL and LL

patients who produce antibodies and have a high antigen load. They manifest with malaise, fever and crops of small pink nodules on the face and limbs. Iritis and episcleritis are common. Other signs are acute neuritis, lymphadenitis, orchitis, bone pain, dactylitis, arthritis and proteinuria. ENL may continue intermittently for several years.

Borderline cases

In borderline tuberculoid (BT) cases, skin lesions are more numerous than in tuberculoid (TT) cases, and there is more severe nerve damage and a risk of type 1 reactions. In borderline leprosy (BB) cases, skin lesions are numerous and vary in size, shape and distribution; annular lesions are characteristic and nerve damage is variable. In borderline lepromatous (BL) cases, there are widespread small macules in the skin and widespread nerve involvement; both type 1 and type 2 reactions occur.

Pure neural leprosy (i.e. without skin lesions) occurs principally in India and accounts for 10% of patients. There is asymmetrical involvement of peripheral nerve trunks and no visible skin lesions. On nerve biopsy, all types of leprosy have been found.

Investigations

The diagnosis is clinical, made by finding a cardinal sign of leprosy and supported by detecting acid-fast bacilli in slit-skin smears or typical histology in a skin biopsy. Slit-skin smears are obtained by scraping dermal material on to a glass slide. The smears are then stained for acid-fast bacilli, the number counted per high-power field and a score derived on a logarithmic scale (0–6): the bacterial index (BI). Smears are useful for confirming the diagnosis and monitoring response to treatment. Neither serology nor PCR is sensitive or specific enough for diagnosis.

Management

The principles of treatment are outlined in Box 13.50. All leprosy patients require MDT with an approved first-line regimen (Box 13.51).

Rifampicin is a potent bactericidal for *M. leprae* but should always be given in combination with other antileprotics, since a single-step mutation can confer resistance. Dapsone is bacteriostatic. It commonly causes mild haemolysis and rarely anaemia. Clofazimine is a red, fat-soluble crystalline dye, weakly bactericidal for *M. leprae*. Skin discoloration (red to purple–black) and ichthyosis are troublesome side-effects, particularly on pale skins. New bactericidal drugs against *M. leprae* have been identified, notably fluoroquinolones (e.g. ofloxacin). Minocycline and clarithromycin may also be used. These agents are second-line drugs. Minocycline causes grey pigmentation of skin lesions.

Single-dose combination treatment (rifampicin ofloxacin and minocycline) is less effective than the conventional 6-month treatment for paucibacillary leprosy and has fallen out of favour.

Lepra reactions are treated as shown in Box 13.49. Chloroquine can also be used.

Patient education

Patient education emphasises that, after 3 days of chemotherapy, they are not infectious, that gross deformities are not inevitable and that they can lead a normal social life.

Patients with anaesthetic hands or feet need to avoid and treat burns or other minor injuries. Good footwear is important. Physiotherapy helps maintain range of movement of affected muscles and neighbouring joints.

Prognosis

Untreated, tuberculoid leprosy has a good prognosis; it may self-heal and peripheral nerve damage is limited. Lepromatous leprosy (LL) is a progressive condition with high morbidity if untreated.

After treatment, the majority of patients, especially those who have no nerve damage at the time of diagnosis, do well, with resolution of skin lesions. Borderline patients are at risk of developing type 1 reactions, which may result in devastating nerve damage.

13

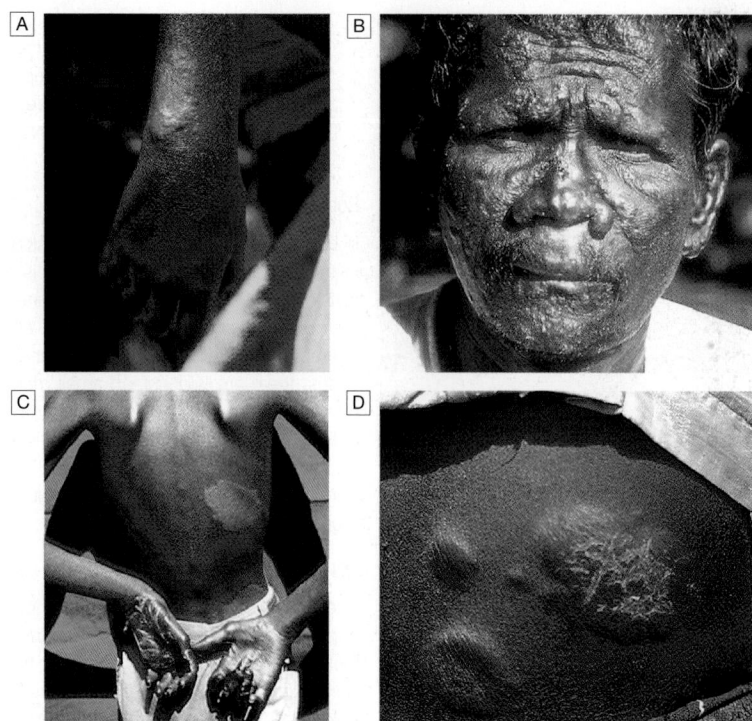

Fig. 13.32 Clinical features of leprosy. [A] Tuberculoid leprosy. Single lesion with a well-defined active edge and anaesthesia within the lesion. [B] Lepromatous leprosy. Widespread nodules and infiltration, with loss of the eyebrows. This man also has early collapse of the nose. [C] Borderline tuberculoid leprosy with severe nerve damage. This boy has several well-defined, hypopigmented, macular, anaesthetic lesions. He has severe nerve damage affecting both ulnar and median nerves bilaterally and has sustained severe burns to his hands. [D] Reversal (type 1) reactions. Erythematous, oedematous lesions.

i · 13.49 Reactions in leprosy

	Lepra reaction type 1 (reversal)	Lepra reaction type 2 (erythema nodosum leprosum)
Mechanism	Cell-mediated hypersensitivity	Immune complexes
Clinical features	Painful tender nerves, loss of function Swollen skin lesions New skin lesions	Tender papules and nodules; may ulcerate Painful tender nerves, loss of function Iritis, orchitis, myositis, lymphadenitis Fever, oedema
Management	Prednisolone 40 mg, reducing over 3–6 months[1]	Moderate: prednisolone 40 mg daily Severe: thalidomide[2] or prednisolone 40–80 mg daily, reducing over 1–6 months; local if eye involved[3]

[1]Indicated for any new impairment of nerve or eye function. [2]Contraindicated in women who may become pregnant. [3]1% hydrocortisone drops or ointment and 1% atropine drops.

i · 13.50 Principles of leprosy treatment

- Stop the infection with chemotherapy
- Treat reactions
- Educate the patient about leprosy
- Prevent disability
- Support the patient socially and psychologically

Prevention and control

The previous strategy of centralised leprosy control campaigns has been superseded by integrated programmes, with primary health-care workers in many countries now responsible for case detection and provision of MDT. It is not yet clear how successful this will be, especially in the time-consuming area of disability prevention.

BCG vaccination offers protection against leprosy; adding killed *M. leprae* to BCG does not further enhance protection.

Rickettsial and related intracellular bacterial infections

Rickettsial fevers

The rickettsial fevers are the most common tick-borne infections. It is important to ask potentially infected patients about contact with ticks, lice or fleas. There are two main groups of rickettsial fevers: spotted fevers and typhus (Box 13.52).

Pathogenesis

The rickettsiae are intracellular Gram-negative organisms that parasitise the intestinal canal of arthropods. Infection of humans through the skin occurs from the excreta of arthropods, but the saliva of some biting vectors is infected. The organisms multiply in capillary endothelial cells, producing lesions in the skin, CNS, heart, lungs, liver, kidneys and skeletal muscles. Endothelial proliferation, associated with a perivascular reaction, may cause thrombosis and purpura. In epidemic typhus, the brain is the target organ; in scrub typhus, the cardiovascular system and lungs in particular are attacked. An eschar, a black necrotic crusted sore, is often found in tick- and mite-borne typhus (see Fig. 13.8C). This is due to vasculitis following immunological recognition of the inoculated organism. Regional lymph nodes often enlarge.

Spotted fever group

Rocky Mountain spotted fever

Rickettsia rickettsii is transmitted by tick bites. It is widely distributed and increasing in western and south-eastern states of the USA and also in Central and South America. The incubation period is about 7 days. The rash appears on about the third or fourth day of illness, looking at first like measles, but in a few hours a typical maculopapular eruption develops. The rash spreads in 24–48 hours from wrists, forearms and ankles to the back, limbs and chest, and then to the abdomen, where it is least pronounced. Larger cutaneous and subcutaneous haemorrhages may appear in severe cases. The liver and spleen become palpable. At the extremes of life, the mortality is 2%–12%.

Other spotted fevers

R. conorii (boutonneuse fever) causes Mediterranean spotted fever, which extends to Africa and India, while *R. africae* (African tick bite fever) causes African tick typhus. The incubation period is approximately 7 days. Infected tick bites result from walking on grasslands or are acquired from pet dogs. Examination may reveal a diagnostic eschar, and the maculopapular rash on the trunk, limbs, palms and soles. There may be delirium and meningeal signs in severe infections, but recovery is usual. *R. africae* may cause multiple eschars. Some cases, particularly those with *R. africae*, present without rash ('spotless spotted fever'). Other spotted fevers are shown in Box 13.52.

Typhus group

Scrub typhus fever

Scrub typhus is caused by *Orientia tsutsugamushi*, transmitted by mites. It occurs in the Far East, Myanmar, Pakistan, Bangladesh, India, Indonesia, the South Pacific islands and Queensland, particularly where patches of forest cleared for plantations have attracted rats and mites.

In many patients, one or more eschars develop, surrounded by cellulitis (see Fig. 13.8C), with regional lymph node enlargement. The incubation period is about 9 days.

Mild or subclinical cases are common. The onset of symptoms is usually sudden, with headache (often retro-orbital), fever, malaise, weakness and cough. In severe illness, the general symptoms increase, with apathy and prostration. An erythematous maculopapular rash often appears on about the 5th–7th day and spreads to the trunk, face and limbs, including the palms and soles, with generalised painless lymphadenopathy. The

---

i | **13.51 World Health Organization 2018 guidelines for multidrug therapy (MDT) regimens in leprosy**

Type of leprosy[1]	Monthly supervised treatment	Daily self-administered treatment	Duration of treatment
Paucibacillary	Rifampicin 600 mg	Dapsone 100 mg	6 months
	Clofazimine 300 mg	Clofazimine 50 mg	
Multibacillary	Rifampicin 600 mg	Dapsone 100 mg	12 months
	Clofazimine 300 mg	Clofazimine 50 mg	
Rifampicin resistant		Clofazimine 50 mg plus two second-line agents[2] ×6 months, then plus one second line ×18 month	24 months

[1]Classification uses the number of skin lesions: paucibacillary (1–5 skin lesions); multibacillary (>5 skin lesions, nerve involvement or positive slit-skin smear). [2]Second-line agents minocycline 100 mg, clarithromycin 500 mg, or a fluoroquinolone (e.g. ofloxacin 400 mg, levofloxacin 500 mg or moxifloxacin 400 mg) but only use a fluoroquinolone if TB excluded and no fluoroquinolone resistance.
From WHO. Guidelines for the Diagnosis, Treatment and Prevention of Leprosy. New Delhi: World Health Organization, Regional Office for South-East Asia; 2018.

---

i | **13.52 Features of rickettsial infections**

Disease	Organism	Reservoir	Vector	Geographical area	Rash	Gangrene	Target organs	Mortality
Spotted fever group								
Rocky Mountain spotted fever	*R. rickettsii*	Rodents, dogs, ticks	*Ixodes* tick	North, Central and South America	Morbilliform Haemorrhagic	Often	Bronchi, myocardium, brain, skin	2%–12%[2]
Boutonneuse fever	*R. conorii*	Rodents, dogs, ticks	*Ixodes* tick	Mediterranean, Africa, South-west Asia, India	Maculopapular	–	Skin, meninges	2.5%[3]
Siberian tick typhus	*R. sibirica*	Rodents, birds, domestic animals, ticks	Various ticks	Siberia, Mongolia, northern China	Maculopapular	–	Skin, meninges	Rare[3]
Australian tick typhus	*R. australis*	Rodents, ticks	Ticks	Australia	Maculopapular	–	Skin, meninges	Rare[3]
Oriental spotted fever	*R. japonica*	Rodents, dogs, ticks	Ticks	Japan	Maculopapular	–	Skin, meninges	Rare[3]
African tick bite fever[1]	*R. africae*	Cattle, game, ticks	*Ixodes* tick	South Africa	Can be spotless	–	Skin, meninges	Rare[3]
Typhus group								
Scrub typhus	*Orientia tsutsugamushi*	Rodents	*Trombicula* mite	South-east Asia	Maculopapular	Unusual	Bronchi, myocardium, brain, skin	Rare[3]
Epidemic typhus	*R. prowazekii*	Humans	Louse	Worldwide	Morbilliform Haemorrhagic	Often	Brain, skin, bronchi, myocardium	Up to 40%
Endemic typhus	*R. typhi*	Rats	Flea	Worldwide	Slight	–	–	Rare[3]

[1]Eschar at bite site and local lymphadenopathy. [2]Highest in adult males. [3]Except in infants, older people and the debilitated.

13

rash fades by the 14th day. The temperature rises rapidly and continues as a remittent fever (i.e. the difference between maximum and minimum temperature exceeds 1°C), remaining above normal with sweating until it falls on the 12th–18th day. In severe infection, the patient is prostrate with cough, pneumonia, delirium and deafness. Cardiac failure, renal failure and haemorrhage may develop. Convalescence is often slow and tachycardia may persist for some weeks.

Epidemic (louse-borne) typhus

Epidemic typhus is caused by *R. prowazekii* and is transmitted by infected faeces of the human body louse, usually through scratching the skin. Patients with epidemic typhus infect lice, which leave when the patient is febrile. In conditions of overcrowding, the disease spreads rapidly. It is prevalent in parts of Africa, especially Ethiopia and Rwanda, and in the South American Andes and Afghanistan. Large epidemics have occurred in Europe, usually during wars. The incubation period is usually 12–14 days.

There may be several days of malaise but the onset is more often sudden, with rigors, fever, frontal headaches, pains in the back and limbs, constipation and bronchitis. The face is flushed and cyanotic, the eyes are congested and the patient becomes confused. The rash appears on the 4th–6th day. In its early stages, it disappears on pressure but soon becomes petechial with subcutaneous mottling. The rash appears first on the anterior folds of the axillae, sides of the abdomen or backs of the hands, then on the trunk and forearms. The neck and face are seldom affected. During the second week, symptoms increase in severity. Sores develop on the lips. The tongue becomes dry, brown, shrunken and tremulous. The spleen is palpable, the pulse feeble and the patient stuporous and delirious. The temperature falls rapidly at the end of the second week and the patient recovers gradually. In fatal cases, the patient usually dies in the second week from toxaemia, cardiac or renal failure, or pneumonia.

Endemic (flea-borne) typhus

Flea-borne or 'endemic' typhus caused by *R. typhi* is endemic worldwide. Humans are infected when the faeces or contents of a crushed flea, which has fed on an infected rat, are introduced into the skin. The incubation period is 8–14 days. The symptoms resemble those of a mild louse-borne typhus. The rash may be scanty and transient.

Investigation of rickettsial infection

Routine blood investigations are not diagnostic. There is usually hepatitis and thrombocytopenia. Diagnosis is made on clinical grounds and response to treatment, and may be confirmed by antibody detection or PCR in specialised laboratories. Differential diagnoses include malaria, typhoid, meningococcal sepsis and leptospirosis.

Management of rickettsial fevers

The rickettsial fevers vary in severity but all respond to tetracycline 500 mg 4 times daily, doxycycline 200 mg daily or chloramphenicol 500 mg 4 times daily for 7 days. Louse-borne typhus and scrub typhus can be treated with a single dose of 200 mg doxycycline, repeated for 2–3 days to prevent relapse. Chloramphenicol- and doxycycline-resistant strains of *O. tsutsugamushi* have been reported from Thailand and patients here may need treatment with rifampicin.

Nursing care is important, especially in epidemic typhus. Sedation may be required for delirium and blood transfusion for haemorrhage. Relapsing fever and typhoid are common intercurrent infections in epidemic typhus, and pneumonia in scrub typhus. Convalescence is usually protracted, especially in older people.

To prevent rickettsial infection, lice, fleas, ticks and mites need to be controlled with insecticides.

▌Q fever

Q fever occurs worldwide and is caused by the rickettsia-like organism *Coxiella burnetii*, an obligate intracellular organism that survives in the extracellular environment. Cattle, sheep and goats are important reservoirs and the organism is transmitted by inhalation of aerosolised particles.

C. burnetii exhibits phase variation, due to antigenic variation resulting from changes to its lipopolysaccharide (LPS). When isolated from animals or humans, *C. burnetii* expresses phase I antigen and is very infectious (a single bacterium is sufficient to infect a human). In culture, there is an antigenic shift to the phase II form, which is not infectious. Measurement of antigenic shift helps differentiate acute and chronic Q fever.

Clinical features

The incubation period is 3–4 weeks. The initial symptoms are non-specific with fever, headache and chills; in 20% of cases, a maculopapular rash occurs. Other presentations include pneumonia and hepatitis. Chronic Q fever may present with osteomyelitis, encephalitis and endocarditis.

Investigations and management

Diagnosis is usually serological and the stage of the infection can be distinguished by isotype tests and phase-specific antigens. Phase I and II IgM titres peak at 4–6 weeks. In chronic infections, IgG titres to phase I and II antigens may be raised. Suspected tissue infection (e.g. endocarditis) can be diagnosed by detection of specific DNA (PCR).

Prompt treatment of acute Q fever with doxycycline reduces fever duration. Treatment of Q fever endocarditis is problematic, requiring prolonged therapy with doxycycline and rifampicin or ciprofloxacin with hydroxychloroquine; even then, organisms are not always eradicated. Valve surgery is often required.

▌Bartonellosis

Bartonellae are intracellular Gram-negative bacilli closely related to the rickettsiae, which are important causes of 'culture-negative' endocarditis. They are found in many domestic pets, such as cats, although for several the host is undefined (Box 13.53). The principal human pathogens are *Bartonella quintana*, *B. henselae* and *B. bacilliformis*. *Bartonella* infections are associated with the following:

- *Trench fever*. This is a relapsing fever with severe leg pain and is caused by *B. quintana*. The disease is not fatal but is very debilitating.
- *Bacteraemia and endocarditis in the homeless*. Endocarditis due to *B. quintana* or *B. henselae* is associated with severe damage to the heart valves.
- *Cat scratch disease*. *B. henselae* causes this common benign lymphadenopathy in children and young adults. A vesicle or papule develops on the head, neck or arms after a cat scratch. The lesion resolves spontaneously but there may be regional lymphadenopathy that persists for up to 4 months before also resolving spontaneously. Rare complications include retinitis and encephalopathy.
- *Bacillary angiomatosis*. This is an HIV-associated disease caused by *B. quintana* or *B. henselae* (see p. 358).
- *Oroya fever and verruga peruana* (*Carrion's disease*). This is endemic in areas of Peru. It is a biphasic disease caused by *B. bacilliformis*, transmitted by sandflies of the genus *Phlebotomus*. Fever, haemolytic anaemia and microvascular thrombosis with end-organ ischaemia are features. It is frequently fatal if untreated.

i	**13.53 Clinical diseases caused by *Bartonella* spp.**		
Reservoir	Vector	Organism	Disease
Cats	Flea	*B. henselae*	Cat scratch disease, bacillary angiomatosis, endocarditis
Undefined	Lice	*B. quintana*	Trench fever, bacillary angiomatosis, endocarditis
Undefined	Sandfly	*B. bacilliformis*	Carrion's disease: Oroya fever and verruga peruana
Undefined	Flea	*B. rochalimae*	Fever, rash, anaemia, splenomegaly

Investigations and management

Bartonellae can be cultured in specialised laboratories but PCR is often used to diagnose infection. Serum antibody detection is possible but cross-reactions occur with *Chlamydia* and *Coxiella* spp.

Bartonella spp. are typically treated with macrolides or tetracyclines. Antibiotic use is guided by clinical need. Cat scratch disease usually resolves spontaneously but *Bartonella* endocarditis requires valve replacement and combination antibiotic therapy with doxycycline and gentamicin.

Chlamydial infections

These are listed in Box 13.54 and are also described on pages 379 and 512.

Trachoma

Trachoma is a chronic keratoconjunctivitis caused by *Chlamydia trachomatis* and is the most common cause of avoidable blindness. The classic trachoma environment is dry and dirty, causing children to have eye and nose discharges. Transmission occurs through flies, on fingers and within families. In endemic areas, the disease is most common in children.

Pathology and clinical features

The onset is usually insidious. Infection may be asymptomatic, last for years with prolonged latency and may recrudesce. The conjunctiva of the upper lid is first affected with vascularisation and cellular infiltration. Early symptoms include conjunctival irritation and blepharospasm. The early follicles are characteristic (Fig. 13.33) but clinical differentiation from conjunctivitis due to other causes may be difficult. Scarring causes inversion of the lids (entropion) so that the lashes rub against the cornea (trichiasis). The cornea becomes vascularised and opaque with detection only when vision begins to fail.

i	13.54 Chlamydial infections	
Organism	**Disease caused**	
Chlamydia trachomatis	Trachoma Lymphogranuloma venereum (see Box 15.12) Cervicitis, urethritis, proctitis (see Ch. 15)	
Chlamydia psittaci	Psittacosis (see Box 17.37)	
Chlamydophila (Chlamydia) pneumoniae	Atypical pneumonia (see Box 17.37) Acute/chronic sinusitis	

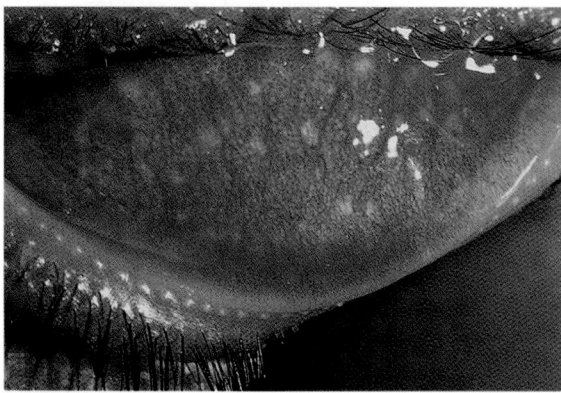

Fig. 13.33 Trachoma. Trachoma is characterised by hyperaemia and numerous pale follicles. *Courtesy of Institute of Ophthalmology, Moorfields Eye Hospital, London.*

Investigations and management

Intracellular inclusions may be demonstrated in conjunctival scrapings by staining with iodine or immunofluorescence. Although chlamydiae may, in theory, be isolated in chick embryo or cell culture or detected by nucleic acid amplification tests, these methods are rarely available in the areas where trachoma is encountered, and in any case their sensitivity and specificity are poorly established. Diagnosis of trachoma is therefore based on clinical and epidemiological features.

A single dose of oral azithromycin (20 mg/kg) is superior to 6 weeks of tetracycline eye ointment twice daily for individuals in mass treatment programmes. Deformity and scarring of the lids, and corneal opacities, ulceration and scarring require surgical treatment after control of local infection.

Prevention

Personal and family hygiene should be improved. Proper care of the eyes of newborn and young children is essential. Family contacts should be examined. The WHO is promoting the SAFE strategy for trachoma control (surgery, antibiotics, facial cleanliness and environmental improvement).

Protozoal infections

Protozoa are important causes of infectious diseases. They can be categorised according to whether they cause systemic or local infection. Trichomoniasis is described on page 374.

Systemic protozoal infections

Malaria

Malaria in humans is caused by *Plasmodium falciparum*, *P. vivax*, *P. ovale* (subspecies *curtisi* and *wallikeri*), *P. malariae* and the zoonotic simian parasite *P. knowlesi*. It is transmitted by the bite of female *Anopheles* mosquitoes and occurs throughout the tropics and subtropics at altitudes below 1500 m (Fig. 13.34). The WHO estimates that 228 million cases of clinical malaria occurred in 2018, 93% of these in Africa, especially among children and pregnant women. The incidence rate of malaria declined globally between 2010 and 2018 due to WHO prevention and treatment campaigns. However, *P. falciparum* has now become resistant to artemisinins as well as chloroquine, mefloquine and sulfadoxine-pyrimethamine, initially in South-east Asia.. The WHO is now planning for elimination of malaria in certain countries by utilising the 'best evidence' in bed nets, rapid diagnostic tests and artemisinin combination therapy (ACT).

Travellers are susceptible to malaria. Most cases are due to *P. falciparum*, usually from Africa, and of these 1% die because of late diagnosis. Migrants from endemic countries who spend long periods of time in non-endemic countries are particularly at risk if they visit friends and family in their country of origin. They have lost their partial immunity and frequently do not take malaria prophylaxis. A few people living near airports in Europe have acquired malaria from accidentally imported mosquitoes.

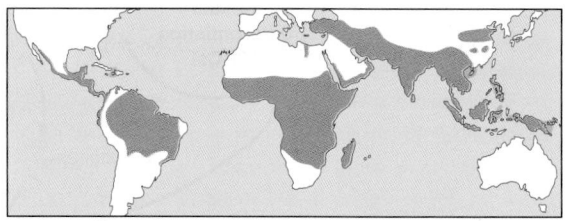

Fig. 13.34 Distribution of malaria. (For up-to-date information see the Malaria Atlas Project (MAP): map.ox.ac.uk.)

Pathogenesis

Life cycle of the malarial parasite

The female anopheline mosquito becomes infected when it feeds on human blood containing gametocytes, the sexual forms of the malarial parasite (Figs. 13.35 and 13.36). Development in the mosquito takes 7–20 days, and results in sporozoites accumulating in the salivary glands and being inoculated into the human blood stream. Sporozoites disappear from human blood within half an hour and enter the liver. After some days, merozoites leave the liver and invade red blood cells, where further asexual cycles of multiplication take place, producing schizonts. Rupture of the schizont releases more merozoites into the blood and causes fever, the periodicity of which depends on the species of parasite.

P. vivax and *P. ovale* may persist in liver cells as dormant forms, hypnozoites, capable of developing into merozoites months or years later. Thus the first attack of clinical malaria may occur long after the patient has left the endemic area, and the disease may relapse after treatment with drugs that only kill the erythrocytic stage of the parasite.

P. falciparum, *P. knowlesi* and *P. malariae* have no persistent exo-erythrocytic phase but recrudescence of fever may result from multiplication of parasites in red cells that have not been eliminated by treatment and immune processes (Box 13.55).

Pathology

Red cells infected with malaria undergo haemolysis. This is most severe with *P. falciparum*, which invades red cells of all ages; *P. vivax* and *P. ovale* preferentially invade younger cells, and *P. malariae* normoblasts, so that infections remain lower. Anaemia may be profound and is worsened by dyserythropoiesis, splenomegaly and depletion of folate stores.

In *P. falciparum* malaria, red cells containing trophozoites adhere to vascular endothelium in post-capillary venules in brain, kidney, liver, lungs and gut by the formation of 'knob' proteins. They also form 'rosettes' and rouleaux with uninfected red cells. Vessel congestion results in organ damage, which is exacerbated by rupture of schizonts, liberating toxic and antigenic substances (Fig. 13.36).

P. falciparum has influenced human evolution, with the appearance of protective mutations such as sickle-cell (Hb), thalassaemia, glucose-6-phosphate dehydrogenase (G6PD) deficiency (see Ch. 25) and HLA-B53. *P. falciparum* does not grow well in red cells that contain haemoglobin F, C or especially S. Haemoglobin S heterozygotes (AS) are protected against the lethal complications of malaria. *P. vivax* cannot enter red cells that lack the Duffy blood group; therefore many West Africans and African Americans are protected.

Clinical features

The clinical features of malaria are non-specific and the diagnosis must be suspected in anyone returning from an endemic area who has features of infection.

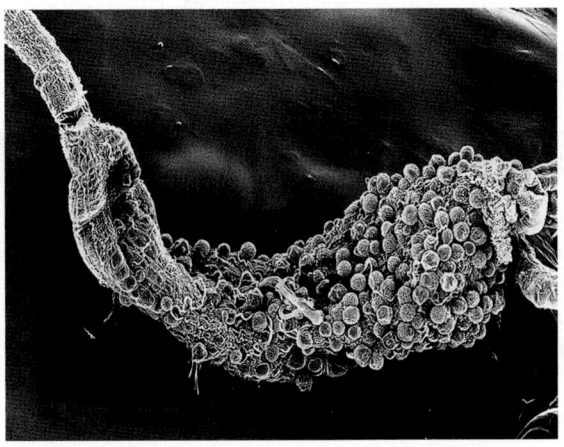

Fig. 13.35 Scanning electron micrograph of *Plasmodium falciparum* oöcysts lining an anopheline mosquito's stomach.

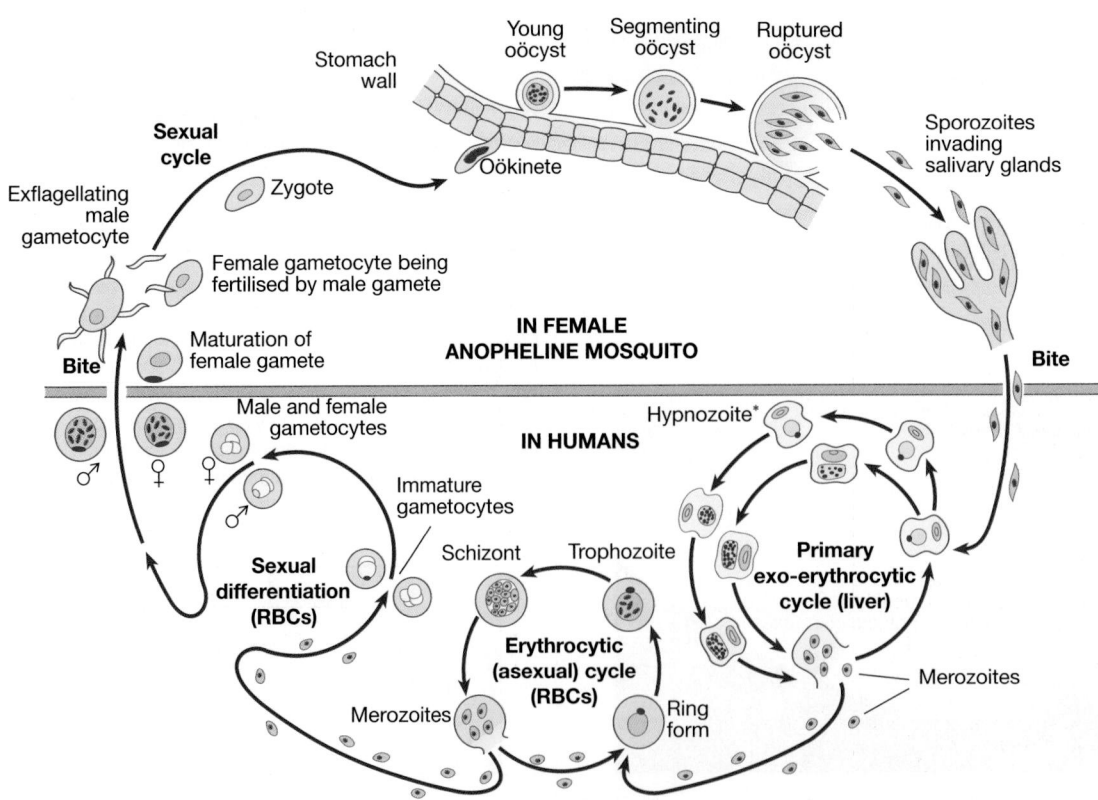

Fig. 13.36 Malarial parasites: life cycle. Hypnozoites (*) are present only in *Plasmodium vivax* and *P. ovale* infections. (RBC = red blood cell)

P. falciparum infection

This is the most dangerous of the malarias. The onset is often insidious, with malaise, headache and vomiting. Cough and mild diarrhoea are also common. The fever has no particular pattern and the classic periodicity is rarely observed. Jaundice is common due to haemolysis and hepatic dysfunction. The liver and spleen enlarge and may become tender. Anaemia develops rapidly, as does thrombocytopenia.

A patient with *falciparum* malaria, apparently not seriously ill, may rapidly develop dangerous complications (Fig. 13.37 and Box 13.56). Cerebral malaria is manifested by delirium, seizures or coma, usually without localising signs. Children die rapidly without any specific symptoms other than fever. Immunity is impaired in pregnancy and the parasite can preferentially bind to the placental protein chondroitin sulphate A. Abortion and intrauterine growth retardation from parasitisation of the maternal side of the placenta are frequent. Previous splenectomy increases the risk of severe malaria. Recurrent infection is rarely associated with later development of endemic Burkitt lymphoma and hyperreactive (tropical) splenomegaly.

Cycle/feature	Plasmodium vivax, P. ovale	P. malariae	P. falciparum
Pre-patent period (minimum incubation)	8–25 days	15–30 days	8–25 days
Exo-erythrocytic cycle	Persistent as hypnozoites	Pre-erythrocytic only	Pre-erythrocytic only
Asexual cycle	48 hrs synchronous	72 hrs synchronous	<48 hrs asynchronous
Fever periodicity	Alternate days	Every third day	None
Delayed onset	Common	Rare	Rare
Relapses	Common up to 2 years	Recrudescence many years later	Recrudescence up to 1 year

13.55 Relationships between life cycle of parasite and clinical features of malaria

P. vivax and P. ovale infection

Illness usually starts with several days of continued fever before the development of classical bouts of fever on alternate days. Fever starts with a rigor. The patient feels cold and the temperature rises to about 40°C. After half an hour to an hour, the hot or flush phase begins. It lasts several hours and gives way to profuse perspiration and a gradual fall in temperature. The cycle is repeated 48 hours later. Gradually, the spleen and liver enlarge and may become tender. Anaemia develops slowly. Relapses are frequent in the first 2 years after leaving the malarious area and infection may be acquired from blood transfusion.

13

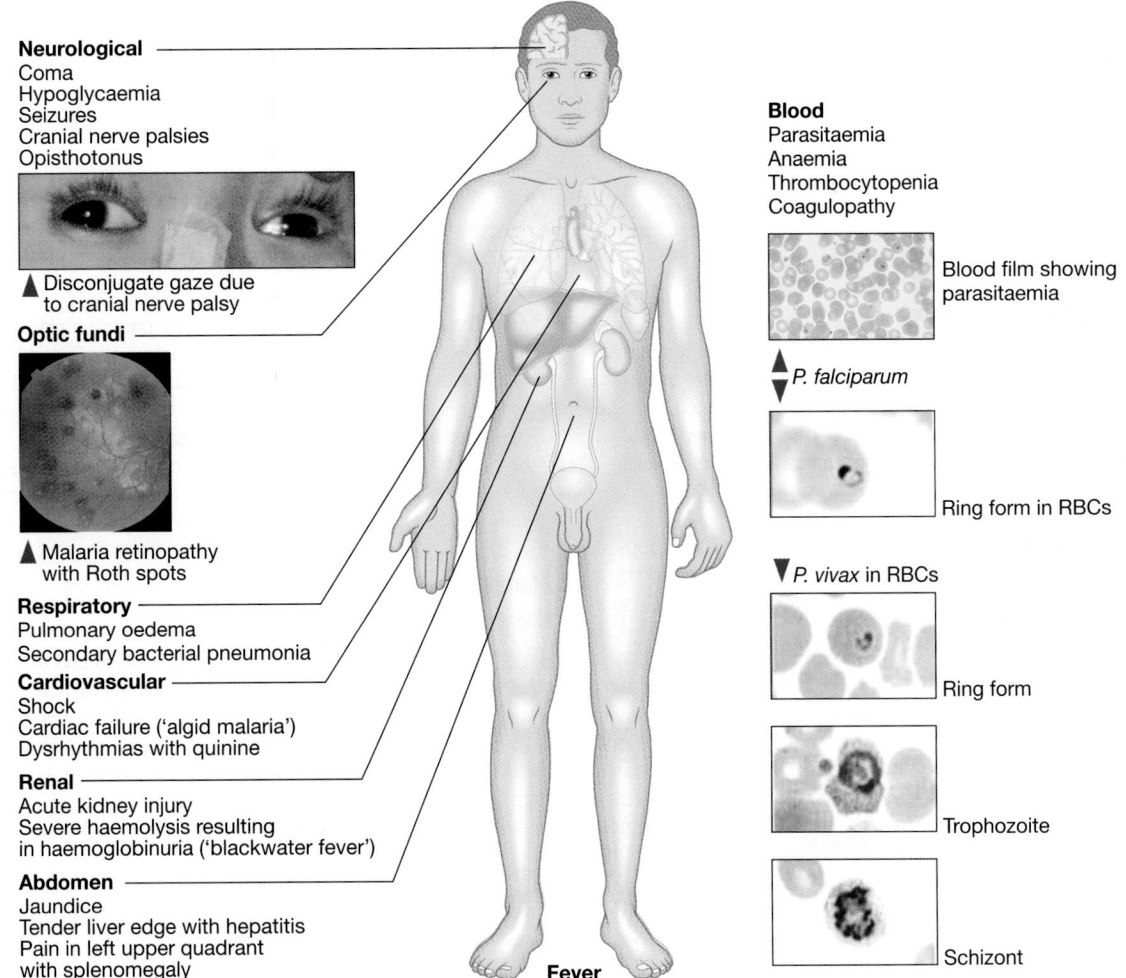

Neurological
Coma
Hypoglycaemia
Seizures
Cranial nerve palsies
Opisthotonus

▲ Disconjugate gaze due to cranial nerve palsy

Optic fundi

▲ Malaria retinopathy with Roth spots

Respiratory
Pulmonary oedema
Secondary bacterial pneumonia

Cardiovascular
Shock
Cardiac failure ('algid malaria')
Dysrhythmias with quinine

Renal
Acute kidney injury
Severe haemolysis resulting in haemoglobinuria ('blackwater fever')

Abdomen
Jaundice
Tender liver edge with hepatitis
Pain in left upper quadrant with splenomegaly

Fever

Blood
Parasitaemia
Anaemia
Thrombocytopenia
Coagulopathy

Blood film showing parasitaemia

▲▼ *P. falciparum*

Ring form in RBCs

▼ *P. vivax* in RBCs

Ring form

Trophozoite

Schizont

Fig. 13.37 Features of *Plasmodium falciparum* infection. (RBC = red blood cell). *Insets (malaria retinopathy) Courtesy of Dr Nicholas Beare, Royal Liverpool University Hospital; (blood films of P. vivax and P. falciparum) Courtesy of Dr Kamolrat Silamut, Mahidol Oxford Research Unit, Bangkok, Thailand.*

13.56 Severe manifestations/complications of *falciparum* malaria and their immediate management

Coma (cerebral malaria)

- Maintain airway
- Nurse on side
- Exclude other treatable causes of coma (e.g. hypoglycaemia, bacterial meningitis)
- Avoid harmful ancillary treatments such as glucocorticoids, heparin and adrenaline (epinephrine)
- Intubate if necessary

Hyperpyrexia

- Tepid sponging, fanning, cooling blanket
- Antipyretic drug (paracetamol)

Convulsions

- Maintain airway
- Treat promptly with diazepam or paraldehyde injection

Hypoglycaemia

- Measure blood glucose
- Give 50% dextrose injection followed by 10% dextrose infusion (glucagon may be ineffective)

Severe anaemia (packed cell volume <15%)

- Transfuse fresh whole blood or packed cells if pathogen screening of donor blood is available

Acute pulmonary oedema

- Nurse at 45°, give oxygen, venesect 250 mL of blood, give diuretic, stop intravenous fluids
- Intubate and add PEEP/CPAP in life-threatening hypoxaemia
- Haemofilter

Acute kidney injury

- Exclude pre-renal causes
- Fluid resuscitation if appropriate
- Peritoneal dialysis (haemofiltration or haemodialysis if available)

Spontaneous bleeding and coagulopathy

- Transfuse screened fresh whole blood (cryoprecipitate/fresh frozen plasma and platelets if available)
- Vitamin K injection

Metabolic acidosis

- Exclude or treat hypoglycaemia, hypovolaemia and Gram-negative sepsis
- Fluid resuscitation
- Give oxygen

Shock ('algid malaria')

- Suspect Gram-negative sepsis
- Take blood cultures
- Give parenteral antimicrobials
- Correct haemodynamic disturbances

Aspiration pneumonia

- Give parenteral antimicrobial drugs
- Change position
- Physiotherapy
- Give oxygen

Hyperparasitaemia

- Consider exchange transfusion (e.g. >10% of circulating erythrocytes parasitised in non-immune patient with severe disease)

Specific therapy

- Intravenous artesunate
- Mefloquine should be avoided due to increased risk of post-malaria neurological syndrome

(CPAP = continuous positive airway pressure; PEEP = positive end-expiratory pressure)
From WHO. Severe falciparum malaria. In: Severe and complicated malaria, 3rd edn. Trans R Soc Trop Med Hyg 2000; 94 (suppl. 1):S1–41.

P. malariae and P. knowlesi infection

This is usually associated with mild symptoms and bouts of fever every third day. Parasitaemia may persist for many years, with the occasional recrudescence of fever or without producing any symptoms. Chronic *P. malariae* infection causes glomerulonephritis and long-term nephrotic syndrome in children. *P. knowlesi* is usually mild but can deteriorate rapidly.

Investigations

WHO recommends prompt malaria diagnosis, either by microscopy or malaria rapid diagnostic test (RDT), whenever malaria is suspected. In a Giemsa-stained thick film, erythrocytes are lysed, releasing all blood stages of the parasite. This, as well as the fact that more blood is used in thick films, facilitates the diagnosis of low-level parasitaemia. A thin film is essential to confirm the diagnosis, species and, in *P. falciparum* infections, to quantify the parasite load (by counting the percentage of infected erythrocytes). *P. falciparum* parasites may be very scanty, especially in patients who have been partially treated. With *P. falciparum*, only ring forms are normally seen in the early stages (see Fig. 13.37); with the other species, all stages of the erythrocytic cycle may be found. Gametocytes appear after about 2 weeks, persist after treatment and are harmless, except that they are the source by which more mosquitoes become infected.

Immunochromatographic RDTs for malaria antigens, such as OptiMAL (which detects the *Plasmodium* LDH of *P. falciparum* and *vivax*) and Parasight-F (which detects the *P. falciparum* histidine-rich protein (HRP) 2), are extremely sensitive and specific for *falciparum* malaria but less so for other species. They are especially useful where the microscopist is less experienced in examining blood films (e.g. in non-endemic or remote areas). They are less sensitive for low-level parasitaemia and positivity may persist for a month or more in some individuals. Dual *pfhrp2/3* gene deletion leads to false-negative HRP2-based tests and is increasingly reported in East Africa. The QBC Malaria Test is a fluorescence microscopy-based malaria diagnostic test that is also used.

Nucleic acid detection (PCR) is used mainly in research and is useful for determining whether a patient has a recrudescence of the same malaria parasite or a reinfection with a new parasite.

Management

Mild P. falciparum malaria

Since *P. falciparum* is widely resistant to chloroquine and sulfadoxine-pyrimethamine (Fansidar) almost worldwide, an artemisinin-based treatment is recommended (Box 13.57). WHO policy recommends always using ACT, e.g. co-artemether or artesunate–amodiaquine. Unfortunately, artemisinin resistance has now been reported in South-east Asia, mandating strict adherence to local guidance on the selection of ACT, e.g. dihydro-artemisinin-piperaquine or pyronaridine-artesunate in Thailand.

Complicated P. falciparum malaria

Severe malaria should be considered in any non-immune patient with a parasite count greater than 2% or with complications, and is a medical emergency (see Box 13.56). Management includes early and appropriate antimalarial chemotherapy, active treatment of complications, correction of fluid, electrolyte and acid–base balance, and avoidance of harmful ancillary treatments.

i 13.57 Malaria treatment

Mild *falciparum* malaria

Preferred therapy

- Co-artemether (CoArtem or Riamet); contains artemether and lumefantrine (4 tablets orally at 0, 8, 24, 36, 48 and 60 hrs)

Alternative therapy

- Quinine (600 mg of quinine salt 3 times daily orally for 5–7 days), together with or followed by doxycycline (200 mg once daily orally for 7 days)
  - Use clindamycin not doxycycline if the patient is a pregnant woman or young child
  or
- Atovaquone–proguanil (Malarone, 4 tablets orally once daily for 3 days)

Pregnancy

- Co-artemether but avoid in early pregnancy
- If not using co-artemether, use quinine plus clindamycin (450 mg 3 times daily orally for 7 days)

Other regimens

- Artesunate (200 mg orally daily for 3 days) and mefloquine (1 g orally on day 2 and 500 mg orally on day 3)

Severe *falciparum* malaria

Preferred therapy

- Artesunate 2.4 mg/kg IV at 0, 12 and 24 hrs and then once daily for 7 days. Once the patient is able to recommence oral intake, switch to 2 mg/kg orally once daily, to complete a total cumulative dose of 17–18 mg/kg

Alternative therapy

- Quinine, loading dose 20 mg/kg IV over 4 hrs, up to a maximum of 1.4 g, then maintenance doses of 10 mg/kg quinine salt given as 4-hr infusions 3 times daily for the first 48 hrs then twice a day, up to a maximum of 700 mg per dose or until the patient can take drugs orally. Combine with doxycycline (or clindamycin if there are contraindications to doxycycline)
- Note the loading dose should not be given if quinine, quinidine or mefloquine has been administered in the previous 24 hrs
- Patients should be monitored by ECG while receiving quinine, with special attention to QRS duration and QT interval

Non-*falciparum* malaria

Preferred therapy

- Chloroquine: 600 mg chloroquine base orally, followed by 300 mg base in 6 hrs, then 150 mg base twice daily for 2 more days plus primaquine (30 mg orally daily (for *P. vivax*) or 15 mg orally daily (for *P. ovale*) for 14 days) after confirming G6PD-negative

Patients with mild to moderate G6PD deficiency and *P. vivax* or *P. ovale*

- Chloroquine plus primaquine 0.75 mg/kg weekly orally for 8 weeks

Chloroquine-resistant *P. vivax*

- Co-artemether as for *P. falciparum*

(ECG = electrocardiogram; G6PD = glucose-6-phosphate dehydrogenase; IV = intravenous)

i 13.58 Chemoprophylaxis of malaria[1]

Antimalarial tablets	Adult prophylactic dose	Regimen
Chloroquine resistance high		
Mefloquine[2]	250 mg weekly	Started 2–3 weeks before travel and continued until 4 weeks after
or Doxycycline[3,4]	100 mg daily	Started 1 week before and continued until 4 weeks after travel
or Atovaquone plus proguanil (Malarone)[4]	1 tablet daily	From 1–2 days before travel until 1 week after return
Chloroquine resistance absent		
Chloroquine[5] *and* proguanil	300 mg base weekly 100–200 mg daily	Started 1 week before and continued until 4 weeks after travel

[1]Choice of regimen is determined by area to be visited, length of stay, level of malaria transmission, level of drug resistance, presence of underlying disease in the traveller and concomitant medication taken. [2]Contraindicated in the first trimester of pregnancy, lactation, cardiac conduction disorders, epilepsy, psychiatric disorders; may cause neuropsychiatric disorders. [3]Causes photosensitisation and sunburn if high-protection sunblock is not used. [4]Avoid in pregnancy. [5]British preparations of chloroquine usually contain 150 mg base, French preparations 100 mg base and American preparations 300 mg base.

13

mefloquine. Box 13.58 gives the recommended doses for protection of the non-immune. The risk of malaria in the area to be visited and the degree of chloroquine resistance guide the recommendations for prophylaxis. Updated recommendations are summarised at fitfortravel.nhs.uk. Mefloquine is useful in areas of multiple drug resistance, such as East and Central Africa and Papua New Guinea. Experience shows it to be safe for at least 2 years but there are several contraindications to its use (see Box 13.58).

Expert advice is required for individuals unable to tolerate the first-line agents listed or in whom they are contraindicated. Mefloquine should be started 2–3 weeks before travel to give time for assessment of side-effects. Chloroquine should not be taken continuously as a prophylactic for more than 5 years without regular ophthalmic examination, as it may cause irreversible retinopathy. Pregnant and lactating women may take proguanil or chloroquine safely.

Prevention also involves advice about the use of high-percentage diethyltoluamide (DEET), covering up extremities when out after dark, and sleeping under permethrin-impregnated mosquito nets.

Malaria control in endemic areas

There are major initiatives to reduce and eliminate malaria in endemic areas, particularly 11 countries with the greatest burden (e.g. the 'High Burden High Impact' approach). Successful programmes combine vector control, including indoor residual spraying, use of long-lasting insecticide-treated bed nets (ITNs) and intermittent preventative therapy (IPT; repeated dose of prophylactic drugs in high-risk groups, such as children and pregnant women, which reduces malaria and anaemia).

Research to produce a fully protective malaria vaccine is ongoing. An adjuvanted vaccine using the R21 vaccine candidate has shown good efficacy in African children under 18 months and has progressed to phase III studies.

Babesiosis

Babesiosis is a tick-borne intra-erythrocytic protozoon parasite. There are more than 100 species of *Babesia*, all of which have an animal reservoir, typically either rodents or cattle. These are transmitted to humans via the tick vector *Ixodes scapularis*. Most American cases of babesiosis are due to *B. microti* and most European cases to *B. divergens*. Patients present

The treatment of choice is intravenous artesunate. Late haemolysis is a treatment side-effect in some patients. Rectal administration of artesunate is also being developed to allow administration in remote rural areas. Quinine salt is the alternative.

Exchange transfusion has not been tested in randomised controlled trials but may be beneficial for non-immune patients with persisting high parasitaemias (>10% circulating erythrocytes).

Non-*falciparum* malaria

P. vivax, *P. ovale*, *P. knowlesi* and *P. malariae* infections should be treated with oral chloroquine but some chloroquine resistance has been reported from Indonesia and all are sensitive to ACTs. 'Radical cure' is essential in patients with *P. vivax* or *P. ovale* malaria using a course of primaquine or tafenoquine, which destroys the hypnozoite phase in the liver. Severe haemolysis may develop in those who are G6PD-deficient. Cyanosis due to the formation of methaemoglobin in the red cells is more common but not dangerous (see Fig. 10.1).

Prevention

Clinical attacks of malaria may be preventable with chemoprophylaxis using chloroquine, atovaquone plus proguanil (Malarone), doxycycline or

with fever and malaise 1–4 weeks after a tick bite. Illness may be complicated by haemolytic anaemia. Severe illness is seen in splenectomised patients. The diagnosis is made by blood-film examination. Treatment is with azithromycin and atovaquone or quinine and clindamycin.

African trypanosomiasis (sleeping sickness)

African sleeping sickness is caused by trypanosomes (Fig. 13.38) carried by tsetse flies, and is unique to sub-Saharan Africa (Fig. 13.39). The incidence of sleeping sickness across Africa has declined 95% since 1999 to <1000 cases per year. It is now on the verge of eradication. *Trypanosoma brucei gambiense* trypanosomiasis is found in West and Central Africa and causes 98% of human African trypanosomiasis (HAT). *T. brucei rhodesiense* trypanosomiasis occurs in East and Central Africa. In West Africa, transmission is mainly at the riverside, where the fly rests in the shade of trees; no animal reservoir has been identified for *T. gambiense*. *T. rhodesiense* has a large reservoir in numerous wild animals and transmission takes place in the shade of woods bordering grasslands. Rural populations employed in agriculture, fishing and animal husbandry are susceptible. Local people and tourists visiting forests infested with tsetse flies and animal reservoirs may become infected.

Clinical features

A bite by a tsetse fly is painful and commonly becomes inflamed; if trypanosomes are introduced, the site may again become painful and swollen about 10 days later ('trypanosomal chancre'), associated with

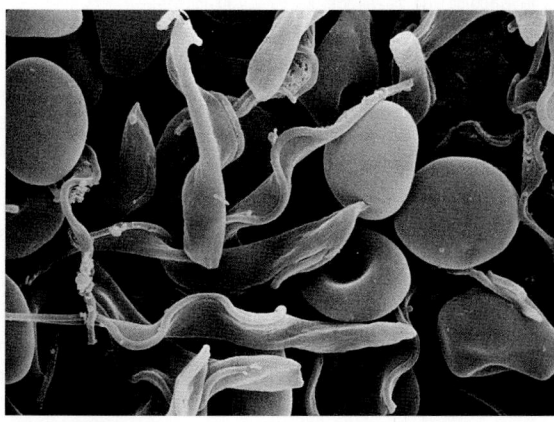

Fig. 13.38 **Trypanosomiasis.** Scanning electron micrograph showing trypanosomes swimming among erythrocytes.

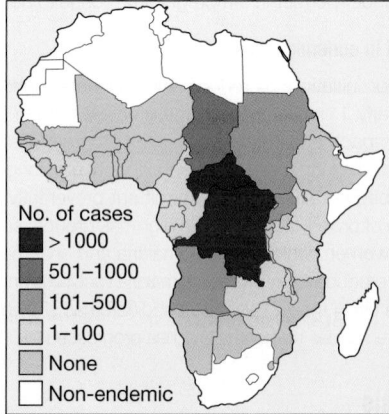

No. of cases
■ >1000
■ 501–1000
■ 101–500
□ 1–100
□ None
□ Non-endemic

Fig. 13.39 **Distribution of human African trypanosomiasis.** Data are from 2009. *From Simarro PP, Diarra A, Ruiz Postigo JA, et al. The human African trypanosomiasis control and surveillance programme of the World Health Organization 2000–2009: the way forward. PLoS Negl Trop Dis 2011; 5(2):e1007.*

regional lymphadenopathy. Within 2–3 weeks of infection, the trypanosomes invade the blood stream. The disease is characterised by an early haematolymphatic (stage 1) and a late chronic encephalopathy phase (stage 2).

Rhodesiense infections

This disease is more acute and severe than in *gambiense* infections. Within days or a few weeks, the patient is usually severely ill and may have developed pleural effusions and signs of myocarditis or hepatitis. There may be a petechial rash. The patient may die before there are signs of involvement of the CNS. If the illness is less acute, drowsiness, tremors and coma develop.

Gambiense infections

The distinction between early and late stages may not be apparent in *gambiense* infections. The disease usually runs a slow course over months or years, with irregular bouts of fever and enlargement of lymph nodes. These are characteristically firm, discrete, rubbery and painless, and are particularly prominent in the posterior triangle of the neck. Hepatosplenomegaly may develop. After some months without treatment, the CNS is invaded. Patients develop headache, altered behaviour, blunting of higher mental functions, insomnia by night and sleepiness by day, delirium and eventually tremors, pareses, wasting, coma and death.

Investigations

Trypanosomiasis should be considered in any febrile patient from an endemic area. In *rhodesiense* infections, thick and thin malaria blood films will reveal trypanosomes. The trypanosomes may be seen in the blood or from puncture of the primary lesion in the earliest stages of *gambiense* infections, but it is usually easier to demonstrate them by aspiration of a lymph node. Concentration methods include buffy coat microscopy and miniature anion exchange chromatography.

Due to the cyclical nature of parasitaemia, the diagnosis is often made by demonstration of antibodies using a simple, rapid screening card agglutination trypanosomiasis test (CATT) for *gambiense* HAT, followed by parasitological confirmation.

No reliable serological test is available for *rhodesiense* HAT. PCR diagnosis is available, although technical requirements limit its availability. If the CNS is affected, the cell count and protein content of the CSF are increased and the glucose is diminished. A very high level of serum IgM or the presence of IgM in the CSF is suggestive of trypanosomiasis. Recognition of CNS involvement is critical, as failure to treat it might be fatal.

Management

The prognosis is good if treatment is begun early, before the brain has been invaded. At this stage, intravenous suramin, after a test dose of 100–200 mg, should be given for *rhodesiense* infections, followed by five injections of 20 mg/kg every 7 days. Fexinidazole, an oral nitroimidazole derivative, acts on the parasite nitroreductase. It is the preferred treatment for stage 1 or stage 2 infections with a CSF white cell count <0.1 ×10⁹/L *gambiense* infections. The adult dose is 1800 mg days 1–4, and 1200 mg days 5–10, taken with food. For adults weighing <35 kg the loading dose is 1200 mg (days 1–4) followed by 600 mg (days 5–10). For *gambiense* infections, deep intramuscular or intravenous pentamidine 4 mg/kg for 7 days is now used mainly in children <6 years of age with stage 1 disease.

For the treatment of stage 2 (nervous system) infection caused by *gambiense* HAT with CSF white cell count ≥0.1 ×10⁹/L or in whom a CSF exam is indicated but not performed, nifurtimox (15 mg/kg daily orally in three divided doses for 10 days) and eflornithine (DFMO; 400 mg/kg in two 2-hour IV infusions for 7 days) combination therapy (NECT) is recommended. DFMO, an irreversible inhibitor of ornithine decarboxylase was formerly given without nifurtimox (100 mg/kg IV 4 times daily for 14 days). This regimen had more side-effects and more injections. Stage 2 *rhodesiense* infection is treated with melarsoprol, an arsenical (2.2 mg/kg IV for 10 days). Treatment-related mortality with melarsoprol is 4–12% due to reactive encephalopathy.

Prevention

In endemic areas, various measures are taken against tsetse flies, and field teams help detect and treat early HAT.

American trypanosomiasis (Chagas' disease)

Chagas' disease occurs widely in South and Central America. The cause is *Trypanosoma cruzi*, transmitted to humans from the faeces of a reduviid (triatomine) bug, in which the trypanosomes develop. These bugs live in wild forests in crevices, burrows and palm trees. The *Triatoma infestans* bug has become domesticated in the Southern Cone countries (Argentina, Brazil, Chile, Paraguay and Uruguay). It lives in the mud and wattle walls and thatched roofs of simple rural houses and emerges at night to feed and defecate on the sleeping occupants. Infected faeces are rubbed in through the conjunctiva, mucosa of mouth or nose, or abrasions of the skin. Over 100 species of mammal – domestic, peridomestic and wild – may serve as reservoirs of infection. In some areas, blood transfusion accounts for about 5% of cases. Congenital transmission occasionally occurs.

Pathology

The trypanosomes migrate via the blood stream, develop into amastigote forms in the tissues and multiply intracellularly by binary fission. In the acute phase, inflammation (primarily cell-mediated) of parasitised, as well as non-parasitised, cardiac muscles and capillaries occurs, resulting in acute myocarditis. In the chronic phase, focal myocardial atrophy, signs of chronic passive congestion and thromboembolic phenomena, cardiomegaly and apical cardiac aneurysm are salient findings. In the digestive form of disease, focal myositis and discontinuous lesions of the intramural myenteric plexus are seen, predominantly in the oesophagus and colon.

Clinical features

Acute phase

Clinical manifestations of the acute phase are seen in only 1%–2% of individuals infected before the age of 15 years. Young children (1–5 years) are most commonly affected. The entrance of *T. cruzi* through an abrasion produces a dusky-red, firm swelling and enlargement of regional lymph nodes. A conjunctival lesion, although less common, is characteristic; the unilateral firm, reddish swelling of the lids may close the eye and constitutes 'Romaña's sign'. In a few patients, an acute generalised infection soon appears, with a transient morbilliform or urticarial rash, fever, lymphadenopathy and enlargement of the spleen and liver. In a small minority of patients, acute myocarditis and heart failure or neurological features, including personality changes and signs of meningoencephalitis, may be seen. The acute infection may be fatal to infants.

Chronic phase

About 50%–70% of infected patients become seropositive and develop an indeterminate form when parasitaemia occurs only at low levels and is not usually detectable. They have a normal lifespan with no symptoms but are a natural reservoir for the disease and maintain the life cycle of parasites in tissues. After a latent period of several years, 10%–30% of chronic cases develop low-grade myocarditis and damage to conducting fibres, which causes cardiomyopathy characterised by cardiac dilatation, arrhythmias, partial or complete heart block and sudden death. In nearly 10% of patients, damage to Auerbach's plexus results in dilatation of various parts of the alimentary canal, especially the colon and oesophagus, so-called 'mega' disease. Dilatation of the bile ducts and bronchi are also recognised sequelae. Autoimmune processes may be responsible for much of the damage. There are geographical variations of the basic pattern of disease. Reactivation of Chagas' disease can occur in patients with HIV if the CD4 count falls lower than 200 cells/mm^3; this can cause space-occupying lesions with a presentation similar to *Toxoplasma gondii* encephalitis in HIV, a more diffuse encephalitis, meningoencephalitis or myocarditis.

Investigations

T. cruzi is easily detectable by direct microscopic examination in a blood film in the acute illness. In chronic disease, antibody detection is highly sensitive, and a positive result with two different serological tests confirms the infection parasite. DNA detection by PCR in the patient's blood is a highly sensitive method for documentation of infection.

Management and prevention

Parasiticidal agents are used to treat the acute phase, congenital disease and early chronic phase (within 10 years of infection). Benznidazole is given at a dose of 5–8mg/kg daily orally, in two divided doses for 60 days. Nifurtimox is an alternative treatment dosed at 8–20mg/kg orally in three divided doses for 60 days. All doses of either treatment are weight adjusted. Treatment with either agent has to be carefully supervised to minimise toxicity while preserving parasiticidal activity. Cure rates of 80% in acute disease are obtained. Both benznidazole and nifurtimox are toxic, with adverse reaction rates of 30%–55%. Parasiticidal treatment of the chronic phase is usually performed but, in the cardiac or digestive 'mega' diseases, does not reverse tissue damage. Surgery may be needed.

Preventative measures include improvement of housing and destruction of reduviid bugs by spraying of houses with insecticides. Blood and organ donors should be screened.

Toxoplasmosis

Toxoplasma gondii is an intracellular parasite. The sexual phase of the parasite's life cycle (Fig. 13.40) occurs in the small intestinal epithelium of the domestic cat. Oöcysts in cat faeces are spread to intermediate hosts (pigs, sheep and also humans) via soil contamination. Oöcysts may survive in moist conditions for weeks or months. After ingestion, the parasite transforms into rapidly dividing tachyzoites through cycles

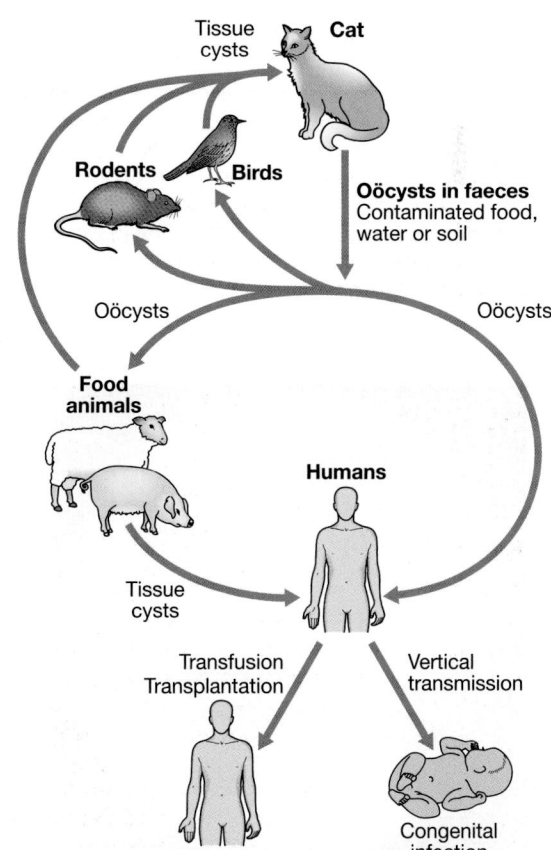

Fig. 13.40 Life cycle of *Toxoplasma gondii*.

of asexual multiplication. Microscopic tissue cysts develop containing bradyzoites, which persist for the lifetime of the host. Cats become infected or reinfected by ingesting tissue cysts in prey such as rodents and birds.

Human infection occurs via oöcyst-contaminated soil, salads and vegetables, or by ingestion of raw or under-cooked meats containing tissue cysts. Sheep, pigs and rabbits are the most common meat sources. Outbreaks of toxoplasmosis have followed consumption of unfiltered water. In high-income countries, toxoplasmosis is the most common protozoal infection; around 22% of adults in the UK are seropositive. Most primary infections are subclinical; however, toxoplasmosis is thought to account for about 15% of heterophile antibody-negative infectious mononucleosis. In India or Brazil, approximately 40%–60% of pregnant females are seropositive for *T. gondii*. Toxoplasmosis is an important opportunistic infection in people with HIV, with considerable morbidity and mortality. Generalised toxoplasmosis has followed occupational exposure of laboratory workers.

Clinical features

In most immunocompetent individuals, including children and pregnant women, the infection goes unnoticed. In approximately 10% of patients, it causes a self-limiting illness, most often in adults aged 25–35 years. The presenting feature is usually localised or generalised painless lymphadenopathy. The cervical nodes are primarily involved but mediastinal, mesenteric or retroperitoneal groups may be affected. The spleen is seldom palpable. Most patients have no systemic symptoms but some complain of malaise, fever, fatigue, muscle pain, sore throat and headache. Complete resolution usually occurs within a few months, although symptoms and lymphadenopathy tend to fluctuate unpredictably and some patients do not recover completely for a year or more. Encephalitis, myocarditis, polymyositis, pneumonitis or hepatitis occasionally occur in immunocompetent patients but are more frequent in immunocompromised hosts. Retinochoroiditis (Fig. 13.41) is usually the result of congenital infection but has also been reported in acquired disease.

Congenital toxoplasmosis

Acute toxoplasmosis, mostly subclinical, affects 0.3%–1% of pregnant women, with approximately 60% transmission rate to the fetus, which rises with increasing gestation. Seropositive females infected 6 months before conception have no risk of fetal transmission. Congenital disease affects approximately 40% of infected fetuses, and is more likely and more severe with infection early in gestation (see Box 13.24). Many fetal infections are subclinical at birth but long-term sequelae include retinochoroiditis, microcephaly and hydrocephalus.

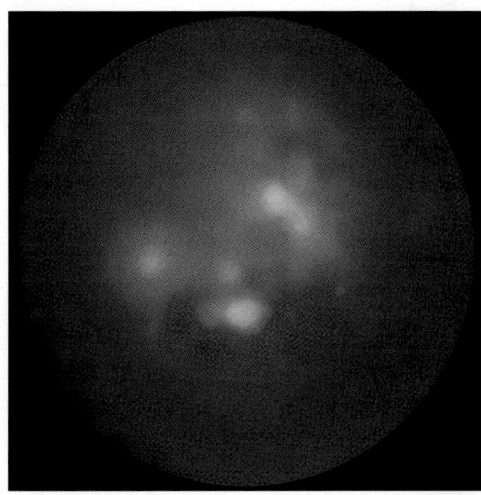

Fig. 13.41 Retinochoroiditis due to toxoplasmosis.

Investigations

In contrast to immunocompromised patients, in whom the diagnosis often requires direct detection of parasites, serology is often used in immunocompetent individuals. The Sabin–Feldman dye test (indirect fluorescent antibody test), which detects IgG antibody, is most commonly used. Recent infection induces a fourfold or greater increase in titre when paired sera are tested. Peak titres ≥1/1000 are reached 1–2 months after infection, and serology then becomes an unreliable indicator of recent infection. The detection of significant levels of *Toxoplasma*-specific IgM antibody may be useful in confirming acute infection. A false-positive result or persistence of IgM antibodies for years after infection makes interpretation difficult; however, negative IgM antibodies virtually rule out acute infection.

During pregnancy, it is critical to differentiate recent from past infection; the presence of high-avidity IgG antibodies excludes infection acquired in the preceding 3–4 months.

If necessary, the presence of *Toxoplasma* organisms in a lymph node biopsy or other tissue can be detected histochemically with *T. gondii* antiserum, or by the use of PCR to detect *Toxoplasma*-specific DNA.

Management

In immunocompetent subjects, uncomplicated toxoplasmosis is self-limiting and responds poorly to antimicrobial therapy. Treatment with sulfadiazine, pyrimethamine and folinic acid is usually reserved for severe or progressive disease, and for infection in immunocompromised patients. Often empirical treatment is initiated in people living with HIV if space-occupying lesions are found in the CNS (see Ch. 14).

In pregnant women with established recent infection, spiramycin (3 g daily in divided doses) is given until term. Once fetal infection is established, treatment with sulfadiazine and pyrimethamine plus calcium folinate is recommended (spiramycin does not cross the placental barrier). The cost/benefit of routine *Toxoplasma* screening and treatment in pregnancy is being debated in many countries. There is insufficient evidence to determine the effects on mother or baby of current antiparasitic treatment for women who seroconvert in pregnancy.

Leishmaniasis

Leishmaniasis is caused by unicellular, flagellate, intracellular protozoa belonging to the genus *Leishmania* (order Kinetoplastidae). The 21 leishmanial species that cause human disease are responsible for three clinical syndromes:

- visceral leishmaniasis (VL, kala-azar)
- cutaneous leishmaniasis (CL)
- mucosal leishmaniasis (ML).

Epidemiology and transmission

Although most clinical syndromes are caused by zoonotic transmission of parasites from animals (chiefly canine and rodent reservoirs) to humans through phlebotomine sandfly vectors (Fig. 13.42A), humans are the only known reservoir (anthroponotic person-to-person transmission) in major VL foci in South Asia and in injection drug-users (Fig. 13.42B and C). Leishmaniasis occurs in approximately 100 countries around the world, with an estimated annual incidence of 1 million new cases, of which VL contributes approximately 20 000 cases.

The life cycle of *Leishmania* is shown in Figure 13.43. Flagellar promastigotes (10–20 μm) are introduced by the feeding female sandfly. The promastigotes are taken up by neutrophils, which undergo apoptosis and are then engulfed by macrophages, in which the parasites transform into amastigotes (2–4 μm; Leishman–Donovan body). These multiply, causing macrophage lysis and infection of other cells. Sandflies pick up amastigotes when feeding on infected patients or animal reservoirs. In the sandfly, the parasite transforms into a flagellar promastigote, which multiplies by binary fission in the gut of the vector and migrates to the proboscis to infect a new host.

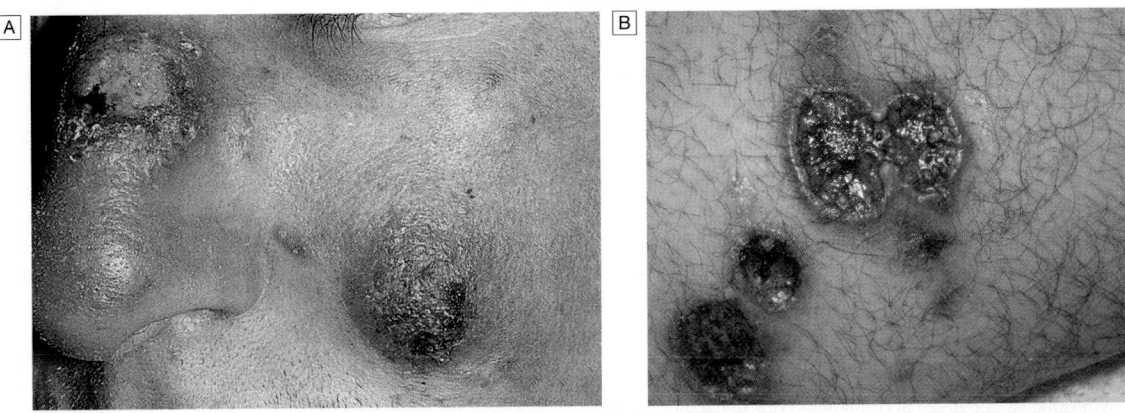

Fig. 13.48 **Cutaneous leishmaniasis.** [A] Papule. [B] Ulcer. *(B) Courtesy of Dr Ravi Gowda, Royal Hallamshire Hospital, Sheffield.*

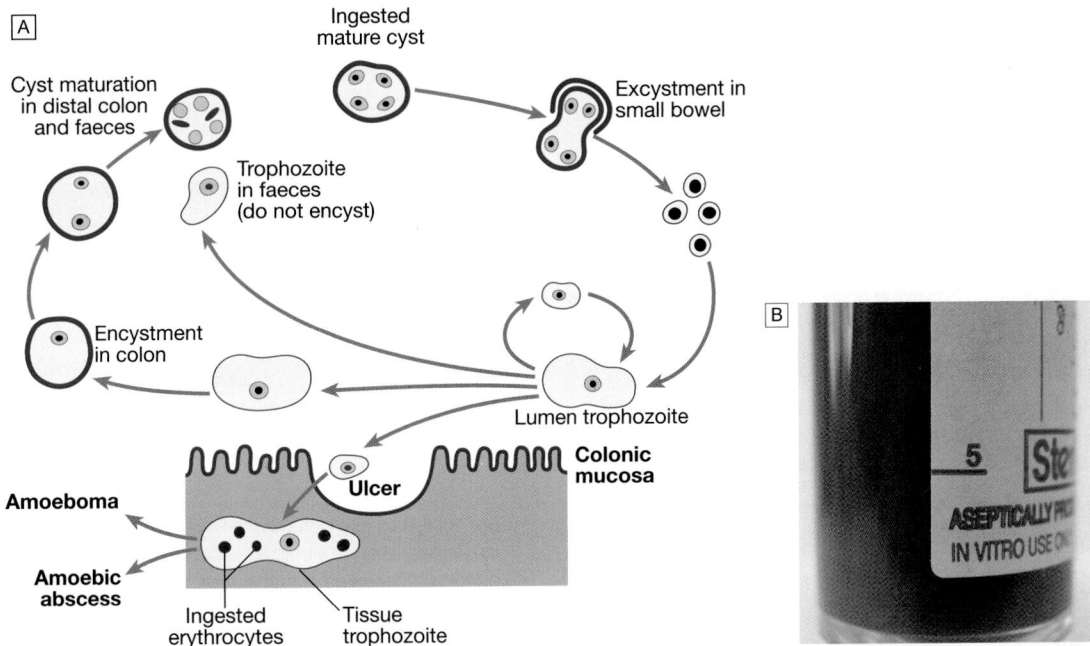

Fig. 13.49 **Amoebiasis.** [A] The life cycle of *Entamoeba histolytica.* [B] The chocolate-brown appearance of aspirated material from an amoebic liver abscess. *(A) From Knight R. Parasitic disease in man. Edinburgh: Churchill Livingstone, Elsevier Ltd; 1982. (B) Courtesy of Dr Ravi Gowda, Royal Hallamshire Hospital, Sheffield.*

Pathology

Cysts of *E. histolytica* are ingested in water or uncooked foods contaminated by human faeces. Infection may also be acquired through anal/oral sexual practices. Trophozoites emerge from the cysts in the small bowel and enter the large bowel. The parasite invades the mucous membrane of the large bowel, producing lesions that are maximal in the caecum but extend to the anal canal. These are flask-shaped ulcers, varying greatly in size and surrounded by healthy mucosa. A rare complication is amoeboma, a localised granuloma that may present as a palpable abdominal mass (usually in the right iliac fossa), a rectal mass (rarely) or a filling defect on colonic radiography. This has to be distinguished from other causes of colonic mass (*e.g.* cancer). Amoebic ulcers may cause severe haemorrhage but rarely perforate the bowel wall.

Amoebic trophozoites can emerge from the vegetative cyst from the bowel and be carried to the liver in a portal venule. They can multiply rapidly and destroy the liver parenchyma, causing an abscess (see also p. 891). The liquid contents at first have a characteristic pinkish colour, which may later change to chocolate-brown (said to resemble anchovy sauce).

Cutaneous amoebiasis, though rare, causes progressive genital, perianal or peri-abdominal surgical wound ulceration.

Clinical features

Intestinal amoebiasis – amoebic dysentery

Most amoebic infections are asymptomatic. The incubation period of amoebiasis ranges from 2 weeks to many years, followed by a chronic course with abdominal pains and two or more unformed stools a day. Offensive diarrhoea, alternating with constipation, and blood or mucus in the stool are common. There may be abdominal pain, especially in the right lower quadrant (which may mimic acute appendicitis). A dysenteric presentation with passage of blood, simulating bacillary dysentery or ulcerative colitis, occurs particularly in older people, in the puerperium and with super-added pyogenic infection of the ulcers.

Amoebic liver abscess

The abscess is usually found in the right hepatic lobe. There may not be associated diarrhoea. Early symptoms may be only local discomfort and malaise; later, a swinging temperature and sweating may develop, usually without marked systemic symptoms or signs. An enlarged, tender liver, cough and pain in the right shoulder are characteristic but symptoms may remain vague and signs minimal. A large abscess may penetrate the diaphragm, rupturing into the lung, and may be coughed up through a hepatobronchial fistula. Rupture into the pleural or peritoneal cavity, or rupture of a left lobe abscess in the pericardial sac, is less common but more serious.

Investigations

Microscopic examination of the stool and exudate can reveal motile trophozoites containing red blood cells. Trophozoite motility decreases rapidly as the stool preparation cools. Several stools may need to be examined in chronic amoebiasis before cysts are found. Sigmoidoscopy may reveal typical flask-shaped ulcers, which should be scraped and examined immediately for E. histolytica. In endemic areas, one-third of the population are symptomless passers of amoebic cysts.

An amoebic abscess of the liver is suspected on clinical grounds; there is often a neutrophil leucocytosis and a raised right hemidiaphragm on chest X-ray. Confirmation is by ultrasonic scanning. Aspirated pus from an amoebic abscess has the characteristic chocolate-brown appearance but rarely contains free amoebae (Fig. 13.49B).

Serum antibodies are detectable by immunofluorescence in over 95% of patients with hepatic amoebiasis and intestinal amoeboma, but in only about 60% of dysenteric amoebiasis. DNA detection by PCR or by loop-mediated isothermal amplification (LAMP) assay have been shown to be useful in diagnosis of E. histolytica infections but are not generally available.

Management

Intestinal and early hepatic amoebiasis responds quickly to oral metronidazole (800 mg 3 times daily for 5–10 days) or other long-acting nitroimidazoles like tinidazole or ornidazole (both in doses of 2 g daily for 3 days). Nitazoxanide (500 mg twice daily for 3 days) is an alternative drug. Either diloxanide furoate or paromomycin, in doses of 500 mg orally 3 times daily for 10 days after treatment, should be given to eliminate luminal cysts.

If a liver abscess is large or threatens to burst, or if the response to chemotherapy is not prompt, aspiration is required and is repeated if necessary. Rupture of an abscess into the pleural cavity, pericardial sac or peritoneal cavity necessitates immediate aspiration or surgical drainage. Small serous effusions resolve without drainage.

Prevention

Personal precautions against contracting amoebiasis include not eating fresh, uncooked vegetables or drinking unclean water.

Giardiasis

Infection with Giardia lamblia (also known as G. intestinalis) is found worldwide and is common in the tropics. It particularly affects children, tourists and immunosuppressed individuals, and is the parasite most commonly imported into the UK. Cysts remain viable in water for up to 3 months and infection usually occurs by ingesting contaminated water. Its flagellar trophozoite form attaches to the duodenal and jejunal mucosa, causing inflammation.

Clinical features and investigations

After an incubation period of 1–3 weeks, there is diarrhoea, abdominal pain, weakness, anorexia, nausea and vomiting. On examination, there may be abdominal distension and tenderness. Chronic diarrhoea and malabsorption may occur, with bulky stools that float.

Stools obtained at 2–3-day intervals should be examined for cysts. Duodenal or jejunal aspiration by endoscopy gives a higher diagnostic yield. A number of stool antigen detection tests are available. Jejunal biopsy specimens may show Giardia on the epithelial surface. PCR/multiplex PCR are increasingly being used in the diagnosis of giardiasis, but may not be freely accessible in low-income countries.

Management

Treatment is with a single dose of tinidazole 2 g, metronidazole 400 mg 3 times daily for 10 days, or nitazoxanide 500 mg orally twice daily for 3 days.

Cryptosporidiosis

Cryptosporidium spp. are coccidian protozoal parasites of humans and domestic animals. Infection is acquired by the faecal–oral route through contaminated water supplies. The incubation period is approximately 7–10 days and is followed by watery diarrhoea and abdominal cramps. The illness is usually self-limiting but in immunocompromised patients, especially those with HIV, the illness can be devastating, with persistent severe diarrhoea and substantial weight loss. Diagnosis is by detection of oöcysts on faecal microscopy or PCR of stool. Treatment is not usually required; nitazoxanide can be used in immunocompromised hosts but efficacy is uncertain.

Cyclosporiasis

Cyclospora cayetanensis is a globally distributed coccidian protozoal parasite of humans. Infection is acquired by ingestion of contaminated water and recent food-borne outbreaks have been associated with raspberries and coriander (cilantro). The incubation period of approximately 2–11 days is followed by diarrhoea with abdominal cramps, which may remit and relapse. Although usually self-limiting, the illness may last as long as 6 weeks, with significant weight loss and malabsorption, and is more severe in immunocompromised individuals. Diagnosis is as for crytosporidiosis. Treatment may be necessary in a few cases, using co-trimoxazole 960 mg twice daily for 7 days.

Infections caused by helminths

Helminths (from the Greek helmins, meaning worm) include three groups of parasitic worm (Box 13.60), large multicellular organisms with complex tissues and organs.

Intestinal human nematodes

Adult nematodes living in the human gut can cause disease. There are two types:

- the hookworms, which have a soil stage in which they develop into larvae that then penetrate the host
- a group of nematodes that survive in the soil merely as eggs, which have to be ingested for their life cycle to continue.

The geographical distribution of hookworms is limited by the larval requirement for warmth and humidity. Soil-transmitted nematode

i 13.60 Classes of helminth that parasitise humans

Nematodes or roundworms

- Intestinal human nematodes: Ancylostoma duodenale, Necator americanus, Strongyloides stercoralis, Ascaris lumbricoides, Enterobius vermicularis, Trichuris trichiura
- Tissue-dwelling human nematodes: Wuchereria bancrofti, Brugia malayi, Loa loa, Onchocerca volvulus, Dracunculus medinensis, Mansonella perstans, Dirofilaria immitis
- Zoonotic nematodes: Trichinella spiralis

Trematodes or flukes

- Blood flukes: Schistosoma haematobium, S. mansoni, S. japonicum, S. mekongi, S. intercalatum
- Lung flukes: Paragonimus spp.
- Hepatobiliary flukes: Clonorchis sinensis, Fasciola hepatica, Opisthorchis felineus
- Intestinal flukes: Fasciolopsis buski

Cestodes or tapeworms

- Intestinal tapeworms: Taenia saginata, T. solium, Diphyllobothrium latum, Hymenolepis nana
- Tissue-dwelling cysts or worms: Taenia solium, Echinococcus granulosus

infections can be prevented by avoidance of faecal soil contamination (adequate sewerage disposal) or skin contact (wearing shoes), and by strict personal hygiene.

Ancylostomiasis (hookworm)

Ancylostomiasis is caused by *Ancylostoma duodenale* or *Necator americanus*. The complex life cycle is shown in Figure 13.50. The adult hookworm is 1 cm long and lives in the duodenum and upper jejunum. Eggs are passed in the faeces. In warm, moist, shady soil, the larvae develop into rhabditiform and then the infective filariform stages; they then penetrate human skin and are carried to the lungs. After entering the alveoli, they ascend the bronchi, are swallowed and mature in the small intestine, reaching maturity 4–7 weeks after infection. The worms attach to the mucosa of the small intestine by their buccal capsule (Fig. 13.51) and withdraw blood. The mean daily blood loss from one *A. duodenale* is 0.15 mL and that from *N. americanus* 0.03 mL.

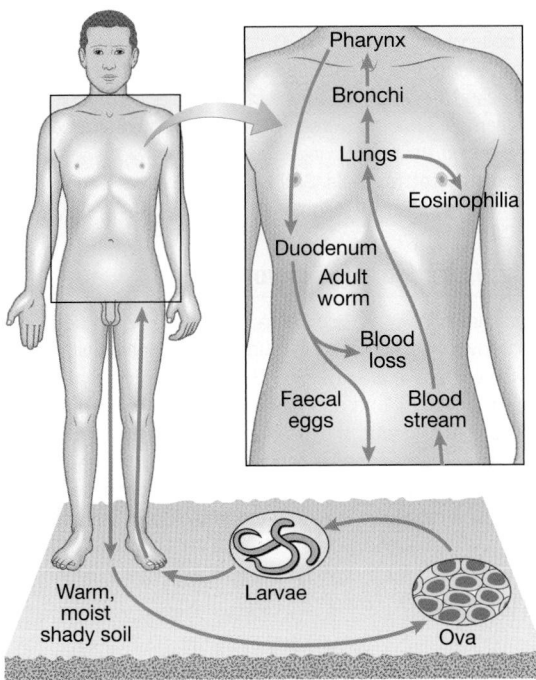

Fig. 13.50 Ancylostomiasis. Life cycle of *Ancylostoma*.

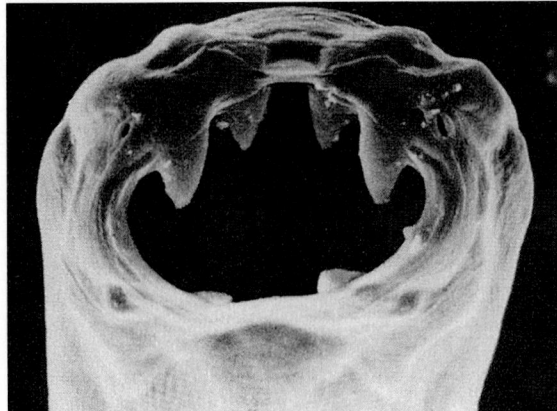

Fig. 13.51 *Ancylostoma duodenale*. Electron micrograph showing the ventral teeth. *From Gibbons LM. SEM guide to the morphology of nematode parasites of vertebrates. Farnham Royal, Slough: Commonwealth Agricultural Bureau International; 1986.*

Hookworm infection is a leading cause of anaemia in the tropics and subtropics. *A. duodenale* is endemic in the Far East and Mediterranean coastal regions, and is also present in Africa, while *N. americanus* is endemic in West, East and Central Africa, and Central and South America, as well as in the Far East.

Clinical features

An allergic dermatitis, usually on the feet (ground itch), may be experienced at the time of infection. The passage of the larvae through the lungs in a heavy infection causes a paroxysmal cough with blood-stained sputum, associated with patchy pulmonary consolidation and eosinophilia. When the worms reach the small intestine, vomiting and epigastric pain resembling peptic ulcer disease may occur. Sometimes, frequent loose stools are passed. The degree of iron and protein deficiency depends on the worm burden, patient nutrition and iron stores. Anaemia with high-output cardiac failure may result. The mental and physical development of children may be delayed in severe infection.

Investigations

There is eosinophilia. The characteristic ovum can be recognised in the stool. If hookworms are present in numbers sufficient to cause anaemia, faecal occult blood testing will be positive.

Management

A single dose of albendazole (400 mg) is the treatment of choice. Alternatively, mebendazole 100 mg twice daily for 3 days may be used. Anaemia and heart failure associated with hookworm infection respond well to oral iron, even when severe; blood transfusion is rarely required.

Strongyloidiasis

Strongyloides stercoralis is a small nematode (2 mm × 0.4 mm) that parasitises the mucosa of the upper part of the small intestine, often in large numbers, causing persistent eosinophilia. The eggs hatch in the bowel but only larvae are passed in the faeces. In moist soil, they moult and become the infective filariform larvae. After penetrating human skin, they undergo a development cycle similar to that of hookworms, except that the female worms burrow into the intestinal mucosa and submucosa. Some larvae in the intestine may develop into filariform larvae, which may then penetrate the mucosa or the perianal skin and lead to autoinfection and persistent infection. Patients with *Strongyloides* infection persisting for more than 35 years have been described. Strongyloidiasis occurs in the tropics and subtropics, and is especially prevalent in the Far East.

Clinical features

These are shown in Box 13.61. The classic triad of symptoms consists of abdominal pain, diarrhoea and urticaria. Cutaneous manifestations, either urticaria or larva currens (a highly characteristic pruritic, elevated, erythematous lesion, rapidly advancing along the course of larval migration), are characteristic and occur in 66% of patients.

i	**13.61 Clinical features of strongyloidiasis**
Penetration of skin by infective larvae	
• Itchy rash	
Presence of worms in gut	
• Abdominal pain, diarrhoea, steatorrhoea, weight loss	
Allergic phenomena	
• Urticarial plaques and papules, wheezing, arthralgia	
Autoinfection	
• Transient itchy, linear, urticarial weals across abdomen and buttocks (larva currens)	
Systemic (super-)infection	
• Diarrhoea, pneumonia, meningoencephalitis, death	

Systemic strongyloidiasis (the *Strongyloides* hyperinfection syndrome), with dissemination of larvae throughout the body, occurs with immune suppression (HIV or HTLV-1 infection, steroid or immunosuppressant treatment). Patients present with severe, generalised abdominal pain, abdominal distension and shock. Massive larval invasion of the lungs causes cough, wheeze and dyspnoea; cerebral involvement has manifestations ranging from subtle neurological signs to coma. Gram-negative sepsis frequently results.

Investigations

There is eosinophilia. Serology (ELISA) is helpful but definitive diagnosis requires microscopic examination of faeces for motile rhabditiform larvae; excretion is intermittent and so repeated examinations are necessary. Larvae may be found in jejunal aspirates or can also be cultured from faeces. PCR can be used for greater specificity and sensitivity.

Management

A course of two doses of ivermectin (200 µg/kg), administered on successive days, is effective. Alternatively, albendazole is given orally (15 mg/kg twice daily for 3 days). A second course may be required. For the *Strongyloides* hyperinfection syndrome, ivermectin is given at 200 µg/kg for 5–7 days.

Ascaris lumbricoides (roundworm)

This pale yellow nematode is 20–35 cm long and the largest of the intestinal nematodes. Humans are infected by eating food contaminated with mature ova. *Ascaris* larvae hatch in the duodenum, migrate through the lungs, ascend the bronchial tree, are swallowed and mature in the small intestine. This tissue migration can provoke both local and general hypersensitivity reactions, with pneumonitis, eosinophilic granulomas, wheezing and urticaria.

Clinical features

Intestinal ascariasis causes symptoms ranging from vague abdominal pain to malnutrition. The large size of the adult worm and its tendency to aggregate and migrate result in obstructive complications. Tropical and subtropical areas are endemic for ascariasis, and here it causes up to 35% of all intestinal obstructions, most commonly in the terminal ileum. Obstruction can be complicated further by intussusception, volvulus, haemorrhagic infarction and perforation. Other complications include blockage of the bile or pancreatic duct and obstruction of the appendix by adult worms. Ascariasis in non-endemic areas has been associated with pig husbandry and may be caused by *Ascaris suum*, which is indistinguishable from *A. lumbricoides*.

Investigations

The diagnosis is made microscopically by finding ova in the faeces. Adult worms are frequently expelled rectally or orally. Occasionally, the worms are demonstrated radiographically by a barium examination. There is eosinophilia.

Management

A single dose of albendazole (400 mg), pyrantel pamoate (11 mg/kg; maximum 1 g), or ivermectin (150–200 µg/kg), or alternatively mebendazole (100 mg twice daily for 3 days) treats intestinal ascariasis. Patients should be warned that they might expel numerous whole, large worms. Obstruction due to ascariasis should be treated with nasogastric suction, piperazine and intravenous fluids. Complete intestinal obstruction and its complications require urgent surgical intervention.

Prevention

Community chemotherapy programmes reduce *Ascaris* infection. The whole community can be treated every 3 months for several years. Alternatively treatment targets schoolchildren to lower the prevalence of ascariasis in the community.

Enterobius vermicularis (threadworm, pinworm)

This helminth is common worldwide and affects mainly children. After the ova are swallowed, development takes place in the small intestine but the adult worms are found chiefly in the colon.

Clinical features

The female lays ova around the anus, causing intense itching, especially at night. The ova are carried to the mouth on the fingers and so reinfection or human-to-human infection occurs (Fig. 13.52). In females, the genitalia may be involved. The adult worms may be seen moving on the buttocks or in the stool.

Investigations

Ova are detected in stool samples or by applying the adhesive surface of cellophane tape to the perianal skin in the morning. This is then examined on a glass slide under the microscope. A perianal swab, moistened with saline, also allows diagnosis.

Management

A single dose of mebendazole (100 mg), albendazole (400 mg), pyrantel pamoate (11 mg/kg) or piperazine (4 g) treats infection and is repeated after 2 weeks to control auto-reinfection. If infection recurs in a family, each member should be treated. All nightclothes and bed linen are laundered during treatment. Fingernails must be kept short and hands washed carefully before meals. Subsequent therapy is reserved for family members with recurrent infection.

Trichuris trichiura (whipworm)

Whipworm infections are common worldwide with poor hygiene. Infection follows ingestion of earth or food contaminated with ova, which have become infective after lying for 3 weeks or more in moist soil. The adult worm is 3–5 cm long and has a coiled anterior end resembling a whip. Whipworms inhabit the caecum, lower ileum, appendix, colon and anal canal. There are usually no symptoms, but intense infections in children may cause persistent diarrhoea or rectal prolapse, and growth retardation. The diagnosis is readily made by identifying ova in faeces. Treatment is with mebendazole in doses of 100 mg twice daily or albendazole 400 mg daily for 3 days for patients with light infections, and for 5–7 days for those with heavy infections.

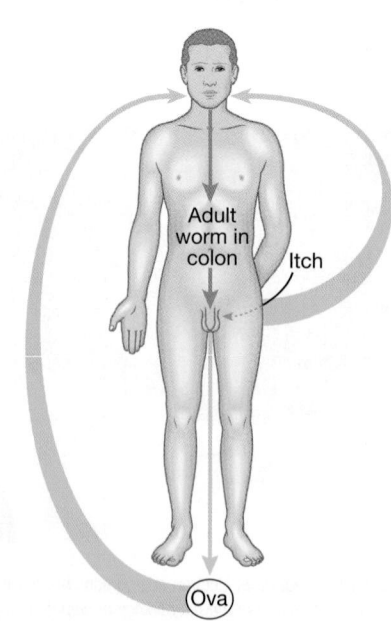

Fig. 13.52 Threadworm. Life cycle of *Enterobius vermicularis*.

Tissue-dwelling human nematodes

Filarial worms are tissue-dwelling nematodes. The larval stages are inoculated by biting mosquitoes or flies, each specific to a particular filarial species. The larvae develop into adult worms (2–50 cm long), which, after mating, produce millions of microfilariae (170–320 μm long) that migrate in blood or skin. The life cycle is completed when the vector takes up microfilariae by biting humans. In the insect, ingested microfilariae develop into infective larvae for inoculation in humans, normally the only host.

Disease is due to the host's immune response to the worms (both adult and microfilariae), particularly dying worms, and its pattern and severity vary with the site and stage of each species (Box 13.62). The worms are long-lived: microfilariae survive 2–3 years and adult worms 10–15 years. The infections are chronic and worst in individuals constantly reinfected.

Lymphatic filariasis

The filarial worms *Wuchereria bancrofti* and *Brugia malayi* infect approximately 120 million people globally whose features range from subclinical infection to hydrocele and elephantiasis.

W. bancrofti is usually transmitted by night-biting culicine or anopheline mosquitoes (Fig. 13.53). The adult worms, 4–10 cm in length, live in the lymphatics, and the females produce microfilariae that circulate in large numbers in the peripheral blood, usually at night. The infection is widespread in tropical Africa, on the North African coast, in coastal areas of Asia, Indonesia and northern Australia, the South Pacific islands, the West Indies and also in North and South America.

B. malayi usually causes less severe disease than *W. bancrofti* and is transmitted by *Mansonia* or *Anopheles* mosquitoes in Indonesia, Borneo, Malaysia, Vietnam, South China, South India and Sri Lanka.

Pathology

Toxins released by adult worms cause lymphangiectasia; this dilatation of the lymphatic vessels leads to lymphatic dysfunction and the chronic clinical manifestations of lymphatic filariasis, lymphoedema and hydrocele. Death of the adult worm results in acute filarial lymphangitis. The filariae are symbiotically infected with rickettsia-like bacteria (*Wolbachia* spp.), and lipopolysaccharide released from *Wolbachia* triggers inflammation. Lymphatic obstruction persists after death of the adult worm. Secondary bacterial infections cause tissue destruction.

Clinical features

Acute filarial lymphangitis presents with fever, pain, tenderness and erythema along the course of inflamed lymphatic vessels. Inflammation of the spermatic cord, epididymis and testis is common. Episodes last a few days but may recur several times a year. Temporary oedema becomes more persistent and regional lymph nodes enlarge. Progressive enlargement, coarsening, corrugation, fissuring and bacterial infection of the skin and subcutaneous tissue develop gradually, causing irreversible 'elephantiasis'. The scrotum may reach an enormous size. Chyluria and chylous effusions are milky and opalescent; on standing, fat globules rise to the top.

Acute lymphatic manifestations of filariasis must be differentiated from thrombophlebitis and infection. Oedema and lymphatic obstructive changes must be distinguished from congestive cardiac failure, malignancy, trauma and idiopathic abnormalities of the lymphatic system. Silicates absorbed from volcanic soil can also cause elephantiasis (podoconiosis).

Tropical pulmonary eosinophilia is a complication, and is the result of the host response to microfilariae. It is seen mainly in India, due to microfilariae trapped in the pulmonary capillaries that are destroyed by allergic inflammation. Patients present with paroxysmal cough, wheeze and fever. If untreated, this may progress to debilitating chronic interstitial lung disease.

13.62 Pathogenicity of filarial infections depending on site and stage of worms		
Worm species	**Adult worm**	**Microfilariae**
Wuchereria bancrofti and *Brugia malayi*	Lymphatic vessels+++	Blood− Pulmonary capillaries++
Loa loa	Subcutaneous+	Blood+
Onchocerca volvulus	Subcutaneous+	Skin+++ Eye+++
Mansonella perstans	Retroperitoneal−	Blood−
Mansonella streptocerca	Skin+	Skin++

(+++ severe; ++ moderate; + mild; − rarely pathogenic)

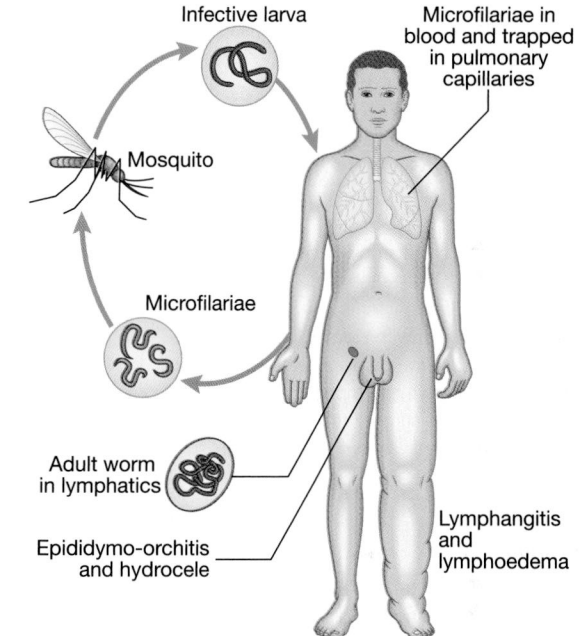

Fig. 13.53 *Wuchereria bancrofti* **and** *Brugia malayi*. Life cycle of organisms and pathogenesis of lymphatic filariasis.

Investigations

Early in filariasis lymphangitis is a clinical diagnosis, supported by eosinophilia and sometimes by positive filarial serology. Filarial infections cause the highest eosinophil counts of all helminthic infections.

Microfilariae can be found in the peripheral blood at night; motile in a wet blood film or detected by microfiltration in lysed blood. They are usually present in hydrocele fluid, which may occasionally yield an adult filaria. By the time elephantiasis develops, microfilariae become difficult to find. Calcified filariae may sometimes be demonstrable by radiography. Movement of adult worms can be seen on scrotal ultrasound. PCR-based tests for detection of *W. bancrofti* and *B. malayi* DNA from blood have been developed.

Indirect fluorescence and ELISA detect antibodies in over 95% of active cases and 70% of established elephantiasis. The test becomes negative 1–2 years after cure. Serological tests cannot distinguish the different filarial infections. Highly sensitive and specific, commercially available, immunochromatographic card tests detect circulating *W. bancrofti* antigen using finger-prick blood samples taken at any time of the day.

In tropical pulmonary eosinophilia, serology is strongly positive and IgE levels are massively elevated but circulating microfilariae are not found. The chest X-ray shows miliary changes or mottled opacities. Pulmonary function tests show a restrictive picture.

13

Management

Treatment is aimed at halting and reversing disease progression. Diethylcarbamazine (DEC, 2 mg/kg orally 3 times daily for 21 days, or 6 mg/kg as a single dose) kills microfilariae and adult worms. Most adverse effects seen with DEC treatment are due to the host response to dying microfilariae, which is directly proportional to the microfilarial load. The main symptoms are fever, headache, nausea, vomiting, arthralgia and prostration, usually within 24–36 hours of the first dose of DEC. Antihistamines or glucocorticoids treat these allergic phenomena. Combining albendazole (400 mg) with ivermectin (200 µg/kg) in a single dose, with or without DEC (300 mg), is also highly effective in clearing the parasites. Treatment of *Wolbachia* with doxycycline (200 mg/day) for 4–8 weeks provides additional benefit by eliminating the bacteria; this leads to interruption of parasite embryogenesis. For tropical pulmonary eosinophilia, DEC for 14 days is the treatment of choice.

Co-infections

Patients co-infected with lymphatic filiariasis and onchocerciasis with eye involvement should be treated with doxycycline before ivermectin. Co-infection with lymphatic filariasis and loaiasis depends on the *Loa loa* microfilarial load. If high ivermectin, doxycycline or albendazole should be given first before DEC to reduce microfilarial load as DEC can result in severe encephalitis/shock.

Chronic lymphatic pathology

Active management of chronic lymphatic pathology can alleviate symptoms. Patients should be taught meticulous skin care for lymphoedema to prevent secondary bacterial and fungal infections. Tight bandaging, massage and bed rest with elevation of the affected limb help to control the lymphoedema. Prompt diagnosis and antibiotic therapy of bacterial cellulitis prevent further lymphatic damage and worsening of existing elephantiasis. Plastic surgery to remove excess tissue may offer relief in established elephantiasis but without establishment of new lymphatic drainage recurrence is likely. Hydroceles and chyluria can be repaired surgically.

Prevention

Treatment of the whole population (mass drug administration, MDA) in endemic areas with annual single-dose DEC (6 mg/kg), either alone or in combination with albendazole and ivermectin (triple drugs), can reduce filarial transmission. MDA should be combined with mosquito control programmes.

█ Loiasis

Loiasis is caused by infection with the filaria *Loa loa*. The disease is endemic in forested and swampy parts of Western and Central Africa. The adult worms, 3–7 cm × 4 mm, chiefly parasitise the subcutaneous tissue of humans, releasing larval microfilariae into the peripheral blood in the daytime. The vector is *Chrysops*, a forest-dwelling, day-biting fly.

The host response to *Loa loa* is usually absent or mild. From time to time a short-lived, inflammatory, oedematous swelling (a Calabar swelling) is produced around an adult worm. Heavy infections, especially when treated, may cause encephalitis.

Clinical features

The infection is often symptomless. The incubation period ranges from 3 months to over a year. The first sign is usually a Calabar swelling: an irritating, tense, localised swelling that may be painful, especially if beside a joint. The swelling is generally on a limb; it measures a few centimetres in diameter but may be diffuse and extensive. It usually disappears after a few days but may persist for 2–3 weeks. Several swellings may appear at irregular intervals, often in adjacent sites. Sometimes, there is urticaria and pruritus elsewhere. Occasionally, a worm may be seen wriggling under the skin, especially that of an eyelid, and may cross the eye under the conjunctiva, taking many minutes to do so.

Investigations

Diagnosis is by demonstrating microfilariae in blood taken during the day, but they may not always be found in patients with Calabar swellings. Antifilarial antibodies are positive in 95% of patients and there is massive eosinophilia. Occasionally, a calcified worm may be seen on X-ray.

Management

DEC (see above) is curative, in a dose of 9–12 mg/kg daily, continued for 21 days. Treatment may precipitate a severe ('Mazzotti') reaction in patients with a heavy microfilaraemia, characterised by fever, joint and muscle pain, and encephalitis; microfilaraemic patients should be given glucocorticoid cover.

Prevention

Building houses away from trees and having dwellings wire-screened reduce infections. Protective clothing and insect repellents are also useful. DEC in a dose of 5 mg/kg daily for 3 days each month is partially protective.

█ Onchocerciasis (river blindness)

Onchocerciasis results from infection by the filarial *Onchocerca volvulus*. The infection is conveyed by flies of the genus *Simulium*, which breed in rapidly flowing, well-aerated water. Adult flies inflict painful bites during the day, both inside and outside houses. While feeding, they pick up the microfilariae, which mature into the infective larva and are transmitted to a new host in subsequent bites. Humans are the only known hosts (Fig. 13.54).

Onchocerciasis is endemic in sub-Saharan Africa, Yemen and a few foci in Central and South America. It is estimated that 21 million people are infected and 1 million have vison loss. Due to onchocerciasis, huge tracts of fertile land lie virtually untilled and individuals and communities are impoverished.

Pathology

After inoculation of larvae by a bite, the worms mature in 2–4 months and live for up to 17 years in subcutaneous and connective tissues. At sites of trauma, over bony prominences and around joints, fibrosis may form nodules around adult worms, which otherwise cause no direct damage. Innumerable microfilariae, discharged by the female *O. volvulus*, move actively in these nodules and in the adjacent tissues. The microfilariae

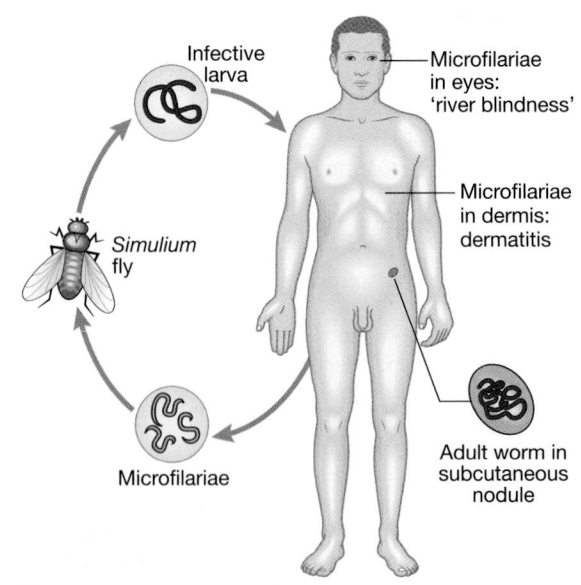

Fig. 13.54 *Onchocerca volvulus*. Life cycle of organism and pathogenesis of onchocerciasis.

are widely distributed in the skin and may invade the eye. Live microfilariae elicit little tissue reaction but dead ones may cause severe allergic inflammation, leading to hyaline necrosis and loss of collagen and elastin. Death of microfilariae in the eye causes inflammation and may lead to blindness.

Clinical features

The infection may remain symptomless for months or years. The first symptom is usually itching, localised to one quadrant of the body and later becoming generalised and involving the eyes. Transient oedema of part or all of a limb is an early sign, followed by papular urticaria, spreading gradually from the site of infection. In dark skins the most common signs are papules excoriated by scratching, spotty hyperpigmentation from resolving inflammation, and chronic changes of a rough, thickened and wrinkled skin. Both infected and uninfected superficial lymph nodes enlarge and may hang down in folds of loose skin in the groin. Hydrocele, femoral hernias and scrotal elephantiasis can occur. Firm subcutaneous nodules ≥1 cm in diameter (onchocercomas) occur in chronic infection.

Eye disease is most common in highly endemic areas and is associated with chronic heavy infections and nodules on the head. Early manifestations include itching, lacrimation and conjunctival injection. These cause conjunctivitis; sclerosing keratitis with pannus formation; uveitis, which may lead to glaucoma and cataract; and, less commonly, choroiditis and optic neuritis. Classically, 'snowflake' deposits are seen in the edges of the cornea.

Investigations

The finding of nodules or characteristic lesions of the skin or eyes in a patient from an endemic area, associated with eosinophilia, is suggestive. Skin snips or shavings, taken with a corneoscleral punch or scalpel blade from calf, buttock and shoulder, are placed in saline under a cover slip on a microscope slide and examined after 4 hours. Microfilariae are seen wriggling free in all but the lightest infections. Slit-lamp examination may reveal microfilariae moving in the anterior chamber of the eye or trapped in the cornea. An excised nodule may reveal a coiled, thread-like adult worm.

Filarial antibodies are positive in up to 95% of patients. Rapid strip tests to detect antibody or antigen are under clinical evaluation. When there is a strong suspicion of onchocerciasis but tests are negative, a provocative Mazzotti test, in which administration of 0.5–1.0 mg/kg of DEC exacerbates pruritus or dermatitis, strongly suggests onchocerciasis. PCR, though highly sensitive and specific, is not available commercially.

Management

Ivermectin is recommended, in a single dose of 100–200 µg/kg, repeated several times at 3-monthly intervals to prevent relapses. It kills microfilariae and has minimal toxicity. In the rare event of a severe reaction causing oedema or postural hypotension, prednisolone 20–30 mg may be given daily for 2 or 3 days. Ivermectin has little macrofilaricidal effect so that, 1 year after ivermectin treatment, skin microfilarial densities regain at least 20% of pre-treatment levels; repeated treatments are required for the lifespan of the adult worm. Eradication of *Wolbachia* with doxycycline (100 mg daily for 6 weeks) prevents worm reproduction.

Prevention

Mass treatment with ivermectin reduces community morbidity and slows the progression of eye disease but it does not clear worm infection. *Simulium* can be destroyed in its larval stage by the application of insecticide to streams. Long trousers, skirts and sleeves discourage the fly from biting.

Dracunculiasis (Guinea worm)

Infestation with the Guinea worm *Dracunculus medinensis* manifests when the female worm, over a metre long, emerges from the skin. Humans are infected by ingesting a small crustacean, *Cyclops*, which inhabits wells and ponds, and contains the infective larval stage of the worm. Global programmes have almost eradicated this disease.

However, recent findings of dracunculiasis in animals pose a challenge to eradication efforts. This is especially the case for dogs in Chad, as 48 of 54 cases in 2019 worldwide were in Chad.

Management and prevention

Traditionally, the protruding worm is extracted by winding it out gently over several days on a matchstick. The worm must never be broken. Antibiotics for secondary infection and prophylaxis of tetanus are also required.

The global eradication campaign aims to provide clean drinking water and eradicate water fleas from drinking water by simple filtration of water through a plastic mesh filter and chemical treatment of water supplies.

Other filariases

Mansonella perstans

This filarial worm is transmitted by the midges *Culicoides austeni* and *C. grahami*. It is common throughout equatorial Africa, as far south as Zambia, and also in Trinidad and parts of northern and eastern South America.

M. perstans has never been proven to cause disease but it may be responsible for a persistent eosinophilia and occasional allergic manifestations. *M. perstans* is resistant to ivermectin and DEC, however, anti-*Wolbachia* treatment (doxycycline 200 mg daily for 6 weeks) can cure this infection.

Dirofilaria immitis

This dog heartworm infects humans, causing skin and lung lesions. It is not uncommon in the USA, Japan and Australia.

Zoonotic nematodes

Trichinosis (trichinellosis)

Trichinella spiralis is a nematode that parasitises rats and pigs, and is transmitted to humans by ingestion of partially cooked infected pork, particularly sausage or ham, or occasionally by bear meat. Symptoms result from invasion of intestinal submucosa by ingested larvae, which develop into adult worms, and the secondary invasion of striated muscle by fresh larvae produced by these adult worms. Outbreaks have occurred in countries where pork is eaten.

Clinical features

The clinical features of trichinosis are determined by the larval numbers. A light infection with a few worms may be asymptomatic; a heavy infection causes nausea and diarrhoea 24–48 hours after the infected meal. A few days later, the symptoms associated with larval invasion predominate: there is fever and oedema of the face, eyelids and conjunctivae; invasion of the diaphragm may cause pain, cough and dyspnoea; and involvement of the muscles of the limbs, chest and mouth causes stiffness, pain and tenderness in affected muscles. Larval migration may cause acute myocarditis and encephalitis. Eosinophilia, which can be very high, is observed after 10 days. An intense infection may prove fatal but those who survive recover completely.

Investigations

Frequently, people who have eaten infected pork from a common source develop symptoms at about the same time. Biopsy from the deltoid or gastrocnemius muscle after the third week of symptoms may reveal encysted larvae. Serological tests are also helpful.

Management

Treatment is with albendazole (400 mg twice daily for 8–14 days) or mebendazole (200–400 mg three times daily for 3 days, followed by 400–500 mg three times daily for 10 days). Treatment commenced early in infection kills newly formed adult worms in the submucosa and reduces the number of larvae reaching the muscles. Glucocorticoids are necessary to control the serious effects of acute inflammation.

Anisakiasis (herring worm)

This infection is caused by the larvae of a fish nematode (*Anisakis simplex* or *Pseudoterranova decipiens*) and is associated with consumption of under-cooked fish or squid. The parasite cannot complete its life cycle in humans but larval ingestion is associated with pharyngeal tingling, abdominal pain, diarrhoea and vomiting. Diagnosis is made by identification of the larva by patients or endoscopists, and albendazole (400 mg twice a day for 5 days) treats larvae that are not manually removed.

Cutaneous larva migrans

Cutaneous larva migrans (CLM) is the most common linear lesion seen in travellers (Fig. 13.55). Intensely pruritic, linear, serpiginous lesions result from the larval migration of the dog hookworm (*Ancylostoma caninum*). The track moves across the skin at a rate of 2–3 cm/day. This contrasts with the fast-moving transient rash of *Strongyloides*. Although the larvae of dog hookworms frequently infect humans, they do not usually develop into the adult form. The most common site for CLM is the foot but elbows, breasts and buttocks may be affected. Most patients with CLM have recently visited a beach where the affected part was exposed. The diagnosis is clinical. Treatment may be local with 12-hourly application of 15% thiabendazole cream, or systemic with a single dose of albendazole (400 mg) or ivermectin (150–200 µg/kg).

Angiostrongylus cantonensis

The rat lungworm infects humans in Asia and the Pacific basin, via ingestion of infected snails or contaminated water. It causes eosinophilic meningitis. The role of combination therapy with glucocorticoids and albendazole remains controversial.

Gnathostomiasis

Gnathostomiasis occurs predominantly in South-east Asia and is due to *Gnathostoma spinigerum*. It also occurs in other parts of Asia, Central and South America, and Africa. Humans are infected by the larvae from intermediate hosts (raw or under-cooked freshwater fish, shrimps and frogs) and are not definitive hosts, so the life cycle is incomplete. Pruritic, painful, migratory nodules appear 3–4 weeks after ingestion due to larval migration. Complications include cough, visual disturbance, eosinophilic meningitis or encephalitis. Serology confirms diagnosis and the preferred

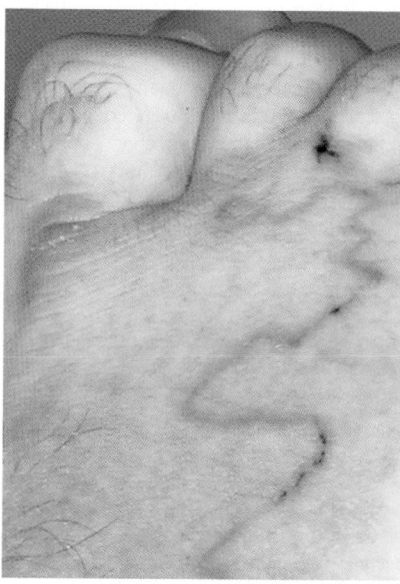

Fig. 13.55 Cutaneous larva migrans. *Courtesy of Dr Ravi Gowda, Royal Hallamshire Hospital, Sheffield.*

treatment is albendazole (400 mg twice daily) for 21 days, but its role in visual or neurological disease is uncertain as it may increase larval migration.

Trematodes (flukes)

These leaf-shaped worms are parasitic to humans and animals. Their complex life cycles may involve one or more intermediate hosts, often freshwater molluscs.

Schistosomiasis

Schistosomiasis is a major cause of morbidity in the tropics. The species commonly causing disease in humans are: *Schistosoma haematobium*, *S. mansoni*, *S. japonicum*, *S. mekongi* and *S. intercalatum*. *S. haematobium* is sometimes called bilharzia or bilharziasis. Schistosome eggs have been found in Egyptian mummies.

The life cycle is shown in Figure 13.56A. The ovum is passed in the urine or faeces of infected individuals and gains access to fresh water, where the ciliated miracidium is liberated; it enters its intermediate host, a species of freshwater snail, and multiplies. Large numbers of fork-tailed cercariae are then liberated into the water, where they may survive for 2–3 days. Cercariae can penetrate the skin or the mucous membrane of the mouth of humans. They transform into schistosomulae and moult as they pass through the lungs; then they are carried by the blood stream to the liver, and so to the portal vein, where they mature. The male worm is up to 20 mm in length and the slenderer cylindrical female, usually enfolded longitudinally by the male, is longer (Fig. 13.56B). Within 4–6 weeks of infection, they migrate to the venules draining the pelvic viscera, where the females deposit ova.

Pathology

The passage of eggs through mucosa and the granulomatous reaction to eggs deposited in tissues causes disease. The eggs of *S. haematobium* pass mainly through the bladder wall but may also involve the rectum, seminal vesicles, vagina, cervix and uterine tubes. *S. mansoni* and *S. japonicum* eggs pass mainly through the wall of the lower bowel or are carried to the liver. The most serious, although rare, site of ectopic egg deposition is the CNS. Granulomas are composed of macrophages, eosinophils, and epithelioid and giant cells around an ovum. Later, there is fibrosis and eggs calcify, which is often visible radiologically. Eggs of *S. haematobium* may leave the vesical plexus and be carried directly to the lung. Those of *S. mansoni* and *S. japonicum* may also reach the lungs after the development of portal hypertension and consequent portasystemic collateral circulation. Egg deposition in the pulmonary vasculature, and the resultant host response, can lead to pulmonary hypertension.

Clinical features

Recent travellers, especially those overlanding through Africa, may present with allergic manifestations and eosinophilia; residents of schistosomiasis-endemic areas are more likely to present with chronic urinary tract pathology or portal hypertension.

During early infection, there may be itching lasting 1–2 days at the site of cercarial penetration ('swimmer's itch'). After a symptom-free period of 3–5 weeks, acute schistosomiasis (Katayama syndrome) may present with allergic manifestations: urticaria, fever, muscle aches, abdominal pain, headaches, cough and sweating. On examination, hepatomegaly, splenomegaly, lymphadenopathy and pneumonia may be present. These allergic phenomena may be severe in infections with *S. mansoni* and *S. japonicum*, but are rare with *S. haematobium*. The features subside after 1–2 weeks.

Chronic schistosomiasis is due to egg deposition and occurs months to years after infection. The symptoms and signs depend on the intensity of infection and the species of infecting schistosome (Box 13.63).

Schistosoma haematobium

Humans are the only natural hosts of *S. haematobium*, which is highly endemic in Egypt and East Africa, and occurs throughout Africa and the

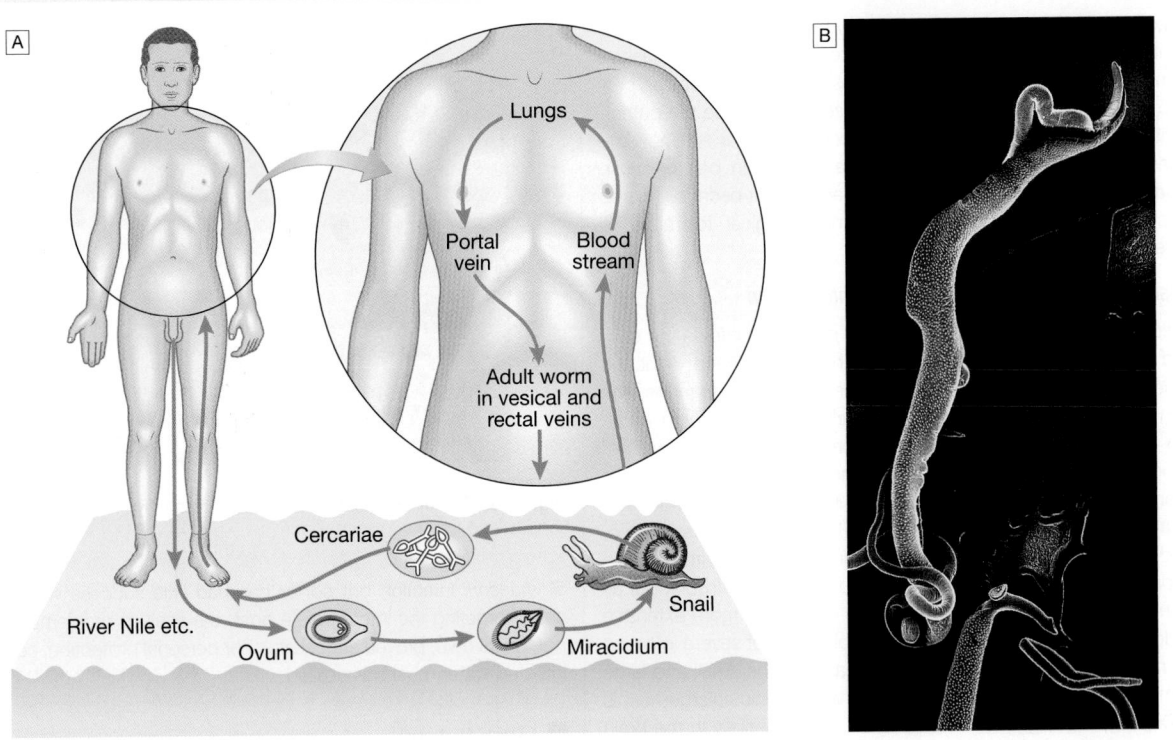

Fig. 13.56 *Schistosoma.* **A** Life cycle. **B** Scanning electron micrograph of adult schistosome worms, showing the larger male worm embracing the thinner female.

i	**13.63 Pathogenesis of schistosomiasis**	
Time	*Schistosoma haematobium*	*S. mansoni* **and** *S. japonicum*
Cercarial penetration		
Days	Papular dermatitis at site of penetration	As for *S. haematobium*
Larval migration and maturation		
Weeks	Pneumonitis, myositis, hepatitis, fever, 'serum sickness', eosinophilia, seroconversion	As for *S. haematobium*
Early egg deposition		
Months	Cystitis, haematuria	Colitis, granulomatous hepatitis, acute portal hypertension
	Ectopic granulomatous lesions: skin, CNS etc. Immune complex glomerulonephritis	As for *S. haematobium*
Late egg deposition		
Years	Fibrosis and calcification of ureters, bladder: bacterial infection, calculi, hydronephrosis, carcinoma	Colonic polyposis and strictures, periportal fibrosis, portal hypertension
	Pulmonary granulomas and pulmonary hypertension	As for *S. haematobium*

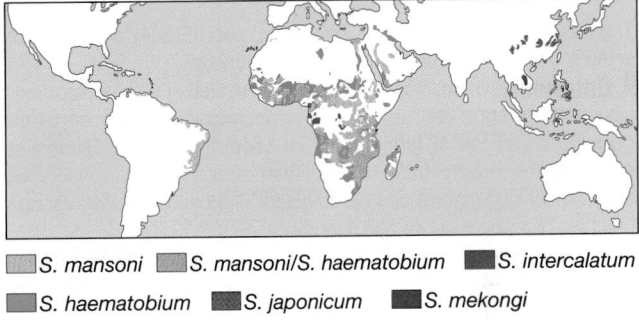

☐ *S. mansoni* ☐ *S. mansoni/S. haematobium* ■ *S. intercalatum*
☐ *S. haematobium* ▨ *S. japonicum* ■ *S. mekongi*

Fig. 13.57 **Geographical distribution of schistosomiasis.** *From Gryseels et al., Lancet 2006; 368:1106–1118.*

obstruction. Later, frequent urinary tract infections, bladder or ureteric stones, hydronephrosis and ultimately renal failure with a contracted calcified bladder may occur. Pain is often felt in the iliac fossa or in the loin, and radiates to the groin. In several endemic areas, there is a strong epidemiological association of *S. haematobium* infection with squamous cell carcinoma of the bladder. Disease of the seminal vesicles may lead to haematospermia. Females may develop schistosomal papillomas of the vulva, and schistosomal lesions of the cervix may be mistaken for cancer. Intestinal symptoms may follow involvement of the bowel wall. Ectopic worms cause skin or spinal cord lesions.

The severity of *S. haematobium* infection varies greatly; light infections are often asymptomatic. However, as adult worms can live for 20 years or more and lesions may progress, these patients should always be treated.

Schistosoma mansoni

S. mansoni is endemic throughout Africa, the Middle East, Venezuela, Brazil and the Caribbean (see Fig. 13.57).

Characteristic symptoms begin from 2 months after infection. They may be minimal (e.g. malaise) or consist of abdominal pain and frequent stools that contain blood-stained mucus. With severe advanced disease,

Middle East (Fig. 13.57). Infection can be acquired after a brief exposure, such as swimming in freshwater lakes in Africa.

Painless terminal haematuria is usually the first and most common symptom. Frequency of micturition follows, due to bladder neck

13

increased discomfort from rectal polyps may be experienced. The early hepatomegaly is reversible but portal hypertension may cause massive splenomegaly, fatal haematemesis from oesophageal varices, or progressive ascites. Liver function is initially preserved because the pathology is fibrotic rather than cirrhotic. *S. mansoni* and other schistosome infections predispose to the carriage of *Salmonella*, in part because *Salmonella* may attach to the schistosomes and in part because shared antigens on schistosomes may induce immunological tolerance to *Salmonella*.

Schistosoma japonicum, S. mekongi and S. intercalatum

In addition to humans, the adult worm of *S. japonicum* infects the dog, rat, field mouse, water buffalo, ox, cat, pig, horse and sheep. Although other *Schistosoma* spp. can infect species other than humans, the non-human reservoir seems to be particularly important only in transmission for *S. japonicum*. *S. japonicum* is prevalent in the Yellow River and Yangtze–Jiang basins in China, where the infection is a major public health problem. It also has a focal distribution in the Philippines, Indonesia and Thailand (see Fig. 13.57). The related *S. mekongi* occurs in Laos, Thailand and Myanmar, and *S. intercalatum* in West and Central Africa.

The pathology of *S. japonicum* is similar to that of *S. mansoni*, but as this worm produces more eggs, the lesions tend to be more extensive and widespread. The clinical features resemble those of severe infection with *S. mansoni*, with added neurological features. The small and large bowel may be affected, and hepatic fibrosis with splenic enlargement is usual. Deposition of eggs or worms in the CNS, especially in the brain or spinal cord, causes symptoms in about 5% of infections, notably epilepsy, blindness, hemiplegia or paraplegia.

Investigations

There is marked eosinophilia. Serological tests (ELISA) are useful as screening tests but remain positive after treatment.

In *S. haematobium* infection, dipstick urine testing shows blood and albumin. The eggs can be found by microscopic examination of the centrifuged deposit of terminal stream urine (Fig. 13.58). Ultrasound assesses the urinary tract; bladder wall thickening, hydronephrosis and bladder calcification can be detected. Cystoscopy reveals 'sandy' patches, bleeding mucosa and later distortion.

In a heavy infection with *S. mansoni* or *S. japonicum*, the characteristic egg with its lateral spine can usually be found in the stool. When the infection is light or of long duration, a rectal biopsy can be examined. Sigmoidoscopy may show inflammation or bleeding. Biopsies should be examined for ova. PCR, though highly sensitive and specific, is not widely available,

Management

Therapy aims to kill the adult schistosomes and stop egg-laying. Praziquantel (20 mg/kg orally twice daily for 1 day) is the drug of choice for all forms of schistosomiasis except *S. japonicum* and *S. mekongi*, for which 20 mg/kg for 3 doses is recommended. The drug produces parasitological cure in 80% of treated individuals and over 90% reduction in egg counts in the remainder. Side-effects are uncommon but include nausea and abdominal pain. Praziquantel therapy in early infection reverses hepatomegaly, bladder wall thickening and granulomas.

Surgery may be required to deal with residual lesions such as ureteric stricture, small fibrotic urinary bladders, or granulomatous masses in the brain or spinal cord. Removal of rectal papillomas by diathermy or by other means may provide symptomatic relief.

Prevention

No single means of controlling schistosomiasis has been established to date. The life cycle is terminated if fresh water containing the snail host is not contaminated by ova-containing urine or faeces. The provision of latrines and of a safe water supply, however, remains challenging in rural areas throughout the tropics. Furthermore, *S. japonicum* has multiple hosts besides humans, therefore latrines would have little impact. Population mass treatment annually helps prevent *S. haematobium* and

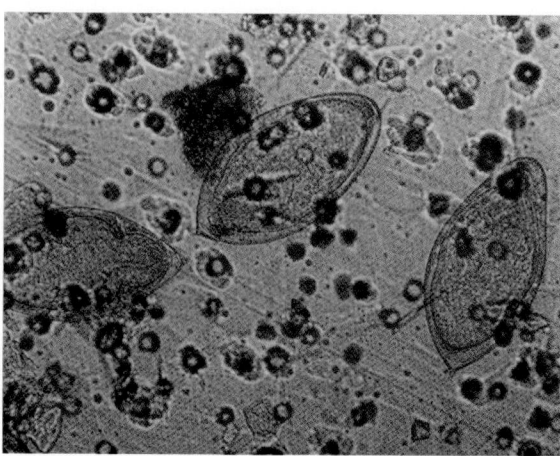

Fig. 13.58 Ova of *Schistosoma haematobium* in urine. Note the terminal spike.

S. mansoni infection but so far has had little success with *S. japonicum*. Targeting the intermediate host, the snail, is problematic and has not, on its own, proved successful. For personal protection, contact with infected water must be avoided.

Liver flukes

Liver flukes infect at least 20 million people and remain public health priorities in endemic areas. Clinical symptoms are abdominal pain, hepatomegaly and relapsing cholangitis. *Clonorchis sinensis* and *Opisthorchis felineus* are major aetiological agents of bile duct cancer. The three major liver flukes have similar life cycles and pathologies, as outlined in Box 13.64.

Other flukes of medical importance include lung and intestinal flukes (see Box 13.60).

Cestodes (tapeworms)

Cestodes are ribbon-shaped worms that inhabit the intestinal tract. They have no alimentary system and absorb nutrients through the tegumental surface. The anterior end, or scolex, has suckers for attaching to the host. From the scolex, a series of progressively developing segments arise, the proglottides, which may continue to show active movements when shed. Cross-fertilisation takes place between segments. Ova, present in large numbers in mature proglottides, remain viable for weeks, and during this period they may be consumed by the intermediate host. Larvae liberated from the ingested ova pass into the tissues of the intermediate host, forming larval cysticerci.

Tapeworms cause two distinct patterns of disease: either intestinal infection or systemic cysticercosis (see Fig. 13.59). *Taenia saginata* (beef tapeworm), *Taenia asiatica* and *Diphyllobothrium latum* (fish tapeworm) cause only intestinal infection in humans, following ingestion of intermediate hosts. *Taenia solium* causes intestinal infection if a cysticerci-containing intermediate host is ingested, and cysticercosis (systemic infection from larval migration) if ova are ingested. *Echinococcus granulosus* (dog tapeworm) does not cause human intestinal infection, but causes hydatid disease (which is analogous to cysticercosis) following ingestion of ova and subsequent larval migration.

Intestinal tapeworm

Humans acquire tapeworm by eating under-cooked beef infected with the larval stage of *T. saginata*, under-cooked pork containing the larval stage of *T. solium* or *T. asiatica*, or under-cooked freshwater fish containing larvae of *D. latum*. Usually, only one adult tapeworm is present in the gut but up to 10 have been reported. The ova of all the three *Taenia* are indistinguishable microscopically. However, examination of scolex

	i	**13.64 Diseases caused by flukes in the bile duct**	

	Clonorchiasis	Opisthorchiasis	Fascioliasis
Parasite	*Clonorchis sinensis*	*Opisthorchis felineus*	*Fasciola hepatica*
Other mammalian hosts	Dogs, cats, pigs	Dogs, cats, foxes, pigs	Sheep, cattle
Mode of spread	Ova in faeces, water	As for *C. sinensis*	Ova in faeces on to wet pasture
1st intermediate host	Snails	Snails	Snails
2nd intermediate host	Freshwater fish	Freshwater fish	Encysts on vegetation
Geographical distribution	Far East, especially South China	Far East, especially North-east Thailand	Cosmopolitan, including UK
Pathology	*Escherichia coli* cholangitis, abscesses, biliary carcinoma	As for *C. sinensis*	Toxaemia, cholangitis, eosinophilia
Symptoms	Often symptom-free, recurrent jaundice	As for *C. sinensis*	Unexplained fever, tender liver, may be ectopic, e.g. subcutaneous fluke
Diagnosis	Ova in stool or duodenal aspirate	As for *C. sinensis*	As for *C. sinensis*, also serology
Prevention	Cook fish	Cook fish	Avoid contaminated watercress
Treatment	Praziquantel 25 mg/kg 3 times daily for 2 days	As for *C. sinensis* but for 1 day only	Triclabendazole 10 mg/kg single dose; repeat treatment may be required*

*In the UK, available from the Hospital for Tropical Diseases, London.

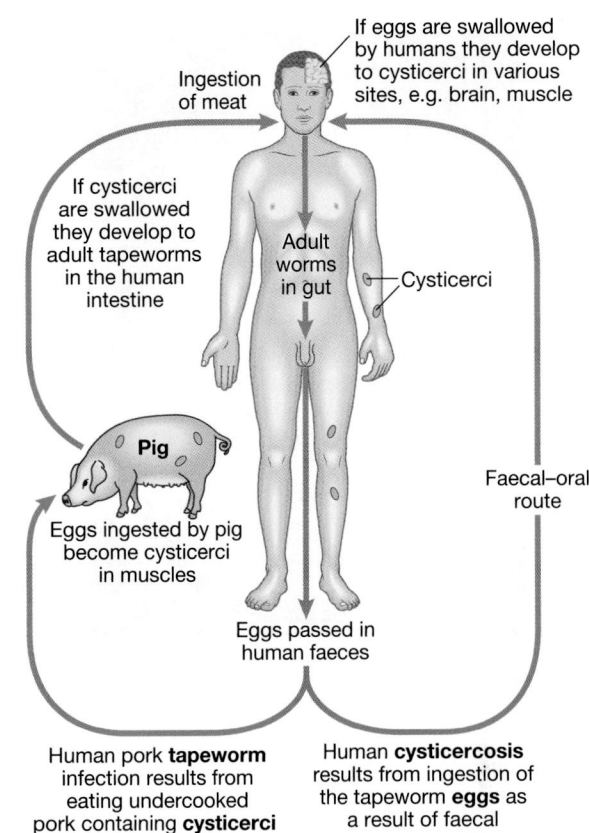

Fig. 13.59 Cysticercosis. Life cycle of *Taenia solium*.

Labels in figure:
Ingestion of meat
If eggs are swallowed by humans they develop to cysticerci in various sites, e.g. brain, muscle
If cysticerci are swallowed they develop to adult tapeworms in the human intestine
Adult worms in gut
Cysticerci
Faecal–oral route
Pig
Eggs ingested by pig become cysticerci in muscles
Eggs passed in human faeces
Human pork **tapeworm** infection results from eating undercooked pork containing **cysticerci**
Human **cysticercosis** results from ingestion of the tapeworm **eggs** as a result of faecal contamination of food

Taenia saginata

Infection with *T. saginata* occurs in all parts of the world. The adult worm may be several metres long and produces minimal intestinal upset in human beings, but identification of segments in the faeces or on under-clothing distresses patients. Ova may be found in the stool. Praziquantel is the drug of choice; niclosamide or nitazoxanide are alternatives. Prevention depends on efficient meat inspection and thorough cooking of beef.

Taenia asiatica

T. asiatica is a newly recognised species of *Taenia*, restricted to Asia. It is acquired by eating uncooked meat or viscera of pigs. Clinical features and treatment are similar to those of *T. saginata*.

Cysticercosis

Human cysticercosis is acquired by ingesting *T. solium* tapeworm ova, from either contaminated fingers or food (Fig. 13.59). The larvae are liberated from eggs in the stomach, penetrate the intestinal mucosa and are carried to many parts of the body, developing into cysticerci, 0.5–1 cm cysts that contain the head of a young worm. They do not grow further or migrate. Common locations are subcutaneous tissue, skeletal muscles and brain (Fig. 13.60).

Clinical features

Superficial cysts can be palpated under the skin or mucosa as pea-like ovoid bodies, but cause few or no symptoms and eventually die and calcify.

Heavy brain infections, especially in children, may cause features of encephalitis. More commonly, however, cerebral signs do not occur until the larvae die, 5–20 years later. Epilepsy, including new-onset focal sei-zures, personality changes, staggering gait and signs of hydrocephalus, are the most common features.

and proglottides can differentiate them: *T. solium* has a rostellum and two rows of hooklets on the scolex, and discharges multiple proglot-tides (3–5) attached together with lower degrees of uterine branching (approximately 10); *T. saginata* has only four suckers in its scolex, and discharges single proglottids with greater uterine branching (up to 30); *T. asiatica* has a rostellum without hooks on its scolex and is difficult to differentiate from *T. saginata*, except that there are fewer uterine branches (16–21).

Taenia solium

T. solium, the pork tapeworm, is common in central Europe, South Africa, South America and parts of Asia. It is smaller than *T. saginata*. The adult worm is found only in humans following the ingestion of pork containing cysticerci. Intestinal infection is treated with praziquantel (5–10 mg/kg) or niclosamide (2 g), both as a single dose, or alternatively with nitazoxanide (500 mg twice daily for 3 days). These are followed by a mild laxative (after 1–2 hours) to prevent retrograde intestinal autoinfection. Cooking pork well prevents intestinal infection. Great care must be taken while attending a patient harbouring an adult worm to avoid ingestion of ova or segments.

13

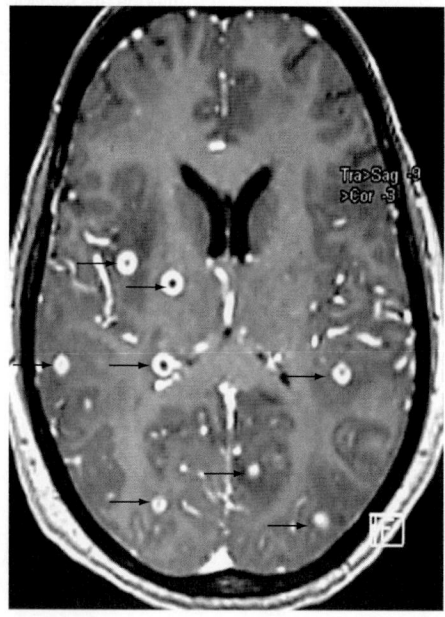

Fig. 13.60 Neurocysticercosis. T2-weighted axial image of the brain showing multiple lesions of neurocysticercosis (arrows show the largest lesions).

Investigations

Calcified cysts in muscles can be recognised radiologically. In the brain, however, less calcification takes place and larvae are only occasionally visible by plain X-ray; CT or magnetic resonance imaging (MRI) will usually show them. Epileptic fits starting in adult life suggest the possibility of cysticercosis if the patient has lived in or travelled to an endemic area. The subcutaneous tissue should be palpated and any nodule excised for histology. Radiological examination of the skeletal muscles may be helpful. Antibody detection is available for serodiagnosis.

Management and prevention

Albendazole (15 mg/kg daily for a minimum of 8 days) is recommended for parenchymal neurocysticercosis. Praziquantel (50 mg/kg in 3 divided doses daily for 10 days) is another option. Prednisolone (10 mg 3 times daily) is also given for 14 days, starting 1 day before anti-cysticercosis therapy. Antiepileptic drugs are often prescribed until the reaction in the brain has subsided. Operative intervention is indicated for hydrocephalus. Studies from India and Peru suggest that most small, solitary cerebral cysts will resolve without treatment.

Echinococcus granulosus (*Taenia echinococcus*) and hydatid disease

Dogs are the definitive hosts of the tiny tapeworm *E. granulosus*. The larval stage, a hydatid cyst, normally occurs in sheep, cattle, camels and other animals exposed to contaminated pastures or water. By handling a dog or drinking contaminated water, humans may ingest eggs (Fig. 13.61). The embryo is liberated from the ovum in the small intestine and invades the blood stream, spreading to the liver. The resultant cyst grows very slowly, sometimes intermittently. It is composed of an enveloping fibrous pericyst, laminated hyaline membrane (ectocyst) and inner germinal layers (endocyst) that give rise to daughter cysts, or a germinating cystic brood capsule in which larvae (protoscolices) develop. Over time, some cysts calcify and become non-viable. The disease is common in the Middle East, North and East Africa, Australia and Argentina. Foci of infection persist in the UK in rural Wales and Scotland. *E. multilocularis*, which has a cycle between foxes and voles, causes a similar but more severe infection, 'alveolar hydatid disease', which invades the liver like cancer.

Clinical features

A hydatid cyst is typically acquired in childhood and, after growing for years, may cause site-specific pressure symptoms. In nearly 75% of patients the right lobe of the liver is invaded and contains a single cyst. In others, a cyst may be found in lung, bone, brain or elsewhere.

Investigations

The diagnosis depends on the clinical, radiological and ultrasound findings in a patient that has close contact with dogs in an endemic area. Complement fixation and ELISA are positive in 70%–90% of patients.

Management and prevention

Hydatid cysts should be excised wherever possible. Great care is taken to avoid spillage and cavities are sterilised with 0.5% silver nitrate or 2.7% sodium chloride. Albendazole (400 mg twice daily for 3 months) should also be used and is often combined with PAIR (percutaneous puncture, aspiration, injection of scolicidal agent and re-aspiration). Praziquantel (20 mg/kg twice daily for 14 days) also kills protoscolices perioperatively.

Prevention is difficult when there is a close association with dogs. Personal hygiene, satisfactory disposal of carcasses, meat inspection and deworming of dogs reduces disease prevalence.

Other tapeworms

Other cestodes' adult or larval stages may infect humans. In sparganosis an immature worm develops, usually subcutaneously, as a result of eating or applying to the skin the secondary or tertiary intermediate host, such as frogs or snakes.

Ectoparasites

Ectoparasites only interact with the outermost surfaces of the host; see also page 1093.

Jiggers (tungiasis)

This is widespread in tropical America and Africa, and is caused by the sand flea *Tunga penetrans*. The pregnant flea burrows into the skin around toes and produces large numbers of eggs. The burrows are intensely irritating and the whole inflammatory nodule should be removed with a sterile needle. Secondary infection of lesions is common.

Myiasis

Myiasis is due to skin infestation with larvae of the South American botfly, *Dermatobia hominis*, or the African tumbu fly, *Cordylobia anthropophaga*. The larvae develop in a subcutaneous space with a central sinus. This orifice is the air source for the larvae, and periodically the larval respiratory spiracles protrude through the sinus. Patients with myiasis feel movement within the larval burrow and can experience intermittent sharp, lancinating pains. Myiasis is diagnosed clinically and should be suspected with any furuncular lesion accompanied by pain and a crawling sensation in the skin. The larva may be suffocated by blocking the respiratory orifice with petroleum jelly and gently removing it with tweezers. Secondary infection of myiasis is rare and rapid healing follows removal of intact larvae.

Fungal infections

Fungal infections, or mycoses, are classified as superficial, subcutaneous or systemic (deep), depending on the degree of tissue invasion.

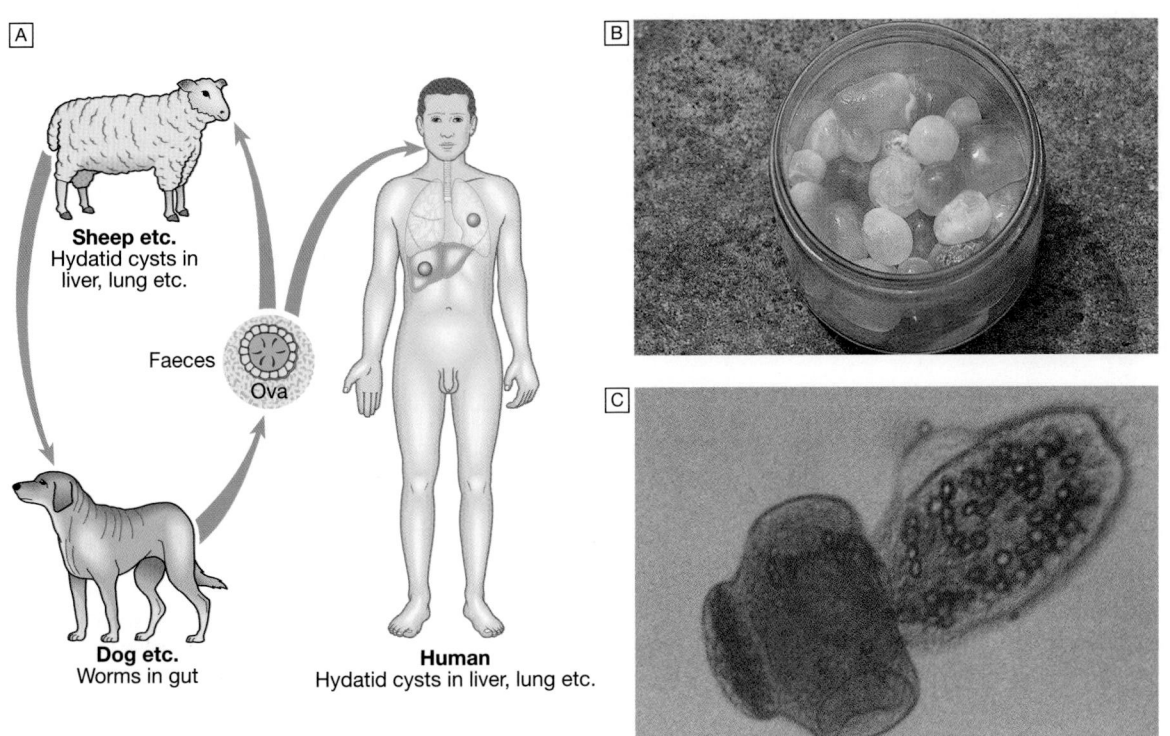

Fig. 13.61 Hydatid disease. [A] Life cycle of *Echinococcus granulosus*. [B] Daughter cysts removed at surgery. [C] Within the daughter cysts are the protoscolices.

Filamentous fungi (moulds)	**Dimorphic fungi**	**Yeasts**
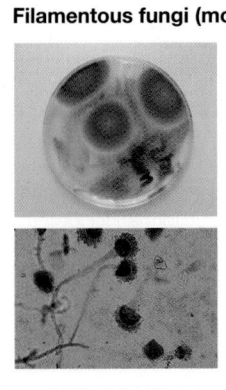	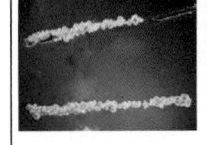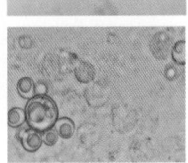	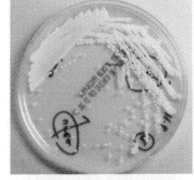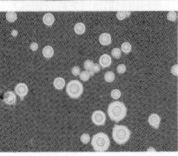
Characterised by the production of elongated, cylindrical, often septate cells (hyphae) and conidia (spores)	Exist in filamentous (top) or yeast (bottom) form, depending on environmental conditions	Characterised by the production of oval or round cells, which reproduce by binary fission (budding)
Examples: • *Aspergillus* spp. (*A. fumigatus* shown here) • *Fusarium* spp. • Dermatophyte fungi (*Tricophyton* spp., *Microsporum* spp. etc.) • Mucorales	Examples: • *Histoplasma capsulatum*, *Coccidioides immitis*, *Paracoccidioides brasiliensis* (shown here), *Blastomyces dermatidis* • *Sporothrix schenkii* • *Talaromyces marneffei* • *Malassezia* spp.	Examples: • *Candida* spp.* • *Cryptococcus* spp. (*C. neoformans* shown here)

Fig. 13.62 Classification of medically important fungi. Fungal classification is based on simple morphological characteristics. *Pneumocystis jirovecii* is morphologically distinct from other fungi and does not fit into this classification. *Although *Candida albicans* exists in a number of forms, including filamentous (hyphae and pseudohyphae), it is generally encountered in its yeast form so is classified in this category. *Insets (dimorphic fungi) Courtesy of Beatriz Gomez and Angela Restrepo, CIB, Medellín, Colombia.*

They are caused by filamentous fungi (moulds), by yeasts or by fungi that vary between these two forms, depending on environmental conditions (dimorphic fungi; Fig. 13.62).

Superficial mycoses

Superficial cutaneous fungal infections caused by dermatophyte fungi are described in Chapter 27.

Candidiasis (thrush)

Superficial candidiasis is caused by *Candida* spp., mainly *C. albicans*. Manifestations include oropharyngeal and vaginal candidiasis ('thrush'), intertrigo and chronic paronychia. Superficial candidiasis often follows antibiotic therapy. Intertrigo is characterised by inflammation in skin folds with surrounding 'satellite lesions'. Chronic paronychia is associated with frequent wetting of the hands. Superficial candidiasis is treated mainly with topical azoles (p. 121), oral azoles being reserved for refractory or recurrent disease. Severe oropharyngeal and oesophageal candidiasis is seen with T-cell immunodeficiency, including HIV infection, and anti-IL-17 therapy. Recurrent vaginal or penile candidiasis may be a manifestation of diabetes mellitus. Rarely, mutations in the autoimmune regulator gene (*AIRE*) or signal transducer and activator of transcription 1 (*STAT1*) cause a syndrome of chronic mucocutaneous candidiasis, resulting in chronic *Candida* infections of skin, mucosa and nails, with hyperkeratotic nails and erythematous periungual skin. Patients have cell-mediated immune defects against *Candida* and may have polyendocrinopathy and autoimmune features.

Subcutaneous mycoses

Chromoblastomycosis

Chromoblastomycosis is a predominantly tropical or subtropical disease caused by environmental dematiaceous (dark-pigmented) fungi, most commonly *Fonsecaea pedrosoi*. Other causes include *F. compacta*, *Cladophialophora carrionii* and *Phialophora verrucosa*. The disease is a cutaneous/subcutaneous mycosis acquired by traumatic inoculation, particularly the foot, ankle and lower leg. Several months after inoculation, lesions develop. Medical attention is often sought several years later. The initial lesion is a papule. Further papules develop and coalesce to form irregular plaques. Nodular lesions may produce a characteristic 'cauliflower' appearance.

Diagnosis is by histopathological examination of infected material, revealing dematiaceous, rounded, thick-walled 'sclerotic bodies' with septa at right-angles to each other. The aetiological agent is confirmed by culture. Therapeutic approaches include antifungal agents, cryosurgery and surgical excision, alone or in combination, but the optimal therapy is unknown. Itraconazole and terbinafine are the most effective antifungal agents. However, posaconazole has also been used with a good outcome.

Mycetoma (eumycetoma and actinomycetoma)

Mycetoma is a chronic suppurative infection of the deep soft tissues and bones, notably the limbs but also the abdominal or chest wall or head. It is caused by either filamentous fungi, Eumyces (eumycetoma – 40%) or aerobic Actinomycetes (actinomycetoma – 60%). Many fungi cause eumycetomas, the most common being *Madurella mycetomatis*, *M. grisea*, *Leptosphaeria senegalensis* and *Scedosporium apiospermum*; causes of actinomycetoma include *Nocardia*, *Streptomyces* and *Actinomadura* spp. Both groups produce characteristically coloured 'grains' (microcolonies), the colour depending on the organism (black grains – eumycetoma, red and yellow grains – actinomycetoma, white grains – either). The disease occurs mostly in the tropics and subtropics.

Clinical features

The disease is acquired by inoculation (e.g. from a thorn), usually of the foot (Madura foot). A painless swelling at the inoculation site becomes chronic and progressive, spreads steadily within the soft tissues, and eventually penetrates bone. Sub-epidermal nodules mature and rupture, revealing sinuses that may discharge grains. Sinuses heal with scarring, while fresh sinuses appear elsewhere. Deeper tissue invasion and bone involvement are less rapid and extensive in eumycetoma than actinomycetoma. There is little pain and usually no fever or lymphadenopathy, but there is progressive disability.

Investigations

Diagnosis of mycetoma involves identification of grains in pus, and/or histopathological examination of tissue. Culture is necessary for species identification and susceptibility testing. Serological tests are not available.

Management

Eumycetoma is usually treated with a combination of surgery and antifungal therapy. Antifungal susceptibility testing, if available, is

recommended, although clinical outcome does not necessarily correspond to in vitro test results. Itraconazole and ketoconazole (both 200–400 mg/day) are used most commonly. Success has also been reported with terbinafine monotherapy, and for some cases with liposomal amphotericin B. Refractory cases have responded to voriconazole or posaconazole. Therapy is continued for 6–12 months or longer. In extreme cases, amputation may be required. Actinomycetoma is treated with prolonged antibiotic combinations, most commonly streptomycin and dapsone. Dapsone is replaced by co-trimoxazole with intolerance or refractory disease. Success has also been reported with co-trimoxazole plus amikacin, with rifampicin added in difficult cases and to prevent recurrence.

Phaeohyphomycosis

Phaeohyphomycoses are a heterogeneous group of fungal diseases caused by a large number (>70) of dematiaceous fungi. In phaeohyphomycosis, the tissue form of the fungus is predominantly mycelial (filamentous), as opposed to eumycetoma (grain) or chromoblastomycosis (sclerotic body). Disease may be superficial, subcutaneous or deep. The most serious manifestation is cerebral phaeohyphomycosis, which presents with a ring-enhancing, space-occupying cerebral lesion. Optimal therapy for this condition is not established but usually includes neurosurgical intervention and antifungal (usually triazole) therapy. Causative agents are *Cladophialophora bantiana*, *Fonsecaea* spp. and *Rhinocladiella mackenziei*, which occurs mainly in the Middle East and is usually fatal.

Sporotrichosis

Sporotrichosis is caused by *Sporothrix schenckii*, a dimorphic fungal saprophyte of plants in tropical and subtropical regions. Disease is caused by dermal inoculation of the fungus, usually from a thorn (occasionally from a cat scratch). A subcutaneous nodule develops at the site of infection and subsequently ulcerates, with a purulent discharge. The disease may then spread along the cutaneous lymphatic channels, resulting in multiple cutaneous nodules that ulcerate and discharge (lymphocutaneous sporotrichosis). Rarer forms include cutaneous disease presenting with arthritis. Later, draining sinuses may form. Pulmonary sporotrichosis occurs as a result of inhalation of the conidia (spores) and causes chronic cavitary fibronodular disease with haemoptysis and constitutional symptoms. Disseminated disease may occur, especially in immuncompromised hosts

Investigations

Typical yeast forms detected on histology confirm diagnosis but are rarely seen; the fungus can also be cultured from biopsy specimens. ELISA detection of antibodies can be helpful.

Management

Cutaneous and lymphocutaneous disease is treated with itraconazole (200–400 mg daily, prescribed as the oral solution, which has better bioavailability than the capsule formulation) for 3–6 months. Alternative agents include a saturated solution of potassium iodide (SSKI, given orally), initiated with 5 drops and increased to 40–50 drops 3 times daily, or terbinafine (500 mg twice daily). Localised hyperthermia may be used in pregnancy (to avoid azole use). Osteoarticular disease requires a longer course of therapy (at least 12 months). Severe or life-threatening disease is treated with amphotericin B (lipid formulation preferred).

Systemic mycoses

Aspergillosis

Aspergillosis is an opportunistic systemic mycosis, which affects the respiratory tract predominantly. It is described on page 525.

Candidiasis

Systemic candidiasis is an opportunistic mycosis caused by *Candida* spp. The most common cause is *C. albicans*. Other agents include *C. dubliniensis*, *C. glabrata*, *C. krusei*, *C. parapsilosis* and *C. tropicalis*. *Candida* species identification often predicts susceptibility to fluconazole: *C. krusei* is universally resistant, many *C. glabrata* isolates have reduced susceptibility or are resistant, and other species are mostly susceptible. Candidiasis is usually an endogenous disease that originates from oropharyngeal, genitourinary or skin colonisation, although nosocomial spread occurs. *C. auris* is an emerging species, which has a particular propensity for nosocomial transmission.

Syndromes of systemic candidiasis

Acute disseminated candidiasis

This usually presents as candidaemia (isolation of *Candida* spp. from the blood). The main predisposing factor is the presence of a central venous catheter. Other major factors include recent abdominal surgery, total parenteral nutrition (TPN), recent antimicrobial therapy and localised *Candida* colonisation. Up to 40% of cases will have ophthalmic involvement, with characteristic retinal 'cotton wool' exudates. As this is a sight-threatening condition, all candidaemic patients should have a full ophthalmoscopy review. Skin lesions (non-tender pink/red nodules) may be seen. Although predominantly a disease of intensive care and surgical patients, acute disseminated candidiasis and/or *Candida* endophthalmitis is seen occasionally in injection drug-users, due to candidal contamination of citric acid or lemon juice used to dissolve heroin.

Chronic disseminated candidiasis (hepatosplenic candidiasis)

Persistent fever in a neutropenic patient, despite antibacterial therapy and neutrophil recovery, associated with the development of abdominal pain, raised alkaline phosphatase and multiple lesions in abdominal organs (e.g. liver, spleen and/or kidneys) on radiological imaging, suggests a diagnosis of hepatosplenic candidiasis. This represents a form of immune reconstitution syndrome in patients recovering from neutropenia and usually lasts for several months, despite appropriate therapy.

Other manifestations

Renal tract candidiasis, osteomyelitis, septic arthritis, peritonitis, meningitis and endocarditis may occur and are usually sequelae of acute disseminated disease. Diagnosis and treatment of these conditions require specialist mycological advice.

Management

Blood cultures positive for *Candida* spp. must never be ignored. Acute disseminated candidiasis is treated with antifungal therapy, removal of any in-dwelling central venous catheter (whether known to be the source of infection or not) and removal of any documented source. Candidaemia should be treated initially with an echinocandin (p. 122), with subsequent adjustment (usually to intravenous or oral fluconazole) guided by clinical response, species identification and susceptibility testing. Treatment should continue for a minimum of 14 days. Alternative therapies include voriconazole and amphotericin B formulations.

Chronic disseminated candidiasis requires prolonged treatment over several months with fluconazole or other agents, depending on species and clinical response. The duration of the condition may be reduced by adjuvant therapy with systemic glucocorticoids.

Cryptococcosis

Cryptococcosis is a systemic mycosis caused by two environmental yeast species, *Cr. neoformans* and *Cr. gattii*. *Cr. neoformans* is distributed worldwide and is primarily an opportunistic pathogen, most commonly associated with HIV infection or other immunocompromised hosts. *Cr. gattii* is a primary pathogen with a widespread distribution, including Australasia, Africa, Canada (Vancouver Island) and the north-western USA.

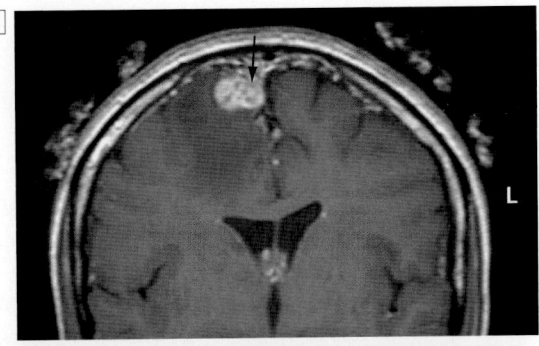

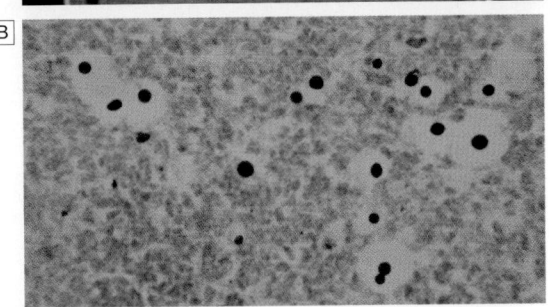

Fig. 13.63 Cryptococcal disease. A 23-year-old HIV-positive male developed headache and left-sided weakness. [A] MRI scan of the brain showed a space-occupying lesion (arrow) with surrounding oedema. [B] Histopathological examination of the lesion stained with Grocott's silver stain showed encapsulated yeasts. *Cryptococcus neoformans* was cultured.

Cryptococcosis is acquired by inhalation of yeasts. These may disseminate to any organ, most commonly the CNS and skin. The manifestations of *Cr. neoformans* are most severe in immunocompromised individuals. Conversely, *Cr. gattii* causes severe disease in immunocompetent hosts. Disseminated cryptococcosis (sepsis with cryptococci present in the blood stream or at multiple sites) is largely restricted to immunocompromised patients. CNS manifestations of cryptococcosis include meningitis and cryptococcoma (Fig. 13.63), the latter more likely with *Cr. gattii* infection. Manifestations of pulmonary cryptococcosis range from severe pneumonia (in more immunocompromised patients) to asymptomatic disease with single or multiple pulmonary nodules, sometimes exhibiting cavitation (in patients with lesser immunosuppression). Cryptococcal nodules may mimic other causes of lung pathology, such as tuberculosis or malignancy, and diagnosis requires histopathology and/or culture.

Treatment of severe cryptococcosis is the same as for cryptococcal meningitis, initially with liposomal amphotericin B. Mild pulmonary disease is usually treated with fluconazole, although for asymptomatic nodules resection of the lesions is likely to be sufficient.

Fusariosis

Fusarium spp. cause disseminated disease in patients with prolonged neutropenia. The disease presents with antibiotic-resistant fever and evidence of dissemination (e.g. skin nodules, endophthalmitis, septic arthritis, pulmonary disease; Fig. 13.64). Unlike *Aspergillus* spp., *Fusarium* spp. are often recovered from blood cultures. Treatment is challenging because of resistance to antifungal agents; voriconazole, posaconazole or lipid-formulated amphotericin B is usually prescribed.

Mucormycosis

Mucormycosis is a severe but uncommon opportunistic systemic mycosis caused by a number of 'mucoraceous' moulds, most commonly *Lichtheimia* spp., *Rhizomucor* spp., *Mucor* spp. and *Rhizopus* spp. Disease patterns include rhinocerebral/craniofacial, pulmonary, cutaneous and systemic disease. All are characterised by the rapid development

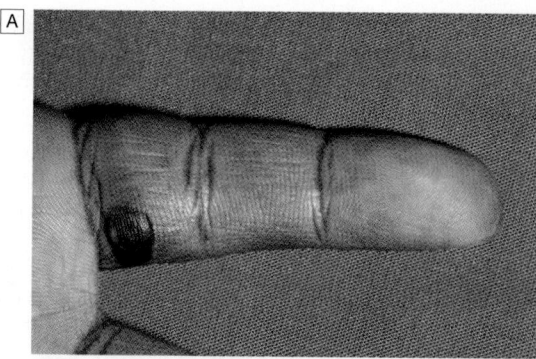
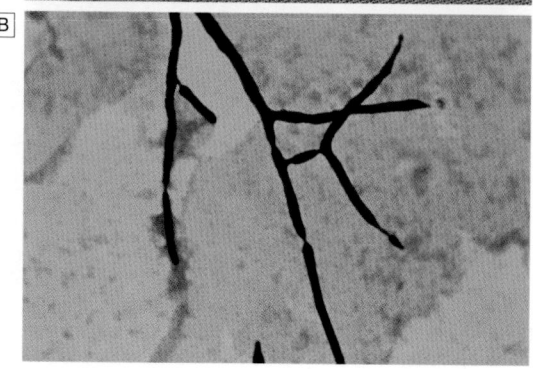

Fig. 13.64 *Fusarium* infection. A patient presented with fever and skin nodules after developing neutropenia secondary to haematopoietic stem cell transplantation and chemotherapy for relapsed leukaemia. *Fusarium solani* was cultured from skin lesions and blood cultures. [A] Tender, erythematous papules/nodules on upper arm. [B] Gram stain of *Fusarium* in blood culture medium.

of severe tissue necrosis, which is usually fatal if left untreated. The most common predisposing factors are profound immunosuppression from neutropenia and/or haematopoietic stem cell transplantation, uncontrolled diabetes mellitus, iron chelation therapy with desferrioxamine and severe burns. During the COVID-19 pandemic mucormycosis emerged as a specific complication of COVID-19, reported mainly from India.

Definitive diagnosis is by culture but histopathological confirmation is required, as the fungi may be environmental contaminants. Treatment requires a combination of antifungal therapy and surgical débridement, with correction of predisposing factor(s) if possible. High-dose lipid-formulated amphotericin B is most commonly used. Posaconazole is active against many mucoraceous moulds in vitro and may be used as a second-line agent or as oral 'step-down' therapy.

Talaromyces marneffei infection

T. marneffei is a thermally dimorphic pathogen (filamentous in environmental conditions and yeast at body temperature), which causes disease in South-east Asia, mainly in association with HIV infection (although immunocompetent patients may also be infected). Acquisition is usually by inhalation of environmental spores, with primary lung infection followed by haematogenous dissemination. A generalised papular rash, which progresses to widespread necrosis and ulceration, is a characteristic feature. Skin lesions may resemble molluscum contagiosum. Diagnosis is by histopathology and/or culture of respiratory secretions, blood or any infected clinical material (e.g. skin lesions, bone marrow, biopsies). Treatment involves an amphotericin B formulation followed by itraconazole (in severe infection), or itraconazole alone.

Histoplasmosis

Histoplasmosis is a primary systemic mycosis caused by the dimorphic fungus *Histoplasma capsulatum*. *H. capsulatum* var. *capsulatum* is endemic to east-central USA (especially the Mississippi and Ohio river valleys), parts of Canada, Latin America, the Caribbean, East and South-east Asia, and Africa. It occurs sporadically in Australia and India, and is very rare in Europe. *H. capsulatum* var. *duboisii* is found in West Africa and Madagascar.

The primary reservoir of *H. capsulatum* is soil enriched by bird and bat droppings, in which the fungus remains viable for many years. Infection is by inhalation of infected dust. Natural infections are found in bats, which represent a secondary reservoir of infection. Histoplasmosis is a specific hazard for explorers of caves and people who clear out bird (including chicken) roosts.

Pathology

The organism is inhaled in the form of conidia or hyphal fragments and transforms to the yeast phase during infection. Conidia or yeasts are phagocytosed by alveolar macrophages and neutrophils, and this may be followed by haematogenous dissemination to any organ. Subsequent development of a T-lymphocyte response brings the infection under control, resulting in a latent state in most exposed individuals.

Clinical features

Disease severity depends on the quantity of spores inhaled and the immune status of the host. In most cases, infection is asymptomatic. Pulmonary symptoms are the most common presentation, with fever, non-productive cough and an influenza-like illness. Erythema nodosum, myalgia and joint pain frequently occur, and chest radiography may reveal a pneumonitis with hilar or mediastinal lymphadenopathy.

Patients with pre-existing lung disease, such as chronic obstructive pulmonary disease (COPD) or emphysema, may develop chronic pulmonary histoplasmosis (CPH). The predominant features of this condition, which mimics tuberculosis, are fever, cough, dyspnoea, weight loss and night sweats. Radiological findings include fibrosis, nodules, cavitation and hilar/mediastinal lymphadenopathy.

Disease caused by *H. capsulatum* var. *duboisii* presents more commonly with papulonodular and ulcerating lesions of the skin and underlying subcutaneous tissue and bone (sometimes referred to as 'African histoplasmosis'). Multiple lesions of the ribs are common and the bones of the limbs may be affected. Lung involvement is relatively rare. Radiological examination may show rounded foci of bone destruction, sometimes associated with abscess formation. Other disease patterns include a visceral form with liver and splenic invasion, and disseminated disease.

Acute disseminated histoplasmosis is seen with immunocompromise, including HIV infection. Features include fever, pancytopenia, hepatosplenomegaly, lymphadenopathy and often a papular skin eruption. Chronic disseminated disease presents with fever, anorexia and weight loss. Cutaneous and mucosal lesions, lymphadenopathy, hepatosplenomegaly and meningitis may develop. *Emergomyces africanus* is a dimorphic fungus described in South Africa, which causes a disseminated histoplasmosis-like illness, mainly associated with HIV infection. Histopathologically, yeast forms appear similar to histoplasmosis and can be distinguished only by PCR.

Investigations

Histoplasmosis should be suspected in endemic areas with every undiagnosed infection in which there are pulmonary signs, enlarged lymph nodes, hepatosplenomegaly or characteristic cutaneous/bony lesions. Radiological examination in long-standing cases may show calcified lesions in the lungs, spleen or other organs. In the more acute phases of the disease, single or multiple soft pulmonary shadows with enlarged tracheobronchial nodes are seen on chest X-ray.

Laboratory diagnosis is by direct detection (histopathology or antigen detection), culture and serology; although antigen detection is the most effective method, it is not widely available. Serology utilises complement fixation testing or immunodiffusion; interpretation is complex and requires a specialist. *Histoplasma* antigen may be detectable in blood or urine. Culture is definitive but slow (up to 12 weeks). Histopathology may show characteristic intracellular yeasts. Diagnosis of subcutaneous or bony infection is mainly by histopathological examination and/or culture.

Management

Mild pulmonary disease does not require treatment. However, if prolonged, it may be treated with itraconazole. More severe pulmonary disease is treated with an amphotericin B formulation for 2 weeks, followed by itraconazole for 12 weeks, with methylprednisolone added for the first 2 weeks of therapy if there is hypoxia or ARDS. CPH is treated with itraconazole oral solution for 12–24 months, and disseminated histoplasmosis with an amphotericin B formulation followed by itraconazole. Lipid formulations of amphotericin B are preferred but their use is subject to availability. In subcutaneous and bone infection, patterns of remission and relapse are more common than cure. A solitary bony lesion may require local surgical treatment only.

▍Coccidioidomycosis

This is a primary systemic mycosis caused by the dimorphic fungi *Coccidioides immitis* and *C. posadasii*, found in the south-western USA and Central and South America. The disease is acquired by inhalation of conidia (arthrospores). In 60% of cases it is asymptomatic but in the remainder it affects the lungs, lymph nodes and skin. Rarely (in approximately 0.5%), it may spread haematogenously to bones, adrenal glands, meninges and other organs, particularly in those with immunocompromise.

Pulmonary coccidioidomycosis has two forms: primary and progressive. If symptomatic, primary coccidioidomycosis presents with cough, fever, chest pain, dyspnoea and (commonly) arthritis and a rash (erythema multiforme). Progressive disease presents with systemic upset (e.g. fever, weight loss, anorexia) and features of lobar pneumonia, and may resemble tuberculosis.

Coccidioides meningitis (which may be associated with CSF eosinophils) is the most severe disease manifestation; it is fatal if untreated and requires life-long suppressive therapy with antifungal azoles.

Investigations and management

Diagnosis is by direct histopathological detection in specimens, culture of infected tissue or fluids, or antibody detection. IgM may be detected after 1–3 weeks of disease by precipitin tests. IgG appears later and is detected with the complement fixation test. Change in IgG titre may be used to monitor clinical progress.

Treatment depends on specific disease manifestations and ranges from regular clinical reassessment without antifungal therapy (in mild pulmonary, asymptomatic cavitary or single nodular disease) to high-dose treatment with an antifungal azole (typically fluconazole), which may be continued indefinitely (e.g. in meningitis). Amphotericin B is used in diffuse pneumonia, disseminated disease and, intrathecally, in meningitis. Posaconazole has been used successfully in refractory disease.

▍Paracoccidioidomycosis

This is a primary systemic mycosis caused by inhalation of the dimorphic fungus *Paracoccidioides brasiliensis*, which is restricted to South America. The disease affects the lungs, mucous membranes (painful destructive ulceration in 50% of cases), skin, lymph nodes and adrenal glands (hypoadrenalism). Diagnosis is by microscopy and culture of lesions, and antibody detection. Oral itraconazole solution (200 mg/day) has demonstrated 98% efficacy and is currently the treatment of choice (mean duration 6 months). Ketoconazole, fluconazole, voriconazole and 2–3-year courses of sulphonamides are alternatives. Amphotericin B is used in severe or refractory disease, followed by an azole or sulphonamide.

▍Blastomycosis

Blastomyces dermatitidis is a dimorphic fungus endemic to restricted parts of North America, mainly around the Mississippi and Ohio rivers. Very occasionally, it is reported from Africa. The disease usually presents as a chronic pneumonia similar to pulmonary tuberculosis. Bones, skin and the genitourinary tract may also be affected. Diagnosis is by culture of the organism or identification of the characteristic yeast form in a clinical specimen. Antibody detection is rarely helpful. Treatment is with amphotericin B (severe disease) or itraconazole.

Further information

Websites

britishinfection.org *British Infection Association; source of general information on communicable diseases.*
cdc.gov *US Centers for Disease Control; source of general information about infectious diseases.*
fitfortravel.nhs.uk *Scottish site with valuable information for travellers.*
gov.uk/government/organisations/public-health-england *Public Health England; information on infectious diseases in the UK.*
idsociety.org *Infectious Diseases Society of America; source of general information relating to infectious diseases and of authoritative practice guidelines.*
who.int; see especially www.who.int/csr/don/en *World Health Organization; invaluable links on travel medicine with updates on outbreaks of infections, changing resistance patterns and vaccination requirements.*

13

G Maartens

14

HIV infection and AIDS

Clinical examination in HIV disease

2 Oropharynx
Mucous membranes

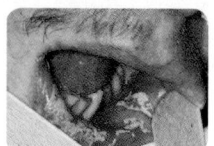

▲ Oropharyngeal candidiasis

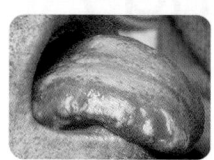

▲ Oral hairy leucoplakia

Herpes simplex
Aphthous ulcers
Kaposi's sarcoma

Teeth

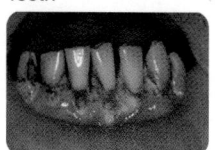

▲ Gingivitis/periodontitis

1 Skin
Papular pruritic eruption

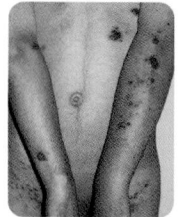

▲ Kaposi's sarcoma

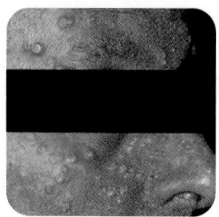

▲ Molluscum contagiosum

Herpes zoster
Seborrhoeic dermatitis

3 Neck
Lymph node enlargement
  Tuberculosis
  Lymphoma
  Kaposi's sarcoma
  Persistent generalised
  lymphadenopathy
Parotidomegaly

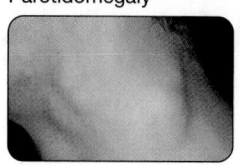

▲ Cervical lymphadenopathy

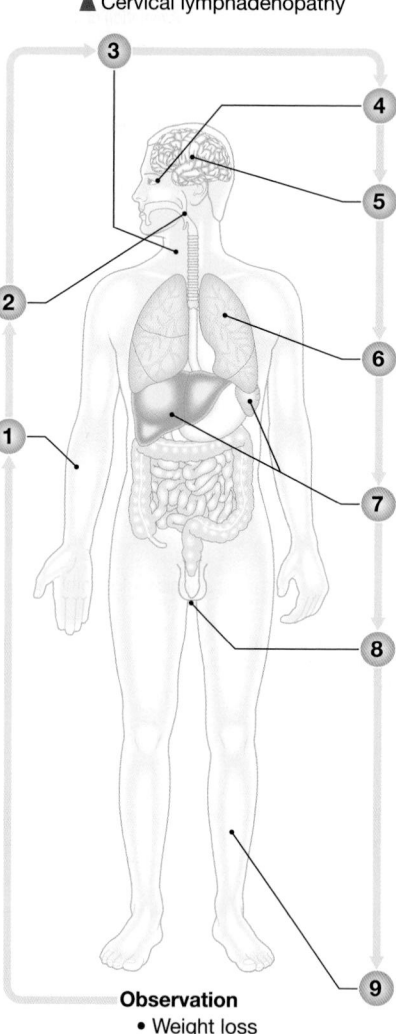

Observation
• Weight loss
• Tachypnoea
• Fevers and sweats

4 Eyes
Retina
  Toxoplasmosis
  HIV retinopathy
  Progressive outer retinal
  necrosis

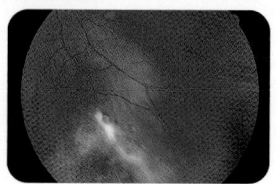

▲ Cytomegalovirus retinitis

5 Central nervous system
Higher mental function
  HIV dementia
  Progressive multifocal
  leucoencephalopathy
Focal signs
  Toxoplasmosis
  Primary CNS lymphoma
Neck stiffness
  Cryptococcal meningitis
  Tuberculous meningitis
  Pneumococcal meningitis

6 Chest
Lungs
  Pleural effusion
  Tuberculosis
  Kaposi's sarcoma
  Parapneumonic

7 Abdomen
Hepatosplenomegaly

8 Anogenital region
Rashes

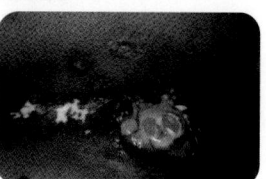

▲ Anal cancer

Condylomas
Herpes simplex
Ulcers

9 Legs
Peripheral nerve examination
  Spastic paraparesis
  Peripheral neuropathy

Inset (oral hairy leucoplakia) Courtesy of Audiovisual Department, St Mary's Hospital, London.

| **i** | **HIV clinical staging classifications** |

World Health Organization (WHO) clinical stage (used in low- and middle-income countries)	Centers for Disease Control (CDC) clinical categories (used in high-income countries)
Stage 1 Asymptomatic Persistent generalised lymphadenopathy	**Category A** Primary HIV infection Asymptomatic Persistent generalised lymphadenopathy
Stage 2 Unexplained moderate weight loss (< 10% of body weight) Recurrent upper respiratory tract infections Herpes zoster Angular cheilitis Recurrent oral ulceration Papular pruritic eruptions Seborrhoeic dermatitis Fungal nail infections	**Category B** Bacillary angiomatosis Candidiasis, oropharyngeal (thrush) Candidiasis, vulvovaginal; persistent, frequent or poorly responsive to therapy Cervical dysplasia (moderate or severe)/cervical carcinoma in situ Constitutional symptoms, such as fever (38.5°C) or diarrhoea lasting > 1 month Oral hairy leucoplakia Herpes zoster, involving two distinct episodes or more than one dermatome Idiopathic thrombocytopenic purpura
Stage 3 Unexplained severe weight loss (> 10% of body weight) Unexplained chronic diarrhoea for > 1 month Unexplained persistent fever (> 37.5°C for > 1 month) Persistent oral candidiasis Oral hairy leucoplakia Pulmonary tuberculosis Severe bacterial infections Acute necrotising ulcerative stomatitis, gingivitis or periodontitis Unexplained anaemia (< 80 g/L), neutropenia (< 0.5 × 10^9/L) and/or chronic thrombocytopenia (< 50 × 10^9/L)	Listeriosis Pelvic inflammatory disease, particularly if complicated by tubo-ovarian abscess Peripheral neuropathy

Stage 4	**Category C**

Candidiasis of oesophagus, trachea, bronchi or lungs
Cervical carcinoma – invasive
Cryptococcosis – extrapulmonary
Cryptosporidiosis, chronic (> 1 month)
Cytomegalovirus disease (outside liver, spleen and nodes)
Herpes simplex chronic (> 1 month) ulcers or visceral
HIV encephalopathy
HIV wasting syndrome
Cystoisosporiasis (formerly known as isosporiasis), chronic (> 1 month)
Kaposi's sarcoma
Lymphoma (cerebral or B-cell non-Hodgkin)
Mycobacterial infection, non-tuberculous, extrapulmonary or disseminated
Mycosis – disseminated endemic (e.g. coccidioidomycosis, talaromycosis (formerly penicilliosis), histoplasmosis)
Pneumocystis pneumonia
Pneumonia, recurrent bacterial
Progressive multifocal leukoencephalopathy
Toxoplasmosis – cerebral
Tuberculosis – extrapulmonary (CDC includes pulmonary)
Sepsis, recurrent (including non-typhoidal *Salmonella*) (CDC only includes *Salmonella*)

Symptomatic HIV-associated nephropathy*
Symptomatic HIV-associated cardiomyopathy*
Leishmaniasis, atypical disseminated*

*These conditions are in WHO stage 4 but not in CDC category C.

14

Epidemiology

The acquired immunodeficiency syndrome (AIDS) was first recognised in 1981, although the earliest documented case of HIV infection has been traced to a blood sample from the Democratic Republic of Congo in 1959. AIDS is caused by the human immunodeficiency virus (HIV), which progressively impairs cellular immunity. HIV is a zoonotic infection with simian immunodeficiency viruses (SIV) from African primates, probably first infecting local hunters. SIVs do not cause disease in their natural primate hosts. HIV-1 was transmitted from chimpanzees and HIV-2 from sooty mangabey monkeys. HIV-1 is the cause of the global HIV pandemic, while HIV-2, which causes a similar illness to HIV-1 but progresses more slowly and is less transmissible, is restricted mainly to western Africa. It has been estimated that both HIV-1 and HIV-2 first infected humans about 100 years ago. HIV-2 will not be discussed further in this chapter.

There are three groups of HIV-1, representing three separate transmission events from chimpanzees: M ('major', worldwide distribution), O ('outlier') and N ('non-major and non-outlier'). Groups O and N are restricted to West Africa. Group M consists of nine subtypes: A–D, F–H, J and K, but recombinants of subtypes occur frequently. Globally, subtype C (which predominates in sub-Saharan Africa and India) accounts for half of infections and appears to be more readily transmitted. Subtype B predominates in Western Europe, the Americas and Australia. In Europe, the prevalence of non-B subtypes is increasing because of migration. Subtypes A and D are associated with slower and faster disease progression, respectively.

Global and regional epidemics

In 2019 it was estimated that there were 38 million people living with HIV (PLWH), 1.7 million new infections and 690 000 AIDS-related deaths. The global epidemiology of HIV has been changed by expanding access to combination antiretroviral therapy (ART), which reached 25.4 million people in 2019: the annual number of AIDS-related deaths has more than halved since the peak in 2004, the number of new infections has decreased by 40% since the peak in 1999, and the number of PLWH has increased. Regions have marked differences in HIV prevalence, incidence and dominant modes of transmission (Box 14.1). HIV has had a devastating impact in sub-Saharan Africa, particularly in southern Africa, where average life expectancy of the general population fell to below 40 years before the introduction of ART.

Modes of transmission

HIV is transmitted by sexual contact, by exposure to blood (e.g. injection drug use, occupational exposure in health-care workers) and blood products, or to infants of HIV-infected mothers, who may be infected in utero (this is uncommon), perinatally or via breastfeeding. The risk of contracting HIV after exposure to infected body fluid is dependent on the integrity of the exposed site, the type and volume of fluid, and the level of viraemia in the source person. The approximate transmission risk after exposure is given in Box 14.2. Factors that increase the risk of transmission are listed in Box 14.3.

A high proportion of patients with haemophilia in high-income countries were infected through contaminated blood products before HIV antibody screening was adopted in 1985. Routine screening of blood and blood products for HIV infection has virtually eliminated this mode of transmission. However, because of the lack of adequate screening facilities in resource-poor countries, it has been estimated that 5%–10% of blood transfusions globally are with HIV-infected blood.

Virology and immunology

HIV is an enveloped ribonucleic acid (RNA) retrovirus from the lentivirus family. After mucosal exposure, HIV is transported via dendritic cells to the lymph nodes, where infection becomes established. This is followed by viraemia and dissemination to lymphoid organs, which are the main sites of viral replication.

Each mature virion has a lipid membrane lined by a matrix protein that is studded with glycoprotein (gp) 120 and gp41 spikes. The inner cone-shaped protein core (p24) houses two copies of the single-stranded RNA genome and viral enzymes. The HIV genome

i 14.2 Risk of HIV transmission after single exposure to an HIV-infected source*	
HIV exposure	**Approximate risk**
Sexual	
Vaginal intercourse: female to male	0.05%
Vaginal intercourse: male to female	0.1%
Anal intercourse: insertive	0.1%
Anal intercourse: receptive	1.4%
Oral intercourse: insertive	<0.01%
Oral intercourse: receptive	<0.01%
Blood exposure	
Blood transfusion	90%
Intravenous drug-users sharing needles	0.67%
Percutaneous needlestick injury	0.3%
Mucous membrane splash	0.09%
Mother to child	
Vaginal delivery	15%
Breastfeeding (per month)	0.5%

*These are approximate estimates and assume that the source person is not being treated with ART.

i 14.1 Regional HIV prevalence in 2019, incidence trend and dominant mode of transmission			
Region	**People living with HIV (millions)**	**HIV incidence trend (2010–2019)**	**Dominant transmission**
Sub-Saharan Africa	25.6	Decreasing	Heterosexual
Asia and Pacific	5.8	Decreasing	MSM, heterosexual
Latin America and Caribbean	2.4	Increasing	MSM, heterosexual
Western and Central Europe, and North America	2.2	Stable	MSM, IDU
Eastern Europe and Central Asia	1.7	Increasing	IDU, MSM
Middle East and North Africa	0.24	Increasing	IDU, MSM

(IDU = injection drug-users; MSM = men who have sex with men)

consists of three characteristic retroviral genes – *gag* (encodes a polyprotein that is processed into structural proteins, including p24), *pol* (codes for the enzymes reverse transcriptase, integrase and protease) and *env* (codes for envelope proteins gp120 and gp41) – as well as six regulatory genes.

HIV infects cells bearing the CD4 receptor; these are T-helper lymphocytes, monocyte–macrophages, dendritic cells, and microglial cells in the central nervous system (CNS). Entry into the cell commences with binding of gp120 to the CD4 receptor (Fig. 14.1), which results in a conformational change in gp120 that permits binding to one of two chemokine co-receptors (CXCR4 or CCR5). The chemokine co-receptor CCR5 is utilised during initial infection, but subsequently the virus may adapt to use CXCR4. Individuals who are homozygous for the CCR5 delta 32 mutation do not express CCR5 on CD4 cells and are immune to HIV infection. Chemokine co-receptor binding is followed by membrane fusion and cellular entry involving gp41. After penetrating the cell and uncoating, a deoxyribonucleic acid (DNA) copy is transcribed from the RNA genome by the reverse transcriptase enzyme, which is carried by the infecting virion. Reverse transcription is an error-prone process and multiple mutations arise with ongoing replication, which results in considerable viral genetic heterogeneity. Viral DNA is transported into the nucleus and integrated within the host cell genome by the integrase enzyme. Integrated virus is known as proviral DNA and persists for the life of the cell. Cells infected with proviral HIV DNA produce new virions only if they undergo cellular activation, resulting in the transcription of viral messenger RNA (mRNA) copies, which are then translated into viral peptide chains. The precursor polyproteins are then cleaved by the viral protease enzyme to form new viral structural proteins and enzymes that migrate to the cell surface and are assembled using the host cellular apparatus to produce infectious viral particles; these bud from the cell surface, incorporating the host cell membrane into the viral envelope. The mature virion then infects other CD4 cells and the process is repeated. CD4 lymphocytes that are replicating HIV have a short survival time of about 1 day. In asymptomatic PLWH it has

14

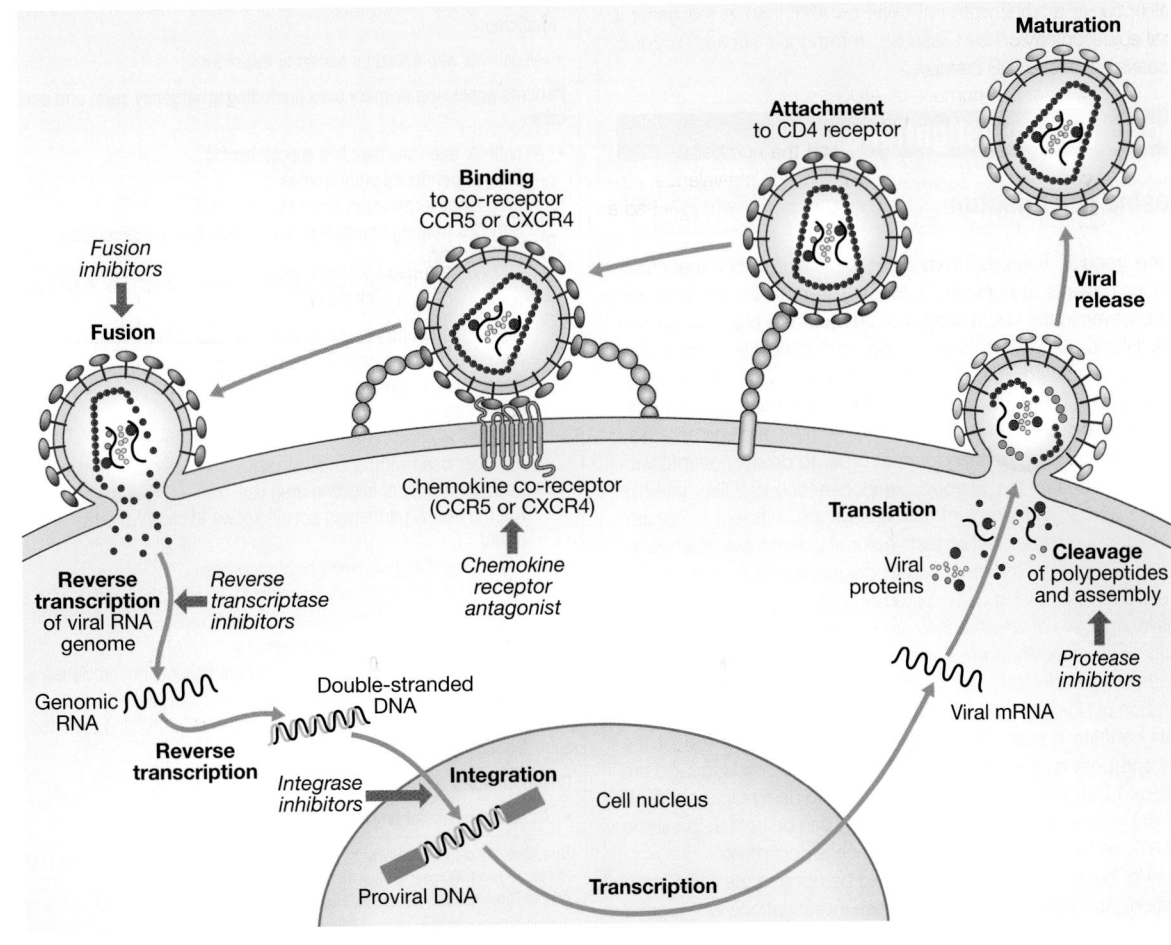

Fig. 14.1 Life cycle of HIV. Red arrows indicate sites of action of antiretroviral drugs.

been estimated that more than 10^{10} virions are produced and 10^9 CD4 lymphocytes destroyed each day. The CD4 lymphocytes are destroyed primarily by the host immune response rather than by cytopathic effects of HIV.

A small population of T-helper lymphocytes enter a post-integration latent phase. Latently infected cells are important as sanctuary sites from antiretroviral drugs, which act only on replicating virus. Current ART is unable to eradicate HIV infection due to the persistence of proviral DNA in long-lived latent CD4 cells.

The host immune response to HIV infection is both humoral, with the development of antibodies to a wide range of antigens, and cellular, with a dramatic expansion of HIV-specific CD8 cytotoxic T lymphocytes, resulting in a CD8 lymphocytosis and reversal of the usual CD4:CD8 ratio. CD8 cytotoxic T lymphocytes kill activated CD4 cells that are replicating HIV, but not latently infected CD4 cells. HIV evades destruction despite this vigorous immune response, in part because the highly conserved regions of gp120 and gp41 that are necessary for viral attachment and entry are covered by highly variable glycoprotein loops that change over time as a result of mutations selected for by the immune response. The initial peak of viraemia in primary infection settles to a plateau phase of persistent chronic viraemia. With time, there is gradual attrition of the T-helper lymphocyte population and, as these cells are pivotal in orchestrating the immune response, the patient becomes susceptible to opportunistic diseases. The predominant opportunist infections in PLWH are the consequences of impaired cell-mediated immunity (e.g. mycobacteria, herpesviruses). However, there is also a B-lymphocyte defect with impaired antibody production to new antigens and dysregulated antibody production, with a polyclonal increase in gamma globulins, resulting in an increased risk of infection with encapsulated bacteria, notably *Streptococcus pneumoniae*.

The immune activation in response to HIV infection does not completely resolve on effective ART. This residual inflammatory state has been implicated in the pathogenesis of several non-communicable diseases that occur at a higher rate in PLWH on ART than in the general population; e.g. ischaemic heart disease, thrombotic strokes, chronic kidney disease and non-AIDS cancers.

Diagnosis and investigations

Diagnosing HIV infection

Globally, the trend is towards universal HIV testing, rather than testing only those patients at high risk or those with manifestations of HIV infection. However, in the UK, testing is still targeted to high-risk groups (Box 14.4). HIV is diagnosed by detecting host antibodies either with rapid point-of-care tests or in the laboratory, where enzyme-linked immunosorbent assay (ELISA) tests are usually done. Most tests detect antibodies to both HIV-1 and HIV-2. Screening tests often include an assay for p24 antigen in addition to antibodies, in order to detect patients with primary infection before the antibody response occurs. Two positive antibody tests from two different immunoassays are sufficient to confirm infection. Nucleic acid amplification tests (usually polymerase chain reaction, PCR) to detect HIV RNA are used to diagnose infections in infants of HIV-positive mothers, who carry maternal antibodies to HIV for up to 15 months irrespective of whether they are HIV-infected, and to diagnose primary infection before antibodies have developed. PCR is more sensitive than p24 antigen detection for diagnosing primary infection.

The purpose of HIV testing is not simply to identify infected individuals, but also to educate people about prevention and transmission of the virus. Pre- and post-test discussions in the client's home language are essential (Box 14.5). There are major advantages to using rapid point-of-care HIV tests as pre- and post-test discussions can be held at the same visit and ART can be initiated if the HIV infection is confirmed.

A number of baseline investigations should be done at the initial medical evaluation (Box 14.6). The extent of these investigations will depend on the resources available.

Viral load and CD4 counts

CD4 counts

CD4 lymphocyte counts are usually determined by flow cytometry but cheaper methods have been developed for low-income countries. The CD4 count is the most clinically useful laboratory indicator of the degree of immune suppression; it is used, together with clinical staging, in decisions to start prophylaxis against opportunistic infections, and is of great value in the differential diagnosis of clinical problems.

The CD4 count varies by up to 20% from day to day and is transiently reduced by intercurrent infections. The normal CD4 count is over 500 cells/mm^3. The rate of decline in CD4 count is highly variable. People with CD4 counts between 200 and 500 cells/mm^3 have a low risk of developing major opportunistic infections. Morbidity due to inflammatory dermatoses, herpes zoster, oral candidiasis, tuberculosis, bacterial pneumonia and HIV-related immune disorders (e.g. immune thrombocytopenia) becomes increasingly common as CD4 counts decline. Once the count is below 200 cells/mm^3, there is severe immune suppression and a high risk of AIDS-defining conditions. It is important to note that patients can be asymptomatic despite very low CD4 counts and that major opportunistic diseases occasionally present with high CD4 counts.

Viral load

The level of viraemia is measured by quantitative PCR of HIV RNA, known as the viral load. Determining the viral load is crucial for monitoring responses to ART (p. 366). People with high viral loads (e.g. > 100 000

14.4 Patients who should be offered and recommended HIV testing in the UK

Patients accessing specialist sexual health services (including genitourinary medicine)

- All patients who attend for testing or treatment

Patients accessing primary care (including emergency care) and secondary care

- All patients attending their first appointment at:
    Drug dependency programmes
    Pregnancy termination services
    Services treating hepatitis B or C, lymphoma or tuberculosis
- All patients who:
    Have symptoms that may indicate HIV or for which HIV is part of the differential diagnosis
    Are from a country or group with high rate of HIV infection
    Are male, or trans women, who have sex with men
    Report sexual contact with someone from a country with a high rate of HIV infection
    Disclose high-risk sexual practices, e.g. 'chemsex'
    Are diagnosed with, or request testing for, a sexually transmitted infection
    Report a history of injecting drug use
    Are the sexual partners of people known to be HIV-positive or at high risk of HIV
- In areas of high[1] and extremely high[2] prevalence:
    All patients not previously diagnosed with HIV who register with a general practice or undergo blood testing for any reason
- In areas of extremely high prevalence[2]:
    All emergency care and secondary care patients not previously diagnosed with HIV
    At each general practice consultation consider offering opportunistic HIV testing

Prison inmates

- All new inmates not previously diagnosed with HIV

[1]Prevalence of diagnosed HIV is 2–5 per 1000 people aged 15–59. [2]Prevalence of diagnosed HIV is ≥ 5 per 1000 people aged 15–59.
Adapted from National Institute for Health and Care Excellence. *HIV testing: increasing uptake among people who may have undiagnosed HIV.* NICE guideline NG60 (Dec. 2016).

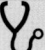

14.5 HIV pre- and post-test discussions*

Pre-test discussion

- Discuss meaning of positive and negative test results
- Realise importance of maintaining confidentiality
- Identify person to whom positive result could be disclosed
- Explore knowledge and explain natural history of HIV
- Discuss transmission and risk reduction
- Assess coping strategy
- Explain test procedure
- Obtain informed consent

Post-test discussion

Test result negative

- Discuss transmission and need for behaviour modification
- Advise second test 3 months after last exposure

Test result positive

- Explain meaning of result
- Organise medical follow-up
- Assess coping strategy
- Stress importance of disclosure
- Explain value of antiretroviral therapy
- Provide written information and useful Internet resources
- Discuss confidentiality issues
- Organise emotional and practical support (names/phone numbers)
- Facilitate notification of sexual partners

*Current UK guidance is that lengthy pre-test discussion is not required; the basic requirement is that individuals should be made aware that they will be tested for HIV and told how they will receive their result.

14.6 Baseline investigations

- CD4 count
- Viral load
- Hepatitis B surface antigen
- Hepatitis C antibody
- Liver function tests
- Full blood count
- Urinalysis, serum creatinine

- Syphilis serology
- Cervical smear in women
- Serum cryptococcal antigen (if CD4 <100)
- Tuberculin skin test or interferon gamma release assay
- Sexually transmitted infection screen

copies/mL) experience more rapid declines in CD4 count, while those with low viral loads (<1000 copies/mL) usually have slow or even no decline in CD4 counts. Viral loads are variable; only changes in viral load of more than 0.5 $\log_{10}$ copies/mL are considered clinically significant.

Clinical manifestations of HIV

Clinical staging of patients should be done at the initial medical examination, as it provides prognostic information and is a key criterion for initiating prophylaxis against opportunistic infections. Two clinical staging systems are used internationally (p. 351). In both, patients are staged according to the most severe manifestation and do not improve their classification. For example, a patient who is asymptomatic following a major opportunistic disease (AIDS) remains at stage 4 or category C of the WHO and CDC systems respectively, and never reverts to earlier stages. Finally, patients do not always progress steadily through all stages and may present with AIDS, having been asymptomatic.

Primary HIV infection

Primary infection is symptomatic in more than 50% of cases but the diagnosis is often missed. The incubation period is usually 2–4 weeks after exposure. The duration of symptoms is variable but is seldom longer than 2 weeks. The clinical manifestations (Box 14.7) resemble those of infectious mononucleosis/glandular fever (p. 285), but the presence of maculopapular rash or mucosal ulceration strongly suggests primary HIV infection rather than the other viral causes of

14.7 Clinical features of primary infection

- Fever
- Maculopapular rash
- Pharyngitis
- Lymphadenopathy
- Myalgia/arthralgia

- Diarrhoea
- Headache
- Oral and genital ulceration
- Meningo-encephalitis
- Bell's palsy

infectious mononucleosis, in which rashes generally occur only if aminopenicillins are given. Atypical lymphocytosis occurs less frequently than in Epstein–Barr (EBV) infection. Transient lymphopenia, including CD4 lymphocytes, is found in most cases (Fig. 14.2), which may result in opportunistic infections, notably oropharyngeal candidiasis. Major opportunistic infections like *Pneumocystis jirovecii* pneumonia (usually referred to as *Pneumocystis* pneumonia, PCP) may rarely occur. Thrombocytopenia and moderate elevation of liver enzymes are commonly present. The differential diagnosis of primary HIV includes acute EBV, primary cytomegalovirus (CMV) infection, rubella, primary toxoplasmosis and secondary syphilis.

Early diagnosis is made by detecting HIV RNA by PCR or p24 antigenaemia. The appearance of specific anti-HIV antibodies in serum (seroconversion) occurs 2–12 weeks after the development of symptoms. The window period, during which antibody tests may be false negative, is prolonged when post-exposure prophylaxis has been used.

Asymptomatic infection

A prolonged period of clinical latency follows primary infection, during which infected individuals are asymptomatic. Persistent generalised lymphadenopathy with nodes typically < 2 cm diameter is a common finding. Eventually, the lymph nodes regress, with destruction of node architecture as disease advances.

Viraemia peaks during primary infection and then drops as the immune response develops, to reach a plateau about 3 months later. The level of viraemia post seroconversion is a predictor of the rate of decline in CD4 counts, which is highly variable and explained in part by genetic factors affecting the immune response. The median time from infection to the development of AIDS in adults is about 9 years (see Fig. 14.2). A small proportion of untreated PLWH are long-term non-progressors, with CD4 counts remaining in the reference range for 10 years or more. Some long-term non-progressors have undetectable viral loads and are known as 'elite controllers'.

Minor HIV-associated disorders

A wide range of disorders indicating some impairment of cellular immunity occur in most patients before they develop AIDS (CDC category B or WHO stages 2 and 3). Careful examination of the mouth is important when patients are being followed up, as oral candidiasis and oral hairy leucoplakia are common conditions that require initiation of prophylaxis against opportunistic infections, irrespective of the CD4 count.

Acquired immunodeficiency syndrome

AIDS is defined by the development of specified opportunistic infections, cancers and severe manifestations of HIV itself (CDC category C or WHO stage 4).

Presenting problems in HIV infection

HIV itself is associated with a wide variety of clinical manifestations, and opportunistic diseases add many more. All body systems can be affected by HIV. The CD4 count is useful in differential diagnosis (Box 14.8). For example, in a patient with a pulmonary infiltrate and a CD4 count of 350 cells/mm³, pulmonary tuberculosis is a likely diagnosis and PCP is very unlikely, but if the patient's CD4 count is 50 cells/mm³, both PCP and tuberculosis are likely.

14

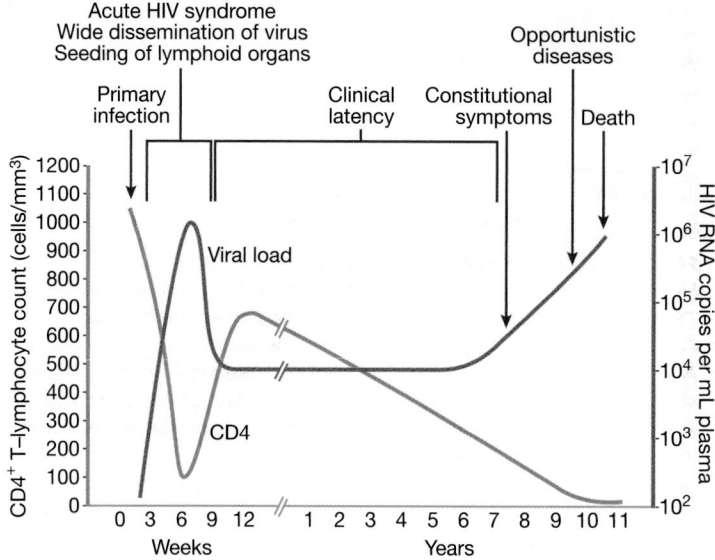

Fig. 14.2 **Virological and immunological progression of untreated HIV infection.**

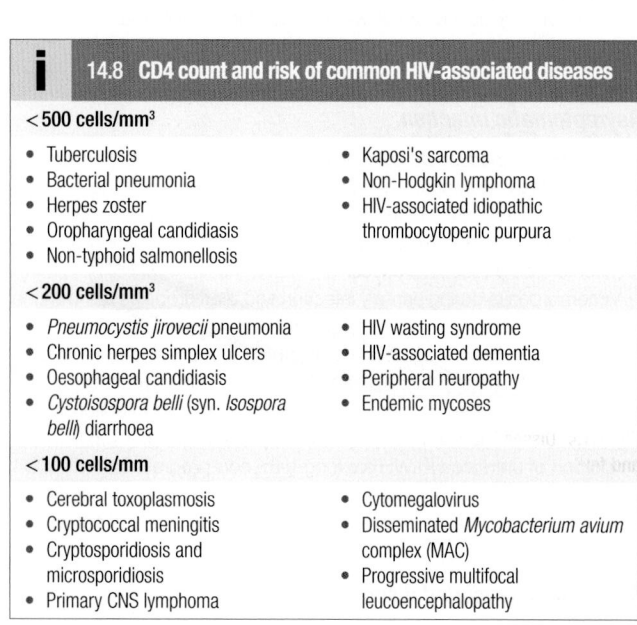

i	14.8 **CD4 count and risk of common HIV-associated diseases**

<500 cells/mm³

- Tuberculosis
- Bacterial pneumonia
- Herpes zoster
- Oropharyngeal candidiasis
- Non-typhoid salmonellosis

- Kaposi's sarcoma
- Non-Hodgkin lymphoma
- HIV-associated idiopathic thrombocytopenic purpura

<200 cells/mm³

- *Pneumocystis jirovecii* pneumonia
- Chronic herpes simplex ulcers
- Oesophageal candidiasis
- *Cystoisospora belli* (syn. *Isospora belli*) diarrhoea

- HIV wasting syndrome
- HIV-associated dementia
- Peripheral neuropathy
- Endemic mycoses

<100 cells/mm

- Cerebral toxoplasmosis
- Cryptococcal meningitis
- Cryptosporidiosis and microsporidiosis
- Primary CNS lymphoma

- Cytomegalovirus
- Disseminated *Mycobacterium avium* complex (MAC)
- Progressive multifocal leucoencephalopathy

Globally, tuberculosis is the most common cause of morbidity and mortality in PLWH. Tuberculosis should be considered in the differential diagnosis of most presenting problems in patients from communities where tuberculosis is common.

Lymphadenopathy

Persistent generalised lymphadenopathy due to HIV is described above under asymptomatic infection. Lymphadenopathy may also be due to malignancy (Kaposi's sarcoma or lymphoma) or infections, especially tuberculosis, which is an extremely common cause in low- and middle-income countries. Tuberculous lymph nodes are often matted and may become fluctuant due to extensive caseous necrosis; inexperienced clinicians often perform incision and drainage inappropriately when aspiration is all that is required. Symmetrical generalised lymphadenopathy may occur in disseminated tuberculosis. Lymphoma typically presents with large, firm, asymmetric nodes. Rapid enlargement of a node, asymmetric enlargement or lymphadenopathy associated with constitutional symptoms (even if the nodes are symmetrical) warrants further investigation. Lymph node needle aspiration should be performed. One portion of the sample should be sent for *Mycobacterium tuberculosis* PCR, which

has about a 70% yield in tuberculosis (or AAFB microscopy if PCR is unavailable). The other portion should be fixed on a slide and sent for cytology. If caseous liquid is aspirated, this should be sent for mycobacterial culture or PCR. If needle aspiration is unhelpful, or if lymphoma or Kaposi's sarcoma is suspected, excision biopsy should be performed.

Weight loss

Weight loss is a common finding in advanced HIV infection. The HIV wasting syndrome is an AIDS-defining condition and is defined as weight loss of more than 10% of body weight, plus either unexplained chronic diarrhoea (lasting over 1 month) or chronic weakness and unexplained prolonged fever (lasting over 1 month). This is a diagnosis of exclusion. If the weight loss is rapid (more than 1 kg a month), then major opportunistic infections or cancers become more likely. Painful oral conditions and nausea from drugs contribute by limiting intake. Depression is common and can cause significant weight loss. Measurement of C-reactive protein is helpful in the work-up of weight loss, as this is markedly raised with most opportunistic diseases but not with HIV itself. Erythrocyte sedimentation rate (ESR) is elevated by HIV infection and is therefore not useful as a screen for opportunistic diseases. The presence of fever or diarrhoea is helpful in the differential diagnosis of weight loss (Fig. 14.3).

Fever

Fever is a common presenting feature. Common causes of prolonged fever with weight loss are listed in Fig. 14.3. Non-typhoid *Salmonella* bacteraemia, which commonly presents with fever in low-income countries, is accompanied by diarrhoea in only about 50% of patients. Pyrexia of unknown origin (PUO) in HIV infection is defined as temperature over 38°C with no cause found after 4 weeks in outpatients or 3 days in inpatients, and initial investigations such as chest X-rays, urinalysis and blood cultures have failed to identify the cause. HIV itself can present with prolonged fever but this is a diagnosis of exclusion, as a treatable cause will be found in most patients. Abdominal imaging, preferably by computed tomography (CT) or magnetic resonance imaging (MRI), should be requested. Abdominal nodes (especially if they are hypodense in the centre) or splenic microabscesses strongly suggest tuberculosis. Mycobacterial blood cultures, which can also detect fungi, should be performed. Bone marrow aspirate and trephine biopsy are helpful if the full blood count shows cytopenias. Liver biopsy may be helpful if the liver enzymes are elevated but is invasive and seldom necessary. Mycobacterial and fungal stains and cultures should be done on all biopsies. Chest X-rays should be repeated after about a week, as micronodular or interstitial infiltrates may have become apparent (see p. 362 for differential diagnosis).

Tuberculosis is by far the most common cause of PUO in low- and middle-income countries, and in these settings a trial of empirical therapy is warranted after cultures have been sent. In high-income countries, disseminated *Mycobacterium avium* complex (MAC) infection is an important cause of PUO, often also presenting with diarrhoea and splenomegaly. Disseminated endemic mycoses (e.g. histoplasmosis, coccidioidomycosis, talaromycosis) present with PUO, often with papular skin eruptions or mucosal ulcerations (Fig. 14.4). Skin biopsy for histology and fungal culture is often diagnostic.

Mucocutaneous disease

The skin and mouth must be carefully examined, as mucocutaneous manifestations are extremely common in advanced HIV infection and many prognostically important conditions can be diagnosed by simple inspection. The differential diagnosis of dermatological conditions is simplified by categorising disorders according to the lesion type (Box 14.9). Some common dermatological diseases, notably psoriasis, are exacerbated by HIV. The risk of many drug rashes is increased in PLWH. Skin biopsy should be taken, and sent for histology and culture for mycobacteria and fungi, in patients with papular rashes or if there are constitutional symptoms coinciding with the development of the rash.

Seborrhoeic dermatitis

Seborrhoeic dermatitis is common in HIV. The severity increases as the CD4 count falls. It presents as scaly red patches, typically in the nasolabial folds and in hairy areas. It is associated with an increased presence of *Malassezia* spp. (dimorphic yeastlike fungi) but the pathogenesis is unknown. It responds well to a combined topical antifungal and glucocorticoid. Selenium sulphide shampoo is helpful for scalp involvement.

Herpes simplex infections

Recurrences of herpes simplex infection are common and primarily affect the nasolabial and anogenital areas (Fig. 14.5). As immune suppression worsens, the ulcers take longer to heal and become more extensive. Ulcers that persist for more than 4 weeks are AIDS-defining. The

diagnosis is based on clinical appearance and PCR of vesicle fluid or from ulcer swabs, although PCR may need to be reserved to resolve atypical presentations if it is not readily available. Response to a course of antiviral drug such as aciclovir is good but relapses are common. Frequent relapses that persist despite ART should be treated with aciclovir 400 mg twice daily long term (Box 14.10).

Herpes zoster

Typically presents with a pathognomonic vesicular rash on an erythematous base in a dermatomal distribution (p. 282). The median CD4 count at the first episode of zoster is 350 cells/mm³. In patients with

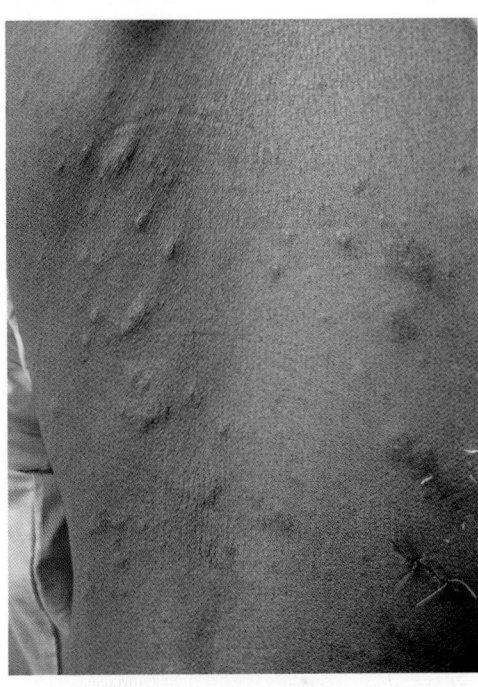

Fig. 14.4 Disseminated histoplasmosis presenting with diffuse papular rash and fever. Skin biopsy was diagnostic. *Courtesy of Professor Graeme Meintjes.*

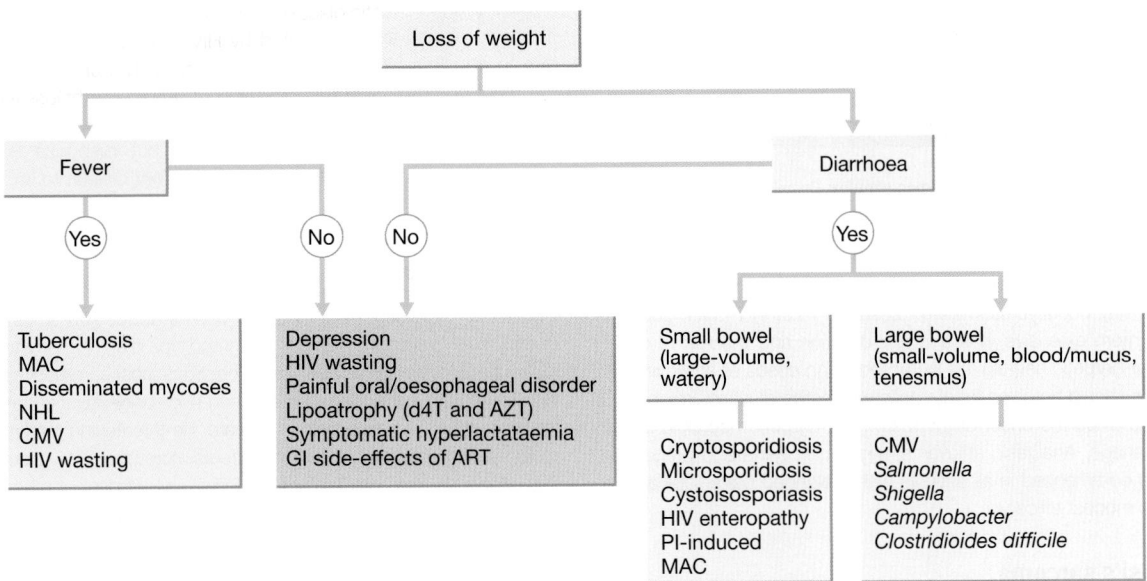

Fig. 14.3 Presentation and differential diagnosis of weight loss. (ART = antiretroviral therapy; AZT = zidovudine; CMV = cytomegalovirus; d4T = stavudine; KS = Kaposi's sarcoma; MAC = *Mycobacterium avium* complex; NHL = non-Hodgkin lymphoma; PI = protease inhibitor)

i 14.9 Differential diagnosis of skin conditions by lesion type

Scaly rashes

- Seborrhoeic dermatitis
- Psoriasis* (exacerbated by HIV)
- Tinea corporis*
- Dry skin/ichthyosis
- Norwegian scabies*
- Drug rashes*

Pruritic papules

- Pruritic papular eruption ('itchy red bump disease')
- Eosinophilic folliculitis
- Scabies*

Papules and nodules (non-pruritic)

- Molluscum contagiosum*
- Secondary syphilis
- Kaposi's sarcoma
- Bacillary angiomatosis
- Cryptococcosis
- Warts*
- Disseminated endemic mycoses (histoplasmosis, coccidioidomycosis, talaromycosis and emergomycosis)

Blisters

- Herpes simplex
- Herpes zoster
- Fixed drug eruptions
- Drug rashes (especially toxic epidermal necrolysis)

Mucocutaneous ulcers

- Ecthyma
- Herpes simplex
- Aphthous ulcers (minor and major)
- Histoplasmosis
- Drug rashes (Stevens–Johnson syndrome)

Hyperpigmentation

- Post-inflammatory (especially pruritic papular eruption)
- Zidovudine
- Emtricitabine (palms and soles)

*See Chapter 27 for more information.

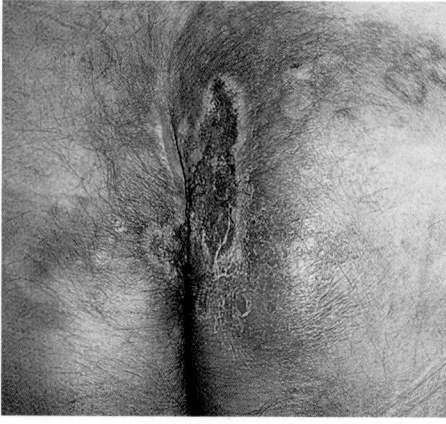

Fig. 14.5 Severe mucocutaneous herpes simplex. Chronic anogenital or perioral ulcers are very common in advanced HIV infection.

advanced HIV disease, the rash may be multidermatomal and recurrent episodes may occur. Disseminated zoster is rare. In PLWH, zoster is generally more extensive, has a longer duration and the risk of developing post-herpetic neuralgia is increased. High doses of aciclovir or its congeners should be given for all cases with active disease, irrespective of the time since the onset of the rash. Post-herpetic neuralgia is difficult to manage. Analgesic adjuvants, e.g. amitriptyline and pregabalin, should be commenced in all patients with prolonged pain. Topical capsaicin has modest efficacy.

Kaposi's sarcoma

Kaposi's sarcoma (KS) is a spindle-cell tumour of lympho-endothelial origin. All forms of KS are due to sexually transmitted human herpesvirus 8, also known as KS-associated herpesvirus. KS occurs in four patterns:

- *classic KS*: rare, indolent and restricted largely to older men of Mediterranean or Jewish origin
- *endemic KS*: occurs in sub-Saharan Africa, is more aggressive, presents at earlier ages than classic KS, and affects men more than women
- *KS in patients on immunosuppressant drugs*: usually transplant recipients, who experience disseminated disease
- *AIDS-associated KS*.

In Africa, the male-to-female ratio of AIDS-associated KS is much lower than is seen with endemic KS, but men are still more affected than women, despite the fact that the seroprevalence of human herpesvirus 8 is the same in both sexes.

AIDS-associated KS is always a multicentric disease. Early mucocutaneous lesions are macular and may be difficult to diagnose. Subsequently, lesions become papular or nodular, and may ulcerate. KS lesions typically have a red–purple colour (Fig. 14.6) but may become hyperpigmented, especially in dark-skinned patients. As the disease progresses, the skin lesions become more numerous and larger. Lymphoedema is common, as lymphatic vessels are infiltrated. KS also commonly spreads to lymph nodes and viscerally, especially to the lungs and gastrointestinal tract. Visceral disease occasionally occurs in the absence of mucocutaneous involvement. B symptoms of fever, night sweats and weight loss may occur.

KS may respond to ART. Chemotherapy should be reserved for those patients who fail to respond to ART, or be given together with ART if there are poor prognostic features such as visceral involvement, oedema, ulcerated lesions and B symptoms.

Bacillary angiomatosis

Bacillary angiomatosis is a bacterial infection caused by *Bartonella henselae* or *B. quintana*. Skin lesions range from solitary superficial red–purple lesions resembling KS or pyogenic granuloma, to multiple subcutaneous nodules or plaques. Lesions are painful and may bleed or ulcerate. The infection may become disseminated with fevers, lymphadenopathy and hepatosplenomegaly. Diagnosis is made by biopsy of a lesion and Warthin–Starry silver staining, which reveals aggregates of bacilli. Treatment with doxycycline or azithromycin is effective.

Papular pruritic eruption

Papular pruritic eruption ('itchy red bump disease') is an intensely itchy, symmetrical rash affecting the trunk and extremities. It is thought to be due to an allergic reaction to insect bites. In sub-Saharan Africa, it is the most common skin manifestation of advanced HIV disease. Post-inflammatory hyperpigmentation is common. Topical glucocorticoids, emollients and antihistamines are useful but response is variable. Measures to reduce insect bites are logical but difficult to implement in low-income settings.

Drug rashes

Cutaneous hypersensitivity to drugs occurs about 100 times more frequently in HIV infection. The most common type is an erythematous maculopapular rash, which may be scaly. The drugs most commonly associated with rashes are sulphonamides and non-nucleoside reverse transcriptase inhibitors (NNRTIs – see below). Severe, life-threatening features of drug rashes include blistering (when this affects more than 30% of surface area it is known as toxic epidermal necrolysis), involvement of mucous membranes (Stevens–Johnson syndrome), or systemic involvement with fever or organ dysfunction (especially hepatitis, which is often delayed for a week or two after the rash develops). Because sulphonamides are important in the treatment and prophylaxis of opportunistic infections, rechallenge or desensitisation is often attempted in patients who have previously experienced rashes, provided the reaction was not life-threatening. Details of rashes caused by ART are given below.

14.10 Treatment of common opportunistic infections in adults with AIDS

Opportunistic infection	Treatment	Alternative treatment	Secondary prophylaxis[1]
Pneumocystis jirovecii pneumonia	Co-trimoxazole 20/100 mg/kg/day IV/PO (in 4 divided doses) for 21 days; maximum per dose 320/1600 mg Early adjunctive prednisone 40 mg twice daily, if hypoxic	Clindamycin 900 mg 3 times daily IV (switch to 600 mg 3 times daily PO once improving) plus primaquine 30 mg PO daily for 21 days	Co-trimoxazole 160/800 mg daily PO
Cerebral toxoplasmosis	Sulfadiazine 15 mg/kg 4 times daily PO plus pyrimethamine 200 mg stat PO, then 75 mg daily plus folinic acid 15–25 mg daily for 6 weeks	Co-trimoxazole 320/1600 mg twice daily IV/PO for 4 weeks, then 160/800 mg twice daily for 3 months	Co-trimoxazole 160/800 mg daily PO
Cryptococcosis	Liposomal amphotericin B 4 mg/kg/day IV plus flucytosine 25 mg/kg 4 times daily PO for 7 days, followed by fluconazole 400 mg daily PO for 8 weeks	Amphotericin B 1 mg/kg/day IV plus fluconazole[2] 800 mg daily IV/PO for 14 days, followed by fluconazole 400 mg daily PO for 8 weeks	Fluconazole 200 mg daily PO (for minimum of 1 year)
Oesophageal candidiasis	Fluconazole 200 mg daily IV/PO for 14 days	Itraconazole 200 mg daily PO for 14–21 days	Not usually recommended
Disseminated *Mycobacterium avium* complex	Clarithromycin 500 mg twice daily PO plus ethambutol 15 mg/kg daily PO	Azithromycin 500 mg daily PO plus ethambutol 15 mg/kg daily PO	Continue treatment for minimum of 1 year
Herpes simplex ulcers	Aciclovir 400 mg 3 times daily PO for 5–10 days	Valaciclovir 500 mg or famciclovir 125 mg twice daily PO for 5–10 days	Aciclovir 400 mg twice daily PO if recurrences are frequent/severe
Cystoisospora belli diarrhoea	Co-trimoxazole 160/800 mg 4 times daily PO for 10 days	Ciprofloxacin 500 mg twice daily PO for 10 days	Co-trimoxazole 160/800 mg daily PO

[1]Secondary prophylaxis may be discontinued once CD4 counts have increased to > 200 cells/mm³ on antiretroviral therapy for at least 3 months. [2]Only if flucytosine is unavailable.
(IV = intravenous; PO = orally)

Oral conditions

Oropharyngeal candidiasis is common in advanced HIV infection. It is nearly always caused by *Candida albicans*, but azole-resistant *Candida* species may be selected for if there have been repeated courses of azole drugs. Pseudomembranous candidiasis is the most common manifestation, with white patches on the buccal mucosa (p. 350) that can be scraped off to reveal a red raw surface. Erythematous candidiasis is more difficult to diagnose and presents with a reddened mucosa and a smooth shiny tongue. Angular cheilitis due to *Candida* is a common manifestation. Topical antifungals are usually effective. Antifungal lozenges are more effective than antifungal solutions. Systemic azole therapy, usually fluconazole, should be given if topical therapy fails or if there are oesophageal symptoms.

Oral hairy leucoplakia (p. 350) appears as corrugated white plaques running vertically on the side of the tongue and is virtually pathognomonic of HIV disease. It is usually asymptomatic and is due to EBV.

Herpetiform oral ulcers occur in primary infection. Herpes simplex typically affects the nasolabial area but may cause oral ulcers. In early disease, minor aphthous ulcers are common. In advanced disease, giant aphthous ulcers occur. These destroy tissue, are painful and need to be differentiated from herpes simplex and CMV ulcers by biopsy. They respond to systemic glucocorticoids and ART. Some disseminated endemic mycoses, notably histoplasmosis (p. 346), may cause oral ulcers, usually associated with constitutional symptoms. Finally, superficial oral ulcers may occur as part of the Stevens–Johnson syndrome, usually caused by sulphonamides or NNRTIs.

KS often involves the mouth, especially the hard palate (see above and Fig. 14.6). Nodular oral lesions are associated with a worse prognosis.

Gingivitis is common in advanced HIV infection. Acute necrotising ulcerative gingivitis and periostitis (p. 350) can result in loss of teeth.

Nail disorders

Fungal infections of the nails (onychomycosis) are common and often involve multiple nails. Blue–black discoloration of nails may be due to HIV or to the antiretroviral drug zidovudine.

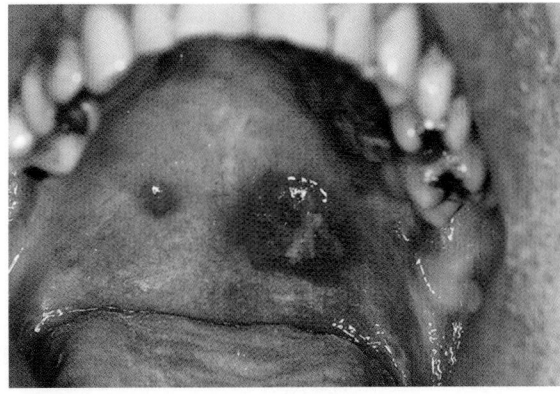

Fig. 14.6 Oral Kaposi's sarcoma. A full examination is important to detect disease that may affect the palate, gums, fauces or tongue.

Gastrointestinal disease

Oesophageal diseases

Oesophageal candidiasis (Fig. 14.7) is the most common cause of pain on swallowing (odynophagia), dysphagia and regurgitation in advanced HIV infection. Concomitant oral candidiasis is present in most patients. Systemic azole therapy, e.g. fluconazole 200 mg daily for 14 days, is usually effective but relapses are common (see Box 14.10). Patients whose oesophageal symptoms fail to respond to azoles should be investigated with oesophagoscopy; major aphthous ulceration and CMV ulcers are the most likely causes and need to be differentiated by biopsy.

Diarrhoea

Chronic diarrhoea is a common presenting problem in patients with advanced HIV, especially in areas where there is no access to safe water. It is a component of the HIV wasting syndrome. The differential diagnosis

14

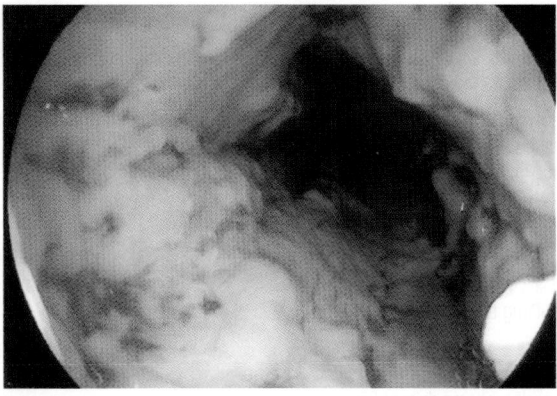

Fig. 14.7 Oesophageal candidiasis. Endoscopy showing typical pseudomembranous candidiasis.

i	14.11 Common causes of chronic watery diarrhoea		
	Cryptosporidiosis	**Microsporidiosis**	**Cystoisosporiasis**
Organism	Protozoan	Fungus	Protozoan
Species	*Cryptosporidium parvum C. hominis*	*Enterozoon bieneusi Encephalitozoon intestinalis* etc.	*Cystoisospora belli*
Animal host	Multiple	Multiple	No
Distribution	Global	Global	Tropics
Stool examination	Acid-fast stain	Trichrome stain Polymerase chain reaction	Acid-fast stain
Specific treatment	No established therapy	Albendazole (some species)	Co-trimoxazole

of diarrhoea depends on whether the presentation is with large or small bowel symptoms (see Fig. 14.3).

Large bowel diarrhoea

Acute diarrhoea caused by the bacterial enteric pathogens *Campylobacter*, *Shigella* and *Salmonella* occurs more frequently than in HIV-negative people and the illness is more severe. Bacteraemia is more common, notably due to non-typhoid *Salmonella*. Diarrhoea caused by *Clostridioides difficile* should be considered if there has been prior exposure to antibiotics, as is often the case in patients with symptomatic HIV.

CMV colitis presents with chronic large bowel symptoms and fever in patients with CD4 counts below 100 cells/mm³. On colonoscopy, ulcers are seen, mostly involving the left side of the colon. Biopsy of ulcers shows typical 'owl's-eye' inclusion bodies.

Small bowel diarrhoea

Chronic small bowel diarrhoea may be due to HIV enteropathy, which is a diagnosis of exclusion. It typically presents with chronic watery diarrhoea and wasting without fever. Infection with one of three unicellular organisms is responsible for most cases: cryptosporidiosis, microsporidiosis and cystoisosporiasis (formerly known as isosporiasis) (Box 14.11). All three organisms are intracellular parasites that invade enterocytes. If the diagnosis is not made by stool microscopy on at least two specimens, a duodenal biopsy should be performed (Fig. 14.8).

About 40% of patients with disseminated MAC infections have watery diarrhoea. Fever is a prominent feature of MAC infection, which helps differentiate it from cryptosporidiosis, microsporidiosis and cystoisosporiasis. Intestinal tuberculosis typically involves the ileocaecal area and may present with fever, weight loss and diarrhoea, but the diarrhoea is seldom profuse.

Hepatobiliary disease

Chronic viral hepatitis

Hepatitis B and/or C (HBV and HCV) co-infection is common in PLWH due to shared risk factors for transmission. The natural history of both HBV and HCV is altered by HIV co-infection. In the ART era, chronic liver disease from viral hepatitis has emerged as a major cause of morbidity and mortality. HBV and HCV are further described in Chapter 24.

Hepatitis B

HBV infection is common in several groups of people at risk of HIV infection: residents of low- and middle-income countries, injection drug-users, people with haemophilia and men who have sex with men (MSM). HBV status should be checked at baseline in all PLWH. HIV co-infection increases HBV viraemia, is associated with less elevation of transaminase, and increases the risk of liver fibrosis and hepatocellular

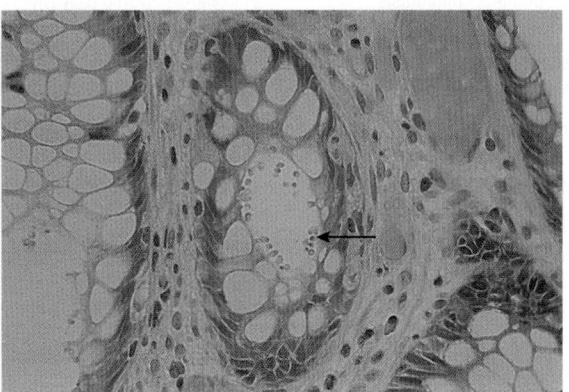

Fig. 14.8 Cryptosporidiosis. Duodenal biopsy may be necessary to confirm cryptosporidiosis or microsporidiosis. The arrow indicates an oöcyst.

carcinoma. All patients with HBV infection should be treated with ART, including the nucleotide reverse transcriptase inhibitor (NRTI) tenofovir, which is also effective for HBV. A flare of hepatitis may be associated with improved immune function after starting ART or discontinuing antiretrovirals that have anti-HBV activity. HBV co-infection increases the risk of antiretroviral hepatotoxicity.

Hepatitis C

HCV infection is common in injection drug-users and people with haemophilia. HIV co-infection increases HCV viraemia and increases the risk of liver fibrosis and hepatocellular carcinoma. Treatment for HCV should be commenced together with ART. As with HBV co-infection, a flare of hepatitis may be associated with improved immune function after starting ART, and there is an increased risk of antiretroviral hepatotoxicity. Response to anti-HCV therapy is similar to that seen in HIV-negative people.

HIV cholangiopathy

HIV cholangiopathy, a form of secondary sclerosing cholangitis, may occur in patients with severe immune suppression. Papillary stenosis is common and is amenable to cautery via endoscopic retrograde cholangiopancreatography (ERCP), which provides symptomatic relief. Acalculous cholecystitis is a common complication of cholangiopathy. ART may improve the condition.

Respiratory disease

Pulmonary disease is common and is the major reason for hospital admission in advanced HIV disease. Influenza and COVID-19 are more severe in PLWH. Most patients who are admitted for respiratory diseases will have either bacterial pneumonia, pulmonary tuberculosis or PCP. PCP is more common in high-income countries, while tuberculosis is more common in low- and middle-income countries. An approach to the differential diagnosis of all three conditions is given in Box 14.12.

Pneumocystis jirovecii pneumonia (Pneumocystis pneumonia, PCP)

The key presenting feature of PCP is progressive dyspnoea with a duration of less than 12 weeks. Dry cough and fever are common. The chest X-ray typically shows a bilateral interstitial infiltrate spreading out from the hilar regions (Fig. 14.9) but may be normal initially. High-resolution CT scan is more sensitive than chest X-ray, usually showing typical 'ground-glass' interstitial infiltrates. Pneumatoceles may occur and may rupture, resulting in a pneumothorax. The diagnosis is made with silver stains, PCR or immunofluorescence of broncho-alveolar lavage or induced sputum (note that spontaneously produced sputum should not be sent, as the yield is low). Treatment is with high-dose co-trimoxazole, together with adjunctive systemic glucocorticoids if the patient is hypoxic (see Box 14.10).

Pulmonary tuberculosis

Tuberculosis is the most common cause of admission in countries with a high tuberculosis incidence. Pulmonary tuberculosis in patients with mild immune suppression typically presents as in HIV-uninfected patients, with a chronic illness and apical pulmonary cavities (p. 518). However, in patients with CD4 counts below 200 cells/mm³, there are four important differences in the clinical presentation of pulmonary tuberculosis:

- Tuberculosis progresses more rapidly, with a subacute or even acute presentation. The diagnosis therefore needs to be made and therapy commenced promptly. A trial of empirical therapy is often justified while awaiting the results of mycobacterial cultures.
- The chest X-ray appearance alters: cavities are rarely seen, pulmonary infiltrates are no longer predominantly in apical areas, and pleural effusions and hilar or mediastinal lymphadenopathy are common (Fig. 14.10). A normal chest X-ray is not unusual in symptomatic patients with tuberculosis confirmed on sputum culture. These atypical findings can result in a delayed or missed diagnosis.
- Sputum smears, which are positive in most HIV-uninfected adults with pulmonary tuberculosis, are negative in more than half of patients. The main reason for this is the absence of pulmonary cavities.
- Many patients have disseminated tuberculosis, sometimes with a classic miliary pattern on chest X-ray, but more commonly

presenting with atypical pulmonary infiltrates together with extrapulmonary tuberculosis. The most common sites of concomitant extrapulmonary tuberculosis are the pleura and lymph nodes. A rapid diagnosis can be made with the urine lipoarabinomannan lateral flow assay.

Tuberculosis in PLWH responds well to standard short-course therapy (p. 522).

Bacterial pneumonia

The incidence of bacterial pneumonia is increased about 100-fold by HIV infection. The severity, likelihood of bacteraemia, risk of recurrent pneumonia and mortality are all increased compared with HIV-negative patients. The aetiology is similar to that of community-acquired pneumonia in HIV-uninfected patients with comorbidity: *S. pneumoniae*

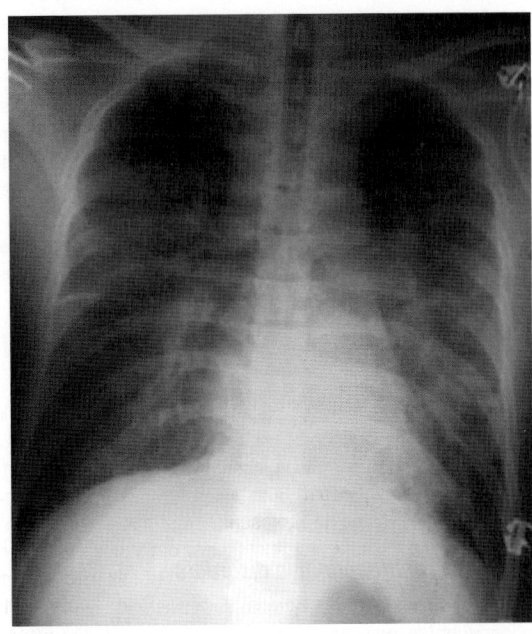

Fig. 14.9 *Pneumocystis* pneumonia: typical chest X-ray appearance. Note the interstitial bilateral infiltrate.

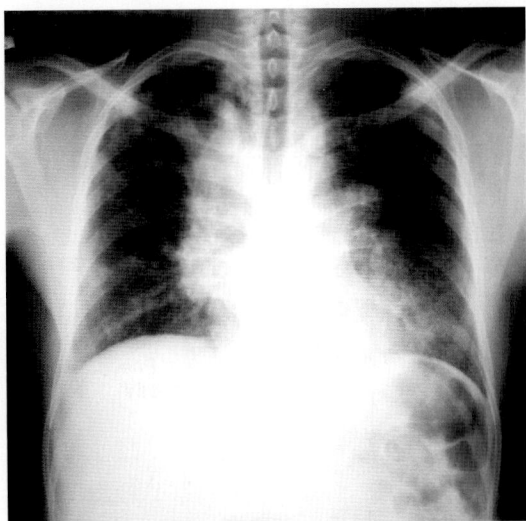

Fig. 14.10 Chest X-ray of pulmonary tuberculosis in advanced HIV infection. Lower-zone infiltrates and hilar or mediastinal nodes in a patient with a CD4 count of <200 cells/mm³.

	Bacterial pneumonia	*Pneumocystis jirovecii* pneumonia (PCP)	Pulmonary tuberculosis
14.12 Comparative features of bacterial pneumonia, *Pneumocystis jirovecii* pneumonia and pulmonary tuberculosis			
Duration	Acute	Subacute	Variable
Dyspnoea	Common	Prominent	Occasional
White cell count	Increased	Normal	Normal/low
Chest X-ray			
Infiltrate	Consolidation	Interstitial	Nodular
Bilateral infiltrate	Occasional	Usual	Common
Effusion	Occasional	No	Common
Nodes	Rare	No	Common

14

is the most common cause, followed by *Haemophilus influenzae*, Enterobacterales (e.g. *Klebsiella pneumoniae*) and *Staphylococcus aureus*. The prevalence of atypical bacteria in PLWH with pneumonia is similar to that in the general population. Treatment is with a broad-spectrum β-lactam (e.g. ceftriaxone, amoxicillin–clavulanate), with the addition of a macrolide if the pneumonia is severe).

Uncommon bacteria causing pneumonia include *Pseudomonas aeruginosa*, *Nocardia* (which mimics tuberculosis) and *Rhodococcus equi* (which can cause pulmonary cavities).

Miscellaneous causes of pulmonary infiltrates

Pulmonary cryptococcosis may present as a component of disseminated disease or be limited to the lungs. The chest X-ray appearances are variable. Cryptococcomas occur less commonly than in HIV-uninfected people. The most common radiographic pattern seen in HIV infection is patchy consolidation, often with small areas of cavitation resembling tuberculosis. Pleural involvement is rare. The disseminated endemic mycoses (histoplasmosis, coccidioidomycosis, emergomycosis and talaromycosis) often cause diffuse pulmonary infiltrates, mimicking miliary tuberculosis.

Lymphoid interstitial pneumonitis is a slowly progressive disorder causing a diffuse reticulonodular infiltrate. It is caused by a benign polyclonal lymphocytic interstitial infiltrate and is part of the diffuse infiltrative lymphocytosis syndrome (DILS), described later in this chapter. Patients may have other features of DILS, notably parotidomegaly.

KS often spreads to the lungs. Typical chest X-ray appearances are large, irregular nodules, linear reticular patterns and pleural effusions. Bronchoscopy is diagnostic.

Nervous system and eye disease

The central and peripheral nervous systems are commonly involved in HIV, either as a direct consequence of HIV infection or due to opportunistic diseases. An approach to common presentations is outlined in Fig. 14.11.

Cognitive impairment

HIV-associated neurocognitive disorders

HIV is a neurotropic virus and invades the CNS early during infection. Meningoencephalitis may occur at seroconversion. PLWH often have abnormalities on neuropsychiatric testing. The term HIV-associated neurocognitive disorder (HAND) describes a spectrum of disorders:

asymptomatic neurocognitive impairment, minor neurocognitive disorder and HIV-associated dementia (also called HIV encephalopathy). The proportion of patients with symptomatic HAND increases with declining CD4 counts. HIV-associated dementia is a subcortical dementia characterised by impairment of executive function, psychomotor retardation and impaired memory. There is no diagnostic test for HIV-associated dementia. CT or MRI shows diffuse cerebral atrophy out of keeping with age. It is important to exclude depression, cryptococcal meningitis and neurosyphilis. ART usually improves HIV-associated dementia but milder forms of HAND often persist.

Progressive multifocal leucoencephalopathy

Progressive multifocal leucoencephalopathy (PML) is a progressive disease that presents with stroke-like episodes and cognitive impairment. Vision is often impaired due to involvement of the occipital cortex. PML is caused by the JC virus. A combination of characteristic appearances on MRI (Fig. 14.12) and detection of JC virus DNA in the cerebrospinal fluid (CSF) by PCR is diagnostic. No specific treatment exists and prognosis remains poor despite ART.

CMV encephalitis

This presents with behavioural disturbance, cognitive impairment and a reduced level of consciousness. Focal signs may also occur. Detection of CMV DNA in the CSF supports the diagnosis. Response to anti-CMV therapy is usually poor.

Space-occupying lesions

Space-occupying lesions in AIDS patients typically present over days to weeks. The most common cause is toxoplasmosis. As toxoplasmosis responds rapidly to therapy, a trial of anti-toxoplasmosis therapy should be given to all patients presenting with space-occupying lesions while the results of diagnostic tests are being awaited.

Cerebral toxoplasmosis

Cerebral toxoplasmosis is caused by reactivation of residual *Toxoplasma gondii* cysts from past infection, which results in the development of space-occupying lesions. The characteristic findings on imaging are multiple space-occupying lesions with ring enhancement on contrast and surrounding oedema (Fig. 14.13). *Toxoplasma* serology shows evidence of previous exposure (positive immunoglobulin (Ig)G antibodies); a negative

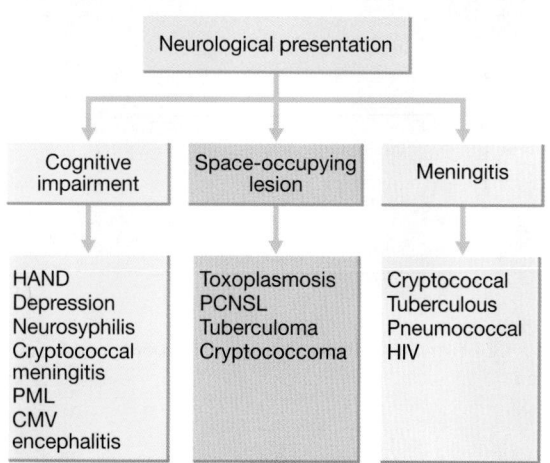

Fig. 14.11 Presentation and differential diagnosis of HIV-related neurological disorders. (CMV = cytomegalovirus; HAND = HIV-associated neurocognitive disorder; PCNSL = primary CNS lymphoma; PML = progressive multifocal leucoencephalopathy)

Neurological presentation

Cognitive impairment	Space-occupying lesion	Meningitis
HAND Depression Neurosyphilis Cryptococcal meningitis PML CMV encephalitis	Toxoplasmosis PCNSL Tuberculoma Cryptococcoma	Cryptococcal Tuberculous Pneumococcal HIV

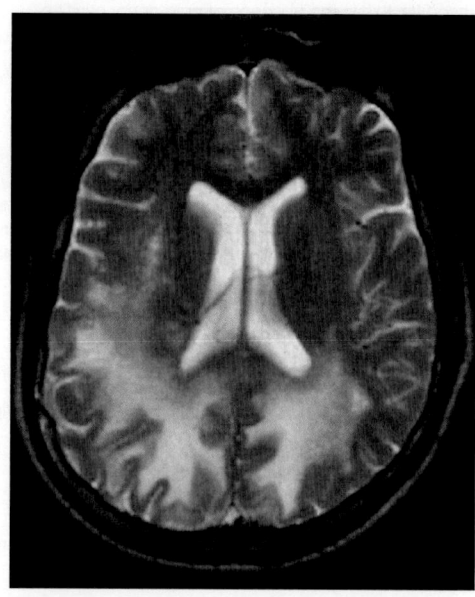

Fig. 14.12 Progressive multifocal leucoencephalopathy. Non-enhancing white-matter lesions without surrounding oedema are seen.

serological test effectively rules out toxoplasmosis but a positive test is not specific. The standard therapy for toxoplasmosis is sulfadiazine with pyrimethamine, together with folinic acid, to reduce the risk of bone marrow suppression (see Box 14.10). However, co-trimoxazole has been shown to be as effective and less toxic, and is also much more widely available. Response to a trial of therapy is usually diagnostic, with clinical improvement in 1–2 weeks and shrinkage of lesions on imaging in 2–4 weeks. Definitive diagnosis is by brain biopsy, but this is seldom necessary.

Primary CNS lymphoma

Primary CNS lymphomas (PCNSLs) are high-grade B-cell lymphomas associated with EBV infection. Characteristically, imaging demonstrates a single homogeneously enhancing, periventricular lesion with surrounding oedema (Fig. 14.14). If it is considered safe to perform a lumbar

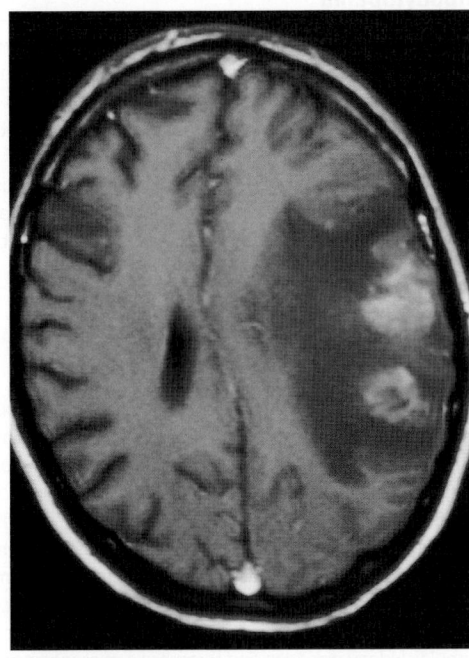

Fig. 14.13 Cerebral toxoplasmosis. Multiple ring-enhancing lesions with surrounding oedema are characteristic.

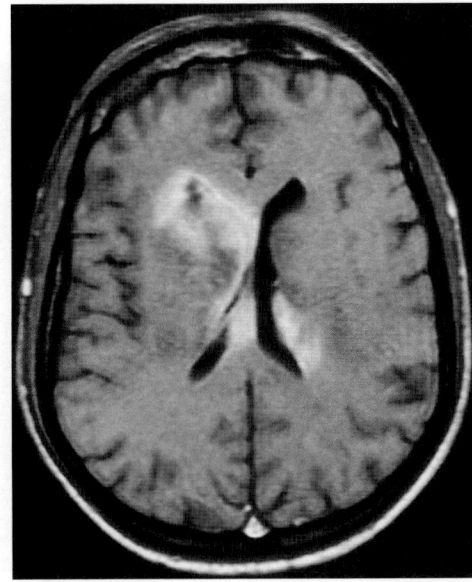

Fig. 14.14 Primary CNS lymphoma. A single enhancing periventricular lesion with moderate oedema is typical.

puncture, PCR for EBV DNA in the CSF has a high sensitivity and specificity for PCNSL. Brain biopsy is definitive but carries a risk of morbidity and may be non-diagnostic in up to one-third. The prognosis is poor.

Tuberculoma

Lesions resemble toxoplasmosis on imaging, except that oedema tends to be less marked and single lesions occur more commonly. There may be evidence of tuberculosis elsewhere. The CSF may show features consistent with tuberculous meningitis. Response to antituberculosis therapy is slow and paradoxical expansion of lesions despite therapy is not uncommon.

Stroke

There is a higher incidence of stroke in patients with HIV disease. Atherosclerosis is accelerated by the presence of inflammation due to the immune response to HIV, which is not completely suppressed by ART, and by dyslipidaemia caused by some antiretroviral drugs. HIV vasculopathy, which is thought to be a vasculitis, can also cause a stroke. It is important to exclude tuberculous meningitis and meningovascular syphilis in all PLWH who present with a stroke.

Meningitis

Cryptococcal meningitis

Cryptococcus neoformans is the most common cause of meningitis in AIDS patients. Patients usually present subacutely with headache, vomiting and decreased level of consciousness. Neck stiffness is present in less than half. CSF pleocytosis is often mild or even absent, and protein and glucose concentrations are variable. It is important to request CSF cryptococcal antigen tests in all PLWH undergoing lumbar puncture, as this test has a high sensitivity and specificity. Treatment is with amphotericin B (liposomal amphotericin B if this is available) plus flucytosine for 1 week, followed by fluconazole (see Box 14.10). Raised intracranial pressure is common and should be treated with repeated therapeutic lumbar punctures, as this is a communicating hydrocephalus, removing sufficient CSF to reduce pressure to less than $20\,\mathrm{cmH_2O}$.

Tuberculous meningitis

The presentation and CSF findings of tuberculous meningitis are similar to those in HIV-negative patients except that concomitant tuberculosis at other sites is more common in HIV infection.

Peripheral nerve disease

HIV infection causes axonal degeneration, resulting in a sensorimotor peripheral neuropathy in about one-third of AIDS patients. The incidence increases with lower CD4 counts, older age and increased height. Sensory symptoms predominate. Treatment involves foot care, analgesia and analgesic adjuvants. ART has minimal effect on halting or reversing the process.

Acute inflammatory demyelinating polyneuropathy is an uncommon manifestation, usually occurring in primary infection. It resembles Guillain–Barré syndrome, except that CSF pleocytosis is more prominent. Mononeuritis may also occur, commonly involving the facial nerve.

Myelopathy and radiculopathy

The most common cause of myelopathy in HIV infection is cord compression from tuberculous spondylitis. Vacuolar myelopathy is seen in advanced disease and is due to HIV. It typically presents with a slowly progressive paraparesis with no sensory level. MRI of the spine is important to exclude other causes. Most patients have concomitant HIV-associated dementia.

CMV polyradiculitis presents with painful legs, progressive flaccid paraparesis, saddle anaesthesia, absent reflexes and sphincter dysfunction. CSF shows a neutrophil pleocytosis (which is unusual for a viral infection), and the detection of CMV DNA by PCR confirms the diagnosis. Functional recovery is poor despite treatment with ganciclovir or valganciclovir.

14

Psychiatric disease

Significant psychiatric morbidity is common and is a major risk factor for poor adherence. Reactive depression is the most common disorder. Diagnosis is often difficult, as many patients have concomitant HAND. Substance misuse is common in many groups of people at risk of HIV. Some of the HIV antiretroviral drugs cause psychiatric adverse effects.

Retinopathy

CMV retinitis presents with painless, progressive visual loss in patients with severe immune suppression. On fundoscopy, the vitreous is clear. Haemorrhages and exudates are seen in the retina (p. 350), often with sheathing of vessels ('frosted branch angiitis'). The disease usually starts unilaterally but progressive bilateral involvement occurs in most untreated patients. Diagnosis is usually clinical, but if there is doubt, demonstrating CMV DNA by PCR of vitreous fluid is diagnostic. Treatment with ganciclovir or valganciclovir stops progression of the disease but lost vision does not recover. Some patients may develop immune recovery uveitis in response to ART, with intraocular inflammation, macular oedema and cataract formation that require prompt treatment with oral and intraocular glucocorticoids to prevent further visual loss.

Three other conditions may mimic CMV retinitis: ocular toxoplasmosis, which typically presents with a vitritis and retinitis without retinal haemorrhages; HIV retinopathy, a microangiopathy that causes cotton wool spots, which are not sight-threatening; and varicella zoster virus, which can cause rapidly progressive outer retinal necrosis.

Rheumatological disease

The immune dysregulation associated with HIV infection may result in autoantibody formation, usually in low titres. Mild arthralgias and a fibromyalgia-like syndrome are common in PLWH.

Arthritis

HIV can cause a seronegative arthritis, which resembles rheumatoid arthritis. A more benign oligoarthritis may also occur. Reactive arthritis is more severe in HIV infection (p. 1035).

Diffuse infiltrative lymphocytosis syndrome

Diffuse infiltrative lymphocytosis syndrome (DILS) is a benign disorder involving polyclonal CD8 lymphocytic infiltration of tissues, which has some features in common with Sjögren syndrome. It is linked to human leucocyte antigen (HLA)-DRB1. Most patients have a marked CD8 lymphocytosis. DILS usually presents in patients with mild immune suppression. The most common manifestation is bilateral parotid gland enlargement; the glands are often massive, with lymphoepithelial cysts on histology (Fig. 14.15). Sicca symptoms are common but usually mild. Lymphocytic interstitial pneumonitis is the most common manifestation outside the salivary glands. Generalised lymphadenopathy may occur, with nodes larger than those seen with persistent generalised lymphadenopathy of HIV. Hepatitis, mononeuritis, polyarthritis and polymyositis may also occur. The manifestations outside the salivary glands usually respond to systemic glucocorticoids. Parotid gland enlargement may be treated by aspiration of parotid cysts and instillation of a sclerosant for cosmetic reasons; surgery is best avoided. DILS may regress on ART but response is variable.

Haematological abnormalities

Disorders of all three major cell lines may occur in HIV. In advanced disease, haematopoiesis is impaired due to the direct effect of HIV and by cytokines. Pancytopenia may occur as a consequence of HIV but it is important to exclude a disorder infiltrating the bone marrow, such as mycobacterial or fungal infections, or lymphoma.

Anaemia

Normochromic, normocytic anaemia is very common in advanced HIV disease. Opportunistic diseases may cause anaemia of chronic disease (e.g. tuberculosis) or marrow infiltration (e.g. MAC, tuberculosis, lymphoma, fungi). Anaemia is a common adverse effect of zidovudine, which also causes a macrocytosis. Red cell aplasia is rare and may be caused either by parvovirus B19 infection or by the NRTIs lamivudine and emtricitabine.

Neutropenia

Isolated neutropenia is occasionally due to HIV but is nearly always caused by drug toxicity (e.g. zidovudine, co-trimoxazole, ganciclovir).

Thrombocytopenia

Mild thrombocytopenia is common in PLWH. Transient thrombocytopenia is frequently found in primary infection. The most common disorder causing severe thrombocytopenia is immune-mediated platelet destruction resembling idiopathic thrombocytopenic purpura (p. 988). This responds to glucocorticoids or intravenous immunoglobulin, together with ART. Splenectomy should be avoided if possible because it further increases the risk of infection with encapsulated bacteria. Severe thrombocytopenia with a microangiopathic anaemia also occurs in a thrombotic thrombocytopenic purpura-like illness, which has a better prognosis and fewer relapses than the classical disease.

Renal disease

Acute kidney injury is common, usually due to acute infection or nephrotoxicity of drugs (e.g. tenofovir (see Box 18.25), amphotericin B). HIV-associated nephropathy (HIVAN) is the most important cause of chronic kidney disease (CKD) and is seen more frequently in patients of African descent and those with low CD4 counts. Progression to end-stage disease is more rapid than with most other causes of CKD, and renal size is usually preserved. HIVAN presents with nephrotic syndrome, CKD or a combination of both. ART has some effect in slowing progression of HIVAN. Other important HIV-associated renal diseases include HIV immune complex kidney diseases and thrombotic microangiopathy. With the overall improvement in life expectancy from ART, conditions such as diabetes mellitus, hypertension and vascular disease add to the burden of CKD. Outcomes of renal transplantation are good in patients on ART.

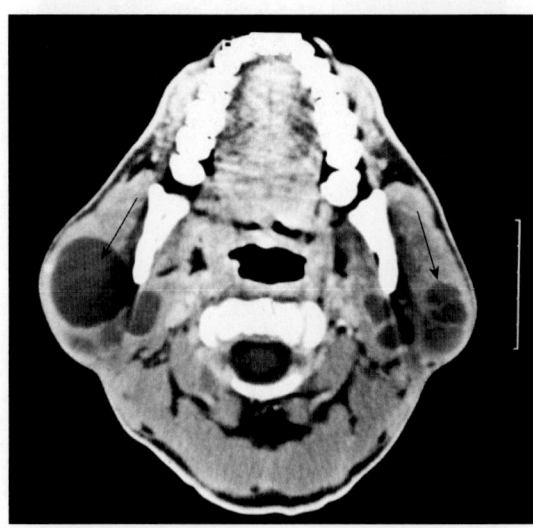

Fig. 14.15 CT scan of parotid glands. Multiple cysts (arrows) seen in a patient with the diffuse infiltrative lymphocytosis syndrome.

Cardiac disease

HIV-associated cardiomyopathy resembles idiopathic dilated cardiomyopathy (p. 474) but progresses more rapidly. ART may improve cardiac failure but does not reverse established cardiomyopathy. Pericardial disease due to opportunistic diseases is not uncommon; globally, the most common cause is tuberculous pericardial effusion. Tuberculous constrictive pericarditis is less common than in HIV-uninfected people. KS and lymphoma may cause pericardial effusions. Septic pericarditis, usually due to *S. pneumoniae*, is uncommon.

HIV is associated with an increased risk of myocardial infarction due to accelerated atherogenesis caused by the inflammatory state, which is not completely suppressed by ART, and by dyslipidaemia caused by some antiretroviral drugs.

HIV-related cancers

The AIDS-defining cancers are KS (see above), cervical cancer and non-Hodgkin lymphoma (NHL). NHL may occur at any CD4 count but is more commonly seen with counts below 200 cells/mm³. Almost all NHLs are B-cell tumours and most are stage 3 or 4. Long-term remission rates similar to those in patients without HIV can be achieved with NHL in AIDS patients using ART and chemotherapy (including the anti-B-cell monoclonal antibody rituximab if it is a B-cell tumour).

The incidence of several other cancers induced by viruses is also increased in PLWH (Box 14.13). Regular cytological examination of the cervix should be performed to detect pre-malignant lesions, which are easier to treat – studies are under way to determine optimal strategies to reduce the risk of anal cancer in people who practise receptive anal sex. In general, the incidence of cancers that are not induced by viruses is similar to that in the general population.

Prevention of opportunistic infections

The best way to prevent opportunistic infections is to improve the CD4 count with ART. However, infections continue to occur in the ART era as CD4 counts take time to improve if ART is initiated in patients with profound immune suppression, immune reconstitution on ART may be suboptimal, and CD4 counts may decline if antiretroviral resistance develops.

Preventing exposure

The best method for avoiding infection is to prevent exposure to the infectious agent. However, this stratgey is possible only for a few opportunistic infections. Many opportunistic infections occur after reactivation of latent/dormant infection after prior exposure; examples include herpes simplex virus, zoster (shingles), CMV, toxoplasmosis, cryptococcosis and the endemic mycoses.

Safe water and food

Cryptosporidiosis, microsporidiosis and cystoisosporiasis may be waterborne. If there is no access to safe water, then water should be boiled before drinking. Food-borne illnesses are also important in HIV infection, notably *Salmonella* species. *Toxoplasma* exposure is related to eating raw or undercooked meat. PLWH should be informed about food hygiene and the importance of adequately cooking meat.

Tuberculosis

Preventing exposure to tuberculosis is important when there is an infectious case in the household, in clinics and in hospitals. Adequate ventilation, masks and safe coughing procedures reduce the risk of exposure.

Malaria vector control

All PLWH living in malarious areas should practise vector control, as malaria occurs more frequently and is more severe in PLWH. The most cost-effective way to achieve this is by using insecticide-impregnated bed nets. Other modalities of vector control that are of benefit to the community, such as reducing standing water and spraying with residual insecticides and larvicides, should also be implemented.

Safer sex

PLWH should practise safer sex to reduce the transmission of HIV. Even if their partners are PLWH, condoms should be used, as HIV mutants that have developed antiretroviral drug resistance can be transmitted. Safer sex will also lower the risk of acquiring herpes simplex virus and human herpesvirus 8.

Pets

Toxoplasma gondii can be acquired from kittens or cat litter, and people living with HIV infection should avoid handling either. Cryptosporidiosis can be transmitted from animals, and patients should be advised to wash their hands after handling animals.

Chemoprophylaxis

Chemoprophylaxis is the use of antimicrobial agents to prevent infections. Primary prophylaxis is used to prevent opportunistic infections that have not yet occurred. Secondary prophylaxis is used to prevent recurrence of opportunistic infections because many may recur after an initial response to therapy (see Box 14.10). Secondary prophylaxis can be discontinued when ART results in immune reconstitution, with CD4 counts increasing to over 200 cells/mm³, but for CMV and MAC, prophylaxis can be stopped if CD4 counts increase to more than 100 cells/mm³.

Co-trimoxazole primary prophylaxis

Co-trimoxazole (sulfamethoxazole–trimethoprim) reduces the incidence of several opportunistic infections (Box 14.14), resulting in lower hospitalisation and mortality rates. The indications for initiating co-trimoxazole are either clinical evidence of immune suppression (WHO clinical stages 3 or 4) or laboratory evidence of immune suppression (CD4 count <200 cells/mm³). In low-income countries where malaria and/or severe bacterial infections are highly prevalent, the WHO recommends initiating co-trimoxazole regardless of CD4 counts or clinical stage. The recommended dose

14.13 Approximate incidence ratio of virus-related cancers compared to the general population	
Viral cancers	**Incidence ratio**
Human herpesvirus 8-related	
Kaposi's sarcoma	3600
Epstein–Barr virus-related	
Non-Hodgkin lymphoma	80
Hodgkin lymphoma	10
Human papillomavirus-related	
Cervical cancer	6
Vulval cancer	6
Anal cancer	30
Penile cancer	4
Hepatitis B/C virus-related	
Hepatocellular carcinoma	5

14

of co-trimoxazole is 960 mg daily. Co-trimoxazole prophylaxis can be discontinued when CD4 counts increase to more than 200 cells/mm³ on ART, except in low-income countries where it should be continued life-long.

Co-trimoxazole prophylaxis is well tolerated. The most common side-effect is hypersensitivity, causing a maculo-papular rash. If therapy is discontinued, desensitisation or rechallenge under antihistamine cover should be attempted, unless the rash was accompanied by systemic symptoms or mucosal involvement. Prophylactic doses of co-trimoxazole can also cause neutropenia, but this is very uncommon and routine monitoring of blood counts is not necessary. If co-trimoxazole cannot be tolerated, then dapsone 100 mg daily should be substituted. Dapsone is equally effective at reducing the incidence of *P. jirovecii* pneumonia (PCP), but has little or no effect on reducing the other opportunistic infections prevented by co-trimoxazole.

Tuberculosis preventive therapy

Trials in patients not on ART showed that preventive therapy, either with isoniazid or combinations of rifamycins with isoniazid, reduces the risk of tuberculosis only in PLWH with a positive tuberculin skin test. However, recent evidence indicates that tuberculin skin tests do not predict benefit in patients starting ART or established on ART in high tuberculosis prevalence settings.

There is no CD4 count or clinical threshold for starting tuberculosis preventive therapy. It is important to rule out active tuberculosis before starting preventive therapy, and symptom screening has been shown to be adequate to achieve this (Box 14.15). The usual duration of isoniazid preventive therapy is 6 months. Rifampicin or rifapentine combined with isoniazid for 12 weeks has been shown to be at least as effective as 6–12 months of isoniazid.

Mycobacterium avium complex prophylaxis

In high-income countries, a macrolide (azithromycin or clarithromycin) is recommended to prevent MAC in patients with a CD4 count below 50 cells/mm³, which can be discontinued once the CD4 count has risen to over 100 cells/mm³ on ART. MAC is uncommon in low- and middle-income countries and primary prophylaxis is thus not warranted.

Preventing cryptococcosis

Serum cryptococcal antigen test should be done in patients with a CD4 count below 100 cells/mm³. If this is positive, pre-emptive therapy with fluconazole should be commenced.

Immunisation

There are significant problems associated with vaccination in HIV infection. First, vaccination with live organisms is contraindicated in patients with severe immune suppression, as this may result in disease from the attenuated organisms. Secondly, immune responses to vaccination are impaired in PLWH. If the CD4 count is below 200 cells/mm³, then immune responses to immunisation are poor. Therefore, it is preferable to wait until the CD4 count has increased to more than 200 cells/mm³ on ART before immunisation is given; this is essential if live virus vaccines are used. All patients should be given a conjugate pneumococcal vaccine and annual influenza vaccination. Hepatitis B vaccination should be given to those who are not immune. In the UK, the following additional vaccines are also recommended:

- *hepatitis A*: in those at risk
- *human papillomavirus*: in people < 40 years old
- *measles, mumps and rubella (MMR)*: in those with negative measles serology
- *meningococcus*: in people < 25 years old, those with asplenia or complement deficiency, during outbreaks
- *diphtheria/tetanus/acellular pertussis (dTaP)/inactivated poliovirus vaccine (IPV)*: meeting general indications
- *chickenpox*: if seronegative; those who are seropositive should receive the shingles vaccine.

Bacille Calmette–Guérin (BCG) is contraindicated in PLWH.

Antiretroviral therapy

ART has transformed HIV from a progressive illness with a fatal outcome into a chronic manageable disease with a near-normal life expectancy.
The goals of ART are to:

- reduce the viral load to an undetectable level for as long as possible
- improve the CD4 count to over 200 cells/mm³ so that severe HIV-related disease is unlikely
- improve the quantity and quality of life without unacceptable drug toxicity
- reduce HIV transmission.

Many of the antiretroviral drugs that were initially used have largely been abandoned because of toxicity or poor efficacy. The pill burden of currently recommended ART is low; the currently recommended first-line regimens are available as a single pill. The drugs that are currently recommended are shown in Box 14.16, and their targets in the HIV life cycle in Fig. 14.1.

Selecting antiretroviral regimens

The standard combination antiretroviral regimens are two NRTIs together with an NNRTI, protease inhibitor (PI) or integrase inhibitor. However, effective combinations have been developed with just two drugs. Currently used PIs are always administered with the pharmacoenhancers ('boosters') ritonavir or cobicistat, which dramatically increase the concentrations of other PIs by inhibiting their metabolism by the cytochrome P450 isoenzyme CYP3A.

 14.14 Opportunistic infections reduced by co-trimoxazole

- *Pneumocystis jirovecii* pneumonia
- Cerebral toxoplasmosis
- Bacterial pneumonia
- Bacteraemia
- Cystoisosporiasis
- Malaria

14.15 Symptom screen for tuberculosis before isoniazid preventive therapy

All of the following must be absent:
- Active cough
- Weight loss
- Night sweats
- Fever

14.16 Currently preferred antiretroviral drugs

Classes	Drugs
Nucleoside reverse transcriptase inhibitors (NRTIs)	Abacavir, emtricitabine, lamivudine, tenofovir
Non-nucleoside reverse transcriptase inhibitors (NNRTIs)	Efavirenz*, rilpivirine (only if viral load < 100 000)
Protease inhibitors (PIs)	Atazanavir*, darunavir, lopinavir*
Integrase inhibitors	Dolutegravir, bictegravir

*These drugs are no longer recommended as first-line options due to their toxicity.

By far the commonest preferred agents for first-line ART globally are a second-generation integrase inhibitor (bictegravir or dolutegravir) combined with the NRTIs tenofovir plus emtricitabine or lamivudine (which have the same mechanism of action and so are never combined).

In high-income countries ART regimen switches for virological failure are guided by the results of resistance testing (see below). In low- and middle-income countries, where resources for resistance testing are limited or absent, a standardised second-line regimen is recommended

Starting ART

Guidelines now recommend starting ART in all people with confirmed HIV infection, irrespective of CD4 count or clinical status. Early initiation of ART, compared with the previous strategy of deferring ART until CD4 thresholds or clinical disease occurs, has been shown to reduce morbidity and mortality, and has the additional benefit of reducing the risk of transmission. In asymptomatic PLWH initiating ART on the same day that the diagnosis is confirmed has been shown to improve retention in care. Disclosure of HIV status, joining support groups and using patient-nominated treatment supporters should be encouraged, as these have been shown to improve adherence. Recognition and management of depression and substance abuse is important.

In patients with major opportunistic infections, ART should generally be started within 2 weeks, with two important exceptions: in cryptococcal meningitis, ART should be deferred for 5 weeks, as earlier initiation increases the risk of death; and in tuberculosis, ART should be deferred until 8 weeks (except if the CD4 count is <50 cells/mm^3), as earlier initiation increases the risk of the immune reconstitution inflammatory syndrome (see below).

Monitoring efficacy

The most important measure of ART efficacy is the viral load. A baseline viral load should be measured prior to initiating treatment. Viral load measurement should be repeated 4 weeks after starting ART, when there should be at least a 10-fold decrease. The viral load should be suppressed after 6 months. Once the viral load is suppressed, measurement should be repeated 6 to 12 monthly. Failure of ART is defined by the viral load becoming detectable after suppression. In most guidelines, a viral load threshold is used to define virological failure, e.g. more than 200 (UK) or more than 1000 (WHO) copies/mL. Adherence support should be enhanced if virological failure is detected.

CD4 counts can be monitored together with the viral load, but there is little point in repeating the CD4 count in patients who maintain virological suppression and whose CD4 count is >350 cells/mm^3. The CD4 count increases rapidly in the first month, followed by a more gradual increase. In the first year, the CD4 count typically increases by 100–150 cells/mm^3, and about 80 cells/mm^3 per annum thereafter until the normal range is reached, provided the viral load is suppressed. However, CD4 responses are highly variable: in about 15%–30% of patients the CD4 count does not increase despite virological suppression, and in a similar proportion of patients the CD4 response is good despite the presence of virological failure. If ART is stopped, the CD4 count rapidly falls to the baseline value before ART was commenced.

Antiretroviral resistance

Reverse transcription is error-prone, generating many mutations. If the viral load is suppressed on ART, viral replication is suppressed and resistance mutations will not be selected. If there is ongoing replication on ART, due to either resistant mutations or suboptimal adherence, mutations conferring resistance to antiretroviral drugs will be selected. Antiretroviral drugs differ in their ability to select for HIV resistance mutations. Some drugs (e.g. emtricitabine, lamivudine, efavirenz, raltegravir) have a low genetic barrier to resistance, rapidly selecting for a single mutation conferring high-level resistance. PIs and the second-generation integrase inhibitors (bictegravir and dolutegravir) select for resistance mutations

slowly, and multiple mutations may need to accumulate before the drug's efficacy is lost. Patients who develop antiretroviral resistance will eventually develop clinical failure if the regimen is not changed, and may transmit resistant virus to others.

Antiretroviral resistance is assessed by sequencing the relevant viral genes to detect mutations that are known to confer resistance. The patient must be taking ART when the test is performed, as otherwise the wild-type virus will predominate and resistant mutations will not be detected. However, the resistant proviral DNA archived in latent CD4 cells will re-emerge rapidly on re-exposure to the antiretroviral. In high-income countries resistance testing is recommended at baseline (to detect primary resistance) and at every confirmed virological failure, in order to select the most appropriate antiretrovirals in a new regimen.

ART complications

Immune reconstitution inflammatory syndrome

Immune reconstitution inflammatory syndrome (IRIS) is a common early complication of ART, especially in patients who start ART with CD4 counts below 50 cells/mm^3. IRIS presents either with paradoxical deterioration of an existing opportunistic disease (including infections that are responding to appropriate therapy) or with the unmasking of a new infection. The clinical presentation of IRIS events is often characterised by an exaggerated immune response, with pronounced inflammatory features. For example, patients with CMV retinitis developing IRIS on ART develop a uveitis; inflammatory haloes occur around KS lesions. Paradoxical tuberculosis IRIS events are common but it is important to exclude multidrug resistance, which could be responsible for the deterioration. IRIS is associated with a mortality of around 5% but this is higher when it complicates CNS infections.

The management of IRIS is to continue ART and to ensure that the opportunistic disease is adequately treated. Symptomatic treatments are helpful. Glucocorticoids are often used for more severe IRIS manifestations but they should not be given to patients with KS, as this can result in rapid progression of KS lesions.

Antiretroviral adverse drug reactions

Currently recommended antiretrovirals are generally well tolerated. Integrase inhibitors may cause insomnia. NNRTIs commonly cause hypersensitivity rashes; efavirenz commonly causes mild neuropsychiatric effects, but tolerance develops in a few weeks in most patients. The NRTI tenofovir occasionally causes nephrotoxicity and loss of bone mineral density, but the newer pro-drug tenofovir alafenamide is less toxic. PIs may cause gastrointestinal symptoms (nausea, vomiting and diarrhoea), and some are associated with dyslipidaemia.

ART in special situations

Pregnancy

All pregnant women should have HIV testing at an early stage in pregnancy. The CD4 count falls by about 25% during pregnancy due to haemodilution. The course of HIV disease progression is not altered by pregnancy. In the pre-ART era, the rate of mother-to-child transmission was 15%–40%, with rates being influenced by several factors (see Box 14.3).

ART has dramatically reduced the risk of mother-to-child transmission of HIV to less than 1%. All pregnant women who are ART-naïve should start ART as soon as possible. Pregnant women on ART may need to have their regimens modified as only a limited number of antiretrovirals are recommended in pregnancy. Close viral load monitoring is essential during pregnancy.

Caesarean section is associated with a lower risk of mother-to-child transmission than vaginal delivery, but the mode of delivery does not affect transmission risk if the viral load is suppressed on ART.

14

14.17 HIV infection in old age

- **Epidemiology**: the HIV-positive population is ageing due to the life-prolonging effects of ART.
- **Immunity**: age-related decline increases the risk of infections. CD4 counts decline more rapidly as age extends beyond 40 years, resulting in faster disease progression. CD4 responses to ART decrease with increasing age.
- **Dementia**: HIV causes cerebral atrophy and neurocognitive disorders; dementia is therefore more common and more severe than in the HIV-uninfected older adults.
- **Vascular disease**: HIV is associated with an increased risk, exacerbated by some antiretrovirals that cause dyslipidaemia or insulin resistance.
- **Fragility fractures**: bone mineral density is lower in PLHW, which can be exacerbated by the NRTI tenofovir.
- **Polypharmacy**: treatment of co-morbidities is complex due to drug–drug interactions with antiretrovirals.

HIV is also transmitted by breastfeeding. In high-income countries, exclusive formula feeding is generally recommended. In resource-poor settings, however, formula feeding is associated with a risk of infant morbidity and mortality, which may negate the benefit of not transmitting HIV to the infant. There is minimal risk of transmitting HIV by breastfeeding in women with a suppressed viral load on ART. Furthermore, providing antiretrovirals to infants (usually nevirapine monotherapy) while they are breastfeeding has been shown to reduce the risk of transmission. Breastfeeding is therefore now encouraged in resource-poor settings. Infants should be exclusively breastfed for the first 6 months, as mixed feeding (with formula or solids) is associated with a higher risk of transmission.

Old age

The specific manifestations of HIV infection in older people are shown in Box 14.17.

Prevention of HIV

An effective HIV vaccine remains elusive due to the extensive genetic diversity of HIV and the lack of a safe attenuated virus. Measures for the prevention of HIV transmission are shown in Box 14.18.

Pre-exposure prophylaxis

Pre-exposure prophylaxis (PrEP) with daily tenofovir plus emtricitabine has been shown to reduce the risk of HIV acquisition in people who are at ongoing high risk (e.g. from sex or injecting drug use) and is well tolerated. Regular HIV testing should be done in people on PrEP.

i **14.18 Prevention measures for HIV transmission**

Sexual

- Sex education programmes in schools
- Easily accessible voluntary counselling and testing centres
- Promotion of safer sex practices (delaying sexual debut, condom use, fewer sexual partners)
- Effective ART for HIV-infected individuals
- Pre-exposure prophylaxis (PrEP) for high-risk groups
- Male circumcision
- Post-exposure prophylaxis

Parenteral

- Blood product transmission: donor questionnaire, routine screening of donated blood
- Injection drug use: education, needle/syringe exchange, avoidance of 'shooting galleries', methadone maintenance programmes

Perinatal

- Routine 'opt-out' antenatal HIV antibody testing
- Measures to reduce vertical transmission (see text)

Occupational

- Education/training: universal precautions, needlestick injury avoidance
- Post-exposure prophylaxis

Post-exposure prophylaxis

Post-exposure prophylaxis (PEP) is recommended after a potential exposure to HIV when the risk is deemed to be significant after a careful risk assessment, in both occupational and non-occupational settings. The first dose should be given as soon as possible. The effectiveness of PEP diminishes with time and it is ineffective (and therefore should not be started) if given more than 72 hours after exposure. Tenofovir together with emtricitabine is the most widely used dual NRTI combination, together with either a PI or an integrase inhibitor depending on ART exposure in the source patient. PEP should not be given if the exposed person is HIV-infected. HIV antibody testing should be performed 3 months after exposure.

Further information

Websites with updated clinical guidelines

aidsinfo.nih.gov *AIDSinfo, a service of the US Department of Health and Human Services (HHS).*
bhiva.org *British HIV Association.*
who.int/health-topics/hiv-aids *World Health Organization.*

DJ Clutterbuck

15

Sexually transmitted infections

Clinical examination in sexually transmitted infection

5 Vagina and cervix
Abnormal discharge
Warts
Ulcers
Inflammation
In women with lower abdominal pain, bimanual examination for adnexal tenderness (pelvic inflammatory disease)

▲ Speculum

4 Labia majora and minora
Ulcers
Vulvitis
Note normal vestibular papillae and sebaceous glands

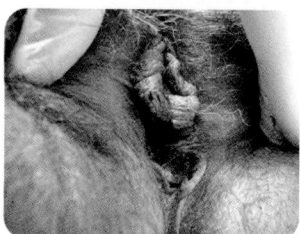

▲ Vulval carcinoma

3 Skin of pubic area
Warts
Tinea cruris

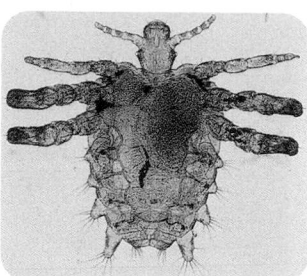

▲ *Pthirus pubis* (crab louse)

2 Inguinal glands
Significant enlargement

1 Abdomen
Abnormal masses or tenderness
Tip: Gentle abdominal palpation is a non-threatening prelude to genital examination in an anxious patient

Consent
Explain what genital examination will involve and confirm informed consent. Presence of a chaperone is routine

Observation
• Mouth
• Eyes
• Joints
• Skin:
  Rash of secondary syphilis
  Scabies
  Manifestations of HIV (Ch. 14)

6 Skin of penis
(Retract foreskin if present)
Genital warts
Ulcers
Be aware of normal anatomical features such as coronal papillae, or prominent sebaceous or parafrenal glands

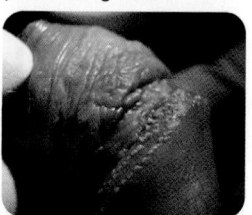

▲ Coronal papillae

7 Urethral meatus

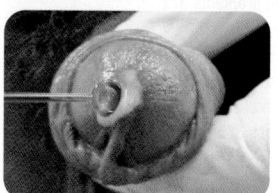

▲ Sampling discharge at urethral meatus

8 Scrotal contents
Abnormal masses or tenderness (epididymo-orchitis)

9 Perineum and perianal skin
Warts
Ulcers
Inflammation

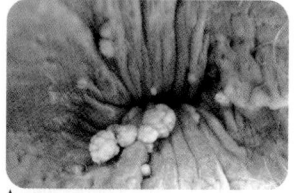

▲ Perianal warts

10 Rectum

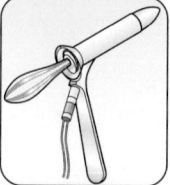

▲ Proctoscope

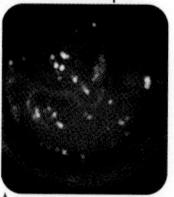

▲ Proctitis

Insets (Coronal papillae, Discharge at urethral meatus, Perianal warts, Vulval carcinoma) From Clutterbuck DJ. Specialist training in sexually transmitted infections and HIV. St Louis: Mosby, Elsevier Inc.; 2004. (Proctitis) From McMillan A, Young H, Ogilvie MM, Scott GR. Clinical practice in sexually transmissible infections. Philadelphia: Saunders, Elsevier Inc.; 2002.

Identifying STIs in the population

- Testing for STIs in those who present with clinical symptoms identifies only a small minority of prevalent infections and other methods of case-finding are widely employed.
- STI testing for asymptomatic individuals is provided through specialist clinics and primary care providers but also directly to populations at risk through screening programmes and opportunistic testing.
- Point-of-care testing (PoCT) in the community, home-based self-testing (where the test is performed at home) and self-sampling (where it is posted to a laboratory) are well proven technologies used internationally for HIV and increasingly for syphilis testing.
- Self-sampling for chlamydia and gonorrhoea testing is widely used in the UK both for home-based testing and in clinics for convenience and efficiency. Technology allows testing for an increasing range of organisms, including *Mycoplasma genitalium*, *Trichomonas vaginalis* and others to be undertaken on the same sample.
- STI testing may be offered remotely from clinical assessment – through online ordering of self-sampling or self-testing kits, or tests provided in non-clinical outreach settings such as youth groups or sex-on-premises venues such as gay saunas.

 Investigations for STIs

- Samples for combined nucleic acid amplification test (NAAT) for gonorrhoea and chlamydia are taken from anatomical sites at risk – these may be identified by face-to-face or online assessment of gender, partner gender and sexual practices.
- First-void urine (FVU) is the specimen of choice to test for infection of the male urethra and a self-taken swab is preferred for vaginal samples. Clinician-obtained urethral, cervical or vaginal swabs are alternatives. Pharyngeal and rectal swabs may be indicated by sexual history and are often offered universally to MSM.
- For gonorrhoea, either as an alternative or adjunct to NAAT testing, swabs from the pharynx, urethra, cervix or rectum plated directly on a selective medium such as modified New York City (MNYC), or sent in an appropriate transport medium, can be cultured for assessment of antimicrobial sensitivities. NAAT-based sensitivity testing is increasingly available.
- Blood for serological tests including syphilis (STS), e.g. enzyme immunoassay (EIA) for antitreponemal immunoglobulin G (IgG) ± IgM antibody. Repeat testing may be necessary in the event of negative test results in the first few weeks following exposure.
- Human immunodeficiency virus (HIV) test. HIV testing should always be offered as part of STI testing. Informed consent is required, but extensive pre-test discussion is not.
- Serological tests for hepatitis B (and sometimes hepatitis A and/or C) are offered to those at epidemiological risk.
- Additional tests routinely used in the investigation of symptomatic patients in sexual health clinics include direct microscopy of Gram-stained samples from the male urethra for the diagnosis of urethritis, or of wet-mount and Gram-stained samples from the vagina for the diagnosis of *Trichomonas vaginalis*, bacterial vaginosis, aerobic vaginitis or candidiasis.

Examples of risk factors for STIs

Demographic factors

- Younger age (<25)*
- Men who have sex with men (MSM)
- Prior STI diagnosis

Behavioural factors

- Frequent partner change or concurrent partners
- Non-use of condoms, condom errors
- Use of drugs during sex ('chemsex')
- Use of geospatial mobile phone dating applications ('dating apps')

*But note that the possibility of STI should never be excluded on the grounds of older age alone.

Sexual health and gender identity

- Medical care in all settings must be inclusive of all patients regardless of sexual orientation or gender identity. This has particular relevance in sexual health.
- Gender identity is a characteristic protected by law in the UK and many other jurisdictions.
- Definitions of terms commonly used:
  - Gender identity: An individual's innate sense of their own gender, which may or may not be congruent with the sex they were assigned at birth.
  - Cisgender/Cis: A cis person's gender identity is generally congruent with the sex they were assigned at birth.
  - Trans: an umbrella term to describe people whose gender identity differs from the sex they were assigned at birth. There is a spectrum of trans identities, including but not limited to: trans woman, trans man, transgender, genderqueer, non-binary, agender.
  - Non-binary (genderqueer): a term for individuals whose gender identity does not align with either of the binary categories of 'man', 'woman', or 'male', 'female'.
- Long-established social norms, health care structures, clinical practice and teaching may create barriers to inclusive care for trans and non-binary individuals (for example by failing to provide cervical screening to trans men who have a cervix, or providing only male and female options in waiting rooms, services or on registration forms).
- Clinicians and services can ensure inclusivity by asking about gender identity, preferred pronouns and gender of partners and providing tests and investigations on the basis of anatomical sites at risk rather than by binary gender.

Tips on sexual history-taking

1. A simple framing statement before taking the sexual history helps avoid any sense of apology or embarrassment. 'So, thinking about your sex life …'; 'Some questions about your sex life …'.
2. Use open language to avoid the impression of being judgemental; inclusive words such as 'partner' rather than 'boyfriend'.
3. Avoid euphemisms ('down below'). Straightforward anatomical terms are advisable (in the UK 'vagina' is generally understood but 'vulva' often is not). 'So, you mean on the lips of your vagina?'
4. Focusing on events helps to avoid labels and generalisations. 'When did you last have sex, any sort of sex …?', 'When did you last have sex with anyone else/any other partner?'
5. Use permission-giving in questioning (explicit permission for a range of answers). 'Have your partners been men, women or both?'
6. Invite the 'non-acceptable' or non-sanctioned answer. 'So was that without a condom …?'
7. Understand and mitigate the ways in which your own values might affect your questioning. 'When was your last previous partner?' (assumes serial monogamy – so avoid).

15

Aetiology

Sexually transmitted infections (STIs) are infections usually but not exclusively transmitted via the moist mucous membranes of the penis, vulva, vagina, cervix, anus, rectum, mouth and pharynx during sexual activity. STIs include syphilis, gonorrhoea, genital herpes, genital warts, chlamydia, *Mycoplasma genitalium*, trichomoniasis and lymphogranuloma venereum (LGV). Chancroid and granuloma inguinale are STIs seen in tropical countries but are rare in the UK. Sexually transmissible blood-borne viruses including human immunodeficiency virus (HIV) and hepatitis B and C (see Ch. 14) are those in which sexual contact is an important, but not the only mode of transmission. Enteric hepatitis virus A and sexually transmitted enteric infections (STEI) including *Salmonella* and *Shigella* may be spread by oro-anal sexual contact, although this is responsible for only a minority of cases. Other viruses, including Zika virus and SARS-CoV-2 (the coronavirus causing COVID-19) (see Ch. 13) are found in semen and may be sexually transmitted, although this is not a commonly recognised route of acquisition. Untreated STIs can lead to chronic pain or infertility and can lead to genital cancers such as cervical and anal carcinoma. Ulcerative STIs increase the risk of transmission of untreated HIV about threefold and up to a third of worldwide HIV transmissions are thought to be attributable to herpes simplex virus (HSV) type 2. STIs in pregnancy can cause serious complications, including stillbirth, neonatal death, prematurity, neonatal sepsis, low birth weight and congenital abnormalities (Box 15.1), or disseminated infection in the mother. Other conditions, including bacterial vaginosis (BV) and genital candidiasis, are not regarded as STIs, although they are common causes of vaginal discharge. Genital itch, discomfort or rash with a wide variety of underlying causes in sexually active individuals also present to sexual health clinicians.

Clinical assessment

The use of a recognisable set of signs and symptoms to identify the likely infective cause and guide antimicrobial treatment without diagnostic testing is termed syndromic management and has been a mainstay of clinical care of STIs worldwide for several decades. The risk of widespread antimicrobial resistance (AMR) is currently one of the greatest challenges in STI control, so syndromic management is increasingly supported by improvements in availability, reliability and speed of diagnostic testing technologies, in particular nucleic acid amplification testing (NAAT). However, diagnosis on the basis of observed syndromes (e.g. vaginal discharge) remains valuable even in resource-rich settings where sophisticated tests are widely available. The majority of those presenting with genital syndromes do not have STI. Conversely, around 50% of all gonorrhoea and syphilis and 80% of chlamydial infections are asymptomatic and many of those who are symptomatic do not seek care. A detailed understanding of symptoms and of social and behavioural risk factors for STI in an individual directs examination, investigations

15.2 History-taking for STI

- **Symptoms**: genital ulceration, rash, irritation, pain, swelling and urinary symptoms, especially dysuria. Urethral discharge, vaginal discharge, pelvic pain or dyspareunia. Testicular pain, abdominal and systemic symptoms.
- **Medical history**: medical problems including previous STI, allergies, medication (prescribed, over the counter, recreational drugs including 'chemsex'), vaccinations (hepatitis A and B, HPV); obstetric and gynaecological history, cervical smears and contraception.*
- **Sexual history**: last sexual contact, partner gender, partner status (one off/regular/other), partner geographical origin, consent to sex, payment/transactional sex. Other recent partners.
- **Sexual practices**: digital or penile insertive or receptive vaginal or anal, orogenital or oro-anal, protection (condoms, PrEP).

*In any sexual health consultation with a woman of reproductive age, contraception should always be discussed and where possible provided.
(HPV = human papilloma virus; PrEP = pre-exposure prophylaxis)

indicated and anatomical sites sampled. For example, rectal samples are indicated in those who have had condomless receptive anal sex. A good sexual history is key to identifying these factors (Box 15.2).

STI in children

The presence of an STI in a child may be indicative of sexual abuse, although vertical transmission may explain some presentations in the first 2 years. In an older child and in adolescents, STI may be the result of voluntary sexual activity. Specific issues regarding the management of STI and other infections in adolescence are discussed in Box 13.23.

Presenting problems

Urethral discharge

Discharge from the male urethra is a very common presenting problem whereas discharge from the female urethra alone is rare. Male urethral discharge caused by gonorrhoea (gonococcal urethritis) is distinguished from the more frequently seen non-gonococcal urethritis (NGU). Causes of NGU include *Chlamydia trachomatis*, *Mycoplasma genitalium* and less frequently *Trichomonas vaginalis*, HSV, other mycoplasmas, urea plasmas or adenoviruses. Some cases are thought not to have an infectious aetiology and are termed non-specific urethritis (NSU).

Gonococcal urethritis usually causes symptoms within 7 days of exposure. The discharge is typically profuse and purulent. Chlamydial urethritis has an incubation period of 1–4 weeks, and tends to result in milder symptoms than gonorrhoea. However, a confirmed microbiological diagnosis should always be the aim.

15.1 Possible outcomes of STI in pregnancy

Organism	Mode of transmission	Outcome for fetus/neonate	Outcome for mother
Treponema pallidum	Transplacental	Ranges from no effect to severe stigmata or miscarriage/stillbirth	None directly relating to the pregnancy
Neisseria gonorrhoeae	Intrapartum	Severe conjunctivitis	Possibility of ascending infection post partum
Chlamydia trachomatis	Intrapartum	Conjunctivitis, pneumonia	Possibility of ascending infection post partum
Herpes simplex	Usually intrapartum, but transplacental infection may occur rarely	Ranges from no effect to severe disseminated infection	Rarely, primary infection during 2nd/3rd trimesters becomes disseminated, with high maternal mortality
Human papillomaviruses	Intrapartum	Anogenital warts or laryngeal papillomas are very rare	Warts may spread and enlarge during pregnancy, but usually regress post partum

Investigations

If microscopy facilities are available, a Gram-stained smear of urethral exudate (Fig. 15.1) reveals significant numbers of polymorphonuclear leucocytes (PMNL). Urethritis is defined as ≥5 PMNL per high-power field in the UK (the US Centers for Disease Control recommends a lower threshold of ≥2). If Gram-negative intracellular diplococci (GNDC) are also seen, a working diagnosis of gonorrhoea is made and further investigations for gonorrhoea are undertaken; if no GNDC are seen, a label of NGU is applied. In all settings, a FVU sample or swab should be taken for a combined nucleic acid amplification test (NAAT) for gonorrhoea, chlamydia and, where available, *M. genitalium*.

Management

Syndromic management with prescription of multiple antimicrobials to cover the possibility of chlamydia, *M. genitalium* and sometimes gonorrhoea may be appropriate where diagnostic tests are unavailable or results delayed. Antibiotic use and selection is influenced by concerns about antibiotic resistance in both *N. gonorrhoeae* and *M. genitalium*. Microscopy findings allow a more accurate presumptive diagnosis. Additional treatment for gonorrhoea may be given on receipt of sensitivity results obtained by culture or NAAT technology (p. 103).

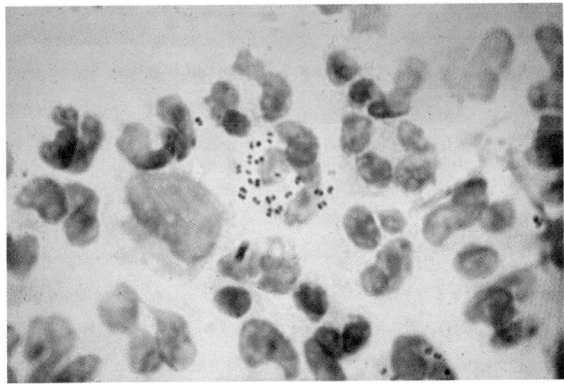

Fig. 15.1 A Gram-stained urethral smear from a man with gonococcal urethritis. Gram-negative diplococci are seen within polymorphonuclear leucocytes.

Genital itch, rash and discomfort

Genital symptoms including itch, irritation or discomfort may present acutely or as chronic problems with or without rash. Causes are infectious, non-infectious or multifactorial. Box 15.3 provides a guide to diagnosis.

Balanitis usually presents acutely and refers to inflammation of the glans penis, often extending to the under-surface of the prepuce (foreskin), in which case it is called balanoposthitis. Candidiasis affecting the glans penis or vulvovagina is sometimes associated with immune deficiency, diabetes mellitus and the use of broad-spectrum antimicrobials,

15

15.3 Differential diagnosis of genital itch and/or rash

Likely diagnosis	Acute or chronic	Itch	Pain	Discharge	Specific characteristics	Diagnostic test	Treatment
Candidiasis	Acute	✓	–	White	Post-coital in men	Microscopy	Antifungal cream, e.g. clotrimazole or single dose oral antifungal, e.g. fluconazole 150 mg
Candidiasis	Chronic/ recurrent	✓	±	White	Usually cyclical, rare in men	Microscopy (culture for yeasts other than *Candida albicans* in recurrent/refractory disease)	Oral antifungal, e.g. fluconazole 150 mg weekly for 6 months
Dermatoses, e.g. eczema or psoriasis	Either	✓	–	–	Similar to lesions elsewhere on skin	Clinical	Mild topical glucocorticoid, e.g. hydrocortisone
Genital herpes	Acute	±	✓	–	Atypical ulcers are not uncommon	Swab for HSV NAAT	Oral antiviral, e.g. aciclovir
Pthirus pubis ('crab lice') infection	Either	✓	–	–	Lice and nits seen attached to pubic hairs	Can be by microscopy but usually visual	According to local sensitivities Often permethrin
Lichen planus (p. 1103)	Either	±	–	–	Violaceous papules ± Wickham's striae	Clinical	None or mild topical glucocorticoid, e.g. hydrocortisone
Lichen sclerosus	Chronic	±	–	–	Ivory–white plaques, scarring	Clinical or biopsy	Strong topical glucocorticoid, e.g. clobetasol
Plasma cell balanitis of Zoon (penis)	Chronic	✓	–	±	Shiny, inflamed circumscribed areas	Clinical or biopsy	Strong topical glucocorticoid, e.g. clobetasol
Circinate balanitis (penis)	Either	–	–	–	Painless erosions with raised edges; usually as part of SARA (p. 1035)	Clinical	Mild topical glucocorticoid, e.g. hydrocortisone
Anaerobic (erosive) balanitis	Acute	±	–	Yellow	Offensive tight prepuce and poor hygiene may be aggravating factors	Clinical	Saline bathing ± metronidazole
Vulvodynia and vulvo vestibulitis	–	✓			Dyspareunia common, pain on touching erythematous area	Clinical	Refer to specialist vulva clinic

(HSV = herpes simplex virus; NAAT = nucleic acid amplification test; SARA = sexually active reactive arthritis)

ℹ 15.4 Infections that cause vaginal discharge

Cause	Clinical features	Treatment (in pregnancy seek specialist advice)
Candidiasis	Vulval and vaginal inflammation	Fluconazole[1] 150 mg orally as a single dose *or*
	Curdy white discharge adherent to walls of vagina	Clotrimazole[2] 500 mg pessary once at night and clotrimazole cream twice daily
	Low vaginal pH	
Trichomoniasis	Vulval and vaginal inflammation	Metronidazole[3] 400 mg orally twice daily for 5–7 days *or*
	Frothy yellow/green discharge	Metronidazole[3] 2 g orally as a single dose
Bacterial vaginosis	No inflammation	Metronidazole[3] 2 g stat or 400 mg twice daily orally for 5–7 days *or*
	White homogeneous discharge	Metronidazole[3] vaginal gel 0.75% daily for 5 days *or*
	High vaginal pH	Clindamycin[1,4] vaginal cream 2% daily for 7 days
Aerobic vaginitis: streptococcal/ staphylococcal infection	Purulent vaginal discharge	Choice of antibiotic depends on sensitivity tests

[1]Avoid in pregnancy and breastfeeding. [2]Clotrimazole, and clindamycin damage latex condoms and diaphragms. [3]Avoid alcoholic drinks until 48 hours after finishing treatment. Avoid high-dose regimens in pregnancy or breastfeeding. [4]*Clostridioides difficile* colitis has been reported with the use of clindamycin cream.

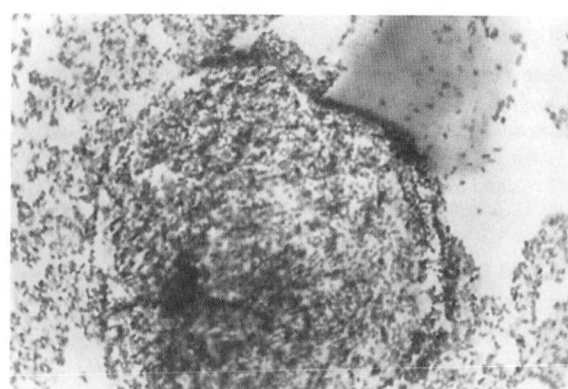

Fig. 15.2 Gram stain of a Clue cell from a patient with bacterial vaginosis. The margin of this vaginal epithelial cell is obscured by a coating of anaerobic organisms. *From McMillan A, Young H, Ogilvie MM, Scott GR. Clinical practice in sexually transmissible infections. Philadelphia: Saunders, Elsevier Inc.; 2002.*

glucocorticoids or antimitotic drugs. Chronic persistent or recurrent itch, commonly affecting the vulva, may be due to recurrent candidiasis with hypersensitivity to candidal antigens. Avoiding irritants such as scented hygiene products, soaps and detergents may be helpful in any case of chronic itch or discomfort.

The importance of psychological issues such as relationship or STI concerns, or a psychiatric diagnosis as a cause or a consequence of chronic or recurrent genital symptoms should always be considered.

Vaginal discharge

The normal physiological vaginal discharge may vary considerably over the menstrual cycle and under the influence of other hormonal changes such as puberty, pregnancy or prescribed contraception. An increase or change in vaginal discharge may also be due to a number of infective and non-infective conditions (Box 15.4). Worldwide, the most common treatable STI causing vaginal discharge is trichomoniasis; other possibilities include gonorrhoea and chlamydia. However, even in areas of high STI prevalence, most of those presenting with vaginal discharge alone will not have STI, so syndromic management of first presentation of vaginal discharge is often appropriate. Symptoms can help to distinguish the causes and anatomical origin of a vaginal discharge including:

- an increased discharge without any itch or irritation accompanied by an unpleasant or fishy odour, worse after sexual intercourse and during menstruation, indicates the possibility of BV
- vulval itching accompanied by a thick, white vaginal discharge, vulval burning, external dysuria and superficial dyspareunia may indicate candidiasis
- a purulent or mucopurulent discharge, with bloodstaining and/or post-coital or intermenstrual bleeding indicates the possibility of a discharge originating from an inflamed cervix, more commonly associated with STI including chlamydia and gonorrhoea.

Testing for STI should usually be decided by risk assessment rather than symptoms and usually includes vulvovaginal swabs for NAAT tests for chlamydia, gonorrhoea and with increasing availability *Trichomonas vaginalis*. Speculum examination, supported in specialist sexual health services by testing with narrow range pH paper and Gram-stain microscopy, allows rapid diagnosis in many cases. A homogeneous off-white discharge, vaginal pH greater than 4.5, and microscopy revealing reduced lactobacilli with Gram-variable organisms coating vaginal squamous cells (so-called Clue cells, Fig. 15.2), suggests BV. If there is vulval and vaginal erythema, a curdy discharge, vaginal pH less than 4.5, and fungal spores and pseudohyphae on microscopy, the diagnosis is candidiasis. A profuse yellow or green discharge with significant vulvovaginal inflammation and a very high pH suggests trichomoniasis, confirmed by finding motile flagellate protozoa on a wet-mount microscopy slide, by culture or by NAAT testing.

A purulent discharge from an inflamed cervix may contain GNDC on Gram-stain microscopy, allowing presumptive treatment for gonorrhoea. However, clinical examination and microscopy has very low sensitivity for *N. gonorrhoeae* in women, so NAAT and/or culture tests for STI should always be taken in women with behavioural or demographic risk factors for STI.

Treatment of infections causing vaginal discharge is shown in Box 15.4.

Genital ulceration

The most common cause of genital ulceration is genital herpes, but the possibility of other diagnoses including syphilis and LGV must be considered in all cases, with a higher index of suspicion if the patient is a MSM or has had a sexual partner from a region where tropical STIs are more common. Clinical signs and symptoms can help to distinguish between herpes and syphilis but certainty requires diagnostic testing. In herpes, multiple painful ulcers typically affect the introitus, labiae and perineum of the female genitalia and the glans, coronal sulcus or shaft of penis (Fig. 15.3). The presence of multiple lesions at different stages (erythematous, vesicular/blistering, ulcerating and resolving) is strongly supportive of a herpes diagnosis. Perianal herpes ulcers may be seen and are usually associated with receptive anal sex. Inguinal lymphadenopathy and systemic features, such as fever and malaise, are more common in women than in men.

In contrast, the classic lesion of primary syphilis (chancre) is single, painless and indurated; however, multiple (usually <5) lesions are commonly seen and anal chancres are often painful. Ulcers also occur in the primary stage of LGV and should be considered in MSM, especially if inguinal lymphadenopathy ensues.

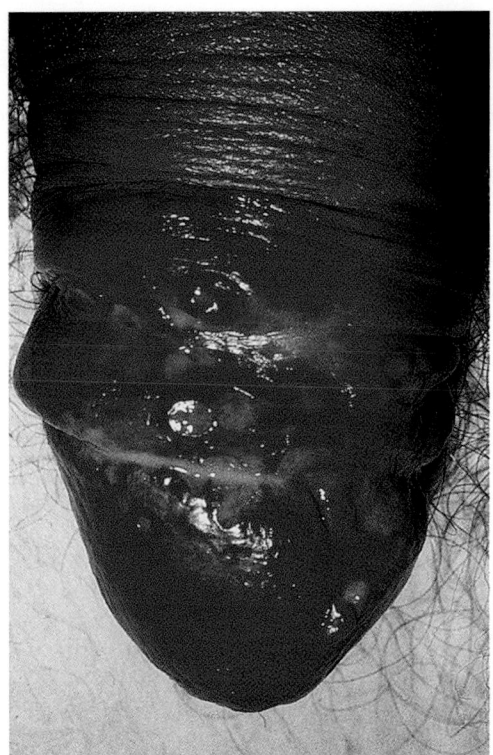

Fig. 15.3 Penile herpes simplex (HSV-2) infection.

Diagnosis is made by gently swabbing the lesion(s) for detection of HSV DNA and increasingly for *Treponema pallidum* by NAAT. A swab for testing for LGV (see Box 15.12) may be taken in MSM. In specialist sexual health services, syphilis may be diagnosed in-clinic by dark-ground microscopy of material obtained from a chancre. Serological tests for syphilis should always be performed in patients presenting with genital ulcer.

Other infective causes seen in the UK include varicella zoster virus (p. 282) and trauma with secondary infection. Tropical STIs, such as chancroid and granuloma inguinale, are rare and are described in Box 15.12.

Non-infective inflammatory causes include lichen sclerosus, aphthosis, Stevens–Johnson syndrome (see Ch. 27), Behçet's disease (p. 1047) and fixed drug reactions. In older patients, squamous cell carcinoma and vulval or penile intra-epithelial neoplasia (VIN and PIN) should be considered and excluded by biopsy in cases of doubt. The possibility of a pre-existing underlying pathology with a co-incident infection should be considered if lesions recur or fail to resolve.

Genital lumps

The most common cause of genital 'lumps' is warts. These are classically found in areas of friction during sex, such as the parafrenal skin and prepuce of the penis, the inner aspect of the vulval labiae, the fourchette and perineum. Warts may also be seen on the keratinised epithelium of the shaft of the penis, pubis or inner thighs and less commonly in the urethral meatus. Perianal warts are relatively common in both men and women even in the absence of a history of receptive anal sex.

The differential diagnosis includes molluscum contagiosum and skin tags. Normal anatomical features may be confused with warts by young men and women and occasionally by clinicians. These include coronal papillae, parafrenal glands or sebaceous glands (Fordyce spots) in men and vulval papillae and sebaceous glands in women.

Proctitis

Proctitis due to STI is almost exclusively diagnosed in MSM, but occasionally presents in women. STIs that may cause proctitis include gonorrhoea, chlamydia, herpes and syphilis. Lymphogranuloma venereum (LGV), caused by sub strains L1–3 of *Chlamydia trachomatis*, is now a common cause of severe proctitis in MSM in the UK.

Symptoms include mucopurulent anal discharge, rectal bleeding, pain and tenesmus. Examination may show mucopus and erythema with contact bleeding (p. 370). In addition to the diagnostic tests listed on page 371, a PCR test for HSV should be performed, with NAAT for LGV subtypes if chlamydia NAAT is positive. Treatment is directed at the individual infections.

Gastrointestinal symptoms including diarrhoea may indicate sexually transmitted enteric infection (STEI) with organisms such as *Salmonella*, *Shigella*, *Campylobacter*, *Cryptosporidium* and *Entamoeba histolytica* (see Ch. 13).

Lower abdominal pain

Lower abdominal and pelvic pain presenting in women of reproductive age has a wide differential diagnosis. In sexually active women, this includes complications of early pregnancy as well as those of STI. Pelvic inflammatory disease (PID) is usually the result of infection ascending from the endocervix to cause inflammation of the endometrium, fallopian tubes and ovaries, sometimes extending to the parametrium and the pelvic peritoneum or causing tubo-ovarian abscess. A diagnosis of chlamydia, gonorrhoea or *M. genitalium* infection supports the diagnosis but PID commonly occurs without STI. A definitive diagnosis of PID can only be made by laparoscopy, which is not practical or appropriate in the majority of cases. Early treatment improves outcomes, so a clinical diagnosis is made with a low threshold for initiating empirical antibiotic treatment. Other symptoms suggesting PID include deep dyspareunia, abnormal vaginal discharge and/or bleeding and symptoms of systemic infection such as fever and malaise. On examination, lower abdominal tenderness is usually bilateral, and bimanual vaginal examination reveals adnexal tenderness with or without cervical motion tenderness. Diagnostic tests (p. 371) should include a pregnancy test because the differential diagnosis includes ectopic pregnancy.

If a clinical diagnosis of PID is thought likely, broad-spectrum antibiotics active against gonorrhoea, chlamydia and Gram-negative organisms, such as ceftriaxone, doxycycline and metronidazole, should be initiated immediately. Hospital admission for intravenous therapy may be required in severe cases. Delaying treatment increases the likelihood of adverse sequelae, such as abscess formation, and tubal scarring that may lead to ectopic pregnancy, infertility or chronic pain.

Acute or chronic pain in the male pelvis may be attributable to infective prostatitis or abacterial prostatic pain syndromes. Infections are usually associated with organisms causing urinary infection and STI is not implicated.

Epidemiology

The World Health Organization (WHO) estimates that there were over 376 million cases of the four major curable STIs (syphilis, gonorrhoea, chlamydia and trichomoniasis) in adults aged 15–49 throughout the world in 2016, with 90% in lower-income countries. Most of the complications of untreated STI, including chronic pain, infertility, genital cancers and the increased risk of acquiring HIV infection, disproportionately affect women.

STI transmission depends partly on the number of sexual partners (high rates of partner change) and concurrency (having sex with more than one partner during the same time period) in any given population. Hence increases in STI prevalence are driven by changes in sexual

i	**15.5** Examples of public health interventions to prevent STI in subpopulations with increased prevalence				
	Primary prevention: Structural/societal	Primary prevention: Biomedical	Primary prevention: Behavioural	Secondary prevention	Tertiary prevention
Syphilis in MSM	Marriage equality Targeted MSM services	Prophylactic antibiotics (research only)	Inclusive schools sex and relationship education (SRE)	Free online syphilis self-testing provision	App-based partner notification, 1-to-1 behaviour change interventions
HPV-related cervical cancer in low-income women	Gender equal pay legislation Countering 'anti-Vacc' propaganda through social media	HPV vaccination Smoking cessation medication	Condom skills demonstration in youth services	Cervical (pre) cancer screening	Surgical treatment for CIN (e.g. loop diathermy)
HIV in transgender women	Hate crime legislation Trans-inclusive health services	Promotion and provision of PrEP	Safer sex advice in holistic gender services	Outreach HIV testing services	Treatment as Prevention (TasP) PrEP for partners

(CIN = cervical intra-epithelial neoplasia; HPV = human papilloma virus; MSM = men who have sex with men; PrEP = pre-exposure prophylaxis)

behaviour, ways of increasing sexual mixing (finding new partners outside a social group or geographical area), such as travel or the use of mobile phone apps, and early sexual debut. Rates of different infections may also be affected by microbiological factors such as the emergence of strains carrying genetic mutations conferring antimicrobial resistance or causing asymptomatic infection. Human biological factors include changes in the prevalence of particular sexual behaviours (such as oral or anal sex), increased geographical mobility within and between countries, or the rates of vaccination and use of protection, for example condoms and pre-exposure HIV prophylaxis (PrEP). Consequently, STI incidence can vary dramatically by geography and over time, affected by structural changes such as economic decline, mass migration, legislation or changes in social mores and sexual behaviour, but also the availability of tests and services, treatment, prevention and vaccination programmes. In common with other infectious diseases, demographic risk factors relating to race, age, gender and sexual orientation combined with geographical and social deprivation ('syndemics') are often associated with increased STI prevalence in subpopulations across the world. These factors are also commonly barriers to access to education, prevention, testing and treatment services. For those affected by multiple risk factors, the population from whom they choose a sexual partner is likely to be a more significant determinant of STI risk than their individual sexual behaviours. The inability of individuals (in particular women) to make choices about consent to sex and reproductive health, including the necessity of transactional sex (exchange of sex for money, goods or protection) is an important additional factor for many such populations.

i	**15.6** Management goals in diagnosed bacterial STI	
Goal		**Interventions**
Prevention of onward transmission		Advice to abstain until treatment completed
		Notification of sexual partners for testing/ epidemiological treatment
Prevention of antimicrobial resistance		Antibiotic selection based on current local resistance data
		Antimicrobial test-of-cure
		Culture/NAAT based antimicrobial resistance testing
Identify other undiagnosed STI/BBV infection		Routine testing for other STIs, including HIV
Prevention of viral STIs for those at increased risk		Vaccination (HPV, hepatitis A, hepatitis B)
		PrEP for HIV
Opportunistic health improvement		Contraceptive advice and provision
		Address problematic alcohol/recreational drug use
		Brief behaviour change interventions

(BBV = blood-borne virus; HPV = human papilloma virus; NAAT = nucleic acid amplification test; PrEP = pre-exposure prophylaxis)

Prevention

STI prevention involves making deliberate changes to affect the epidemiological factors described above at all levels to reduce the risk of acquisition of infection (Box 15.5). This may involve structural and legislative interventions (such as UK marriage equality, gender recognition laws) and deliberate social influencing (such as addressing HIV or trans stigma through TV drama). Primary biomedical and behavioural interventions (to prevent acquisition of infection) such as hepatitis B vaccination for MSM may be applied to populations or individuals at risk. Secondary prevention includes the early detection of infection to reduce the spread of infection by limiting the period of infectivity and mitigate harm and often involves designing services to provide equity of access

to groups affected by higher prevalence of infection (e.g. chlamydia screening for young people, antenatal HIV testing in maternity services). Tertiary prevention includes biomedical interventions such as ensuring access to effective early treatment for the individual to prevent onward transmission. Partner notification (contact tracing) is a cornerstone of STI prevention (Box 15.6). It involves identifying recent sexual contacts at risk of infection to allow testing and in some cases the provision of treatment without confirming the individual is infected (termed epidemiological treatment). Partner notification may be undertaken by the patient, sometimes with professional help, or by the provider (clinician), requiring high levels of sensitivity and respect for confidentiality and anonymity. It is increasingly supported by technology such as dedicated partner notification apps and online systems. The benefits of provision of antibiotics for partners without a confirmed diagnosis must be carefully weighed against the risks of antibiotic resistance in the community. Behaviour change interventions, applied to populations or individuals at increased STI risk, sometimes following an initial STI diagnosis, have a good evidence base. However, proving or excluding a direct effect of population interventions that are 'distal' to the outcome measure (i.e. STI rates), such as schools sex and relationships education (SRE) or mass media campaigns, is extremely challenging due to multiple confounding factors.

Sexually transmitted bacterial infections

Syphilis

Syphilis is caused by infection, through abrasions in the skin or mucous membranes, with the spirochaete *Treponema pallidum* subspecies *pallidum*. In adults the infection is usually sexually acquired; however, transmission by kissing, blood transfusion and percutaneous injury has been reported. Congenital syphilis, caused by transplacental infection of the fetus, remains rare in the UK, but an estimated one million pregnant women worldwide had active syphilis in 2016, causing about 200 000 stillbirths or neonatal deaths. Rates of infectious syphilis have risen in the UK over the last decade to levels last seen in the 1940s. About 75% of syphilis cases in the UK are in MSM.

The natural history of untreated syphilis is variable. Primary and secondary syphilis symptoms resolve spontaneously without treatment, meaning that the disease may go unrecognised and untreated with a risk of late complications. Infection may remain latent throughout, or clinical features may develop at any time.

Acquired syphilis

Early syphilis

Primary syphilis

Following exposure, the incubation period is typically around 21 days, with a range of 9–90 days. A primary lesion or chancre (Fig. 15.4) develops at the site of infection, usually in the genital area. A dull red macule develops, becomes papular and then erodes to form an indurated ulcer (chancre). Chancres may be multiple or atypical. The draining inguinal lymph nodes may become moderately enlarged, mobile, discrete and rubbery. The chancre and the lymph nodes are both painless and non-tender, unless there is concurrent or secondary infection. Without treatment, the chancre will resolve within 2–6 weeks to leave a thin atrophic scar.

Chancres may develop on the vaginal wall and on the cervix. Extragenital chancres are found in up to a third of MSM, affecting sites such as the finger, lip, tongue, tonsil, nipple, anus or rectum. Anal chancres often resemble fissures and may be painful.

Secondary syphilis

This occurs 6–8 weeks after the development of the chancre, when treponemes disseminate to produce a multisystem disease. Constitutional symptoms, such as mild fever, malaise and headache, are common. Over 75% of patients present with a rash on the trunk and limbs that may later involve the palms and soles; this is initially macular but evolves to maculopapular or papular forms, which are generalised, symmetrical and non-irritable. Scales may form on the papules later. Lesions are red, changing to a 'gun-metal' grey as they resolve. Without treatment, the rash may last for up to 12 weeks and is easily confused with psoriasis, pityriasis rosea, scabies, allergic drug reaction, erythema multiforme or pityriasis (tinea) versicolor, particularly if risk factors for syphilis infection have not been identified. Primary HIV infection (Ch. 14) is an important differential diagnosis.

Condylomata lata (papules coalescing to plaques) may develop in warm, moist sites such as the vulva or perianal area. Generalised non-tender lymphadenopathy is present in over 50% of patients.

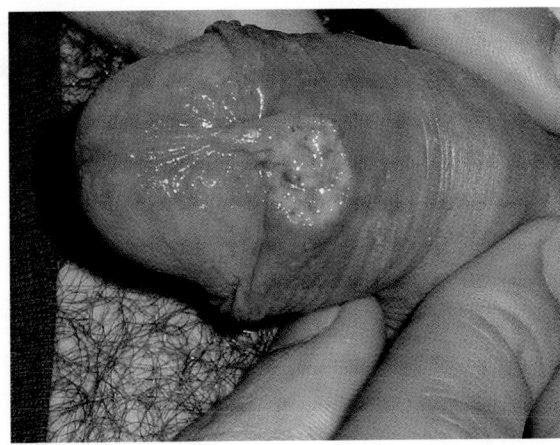

Fig. 15.4 Primary syphilis. A painless ulcer (chancre) is shown in the coronal sulcus of the penis. This is usually associated with inguinal lymphadenopathy. *From Clutterbuck DJ. Specialist training in sexually transmitted infections and HIV. St Louis: Mosby, Elsevier Inc.; 2004.*

Mucosal lesions, known as mucous patches, may affect the genitalia, mouth, pharynx or larynx. Rarely, confluence produces characteristic 'snail track ulcers' in the mouth.

Other features of secondary syphilis may present with or without rash; these include meningitis, cranial nerve palsies, anterior or posterior uveitis, hepatitis, gastritis, glomerulonephritis or periostitis. Although neurosyphilis has often been regarded as a manifestation of late syphilis, the commonest presentation of neurosyphilis in the UK is neurovascular syphilis presenting in the secondary stage.

The clinical manifestations of secondary syphilis will resolve without treatment but relapse occurs in up to 25% of cases within the 2 years of infection. The disease then enters the phase of latency.

Latent syphilis

This phase is characterised by the presence of positive syphilis serology or the diagnostic cerebrospinal fluid (CSF) abnormalities of neurosyphilis in an untreated patient with no evidence of clinical disease. In early latency (within 2 years of infection), syphilis may be transmitted sexually. In late latent syphilis the patient is no longer sexually infectious. Transmission of syphilis from a pregnant woman to her fetus, and rarely by blood transfusion, is possible for several years following infection.

Late syphilis

Late latent syphilis

Without treatment, over 60% of patients will suffer little or no ill health from untreated syphilis, although many of these have asymptomatic pathological changes identifiable at autopsy. This is termed late latent syphilis. Other manifestations of late syphilis are now rarely seen in the UK, partly because of the prescription of antibiotics for other illnesses, such as respiratory tract or skin infections, may treat syphilis serendipitously.

Cardiovascular syphilis

The commonest late manifestation of untreated syphilis is involvement of the ascending aorta and sometimes the aortic arch, presenting between 10 and 30 years after infection as aortic incompetence, angina and aortic aneurysm (p. 442).

Benign tertiary syphilis

A chronic granulomatous lesion called a gumma is characteristic and may be single or multiple, developing 3–10 years after infection. It is rarely seen in the UK. Mucosal lesions may occur in the mouth, pharynx, larynx or nasal septum, appearing as punched-out ulcers. Gummas of the tibia, skull, clavicle and sternum have been described, as has involvement of

15

---

i | 15.7 Clinical features of congenital syphilis

Early congenital syphilis (neonatal period)

- Maculopapular rash
- Condylomata lata
- Mucous patches
- Fissures around mouth, nose and anus
- Rhinitis with nasal discharge (snuffles)
- Hepatosplenomegaly
- Osteochondritis/periostitis
- Generalised lymphadenopathy
- Choroiditis
- Meningitis
- Anaemia/thrombocytopenia

Late congenital syphilis

- Benign tertiary syphilis
- Periostitis
- Paroxysmal cold haemoglobinuria
- Neurosyphilis
- 8th nerve deafness
- Interstitial keratitis
- Clutton's joints (painless effusion into knee joints)

Stigmata

- Hutchinson's incisors (anterior–posterior thickening with notch on narrowed cutting edge)
- Mulberry molars (imperfectly formed cusps/deficient dental enamel)
- High arched palate
- Maxillary hypoplasia
- Saddle nose (following snuffles)
- Rhagades (radiating scars around mouth, nose and anus following rash)
- Salt and pepper scars on retina (from choroiditis)
- Corneal scars (from interstitial keratitis)
- Sabre tibia (from periostitis)
- Bossing of frontal and parietal bones (healed periosteal nodes)

---

i | 15.8 Serological tests for syphilis

Non-treponemal tests: detect antibodies non-specific to syphilis antigens

- Venereal Diseases Research Laboratory (VDRL) test
- Rapid plasma reagin (RPR) test

Treponemal antibody tests: specific for antibody to syphilis antigens

- Treponemal antigen-based enzyme immunoassay (EIA) for IgG and IgM
- *Treponema pallidum* haemagglutination assay (TPHA)
- *T. pallidum* particle agglutination assay (TPPA)
- Fluorescent treponemal antibody-absorbed (FTA-ABS) test

---

the brain, spinal cord, liver, testis and, rarely, other organs. Resolution of active disease should follow treatment, though some tissue damage may be permanent. Paroxysmal cold haemoglobinuria (p. 959) may be seen.

Neurosyphilis

This may also take years to develop. Asymptomatic infection is associated with CSF abnormalities in the absence of clinical signs. Meningovascular disease, tabes dorsalis and general paralysis of the insane constitute the symptomatic forms (p. 1178).

Congenital syphilis

Where antenatal serological screening is routinely practised with high uptake, including the UK, congenital syphilis is rare. Antisyphilitic treatment in pregnancy treats the fetus, if infected, as well as the mother.

Treponemal infection may give rise to a variety of outcomes after 4 months of gestation, when the fetus becomes immunocompetent:

- miscarriage or stillbirth, prematurely or at term
- birth of a syphilitic baby (a very sick baby with hepatosplenomegaly, bullous rash and perhaps pneumonia)
- birth of a baby who develops signs of early congenital syphilis during the first few weeks of life (Box 15.7)
- birth of a baby with latent infection who either remains well or develops congenital syphilis/stigmata later in life (see Box 15.7).

Investigations in adult cases

Nucleic acid testing such as PCR for *Treponema pallidum* is available increasingly routinely for the diagnosis of early syphilis in samples of serum collected from chancres, or from moist or eroded lesions in secondary syphilis. Dark field microscopy remains in use as the fastest near patient test in many specialist sexual health services.

Serological tests for syphilis (STS) such as treponemal enzyme immunoassays (EIAs) for IgG and IgM antibodies are more commonly used for routine testing in most settings and for antenatal screening. Other treponemal and non-treponemal tests are usually done if an initial screening test is positive or for follow up for positive cases and are listed in Box 15.8. Syphilis IgM becomes positive at approximately 2 weeks, while non-treponemal tests become positive about 4 weeks after primary syphilis.

Following treatment, non-treponemal tests are routinely monitored for declining titres, usually to low or undetectable levels within 12–18 months for primary or secondary syphilis. In patients with longstanding untreated late syphilis there may be high antibody titres with little change even after adequate treatment. Consequently, positive syphilis serology may be found during the investigation of other conditions (e.g. dementia), reflecting infection that has been treated deliberately or by accident, many years previously. Interpretation of results requires knowledge of any treatment, which may include antibiotics given for other indications.

Biological false-positive reactions occur occasionally; these are most commonly seen with Venereal Diseases Research Laboratory (VDRL) or rapid plasma reagin (RPR) tests, which do not require laboratory facilities so are used as screening tests in many countries. False positives are identified when treponemal tests are negative. Acute false-positive reactions may be associated with infections, such as infectious mononucleosis, chickenpox and malaria, and may also occur in pregnancy. Chronic false-positive reactions may be associated with autoimmune diseases.

The CSF should also be examined in patients with clinical signs of neurosyphilis (p. 1178) and in both early and late congenital syphilis.

Chest X-ray, electrocardiogram (ECG) and echocardiogram are useful in the investigation of cardiovascular syphilis. Biopsy may be required to diagnose gumma.

Endemic treponematoses, such as yaws, endemic (non-venereal) syphilis (bejel) and pinta (see Ch. 13), are caused by treponemes that are morphologically indistinguishable from *T. pallidum* and cannot be reliably differentiated by serological tests.

Investigations in suspected congenital syphilis

A newborn baby may have positive serological tests due to passively transferred maternal antibodies, but non-treponemal tests should become negative within 3–6 months of birth if the mother is adequately treated and child is uninfected. A neonate with a positive EIA test for antitreponemal IgM suggests early congenital syphilis. A diagnosis of congenital syphilis mandates investigation of the mother, her partner and any siblings.

Management

Penicillin remains the drug of choice for all stages of infection almost 80 years after its introduction. A single dose of 2.4 megaunits of long-acting intramuscular benzathine benzylpenicillin is recommended for early syphilis (<2 years' duration), or three doses at weekly intervals for late syphilis. A 14-day course of intramuscular procaine penicillin 2.4 megaunits once daily with oral probenecid 500 mg 4 times daily is recommended for the treatment of neurosyphilis, supplemented by a 3-day course of prednisolone (see below). Oral doxycycline is indicated for patients allergic to penicillin, except in pregnancy (see below). Azithromycin showed promise as an alternative treatment but resistance has been reported. All patients must be followed up until clinical signs have resolved and for partner notification. Serology is usually repeated for a year following treatment.

Pregnancy

Penicillin is the treatment of choice in pregnancy. If there is penicillin hypersensitivity, options include penicillin desensitisation, treatment with

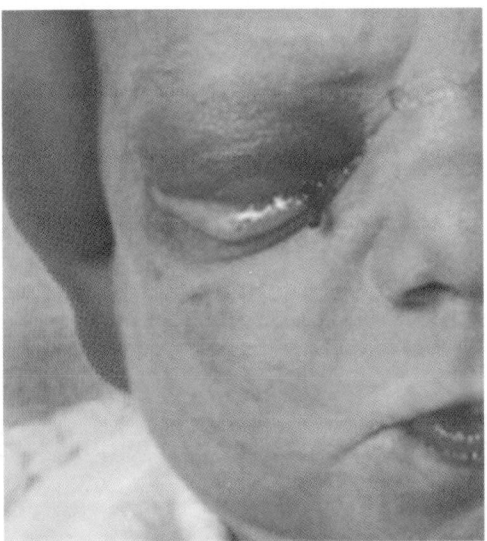

Fig. 15.5 Gonococcal ophthalmia neonatorum. *From McMillan A, Scott GR. Sexually transmitted infections: a colour guide. Edinburgh: Churchill Livingstone, Elsevier Ltd; 2000.*

- Acute prostatitis
- Epididymo-orchitis
- Bartholin's gland abscess
- Pelvic inflammatory disease (may lead to infertility or ectopic pregnancy)
- Disseminated gonococcal infection

erythromycin (with penicillin for the baby at birth because it crosses the placenta poorly), or intramuscular ceftriaxone 500 mg daily for 10 days (2 g daily for late infection/neurosyphilis).

Treatment reactions

- *Anaphylaxis.* Penicillin is a common cause; adrenaline and resuscitation equipment should be immediately to hand (p. 183).
- *Jarisch–Herxheimer reaction.* This is an acute febrile reaction that follows treatment and is characterised by headache, malaise and myalgia; it resolves within 24 hours. It is common in early syphilis and rare in late syphilis. Fetal distress or premature labour can occur in pregnancy. The reaction may also cause worsening of neurological (cerebral artery occlusion) or ophthalmic (uveitis, optic neuritis) disease, myocardial ischaemia (inflammation of the coronary ostia) and laryngeal stenosis (swelling of a gumma). Prednisolone 40–60 mg daily for 3 days is recommended to prevent the reaction in patients with these forms of the disease; antibiotic treatment can be started 24 hours after the first steroid dose. In high-risk situations the first antibiotic dose should be given in hospital.
- *Procaine reaction.* Fear of impending death occurs immediately after the accidental intravenous injection of procaine penicillin and may be associated with short-lived hallucinations or fits. Aspiration before any intramuscular injection is mandatory.

Gonorrhoea

Gonorrhoea is caused by the Gram-negative diplococcus *Neisseria gonorrhoeae* and usually involves columnar epithelium in the lower genital tract, rectum, pharynx and eyes. Transmission is usually the result of vaginal, anal or oral sex. Gonococcal conjunctivitis may be caused by accidental infection from contaminated fingers. Untreated mothers may infect babies during delivery, resulting in ophthalmia neonatorum (Fig. 15.5).

Clinical features

The incubation period is usually 2–10 days. Infection of the male urethra causes urethral discharge and dysuria; only a minority are asymptomatic. The female urethra, paraurethral glands/ducts, Bartholin's glands/ducts or endocervical canal may be infected, but about 80% of women are asymptomatic. There may be vaginal discharge or dysuria but these symptoms may be due to co-existing infections, such as chlamydia (see below), trichomoniasis or candidiasis. Intermenstrual or post-coital

bleeding suggests involvement of the cervix and lower abdominal/pelvic pain and dyspareunia suggests that the infection has ascended to the upper genital tract (PID)

Rectal infection is seen in MSM and in women due either to anal sex or to contamination from a urogenital site. It is usually asymptomatic but may present with anal discomfort, discharge or rectal bleeding.

Clinical examination may show no abnormality, but mucopurulent or purulent urethral discharge may be seen at infected sites. This is often obvious at the male urethra (p. 372). Discharge may be expressed from the female urethra, paraurethral ducts or Bartholin's ducts. The cervix may be inflamed, with mucopurulent discharge and contact bleeding. Proctoscopy may reveal either no abnormality, or clinical evidence of proctitis (p. 375) such as inflamed rectal mucosa and mucopus.

Pharyngeal gonorrhoea is usually symptomless and is largely attributed to receptive orogenital sex. Gonococcal conjunctivitis is an uncommon complication of adults and neonates, presenting with purulent discharge from the eye(s), severe inflammation of the conjunctivae and oedema of the eyelids, pain and photophobia. Conjunctivitis must be treated urgently to prevent corneal damage.

Other complications arise if diagnosis or treatment is delayed (Box 15.9). Disseminated gonococcal infection (DGI) is rare. Symptoms include arthritis of one or more joints, pustular skin lesions, tenosynovitis and fever. Gonococcal endocarditis has been described.

Investigations

Gram-negative diplococci may be seen on microscopy of smears from infected sites (see Fig. 15.1). Pharyngeal smears are not helpful due to the presence of commensal *Neisseria* spp., which have the same microscopic appearance. Nucleic acid amplification tests (NAAT) are a widely used diagnostic test (see Box 15.1), with culture on selective medium in positive cases for antibiotic sensitivity surveillance. Nucleic acid probes for specific antibody resistance mutations (e.g. to ciprofloxacin) are increasingly available, with the prospect of whole-genome sequencing in the near future.

Management of adults

Neisseria gonorrhoeae is a highly adaptable organism and has developed high-level resistance to a range of antibiotics over time, with frequent changes to recommended antibiotics and dosage. Multi-drug-resistant gonorrhoea (MDRGC) has emerged as a significant concern in recent years. Current UK treatment recommendations are for a single 1 g dose of IM ceftriaxone. Longer courses of antibiotics are required for complicated infection. NAAT-based antibiotic sensitivity testing available at the time of diagnosis offers the possibility of selective use of antibiotics previously rendered unsuitable for blind treatment (see Box 15.10).

The partner(s) of patients with gonorrhoea should be seen as soon as possible.

Chlamydial infection

Chlamydia is transmitted and presents in a similar way to gonorrhoea. In women, the cervix and urethra are commonly involved. Infection is asymptomatic in about 80%, but may cause intermenstrual and/or post-coital bleeding, dysuria or vaginal discharge. Lower abdominal pain and dyspareunia are features of PID. Examination may reveal mucopurulent cervicitis, contact bleeding from the cervix, evidence of PID or no obvious clinical signs.

15

15.10 Treatment of uncomplicated anogenital gonorrhoea

Uncomplicated anogenital or pharyngeal infection

- Ceftriaxone 1 g IM as a single dose
- Ciprofloxacin 500 mg orally as a single dose[1,2]

Pregnancy and breastfeeding

- Ceftriaxone 1 g IM as a single dose
- Spectinomycin 2 g IM stat[3]

Disseminated gonorrhoea

- Ceftriaxone 1 g IM or IV once daily or
- Cefotaxime 1 g IV 3 times daily
- Switched to an oral alternative according to sensitivities after 48 hrs and continued for 7 days

[1]Contraindicated in pregnancy and breastfeeding. [2]Only where nucleic acid amplification test (NAAT) or culture-based sensitivity testing shows sensitivity at all sites. [3]Not routinely available. (IM = intramuscular; IV = intravenous)

15.11 Treatment of chlamydial infection

Uncomplicated infection

- First choice: Doxycycline 100 mg orally twice daily for 7 days[1]
- Second choice: Azithromycin 1 g orally as a single dose followed by 500 mg once daily for 2 days

Infection with possible complications (epididymo-orchitis, PID, SARA)[2]

- First choice: Doxycycline 100 mg orally twice daily for 14 days[1]
- Second choice: Ofloxacin 400 mg orally twice daily for 14 days[3]

[1]Contraindicated in pregnancy and breastfeeding. [2]With additional antibiotics to cover other possible organisms. [3]Quinolones are now less commonly used first line because of concerns about rare permanent and disabling side-effects. (PID = pelvic inflammatory disease; SARA = sexually acquired reactive arthritis)

Other complications include perihepatitis (Fitz-Hugh–Curtis syndrome, p. 856), chronic pelvic pain, conjunctivitis and sexually acquired reactive arthritis (SARA) (p. 1035). Perinatal transmission may lead to ophthalmia neonatorum and/or pneumonia in the neonate. The majority of chlamydial infections clear spontaneously without treatment but others persist. The individual's risk of 'silent' tubal damage and subsequent infertility or ectopic pregnancy following asymptomatic chlamydial infection is low, but is a concern because of the high prevalence of chlamydial infection in the sexually active population.

In men, urethral symptoms are usually milder than those of gonorrhoea and may be absent in over 50% of cases. Conjunctivitis is also milder than in gonorrhoea; pharyngitis does not occur, although chlamydia is detected in pharyngeal samples in a small proportion of individuals. The incubation period varies from 1 week to a few months. Without treatment, symptoms may resolve but the patient remains infectious for several months. Complications, such as epididymo-orchitis and SARA are rare. Sexually transmitted pathogens, such as chlamydia or gonococci, are usually responsible for epididymo-orchitis in men aged less than 35 years, whereas bacteria such as Gram-negative enteric organisms are more commonly implicated in older men.

Treatments for chlamydia (Box 15.11) are also used for empirical treatment of NGU. Antibiotic resistance has not yet been a significant issue. Sexual partners should be traced and may be tested and/or treated epidemiologically depending on circumstances. Technologies supporting testing, treatment and partner notification for chlamydia include app-based notification systems and electronic treatment vouchers which can be redeemed at community pharmacies.

Mycoplasma genitalium

Mycoplasma genitalium is strongly associated with NGU (p. 372) and is implicated in the pathogenesis of PID. Its role in the development of other STI syndromes is not clear. A very high proportion of *M. genitalium* isolates in the UK are resistant to macrolides. This has led to doxycycline replacing azithromycin as the first choice empirical treatment of chlamydial infection and NGU. Where azithromycin is used, the multiple-dose regimen shown in Box 15.11 is preferred over a single dose because this may be both more effective and reduce the risk of macrolide resistance developing in *M. genitalium*.

Other sexually transmitted bacterial infections

Chancroid, granuloma inguinale and LGV as causes of genital ulcers in the tropics are described in Box 15.12. LGV now much more commonly presents as proctitis in MSM, having been acquired in Europe (p. 375).

Sexually transmitted viral infections

Genital herpes simplex

Infection with herpes simplex virus type 1 (HSV-1) or type 2 (HSV-2) produces a wide spectrum of clinical problems (p. 290), and facilitates the transmission of untreated HIV. Herpes is usually acquired sexually (vaginal, anal, orogenital or oro-anal), but perinatal transmission to the neonate may also occur. Primary infection at the site of HSV entry may be symptomatic or asymptomatic. HSV then establishes latency in local sensory ganglia, intermittently reactivating to cause either symptomatic or asymptomatic recurrences at the same site with viral shedding, during which transmission may occur. Most transmissions are thought to originate from people unaware of their infection. Although HSV-1 is classically associated with orolabial herpes and HSV-2 with anogenital herpes, HSV-1 accounts for more than 50% of anogenital infections in the UK.

Clinical features

Symptomatic episodes usually involve the external genitalia with irritable vesicles that soon rupture to form small, tender ulcers which scab and heal without scarring (Fig. 15.6 and see Fig. 15.3). A symptomatic episode at the time of acquisition is usually the most severe, but may occasionally be delayed following asymptomatic primary infection. Constitutional symptoms such as fever, headache and malaise are common. Complications, such as urinary retention due to autonomic neuropathy, and aseptic meningitis, are occasionally seen. Inguinal lymph nodes become enlarged and tender, and there may be nerve root pain in the 2nd and 3rd sacral dermatomes. Lesions at other sites (e.g. urethra, vagina, cervix, perianal area, anus or rectum) may cause dysuria, urethral or vaginal discharge, or anal, perianal or rectal pain. First episodes usually heal within 2–4 weeks without treatment; recurrences are similar but usually milder and of shorter duration than the initial attack

Extragenital lesions may develop at other sites, such as the buttock, finger or eye, due to auto-inoculation.

HSV-1 and HSV-2 episodes are clinically identical, but recurrences occur more often in HSV-2 infection and their frequency tends to decrease more slowly with time. Prodromal symptoms, such as irritation or burning at the affected site, or neuralgic pain affecting buttocks, legs or hips often occur prior to a symptomatic recurrence.

Diagnosis

Swabs are taken from vesicular fluid or ulcers for detection of HSV-1 and 2 DNA by NAAT. Type-specific antibody tests for HSV-1 and 2 are available but not routinely used for diagnosis.

Management

First episode

Oral antiviral treatment will shorten the duration of symptoms if started within 5 days of the beginning of the episode, or while lesions are still forming. Occasionally, intravenous therapy may be indicated if oral

i | **15.12** Salient features of lymphogranuloma venereum, chancroid and granuloma inguinale (Donovanosis)

Infection and distribution	Organism	Incubation period	Genital lesion	Lymph nodes	Diagnosis	Management
Lymphogranuloma venereum (LGV)						
E/W Africa, India, SE Asia, S America, Caribbean	*Chlamydia trachomatis* types L1, 2, 3	3–30 days	Small, transient, painless ulcer, vesicle, papule; often unnoticed	Tender, usually unilateral, matted, suppurative bubo; inguinal/femoral nodes involved[1]	Swab from ulcer or bubo pus for *Chlamydia*, NAAT with LGV subtypes if positive	Doxycycline[2] 100 mg twice daily orally for 21 days *or* Erythromycin 500 mg orally 4 times daily
Chancroid						
Africa, Asia, Central and S America	*Haemophilus ducreyi* (short Gram-negative bacillus)	3–10 days	Single or multiple painful ulcers with ragged undermined edges	As above but unilocular, suppurative bubo; inguinal nodes involved in ~50%	Microscopy and culture of scrapings from ulcer or pus from bubo	Azithromycin[3] 1 g orally once *or* Ceftriaxone 250 mg IM once *or* Ciprofloxacin[2] 500 mg orally twice daily for 3 days
Granuloma inguinale						
Australia, India, Caribbean, S Africa, S America, Papua New Guinea	*Klebsiella granulomatis* (Donovan bodies)	3–40 days	Ulcers or hypertrophic granulomatous lesions; usually painless[4]	Initial swelling of inguinal nodes, then spread of infection to form abscess or ulceration through adjacent skin	Microscopy of cellular material for intracellular bipolar-staining Donovan bodies	Azithromycin[3] 1 g orally weekly or 500 mg orally daily *or* Doxycycline[2] 100 mg orally twice daily *or* Ceftriaxone 1 g IM daily

N.B. Partners of patients with LGV, chancroid and granuloma inguinale should be investigated and treated, even if asymptomatic.
[1]LGV acquired as a rectal infection in MSM commonly presents as proctitis. [2]Doxycycline and ciprofloxacin are contraindicated in pregnancy and breastfeeding. [3]The safety of azithromycin in pregnancy and breastfeeding has not been fully assessed. [4]Mother-to-baby transmission of granuloma inguinale may rarely occur.
(IM = intramuscular; NAAT = nucleic acid amplification test)

15

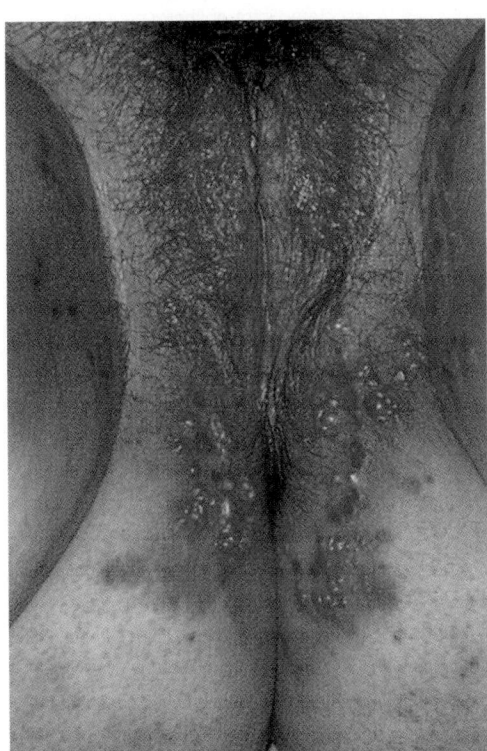

Fig. 15.6 Herpetic ulceration of the vulva. *From McMillan A, Scott GR. Sexually transmitted infections: a colour guide. Edinburgh: Churchill Livingstone, Elsevier Ltd; 2000.*

therapy is poorly tolerated or aseptic meningitis occurs. Many possible oral dosage regimens are used, including:

- aciclovir 400 mg 3 times daily for 5 days
- valaciclovir 500 mg twice daily for 5 days.

Topical and oral analgesia is helpful and patients are advised to use a warm shower spray to ease urination. Catheterisation via the suprapubic route is occasionally required for urinary retention. Treatment may be continued for longer than 5 days if new lesions develop.

Recurrent genital herpes

Symptomatic recurrences are usually mild and may require no specific treatment other than saline bathing, although the psychosexual impact of herpes stigma in a minority of patients should be considered. For more severe or prolonged episodes, patient-initiated treatment within 24 hours of onset, with one of the following oral regimens, should reduce the duration of the recurrence:

- aciclovir 800 mg 3 times daily for 2 days
- valaciclovir 500 mg twice daily for 5 days.

In a few patients, treatment started at the onset of prodromal symptoms may abort recurrence.

Those with recurrences that are severe and/or frequent may benefit from suppressive therapy. Daily treatment should be given for a minimum of 1 year before stopping to assess recurrence rate. The rate of decay in frequency of recurrence is low, so only about 20% of patients will experience significantly reduced rates. For others, resumption of suppressive therapy is justified. Aciclovir 400 mg twice daily is most commonly prescribed.

Management in pregnancy

The risk of disseminated infection is increased in pregnancy, particularly in the third trimester. A pregnant woman with no previous anogenital herpes and a partner with a history of HSV infection should be advised on avoiding acquisition, which may include consistent condom use during pregnancy to reduce genital-to-genital transmission. Antibody testing can identify the type-specific HSV serostatus of a woman and her partner and inform the advice given. Treatment with aciclovir is usually offered for genital herpes acquired during pregnancy after appropriate discussion; although aciclovir is not licensed for use in pregnancy in the UK, there is considerable clinical evidence to support its safety.

Vaginal delivery is routine in most women with herpes in pregnancy. Caesarean section is sometimes considered if there is a recurrence at the beginning of labour, although the risk of neonatal herpes through vaginal transmission is very low. Caesarean section is often recommended if primary infection occurs after 34 weeks because the risk of viral shedding in labour is very high and the antibody response to HSV which develops in the mother and protects the neonate by transplacental transmission may not have fully developed.

Human papillomavirus and anogenital warts

Human papillomavirus (HPV) subtypes (p. 1091) that preferentially infect the genital skin and are mainly sexually transmitted include benign genotypes (HPV-6 and 11) causing anogenital warts as well as genotypes such as 16 and 18, which do not cause genital warts but are associated with cervical, vulval, penile and anal intra-epithelial neoplasia (CIN, VIN, PIN and AIN) and the associated invasive cancers, as well as with cancers of the oropharynx. HPV is commonly transmitted through non-penetrative sex so affects individuals from the early years of adolescence onwards. Asymptomatic infection without any clinical sequelae is usual with all subtypes and infection with multiple subtypes is common.

Clinical features

Anogenital warts caused by HPV may be single or multiple, exophytic, papular or flat. Rarely, a giant condyloma (Buschke–Löwenstein tumour) develops, with local tissue destruction. Because of the association with intra-epithelial neoplasia, warts with an atypical appearance should be biopsied. Perianal warts (p. 370) are more common in MSM, but are also found in women and in heterosexual men. In pregnancy, warts may dramatically increase in size and number, making treatment difficult. Rarely, they are large enough to obstruct labour so delivery by caesarean section is required. Perinatal transmission of HPV occasionally leads to anogenital warts and rarely to laryngeal papillomas in the neonate.

Management

The use of condoms can help prevent the transmission of HPV to non-infected partners, but as condoms do not cover all of the genital skin, protection is incomplete. Vaccination against genital HPV infection is routine in many countries. There are three types of vaccine:

- A bivalent vaccine offers protection against HPV types 16 and 18, which account for approximately 75% of cervical cancers in the UK.
- A quadrivalent vaccine offers additional protection against HPV types 6 and 11, which account for over 90% of genital warts.
- A nonavalent vaccine protects against five additional high-risk types (31, 33, 45, 52 and 58).

All vaccines have been shown to be highly effective in the prevention of cervical intra-epithelial neoplasia in young women, and the quadrivalent and nonavalent vaccines have also been demonstrated to be highly effective in protecting against HPV-associated genital warts. HPV vaccination is usually administered prior to the onset of sexual activity, typically at age 11–13, in a course of three injections. In the UK, vaccination has

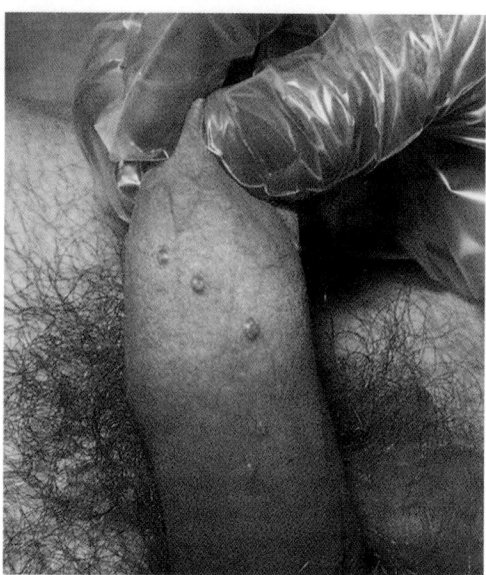

Fig. 15.7 **Molluscum contagiosum of the shaft of the penis.** *From McMillan A, Scott GR. Sexually transmitted infections: a colour guide. Edinburgh: Churchill Livingstone, Elsevier Ltd; 2000.*

been offered to girls since 2007 (with quadrivalent vaccine from 2012) and the recommendation was extended to boys from 2020.

Benign anogenital warts sometimes resolve spontaneously without treatment and in the vast majority of cases are a harmless, if sometimes distressing, inconvenience. Topical self-administered treatments commonly prescribed for use at home include:

- Podophyllotoxin, 0.5% solution or 0.15% cream (contraindicated in pregnancy)
- Imiquimod cream (contraindicated in pregnancy), also used in the treatment of HPV-associated intra-epithelial neoplasia
- Catephen, an extract of the green tea plant, *Camellia sinensis*.

Ablative therapies, usually performed by a clinician, are sometimes used first line or for warts that are keratinised, extensive or resistant to topical treatment.

- *Cryotherapy* using liquid nitrogen to freeze warty tissue often requires repeated clinic visits, although home cryotherapy is available. It is one of the few options for treatment of warts in pregnancy.
- *Hyfrecation* – surgical electrofulguration using the heat from an electric current to destroy tissue – is suitable for external and internal warts.
- *Surgical removal* may be used to excise extensive and/or refractory warts, especially pedunculated perianal lesions, under local or general anaesthesia.

Molluscum contagiosum

Infection by molluscum contagiosum virus, both sexual and non-sexual, produces flesh-coloured, umbilicated, hemispherical papules usually up to 5 mm in diameter after an incubation period of 3–12 weeks (Fig. 15.7). Lesions are often multiple and, once established in an individual, may spread by auto-inoculation. Infection in childhood is common; many individuals are immune by adulthood. If not, sexually acquired infection causes lesions on the genitalia, lower abdomen and upper thighs. The diagnosis is usually clinical. Typically, lesions persist for several months before spontaneous resolution occurs. Treatment regimens are therefore cosmetic; they include cryotherapy, hyfrecation or topical applications of 0.15% podophyllotoxin cream (contraindicated in pregnancy). The hard, pearly central core of each lesion can be removed using a needle and results in resolution, but this carries a risk of scarring.

Viral hepatitis

The hepatitis viruses A–D (p. 884) may be sexually transmitted:

- *Hepatitis A (HAV)*. Enteric infection may be transmitted through insertive oro-anal, digital-anal sex or peno-anal sex. Outbreaks of hepatitis A occur in MSM populations, most recently across Europe in 2016–18.
- *Hepatitis B (HBV)*. Hepatitis B is highly transmissible through all forms of penetrative sex, including oral sex, and is seen more commonly in groups with higher rates of partner change including sex workers and MSM, or with partners from endemic areas. Hepatitis D (HDV) may also be sexually transmitted.
- *Hepatitis C (HCV)*. Hepatitis C is much less transmissible through sex than HBV. Sex involving mucosal trauma (such as anal sex) carries a higher risk and sexually transmitted HCV is seen more commonly in MSM, particularly those co-infected with HIV, than in other populations.

Active immunisation against HAV and HBV should be offered to susceptible people at risk of infection. Many STI clinics offer a combined HAV and HBV vaccine to all MSM.

Partner notification, for testing and advice on preventing onward transmission, is offered to all those diagnosed with sexually transmitted viral hepatitis, with vaccination for HAV and HBV. No active or passive immunisation is available for protection against HCV but the consistent use of condoms is likely to protect susceptible partners until the index patient is able to complete treatment.

Further information

Books and journal articles

Mitchell L, Howe B, Ashley Price D, eds. Oxford handbook of genitourinary medicine, HIV, and sexual health, 3rd edn. Oxford: Oxford University Press; 2018.

Website

bashh.org/guidelines *British Association for Sexual Health and HIV; updates on treatment of all STIs.*

15

DE Newby
NR Grubb

16

Cardiology

Clinical examination of the cardiovascular system

6 **Face, mouth and eyes**
Pallor
Central cyanosis
Dental caries
Fundi (retinopathy)
Stigmata of
hyperlipidaemia
and thyroid disease

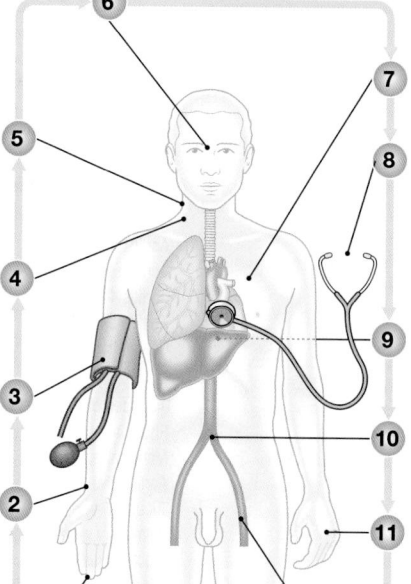

▲ Malar flush

▲ Poor oral hygiene in a
patient with infective
endocarditis

▲ Xanthelasma

5 **Jugular venous pulse**
(see opposite)
Height
Waveform

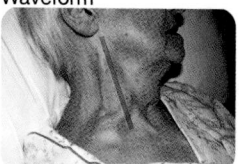

▲ Jugular venous pulse

4 **Carotid pulses**
Volume
Character
Bruits
(see opposite)

3 **Blood pressure**

2 **Radial pulse**
Rate
Rhythm

1 **Hands**
Clubbing
Splinter haemorrhages
and other stigmata of
infective endocarditis

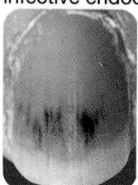

▲ Splinter haemorrhage

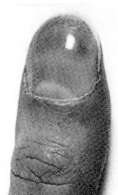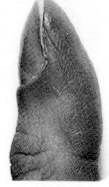

▲ Cyanosis and clubbing in a
patient with complex cyanotic
congenital heart disease

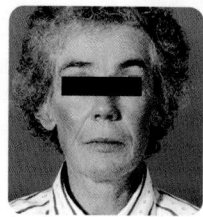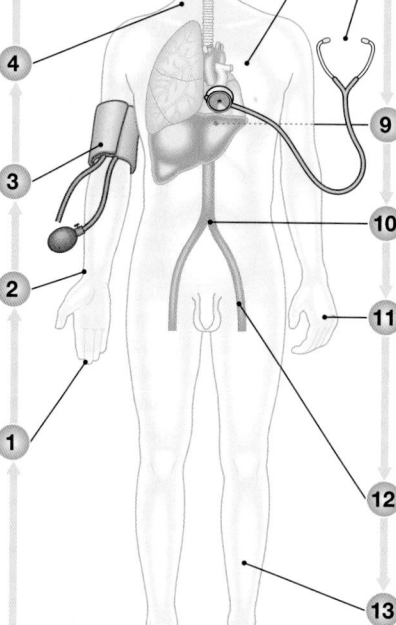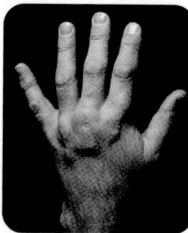

7 **Precordium**
Inspect
Palpate
(see opposite)

8 **Auscultation**
(see opposite)

9 **Back**
Lung crepitations
Sacral oedema

10 **Abdomen**
Hepatomegaly
Ascites
Aortic aneurysm
Bruits

11 **Tendon xanthomas**
(hyperlipidaemia)

▲ Vasculitis in a
patient with
infective
endocarditis

▲ Peripheral
oedema in a
patient with
congestive
cardiac failure

12 **Femoral pulses**
Radio-femoral delay
Bruits

13 **Legs**
Peripheral pulses
Oedema

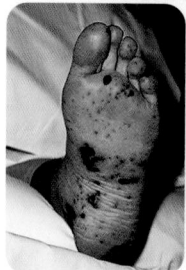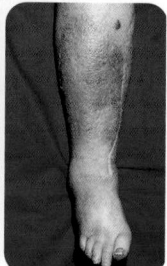

Observation
Symptoms and well-being
• Breathlessness
• Distress etc.
Body habitus
• Body mass (obesity, cachexia)
• Marfan and other syndromes
Tissue perfusion
• Skin temperature
• Sweating
• Urine output

Insets (Splinter haemorrhage, jugular venous pulse, malar flush, tendon xanthomas) From Newby D, Grubb N. Cardiology: an illustrated colour text. Edinburgh: Churchill Livingstone, Elsevier Ltd; 2005.

4 Examination of the arterial pulse

- The character of the pulse is determined by stroke volume and arterial compliance, and is best assessed by palpating a major artery, such as the carotid or brachial artery.
- Aortic regurgitation, anaemia, sepsis and other causes of a large stroke volume typically produce a bounding pulse with a high amplitude and wide pulse pressure (panel A).
- Aortic stenosis impedes ventricular emptying. If severe, it causes a slow-rising, weak and delayed pulse (panel A).
- Sinus rhythm produces a pulse that is regular in time and volume. Arrhythmias may cause irregularity. Atrial fibrillation produces a pulse that is irregular in time and volume (panel B).

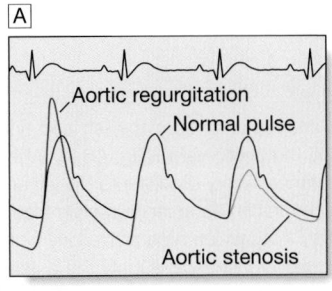

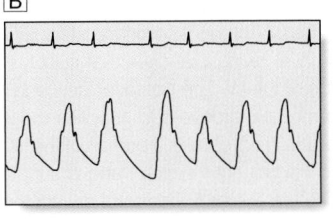

5 Examination of the jugular venous pulse

The internal jugular vein, superior vena cava and right atrium are in continuity, so the height of the jugular venous pulsation reflects right atrial pressure. When the patient is placed at 45°, with the head supported and turned to the left, the jugular venous pulse is visible along the line of the sternocleidomastoid muscle (see opposite). In health it is normally just visible above the clavicle.

- The height of the jugular venous pulse is determined by right atrial pressure and is therefore elevated in right heart failure and reduced in hypovolaemia.
- If the jugular venous pulse is not easily seen, it may be exposed by applying firm pressure over the abdomen.
- In sinus rhythm, the two venous peaks, the *a* and *v* waves, approximate to atrial and ventricular systole, respectively.
- The *x* descent reflects atrial relaxation and apical displacement of the tricuspid valve ring. The *y* descent reflects atrial emptying early in diastole. These signs are subtle.
- Tricuspid regurgitation produces giant *v* waves that coincide with ventricular systole.

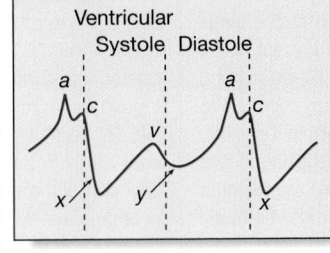

 Distinguishing venous/arterial pulsation in the neck

- The venous pulse has two peaks in each cardiac cycle; the arterial pulse has one peak.
- The height of the venous pulse varies with respiration (falls on inspiration) and position.
- Abdominal compression causes the venous pulse to rise.
- The venous pulse is not easily palpable and can be occluded with light pressure.

7 Palpation of the precordium

Technique

- Place fingertips over apex (1) to assess for position and character. Place heel of hand over left sternal border (2) for a parasternal heave or 'lift'. Assess for thrills in all areas, including the aortic and pulmonary areas (3). Normal position is the 5th or 6th intercostal space, at the mid-clavicular line.

Common abnormalities of the apex beat

- Volume overload, such as mitral or aortic regurgitation: displaced, thrusting
- Pressure overload, such as aortic stenosis, hypertension: discrete, heaving
- Dyskinetic, such as left ventricular aneurysm: displaced, incoordinate

Other abnormalities

- Palpable S1 (tapping apex beat: mitral stenosis)
- Palpable P2 (severe pulmonary hypertension)
- Left parasternal heave or 'lift' felt by heel of hand (right ventricular hypertrophy)
- Palpable thrill (aortic stenosis)

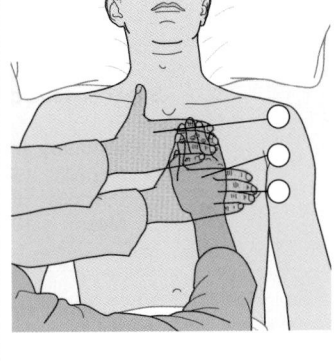

8 Auscultation of the heart

- Use the diaphragm to examine at the apex, lower left sternal border (tricuspid area) and upper left (pulmonary area) and right (aortic area) sternal borders.
- Use the bell to examine low-pitched noises, particularly at the apex for the mid-diastolic murmur of mitral stenosis.
- Time the sounds and murmurs by feeling the carotid pulse; the first heart sound (S1) just precedes the upstroke of the pulse and the second heart sound (S2) is out of step with it. If present, a third heart sound (S3) immediately follows S2, and a fourth heart sound (S4) just precedes S1. Systolic murmurs are synchronous with the pulse.
- Listen for radiation of systolic murmurs, over the base of the neck (aortic stenosis) and in the axilla (mitral incompetence).
- Listen over the left sternal border with the patient sitting forward (aortic incompetence), then at the apex with the patient rolled on to the left side (mitral stenosis).

16

The haemodynamic effects of respiration are discussed on page 391, and the analysis and interpretation of heart sounds and murmurs on page 400.

Cardiovascular disease is the commonest cause of death worldwide. The World Health Organization estimates that more people have died from cardiovascular disease since 1990 than any other category of illness, including infectious diseases. Strategies for the treatment and prevention of heart disease can be highly effective and have been subjected to rigorous evaluation by randomised trials. The evidence base for the treatment of cardiovascular disease is stronger than for almost any other disease group.

Coronary heart disease is the leading cause of death, with 3.8 million men and 3.4 million women dying each year. Although the incidence has been falling in some countries, it is rising in lower-income countries, where it accounts for more than 60% of the global burden of coronary heart disease. Valvular heart disease is also common but the aetiology varies in different parts of the world. In South Asia and in Africa it is predominantly due to rheumatic fever, whereas calcific aortic valve disease is the commonest problem in high-income countries.

Prompt recognition of the development of heart disease is limited by two key factors. First, it is often clinically silent for prolonged periods and coronary heart disease can proceed to an advanced stage before the patient notices any symptoms. Second, the diversity of symptoms attributable to heart disease is limited, so different pathologies may frequently present with the same symptoms.

Functional anatomy and physiology

Anatomy

The heart acts as two serial pumps that share several electrical and mechanical components. The right heart circulates blood to the lungs where it is oxygenated, and the left heart circulates it to the rest of the body (Fig. 16.1). The atria are thin-walled structures that act as priming pumps for the ventricles which provide most of the energy required to maintain the circulation. The atria are situated posteriorly within the mediastinum where the left atrium (LA) sits anterior to the oesophagus and descending aorta. The right atrium (RA) receives blood from the superior and inferior venae cavae and the coronary sinus. The LA receives blood from four pulmonary veins, two from each of the left and right lungs. The ventricles are thick-walled structures that pump blood through large vascular beds under pressure. The atria and ventricles are separated by the annulus fibrosus, which forms the skeleton for the atrioventricular (AV) valves and electrically insulates the atria from the ventricles. The right ventricle (RV) is about 2–3mm thick and triangular in shape. It extends from the annulus fibrosus to near the cardiac apex and sits anterior and to the right of the left ventricle (LV). The anterosuperior surface of the RV is rounded and convex, and its posterior extent is bounded by the interventricular septum, which bulges into the chamber. Its upper extent forms the conus arteriosus or outflow tract, from which the pulmonary artery arises. The LV is more conical in shape and in cross-section is nearly circular. It extends from the LA to the apex of the heart. The LV myocardium is approximately 10mm thick because it pumps blood at a higher pressure than the RV.

Normally, the heart occupies less than 50% of the transthoracic diameter in the frontal plane, as seen on a chest X-ray. On the patient's left, the cardiac silhouette is formed by the aortic arch, the pulmonary trunk, the left atrial appendage and the LV. On the right, the silhouette is formed by the RA and the superior and inferior venae cavae, and the lower right border is formed by the RV (Fig. 16.2). In disease states or congenital cardiac abnormalities, the silhouette may change as a result of hypertrophy or dilatation.

Coronary circulation

The left main and right coronary arteries arise from the left and right sinuses of the aortic root, distal to the aortic valve (Fig. 16.3). Within 2.5cm of its origin, the left main coronary artery divides into the left anterior descending artery (LAD), which runs in the anterior interventricular groove, and the left circumflex artery (CX), which runs posteriorly in the atrioventricular groove. The LAD gives branches to supply the anterior part of the septum (septal perforators) and the anterior, lateral and apical walls of the LV. The CX gives marginal branches that supply the lateral, posterior and inferior segments of the LV. The right coronary artery (RCA) runs in the right atrioventricular groove, giving branches that supply the RA, RV and inferoposterior aspects of the LV. The posterior descending artery runs in the posterior interventricular groove and supplies the inferior part of the interventricular septum. This vessel is a branch of the RCA in approximately 90% of people (dominant right system) and is supplied by the CX in the remainder (dominant left system). The coronary anatomy varies greatly from person to person and there are many normal variants.

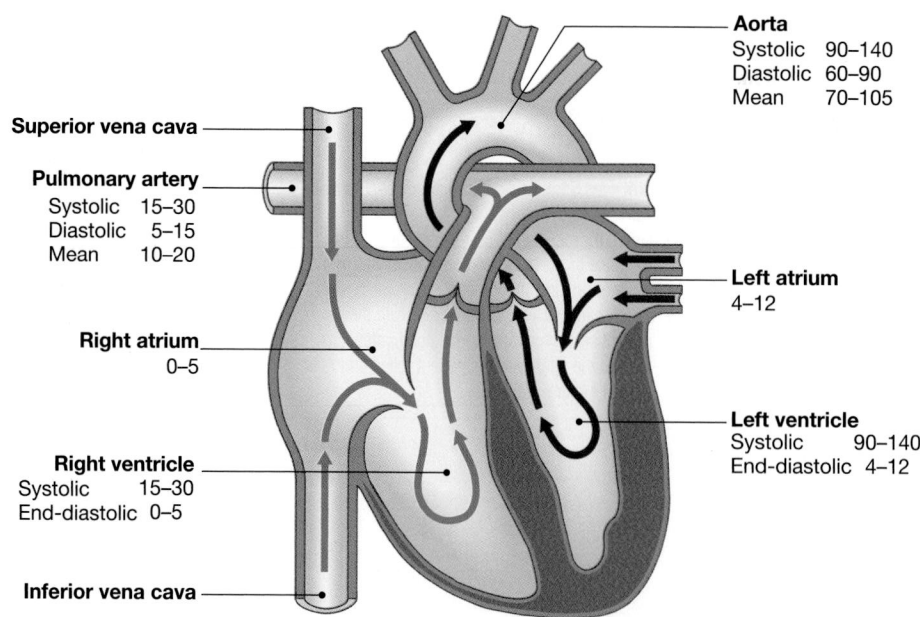

Aorta
Systolic 90–140
Diastolic 60–90
Mean 70–105

Superior vena cava

Pulmonary artery
Systolic 15–30
Diastolic 5–15
Mean 10–20

Left atrium
4–12

Right atrium
0–5

Left ventricle
Systolic 90–140
End-diastolic 4–12

Right ventricle
Systolic 15–30
End-diastolic 0–5

Inferior vena cava

Fig. 16.1 Direction of blood flow through the heart. The blue arrows show deoxygenated blood moving through the right heart to the lungs. The red arrows show oxygenated blood moving from the lungs to the systemic circulation. The normal pressures are shown for each chamber in mmHg.

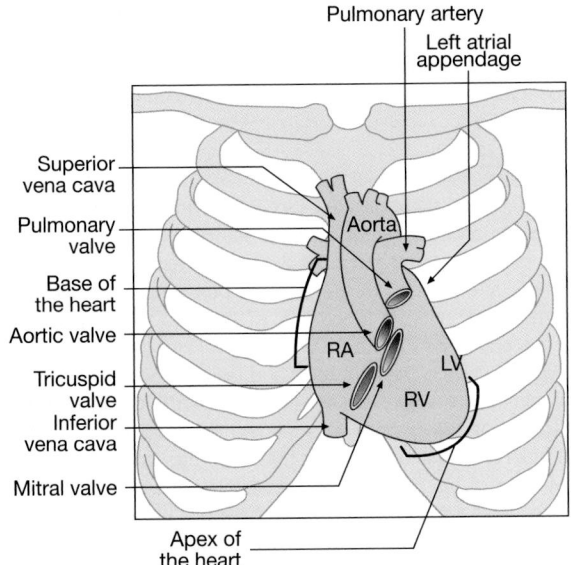

Fig. 16.2 Surface anatomy of the heart. The positions of the major cardiac chambers and heart valves are shown. (LV = left ventricle; RA = right atrium; RV = right ventricle)

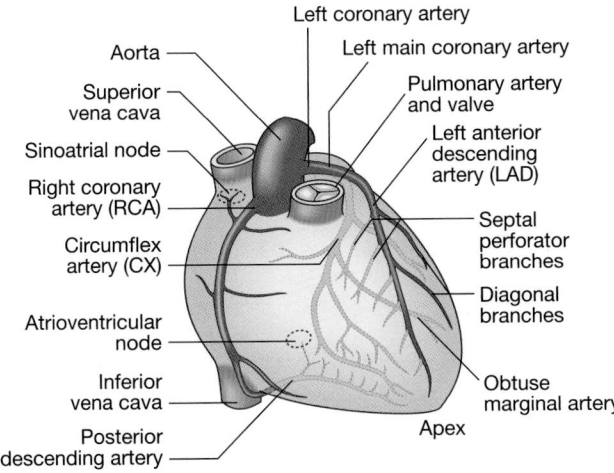

Fig. 16.3 The coronary arteries: anterior view.

The RCA supplies the sinoatrial (SA) node in about 60% of individuals and the AV node in about 90%. Proximal occlusion of the RCA therefore often results in sinus bradycardia and may also cause AV nodal block. Abrupt occlusion of the RCA, due to coronary thrombosis, results in infarction of the inferior part of the LV and often the RV. Abrupt occlusion of the LAD or CX causes infarction in the corresponding territory of the LV, and occlusion of the left main coronary artery is usually fatal.

The venous system follows the coronary arteries but drains into the coronary sinus in the atrioventricular groove, and then to the RA. An extensive lymphatic system drains into vessels that travel with the coronary vessels and then into the thoracic duct.

Conduction system

The SA node is situated at the junction of the superior vena cava and RA (Fig. 16.4). It comprises specialised atrial cells that depolarise at a rate influenced by the autonomic nervous system and by circulating catecholamines. During normal (sinus) rhythm, this depolarisation wave propagates through the atria via sheets of atrial myocytes. The annulus fibrosus

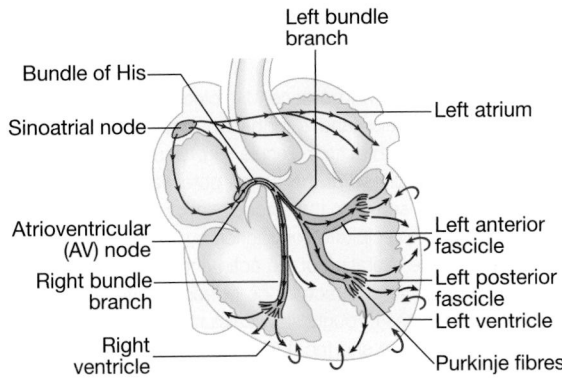

Fig. 16.4 The cardiac conduction system. Depolarisation starts in the sinoatrial node and spreads through the atria (blue arrows), and then through the atrioventricular node (black arrows). Depolarisation then spreads through the bundle of His and the bundle branches to reach the ventricular muscle (red arrows). Repolarisation spreads from epicardium to endocardium (green arrows).

forms a conduction barrier between atria and ventricles, preventing transmission of conduction except through the AV node. The AV node is a midline structure, extending from the right side of the interatrial septum, penetrating the annulus fibrosus anteriorly. It conducts relatively slowly, producing a necessary time delay between atrial and ventricular contraction. The His–Purkinje system is composed of the bundle of His extending from the AV node into the interventricular septum, the right and left bundle branches passing along the ventricular septum and into the respective ventricles, the anterior and posterior fascicles of the left bundle branch, and the smaller Purkinje fibres that ramify through the ventricular myocardium. The tissues of the His–Purkinje system conduct very rapidly and allow near-simultaneous depolarisation of the entire ventricular myocardium.

Nerve supply of the heart

The heart is innervated by both sympathetic and parasympathetic fibres. Adrenergic nerves from the cervical sympathetic chain supply muscle fibres in the atria and ventricles, and the electrical conducting system. Activation of β_1-adrenoceptors in the heart results in positive inotropic and chronotropic effects, whereas activation of β_2-adrenoceptors in vascular smooth muscle causes vasodilatation. Parasympathetic preganglionic fibres and sensory fibres reach the heart through the vagus nerves. Cholinergic nerves supply the AV and SA nodes via muscarinic (M2) receptors. Under resting conditions, vagal inhibitory activity predominates and the heart rate is slow. Adrenergic stimulation, associated with exercise, emotional stress, fever and so on, causes the heart rate to increase. In disease states, the nerve supply to the heart may be affected. For example, in heart failure the sympathetic system may be up-regulated, and in diabetes mellitus the nerves themselves may be damaged by autonomic neuropathy so that there is little variation in heart rate.

Physiology

Myocardial contraction

Myocardial cells (myocytes) are about 50–100 μm long; each cell branches and interdigitates with adjacent cells. An intercalated disc permits electrical conduction via gap junctions, and mechanical conduction via the fascia adherens, to adjacent cells (Fig. 16.5A). The basic unit of contraction is the sarcomere (2 μm long), which is aligned to those of adjacent myofibrils, giving a striated appearance due to the Z-lines (Fig. 16.5B and C). Actin filaments are attached at right angles to the Z-lines and interdigitate with thicker parallel myosin filaments. The cross-links between actin

16

and myosin molecules contain myofibrillar adenosine triphosphatase (ATPase), which breaks down adenosine triphosphate (ATP) to provide the energy for contraction (Fig. 16.5E). Two chains of actin molecules form a helical structure, with a second molecule, tropomyosin, in the grooves of the actin helix, and a further molecule complex, troponin, attached to every seventh actin molecule (Fig. 16.5D).

During the plateau phase of the action potential, calcium ions enter the cell and are mobilised from the sarcoplasmic reticulum. They bind to troponin and thereby precipitate contraction by shortening of the sarcomere through the interdigitation of the actin and myosin molecules. The force of cardiac muscle contraction, or inotropic state, is regulated by the influx of calcium ions through 'slow calcium channels'. The extent to which the sarcomere can shorten determines stroke volume of the ventricle. It is maximally shortened in response to powerful inotropic drugs or marked exercise. However, the enlargement of the heart seen in heart failure is due to slippage of the myofibrils and adjacent cells rather than lengthening of the sarcomere.

Cardiac peptides

Cardiomyocytes secrete peptides that have humoral effects on the vasculature and kidneys. Atrial natriuretic peptide (ANP) is a 28-amino acid peptide that acts as a vasodilator, reducing blood pressure (BP), and as a diuretic, promoting renal excretion of water and sodium. It is released by atrial myocytes in response to stretch. Brain natriuretic peptide (BNP; originally identified in extracts of porcine brain) is a 32-amino acid peptide produced by ventricular cardiomyocytes in response to

stretch, as occurs in heart failure. Like ANP, it has diuretic properties. Neprilysin, an enzyme produced by the kidney and other tissues, breaks down ANP, BNP and other proteins and, in so doing, acts as a vasoconstrictor. It forms a therapeutic target in patients with heart failure.

Circulation

The RA receives deoxygenated blood from the superior and inferior venae cavae and discharges blood to the RV, which in turn pumps it into the pulmonary artery. Blood is oxygenated as it passes through the pulmonary arterial and alveolar capillary bed before draining into the pulmonary veins and LA. Blood then passes into the LV which pumps it into the aorta (see Fig. 16.1). During ventricular contraction (systole), the tricuspid valve in the right heart and the mitral valve in the left heart close, and the pulmonary and aortic valves open. In diastole, the pulmonary and aortic valves close, and the two AV valves open. Collectively, these atrial and ventricular events constitute the cardiac cycle of filling and ejection of blood from one heart beat to the next. Blood passes from the heart through the large central elastic arteries into muscular arteries before encountering the resistance vessels, and ultimately the capillary bed, where there is exchange of nutrients, oxygen and waste products of metabolism. The central arteries, such as the aorta, are predominantly composed of elastic tissue with little or no vascular smooth muscle cells. When blood is ejected from the heart, the compliant aorta expands to accommodate the volume of blood before the elastic recoil sustains BP and blood flow following cessation of cardiac contraction. This 'Windkessel' effect prevents excessive rises in systolic

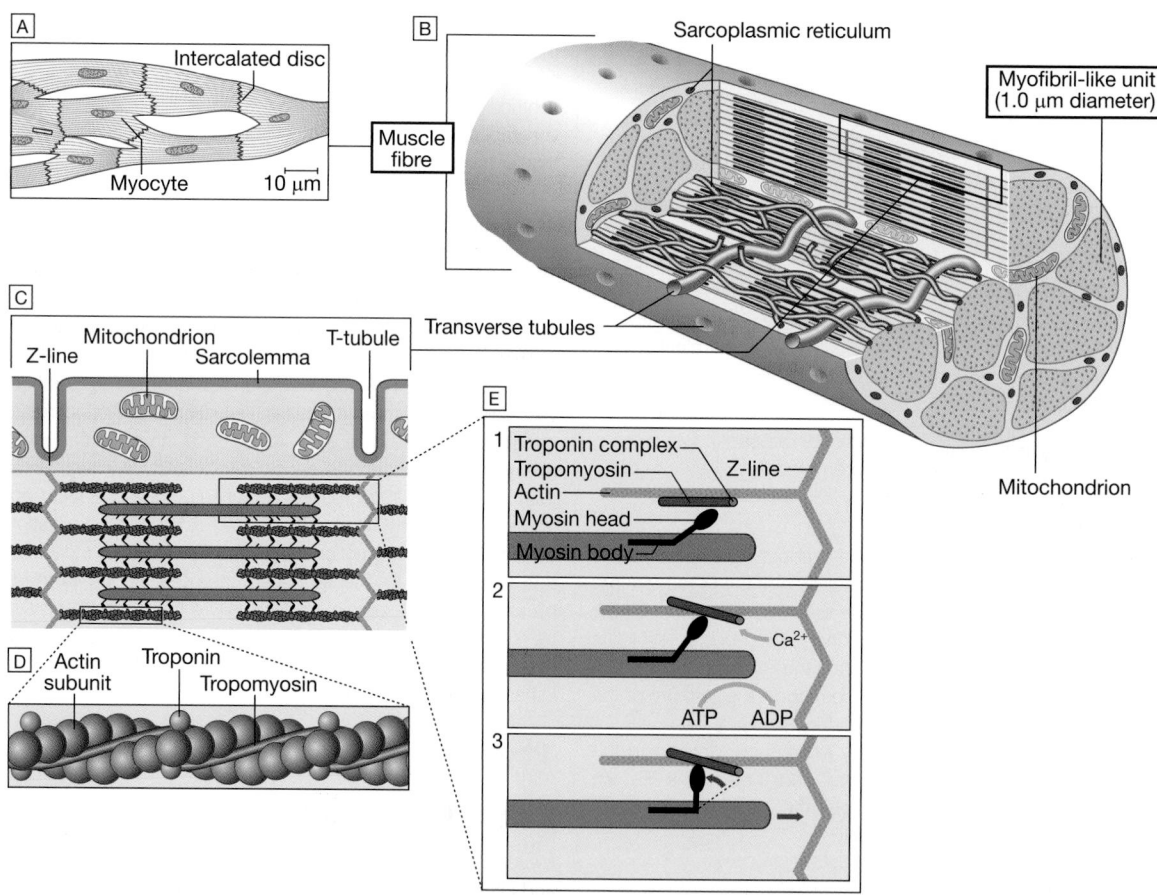

Fig. 16.5 Schematic of myocytes and the contraction process within a muscle fibre. [A] Myocytes are joined together through intercalated discs. [B] Within the myocytes, myofibrils are composed of longitudinal and transverse tubules extending from the sarcoplasmic reticulum. [C] The expanded section shows a schematic of an individual sarcomere with thick filaments composed of myosin and thin filaments composed primarily of actin. [D] Actin filaments are composed of troponin, tropomyosin and actin subunits. [E] The three stages of contraction, resulting in shortening of the sarcomere. (1) The actin-binding site is blocked by tropomyosin. (2) ATP-dependent release of calcium ions, which bind to troponin, displacing tropomyosin. The binding site is exposed. (3) Tilting of the angle of attachment of the myosin head, resulting in fibre shortening. (ADP = adenosine diphosphate; ATP = adenosine triphosphate)

BP while sustaining diastolic BP, thereby reducing cardiac afterload and maintaining coronary perfusion. These benefits are lost with progressive arterial stiffening, which occurs with ageing and advanced renal disease. Passing down the arterial tree, vascular smooth muscle cells progressively play a greater role until the resistance arterioles are encountered. Although all vessels contribute, the resistance vessels (diameter 50–200 μm) provide the greatest contribution to systemic vascular resistance, with small changes in radius having a marked influence on blood flow; resistance is inversely proportional to the fourth power of the radius (Poiseuille's Law). The tone of these resistance vessels is tightly regulated by humoral, neuronal and mechanical factors. Neurogenic constriction operates via α-adrenoceptors on vascular smooth muscle, and dilatation via muscarinic and β₂-adrenoceptors. In addition, systemic and locally released vasoactive substances influence tone; vasoconstrictors include noradrenaline (norepinephrine), angiotensin II and endothelin-1, whereas adenosine, bradykinin, prostaglandins and nitric oxide are vasodilators. Resistance to blood flow rises with viscosity and is mainly influenced by the haematocrit.

Coronary blood vessels receive sympathetic and parasympathetic innervation. While stimulation of α-adrenoceptors causes vasoconstriction and stimulation of β₂-adrenoceptors causes vasodilatation, the predominant effect of sympathetic stimulation in coronary arteries is vasodilatation. Parasympathetic stimulation also causes modest dilatation of normal coronary arteries. Because of these homeostatic mechanisms that regulate vessel tone, narrowing or stenosis in a coronary artery does not limit flow, even during exercise, until the cross-sectional area of the vessel is reduced by at least 70%.

Endothelium

The endothelium plays a vital role in the control of vascular homeostasis. It synthesises and releases many vasoactive mediators that cause vasodilatation, including nitric oxide, prostacyclin and endothelium-derived hyperpolarising factor, and vasoconstriction, including endothelin-1 and angiotensin II. A balance exists whereby the release of such factors contributes to the maintenance and regulation of vascular tone and BP. Damage to the endothelium may disrupt this balance and lead to vascular dysfunction, tissue ischaemia and hypertension.

The endothelium has a major influence on key regulatory steps in the recruitment of inflammatory cells and on the formation and dissolution of thrombus. Once activated, the endothelium expresses surface receptors such as E-selectin, intercellular adhesion molecule type 1 (ICAM-1) and platelet–endothelial cell adhesion molecule type 1 (PECAM-1), which mediate rolling, adhesion and migration of inflammatory leucocytes into the subintima. The endothelium also stores and releases the multimeric glycoprotein von Willebrand factor, which promotes thrombus formation by linking platelet adhesion to denuded surfaces, especially in the arterial vasculature. In contrast, once intravascular thrombus forms, tissue plasminogen activator is rapidly released from a dynamic storage pool within the endothelium to induce fibrinolysis and thrombus dissolution. These processes are critically involved in the development and progression of atherosclerosis, and endothelial function and injury are seen as central to the pathogenesis of many cardiovascular disease states.

Respiration

Cardiac output, BP and pulse rate change with respiration as the result of changes in blood flow to the right and left heart, as summarised in Box 16.1. During inspiration, the fall in intrathoracic pressure causes increased return of venous blood into the chest and right side of the heart, which increases cardiac output from the RV. However, blood is sequestered in the lungs due to the increased capacitance of the pulmonary vascular bed, leading to a reduction in blood flow to the LV and a slight fall in BP. With expiration the opposite sequence of events occurs; there is a fall in venous return to the right heart with a reduction in RV output, and a rise in the venous return to the left side of the heart with an increase in LV output. As the result of these changes, BP normally falls

16.1 Haemodynamic effects of respiration

	Inspiration	Expiration
Jugular venous pressure	Falls	Rises
Blood pressure	Falls (up to 10 mmHg)	Rises
Heart rate	Accelerates	Slows
Second heart sound	Splits*	Fuses*

*Inspiration prolongs right ventricular ejection, delaying P₂, and shortens left ventricular ejection, bringing forward A₂; expiration produces the opposite effects.

during inspiration but rises during expiration. These changes are exaggerated in patients with severe airways obstruction secondary to asthma or chronic obstructive pulmonary disease (COPD) leading to pulsus paradoxus, which describes an exaggerated fall in BP during inspiration. As well as being found in airways obstruction, pulsus paradoxus is also characteristic of cardiac tamponade. Here, cardiac filling is constrained by external pressure, and on inspiration, compression of the RV impedes the normal increase in flow during inspiration. The interventricular septum then moves to the left, impeding left ventricular filling and cardiac output. This produces an exaggerated fall in BP (> 10 mmHg fall during inspiration).

Investigation of cardiovascular disease

Several investigations may be required in the diagnosis of cardiac disease and assessment of its severity. Basic tests, such as electrocardiography, chest X-ray and echocardiography, can be performed in an outpatient clinic or at the bedside, whereas more complex procedures such as cardiac catheterisation, radionuclide imaging, computed tomography (CT) and magnetic resonance imaging (MRI) require specialised facilities.

Electrocardiogram

The electrocardiogram (ECG) is used to assess cardiac rhythm and conduction as well as the diagnosis of myocardial ischaemia and infarction.

The ECG is recorded by electrodes on the body surface which detect the electrical depolarisation of myocardial tissue produced from a small dipole current. These signals are amplified and either printed or displayed on a monitor (Fig. 16.6). During sinus rhythm, the SA node triggers atrial depolarisation, producing a P wave. Depolarisation proceeds slowly

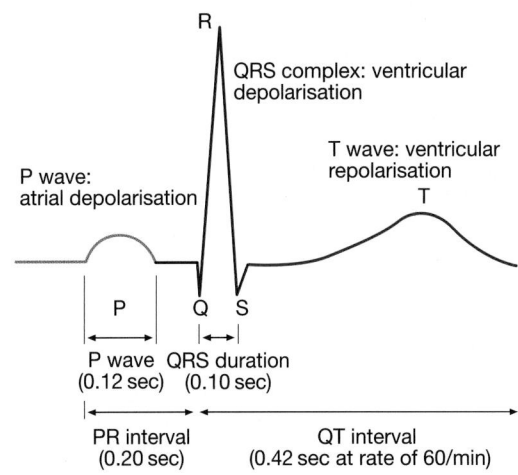

Fig. 16.6 The electrocardiogram. The components correspond to depolarisation and repolarisation, as depicted in Fig. 16.4. The upper limit of the normal range for each interval is given in brackets.

16

16.2 How to read a 12-lead electrocardiogram: examination sequence

Rhythm strip (lead II)	To determine heart rate and rhythm
Cardiac axis	Normal if QRS complexes +ve in leads I and II
P-wave shape	Tall P waves denote right atrial enlargement (P pulmonale) and notched P waves denote left atrial enlargement (P mitrale)
PR interval	Normal = 0.12–0.20 sec. Prolongation denotes impaired atrioventricular nodal conduction. A short PR interval occurs in Wolff–Parkinson–White syndrome
QRS duration	If > 0.12 sec, ventricular conduction is abnormal (left or right bundle branch block)
QRS amplitude	Large QRS complexes occur in slim young patients and in patients with left ventricular hypertrophy
Q waves	May signify previous myocardial infarction
ST segment	ST elevation may signify myocardial infarction, pericarditis or left ventricular aneurysm; ST depression may signify ischaemia or infarction
T waves	T-wave inversion has many causes, including myocardial ischaemia or infarction, and electrolyte disturbances
QT interval	Normal < 0.44 sec (male), 0.46 sec (female) corrected for heart rate. QT prolongation may occur with congenital long QT syndrome, low K^+, Mg^{2+} or Ca^{2+}, and some drugs (see Box 16.28)
ECG conventions	Depolarisation towards electrode: +ve deflection Depolarisation away from electrode: −ve deflection Sensitivity: 10 mm = 1 mV Paper speed: 25 mm per sec Each large (5 mm) square = 0.2 sec Each small (1 mm) square = 0.04 sec Heart rate = 1500/RR interval (mm) (i.e. 300 ÷ number of large squares between beats)

through the AV node, which is too small to produce a depolarisation wave detectable from the body surface. The bundle of His, bundle branches and Purkinje system are then activated, initiating ventricular myocardial depolarisation, which produces the QRS complex. The muscle mass of the ventricles is much larger than that of the atria, so the QRS complex is larger than the P wave. The interval between the onset of the P wave and the onset of the QRS complex is termed the 'PR interval' and largely reflects the duration of AV nodal conduction. Injury to the left or right bundle branch delays ventricular depolarisation, widening the QRS complex. Selective injury of one of the left fascicles (hemiblock) affects the electrical axis. Repolarisation is slower and spreads from the epicardium to the endocardium. Atrial repolarisation does not cause a detectable signal but ventricular repolarisation produces the T wave. The QT interval represents the total duration of ventricular depolarisation and repolarisation.

The 12-lead ECG

The 12-lead ECG (Box 16.2) is generated from 10 electrodes that are attached to the skin. One electrode is attached to each limb and six electrodes are attached to the chest. In addition, the left arm, right arm and left leg electrodes are attached to a central terminal acting as an additional virtual electrode in the centre of the chest (the right leg electrode acts as an earthing electrode). The 12 'leads' of the ECG refer to recordings made from pairs or sets of these electrodes. They comprise three

groups: three dipole limb leads, three augmented voltage limb leads and six unipole chest leads.

Leads I, II and III are the dipole limb leads and refer to recordings obtained from pairs of limb electrodes. Lead I records the signal between the right (negative) and left (positive) arms. Lead II records the signal between the right arm (negative) and left leg (positive). Lead III records the signal between the left arm (negative) and left leg (positive). These three leads thus record electrical activity along three different axes in the frontal plane. Leads aVR, aVL and aVF are the augmented voltage limb leads. These record electrical activity between a limb electrode and a modified central terminal. For example, lead aVL records the signal between the left arm (positive) and a central (negative) terminal, formed by connecting the right arm and left leg electrodes (Fig. 16.7). Similarly augmented signals are obtained from the right arm (aVR) and left leg (aVF). These leads also record electrical activity in the frontal plane, with each lead 120° apart. Lead aVF thus examines activity along the axis +90°, and lead aVL along the axis −30°, and so on.

When depolarisation moves towards a positive electrode, it produces a positive deflection in the ECG; depolarisation in the opposite direction produces a negative deflection. The average vector of ventricular depolarisation is known as the frontal cardiac axis. When the vector is at right

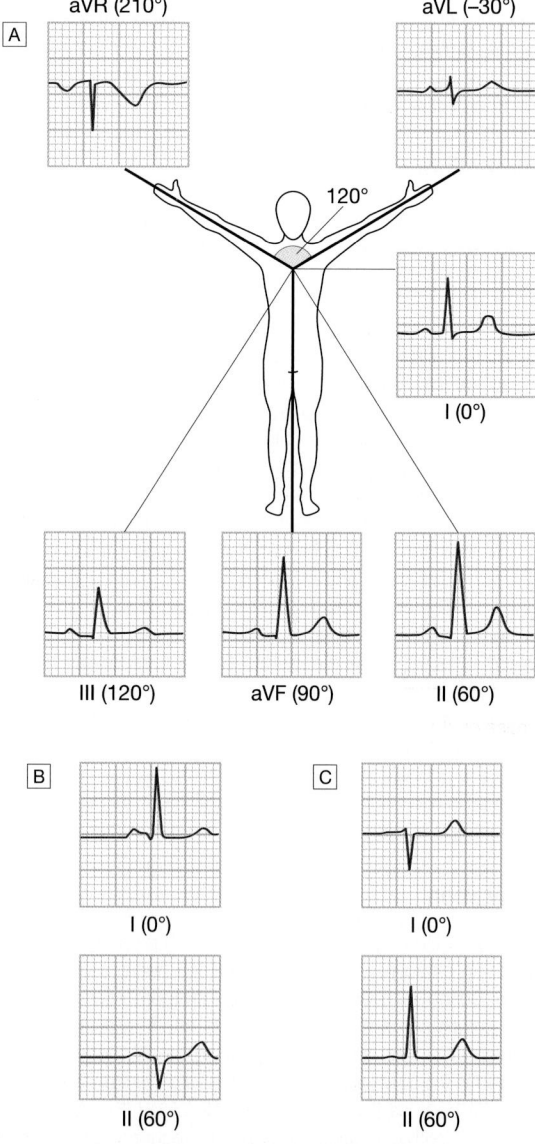

Fig. 16.7 The appearance of the ECG from different leads in the frontal plane. **A** Normal. **B** Left axis deviation, with negative deflection in lead II and positive in lead I. **C** Right axis deviation, with negative deflection in lead I and positive in lead II.

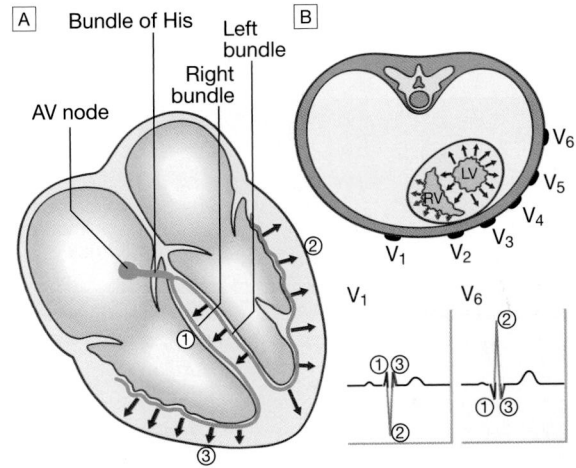

Fig. 16.8 The sequence of activation of the ventricles. $\boxed{A}$ Activation of the septum occurs first (red arrows), followed by spreading of the impulse through the left ventricle (LV, blue arrows) and then the right ventricle (RV, green arrows). $\boxed{B}$ Normal electrocardiographic complexes from leads V_1 and V_6. (AV = atrioventricular)

angles to a lead, the depolarisation in that lead is equally negative and positive (isoelectric). In Fig. 16.7A, the QRS complex is isoelectric in aVL, negative in aVR and most strongly positive in lead II; the main vector or axis of depolarisation is therefore 60°. The normal cardiac axis lies between −30° and +90°. Examples of left and right axis deviation are shown in Fig. 16.7B and C.

There are six chest leads, V_1–V_6, derived from electrodes placed on the anterior and lateral left side of the chest, over the heart. Each lead records the signal between the corresponding chest electrode (positive) and the central terminal (negative). Leads V_1 and V_2 lie approximately over the RV, V_3 and V_4 over the interventricular septum, and V_5 and V_6 over the LV (Fig. 16.8). The LV has the greater muscle mass and contributes the major component of the QRS complex.

The shape of the QRS complex varies across the chest leads. Depolarisation of the interventricular septum occurs first and moves from left to right; this generates a small initial negative deflection in lead V_6 (Q wave) and an initial positive deflection in lead V_1 (R wave). The second phase of depolarisation is activation of the body of the LV, which creates a large positive deflection or R wave in V_6 (with reciprocal changes in V_1). The third and final phase involves the RV and produces a small negative deflection or S wave in V_6.

Exercise ECG

In exercise or stress electrocardiography, a 12-lead ECG is recorded during exercise on a treadmill or bicycle ergometer. It is similar to a resting ECG, except that the limb electrodes are placed on the shoulders and hips rather than the wrists and ankles. The Bruce Protocol is the most commonly used. During an exercise ECG, BP is recorded and symptoms are assessed. Common indications for exercise testing are shown in Box 16.3. The test is considered positive if angina occurs, BP falls or fails to increase, or if there are ST segment shifts of more than 1 mm (see Fig. 16.57). Exercise testing is useful in confirming the diagnosis of coronary artery disease in patients with suspected angina, and under these circumstances has reasonable sensitivity and excellent specificity (see Box 16.3). False-negative results can occur in patients with coronary artery disease, and not all patients with a positive test have coronary disease. This is especially true in low-risk individuals, such as asymptomatic young or middle-aged women, in whom an abnormal response is more likely to represent a false-positive than a true-positive test. Stress testing is contraindicated in the presence of acute coronary syndrome, decompensated heart failure and severe hypertension.

Ambulatory ECG

Ambulatory ECG recordings can be obtained using a portable digital recorder. These devices usually provide limb lead ECG recordings only, on a continuous basis for periods of between 1 and 7 days. The main indication for ambulatory ECG is in the investigation of patients with suspected arrhythmia, such as those with intermittent palpitation, dizziness or syncope. In this situation, a standard ECG provides only a snapshot of the cardiac rhythm and is unlikely to detect an intermittent arrhythmia, so a longer period of recording is required (see Fig. 16.30). Ambulatory ECG can also be used to assess rate control in patients with atrial fibrillation, and to detect transient myocardial ischaemia using ST segment analysis. If symptoms are infrequent, special recorders can be issued that can be activated by the patient when a symptom episode occurs and placed on the chest wall to record the cardiac rhythm at that point in time. With some devices, the recording can be transmitted to hospital electronically. If the symptoms are very infrequent but potentially serious, such as syncope, implantable 'loop recorders' resembling a leadless pacemaker can be used and implanted subcutaneously to record cardiac rhythm for prolonged periods of between 1 and 3 years (see Fig. 16.51).

Cardiac biomarkers

Several biomarkers are available that can be measured in peripheral blood to assess myocardial dysfunction and ischaemia.

Brain natriuretic peptide

Brain natriuretic peptide (BNP) is a peptide hormone of 32 amino acids with diuretic properties. It is secreted by the LV as a 108-amino acid prohormone, which is cleaved to produce active BNP, and an inactive 76-amino acid N-terminal fragment (NT-proBNP). Serum concentrations are elevated in conditions associated with LV systolic dysfunction. Generally, NT-proBNP is measured in preference to BNP since it is more stable. Measurements of NT-proBNP are indicated for the diagnosis of LV dysfunction and to assess prognosis and response to therapy in patients with heart failure.

Cardiac troponins

Troponin I and troponin T are structural cardiac muscle proteins (see Fig. 16.5) that are released during myocyte damage and necrosis, and represent the cornerstone of the diagnosis of acute myocardial infarction (MI, see Box 16.47). Modern assays are extremely sensitive and can detect minor degrees of myocardial damage, so that elevated plasma troponin concentrations may be observed in conditions other than acute MI, such as pulmonary embolus, septic shock and pulmonary oedema.

16

Chest X-ray

This is useful for determining the size and shape of the heart, and the state of the pulmonary blood vessels and lung fields. Most information is given by a postero-anterior (PA) projection taken in full inspiration. Anteroposterior (AP) projections can be performed when patient movement is restricted but result in magnification of the cardiac silhouette.

An estimate of overall heart size can be made by comparing the maximum width of the cardiac outline with the maximum internal transverse diameter of the thoracic cavity. The term cardiomegaly is used to describe an enlarged cardiac silhouette when the ratio of cardiac width to the width of the lung fields is greater than 0.5. Cardiomegaly can be caused by chamber dilatation, especially left ventricular dilatation, or by a pericardial effusion, but may also be due to a mediastinal mass or pectus excavatum. Cardiomegaly is not a sensitive indicator of left ventricular systolic dysfunction since the cardiothoracic ratio is normal in many patients with poor left ventricular function and is not specific, since many patients with cardiomegaly on chest X-ray have normal echocardiograms.

Dilatation of individual cardiac chambers can be recognised by the characteristic alterations to the cardiac silhouette (Fig. 16.9):

- Left atrial dilatation results in prominence of the left atrial appendage, creating the appearance of a straight left heart border, a double cardiac shadow to the right of the sternum, and widening of the angle of the carina (bifurcation of the trachea) as the left main bronchus is pushed upwards.
- Right atrial enlargement projects from the right heart border towards the right lower lung field.
- Left ventricular dilatation causes prominence of the left heart border and enlargement of the cardiac silhouette. Left ventricular hypertrophy produces rounding of the left heart border (Fig. 16.10).
- Right ventricular dilatation increases heart size, displaces the apex upwards and straightens the left heart border.

Lateral or oblique projections may be useful for detecting pericardial calcification in patients with constrictive pericarditis or a calcified thoracic aortic aneurysm, as these abnormalities may be obscured by the spine on the PA view.

The lung fields on the chest X-ray may show congestion and oedema in patients with heart failure (see Fig. 16.25), and an increase in pulmonary blood flow ('pulmonary plethora') in those with left-to-right shunt. Pleural effusions may also occur in heart failure.

Echocardiography

Transthoracic echocardiography

Transthoracic echocardiography, commonly referred to as 'echo', is obtained by placing an ultrasound transducer on the chest wall to image the heart structures as a real-time two-dimensional 'slice'. This can be used for rapid evaluation of various aspects of cardiac structure and function (Box 16.4).

Doppler echocardiography

Doppler echocardiography provides information on blood flow within the heart and the great vessels. It is based on the Doppler principle that sound waves reflected from moving objects, such as red blood cells, undergo a frequency shift. Doppler echocardiography can therefore detect the speed and direction of blood flow in the heart chambers and great vessels. The information can be presented either as a plot of blood velocity against time for a particular point in the heart (Fig. 16.11) or as a colour overlay on a two-dimensional real-time echo picture (colour-flow Doppler, Fig. 16.12). Doppler echocardiography is useful in the detection

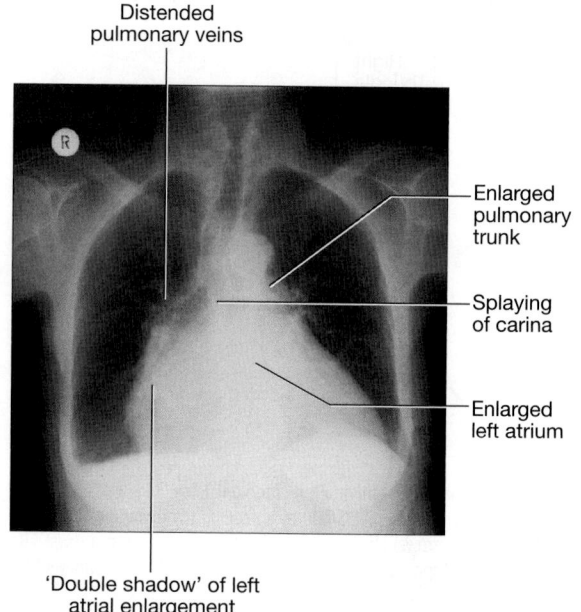

Fig. 16.9 Chest X-ray of a patient with mitral stenosis and regurgitation indicating enlargement of the LA and prominence of the pulmonary artery trunk.

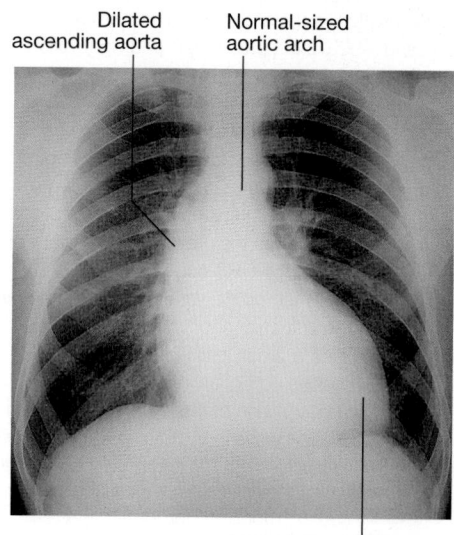

Fig. 16.10 Chest X-ray of a patient with aortic regurgitation, left ventricular enlargement and dilatation of the ascending aorta.

i | 16.4 Common indications for echocardiography

- Assessment of left ventricular function
- Diagnosis and quantification of severity of valve disease
- Identification of vegetations in endocarditis
- Identification of structural heart disease in atrial fibrillation, cardiomyopathies or congenital heart disease
- Detection of pericardial effusion
- Identification of structural heart disease or intracardiac thrombus in systemic embolism

of valvular regurgitation, where the direction of blood flow is reversed and turbulence is seen, and is also used to detect pressure gradients across stenosed valves. For example, the normal resting systolic flow velocity across the aortic valve is approximately 1 m/sec; in the presence of aortic

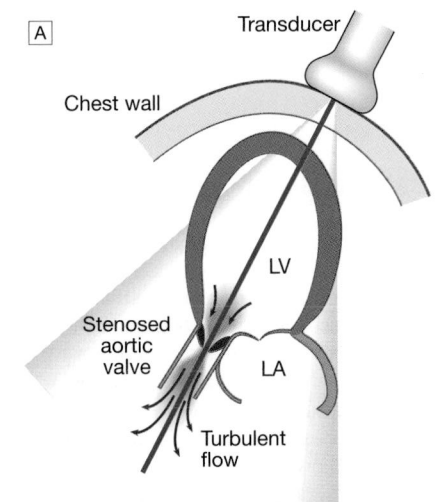

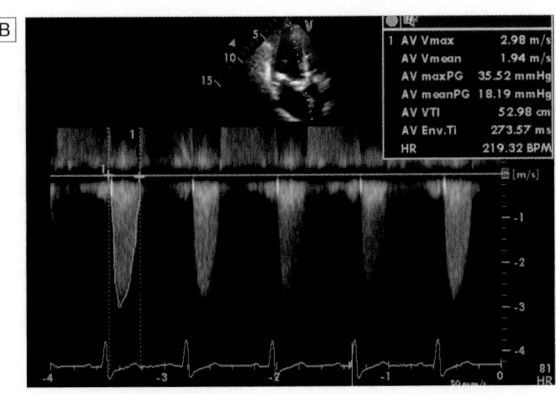

Fig. 16.11 **Doppler echocardiography in aortic stenosis.** ⒜ The aortic valve is imaged and a Doppler beam passed directly through the left ventricular outflow tract and the aorta into the turbulent flow beyond the stenosed valve. ⒝ The velocity of the blood cells is recorded to determine the maximum velocity and hence the pressure gradient across the valve. In this example, the peak velocity is approximately 450 cm/sec (4.5 m/sec), indicating severe aortic stenosis (peak gradient of 81 mmHg). (LA = left atrium; LV = left ventricle)

stenosis, this is increased as blood accelerates through the narrow orifice. In severe aortic stenosis, the peak aortic velocity may be increased to 5 m/sec (see Fig. 16.11). An estimate of the pressure gradient across a valve or lesion is given by the modified Bernoulli equation:

$$\text{Pressure gradient (mmHg)} = 4 \times (\text{peak velocity (m/sec)})^2$$

Advanced techniques include three-dimensional echocardiography, intravascular ultrasound (defines vessel wall abnormalities and guides coronary intervention), intracardiac ultrasound (provides high-resolution images), tissue Doppler imaging (quantifies myocardial contractility and diastolic function) and speckle tracking (assesses myocardial motion and strain).

Transoesophageal echocardiography

Transoesophageal echocardiography (TOE) involves passing an endoscope-like ultrasound probe into the oesophagus and upper stomach under light sedation and positioning it behind the LA. It is particularly useful for imaging structures such as the left atrial appendage, pulmonary veins, thoracic aorta and interatrial septum, which may be poorly visualised by transthoracic echocardiography, especially if the patient is overweight or has obstructive airways disease. The high-resolution

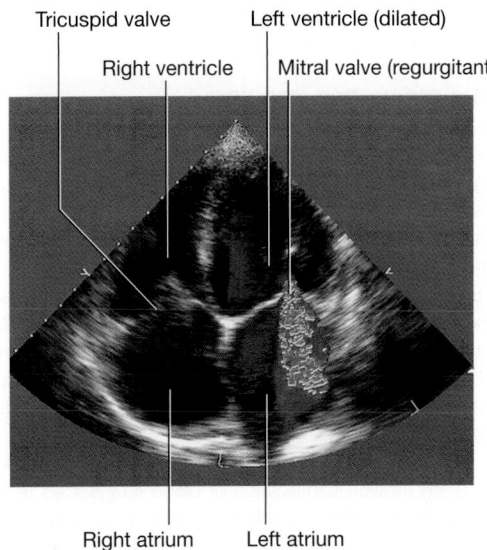

Fig. 16.12 **Echocardiographic illustration of the principal cardiac structures in the 'four-chamber' view.** Colour-flow Doppler has been used to demonstrate mitral regurgitation: a flame-shaped (yellow/blue) turbulent jet into the left atrium.

images that can be obtained makes TOE particularly valuable for investigating patients with prosthetic (especially mitral) valve dysfunction, congenital abnormalities such as atrial septal defects, aortic dissection, infective endocarditis (vegetations that are too small to be detected by transthoracic echocardiography) and systemic embolism (intracardiac thrombus or masses).

Stress echocardiography

Stress echocardiography is used to investigate patients with suspected coronary artery disease who are unsuitable for exercise stress testing, such as those with mobility problems or pre-existing bundle branch block. A two-dimensional echo is performed before and during infusion of a moderate to high dose of an inotrope, such as dobutamine. Myocardial segments with poor perfusion become ischaemic and contract poorly under stress, manifesting as a wall motion abnormality on the scan. Stress echocardiography is sometimes used to examine myocardial viability in patients with impaired left ventricular function. Low-dose dobutamine can induce contraction in 'hibernating' myocardium; such patients may benefit from bypass surgery or percutaneous coronary intervention.

Computed tomography

Computed tomography (CT) is useful for imaging the cardiac chambers, great vessels, pericardium, and mediastinal structures and masses. Multidetector scanners can acquire up to 320 slices per rotation, allowing very high-resolution imaging in a single heartbeat. CT is often performed using a timed injection of X-ray contrast to produce clear images of blood vessels and associated pathologies. Contrast scans are very useful for imaging the aorta in suspected aortic dissection (see Fig. 16.73), and the pulmonary arteries and branches in suspected pulmonary embolism.

Some centres use cardiac CT scans for quantification of coronary artery calcification, which may serve as an index of cardiovascular risk. However, modern multidetector scanning allows non-invasive coronary angiography (Fig. 16.13) with a spatial resolution approaching that of conventional coronary arteriography and at a lower radiation dose. CT coronary angiography is particularly useful in the initial assessment of patients with chest pain and a low or intermediate likelihood of disease, since it has a high negative predictive value in excluding coronary artery

16

disease. Modern volume scanners are also able to assess myocardial perfusion, often at the same sitting.

Magnetic resonance imaging

Magnetic resonance imaging (MRI) can be used to generate cross-sectional images of the heart, lungs and mediastinal structures. It provides better differentiation of soft tissue structures than CT but is poor at demonstrating calcification. MRI scans need to be 'gated' to the ECG, allowing the scanner to produce moving images of the heart and mediastinal structures throughout the cardiac cycle. MRI is very useful for imaging the aorta, including suspected dissection (see Fig. 16.72), and can define the anatomy of the heart and great vessels in patients with congenital heart disease. It is also useful for detecting infiltrative conditions affecting the heart and for evaluation of the RV that is difficult to image by echocardiography.

Physiological data can be obtained from the signal returned from moving blood, which allows quantification of blood flow across regurgitant or stenotic valves. It is also possible to analyse regional wall motion in patients with suspected coronary disease or cardiomyopathy.

Myocardial perfusion and viability can also be readily assessed by MRI. When enhanced by gadolinium-based contrast media, areas of myocardial hypoperfusion can be identified with better spatial resolution than nuclear medicine techniques. Later redistribution of this contrast, so-called delayed enhancement, can be used to identify myocardial scarring and fibrosis: this is a particular strength of cardiac MRI (Fig. 16.14). This can help in selecting patients for revascularisation procedures, or in identifying those with myocardial infiltration, such as that seen with sarcoid heart disease and arrhythmogenic right ventricular cardiomyopathy.

Cardiac catheterisation

This involves passing a specialised catheter through a peripheral vein or artery into the heart under X-ray guidance. Cardiac catheterisation allows BP and oxygen saturation to be measured in the cardiac chambers and great vessels, and is used to perform angiograms by injecting contrast media into a chamber or blood vessel.

Left heart catheterisation involves accessing the arterial circulation, usually through the radial artery, to allow catheterisation of the aorta, LV and coronary arteries. Coronary angiography is the most widely performed procedure, in which the left and right coronary arteries are selectively imaged, providing information about the extent and severity of coronary stenoses, thrombus and calcification (Fig. 16.15). Additional anatomical (intravascular ultrasound, optical coherence tomography) or functional (pressure wire) assessments are sometimes used to define plaque characteristics and severity more precisely. This permits planning of percutaneous coronary intervention and coronary artery bypass graft surgery. Left ventriculography can be performed during the procedure to determine the size and function of the LV (Fig. 16.16) and to demonstrate mitral regurgitation. Aortography defines the size of the aortic root and thoracic aorta, and can help quantify aortic regurgitation. Left heart catheterisation is a day-case procedure and is relatively safe, with serious complications occurring in only approximately 1 in 1000 cases.

Right heart catheterisation is used to assess right heart and pulmonary artery pressures, and to detect intracardiac shunts by measuring oxygen saturations in different chambers. For example, a step up in oxygen saturation from 65% in the RA to 80% in the pulmonary artery is indicative of a large left-to-right shunt that might be due to a ventricular septal defect. Cardiac output can also be measured using thermodilution techniques. Left atrial pressure can be measured directly by puncturing the interatrial septum from the RA with a special catheter. For most purposes, a satisfactory approximation to left atrial pressure can be obtained by 'wedging' an end-hole or balloon catheter in a branch of the pulmonary artery. Swan–Ganz balloon catheters are often used to monitor pulmonary 'wedge' pressure as a guide to left heart filling pressure in critically ill patients (see Fig. 9.25).

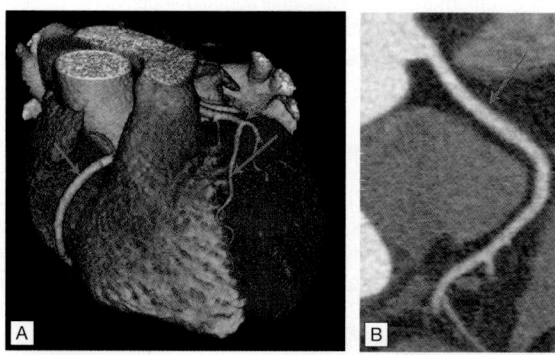

Fig. 16.13 **Computed tomography coronary angiography, demonstrating normal coronary arteries (arrows).** [A] Three-dimensional image. [B] Two-dimensional image.

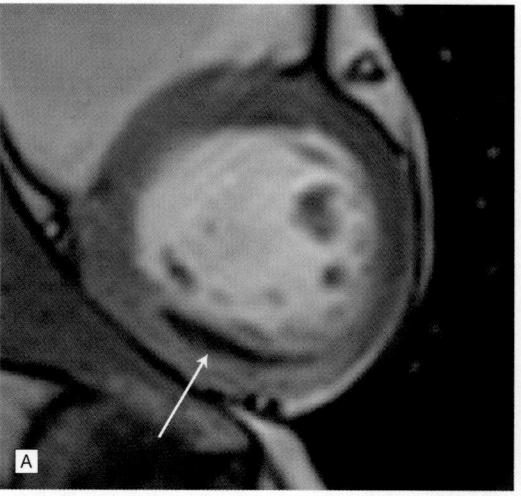
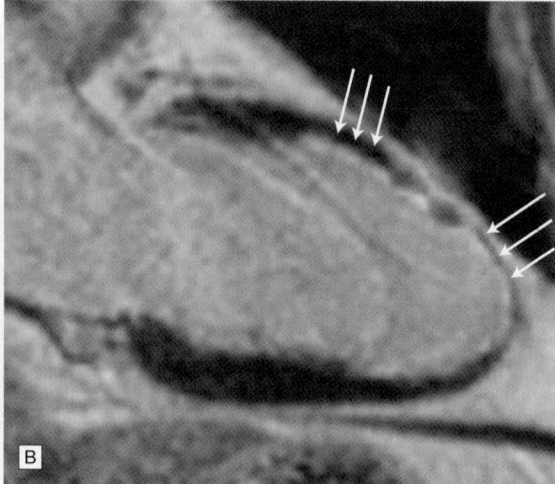

Fig. 16.14 **Cardiac magnetic resonance imaging.** [A] Recent inferior myocardial infarction with black area of microvascular obstruction (arrow). [B] Old anterior myocardial infarction with large area of subendocardial delayed gadolinium enhancement (white area, arrows).

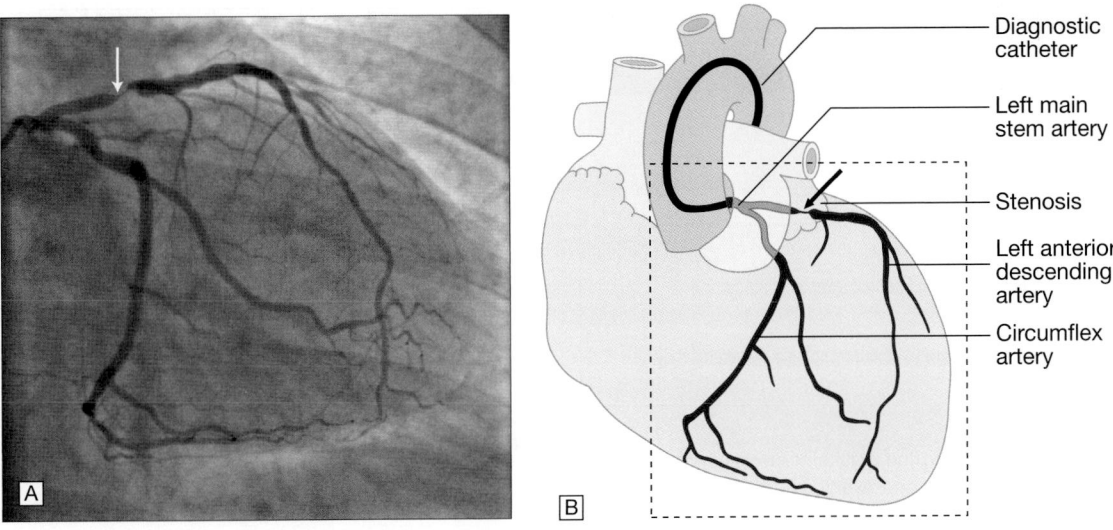

Fig. 16.15 The left anterior descending and circumflex coronary arteries with a stenosis (arrow) in the left anterior descending vessel. [A] Coronary artery angiogram. [B] Schematic of the vessels and branches.

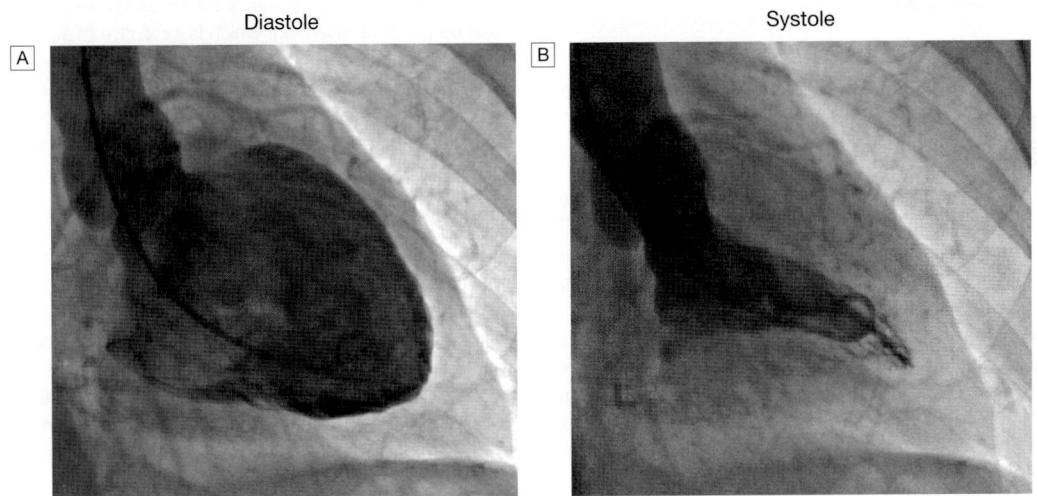

Fig. 16.16 Left ventriculograms in diastole [A] and systole [B] in a patient with normal left ventricular contraction.

Electrophysiology

Patients with known or suspected arrhythmia are investigated by percutaneous placement of electrode catheters into the heart via the femoral and neck veins. An electrophysiology study (EPS) is most commonly performed to evaluate patients for catheter ablation and is normally done at the same time as the ablation procedure. EPS is occasionally used for risk stratification of patients suspected of being at risk of ventricular arrhythmias.

Radionuclide imaging

Radionuclide imaging can be used to evaluate cardiac function but is declining in popularity due to the availability of alternative techniques, such as MRI and CT, that either do not involve exposure to radiation or provide superior quality data to radionuclide imaging.

Blood pool imaging

The patient is given an intravenous injection of radioisotope-labelled blood cells, and after 4–5 minutes, the distribution of isotope in the heart is evaluated by a gamma camera at different phases of the cardiac cycle, thereby permitting the calculation of ventricular ejection fractions. It can also assess the size and 'shape' of the cardiac chambers.

Myocardial perfusion scanning

The patient is given an intravenous injection of a radioactive isotope, such as ^{99}technetium-tetrofosmin, and scintiscans of the myocardium are subsequently obtained by gamma camera at rest and during stress (see Fig. 16.57). Either exercise stress or pharmacological stress (using the inotrope dobutamine or the vasodilator dipyridamole) can be used. More sophisticated quantitative information can be obtained with positron emission tomography (PET), which can also be used to assess myocardial metabolism, but this is available in only a few centres.

Presenting problems in cardiovascular disease

Cardiovascular disease gives rise to several symptoms, which may overlap those caused by pathologies of other systems. Making the correct diagnosis depends on careful analysis of the factors that provoke symptoms, the subtle differences in how they are described by the

16.5 New York Heart Association (NYHA) functional classification

Class I
- No limitation during ordinary activity

Class II
- Slight limitation during ordinary activity

Class III
- Marked limitation of normal activities without symptoms at rest

Class IV
- Unable to undertake physical activity without symptoms; symptoms may be present at rest

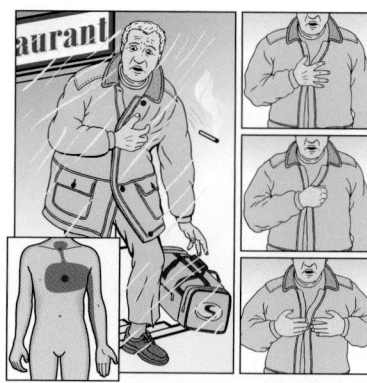

Fig. 16.17 Typical ischaemic cardiac pain. Characteristic hand gestures used to describe cardiac pain. Typical radiation of pain is shown in the schematic.

patient, the clinical findings and the results of investigations. A close relationship between symptoms and exertion is usually suggestive of heart disease. The New York Heart Association (NYHA) functional classification is used to grade the degree of disability caused by cardiac symptoms (Box 16.5).

Chest pain on exertion

There are many other non-cardiac causes of chest pain, as discussed in Chapter 9. This section will focus on exertional chest pain (or discomfort), which is a typical presenting symptom of coronary artery disease.

Clinical assessment

Detailed history taking is crucial in determining the likely cause of chest pain. Chest pain on exertion suggests angina pectoris (Fig. 16.17). The reproducibility, predictability and relationship to physical exertion (and occasionally emotion) of the chest pain are the most important features. The duration of symptoms should be noted because patients with recent-onset angina are at greater risk than those with long-standing and unchanged symptoms. Physical examination is often normal but may reveal evidence of risk factors for cardiovascular disease, such as xanthoma or xanthelasma indicating hyperlipidaemia. Signs of anaemia or thyrotoxicosis may be identified, both of which can exacerbate angina. Cardiovascular examination may reveal evidence of left ventricular dysfunction or cardiac murmurs in patients with aortic valve disease and hypertrophic cardiomyopathy. Other manifestations of arterial disease, such as bruits and loss of peripheral pulses, may also be observed.

Investigations

A full blood count, fasting blood glucose, lipids, thyroid function tests and a 12-lead ECG are the most important baseline investigations. Stress testing, including exercise ECG, stress echocardiography and magnetic resonance perfusion imaging, can be helpful in confirming anginal symptoms and identifying high-risk patients who require further investigation and treatment but cannot reliably exclude the presence of coronary artery disease. However, CT coronary angiography is the first-line test of choice to diagnose angina due to coronary artery disease. If a murmur is found, echocardiography should be performed to check for valve disease or hypertrophic cardiomyopathy.

Severe prolonged chest pain

Severe prolonged cardiac chest pain may be due to acute myocardial infarction or to unstable angina – known collectively as acute coronary syndrome.

Clinical assessment

Acute coronary syndrome is suggested by a previous history of stable angina but an episode of acute severe chest pain at rest can also be the

first presentation of coronary artery disease. Making the correct diagnosis depends on analysing the character of the pain and its associated features. Physical examination may reveal signs of risk factors for coronary artery disease as described for exertional chest pain. There may also be pallor or sweating, which is indicative of autonomic disturbance and typical of acute coronary syndrome. Other features, such as arrhythmia, hypotension and heart failure, may occur. Patients presenting with symptoms consistent with an acute coronary syndrome require hospitalisation and urgent investigation, because there is a high risk of avoidable complications.

Investigations

A 12-lead ECG is mandatory and is the most useful method of initial triage, along with measurement of cardiac troponin I or T. The diagnosis of an acute coronary syndrome is supported by ST segment elevation or depression on ECG and an elevated level of troponin I or T, which demonstrates that there has been myocardial damage.

If the diagnosis remains unclear after initial investigation, repeat ECG recordings should be performed and are particularly useful if they can be obtained during an episode of pain. If the plasma troponin concentrations are normal at baseline, repeat measurements should be made 6–12 hours after the onset of symptoms or admission to hospital. New ECG changes or an elevated plasma troponin concentration usually confirm the diagnosis of an acute coronary syndrome. If the pain settles and does not recur, there are no new ECG changes and troponin concentrations remain normal, the patient can be discharged from hospital but further investigations may be indicated to look for evidence of coronary artery disease, as discussed on page 424.

Management

The differential diagnosis and management of acute coronary syndrome are described in more detail later in this chapter.

Breathlessness

Cardiac causes of breathlessness include cardiac arrhythmias, acute and chronic heart failure, acute coronary syndrome, valvular disease, cardiomyopathy and constrictive pericarditis, all discussed later in this chapter. The differential diagnosis of breathlessness is wide, however, and has many other non-cardiac causes. These are discussed in more detail on pages 181 and 489.

Syncope

The term 'syncope' refers to loss of consciousness due to reduced cerebral perfusion. The differential diagnosis, investigation and management of syncope are discussed on page 184.

Palpitation

Palpitation is a common and sometimes frightening symptom that is usually due to a disorder of cardiac rhythm. Patients use the term to describe many sensations, including an unusually erratic, fast, slow or forceful heart beat, or even chest pain or breathlessness.

Clinical assessment

Initial evaluation should concentrate on determining the likely mechanism of palpitation and whether or not there is significant underlying heart disease. A detailed description of the sensation is essential and patients should be asked to describe their symptoms clearly, or to demonstrate the sensation of rhythm by tapping with their hand. A provisional diagnosis can usually be made on the basis of the history (Box 16.6 and Fig. 16.18). Recurrent but short-lived bouts of an irregular heart rhythm are usually due to atrial or ventricular extrasystoles (ectopic beats). Some patients will describe the experience as a 'flip' or a 'jump' in the chest, while others report dropped or missed beats. Extrasystoles are often more frequent during periods of stress or debility; they can be triggered by alcohol or nicotine.

Episodes of a pounding, forceful and relatively fast (90–120/min) heart beat are a common manifestation of anxiety. These may also reflect a hyperdynamic circulation, such as anaemia, pregnancy and thyrotoxicosis, and can occur in some forms of valve disease such as aortic regurgitation. Discrete bouts of more rapid (over 120/min) heart beats are more likely to be due to a paroxysmal supraventricular or ventricular tachycardia. In contrast, episodes of atrial fibrillation typically present with irregular and usually rapid palpitation.

Investigation

If initial assessment suggests that the palpitation is due to an arrhythmia, the diagnosis should be confirmed by an ECG recording during an episode using an ambulatory ECG monitor. Smartphones and smart watches with additional hardware and apps are extremely helpful in capturing the ECG during episodes. Additional investigations may be required depending on the nature of the arrhythmia, as discussed later in this chapter.

Management

Palpitation is usually benign and even if the patient's symptoms are due to an arrhythmia, the outlook is good if there is no underlying structural heart disease. Most cases are due to an awareness of the normal heart beat, a sinus tachycardia or benign extrasystoles, in which case an explanation and reassurance may be all that is required. Palpitation associated with pre-syncope or syncope (p. 184) may reflect more serious structural or electrical disease and should be investigated without delay. Other arrhythmias may require treatment, such as drugs or ablation, and are discussed in more detail in the section on cardiac arrythmias

Cardiac arrest

Cardiac arrest describes the sudden and complete loss of cardiac output due to asystole, ventricular tachycardia or ventricular fibrillation

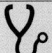

16.6 How to evaluate palpitation

- Is the palpitation continuous or intermittent?
- Is the heart beat regular or irregular?
- What is the approximate heart rate?
- Do symptoms occur in discrete attacks?
   - Is the onset abrupt? How do attacks terminate?
- Are there any associated symptoms?
   - Chest pain, lightheadedness, polyuria (a feature of supraventricular tachycardia)
- Are there any precipitating factors, such as exercise or alcohol excess?
- Is there a history of structural heart disease, such as coronary artery disease or valvular heart disease?

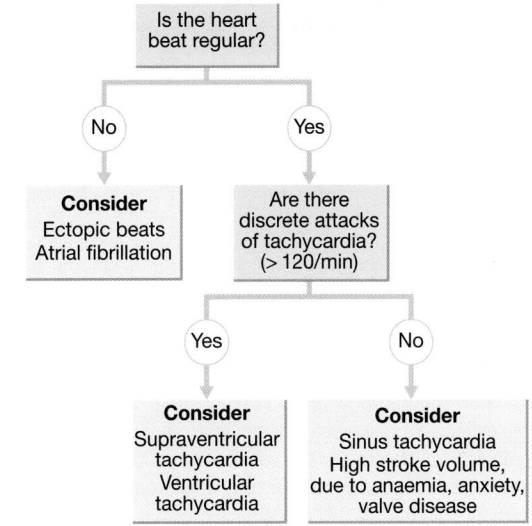

Fig. 16.18 A simple approach to the diagnosis of palpitation.

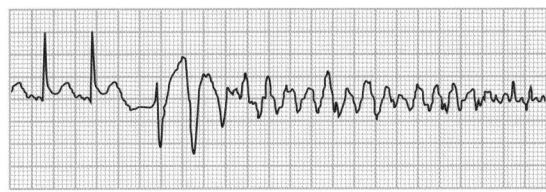

Fig. 16.19 Ventricular fibrillation. A bizarre chaotic rhythm, initiated in this case by two ventricular ectopic beats in rapid succession.

(Fig. 16.19), or loss of mechanical cardiac contraction (pulseless electrical activity). The causes of sudden arrhythmic death are summarised in Box 16.7. The clinical diagnosis is based on the victim being unconscious and pulseless; breathing may take some time to stop completely after cardiac arrest. Death is virtually inevitable, unless effective treatment is given promptly. Sudden cardiac death is usually caused by a catastrophic arrhythmia and accounts for 25%–30% of all deaths from cardiovascular disease, claiming an estimated 70000 to 90000 lives each year in the UK. Many of these deaths are potentially preventable. Management of cardiac arrest is further discussed in detail on page 202.

16.7 Causes of sudden arrhythmic death

Coronary artery disease (85%)

- Myocardial ischaemia
- Acute myocardial infarction
- Prior myocardial infarction with myocardial scarring

Structural heart disease (10%)

- Aortic stenosis
- Hypertrophic cardiomyopathy
- Dilated cardiomyopathy
- Arrhythmogenic right ventricular cardiomyopathy
- Congenital heart disease

No structural heart disease (5%)

- Long QT syndrome
- Brugada syndrome
- Wolff–Parkinson–White syndrome
- Adverse drug reactions (torsades de pointes)
- Severe electrolyte abnormalities

16

Abnormal heart sounds

The first indication of heart disease may be the discovery of an abnormal sound on auscultation (Box 16.8). This may be incidental – for example, during a routine examination – or may be prompted by symptoms of heart disease.

Clinical assessment

The aims of clinical assessment are, first, to determine if the abnormal sound is cardiac; second, to determine if it is pathological; and third, to try to determine its cause.

Is the sound cardiac?

Additional heart sounds and murmurs demonstrate a consistent relationship to the cardiac cycle, whereas extracardiac sounds, such as a pleural rub or venous hum, do not. Pericardial friction produces a characteristic scratching noise termed a pericardial rub, which may have two components corresponding to atrial and ventricular systole, and may vary with posture and respiration.

Is the sound pathological?

Pathological sounds and murmurs are the product of turbulent blood flow or rapid ventricular filling due to abnormal loading conditions. Some added sounds are physiological but may also occur in pathological conditions; for example, a third sound is common in young people and in pregnancy but is also a feature of heart failure (see Box 16.8). Similarly, a systolic murmur due to turbulence across the right ventricular outflow tract may occur in hyperdynamic states such as anaemia or pregnancy, but may also be due to pulmonary stenosis or an intracardiac shunt leading to volume overload of the RV, such as an atrial septal defect. Benign murmurs do not occur in diastole (Box 16.9), and systolic murmurs that radiate or are associated with a thrill are almost always pathological.

i	**16.9 Features of a benign or innocent heart murmur**

- Soft
- Mid-systolic
- Heard at left sternal border
- No radiation
- No other cardiac abnormalities

What is the origin of the sound?

Timing, intensity, location, radiation and quality are all useful clues to the origin and nature of an additional sound or murmur (Box 16.10). Radiation of a murmur is determined by the direction of turbulent blood flow and is detectable only when there is a high-velocity jet, such as in mitral regurgitation (radiation from apex to axilla) or aortic stenosis (radiation from base to neck). Similarly, the pitch and quality of the sound can help to distinguish the murmur, such as the 'blowing' murmur of mitral regurgitation or the 'rasping' murmur of aortic stenosis. The position of a murmur in relation to the cardiac cycle is crucial and should be assessed by timing it with the heart sounds, carotid pulse and apex beat (Figs. 16.20 and 16.21).

Systolic murmurs

Ejection systolic murmurs are associated with ventricular outflow tract obstruction and occur in mid-systole with a crescendo–decrescendo pattern, reflecting the changing velocity of blood flow (Box 16.11). Pansystolic murmurs maintain a constant intensity and extend from the first heart sound throughout systole to the second heart sound, sometimes obscuring it. They occur when blood leaks from a ventricle into a low-pressure chamber at an even or constant velocity. Mitral regurgitation, tricuspid regurgitation and ventricular septal defect are the only causes of a pansystolic murmur. Late systolic murmurs are unusual but may occur in mitral valve prolapse, if the mitral regurgitation is confined to late systole, and hypertrophic obstructive cardiomyopathy, if dynamic obstruction occurs late in systole.

i	**16.8 Normal and abnormal heart sounds**				
Sound	**Timing**	**Characteristics**	**Mechanisms**	**Variable features**
First heart sound (S1)	Onset of systole	Usually single or narrowly split	Closure of mitral and tricuspid valves	Loud: hyperdynamic circulation (anaemia, pregnancy, thyrotoxicosis); mitral stenosis
				Soft: heart failure; mitral regurgitation
Second heart sound (S2)	End of systole	Split on inspiration Single on expiration	Closure of aortic and pulmonary valve	Fixed wide splitting with atrial septal defect
			A_2 first	Wide but variable splitting with delayed right heart emptying (right bundle branch block)
			P_2 second	Reversed splitting due to delayed left heart emptying (left bundle branch block)
Third heart sound (S3)	Early in diastole, just after S2	Low pitch, often heard as 'gallop'	From ventricular wall due to abrupt cessation of rapid filling	Physiological: young people, pregnancy
				Pathological: heart failure, mitral regurgitation
Fourth heart sound (S4)	End of diastole, just before S1	Low pitch	Ventricular origin (stiff ventricle and augmented atrial contraction) related to atrial filling	Absent in atrial fibrillation
				A feature of severe left ventricular hypertrophy
Systolic clicks	Early or mid-systole	Brief, high-intensity sound	Valvular aortic stenosis	Click may be lost when stenotic valve becomes thickened or calcified
			Valvular pulmonary stenosis	
			Floppy mitral valve	Prosthetic clicks lost when valve obstructed by thrombus or vegetations
			Prosthetic heart sounds from opening and closing of normally functioning mechanical valves	
Opening snap (OS)	Early in diastole	High pitch, brief duration	Opening of stenosed leaflets of mitral valve	Moves closer to S2 as mitral stenosis becomes more severe. May be absent in calcific mitral stenosis
			Prosthetic heart sounds	

16.10 How to assess a heart murmur

When does it occur?

- Time the murmur using heart sounds, carotid pulse and the apex beat. Is it systolic or diastolic?
- Does the murmur extend throughout systole or diastole or is it confined to a shorter part of the cardiac cycle?

How loud is it?

- Grade 1: very soft (audible only in ideal conditions)
- Grade 2: soft
- Grade 3: moderate
- Grade 4: loud with associated thrill
- Grade 5: very loud
- Grade 6: heard without stethoscope

   Note: Diastolic murmurs are very rarely above grade 4

Where is it heard best?

- Listen over the apex and base of the heart, including the aortic and pulmonary areas

Where does it radiate?

- Listen at the neck, axilla or back

What does it sound like?

- Pitch is determined by flow (high pitch indicates high-velocity flow)
- Is the intensity constant or variable?

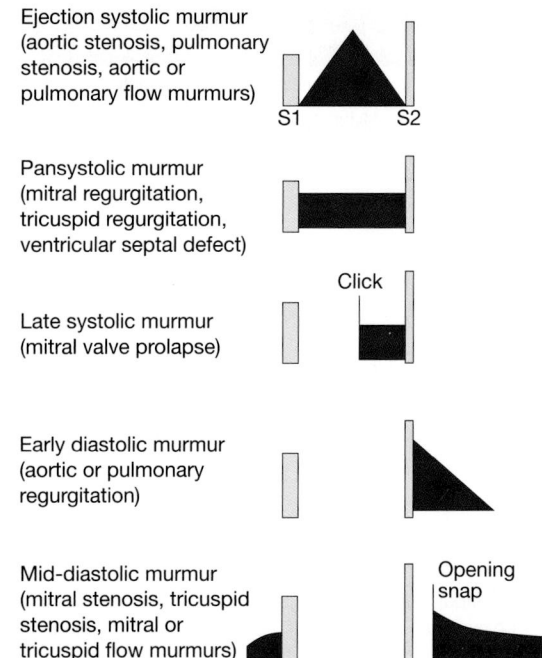

Fig. 16.21 **The timing and pattern of cardiac murmurs.**

Diastolic murmurs

These are due to accelerated or turbulent flow across the mitral or tricuspid valves. They are low-pitched noises that are often difficult to hear and should be evaluated with the bell of the stethoscope. A mid-diastolic murmur may be due to mitral stenosis (located at the apex and axilla), tricuspid stenosis (located at the left sternal border), increased flow across the mitral valve (for example, the to-and-fro murmur of severe mitral regurgitation) or increased flow across the tricuspid valve (for example, a left-to-right shunt through a large atrial septal defect). Early diastolic murmurs have a soft, blowing quality with a decrescendo pattern and should be evaluated with the diaphragm of the stethoscope. They are due to regurgitation across the aortic or pulmonary valves and are best heard at the left sternal border, with the patient sitting forwards in held expiration.

Continuous murmurs

These result from a combination of systolic and diastolic flow, such as occurs with a persistent ductus arteriosus, and must be distinguished from extracardiac noises such as bruits from arterial shunts, venous hums (high rates of venous flow in children) and pericardial friction rubs.

Investigations

If clinical evaluation suggests that the additional sound is cardiac and likely to be pathological, then echocardiography is indicated to determine the underlying cause.

Management

Management of patients with additional heart sounds or murmurs depends on the underlying cause. More details are provided in the sections on specific valve defects and congenital anomalies later in this chapter.

Heart failure

Heart failure describes the clinical syndrome that develops when the heart cannot maintain adequate output, or can do so only at the expense of elevated ventricular filling pressure. In mild to moderate forms of heart failure, symptoms occur only when the metabolic demand increases during exercise or some other form of stress. In severe heart failure, symptoms may be

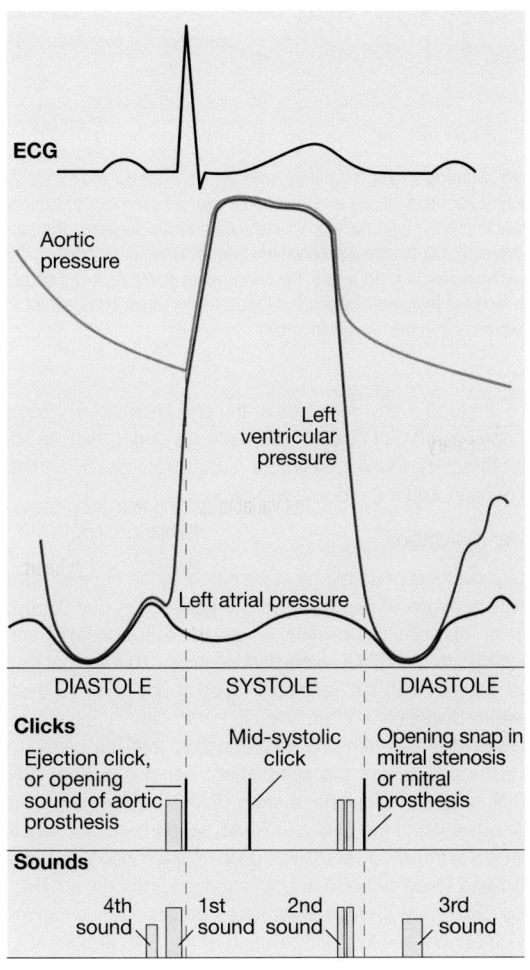

Fig. 16.20 **The relationship of the cardiac cycle to the ECG, the left ventricular pressure wave and the position of heart sounds.**

i 16.11 Features of some common systolic murmurs				
Condition	**Timing and duration**	**Quality**	**Location and radiation**	**Associated features**
Aortic stenosis	Mid-systolic	Loud, rasping	Base and left sternal border, radiating to suprasternal notch and carotids	Single second heart sound Ejection click (in young patients) Slow-rising pulse Left ventricular hypertrophy (pressure overload)
Mitral regurgitation	Pansystolic	Blowing	Apex, radiating to axilla	Soft first heart sound Third heart sound Left ventricular hypertrophy (volume overload)
Ventricular septal defect	Pansystolic	Harsh	Lower left sternal border, radiating to whole precordium	Thrill Biventricular hypertrophy
Benign	Mid-systolic	Soft	Left sternal border, no radiation	No other signs of heart disease

present at rest. In clinical practice, heart failure may be diagnosed when a patient with significant heart disease develops the signs or symptoms of a low cardiac output, pulmonary congestion or systemic venous congestion at rest or on exercise. Three types of heart failure are recognised.

Left heart failure

This is characterised by a reduction in left ventricular output and an increase in left atrial and pulmonary venous pressure. If left heart failure occurs suddenly – for example, as the result of an acute MI – the rapid increase in left atrial pressure causes pulmonary oedema. If the rise in atrial pressure is more gradual, as occurs with mitral stenosis, there is reflex pulmonary vasoconstriction, which protects the patient from pulmonary oedema. However, the resulting increase in pulmonary vascular resistance causes pulmonary hypertension, which in turn impairs right ventricular function.

Right heart failure

This is characterised by a reduction in right ventricular output and an increase in right atrial and systemic venous pressure. The most common causes are chronic lung disease, pulmonary embolism and pulmonary valvular stenosis. The term 'cor pulmonale' is used to describe right heart failure that is secondary to chronic lung disease.

Biventricular heart failure

In biventricular failure, both sides of the heart are affected. This may occur because the disease process, such as dilated cardiomyopathy or coronary heart disease, affects both ventricles or because disease of the left heart leads to chronic elevation of the left atrial pressure, pulmonary hypertension and right heart failure.

Epidemiology

Heart failure predominantly affects older people; the prevalence is 1.6% in the UK adult population but affects more than 10% in those aged 80–89 years. In the UK, most patients admitted to hospital with heart failure are more than 70 years old; they typically remain hospitalised for a week or more and may be left with chronic disability. Although the outlook depends, to some extent, on the underlying cause of the problem, untreated heart failure generally carries a poor prognosis; approximately 50% of patients with severe heart failure due to left ventricular dysfunction will die within 2 years because of either pump failure or malignant ventricular arrhythmias. The most common causes are coronary artery disease and myocardial infarction but almost all forms of heart disease can lead to heart failure, as summarised in Box 16.12. An accurate diagnosis is important because treatment of the underlying cause may reverse heart failure or prevent its progression.

Pathogenesis

Heart failure occurs when cardiac output fails to meet the demands of the circulation. Cardiac output is determined by preload (the volume and

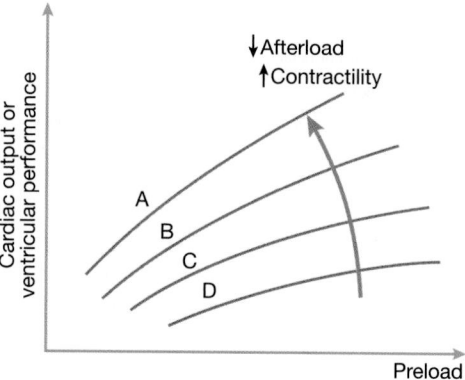

Fig. 16.22 Starling's Law. Normal (A), mild (B), moderate (C) and severe (D) heart failure. Ventricular performance is related to the degree of myocardial stretching. An increase in preload (end-diastolic volume, end-diastolic pressure, filling pressure or atrial pressure) will therefore enhance function; however, overstretching causes marked deterioration. In heart failure, the curve moves to the right and becomes flatter. An increase in myocardial contractility or a reduction in afterload will shift the curve upwards and to the left (green arrow).

pressure of blood in the ventricles at the end of diastole), afterload (the volume and pressure of blood in the ventricles during systole) and myocardial contractility, forming the basis of Starling's Law (Fig. 16.22). The causes of heart failure are discussed below.

Ventricular dysfunction

Ventricular dysfunction is the most common cause of heart failure. This can occur because of impaired systolic contraction due to myocardial disease, or diastolic dysfunction where there is abnormal ventricular relaxation due to a stiff, non-compliant ventricle. This is most commonly found in patients with left ventricular hypertrophy. Systolic dysfunction and diastolic dysfunction often coexist, particularly in patients with coronary artery disease. Ventricular dysfunction reduces cardiac output, which, in turn, activates the sympathetic nervous system (SNS) and renin–angiotensin–aldosterone system (RAAS). Under normal circumstances, activation of the SNS and RAAS supports cardiac function but, in the setting of impaired ventricular function, the consequences are negative and lead to an increase in both afterload and preload (Fig. 16.23). A vicious circle may then be established because any additional fall in cardiac output causes further activation of the SNS and RAAS, and an additional increase in peripheral vascular resistance.

Activation of the RAAS causes vasoconstriction and sodium and water retention. This is primarily mediated by angiotensin II, a potent constrictor of arterioles, in both the kidney and the systemic circulation (see Fig. 16.23). Activation of the SNS also occurs and can initially sustain cardiac output through increased myocardial contractility and heart

	16.12	Mechanisms of heart failure

Cause	Examples	Features
Reduced ventricular contractility	Myocardial infarction (segmental dysfunction)	In coronary artery disease, 'akinetic' or 'dyskinetic' segments contract poorly and may impede the function of normal segments by distorting their contraction and relaxation patterns
	Myocarditis/cardiomyopathy (global dysfunction)	Progressive ventricular dilatation
Ventricular outflow obstruction (pressure overload)	Hypertension, aortic stenosis (left heart failure)	Initially, concentric ventricular hypertrophy allows the ventricle to maintain a normal output by generating a high systolic pressure. Later, secondary changes in the myocardium and increasing obstruction lead to failure with ventricular dilatation and rapid clinical deterioration
	Pulmonary hypertension, pulmonary valve stenosis (right heart failure)	
Ventricular inflow obstruction	Mitral stenosis, tricuspid stenosis	Small, vigorous ventricle; dilated, hypertrophied atrium. Atrial fibrillation is common and often causes marked deterioration because ventricular filling depends heavily on atrial contraction
Ventricular volume overload	Left ventricular volume overload (mitral or aortic regurgitation)	Dilatation and hypertrophy allow the ventricle to generate a high stroke volume and help to maintain a normal cardiac output. However, secondary changes in the myocardium lead to impaired contractility and worsening heart failure
	Ventricular septal defect	
	Right ventricular volume overload (atrial septal defect)	
	Increased metabolic demand (high output)	
Arrhythmia	Atrial fibrillation	Tachycardia does not allow for adequate filling of the heart, resulting in reduced cardiac output and back pressure
	Tachycardia	Prolonged tachycardia causes myocardial fatigue
	Complete heart block	Bradycardia limits cardiac output, even if stroke volume is normal
Diastolic dysfunction	Constrictive pericarditis	Marked fluid retention and peripheral oedema, ascites, pleural effusions and elevated jugular veins
	Restrictive cardiomyopathy	Bi-atrial enlargement (restrictive filling pattern and high atrial pressures). Atrial fibrillation may cause deterioration
	Left ventricular hypertrophy and fibrosis	Good systolic function but poor diastolic filling
	Cardiac tamponade	Hypotension, elevated jugular veins, pulsus paradoxus, poor urine output

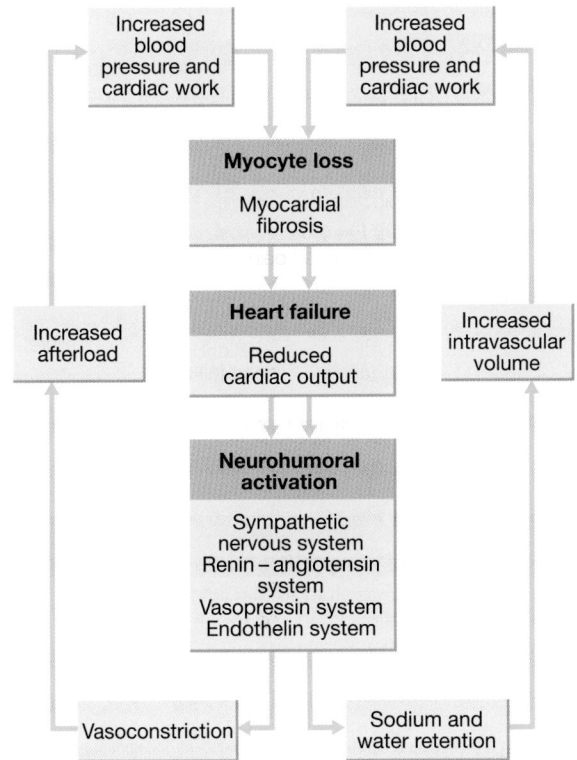

Fig. 16.23 Neurohumoral activation and compensatory mechanisms in heart failure. There is a vicious circle in progressive heart failure.

rate. Prolonged sympathetic stimulation has negative effects, however, causing cardiac myocyte apoptosis, cardiac hypertrophy and focal myocardial necrosis. Sympathetic stimulation also contributes to vasoconstriction and predisposes to arrhythmias. Sodium and water retention is further enhanced by the release of aldosterone, endothelin-1 (a potent vasoconstrictor peptide with marked effects on the renal vasculature) and, in severe heart failure, vasopressin (antidiuretic hormone, ADH). Natriuretic peptides are released from the atria in response to atrial dilatation and compensate to an extent for the sodium-conserving effect of aldosterone, but this mechanism is overwhelmed in heart failure. Pulmonary and peripheral oedema occur because of high left and right atrial pressures, and are compounded by sodium and water retention, caused by impairment of renal perfusion and by secondary hyperaldosteronism. If the underlying cause is a myocardial infarction, cardiac contractility is impaired and SNS and RAAS activation causes hypertrophy of non-infarcted segments, with thinning, dilatation and expansion of the infarcted segment (see Fig. 16.63). This leads to further deterioration in ventricular function and worsening heart failure.

High-output failure

Sometimes cardiac failure can occur in patients without heart disease due to a large arteriovenous shunt, or where there is an excessively high cardiac output due to beri-beri, severe anaemia or thyrotoxicosis.

Valvular disease

Heart failure can also be caused by valvular disease in which there is impaired filling of the ventricles due to mitral or tricuspid stenosis; where there is obstruction to ventricular outflow, as occurs in aortic and pulmonary stenosis and hypertrophic cardiomyopathy; or as the result of ventricular overload secondary to valvular regurgitation.

Clinical assessment

Heart failure may develop suddenly, as in MI, or gradually, as in valvular heart disease. When there is gradual impairment of cardiac function, several compensatory changes take place. The term compensated heart failure is sometimes used to describe the condition of those with impaired cardiac function, in whom adaptive changes have prevented the development of overt heart failure. However, a minor event, such as an intercurrent infection or development of atrial fibrillation, may precipitate acute heart failure in these circumstances (Box 16.13). Similarly, acute heart failure sometimes supervenes as the result of a decompensating episode, on a background of chronic heart failure; this is called acute-on-chronic heart failure.

Acute left heart failure

Acute left heart failure presents with a sudden onset of dyspnoea at rest that rapidly progresses to acute respiratory distress, orthopnoea and ultimately respiratory failure. Often there is a clear precipitating factor, such as an acute MI, which may be apparent from the history. The patient appears agitated, pale and clammy. The peripheries are cool to the touch and the pulse is rapid, but in some cases there may be an inappropriate bradycardia that aggravates the acute episode of heart failure. The BP is usually high because of SNS activation, but may be normal or low if the patient is in cardiogenic shock.

The jugular venous pressure (JVP) is usually elevated, particularly with associated fluid overload or right heart failure. In acute heart failure, there has been no time for ventricular dilatation and the apex is not displaced. A 'gallop' rhythm, with a third heart sound, is heard quite early in the development of acute left-sided heart failure. A new systolic murmur may signify acute mitral regurgitation or ventricular septal rupture. Chest examination may reveal crepitations at the lung bases if there is pulmonary oedema, or

---

i **16.13 Factors that may precipitate or aggravate heart failure in pre-existing heart disease**

- Myocardial ischaemia or infarction
- Intercurrent illness
- Arrhythmia
- Inappropriate reduction of therapy
- Administration of a drug with negative inotropic (β-blocker) or fluid-retaining properties (non-steroidal anti-inflammatory drugs, glucocorticoids)
- Pulmonary embolism
- Conditions associated with increased metabolic demand (pregnancy, thyrotoxicosis, anaemia)
- Intravenous fluid overload

---

crepitations throughout the lungs if this is severe. There may be expiratory wheeze. Patients with acute-on-chronic heart failure may have additional features of chronic heart failure (see below). Potential precipitants, such as an upper respiratory tract infection or inappropriate cessation of diuretic medication, may be identified on clinical examination or history-taking.

Chronic heart failure

Patients with chronic heart failure commonly follow a relapsing and remitting course, with periods of stability and episodes of decompensation, leading to worsening symptoms that may necessitate hospitalisation. The clinical picture depends on the nature of the underlying heart disease, the type of heart failure that it has evoked, and the changes in the SNS and RAAS that have developed (see Box 16.12 and Fig. 16.24).

Low cardiac output causes fatigue and poor effort tolerance; the peripheries are cold and the BP is low. To maintain perfusion of vital organs, blood flow is diverted away from skeletal muscle and this may contribute to fatigue and weakness. Poor renal perfusion leads to oliguria and uraemia.

Pulmonary oedema due to left heart failure presents with dyspnoea and inspiratory crepitations over the lung bases. In contrast, right heart

failure produces a high JVP with hepatic congestion and dependent peripheral oedema. In ambulant patients the oedema affects the lower legs, whereas in bed-bound patients it collects around the thighs and sacrum. Ascites or pleural effusion may occur (Fig. 16.24). Heart failure is not the only cause of oedema (see Box 16.14).

Chronic heart failure is sometimes associated with marked weight loss (cardiac cachexia), caused by a combination of anorexia and impaired absorption due to gastrointestinal congestion, poor tissue perfusion due to a low cardiac output, and skeletal muscle atrophy due to immobility.

Complications of heart failure

Several complications may occur in advanced heart failure, as described below.

- *Renal failure* is caused by poor renal perfusion due to low cardiac output and may be exacerbated by diuretic, ACE inhibitor and angiotensin receptor blocker (ARB) therapies.
- *Hypokalaemia* may be caused by potassium-losing diuretics, and also by hyperaldosteronism due to activation of the renin–angiotensin system and impairment of aldosterone metabolism from hepatic congestion. Most of the body's potassium is intracellular and there may be substantial depletion of potassium stores, even when the plasma concentration is in the reference range.
- *Hyperkalaemia* may be due to the effects of drugs that promote renal resorption of potassium, in particular the combination of ACE inhibitors, ARBs and mineralocorticoid receptor antagonists. These effects are amplified if there is renal dysfunction due to low cardiac output or atherosclerotic renal vascular disease.
- *Hyponatraemia* is a feature of severe heart failure and is a poor prognostic sign. It may be caused by diuretic therapy, inappropriate water retention due to high vasopressin secretion, or failure of the cell membrane ion pump due to intracellular energy depletion.

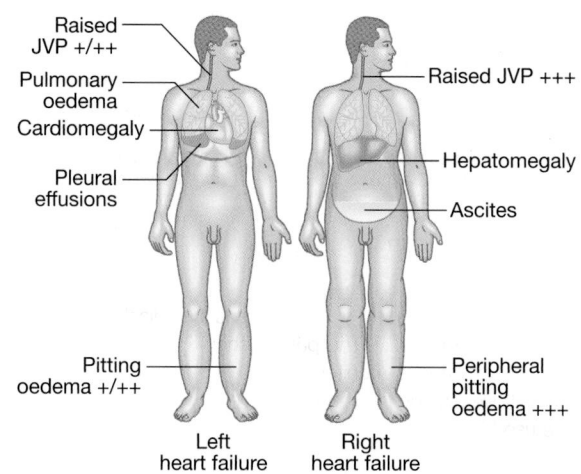

Fig. 16.24 Clinical features of left and right heart failure. (JVP = jugular venous pressure)

---

i **16.14 Differential diagnosis of peripheral oedema**

- Cardiac failure: right or combined left and right heart failure, pericardial constriction, cardiomyopathy
- Chronic venous insufficiency: varicose veins
- Hypoalbuminaemia: nephrotic syndrome, liver disease, protein-losing enteropathy; often widespread, can affect arms and face
- Drugs:
  Sodium retention: fludrocortisone, non-steroidal anti-inflammatory drugs
  Increasing capillary permeability: nifedipine, amlodipine
- Idiopathic: women > men
- Chronic lymphatic obstruction

- *Impaired liver function* is caused by hepatic venous congestion and poor arterial perfusion, which frequently cause mild jaundice and abnormal liver function tests; reduced synthesis of clotting factors can make anticoagulant control difficult.
- *Thromboembolism*. Deep vein thrombosis and pulmonary embolism may occur due to the effects of low cardiac output and enforced immobility. Systemic embolism, including stroke, occurs in patients with atrial fibrillation or flutter, or with intracardiac thrombus complicating mitral stenosis, MI or left ventricular aneurysm.
- *Atrial and ventricular arrhythmias* are very common and may be related to electrolyte changes such as hypokalaemia and hypomagnesaemia, myocardial fibrosis and the pro-arrhythmic effects of sympathetic activation. Atrial fibrillation occurs in approximately 20% of patients with heart failure and causes further impairment of cardiac function. Ventricular ectopic beats and non-sustained ventricular tachycardia are common findings in patients with heart failure and are associated with an adverse prognosis.
- *Sudden death* occurs in up to 50% of patients with heart failure and is most often due to ventricular fibrillation.

Investigations

An erect chest X-ray should be performed in all cases. This may show abnormal distension of the upper lobe pulmonary veins (Fig. 16.25). Vascularity of the lung fields becomes more prominent and the pulmonary arteries dilate. Subsequently, interstitial oedema causes thickened interlobular septa and dilated lymphatics. These are evident as horizontal lines in the costophrenic angles (septal or 'Kerley B' lines). More advanced changes due to alveolar oedema cause a hazy opacification spreading from the hila, and pleural effusions. Echocardiography should be considered in all patients with heart failure in order to:

- determine the aetiology
- detect valvular heart disease, such as occult mitral or aortic stenosis, and other conditions that may be amenable to treatment
- identify patients who will benefit from long-term drug therapy and cardiac device implantation.

Serum urea, creatinine and electrolytes, haemoglobin and thyroid function may help to establish the nature and severity of the underlying heart disease and detect any complications. BNP is elevated in heart failure and is a prognostic marker, as well as being useful in differentiating heart failure from other causes of breathlessness or peripheral oedema.

Management of acute heart failure

Acute heart failure with pulmonary oedema is a medical emergency that should be treated urgently. The patient should initially be kept rested upright, with continuous monitoring of cardiac rhythm, BP and pulse oximetry. Intravenous opiates can be of value in distressed patients but must be used sparingly, as they may cause respiratory depression and exacerbation of hypoxaemia and hypercapnia. The key elements of management are summarised in Box 16.15.

If these measures prove ineffective, inotropic agents such as dobutamine (2.5–10 µg/kg/min) may be required to augment cardiac output, particularly in hypotensive patients. An intra-aortic balloon pump may be beneficial in patients with acute cardiogenic pulmonary oedema and shock. Following management of the acute episode, additional measures must be used to control heart failure in the longer term, as discussed below.

Management of chronic heart failure

The aims of treatment in chronic heart failure are to improve cardiac function by increasing contractility and coordination of the myocardium, by optimising preload or decreasing afterload, and controlling cardiac rate and rhythm (see Fig. 16.23). This can be achieved by using drug treatments, implantable device therapy, coronary revascularisation, and in resistant cases, mechanical assist devices or cardiac transplantation.

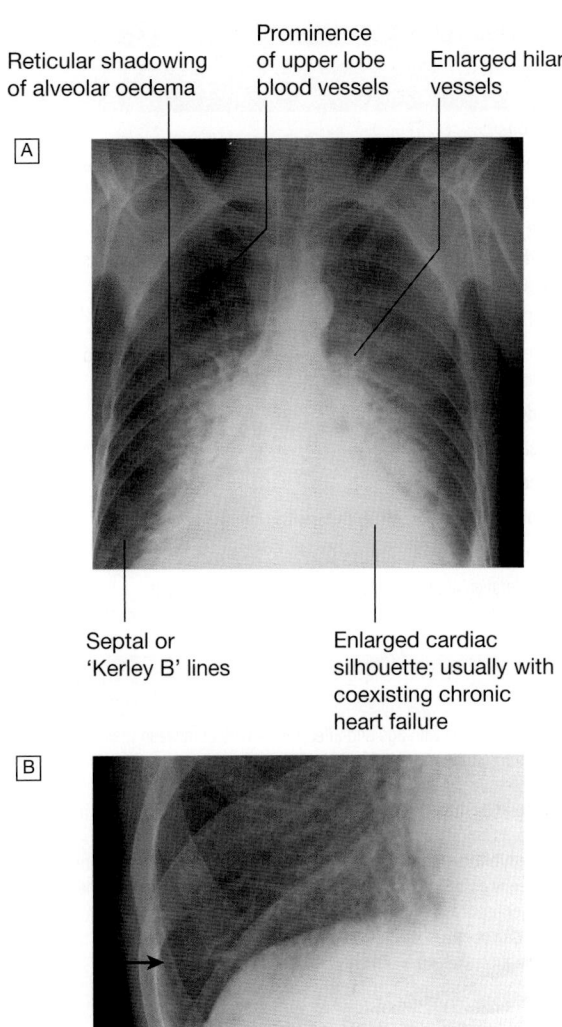

Reticular shadowing of alveolar oedema

Prominence of upper lobe blood vessels

Enlarged hilar vessels

Septal or 'Kerley B' lines

Enlarged cardiac silhouette; usually with coexisting chronic heart failure

Fig. 16.25 Radiological features of heart failure. [A] Chest X-ray of a patient with pulmonary oedema. [B] Enlargement of lung base showing septal or 'Kerley B' lines (arrow).

16.15 Management of acute pulmonary oedema

Action	Effect
Sit the patient up	Reduces preload
Give high-flow oxygen	Corrects hypoxia
Ensure continuous positive airway pressure (CPAP) of 5–10 mmHg by tight-fitting mask	Reduces preload and pulmonary capillary hydraulic gradient
Administer nitrates:* IV glyceryl trinitrate (10–200 µg/min) Buccal glyceryl trinitrate 2–5 mg	Reduces preload and afterload
Administer a loop diuretic: Furosemide (50–100 mg IV)	Combats fluid overload

*The dose of nitrate should be titrated upwards every 10 minutes until there is an improvement or systolic blood pressure is <110 mmHg.
(IV = intravenous)

Education

Education of patients and their relatives about the causes and treatment of heart failure can improve adherence to a management plan (Box 16.16). Some patients may need to weigh themselves daily, as a measure of fluid load, and adjust their diuretic therapy accordingly.

16

16.16 General measures for the management of heart failure

Education

- Explanation of nature of disease, treatment and self-help strategies

Diet

- Good general nutrition and weight reduction for the obese
- Avoidance of high-salt foods and added salt, especially for patients with severe congestive heart failure

Alcohol

- Moderation or elimination of alcohol consumption; alcohol-induced cardiomyopathy requires abstinence

Smoking

- Cessation

Exercise

- Regular moderate aerobic exercise within limits of symptoms

Vaccination

- Consideration of influenza and pneumococcal vaccination

16.17 Congestive cardiac failure in old age

- **Incidence**: rises with age and affects 5%–10% of those in their eighties.
- **Common causes**: coronary artery disease, hypertension and calcific degenerative valvular disease.
- **Diastolic dysfunction**: often prominent, particularly in those with a history of hypertension.
- **ACE inhibitors and ARBs**: improve symptoms and mortality but are more frequently associated with postural hypotension and renal impairment than in younger patients.
- **Loop diuretics**: usually required but may be poorly tolerated in those with urinary incontinence and men with prostate enlargement.

Drug treatment

Many drug treatments are now available for heart failure. Drugs that reduce preload are appropriate in patients with high end-diastolic filling pressures and evidence of pulmonary or systemic venous congestion, whereas those that reduce afterload or increase myocardial contractility are more useful in patients with signs and symptoms of a low cardiac output. Some considerations specific to management of older patients are given in Box 16.17.

Diuretics Diuretics promote urinary sodium and water excretion, leading to a reduction in blood plasma volume, which in turn reduces preload and improves pulmonary and systemic venous congestion. They may also reduce afterload and ventricular volume, leading to a fall in ventricular wall tension and increased cardiac efficiency. Although a fall in preload (ventricular filling pressure) normally reduces cardiac output, patients with heart failure are beyond the apex of the Starling curve, so there may be a substantial and beneficial fall in filling pressure with either no change or an improvement in cardiac output (see Figs. 16.22 and 16.26). Over-diuresis can cause excessive volume depletion, resulting in a fall in cardiac output with hypotension, lethargy and renal failure. This is especially likely in patients with a marked diastolic component to their heart failure.

Oedema may persist, despite oral loop diuretic therapy, in some patients with severe chronic heart failure, particularly if there is renal impairment. Under these circumstances an intravenous infusion of a loop diuretic, such as furosemide (5–10 mg/hr), may initiate a diuresis. Combining this with a thiazide diuretic, such as bendroflumethiazide (5 mg daily), may augment the diuresis but care must be taken to avoid an excessive fluid loss, hyponatraemia and hypokalaemia.

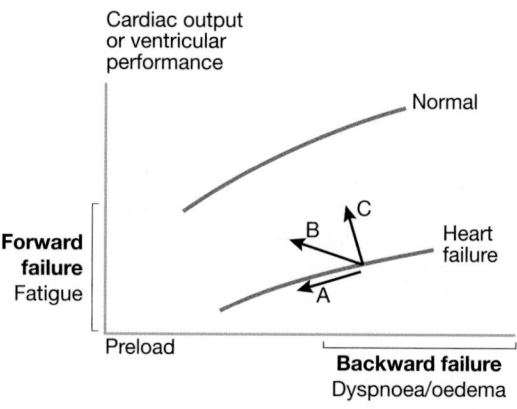

Fig. 16.26 The effect of treatment on ventricular performance curves in heart failure. Diuretics and venodilators (A), angiotensin-converting enzyme (ACE) inhibitors and mixed vasodilators (B), and positive inotropic agents (C).

Mineralocorticoid receptor antagonists, such as spironolactone and eplerenone, are potassium-sparing diuretics that are of particular benefit in patients with heart failure with severe left ventricular systolic dysfunction. They improve long-term clinical outcome in individuals with severe heart failure or heart failure following acute MI but may cause hyperkalaemia, particularly when used with an ACE inhibitor.

Originally developed as a treatment for type 2 diabetes mellitus, sodium-glucose co-transporter 2 (SGLT-2) inhibitors block the resorption of glucose in the nephron of the kidney to cause an osmotic diuresis. Their use is associated with reduced hospitalisations for heart failure and lower mortality in patients with heart failure irrespective of the presence of diabetes. However, they are associated with an increased risk of genitourinary tract infections and diabetic ketoacidosis.

Angiotensin-converting enzyme inhibitors Angiotensin-converting enzyme (ACE) inhibitors play a central role in the management of heart failure since they interrupt the vicious circle of neurohumoral activation that is characteristic of the disease by preventing the conversion of angiotensin I to angiotensin II. This, in turn, reduces peripheral vasoconstriction, activation of the sympathetic nervous system (Fig. 16.27), and salt and water retention due to aldosterone release, as well as preventing the activation of the renin–angiotensin system caused by diuretic therapy.

In moderate and severe heart failure, ACE inhibitors can produce a substantial improvement in effort tolerance and in mortality. They can also improve outcome and prevent the onset of overt heart failure in patients with poor residual left ventricular function following MI.

Adverse effects of ACE inhibitors include hypotension and renal impairment, especially in patients with bilateral renal artery stenosis or those with pre-existing renal disease. An increase in serum potassium concentration may also occur, which can be beneficial in offsetting the hypokalaemia associated with loop diuretic therapy. In stable patients without hypotension (systolic BP over 100 mmHg), ACE inhibitors can usually be safely started in the community. In other patients, however, it is usually advisable to withhold diuretics for 24 hours before starting treatment with a small dose of a long-acting agent, preferably given at night (Box 16.18). Renal function and serum potassium must be monitored and should be checked 1–2 weeks after starting therapy.

Angiotensin receptor blockers Angiotensin receptor blockers (ARBs) act by blocking the action of angiotensin II on the heart, peripheral vasculature and kidneys. In heart failure they produce beneficial haemodynamic changes similar to those of ACE inhibitors (see Fig. 16.27) but are generally better tolerated. They have comparable effects on mortality and are a useful alternative for patients who cannot tolerate ACE inhibitors. They should be started at a low dose and titrated upwards, depending on response (see Box 16.18). Unfortunately, they share all the more

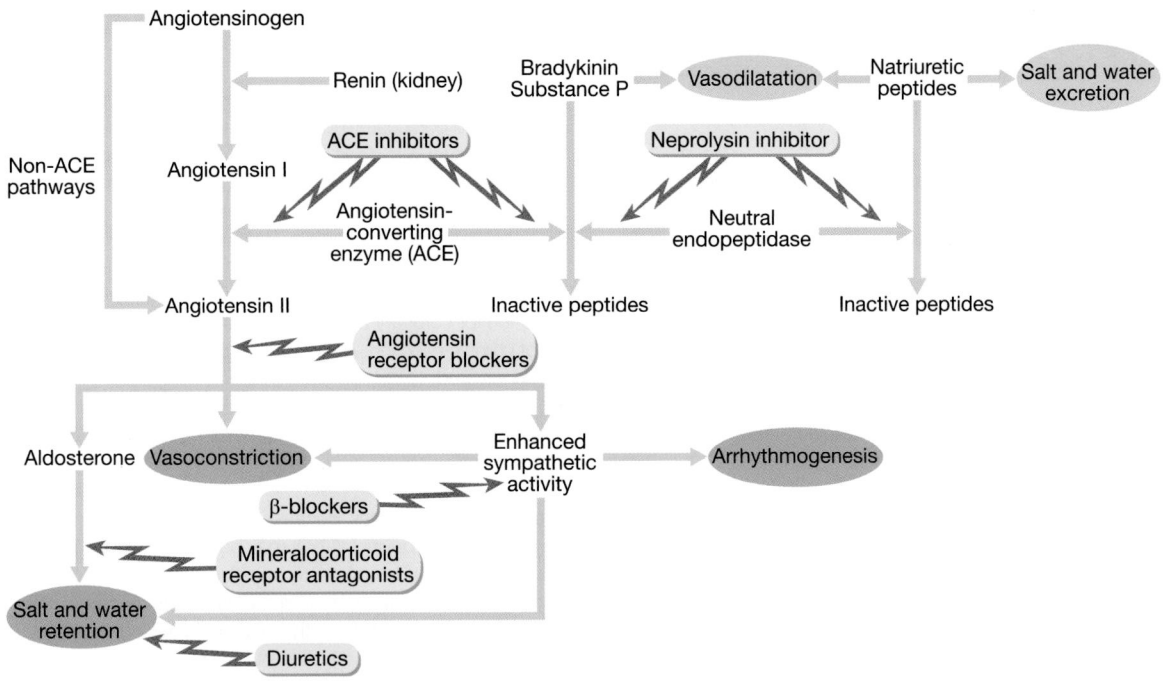

Fig. 16.27 Neurohumoral activation of the renin–angiotensin and sympathetic nervous systems have adverse (red) effects on the cardiovascular system which are counterbalanced by beneficial effects of endogenous natriuretic and vasoactive peptide systems (yellow). Heart failure treatments are targeted at inhibiting the detrimental pathways and enhancing the beneficial compensatory systems.

16

i	**16.18 Dosages of ACE inhibitors, angiotensin receptor blockers, β-blockers and neprilysin inhibitors in heart failure**	
	Starting dose	**Target dose**
ACE inhibitors		
Enalapril	2.5 mg twice daily	10 mg twice daily
Lisinopril	2.5 mg daily	20 mg daily
Ramipril	1.25 mg daily	10 mg daily
Angiotensin receptor blockers		
Losartan	25 mg daily	100 mg daily
Candesartan	4 mg daily	32 mg daily
Valsartan	40 mg daily	160 mg daily
β-blockers		
Bisoprolol	1.25 mg daily	10 mg daily
Metoprolol	25 mg twice daily	100 mg twice daily
Carvedilol	3.125 mg twice daily	25 mg twice daily
Neprilysin inhibitor-ARB		
Sacubitril–valsartan	24/26 mg twice daily	97/103 mg twice daily

serious adverse effects of ACE inhibitors, including renal dysfunction and hyperkalaemia. While ARB are normally used as an alternative to ACE inhibitors, they can be combined in patients with resistant or recurrent heart failure.

Neprilysin inhibitors The only drug currently in this class is sacubitril, a small-molecule inhibitor of neutral endopeptidase, or neprilysin, which is responsible for the breakdown of the endogenous diuretics ANP and BNP as well as vasoactive peptides such as bradykinin and substance P (see Fig. 16.27). If used in combination with the ARB in an initial oral dose of 24 mg sacubitril and 26 mg valsartan daily, it produces additional symptomatic and mortality benefit over ACE inhibition and is increasingly being used in preference to ACE inhibitors in patients with chronic heart failure.

Vasodilators These drugs are valuable in chronic heart failure, when ACE inhibitors or ARBs are contraindicated. Venodilators, such as nitrates, reduce preload. Arterial dilators, such as hydralazine, reduce afterload (see Fig. 16.26). Their use is limited by pharmacological tolerance and hypotension.

Beta-adrenoceptor antagonists (β-blockers) Beta-blockade helps to counteract the deleterious effects of enhanced sympathetic stimulation and reduces the risk of arrhythmias and sudden death. When initiated in standard doses β-blockers may precipitate acute-on-chronic heart failure, but when given in small incremental doses they can increase ejection fraction, improve symptoms, reduce the frequency of hospitalisation and reduce mortality in patients with chronic heart failure. A typical regimen is bisoprolol, starting at 1.25 mg daily and increased gradually over 12 weeks to a target maintenance dose of 10 mg daily. Beta-blockers are more effective at reducing mortality than ACE inhibitors, with a relative risk reduction of 33% versus 20%, respectively.

Ivabradine Ivabradine acts on the I_f inward current in the SA node, resulting in reduction of heart rate. Typical dosages are 2.5–5 mg twice daily, increasing to 7.5 mg twice daily if necessary. It reduces hospital admission and mortality rates in patients with heart failure due to moderate or severe left ventricular systolic impairment. In trials, its effects were most marked in patients with a relatively high heart rate (over 77/min), so ivabradine is best suited to patients who cannot take β-blockers or whose heart rate remains high despite β-blockade. It is ineffective in patients with atrial fibrillation.

Digoxin Digoxin in maintenance doses of 0.0625–0.25 mg daily can be used to provide rate control in patients with heart failure and atrial fibrillation. In patients with severe heart failure (NYHA class III–IV, see Box 16.5), digoxin reduces the likelihood of hospitalisation for heart failure, although it has no effect on long-term survival.

Amiodarone This is a potent anti-arrhythmic drug that has little negative inotropic effect and may be valuable in patients with poor left ventricular function. It is effective only in the treatment of symptomatic arrhythmias and should not be used as a preventative agent in asymptomatic patients. Amiodarone is used for prevention of symptomatic atrial arrhythmias and of ventricular arrhythmias when other pharmacological options have been exhausted.

Non-pharmacological treatments

Implantable cardiac defibrillators These devices are indicated in patients with heart failure who have had, or who are at high risk of, life-threatening ventricular arrhythmias, since they reduce the risk of sudden death.

Cardiac resynchronisation therapy devices In patients with marked conduction system disease, especially left bundle branch block, there is uncoordinated left ventricular contraction which exacerbates heart failure. Cardiac resynchronisation therapy (CRT) uses pacemaker technology to overcome dyssynchronous contraction by pacing the LV and RV simultaneously (Fig. 16.28). This improves cardiac output and is associated with improved symptoms and reduced mortality.

Coronary revascularisation Coronary artery bypass surgery or percutaneous coronary intervention may improve function in areas of the myocardium that are 'hibernating' because of inadequate blood supply, and can be used to treat carefully selected patients with heart failure and coronary artery disease. If necessary, 'hibernating' myocardium can be identified by stress echocardiography and specialised nuclear or magnetic resonance imaging.

Cardiac transplantation Cardiac transplantation is an established and successful treatment for patients with intractable heart failure. Coronary artery disease and dilated cardiomyopathy are the most common indications. The use of transplantation is limited by the efficacy of modern drug and device therapies, as well as the availability of donor hearts, so it is generally reserved for young patients with severe symptoms despite optimal therapy.

Conventional heart transplantation is contraindicated in patients with pulmonary vascular disease due to long-standing left heart failure, complex congenital heart disease such as Eisenmenger syndrome, or primary pulmonary hypertension because the RV of the donor heart may fail in the face of high pulmonary vascular resistance. However, heart–lung transplantation can be successful in patients with Eisenmenger syndrome, and lung transplantation has been used for primary pulmonary hypertension.

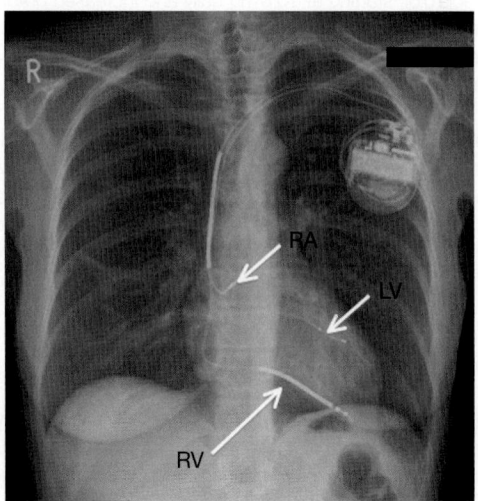

Fig. 16.28 Chest X-ray of a biventricular pacemaker and defibrillator (cardiac resynchronisation therapy). The right ventricular lead (RV) is in position in the ventricular apex and is used for both pacing and defibrillation. The left ventricular lead (LV) is placed via the coronary sinus, and the right atrial lead (RA) is placed in the right atrial appendage; both are used for pacing only.

Although cardiac transplantation usually produces a dramatic improvement in the recipient's quality of life, serious complications may occur:

- *Rejection.* In spite of routine therapy with ciclosporin A, azathioprine and corticosteroids, episodes of rejection are common and may present with heart failure, arrhythmias or subtle ECG changes. Cardiac biopsy is often used to confirm the diagnosis before starting treatment with high-dose corticosteroids.
- *Accelerated atherosclerosis.* Recurrent heart failure is often due to progressive atherosclerosis in the coronary arteries of the donor heart. This is not confined to patients who underwent transplantation for coronary artery disease and is probably a manifestation of chronic rejection. Angina is rare because the heart has been denervated.
- *Infection.* Opportunistic infection with organisms such as cytomegalovirus or *Aspergillus* remains a major cause of death in transplant recipients.

Ventricular assist devices Because of the limited supply of donor organs, ventricular assist devices (VAD) may be employed as a bridge to cardiac transplantation and as short-term restoration therapy following a potentially reversible insult such as viral myocarditis. In some patients, VADs may be used as a long-term therapy if no other options exist.

These devices assist cardiac output by using a roller, centrifugal or pulsatile pump that, in some cases, is implantable and portable. They withdraw blood through cannulae inserted in the atria or ventricular apex and pump it into the pulmonary artery or aorta. They are designed not only to unload the ventricles but also to provide support to the pulmonary and systemic circulations. Their more widespread application is limited by high complication rates (haemorrhage, systemic embolism, infection, neurological and renal sequelae), although some improvements in survival and quality of life have been demonstrated in patients with severe heart failure.

Cardiac arrhythmias

A cardiac arrhythmia is defined as a disturbance of the electrical rhythm of the heart. Arrhythmias are often a manifestation of structural heart disease but may also occur because of abnormal conduction or depolarisation in an otherwise healthy heart. There are many types of cardiac arrhythmia, as discussed later in this section. By convention, however, a heart rate of more than 100/min is a tachycardia, and a heart rate of less than 60/min is a bradycardia.

Pathogenesis

Arrhythmias usually occur as the result of pathology affecting the conduction system of the heart. The cardiac cycle is normally initiated by spontaneous depolarisation in the SA node. The atria and ventricles then activate sequentially as the depolarisation wave passes through specialised conducting tissues (see Fig. 16.4). The SA node acts as a pacemaker and its intrinsic rate is regulated by the autonomic nervous system; parasympathetic (vagal) activity decreases the heart rate and sympathetic activity increases it via cardiac sympathetic nerves and circulating catecholamines.

There are three main mechanisms of tachycardia:
- *Increased automaticity.* The tachycardia is produced by spontaneous depolarisation of an ectopic focus in the atria, atrioventricular junction or ventricles, often in response to catecholamines. Single depolarisations lead to atrial, junctional or ventricular premature (ectopic) beats. Repeated depolarisation leads to atrial, junctional or ventricular tachycardia.
- *Re-entry.* The tachycardia is initiated by an ectopic beat and sustained by a re-entry circuit (Fig. 16.29). Most tachyarrhythmias are caused by re-entry.
- *Triggered activity.* This can cause ventricular arrhythmias in patients with coronary artery disease. It is a form of secondary depolarisation

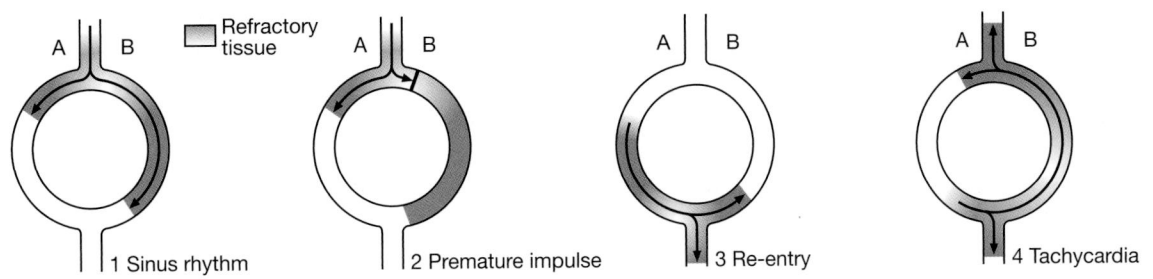

Fig. 16.29 The mechanism of re-entry. Re-entry can occur when there are two alternative pathways with different conducting properties, such as the atrioventricular node and an accessory pathway, or an area of normal and an area of ischaemic tissue. Here, pathway A conducts slowly and recovers quickly, while pathway B conducts rapidly and recovers slowly. (1) In sinus rhythm, each impulse passes down both pathways before entering a common distal pathway. (2) As the pathways recover at different rates, a premature impulse may find pathway A open and B closed. (3) Pathway B may recover while the premature impulse is travelling selectively down pathway A. The impulse can then travel retrogradely up pathway B, setting up a closed loop or re-entry circuit. (4) This may initiate a tachycardia that continues until the circuit is interrupted by a change in conduction rates or electrical depolarisation.

arising from an incompletely repolarised cell membrane. Arrhythmias may be supraventricular (sinus, atrial or junctional) or ventricular in origin.

Supraventricular rhythms usually produce narrow QRS complexes because the ventricles are depolarised in their normal sequence via the AV node, the bundle of His, bundle branches and Purkinje fibres. In contrast, ventricular arrhythmias often produce broad, bizarre QRS complexes because the ventricles are activated in sequence rather than in parallel, and activation occurs via myocardial cells rather than the rapidly conducting Purkinje fibres. Occasionally, supraventricular tachycardia can mimic ventricular tachycardia and present as a broad-complex tachycardia due to coexisting bundle branch block or the presence of an additional atrioventricular connection (accessory pathway, see below).

Bradycardia is caused by either reduced automaticity of the SA node or impaired conduction through the AV node or His–Purkinje system. If the sinus rate becomes unduly slow, another, more distal part of the conducting system may assume the role of pacemaker. This is known as an escape rhythm and may arise in the AV node or His bundle (junctional rhythm) or in the ventricles (idioventricular rhythm).

Clinical features

Many arrhythmias are asymptomatic but sustained tachycardias typically present with rapid palpitation. Dizziness, chest discomfort or breathlessness may also occur. Extreme tachycardias can also cause syncope because the heart is unable to fill properly at extreme rates. Bradycardias tend to cause symptoms of low cardiac output, including fatigue, lightheadedness and syncope. Extreme bradycardias or tachycardias can precipitate sudden death or cardiac arrest.

Investigations

The first-line investigation is a 12-lead ECG, which can be diagnostic in many cases. If arrhythmias are intermittent and the resting ECG is normal, an attempt should be made to capture the abnormal rhythm using an ambulatory ECG or a patient-activated ECG.

Management

Features of individual arrhythmias are discussed below. Management depends on the nature of the arrhythmia and the general principles of medical management are discussed later in this chapter.

Sinus arrhythmia

This is defined as a cyclical alteration of the heart rate during respiration, with an increase during inspiration and a decrease during expiration. Sinus arrhythmia is a normal phenomenon and can be quite pronounced in children. Absence of heart rate variation with breathing or with changes in

posture may be a feature of diabetic neuropathy autonomic neuropathy or increased sympathetic drive. Sinus arrhythmia does not require treatment.

Sinus bradycardia

This may occur in healthy people at rest and is a common finding in athletes. Some pathological causes are listed in Box 16.19. If sinus bradycardia is asymptomatic, then no treatment is required. Symptomatic sinus bradycardia may occur acutely during an MI and can be treated with intravenous atropine (0.6–1.2 mg). Patients with recurrent or persistent symptomatic sinus bradycardia should be considered for permanent pacemaker implantation.

Sinus tachycardia

Sinus tachycardia is usually due to an increase in sympathetic activity associated with exercise or emotion. Healthy young adults can produce a rapid sinus rate, up to 200/min, during intense exercise. Sinus tachycardia usually does not require treatment but sometimes may reflect an underlying disease, as summarised in Box 16.19.

Sinoatrial disease

Sinoatrial disease or 'sick sinus syndrome' can occur at any age but is most common in older people. It is caused by degenerative changes in the SA node and is characterised by a variety of arrhythmias (Box 16.20). The typical presentation is with palpitation, dizzy spells or syncope, due to intermittent tachycardia, bradycardia, or pauses in sinus rhythm with no atrial or ventricular activity (Fig. 16.30).

In sinoatrial disease, a permanent pacemaker improves symptoms but not prognosis so is not indicated in asymptomatic patients. It is used in

16.19 Some pathological causes of sinus bradycardia and tachycardia

Sinus bradycardia
- Myocardial infarction
- Sinus node disease (sick sinus syndrome)
- Hypothermia
- Hypothyroidism

- Cholestatic jaundice
- Raised intracranial pressure
- Drugs (β-blockers, digoxin, verapamil)

Sinus tachycardia
- Anxiety
- Fever
- Anaemia
- Heart failure

- Thyrotoxicosis
- Phaeochromocytoma
- Drugs (β-agonists)

16

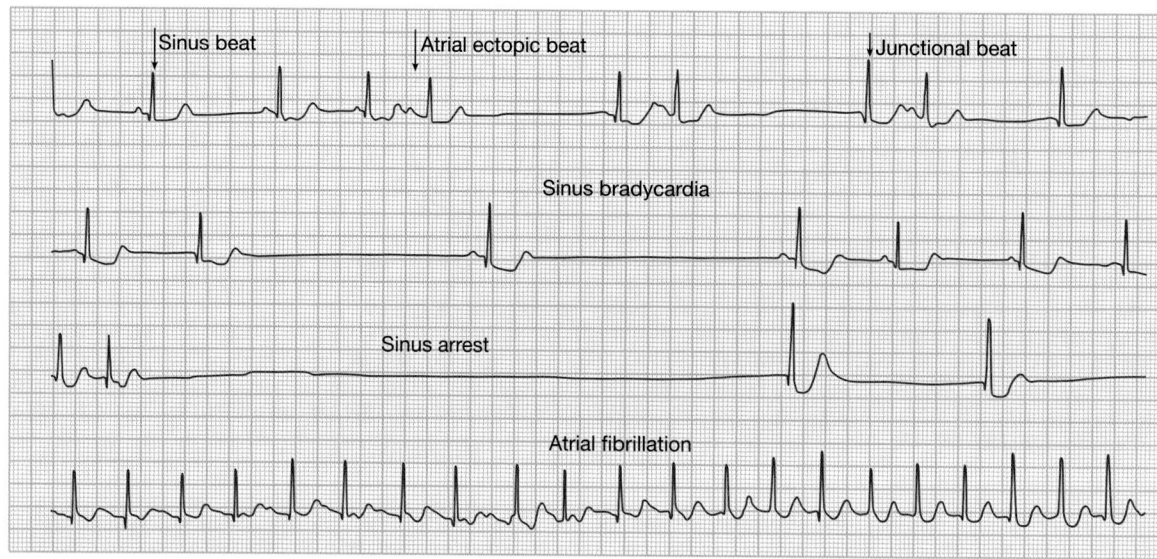

Fig. 16.30 Sinoatrial disease (sick sinus syndrome). A continuous rhythm strip from a 24-hour ECG tape recording illustrating periods of sinus rhythm, atrial ectopics, junctional beats, sinus bradycardia, sinus arrest and paroxysmal atrial fibrillation.

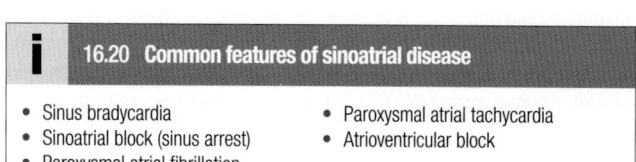

i	**16.20 Common features of sinoatrial disease**

- Sinus bradycardia
- Sinoatrial block (sinus arrest)
- Paroxysmal atrial fibrillation
- Paroxysmal atrial tachycardia
- Atrioventricular block

patients with symptomatic bradycardia, including bradycardia induced by drugs required to prevent tachyarrhythmias. A dual-chamber pacemaker is normally used (see p. 422). The right atrial lead is used to assist the SA node, and the right ventricular lead is a backup in case AV nodal block occurs later on.

Atrioventricular block

This usually occurs as the result of disease affecting the AV node. AV block can be intermittent, however, and may become evident only when the conducting tissue is stressed by a rapid atrial rate. Reflecting this fact, atrial tachyarrhythmias are often associated with AV block (see Fig. 16.36). Episodes of ventricular asystole may also complicate complete heart block or Mobitz type II second-degree AV block. Several types of AV block are recognised.

First-degree atrioventricular block

In this condition, AV conduction is delayed and so the PR interval is prolonged (> 0.20 sec; Fig. 16.31). It rarely causes symptoms and does not usually require treatment.

Second-degree atrioventricular block

Here dropped beats occur because some impulses from the atria fail to conduct to the ventricles. Two subtypes are recognised. In Mobitz type I second-degree AV block (Fig. 16.32), there is progressive lengthening of successive PR intervals, culminating in a dropped beat. The cycle then repeats itself. This is known as the Wenckebach phenomenon and is usually due to impaired conduction in the AV node itself. The phenomenon may be physiological and is sometimes observed at rest or during sleep in athletic young adults with high vagal tone.

In Mobitz type II second-degree AV block (Fig. 16.33), the PR interval of the conducted impulses remains constant but some P waves are not conducted. This is usually caused by disease of the His–Purkinje system and carries a risk of asystole.

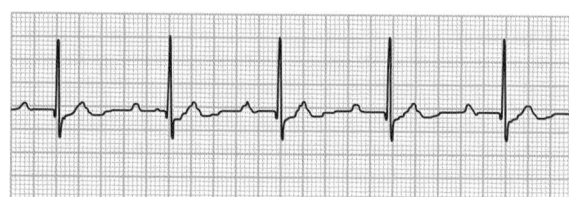

Fig. 16.31 First-degree atrioventricular block. The PR interval is prolonged and measures 0.32 sec.

In 2:1 AV block (Fig. 16.34), alternate P waves are not conducted, so it is impossible to distinguish between Mobitz type I and type II block.

Third-degree atrioventricular block

In third-degree AV block, conduction fails completely and the atria and ventricles beat independently. This is known as AV dissociation, as shown in Fig. 16.35. Ventricular activity is maintained by an escape rhythm arising in the AV node or bundle of His (narrow QRS complexes) or the distal Purkinje tissues (broad QRS complexes). Distal escape rhythms tend to be slower and less reliable. Complete AV block (Box 16.21) produces a slow (25–50/min), regular pulse that does not vary with exercise, except in the case of congenital complete AV block. There is usually a compensatory increase in stroke volume, producing a large-volume pulse. Cannon waves may be visible in the neck and the intensity of the first heart sound varies due to the loss of AV synchrony.

Clinical features

The typical presentation is with recurrent syncope or 'Stokes–Adams' attacks. These episodes are characterised by sudden loss of consciousness that occurs without warning and results in collapse. A brief anoxic seizure (due to cerebral ischaemia) may occur if there is prolonged asystole. There is pallor and a death-like appearance during the attack, but when the heart starts beating again there is a characteristic flush. In distinction to epilepsy, recovery is rapid. Sinoatrial disease and neurocardiogenic syncope (p. 184) may cause similar symptoms.

Management

This depends on the clinical circumstances. Inferior ST elevation MI is sometimes complicated by transient AV block because the right coronary artery (RCA) supplies the AV node. There is usually a reliable

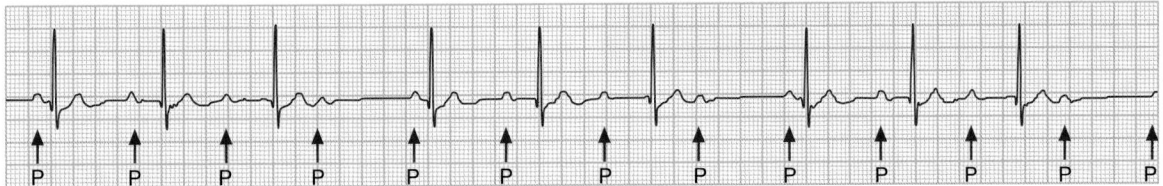

Fig. 16.32 Second-degree atrioventricular block (Mobitz type I – the Wenckebach phenomenon). The PR interval progressively increases until a P wave is not conducted. The cycle then repeats itself. In this example, conduction is at a ratio of 4:3, leading to groupings of three ventricular complexes in a row.

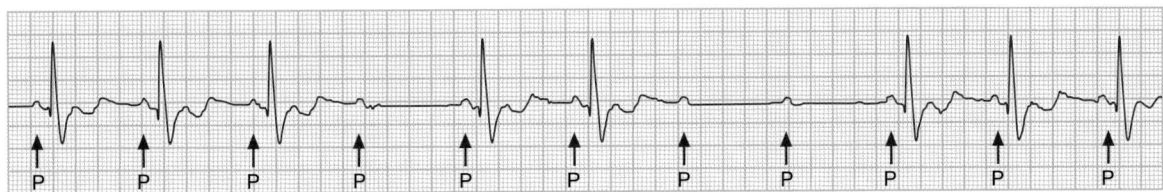

Fig. 16.33 Second-degree atrioventricular block (Mobitz type II). The PR interval of conducted beats is normal but some P waves are not conducted. The constant PR interval distinguishes this from the Wenckebach phenomenon.

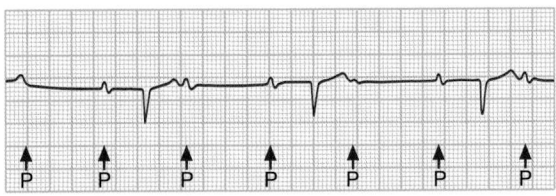

Fig. 16.34 Second-degree atrioventricular block with fixed 2:1 block. Alternate P waves are not conducted. This may be due to Mobitz type I or II block.

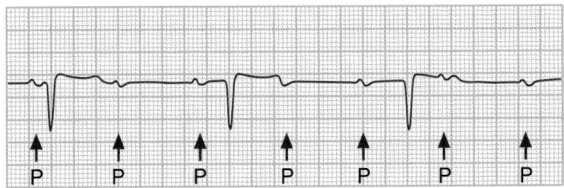

Fig. 16.35 Complete (third-degree) atrioventricular block. There is complete dissociation of atrial and ventricular complexes. The atrial rate is 80/min and the ventricular rate is 38/min.

> **i 16.21 Causes of complete atrioventricular block**
>
> **Congenital**
> **Acquired**
> - Idiopathic fibrosis
> - Myocardial infarction/ischaemia
> - Inflammation:
>   Infective endocarditis
>   Sarcoidosis
>   Chagas' disease
> - Trauma
> - Drugs:
>   Digoxin
>   β-blockers
>   Calcium antagonists

escape rhythm and, if the patient remains well, no treatment is required. Symptomatic second- or third-degree AV block may respond to atropine (0.6 mg IV, repeated as necessary) or, if this fails, a temporary pacemaker. In most cases, the AV block will resolve within 7–10 days.

Second- or third-degree AV heart block complicating acute anterior MI indicates extensive ventricular damage involving both bundle branches and carries a poor prognosis. Asystole may ensue and a temporary pacemaker should be inserted promptly. If the patient presents with asystole, intravenous atropine (3 mg) or intravenous isoprenaline (2 mg in 500 mL 5% dextrose, infused at 10–60 mL/hr) may help to maintain the circulation until a temporary pacing electrode can be inserted. Temporary pacing can provide effective rhythm support in the short term.

Patients with symptomatic bradyarrhythmias associated with AV block should be treated with a permanent pacemaker. Asymptomatic first-degree or Mobitz type I second-degree AV block (Wenckebach phenomenon) does not require treatment but may be an indication of underlying heart disease. A permanent pacemaker is usually indicated in patients with asymptomatic Mobitz type II second-degree AV block or third-degree AV heart block because of the risk of asystole and sudden death. Pacing improves prognosis.

Bundle branch block

Damage to the right or left bundle branch of the conducting system can occur as a result of many pathologies, including ischaemic heart disease, hypertensive heart disease and cardiomyopathy. However, right bundle branch block (RBBB) can occur as a normal variant in healthy individuals (Box 16.22). In left bundle branch block (LBBB) and RBBB, depolarisation proceeds through a slow myocardial route in the affected ventricle rather than through the rapidly conducting Purkinje tissues that constitute the bundle branches. This causes delayed conduction into the LV or RV, broadens the QRS complex (≥0.12 sec) and produces characteristic alterations in QRS morphology (Figs. 16.36 and 16.37). Damage to the left bundle can also occur after it divides into anterior and posterior fascicles, when it is called hemiblock. In this case, the QRS complex is not broad but the direction of ventricular depolarisation is changed, causing left axis deviation in left anterior hemiblock and right axis deviation in left posterior hemiblock (see Fig. 16.7). The combination of RBBB and left anterior or posterior hemiblock is known as bifascicular block. LBBB usually signifies important underlying heart disease and also causes ventricular incoordination, which may aggravate symptoms in patients with heart failure. This can be treated in selected patients by cardiac resynchronisation therapy.

Atrial ectopic beats

Atrial ectopic beats usually cause no symptoms but can give the sensation of a missed beat or an abnormally strong beat. The ECG (Fig. 16.39)

| | 16.22 Common causes of bundle branch block |

Right bundle branch block

- Normal variant
- Right ventricular hypertrophy or strain, e.g. pulmonary embolism
- Congenital heart disease, e.g. atrial septal defect
- Coronary artery disease

Left bundle branch block

- Coronary artery disease
- Hypertension
- Aortic valve disease
- Cardiomyopathy

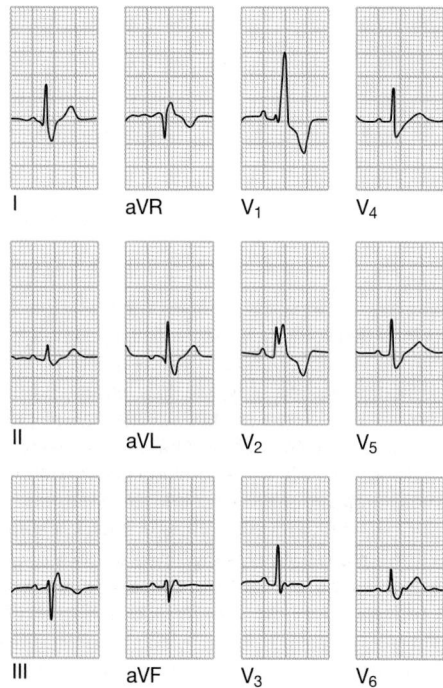

I aVR V₁ V₄

II aVL V₂ V₅

III aVF V₃ V₆

Fig. 16.36 Right bundle branch block. Note the wide QRS complexes with 'M'-shaped configuration in leads V₁ and V₂ and a wide S wave in lead I.

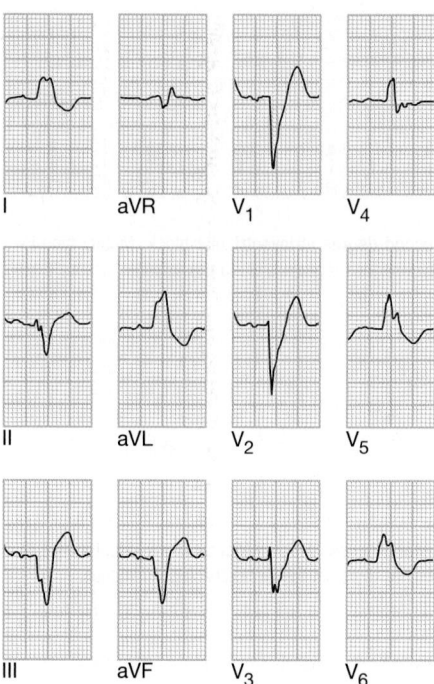

I aVR V₁ V₄

II aVL V₂ V₅

III aVF V₃ V₆

Fig. 16.37 Left bundle branch block. Note the wide QRS complexes with loss of the Q wave or septal vector in lead I and 'M'-shaped QRS complexes in V₅ and V₆.

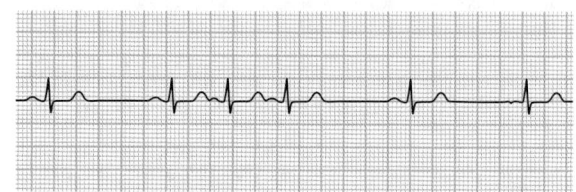

Fig. 16.38 Atrial ectopic beats. The first, second and fifth complexes are normal sinus beats. The third, fourth and sixth complexes are atrial ectopic beats with identical QRS complexes and abnormal (sometimes barely visible) P waves.

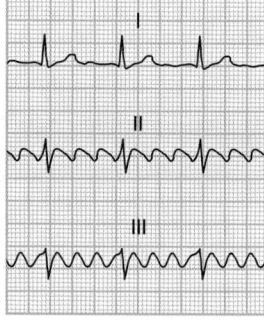

Fig. 16.39 Atrial flutter. Simultaneous recording showing atrial flutter with 4:1 atrioventricular block. Flutter waves are visible only in leads II and III.

shows a premature but otherwise normal QRS complex; if visible, the preceding P wave has a different morphology because the atria activate from an abnormal site. In most cases these are of no consequence, although very frequent atrial ectopic beats may herald the onset of atrial fibrillation. Treatment is rarely necessary but β-blockers can be used if symptoms are intrusive.

Atrial tachycardia

Atrial tachycardia may be a manifestation of increased atrial automaticity, sinoatrial disease or digoxin toxicity. It produces a narrow-complex tachycardia with abnormal P-wave morphology, sometimes associated with AV block if the atrial rate is rapid. It may respond to β-blockers, which reduce automaticity, or class I or III anti-arrhythmic drugs (see Box 16.30). The ventricular response in rapid atrial tachycardias may be controlled by AV node-blocking drugs. Catheter ablation (p. 423) can be used to target the ectopic site and should be offered as an alternative to anti-arrhythmic drugs in patients with recurrent atrial tachycardia.

Atrial flutter

Atrial flutter is characterised by a large (macro) re-entry circuit, usually within the right atrium encircling the tricuspid annulus. The atrial rate is approximately 300/min, and is usually associated with 2:1, 3:1 or 4:1 AV block (with corresponding heart rates of 150, 100 or 75/min). Rarely, in young patients, every flutter wave is conducted, producing a rate of 300/min and, potentially, haemodynamic compromise. The ECG shows sawtooth flutter waves (Fig. 16.39). When there is regular 2:1 AV block, it may be difficult to identify flutter waves that are buried in QRS complexes and T waves. Atrial flutter should be suspected when there is a narrow-complex tachycardia of 150/min. Carotid sinus pressure or intravenous adenosine may help to establish the diagnosis by temporarily increasing the degree of AV block and revealing flutter waves (Fig. 16.40).

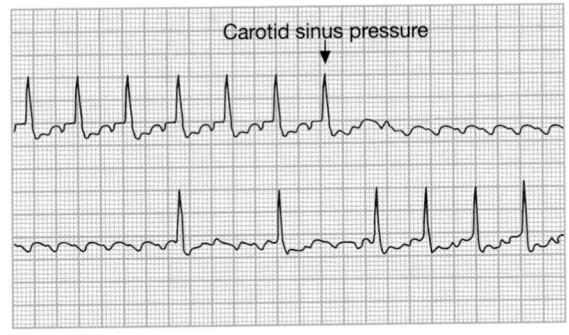

Fig. 16.40 Carotid sinus pressure in atrial flutter: continuous trace. The diagnosis of atrial flutter with 2:1 block was established when carotid sinus pressure produced temporary atrioventricular block, revealing the flutter waves.

Management

Atrial flutter can be managed by either 'rate control' or 'rhythm control'. Rate control uses AV node-blocking drugs, such as β-blockers, verapamil or digoxin at the dosages shown in Box 16.30, to control the ventricular rate. In most cases rhythm control is preferable. This can be achieved by either direct current (DC) cardioversion, or catheter ablation. DC cardioversion is associated with a high recurrence rate even when drugs, such as β-blockers or amiodarone, are used afterwards. Class Ic anti-arrhythmic drugs, such as flecainide, are contraindicated because they can produce a paradoxical extreme tachycardia and haemodynamic compromise. Catheter ablation offers a greater than 90% chance of permanent cure and is the treatment of choice for patients with persistent symptoms. Anticoagulant management in patients with atrial flutter, including management around cardioversion, is identical to that of patients with atrial fibrillation.

▌Atrial fibrillation

Atrial fibrillation (AF) is the most common sustained cardiac arrhythmia, with an overall prevalence of 0.5% in the adult population of the UK. The prevalence rises with age, affecting 1% of those aged 60–64 years, increasing to 9% of those aged over 80 years. It is associated with significant morbidity and a twofold increase in mortality. This is mainly because of its association with underlying heart disease but also because of its association with systemic embolism and stroke.

Pathogenesis

AF is a complex arrhythmia characterised by both abnormal automatic firing and the presence of multiple interacting re-entry circuits within the atria. Episodes of AF are initiated by rapid bursts of ectopic beats arising from conducting tissue in the pulmonary veins or from diseased atrial tissue. It becomes sustained because of re-entrant conduction within the atria or sometimes because of continuous ectopic firing (Fig. 16.41). Re-entry is more likely to occur in atria that are enlarged or in which conduction is slow, as is the case in many forms of heart disease. During episodes of AF, the atria beat rapidly but in an uncoordinated and ineffective manner. The ventricles are activated irregularly at a rate determined by conduction through the AV node. This produces the characteristic 'irregularly irregular' pulse. The ECG (Fig. 16.42) shows normal but irregular QRS complexes; there are no P waves but the baseline may show irregular fibrillation waves. Commonly, AF is classified as paroxysmal (intermittent episodes that self-terminate within 7 days), persistent (prolonged episodes that can be terminated by electrical or pharmacological cardioversion) or permanent. It can be difficult to identify what type of AF patients have at first presentation but this usually becomes clearer as time progresses. Unfortunately for many patients, paroxysmal AF becomes permanent as the underlying disease process progresses. This is partly because of electrophysiological changes that occur in the atria within a few hours of the onset of AF and which tend to maintain fibrillation: a

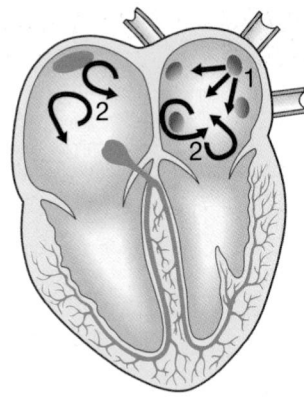

Fig. 16.41 Mechanisms initiating atrial fibrillation. (1) Ectopic beats, often arising from the pulmonary veins, trigger atrial fibrillation. (2) Re-entry within the atria maintains atrial fibrillation, with multiple interacting re-entry circuits operating simultaneously.

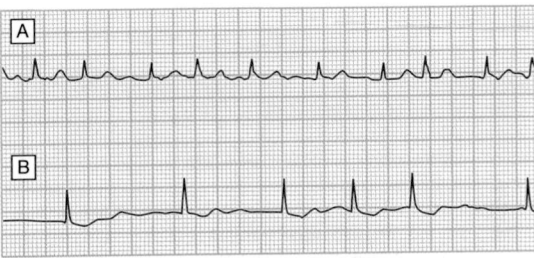

Fig. 16.42 Two examples of atrial fibrillation. The QRS complexes are irregular and there are no P waves. [A] There is usually a fast ventricular rate, between 120 and 160/min, at the onset of atrial fibrillation. [B] In chronic atrial fibrillation, the ventricular rate may be much slower, due to the effects of medication and AV nodal fatigue.

process called electrical remodelling. When AF persists for a period of months, structural remodelling also occurs, leading to atrial fibrosis and dilatation that predispose to chronicity of the AF. Early treatment of AF can sometimes prevent the arrhythmia from becoming persistent.

Many forms of heart disease can present with AF (Box 16.23), particularly those that are associated with enlargement or dilatation of the atria. Alcohol excess, hyperthyroidism and chronic lung disease are also common causes of AF, although multiple predisposing factors may coexist, such as the combination of alcohol, hypertension and coronary artery disease. About 50% of all patients with paroxysmal AF and 20% of patients with persistent or permanent AF have structurally normal hearts; this is known as 'lone atrial fibrillation'. Aspects of atrial fibrillation that pertain particularly to old age are listed in Box 16.24.

Clinical features

The typical presentation is with palpitation, breathlessness and fatigue. In patients with poor ventricular function or valve disease, AF may precipitate or aggravate cardiac failure because of loss of atrial function and heart rate control. A fall in BP may cause lightheadedness, and chest pain may occur with underlying coronary artery disease, sometimes accompanied by ST segment and T-wave abnormalities on the ECG, and troponin elevation. In older patients, AF may not be associated with a rapid ventricular rate and may be asymptomatic, only to be discovered as a result of a routine examination or an ECG. Asymptomatic AF may also present with systemic embolism and is a major cause of stroke in older people.

Investigations

Assessment of patients with newly diagnosed AF should include a full history, physical examination, a 12-lead ECG, echocardiogram and thyroid function tests to exclude thyrotoxicosis. The echocardiogram is used to identify any structural heart disease, particularly mitral valve disease.

16

16.23 Common causes of atrial fibrillation

- Coronary artery disease (including acute MI)
- Valvular heart disease, especially rheumatic mitral valve disease
- Hypertension
- Sinoatrial disease
- Hyperthyroidism
- Alcohol
- Cardiomyopathy
- Congenital heart disease
- Chest infection
- Pulmonary embolism
- Pericardial disease
- Idiopathic (lone atrial fibrillation)

16.24 Atrial fibrillation in old age

- **Prevalence:** rises with age, reaching 9% in those over 80 years.
- **Symptoms:** sometimes asymptomatic but often accompanied by diastolic heart failure.
- **Hyperthyroidism:** atrial fibrillation may emerge as the dominant feature of otherwise silent or occult hyperthyroidism.
- **Cardioversion:** followed by high rates (~70% at 1 year) of recurrent atrial fibrillation.
- **Stroke:** atrial fibrillation is an important cause of cerebral embolism, found in 15% of all stroke patients and 2%–8% of those with transient ischaemic attacks (TIAs).
- **Anticoagulation:** although the risk of thromboembolism rises, the hazards of anticoagulation also become greater with age because of increased comorbidity, particularly cognitive impairment and falls.
- **Direct oral anticoagulants:** alternatives to warfarin. No blood monitoring is required, there are fewer drug interactions, and fixed dosing may aid adherence. Renal impairment affects dosing, for example apixaban dose is reduced from 5 mg twice daily to 2.5 mg twice daily if two or more of the following apply: serum creatinine more than 132 μmol/L, age 80 years or greater, weight 60 kg or less.
- **Warfarin:** in those over 75 years, care should be taken to maintain an INR (International Normalised Ratio) below 3.0 because of the increased risk of intracranial haemorrhage.

Management

Management depends on whether the AF is transient or persistent and whether there is a clear precipitating factor. When AF complicates an acute illness such as a chest infection or pulmonary embolism, treatment of the underlying disorder will often restore sinus rhythm. Where AF does not resolve, the choice lies between rate control or rhythm control. Stroke risk stratification and prevention are the most important issues in managing atrial fibrillation. Management of paroxysmal and persistent AF is discussed below.

Paroxysmal atrial fibrillation

Occasional attacks of AF that are well tolerated do not require treatment. Beta-blockers are normally used as first-line therapy if symptoms are troublesome, since they reduce the ectopic firing that normally initiates the arrhythmia. They are particularly useful for treating patients with AF associated with coronary artery disease, hypertension and cardiac failure. Class Ic drugs (see Box 16.30), such as propafenone or flecainide, are also effective at preventing episodes but should not be given to patients with coronary artery disease or left ventricular dysfunction. Flecainide is seldom used alone, since it can precipitate atrial flutter, and is usually prescribed with a rate-limiting β-blocker. Class III drugs can also be used; amiodarone is the most effective agent for preventing AF but side-effects restrict its use to when other measures fail. Dronedarone is an effective alternative but is contraindicated in patients with heart failure or significant left ventricular impairment. Calcium channel blockers, such as diltiazem (200-400 mg daily), are sometimes used to prevent atrial fibrillation but they are not as effective.

Catheter ablation can be considered as an alternative to anti-arrhythmic drug therapy. Ablation targets the left atrial to pulmonary venous connections, preventing ectopic triggering of AF. In addition, lines of conduction block can be created within the atria to prevent re-entry. Ablation

prevents AF in approximately 75% of patients, although a repeat procedure is sometimes required before this is achieved. There is emerging evidence that ablation may improve prognosis in some patients with AF and heart failure. Ablation for AF is an attractive treatment but is not risk-free, and may be complicated by cardiac tamponade, stroke, phrenic nerve injury and, rarely, pulmonary vein stenosis.

Persistent atrial fibrillation

There are two options for treating persistent AF – rate control or rhythm control. With both options prophylaxis against thromboembolism is required on either a short-term or long-term basis.

Rhythm control Restoration of sinus rhythm is appropriate if the arrhythmia causes troublesome symptoms and if there is a treatable underlying cause. Electrical DC cardioversion or pharmacological cardioversion may be used. Cardioversion is initially successful in most patients but relapse is frequent (25%–50% at 1 month and 70%–90% at 1 year). Attempts to restore and maintain sinus rhythm are most successful if AF has been present for less than 3 months, the patient is young and there is no important structural heart disease.

Immediate cardioversion is appropriate if AF has been present for less than 48 hours. In stable patients with no history of structural heart disease, intravenous flecainide (2 mg/kg over 30 mins, maximum dose 150 mg) can be used and will restore sinus rhythm in 75% of patients within 8 hours. In patients with structural or ischaemic heart disease, intravenous amiodarone can be given through a central venous catheter. DC cardioversion may also be used but requires deep sedation or general anaesthesia. If AF has been present for 48 hours or longer, or if there is doubt about its duration, DC cardioversion should be deferred until the patient has been established on effective oral anticoagulation for a minimum of 4 weeks and any underlying problems, such as hypertension or alcohol excess, have been corrected. Prophylactic treatment with amiodarone can reduce the risk of recurrence. Catheter ablation is sometimes used to restore and to maintain sinus rhythm in persistant AF but is a less effective treatment than for paroxysmal AF.

Rate control If sinus rhythm cannot be restored, treatment should be directed at controlling the heart rate. Beta-blockers, rate-limiting calcium antagonists, such as verapamil or diltiazem (see Box 16.29 and Fig. 16.49), and digoxin all reduce the ventricular rate by slowing AV conduction. This alone may produce a striking improvement in cardiac function, particularly in patients with mitral stenosis. Beta-blockers and rate-limiting calcium antagonists are more effective than digoxin at controlling the heart rate during exercise and have additional benefits in patients with hypertension or structural heart disease. Combination therapy with digoxin and a β-blocker can help with rate control but calcium channel antagonists should not be used with β-blockers because of the risk of bradycardia.

In exceptional cases, poorly controlled and symptomatic AF can be treated by implanting a permanent pacemaker and then deliberately inducing complete AV nodal block with catheter ablation. This is known as the 'pace and ablate' strategy.

Prevention of thromboembolism and stroke Loss of atrial contraction and left atrial dilatation cause stasis of blood in the LA and may lead to thrombus formation in the left atrial appendage. This predisposes patients to stroke and systemic embolism. Patients undergoing cardioversion for AF of greater than 48 hours' duration require temporary anticoagulation to reduce these risks. Direct oral anticoagulants or warfarin may be used. Anticoagulation should be started for at least 4 weeks before cardioversion and should be maintained for at least 3 months following successful cardioversion.

In patients with AF, the annual risk of stroke is influenced by many factors and a decision has to be made in which the risk of stroke is balanced against the risk of bleeding with anticoagulation. Patients with AF secondary to mitral valve disease should always be anticoagulated because the risk is so high. In other patients, clinical scoring systems can be used to assess the risk of stroke and bleeding. The risk of stroke is usually assessed by the CHA_2DS_2-VASc score (Box 16.25), and the HAS-BLED score can be used to estimate the bleeding risk (Box 16.26). Patients with a HAS-BLED score of 3 or more points may require more careful monitoring if anticoagulated.

In patients with paroxysmal AF, stroke risk is similar to that in patients with persistent AF when adjusted for CHA_2DS_2-VASc score. The risk of embolism is only weakly related to the frequency and duration of AF episodes, so stroke prevention guidelines do not distinguish between those with paroxysmal, persistent and permanent AF.

Several agents can be used to reduce stroke risk in AF. The factor Xa inhibitors rivaroxaban, apixaban and edoxaban, and the direct thrombin inhibitor dabigatran (collectively referred to as direct-acting oral anticoagulants, or DOACs) have largely replaced warfarin for stroke prevention in AF. These drugs are described in more detail in Chapter 25. They are at least as effective at preventing thrombotic stroke and are generally associated with a lower risk of intracranial haemorrhage. Other advantages include the lack of requirement for monitoring and the fact that they have fewer drug and food interactions. They should be considered in patients with AF and CHA_2DS_2-VASc score of 1 or more (male), or 2 or more (female). Stroke risk is reduced by around two-thirds, with an annual major bleeding risk of around 1%. Risk factors for bleeding include active peptic ulcer disease, uncontrolled hypertension, alcohol misuse and frequent falls. Agents that reverse the effects of DOACs have been developed. These include idarucizumab, which binds to dabigatran, and andexanet alfa, which binds to apixaban and rivaroxaban.

Warfarin can be used, adjusted to a target INR (International Normalised Ratio) of 2.0–3.0. If bleeding does occur in warfarin-treated patients, anticoagulation can be reversed by administering vitamin K or clotting factors.

Aspirin should not be used since it has little or no effect on embolic stroke and is associated with significant bleeding risk.

Supraventricular tachycardia

The term supraventricular tachycardia (SVT) describes a group of regular tachycardias that have a similar appearance on ECG. These are usually narrow-complex tachycardias and are characterised by a re-entry circuit or automatic focus involving the atria. The three principal types are atrioventricular nodal re-entrant tachycardia (AVNRT), atrioventricular re-entrant tachycardia (AVRT) and atrial tachycardia. The term SVT is not strictly accurate as, in many cases, the ventricles also form part of the re-entry circuit.

Atrioventricular nodal re-entrant tachycardia

Atrioventricular nodal re-entrant tachycardia (AVNRT) is a type of SVT caused by re-entry in a circuit involving the AV node and its two right atrial input pathways: a superior 'fast' pathway and an inferior 'slow' pathway (see Fig. 16.44A). This produces a regular tachycardia with a rate of 120–240/min. It tends to occur in the absence of structural heart disease and episodes may last from a few seconds to many hours. The patient is usually aware of a rapid, very forceful, regular heart beat and may experience chest discomfort, lightheadedness or breathlessness. Polyuria, mainly due to the release of ANP, is sometimes a feature. The ECG (Fig. 16.43) usually shows a tachycardia with normal QRS complexes but occasionally there may be rate-dependent bundle branch block.

Management

Treatment is not always necessary. However, an acute episode may be terminated by carotid sinus pressure or by the Valsalva manoeuvre. Adenosine (3–12 mg rapidly IV in incremental doses until tachycardia stops) or verapamil (5 mg IV over 1 min) will restore sinus rhythm in most cases. Intravenous β-blocker or flecainide can also be used. In rare

	16.25 CHA_2DS_2-VASc stroke risk scoring system for non-valvular atrial fibrillation	
	Parameter	**Score**
C	Congestive heart failure	1 point
H	Hypertension history	1 point
A_2	Age $\geq$ 75 years	2 points
D	Diabetes mellitus	1 point
S_2	Previous stroke or transient ischaemic attack (TIA)	2 points
V	Vascular disease	1 point
A	Age 65–74 years	1 point
Sc	Sex category female	1 point
	Maximum total score	9 points

Annual stroke risk
0 points = 0% (no prophylaxis required)
1 point = 1.3% (oral anticoagulant recommended in males only)
2+ points = > 2.2% (oral anticoagulant recommended)

From European Society of Cardiology clinical practice guidelines: atrial fibrillation (management of) 2010 and focused update (2012). Eur Heart J 2012; 33:2719–2747.

	16.26 HAS-BLED bleeding risk scoring system for patients receiving oral anticoagulation	
	Parameter	**Score**
H	Hypertension; current systolic blood pressure > 160 mmHg	1 point
A	Abnormal liver function (cirrhosis OR bilirubin > twice upper limit of reference range or transaminases > three times upper limit of reference range)	1 point
	Abnormal renal function (creatinine > 200 µmol/L (2.26 mg/dL)	1 point
S	Stroke history	1 point
B	Bleeding: prior major event	1 point
L	Labile INR on warfarin	1 point
E	Elderly: age $\geq$ 65 years	1 point
D	Drugs:	
	Use of antiplatelet drug	1 point
	High alcohol consumption	1 point
	Maximum total score	9 points

HAS-BLED score of $\geq$ 3 points requires close patient monitoring

cases, when there is severe haemodynamic compromise, the tachycardia should be terminated by DC cardioversion.

In patients with recurrent SVT, catheter ablation is the most effective therapy and will permanently prevent SVT in more than 90% of cases. Alternatively, prophylaxis with oral β-blocker, verapamil or flecainide may be used but commits predominantly young patients to long-term drug therapy and can create difficulty in female patients, as these drugs should be avoided during pregnancy where possible.

Atrioventricular re-entrant tachycardia

In this condition there is an abnormal band of conducting tissue that connects the atria and ventricles. This so-called accessory pathway comprises rapidly conducting fibres that resemble Purkinje tissue, in that they conduct very rapidly and are rich in sodium channels. In about 50% of cases, this pathway conducts only in the retrograde direction (from ventricles to atria) and thus does not alter the appearance of the ECG in sinus rhythm. This is known as a concealed accessory pathway. In the rest, the pathway also conducts in an antegrade direction (from atria to ventricles), so AV conduction in sinus rhythm is mediated via both the AV node and the accessory pathway, distorting the QRS complex. Premature ventricular activation via the pathway shortens the PR interval and produces a 'slurred' initial deflection of the QRS complex, called a delta wave (Fig. 16.44B). This is known as a manifest accessory pathway. As the AV node and accessory pathway have different conduction speeds and refractory periods, a re-entry circuit can develop, causing tachycardia (Fig. 16.44C); when associated with symptoms, the condition is known as Wolff–Parkinson–White (WPW) syndrome. The ECG during this tachycardia is almost indistinguishable from that of AVNRT (Fig. 16.44A).

Management

Carotid sinus pressure or intravenous adenosine can terminate the tachycardia. If AF occurs, it may produce a dangerously rapid ventricular rate because the accessory pathway lacks the rate-limiting properties of

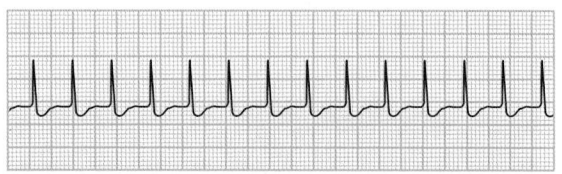

Fig. 16.43 Supraventricular tachycardia. The rate is 180/min and the QRS complexes are normal.

the AV node (Fig. 16.44D). This is known as pre-excited atrial fibrillation and may cause collapse, syncope and even death. It should be treated as an emergency, usually with DC cardioversion.

Catheter ablation is first-line treatment in symptomatic patients and is nearly always curative. Alternatively, prophylactic anti-arrhythmic drugs, such as flecainide or propafenone (see Box 16.30) can be used to slow conduction in, and prolong the refractory period of, the accessory pathway. Long-term drug therapy is not the preferred treatment for most patients and amiodarone should not be used, as its side-effect profile cannot be justified and ablation is safer and more effective. Digoxin and verapamil shorten the refractory period of the accessory pathway and should not be used.

Ventricular premature beats

Ventricular premature beats (VPBs) are frequently found in healthy people and their prevalence increases with age. Ectopic beats in patients with otherwise normal hearts are more prominent at rest and disappear with exercise. Sometimes VPBs are a manifestation of subclinical coronary artery disease or cardiomyopathy but also may occur in patients with established heart disease following an MI. Most patients with VPBs are asymptomatic but some present with an irregular heart beat, missed beats or abnormally strong beats, due to increased cardiac output of the post-ectopic sinus beat. On examination the pulse is irregular, with weak or missed beats as a result of the fact that the stroke volume is low because left ventricular contraction occurs before filling is complete (Fig. 16.45). The ECG shows broad and bizarre complexes because the ventricles are activated sequentially rather than simultaneously. The complexes may be unifocal (identical beats arising from a single ectopic focus) or multifocal (varying morphology with multiple foci, see Fig. 16.46). 'Couplet' and 'triplet' are the terms used to describe two or three successive ectopic beats. A run of alternating

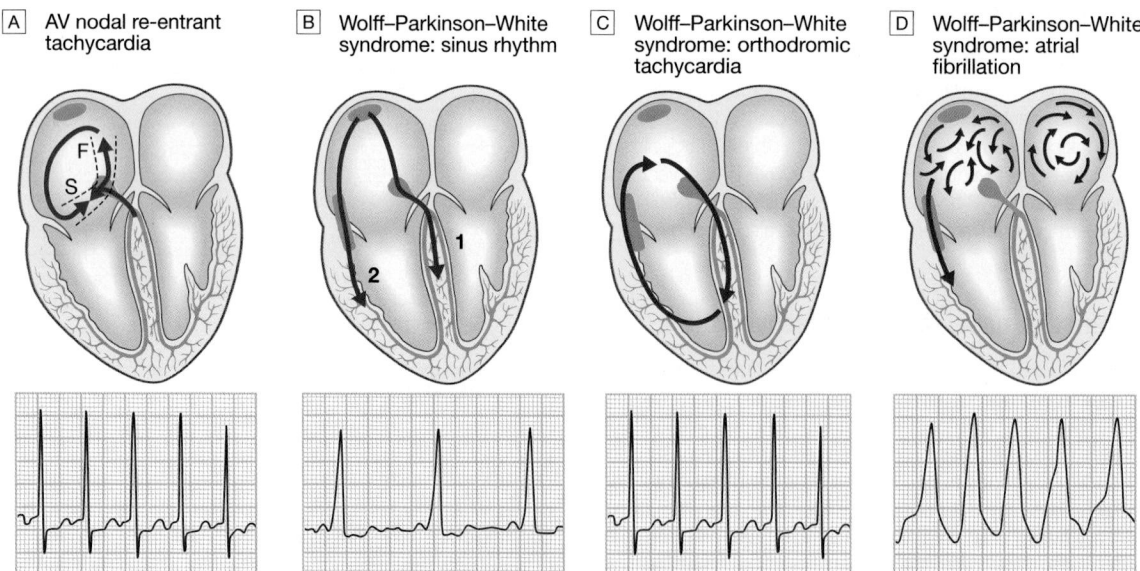

Fig. 16.44 Atrioventricular nodal re-entrant tachycardia (AVNRT) and Wolff–Parkinson–White (WPW) syndrome. [A] Atrioventricular (AV) nodal re-entrant tachycardia. The mechanism of AVNRT occurs via two right atrial AV nodal input pathways: the slow (S) and fast (F) pathways. Antegrade conduction occurs via the slow pathway; the wavefront enters the AV node and passes into the ventricles, at the same time re-entering the atria via the fast pathway. In WPW syndrome, there is a strip of accessory conducting tissue that allows electricity to bypass the AV node and spread from the atria to the ventricles rapidly and without delay. When the ventricles are depolarised through the AV node the ECG is normal, but when the ventricles are depolarised through the accessory conducting tissue the ECG shows a very short PR interval and a broad QRS complex. [B] Sinus rhythm. In sinus rhythm, the ventricles are depolarised through (1) the AV node and (2) the accessory pathway, producing an ECG with a short PR interval and broadened QRS complexes; the characteristic slurring of the upstroke of the QRS complex is known as a delta wave. The degree of pre-excitation (the proportion of activation passing down the accessory pathway) and therefore the ECG appearances may vary a lot, and at times the ECG can look normal. [C] Orthodromic tachycardia. This is the most common form of tachycardia in WPW. The re-entry circuit passes antegradely through the AV node and retrogradely through the accessory pathway. The ventricles are therefore depolarised in the normal way, producing a narrow-complex tachycardia that is indistinguishable from other forms of supraventricular tachycardia. [D] Atrial fibrillation. In this rhythm, the ventricles are largely depolarised through the accessory pathway, producing an irregular broad-complex tachycardia that is often more rapid than the example shown.

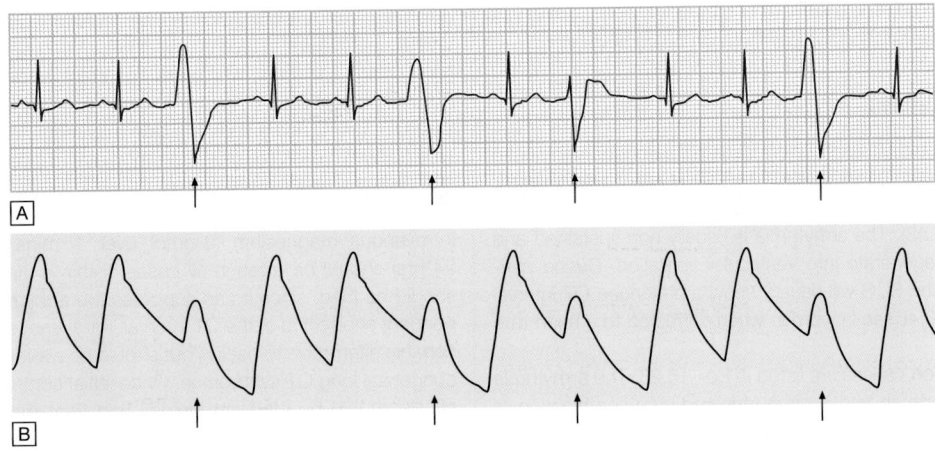

Fig. 16.45 Ventricular ectopic beats. [A] There are broad, bizarre QRS complexes (arrows) with no preceding P wave in between normal sinus beats. Their configuration varies, so these are multifocal ectopics. [B] A simultaneous arterial pressure trace is shown. The ectopic beats result in a weaker pulse (arrows), which may be perceived as a 'dropped beat'.

sinus and ventricular ectopic beats is known as ventricular 'bigeminy'. The significance depends on the presence or absence of underlying heart disease.

Management

Treatment may not be necessary, unless the patient is highly symptomatic, in which case β-blockers or, in some situations, catheter ablation can be used. There is no evidence that anti-arrhythmic therapy improves prognosis but the discovery of very frequent VPBs in a patient not known to have heart disease should prompt further investigations with echocardiography and an exercise ECG to screen for structural heart disease and ischaemic heart disease. It is common for VPBs to occur during the course of an acute MI. Persistent, frequent VPBs (over 10/hr) in patients who have survived the acute phase of MI indicate a poorer long-term outcome. In this situation, anti-arrhythmic drugs do not improve and may even worsen prognosis. The exception is β-blockers, which should be prescribed for other reasons following MI. Similarly, heart failure of any cause is associated with VPBs. While they indicate an adverse prognosis, this is not improved by anti-arrhythmic drugs. Effective treatment of the heart failure may suppress the ectopic beats.

Ventricular tachycardia

Ventricular tachycardia (VT) occurs most commonly in the settings of acute MI, chronic coronary artery disease and cardiomyopathy. It is associated with extensive ventricular disease, impaired left ventricular function and ventricular aneurysm. In these settings, VT may cause haemodynamic compromise or degenerate into ventricular fibrillation (see Fig. 16.19). VT is most often caused by re-entry within scarred ventricular tissue, and less often by abnormal automaticity or triggered activity in ischaemic tissue. Patients may experience palpitation, dyspnoea, lightheadedness and syncope. The ECG shows tachycardia and broad, abnormal QRS complexes with a rate of more than 120/min (Fig. 16.46). It may be difficult to distinguish VT from SVT with bundle branch block or pre-excitation (WPW syndrome) on ECG but features in favour of VT are listed in Box 16.27. A 12-lead ECG (Fig. 16.47) or electrophysiology study may help establish the diagnosis. When there is doubt, it is safer to manage the problem as VT.

Patients recovering from MI sometimes have periods of idioventricular rhythm ('slow' VT) at a rate only slightly above the preceding sinus rate and below 120/min. These episodes often reflect reperfusion of the infarct territory and may be a good sign. They are usually self-limiting and asymptomatic, and do not require treatment. Other forms of sustained VT require treatment, often as an emergency.

Occasionally, VT occurs in patients with otherwise healthy hearts ('normal heart VT'), usually because of abnormal automaticity in the right ventricular outflow tract or one of the fascicles of the left bundle branch.

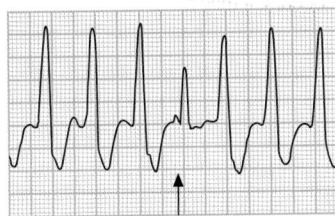

Fig. 16.46 Ventricular tachycardia: fusion beat. In ventricular tachycardia, there is independent atrial and ventricular activity. Occasionally, a P wave is conducted to the ventricles through the AV node, producing a normal sinus beat in the middle of the tachycardia (a capture beat); more commonly, however, the conducted impulse fuses with an impulse from the tachycardia (a fusion beat, arrow). This can occur only when there is atrioventricular dissociation and is therefore diagnostic of ventricular tachycardia.

---

i   16.27 Features more in keeping with ventricular tachycardia

- History of myocardial infarction
- Atrioventricular dissociation (pathognomonic)
- Capture/fusion beats (pathognomonic; see Fig. 16.40)
- Extreme left axis deviation
- Very broad QRS complexes (> 140 msecs)
- No response to carotid sinus massage or intravenous adenosine

---

Management

Prompt action to restore sinus rhythm is required and should usually be followed by prophylactic therapy. Synchronised DC cardioversion is the treatment of choice if systolic BP is less than 90 mmHg. If the arrhythmia is well tolerated, intravenous amiodarone may be given as a bolus, followed by a continuous infusion (see Box 16.30). Intravenous lidocaine can also be used but may depress left ventricular function, causing hypotension or acute heart failure. Hypokalaemia, hypomagnesaemia, acidosis and hypoxia should be corrected if present.

Beta-blockers are effective at preventing VT by reducing ventricular automaticity. Amiodarone can be added if additional control is needed. Class Ic anti-arrhythmic drugs should not be used for prevention of VT in patients with coronary artery disease or heart failure because they depress myocardial function and can increase the likelihood of a dangerous arrhythmia. In patients with poor left ventricular function or where VT is associated with haemodynamic compromise, the use of an implantable cardiac defibrillator is recommended. In resistant cases of focal or infarct scar-mediated VT, catheter ablation can be used to interrupt the

16

arrhythmia focus or circuit. The treatment of choice for VT occurring in a normal heart is catheter ablation, which often can be curative.

Torsades de pointes

This form of polymorphic VT is a complication of prolonged ventricular repolarisation (prolonged QT interval). The ECG shows rapid irregular complexes that seem to twist around the baseline as the mean QRS axis changes (Fig. 16.48). The arrhythmia is usually non-sustained and repetitive, but may degenerate into ventricular fibrillation. During periods of sinus rhythm, the ECG will usually show a prolonged QT interval (> 0.44 sec in men, > 0.46 sec in women when corrected to a heart rate of 60/min).

Some of the common causes are listed in Box 16.28. The arrhythmia is more common in women and is often triggered by a combination of factors, such as administration of QT-prolonging medications and hypokalaemia. The congenital long QT syndromes are a family of genetic disorders that are characterised by mutations in genes that code for cardiac potassium or sodium channels. Long QT syndrome subtypes have different triggers, which are important when counselling patients. Adrenergic stimulation through vigorous exercise is a common trigger in long QT type 1, and a sudden noise may trigger arrhythmias in long QT type 2. Arrhythmias are more common during sleep in type 3.

Management

Intravenous magnesium (8 mmol over 15 mins, then 72 mmol over 24 hrs) should be given in all cases. If this is ineffective, atrial pacing should be tried, since it can suppress the arrhythmia through rate-dependent shortening of the QT interval. Intravenous isoprenaline is a reasonable alternative to pacing but should be avoided in patients with congenital long QT syndromes. Once initial control has been achieved, efforts should be made to identify and treat the underlying cause or stop medications that predispose to the arrhythmia. If the underlying cause cannot be corrected or the arrhythmia is the result of an inherited syndrome, then long-term pharmacological therapy may be necessary. Beta-blockers are effective at preventing syncope in patients with congenital long QT syndrome. Some patients, particularly those with extreme QT interval prolongation (> 500 msecs) or certain high-risk genotypes, should be considered for an implantable defibrillator. Left stellate ganglion block may be of value in patients with resistant arrhythmias.

Brugada syndrome is a related genetic disorder that may present with polymorphic VT or sudden death. It is most commonly caused by mutations in the *SCN5A* gene which encodes a sodium channel expressed in cardiac myocytes. It is characterised by an abnormal ECG (right bundle branch block and ST elevation in V_1 and V_2 but not usually prolongation of the QT interval). The only known effective treatment is an implantable defibrillator.

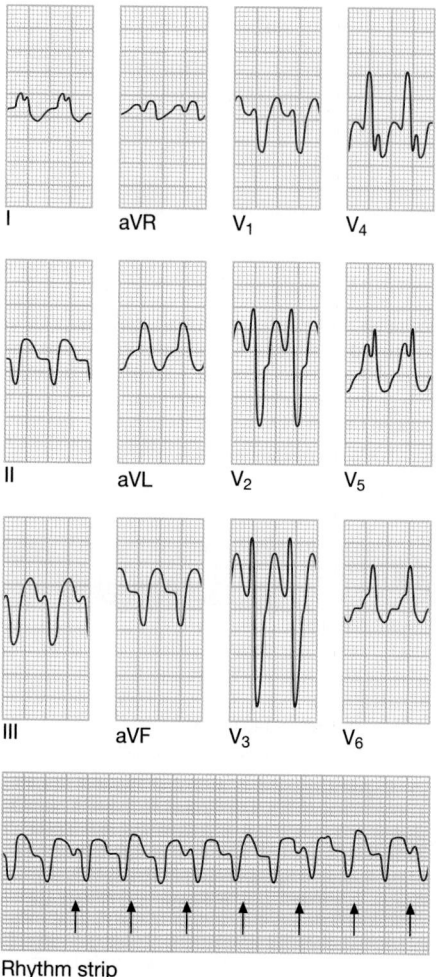

I   aVR V_1 V_4

II   aVL V_2 V_5

III   aVF V_3 V_6

Rhythm strip

Fig. 16.47 Ventricular tachycardia: 12-lead ECG. There are typically very broad QRS complexes and marked left axis deviation. There is also atrioventricular dissociation; some P waves are visible and others are buried in the QRS complexes (arrows).

i	**16.28 Causes of long QT interval and torsades de pointes**

Bradycardia

- Bradycardia potentiates other factors that cause torsades de pointes

Electrolyte disturbance

- Hypokalaemia
- Hypomagnesaemia
- Hypocalcaemia

Drugs*

- Disopyramide, flecainide and other class Ia, Ic anti-arrhythmic drugs (Box 16.29 and Fig. 16.49)
- Sotalol, amiodarone and other class III anti-arrhythmic drugs
- Amitriptyline and other tricyclic antidepressants
- Chlorpromazine and other phenothiazines
- Erythromycin and other macrolides
- Hydroxychloroquine and chloroquine

Congenital syndromes

- Long QT1: gene affected *KCNQ1*: K+ channel, 30%–35%
- Long QT2: gene affected *HERG*: K+ channel, 25%–30%
- Long QT3: gene affected *SCN5A*: Na+ channel, 5%–10%
- Long QT4–12: rare; various genes implicated

*Many other drugs that are not shown can be associated with prolongation of the QT interval. See www.crediblemeds.org for a complete list.

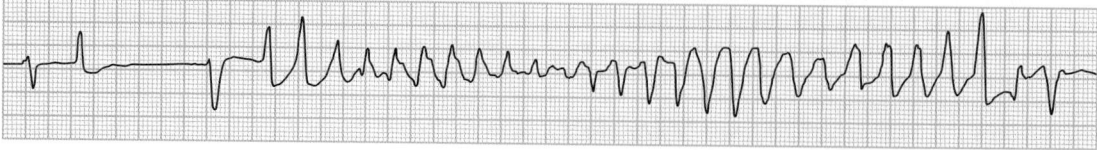

Fig. 16.48 Torsades de pointes. A bradycardia with a long QT interval is followed by polymorphic ventricular tachycardia that is triggered by an R on T ectopic.

Principles of management of cardiac arrhythmias

Cardiac arrhythmias can be managed with anti-arrhythmic drug therapy, cardiac implantable electronic devices (CIEDs), or catheter ablation.

Anti-arrhythmic drugs

Traditionally, the Vaughan Williams system has been used to categorise anti-arrhythmic drugs based on their effects on the action potential. Increased understanding of the mechanisms of action has allowed further subclassification, based on the cardiac ion channels and receptors on which they act see (Box 16.29 and Fig. 16.49). The individual agents, dosages and most common side-effects are summarised in Box 16.30 and the general principles of use are summarised in Box 16.31.

Class I drugs

Class I drugs act principally by suppressing excitability and slowing conduction in atrial or ventricular muscle. They block sodium channels, of which there are several types in cardiac tissue. These drugs should generally be avoided in patients with heart failure because they depress myocardial function, and class Ia and Ic drugs are often pro-arrhythmic.

Class Ia drugs

These prolong cardiac action potential duration and increase the tissue refractory period. They are used to prevent both atrial and ventricular arrhythmias.

Disopyramide

This is an effective drug but causes anticholinergic side-effects, such as urinary retention, and can precipitate glaucoma. It can depress myocardial function and should be avoided in cardiac failure.

Quinidine

This drug is effective at preventing AF and is occasionally used in Brugada syndrome. It is strongly pro-arrhythmic and can cause gastrointestinal upset.

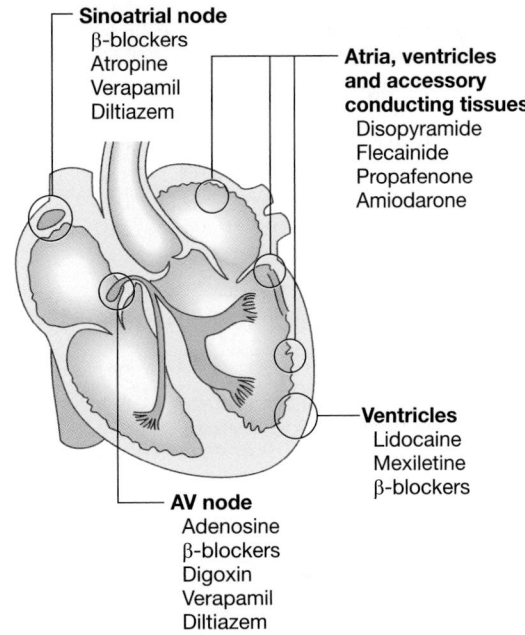

Sinoatrial node
β-blockers
Atropine
Verapamil
Diltiazem

Atria, ventricles and accessory conducting tissues
Disopyramide
Flecainide
Propafenone
Amiodarone

Ventricles
Lidocaine
Mexiletine
β-blockers

AV node
Adenosine
β-blockers
Digoxin
Verapamil
Diltiazem

Fig. 16.49 Classification of anti-arrhythmic drugs by site of action. (AV = atrioventricular)

Class Ib drugs

These shorten the action potential and tissue refractory period. They act on channels found predominantly in ventricular myocardium and so are used to treat or prevent VT and VF.

Lidocaine

This must be given intravenously and has a very short plasma half-life.

Mexiletine

This can be given intravenously or orally but has many side-effects.

Class Ic drugs

These affect the slope of the action potential without altering its duration or refractory period. They are used mainly for prophylaxis of AF but are effective in prophylaxis and treatment of supraventricular or ventricular arrhythmias. They are useful for WPW syndrome because they block conduction in accessory pathways. They should not be used in patients with previous MI because they increase the risk of arrhythmia in this setting.

Flecainide

This is effective for prevention of AF, and an intravenous infusion may be used for pharmacological cardioversion of AF of less than 24 hours' duration. Since flecainide can cause slow atrial flutter with a paradoxically rapid ventricular rate, it should be prescribed along with an AV node-blocking drug such as a β-blocker to control the ventricular rate.

Propafenone

This also has some β-blocker (class II) properties. Important interactions with digoxin, warfarin and cimetidine have been described.

Class II drugs

This group comprises the β-adrenoceptor antagonists (β-blockers). These agents reduce the rate of SA node depolarisation and cause relative block in the AV node, making them useful for rate control in atrial flutter and AF. They can be used to prevent VT and SVT. They reduce myocardial excitability and the risk of arrhythmic death in patients with coronary artery disease and heart failure.

16.29 Classification of anti-arrhythmic drugs by effect on the intracellular action potential*

Class I: membrane-stabilising agents (sodium channel blockers)

(a) Block Na+ channel and prolong action potential
- Quinidine, disopyramide

(b) Block Na+ channel and shorten action potential
- Lidocaine, mexiletine

(c) Block Na+ channel with no effect on action potential
- Flecainide, propafenone

Class II: β-adrenoceptor antagonists (β-blockers)
- Atenolol, bisoprolol, metoprolol

Class III: drugs whose main effect is to prolong the action potential
- Amiodarone, dronedarone, sotalol

Class IV: slow calcium channel blockers
- Verapamil, diltiazem

*Some drugs such as digoxin, ivabradine and adenosine have no place in this classification, while others such as amiodarone have properties in more than one class.

i 16.30 Uses, dosage and side-effects of anti-arrhythmic drugs

Drug	Main uses	Route	Dosage (adult)	Important side-effects
Class I				
Disopyramide	Prevention and treatment of atrial and ventricular tachyarrhythmias	IV	2 mg/kg at 30 mg/min, then 0.4 mg/kg/hr (max 800 mg/day)	Myocardial depression, hypotension, dry mouth, urinary retention
Lidocaine	Treatment and short-term prevention of VT and VF	Oral	300–800 mg daily in divided dosage	Myocardial depression, delirium, convulsions
		IV	Bolus 50–100 mg, 4 mg/min for 30 mins, then 2 mg/min for 2 hrs, then 1 mg/min for 24 hrs	
Mexiletine	Prevention and treatment of ventricular tachyarrhythmias	IV	Loading dose: 100–250 mg at 25 mg/min, then 250 mg in 1 hr, then 250 mg in 2 hrs Maintenance therapy: 0.5 mg/min	Myocardial depression, gastrointestinal irritation, delirium, dizziness, tremor, nystagmus, ataxia
		Oral	167–500 mg daily	
Flecainide	Prevention and treatment of atrial and ventricular tachyarrhythmias	IV	2 mg/kg over 10 mins, then if required 1.5 mg/kg/hr for 1 hr, then 0.1 mg/kg/hr	Myocardial depression, dizziness
		Oral	50–150 mg twice daily	
Propafenone	Prevention and treatment of atrial and ventricular tachyarrhythmias	Oral	150 mg 3 times daily for 1 week, then 300 mg twice daily	Myocardial depression, dizziness
Class II				
Atenolol	Treatment and prevention of SVT and AF, prevention of VEs and exercise-induced VF	IV	2.5 mg at 1 mg/min, repeated at 5-min intervals (max 10 mg)	Myocardial depression, bradycardia, bronchospasm, fatigue, depression, nightmares, cold peripheries
		Oral	25–100 mg daily	
Bisoprolol		Oral	2.5–10 mg daily	
Metoprolol		IV	5 mg over 2 mins to a maximum of 15 mg	
Class III				
Amiodarone	Serious or resistant atrial and ventricular tachyarrhythmias	IV	5 mg/kg over 20–120 mins, then up to 15 mg/kg/24 hrs	Photosentivity skin discoloration, corneal deposits, thyroid dysfunction, alveolitis, nausea and vomiting, hepatotoxicity, peripheral neuropathy, torsades de pointes; potentiates digoxin and warfarin
		Oral	Initially 600–1200 mg/day, then 100–400 mg daily	
Dronedarone	Paroxysmal atrial fibrillation	Oral	400 mg twice daily	Renal and hepatic dysfunction requiring regular blood monitoring
Sotalol*	AF, rarely ventricular tachyarrhythmias	IV	10–20 mg slowly	Can cause torsade de pointes
		Oral	40–160 mg twice daily	
Class IV				
Verapamil	Treatment of SVT, control of AF	IV	5–10 mg over 30 secs	Myocardial depression, hypotension, bradycardia, constipation
		Oral	40–120 mg 3 times daily or 240 mg SR daily	
Other				
Atropine	Treatment of bradycardia and/or hypotension due to vagal over-activity (see Box 16.32)	IV	0.6–3 mg	Dry mouth, thirst, blurred vision, atrial and ventricular extrasystoles
Adenosine	Treatment of SVT, aid to diagnosis in unidentified tachycardia	IV	3 mg over 2 secs, followed if necessary by 6 mg, then 12 mg at intervals of 1–2 mins	Flushing, dyspnoea, chest pain Avoid in asthma
Digoxin	Rate control of AF	IV	Loading dose: 0.5–1 mg (total), 0.5 mg over 30 mins, then 0.25–0.5 mg after 4–6 hrs	Gastrointestinal disturbance, xanthopsia, arrhythmias
		Oral	0.5 mg repeated after 6 hrs, then 0.0625–0.25 mg daily	

*Sotalol also has class II activity as a β-blocker.
(AF = atrial fibrillation; IV = intravenous; SR = sustained-release formulation; SVT = supraventricular tachycardia; VE = ventricular ectopic; VF = ventricular fibrillation; VT = ventricular tachycardia)

Non-selective β-blockers

These act on both β_1 and β_2 receptors. Beta$_2$-blockade causes side-effects, such as bronchospasm and peripheral vasoconstriction. Propranolol is non-selective and is subject to extensive first-pass metabolism in the liver. The effective oral dose is therefore unpredictable and must be titrated after treatment is started with a small dose. Other non-selective drugs include nadolol and carvedilol.

Cardioselective β-blockers

These act mainly on myocardial β_1 receptors and are relatively well tolerated. Bisoprolol and metoprolol are examples of cardioselective β-blockers.

Sotalol

This is a racemic mixture of two isomers with non-selective β-blocker (mainly l-sotalol) and class III (mainly d-sotalol) activity. It may cause torsades de pointes.

Class III drugs

Class III drugs act by prolonging the plateau phase of the action potential, thus lengthening the refractory period. These drugs are very effective at preventing atrial and ventricular tachyarrhythmias. They cause QT interval prolongation and can predispose to torsades de pointes and VT, especially in patients with other predisposing risk factors (see Box 16.28). Disopyramide and sotalol have some class III activity but the main drug in this class is amiodarone, as discussed below.

Amiodarone

While amiodarone is primarily considered a class III drug, it also has class I, II and IV activity. It is probably the most effective drug currently available for controlling paroxysmal AF. It is also used to prevent episodes of recurrent VT, particularly in patients with poor left ventricular function or those with implantable defibrillators (to prevent unnecessary DC shocks). Amiodarone has a very long tissue half-life (25–110 days). An intravenous or oral loading regime is often used to achieve therapeutic tissue concentrations. The drug's effects may last for weeks or months after treatment has been stopped. Side-effects are common (up to one-third of patients), numerous and potentially serious. Drug interactions are also common (see Box 16.30).

Dronedarone

Dronedarone is related to amiodarone but has a short tissue half-life and fewer side-effects. It has recently been shown to be effective at preventing episodes of atrial flutter and AF. It is contraindicated in patients with permanent AF, or if there is heart failure or left ventricular impairment, because it increases mortality. Regular liver and renal function test monitoring is required.

Class IV drugs

These block the 'slow calcium channel', which is important for impulse generation and conduction in atrial and nodal tissue, although it is also present in ventricular muscle. Their main indications are prevention of SVT (by blocking the AV node) and rate control in patients with AF.

Verapamil

This is the most widely used drug in this class. Intravenous verapamil may cause profound bradycardia or hypotension, and should not be used in conjunction with β-blockers.

Diltiazem

This has similar properties to verapamil.

Other anti-arrhythmic drugs

Atropine sulphate

Atropine is a muscarinic receptor antagonist that increases the sinus rate and SA and AV conduction. It is the treatment of choice for severe bradycardia or hypotension due to vagal over-activity. It is used for initial management of symptomatic bradyarrhythmias complicating inferior MI, and in cardiac arrest due to asystole. The usual dose is 0.6 mg IV, repeated if necessary to a maximum of 3 mg. Repeat dosing may be necessary because the drug disappears rapidly from the circulation after parenteral administration. Side-effects are listed in Box 16.30.

Adenosine

This works by binding to A1 receptors in conducting tissue, producing a transient AV block lasting a few seconds. It is used to terminate SVTs when the AV node is part of the re-entry circuit, or to help establish the diagnosis in difficult arrhythmias, such as atrial flutter with 2:1 AV block (see Fig. 16.40) or broad-complex tachycardia (see Boxes 16.30 and 16.32). Adenosine is given as an intravenous bolus, initially 3 mg over 2 seconds (see Box 16.30). If there is no response after 1–2 minutes, 6 mg should be given; if necessary, after another 1–2 minutes the maximum dose of 12 mg may be given. Patients should be warned to expect short-lived and sometimes distressing flushing, breathlessness and chest pain. Adenosine can cause bronchospasm and should be avoided in patients with asthma; its effects are greatly potentiated by dipyridamole and inhibited by theophylline and other xanthines.

Digoxin

Digoxin is a glycoside purified from the European foxglove, *Digitalis lanata*, which slows conduction and prolongs the refractory period in the AV node. This effect helps to control the ventricular rate in AF. Digoxin also shortens refractory periods and enhances excitability and conduction in other parts of the heart, including accessory pathways. It may therefore increase atrial and ventricular ectopic activity and can lead to more complex atrial and ventricular tachyarrhythmias. Digoxin is largely excreted by the kidneys, and the maintenance dose (see Box 16.30) should be reduced in children, older people and those with renal impairment. It is widely distributed and has a long tissue half-life (36 hours), so that effects may persist for several days. Measurement of plasma digoxin concentration helps identify digoxin toxicity or under-treatment (Box 16.33).

Non-pharmacological treatments

Electrical cardioversion

Electrical cardioversion, also known as direct current (DC) cardioversion, is useful for terminating an organised rhythm, such as AF or VT. The shock depolarises the myocardium, interrupts the arrhythmia and produces a brief period of asystole, followed by the resumption of sinus rhythm. Cardioversion is usually carried out as an elective procedure under general anaesthesia. The shock is delivered immediately after the R wave because, if it is applied during ventricular repolarisation (on the T wave), it may provoke VF. A 100–150 Joule shock is normally used.

16

16.33 Digoxin toxicity

Extracardiac manifestations

- Anorexia, nausea, vomiting
- Diarrhoea
- Altered colour vision (xanthopsia)

Cardiac manifestations

- Bradycardia
- Multiple ventricular ectopics
- Ventricular bigeminy (alternate ventricular ectopics)
- Atrial tachycardia (with variable block)
- Ventricular tachycardia
- Ventricular fibrillation

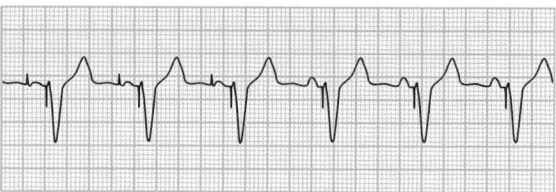

Fig. 16.50 Dual-chamber pacing. The first three beats show atrial and ventricular pacing with narrow pacing spikes in front of each P wave and QRS complex. The last four beats show spontaneous P waves with a different morphology and no pacing spike; the pacemaker senses or tracks these P waves and maintains atrioventricular synchrony by pacing the ventricle after an appropriate interval.

Defibrillation

Defibrillators deliver a DC, high-energy, short-duration shock via two large electrodes or paddles coated with conducting jelly or a gel pad, positioned over the upper right sternal border and the apex. Defibrillators are primarily used in the management of cardiac arrest due to VF and deliver an unsynchronised shock, since the precise timing of the discharge is not important in this situation. A biphasic shock is used during which the shock polarity is reversed mid-shock. This reduces the total shock energy required to depolarise the heart. In VF and other emergencies, the energy of the first and second shocks should be 150 Joules and thereafter up to 200 Joules; there is no need for an anaesthetic, as the patient is unconscious.

Temporary pacemakers

Temporary pacing involves delivery of an electrical impulse into the heart to initiate tissue depolarisation and to trigger cardiac contraction. This is achieved by inserting a bipolar pacing electrode through the internal jugular, subclavian or femoral vein and positioning it at the apex of the RV, using fluoroscopic imaging. The electrode is connected to an external pacemaker with an adjustable energy output and pacing rate. The ECG of right ventricular pacing is characterised by regular broad QRS complexes with a left bundle branch block pattern. Each complex is immediately preceded by a 'pacing spike' (Fig. 16.50). The pacemaker will operate only if the heart rate falls below a preset level. Occasionally, temporary atrial or dual-chamber pacing (see below) is used.

Temporary pacing is indicated for transient AV block and other arrhythmias complicating acute MI or cardiac surgery, to maintain the rhythm in other situations of reversible bradycardia (such as metabolic disturbance or drug overdose), or as a bridge to permanent pacing. Complications include pneumothorax, brachial plexus or subclavian artery injury, local infection or sepsis (usually with *Staphylococcus aureus*), and pericarditis. Failure of the system may be due to lead displacement or a progressive increase in the threshold (exit block) caused by tissue oedema. Complication rates increase with time and so a temporary pacing system should ideally not be used for more than 7 days.

Transcutaneous pacing is administered by delivering an electrical stimulus through two large adhesive gel pad electrodes placed over the apex and upper right sternal border, or over the anterior and posterior chest. It is easy and quick to set up, but causes discomfort because it induces forceful pectoral and intercostal muscle contraction. Modern external defibrillators often incorporate a transcutaneous pacing system that can be used until transvenous pacing is established.

Permanent pacemakers

Permanent pacemakers are small, flat, metal devices that are implanted under the skin, usually in the pectoral area (Fig. 16.51). They contain a battery, a pulse generator, and programmable electronics that allow adjustment of pacing and memory functions. Pacing electrodes (leads) can be placed via the subclavian or cephalic veins into the RV (usually at the apex), the right atrial appendage or, to maintain AV synchrony, both.

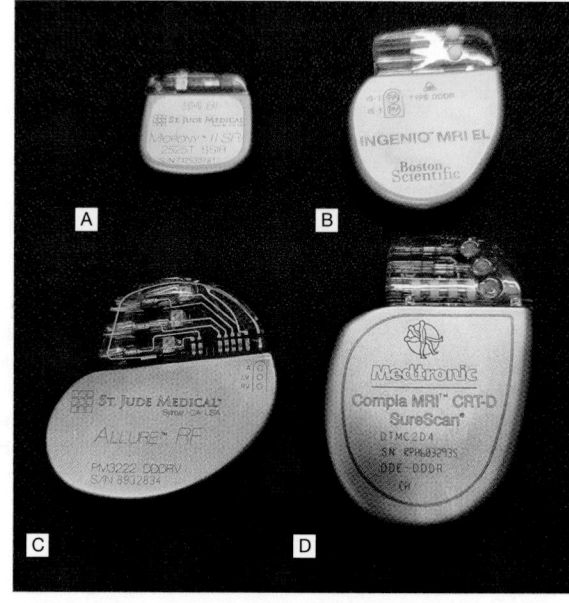

Fig. 16.51 Cardiac implantable electronic devices. [A] Single-chamber pacemaker. [B] Dual-chamber pacemaker. [C] Cardiac resynchronisation therapy pacemaker (CRT-P). [D] Cardiac resynchronisation therapy defibrillator (CRT-D).

Permanent pacemakers are controlled using an external programmer through a wireless telemetry system, allowing rate, output, timing and other parameters to be adjusted. This allows the device settings to be tailored to the patient's needs. Aside from their therapeutic role, pacemakers store useful diagnostic data about the patient's heart rate trends and the occurrence of tachyarrhythmias, such as VT.

Single-chamber atrial pacing is indicated in patients with SA disease without AV block and ventricular pacing in patients with continuous AF and bradycardia. Here the pacemaker acts as an external sinus node. Dual-chamber pacing is most often used in patients with second- or third-degree AV block. Here, the atrial electrode is used to detect spontaneous atrial activity and trigger ventricular pacing (see Fig. 16.50), thereby preserving AV synchrony and allowing the ventricular rate to increase, together with the sinus node rate, during exercise and other forms of stress. Dual-chamber pacing has many advantages over single-chamber ventricular pacing, including superior haemodynamics and better effort tolerance; a lower prevalence of atrial arrhythmias in patients with SA disease; and avoidance of 'pacemaker syndrome', in which a fall in BP and dizziness occur due to loss of AV synchrony.

A code is used to signify the pacing mode (Box 16.34). For example, a system that paces the atrium, senses the atrium and is inhibited if it senses spontaneous activity is designated AAI. Most dual-chamber pacemakers are programmed to a mode termed DDD; in this case, ventricular pacing is triggered by a sensed sinus P wave and inhibited by a sensed spontaneous QRS complex. A fourth letter, 'R', is added if the pacemaker has a rate response function. For example, the letters

16

16.34 International generic pacemaker code		
Chamber paced	**Chamber sensed**	**Response to sensing**
O = none	O = none	O = none
A = atrium	A = atrium	T = triggered
V = ventricle	V = ventricle	I = inhibited
D = both	D = both	D = both

---

i 16.35 Key indications for implantable cardiac defibrillator therapy

Primary prevention

- After myocardial infarction, if the left ventricular ejection fraction is < 30%
- Mild to moderate symptomatic heart failure on optimal drug therapy, with left ventricular ejection fraction < 35%
- Some patients with inherited cardiac conditions (long QT syndrome, cardiomyopathy)

Secondary prevention

- Survivors of ventricular fibrillation or ventricular tachycardia cardiac arrest not having a transient or reversible cause
- Ventricular tachycardia with haemodynamic compromise or significant left ventricular impairment (left ventricular ejection fraction < 35%)

AAIR indicate an atrial demand pacemaker with a rate response function. Rate-responsive pacemakers are used in patients with chronotropic incompetence, who are unable to increase their heart rate during exercise. These devices have a sensor that triggers an increase in heart rate in response to movement or increased respiratory rate. The sensitivity of the sensor is programmable, as is the maximum paced heart rate.

Early complications of permanent pacing include pneumothorax, cardiac tamponade, infection and lead displacement. Late complications include infection (which usually necessitates removing the pacing system), erosion of the generator or lead, chronic pain related to the implant site, and lead fracture due to mechanical fatigue.

Implantable cardiac defibrillators

In addition to the functions of a permanent pacemaker, implantable cardiac defibrillators (ICDs) can also detect and terminate life-threatening ventricular tachyarrhythmias. ICDs are larger than pacemakers mainly because of the need for a large battery and capacitor to enable cardioversion or defibrillation. ICD leads are similar to pacing leads but have one or two shock coils along the length of the lead, used for delivering defibrillation. ICDs treat ventricular tachyarrhythmias using overdrive pacing, cardioversion or defibrillation. They are implanted in a similar manner to pacemakers and carry a similar risk of complications. In addition, patients can be prone to psychological problems and anxiety, particularly if they have experienced repeated shocks from their device.

The evidence-based indications for ICD implantation are shown in Box 16.35. These can be divided into secondary prevention indications, when patients have already had a potentially life-threatening ventricular arrhythmia, and primary prevention indications, when patients are considered to be at significant future risk of arrhythmic death. A common primary prevention indication is in patients with inherited conditions associated with a high risk of sudden cardiac death, such as long QT syndrome, hypertrophic cardiomyopathy and arrhythmogenic right ventricular cardiomyopathy. Treatment with ICDs is expensive and so the indications for which the devices are routinely implanted depend on the health-care resources available.

Cardiac resynchronisation therapy

Cardiac resynchronisation therapy (CRT) is a useful treatment for selected patients with heart failure, in whom cardiac function is impaired by the presence of left bundle branch block. This conduction defect is associated with poorly coordinated left ventricular contraction that can aggravate heart failure in susceptible patients. The systems used to deliver CRT comprise a right atrial lead, a right ventricular lead and a third lead that is placed via the coronary sinus into one of the veins on the epicardial surface of the LV (see Fig. 16.28). Simultaneous septal and left ventricular epicardial pacing resynchronises left ventricular contraction.

CRT improves symptoms and quality of life, and reduces mortality in patients with moderate to severe (NYHA class III–IV) heart failure who are in sinus rhythm, with left bundle branch block and left ventricular ejection fraction of 35% or less. CRT also prevents heart failure progression in similar patients with mild (NYHA class I–II) heart failure symptoms. These devices are more effective in patients in sinus rhythm than in those with AF. Most devices are also defibrillators (CRT-D) because many patients with heart failure are predisposed to ventricular arrhythmias. CRT pacemakers (CRT-P) are used when the focus is palliation of symptoms rather than prolonging life.

Catheter ablation therapy

Catheter ablation therapy is the treatment of choice for patients with SVT or atrial flutter, and is a useful treatment for some patients with AF or ventricular arrhythmias (Fig. 16.52). It involves inserting a series of catheter

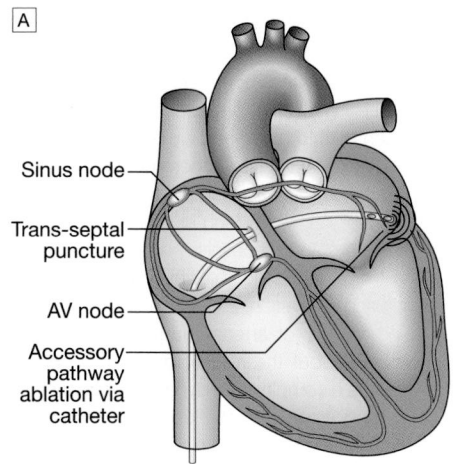

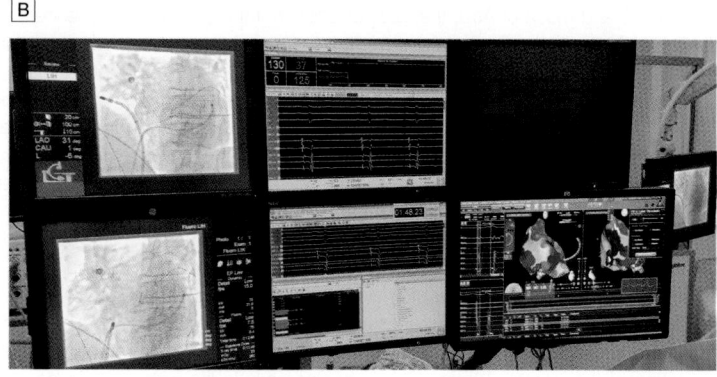

Fig. 16.52 Radiofrequency ablation. [A] Schematic of an ablation of the accessory conducting pathway in Wolff–Parkinson–White syndrome (see text for details). [B] Fluoroscopy and mapping for an ablation procedure. (AV = atrioventricular)

electrodes into the heart through the venous system. These are used to record the activation sequence of the heart in sinus rhythm, during tachycardia and after pacing manoeuvres. Once the arrhythmia focus or circuit, such as an accessory pathway in WPW syndrome, has been identified, a catheter is used to ablate the culprit tissue. This can be done either by using heat, which is termed radiofrequency ablation, or by freezing, which is termed cryoablation. The procedure takes approximately 1–4 hours and does not require a general anaesthetic, although the patient may experience some discomfort during the ablation procedure. Serious complications are rare (< 1%) but include complete heart block requiring pacemaker implantation, and cardiac tamponade. For many arrhythmias, radiofrequency ablation is very attractive because it offers the prospect of a lifetime cure, thereby eliminating the need for long-term drug therapy.

The technique has revolutionised the management of many arrhythmias and is now the treatment of choice for AVNRT and AV re-entrant (accessory pathway) tachycardias, when it is curative in over 90% of cases. Focal atrial tachycardias and atrial flutter can also be treated by radiofrequency ablation, although some patients subsequently experience episodes of AF. Ablation is highly effective in patients with VT occurring in a structurally normal heart, and can be life-saving in patients with refractory VT due to ventricular scar or structural disease. Catheter ablation techniques are also employed to prevent AF. This involves ablation at two sites: the ostia of the pulmonary veins, from which ectopic beats may trigger paroxysms of arrhythmia, and in the LA itself, where re-entry circuits maintain AF, once established. This is effective at reducing episodes of AF in around 70%–80% of younger patients with structurally normal hearts.

In patients with permanent AF and poor rate control, in whom drugs are ineffective or are not tolerated, rate control can be achieved by implantation of a permanent pacemaker, followed by ablation of the AV node to induce complete AV block and bradycardia, thus allowing the pacemaker to assume control of the heart rate.

Coronary artery disease

Coronary artery disease (CAD) is the commonest cause of angina and acute coronary syndrome and the leading cause of death worldwide. It also has a devastating effect on quality of life. Disability-adjusted life years, a measure of healthy years of life lost, can be used to indicate the burden of disease rather than the resulting deaths. It has been estimated that CAD is responsible for 10% of disability-adjusted life years in low-income countries and 18% in high-income ones. In the UK, 1 in 3 men and 1 in 4 women die from CAD, an estimated 188 000 people have a myocardial infarct each year, and approximately 2.3 million people are living with CAD. The death rates from CAD in the UK are among the highest in Western Europe (more than 70 000 people) but are falling, particularly in younger age groups; over the last 50 years, CAD mortality has more than halved. In Eastern Europe and much of Asia, the rates of CAD are rapidly rising. Occult CAD is common in those who present with other forms of atherosclerotic vascular disease, such as intermittent claudication or stroke, and is an important cause of morbidity and mortality in these patients.

Pathogenesis

In the vast majority of patients, CAD is caused by atherosclerosis (Box 16.36) but rarely it can occur as the result of aortitis, vasculitis and autoimmune connective tissue diseases. Atherosclerosis is a progressive inflammatory disorder of the arterial wall that is characterised by focal lipid-rich deposits of atheroma that remain clinically silent until they become large enough to impair tissue perfusion, or until ulceration and disruption of the lesion occurs resulting in thrombotic occlusion or distal embolisation of the vessel. Atherosclerosis begins early in life with deposits of lipids in the vessel wall, which tend to occur at sites of altered arterial shear stress, such as bifurcations, and are associated with abnormalities of endothelial function at that site. Abnormalities of arterial function have been detected among high-risk children and adolescents, such as cigarette smokers and those with familial hyperlipidaemia or

16.36 Coronary artery disease: clinical manifestations and pathology	
Clinical problem	**Pathology**
Stable angina	Ischaemia due to fixed atheromatous stenosis of one or more coronary arteries
Unstable angina	Ischaemia caused by dynamic complete or partial obstruction of a coronary artery due to plaque rupture or erosion with superimposed thrombosis
Myocardial infarction (type 1)	Myocardial necrosis caused by acute occlusion of a coronary artery due to plaque rupture or erosion with superimposed thrombosis
Myocardial infarction (type 2)	Supply demand imbalance where blood flow cannot meet the needs of the myocardium. This may be caused by fixed atheromatous obstruction with high myocardial demand for blood
Heart failure	Myocardial dysfunction due to infarction or ischaemia
Arrhythmia	Altered conduction due to ischaemia or infarction
Sudden death	Ventricular arrhythmia, asystole or massive myocardial infarction

hypertension. Early lesions have been found in the arteries of victims of accidental death in the second and third decades of life but clinical manifestations often do not appear until the sixth, seventh or eighth decade. During evolution of an atherosclerotic plaque, monocytes and other inflammatory cells bind to receptors expressed by endothelial cells. Subsequently, they migrate into the intima, and take up oxidised low-density lipoprotein (LDL) particles by phagocytosis to become lipid-laden macrophages or foam cells. Extracellular lipid pools appear in the intimal space when foam cells die and release their contents (Fig. 16.53). In response to cytokines and growth factors produced by activated macrophages, smooth muscle cells migrate from the media of the arterial wall into the intima, and change from a contractile to a fibroblastic phenotype, which can stabilise the atherosclerotic lesion. If this is successful, the lipid core will be covered by smooth muscle cells and matrix, producing a stable atherosclerotic plaque that will remain asymptomatic until it becomes large enough to obstruct arterial flow.

In an established atherosclerotic plaque, macrophages mediate inflammation and smooth muscle cells promote repair. If inflammation predominates, the plaque becomes active or unstable and may be complicated by ulceration and thrombosis. Cytokines, such as interleukin-1, tumour necrosis factor-alpha, interferon-gamma, platelet-derived growth factors and matrix metalloproteinases, are released by activated macrophages. They cause the intimal smooth muscle cells overlying the plaque to become senescent and the collagen cross-links within the plaque to degrade. This results in thinning of the protective fibrous cap, making the lesion vulnerable to mechanical stress that ultimately causes erosion, fissuring or rupture of the plaque surface (see Fig. 16.53). Any breach in the integrity of the plaque will expose its contents to blood and will trigger platelet aggregation and thrombosis that extend into the atheromatous plaque and the arterial lumen. This may cause partial or complete obstruction at the site of the lesion or distal embolisation, resulting in infarction or ischaemia of the affected organ. This common mechanism underlies acute coronary syndromes, as well as other manifestations of atherosclerotic disease such as lower limb ischaemia and stroke (Ch. 29).

The number and complexity of arterial plaques increase with age and risk factors (see below) but the rate of progression of individual plaques is variable. There is a complex and dynamic interaction between mechanical wall stress and atherosclerotic lesions. Vulnerable plaques are characterised by a lipid-rich core, a thin fibrocellular cap, speckled calcification and an increase in inflammatory cells that release specific enzymes to degrade matrix proteins. In contrast, stable plaques are typified by a small lipid pool, a thick fibrous cap, heavy calcification and

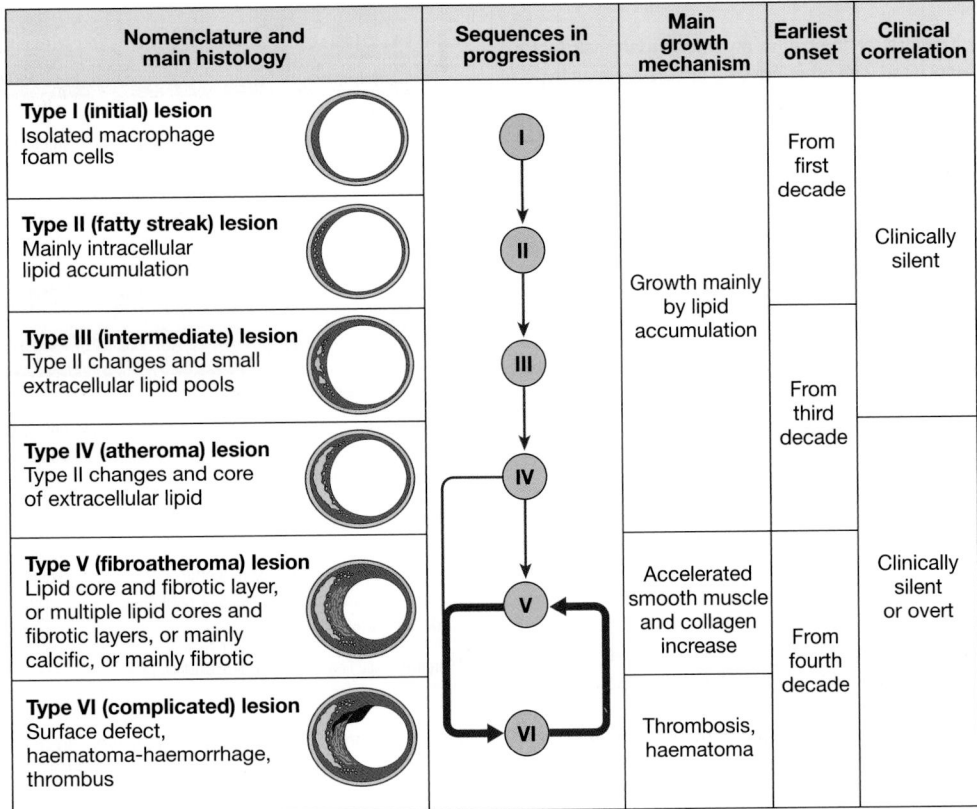

Nomenclature and main histology	Sequences in progression	Main growth mechanism	Earliest onset	Clinical correlation
Type I (initial) lesion Isolated macrophage foam cells	I	Growth mainly by lipid accumulation	From first decade	Clinically silent
Type II (fatty streak) lesion Mainly intracellular lipid accumulation	II			
Type III (intermediate) lesion Type II changes and small extracellular lipid pools	III		From third decade	
Type IV (atheroma) lesion Type II changes and core of extracellular lipid	IV			Clinically silent or overt
Type V (fibroatheroma) lesion Lipid core and fibrotic layer, or multiple lipid cores and fibrotic layers, or mainly calcific, or mainly fibrotic	V	Accelerated smooth muscle and collagen increase	From fourth decade	
Type VI (complicated) lesion Surface defect, haematoma-haemorrhage, thrombus	VI	Thrombosis, haematoma		

Fig. 16.53 The six stages of atherosclerosis: American Heart Association classification. *From Stary HC, Chandler B, Dinsmore RE, et al. A definition of advanced types of atherosclerotic lesions and a histological classification of atherosclerosis. Circulation 1995; 92:1355–1374. © 1995 American Heart Association.*

16

plentiful collagenous cross-links. Fissuring or rupture tends to occur at sites of maximal mechanical stress, particularly the margins of an eccentric plaque, and may be triggered by a surge in BP, such as during exercise or emotional stress. Surprisingly, most plaque events are subclinical and heal spontaneously, although this may allow thrombus to be incorporated into the lesion, producing plaque growth and further obstruction to flow.

Atherosclerosis may induce complex changes in the media that lead to arterial remodelling. Some arterial segments may slowly constrict (negative remodelling), while others may gradually enlarge (positive remodelling). These changes are important because they may amplify or minimise the degree to which atheroma encroaches into the arterial lumen.

Many risk factors have been identified for atherosclerosis but the causes are incompletely understood, since unknown factors account for up to 40% of the variation in risk from one person to the next.

Age and sex

Age is the most powerful independent risk factor for atherosclerosis and sex also plays a role. Pre-menopausal women have lower rates of disease than men, although the sex difference disappears after the menopause. Hormone replacement therapy (HRT) is not effective in the prevention of CAD, and HRT in post-menopausal women is associated with an increased risk of cardiovascular events.

Genetics

Atherosclerotic CAD often runs in families and a positive family history is common in patients with early-onset disease (age <50 in men and <55 in women). Twin studies have shown that a monozygotic twin of an affected individual has an eightfold increased risk and a dizygotic twin a fourfold increased risk of dying from CAD, compared to the general population due to a combination of shared genetic, environmental and lifestyle factors. The most common risk factors, such as hypertension, hyperlipidaemia and diabetes mellitus, are inherited in a polygenic manner.

Smoking

There is a strong relationship between cigarette smoking and CAD, especially in younger (<70 years) individuals, and this is the most important modifiable risk factor.

Hypertension

The incidence of atherosclerosis increases as BP rises, and this is related to systolic and diastolic BP, as well as pulse pressure. Antihypertensive therapy reduces cardiovascular mortality, stroke and heart failure.

Hypercholesterolaemia

The risk of atherosclerosis rises with serum cholesterol concentrations and lowering serum total and LDL cholesterol concentrations reduces the risk of cardiovascular events.

Diabetes mellitus

This is a potent risk factor for all forms of atherosclerosis, especially type 2 diabetes mellitus. It is often associated with diffuse disease that is difficult to treat. Insulin resistance (normal glucose homeostasis with high levels of insulin) is associated with obesity and physical inactivity, and is also a risk factor for CAD. Glucose intolerance makes a major contribution to the high incidence of CAD in people from South Asia and some other ethnic groups.

Haemostatic factors

Platelet activation and high plasma fibrinogen concentrations are associated with an increased risk of coronary thrombosis, whereas antiphospholipid antibodies are associated with recurrent arterial thromboses.

Physical activity

Regular exercise (brisk walking, cycling or swimming for 20 minutes two or three times a week) has a protective effect, whereas inactivity roughly doubles the risk of CAD and is a major risk factor for stroke.

Obesity

Obesity, particularly if central or truncal, is an independent risk factor, although it is often associated with other adverse factors such as hypertension, diabetes mellitus and physical inactivity.

Alcohol

Excess alcohol consumption is associated with hypertension and cerebrovascular disease.

Diet

Diets deficient in fresh fruit, vegetables and polyunsaturated fatty acids are associated with an increased risk of cardiovascular disease. The introduction of a Mediterranean-style diet reduces cardiovascular events. However, dietary supplements, such as vitamins C and E, beta-carotene, folate and fish oils, do not reduce cardiovascular events and, in some cases, have been associated with harm.

Personality

While certain personality traits are associated with an increased risk, there is no evidence to support the popular belief that stress is a major cause of CAD.

Social deprivation

Social deprivation is strongly associated with cardiovascular disease. This may be partly due to associations with lifestyle risk factors, such as smoking and alcohol excess, which are more common in socially deprived individuals. Current guidelines recommend that treatment thresholds should be lowered for patients from socially deprived areas.

The effect of risk factors can be multiplicative rather than additive. People with a combination of risk factors are at greatest risk and so assessment should take account of all identifiable risk factors. It is important to distinguish between relative risk (the proportional increase in risk) and absolute risk (the actual chance of an event). For example, a man of 35 years with a plasma cholesterol of 7 mmol/L (approximately 170 mg/dL), who smokes 40 cigarettes a day, is much more likely to die from CAD within the next decade than a non-smoking man of the same age with a normal cholesterol, but the absolute likelihood of his dying during this time is small (high relative risk, low absolute risk).

Management

Two approaches can be employed. Primary prevention aims to introduce lifestyle changes or therapeutic interventions to prevent CAD and other forms of atherosclerosis in the whole population or in healthy individuals with an elevated risk of disease. Secondary prevention involves initiating treatment in patients who already have had an event, with the aim of reducing the risk of subsequent events. The distinction between primary and secondary prevention is increasingly seen as arbitrary since many people will have CAD despite having no symptoms or experienced any clinical events.

Primary prevention

The population-based strategy aims to modify the risk factors of the whole population through diet and lifestyle advice, on the basis that even a small reduction in smoking or average cholesterol, or modification of exercise and diet, will produce worthwhile benefits (Box 16.37). Some risk factors, such as obesity and smoking, are also associated with a higher risk of other diseases and should be actively discouraged through public health measures. The effectiveness of this approach has been demonstrated by introduction of legislation to restrict smoking in public places, which has been associated with reductions in rates of MI.

The targeted strategy aims to identify and to treat high-risk individuals who have a combination of risk factors that can be quantified by composite scoring systems. It is important to consider the absolute risk of atheromatous cardiovascular disease that an individual is facing before initiating treatment since this will help to determine whether the potential benefits of intervention are likely to outweigh the expense, inconvenience and possible side-effects of treatment. For example, a 65-year-old man

16.37 Population-based strategies to prevent coronary disease

- Do not smoke
- Take regular exercise (minimum of 20 mins, three times per week)
- Maintain an 'ideal' body weight
- Eat a mixed diet rich in fresh fruit and vegetables
- Aim to get no more than 10% of energy intake from saturated fat

16.38 Factors influencing myocardial oxygen supply and demand

Oxygen demand: cardiac work

- Heart rate
- Blood pressure
- Myocardial contractility
- Left ventricular hypertrophy
- Valve disease

Oxygen supply: coronary blood flow*

- Duration of diastole
- Coronary perfusion pressure (aortic diastolic minus coronary sinus or right atrial diastolic pressure)
- Coronary vasomotor tone
- Oxygenation:
  Haemoglobin
  Oxygen saturation

*Coronary blood flow occurs mainly in diastole.

with an average BP of 150/90 mmHg, who smokes and has diabetes mellitus with a total:high-density lipoprotein (HDL) cholesterol ratio of 8, has a 10-year risk of MI or stroke of 56%. Conversely, a 55-year-old woman who has an identical BP, is a non-smoker, does not have diabetes mellitus, and has a total:HDL cholesterol ratio of 6 has a much better outlook, with a 10-year coronary MI or stroke risk of 5.7%. Lowering cholesterol will reduce the risk in both of these individuals by 30% and lowering BP will produce a further 20% reduction. In combination, both strategies would reduce the risk of an event from 56% to 25% in the male patient (treat 4 patients to prevent one event) and from 5.7% to 2.5% in the female patient (treat 40 patients to prevent one event). Thresholds for treatment vary in different countries. In the UK and North America, current guidelines recommend initiation of cholesterol and BP-lowering therapies in individuals with a 10-year cardiovascular risk of 7.5%–10%.

Secondary prevention

This involves targeting interventions at individuals who have had cardiovascular disease. Patients who recover from a clinical event such as an MI are usually keen to help themselves and are particularly receptive to lifestyle advice, such as dietary modification and smoking cessation. Additional interventions that should be introduced in patients with angina pectoris or an acute coronary syndrome are discussed in more detail below.

Angina pectoris

Angina pectoris is a symptom complex caused by transient myocardial ischaemia, which occurs whenever there is an imbalance between myocardial oxygen supply and demand (Box 16.38).

Pathogenesis

Coronary atherosclerosis is by far the most common cause of angina pectoris. Angina may also occur in aortic valve disease and hypertrophic cardiomyopathy, and when the coronary arteries are involved with vasculitis or aortitis. The underlying mechanisms and risk factors for atherosclerosis have already been discussed. Approximately 10% of patients who report stable angina on effort have normal coronary arteries on angiography. The main causes are discussed in more detail below.

Coronary artery spasm

Angina may result from vasospasm of the coronary arteries. This may coexist with atherosclerosis, especially in unstable angina (see below),

16.39 Classification of angina pectoris and chest pain

Three characteristic features of angina

1. Constricting discomfort in the centre of the chest, or in the neck, shoulders, jaw or arms
2. Precipitated by physical exertion
3. Relieved by rest (or GTN) within 5 minutes

Classification

- **Typical angina**: All three features
- **Atypical angina**: Two features
- **Non-anginal chest pain**: One or no features

NICE classification

- **Possible angina**: Typical angina, atypical angina or non-anginal chest pain with an abnormal resting 12-lead ECG
- **Non-anginal chest pain**: Non-anginal chest pain with a normal resting 12-lead ECG

(ECG = electrocardiogram; GTN = glyceryl trinitrate; NICE = National Institute for Health and Care Excellence)

16.40 Canadian Cardiovascular Society (CCS) angina score

Class I

- Angina only during strenuous or prolonged physical activity

Class II

- Slight limitation, with angina only during vigorous physical activity

Class III

- Moderate limitation where symptoms occur with everyday activities

Class IV

- Inability to perform any activity without angina or angina at rest, i.e. severe limitation

---

but may rarely occur as an isolated phenomenon in patients with normal coronary arteries on angiography. This is sometimes known as variant angina; when it is accompanied by transient ST elevation on the ECG, it is termed Prinzmetal's angina.

Syndrome X and microvascular angina

The constellation of typical angina on effort and normal coronary arteries on angiography with objective evidence of myocardial ischaemia on stress testing is sometimes known as Syndrome X. Many of these patients are women and the mechanisms of their symptoms are unclear. In a subset of patients, there is evidence of impaired myocardial vasodilatory reserve giving rise to the term microvascular angina. These disorders are poorly understood but carry a good prognosis and respond variably to anti-anginal therapy.

Other causes

Angina can occur in association with aortic stenosis, hypertrophic obstructive cardiomyopathy and aortitis, all of which are discussed in more detail later in this chapter. It may also rarely be found in association with some types of systemic vasculitis (Ch. 26).

Clinical features

The history is the most important factor in making the diagnosis. Stable angina is categorised as typical angina, atypical angina or non-anginal chest pain (Box 16.39; see also Fig. 9.1). Some patients find the discomfort comes when they start walking and that later it does not return despite greater effort ('warm-up angina'). The Canadian Cardiovascular Society (CCS) scoring system is commonly used to grade the severity of angina (Box 16.40). This is of clinical value, not only in documenting the severity of angina but also in assessing prognosis.

Physical examination is frequently unremarkable but should include a careful search for an ejection systolic murmur (particularly aortic stenosis and hypertrophic obstructive cardiomyopathy), important risk factors (hypertension, diabetes mellitus), left ventricular dysfunction (cardiomegaly, gallop rhythm), other manifestations of arterial disease (carotid bruits, peripheral arterial disease), and unrelated conditions that may exacerbate angina (anaemia, thyrotoxicosis).

Investigations

Stress testing and non-invasive imaging are advisable to confirm the diagnosis and to risk stratify patients with possible angina (see Box 16.39). An algorithm for the investigation and treatment of patients with stable angina is shown in Fig. 16.54. An exercise ECG is commonly performed using a standard treadmill or bicycle ergometer protocol. while monitoring the patient's pulse, BP and general condition. Planar or down-sloping ST segment depression of 1 mm or more is indicative of ischaemia (Fig. 16.55). Up-sloping ST depression is less specific; it often occurs in normal individuals and false-positive results can occur with digoxin therapy, left ventricular hypertrophy, bundle branch block and WPW syndrome. Overall, the exercise ECG confirms the history of exertional angina, provides an objective measure of the patient's exercise tolerance and is indicative of the underlying disease severity (Fig. 16.56) that can identify high-risk individuals with severe coronary disease in combination with other clinical features (Box 16.41). However, exercise testing may be normal in a substantial proportion of patients with CAD or may be inconclusive because of inadequate exercise tolerance due to reduced mobility or other non-cardiac problems.

If the diagnosis is unclear following the investigations listed above, CT coronary angiography is the imaging investigation of first choice. It clarifies the diagnosis and guides the use of preventative and anti-anginal therapies. It also serves as an excellent guide to the appropriate use of invasive cardiac catheterisation, reducing its use in those with normal coronary arteries (see Fig. 16.13) and targeting it to those with significant disease (see Fig. 16.54). Its use is also associated with a marked reduction in the future risk of MI, likely due to better targeted preventative interventions in those with previously unrecognised CAD.

In patients with known CAD, further imaging with myocardial perfusion scanning or stress echocardiography is indicated. A perfusion defect present during stress but not at rest provides evidence of reversible myocardial ischaemia (Fig. 16.57), whereas a persistent perfusion defect seen during both phases of the study is usually indicative of previous MI.

Coronary angiography provides detailed anatomical information about the extent and nature of CAD (see Fig. 16.15). It is usually performed when coronary artery bypass graft surgery or percutaneous coronary intervention is being considered.

Management

This should begin with a careful explanation of the problem and a discussion of the lifestyle and medical interventions that can be deployed to relieve symptoms and improve prognosis (Box 16.42). Anxiety and misconceptions often contribute to disability. For example, some patients avoid all forms of exertion because they believe that each attack of angina is a 'mini-heart attack' that results in permanent damage. Education and reassurance can dispel these misconceptions and make a huge difference to the patient's quality of life.

The principles of management involve:

- identification and treatment of risk factors
- advice on smoking cessation
- introduction of drug treatment for symptom control
- a careful assessment of the extent and severity of CAD
- identification of high-risk patients for treatment to improve life expectancy.

All patients with angina secondary to CAD should receive antiplatelet therapy. Low-dose (75 mg) aspirin should be prescribed and continued

16

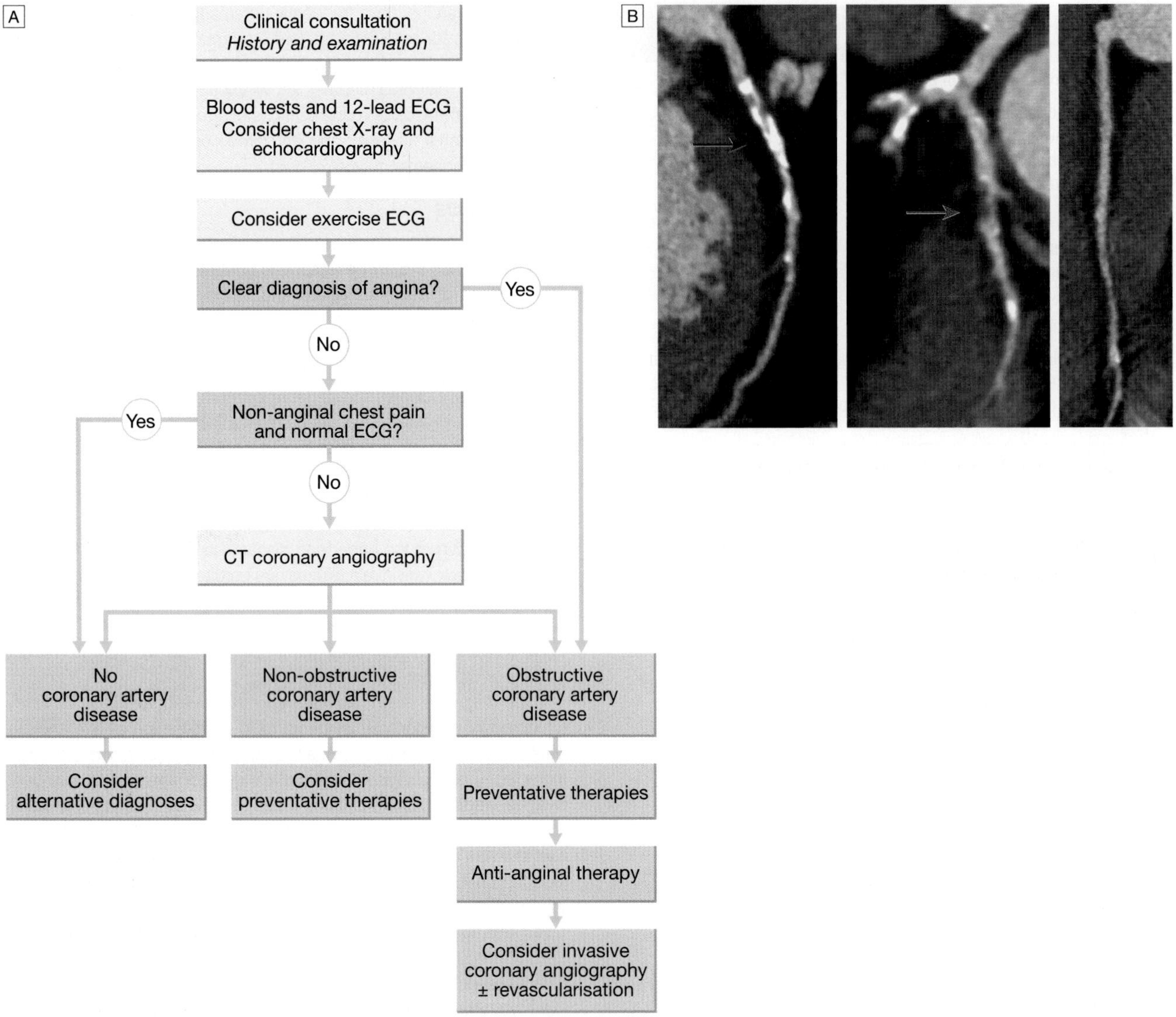

A

```
Clinical consultation
History and examination
        │
        ▼
Blood tests and 12-lead ECG
Consider chest X-ray and
echocardiography
        │
        ▼
Consider exercise ECG
        │
        ▼
Clear diagnosis of angina? ──── Yes
        │
        No
        │
        ▼
Non-anginal chest pain ──── Yes
and normal ECG?
        │
        No
        │
        ▼
CT coronary angiography
```

No coronary artery disease	Non-obstructive coronary artery disease	Obstructive coronary artery disease
Consider alternative diagnoses	Consider preventative therapies	Preventative therapies
		Anti-anginal therapy
		Consider invasive coronary angiography ± revascularisation

B

Fig. 16.54 [A] A scheme for the investigation and treatment of stable angina on effort. This scheme is best adopted for patients without prior known coronary artery disease and possible angina. For patients with known coronary artery disease, further stress imaging (echocardiography, radionuclide perfusion or magnetic resonance perfusion) rather than computed tomography coronary angiography is recommended. [B] An example CT coronary angiogram showing coronary artery disease in all three vessels with evidence of 'soft' lipid-rich plaque (yellow arrow) and extensive calcified coronary atheroma (red arrow).

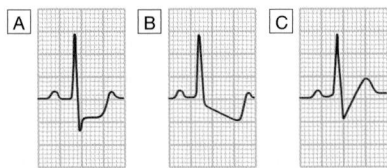

Fig. 16.55 Forms of exercise-induced ST depression. [A] Planar ST depression is usually indicative of myocardial ischaemia. [B] Down-sloping depression also usually indicates myocardial ischaemia. [C] Up-sloping depression may be a normal finding.

indefinitely since it reduces the risk of MI. Clopidogrel (75 mg daily) is an equally effective alternative if aspirin causes dyspepsia or other side-effects. Similarly, all patients should be prescribed a statin, even if the serum cholesterol concentration is normal.

Anti-anginal drug therapy

The goal of anti-anginal therapy is to control symptoms using a regimen that is as simple as possible and does not cause side-effects. Five main groups of drug are used in the treatment of angina but there is

little evidence that one group is more effective than another. It is conventional to start therapy with sublingual glyceryl trinitrate (GTN) and a β-blocker, and then add a calcium channel antagonist or a long-acting nitrate if needed. If the combination of two drugs fails to achieve an acceptable symptomatic response, the addition of further classes of drug has modest additional benefits and coronary revascularisation should be considered.

Nitrates

Nitrates act directly on vascular smooth muscle to produce venous and arteriolar dilatation. Several preparations are available, as shown in Box 16.43. They help angina by lowering preload and afterload, which reduces myocardial oxygen demand, and by increasing myocardial oxygen supply through coronary vasodilatation. Sublingual GTN, administered from a metered-dose aerosol (400 μg per spray) or as a tablet (300 or 500 μg), is indicated for acute attacks and relieves symptoms in 2–3 minutes. It can also be used before taking exercise to avoid provoking symptoms. Sublingual GTN has a short duration of action and side-effects include headache, symptomatic hypotension and, rarely, syncope. A more prolonged therapeutic effect can be achieved by giving GTN transcutaneously as a patch (5–10 mg daily) or as a slow-release

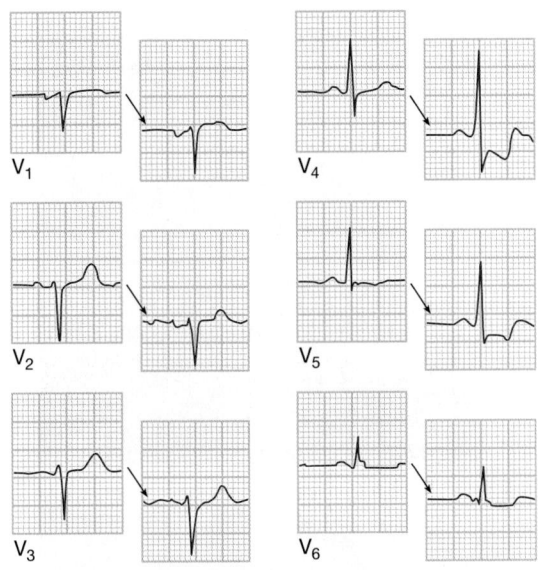

Fig. 16.56 A positive exercise test (chest leads only). The resting 12-lead ECG shows some minor T-wave changes in the inferolateral leads but is otherwise normal. After 3 minutes' exercise on a treadmill, there is marked planar ST depression in leads V_4 and V_5 (right-hand offset). Subsequent coronary angiography revealed critical three-vessel coronary artery disease.

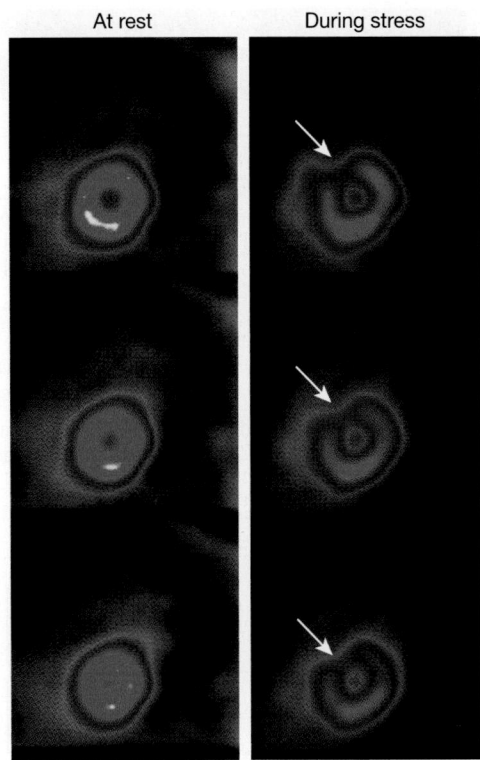

Fig. 16.57 A myocardial perfusion scan showing reversible anterior myocardial ischaemia. The images are cross-sectional tomograms of the left ventricle. The resting scans (left) show even uptake of the ^{99}technetium-labelled tetrofosmin and look like doughnuts. During stress there is reduced uptake of technetium, particularly along the anterior wall (arrows), and the scans look like crescents (right).

16

ⓘ 16.41 Risk stratification in patients with stable angina[1]	
High risk	**Low risk**
Recent-onset symptoms (< 6 months)	Long-standing symptoms
Class II to IV symptoms†	Class I symptoms[2]
Diabetes mellitus	
Comorbidity	
Post-infarct angina	Predictable exertional angina
Ischaemia at low workload	Ischaemia only at high workload
Left main or three-vessel disease	Single-vessel or two-vessel disease
Poor left ventricular function	Good left ventricular function

[1]Patients may fall between these two categories. [2]Canadian Cardiovascular Society Classification.

ⓘ 16.42 Advice to patients with stable angina
• Do not smoke
• Aim for an ideal body weight
• Take regular exercise (exercise up to, but not beyond, the point of chest discomfort is beneficial and may promote collateral vessels)
• Avoid severe unaccustomed exertion, and vigorous exercise after a heavy meal or in very cold weather
• Take sublingual nitrate before undertaking exertion that may induce angina

buccal tablet (1–5 mg 4 times daily). Isosorbide dinitrate (10–20 mg 3 times daily) and isosorbide mononitrate (20–60 mg once or twice daily) can be given by mouth, unlike GTN, which undergoes extensive metabolism in the liver. Headache is common with oral nitrates but tends to diminish if the patient perseveres with the treatment. Continuous nitrate therapy can cause pharmacological tolerance but this can be avoided by a 6–8-hour nitrate-free period, best achieved at night when the patient is inactive. If nocturnal angina is a predominant symptom, long-acting nitrates can be taken at the end of the day.

Beta-blockers

These lower myocardial oxygen demand by reducing heart rate, BP and myocardial contractility, but they may provoke bronchospasm in patients with asthma. Dosages of commonly used beta-blockers are shown in Box 16.18. In theory, non-selective β-blockers may aggravate coronary vasospasm by blocking coronary artery $β_2$-adrenoceptors, and so a once-daily cardioselective preparation such as slow-release metoprolol (50–200 mg daily) or bisoprolol (5–15 mg daily) is preferable. Beta-blockers should not be withdrawn abruptly, as rebound effects may precipitate dangerous arrhythmias, worsening angina or precipitate MI: the β-blocker withdrawal syndrome.

ⓘ 16.43 Duration of action of some nitrate preparations		
Preparation	**Peak action**	**Duration of action**
Sublingual GTN	4–8 mins	10–30 mins
Buccal GTN	4–10 mins	30–300 mins
Transdermal GTN	1–3 hrs	Up to 24 hrs
Oral isosorbide dinitrate	45–120 mins	2–6 hrs
Oral isosorbide mononitrate	45–120 mins	6–10 hrs

(GTN = glyceryl trinitrate)

Calcium channel antagonists

These drugs lower myocardial oxygen demand by reducing BP and myocardial contractility. Since dihydropyridine calcium antagonists, such as nifedipine and amlodipine, may cause a reflex tachycardia, it is best to use them in combination with a β-blocker. In contrast, verapamil and diltiazem can be used as monotherapy because they slow SA node

16.44 Calcium channel antagonists used for the treatment of angina

Drug	Dose	Feature
Nifedipine	5–20 mg 3 times daily*	May cause marked tachycardia
Nicardipine	20–40 mg 3 times daily	May cause less myocardial depression than the other calcium antagonists
Amlodipine	2.5–10 mg daily	Long-acting
Verapamil	40–80 mg 3 times daily*	Commonly causes constipation; useful anti-arrhythmic properties
Diltiazem	60–120 mg 3 times daily*	Similar anti-arrhythmic properties to verapamil

*Once- or twice-daily sustained-release preparations are available.

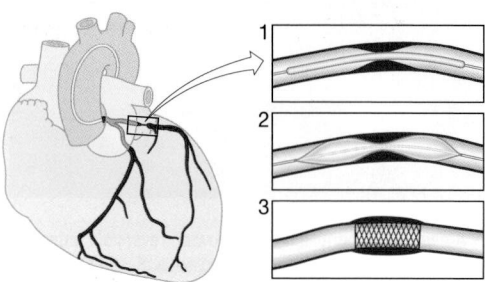

Fig. 16.58 Percutaneous coronary intervention. A guidewire is advanced from the radial (or femoral) artery to the coronary artery under radiographic control (1). A fine balloon catheter is then advanced over the guidewire to the stenotic coronary artery and the balloon is inflated to dilate the stenosis (2). When this has been achieved, a stent is usually placed at the site of the stenosis to maintain patency of the artery (3) (see text for more details).

firing, inhibit conduction through the AV node and tend to cause brady-cardia. They are particularly useful when β-blockers are contraindicated. Calcium channel antagonists reduce myocardial contractility and must be used with care in patients with poor LV function, since they can aggra-vate or precipitate heart failure. Other unwanted effects include periph-eral oedema, flushing, headache and dizziness (Box 16.44).

Potassium channel activators

Nicorandil (10–30 mg twice daily orally) is the only drug in this class that is currently available for clinical use. It acts as a vasodilator with effects on the arterial and venous systems, and has the advantage that it does not exhibit the tolerance seen with nitrates.

I_f channel antagonist

Ivabradine (initial dose 2.5–5 mg twice daily orally) is the first in this class of drug. It induces bradycardia by modulating ion channels in the sinus node. It does not inhibit myocardial contractility and appears to be safe in patients with heart failure.

Ranolazine

Ranolazine (initial dose 375 mg twice daily) inhibits the late inward sodium current in coronary artery smooth muscle cells, with a secondary effect on calcium flux and vascular tone, reducing angina symptoms.

Non-pharmacological treatments

Percutaneous coronary intervention

Percutaneous coronary intervention (PCI) involves passing a fine guide-wire across a coronary stenosis under radiographic control and using

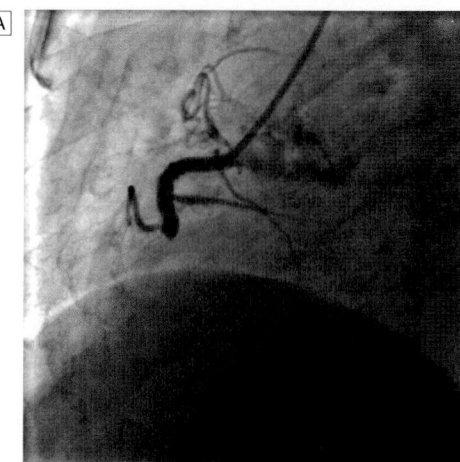

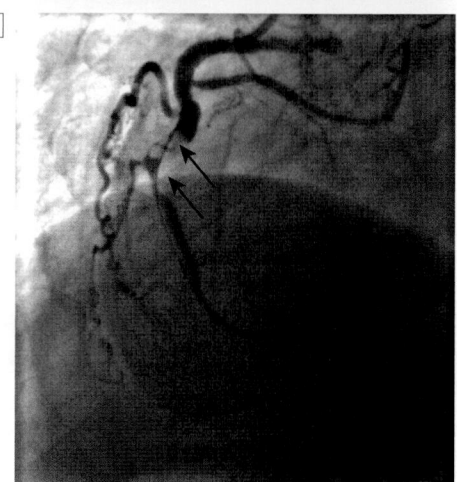

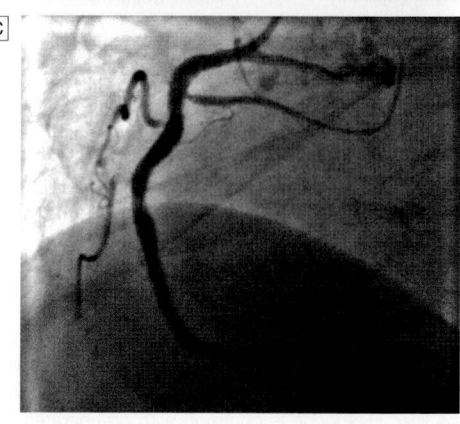

Fig. 16.59 Primary percutaneous coronary intervention. [A] Acute right coronary artery occlusion. [B] Initial angioplasty demonstrates a large thrombus filling defect (arrows). [C] Complete restoration of normal flow following intracoronary stenting.

it to position a balloon, which is then inflated to dilate the stenosis (Fig. 16.58). This can be combined with deployment of a coronary stent, which is a piece of metallic 'scaffolding' that can be impregnated with drugs with antiproliferative properties and that helps to maximise and maintain dilatation of a stenosed vessel. The routine use of stents in appropriate vessels reduces both acute complications and the incidence of clinically important restenosis (Fig. 16.59).

Treatment with PCI often provides excellent symptom control but it does not reduce MI or improve survival in patients with chronic stable angina. It is mainly used in single- or two-vessel disease. Stenoses in bypass grafts can be dilated, as well as those in the native coronary arteries. The technique is often used to provide

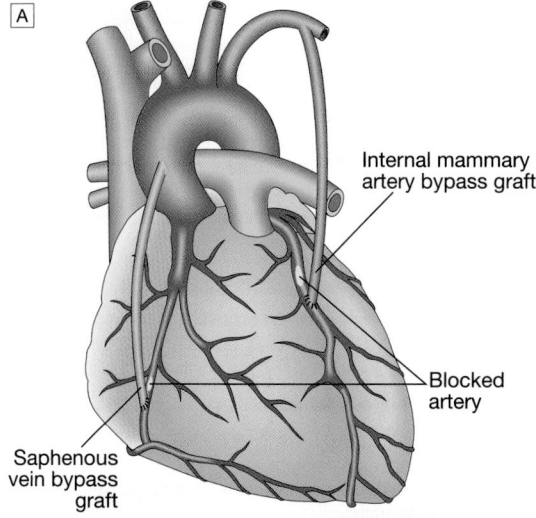

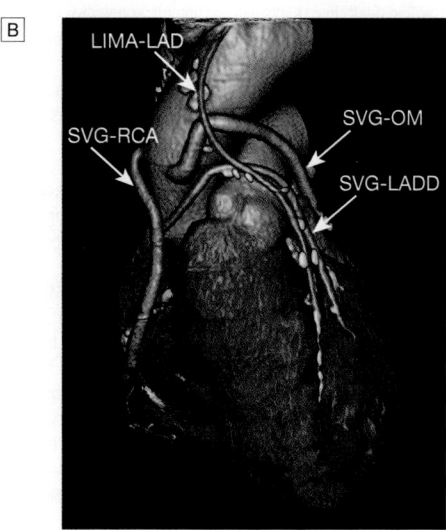

Fig. 16.60 Coronary artery bypass graft surgery. [A] Narrowed or stenosed arteries are bypassed using saphenous vein grafts connected to the aorta or by utilising the internal mammary artery. [B] Three-dimensional reconstruction of multidetector CT of the heart. The image shows the patent saphenous vein grafts (SVG) to the right coronary artery (RCA), obtuse marginal branch (OM) and diagonal branch (LADD), and left internal mammary artery graft (LIMA) to the left anterior descending (LAD) coronary artery.

palliative therapy for patients with recurrent angina after coronary artery bypass grafting.

The main acute complications of PCI are occlusion of the coronary artery by thrombus or a loose flap of intima (coronary artery dissection), and consequent MI. This occurs in about 2%–5% of procedures and can often be corrected by further intervention, although emergency coronary artery bypass grafting may occasionally be required. Mild myocardial damage, as indicated by elevation of cardiac troponin, occurs in up to 25%–30% of cases. The main long-term complication of PCI is restenosis, in up to one-third of cases. This is due to a combination of elastic recoil and smooth muscle proliferation and tends to occur within 3 months. Stenting substantially reduces the risk of restenosis, probably because it allows the operator to achieve more complete dilatation. Drug-eluting stents reduce this risk further by allowing an antiproliferative drug, such as sirolimus or paclitaxel, to elute slowly from the coating and prevent neo-intimal hyperplasia and in-stent restenosis. These are especially indicated in patients with diabetes, or in arteries with long calcific lesions or small diameters. Recurrent angina (affecting up to 5%–10% of patients at 6 months) may require further PCI or bypass grafting.

The risk of complications and the likely success of the procedure are closely related to the complexity of the disease, the experience of the operator and the presence of important comorbidity, such as diabetes and peripheral arterial disease. A good outcome is less likely if the target lesion is complex, long, eccentric or calcified, lies on a bend or within a tortuous vessel, involves a branch or contains thrombus.

Adjunctive therapy with a potent platelet inhibitor such as the P2Y12 receptor antagonists (clopidogrel, prasugrel or ticagrelor) in combination with aspirin and heparin improves the outcome following PCI.

Coronary artery bypass grafting

The internal mammary arteries, radial arteries or reversed segments of the patient's own saphenous vein can be used to bypass coronary artery stenoses (Fig. 16.60). This usually involves major surgery under cardiopulmonary bypass but, in some cases, grafts can be applied to the beating heart: 'off-pump' surgery. The operative mortality is approximately 1.5% but risks are higher in older patients, those with poor left ventricular function and those with significant comorbidity, such as renal failure.

Approximately 90% of patients are free of angina 1 year after coronary artery bypass grafting (CABG), but fewer than 60% of patients are asymptomatic after 5 or more years. Early post-operative angina is usually due to graft failure arising from technical problems during the operation, or poor 'run-off' due to disease in the distal native coronary vessels. Late recurrence of angina may be caused by progressive disease in the native coronary arteries or graft degeneration. Fewer than 50% of vein grafts are patent 10 years after surgery. Arterial grafts have a much better long-term patency rate with more than 80% of internal mammary artery grafts patent at 10 years. This has led many surgeons to consider total arterial revascularisation during CABG surgery. Aspirin (75–150 mg daily) and clopidogrel (75 mg daily) both improve graft patency, and one or the other should be prescribed indefinitely. Intensive lipid-lowering therapy slows the progression of disease in the native coronary arteries and bypass grafts and reduces clinical cardiovascular events. There is substantial excess cardiovascular morbidity and mortality in patients who continue to smoke after bypass grafting. Persistent smokers are twice as likely to die in the 10 years following surgery than those who give up at surgery.

Survival is improved by CABG in symptomatic patients with left main stem stenosis or three-vessel coronary disease when the LAD, CX and right coronary arteries are involved, or two-vessel disease involving the proximal LAD coronary artery. Improvement in survival is most marked in those with impaired left ventricular function or positive stress testing prior to surgery and in those who have undergone left internal mammary artery grafting.

Neurological complications are common, with a 1%–5% risk of perioperative stroke. Between 30% and 80% of patients develop short-term cognitive impairment that typically resolves within 6 months. There are also reports of long-term cognitive decline that may be evident in more than 30% of patients at 5 years. PCI and CABG are compared in Box 16.45.

Prognosis

The prognosis of CAD is related to the burden of CAD and the degree of left ventricular dysfunction. A patient with single-vessel disease and good left ventricular function has a 5-year survival of more than 90%. In contrast, a patient with severe left ventricular dysfunction and extensive three-vessel disease has a 5-year survival of less than 30% unless revascularisation is performed. Although symptoms are a poor guide to prognosis, the 5-year mortality of patients with severe angina (CCS angina scale III or IV, see Box 16.40) is nearly double that of patients with mild symptoms.

Some considerations specific to angina in old age are listed in Box 16.46.

Acute coronary syndrome

Acute coronary syndrome is a term that encompasses both unstable angina and myocardial infarction. Unstable angina is characterised by

16

16.45 Comparison of percutaneous coronary intervention (PCI) and coronary artery bypass grafting (CABG)

	PCI	CABG
Death	<0.5%	<1.5%
Myocardial infarction*	2%	10%
Hospital stay	6–18 hrs	5–8 days
Return to work	2–5 days	6–12 weeks
Recurrent angina	15%–20% at 6 months	10% at 1 year
Repeat revascularisation	10%–20% at 2 years	2% at 2 years
Neurological complications	Rare	Common (see text)
Other complications	Emergency CABG Vascular damage related to access site	Diffuse myocardial damage Infection (chest, wound) Wound pain

*Defined as CK-MB > 2× normal

16.46 Angina in old age

- **Incidence**: coronary artery disease increases in old age and affects women almost as often as men.
- **Comorbid conditions**: anaemia and thyroid disease are common and may worsen angina.
- **Calcific aortic stenosis**: common and should be sought in all older people with angina.
- **Atypical presentations**: when myocardial ischaemia occurs, age-related changes in myocardial compliance and diastolic relaxation can cause the presentation to be with symptoms of heart failure, such as breathlessness, rather than with chest discomfort.
- **Angioplasty and coronary artery bypass surgery**: provide symptomatic relief, although with increased procedure-related morbidity and mortality. Outcome is determined by the number of diseased vessels, severity of cardiac dysfunction and the number of concomitant diseases, as much as by age itself.

new-onset or rapidly worsening angina (crescendo angina), angina on minimal exertion or angina at rest in the absence of myocardial injury. Myocardial infarction (MI) is distinguished from unstable angina by the occurrence of myocardial necrosis and is diagnosed when myocardial injury occurs in the presence of clinical evidence of acute myocardial ischaemia (Box 16.47). The diagnosis of a prior MI can be made when any one of the features shown in Box 16.48 is present.

Acute coronary syndrome may present as a new phenomenon in patients with no previous history of heart disease or against a background of chronic stable angina. Approximately 12% of patients with acute coronary syndrome die within 1 month and 20% within 6 months of the index event. The risk markers that are indicative of an adverse prognosis include recurrent ischaemia, extensive ECG changes at rest or during pain, raised plasma troponin I or T concentrations, arrhythmias and haemodynamic complications (hypotension, mitral regurgitation) during episodes of ischaemia. Careful assessment and risk stratification are important because these guide the use of more complex pharmacological and interventional treatments (Fig. 16.61 and see Fig. 16.69), which can improve outcome.

Pathogenesis

Acute coronary syndrome almost always occurs in patients who have coronary atherosclerosis. The culprit lesion that precipitates the acute event is usually a complex ulcerated or fissured atheromatous plaque with adherent platelet-rich thrombus and local coronary artery spasm

16.47 Classification and criteria for diagnosis of acute myocardial infarction

Criteria for acute myocardial infarction

The term acute myocardial infarction (MI) should be used when there is acute myocardial injury with clinical evidence of acute myocardial ischaemia and with detection of a rise and/or fall of cardiac troponin values with at least one value above the 99th centile upper reference limit and at least one of the following:

- Symptoms of myocardial ischaemia
- New ischaemic ECG changes
- Development of pathological Q waves
- Imaging evidence of new loss of viable myocardium or new regional wall motion abnormality in a pattern consistent with an ischaemic aetiology
- Identification of a coronary thrombus by angiography or autopsy

Classification of acute myocardial infarction

- **Type 1 MI:** Acute atherothrombosis in the artery supplying the infarcted myocardium
- **Type 2 MI:** An imbalance between myocardial oxygen supply and demand unrelated to acute atherothrombosis
- **Type 3 MI:** Cardiac death in patients with symptoms suggestive of myocardial ischaemia and presumed new ischaemic ECG changes before cardiac troponin values become available or abnormal
- **Type 4 MI:** MI caused during percutaneous coronary intervention (PCI; type 4a). Other types include stent thrombosis (type 4b) and restenosis (type 4c) and consistent with type 1 MI
- **Type 5 MI:** MI caused during coronary artery bypass grafting
  Coronary procedure-related MI ≤ 48 hours after the index procedure is arbitrarily defined by an elevation of cardiac troponin values > 5× for type 4a MI and > 10× for type 5 MI of the 99th centile upper reference limit in patients with normal baseline values together with at least one of the following:
- New ischaemic ECG changes (this criterion is related to type 4a MI only)
- Development of new pathological Q waves
- Imaging evidence of loss of viable myocardium that is presumed to be new and consistent with an ischaemic aetiology
- Angiographic findings consistent with a procedural flow-limiting complication such as coronary dissection, occlusion of a major epicardial artery or graft, side-branch occlusion-thrombus, disruption of collateral flow or distal embolisation

Adapted from Thygesen K, Alpert JS, Jaffe AS, et al. Fourth universal definition of myocardial infarction. Eur Heart J 2019; 40: 237–269.

16.48 Criteria for diagnosis of a previously unrecognised myocardial infarction

- Abnormal Q waves with or without symptoms in the absence of non-ischaemic causes
- Imaging evidence of loss of viable myocardium in a pattern consistent with ischaemic aetiology
- Patho-anatomical findings of a prior MI

Adapted from Thygesen K, Alpert JS, Jaffe AS, et al. Fourth universal definition of myocardial infarction. Eur Heart J 2019; 40: 237–269.

(see Fig. 16.53). These vascular changes during an acute coronary syndrome are dynamic, such that the degree of obstruction may either increase, leading to complete vessel occlusion, or regress due to the effects of platelet disaggregation and endogenous fibrinolysis.

Myocardial infarction

The criteria for diagnosis classification of acute MI and classification of subtypes of MI are shown in Box 16.47. In acute type 1 MI, occlusive thrombus is present at the site of rupture or erosion of an atheromatous plaque; so-called atherothrombosis. The thrombus may undergo spontaneous lysis over the course of the next few days, although irreversible myocardial damage will have occurred. Without treatment, the artery responsible for the type 1 MI remains permanently occluded in 20%–30% of patients. Since the process of infarction progresses over several hours (Fig. 16.62), most patients present when it is still possible to salvage myocardium and improve outcome.

1. Find points for each predictive factor

Killip class	Points	SBP (mmHg)	Points	Heart rate (beats/min)	Points	Age (years)	Points	Serum creatinine level (µmol/L)	Points	Other risk factors	Points
I	0	≤ 80	58	≤ 50	0	≤ 30	0	0–34	1		
II	20	80–99	53	50–69	3	30–39	8	35–70	4	Cardiac arrest at admission	39
III	39	100–119	43	70–89	9	40–49	25	71–105	7		
IV	59	120–139	34	90–109	15	50–59	41	106–140	10	ST-segment deviation	28
		140–159	24	110–149	24	60–69	58	141–176	13		
		160–199	10	150–199	38	70–79	75	177–353	21	Elevated cardiac biomarker concentrations	14
		≥ 200	0	≥ 200	46	80–89	91	≥ 353	28		
						≥ 90	100				

2. Sum points for all predictive factors

Killip class	+	SBP	+	Heart rate	+	Age	+	Creatinine level	+	Cardiac arrest at admission	+	ST-segment deviation	+	Elevated cardiac biomarker concentrations	=	Total points

3. Look up risk corresponding to total points

Total points	≤ 60	70	80	90	100	110	120	130	140	150	160	170	180	190	200	210	220	230	240	≥ 250
Probability of in-hospital death (%)	≤ 0.2	0.3	0.4	0.6	0.8	1.1	1.6	2.1	2.9	3.9	5.4	7.3	9.8	13	18	23	29	36	44	≥ 52

Examples
A patient has Killip class II, SBP of 99 mmHg, heart rate of 100 beats/min, is 65 years of age, has a serum creatinine level of 76 µmol/L, did not have a cardiac arrest at admission but did have ST-segment deviation and elevated cardiac troponin. His score would be: 20 + 53 + 15 + 58 + 7 + 0 + 28 + 14 = 195. This gives about a 16% risk of having an in-hospital death.

Similarly, a patient with Killip class I, SBP of 80 mmHg, heart rate of 60 beats/min, who is 55 years of age, has a serum creatinine level of 30 µmol/L, and no risk factors would have the following score: 0 + 58 + 3 + 41 + 1 = 103. This gives about a 0.9% risk of having an in-hospital death.

Fig. 16.61 Risk stratification in the acute coronary syndrome: the GRACE score. Killip class refers to a categorisation of the severity of heart failure based on easily obtained clinical signs. The main clinical features are as follows: class I = no heart failure; class II = crackles audible halfway up the chest; class III = crackles heard in all the lung fields; class IV = cardiogenic shock. To convert creatinine in µmol/L to mg/dL, divide by 88.4. (SBP = systolic blood pressure) *From Scottish Intercollegiate Guidelines Network (SIGN) Guideline no. 93 – Acute coronary syndromes; updated February 2013.*

16

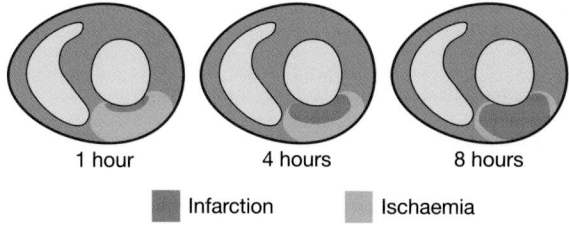

| 1 hour | 4 hours | 8 hours |

■ Infarction   ■ Ischaemia

Fig. 16.62 The time course of myocardial infarction. The relative proportion of ischaemic, infarcting and infarcted tissue slowly changes over a period of 12 hours. In the early stages of myocardial infarction, a significant proportion of the myocardium in jeopardy is potentially salvageable.

Myocardial infarction may also occur as the result of an imbalance between the blood supply and metabolic demands of the heart (type 2 MI). This may occur because of the presence of CAD and major non-cardiac stress, such as sepsis in a patient with three-vessel CAD, or because there is overwhelming demand in the presence of unobstructed coronary arteries, such as an excessively fast heart rate from a primary arrhythmia. For the diagnosis of type 2 MI, there needs to be clinical evidence of ischaemia, such as ECG changes or symptoms of chest pain. This should be distinguished from myocardial injury where there is evidence of elevated cardiac troponin concentration

(myocardial necrosis) without evidence of myocardial ischaemia, such as occurs in myocarditis. Myocardial injury can be acute or chronic depending upon its underlying cause.

The term type 3 MI is used to describe the situation where there is sudden death presumed to be due to MI. The terms type 4 and type 5 MI are used to describe the situations where MI occurs during or following the conduct of the coronary revascularisation procedures PCI and CABG, respectively. In these situations, clinical evidence of ischaemia is required to distinguish MI from procedure-related myocardial injury.

Clinical features

The differential diagnosis of acute coronary syndrome is wide and includes most causes of central chest pain or collapse. Chest pain at rest is the cardinal symptom but breathlessness, vomiting and collapse are also common features (Box 16.49). The pain occurs in the same sites as angina but is usually more severe and lasts longer; it is often described as a tightness, heaviness or constriction in the chest. In acute MI, the pain can be excruciating, and the patient's expression and pallor may vividly convey the seriousness of the situation. Most patients are breathless and, in some, this is the only symptom. Painless or 'silent' MI may also occur and is particularly common in older patients or those with diabetes mellitus. If syncope occurs, it is usually caused by an arrhythmia or profound hypotension. Vomiting and sinus bradycardia are often due to vagal stimulation and are particularly common in patients with inferior MI. Nausea and vomiting may also be caused or aggravated by opiates given for pain relief. Sometimes

16.49 Clinical features of acute coronary syndromes

Symptoms

- Prolonged cardiac pain: chest, throat, arms, epigastrium or back
- Anxiety and fear of impending death
- Nausea and vomiting
- Breathlessness
- Collapse/syncope

Physical signs

Signs of sympathetic activation

- Pallor
- Sweating
- Tachycardia

Signs of vagal activation

- Vomiting
- Bradycardia

Signs of impaired myocardial function

- Hypotension, oliguria, cold peripheries
- Narrow pulse pressure
- Raised jugular venous pressure
- Third heart sound
- Quiet first heart sound
- Diffuse apical impulse
- Lung crepitations

Low-grade fever

16.50 Common arrhythmias in acute coronary syndrome

- Ventricular fibrillation
- Ventricular tachycardia
- Accelerated idioventricular rhythm
- Ventricular ectopics
- Atrial fibrillation
- Sinus bradycardia (particularly after inferior myocardial infarction)
- Atrioventricular block

infarction occurs in the absence of physical signs. Sudden death, from ventricular fibrillation or asystole, may occur immediately and often within the first hour. If the patient survives this most critical stage, the liability to dangerous arrhythmias remains, but diminishes as each hour goes by. It is vital that patients know not to delay calling for help if symptoms occur. Complications may occur in all forms of acute coronary syndrome but have become less frequent in the modern era of immediate or early coronary revascularisation. Specific complications of acute coronary syndromes and their management are discussed below.

Arrhythmias

Arrhythmias are common in patients with acute coronary syndrome (Box 16.50) but are often transient and of no haemodynamic or prognostic importance. The risk of arrhythmia can be minimised by adequate pain relief, rest and the correction of hypokalaemia. VF occurs in 5%–10% of patients who reach hospital and is thought to be the major cause of death in those who die before receiving medical attention. Prompt defibrillation restores sinus rhythm and is life-saving. The prognosis of patients with early VF (within the first 48 hours) who are successfully and promptly resuscitated is identical to that of patients who do not suffer VF. The presence of ventricular arrhythmias during the convalescent phase of acute coronary syndrome may be a marker of poor ventricular function and may herald sudden death. Selected patients may benefit from electrophysiological testing and specific anti-arrhythmic therapy, including ICDs, as discussed in the previous section on cardiac arrhythmias. AF is a common but frequently transient arrhythmia, and usually does not require emergency treatment. However, if it causes a rapid ventricular rate with hypotension or circulatory collapse, prompt cardioversion is essential. In other situations, digoxin or a β-blocker is usually the treatment of choice. AF may be a feature of impending or overt left ventricular failure, and therapy may be ineffective if heart failure is not recognised and treated appropriately. Anticoagulation is required if AF persists. Bradycardia may occur but does not require treatment unless there is hypotension or haemodynamic deterioration, in which case atropine (0.6–1.2 mg IV) may be given. Inferior MI may be complicated by AV block, which is usually

temporary and often resolves following reperfusion therapy. If there is clinical deterioration due to second-degree or complete AV block, a temporary pacemaker should be considered. AV block complicating anterior infarction is more serious because asystole may suddenly supervene. A prophylactic temporary pacemaker should be inserted in these patients.

Recurrent angina

Patients who develop recurrent angina at rest or on minimal exertion following an acute coronary syndrome are at high risk and should be considered for prompt coronary angiography with a view to revascularisation. Patients with dynamic ECG changes and ongoing pain should be treated with intravenous glycoprotein IIb/IIIa receptor antagonists (tirofiban 400 ng/kg/min for 30 min, then 100 ng/kg/min for 48 hrs, or abciximab, initially 180 µg/kg, then 2 µg/kg/min for up to 72 hrs). Patients with resistant pain or marked haemodynamic changes should be considered for intra-aortic balloon counterpulsation and emergency coronary revascularisation. Post-infarct angina occurs in up to 50% of patients treated with thrombolysis. Most patients have a residual stenosis in the infarct-related vessel, despite successful thrombolysis, and this may cause angina if there is still viable myocardium downstream. For this reason, all patients who have received successful thrombolysis should be considered for early (within the first 24 hours) coronary angiography with a view to coronary revascularisation.

Acute heart failure

Acute heart failure usually reflects extensive myocardial damage and is associated with a poor prognosis. All the other complications of MI are more likely to occur when acute heart failure is present. The assessment and management of heart failure is discussed in more detail earlier in this chapter.

Pericarditis

This only occurs following infarction and is particularly common on the second and third days. The patient may recognise that a different pain has developed, even though it is at the same site, and that it is positional and tends to be worse or sometimes present only on inspiration. A pericardial rub may be audible. Opiate-based analgesia should be used. Non-steroidal (NSAIDs) and steroidal anti-inflammatory drugs may increase the risk of aneurysm formation and myocardial rupture in the early recovery period, and should be avoided.

Dressler syndrome

This syndrome is characterised by persistent fever, pericarditis and pleurisy, and is probably due to autoimmunity. The symptoms tend to occur a few weeks or even months after MI and often subside after a few days. If the symptoms are prolonged or severe, treatment with high-dose aspirin, NSAIDs or even glucocorticoid steroids may be required.

Papillary muscle rupture

This typically presents with acute pulmonary oedema and shock due to the sudden onset of severe mitral regurgitation. Examination usually reveals a pansystolic murmur and third heart sound but the murmur may be quiet or absent in patients with severe regurgitation. The diagnosis is confirmed by echocardiography, and emergency valve replacement may be necessary. Lesser degrees of mitral regurgitation due to papillary muscle dysfunction are common and may be transient.

Ventricular septal rupture

This usually presents with sudden haemodynamic deterioration accompanied by a new loud pansystolic murmur radiating to the right sternal border, which may be difficult to distinguish from acute mitral regurgitation. Rupture of the intraventricular septum causes left-to-right shunting through a ventricular septal defect, which tends to cause acute right heart failure rather than pulmonary oedema. Doppler echocardiography and right heart catheterisation will confirm the diagnosis. Treatment is by emergency surgical repair; without this, the condition is usually fatal.

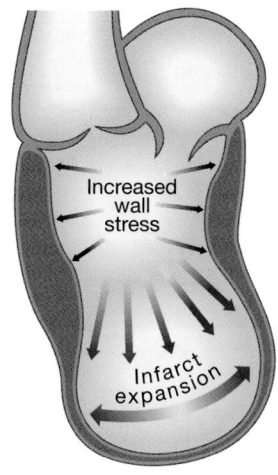

Fig. 16.63 Infarct expansion and ventricular remodelling. Full-thickness myocardial infarction causes thinning and stretching of the infarcted segment (infarct expansion), which leads to increased wall stress with progressive dilatation and hypertrophy of the remaining ventricle (ventricular remodelling).

Ventricular rupture

Rupture of the ventricle may lead to cardiac tamponade and is usually fatal, although it is occasionally possible to support a patient with an incomplete rupture until emergency surgery can be performed.

Embolism

Thrombus often forms on the endocardial surface of freshly infarcted myocardium. This can lead to systemic embolism and occasionally causes a stroke or ischaemic limb. Venous thrombosis and pulmonary embolism may occur but have become less common with the use of prophylactic anticoagulants and early mobilisation.

Ventricular remodelling

This is a potential complication of an acute transmural MI due to thinning and stretching of the infarcted segment. This leads to an increase in wall stress with progressive dilatation and hypertrophy of the remaining ventricle (ventricular remodelling, Fig. 16.63). As the ventricle dilates, it becomes less efficient and heart failure may supervene. Infarct expansion occurs over a few days and weeks but ventricular remodelling can take years. Beta-blocker, ACE inhibitor and mineralocorticoid receptor antagonist therapies can reduce late ventricular remodelling and prevent the onset of heart failure.

Ventricular aneurysm

Ventricular aneurysm develops in approximately 10% of patients with MI and is particularly common when there is persistent occlusion of the infarct-related vessel. Heart failure, ventricular arrhythmias, mural thrombus and systemic embolism are all recognised complications of aneurysm formation. Other features include a paradoxical impulse on the chest wall, persistent ST elevation on the ECG, and sometimes an unusual bulge from the cardiac silhouette on the chest X-ray. Echocardiography is diagnostic. Surgical removal of a left ventricular aneurysm carries a high morbidity and mortality but is sometimes necessary.

Investigations

Electrocardiogram

The standard 12-lead ECG is central to confirming the diagnosis and deciding immediate management but may be difficult to interpret if there is bundle branch block or previous MI. The initial ECG may be normal or non-diagnostic in one-third of cases. Repeated ECGs are important, especially where the diagnosis is uncertain or the patient has recurrent or persistent symptoms. The earliest ECG change is usually ST-segment deviation. With proximal occlusion of a major coronary artery, ST-segment elevation

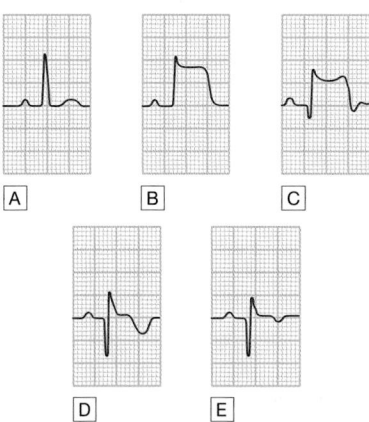

Fig. 16.64 The serial evolution of ECG changes in transmural myocardial infarction. [A] Normal ECG complex. [B] Acute ST elevation ('the current of injury'). [C] Progressive loss of the R wave, developing Q wave, resolution of the ST elevation and terminal T-wave inversion. [D] Deep Q wave and T-wave inversion. [E] Old or established infarct pattern; the Q wave tends to persist but the T-wave changes become less marked. The rate of evolution is very variable but, in general, stage B appears within minutes, stage C within hours, stage D within days and stage E after several weeks or months. This should be compared with the 12-lead ECGs in Figs. 16.65–16.67.

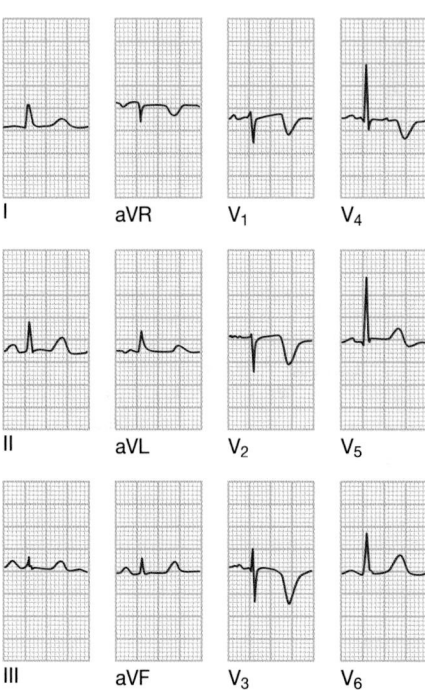

Fig. 16.65 Recent anterior non-ST elevation (subendocardial) myocardial infarction. This ECG demonstrates deep symmetrical T-wave inversion, together with a reduction in the height of the R wave in leads V_1, V_2, V_3 and V_4.

(or new bundle branch block) is seen initially, with later diminution in the size of the R wave and, in transmural (full-thickness) infarction, development of a Q wave. Subsequently, the T wave becomes inverted because of a change in ventricular repolarisation; this change persists after the ST segment has returned to normal. These sequential features (Fig. 16.64) are sufficiently reliable for the approximate age of the infarct to be deduced.

In non-ST segment elevation acute coronary syndrome, there is partial occlusion of a major vessel or complete occlusion of a minor vessel, causing unstable angina or partial-thickness (subendocardial) MI. This is usually associated with ST-segment depression and T-wave changes. In the presence of infarction, this may be accompanied by some loss of R waves in the absence of Q waves (Fig. 16.65).

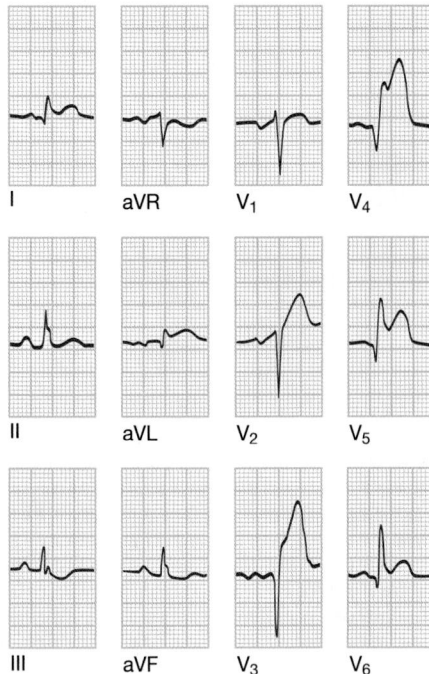

Fig. 16.66 Acute transmural anterior myocardial infarction. This ECG was recorded from a patient who had developed severe chest pain 6 hours earlier. There is ST elevation in leads I, aVL, V_2, V_3, V_4, V_5 and V_6, and there are Q waves in leads V_3, V_4 and V_5. Anterior infarcts with prominent changes in leads V_2, V_3 and V_4 are sometimes called 'anteroseptal' infarcts, as opposed to 'anterolateral' infarcts, in which the ECG changes are predominantly found in V_4, V_5 and V_6.

The ECG changes are best seen in the leads that 'face' the ischaemic or infarcted area. When there has been anteroseptal infarction, abnormalities are found in one or more leads from V_1 to V_4, while anterolateral infarction produces changes from V_4 to V_6, in aVL and in lead I. Inferior infarction is best shown in leads II, III and aVF, while, at the same time, leads I, aVL and the anterior chest leads may show 'reciprocal' changes of ST depression (Figs. 16.66 and 16.67). Infarction of the posterior wall of the LV does not cause ST elevation or Q waves in the standard leads, but can be diagnosed by the presence of reciprocal changes (ST depression and a tall R wave in leads V_1–V_4). Some infarctions (especially inferior) also involve the RV. This may be identified by recording from additional leads placed over the right precordium.

Cardiac biomarkers

Serial measurements of cardiac troponin concentration should be taken. In unstable angina, there is no detectable rise in troponin and the diagnosis is made on the basis of the clinical features and investigations such as ECG or coronary angiography. In contrast, MI causes a rise in plasma concentrations of troponin T and I and other cardiac muscle enzymes (Fig. 16.68 and see Box 16.47). Levels of troponins T and I increase within 3–6 hours, peak at about 36 hours and remain elevated for up to 2 weeks. A full blood count may reveal the presence of a leucocytosis, which reaches a peak on the first day. The erythrocyte sedimentation rate (ESR) and C-reactive protein (CRP) are also elevated. Lipids should be measured within 24 hours of presentation because there is often a transient fall in cholesterol in the 3 months following infarction.

Radiography

A chest X-ray should be performed since this may demonstrate pulmonary oedema that is not evident on clinical examination (see Fig. 16.25). The heart size is often normal but there may be cardiomegaly due to pre-existing myocardial damage.

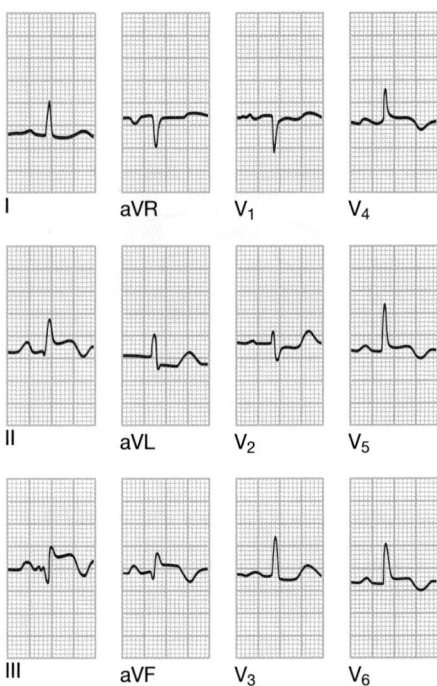

Fig. 16.67 Acute transmural inferolateral myocardial infarction. This ECG was recorded from a patient who had developed severe chest pain 4 hours earlier. There is ST elevation in inferior leads II, III and aVF and lateral leads V_4, V_5 and V_6. There is also 'reciprocal' ST depression in leads aVL and V_2.

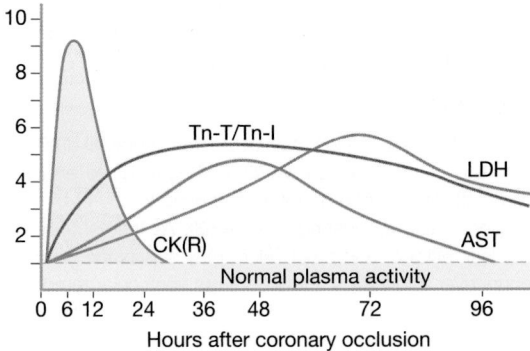

Fig. 16.68 Changes in plasma cardiac biomarker concentrations after myocardial infarction. Creatine kinase (CK) and troponins T (Tn-T) and I (Tn-I) are the first to rise, followed by aspartate aminotransferase (AST) and then lactate (hydroxybutyrate) dehydrogenase (LDH). In patients treated with reperfusion therapy, a rapid rise in plasma creatine kinase (curve CK(R)) occurs, due to a washout effect.

Echocardiography

Echocardiography is normally performed before discharge from hospital and is useful for assessing ventricular function and for detecting important complications, such as mural thrombus, cardiac rupture, ventricular septal defect, mitral regurgitation and pericardial effusion.

Coronary angiography

Coronary arteriography should be considered with a view to revascularisation in all patients at moderate or high risk of a further event, including those who fail to settle on medical therapy, those with extensive ECG changes, those with an elevated cardiac troponin and those with severe pre-existing stable angina (see Fig. 16.69). This often reveals disease that is amenable to PCI or urgent CABG (see below).

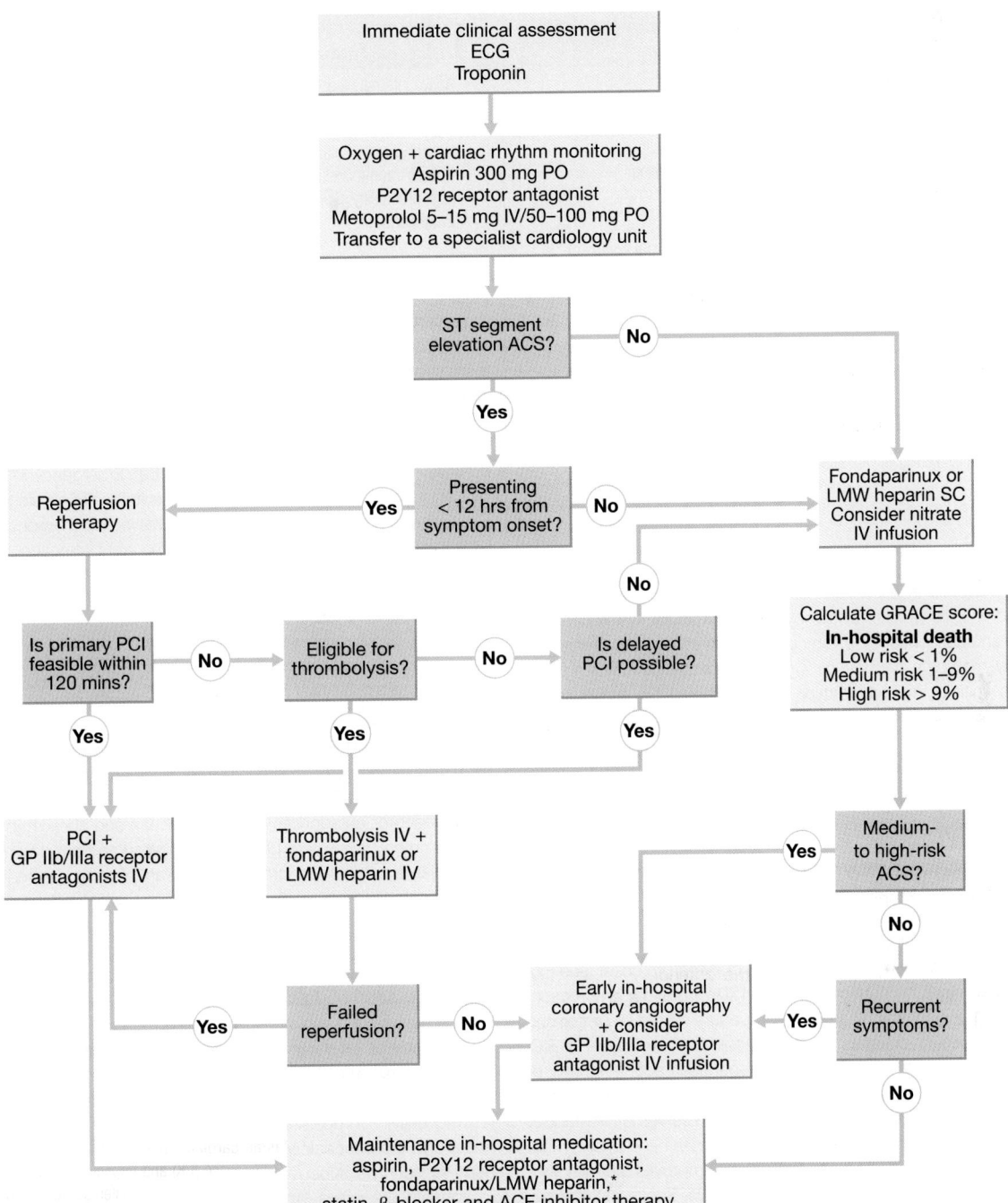

Fig. 16.69 Summary of treatment for acute coronary syndrome (ACS). *Not required following PCI. For details of the GRACE score, see Fig. 16.61. (ACE = angiotensin-converting enzyme; ECG = electrocardiogram; GP = glycoprotein; IV = intravenous; LMW = low-molecular-weight; PCI = percutaneous coronary intervention; PO = by mouth; SC = subcutaneous) Adapted from Scottish Intercollegiate Guidelines Network (SIGN) Guideline no. 93 – Acute coronary syndromes, February 2007 and updated in SIGN 148, April 2016.*

Management

All patients with suspected acute coronary syndrome should be admitted urgently to hospital because there is a risk of death or recurrent myocardial ischaemia during the early unstable phase. Appropriate medical therapy can reduce the incidence of these complications by at least 60%. The key elements of immediate in-hospital management are shown in Fig. 16.69. Patients should ideally be managed in a dedicated cardiac unit, where the necessary expertise, monitoring and resuscitation facilities are available. Clinical risk factor analysis using tools such as the GRACE score (see Fig. 16.61) should be performed to identify patients that should be selected for intensive therapy, and

specifically early inpatient coronary angiography (thresholds vary, but a score of 140 points or more supports early intervention). If there are no complications and risk factor analysis shows that angiography is not required, the patient can be mobilised from the second day and discharged after 2–3 days. Low-risk patients without spontaneous angina may be considered for an exercise tolerance test 4-6 weeks after the acute coronary syndrome. This will help to identify those individuals who may require further investigation, and may help to boost the confidence of the remainder. Management of the acute event is discussed below and the principles of long-term management are summarised in Box 16.51.

16.51 Late management of myocardial infarction

Risk stratification and further investigation
See text for details

Lifestyle modification

- Diet (weight control, lipid-lowering, 'Mediterranean diet')
- Cessation of smoking
- Regular exercise

Secondary prevention drug therapy

- Antiplatelet therapy (aspirin and/or clopidogrel)
- β-blocker
- ACE inhibitor/ARB
- Statin
- Additional therapy for control of diabetes and hypertension
- Mineralocorticoid receptor antagonist

Rehabilitation

Devices

- Implantable cardiac defibrillator (high-risk patients)

(ACE = angiotensin-converting enzyme; ARB = angiotensin receptor blocker)

16.52 Relative contraindications to thrombolytic therapy

- Active internal bleeding
- Previous subarachnoid or intracerebral haemorrhage
- Uncontrolled hypertension
- Recent surgery (within 1 month)
- Recent trauma (including traumatic resuscitation)
- High probability of active peptic ulcer
- Pregnancy

Analgesia

Adequate analgesia is essential, not only to relieve distress but also to lower adrenergic drive and thereby reduce vascular resistance, BP, infarct size and susceptibility to ventricular arrhythmias. Intravenous opiates (initially, morphine sulphate 5–10 mg or diamorphine 2.5–5 mg) and antiemetics (initially, metoclopramide 10 mg) should be administered, and titrated until the patient is comfortable. Intramuscular injections should be avoided because the clinical effect may be delayed by poor skeletal muscle perfusion, and a painful haematoma may form following thrombolytic or antithrombotic therapy.

Reperfusion therapy

Immediate reperfusion therapy with PCI (see Fig. 16.59) is indicated when the ECG shows new bundle branch block or characteristic ST-segment elevation in two contiguous leads of 1 mm or more in the limb leads or 2 mm or more in the chest leads. This is the treatment of choice for those presenting within 12 hours of symptom onset (see Fig. 16.69). If PCI cannot be performed within 120 minutes for any reason, and thrombolysis is contraindicated, the procedure should be performed as soon as practically possible. Patients should be considered for PCI within the first 24 hours, even if they have reperfused spontaneously or with thrombolytic therapy. Coronary artery patency is restored in over 95% of patients undergoing PCI. The procedure preserves left ventricular function with a marked reduction in the progression to heart failure, more than halves rates of recurrent MI and dramatically improves mortality with more than 95% 1-year survival rates in clinical trials. Successful therapy is also associated with rapid pain relief, resolution of acute ST elevation and occasional transient arrhythmias.

Reperfusion therapy with PCI confers no immediate mortality benefit in patients with non-ST segment elevation acute coronary syndrome. Selected medium- to high-risk patients do benefit from in-hospital coronary angiography and coronary revascularisation but this does not need to take place in the first 12 hours unless there are high-risk features, such as ongoing chest pain or ECG changes.

Thrombolytic therapy

If primary PCI cannot be achieved in a timely manner in patients with ST-segment elevation MI (see Fig. 16.69), thrombolytic therapy should be administered. Although the survival advantage is not as good as primary PCI, mortality is reduced and this is maintained for at least 10 years. The benefit of thrombolytic therapy is greatest in those patients who receive treatment within the first 12 hours and especially the first 2 hours. Modern thrombolytic agents, such as tenecteplase (TNK) and reteplase (rPA), are analogues of human tissue plasminogen activator and can be given as an intravenous bolus, allowing prompt treatment to be given in

the emergency department or in the pre-hospital setting. The major hazard of thrombolytic therapy is bleeding. Cerebral haemorrhage causes 4 extra strokes per 1000 patients treated, and the incidence of other major bleeds is between 0.5% and 1%. Accordingly, the treatment should be withheld if there is a significant risk of serious bleeding (Box 16.52). For some patients, thrombolytic therapy is contraindicated or fails to achieve coronary arterial reperfusion (see Fig. 16.69). Emergency PCI may then be considered, particularly where there is evidence of cardiogenic shock. Even where thrombolysis successfully achieves reperfusion, PCI should be considered within 24 hours to prevent recurrent infarction and improve outcome.

Antithrombotic therapy

Oral administration of 75–325 mg aspirin daily improves survival, with a 25% relative risk reduction in mortality. The first tablet (300 mg) should be given orally within the first 12 hours and therapy should be continued indefinitely if there are no side-effects. A P2Y12 receptor antagonist (ticagrelor (180 mg, followed by 90 mg twice daily), prasugrel (60 mg, followed by 10 mg daily) or clopidogrel (300 mg, followed by 75 mg daily)) should be given in combination with aspirin for up to 12 months. Glycoprotein IIb/IIIa receptor antagonists, such as tirofiban and abciximab, block the final common pathway of platelet aggregation and are potent inhibitors of platelet-rich thrombus formation. They are of particular benefit in high-risk patients with acute coronary syndromes who undergo PCI, especially those with a high thrombus burden at angiography or who have received inadequate prior antiplatelet therapy. These intravenous agents should be administered in addition to oral aspirin and a P2Y12 receptor antagonist. Anticoagulation further reduces the risk of thromboembolic complications, and prevents re-infarction in the absence of reperfusion therapy or after successful thrombolysis. Anticoagulation can be achieved using unfractionated heparin, fractioned (low-molecular-weight) heparin or a pentasaccharide, such as subcutaneous fondaparinux (2.5 mg daily). Comparative clinical trials show that the pentasaccharides have the best safety and efficacy profile but low-molecular-weight heparin, such as subcutaneous enoxaparin (1 mg/kg twice daily), is a reasonable alternative. Anticoagulation should be continued for 8 days or until discharge from hospital or coronary revascularisation has been completed. A period of treatment with an oral anticoagulant should be considered if there is persistent AF or evidence of extensive anterior infarction with mural thrombus because these patients are at increased risk of systemic thromboembolism.

Anti-anginal therapy

Sublingual glyceryl trinitrate (300–500 μg) is a valuable first-aid measure in unstable angina or threatened infarction, and intravenous nitrates (glyceryl trinitrate 0.6–1.2 mg/hr or isosorbide dinitrate 1–2 mg/hr) are useful for the treatment of left ventricular failure and the relief of recurrent or persistent ischaemic pain. Intravenous β-blockade (atenolol 5–10 mg or metoprolol 5–15 mg given over 5 min) relieves pain, reduces arrhythmias and improves short-term mortality in patients who present within 12 hours of symptom onset (see Fig. 16.69). However, they should be avoided if there is heart failure (pulmonary oedema), hypotension (systolic BP <105 mmHg) or bradycardia (heart rate <65/min). Nifedipine or amlodipine can be added if there is persistent chest discomfort but these drugs may cause tachycardia if used alone. Verapamil and diltiazem should be used if β-blockade is contraindicated. In the longer term, treatment with an oral β-blocker reduces long-term mortality by approximately 25% among the survivors of an acute MI, especially those with left ventricular systolic dysfunction. Patients with heart failure, COPD or peripheral arterial disease appear to derive similar secondary preventative benefits from β-blocker therapy and should receive maintenance therapy unless poorly tolerated. Unfortunately, a minority of patients do not tolerate β-blockade because of bradycardia, AV block, hypotension or asthma.

Renin–angiotensin blockade

Long-term treatment with ACE inhibitors such as enalapril (10 mg twice daily) or ramipril (2.5–5 mg twice daily) can counteract ventricular remodelling, prevent the onset of heart failure, improve survival, reduce recurrent MI and avoid rehospitalisation. The benefits are greatest in those with overt heart failure (clinical or radiological) but extend to patients with asymptomatic left ventricular systolic dysfunction and those with preserved left ventricular function. They should be considered in all patients with acute coronary syndrome. Caution must be exercised in hypovolaemic or hypotensive patients because ACE inhibition may exacerbate hypotension and impair coronary perfusion. In patients intolerant of ACE inhibitors, ARBs such as valsartan (40–160 mg twice daily) or candesartan (4–16 mg daily) are alternatives that are better tolerated.

Mineralocorticoid receptor antagonists

Patients with acute MI and left ventricular dysfunction (ejection fraction <35%) and either pulmonary oedema or diabetes mellitus further benefit from additional mineralocorticoid receptor antagonists (eplerenone 25–50 mg daily, or spironolactone 25–50 mg daily).

Lipid-lowering therapy

The benefits of lowering serum cholesterol following acute coronary syndrome have been demonstrated in several large-scale randomised trials. All patients should receive therapy with HMG CoA reductase enzyme inhibitors (statins) after acute coronary syndrome, irrespective of serum cholesterol concentrations. Patients with serum LDL cholesterol concentrations above 3.2 mmol/L (approximately 120 mg/dL) benefit from more intensive therapy, such as atorvastatin (80 mg daily). Other agents, such as ezetimibe, fibrates, anion exchange resins and injectable PCSK9 inhibitors, may be used in cases where total cholesterol or LDL cholesterol cannot be lowered adequately using statins alone.

Smoking cessation

The 5-year mortality of patients who continue to smoke cigarettes is double that of those who quit smoking at the time of their acute coronary syndrome. Giving up smoking is the single most effective contribution a patient can make to their future. The success of smoking cessation can be increased by supportive advice and pharmacological therapy.

Diet and exercise

Maintaining an ideal body weight, eating a Mediterranean-style diet, taking regular exercise, and achieving good control of hypertension and diabetes mellitus may all improve the long-term outlook.

Rehabilitation

When there are no complications, the patient can mobilise on the second day, return home in 2–3 days and gradually increase activity, with the aim of returning to work in 4 weeks. The majority of patients may resume driving after 1–4 weeks, although, in most countries, drivers of heavy goods and public service vehicles require special assessment before returning to work. Emotional problems, such as denial, anxiety and depression, are common and must be addressed. Some patients are severely and even permanently incapacitated as a result of the psychological effects of acute coronary syndrome rather than the physical ones, and all benefit from thoughtful explanation, counselling and reassurance. Many patients

16.53 Myocardial infarction in old age

- **Atypical presentation**: often with anorexia, fatigue, weakness, delirium or falls rather than chest pain.
- **Case fatality**: rises steeply. Hospital mortality exceeds 25% in those over 75 years old, which is five times greater than that seen in those aged less than 55 years.
- **Survival benefit of treatments**: not influenced by age. The absolute benefit of evidence-based treatments may therefore be greatest in older people.
- **Hazards of treatments**: rise with age (for example, increased risk of intracerebral bleeding after thrombolysis) and are due partly to increased comorbidity.
- **Quality of evidence**: older patients, particularly those with significant comorbidity, were under-represented in many of the randomised controlled clinical trials that helped to establish the treatment of myocardial infarction. The balance of risk and benefit for many treatments, such as thrombolysis and primary percutaneous transluminal coronary angiography, in frail older people is uncertain.

mistakenly believe that stress was the cause of their heart attack and may restrict their activity inappropriately. The patient's spouse or partner will also require emotional support, information and counselling. Formal rehabilitation programmes, based on graded exercise protocols with individual and group counselling, are often very successful and, in some cases, have been shown to improve quality of life and long-term outcome.

Implantable defibrillators

These devices are of benefit in preventing sudden cardiac death in patients who have severe left ventricular impairment (ejection fraction ≤30%) after MI. More details are provided in the section on treatment of cardiac arrhythmias.

Type 2 myocardial infarction

The optimal management and treatment of patients with type 2 MI has yet to be established. There is currently no evidence that treatments for type 1 MI are effective in the setting of type 2 MI. The focus for patients with type 2 MI should be on treating the underlying cause of their presentation and, where applicable, their previously undiagnosed concomitant CAD.

Prognosis

The prognosis of patients who have survived an acute coronary syndrome is related to the extent of residual myocardial ischaemia, the degree of myocardial damage and the presence of ventricular arrhythmias. In almost one-quarter of all cases of MI, death occurs within a few minutes without medical care. Half the deaths occur within 24 hours of the onset of symptoms and about 40% of all affected patients die within the first month. The prognosis of those who survive to reach hospital is much better, with a 28-day survival of more than 85%. Patients with unstable angina have a mortality of approximately half that of patients with MI. Early death is usually due to an arrhythmia and is independent of the extent of MI. However, late outcomes are determined by the extent of myocardial damage, and unfavourable features include poor left ventricular function, AV block and persistent ventricular arrhythmias. The prognosis is worse for anterior than for inferior infarcts. Bundle branch block and high cardiac marker concentrations both indicate extensive myocardial damage. Old age, depression and social isolation are also associated with a higher mortality. Of those who survive an acute attack, more than 80% live for a further year, about 75% for 5 years, 50% for 10 years and 25% for 20 years.

Some considerations specific to myocardial infarction in old age are listed in Box 16.53.

Non-cardiac surgery in patients with heart disease

Non-cardiac surgery, particularly major vascular, abdominal or thoracic surgery, can precipitate serious perioperative cardiac complications,

16.54 Major risk factors for cardiac complications of non-cardiac surgery

- Recent (< 6 months) myocardial infarction or unstable angina
- Severe coronary artery disease: left main stem or three-vessel disease
- Severe stable angina on effort
- Severe left ventricular dysfunction
- Severe valvular heart disease (especially aortic stenosis)

such as MI and death, in patients with CAD and other forms of heart disease. Careful pre-operative cardiac assessment may help to determine the balance of benefit versus risk on an individual basis, and identify measures that minimise the operative risk (Box 16.54).

A hypercoagulable state is part of the normal physiological response to surgery, and may promote coronary thrombosis leading to an acute coronary syndrome in the early post-operative period. Patients with a history of recent PCI or acute coronary syndrome are at greatest risk and, whenever possible, elective non-cardiac surgery should be avoided for 3 months after such an event. Where possible, antiplatelet, statin and β-blocker therapies should be continued throughout the perioperative period.

Careful attention to fluid balance during and after surgery is particularly important in patients with impaired left ventricular function and valvular heart disease because vasopressin is released as part of the normal physiological response to surgery and, in these circumstances, the over-zealous administration of intravenous fluids can easily precipitate heart failure. Patients with severe valvular heart disease, particularly aortic stenosis and mitral stenosis, are also at increased risk because they may not be able to increase their cardiac output in response to the stress of surgery.

Atrial fibrillation is a common post-operative complication in patients with pre-existing heart disease which may be triggered by hypoxia, myocardial ischaemia or heart failure. It usually terminates spontaneously when the precipitating factors have been eliminated, but digoxin or β-blockers can be prescribed to control the heart rate if necessary.

Peripheral arterial disease

Peripheral arterial disease (PAD) has been estimated to affect about 20% of individuals aged 55–75 years in the UK. Only 25% of patients present with symptoms, the commonest of which is intermittent claudication (IC). About 1%–2% of patients with IC per year progress to a point where amputation or revascularisation is required. However, the annual mortality rate of people with IC is about 5%, which is 2–3 times higher than the general population of the same age and sex. The cause of death is typically an MI or stroke, reflecting the fact that IC nearly always occurs in association with widespread atherosclerosis.

Pathogenesis

In developed countries, almost all PAD is due to atherosclerosis and the risk factors are the same as described in patients with CAD. As with CAD, plaque rupture is responsible for the most serious manifestations of PAD, and not infrequently occurs in a plaque that hitherto has been asymptomatic. The clinical manifestations depend on the anatomical site, the presence or absence of a collateral supply, the speed of onset and the mechanism of injury (Box 16.55). Approximately 5%–10% of patients with PAD have diabetes but this proportion increases to 30%–40% in those with severe limb ischaemia. The mechanism of PAD in diabetes is atheroma affecting the medium to large-sized arteries rather than obstructive microangiopathy and so diabetes is not a contraindication to lower limb revascularisation. Nevertheless, patients with diabetes and PAD pose a number of particular problems (Box 16.56).

16.55 Factors influencing the clinical manifestations of peripheral arterial disease (PAD)

Anatomical site

Cerebral circulation
- TIA, amaurosis fugax, vertebrobasilar insufficiency

Renal arteries
- Hypertension and renal failure

Mesenteric arteries
- Mesenteric angina, acute intestinal ischaemia

Limbs (legs >> arms)
- Intermittent claudication, critical limb ischaemia, acute limb ischaemia

Collateral supply
- In a patient with a complete circle of Willis, occlusion of one carotid artery may be asymptomatic
- In a patient without cross-circulation, stroke is likely

Speed of onset
- Where PAD develops slowly, a collateral supply will develop
- Sudden occlusion of a previously normal artery is likely to cause severe distal ischaemia

Mechanism of injury

Haemodynamic
- Plaque must reduce arterial diameter by 70% ('critical stenosis') to reduce flow and pressure at rest. On exertion a moderate stenosis may become 'critical'. This mechanism tends to have a relatively benign course due to collateralisation

Thrombotic
- Occlusion of a long-standing critical stenosis may be asymptomatic due to collateralisation. However, acute rupture and thrombosis of a non-haemodynamically significant plaque usually has severe consequences

Atheroembolic
- Symptoms depend on embolic load and size
- Carotid (TIA, amaurosis fugax or stroke) and peripheral arterial (blue toe/finger syndrome) plaque are common examples

Thromboembolic
- Usually secondary to atrial fibrillation
- The consequences are usually dramatic, as the thrombus load is often large and occludes a major, previously healthy, non-collateralised artery suddenly and completely

(TIA = transient ischaemic attack)

Clinical features

Symptomatic PAD affects the legs about eight times more commonly than the arms. Several locations may be affected, including the aortoiliac vessels, the femoropopliteal vessels and the infrapopliteal vessels. One or more of these segments may be affected in a variable and asymmetric manner. In the arm, the subclavian artery is the most common site of disease. Peripheral artery disease can present clinically in a variety of ways, as detailed below.

Intermittent claudication

This is the most common presentation of PAD affecting the lower limbs. It is characterised by ischaemic pain affecting the muscles of the leg. The pain is usually felt in the calf because the disease most commonly affects the superficial femoral artery, but it may be felt in the thigh or buttock if the iliac arteries are involved. Typically, the pain comes on after walking, often once a specific distance has been covered, and rapidly subsides on resting. Resumption of walking leads to a return of the pain. Most patients describe a cyclical pattern of exacerbation and resolution due to the progression of disease and the subsequent development of collaterals. When PAD affects the upper limbs, arm claudication may occur, although this is uncommon.

Critical limb ischaemia

Critical limb ischaemia (CLI) is defined as rest pain requiring opiate analgesia, or ulceration or gangrene that has been present for more than

16.56 Peripheral vascular disease in diabetes

Feature	Difficulty
Arterial calcification	Spuriously high ABPI due to incompressible ankle vessels. Inability to clamp arteries for the purposes of bypass surgery. Resistant to angioplasty
Immunocompromise	Prone to rapidly spreading cellulitis, gangrene and osteomyelitis
Multisystem arterial disease	Coronary and cerebral arterial disease increase the risks of intervention
Distal disease	Diabetic vascular disease has a predilection for the calf vessels. Although vessels in the foot are often spared, performing a satisfactory bypass or angioplasty to these small vessels is a technical challenge
Sensory neuropathy	Even severe ischaemia and/or tissue loss may be completely painless. Diabetic patients often present late with extensive destruction of the foot. Loss of proprioception leads to abnormal pressure loads and worsens joint destruction (Charcot joints)
Motor neuropathy	Weakness of the long and short flexors and extensors leads to abnormal foot architecture, abnormal pressure loads, callus formation and ulceration
Autonomic neuropathy	Leads to a dry foot deficient in sweat that normally lubricates the skin and is antibacterial. Scaling and fissuring create a portal of entry for bacteria. Abnormal blood flow in the bones of the ankle and foot may also contribute to osteopenia and bony collapse

(ABPI = ankle–brachial pressure index)

2 weeks, in the presence of an ankle BP of less than 50mmHg. The typical progression of symptoms in CLI is summarised in Fig. 16.70. Rest pain only, with ankle pressures above 50mmHg, is known as subcritical limb ischaemia (SCLI). The term severe limb ischaemia (SLI) is used to describe the situation where either CLI and SCLI occurs. Whereas IC is usually due to single-segment plaque, SLI is always due to multilevel disease. Many patients with SLI have not previously sought medical advice, principally because they have other comorbidity that prevents them from walking to a point where IC develops. Patients with SLI are at high risk of losing their limb, and sometimes their life, in a matter of weeks or months without surgical bypass or endovascular revascularisation by angioplasty or stenting. Treatment of these patients is difficult because most are older adults with extensive and severe disease and major multisystem comorbidities.

Acute limb ischaemia

This is most frequently caused by acute thrombotic occlusion of a pre-existing stenotic arterial segment, thromboembolism and trauma that may be iatrogenic. The typical presentation is with paralysis (inability to wiggle toes or fingers) and paraesthesia (loss of light touch over the dorsum of the foot or hand); the so-called 'Ps of acute ischaemia' (Box 16.57). These features are non-specific and inconsistently related to its severity. Pain on squeezing the calf indicates muscle infarction and impending irreversible ischaemia. All patients with suspected acutely ischaemic limbs must be discussed immediately with a vascular surgeon; a few hours can make the difference between death/amputation and complete recovery of limb function. If there are no contraindications (acute aortic dissection or trauma, particularly head injury), an intravenous bolus of heparin (3000–5000 U) should be administered to limit propagation of thrombus and protect the collateral circulation. Distinguishing thrombosis from embolism is frequently difficult but is important because

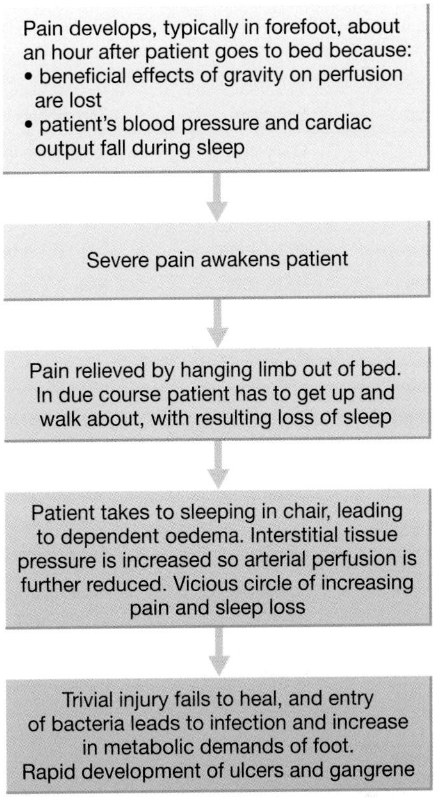

Fig. 16.70 Progressive night pain and the development of tissue loss.

16.57 Symptoms *and* signs of acute limb ischaemia

Symptoms/signs	Comment
Pain Pallor Pulselessness	May be absent in complete acute ischaemia, and can be present in chronic ischaemia
Perishing cold	Unreliable, as the ischaemic limb takes on the ambient temperature
Paraesthesia Paralysis	Important features of impending irreversible ischaemia

treatment and prognosis are different (Box 16.58). Acute limb ischaemia due to thrombosis in situ can usually be treated medically in the first instance with intravenous heparin (target activated partial thromboplastin time (APTT) 2.0–3.0), antiplatelet agents, high-dose statins, intravenous fluids to avoid dehydration, correction of anaemia, oxygen and sometimes prostaglandins, such as iloprost. Embolism will normally result in extensive tissue necrosis within 6 hours unless the limb is revascularised. The indications for thrombolysis, if any, remain controversial. Irreversible ischaemia mandates early amputation or palliative care.

Atheroembolism

This may be a presenting feature of PAD affecting the subclavian arteries. The presentation is with blue fingers, which are due to small emboli lodging in digital arteries. This may be confused with Raynaud's phenomenon but the symptoms of atheroembolism are typically unilateral rather than bilateral as in Raynaud's.

Subclavian steal

This can be a feature of PAD affecting the upper limbs. The presentation is with dizziness, cortical blindness and/or collapse, which occurs when the arm is used and is thought to be caused by diversion (or steal) of blood from the brain to the limbs via the vertebral artery.

16.58 Distinguishing features of embolism and thrombosis in peripheral arteries

Clinical features	Embolism	Thrombosis
Severity	Complete (no collaterals)	Incomplete (collaterals)
Onset	Seconds or minutes	Hours or days
Limb	Leg 3:1 arm	Leg 10:1 arm
Multiple sites	Up to 15%	Rare
Embolic source	Present (usually atrial fibrillation)	Absent
Previous claudication	Absent	Present
Palpation of artery	Soft, tender	Hard, calcified
Bruits	Absent	Present
Contralateral leg pulses	Present	Absent
Diagnosis	Clinical	Angiography
Treatment	Embolectomy, warfarin	Medical, bypass, thrombolysis
Prognosis	Loss of life > loss of limb	Loss of limb > loss of life

Investigations

The presence and severity of ischaemia can usually be determined by clinical examination (Box 16.59) and measurement of the ankle–brachial pressure index (ABPI), which is the ratio between the highest systolic ankle and brachial blood pressures. In health, the ABPI is over 1.0, in IC typically 0.5–0.9 and in CLI usually less than 0.5. Further investigation with duplex ultrasonography, MRI or CT with intravenous injection of contrast agents may be used to characterise the sites of involvement further. Intra-arterial digital subtraction angiography (IA-DSA) is used for those undergoing endovascular revascularisation. Other investigations should look for evidence of treatable secondary causes including a full blood count (for thrombocythaemia), lipids (for hyperlipidaemia) and blood glucose (for diabetes mellitus).

Management

Key elements of medical management are summarised in Box 16.60. This consists of smoking cessation (if applicable), taking regular exercise, antiplatelet therapy with low-dose aspirin or clopidogrel, therapy with a statin, and treatment of coexisting disease such as diabetes, hypertension or polycythaemia. Recent evidence suggests that low-dose factor Xa inhibition (rivaroxaban 2.5 mg twice daily) when used in combination with aspirin can further reduce cardiovascular events, ischaemic limb events and mortality in patients with PAD although there is a modest increase in bleeding risk. The peripheral vasodilator cilostazol has been shown to improve walking distance and should be considered in patients who do not respond adequately to best medical therapy. Intervention with angioplasty, stenting, endarterectomy or bypass is usually considered only after medical therapy has been given for at least 6 months to effect symptomatic improvement, and then just in patients who are severely disabled or whose livelihood is threatened by their disability. Subclavian artery disease is usually treated by means of angioplasty and stenting, as carotid–subclavian bypass surgery can be technically difficult.

Some considerations specific to atherosclerotic vascular disease in old age are listed in Box 16.61.

Buerger's disease

Buerger's disease or thromboangiitis obliterans is an inflammatory disease of the arteries that is distinct from atherosclerosis and usually presents in young (20–30 years) male smokers. It is most common in those from the Mediterranean and North Africa. It characteristically affects distal

16.59 Clinical features of chronic lower limb ischaemia

- Pulses: diminished or absent
- Bruits: denote turbulent flow but bear no relationship to the severity of the underlying disease
- Reduced skin temperature
- Pallor on elevation and rubor on dependency (Buerger's sign)
- Superficial veins that fill sluggishly and empty ('gutter') on minimal elevation
- Muscle-wasting
- Skin and nails: dry, thin and brittle
- Loss of hair

Box 16.60 Medical therapy for peripheral arterial disease

- Smoking cessation
- Regular exercise (30 mins of walking, three times per week)
- Antiplatelet agent (aspirin 75 mg or clopidogrel 75 mg daily)
- Consider low-dose factor Xa inhibitor (rivaroxaban 2.5 mg twice daily)
- Reduction of cholesterol: statins
- Diet and weight loss
- Diagnosis and treatment of diabetes mellitus
- Diagnosis and treatment of associated conditions:
  Hypertension
  Anaemia
  Heart failure

16.61 Atherosclerotic vascular disease in old age

- **Prevalence**: related almost exponentially to age in developed countries, although atherosclerosis is not considered part of the normal ageing process.
- **Statin therapy**: no role in the primary prevention of atherosclerotic disease in those over 75 years but reduces cardiovascular events in those with established vascular disease, albeit with no reduction in overall mortality.
- **Presentation in the frail**: frequently with advanced multisystem arterial disease, along with a host of other comorbidities.
- **Intervention in the frail**: in those with extensive disease and limited life expectancy, the risks of surgery may outweigh the benefits, and symptomatic care is all that should be offered.

arteries, giving rise to claudication in the feet or rest pain in the fingers or toes. Wrist and ankle pulses are absent but brachial and popliteal pulses are present. It may also affect the veins, giving rise to superficial thrombophlebitis. It often remits if the patient stops smoking. Symptomatic therapy with vasodilators such as prostacyclin and calcium antagonists or sympathectomy may also be helpful. Major limb amputation is the most frequent outcome if patients continue to smoke.

Raynaud's syndrome

This common disorder affects 5%–10% of young women aged 15–30 years in temperate climates. It does not progress to ulceration or infarction, and significant pain is unusual. The underlying cause is unclear and no investigation is necessary. The patient should be reassured and advised to avoid exposure to cold. Usually, no other treatment is required, although vasodilators such as nifedipine can may be helpful if symptoms are troublesome. More severe Raynaud's syndrome can also occur in association with digital ulceration in patients with connective tissue disease.

Diseases of the aorta

Aortic aneurysm

Aortic aneurysm is defined as an abnormal dilatation of the aortic lumen. The most common site is the infrarenal abdominal aorta. The suprarenal abdominal aorta and a variable length of the descending thoracic aorta

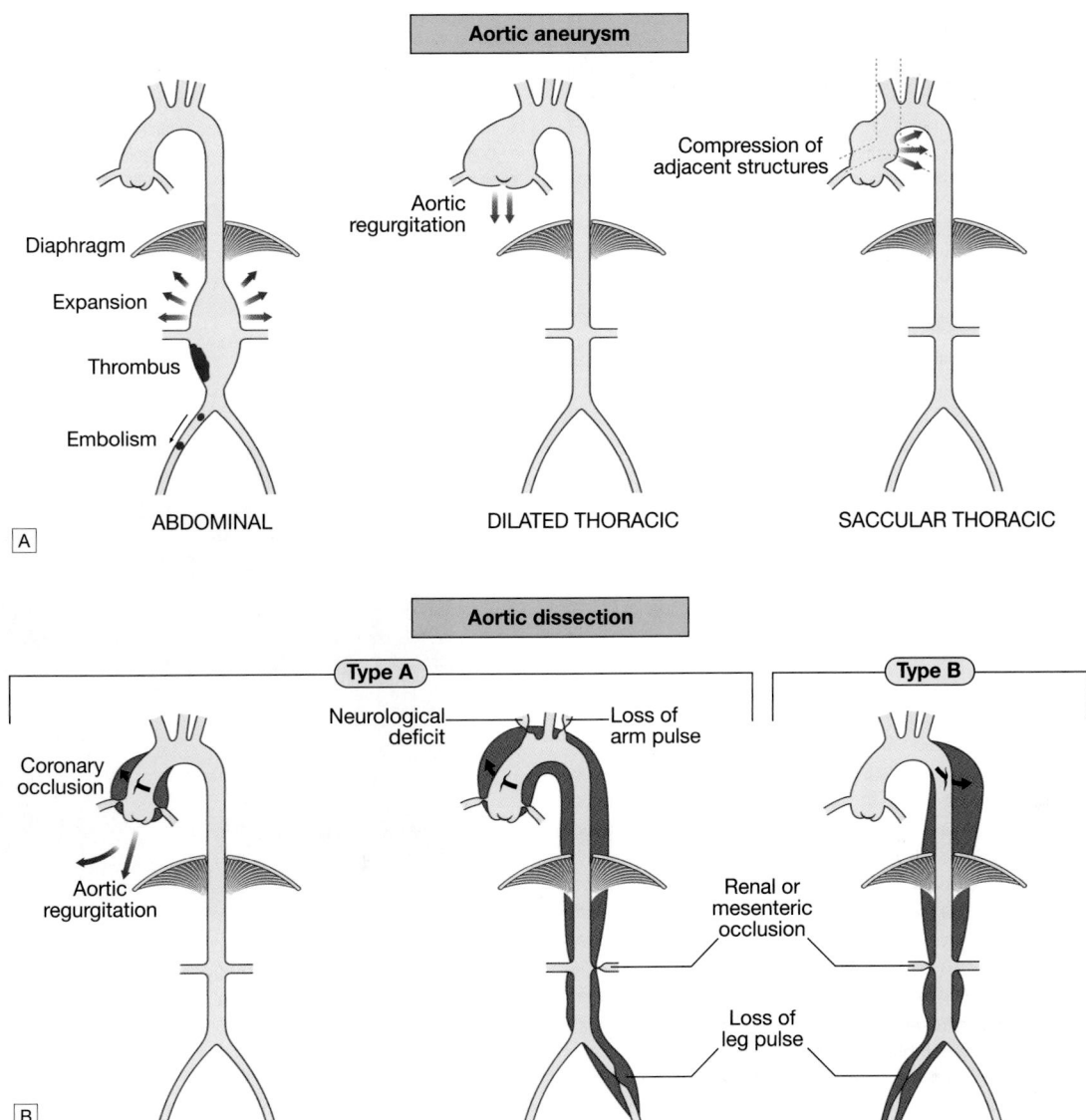

Aortic aneurysm

Diaphragm

Aortic
regurgitation

Compression of
adjacent structures

Expansion

Thrombus

Embolism

ABDOMINAL

DILATED THORACIC

SACCULAR THORACIC

A

Aortic dissection

Type A

Type B

Coronary
occlusion

Neurological
deficit

Loss of
arm pulse

Aortic
regurgitation

Renal or
mesenteric
occlusion

Loss of
leg pulse

B

Fig. 16.71 Types of aortic disease and their complications. A Types of aortic aneurysm. B Types of aortic dissection.

16

may be affected in 10%–20% of patients but the ascending aorta is usually spared. Abdominal aortic aneurysms (AAAs) affect men three times more commonly than women and are estimated to occur in about 5% of men over the age of 60 years.

Pathogenesis

The most common cause of aortic aneurysm is atherosclerosis, the risk factors for which have previously been described. However, smoking and hypertension predominate with 90%–95% of patients having one or both of these risk factors. There also appears to be an additional and specific genetic component since aortic aneurysm tends to run in families. This may explain in part why only some patients with risk factors for atheroma develop aneurysmal disease. Marfan syndrome is an inherited disorder of connective tissue that is associated with aortic aneurysm and aortic dissection.

Clinical features

The clinical presentation is dependent on the site of the aneurysm. Thoracic aneurysms may typically present with acute severe chest pain but other features, including aortic regurgitation, compressive symptoms such as stridor (trachea, bronchus), hoarseness (recurrent laryngeal nerve) and superior vena cava syndrome, may occur (Fig. 16.71A). If the aneurysm erodes into an adjacent structure, such as the oesophagus or

bronchus, the presentation may be with massive bleeding. AAAs affect the infrarenal segment of the aorta. They can present in a number of ways, as summarised in Box 16.62. The usual age at presentation is 65–75 years for elective presentations and 75–85 years for emergency presentations.

Investigations

Ultrasound is the best way of establishing the diagnosis of an abdominal aneurysm and of following up patients with asymptomatic aneurysms that are not yet large enough to warrant surgical repair. In the UK, a national screening programme for men over 65 years of age has been introduced using ultrasound scanning. For every 10 000 men scanned, 65 ruptures are prevented and 52 lives saved. CT provides more accurate information about the size and extent of the aneurysm, the surrounding structures and the presence of any other intra-abdominal pathology. It is the standard pre-operative investigation but is not suitable for surveillance because of the high cost and radiation dose.

Management

The risks of surgery generally outweigh the risks of rupture until an asymptomatic AAA has reached a maximum of 5.5 cm in diameter. All symptomatic AAAs should be considered for repair, not only to rid the patient of symptoms but also because pain often predates rupture. Distal

16.62 Abdominal aortic aneurysm (AAA): common presentations

Incidental

- On physical examination, plain X-ray or, most commonly, abdominal ultrasound
- Even large AAAs can be difficult to feel, so many remain undetected until they rupture
- Studies are currently under way to determine whether screening will reduce the number of deaths from rupture

Pain

- In the central abdomen, back, loin, iliac fossa or groin

Thromboembolic complications

- Thrombus within the aneurysm sac may be a source of emboli to the lower limbs
- Less commonly, the aorta may undergo thrombotic occlusion

Compression

- Surrounding structures such as the duodenum (obstruction and vomiting) and the inferior vena cava (oedema and deep vein thrombosis)

Rupture

- Into the retroperitoneum, the peritoneal cavity or surrounding structures (most commonly the inferior vena cava, leading to an aortocaval fistula)

16.63 Risk factors for aortic dissection

- Hypertension (in 80%)
- Atherosclerosis
- Coarctation
- Genetic:
  Marfan syndrome
  Ehlers–Danlos syndrome
- Fibromuscular dysplasia
- Previous cardiac surgery:
  CABG
  Aortic valve replacement
- Pregnancy (usually third trimester)
- Trauma
- Iatrogenic:
  Cardiac catheterisation
  Intra-aortic balloon pumping

(CABG = coronary artery bypass grafting)

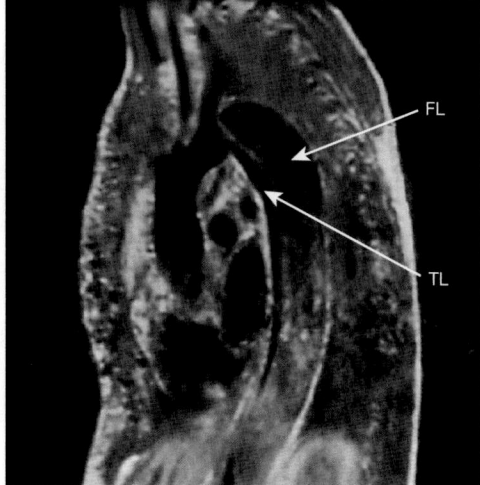

Fig. 16.72 Sagittal view of an MRI scan from a patient with long-standing aortic dissection, illustrating a biluminal aorta. There is sluggish flow in the false lumen (FL), accounting for its grey appearance. (TL = true lumen)

embolisation is a strong indication for repair, regardless of size, because otherwise limb loss is common. Most patients with a ruptured AAA do not survive to reach hospital, but if they do and surgery is thought to be appropriate, there must be no delay in getting them to the operating theatre to clamp the aorta.

Open AAA repair has been the treatment of choice in both the elective and the emergency settings, and entails replacing the aneurysmal segment with a prosthetic (usually Dacron) graft. The 30-day mortality for this procedure is approximately 5%–8% for elective asymptomatic AAA, 10%–20% for emergency symptomatic AAA and 50% for ruptured AAA. However, patients who survive the operation to leave hospital have a long-term survival approaching that of the normal population. Increasingly, endovascular aneurysm repair (EVAR), using a stent graft introduced via the femoral arteries in the groin, is replacing open surgery. It is cost-effective and likely to become the treatment of choice for infrarenal AAA. It is possible to treat many suprarenal and thoraco-abdominal aneurysms by EVAR too. If the aneurysm is secondary to Marfan syndrome, treatment with β-blockers reduces the rate of aortic dilatation and the risk of rupture. Elective replacement of the ascending aorta may also be considered in patients with evidence of progressive aortic dilatation but carries a mortality of 5%–10%.

Aortic dissection

Aortic dissection occurs when a breach in the integrity of the aortic wall allows arterial blood to enter the media, which is then split into two layers, creating a false lumen alongside the existing or true lumen (Fig. 16.71B). The aortic valve may be damaged and the branches of the aorta may be compromised. Typically, the false lumen eventually re-enters the true lumen, creating a double-barrelled aorta, but it may also rupture into the left pleural space or pericardium with fatal consequences. The peak incidence is in the sixth and seventh decades but dissection can occur in younger patients, usually in association with Marfan syndrome, pregnancy or trauma; men are affected twice as frequently as women.

Pathogenesis

The primary event is often a spontaneous or iatrogenic tear in the intima of the aorta; multiple tears or entry points are common. Other dissections are triggered by primary haemorrhage in the media of the aorta, which then ruptures through the intima into the true lumen. This form of spontaneous bleeding from the vasa vasorum is sometimes confined to the aortic wall, when it may present as a painful intramural haematoma.

Aortic disease and hypertension are the most important aetiological factors but other conditions may also be implicated (Box 16.63). Chronic dissections may lead to aneurysmal dilatation of the aorta, and thoracic aneurysms may be complicated by dissection. It can therefore be difficult to identify the primary pathology.

Aortic dissection is classified anatomically and for management purposes into type A and type B (see Fig. 16.71B), involving or sparing the ascending aorta, respectively. Type A dissections account for two-thirds of cases and frequently also extend into the descending aorta.

Clinical features

Involvement of the ascending aorta typically gives rise to anterior chest pain, and involvement of the descending aorta to intrascapular back pain. The pain is typically described as 'tearing' and very abrupt in onset; collapse is common. Unless there is major haemorrhage, the patient is invariably hypertensive. There may be asymmetry of the brachial, carotid or femoral pulses and signs of aortic regurgitation. Occlusion of aortic branches may cause MI (coronary), stroke (carotid), paraplegia (spinal), mesenteric infarction with an acute abdomen (coeliac and superior mesenteric), renal failure (renal) and acute limb (usually leg) ischaemia.

Investigations

The investigations of choice are CT or MR angiography (Figs. 16.72 and 16.73), both of which are highly specific and sensitive. A chest X-ray should be performed. It characteristically shows broadening of the upper mediastinum and distortion of the aortic 'knuckle' but these findings are absent in 10% of cases. A left-sided pleural effusion is common. The

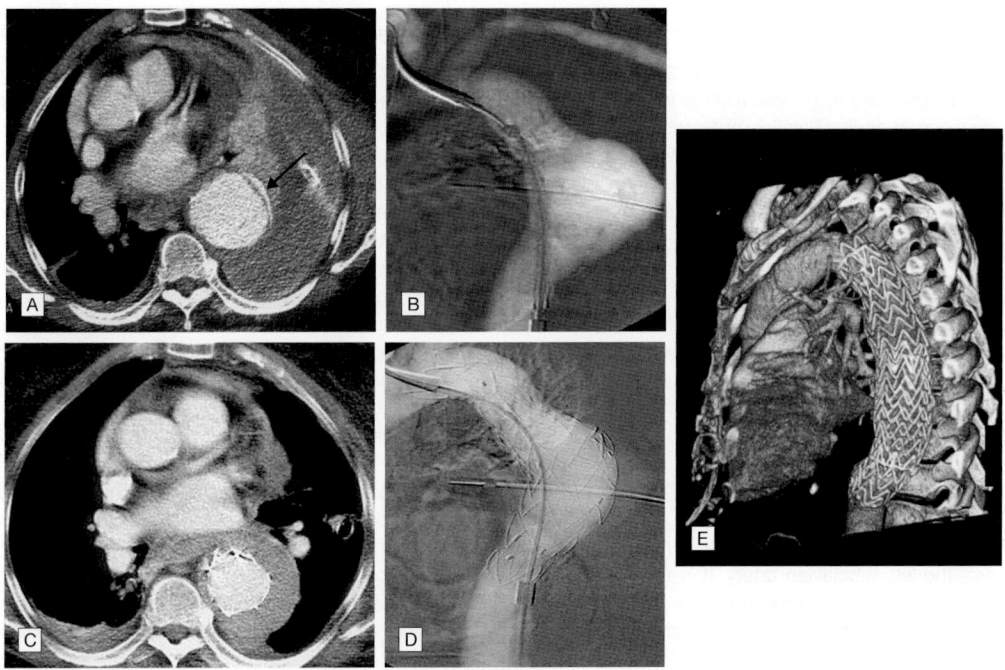

Fig. 16.73 Images from a patient with an acute type B aortic dissection that had ruptured into the left pleural space and was repaired by deploying an endoluminal stent graft. [A] CT scan illustrating an intimal flap (arrow) in the descending aorta and a large pleural effusion. [B] Aortogram illustrating aneurysmal dilatation; a stent graft has been introduced from the right femoral artery and is about to be deployed. [C] CT scan after endoluminal repair. The pleural effusion has been drained but there is a haematoma around the descending aorta. [D] Aortogram illustrating the stent graft. [E] Three-dimensional reconstruction of an aortic stent graft. *(E) Courtesy of Dr T. Lawton.*

16

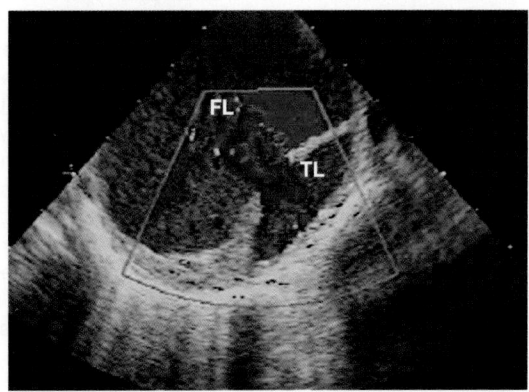

Fig. 16.74 Echocardiograms from a patient with a chronic aortic dissection. Colour-flow Doppler shows flow from the larger false lumen (FL) into the true lumen (TL), characteristic of chronic disease.

ECG may show left ventricular hypertrophy in patients with hypertension or, rarely, changes of acute MI (usually inferior). Doppler echocardiography may show aortic regurgitation, a dilated aortic root and, occasionally, the flap of the dissection. TOE is particularly helpful because transthoracic echocardiography can provide images of the first 3–4 cm of the ascending aorta only (Fig. 16.74).

Management

The early mortality of acute dissection is approximately 1%–5% per hour and so treatment is urgently required. Initial management comprises pain control and antihypertensive treatment. Type A dissections require emergency surgery to replace the ascending aorta. Type B dissections are treated medically unless there is actual or impending external rupture, or vital organ (gut, kidneys) or limb ischaemia, as the morbidity and mortality associated with surgery are very high. The aim of medical management is to maintain a mean arterial pressure (MAP) of 60–75 mmHg to reduce the force of the ejection of blood from the

LV. First-line therapy is with β-blockers; the additional α-blocking properties of labetalol make it especially useful. Rate-limiting calcium channel blockers, such as verapamil or diltiazem, are used if β-blockers are contraindicated. Sodium nitroprusside may be considered if these fail to control BP adequately.

Percutaneous or minimal access endoluminal repair is sometimes possible and involves either 'fenestrating' (perforating) the intimal flap so that blood can return from the false to the true lumen (so decompressing the former), or implanting a stent graft placed from the femoral artery (see Fig. 16.73).

Aortitis

Syphilis is a rare cause of aortitis that characteristically produces saccular aneurysms of the ascending aorta containing calcification. Other conditions that may be associated with aortitis include Takayasu's disease, giant cell arteritis and axial spondyloarthritis, all of which are discussed in more detail in Chapter 26.

Marfan syndrome

Marfan syndrome is a rare (0.02% of the population) inherited autosomal dominant disorder of connective tissue with a high risk of aortic aneurysm and dissection. It is caused by mutations of the *FBN1* gene which leads to deficiency of fibrillin-1 leading to reduced microfibril formation. This disrupts the mechanical integrity of connective tissue, giving rise to a wide range of clinical features.

Clinical features

Aortic dissection and aneurysm are the most serious complications of Marfan syndrome but many other clinical manifestations may be observed. These include aortic and mitral valve regurgitation; skin laxity and joint hypermobility; abnormalities of body habitus, including long arms, legs and fingers (arachnodactyly), scoliosis, pectus excavatum and a high-arched palate; ocular abnormalities, such as lens dislocation and retinal detachment; and an increased risk of pneumothorax.

Investigations

The diagnosis is usually suspected on the basis of the characteristic clinical features and can be confirmed by genetic testing. Imaging by chest X-ray may reveal evidence of aortic dilatation but echocardiography is more sensitive and can also demonstrate valvular disease, if present. Patients with Marfan syndrome should undergo serial monitoring of the aortic root by echocardiography; if evidence of dilatation is observed, then elective surgery should be considered.

Management

Treatment with β-blockers or angiotensin receptor blockers may reduce the risk of aortic dilatation and should be given in all patients with Marfan syndrome. Activities that are associated with increases in cardiac output are best avoided. Surgery to replace the aortic root can be performed in patients with progressive aortic dilatation.

Coarctation of the aorta

Coarctation of the aorta is the term used to describe a narrowing distal to the origin of the left subclavian artery. It is most commonly due to congenital heart disease, but narrowing of the aorta leading to similar symptoms can occur in other conditions such as Takayasu's arteritis and trauma. Diagnosis and management of coarctation are discussed later in this chapter in the section on congenital heart disease.

Hypertension

The risk of cardiovascular diseases such as stroke and CAD is closely related to levels of BP, which follows a normal distribution in the general population. Although there is no specific cut-off above which the risk of cardiovascular risk suddenly increases, the diagnosis of hypertension is made when systolic and diastolic values rise above a specific threshold that corresponds to the level of BP at which the risk of cardiovascular complications and benefits of treatment outweigh the treatment costs and potential side-effects of therapy. The British Hypertension Society classification, provided in Box 16.64, defines mild hypertension as existing when the BP is above 140/90 mmHg. Similar thresholds have been published by the European Society of Hypertension and the WHO–International Society of Hypertension. The cardiovascular risks associated with high BP depend on the combination of risk factors in an individual, such as age, sex, weight, physical activity, smoking, family history, serum cholesterol, diabetes mellitus and pre-existing vascular disease.

Pathogenesis

Many factors may contribute to the regulation of BP and the development of hypertension, including renal dysfunction, peripheral resistance, vessel tone, endothelial dysfunction, autonomic tone, insulin resistance and neurohumoral factors. In more than 95% of cases, no specific underlying cause of hypertension can be found. Such patients are said to have essential hypertension. Hypertension is more common in some ethnic groups, particularly African Americans and Japanese, and approximately 40%–60% is explained by genetic factors. Age is a strong risk factor in all ethnic groups. Important environmental factors include a high salt intake, heavy consumption of alcohol, obesity and lack of exercise. Impaired intrauterine growth and low birth weight are associated with an increased risk of hypertension later in life. In about 5% of cases, hypertension is secondary to a specific disease, as summarised in Box 16.65.

Hypertension has a number of adverse effects on the cardiovascular system. In larger arteries (> 1 mm in diameter), the internal elastic lamina is thickened, smooth muscle is hypertrophied and fibrous tissue is deposited. The vessels dilate and become tortuous, and their walls become less compliant. In smaller arteries (< 1 mm), hyaline arteriosclerosis occurs in the wall, the lumen narrows and aneurysms may develop. Widespread atheroma develops and may lead to coronary and cerebrovascular disease, particularly if other risk factors are present. These structural changes in the vasculature often perpetuate and aggravate hypertension by increasing peripheral vascular resistance and reducing renal blood flow, thereby activating the renin–angiotensin–aldosterone axis.

Clinical features

Hypertension is usually asymptomatic until the diagnosis is made at a routine physical examination or when a complication arises. Reflecting this fact, a BP check is advisable every 5 years in adults over 40 years of age to pick up occult hypertension. Sometimes clinical features may be observed that can give a clue to the underlying cause of hypertension. These include radio-femoral delay in patients with coarctation of the aorta (see Fig. 16.93), enlarged kidneys in patients with polycystic kidney disease, abdominal bruits that may suggest renal artery stenosis and the characteristic facies and habitus of Cushing's syndrome (see Box 16.65). Examination may also reveal evidence of risk factors for hypertension, such as central obesity and hyperlipidaemia. Other signs may be observed that are due to the complications of hypertension. These include signs of left ventricular hypertrophy, accentuation of the aortic component of the second heart sound, and a fourth heart sound.

---

i · 16.64 Definition of hypertension

Category	Systolic blood pressure (mmHg)	Diastolic blood pressure (mmHg)
Blood pressure		
Optimal	< 120	< 80
Normal	< 130	85
High normal	130–139	85–89
Hypertension		
Grade 1 (mild)	140–159	90–99
Grade 2 (moderate)	160–179	100–109
Grade 3 (severe)	≥ 180	> 110
Isolated systolic hypertension		
Grade 1	140–159	< 90
Grade 2	≥ 160	< 90

---

i · 16.65 Causes of secondary hypertension

Alcohol

Obesity

Pregnancy

Renal disease
- Parenchymal renal disease, particularly glomerulonephritis
- Renal vascular disease
- Polycystic kidney disease

Endocrine disease
- Phaeochromocytoma
- Cushing's syndrome
- Primary hyperaldosteronism (Conn syndrome)
- Glucocorticoid-suppressible hyperaldosteronism
- Hyperparathyroidism
- Acromegaly
- Primary hypothyroidism
- Thyrotoxicosis
- Congenital adrenal hyperplasia due to 11β-hydroxylase or 17α-hydroxylase deficiency
- Liddle syndrome
- 11β-hydroxysteroid dehydrogenase deficiency

Drugs

Coarctation of the aorta

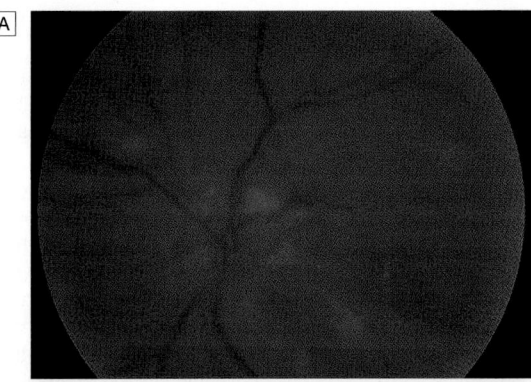

Fig. 16.75 Retinal changes in hypertension. [A] Grade 4 hypertensive retinopathy showing swollen optic disc, retinal haemorrhages and multiple cotton wool spots (infarcts). [B] Central retinal vein thrombosis showing swollen optic disc and widespread fundal haemorrhage, commonly associated with systemic hypertension. *(A and B) Courtesy of Dr B. Cullen.*

16.66 Hypertensive retinopathy

Grade 1

• Arteriolar thickening, tortuosity and increased reflectiveness ('silver wiring')

Grade 2

• Grade 1 plus constriction of veins at arterial crossings ('arteriovenous nipping')

Grade 3

• Grade 2 plus evidence of retinal ischaemia (flame-shaped or blot haemorrhages and 'cotton wool' exudates)

Grade 4

• Grade 3 plus papilloedema

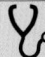

16.67 How to measure blood pressure

• Use a machine that has been validated, well maintained and properly calibrated
• Measure sitting BP routinely, with additional standing BP in older and diabetic patients and those with possible postural hypotension; rest the patient for 2 minutes
• Remove tight clothing from the arm
• Support the arm at the level of the heart
• Use a cuff of appropriate size (the bladder must encompass more than two-thirds of the arm)
• Lower the pressure slowly (2 mmHg per second)
• Read the BP to the nearest 2 mmHg
• Use phase V (disappearance of sounds) to measure diastolic BP
• Take two measurements at each visit

AF is common and may be due to diastolic dysfunction caused by left ventricular hypertrophy or the effects of CAD.

Severe hypertension can cause left ventricular failure in the absence of CAD, particularly when there is an impairment of renal function. The optic fundi are often abnormal (see Fig. 16.75 below) and there may be evidence of generalised atheroma or specific complications, such as aortic aneurysm, PAD or stroke. Examination of the optic fundi reveals a gradation of changes linked to the severity of hypertension; fundoscopy can provide an indication of the arteriolar damage occurring elsewhere (Box 16.66). 'Cotton wool' exudates are associated with retinal ischaemia or infarction, and fade in a few weeks (Fig. 16.75A). 'Hard' exudates (small, white, dense deposits of lipid) and microaneurysms ('dot' haemorrhages) are more characteristic of diabetic retinopathy (see Fig. 30.12A). Hypertension is also associated with central retinal vein thrombosis (Fig. 16.75B).

Investigations

A decision to embark on antihypertensive therapy effectively commits the patient to life-long treatment, so readings must be as accurate as possible. The objectives are to:

• confirm the diagnosis by obtaining accurate, representative BP measurements
• identify contributory factors and any underlying causes
• assess other risk factors and quantify cardiovascular risk
• detect any complications that are already present
• identify comorbidity that may influence the choice of antihypertensive therapy.

Blood pressure measurements

Measurements should be made to the nearest 2 mmHg, in the sitting position with the arm supported, and repeated after 5 minutes' rest if

the first recording is high (Box 16.67). To avoid spuriously high readings in obese subjects, the cuff should contain a bladder that encompasses at least two-thirds of the arm circumference. Exercise, anxiety, discomfort and unfamiliar surroundings can all lead to a transient rise in BP. Sphygmomanometry, particularly when performed by a doctor, can cause a transient elevation in BP, which has been termed 'white coat' hypertension. It has been estimated that up to 20% of patients with a raised BP at outpatient clinics have a normal BP when it is recorded by automated devices used at home. The risk of cardiovascular disease in these patients is less than that in patients with sustained hypertension but greater than that in normotensive subjects. If clinic BP measurements show borderline levels or if white coat hypertension is suspected, then ambulatory measurement or home-based measurements are of value in confirming the diagnosis.

Ambulatory blood pressure measurements

A series of automated ambulatory BP measurements obtained over 24 hours or longer provide a better profile than a limited number of clinic readings and correlate more closely with evidence of target organ damage than casual BP measurements. Treatment thresholds and targets (see Box 16.71) must be adjusted downwards, because ambulatory BP readings are systematically lower (approximately 12/7 mmHg) than clinic measurements. The average ambulatory daytime (not 24-hour or night-time) BP should be used to guide management decisions.

Home blood pressure measurements

Patients can measure their own BP at home using a range of commercially available semi-automatic devices. The value of such measurements is dependent on the environment and timing of the readings measured. Home or ambulatory BP measurements are particularly helpful in patients with unusually labile BP, those with refractory hypertension, those who may have symptomatic hypotension, and those in whom white coat hypertension is suspected.

16

16.68 Investigation of hypertension

- Urinalysis for blood, protein and glucose
- Blood urea, electrolytes and creatinine
    Hypokalaemic alkalosis may indicate primary hyperaldosteronism but is usually due to diuretic therapy
- Blood glucose
- Serum total and HDL cholesterol
- Thyroid function tests
- 12-lead ECG (left ventricular hypertrophy, coronary artery disease)

(HDL = high-density lipoprotein)

16.69 Specialised investigation of hypertension

- Chest X-ray: to detect cardiomegaly, heart failure, coarctation of the aorta
- Ambulatory BP recording: to assess borderline or 'white coat' hypertension
- Echocardiogram: to detect or quantify left ventricular hypertrophy
- Renal ultrasound: to detect possible renal disease
- Renal angiography: to detect or confirm the presence of renal artery stenosis
- Urinary catecholamines: to detect possible phaeochromocytoma)
- Urinary cortisol and dexamethasone suppression test: to detect possible Cushing's syndrome
- Plasma renin activity and aldosterone: to detect possible primary aldosteronism

Other investigations

All hypertensive patients should undergo a limited number of investigations (Box 16.68) but additional investigations are appropriate in patients younger than 40 years of age or those with resistant hypertension (Box 16.69). Family history, lifestyle (exercise, salt intake, smoking habit) and other risk factors should also be recorded. A careful history will identify those patients with drug- or alcohol-induced hypertension and may elicit the symptoms of other causes of secondary hypertension, such as phaeochromocytoma (paroxysmal headache, palpitation and sweating) or complications such as CAD.

Management

The objective of antihypertensive therapy is to reduce the incidence of adverse cardiovascular events, particularly CAD, stroke and heart failure. Randomised controlled trials have demonstrated that antihypertensive therapy can reduce the incidence of stroke and, to a lesser extent, CAD. The relative benefits (approximately 30% reduction in risk of stroke and 20% reduction in risk of CAD) are similar in all patient groups, so the absolute benefit of treatment (total number of events prevented) is greatest in those at highest risk. For example, to extrapolate from the Medical Research Council (MRC) Mild Hypertension Trial (1985), 566 young patients would have to be treated with bendroflumethiazide for 1 year to prevent 1 stroke, while in the MRC trial of antihypertensive treatment in older adults (1992), 1 stroke was prevented for every 286 patients treated for 1 year.

A formal estimate of absolute cardiovascular risk, which takes account of all the relevant risk factors, may help to determine whether the likely benefits of therapy will outweigh its costs and hazards. Several online risk calculators are available for this purpose, such as the Joint British Societies risk calculator (http://www.jbs3risk.com and see 'Further information'). Most of the excess morbidity and mortality associated with hypertension are attributable to CAD and many treatment guidelines are therefore based on estimates of the 10-year CAD risk. Total cardiovascular risk can be estimated by multiplying CAD risk by 4/3 (i.e. if CAD risk is 30%, cardiovascular risk is 40%). The value of this approach can be illustrated by comparing the two hypothetical cases on page 426.

Intervention thresholds

Systolic BP and diastolic BP are both powerful predictors of cardiovascular risk. The British Hypertension Society management guidelines use both readings, and treatment should be initiated if they exceed the given threshold (Fig. 16.76).

Patients with diabetes or cardiovascular disease are at particularly high risk and the threshold for initiating antihypertensive therapy is therefore lower (≤ 130/80) in these patient groups. The thresholds for treatment in older adults are the same as for younger patients (Box 16.70).

Treatment targets

The optimum BP for reduction of major cardiovascular events has been found to be 139/83 mmHg, and even lower in patients with diabetes mellitus. The targets suggested by the British Hypertension Society (Box 16.71) are ambitious. Primary care strategies have been devised to improve screening and detection of hypertension that, in the past, remained undetected in up to half of affected individuals. Application of new guidelines should help establish patients on appropriate treatment, and allow step-up if lifestyle modification and first-line drug therapy fail to control hypertension.

Patients taking antihypertensive therapy require follow-up at regular intervals to monitor BP, minimise side-effects and reinforce lifestyle advice.

Non-drug therapy

Appropriate lifestyle measures may obviate the need for drug therapy in patients with borderline hypertension, reduce the dose or the number of drugs required in patients with established hypertension, and directly reduce cardiovascular risk.

Correcting obesity, reducing alcohol intake, restricting salt intake, taking regular physical exercise and increasing consumption of fruit and vegetables can all lower BP. Moreover, stopping smoking, eating oily fish and adopting a diet that is low in saturated fat may produce further reductions in cardiovascular risk that are independent of changes in BP.

Drug therapy

Thiazides The mechanism of action of these drugs is incompletely understood and it may take up to a month for the maximum effect to be observed. An appropriate daily dose is 2.5 mg bendroflumethiazide or 0.5 mg cyclopenthiazide. More potent loop diuretics, such as furosemide (40 mg daily) or bumetanide (1 mg daily), have few advantages over thiazides in the treatment of hypertension, unless there is substantial renal impairment or they are used in conjunction with an ACE inhibitor.

ACE inhibitors ACE inhibitors (enalapril 5–40 mg daily, ramipril 5–10 mg daily or lisinopril 10–40 mg daily) are effective and usually well tolerated. They should be used with care in patients with impaired renal function or renal artery stenosis because they can reduce glomerular filtration rate and precipitate renal failure. Electrolytes and creatinine should be checked before and 1–2 weeks after commencing therapy. Side-effects include first-dose hypotension, cough, rash, hyperkalaemia and renal dysfunction.

Angiotensin receptor blockers ARBs (irbesartan 75–300 mg daily, valsartan 40–160 mg daily) have similar efficacy to ACE inhibitors but they do not cause cough and are better tolerated.

Calcium channel antagonists Amlodipine (5–10 mg daily) and nifedipine (30–90 mg daily) are effective and usually well tolerated antihypertensive drugs that are particularly useful in older people. Side-effects include flushing, palpitations and fluid retention. The rate-limiting calcium channel antagonists (diltiazem 200–500 mg daily, verapamil 240–480 mg daily in divided doses) can be useful when hypertension coexists with angina but may cause bradycardia. The main side-effect of verapamil is constipation.

Beta-blockers These are no longer used as first-line antihypertensive therapy, except in patients with another indication for the drug such as angina. Metoprolol (100–200 mg daily), atenolol (50–100 mg daily) and bisoprolol (5–10 mg daily), which preferentially block cardiac

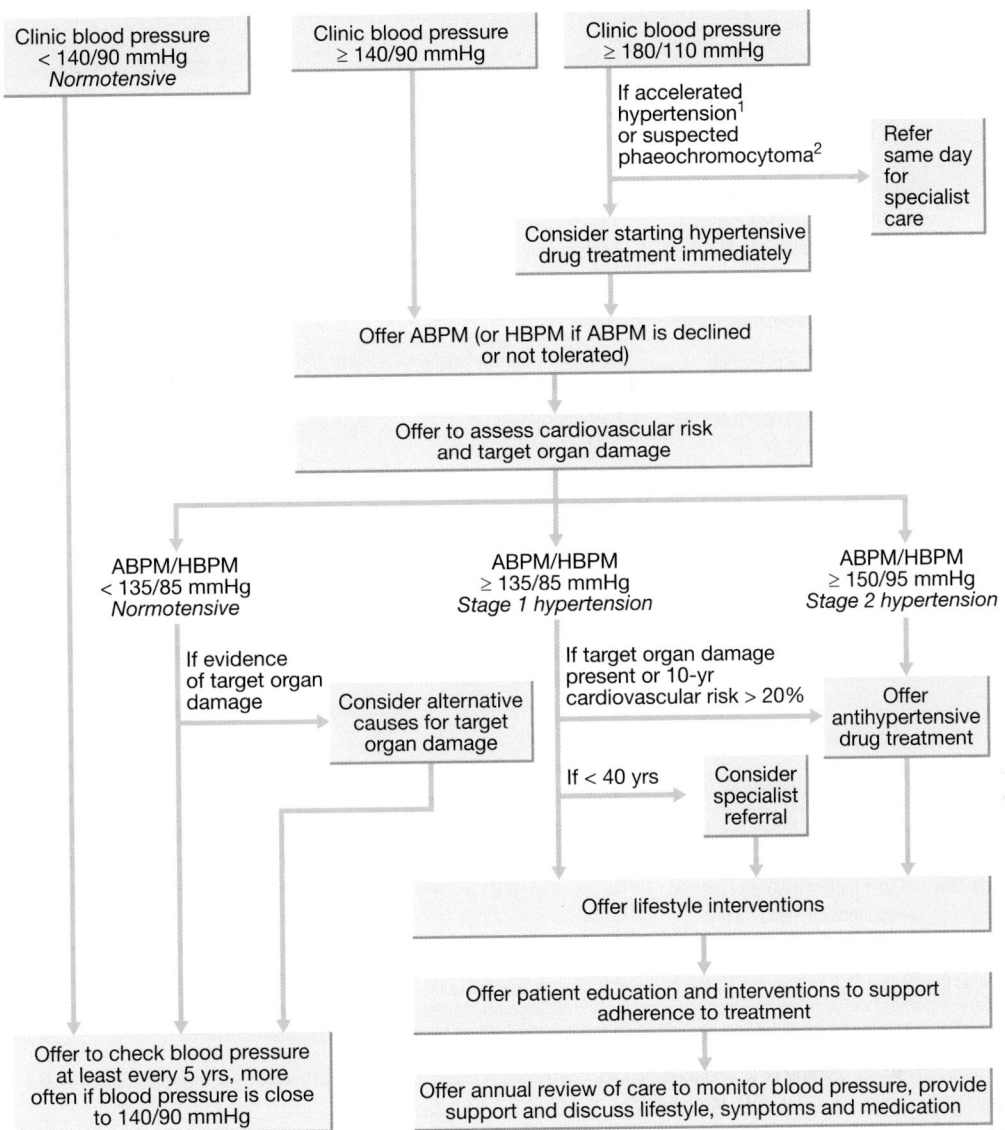

Fig. 16.76 Management of hypertension. [1]Signs of papilloedema or retinal haemorrhage. [2]Labile or postural hypotension, headache, palpitations, pallor and diaphoresis. (ABPM = ambulatory blood pressure monitoring; HBPM = home blood pressure monitoring). *Adapted from 2020 International Society of Hypertension Global Hypertension Practice Guidelines.*

16

16.70 Hypertension in old age

- **Prevalence**: hypertension affects more than half of all people over the age of 60 years (including isolated systolic hypertension).
- **Risks**: hypertension is the most important risk factor for myocardial infarction, heart failure and stroke in older people.
- **Benefit of treatment**: absolute benefit from therapy is greatest in older people (at least up to age 80 years).
- **Target blood pressure**: targets may be relaxed in older people to 150/90 mmHg.
- **Tolerance of treatment**: antihypertensives are tolerated as well as in younger patients.
- **Drug of choice**: low-dose thiazides but, in the presence of coexistent disease such as gout or diabetes, other agents may be more appropriate.

16.71 Optimal target blood pressures[1]

Age	Clinic BP (mmHg)	Ambulatory or home BP (mmHg)[2]
< 80 years	< 140/90	< 135/85
≥ 80 years	< 150/90	< 140/85

[1]Both systolic and diastolic values should be attained. [2]Average BP during waking hours.

β_1-adrenoceptors, should be used rather than non-selective agents that also block β_2-adrenoceptors, which mediate vasodilatation and bronchodilatation.

Combined β- and α-blockers Labetalol (200 mg–2.4 g daily in divided doses) and carvedilol (6.25–25 mg twice daily) are combined β- and

α-adrenoceptor antagonists that are sometimes more effective than pure β-blockers. Labetalol can be used as an infusion in malignant phase hypertension (see below).

Other vasodilators A variety of other vasodilators may be used. These include the α_1-adrenoceptor antagonists prazosin (0.5–20 mg daily in divided doses), indoramin (25–100 mg twice daily) and doxazosin (1–16 mg daily), and drugs that act directly on vascular smooth muscle, such as hydralazine (25–100 mg twice daily) and minoxidil (10–50 mg daily). Side-effects include first-dose and postural hypotension,

| i | 16.72 The influence of comorbidity on choice of antihypertensive drug therapy |

Class of drug	Compelling indications	Possible indications	Caution	Compelling contraindications
α-blockers	Benign prostatic hypertrophy	–	Postural hypotension, heart failure[1]	Urinary incontinence
ACE inhibitors	Heart failure	Chronic renal disease[2]	Renal impairment[2]	Pregnancy
	Left ventricular dysfunction, post-MI or established CAD	Type 2 diabetic nephropathy	PAD[3]	Renovascular disease[2]
	Type 1 diabetic nephropathy			
	Secondary stroke prevention[4]			
Angiotensin II receptor blockers	ACE inhibitor intolerance	Left ventricular dysfunction after MI	Renal impairment[2]	Pregnancy
	Type 2 diabetic nephropathy	Intolerance of other antihypertensive drugs	PAD[3]	
	Hypertension with left ventricular hypertrophy	Proteinuric or chronic renal disease[2]		
	Heart failure in ACE-intolerant patients, after MI	Heart failure		
β-blockers	MI, angina	–	Heart failure[5]	Asthma or chronic obstructive pulmonary disease
	Heart failure[5]		PAD	Heart block
			Diabetes (except with CAD)	
Calcium channel blockers (dihydropyridine)	Older patients, isolated systolic hypertension	Angina	–	–
Calcium channel blockers (rate-limiting)	Angina	Older patients	Combination with β-blockade	Atrioventricular block, heart failure
Thiazides or thiazide-like diuretics	Older patients, isolated systolic hypertension, heart failure, secondary stroke prevention	–	–	Gout[6]

[1]In heart failure when used as monotherapy. [2]ACE inhibitors or ARBs may be beneficial in chronic renal failure and renovascular disease but should be used with caution, close supervision and specialist advice when there is established and significant renal impairment. [3]Caution with ACE inhibitors and ARBs in PAD because of association with renovascular disease. [4]In combination with a thiazide or thiazide-like diuretic. [5]β-blockers are used increasingly to treat stable heart failure but may worsen acute heart failure. [6]Thiazides or thiazide-like diuretics may sometimes be necessary to control BP in people with a history of gout, ideally used in combination with allopurinol.
(ACE = angiotensin-converting enzyme; ARBs = angiotensin II receptor blockers; CAD = coronary artery disease; MI = myocardial infarction; PAD = peripheral arterial disease)

headache, tachycardia and fluid retention. Minoxidil also causes increased facial hair and is therefore unsuitable for female patients.

Aspirin Antiplatelet therapy is a powerful means of reducing cardiovascular risk but may cause bleeding, particularly intracerebral haemorrhage, in a small number of patients. The benefits are thought to outweigh the risks in hypertensive patients aged 50 years or over who have well-controlled BP and either target organ damage or diabetes or a 10-year CAD risk of at least 15% (or 10-year cardiovascular disease risk of at least 20%).

Statins Treating hyperlipidaemia can produce a substantial reduction in cardiovascular risk. These drugs are strongly indicated in patients who have established vascular disease, or hypertension with a high (at least 10% in 10 years) risk of developing cardiovascular disease.

Choice of antihypertensive drug

Trials that have compared thiazides, calcium antagonists, ACE inhibitors and ARBs have not shown consistent differences in outcome, efficacy, side-effects or quality of life. Beta-blockers, which previously featured as first-line therapy in guidelines, have a weaker evidence base. The choice of antihypertensive therapy is initially dictated by the patient's age and ethnic background, although cost and convenience will influence the exact drug and preparation used. Response to initial therapy and side-effects guide subsequent treatment. Comorbid conditions also have an influence on initial drug selection (Box 16.72); for example, a β-blocker might be the most appropriate treatment for a patient with angina. Thiazide diuretics and dihydropyridine calcium channel antagonists are the most suitable drugs for treatment in older people.

Combination therapy

Although some patients can be treated with a single antihypertensive drug, a combination of drugs is often required to achieve optimal control (Fig. 16.77). Combination therapy may be desirable for other reasons; for example, low-dose therapy with two drugs may produce fewer unwanted effects than treatment with the maximum dose of a single drug. Some drug combinations have complementary or synergistic actions; for example, thiazides increase activity of the renin–angiotensin system, while ACE inhibitors block it.

Refractory hypertension

Refractory hypertension refers to the situation where multiple drug treatments do not give adequate control of BP. Although this may be due to genuine resistance to therapy in some cases, a more common cause of treatment failure is non-adherence to drug therapy. Resistant hypertension can also be caused by failure to recognise an underlying cause, such as renal artery stenosis or phaeochromocytoma. There is no easy solution to problems with adherence, but simple treatment regimens,

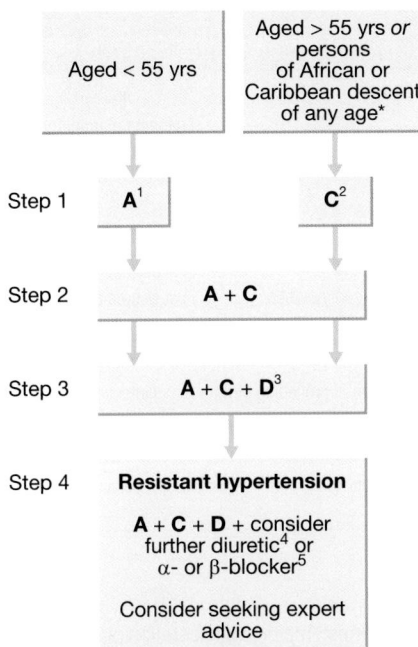

Fig. 16.77 Antihypertensive drug combinations. *Does not apply to those who are of mixed race. [1]A = Angiotensin-converting enzyme (ACE) inhibitor or consider angiotensin II receptor blocker (ARB); choose a low-cost ARB. [2]C = calcium channel blocker (CCB); a CCB is preferred but consider a thiazide-like diuretic if a CCB is not tolerated or the person has oedema, evidence of heart failure or a high risk of heart failure. [3]D = thiazide-type diuretic. [4]Consider a low dose of spironolactone or higher doses of a thiazide-like diuretic. [5]Consider an α- or β-blocker if further diuretic therapy is not tolerated, or is contraindicated or ineffective. *Adapted from 2020 International Society of Hypertension Global Hypertension Practice Guidelines.*

attempts to improve rapport with the patient and careful supervision can all help. Spironolactone is a particularly useful addition in patients with treatment-resistant hypertension.

Accelerated hypertension

Accelerated or malignant hypertension is a rare condition that can complicate hypertension of any aetiology. It is characterised by accelerated microvascular damage with necrosis in the walls of small arteries and arterioles (fibrinoid necrosis) and by intravascular thrombosis. The diagnosis is based on evidence of high BP and rapidly progressive end-organ damage, such as retinopathy (grade 3 or 4), renal dysfunction (especially proteinuria) and hypertensive encephalopathy (see above). Left ventricular failure may occur and death occurs within months if untreated.

Management

In accelerated phase hypertension, lowering BP too quickly may compromise tissue perfusion due to altered autoregulation and can cause cerebral damage, including occipital blindness, and precipitate coronary or renal insufficiency. Even in the presence of cardiac failure or hypertensive encephalopathy, a controlled reduction to a level of about 150/90 mmHg over a period of 24–48 hours is ideal.

In most patients, it is possible to avoid parenteral therapy and bring BP under control with bed rest and oral drug therapy. Intravenous or intramuscular labetalol (2 mg/min to a maximum of 200 mg), intravenous GTN (0.6–1.2 mg/hr), intramuscular hydralazine (5 or 10 mg aliquots repeated at half-hourly intervals) and intravenous sodium nitroprusside (0.3–1.0 µg/kg body weight/min) are all effective but require careful supervision, preferably in a high-dependency unit.

Diseases of the heart valves

The heart valves allow forward movement of blood through the cardiac chambers when they are open and prevent backward flow when they are closed. A diseased valve may become narrowed, obstructing forward flow, or become leaky, causing backward flow or regurgitation. Breathlessness is a common symptom of valve disease, and acute severe breathlessness may be a presenting symptom of valve failure. The causes of this are shown in Box 16.73. Predisposition to valvular disease may be genetically determined, can arise as the result of rheumatic fever or infections, or can occur in association with dilatation of the cardiac chambers in heart failure. The principal causes of valvular disease are summarised in Box 16.74.

Rheumatic heart disease

Acute rheumatic fever

Acute rheumatic fever usually affects children and young adults between the ages of 5 and 15 years. It is now rare in high-income countries in Western Europe and North America, where the incidence is about 0.5 cases per 100000, but remains endemic in South Asia, Africa and South America. Recent studies indicate that the current incidence of rheumatic heart disease in India ranges between 13 and 150 cases per 100000 population per year, where it is the commonest cause of acquired heart disease in childhood and adolescence.

Pathogenesis

The condition is triggered by an immune-mediated delayed response to infection with specific strains of group A streptococci, which have antigens that cross-react with cardiac myosin and sarcolemmal membrane proteins. Antibodies produced against the streptococcal antigens cause inflammation in the endocardium, myocardium and pericardium, as well as the joints and skin. Histologically, fibrinoid degeneration is seen in the collagen of connective tissues. Aschoff nodules are pathognomonic and

16.73 Causes of acute valve failure

Aortic regurgitation
- Aortic dissection
- Infective endocarditis

Mitral regurgitation
- Papillary muscle rupture due to acute myocardial infarction
- Infective endocarditis
- Rupture of chordae due to myxomatous degeneration

Prosthetic valve failure
- Mechanical valves: fracture, jamming, thrombosis, dehiscence
- Biological valves: degeneration with cusp tear

 16.74 Principal causes of valve disease

Valve regurgitation
- Congenital
- Acute rheumatic carditis
- Chronic rheumatic carditis
- Infective endocarditis
- Cardiac failure*
- Syphilitic aortitis
- Traumatic valve rupture
- Senile degeneration
- Damage to chordae and papillary muscles

Valve stenosis
- Congenital
- Rheumatic carditis
- Senile degeneration

*Causes dilatation of the valve ring.

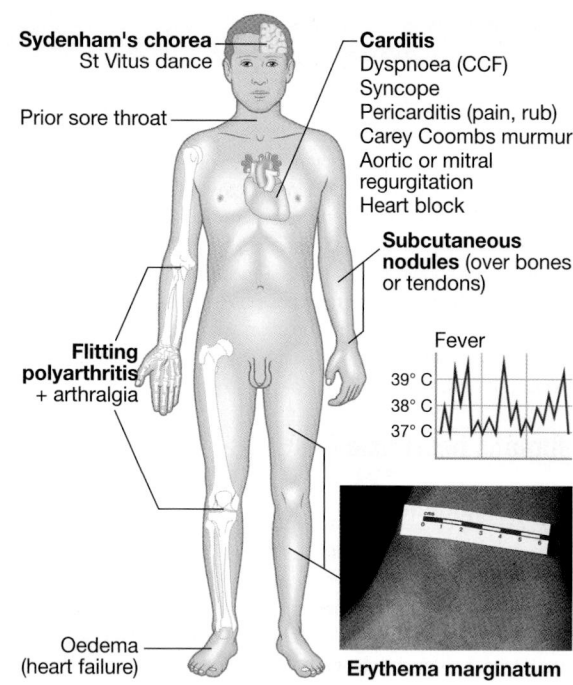

Sydenham's chorea
St Vitus dance

Prior sore throat

Carditis
Dyspnoea (CCF)
Syncope
Pericarditis (pain, rub)
Carey Coombs murmur
Aortic or mitral
regurgitation
Heart block

Subcutaneous nodules (over bones or tendons)

Flitting polyarthritis
+ arthralgia

Fever
39° C
38° C
37° C

Oedema
(heart failure)

Erythema marginatum

Fig. 16.78 Clinical features of rheumatic fever. Bold labels indicate Jones major criteria. (CCF = congestive cardiac failure) *Inset (Erythema marginatum) From Savin JA, Hunter JAA, Hepburn NC. Skin signs in clinical medicine. London: Mosby–Wolfe, Elsevier; 1997.*

i	16.75 Jones criteria for the diagnosis of rheumatic fever

Major manifestations
- Carditis
- Polyarthritis
- Chorea
- Erythema marginatum
- Subcutaneous nodules

Minor manifestations
- Fever
- Arthralgia
- Raised erythrocyte sedimentation rate or C-reactive protein
- Previous rheumatic fever
- Leucocytosis
- First-degree atrioventricular block

Plus
- Supporting evidence of preceding streptococcal infection: recent scarlet fever, raised antistreptolysin O or other streptococcal antibody titre, positive throat culture*

*Evidence of recent streptococcal infection is particularly important if there is only one major manifestation.

occur only in the heart. They are composed of multinucleated giant cells surrounded by macrophages and T lymphocytes, and are not seen until the subacute or chronic phases of rheumatic carditis.

Clinical features

Acute rheumatic fever is a multisystem disorder that usually presents with fever, anorexia, lethargy and joint pain, 2–3 weeks after an episode of streptococcal pharyngitis although there may be no history of sore throat. Arthritis occurs in approximately 75% of patients. Other features include rashes, subcutaneous nodules, carditis and neurological changes (Fig. 16.78). Using the revised Jones criteria (Box 16.75), the diagnosis is based on two or more major manifestations, or one major and two or more minor manifestations, along with evidence of preceding streptococcal infection. A presumptive diagnosis of acute rheumatic fever can be made without evidence of preceding streptococcal infection in cases of isolated chorea or pancarditis, if other causes have been excluded. In cases of established rheumatic heart disease or prior rheumatic fever, acute rheumatic fever can be diagnosed based only on the presence of multiple minor criteria and evidence of preceding group A streptococcal pharyngitis.

Carditis

Rheumatic fever causes a pancarditis involving the endocardium, myocardium and pericardium to varying degrees. Its incidence declines with increasing age, ranging from 90% at 3 years to around 30% in adolescence. It may manifest as breathlessness (due to heart failure or pericardial effusion), palpitations or chest pain (usually due to pericarditis or pancarditis). Other features include tachycardia, cardiac enlargement and new or changed murmurs. A soft systolic murmur due to mitral regurgitation is very common. A soft mid-diastolic murmur (the Carey Coombs murmur) is typically due to valvulitis, with nodules forming on the mitral valve leaflets. Aortic regurgitation occurs in 50% of cases but the tricuspid and pulmonary valves are rarely involved. Pericarditis may cause chest pain, a pericardial friction rub and precordial tenderness. Cardiac failure may be due to myocardial dysfunction or valvular regurgitation. ECG evidence commonly includes ST and T wave changes. Conduction defects, including AV block, sometimes occur and may cause syncope.

Arthritis

This is the commonest major manifestation and occurs early when streptococcal antibody titres are high. An acute painful, asymmetric and migratory inflammation of the large joints typically affects the knees, ankles, elbows and wrists. The joints are involved in quick succession and are usually red, swollen and tender for between a day and 4 weeks.

Skin lesions

Erythema marginatum occurs in less than 5% of patients. The lesions start as red macules that fade in the centre but remain red at the edges, and occur mainly on the trunk and proximal extremities but not the face. The resulting red rings or 'margins' may coalesce or overlap (see Fig. 16.78). Subcutaneous nodules occur in 5%–7% of patients. They are small (0.5–2.0 cm), firm and painless, and are best felt over extensor surfaces of bone or tendons. They typically appear more than 3 weeks after the onset of other manifestations and therefore help to confirm rather than make the diagnosis.

Sydenham's chorea

Sydenham's chorea, also known as St Vitus dance, is a late neurological manifestation that appears at least 3 months after the episode of acute rheumatic fever, when all the other signs may have disappeared. It occurs in up to one-third of cases and is more common in females. Emotional lability may be the first feature and is typically followed by purposeless, involuntary, choreiform movements of the hands, feet or face. Speech may be explosive and halting. Spontaneous recovery usually occurs within a few months. Approximately one-quarter of affected patients will go on to develop chronic rheumatic valve disease.

Other features

Other systemic manifestations, such as pleurisy, pleural effusion and pneumonia, may occur but are rare.

Investigations

Blood should be taken for measurement of ESR and CRP since these are useful for monitoring progress of the disease (Box 16.76). Throat cultures should be taken but positive results are obtained in only 10%–25% of cases since the infection has often resolved by the time of presentation. Serology for antistreptolysin O antibodies (ASO) should be performed and provide supportive evidence for the diagnosis but are normal in one-fifth of adult cases of rheumatic fever and most cases of chorea. Echocardiography should be carried out and typically shows mitral regurgitation with dilatation of the mitral annulus and prolapse of the anterior mitral leaflet; it may also demonstrate aortic regurgitation and pericardial effusion.

Management

The aims of management are to limit cardiac damage and relieve symptoms.

Bed rest

Bed rest is important, as it lessens joint pain and reduces cardiac workload. The duration should be guided by symptoms, along with temperature, leucocyte count and ESR, and should be continued until these have settled. Patients can then return to normal physical activity but strenuous exercise should be avoided in those who have had carditis.

Treatment of cardiac failure

Some patients, particularly those in early adolescence, can develop a fulminant form of the disease with severe mitral regurgitation and, sometimes, concomitant aortic regurgitation. If heart failure does not respond to medical treatment, valve replacement may be necessary and is often associated with a dramatic decline in rheumatic activity. Occasionally, AV block may occur but is seldom progressive and usually resolves spontaneously. Rarely, pacemaker insertion may be required.

Antibiotic therapy

A single dose of benzathine benzylpenicillin (1.2 million U IM) or oral phenoxymethylpenicillin (250 mg 4 times daily for 10 days) should be given on diagnosis to eliminate any residual streptococcal infection. If the patient is penicillin-allergic, erythromycin or a cephalosporin can be used. Patients are susceptible to further attacks of rheumatic fever if another streptococcal infection occurs, and long-term prophylaxis with penicillin should be given with oral phenoxymethylpenicillin (250 mg twice daily) or as benzathine benzylpenicillin (1.2 million U IM monthly), if adherence is in doubt. Sulfadiazine or erythromycin may be used if the patient is allergic to penicillin; sulphonamides prevent infection but are not effective in the eradication of group A streptococci. Further attacks of rheumatic fever are unusual after the age of 21, when antibiotic treatment can usually be stopped. The duration of prophylaxis should be extended if an attack has occurred in the last 5 years, or if the patient lives in an area of high prevalence and has an occupation (such as teaching) with a high risk of exposure to streptococcal infection. In those with residual heart disease, prophylaxis should continue until 10 years after the last episode or 40 years of age, whichever is later. While long-term antibiotic prophylaxis prevents further attacks of acute rheumatic fever, it does not protect against infective endocarditis.

Aspirin

This usually relieves the symptoms of arthritis rapidly and a response within 24 hours helps confirm the diagnosis. A reasonable starting dose is 60 mg/kg body weight/day, divided into six doses. In adults, 100 mg/kg per day may be needed up to the limits of tolerance or a maximum of 8 g per day. Mild toxicity includes nausea, tinnitus and deafness; vomiting, tachypnoea and acidosis are more serious. Aspirin should be continued until the ESR has fallen and then gradually tailed off.

Glucocorticoid steroids

These produce more rapid symptomatic relief than aspirin and are indicated in cases with carditis or severe arthritis. There is no evidence that long-term steroids are beneficial. Prednisolone (1.0–2.0 mg/kg per day in divided doses) should be continued until the ESR is normal and then gradually reduced.

Chronic rheumatic heart disease

Chronic valvular heart disease develops in at least half of those affected by rheumatic fever with carditis. Two-thirds of cases occur in women. Some episodes of rheumatic fever pass unrecognised and it is possible to elicit a history of rheumatic fever or chorea in only about half of all patients with chronic rheumatic heart disease.

The mitral valve is affected in more than 90% of cases; the aortic valve is the next most frequently involved, followed by the tricuspid and then the pulmonary valve. Isolated mitral stenosis accounts for about 25% of all cases, and an additional 40% have mixed mitral stenosis and regurgitation.

Pathogenesis

The main pathological process in chronic rheumatic heart disease is progressive fibrosis. The heart valves are predominantly affected but involvement of the pericardium and myocardium also occurs and may contribute to heart failure and conduction disorders. Fusion of the mitral valve commissures and shortening of the chordae tendineae may lead to mitral stenosis with or without regurgitation. Similar changes in the aortic and tricuspid valves produce distortion and rigidity of the cusps, leading to stenosis and regurgitation. Once a valve has been damaged, the altered haemodynamic stresses perpetuate and extend the damage, even in the absence of a continuing rheumatic process.

Mitral valve disease

Mitral stenosis

Mitral stenosis is almost always rheumatic in origin, although in older people it can be caused by heavy calcification of the mitral valve. There is also a rare form of congenital mitral stenosis.

Pathogenesis

In rheumatic mitral stenosis, the mitral valve orifice is slowly diminished by progressive fibrosis, calcification of the valve leaflets, and fusion of the cusps and subvalvular apparatus. The mitral valve orifice is normally about 5 cm^2 in diastole but can be reduced to < 1 cm^2 in severe mitral stenosis. The patient is usually asymptomatic until the orifice is < 2 cm^2. As stenosis progresses, left ventricular filling becomes more dependent on left atrial contraction. There is dilatation and hypertrophy of the LA and left atrial pressure rises, leading to pulmonary venous congestion and breathlessness. Any increase in heart rate shortens diastole when the mitral valve is open and produces a further rise in left atrial pressure. Situations that demand an increase in cardiac output, such as pregnancy and exercise, also increase left atrial pressure and are poorly tolerated.

Atrial fibrillation is very common due to progressive dilatation of the LA. Its onset often precipitates pulmonary oedema because the accompanying tachycardia and loss of atrial contraction lead to haemodynamic deterioration and a rapid rise in left atrial pressure. In the absence of AF, a more gradual rise in left atrial pressure may occur. Irrespective of AF, pulmonary hypertension may occur, which can protect the patient from pulmonary oedema. Pulmonary hypertension leads to right ventricular hypertrophy and dilatation, tricuspid regurgitation and right heart failure. Fewer than 20% of patients remain in sinus rhythm but many of these have a small fibrotic LA and severe pulmonary hypertension.

16

16.77	Clinical features of mitral stenosis
Clinical feature	**Cause**
Symptoms	
Breathlessness	Pulmonary congestion, low cardiac output
Fatigue	Low cardiac output
Oedema, ascites	Right heart failure
Palpitation	Atrial fibrillation
Haemoptysis	Pulmonary congestion
Cough	Pulmonary congestion
Chest pain	Pulmonary hypertension
Thromboembolism	Atrial stasis and atrial fibrillation
Signs	
Atrial fibrillation	Atrial dilatation
Mitral facies	Low cardiac output
Auscultation:	
Loud first heart sound, opening snap	Non-compliant, stenotic valve
Mid-diastolic murmur	
Crepitations	Left heart failure
Pulmonary oedema	
Pleural effusions	
Right ventricular heave, loud P_2	Pulmonary hypertension

Clinical features

Effort-related dyspnoea is usually the dominant symptom (Box 16.77). Typically, exercise tolerance diminishes very slowly over many years until symptoms eventually occur at rest. Patients frequently do not appreciate the extent of their disability until the diagnosis is made and their valve disease is treated. Acute pulmonary oedema or pulmonary hypertension can lead to haemoptysis. Fatigue is a common symptom due to a low cardiac output. Thromboembolism is a common complication, especially in patients with AF. Prior to the advent of anticoagulant therapy, emboli caused one-quarter of all deaths.

The physical signs of mitral stenosis are often found before symptoms develop and their recognition is of particular importance in pregnancy. The forces that open and close the mitral valve increase as left atrial pressure rises. The first heart sound (S1) is therefore loud and can be palpable (tapping apex beat). An opening snap may be audible and moves closer to the second sound (S2) as the stenosis becomes more severe and left atrial pressure rises. However, the first heart sound and opening snap may be inaudible if the valve is heavily calcified.

Turbulent flow produces the characteristic low-pitched mid-diastolic murmur and sometimes a thrill (Fig. 16.79). The murmur is accentuated by exercise and during atrial systole (pre-systolic accentuation). Early in the disease a pre-systolic murmur may be the only auscultatory abnormality, but in patients with symptoms, the murmur extends from the opening snap to the first heart sound. Coexisting mitral regurgitation causes a pansystolic murmur that radiates towards the axilla.

Pulmonary hypertension may ultimately lead to right ventricular hypertrophy and dilatation with secondary tricuspid regurgitation, which causes a parasternal lift, and a systolic murmur and giant 'v waves' in the venous pulse.

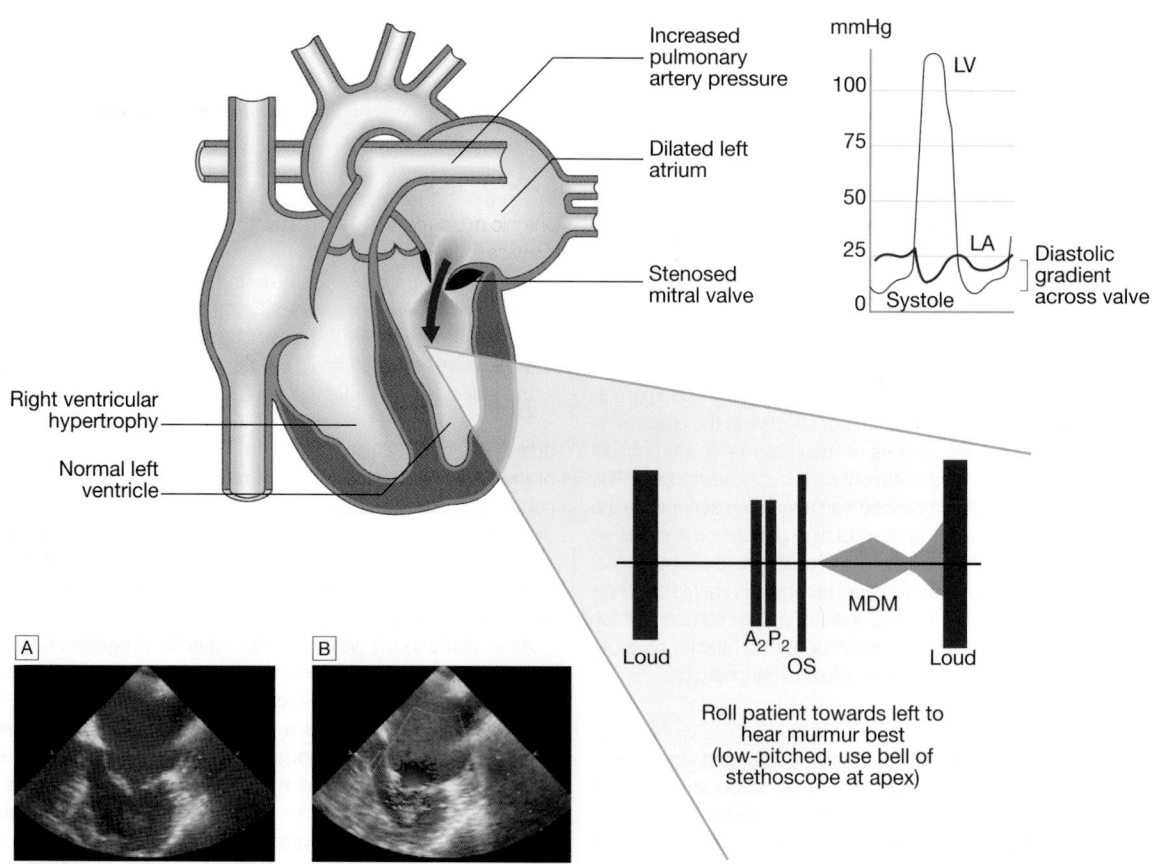

Fig. 16.79 Mitral stenosis: murmur and the diastolic pressure gradient between left atrium (LA) and left ventricle (LV). (Mean gradient is reflected by the area between LA and LV in diastole.) The first heart sound is loud, and there is an opening snap (OS) and mid-diastolic murmur (MDM) with pre-systolic accentuation. **A** Echocardiogram showing reduced opening of the mitral valve in diastole. **B** Colour Doppler showing turbulent flow.

Investigations

Doppler echocardiography is the investigation of choice for evaluation of suspected mitral stenosis (see Fig. 16.79). Cardiac catheterisation may also be required if surgery or valvuloplasty is being considered, to screen for coexisting conditions such as CAD. The ECG may show either AF or bifid P waves (P mitrale) associated with left atrial hypertrophy (Box 16.78). A typical chest X-ray is shown in Fig. 16.9.

Management

Patients with mild symptoms can be treated medically but intervention by balloon valvuloplasty, mitral valvotomy or mitral valve replacement should be considered if the patient remains symptomatic despite medical treatment or if pulmonary hypertension develops.

Medical management

This consists of anticoagulation to reduce the risk of systemic embolism, ventricular rate control with digoxin, β-blockers or rate-limiting calcium antagonists for AF, and diuretic to control pulmonary congestion. Antibiotic prophylaxis against infective endocarditis is no longer routinely recommended.

Mitral balloon valvuloplasty and valve replacement

Valvuloplasty is the treatment of choice if specific criteria are fulfilled (Box 16.79 and Fig. 16.80), although surgical closed or open mitral valvotomy is an acceptable alternative. Patients who have undergone mitral valvuloplasty or valvotomy should be followed up at 1–2-yearly intervals because restenosis may occur. Clinical symptoms and signs are a guide to the severity of mitral restenosis but Doppler echocardiography provides a more accurate assessment.

Valve replacement is indicated if there is substantial mitral reflux or if the valve is rigid and calcified.

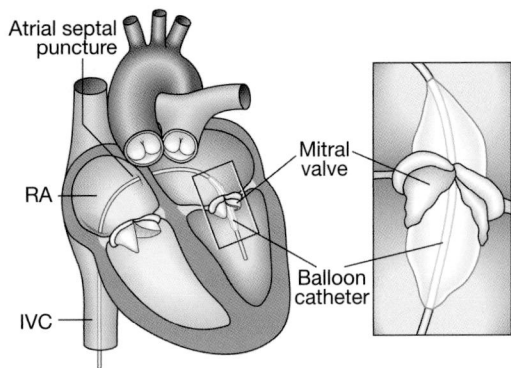

Fig. 16.80 Mitral valvuloplasty. A guidewire is introduced into the right atrium (RA) from the femoral vein and the inferior vena cava (IVC). The interatrial septum is punctured, providing access to the left atrium and mitral valve. A balloon catheter is then advanced over the guidewire across the mitral valve and the balloon dilated to stretch the valve and reduce the degree of stenosis.

16.80 Causes of mitral regurgitation
• Mitral valve prolapse
• Dilatation of the left ventricle and mitral valve ring (coronary artery disease, cardiomyopathy)
• Damage to valve cusps and chordae (rheumatic heart disease, endocarditis)
• Ischaemia or infarction of the papillary muscle
• Myocardial infarction

16

Mitral regurgitation

Rheumatic disease is the principal cause in countries where rheumatic fever is common but elsewhere, including in the UK, other causes are more important (Box 16.80). Mitral regurgitation may also follow mitral valvotomy or valvuloplasty.

Pathogenesis

Chronic mitral regurgitation causes gradual dilatation of the LA with little increase in pressure and relatively few symptoms. Nevertheless, the LV dilates slowly and the left ventricular diastolic and left atrial pressures gradually increase as a result of chronic volume overload of the LV. In contrast, acute mitral regurgitation causes a rapid rise in left atrial pressure (because left atrial compliance is normal) and marked symptomatic deterioration.

Mitral valve prolapse

This is also known as 'floppy' mitral valve and is a common cause of mild mitral regurgitation (Fig. 16.81). Some cases are thought to be due to a developmental abnormality of the mitral valve and others due to degenerative myxomatous change in a normal mitral valve. Rarely, mitral valve prolapse may occur in association with Marfan syndrome.

In its mildest forms, the valve remains competent but bulges back into the atrium during systole, causing a mid-systolic click but no murmur. In the presence of a regurgitant valve, the click is followed by a late systolic murmur, which lengthens as the regurgitation becomes more severe. A click is not always audible and the physical signs may vary with both posture and respiration. Progressive elongation of the chordae tendineae leads to increasing mitral regurgitation, and if chordal rupture occurs, regurgitation suddenly becomes severe. This is rare before the fifth or sixth decade of life.

Mitral valve prolapse is associated with a variety of typically benign arrhythmias, atypical chest pain and a very small risk of embolic stroke or transient ischaemic attack (TIA). Nevertheless, the overall long-term prognosis is good.

16.78 Investigations in mitral stenosis

ECG

• Right ventricular hypertrophy: tall R waves in V_1–V_3	• P mitrale or atrial fibrillation

Chest X-ray

Enlarged left atrium and appendage	Signs of pulmonary venous congestion

Echo

• Thickened immobile cusps	• Reduced rate of diastolic filling
• Reduced valve area	of left ventricle
• Enlarged left atrium	

Doppler

• Pressure gradient across mitral valve	• Left ventricular function
• Pulmonary artery pressure	

Cardiac catheterisation

• Coronary artery disease	• Mitral stenosis and regurgitation
• Pulmonary artery pressure	

16.79 Criteria for mitral valvuloplasty*
• Significant symptoms
• Isolated mitral stenosis
• No (or trivial) mitral regurgitation
• Mobile, non-calcified valve/subvalve apparatus on echo
• Left atrium free of thrombus

*For comprehensive guidelines on valvular heart disease, see www.acc.org.

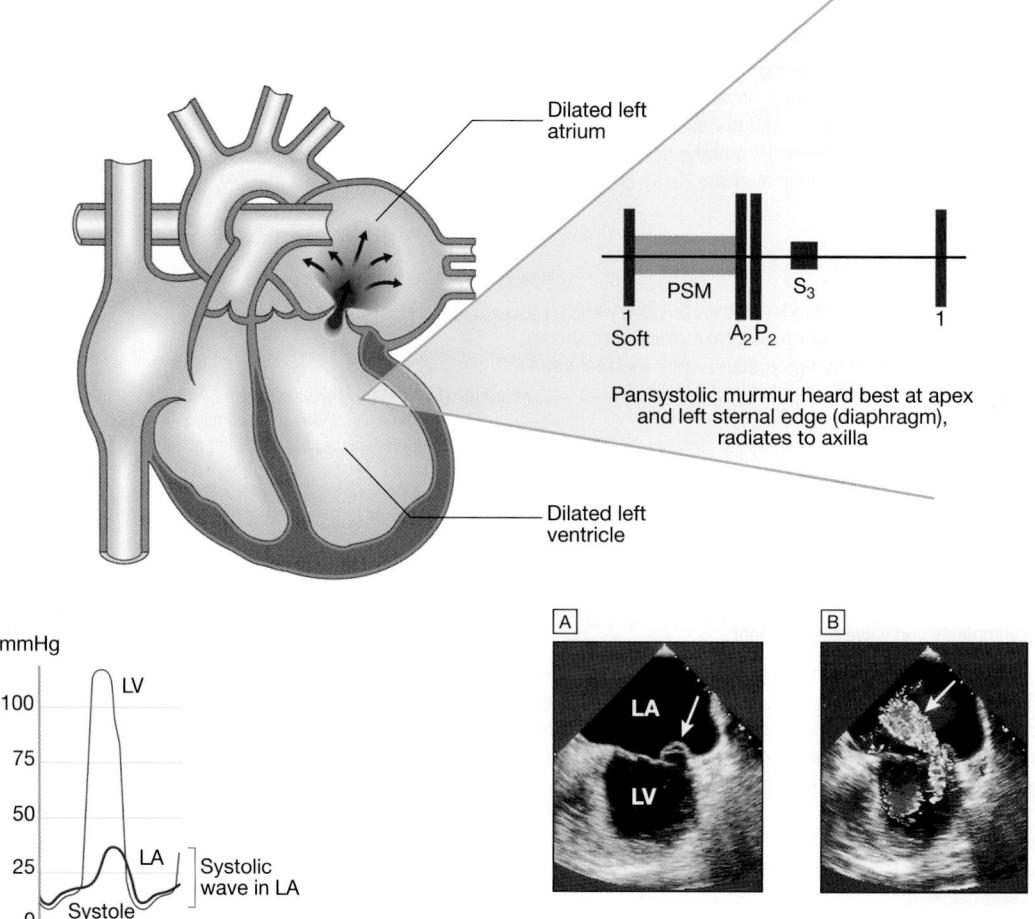

Fig. 16.81 Mitral regurgitation: murmur and systolic wave in left atrial pressure. The first sound is normal or soft and merges with a pansystolic murmur (PSM) extending to the second heart sound. A third heart sound occurs with severe regurgitation. **A** A transoesophageal echocardiogram shows mitral valve prolapse, with one leaflet bulging towards the left atrium (LA, arrow). **B** This results in a jet of mitral regurgitation on colour Doppler (arrow). (LV = left ventricle)

Other causes of mitral regurgitation

Mitral valve function depends on the chordae tendineae and their papillary muscles; dilatation of the LV distorts the geometry of these and may cause mitral regurgitation (see Box 16.80). Dilated cardiomyopathy and heart failure from CAD are common causes of so-called 'functional' mitral regurgitation. Endocarditis is an important cause of acute mitral regurgitation.

Clinical features

Symptoms and signs depend on the underlying cause and how suddenly the regurgitation develops (Box 16.81). Chronic mitral regurgitation produces a symptom complex that is similar to that of mitral stenosis but sudden-onset mitral regurgitation usually presents with acute pulmonary oedema.

The regurgitant jet causes an apical systolic murmur (Fig. 16.82), which radiates into the axilla and may be accompanied by a thrill. Increased forward flow through the mitral valve causes a loud third heart sound and even a short mid-diastolic murmur. The apex beat feels active and rocking due to left ventricular volume overload and is usually displaced to the left as a result of left ventricular dilatation.

Investigations

Echocardiography is a pivotal investigation. The severity of regurgitation can be assessed by Doppler and information may also be gained on papillary muscle function and valve prolapse. An ECG should be performed and commonly shows AF, as a consequence of atrial dilatation.

16.81 Clinical features of mitral regurgitation	
Clinical feature	**Cause**
Symptoms	
Breathlessness	Pulmonary congestion
Fatigue	Low cardiac output
Oedema, ascites	Right heart failure
Palpitation	Atrial fibrillation
Signs	
Atrial fibrillation	Atrial dilatation
Displaced apex beat	Cardiomegaly
Auscultation:	
Apical pansystolic murmur	Regurgitation of blood from left ventricle to left atrium
Soft S1	Valve does not close properly
Apical S3	Rapid flow of blood into left ventricle
Crepitations	
Pulmonary oedema	} Left heart failure
Pleural effusions	
Right ventricular heave	Pulmonary hypertension
Raised jugular venous pressure	Right heart failure
Oedema	Right heart failure

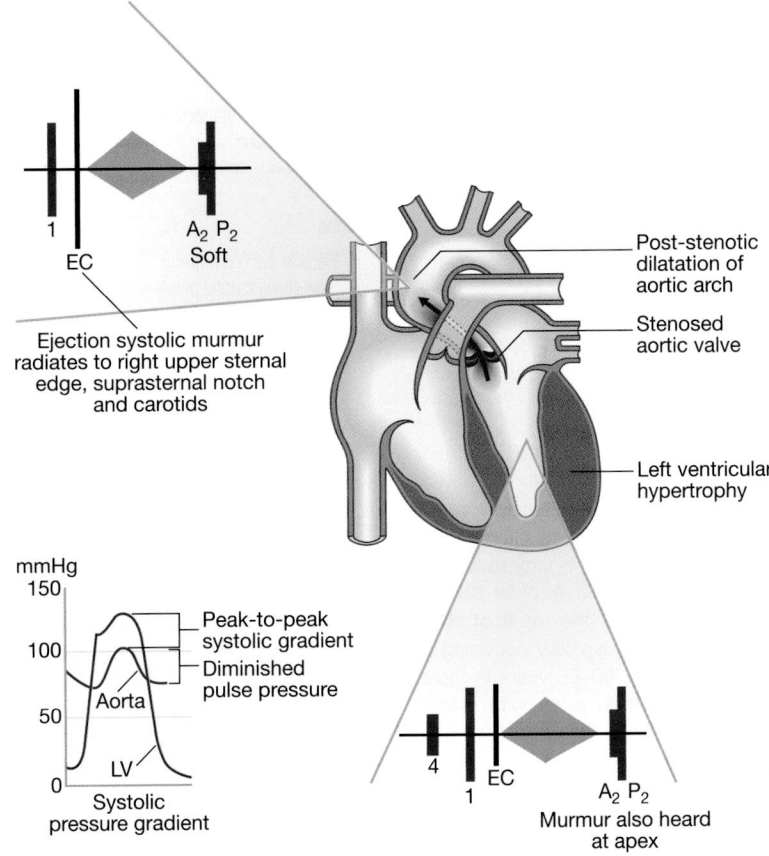

Fig. 16.82 Aortic stenosis. Pressure traces show the systolic gradient between left ventricle (LV) and aorta. The 'diamond-shaped' murmur is heard best with the diaphragm in the aortic outflow and also at the apex. An ejection click (EC) may be present in young patients with a bicuspid aortic valve but not in older patients with calcified valves. Aortic stenosis may lead to left ventricular hypertrophy with a fourth sound at the apex and post-stenotic dilatation of the aortic arch. Fig. 16.11 shows the typical Doppler signal with aortic stenosis.

Cardiac catheterisation is indicated when surgery is being considered (Box 16.82). During catheterisation, the severity of mitral regurgitation can be assessed by left ventriculography and by the size of the *v* (systolic) waves in the left atrial or pulmonary artery wedge pressure trace.

Management

Mitral regurgitation of moderate severity can be treated medically with diuretics and vasodilators. Digoxin and anticoagulants should be given if AF is present (Box 16.83). If systemic hypertension is present, it should be treated with vasodilators such as ACE inhibitors or ARBs, since high

i	16.82 Investigations in mitral regurgitation

ECG

• P-mitrale	• Atrial fibrillation

Chest X-ray

• Enlarged left atrium	• Pulmonary venous congestion
• Enlarged left ventricle	• Pulmonary oedema (if acute)

Echo

• Dilated left atrium, left ventricle	• Structural abnormalities of mitral valve
• Dynamic left ventricle (unless myocardial dysfunction predominates)	

Doppler

• Detects and quantifies regurgitation

Cardiac catheterisation

• Dilated left atrium, dilated left ventricle, mitral regurgitation	• Coexisting coronary artery disease
• Pulmonary hypertension	

i	16.83 Medical management of mitral regurgitation

- Diuretics
- Vasodilators if hypertension is present
- Digoxin if atrial fibrillation is present
- Anticoagulants if atrial fibrillation is present

afterload may worsen the degree of regurgitation. All patients should be reviewed at regular intervals, both clinically and by echocardiography. Worsening symptoms, progressive cardiomegaly or echocardiographic evidence of deteriorating left ventricular function are indications for mitral valve replacement or repair. Mitral valve repair is now the treatment of choice for severe mitral regurgitation, because early repair appears to prevent irreversible left ventricular damage. Mitral regurgitation often accompanies left ventricular failure associated with CAD. If such patients are to undergo CABG surgery, it is common practice to repair the valve and restore mitral valve function by inserting an annuloplasty ring to overcome annular dilatation and to bring the valve leaflets closer together. Unfortunately, it can be difficult to determine whether it is the ventricular dilatation or the mitral regurgitation that is the predominant problem. If ventricular dilatation is the underlying cause of mitral regurgitation, then mitral valve repair or replacement may actually worsen ventricular function, as the ventricle can no longer empty into the low-pressure LA.

Aortic valve disease

Aortic stenosis

There are several causes of aortic stenosis but the age at which patients present can give a clue to the most likely diagnosis (Box 16.84).

16

> **i 16.84 Causes of aortic stenosis**

Infants, children, adolescents
- Congenital aortic stenosis
- Congenital subvalvular aortic stenosis
- Congenital supravalvular aortic stenosis

Young to middle-aged adults
- Calcification and fibrosis of congenitally bicuspid aortic valve
- Rheumatic aortic stenosis

Middle-aged to older adults
- Senile degenerative aortic stenosis
- Calcification of bicuspid valve
- Rheumatic aortic stenosis

> **i 16.85 Clinical features of aortic stenosis**

Symptoms
- Mild or moderate stenosis: usually asymptomatic
- Exertional dyspnoea
- Angina
- Exertional syncope
- Sudden death
- Episodes of acute pulmonary oedema

Signs
- Ejection systolic murmur
- Slow-rising carotid pulse
- Heaving apex beat (left ventricular pressure overload)
- Narrow pulse pressure
- Signs of pulmonary venous congestion

In congenital aortic stenosis, obstruction is present from birth or becomes apparent during infancy. With bicuspid aortic valves, obstruction may take years to develop as the valve becomes fibrotic and calcified, and these patients present as young to middle-aged adults. Rheumatic disease of the aortic valve presents at a similar age but is usually accompanied by mitral valve disease. In older people, tricuspid aortic valves may become stenotic as the result of fibrosis and calcification. Stenosis develops slowly, typically occurring at 30–60 years in those with rheumatic disease, 50–60 years in those with bicuspid aortic valves and 70–90 years in those with calcific aortic disease.

Pathogenesis

Cardiac output is initially maintained in patients with aortic stenosis at the cost of a steadily increasing pressure gradient across the aortic valve. With progression of the stenosis, the LV becomes increasingly hypertrophied and coronary blood flow may be inadequate to supply the myocardium, such that angina can develop even in the absence of coexisting CAD. The fixed outflow obstruction limits the increase in cardiac output required on exercise. Eventually, the LV can no longer overcome the outflow tract obstruction and LV failure results, leading to pulmonary oedema.

Clinical features

Aortic stenosis is commonly picked up in asymptomatic patients at routine clinical examination but the three cardinal symptoms are angina, breathlessness and syncope (Box 16.85). Angina arises either because of the increased demands of the hypertrophied LV working against the high-pressure outflow tract obstruction, or the presence of coexisting CAD, which affects over 50% of patients. Exertional breathlessness suggests cardiac decompensation as a consequence of the excessive pressure overload placed on the LV. Syncope usually occurs on exertion when cardiac output fails to rise to meet demand, leading to a fall in BP. Sometimes patients with severe aortic stenosis do not complain of symptoms. If, on clinical evaluation, this appears to be due to a sedentary lifestyle, a careful exercise test may reveal symptoms on modest exertion.

The characteristic clinical signs of severe aortic stenosis are shown in Box 16.85. A harsh ejection systolic murmur radiates to the neck, with a soft second heart sound, particularly in those with calcific valves. The murmur is often likened to a saw cutting wood and may (especially in older patients) have a musical quality like the 'mew' of a seagull (see Fig. 16.82). The severity of aortic stenosis may be difficult to gauge clinically, as older patients with a non-compliant 'stiff' arterial system may have an apparently normal carotid upstroke in the presence of severe aortic stenosis. Milder degrees of stenosis may be difficult to distinguish from aortic sclerosis, in which the valve is thickened or calcified but not obstructed. A careful examination should be made for other valve lesions, particularly in rheumatic heart disease, when there is frequently concomitant mitral valve disease. In contrast to patients with mitral stenosis, which tends to progress very slowly, patients with aortic stenosis typically remain asymptomatic for many years but deteriorate rapidly when symptoms develop; if otherwise untreated, they usually die within 3–5 years of presentation.

Investigations

Echocardiography is a pivotal investigation in patients suspected of having aortic stenosis. It can demonstrate restricted valve opening (Fig. 16.83) and Doppler assessment permits calculation of the systolic gradient across the aortic valve, from which the severity of stenosis can be assessed (see Fig. 16.11). In patients with impaired left ventricular function, velocities across the aortic valve may be diminished because of a reduced stroke volume; this is called low-flow aortic stenosis. When marked aortic regurgitation or elevated cardiac output is present, velocities are increased because of an increased stroke volume and this may overestimate stenosis severity on Doppler echocardiography. In advanced cases, ECG features of LV hypertrophy (Box 16.86) are often pronounced (Fig. 16.84), and down-sloping ST segments and T inversion ('strain pattern') are seen in the lateral leads, reflecting left ventricular fibrosis. Nevertheless, the ECG can be normal, despite severe stenosis. Occasionally, there is evidence of AV block due to the encroachment of the fibrocalcific process on the adjacent AV node and His–Purkinje system; an occasional cause of syncope in these patients. Imaging with CT may be useful in assessing the degree of valve calcification where there is uncertainty of disease severity.

Management

Irrespective of the severity of valve stenosis, patients with asymptomatic aortic stenosis have a good immediate prognosis and conservative management is appropriate. Such patients should be kept under review, as the development of angina, syncope, symptoms of low cardiac output or heart failure has a poor prognosis and is an indication for prompt surgery. In practice, patients with moderate or severe stenosis should be evaluated every 1–2 years with Doppler echocardiography to detect evidence of progression in severity. The intervals between reviews should be more frequent (typically 3–6-monthly) in older patients with heavily calcified valves.

Patients with symptomatic severe aortic stenosis should have prompt aortic valve replacement. Delay exposes the patient to the risk of sudden death or irreversible deterioration in ventricular function. Old age is not a contraindication to valve replacement and results are very good in experienced centres, even for those in their eighties (Box 16.87). This is especially the case with transcatheter aortic valve implantation (TAVI, see Fig. 16.86). Aortic balloon valvuloplasty is useful in congenital aortic stenosis but has limited value in older patients with calcific aortic stenosis.

Anticoagulants are required only in patients who have AF or those who have had a valve replacement with a mechanical prosthesis.

Aortic regurgitation

This condition can result from either disease of the aortic valve cusps, infection, trauma or dilatation of the aortic root. The causes are summarised in Box 16.88.

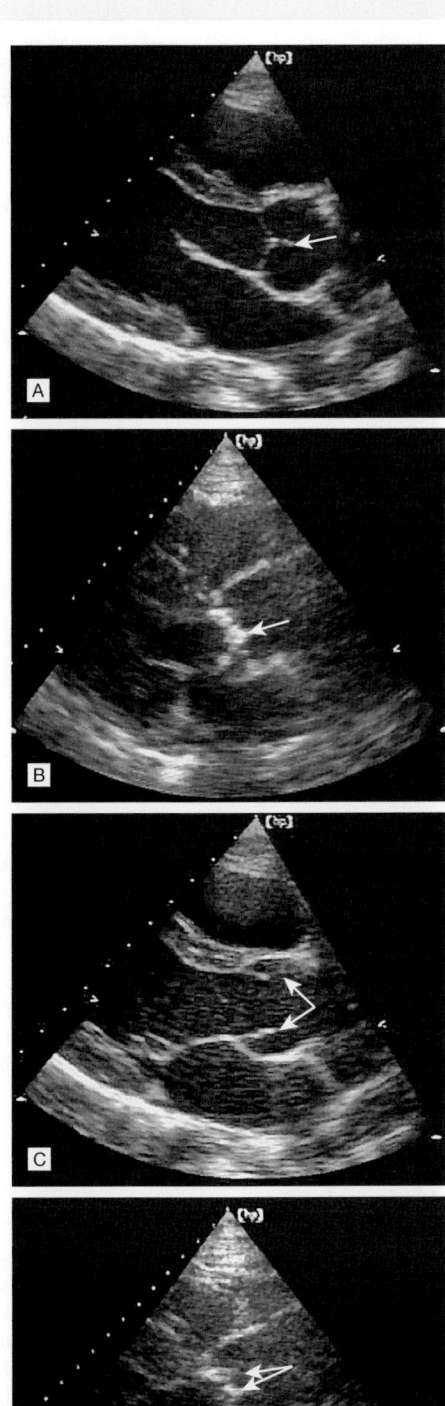

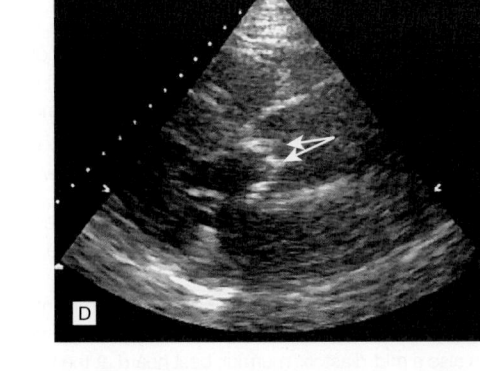

Fig. 16.83 Two-dimensional echocardiogram comparing a normal individual and a patient with calcific aortic stenosis. [A] Normal individual in diastole; the aortic leaflets are closed and thin, and a point of coaptation is seen (arrow). [B] Calcific aortic stenosis in diastole; the aortic leaflets are thick and calcified (arrow). [C] Normal in systole; the aortic leaflets are open (arrows). [D] Calcific aortic stenosis in systole; the thickened leaflets have barely moved (arrows). *From Newby D, Grubb N. Cardiology: an illustrated colour text. Edinburgh: Churchill Livingstone, Elsevier Ltd; 2005.*

Pathogenesis

Regurgitation of blood through the aortic valve causes the LV to dilate as cardiac output increases to maintain the demands of the circulation.

<table><tr><td>i</td><td>**16.86 Investigations in aortic stenosis**</td></tr></table>

ECG

- Left ventricular hypertrophy
- Left bundle branch block

Chest X-ray

- May be normal; sometimes enlarged left ventricle and dilated ascending aorta on postero-anterior view, calcified valve on lateral view

Echo

- Calcified valve with restricted opening, hypertrophied left ventricle

Doppler

- Measurement of severity of stenosis
- Detection of associated aortic regurgitation

Cardiac catheterisation

- Mainly to identify associated coronary artery disease
- May be used to measure gradient between left ventricle and aorta

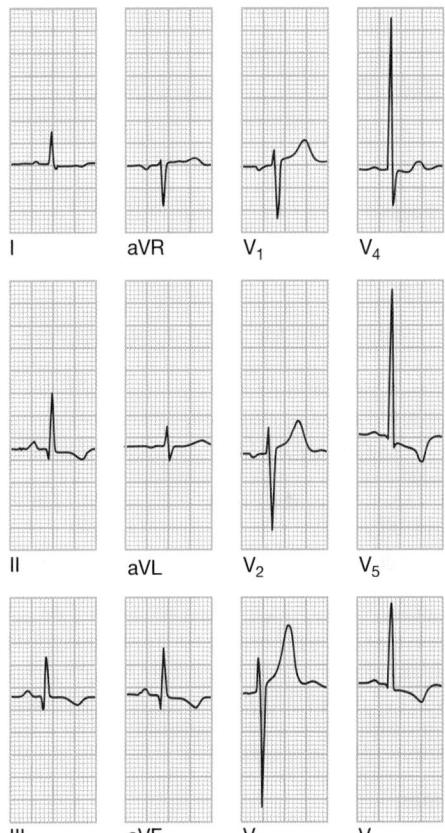

Fig. 16.84 Left ventricular hypertrophy. QRS complexes in limb leads have increased amplitude with very large R waves in V_4 and V_5 and a deep S wave in V_3. There is ST depression and T-wave inversion in leads II, III, aVF, V_5 and V_6: a 'left ventricular strain' pattern.

The stroke volume of the LV may eventually be doubled and the major arteries are then conspicuously pulsatile. As the disease progresses, left ventricular failure develops, leading to a rise in left ventricular end-diastolic pressure and pulmonary oedema.

Clinical features

Until the onset of breathlessness, the only symptom may be an awareness of the heart beat (Box 16.89), particularly when lying on the left side, which results from the increased stroke volume. Paroxysmal nocturnal

16.87 Aortic stenosis in old age

- **Incidence**: the most common form of valve disease affecting the very old.
- **Symptoms**: a common cause of syncope, angina and heart failure in the very old.
- **Signs**: because of increasing stiffening in the central arteries, low pulse pressure and a slow-rising pulse may not be present.
- **Transcatheter aortic valve implantation (TAVI)**: a good option in older individuals because less invasive than surgery.
- **Surgery**: can be successful in those aged 80 years or more in the absence of comorbidity, but with a higher operative mortality. The prognosis without surgery is poor once symptoms have developed.
- **Valve replacement type**: a biological valve is often preferable to a mechanical one because this obviates the need for anticoagulation, and the durability of biological valves usually exceeds the patient's anticipated life expectancy.

16.88 Causes of aortic regurgitation

Congenital

- Bicuspid valve or disproportionate cusps

Acquired

- Rheumatic disease
- Infective endocarditis
- Trauma
- Causes of aortic dilatation:
    Marfan syndrome
    Aneurysm
    Aortic dissection
    Syphilis
    Ankylosing spondylitis

16.89 Clinical features of aortic regurgitation

Symptoms

Mild to moderate aortic regurgitation

- Often asymptomatic
- Palpitations

Severe aortic regurgitation

- Breathlessness
- Angina

Signs

Pulses

- Large-volume or 'collapsing' pulse
- Low diastolic and increased pulse pressure
- Bounding peripheral pulses
- Capillary pulsation in nail beds: Quincke's sign
- Femoral bruit ('pistol shot'): Duroziez's sign
- Head nodding with pulse: de Musset's sign

Murmurs

- Early diastolic murmur
- Systolic murmur (increased stroke volume)
- Austin Flint murmur (soft mid-diastolic)

Other signs

- Displaced, thrusting apex beat (volume overload)
- Pre-systolic impulse
- Third heart sound
- Fourth heart sound
- Crepitations (pulmonary venous congestion)

dyspnoea is sometimes the first symptom, and peripheral oedema or angina may occur. The characteristic murmur is best heard to the left of the sternum during held expiration (Fig. 16.85); a thrill is rare. A systolic murmur due to the increased stroke volume is common and does not necessarily indicate stenosis. The regurgitant jet causes fluttering of the mitral valve and, if severe, causes partial closure of the anterior mitral leaflet, leading to functional mitral stenosis and a soft mid-diastolic (Austin Flint) murmur.

Acute severe regurgitation may occur as the result of perforation or tear of an aortic cusp in endocarditis. In this circumstance there may be no time for compensatory left ventricular hypertrophy and dilatation to develop and the features of heart failure may predominate. The classical signs of aortic regurgitation in such patients may be masked by tachycardia and an abrupt rise in left ventricular end-diastolic pressure. The pulse pressure may also be normal or near-normal and the diastolic murmur may be short or even absent.

Investigations

Doppler echocardiography is the investigation of first choice for detecting regurgitation (Box 16.90). In severe acute aortic regurgitation the rapid rise in left ventricular diastolic pressure may cause premature mitral valve closure. Cardiac catheterisation and aortography are usually performed to assess the severity of regurgitation, to determine if there is dilatation of the aorta and to screen for the presence of coexisting CAD. MRI can also be useful in assessing the degree and extent of aortic dilatation if this is suspected on chest X-ray or echocardiography.

Management

Treatment may be required for underlying conditions, such as endocarditis or syphilis. Aortic valve replacement is indicated if aortic regurgitation causes symptoms, and this may need to be combined with aortic root replacement and coronary bypass surgery. Those with chronic aortic regurgitation can remain asymptomatic for many years because compensatory ventricular dilatation and hypertrophy occur, but should be advised to report the development of any symptoms of breathlessness

or angina. Asymptomatic patients should also be followed up annually with echocardiography for evidence of increasing ventricular size. If this occurs or if the end-systolic dimension increases to 55 mm or more, then aortic valve replacement should be undertaken. If systemic hypertension is present, non-rate-limiting vasodilators, such as nifedipine, should be used to control systolic BP. There is conflicting evidence regarding the need for aortic valve replacement in asymptomatic patients with severe aortic regurgitation. When aortic root dilatation is the cause of aortic regurgitation, as can occur in Marfan syndrome, aortic root replacement is usually necessary.

Tricuspid valve disease

Tricuspid stenosis

Tricuspid stenosis is usually rheumatic in origin and is rare in higher-income countries. Tricuspid disease occurs in fewer than 5% of patients with rheumatic heart disease and then nearly always occurs in association with mitral and aortic valve disease. Tricuspid stenosis and regurgitation may also occur in the carcinoid syndrome.

Clinical features and investigations

Although the symptoms of mitral and aortic valve disease predominate, tricuspid stenosis may cause symptoms of right heart failure, including hepatic discomfort and peripheral oedema.

The main clinical feature is a raised JVP with a prominent *a* wave, and a slow *y* descent due to the loss of normal rapid right ventricular filling. There is also a mid-diastolic murmur, best heard at the lower left or right sternal border. This is generally higher-pitched than the murmur of mitral stenosis and is increased by inspiration. Right heart failure causes hepatomegaly with pre-systolic pulsation (large *a* wave), ascites and peripheral oedema. The diagnosis can be confirmed by Doppler echocardiography, which shows similar appearances to those of rheumatic mitral stenosis.

Management

In patients who require surgery to other valves, the tricuspid valve can either be replaced or treated with valvotomy. Balloon valvuloplasty can be used to treat rare cases of isolated tricuspid stenosis.

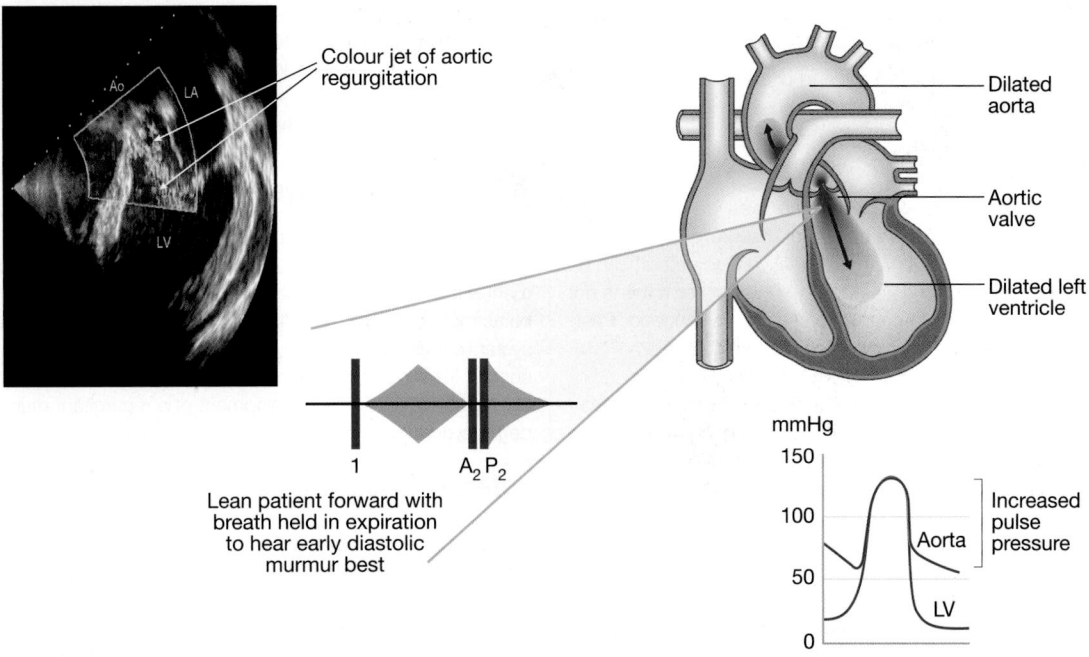

Fig. 16.85 Aortic regurgitation. The early diastolic murmur is best heard at the left sternal border and may be accompanied by an ejection systolic ('to-and-fro') murmur. The aortic arch and left ventricle (LV) may become dilated. The inset shows a Doppler echocardiogram with the regurgitant jet (arrows). *Inset (Colour Doppler echo) From Newby D, Grubb N. Cardiology: an illustrated colour text. Edinburgh: Churchill Livingstone, Elsevier Ltd; 2005.*

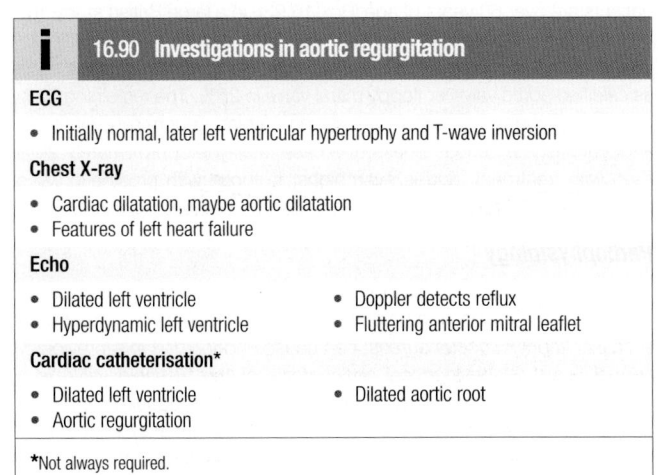

i 16.90 Investigations in aortic regurgitation

ECG

- Initially normal, later left ventricular hypertrophy and T-wave inversion

Chest X-ray

- Cardiac dilatation, maybe aortic dilatation
- Features of left heart failure

Echo

- Dilated left ventricle
- Hyperdynamic left ventricle
- Doppler detects reflux
- Fluttering anterior mitral leaflet

Cardiac catheterisation*

- Dilated left ventricle
- Aortic regurgitation
- Dilated aortic root

*Not always required.

i 16.91 Causes of tricuspid regurgitation

Primary

- Rheumatic heart disease
- Endocarditis, particularly in intravenous drug users
- Ebstein's congenital anomaly (see Box 16.102)

Secondary

- Right ventricular failure
- Right ventricular infarction
- Pulmonary hypertension, secondary to chronic pulmonary disease

artery pressure tolerate isolated tricuspid reflux well, and valves damaged by endocarditis do not usually need to be replaced. Patients undergoing mitral valve replacement, who have tricuspid regurgitation due to marked dilatation of the tricuspid annulus, benefit from valve repair with an annuloplasty ring to bring the leaflets closer together. Those with rheumatic damage may require tricuspid valve replacement.

Pulmonary valve disease

Pulmonary stenosis

This can occur in the carcinoid syndrome but is usually congenital, in which case it may be isolated or associated with other abnormalities, such as Fallot's tetralogy.

Clinical features

The principal finding on examination is an ejection systolic murmur, loudest at the left upper sternum and radiating towards the left shoulder. There may be a thrill, best felt when the patient leans forwards and breathes out. The murmur is often preceded by an ejection sound (click). Delay in right ventricular ejection may cause wide splitting of the second heart sound. Severe pulmonary stenosis is characterised by a loud, harsh murmur, an inaudible pulmonary closure sound (P_2), an increased right ventricular heave, and prominent *a* waves in the jugular pulse.

Tricuspid regurgitation

Tricuspid regurgitation is common, and is most frequently functional, occurring as a result of right ventricular dilatation due to right heart failure or biventricular failure. It may also be the result of other conditions, as summarised in Box 16.91.

Clinical features

Symptoms are usually non-specific, with tiredness related to reduced cardiac output, and oedema and hepatic enlargement due to venous congestion. The most prominent sign is a 'giant' *v* wave in the jugular venous pulse (a *cv* wave replaces the normal *x* descent). Other features include a pansystolic murmur at the left sternal border and a pulsatile liver. Echocardiography may reveal dilatation of the RV. If the valve has been affected by rheumatic disease, the leaflets will appear thickened and, in endocarditis, vegetations may be seen.

Management

Tricuspid regurgitation due to right ventricular dilatation often improves when the cardiac failure is treated. Patients with a normal pulmonary

16

Investigations

Doppler echocardiography is the definitive investigation. ECG may show evidence of right ventricular hypertrophy, and post-stenotic dilatation in the pulmonary artery may be observed on the chest X-ray.

Management

Mild to moderate isolated pulmonary stenosis is relatively common and does not usually progress or require treatment. Severe pulmonary stenosis (resting gradient > 50 mmHg with a normal cardiac output) can be treated by percutaneous pulmonary balloon valvuloplasty or, if this is not available, by surgical valvotomy. Long-term results are very good. Post-operative pulmonary regurgitation is common but benign.

Pulmonary regurgitation

This is rare in isolation and is usually associated with pulmonary artery dilatation due to pulmonary hypertension. It may complicate mitral stenosis, producing an early diastolic decrescendo murmur at the left sternal border that is difficult to distinguish from aortic regurgitation (Graham Steell murmur). The pulmonary hypertension may be secondary to other disease of the left side of the heart, primary pulmonary vascular disease or Eisenmenger syndrome. Trivial pulmonary regurgitation is a frequent finding in normal individuals and has no clinical significance.

Prosthetic valves

Diseased heart valves can be replaced with mechanical or biological prostheses. The three main types of mechanical prosthesis are the ball and cage, tilting single disc and tilting bi-leaflet valves. All generate prosthetic sounds or clicks on auscultation. Pig or allograft valves mounted on a supporting stent are the most commonly used biological valves. They generate normal heart sounds. All prosthetic valves used in the aortic position produce a systolic flow murmur.

All mechanical valves require long-term anticoagulation because they can cause systemic thromboembolism or may develop valve thrombosis or obstruction (Box 16.92); the prosthetic clicks may become inaudible if the valve malfunctions. Biological valves have the advantage of not requiring anticoagulants to maintain proper function although many patients undergoing valve replacement surgery, especially mitral valve replacement, will have AF that requires anticoagulation anyway. Biological valves are less durable than mechanical valves and may degenerate 7 or more years after implantation, particularly when used in the mitral position. They are more durable in the aortic position and in older patients, so are particularly appropriate for patients over 65 undergoing aortic valve replacement.

Transcatheter aortic valve implantation

For patients being considered for aortic valve surgery, especially due to aortic stenosis, transcatheter aortic valve implantation (TAVI) is an alternative to surgical aortic valve replacement. The native valve is not removed but is compressed by the new bioprosthetic valve, which is implanted within it. The bioprosthetic valve is mounted on a large stent-like structure and is implanted through a catheter inserted in the femoral artery (Fig. 16.86). TAVI has several major advantages. It avoids the need for a sternotomy, is associated with a short recovery period, can be used in high-risk and otherwise inoperable patients, and is much better tolerated by older patients. Complications include stroke (2%) and heart block necessitating pacemaker implantation (5%–15%).

Prosthetic valve dysfunction

Symptoms or signs of unexplained heart failure in a patient with a prosthetic heart valve may be due to valve dysfunction, and urgent assessment is required. Metallic valves can suffer strut fracture and fail, causing catastrophic regurgitation. Alternatively, they may thrombose and cause systemic thromboembolism or valve obstruction, especially in the presence of inadequate anticoagulation. Biological valve dysfunction is usually associated with the development of a regurgitant murmur and may begin to develop 8–10 years after implantation.

Infective endocarditis

This is caused by microbial infection of a heart valve, the lining of a cardiac chamber or blood vessel, or a congenital anomaly. Both native and prosthetic valves can be affected. The most common causes of infective endocarditis are streptococci and staphylococci but other organisms may also be involved.

Epidemiology

The incidence of infective endocarditis in community-based studies ranges from 5 to 15 cases per 100 000 per annum. More than 50% of patients are over 60 years of age (Box 16.93). In a large British study, the underlying condition was rheumatic heart disease in 24% of patients, congenital heart disease in 19%, and other cardiac abnormalities such as calcified aortic valve or floppy mitral valve in 25%. The remaining 32% were not thought to have a pre-existing cardiac abnormality. Bacterial endocarditis is a serious illness; the case fatality is approximately 20% even with treatment, and is even higher in those with prosthetic valve endocarditis and those infected with antibiotic-resistant organisms.

Pathophysiology

Infective endocarditis typically occurs at sites of pre-existing endocardial damage, but infection with particularly virulent or aggressive organisms, such as *Staphylococcus aureus*, can cause endocarditis in a previously normal heart. Staphylococcal endocarditis of the tricuspid valve is a common complication of intravenous drug use. Many acquired and congenital cardiac lesions are vulnerable, particularly areas of endocardial damage caused by a high-pressure jet of blood, such as ventricular septal defect, mitral regurgitation and aortic regurgitation, many of which are haemodynamically insignificant. In contrast, the risk of endocarditis at the site of haemodynamically important low-pressure lesions, such as a large atrial septal defect, is minimal.

Infection tends to occur at sites of endothelial damage because they attract deposits of platelets and fibrin that are vulnerable to colonisation by blood-borne organisms. The avascular valve tissue and presence of fibrin and platelet aggregates help to protect proliferating organisms from host defence mechanisms. When the infection is established, vegetations composed of organisms, fibrin and platelets grow and may become large enough to cause obstruction or embolism. Adjacent tissues are destroyed and abscesses may form. Valve regurgitation may develop or increase if the affected valve is damaged by tissue distortion, cusp perforation or disruption of chordae. Extracardiac manifestations, such as vasculitis and skin lesions, may occur as the result of either emboli or immune complex deposition. Mycotic aneurysms may develop in arteries at the site of infected emboli. In fatal cases, infarction of the spleen and kidneys and, sometimes, an immune glomerulonephritis may be found at postmortem.

Microbiology

Over three-quarters of cases are caused by streptococci or staphylococci. Viridans streptococci, such as *Streptococcus mitis* and *Strep.*

ℹ 16.92 Anticoagulation targets and prosthetic heart valves	
Mechanical valves	Target INR
Ball and cage (e.g. Starr–Edwards)	3.0–4.0
Tilting disc (e.g. Bjork–Shiley)	
Bi-leaflet (e.g. St Jude)	2.5–3.0
Biological valves with atrial fibrillation	2.0–3.0
(INR = International Normalised Ratio)	

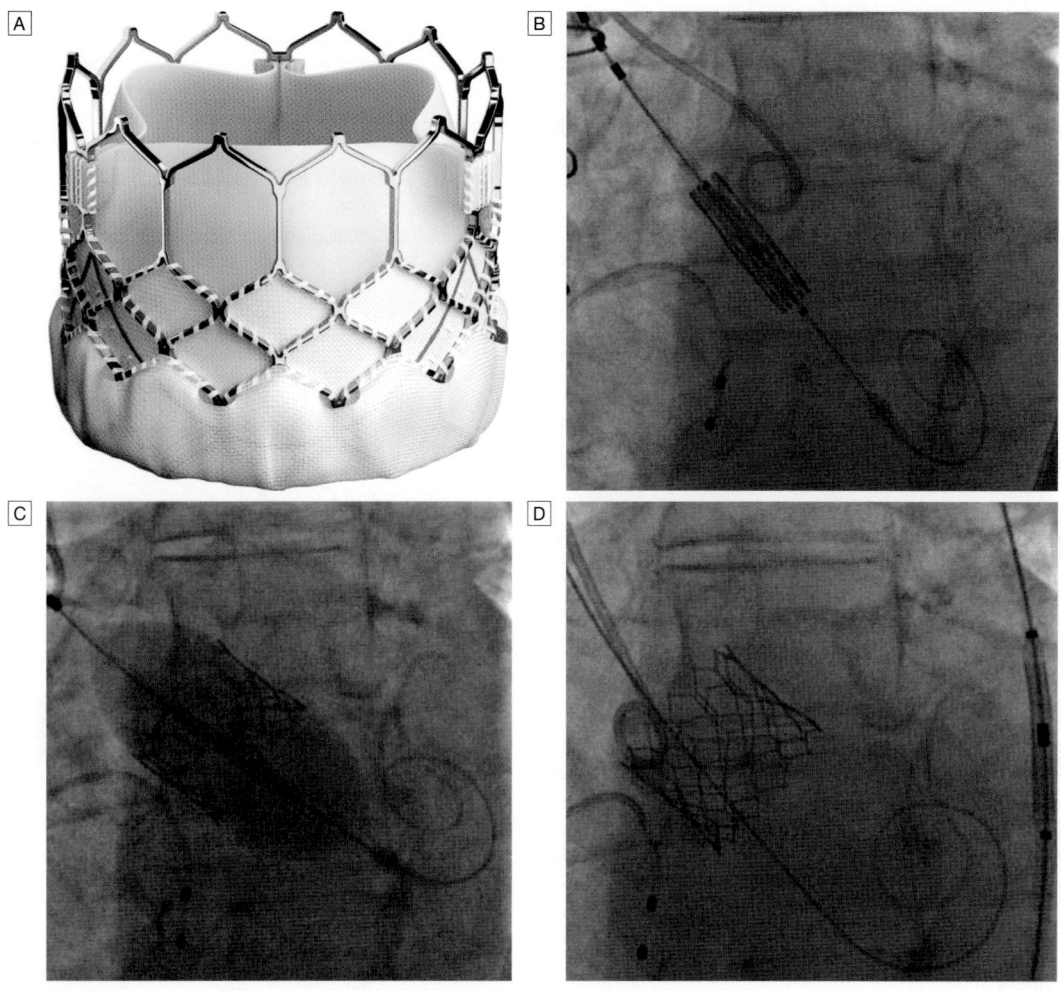

Fig. 16.86 Transcatheter aortic valve implantation (TAVI). Appearance of an expanded bioprosthetic valve A, which is positioned through a large femoral catheter in an unexpanded form B, before the valve is deployed by a balloon C during rapid ventricular pacing, to leave behind the fully expanded valve D.

 16.93 Endocarditis in old age

- **Symptoms and signs**: may be non-specific, with delirium, weight loss, malaise and weakness, and the diagnosis may not be suspected.
- **Common causative organisms**: often enterococci (from the urinary tract) and *Streptococcus gallolyticus* subsp. *gallolyticus* (from a colonic source).
- **Morbidity and mortality**: much higher.

sanguis, which are commensals in the oral cavity, can enter the blood stream on chewing or tooth-brushing, or at the time of dental treatment, and are common causes of subacute endocarditis (Box 16.94). Other organisms, including *Enterococcus faecalis, E. faecium* and *Strep. gallolyticus* subsp. *gallolyticus* (previously known as *Strep. bovis*), may enter the blood from the bowel or urinary tract. Patients who are found to have endocarditis caused by *Strep. gallolyticus* should undergo colonoscopy, since this organism is associated with large-bowel malignancy.

Staph. aureus has now overtaken streptococci as the most common cause of acute endocarditis. It originates from skin infections, abscesses or vascular access sites such as intravenous and central lines, or from intravenous drug use. It is highly virulent and invasive, usually producing florid vegetations, rapid valve destruction and abscess formation. Other causes of acute endocarditis include *Strep. pneumoniae* and *Strep. pyogenes*.

Post-operative endocarditis after cardiac surgery may affect native or prosthetic heart valves or other prosthetic materials. The most common organisms are coagulase-negative staphylococci such as *Staph. epidermidis*, which are part of the normal skin flora. There is frequently a history of wound infection with the same organism. Coagulase-negative staphylococci cause native valve endocarditis in approximately 5% of cases and this possibility should always be considered before they are dismissed as blood culture contaminants. Another coagulase-negative staphylococcus, *Staph. lugdenensis*, causes a rapidly destructive acute endocarditis that is associated with previously normal valves and multiple emboli. Unless accurately identified, it may also be overlooked as a contaminant.

In Q fever endocarditis due to *Coxiella burnetii*, the patient often has a history of contact with farm animals. The aortic valve is usually affected and there may also be hepatitis, pneumonia and purpura. Life-long antibiotic therapy may be required.

In about 3%–4% of cases, endocarditis may be caused by Gramnegative bacteria of the so-called HACEK group (*Haemophilus aprophilus* – now known as *Aggregatibacter aprophilus–Aggregatibacter actinomycetemcomitans*; *Cardiobacterium hominis*; *Eikenella corrodens*; and *Kingella kingae*). These are slow-growing, fastidious Gram-negative organisms that are oropharyngeal commensals. The diagnosis may be revealed only after prolonged culture and the organisms may be resistant to penicillin.

Brucella endocarditis is associated with a history of contact with goats or cattle and often affects the aortic valve.

Yeasts and fungi, such as *Candida* and *Aspergillus*, may attack previously normal or prosthetic valves, particularly in immunocompromised patients or those with in-dwelling intravenous catheters. Abscesses and emboli are common, therapy is difficult, surgery is often required and mortality is high. Concomitant bacterial infection may be present.

16.94 Microbiology of infective endocarditis

Pathogen	Of native valve (n = 280)	In injection drug users (n = 87)	Of prosthetic valve Early (n = 15)	Of prosthetic valve Late (n = 72)
Staphylococci	124 (44%)	60 (69%)	10 (67%)	33 (46%)
Staph. aureus	106 (38%)	60 (69%)	3 (20%)	15 (21%)
Coagulase-negative	18 (6%)	0	7 (47%)	18 (25%)
Streptococci	86 (31%)	7 (8%)	0	25 (35%)
Oral	59 (21%)	3 (3%)	0	19 (26%)
Others (non-enterococcal)	27 (10%)	4 (5%)	0	6 (8%)
Enterococcus spp.	21 (8%)	2 (2%)	1 (7%)	5 (7%)
HACEK	12 (4%)	0	0	1 (1%)
Polymicrobial	6 (2%)	8 (9%)	0	1 (1%)
Other bacteria	12 (4%)	4 (5%)	0	2 (3%)
Fungi	3 (1%)	2 (2%)	0	0
Negative blood culture	16 (6%)	4 (5%)	4 (27%)	5 (7%)

(HACEK = Haemophilus aphrophilus – now known as Aggregatibacter aphrophilus–Aggregatibacter actinomycetemcomitans; Cardiobacterium hominis; Eikenella corrodens; and Kingella kingae)
Adapted from Moreillon P, Que YA. Infective endocarditis. Lancet 2004; 363:139–149.

Clinical features

Endocarditis can take either an acute or a more insidious 'subacute' form; the latter often passes undetected initially. There is considerable overlap because the clinical pattern is influenced not only by the organism but also by the site of infection, prior antibiotic therapy and the presence of a valve or shunt prosthesis. The subacute form may abruptly develop acute life-threatening complications, such as valve disruption or emboli. The Duke criteria for diagnosis of infective endocarditis are shown in Box 16.95.

Subacute endocarditis

This should be suspected when a patient with congenital or valvular heart disease develops a persistent fever, complains of unusual tiredness, night sweats or weight loss, or develops new signs of valve dysfunction or heart failure. Less often, it presents as an embolic stroke or peripheral arterial embolism. Other features (Fig. 16.87) include purpura and petechial haemorrhages in the skin and mucous membranes, and splinter haemorrhages under the fingernails or toenails. Osler's nodes are painful, tender swellings at the fingertips that are probably the product of vasculitis; they are rare. Digital clubbing is a late sign. The spleen is frequently palpable; in Coxiella infections, the spleen and the liver may be considerably enlarged. Non-visible haematuria is common. The finding of any of these features in a patient with persistent fever or malaise is an indication for re-examination to detect hitherto unrecognised heart disease.

Acute endocarditis

This presents as a severe febrile illness with prominent and changing heart murmurs and petechiae. Clinical stigmata of chronic endocarditis are usually absent. Embolic events are common, and cardiac or renal failure may develop rapidly. Abscesses may be detected on echocardiography. Partially treated acute endocarditis behaves like subacute endocarditis.

Post-operative endocarditis

This may present as an unexplained fever in a patient who has had heart valve surgery. The infection usually involves the valve ring and may resemble subacute or acute endocarditis, depending on the virulence of the organism. Morbidity and mortality are high and revision surgery is often required. The range of organisms is similar to that seen in native valve disease, but when endocarditis occurs during the first few weeks after surgery it is usually due to infection with a coagulase-negative staphylococcus that was introduced during the perioperative period.

16.95 Diagnosis of infective endocarditis*

Major criteria

Positive blood culture
- Typical organism from two cultures
- Persistent positive blood cultures taken > 12 hrs apart
- Three or more positive cultures taken over > 1 hr

Endocardial involvement
- Positive echocardiographic findings of vegetations
- New valvular regurgitation

Minor criteria
- Predisposing valvular or cardiac abnormality
- Intravenous drug misuse
- Pyrexia ≥ 38°C
- Embolic phenomenon
- Vasculitic phenomenon
- Blood cultures suggestive: organism grown but not achieving major criteria
- Suggestive echocardiographic findings

*Modified Duke criteria. Patients with two major, or one major and three minor, or five minor have definite endocarditis. Patients with one major and one minor, or three minor have possible endocarditis.

Investigations

Blood culture (see Fig. 6.6) is the pivotal investigation to identify the organism that is the cause of the infection and to guide antibiotic therapy. Three to six sets of blood cultures should be taken prior to commencing therapy and should not wait for episodes of pyrexia. The first two specimens will detect bacteraemia in 90% of culture-positive cases. A meticulous aseptic technique is essential. Taking discrete sets of blood cultures from peripheral sites at intervals of ≥6 hours reduces the risk of misdiagnosis due to contamination with skin commensals. Isolation of a typical organism in more than one culture provides strong evidence in favour of the diagnosis (see Box 16.95). An in-dwelling line should not be used to take cultures. Both aerobic and anaerobic cultures are required.

Echocardiography is key for detecting and following the progress of vegetations, for assessing valve damage and for detecting abscess formation. Vegetations as small as 2–4 mm can be detected by transthoracic echocardiography, and even smaller ones (1–1.5 mm) can be visualised by TOE, which is particularly valuable for identifying abscess formation and investigating patients with prosthetic heart valves. Vegetations may be difficult to distinguish in the presence of an abnormal

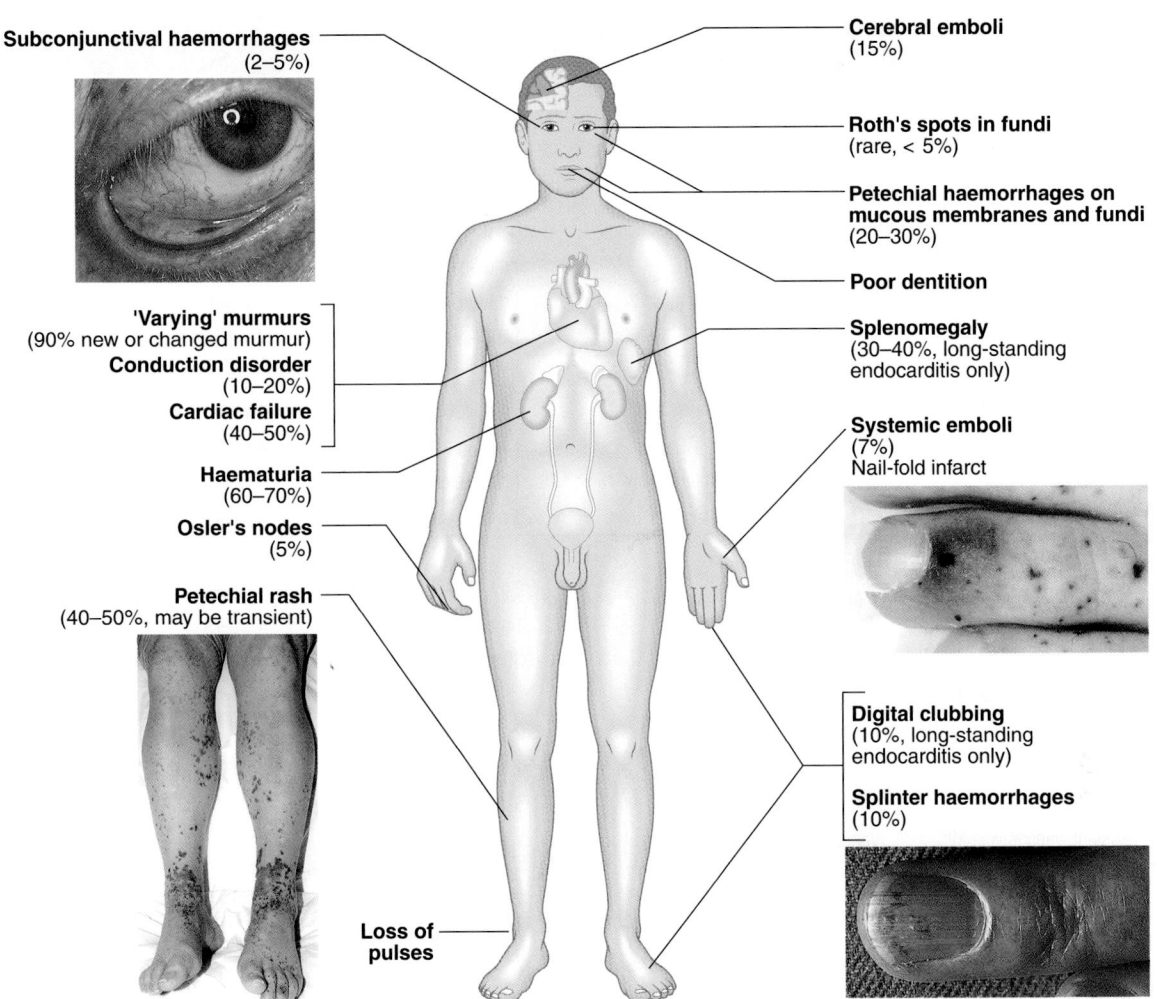

Subconjunctival haemorrhages
(2–5%)

Cerebral emboli
(15%)

Roth's spots in fundi
(rare, < 5%)

**Petechial haemorrhages on
mucous membranes and fundi**
(20–30%)

Poor dentition

'Varying' murmurs
(90% new or changed murmur)
Conduction disorder
(10–20%)
Cardiac failure
(40–50%)

Haematuria
(60–70%)

Osler's nodes
(5%)

Petechial rash
(40–50%, may be transient)

Splenomegaly
(30–40%, long-standing
endocarditis only)

Systemic emboli
(7%)
Nail-fold infarct

Digital clubbing
(10%, long-standing
endocarditis only)

Splinter haemorrhages
(10%)

**Loss of
pulses**

Fig. 16.87 Clinical features that may be present in endocarditis. *Insets (Petechial rash, nail-fold infarct) From Newby D, Grubb N. Cardiology: an illustrated colour text. Edinburgh: Churchill Livingstone, Elsevier Ltd; 2005.*

valve; the sensitivity of transthoracic echo is approximately 65% but that of TOE is more than 90%. Failure to detect vegetations does not exclude the diagnosis.

Elevation of the ESR, a normocytic normochromic anaemia, and leucocytosis are common but not invariable. Measurement of serum CRP is more reliable than the ESR in monitoring progress. Proteinuria may occur and non-visible haematuria is usually present.

The ECG may show the development of AV block (due to aortic root abscess formation) and occasionally infarction due to emboli. The chest X-ray may show evidence of cardiac failure and cardiomegaly.

Management

A multidisciplinary approach, with cooperation between the physician, surgeon and microbiologist, increases the chance of a successful outcome. Any source of infection should be removed as soon as possible; for example, a tooth with an apical abscess should be extracted, or an in-dwelling catheter or device removed.

Empirical treatment depends on the mode of presentation, the suspected organism and the presence of a prosthetic valve or penicillin allergy. If the presentation is subacute, antibiotic treatment should ideally be withheld until the results of blood cultures are available. However, if empirical antibiotic treatment is considered necessary, amoxicillin (2 g IV 6 times daily) should be considered (with or without gentamicin). If the presentation is acute, empirical therapy should be started with vancomycin (1 g IV twice daily) and gentamicin (1 mg/kg IV twice daily), with dose adjustment based on antibiotic levels. The same regimen is used in true penicillin allergy. Patients with suspected prosthetic valve

endocarditis should be treated with vancomycin and gentamicin at the above-mentioned doses, plus rifampicin orally in a dose of 300–600 mg twice daily. Following identification of the causal organism, determination of the minimum inhibitory concentration (MIC) for the organism helps guide antibiotic therapy. Recommended regimens for some of the most common scenarios are shown in Box 16.96. More detailed information can be found in the 2012 British Society for Antimicrobial Chemotherapy guidelines (see 'Further reading').

A 2-week treatment regimen may be sufficient for fully sensitive strains of streptococci, provided specific conditions are met (Box 16.97).

Cardiac surgery with débridement of infected material and valve replacement may be required in a substantial proportion of patients, particularly those with *Staph. aureus* and fungal infections (Box 16.98). Antimicrobial therapy must be started before surgery.

Prevention

Antibiotic prophylaxis is no longer routinely given to people at risk of infective endocarditis undergoing interventional procedures. It can be considered in those at the highest risk of endocarditis.

Congenital heart disease

Congenital heart disease can be the result of defects in the formation of the heart or great vessels or can arise because the anatomical changes that occur during transition between the fetus and the newborn child fail to proceed normally. Congenital heart disease usually presents in

16

16.96 Antimicrobial treatment of common causative organisms in infective endocarditis

Antimicrobial susceptibility	Antimicrobial	Dose	Duration	
			Native valve	Prosthetic valve
Streptococci				
Penicillin MIC ≤ 0.125 mg/L	Benzylpenicillin IV	1.2 g 6 times daily	4 weeks[1]	6 weeks
Penicillin MIC > 0.125, ≤ 0.5 mg/L	Benzylpenicillin IV and gentamicin IV	2.4 g 6 times daily	4 weeks	6 weeks
		1 mg/kg twice daily[2]	2 weeks	2 weeks
Penicillin MIC > 0.5 mg/L	Vancomycin IV and gentamicin IV	1 g twice daily[3]	4 weeks	6 weeks
		1 mg/kg twice daily[2]	4 weeks	6 weeks
Enterococci				
Amoxicillin MIC ≤ 4 mg/L and gentamicin MIC ≤ 128 mg/L	Amoxicillin IV and gentamicin IV[2]	2 g 6 times daily	4 weeks	6 weeks
		1 mg/kg twice daily[2]	4 weeks	6 weeks
Amoxicillin MIC > 4 mg/L and gentamicin MIC ≤ 128 mg/L	Vancomycin IV and gentamicin IV[2]	1 g twice daily[3]	4 weeks	6 weeks
		1 mg/kg twice daily[2]	4 weeks	6 weeks
Staphylococci – native valve				
Meticillin-sensitive	Flucloxacillin IV	2 g 4–6 times daily[4]	4 weeks	–
Meticillin-resistant, vancomycin MIC ≤ 2 mg/L, rifampicin-sensitive	Vancomycin IV	1 g twice daily[3]	4 weeks	–
	Rifampicin orally	300–600 mg twice daily	4 weeks	–
Staphylococci – prosthetic valve				
Meticillin-sensitive	Flucloxacillin IV	2 g 4–6 times daily	–	6 weeks
	and gentamicin IV	1 mg/kg twice daily[2]	–	6 weeks
	and rifampicin orally	300–600 mg twice daily	–	6 weeks
Meticillin-resistant, vancomycin MIC ≤ 2 mg/L, rifampicin-sensitive	Vancomycin IV	1 g twice daily[3]	–	6 weeks
	and rifampicin orally	300–600 mg twice daily	–	6 weeks

[1]When conditions in Box 16.97 are met, 2 weeks of benzylpenicillin and gentamicin (1 mg/kg twice daily) may be sufficient. Ceftriaxone 2 g once daily IV/IM can be used instead of benzylpenicillin for those with non-severe penicillin allergy. [2]Pre-dose gentamicin level should be ≤ 1 mg/L, post-dose 3–5 mg/L. Adjust dose according to levels and renal function. [3]Pre-dose vancomycin level should be 15–20 mg/L. Adjust dose according to levels and renal function. [4]Use 6 times daily if weight > 85 kg.
(IM = intramuscular; IV = intravenous; MIC = minimum inhibitory concentration)
Adapted from Gould FK, Denning DW, Elliott TS, et al. Guidelines for the diagnosis and antibiotic treatment of endocarditis in adults: a report of the working party of the British Society for Antimicrobial Chemotherapy. J Antimicrob Chemother 2012; 67:269–289.

16.97 Conditions for the short-course treatment of endocarditis caused by fully sensitive streptococci

- Native valve infection
- Minimum inhibitory concentration (MIC) ≤ 0.125 mg/L
- No adverse prognostic factors (heart failure, aortic regurgitation, conduction defect)
- No evidence of thromboembolic disease
- No vegetations > 5 mm diameter
  Clinical response within 7 days

16.98 Indications for cardiac surgery in infective endocarditis*

- Heart failure due to valve damage
- Failure of antibiotic therapy (persistent/uncontrolled infection)
- Large vegetations on left-sided heart valves with echo appearance suggesting high risk of emboli
- Previous evidence of systemic emboli
- Abscess formation

*Patients with prosthetic valve endocarditis or fungal endocarditis often require cardiac surgery.

---

childhood but some patients do not present until adult life. It has been estimated that the incidence of haemodynamically significant congenital cardiac abnormalities is about 0.8% of live births (Box 16.99). Defects that are well tolerated, such as atrial septal defect, may cause no symptoms until adult life or may be detected incidentally on routine examination or chest X-ray. Congenital defects that were previously fatal in childhood can now be corrected, or at least partially, so that survival to adult life is the norm. Such patients remain well for many years but subsequently re-present in later life with related problems, such as arrhythmia or heart failure (Box 16.100).

Pathophysiology

Understanding the fetal circulation helps clarify how some forms of congenital heart disease occur. Fig. 16.88 shows the fetal circulation

and the changes that normally occur immediately after birth. In the fetus there is little blood flow through the lungs, which are collapsed because they are not required for gas exchange. Instead, oxygenated blood from the placenta passes directly from the right atrium to the left side of the heart through the foramen ovale without having to flow through the lungs, and also from the pulmonary artery into the aorta via the ductus arteriosus.

During early embryonic life, the heart develops as a single tube that folds back on itself and then divides into two separate circulations. Failure of septation can cause some forms of atrial and ventricular septal defect, whereas failure of alignment of the great vessels with the ventricles contributes to transposition of the great arteries, tetralogy of Fallot and truncus arteriosus. Atrial septal defects occur because the foramen ovale fails to close at birth, as is normal. Similarly, a persistent ductus arteriosus will remain if it fails to close after birth. Failure of the aorta to develop at the point of the aortic isthmus and where the ductus arteriosus attaches can lead to coarctation of the aorta. Maternal infection and exposure to drugs or toxins are important causes of congenital heart disease. Maternal rubella infection is associated with persistent ductus arteriosus, pulmonary valvular and/or artery stenosis, and atrial septal defect. Maternal alcohol misuse is associated with septal defects, and maternal lupus erythematosus with congenital complete heart block. Genetic or chromosomal abnormalities, such as Down syndrome, may cause septal defects, and gene defects have also been identified as leading to specific abnormalities, such as Marfan syndrome and Turner syndrome (karyotype XO).

Clinical features

Symptoms may be absent, or the child may be breathless or fail to attain normal growth and development. Some defects are not compatible with extrauterine life and lead to neonatal death. Clinical signs vary with the anatomical lesion. Murmurs, thrills or signs of cardiomegaly may be present. In coarctation of the aorta, radio-femoral delay may be noted (Fig. 16.89) and some female patients have the features of Turner syndrome (p. 674). Features of other congenital conditions, such as Marfan syndrome or Down syndrome, may also be apparent. Cerebrovascular events and cerebral abscesses may complicate severe cyanotic congenital disease.

Early diagnosis is important because many types of congenital heart disease are amenable to surgery, but this opportunity is lost if secondary changes, such as irreversible pulmonary hypertension, occur.

Central cyanosis and digital clubbing

Central cyanosis of cardiac origin occurs when desaturated blood enters the systemic circulation without passing through the lungs (right-to-left

shunting). In the neonate, the most common cause is transposition of the great arteries, in which the aorta arises from the RV and the pulmonary artery from the LV in association with a ventricular septal defect. In older children, cyanosis is usually the consequence of a ventricular septal defect combined with severe pulmonary stenosis (as in tetralogy of Fallot) or with pulmonary vascular disease (Eisenmenger syndrome). Chronic cyanosis is associated with finger and toe clubbing.

Growth retardation and learning difficulties

These may occur with large left-to-right shunts at ventricular or great arterial level, and also with other defects, especially if they form part of a genetic syndrome. Major intellectual impairment is uncommon in children with isolated congenital heart disease but minor learning difficulties can occur. Cerebral function can also be affected after cardiac surgery if cerebral perfusion is compromised.

Syncope

In the presence of increased pulmonary vascular resistance or severe left or right ventricular outflow obstruction, exercise may provoke syncope as systemic vascular resistance falls but pulmonary vascular resistance rises, worsening right-to-left shunting and cerebral oxygenation. Syncope can also occur because of associated arrhythmias.

Pulmonary hypertension

Persistently raised pulmonary flow with a left-to-right shunt causes increased pulmonary vascular resistance followed by pulmonary hypertension. Progressive changes, including obliteration of distal arterioles, take place and are irreversible. At this stage, central cyanosis occurs and digital clubbing develops. The chest X-ray shows enlarged central pulmonary arteries and peripheral 'pruning' of the pulmonary vessels. The ECG shows features of right ventricular hypertrophy.

Eisenmenger syndrome

In patients with severe and prolonged pulmonary hypertension the left-to-right shunt may reverse, resulting in right-to-left shunt and marked cyanosis. This is termed Eisenmenger syndrome. The cyanosis in Eisenmenger syndrome may be more apparent in the feet and toes than in the upper part of the body, resulting in so-called differential cyanosis. Eisenmenger syndrome is more common with large ventricular septal defects or persistent ductus arteriosus than with atrial septal defects. Patients with Eisenmenger syndrome are at particular risk from abrupt changes in afterload that exacerbate right-to-left shunting, such as vasodilatation, anaesthesia and pregnancy. The long-term prognosis is poor with around 50% of young adults surviving 10 years from diagnosis.

Congenital heart disease in pregnancy

During pregnancy, there is a 50% increase in plasma volume, a 40% increase in whole blood volume and a similar increase in cardiac output, so problems may arise in women with congenital heart disease (Box 16.101). Many with palliated or untreated disease will tolerate pregnancy well, however. Pregnancy is particularly hazardous in the presence of conditions associated with cyanosis or severe pulmonary hypertension; maternal mortality in patients with Eisenmenger syndrome is more than 50%.

Persistent ductus arteriosus

Normally, the ductus arteriosus closes soon after birth but in this anomaly it fails to do so. Persistence of the ductus is often associated with other abnormalities and is more common in females.

Pathophysiology

During fetal life, before the lungs begin to function, most of the blood from the pulmonary artery passes through the ductus arteriosus into the aorta (see Fig. 16.88). Persistence of the ductus causes a continuous AV shunt from the aorta to the pulmonary artery since pressure in the aorta is higher than that in the pulmonary artery. The volume of

16

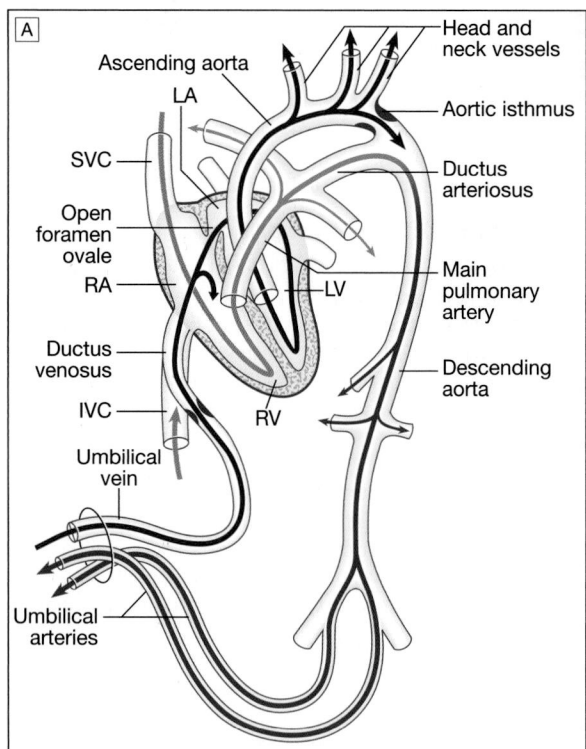
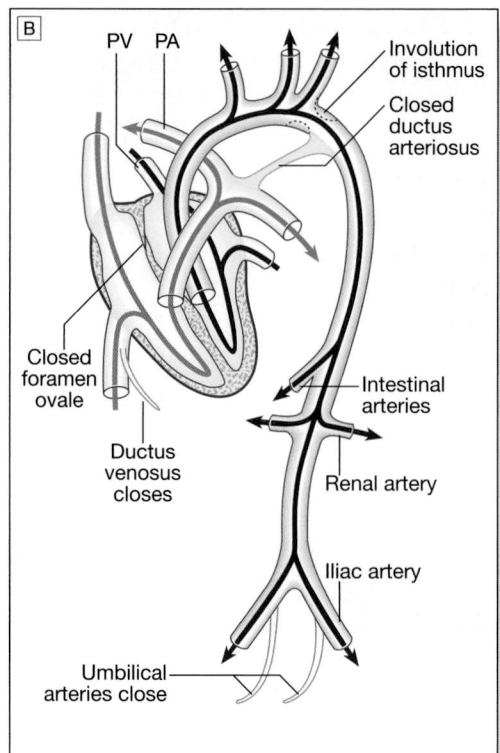

Fig. 16.88 Changes in the circulation at birth. [A] In the fetus, oxygenated blood comes through the umbilical vein where it enters the inferior vena cava (IVC) via the ductus venosus (red). The oxygenated blood streams from the right atrium (RA) through the open foramen ovale to the left atrium (LA) and via the left ventricle (LV) into the aorta. Venous blood from the superior vena cava (SVC, blue) crosses under the main blood stream into the RA and then, partly mixed with oxygenated blood (purple), into the right ventricle (RV) and pulmonary artery (PA). The pulmonary vasculature has a high resistance and so little blood passes to the lungs; most blood passes through the ductus arteriosus to the descending aorta. The aortic isthmus is a constriction in the aorta that lies in the aortic arch before the junction with the ductus arteriosus and limits the flow of oxygen-rich blood to the descending aorta. This configuration means that less oxygen-rich blood is supplied to organ systems that take up their function mainly after birth, e.g. the kidneys and intestinal tract. [B] At birth, the lungs expand with air and pulmonary vascular resistance falls, so that blood now flows to the lungs and back to the LA. The left atrial pressure rises above right atrial pressure and the flap valve of the foramen ovale closes. The umbilical arteries and the ductus venosus close. In the next few days, the ductus arteriosus closes under the influence of hormonal changes (particularly prostaglandins) and the aortic isthmus expands. (PV = pulmonary vein) *Adapted from Drews U. Colour atlas of embryology. Stuttgart: Georg Thieme; 1995.*

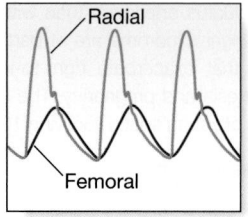

Fig. 16.89 Radio-femoral delay. The difference in pulse pressures is shown.

 16.101 Pregnancy in women with congenital heart disease

- **Obstructive lesions**: poorly tolerated and associated with significant maternal morbidity and mortality.
- **Cyanotic conditions**: especially poorly tolerated. Specialised pre-conception counselling should explain the increased risks.
- **Surgically corrected disease**: patients often tolerate pregnancy well.
- **Children of patients with congenital heart disease**: 2%–5% will be born with cardiac abnormalities, especially if the mother is affected. The risk may be up to 20% in babies born of women with left-sided lesions.

the shunt depends on the size of the ductus but as much as 50% of the left ventricular output may be recirculated through the lungs, with a consequent increase in the work of the heart (Fig. 16.90). A large left-to-right shunt in infancy may cause a considerable rise in pulmonary artery pressure and sometimes this leads to progressive pulmonary vascular damage.

Clinical features

With small shunts there may be no symptoms for years, but when the ductus is large, growth and development may be retarded. Usually, there is no disability in infancy but cardiac failure may eventually ensue, dyspnoea being the first symptom. A continuous 'machinery' murmur is heard with late systolic accentuation, maximal in the second left intercostal space below the clavicle (see Fig. 16.90). It is often accompanied by a thrill. Pulses are increased in volume.

Enlargement of the pulmonary artery may be detected radiologically. The ECG is usually normal. If pulmonary vascular resistance increases, pulmonary artery pressure may rise until it equals or exceeds aortic pressure. The shunt through the defect may then reverse, causing Eisenmenger syndrome. The murmur becomes quieter, may be confined to systole or may disappear.

Investigations

Echocardiography is the investigation of choice although the persistent ductus requires specific echocardiographic views, such as from the suprasternal notch, to reveal it. The ECG shows evidence of right ventricular hypertrophy.

Management

A persistent ductus can be closed at cardiac catheterisation with an implantable occlusive device. Closure should be undertaken in infancy if the shunt is significant and pulmonary resistance not elevated, but this

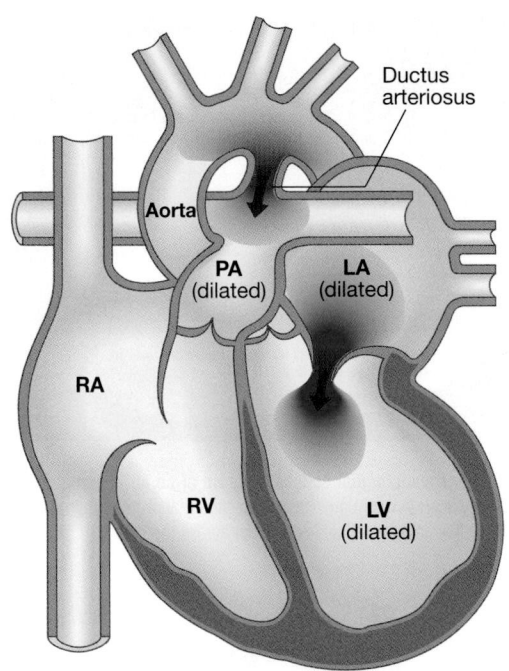

Fig. 16.90 Persistent ductus arteriosus. There is a connection between the aorta and the pulmonary artery with left-to-right shunting. (LA = left atrium; LV = left ventricle; PA = pulmonary artery; RA = right atrium; RV = right ventricle)

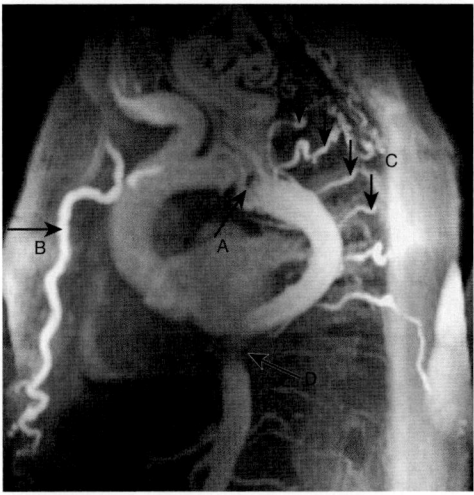

Fig. 16.91 MRI scan of coarctation of the aorta. The aorta is severely narrowed just beyond the arch at the start of the descending aorta (arrow A). Extensive collaterals have developed; a large internal mammary artery (arrow B) and several intercostal arteries (arrows C) are shown. Unusually, in this case, there is also a coarctation of the abdominal aorta (arrow D).

may be delayed until later childhood in those with smaller shunts, for whom closure remains advisable to reduce the risk of endocarditis. When the ductus is structurally intact, a prostaglandin synthetase inhibitor (indometacin or ibuprofen) may be used in the first week of life to induce closure. However, in the presence of a congenital defect with impaired lung perfusion, such as occurs in severe pulmonary stenosis and left-to-right shunt through the ductus, it may be advisable to improve oxygenation by keeping the ductus open with prostaglandin treatment. Unfortunately, these treatments do not work if the ductus is intrinsically abnormal.

Coarctation of the aorta

This condition is twice as common in males and occurs in 1 in 4000 children. It is associated with other abnormalities, most frequently bicuspid aortic valve and 'berry' aneurysms of the cerebral circulation. Acquired coarctation of the aorta is rare but may follow trauma or occur as a complication of Takayasu's disease.

Pathogenesis

Narrowing of the aorta occurs in the region where the ductus arteriosus joins the aorta, at the isthmus just below the origin of the left subclavian artery (see Fig. 16.88). This causes raised BP affecting vessels of the head and neck proximal to the coarctation, and reduced BP and impaired circulation distally.

Clinical features

Aortic coarctation is an important cause of cardiac failure in the newborn but symptoms are often absent in older children or in adults. Headaches may occur from hypertension proximal to the coarctation, and occasionally weakness or cramps in the legs may result from decreased circulation in the lower part of the body. The BP is raised in the upper body but normal or low in the legs. The femoral pulses are weak and delayed in comparison with the radial pulse (see Fig. 16.89). A systolic murmur is usually heard posteriorly, over the coarctation. There may also be an ejection click and systolic murmur in the aortic area due to a bicuspid aortic valve. As a result of the aortic narrowing, collaterals form; they mainly involve the periscapular, internal mammary and intercostal arteries, and may result in localised bruits.

Investigations

Imaging by MRI is the investigation of choice (Fig. 16.91). The chest X-ray in early childhood is often normal but later may show changes in the contour of the aorta (indentation of the descending aorta, '3 sign') and notching of the under-surfaces of the ribs from collaterals. The ECG may show evidence of left ventricular hypertrophy, which can be confirmed by echocardiography.

Management

In untreated cases death may occur from left ventricular failure, dissection of the aorta or cerebral haemorrhage. Surgical correction is advisable in all but the mildest cases. If this is carried out sufficiently early in childhood, persistent hypertension can be avoided. Patients repaired in late childhood or adult life often remain hypertensive or develop recurrent hypertension later on. Recurrence of stenosis may occur as the child grows and this may be managed by balloon dilatation and sometimes stenting. The latter may be used as the primary treatment. Coexistent bicuspid aortic valve, which occurs in over 50% of cases, may lead to progressive aortic stenosis or regurgitation, and also requires long-term follow-up.

Atrial septal defect

Atrial septal defect is one of the most common congenital heart defects and occurs twice as frequently in females. Most are 'ostium secundum' defects, involving the fossa ovalis that, in utero, was the foramen ovale (see Fig. 16.88). 'Ostium primum' defects result from a defect in the atrioventricular septum and are associated with a 'cleft mitral valve' (split anterior leaflet).

Pathogenesis

Since the normal RV is more compliant than the LV, a patent foramen ovale is associated with shunting of blood from the LA to the RA, and then to the RV and pulmonary arteries (Fig. 16.92). As a result, there is gradual enlargement of the right side of the heart and of the pulmonary arteries. Pulmonary hypertension and shunt reversal sometimes complicate atrial septal defect, but are less common and tend to occur later in life than with other types of left-to-right shunt.

Clinical features

Most children are asymptomatic for many years and the condition is often detected at routine examination or following a chest X-ray. Symptoms include dyspnoea, cardiac failure and arrhythmias, especially AF. The characteristic physical signs are the result of the volume overload of the RV:

16

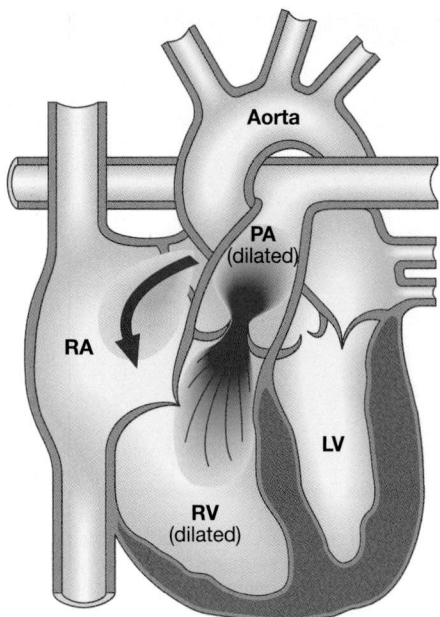

Fig. 16.92 Atrial septal defect. Blood flows across the atrial septum (arrow) from left to right. The murmur is produced by increased flow velocity across the pulmonary valve, as a result of left-to-right shunting and a large stroke volume. The density of shading is proportional to velocity of blood flow. (LV = left ventricle; PA = pulmonary artery; RA = right atrium; RV = right ventricle)

- wide, fixed splitting of the second heart sound: wide because of delay in right ventricular ejection (increased stroke volume and RBBB), and fixed because the septal defect equalises left and right atrial pressures throughout the respiratory cycle
- a systolic flow murmur over the pulmonary valve.

In children with a large shunt, there may be a diastolic flow murmur over the tricuspid valve. Unlike a mitral flow murmur, this is usually high-pitched.

Investigations

Echocardiography is diagnostic. It directly demonstrates the defect and typically shows right ventricular dilatation, right ventricular hypertrophy and pulmonary artery dilatation. The precise size and location of the defect are best defined by TOE (Fig. 16.93). The chest X-ray typically shows enlargement of the heart and the pulmonary artery, as well as pulmonary plethora. The ECG usually demonstrates incomplete RBBB because right ventricular depolarisation is delayed as a result of ventricular dilatation (with a 'primum' defect, there is also left axis deviation).

Management

Atrial septal defects in which pulmonary flow is increased 50% above systemic flow (i.e. a flow ratio of 1.5:1) are often large enough to be clinically recognisable and should be closed surgically. Smaller defects may be managed conservatively and patients monitored periodically with echocardiography. Closure can also be accomplished at cardiac catheterisation using implantable closure devices (Fig. 16.94). The long-term prognosis thereafter is excellent, unless pulmonary hypertension has developed. Severe pulmonary hypertension and shunt reversal are both contraindications to surgery.

▌ Ventricular septal defect

Ventricular septal defect is the most common congenital cardiac defect, occurring once in 500 live births. The defect may be isolated or part of complex congenital heart disease.

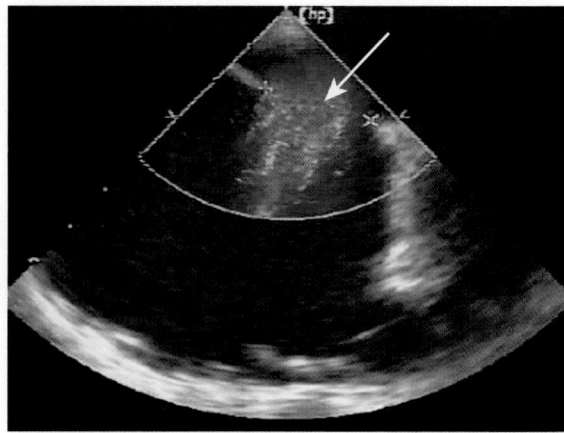

Fig. 16.93 Transoesophageal echocardiogram of an atrial septal defect. The defect is clearly seen (arrow) between the left atrium above and right atrium below. Doppler colour-flow imaging shows flow (blue) across the defect.

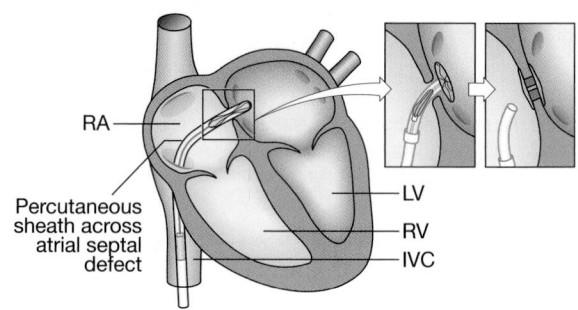

Fig. 16.94 Percutaneous closure of atrial septal defect. The closure device is delivered across the interatrial septum and a disc deployed on either side to seal the defect. (IVC = inferior vena cava; LV = left ventricle; PA = pulmonary artery; RA = right atrium; RV = right ventricle)

Pathogenesis

Congenital ventricular septal defect occurs as a result of incomplete septation of the ventricles. Embryologically, the interventricular septum has a membranous and a muscular portion, and the latter is further divided into inflow, trabecular and outflow portions. Most congenital defects are 'perimembranous', occurring at the junction of the membranous and muscular portions of the septum.

Clinical features

Flow from the high-pressure LV to the low-pressure RV during systole produces a pansystolic murmur, usually heard best at the left sternal border but radiating all over the precordium (Fig. 16.95). A small defect often produces a loud murmur (maladie de Roger) in the absence of other haemodynamic disturbance. Conversely, a large defect produces a quieter murmur, particularly if pressure in the RV is elevated. This may be found immediately after birth, while pulmonary vascular resistance remains high, or when the shunt is reversed in Eisenmenger syndrome. Congenital ventricular septal defect may present with cardiac failure in infants, as a murmur with only minor haemodynamic disturbance in older children or adults, or, rarely, as Eisenmenger syndrome. In some infants, the murmur becomes quieter or disappears due to spontaneous closure of the defect.

If cardiac failure complicates a large defect, it is usually absent in the immediate postnatal period and becomes apparent only in the first 4–6 weeks of life. In addition to the murmur, there is prominent parasternal pulsation, tachypnoea and indrawing of the lower ribs on inspiration.

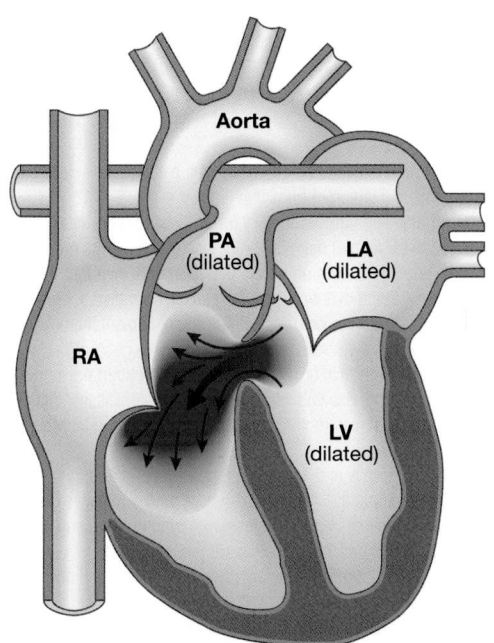

Fig. 16.95 Ventricular septal defect. In this example, a large left-to-right shunt (arrows) has resulted in chamber enlargement. (LA = left atrium; LV = left ventricle; PA = pulmonary artery; RA = right atrium)

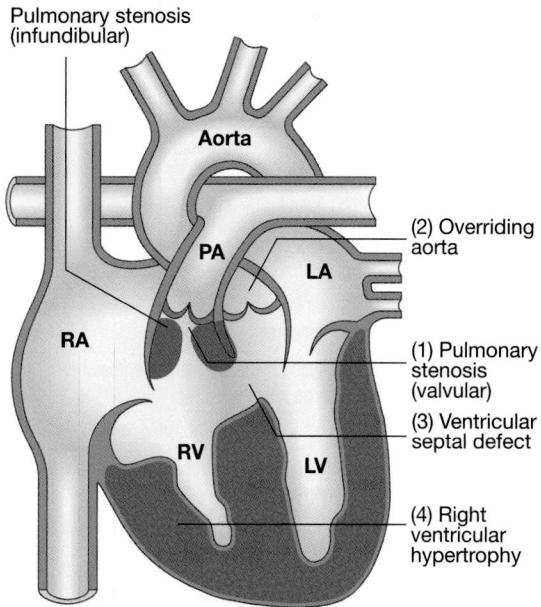

Fig. 16.96 Tetralogy of Fallot. The tetralogy comprises (1) pulmonary stenosis, (2) overriding of the ventricular septal defect by the aorta, (3) a ventricular septal defect and (4) right ventricular hypertrophy. (LA = left atrium; LV = left ventricle; PA = pulmonary artery; RA = right atrium; RV = right ventricle)

16

Investigations

Echocardiography should be performed since it helps to identify the small septal defects that are not haemodynamically significant and are likely to close spontaneously. Patients with larger defects should be monitored by serial echocardiography to check for signs of pulmonary hypertension. With larger defects, the chest X-ray shows pulmonary congestion and the ECG shows bilateral ventricular hypertrophy.

Management

Small ventricular septal defects require no specific treatment. If there is cardiac failure in infancy, this should initially be treated with digoxin, diuretics and sometimes ACE inhibitors. Persisting failure is an indication for surgical repair of the defect. Percutaneous closure devices are under development.

If serial ECG and echocardiography suggest that pulmonary hypertension is developing, surgical repair should be performed. Surgical closure is contraindicated in Eisenmenger syndrome, and heart–lung transplantation is the only effective treatment. The long-term prognosis is generally very good unless Eisenmenger syndrome develops, when death occurs in the second or third decade of life, but a few individuals survive to the fifth decade without transplantation.

Tetralogy of Fallot

This is a complex defect consisting of right ventricular outflow tract obstruction and right ventricular hypertrophy, a large ventricular septal defect and an overriding aorta that, when combined with the septal defect, allows blood to be pumped directly from the RV into the aorta. It occurs in about 1 in 2000 births and is the most common cause of cyanosis in infancy after the first year of life.

Pathogenesis

Tetralogy of Fallot occurs as the result of abnormal development of the bulbar septum that separates the ascending aorta from the pulmonary artery, and which normally aligns and fuses with the outflow part of the interventricular septum. The right ventricular outflow obstruction is most often subvalvular (muscular) but may be valvular, supravalvular or a combination of these (Fig. 16.96). The subvalvular component of the right

ventricular outflow obstruction is dynamic and may increase suddenly with sympathetic stimulation. The ventricular septal defect is usually large and similar in aperture to the aortic orifice. The combination results in elevated right ventricular pressure and right-to-left shunting of cyanotic blood across the ventricular septal defect into the aorta.

Clinical features

Children are usually cyanosed but this may not be the case in the neonate because it is only when right ventricular pressure rises to equal or exceed left ventricular pressure that a large right-to-left shunt develops. The affected child may suddenly become increasingly cyanosed, often after feeding or a crying attack, and may become apnoeic and unconscious. In older children, cyanotic spells are uncommon but cyanosis becomes increasingly apparent, with stunting of growth, digital clubbing and polycythaemia. Some children characteristically obtain relief by squatting after exertion, which increases the afterload of the left heart and reduces the right-to-left shunting. This is called Fallot's sign. The natural history before the development of surgical correction was variable but most patients died in infancy or childhood.

On examination, the most characteristic feature is the combination of cyanosis with a loud ejection systolic murmur in the pulmonary area (as for pulmonary stenosis). Cyanosis may be absent in the newborn or in patients with only mild right ventricular outflow obstruction, however. This is called acyanotic tetralogy of Fallot.

Investigations

Echocardiography is diagnostic and demonstrates that the aorta is not continuous with the anterior ventricular septum. The ECG shows right ventricular hypertrophy and the chest X-ray shows an abnormally small pulmonary artery and a 'boot-shaped' heart.

Management

The definitive management is total correction of the defect by surgical relief of the pulmonary stenosis and closure of the ventricular septal defect. Primary surgical correction may be undertaken prior to the age of 5 years. If the pulmonary arteries are too hypoplastic for surgical repair, then palliation in the form of a Blalock–Taussig shunt may be performed, where an anastomosis is created between the pulmonary artery and

16.102 Other causes of cyanotic congenital heart disease

Defect	Features
Tricuspid atresia	Absent tricuspid orifice, hypoplastic RV, RA-to-LA shunt, ventricular septal defect shunt, other anomalies
	Surgical correction may be possible
Transposition of the great arteries	Aorta arises from the morphological RV, pulmonary artery from LV
	Shunt via atria, ductus and possibly ventricular septal defect
	Palliation by balloon atrial septostomy/enlargement
	Surgical correction possible
Pulmonary atresia	Pulmonary valve atretic and pulmonary artery hypoplastic
	RA-to-LA shunt, pulmonary flow via ductus
	Palliation by balloon atrial septostomy
	Surgical correction may be possible
Ebstein's anomaly	Tricuspid valve is dysplastic and displaced into RV, RV 'atrialised'
	Tricuspid regurgitation and RA-to-LA shunt
	Wide spectrum of severity
	Arrhythmias
	Surgical repair possible but significant risk

(LA = left atrium; LV = left ventricle; RA = right atrium; RV = right ventricle)

16.103 Congenital heart disease in adolescence

- **Patients**: a heterogeneous population with residual disease and sequelae that vary according to the underlying lesion and in severity; each patient must be assessed individually.
- **Management plan**: should be agreed with the patient and include short- and long-term goals and timing of transition to adult care.
- **Risks of surgery**: non-cardiac surgery for associated congenital abnormalities carries increased risks and needs to be planned, with careful pre-operative assessment. Risks include thrombosis, embolism from synthetic shunts or patches, and volume overload from fluid shifts. Operative approaches should address cosmetic concerns, such as site of implantation of abdominal generator.
- **Exercise**: patients with mild or repaired defects can undertake moderately vigorous exercise but those with complex defects, cyanosis, ventricular dysfunction or arrhythmias require specialist evaluation and individualised advice regarding exercise.
- **Genetics**: Between 10% and 15% have a genetic basis and this should be assessed to understand the impact it may have for the patient's own future children. A family history, genetic evaluation of syndromic versus non-syndromic disorders and, sometimes, cytogenetics are required.
- **Education and employment**: may be adversely affected and occupational activity levels need to be assessed.
- **End of life**: some adolescents with complex disorders may misperceive and think they have been cured; transition to adult services may be the first time they receive information about mortality. Expectations on life expectancy need to be managed and adolescents are often willing to engage with this and play a role in decision-making.

subclavian artery. This improves pulmonary blood flow and pulmonary artery development, and may facilitate later definitive correction.

The prognosis after total correction is good, especially if the operation is performed in childhood. Follow-up is needed to identify residual shunting, recurrent pulmonary stenosis and arrhythmias. An implantable defibrillator is sometimes recommended in adulthood.

Other causes of cyanotic congenital heart disease

Other types of cyanotic congenital heart disease are summarised in Box 16.102.

Grown-up congenital heart disease

There are increasing numbers of children who have had surgical correction of congenital defects and who may have further problems as adults. The transition period between paediatric and adult care needs to be managed in a carefully planned manner, addressing many diverse aspects of care (Box 16.103). Those who have undergone correction of coarctation of the aorta may develop hypertension in adult life. Those with transposition of the great arteries who have had a 'Mustard' repair, in which blood is redirected at atrial level leaving the RV connected to the aorta, may develop right ventricular failure in adult life. This is because the RV is unsuited for function at systemic pressures and may begin to dilate and fail when patients are in their twenties or thirties.

Those who have had surgery involving the atria may develop atrial arrhythmias, and those who have VSD repair (and consequent ventricular scar) may develop ventricular arrhythmias. Anti-arrhythmic drugs and an ICD may be required. Such patients require careful follow-up from adolescence throughout adult life, so that problems can be identified early and appropriate medical or surgical treatment instituted. The management of patients with grown-up congenital heart disease (GUCH) is complex and has developed as a cardiological subspecialty.

Diseases of the myocardium

The myocardium can be injured secondary to ischaemia in CAD and to pressure or volume overload in hypertension or valvular heart disease. The heart muscle can be directly affected by primary heart muscle diseases.

Myocarditis

This is an acute inflammatory condition that can have an infectious, toxic or autoimmune aetiology (Box 16.104). Myocarditis can complicate many infections in which inflammation may be due directly to infection of the myocardium or the effects of circulating toxins. Viral infections are the most common causes, such as Coxsackie (35 cases per 1000 infections), influenza A and B (25 cases per 1000 infections) and, more recently, SARS-CoV-2 infection. Myocarditis may occur several weeks after the initial viral symptoms, and susceptibility is increased by glucocorticoid treatment, immunosuppression, radiation, previous myocardial damage and exercise. Some bacterial and protozoal infections may be complicated by myocarditis; for example, approximately 5% of patients with Lyme disease (*Borrelia burgdorferi*) develop myopericarditis, which is often associated with AV block. Toxins such as alcohol and drugs such as cocaine, lithium and doxorubicin may directly injure the myocardium. Other drugs, including penicillins and sulphonamides, and poisons such as lead and carbon monoxide, may cause a hypersensitivity reaction and associated myocarditis. Occasionally, autoimmune conditions, such as systemic lupus erythematosus and rheumatoid arthritis, are associated with myocarditis.

Clinical features

Myocarditis may present in one of four ways:

- *Fulminant myocarditis* follows a viral prodrome or influenza-like illness and results in severe heart failure or cardiogenic shock.
- *Acute myocarditis* presents over a longer period with heart failure; it can lead to dilated cardiomyopathy.

- *Chronic active myocarditis* is rare and associated with chronic myocardial inflammation.
- *Chronic persistent myocarditis* is characterised by focal myocardial infiltrates and can cause chest pain and arrhythmia without necessarily causing ventricular dysfunction.

Myocarditis is self-limiting in most patients and the immediate prognosis is good. Death may, however, occur due to a ventricular arrhythmia or rapidly progressive heart failure. Myocarditis has been reported as a cause of sudden and unexpected death in young athletes. Some forms of myocarditis may lead to chronic low-grade myocarditis or dilated cardiomyopathy (see below). For example, in Chagas' disease, the patient frequently recovers from the acute infection but goes on to develop a chronic dilated cardiomyopathy 10 or 20 years later.

Investigations

The diagnosis of myocarditis is often made after other more common causes of cardiac dysfunction have been excluded. Echocardiography should be performed and may reveal left ventricular dysfunction that is sometimes regional (due to focal myocarditis). Cardiac MRI is also useful since it may show diagnostic patterns of myocardial inflammation or infiltration. The ECG is frequently abnormal but the changes are non-specific. Blood should be taken to assess for cardiac troponin I or T which can be used to monitor severity and progression of cardiac injury and myocarditis. Occasionally, endomyocardial biopsy may be required to confirm the diagnosis.

Management

Treatment of myocarditis is primarily supportive. Treatment for cardiac failure or arrhythmias should be given and patients should be advised to avoid intense physical exertion because there is some evidence that this can induce potentially fatal ventricular arrhythmias. There is no evidence of benefit from treatment with glucocorticoids and immunosuppressive agents.

Specific antimicrobial therapy may be used if a causative organism has been identified but this is rare. Patients who do not respond adequately to medical treatment may temporarily require circulatory support with a mechanical ventricular assist device. Rarely, cardiac transplantation may be required.

Cardiomyopathy

Cardiomyopathies are primary diseases of the myocardium, which are classified according to their effects on cardiac structure and function (Fig. 16.97). They can be inherited or be caused by infections or exposure to toxins. In some cases no cause is identified.

i	**16.104**	**Some causes of myocarditis**

Infections

Viral
- Coxsackie
- Adenovirus
- Influenza A
- Human immunodeficiency virus (HIV)
- Influenza B
- SARS-CoV-2

Bacterial
- *Borrelia burgdorferi* (Lyme disease)
- *Mycoplasma pneumoniae*

Protozoal
- *Trypanosoma cruzi* (Chagas' disease)
- *Toxoplasma gondii*

Fungal
- *Aspergillus*

Parasitic
- *Shistosoma*

Drugs/Toxins
- Alcohol
- Anthracyclines
- Clozapine
- Cocaine
- Lithium

Autoimmune
- Systemic lupus erythematosus
- Systemic sclerosis
- Rheumatoid arthritis
- Sarcoidosis
- Hypersensitivity reaction to penicillins, sulphonamides, lead, carbon monoxide

16

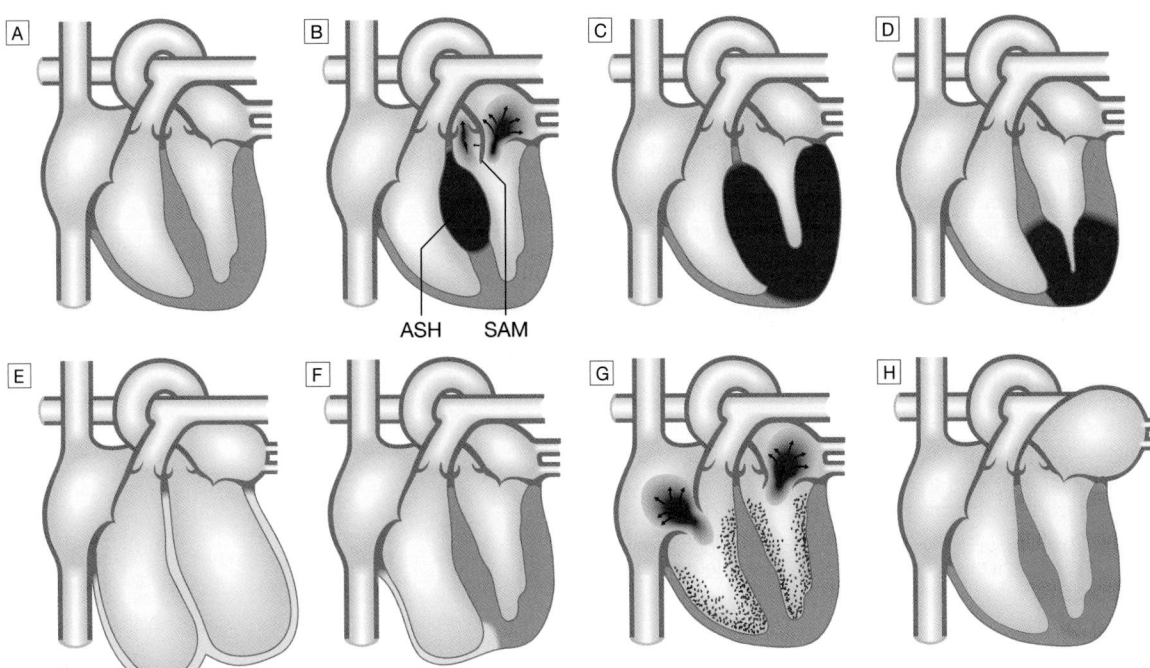

Fig. 16.97 Types of cardiomyopathy. ⒶNormaI heart. ⒷHypertrophic cardiomyopathy: asymmetric septal hypertrophy (ASH) with systolic anterior motion of the mitral valve (SAM), causing mitral reflux and dynamic left ventricular outflow tract obstruction. ⒸHypertrophic cardiomyopathy: concentric hypertrophy. ⒹHypertrophic cardiomyopathy: apical hypertrophy. ⒺDilated cardiomyopathy. ⒻArrhythmogenic right ventricular cardiomyopathy. ⒼObliterative cardiomyopathy. ⒽRestrictive cardiomyopathy.

Dilated cardiomyopathy

In North America and Europe, symptomatic dilated cardiomyopathy has an incidence of 20 per 100 000 and a prevalence of 38 per 100 000. Men are affected more than twice as often as women.

Pathogenesis

Cardiomyopathy is characterised by dilatation and impaired contraction of the LV and often the RV. Left ventricular mass is increased but wall thickness is normal or reduced (see Fig. 16.97). Dilatation of the valve rings can lead to functional mitral and tricuspid incompetence. Histological changes are variable but include myofibrillary loss, interstitial fibrosis and T-cell infiltrates. The term 'dilated cardiomyopathy' encompasses a heterogeneous group of conditions. Alcohol may be an important cause in some patients. At least 25% of cases are inherited as an autosomal dominant trait and a variety of single-gene mutations have been identified. Most of these mutations affect proteins in the cytoskeleton of the myocytes, such as dystrophin, lamin A and C, titan, emerin and metavinculin. Many are also associated with abnormalities of skeletal muscle. The X-linked inherited skeletal muscular dystrophies, such as Becker and Duchenne, are also associated with cardiomyopathy. Finally, a late autoimmune reaction to viral myocarditis is thought to be the cause in a substantial subgroup of patients with dilated cardiomyopathy; a similar mechanism is believed to be responsible for the myocardial involvement that occurs in up to 10% of patients with advanced human immunodeficiency virus (HIV) infection.

Clinical features

Most patients present with heart failure or are found to have the condition during routine investigation. Arrhythmia, thromboembolism and sudden death may occur at any stage but these are more common in advanced disease; non-exertional chest pain is surprisingly common. The differential diagnosis includes ventricular dysfunction due to CAD, and a diagnosis of dilated cardiomyopathy should be made only when this has been excluded.

Investigations

Echocardiography and cardiac MRI are the most useful investigations. Although ECG changes are common, they are non-specific. Genetic testing is indicated if more than one family member is diagnosed with the condition.

Management

The focus of management is to control heart failure using the strategies described earlier in this chapter. Although some patients remain well for many years, the prognosis is variable and cardiac transplantation may be indicated. Patients with dilated cardiomyopathy and moderate or severe heart failure are at risk of sudden arrhythmic death and this can be reduced by rigorous medical therapy with β-blockers and either ACE inhibitors or ARBs. Some patients may be considered for implantation of a cardiac defibrillator and/or cardiac resynchronisation therapy.

Hypertrophic cardiomyopathy

This is the most common form of cardiomyopathy, with a prevalence of approximately 100 per 100 000. It is characterised by inappropriate left ventricular hypertrophy with malalignment of the myocardial fibres and myocardial fibrosis. The hypertrophy may be generalised or confined largely to the interventricular septum (asymmetric septal hypertrophy, see Fig. 16.97) or other regions of the heart. A specific variant termed apical hypertrophic cardiomyopathy is common in the Far East.

Pathogenesis

Hypertrophic cardiomyopathy is a genetic disorder, usually with autosomal dominant transmission, a high degree of penetrance and variable expression. In most patients, it is due to a single-point mutation in one of the genes that encode sarcomeric contractile proteins. There are three common

groups of mutation with different phenotypes. Beta-myosin heavy-chain mutations are associated with marked ventricular hypertrophy. In contrast, troponin mutations are associated with little, if any, hypertrophy but are characterised by marked myocardial fibre disarray, exercise-induced hypotension and a high risk of sudden death. Myosin-binding protein C mutations tend to present late in life and are often associated with hypertension and arrhythmia. In all subtypes, heart failure may develop because the stiff, non-compliant LV impedes diastolic filling. Septal hypertrophy may also cause dynamic left ventricular outflow tract obstruction (hypertrophic obstructive cardiomyopathy, HOCM) and mitral regurgitation due to abnormal systolic anterior motion of the anterior mitral valve leaflet.

Clinical features

Effort-related symptoms, such as angina, breathlessness, arrhythmia and sudden death, are the dominant clinical presentations. The symptoms and signs are similar to those of aortic stenosis, except that, in hypertrophic cardiomyopathy, the character of the arterial pulse is jerky (Box 16.105). The annual mortality from sudden death is 2%–3% among adults and 4%–6% in children and adolescents (Box 16.106). Sudden death typically occurs during or just after vigorous physical activity and is thought to be due to ventricular arrhythmias. Hypertrophic cardiomyopathy is the most common cause of sudden death in young athletes. In patients who do not suffer fatal arrhythmias, the natural history is variable but clinical deterioration is often slow.

Investigations

Echocardiography is the investigation of choice and is usually diagnostic. Sometimes the diagnosis is more difficult when another cause of left ventricular hypertrophy is present but the degree of hypertrophy in hypertrophic cardiomyopathy is usually greater than in physiological hypertrophy and the pattern is asymmetrical. The ECG is abnormal and shows features of left ventricular hypertrophy with a wide variety of often bizarre abnormalities, including deep T-wave inversion. Genetic testing can be performed and is helpful in screening relatives of affected individuals.

Management

Beta-blockers, rate-limiting calcium antagonists and disopyramide can help to relieve symptoms and prevent syncopal attacks. Arrhythmias often respond to treatment with amiodarone. No pharmacological

16.105 Clinical features of hypertrophic cardiomyopathy

Symptoms

- Angina on effort
- Dyspnoea on effort
- Syncope on effort
- Sudden death

Signs

- Jerky pulse*
- Palpable left ventricular hypertrophy
- Double impulse at the apex (palpable fourth heart sound due to left atrial hypertrophy)
- Mid-systolic murmur at the base*
- Pansystolic murmur (due to mitral regurgitation) at the apex

*Signs of left ventricular outflow tract obstruction may be augmented by standing up (reduced venous return), inotropes and vasodilators

16.106 Risk factors for sudden death in hypertrophic cardiomyopathy

- A history of previous cardiac arrest or sustained ventricular tachycardia
- Recurrent syncope
- An adverse genotype and/or family history
- Exercise-induced hypotension
- Non-sustained ventricular tachycardia on ambulatory ECG monitoring
- Marked increase in left ventricular wall thickness

treatment has been identified that can improve prognosis, however. Outflow tract obstruction can be improved by partial surgical resection (myectomy) or by iatrogenic infarction of the basal septum (septal ablation) using a catheter-delivered alcohol solution. An ICD should be considered in patients with clinical risk factors for sudden death (see Box 16.106). Digoxin and vasodilators may increase outflow tract obstruction and should be avoided.

Arrhythmogenic ventricular cardiomyopathy

Arrhythmogenic ventricular cardiomyopathy (AVC) predominantly affects the myocardium of the right ventricle. It is inherited in an autosomal dominant manner and has a prevalence of approximately 10 per 100 000. The genetic defect involves desmosomal protein genes, most commonly plakophilin 2 (*PKP-2*), although current genetic testing protocols will not identify the culprit gene in many cases. It is characterised by replacement of patches of the right ventricular myocardium with fibrous and fatty tissue (see Fig. 16.97). In some cases, the LV is also involved and this is associated with a poorer prognosis. The diagnosis is based on a complex set of criteria that take account of the ECG, structural assessment, genetics and arrhythmias. The dominant clinical problems are ventricular arrhythmias, sudden death and right-sided cardiac failure. The ECG typically shows a slightly broadened QRS complex and inverted T waves in the right precordial leads. MRI is a helpful diagnostic tool and is used, along with the 12-lead ECG and ambulatory ECG monitoring, to screen the first-degree relatives of affected individuals. Management is based on treating right-sided cardiac failure with diuretics and cardiac arrhythmias with β-blockers or, in patients at high risk of sudden death, an implantable defibrillator can be offered.

Restrictive cardiomyopathy

In this rare condition, ventricular filling is impaired because the ventricles are 'stiff' (see Fig. 16.97). This leads to high atrial pressures with atrial hypertrophy, dilatation and, later, AF. Amyloidosis is the most common cause in the UK, although other forms of infiltration due to glycogen storage diseases, idiopathic perimyocyte fibrosis and a familial form of restrictive cardiomyopathy can also occur. The diagnosis can be difficult and requires assessment with Doppler echocardiography, CT or MRI, and endomyocardial biopsy. Treatment is symptomatic but the prognosis is usually poor and cardiac transplantation may be indicated.

Obliterative cardiomyopathy

This is a rare form of restrictive cardiomyopathy, involving the endocardium of one or both ventricles; it is characterised by thrombosis and fibrosis, with gradual obliteration of the ventricular cavities by fibrous tissue (see Fig. 16.97). The mitral and tricuspid valves become regurgitant. Heart failure and pulmonary and systemic embolism are prominent features. It can sometimes be associated with eosinophilia and can occur in eosinophilic leukaemia and eosinophilic granulomatosis with polyangiitis (formerly known as Churg–Strauss syndrome). In tropical countries, the disease may be responsible for up to 10% of cardiac deaths. Prognosis is poor, with a 50% mortality within 2 years of diagnosis. Anticoagulation and antiplatelet therapy are used to reduce the risk of embolism, and diuretics to treat heart failure. Surgery (tricuspid and/or mitral valve replacement with decortication of the endocardium) may be helpful in selected cases.

Takotsubo cardiomyopathy

Takotsubo cardiomyopathy (Takotsubo syndrome) is a form of acute left ventricular dysfunction characterised by dilatation of the left ventricular apex and adjacent myocardium, with associated left ventricular impairment. The mechanism is poorly understood. It is often associated with acute environmental or emotional stress (such as a bereavement) and presents with chest pain, breathlessness and sometimes cardiac failure. It occurs more frequently in women than in men and there is a high prevalence of neurological and psychiatric disorders. The symptoms and ECG often mimic acute ST elevation acute coronary syndrome. The diagnosis is usually made at coronary angiography, when CAD is found to be absent or minimal. Echocardiography or left ventriculography then shows characteristic 'apical ballooning' of the LV. The dilated apex and narrow outflow of the LV resemble a Japanese octopus trap, or takotsubo (Fig. 16.98).

Left ventricular ejection fraction returns to normal within days to weeks. Although commonly thought to be a benign condition, it is associated with a recurrence rate of 10% and a mortality of 20% at 5 years. There are no known treatments that have been shown to influence clinical outcome.

Secondary causes of cardiomyopathy

Many systemic conditions can produce a picture that is indistinguishable from dilated cardiomyopathy, including connective tissue disorders, sarcoidosis, haemochromatosis and alcoholic heart muscle disease (Box 16.107). In contrast, amyloidosis and eosinophilic heart disease produce symptoms and signs similar to those found in restrictive or obliterative cardiomyopathy, whereas the heart disease associated with Friedreich's ataxia can mimic hypertrophic cardiomyopathy.

16

Diastole	Systole
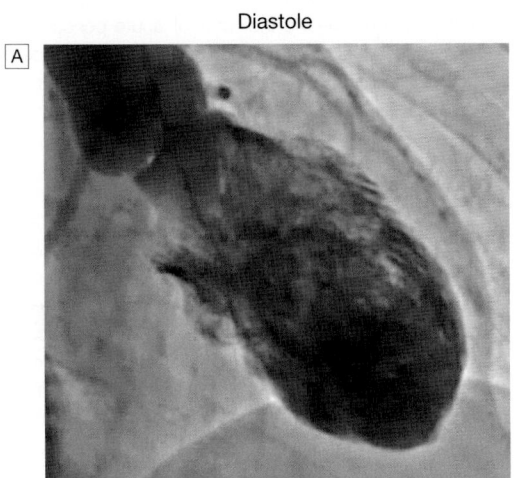	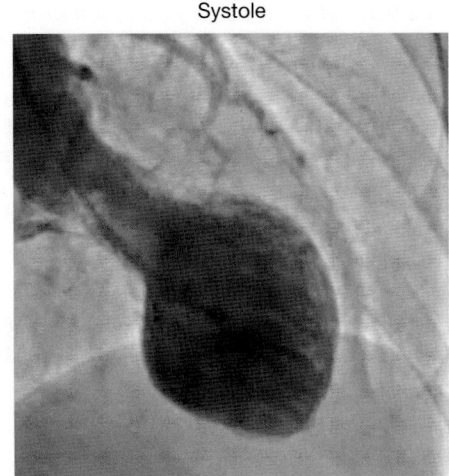

Fig. 16.98 Left ventriculograms in diastole A and systole B in a patient with Takotsubo cardiomyopathy. Note the ballooning of the left ventricular apex in systole which is characteristic of this condition (compare with Fig. 16.16).

---

i **16.107 Specific diseases of heart muscle**

Infections

Viral
- Coxsackie A and B
- Influenza
- HIV
- SARS-CoV-2

Bacterial
- Diphtheria
- *Borrelia burgdorferi*

Protozoal
- Trypanosomiasis
- *Toxoplasma gondii*

Endocrine and metabolic disorders
- Diabetes
- Hypo- and hyperthyroidism
- Acromegaly
- Carcinoid syndrome
- Phaeochromocytoma
- Inherited storage diseases

Connective tissue diseases
- Systemic sclerosis
- Systemic lupus erythematosus
- Polyarteritis nodosa

Infiltrative disorders
- Haemochromatosis
- Haemosiderosis
- Sarcoidosis
- Amyloidosis

Toxins
- Doxorubicin
- Alcohol
- Cocaine
- Irradiation

Neuromuscular disorders
- Dystrophia myotonica
- Friedreich's ataxia

---

i **16.108 Causes of acute pericarditis and pericardial effusion**

Infection
- Viral
- Bacterial
- Tuberculosis

Inflammatory
- Rheumatoid arthritis
- Systemic lupus erythematosus
- Rheumatic fever

Other
- Post-myocardial infarction
- Uraemia
- Malignancy
- Trauma

Treatment and prognosis are determined by the underlying disorder. Abstention from alcohol may lead to a dramatic improvement in patients with alcoholic heart muscle disease.

Cardiac tumours

Primary cardiac tumours are rare (<0.2% of autopsies) but the heart and mediastinum may be the sites of metastases. Most primary tumours are benign (75%) and, of these, the majority are myxomas. The remainder are fibromas, lipomas, fibroelastomas and haemangiomas.

Atrial myxoma

Myxomas most commonly arise in the LA as single or multiple polypoid tumours, attached by a pedicle to the interatrial septum. They are usually gelatinous but may be solid and even calcified, with superimposed thrombus.

On examination, the first heart sound is usually loud, and there may be a murmur of mitral stenosis with a variable diastolic sound (tumour 'plop') due to prolapse of the mass through the mitral valve. The tumour can be detected incidentally on echocardiography, or following investigation of pyrexia, syncope, arrhythmias or emboli. Occasionally, the condition presents with malaise and features suggestive of a connective tissue disorder, including a raised ESR.

Treatment is by surgical excision. If the pedicle is removed, fewer than 5% of tumours recur.

Diseases of the pericardium

The normal pericardial sac contains about 50 mL of fluid, similar to lymph, which lubricates the surface of the heart. The pericardium limits distension of the heart, contributes to the haemodynamic interdependence of the ventricles, and acts as a barrier to infection. Nevertheless, congenital absence of the pericardium does not result in significant clinical or functional limitations.

Acute pericarditis

This is due to an acute inflammatory process affecting the pericardium, which may coexist with myocarditis.

Pathogenesis

A number of causes are recognised (Box 16.108), but in some cases the cause is unclear. All forms of pericarditis may produce a pericardial effusion that, depending on the aetiology, may be fibrinous, serous, haemorrhagic or purulent. A fibrinous exudate may eventually lead to varying degrees of adhesion formation, whereas serous pericarditis often produces a large effusion of turbid, straw-coloured fluid with a high protein content. A haemorrhagic effusion is often due to malignant disease, particularly carcinoma of the breast or bronchus, and lymphoma. Purulent pericarditis is rare and may occur as a complication of sepsis, by direct spread from an intrathoracic infection, or from a penetrating injury.

Clinical features

The typical presentation is with chest pain that is retrosternal, radiates to the shoulders and neck, and is typically aggravated by deep breathing, movement, a change of position, exercise and swallowing. A low-grade fever is common. A pericardial friction rub is a high-pitched, superficial scratching or crunching noise, produced by movement of the inflamed pericardium, and is diagnostic of pericarditis; it is usually heard in systole but may also be audible in diastole and frequently has a 'to-and-fro' quality.

Investigations

The diagnosis can often be made on the basis of clinical features and the ECG; the latter shows ST elevation with upward concavity (Fig. 16.99) over the affected area, which may be widespread. PR interval depression is a very specific indicator of acute pericarditis. Later, there may be T-wave inversion, particularly if there is a degree of myocarditis. Echocardiography may be normal or may reveal pericardial effusion, in which case regular echocardiographic monitoring is recommended.

Management

The pain usually responds to aspirin (600 mg 6 times daily) but a more potent anti-inflammatory agent, such as indometacin (500 mg 3 times daily), may be required. Colchicine is very effective at relieving symptoms and also prevents relapsing episodes if taken for 3 months from symptom onset. Glucocorticoids are no longer recommended for this condition. In viral pericarditis, recovery usually occurs within a few days or weeks but there may be recurrences (chronic relapsing pericarditis). Purulent pericarditis requires treatment with antimicrobial therapy, pericardiocentesis and, if necessary, surgical drainage.

Pericardial effusion

Pericardial effusion often accompanies pericarditis and can have a number of causes, as shown in Box 16.108.

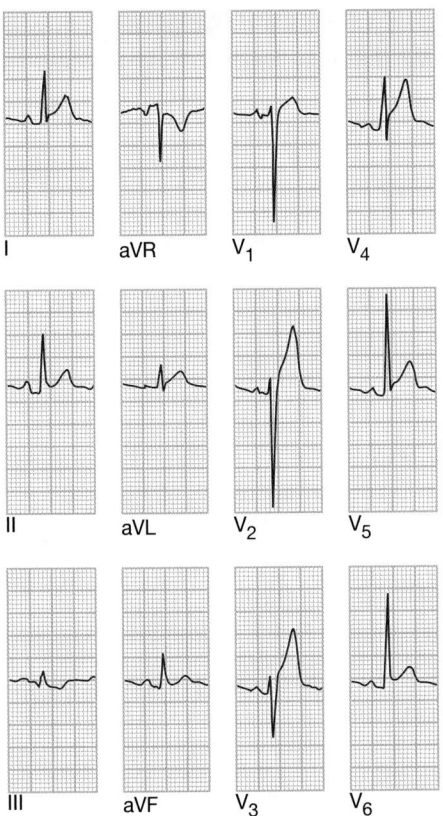

Fig. 16.99 ECG in viral pericarditis. Widespread ST elevation (leads I, II, aVL and V$_1$–V$_6$) is shown. The upward concave shape of the ST segments (see leads II and V$_6$) and the unusual distribution of changes (involving anterior and inferior leads) help to distinguish pericarditis from acute myocardial infarction.

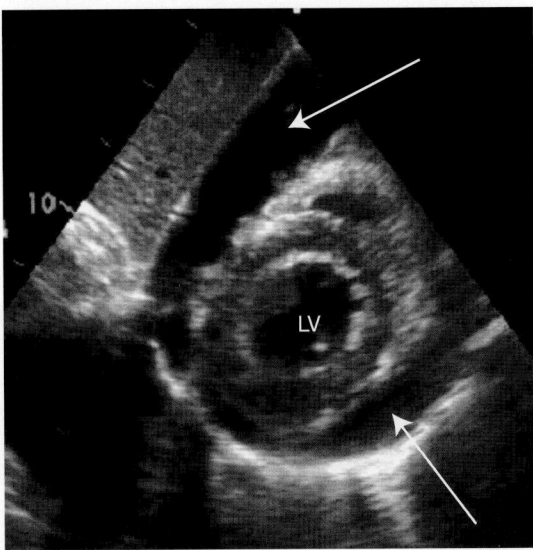

Fig. 16.100 Pericardial effusion: echocardiogram (apical view). Short-axis view of the heart showing a large circumferential pericardial effusion (arrows). (LV = left ventricle)

Clinical features

With the onset of an effusion the heart sounds may become quieter, and a friction rub, if present, may diminish in intensity but is not always abolished. Larger effusions may be accompanied by a sensation of retrosternal oppression. While most effusions do not have significant haemodynamic effects, large or rapidly developing effusions may cause cardiac tamponade. This term is used to describe acute heart failure due to compression of the heart and is described in detail below. Typical physical findings are a markedly raised JVP, hypotension, pulsus paradoxus and oliguria. Atypical presentations may occur when the effusion is loculated as a result of previous pericarditis or cardiac surgery.

Investigations

Echocardiography is the definitive investigation and is helpful in monitoring the size of the effusion and its effect on cardiac function (Fig. 16.100). The QRS voltages on the ECG are often reduced in the presence of a large effusion. The QRS complexes may alternate in amplitude due to a to-and-fro motion of the heart within the fluid-filled pericardial sac (electrical alternans). The chest X-ray may show an increase in the size of the cardiac silhouette and, when there is a large effusion, this has a globular appearance. Aspiration of the effusion may be required for diagnostic purposes and, if necessary, for treatment of large effusions, as described below.

Management

Patients with large effusions that are causing haemodynamic compromise or cardiac tamponade should undergo aspiration of the effusion. This involves inserting a needle under echocardiographic guidance medial to the cardiac apex or below the xiphoid process, directed upwards towards the left shoulder. The route of choice will depend on

the experience of the operator, the shape of the patient and the position of the effusion. A pericardial drain may be placed to provide symptomatic relief. Complications of pericardiocentesis include arrhythmias, damage to a coronary artery and bleeding, with exacerbation of tamponade as a result of injury to the RV. When tamponade is due to cardiac rupture or aortic dissection, pericardial aspiration may precipitate further potentially fatal bleeding and, in these situations, emergency surgery is the treatment of choice. A viscous, loculated or recurrent effusion may also require formal surgical drainage.

Tuberculous pericarditis

Tuberculous pericarditis may complicate pulmonary tuberculosis but may also be the first manifestation of the infection. In Africa, a tuberculous pericardial effusion is a common feature of AIDS. The condition typically presents with chronic malaise, weight loss and a low-grade fever. An effusion usually develops and the pericardium may become thick and unyielding, leading to pericardial constriction or tamponade. An associated pleural effusion is often present.

The diagnosis may be confirmed by aspiration of the fluid and direct examination or culture for tubercle bacilli. Treatment requires specific antituberculous chemotherapy (p. 522); in addition, a 3-month course of prednisolone (initial dose 60 mg a day, tapering down rapidly) improves outcome.

Chronic constrictive pericarditis

Constrictive pericarditis is due to progressive thickening, fibrosis and calcification of the pericardium. In effect, the heart is encased in a solid shell and cannot fill properly. The calcification may extend into the myocardium, so there may also be impaired myocardial contraction. The condition often follows an attack of tuberculous pericarditis but can also complicate haemopericardium, viral pericarditis, rheumatoid arthritis and purulent pericarditis. It is often impossible to identify the original insult.

Clinical features

The symptoms and signs of systemic venous congestion are the hallmarks of constrictive pericarditis. AF is common and there is often dramatic ascites and hepatomegaly (Box 16.109). Breathlessness is not a prominent symptom because the lungs are seldom congested. The condition is sometimes overlooked but should be suspected in any patient

---

i | **16.109** Clinical features of constrictive pericarditis

- Fatigue
- Rapid, low-volume pulse
- Elevated JVP with a rapid *y* descent
- Loud early third heart sound or 'pericardial knock'

- Kussmaul's sign
- Hepatomegaly
- Ascites
- Peripheral oedema
- Pulsus paradoxus

(JVP = jugular venous pressure)

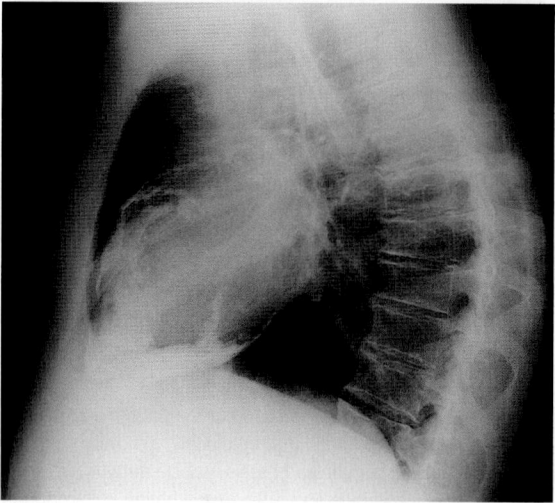

Fig. 16.101 Lateral chest X-ray from a patient with severe heart failure due to chronic constrictive pericarditis. There is heavy calcification of the pericardium.

with unexplained right heart failure and apparently normal heart size and function on echocardiography.

Investigations

A chest X-ray, which may show pericardial calcification (Fig. 16.101), and echocardiography often help to establish the diagnosis. CT scanning is useful for imaging the pericardial calcification. Constrictive pericarditis is often difficult to distinguish from restrictive cardiomyopathy and in such cases complex echo–Doppler studies and cardiac catheterisation may be required.

Management

The resulting diastolic heart failure is treated using loop diuretics and aldosterone antagonists, such as spironolactone. Surgical resection of the diseased pericardium can lead to a dramatic improvement but carries a high morbidity, especially if performed late in the disease course, as the pericardium becomes heavily bound to the myocardium.

Cardiac tamponade

This term is used to describe acute heart failure due to compression of the heart as the result of a large pericardial effusion. Tamponade may complicate any form of pericarditis but can be caused by malignant disease, by blood in the pericardial space following trauma, or by rupture of the free wall of the myocardium following MI.

---

i | **16.110** Clinical features of cardiac tamponade

- Dyspnoea
- Collapse
- Tachycardia
- Hypotension
- Gross elevation of the JVP
- Soft heart sounds with an early third heart sound
- Pulsus paradoxus (a large fall in BP during inspiration, when the pulse may be impalpable)
- Kussmaul's sign (a paradoxical rise in JVP during inspiration)

(JVP = jugular venous pressure)

Clinical features

Patients with tamponade are unwell, with hypotension, tachycardia and a markedly raised JVP. Other clinical features are summarised in Box 16.110.

Investigations

The pivotal investigation is echocardiography, which can confirm the diagnosis and also helps to identify the optimum site for aspiration of the fluid. The ECG may show features of the underlying disease, such as pericarditis or acute MI. When there is a large pericardial effusion, the ECG complexes are small and there may be electrical alternans: a changing axis with alternate beats caused by the heart swinging from side to side in the pericardial fluid. A chest X-ray shows an enlarged globular heart but can look normal.

Management

Cardiac tamponade is a medical emergency. When the diagnosis is confirmed, percutaneous pericardiocentesis should be performed as soon as possible, which usually results in a dramatic improvement. In some cases, surgical drainage may be required.

Further information

Journal article

Gould FK, Denning DW, Elliott TS, et al. Guidelines for the diagnosis and antibiotic treatment of endocarditis in adults: a report of the working party of the British Society for Antimicrobial Chemotherapy. J Antimicrob Chemother. 2012;67:269–289.

Websites

acc.org *American College of Cardiology (ACC): free access to guidelines for the evaluation and management of many cardiac conditions.*

americanheart.org *American Heart Association (AHA): free access to all the ACC/AHA/ESC guidelines, AHA scientific statements and fact sheets for patients.*

americanheart.org *European Society of Cardiology (ESC): free access to guidelines for the diagnosis and management of many cardiac conditions, and to educational modules.*

jbs3risk.com *Joint British Societies for the Prevention of Cardiovascular Disease: risk calculator.*

IJ Clifton
DAB Ellames

Respiratory medicine

Clinical examination of the respiratory system

6 — 9 Thorax
(see opposite)

5 Face, mouth and eyes
Pursed lips
Central cyanosis
Anaemia
Horner syndrome
(Ch. 28)

4 Jugular venous pulse
Elevated
Pulsatile

3 Blood pressure
Arterial paradox

2 Radial pulse
Rate
Rhythm

1 Hands
Digital clubbing
Tar staining
Peripheral cyanosis
Signs of occupation
CO_2 retention flap

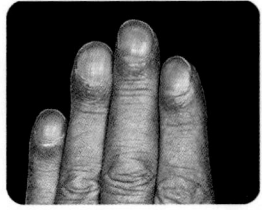

▲ Finger clubbing

6 Inspection
Deformity
(e.g. pectus excavatum)
Scars
Intercostal indrawing
Symmetry of expansion
Hyperinflation
Paradoxical rib movement
(low flat diaphragm)

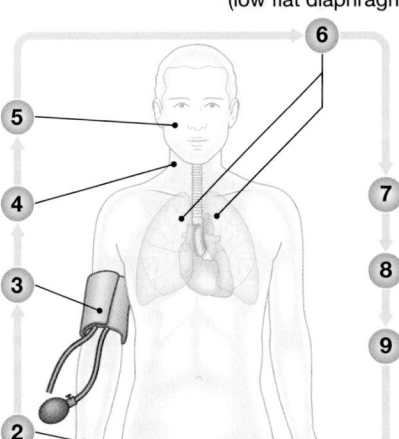

▲ Idiopathic kyphoscoliosis

7 Palpation
From the front:
  Trachea central
  Cricosternal distance
  Cardiac apex displaced
  Expansion
From behind:
  Cervical lymphadenopathy
  Expansion

8 Percussion
Resonant or dull
'Stony dull' (effusion)

9 Auscultation
Breath sounds:
normal, bronchial, louder or softer
Added sounds:
wheezes, crackles, rubs
Spoken voice (vocal resonance):
absent (effusion), increased
(consolidation)
Whispered voice:
whispering pectoriloquy

10 Leg oedema
Salt and water retention
Cor pulmonale
Venous thrombosis

Observation
- Respiratory rate
- Cachexia, fever, rash
- Sputum (see below)
- Fetor
- Locale:
  Oxygen delivery
  (mask, cannulae)
  Nebulisers
  Inhalers

Sputum

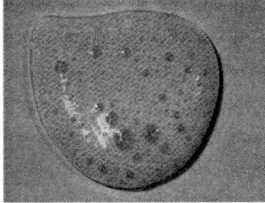

▲ Serous/frothy/pink
Pulmonary oedema

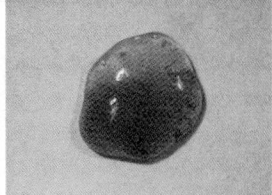

▲ Mucopurulent
Bronchial or pneumonic
infection

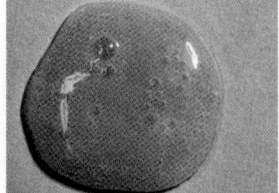

▲ Purulent
Bronchial or pneumonic
infection

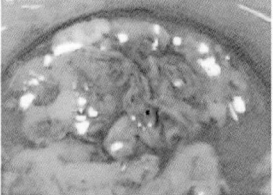

▲ Blood-stained
Cancer, tuberculosis,
bronchiectasis,
pulmonary embolism

Insets (idiopathic kyphoscoliosis) Courtesy of Dr I. Smith, Papworth Hospital, Cambridge; (serous, mucopurulent and purulent sputum) Courtesy of Dr J. Foweraker, Papworth Hospital, Cambridge.

Chronic obstructive pulmonary disease

Pulmonary fibrosis

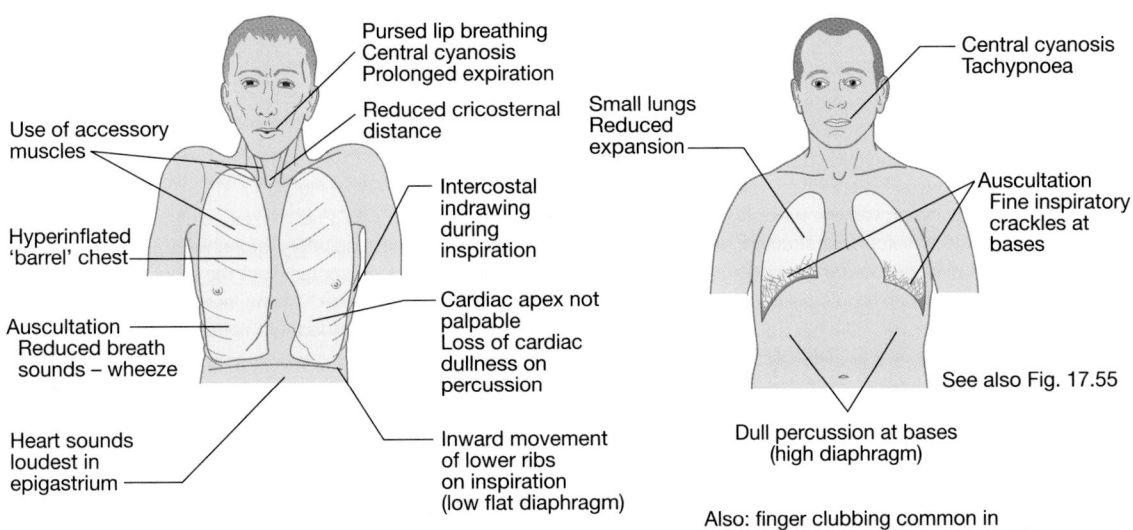

Pursed lip breathing
Central cyanosis
Prolonged expiration

Reduced cricosternal distance

Use of accessory muscles

Hyperinflated 'barrel' chest

Auscultation
Reduced breath sounds – wheeze

Heart sounds loudest in epigastrium

Intercostal indrawing during inspiration

Cardiac apex not palpable
Loss of cardiac dullness on percussion

Inward movement of lower ribs on inspiration (low flat diaphragm)

Also: raised jugular venous pressure (JVP), peripheral oedema from salt and water retention and/or cor pulmonale

Central cyanosis
Tachypnoea

Small lungs
Reduced expansion

Auscultation
Fine inspiratory crackles at bases

See also Fig. 17.55

Dull percussion at bases (high diaphragm)

Also: finger clubbing common in idiopathic pulmonary fibrosis; raised JVP and peripheral oedema if cor pulmonale

Right middle lobe pneumonia

Right upper lobe collapse

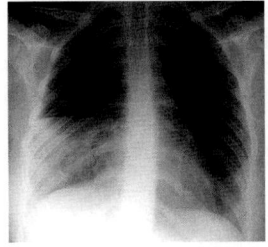

Obscures R heart border on X-ray

Inspection
  Tachypnoea
  Central cyanosis (if severe)
Palpation
  ↓Expansion on R
Percussion
  Dull R mid-zone and axilla
Auscultation
  Bronchial breath sounds and ↑vocal resonance over consolidation and whispering pectoriloquy
  Pleural rub if pleurisy

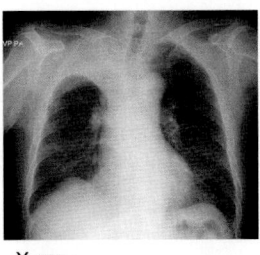

Inspection
  ↓Volume R upper zone
Palpation
  Trachea deviated to R
  ↓Expansion R upper zone
Percussion
  Dull R upper zone
Auscultation
  ↓Breath sounds with central obstruction

X-ray
  Deviated trachea (to R)
  Elevated horizontal fissure
  ↓Volume R hemithorax
  Central (hilar) mass may be seen

Right pneumothorax

Large right pleural effusion

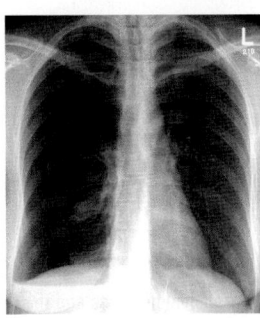

Inspection
  Tachypnoea (pain, deflation reflex)
Palpation
  ↓Expansion R side
Percussion
  Resonant or hyper-resonant on R
Auscultation
  Absent breath sounds on R

Tension pneumothorax also causes
  Deviation of trachea to opposite side
  Tachycardia and hypotension

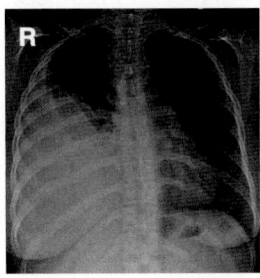

Inspection
  Tachypnoea
Palpation
  ↓Expansion on R
  Trachea and apex may be moved to L
Percussion
  Stony dull
  R mid- and lower zones
Auscultation
  Absent breath sounds and vocal resonance R base
  Bronchial breathing or crackles above effusion

17

Insets (upper lobe collapse) From http://3.bp.blogspot.com; (pneumothorax) http://chestatlas.com; (pleural effusion) www.ispub.com.

Respiratory infections such as tuberculosis, pneumonia and virus infections (e.g. influenza, COVID-19) represent a major burden of morbidity and mortality globally. The increasing prevalence of allergy, asthma and chronic obstructive pulmonary disease (COPD) contributes to the burden of chronic disease in the community. By 2025, the number of cigarette smokers worldwide is anticipated to increase to 1.5 billion, ensuring a growing burden of tobacco-related respiratory conditions.

Respiratory disease covers many pathologies, including infectious, inflammatory, neoplastic and degenerative processes. The practice of respiratory medicine thus requires collaboration with a range of disciplines. Recent advances have improved the lives of many patients with obstructive lung disease, cystic fibrosis, obstructive sleep apnoea and pulmonary hypertension, but the outlook remains poor for lung and other respiratory cancers and for some of the interstitial lung diseases.

Functional anatomy and physiology

The lungs occupy the upper two-thirds of the bony thorax, bounded medially by the spine, the heart and the mediastinum and inferiorly by the diaphragm. During breathing, free movement of the lung surface relative to the chest wall is facilitated by sliding contact between the parietal and visceral pleura, which cover the inner surface of the chest wall and the lung respectively, and are normally closely apposed. Inspiration involves downward contraction of the diaphragm (innervated by the phrenic nerves originating from C3, 4 and 5) and upward, outward movement of the ribs, caused by contraction of the external intercostal muscles (innervated by intercostal nerves originating from the thoracic spinal cord). Expiration is largely passive, driven by elastic recoil of the lungs.

The conducting airways from the nose to the alveoli connect the external environment with the alveolar surface. As air is inhaled through the upper airways it is filtered in the nose, heated to body temperature and fully saturated with water vapour; partial recovery of this heat and moisture occurs on expiration. Total airway cross-section is smallest in the glottis and trachea, making the central airway particularly vulnerable to obstruction. Normal breath sounds originate mainly from the rapid turbulent airflow in the larynx, trachea and main bronchi.

The multitude of small airways within the lung parenchyma has a very large combined cross-sectional area (over $300\,cm^2$ in the third-generation respiratory bronchioles), resulting in very slow flow rates. Airflow is virtually silent here and gas transport occurs largely by diffusion in the final generations. Major bronchial and pulmonary divisions are shown in Figure 17.1.

The acinus (Fig. 17.2) is the gas exchange unit of the lung and comprises branching respiratory bronchioles and clusters of alveoli. Here the air makes close contact with the blood in the pulmonary capillaries (gas-to-blood distance $< 0.4\,\mu m$), and oxygen uptake and CO_2 excretion occur. The alveoli are lined with flattened epithelial cells (type I pneumocytes) and a few, more cuboidal, type II pneumocytes. The latter produce surfactant, which is a phospholipid mixture that reduces surface tension and thereby counteracts the tendency of alveoli to collapse. Type II pneumocytes can divide to reconstitute type I pneumocytes after lung injury.

Lung mechanics

Healthy alveolar walls contain a fine network of elastin and collagen fibres (see Fig. 17.2). The volume of the lungs at the end of a tidal ('normal') breath out is called the functional residual capacity (FRC). At this volume, the inward elastic recoil of the lungs (resulting from elastin fibres and surface tension in the alveolar lining fluid) is balanced by the resistance of the chest wall to inward distortion from its resting shape, causing negative pressure in the pleural space. Elastin fibres allow the lung to be easily distended at physiological lung volumes, but collagen fibres cause increasing stiffness as full inflation is approached, so that, in health, the maximum inspiratory volume is limited by the lung (rather than the chest wall). The weight of lung tissue compresses the dependent regions and

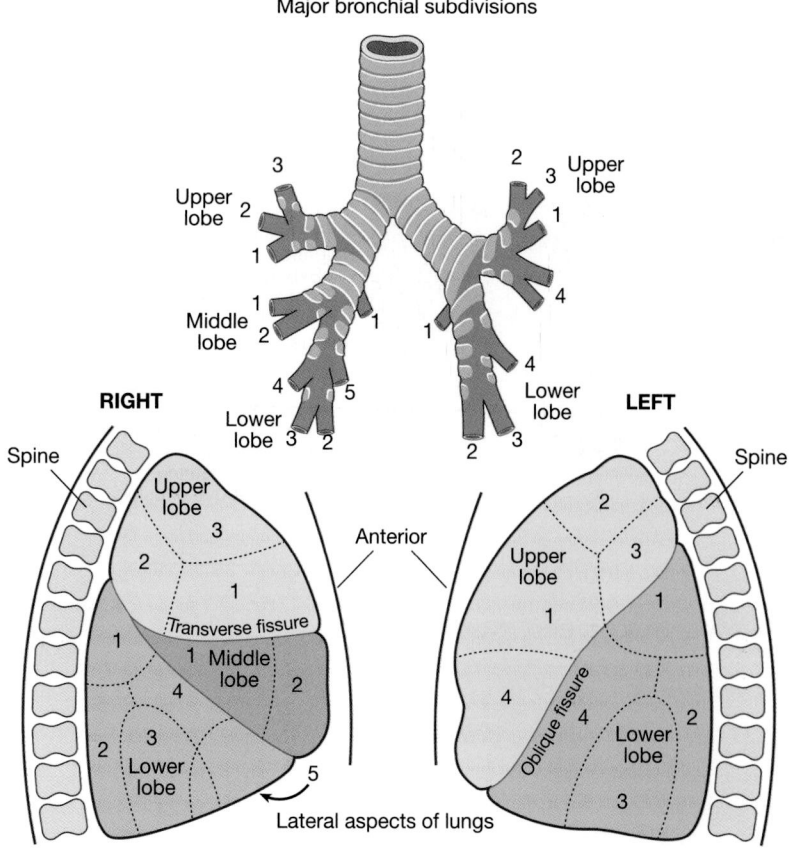

Major bronchial subdivisions

RIGHT

LEFT

Spine

Spine

Lateral aspects of lungs

Fig. 17.1 The major bronchial divisions and the fissures, lobes and segments of the lungs. The angle of the oblique fissure means that the left upper lobe is largely anterior to the lower lobe. On the right, the transverse fissure separates the upper from the anteriorly placed middle lobe, which is matched by the lingular segment on the left side. The site of a lobe determines whether physical signs are mainly anterior or posterior. Each lobe is composed of two or more bronchopulmonary segments that are supplied by the main branches of each lobar bronchus. *Bronchopulmonary segments*: **Right** *Upper lobe*: (1) Anterior, (2) Posterior, (3) Apical. *Middle lobe*: (1) Lateral, (2) Medial. *Lower lobe*: (1) Apical, (2) Posterior basal, (3) Lateral basal, (4) Anterior basal, (5) Medial basal. **Left** *Upper lobe*: (1) Anterior, (2) Apical, (3) Posterior, (4) Lingular. *Lower lobe*: (1) Apical, (2) Posterior basal, (3) Lateral basal, (4) Anterior basal.

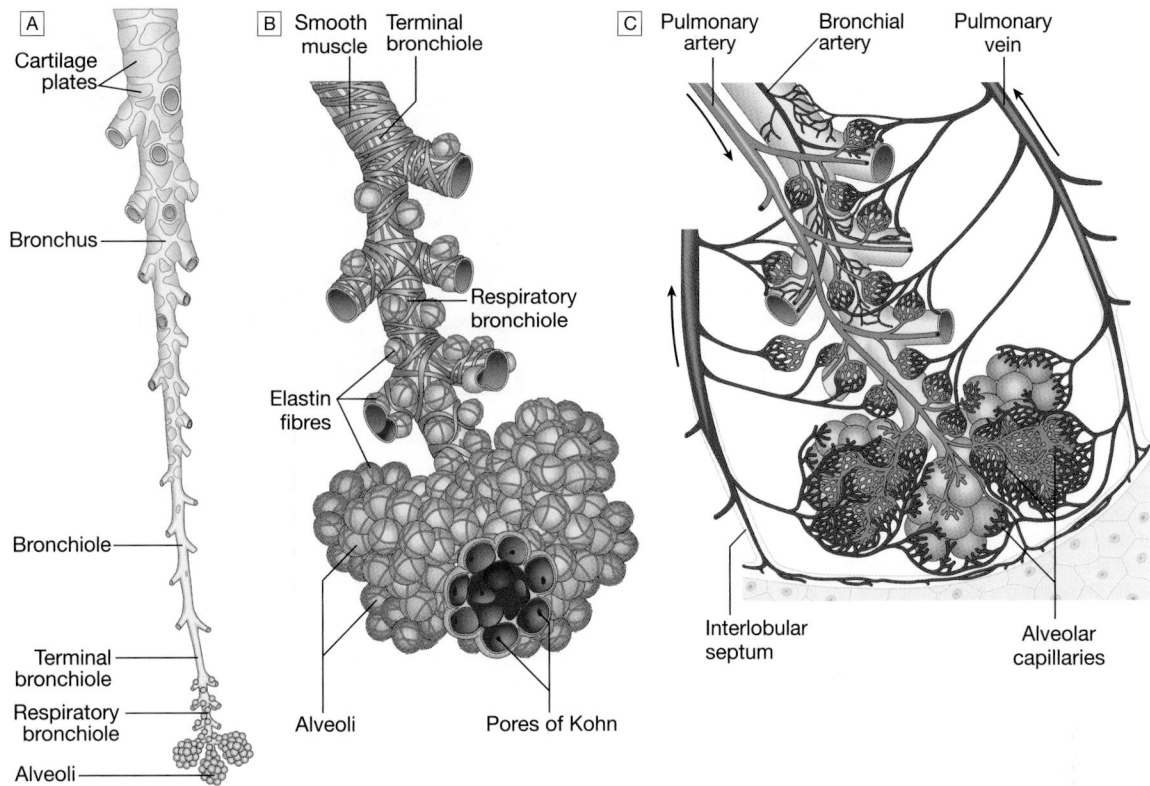

Fig. 17.2 Functional anatomy of the lung. **A** The tapering, branching bronchus is armoured against compression by plates of cartilage. The more distal bronchioles are collapsible, but held patent by surrounding elastic tissue. **B** The unit of lung supplied by a terminal bronchiole is called an acinus. The bronchiolar wall contains smooth muscle and elastin fibres. The latter also run through the alveolar walls. Gas exchange occurs in the alveoli, which are connected to each other by the pores of Kohn. **C** Vascular anatomy of an acinus. Both the pulmonary artery (carrying desaturated blood) and the bronchial artery (systemic supply to airway tissue) run along the bronchus. The venous drainage to the left atrium follows the interlobular septa. *From www.Netter.com: Illustrations 155 (bronchus, acinus) and 191 (circulation), Elsevier.*

distends the uppermost parts, so a greater portion of an inhaled breath passes to the basal regions, which also receive the greatest blood flow as a result of gravity. Elastin fibres in alveolar walls maintain small airway patency by radial traction on the airway walls. Even in health, however, these small airways narrow during expiration because they are surrounded by alveoli at higher pressure, but are prevented from collapsing by radial elastic traction. The volume that can be exhaled is thus limited purely by the capacity of the expiratory muscles to distort the chest wall inwards. In emphysema, loss of alveolar walls leaves the small airways unsupported, and their collapse on expiration causes air trapping and limits expiration at a high end-expiratory volume.

Control of breathing

The respiratory motor neurons in the posterior medulla oblongata are the origin of the respiratory cycle. Their activity is modulated by multiple external inputs in health and in disease (see Fig. 17.9):

- Central chemoreceptors in the ventrolateral medulla sense the pH of the cerebrospinal fluid (CSF) and are indirectly stimulated by a rise in arterial PCO_2.
- The carotid bodies sense hypoxaemia but are mainly activated by arterial PO_2 values below 8 kPa (60 mmHg). They are also sensitised to hypoxia by raised arterial PCO_2.
- Muscle spindles in the respiratory muscles sense changes in mechanical load.
- Vagal sensory fibres in the lung may be stimulated by stretch, inhaled toxins or disease processes in the interstitium.
- Cortical (volitional) and limbic (emotional) influences can override the automatic control of breathing.

Ventilation/perfusion matching and the pulmonary circulation

The regional distribution of ventilation and perfusion must be matched for optimal gas exchange within the lungs. At segmental and subsegmental level, hypoxia constricts pulmonary arterioles and airway CO_2 dilates bronchi, helping to maintain good regional matching of ventilation and perfusion. Lung disease may create regions of relative under-ventilation or under-perfusion, which disturb this regional matching, causing respiratory failure. In addition to causing ventilation–perfusion mismatch, diseases that destroy capillaries or thicken the alveolar capillary membrane (e.g. emphysema or fibrosis) can impair gas diffusion directly.

The pulmonary circulation in health operates at low pressure (approximately 24/9 mmHg) and can accommodate large increases in flow with minimal rise in pressure, e.g. during exercise. Pulmonary hypertension occurs when vessels are destroyed by emphysema, obstructed by thrombus, involved in interstitial inflammation or thickened by pulmonary vascular disease. The right ventricle responds by hypertrophy, with right axis deviation and P pulmonale (tall, peaked p waves) on the electrocardiogram (ECG), and clinical features of right heart failure; the term 'cor pulmonale' is often used for these findings.

Changes in respiratory function associated with old age are shown in Box 17.1.

Lung defences

Upper airway defences

Large airborne particles are trapped by nasal hairs, and smaller particles settling on the mucosa are cleared towards the oropharynx by the columnar ciliated epithelium that covers the turbinates and septum

17.1 Respiratory function in old age

- **Reserve capacity**: a significant reduction in function can occur with ageing with only minimal effect on normal breathing, but the ability to combat acute disease is reduced.
- **Decline in FEV$_1$**: the FEV$_1$/FVC (forced expiratory volume/forced vital capacity) ratio falls by around 0.2% per year from 70% at the age of 40–45 years, due to a decline in elastic recoil in the small airways with age. Smoking accelerates this decline threefold on average. Symptoms usually occur only when FEV$_1$ drops below 50% of predicted.
- **Increasing ventilation–perfusion mismatch**: the reduction in elastic recoil causes a tendency for the small airways to collapse during expiration, particularly in dependent areas of the lungs, thus reducing ventilation.
- **Reduced ventilatory responses to hypoxia and hypercapnia**: older people may be less tachypnoeic for any given fall in PaO_2 or rise in $PaCO_2$.
- **Impaired defences against infection**: due to reduced numbers of glandular epithelial cells, which lead to a reduction in protective mucus.
- **Decline in maximum oxygen uptake**: due to a combination of impairments in muscle, and the respiratory and cardiovascular systems. This leads to a reduction in cardiorespiratory reserve and exercise capacity.
- **Loss of chest wall compliance**: due to reduced intervertebral disc spaces and ossification of the costal cartilages; respiratory muscle strength and endurance also decline. These changes become important only in the presence of other respiratory disease.

(Fig. 17.3). During cough, expiratory muscle effort against a closed glottis results in high intrathoracic pressure, which is then released explosively. The flexible posterior tracheal wall is pushed inwards by the high surrounding pressure, which reduces tracheal cross-section and thus maximises the airspeed to achieve effective expectoration. The larynx also acts as a sphincter, closing to protect the airway during swallowing and vomiting.

Lower airway defences

The structure and function of the lower airways are maintained by close cooperation between the innate and adaptive immune responses. Traditionally, the healthy lower respiratory tract was considered to be sterile. However, molecular analysis has established that it harbours a diverse resident microbial population (the lung microbiome); understanding of the interactions between the immune system and the lung microbiome, and its role in health and disease, is in its infancy.

The innate response in the lungs is characterised by a number of non-specific defence mechanisms. Inhaled particulate matter is trapped in airway mucus and cleared by the mucociliary escalator. Tobacco smoke increases mucus secretion but reduces mucociliary clearance and predisposes towards lower respiratory tract infections, including pneumonia. Defective mucociliary transport is also a feature of several rare diseases including cystic fibrosis, primary ciliary dyskinesia and Young syndrome, which are characterised by repeated sino-pulmonary infections and bronchiectasis.

Airway secretions contain an array of antimicrobial peptides (AMPs), such as defensins and lysozyme), immunoglobulin A (IgA), antiproteinases and antioxidants. Many assist with the opsonisation and killing of bacteria and the regulation of the proteolytic enzymes secreted by inflammatory cells. In particular, α_1-antitrypsin regulates neutrophil elastase, and deficiency of this may be associated with premature emphysema.

Macrophages engulf microbes, organic dusts and other particulate matter. They cannot digest inorganic agents such as asbestos or silica, which cause their death and lead to the release of powerful proteolytic enzymes that damage the lung. Neutrophil numbers in the airway are low but the pulmonary circulation contains a marginated pool that may be recruited rapidly in response to bacterial infection.

Adaptive immunity is characterised by a specific response and immunological memory. Lung dendritic cells facilitate antigen presentation to T and B lymphocytes.

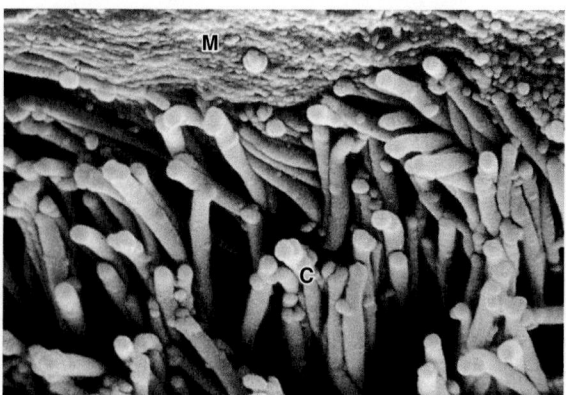

Fig. 17.3 The mucociliary escalator. Scanning electron micrograph of the respiratory epithelium showing large numbers of cilia (C) overlaid by the mucus 'raft' (M).

Investigation of respiratory disease

A detailed history, thorough examination and basic haematological and biochemical tests usually indicate the likely diagnosis and differential. A number of other investigations are normally required to confirm the diagnosis and/or monitor disease activity.

Imaging

The 'plain' chest X-ray

The chest X-ray (CXR) is one of the initial investigations performed on the majority of patients suspected of having respiratory disease. A posteroanterior (PA) film provides information on the lung fields, heart, mediastinum, vascular structures and thoracic cage (Fig. 17.4). A lateral film may provide additional information, particularly if pathology is suspected behind the heart or deep in the diaphragmatic sulci. An approach to interpreting the chest X-ray is given in Box 17.2; common abnormalities are listed in Box 17.3.

Increased shadowing may represent accumulation of fluid, lobar collapse or consolidation. Uncomplicated consolidation should not change the position of the mediastinum and the presence of an air bronchogram means that proximal bronchi are patent. Collapse (implying obstruction of the lobar bronchus) is accompanied by loss of volume and displacement of the mediastinum towards the affected side (Fig. 17.5).

The presence of ring shadows (thickened bronchi seen end-on), tramline shadows (thickened bronchi side-on) or tubular shadows (bronchi filled with secretions) suggests bronchiectasis. The presence of pleural fluid is suggested by a dense basal shadow, which, in the erect patient, ascends towards the axilla. In a large pulmonary embolism, relative oligaemia may cause a lung field to appear abnormally dark.

Computed tomography

Computed tomography (CT) provides detailed images of the pulmonary parenchyma, mediastinum, pleura and bony structures. The displayed range of densities can be adjusted to highlight different structures such as the lung parenchyma, the mediastinal vascular structures or bone. Cross-sectional formatting allows recognition of the axial distribution of the disease, while coronal reformation displays the craniocaudal distribution. In cases of suspected lung cancer, CT is central to both diagnosis and staging, and facilitates percutaneous needle biopsy. CT identifies the extent and appearance of pleural thickening (see Fig. 17.64) and reliably differentiates pleural and pericardial fat from pathology. High-resolution thin-section scanning provides detailed images of the pulmonary parenchyma and is superior to chest X-ray for assessment of diffuse parenchymal lung disease (see Fig. 17.55), identifying airway thickening, bronchiectasis (see Fig. 17.29) and emphysema (see Fig. 17.27). The relative contribution of competing pathologies to a breathless patient may be assessed. Prone imaging may be used to differentiate the gravity-induced posterobasal attenuation seen in supine scans. CT pulmonary angiography (CTPA) has become the investigation of choice in the diagnosis of pulmonary thromboembolism (see Fig. 17.67), when it may either confirm the suspected embolism or highlight an alternative diagnosis. CTPA has largely replaced the radioisotope-based ventilation–perfusion ($\dot{V}/\dot{Q}$) scan for this purpose. CT may assist in identifying cavitation and other features of infection (e.g. air creascent and halo signs in aspergillosis). Finally, CT may be used to monitor disease progression in established disease and for screening in certain high-risk populations.

Positron emission tomography

Positron emission tomography (PET) scanners employ the radiotracer ¹⁸F-fluorodeoxyglucose (FDG) to quantify the rate of glucose metabolism by cells. The ¹⁸FDG is rapidly taken up by metabolically active tissue, where it is phosphorylated and 'trapped' in the cell. The assessment of ¹⁸FDG uptake may be qualitative (visual analysis) or semi-quantitative, using the standardised uptake value (SUV) (Fig. 17.6). FDG-PET is useful in the staging of mediastinal lymph nodes and distal metastatic disease in patients with lung cancer and in the investigation of pulmonary nodules. Co-registration of PET and CT (PET-CT) enhances localisation and characterisation of metabolically active deposits (see Fig. 17.6). FDG-PET may also differentiate benign from malignant pleural disease and can be used to assess the extent of extrapulmonary disease in sarcoidosis. However, ¹⁸FDG uptake by a lesion is affected by a large number of parameters, including equipment used, the physics, and biological factors such as amount of body fat and brown fat uptake and the blood glucose level.

17.2 How to interpret a chest X-ray

Name, date, orientation	Films are posteroanterior (PA) unless marked AP to denote that they are anteroposterior
Lung fields	Equal translucency? Check horizontal fissure from right hilum to sixth rib at the anterior axillary line Masses? Consolidation? Cavitation?
Lung apices	Check behind the clavicles. Masses? Consolidation? Cavitation?
Trachea	Central (midway between the clavicular heads)? Paratracheal mass? Goitre?
Heart	Normal shape? Cardiothoracic ratio (should be < half the intrathoracic diameter) Retrocardiac mass?
Hila	Left should be higher than right Shape (should be concave laterally; if convex, consider mass or lymphadenopathy)? Density?
Diaphragm	Right should be higher than left Hyperinflation (no more than 10 ribs should be visible posteriorly above the diaphragm)?
Costophrenic angles	Acute and well defined (pleural fluid or thickening, if not)?
Soft tissues	Breast shadows in females Chest wall for masses or subcutaneous emphysema
Bones	Ribs, vertebrae, scapulae and clavicles Any fracture visible at bone margins or lucencies?

17

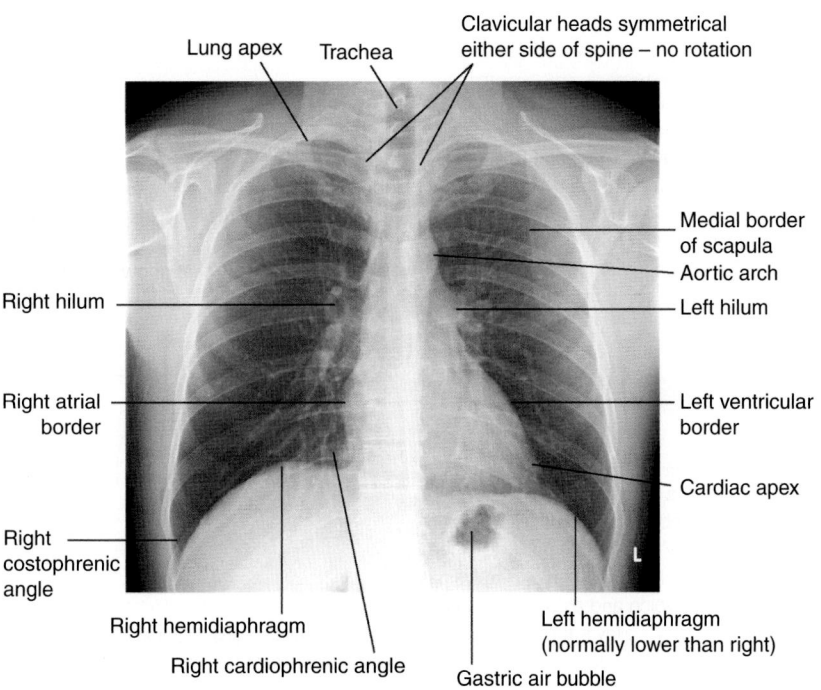

Fig. 17.4 **The normal chest X-ray.** The lung markings consist of branching and tapering lines radiating out from the hila. Where airways and vessels turn towards the film, they can appear as open or filled circles (see upper pole of right hilum). The scapulae may overlie the lung fields; trace the edge of bony structures to avoid mistaking them for pleural or pulmonary shadows. To check for hyperinflation, count the ribs; if more than 10 are visible posteriorly above the diaphragm, the lungs are hyperinflated. *From Innes JA. Davidson's Essentials of medicine. Edinburgh: Churchill Livingstone, Elsevier Ltd; 2009.*

17.3 Common chest X-ray abnormalities

Pulmonary and pleural shadowing

- Consolidation: infection, infarction, inflammation and, rarely, bronchoalveolar cell carcinoma
- Lobar collapse: mucus plugging, tumour, compression by lymph nodes
- Solitary nodule
- Multiple nodules: miliary tuberculosis (TB), dust inhalation, metastatic malignancy, healed varicella pneumonia, rheumatoid disease
- Ring shadows, tramlines and tubular shadows: bronchiectasis
- Cavitating lesions: tumour, abscess, infarct, pneumonia (*Staphylococcus/Klebsiella*), granulomatosis with polyangiitis (GPA)
- Reticular, nodular and reticulonodular shadows: diffuse parenchymal lung disease, infection
- Pleural abnormalities: fluid, plaques, tumour

Increased translucency

- Bullae
- Pneumothorax
- Oligaemia

Hilar abnormalities

- Unilateral hilar enlargement: TB, lung cancer, lymphoma
- Bilateral hilar enlargement: sarcoidosis, lymphoma, TB, silicosis

Other abnormalities

- Hiatus hernia
- Surgical emphysema

Magnetic resonance imaging

Conventional magnetic resonance imaging (MRI) of the lung parenchyma is seldom useful, although the technique is being used increasingly in distinguishing benign from malignant pleural disease and in delineating invasion of the chest wall or diaphragm by tumour.

The use of hyperpolarized ³He MRI is a developing method of assessing the distribution of ventilation within the lung.

Ultrasound

Transthoracic ultrasound is a point-of-care investigation used to assess the pleural space (see Fig. 17.15). In the hands of an experienced operator it can distinguish pleural fluid from pleural thickening, identify a pneumothorax and, by directly visualising the diaphragm and solid organs such as the liver, spleen and kidneys, may be used to guide pleural aspiration, biopsy and intercostal chest drain insertion. It is also used to guide needle biopsy of superficial lymph node or chest wall masses and provides useful information on the shape and movement of the diaphragm.

Endoscopic examination

Laryngoscopy

The larynx may be inspected directly with a fibreoptic laryngoscope in cases of suspected intermittent laryngeal obstruction (ILO), when paradoxical movement of the vocal cords may mimic asthma. Left-sided lung tumours may involve the left recurrent laryngeal nerve, paralysing the left vocal cord and leading to a hoarse voice and a 'bovine' cough. Continuous laryngoscopy during exercise tests allows the identification of exercise-induced ILO.

Bronchoscopy

The trachea and the first 3–4 generations of bronchi may be inspected using a flexible fibreoptic bronchoscope. This is usually performed under local anaesthesia with sedation, on an outpatient basis. Abnormal tissue

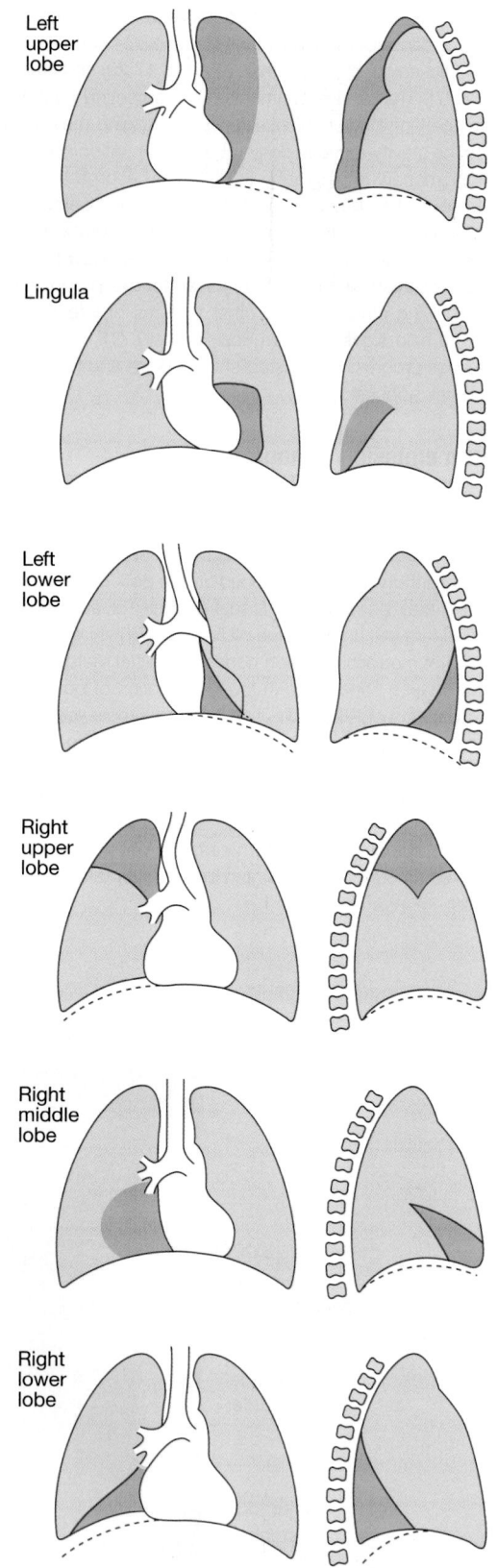

Fig. 17.5 Radiological features of lobar collapse caused by bronchial obstruction. The dotted line in the drawings represents the normal position of the diaphragm. The dark pink area represents the extent of shadowing seen on the X-ray.

in the bronchial lumen or wall can be biopsied, and bronchial brushings, washings or aspirates can be taken for cytological or bacteriological examination. Small biopsy specimens of lung tissue, taken by forceps passed through the bronchial wall (transbronchial biopsies), may be

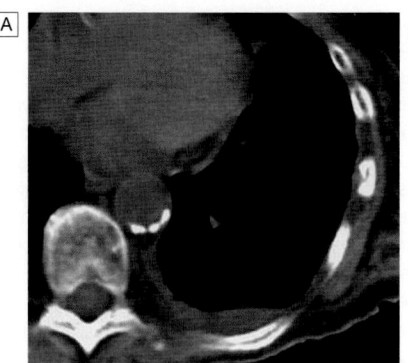 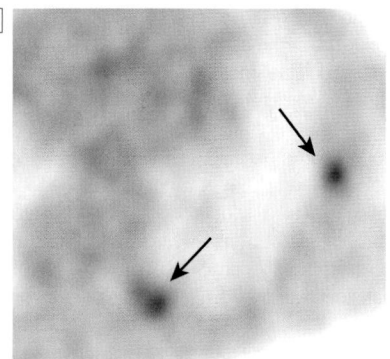 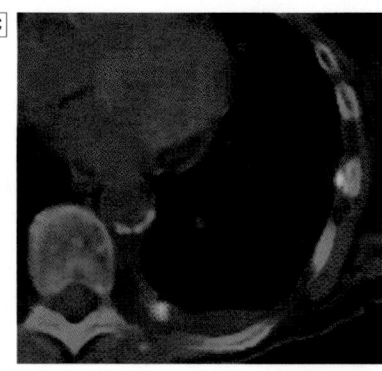

Fig. 17.6 Computed tomography and positron emission tomography combined to reveal intrathoracic metastases. A In a patient with lung cancer, CT shows some posterior pleural thickening. B FDG-PET scanning reveals FDG uptake in two pleural lesions (arrows). C The lesions are highlighted in yellow in the combined PET-CT image. (CT = computed tomography; FDG = ¹⁸F-fluorodeoxyglucose; PET = positron emission tomography) *(A–C) From http://radiology.rsnajnls.org.*

helpful in the diagnosis of bronchocentric disorders such as sarcoidosis and diffuse malignancy but are generally too small to be of diagnostic value in other diffuse parenchymal pulmonary disease.

Rigid bronchoscopy requires general anaesthesia and is reserved for specific situations, such as massive haemoptysis or removal of a foreign body (see Fig. 9.2), and can facilitate endobronchial laser therapy and stenting.

Endobronchial ultrasound

Endobronchial ultrasound (EBUS) allows directed needle aspiration from peribronchial nodes and is used increasingly to stage lung cancer. It may also be useful in non-malignant conditions, such as mediastinal lymphadenopathy caused by tuberculosis or sarcoidosis. Lymph nodes down to the main carina can also be sampled using a mediastinoscope passed through a small incision at the suprasternal notch under general anaesthetic. Lymph nodes in the lower mediastinum may be biopsied via the oesophagus using an oesophageal endoscope equipped with an ultrasound transducer and biopsy needle (endoscopic ultrasound).

Thoracoscopy

Thoracoscopy, which involves the insertion of an endoscope through the chest wall, facilitates biopsy under direct vision and is the gold standard for the evaluation of the pleural surfaces, characterisation of complex pleural effusion, and identification of exudate and haemorrhage. It is also used for accurate staging of apical tumours.

Microbiological investigations

Sputum, pleural fluid, throat swabs, blood, and bronchial washings and aspirates can be examined for bacteria, fungi and viruses. The use of hypertonic saline to induce expectoration of sputum may obviate the need for more invasive procedures such as bronchoscopy. Molecular tests (nucleic acid amplification tests, NAATs) are being used increasingly as first-line diagnostic tests for respiratory viruses (including influenza and coronaviruses such as SARS-CoV-2), as well as bacterial pathogens (e.g. *Legionella*, *Mycoplasma*), for which they have largely replaced paired serology and antigen-based tests. NAATs are also gaining an increased role as first-line diagnostic tests for tuberculosis and for rapid identification of antimicrobial drug resistance.

Immunological and serological tests

The presence of atopy can be detected by demonstrating an elevated level of immunoglobulin E (IgE), and the measurement of IgE directed against specific antigens. This can be useful to support the diagnosis of asthma and in identifying triggers. Many autoimmune diseases present with pulmonary involvement and autoantibodies may be identified in the serum. IgG enzyme immunoassay or identification of serum precipitins (antibodies that form visible lines of precipitated glycoprotein when they encounter their specific antigen in an agarose gel) can be used to identify a reaction to fungi such as *Aspergillus* or to antigens involved in hypersensitivity pneumonitis, such as farmer's lung or bird fancier's lung. The presence of pneumococcal antigen in sputum, blood or urine may be of diagnostic importance in pneumonia. Respiratory viruses can be detected in nose/throat swabs by immunofluorescence and *Legionella* infection may diagnosed by detection of a *Legionella* antigen in urine. ß-1,3-D-glucan detection (in blood) is a marker of fungal infection (see Chapter 13) and *Aspergillus* galactomannan (in blood and bronchial lavage fluid) is used to diagnose invasive aspergillosis. Interferon-gamma release assays are useful in the detection of latent tuberculosis.

Cytology and histopathology

Cytological examination of exfoliated cells in pleural fluid or bronchial brushings and washings, or of fine needle aspirates from lymph nodes or pulmonary lesions, can support a diagnosis of malignancy. A larger tissue biopsy is often necessary, however, as this allows immunohistochemistry and genetic testing to characterise the tumor and guide variant-specific therapy. Histopathology may also allow identification of microorganisms using conventional staining or NAATs. Differential cell counts in bronchial lavage fluid may help to distinguish pulmonary changes due to sarcoidosis, idiopathic pulmonary fibrosis or hypersensitivity pneumonitis.

Respiratory function testing

Respiratory function tests are used to aid diagnosis, quantify functional impairment and monitor treatment or progression of disease. Airway narrowing, lung volume and gas exchange capacity are quantified and compared with normal values adjusted for age, gender, height and ethnic origin. In diseases characterised by airway narrowing (e.g. asthma, bronchitis and emphysema), maximum expiratory flow is limited by dynamic compression of small intrathoracic airways, some of which may close completely during expiration, limiting the volume that can be expired ('obstructive' defect). This causes hyperinflation of the chest, which can become extreme if elastic recoil is also lost due to parenchymal destruction, as in emphysema. In contrast, diseases that cause interstitial inflammation and/or fibrosis lead to progressive loss of lung volume ('restrictive' defect) with normal expiratory flow rates. Typical laboratory traces are illustrated in Figure 17.7.

Measurement of airway obstruction

Airway narrowing is assessed by asking patients to breathe in fully, then blow out as hard and fast as they can into a peak flow meter or

17

a spirometer. Peak flow meters are useful for home monitoring of peak expiratory flow (PEF) in the detection and monitoring of asthma but results are effort-dependent. More accurate and reproducible measures are obtained by maximum forced expiration into a spirometer. The forced expired volume in 1 second (FEV_1) is the volume exhaled in the first second, and the forced vital capacity (FVC) is the total volume exhaled. Airflow obstruction is defined as a FEV_1/FVC ratio of less than 70%. In this situation, spirometry should be repeated following inhaled short-acting β_2-adrenoceptor agonists (e.g. salbutamol); an increase of > 12% and > 200 mL in FEV_1 or FVC indicates significant reversibility. A large improvement in FEV_1 (> 400 mL) and variability in peak flow over time are features of asthma.

Large airway narrowing (e.g. tracheal stenosis or compression; see Fig. 20.12) can be distinguished from small airway narrowing through plotting spirometry data as flow/volume loops. These display flow in relation to lung volume (rather than time) during maximum expiration and inspiration, and the pattern of flow reveals the site of airflow obstruction (Fig. 17.7B).

Lung volumes

Spirometry can measure only the volume of gas that can be exhaled; it cannot measure the gas remaining in the lungs after a maximal expiration. All the gas in the lungs can be measured by rebreathing an inert non-absorbed gas (usually helium) and recording how much the test gas is diluted by lung gas at equilibrium. This measures the volume of intrathoracic gas that mixes freely with tidal breaths. Alternatively, lung volume may be measured by body plethysmography (see Chapter 9), which determines the pressure/volume relationship of the thorax. This method measures total intrathoracic gas volume, including poorly ventilated areas such as bullae. The terms used to describe lung volume are shown in Figure 17.7C.

Transfer factor

To measure the capacity of the lungs to exchange gas, patients inhale a test mixture of 0.3% carbon monoxide, which is taken up avidly by haemoglobin in pulmonary capillaries. After a short breath-hold, the rate of disappearance of CO into the circulation is calculated from a sample of expirate, and expressed as the TL_{CO} or carbon monoxide transfer factor. Helium is also included in the test breath to allow calculation of the volume of lung examined by the test breath. Transfer factor expressed per unit lung volume is termed K_{CO}. Common respiratory function abnormalities are summarised in Box 17.4.

Arterial blood gases and oximetry

The measurement of hydrogen ion concentration, PaO_2 and $PaCO_2$, and derived bicarbonate concentration in an arterial blood sample is essential for assessing the degree and type of respiratory failure and for measuring acid–base status. This is discussed in detail on pages 496 and 630 (see Box 17.16). Interpretation of results is facilitated by blood gas diagrams (Fig. 17.8), which indicate whether any acidosis or alkalosis is due to acute or chronic respiratory derangements of $PaCO_2$ or to metabolic causes.

Pulse oximeters provide a continuous estimation of arterial oxygen saturation (SaO_2, or SpO_2 if measured by pulse oximetry) (see p.177), thus allowing a real-time assessment of a patient's response to oxygen therapy.

Exercise tests

Resting measurements may be unhelpful in early disease or in patients complaining only of exercise-induced symptoms. Spirometry testing before and after exercise can help to reveal exercise-induced asthma. Walk tests include the self-paced 6-minute walk and the externally

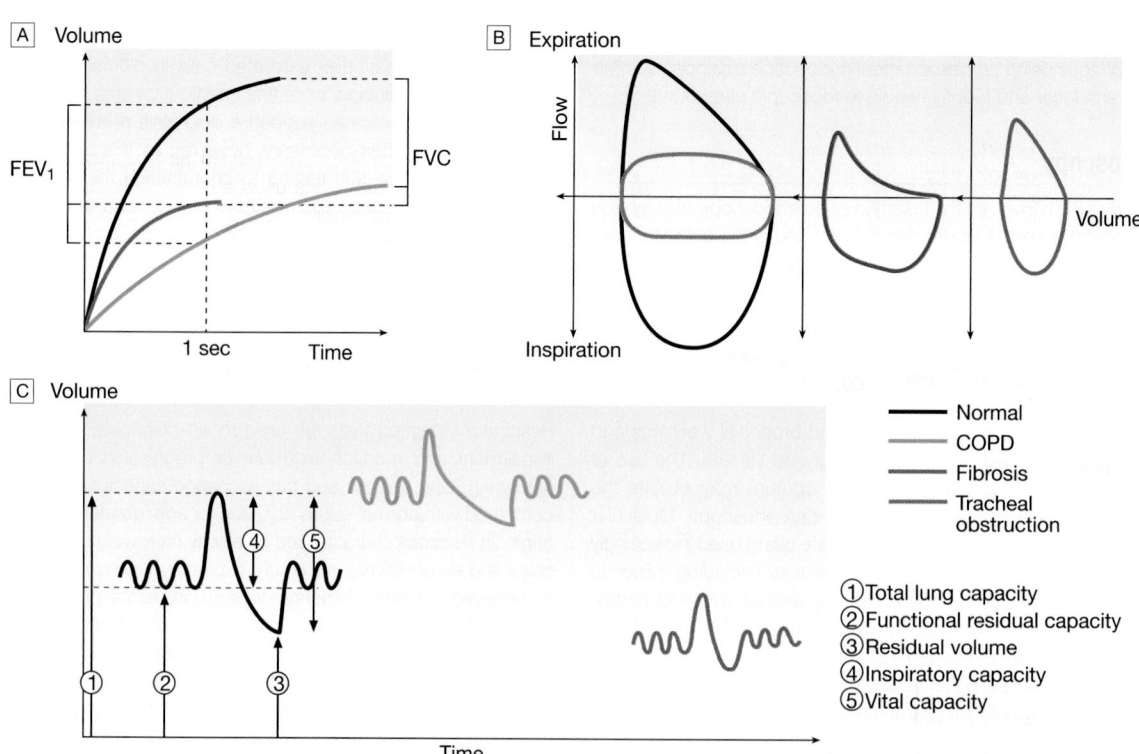

Fig. 17.7 Respiratory function tests in health and disease. [A] Volume/time traces from forced expiration in health, chronic obstructive pulmonary disease (COPD) and fibrosis. COPD causes slow, prolonged and limited exhalation. In fibrosis, forced expiration results in rapid expulsion of a reduced forced vital capacity (FVC). Forced expiratory volume (FEV_1) is reduced in both diseases but disproportionately so, compared to FVC, in COPD. [B] The same data plotted as flow/volume loops. In COPD, collapse of intrathoracic airways limits flow, particularly during mid- and late expiration. The blue trace illustrates large airway obstruction, which particularly limits peak flow rates. [C] Lung volume measurement. Volume/time graphs during quiet breathing with a single maximal breath in and out. COPD causes hyperinflation with increased residual volume. Fibrosis causes a proportional reduction in all lung volumes.

17.4 How to interpret respiratory function abnormalities

	Asthma	Chronic bronchitis	Emphysema	Pulmonary fibrosis
FEV$_1$	↓↓	↓↓	↓↓	↓
FVC	↓	↓	↓	↓↓
FEV$_1$/FVC	↓	↓	↓	→/↑
TL$_{CO}$	→	→	↓↓	↓↓
K$_{CO}$	→/↑	→	↓	→/↓
TLC	→/↑	↑	↑↑	↓
RV	→/↑	↑	↑↑	↓

(RV = residual volume; TLC = total lung capacity; see text for other abbreviations)

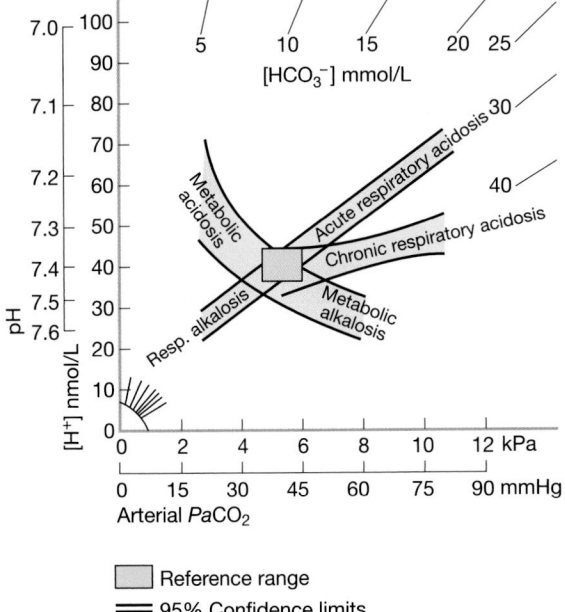

Reference range
95% Confidence limits

Fig. 17.8 Changes in blood [H$^+$], *Pa*CO$_2$ and plasma [HCO3$^-$] in acid–base disorders. The rectangle indicates normal limits for [H$^+$] and *Pa*CO$_2$. The bands represent 95% confidence limits of single disturbances in human blood. To determine the likely cause of an acid–base disorder, plot the values of [H$^+$] and *Pa*CO$_2$ from an arterial blood gas measurement. The diagram indicates whether any acidosis or alkalosis results primarily from a respiratory disorder of *Pa*CO$_2$ or from a metabolic derangement. *From Flenley D. Lancet 1971; 1:1921, with permission from Elsevier.*

paced incremental 'shuttle' test, where patients walk at increasing pace between two cones 10 m apart. These provide simple, repeatable assessments of disability and response to treatment. Cardiopulmonary bicycle exercise testing, with measurement of metabolic gas exchange, ventilation and ECG changes, is useful for quantifying exercise limitation and detecting occult cardiovascular or respiratory limitation in a breathless patient.

Presenting problems in respiratory disease

Cough

Cough is the most frequent symptom of respiratory disease and is caused by stimulation of sensory nerves in the mucosa of the pharynx, larynx, trachea and bronchi. Acute sensitisation of the normal cough reflex occurs in a number of conditions and it is typically induced by changes in air temperature or exposure to irritants, such as cigarette smoke or perfumes. Distinguishing characteristics of various causes of cough are detailed in Box 17.5.

The explosive quality of a normal cough is lost in patients with respiratory muscle paralysis or vocal cord palsy. Paralysis of a single vocal cord gives rise to a prolonged, low-pitched, inefficient 'bovine' cough accompanied by hoarseness. Coexistence of an inspiratory noise (stridor) indicates partial obstruction of a major airway (e.g. laryngeal oedema, tracheal tumour, scarring, compression or inhaled foreign body) and requires urgent investigation and treatment. Sputum production is common in patients with acute or chronic cough, and its nature and appearance can provide clues to the aetiology.

Aetiology

Acute transient cough is most commonly caused by viral tracheobronchial infection, post-nasal drip resulting from rhinitis or sinusitis, aspiration of a foreign body, or throat-clearing secondary to laryngitis or pharyngitis. When cough occurs in the context of more serious diseases, such as pneumonia, aspiration, congestive heart failure or pulmonary embolism, it is usually easy to diagnose from other clinical features.

Patients with chronic cough present more of a challenge and should be assessed with history, physical examination, chest X-ray and lung function studies.

Adults with chronic cough and a history of tobacco exposure should be considered for CT scanning if they have either an abnormal chest X-ray or a normal X-ray and other symptoms that might suggest lung cancer.

In the context of normal respiratory examination and investigations, extra-thoracic causes of cough need to be considered such as post-nasal drip secondary to nasal or sinus disease, gastro-oesophageal reflux disease or cough hypersensitivity. Use of angiotensin-converting enzyme (ACE) inhibitors can result in a chronic dry cough, taking up to 6 months to resolve following cessation. *Bordetella pertussis* infection in adults can result in cough lasting up to 3 months.

The prescence of fine inspiratory crackles and a dry cough should prompt investigation for the possibility of an interstitial lung disease.

Breathlessness

Breathlessness or dyspnoea is defined as the feeling of an uncomfortable need to breathe. It is unusual among sensations, as it has no defined receptors, no localised representation in the brain, and multiple causes both in health (e.g. exercise) and in diseases of the lungs, heart or muscles.

Pathophysiology

Stimuli to breathing resulting from disease processes are shown in Figure 17.9. Respiratory diseases can stimulate breathing and dyspnoea by:

- stimulating intrapulmonary sensory nerves (e.g. pneumothorax, interstitial inflammation and pulmonary embolus)
- increasing the mechanical load on the respiratory muscles (e.g. airflow obstruction or pulmonary fibrosis)
- causing hypoxia, hypercapnia or acidosis, which stimulate chemoreceptors.

In cardiac failure, pulmonary congestion reduces lung compliance and can also obstruct the small airways. Reduced cardiac output also limits oxygen supply to the skeletal muscles during exercise, causing early lactic acidaemia and further stimulating breathing via the central chemoreceptors.

Breathlessness and the effects of treatment can be quantified using a symptom scale. Patients tend to report breathlessness in proportion to the sum of the above stimuli to breathing. Individual patients differ greatly in the intensity of breathlessness reported for a given set of circumstances, but breathlessness scores during exercise within individuals are reproducible and can be used to monitor the effects of therapy.

17

	17.5 **Cough**	
Origin	**Common causes**	**Clinical features**
Pharynx	Post-nasal drip	History of chronic rhinitis
Larynx	Laryngitis, tumour, whooping cough, croup	Voice or swallowing altered, harsh or painful cough Paroxysms of cough, often associated with stridor
Trachea	Tracheitis	Raw retrosternal pain with cough
Bronchi	Bronchitis (acute) and chronic obstructive pulmonary disease (COPD)	Dry or productive, worse in mornings
	Asthma	Usually dry, worse at night
	Eosinophilic bronchitis	Features similar to asthma but airway hyper-reactivity absent
	Lung cancer	Persistent (often with haemoptysis)
Lung parenchyma	Tuberculosis	Productive (often with haemoptysis)
	Pneumonia	Dry initially, productive later Atypical pneumonias including COVID-19 often present with a dry cough
	Bronchiectasis	Productive, changes in posture induce sputum production
	Pulmonary oedema	Often at night (may be productive of pink, frothy sputum)
	Interstitial fibrosis	Dry and distressing
Drug side-effect	Angiotensin-converting enzyme (ACE) inhibitors	Dry cough
Aspiration	Gastro-oesophageal reflux disease (GORD)	History of acid reflux, heartburn, hiatus hernia Obesity

Adapted from Munro JF, Campbell IW. Macleod's Clinical examination, 10th edn. Edinburgh: Churchill Livingstone, Elsevier Ltd; 2000.

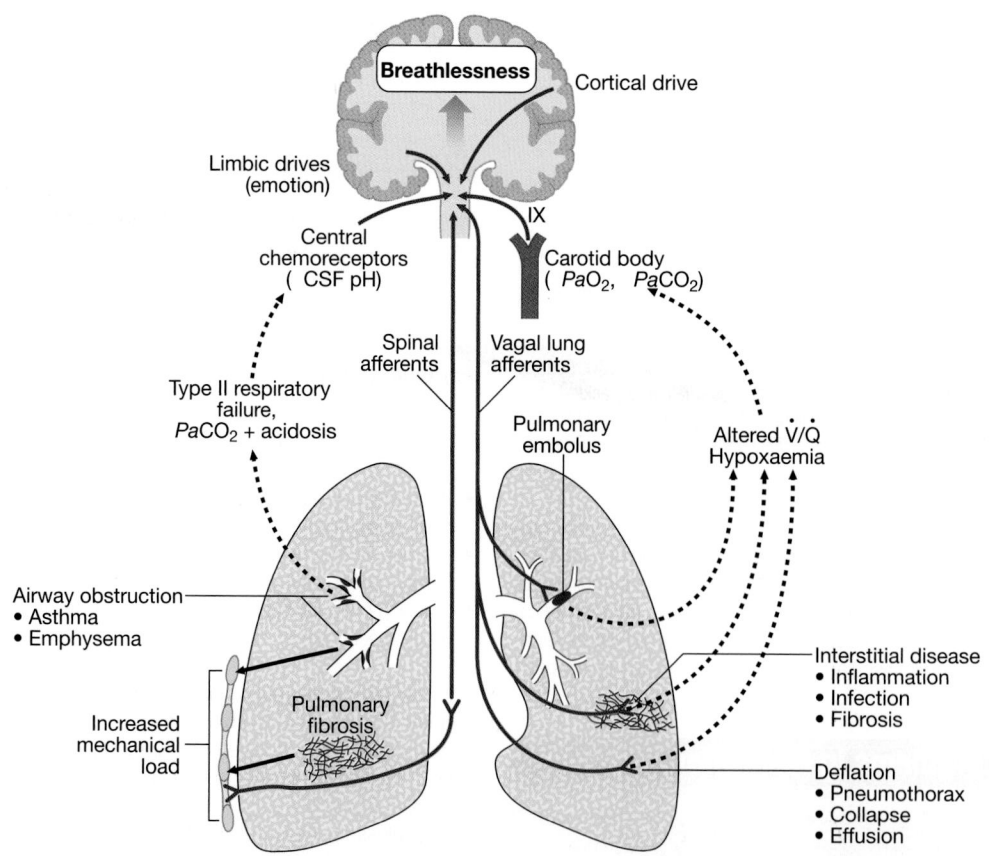

Fig. 17.9 Respiratory stimuli contributing to breathlessness. Mechanisms by which disease can stimulate the respiratory motor neurons in the medulla. Breathlessness is usually felt in proportion to the sum of these stimuli. Further explanation is given on page 181. (CSF = cerebrospinal fluid; V̇/Q̇ = ventilation/perfusion ratio; IX = glosso-pharyngeal nerve)

Differential diagnosis

Patients may present with either chronic exertional breathlessness or as an emergency with acute breathlessness, with prominent symptoms even at rest. The causes are classified in Box 17.6.

Chronic exertional breathlessness

The cause of breathlessness is often apparent from the clinical history. Key questions are detailed below.

How is your breathing at rest and overnight?

In COPD, there is a fixed, structural limit to maximum ventilation, and a tendency for progressive hyperinflation during exercise. Breathlessness is apparent mainly when walking and patients usually report minimal symptoms at rest and overnight. In contrast, patients with significant asthma are often woken from their sleep by breathlessness with chest tightness and wheeze.

Orthopnoea is common in COPD, as well as in heart disease, because airflow obstruction is made worse by cranial displacement of the diaphragm by the abdominal contents when recumbent, so many patients choose to sleep propped up. Thus it is not a useful differentiating symptom unless there is a clear history of previous angina or infarction to suggest cardiac disease.

How much can you do on a good day?

Noting 'breathless on exertion' is not enough; the approximate distance the patient can walk on the level should be documented, along with capacity to climb inclines or stairs. Variability within and between days is a hallmark of asthma; in mild asthma, the patient may be free of symptoms and signs when well. Gradual, progressive loss of exercise capacity over months and years, with consistent disability over days, is typical of COPD. When asthma is suspected, the degree of variability can be detected by home peak flow monitoring.

Relentless, progressive breathlessness that is also present at rest, often accompanied by a dry cough, suggests interstitial lung disease. Impaired left ventricular function can also cause chronic exertional breathlessness, cough and wheeze. A history of angina, hypertension or myocardial infarction raises the possibility of a cardiac cause. This may be confirmed by a displaced apex beat, a raised JVP and cardiac murmurs (although these signs can occur in severe hypoxic lung disease with fluid retention). The chest X-ray may show cardiomegaly and an ECG and echocardiogram may provide evidence of left ventricular disease. Measurement of arterial blood gases may help, as, in the absence of an intracardiac shunt or pulmonary oedema, the PaO_2 in cardiac disease is normal and the $PaCO_2$ is low or normal.

Did you have breathing problems in childhood or at school?

When present, a history of childhood wheeze increases the likelihood of asthma, although this history may be absent in late-onset asthma. A history of atopic disease also increases the likelihood of asthma.

Do you have other symptoms along with your breathlessness?

Digital or perioral paraesthesiae and a feeling that 'I cannot get a deep enough breath in' are typical features of breathing pattern disorders but this cannot be diagnosed until other potential causes have been excluded. Additional symptoms include lightheadedness, central chest discomfort and occasionally carpopedal spasm due to acute respiratory alkalosis. These alarming symptoms may provoke further anxiety and exacerbate hyperventilation. Breathing pattern disorders rarely disturb sleep, can occur at rest, and may be provoked by stress. The Nijmegen questionnaire can be used to score some of the typical symptoms of breathing pattern disorders (Box 17.7). Arterial blood gases show normal (or high) PO_2, low PCO_2 and alkalosis.

Pleuritic chest pain in a patient with chronic breathlessness, particularly if it occurs in more than one site over time, should raise suspicion of thromboembolic disease, which can occasionally present as chronic breathlessness with no other specific features and should always be considered before a diagnosis of breathing pattern disorder is made.

Morning headache is an important symptom in patients with breathlessness, as it may signal the onset of carbon dioxide retention and respiratory failure. This is particularly significant in patients with musculoskeletal disease impairing respiratory function (e.g. kyphoscoliosis or muscular dystrophy).

Acute severe breathlessness

This is one of the most common and dramatic medical emergencies. Although respiratory causes are common, it can result from cardiac disease, metabolic disease or poisoning causing acidosis, or from psychogenic causes. The approach to patients with acute severe breathlessness is covered on page 181.

17

i | 17.6 Causes of breathlessness

System	Acute dyspnoea	Chronic exertional dyspnoea
Cardiovascular	Acute pulmonary oedema*	Chronic heart failure Myocardial ischaemia (angina equivalent)
Respiratory	Acute severe asthma* Acute exacerbation of COPD* Pneumothorax* Bacterial and viral pneumonias* Pulmonary embolus* ARDS Inhaled foreign body (especially in children) Lobar collapse Laryngeal oedema (e.g. anaphylaxis)	COPD* Chronic asthma* Lung cancer Interstitial lung disease (sarcoidosis, fibrosing alveolitis, extrinsic allergic alveolitis, pneumoconiosis) Chronic pulmonary thromboembolism Lymphangitis carcinomatosis (may cause intolerable breathlessness) Large pleural effusion(s)
Others	Metabolic acidosis (e.g. diabetic ketoacidosis, lactic acidosis, uraemia, overdose of salicylates, ethylene glycol poisoning) Psychogenic hyperventilation (anxiety- or panic-related)	Severe anaemia Obesity Deconditioning

*Denotes a common cause.
(ARDS = acute respiratory distress syndrome; COPD = chronic obstructive pulmonary disease)

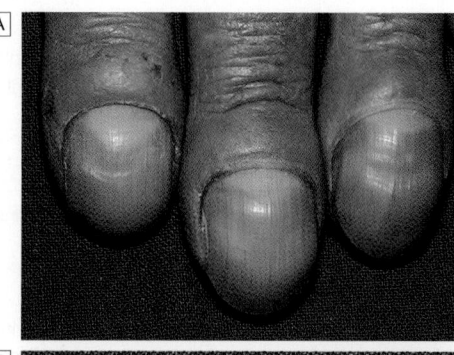
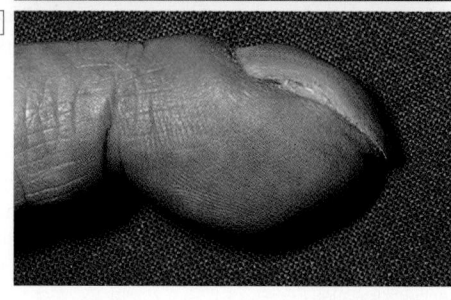

Fig. 17.10 Finger clubbing. A Anterior view. B Lateral view. *From Douglas G, Nicol F, Robertson C. Macleod's Clinical examination, 13th edn. Edinburgh: Churchill Livingstone, Elsevier Ltd; 2013.*

Chest pain

Chest pain can result from cardiac, respiratory, oesophageal or musculoskeletal disorders. The approach to this common symptom is covered on page 179.

Finger clubbing

Finger clubbing describes painless swelling of the soft tissues of the terminal phalanges, causing increased longitudinal and lateral convexity of the nail (Fig. 17.10). Upward displacement of the proximal nail margin causes the anteroposterior diameter of the finger at that point to exceed that at the distal interphalangeal joint. It also removes the normal hyponychial angle between the proximal part of the nail and the adjoining skin. Clubbing usually affects the fingers symmetrically and commonly also involves the toes, but can be unilateral if caused by a proximal vascular condition, e.g. arteriovenous shunts for dialysis. Although clubbing is usually idiopathic, it can be associated with suppurative or malignant lung conditions (Box 17.8). Clubbing may recede if the underlying condition resolves, e.g. following lung transplantation for cystic fibrosis.

Haemoptysis

Coughing up blood is an alarming symptom and patients nearly always seek medical advice. Care should be taken to establish that it is true haemoptysis and not haematemesis, or gum or nose bleeding. Haemoptysis must always be assumed to have a serious cause until this is excluded (Box 17.9).

Many episodes of haemoptysis remain unexplained, even after full investigation, and are likely to be due to simple bronchial infection. A history of repeated small haemoptysis, or blood-streaking of sputum, is highly suggestive of lung cancer. Fever, night sweats and weight loss suggest tuberculosis. Pneumococcal pneumonia often causes 'rusty'-coloured sputum but can cause frank haemoptysis, as can all suppurative respiratory infections. Lung abscess, bronchiectasis and intracavitary mycetoma can cause catastrophic bronchial haemorrhage. Finally, pulmonary thromboembolism is a common cause of haemoptysis and should always be considered.

Physical examination may reveal additional clues. Finger clubbing suggests lung cancer or bronchiectasis; other signs of malignancy, such as cachexia, hepatomegaly and lymphadenopathy, should also be sought. Fever, pleural rub and signs of consolidation occur in pneumonia or pulmonary infarction; a minority of patients with pulmonary infarction also have unilateral leg swelling or pain suggestive of deep venous thrombosis. Rashes, haematuria and digital infarcts point to an underlying systemic disease such as a vasculitis, which may cause haemoptysis.

Management

In severe acute haemoptysis the patient should be nursed upright (or on the side of the bleeding, if this is known), given high-flow oxygen and resuscitated as required. Bronchoscopy in the acute phase is difficult and often merely shows blood throughout the bronchial tree. Infusions of the antifibrinolytic agent tranexamic acid or the vasopressin precursor terlipressin may help to limit bleeding but evidence of efficacy is limited. If radiology shows an obvious central cause, then rigid bronchoscopy under general anaesthesia may allow intervention to stop bleeding; however, the

source often cannot be visualised. Intubation with a divided endotracheal tube may allow protected ventilation of the unaffected lung to stabilise the patient. Bronchial arteriography and embolisation (Fig. 17.11), or even emergency surgery, can be life-saving in the acute situation.

In the vast majority of cases, however, the haemoptysis itself is not life-threatening and a logical sequence of investigations can be followed:

- Chest X-ray may provide evidence of a localised lesion such as tumour, pneumonia, mycetoma or tuberculosis
- Full blood count (FBC) and clotting screen
- CTPA may show underlying pulmonary thromboembolic disease or alternative causes not seen on the chest X-ray (e.g. pulmonary arteriovenous malformation or small or hidden tumours)
- Bronchoscopic biopsy (after acute bleeding has settled) if the CT scan suggests an abnormality that needs biopsy.

'Incidental' pulmonary nodule

A pulmonary nodule may be defined as a well or poorly circumscribed, approximately rounded structure that appears on imaging as a focal opacity less than 3 cm in diameter that is surrounded by aerated lung. 'Incidental' pulmonary nodules have become increasingly common with the increased use of CT scanning (Fig. 17.12). Nodules must not be dismissed as 'incidental', however, until either a treatable condition has been excluded or stability has been demonstrated for at least 2 years.

The list of potential causes of pulmonary nodules is extensive and most are benign (Box 17.10). Features on a CT scan consistent with a benign lesion include being less than 5 mm in diameter or less than 80 mm³ in volume; diffuse, central, laminated or popcorn calcification; or the presence of macroscopic fat. In addition, perifissural lymph nodes and subpleural nodules with a lentiform or triangular shape do not require any further investigation.

In cases where a benign lesion cannot be confidently assumed, further assessment depends on both the appearance of the nodule and the clinical context. These assessments may be aided by the use of computer prediction models (Box 17.11).

A variety of diagnostic approaches may be considered, including bronchoscopy, percutaneous needle biopsy, FDG-PET, interval CT scanning or surgical resection of the lesion. Pulmonary nodules are invariably beyond the vision of the bronchoscope and, with the notable exception of pulmonary infection (e.g. tuberculosis), the yield from blind washings is low. If the nodule is favourably located and of sufficient size, percutaneous needle biopsy under ultrasound or CT guidance may be employed. The risk of pneumothorax is approximately 15% and around 7% require intercostal drainage, so this should be contemplated only in individuals with an FEV_1 of more than 35% predicted. Haemorrhage into the lung or pleural space, air embolism and tumour seeding are rare but recognised complications.

PET-CT scanning provides useful information about nodules of at least 1 cm in diameter. The presence of high metabolic activity is strongly suggestive of malignancy, while an inactive 'cold' nodule suggests benign disease. However, a high SUV is a marker of glucose metabolism, not malignancy, and PET-CT has significant limitations in regions with high endemic rates of infectious or granulomatous disease. False-negative results may occur with neuro-endocrine tumours and minimally invasive lepidic adenocarcinoma. Detection of neuro-endocrine tumours may be improved by the use of ⁶⁸Ga-DOTATOC in place of FDG.

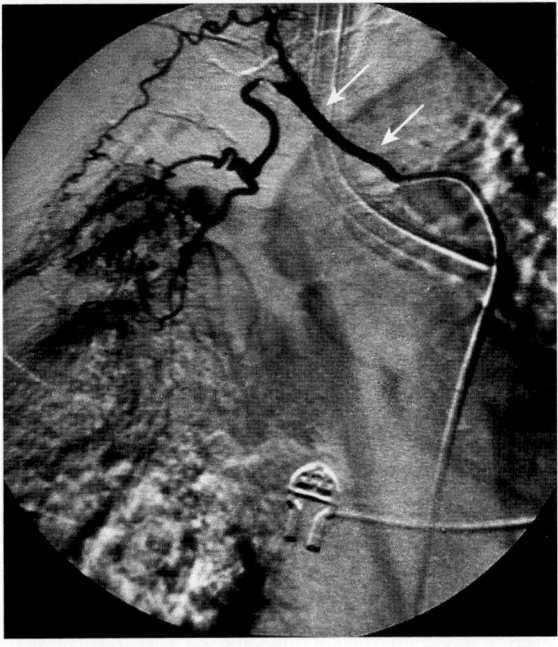

Fig. 17.11 Bronchial artery angiography. An angiography catheter has been passed via the femoral artery and aorta into an abnormally dilated right bronchial artery (arrows). Contrast is seen flowing into the lung. This patient had post-tuberculous bronchiectasis and presented with massive haemoptysis. Bronchial artery embolisation was successfully performed.

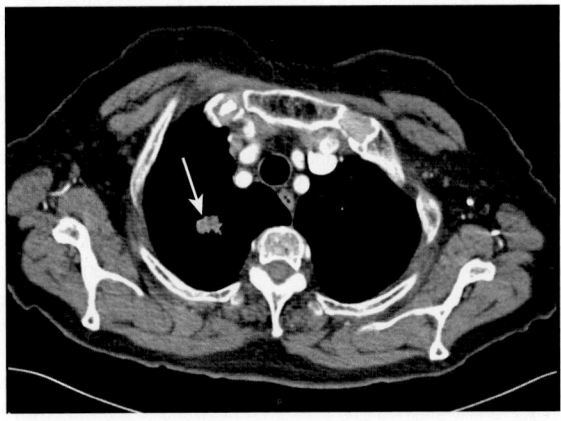

Fig. 17.12 Thoracic CT scan showing a solitary pulmonary nodule identified in the right upper lobe (arrow).

---

i 17.9 Causes of haemoptysis

Bronchial disease

- Cancer*
- Bronchiectasis*
- Acute bronchitis*
- Bronchial adenoma
- Foreign body

Parenchymal disease

- Tuberculosis*
- Suppurative pneumonia
- Parasites (e.g. hydatid disease, flukes)
- Lung abscess
- Trauma
- Actinomycosis
- Mycetoma

Lung vascular disease

- Pulmonary infarction*
- Goodpastur's disease
- Polyarteritis nodosa
- Idiopathic pulmonary haemosiderosis

Cardiovascular disease

- Acute left ventricular failure*
- Mitral stenosis
- Aortic aneurysm

Blood disorders

- Leukaemia
- Haemophilia
- Anticoagulants

*More common causes.

---

i 17.10 Causes of pulmonary nodules

Common causes

- Lung cancer
- Single metastasis
- Localised pneumonia
- Lung abscess
- Tuberculoma
- Pulmonary infarct

Uncommon causes

- Benign tumour
- Lymphoma
- Arteriovenous malformation
- Hydatid cyst
- Bronchogenic cyst
- Rheumatoid nodule
- Granulomatosis with polyangiitis (GPA)
- Pulmonary sequestration
- Pulmonary haematoma
- 'Pseudotumour' – fluid collection in a fissure
- Aspergilloma (usually surrounded by air crescent)
- *Cryptococcus*
- *Aspergillus* nodule

| i | 17.11 | Clinical and radiographic features distinguishing benign from malignant nodules* | | |

Feature	Risk of malignancy	Feature	Risk of malignancy
Characteristics of nodule		**Characteristics of patient**	
Size	Nearly all >3 cm but fewer than 1% <4 mm are malignant	Age	Increases with age and is uncommon below age of 40
Margin	Usually smooth in benign lesions	Smoking history	Increases in proportion to duration and amount smoked
	Spiculated suggests malignancy	Other	Increased by history of lung cancer in first-degree
Calcification or fat	Laminated or central deposition of calcification		relative and by exposure to asbestos, silica, uranium
	suggests granuloma		and radon
	'Popcorn' pattern suggests hamartoma		
	Fat may suggest hamartoma or lipoid granuloma		
Location	70% of lung cancers occur in upper lobes		
	Benign lesions are equally distributed throughout upper and lower lobes		

*Linear or sheet-like lung opacities are unlikely to represent neoplasms and do not require follow-up. Some nodular opacities may be sufficiently typical of scarring for follow-up not to be warranted.
Adapted from MacMahon H, Austin JH, Gamsu G, et al. Guidelines for management of small pulmonary nodules detected on CT scans: a statement from the Fleischner Society. Radiology 2005; 237:395–400.

If the nodule is small and inaccessible, interval CT scanning may be employed. A repeat CT scan at 3 months will reliably detect growth in larger nodules and may also demonstrate resolution. Further interval scans may be arranged depending on the clinical context (Fig. 17.13). Particular care must be taken with subsolid nodules, particularly if further imaging demonstrates the development of a new solid component, as these may represent a pre-malignant or an early invasive form of adenocarcinoma.

Nodules with a high clinical suspicion for malignancy despite benign or indeterminate biopsies may merit proceeding straight to surgical resection, as this represents the best chance of curative therapy for lung cancer. It is important for the logic underlying this approach to be discussed with the patient, consideration of frozen intra-operative histology, and the consequences of resection of a benign lesion explained.

Where the probability of cancer is low, the potential risk of further scanning must be considered. Subsequent scans often detect further nodules, increase the risk of false-positive findings and lead to unnecessary patient anxiety while exposing the individual to increased radiation.

Pleural effusion

The accumulation of serous fluid within the pleural space is termed pleural effusion. Accumulations of pus, blood and chyle are termed empyema, haemothorax and chylothorax respectively. In general, pleural fluid accumulates because of either increased hydrostatic pressure or decreased osmotic pressure ('transudative' effusion, as seen in cardiac, liver or renal failure), or from increased microvascular pressure due to disease of the pleura or injury in the adjacent lung ('exudative' effusion). The causes of the majority of pleural effusions (Boxes 17.12 and 17.13) are identified by a thorough history, examination and relevant investigations.

Clinical assessment

Symptoms (pain on inspiration and coughing) and signs of pleurisy (a pleural rub) often precede the development of an effusion, especially in patients with underlying pneumonia, pulmonary infarction or connective tissue disease. When breathlessness is the only symptom, however, the onset may be insidious, depending on the size and rate of accumulation. The physical signs are detailed on page 481.

Investigations

Radiological investigations

The classical appearance of pleural fluid on the erect PA chest X-ray is of a curved shadow at the lung base, blunting the costophrenic angle and ascending towards the axilla. Fluid appears to track up the lateral chest wall. In fact, fluid surrounds the whole lung at this level but casts a radiological shadow only where the X-ray beam passes tangentially across the fluid against the lateral chest wall. Around 200 mL of fluid is required in order for it to be detectable on a PA chest X-ray. Previous scarring or adhesions in the pleural space can cause localised effusions. Pleural fluid localised below the lower lobe ('subpulmonary effusion') simulates an elevated hemidiaphragm. Pleural fluid localised within an oblique fissure may produce a rounded opacity that may be mistaken for a tumour.

Ultrasound is more accurate than plain chest X-ray for determining the presence of fluid. A clear hypoechoic space is consistent with a transudate and the presence of moving, floating densities suggests an exudate. The presence of septation most likely indicates an evolving empyema or resolving haemothorax. CT scanning is indicated where there is concern for malignant disease or loculation is suspected.

Pleural aspiration and biopsy

In some conditions (e.g. left ventricular failure), it should not be necessary to sample fluid unless atypical features are present; appropriate treatment should be administered and the effusion re-evaluated. In most other circumstances, however, diagnostic sampling is required. Simple aspiration provides information on the colour and texture of fluid and these alone may immediately suggest an empyema or chylothorax. The presence of blood is consistent with pulmonary infarction or malignancy but may result from a traumatic tap. Biochemical analysis allows classification into transudate or exudate (Box 17.14). Cytological examination can characterize the presence of inflammatory or malignant cells. Microbiological staining can dectect bacteria and mycobacteria. If a diagnosis of tuberculosis is being considered, adenosine deaminase (ADA) should be measured (see p. 520). A low pH suggests infection but may also be seen in rheumatoid arthritis, ruptured oesophagus or advanced malignancy.

Ultrasound- or CT-guided pleural biopsy provides tissue for pathological and microbiological analysis. Where necessary, video-assisted thoracoscopy allows visualisation of the pleura and direct guidance of a biopsy.

Management

Therapeutic aspiration may be required to palliate breathlessness but removing more than 1.5 L at a time is associated with a small risk of re-expansion pulmonary oedema. An effusion should never be drained to dryness before establishing a diagnosis, as biopsy may be precluded until further fluid accumulates. Treatment of an underlying cause such as heart failure, pneumonia, pulmonary embolism or subphrenic abscess will often be followed by resolution of the effusion. The management of pleural effusion in pneumonia, tuberculosis and malignancy is dealt with below.

Empyema

An empyema is a collection of pus within the pleural space. Microscopically, neutrophil leucocytes are present in large numbers and bacteria may be identified on Gram's stain. An empyema may involve the whole pleural space or only part of it ('loculated' or 'encysted' empyema) and is usually unilateral. It is usually secondary to infection in a neighbouring structure, usually the lung, most commonly due to the bacterial pneumonia or tuberculosis. Over 40% of patients with community-acquired pneumonia develop an associated pleural effusion ('parapneumonic' effusion) and about 15% of these become secondarily infected. Other causes are infection of a haemothorax following trauma or surgery, oesophageal rupture, and rupture of a subphrenic abscess through the diaphragm.

Macroscopically, the pleural surfaces are covered with an inflammatory exudate. The pus can be under considerable pressure. Inadequate treatment can result in rupture into a bronchus, causing a bronchopleural fistula and pyopneumothorax, or tracking through the chest wall forming a subcutaneous abscess or sinus ('empyema necessitans').

Clinical assessment

An empyema should be suspected in patients with pulmonary infection if there is severe pleuritic chest pain or persisting or recurrent pyrexia despite appropriate antimicrobial treatment. In other cases, the primary infection may be so mild that it passes unrecognised and the first definite clinical features are due to the empyema itself. Once an empyema has developed, systemic features are prominent (Box 17.15).

Investigations

Chest X-ray appearances may be indistinguishable from those of pleural effusion, although pleural adhesions may confine the empyema to form a 'D'-shaped shadow against the inside of the chest wall (Fig. 17.14). When air is present as well as pus (pyopneumothorax), a horizontal 'fluid level' marks the air/liquid interface. Ultrasound shows the position of the fluid, the extent of pleural thickening and whether fluid is in a single collection or multiloculated, containing fibrin and debris (Fig. 17.15). CT provides information on the pleura, underlying lung parenchyma and patency of the major bronchi.

Ultrasound or CT is used to identify the optimal site for aspiration, which is best performed using a wide-bore needle. If the fluid is thick and turbid pus, empyema is confirmed. Other features suggesting empyema are a fluid glucose of less than 3.3 mmol/L (60 mg/dL), lactate dehydrogenase (LDH) of more than 1000 IU/L, or a fluid pH of less than 7.2. However, pH measurement should be avoided if pus is thick, as it damages blood gas machines. Bacterial culture may be negative if

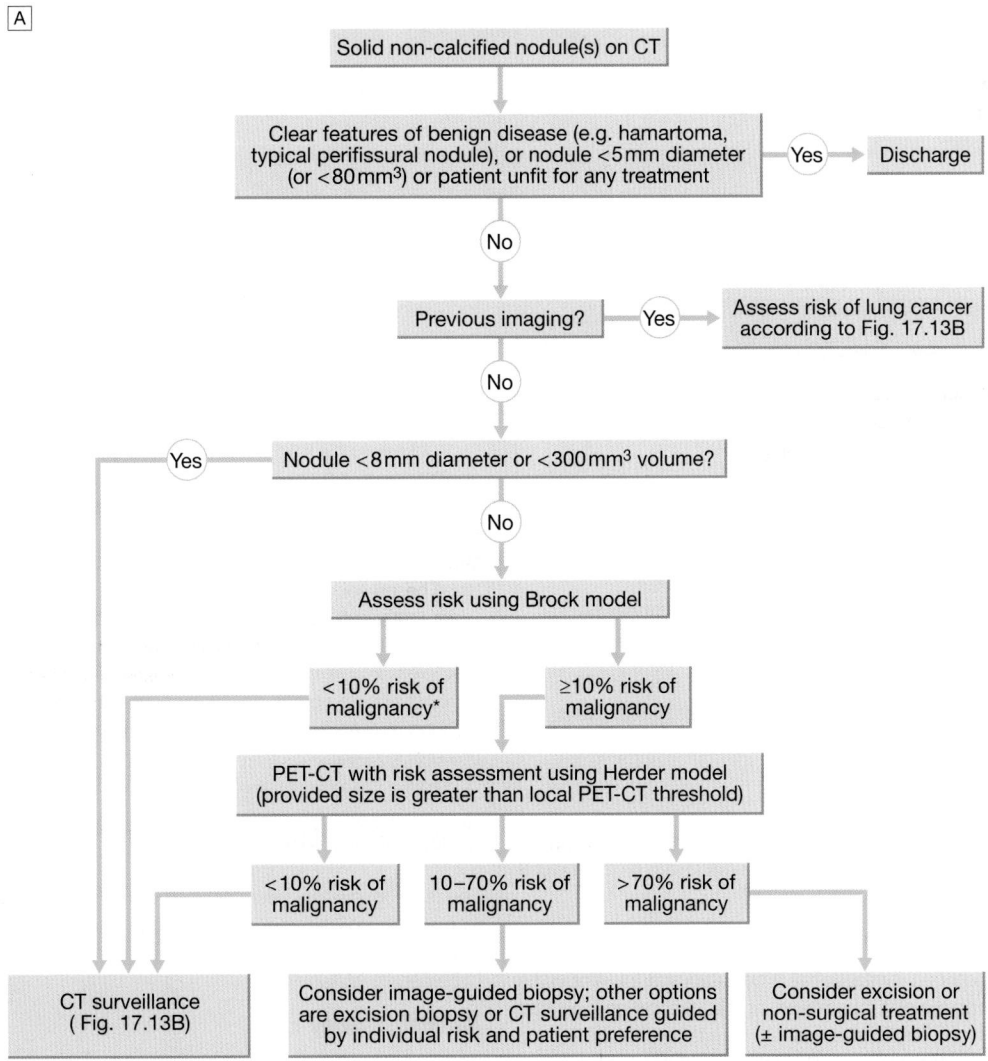

Fig. 17.13 Recommendations on the assessment of a solid pulmonary nodule. [A] Initial approach to solid pulmonary nodules. The Brock model is an online calculator that can also be downloaded as an app (https://brocku.ca/lung-cancer-risk-calculator). The model integrates data on age, sex, family history of cancer, the presence of emphysema, nodule size, nodule type, nodule position, nodule count and speculation, and calculates the probability that a nodule will become malignant within a 2- to 4-year follow-up period. Herder is a similar model. *Consider positron emission tomography–computed tomography (PET-CT) for larger nodules in young patients with low risk by Brock score, as this score was developed in a screening cohort (50–75 years) and so performance in younger patients is unproven. *Continues overleaf*

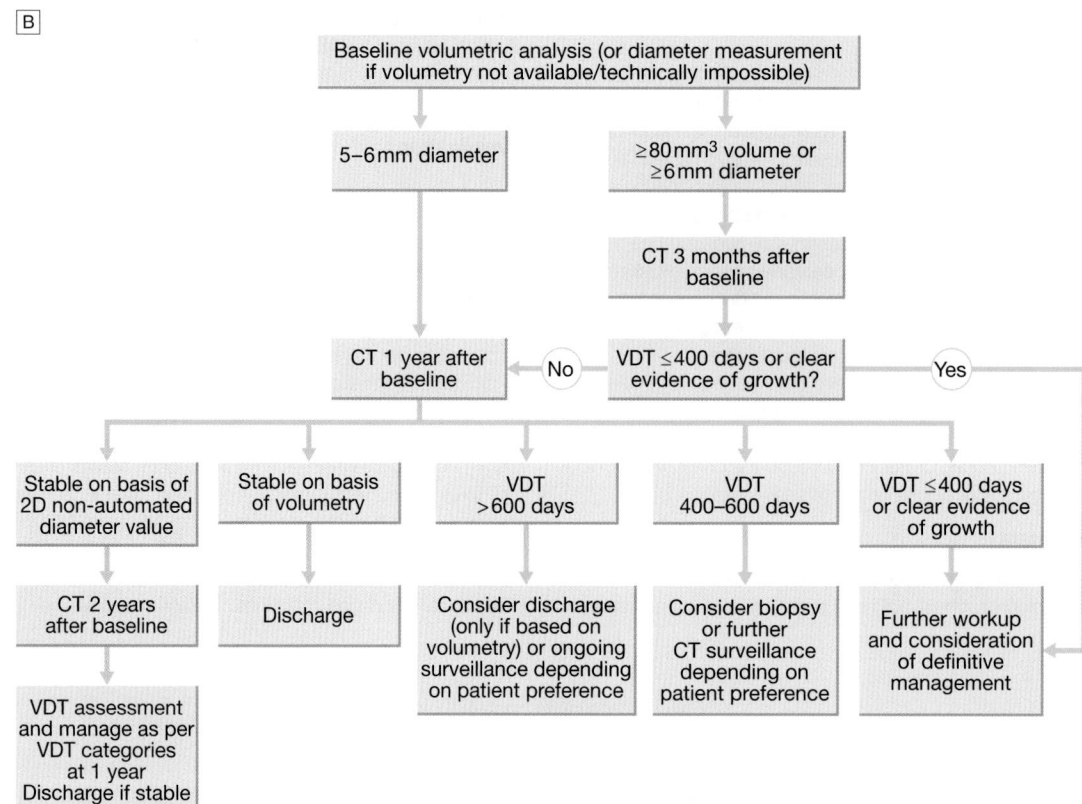

Fig. 17.13, cont'd [B] Solid pulmonary nodule surveillance algorithm. (VDT = volume doubling time) *From Callister ME, Baldwin DR, Akram AR, et al. British Thoracic Society Guidelines on the investigation and management of pulmonary nodules. Thorax 2015; Suppl. 2:ii1–ii54.*

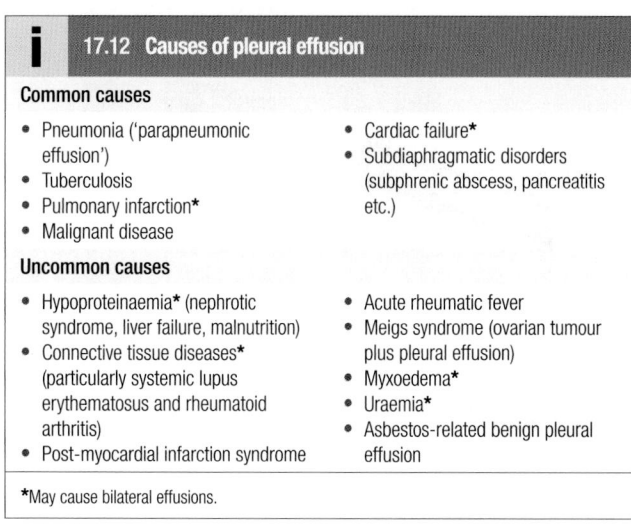

i 17.12 Causes of pleural effusion

Common causes

- Pneumonia ('parapneumonic effusion')
- Tuberculosis
- Pulmonary infarction*
- Malignant disease
- Cardiac failure*
- Subdiaphragmatic disorders (subphrenic abscess, pancreatitis etc.)

Uncommon causes

- Hypoproteinaemia* (nephrotic syndrome, liver failure, malnutrition)
- Connective tissue diseases* (particularly systemic lupus erythematosus and rheumatoid arthritis)
- Post-myocardial infarction syndrome
- Acute rheumatic fever
- Meigs syndrome (ovarian tumour plus pleural effusion)
- Myxoedema*
- Uraemia*
- Asbestos-related benign pleural effusion

*May cause bilateral effusions.

antibiotics have already been given. The distinction between tuberculous and non-tuberculous disease can be difficult and may require pleural biopsy, histology and microbiological tests.

Management

An empyema will heal only if infection is eradicated and the empyema space is obliterated, allowing apposition of the visceral and parietal pleural layers. This can only occur if all the pus is removed from the pleural space. When the pus is sufficiently thin this is most easily achieved by the insertion of a wide-bore intercostal tube into the most dependent part of the empyema space. If the initial aspirate reveals turbid fluid or frank pus, or if loculations are seen on ultrasound, the tube should be put on suction (−5 to −10 cmH$_2$O) and flushed regularly with 20 mL normal saline. Antibiotics should not be started until

they are deemed clinically necessary, and ideally not until a sample has been taken and the causative organism identified. If an organism is identified, the narrowest spectrum antibiotic that will cover that organism should be used. If not, empirical antibiotic treatment (e.g. intravenous co-amoxiclav 1.2 g 8-hourly or cefuroxime 1.5 g 12-hourly plus metronidazole 500 mg 8-hourly) should be used. Antibiotics should be continued until the infection has resolved and inflammatory markers have normalised, usually about 2–4 weeks. There is no consensus on the optimum duration of intravenous vs. oral antibiotics. The use of intrapleural fibrinolytics in combination with DNAase has been shown to be beneficial.

An empyema can be sucessfully treated with a combination of antibiotics and pleual drainage, but delays can result in a failure of these therapies, and a need for surgical intervention to clear the empyema cavity of pus and break down any adhesions. Surgical 'decortication' of the lung may also be required if gross thickening of the visceral pleura is preventing re-expansion of the lung. Surgery is also necessary if a bronchopleural fistula or empyema necessitans develops.

Respiratory failure

The term 'respiratory failure' is used when pulmonary gas exchange fails to maintain normal arterial oxygen and carbon dioxide levels. Its classification into types I and II is defined by the absence or presence of hypercapnia (raised $PaCO_2$).

Pathophysiology

When disease impairs ventilation of part of a lung (e.g. in asthma or pneumonia), perfusion of that region results in hypoxic and CO_2-laden blood entering the pulmonary veins. Increased ventilation of neighbouring regions of normal lung can increase CO_2 excretion, correcting arterial CO_2 to normal, but cannot augment oxygen uptake because the haemoglobin flowing through these normal regions is already fully saturated.

17.13 Pleural effusion: main causes and features

Cause	Appearance of fluid	Type of fluid	Predominant cells in fluid	Other diagnostic features
Tuberculosis	Serous, usually amber-coloured	Exudate	Lymphocytes (occasionally polymorphs)	Positive tuberculin test Isolation of *Mycobacterium tuberculosis* from pleural fluid (20%) Positive pleural biopsy (80%) Raised adenosine deaminase
Malignant disease	Serous, often blood-stained	Exudate	Serosal cells and lymphocytes Often clumps of malignant cells	Positive pleural biopsy (40%) Evidence of malignancy elsewhere
Cardiac failure	Serous, straw-coloured	Transudate	Few serosal cells	Other signs of cardiac failure Response to diuretics
Pulmonary infarction	Serous or blood-stained	Exudate (rarely transudate)	Red blood cells Eosinophils	Evidence of pulmonary infarction Obvious source of embolism Factors predisposing to venous thrombosis
Rheumatoid disease	Serous Turbid if chronic	Exudate	Lymphocytes (occasionally polymorphs)	Rheumatoid arthritis: rheumatoid factor and anti-cyclic citrullinated peptide (anti-CCP) antibodies Cholesterol in chronic effusion; very low glucose in pleural fluid
Systemic lupus erythematosus (SLE)	Serous	Exudate	Lymphocytes and serosal cells	Other signs of SLE Antinuclear factor or anti-DNA positive
Acute pancreatitis	Serous or blood-stained	Exudate	No cells predominate	Higher amylase in pleural fluid than in serum
Obstruction of thoracic duct	Milky	Chyle	None	Chylomicrons

17.14 Light's criteria for distinguishing pleural transudate from exudate

Exudate is likely if one or more of the following criteria are met:
- Pleural fluid protein:serum protein ratio >0.5
- Pleural fluid LDH:serum LDH ratio >0.6
- Pleural fluid LDH > two-thirds of the upper limit of normal serum LDH

(LDH = lactate dehydrogenase)

17.15 Clinical features of empyema

Systemic features
- Pyrexia, usually high and remittent
- Rigors, sweating, malaise and weight loss
- Polymorphonuclear leucocytosis, high C-reactive protein

Local features
- Pleural pain; breathlessness; cough and sputum, usually because of underlying lung disease; copious purulent sputum if empyema ruptures into a bronchus (bronchopleural fistula)
- Clinical signs of pleural effusion

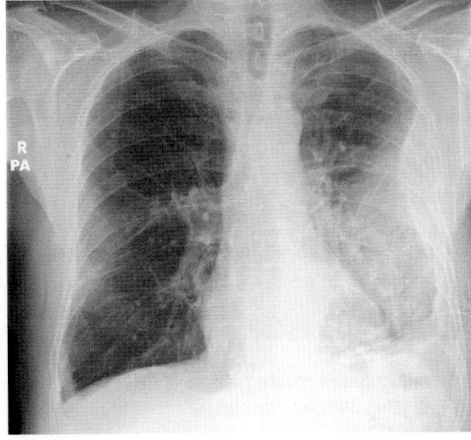

Fig. 17.14 Chest X-ray showing a 'D'-shaped shadow in the left mid-zone, consistent with an empyema. In this case, an intercostal chest drain has been inserted but the loculated collection of pus remains.

Admixture of blood from the under-ventilated and normal regions thus results in hypoxia with normocapnia, which is called 'type I respiratory failure'. Diseases causing this include all those that impair ventilation locally with sparing of other regions (Box 17.16).

Arterial hypoxia with hypercapnia (type II respiratory failure) is seen in conditions that cause generalised, severe ventilation–perfusion mismatch, leaving insufficient normal lung to correct $PaCO_2$, or any disease that reduces total ventilation. The latter includes not just diseases of the lung but also disorders affecting any part of the neuromuscular mechanism of ventilation (see Box 17.16). Acute type II respiratory failure is an emergency requiring immediate intervention. It is useful to distinguish between patients with high ventilatory drive (rapid respiratory rate and accessory muscle recruitment) who cannot move sufficient air, and those with reduced or inadequate respiratory effort.

Management of acute respiratory failure

Prompt diagnosis and management of the underlying cause is crucial. In type I respiratory failure, oxygen should be administed and titrated to maintain a normal arterial oxygen saturation (SaO_2), which will usually relieve hypoxia by increasing the alveolar PO_2 in poorly ventilated lung units. Occasionally, however (e.g. severe pneumonia affecting several lobes), mechanical ventilation may be needed to relieve hypoxia.

If inspiratory stridor is present then an upper or large airway issue should be considered. This can include acute upper airway obstruction, foreign body inhalation or laryngeal obstruction (angioedema, carcinoma or vocal cord paralysis). Depending on cause, the Heimlich manoeuvre, immediate intubation or emergency tracheostomy may be required.

More commonly, the problem is within the lungs, with severe generalised bronchial obstruction from COPD or asthma, acute respiratory distress syndrome (ARDS), or tension pneumothorax. Oxygen should be administered to maintain the SaO_2 within the target range of 94%–98%, or 88%–92% for those patients at risk of type II respiratory failure, pending a rapid examination of the respiratory system and measurement of arterial blood gases. Patients with the trachea deviated away from a silent and resonant hemithorax are likely to have tension pneumothorax, and air should be aspirated from the pleural space and a chest drain inserted as soon as possible. Patients with generalised wheeze, scanty breath sounds bilaterally or a history of asthma or COPD should be treated with salbutamol 2.5 mg nebulised with oxygen, repeated until bronchospasm is relieved. Failure to respond to initial treatment, declining conscious level and worsening respiratory acidosis (pH <7.35), $PaCO_2$ >6.6 kPa) on blood gases are all indications that supported ventilation is required.

A small proportion of patients with severe chronic lung disease and type II respiratory failure develop abnormal tolerance to raised $PaCO_2$ and may become dependent on hypoxic drive to breathe. In these patients only, lower concentrations of oxygen (24%–28% by Venturi mask) should be used to avoid precipitating worsening respiratory depression (see below). In all cases, regular monitoring of arterial blood gases is important to assess progress.

Patients with acute type II respiratory failure who have reduced drive or conscious level may be suffering from sedative poisoning, CO_2 narcosis or a primary failure of neurological drive (e.g. following intracerebral haemorrhage or head injury). History from a witness may be invaluable, and reversal of specific drugs with (for example) opiate antagonists is occasionally successful, but should not delay intubation and supported mechanical ventilation in appropriate cases.

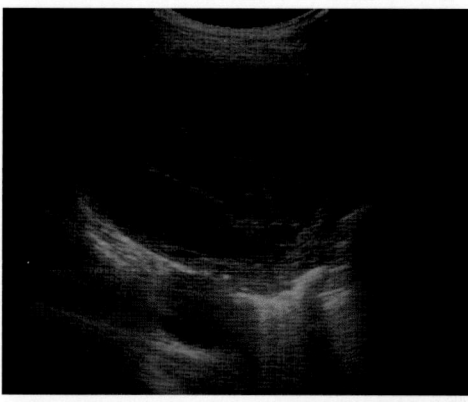

Fig. 17.15 Pleural ultrasound showing septation. *Courtesy of Dr P. Sivasothy, Department of Respiratory Medicine, Addenbrooke's Hospital, Cambridge.*

Chronic and 'acute on chronic' type II respiratory failure

The most common cause of chronic type II respiratory failure is severe COPD. Although $PaCO_2$ may be persistently raised, there is no persisting acidaemia because the kidneys retain bicarbonate, correcting arterial pH to normal. This 'compensated' pattern, which may also occur in chronic neuromuscular disease, kyphoscoliosis or other end-stage respiratory diseases, is maintained until there is a further acute illness (see Box 17.16), such as an exacerbation of COPD that precipitates an episode of 'acute on chronic' respiratory failure, with acidaemia and initial respiratory distress followed by drowsiness and eventually coma. These patients have lost their chemosensitivity to elevated $PaCO_2$, and so they may paradoxically depend on hypoxia for respiratory drive and are at risk of respiratory depression if given high concentrations of oxygen, e.g. during ambulance transfers or in emergency departments. Moreover, in contrast to acute severe asthma, some patients with 'acute on chronic' type II respiratory failure due to COPD may not appear distressed, despite being critically ill with severe hypoxaemia, hypercapnia and acidaemia. While the physical signs of CO_2 retention (delirium, flapping tremor, bounding pulses and so on) can be helpful if present, they may not be, so measurement of arterial blood gases is mandatory in the assessment of initial severity and response to treatment.

Management

The principal aims of treatment in acute on chronic type II respiratory failure are to achieve a safe PaO_2 (>7.0 kPa (52 mmHg)) without increasing $PaCO_2$ and acidosis, while identifying and treating the precipitating condition. In these patients, it is not necessary to achieve a normal PaO_2; even a small increase will greatly improve tissue oxygen delivery, since their PaO_2 values are often on the steep part of the oxygen dissociation curve (see Fig. 9.10). The risks of worsening hypercapnia and coma must be balanced against those of severe hypoxaemia, which include potentially fatal arrhythmias and hypoxic brain damage. Immediate treatment is shown in Box 17.17. Patients who are conscious and have adequate respiratory drive may benefit from non-invasive ventilation (NIV), which has been shown to reduce mortality and the requirement for intubation, and shorten hospital stay in acidotic exacerbations of COPD. Patients who are drowsy and have low respiratory drive require an urgent decision regarding intubation and ventilation, as this is likely to be the only effective treatment, even though weaning off the ventilator may be difficult in severe disease. The decision is challenging, and important factors to consider include patient wishes, presence of a potentially remediable precipitating condition, prior functional capacity and quality of life. The

17.16	How to interpret blood gas abnormalities in respiratory failure				
	Type I		**Type II**	
	Hypoxia (PaO_2 <8.0 kPa (60 mmHg)) Normal or low $PaCO_2$ ($\leq$ 6 kPa (45 mmHg))		Hypoxia (PaO_2 <8.0 kPa (60 mmHg)) Raised $PaCO_2$ (>6 kPa (45 mmHg))	
	Acute	Chronic	Acute	Chronic
H⁺	→	→	↑	→ or ↑
Bicarbonate	→	→	→	↑
Causes	Acute asthma Pulmonary oedema Pneumonia Lobar collapse Pneumothorax Pulmonary embolus ARDS	COPD Lung fibrosis Lymphangitic carcinomatosis Right-to-left shunts	Acute severe asthma Acute exacerbation of COPD Upper airway obstruction Acute neuropathies/paralysis Narcotic drugs Primary alveolar hypoventilation Flail chest injury	COPD Sleep apnoea Kyphoscoliosis Myopathies/muscular dystrophy Ankylosing spondylitis

(ARDS = acute respiratory distress syndrome; COPD = chronic obstructive pulmonary disease)

various types of non-invasive (via a face or nasal mask) or invasive (via an endotracheal tube) ventilation are detailed on page 207. Respiratory stimulant drugs, such as doxapram, have been superseded by non-invasive or invasive ventilation.

Home ventilation for chronic respiratory failure

NIV is of significant benefit in the long-term treatment of respiratory failure due to spinal deformity, neuromuscular disease and central alveolar hypoventilation. Some patients with advanced lung disease, e.g. COPD and cystic fibrosis, also benefit from NIV for respiratory failure. In these conditions, type II respiratory failure can develop slowly and insidiously. Morning headache (due to elevated $PaCO_2$) and fatigue are common symptoms but, in many cases, the diagnosis is revealed only by sleep studies or morning blood gas analysis. In the initial stages, ventilation is insufficient for metabolic needs only during sleep, when there is a physiological decline in ventilatory drive. Over time, however, CO_2 retention becomes chronic, with renal compensation of acidosis. Treatment by home-based NIV overnight is often sufficient to restore the daytime PCO_2 to normal, and to relieve fatigue and headache. In advanced disease (e.g. muscular dystrophies or cystic fibrosis), daytime NIV may also be required.

Lung transplantation

Lung transplantation is an established treatment for carefully selected patients with advanced lung disease unresponsive to medical treatment (Box 17.18). Single-lung transplantation may be used for selected patients with advanced emphysema or lung fibrosis. This is contraindicated in patients with chronic bilateral pulmonary infection, such as cystic fibrosis and bronchiectasis, because the transplanted lung is vulnerable to cross-infection in the context of post-transplant immunosuppression, and for these individuals bilateral lung transplantation is the standard procedure. Combined heart–lung transplantation is still occasionally needed for patients with advanced congenital heart disease, such as Eisenmenger syndrome, and is preferred by some surgeons for the treatment of primary pulmonary hypertension unresponsive to medical therapy.

The prognosis following lung transplantation is improving steadily with modern immunosuppressive drugs: According to the International Society for Heart and Lung Transplantation median survival for double lung transplantation is 7.8 years. Chronic rejection with obliterative bronchiolitis continues to afflict some recipients, however. Glucocorticoids are used to manage acute rejection, but drugs that inhibit cell-mediated immunity specifically, such as ciclosporin, mycophenolate and tacrolimus, are used to prevent chronic lung allograft dysfunction (CLAD). Azithromycin, statins and total lymphoid irradiation are employed to treat progressive CLAD, but late organ failure remains a significant problem.

The major factor limiting the availability of lung transplantation is the shortage of donor lungs.

Obstructive pulmonary diseases

Asthma

Asthma is a chronic inflammatory disorder of the airways, in which many cells and cellular elements play a role. Chronic inflammation is associated with airway hyper-responsiveness that leads to recurrent episodes of wheezing, breathlessness, chest tightness and coughing, particularly at night and in the early morning. These episodes are usually associated with widespread but variable airflow obstruction within the lung that is often reversible, either spontaneously or with treatment.

The prevalence of asthma increased steadily over the latter part of last century. As asthma affects all age groups, it is one of the most common and important long-term respiratory conditions in terms of global years lived with disability (Fig. 17.16).

The development and course of asthma and the response to treatment are influenced by genetic determinants, while the rapid rise in prevalence implies that environmental factors are critically important in the development and expression of the disease. The potential role of indoor and outdoor allergens, microbial exposure, diet, vitamins, breast-feeding, tobacco smoke, air pollution and obesity have been explored but no clear consensus has emerged.

Pathophysiology

Airway hyper-reactivity (AHR) – the tendency for airways to narrow excessively in response to triggers that have little or no effect in normal individuals – is integral to the diagnosis of asthma and appears to be related, although not exclusively, to airway inflammation (Fig. 17.17). Other factors likely to be important in the behaviour of airway smooth muscle include the degree of airway narrowing and neurogenic mechanisms.

The relationship between atopy (the propensity to produce IgE) and asthma is well established and in many individuals there is a clear relationship between sensitisation and allergen exposure, as demonstrated by skin-prick reactivity or elevated serum-specific IgE. Common examples of allergens include house dust mites, pets, insect pests and fungi. Inhalation of an allergen into the airway is followed by early and late-phase bronchoconstrictor responses (Fig. 17.18). Allergic mechanisms are also implicated in some cases of occupational asthma.

In cases of NSAID-induced asthma, the ingestion of salicylates results in inhibition of the cyclo-oxygenase enzymes, preferentially shunting the metabolism of arachidonic acid through the lipoxygenase pathway with resultant production of the asthmogenic cysteinyl leukotrienes. In exercise-induced asthma, hyperventilation results in water loss from the pericellular lining fluid of the respiratory mucosa, which, in turn, triggers mediator release. Heat loss from the respiratory mucosa may also be important.

In persistent asthma, a chronic and complex inflammatory response ensues, characterised by an influx of numerous inflammatory cells, the transformation and participation of airway structural cells, and the secretion of an array of cytokines, chemokines and growth factors. Examination of the inflammatory cell profile in induced sputum samples demonstrates that, although asthma is predominantly characterised by

17

✚ 17.17 Assessment and management of 'acute on chronic' type II respiratory failure

Initial assessment

Patient may not appear distressed, despite being critically ill
- Conscious level (response to commands, ability to cough)
- CO_2 retention (warm periphery, bounding pulses, flapping tremor)
- Airways obstruction (wheeze, prolonged expiration, hyperinflation, intercostal indrawing, pursed lips)
- Cor pulmonale (peripheral oedema, raised jugular venous pressure, hepatomegaly, ascites)
- Background functional status and quality of life
- Signs of precipitating cause (see Box 17.16)

Investigations

- Arterial blood gases (severity of hypoxaemia, hypercapnia, acidaemia, bicarbonate)
- Chest X-ray

Management

- Maintenance of airway
- Treatment of specific precipitating cause
- Frequent physiotherapy ± pharyngeal suction
- Nebulised bronchodilators
- Controlled oxygen therapy:
  Start with 24% Venturi mask
  Aim for a PaO_2 >7 kPa (52 mmHg) (a PaO_2 <5 (37 mmHg) is dangerous)
- Antibiotics if evidence of infection
- Diuretics if evidence of fluid overload

Progress

- If $PaCO_2$ continues to rise or a safe PaO_2 cannot be achieved without severe hypercapnia and acidaemia, mechanical ventilatory support may be required

airway eosinophilia, neutrophilic inflammation predominates in some patients while in others scant inflammation is observed ('pauci-granu-locytic' asthma).

With increasing severity and chronicity of the disease, remodelling of the airway may occur, leading to fibrosis of the airway wall, fixed narrowing of the airway and a reduced response to bronchodilator medication.

Clinical features

Typical symptoms include recurrent episodes of wheezing, chest tightness, breathlessness and cough. Asthma is commonly mistaken for a cold or a persistent chest infection (e.g. longer than 10 days). Classical precipitants include exercise, particularly in cold weather, exposure to airborne allergens or pollutants, and viral upper respiratory tract infections. Wheeze apart, there is often very little to find on examination. An inspection for nasal polyps and eczema should be performed. Rarely, a vasculitic rash may suggest eosinophilic granulomatosis with polyangiitis (EGPA, formerly known as Churg–Strauss syndrome).

Patients with mild intermittent asthma are usually asymptomatic between exacerbations. Individuals with persistent asthma report ongoing breathlessness and wheeze but these are variable, with symptoms fluctuating over the course of one day, or from day to day or month to month.

Asthma characteristically displays a diurnal pattern, with symptoms and lung function being worse in the early morning. Particularly when poorly controlled, symptoms such as cough and wheeze disturb sleep. Cough may be the dominant symptom in some patients, and the lack of wheeze or breathlessness may lead to a delay in reaching the diagnosis of so-called 'cough-variant asthma'.

Some patients with asthma have a similar inflammatory response in the upper airway. Careful enquiry should be made as to a history of sinusitis, sinus headache, a blocked or runny nose and loss of sense of smell.

Although the aetiology of asthma is often elusive, an attempt should be made to identify any agents that may contribute to the appearance or aggravation of the condition. Particular enquiry should be made about potential allergens, such as exposure to pets or other animals, pest infestation, exposure to moulds following water damage to a home or building, and any potential occupational agents.

In some circumstances, asthma is triggered by prescription drugs. Beta-adrenoceptor antagonists (β-blockers), even when administered topically as eye drops, may induce bronchospasm, as may aspirin and

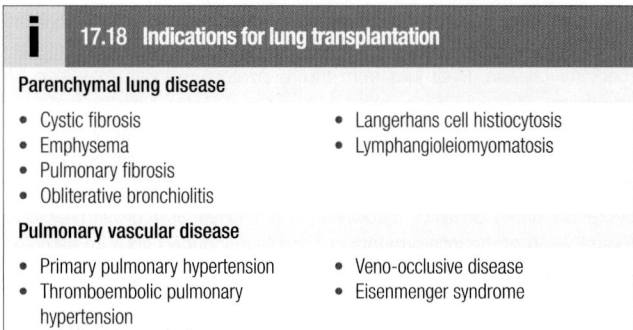

i | **17.18 Indications for lung transplantation**

Parenchymal lung disease

- Cystic fibrosis
- Emphysema
- Pulmonary fibrosis
- Obliterative bronchiolitis
- Langerhans cell histiocytosis
- Lymphangioleiomyomatosis

Pulmonary vascular disease

- Primary pulmonary hypertension
- Thromboembolic pulmonary hypertension
- Veno-occlusive disease
- Eisenmenger syndrome

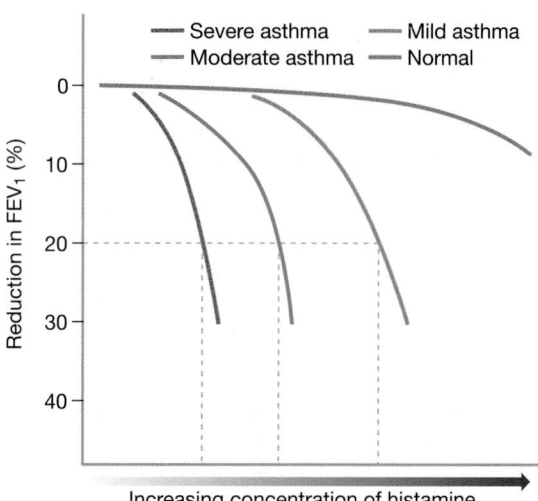

Fig. 17.17 Airway hyper-reactivity in asthma. This is demonstrated by bronchial challenge tests with sequentially increasing concentrations of either histamine, or methacholine or mannitol. The reactivity of the airways is expressed as the concentration or dose of either chemical required to produce a specific decrease (usually 20% or 15%) in the forced expired volume in 1 second (FEV_1) (PC_{20} [histamine and methacholine challenges] or PD_{15} [mannitol challenges], respectively). (PC = concentration of drug; PD = dose of drug)

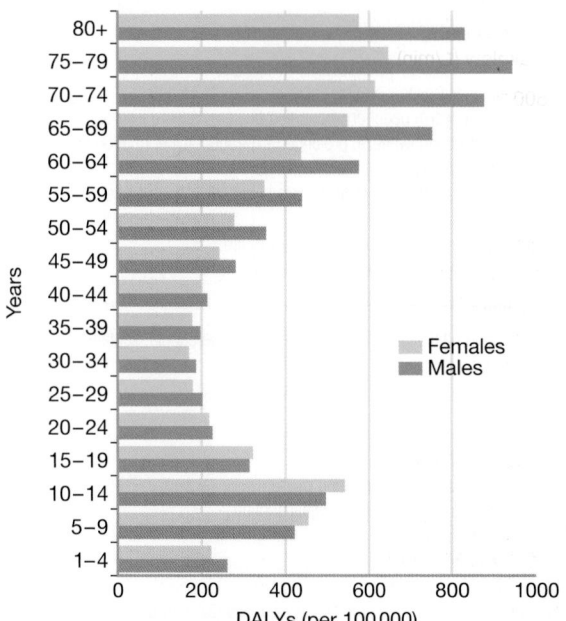

Fig. 17.16 The burden of asthma, measured by disability life years (DALYs) per 100 000 population. The burden of asthma is greatest in children approaching adolescence and in old age. The burden is similar in males and females at ages below 30–34 but at older ages the burden is higher in males. *From The Global Asthma Report 2014. Copyright 2014 The Global Asthma Network.*

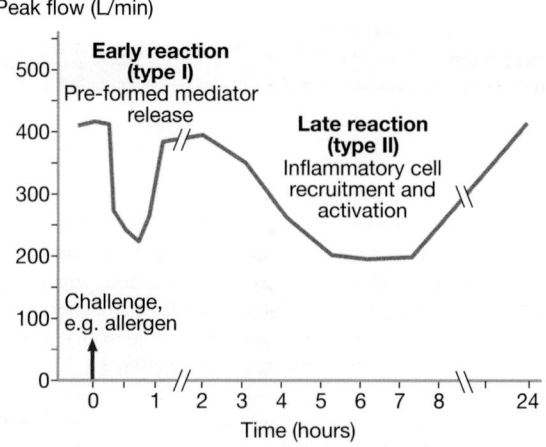

Fig. 17.18 Changes in peak flow following allergen challenge. A similar biphasic response is observed following a variety of different challenges. Occasionally, an isolated late response is seen with no early reaction.

other non-steroidal anti-inflammatory drugs (NSAIDs). The classical NSAID-induced asthma patient is female and presents in middle age with asthma, rhinosinusitis and nasal polyps. Aspirin-sensitive patients may also report symptoms following alcohol and foods containing salicylates. Other medications implicated include the oral contraceptive pill, cholinergic agents and prostaglandin $F_{2\alpha}$. Betel nuts contain arecoline, which is structurally similar to methacholine and can aggravate asthma. An important minority of patients develop a particularly severe form of asthma and this appears to be more common in women. Allergic triggers are less important and airway neutrophilia predominates.

Diagnosis

The diagnosis of asthma is predominantly clinical and is based on the combination of history, lung function and 'other' tests, which allows high, intermediate or low probability of asthma to emerge. The approach may vary from patient to patient and may need to be re-evaluated following the introduction of treatment.

Supportive evidence is provided by the demonstration of variable airflow obstruction, preferably by using spirometry (Box 17.19) to measure FEV_1 and FVC. This identifies the obstructive defect, defines its severity, and provides a baseline for bronchodilator reversibility (Fig. 17.19). If spirometry is not available, a peak flow meter may be used. Symptomatic patients should be instructed to record peak flow readings after rising in the morning and before retiring in the evening. A diurnal variation in PEF of more than 20% (the lowest values typically being recorded in the morning) is considered diagnostic and the magnitude of variability provides some indication of disease severity (Fig. 17.20).

It is not uncommon for patients whose symptoms are suggestive of asthma to have normal lung function. In these circumstances, the demonstration of AHR by challenge tests may be useful to confirm the diagnosis (see Fig. 17.17). AHR has a high negative predictive value but positive results may be seen in other conditions such as COPD, bronchiectasis and cystic fibrosis. Exercise tests are useful when symptoms are predominantly related to exercise (Fig. 17.21). Measurement of exhaled nitric oxide (FeNO) is a useful test for glucocorticoid-naïve patients as a measure of eosinophilic airways inflammation. An elevated FeNO value (adults >50 ppb; children >35 ppb) supports the diagnosis of asthma and suggests that the patient's symptoms are highly likely to respond to glucocorticoids.

The diagnosis may be supported by the presence of peripheral blood eosinophilia or atopy demonstrated by skin-prick tests or measurement of total and allergen-specific IgE. X-ray appearances are often normal, but lobar collapse may be seen if mucus occludes a large bronchus and, if accompanied by the presence of flitting infiltrates, may suggest that asthma has been complicated by allergic bronchopulmonary aspergillosis.

Management

Setting goals

Asthma is a chronic condition but may be controlled with appropriate treatment in the majority of patients. The goal of treatment should be to obtain and maintain complete control (Box 17.20) but aims may be modified according to the circumstances and the patient. Unfortunately, surveys consistently demonstrate that the majority of individuals with asthma report suboptimal control, perhaps reflecting the poor expectations of

patients and their clinicians. Pregnancy raises some issues in asthma management, which are shown in Box 17.21.

Self-management

Patients should be encouraged to take responsibility for managing their own disease. A key aspect of self-management is education, ensuring that the patient understands the relationship between symptoms and inflammation, key symptoms such as nocturnal waking and the indications for medication. The patient must also be able to use the prescribed inhalers and understand the importance of concordance with therapy. Written action plans can be helpful in developing self-management skills and they can be guided by symptoms or PEF.

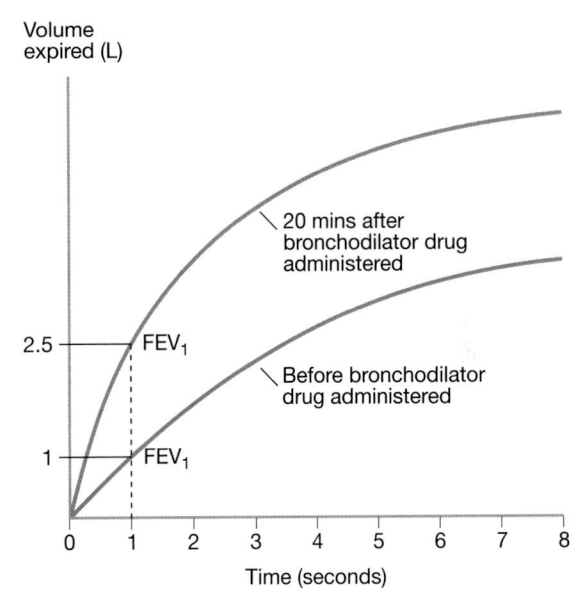

Fig. 17.19 **Reversibility test.** Forced expiratory manoeuvres before and 20 minutes after inhalation of a β_2-adrenoceptor agonist. Note the increase in forced expiratory volume in 1 second (FEV_1) from 1.0 to 2.5 L.

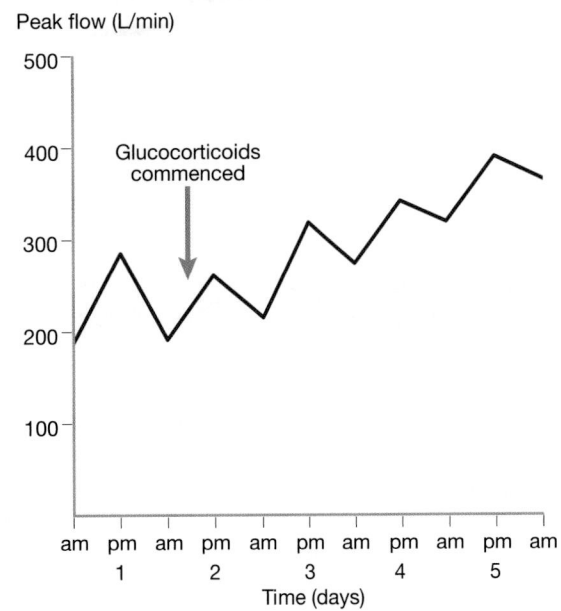

Fig. 17.20 **Serial recordings of peak expiratory flow (PEF) in a patient with asthma.** Note the sharp overnight fall (morning dip) and subsequent rise during the day. Following the introduction of glucocorticoids, there is an improvement in PEF rate and reduction of morning dipping.

17.19 How to make a diagnosis of asthma

Compatible clinical history *plus either/or*:
- FEV_1 ≥12% (and 200 mL) increase following administration of a bronchodilator/ trial of glucocorticoids. Greater confidence is gained if the increase is >15% and >400 mL
- >20% diurnal variation on ≥3 days in a week for 2 weeks on PEF diary
- FEV_1 ≥15% decrease after 6 mins of exercise

(FEV_1 = forced expiratory volume in 1 sec; PEF = peak expiratory flow)

17

Avoidance of aggravating factors

This is particularly important in the management of occupational asthma but may also be relevant in atopic patients, for whom removing or reducing exposure to relevant antigens may effect improvement. House dust mite exposure may be reduced by replacing carpets with floorboards and using mite-impermeable bedding, but these measures have not demonstrated major improvements in asthma control. Many patients are sensitised to several ubiquitous aeroallergens, making avoidance strategies impracticable. Measures to reduce fungal exposure may be applicable in specific circumstances and medications known to precipitate or aggravate asthma should be avoided. Smoking cessation (p.90) is particularly important, as smoking not only encourages sensitisation but also induces a relative glucocorticoid resistance in the airway.

The stepwise approach to the management of asthma

Prior to any step up in a patient's asthma therapy they should be reviewed to ensure that aggravating factors have been addressed, concordance assessed and inhaler technique checked.

Once asthma control is established, the dose of inhaled (or oral) glucocorticoid should be titrated to the lowest dose at which effective control is maintained. Decreasing the dose of glucocorticoid by around 25%–50% every 3 months is a reasonable strategy for most patients.

The stepwise approach is summarized in Figure 17.22.

Step 1: Regular preventer

The initial therapy for a patient diagnosed with asthma would be a low-dose inhaled glucocorticoid (ICS). For adults, a starting dose equivalent to beclometasone dipropionate (BDP) 400 μg per day is reasonable, although higher doses may be required in smokers.

A variety of different inhaled devices are available and the choice of device should be guided by patient preference and competence in its use. The metered-dose inhaler remains the most widely prescribed (Fig. 17.23).

Step 2: Initial add-on therapy

If the asthma remains poorly controlled despite regular preventer therapy, the next step should be addition of a long-acting beta agonist (LABA). This should be done via a combination ICS/LABA inhaler to prevent inadvertent administration of LABA monotherapy and risk of asthma death.

Combination ICS/LABA inhalers containing the fast-acting LABA formoterol can be used as a maintenance and reliever (MART) inhaler allowing for auto-titration of therapy in response to symptoms.

Step 3: Additional add-on therapies

If asthma control remains poor despite initial add-on therapy, the patient should have a detailed asthma review. There are a number of options to consider at this stage:

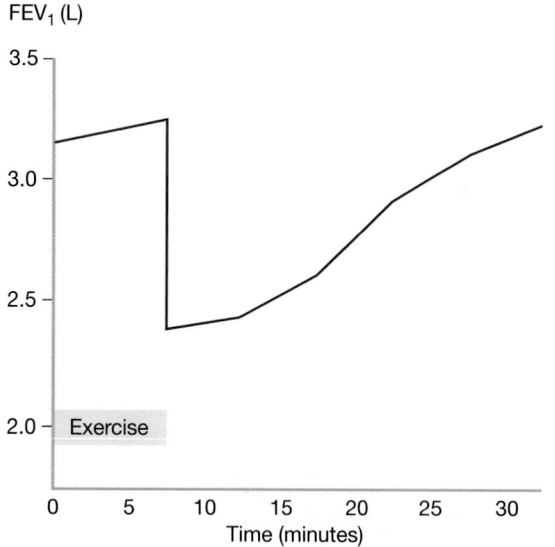

FEV$_1$ (L)

Fig. 17.21 Exercise-induced asthma. Serial recordings of forced expiratory volume in 1 second (FEV$_1$) in a patient with bronchial asthma before and after 6 minutes of strenuous exercise. Note initial rise on completion of exercise, followed by sudden fall and gradual recovery. Adequate warm-up exercise or pre-treatment with a β$_2$-adrenoceptor agonist, nedocromil sodium or a leukotriene antagonist can protect against exercise-induced symptoms.

17.21 Asthma in pregnancy

- **Clinical course**: women with well-controlled asthma usually have good pregnancy outcomes. Pregnancy in women with more severe asthma can precipitate worsening control and lead to increased maternal and neonatal morbidity.
- **Labour and delivery**: 90% have no symptoms.
- **Safety data**: good for β$_2$-agonists, inhaled glucocorticoids, theophyllines, oral prednisolone and chromones.
- **Oral leukotriene receptor antagonists**: no evidence that these harm the fetus and they should not be stopped in women who have previously demonstrated significant improvement in asthma control prior to pregnancy.
- **Glucocorticoids**: women on maintenance prednisolone >7.5 mg/day should receive hydrocortisone 100 mg 3–4 times daily during labour.
- **Prostaglandin F$_{2\alpha}$**: may induce bronchospasm and should be used with extreme caution.
- **Breastfeeding**: use medications as normal.
- **Uncontrolled asthma**: associated with maternal (hyperemesis, hypertension, pre-eclampsia, vaginal haemorrhage, complicated labour) and fetal (intrauterine growth restriction and low birth weight, preterm birth, increased perinatal mortality, neonatal hypoxia) complications.

17.20 Levels of asthma control

Characteristic	Controlled	Partly controlled (any present in any week)	Uncontrolled
Daytime symptoms	None (≤twice/week)	>twice/week	
Limitations of activities	None	Any	
Nocturnal symptoms/awakening	None	Any	≥3 features of partly controlled asthma present in any week
Need for rescue/'reliever' treatment	None (≤twice/week)	>twice/week	
Lung function (PEF or FEV$_1$)	Normal	<80% predicted or personal best (if known) on any day	
Exacerbation	None	≥1/year	1 in any week

(FEV$_1$ = forced expiratory volume in 1 sec; PEF = peak expiratory flow)

- If there has been no response to the LABA, then it should be stopped and an increase of the ICS to a medium dose (800 µg) considered.
- If there is benefit from the LABA, but control is poor then the ICS should be increased to a medium dose, alternatively trial of a leukotriene antagonist (LTRA) or a slow-release theophylline preparation should be considered.

Step 4: High-dose therapies

In adults, the dose of inhaled glucocorticoid should be trialled up to a high dose (2000 µg BDP) (or equivalent) daily. Trials of LTRA, long-acting antimuscarinic agents (LAMA), theophyllines or a slow-release oral β_2-agonist may be considered. If the trial of add-on therapy is ineffective, it should be discontinued.

Step 5: Continuous or frequent use of oral glucocorticoids

At this stage, oral prednisolone (usually administered as a single daily dose in the morning) should be prescribed at the lowest dose necessary to control symptoms and the patients should be referred for specialist severe asthma assessment. Patients who are on long-term glucocorticoid tablets (>3 months) or are receiving more than three or four courses per year will be at risk of systemic side-effects (p. 684). The risk of osteoporosis in this group can be reduced by giving bisphosphonates. These patients should be considered for biologic therapy to minimise long-term harm from oral glucocorticoids.

Omalizumab (anti-IgE) therapy may be considered for those patients with severe IgE-driven atopic asthma. Benralizumab (anti-IL5r), mepolizumab (anti-IL5), reslizumab (anti-IL5) or dupiliumab (anti-IL4/13) could be considered for patients with eosinophilic forms of asthma.

Exacerbations of asthma

The course of asthma may be punctuated by exacerbations with increased symptoms, deterioration in lung function, and an increase in airway inflammation. Exacerbations are most commonly precipitated by viral infections but moulds, pollens (particularly following thunderstorms) and air pollution are also implicated. Most attacks are characterised by a gradual deterioration over several hours to days but some appear to occur with little or no warning: so-called brittle asthma. An important minority of patients appear to have a blunted perception of airway narrowing and fail to appreciate the early signs of deterioration.

Management of mild to moderate exacerbations

Doubling the dose of inhaled glucocorticoids does not prevent an impending exacerbation. Short courses of at least 5 days of 'rescue' glucocorticoids (prednisolone 40–50 mg/day) are therefore often required to regain control. Tapering of the glucocorticoid dose to withdraw treatment is not necessary, unless it has been given for more than 3 weeks.

Indications for 'rescue' courses include:

- symptoms and PEF progressively worsening day by day, with a fall of PEF below 75% of the patient's personal best recording
- onset or worsening of sleep disturbance by asthma
- persistence of morning symptoms until midday

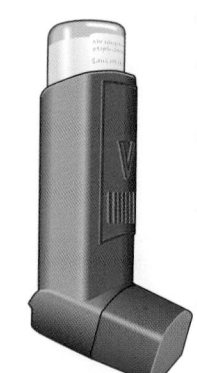

- Remove the cap and shake the inhaler
- Breathe out gently and place the mouthpiece into the mouth
- Incline the head backwards to minimise oropharyngeal deposition
- Simultaneously, begin a slow deep inspiration, depress the canister and continue to inhale
- Hold the breath for 10 seconds

Fig. 17.23 How to use a metered-dose inhaler.

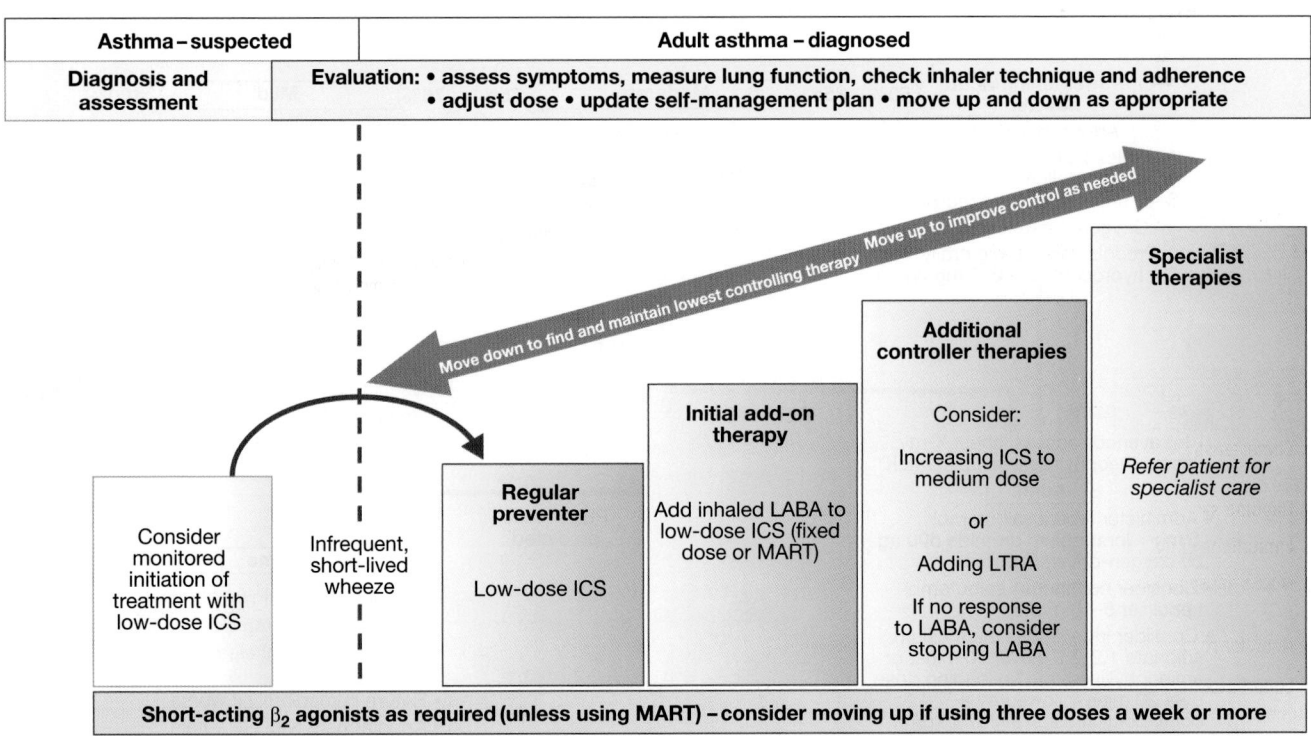

Fig. 17.22 Management approach in adults based on asthma control. (ICS = inhaled corticosteroids (glucocorticoids); LABA = long-acting β_2-agonist; MART = maintenance and reliever therapy; LTRA = leukotriene receptor antagonist; SR = sustained-release) *From British Thoracic Society and Scottish Intercollegiate Guidelines Network (SIGN). British Guideline on the Management of Asthma: SIGN 158. Edinburgh: SIGN; 2019. http://www.sign.ac.uk.*

- progressively diminishing response to an inhaled bronchodilator
- symptoms that are sufficiently severe to require treatment with nebulised bronchodilators

Management of acute severe asthma

Box 17.22 highlights the immediate assessment requirements in acute asthma. Measurement of PEF is mandatory, unless the patient is too ill to cooperate, and is most easily interpreted when expressed as a percentage of the predicted normal or of the previous best value obtained on optimal treatment (Fig. 17.24). Arterial blood gas analysis is essential for those patients with life-threatening or near-fatal asthma to determine the $PaCO_2$, a normal or elevated level being particularly dangerous. A chest X-ray is not immediately necessary, unless pneumothorax is suspected. Treatment includes the following measures:

- *Oxygen.* Controlled supplemental oxygen should be administered to maintain SaO_2 94%–98%. The presence of a high $PaCO_2$ should not be taken as an indication to reduce oxygen concentration but as a warning sign of a severe or life-threatening attack. Failure to achieve appropriate oxygenation is an indication for assisted ventilation.
- *High doses of inhaled bronchodilators.* Short-acting β_2-agonists are the agent of choice. They can be administered either via multiple doses of a metered-dose inhaler via a spacer device, or via a nebuliser driven by oxygen. Ipratropium bromide provides further bronchodilator therapy and should be added to if there is a failure to respond to salbutamol or in life-threatening attacks.
- *Systemic glucocorticoids.* These reduce the inflammatory response, reduce mortality, subsequent hospital admission and requirement for bronchodilators. They should be administered to all patients with an acute severe attack. They can usually be administered orally as prednisolone but intravenous hydrocortisone may be used in patients who are vomiting or unable to swallow.

There is no evidence base for the use of intravenous fluids but many patients are dehydrated due to high insensible water loss and may benefit. Potassium supplements may be necessary to counteract hypokalaemia caused by repeated doses of beta-agonists.

If patients fail to improve, a number of further options may be considered, including intravenous magnesium for patients with life-threatening or near-fatal attacks and intravenous aminophylline, although cardiac and therapeutic drug level monitoring is recommended.

PEF should be recorded 15–30 minutes after starting therapy and thereafter according to response every 4–6 hours and pulse oximetry should be monitored to ensure that SaO_2 94%–98% is maintained.

✚ 17.22 Immediate assessment of acute severe asthma

Acute severe asthma

- PEF 33%–50% predicted (<200 L/min)
- Heart rate ≥ 110 beats/min
- Respiratory rate ≥ 25 breaths/min
- Inability to complete sentences in 1 breath

Life-threatening features

- PEF <33% predicted (<100 L/min)
- SpO_2 <92% or PaO_2 <8 kPa (60 mmHg) (especially if being treated with oxygen)
- Normal or raised $PaCO_2$
- Silent chest
- Cyanosis
- Feeble respiratory effort
- Bradycardia or arrhythmias
- Hypotension
- Exhaustion
- Delirium
- Coma

Near-fatal asthma

- Raised $PaCO_2$ and/or requiring mechanical ventilation with raised inflation pressures

(PEF = peak expiratory flow)

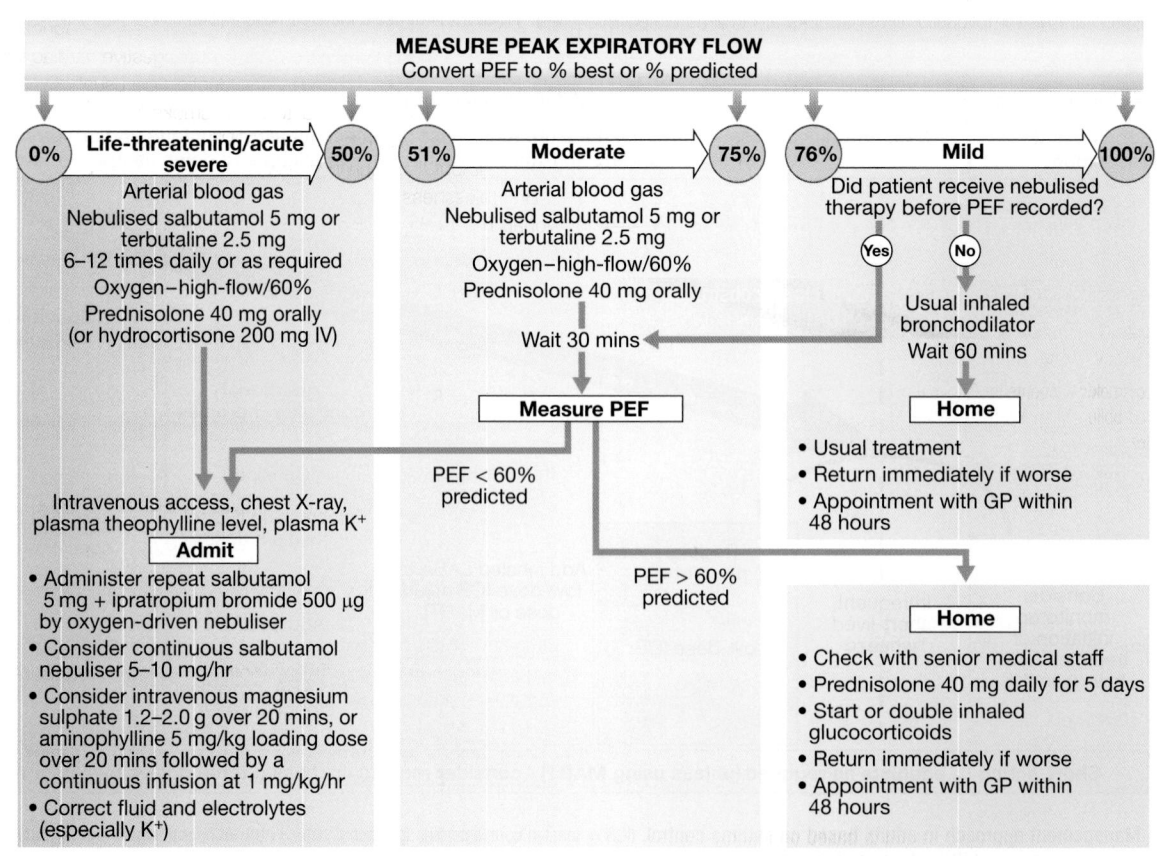

Fig. 17.24 Immediate treatment of patients with acute severe asthma. (GP = general practitioner; IV = intravenous; PEF = peak expiratory flow)

Repeat arterial blood gases are necessary if the initial $PaCO_2$ measurements were normal or raised, the PaO_2 was below 8 kPa (60 mmHg) or the patient deteriorates. Box 17.23 lists the indications for endotracheal intubation and intermittent positive pressure ventilation (IPPV).

Prognosis

The outcome from acute severe asthma is generally good but a considerable number of deaths occur in young people and many are preventable. Failure to recognise the severity of an attack, on the part of either the assessing physician or the patient, contributes to delay in delivering appropriate therapy and to under-treatment.

Prior to discharge, patients should be stable on discharge medication (nebulised therapy should have been discontinued for at least 24 hours) and the PEF should have reached 75% of predicted or personal best. The acute attack should prompt a look for and avoidance of any trigger factors, the delivery of asthma education and the provision of a written self-management plan. The patient should be offered an appointment with a general practitioner or asthma nurse within 2 working days of discharge, and follow-up at a specialist hospital clinic within a month.

Chronic obstructive pulmonary disease

Chronic obstructive pulmonary disease (COPD) is defined as a preventable and treatable disease characterised by persistent respiratory symptoms and airflow limitation that is due to airway and/or alveolar abnormalities, usually caused by significant exposure to noxious particles or gases. The spectrum of COPD includes chronic bronchitis and emphysema. Chronic bronchitis is defined as cough and sputum for at least 3 consecutive months in each of 2 consecutive years. Emphysema is abnormal permanent enlargement of the airspaces distal to the terminal bronchioles, accompanied by destruction of their walls. Exacerbations and comorbidities contribute to the overall severity in individual patients. Extrapulmonary effects include weight loss and skeletal muscle dysfunction (see Fig. 17.25). Commonly associated comorbid conditions include cardiovascular disease, cerebrovascular disease, the metabolic syndrome, osteoporosis, depression and lung cancer.

COPD prevalence is directly related to the prevalence of risk factors in the community, such as tobacco smoking, coal dust exposure or the use of biomass fuels, and to the age of the population being studied.

Risk factors are shown in Box 17.24. Cigarette smoking represents the most significant risk factor for COPD and the risk of developing the condition relates to both the amount and duration of smoking. It is unusual to develop COPD with less than 10 pack years (1 pack year=20 cigarettes daily per year) and not all smokers develop the condition, suggesting that individual susceptibility factors are important.

Pathophysiology

COPD has both pulmonary and systemic components (Fig. 17.25). The presence of airflow limitation combined with premature airway closure leads to gas trapping and hyperinflation, adversely affecting pulmonary and chest wall compliance. Pulmonary hyperinflation also results, which flattens the diaphragmatic muscles and leads to an increasingly horizontal alignment of the intercostal muscles, placing the respiratory muscles at a mechanical disadvantage. The work of breathing is therefore markedly increased – first on exercise, when the time for expiration is further shortened, but then, as the disease advances, at rest.

Emphysema (Fig. 17.26) may be classified by the pattern of the enlarged airspaces: centriacinar, panacinar and paraseptal. Some individuals develop bullae; permanent air-filled spaces within the lung that are more than 1 cm in diameter. This results in impaired gas exchange and respiratory failure.

Clinical features

COPD should be suspected in any patient over 40 years old who presents with symptoms of chronic bronchitis and/or breathlessness. Depending on the presentation, important differential diagnoses include asthma, tuberculosis, bronchiectasis and congestive cardiac failure.

Cough and associated sputum production are usually the first symptoms, and are often referred to as a 'smoker's cough'. Haemoptysis may complicate exacerbations of COPD but should not be attributed to COPD without thorough investigation.

Breathlessness usually prompts presentation to a health professional. The level should be quantified for future reference, often by documenting what the patient can manage before stopping; scales such as the modified Medical Research Council (mMRC) dyspnoea scale may be useful (Box 17.25). In advanced disease, enquiry should be made as to the presence of oedema (which may be seen for the first time during an exacerbation) and morning headaches (which may suggest hypercapnia).

Physical signs are non-specific, correlate poorly with lung function, and are seldom obvious until the disease is advanced. Breath sounds are typically quiet; crackles may accompany infection but, if persistent, raise the possibility of bronchiectasis. Finger clubbing is not a feature of COPD and should trigger further investigation for lung cancer or fibrosis. Right heart failure may develop in patients with advanced COPD, particularly if there is coexisting sleep apnoea or thromboembolic disease. However, even in the absence of right heart failure, COPD patients often have pitting oedema from salt and water retention caused by renal hypoxia and hypercapnia. This is known as 'cor pulmonale', but the term is a misnomer in such patients, as they do not have heart failure. Fatigue, anorexia and weight loss may point to the development of lung cancer or tuberculosis, but are common in patients with severe COPD. Body mass index (BMI) is of prognostic significance. Depression and anxiety are also common.

Two classical phenotypes have been described: 'pink puffers' and 'blue bloaters'. The former are typically thin and breathless, and maintain a normal $PaCO_2$ until the late stage of disease. The latter develop

---

17.23 Indications for assisted ventilation in acute severe asthma

- Coma
- Respiratory arrest
- Deterioration of arterial blood gas tensions despite optimal therapy:
  - PaO_2 <8 kPa (60 mmHg) and falling
  - $PaCO_2$ >6 kPa (45 mmHg) and rising
  - pH low and falling (H^+ high and rising)
- Exhaustion, delirium, drowsiness

17.24 Risk factors for development of chronic obstructive pulmonary disease

Environmental factors

- Tobacco smoke: accounts for 95% of cases in the UK
- Indoor air pollution: cooking with biomass fuels in confined areas in low-income countries
- Occupational exposures, such as coal dust, silica and cadmium
- Low birth weight: may reduce maximally attained lung function in young adult life
- Lung growth: childhood infections or maternal smoking may affect growth of lung during childhood, resulting in a lower maximally attained lung function in adult life
- Infections: recurrent infection may accelerate decline in FEV_1; persistence of adenovirus in lung tissue may alter local inflammatory response, predisposing to lung damage; HIV infection is associated with emphysema
- Low socioeconomic status
- Cannabis smoking

Host factors

- Genetic factors: alpha-1-antitrypsin deficiency; other COPD susceptibility genes are likely to be identified
- Airway hyper-reactivity

(FEV_1 = forced expiratory volume in 1 sec)

17

Enlargement of mucus-secreting glands and increase in number of goblet cells, accompanied by an inflammatory cell infiltrate, result in increased sputum production leading to chronic bronchitis

Loss of elastic tissue, inflammation and fibrosis in airway wall result in premature airway closure, gas trapping and dynamic hyperinflation leading to changes in pulmonary and chest wall compliance

Pulmonary vascular remodelling and impaired cardiac performance

Unopposed action of proteases and oxidants leading to destruction of alveoli and appearance of emphysema

Pulmonary

Systemic

Muscular weakness reflecting deconditioning and cellular changes in skeletal muscles

Increased circulating inflammatory markers

Impaired salt and water excretion leading to peripheral oedema

Altered fat metabolism contributing to weight loss

↑ Prevalence of osteoporosis

Fig. 17.25 The pulmonary and systemic features of chronic obstructive pulmonary disease.

(or tolerate) hypercapnia earlier and may develop oedema and secondary polycythaemia. In practice, these phenotypes often overlap.

Investigations

Although there are no reliable radiographic signs that correlate with the severity of airflow limitation, a chest X-ray is essential to identify alternative diagnoses such as cardiac failure, lung cancer and the presence of bullae. A blood count is useful to exclude anaemia or document polycythaemia, and all patients should be tested for alpha-1-antitrypsin deficiency.

The diagnosis requires objective demonstration of airflow obstruction by spirometry and is established when the post-bronchodilator FEV_1/FVC is <70%. The severity of COPD may be defined in relation to the post-bronchodilator FEV_1 (Box 17.26).

Measurement of lung volumes provides an assessment of hyperinflation. This is generally performed by helium dilution technique (p. 488); however, in patients with severe COPD, and in particular large bullae, body plethysmography is preferred because the use of helium may under-estimate lung volumes. The presence of emphysema is suggested by a low gas transfer. Exercise tests provide an objective assessment of exercise tolerance and provide a baseline on which to judge the response to bronchodilator therapy or rehabilitation programmes; they may also be valuable when assessing prognosis. Pulse oximetry may prompt referral for a domiciliary oxygen assessment if less than 93%.

The assessment of health status by the St George's Respiratory Questionnaire (SGRQ) is commonly used for research. In practice, the COPD Assessment Test and the COPD Control Questionnaire are easier to administer. High-resolution computed tomography (HRCT) is likely to play an increasing role in the assessment of COPD, as it allows the detection, characterisation and quantification of emphysema (Fig. 17.27) and is more sensitive than the chest X-ray at detecting bullae. It is also used to guide lung volume reduction surgery.

Assessment of severity

The severity of COPD has traditionally been defined in relation to the FEV% predicted. However, assessing the impact of COPD on individual

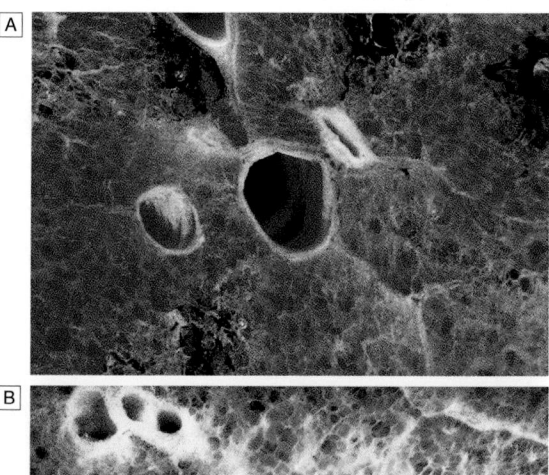

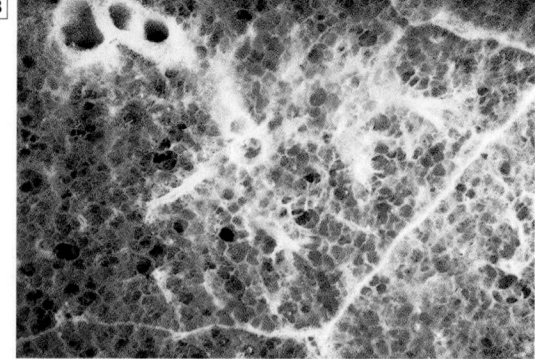

Fig. 17.26 The pathology of emphysema. [A] Normal lung. [B] Emphysematous lung, showing gross loss of the normal surface area available for gas exchange. *(B) Courtesy of the British Lung Foundation.*

patients in terms of the symptoms and limitations in activity that they experience and whether they suffer frequent or significant exacerbations may provide a more clinically relevant assessment and help guide management.

	17.25 Modified Medical Research Council (mMRC) dyspnoea scale	

Grade	Degree of breathlessness related to activities
0	No breathlessness, except with strenuous exercise
1	Breathlessness when hurrying on the level or walking up a slight hill
2	Walks slower than contemporaries on level ground because of breathlessness or has to stop for breath when walking at own pace
3	Stops for breath after walking about 100 m or after a few minutes on level ground
4	Too breathless to leave the house, or breathless when dressing or undressing

	17.26 Spirometric classification of COPD severity based on post-bronchodilator FEV_1			

| PD FEV_1/ FVC | FEV_1% predicted | Severity of airflow obstruction post-bronchodilator | | |
		ATS/ERS (2004)	GOLD (2020)	NICE Clinical Guideline 101 (2010)
<0.7	≥80%	Mild	Stage I – mild	Stage I – mild[1]
<0.7	50%–79%	Moderate	Stage II – moderate	Stage II – moderate
<0.7	30%–49%	Severe	Stage III – severe	Stage III – severe
<0.7	<30%	Very severe	Stage IV – very severe	Stage IV – very severe[2]

[1]Mild COPD should not be diagnosed on lung function alone if the patient is asymptomatic. [2]Or FEV_1 <50% with respiratory failure.
(ATS/ERS = American Thoracic Society/European Respiratory Journal; FEV_1 = forced expiratory volume in 1 sec; GOLD = Global Initiative for Chronic Obstructive Lung Disease; PD = post-bronchodilator)

Adapted from National Institute for Health and Care Excellence (NICE). Chronic obstructive pulmonary disease in over 16s: diagnosis and management. NICE Guideline [NG115], July 2019. http://www.nice.org.uk/guidance/ng115/

Management

The management of COPD focuses on improving breathlessness, reducing the frequency and severity of exacerbations, and improving health status and prognosis.

Reducing exposure to noxious particles and gases

Sustained smoking cessation in mild to moderate COPD is accompanied by a reduced decline in FEV_1 compared to persistent smokers, and cessation remains the only strategy that impacts favourably on the natural history of COPD. Complete cessation is accompanied by an improvement in lung function and deceleration in the rate of FEV_1 decline (Fig. 17.28). In regions where the indoor burning of biomass fuels is important, the introduction of non-smoking cooking devices or alternative fuels should be encouraged.

Pulmonary rehabilitation

Exercise should be encouraged at all stages and patients should be reassured that breathlessness, while distressing, is not dangerous.

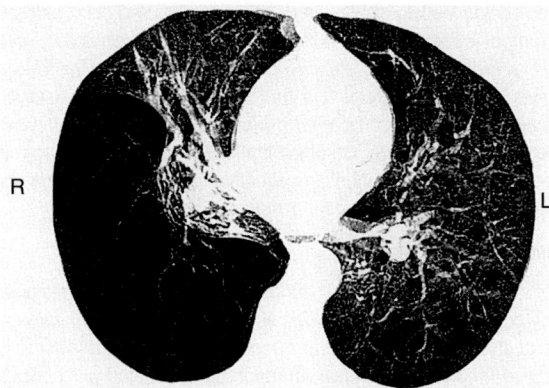

Fig. 17.27 Gross emphysema. High-resolution computed tomogram showing emphysema, most evident in the right lower lobe.

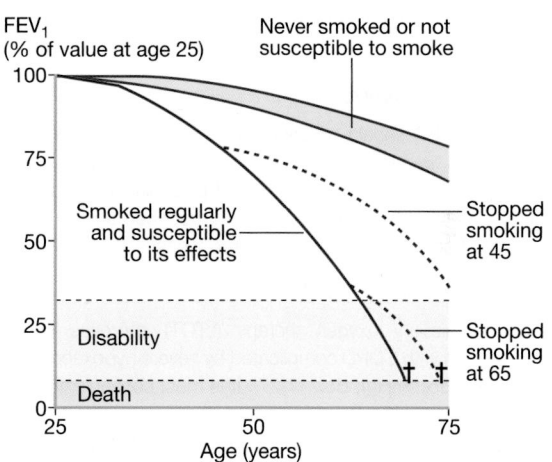

Fig. 17.28 Model of annual decline in FEV1 with accelerated decline in susceptible smokers. When smoking is stopped, subsequent loss is similar to that in healthy non-smokers. (FEV_1 = forced expiratory volume in 1 second)

Multidisciplinary programmes that incorporate physical training, disease education and nutritional counselling reduce symptoms, improve health status and enhance confidence. Most programmes include two to three sessions per week, last between 6 and 12 weeks, and are accompanied by demonstrable and sustained improvements in exercise tolerance and health status.

Bronchodilators

Bronchodilator therapy is central to the management of breathlessness. Choice should be informed by patient preference and inhaler assessment. Short-acting bronchodilators are used as relievers and may be used as sole treatment for patients with very mild disease but combination longer-acting bronchodilators are preferred. Long-acting beta-agonists (LABA) and long-acting muscarinic-antagonists (LAMA) are available in single agent or combination inhalers. Nebulised short-acting bronchodilators can be used in those unable to take inhalers. Significant improvements in breathlessness may be reported despite minimal changes in FEV_1, probably reflecting improvements in lung emptying that reduce dynamic hyperinflation and ease the work of breathing. Oral bronchodilator therapy, such as theophylline, is only recommended when other long-acting bronchodilators are not available. Their use is limited by side-effects, unpredictable metabolism and drug interactions; hence the requirement to monitor plasma levels.

Combined inhaled glucocorticoids and bronchodilators

Those with frequent exacerbations and/or persistent breathlessness despite long-acting bronchodilators, may benefit from inhaled glucocorticoids (usually abbreviated to ICS, for 'inhaled corticosteroids'), in the form of either a LABA/LAMA/ICS or LABA/ICS combination inhaler. These combined therapies improve lung function, reduce the frequency and severity of exacerbations and improve quality of life. However, these advantages may be accompanied by an increased risk of pneumonia, particularly in older people. Combination ICS inhalers are likely to reduce the frequency of exacerbations in patients with eosinophilia, and should be used in patients with a history of asthma.

Oral anti-inflammatories

Oral glucocorticoids are useful during exacerbations but maintenance therapy contributes to osteoporosis and impaired skeletal muscle function, and should be avoided. Oral glucocorticoid trials assist in the diagnosis of asthma but do not predict response to inhaled glucocorticoids in COPD. Roflumilast, a phosphodiesterase-4 inhibitor, improves lung function and reduces moderate to severe exacerbations in patients with severe or very severe COPD. Azithromycin 500 mg three times weekly can reduce the number of exacerbations, but non-tuberculous mycobacterial infections must first be excluded, and LFTs, QTC and hearing should be monitored.

Other maintenance measures

Patients with COPD should be offered pneumococcal vaccination and annual influenza vaccination. Obesity, poor nutrition, depression and social isolation should be identified and, if possible, addressed. Chest physiotherapy techniques and devices and mucolytic agents ease sputum expectoration and may reduce exacerbations.

Oxygen therapy and home ventilation

Long-term domiciliary oxygen therapy (LTOT) improves survival in selected patients with COPD complicated by severe hypoxaemia (arterial PaO_2 <7.3 kPa (55 mmHg); Box 17.27). It is most conveniently provided by an oxygen concentrator and patients should be instructed to use oxygen for a minimum of 15 hours a day; greater benefits are seen in those who use it for more than 20 hours a day. The aim of therapy is to increase the PaO_2 to at least 8 kPa (60 mmHg) or SaO_2 to at least 90%. Ambulatory oxygen therapy should be considered in patients who desaturate on exercise and show objective improvement in exercise capacity and/or dyspnoea with oxygen. Oxygen flow rates should be adjusted to maintain SaO_2 above 90%. Home non-invasive ventilation improves quality of life and prolongs time to readmission in patients with persistent hypercapnia.

Surgical intervention

Bullectomy may be considered when large bullae compress surrounding normal lung tissue. Patients with predominantly upper lobe emphysema, preserved gas transfer and no evidence of pulmonary hypertension may benefit from lung volume reduction surgery (LVRS). LVRS involves resection of peripheral emphysematous lung tissue with the aim of reducing hyperinflation and decreasing the work of breathing. Both bullectomy and LVRS can be performed thoracoscopically, minimising morbidity. Bronchoscopic LVRS involves the use of one-way valves, lung coils or thermal ablation to collapse down areas of ineffective emphysematous lung. This enables the neighbouring areas of healthier lung to expand

and work more efficiently. Lung transplantation may benefit carefully selected patients with advanced disease.

Palliative care

Addressing end-of-life needs is an important aspect of care in advanced COPD. Hand-held electric fans and morphine preparations may be used for palliation of breathlessness and low-dose benzodiazepines may reduce anxiety. Decisions regarding resuscitation and escalation of care should be addressed in advance of critical illness.

Prognosis

COPD has a variable natural history but is usually progressive. The prognosis is inversely related to age and directly related to the post-bronchodilator FEV_1. Additional poor prognostic indicators include weight loss and pulmonary hypertension. A composite score comprising the body mass index (B), the degree of airflow obstruction (O), a measurement of dyspnoea (D) and exercise capacity (E) (BODE index) may assist in predicting death from respiratory and other causes (Box 17.28). Respiratory failure, pneumonia, cardiac disease and lung cancer represent common modes of death.

Specific challenges with the diagnosis and management of obstructive pulmonary disease in older people are shown in Box 17.29.

Acute exacerbations of COPD

Acute exacerbations of COPD (AECOPD) are characterised by an increase in symptoms and deterioration in lung function and health status. They become more frequent as the disease progresses and are usually triggered by infection or a change in air quality. They may be

---

i | **17.28 Calculation of the BODE index**

	Points on BODE index			
Variable	0	1	2	3
FEV_1	≥65	50–64	36–49	≤35
Distance walked in 6 mins (m)	≥350	250–349	150–249	≤149
mMRC dyspnoea scale*	0–1	2	3	4
Body mass index	>21	≤21		

A patient with a BODE index of 0–2 has a mortality rate of 20% at 4 years, whereas a patient with a BODE index of 7–10 has a mortality rate of 82% at 4 years.

*See Box 17.25.
(BODE – see text; FEV_1 = forced expiratory volume in 1 sec)

 | **17.29 Obstructive pulmonary disease in old age**

- **Asthma**: may appear de novo in old age, so airflow obstruction should not always be assumed to be due to COPD.
- **Peak expiratory flow recordings**: older people with poor vision have difficulty reading PEF meters.
- **Perception of bronchoconstriction**: impaired by age, so an older patient's description of symptoms may not be a reliable indicator of severity.
- **Stopping smoking**: the benefits on the rate of loss of lung function decline with age but remain valuable up to the age of 80.
- **Metered-dose inhalers**: many older people cannot use these because of difficulty coordinating and triggering the device. Aids are available, and frequent demonstration and re-instruction in the use of all devices are required.
- **Mortality rates for acute asthma**: higher in old age, partly because patients under-estimate the severity of bronchoconstriction and also develop a lower degree of tachycardia and pulsus paradoxus for the same degree of bronchoconstriction.
- **Treatment decisions**: advanced age in itself is not a barrier to intensive care or mechanical ventilation in an acute episode of asthma or COPD, but this decision may be difficult and should be shared with the patient (if possible), the relatives and the wider medical team.

---

i | **17.27 Prescription of long-term oxygen therapy in COPD**

Arterial blood gases are measured in clinically stable patients on optimal medical therapy on at least two occasions 3 weeks apart:

- PaO_2 <7.3 kPa (55 mmHg) irrespective of $PaCO_2$
- PaO_2 7.3–8 kPa (55–60 mmHg) plus pulmonary hypertension, peripheral oedema or polycythaemia (haematocrit >55%)
- the patient has stopped smoking

Use at least 15 hrs/day at the necessary flow rate to achieve a PaO_2 >8 kPa (60 mmHg) without unacceptable rise in $PaCO_2$

accompanied by the development of respiratory failure and/or fluid retention and represent an important cause of death.

Many patients can be managed at home with the use of increased bronchodilator therapy, a short course of oral glucocorticoids and, if appropriate, antibiotics. The presence of cyanosis, peripheral oedema or an alteration in consciousness should prompt referral to hospital. In other patients, consideration of comorbidity and social circumstances may influence decisions regarding hospital admission.

Oxygen therapy

In patients with an exacerbation of severe COPD, high concentrations of oxygen may cause respiratory depression and worsening acidosis. Controlled oxygen at 24% or 28% should be used with the aim of maintaining SaO_2 of 88%–92% or PaO_2 of more than 8 kPa (60 mmHg) without worsening acidosis.

Bronchodilators

Nebulised short-acting β_2-agonists combined with an anticholinergic agent (e.g. salbutamol and ipratropium) are routinely administered. However, the latter is only appropriate if the patient is unable to take their LAMA inhaler. Nebulisers can be driven with oxygen, but due to concern regarding oxygen sensitivity, they are more safely driven by compressed air with supplemental oxygen delivered by nasal cannula.

Glucocorticoids

Oral prednisolone reduces symptoms and improves lung function. Doses of 30 mg for 5 days are currently recommended but weaning courses are required if the patient has had a recent course of steroids. Prophylaxis against osteoporosis should be considered in patients who receive repeated courses of glucocorticoids.

Antibiotic therapy

The role of bacteria in exacerbations remains controversial. There is little evidence for the routine administration of antibiotics, but they are recommended for patients reporting an increase in sputum purulence, sputum volume or breathlessness. In most cases simple regimens are advised, such as an aminopenicillin, a tetracycline or a macrolide. However, local practice will depend on local guidance and epidemiology.

Non-invasive ventilation

Non-invasive ventilation (NIV) reduces mortality and invasive ventilation rates in patients with an acute exacerbation of COPD complicated by mild to moderate respiratory acidosis (pH <7.35 and $PaCO_2$ >6.5 kPa). It should be considered when respiratory acidosis is not corrected within an hour of identification, despite optimal medical therapy, including controlled oxygen therapy with a target saturation of 88%–92%. Invasive ventilation should be considered in patients with deteriorating acidosis despite optimal NIV settings, those unable to tolerate or wear the interface (e.g. due to facial injury) and those who cannot protect their airway.

Additional therapy

Exacerbations may be accompanied by the development of peripheral oedema; this usually responds to diuretics. Hospital admission provides a good opportunity to address smoking cessation, mobility and sputum clearance, inhaler technique and concordance, nutrition and swallowing concerns.

Discharge

Discharge from hospital may be contemplated once patients are clinically stable on their usual maintenance medication. Hospital-at-home teams may provide short-term nebuliser loan, improving discharge rates and providing additional support for the patient.

Bronchiectasis

Bronchiectasis means abnormal dilatation of the bronchi. Chronic suppurative airway infection with sputum production, progressive scarring and lung damage occur, whatever the cause.

Aetiology and pathology

Bronchiectasis may result from a congenital defect affecting airway ion transport or ciliary function, such as cystic fibrosis (see below), or may be acquired secondary to damage to the airways by a destructive infection, inhaled toxin or foreign body. The result is chronic inflammation and infection in the airways. Box 17.30 shows the common causes, of which tuberculosis is the most common worldwide.

Localised bronchiectasis may occur due to the accumulation of pus beyond an obstructing bronchial lesion, such as enlarged tuberculous hilar lymph nodes, a bronchial tumour or an inhaled foreign body.

The bronchiectatic cavities may be lined by granulation tissue, squamous epithelium or normal ciliated epithelium. There may also be inflammatory changes in the deeper layers of the bronchial wall and hypertrophy of the bronchial arteries. Chronic inflammatory and fibrotic changes are usually found in the surrounding lung tissue, causing progressive destruction of the normal lung architecture in advanced cases.

Clinical features

The symptoms are shown in Box 17.31.

Physical signs in the chest may be unilateral or bilateral. If the bronchiectatic airways do not contain secretions and there is no associated lobar collapse, there are no abnormal physical signs. When there are large amounts of sputum in the bronchiectatic spaces, numerous coarse crackles may be heard over the affected areas. Collapse with retained secretions blocking a proximal bronchus may lead to locally diminished breath sounds, while advanced disease may cause scarring and overlying bronchial breathing. Acute haemoptysis is an important complication of bronchiectasis; management is described on page 492.

17.30 Causes of bronchiectasis

Congenital
- Cystic fibrosis
- Ciliary dysfunction syndromes:
  Primary ciliary dyskinesia (immotile cilia syndrome)
  Kartagener syndrome (sinusitis and transposition of the viscera)
- Primary hypogammaglobulinaemia

Acquired: children
- Severe infections in infancy (especially whooping cough, measles)
- Primary tuberculosis
- Inhaled foreign body

Acquired: adults
- Suppurative pneumonia
- Pulmonary tuberculosis
- Allergic bronchopulmonary aspergillosis complicating asthma
- Bronchial tumours

17.31 Symptoms of bronchiectasis

- **Cough**: chronic, daily, persistent
- **Sputum**: copious, continuously purulent
- **Pleuritic pain**: when infection spreads to involve pleura, or with segmental collapse due to retained secretions
- **Haemoptysis**:
  Streaks of blood common, larger volumes with exacerbations of infection
  Massive haemoptysis requiring bronchial artery embolisation sometimes occurs
- **Infective exacerbation**: increased sputum volume with fever, malaise, anorexia
- **Halitosis**: frequently accompanies purulent sputum
- **General debility**: difficulty maintaining weight, anorexia, exertional breathlessness

Investigations

In addition to common respiratory pathogens, sputum culture may reveal *Pseudomonas aeruginosa* and *Staphylococcus aureus*, fungi such as *Aspergillus* and non-tuberculous mycobacteria.

Mild bronchiectasis may not be apparent on a plain chest X-ray. In advanced disease, thickened airway walls, cystic bronchiectatic spaces and associated areas of pneumonic consolidation or collapse may be visible. CT is much more sensitive and shows thickened, dilated airways (Fig. 17.29).

If the patient is suspected of having a ciliary dysfunction syndrome a nasal FeNO sample should be taken as a screening test, then consideration of nasal brush biopsy and genetic testing. The nasal biopsies shoud be assessed for cilary beat frequency and structural ciliary abnormalities assessed by electron microscopy.

Management

Physiotherapy

Patients should be shown how to perform regular daily physiotherapy to assist the drainage of excess bronchial secretions. This reduces the amount of cough and sputum and prevents recurrent episodes of bronchopulmonary infection. Patients should lie in a position in which the lobe to be drained is uppermost. Deep breathing, followed by forced expiratory manoeuvres (the 'active cycle of breathing' technique), helps to move secretions in the dilated bronchi towards the trachea, from which they can be cleared by vigorous coughing. Devices that increase airway pressure either by a constant amount (positive expiratory pressure mask) or in an oscillatory manner (flutter valve) aid sputum clearance in some patients and a variety of techniques should be tried to find the one that suits the individual. The optimum duration and frequency of physiotherapy depend on the amount of sputum but 5–10 minutes twice daily is a minimum for most patients.

Antibiotic therapy

For most patients with bronchiectasis, the appropriate antibiotics are the same as those used in COPD but larger doses and longer courses are required. When secondary infection occurs with staphylococci and Gram-negative bacilli, in particular *Pseudomonas* species, antibiotic therapy becomes more challenging and should be guided by microbiological sensitivities. For *Pseudomonas*, oral ciprofloxacin (500–750 mg twice daily) or an intravenous anti-pseudomonal β-lactam (e.g. piperacillin–tazobactam or ceftazidime) will be required. Haemoptysis in bronchiectasis often responds to treatment of the underlying infection, although percutaneous embolisation of the bronchial circulation by an interventional radiologist may be necessary in the event of massive or repeated haemoptysis.

Surgical treatment

Excision of bronchiectatic areas is indicated in only a small proportion of cases. These are usually patients in whom the bronchiectasis is confined to a single lobe or segment on CT. Unfortunately, many of those in whom medical treatment proves unsuccessful are also unsuitable for surgery because of either extensive bilateral bronchiectasis or coexisting severe airflow obstruction. In progressive forms of bronchiectasis, resection of destroyed areas of lung that are acting as a reservoir of infection should be considered only as a last resort.

Prognosis

The disease is progressive when associated with ciliary dysfunction or cystic fibrosis, and eventually causes respiratory failure. In other patients, the prognosis can be relatively good if physiotherapy is performed regularly and antibiotics are used aggressively.

Prevention

As bronchiectasis commonly starts in childhood following measles, whooping cough or a primary tuberculous infection, adequate prevention and treatment of these conditions is essential. Early recognition and treatment of bronchial obstruction is also important.

Cystic fibrosis

Genetics, pathogenesis and epidemiology

Cystic fibrosis (CF) is the most common life-limiting genetic disease in people of predominantly European descent, with autosomal recessive inheritance, a carrier rate of 1 in 25, and an incidence of about 1 in 2500 live births in this population, although worldwide the incidence of CF varies widely. CF is the result of pathogenic variants affecting a gene on the long arm of chromosome 7, which codes for a chloride channel known as cystic fibrosis transmembrane conductance regulator (*CFTR*); this influences salt and water movement across epithelial cell membranes. The most common pathogenic *CFTR* variant in northern European and American populations is ΔF508, but over 2000 pathogenic variants of this gene have now been identified. The genetic defect causes increased sodium and chloride content in sweat and increased resorption of sodium and water from respiratory epithelium (Fig. 17.30). Relative dehydration of the airway epithelium is thought to predispose to chronic bacterial infection, ciliary dysfunction and bronchiectasis. The gene defect also causes disorders in the gut epithelium, pancreas, liver and reproductive tract (see below).

In the 1960s, few patients with CF survived infancy. In modern practice, however, life expectancy has been increased by aggressive treatment of airway infection and nutritional support and in many high income countries there are now more adults than children with CF. Until recently, the diagnosis was most commonly made from the clinical picture (bowel obstruction, failure to thrive, steatorrhoea and/or chest symptoms in a young child), supported by sweat electrolyte testing and genotyping. Patients with unusual phenotypes were commonly missed, however, and late diagnosis led to poorer outcomes. Neonatal screening for CF using immunoreactive trypsin and genetic testing of newborn blood samples is now routine in the UK and should reduce delayed diagnosis and improve outcomes. Pre-implantation and/or prenatal testing may be offered to those known to be at high risk.

Clinical features

The lungs are macroscopically normal at birth, but bronchiolar inflammation and infections usually lead to bronchiectasis in childhood. At this stage, the lungs are most commonly infected with *Staph. aureus*, while in adulthood, many patients become colonised with antibiotic resistant Gram-negative bacilli. Recurrent exacerbations of bronchiectasis, initially in the upper lobes but subsequently throughout both lungs, cause progressive lung damage, resulting ultimately in death from respiratory failure.

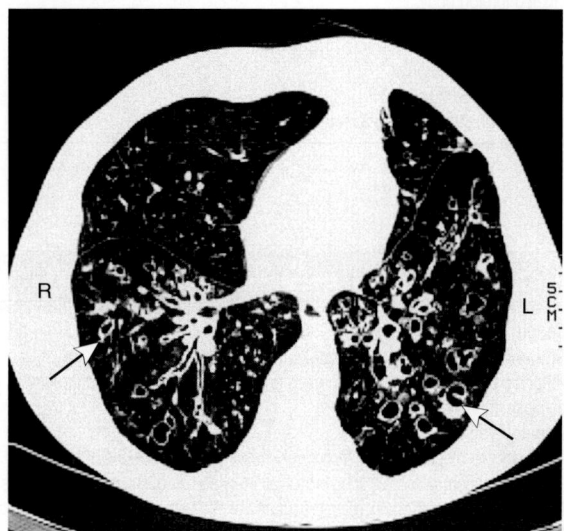

Fig. 17.29 Computed tomogram of bronchiectasis. Extensive dilatation of the bronchi, with thickened walls (arrows) in both lower lobes.

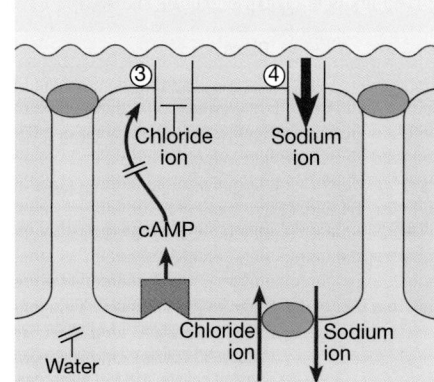

 β₂-adrenoceptor

Fig. 17.30 Cystic fibrosis: basic defect in the pulmonary epithelium. [A] The cystic fibrosis gene (*CFTR*) codes for a chloride channel (1) in the apical (luminal) membrane of epithelial cells in the conducting airways. This is normally controlled by cyclic adenosine monophosphate (cAMP) and indirectly by β-adrenoceptor stimulation, and is one of several apical ion channels that control the quantity and solute content of airway-lining fluid. Normal channels appear to inhibit the adjacent epithelial sodium channels (2). [B] In cystic fibrosis, one of many cystic fibrosis gene defects causes absence or defective function of this chloride channel (3). This leads to reduced chloride secretion and loss of inhibition of sodium channels, with excessive sodium resorption (4) and dehydration of the airway lining. The resulting abnormal airway-lining fluid predisposes to infection by mechanisms still to be fully explained.

Other clinical manifestations are shown in Box 17.32. Most men with CF are infertile due to failure of development of the vas deferens, but microsurgical sperm aspiration and in vitro fertilisation are possible. Genotype is a poor predictor of disease severity in individuals; even siblings with matching genotypes may have different phenotypes. This suggests that other 'modifier genes', as yet unidentified, influence clinical outcome.

Management

Treatment of CF lung disease

The management of CF lung disease is that of severe bronchiectasis. All patients with CF who produce sputum should perform chest physiotherapy daily, and more frequently during exacerbations. While infections with *Staph. aureus* can often be managed with oral antibiotics, intravenous treatment (frequently self-administered at home through an implanted subcutaneous vascular access device) is usually needed for *Pseudomonas* infections.

Over time patients with CF become chronically infected with antibiotic-resistant organisms. These include *P. aeruginosa*, *Stenotrophomonas maltophilia* and *Burkholderia cepacia* complex, which may require prolonged treatment with combinations of intravenous antibiotics. The impact of non-tuberculous mycobacteria is less clear, with the exception of *Mycobacterium abscessus*. This organism, which is often pan-resistant, may be transmitted between patients with CF causing progressive lung destruction and potentially precluding lung transplantation. Fungi such as *Aspergillus fumigatus* may cause infection or allergic bronchopulmonary aspergillosis.

There has been a rapid advance in the maintenance therapies for patients with CF, including mucolytic therapies, long-term inhaled antibiotics, anti-inflammatory agents and more recently CFTR modulator therapies (Box 17.33) (see below).

For advanced CF lung disease, home oxygen and NIV may be necessary to treat respiratory failure. Ultimately, lung transplantation can produce dramatic improvements but is limited by donor organ availability and the long-term issues associated with CLAD.

The transition from paediatric to adult CF care raises specific management issues in adolescence, which are summarized in Box 17.34.

Treatment of non-respiratory manifestations of CF

There is a clear link between good nutrition and prognosis in CF. Malabsorption occurs in 85% of patients due to exocrine pancreatic failure and is treated with oral pancreatic enzymes and vitamin supplements.

> ### i 17.32 Clinical features and complications of cystic fibrosis
>
> **Respiratory**
> - Progressive airway obstruction
> - Infective exacerbations of bronchiectasis
> - Respiratory failure
> - Spontaneous pneumothorax
> - Allergic bronchopulmonary aspergillosis
> - Haemoptysis
> - Lobar collapse due to secretions
> - Pulmonary hypertension
> - Nasal polyps
>
> **Gastrointestinal and hepatic**
> - Malabsorption and steatorrhoea
> - Distal intestinal obstruction syndrome
> - Increased risk of gastrointestinal malignancy
> - Cystic fibrosis-associated liver disease (CFLD), including biliary cirrhosis, portal hypertension, varices and splenomegaly
> - Gallstones
>
> **Others**
> - Diabetes (25% of adults)
> - Delayed puberty
> - Male infertility
> - Stress incontinence due to repeated forced cough
> - Psychosocial problems
> - Osteoporosis
> - Arthropathy
> - Cutaneous vasculitis

The increased calorie requirements of patients with CF are met by supplemental feeding, including nasogastric or gastrostomy tube feeding if required. Diabetes eventually develops in over 25% of patients and needs insulin therapy. Osteoporosis secondary to malabsorption and chronic ill health should be sought and treated.

CFTR modulator therapies

CFTR modulators are small molecules designed to target specific *CFTR* variants. 'Correctors' act by correcting CFTR misfolding, thereby improving trafficking to the cell surface; and 'potentiators' act by improving the function of CFTR that is already at the cell surface.

Ivacaftor, a CFTR potentiator, is an oral treatment for the 5% of patients with the G551D variant and a number of other gating variants. It causes sustained improvements in FEV₁ and weight, and normalization of the sweat chloride levels. Newer combinations of CFTR correctors and potentiators (lumacaftor/ivacaftor and elexacaftor/tezacaftor/ivacaftor) are now treating patients with the more common ΔF 508 variant and represent a

17

17.33 Treatments that reduce chest exacerbations and/or improve lung function in cystic fibrosis

Therapy	Drugs
Mucolytic therapies	Nebulised recombinant human DNase 2.5 mg daily Nebulised hypertonic saline (7%) 4 mL twice daily Inhaled mannitol 400 mg twice daily
Inhaled antibiotics	Nebulised tobramycin 300 mg twice daily, alternate months Inhaled powder tobramycin 28 mg twice daily, given alternate months Nebulised colistin 1 MU twice daily Nebulised colistin 2 MU twice daily Inhaled colistin 1.6 MU twice daily Nebulised aztreonam 75 mg three times daily alternate months Nebulised levofloxacin 240 mg twice daily, alternate months
Anti-inflammatory therapy	Azithromycin 250 mg/500 mg once a day three times weekly
CFTR modulator therapy	Ivacaftor Ivacaftor/lumacaftor Ivacaftor/tezacaftor Ivacaftor/tezacaftor/elexacaftor

(CFTR = cystic fibrosis transmembrane conductance regulator; FEV$_1$ = forced expiratory volume in 1 sec; FVC = forced vital capacity)

17.34 Cystic fibrosis (CF) in adolescence

Issues for the patient

- Move to adult CF centre – loss of trusted paediatric team
- Feelings of being different from peers due to chronic illness
- Demanding treatments that conflict with social and school life
- Pressure to take responsibility for self-care
- Relationship/fertility concerns

Issues for the patient's parents

- Loss of control over patient's treatment – feeling excluded
- Loss of trusted paediatric team
- Need to develop trust in adult team
- Feelings of helplessness when adolescent rebels or will not take treatment

Issues for the CF team

- Reluctance or refusal by patient to engage with transition
- Management of deterioration due to non-adherence
- Motivation of adolescents to self-care
- Provision of adolescent-friendly health-care environment

step forward in therapy. Other strategies under development for the treatment of CF including delivery of somatic gene therapy via liposome or viral vectors, and the use of gene-editing technology such as CRISPR.

Infections of the respiratory system

Infections of the upper and lower respiratory tract are a major cause of morbidity and mortality, particularly in patients at the extremes of age and those with pre-existing lung disease or immune suppression. Features that are specific to older people are shown in Box 17.35.

Upper respiratory tract infection

Upper respiratory tract infections (URTIs), such as coryza (the common cold), acute pharyngitis and acute tracheobronchitis, are the most

17.35 Respiratory infection in old age

- **Increased risk of and from respiratory infection**: because of reduced immune responses, increased closing volumes, reduced respiratory muscle strength and endurance, altered mucus layer, poor nutritional status and the increased prevalence of chronic lung disease.
- **Predisposing factors**: other medical conditions may predispose to infection, e.g. swallowing difficulties due to stroke increase the risk of aspiration pneumonia.
- **Atypical presentation**: older patients often present with delirium, rather than breathlessness or cough.
- **Mortality**: the vast majority of deaths from pneumonia in high-income countries occur in older people.
- **Influenza**: has a much higher morbidity and mortality rate. Vaccination significantly reduces morbidity and mortality in old age but uptake is poor.
- **COVID-19**: increasing age is recognized as a highly significant risk factor for morbidity and mortality.
- **Tuberculosis**: most cases in old age represent reactivation of previous, often unrecognised, disease and may be precipitated by glucocorticoid therapy, diabetes mellitus and the factors above. Cryptic miliary tuberculosis is an occasional alternative presentation. Older people more commonly suffer adverse effects from antituberculous chemotherapy and require close monitoring.

common of all communicable diseases and represent the most frequent cause of short-term absenteeism from work and school. The vast majority of such infections are caused by viruses and, in adults, are usually short-lived and rarely serious.

Acute coryza is the most common URTI and is usually caused by rhinovirus infection. The usual symptoms are general malaise, nasal discharge, sneezing and cough. Involvement of the pharynx causes a sore throat, and that of the larynx a hoarse or 'lost' voice. If complicated by tracheitis or bronchitis, chest tightness and wheeze typical of asthma occur. Specific investigation is rarely warranted and treatment is symptomatic. Symptoms usually resolve quickly, but if repeated URTIs 'go to the chest', a more formal diagnosis of asthma ought to be considered. A variety of viruses causing URTI may also trigger exacerbations of asthma or COPD and aggravate other lung diseases.

Bordetella pertussis, the cause of whooping cough (pertussis), is an important cause of URTI. Vaccination confers protection and is usually offered in infancy, but its efficacy wanes in adult life and the infection is easily spread. Adults usually experience a mild illness similar to acute coryza but some individuals develop paroxysms of coughing that can persist for weeks to months, earning whooping cough the designation of 'the cough of 100 days'. The diagnosis may be confirmed by bacterial culture, polymerase chain reaction (PCR) from a nasopharyngeal swab or serological testing. If the illness is recognised early in the clinical course, macrolide antibiotics may ameliorate the course. Pertussis is a reportable disease in the UK.

Rhinosinusitis typically manifests as a combination of nasal congestion, blockage or discharge and may be accompanied by facial pain/pressure or loss of smell. Examination usually confirms erythematous swollen nasal mucosa and pus may be evident. Nasal polyps should be sought and dental infection excluded. Treatment with topical glucocorticoids, nasal decongestants and regular nasal douching is usually sufficient and, although bacterial infection is often present, antibiotics are indicated only if symptoms persist for more than 5 days. Persistent symptoms or recurrent episodes should prompt a referral to an ear, nose and throat specialist.

Viral respiratory tract infections with the potential to cause more severe disease (including COVID-19) are discussed in Chapter 13.

Pneumonia

Pneumonia is as an acute respiratory illness associated with recently developed radiological pulmonary shadowing that may be segmental, lobar or multilobar. The context in which pneumonia develops is highly suggestive of the likely organism(s) involved; therefore, pneumonias are usually classified as community- or hospital-acquired, or those occurring in immunocompromised hosts. 'Lobar pneumonia' is a radiological and pathological term referring to homogeneous consolidation of one or more lung lobes, often with associated pleural inflammation; bronchopneumonia refers to more patchy alveolar consolidation associated with bronchial and bronchiolar inflammation, often affecting both lower lobes.

Community-acquired pneumonia

Figures from the UK suggest that an estimated 5–11/1000 adults suffer from community-acquired pneumonia (CAP) each year, accounting for around 5%–12% of all lower respiratory tract infections. CAP may affect all age groups but is commonest at the extremities of age.

Most cases are spread by droplet infection, and while CAP may occur in previously healthy individuals, several factors may impair the effectiveness of local defences and predispose to CAP (Box 17.36). *Streptococcus pneumoniae* (Fig. 17.31) remains the most common infecting agent, and thereafter the likelihood that other organisms may be involved depends on the age of the patient and the clinical context. Viral infections are recognised as important causes of CAP in children and their contribution to adult CAP is increasingly recognized. The common causative organisms are shown in Box 17.37.

Clinical features

Pneumonia, particularly lobar pneumonia, usually presents as an acute illness. Systemic features, such as fever, rigors, shivering and malaise, predominate and delirium may be present. The appetite is invariably lost and headache frequently reported.

Pulmonary symptoms include cough, which at first is characteristically short, painful and dry, but later is accompanied by the expectoration of mucopurulent sputum. Rust-coloured sputum may be produced by patients with *Strep. pneumoniae* infection and the occasional patient may report haemoptysis. Pleuritic chest pain may be a presenting feature and on occasion may be referred to the shoulder or anterior abdominal wall. Upper abdominal tenderness is sometimes apparent in patients with lower lobe pneumonia or those with associated hepatitis. Less typical presentations may be seen in childhood and old age.

While different organisms often give rise to a similar clinical and radiological picture, it may be possible to infer the likely agent from the clinical context. *Mycoplasma pneumoniae* is more common in young people and rare in old age, whereas *Haemophilus influenzae* is more common in older people, particularly those with underlying lung disease. *Legionella pneumophila* occurs in local outbreaks centred on contaminated cooling towers in hotels, hospitals and other industries. *Staphylococcus aureus* is more common following an episode of influenza. *Klebsiella* pneumonia has a specific association with alcohol abuse and often presents with a particularly severe bacteraemic illness and cavitation on the chest X-ray. Recent foreign travel raises the possibility of infections that may otherwise be unusual in the UK, e.g. Middle East respiratory syndrome (MERS), melioidosis (South-east Asia and northern Australia) and endemic fungal infection (North, Central or South America). Certain occupations may be associated with exposure to specific bacteria (p. 546).

Clinical examination should first focus on the respiratory and pulse rates, blood pressure and an assessment of the mental state, as these are important in assessing the severity of the illness. In the UK, severity is assessed using the CURB-65 score, which takes into account both examination and investigation findings (Fig. 17.32). Chest signs vary, depending on the inflammatory response, which proceeds through stages of acute exudation, red and then grey hepatisation, and finally resolution. When consolidated, the lung is typically dull to percussion and, as conduction of sound is enhanced, auscultation reveals bronchial breathing and whispering pectoriloquy; crackles are heard throughout. An assessment of the state of nutrition is important, particularly in old age and frailty. The presence of herpes labialis may point to streptococcal infection, as may the finding of 'rusty' sputum. The differential diagnosis of pneumonia is shown in Box 17.38.

Investigations

The object of investigations, which are summarised in Box 17.39, is to confirm the diagnosis, assess severity and identify the development of complications.

Management

The most important aspects of management are oxygenation, fluid balance and antibiotic therapy. In severe or prolonged illness, nutritional support may be required.

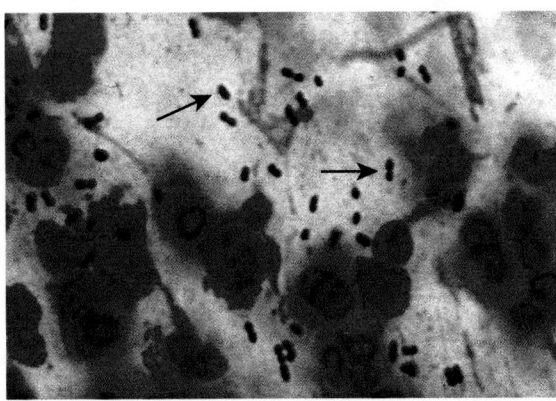

Fig. 17.31 Gram stain of sputum showing Gram-positive diplococci characteristic of *Streptococcus pneumoniae* (arrows).

 17.36 Factors that predispose to pneumonia

- Cigarette smoking
- Upper respiratory tract infections
- Alcohol
- Glucocorticoid therapy
- Old age
- Recent influenza infection
- Pre-existing lung disease
- HIV
- Indoor air pollution

17.37 Organisms causing community-acquired pneumonia

Bacteria

- *Streptococcus pneumoniae*
- *Mycoplasma pneumoniae*
- *Legionella pneumophila*
- *Chlamydia pneumoniae*
- *Haemophilus influenzae*
- *Staphylococcus aureus*
- *Chlamydia psittaci*
- *Coxiella burnetii* (Q fever)
- *Klebsiella pneumoniae* (Freidländer's bacillus)

Viruses

- Influenza, parainfluenza
- Measles
- Herpes simplex
- Varicella
- Adenovirus
- Cytomegalovirus
- Coronaviruses (SARS-CoV-2 and MERS-CoV)

(MERS = Middle East respiratory syndrome; SARS = severe acute respiratory syndrome)

17.38 Differential diagnosis of pneumonia

- Pulmonary infarction
- Pulmonary/pleural tuberculosis
- Pulmonary oedema (can be unilateral)
- Pulmonary eosinophilia
- Malignancy: bronchoalveolar cell carcinoma
- Cryptogenic organising pneumonia/bronchiolitis obliterans organising pneumonia (COP/BOOP)

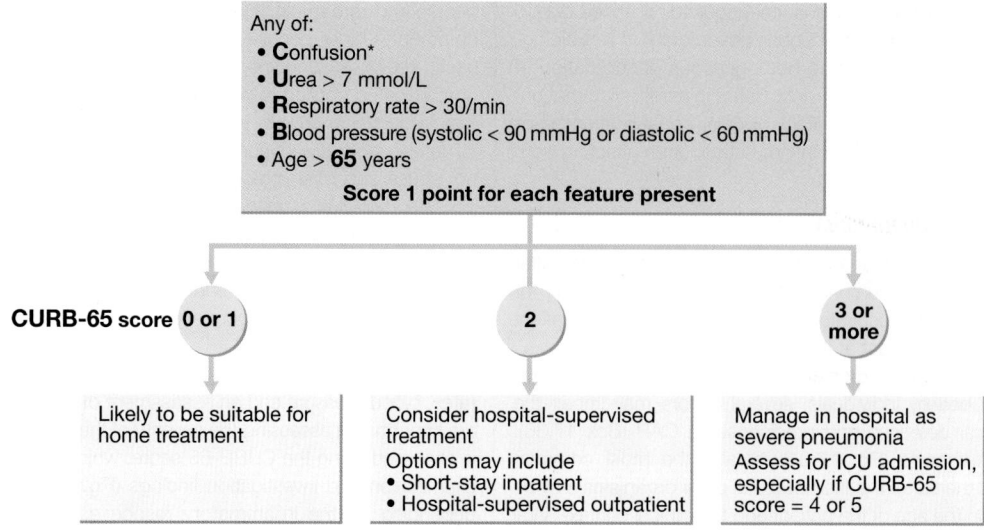

Fig. 17.32 **Hospital CURB-65.** *Defined as a mental test score of 8 or less, or new disorientation in person, place or time. (ICU = intensive care unit; urea of 7 mmol/L ≅ 20 mg/dL)

Oxygen

Oxygen should be administered to all patients with tachypnoea, hypox-aemia, hypotension or acidosis to maintain the target oxygen saturations specified on p. 195. Continuous positive airway pressure (CPAP) should be considered in those who remain hypoxic despite high-concentration oxygen therapy, and these patients should be managed in a high-dependency or intensive care environment where mechanical ventilation is available. Indications for referral to an intensive care unit are summarised in Box 17.40.

Fluid balance

Intravenous fluids should be considered in those with severe illness, in older patients and those with vomiting. It may be appropriate to discontinue hypertensive agents temporarily, particularly if there is evidence of acute kidney injury secondary to sepsis. Otherwise, an adequate oral intake of fluid should be encouraged. Vasopressor support may be required in patients with shock.

Antibiotic treatment

Prompt administration of appropriate antibiotics improves the outcome. The initial choice of antibiotic is guided by clinical context, severity assessment, local knowledge of antibiotic resistance patterns and antibiotic guidelines. Current regimens are detailed in Box 17.41. In most patients with uncomplicated pneumonia a 5-day course is adequate, although treatment is usually required for longer in patients with pneumonia due to *Legionella pneumophila*, *Staph. aureus* or *Klebsiella pneumoniae*.

Treatment of pleural pain

It is important to relieve pleural pain in order to allow the patient to breathe normally and cough efficiently. For the majority, simple analgesia with paracetamol, co-codamol or NSAIDs is sufficient. In some patients, opiates may be required but must be used with extreme caution in individuals with poor respiratory function.

Physiotherapy

Physiotherapy is not usually indicated in patients with CAP, although it may be helpful to assist expectoration in patients who suppress cough because of pleural pain.

Prognosis

Most patients respond promptly to antibiotic therapy. Fever may persist for several days, however, and the chest X-ray often takes several weeks or even months to resolve, especially in old age. Delayed recovery

suggests either that a complication has occurred (Box 17.42) or that the diagnosis is incorrect (see Box 17.38). Alternatively, the pneumonia may be secondary to a proximal bronchial obstruction or recurrent aspiration. The mortality rate of adults with non-severe pneumonia is very low (<1%); hospital death rates are typically between 5% and 10% but may be as high as 50% in severe illness.

Discharge and follow-up

The decision to discharge a hospitalised patient depends on the home circumstances and the likelihood of complications. A chest X-ray need not be repeated before discharge in patients making a satisfactory clinical recovery. Clinical review by general practitioner or hospital should be arranged around 6 weeks later and a chest X-ray obtained if there are persistent symptoms, physical signs or reasons to suspect underlying malignancy, such as tobacco exposure.

Prevention

Current smokers should be advised to stop. Influenza and pneumococcal vaccination should be offered to patients at highest risk of pneumonia (e.g. those over 65 or with chronic lung, heart, liver or kidney disease, diabetes or immunosuppression). Causes of pneumonia that have important public health implications must be notified to the appropriate health authority for appropriate investigation and follow-up (see Box 6.11). In resource-poor settings, tackling malnourishment and indoor air pollution, and encouraging immunisation against measles, pertussis and *Haemophilus influenzae* type b, are particularly important in children.

Hospital-acquired pneumonia

Hospital-acquired pneumonia (HAP) is defined as an episode of pneumonia that presents at least 48 hours after admission to hospital and was not incubating at the time of admission. It is the second most common healthcare-associated infection (HAI) after surgical-site infections and the leading cause of HAI-associated death. Older patients are particularly at risk, as are patients in intensive care units. The term ventilator-associated pneumonia (VAP) is used to describe pneumonia that develops in a person who is mechanically ventilated. The factors predisposing to the development of HAP are listed in Box 17.43.

Clinical features and investigation

The diagnosis should be considered in any hospitalised patient who develops purulent sputum (or endotracheal secretions), new radiological infiltrates, an otherwise unexplained increase in oxygen requirement, a core temperature >38.3°C, and a leucocytosis or leucopenia. The clinical

17.39 Investigations in community-acquired pneumonia*

Blood

Full blood count

- Very high (>20 × 10⁹/L) or low (<4 × 10⁹/L) white cell count: marker of severity
- Neutrophil leucocytosis >15 × 10⁹/L: suggests bacterial aetiology
- Haemolytic anaemia: occasional complication of *Mycoplasma*

Urea and electrolytes

- Urea >7 mmol/L (~20 mg/dL): marker of severity
- Hyponatraemia: marker of severity

Liver function tests

- Abnormal if basal pneumonia inflames liver
- Hypoalbuminaemia: marker of severity

Procalcitonin

- A high procalcitonin is more suggestive of bacterial than viral infection (see Ch. 6)

C-reactive protein/erythrocyte sedimentation rate

- Non-specifically elevated

Blood culture

- Bacteraemia: marker of severity

Arterial blood gases

- Measure when SpO_2 <93% or when clinical features are severe, to assess ventilatory failure or acidosis

Sputum

Sputum samples

- Gram stain (see Fig. 17.31), culture and antimicrobial sensitivity testing

Pharyngeal swab

- NAAT for respiratory viruses (e.g. influenza, parainfluenza, coronaviruses) and bacteria (e.g. *Mycoplasma pneumoniae*)

Urine

- Pneumococcal and/or *Legionella* antigen

Chest X-ray

Lobar pneumonia

- Patchy opacification evolves into homogeneous consolidation of affected lobe
- Air bronchogram (air-filled bronchi appear lucent against consolidated lung tissue) may be present (Fig. 17.33)

Bronchopneumonia

- Typically patchy and segmental shadowing

Complications

- Para-pneumonic effusion, intrapulmonary abscess or empyema

Staphylococcus aureus

- Suggested by multilobar shadowing, cavitation, pneumatoceles and abscesses

Pleural fluid

- Always aspirate and culture when present in more than trivial amounts, preferably with ultrasound guidance

*These investigations are for moderate- to high-severity community-acquired ammonia (CAP). Low-severity CAP is usually managed empirically without the need for blood tests and microbiological investigations, unless the patient has risk factors for underlying disease or an atypical clinical course.
(NAAT = nucleic acid amplification test)

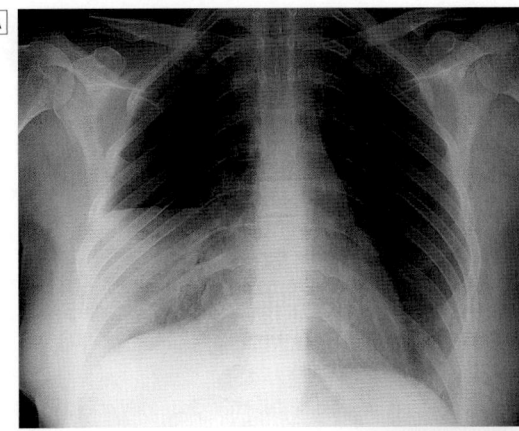
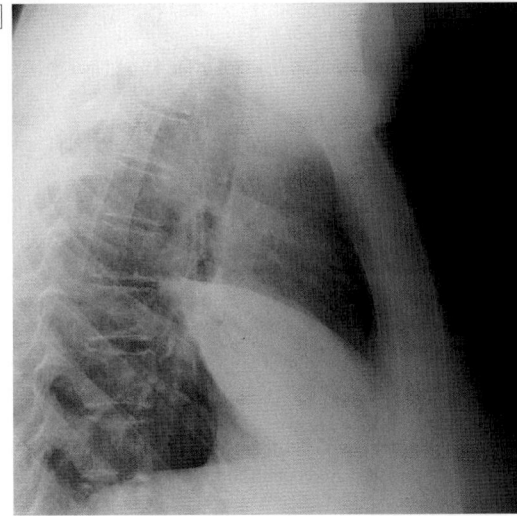

Fig. 17.33 Pneumonia of the right middle lobe. [A] Posteroanterior view: consolidation in the right middle lobe with characteristic opacification beneath the horizontal fissure and loss of normal contrast between the right heart border and lung. [B] Lateral view: consolidation confined to the anteriorly situated middle lobe.

17.40 Indications for referral to intensive care

- CURB score of 4–5 (see Fig. 17.32), failing to respond rapidly to initial management
- Persisting hypoxia (PaO_2 <8 kPa (60 mmHg)), despite high concentrations of oxygen
- Progressive hypercapnia
- Severe acidosis
- Circulatory shock
- Reduced conscious level

Management

The principles of management are similar to those of CAP, focusing on adequate oxygenation, appropriate fluid balance and antibiotics. The choice of empirical antibiotic therapy is considerably more challenging, however, given the diversity of pathogens and the potential for drug resistance.

The organisms implicated in early-onset HAP (occurring within 4–5 days of admission) are similar to those involved in CAP. The initial choice of agents is most appropriately guided by knowledge of local patterns of microbiology and antibiotic resistance (Box 17.44). If the infecting organism is identified, antibiotic therapy should be refined, with the narrowest possible spectrum agent(s) being used. The most appropriate duration of antibiotic therapy has not been established and is a matter of clinical judgement. Physiotherapy is important to aid expectoration in less mobile patients and adequate nutritional support is often required.

features and radiographic signs are variable and non-specific, however, raising a broad differential diagnosis that includes pulmonary embolism, ARDS, pulmonary oedema, pulmonary haemorrhage and drug toxicity. Therefore, in contrast to CAP, microbiological confirmation should be sought whenever possible. Adequate sputum samples may be difficult to obtain and physiotherapy should be considered to aid expectoration. In patients who are mechanically ventilated, bronchoscopy-directed protected brush specimens, bronchoalveolar lavage (BAL) or endotracheal aspirates may be obtained.

Prevention

Despite appropriate management, the mortality from HAP is high (approximately 30%), mandating prevention whenever possible. Good hygiene is paramount, particularly with regard to hand-washing and any equipment used. Steps should be taken to minimise the chances of aspiration and to limit the use of stress ulcer prophylaxis with proton pump inhibitors. Oral antiseptic (chlorhexidine 2%) may be used to decontaminate the upper airway and some intensive care units employ selective decontamination of the digestive tract when the anticipated requirement for ventilation will exceed 48 hours.

Suppurative pneumonia, aspiration pneumonia and pulmonary abscess

These conditions are considered together, as their aetiology and clinical features overlap. Suppurative pneumonia is characterised by destruction of the lung parenchyma by the inflammatory process. Although micro-abscess formation is a characteristic histological feature, 'pulmonary abscess' is usually taken to refer to lesions in which there is a large localised collection of pus, or a cavity lined by chronic inflammatory tissue, from which pus has escaped by rupture into a bronchus.

Suppurative pneumonia and pulmonary abscess often develop after the inhalation of septic material during operations on the nose, mouth or throat, under general anaesthesia, or of vomitus during anaesthesia or coma, particularly if oral hygiene is poor. Additional risk factors for aspiration pneumonia include bulbar or vocal cord palsy, achalasia or oesophageal reflux, and alcoholism. Aspiration tends to localise to dependent areas of the lung, such as the apical segment of the lower lobe in a supine patient. These conditions may also complicate local bronchial obstruction from a neoplasm or foreign body.

Infections are usually due to a mixture of anaerobes and aerobes in common with the typical flora encountered in the mouth and upper respiratory tract. Isolates of *Prevotella melaninogenica*, *Fusobacterium necrophorum*, anaerobic or microaerophilic cocci and *Bacteroides fragilis* may be identified. When suppurative pneumonia or a pulmonary abscess occurs in a previously healthy lung, the most likely infecting organisms are *Staph. aureus* or *K. pneumoniae*. *Actinomyces* spp. cause chronic suppurative pulmonary infections, which may be associated with poor dental hygiene.

Bacterial infection of a pulmonary infarct or a collapsed lobe may also produce a suppurative pneumonia or lung abscess. The organism(s) isolated from the sputum include *Strep. pneumoniae*, *Staph. aureus*, *Streptococcus pyogenes*, *H. influenzae* and, in some cases, anaerobic bacteria. In many cases, however, no pathogen can be isolated, particularly when antibiotics have been given.

Some strains of *Staph. aureus*, often community-acquired MRSA (CA-MRSA), produce the cytotoxin Panton–Valentine leukocidin (PVL). PVL-producing strains are mainly responsible for suppurative skin infection but also cause a rapidly progressive severe necrotising pneumonia.

Lemierre syndrome is a rare cause of pulmonary abscesses. The usual causative agent is the anaerobe *Fusobacterium necrophorum*. The illness typically commences as a sore throat, painful swollen neck, fever, rigor, haemoptysis and dyspnoea; spread into the jugular veins leads to thrombosis and metastatic dispersal of the organisms.

Injection drug-users are at particular risk of developing haematogenous lung abscess, often in association with endocarditis affecting the pulmonary and tricuspid valves. These abcesses are usually caused by staphylococci and streptococci, and occasionally by fungi such as *Candida* spp.

A non-infective form of aspiration pneumonia – exogenous lipid pneumonia – may follow the aspiration of animal, vegetable or mineral oils.

The clinical features of suppurative pneumonia are summarised in Box 17.45.

Investigations

Radiological features of suppurative pneumonia include homogeneous lobar or segmental opacity consistent with consolidation or collapse. Abscesses are characterised by cavitation and a fluid level. Occasionally, a pre-existing emphysematous bulla becomes infected and appears as a cavity containing an air–fluid level.

i	17.44 Antibiotics for adults aged 18 years and over with hospital-acquired pneumonia	
Antibiotic	**Dosage and course length**	
First-choice oral antibiotic for non-severe symptoms or signs and not at higher risk of resistance[1]		
Co-amoxiclav	500/125 mg 8-hourly for 5 days then review	
Alternative oral antibiotics for non-severe symptoms or signs and not at higher risk of resistance, if penicillin allergy or if co-amoxiclav unsuitable[2]		
Options include:		
Doxycycline	200 mg on first day, then 100 mg daily for 4 days (5-day course) then review	
Cefalexin (caution in penicillin allergy)	500 mg 3 times or twice daily (can be increased to 1 g to 1.5 g 4 or 3 times daily) for 5 days then review	
Co-trimoxazole	960 mg twice daily for 5 days then review	
Levofloxacin (only if switching from IV levofloxacin with specialist advice; consider safety issues)	500 mg daily or twice daily for 5 days then review	
First-choice IV antibiotics if severe symptoms or signs (e.g. of sepsis) or at higher risk of resistance. Review IV antibiotics by 48 hrs and consider switching to oral antibiotics as above for a total of 5 days then review[2]		
Options include:		
Piperacillin with tazobactam	4.5 g 3 times daily (increased to 4.5 g 4 times daily if severe infection)	
Ceftazidime	2 g 3 times daily	
Ceftriaxone	2 g once daily	
Cefuroxime	750 mg 4 or 3 times daily (increased to 1.5 g 4 or 3 times daily if severe infection)	
Meropenem	0.5 g to 1 g 3 times daily	
Ceftazidime with avibactam	2/0.5 g 3 times daily	
Levofloxacin (consider safety issues)	500 mg daily or twice daily (use higher dosage if severe infection)	
Antibiotics to be added if suspected or confirmed MRSA infection (dual therapy with an IV antibiotic listed above)		
Vancomycin	15 mg/kg to 20 mg/kg 3 times or twice daily IV, adjusted according to serum vancomycin concentration (a loading dose of 25 mg/kg to 30 mg/kg can be used in seriously ill people); maximum 2 g per dose	
Teicoplanin	Initially 6 mg/kg twice daily for 3 doses, then 6 mg/kg daily	
Linezolid (if vancomycin cannot be used; specialist advice only)	600 mg twice daily or IV	

[1]Guided by microbiological results when available. [2]Choice should be based on specialist microbiological advice and local resistance data.
Adapted from National Institute for Health and Care Excellence (NICE). Pneumonia (hospital-acquired): antimicrobial prescribing. NICE Guideline [NG139], September 2019. https://www.nice.org.uk/guidance/ng139.

Management

Aspiration pneumonia can usually be treated with amoxicillin and metronidazole. Further modification of antibiotics should be informed by clinical response and microbiological results. CA-MRSA is usually susceptible to a variety of oral non-β-lactam antibiotics, such as trimethoprim–sulfamethoxazole, clindamycin, tetracyclines and linezolid. Parenteral therapy with vancomycin or linezolid can also be considered. *Fusobacterium necrophorum* is highly susceptible to β-lactam antibiotics and to metronidazole, clindamycin and third-generation cephalosporins. Prolonged treatment for 4–6 weeks may be required in some patients with lung abscess. Established pulmonary actinomycosis requires 6–12 months' treatment with intravenous or oral penicillin, or with a tetracycline in penicillin-allergic patients.

Physiotherapy is of great value, especially when suppuration is present in the lower lobes or when a large abscess cavity has formed. In most patients there is a good response to treatment, and although residual fibrosis and bronchiectasis are common sequelae, these seldom give rise to serious morbidity. Surgery should be contemplated if no improvement occurs despite optimal medical therapy. Removal or treatment of any obstructing endobronchial lesion is essential.

i	17.45 Clinical features of suppurative pneumonia

Symptoms

- Cough with large amounts of sputum, sometimes fetid and blood-stained
- Pleural pain common
- Sudden expectoration of copious amounts of foul sputum if abscess ruptures into a bronchus

Clinical signs

- High remittent pyrexia
- Profound systemic upset
- Digital clubbing may develop quickly (10–14 days)
- Consolidation on chest examination; signs of cavitation rarely found
- Pleural rub common
- Rapid deterioration in general health, with marked weight loss if not adequately treated

Pneumonia in the immunocompromised patient

Patients immunocompromised by drugs or disease (particularly human immunodeficiency virus (HIV) infection) are at increased risk of pulmonary infection and pneumonia is the most common cause of death in this group. The majority of infections are caused by the same pathogens that cause pneumonia in immunocompetent individuals, but in patients with more profound immunosuppression less common organisms, or those normally considered to be of low virulence or non-pathogenic, may become 'opportunistic' pathogens. Depending on the clinical context, clinicians should consider the possibility of Gram-negative bacteria, especially *P. aeruginosa*, viruses, fungi, mycobacteria, and less common organisms such as *Nocardia* spp. Infection is often due to more than one organism.

Clinical features

These typically include fever, cough and breathlessness but are influenced by the degree of immunosuppression, and the presentation may be less specific in the more profoundly immunosuppressed. The onset of symptoms tends to be swift in those with a bacterial infection but more gradual in patients with opportunistic organisms such as *Pneumocystis jirovecii* and mycobacterial infections. In *P. jirovecii* pneumonia, symptoms of cough and breathlessness can be present several days or weeks before the onset of systemic symptoms or the appearance of radiographic abnormality. The clinical features of invasive pulmonary aspergillosis are dealt with on p. 525.

Investigations

The approach is informed by the clinical context and severity of the illness. Invasive investigations, such as bronchoscopy, BAL, trans-bronchial biopsy or surgical lung biopsy, are often impractical, as many patients are too ill to undergo these safely; however, 'induced sputum' (p. 487) offers a relatively safe method of obtaining microbiological samples. HRCT can be helpful:

- focal unilateral airspace opacification favours bacterial infection, mycobacteria or *Nocardia*
- bilateral opacification favours *P. jirovecii* pneumonia, fungi, viruses and unusual bacteria, e.g. *Nocardia*
- cavitation may be seen with *N. asteroides*, mycobacteria and fungi
- the presence of a 'halo sign' (a zone of intermediate attenuation between the nodule and the lung parenchyma) may suggest aspergillosis or other invasive fungal infection
- pleural effusions suggest pyogenic bacterial infections and are uncommon in *P. jirovecii* pneumonia.

ß-1,3-D-glucan levels are characteristically elevated in *P. jirovecii* pneumonia.

Management

In theory, treatment should be based on an established aetiological diagnosis; in practice, however, the causative agent is frequently unknown. Factors that favour a bacterial aetiology include neutropenia, rapid onset and deterioration. In these circumstances, broad-spectrum antibiotic therapy should be commenced immediately, e.g. a third-generation cephalosporin, or a quinolone, plus an antistaphylococcal antibiotic, or an antipseudomonal penicillin plus an aminoglycoside. Thereafter, treatment may be tailored according to the results of investigations and the clinical response. Depending on the clinical context and response to treatment, antifungal or antiviral therapies may be added. The management of *P. jirovecii* infection is detailed on page 361 and that of invasive aspergillosis on page 527.

Tuberculosis

Epidemiology

Tuberculosis (TB) is caused by infection with *Mycobacterium tuberculosis* (MTB), which is part of a complex of organisms including *M. bovis* (reservoir cattle) and *M. africanum* (reservoir humans). The resurgence in TB in the UK observed over the latter part of the 20th century has been reversed. Following a 44% drop between 2011 and 2018, the number of new cases of TB in England has dropped to the lowest levels since records began in 1960. Nevertheless, its impact on world health remains significant. An estimated 10 million new cases were recorded in 2018, with the majority of these presenting in the world's poorest nations, which struggle to cover the costs associated with management and control

programmes (Fig. 17.34). In the same year, 1.5 million men, women and children died of TB, compared to 1 million of HIV/AIDS, making TB the worldwide leading cause of death from a single infectious agent that year.

Pathology and pathogenesis

M. tuberculosis is spread by the inhalation of aerosolised droplet nuclei from other infected patients. Once inhaled, the organisms lodge in the alveoli and initiate the recruitment of macrophages and lymphocytes. Macrophages undergo transformation into epithelioid and Langhans cells, which aggregate with the lymphocytes to form the classical tuberculous granuloma (Fig. 17.35). Numerous granulomas aggregate to form a primary lesion or 'Ghon focus' (a pale yellow, caseous nodule, usually a few millimetres to 1–2 cm in diameter), which is characteristically situated in the periphery of the lung. Spread of organisms to the hilar lymph nodes is followed by a similar pathological reaction, and the combination of the primary lesion and regional lymph nodes is referred to as the 'primary complex of Ranke'. Reparative processes encase the primary complex in a fibrous capsule, limiting the spread of bacilli. If no further complications ensue, this lesion eventually calcifies and is clearly seen on a chest X-ray. Lymphatic or haematogenous spread may occur before containment is established, however, seeding secondary foci in other organs, including lymph nodes, serous membranes, meninges, bones, liver, kidneys and lungs, which may lie dormant for years. The only clue that infection is

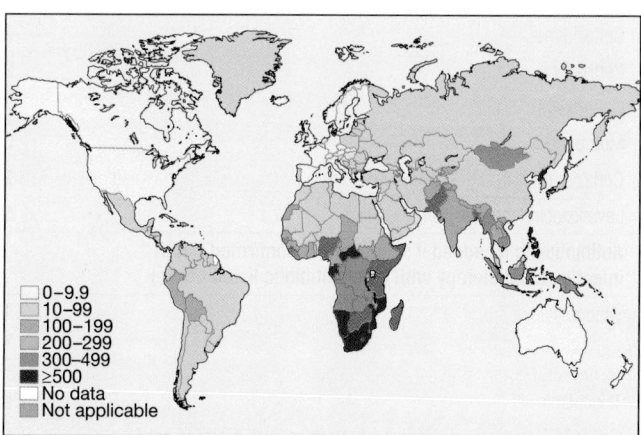

Fig. 17.34 Worldwide incidence of tuberculosis (2019). Estimated new cases (all forms) per 100 000 population. *From Global tuberculosis report 2020. Geneva: World Health Organization; 2020.*

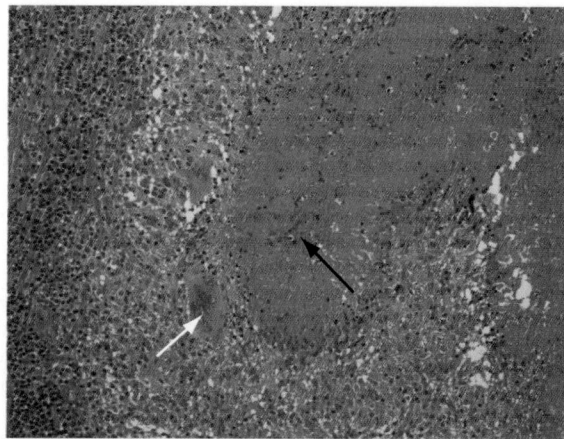

Fig. 17.35 Tuberculous granuloma. Normal lung tissue is lost and replaced by a mass of fibrous tissue with granulomatous inflammation characterised by large numbers of macrophages and multinucleate giant cells (white arrow). The central area of this focus shows caseous degeneration (black arrow). *Courtesy of Dr William Wallace, Department of Pathology, Royal Infirmary of Edinburgh.*

present may be the appearance of a cell-mediated, delayed-type hypersensitivity reaction to tuberculin, demonstrated by tuberculin skin testing or an interferon-gamma release assay (IGRA): so-called latent TB infection (LTBI). If these controlling processes fail, primary progressive disease ensues (Fig. 17.36). The estimated lifetime risk of developing active disease after infection is 10%, with roughly half of this risk occurring in the first 2 years after infection. Factors predisposing to TB are summarised in Box 17.46 and the natural history of infection with TB is summarised in Box 17.47.

Clinical features: pulmonary disease

Primary pulmonary TB

Primary TB refers to the infection of a previously uninfected (tuberculin-negative) individual. A few patients develop a self-limiting febrile illness but clinical disease occurs only if there is a hypersensitivity reaction or progressive infection (Box 17.48). Progressive primary disease may appear during the course of the initial illness or after a latent period of weeks or months.

Miliary TB

Blood-borne dissemination gives rise to miliary TB, which may present acutely but more frequently is characterised by 2–3 weeks of fever, night sweats, anorexia, weight loss and a dry cough. Hepatosplenomegaly may develop and the presence of a headache may indicate coexistent tuberculous meningitis. Auscultation of the chest is frequently normal but in more advanced disease widespread crackles are evident. Fundoscopy may show choroidal tubercles. The classical appearances on chest X-ray are of fine 1–2 mm lesions ('millet seed') distributed throughout the lung fields, although occasionally the appearances are coarser. Anaemia and leucopenia reflect bone marrow involvement.

Post-primary pulmonary TB

Post-primary disease refers to exogenous ('new' infection) or endogenous (reactivation of a dormant primary lesion) infection in a person who has been sensitised by earlier exposure. It is most frequently pulmonary and characteristically occurs in the apex of an upper lobe, where the oxygen tension favours survival of the strictly aerobic organism. The onset is usually insidious, developing slowly over several weeks. Systemic symptoms include fever, night sweats, malaise and loss of appetite and weight, and are accompanied by progressive pulmonary symptoms (Box 17.49). Radiological changes include ill-defined opacification in one

or both of the upper lobes, and as progression occurs, consolidation, collapse and cavitation develop to varying degrees (Fig. 17.37). It is often difficult to distinguish active from quiescent disease on radiological criteria alone but the presence of a miliary pattern or cavitation favours active disease. In extensive disease, collapse may be marked and results in significant displacement of the trachea and mediastinum. Occasionally, a caseous lymph node may drain into an adjoining bronchus, leading to tuberculous pneumonia.

Clinical features: extrapulmonary disease

Extrapulmonary TB accounts for 20% of cases in those who are HIV-negative but is more common in HIV-positive patients.

Lymphadenitis

Lymph nodes are the most common extrapulmonary site of disease. Cervical and mediastinal glands are affected most frequently, followed by axillary and inguinal, and more than one region may be involved. Disease may represent primary infection, spread from contiguous sites or reactivation. Supraclavicular lymphadenopathy is often the result of spread from mediastinal disease. The nodes are usually painless and initially mobile but become matted together with time. When caseation and liquefaction occur, the swelling becomes fluctuant and may discharge through the skin with the formation of a 'collar-stud' abscess and sinus formation. Approximately half of cases fail to show any constitutional features, such as fevers or night sweats. During or after treatment, paradoxical enlargement, development of new nodes and suppuration may all occur but without evidence of continued infection; surgical excision is

| i | 17.46 Factors increasing the risk of tuberculosis |

Patient-related
- Age (children > young adults < old age)
- First-generation immigrants from high-prevalence countries
- Close contacts of patients with smear-positive pulmonary TB
- Overcrowding (prisons, collective dormitories); homelessness (shelters and hostels)
- Chest X-ray evidence of primary TB infection
- Primary infection <1 year previously
- Smoking: cigarettes, bidis (Indian cigarettes made of tobacco wrapped in tembhurni leaves) and cannabis

Associated diseases
- Immunosuppression: HIV (reduced by ART), anti-tumour necrosis factor (TNF) and other biologic therapies, high-dose glucocorticoids, cytotoxic agents
- Malignancy (especially lymphoma and leukaemia)
- Diabetes mellitus
- Chronic kidney disease
- Silicosis
- Gastrointestinal disease associated with malnutrition (gastrectomy, jejuno-ileal bypass, cancer of the pancreas, malabsorption)
- Deficiency of vitamin D or A
- Recent measles in children

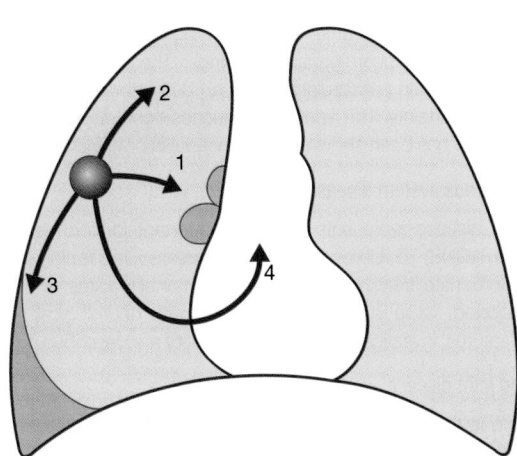

Fig. 17.36 Primary pulmonary tuberculosis. (1) Spread from the primary focus to hilar and mediastinal lymph glands to form the 'primary complex', which heals spontaneously in most cases. (2) Direct extension of the primary focus – progressive pulmonary tuberculosis. (3) Spread to the pleura – tuberculous pleurisy and pleural effusion. (4) Blood-borne spread: *few bacilli* – pulmonary, skeletal, renal, genitourinary infection, often months or years later; *massive spread* – miliary pulmonary tuberculosis and meningitis.

| i | 17.47 Natural history of untreated primary tuberculosis |

Time from infection	Manifestations
3–8 weeks	Primary complex, positive tuberculin skin test
3–6 months	Meningeal, miliary and pleural disease
Up to 3 years	Gastrointestinal, bone and joint, and lymph node disease
Around 8 years	Renal tract disease
From 3 years onwards	Post-primary disease due to reactivation or re-infection

Adapted from Davies PDO, ed. Clinical tuberculosis. London: Hodder Arnold; 1998.

17

---

i 17.48 Features of primary tuberculosis

Infection (4–8 weeks)

- Influenza-like illness
- Skin test conversion
- Primary complex

Disease

- Lymphadenopathy: hilar (often unilateral), paratracheal or mediastinal
- Collapse (especially right middle lobe)
- Consolidation (especially right middle lobe)
- Obstructive emphysema
- Cavitation (rare)
- Pleural effusion
- Miliary disease
- Meningitis
- Pericarditis

Hypersensitivity

- Erythema nodosum
- Phlyctenular conjunctivitis
- Dactylitis

---

i 17.49 Clinical presentations of pulmonary tuberculosis

- Chronic cough, often with haemoptysis
- Pyrexia of unknown origin
- Unresolved pneumonia
- Exudative pleural effusion
- Asymptomatic (diagnosis on chest X-ray)
- Weight loss, general debility
- Spontaneous pneumothorax

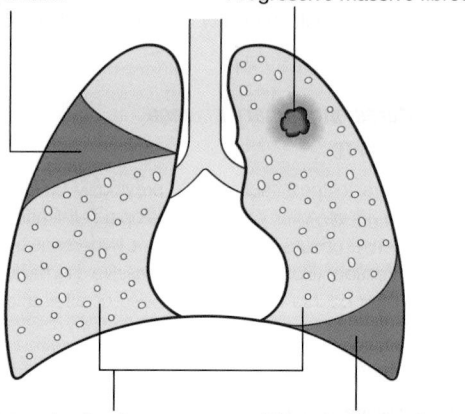

Consolidation/collapse
Differential diagnosis
- Pneumonia
- Bronchial carcinoma
- Pulmonary infarct

Cavitation
Differential diagnosis
- Pneumonia/lung abscess
- Lung cancer
- Pulmonary infarct
- Granulomatosis with polyangiitis (Wegener's granulomatosis)
- Progressive massive fibrosis

'Miliary' diffuse shadowing
Differential diagnosis
- Sarcoidosis
- Malignancy
- Pneumoconiosis
- Infection (e.g. histoplasmosis, melioidosis)
- Tropical pulmonary eosinophilia (TPE)

Pleural effusion/empyema
Differential diagnosis
- Bacterial pneumonia
- Pulmonary infarction
- Carcinoma
- Connective tissue disorder

Fig. 17.37 Chest X-ray: major manifestations and differential diagnosis of pulmonary tuberculosis. Less common manifestations include pneumothorax, acute respiratory distress syndrome (ARDS), cor pulmonale and localised emphysema.

---

rarely necessary. In non-immigrant children in the UK, most mycobacterial lymphadenitis is caused by opportunistic mycobacteria, especially of the *M. avium* complex.

Pleural tuberculosis

Tuberculous pleural effusions are common. Patients present with pleuritic chest pain in addition to the classic clinical features of pulmonary TB. Effusions are caused by both primary and reactivated TB, but can also result from a delayed hypersensitivity reaction to TB in the pleural cavity. Pseudochylothorax, due to compression from TB lymphadenitis, and empyema occur infrequently. Pleural fluid analysis demonstrates a lymphocytic exudate, with low glucose and pH. Pleural fluid smear and culture have sensitivities of only 10% and 25% respectively, however pleural tissue culture increases this to 80%. Raised adenosine deaminase has high sensitivity but low specificity as it occurs in malignancy and empyema also. Effusion volume fluctuates during treatment, even when successful. Therapeutic drainage is performed when necessary and steroids are sometimes used as an alternative.

Gastrointestinal tuberculosis

TB can affect any part of the bowel and patients may present with a wide range of symptoms and signs (Fig. 17.38). Upper gastrointestinal tract involvement is rare and is usually an unexpected histological finding in an endoscopic or laparotomy specimen. Ileocaecal disease accounts for approximately half of abdominal TB cases. Fever, night sweats, anorexia and weight loss are usually prominent and a right iliac fossa mass may be palpable. Up to 30% of cases present with an acute abdomen. Ultrasound or CT may reveal thickened bowel wall, abdominal lymphadenopathy, mesenteric thickening or ascites. Diagnosis rests on obtaining histology by either colonoscopy or mini-laparotomy. The main differential diagnosis is Crohn's disease. Tuberculous peritonitis is characterised by abdominal distension, pain and constitutional symptoms. The ascitic fluid is exudative and cellular, with a predominance of lymphocytes. Laparoscopy reveals multiple white 'tubercles' over the peritoneal and omental surfaces. Low-grade hepatic dysfunction is common in miliary disease, in which biopsy reveals granulomas.

Pericardial disease

Disease occurs in two forms: pericardial effusion and constrictive pericarditis (see Fig. 17.38 and p. 476). Fever and night sweats are rarely prominent and the presentation is usually insidious, with breathlessness and abdominal swelling. Coexistent pulmonary disease is very rare, with the exception of pleural effusion. Pulsus paradoxus, a raised JVP, hepatomegaly, prominent ascites and peripheral oedema are common to both types. Pericardial effusion is associated with increased pericardial dullness and a globular enlarged heart on chest X-ray, and pericardial calcification occurs in around 25% of cases. Constriction is associated with an early third heart sound and, occasionally, atrial fibrillation. Diagnosis is based on clinical, radiological and echocardiographic findings. The effusion is frequently blood-stained. Open pericardial biopsy can be performed where there is diagnostic uncertainty. The addition of glucocorticoids to antituberculous chemotherapy has been shown to be beneficial in constrictive pericarditis.

Central nervous system disease

Meningeal disease represents the most important form of central nervous system (CNS) TB. Unrecognised and untreated, it is rapidly fatal. Even when appropriate treatment is prescribed, mortality rates of 30% have been reported, while survivors may be left with neurological sequelae. Clinical features, investigations and management are described on p.1173.

Bone and joint disease

The spine is the most common site for bony TB (Pott disease), which usually presents with chronic back pain and typically involves the lower thoracic and lumbar spine (see Fig. 17.38). The infection starts as a discitis and then spreads along the spinal ligaments to involve the adjacent anterior vertebral bodies, causing angulation of the vertebrae with subsequent kyphosis. Paravertebral and psoas abscess formation is common and the disease may present with a large (cold) abscess in the inguinal region. CT or MRI is valuable in gauging the extent of disease, the degree of cord compression, and the site for needle biopsy or open exploration,

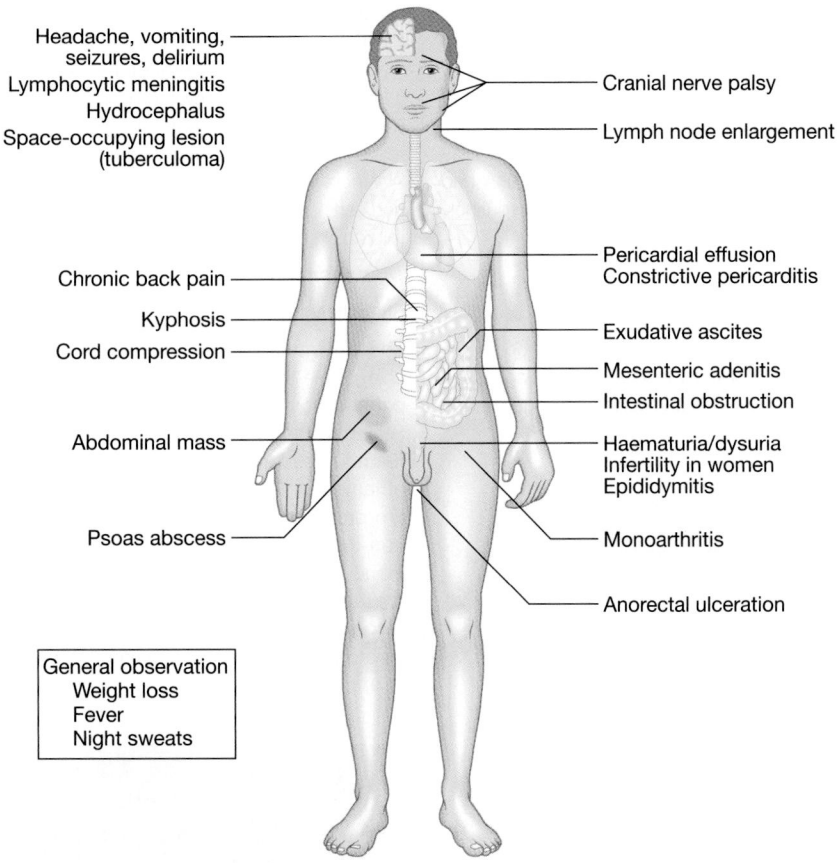

Headache, vomiting, seizures, delirium
Lymphocytic meningitis
Hydrocephalus
Space-occupying lesion (tuberculoma)

Cranial nerve palsy

Lymph node enlargement

Chronic back pain

Pericardial effusion
Constrictive pericarditis

Kyphosis

Exudative ascites

Cord compression

Mesenteric adenitis
Intestinal obstruction

Abdominal mass

Haematuria/dysuria
Infertility in women
Epididymitis

Psoas abscess

Monoarthritis

Anorectal ulceration

General observation
Weight loss
Fever
Night sweats

Fig. 17.38 Systemic presentations of extrapulmonary tuberculosis.

if required. The major differential diagnosis is malignancy, which tends to affect the vertebral body and leave the disc intact. Important complications include spinal instability or cord compression.

TB can affect any joint but most frequently involves the hip or knee. Presentation is usually insidious, with pain and swelling; fever and night sweats are uncommon. Radiological changes are often non-specific but, as disease progresses, reduction in joint space and erosions appear. Poncet arthropathy is an immunologically mediated polyarthritis that usually resolves within 2 months of starting treatment.

Genitourinary disease

Fever and night sweats are rare with renal tract TB and patients are often only mildly symptomatic for many years. Haematuria, frequency and dysuria are often present, with sterile pyuria found on urine microscopy and culture. In women, infertility from endometritis, or pelvic pain and swelling from salpingitis or a tubo-ovarian abscess occurs occasionally. In men, genitourinary TB may present as epididymitis or prostatitis.

Investigations

The presence of an otherwise unexplained cough for more than 3 weeks, particularly in regions where TB is prevalent, or typical chest X-ray or CT changes (Fig. 17.39) should prompt further investigation (Box 17.50). Direct microscopy of a sputum smear remains the most important first step. At least two sputum samples (including at least one obtained in the early morning) from a spontaneously produced deep cough should be obtained. Induced sputum may be used in those unable to expectorate. In selected cases, bronchoscopy and lavage or aspiration of a lymph node by EBUS may be used.

Light-emitting diode fluorescent microscopy with auramine staining (Fig. 17.40) is increasingly replacing the more traditional standard light microscopy and Ziehl–Neelsen stain. A positive smear is sufficient for the presumptive diagnosis of TB but definitive diagnosis requires either

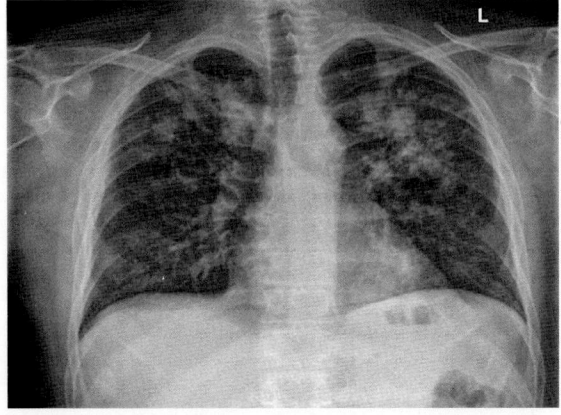

Fig. 17.39 Typical changes of tuberculosis. The chest X-ray shows bilateral upper lobe airspace shadowing with cavitation.

culture or the detection of *M. tuberculosis* DNA. The probability of visualising acid-fast bacilli is proportional to the bacillary burden in the sputum. Smear-negative sputum should also be cultured, as only 10–100 viable organisms are required for sputum to be culture-positive. A diagnosis of smear-negative TB may be considered in advance of culture if the chest X-ray appearances are typical of TB.

The slow growth of MTB on solid (typically between 4 and 6 weeks) and liquid (typically around 2 weeks) culture media has prompted the development of rapid NAATs. For example, the Cepheid GeneXpert MTB/RIF has the capacity to detect MTB (and certain molecular markers of rifampicin resistance) in less than 2 hours. However, while it is specific to MTB, it is not sufficiently sensitive to have replaced culture.

17

The diagnosis of extrapulmonary TB can be more challenging. There are generally fewer organisms (particularly in meningeal or pleural fluid), so culture, histopathological examination of tissue and/or NAAT may be required. Stimulation of T cells by mycobacterial antigens leads to increased levels of adenosine deaminase (ADA) in pleural, pericardial, cerebrospinal and ascitic fluid, so measuring ADA in these fluids may support a diagnosis of TB, but should not replace culture. IGRA and tuberculin skin tests have low sensitivity and specificity, are not routinely used in the diagnosis of active TB infection.

Drug sensitivity testing

The rapid detection of drug resistance is central both to the management of the individual with TB and to control of the disease in the population. The gold standard remains culture. Molecular tests are increasingly used to provide rapid drug sensitivity testing (DST), particularly with regard to the detection of rifampicin resistance, which is important because rifampicin forms the cornerstone of 6-month chemotherapy. Rapid identification of rifampicin resistance is provided by Xpert MTB/RIF. Line probe assays (LPAs) use PCR and reverse hybridisation to detect genetic sequences linked to resistance to both rifampicin and isoniazid, and increasingly to resistance to pyrazinamide, ethambutol and second-line agents.

Whole genome sequencing is now being used routinely in resource-rich settings both for identification of mycobacterium and to predict anti-microbial susceptibility, at least to first-line agents.

Management

Chemotherapy

The treatment of TB is based on the principle of an initial intensive phase to reduce the bacterial population rapidly, followed by a continuation phase to destroy any remaining bacteria (Box 17.51). Standard treatment involves 6 months' treatment with isoniazid and rifampicin, supplemented in the first 2 months with pyrazinamide and ethambutol. Fixed-dose tablets combining two, three or four drugs are preferred. Unless there is reason to suspect drug resistance or non-tuberculous mycobacterium, treatment should be commenced immediately in any patient who is smear-positive, and in those who are smear-negative but with typical chest X-ray changes and no response to standard antibiotics. Where drug resistance is not anticipated, patients can be assumed to be non-infectious after 2 weeks of appropriate therapy.

 17.50 Diagnosis of tuberculosis

Specimens required

Pulmonary

- Sputum* (induced with nebulised hypertonic saline if patient not expectorating)
- Bronchoscopy with washings or BAL
- Gastric washing* (mainly used for children)

Extrapulmonary

- Fluid examination (cerebrospinal, ascitic, pleural, pericardial, joint): yield classically very low
- Tissue biopsy (from affected site or enlarged lymph node): bone marrow/liver may be diagnostic in disseminated disease

Diagnostic tests

- Stain
  Auramine fluorescence
  Ziehl–Neelsen
- Nucleic acid amplification
- Culture
  Solid media (Löwenstein–Jensen, Middlebrook)
  Liquid media (e.g. MGIT)
- Pleural fluid: adenosine deaminase
- Response to empirical antituberculous drugs

Baseline blood tests

- Full blood count, C-reactive protein, urea and electrolytes, liver function tests

*Preferably three early morning samples.
(BAL = bronchoalveolar lavage; MGIT = mycobacteria growth indicator tube)

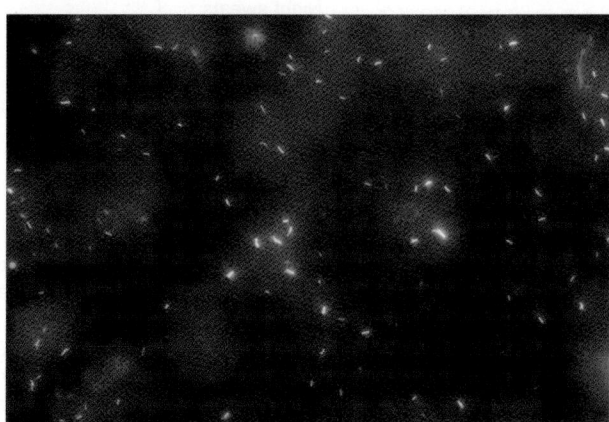

Fig. 17.40 Auramine-stained sputum sample. *Mycobacterium tuberculosis* and other mycobacteria retain the auramine stain after washing with acid and alcohol and are therefore seen as fluorescent organisms against a dark background. *Courtesy of Richard Hobson.*

17.51 Treatment of new tuberculosis (TB) patients (World Health Organization recommendations)

Intensive phase	Continuation phase	Comments
Standard regimen		
2 months of HRZE	4 months of HR	
2 months of HRZE	4 months of HRE	Applies only in countries with high levels of isoniazid resistance in new TB patients, and where isoniazid drug susceptibility testing in new patients is not done (or results are unavailable) before the continuation phase begins
Dosing frequency		
Daily*	Daily	Optimal
Daily*	3 times/week	No longer recommended but sometimes used in practice for patients receiving directly observed therapy
3 times/week	3 times/week	No longer recommended but sometimes used in practice for patients receiving directly observed therapy, provided the patient is *not* living with HIV or living in an HIV-prevalent setting

*Daily (rather than 3 times weekly) intensive-phase dosing may help to prevent acquired drug resistance in TB patients starting treatment with isoniazid resistance. (H = isoniazid; R = rifampicin; Z = pyrazinamide; E = ethambutol; HIV = human immunodeficiency virus)
Adapted from World Health Organization. Guidelines for treatment of drug-susceptible tuberculosis and patient care, 2017 update.

i	**17.52 Main adverse reactions of first-line antituberculous drugs**			
	Isoniazid	**Rifampicin**	**Pyrazinamide**	**Ethambutol**
Mode of action	Cell wall synthesis	DNA transcription	Unknown	Cell wall synthesis
Major adverse reaction	Peripheral neuropathy[1] Hepatitis[2] Rash	Febrile reactions Hepatitis Rash Gastrointestinal disturbance	Hepatitis Gastrointestinal disturbance Hyperuricaemia	Retrobulbar neuritis[3] Arthralgia
Less common adverse reaction	Lupoid reactions Seizures Psychoses	Interstitial nephritis Thrombocytopenia Haemolytic anaemia	Rash Photosensitisation Gout	Peripheral neuropathy Rash

[1]The risk may be reduced by prescribing pyridoxine. [2]More common in patients with a slow acetylator status and in alcoholics. [3]Reduced visual acuity and colour vision may be reported with higher doses and are usually reversible.

Six months of therapy is appropriate for all patients with pulmonary TB and most cases of extrapulmonary TB. However, 12 months of therapy is recommended for CNS TB. Most patients can be treated at home. Admission to a hospital unit with appropriate isolation facilities should be considered where there is uncertainty about the diagnosis, intolerance of medication, questionable treatment adherence, adverse social conditions or a significant risk of multidrug-resistant TB.

Adverse drug reactions occur in about 10% of patients (Box 17.52). Patients treated with rifampicin should be advised that their urine, tears and other secretions will develop a bright, orange/red coloration. Rifampicin is a cytochrome P450 inducer, it accelerates the metabolism of several drugs, thereby reducing their effective dose. These medications include steroids, oral hypoglycaemics, antiretrovirals, warfarin, opiates (including methadone) and contraceptives. Women taking oral or depot hormonal contraceptives must be warned that their efficacy, and that of emergency hormonal contraception, will be reduced and alternative contraception may be necessary. Standard TB medication is safe during pregnancy, however pregnant women experience an increased rate of side-effects, so conception is not advised. Pyridoxine should be prescribed in pregnant women and malnourished patients to reduce the risk of peripheral neuropathy with isoniazid. Ethambutol should be used with caution in severe renal impairment, with appropriate dose reduction and monitoring of drug levels. Visual acuity and colour vision should be assessed before commencing ethambutol.

Baseline liver function and regular monitoring are important for patients treated with standard therapy. Rifampicin may cause asymptomatic hyperbilirubinaemia but, along with isoniazid and pyrazinamide, may also cause hepatitis. Mild asymptomatic increases in transaminases are common but significant hepatotoxicity occurs in only 2%–5%. It is important to stop treatment and allow any symptoms to subside and the liver function tests to recover before commencing a stepwise re-introduction of the individual drugs. Less hepatotoxic regimens may be considered, including streptomycin, ethambutol and fluoroquinolones.

Glucocorticoids reduce inflammation and limit tissue damage; they are currently recommended when treating constrictive pericarditis or CNS disease, and in children with endobronchial disease. They may confer benefit in TB of the ureter, pleural effusions and extensive pulmonary disease, and can suppress hypersensitivity drug reactions. Embolization should be considered for treatment of massive haemoptysis. Surgery is required for patients with spinal TB causing spinal cord compression.

The effectiveness of therapy for pulmonary TB is assessed by further sputum analysis at 2 months to ensure sputum culture conversion, if the patient is still producing sputum. If sputum is culture-positive at 2 months, repeat sputum should be obtained at month 3. If this sample is culture-positive then DST should be repeated. Treatment failure is defined as a positive sputum culture at 5 months or any patient with a newly converted multidrug-resistant strain, regardless of whether they are smear-positive or negative. Extrapulmonary TB must be assessed clinically or radiographically, as appropriate.

Control and prevention

Active TB is preventable, particularly so in those with latent TB. Supporting the development of laboratory and health-care services to improve detection and treatment of active and latent TB is an important component of this goal.

Latent TB infection (LTBI)

The majority of individuals exposed to MTB harbour the bacteria, which remain dormant. They do not develop any signs of active disease and are non-infectious. They are, however, at risk of developing active TB disease and becoming infectious. The lifetime risk of TB disease for a person with documented LTBI is estimated at 5%–15%, with the majority of cases occurring within the first 5 years after initial infection.

LTBI may be identified by the presence of immune responses to M. tuberculosis antigens. Contact tracing is a legal requirement in many countries. It has the potential to identify the probable index case, other cases infected by the same index patient (with or without evidence of disease), and close contacts who should receive BCG vaccination (see below) or chemotherapy. Approximately 10%–20% of close contacts of patients with smear-positive pulmonary TB and 2%–5% of those with smear-negative, culture-positive disease have evidence of TB infection.

Cases are commonly identified using the tuberculin skin test (TST; Fig. 17.41) or an IGRA (Fig. 17.42). An otherwise asymptomatic contact who tests positive but has a normal chest X-ray may be treated with chemoprophylaxis to prevent infection from progressing to clinical disease. Chemoprophylaxis should be offered to adults up to the age of 65 (although age-specific cut-off varies by country). It should also be considered for HIV-infected close contacts of a patient with smear-positive disease. A course of rifampicin and isoniazid for 3 months or isoniazid for 6 months is effective.

Tuberculin skin testing may be associated with false-positive reactions in those who have had a BCG vaccination and in areas where exposure to non-tuberculous mycobacteria is high. The skin tests may also be falsely negative in the setting of immunosuppression or overwhelming TB infection.

IGRAs detect the release of interferon-gamma (IFN-γ) from sensitised T cells in response to antigens, such as early secretory antigenic target (ESAT)-6 or culture filtrate protein (CFP)-10, which are encoded by genes specific to M. tuberculosis and are not shared with BCG or opportunistic mycobacteria (see Fig. 17.42). IGRAs are more specific than skin testing and logistically more convenient, as they require a single blood test rather than two clinic visits. In the UK, IGRA represents the first choice investigation, except in children, for whom TST is recommended.

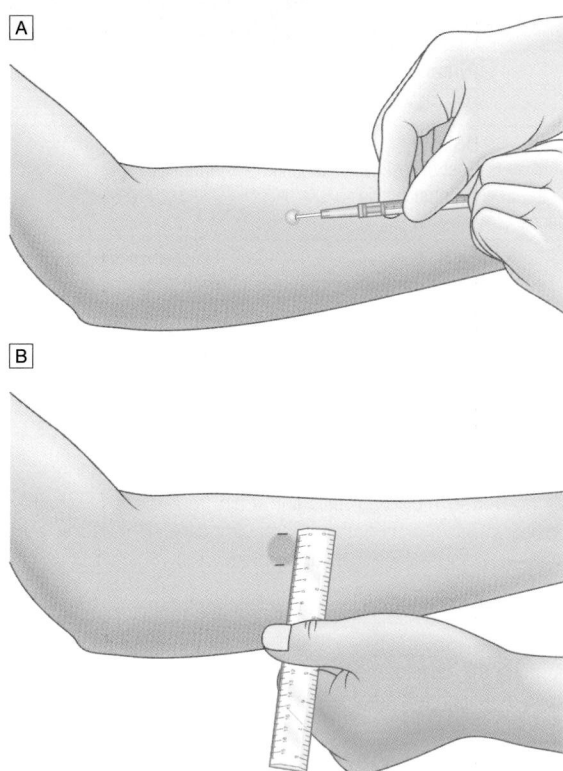

Fig. 17.41 The tuberculin skin test. [A] The reaction to the intradermal injection of tuberculin purified protein derivative (PPD) on the inner surface of the forearm is read between 48 and 72 hours. [B] The diameter of the indurated area should be measured across the forearm and is positive when ≥5 mm.

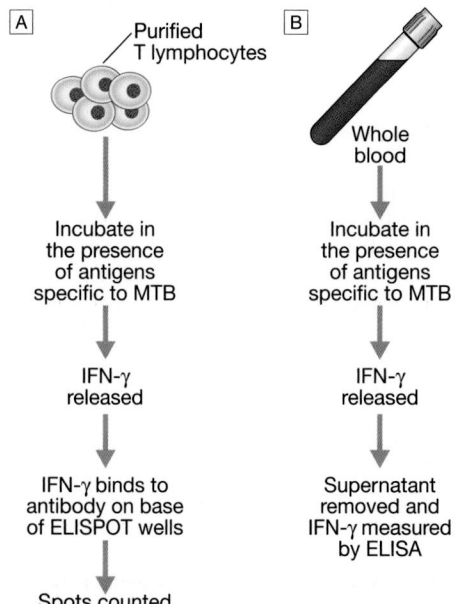

Fig. 17.42 The principles of interferon-gamma release assays (IGRAs). A sample of either [A] purified T cells (T-SPOT.TB test) or [B] whole blood (QuantiFERON–TB Gold test) is incubated in the presence of antigens specific to *Mycobacterium tuberculosis* (MTB). The release of interferon-gamma (IFN-γ) by the cells is measured by enzyme-linked immunosorbent assay (ELISA). (ELISPOT = enzyme-linked immunosorbent spot assay)

Directly observed therapy

Poor adherence to therapy is a major factor in prolonged illness, risk of relapse and the emergence of drug resistance. Directly observed therapy (DOT) involves the supervised administration of therapy three times weekly to improve adherence. DOT has become an important control strategy in resource-poor nations. In the UK, it is currently recommended for patients with previous TB, multidrug-resistant TB, poor adherence to treatment, denial of the diagnosis, those with a history of homelessness, alcohol or drug misuse, those currently or recently in prison, and those with major psychiatric, memory or cognitive disorders. DOT can be replaced by video-observed consultation (VOT) if appropriate facilities are available.

TB and HIV/AIDS

The close links between HIV and TB, particularly in sub-Saharan Africa, and the potential for both diseases to overwhelm health-care funding in resource-poor nations, have been recognised, with the promotion of programmes that link detection and treatment of TB with detection and treatment of HIV. It is recommended that all patients with TB should be tested for HIV infection, in addition to hepatits B and C. Mortality is high and TB is a leading cause of death in HIV-positive patients. Full discussion of its presentation and management with antiretroviral therapy (ART) is given in Chapter 14.

ART should be initiated for all HIV-positive patients with TB. ART is usually initiated after 2 weeks of tuberculous therapy, but in patients with a CD4 count under 50 cells/µL or CNS TB is often delayed until 8 weeks of TB therapy has been completed to reduced the risk of IRIS/paradoxical reaction. TB-associated immune reconstitution inflammatory syndrome (TB-IRIS) is a paradoxical increase in pre-existing, or development of new, TB signs or symptoms, due to ART reviving the immune system. TB-IRIS may be self-limiting, but in severe cases steroids are used to reduce symptoms, and patients are advised to continue TB chemotherapy and ART. Choice of initial ART or change in ART should reflect the need to avoid drug interactions.

Drug-resistant TB

Drug-resistant TB is defined by the presence of resistance to any first-line agent. Multidrug-resistant tuberculosis (MDR-TB) is defined by resistance to at least rifampicin and isoniazid, with or without other drug resistance. Globally, an estimated 3.5% of new TB cases and 18% of previously treated cases have MDR-TB. In 2017, an estimated 230000 people died of MDR-TB. Extensively drug-resistant tuberculosis (XDR-TB) is defined as resistance to at least rifampicin and isoniazid, in addition to any quinolone and at least one injectable second-line agent. An estimated 8.5% of people with MDR-TB have XDR-TB. The prevalence of MDR-TB is rising, particularly in post-Soviet states, Central Asia and South Africa. It is more common in individuals with a prior history of TB, particularly if treatment has been inadequate. Box 17.53 lists the factors contributing to the emergence of drug-resistant TB. Diagnosis is challenging, especially in resource-poor settings, and although cure is possible, it requires prolonged treatment with less effective, more toxic and more expensive second-line therapies. These include injectable drugs (aminoglycosides), fluoroquinolones and various other antibiotics and TB-specific agents (see p. 315). The mortality rate from tuberculosis increases with the level of drug resistance.

Vaccines

BCG (bacille Calmette–Guérin), a live attenuated vaccine derived from *M. bovis*, is the most established TB vaccine. It is administered by intradermal injection and is highly immunogenic. BCG appears to be effective in preventing disseminated disease, including tuberculous meningitis, in children, but its efficacy in adults is inconsistent and new vaccines are urgently needed. Current vaccination policies vary worldwide according to incidence and health-care resources, but usually target children and other high-risk individuals. BCG is very safe, with the occasional complication of local abscess formation. It should not be administered to those who are immunocompromised (e.g. by HIV) or pregnant.

Prognosis

Following successful completion of chemotherapy, cure should be anticipated in the majority of patients, though complications such as lung scarring and bronchiectasis are not uncommon (Box 17.54). There is a small (<5%) and unavoidable risk of relapse. Most relapses occur within 5 months and usually have the same drug susceptibility. In the absence of treatment, a patient with smear-positive TB will remain infectious for an average of 2 years; in 1 year, 25% of untreated cases will die. Death is more likely in those who are smear-positive and those who smoke. A few patients die unexpectedly soon after commencing therapy and it is possible that some have subclinical hypoadrenalism that is unmasked by a rifampicin-induced increase in glucocorticoid metabolism. HIV-positive patients have higher mortality rates and a modestly increased risk of relapse.

Non-tuberculous mycobacterial infection

Other species of environmental mycobacteria (termed 'non-tuberculous') may cause human disease (Box 17.55). The sites commonly involved are the lungs, lymph nodes, skin and soft tissues. The most widely recognised of these mycobacteria, *M. avium* complex (MAC), is well described in severe HIV disease (CD4 count <50 cells/µL). However, several others (including MAC) colonise and/or infect apparently immunocompetent patients with chronic lung diseases such as COPD, bronchiectasis, pneumoconiosis, old TB, or cystic fibrosis. The clinical presentation varies from a relatively indolent course in some to an aggressive course characterised by cavitatory or nodular disease in others. Radiological appearances may be similar to classical TB, but in patients with bronchiectasis, opportunistic infection may present with lower-zone nodules. The most commonly reported organisms include *M. kansasii*, *M. malmoense*, *M. xenopi* and *M. abscessus* but geographical variation is marked. *M. abscessus* and *M. fortuitum* grow rapidly but the majority of others grow slowly. More rapid diagnostic systems are under development, including DNA probes, high-performance liquid chromatography (HPLC), PCR restriction enzyme analysis (PRA) and 16S rRNA gene sequence analysis. Drug sensitivity testing is often unhelpful in predicting treatment response, with the exception of macrolide susceptibility for MAC and rifampicin sensitivity for *M. kansasii*. In the UK, these organisms are not

<table>
<tr><td>i</td><td>17.53 Factors contributing to the emergence of drug-resistant tuberculosis</td></tr>
</table>

- Drug shortages
- Poor-quality drugs
- Poor concordance with drugs
- Lack of appropriate supervision
- Transmission of drug-resistant strains
- Prior antituberculosis treatment
- Treatment failure (culture-positive at 5 months)

<table>
<tr><td>i</td><td>17.54 Complications of pulmonary tuberculosis</td></tr>
</table>

- Bronchiectasis
- Massive haemoptysis
- Cor pulmonale
- Fibrosis/emphysema
- Atypical mycobacterial infection
- Aspergilloma/chronic pulmonary aspergillosis
- Obstructive airways disease
- Bronchopleural fistula
- Lung/pleural calcification and pleural thickening

Non-pulmonary complications

- Empyema necessitans
- Laryngitis
- Enteritis*
- Anorectal disease*
- Amyloidosis
- Poncet's polyarthritis

*From swallowed sputum.

notifiable to local public health departments as they are not normally communicable; patient-to-patient transmission of *M. abscessus* in cystic fibrosis is a key exception.

Respiratory diseases caused by fungi

The majority of fungi encountered by humans are harmless saprophytes but in certain circumstances (Box 17.56) some species may cause disease by infecting human tissue, promoting damaging allergic reactions or producing toxins. 'Mycosis' is the term applied to disease caused by fungal infection. The conditions associated with *Aspergillus* species are listed in Box 17.57.

Allergic bronchopulmonary aspergillosis

Allergic bronchopulmonary aspergillosis (ABPA) occurs as a result of a hypersensitivity reaction to germinating fungal spores in the airway wall. The condition may complicate the course of asthma and cystic fibrosis, and is a recognised cause of pulmonary eosinophilia. The prevalence of ABPA is approximately 1%–2% in asthma and 5%–10% in patients with CF. A variety of human leucocyte antigens (HLAs) convey both an increased and a decreased risk of developing the condition, suggesting that genetic susceptibility is important.

Clinical features

Clinical features depend on the stage of the disease. Common manifestations in the early phases include fever, breathlessness, cough

<table>
<tr><td>i</td><td colspan="2"> 17.55 Site-specific opportunistic mycobacterial disease</td></tr>
</table>

Pulmonary

- *M. xenopi*
- *M. kansasii*
- *M. malmoense*
- MAC
- *M. abscessus* (in cystic fibrosis)

Lymph node

- MAC
- *M. malmoense*
- *M. fortuitum*
- *M. chelonei*

Soft tissue/skin

- *M. leprae*
- *M. ulcerans* (prevalent in Africa, northern Australia and South-east Asia)
- *M. marinum*
- *M. fortuitum*
- *M. chelonae*

Disseminated

- MAC (HIV-associated)
- *M. haemophilum*
- *M. genavense*
- *M. chimera* (cardiopulmonary bypass-associated)
- *M. fortuitum*
- *M. chelonae*
- BCG

(BCG = bacille Calmette–Guérin; MAC = *Mycobacterium avium* complex – *M. scrofulaceum*, *M. intracellulare* and *M. avium*)

<table>
<tr><td>i</td><td colspan="2"> 17.56 Factors predisposing to pulmonary fungal disease</td></tr>
</table>

Systemic factors

- Haematological malignancy
- HIV
- Diabetes mellitus
- Chronic alcoholism
- Radiotherapy
- Glucocorticoids, cytotoxic chemotherapy, biologic therapies and other immunosuppressant medication

Local factors

- Tissue damage by suppuration or necrosis
- Alteration of normal bacterial flora by antibiotic therapy

17

productive of bronchial casts and worsening of asthmatic symptoms. The appearance of radiographic infiltrates may cause ABPA to be mistaken for pneumonia but the diagnosis may also be suggested by segmental or lobar collapse on chest X-rays of patients whose asthma symptoms are stable. Diagnostic features are shown in Box 17.58. If bronchiectasis develops, the symptoms and complications of that disease often overshadow those of asthma.

Management

ABPA is generally considered an indication for regular therapy with low-dose oral glucocorticoids (prednisolone 7.5–10 mg/day) with the aim of suppressing the immunopathological responses and preventing progressive tissue damage. In some patients, itraconazole (400 mg/day) facilitates a reduction in oral glucocorticoids; a 4-month trial is usually recommended to assess its efficacy, but there needs to be consideration for the interactions with inhaled glucocorticoids. The use of specific anti-IgE monoclonal antibodies is under consideration. Exacerbations, particularly when associated with new chest X-ray changes, should be treated promptly with prednisolone (40–60 mg/day) and physiotherapy. If persistent lobar collapse occurs, bronchoscopy (usually under general anaesthetic) should be performed to remove impacted mucus and ensure prompt re-inflation.

Chronic pulmonary aspergillosis

The term chronic pulmonary aspergillosis (CPA) encompasses simple aspergilloma, chronic cavitary pulmonary aspergillosis, chronic fibrosing pulmonary aspergillosis, *Aspergillus* nodule and semi-invasive aspergillosis. They are uncommon conditions and challenging to diagnose and treat.

Simple aspergilloma

Cavities left by diseases such as TB or by damaged bronchi provide favourable conditions in which inhaled *Aspergillus* may lodge and germinate. At the earliest stage, CT scanning may identify an irregular mucosal wall and, as fungal growth progresses, this finally collapses into the cavity, forming a fungal ball that may be identified on imaging (Fig. 17.43).

Simple aspergillomas are often asymptomatic. They can, however, give rise to a variety of non-specific symptoms, such as lethargy and weight loss, and may cause recurrent haemoptysis, which may be life-threatening.

The typical radiological picture is invariably accompanied by elevated serum IgG/precipitins to *A. fumigatus*. Sputum microscopy typically demonstrates scanty hyphal fragments and is usually positive on culture. Less than half exhibit skin hypersensitivity to extracts of *A. fumigatus*.

Rarely, other filamentous fungi can cause intracavity mycetoma and are identified by culture.

Asymptomatic cases do not require treatment but haemoptysis should be controlled by surgery. Tranexamic acid or bronchial artery embolisation may provide a bridge to surgery or palliate haemoptysis when surgery is not possible. Antifungal agents are usually not benefical due to poor penetration into the mycetoma, and generally surgical resection is the treatment of choice. Antifungals can be trialled in those patients with multiple mycetomas or who are not fit enough for surgical resection. Instillation of antifungal agents, such as amphotericin B, via a catheter placed into the cavity has been reported but is rarely used in the UK.

Chronic cavitary pulmonary aspergillosis and chronic fibrosing pulmonary aspergillosis

The features of chronic cavitary pulmonary aspergillosis (CCPA) include cough (with or without haemoptysis), weight loss, anorexia and fatigue over months or years, with associated fever, night sweats and elevated inflammatory markers. Radiological features include thick-walled cavities (predominantly apical), pulmonary infiltrates and pleural thickening (Fig. 17.44). Once again, diagnosis rests on a combination of radiological examination, histopathology, isolation of fungus from the respiratory tract and detection of *Aspergillus* IgG in serum. Treatment usually involves prolonged courses of itraconazole or voriconazole. Cure is unusual and the most frequent pattern is chronic relapse/remission with gradual deterioration. Surgical intervention is fraught with complications and should be avoided. Many patients are malnourished and require nutritional support. Glucocorticoids should be avoided. As CCPA progresses, fibrotic destruction of the lung results and the condition may then be referred to as chronic fibrosing pulmonary aspergillosis (CFPA).

Aspergillus nodule

The formation of one or more nodules is a less common manifestation of *Aspergillus* infection. In addition to lung cancer, the *Aspergillus* nodule may mimic TB but cavitation is unusual. Cryptococcosis or coccidioidomycosis should be considered in areas where these conditions are endemic.

Subacute invasive aspergillosis

Subacute invasive aspergillosis (SIA) was previously referred to as chronic necrotising or semi-invasive pulmonary aspergillosis. The clinical and radiological picture is similar to CCPA but lung biopsy demonstrates invasion of lung tissue by hyphae. The development of SIA is favoured by mild immunocompromise and should be suspected in patients with diabetes mellitus, malnutrition or alcoholism, or with advanced age and in prolonged glucocorticoid use. It is also seen in the presence of COPD, non-tuberculous mycobacteria or HIV infection. SIA should be treated in a similar manner to invasive pulmonary aspergillosis.

> **i** | **17.57 Classification of bronchopulmonary aspergillosis**
>
> - Allergic bronchopulmonary aspergillosis (asthmatic pulmonary eosinophilia)
> - Hypersensitivity pneumonitis (*Aspergillus clavatus*)
> - Intracavitary aspergilloma
> - Invasive pulmonary aspergillosis
> - Chronic and subacute pulmonary aspergillosis

> **i** | **17.58 Features of allergic bronchopulmonary aspergillosis**
>
> - Asthma (in the majority of cases)
> - Proximal bronchiectasis (inner two-thirds of chest CT field)
> - Positive skin test to an extract of *Aspergillus fumigatus*
> - Elevated total serum IgE >417 kU/L (1000 ng/mL)
> - Elevated *A. fumigatus*-specific IgE or IgG
> - Peripheral blood eosinophilia >0.5 ×10^9/L
> - Presence or history of chest X-ray abnormalities
> - Recovery of *A. fumigatus* from sputum
>
> (CT = computed tomography; Ig = immunoglobulin)

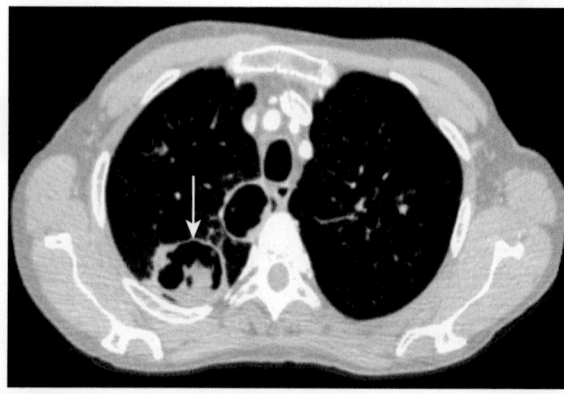

Fig. 17.43 Computed tomogram of aspergilloma in the left upper lobe. The rounded fungal ball is separated from the wall of the cavity by an 'air crescent' (arrow).

Invasive pulmonary aspergillosis

Invasive pulmonary aspergillosis (IPA) is most commonly a complication of profound neutropenia caused by drugs (especially immunosuppressive agents) and/or disease (Box 17.59).

Clinical features

Acute IPA causes a severe necrotising pneumonia and must be considered in any immunocompromised patient who develops fever, new respiratory symptoms (particularly pleural pain or haemoptysis) or a pleural rub. Invasion of pulmonary vessels causes thrombosis and infarction, and systemic spread may occur to the brain, heart, kidneys and others organs. Tracheobronchial aspergillosis involvement is characterised by the formation of fungal plaques and ulceration.

HRCT characteristically shows macronodules (usually ≥ 1 cm), which may be surrounded by a 'halo' of intermediate attenuation if captured early (<5 days). Culture or histopathological evidence of *Aspergillus* in diseased tissues provides a definitive diagnosis but the majority of patients are too ill for invasive tests, such as bronchoscopy or lung biopsy. Other investigations include detection of *Aspergillus* galactomannan in blood or BAL fluid, β-1,3-D-glucan in blood and (where available) *Aspergillus* DNA in blood. Diagnosis is often inferred from a combination of features (Box 17.60).

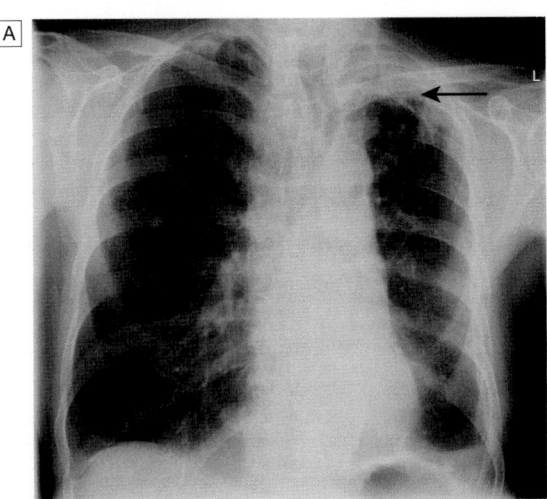

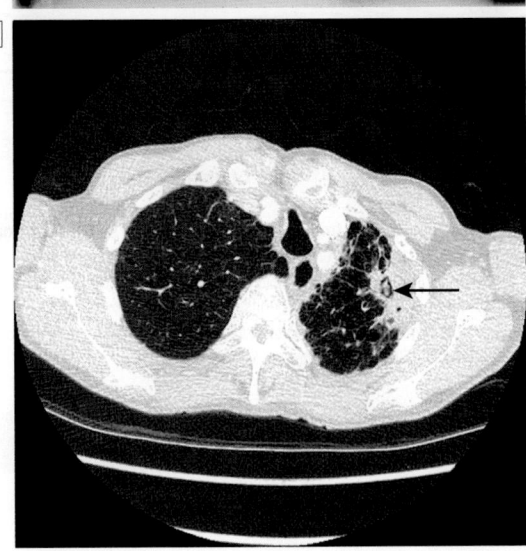

Fig. 17.44 Chronic pulmonary aspergillosis. **A** The chest X-ray shows pleural thickening with loss of lung volume at the left apex (arrow). **B** High-resolution computed tomography reveals multiple small cavities and pleural thickening with an aspergilloma and surrounding air crescent (arrow) in one of the cavities. *Courtesy of Professor David Denning, National Aspergillosis Centre, Manchester, UK.*

Management and prevention

IPA carries a high mortality rate, especially if treatment is delayed. The drug of choice is voriconazole. Second-line agents include liposomal amphotericin, caspofungin, posaconazole and isavuconazole. Response may be assessed clinically, radiologically and serologically (by estimation of the circulating galactomannan level). Recovery is dependent on immune reconstitution, which may be accompanied by enlargement and/or cavitation of pulmonary nodules.

Patients at risk of *Aspergillus* (and other fungal infections) should be managed in rooms with high-efficiency particulate air (HEPA) filters and laminar airflow. In areas with high spore counts, patients are advised to wear a mask if venturing outside their hospital room. Posaconazole (200 mg 3 times daily) or itraconazole (200 mg/day) may be prescribed for primary prophylaxis, and patients with a history of definite or probable IPA should be considered for secondary prophylaxis before further immunosuppression.

---

i | 17.59 Risk factors for invasive aspergillosis

- Neutropenia: risk related to duration and degree
- Solid organ or allogeneic stem cell transplantation
- Prolonged high-dose glucocorticoid therapy
- Leukaemia and other haematological malignancies
- Cytotoxic chemotherapy
- Advanced HIV disease
- Severe chronic obstructive pulmonary disease
- Critically ill patients on intensive care units
- Chronic granulomatous disease

---

i | 17.60 Criteria for the diagnosis of probable invasive pulmonary aspergillosis

Host factors

- Recent history of neutropenia (<0.5 ×10⁹/L for ≥10 days) temporally related to the onset of fungal disease
- Recipient of allogeneic stem cell transplant
- Prolonged use of glucocorticoids (average minimum 0.3 mg/kg daily prednisolone or equivalent) for >3 weeks (excludes allergic bronchopulmonary aspergillosis)
- Treatment with other recognised T-cell immune suppressants, such as ciclosporin, tumour necrosis factor alpha-blockers, specific monoclonal antibodies (e.g. alemtuzumab) or nucleoside analogues during the last 90 days
- Inherited severe immune deficiency, e.g. chronic granulomatous disease or severe combined immune deficiency

Clinical criteria[1]

- The presence of one of the following on CT:
  Dense, well-circumscribed lesion(s) with or without a halo sign
  Air crescent sign
  Cavity

Tracheobronchitis

- Tracheobronchial ulceration, nodule, pseudomembrane, plaque or eschar seen on bronchoscopy

Mycological criteria

- Mould in sputum, BAL fluid or bronchial brush, indicated by one of the following:
  Recovery of fungal elements indicating a mould of *Aspergillus*
  Recovery by culture of a mould of *Aspergillus*
- Indirect tests (detection of antigen or cell wall constituents)
  Galactomannan antigen in plasma, serum or BAL fluid
  β-1,3-glucan detected in serum (detects other species of fungi, as well as *Aspergillus*)[2]

---

[1]Must be consistent with the mycological findings and temporally related to current episode. [2]May be useful as a preliminary screening tool for invasive aspergillosis. (BAL = bronchoalveolar lavage)

Adapted from De Pauw B, Walsh TJ, Donnelly JP, et al. Revised definitions of invasive fungal disease from the European Organisation for Research and Treatment of Cancer/Mycoses Study Group. Clin Infect Dis 2008; 46:1813–1821.

17

Other fungal infections

Mucormycosis may present with a pulmonary syndrome that is clinically indistinguishable from acute IPA. Diagnosis relies on histopathology (where available) and/or culture of the organism from diseased tissue. The principles of treatment are as for other forms of mucormycosis: correction of predisposing factors, antifungal therapy with high-dose lipid amphotericin B or posaconazole (second line), and surgical débridement.

The endemic mycoses (histoplasmosis, coccidioidomycosis, blastomycosis and emergomycosis) and cryptococcosis are discussed on pages 345–347. *Pneumocystis jirovecii* pneumonia is described on page 361.

Tumours of the bronchus and lung

Lung cancer is the most common cause of death from cancer worldwide, causing 2 million deaths per year (Box 17.61). Tobacco use is the major preventable cause. Just as tobacco use and cancer rates are falling in some high-income countries, both smoking and lung cancer are rising in many low- and middle-income countries. The great majority of tumours in the lung are primary lung cancers and, in contrast to many other tumours, the prognosis remains poor, with approximately 40% and 16% of patients surviving at 1 and 5 years respectively.

Primary tumours of the lung

Aetiology

Cigarette smoking is by far the most important cause of lung cancer. It is thought to be directly responsible for at least 85% of cases in the UK, the risk being proportional to the amount smoked and the tar content of cigarettes. but the proportion of cases not related to tobacco exposure is rising. The death rate from the disease in heavy smokers is 40 times that in non-smokers. Risk falls slowly after smoking cessation but remains above that in non-smokers for many years. It is estimated that 1 in 2 smokers dies from a smoking-related disease, about half in middle age. The effect of 'passive' smoking is more difficult to quantify but is currently thought to be a factor in 5% of all lung cancer deaths. Exposure to naturally occurring radon is another risk. The incidence of lung cancer is slightly higher in urban than in rural dwellers, which may reflect differences in atmospheric pollution (including tobacco smoke) or occupation, since a number of industrial materials are associated with lung cancer, such as asbestos, arsenicals and beryllium-containing compounds. In recent years, the strong link between smoking and ill health has led many governments to legislate against smoking in public places, and smoking prevalence and some smoking-related diseases are already declining in these countries.

Lung cancer

The incidence of lung cancer increased dramatically during the 20th century as a direct result of the tobacco epidemic (Fig. 17.45). In women, smoking prevalence and deaths from lung cancer continue to increase, and more women now die of lung cancer than breast cancer in the United States and the UK.

<table>
<tr><td>**i**</td><td>**17.61 The burden of lung cancer**</td></tr>
</table>

- 1.8 million new cases worldwide each year
- Most common cancer in men
- Rates rising in women:
  - Female lung cancer deaths outnumber male in some Nordic countries
  - Has overtaken breast cancer in several countries
- More than a threefold increase in deaths since 1950
- More than 50% of cases have metastatic disease at diagnosis

Pathology

Lung cancers arise from the bronchial epithelium or mucous glands. The common cell types are listed in Box 17.62. When the tumour occurs in a large bronchus, symptoms arise early but tumours originating in a peripheral bronchus can grow very large without producing symptoms, resulting in delayed diagnosis. Peripheral squamous tumours may undergo central necrosis and cavitation and may resemble a lung abscess on X-ray (Fig. 17.46). Lung cancer may involve the pleura directly or by lymphatic spread and may extend into the chest wall, invading the intercostal nerves or the brachial plexus and causing pain. Lymphatic spread to mediastinal and supraclavicular lymph nodes often occurs before diagnosis. Blood-borne metastases occur most commonly in liver, bone, brain, adrenals and skin. Even a small primary tumour may cause widespread metastatic deposits and this is a particular characteristic of small-cell lung cancers.

Clinical features

Lung cancer presents in many different ways, reflecting local, metastatic or paraneoplastic tumour effects.

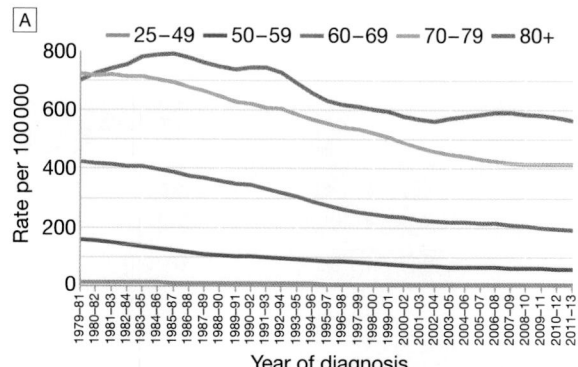

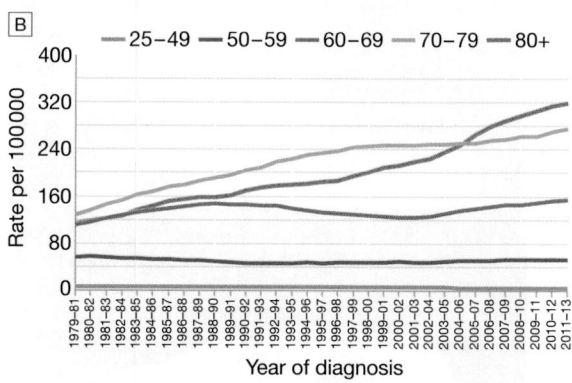

Fig. 17.45 Mortality trends from lung cancer in UK, 1979–2013, by age and year of death. [A] Males. [B] Females. Note the decline in mortality from lung cancer in men and increase in mortality in older women towards the end of this period, reflecting changes in smoking habits. *From Cancer Research UK: http://www.cancerresearchuk.org/health-professional/cancer-statistics/statistics-by-cancer-type/lung-cancer/mortality. Accessed January 2017.*

<table>
<tr><td>**i**</td><td colspan="2">**17.62 Common cell types in lung cancer**</td></tr>
<tr><td colspan="2">**Cell type**</td><td>**%**</td></tr>
<tr><td colspan="2">Adenocarcinoma</td><td>35–40</td></tr>
<tr><td colspan="2">Squamous</td><td>25–30</td></tr>
<tr><td colspan="2">Small-cell</td><td>15</td></tr>
<tr><td colspan="2">Large-cell</td><td>10–15</td></tr>
</table>

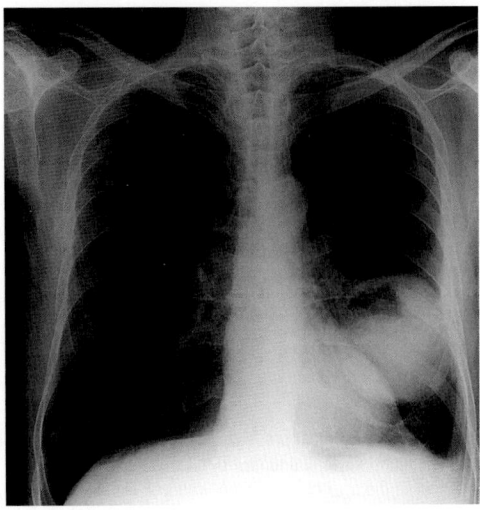

Fig. 17.46 Large cavitated lung cancer in left lower lobe.

Cough This is the most common early symptom. It is often dry, but secondary infection may cause purulent sputum. A change in the character of a smoker's cough, particularly if associated with other new symptoms, should always raise suspicion of lung cancer.

Haemoptysis Haemoptysis is common, especially with central bronchial tumours. Although it may be caused by bronchitic infection, haemoptysis in a smoker should always be investigated to exclude a lung cancer. Occasionally, central tumours invade large vessels, causing sudden massive haemoptysis which is invariably a terminal event.

Bronchial obstruction This is another common presentation. The clinical and radiological manifestations (Fig. 17.47 and see Fig. 17.5, and Box 17.63) depend on the site and extent of the obstruction, any secondary infection and the extent of coexisting lung disease. Complete obstruction causes collapse of a lobe or lung, with breathlessness, mediastinal displacement and dullness to percussion with reduced breath sounds. Partial bronchial obstruction may cause a monophonic, unilateral wheeze that fails to clear with coughing, and may also impair the drainage of secretions to cause pneumonia or lung abscess as a presenting problem. Pneumonia that recurs at the same site or responds slowly to treatment, particularly in a smoker, should always suggest an underlying lung cancer. Stridor (a harsh inspiratory noise) occurs when the larynx, trachea or a main bronchus is narrowed by the primary tumour or by compression from malignant enlargement of the subcarinal and paratracheal lymph nodes.

Breathlessness Breathlessness may be caused by collapse or pneumonia, or by tumour causing a large pleural effusion or compressing a phrenic nerve and leading to diaphragmatic paralysis.

Pain and nerve entrapment Pleural pain may indicate malignant pleural invasion, although it can occur with distal infection. Intercostal nerve involvement causes pain in the distribution of a thoracic dermatome. Cancer in the lung apex may cause Horner syndrome (ipsilateral partial ptosis, enophthalmos, miosis and hypohidrosis of the face) due to involvement of the sympathetic nerves to the eye at or above the stellate ganglion. Pancoast syndrome (pain in the inner aspect of the arm, sometimes with small muscle wasting in the hand) indicates malignant destruction of the T1 and C8 roots in the lower part of the brachial plexus by an apical lung tumour.

Mediastinal spread Involvement of the oesophagus may cause dysphagia. If the pericardium is invaded, arrhythmia or pericardial effusion may occur. Superior vena cava obstruction by malignant nodes causes

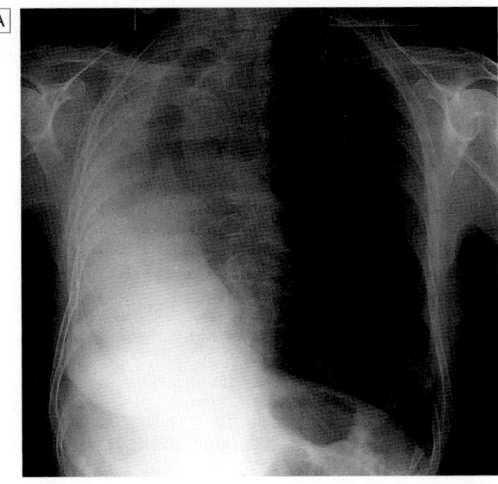

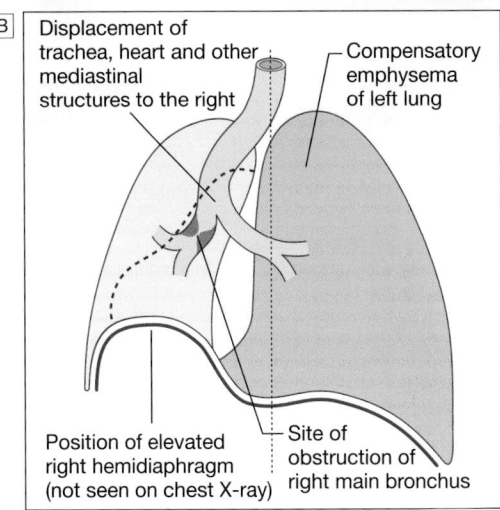

Fig. 17.47 Collapse of the right lung: effects on neighbouring structures. [A] Chest X-ray. [B] The typical abnormalities are highlighted.

suffusion and swelling of the neck and face, conjunctival oedema, headache and dilated veins on the chest wall and is most commonly due to lung cancer. Involvement of the left recurrent laryngeal nerve by tumours at the left hilum causes vocal cord paralysis, voice alteration and a 'bovine' cough (lacking the normal explosive character). Supraclavicular lymph nodes may be palpably enlarged or identified using ultrasound; if so, a needle aspirate may provide a simple means of cytological diagnosis.

Metastatic spread This may lead to focal neurological defects, epileptic seizures, personality change, jaundice, bone pain or skin nodules. Lassitude, anorexia and weight loss usually indicate metastatic spread.

Finger clubbing Overgrowth of the soft tissue of the terminal phalanx, leading to increased nail curvature and nail bed fluctuation, is often seen.

Hypertrophic pulmonary osteoarthropathy (HPOA) This is a painful periostitis of the distal tibia, fibula, radius and ulna, with local tenderness and sometimes pitting oedema over the anterior shin. X-rays reveal subperiosteal new bone formation. While most frequently associated with lung cancer, HPOA can occur with other tumours.

Non-metastatic extrapulmonary effects (Box 17.64) The syndrome of inappropriate antidiuretic hormone secretion (SIADH, p. 624) and ectopic adrenocorticotrophic hormone secretion (p. 684) are usually associated with small-cell lung cancer. Hypercalcaemia may indicate malignant

17

17.63 Causes of large bronchus obstruction

Common

- Lung cancer or adenoma
- Enlarged tracheobronchial lymph nodes (malignant or tuberculous)
- Inhaled foreign bodies (especially right lung)
- Bronchial casts or plugs consisting of inspissated mucus or blood clot (especially asthma, cystic fibrosis, haemoptysis, debility)
- Collections of mucus or mucopus retained in the bronchi as a result of ineffective expectoration (especially post-operative following abdominal surgery)

Rare

- Aortic aneurysm
- Giant left atrium
- Pericardial effusion
- Congenital bronchial atresia
- Fibrous bronchial stricture (e.g. following tuberculosis or bronchial surgery/lung transplant)

17.64 Non-metastatic extrapulmonary manifestations of lung cancer

Endocrine (Ch. 20)

- Inappropriate antidiuretic hormone (ADH, vasopressin) secretion, causing hyponatraemia
- Ectopic adrenocorticotrophic hormone secretion
- Hypercalcaemia due to secretion of parathyroid hormone-related peptides
- Carcinoid syndrome
- Gynaecomastia

Neurological (Ch. 28)

- Polyneuropathy
- Myelopathy
- Cerebellar degeneration
- Myasthenia (Lambert–Eaton syndrome

Other

- Digital clubbing
- Hypertrophic pulmonary osteoarthropathy
- Nephrotic syndrome
- Polymyositis and dermatomyositis
- Eosinophilia

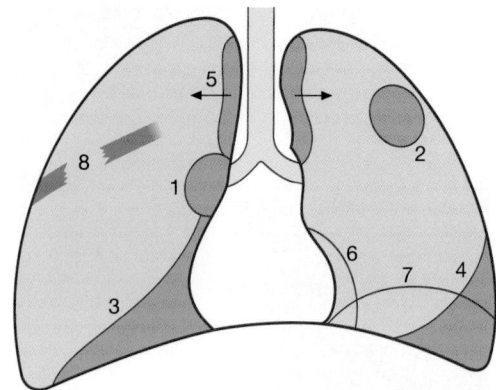

Fig. 17.48 Common radiological presentations of lung cancer. (1) Unilateral hilar enlargement suggests a central tumour or hilar glandular involvement. However, a peripheral tumour in the apex of a lower lobe can look like an enlarged hilar shadow on the posteroanterior X-ray. (2) Peripheral pulmonary opacity is usually irregular but well circumscribed, and may contain irregular cavitation. It can be very large. (3) Lung, lobe or segmental collapse is usually caused by tumour occluding a proximal bronchus. Collapse may also be due to compression of a bronchus by enlarged lymph glands. (4) Pleural effusion usually indicates tumour invasion of the pleural space or, very rarely, infection in collapsed lung tissue distal to a lung cancer. (5) Paratracheal lymphadenopathy may cause widening of the upper mediastinum. (6) A malignant pericardial effusion may cause enlargement of the cardiac shadow. (7) A raised hemidiaphragm may be caused by phrenic nerve palsy. Screening will show paradoxical upward movement when the patient sniffs. (8) Osteolytic rib destruction indicates direct invasion of the chest wall or metastatic spread.

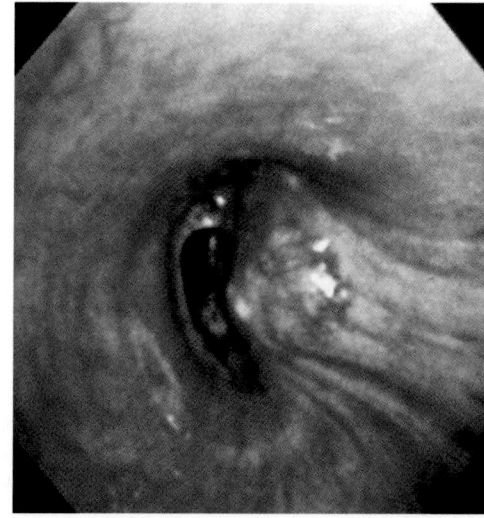

Fig. 17.49 Bronchoscopic view of a lung cancer. There is distortion of mucosal folds, partial occlusion of the airway lumen and abnormal tumour tissue.

bone destruction or production of hormone-like peptides by a tumour. Associated neurological syndromes may occur with any type of lung cancer.

Investigations

The main aims of investigation are to confirm the diagnosis, establish the histological cell type and define the extent of the disease.

Imaging

Lung cancer produces a range of appearances on chest X-ray, from lobar collapse (see Fig. 17.5) to mass lesions, effusion or malignant rib destruction (Fig. 17.48). CT should be performed early, as it may reveal mediastinal or metastatic spread and is helpful for planning biopsy procedures, e.g. in establishing whether a tumour is accessible by bronchoscopy or percutaneous CT-guided biopsy.

Biopsy and histopathology

Over half of primary lung tumours can be visualised and sampled directly by biopsy and brushing using a flexible bronchoscope. Bronchoscopy also allows an assessment of operability, from the proximity of central tumours to the main carina (Fig. 17.49).

For tumours that are too peripheral to be accessible by bronchoscope, the yield of 'blind' bronchoscopic washings and brushings from the radiologically affected area is low and percutaneous needle biopsy under CT

(or less commonly ultrasound) guidance is a more reliable way to obtain a histological diagnosis. There is a risk of iatrogenic pneumothorax, which may preclude the procedure if there is extensive coexisting emphysema. In patients with a peripheral tumour and enlarged hilar or paratracheal lymph nodes on CT, bronchoscopy with EBUS-guided node sampling may allow both diagnosis and staging.

In patients with pleural effusions, pleural aspiration and biopsy is the preferred investigation. Where facilities exist, thoracoscopy increases yield by allowing targeted biopsies under direct vision. In patients with metastatic disease, the diagnosis can often be confirmed by needle aspiration or biopsy of affected lymph nodes, skin lesions, liver or bone marrow.

Staging to guide treatment

The propensity of small-cell lung cancer to metastasise early means these patients are usually not suitable for surgical intervention. In non-small-cell lung cancer (NSCLC), treatment and prognosis are determined by disease extent, so careful staging is required. CT is used early to detect obvious local or distant spread. Enlarged upper mediastinal nodes may be sampled using an EBUS-equipped bronchoscope or by mediastinoscopy. Nodes in the lower mediastinum can be sampled through the oesophageal wall using endoscopic ultrasound. Combined CT and whole-body FDG-PET (see Fig. 17.6) is commonly used to detect occult but metabolically active metastases. Head CT, radionuclide bone scanning, liver ultrasound and bone marrow biopsy are generally reserved for patients with clinical, haematological or biochemical evidence of tumour spread to these sites. Information on tumour size and nodal and metastatic spread is then collated to assign the patient to one of nine staging groups that determine optimal management and prognosis (Fig. 17.50). Detailed physiological testing is required to assess whether respiratory and cardiac function is sufficient to allow aggressive treatment.

Management

Surgical resection carries the best hope of long-term survival but some patients treated with radical radiotherapy and chemotherapy also achieve prolonged remission or cure. In over 75% of cases, treatment with the aim of cure is not possible or is inappropriate due to extensive spread or comorbidity. Such patients are offered palliative therapy and best supportive care. Radiotherapy and, in some cases, chemotherapy can relieve symptoms.

Surgical treatment

Accurate preoperative staging, coupled with improvements in surgical and postoperative care, now offers 5-year survival rates of over 80% in stage I disease (N0, tumour confined within visceral pleura) and over 70% in stage II disease, which includes resection in patients with ipsilateral peribronchial or hilar node involvement.

Radiotherapy

While much less effective than surgery, radical radiotherapy can offer long-term survival in selected patients with localised disease in whom comorbidity precludes surgery. Radical radiotherapy is usually combined with chemotherapy when lymph nodes are involved (stage III). Highly targeted (stereotactic) radiotherapy may be given in 3–5 treatments for small lesions.

The greatest value of radiotherapy, however, is in the palliation of distressing complications, such as superior vena cava obstruction, recurrent haemoptysis and pain caused by chest wall invasion or by skeletal metastatic deposits. Obstruction of the trachea and main bronchi can also be relieved temporarily. Radiotherapy can be used in conjunction with chemotherapy in the treatment of small-cell carcinoma and is particularly efficient at preventing the development of brain metastases in patients who have had a complete response to chemotherapy.

Chemotherapy

The treatment of small-cell carcinoma with combinations of cytotoxic drugs, sometimes with radiotherapy, can increase median survival from 3 months to well over a year. The use of combinations of chemotherapeutic drugs requires considerable skill and should be overseen by multidisciplinary teams of clinical oncologists and specialist nurses. Combination chemotherapy leads to better outcomes than single-agent treatment. Regular cycles of therapy, including combinations of intravenous cyclophosphamide, doxorubicin and vincristine or intravenous cisplatin and etoposide, are commonly used.

In NSCLC chemotherapy is less effective, though platinum-based chemotherapy regimens offer 30% response rates and a modest increase in survival, and are widely used. Some non-small-cell lung tumours, particularly adenocarcinomas in non-smokers, carry detectable pathogenic variants, e.g. in the epidermal growth factor receptor (*EGFR*) gene. Tyrosine kinase inhibitors, such as erlotinib and monoclonal antibodies to EGFR (e.g. bevacizumab), show improved treatment responses in metastatic NSCLC and *EGFR* variants, and similar approaches are being developed to target other known genetic abnormalities.

In NSCLC there is some evidence that chemotherapy given before surgery may increase survival and can effectively 'down-stage' disease with limited nodal spread. Post-operative chemotherapy is now proven to enhance survival rates when operative samples show nodal involvement by tumour.

Nausea and vomiting are common side-effects of chemotherapy and are best treated with 5-HT$_3$ receptor antagonists.

Laser therapy and stenting

Palliation of symptoms caused by major airway obstruction can be achieved in selected patients using bronchoscopic laser treatment to

17

Tumour stage	Lymph node spread			
	N0 (None)	N1 (Ipsilateral hilar)	N2 (Ipsilateral mediastinal or subcarinal)	N3 (Contralateral or supraclavicular)
T1a (≤1 cm)	IA1 (92%)	IIB (53%)	IIIA (36%)	IIIB (26%)
T1b (>1 to ≤2 cm)	IA2 (83%)	IIB (53%)	IIIA (36%)	IIIB (26%)
T1c (>2 to ≤3 cm)	IA3 (77%)	IIB (53%)	IIIA (36%)	IIIB (26%)
T2a (>3 to ≤4 cm)	IB (68%)	IIB (53%)	IIIA (36%)	IIIB (26%)
T2b (>4 cm to ≤5 cm)	IIA (60%)	IIB (53%)	IIIA (36%)	IIIB (26%)
T3 (>5 cm)	IIB (53%)	IIIA (36%)	IIIB (26%)	IIIC (13%)
T4 (>7 cm or invading heart, vessels, oesophagus, carina etc.)	IIIA (36%)	IIIA (36%)	IIIB (26%)	IIIC (13%)
M1a Lung metastasis/effusion	IVA (10%)			
M1b Single extrathoracic metastasis	IVA (10%)			
M1c Multiple extrathoracic metastases	IVB (0%)			

Fig. 17.50 Tumour stage and 5-year survival in non-small-cell lung cancer. The figure shows the relationship between tumour extent (size, lymph node status and metastases) and prognosis (% survival at 5 years for each clinical stage). *Based on data from Detterbeck FC, Boffa DJ, Kim AW, Tanoue T. The eighth edition lung cancer stage classification. Chest 2017; 151:193–203.*

clear tumour tissue and allow re-aeration of collapsed lung. The best results are achieved in tumours of the main bronchi. Endobronchial stents can be used to maintain airway patency in the face of extrinsic compression by malignant nodes.

General aspects of management

The best outcomes are obtained when lung cancer is managed in specialist centres by multidisciplinary teams, including oncologists, thoracic surgeons, respiratory physicians and specialist nurses. Effective communication, pain relief and attention to diet are important. Lung tumours can cause clinically significant depression and anxiety, and these may need specific therapy. The management of non-metastatic endocrine manifestations is described in Chapter 20. When a malignant pleural effusion is present, an attempt should be made to drain the pleural cavity using an intercostal drain; depending upon response to initial drainage, subsequent fluid acculumlations can be managed with long-term indwelling pleural catheters or pleuredesis with sclerosing agents such as talc.

Prognosis

The overall prognosis in lung cancer is very poor, approximately 60% and over 80% of patients dying within 1 and 5 years respectively of diagnosis. The best prognosis is with well-differentiated squamous cell tumours that have not metastasised and are amenable to surgical resection. The clinical features and prognosis of some less common tumours are given in Box 17.65.

Secondary tumours of the lung

Blood-borne metastatic deposits in the lungs may be derived from many primary carcinomas, in particular breast, kidney, uterus, ovary, testes and thyroid, and also from osteogenic and other sarcomas. These secondary deposits are usually multiple and bilateral. Often there are no respiratory symptoms and the diagnosis is incidental on X-ray. Breathlessness may occur if a considerable amount of lung tissue has been replaced by metastatic tumour. Endobronchial deposits are uncommon but can cause haemoptysis and lobar collapse.

Lymphatic infiltration may develop in carcinoma of the breast, stomach, bowel, pancreas or bronchus. 'Lymphangitic carcinomatosis' causes severe, rapidly progressive breathlessness with marked hypoxaemia. The chest X-ray shows diffuse pulmonary shadowing radiating from the hilar regions, often with septal lines, and CT shows characteristic polygonal thickened interlobular septa. Palliation of breathlessness with opiates may help.

Tumours of the mediastinum

Figure 17.51 shows the major compartments of the mediastinum and Box 17.66 lists likely causes of a mediastinal mass.

Benign tumours and cysts in the mediastinum are often diagnosed when a chest X-ray is undertaken for some other reason. In general, they do not invade vital structures but may cause symptoms by compressing

i	**17.65 Rare types of lung tumour**				
Tumour	**Status**	**Histology**	**Typical presentation**	**Prognosis**
Adenosquamous carcinoma	Malignant	Tumours with areas of unequivocal squamous and adeno-differentiation	Peripheral or central lung mass	Stage-dependent
Neuro-endocrine (carcinoid) tumour	Low-grade malignant	Neuro-endocrine differentiation	Bronchial obstruction, cough	95% 5-year survival with resection
Bronchial gland adenoma	Benign	Salivary gland differentiation	Tracheobronchial irritation/obstruction	Local resection curative
Bronchial gland carcinoma	Low-grade malignant	Salivary gland differentiation	Tracheobronchial irritation/obstruction	Local recurrence
Hamartoma	Benign	Mesenchymal cells, cartilage	Peripheral lung nodule	Local resection curative
Bronchoalveolar carcinoma	Malignant	Tumour cells line alveolar spaces	Alveolar shadowing, productive cough	Variable, worse if multifocal

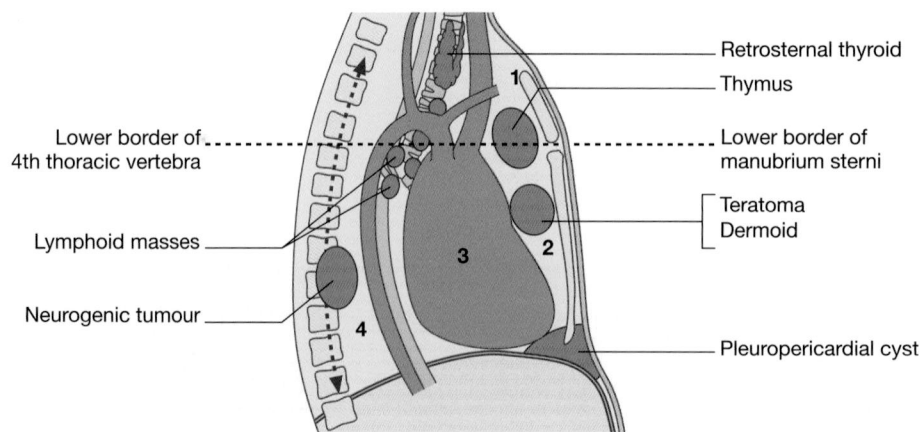

Fig. 17.51 The divisions of the mediastinum. (1) Superior mediastinum. (2) Anterior mediastinum. (3) Middle mediastinum. (4) Posterior mediastinum. Sites of the more common mediastinal tumours are also illustrated. *From Johnson N McL. Respiratory medicine. Oxford: Blackwell Science; 1986.*

the trachea or the superior vena cava. A dermoid cyst may very occasionally rupture into a bronchus.

Malignant mediastinal tumours are distinguished by their power to invade, as well as compress, surrounding structures. As a result, even a small malignant tumour can produce symptoms, although, more commonly, the tumour has attained a considerable size before this happens (Box 17.67). The most common cause is mediastinal lymph node metastasis from lung cancer but lymphomas, leukaemia, malignant thymic tumours and germ-cell tumours can cause similar features. Aortic and innominate aneurysms have destructive features resembling those of malignant mediastinal tumours.

Investigations

A benign mediastinal tumour generally appears on chest X-ray as a sharply circumscribed mediastinal opacity encroaching on one or both lung fields (as shown in Fig. 17.52). CT (or MRI) is the investigation of choice for mediastinal tumours (e.g. see Fig. 20.12). A malignant mediastinal tumour seldom has a clearly defined margin and often presents as a general broadening of the mediastinum.

Bronchoscopy may reveal a primary lung cancer causing mediastinal lymphadenopathy. EBUS may be used to guide sampling of peribronchial masses. The posterior mediastinum can be imaged and biopsied via the oesophagus using endoscopic ultrasound.

Mediastinoscopy under general anaesthetic can be used to visualise and biopsy masses in the superior and anterior mediastinum but surgical exploration of the chest, with removal of part or all of the tumour, is often required to obtain a histological diagnosis.

Management

Benign mediastinal tumours should be removed surgically because most produce symptoms sooner or later. Cysts may become infected, while neural tumours have the potential to undergo malignant transformation. The operative mortality is low in the absence of coexisting cardiovascular disease, COPD or extreme age.

Interstitial and infiltrative pulmonary diseases

Diffuse parenchymal lung disease

The diffuse parenchymal lung diseases (DPLDs) are a heterogeneous group of conditions affecting the pulmonary parenchyma (interstitium)

and/or alveolar lumen, which are frequently considered collectively as they share a sufficient number of clinical physiological and radiographic similarities (Box 17.68). They often present with cough, which is typically dry and distressing, and breathlessness, which is often insidious in onset but thereafter relentlessly progressive. Physical examination reveals the presence of inspiratory crackles and in many cases digital clubbing develops. Pulmonary function tests typically show a restrictive ventilatory defect in the presence of small lung volumes and reduced gas transfer. The typical radiographic findings include, in the earliest stages, ground glass and reticulonodular shadowing, with progression to honeycomb cysts and traction bronchiectasis. While these appearances may be seen on a 'plain' chest X-ray, they are most easily appreciated on HRCT, which has assumed a central role in the evaluation of DPLD (Fig. 17.53). The current classification is shown in Figure 17.54 and the potential differential diagnoses in Box 17.69. Common features of interstitial lung disease in old age are shown in Box 17.70.

17.67 Clinical features of malignant mediastinal invasion

Trachea and main bronchi
- Stridor, breathlessness, cough, pulmonary collapse

Oesophagus
- Dysphagia, oesophageal displacement or obstruction on barium swallow examination

Phrenic nerve
- Diaphragmatic paralysis

Left recurrent laryngeal nerve
- Paralysis of left vocal cord with hoarseness and 'bovine' cough

Sympathetic trunk
- Horner syndrome

Superior vena cava
- SVC obstruction: non-pulsatile distension of neck veins, subconjunctival oedema, and oedema and cyanosis of head, neck, hands and arms; dilated anastomotic veins on chest wall

Pericardium
- Pericarditis and/or pericardial effusion

17.66 Causes of a mediastinal mass

Superior mediastinum
- Retrosternal goitre
- Persistent left superior vena cava
- Prominent left subclavian artery
- Thymic tumour
- Dermoid cyst
- Lymphoma
- Aortic aneurysm

Anterior mediastinum
- Retrosternal goitre
- Dermoid cyst
- Thymic tumour
- Lymphoma
- Aortic aneurysm
- Germ cell tumour
- Pericardial cyst
- Hiatus hernia through the diaphragmatic foramen of Morgagni

Posterior mediastinum
- Neurogenic tumour
- Paravertebral abscess
- Oesophageal lesion
- Aortic aneurysm
- Foregut duplication

Middle mediastinum
- Lung cancer
- Lymphoma
- Sarcoidosis
- Bronchogenic cyst
- Hiatus hernia

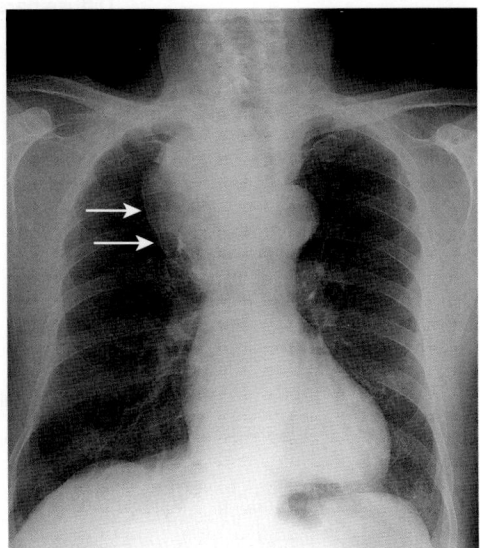

Fig. 17.52 Intrathoracic goitre (arrows) extending from right upper mediastinum.

Idiopathic interstitial pneumonias

The idiopathic interstitial pneumonias represent a major subgroup of DPLD that are grouped together as a result of their unknown aetiology (Box 17.71). They are often distinguished by the predominant histological pattern on tissue biopsy; hence they are frequently referred to by their pathological description, e.g. usual interstitial pneumonia (UIP) or non-specific interstitial pneumonia (NSIP). The most important of these is idiopathic pulmonary fibrosis.

Idiopathic pulmonary fibrosis

Idiopathic pulmonary fibrosis (IPF) is defined as a progressive fibrosing interstitial pneumonia of unknown cause, occurring in adults and associated with the histological or radiological pattern of UIP. Important differentials include fibrosing diseases caused by occupational exposure, medication or connective tissue diseases, which must be excluded by careful history, examination and investigation.

The histological features of the condition are suggestive of repeated episodes of focal damage to the alveolar epithelium consistent with an autoimmune process but the aetiology remains elusive: speculation has included exposure to viruses (e.g. Epstein–Barr virus), occupational dusts (metal or wood), drugs (antidepressants) or chronic gastro-oesophageal

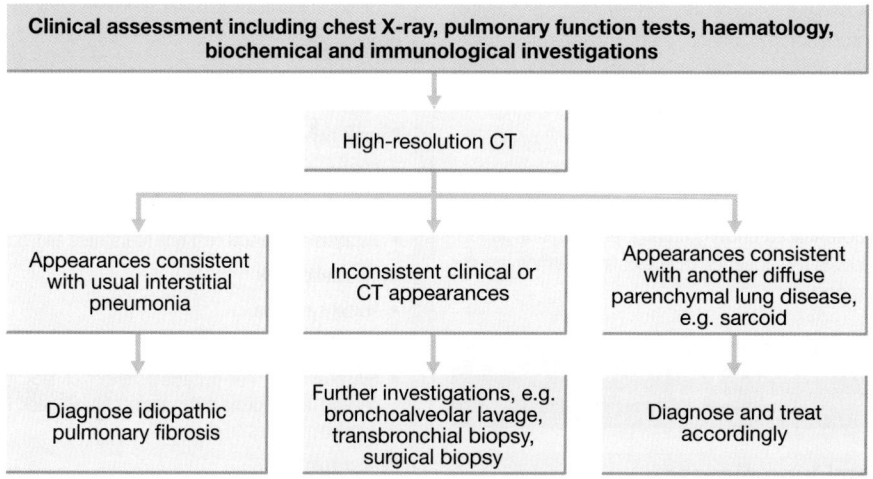

Fig. 17.53 Algorithm for the investigation of patients with interstitial lung disease following initial clinical and chest X-ray examination.

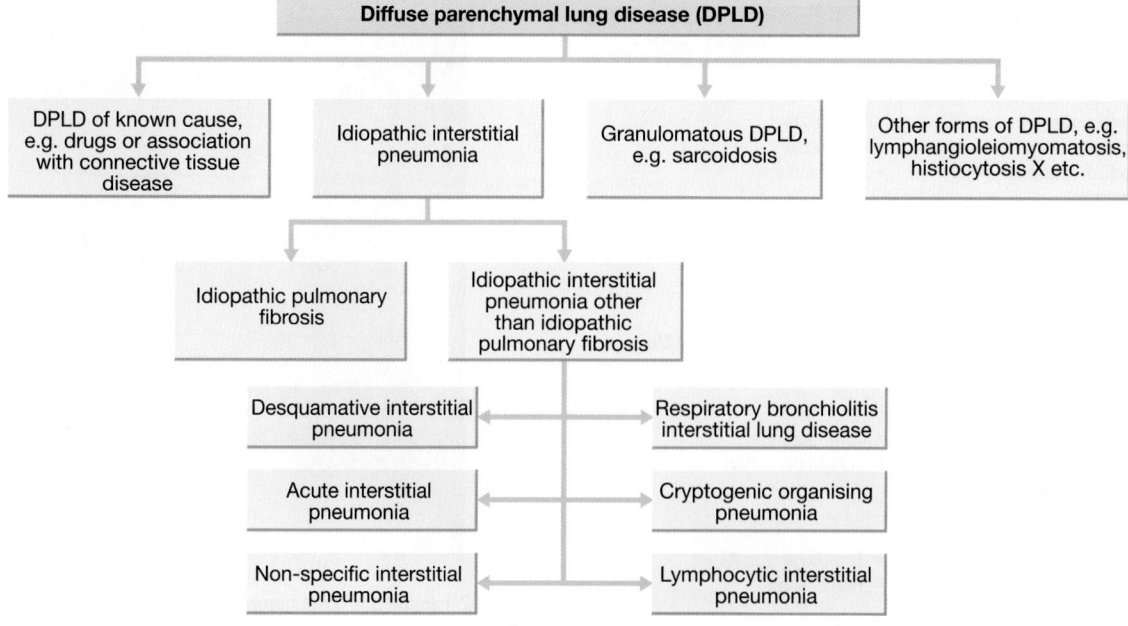

Fig. 17.54 Classification of diffuse parenchymal lung disease.

---

i | **17.69 Conditions that mimic diffuse parenchymal lung disease**

Infection

- Viral pneumonia
- *Pneumocystis jirovecii*
- *Mycoplasma pneumoniae*
- Tuberculosis
- Parasite, e.g. filariasis
- Fungal infection

Malignancy

- Leukaemia and lymphoma
- Lymphangitic carcinomatosis
- Multiple metastases
- Bronchoalveolar carcinoma

Pulmonary oedema

Aspiration pneumonitis

17.70 Interstitial lung disease in old age

- **Idiopathic pulmonary fibrosis**: the most common interstitial lung disease, with a poor prognosis.
- **Chronic aspiration pneumonitis**: must always be considered in older patients presenting with bilateral basal shadowing on a chest X-ray.
- **Granulomatosis with polyangiitis (GPA)**: a rare condition but more common in old age. Renal involvement is more common at presentation and upper respiratory problems are fewer.
- **Asbestosis**: symptoms may appear only in old age because of the prolonged latent period between exposure and disease.
- **Drug-induced interstitial lung disease**: more common, presumably because of the increased chance of exposure to multiple drugs.
- **Rarer interstitial disease**: sarcoidosis, idiopathic pulmonary haemosiderosis, alveolar proteinosis and eosinophilic pneumonia rarely present.
- **Increased dyspnoea**: coexistent muscle weakness, chest wall deformity (e.g. thoracic kyphosis) and deconditioning may all exacerbate dyspnoea associated with interstitial lung disease.
- **Surgical lung biopsy**: often inappropriate in the very frail. A diagnosis therefore frequently depends on clinical and high-resolution computed tomography findings alone.

---

reflux. Familial cases are rare but genetic factors that control the inflammatory and fibrotic response are likely to be important. There is a strong association with cigarette smoking.

Clinical features

IPF usually presents in the older adult and is uncommon before the age of 50 years. With the advent of widespread CT scanning it may present as an incidental finding in an otherwise asymptomatic individual but more typically presents with progressive breathlessness (which may have been insidious) and a non-productive cough. Constitutional symptoms are unusual. Clinical findings include finger clubbing and the presence of bi-basal fine late inspiratory crackles likened to the unfastening of Velcro.

Investigations

These are summarised in Box 17.72. Established IPF will be apparent on chest X-ray as a bilateral lower lobe and subpleural reticular shadowing. The chest X-ray may be normal in individuals with early or limited disease, however. HRCT typically demonstrates a patchy, predominantly peripheral, subpleural and basal reticular pattern and, in more advanced disease, the presence of honeycombing cysts and traction bronchiectasis (Fig. 17.55). When these features are present, HRCT has a high positive predictive value for the diagnosis of IPF and recourse to biopsy is seldom necessary. HRCT appearances may also be sufficiently characteristic to suggest an alternative diagnosis such as hypersensitivity pneumonitis or sarcoidosis. The presence of pleural plaques may suggest asbestosis.

Pulmonary function tests classically show a restrictive defect with reduced lung volumes and gas transfer. However, lung volumes may be preserved in patients with concomitant emphysema. Dynamic tests are useful to document exercise tolerance and demonstrate exercise-induced arterial hypoxaemia, but as IPF advances, arterial hypoxaemia and hypocapnia are present at rest.

---

i | **17.71 Idiopathic interstitial pneumonias**

Clinical diagnosis	Notes
Usual interstitial pneumonia (UIP)	Idiopathic pulmonary fibrosis – see text
Non-specific interstitial pneumonia (NSIP)	See page 537
Respiratory bronchiolitis–interstitial lung disease	More common in men and smokers. Usually presents at age 40–60 years. Smoking cessation may lead to improvement. Natural history unclear
Acute interstitial pneumonia	Often preceded by viral upper respiratory tract infection. Severe exertional dyspnoea, widespread pneumonic consolidation and diffuse alveolar damage on biopsy. Prognosis often poor
Desquamative interstitial pneumonia (DIP)	More common in men and smokers. Presents at age 40–60 years. Insidious onset of dyspnoea. Clubbing in 50%. Biopsy shows increased macrophages in alveolar space, septal thickening and type II pneumocyte hyperplasia. Prognosis generally good
Cryptogenic organising pneumonia ('bronchiolitis obliterans organising pneumonia' – BOOP)	Presents as clinical and radiological pneumonia. Systemic features and markedly raised erythrocyte sedimentation rate common. Finger clubbing absent. Biopsy shows florid proliferation of immature collagen (Masson bodies) and fibrous tissue. Response to glucocorticoids classically excellent
Lymphocytic interstitial pneumonia (LIP)	More common in women, slow onset over years. Investigate for associations with connective tissue disease or HIV. Unclear whether glucocorticoids are helpful

---

17

Bronchoscopy is seldom indicated unless there is serious consideration of differential diagnoses of infection or a malignant process; lymphocytosis may suggest chronic hypersensitivity pneumonitis. The tissue samples obtained by transbronchial lung biopsy are invariably insufficient to be of value, and if tissue is required, a surgical lung biopsy should be sought. Lung biopsy should be considered in cases of diagnostic uncertainty or with atypical features. UIP is the histological pattern predominantly encountered in IPF (Fig. 17.56); however, it is also found in asbestosis, hypersensitivity pneumonitis, connective tissue diseases and drug reactions.

It is not uncommon to identify a mildly positive antinuclear antibody (ANA) or anti-cyclic citrullinated peptide 2 (anti-CCP2) and repeat serological testing may be performed, as lung disease may precede the appearance of connective tissue disease.

Management

The management options for IPF are improving. If the vital capacity is between 50% and 80% predicted, patients may be offered either pirfenidone (an antifibrotic agent) or nintedanib (a tyrosine kinase inhibitor). Both of these agents have been shown to reduce the rate of decline in lung function. Patients taking pirfenidone should be advised to avoid direct exposure to sunlight and use photoprotective clothing and high-protection sunscreens. Nintedanib may be accompanied by diarrhoea. Neither drug improves cough or breathlessness and treatment should be discontinued if lung function declines by more than 10% over the first year of treatment. Medication to control gastro-oesophageal reflux may improve the cough. Current smokers should be apprised of the increased risk of lung cancer and advised to stop. Influenza and pneumococcal vaccination should be recommended. Patients should be encouraged to exercise and participate in pulmonary rehabilitation using ambulatory oxygen if appropriate. Domiciliary oxygen should be considered for palliation of breathlessness in severe cases. Where appropriate, lung transplantation should be considered. The optimum treatment for acute exacerbations is unknown. Treatment is largely supportive. Broad-spectrum antibiotics may be combined with glucocorticoids and sometimes additional immunosuppression but there are few data to support this approach.

Prognosis

The natural history is usually one of steady decline; however, some patients are prone to exacerbations accompanied by an acute deterioration in

 17.72 Investigations in diffuse parenchymal lung disease

Laboratory investigations

- Full blood count: lymphopenia in sarcoidosis; eosinophilia in pulmonary eosinophilias and drug reactions; neutrophilia in hypersensitivity pneumonitis
- Ca^{2+}: may be elevated in sarcoidosis
- Lactate dehydrogenase: may be elevated in active alveolitis
- Serum angiotensin-converting enzyme: non-specific indicator of disease activity in sarcoidosis
- Erythrocyte sedimentation rate and C-reactive protein: non-specifically raised
- Autoimmune screen: anti-cyclic citrullinated peptide (anti-CCP) and other autoantibodies may suggest connective tissue disease

Radiology

- See Box 17.68

Pulmonary function

- See Box 17.68

Bronchoscopy

- Bronchoalveolar lavage: differential cell counts may point to sarcoidosis and drug-induced pneumonitis, pulmonary eosinophilias, hypersensitivity pneumonitis or cryptogenic organising pneumonia; useful to exclude infection
- Transbronchial biopsy: useful in sarcoidosis and differential of malignancy or infection
- Bronchial biopsy: occasionally useful in sarcoidosis

Video-assisted thoracoscopic lung biopsy (in selected cases)

- Allows pathological classification: presence of asbestos bodies may suggest asbestosis; silica in occupational fibrosing lung disease

Others

- Liver biopsy: may be useful in sarcoidosis
- Urinary calcium excretion: may be useful in sarcoidosis

breathlessness, disturbed gas exchange, and new ground glass changes or consolidation on HRCT. In advanced disease, central cyanosis is detectable and patients may develop pulmonary hypertension and features of right heart failure. A median survival of 3 years is widely quoted; the rate of disease progression varies considerably, however, from death

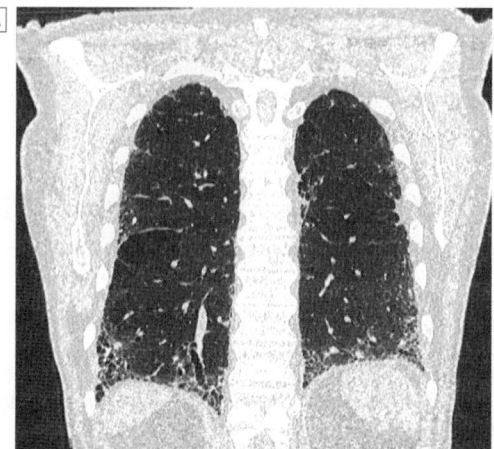
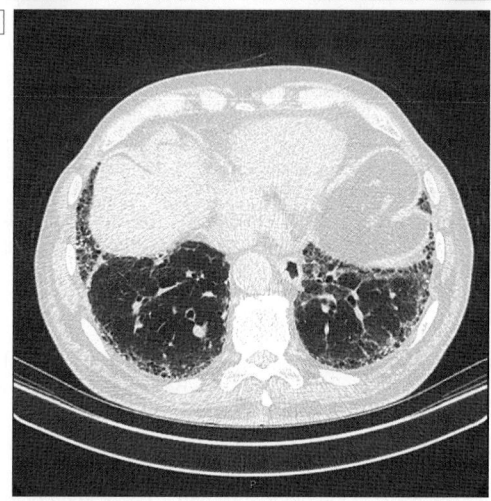

Fig. 17.55 Idiopathic pulmonary fibrosis. Typical high-resolution CT images demonstrate the bilateral, predominantly basal and peripheral reticular opacities, accompanied by honeycombing in the later stages. **A** Anteroposterior view. **B** Transverse section. *Courtesy of Dr Andrew Baird, Consultant Radiologist, NHS Lothian, Edinburgh, UK.*

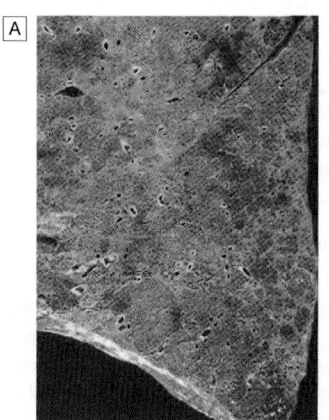
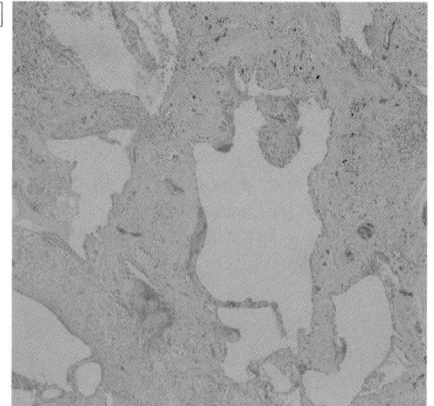

Fig. 17.56 Pathology of usual interstitial pneumonia (UIP). **A** Lung tissue showing subpleural scarring, most prominently down the posterior edge of the lower lobe. This distribution of fibrosis is typical of usual interstitial pneumonitis. The fibrosis may be associated with prominent cystic change known as 'honeycomb lung'. **B** Histology showing severe interstitial fibrosis with loss of the normal alveolar architecture and the development of 'honeycomb' cysts. *Courtesy of Dr William Wallace, Department of Pathology, Royal Infirmary of Edinburgh.*

within a few months to survival with minimal symptoms for many years. Serial lung function testing may provide useful prognostic information, relative preservation of lung function suggesting longer survival and significantly impaired gas transfer and/or desaturation on exercise heralding a poorer prognosis. The finding of high numbers of fibroblastic foci on biopsy suggests a more rapid deterioration.

Non-specific interstitial pneumonia

The clinical picture of fibrotic NSIP is similar to that of IPF, although patients tend to be women and younger in age. As with UIP, the condition may present as an isolated idiopathic pulmonary condition, but an NSIP pattern is often associated with connective tissue disease, certain drugs, chronic hypersensitivity pneumonitis or HIV infection and care must be taken to exclude these possibilities. As with UIP, the pulmonary condition may precede the appearance of connective tissue disease. HRCT findings are less specific than with IPF and lung biopsy may be required. The prognosis is significantly better than that of IPF, particularly in the cellular form of the condition, and the 5-year mortality rate is typically less than 15%.

Sarcoidosis

Sarcoidosis is a multisystem granulomatous disorder of unknown aetiology that is characterised by the presence of non-caseating granulomas (Fig. 17.57). The condition is more frequently described in colder parts of northern Europe. It also appears to be more common and more severe in those from an African Caribbean background. The tendency for sarcoidosis to present in the spring and summer has led to speculation about the role of infective agents, including mycobacteria, propionibacteria and viruses, but the cause remains elusive. Genetic susceptibility is supported by familial clustering; a range of class II HLA alleles confer protection from,

or susceptibility to, the condition. Sarcoidosis occurs less frequently in smokers. It may be associated with common variable immunodeficiency.

Clinical features

Sarcoidosis is considered with other DPLDs, as over 90% of cases affect the lungs, but the condition can involve almost any organ (Fig. 17.58 and Box 17.73). Löfgren syndrome – an acute illness characterised by

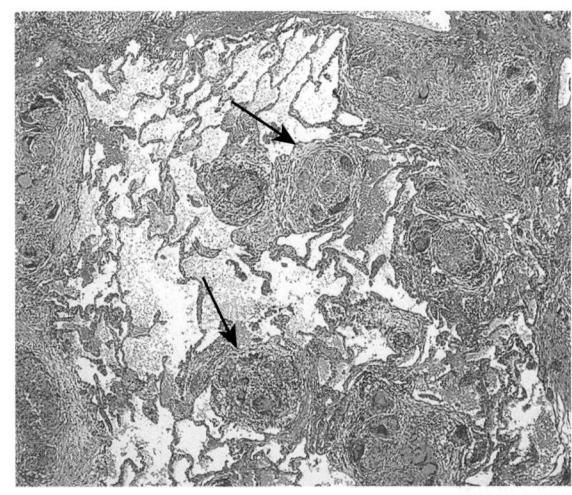

Fig. 17.57 Sarcoidosis of the lung. Histology showing non-caseating granulomas (arrows). *Courtesy of Dr William Wallace, Department of Pathology, Royal Infirmary of Edinburgh.*

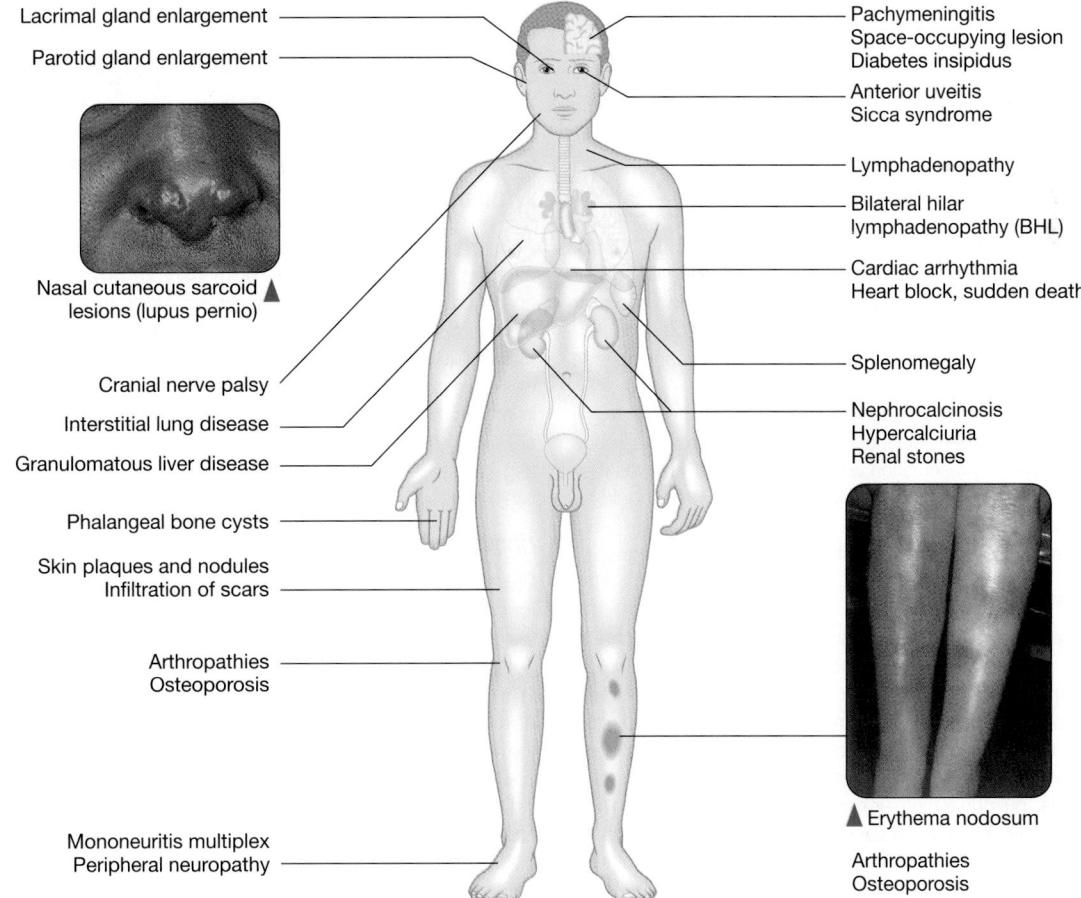

Lacrimal gland enlargement

Parotid gland enlargement

Nasal cutaneous sarcoid lesions (lupus pernio) ▲

Cranial nerve palsy

Interstitial lung disease

Granulomatous liver disease

Phalangeal bone cysts

Skin plaques and nodules
Infiltration of scars

Arthropathies
Osteoporosis

Mononeuritis multiplex
Peripheral neuropathy

Pachymeningitis
Space-occupying lesion
Diabetes insipidus

Anterior uveitis
Sicca syndrome

Lymphadenopathy

Bilateral hilar
lymphadenopathy (BHL)

Cardiac arrhythmia
Heart block, sudden death

Splenomegaly

Nephrocalcinosis
Hypercalciuria
Renal stones

▲ Erythema nodosum

Arthropathies
Osteoporosis

Fig. 17.58 Possible systemic involvement in sarcoidosis. *Inset (Erythema nodosum): From Savin JA, Hunter JAA, Hepburn NC. Skin signs in clinical medicine. London: Mosby–Wolfe; 1997.*

erythema nodosum, peripheral arthropathy, uveitis, bilateral hilar lymphadenopathy (BHL), lethargy and occasionally fever – is often seen in young women. Alternatively, BHL may be detected in an otherwise asymptomatic individual undergoing a chest X-ray for other purposes. Pulmonary disease may also present in a more insidious manner with cough, exertional breathlessness and radiographic infiltrates; chest auscultation is often surprisingly unremarkable. Fibrosis occurs in around 20% of cases of pulmonary sarcoidosis and may cause a silent loss of lung function. Pleural disease is uncommon and finger clubbing is not a feature. Complications such as bronchiectasis, aspergilloma, pneumothorax, pulmonary hypertension and cor pulmonale have been reported but are rare.

Investigations

Lymphopenia is characteristic and liver function tests may be mildly deranged. Hypercalcaemia may be present (reflecting increased formation of calcitriol – 1,25-dihydroxyvitamin D – by alveolar macrophages), particularly if the patient has been exposed to strong sunlight. Hypercalciuria may also be seen and may lead to nephrocalcinosis. Serum angiotensin-converting enzyme (ACE) may provide a non-specific marker of disease activity and can assist in monitoring the clinical course. Chest radiography has been used to stage sarcoidosis (Box 17.74). In patients with pulmonary infiltrates, pulmonary function testing may show a restrictive defect accompanied by impaired gas exchange. Exercise tests may reveal oxygen desaturation. Bronchoscopy may demonstrate a 'cobblestone' appearance of the mucosa, and bronchial and transbronchial biopsies usually show non-caseating granulomas, as may samples from the mediastinal nodes obtained by EBUS. Bronchoalveolar lavage fluid typically contains an increased CD4:CD8 T-cell ratio. Characteristic HRCT appearances include reticulonodular opacities that follow a perilymphatic distribution centred on bronchovascular bundles and the subpleural areas. FDG-PET scanning can detect extrapulmonary disease.

The occurrence of erythema nodosum with BHL on chest X-ray is often sufficient for a confident diagnosis, without recourse to a tissue biopsy. Similarly, a typical presentation with classical HRCT features may also be accepted. In other instances, however, the diagnosis should be confirmed by histological examination of the involved organ. The presence of anergy (e.g. to tuberculin skin tests) may support the diagnosis.

Management

Patients who present with acute illness and erythema nodosum should receive NSAIDs and, on occasion, a short course of glucocorticoids. The majority of patients enjoy spontaneous remission and so, if there is no evidence of organ damage, systemic glucocorticoid therapy can be withheld for 6 months. However, prednisolone (at a starting dose of 20–40 mg/day) should be commenced immediately in the presence of hypercalcaemia, pulmonary impairment, renal impairment and uveitis. Topical glucocorticoids may be useful in cases of mild uveitis, and inhaled glucocorticoids have been used to shorten the duration of systemic glucocorticoid use in asymptomatic parenchymal sarcoidosis. Patients should be warned that strong sunlight may precipitate hypercalcaemia and endanger renal function.

Features suggesting a less favourable outlook include age over 40, African Caribbean ancestry, persistent symptoms for more than 6 months, the involvement of more than three organs, lupus pernio (see Fig. 17.58) and a stage III/IV chest X-ray. In patients with severe disease, methotrexate (10–20 mg/week), azathioprine (50–150 mg/day) and specific tumour necrosis factor alpha (TNF-α) inhibitors have been effective. Chloroquine, hydroxychloroquine and low-dose thalidomide may be useful in cutaneous sarcoidosis with limited pulmonary involvement. Selected patients may be referred for consideration of single lung transplantation. The overall mortality is low (1%–5%) and usually reflects cardiac involvement or pulmonary fibrosis.

Lung diseases due to systemic inflammatory disease

The acute respiratory distress syndrome

See page 201.

Respiratory involvement in connective tissue disorders

Pulmonary complications of connective tissue disease are common, affecting the airways, alveoli, pulmonary vasculature, diaphragm and chest wall muscles, and the chest wall itself. In some instances, pulmonary disease may precede the appearance of the connective tissue disorder (Box 17.75). Indirect associations between connective tissue disorders and respiratory complications include those due to disease in other organs, e.g. thrombocytopenia causing haemoptysis; pulmonary toxic effects of drugs used to treat the connective tissue disorder (e.g. gold and methotrexate); and secondary infection due to the disease itself, neutropenia or immunosuppressive drug regimens.

Rheumatoid disease

Pulmonary involvement in rheumatoid disease is important, accounting for around 10%–20% of the mortality associated with the condition. The majority of cases occur within 5 years of the rheumatological diagnosis but pulmonary manifestations may precede joint involvement in 10%–20%. Pulmonary fibrosis is the most common pulmonary manifestation. All forms of interstitial disease have been described but NSIP is probably the most common. A rare variant of localised upper lobe fibrosis and cavitation is occasionally seen.

Pleural effusion is common, especially in men with seropositive disease. Effusions are usually small and unilateral, but can be large and bilateral. Most resolve spontaneously. Biochemical testing shows an exudate with markedly reduced glucose levels and raised lactate dehydrogenase (LDH). Effusions that fail to resolve spontaneously may respond to a short course of oral prednisolone (30–40 mg/day) but some become chronic.

i	**17.75 Respiratory complications of connective tissue disorders**			
Disorder	**Airways**	**Parenchyma**	**Pleura**	**Diaphragm and chest wall**
Rheumatoid arthritis	Bronchitis, obliterative bronchiolitis, bronchiectasis, crico-arytenoid arthritis, stridor	Pulmonary fibrosis, nodules, upper lobe fibrosis, infections	Pleurisy, effusion, pneumothorax	Poor healing of intercostal drain sites
Systemic lupus erythematosus	–	Pulmonary fibrosis, 'vasculitic' infarcts	Pleurisy, effusion	Diaphragmatic weakness (shrinking lungs)
Systemic sclerosis	Bronchiectasis	Pulmonary fibrosis, aspiration pneumonia	–	Cutaneous thoracic restriction (hidebound chest)
Dermatomyositis/ polymyositis	Lung cancer	Pulmonary fibrosis	–	Intercostal and diaphragmatic myopathy
Granulomatosis with polyangiitis (GPA)	Epistaxis, nasal discharge crusting, subglottic stenosis	Pulmonary nodules that may cavitate	Pleurisy, effusion	–

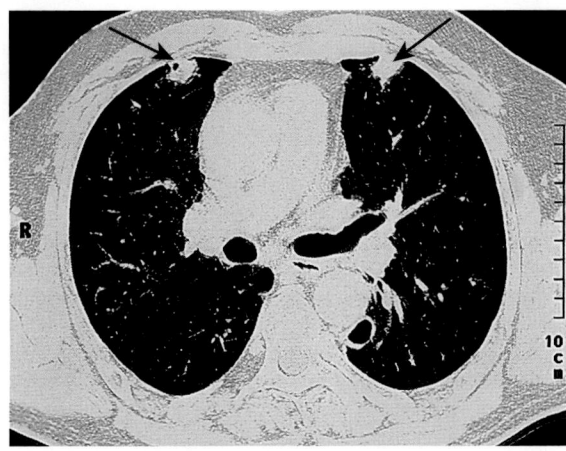

Fig. 17.59 Rheumatoid (necrobiotic) nodules. Thoracic CT just below the level of the main carina, showing the typical appearance of peripheral pleural-based nodules (arrows). The nodule in the left lower lobe shows characteristic cavitation.

Rheumatoid pulmonary nodules are usually asymptomatic and detected incidentally on imaging. They are most often multiple and subpleural in site (Fig. 17.59). Solitary nodules can mimic primary lung cancer; when multiple, the differential diagnoses include pulmonary metastatic disease. Cavitation raises the possibility of TB and predisposes to pneumothorax. The combination of rheumatoid nodules and pneumoconiosis is known as Caplan syndrome.

Bronchitis and bronchiectasis are both more common in rheumatoid patients. Rarely, the potentially fatal condition called obliterative bronchiolitis may develop. Bacterial lower respiratory tract infections are frequent. Treatments given for rheumatoid arthritis may also be relevant: glucocorticoid therapy predisposes to infections, methotrexate may cause pulmonary fibrosis, and anti-TNF therapy has been associated with the reactivation of TB.

Systemic lupus erythematosus

Pleuropulmonary involvement is more common in lupus than in any other connective tissue disorder and may be a presenting problem, when it is sometimes attributed incorrectly to infection or pulmonary embolism. Up to two-thirds of patients have repeated episodes of pleurisy, with or without effusions. Effusions may be bilateral and may also involve the pericardium.

The most serious manifestation of lupus is an acute pneumonitis that may be associated with diffuse alveolar haemorrhage. This condition is life-threatening and requires either immediate immunosuppression with glucocorticoids or a step-up in immunosuppressive treatment, if already started.

Pulmonary fibrosis is a relatively uncommon manifestation of systemic lupus erythematosus (SLE). Some patients with SLE present with exertional dyspnoea and orthopnoea but without overt signs of pulmonary fibrosis. The chest X-ray reveals elevated diaphragms and pulmonary function testing shows reduced lung volumes. This condition has been described as 'shrinking lungs' and has been attributed to diaphragmatic myopathy.

SLE patients with antiphospholipid antibodies are at increased risk of venous and pulmonary thromboembolism and require life-long anticoagulation.

Systemic sclerosis

Most patients with systemic sclerosis eventually develop diffuse pulmonary fibrosis; at necropsy more than 90% have evidence of lung fibrosis. In some patients it is indolent, but when progressive, as in IPF, the median survival time is around 4 years. Pulmonary fibrosis is rare in CREST syndrome but isolated pulmonary hypertension may develop.

Other pulmonary complications include recurrent aspiration pneumonias secondary to oesophageal disease. Rarely, sclerosis of the skin of the chest wall may be so extensive and cicatrising as to restrict chest wall movement – the so-called 'hidebound chest'.

Pulmonary eosinophilia and vasculitides

Pulmonary eosinophilia refers to the association of radiographic (usually pneumonic) abnormalities and peripheral blood eosinophilia. The term encompasses a group of disorders of different aetiology (Box 17.76). Eosinophils are the predominant cell recovered in sputum or BAL, and eosinophil products are likely to the prime mediators of tissue damage.

Acute eosinophilic pneumonia

Acute eosinophilic pneumonia is an acute febrile illness (of less than 5 days' duration), characterised by diffuse pulmonary infiltrates and hypoxic respiratory failure. The pathology is usually that of diffuse alveolar damage. Diagnosis is confirmed by BAL, which characteristically demonstrates >25% eosinophils. The condition is usually idiopathic but drug reactions should be considered. Glucocorticoids invariably induce prompt and complete resolution.

Chronic eosinophilic pneumonia

Chronic eosinophilic pneumonia typically presents in an insidious manner with malaise, fever, weight loss, breathlessness and unproductive cough. It is more common in middle-aged females. The classical chest X-ray appearance has been likened to the photographic negative of pulmonary oedema with bilateral, peripheral and predominantly upper lobe

17

parenchymal shadowing. The peripheral blood eosinophil count is almost always very high, and the erythrocyte sedimentation rate (ESR) and total serum IgE are elevated. BAL reveals a high proportion of eosinophils in the lavage fluid. Response to prednisolone (20–40 mg/day) is usually dramatic. Prednisolone can usually be withdrawn after a few weeks without relapse but long-term, low-dose therapy is occasionally necessary.

Tropical pulmonary eosinophilia

Tropical pulmonary eosinophilia occurs as a result of a mosquito-borne filarial infection with *Wuchereria bancrofti* or *Brugia malayi* (p. 335). The condition presents with fever, weight loss, dyspnoea and asthma-like symptoms. The peripheral blood eosinophilia is marked, as is the elevation of total IgE. High antifilarial antibody titres are seen. The diagnosis may be confirmed by a response to treatment with diethylcarbamazine (6 mg/kg daily for 3 weeks). Tropical pulmonary eosinophilia must be distinguished from infection with *Strongyloides stercoralis*, in which glucocorticoids may cause a life-threatening hyperinfection syndrome. Ascariasis ('larva migrans') and other hookworm infestations are covered in Chapter 13.

Granulomatosis with polyangiitis

Granulomatosis with polyangiitis (GPA, formerly referred to as Wegener's granulomatosis) is a rare vasculitic and granulomatous condition described in Chapter 26. The lung is commonly involved in systemic forms of the disease but a limited pulmonary form may also occur. Respiratory symptoms include cough, haemoptysis and chest pain. Associated upper respiratory tract manifestations include nasal discharge and crusting, and otitis media. Fever, weight loss and anaemia are common. Radiological features include multiple nodules and cavitation that may resemble primary or metastatic carcinoma, or a pulmonary abscess. Tissue biopsy confirms the distinctive pattern of necrotising granulomas and necrotising vasculitis. Other respiratory complications include tracheal subglottic stenosis and saddle nose deformity. The differential diagnoses include mycobacterial and fungal infection and other forms of pulmonary vasculitis, including polyarteritis nodosa (pulmonary infarction), microscopic polyangiitis, eosinophilic granulomatosis with polyangiitis (EGPA: marked tissue eosinophilia and association with asthma), necrotising sarcoidosis, bronchocentric granulomatosis and lymphomatoid granulomatosis.

Goodpasture's disease

This describes the association of pulmonary haemorrhage and glomerulonephritis, in which IgG antibodies bind to the glomerular or alveolar basement membranes. Pulmonary disease usually precedes renal involvement and includes radiographic infiltrates and hypoxia with or without haemoptysis. It occurs more commonly in men and almost exclusively in smokers.

Lung diseases due to irradiation and drugs

Radiotherapy

Targeting radiotherapy to certain tumours is inevitably accompanied by irradiation of normal lung tissue. Although delivered in divided doses, the effects are cumulative. Acute radiation pneumonitis is typically seen within 6–12 weeks and presents with cough and dyspnoea. This may resolve spontaneously but responds to glucocorticoid treatment. Chronic interstitial fibrosis may present several months later with symptoms of exertional dyspnoea and cough. Changes are often confined to the area irradiated but may be bilateral. Established post-irradiation fibrosis does not usually respond to glucocorticoid treatment. The pulmonary effects of radiation are exacerbated by treatment with cytotoxic drugs, and the phenomenon of 'recall pneumonitis' describes the appearance of radiation injury in a previously irradiated area when chemotherapy follows radiotherapy. If the patient survives, there are long-term risks of lung cancer.

Drugs

Drugs may cause a variety of pulmonary conditions (Box 17.77). Pulmonary fibrosis may occur in response to a variety of drugs but is seen most frequently with bleomycin, methotrexate, amiodarone and nitrofurantoin. Eosinophilic pulmonary reactions can also be caused by drugs. The pathogenesis may be an immune reaction similar to that in hypersensitivity pneumonitis, which specifically attracts large numbers of eosinophils into the lungs. This type of reaction is well described as a rare reaction to a variety of antineoplastic agents (e.g. bleomycin), antibiotics (e.g. sulphonamides), sulfasalazine and the anticonvulsants phenytoin and carbamazepine. Patients usually present with breathlessness, cough and fever. The chest X-ray characteristically shows

---

17.76 Pulmonary eosinophilia

Extrinsic (cause known)

- Helminths: e.g. *Ascaris, Toxocara, Filaria*
- Drugs: nitrofurantoin, para-aminosalicylic acid (PAS), sulfasalazine, imipramine, chlorpropamide, phenylbutazone
- Fungi: e.g. *Aspergillus fumigatus* causing allergic bronchopulmonary aspergillosis

Intrinsic (cause unknown)

- Cryptogenic eosinophilic pneumonia
- Eosinophilic granulomatosis with polyangiitis (EGPA, formerly Churg–Strauss syndrome), diagnosed on the basis of four or more of the following features:
    - Asthma
    - Peripheral blood eosinophilia >1.5×10⁹/L (or >10% of a total white cell count)
    - Mononeuropathy or polyneuropathy
    - Pulmonary infiltrates
    - Paranasal sinus disease
    - Eosinophilic vasculitis on biopsy of an affected site
- Hypereosinophilic syndrome
- Polyarteritis nodosa

17.77 Drug-induced respiratory disease

Non-cardiogenic pulmonary oedema (ARDS)

- Hydrochlorothiazide
- Thrombolytics (streptokinase)
- Intravenous β-adrenoceptor agonists (e.g. for premature labour)
- Aspirin and opiates (in overdose)

Non-eosinophilic alveolitis

- Amiodarone, flecainide, gold, nitrofurantoin, cytotoxic agents – especially bleomycin, busulfan, mitomycin C, methotrexate, sulfasalazine

Pulmonary eosinophilia

- Antimicrobials (nitrofurantoin, penicillin, tetracyclines, sulphonamides, nalidixic acid)
- Drugs used in joint disease (gold, aspirin, penicillamine, naproxen)
- Cytotoxic drugs (bleomycin, methotrexate, procarbazine)
- Psychotropic drugs (chlorpromazine, dosulepin, imipramine)
- Anticonvulsants (carbamazepine, phenytoin)
- Others (sulfasalazine, nadolol)

Pleural disease

- Bromocriptine, amiodarone, methotrexate, methysergide
- Induction of systemic lupus erythematosus – phenytoin, hydralazine, isoniazid

Asthma

- Pharmacological mechanisms (β-blockers, cholinergic agonists, aspirin and NSAIDs)
- Idiosyncratic reactions (tamoxifen, dipyridamole)

(ARDS = acute respiratory distress syndrome; NSAIDs = non-steroidal anti-inflammatory drugs)

patchy shadowing. Most cases resolve completely on withdrawal of the drug, but if the reaction is severe, rapid resolution can be obtained with glucocorticoids.

Drugs may also cause other lung diseases, such as asthma, pulmonary haemorrhage, pleural effusion and, rarely, pleural thickening. An ARDS-like syndrome of acute non-cardiogenic pulmonary oedema may present with dramatic onset of breathlessness, severe hypoxaemia and signs of alveolar oedema on the chest X-ray. This syndrome has been reported most frequently in cases of opiate overdose in injection drug users but also after salicylate overdose, and there are occasional reports of its occurrence after therapeutic doses of drugs, including hydrochlorothiazides and some cytotoxic agents.

Rare interstitial lung diseases

See Box 17.78.

Occupational and environmental lung disease

The role of occupation and environmental exposure in lung disease is a particularly important area of respiratory medicine. Occupational lung disease is common and, in addition to the challenges of its diagnosis and management, often involves discussions about the workplace and, in some circumstances, litigation. Many countries encourage the registration of cases of occupational lung disease.

Occupational airway disease

Occupational asthma

Occupational asthma is asthma that results from specific workplace sensitizers and not asthma exacerbated by occupational irritants. It is responsible for 10% of adult-onset asthma and should be considered in any individual of working age who develops new-onset asthma, particularly if the individual reports improvement in asthma symptoms during periods away from work, e.g. at weekends and on holidays. Workers in certain occupations appear to be at particularly high risk (Box 17.79) and the condition is more common in smokers and atopic individuals. Depending on the intensity of exposure, asthmatic symptoms usually develop within the first few years of employment but are classically preceded by a latent period. Symptoms of rhinoconjunctivitis often precede the development of asthma. When occupational asthma follows exposure to high-molecular-weight proteins, sensitisation may be demonstrated by skin testing or measurement of specific IgE to the agent in question. Confirmation of occupational asthma should be sought from lung function tests. This usually involves serial recording of peak flow at work and home at least four times per day for a minimum of 3 weeks and, if possible, including a holiday period away from work (Fig. 17.60). In certain circumstances, specific challenge tests are required to confirm the diagnosis.

It may be possible to remove the worker from the implicated agent, but when this cannot be done, consideration of personal protective equipment and workplace hygiene may allow the worker to retain their job

i	**17.79 Occupational asthma**

Most frequently reported causative agents

• Isocyanates	• Animals
• Flour and grain dust	• Aldehydes
• Colophony and fluxes	• Wood dust
• Latex	

Workers most commonly reported to occupational asthma schemes

• Paint sprayers	• Nurses
• Bakers and pastry-makers	• Chemical workers

17

i	**17.78 Rare interstitial lung diseases**			
Disease	**Presentation**	**Chest X-ray**	**Course**	
Idiopathic pulmonary haemosiderosis	Haemoptysis, breathlessness, anaemia	Bilateral infiltrates, often perihilar Diffuse pulmonary fibrosis	Rapidly progressive in children Slow progression or remission in adults Death from massive pulmonary haemorrhage or cor pulmonale and respiratory failure	
Alveolar proteinosis	Breathlessness and cough Occasionally fever, chest pain and haemoptysis	Diffuse bilateral shadowing, often more pronounced in the hilar regions Air bronchogram	Spontaneous remission in one-third Whole-lung lavage or granulocyte–macrophage colony-stimulating factor (GM–CSF) therapy may be effective	
Langerhans cell histiocytosis (histiocytosis X)	Breathlessness, cough, pneumothorax	Diffuse interstitial shadowing progressing to honeycombing	Course unpredictable but may progress to respiratory failure Smoking cessation may be followed by significant improvement Poor response to immunosuppressive treatment	
Neurofibromatosis	Breathlessness and cough in a patient with multiple organ involvement with neurofibromas, including skin	Bilateral reticulonodular shadowing of diffuse interstitial fibrosis	Slow progression to death from respiratory failure Poor response to glucocorticoid therapy	
Alveolar microlithiasis	May be asymptomatic Breathlessness and cough	Diffuse calcified micronodular shadowing more pronounced in the lower zones	Slowly progressive to cor pulmonale and respiratory failure May stabilise in some	
Lymphangioleiomyomatosis (LAM)	Haemoptysis, breathlessness, pneumothorax and chylous effusion in females	Diffuse bilateral shadowing CT shows characteristic thin-walled cysts with well-defined walls throughout both lungs	Progressive to death within 10 years Oestrogen ablation and progesterone therapy of doubtful value Consider lung transplantation	
Pulmonary tuberous sclerosis	Very similar to lymphangioleiomyomatosis, except occasionally occurs in men			

and livelihood. Specialist follow-up in such situations is highly advisable. Where reduction or avoidance of exposure fails to bring about resolution, the management is identical to that of any patient with asthma.

Irritant-induced asthma

Irritant-induced asthma (previously called reactive airways dysfunction syndrome) refers to the development of a persistent asthma-like syndrome following the inhalation of an airway irritant: typically, a single, specific exposure to a gas, smoke, fume or vapour in very high concentrations. Pulmonary function tests show airflow obstruction and airway hyper-reactivity, and the management is similar to that of asthma. Once developed, the condition often persists but it is common for symptoms to improve over years.

Chronic obstructive pulmonary disease

While tobacco smoking remains the most important preventable cause of COPD, there is increasing recognition that other noxious particles and gases can cause, or aggravate, the condition. Occupational COPD is recognised in workers exposed to coal dust, crystalline silica and cadmium. In many low-income countries, indoor air pollution from the burning of biomass fuels in confined spaces used for cooking contributes to the development of COPD.

Byssinosis

Byssinosis occurs in workers of cotton and flax mills exposed to cotton brack (dried leaf and plant debris). An acute form of the disease may occur, but more typically, byssinosis develops after 20–30 years' exposure. Typical symptoms include chest tightness or breathlessness accompanied by a drop in lung function; classically, these are most severe on the first day of the working week ('Monday fever') or on return to work following a period away. As the week progresses, symptoms improve and the fall in lung function becomes less dramatic. Continued exposure leads to the development of persistent symptoms and a progressive decline in FEV_1, similar to that observed in COPD.

Pneumoconiosis

Pneumoconiosis may be defined as a permanent alteration of lung structure due to the inhalation of mineral dust and the tissue reactions of the lung to its presence, excluding bronchitis and emphysema (Box 17.80).

Not all dusts are pathogenic. For example, silica is highly fibrogenic, whereas iron (siderosis), tin (stannosis) and barium (baritosis) are almost inert. Beryllium causes an interstitial granulomatous disease similar to sarcoidosis. In many types of pneumoconiosis, a long period of dust exposure is required before radiological changes appear and these may precede clinical symptoms. The most important pneumoconioses include coal worker's pneumoconiosis, silicosis and asbestosis.

Coal worker's pneumoconiosis

Coal worker's pneumoconiosis (CWP) follows prolonged inhalation of coal dust. Dust-laden alveolar macrophages aggregate to form macules in or near the centre of the secondary pulmonary lobule and a fibrotic reaction ensues, resulting in the appearance of scattered discrete fibrotic lesions. Classification is based on the size and extent of radiographic nodularity. Simple coal worker's pneumoconiosis (SCWP) refers to the appearance of small radiographic nodules in an otherwise asymptomatic individual. SCWP does not impair lung function and, once exposure ceases, will seldom progress. Progressive massive fibrosis (PMF) refers to the formation of one or more conglomerate masses more than 1 cm in diameter (mainly in the upper lobes), which may calcify, cavitate, or undergo necrosis. The development of PMF is usually associated with cough, sputum that may be black (melanoptysis) and breathlessness. Despite the term fibrosis, examination is unremarkable, and the identification of clubbing or crepitations suggests an alternative diagnosis. The chest X-ray appearances may be confused with lung cancer, TB and granulomatosis with polyangiitis (GPA). Management involves removing or reducing coal dust exposure, and is otherwise supportive treatment. PMF may progress, even after coal dust exposure ceases, and in extreme cases leads to respiratory failure and right ventricular failure. CWP is not associated with increased risk of lung cancer.

Caplan syndrome describes the coexistence of rheumatoid arthritis and rounded fibrotic nodules 0.5–5 cm in diameter. They show pathological features similar to a rheumatoid nodule, including central necrosis, palisading histiocytes, and a peripheral rim of lymphocytes and plasma cells. This syndrome may also occur in other types of pneumoconiosis.

Silicosis

Silicosis results from the inhalation of crystalline silica, usually in the form of quartz, by workers cutting, grinding and polishing stone. Patients experience dry cough and breathlessness, with the sensation of chest restriction

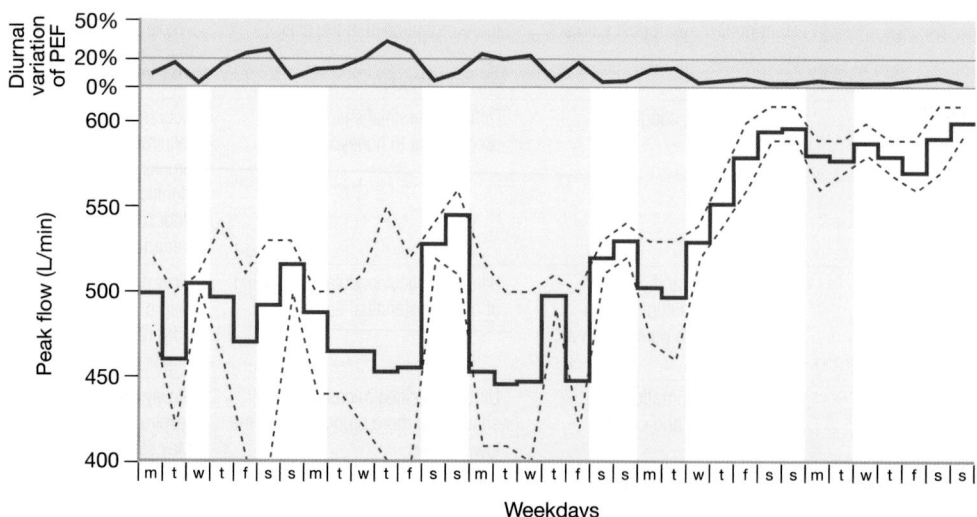

Fig. 17.60 Peak flow readings in occupational asthma. In this example, an individual with suspected occupational asthma has performed serial peak flow recording both at and away from work. The maximum, mean and minimum values are plotted daily. Days at work are indicated by the shaded areas. The diurnal variation is displayed at the top. Here, a period away from work is followed by a marked improvement in peak flow readings and a reduction in diurnal variation. (PEF = peak expiratory flow)

	17.80	Lung diseases caused by exposure to inorganic dusts		
Cause		**Occupation**	**Description**	**Characteristic pathological features**
Coal dust		Coal mining	Coal worker's pneumoconiosis	Focal and interstitial fibrosis, centrilobular emphysema, progressive massive fibrosis
Silica		Mining, quarrying, stone dressing, metal grinding, pottery, boiler scaling	Silicosis	
Asbestos		Demolition, ship breaking, manufacture of fireproof insulating materials, pipe and boiler lagging	Asbestos-related disease	Pleural plaques, diffuse pleural thickening, acute benign pleurisy, carcinoma of lung, interstitial fibrosis, mesothelioma
Iron oxide		Arc welding	Siderosis	Mineral deposition only
Tin oxide		Tin mining	Stannosis	Tin-laden macrophages
Beryllium		Aircraft, atomic energy and electronics industries	Berylliosis	Granulomas, interstitial fibrosis

replicated on spirometry. Classic or sub-acute silicosis is most common and usually manifests after 10–20 years of continuous silica exposure, during which time the patient remains asymptomatic. Accelerated silicosis is associated with a much shorter duration of dust exposure (typically 5–10 years), may present as early as after 1 year of exposure and, as the name suggests, follows a more aggressive course. Intense exposure to very fine crystalline silica dust can cause a more acute disease: silicoproteinosis, similar to alveolar proteinosis (see Box 17.78). Chronic silicosis can develop after 10–30 years of continuous exposure to lower concentrations of silica dust.

Radiological features are similar to those of CWP, with multiple well-circumscribed 3–5mm nodular opacities predominantly in the mid- and upper zones. As the disease progresses, PMF may develop (Fig. 17.61), and often does so more rapidly than in CWP and with larger opacities. Enlargement of the hilar glands with an 'egg-shell' pattern of calcification is said to be characteristic but is non-specific. Silica is highly fibrogenic and the disease is usually progressive, even when exposure ceases; hence the affected worker should invariably be removed from further exposure. Individuals with silicosis are at increased risk of TB (silicotuberculosis), non-tuberculous mycobacterial infection, lung cancer and COPD; associations with renal and connective tissue disease have also been described. Treatment, aside from stopping exposure, is mainly supportive, though some individuals benefit from inhaled bronchodilators, and transplant is occasionally appropriate.

Berylliosis

Exposure to beryllium is encountered in the aerospace, engineering, telecommunications and biomedical industries. The presence of cough, progressive breathlessness, night sweats and arthralgia in a worker exposed to dusts, fumes or vapours containing beryllium should raise suspicion of berylliosis. Berylliosis is a delayed hypersensitivity-type reaction with a symptom latency ranging from months to more than 10 years. The radiographic appearances are similar in type and distribution to those of sarcoidosis, with nodules and then progression to interstitial fibrosis predominantly in the upper lobes. Bronchoalveolar lavage reveals lymphocytes, biopsy shows sarcoid-like granulomas, and spirometry is restrictive. The diagnosis may be confirmed by the beryllium lymphocyte proliferation test, which indicates sensitization to beryllium. Treatment is with long-term steroids to delay or prevent progression to fibrosis. As with sarcoidosis, complications can occur as a result of hypercalcaemia.

Less common pneumoconioses

Siderosis refers to the development of a benign iron oxide pneumoconiosis in welders and other iron foundry workers. Baritosis may be seen

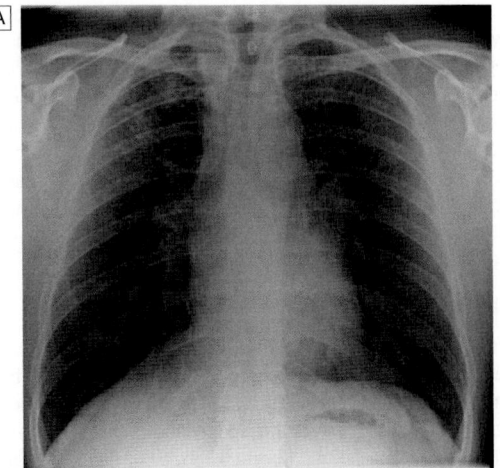

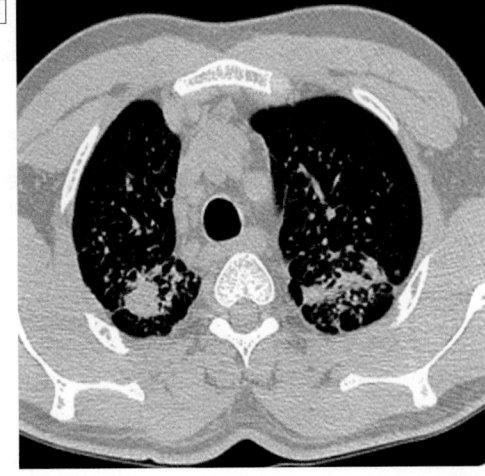

Fig. 17.61 Silicosis. [A] A chest X-ray from a patient with silicosis, showing the presence of small rounded nodules, predominantly seen in the upper zones. [B] High-resolution computed tomogram from the same patient, demonstrating conglomeration of nodules with posterior bias.

in barium process workers and stannosis in tin refining. Haematite lung occurs in iron ore miners and resembles silicosis but stains the lung red. Diamond polishers may develop hard metal disease, which is similar to UIP but the pathology shows a giant-cell interstitial pneumonia. Workers exposed to aluminium oxide develop bauxite pneumoconiosis, sometimes referred to as Shaver disease. Popcorn worker's lung is a form

17

of obliterative bronchiolitis following ingestion of diacetyl, used in butter flavouring.

Lung diseases due to organic dusts

A wide range of organic agents may cause respiratory disorders (Box 17.81). Disease results from a local immune response to animal proteins or fungal antigens in mouldy vegetable matter. Hypersensitivity pneumonitis is the most common of these conditions.

Hypersensitivity pneumonitis

Hypersensitivity pneumonitis (HP; previously called extrinsic allergic alveolitis) results from the inhalation of a wide variety of organic antigens that give rise to a diffuse immune complex reaction in the walls of alveoli and bronchioles. Common causes include farmer's lung and bird fancier's lung. Other examples are shown in Box 17.81. HP is not exclusively occupational or environmental and other important causes include medications (see Box 17.77).

The pathology of HP is consistent with both type III and type IV immunological mechanisms. Precipitating IgG antibodies may be detected in the serum and a type III Arthus reaction is believed to occur in the lung, where the precipitation of immune complexes results in activation of complement and an inflammatory response in the alveolar walls, characterised by the influx of mononuclear cells and foamy histiocytes. The presence of poorly formed non-caseating granulomas in the alveolar walls suggests that type IV responses are also important. The distribution of the inflammatory infiltrate is predominantly peribronchiolar. Chronic forms of the disease may be accompanied by fibrosis. For reasons that remain uncertain, there is a lower incidence of HP in smokers compared to non-smokers.

Clinical features

The presentation of HP varies from an acute form to a more indolent pattern in accordance with the antigen load. For example, the farmer exposed to mouldy hay, as occurs when the hay is gathered and stored damp during a wet summer, or the pigeon fancier cleaning a large pigeon loft, will, within a few hours, report influenza-like symptoms accompanied by cough, breathlessness and wheeze. The individual with low-level antigen exposure, however, such as the owner of an indoor pet bird, will typically present in a more indolent fashion with slowly progressive breathlessness; in some cases, established fibrosis may be present by the time the disease is recognised. Chest auscultation typically reveals widespread end-inspiratory crackles and squeaks.

Investigations

In cases of acute HP, the chest X-ray typically shows ill-defined patchy airspace shadowing, which, given the systemic features, may be confused with pneumonia. HRCT is more likely to show bilateral ground-glass shadowing and areas of consolidation superimposed on small centrilobar nodular opacities with an upper and middle lobe predominance and mosaicism (areas of increased lucency due to air-trapping) (Fig. 17.62). In more chronic disease, features of fibrosis, such as volume loss, traction bronchiectasis and honeycombing, appear. In common with other fibrotic diseases, pulmonary function tests show a restrictive ventilatory defect with reduced lung volumes and impaired gas transfer, dynamic tests may detect oxygen desaturation and, in more advanced disease, type I respiratory failure is present at rest.

Diagnosis

The diagnosis of HP is usually based on the characteristic clinical and radiological features, together with the identification of a potential source of antigen at the patient's home or place of work (Box 17.82). It may be supported by a positive serum antibody (IgG) or precipitin test or by more sensitive serological investigations. It is important, however, to be aware that the presence of antibodies in the absence of other features does not make the diagnosis; the great majority of farmers with positive precipitins do not have farmer's lung, and up to 15% of pigeon breeders may have positive serum precipitins yet remain healthy.

Where HP is suspected but the cause is not readily apparent, a visit to the patient's home or workplace should be arranged. Occasionally,

i	17.81 Examples of lung diseases caused by organic dusts		
Disorder	**Source**	**Antigen/agent**	
Farmer's lung*	Mouldy hay, straw, grain	*Saccharopolyspora rectivirgula* (formerly *Micropolyspora faeni*) *Aspergillus fumigatus*	
Bird fancier's lung*	Avian excreta, proteins and feathers	Avian serum proteins	
Malt worker's lung*	Mouldy maltings	*Aspergillus clavatus*	
Cheese worker's lung*	Mouldy cheese	*Aspergillus clavatus* *Penicillium casei*	
Maple bark stripper's lung*	Bark from stored maple	*Cryptostroma corticale*	
Saxophone player's lung*	Reed of any wind instrument	*Fusarium* spp. *Penicillium* spp. *Cladosporium* spp.	
Byssinosis	Textile industries	Cotton, flax, hemp dust	
Inhalation ('humidifier') fever	Contamination of air conditioning	Thermophilic actinomycetes	

*Presents as hypersensitivity pneumonitis.

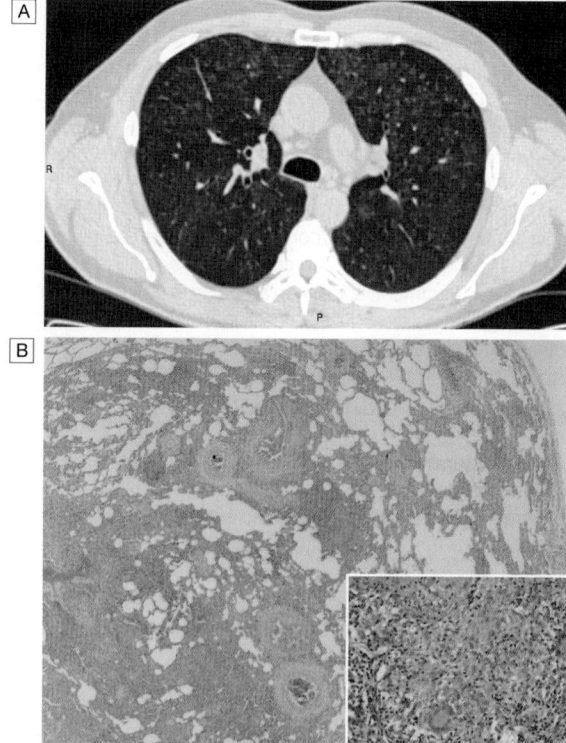

Fig. 17.62 Hypersensitivity pneumonitis. A High-resolution computed tomogram showing typical patchy ground-glass opacification. B Histology shows evidence of an interstitial inflammatory infiltrate in the lung, and expanding alveolar walls, with a peribronchial distribution. Within the infiltrate, there are foci of small, poorly defined non-caseating granulomas *(inset)*, which often lie adjacent to the airways. In this case, there is little in the way of established lung fibrosis but this can be marked. *(A) Courtesy of Dr S. Jackson, Western General Hospital, Edinburgh. (B) Courtesy of Dr William Wallace, Department of Pathology, Royal Infirmary of Edinburgh.*

such as when an agent previously unrecognised as causing HP is suspected, provocation testing may be necessary to prove the diagnosis; if positive, inhalation of the relevant antigen is followed after 3–6 hours by pyrexia and a reduction in vital capacity and gas transfer factor. BAL fluid usually shows an increase in the number of $CD8^+$ T lymphocytes and transbronchial biopsy can occasionally provide sufficient tissue for a confident diagnosis; however, open lung biopsy may be necessary. In up to 40% of patients with HP, the causative antigen remains unknown despite extensive investigation.

Management

If it is practical, the patient should cease exposure to the inciting agent. In some cases this may be difficult, however, because of either implications for livelihood (e.g. farmers) or addiction to hobbies (e.g. pigeon breeders). Dust masks with appropriate filters may minimise exposure and may be combined with methods of reducing levels of antigen (e.g. drying hay before storage). In acute cases, prednisolone 0.5 mg/kg is given daily until clinical and radiological resolution, before slowly weaning over several months down to 10 mg/day for a further few months. Severely hypoxaemic patients may require high-concentration oxygen therapy initially. Most patients recover completely, but if unchecked, fibrosis may progress to cause severe respiratory disability, hypoxaemia, pulmonary hypertension, cor pulmonale and eventually death.

Inhalation ('humidifier') fever

Inhalation fever shares similarities with HP. It occurs as a result of contaminated humidifiers or air-conditioning units that release a fine spray of microorganisms into the atmosphere. The illness is characterised by self-limiting fever and breathlessness; permanent sequelae are unusual. An identical syndrome can also develop after disturbing an accumulation of mouldy hay, compost or mulch. So-called 'hot tub lung' appears to be attributable to *Mycobacterium avium*. Outbreaks of HP in workers using metalworking fluids appear to be linked to *Acinetobacter* or *Ochrobactrum*.

Asbestos-related lung and pleural diseases

Asbestos is a naturally occurring silicate. Asbestos fibres may be classified as either serpentine (chrysotile or white asbestos), which accounts for 95% of the world's production, or amphibole serpentine (crocidolite or blue asbestos, and amosite or brown asbestos). The favourable thermal and chemical insulation properties led to its extensive use by the shipbuilding and construction industries throughout the latter part of the 20th century. Exposure to asbestos may be followed, after a lengthy latent period, by the development of both pleural and pulmonary disease. With the exception of an increased risk of lung cancer in asbestosis, benign asbestos-related diseases do not increase the risk of malignancy beyond that already resulting from exposure to asbestos.

Pleural plaques

Pleural plaques are the most common manifestation of previous asbestos exposure, being discrete circumscribed areas of hyaline fibrosis situated on the parietal pleura of the chest wall, diaphragm, pericardium or mediastinum. They are virtually always asymptomatic, usually being identified as an incidental finding on a chest X-ray (Fig. 17.63) or thoracic

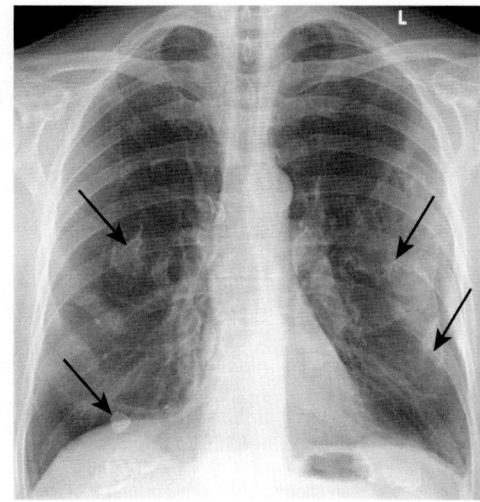

Fig. 17.63 Asbestos-related benign pleural plaques. Chest X-ray showing extensive calcified pleural plaques ('candle wax' appearance – arrows), particularly marked on the diaphragm and lateral pleural surfaces.

CT scan, particularly when partially calcified. They do not cause impairment of lung function and are benign.

Acute benign asbestos pleurisy

Benign asbestos pleurisy is estimated to occur in around 20% of asbestos workers but many episodes are subclinical and pass unreported. When symptomatic, patients present with features of pleurisy, including mild fever and systemic disturbance. The diagnosis requires the exclusion of other causes of pleurisy, and treatment is with NSAIDs. Repeated episodes may be followed by the development of diffuse (visceral) pleural thickening.

Benign asbestos-related pleural effusion

Benign asbestos-related pleural effusions are usually small and unilateral. The patient is commonly asymptomatic, though some have symptoms of pleurisy or breathlessness, especially if the effusion is moderate to large. Diagnosis requires the exclusion of mesothelioma, usually by thoracoscopy. Pleural fluid analysis demonstrates an exudate that is often haemorrhagic. Treatment is with drainage if symptomatic.

Diffuse pleural thickening

Diffuse pleural thickening (DPT) refers to thickening of the visceral pleura. In contrast to pleural plaques, if this is sufficiently extensive, it may cause restrictive lung function impairment, exertional breathlessness and, occasionally, persistent chest pain. The typical appearances of DPT on chest X-ray include thickening of the pleura along the chest wall and obliteration of the costophrenic angles. Earlier manifestations detected by CT scanning include parenchymal bands (Fig. 17.64) and 'rounded atelectasis'. There is no treatment and the condition may be progressive in around one-third of individuals. A pleural biopsy may be required to exclude mesothelioma.

Asbestosis

Fibrosis of the lung following asbestos exposure generally requires substantial exposure over several years and is rarely associated with low-level or bystander exposure (unlike other asbestos-related diseases). In common with other fibrosing lung diseases, asbestosis usually presents with exertional breathlessness and fine, late inspiratory crackles over the lower zones. Finger clubbing may be present. Pulmonary function tests and HRCT appearances are similar to those of UIP. These features,

17

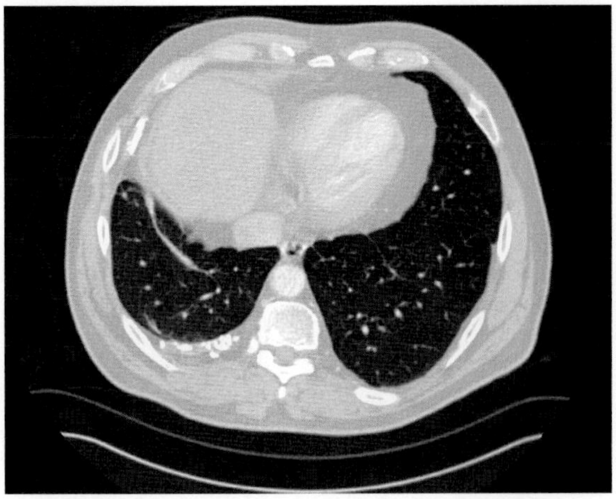

Fig. 17.64 Thoracic CT scan showing right-sided pleural thickening and an associated parenchymal band.

accompanied by a history of substantial asbestos exposure, are generally sufficient to establish the diagnosis. In some cases, asbestos fibre counts may be performed on lung biopsy material to establish the diagnosis, but this is rarely appropriate pre-mortem.

Asbestosis is usually slowly progressive and has a better prognosis than untreated IPF. In advanced cases respiratory failure, pulmonary hypertension and cor pulmonale may still develop, and treatment is supportive. Those with asbestosis have a 10-fold increased risk of developing lung cancer, with rates even higher amongst those with additional smoking history.

Mesothelioma

Mesothelioma is a malignant tumour affecting the pleura or, less commonly, the peritoneum. Its occurrence almost invariably suggests past asbestos exposure, which may be low-level. There is typically a long latent interval between first exposure and the onset of clinical manifestations, and this accounts for the continued increasing incidence many years after control measures have been implemented. Despite regulations, 125 million people are exposed to asbestos in the workplace. Around 1 in 170 of all British men born in the 1940s will die of mesothelioma.

Pleural mesothelioma typically presents with increasing breathlessness resulting from pleural effusion or unremitting chest pain, reflecting involvement of the chest wall. As the tumour progresses, it encases the underlying lung and may invade the parenchyma, the mediastinum and the pericardium. Metastatic disease, although not often clinically detectable in life, is a common finding on postmortem examination.

Mesothelioma is almost invariably fatal. The use of chemotherapy may improve quality of life and is accompanied by a small survival benefit, typically regarded as being around 3 months. Radiotherapy can be used to control pain. A variety of surgical techniques have been trialled, but to date these have shown no benefit and even possible harm to patients. Pleural effusions are managed with drainage (preferably with indwelling pleural catheters) with or without pleurodesis. Typical figures for survival from onset of symptoms are around 16 months for epithelioid tumours, 10 months for sarcomatoid tumours and 15 months for biphasic tumours, with only a minority of patients surviving for longer periods.

Occupational lung cancer

Individuals exposed to substantial quantities of asbestos are at increased risk of lung cancer, particularly if they smoke tobacco. Increased risks of lung cancer have also been reported in workers who develop silicosis and those exposed to radon gas, beryllium, diesel exhaust fumes, cadmium, chromium, and dust and fumes from coke plants.

Occupational pneumonia

Occupational and environmental exposures may be linked to the development of pneumonia. Pneumococcal vaccine is recommended for welders and metal workers. Farm workers, abattoir workers and hide factory workers may be exposed to *Coxiella burnetii*, the causative agent of Q fever. The organisms are excreted from milk, urine, faeces and amniotic fluid; they may be transmitted by cattle ticks or contaminated dust from the milking floor, or by drinking milk that is inadequately pasteurised. Birds (often parrots) or budgerigars infected with *Chlamydophila psittaci* can cause psittacosis. Sewage workers, farmers, animal handlers and vets run an increased risk of leptospirosis and leptospiral pneumonia, due to their exposure to *Leptospira interrogans* in rodent urine. Contact with rabbits, hares, muskrats and ground squirrels is associated with tularaemic pneumonia, caused by *Francisella tularensis*. Anthrax (wool-sorter's disease) may occur in workers exposed to hides, hair, bristle, bonemeal and animal carcases that are contaminated with *Bacillus anthracis* spores. In some countries, COVID-19 is classified as an occupational disease of people whose occupations cause them to come into close contact with other people (e.g. medical staff, taxi drivers, retail workers etc.). This is potentially a contentious issue, however, as the high prevalance of the disease in the community makes it difficult to establish the specific source of a COVID-19 infection.

Pulmonary vascular disease

Pulmonary embolism

The majority of pulmonary emboli arise from the propagation of lower limb deep vein thrombosis (venous thromboembolism, VTE). Rare causes include septic emboli (from endocarditis affecting the tricuspid or pulmonary valves), tumour (especially choriocarcinoma), fat following fracture of long bones (such as the femur), air, and amniotic fluid (which may enter the mother's circulation following delivery).

Clinical features

The diagnosis of pulmonary embolism (PE) may be aided by asking three questions:

- Is the clinical presentation consistent with PE?
- Does the patient have risk factors for PE?
- Are there any alternative diagnoses that can explain the patient's presentation?

Clinical presentation varies, depending on number, size and distribution of emboli and on underlying cardiorespiratory reserve (Box 17.83). A recognised risk factor for VTE is present in 80%–90% (see Box 25.67). The presence of one or more risk factors increases the risk further still.

Investigations

A variety of non-specific radiographic appearances have been described (Fig. 17.65) but the chest X-ray is most useful in excluding key differential diagnoses, e.g. pneumonia or pneumothorax. Normal appearances in an acutely breathless and hypoxaemic patient should raise the suspicion of PE, as should bilateral changes in anyone presenting with unilateral pleuritic chest pain.

The ECG is often normal but is useful in excluding other important differential diagnoses, such as acute myocardial infarction and pericarditis. The most common findings in PE include sinus tachycardia and anterior T-wave inversion but these are non-specific; larger emboli may cause right heart strain revealed by an $S_1Q_3T_3$ pattern, ST-segment and T-wave changes, or the appearance of right bundle branch block.

Arterial blood gases typically show a reduced PaO_2 and a normal or low $PaCO_2$, and an increased alveolar–arterial oxygen gradient, but may

i 17.83 Features of pulmonary thromboemboli			
	Acute massive PE	Acute small/medium PE	Chronic PE
Pathophysiology	Major haemodynamic effects: ↓cardiac output; acute right heart failure	Occlusion of segmental pulmonary artery → infarction ± effusion	Chronic occlusion of pulmonary microvasculature, right heart failure
Symptoms	Faintness or collapse, crushing central chest pain, apprehension, severe dyspnoea	Pleuritic chest pain, restricted breathing, haemoptysis	Exertional dyspnoea Late: symptoms of pulmonary hypertension or right heart failure
Signs	Major circulatory collapse: tachycardia, hypotension, ↑JVP, RV gallop rhythm, loud P_2, severe cyanosis, ↓urinary output	Tachycardia, pleural rub, raised hemidiaphragm, crackles, effusion (often blood-stained), low-grade fever	Early: may be minimal Later: RV heave, loud P_2 Terminal: signs of right heart failure
Chest X-ray	Usually normal; may be subtle oligaemia	Pleuropulmonary opacities, pleural effusion, linear shadows, raised hemidiaphragm	Enlarged pulmonary artery trunk, enlarged heart, prominent right ventricle
Electrocardiogram	$S_1Q_3T_3$ anterior T-wave inversion, RBBB	Sinus tachycardia	RV hypertrophy and strain
Arterial blood gases	Markedly abnormal with ↓PaO_2 and ↓$PaCO_2$, metabolic acidosis	May be normal or ↓PaO_2 or ↓$PaCO_2$	Exertional ↓PaO_2 or desaturation on formal exercise testing
Alternative diagnoses	Myocardial infarction, pericardial tamponade, aortic dissection	Pneumonia, pneumothorax, musculoskeletal chest pain	Other causes of pulmonary hypertension

(JVP = jugular venous pressure; PE = pulmonary embolism; RBBB = right bundle branch block; RV = right ventricular)

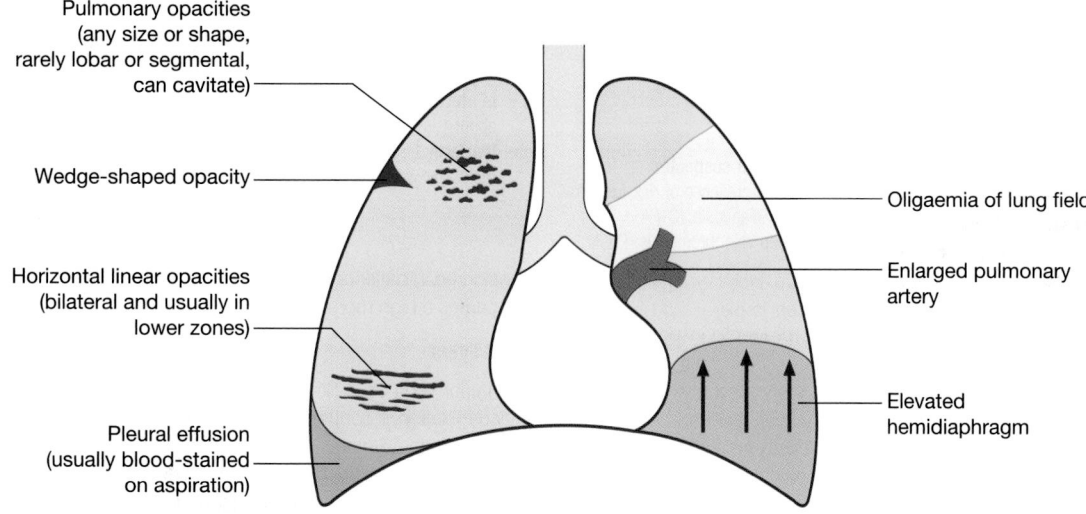

Pulmonary opacities (any size or shape, rarely lobar or segmental, can cavitate)

Wedge-shaped opacity

Horizontal linear opacities (bilateral and usually in lower zones)

Pleural effusion (usually blood-stained on aspiration)

Oligaemia of lung field

Enlarged pulmonary artery

Elevated hemidiaphragm

Fig. 17.65 Features of pulmonary thromboembolism/infarction on chest X-ray.

be normal in a significant minority. A metabolic acidosis may be seen in acute massive PE with cardiovascular collapse.

The 2-level PE Wells score is used to estimate the likelihood of PE (Fig. 17.66). If a PE is likely, the patient should have definitive imaging (as below). If a PE is unlikely, a D-dimer test is performed. An elevated D-dimer (see Fig. 9.6) is of limited value, as it may be raised in a variety of other conditions, including myocardial infarction, pneumonia and sepsis. However, low levels, particularly in the context of a low clinical risk, have a high negative predictive value and further investigation is usually unnecessary (Fig. 17.66). The serum troponin I (see Box 9.3) may be elevated, reflecting right heart strain.

CTPA is the first-line diagnostic test (Fig. 17.67). It has the advantage of visualising the distribution and extent of the emboli or highlighting an alternative diagnosis, such as consolidation, pneumothorax or aortic dissection. The sensitivity of CT scanning may be increased by simultaneous visualisation of the femoral and popliteal veins, although this is not

widely practised. As the contrast media may be nephrotoxic, care should be taken in patients with renal impairment, and CTPA avoided in those with a history of allergy to iodinated contrast media. In these cases, either V̇/Q̇ scanning or ventilation/perfusion single photon emission computed tomography (V̇/Q̇ SPECT) may be considered. V̇/Q̇ scanning is of little benefit in patients with an abnormal chest X-ray, as perfusion abnormalities are likely due to underlying lung disease rather than PE. Specific diagnostic and management considerations for PE in pregnancy are shown in Box 17.84.

Colour Doppler ultrasound of the leg veins may be used in patients with suspected PE, particularly if there are clinical signs in a limb, as many will have identifiable proximal thrombus in the leg veins.

Bedside echocardiography is extremely helpful in the differential diagnosis and assessment of acute circulatory collapse. Acute dilatation of the right heart is usually present in massive PE, and thrombus (embolism in transit) may be visible. Important differential diagnoses, including left

17

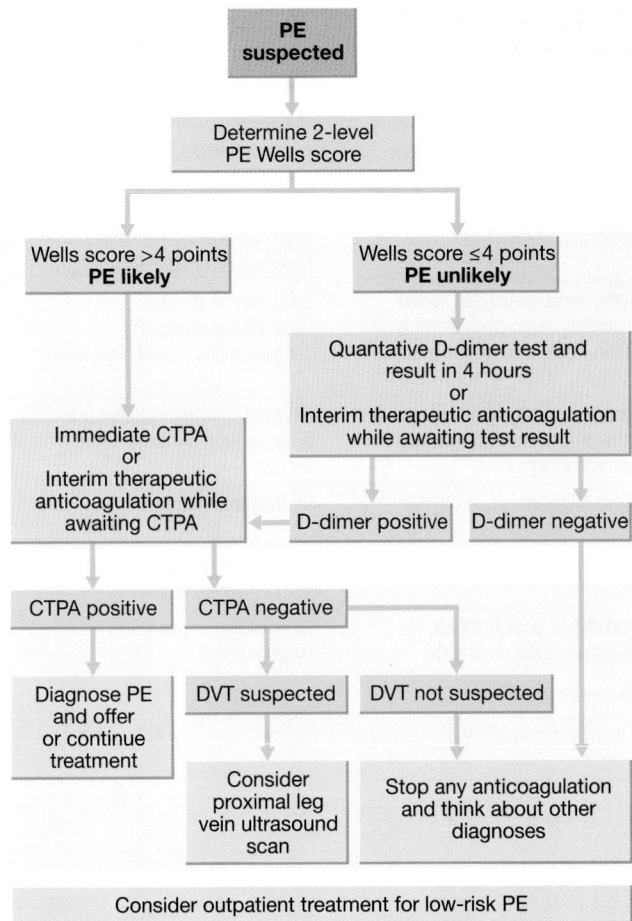

Fig. 17.66 **Algorithm for the investigation of patients with suspected pulmonary thromboembolism.** Clinical risk is based on the presence of risk factors for venous thromboembolism and the probability of another diagnosis. (CTPA = computed tomography pulmonary angiography; DVT = deep vein thrombosis; PE = pulmonary embolism)

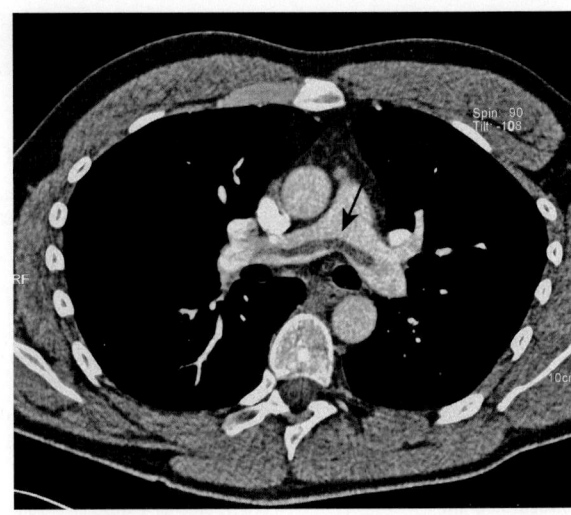

Fig. 17.67 **CT pulmonary angiogram.** The arrow points to a saddle embolism in the bifurcation of the pulmonary artery.

17.84 Pulmonary embolism in pregnancy

- **Maternal mortality**: venous thromboembolism is the leading direct cause in the UK.
- **CT pulmonary angiography**: may be performed safely (0.01–0.06 mGy). It is important to consider the risk of radiation to breast tissue (particularly if there is a family history of breast carcinoma).
- **V̇/Q̇ scanning**: greater radiation dose to fetus (0.11–0.22 mGy) but significantly less to maternal breast tissue.
- **In utero radiation exposure**: estimated incidence of childhood malignancy is about 1 in 16 000 per mGy.
- **Warfarin**: teratogenic, so pulmonary embolism should be treated with low-molecular-weight heparin during pregnancy.

ventricular failure, aortic dissection and pericardial tamponade, can also be identified.

In the absence of haemodynamic instability and hypoxia, most patients can have outpatient investigations for PE, providing they receive anticoagulation. The Pulmonary Embolism Severity Index (PESI) predicts 30-day outcome, and those with a low risk of morbidity and mortality can be considered for outpatient management.

Management

General measures

Prompt recognition and treatment are potentially life-saving. Sufficient oxygen should be given to hypoxaemic patients to maintain the target oxygen saturations specified on p. 195. Opiates may be necessary to relieve pain and distress but should be used with caution in the hypotensive patient.

Anticoagulation

The main principle of treatment for PE is anticoagulation, which is discussed for PE and other forms of venous thromboembolism (VTE) on page 985.

Thrombolytic and surgical therapy

Thrombolysis is indicated in any patient presenting with acute massive PE accompanied by haemodynamic instability. Patients must be screened carefully for haemorrhage risk, as there is a high risk of intracranial haemorrhage. Surgical or percutaneous pulmonary embolectomy may be considered in patients with an absolute contraindication to thrombolysis, but carries a high mortality.

Caval filters

An inferior vena cava filter should be considered in any patient in whom anticoagulation is contraindicated or who has had recurrent VTE despite anticoagulation. Retrievable caval filters are particularly useful in individuals with temporary risk factors. The caval filter should be used only until anticoagulation can be safely initiated, at which time the filter should be removed if possible.

Further investigations

All patients with an unprovoked PE (those with no risk factors) should be assessed for underlying malignancy. A detailed history, examination (including breast and rectal examination) and review of baseline bloods, should elicit any red-flag symptoms, signs or results. Further focused investigation is required only if there are any positive findings.

Thrombophilia screening is only considered for patients with an unprovoked PE and a plan to stop anticoagulation. Specialist advice is recommended as test results can be affected by anticoagulation.

Prognosis

Immediate mortality is greatest in those with echocardiographic evidence of right ventricular dysfunction or cardiogenic shock. Once anticoagulation is commenced, however, the risk of mortality falls rapidly. The risk of recurrence is highest in the first 6–12 months after the initial event, and at 10 years around one-third of individuals will have suffered a further event. Patients with right ventricular dysfunction at presentation should have a repeat echocardiogram at 3 months to assess for evidence of chronic thromboembolic pulmonary hypertension (CTEPH).

Pulmonary hypertension

Pulmonary hypertension (PH) is defined as a mean pulmonary artery pressure (PAP) of at least 25 mmHg at rest, as measured by right heart catheterisation. The definition may be further refined by consideration of the pulmonary wedge pressure (PWP), the cardiac output and the transpulmonary pressure gradient (mean PAP – mean PWP). The clinical classification of PH is shown in Box 17.85. Further classification is based on the degree of functional disturbance, assessed using the New York Heart Association (NYHA) grades I–IV. Although respiratory failure due to intrinsic pulmonary disease is the most common cause of PH, severe PH may occur as a primary disorder, as a complication of connective tissue disease (e.g. systemic sclerosis), left heart disease, or as a result of CTEPH.

Primary pulmonary hypertension (PPH) is a rare but important disease that predominantly affects women aged between 20 and 30 years. Familial disease is rarer still but is known to be associated with pathogenic variants in the gene encoding type II bone morphogenetic protein receptor (*BMPR2*), a member of the transforming growth factor beta (TGF-β) superfamily. Variants in this gene have been identified in some patients with sporadic PH. Pathological features include hypertrophy of both the media and the intima of the vessel wall and a clonal expansion of endothelial cells, which take on the appearance of plexiform lesions. There is marked narrowing of the vessel lumen and this, together with the frequently observed in situ thrombosis, leads to an increase in pulmonary vascular resistance and PH.

Clinical features

PH presents insidiously and is often diagnosed late. Typical symptoms include breathlessness, chest pain, fatigue, palpitations, exertional dizziness and syncope. Important signs include elevation of the JVP (with a prominent 'a' wave if in sinus rhythm), a parasternal heave (right ventricular hypertrophy), accentuation of the pulmonary component of the second heart sound, a right ventricular third heart sound, peripheral oedema and ascites. Signs of interstitial lung disease or cardiac, liver or connective tissue disease may suggest the underlying cause.

Investigations

PH is suspected if an ECG shows a right ventricular 'strain' pattern or a chest X-ray shows enlarged pulmonary arteries, peripheral pruning and right ventricle enlargement (Fig. 17.68). Doppler assessment of the tricuspid regurgitant jet by transthoracic echocardiography provides a non-invasive estimate of the PAP, which is equal to 4×(tricuspid regurgitation velocity)^2. Further assessment should be by right heart catheterisation to assess pulmonary haemodynamics, measure vasodilator responsiveness and thus guide further therapy. Additional investigations are performed to identify the cause of PH, including pulmonary function tests, V̇/Q̇ scan, CT thorax, CTPA, MRI, overnight oximetry and exercise testing.

Management

Specialist centres should direct the management of PH. Diuretic therapy should be prescribed for patients with right heart failure. Supplemental oxygen should be given to maintain resting PaO_2 above 8 kPa (60 mmHg). Anticoagulation should be considered unless there is an increased risk of bleeding. Digoxin may be useful in patients who develop atrial tachyarrhythmias. Pregnancy carries a very high risk of death and women of child-bearing age should be counselled appropriately. Excessive physical activity that leads to distressing symptoms should be avoided but otherwise patients should be encouraged to remain active. Pneumococcal and influenza vaccination should be offered. Nitrates should be avoided owing to the risk of hypotension, and β-blockers are poorly tolerated. Cyclizine can aggravate PH and should also be avoided.

Disease-targeted strategies have focused on replacing endogenous prostacyclins with epoprostenol, treprostinil or iloprost; blocking endothelin-mediated vasoconstriction with agents such as bosentan,

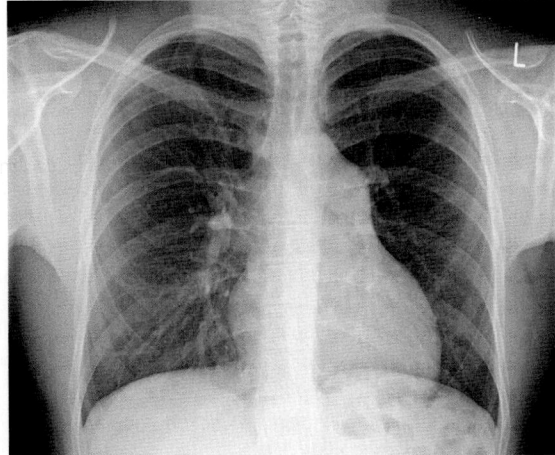

Fig. 17.68 Chest X-ray showing the typical appearance in pulmonary hypertension.

ambrisentan or macitentan; or enhancing endogenous nitric oxide-mediated vasodilatation with phosphodiesterase V inhibitors such as sildenafil or tadalafil, or the guanylate cyclase stimulator riociguat. High-dose calcium channel blockers may be appropriate in those with an acute vasodilator response.

Selected patients are referred for double-lung transplantation, and pulmonary thrombo-endarterectomy may be contemplated in those with CTEPH. Atrial septostomy (the creation of a right-to-left shunt) decompresses the right ventricle and improves haemodynamic performance; it may be used as a bridge to transplantation.

Diseases of the upper airway

Diseases of the nasopharynx

Allergic rhinitis

This is a disorder in which there are episodes of nasal congestion, watery nasal discharge and sneezing. It may be seasonal or perennial, and is due to an immediate hypersensitivity reaction in the nasal mucosa. Seasonal antigens include pollens from grasses, flowers, weeds or trees. Grass pollen is responsible for hay fever, the most common type of seasonal allergic rhinitis in northern Europe, which is at its peak between May and July. This is a worldwide problem, however, which may be aggravated during harvest seasons.

Perennial allergic rhinitis may be a specific reaction to antigens derived from house dust, fungal spores or animal dander, but similar symptoms can be caused by physical or chemical irritants, e.g. pungent odours or fumes, including strong perfumes, cold air and dry atmospheres. The phrase 'vasomotor rhinitis' is often used in this context, as the term 'allergic' is a misnomer.

Clinical features

In the seasonal type, there are frequent sudden attacks of sneezing, with profuse watery nasal discharge and nasal obstruction. These attacks last for a few hours and are often accompanied by pruritus, watering of the eyes and conjunctival irritation. In perennial rhinitis, the symptoms are similar but more continuous and usually less severe. Skin hypersensitivity tests with the relevant antigen are usually positive in seasonal allergic rhinitis but are less useful in perennial rhinitis.

Management

In those sensitised to house dust, simple measures, such as thorough dust removal from the bed area, leaving a window open and washing all bedding once weekly, are often helpful. Avoidance of pollen and antigens from domestic pets, however desirable and beneficial, is usually impractical.

The following medications, singly or in combination, are usually effective in both seasonal and perennial allergic rhinitis:

- an antihistamine (such as loratadine or cetirizine)
- sodium cromoglicate nasal spray
- glucocorticoid nasal spray, e.g. beclometasone dipropionate, fluticasone, mometasone or budesonide.

When symptoms are very severe, resistant to usual treatments and seriously interfering with school, business or social activities, immunotherapy (desensitisation) is also used but carries the risk of serious reactions and must be managed in specialist centres. Vasomotor rhinitis is often difficult to treat but may respond to ipratropium bromide, administered into each nostril 3 times daily.

Sleep-disordered breathing

A variety of respiratory disorders affect sleep or are affected by sleep. Cough and wheeze disturbing sleep are characteristic of asthma, while the hypoventilation that accompanies normal sleep can precipitate respiratory failure in patients with disordered ventilation due to chest wall restrictive diseases, neuromuscular diseases, or diaphragmatic paralysis.

In contrast, a small but important group of disorders cause problems only during sleep. Patients may have normal lungs and daytime respiratory function, but during sleep have either abnormalities of ventilatory drive (central sleep apnoea) or upper airway obstruction (obstructive sleep apnoea). Of these, the obstructive sleep apnoea/hypopnoea syndrome is by far the most common and important. When this coexists with COPD (overlap syndrome), severe respiratory failure can result, even if the COPD is mild.

The obstructive sleep apnoea/hypopnoea syndrome

Recurrent upper airway obstruction during sleep, sufficient to cause sleep fragmentation and daytime sleepiness, is thought to affect 2% of women and 4% of men aged 30–60 in populations of predominantly European descent. Daytime sleepiness, especially in monotonous situations, results in a threefold increased risk of road traffic accidents and a ninefold increased risk of single-vehicle accidents.

Aetiology

Sleep apnoea results from recurrent occlusion of the pharynx during sleep, usually at the level of the soft palate. Inspiration results in negative pressure within the pharynx. During wakefulness, upper airway dilating muscles, including palatoglossus and genioglossus, contract actively during inspiration to preserve airway patency. During sleep, muscle tone declines, impairing the ability of these muscles to maintain pharyngeal patency. In a minority of people, a combination of an anatomically narrow palatopharynx and under-activity of the dilating muscles during sleep results in inspiratory airway obstruction. Incomplete obstruction causes turbulent flow, resulting in snoring (44% of men and 28% of women aged 30–60 snore). More severe obstruction triggers increased inspiratory effort and transiently wakes the patient, allowing the dilating muscles to re-open the airway. These awakenings are so brief that patients have no recollection of them. After a series of loud deep breaths that may wake their bed partner, the patient rapidly returns to sleep, snores and becomes apnoeic once more. This cycle of apnoea and awakening may repeat itself many hundreds of times per night and results in severe sleep fragmentation and secondary variations in blood pressure, which may predispose over time to cardiovascular disease.

Factors that predispose to the obstructive sleep apnoea/hypopnoea syndrome (OSAHS) include male gender, which doubles the risk, and obesity, which is found in about 70% because parapharyngeal fat deposits tend to narrow the pharynx. Nasal obstruction or a recessed mandible can further exacerbate the problem. Acromegaly and hypothyroidism also predispose by causing submucosal infiltration and narrowing of the upper airway. Sleep apnoea is often familial, where the maxilla and mandible are back-set, narrowing the upper airway. Alcohol and sedatives predispose to snoring and apnoea by relaxing the upper airway dilating muscles. As a result of marked sympathetic activation during apnoea, sleep-disordered breathing is associated over time with sustained hypertension and an increased risk of coronary events and stroke. Associations have also been described with insulin resistance, the metabolic syndrome and type 2 diabetes. In addition to improving symptoms and reducing vehicular risk, treatment of sleep apnoea reduces sympathetic drive and blood pressure and may also improve these associated metabolic disorders.

Clinical features

Excessive daytime sleepiness is the principal symptom and snoring is virtually universal. The patient usually feels that he or she has been asleep all night but wakes unrefreshed, though may recall waking with choking/gasping episodes. Bed partners report loud snoring in all body positions and often have noticed multiple breathing pauses (apnoeas). Difficulty with concentration, impaired cognitive function and work performance, depression, irritability and nocturia are other features. Early morning headaches may be a sign of more severe OSAHS.

Investigations

Provided that the sleepiness does not result from inadequate time in bed or from shift work, anyone who repeatedly falls asleep during the day when not in bed, who complains that their work is impaired by sleepiness, or who is a habitual snorer with multiple witnessed apnoeas should be referred for a sleep assessment. A more quantitative assessment of daytime tendency to fall asleep can be obtained by questionnaire (Box 17.86). Overnight studies of breathing, oxygenation and sleep quality are diagnostic (Fig. 17.69) but the level of investigation depends on local resources and the probability of the diagnosis. The severity of OSAHS

i **17.86 Epworth sleepiness scale**

How likely are you to doze off or fall asleep in the situations described below? Choose the most appropriate number for each situation from the following scale:

0 = would never doze
1 = slight chance of dozing
2 = moderate chance of dozing
3 = high chance of dozing

- Sitting and reading
- Watching TV
- Sitting inactive in a public place (e.g. a theatre or a meeting)
- As a passenger in a car for an hour without a break
- Lying down to rest in the afternoon when circumstances permit
- Sitting and talking to someone
- Sitting quietly after a lunch without alcohol
- In a car, while stopped for a few minutes in the traffic

Normal subjects average 5.9 (SD 2.2) and patients with severe obstructive sleep apnoea average 16.0 (SD 4.4).

17.87 Differential diagnosis of persistent sleepiness

Lack of sleep

- Inadequate time in bed
- Extraneous sleep disruption (e.g. babies/children)
- Shift work
- Excessive caffeine intake
- Physical illness (e.g. pain)

Sleep disruption

- Sleep apnoea/hypopnoea syndrome
- Periodic limb movement disorder (recurrent limb movements during non-REM sleep, frequent nocturnal awakenings)

Sleepiness with relatively normal sleep

- Narcolepsy
- Idiopathic hypersomnolence (rare)
- Neurological lesions (e.g. hypothalamic or upper brainstem infarcts or tumours)
- Drugs

Psychological/psychiatric

- Depression

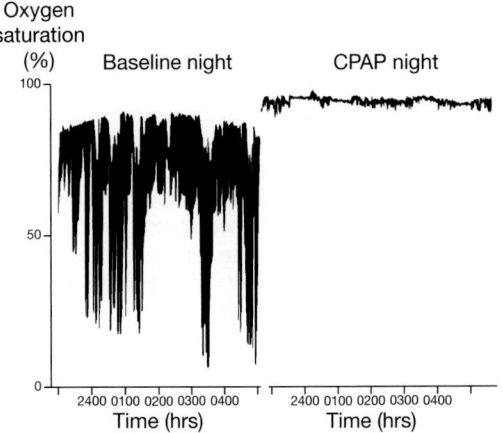

Fig. 17.69 Sleep apnoea/hypopnoea syndrome: overnight oxygen saturation trace. The left-hand panel shows the trace of a patient who had 53 apnoeas plus hypopnoeas/hour, 55 brief awakenings/hour and marked oxygen desaturation. The right-hand panel shows the effect of continuous positive airway pressure (CPAP) of 10 cm H_2O delivered through a tight-fitting nasal mask: it abolished his breathing irregularity and awakenings, and improved oxygenation. *Courtesy of Professor N.J. Douglas.*

is determined by the number of apnoeas/hypopnoeas per hour of sleep (apnoea/hypopnoea index, AHI). An apnoea is defined as a 10-second or longer breathing pause and a hypopnoea is a 10-second or longer 50% reduction in ventilation that results in a 4% drop in arterial oxygen saturation. An AHI of 5–14 indicates mild OSAHS, 15–30 is moderate and more than 30 is severe.

Several other conditions can cause daytime sleepiness but can usually be excluded by a careful history (Box 17.87). Narcolepsy is a rare cause of sudden-onset sleepiness, occurring in 0.05% of the population. Idiopathic hypersomnolence occurs in younger individuals and is characterised by long nocturnal sleeps.

Management

The major hazard to patients and those around them is traffic accidents. Drivers must be strongly advised not to drive until treatment has relieved their sleepiness, and have a responsibility to inform their driving licence authority if there is sleepiness sufficient to impair driving. Overweight or obese patients should be encouraged to lose weight, and be considered for bariatric surgery if appropriate. Though rarely resulting in complete remission of OSAHS, weight loss decreases the AHI and blood pressure, and improves overall health and quality of life. In a minority, relief of nasal obstruction or the avoidance of alcohol or sedating medication

may prevent obstruction. Mandibular advancement devices that fit over the teeth and hold the mandible forward, thus opening the pharynx, are an alternative that is effective in some patients. There is no evidence that palatal surgery is of benefit. The gold standard therapy for the majority of patients is continuous positive airway pressure (CPAP) delivered by a mask every night to splint the upper airway open. When CPAP is tolerated, the effect is often dramatic (see Fig. 17.69), with relief of somnolence and improved daytime performance, quality of life and survival. Unfortunately, 30%–50% of patients do not tolerate CPAP or have poor adherence. Increasing use of telemedicine to remotely monitor CPAP use and overnight oximetry will enable non-adherers to be identified and supported to improve adherence. Interventions to promote adherence include improving mask fit, pressure modification and humidification, education and behavioural therapy.

Central sleep apnoea and nocturnal hypoventilation

Episodic reduced ventilation during sleep in the absence of upper airway obstruction is called central sleep apnoea (CSA) or nocturnal hypoventilation. CSA is much less prevalent than OSAHS.

Aetiology

CSA or nocturnal hypoventilation occur when there is an altered ventilatory drive and/or an inability to adequately expand the chest. Loss of drive can be a result of brainstem abnormality, such as in post-polio syndrome and brainstem stroke, or ventilatory suppression, such as by opiates and alcohol. Cheyne–Stokes breathing is a sinusoidal cycling between hypoventilation and compensatory hyperventilation, that occurs most often when left ventricular failure influences ventilatory drive. The normal ventilatory mechanism can be impaired by neurological conditions, including myopathies (e.g. Duchenne muscular dystrophy, myotonic dystrophy), neuropathies (e.g. motor neurone disease, Guillain–Barré syndrome), and neuromuscular junction abnormalities (e.g. myasthenia gravis). Chest wall expansion is reduced by conditions such as scoliosis and severe ankylosing spondylitis. Severe obstructive airways disease also impairs ventilation, and the effect is exacerbated by coexisting OSA, obesity and/or muscle weakness.

Clinical features

Patients may present with the same signs and symptoms as those with OSAHS, in addition to features of the condition that has caused their CSA or hypoventilation. Patients can also present in acute type II respiratory failure or with features of cor pulmonale (fluid retention due to chronic hypoxia). Early morning headaches are common.

17

Investigations

Sleep studies are used to differentiate between OSAHS, CSA and nocturnal hypoventilation. Blood gases can demonstrate the presence of type II respiratory failure, and PFTs can assess ventilatory muscle strength. History and examination will often reveal the underlying cause for CSA or hypoventilation, but further targeted investigations may be necessary.

Management

Overnight home NIV improves symptoms and, in many conditions, prognosis. Sedating medications (unless palliative) and excessive alcohol should be stopped. Optimizing heart failure treatment can reduce Cheyne–Stokes breathing, but patients who remain symptomatic may benefit from CPAP or nocturnal oxygen.

Laryngeal disorders

The larynx is commonly affected by acute self-limiting infections. Other disorders include chronic laryngitis, laryngeal tuberculosis, laryngeal paralysis and laryngeal obstruction. Tumours of the larynx are relatively common, particularly in smokers. For further details, the reader should refer to an otolaryngology text.

Chronic laryngitis

The common causes are listed in Box 17.88. The chief symptoms are hoarseness or loss of voice (aphonia). There is irritation of the throat and a spasmodic cough. The disease pursues a chronic course, frequently uninfluenced by treatment, and the voice may become permanently impaired. Other causes of chronic hoarseness include use of inhaled glucocorticoid treatment, tuberculosis, laryngeal paralysis or tumour.

In some patients, a chest X-ray may reveal an unsuspected lung cancer or pulmonary tuberculosis. If these are not found, laryngoscopy should be performed to exclude a local structural cause.

When no specific treatable cause is found, the voice must be rested completely. This is particularly important for public speakers and singers. Smoking should be avoided. Some benefit may be obtained from frequent inhalations of steam.

Laryngeal paralysis

Interruption of the motor nerve supply of the larynx is nearly always unilateral and, because of the intrathoracic course of the left recurrent laryngeal nerve, usually left-sided. One or both recurrent laryngeal nerves may be damaged by thyroidectomy, carcinoma of the thyroid or anterior neck injury. Rarely, the vagal trunk itself is involved by tumour, aneurysm or trauma.

Clinical features and management

Hoarseness always accompanies laryngeal paralysis, whatever its cause. Paralysis of organic origin is seldom reversible, but when only one vocal cord is affected, hoarseness may improve or even disappear after a few weeks, as the normal cord compensates by crossing the midline to approximate with the paralysed cord on phonation.

'Bovine cough' is a characteristic feature of organic laryngeal paralysis, and lacks the explosive quality of normal coughing because the cords fail to close the glottis. Sputum clearance may also be impaired. A normal cough in patients with partial loss of voice or aphonia virtually excludes laryngeal paralysis. Stridor is occasionally present but seldom severe, except when laryngeal paralysis is bilateral.

Laryngoscopy is required to establish the diagnosis of laryngeal paralysis. The paralysed cord lies in a paramedian position, midway between abduction and adduction.

The cause of laryngeal paralysis should be treated, if possible, and speech and language therapy offered. In unilateral paralysis, persistent dysphonia may be improved by the injection of bulking agents into the affected vocal cord. In bilateral organic paralysis, tracheal intubation, tracheostomy or surgery to reposition and/or reshape the larynx may be necessary.

Psychogenic hoarseness and aphonia

Psychogenic causes of hoarseness or aphonia may be suggested by associated symptoms in the history (p. 1242). Laryngoscopy may be necessary, however, to exclude a physical cause. In psychogenic aphonia, only the voluntary movement of adduction of the vocal cords is seen to be impaired. Speech therapy may be helpful.

Laryngeal obstruction

Laryngeal obstruction is more liable to occur in children than in adults because of the smaller size of the glottis. Important causes are given in Box 17.89. Sudden complete laryngeal obstruction by a foreign body produces the clinical picture of acute asphyxia: violent but ineffective inspiratory efforts with indrawing of the intercostal spaces and the unsupported lower ribs, accompanied by cyanosis. Unrelieved, the condition progresses to coma and death within a few minutes. When, as in most cases, the obstruction is incomplete at first, the main clinical features are progressive breathlessness accompanied by stridor and cyanosis. Urgent treatment to prevent complete obstruction is needed.

Management

Laryngeal obstruction carries a high mortality and demands prompt treatment. When a foreign body causes laryngeal obstruction, give up to five sharp back blows using the heel of the hand between the scapulae. If this is ineffective use abdominal thrusts, or, in those aged under 12 months old or pregnant, give chest thrusts. Tracheostomy must be performed without delay if these procedures fail to relieve complete obstruction. If the adult patient is stable with only partial obstruction, direct laryngoscopy can be used to remove the foreign body or insert a tube past the obstruction into the trachea to maintain the airway.

In diphtheria, antitoxin should be administered, and for other infections the appropriate antibiotic should be given. In angioedema, complete laryngeal occlusion can usually be prevented by treatment with adrenaline (epinephrine; 0.5–1 mg (0.5–1 mL of 1 : 1000) IM), chlorphenamine (10 mg by slow intravenous injection) and intravenous hydrocortisone sodium succinate (200 mg).

---

i | **17.88 Causes of chronic laryngitis**

- Excessive use of the voice
- Heavy tobacco smoking
- Heavy alcohol intake
- Gastroesophageal reflux disease
- Repeated attacks of acute laryngitis
- Chronic sinusitis with post-nasal drip
- Occupational exposure to irritating chemicals or dusts
- Sarcoidosis

---

i | **17.89 Causes of laryngeal obstruction**

- Inflammatory or allergic oedema, or exudate
- Spasm of laryngeal muscles
- Inhaled foreign body
- Inhaled blood clot or vomitus in an unconscious patient
- Tumours of the larynx
- Bilateral vocal cord paralysis
- Fixation of both cords in rheumatoid disease

Tracheal disorders

Tracheal obstruction

External compression by lymph nodes containing metastases, usually due to lung cancer, is a more frequent cause of tracheal obstruction than primary benign or malignant tumours. The trachea may also be compressed by a retrosternal goitre (see Fig. 20.12). Rare causes include an aneurysm of the aortic arch and (in children) tuberculous mediastinal lymph nodes. Tracheal stenosis is an occasional complication of tracheostomy, prolonged intubation, granulomatosis with polyangiitis (GPA) or trauma.

Clinical features and management

Stridor can be detected in every patient with severe tracheal narrowing. CT will usually enable the cause to be identified, and bronchoscopic examination (if safe) can determine the degree and nature of the obstruction and enable biopsy.

Localised tumours of the trachea can be resected but reconstruction after resection may be technically difficult. Endobronchial laser therapy, bronchoscopically placed tracheal stents, chemotherapy and radiotherapy are alternatives to surgery. The choice of treatment depends on the nature of the tumour and the general health of the patient. Benign tracheal strictures can sometimes be dilated but may require resection.

Tracheo-oesophageal fistula

Tracheo-oesophageal fistula may be present in newborn infants as a congenital abnormality. In adults, it is usually due to malignant lesions in the mediastinum, such as carcinoma or lymphoma, eroding both the trachea and oesophagus to produce a communication between them. Swallowed liquids enter the trachea and bronchi through the fistula and provoke coughing.

Surgical closure of a congenital fistula, if undertaken promptly, is usually successful. There is usually no curative treatment for malignant fistulae, and death from overwhelming pulmonary infection rapidly supervenes.

Pleural disease

Pleurisy, pleural effusion, empyema and asbestos-associated pleural disease have been described above. Specific features of pleural disease in old age are shown in Box 17.90.

Pneumothorax

Pneumothorax is the presence of air in the pleural space, which can either occur spontaneously, or result from iatrogenic injury or trauma to the lung or chest wall (Box 17.91). Primary spontaneous pneumothorax occurs in patients with no history of lung disease. Smoking, tall stature and the presence of apical subpleural blebs are risk factors. Secondary

17.90 Pleural disease in old age

- **Spontaneous pneumothorax**: invariably associated with underlying lung disease in old age and has a significant mortality.
- **Rib fracture**: common cause of pleural-type pain; may be spontaneous (due to coughing), traumatic or pathological. Underlying osteomalacia may contribute to poor healing, especially in the housebound with no exposure to sunlight.
- **Tuberculosis**: should always be considered and actively excluded in older patients presenting with a unilateral pleural effusion.
- **Mesothelioma**: more common in older individuals than younger people due to a long latency period between asbestos exposure (often more than 20 years) and the development of disease.
- **Analgesia**: frail older people are particularly sensitive to the respiratory depressant effects of opiate-based analgesia and careful monitoring is required when using these agents for pleural pain.

pneumothorax affects patients with pre-existing lung disease and is associated with higher mortality rates (Fig. 17.70).

Where the communication between the airway and the pleural space seals off as the lung deflates and does not re-open, the pneumothorax is referred to as 'closed' (Fig. 17.71A). The mean pleural pressure remains negative, spontaneous re-absorption of air and re-expansion of the lung occur over a few days or weeks, and infection is uncommon. This contrasts with an 'open' pneumothorax, where the communication fails to seal and air continues to pass freely between the bronchial tree and pleural space (Fig. 17.71B). An example of the latter is a bronchopleural fistula, which can facilitate the transmission of infection from the airways into the pleural space, leading to empyema. An open pneumothorax is commonly seen following rupture of an emphysematous bulla, tuberculous cavity or lung abscess into the pleural space.

Occasionally, the communication between the airway and the pleural space acts as a one-way valve, allowing air to enter the pleural space during inspiration but not to escape on expiration. This is a tension pneumothorax. Large amounts of trapped air accumulate progressively in the pleural space and the intrapleural pressure rises to well above atmospheric levels. This causes mediastinal displacement towards the opposite side, with compression of the opposite normal lung and impairment of systemic venous return, causing cardiovascular compromise (Fig. 17.71C).

Clinical features

The most common symptoms are sudden-onset unilateral pleuritic chest pain and/or breathlessness. In those individuals with underlying lung disease, breathlessness can be severe and may not resolve spontaneously. In patients with a small pneumothorax, physical examination may be normal. A larger pneumothorax (>15% of the hemithorax) results in decreased or absent breath sounds. The combination of absent breath sounds and a resonant percussion note is diagnostic of pneumothorax.

17.91 Classification of pneumothorax

Spontaneous

Primary
- No evidence of overt lung disease; air escapes from the lung into the pleural space through rupture of a small pleural bleb, or the pulmonary end of a pleural adhesion

Secondary
- Underlying lung disease, most commonly chronic obstructive pulmonary disease and tuberculosis; also seen in asthma, lung abscess, pulmonary infarcts, lung cancer and all forms of fibrotic and cystic lung disease

Traumatic
- Iatrogenic (e.g. following thoracic surgery or biopsy) or chest wall injury

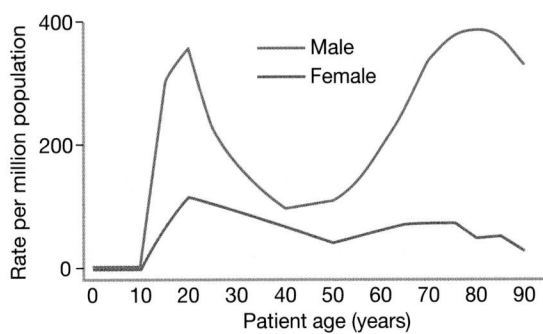

Fig. 17.70 Bimodal age distribution for hospital admissions for pneumothorax in England. The incidence of primary spontaneous pneumothorax peaks in males aged 15–30 years. Secondary spontaneous pneumothorax occurs mainly in males over 55 years.

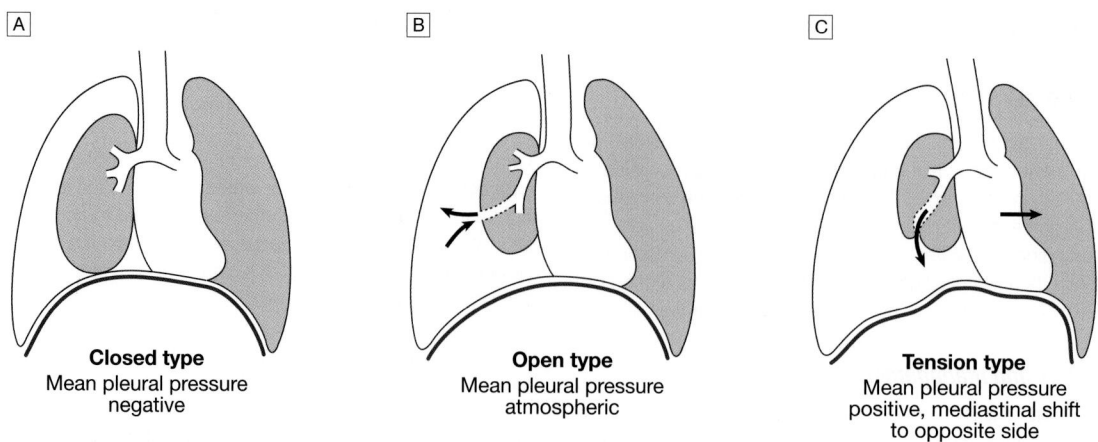

Fig. 17.71 Types of spontaneous pneumothorax. A Closed type. B Open type. C Tension (valvular) type.

By contrast, in tension pneumothorax there is rapidly progressive breathlessness, associated with a marked tachycardia, hypotension, cyanosis and tracheal displacement away from the side of the silent hemithorax. Occasionally, tension pneumothorax may occur without mediastinal shift, if malignant disease or scarring has splinted the mediastinum.

Investigations

The chest X-ray shows the sharply defined edge of the deflated lung with complete translucency (no lung markings) between this and the chest wall. Care must be taken to differentiate between a large pre-existing emphysematous bulla and a pneumothorax. In general, the lung edge is convex in a pneumothorax, whereas the edge of a bulla is concave. X-ray findings should be correlated with the patient's clinical condition. CT is used in difficult cases to avoid iatrogenic bronchopleural fistula, caused by misdirected attempts at aspiration. X-rays may also show the extent of any mediastinal displacement and reveal any pleural fluid or underlying pulmonary disease.

Management

Spontaneous pneumothoraces are classified as large or small on account of the distance between the lung edge and chest wall being greater or less than 2 cm (this equates to approximately half the volume of the hemithorax). Small primary pneumothoraces usually resolve spontaneously, and only require intervention if the patient is breathless. For these patients, and those with large primary pneumothoraces, percutaneous needle aspiration of air is a simple and well-tolerated alternative to intercostal tube drainage, with a 60%–80% chance of avoiding the need for a chest drain (Fig. 17.72). Patients who remain breathless or have a persistent large pneumothorax despite aspiration will require a chest drain. In patients with significant underlying chronic lung disease, however, secondary pneumothorax may cause respiratory distress. In these individuals, the success rate of aspiration is much lower, and this should therefore be attempted only for 1–2 cm pneumothoraces in patients who are not breathless. A chest drain is required if the pneumothorax remains greater than 1 cm, and in patients who are breathless or have a large pneumothorax. All patients with a secondary pneumothorax require admission for observation. If there is a tension pneumothorax, life-saving immediate release of the positive pressure by insertion of a cannula into the pleural space is performed, allowing time to prepare for chest drain insertion.

When needed, intercostal drains are inserted in the triangle of safety (Fig. 17.73), connected to an underwater seal or one-way Heimlich valve, and secured firmly to the chest wall with stitches. Clamping of an intercostal drain is potentially dangerous and rarely indicated. The drain should be removed the morning after the lung has fully re-inflated and bubbling has stopped. Continued bubbling after 5–7 days is an

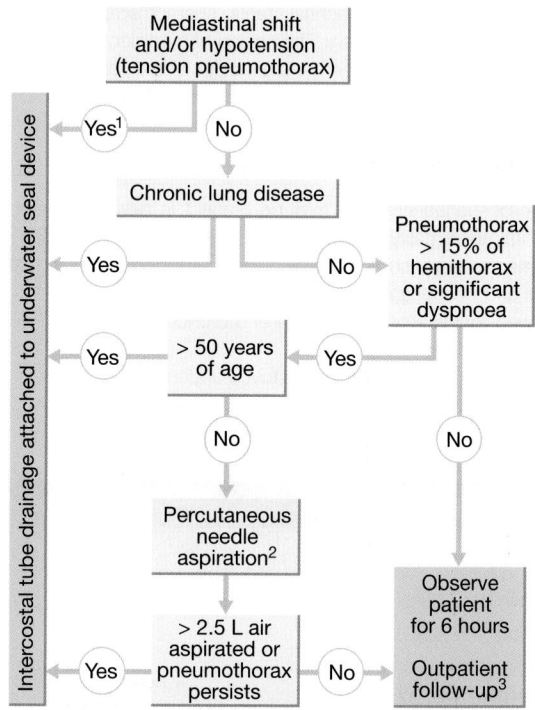

Fig. 17.72 Management of spontaneous pneumothorax. (1) Immediate decompression prior to insertion of the intercostal drain. (2) Aspirate in the second intercostal space anteriorly in the mid-clavicular line using a 16 F cannula; discontinue if resistance is felt, the patient coughs excessively, or more than 2.5 L of air are removed. (3) The post-aspiration chest X-ray is not a reliable indicator of whether a pleural leak remains, and all patients should be told to attend again immediately in the event of deterioration.

indication for surgery, though in practice CT and surgical referral occurs after 48 hours. If bubbling in the drainage bottle stops before full re-inflation, the tube is either blocked or kinked or displaced. Supplemental oxygen may speed resolution, as it accelerates the rate at which nitrogen is reabsorbed by the pleura.

Patients with a closed pneumothorax should be advised not to fly, as the trapped gas expands at altitude. After complete resolution, there is no clear evidence to indicate how long patients should avoid flying. British Thoracic Society guidelines suggest that flying should be delayed until 7 days after X-ray confirmation of full inflation. Patients should also be advised to stop smoking and informed about the risks of a recurrent pneumothorax, which is significantly reduced by smoking cessation.

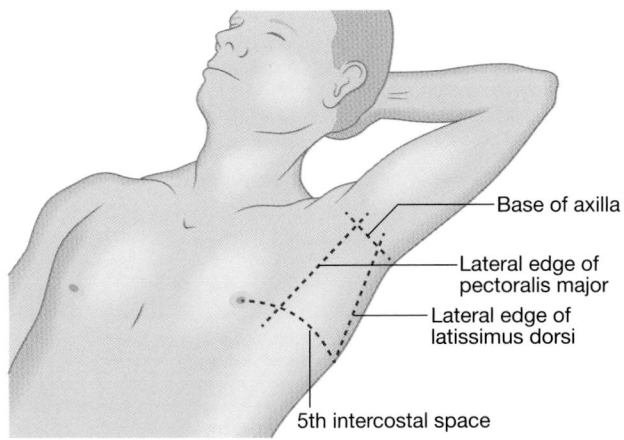

— Base of axilla

— Lateral edge of pectoralis major

— Lateral edge of latissimus dorsi

5th intercostal space

Fig. 17.73 The triangle of safety. The triangle of safety is the anatomical region that has the axilla as the apex, the lateral border of the pectoralis major anteriorly, the lateral border of the latissimus dorsi posteriorly and, inferiorly, the 5th intercostal space.

Diving is contraindicated following a pneumothorax, unless a surgical pleurodesis has sealed the lung to the chest wall.

Recurrent spontaneous pneumothorax

After primary spontaneous pneumothorax, recurrence occurs within a year of either aspiration or tube drainage in approximately 25% of patients and should prompt definitive treatment. Surgical pleurodesis is recommended in all patients following a second pneumothorax and should be considered following the first episode of secondary pneumothorax if low respiratory reserve makes recurrence hazardous. Pleurodesis can be achieved by pleural abrasion or parietal pleurectomy at thoracotomy or thoracoscopy.

Diseases of the diaphragm and chest wall

Disorders of the diaphragm

Congenital disorders

Diaphragmatic hernias

Congenital defects of the diaphragm can allow herniation of abdominal viscera. Posteriorly situated hernias through the foramen of Bochdalek are more common than anterior hernias through the foramen of Morgagni.

Eventration of the diaphragm

Abnormal elevation or bulging of one hemidiaphragm, more often the left, results from total or partial absence of muscular development of the septum transversum. Most eventrations are asymptomatic and are detected by chance on X-ray in adult life but severe respiratory distress can be caused in infancy if the diaphragmatic muscular defect is extensive.

Acquired disorders

Elevation of a hemidiaphragm may result from paralysis or other structural causes (Box 17.92). The phrenic nerve may be damaged by lung cancer, disease of cervical vertebrae, tumours of the cervical cord, shingles, trauma (including road traffic and birth injuries), surgery, and stretching of the nerve by mediastinal masses and aortic aneurysms. Idiopathic diaphragmatic paralysis occasionally occurs in otherwise fit patients. Paralysis of one hemidiaphragm results in loss of around 20% of ventilatory capacity but may not be noticed by otherwise healthy

| **i** | **17.92 Causes of elevation of a hemidiaphragm** |

- Phrenic nerve paralysis
- Eventration of the diaphragm
- Decrease in volume of one lung (e.g. lobectomy, unilateral pulmonary fibrosis)
- Severe pleuritic pain
- Pulmonary infarction
- Subphrenic abscess
- Large volume of gas in the stomach or colon
- Large tumours or cysts of the liver

individuals. Supine vital capacity is significantly reduced compared to erect. Ultrasound screening can be used to demonstrate paradoxical upward movement of the paralysed hemidiaphragm on sniffing. CT of the chest and neck is the best way to exclude occult disease affecting the phrenic nerve.

Bilateral diaphragmatic weakness occurs in peripheral neuropathies of any type, including Guillain–Barré syndrome; in disorders affecting the anterior horn cells, e.g. poliomyelitis; in muscular dystrophies; and in connective tissue disorders, such as SLE and polymyositis.

Hiatus hernia is common. Diaphragmatic rupture is usually caused by a crush injury and may not be detected until years later. Respiratory disorders that cause pulmonary hyperinflation (e.g. emphysema), and those that result in small stiff lungs (e.g. diffuse pulmonary fibrosis), compromise diaphragmatic function and predispose to fatigue.

Deformities of the chest wall

Thoracic kyphoscoliosis

Abnormalities of alignment of the dorsal spine and their consequent effects on thoracic shape may be caused by:

- congenital abnormality
- vertebral disease, including tuberculosis, osteoporosis and ankylosing spondylitis
- trauma
- neuromuscular disease, such as poliomyelitis.

Simple kyphosis (increased anterior curvature of the thoracic spine) causes less pulmonary embarrassment than kyphoscoliosis (anteroposterior and lateral curvature). Kyphoscoliosis, if severe, restricts and distorts expansion of the chest wall and impairs diaphragmatic function, causing ventilation–perfusion mismatch in the lungs. Patients with severe deformity may develop type II respiratory failure (initially manifest during sleep), pulmonary hypertension and right ventricular failure. They can often be successfully treated with non-invasive ventilatory support.

Pectus

Pectus is the result of abnormal costal cartilage growth, causing the sternum to protrude (carinatum), or more commonly, to be depressed (excavatum). In patients with pectus excavatum the heart is displaced to the left and may be compressed between the sternum and the vertebral column but only rarely is there associated disturbance of cardiac function. The deformity may restrict chest expansion and reduce vital capacity. Operative correction is rarely performed, and then only for cosmetic reasons. Although no associated gene has yet been identified, pectus is likely genetic, and a quarter of those affected have a family history of chest wall deformity. Pectus can be associated with kyphoscoliosis and is a feature of certain syndromes (including Marfan and Poland syndromes).

17

Further information

Websites

brit-thoracic.org.uk *British Thoracic Society: access to guidelines on a range of respiratory conditions.*

ersnet.org *European Respiratory Society: provides information on education and research, and patient information.*

ginasthma.com *Global Initiative for Asthma: comprehensive overview of asthma.*

goldcopd.org *Global Initiative for Chronic Obstructive Lung Disease: comprehensive overview of COPD.*

thoracic.org *American Thoracic Society: provides information on education and research, and patient information.*

B Conway
PJ Phelan
GD Stewart

18

Nephrology and urology

Clinical examination of the kidney and urinary tract

Many diseases of the kidney and urinary tract are clinically silent, at least in the early stages. Accordingly, it is common for these conditions to be detected first by routine blood tests or on dipstick testing of the urine. Several important abnormalities can also be picked up on physical examination and these are summarised below.

5 Fundoscopy

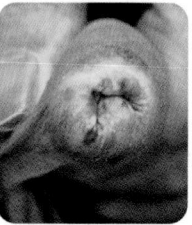

▲ Hypertensive changes

4 Jugular venous pressure
Elevated in fluid overload

3 Blood pressure
Often elevated

2 Skin
Yellow complexion*
Bruising*
Excoriation of pruritus*
Reduced skin turgor in fluid depletion

1 Hands

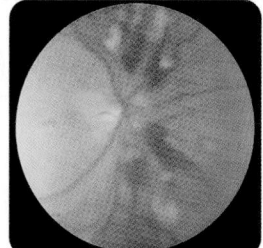

▲ Splinter haemorrhages

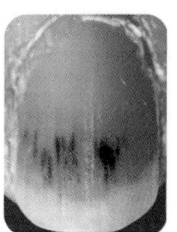

▲ 'Brown line' pigmentation of nails

6 Lungs
Crepitations in fluid overload

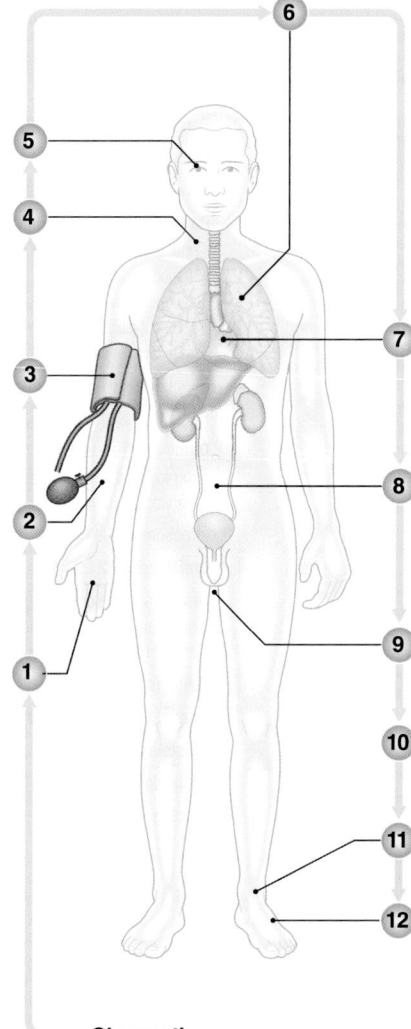

Observation
• Tiredness
• Respiratory rate and depth increased in metabolic acidosis
• Pallor*

*Features of advanced chronic kidney disease (see also Fig. 18.22)

7 Heart
Extra heart sounds in fluid overload
Pericardial friction rub*

8 Abdomen
Renal mass
Local tenderness
Renal or other arterial bruits in renal vascular disease
Rectal examination — prostate

9 Genitalia
Scrotal swellings

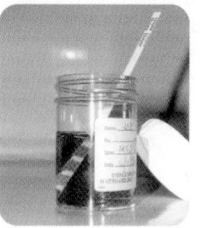

▲ Phimosis

10 Sacral oedema

11 Ankle oedema

12 Peripheral neuropathy*

13 Urinalysis for blood and protein

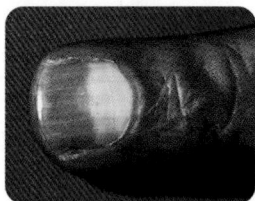

14 Urine microscopy
See Fig. 18.3

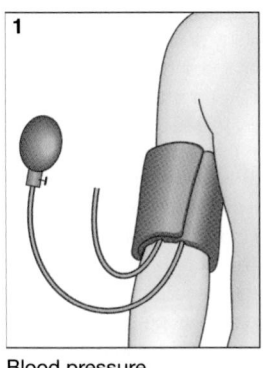

Blood pressure measurements

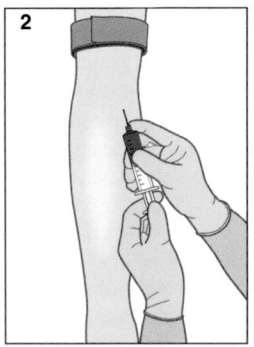

Blood tests for abnormal creatinine and electrolytes

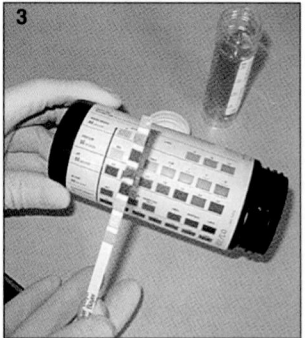

Urinalysis for protein, blood, nitrites and leucocytes

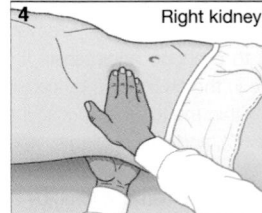

Abdominal examination for palpable kidneys

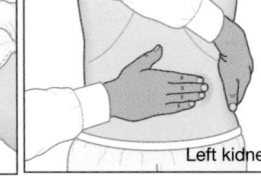

Percussing for tenderness in renal angle

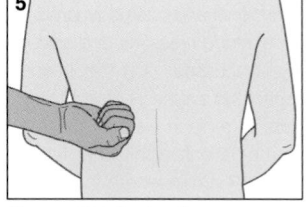

Digital rectal examination for prostate assessment

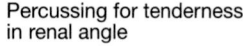

Checking sacrum and ankles for pitting oedema

Clinical examination techniques to evaluate urological and renal abnormalities. *Inset (Dipstick): From Pitkin J, Peattie AB, Magowan BA. Obstetrics and gynaecology: An illustrated colour text. Edinburgh: Churchill Livingstone, Elsevier Ltd; 2003.*

18

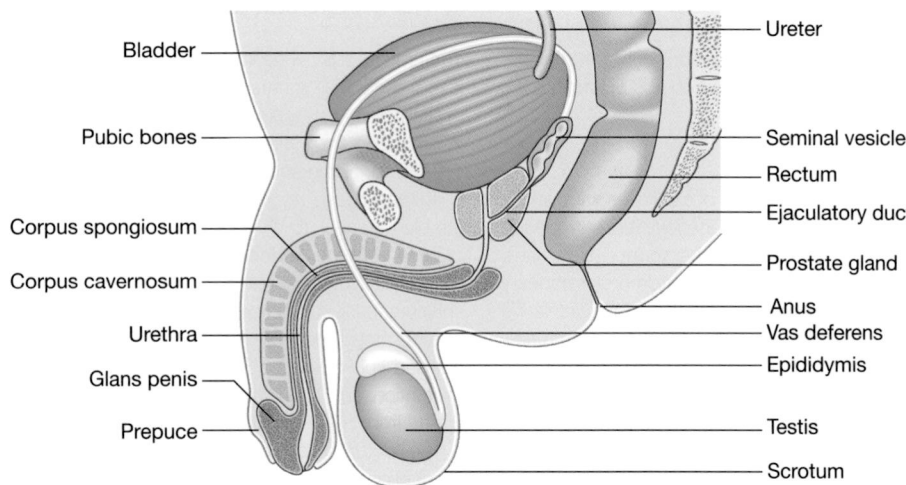

Male lower urinary tract demonstrating the relationship of the bladder, urethra, vas deferens and testes.

This chapter describes the disorders of the kidneys and urinary tract that are commonly encountered in routine practice, as well as giving an overview of the highly specialised field of renal replacement therapy. Disorders of renal tubular function, which may cause alterations in electrolyte and acid–base balance, are described in Chapter 19.

Functional anatomy and physiology

The kidneys

The kidneys play a central role in excretion of many metabolic breakdown products, including ammonia and urea from protein, creatinine from muscle, uric acid from nucleic acids, drugs and toxins. They achieve this by making large volumes of an ultrafiltrate of plasma (125 mL/min, 180 L/24 hrs) at the glomerulus, and selectively reabsorbing components of this ultrafiltrate at points along the nephron. The rates of filtration and reabsorption are controlled by many hormonal and haemodynamic signals to regulate fluid and electrolyte balance, blood pressure, and acid–base and calcium–phosphate homeostasis (all discussed in Ch. 19). In addition, the kidneys activate vitamin D and control the synthesis of red blood cells by producing erythropoietin. Strategies to replace each of these important functions are required when managing patients with kidney failure.

Each kidney is approximately 10–13 cm in length in healthy adults; they are located retroperitoneally on either side of the aorta and inferior vena cava between the 12th thoracic and 3rd lumbar vertebrae (Fig. 18.1A). The right kidney is usually a few centimetres lower because the liver lies above it. Both kidneys rise and descend several centimetres with respiration.

In keeping with their role as efficient blood filters, the kidneys have a rich blood supply and receive approximately 20%–25% of cardiac output through the renal arteries, which arise from the abdominal aorta. The renal arteries undergo various subdivisions within the kidney, eventually forming interlobular arteries that run through the renal cortex. These eventually give rise to afferent glomerular arterioles that supply the glomeruli. The efferent arteriole, leading from the glomerulus, supplies the distal nephron and medulla (Fig. 18.1B). This unique arrangement of two serial capillary beds reflects the role of the afferent and efferent arterioles in autoregulation of glomerular filtration.

The nephron

Each kidney contains approximately 1 million individual functional units, called nephrons. Each nephron consists of a glomerulus, which is responsible for ultrafiltration of blood, a proximal renal tubule, a loop of Henle, a distal renal tubule and a collecting duct, which together are responsible for selective reabsorption of water and electrolytes that have been filtered at the glomerulus (see Fig. 19.2 and Fig. 18.1B). Under normal circumstances, approximately 99% of the 180 L of glomerular filtrate that is produced each day is reabsorbed in the tubules. The remainder passes through the collecting ducts of each nephron and drains into the renal pelvis and ureters.

The glomerulus

The glomerulus comprises a tightly packed loop of capillaries supplied by an afferent arteriole and drained by an efferent arteriole. It is surrounded by a cup-shaped extension of the proximal tubule termed Bowman's capsule, which is composed of epithelial cells. The glomerular capillary endothelial cells contain pores (fenestrae), through which circulating molecules can pass to reach the underlying glomerular basement membrane (GBM), which is formed by fusion of the basement membranes of tubular epithelial and vascular endothelial cells (Fig. 18.1C and D). Glomerular epithelial cells (podocytes) have multiple long foot processes that interdigitate with those of the adjacent epithelial cells, thereby maintaining a selective barrier to filtration (Fig. 18.1E). Mesangial cells lie in the central region of the glomerulus. They have contractile properties similar to those of vascular smooth muscle cells and play a role in regulating glomerular filtration rate.

Under normal circumstances, the glomerulus is impermeable to proteins the size of albumin (67 kDa) or larger, while proteins of 20 kDa or smaller are filtered freely. The ability of molecules between 20 and 67 kDa to pass through the GBM is variable and depends on the size (smaller molecules are filtered more easily) and charge (positively charged molecules are filtered more easily). Very little lipid is filtered by the glomerulus.

Filtration pressure in the glomerulus is normally maintained at a constant level in the face of wide variations in systemic blood pressure and cardiac output, by alterations in muscle tone within the afferent and efferent arterioles and mesangial cells. This is known as autoregulation. Reduced renal perfusion pressure increases local production of prostaglandins that mediate vasodilatation of the afferent arteriole, thereby increasing the intraglomerular pressure (see Fig. 18.1D). In addition, renin is released by specialised smooth muscle cells in the juxtaglomerular apparatus in response to reduced perfusion pressure, stimulation of sympathetic nerves or low sodium concentration of fluid in the distal convoluted tubule at the macula densa. Renin cleaves angiotensinogen to release angiotensin I, which is further cleaved by angiotensin-converting enzyme (ACE) to produce angiotensin II. This restores glomerular perfusion pressure in the short term by causing vasoconstriction of the efferent arterioles within the kidney to raise intraglomerular pressure selectively (see Fig. 18.1D), and by inducing systemic vasoconstriction to increase blood pressure and thus renal perfusion pressure. In the longer term, angiotensin II increases plasma volume by stimulating aldosterone release, which enhances sodium reabsorption by the renal tubules (see Fig. 20.19). Consumption of non-steroidal anti-inflammatory preparations and renin–angiotensin system inhibitors in the context of volume depletion may impair the ability of the kidney to maintain glomerular filtration and exacerbate pre-renal failure (see Fig. 18.19).

Renal tubules, loop of Henle and collecting ducts

The proximal renal tubule, loop of Henle, distal renal tubule and collecting ducts are responsible for reabsorption of water, electrolytes and other solutes, as well as regulating acid–base balance, as described in detail on page 618 and in Figure 19.2. They also play a key role in regulating calcium homeostasis by converting 25-hydroxyvitamin D to the active metabolite 1,25-dihydroxyvitamin D Fig. 26.62. Failure of this process contributes to the pathogenesis of hypocalcaemia and hyperparathyroidism that occurs in chronic kidney disease (CKD). Fibroblast-like cells that lie in the interstitium of the renal cortex are responsible for production of erythropoietin, which is required for production of red blood cells. Erythropoietin synthesis is regulated by oxygen tension; anaemia and hypoxia increase production, whereas polycythaemia and hyperoxia inhibit it. Failure of erythropoietin production plays an important role in the pathogenesis of anaemia in CKD.

The ureters and bladder

The ureters drain urine from the renal pelvis (see Fig. 18.1A) and deliver it to the bladder, a muscular organ that lies anteriorly in the lower part of the pelvis, just behind the pubic bone. The function of the bladder is to store and then release urine during micturition. The bladder is richly innervated. Sympathetic nerves arising from T10–L2 relay in the pelvic ganglia to cause relaxation of the detrusor muscle and contraction of the bladder neck (both via α-adrenoceptors), thereby preventing release of urine from the bladder. The distal sphincter mechanism is innervated by somatic motor fibres from sacral segments S2–4, which reach the sphincter either by the pelvic plexus or via the pudendal nerves. Afferent sensory impulses pass to the cerebral cortex, from where reflex-increased sphincter tone and suppression of detrusor contraction inhibit micturition until it is appropriate. Conversely, parasympathetic nerves arising from S2–4 stimulate detrusor contraction, promoting micturition.

The micturition cycle has a storage (filling) phase and a voiding (micturition) phase. During the filling phase, the high compliance of the detrusor muscle allows the bladder to fill steadily without a rise in intravesical pressure. As bladder volume increases, stretch receptors in its wall cause reflex bladder relaxation and increased sphincter tone. The act of micturition is initiated first by voluntary and then by reflex relaxation of the pelvic floor and distal sphincter mechanism, followed by reflex detrusor contraction. These actions are coordinated by the pontine micturition centre. Intravesical pressure remains greater than urethral pressure until the bladder is empty.

The prostate gland

The prostate gland is situated at the base of the bladder, surrounding the proximal urethra (p. 559). Exocrine glands within the prostate produce fluid, which comprises about 20% of the volume of ejaculated seminal

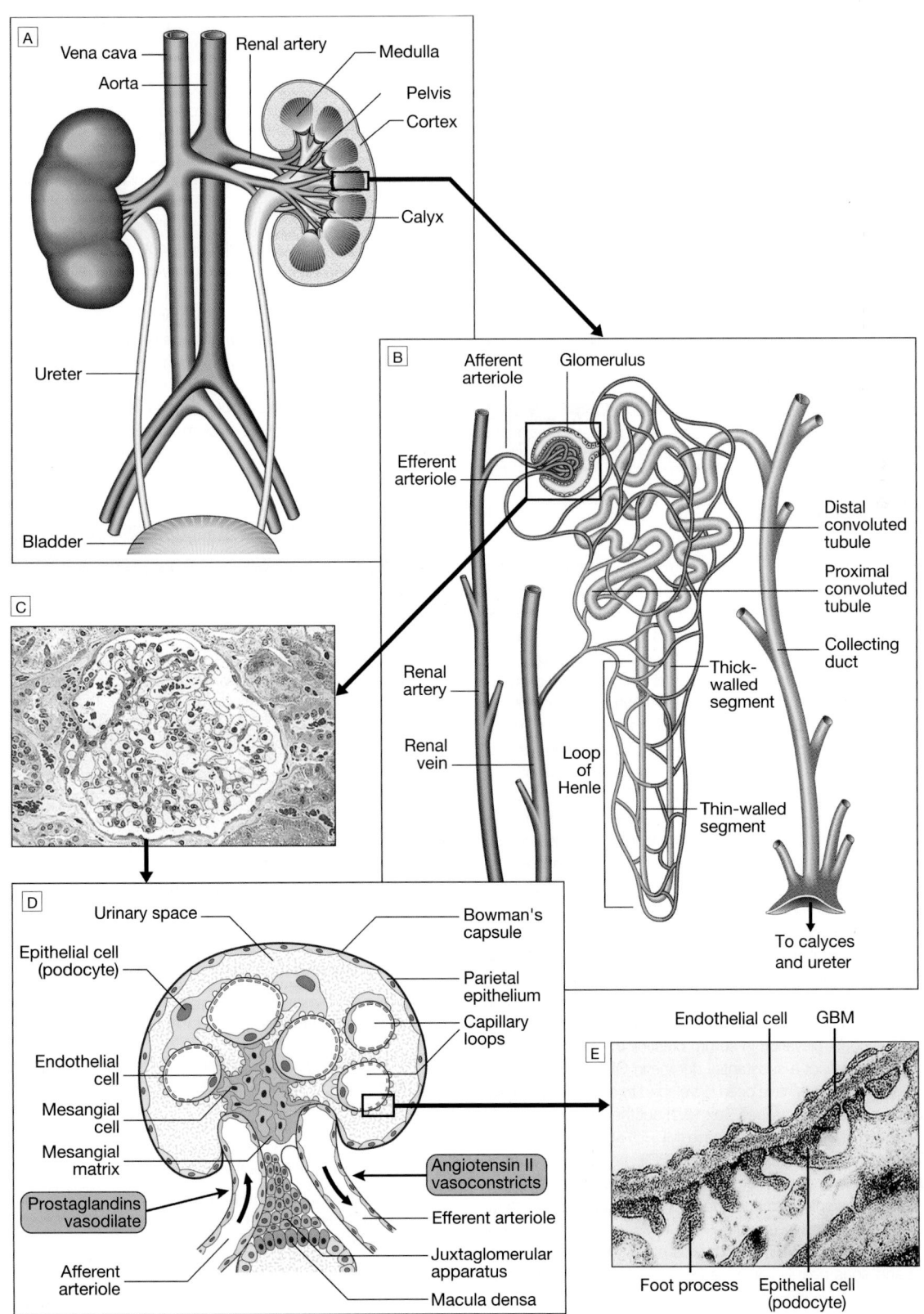

Fig. 18.1 Functional anatomy of the kidney. **A** Anatomical relationships of the kidney. **B** A single nephron. For the functions of different segments, see Fig. 19.2. **C** Histology of a normal glomerulus. **D** Schematic cross-section of a glomerulus, showing five capillary loops, to illustrate structure and show cell types. **E** Electron micrograph of the filtration barrier. (GBM = glomerular basement membrane) *(C) Courtesy of Dr J.G. Simpson, Aberdeen Royal Infirmary.*

fluid and is rich in zinc and proteolytic enzymes. The remainder of the ejaculate is formed in the seminal vesicles and bulbo-urethral glands, with spermatozoa arising from the testes.

Smooth muscle fibres within the prostate, which are under sympathetic control, play a role in controlling urine flow through the bulbar urethra, and also contract at orgasm to move seminal fluid through ejaculatory ducts into the bulbar urethra (emission). Contraction of the bulbocavernosus muscle (via a spinal muscle reflex) then ejaculates the semen out of the urethra.

The penis

Blood flow into the corpus cavernosum of the penis is controlled by sympathetic nerves from the thoracolumbar plexus, which maintain smooth muscle contraction (p. 559). In response to afferent input from the glans penis and from higher centres, pelvic splanchnic parasympathetic nerves actively relax the cavernosal smooth muscle via neurotransmitters such as nitric oxide, acetylcholine, vasoactive intestinal polypeptide (VIP) and prostacyclin, with consequent dilatation of the lacunar space. At the same time, draining venules are compressed, trapping blood in the lacunar space with consequent elevation of pressure and erection (tumescence) of the penis.

Investigation of renal and urinary tract disease

Glomerular filtration rate

The glomerular filtration rate (GFR) is the sum of the ultrafiltration rates from plasma into the Bowman's space in each nephron and is a measure of renal excretory function. It is proportionate to body size and the reference value is usually expressed after correction for body surface area as 150 ± 25 mL/min/1.73 m². The GFR may be measured directly by injecting and measuring the clearance of compounds such as inulin or radiolabelled ethylenediamine-tetra-acetic acid (EDTA), which are completely filtered at the glomerulus and are not secreted or reabsorbed by the renal tubules (Box 18.1). This is not performed routinely, however, and is usually reserved for special circumstances, such as the assessment of renal function in potential live kidney donors. Instead, GFR is usually assessed indirectly in clinical practice by measuring serum levels of endogenously produced compounds that are excreted by the kidney. The most widely used is serum creatinine, which is produced by muscle at a constant rate, is almost completely filtered at the glomerulus, and is not reabsorbed. Although creatinine is secreted to a small degree by the proximal tubule, this is only usually significant in terms of GFR estimation in severe renal impairment, where it accounts for a larger proportion of the creatinine excreted. Accordingly, provided muscle mass remains constant, changes in serum creatinine concentrations closely reflect changes in GFR. The relationship between serum creatinine and GFR is not linear, however, and a modest elevation in serum creatinine above the normal range may therefore reflect a substantial decline in GFR (Fig. 18.2). For this reason, several methods have been developed to estimate GFR from serum creatinine measurements (see Box 18.1) but the most widely used are the Modification of Diet in Renal Disease (MDRD) and Chronic Kidney Disease Epidemiology Collaboration (CKD-EPI) equations. Routine reporting by laboratories of estimated GFR (eGFR) has increased recognition of moderate kidney damage and encouraged early deployment of protective therapies; however, some limitations remain (Boxes 18.2 and 18.3). In particular, the MDRD formula is based on the serum creatinine value and so is heavily influenced by muscle mass; eGFR may therefore be misleading in individuals whose muscle bulk is outside the normal range for their sex and age. Measurement of other endogenous metabolites, such as cystatin C, may provide a more accurate estimate of GFR in this setting, though this test is not yet widely available in routine clinical practice.

Direct measurement of creatinine clearance by collecting a 24-hour urine sample and relating serum creatinine levels to urinary creatinine excretion (see Box 18.1) is now less commonly performed due to the difficulty in obtaining accurate 24-hour urine collections. It may still have a role in assessing renal function in patients at extremes of muscle mass, where the creatinine-based equations perform poorly.

Urine investigations

Screening for the presence of blood, protein, glucose, ketones, nitrates and leucocytes, and assessment of urinary pH and osmolality can be achieved by dipstick testing. The presence of leucocytes and nitrites in urine is indicative of renal tract infection. Urine pH can provide diagnostic information in the assessment of renal tubular acidosis and urinary tract stones (p. 630).

Urine microscopy (Fig. 18.3) may detect dysmorphic erythrocytes or red cell casts, which suggest the presence of glomerular disease. White cell casts are strongly suggestive of pyelonephritis but may also occur in other forms of inflammation such as interstitial nephritis. Microscopy may also detect the presence of bacteria in those with urinary infection and crystals in patients with renal stone disease. It should be noted that calcium oxalate and urate crystals can sometimes be found in normal urine that has been left to stand, due to crystal formation ex vivo.

Urine collection over a 24-hour period may be performed to measure excretion of solutes, such as calcium, oxalate and urate, in patients with recurrent renal stone disease (p. 602). Proteinuria can also be measured

---

🩺 18.1 How to estimate glomerular filtration rate (GFR)

Measuring GFR

- Direct measurement using labelled ethylenediamine-tetra-acetic acid (EDTA) or inulin
- Creatinine clearance (CrCl):
    - Minor tubular secretion of creatinine causes CrCl to exaggerate GFR when renal function is poor; can be affected by drugs (e.g. trimethoprim, cimetidine)
    - Needs 24-hr urine collection (inconvenient and often unreliable)

$$CrCl(mL/min) = \frac{\text{urine creatinine concentration (micromol/L)} \times \text{volume (mL)}}{\text{plasma creatinine concentration (micromol/L)} \times \text{time (min)}}$$

Estimating GFR with equations

- The Modification of Diet in Renal Disease (MDRD) study equation (see www.renal.org/eGFR):
    - Requires knowledge of age and sex only; it can therefore be reported automatically by laboratories
    - For limitations, see Box 18.2

$$eGFR = 175^* \times (\text{creatinine in micromol/L } 88.4)^{-1.154} \times (\text{age in yrs})^{-0.203} \times (0.742 \text{ if female}) \times (1.21 \text{ if Black})$$

- The Chronic Kidney Disease Epidemiology Collaboration (CKD-EPI) equation:
    - More accurately estimates the actual GFR than the MDRD eGFR in those with relatively preserved renal function

$$eGFR = 141 \times \min(SCr/\kappa, 1)^{\alpha} \times \max(SCr/\kappa, 1)^{-1.206} \times 0.993^{Age} \times (1.018 \text{ if female}) \times (1.21 \text{ if Black})$$

Where SCr = serum creatinine in micromol/L
κ = 61.9 if female and 79.6 if male
α = − 0.329 if female and − 0.411 if male
min = whichever is the minimum of serum creatinine/κ or 1
max = whichever is the maximum of serum creatinine/κ or 1

- No equations perform well in unusual circumstances, such as extremes of body (and muscle) mass or in acutely unwell patients (see Box 18.2)

*A correction factor of 175 is used for isotope dilution mass spectrometry traceable creatinine measurements. To convert creatinine in mg/dL to μmol/L, multiply by 88.4.

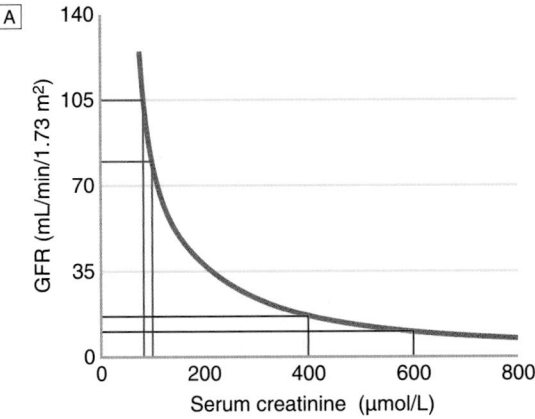

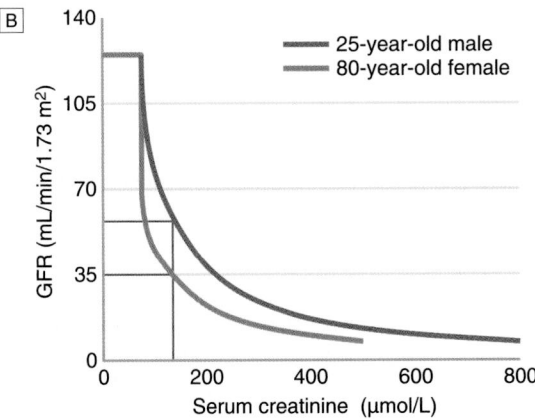

Fig. 18.2 Serum creatinine and the glomerular filtration rate (GFR). [A] The relationship between serum creatinine and estimated GFR (eGFR) is non-linear: small increases above the normal range (e.g. 80–100 μmol/L; green lines) can indicate a substantial decline in renal function (e.g. 105–80 mL/min/1.73 m²); conversely, in the high range, large changes in creatinine (e.g. 400–600 μmol/L; blue lines) can occur with only small declines in renal function (e.g. 20–15 mL/min/1.73 m²). [B] Creatinine is dependent on muscle mass; the same creatinine value may therefore reflect very different levels of renal function depending on the age and sex of the individual. To convert creatinine in mg/dL to μmol/L, multiply by 88.4.

on 24-hour collections but is usually now quantified by protein:creatinine ratio on single urine samples.

Other dynamic tests of tubular function, including concentrating ability (p. 700), ability to excrete a water load (p. 624), ability to excrete acid (p. 588) and calculation of fractional calcium, phosphate or sodium excretion are valuable in some circumstances but are usually performed in very specific contexts. The fractional excretion of these ions can be calculated by the general formula: 100× (urine concentration of analyte×serum creatinine) / (serum concentration of analyte×urinary creatinine). Calculation of fractional excretion of sodium (FENa) can help in the setting of acute kidney injury (AKI) to differentiate pre-renal failure, when the intact tubules are avidly conserving sodium in response to volume depletion (FENa typically <1.0%), from acute tubular necrosis, when the tubules are damaged and are less able to conserve sodium (FENa typically >1.0%). In clinical practice this is seldom required.

Blood tests

Haematology

A normochromic normocytic anaemia is common in CKD and is due in part to deficiency of erythropoietin and bone marrow suppression secondary to toxins retained in CKD. Other causes of anaemia include iron deficiency from urinary tract bleeding, and haemolytic anaemia

---

- It is only an estimate, with wide confidence intervals (90% of patients will have eGFR within 30% of their measured GFR, and 98% within 50%)
- It is based on serum creatinine, and so may overestimate actual GFR in patients with low muscle mass (e.g. those with cachexia, amputees) and underestimate actual GFR in individuals taking creatine supplements (creatinine is a metabolite of creatine) or trimethoprim (inhibits secretion of creatinine)
- Creatinine level must be stable over days; eGFR is not valid in assessing acute kidney injury
- It tends to underestimate true GFR at normal or near-normal function, so slightly low values should not be over-interpreted
- In older adults, who constitute the majority of those with low eGFR, there is controversy about categorising people as having chronic kidney disease (see Box 18.3) on the basis of eGFR alone, particularly at stage 3A, since there is little evidence of adverse outcomes when eGFR is >45 mL/min/1.73 m² unless there is also proteinuria
- eGFR is not valid in under-18s or during pregnancy
- Ethnicity is not taken into account in routine laboratory reporting; the laboratory eGFR value should therefore be multiplied by 1.21 for Black people
- Few patients will understand eGFR in terms of mL/min/1.73 m²; it may therefore be helpful to assume that a GFR of 100 mL/min/1.73 m² is approximately normal and to discuss eGFR values in terms of a percentage of normal, e.g. 25 mL/min/1.73 m² = 25% of normal kidney function

secondary to disorders such as haemolytic uraemic syndrome (HUS) and thrombotic thrombocytopenic purpura (TTP). Other abnormalities may be observed that reflect underlying disease processes, such as neutrophilia and raised erythrocyte sedimentation rate (ESR) in vasculitis or sepsis, and lymphopenia and raised ESR in systemic lupus erythematosus (SLE). Fragmented red cells on blood film and low platelets may be observed in thrombotic microangiopathies such as HUS/TTP and malignant hypertension. Pancytopenia may occur in SLE or bone marrow suppression due to myeloma.

Biochemistry

Abnormalities of routine biochemistry are common in renal disease. Serum levels of creatinine may be raised, reflecting reduced GFR (see above), as may serum potassium. Serum levels of urea are often increased in kidney disease but this analyte has limited value as a measure of GFR since levels are dependent on factors other than renal function. Serum urea increases with high protein intake, following gastrointestinal haemorrhage and in catabolic states. Conversely, urea levels may be reduced in patients with chronic liver disease and in patients who are anorexic or malnourished. In the absence of the other causes mentioned above, an elevated urea:creatinine ratio is indicative of volume depletion and pre-renal failure (see AKI section). Serum calcium tends to be reduced and phosphate increased in CKD, in association with high parathyroid hormone (PTH) levels caused by reduced production of 1,25-dihydroxy-vitamin D (1,25(OH)$_2$D) by the kidney (secondary hyperparathyroidism). In some patients, this may be accompanied by raised serum alkaline phosphatase levels, which are indicative of renal osteodystrophy. Serum bicarbonate may be low in renal failure and also in renal tubular acidosis independently of renal function. Serum albumin may be low in malnutrition/malabsorption, in liver disease, or as a negative acute phase response, however, if it is a new finding it should prompt urinalysis to exclude nephrotic syndrome. Other biochemical abnormalities that may reflect underlying disease processes include: raised glucose and HbA$_{1c}$ in diabetes mellitus (p. 711) and raised serum C-reactive protein (CRP) in sepsis and vasculitis.

Immunology

Antinuclear antibodies, antibodies to extractable nuclear antigens and anti-double-stranded DNA antibodies may be detected in patients with renal disease secondary to SLE (Ch. 26). Antineutrophil cytoplasmic antibodies

18

i | **18.3 Stages of chronic kidney disease (CKD)**

Stage[1]	Definition[2]	Description	Prevalence[4]	Clinical presentation[5]
1	Kidney damage[3] with normal or high GFR (>90)	Normal function	3.5%	Asymptomatic
2	Kidney damage and GFR 60–89	Mild CKD	3.9%	Asymptomatic
3A	GFR 45–59	Mild to moderate CKD	7.6% (3A and 3B combined)	Usually asymptomatic
3B	GFR 30–44	Moderate to severe CKD		Anaemia in some patients at 3B Most are non-progressive or progress very slowly
4	GFR 15–29	Severe CKD	0.4%	First symptoms often at GFR <20 Electrolyte problems likely as GFR falls
5	GFR <15 or on dialysis	Kidney failure	0.1%	Significant symptoms and complications usually present Dialysis initiation varies but usually at GFR <10

[1]Stages of CKD 1–5 were originally defined by the US National Kidney Foundation Kidney Disease Quality Outcomes Initiative 2002. In the 2013 Kidney Disease Outcomes Quality Initiative (K/DOQI) CKD guideline update, the suffices A1, A2 and A3 are recommended, indicating the presence of albuminuria of <30, 30–300 and >300 mg/24 hrs respectively, in view of the prognostic importance of albuminuria. [2]Two glomerular filtration rate (GFR) values 3 months apart are required to assign a stage. All GFR values are in mL/min/1.73 m². [3]Kidney damage means pathological abnormalities or markers of damage, including abnormalities in urine tests or imaging studies. [4]From Hill NR, Fatoba ST, Oke JL, et al. Global prevalence of chronic kidney disease – a systematic review and meta-analysis. PLoS One 2016; 11:e0158765. [5]For further information, see page 588.

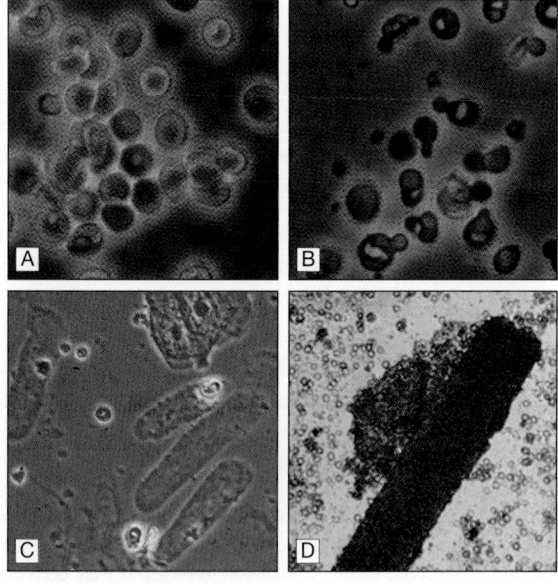

Fig. 18.3 Urine microscopy. [A] Intact erythrocytes due to bleeding from lower in the urinary tract (×400). [B] Dysmorphic erythrocytes due to glomerular inflammation (×400). [C] Hyaline casts in normal urine. [D] Erythrocytes and a red cell cast in glomerulonephritis (×100). Panels A–C are phase contrast images; D is a bright field image. *(A, B) Courtesy of Dr G.M. Iadorola and Dr F. Quarello, B. Bosco Hospital, Turin (from www.sin-italia.org/imago/sediment/sed.htm).*

(ANCAs) may be detected in patients with glomerulonephritis secondary to systemic vasculitis (Ch. 26), as may antibodies to GBM in patients with Goodpasture's disease, and low levels of complement may be observed in a number of kidney diseases (see Box 18.17). Antibodies directed against M-type phospholipase A_2 receptor (anti-PLA2R) are positive in about 70%–80% of cases of primary membranous nephropathy.

Imaging

Ultrasound

Renal ultrasound is a valuable non-invasive technique that may be performed to assess renal size and to investigate patients suspected of having urinary tract obstruction (Fig. 18.4), renal tumours, cysts or stones. Ultrasound can also be used to provide images of the prostate gland

and bladder, and to estimate the completeness of bladder emptying in patients with suspected bladder outflow obstruction. Increased echogenic signal in the renal cortex on ultrasonography with loss of distinction between cortex and medulla is characteristic of intrinsic renal disease, but not specific for any particular pathology. Doppler imaging can be used to study blood flow in extrarenal and larger intrarenal vessels, and to assess the resistivity index (peak systolic velocity – end-diastolic velocity/peak systolic velocity in the intrarenal arteries), which may be elevated (>0.7) in various diseases, including acute tubular necrosis and rejection of a renal transplant. However, renal ultrasound is operator-dependent and the results are often less clear in obese patients.

Computed tomography

Computed tomography urography (CTU) is used to evaluate cysts and mass lesions in the kidney or filling defects within the collecting system. It usually entails an initial scan without contrast medium, and subsequent scans following injection of contrast to obtain a nephrogram image and images during the excretory phases. CTU has largely replaced the previous gold-standard investigation of intravenous urography (IVU) for investigation of the upper urinary tract, having the advantage of providing complete staging information and details of surrounding organs. Contrast enhancement is particularly useful for characterising mass lesions within the kidney and differentiating benign from malignant lesions (see Fig. 18.32A). CT without contrast gives clear definition of retroperitoneal anatomy regardless of obesity and is superior to ultrasound in this respect. Non-contrast CT of kidneys, ureters and bladder (CTKUB) is the method of choice for demonstrating stones within the kidney or ureter (see Fig. 18.28). For investigation of patients with renal trauma, a triple-phase CT scan with a delayed phase, to assess the integrity of the collecting system, is performed. Drawbacks of contrast-enhanced CT scans include the significant radiation dose required and the fact that contrast medium may cause AKI. The incidence of contrast nephropathy is probably lower than previously thought and the AKI is typically mild and reversible, therefore this potential risk should not preclude CT scanning when indicated (Box 18.4).

Magnetic resonance imaging

Magnetic resonance imaging (MRI) offers excellent resolution and distinction between different tissue types (see Fig. 18.15). It is very useful for local staging of prostate, bladder and penile cancers. Magnetic resonance angiography (MRA) provides an alternative to CT for imaging renal vessels but involves administration of gadolinium-based contrast media, which may carry risks for patients with impaired renal function

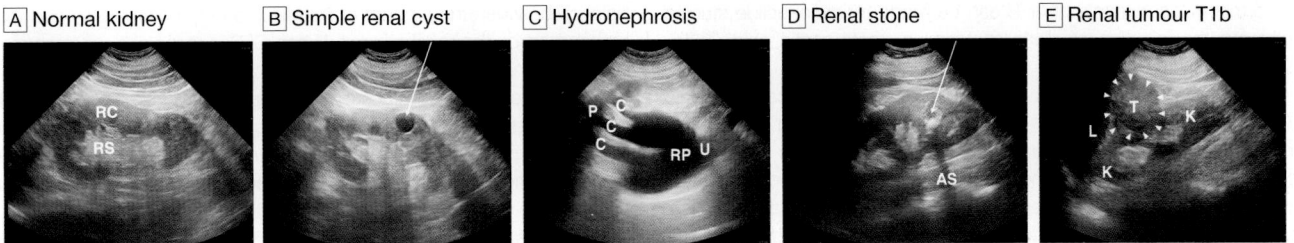

A Normal kidney   B Simple renal cyst   C Hydronephrosis   D Renal stone   E Renal tumour T1b

Fig. 18.4 Renal ultrasound. A Normal kidney. The normal cortex is less echo-dense (blacker) than the adjacent liver. B Simple renal cyst: round, echo-free fluid content, no septa, posterior acoustic enhancement. C The renal pelvis and calyces are dilated due to obstruction. The thinness of the parenchyma (P) indicates chronic obstruction. D A typical renal stone with posterior shadowing. E A T1b renal tumour arising from the renal cortex. (AS = posterior acoustic shadow; C = calyx; K = kidney; L = liver; RC = renal cortex; RP = renal pelvis; RS = renal sinus – calyx, renal pelvis, blood vessels, sinus fat; T = tumour; U = ureter) *(A–E) Courtesy of Dr Tobias Klatte, Addenbrooke's Hospital, Cambridge.*

---

i 18.4 Renal complications of radiological investigations

Contrast nephrotoxicity

- Acute deterioration in renal function commencing <48 hrs after administration of IV radiographic contrast media. Typically modest and reversible AKI

Risk factors

- Pre-existing renal impairment (eGFR <45 mL/min/1.73m^2)
- Use of ionic contrast media and repetitive dosing in short time periods
- Diabetes mellitus and myeloma

Prevention

- Provide hydration with free oral fluids plus IV isotonic saline 500 mL, then 250 mL/hr during procedure
- Withhold NSAIDs. Omit metformin for 48 hrs after the procedure, in moderate or high-risk patients
- If the risks are high (eGFR <30mL/min/1.73m^2), consider alternative methods of imaging, but proceed if benefit of imaging exceeds risk of nephropathy, which is often the case

Cholesterol atheroembolism

- Typically follows days to weeks after intra-arterial investigations or interventions

Nephrogenic sclerosing fibrosis after MRI contrast agents

- Chronic progressive sclerosis of skin, deeper tissues and other organs, associated with gadolinium-based contrast agents
- Only reported in patients with renal impairment, typically on dialysis or with GFR <15 mL/min/1.73 m^2, but caution is advised in patients with GFR <30 mL/min/1.73 m^2
- Rare since switch to more stable gadolinium-based agents

(AKI = acute kidney injury; eGFR = estimated glomerular filtration rate; IV = intravenous; NSAIDs = non-steroidal anti-inflammatory drugs)

(see Box 18.4). Whilst MRA provides good images of the main renal vessels, stenosis of small branch arteries may be missed.

Renal arteriography

Renal arteriography involves obtaining X-rays following an injection of contrast medium directly into the renal artery via a catheter that is usually inserted into the femoral artery. The main indication is to investigate renal artery stenosis (p. 580) or haemorrhage following renal trauma. Renal angiography can be combined with therapeutic balloon dilatation or stenting of the renal artery. It can be used to occlude bleeding vessels and arteriovenous fistulae by the insertion of thin platinum wires (coils), which promote thrombosis, thereby securing haemostasis.

Pyelography

Pyelography involves direct injection of contrast medium into the collecting system from above (antegrade) or below (retrograde). It offers the best views of the collecting system and upper tract, and is often

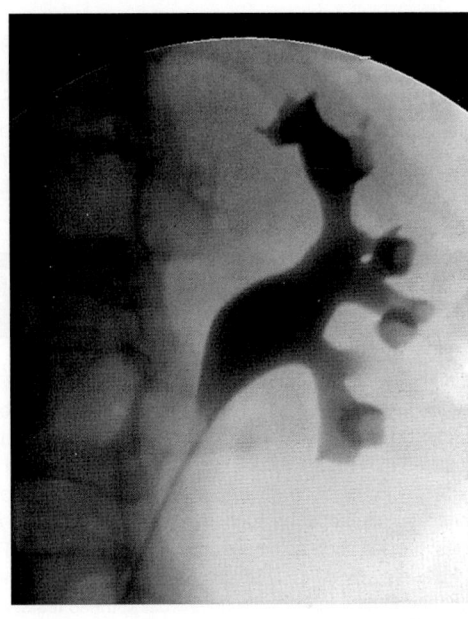

Fig. 18.5 Retrograde pyelography. The best views of the collecting system are obtained by pyelography. A catheter has been passed into the left renal pelvis at cystoscopy. In the image shown the calyces are sharp-edged and normal. *Courtesy of Dr A.P. Bayliss and Dr P. Thorpe, Aberdeen Royal Infirmary.*

used to identify the cause of urinary tract obstruction. Antegrade pyelography requires the insertion of a fine needle into the pelvicalyceal system under ultrasound or radiographic control. In addition to visualising the cause of obstruction, percutaneous nephrostomy drainage can be established and an antegrade stent can be passed through any obstruction. Retrograde pyelography can be performed by inserting a ureteric catheter into the ureteric orifice at cystoscopy (Fig. 18.5) and again a stent can be inserted to bypass any obstruction.

Radionuclide studies

These are functional studies requiring the injection of gamma ray-emitting radiopharmaceuticals that are taken up and excreted by the kidney, a process that can be monitored by an external gamma camera.

Dynamic radionuclide studies are performed with mercaptoacetyltriglycine labelled with technetium (^{99m}Tc-MAG3), which is filtered by the glomerulus and excreted into the urine. Imaging following ^{99m}Tc-MAG3 injection can provide valuable information about the perfusion of each kidney but is not a reliable method for identifying renal artery stenosis. In patients with significant obstruction of the outflow tract, ^{99m}Tc-MAG3 persists in the renal pelvis and a loop diuretic fails to accelerate its disappearance. This study can be useful in determining the functional significance of a collecting system that appears obstructed on imaging.

18

Formal measurements of GFR can be made by radionuclide studies following the injection of diethylenetriamine penta-acetic acid (^{99m}Tc-DPTA) or ^{51}Cr-EDTA.

Static radionuclide studies are performed with dimercaptosuccinic acid labelled with technetium (^{99m}Tc-DMSA), which is taken up by proximal tubular cells. Following intravenous injection, images of the renal cortex are obtained to show the shape, size and relative function of each kidney (Fig. 18.6). This is a sensitive method for demonstrating cortical scarring in reflux nephropathy and a way of assessing the individual function of each kidney.

Radionuclide bone scanning following the injection of methylene diphosphonate (^{99m}Tc-MDP) can assess the presence and extent of bone metastases in men with prostate cancer (p. 610).

Renal biopsy

Renal biopsy is used to establish the diagnosis and severity of renal disease in order to judge the prognosis and need for treatment (Box 18.5). Renal tumour biopsy may be performed to determine the aetiology of a renal mass. The procedure is performed percutaneously under local anaesthetic with ultrasound guidance to ensure accurate needle placement into a renal pole. Light microscopy, electron microscopy and immunohistological assessment of the specimen may all be required.

Presenting problems in renal and urinary tract disease

It is important to recognise that many forms of kidney disease and urological diseases are asymptomatic. For example, most causes of chronic kidney disease do not present with symptoms until kidney function is severely impaired (GFR <20 mL/min/1.73 m²), and even then the symptoms are non-specific, such as lethargy, swelling and loss of appetite and weight. Hence, for many patients kidney disease will only be detected through investigations such as serum creatinine or urinalysis. People at high risk of disease, for example those with diabetes, hypertension or SLE, should therefore be screened regularly using these tests, as should people presenting with symptoms such as oedema. Patients with renal or prostate cancer often have no relevant symptoms and the diagnosis is made serendipitously.

Oliguria/anuria

Oliguria and anuria are defined as a urine output of less than 400 mL/day or 100 mL/day, respectively. The volume of urine produced represents a balance between the amount of fluid filtered at the glomerulus and that reabsorbed by the renal tubules. When GFR is low, urine volumes may still be normal if tubular reabsorption is also reduced; hence patients with advanced kidney disease may not report a reduction in urinary output. Complete anuria, particularly when sudden in onset, may indicate a structural problem such as complete urinary obstruction or vascular occlusion, though it may occur with severe renal disease of any cause (Box 18.6).

Oliguria is common in pre-renal AKI, as the intravascular volume depletion activates the renin–angiotensin–aldosterone system to promote sodium retention and stimulates release of ADH to promote water retention. Indeed, oliguria may precede and predict the onset of AKI and hence urinary output <0.5 mL/kg/hr should prompt assessment of fluid status and correction of volume depletion where present. Urine volume may remain normal in pre-renal failure when there is an osmotic diuresis as occurs in diabetic ketoacidosis with marked glycosuria.

Urine volumes are variable in AKI due to intrinsic renal disease, but a rapid decline in urine volume may be observed. Marked oliguria predicts

---

i   18.5 Renal biopsy

Indications

- Acute kidney injury and chronic kidney disease of uncertain aetiology
- Nephrotic syndrome or glomerular proteinuria (protein:creatinine ratio >100 mg/mol) in adults
- Nephrotic syndrome in children that has atypical features or is not responding to treatment
- Nephritic syndrome
- Renal transplant dysfunction
- Rarely performed for isolated haematuria or isolated low-grade proteinuria in the absence of impaired renal function or evidence of a multisystem disorder

Contraindications

- Disordered coagulation or thrombocytopenia. Aspirin and other antiplatelet agents increase bleeding risk
- Uncontrolled hypertension
- Kidneys <60% predicted size
- Solitary kidney* (except transplants)

Complications

- Pain, usually mild
- Bleeding into urine, usually minor but may produce clot colic and obstruction
- Bleeding around the kidney, occasionally massive and requiring angiography with intervention, or surgery
- Arteriovenous fistula, rarely significant clinically

*Relative contraindication.

---

i   18.6 Causes of anuria (<100 mL urine output per day)

Condition	Examples
Urinary obstruction (complete)	Urinary retention due to prostatic enlargement, urethral stenosis, bladder tumour Bilateral ureteric obstruction due to retroperitoneal fibrosis, cancer, bilateral ureteric stones, radiation injury Bilateral renal stones (usually staghorn calculi) Massive crystalluria obstruction of tubules (rare)
Lack of renal perfusion (bilateral)	Aortic dissection involving renal arteries Severe acute tubular necrosis Severe functional hypoperfusion (cardiorenal, hepatorenal)
Rapidly progressive glomerulonephritis	Anti-glomerular basement membrane disease, severe antineutrophil cytoplasmic antibody (ANCA) vasculitis (100% glomerular crescents on biopsy)

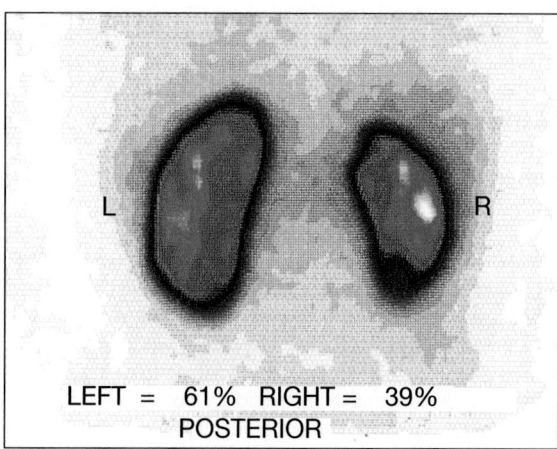

LEFT = 61% RIGHT = 39%
POSTERIOR

Fig. 18.6 DMSA radionuclide scan. A posterior view is shown of a normal left kidney and a small right kidney (with evidence of cortical scarring at upper and lower poles) that contributes only 39% of total renal function.

poor renal outcome in those with glomerulonephritis and poor patient survival in those with acute tubular necrosis in ICU.

Obstruction of the renal tract can result in oliguria and anuria; however, for this to occur the obstruction must be complete and affect both kidneys, unless the patient has a single functioning kidney. Hence, the obstruction is most likely to occur at the level of the bladder outlet, for example in benign prostatic hypertrophy (see Fig. 18.18). It is less common for both ureters to become obstructed simultaneously, though this can occur with retroperitoneal fibrosis or bilateral renal calculi. Partial obstruction can be associated with normal or even high urine volume due to chronic tubular injury, which causes loss of tubular concentrating ability.

Polyuria

Polyuria is defined as a urine volume in excess of 3L/24hrs. Various underlying conditions, both renal and extrarenal, may be responsible, as outlined in Box 18.7.

Investigation of polyuria includes measurement of urea, creatinine, sodium, potassium, osmolarity, glucose and calcium. A 24-hour urine collection may be helpful to confirm the severity of polyuria. The presence of nocturnal polyuria suggests a pathological cause. Investigation and management of suspected diabetes insipidus are described in Chapter 20.

Frequency

Frequency describes daytime micturition more often than a patient would expect. It may be a consequence of polyuria, when urine volume is normal or high, but is also found in patients with urinary infection and prostatic diseases, when small amounts of urine are passed each time and the total daily urine volume is normal.

Nocturia

Nocturia is defined as waking to pass urine during the main sleep period. Nocturia occurs in the recovery phase of AKI and in many patients with CKD due to loss of urine-concentrating ability due to tubular injury. It may also be due to prostatic enlargement when it is associated with other lower urinary tract symptoms such as poor stream, hesitancy, incomplete bladder emptying, terminal dribbling and urinary frequency due to partial urethral obstruction (p. 609). Nocturia may be exacerbated by increased fluid intake or diuretic use in the late evening (including caffeine). It may also occur due to sleep disturbance without any functional abnormalities of the urinary tract.

Urinary incontinence

Urinary incontinence is defined as any involuntary leakage of urine. It may occur in patients with a normal urinary tract, as the result of dementia or poor mobility, or transiently during an acute illness or hospitalisation, especially in older people (see Box 18.52). The pathophysiology,

investigation and management of urinary incontinence are discussed in detail later in the chapter.

Abdominal pain

Loin pain is more often musculoskeletal in origin but can be a manifestation of urinary tract disease; in the latter case, it may arise from renal stones, ureteric stones, renal tumours, acute pyelonephritis and urinary tract obstruction. Acute loin pain radiating to the groin is termed renal colic. This is typical of ureteric obstruction due to calculi and is often accompanied by haematuria. Precipitation of dull loin pain by a large fluid intake (Dietl's crisis) suggests upper urinary tract obstruction such as caused by a congenital pelvi-ureteric junction obstruction (p. 604). Obstruction at the bladder neck is associated with lower midline abdominal discomfort. Chronic obstruction rarely produces pain but may give rise to a dull ache.

Dysuria

Dysuria refers to painful urination, often described as burning or stinging, and is commonly accompanied by suprapubic pain. It is often associated with frequency of micturition and a feeling of incomplete emptying of the bladder. By far the most common cause is urinary tract infection, as described on page 599. Other diagnoses that need to be considered in patients with dysuria include sexually transmitted infections (Ch. 15) and bladder stones (p. 602).

Oedema

Oedema is caused by an excessive accumulation of fluid within the interstitial space. Clinically, this can be detected by persistence of an indentation in tissue following pressure on the affected area (pitting oedema). Non-pitting oedema is typical of lymphatic obstruction and may also occur as the result of excessive matrix deposition in tissues: for example, in hypothyroidism (Ch. 20) or systemic sclerosis (Ch. 26). Oedema may be due to a number of causes (Box 18.8).

Clinical assessment

Dependent areas, such as the ankles and lower legs, are typically affected first but oedema can be restricted to the sacrum in bed-bound

18

18.7 Causes of polyuria

- Excess fluid intake (characterised by low serum osmolarity)
- Osmotic diuresis: hyperglycaemia, hypercalcaemia, sodium-glucose transporter inhibitors
- Cranial diabetes insipidus
- Nephrogenic diabetes insipidus:
  - Rare inherited mutations in vasopressin receptor or aquaporin 2 genes
  - Vasopressin receptor antagonists (tolvaptan)
  - Lithium
  - Interstitial nephritis
  - Hypokalaemia
  - Transiently following recovery from acute tubular necrosis (ATN) or relief of urinary obstruction

---

18.8 Causes of oedema

Increased total extracellular fluid

- Congestive heart failure
- Renal failure
- Liver disease

High local venous pressure

- Deep venous thrombosis or venous insufficiency
- Pregnancy
- Pelvic tumour

Low plasma oncotic pressure/serum albumin

- Nephrotic syndrome
- Liver failure
- Malnutrition/malabsorption

Increased capillary permeability

- Local infection/inflammation
- Severe sepsis
- Calcium channel blockers

Lymphatic obstruction

- Infection: filariasis, lymphogranuloma venereum
- Malignancy
- Radiation injury
- Congenital abnormality

patients. Pitting oedema tends to accumulate in the ankles during the day and improves overnight as the interstitial fluid is reabsorbed. Conversely, facial oedema on waking is common. With increasing severity, oedema spreads to affect the upper parts of the legs, the genitalia and abdomen. Ascites is common and often an earlier feature in children or young adults, and in liver disease. Pleural effusions are common, particularly on the right side. Raised JVP and pulmonary oedema are uncommon in patients with low oncotic pressure such as nephrotic syndrome, but common in the context of increased total extracellular fluid such as in cardiac and renal failure. Features of intravascular volume depletion (tachycardia, postural hypotension) may occur when oedema is due to decreased oncotic pressure or increased capillary permeability. If oedema is localised – for example, to one ankle but not the other – then local inflammation, venous thrombosis or lymphatic disease should be suspected.

Investigations

Blood should be taken for measurement of creatinine and electrolytes, liver function and serum albumin, and the urine tested for protein. Further imaging of the liver, heart or kidneys may be indicated, based on history and clinical examination. Where ascites or pleural effusions occur in isolation, measurement of protein, glucose and LDH, and microscopy for cells in the aspirate will usually differentiate a transudate (typical of oedema) from an exudate (more suggestive of local pathology, p. 494).

Management

Mild oedema usually responds to elevation of the legs, compression stockings, or a thiazide or a low dose of a loop diuretic. In nephrotic syndrome, renal failure and severe cardiac failure, very large doses of diuretics, sometimes in combination, may be required to achieve a negative sodium and fluid balance. Restriction of sodium and fluid intake may be required. Diuretics are not helpful in the treatment of oedema caused by increased capillary permeability or by venous or lymphatic obstruction. Specific causes of oedema, such as venous thrombosis, should be treated.

Hypertension

Hypertension is a very common feature of renal disease. Additionally, the presence of hypertension identifies a population at risk of developing CKD and current recommendations are that hypertensive patients should have renal function checked annually. Control of hypertension is very important in patients with renal impairment because of its close relationship with further decline of renal function (p. 593) and increased cardiovascular risk. Pathophysiology and management are discussed in Chapter 16.

Haematuria

Healthy individuals may have occasional red blood cells in the urine (<3 red blood cells/high power field), but the presence of visible (macroscopic) haematuria or non-visible (microscopic, only detectable on dipstick testing) haematuria is indicative of bleeding from somewhere in the urinary tract (Fig. 18.7). Once infection, menstruation and causes of a positive urinary dipstick in the absence of red cells (haemoglobinuria/myoglobinuria) have been excluded (Box 18.9), both visible and persistent non-visible haematuria require investigation, as they may be caused by malignancy or indicate glomerulonephritis.

Visible haematuria is most likely to be caused by malignancy (14% of patients present with visible haematuria), which can affect any part of the urogenital tract (see Fig. 18.7). Patients with visible haematuria must therefore be referred to urology for imaging (ultrasound or CT scan) and cystoscopy (Fig. 18.8). Other common causes of visible haematuria are urine infection and stones. Visible haematuria may also be encountered in patients with IgA nephropathy, typically following an upper respiratory tract infection.

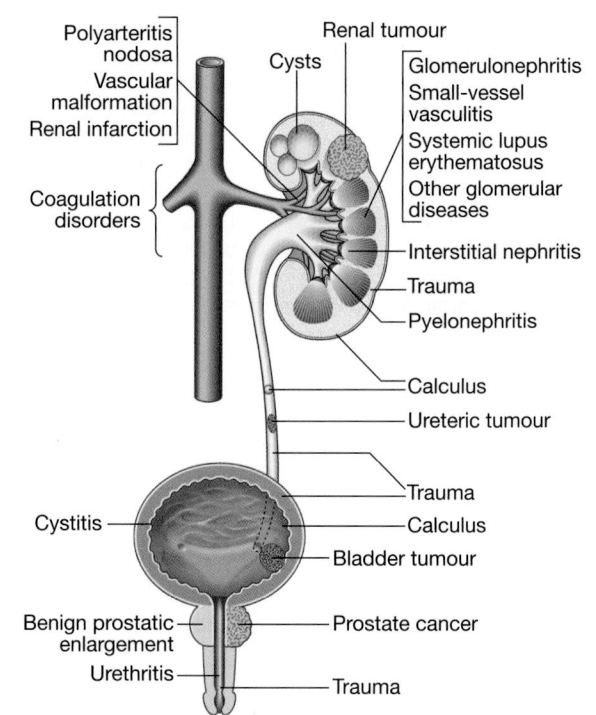

Fig. 18.7 Causes of haematuria.

<table>
<tr><td colspan="3">i 18.9 Interpretation of non-visible haematuria</td></tr>
<tr><th>Dipstick test positive</th><th>Urine microscopy</th><th>Suggested cause</th></tr>
<tr><td>Haematuria</td><td>White blood cells
Abnormal epithelial cells
Red cell casts
Dysmorphic erythrocytes (phase contrast microscopy)</td><td>Infection
Tumour
Glomerular bleeding*</td></tr>
<tr><td>Haemoglobinuria</td><td>No red cells</td><td>Intravascular haemolysis</td></tr>
<tr><td>Myoglobinuria (brown urine)</td><td>No red cells</td><td>Rhabdomyolysis</td></tr>
</table>

*Glomerular bleeding implies that the glomerular basement membrane (GBM) is ruptured. It can occur physiologically following very strenuous exertion but usually indicates intrinsic renal disease and is an important feature of the nephritic syndrome.

Non-visible haematuria may also indicate an underlying cancer, and although guidelines vary, current UK guidelines are that all patients over 60 years old with persistent (detected on at least two of three consecutive dipstick tests) non-visible haematuria and either dysuria or an elevated serum white cell count should therefore undergo imaging and cystoscopy. In younger patients, an underlying tumour is much less likely, and if a glomerular cause is not suspected (see below), it may be appropriate to manage them by periodic observation in primary care, although occasionally these individuals develop significant overt renal disease during follow-up.

Glomerular bleeding occurs when inflammatory, destructive or degenerative processes disrupt the GBM, permitting passage of red blood cells into the urine. A characteristic feature of glomerular bleeding is an 'active urinary sediment' (the presence of dysmorphic red blood cells or red cell casts on microscopy); this is not always present, however. Patients with visible and non-visible haematuria should also be assessed for hypertension, proteinuria, reduced/declining renal function, family history of renal

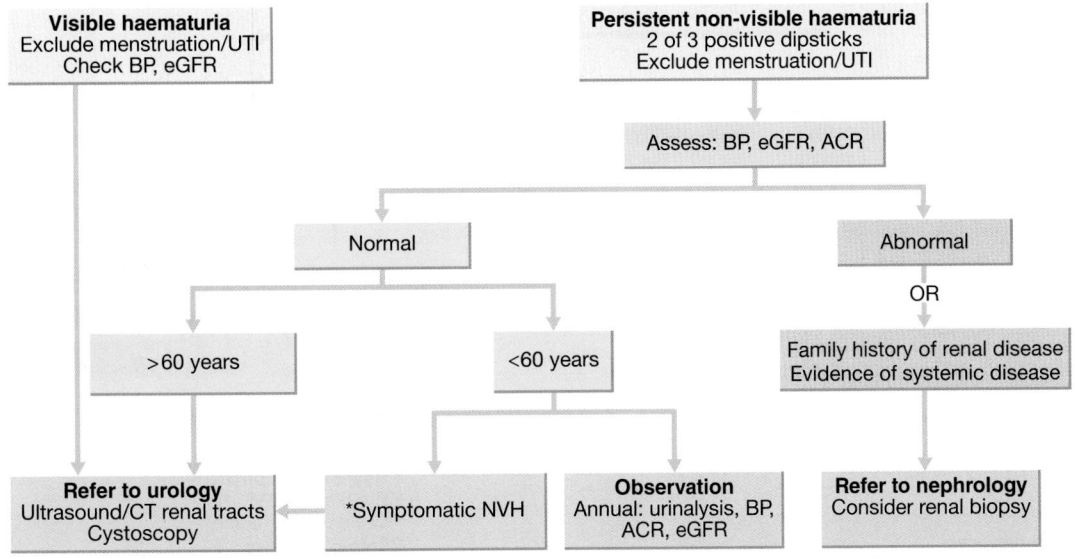

Fig. 18.8 Investigation of haematuria. *Symptomatic: lower urinary tract voiding symptoms such as hesitancy, frequency, urgency and dysuria. (ACR = albumin:creatinine ratio; BP = blood pressure; CT = computed tomography; eGFR = estimated glomerular filtration rate; NVH = non-visible haematuria; UTI = urinary tract infection)

disease or features of systemic disease (see Fig. 18.8). The presence of any of these features raises the possibility of intrinsic renal pathology and warrants referral to nephrology for further investigation, including consideration of renal biopsy.

Nephritic syndrome

The nephritic syndrome is characterised by the presence of haematuria in association with hypertension, oliguria, fluid retention and reduced/declining renal function. Many patients with glomerulonephritis, particularly those with milder disease, do not exhibit all of these features; however, their combined presence is typical of a rapidly progressive glomerulonephritis and warrants urgent investigation. In many cases, investigation will include a renal biopsy to confirm diagnosis and guide management, but less invasive investigations may also be useful (Box 18.10).

Patients with nephritic syndrome may also exhibit varying degrees of proteinuria, including nephrotic-range proteinuria; the prominence of haematuria on dipstick should, however, alert the physician to the possibility of a glomerulonephritis. Indeed, it is important to recognise that the characteristic features of nephritic syndrome and nephrotic syndrome do not always present in isolation, but should be considered to be the extreme phenotypes at either end of a spectrum of presentations (Fig. 18.9).

Proteinuria

While small amounts of high-molecular-weight proteins and moderate amounts of low-molecular-weight proteins pass through the healthy GBM, these proteins normally are completely reabsorbed by tubular cells. Hence, in healthy individuals, less than 150 mg of protein is excreted in the urine each day, much of which is derived from tubular cells. This includes Tamm–Horsfall protein (uromodulin), encoded by the *UMOD* gene, mutations in which have been linked to tubulo-interstitial disease (see Box 18.20). The presence of larger amounts of proteinuria indicates significant renal disease, with greater than 1 g/day indicative of glomerular pathology.

Proteinuria is usually asymptomatic and is often picked up by urinalysis, although large amounts of protein may make the urine frothy. Transient proteinuria can occur after vigorous exercise, during fever, in heart failure and in people with urinary tract infection. Patients should be assessed for the presence of these conditions and urine testing repeated once the potential trigger has been treated or resolved.

18.10 Investigation of nephritic syndrome

Cause	Investigations
Rapidly progressive glomerulonephritis (RPGN)	
Post-infectious glomerulonephritis	ASOT, C3, C4
Anti-GBM disease	Anti-GBM antibody
Small-vessel vasculitis	p-ANCA, c-ANCA
Lupus nephritis	ANA, dsDNA, C3, C4
Mild glomerulonephritic presentation	
IgA nephropathy	Serum IgA (polyclonal rise in 50% of patients)
Mesangioproliferative glomerulonephritis	C3, C4, hepatitis B, C + HIV serology, ANA, dsDNA, immunoglobulins, PPE
Alport syndrome*	Genetic screening, hearing test

*Not a glomerulonephritis but may present in a similar manner with haematuria, variable proteinuria, hypertension and slowly declining renal function.
(ANA = antinuclear antibody; ANCA = antineutrophil cytoplasmic antibody; ASOT = anti-streptolysin O titre; C3, C4 = complement proteins 3, 4; dsDNA = double-stranded DNA; GBM = glomerular basement membrane; HIV = human immunodeficiency virus; IgA = immunoglobulin A; PPE = plasma protein electrophoresis)

Testing for proteinuria is best done on an early morning sample, as some individuals exhibit orthostatic proteinuria. In these patients, urinary dipstick is positive only when upright, with the first morning sample being negative. Orthostatic proteinuria is regarded as a benign disorder that does not require treatment.

Moderately elevated albuminuria (microalbuminuria)

In healthy individuals, there is virtually no urinary excretion of large-molecular-weight serum proteins, such as albumin, in contrast to modest urinary excretion of tubule-derived proteins. The presence of even moderate amounts of albuminuria (previously referred to as microalbuminuria) is therefore abnormal, and is the most sensitive marker of early glomerular pathology, when the standard dipstick test remains negative (Box 18.11). Screening for moderately elevated albuminuria should be performed regularly in patients with diabetes, as persistently high levels warrant therapy with inhibitors of the renin–angiotensin–aldosterone system,

18

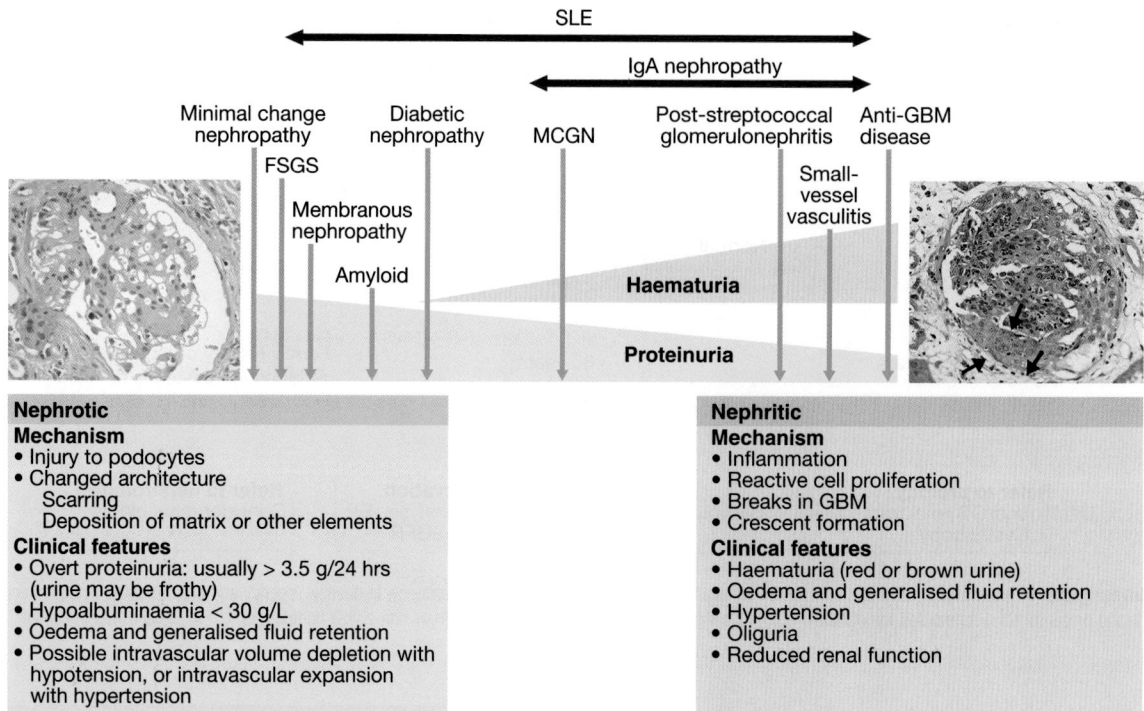

Fig. 18.9 Nephritic and nephrotic syndrome. At one extreme, specific injury to podocytes causes proteinuria and nephrotic syndrome. The histology to the left shows diabetic nephropathy. At the other end of the spectrum, inflammation leads to cell damage and proliferation, breaks form in the glomerular basement membrane (GBM) and blood leaks into urine. In its extreme form, with acute sodium retention and hypertension, such disease is labelled nephritic syndrome. The histology to the right shows a glomerulus with many extra nuclei from proliferating intrinsic cells, and influx of inflammatory cells leading to crescent formation (arrows) in response to severe post-infectious glomerulonephritis. (FSGS = focal and segmental glomerulosclerosis; IgA = immunoglobulin A; MCGN = mesangiocapillary glomerulonephritis; SLE = systemic lupus erythematosus)

i	**18.11**	**Quantifying proteinuria in random urine samples**		
ACR[1] mg/mmol	**PCR[1] mg/mmol**	**Typical dipstick results[2]**	**Significance**	
<3.5 (female) <2.5 (male)	< 25	–	Normal	
3.5–30	25–50	–	Moderately elevated	
30–70	50–100	+ to ++	Dipstick positive	
70–300	100–350	++ to +++	Glomerular disease more likely; equivalent to >1 g/24 hrs	
>300	>350	+++ to ++++	Nephrotic range: almost always glomerular disease, equivalent to >3.5 g/24 hrs	

[1]Values are given for mg/mmol; if urine creatinine is measured in mg/dL, reference values for PCR and ACR can be derived by dividing by 11.31. [2]Dipstick results are affected by urine concentration and are occasionally weakly positive on concentrated samples from healthy individuals.

even in normotensive individuals (see Box 21.30). Persistent moderately increased albuminuria has also been associated with cardiovascular mortality.

Overt (dipstick-positive) proteinuria

Urinary dipstick testing is a valuable screening tool for the detection of proteinuria; it is only semi-quantitative, however, as it is highly dependent on the concentration of the urine. Typically, standard dipsticks test positive for protein once the urinary protein exceeds approximately 0.5 g/24 hrs; however, trace to 1+ may be observed on dipstick in very concentrated urine from healthy individuals. After urinary tract infection has been excluded, all patients with persistent proteinuria on dipstick should have the amount of protein quantified to guide further investigations (Fig. 18.10). When more than 1 g of protein per day is excreted, glomerular disease is likely and this is an indication for renal biopsy. Since 24-hour urine collection is often inaccurate, the protein:creatinine ratio (PCR) in a single sample of urine is preferred. This makes an allowance for the variable degree of urinary dilution and can be used to extrapolate to 24-hour values (see Box 18.11). Changes in PCR also give valuable information about the progression of

renal disease and response to therapy in CKD. It is possible to measure albumin:creatinine ratio (ACR), but this requires a more expensive immunoassay and is usually reserved for situations when high sensitivity is required, such as detection of moderately elevated albuminuria in the early stages of diabetic nephropathy (p. 749).

It is sometimes helpful to identify the type of protein in the urine. Large amounts of low-molecular-weight proteins, such as β_2-microglobulin (molecular weight 12 kDa), in the urine suggest renal tubular damage and are referred to as tubular proteinuria. This rarely exceeds 1.5–2 g/24 hrs (maximum PCR 150–200 mg/mmol; see Box 18.11 for conversion of mg/mmol to mg/dL).

Free immunoglobulin light chains (molecular weight 25 kDa) are filtered freely at the glomerulus but are poorly identified by dipstick tests. Their presence may also be indicated by a 'protein gap', where the PCR is markedly greater than the ACR (i.e. by more than the normal gap of 30 mg/mmol, see Box 18.11). In this context, electrophoresis of the urine and specific immunodetection methods are required to detect immunoglobulin light chains, known as 'Bence Jones protein'. This may occur in AL amyloidosis (Ch. 4) and in plasma-cell dyscrasias such as myeloma (Ch. 25).

Nephrotic syndrome

Nephrotic syndrome is characterised by very heavy proteinuria (>3.5 g/24 hrs), hypoalbuminaemia and oedema. Blood volume may be normal, reduced or increased. Renal sodium retention is an early and universal feature; the mechanisms of this are shown in Figure 19.4. The diseases that cause nephrotic syndrome all affect the glomerulus (see Fig. 18.9), either directly, by damaging podocytes, or indirectly, by causing scarring or deposition of exogenous material such as amyloid into the glomerulus.

Investigation of nephrotic syndrome usually involves renal biopsy, although non-invasive tests may also be helpful in suggesting the underlying cause (Box 18.12). In children, minimal change disease is by far the most common cause of nephrotic syndrome and therefore renal biopsy is not usually required unless the patient fails to respond to high-dose glucocorticoid therapy. Similarly, most patients with diabetes presenting with nephrotic syndrome will have diabetic nephropathy, and so renal biopsy is usually not performed unless the course of the disease is atypical (rapidly increasing proteinuria or rapid decline in renal function; p. 749).

Management of nephrotic syndrome should be directed at the underlying cause. In addition, nephrotic syndrome is associated with a number of complications (Box 18.13), which may require supportive management unless the nephrosis is expected to resolve rapidly, such as in glucocorticoid-responsive minimal change disease. Diuretics are often required to reduce oedema. ACE inhibitors or angiotensin receptor blockade are indicated to reduce intraglomerular pressure and proteinuria, which may lead to an increase in serum albumin concentration.

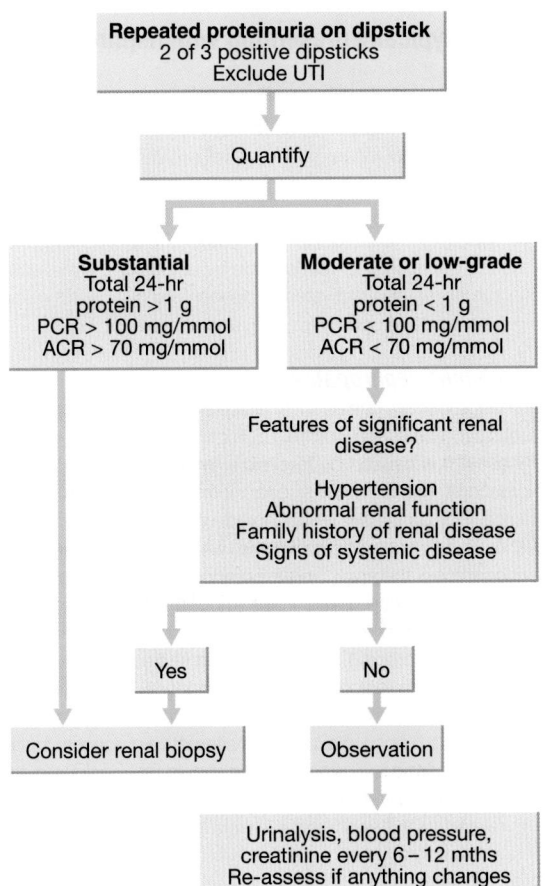

Fig. 18.10 Investigation of proteinuria. (ACR = albumin:creatinine ratio; PCR = protein:creatinine ratio; UTI = urinary tract infection)

Glomerular diseases

Glomerular diseases account for a significant proportion of acute and chronic kidney disease. Most patients with glomerular disease do not present acutely and are asymptomatic until abnormalities are detected on routine screening of blood or urine samples.

There are many causes of glomerular damage, including immunological injury, inherited diseases such as Alport syndrome (p. 577), metabolic diseases such as diabetes mellitus (Ch. 21), and deposition of abnormal proteins such as amyloid in the glomeruli (Ch. 4). The glomerular cell types that may be the target of injury are shown in Fig. 18.11. Proteinuria is the hallmark of glomerular disease; however, the response of the glomerulus to injury and hence the predominant clinical features vary according to the nature of the insult, ranging from fulminant nephrotic syndrome when the primary target is usually the podocyte to rapidly progressive glomerulonephritis (see Fig. 18.9). Several prognostic indicators are common to all causes of glomerulonephritis (Box 18.14) and may be helpful in assessing the need for immunosuppressive therapy.

Glomerulonephritis

While glomerulonephritis literally means 'inflammation of glomeruli', the term is often used more broadly to describe all types of glomerular disease, even though some of these (e.g. minimal change nephropathy) are not associated with inflammation.

Most types of glomerulonephritis are immunologically mediated and several respond to immunosuppressive drugs. Deposition of antibody occurs in many types of glomerulonephritis and testing for circulating or glomerular deposition of antibodies may aid diagnosis (see Fig. 18.11 and Boxes 18.10 and 18.12). In small-vessel vasculitis, no glomerular antibody deposition is observed (pauci-immune), but the antibodies may be indirectly pathogenic by activating neutrophils to promote endothelial injury (see Fig. 18.11).

Glomerulonephritis is generally classified in terms of the histopathological appearances, as summarised in Box 18.15 and Fig. 18.12. Many non-specialists find the terminology used in describing glomerulonephritis confusing, therefore some definitions are provided in Box 18.16. It is important to stress that the histological appearance rarely confirms a specific renal disease but rather suggests a limited range of

18

i 18.12 Investigation of nephrotic syndrome		
Cause	**Typical age group**	**Investigations**
Minimal change disease	Children, young adults, occasionally seen in older patients	None specific
Primary focal segmental glomerulosclerosis	Young adults	None specific
Membranous nephropathy	Middle-aged to older patients	Anti-phospholipase A2 receptor antibody (primary disease) Hepatitis B, C + HIV serology, ANA, dsDNA
Amyloid	Older patients	Immunoglobulins, PPE, Bence Jones protein, serum free light chains
Diabetic nephropathy	Any age, but rarely <10 years from diagnosis of type 1 diabetes	Glucose, glycosylated haemoglobin

(ANA = antinuclear antibody; dsDNA = double-stranded DNA; HIV = human immunodeficiency virus; PPE = plasma protein electrophoresis)

	18.13 Consequences of the nephrotic syndrome and their management			
Feature	**Mechanism**	**Consequence**	**Management**
Hypoalbuminaemia	Urinary protein losses exceed synthetic capacity of liver	Reduced oncotic pressure Oedema	Treatment of underlying cause
Avid sodium retention	Secondary hyperaldosteronism Additional poorly characterised intrarenal mechanisms	Oedema	Diuretics and a low-sodium diet*
Hypercholesterolaemia	Non-specific increase in lipoprotein synthesis by liver in response to low oncotic pressure	High rate of atherosclerosis	Statins, ezetimibe
Hypercoagulability	Relative loss of inhibitors of coagulation (antithrombin III, protein C and S) and increase in liver synthesis of procoagulant factors	Venous thromboembolism	Consideration of prophylaxis in chronic or severe nephrotic syndrome
Infection	Hypogammaglobulinaemia due to urinary loss of immunoglobulins	Pneumococcal and meningococcal infection	Consideration of vaccination

*Severe nephrotic syndrome may need very large doses of combinations of diuretics acting on different parts of the nephron (e.g. loop diuretic plus thiazide plus amiloride). Over-diuresis risks secondary impairment of renal function through hypovolaemia.

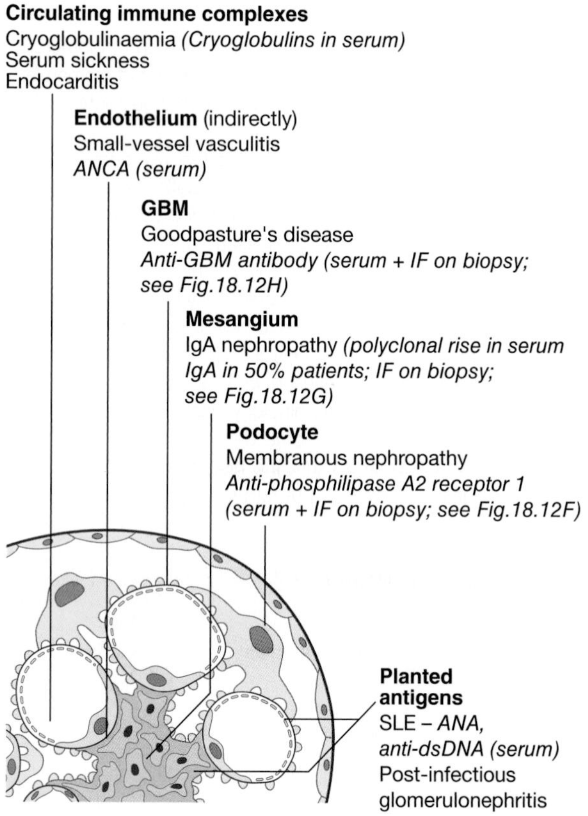

Circulating immune complexes
Cryoglobulinaemia (Cryoglobulins in serum)
Serum sickness
Endocarditis

Endothelium (indirectly)
Small-vessel vasculitis
ANCA (serum)

GBM
Goodpasture's disease
Anti-GBM antibody (serum + IF on biopsy; see Fig.18.12H)

Mesangium
IgA nephropathy (polyclonal rise in serum IgA in 50% patients; IF on biopsy; see Fig.18.12G)

Podocyte
Membranous nephropathy
Anti-phospholipase A2 receptor 1 (serum + IF on biopsy; see Fig.18.12F)

Planted antigens
SLE – ANA, anti-dsDNA (serum)
Post-infectious glomerulonephritis

Fig. 18.11 Glomerulonephritis associated with antibody production. Antibodies and antigen–antibody (immune) complexes may target or be deposited in specific components of the glomerulus, resulting in different patterns of histological injury and clinical presentation. Testing for antibody deposition in the glomerulus by immunofluorescence (IF) on renal biopsy tissue or for antibodies in the serum may aid diagnosis. Diagnostic tests are shown in italics. (ANA = antinuclear antibody; ANCA = antineutrophil cytoplasmic antibody; dsDNA = double-stranded DNA; GBM = glomerular basement membrane; IgA = immunoglobulin A; SLE = systemic lupus erythematosus)

diagnoses, which may be confirmed by further investigation. Conversely, some diseases, such as lupus, are associated with more than one histological pattern of injury. The most common histological subtypes may be categorised according to their typical clinical presentation, as discussed below. Genetic disorders associated with glomerular disease are described later in this chapter.

	18.14 Poor prognostic indicators in glomerular disease

- Male sex
- Hypertension
- Persistent and severe proteinuria
- Elevated creatinine at time of presentation
- Rapid rate of decline in renal function
- Tubulo-interstitial fibrosis observed on renal biopsy

Diseases typically presenting with nephrotic syndrome

In these diseases, the injury is focused on the podocyte and there is little histological evidence of inflammation or cell proliferation in the glomerulus (non-proliferative, see Fig. 18.12). Minimal change and primary focal segmental glomerulosclerosis (FSGS) typically present with fulminant nephrotic syndrome, whereas in membranous nephropathy and secondary FSGS, the nephrosis tends to be more indolent. Other causes of nephrotic syndrome due to systemic disease are discussed elsewhere, including diabetic nephropathy (p. 749) and amyloid (p. 77).

Minimal change nephropathy
Minimal change disease can occur at all ages but accounts for most cases of nephrotic syndrome (see Box 18.15) in children and about one-quarter of adult cases. It is caused by reversible dysfunction of podocytes. On light microscopy, the glomeruli appear normal (Fig. 18.12A), but fusion of podocyte foot processes is observed on electron microscopy. The presentation is with nephrotic syndrome, which typically is severe. High-dose glucocorticoid therapy (1 mg/kg prednisolone for 6 weeks) usually promotes rapid remission of nephrosis, though the response to therapy is often less satisfactory in older patients. Some patients who respond incompletely (glucocorticoid-resistant) or relapse frequently need maintenance glucocorticoids (glucocorticoid dependence) or additional agents such as cytotoxics or calcineurin inhibitors. Glucocorticoid resistance in children warrants a biopsy to exclude an alternative diagnosis, but if minimal change is confirmed, a genetic cause should be considered. Minimal change disease typically does not progress to CKD but can present with problems related to the nephrotic syndrome (see Box 18.11) and complications of treatment.

Focal segmental glomerulosclerosis
Primary focal segmental glomerulosclerosis (FSGS) (Fig. 18.12B) can occur in all age groups and is thought to be due to an as yet undiscovered circulating factor. Histological analysis shows sclerosis initially

Histology	Immune deposits	Pathogenesis	Associations	Comments
i 18.15 Glomerulonephritis categorised by clinical presentation and histological classification				
Nephrotic presentation				
Minimal change				
Normal, except on electron microscopy, where fusion of podocyte foot processes is observed (non-specific finding)	None	Unknown; probable circulating factor promoting podocyte injury. Some cases are genetic (p. 577)	Atopy. Drugs, most commonly NSAIDs. Haematological malignancies	Acute and often severe nephrotic syndrome. Good response to glucocorticoids. Dominant cause of idiopathic nephrotic syndrome in childhood
Focal segmental glomerulosclerosis (FSGS)				
Segmental scars in some glomeruli. No acute inflammation. Podocyte foot process fusion seen in primary FSGS	Non-specific trapping in focal scars	Unknown; circulating factors may increase glomerular permeability. Injury to podocytes may be common feature. Some cases are genetic (p. 577)	*APOL1* variant in people of West African descent. Causes of secondary FSGS include: Healing of previous local glomerular injury; HIV infection; Heroin misuse; Morbid obesity; Chronic hypertension	*Primary FSGS* presents as idiopathic nephrotic syndrome but is less responsive to treatment than minimal change; may progress to renal impairment, and can recur after transplantation. *Secondary FSGS* presents with variable proteinuria and outcome
Membranous nephropathy				
Thickening of GBM. Progressing to increased matrix deposition and glomerulosclerosis	Granular subepithelial IgG	Antibodies to a podocyte surface antigen (commonly phospholipase A_2 receptor 1), with complement-dependent podocyte injury	*HLA-DQA1* (for idiopathic). Drugs: Penicillamine, NSAIDs, heavy metals. Hepatitis B virus. Malignancy. Lupus[1]	Common cause of adult idiopathic nephrotic syndrome. One-third progress, one-third spontaneously remit and one-third remain stable; may respond to glucocorticoids and immunosuppressants
Mild glomerulonephritic presentation				
IgA nephropathy				
Increased mesangial matrix and cells. Focal segmental nephritis in acute disease	Mesangial IgA (and C3)	Unknown. Mucosal infections (e.g. helminths) may be involved	Usually idiopathic, flares triggered by upper respiratory infection. Liver disease. Coeliac disease	Common disease with range of presentations, usually including haematuria and hypertension. Henoch–Schönlein purpura is an acute IgA variant common in children
Mesangiocapillary glomerulonephritis				
Immunoglobulin type	Immunoglobulins	Deposition of circulating immune complexes or 'planted' antigens	Infections, autoimmunity or monoclonal gammopathies	Most common pattern found in association with subacute bacterial infection, but also with cryoglobulinaemia ± hepatitis C virus, and others
Complement type	Complement components	Complement abnormalities, inherited or acquired. Dense deposit disease is associated with abnormal activation of alternative complement pathway	Complement gene mutations. C3 nephritic factor and partial lipodystrophy	In dense deposit disease, intramembranous deposits. No proven treatments
Rapidly progressive glomerulonephritis presentation				
Focal necrotising glomerulonephritis				
Segmental inflammation and/or necrosis in some glomeruli ± crescent formation	Variable according to cause but typically negative (or 'pauci-immune')	Small-vessel vasculitis, often ANCA-mediated	Primary or secondary small-vessel vasculitis	Often occurs in systemic disease. Responds to treatment with glucocorticoids and immunosuppressants
Diffuse proliferative glomerulonephritis[2]				
Infection-related diffuse proliferative glomerulonephritis[3]				
Diffuse proliferation of endothelial and mesangial cells. Infiltration by neutrophils and macrophages ± crescent formation	Subendothelial and subepithelial	Immune complex-mediated (e.g. to streptococcal infection with presumed cross-reactive epitopes)	Post-streptococcal. Concurrent infection with staphylococci, endocarditis	Presents with severe sodium and fluid retention, hypertension, haematuria, oliguria. Usually resolves spontaneously

18

Histology	Immune deposits	Pathogenesis	Associations	Comments
Anti-glomerular basement membrane disease				
Usually crescentic nephritis	Linear IgG along GBM	Autoantibodies to α3 chain of type IV collagen in GBM	*HLA-DR15* (previously known as *DR2*)	Associated with lung haemorrhage but renal or lung disease may occur alone. Treat with glucocorticoids, cyclophosphamide and plasma exchange

i 18.15 Glomerulonephritis categorised by clinical presentation and histological classification—continued

[1]Systemic lupus erythematosus can cause almost any histological injury pattern, most commonly membranous nephropathy or diffuse proliferative glomerulonephritis. [2]In addition to the association with infection and anti-GBM disease, a diffuse proliferative glomerulonephritis picture may also be seen with lupus and occasionally IgA nephropathy. [3]Infection may also present with mesangioproliferative glomerulonephritis and membranous nephropathy (HIV).
(ANA = antinuclear antibody; ANCA = antineutrophil cytoplasmic antibody; APOL1 = apolipoprotein L1; FSGS = focal segmental glomerulosclerosis; GBM = glomerular basement membrane; HLA = human leucocyte antigen; IgA = immunoglobulin A; NSAIDs = non-steroidal anti-inflammatory drugs)

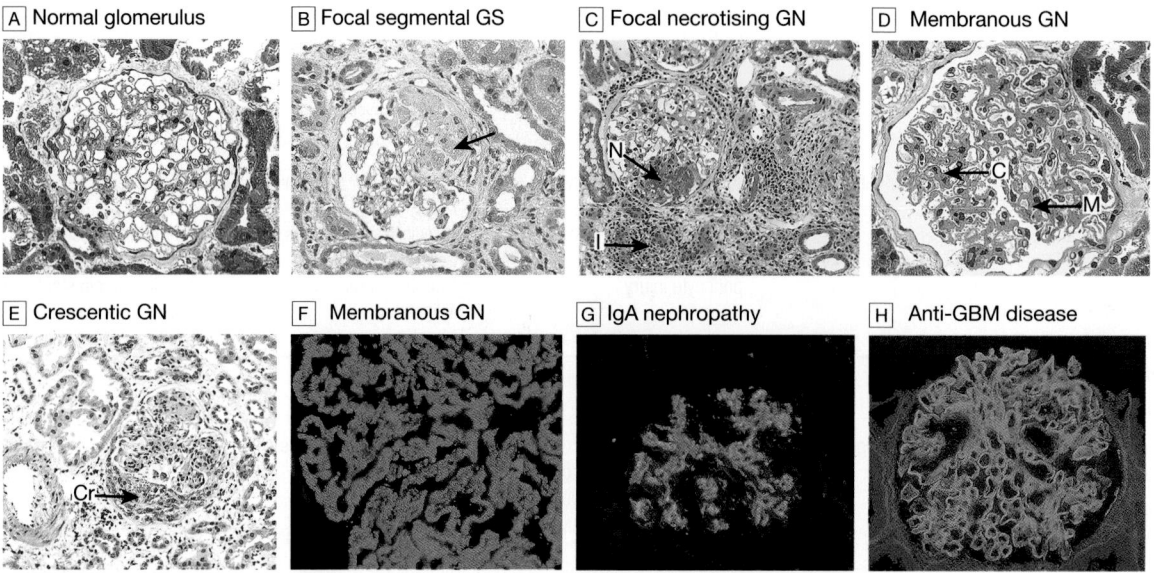

Fig. 18.12 Histopathology of glomerular disease. (**A** – **E** *Light microscopy*) **A** A normal glomerulus. Note the open capillary loops and thinness of their walls. **B** Focal segmental glomerulosclerosis (GS). The portion of the glomerulus arrowed shows loss of capillary loops and cells, which are replaced by matrix. **C** Focal necrotising glomerulonephritis (GN). A portion of the glomerulus (N = focal necrotising lesion) is replaced by bright pink material with some 'nuclear dust'. Neutrophils may be seen elsewhere in the glomerulus. There is surrounding interstitial inflammation (I). This is most commonly associated with small-vessel vasculitis and may progress to crescentic nephritis (see **E**). **D** Membranous glomerulonephritis. The capillary loops (C) are thickened (compare with the normal glomerulus) and there is expansion of the mesangial regions by matrix deposition (M). However, there is no gross cellular proliferation or excess of inflammatory cells. **E** Crescentic glomerulonephritis. The lower part of Bowman's space is occupied by a semicircular formation ('crescent', Cr) of large pale cells, compressing the glomerular tuft. This is seen in aggressive inflammatory glomerulonephritis. *Antibody deposition in the glomerulus* (**F** – **H** *Direct immunofluorescence*). **F** Granular deposits of IgG along the basement membrane in a subepithelial pattern, typical of membranous GN. **G** Immunoglobulin A (IgA) deposits in the mesangium, as seen in IgA nephropathy. **H** Ribbon-like linear deposits of anti-GBM antibodies along the glomerular basement membrane in Goodpasture's disease. The glomerular structure is well preserved in all of these examples. *(A, C, D, E) Courtesy of Dr J.G. Simpson, Aberdeen Royal Infirmary; (F, G, H) Courtesy of Dr R. Herriot.*

limited to segments of the glomeruli, which may also show positive staining for deposits of C3 and IgM on immunofluorescence. Since FSGS is a focal process, abnormal glomeruli may not be detected on renal biopsy if only a few are sampled, leading to an initial diagnosis of minimal change nephropathy.

In most cases the underlying cause is unknown (primary FSGS) and these patients typically present with abrupt onset of severe nephrotic syndrome. Primary FSGS may respond to high-dose glucocorticoid therapy (0.5–2.0 mg/kg/day) but the response is rarely as rapid as in minimal change disease. Immunosuppressive drugs, such as calcineurin inhibitors, cyclophosphamide and mycophenolate mofetil, have also been used but their efficacy is uncertain. Progression to CKD is common in patients who do not respond to glucocorticoids and the disease frequently recurs after renal transplantation.

FSGS is particularly common in people of West African descent, who, compared with other ethnicities, have a much higher carriage rate

of apolipoprotein L1 (*APOL1*) gene variants that are associated with increased risk of FSGS. In addition, mutations in other podocyte proteins may cause FSGS (see Genetic renal diseases section below). FSGS may also be secondary to other diseases such as human immunodeficiency virus (HIV) renal disease (particularly in African Americans), morbid obesity or chronic hypertension. In addition, it may reflect scarring from previous focal glomerular injury resulting from HUS, cholesterol embolism or vasculitis. Patients with secondary FSGS typically present with more modest proteinuria than those with primary disease and rarely exhibit full-blown nephrotic syndrome. Management of secondary FSGS is focused on treating the underlying cause and reducing proteinuria by inhibiting the renin–angiotensin system.

Membranous nephropathy

Membranous nephropathy is the most common cause of nephrotic syndrome in people of European descent. It is caused by antibodies

---

18.16 Terminology used in glomerulonephritis

Light microscopy

- *Focal*: affecting some but not all glomeruli
- *Diffuse*: affecting > 50% of glomeruli
- *Segmental*: affecting a portion of a glomerulus
- *Global*: affecting all of the glomerulus
- *Necrotising*: severe injury leading to an area of necrosis, usually associated with vasculitis
- *Crescentic*: a crescent-shaped area of inflammatory cells responding to severe glomerular injury

Electron microscopy

- *Subendothelial immune deposits*: found between the endothelial cell and the GBM – often found in nephritic presentations
- *Intramembranous immune deposits*: found within the GBM – found in the dense deposit variant of mesangiocapillary glomerulonephritis
- *Subepithelial immune deposits*: found between the epithelial cell and the GBM – often found in nephrotic presentations, including membranous presentation of lupus

(GBM = glomerular basement membrane)

(usually autoantibodies) directed at antigen(s) expressed on the surface of podocytes, including the M-type phospholipase A_2 receptor 1, and is characterised by thickening of the glomerular basement membrane on light microscopy (see Fig. 18.12). While most cases are idiopathic, a proportion are associated with other causes, such as heavy metal poisoning, drugs, infections, lupus and tumours (see Box 18.15). Approximately one-third of patients with idiopathic membranous nephropathy undergo spontaneous remission, one-third remain in a nephrotic state, and one-third develop progressive CKD. Management includes tight blood pressure control, in particular with inhibitors of the renin–angiotensin–aldosterone system. In idiopathic disease immunosuppression treatment may improve both the nephrotic syndrome and the long-term prognosis and regimens include steroids with either cyclophosphamide or rituximab. However, because of the toxicity of these regimens, many nephrologists reserve such treatment for those with severe nephrotic syndrome or deteriorating renal function. Treatment of secondary membranous nephropathy is directed at the underlying cause.

Diseases typically presenting with mild nephritic syndrome

Patients with mild glomerulonephritis typically present with non-visible haematuria and modest proteinuria, and their renal disease tends to follow a slowly progressive course. IgA nephropathy and mesangiocapillary glomerulonephritis (MCGN) typically fall in this category. However, their presentation is highly variable: IgA nephropathy occasionally presents with rapidly progressive glomerulonephritis while MCGN may present with nephrotic syndrome. Other diseases that present with haematuria, modest proteinuria and slow progression include Alport syndrome.

IgA nephropathy

This is one of the most common types of glomerulonephritis and can present in many ways. Haematuria is the earliest sign and non-visible haematuria is almost universal, while hypertension is also very common. These are often detected during routine screening: for example, at occupational medical examinations. Proteinuria can also occur but is usually a later feature. In many cases, there is slowly progressive loss of renal function leading to end-stage renal disease (ESRD), though in others, renal function is persistently normal. A particular hallmark of IgA nephropathy in young adults is the occurrence of acute self-limiting exacerbations, often with visible haematuria, in association with minor respiratory infections. This may be so acute as to resemble acute post-infectious glomerulonephritis, with fluid retention, hypertension and oliguria with dark or red urine. Characteristically, the latency from clinical infection to

nephritis is short, in contrast to post-infectious glomerulonephritis, which typically occurs after the infection has resolved. Asymptomatic presentations dominate in older adults, with non-visible haematuria, hypertension and reduced GFR. Occasionally, IgA nephropathy progresses rapidly in association with crescent formation on biopsy. Management is largely directed towards the control of blood pressure, with renin–angiotensin system inhibitors preferable in those with proteinuria. There is some evidence for additional benefit from several months of high-dose glucocorticoid treatment in those at high risk of progressive disease (see Box 18.14), but no strong evidence for other immunosuppressive agents. A role for other therapies, such as fish oil, remains uncertain.

Henoch–Schönlein purpura

This condition most commonly occurs in children but can also be observed in adults. It is a systemic vasculitis that often arises in response to an infectious trigger. It presents with a tetrad of features:

- a characteristic petechial rash typically affecting buttocks and lower legs
- abdominal pain due to vasculitis involving the gastrointestinal tract
- arthralgia
- renal disease characterised by visible or non-visible haematuria, with or without proteinuria.

Renal biopsy shows mesangial IgA deposition and appearances that are indistinguishable from acute IgA nephropathy (Fig. 18.12G). Treatment is supportive in nature; in most patients, the prognosis is good, with spontaneous resolution, though relapses are common. Some patients, particularly adults and those with severe or persistent proteinuria, progress to develop ESRD.

Mesangiocapillary glomerulonephritis

Mesangiocapillary glomerulonephritis (MCGN), also known as membranoproliferative glomerulonephritis, is a pattern of injury seen on renal biopsy that is characterised by an increase in mesangial cellularity with thickening of glomerular capillary walls. The typical presentation is with proteinuria and haematuria. Several underlying causes have been identified, as summarised in Box 18.15. It can be classified into two main subtypes. The first is characterised by deposition of immunoglobulins within the glomeruli. This subtype is associated with chronic infections, autoimmune diseases and monoclonal gammopathy. The second is characterised by deposition of complement in the glomeruli and is associated with inherited or acquired abnormalities in the complement pathway. This category comprises 'dense deposit disease', which is typified by electron-dense deposits within the GBM, and C3 glomerulonephritis that shows deposits of C3 in the glomerulus.

Treatment of MCGN associated with immunoglobulin deposits consists of the identification and treatment of the underlying disease, if possible, and the use of immunosuppressive drugs such as mycophenolate mofetil or cyclophosphamide. There are few specific treatments for MCGN associated with complement dysregulation, although eculizumab, the anti-C5 inhibitor that prevents formation of the membrane attack complex, has shown promise.

Diseases typically presenting with rapidly progressive glomerulonephritis

Rapidly progressive glomerulonephritis (RPGN) is characterised by rapid loss of renal function over days to weeks, usually in association with hypertension and oedema. Non-visible haematuria is almost always present, with variable amounts of proteinuria, while characteristic red cell casts and dysmorphic red cells may be observed on urine microscopy (see Fig. 18.3). Renal biopsy typically shows crescentic lesions (Fig. 18.12E), often associated with necrotising lesions within the glomerulus (Fig. 18.12C), particularly in small-vessel vasculitides.

This pattern of presentation is typical of post-infectious glomerulonephritis, anti-GBM disease and small-vessel vasculitides (Ch. 26). It can also be observed in SLE and occasionally in IgA and other nephropathies (see Fig. 18.9).

Anti-glomerular basement membrane disease

Anti-GBM disease is a rare autoimmune disease in which antibodies develop against the α3 chain of type 4 collagen in the GBM. Expression of the α3 chain is largely restricted to the basement membranes of glomeruli and lungs, and hence the disease may present with rapidly progressive glomerulonephritis, lung haemorrhage, or disease of both organs, when it is known as Goodpasture's disease. Goodpasture's disease is more common in younger patients, while older adult patients often present with renal-limited disease. Patients with anti-GBM disease should be treated with plasma exchange combined with glucocorticoids and immunosuppressants, but early diagnosis is essential, as renal function is rarely recoverable in those requiring dialysis at presentation.

The combination of glomerulonephritis and pulmonary haemorrhage may also be observed with small-vessel vasculitis (particularly granulomatosis with polyangiitis, previously known as Wegener's granulomatosis) and lupus.

Infection-related glomerulonephritis

RPGN may occur either during or following an infection. In both cases, circulating immune complexes are present and activation of the complement system promotes consumption of complement factors, resulting in low serum C3 and C4 concentration, as observed in many causes of glomerulonephritis (Box 18.17).

Post-infectious glomerulonephritis is observed most commonly in children and young adults, and typically presents 10 days *after* a streptococcal throat infection or longer after a skin infection. The clinical presentation ranges from mild abnormalities on urinalysis to RPGN with severe AKI. The anti-streptolysin (ASO) test is positive in up to 95% of patients with streptococcal throat infections. Treatment is supportive, with control of blood pressure and fluid overload with salt restriction, diuretics and dialysis if required. Antibiotic therapy is rarely needed, as the renal disease occurs after the infection has subsided. The medium-term prognosis for children and most adults is good, with recovery of renal function typical even in those requiring dialysis therapy. Some patients may develop CKD 20–30 years after the original presentation.

An immune complex-mediated disease may also be observed *during* an infection, typically a staphylococcal infection such as endocarditis, skin infection or pneumonia, but also with subacute endocarditis due to *Streptococcus viridans*. This occurs more commonly in older adults and the presentation tends not to be as fulminant as with post-streptococcal disease. In addition to supportive measures, antibiotic therapy is required, as infection is usually concurrent with renal disease.

Tubulo-interstitial diseases

These diseases primarily affect the renal tubules and interstitial components of the renal parenchyma. They are characterised by tubular dysfunction with electrolyte abnormalities, moderate levels of proteinuria and varying degrees of renal impairment. Often the urinary output may be relatively preserved for any given GFR, and indeed there may be polyuria and nocturia due to loss of concentrating ability in damaged tubules.

Acute interstitial nephritis

Acute interstitial nephritis (AIN) is an immune-mediated disorder, characterised by acute inflammation affecting the tubulo-interstitium of the kidney. It is commonly drug-induced, typically due to antibiotics and proton pump inhibitors (PPIs), but can be caused by other toxins, and can complicate a variety of systemic diseases and infections (Box 18.18). Ingestion of mushrooms within the *Cortinarius* genus can cause a devastating and irreversible AIN. It is encountered occasionally in Scandinavia and Scotland.

18.17	**Causes of glomerulonephritis associated with low serum complement**

- Post-infectious glomerulonephritis
- Subacute bacterial infection, especially endocarditis
- Systemic lupus erythematosus
- Cryoglobulinaemia
- Mesangiocapillary glomerulonephritis, usually complement type

18.18	**Causes of acute interstitial nephritis**

Allergic

Many drugs but particularly:

- Penicillins
- Non-steroidal anti-inflammatory drugs (NSAIDs)
- Proton pump inhibitors
- Mesalazine (delayed)

Immune

- Autoimmune nephritis ± uveitis
- Transplant rejection

Infections

- Acute bacterial pyelonephritis
- Leptospirosis
- Tuberculosis
- Hantavirus

Toxic

- Myeloma light chains
- Mushrooms (*Cortinarius*)

Clinical features

The clinical presentation is typically with AKI and it may cause a rapid deterioration in renal function. AIN should always be considered in patients with non-oliguric AKI. In some patients with drug-induced AIN there may be signs of a generalised drug hypersensitivity reaction with fever and rash. Eosinophilia occurs in 20%–30% of cases, so its absence does not rule out AIN, but its presence should prompt a drug history. Proteinuria is generally modest (PCR <100 mg/mmol; see Box 18.11 for conversion of mg/mmol to mg/dL). The urine may contain white blood cells and white cell casts but is sterile on culture. Leucocytes are commonly present on urinalysis.

Investigations

Renal biopsy is usually required to confirm the diagnosis (Fig. 18.13D). This typically shows evidence of intense inflammation, with infiltration of the tubules and interstitium by lymphocytes. The presence of eosinophils may suggest drug-induced AIN and a predominant neutrophil infiltration suggests infection. Often granulomas may be evident, especially in drug-induced AIN. The degree of chronic inflammation in a biopsy is a useful predictor of long-term renal function. Eosinophiluria may be present but is not a good discriminator for AIN.

Management

Some patients with drug-induced AIN recover following withdrawal of the drug alone, but high-dose glucocorticoids (prednisolone 1 mg/kg/day) may accelerate recovery and prevent long-term scarring. Other specific causes (see Box 18.18) should be treated, if possible.

Chronic interstitial nephritis

Chronic interstitial nephritis (CIN) is characterised by renal dysfunction. It may follow on from AIN that does not resolve, or may be associated with ingestion of various toxins and drugs, particularly those taken chronically, such as lithium or non-steroidal anti-inflammatory drugs (NSAIDs). In addition, it is associated with metabolic and chronic inflammatory diseases, as summarised in Box 18.19. In many patients, CIN presents at a late stage and no underlying cause can be identified.

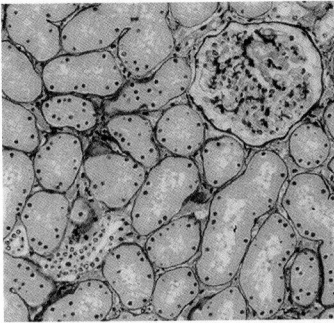

A Normal tubular histology

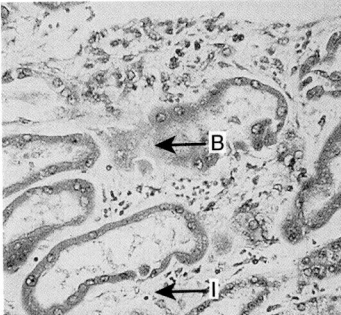

B Acute tubular necrosis

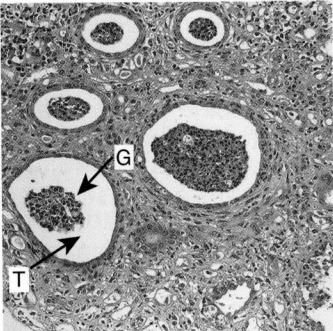

C Acute pyelonephritis

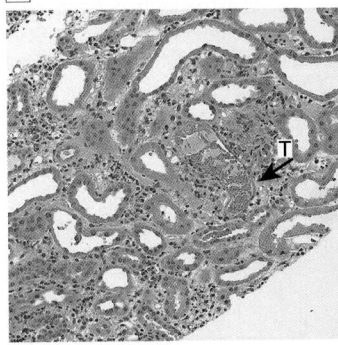

D Acute interstitial nephritis

Fig. 18.13 Tubular histopathology. A Normal tubular histology. The tubules are densely packed with minimal space between. Brush borders can be seen on the luminal borders of cells in the proximal tubule. B Acute tubular necrosis. There are scattered breaks (B) in tubular basement membranes, swelling and vacuolation of tubular cells, and, in places, apoptosis and necrosis of tubular cells with shedding of cells into the lumen. During the regenerative phase, there is increased tubular mitotic activity. The interstitium (I) is oedematous and infiltrated by inflammatory cells. C Acute bacterial pyelonephritis. There is a widespread inflammatory infiltrate that includes many neutrophils. Granulocyte casts (G) are forming within some dilated tubules (T). Other tubules are scarcely visible because of the extent of the inflammation and damage. D Acute (allergic) interstitial nephritis. In this patient who received a non-steroidal anti-inflammatory drug (NSAID), an extensive mononuclear cell infiltrate (no neutrophils) in the tubule-interstitium (T) is seen. Sometimes eosinophils are prominent.

Pathophysiology

Genetic causes may underlie many of these cases (p. 577) while autoimmune mechanisms are also common. Toxins that have been associated with CIN include those contained within the plant *Aristolochia clematitis* (birthwort). These are probably responsible for the severe nephrotoxicity that can be associated with treatment with herbal medicines in Asia and for Balkan nephropathy, which affects isolated rural communities in Bosnia, Bulgaria, Croatia, Romania and Serbia, possibly through contaminated flour. The nephropathy is commonly linked with tumours of the collecting system and is probably due to the mutagenic effects of the plant toxin on the urothelial epithelium. Chronic interstitial nephritis in agricultural communities (also known as CKD of unknown cause, CKDu) is observed in central American countries and Sri Lanka. The cause is unknown, but is likely to reflect a toxin used in agriculture exacerbated by episodes of dehydration due to heat exposure.

Clinical features

Most patients with CIN present in adult life with CKD. A minority have salt-losing nephropathy due to impairment of urine-concentrating ability and sodium conservation. This presents with polyuria, nocturia and hypotension and puts them at risk of AKI during an acute illness. Renal tubular acidosis (p. 631) may complicate CIN but is seen most often in myeloma, sarcoidosis, cystinosis, amyloidosis and Sjögren syndrome. Typically, urinalysis is unremarkable and small kidneys are observed on ultrasound scan. Renal biopsy demonstrates infiltration of the renal parenchyma by lymphocytes, plasma cells and macrophages, in association with tubular atrophy and interstitial fibrosis.

Management

Management is to identify and withdraw or treat the primary cause. Otherwise, treatment is supportive in nature, with correction of acidosis and hyperkalaemia; replacement of fluid and electrolytes, as required; and renal replacement therapy if irreversible renal damage has occurred.

Papillary necrosis

The renal papillae lie within a hypoxic and hypertonic environment in the renal medulla, at the end of the vasa recta. They are susceptible to ischaemic damage because of this and can undergo necrosis when their vascular supply is impaired as the result of diabetes mellitus, sickle-cell disease or long-term ingestion of NSAIDs. The condition may occasionally occur in other diseases. There is an association with pyelonephritis but it is difficult to determine whether this is a cause of papillary necrosis or a complication. The clinical presentation is variable. Some patients are asymptomatic and clinically silent, whereas others present with renal colic and renal impairment as necrosed papillae slough off and cause ureteric obstruction. Urinalysis may be normal but more frequently haematuria and sterile pyuria are present. Significant proteinuria is unusual. The imaging method of choice to make the diagnosis is CTU or intravenous pyelography. Management is based on relieving obstruction, where present, and withdrawal of the offending drugs.

Genetic renal diseases

The advent of modern genetic techniques such as next-generation sequencing has allowed us to understand the breadth of inherited renal diseases on a much deeper level than before.

Inherited glomerular diseases

Alport syndrome

A number of uncommon diseases may involve the glomerulus in childhood but the most important one affecting adults is Alport syndrome. Most cases arise from a mutation or deletion of the *COL4A5* gene on the X chromosome, which encodes the alpha 5 subunit of type IV collagen, resulting in inheritance as an X-linked recessive disorder (Ch. 3). Mutations in *COL4A3* or *COL4A4* genes are less common and cause autosomal disease, which may be recessive or dominant and affect males and females equally. The accumulation of abnormal collagen results in a progressive degeneration of the GBM (Fig. 18.14). Affected patients progress from haematuria to ESRD in late adolescence or their twenties. Female carriers of *COL4A5* mutations usually have haematuria but less commonly develop significant renal disease. Some other

18

basement membranes containing the same collagen isoforms are similarly involved, notably in the cochlea, so that Alport syndrome is associated with sensorineural deafness and ocular abnormalities.

Angiotensin-converting enzyme (ACE) inhibitors may slow but not prevent loss of kidney function. Patients with Alport syndrome are good candidates for renal replacement therapy (RRT), as they are young and usually otherwise healthy. They can develop an immune response to the normal collagen antigens present in the GBM of the donor kidney and, in a small minority, anti-GBM disease develops and destroys the allograft.

---

i 18.19 Causes of chronic interstitial nephritis

Acute interstitial nephritis

- Any of the causes of acute interstitial nephritis, if persistent (see Box 18.18)

Glomerulonephritis

- Varying degrees of interstitial inflammation occur in association with most types of inflammatory glomerulonephritis

Immune/inflammatory

- Sarcoidosis
- Sjögren syndrome
- Chronic transplant rejection
- Systemic lupus erythematosus, primary autoimmune

Toxic

- *Aristolochia* in herbal medicines
- Lead
- Balkan nephropathy
- Chronic interstitial nephritis in agriculture communities (CKDu)

Drugs

- All drugs causing acute interstitial nephritis
- Tenofovir
- Lithium toxicity
- Analgesic nephropathy
- Ciclosporin, tacrolimus

Infection

- Consequence of severe pyelonephritis

Congenital/developmental

- Vesico-ureteric reflux: associated but causation not clear
- Renal dysplasias: often associated with reflux
- Inherited: now well recognised but mechanisms unclear
- Other: Wilson's disease, sickle-cell nephropathy, medullary sponge kidney (nephrocalcinosis)

Metabolic and systemic diseases

- Calcium phosphate crystallisation after excessive phosphate administration (e.g. phosphate enemas in patients with chronic kidney disease)
- Hypokalaemia
- Hyperoxaluria

Thin glomerular basement membrane disease

In thin glomerular basement membrane disease there is non-visible haematuria without associated hypertension, proteinuria or a reduction in GFR. The glomeruli appear normal by light microscopy but, on electron microscopy, the GBM is abnormally thin. The condition may be familial and some patients are carriers of Alport mutations. This does not appear to account for all cases, and in many patients the cause is unclear. Monitoring of these patients is advisable, as proteinuria may develop in some and there appears to be an increased rate of progressive CKD in the long term.

Hereditary nephrotic syndrome

Many genes have been discovered that cause early-onset nephrotic syndrome, often with an FSGS pattern of injury on histology. Inheritance may be autosomal dominant or recessive, the former conditions having a less severe and later-onset phenotype and often exhibiting incomplete penetrance. The involved genes almost all code for podocyte proteins, including nephrin ('Finnish-type' nephropathy) and podocin, which both cause early congenital nephrotic syndrome. Autosomal dominant mutations in various genes may cause FSGS as part of systemic syndromes; the genes include *INF2* (Charcot–Marie–Tooth disease), *LMX1B* (nail-patella syndrome) and *WT1* (abnormal genitalia, Wilms' tumour, mental retardation).

Inheriting certain polymorphisms in the *APOL1* gene, which occur predominantly in people of West African ancestry, leads to a greatly increased risk of kidney disease in adults, including FSGS.

Inherited tubulo-interstitial diseases

It has become evident in recent years that a significant number of cases of CKD with low or absent proteinuria have genetic causes, which may be inherited in an autosomal dominant or recessive pattern and include genes predominantly expressed in tubular cells (Box 18.20). This is a heterogeneous group of inherited disorders. Small cysts are sometimes evident, explaining the previous name of medullary cystic kidney disease, but tubulo-interstitial nephritis is the predominant pattern of injury. Many of these conditions, especially those formerly known as nephronophthisis, are associated with retinal dystrophies and brain or other abnormalities, and some may be associated with hyperuricaemia or gout (*UMOD* or *HNF1-beta* mutations). Many patients will progress to ESRD in later life. Modern genetics have brought clarity to a disease spectrum comprising many different conditions with previous descriptive names.

Isolated defects of tubular function

An increasing number of disorders have been identified that are caused by specific defects in transporter molecules expressed in renal tubular cells. Only the most common are mentioned here. Renal glycosuria is a

---

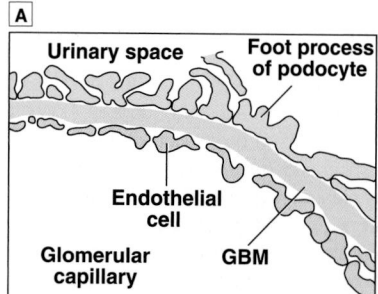 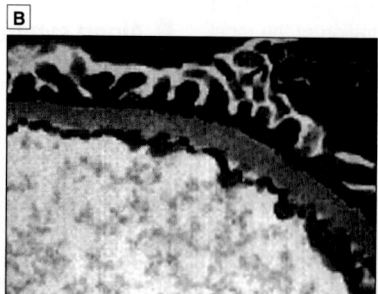 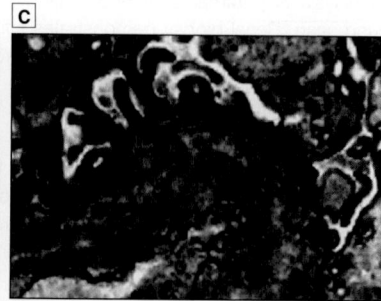

Fig. 18.14 Alport syndrome. A Diagrammatic structure of the normal glomerular basement membrane (GBM). B The normal GBM (electron micrograph) contains mostly the tissue-specific ($\alpha 3$, $\alpha 4$ and $\alpha 5$) chains of type IV collagen. C In Alport syndrome, this network is disrupted and replaced by $\alpha 1$ and $\alpha 2$ chains. Although the GBM appears structurally normal in early life, in time thinning appears, progressing to thickening, splitting and degeneration. *(B, C) Courtesy of Dr J. Collar, St Mary's Hospital, London.*

benign autosomal recessive defect of tubular reabsorption of glucose, caused by mutations of the sodium/glucose co-transporter *SGLT2*. Glucose appears in the urine in the presence of a normal blood glucose concentration. Notably, *SGLT2* inhibitors have been developed as a treatment for diabetes mellitus.

Cystinuria is a rare condition, in which reabsorption of filtered cystine, ornithine, arginine and lysine is defective. It is caused by mutations in the *SLC3A1* amino acid transporter gene. The high concentration of cystine in urine leads to cystine stone formation (p. 602).

Other uncommon tubular disorders include hereditary hypophosphataemic rickets, in which reabsorption of filtered phosphate is reduced; nephrogenic diabetes insipidus (Ch. 20), in which the tubules are resistant to the effects of vasopressin (antidiuretic hormone, ADH). In Bartter and Gitelman syndromes, there are inactivating mutations in the genes that encode the Na-K-2Cl and NaCl transporters, the targets of loop and thiazide diuretics respectively. Hence, both disorders present with sodium-wasting and hypokalaemia (Ch. 19).

The term 'Fanconi syndrome' is used to describe generalised proximal tubular dysfunction. The condition typically presents with low blood phosphate and uric acid concentrations, glycosuria, aminoaciduria and proximal renal tubular acidosis. In addition to the causes of interstitial nephritis described above, some congenital metabolic disorders are associated with Fanconi syndrome, notably Wilson's disease, cystinosis and hereditary fructose intolerance.

Renal tubular acidosis describes the common end-point of a variety of diseases affecting distal (classical or type 1) or proximal (type 2) renal tubular function. These syndromes may also be inherited and are described in Chapter 19.

Cystic diseases of the kidney

It is common to encounter patients with a single renal cyst or even multiple cysts as an incidental finding, especially in those aged 50 years and over. Usually, these cysts are of no clinical consequence and are asymptomatic, but occasionally they can cause pain or haematuria. In addition, several specific diseases are recognised as being caused by the formation of multiple renal cysts. These are discussed in more detail below.

Autosomal dominant polycystic kidney disease

Autosomal dominant polycystic kidney disease (PKD) is a common condition, with a prevalence of approximately 1:1000. Small cysts lined by tubular epithelium develop from infancy or childhood and enlarge slowly and irregularly. The surrounding normal kidney tissue is compressed and progressively damaged. Mutations in the *PKD1* gene account for 80% of cases and those in *PKD2* for about 15% (coding for polycystin 1 and 2 genes, respectively) with some other rare genes

accounting for the remainder. The median age of ESRD is approximately 52 years with a *PKD1* mutation and 70 years with a *PKD2* mutation. It has been estimated that between 5% and 10% of patients with ESRD have PKD.

Clinical features

Common clinical features are shown in Box 18.21. Affected people are usually asymptomatic until later life but hypertension occurs from the age of 20 onwards. One or both kidneys may be palpable and the surface may feel nodular. About 30% of patients with PKD also have hepatic cysts (see Fig. 24.39) but disturbance of liver function is rare. Sometimes (almost always in women) the cysts cause massive and symptomatic hepatomegaly, usually concurrent with renal enlargement but occasionally with only minor renal involvement. Berry aneurysms of cerebral vessels are an associated feature in about 5% of patients with PKD. This feature appears to be largely restricted to certain families (and presumably specific mutations). Mitral and aortic regurgitation is frequent but rarely severe, and colonic diverticula and abdominal wall hernias may occur.

Investigations

The diagnosis is usually based on family history, clinical findings and ultrasound examination. Ultrasound demonstrates cysts in approximately 95% of affected patients over the age of 20 and is the screening method of choice, but may not detect small developing cysts in younger subjects. Cysts may also be identified by other imaging modalities, such as MRI (Fig. 18.15). Simple renal cysts may occur in normal individuals but are uncommon below the age of 30. The following criteria exist for an ultrasound diagnosis of PKD in patients with a family history but unknown genotype:

- 15–39 years of age: at least three unilateral or bilateral kidney cysts
- 40–59 years of age: at least two cysts in each kidney
- 60 years or older: at least four cysts in each kidney.

It is possible to make a molecular diagnosis by next-generation sequencing of *PKD1* or *PKD2*. This is used in cases with an uncertain

18

> **i 18.21 Autosomal dominant polycystic kidney disease: common clinical features**
>
> - Vague discomfort in loin or abdomen due to increasing mass of renal tissue
> - Acute loin pain or renal colic due to cyst rupture, haemorrhage into a cyst or ureteric stones
> - Hypertension
> - Haematuria – often visible, but with little or no proteinuria
> - Urinary tract or cyst infections
> - Renal failure

> **i 18.20 Hereditary tubulo-interstitial kidney diseases**

Inheritance	Gene(s)	Other name(s)	Clinical features
Autosomal dominant	*UMOD*	MCKD type 2 Juvenile hyperuricaemic nephropathy	Gout
	MUC1	MCKD type 1	Progressive CKD without other manifestations
	HNF1-beta	Juvenile hyperuricaemic nephropathy	Cystic kidneys, solitary kidney; gout; MODY; abnormal LFTs; pancreatic atrophy; hypomagnesaemia
	REN (codes for renin)	Juvenile hyperuricaemic nephropathy	Gout; hyperkalaemia; salt-losing nephropathy
Autosomal recessive	*NPHP* genes (>20 genes discovered so far)	Nephronophthisis Part of many syndromes (Bardet–Biedl)	Common cause of paediatric ESRD Occurs earlier than AD interstitial nephritis Extrarenal manifestation common (learning difficulty, eye/limb problems)

(AD = autosomal dominant; CKD = chronic kidney disease; ESRD = end-stage renal disease; LFTs = liver function tests; MCKD = medullary cystic kidney disease; MODY = maturity-onset diabetes of the young)

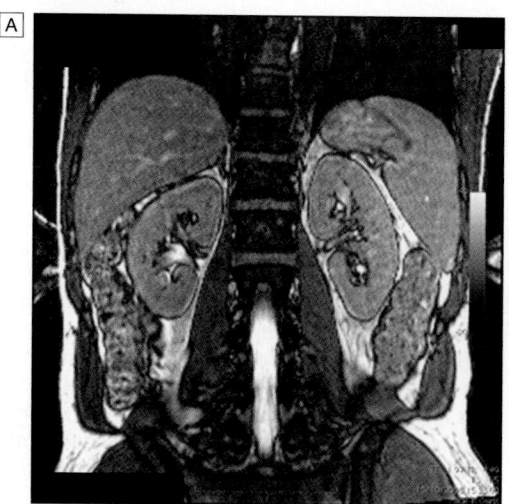
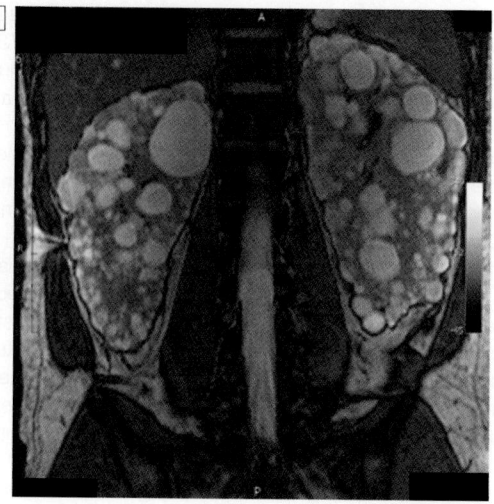

Fig. 18.15 **MRI images of the kidneys.** [A] Normal kidneys. [B] Polycystic kidneys; although the kidney enlargement is extreme, this patient had only slightly reduced GFR.

diagnosis (young patients, few cysts, lack of family history), for workup of living kidney donors, or for screening for mutations associated with a worse prognosis (see below). Screening for intracranial aneurysms is not generally indicated but can be done by MR angiography in families with a history of subarachnoid haemorrhage. The yield of screening is low, however, and the risk:benefit ratio of intervention in asymptomatic aneurysms in this disease is not clear.

Management

Blood pressure control is important because cardiovascular morbidity and mortality are so common in renal disease, but evidence is lacking that controlling blood pressure to generally recommended CKD targets (e.g. <130/80 mmHg) influences renal outcomes. There are data suggesting that targeting a very low blood pressure (<110/75 mmHg) with ACE inhibitors or angiotensin II receptor blocker (ARBs) leads to slower increases in kidney volume, but no improvements in eGFR decline were observed and these targets are often not tolerated. This tight blood pressure target did lead to a greater decline in left ventricular mass index, which may have implications for improved cardiovascular risk later in life.

The vasopressin V2 receptor antagonist tolvaptan slows the increase in kidney volume and the rate of GFR decline. It has been licensed in many countries for patients at high risk of progression. Risk factors for progression include large kidneys (more specifically height-adjusted kidney volume), truncating *PKD1* mutations, and family history of early progression, as well as male sex, hypertension, proteinuria and development of early symptomatic cysts.

Patients with PKD are usually good candidates for dialysis and transplantation. Sometimes kidneys are so large that one or both have to be removed to make space for a renal transplant. Otherwise, they are usually left in situ unless they are a source of pain or infection.

Other cystic diseases

Renal cysts and diabetes syndrome is caused by *HNF1-beta* mutations; it has a varying renal phenotype that often causes cysts but also may cause a tubulo-interstitial pattern of injury or congenital anomalies of the kidneys. It also causes a form of maturity-onset diabetes of the young (MODY).

Autosomal recessive PKD is caused by mutations in the *PKHD1* gene, encoding fibrocystin. It is less common than autosomal dominant PKD (about 1:20000 live births). Patients often present in infancy or young childhood with renal cysts and congenital hepatic fibrosis.

Some uncommon autosomal dominantly inherited conditions are associated with multiple renal cysts and tumours in adult life. In tuberous sclerosis, replacement of renal tissue by multiple angiomyolipomas

may occasionally cause renal failure in adults. Patients may also develop renal cysts and have a higher risk of renal cell carcinoma. Other organs affected include the skin (adenoma sebaceum on the face) and brain (causing seizures and mental retardation). von Hippel–Lindau syndrome is associated with multiple renal cysts, renal adenomas and renal cell carcinoma. Other involved organs include the central nervous system (haemangioblastomas), pancreas (serous cystadenomas) and adrenals (phaeochromocytoma).

A number of other rarer inherited cystic diseases are recognised that have some similarities to PKD but distinct genetic causes. Multicystic dysplastic kidneys are often unilateral and are a developmental abnormality found in children. Most of these seem to involute during growth, leaving a solitary kidney in adults.

Acquired cystic kidney disease can develop in patients with a very long history of renal failure, so it is not an inherited cystic disease. It is associated with increased erythropoietin production and sometimes with the development of renal cell carcinoma. The kidneys are usually normal or small in size and with a smooth outline, which can be useful to distinguish acquired from genetic disease.

Renal vascular diseases

Diseases that affect renal blood vessels may cause renal ischaemia, leading to acute or chronic kidney disease or secondary hypertension. The rising prevalence of atherosclerosis and diabetes mellitus in ageing populations has made renovascular disease an important cause of ESRD.

Renal artery stenosis

A stenosis of more than 50% may be observed on imaging of the renal arteries in up to 20% of older patients with advanced kidney disease; however, a haemodynamically significant effect will be present in only a relatively small proportion. Renal artery stenosis is the most common cause of secondary hypertension, with an estimated prevalence of about 2% in unselected patients, but this may increase to 4% in older patients who have evidence of atherosclerotic disease elsewhere. Most cases of renal artery stenosis are caused by atherosclerosis but fibromuscular dysplasia involving the vessel wall may be responsible in younger patients. Rare causes include vasculitis, thromboembolism and aneurysms of the renal artery.

Pathophysiology

Renal artery stenosis results in a reduction in renal perfusion pressure, which activates the renin–angiotensin system, leading to increased circulating levels of angiotensin II. This results in hypertension by provoking vasoconstriction and increasing aldosterone production by the adrenal, causing sodium retention by the renal tubules (p. 619). Significant reduction of renal blood flow occurs when there is more than 70% narrowing of the artery, and this is commonly associated with distal, post-stenotic dilatation. Atherosclerotic lesions are typically ostial and are associated with more widespread atherosclerosis within the aorta and other vessels, particularly the iliac vessels. There is often concurrent small-vessel disease in affected kidneys, due to subclinical atheroemboli. As the stenosis becomes more severe, global renal ischaemia leads to shrinkage of the affected kidney and may cause renal failure if bilateral or if unilateral in the presence of a single kidney (ischaemic nephropathy).

In younger patients, fibromuscular dysplasia is a more likely cause of renal artery stenosis. This is an uncommon disorder of unknown cause. It is characterised by hypertrophy of the media (medial fibroplasia), which narrows the artery but rarely leads to total occlusion. It may be associated with disease in other arteries; for example, those who have carotid artery dissections are more likely to have renal arteries with this appearance. It most commonly presents with hypertension in patients aged 15–30 years, and women are affected more frequently than men. Irregular narrowing (beading) may occur in the distal renal artery and this sometimes extends into the intrarenal branches of the vessel. Rarely, renal artery stenosis may occur as a complication of large-vessel vasculitis, such as Takayasu's arteritis and polyarteritis nodosa (see Ch. 26).

Untreated, atheromatous renal artery stenosis is thought to progress to complete arterial occlusion in about 15% of cases. This figure increases with more severe degrees of stenosis. If the progression is gradual, collateral vessels may develop and some function may be preserved, preventing infarction and loss of kidney structure. Conversely, at least 85% of patients with renal artery stenosis will not develop progressive renal impairment, and many patients die from coronary, cerebral or other vascular disease rather than renal failure. Unfortunately, methods of predicting which patients are at risk of progression or who will respond to treatment are still imperfect.

Clinical features

Renal artery stenosis can present in various ways, including hypertension, acute pulmonary oedema, progressive renal failure (with bilateral disease) or a deterioration in renal function when ACE inhibitors or ARBs are administered. Although many patients experience a slight drop in GFR when commencing these drugs, an increase in serum creatinine of 30% or more raises the possibility of renal artery stenosis. Acute pulmonary oedema is particularly characteristic of bilateral renovascular disease. It typically occurs at night and is associated with severe hypertension, often in the context of normal or only mildly impaired renal and cardiac function. Clinical evidence of generalised vascular disease may be observed, particularly in the legs and in older patients with atherosclerotic renal artery stenosis. Clinical features associated with an increased risk of renal artery stenosis in hypertensive patients are summarised in Box 18.22. However, given the risk of imaging and angiography in patients with renal disease (see Box 18.4), further investigation should be performed only if intervention is being contemplated (see below).

Investigations

When appropriate, imaging of the renal vasculature with either CT angiography or MR angiography should be performed to confirm the diagnosis (Fig. 18.16). Both give good views of the main renal arteries, the vessels most amenable to intervention. Biochemical testing may reveal impaired renal function and an elevated plasma renin activity, sometimes with hypokalaemia due to hyperaldosteronism. Ultrasound may also reveal a discrepancy in size between the two kidneys, although this is insufficiently sensitive or specific to be of value in diagnosis of renovascular disease in hypertensive patients.

Management

The first-line management in patients with renal artery stenosis is medical therapy with antihypertensive drugs, supplemented, where appropriate,

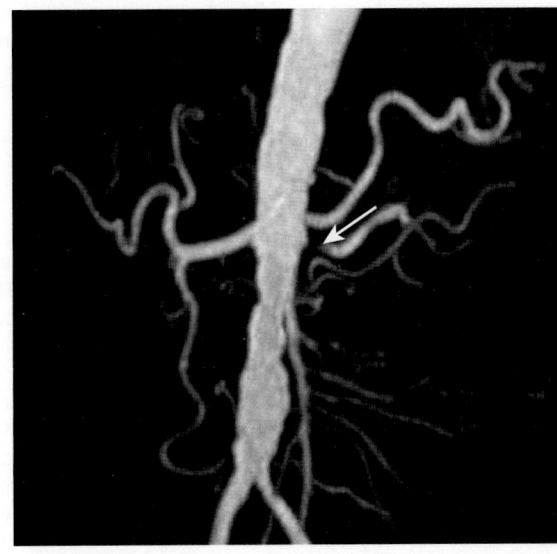

Fig. 18.16 Renal artery stenosis. A magnetic resonance angiogram following injection of contrast. The abdominal aorta is severely irregular and atheromatous. The left renal artery is stenosed (arrow).

by statins and low-dose aspirin in those with atherosclerotic disease. Interventions to correct the vessel narrowing should be considered in:

- young patients (age below 40) suspected of having renal artery stenosis
- those whose blood pressure cannot easily be controlled with antihypertensive agents
- those who have a history of 'flash' pulmonary oedema
- those with accelerated phase (malignant) hypertension
- those whose renal function is deteriorating.

The most commonly used technique is angioplasty. The best results are obtained in non-atheromatous fibromuscular dysplasia, where correction of the stenosis has a high chance of success in improving blood pressure and protecting renal function. Beyond the indications above, angioplasty and stenting is now rarely performed in atherosclerotic disease, as randomised trials such as ASTRAL and CORAL have produced no convincing evidence for overall benefit in terms of renal function, blood pressure control or cardiovascular outcomes. The risks of angioplasty and stenting include renal artery occlusion, renal infarction and atheroemboli (see below) from manipulations in a severely diseased aorta. Small-vessel disease distal to the stenosis may preclude substantial functional recovery.

Acute renal infarction

This is an uncommon condition that occurs as the result of sudden occlusion of the renal artery. The presentation is typically with loin pain of acute onset, usually in association with non-visible haematuria, but pain may be absent in some cases. Severe hypertension is common but not universal. Blood levels of lactate dehydrogenase (LDH) and CRP are commonly raised. The condition may be caused by thrombosis of a renal artery or by thromboemboli from a distant source, when occlusion may occur in branch arteries distal to the main renal artery. This can cause multiple infarcts within the renal parenchyma of both kidneys, which may be visualised by CT scanning. If occlusion of the main renal arteries is bilateral or if there is occlusion in a single functioning kidney, the presentation is with AKI and the patient is typically anuric. Patients with bilateral occlusion usually have evidence of widespread vascular disease and may show evidence of aortic occlusion, with absent femoral pulses and reduced lower limb perfusion. Management is largely supportive, and includes anticoagulation if a source of thromboembolism is identified. It is sometimes possible to perform stenting of an acutely blocked main renal artery to try to restore renal blood flow; in most cases, however, presentation is too late to salvage renal function.

Diseases of small intrarenal vessels

Thrombotic microangiopathies

A number of conditions are associated with acute damage and occlusion of small blood vessels (arterioles and capillaries) in the kidney (Box 18.23) and other organs. A common feature of these syndromes is microangiopathic haemolytic anaemia (MAHA), in which haemolysis and red cell fragmentation arise as a consequence of damage incurred to red blood cells during passage through the abnormal vessels. The red blood cell fragments (schistocytes) may be observed on blood films, together with laboratory features of intravascular haemolysis (p. 955), including an elevated unconjugated bilirubin level, raised serum LDH concentration and decreased circulating levels of haptoglobin. A reticulocytosis is often seen. Endothelial injury is pronounced, leading to increased platelet adherence and a marked reduction in the platelet count. These abnormal blood parameters should alert the physician to the possibility of a thrombotic microangiopathy and may also be useful in monitoring response to treatment. The key is to distinguish between the various aetiologies, as the management differs according to the primary cause (see Box 18.23).

Haemolytic uraemic syndrome

Haemolytic uraemic syndrome (HUS) is characterised by thrombotic microangiopathy that predominantly affects the renal microcirculation, with involvement of other organs (including the brain) observed in more severe cases.

The most common cause of HUS is infection with organisms that produce enterotoxins called Shiga-like toxin or verotoxins. The organisms most commonly implicated are enterohaemorrhagic *Escherichia coli* and *Shigella dysenteriae*. The *E. coli* O157:H7 serotype is the best known but other serotypes that produce verotoxins may also be responsible. Although these bacteria live as commensals in the gut of cattle and other livestock, they can cause haemorrhagic diarrhoea in humans when the infection is contracted from contaminated food products, water or other infected individuals. In a proportion of cases, verotoxin produced by the organisms enters the circulation and binds to specific glycolipid receptors that are expressed on the surface of microvascular endothelial cells. Most cases are sporadic but large outbreaks related to poor sanitation may occur. In developed countries, Shiga-like toxin-associated HUS is now the most common cause of AKI in children. Recovery is good in most patients but sometimes RRT may be required, usually temporarily. Some patients may initially recover, but develop CKD in later life. No specific treatments have been shown to accelerate renal recovery.

In the absence of bloody diarrhoea, other (atypical) causes of HUS should be considered, in particular, abnormalities of the complement system. Familial forms are due to mutations in various genes that encode components or regulators of the complement cascade, including factor H (*CFH*), factor I (CFI), factor B (*CFB*), membrane co-factor protein (*MCP*) and complement component 3 (*C3*). The penetrance of familial HUS is incomplete, indicating that environmental triggers are also involved: often infection, including diarrhoea. Sporadic cases may be associated with the development of autoantibodies to complement factor H. In addition to supportive care, including RRT if necessary, management of complement-mediated HUS includes plasma exchange to replace complement

i	18.23 Thrombotic microangiopathies associated with acute renal damage		
Condition	**Typical features**		**Management**
Primary thrombotic microangiopathies			
Haemolytic uraemic syndrome:	Renal failure prominent in all causes		
Shiga toxin +ve HUS	Bloody diarrhoea; check stool for *Escherichia coli* O157:H7		Supportive therapy
Complement-mediated	Positive family history; screen for complement factor mutations		Plasma exchange, eculizumab
Drug-induced: quinine, calcineurin and VEGF-A inhibitors	Drug exposure, fever with quinine		Cessation of offending drug
Thrombotic thrombocytopenic purpura	Neurological manifestations prominent; check ADAMTS-13 activity		Plasma exchange
Thrombotic microangiopathy associated with systemic disorders			
Disseminated intravascular coagulation (DIC)	Clotting system involvement: elevated D-dimers, low fibrinogen, prolonged PT and APTT		Treatment of primary cause
Malignancy	May occur with breast, prostate, lung, pancreas and GI tumours		Treatment of tumour where possible
Systemic sclerosis	Cutaneous features of systemic sclerosis		Blood pressure control with ACE inhibitors
Pre-eclampsia and HELLP syndrome	Typically in third trimester; abnormal LFTs		Resolution with delivery
Malignant hypertension	Blood pressure typically very high; evidence of hypertensive retinopathy including papilloedema		Blood pressure control

(ACE = angiotensin-converting enzyme; ADAMTS-13 = a disintegrin and metalloproteinase with a thrombospondin type 1 motif, member 13; APTT = activated partial thromboplastin time; GI = gastrointestinal; HELLP = haemolysis, elevated liver enzymes and low platelets; HUS = haemolytic uraemic syndrome; LFTs = liver function tests; PT = prothrombin time; VEGF = vascular endothelial growth factor)

components and remove pathogenic autoantibodies. Impressive results have been reported with the anti-C5 monoclonal antibody, eculizumab, which binds to C5, thereby preventing activation of the terminal complement cascade.

Thrombotic thrombocytopenic purpura

Like HUS, thrombotic thrombocytopenic purpura (TTP) is characterised by microangiopathic haemolytic anaemia and thrombocytopenia; in contrast, however, the brain is more commonly affected in TTP and involvement of the kidney is usually less prominent. TTP is an autoimmune disorder caused by antibodies against ADAMTS-13, which is involved in regulating platelet aggregation, and a low (<10%) serum ADAMTS-13 activity level may be useful in distinguishing TTP from HUS. This distinction is important, as early therapy with plasma exchange is crucial in TTP. More details are provided on page 988.

Cholesterol emboli

These present with renal impairment, haematuria, proteinuria and sometimes eosinophilia with inflammatory features that can mimic a small-vessel vasculitis. The symptoms are provoked by showers of cholesterol-containing microemboli, arising in atheromatous plaques in major arteries. The diagnosis should be suspected when these clinical features occur in patients with widespread atheromatous disease, who have undergone interventions such as surgery or arteriography. They may also be precipitated by anticoagulants and thrombolytic agents. On clinical examination, signs of large-vessel disease and microvascular occlusion in the lower limbs (ischaemic toes, livedo reticularis) are common but not invariable (Fig. 18.17). There is no specific treatment.

Small-vessel vasculitis

Renal disease caused by small-vessel vasculitis usually presents with a clinical picture typical of a glomerulonephritis (see Figs. 18.9 and 18.12C). More information is given below.

Renal involvement in systemic conditions

The kidneys may be directly involved in a number of multisystem diseases or secondarily affected by diseases of other organs. Involvement may be at a pre-renal, renal (glomerular or interstitial) or post-renal level. Many of the diseases are described in other sections of this chapter or in other chapters of the book.

Diabetes mellitus

Diabetic nephropathy is the most common cause of CKD in developed countries. In patients with diabetes, there is a steady advance from moderately elevated albuminuria (microalbuminuria) to dipstick-positive proteinuria, in association with evolving hypertension and progressive renal failure, as described on page 749. Few patients require renal biopsy to establish the diagnosis, but atypical features such as very rapid

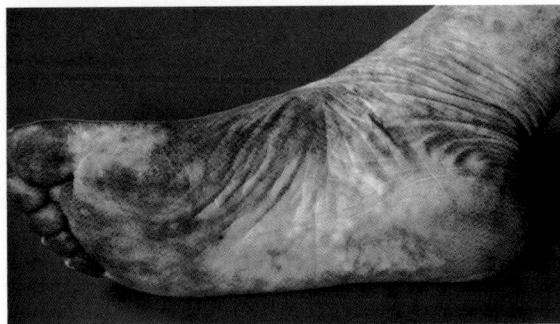

Fig. 18.17 The foot of a patient who suffered extensive atheroembolism following coronary artery stenting.

progression of proteinuria/decline in renal function or the absence of microvascular disease in other organs, including retinopathy, should lead to suspicion that an alternative condition could be present.

Management with ACE inhibitors and ARBs to slow progression is described on page 749. In some patients, proteinuria may be eradicated and progression completely halted, although most still have progressive disease, albeit at a slower rate. SGLT2 inhibitors, reduce cardiovascular mortality and progression of kidney disease at the expense of increased risk of genital infections.

Multiple myeloma

In myeloma, a malignant clone of plasma cells produces a paraprotein, often a monoclonal light chain. Renal manifestations are dominated by these toxic light chains, which may cause a variety of insults (Box 18.24). Hypercalcaemia may also occur due to bony metastases.

Hepatic–renal disease

Severe hepatic dysfunction may cause a haemodynamically mediated type of renal failure, hepatorenal syndrome (HRS), described on page 877. Patients with chronic liver disease are also predisposed to develop AKI (acute tubular necrosis) in response to relatively minor insults, including bleeding, diuretic therapy and infection. Differentiating true HRS from acute tubular necrosis (ATN) can be difficult, but in HRS the urinary sodium is typically low. Patients with true HRS are often difficult to treat by dialysis and have a poor prognosis. Where treatment is justified – for example, if there is a good chance of recovery or of a liver transplant – slow or continuous renal replacement therapy treatments are less likely to precipitate or exacerbate hepatic encephalopathy. IgA nephropathy (p. 575) is more common in patients with chronic liver disease.

Sarcoidosis

Sarcoidosis may lead to a granulomatous interstitial nephritis, sometimes presenting acutely, where renal function may improve with glucocorticoid therapy. Postmortem examinations reveal a chronic interstitial nephritis in 15%–30% of patients with sarcoidosis but clinically relevant disease appears to be much less common.

18.24 Renal manifestations of multiple myeloma

Condition	Presentation	Pathogenesis
Cast nephropathy ('myeloma kidney')	AKI Little/no proteinuria	Light chains combine with Tamm–Horsfall protein precipitating in tubules
Fanconi syndrome	Aminoaciduria, phosphaturia, glycosuria Proximal (type II) RTA	Proximal tubular injury due to light chain deposition in tubular epithelium
AL (primary) amyloidosis*	Proteinuria/nephrotic syndrome Renal impairment	Misfolded light chains (usually lambda) form amyloid, which is deposited in glomeruli
Monoclonal immunoglobulin deposition disease*	Proteinuria (may be in nephrotic range) Renal impairment	Usually light chains (frequently kappa) are deposited in glomeruli, causing a nodular glomerulosclerosis
Hypercalcaemia	Thirst, polyuria, bony and abdominal pain, headache	Bony destruction from metastases

*These may also occur as primary conditions without myeloma being present.
(AKI = acute kidney injury; RTA = renal tubular acidosis)

Systemic vasculitis

Small-vessel vasculitis (Ch. 26) commonly affects the kidneys, with rapid and profound impairment of glomerular function. Histologically, there is a focal inflammatory glomerulonephritis, usually with focal necrosis (see Box 18.15 and Fig. 18.12C) and often with crescentic changes (see Fig. 18.12C). Typically, the patient is systemically unwell with an acute phase response, weight loss and arthralgia. In some patients, it presents as a kidney-limited disorder, with rapidly deteriorating renal function and crescentic nephritis (a rapidly progressive glomerulonephritis). In others, pulmonary haemorrhage may occur, which can be life-threatening.

The most important cause is ANCA vasculitis (Ch. 26). Two subtypes are recognized: microscopic polyangiitis (MPA) and granulomatosis with polyangiitis. Both may present with constitutional symptoms and glomerulonephritis, though lung and ENT involvement is more common with granulomatosis with polyangiitis. Gastrointestinal involvement, arthritis, scleritis/uveitis, purpuric rash and neuropathy may also occur. Serological testing for antibodies to myeloperoxidase (MPO) and proteinase 3 (PR3) is usually positive (see Box 18.10) but these are not specific and a biopsy of affected tissue should be obtained, if possible, to confirm the diagnosis.

The standard treatment of glomerulonephritis associated with systemic vasculitis is high-dose glucocorticoids combined with cyclophosphamide, or mycophenolate mofetil (p. 1012). Recent studies indicate that rituximab is as effective as oral cyclophosphamide, when combined with high-dose glucocorticoids. Plasma exchange can offer additional benefit in patients with progressive renal damage who are not responding adequately to immunosuppressive therapy.

Glomerulonephritis secondary to vasculitis may rarely be seen in rheumatoid arthritis, SLE and cryoglobulinaemia, although SLE can affect the kidney in several different ways (see below).

Medium- to large-vessel vasculitis, such as polyarteritis nodosa (Ch. 26), does not cause glomerulonephritis but can cause hypertension, renal aneurysms and infarction if the renal vessels are involved.

Systemic sclerosis

Renal involvement is a serious complication of systemic sclerosis, which is more likely to occur in diffuse cutaneous systemic sclerosis (DCSS) than in limited cutaneous systemic sclerosis (LCSS). The renal lesion is caused by intimal cell proliferation and luminal narrowing of intrarenal arteries and arterioles. There is intense intrarenal vasospasm and plasma renin activity is markedly elevated. Renal involvement usually presents clinically with severe hypertension, microangiopathic features and progressive oliguric renal failure ('scleroderma renal crisis'). Use of ACE inhibitors to control the hypertension has improved the 1-year survival from 20% to 75% but about 50% of patients continue to require RRT. Onset or acceleration of the syndrome after glucocorticoid use or cessation of ACE inhibitors is well described.

Systemic lupus erythematosus

Subclinical renal involvement, with non-visible haematuria and proteinuria but minimally impaired or normal renal function, is common in systemic lupus erythematosus (SLE). Usually, this is due to glomerular disease, although interstitial nephritis may also occur, particularly in patients with overlap syndromes such as mixed connective tissue disease and Sjögren syndrome.

Almost any histological pattern of glomerular disease can be observed in SLE and the clinical presentation ranges from florid, rapidly progressive glomerulonephritis to nephrotic syndrome (see Fig. 18.9). The most common presentation is with subacute disease and inflammatory features (haematuria, hypertension, variable renal impairment), accompanied by heavy proteinuria that often reaches nephrotic levels. In severely affected patients, the most common histological pattern is a proliferative glomerulonephritis with substantial deposits of immunoglobulins and complement on immunofluorescence. Randomised controlled trials have shown that high-dose glucocorticoids administered in combination with

either cyclophosphamide or mycophenolate mofetil is effective in both induction and maintenance treatment of lupus nephritis and lowers the risk of progression to ESRD.

Many patients with SLE who develop ESRD go into remission, possibly because of immunosuppression related to the ESRD. Patients with ESRD caused by SLE are usually good candidates for dialysis and transplantation. Although it may recur in renal allografts, the immunosuppression required to prevent allograft rejection usually controls SLE.

Sickle-cell nephropathy

Improved survival of patients with sickle-cell disease means that a high proportion now live to develop chronic complications of microvascular occlusion. In the kidney, these changes are most pronounced in the medulla, where the vasa recta are the site of sickling because of hypoxia and hypertonicity. Loss of urinary concentrating ability and polyuria are the earliest changes; distal renal tubular acidosis and impaired potassium excretion are typical. Papillary necrosis may also occur (p. 577). A minority of patients develop ESRD. This is managed according to the usual principles, but response to recombinant erythropoietin is poor because of the haemoglobinopathy. Patients with sickle trait have an increased incidence of unexplained non-visible haematuria.

Acute kidney injury

Acute kidney injury (AKI) is not a diagnosis, rather it describes the situation where there is a sudden and often reversible loss of renal function, which develops over days or weeks and is often accompanied by a reduction in urine volume. Approximately 7% of all hospitalised patients and 20% of acutely ill patients develop AKI. In uncomplicated AKI mortality is low, however when it is associated with sepsis and multiple organ failure mortality is 50%–70% and the outcome is usually determined by the severity of the underlying disorder and other complications, rather than by kidney injury itself. Older patients are at higher risk of developing AKI and have a worse outcome (Box 18.25).

Pathophysiology

There are many causes of AKI and it is frequently multifactorial. It is helpful to classify it into three subtypes as these have different presentations and treatment (Fig. 18.18):

- 'pre-renal', when perfusion to the kidney is reduced
- 'renal', when the primary insult affects the kidney itself
- 'post-renal', when there is obstruction to urine flow at any point from the tubule to the urethra.

Pre-renal AKI results from a reduction in renal perfusion, typically due to a reduction in systemic blood pressure. The drop in renal perfusion activates the renin–angiotensin–aldosterone system, which promotes

---

18.25 Acute kidney injury in old age

- **Physiological change**: nephrons decline in number with age and average GFR falls progressively, so many older patients will have established CKD and less functional reserve. Small acute declines in renal function may therefore have a significant impact.
- **Creatinine**: as muscle mass falls with age, less creatinine is produced each day. Serum creatinine can therefore underestimate the severity of renal failure.
- **Renal tubular function**: declines with age, leading to loss of urinary concentrating ability.
- **Drugs**: increased drug prescription in older people (diuretics, ACE inhibitors and NSAIDs) may contribute to the risk of AKI.
- **Causes**: infection, renal vascular disease, prostatic obstruction, myeloma and severe cardiac dysfunction are common.
- **Mortality**: rises with age, primarily because of comorbid conditions.

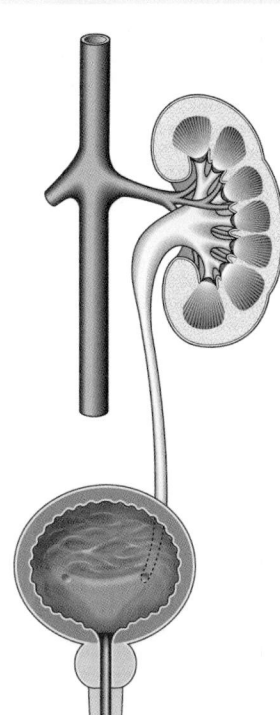

PRE-RENAL

Impaired perfusion:
• Cardiac failure
• Sepsis
• Blood loss
• Dehydration
• Vascular occlusion

RENAL

Glomerulonephritis
Small-vessel vasculitis
Acute tubular necrosis
• Drugs
• Toxins
• Prolonged hypotension
Interstitial nephritis
• Drugs
• Toxins
• Inflammatory disease
• Infection, including COVID-19

POST-RENAL

Urinary calculi (bilateral)
Retroperitoneal fibrosis
Benign prostatic
hypertrophy
Bladder cancer
Prostate cancer
Cervical cancer
Urethral stricture/valves
Meatal stenosis/phimosis

Fig. 18.18 Causes of acute kidney injury.

sodium retention in the kidney and systemic vasoconstriction (see Fig. 20.19), in order to restore blood pressure. Angiotensin also preferentially constricts the glomerular efferent arteriole, while prostaglandins are released locally to vasodilate the afferent arteriole (see Figs. 18.1D and 18.19). The combined effect increases glomerular pressure to maintain GFR, however if the blood pressure is very low, autoregulation fails and the GFR falls. Importantly, in pre-renal AKI, the kidney is not damaged, therefore GFR can improve rapidly if the renal perfusion is restored.

If the drop in renal perfusion is severe or sustained, pre-renal AKI may progress to renal AKI as ischaemic injury causes ATN, the most extreme example being with renal arterial or venous occlusion. Histologically, the kidney shows inflammatory changes, focal breaks in the tubular basement membrane and interstitial oedema (see Fig. 18.13B). Dead tubular cells may also be shed into the tubular lumen, leading to tubular obstruction. While ischaemia is the most common cause of ATN in hospital, it may also be caused by toxins and nephrotoxic drugs (see Boxes 18.26 and 18.42). Drugs can also cause allergic interstitial nephritis. The other common 'renal' cause of AKI is glomerulonephritis, in which there is direct inflammatory damage to the glomeruli. COVID-19 infection is also associated with AKI in a significant proportion of patients.

Post-renal AKI occurs as the result of obstruction to the renal tract (see Box 18.6). This leads to elevation of intraluminal ureteral pressure transmitted to the nephrons, with a subsequent fall in GFR. The obstruction needs to be bilateral to cause renal failure, therefore it is unusual for renal stones to cause AKI, while obstruction of the bladder outlet is a much more common cause. If the obstruction is not relieved, the low GFR is maintained by a drop in renal perfusion via thromboxane A_2 and angiotensin II. This leads to chronic renal injury over several weeks. If obstruction is reversed, the extent of recovery of renal function is dependent on the duration of obstruction and the pre-morbid GFR.

Clinical features

All emergency admissions to hospital should have renal function, blood pressure, temperature and pulse checked on arrival and undergo risk assessment for the likelihood of developing AKI. Those with coexisting diseases such as diabetes, cardiovascular, liver disease and existing CKD are at greater risk and need more regular assessment of renal function. If a patient is found to have a high serum creatinine, it is important to establish whether this is an acute or acute-on-chronic phenomenon, or a sign of CKD. Previous measurements of renal function are the best guide, but clinical features of AKI include short duration of symptoms, and an absence of markers of CKD such as anaemia, elevated PTH and small kidneys observed on imaging (see Fig. 18.22). Early recognition of AKI, assessment of volume status and prompt action to treat the underlying cause is required to prevent rapid progression of renal injury and to facilitate recovery as the damage may be potentially reversible if detected at an early stage. Importantly, eGFR is not accurate in AKI (see Box 18.2) and it may overestimate renal function in early AKI when creatinine is increasing rapidly.

Clinical features and pertinent investigations for the different causes of AKI are shown in Box 18.26 and are discussed below.

Pre-renal AKI

Tachycardia and postural hypotension (a fall in blood pressure of >20/10 mmHg from lying to standing) are valuable early signs of intravascular volume depletion. More significant hypovolaemia is associated with hypotension and signs of poor peripheral perfusion, such as cold peripheries and delayed capillary return. Warm peripheries in the presence of hypotension may indicate sepsis, as peripheral vasodilatation may be triggered by bacterial toxins and immune mediators. Pre-renal AKI may also occur without systemic hypotension, particularly in patients who are dehydrated or who are taking NSAIDs or ACE inhibitors (Fig. 18.19).

The cause of hypotension is often obvious, but concealed blood loss can occur into the gastrointestinal tract, retroperitoneum, following trauma (particularly with pelvic and femoral fractures) and into the pregnant uterus. Large volumes of intravascular fluid may also be lost into tissues after crush injuries or burns, following abdominal surgery, in severe inflammatory skin diseases or sepsis.

While diagnosis of pre-renal failure is usually based on history and assessment of volume status, the most helpful investigations reflect activation of hormonal systems due to intravascular volume depletion. Activation of the renin–angiotensin–aldosterone system promotes sodium and urea reabsorption in the proximal tubule, leading to a low urinary sodium and a high serum urea:creatinine ratio; ADH release promotes water reabsorption leading to a high specific gravity on urinalysis.

Renal AKI

Factors that can help differentiate the various causes of intrinsic renal AKI are summarised in Box 18.26. Patients with glomerulonephritis demonstrate haematuria and proteinuria, and may have clinical manifestations of an underlying disease, such as SLE or systemic vasculitis. Although blood tests, including an immunological screen, should be performed to clarify the diagnosis in glomerulonephritis, a renal biopsy is usually required. Drug-induced acute interstitial nephritis should be suspected in a previously well patient if there is an acute deterioration of renal function coinciding with introduction of a new drug treatment. Drugs that are commonly implicated include PPIs, NSAIDs and many antibiotics. Vascular disease is included here as diseases of the large and small renal vessels typically present with hypertension and volume expansion, in contrast to the volume depletion observed in pre-renal failure.

Post-renal AKI

Patients should be examined clinically to look for evidence of a distended bladder and should also undergo imaging with ultrasound to detect evidence of obstruction above the level of the bladder. Post-renal AKI is usually accompanied by hydronephrosis.

Management

Management options common to all forms of AKI are discussed in more detail below and summarised in Box 18.27.

18

	18.26	Categorising acute kidney injury based on history, examination and investigations

Type of AKI	History	Examination	Investigations
Pre-renal	Volume depletion (vomiting, diarrhoea, burns, haemorrhage) Sepsis Cardiac disease Liver disease Drugs (diuretics, ACE inhibitors, ARBs, NSAIDs, calcineurin inhibitors, iodinated contrast)	Low BP relative to normal for patient (including postural drop) Tachycardia Weight decrease Dry mucous membranes Decreased skin turgor JVP not visible even when lying down	Urine Na <20 mmol/L Fractional excretion Na < 1% High serum urea:creatinine ratio Urinalysis bland
Renal ATN	Ischaemic injury due to severe or prolonged pre-renal state Toxic ATN: drugs (aminoglycosides, cisplatin, tenofovir, methotrexate, iodinated contrast) Other (rhabdomyolysis, snake bite, *Amanita* mushrooms)	Vital signs Fluid assessment Limbs for compartment syndrome	Urine Na >40 mmol/L Fractional excretion Na ≥ 1% Dense granular ('muddy brown') casts Creatine kinase
Glomerular	Rash, weight loss, arthralgia, ENT and chest symptoms (pulmonary renal syndromes) IV drug use Recent infection	Hypertension Oedema Purpuric rash, uveitis, arthritis	Proteinuria, haematuria Red cell casts, dysmorphic red cells ANCA, anti-GBM, ANA, C3 and C4 Viral hepatitis screen, HIV Renal biopsy
Tubulo-interstitial	Interstitial nephritis: drugs (PPIs, penicillins, NSAIDs) Sarcoidosis	Fever Rash	Leucocyturia White cell casts Minimal proteinuria
	Tubular obstruction: Myeloma (cast nephropathy)		Paraprotein, Bence Jones protein Calcium (myeloma, sarcoidosis)
	Tubular crystal nephropathy: Drugs (aciclovir, indinavir, triamterene, methotrexate) Oxalate (fat malabsorption, ethylene glycol) Urate (tumour lysis)		Urine microscopy for crystals Serum urate Urine collection for oxalate
Vascular (including renal infarction, renal vein thrombosis, cholesterol emboli, malignant hypertension)	Flank pain, trauma Anticoagulation Recent angiography (cholesterol emboli) Nephrotic syndrome (renal vein thrombosis) Systemic sclerosis (renal crisis) Diarrhoea (HUS)	Hypertension Hypertensive changes on fundoscopy Livedo reticularis (cholesterol emboli) Sclerodactyly	Normal urinalysis or some haematuria CT angiography Doppler renal ultrasound C3 and C4 (cholesterol emboli) Platelets, haemolytic screen, LDH (HUS) Consider ADAMTS13 and complement genetics (if TMA)
Post-renal	Bladder outlet symptoms History of BPH or prostate, bladder or cervical cancer Retroperitoneal fibrosis Neurogenic bladder	Rectal examination (prostate and anal tone) Distended bladder Pelvic mass	Urinalysis frequently normal (may reveal haematuria depending on cause) Renal ultrasound (hydronephrosis) Isotope renogram (delayed excretion) if ultrasound inconclusive

(ACE = angiotensin-converting enzyme; ANA = antinuclear antibody; ANCA = antineutrophil cytoplasmic antibody; ARBs = angiotensin receptor blockers; ATN = acute tubular necrosis; BP = blood pressure; BPH = benign prostatic hypertrophy; GBM = glomerular basement membrane; HIV = human immunodeficiency virus; HUS = haemolytic uraemic syndrome; IV = intravenous; JVP = jugular venous pulse; LDH = lactate dehydrogenase; NSAIDs = non-steroidal anti-inflammatory drugs; PPIs = proton pump inhibitors; TMA = thrombotic microangiopathy)

Optimisation of volume status

Regular assessment of volume status is essential to guide ongoing fluid requirements. Where clinical assessment is challenging, such as in obesity, invasive monitoring of central venous pressure may be of value. If hypovolaemia is present, it should be corrected by prompt replacement of intravenous fluid or blood. When large volumes of fluid are required, balanced crystalloid solutions, such as Plasma-Lyte or Hartmann's, may be preferable to isotonic saline (0.9% NaCl) in order to avoid hyperchloraemic acidosis. Once the patient is volume replete, fluid intake should be matched to urine output plus 500 mL per day to cover insensible losses, unless additional losses are anticipated, such as with diarrhoea or high nasogastric aspirates. Excessive administration of fluid should be avoided, since this can provoke pulmonary oedema. In situations where vasodilatation is a prominent cause of relative intravascular volume depletion, such as sepsis or liver failure, inotropes may be required to restore an effective blood pressure.

In patients with volume expansion, diuretics may be used, but in those with AKI high doses may be required and they are not always effective. If pulmonary oedema (Fig. 18.20) is present and urine output cannot be rapidly restored, treatment with dialysis may be required to remove excess fluid.

Treatment of underlying cause

In pre-renal failure, rapid fluid resuscitation may be sufficient for resolution of AKI, though it is important to identify and manage underlying causes such as blood loss, sepsis and cardiac events.

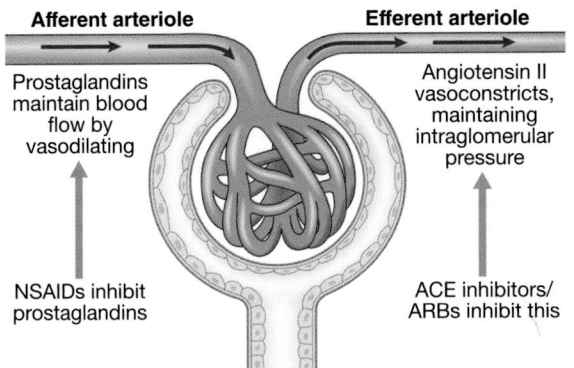

Fig. 18.19 Renal haemodynamics and autoregulation of glomerular filtration rate (GFR). It is evident from this figure how angiotensin-converting enzyme (ACE) inhibitors/angiotensin receptor blockers (ARBs) may be associated with profound drops in GFR in the context of bilateral renal artery stenosis or intravascular volume depletion (which decrease perfusion to afferent arterioles). (NSAIDs = non-steroidal anti-inflammatory drugs)

18.27 Management of acute kidney injury

- Assess fluid status as this will determine fluid prescription:
  If hypovolaemic: optimise systemic haemodynamic status with fluid challenge and inotropes if necessary
  Once euvolaemic, match fluid intake to urine output plus an additional 500 mL/24 hrs to cover insensible losses
  If fluid-overloaded, prescribe diuretics (loop diuretics at high dose will often be required); if the response is unsatisfactory, dialysis may be required
- Treat underlying cause
- If K⁺ > 6.5 mmol/L and ECG changes of hyperkalaemia are present administer calcium gluconate to stabilise myocardium, lower potassium by oral potassium exchange resin to prevent potassium absorption, or administering intravenous glucose/insulin or sodium bicarbonate to move potassium intracellularly (see Box 19.17). These are holding measures until a definitive method of removing potassium is achieved (restoration of renal function or dialysis)
- Discontinue potentially nephrotoxic drugs and reduce doses of therapeutic drugs according to level of renal function
- Ensure adequate nutritional support
- Consider proton pump inhibitors to reduce the risk of upper gastrointestinal bleeding
- Screen for intercurrent infections and treat promptly if present

(ECG = electrocardiogram)

In those with suspected ATN, volume status should be optimised, offending drugs should be discontinued, conditions such as sepsis, compartment syndrome or myeloma identified and treated. However, once ATN is established, even if the underlying cause has been corrected, regeneration of necrotic tubules and recovery of renal function may take days or even weeks and the patient may need support with renal replacement therapy in the interim.

In post-renal AKI, the obstruction should be relieved as soon as possible. This may involve urinary catheterisation for bladder outflow obstruction, or relief of ureteric obstruction with ureteric stents or percutaneous nephrostomies.

Electrolyte and acid–base disturbances

Hyperkalaemia is common, particularly in patients with rhabdomyolysis, burns, haemolysis or metabolic acidosis or in those taking medications that inhibit the renin–angiotensin–aldosterone system. If serum K⁺ concentration is >6.5 mmol/L, an electrocardiogram (ECG) should be performed, and if there are changes consistent with hyperkalaemia, this should be treated immediately, as described in Box 19.17, to prevent life-threatening cardiac arrhythmias.

Severe acidosis can be ameliorated by treatment with sodium bicarbonate if volume status allows. This may also be helpful in lowering serum potassium.

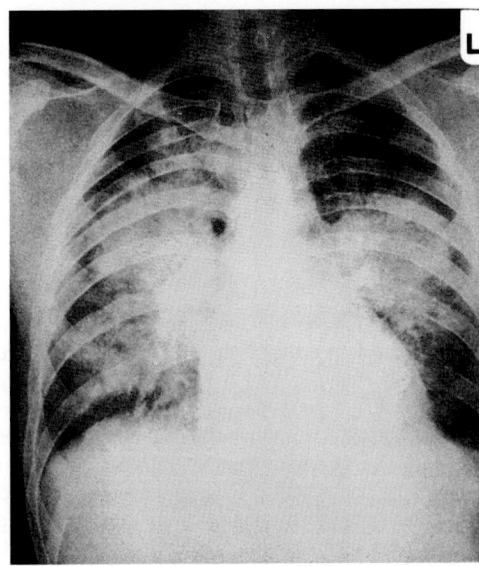

Fig. 18.20 Pulmonary oedema in acute kidney injury. The appearances are indistinguishable from left ventricular failure but the heart size is usually normal. Blood pressure is often high.

Dilutional hyponatraemia may occur if the patient has continued to drink freely despite oliguria or has received inappropriate amounts of intravenous dextrose. This can be corrected by fluid restriction. Modest hypocalcaemia is common but rarely requires treatment. Serum phosphate levels are usually high but may fall in patients on daily or continuous renal replacement therapy (CRRT), necessitating phosphate replacement.

Dietary measures

Adequate nutritional support may be required to ensure sufficient calorie and protein intake. This is particularly important in patients in catabolic states such as with sepsis and burns. Enteral or parenteral nutrition may be required.

Infection

Sepsis may either be the cause of AKI or a consequence of the depression of humoral and cellular immune mechanisms found in patients with AKI. Regular clinical examination, supplemented by microbiological investigation where appropriate, is required to diagnose infection. If infection is discovered, it should be treated promptly according to standard principles (see Ch. 6).

Medications

Patients with drug-induced kidney injury (see Box 18.42) should have the offending drug withdrawn. Additionally, NSAIDs and drugs that block the renin–angiotensin–aldosterone system should be discontinued, as they may reduce GFR (see Fig. 18.19) and exacerbate hyperkalaemia. Other drug treatments should be reviewed and the doses adjusted if necessary, to take account of reduced renal function (see p. 31). Non-essential drug treatments should be stopped.

Renal replacement therapy (RRT)

Conservative management can be successful in AKI with meticulous attention to fluid balance, electrolytes and nutrition, but RRT may be required in patients who are not showing signs of recovery with these measures (see Box 18.27). No specific cut-off values for serum urea or creatinine have been identified at which RRT should be commenced, and clinical trials of earlier versus later initiation of RRT have not shown differences in outcome in patients with AKI. Furthermore, RRT can be a risky intervention, since it requires the placement of central venous catheters that may become infected and it may represent a major haemodynamic

18

challenge in unstable patients. Accordingly, the decision to institute RRT should be made on an individual basis, taking account of the potential risks and benefits, comorbidity and an assessment of whether early or delayed recovery is likely. Severe uraemia with pericarditis and neurological signs (uraemic encephalopathy) are uncommon in AKI but, when present, are strong indications for RRT; other indications are given in Box 18.35. The two main options for RRT in AKI are intermittent haemodialysis and continuous renal replacement therapy. Peritoneal dialysis is also an option if haemodialysis is not available (p. 595).

Recovery from AKI

Most cases of AKI will recover after the insult resolves but recovery may be impaired in those with pre-existing CKD or following a prolonged, severe or irreversible insult (Fig. 18.21). Recovery is heralded by a gradual return of urine output and a steady reduction in serum creatinine. There is often a diuretic phase in which urine output increases rapidly and remains excessive for several days before returning to normal. This is due to loss of the concentrating ability of the kidneys due to tubular damage and to temporary loss of the medullary concentration gradient. After a few days, urine volume falls to normal as the concentrating mechanism and tubular reabsorption are restored. During the recovery phase of AKI, it may be necessary to provide temporary supplementation of fluid, potassium and sometimes calcium, phosphate and magnesium.

Chronic kidney disease

Chronic kidney disease (CKD) refers to an irreversible deterioration in renal function that usually develops over a period of years (see Box 18.3). Initially, it manifests only as a biochemical abnormality but, eventually, loss of the excretory, metabolic and endocrine functions of the kidney leads to the clinical symptoms and signs of renal failure, collectively referred to as uraemia. When death is likely without RRT (CKD stage 5), it is called end-stage renal disease (ESRD).

Epidemiology

The social and economic consequences of CKD are considerable. In many countries, estimates of the prevalence of CKD stages 3–5 (eGFR <60 mL/min/1.73 m^2) are around 5%–7%, mostly affecting people aged 65 years and above (see Box 18.3). The prevalence of CKD in patients with hypertension, diabetes and vascular disease is substantially higher, and targeted screening for CKD should be considered in these and other high-risk groups. More than 25% of the population aged over 75

years have an eGFR of <60 mL/min/1.73 m^2, mostly stage 3A CKD (see Box 18.3). In these patients, investigation and management should be focused on cardiovascular risk prevention, as very few will ever develop ESRD. Many primary renal diseases, however, are more common in older people, so investigation is warranted for those with declining renal function or with haematuria/proteinuria on dipstick.

Pathophysiology

Common causes of CKD are shown in Box 18.28. In many cases the underlying diagnosis is unclear, especially among the large number of older patients with stage 3 CKD. Many patients diagnosed at a late stage have bilateral small kidneys. Renal biopsy is rarely undertaken in this group since it is more risky, less likely to provide a histological diagnosis because of the severity of damage, and unlikely to alter management.

Clinical features

The typical presentation is for a reduced eGFR to be found incidentally during routine blood tests, often during screening of high-risk patients, such as those with diabetes or hypertension. Most patients with slowly progressive disease are asymptomatic until GFR falls below 30 mL/min/1.73 m^2 and some can remain asymptomatic with much lower GFR values than this. An early symptom is nocturia, due to the loss of concentrating ability, but this is non-specific. When GFR falls below 15–20 mL/min/1.73 m^2, symptoms and signs are common and can affect almost all body systems, but are often non-specific and may not immediately raise suspicion of kidney disease (Fig. 18.22). They typically include tiredness or breathlessness, which may, in part, be related to renal anaemia or fluid overload. With further deterioration in renal function, patients may suffer pruritus, anorexia, weight loss, nausea, vomiting and hiccups. In very advanced renal failure, respiration may be particularly deep (Kussmaul breathing) due to profound metabolic acidosis, and patients may develop muscular twitching, fits, drowsiness and coma.

Investigations

The recommended investigations in patients with CKD are shown in Box 18.29. Their main aims are:

- to exclude AKI requiring rapid investigation; in patients with unexpectedly high urea and creatinine (when there is an increase from previous results or no prior results are available), renal function should be retested within 2 weeks to avoid missing AKI
- to identify the underlying cause where possible, since this may influence the treatment

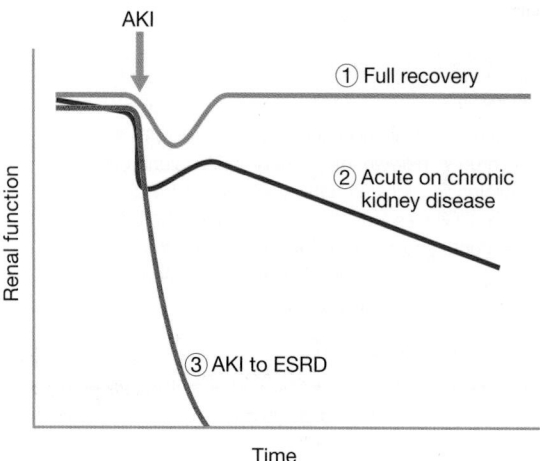

Fig. 18.21 Recovery from acute kidney injury (AKI). Many patients make a full recovery of renal function (1). If the insult is prolonged or prior renal function not normal, however, patients may develop progressive chronic kidney disease (2) or, rarely, irreversible, complete loss of renal function (3). (ESRD = end-stage renal disease)

i	18.28	Common causes of chronic kidney disease	
Disease	**Proportion**	**Comments**	
Diabetes mellitus	20%–45%	Large racial and geographical differences	
Interstitial diseases	20%–30%	Drug-induced, reflux nephropathy	
Glomerular diseases	10%–20%	IgA nephropathy is most common	
Hypertension	5%–20%	Causality controversial, much may be secondary to another primary renal disease	
Systemic inflammatory diseases	5%–10%	Systemic lupus erythematosus, vasculitis	
Renovascular disease	5%	Mostly atheromatous, may be more common	
Congenital and inherited	10%	Polycystic kidney disease, Alport syndrome	
Unknown	5%–10%		

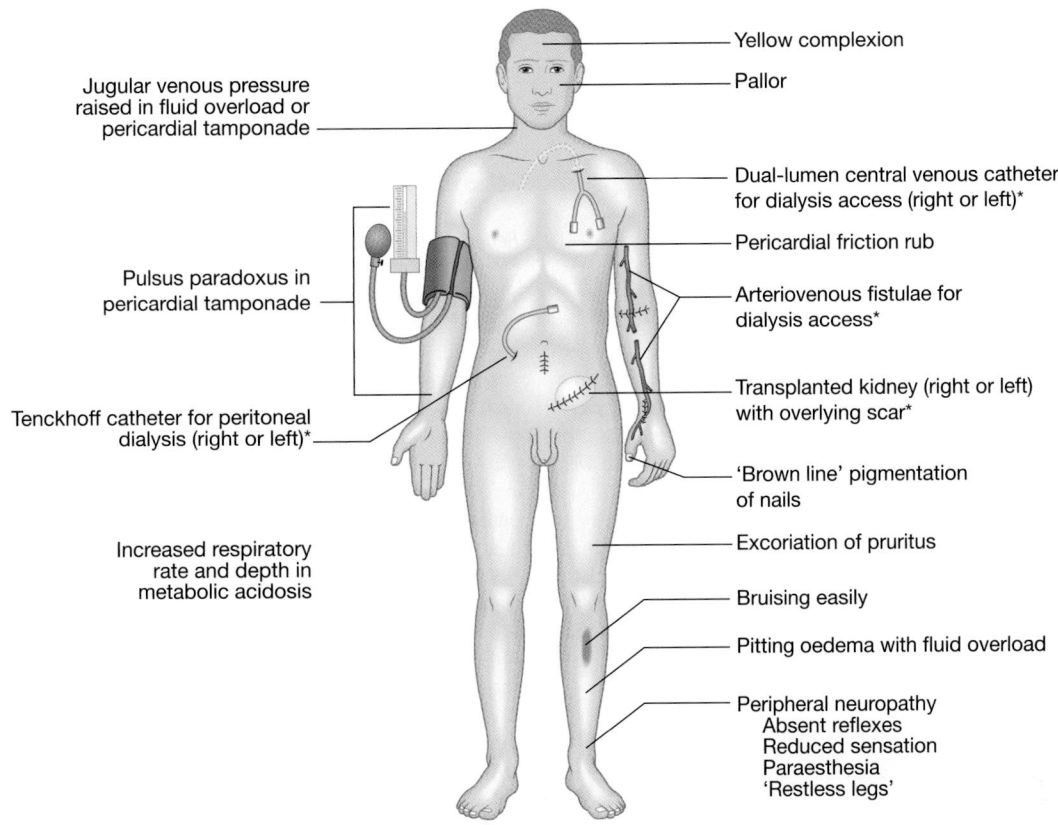

Fig. 18.22 Physical signs in advanced chronic kidney disease. (*Features of renal replacement therapy.)

The figure shows labels pointing to a human body:
- Yellow complexion
- Pallor
- Jugular venous pressure raised in fluid overload or pericardial tamponade
- Dual-lumen central venous catheter for dialysis access (right or left)*
- Pericardial friction rub
- Pulsus paradoxus in pericardial tamponade
- Arteriovenous fistulae for dialysis access*
- Transplanted kidney (right or left) with overlying scar*
- Tenckhoff catheter for peritoneal dialysis (right or left)*
- 'Brown line' pigmentation of nails
- Excoriation of pruritus
- Increased respiratory rate and depth in metabolic acidosis
- Bruising easily
- Pitting oedema with fluid overload
- Peripheral neuropathy / Absent reflexes / Reduced sensation / Paraesthesia / 'Restless legs'

18

i	18.29 Suggested investigations in chronic kidney disease	
Initial tests	**Interpretation**	
Creatinine, eGFR	To assess stability/progression: compare to previous results	
Urinalysis and quantification of proteinuria	Haematuria and proteinuria may indicate glomerular disease and need for biopsy (p. 566). Proteinuria indicates risk of progressive CKD requiring preventive ACE inhibitor or ARB therapy	
Electrolytes	To identify hyperkalaemia and acidosis	
Calcium, phosphate, parathyroid hormone and 25(OH)D	Assessment of renal osteodystrophy	
Albumin	Low albumin: consider malnutrition, inflammation, nephrotic syndrome	
Full blood count (± Fe, ferritin, folate, B_{12})	If anaemic, exclude common non-renal explanations, then manage as renal anaemia	
Lipids, glucose ± HbA_{1c}	Cardiovascular risk high in CKD: treat risk factors aggressively	
Renal ultrasound	Consider with obstructive urinary symptoms, persistent haematuria, family history of polycystic kidney disease or progressive CKD. Small kidneys suggest chronicity. Asymmetric renal size suggests renovascular or congenital disease	
Hepatitis and HIV serology	If dialysis or transplant is planned. Hepatitis B vaccination recommended if seronegative	
Other tests	Consider relevant tests from Box 18.26, especially if the cause of CKD is unknown	

(ACE = angiotensin-converting enzyme; ARB = angiotensin II receptor blocker; CKD = chronic kidney disease; HIV = human immunodeficiency virus; 25(OH)D = 25-hydroxyvitamin D)

- to identify reversible factors that may worsen renal function, such as hypertension or urinary tract obstruction
- to screen for complications of CKD, such as anaemia and renal osteodystrophy
- to screen for cardiovascular risk factors.

Referral to a nephrologist is appropriate for patients with potentially treatable underlying disease and those who are likely to progress to ESRD. Suggested referral criteria are listed in Box 18.30.

Management

The aims of management in CKD are to:

- monitor renal function
- prevent or slow further renal damage
- limit complications of renal failure
- treat risk factors for cardiovascular disease
- prepare for RRT, if appropriate (p. 593).

Monitoring of renal function

The rate of change in renal function varies between patients and may vary over time in each individual. Renal function should therefore be monitored every 6 months in patients with stage 3 CKD, but more frequently in patients who are deteriorating rapidly or have stage 4 or 5 CKD. A plot of GFR against time (Fig. 18.23) can demonstrate whether therapy has been successful in slowing progression, detect any unexpected increase in the rate of decline that may warrant further investigation, and help predict when ESRD will be reached to facilitate timely planning for RRT.

Reduction of rate of progression

Slowing the rate of progression of CKD may reduce complications and delay symptom onset and the need for RRT (see Fig. 18.23). Therapies directed towards the primary cause of CKD should be employed where possible; tight blood pressure control is applicable to CKD regardless of cause, however, and reducing proteinuria is a key target in those with glomerular disease.

Antihypertensive therapy Lowering of blood pressure slows the rate at which renal function declines in CKD, independently of the agent used (apart from those with proteinuria; see below) and has additional benefits in lowering the risk of hypertensive heart failure and cardiovascular disease. No threshold for beneficial effects has been identified and any reduction of blood pressure appears to be beneficial. A target blood pressure of less than 140/90 mmHg is recommended for patients with CKD and no albuminuria (ACR <3 mg/mmol; see Box 18.11 for conversion of mg/mmol to mg/dL). A lower target of 130/80 mmHg is recommended for those with diabetes or an ACR of more than 70 mg/mmol. Achieving these blood pressure targets often requires multiple drugs, and therapeutic success may be limited by adverse effects and poor adherence.

Reduction of proteinuria Patients with proteinuria are at higher risk of progression of renal disease, and there is strong evidence that reducing proteinuria reduces the risk of progression. ACE inhibitors and ARBs reduce proteinuria and retard the progression of CKD. These effects are partly due to the reduction in blood pressure but there is evidence for a specific beneficial effect in patients with proteinuria (PCR >50 mg/mmol or ACR >30 mg/mmol; see Box 18.11) through a reduction in glomerular perfusion pressure (see Fig. 18.19). In addition, ACE inhibitors have been shown to reduce the risk of cardiovascular events and all-cause mortality in CKD. Accordingly, ACE inhibitors or ARBs should be prescribed to all patients with diabetic nephropathy and patients with CKD and proteinuria, irrespective of whether or not hypertension is present.

While ACE inhibitors and ARBs are excellent drugs for patients with diabetes or CKD and proteinuria, they need to be prescribed with care in certain circumstances. Initiation of treatment with ACE inhibitors and ARBs may be accompanied by an immediate reduction in GFR; patients should therefore have their renal function checked within 7–10 days of initiating or increasing the dose of an ACE inhibitor or ARB. Treatment can be continued so long as the reduction in GFR is not greater than 25% and is not progressive. Angiotensin II is critical for autoregulation of GFR in the context of low renal perfusion (see Fig. 18.1D), and so ACE inhibitors or ARBs may exacerbate pre-renal failure (see Fig. 18.19). Patients on ACE inhibitors/ARBs should therefore be warned to stop taking the medication if they become unwell, such as with fever, vomiting or diarrhoea, restarting once they are better. This also applies to other common medications used in patients with CKD, such as diuretics, metformin and NSAIDs, and this advice may be reinforced by providing written information such as 'sick-day rule' cards (Box 18.31). ACE inhibitors and ARBs increase serum potassium and should not be commenced in patients with baseline potassium >5.5 mmol/L. In patients with serum potassium >6.0 mmol/L, the dose of ACE inhibitors or ARBs should be reduced or discontinued entirely, but only after all other measures to

 18.30 Criteria for referral of chronic kidney disease patients to a nephrologist

- eGFR <30 mL/min/1.73 m²
- Rapid deterioration in renal function (>25% from previous or >15 mL/min/1.73 m²/year)
- Significant proteinuria (PCR >100 mg/mmol or ACR >70 mg/mmol*), unless known to be due to diabetes and patient is already on appropriate medications
- ACR >30 mg/mmol* with non-visible haematuria
- Hypertension that remains poorly controlled despite at least four antihypertensive medications
- Suspicion of renal involvement in multisystem disease

*See Box 18.11 for conversion of mg/mmol to mg/dL.
(ACR = albumin:creatinine ratio; eGFR = estimated glomerular filtration rate; PCR = protein:creatinine ratio)

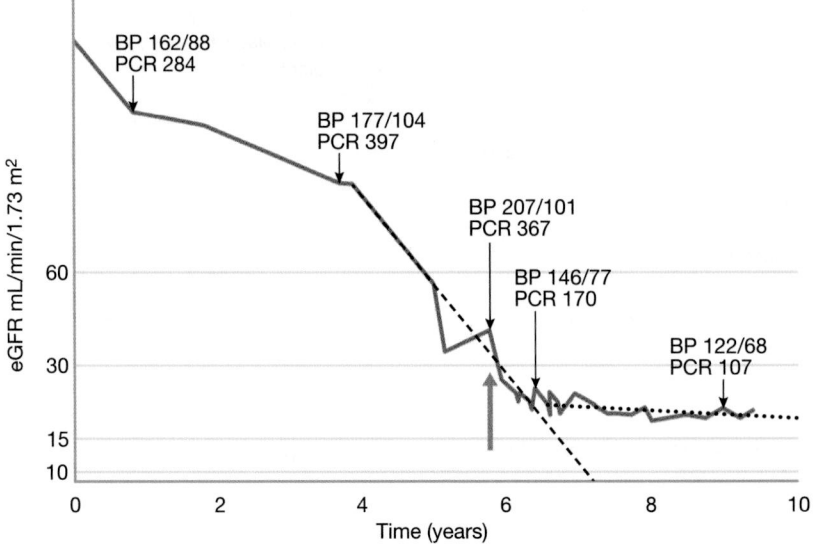

Fig. 18.23 Plot of estimated glomerular filtration rate (eGFR) against time in a patient with type 1 diabetes mellitus. After approximately 6 years of monitoring (blue arrow), this patient entered an aggressive treatment programme aimed at optimising blood pressure (BP) and glycaemic control. The reduction in BP was accompanied by a fall in proteinuria (protein:creatinine ratio, PCR; shown in mg/mmol). At the previous rate of decline in renal function (dashed line), he was likely to reach the level of renal function at which dialysis therapy is typically required (eGFR = 10 mL/min/1.73 m²) within 18 months; however, the relative stabilisation in his renal function (dotted line) means that this has been deferred, potentially for several years.

reduce potassium have been considered (see below). Combination therapy with ACE inhibitors and ARBs or direct renin inhibitors has not been shown to reduce progression of kidney disease but is associated with higher rates of hyperkalaemia and AKI, and is therefore to be avoided.

Treatment of complications

The kidneys have many functions in addition to excretion of waste (p. 560). Treatments that substitute for all of the normal roles of the kidneys must therefore be instigated to maintain normal body homeostasis and prevent complications.

Maintenance of fluid and electrolyte balance The kidneys excrete waste and regulate many electrolytes, and so patients with CKD may accumulate waste products and develop electrolyte abnormalities.

Urea is a key product of protein degradation and accumulates with progressive CKD. All patients with stages 4 and 5 CKD should be given dietetic advice aimed at preventing excessive consumption of protein. Severe protein restriction is not recommended, however; there is no evidence that this reduces the rate of decline in renal function but may lead to malnutrition.

Potassium often accumulates in patients with advanced CKD, who should be provided with dietary advice to reduce daily potassium intake to below 70 mmol (Box 18.32). Potassium-binding compounds limit absorption of potassium from the gut and may be a useful adjunctive therapy. Calcium resonium is not recommended, other than as a very short-term measure, as it can be associated with bowel necrosis; however, newer agents, such as sodium zirconium cyclosilicate and patiromer, appear promising for chronic use. Other measures that may help regulate potassium include diuretic therapy and control of acidosis with sodium bicarbonate (see below). Consideration should be given to stopping or reducing drugs that elevate potassium, such as potassium-sparing diuretics and ACE inhibitors/ARBs; however, this has to be balanced against the potential benefit that such drugs may have on retarding progression of renal and cardiovascular disease, and hence withdrawal should be reserved for when other measures have failed.

The inability of the failing kidney to excrete sodium and water commonly leads to their accumulation, which may manifest as oedema and drive hypertension. Patients with evidence of volume expansion should be instructed to consume a low-sodium diet (< 100 mmol/24 hrs) and in severe cases fluid intake should also be restricted. Diuretics are commonly required, and as renal function deteriorates, increasing doses of potent loop diuretics or synergistic combinations of loop, thiazide and potassium-sparing diuretics may be necessary.

Occasionally, some patients with tubulo-interstitial disease can develop 'salt-wasting' disease and may require a high sodium and water intake, including supplements of sodium salts, to prevent fluid depletion and worsening of renal function.

Acid–base balance Reduced ability to excrete organic acids in patients with CKD may lead to an anion-gap metabolic acidosis. In addition, in patients with tubulo-interstitial disease or diabetic nephropathy, there may be specific defects in acid–base regulation within the kidney, causing a non-anion-gap renal tubular acidosis (p. 631). Although acidosis is usually asymptomatic, it may be associated with increased tissue catabolism and decreased protein synthesis, and may exacerbate bone disease and the rate of decline in renal function. Hence, plasma bicarbonate concentrations should be maintained above 22 mmol/L by prescribing sodium bicarbonate supplements (starting dose of 1 g 3 times daily, increasing as required). There is some evidence that correcting acidosis may reduce the rate of decline in renal function.

Renal bone disease Disturbances of calcium and phosphate metabolism are almost universal in advanced CKD (Fig. 18.24). The sequence of events that leads to renal bone disease is complex, but two primary factors are: impaired excretion of phosphate and failure of the renal tubular cells to convert 25-hydroxyvitamin D to its active metabolite 1,25-dihydroxyvitamin D. A rise in serum phosphate levels promotes production of the hormone fibroblast growth factor 23 (FGF23) from osteocytes (see Fig. 26.3) and stimulates parathyroid hormone (PTH) release and hyperplasia of the parathyroid glands. The FGF23 and PTH promote tubular phosphate excretion, thereby partly compensating for the reduced glomerular filtration of phosphate. The reduced 1,25-dihydroxyvitamin D level stimulates PTH release and reduces intestinal absorption of calcium. In addition, raised levels of serum phosphate complex with calcium in the extracellular space, leading to calcium phosphate deposition in tissues including the cardiovascular system. The combination of reduced absorption and increased deposition of calcium promotes hypocalcaemia, which also stimulates PTH production by the parathyroid glands. Hence in many patients with CKD, compensatory responses initially maintain phosphate and calcium levels at the upper and lower ends of their respective normal ranges, at the expense of an elevated PTH level (secondary hyperparathyroidism). This is associated with bone resorption (osteitis fibrosa cystica), and in severe cases this may result in bony pain and increased risk of fractures. Conversely there is increased deposition of calcium phosphate in many tissues, most notably blood vessels and heart valves, which may contribute to the increased risk of cardiovascular disease in patients with CKD (see below). In some cases, tertiary hyperparathyroidism supervenes, due to autonomous production of PTH by the enlarged parathyroid glands; this presents with hypercalcaemia. Additional problems in bone metabolism include low bone turnover (adynamic bone disease) in patients who have been over-treated with vitamin D metabolites and osteoporosis in patients with poor nutritional intake.

The key focus in the management of renal bone disease should be directed towards the two main driving factors, hyperphosphataemia and inadequate activation of vitamin D. Hyperphosphataemia should be treated by dietary restriction of foods with high phosphate content (milk, cheese, eggs and protein-rich foods) and by the use of phosphate-binding drugs that inhibit phosphate reabsorption in the gut. Various drugs are available, including calcium carbonate, aluminium hydroxide, lanthanum carbonate and polymer-based phosphate binders such as sevelamer. The aim is to maintain serum phosphate values below 1.5 mmol/L (4.6 mg/dL) if possible, but many of these drugs are difficult to take and adherence can be a problem. Active vitamin D metabolites (either 1-α-hydroxyvitamin D or 1,25-dihydroxyvitamin D) should be administered in patients who are hypocalcaemic or have serum PTH levels more than twice the upper limit of normal. The dose should be adjusted to try to reduce PTH levels to between 2 and 4 times the upper limit of

18

18.31 Exemplar medicine sick-day card

When you are unwell with vomiting, diarrhoea or fever, stop taking the following medications:

- ACE inhibitors: medicines ending in '-pril', e.g. lisinopril, ramipril
- Angiotensin receptor blockers: medicines ending in '-sartan', e.g. irbesartan, losartan, candesartan
- Non-steroidal anti-inflammatory painkillers: e.g. ibuprofen (Brufen), diclofenac (Voltarol)
- Diuretics: e.g. furosemide, bendroflumethiazide, indapamide, spironolactone
- Metformin: a medicine for diabetes.

Restart when you are well again (after 24–48 hours of eating and drinking normally).

18.32 Foods high in potassium

- Fruit: bananas, avocados, figs, rhubarb
- Vegetables: tomatoes, spinach, parsnips, courgettes, sprouts, potatoes (including baked, fries, wedges; boiling vegetables reduces potassium content)
- Sweets/snacks: crisps, chocolate, toffee, nuts (including peanut butter)
- Drinks: beer, cider, wine (spirits contain less potassium), hot chocolate, fruit juice, milk, yoghurt
- Some salt substitutes, such as Lo-Salt: sodium chloride is substituted with potassium chloride

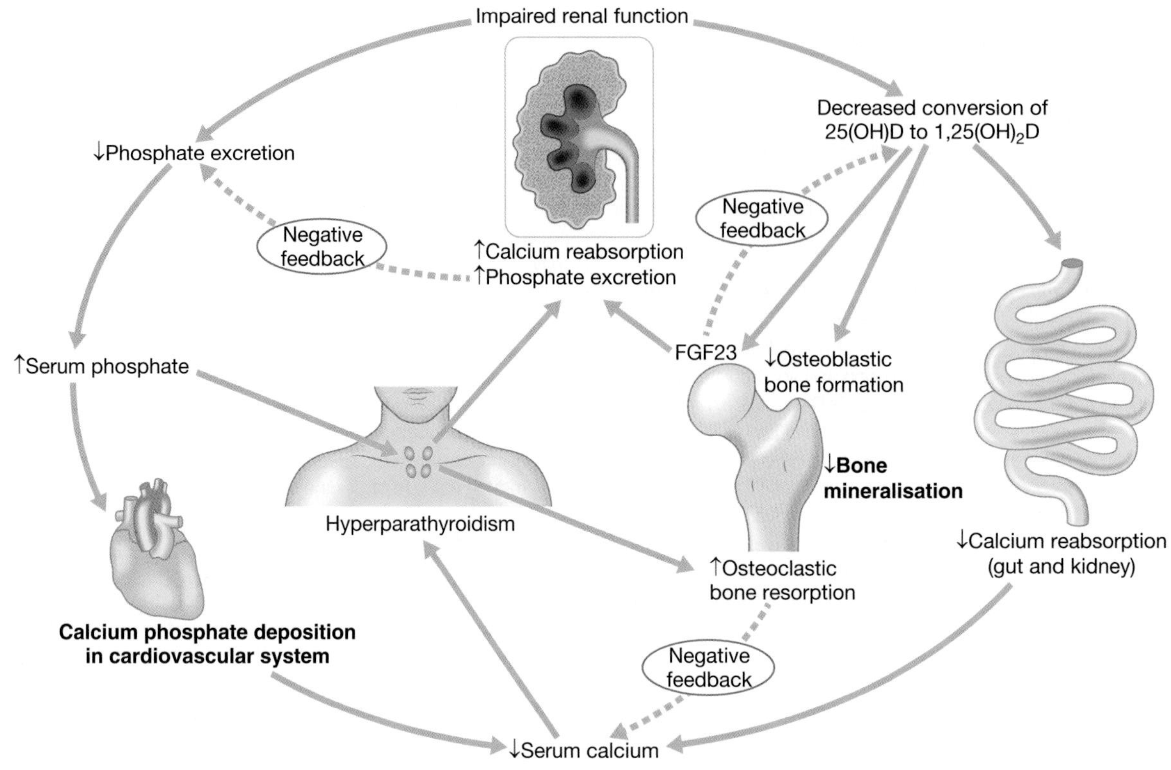

Fig. 18.24 Pathogenesis of renal osteodystrophy. Impaired renal clearance of phosphate promotes elevated serum phosphate, which binds to calcium, lowering the serum calcium and leading to calcium phosphate deposition in tissues including the cardiovascular system. Low 1,25-dihydroxyvitamin D (1,25(OH)$_2$D) levels reduce calcium absorption from gut and kidney exacerbating hypocalcaemia. Low serum calcium and 1,25(OH)$_2$D levels (arrow not shown in figure for ease of reading) and high phosphate stimulate release of parathyroid hormone (PTH) which increases osteoclastic bone resorption, contributing to renal osteodystrophy. The elevated PTH and production of fibroblast growth factor 23 (FGF23) from osteocytes promotes phosphate excretion, however this is insufficient to prevent hyperphosphataemia in advanced chronic kidney disease.

normal to limit hyperparathyroidism while avoiding over-suppression of bone turnover and adynamic bone disease, but care must be exercised in order to avoid hypercalcaemia. In patients with persistent hypercalcaemia (tertiary hyperparathyroidism), parathyroidectomy may be required. If parathyroidectomy is unsuccessful or not possible, calcimimetic agents, such as cinacalcet, may be used. These bind to the calcium-sensing receptor in the parathyroid glands and reduce PTH secretion.

Anaemia Anaemia is common in patients with CKD and contributes to many of the non-specific symptoms, including fatigue and shortness of breath. Haemoglobin can be as low as 50–70 g/L in CKD stage 5, although it is often less severe or absent in patients with polycystic kidney disease. Several mechanisms are implicated, as summarised in Box 18.33. Iron deficiency is common in patients with CKD, and even more prevalent in those on haemodialysis as a result of haemolysis in the dialysis circuit. Hence many patients require iron supplements, which may be given intravenously for those with iron intolerance or in situations where adherence may be difficult. Once iron deficiency and other causes of anaemia have been excluded or corrected, recombinant human erythropoietin is very effective in correcting the anaemia of CKD and improving symptoms. However, correcting haemoglobin to normal levels confers higher risk of hypertension and thrombosis, therefore the target haemoglobin is usually between 100 and 120 g/L or avoidance of blood transfusions. Erythropoietin is less effective in the presence of iron deficiency, active inflammation or malignancy, in particular myeloma.

Treatment of risk factors for cardiovascular disease

The risk of cardiovascular disease is substantially increased in patients with a GFR below 60 mL/min/1.73 m^2 and in those with proteinuria, the

i	**18.33 Causes of anaemia in chronic kidney disease**

- Deficiency of erythropoietin
- Toxic effects of uraemia on marrow precursor cells
- Reduced intake, absorption and utilisation of dietary iron
- Reduced red cell survival
- Blood loss due to capillary fragility and poor platelet function

combination of reduced eGFR and proteinuria being particularly unfavourable. Patients with CKD have a higher prevalence of traditional risk factors for atherosclerosis, such as hypertension, hyperlipidaemia and diabetes; however, additional mechanisms of cardiovascular disease may also be implicated. Left ventricular hypertrophy is commonly found in patients with CKD, secondary to hypertension or anaemia. Calcification of the media of blood vessels, heart valves, myocardium and the conduction system of the heart is also common and may be due, in part, to the high serum phosphate levels. Reflecting this fact, serum FGF23 levels, which increase in response to serum phosphate, are an independent predictor of mortality in CKD. Both left ventricular hypertrophy and cardiac calcification may increase the risk of arrhythmias and sudden cardiac death, which is a much more common mode of death in patients with CKD than in the general population, particularly in those with more advanced disease and those on dialysis.

To reduce vascular risk, patients with CKD should be encouraged to adopt a healthy lifestyle, including regular exercise, and weight loss and smoking cessation where appropriate. Lipid-lowering drugs reduce cardiovascular events in patients with CKD, although their efficacy may be lower once patients require dialysis.

Preparing for renal replacement therapy

It is crucial for patients who are known to have progressive CKD to be prepared well in advance for the institution of RRT. They should be referred to a nephrologist in a timely manner, as those who are referred late, when they are very close to requiring dialysis, tend to have poorer outcomes.

Several decisions need to be taken in discussion with the patient and family. The first is to decide whether RRT is an appropriate choice or whether conservative treatment might be preferable (see the next section). This is especially relevant in patients with significant comorbidity. For those who decide to go ahead with RRT, there are further choices between haemodialysis and peritoneal dialysis (Box 18.34), between hospital and home treatment, and on referral for renal transplantation.

Since there is no evidence that early initiation of RRT improves outcome, the overall aim is to commence RRT when symptoms of CKD begin to impact on quality of life but before serious complications have occurred. While there is wide variation between patients, this typically occurs when the eGFR approaches $10\,mL/min/1.73\,m^2$. This may be a useful marker to predict the timing of initiation of RRT by extrapolating from a plot of serial eGFR measurements over time (see Fig. 18.23).

Preparations for starting RRT should begin at least 12 months before the predicted start date. This involves providing the patient with psychological and social support, assessing home circumstances and discussing the various choices of treatment (Fig. 18.25). Depression is common in patients who are on or approaching RRT, and support from the renal multidisciplinary team should be provided both for them and for their relatives, to explain and help them adapt to the changes to lifestyle that may be necessary once RRT starts; this may help to reduce their anxieties about these changes. Physical preparations include establishment of timely access for haemodialysis or peritoneal dialysis and vaccination against hepatitis B.

Renal replacement therapy

Renal replacement therapy (RRT) may be required on a temporary basis in patients with AKI or on a permanent basis for those with advanced CKD. Since the advent of long-term RRT in the 1960s, the number of patients with ESRD who are kept alive by dialysis and transplantation has increased considerably. By the end of 2017, almost 65 000 patients were on RRT in the UK, with a median age of 59 years. After a long period of expansion, the number of patients on dialysis in the UK and the United States has begun to stabilise; however, the total number of patients on RRT continues to expand, due to an increasing proportion (55%) of patients with a functional transplant. The remaining patients were on haemodialysis (39%) and peritoneal dialysis (6%).

There are variations in the number of patients receiving RRT in different countries because of differences in the incidence of predisposing disease, as well as differences in medical practice. For example, the incidence rate for RRT in the United States in 2017 was three times higher than in the UK (370 versus 121 patients per million population), and the prevalence rate at the end of 2017 was more than twice as high (2204 versus 983 per million population). Diabetic kidney disease is the most common cause of ESRD in many countries, accounting for 29% of all ESRD in the UK and almost 50% in the United States. The large increase in the prevalence of type 2 diabetes in developing countries is resulting in a predictable rise in cases of ESRD, which is challenging already stretched health-care resources.

Survival on dialysis is strongly influenced by age and presence of complications such as diabetes (Fig. 18.26). For this reason, conservative care rather than RRT may be a more appropriate option for older patients or those with extensive comorbidities. Although many young patients without extrarenal disease lead normal and active lives on RRT, those aged 30–34 have a mortality rate 25 times higher than that of age-matched controls.

The aim of RRT is to replace the excretory functions of the kidney and to maintain normal electrolyte concentrations and fluid balance. Various

i 18.34 Comparison of haemodialysis and peritoneal dialysis	
Haemodialysis	**Peritoneal dialysis**
Efficient; 4 hrs three times per week is usually adequate	Less efficient; four exchanges per day are usually required, each taking 30–60 mins (continuous ambulatory peritoneal dialysis) or 8–10 hrs each night (automated peritoneal dialysis)
2–3 days between treatments	A few hours between treatments
Requires visits to hospital (although home treatment is possible with adaptations for some patients)	Performed at home
Requires adequate vascular access	Requires an intact peritoneal cavity without major scarring from previous surgery
Careful adherence to diet and fluid restrictions required between treatments	Diet and fluid less restricted
Fluid removal compressed into treatment periods; may cause symptoms and haemodynamic instability	Slow continuous fluid removal, usually asymptomatic
Infections related to vascular access may occur	Peritonitis and catheter-related infections may occur
Patients are usually dependent on others	Patients can take full responsibility for their treatment

options are available, including haemodialysis, haemofiltration, haemodiafiltration, peritoneal dialysis and renal transplantation, and each of these is discussed in more detail below. Indications for starting RRT in both AKI and CKD may be found in Box 18.35.

Conservative treatment

In older patients and those with multiple comorbidities, conservative treatment of stage 5 CKD, aimed at limiting the adverse symptoms of ESRD without commencing RRT, is increasingly viewed as a positive choice (see Box 18.36). Current evidence suggests that survival of these patients without dialysis can be similar or only slightly shorter than that of patients who undergo RRT, but they avoid the hospitalisation and interventions associated with dialysis. Patients are offered full medical, psychological and social support to optimise and sustain their existing renal function and to treat complications, such as anaemia, for as long as possible, with appropriate palliative care in the terminal phase of their disease. Many of these patients enjoy a good quality of life for several years. When quality of life on dialysis is poor, it is appropriate to consider discontinuing it, following discussion with the patient and family, and to offer palliative care.

Haemodialysis

Haemodialysis is the most common form of dialysis employed in ESRD and is also used in AKI. Haemodialysis involves gaining access to the circulation, either through a central venous catheter or an arteriovenous fistula or graft. The patient's blood is pumped through a haemodialyser, which allows bidirectional diffusion of solutes between blood and the dialysate across a semipermeable membrane down a concentration gradient (see Fig. 18.25A). The composition of the dialysate can be varied to achieve the desired solute gradient, and fluid can be removed by applying negative pressure to the dialysate side.

Haemodialysis in AKI

Haemodialysis offers the best rate of small-solute clearance in AKI, compared with other techniques such as haemofiltration, but should be

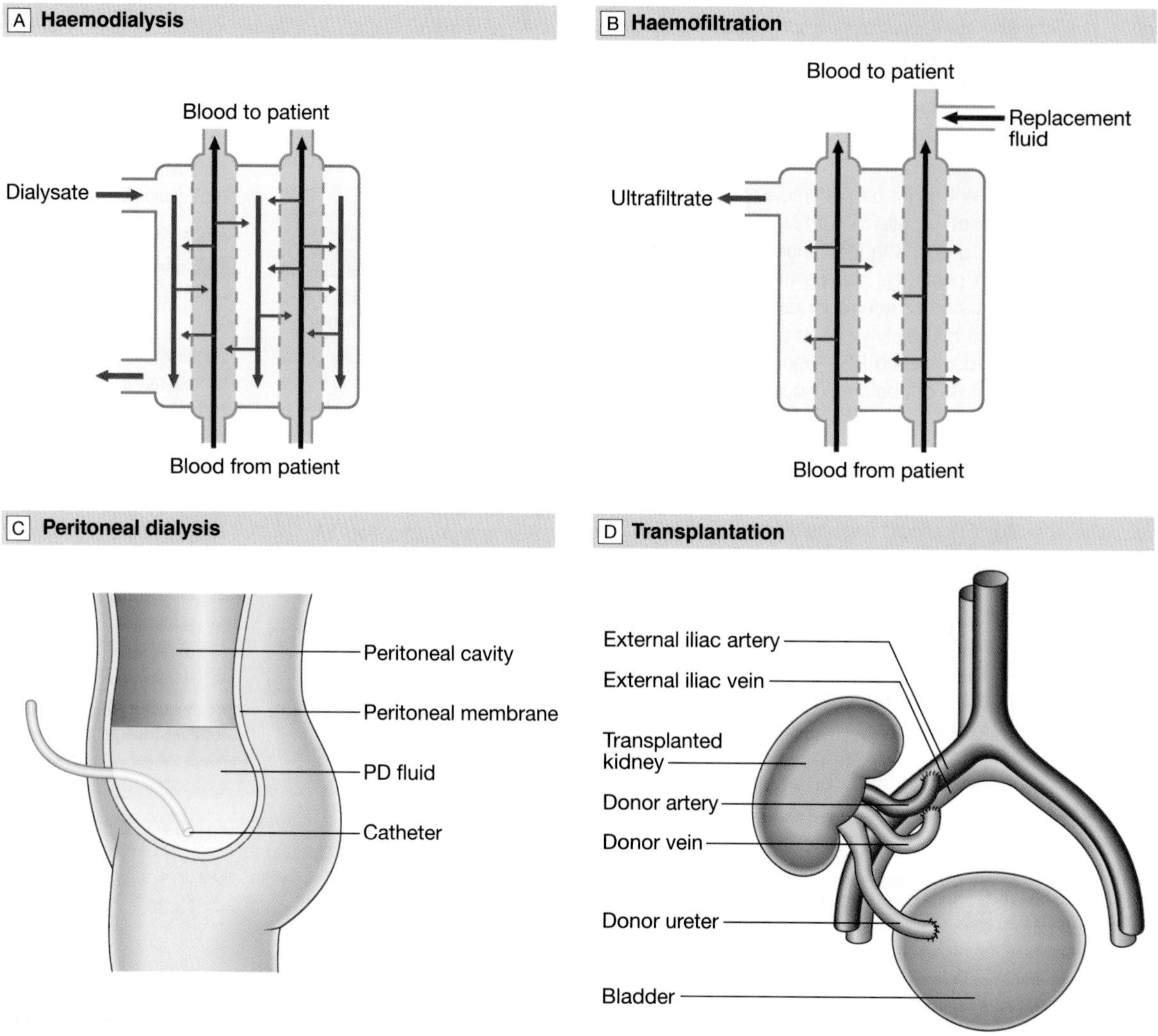

A **Haemodialysis**

Blood to patient

Dialysate →

Blood from patient

B **Haemofiltration**

Blood to patient

→ Replacement fluid

Ultrafiltrate ←

Blood from patient

C **Peritoneal dialysis**

Peritoneal cavity
Peritoneal membrane
PD fluid
Catheter

D **Transplantation**

External iliac artery
External iliac vein
Transplanted kidney
Donor artery
Donor vein
Donor ureter
Bladder

Fig. 18.25 Options for renal replacement therapy. A In haemodialysis, there is diffusion of solutes from blood to dialysate across a semipermeable membrane down a concentration gradient. B In haemofiltration, both water and solutes are filtered across a porous semipermeable membrane by a pressure gradient. Replacement fluid is added to the filtered blood before it is returned to the patient. C In peritoneal dialysis (PD), fluid is introduced into the abdominal cavity using a catheter. Solutes diffuse from blood across the peritoneal membrane to PD fluid down a concentration gradient, and water diffuses through osmosis (see text for details). D In transplantation, the blood supply of the transplanted kidney is generally anastomosed to the external iliac vessels and the ureter to the bladder. The transplanted kidney replaces all functions of the failed kidney.

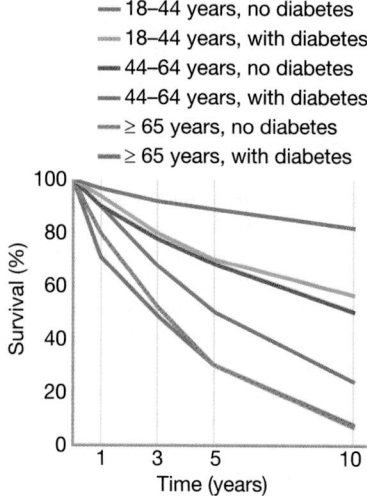

— 18–44 years, no diabetes
— 18–44 years, with diabetes
— 44–64 years, no diabetes
— 44–64 years, with diabetes
— ≥ 65 years, no diabetes
— ≥ 65 years, with diabetes

Fig. 18.26 Percentage survival after commencing renal replacement therapy according to age group and presence of diabetes.

started gradually because of the risk of delirium and convulsions due to cerebral oedema (dialysis disequilibrium). Typically, 1–2 hours of dialysis is prescribed initially but, subsequently, patients with AKI who are haemodynamically stable can be treated by 4–5 hours of haemodialysis on alternate days, or 2–3 hours every day. During dialysis, it is standard practice to anticoagulate patients, typically using heparin but the dose may be reduced if there is a bleeding risk. In patients undergoing short treatments and in those with abnormal clotting, it may be possible to avoid anticoagulation altogether. In AKI, dialysis is performed through a large-bore, dual-lumen catheter inserted into the femoral or internal jugular vein (Fig. 18.27A).

Haemodialysis in ESRD

In ESRD, vascular access for haemodialysis is gained by formation of an arteriovenous fistula (AVF), usually in the forearm, up to a year before dialysis is contemplated (Fig. 18.27B). After 4–6 weeks, increased pressure transmitted from the artery to the vein leading from the fistula causes distension and thickening of the vessel wall (arterialisation). Large-bore needles can then be inserted into the vein to provide access for each haemodialysis treatment.

18.35 Indications for dialysis with examples for AKI and CKD		
Indication*	Acute examples	Chronic examples
Uraemia	Pericarditis Encephalopathy	Uraemic syndrome including anorexia, nausea, lethargy (generally not seen until eGFR <10 mL/min/1.73 m^2)
Fluid overload	Acute pulmonary oedema	Intractable dependent oedema resistant to diuretics Pulmonary oedema Severe hypertension
Hyperkalaemia	High potassium (generally >6.5 mmol/L) with ECG changes (especially broad QRS)	Potassium resistant to dietary control and medical intervention
Metabolic acidosis	Severe acidosis (H$^+$ >79 nmol/L; pH <7.1)	Chronic acidosis resistant to bicarbonate therapy
Other (often relative indications)	Bleeding diathesis considered due to uraemia-induced platelet dysfunction	Intractable anaemia despite erythropoietin and iron Hyperphosphataemia despite binders

*The presence of anuria in AKI will modify the above indications, as these complications will not resolve if the patient is persistently anuric. Most indications to commence chronic dialysis are relative indications; a holistic approach is taken to making this decision.
(AKI = acute kidney injury; CKD = chronic kidney disease; ECG = electrocardiogram; eGFR = estimated glomerular filtration rate)

18.36 Renal replacement therapy in old age

- **Quality of life**: age itself is not a barrier to good quality of life on RRT.
- **Coexisting cardiovascular disease**: older people are more sensitive to fluid balance changes, predisposing to hypotension during dialysis with rebound hypertension between dialysis sessions. A failing heart cannot cope with fluid overload, and pulmonary oedema develops easily.
- **Confusion**: sudden changes in serum electrolyte composition during dialysis may exacerbate confusion in patients with early dementia.
- **Provision of treatment**: peritoneal dialysis may avoid the problems due to sudden changes in fluid and electrolyte status; however, older patients often require assistance with performing peritoneal dialysis, typically assistance setting up fluids and connecting/disconnecting to automated peritoneal dialysis.
- **Survival on dialysis**: difficult to predict for an individual patient, but old age plus substantial comorbidity are associated with poor survival. In such patients similar survival may be achieved through conservative care, without the complications associated with dialysis.
- **Withdrawal from dialysis**: may be appropriate whenever quality of life deteriorates irreversibly, usually in the context of severe comorbidity.
- **Transplantation**: relative risks of surgery and immunosuppression exclude many older people from transplantation.
- **Conservative therapy**: without dialysis but with adequate support. This is an appropriate option for patients at high risk of complications from dialysis who have a limited prognosis.

Preservation of arm veins is thus very important in patients with progressive renal disease who may require haemodialysis in the future. If creation of an AVF is not possible, synthetic polytetrafluoroethylene (PTFE) grafts may be fashioned between an artery and a vein, or central venous catheters may be used for short-term access (Fig. 18.27C). These are tunnelled under the skin to reduce infection risk.

All patients starting dialysis must be screened in advance for hepatitis B, hepatitis C and HIV, and vaccinated against hepatitis B if they are not immune. All dialysis units should have segregation facilities for hepatitis B-positive patients, given its easy transmissibility. Patients with hepatitis C and HIV are less infectious and can be treated satisfactorily using machine segregation and standard infection control measures.

Haemodialysis is usually carried out for 3–5 hours three times weekly, either at home or in an outpatient dialysis unit. The intensity and frequency of dialysis should be adjusted to achieve a reduction in urea during dialysis (urea reduction ratio) of over 65%; below this level there is an increase in mortality. Most patients notice an improvement in symptoms during the first 6 weeks of treatment. The intensity of dialysis can be increased by:

- escalating the number of standard sessions to four or more per week
- performing short, frequent dialysis sessions of 2–3 hours 5–7 times per week

- performing nocturnal haemodialysis, when low blood-pump speeds are used for approximately 8 hours overnight 5–6 times per week
- including a filtration component (haemodiafiltration) to achieve greater clearance of larger molecules.

More frequent dialysis and nocturnal dialysis can achieve better fluid balance and phosphate control, improve left ventricular mass and possibly improve mortality, although the latter has not yet been robustly demonstrated. Box 18.37 summarises some of the problems related to haemodialysis.

Haemofiltration

Haemofiltration is employed continuously for long periods daily using a dual-lumen intravenous catheter and is hence termed continuous venovenous haemofiltration (CVVH). This technique is principally used in the treatment of AKI in patients who are haemodynamically unstable and who therefore may not tolerate the rapid fluid and electrolyte changes associated with intermittent haemodialysis. Large volumes of water are filtered from blood across a porous semipermeable membrane under a pressure gradient. Solutes are removed via 'solvent drag' rather than by diffusion, therefore this method is less efficient at clearing urea and potassium than haemodialysis. Replacement fluid of a suitable electrolyte composition is added to the blood after it exits the haemofilter. If removal of fluid is required, then less fluid is added back than is removed (see Fig. 18.25B). Typically 1–2 L of filtrate is replaced per hour (equivalent to a GFR of 15–30 mL/min/1.73 m^2); higher rates of filtration may be of benefit in patients with sepsis and multi-organ failure. Issues concerning anticoagulation are similar to those for haemodialysis, but may be more problematic because longer or continuous anticoagulation is necessary.

Haemodiafiltration combines haemodialysis with approximately 20–30 L of ultrafiltration (with replacement of filtrate) over a 3–5-hour treatment. It uses a large-pore membrane and combines the improved clearance of medium-sized molecules observed in haemofiltration with the higher small-solute clearance of haemodialysis. It is sometimes used in the treatment of AKI, often as continuous therapy. It is increasingly employed in patients on chronic dialysis but is more expensive than haemodialysis and the long-term benefits are not yet established.

Peritoneal dialysis

Peritoneal dialysis is principally used in the treatment of CKD, though it may occasionally be employed in AKI. It requires the insertion of a permanent Silastic catheter into the peritoneal cavity (see Fig. 18.25C). Two types are in common use. In continuous ambulatory peritoneal dialysis (CAPD), about 2 L of sterile dialysis fluid are introduced and left in place

18

for approximately 4–6 hours. Metabolic waste products diffuse from peritoneal capillaries into the dialysis fluid down a concentration gradient. The fluid is then drained and fresh dialysis fluid introduced, in a continuous four-times-daily cycle. The inflow fluid is rendered hyperosmolar by the addition of glucose or glucose polymer; this results in net removal of fluid from the patient during each cycle, due to diffusion of water from the blood through the peritoneal membrane down an osmotic gradient (ultrafiltration). The patient is mobile and able to undertake normal daily activities. Automated peritoneal dialysis (APD) is similar to CAPD but uses a machine to perform the fluid exchanges during the night, typically leaving some fluid in the peritoneum during the day for ongoing dialysis.

CAPD is particularly useful in children, as a first treatment in adults with some residual renal function, and as a treatment for older patients with cardiovascular instability. The long-term use of peritoneal dialysis may be limited by episodes of bacterial peritonitis and damage to the peritoneal membrane, including encapsulating peritoneal sclerosis, but some patients have been treated successfully for more than 10 years. Box 18.38 summarises some of the problems related to CAPD treatment.

Renal transplantation

Renal transplantation offers the best chance of long-term survival in ESRD and is the most cost-effective treatment. All patients with ESRD should be considered for transplantation but many are not suitable due to a combination of comorbidity and advanced age (although no absolute age limit applies). Active malignancy, vasculitis and cardiovascular comorbidity are common contraindications to transplantation, with risk of recurrence of the original renal disease (generally glomerulonephritides) being a less common problem.

Kidney grafts may be taken from a deceased donor in the UK after brain death (37%) or circulatory death (25%), or from a living donor (38%). As described in the section on transplantation and graft rejection in Chapter 4, matching of a donor to a specific recipient is strongly influenced by immunological factors, since graft rejection is the major cause of transplant failure. Compatibility of ABO blood group between donor and recipient is usually required and the degree of matching for major histocompatibility (MHC) antigens, particularly human leucocyte antigens (HLA) A, B and DR, influences the incidence of rejection. Immediately prior to transplantation, cross-matching should be performed for anti-HLA antibodies (traditionally mixing of recipient serum with donor lymphocytes) (Ch. 4). Positive tests predict early rejection and worse graft survival. Although some ABO- and HLA-incompatible transplants are now possible, this involves appropriate preparation with pre-transplant plasma exchange and/or immunosuppression, so that recipient antibodies to the donor's tissue are reduced to acceptably low levels. This option is generally only available for living donor transplants because of the preparation required. Paired exchanges, in which a donor–recipient pair who are incompatible, either due to blood group or anti-HLA antibodies, are computer-matched with another pair to overcome the mismatch, are also used to increase the number of successful transplants that can be performed.

During the transplant operation, the kidney is placed in the pelvis; the donor vessels are usually anastomosed to the recipient's external iliac artery and vein, and the donor ureter to the bladder (see Fig. 18.25D). The native kidneys are typically left in place but may be removed pre-transplant if they are a source of repeated sepsis or to make room for a transplant kidney in patients with very large kidneys due to adult polycystic kidney disease.

All transplant patients require regular life-long follow-up to monitor renal function and complications of immunosuppression. Allograft dysfunction is often asymptomatic and picked up during routine surveillance blood tests. The common causes at different time points post transplant are summarised in Box 18.39. Immunosuppressive therapy (see Box 4.21) is required to prevent rejection and is more intensive in the early post-transplantation period, when rejection risk is highest. A common regimen is triple therapy with prednisolone; ciclosporin or tacrolimus; and azathioprine or mycophenolate mofetil. Sirolimus is an alternative that can be introduced later but is generally not used initially due to impaired wound healing. Basiliximab, an interleukin (IL)-2 receptor antagonist, is frequently used at induction to lower rates of rejection. Anti-lymphocyte preparations (e.g. anti-thymocyte globulin, ATG) may also be used as induction, especially in higher risk cases. Acute cellular rejection is usually treated, in the first instance, by high-dose glucocorticoids, such as intravenous methylprednisolone on three consecutive days. ATG is also used for glucocorticoid-resistant rejection. Antibody-mediated rejection is more difficult to treat and usually requires plasma exchange and intravenous immunoglobulin (Ch. 4). Complications of immunosuppression include infections and malignancy (Ch. 4).

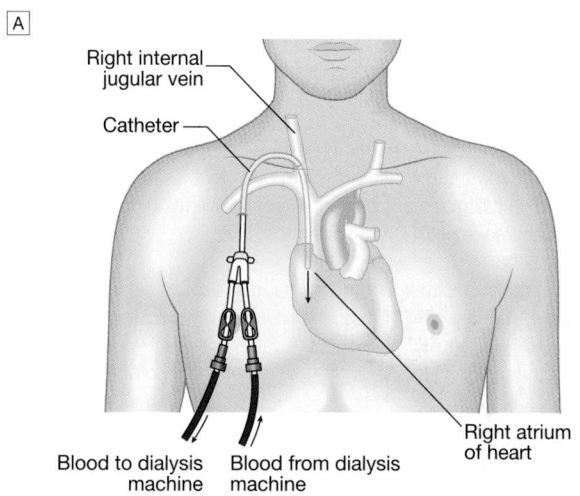

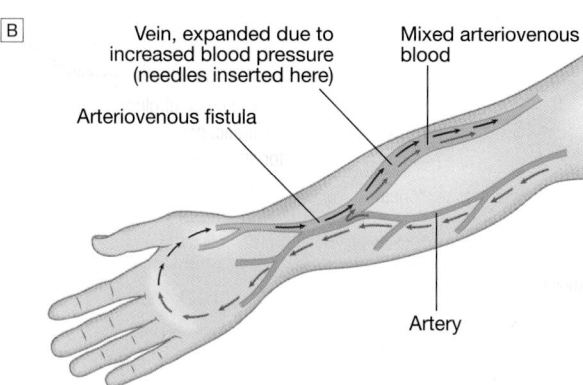

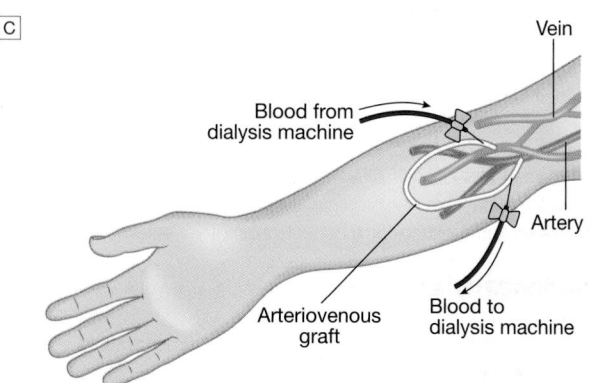

Fig. 18.27 Haemodialysis access. [A] A tunnelled cuffed dialysis catheter. [B] An arteriovenous fistula. [C] An arteriovenous graft.

18.37 Problems with haemodialysis

Problem	Clinical features	Cause	Treatment
During treatments			
Hypotension	Sudden ↓BP; often leg cramps; sometimes chest pain	Fluid removal and hypovolaemia	Saline infusion; exclude cardiac ischaemia; quinine may help cramp
Cardiac arrhythmias	Hypotension; sometimes chest pain	Potassium and acid–base shifts	Check K⁺; review dialysis prescription; stop dialysis
Haemorrhage	Blood loss (overt or occult); hypotension	Anticoagulation Venous needle disconnection	Stop dialysis; seek source; consider heparin-free treatment
Air embolism	Circulatory collapse; cardiac arrest	Disconnected or faulty lines and equipment malfunction	Stop dialysis
Dialyser hypersensitivity	Acute circulatory collapse	Allergic reaction to dialysis membrane or sterilisant	Stop dialysis; change to different artificial kidney
Systemic sepsis	Rigors; fever; ↓BP	Usually involves vascular access devices (catheter or fistula)	Blood cultures; antibiotics
Between treatments			
Pulmonary oedema	Breathlessness	Fluid overload	Ultrafiltration, fluid restriction, lower dry weight

(BP = blood pressure)

18.38 Problems with continuous ambulatory peritoneal dialysis

Problem	Clinical features	Cause	Treatment
Peritonitis	Cloudy drainage fluid; abdominal pain and systemic sepsis are variable	Usually entry of skin contaminants via catheter; bowel organisms less common	Culture of peritoneal dialysis fluid Intraperitoneal antibiotics Catheter removal sometimes required
Catheter exit site infection	Erythema and pus around exit site	Usually skin organisms	Antibiotics; sometimes surgical drainage
Peritoneal membrane leaks	Fluid leak from tunnel or pleural effusion (typically unilateral and right-sided)	Leak adjacent to catheter or via congenital pleuroperitoneal communication	Temporary reduction in volume of dialysis fluid. However, pleuroperitoneal leaks are likely to require switch to haemodialysis
Ultrafiltration failure	Fluid overload	Damage to peritoneal membrane, leading to rapid transport of glucose and loss of osmotic gradient	Replacement of glucose with synthetic, poorly absorbed polymers for some exchanges (icodextrin)
Peritoneal membrane failure	Inadequate clearance of urea etc.	Scarring/damage to peritoneal membrane	Increase in exchange volumes; consideration of automated peritoneal dialysis or switch to haemodialysis
Sclerosing peritonitis	Intermittent bowel obstruction Malnutrition	Unknown; typically occurs after many years on peritoneal dialysis	Switch to haemodialysis (may still progress) Surgery and tamoxifen may be used

Approximately 50% of patients of European descent develop skin malignancy by 15 years after transplantation.

The prognosis after kidney transplantation is good. Recent UK statistics for transplants from deceased donors indicate 97% patient survival and 94% graft survival at 1 year, and 87% patient and 87% graft survival at 5 years. Even better figures are obtained with living donor transplantation (92% graft survival and 94% patient survival at 5 years).

Renal disease in pregnancy

Pregnancy has important physiological effects on the renal system. Some diseases are more common in pregnancy (Box 18.40), the manifestations of others are modified during pregnancy, and a few diseases, such as pre-eclampsia (see Box 32.8), are unique to pregnancy. These are discussed in detail in Chapter 32.

Renal disease in adolescence

Many causes of renal failure present during infancy or childhood, such as congenital urological malformations and inherited disorders like cystinosis and autosomal recessive polycystic kidney disease. The consequences continue throughout the patient's life and the situation often arises whereby patients transition from paediatric to adult nephrology services. Some of the issues and challenges surrounding this transition are summarised in Box 18.41.

Drugs and the kidney

Drug-induced renal disease

The kidney is susceptible to damage by drugs because it is the route of excretion of many water-soluble compounds, including drugs and

i 18.39 Common causes of renal allograft dysfunction

Time post transplant	Cause	Risk factors
Hours to days	Renal artery/vein thrombosis	Technically difficult surgery Thrombophilia/SLE
	Ureteric anastomotic leak	Small bladder/anuria pre-transplant
	Delayed graft function (i.e. transplant does not start working immediately)	Prolonged cold ischaemia time* Donation after circulatory death Older, hypertensive donor with stroke as cause of death, high tacrolimus level
	Hyperacute rejection	Pre-formed anti-HLA antibodies HLA mismatch Previous transplant
Weeks	Acute rejection (especially <3 months; can occur later with non-adherence/insufficient immunosuppression)	Pre-formed anti-HLA antibodies HLA mismatch Previous transplant
Months	BK virus nephropathy	Intensive immunosuppression Ureteric stent use
	Renal artery stenosis	Donor disease Injury at organ retrieval
Years	Chronic allograft injury (often antibody-mediated)	Previous acute rejections Non-adherence/insufficient immunosuppression
Any time	Tacrolimus/ciclosporin toxicity	High doses/serum levels Concurrent use of drugs that inhibit cytochrome P450 system

	Sepsis (opportunistic and conventional)
	Recurrence of disease:
	  Early (FSGS/MCGN/aHUS)
	  Later (IgA nephropathy/membranous glomerulonephritis)
		Primary FSGS and MCGN
		Previous transplant recurrence

*Time from organ retrieval in the donor until implantation into the recipient.
(aHUS = atypical haemolytic uraemic syndrome; FSGS = focal segmental glomerulosclerosis; HLA = human leucocyte antigen; IgA = immunoglobulin A; MCGN = mesangiocapillary glomerulonephritis; SLE = systemic lupus erythematosus)

 18.40 Renal diseases in pregnancy

- **Eclampsia**: severe hypertension, encephalopathy and fits
- **Disseminated intravascular coagulation**
- **Thrombotic microangiopathy**: may be part of pre-eclampsia spectrum and can also occur post-partum (including thrombotic thrombocytopenic purpura/haemolytic uraemic syndrome)
- **Acute fatty liver of pregnancy**
- **'HELLP' syndrome**: haemolysis, elevated liver enzymes, low platelets (thrombotic microangiopathy with abnormal liver function)

 18.41 Kidney disease in adolescence

- **Adherence**: young adults moving from parental supervision may become disengaged. There may also be reduced adherence to prophylactic and therapeutic treatment, including immunosuppressive medications, diet and fluid restrictions and dialysis.
- **Adverse events**: there is an increased risk of transplant loss and other adverse events in young adults on renal replacement therapy.
- **Management**: joint transition clinics should be established with the paediatric team to facilitate transfer to adult specialist clinics.

their metabolites. Some may reach high concentrations in the renal cortex as a result of proximal tubular transport mechanisms. Others are concentrated in the medulla by the operation of the countercurrent system.

Toxic renal damage may occur by a variety of mechanisms (Box 18.42). Very commonly, drugs contribute to the development of acute tubular necrosis as one of multiple insults. Numerically, reactions to NSAIDs and ACE inhibitors are the most important. Haemodynamic renal impairment, acute tubular necrosis and allergic reactions are usually reversible if recognised early enough. Other types, however, especially those associated with extensive fibrosis, are less likely to be reversible.

Non-steroidal anti-inflammatory drugs

Impairment of renal function may develop in patients on NSAIDs, since prostaglandins play an important role in regulating renal blood flow by vasodilating afferent arterioles (see Fig. 18.19). This is particularly likely in patients with other disorders, such as volume depletion, heart failure, cirrhosis, sepsis and pre-existing renal impairment. In addition, idiosyncratic immune reactions may occur, causing minimal change nephrotic syndrome, membranous nephropathy (p. 574) and acute interstitial nephritis (p. 576). Analgesic nephropathy (see Box 18.19) is now a rare complication of long-term use.

ACE inhibitors

These abolish the compensatory angiotensin II-mediated vasoconstriction of the glomerular efferent arteriole that takes place in order to maintain glomerular perfusion pressure distal to a renal artery stenosis and in renal hypoperfusion (see Figs. 18.1 and 18.19). Monitoring of renal function before and after initiation of therapy is essential and an expected rise in creatinine of about 20% is frequently observed.

Prescribing in renal disease

Many drugs and drug metabolites are excreted by the kidney and so the presence of renal impairment alters the required dose and frequency (p. 31). Immunosuppressive medications such as tacrolimus or ciclosporin are metabolised by the cytochrome P450 system, hence drug interactions need to be considered before prescribing other medications.

i	18.42 Mechanisms and examples of drug-induced renal disease/dysfunction		
Mechanism	**Drug or toxin**	**Comments**	
Haemodynamic	NSAIDs	Reduce renal blood flow due to inhibition of prostaglandin synthesis causing afferent arteriolar vasoconstriction	
	ACE inhibitors	Reduce efferent glomerular arteriolar tone, so especially problematic in the presence of renal artery stenosis and other causes of renal hypoperfusion (e.g. sepsis)	
	Radiographic contrast media	Multifactorial aetiology may include intense vasoconstriction	
Acute tubular necrosis	Aminoglycosides, amphotericin	In most examples there is evidence of direct tubular toxicity but haemodynamic and other factors probably contribute	
	Paracetamol overdose	May occur with or without serious hepatotoxicity	
	Radiographic contrast media	Directly toxic to proximal tubular cells	
Loss of tubular/collecting duct function	Lithium Cisplatin Aminoglycosides, amphotericin	Dose-related, partially reversible loss of concentrating ability Occurs at lower exposures than cause acute tubular necrosis	
Glomerulonephritis (immune-mediated)	Penicillamine, gold	Membranous nephropathy	
	Penicillamine, propylthiouracil, hydralazine	Crescentic or focal necrotising glomerulonephritis in association with ANCA and systemic small-vessel vasculitis	
	NSAIDs	Minimal change nephropathy, membranous nephropathy	
Interstitial nephritis (immune-mediated)	NSAIDs, penicillins, proton pump inhibitors, many others	Acute interstitial nephritis	
Interstitial nephritis (toxicity)	Lithium	As a consequence of acute toxicity Chronic interstitial nephritis	
	Ciclosporin, tacrolimus		
Papillary necrosis	Various NSAIDs	Ischaemic damage secondary to NSAID effects on renal blood flow	
Tubular obstruction (crystal formation)	Aciclovir	Crystals of the drug form in tubules Aciclovir is now more common than the original example of sulphonamides	
	Chemotherapy	Uric acid crystals form as a consequence of tumour lysis (typically, a first-dose effect in haematological malignancy)	
Nephrocalcinosis	Oral sodium phosphate-containing bowel cleansing agents	Precipitation of calcium phosphate occurring in 1%–4% and exacerbated by volume depletion Usually mild but damage can be irreversible	
Retroperitoneal fibrosis	Ergolinic dopamine agonists (cabergoline),	Idiopathic retroperitoneal fibrosis is more common	

(ACE = angiotensin-converting enzyme; ANCA = antineutrophil cytoplasmic antibody; NSAIDs = non-steroidal anti-inflammatory drugs)

Infections of the urinary tract

In health, bacterial colonisation is confined to the lower end of the urethra and the remainder of the urinary tract is sterile (see Ch. 6). The urinary tract can become infected with various bacteria but the most common is *E. coli* derived from the gastrointestinal tract. The most common presenting problem is cystitis with urethritis (generally referred to as urinary tract infection (UTI)).

Urinary tract infection

UTI is a common disorder, accounting for 1%–3% of consultations in general medical practice. The prevalence of UTI in women is about 3% at the age of 20, increasing by about 1% in each subsequent decade. In males, UTI is uncommon, except in the first year of life and in men over 60, when it may complicate bladder outflow obstruction.

Pathophysiology

Urine is an excellent culture medium for bacteria; in addition, the urothelium of susceptible persons may have more receptors, to which virulent strains of *E. coli* become adherent. In women, the ascent of organisms into the bladder is easier than in men; the urethra is shorter and the absence of bactericidal prostatic secretions may be relevant. Sexual intercourse may cause minor urethral trauma and transfer bacteria from the perineum into the bladder. Instrumentation of the bladder may also introduce organisms. Multiplication of organisms then depends on a number of factors, including the size of the inoculum and virulence of the bacteria. Conditions that predispose to UTI are shown in Box 18.43.

Clinical features

Typical features of cystitis and urethritis include:

- abrupt onset of frequency of micturition and urgency
- burning pain in the urethra during micturition (dysuria)
- suprapubic pain during and after voiding
- intense desire to pass more urine after micturition, due to spasm of the inflamed bladder wall (strangury)
- urine that may appear cloudy and have an unpleasant odour
- non-visible or visible haematuria.

Systemic symptoms are usually slight or absent. However, infection in the lower urinary tract can spread to cause acute pyelonephritis. This is suggested by prominent systemic symptoms with fever, rigors, vomiting, hypotension and loin pain, guarding or tenderness, and may be an indication for hospitalisation. Only about 30% of patients with acute pyelonephritis have associated symptoms of cystitis or urethritis. Prostatitis is suggested by perineal or suprapubic pain, pain on ejaculation and prostatic tenderness on rectal examination.

The differential diagnosis of lower urinary tract symptoms includes urethritis due to sexually transmitted disease, notably chlamydia (Ch. 15) and urethritis associated with reactive arthritis (Ch. 26). Some patients, usually female, have symptoms suggestive of urethritis and cystitis but no bacteria are cultured from the urine ('urethral syndrome'). Possible explanations include infection with organisms not readily cultured by ordinary methods (such as *Chlamydia* and certain anaerobes), intermittent or low-count bacteriuria, reaction to toiletries or disinfectants, symptoms related to sexual intercourse, or post-menopausal atrophic vaginitis.

The differential diagnosis of acute pyelonephritis includes pyonephrosis, acute appendicitis, diverticulitis, cholecystitis, salpingitis, ruptured ovarian cyst or ectopic pregnancy. In pyonephrosis due to an infected and obstructed upper urinary tract, patients may become extremely ill, with fever, leucocytosis and positive blood cultures. With a perinephric abscess, there is marked pain and tenderness, and often bulging of the loin on the affected side. Urinary symptoms may be absent in this situation and urine testing negative, containing neither pus cells nor organisms.

Investigations

An approach to investigation is shown in Box 18.44. In an otherwise healthy woman with a single lower urinary tract infection, urine culture prior to treatment is not mandatory. Investigation is necessary, however, in patients with recurrent infection or after failure of initial treatment, during pregnancy, or in patients susceptible to serious infection, such as the immunocompromised, those with diabetes or an indwelling catheter, and older people (Box 18.45). The diagnosis can be made from the combination of typical clinical features and abnormalities on urinalysis. In symptomatic infections, urine dipstick tests may be positive for leucocyte esterase released from neutrophils and nitrites, due to conversion of nitrates to nitrites by urinary pathogens. The absence of both nitrites and leucocyte esterase in the urine makes UTI unlikely. Interpretation of bacterial counts in the urine, and of what is a 'significant' culture result, is based on probabilities. Urine taken by suprapubic aspiration should be sterile, so the presence of any organisms is significant. If the patient has symptoms and there are neutrophils in the urine, a small number of organisms is significant. In asymptomatic patients, more than 10^5 organisms/mL is usually regarded as significant (asymptomatic bacteriuria; see below).

Typical organisms causing UTI in the community include *E. coli* derived from the gastrointestinal tract (about 75% of infections), *Proteus* spp., *Pseudomonas* spp., streptococci and *Staphylococcus epidermidis*. In hospital, *E. coli* still predominates but *Klebsiella* and streptococci are becoming more common. Certain strains of *E. coli* have a particular propensity to invade the urinary tract.

Investigations to detect underlying predisposing factors for UTI are used selectively, most commonly in children, men or patients with recurrent infections (see Box 18.44).

Management

Antibiotics are recommended in all cases of proven UTI (Box 18.46), but not asymptomatic bacteriuria (see below). If urine culture has been

---

18.44 Investigation of patients with urinary tract infection

All patients

- Dipstick* estimation of nitrite, leucocyte esterase and glucose
- Microscopy/cytometry of urine for white blood cells, organisms
- Urine culture

Infants, children, anyone with fever or complicated infection

- Full blood count; creatinine, eGFR
- Blood cultures

Pyelonephritis: men, children, women with recurrent infections

- Renal tract ultrasound or CT
- Pelvic examination in women, rectal examination in men

Continuing haematuria or other suspicion of bladder lesion

- Cystoscopy

*May substitute for microscopy and culture in simple uncomplicated infection.

18.45 Urinary infection in old age

- **Prevalence of asymptomatic bacteriuria**: rises with age. Among the most frail in institutional care it rises to 40% in women and 30% in men.
- **Decision to treat**: treating asymptomatic bacteriuria does not improve chronic incontinence or decrease mortality or morbidity from symptomatic urinary infection. It risks adverse effects from the antibiotic and the emergence of resistant organisms. Bacteriuria should not be treated in the absence of urinary symptoms.
- **Source of infection**: the urinary tract is the most frequent source of bacteraemia in older patients admitted to hospital. It may present with an acute confusional state.
- **Incontinence**: new or increased incontinence is a common presentation of UTI in older women.
- **Treatment**: post-menopausal women with acute lower urinary tract symptoms may require longer than 3 days' therapy.

18.43 Risk factors for urinary tract infection

Bladder outflow obstruction

- Benign prostatic enlargement
- Prostate cancer
- Urethral stricture

Anatomical abnormalities

- Vesico-ureteric reflux
- Uterine prolapse
- Bladder fistula

Neurological problems

- Multiple sclerosis
- Spina bifida
- Diabetic neuropathy

Foreign bodies

- Urethral or suprapubic catheter
- Ureteric stent
- Nephrostomy tube
- Urolithiasis

Loss of host defences

- Atrophic urethritis and vaginitis in post-menopausal women

18.46 Antibiotic regimens for urinary tract infection in adults[1]				
Scenario	Drug	Regimen	Duration	Comment
Cystitis				
First choices	Trimethoprim	200 mg twice daily	3 days	7–10 days in men
	Nitrofurantoin	50 mg 4 times daily		
Second choices[1]	Cefalexin	250 mg 4 times daily		
	Ciprofloxacin	250 mg twice daily		
	Pivmecillinam	400 mg 3 times daily		
In pregnancy	Nitrofurantoin	50 mg 4 times daily	7 days	Avoid trimethoprim and quinolones during pregnancy; avoid nitrofurantoin at term
	Cefalexin	250 mg 4 times daily		
Prophylactic therapy				
First choice	Trimethoprim	100 mg at night	Continuous	
Second choice[1]	Nitrofurantoin	50 mg at night		
Pyelonephritis				
First choices	Cefalexin	1 g 4 times daily	14 days	Admit to hospital if no response within 24 hrs
	Ciprofloxacin	500 mg twice daily	7 days	
Second choices	Gentamicin[2]	Adjust dose according to renal function and serum levels	14 days	Switch to appropriate oral agent as soon as possible
	Cefuroxime	750–1500 mg 3 times daily		
Epididymo-orchitis				
Young men	Ciprofloxacin	100 mg twice daily	14 days	Refer young men to genito-urinary department to check for *Chlamydia trichomatis* and *Neisseria gonorrhoeae*, which requires addition of a single dose of ceftriaxone 500 mg IM
Older men	Ciprofloxacin	500 mg twice daily		
Acute prostatitis				
First choice	Ciprofloxacin	500 mg twice daily	14 days	
Second choice	Trimethoprim	200 mg twice daily		

[1]In all cases, the choice of drug should take locally determined antibiotic resistance patterns into account. [2]See Hartford nomogram (Fig. 6.18).
(IM = intramuscular)

18

performed, treatment may be started while awaiting the result. For infection of the lower urinary tract, treatment for 3 days is the norm and is less likely to induce significant alterations in bowel flora, including *Clostridioides* (formerly *Clostridium*) *difficile*, than more prolonged therapy. Trimethoprim or nitrofurantoin is the usual first choice of drug for initial treatment; however, between 10% and 40% of organisms causing UTI are resistant to trimethoprim, the lower rates being seen in community-based practice. Trimethoprim and nitrofurantoin are not recommended if eGFR is <30 mL/min/1.73m² due to reduced efficacy/increased risk of toxicity. In addition, trimethoprim may increase serum potassium and creatinine levels and lead to artefactual reductions in eGFR, which resolve once the drug is discontinued. Quinolone antibiotics such as ciprofloxacin and norfloxacin, and cephalosporins such as cefalexin are also generally effective. Co-amoxiclav and amoxicillin are no longer recommended as blind therapy, as up to 30% of organisms are resistant. They may be used once cultures confirm that the organism is sensitive. Penicillins and cephalosporins are safe to use in pregnancy but trimethoprim, sulphonamides, quinolones and tetracyclines should be avoided.

In more severe infection, antibiotics should be continued for 7–14 days. Seriously ill patients may require intravenous therapy with gentamicin for a few days (see Box 18.46), later switching to an oral agent.

A fluid intake of at least 2 L/day is usually recommended, although this is not based on evidence and may exacerbate symptoms of dysuria.

Persistent or recurrent UTI

If the causative organism persists on repeat culture despite treatment, or if there is reinfection with any organism after an interval, then an underlying cause is more likely to be present (see Box 18.43) and more

18.47 Prophylactic measures to be adopted by women with recurrent urinary infections
• Fluid intake of at least 2 L/day
• Regular complete emptying of bladder
• Good personal hygiene
• Emptying of bladder before and after sexual intercourse
• Cranberry juice/tablets and/or D-mannose may be effective

detailed investigation is justified (see Box 18.44). In women, recurrent infections are common and investigation is justified only if infections are frequent (three or more per year) or unusually severe. Recurrent UTI, particularly in the presence of an underlying cause, may result in permanent renal damage, whereas uncomplicated infections rarely (if ever) do so (see chronic reflux nephropathy below).

If an underlying cause cannot be treated, suppressive antibiotic therapy (see Box 18.46) can be used to prevent recurrence and reduce the risk of sepsis and renal damage. Urine should be cultured at regular intervals; a regimen of two or three antibiotics in sequence, rotating every 6 months, is often used in an attempt to reduce the emergence of resistant organisms. Other simple measures may help to prevent recurrence (Box 18.47). Trimethoprim or nitrofurantoin is recommended for prophylaxis. Alternative antibiotics include cefalexin, co-amoxiclav and ciprofloxacin, but these should be avoided if possible because of adverse effects and the generation of resistance.

Asymptomatic bacteriuria

This is defined as more than 10⁵ organisms/mL in the urine of apparently healthy asymptomatic patients. Approximately 1% of children under the age of 1 year, 1% of schoolgirls, 0.03% of schoolboys and men, 3% of non-pregnant adult women and 5% of pregnant women have asymptomatic bacteriuria. It is increasingly common in those aged over 65. There is no evidence that this condition causes renal scarring in adults who are not pregnant and have a normal urinary tract, and, in general, treatment is not indicated. Up to 30% will develop symptomatic infection within 1 year, however. Treatment is required in infants, pregnant women and those with urinary tract abnormalities.

Catheter-related bacteriuria

In patients with a urinary catheter, bacteriuria increases the risk of Gram-negative bacteraemia fivefold. Bacteriuria is common, however, and almost universal during long-term catheterisation. Treatment is usually avoided in asymptomatic patients, as this may promote antibiotic resistance. Careful sterile insertion technique is important and the catheter should be removed as soon as it is not required.

Acute pyelonephritis

The kidneys are infected in a minority of patients with UTI. Acute renal infection (pyelonephritis) presents as a classic triad of loin pain, fever and tenderness over the kidneys. The renal pelvis is inflamed and small abscesses are often evident in the renal parenchyma (see Fig. 18.13C).

Renal infection is almost always caused by organisms ascending from the bladder, and the bacterial profile is the same as for lower urinary tract infection (see above). Rarely, bacteraemia may give rise to renal or perinephric abscesses, most commonly due to staphylococci. Predisposing factors may facilitate infection, such as cysts or renal scarring.

Rarely, acute pyelonephritis is associated with papillary necrosis. Fragments of renal papillary tissue are passed per urethra and can be identified histologically. They may cause ureteric obstruction and, if this occurs bilaterally or in a single kidney, it may lead to AKI. Predisposing factors include diabetes mellitus, chronic urinary obstruction, analgesic nephropathy and sickle-cell disease. A necrotising form of pyelonephritis with gas formation, emphysematous pyelonephritis, is occasionally seen in patients with diabetes mellitus. Xanthogranulomatous pyelonephritis is a chronic infection that can resemble renal cell cancer. It is usually associated with obstruction, is characterised by accumulation of foamy macrophages and generally requires nephrectomy. Infection of cysts in polycystic kidney disease (p. 579) requires prolonged antibiotic treatment.

Appropriate investigations are shown in Box 18.44 and management is described above and in Box 18.46. Intravenous rehydration may be needed in severe cases. If complicated infection is suspected or response to treatment is not prompt, urine should be re-cultured and renal tract ultrasound performed to exclude urinary tract obstruction or a perinephric collection. If obstruction is present, drainage by a percutaneous nephrostomy or ureteric stent should be considered and the underlying cause treated.

Tuberculosis

Tuberculosis of the kidney and renal tract is secondary to tuberculosis elsewhere and is the result of blood-borne infection. Initially, lesions develop in the renal cortex; these may ulcerate into the renal pelvis and involve the ureters, bladder, epididymis, seminal vesicles and prostate. Calcification in the kidney and stricture formation in the ureter are typical.

Clinical features may include symptoms of bladder involvement (frequency, dysuria); haematuria (sometimes macroscopic); malaise, fever, night sweats, lassitude and weight loss; loin pain; associated genital disease; and chronic renal failure as a result of urinary tract obstruction or destruction of kidney tissue.

Neutrophils are present in the urine but routine urine culture may be negative (sterile pyuria). Special techniques of microscopy and culture may be required to identify tubercle bacilli and are most usefully performed on early morning urine specimens. Bladder involvement should be assessed by cystoscopy. Radiology of the urinary tract and a chest X-ray to look for pulmonary tuberculosis are mandatory. Anti-tuberculous chemotherapy follows standard regimens (see Box 17.52). Surgery to relieve urinary tract obstruction or to remove a very severely infected kidney may be required.

Urolithiasis

Renal stone disease is common, affecting people of all countries and ethnic groups. In the UK, the prevalence is about 1.2%, with a lifetime risk of developing a renal stone by age 60–70 of approximately 7% in men. In some regions, the risk is higher, most notably in Saudi Arabia, where the lifetime risk of developing a renal stone in men aged 60–70 is just over 20%.

Pathophysiology

Urinary calculi consist of aggregates of crystals, usually containing calcium or phosphate in combination with small amounts of proteins and glycoproteins. The most common types are summarised in Box 18.48. A number of risk factors have been identified for renal stone formation (Box 18.49), however in developed countries most calculi occur in healthy young men, in whom investigations reveal no clear predisposing cause. Renal stones vary greatly in size, from sand-like particles anywhere in the urinary tract to large, round stones in the bladder. In developing countries, bladder stones are common, particularly in children, whereas in developed countries, renal stones are more common. Staghorn calculi fill the whole renal pelvis and branch into the calyces (Fig. 18.28); they are usually associated with infection and composed largely of struvite. Deposits of calcium may be present throughout the renal parenchyma, giving rise to fine calcification within it (nephrocalcinosis), especially in patients with renal tubular acidosis, hyperparathyroidism, vitamin D intoxication and healed renal tuberculosis. Cortical nephrocalcinosis may occur in areas of cortical necrosis, typically after AKI in pregnancy or other severe AKI.

Clinical features

The clinical presentation is highly variable. Many patients with renal stone disease are asymptomatic, whereas others present with pain, haematuria, UTI or urinary tract obstruction. A common presentation is with acute loin pain together with haematuria: a symptom complex termed renal or ureteric colic. This is most commonly caused by ureteric obstruction by a calculus but the same symptoms can occur in association with a sloughed renal papilla, tumour or blood clot. The patient is suddenly aware of pain in the loin, which radiates round the flank to the groin and often into the testis or labium, in the sensory distribution of the first lumbar nerve. The pain steadily increases in intensity to reach a peak in a few minutes. The patient is restless and generally tries unsuccessfully to obtain relief by changing position or pacing the room. There is pallor, sweating and often vomiting.

i 18.48 Composition of renal stones

Composition	Percentage
Calcium oxalate[1]	60%
Calcium phosphate	15%
Uric acid	10%
Magnesium ammonium phosphate (struvite)[2]	15%
Cystine and others	1%

[1]Stones often contain small amounts of calcium phosphate. [2]Associated with urine infection.

i 18.49 Predisposing factors for kidney stones

General factors

- Early onset of urolithiasis (especially children and adolescents)
- Familial stone formation
- Uric acid and urate-containing stones
- Infection stones

Diseases associated with stone formation

- Hyperparathyroidism
- Metabolic syndrome
- Nephrocalcinosis
- Ileal disease or resection (increases oxalate absorption and urinary excretion)
- Polycystic kidney disease (PKD)
- Increased levels of vitamin D
- Sarcoidosis
- Spinal cord injury, neurogenic bladder

Environmental and dietary causes

- Low urine volumes: high ambient temperatures, low fluid intake
- Chronic lead and cadmium exposure

Congenital and inherited causes

- Cystinuria (type A, B and AB)
- Renal tubular acidosis type I (distal)
- Primary hyperoxaluria
- Xanthinuria
- Lesch–Nyhan syndrome
- Cystic fibrosis

Anatomical abnormalities associated with stone formation

- Medullary sponge kidney
- Pelvi-ureteric junction obstruction
- Calyceal diverticulum
- Ureteric stricture
- Ureteric reflux
- Horseshoe kidney
- Ureterocele

From EAU guidelines 2019. https://uroweb.org/guideline/urolithiasis/.

Frequency, dysuria and haematuria may occur. The intense pain usually subsides within 2 hours but may continue unabated for hours or days. It is usually constant during attacks, although slight fluctuations in severity may be seen. Subsequent to an attack of renal colic, intermittent dull pain in the loin or back may persist for several hours.

Investigations

Patients with symptoms of renal colic should be investigated to determine whether or not a stone is present, to identify its location and to assess whether it is causing obstruction. About 90% of stones contain calcium and these can be visualised on plain abdominal X-ray (radio-opaque stones) but non-contrast CTKUB (see Fig. 18.28) is the gold standard for diagnosing a stone within the kidney or ureter, as 99% of stones are visible using this method. Ultrasound can show stones within the kidney and dilatation of the renal pelvis and ureter if the stone is obstructing urine flow; it is useful in unstable patients or young women, in whom exposure to ionising radiation is particularly undesirable.

A minimum set of investigations (Box 18.50) should be performed in patients with a first renal stone. The yield of more detailed investigation is low, and hence is usually reserved for those at high risk for further stone formation (see Box 18.50). Chemical analysis of stones is often helpful in defining the underlying cause. Since most stones pass spontaneously through the urinary tract, ideally the urine should be sieved for a few days after an episode of colic in order to collect the calculus for analysis.

Management

The immediate treatment of renal colic is with analgesia and antiemetics. Renal colic is often unbearably painful and demands powerful analgesia; a non-steroidal anti-inflammatory drug (NSAID), e.g. diclofenac, given by any route is first-line treatment and is often very effective. Intravenous paracetamol should be given if NSAIDs are contraindicated or are not giving sufficient pain relief. An opioid should then be considered, e.g. morphine (10–20 mg) or pethidine (100 mg) intramuscularly.

i 18.50 Investigations for renal stones

Sample	Test	First stone	High-risk stone formers
Stone	Chemical composition[1]	✓	✓
Blood	Calcium	✓	✓
	Uric acid	✓	✓
	Urea and electrolytes	✓	✓
	Bicarbonate	✓	✓
	Parathyroid hormone[2]		(✓)
Urine	Dipstick test for protein, blood, nitrites, leucocytes, urine pH	✓	✓
	Amino acids		✓
24-hr urine	Urea		✓
	Creatinine clearance		✓
	Sodium		✓
	Calcium		✓
	Oxalate		✓
	Uric acid		✓

[1]The most valuable test if a stone can be obtained. [2]Only if serum calcium or urinary calcium excretion is high.

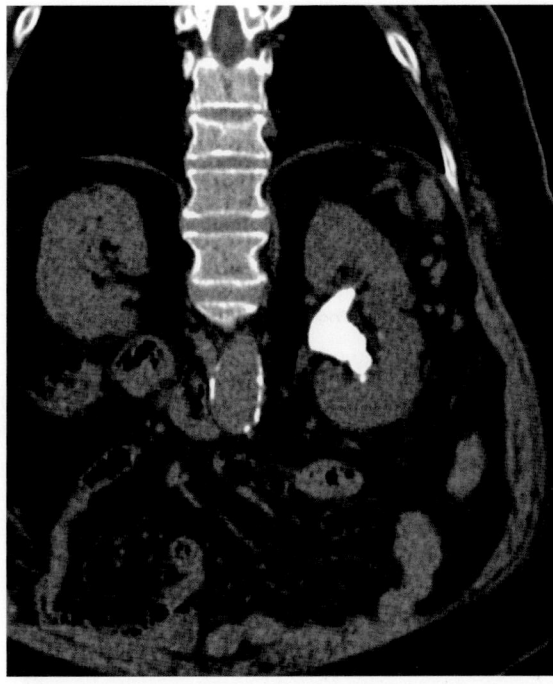

Fig. 18.28 Non-contrast computed tomogram of the kidneys, ureters and bladder (CTKUB). Coronal view showing a staghorn calculus in the left kidney. *Courtesy of Dr I. Mendichovszky, University of Cambridge.*

Patients with renal or ureteric stones are at high risk of infection; if surgery is contemplated, the patient should be covered with appropriate antibiotics. Urgent drainage of the affected collecting system with a ureteric stent or percutaneous nephrostomy is required if infection occurs in the stagnant urine proximal to the stone (pyonephrosis), and in patients with a solitary kidney who develop anuria in association with a stone in the ureter.

Asymptomatic stones less than 5 mm in diameter can be observed as they are not likely to affect quality of life and up to 90% may pass spontaneously without intervention. Conversely, only 10% of stones >6 mm in diameter pass spontaneously through the urinary tract and hence these may need an intervention. Stones can be fragmented by extracorporeal shock wave lithotripsy (ESWL), in which shock waves generated outside the body are focused on the stone, breaking it into small pieces that can pass easily down the ureter (Fig. 18.29). Surgical options are ureteroscopy and stone fragmentation, usually with a laser, or percutaneous nephrolithotomy (PCNL) and fragmentation with an ultrasonic disaggregator. The recommended treatment depends on stone size, location and patient characteristics. Figure 18.29 details options by stone location.

Measures to prevent further stone formation are guided by the investigations in Box 18.50. Some general principles apply to almost every patient with calcium-containing stones (Box 18.51), while other measures apply to specific stone types. Urate stones can be prevented by allopurinol but its role in patients with calcium stones and high urate excretion is uncertain. Stones formed in cystinuria can be reduced by penicillamine therapy. It may also be helpful to attempt to alkalinise the urine with sodium bicarbonate, as a high pH discourages urate and cystine stone formation.

Diseases of the collecting system and ureters

Congenital abnormalities

Various congenital anomalies of the kidney and urinary tract (often abbreviated as CAKUT) can occur (Fig. 18.30); they affect more than 10% of infants. If not immediately lethal, they can lead to complications in later life, including obstructive nephropathy and CKD.

Single kidneys

About 1 in 500 infants is born with only one kidney. In isolation this is usually compatible with normal life, although it may be associated with other developmental abnormalities.

Medullary sponge kidney disease

Medullary sponge kidney is a congenital disorder characterised by malformation of the papillary collecting ducts in the pericalyceal region of the renal pyramids. This leads to the formation of microscopic and large medullary cysts. Patients often present as adults with renal stones but the renal function usually remains adequate. The diagnosis is made by ultrasound, CT or intravenous urography, where contrast medium is seen to fill dilated or cystic tubules, which are sometimes calcified.

Ureterocele

A ureterocele occurs behind a pin-hole ureteric orifice when the intramural part of the ureter dilates and bulges into the bladder. It can become very large and cause lower urinary tract obstruction. Incision of the pin-hole opening relieves the obstruction.

Ectopic ureters and duplex kidneys

Ectopic ureters occur with congenital duplication of one or both kidneys (duplex kidneys). Developmentally, the ureter has two main branches and, if this arrangement persists, the two ureters of the duplex kidneys may drain separately into the bladder. The lower pole moiety enters the bladder superiorly and laterally, while the upper pole moiety enters the bladder inferomedially to the lower pole moiety ureter or, more rarely, enters the vagina or seminal vesicle. The lower pole moiety has an ineffective valve mechanism, so that urine passes up the ureter on voiding (vesico-ureteric reflux, see below), whereas the upper pole moiety is often associated with a ureterocele.

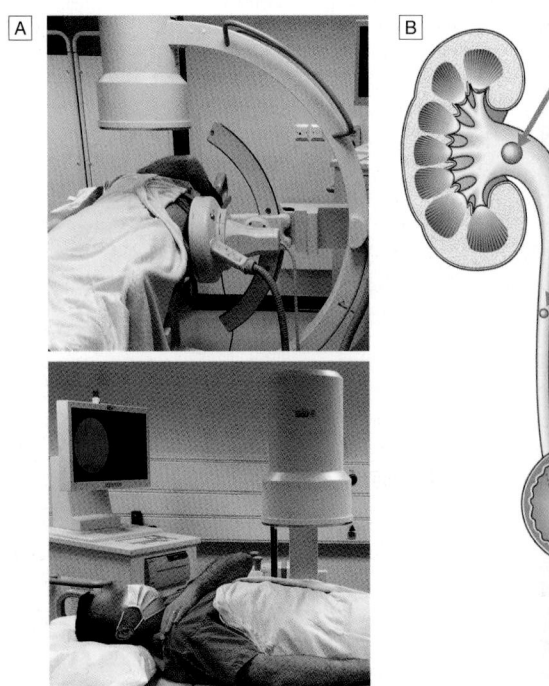
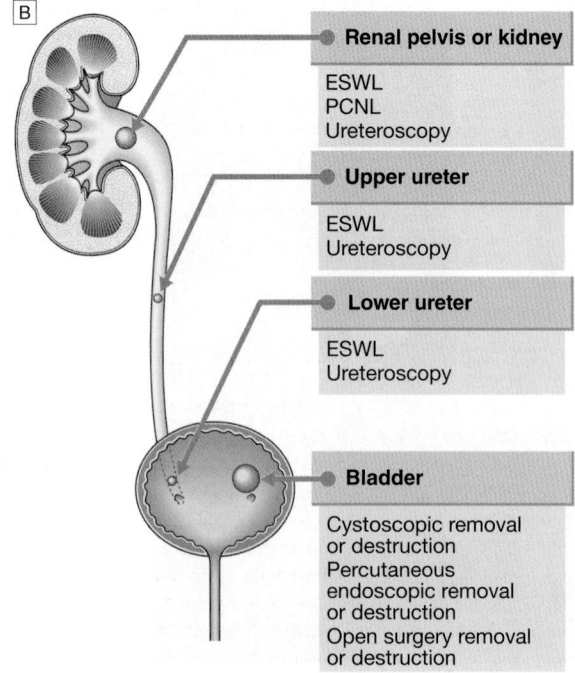

A

B

● **Renal pelvis or kidney**

ESWL
PCNL
Ureteroscopy

● **Upper ureter**

ESWL
Ureteroscopy

● **Lower ureter**

ESWL
Ureteroscopy

● **Bladder**

Cystoscopic removal
or destruction
Percutaneous
endoscopic removal
or destruction
Open surgery removal
or destruction

Fig. 18.29 Options for removal of urinary stones. **A** A patient undergoing extracorporeal shock wave lithotripsy (ESWL). **B** The procedures that are used for removal of stones in the urinary tract, shown in relation to the site of the stone. (PCNL = percutaneous nephrolithotomy) *(A) Images courtesy of Mr Laurian Dragos, Addenbroke's Hospital, Cambridge.*

Megaureter

A megaureter is a ureter dilated to more than 5 mm in diameter. It may be obstructed or non-obstructed and refluxing or non-refluxing. Some 50% of cases are asymptomatic but patients may present with pain, haematuria or infection. Radiographic and pressure/flow studies may be needed to determine whether there is obstruction to urine flow. Patients with symptoms or reduced renal function are treated. Ideally, treatment is expectant with antibiotic prophylaxis. Surgery (narrowing of the ureter and/or reimplantation) may, however, be needed for recurrent symptoms, reduction of more than 10% in renal function or complications (i.e. stones).

Pelvi-ureteric junction obstruction

Pelvi-ureteric junction obstruction (PUJO) causes idiopathic hydronephrosis and results from a functional obstruction at the junction of the ureter and renal pelvis. The abnormality is likely to be congenital and is often bilateral. It can be seen in very young children but gross hydronephrosis may present at any age. The common presentation is ill-defined renal pain or ache, exacerbated by drinking large volumes of liquid (Dietl's crisis). Rarely, it is asymptomatic. The diagnosis is often suspected after ultrasound or CT scan, and can be confirmed with a ^{99m}Tc-MAG3 renogram followed by diuretic. In a PUJO, the MAG3 renogram shows a pathognomonic 'rising curve' as the radioisotope accumulates in the renal pelvis and still does not drain following the diuretic injection. Treatment is surgical excision of the pelvi-ureteric junction and reanastomosis (pyeloplasty), which can now be performed laparoscopically or

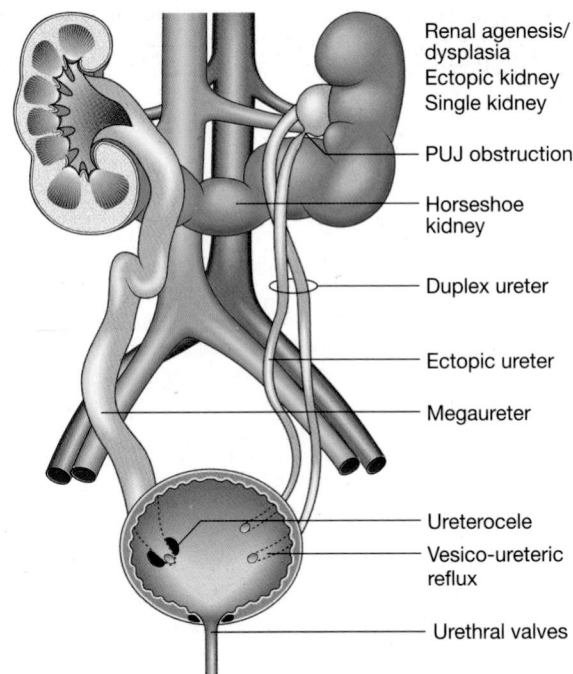

Renal agenesis/
dysplasia
Ectopic kidney
Single kidney

PUJ obstruction

Horseshoe kidney

Duplex ureter

Ectopic ureter

Megaureter

Ureterocele
Vesico-ureteric reflux

Urethral valves

Fig. 18.30 Congenital abnormalities of the urinary tract. (PUJ = pelvi-ureteric junction)

by robot-assisted surgery. Less invasive alternatives are also possible, including balloon dilatation and endoscopic pyelotomy, but are generally less effective.

Reflux nephropathy

This condition, which was previously known as chronic pyelonephritis, is a specific type of chronic interstitial nephritis associated with vesico-ureteric reflux (VUR) in early life and with the appearance of scars in the kidney, as demonstrated by various imaging techniques. About 12% of patients in Europe requiring treatment for ESRD may have this disorder but diagnostic criteria are imprecise.

Pathophysiology

Reflux nephropathy is thought to be due to chronic reflux of urine from the bladder into the ureters, in association with recurrent UTI in childhood. It was previously assumed that ascending infection was necessary for progressive renal damage in patients with VUR but there is evidence to suggest that renal scars can occur, even in the absence of infection. Furthermore, studies have found that efforts to surgically correct VUR or use prophylactic antibiotics to prevent the UTIs are ineffective in halting progression of the disease.

Susceptibility to VUR has a genetic component and may be associated with renal dysplasia and other congenital abnormalities of the urinary tract. It can be connected with outflow obstruction, usually caused by urethral valves, but usually occurs with an apparently normal bladder.

Clinical features

Usually, the renal scarring and dilatation are asymptomatic and the patient may present at any age with hypertension (sometimes severe), proteinuria or features of CKD. There may be no history of overt UTI. However, symptoms arising from the urinary tract may be present and include frequency of micturition, dysuria and aching lumbar pain. VUR may occur in children but diminishes as the child grows, and usually has disappeared by adulthood. Urinalysis often shows the presence of leucocytes and moderate proteinuria (usually <1 g/24 hrs) but these are not always present. The risk of renal stone formation is increased. A number of women first present with hypertension and/or proteinuria in pregnancy. Children and adults with small or unilateral renal scars have a

18

good prognosis, provided renal growth is normal. With significant unilateral scars there is usually compensatory hypertrophy of the contralateral kidney. In patients with more severe bilateral disease, prognosis is related to the severity of renal dysfunction, hypertension and proteinuria. If the serum creatinine is normal and hypertension and proteinuria are absent, then the long-term prognosis is usually good.

Investigations

Renal scarring can be detected by ultrasound but it has poor sensitivity and is only capable of detecting major defects and excluding significant obstruction. Radionuclide DMSA scans are more sensitive (see Fig. 18.6), and serial imaging by MRI or CT may be useful in assessing progression. Abnormalities may be unilateral or bilateral and of any grade of severity. Gross scarring of the kidneys, commonly at the poles, is seen, with reduced kidney size and narrowing of the cortex and medulla. Renal scars may be juxtaposed to dilated calyces. In patients who develop heavy proteinuria and hypertension, renal biopsies show glomerulomegaly and focal glomerulosclerosis, probably as a secondary response to reduced nephron numbers. Radionuclide techniques can also be used to demonstrate VUR as a non-invasive alternative to micturating cystourethrography (MCUG; the bladder is filled with contrast media through a urinary catheter and images are taken during and after micturition; Fig. 18.31). As surgical intervention for VUR has declined in popularity (see below), however, this type of imaging is used less often.

Management

Infection, if present, should be treated; if recurrent, it should be prevented with prophylactic therapy, as described above in this chapter for UTI, although as mentioned above this does not prevent CKD. If recurrent pyelonephritis occurs in an abnormal kidney with minimal function, nephrectomy may be indicated. Occasionally, hypertension is cured by the removal of a diseased kidney when the disease is predominantly or entirely unilateral.

As most childhood reflux tends to disappear spontaneously and trials have shown small or no benefits from anti-reflux surgery, such intervention is now less common. Severe reflux may be managed by ureteric reimplantation or subtrigonal injection of Teflon or polysaccharide (STING) beneath the ureteric orifice.

Retroperitoneal fibrosis

Fibrosis of the retroperitoneal connective tissues may encircle and compress the ureter(s), causing obstruction. The fibrosis is most commonly idiopathic but can represent a reaction to infection, radiation or aortic aneurysm, or be caused by metastatic cancer. It is recognised as part of the spectrum of disorders associated with elevated IgG4 levels. Rarely, it can be associated with inflammatory bowel disease. Patients usually present with ill-defined symptoms of ureteric obstruction. Typically, there is an acute phase response (high CRP and ESR, and polyclonal hypergammaglobulinaemia). Imaging with CT or IVU shows ureteric obstruction with medial deviation of the ureters. Idiopathic retroperitoneal fibrosis may respond well to glucocorticoids (with a reduction in inflammatory marker levels) but ureteric stenting is often necessary to relieve obstruction and preserve renal function. Failure to improve indicates the need for surgery (ureterolysis), both to relieve obstruction and to exclude malignancy.

Tumours of the kidney and urinary tract

Several malignant tumours can affect the kidney and urinary tract, including renal cell cancer, upper urinary tract urothelial cancers, bladder cancer, prostate cancer and cancers of the testis and penis. The urogenital tract can also be affected by benign tumours and secondary tumour deposits, which can cause obstructive uropathy. Renal cell cancer and bladder cancer are described here, while prostate cancer and testicular tumours are covered later in this chapter.

Renal cell cancer

Renal cell cancer (RCC) is by far the most common malignant tumour of the kidney in adults, making up 2.5% of all adult cancers, with a prevalence of 16 cases per 100 000 population. It is twice as common in males. The peak incidence is between 65 and 75 years of age and it is uncommon before 40. RCCs of differing histological subtype arise from different parts of the nephron or collecting duct. Haemorrhage and necrosis give the cut surface a characteristic mixed golden-yellow and red appearance (Fig. 18.32B). Microscopically, clear cell RCCs are the most common histological subtype (85%), with papillary, chromophobe and collecting duct tumours comprising the majority of the remainder. In RCC, there is potentially spread along the renal vein and the inferior vena cava. Direct invasion of perinephric tissues is common. Lymphatic spread occurs to para-aortic nodes, while distant metastases (which may be solitary) most commonly develop in the lungs, bone and brain.

Clinical features

In 50% of patients, asymptomatic renal tumours are identified as an incidental finding during imaging investigations carried out for other reasons. Among symptomatic patients, about 60% present with haematuria, 40% with loin pain and a few with a palpable mass. About 10% present with a triad of pain, haematuria and a mass; this usually represents advanced disease. RCC is one of the great mimics of medicine as patients may present with a remarkable range of systemic effects, including fever, raised ESR, polycythaemia, disorders of coagulation, hypercalcaemia, and abnormalities of plasma proteins and liver function tests. The patient may present with pyrexia of unknown origin (PUO) or, rarely, with neuropathy. Some of these systemic effects are caused by secretion of products by the tumour, such as renin, erythropoietin, parathyroid hormone-related protein (PTHrP) and gonadotrophins. The effects disappear when the tumour is removed but may reappear when metastases develop.

Investigations

Ultrasound is often the initial investigation and allows differentiation between solid tumour and simple renal cysts. If the results are suggestive of a tumour, contrast-enhanced CT of the abdomen and chest should be

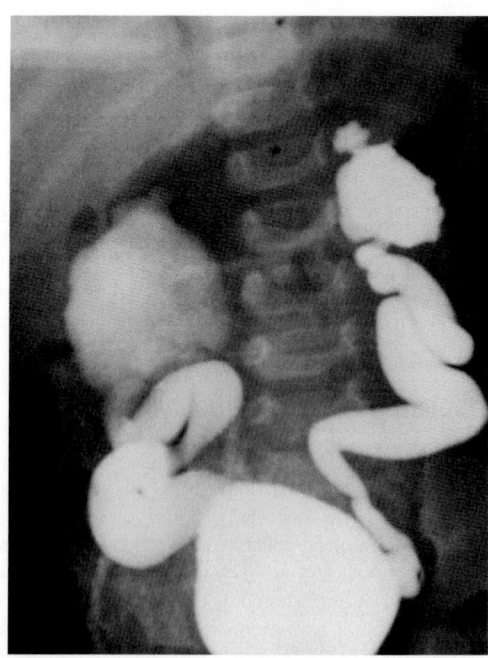

Fig. 18.31 Vesico-ureteric reflux (grade IV) shown by micturating cystogram. The bladder has been filled with contrast medium through a urinary catheter. After micturition, there was gross vesico-ureteric reflux into widely distended ureters and pelvicalyceal systems. *Courtesy of Dr A.P. Bayliss and Dr P. Thorpe, Aberdeen Royal Infirmary.*

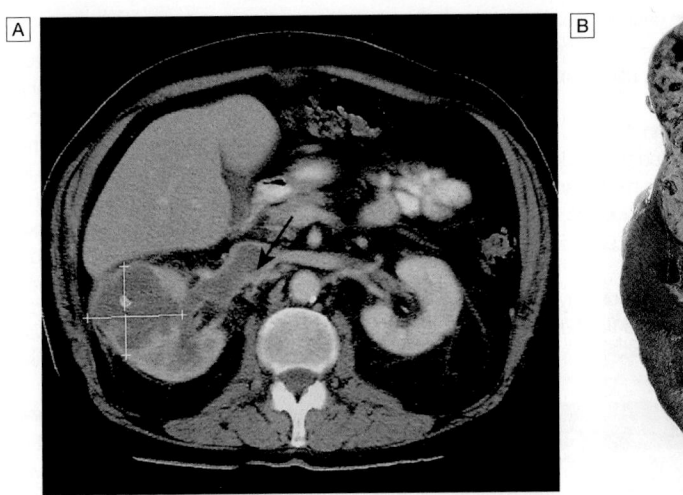

Fig. 18.32 Renal cell cancer. A In this CT, the right kidney is expanded by a low-density tumour, which fails to take up contrast material. Tumour is shown extending into the renal vein and inferior vena cava (arrow). B Pathology specimen showing typical necrosis of a renal cell cancer. *(A, B) Courtesy of Dr A.P. Bayliss and Dr P. Thorpe, Aberdeen Royal Infirmary.*

performed for staging (Fig. 18.32A). For tumours with no evidence of metastatic spread and when the nature of the lesion is uncertain, ultrasound or CT-guided biopsy may be used to avoid nephrectomy for benign disease.

Management

Radical nephrectomy that includes the perirenal fascial envelope is the treatment of choice. Nephrectomy is commonly performed laparoscopically, with equivalent outcomes to open surgery. Partial nephrectomy, which may be carried out by open but increasingly by minimally invasive robot-assisted or laparoscopic surgery, is recommended, where possible, for tumours of 7 cm or less, as there is a lower incidence of long-term cardiac- and renal-related morbidity. Patients at high operative risk who have small tumours may also be treated percutaneously by cryotherapy or radiofrequency ablation. Active surveillance with serial imaging in those with renal masses <4 cm is a management option that should also be discussed with patients. Surgery may also play a role in the treatment of solitary metastases, since these can remain single for long periods and excision may be curative.

RCC is resistant to most chemotherapeutic agents. Tyrosine kinase inhibitors (TKIs) such as sunitinib and pazopanib are the mainstay of treatment. Recently, T-cell checkpoint inhibitors such as PD-L1, PD-1 and CTLA-4 inhibitors have been licensed for use as single agents or in combination (PD-L1/PD-1 with CTLA-4 inhibitor or TKI) as first-line treatment options for metastatic RCC.

In previous years, patients who presented with distant metastases were treated with cytoreductive nephrectomy, in which nephrectomy was coupled with systemic cytokine treatment, since this was shown to improve survival as compared with either treatment in isolation. The benefit of cytoreductive nephrectomy is less clear with TKIs and hence is used sparingly; the benefit is unknown for T-cell checkpoint inhibitors.

Current survival data indicate that, if RCC is confined to the kidney, 5-year survival is 75%, but this falls to 12% when there are distant metastases.

Urothelial tumours

Tumours arising from the transitional epithelium of the renal tract can affect the renal pelvis, ureter, bladder or urethra. They are rare under the age of 40, affect men 3–4 times more often than women, and account for about 3% of all malignant tumours. The bladder is by far the most frequently affected site. Although almost all tumours are urothelial cell cancer (previously known as transitional cell cancers), squamous cell cancer may occur in urothelium that has undergone metaplasia, usually following chronic inflammation due to stones or schistosomiasis. The appearance of a urothelial cell cancer ranges from a delicate papillary structure with a relatively good prognosis to a solid ulcerating mass in more aggressive disease.

Pathophysiology

Risk factors include cigarette smoking and exposure to industrial carcinogens such as aromatic amines, aniline dyes and aldehydes.

Clinical features

More than 80% of patients present with painless, visible haematuria. It should be assumed that such bleeding is from a tumour until proven otherwise (p. 568). Tumours of the ureter or bladder may also cause symptoms of obstruction, depending on the site of involvement, and tumours of the bladder present with dysuria or storage symptoms. Physical examination is usually unremarkable, except in patients with very advanced disease, when bimanual examination may reveal a palpable mass.

Investigations

Cystoscopy (usually flexible cystoscopy under a local anaesthetic) is used to evaluate the bladder in cases of haematuria or suspected bladder cancer. Imaging of the upper urinary tract (CT urogram is the gold standard but IVU combined with renal ultrasound is also acceptable) is also important to rule out abnormalities of the kidney, ureters and renal pelvis in patients with haematuria. If a suspicious defect is seen on CT urography or IVU in the ureter or renal pelvis, a retrograde ureteropyelogram, ureteroscopy and biopsy are required. If evidence of a solid invasive urothelial tumour is found, CT of the abdomen, pelvis and chest should be performed to define tumour stage.

Management

Most bladder tumours are low-grade, non-muscle-invasive lesions that can be successfully treated endoscopically by transurethral resection of the tumour. Intravesical chemotherapy with mitomycin C is usually administered as a one-off treatment post resection to prevent tumour recurrence, or may be given as a prolonged course to treat multiple low-grade bladder tumours. Patients with carcinoma in situ have a high risk of progression to invasive cancer. These patients often respond well to intravesical bacille Calmette–Guérin (BCG) treatment but more radical treatment by cystectomy may be required if this is unsuccessful. Following initial treatment and endoscopic clearance of bladder tumours, regular check cystoscopies are required to look for evidence of recurrence. Patients with recurrences of non-muscle-invasive disease can usually be treated by further resection and diathermy, but if this is unsuccessful, a cystectomy may be needed.

18

The management of muscle-invasive bladder cancer involves radical cystectomy with urinary diversion into an incontinent ileal conduit or a continent catheterisable bowel pouch; the latter is usually reserved for patients under the age of 70 years.

The prognosis of bladder cancer depends on tumour stage and grade. In patients where the cancer has not invaded the bladder muscle at diagnosis, 5% of low-grade tumours and 50% of high-grade tumours progress to develop invasion of the bladder muscle. Overall, the 5-year survival for patients with muscle-invasive bladder cancer of either grade is 50%–70%.

Urothelial cell cancer of the renal pelvis and ureter is usually treated by laparoscopic or open nephro-ureterectomy, but if the tumour is solitary and low-grade, it may be treated endoscopically.

Urinary incontinence

Urinary incontinence is defined as any involuntary leakage of urine. It may occur in patients with a normal urinary tract, as the result of dementia or poor mobility, or transiently during an acute illness or hospitalisation, especially in older people (Box 18.52). The prevalence of any form of incontinence in all females is 25%–45%, with a concomitant socioeconomic burden. Childbirth, hysterectomy, obesity, recurrent UTI, smoking, caffeine and constipation are risk factors for incontinence.

Pathophysiology

In the normal micturition cycle, urine accumulates in the bladder during the storage phase, the sphincter tone gradually increases, but there are no significant changes in vesical pressure, detrusor pressure or intra-abdominal pressure. During voiding, intravesical pressure increases as a result of detrusor contraction and the sphincter relaxes, allowing urine to flow from the bladder until it is empty. Clinical disorders associated with incontinence are connected with various abnormalities in this cycle and these are discussed in more detail below.

Stress incontinence

This occurs because passive bladder pressure exceeds the urethral pressure, due either to poor pelvic floor support or a weak urethral sphincter. Usually there is an element of both these factors. Stress incontinence is very common in women and seen most frequently following childbirth. It is rare in men and usually follows surgery to the prostate. The presentation is with incontinence during coughing, sneezing or exertion. In women, perineal inspection may reveal leakage of urine when the patient coughs.

Urge incontinence

This usually occurs because of detrusor over-activity, which produces an increased bladder pressure that overcomes the urethral sphincter. Urgency with or without incontinence may also be driven by a hypersensitive bladder resulting from UTI or a bladder stone. Detrusor over-activity is usually idiopathic, other than in patients with neurological conditions such as spina bifida or multiple sclerosis, in whom it is neurogenic. The incidence of urge incontinence increases with age, occurring in 10%–15% of the population aged over 65 years and in approximately 50% of patients requiring nursing home care. It is more common in women, but is also seen in men with lower urinary tract obstruction and most often remits after the obstruction is relieved.

Continual incontinence

This is suggestive of a fistula, usually between the bladder and vagina (vesicovaginal), or the ureter and vagina (ureterovaginal). It is most common following gynaecological surgery but is also seen in patients with gynaecological malignancy or post radiotherapy. In parts of the world where obstetric services are scarce, prolonged obstructed labour can be a common cause of vesicovaginal fistulae. Continual incontinence may also be seen in infants with congenital ectopic ureters. Occasionally, stress incontinence is so severe that the patient leaks continuously.

Overflow incontinence

This occurs when the bladder becomes chronically over-distended and may lead to AKI (high-pressure chronic urinary retention). It is most commonly seen in men with benign prostatic enlargement or bladder neck obstruction (see below) but may arise in either sex as a result of failure of the detrusor muscle (atonic bladder). The latter may be idiopathic but more commonly is the result of damage to the pelvic nerves, either from surgery (commonly, hysterectomy or rectal excision), trauma or infection, or from compression of the cauda equina by disc prolapse, trauma or tumour. Incontinence due to prostatic enlargement can be regarded as a type of overflow incontinence.

Post-micturition dribble

This is very common in men, even in the relatively young. It is due to a small amount of urine becoming trapped in the U-bend of the bulbar urethra, which leaks out when the patient moves. Post-micturition dribble is more pronounced if associated with a urethral diverticulum or urethral stricture. It may occur in women with a urethral diverticulum and may mimic stress incontinence.

Clinical assessment

Patients should be encouraged to keep a voiding diary, including the measured volume voided, frequency of voiding, a note of incontinence pad usage, precipitating factors and associated features, such as urgency, since this can be of diagnostic value. Structured questionnaires may help objectively quantify symptoms. The patient should be assessed for evidence of cognitive impairment and impaired mobility. A neurological assessment should be performed to detect disorders such as multiple sclerosis that may affect the nervous supply of the bladder, and the lumbar spine should be inspected for features of spina bifida occulta. Perineal sensation and anal sphincter tone should be assessed. Rectal examination is needed to assess the prostate in men and to exclude faecal impaction as a cause of incontinence. Genital examination should be done to identify phimosis or paraphimosis in men, and vaginal mucosal atrophy, cystoceles or rectoceles in women.

Investigations

Urinalysis and culture should be performed in all patients. Ultrasound examination can be helpful in identifying patients with overflow incontinence who have incomplete bladder emptying, as it may reveal a significant amount of fluid in the bladder (>100 mL) post-micturition. Urine flow rates and full urodynamic assessment by cystometrography may be required to diagnose the type of incontinence and are indicated in selected cases when the diagnosis is unclear on clinical grounds. A CT scan and cystoscopy should be performed in patients with continual incontinence who are suspected of having a fistula. Imaging with MRI is indicated when a urethral diverticulum is suspected.

Management

Weight reduction in obese patients will aid resolution of incontinence. Women with stress incontinence respond well to physiotherapy. The

18.52 Incontinence in old age

- **Prevalence**: urinary incontinence affects 15% of women and 10% of men aged over 65 years.
- **Cause**: incontinence may be transient and due to delirium, urinary infection, medication (such as diuretics), faecal impaction or restricted mobility, and these should be treated before embarking on further specific investigation. Routine urinalysis is rarely helpful and can be misleading.
- **Detrusor over-activity**: established incontinence in old age is most commonly due to detrusor over-activity, which may be caused by damage to central inhibitory centres or local detrusor muscle abnormalities.
- **Catheterisation**: poor manual dexterity or cognitive impairment may necessitate the help of a carer to assist with intermittent catheterisation.

mainstay of treatment for urge incontinence is bladder retraining, which involves teaching patients to hold more urine voluntarily in their bladder, assisted by anticholinergic medication.

Surgery may be required in patients who have severe daytime incontinence despite conservative treatment. In neurologically intact patients, stress urinary incontinence in males is treated surgically by artificial urinary sphincter and in females by returning the urethra and bladder neck to their normal position with a pubovaginal sling or colposuspension. For urge incontinence intravesical injection of botulinum neurotoxin type A has excellent results. Further surgical options are sacral nerve stimulation, detrusor myectomy or bladder augmentation.

The treatment of incontinence secondary to fistula formation is surgical. Patients with overflow incontinence due to bladder obstruction should be treated surgically or with long-term catheterisation (intermittent or continuous). Incontinence secondary to neurological diseases can be managed by intermittent self-catheterisation.

Prostate disease

Prostatitis

This results from inflammation of the prostate gland. Acute or chronic bacterial prostatitis can be caused by infection with the same bacteria that are associated with UTI (p. 599) but chronic prostatitis can also be 'non-bacterial', in which case no organism can be cultured from the urine. This is also known as chronic pelvic pain syndrome. Clinical features of prostatitis include frequency, dysuria, painful ejaculation, perineal or groin pain, difficulty passing urine and, in acute disease, considerable systemic disturbance. The prostate is enlarged and tender. Bacterial prostatitis is confirmed by a positive culture from urine or from urethral discharge obtained after prostatic massage, and the treatment of choice is a quinolone antibiotic. A 6-week course of antibiotics is required (see Box 18.46). Treatment of chronic pelvic pain syndrome is challenging but some patients respond to a combination of α-adrenoceptor antagonists (α-blockers), NSAIDs and amitriptyline.

Benign prostatic enlargement

Benign prostatic enlargement (BPE) is extremely common. It has been estimated that about half of all men aged 80 years and over will have lower urinary tract symptoms associated with bladder outlet obstruction (BOO) due to BPE. Benign prostatic hyperplasia (BPH) is the histological abnormality that underlies BPE.

Pathophysiology

The prostate gland increases in volume by 2.4 cm^3 per year on average from 40 years of age. The process begins in the periurethral (transitional) zone and involves both glandular and stromal tissue to a variable degree. The cause is unknown, although BPE does not occur in patients with hypogonadism, suggesting that hormonal factors may be important.

Clinical features

The primary symptoms of BPE arise because of difficulty in voiding urine due to obstruction of the urethra by the prostate; these voiding symptoms consist of hesitancy, poor urinary flow and a sensation of incomplete emptying. Other storage symptoms include urinary frequency, urgency of micturition and urge incontinence, although these are not specific to BPE. Some patients present suddenly with acute urinary retention, when they are unable to micturate and develop a painful, distended bladder. This is often precipitated by excessive alcohol intake, constipation or prostatic infection. Severity of symptoms can be ascertained by using the International Prostate Symptom Score (IPSS) questionnaire (Box 18.53), which serves as a valuable starting point for assessment of the patient. Once a baseline value is established, any improvement or deterioration may be monitored on subsequent visits. The IPSS is combined with a quality-of-life score, in which patients are asked the following question:

18.53 The International Prostate Symptom Score (IPSS)

Symptom	Question	Example score
Straining	How often have you had to push or strain to begin urination?	1
Urgency	How often have you found it difficult to postpone urination?	2
Intermittency	How often have you found that you stopped and started again several times when you urinated?	1
Emptying	How often have you had a sensation of not emptying your bladder completely after you finished urinating?	3
Frequency	How often have you had to urinate again less than 2 hours after you finished urinating?	1
Weak stream	How often have you had a weak urinary stream?	2
Nocturia	How many times did you most typically get up to urinate from the time you went to bed at night until the time you got up in the morning?	1
Total score		11

0 = not at all; 1 = less than one-fifth of the time; 2 = less than half the time; 3 = about half of the time; 4 = more than half of the time; 5 = almost always.
A score of 0–7 indicates mild symptoms, 8–19 moderate symptoms and 20–35 severe symptoms. In the example shown, the patient had moderate symptoms.

'If you were to spend the rest of your life with your urinary condition the way it is now, how would you feel about that?' Responses range from 0 (delighted) to 6 (terrible).

Patients may also present with chronic urinary retention. Here, the bladder slowly distends due to inadequate emptying over a long period of time. Patients with chronic retention can also develop acute retention: so-called acute-on-chronic retention. This condition is characterised by pain-free bladder distension, which may result in hydroureter, hydronephrosis and renal failure (high-pressure chronic retention, of which nocturnal incontinence is a pathognomonic symptom). On digital rectal examination (DRE), patients with BPE have evidence of prostatic enlargement with a smooth prostate gland. Abdominal examination may also reveal evidence of bladder enlargement in patients with urinary retention.

Investigations

The diagnosis of BOO secondary to BPE is a clinical one but flow rates can be accurately measured with a flow meter, post-void residual volume of urine assessed with ultrasound, and prostate volume by transrectal ultrasound scan (TRUS). Objective assessment of obstruction is possible by urodynamics and should be undertaken if symptoms are mixed, with both voiding and storage making underlying pathophysiology uncertain and/or flow test equivocal for obstruction (<150 ml voided or >10 mL/s). If symptoms or signs, such as a palpable bladder, nocturnal enuresis, recurrent UTI or a history of renal stones, are present, renal function should be assessed; if it is abnormal, screening should be conducted for evidence of obstructive uropathy by ultrasound examination.

Management

Patients who present with acute retention require urgent treatment and should undergo immediate catheterisation to relieve the obstruction. Those with mild to moderate symptoms can be treated by medication (Box 18.54). The first-line treatments are α_{1A}-adrenoceptor blockers such as tamsulosin, which reduce the tone of smooth muscle cells in the prostate and bladder neck, thereby reducing the obstruction. The 5α-reductase inhibitors finasteride and dutasteride inhibit conversion of testosterone to the nine times more potent dihydrotestosterone in the prostate and so cause the prostate to reduce in size. This class of drugs is indicated in patients with an estimated prostate size of more than 30 g or a prostate-specific antigen (PSA) level of more than 1.4 ng/mL. Patients who fail to respond to a single drug may be treated with a combination of α-blockers and 5α-reductase inhibitors, since this is more efficacious than either agent alone. Symptoms that are resistant to medical therapy require surgical treatment to remove some of the prostate tissue that is causing urethral obstruction. This is usually achieved by transurethral resection of the prostate (TURP) but enucleation of the prostate by holmium laser or vaporisation by potassium-titanyl-phosphate (KTP) laser (Greenlight laser) is equally effective and has potentially fewer complications. Open surgery is very rarely needed, as very large glands can be treated with holmium laser treatment.

Prostate cancer

Prostate cancer is the most common malignancy in men in the UK, with an incidence of ~170 per 100 000 population. It is also common in northern Europe and the United States (particularly in the African American population) but is rare in China and Japan. It is uncommon in India but the incidence is increasing. Prostate cancer rarely occurs before the age of 50 and has a mean age at presentation of 70 years.

Pathophysiology

Prostate cancers tend to arise within the peripheral zone of the prostate and almost all are adenocarcinomas. Metastatic spread to pelvic lymph nodes occurs early and metastases to bone, mainly the lumbar spine and pelvis, are common. Genetic factors are known to play an important role in pathogenesis, and multiple genetic loci have been found to predispose to the disease in genome-wide association studies. A family history of prostate cancer greatly increases a man's chances of developing the disease.

Clinical features

Most patients either are asymptomatic or present with lower urinary tract symptoms indistinguishable from BPE. On DRE the prostate may feel nodular and stony-hard, and the median sulcus may be lost, but up to 45% of cancers are impalpable. Symptoms and signs due to metastases are much less common at the initial presentation but may include back pain, weight loss, anaemia and obstruction of the ureters.

Investigations

Measurement of PSA levels in a peripheral blood sample, together with DRE, is the cornerstone of diagnosis. Prior to a PSA test, men should be given careful counselling about the limitations of the test: namely, a normal level does not exclude prostate cancer, while a high value does not confirm the diagnosis but will open a discussion about biopsy and possible future treatments with potential side-effects (Box 18.55). The need for radical treatment of localised prostate cancer is still not established; radical treatments have significant potential morbidity and mortality, yet early identification and treatment of prostate cancer may save lives. Current evidence suggests that population-based screening for prostate cancer with PSA is of limited value, due in part to the fact that over 700 patients would need to be screened to cure 1 man of prostate cancer. Individuals suspected of having prostate cancer, based on an elevated PSA and/or abnormal DRE,

18.54 Treatment for benign prostatic enlargement

Medical

- Prostate <30 g: α-blockers
- Prostate > 30 g: 5α-reductase inhibitors ± α-blockers

Surgical

- Transurethral resection of the prostate (TURP)
- Laser enucleation
- Laser vaporisation
- Open prostatectomy

18.55 Advantages and disadvantages of prostate-specific antigen (PSA) testing in order to identify men with prostate cancer

Advantages

- Identification of prostate cancer at a treatable stage, which otherwise may not have been identified*

Disadvantages

- High false-positive rate: 50%–60% of men with an elevated PSA will not have prostate cancer
- High false-negative rate: 25% of men with a normal PSA have prostate cancer
- Leads to further invasive tests (biopsy) with morbidity (e.g. sepsis or bleeding)
- May lead to diagnosis of prostate cancer, which is often over-treated by surgery or radiotherapy with associated side-effects (e.g. impotence or incontinence)
- If PSA is elevated but biopsy is normal, there is a potential need for further testing and associated anxiety

*The advantages of identifying prostate cancer earlier than would be the case if the man developed symptomatic disease must be considered against the limitations of PSA testing.

should undergo transrectal or transperineal ultrasound-guided prostate biopsies. About 40% of patients with a serum PSA of 4.0–10 ng/mL or more will have prostate cancer on biopsy, although 25% of patients with a PSA of less than 4 ng/mL may also have prostate cancer. Occasionally, a small focus of tumour is found incidentally in patients undergoing TURP for benign hyperplasia. If the diagnosis of prostate cancer is confirmed, staging should be performed by pelvic MRI to assess the presence and extent of local involvement. An isotope bone scan should be carried out if distant metastases are suspected (rare if the PSA is below 20 ng/mL); very high levels of serum PSA (>100 ng/mL) almost always indicate distant bone metastases. Following diagnosis, serial assessment of PSA levels is useful for monitoring response to treatment and disease progression.

Management

Tumour confined to the prostate is potentially curable by radical prostatectomy, radical radiotherapy or brachytherapy (implantation of small radioactive particles into the prostate). These options should be considered only in patients with more than 10 years' life expectancy. Patients who are found to have small-volume, low-grade disease do not appear to require specific treatment but should be followed up periodically with PSA testing, DRE and a schedule of biopsies; this is known as active surveillance. Prostate cancer, like breast cancer, is sensitive to steroid hormones; metastatic prostate cancer is treated by androgen depletion, involving either surgery (orchidectomy) or, more commonly, androgen-suppressing drugs. Androgen receptor blockers, such as bicalutamide or cyproterone acetate, may also prevent tumour cell growth. Gonadotrophin-releasing hormone (GnRH) analogues, such as goserelin, continuously occupy pituitary receptors, preventing them from responding to the GnRH pulses that normally stimulate luteinising hormone (LH) and follicle-stimulating hormone (FSH) release. This initially causes an increase in testosterone before producing a prolonged reduction, and for this reason the initial dose must be covered with an androgen receptor blocker to prevent a tumour flare.

A small proportion of patients fail to respond to endocrine treatment. A larger number respond for a year or two but then the disease progresses.

Chemotherapy with docetaxel can then be effective and provide a modest (around 3 months) survival advantage. Newer hormonal agents such as enzalutamide and abiraterone acetate also provide some survival benefit. There is also a role for initial prostate radiotherapy in those with low volume metastatic prostate cancer. Radiotherapy is useful for localised bone pain but the basis of treatment remains pain control by analgesia (p. 145). Provided that patients do not die of another cause, the 10-year survival rate of patients with tumours localised to the prostate is 95%, but if metastases are present, this falls to 10%. Life expectancy is not reduced in patients with small foci of tumour.

Testicular tumours

Testicular tumours are uncommon, with a prevalence of 5 cases per 100 000 population. They occur mainly in young men aged between 20 and 40 years. They often secrete α-fetoprotein (AFP) and β-human chorionic gonadotrophin (β-hCG), which are useful biochemical markers for both diagnosis and prognosis. Seminoma and non-seminomatous germ cell tumours (NSGCT) account for ~85% of all tumours of the testis. Leydig cell tumours are less common.

Seminomas arise from seminiferous tubules and represent a relatively low-grade malignancy. Metastases can occur through lymphatic spread, however, and typically involve the lungs.

NSGCTs arise from primitive germinal cells and tend to occur at a younger age than seminomas. They may contain cartilage, bone, muscle, fat and a variety of other tissues, and are classified according to the degree of differentiation. Well-differentiated tumours are the least aggressive; at the other extreme, trophoblastic teratoma is highly malignant. Occasionally, teratoma and seminoma occur together.

Leydig cell tumours are usually small and benign but secrete oestrogens, leading to presentation with gynaecomastia.

Clinical features and investigations

The common presentation is incidental discovery of a painless testicular lump, although some patients complain of a testicular ache.

All suspicious scrotal lumps should be imaged by ultrasound. Serum levels of AFP and β-hCG are elevated in extensive disease. Oestradiol may be elevated, suppressing LH, FSH and testosterone. Accurate staging is based on CT of the lungs, liver and retroperitoneal area.

Management and prognosis

The primary treatment is surgical inguinal orchidectomy. Subsequent adjuvant treatment depends on the histological type and stage. Adjuvant chemotherapy with carboplatin is the treatment of choice for early-stage but high-risk seminoma. NSGCTs confined to the testes may be managed conservatively, but more advanced cancers are treated with chemotherapy, usually the combination of bleomycin, etoposide and cisplatin. Follow-up is by CT and assessment of LDH, AFP and β-hCG. Retroperitoneal lymph node dissection is performed for residual or recurrent nodal masses.

The 5-year survival rate for patients with seminoma is 90%–95%. For NSGCT, the 5-year survival varies between 60% and 95%, depending on tumour type, stage and volume.

Erectile dysfunction

Causes of erectile failure are shown in Box 18.56. Vascular, neuropathic and psychological causes are most common. Exclusion of previously unrecognised cardiovascular disease is important in men presenting with erectile dysfunction. With the exception of diabetes mellitus, endocrine causes are relatively uncommon and are characterised by loss of libido,

 18.56 Causes of erectile dysfunction

With reduced libido
- Hypogonadism
- Depression

With intact libido
- Psychological problems, including anxiety
- Vascular insufficiency (atheroma)
- Neuropathic causes (diabetes mellitus, alcohol excess, multiple sclerosis)
- Drugs (β-blockers, thiazide diuretics)

as well as erectile dysfunction. Erectile dysfunction and reduced libido occur in over 50% of men with advanced CKD or those on dialysis, and is a markedly under-diagnosed problem. It is important to discuss matters frankly with the patient, and to establish whether there are associated features of hypogonadism and if erections occur at any other time. If the patient has erections on wakening, vascular and neuropathic causes are much less likely and a psychological cause should be suspected.

Investigations

Blood should be taken for glucose, lipids, prolactin, testosterone, LH and FSH. A number of further tests are available but are rarely employed because they do not usually influence management. These include nocturnal tumescence monitoring (using a plethysmograph placed around the shaft of the penis overnight) to establish whether blood supply and nerve function are sufficient to allow erections to occur during sleep; intracavernosal injection of prostaglandin E_1 to test the adequacy of blood supply; and internal pudendal artery angiography.

Management

First-line therapy is usually with oral phosphodiesterase type 5 inhibitors, such as sildenafil, which elevate cyclic guanosine monophosphate (cGMP) levels in vascular smooth muscle cells of the corpus cavernosum, causing vasodilatation and penile erection. Co-administration of these drugs with nitric oxide donors, such as glycerol trinitrate, is contraindicated because of the risk of severe hypotension. Other treatments for impotence include self-administered intracavernosal injection or urethral administration of prostaglandin E1; vacuum devices that achieve an erection maintained by a tourniquet around the base of the penis; and prosthetic implants, either of a fixed rod or an inflatable reservoir. Psychotherapy involving the patient and sexual partner may be helpful for psychological problems. Erectile dysfunction associated with peripheral neuropathy and vascular disease is difficult to treat. If hypogonadism is detected, it should be managed as described on page 670.

Further information

Websites

edren.org *Renal Unit, Royal Infirmary of Edinburgh; information about individual diseases, protocols for immediate in-hospital management and more.*
edrep.org/resources *Educational resources.*
nephjc.com *Online journal club, blog and resource for those interested in nephrology.*
ukidney.com *Educational resource with calculators, case presentations, videos and seminal papers.*
renalfellow.org *Educational blog written by renal trainees for trainees.*
nice.org.uk/guidance/cg182 *National Institute of Health and Care Excellence CKD Guidelines.*
uroweb.org/guidelines *European Association of Urology guidelines; current European guidelines on the management of all common urological conditions.*

18

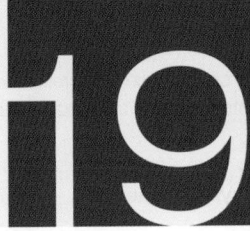

Clinical biochemistry and metabolic medicine

Clinical examination in biochemical and metabolic disorders

Many biochemical and metabolic disorders are clinically silent or present with non-specific manifestations, and are first detected by laboratory testing. Several abnormalities can be picked up by history and physical examination, however, as summarised below.

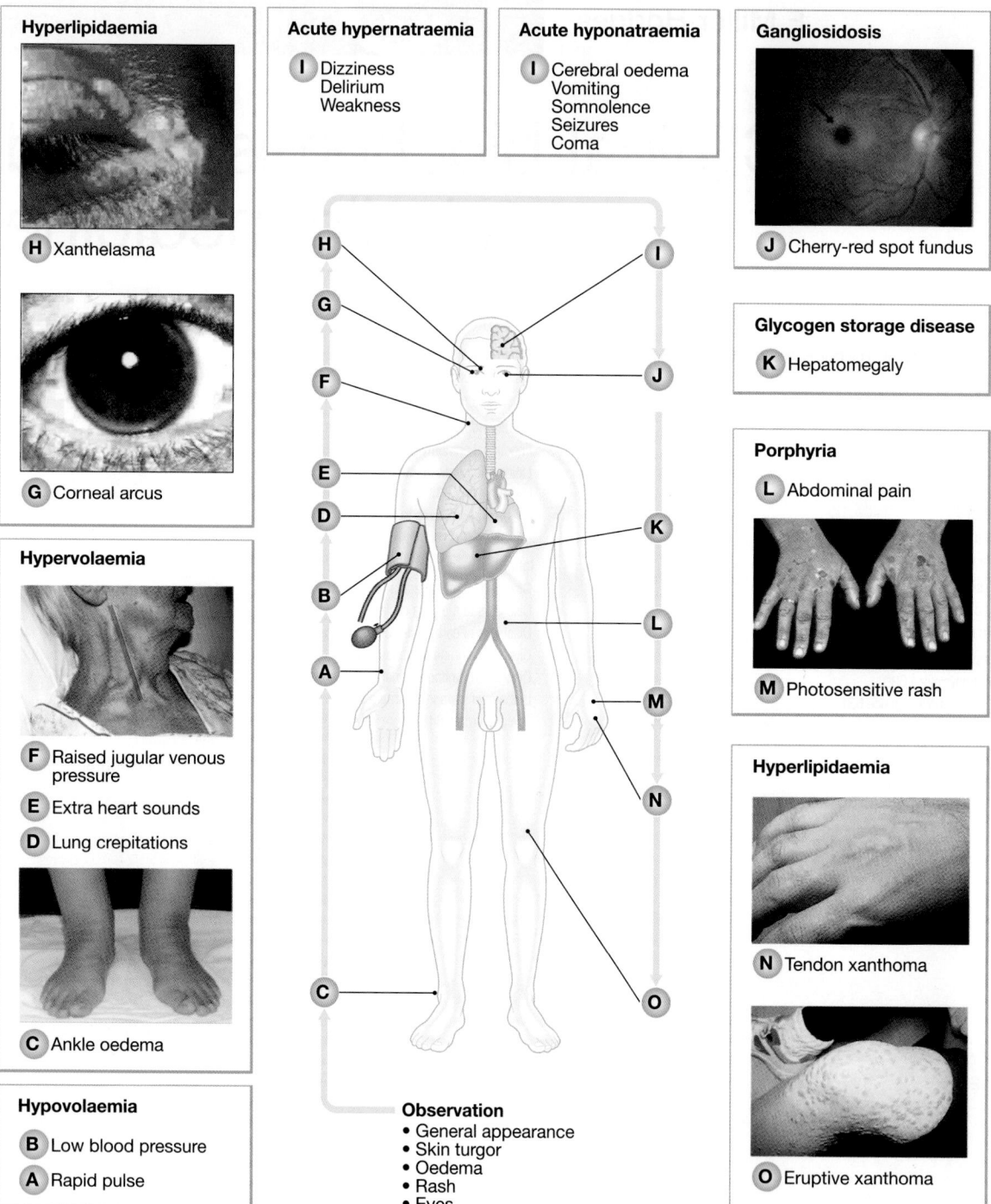

Hyperlipidaemia

H Xanthelasma

G Corneal arcus

Hypervolaemia

F Raised jugular venous pressure

E Extra heart sounds

D Lung crepitations

C Ankle oedema

Hypovolaemia

B Low blood pressure

A Rapid pulse

Acute hypernatraemia

I Dizziness
Delirium
Weakness

Acute hyponatraemia

I Cerebral oedema
Vomiting
Somnolence
Seizures
Coma

Observation
- General appearance
- Skin turgor
- Oedema
- Rash
- Eyes

Gangliosidosis

J Cherry-red spot fundus

Glycogen storage disease

K Hepatomegaly

Porphyria

L Abdominal pain

M Photosensitive rash

Hyperlipidaemia

N Tendon xanthoma

O Eruptive xanthoma

Insets: (ankle oedema) From Huang H-W, Wong L-S, Lee C-H. Sarcoidosis with bilateral leg lymphedema as the initial presentation: a review of the literature. Dermatologica Sinica 2016; 34:29–32; (raised jugular venous pressure) Newby D, Grubb N. Cardiology: an illustrated colour text. Edinburgh: Churchill Livingstone, Elsevier Ltd; 2005; (cherry-red spots) Vieira de Rezende Pinto WB, Sgobbi de Souza PV, Pedroso JL, et al. Variable phenotype and severity of sialidosis expressed in two siblings presenting with ataxia and macular cherry-red spots. J Clin Neurosci 2013; 20:1327–1328; (photosensitive rash) Ferri FF. Ferri's Color atlas and text of clinical medicine. Philadelphia: Saunders, Elsevier Inc.; 2009; courtesy of the Institute of Dermatology, London.

Assessment of volume status and electrolyte disturbances

Check blood pressure, pulse and jugular venous pressure

Check skin turgor

Check for dry mouth

Check for sacral and ankle oedema

Examine chest for pleural effusion

Examine abdomen for hepatomegaly and ascites

Check bloods

Review results

Check ECG

U wave

ST depression

Hypokalaemia

Peaked T wave

Hyperkalaemia

19

Check for signs of hyperlipidaemia

Check skin and tendons for xanthomas

Check eyes for arcus and xanthelasma

Examine for signs of multi-system disease

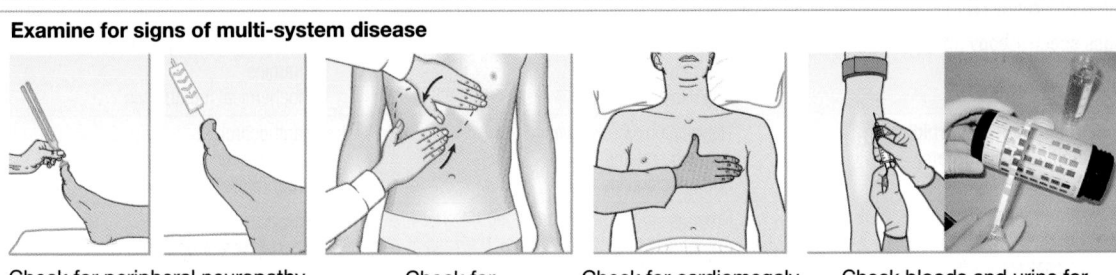

Check for peripheral neuropathy and for muscle tenderness or weakness

Check for hepato-splenomegaly

Check for cardiomegaly and arrhythmias

Check bloods and urine for metabolic biochemistry

There is a worldwide trend towards increased use of laboratory-based diagnostic investigations, and biochemical investigations in particular. In the health-care systems of higher-income countries, it has been estimated that 60%–70% of all critical decisions taken in regard to patients, and over 90% of data stored in electronic medical records systems, involve a laboratory service or result.

This chapter covers a diverse group of disorders affecting adults that are not considered elsewhere in this book, whose primary manifestation is in abnormalities of biochemistry laboratory results, or whose underlying pathophysiology involves disturbance in specific biochemical pathways.

Biochemical investigations

There are three broad reasons why a clinician may request a biochemical laboratory investigation:

- to screen an asymptomatic subject for the presence of disease
- to assist in diagnosis of a patient's presenting complaint
- to monitor changes in test results, as a marker of disease progression or response to treatment.

Contemporary medical practice has become increasingly reliant on laboratory investigation and, in particular, on biochemical investigation. This has been associated with extraordinary improvements in the analytical capacity and speed of laboratory instrumentation and the following operational trends:

- Large central biochemistry laboratories feature extensive use of automation and information technology. Specimens are transported from clinical areas to the laboratory using high-speed transport systems (such as pneumatic tubes) and identified with machine-readable labels (such as bar codes). Laboratory instruments have been miniaturised and integrated with robot transport systems to enable multiple rapid analyses of a single sample. Statistical process control techniques are used to assure the quality of analytical results, and increasingly to monitor other aspects of the laboratory, such as the time taken to complete the analysis ('turn-around time').
- Point-of-care testing (POCT) brings selected laboratory analytical systems into clinical areas, to the patient's bedside or even connected to an individual patient. These systems allow the clinician to receive results almost instantaneously for immediate treatment of the patient, although often with lesser precision or at greater cost than using a central laboratory.
- The diversity of analyses has widened considerably with the introduction of many techniques borrowed from the chemical or other industries (Box 19.1).

Good medical practice involves the appropriate ordering of laboratory investigations and correct interpretation of test results (Box 19.2). The key principles, including the concepts of sensitivity and specificity, are described in Chapter 1. Reference intervals for laboratory results are provided in Chapter 35. Many laboratory investigations can be subject to variability arising from whether the sample is being taken in the fed or fasted state; the timing of sample collection, in relation to diurnal variation of analytes; dosage intervals for therapeutic drug monitoring; sample type, such as serum, plasma; use of anticoagulants, such as EDTA, which can interfere with some assays; or artefacts, such as taking a venous sample proximal to the site of an intravenous infusion. It is therefore important for clinical and laboratory staff to communicate effectively and for clinicians to follow local recommendations concerning collection and transport of samples in the appropriate container and with appropriate labelling.

i	19.1 Range of analytical modalities used in the clinical biochemistry laboratory

Analytical modality	Analyte	Typical applications
Ion-selective electrodes	Blood gases, electrolytes (Na, K, Cl)	Point-of-care testing (POCT) High-throughput analysers
Colorimetric chemical reaction or coupled enzymatic reaction	Simple mass or concentration measurement (creatinine, phosphate) Simple enzyme activity	High-throughput analysers
Ligand assay (usually immunoassay)	Specific proteins Hormones Drugs	Increasingly available for POCT or high-throughput analysers
Chromatography: gas chromatography (GC), high-performance liquid chromatography (HPLC), thin-layer chromatography (TLC)	Organic compounds	Therapeutic drug monitoring (TDM)
Mass spectroscopy (MS)	Drugs Vitamins Organic compounds	Screening for drugs of misuse Vitamins Biochemical metabolites
Spectrophotometry, turbidimetry, nephelometry, fluorimetry	Haemoglobin derivatives Specific proteins Immunoglobulins	Xanthochromia Lipoproteins Paraproteins
Electrophoresis	Proteins Some enzymes	Paraproteins Isoenzyme analysis
Atomic absorption (AA) Inductively coupled plasma/mass spectroscopy (ICP-MS)	Trace elements and metals	Quantitation of heavy metals
Molecular diagnostics	Nucleic acid quantification and/or sequence	Inherited and somatic cell variants (Ch. 3) Genetic polymorphisms (Ch. 3) Variations in rates of drug metabolism (Ch. 2) Microbial diagnosis (Ch. 6)

19.2 How to interpret urea and electrolytes results*

Sodium

- Largely reflects changes in water balance
- See 'Hypernatraemia' and 'Hyponatraemia'

Potassium

- May reflect K shifts in and out of cells
- Low levels usually mean excessive losses (gastrointestinal or renal)
- High levels usually mean renal dysfunction
- See 'Hypokalaemia' and 'Hyperkalaemia'

Chloride

- Generally changes in parallel with plasma Na
- Low in metabolic alkalosis
- High in some forms of metabolic acidosis

Bicarbonate

- Abnormal in acid–base disorders
- See Box 19.18

Urea

- Increased with a fall in glomerular filtration rate (GFR), reduced renal perfusion or urine flow rate, and in high protein intake or catabolic states

Creatinine

- Increased with a fall in GFR, in individuals with high muscle mass, and with some drugs
- See Figure 18.2

*The term urea and electrolytes (U&Es) refers to urea, electrolyes and creatinine. In some countries this is abbreviated to EUC (electrolytes/urea/creatinine).

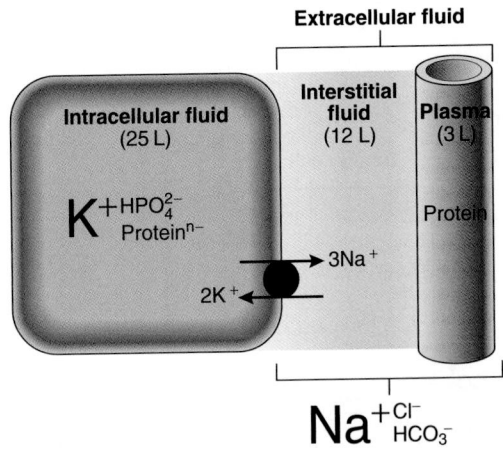

Fig. 19.1 Normal distribution of body water and electrolytes. Schematic representation of volume (L = litres) and composition (dominant ionic species only shown) of the intracellular fluid (ICF) and extracellular fluid (ECF) in a 70 kg male. The main difference in composition between the plasma and interstitial fluid (ISF) is the presence of appreciable concentrations of protein in the plasma but not the ISF. The Na/K differential is maintained by the Na,K-adenosine triphosphatase (ATPase) pump.

Water and electrolyte homeostasis

Total body water (TBW) is approximately 60% of body weight in an adult male, although the proportion is somewhat more for infants and less for women. In a 70 kg man TBW is therefore about 40 L. Approximately 25 L is located inside cells (the intracellular fluid or ICF), while the remaining 15 L is in the extracellular fluid (ECF) compartment (see Fig. 19.1). Most of the ECF (approximately 12 L) is interstitial fluid, which is within the tissues but outside cells, whereas the remainder (about 3 L) is in the plasma compartment.

The ion composition between the main body fluid compartments intracellularly and extracellularly is illustrated in Figure 19.1. The dominant positively charged ion (cation) within cells is potassium, whereas phosphates and negatively charged proteins constitute the major intracellular negatively charged ions (anions). In the ECF the dominant cation is sodium, while chloride and, to a lesser extent, bicarbonate are the most important ECF anions. An important difference between the intravascular (plasma) and interstitial compartments of the ECF is that only plasma contains significant concentrations of protein.

The major force maintaining the difference in cation concentrations between the ICF and ECF is the sodium–potassium pump (Na,K-activated adenosine triphosphatase – ATPase), which is present in all cell membranes. Maintenance of these gradients is essential for many cell processes, including the excitability of conducting tissues such as nerve and muscle. The difference in protein content between the plasma and the interstitial fluid compartment is maintained by the impermeability of the capillary wall to protein. This protein concentration gradient (the colloid osmotic, or oncotic, pressure of the plasma) contributes to the balance of forces across the capillary wall that favour fluid retention within the plasma compartment.

The concentration of sodium in the ECF plays a pivotal role in determining plasma osmolality and thereby controlling intracellular volume through changes in water balance between the intracellular and extracellular space. In contrast, plasma volume is largely controlled by total body sodium, which determines volume change. Therefore, disturbances in

water homeostasis typically present with biochemical abnormalities such as hyponatraemia or hypernatraemia, whereas disturbances in sodium homeostasis present with hypervolaemia or hypovolaemia as the result of expansion or contraction of ECF volume, respectively.

Sodium homeostasis

Most of the body's sodium is located in the ECF, where it is by far the most abundant cation. Accordingly, total body sodium is the principal determinant of ECF volume. Sodium intake varies widely between individuals, ranging between 50 and 250 mmol/24 hr. The kidneys can compensate for these wide variations in sodium intake by increasing excretion of sodium when there is sodium overload, and retaining sodium in the presence of sodium depletion, to maintain normal ECF volume and plasma volume.

Functional anatomy and physiology

The functional unit for renal excretion is the nephron, which is illustrated in Figure 19.2. Blood undergoes ultrafiltration in the glomerulus, generating a fluid that is free from cells and protein and which resembles plasma in its electrolyte composition. This is delivered into the renal tubules, where reabsorption of water and various electrolytes occurs. (More detail on the structure and function of the glomerulus is given in Ch. 18.) The glomerular filtration rate (GFR) is approximately 125 mL/min (equivalent to 180 L/24 hr) in a normal adult. Over 99% of the filtered fluid is reabsorbed into the blood in the peritubular capillaries during its passage through successive segments of the nephron, mainly as a result of tubular reabsorption of sodium. The processes mediating sodium reabsorption, and the factors that regulate it, are key to understanding clinical disturbances and pharmacological interventions of sodium and fluid balance.

The nephron can be divided into four different functional segments in terms of sodium and water reabsorption (see Fig. 19.2).

Proximal renal tubule

About 65% of the filtered sodium load is reabsorbed in the proximal renal tubule. The cellular mechanisms are complex but some of the key features are shown in panel (A) of Figure 19.2. The key to sodium reabsorption from the luminal fluid rests on the basolateral (blood-side) of the cell where large numbers of Na,K-ATPase pumps are present (black circle)

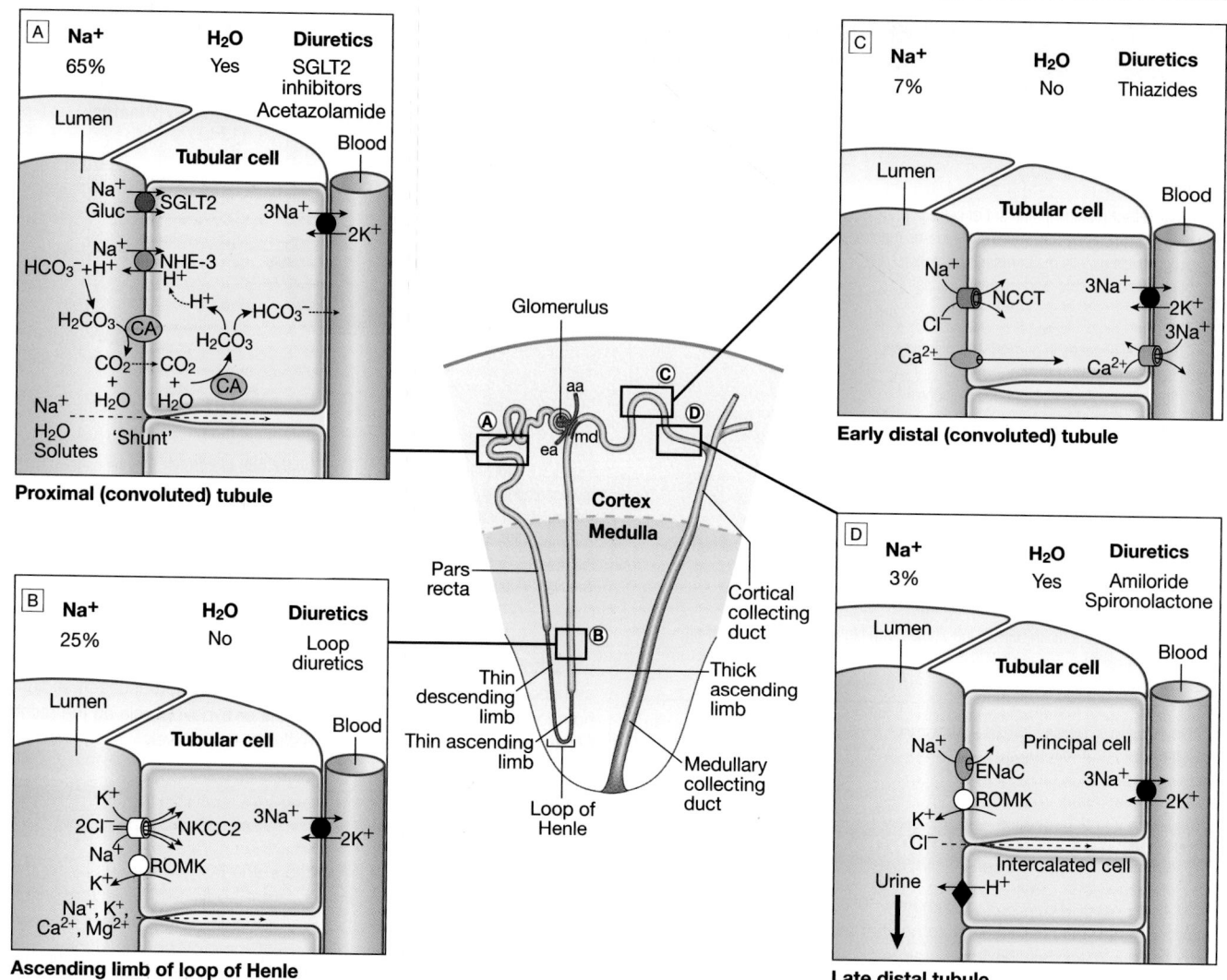

Fig. 19.2 Anatomy of the nephron and principal transport mechanisms in different parts of the renal tubule. The apical membrane of tubular cells is the side facing the lumen and the basolateral membrane is the side facing the blood. Black circles indicate active transport pumps linked to ATP hydrolysis and other symbols indicate ion channels and transporter molecules (see text for more details). Details of the proportion of sodium reabsorbed, water permeability and sites of action for different classes of diuretics are shown. The SGLT2 inhibitors are primarily used for the treatment of diabetes but have diuretic properties by blocking SGLT2 (yellow circle) in the proximal tubule [A]. At the same site, acetazolamide inhibits carbonic anhydrase (CA), which, by reducing production of hydrogen ions by proximal tubular cells, inhibits sodium–hydrogen exchange through the NHE-3 transporter (pink circle). Loop diuretics block the NKCC2 transporter (white cylinder) in the loop of Henle [B], whereas thiazide diuretics block the NCCT channel (orange cylinder) in the early distal tubule [C]. Amiloride and spironolactone block the ENaC channel (blue doughnut) in the late distal tubule and collecting ducts [D]. See text for further details and abbreviations. (aa = afferent arteriole; ea = efferent arteriole; md = macula densa)

which transport sodium from the cells into the blood. This creates a low concentration of sodium within the cell that drives the passive reabsorption of sodium from the lumen into the epithelial cell. Transporters in the apical membrane are then able to couple sodium transport to the entry of various organic molecules, including glucose, amino acids, phosphate and others. An example of this is shown in Figure 19.2 where the reabsorption of Na is coupled to the reabsorption of glucose via the SGLT2 transport protein (yellow circle). Entry of sodium into the tubular cells at this site is also linked to secretion of H+ ions, through the sodium–hydrogen exchanger (NHE-3) (pink circle). This relates to a complicated system responsible for bicarbonate reabsorption where HCO_3 ions in the lumen are combined with H+ ions to form carbonic acid (H_2CO_3). The H_2CO_3 is broken down to form H_2O and CO_2 in a reaction catalysed by carbonic anhydrase (CA) present on the luminal membrane of the tubular cell. The CO_2 and H_2O are then freely able to diffuse into the tubular cell. Within the tubular cell, H_2CO_3 is generated from H_2O and CO_2 by intracellular CA. The H_2CO_3 then dissociates spontaneously to produce H+ ions which are transported into the lumen by the NHE-3 transporter and

HCO_3- ions which are transported into the blood. This allows for almost complete reabsorption of bicarbonate in the proximal tubule. In addition, a large component of the transepithelial flux of sodium, water and other dissolved solutes occurs through gaps *between* the cells (the 'shunt' pathway). Overall, fluid and electrolyte reabsorption is almost isotonic in this segment, as water reabsorption is matched very closely to sodium fluxes, such that the osmolality of fluid passing into the loop of Henle is very similar to that of plasma. A component of this water flow also passes *through* the cells, via aquaporin-1 (AQP-1) water channels (see Fig. 19.5), which are not sensitive to hormonal regulation. Acetazolamide and SGLT2 inhibitors both act on this segment to promote sodium excretion by their effects on carbonic anhydrase and the SLGT2 protein, respectively.

Loop of Henle

The thick ascending limb of the loop of Henle reabsorbs a further 25% of the filtered sodium but is impermeable to water, resulting in dilution of the luminal fluid as illustrated in panel (B) in Figure 19.2. Again, the primary driving force is the Na,K-ATPase on the basolateral cell membrane (black circle) which creates a low intracellular concentration of sodium, but in this segment, sodium entry through the Na,K,2Cl (NKCC2, white cylinder) allows electroneutral entry of these ions into the renal tubular cell by balancing transport of cations (Na+/K+) with anions (Cl-). Some of the potassium accumulated inside the cell recirculates across the apical membrane back into the lumen through the ROMK potassium channel (white circle), providing a continuing supply of potassium to match the high concentrations of sodium and chloride in the lumen. Due to this, a small positive transepithelial potential difference exists in the lumen of this segment relative to the interstitium, and this serves to drive cations such as sodium, potassium, calcium and magnesium between the cells, forming a reabsorptive shunt pathway. Loop diuretics like furosemide inhibit sodium reabsorption in this segment by inhibiting the NKCC2 transporter.

Early distal renal tubule

The early distal tubule (also called distal convoluted tubule) is responsible for reabsorption of about 7% of the filtered sodium load, as shown in panel (C) in Figure 19.2. This is again primarily driven by the activity of the basolateral Na,K-ATPase (black circle). In this segment, entry of sodium into the cell from the luminal fluid occurs via the NCCT sodium–chloride co-transport carrier (orange cylinder). This segment is also impermeable to water, resulting in further dilution of the luminal fluid. There is no significant transepithelial flux of potassium in this segment, but calcium is reabsorbed in exchange for sodium, where a basolateral sodium–calcium exchanger (blue cylinder) leads to low intracellular concentrations of calcium, promoting calcium entry from the luminal fluid through a calcium channel (blue ellipse). Thiazide diuretics inhibit sodium reabsorption in this segment by inhibiting the NCCT transporter.

Late distal renal tubule and collecting ducts

The late distal tubule and cortical collecting duct are anatomically and functionally continuous (panel (D) in Fig. 19.2). Here, sodium entry from the luminal fluid into principal cells occurs through the epithelial sodium channel (ENaC), generating a substantial lumen-negative transepithelial potential difference. This sodium flux into the tubular cells is balanced by secretion of potassium and hydrogen ions into the lumen and by reabsorption of chloride ions. Potassium passes into the luminal fluid down its electrochemical gradient, through an apical potassium channel (ROMK) in the principal cells (white circle). Hydrogen ion secretion is mediated by an H+-ATPase (black triangle) located on the luminal membrane of the alpha intercalated cells. Beta intercalated cells secrete bicarbonate and both cell types participate in the excretion of ammonia and ammonium. The distal tubule and collecting duct have a variable permeability to water, depending on circulating levels of vasopressin (antidiuretic hormone, ADH). All ion transport processes in this segment are stimulated by the steroid hormone aldosterone, which can increase sodium reabsorption to a maximum of 2%–3% of the filtered sodium load. Amiloride and spironolactone both reduce sodium reabsorption in this segment by inhibiting the activity of the ENaC transporter (blue doughnut), either directly, as in the case of amiloride, or by inhibiting the effects of aldosterone, as is the case with spironolactone.

Less than 1% of sodium reabsorption occurs in the medullary collecting duct, where it is inhibited by atrial natriuretic peptide (ANP) and brain natriuretic peptide (BNP).

Regulation of sodium transport

The amount of sodium excreted by the kidney is dependent on the filtered load of sodium (which is principally determined by GFR) and the control of tubular sodium reabsorption. A number of interrelated mechanisms serve to maintain whole-body sodium balance, and hence ECF volume, by matching urinary sodium excretion to sodium intake (Fig. 19.3), and controlling those two processes.

Important sensing mechanisms include volume receptors in the cardiac atria and the intrathoracic veins, as well as pressure receptors

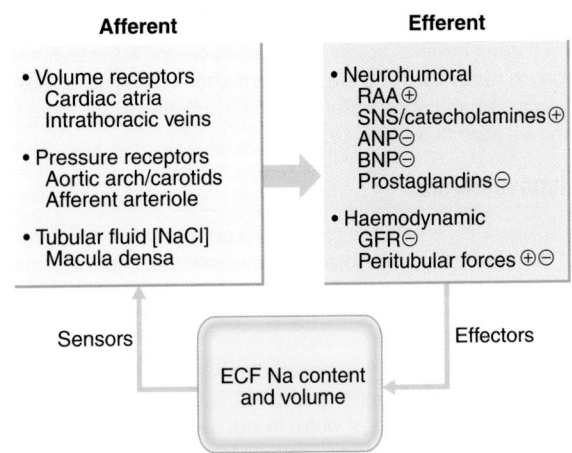

Fig. 19.3 Mechanisms involved in the regulation of sodium transport. ANP = atrial natriuretic peptide; BNP = brain natriuretic peptide; ECF = extracellular fluid; GFR = glomerular filtration rate; RAA = renin–angiotensin–aldosterone system; SNS = sympathetic nervous system. ⊕ indicates an effect to stimulate Na reabsorption and hence reduce Na excretion, while ⊖ indicates an effect to inhibit Na reabsorption and hence increase Na excretion.

located in the central arterial tree (aortic arch and carotid sinus) and the afferent arterioles within the kidney. A further afferent signal is generated within the kidney itself: the enzyme renin is released from specialised smooth muscle cells in the walls of the afferent and efferent arterioles, at the point where they make contact with the early distal tubular cells of the macula densa to form the juxtaglomerular apparatus (see Fig. 19.2). Renin release is stimulated by:

- reduced perfusion pressure in the afferent arteriole
- increased sympathetic nerve activity
- decreased sodium chloride concentration in the distal tubular fluid.

Renin acts on the peptide substrate, angiotensinogen (which is produced by the liver), to produce angiotensin I, which is cleaved by angiotensin-converting enzyme (ACE), largely in the pulmonary capillary bed, to produce angiotensin II (see Fig. 20.19). Angiotensin II has multiple actions: it stimulates proximal tubular sodium reabsorption and release of aldosterone from the zona glomerulosa of the adrenal cortex, and causes vasoconstriction of small arterioles. Aldosterone amplifies sodium retention by its action on the cortical collecting duct. The net effect of activation of the renin–angiotensin system is to raise blood pressure and cause sodium and water retention, thereby correcting hypovolaemia.

Changes in GFR alter peritubular hydrostatic pressure and oncotic pressure in opposite directions, resulting in a change in sodium reabsorption. In particular, with hypovolaemia, and a reduction in hydrostatic pressure and an increase in oncotic pressure, there is an increase in sodium reabsorption.

The sympathetic nervous system also acts to increase sodium retention, both through haemodynamic mechanisms (afferent arteriolar vasoconstriction and GFR reduction) and by direct stimulation of proximal tubular sodium reabsorption. In contrast, other humoral mediators, such as the natriuretic peptides, which inhibit sodium reabsorption, contribute to natriuresis during periods of sodium and volume excess.

Increases in sodium intake cause hypervolaemia, which increases renal perfusion and GFR and suppresses renin production through increased delivery of sodium into the macula densa. This sets in motion a train of events opposite to those that occur in hypovolaemia, to cause an increase in sodium excretion.

Presenting problems in sodium balance

When the balance of sodium intake and excretion is disturbed, any tendency for plasma sodium concentration to change is usually corrected by the osmotic mechanisms controlling water balance. As a result, disorders in sodium balance present chiefly as alterations in the ECF volume, resulting in hypovolaemia or hypervolaemia, rather than as an alteration in plasma sodium concentration. Clinical manifestations of altered ECF volume are illustrated in Box 19.3.

Hypovolaemia

Hypovolaemia is defined as a reduction in circulating blood volume. The most common causes are loss or sequestration of sodium-containing fluids or acute blood loss, as summarised in Box 19.4.

Pathogenesis

Loss of sodium-containing fluid triggers the changes in renal sodium handling and activation of the renin–angiotensin system that were described earlier in this chapter. Loss of whole blood, as in acute haemorrhage, is another cause of hypovolaemia, and elicits the same mechanisms for the conservation of sodium and water as loss of sodium-containing fluid.

Clinical features

Hypovolaemia is primarily a clinical diagnosis, based on characteristic symptoms such as thirst, dizziness and weakness along with characteristic clinical signs (see Box 19.3) in the context of a relevant precipitating illness.

Investigations

Serum sodium concentrations do not reflect total body sodium and are therefore not helpful in making the diagnosis of hypovolaemia. The GFR is usually maintained unless the hypovolaemia is very severe or prolonged, but urinary flow rate is reduced as a consequence of activation of sodium- and water-retaining mechanisms in the nephron. Serum creatinine, which reflects GFR, is usually normal, but serum urea concentration is typically elevated due to a low urine flow rate, which is accompanied by increased tubular reabsorption of urea. Similarly, serum uric acid may also rise, reflecting increased reabsorption in the proximal renal tubule. The urine sodium concentration appropriately falls and sodium excretion may reduce to less than 0.1% of the filtered sodium load.

Management

Management of sodium and volume depletion has two main components:

- treat the cause where possible, to stop ongoing salt and volume losses
- replace the salt and water deficits, and provide ongoing maintenance requirements, usually by intravenous fluid replacement when depletion is severe.

Intravenous fluid therapy

Intravenous fluid therapy can be used to maintain water, sodium and potassium intake when the patient is fasting, such as during an acute illness or post-operatively. If any deficits or continuing pathological losses are identified, additional fluid and electrolytes will be required. In prolonged periods of fasting (more than a few days), attention also needs to be given to providing sufficient caloric and nutritional intake to prevent excessive catabolism of body energy stores. The daily maintenance requirements for water and electrolytes in a typical adult are shown in Box 19.5 and the composition of some widely available intravenous fluids are given in Box 19.6. The choice of fluid and the rate of administration depend on the clinical circumstances, as assessed at the bedside and from laboratory data, as described in Box 19.7.

The choice of intravenous fluid therapy in the treatment of significant hypovolaemia relates to the concepts in Figure 19.1. If fluid containing neither sodium nor protein is given, it will distribute in the body fluid compartments in proportion to the normal distribution of total body water. For example, administration of 1 L of 5% dextrose contributes little (approximately 3/40 of the infused volume) towards expansion of the plasma volume, which makes this fluid unsuitable for restoring the circulation and perfusion of vital organs. Intravenous infusion of an isotonic (normal) saline solution, on the other hand, is more effective at expanding the ECF, although only a small proportion (about 3/15) of the infused volume actually contributes to plasma volume.

Whilst it would appear that solutions containing plasma proteins (colloids) would be better retained within the vascular space and be more effective at correcting hypovolaemia than protein-free fluids (crystalloids), clinical studies have not shown any advantage of giving albumin-containing infusions in the treatment of acute hypovolaemia and indeed have demonstrated increased morbidity related to their use. Therefore, crystalloids are the fluid of choice for resuscitation in acute hypovolaemia. More studies, however, are required to clarify the most appropriate crystalloid in this situation, given that normal saline can cause a mild metabolic acidosis, perhaps related to excessive chloride loading, whereas 'balanced solutions', such as Hartmann's, may cause a mild hyponatraemia, as their composition is slightly hypotonic.

Hypervolaemia

Hypervolaemia is the result of sodium and water excess and is rare in patients with normal cardiac and renal function, since the kidney has a

---

i | 19.3 Clinical features of hypovolaemia and hypervolaemia

	Hypovolaemia	Hypervolaemia
Symptoms	Thirst Dizziness on standing Weakness	Ankle swelling Abdominal swelling Breathlessness
Signs	Postural hypotension Tachycardia Dry mouth Reduced skin turgor Reduced urine output Weight loss Delirium, stupor	Peripheral oedema Raised JVP Pulmonary crepitations Pleural effusion Ascites Weight gain Hypertension (sometimes)

(JVP = jugular venous pressure)

---

i | 19.4 Causes of hypovolaemia

Mechanism	Examples
Inadequate sodium intake	Environmental deprivation, inadequate therapeutic replacement
Gastrointestinal sodium loss	Vomiting, diarrhoea, nasogastric suction, external fistula
Skin sodium loss	Excessive sweating, burns
Renal sodium loss	Diuretic therapy, mineralocorticoid deficiency, tubulointerstitial disease
Internal sequestration*	Bowel obstruction, peritonitis, pancreatitis, crush injury
Reduced blood volume	Acute blood loss

*A cause of circulatory volume depletion, although total body sodium and water may be normal or increased.

---

i | 19.5 Basic daily water and electrolyte requirements

	Requirement per kg	Typical 70 kg adult
Water	35–45 mL/kg	2.45–3.15 L/24 hrs
Sodium	1.5–2 mmol/kg	105–140 mmol/24 hrs
Potassium	1.0–1.5 mmol/kg	70–105 mmol/24 hrs

i	**19.6 Composition of some isotonic intravenous fluids**					
Fluid	D-glucose	Calories	Na⁺ (mmol/L)	Cl⁻ (mmol/L)	Other (mmol/L)
5% dextrose	50 g	200	0	0	0
Normal (0.9%) saline	0	0	154	154	0
Hartmann's solution	0	0	131	111	K⁺ 5 Ca²⁺ 2 Lactate⁻ 29

⚕	**19.7 How to assess fluid and electrolyte balance in hospitalised patients**

Step 1: assess clinical volume status

- Examine patient for signs of hypovolaemia or hypervolaemia (see Box 19.3)
- Check daily weight change

Step 2: review fluid balance chart

- Check total volumes IN and OUT on previous day (IN–OUT is positive by ~400 mL in normal balance, reflecting insensible fluid losses of ~800 mL and metabolic water generation of ~400 mL)
- Check cumulative change in daily fluid balance over previous 3–5 days
- Correlate chart figures with weight change and clinical volume status to estimate net fluid balance

Step 3: assess ongoing fluid losses

- Check losses from gastrointestinal tract and surgical drains
- Estimate increased insensible losses (e.g. in fever) and internal sequestration ('third space')

Step 4: check plasma U&Es (see Box 19.2)

- Check plasma Na as marker of relative water balance
- Check plasma K as a guide to extracellular K balance
- Check HCO₃ as a clue to acid–base disorder
- Check urea and creatinine to monitor renal function

Step 5: prescribe appropriate intravenous fluid replacement therapy

- Replace basic water and electrolytes each day (see Box 19.5)
- Allow for anticipated oral intake and pathological fluid loss
- Adjust amounts of water (if IV, usually given as isotonic 5% dextrose), sodium and potassium according to plasma electrolyte results

(IV = intravenous; U&Es = urea and electrolytes)

i	**19.8 Causes of sodium and water excess**	
Mechanism	Examples
Impaired renal function	Primary renal disease
Primary hyperaldosteronism*	Conn syndrome
Secondary hyperaldosteronism (see Fig. 19.5)	Congestive cardiac failure Cirrhotic liver disease Nephrotic syndrome Protein-losing enteropathy Malnutrition Idiopathic/cyclical oedema Renal artery stenosis*

*Conditions in this box *other than* primary hyperaldosteronism and renal artery stenosis are typically associated with generalised oedema.

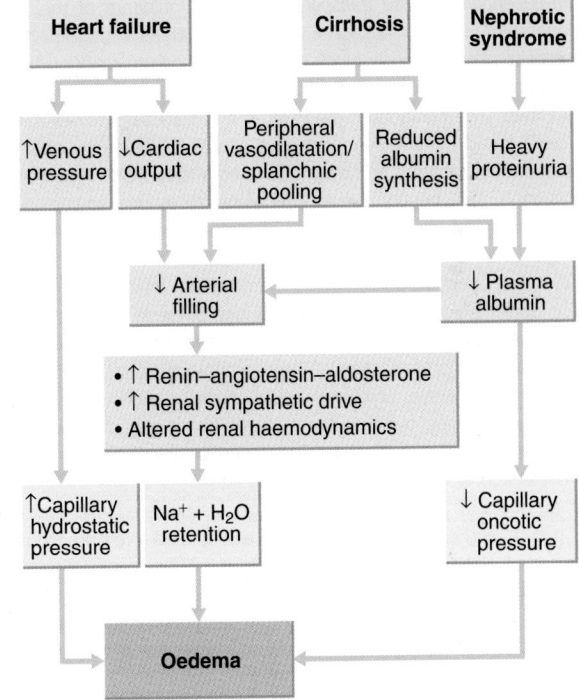

Fig. 19.4 Secondary mechanisms causing sodium excess and oedema in cardiac failure, cirrhosis and nephrotic syndrome. Primary renal retention of Na and water may also contribute to oedema formation when glomerular filtration rate is significantly reduced (see Box 19.8).

large capacity to increase renal excretion of sodium and water via the homeostatic mechanisms described earlier in the chapter.

Pathogenesis

The most common systemic disorders responsible for hypervolaemia are outlined in Box 19.8. In cardiac failure, cirrhosis and nephrotic syndrome, sodium retention occurs in response to circulatory insufficiency caused by the primary disorder, as illustrated in Figure 19.4. The pathophysiology is different in kidney failure, when the primary cause of volume expansion is the profound reduction in GFR impairing sodium and water excretion, while secondary tubular mechanisms are of lesser importance. In primary hyperaldosteronism (Conn syndrome) the pathophysiology also differs, in that increased secretion of aldosterone directly stimulates sodium reabsorption.

Clinical features

Peripheral oedema is the most common physical sign of hypervolaemia since the excess fluid leaks out of the capillaries to expand the interstitial compartment of the ECF. This is particularly the case in nephrotic syndrome and chronic liver disease, in which hypoalbuminaemia is a prominent feature. The main exception is Conn syndrome, which presents with hypertension and often hypokalaemia, but in which peripheral oedema is unusual.

Investigations

Although hypervolaemia is accompanied by an excess of total body sodium, serum sodium concentrations tend to be normal due to the accompanying water retention. Serum concentrations of potassium are normal except in

19

Conn syndrome, where there is hypokalaemia due to the increased aldosterone production. Creatinine, GFR and urea are usually normal, unless the underlying cause of hypervolaemia is renal failure. General investigations may reveal evidence of cardiac, renal or liver disease.

Management

The management of hypervolaemia involves a number of components:

- specific treatment directed at the underlying cause, such as ACE inhibitors in heart failure and glucocorticoids in minimal change nephropathy
- restriction of dietary sodium (to 50–80 mmol/24 hr) to match the diminished excretory capacity
- fluid restriction

Diuretic therapy

Diuretics play a pivotal role in the treatment of hypervolaemia due to salt and water retention and in hypertension. They act by inhibiting sodium reabsorption at various locations along the nephron (see Fig. 19.2). Their potency and adverse effects relate to their mechanism and site of action.

Carbonic anhydrase inhibitors Acetazolamide is a carbonic anhydrase inhibitor that inhibits intracellular production of H^+ ions in the proximal tubule, reducing the fraction of sodium reabsorption that is exchanged for H^+ by the apical membrane sodium–hydrogen exchanger. It is a weak diuretic but is seldom used clinically for this purpose, since only a small fraction of proximal sodium reabsorption uses this mechanism, and much of the sodium that is not reabsorbed in the proximal tubule can be reabsorbed by downstream segments of the nephron. Its use is also complicated by metabolic acidosis due to reduction in proximal bicarbonate reabsorption.

Sodium-dependent glucose transporter inhibitors Inhibitors of the sodium-dependent glucose transporter 2 (SGLT2), such as dapagliflozin and canagliflozin, simultaneously block glucose and sodium reabsorption in the proximal tubule. They have mild diuretic properties but are principally used to lower blood glucose in the treatment of diabetes. However, they have been found to have renoprotective effects beyond their ability to improve diabetic control, probably related to a reduction in glomerular hyperfiltration. This occurs due to their ability to reduce sodium reabsorption and thereby a reduction in tubuloglomerular feedback.

Loop diuretics Loop diuretics, such as furosemide, inhibit sodium reabsorption in the thick ascending limb of the loop of Henle, by blocking the action of the apical membrane NKCC2 co-transporter. Because this segment reabsorbs a large fraction of the filtered sodium, these drugs are potent diuretics, and are commonly used in diseases associated with significant oedema. Loop diuretics cause excretion not only of sodium (and with it water) but also of potassium. This occurs chiefly as a result of delivery of increased amounts of sodium to the late distal tubule and cortical collecting ducts, where sodium reabsorption is associated with secretion of potassium, and is amplified if circulating aldosterone levels are high.

Thiazide diuretics Thiazide diuretics inhibit sodium reabsorption in the early distal tubule, by blocking the NCCT co-transporter in the apical membrane. Since this segment reabsorbs a much smaller fraction of the filtered sodium, these are less potent than loop diuretics, but are widely used in the treatment of hypertension and less severe oedema. Like loop diuretics, thiazides increase excretion of potassium through delivery of increased amounts of sodium to the late distal tubule and collecting duct. They are the diuretics that are most likely to be complicated by the development of hyponatraemia.

Potassium-sparing diuretics Potassium-sparing diuretics act on the late distal renal tubule and cortical collecting duct segment to inhibit sodium reabsorption. Since sodium reabsorption and potassium secretion are linked at this site, the reduced sodium reabsorption is accompanied by reduced potassium secretion. The apical sodium channel ENaC (see Fig. 19.2) is blocked by amiloride and triamterene, while spironolactone and eplerenone also act at this site by blocking binding of aldosterone to mineralocorticoid receptors thereby blocking ENaC activity.

Osmotic diuretics These act independently of a specific transport mechanism. As they are freely filtered at the glomerulus but not reabsorbed by any part of the tubular system, they retain fluid osmotically within the tubular lumen and limit the extent of sodium reabsorption in multiple segments. Mannitol is the most commonly used osmotic diuretic. It is given by intravenous infusion to achieve short-term diuresis in conditions such as cerebral oedema.

Clinical use of diuretics

The following principles should be observed when using diuretics:

- Use the minimum effective dose.
- Use for as short a period of time as necessary.
- Monitor regularly for adverse effects.

The choice of diuretic is determined by the potency required, the presence of coexistent conditions and the side-effect profile.

Adverse effects encountered with the most frequently used classes of diuretic (loop drugs and thiazide drugs) are summarised in Box 19.9. Volume depletion and electrolyte disorders are the most common, as predicted from their mechanism of action. The metabolic side-effects listed are rarely of clinical significance and may reflect effects on K^+ channels that influence insulin secretion. Since most drugs from these classes are sulphonamides, there is a relatively high incidence of hypersensitivity reactions, and occasional idiosyncratic side-effects in a variety of organ systems.

The side-effect profile of the potassium-sparing diuretics differs in a number of important respects from that of other diuretics. The disturbances in potassium, magnesium and acid–base balance are in the opposite direction, so that normal or increased levels of potassium and magnesium are found in the blood, and there is a tendency to metabolic acidosis, especially when renal function is impaired.

An important feature of the most commonly used diuretic drugs (furosemide, thiazides and amiloride) is that they act on their target molecules from the luminal side of the tubular epithelium. Since they are highly protein-bound in the plasma, very little reaches the urinary fluid by glomerular filtration, but there are active transport mechanisms for secreting organic acids and bases, including these drugs, across the proximal tubular wall into the lumen, resulting in adequate drug concentrations being delivered to later tubular segments. This secretory process may be impaired by certain other drugs, and also by accumulated organic anions as occurs in chronic kidney disease and chronic liver failure, leading to resistance to diuretics. The transport protein is also responsible for the secretion of uric acid so the use of these diuretics can competitively inhibit this process and result in gout.

Diuretic resistance is encountered under a variety of circumstances, including impaired renal function, activation of sodium-retaining mechanisms, impaired oral bioavailability (such as in patients with gastrointestinal disease) and decreased renal blood flow. In these circumstances,

---

i	19.9 Adverse effects of loop-acting and thiazide diuretics	
Renal side-effects		
• Hypovolaemia		• Hyperuricaemia
• Hyponatraemia		• Hypomagnesaemia
• Hypokalaemia		• Hypercalciuria (loop)
• Metabolic alkalosis		• Hypocalciuria (thiazide)
Metabolic side-effects		
• Glucose intolerance/hyperglycaemia		• Hyperlipidaemia
Miscellaneous side-effects		
• Hypersensitivity reactions		• Acute pancreatitis/
• Erectile dysfunction		cholecystitis (thiazide)

short-term intravenous therapy with a loop-acting agent such as furosemide may be useful. Combinations of diuretics administered orally may also increase potency. Either a loop or a thiazide drug can be combined with a potassium-sparing drug, and all three classes can be used together for short periods, with carefully supervised clinical and laboratory monitoring.

Water homeostasis

Daily water intake can vary from about 500 mL to several litres a day. About 800 mL of water is lost daily through the stool, sweat and the respiratory tract (insensible losses) and about 400 mL is generated daily through oxidative metabolism (metabolic water). The kidneys are chiefly responsible for adjusting water excretion to balance intake, endogenous production and losses so as to maintain total body water content and serum osmolality within the reference range of 280–296 mOsmol/kg.

Functional anatomy and physiology

While regulation of total ECF volume is principally achieved through renal control of sodium excretion, mechanisms exist to allow for the excretion of urine that is hypertonic or hypotonic in relation to plasma to maintain constant plasma osmolality.

These functions are largely achieved by the loop of Henle and the collecting ducts (see Fig. 19.2). The countercurrent configuration of flow in adjacent limbs of the loop (Fig. 19.5) involves osmotic movement of water from the descending limbs and reabsorption of solute from neighbouring ascending limbs, to set up a gradient of osmolality from isotonic (like plasma) in the renal cortex to hypertonic (around 1200 mOsmol/kg) in the inner part of the medulla. At the same time, the fluid emerging from the thick ascending limb is hypotonic compared to plasma because it

has been diluted by the reabsorption of sodium, but not water, from the thick ascending limb and is further diluted in the early distal tubule. As this dilute fluid passes from the cortex through the collecting duct system to the renal pelvis, it traverses the medullary interstitial gradient of osmolality set up by the operation of the loop of Henle, and water is able to be reabsorbed. Whether water is reabsorbed at this point to concentrate the urine or whether the duct becomes impermeable to water allowing for dilute urine to be excreted depends on the presence or absence of the circulating level of vasopressin respectively. Vasopressin is released by the posterior pituitary gland under conditions of increased plasma osmolality or hypovolaemia.

- When water intake is high and plasma osmolality is normal or low–normal (Fig. 19.5B), vasopressin levels are suppressed and the collecting ducts remain impermeable to water. The luminal fluid osmolality remains low, resulting in the excretion of a dilute urine (minimum osmolality approximately 50 mOsmol/kg in a healthy young person).
- When water intake is restricted and plasma osmolality is high (Fig. 19.5A), or in the presence of significant plasma volume depletion, vasopressin levels rise. This causes water permeability of the collecting ducts to increase through binding of vasopressin to the V2 receptor, which enhances collecting duct water permeability through the insertion of AQP-2 channels into the luminal cell membrane. This results in osmotic reabsorption of water along the entire length of the collecting duct, with maximum urine osmolality approaching that in the medullary tip (up to 1200 mOsmol/kg).

Parallel to these changes in vasopressin release are changes in water-seeking behaviour triggered by the sensation of thirst, which also becomes activated as plasma osmolality rises.

In summary, for adequate dilution of the urine there must be:
- adequate solute delivery to the loop of Henle and early distal tubule
- normal function of the loop of Henle and early distal tubule

19

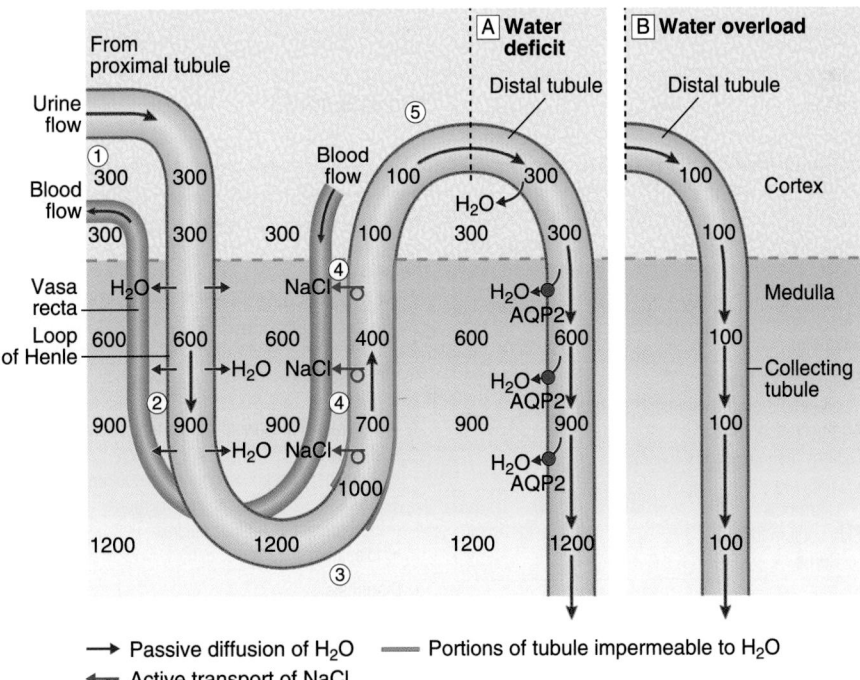

Fig. 19.5 Mechanisms of renal water handling. (1) Filtrate from the proximal tubule is isosmotic to plasma and cortical interstitial fluid. (2) Water moves down its osmotic gradient, concentrating the filtrate but not diluting the interstitium, as the vasa recta carries away the water. (3) The filtrate is at its highest concentration at the bend of the loop and therefore the surrounding medulla is also concentrated. (4) NaCl is pumped out of the filtrate in the thick ascending limb and early distal tubule, increasing the interstitial fluid osmolality. (5) The filtrate has a concentration of 100 mOsmol/kg as it leaves the early distal tubule. [A] In the face of water deficit, vasopressin levels rise, causing AQP2 channels to migrate to the luminal side of the cell membrane increasing water permeability of the collecting ducts, resulting in osmotic reabsorption of water. [B] In the situation of water overload, vasopressin secretion is suppressed, AQP2 channels are held intracellularly, rendering the collecting ducts impermeable to water, resulting in production of a dilute urine.

- absence of vasopressin in the circulation.

If any of these processes is faulty, water retention and hyponatraemia may result.

Conversely, to achieve concentration of the urine there must be:

- adequate solute delivery to the loop of Henle
- normal function of the loop of Henle
- vasopressin release into the circulation
- vasopressin action on the collecting ducts.

Failure of any of these steps may result in inappropriate water loss and hypernatraemia.

Presenting problems in regulation of osmolality

Changes in plasma osmolality are mainly determined by changes in serum sodium concentration and its associated anions. As outlined above, changes in sodium concentration usually occur because of disturbances in water balance, either because there is a relative excess of body water compared to total body sodium (hyponatraemia) or a relative lack of body water compared to total body sodium (hypernatraemia). Abnormalities of water balance can result from disturbances in urinary concentration or dilution.

If extracellular osmolality falls, water flows across cell membranes, causing cell swelling, whereas cell shrinkage occurs when osmolality rises. Brain cells and therefore cerebral function are particularly sensitive to such volume changes and can result in increased intracerebral pressure and reduced cerebral perfusion.

Hyponatraemia

Hyponatraemia is defined as a serum Na <135 mmol/L. It is a common electrolyte abnormality with many potential underlying causes, as summarised in Box 19.10.

Pathophysiology

In all cases, hyponatraemia is caused by greater retention of water relative to sodium. The causes are best categorised according to associated changes in the ECF volume (see Box 19.10).

Hyponatraemia with hypovolaemia

In this situation there is depletion of sodium and water but the sodium deficit exceeds the water deficit, causing hypovolaemia and hyponatraemia (see Box 19.3). The cause of sodium loss is usually apparent and common examples are shown in Box 19.10.

Hyponatraemia with euvolaemia

In this situation there are no major disturbances of body sodium content and the patient is clinically euvolaemic. Excess body water may be the result of abnormally high intake, either orally (primary polydipsia) or as a result of medically infused fluids (as intravenous dextrose solutions, or by absorption of sodium-free bladder irrigation fluid after prostatectomy).

Water retention also occurs in the syndrome of inappropriate secretion of antidiuretic hormone, or vasopressin (SIADH). In this condition, an endogenous source of vasopressin (either cerebral or tumour-derived) promotes water retention by the kidney in the absence of an appropriate physiological stimulus (Box 19.11). The clinical diagnosis requires the patient to be euvolaemic, with no evidence of cardiac, renal or hepatic disease potentially associated with hyponatraemia. Other non-osmotic stimuli that cause release of vasopressin (pain, stress, nausea) should also be excluded. Supportive laboratory findings are shown in Box 19.11.

Hyponatraemia with hypervolaemia

In this situation, excess water retention is associated with sodium retention and volume expansion, as in heart failure, liver disease or kidney disease.

Clinical features

Hyponatraemia is often asymptomatic but can also be associated with profound disturbances of cerebral function, manifesting as anorexia, nausea, vomiting, delirium, lethargy, seizures and coma. The likelihood of symptoms occurring is related to the speed at which hyponatraemia develops rather than the severity of hyponatraemia. This is because water rapidly flows into cerebral cells when plasma osmolality falls acutely, causing them to become swollen and ischaemic. However, when hyponatraemia develops gradually, cerebral neurons have time to respond by reducing intracellular osmolality, through excreting potassium and reducing synthesis of intracellular organic osmolytes (Fig. 19.6). The osmotic gradient favouring water movement into the cells is thus reduced and symptoms are avoided. This process takes about 24–48 hours and hyponatraemia is therefore classified as acute (<48 hrs) and chronic (>48 hrs). Hyponatraemia can also be defined as mild (130–135 mmol/L), moderate (125–129 mmol/L) or severe (<124 mmol/L), based on biochemical findings or on the degree of severity of symptoms (Box 19.12).

Investigations

An algorithm for the clinical assessment of patients with hyponatraemia is shown in Figure 19.7. Artefactual causes of hyponatraemia should be considered in all cases. These include severe hyperlipidaemia or hyperproteinaemia, when the aqueous fraction of the serum specimen

---

i | **19.10 Causes of hyponatraemia**

Volume status	Examples
Hypovolaemic	Renal sodium losses:
	Diuretic therapy (especially thiazides)
	Adrenocortical failure
	Gastrointestinal sodium losses:
	Vomiting
	Diarrhoea
	Skin sodium losses:
	Burns
Euvolaemic	Primary polydipsia
	Excessive electrolyte-free water infusion
	SIADH
	Hypothyroidism
Hypervolaemic	Congestive cardiac failure
	Cirrhosis
	Nephrotic syndrome
	Chronic kidney disease (during free water intake)

(SIADH = syndrome of inappropriate antidiuretic hormone (vasopressin) secretion; see Box 19.11).

---

i | **19.11 Causes and diagnosis of syndrome of inappropriate antidiuretic hormone secretion (SIADH)**

Causes

- Tumours
- Central nervous system disorders: stroke, trauma, infection, psychosis, porphyria
- Pulmonary disorders: pneumonia, tuberculosis, obstructive lung disease
- Drugs: anticonvulsants, psychotropics, antidepressants, cytotoxics, oral hypoglycaemic agents, opiates
- Idiopathic

Diagnosis

- Low plasma sodium concentration (typically <130 mmol/L)
- Low plasma osmolality (<275 mOsmol/kg)
- Urine osmolality not minimally low (typically >100 mOsmol/kg)
- Urine sodium concentration not minimally low (>30 mmol/L)
- Low–normal plasma urea, creatinine, uric acid
- Clinical euvolaemia
- Absence of adrenal, thyroid, pituitary or renal insufficiency
- No recent use of diuretics
- Exclusion of other causes of hyponatraemia (see Box 19.10)
- Appropriate clinical context (above)

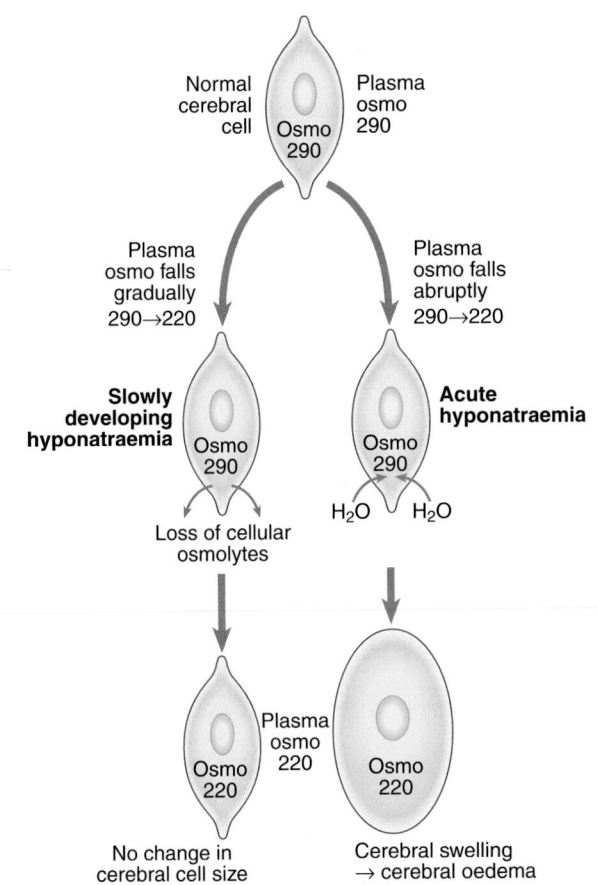

Fig. 19.6 Hyponatraemia and the brain. Numbers represent osmolality (osmo) in mOsmol/kg.

ℹ️	**19.12**	**Symptoms and severity of hyponatraemia**

Severity	Serum sodium	Symptoms
Mild	130–135 mmol/L	None
Moderate	125–129 mmol/L	Nausea Delirium Headache
Severe	<124 mmol/L	Vomiting Somnolence Seizures Coma Cardiorespiratory arrest

is reduced because of the volume occupied by the macromolecules (although this artefact is dependent on the assay technology). Transient hyponatraemia may also occur due to osmotic shifts of water out of cells during hyperosmolar states caused by acute hyperglycaemia or by mannitol infusion, but in these cases plasma osmolality is normal.

When these conditions have been excluded, serum and urine electrolytes and osmolality (Fig. 19.7) are usually the only tests required to clarify the underlying cause. Hypovolaemic hyponatraemia is characterised by a low urinary sodium concentration (<30 mmol/L) when there are extrarenal causes of sodium loss and high urinary sodium concentration (>30 mmol/L) in patients with excessive renal sodium loss.

Measurement of vasopressin is not generally helpful in distinguishing between different categories of hyponatraemia. This is because concentrations of vasopressin are raised both in hypovolaemic states and in most chronic hypervolaemic states, as the impaired circulation in those disorders activates vasopressin release through non-osmotic mechanisms. Indeed, patients with these disorders may have higher circulating vasopressin (ADH) levels than patients with SIADH. The only disorders listed in Box 19.10 in which vasopressin is suppressed are primary polydipsia and iatrogenic water intoxication, where the hypo-osmolar state inhibits vasopressin release from the pituitary. Plasma vasopressin measurements are no longer used in routine practice since it is unstable and have been replaced by measurements of copeptin. This is a peptide derived from the carboxyl terminal of the vasopressin precursor and acts as a surrogate for vasopressin. Copeptin measurements can be useful in the differential diagnosis of patients with the combination of hyponatraemia and polyuria.

Management

The treatment of hyponatraemia is critically dependent on its rate of development, severity, presence of symptoms and underlying cause. If hyponatraemia has developed rapidly (<48 hrs) and there are signs of cerebral oedema, such as obtundation or convulsions, sodium levels should be restored rapidly to normal by infusion of hypertonic (3%) sodium chloride. A common approach is to give an initial bolus of 150 mL over 20 minutes, which may be repeated once or twice over the initial hours of observation, depending on the neurological response and rise in plasma sodium.

Rapid correction of hyponatraemia that has developed more slowly (>48 hrs) can be hazardous, since brain cells adapt to slowly developing hypo-osmolality by reducing the intracellular osmolality, thus maintaining normal cell volume (see Fig. 19.6). Under these conditions, an abrupt increase in extracellular osmolality can lead to water shifting out of neurons, abruptly reducing their volume and causing them to detach from their myelin sheaths. The resulting 'myelinolysis' can produce permanent structural and functional damage to mid-brain structures, and is generally fatal. The rate of correction of the plasma Na concentration in chronic asymptomatic hyponatraemia should not exceed 10 mmol/L/24 hrs, and an even slower rate is generally safer.

The underlying cause should also be treated. For hypovolaemic patients, this involves controlling the source of sodium loss, and administering intravenous saline if clinically warranted. Patients with euvolaemic hyponatraemia generally respond to fluid restriction in the range of 600–1000 mL/24 hrs, accompanied where possible by withdrawal of the precipitating stimulus (such as drugs causing SIADH). In patients with persistent hyponatraemia due to prolonged SIADH, oral urea therapy (30–45 g/day) can be used, which provides a solute load to promote water excretion. Oral vasopressin receptor antagonists such as tolvaptan may also be used to block the vasopressin-mediated component of water retention in a range of hyponatraemic conditions, but concerns exist with regard to the risk of overly rapid correction of hyponatraemia with these agents. Hypervolaemic patients with hyponatraemia need treatment of the underlying condition, accompanied by cautious use of diuretics in conjunction with strict fluid restriction. Potassium-sparing diuretics may be particularly useful in this context when there is significant secondary hyperaldosteronism.

Hypernatraemia

Hypernatraemia is defined to exist when the serum Na is >145 mmol/L. The causes are summarised in Box 19.13, grouped according to any associated disturbance in total body sodium content.

Pathophysiology

Hypernatraemia occurs due to inadequate concentration of the urine in the face of restricted water intake. This can arise because of failure to generate an adequate medullary concentration gradient in the kidney due to low GFR or loop diuretic therapy, but more commonly is caused by failure of the vasopressin system. This can occur because of pituitary damage (cranial diabetes insipidus) or because the collecting duct cells are

19

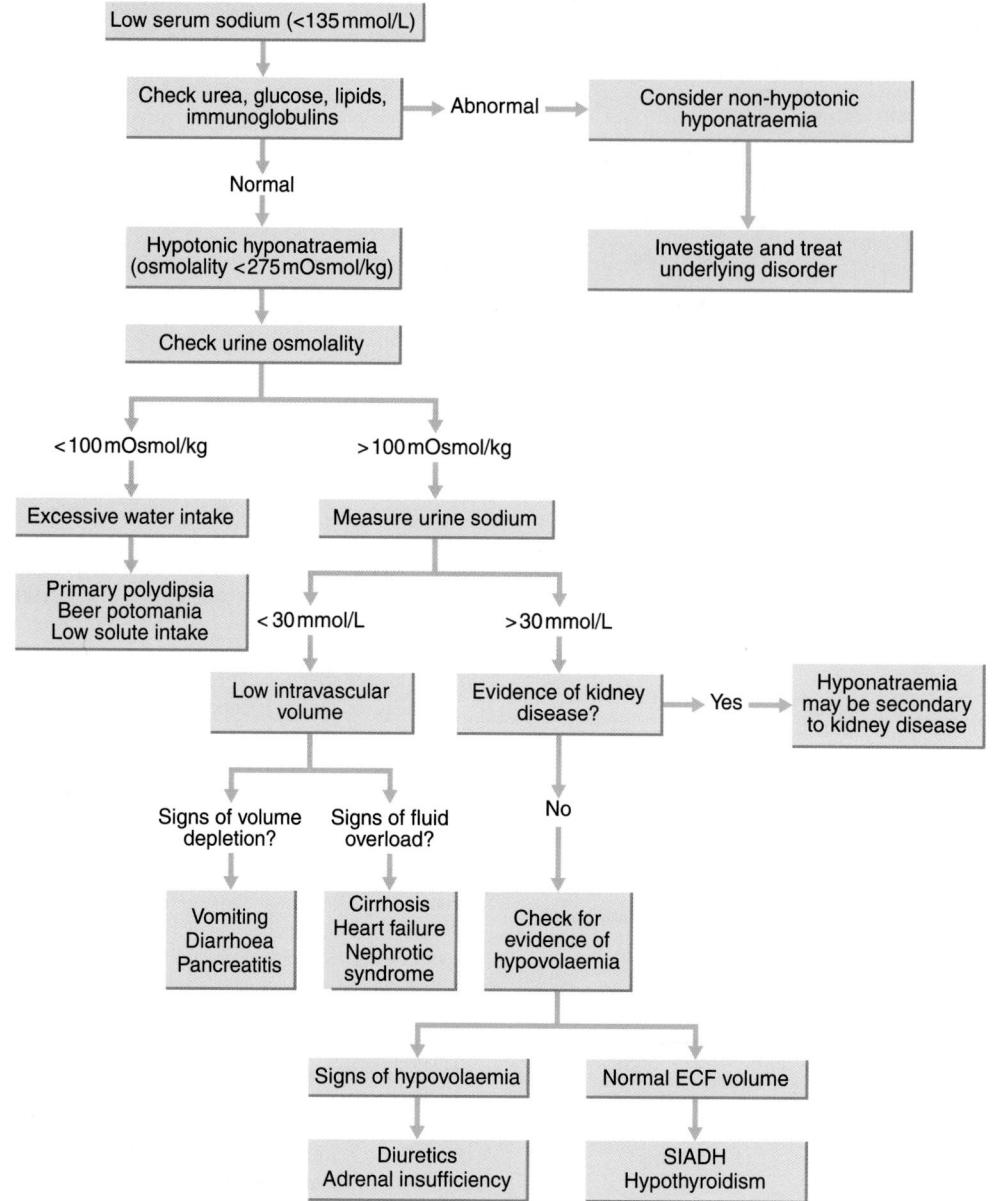

Fig. 19.7 Algorithm for the diagnosis of hyponatraemia. (ECF = extracellular fluid; SIADH = syndrome of inappropriate antidiuretic hormone (vasopressin) secretion)

i	19.13 Causes of hypernatraemia	
Volume status	**Examples**	

Hypovolaemic	Renal sodium losses:
	   Diuretic therapy (especially osmotic diuretic, or
	   loop diuretic during water restriction)
	   Glycosuria (hyperglycaemic hyperosmolar state)
	 Gastrointestinal sodium losses:
	   Colonic diarrhoea
	 Skin sodium losses:
	   Excessive sweating	

Euvolaemic	Diabetes insipidus (central or nephrogenic)	
Hypervolaemic	Enteral or parenteral feeding Intravenous or oral salt administration Chronic kidney disease (during water restriction)	

Clinical features

Patients with hypernatraemia generally have reduced cerebral function, either as a primary problem or as a consequence of the hypernatraemia itself, which results in dehydration of neurons and brain shrinkage. In the presence of an intact thirst mechanism and preserved capacity to obtain and ingest water, hypernatraemia may not progress very far. If adequate water is not obtained, dizziness, delirium, weakness and, ultimately, coma and death can result.

As outlined above, copeptin can be used in the diagnosis of water regulation disorders as a surrogate marker of vasopressin release. It is used in this regard to distinguish between central and nephrogenic diabetes insipidus.

Management

Treatment of hypernatraemia depends on both the rate of development and the underlying cause. If there is reason to think that the condition has developed rapidly, neuronal shrinkage may be acute and relatively rapid correction may be attempted. This can be achieved by infusing an appropriate volume of intravenous fluid (isotonic 5% dextrose or hypotonic 0.45% saline) at an initial rate of 50–70 mL/hr. In older, institutionalised patients, however, it is more likely that the disorder has developed slowly, and extreme caution should be exercised in lowering plasma sodium to

unable to respond to circulating vasopressin concentrations in the face of restricted water intake (nephrogenic diabetes insipidus). Whatever the underlying cause, sustained or severe hypernatraemia generally reflects an impaired thirst mechanism or responsiveness to thirst.

19.14 Hyponatraemia and hypernatraemia in old age

- **Decline in GFR**: older patients are predisposed to both hyponatraemia and hypernatraemia, mainly because, as glomerular filtration rate declines with age, the capacity of the kidney to dilute or concentrate the urine is impaired.
- **Hyponatraemia**: occurs when free water intake continues in the presence of a low dietary salt intake and/or diuretic drugs (particularly thiazides).
- **Vasopressin release**: water retention is aggravated by any condition that stimulates vasopressin release, especially heart failure. Moreover, the vasopressin response to non-osmotic stimuli may be brisker in older subjects. Appropriate water restriction may be a key part of management.
- **Hypernatraemia**: occurs when water intake is inadequate, due to physical restrictions preventing access to drinks and/or blunted thirst. Both are frequently present in patients with advanced dementia or following a severe stroke.
- **Dietary salt**: hypernatraemia is aggravated if dietary supplements or medications with a high sodium content (especially effervescent preparations) are administered. Appropriate prescription of fluids is a key part of management.

avoid the risk of cerebral oedema. Where possible, the underlying cause should also be addressed (see Box 19.13).

Older adult patients are predisposed, in different circumstances, to both hyponatraemia and hypernatraemia, and a high index of suspicion of these electrolyte disturbances is appropriate in older patients with recent alterations in behaviour (Box 19.14).

Potassium homeostasis

Potassium is the major intracellular cation (see Fig. 19.1), and the steep concentration gradient for potassium across the cell membrane of excitable cells plays an important part in generating the resting membrane potential and allowing the propagation of the action potential that is crucial to normal functioning of nerve, muscle and cardiac tissues. Control of body potassium balance is described below.

Functional anatomy and physiology

The kidneys normally excrete some 90% of the daily intake of potassium, typically 80–100 mmol/24 hrs. Potassium is freely filtered at the glomerulus; around 65% is reabsorbed in the proximal tubule and a further 25% in the thick ascending limb of the loop of Henle. Little potassium is transported in the early distal tubule but a significant secretory flux of potassium into the urine occurs in the late distal tubule and cortical collecting duct to ensure that the amount removed from the blood is proportional to the ingested load.

The mechanism for potassium secretion in the distal parts of the nephron is shown in panel (D) of Figure 19.2. Movement of potassium from blood to lumen is dependent on active uptake across the basal cell membrane by the Na,K-ATPase, followed by diffusion of potassium through the ROMK channel into the tubular fluid. The electrochemical gradient for potassium movement into the lumen is contributed to both by the high intracellular potassium concentration and by the negative luminal potential difference relative to the blood.

A number of factors influence the rate of potassium secretion. Luminal influences include the rate of sodium delivery and fluid flow through the late distal tubule and cortical collecting ducts. This is a major factor responsible for the increased potassium loss that accompanies diuretic treatment. Agents interfering with the generation of the negative luminal potential also impair potassium secretion, and this is the basis of reduced potassium secretion associated with potassium-sparing diuretics such as amiloride. Factors acting on the blood side of this tubular segment include plasma potassium and pH, such that hyperkalaemia and alkalosis both enhance potassium secretion directly. However, the most important factor in the acute and chronic adjustment of potassium secretion to match metabolic potassium load is aldosterone.

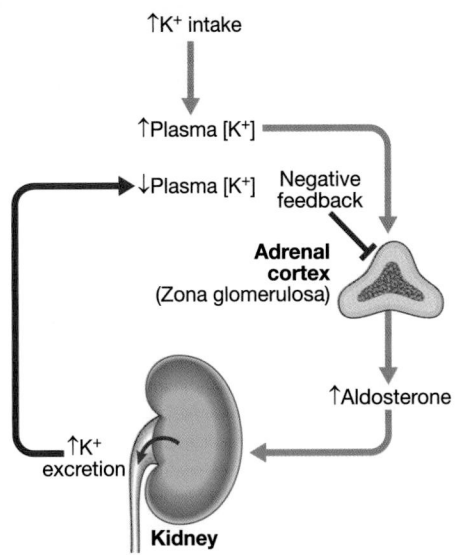

Fig. 19.8 Feedback control of plasma potassium concentration.

As shown in Figure 19.8, a negative feedback relationship exists between the plasma potassium concentration and aldosterone. In addition to its regulation by the renin–angiotensin system (see Fig. 20.19), aldosterone is released from the adrenal cortex in direct response to an elevated plasma potassium. Aldosterone then acts on the kidney to enhance potassium secretion, hydrogen secretion and sodium reabsorption, in the late distal tubule and cortical collecting ducts. The resulting increase in excretion of potassium maintains plasma potassium within a narrow range (3.5–5.0 mmol/L). Factors that reduce angiotensin II levels may indirectly affect potassium balance by blunting the rise in aldosterone that would otherwise be provoked by hyperkalaemia. This accounts for the increased risk of hyperkalaemia during therapy with ACE inhibitors and related drugs.

Presenting problems in potassium homeostasis

Changes in the distribution of potassium between the ICF and ECF compartments can alter plasma potassium concentration, without any overall change in total body potassium content. Potassium is driven into the cells by extracellular alkalosis and by a number of hormones, including insulin, catecholamines (through the β_2-receptor) and aldosterone. Any of these factors can produce hypokalaemia, whereas extracellular acidosis, lack of insulin and insufficiency or blockade of catecholamines or aldosterone can cause hyperkalaemia due to efflux of potassium from the intracellular compartment.

Hypokalaemia

Hypokalaemia is a common electrolyte disturbance and is defined as existing when serum K^+ falls below 3.5 mmol/L. The main causes of hypokalaemia are shown in Box 19.15.

Pathophysiology

Hypokalaemia is generally indicative of abnormal potassium loss from the body, through either the kidney or the gastrointestinal tract. Renal causes of hypokalaemia can be divided into those with and those without hypertension. Hypokalaemia in the presence of hypertension may be due to increased aldosterone secretion in Conn syndrome or a genetic defect affecting sodium channels in the distal nephron (Liddle syndrome). Excessive intake of liquorice or treatment with carbenoxolone may result in a similar clinical picture, due to inhibition of the renal 11βHSD2 enzyme, which inactivates cortisol in peripheral tissues.

If blood pressure is normal or low, hypokalaemia can be classified according to the associated change in acid–base balance. Inherited

19

628 • CLINICAL BIOCHEMISTRY AND METABOLIC MEDICINE

19.15 Causes of hypokalaemia

Cause	Other features and comment
Reduced intake Dietary deficiency Potassium-free intravenous fluids	Urine K+ <20–30 mmol/24 hrs
Redistribution into cells Alkalosis Insulin Catecholamines β-adrenergic agonists Hypokalaemic periodic paralysis	Caused by flux of K+ into cells
Increased urinary excretion Activation of mineralocorticoid receptor: Conn syndrome Cushing's syndrome Glucocorticoid excess Carbenoxolone/liquorice	Urine K+ > 20–30 mmol/24 hrs Associated with hypertension with alkalosis
Genetic disorders: Liddle syndrome	Associated with hypertension with alkalosis
Bartter syndrome Gitelman syndrome	Associated with alkalosis and hypomagnesaemia
Renal tubular acidosis Type 1 (distal) Type 2 (proximal)	Inherited and acquired forms; associated with high serum chloride. Type 2 associated with glycosuria, aminoaciduria and phosphaturia
Acetazolamide	Associated with acidosis
Diuresis: Loop diuretics Thiazides Recovery from acute tubular necrosis Recovery from renal obstruction	Increased sodium delivery to distal tubule
Increased gastrointestinal loss Upper gastrointestinal tract: Vomiting Nasogastric aspiration	Urine K+ <20–30 mmol/L Loss of gastric acid Associated with metabolic alkalosis
Lower gastrointestinal tract: Diarrhoea Laxative abuse Villous adenoma Bowel obstruction/fistula Ureterosigmoidostomy	Associated with metabolic acidosis

defects in tubular transport should be suspected when hypokalaemia occurs in association with hypotension and alkalosis, provided that diuretic use has been excluded. One such disease is Bartter syndrome, in which sodium reabsorption in the thick ascending limb of Henle is defective, usually due to a loss-of-function variant of the NKCC2 transporter. The clinical and biochemical features are similar to those in chronic treatment with furosemide. In Gitelman syndrome there is a loss-of-function variant affecting the NCCT transporter in the early distal tubule. The clinical and biochemical features are similar to chronic thiazide treatment. Note that while both Bartter and Gitelman syndromes are characterised by hypokalaemia and hypomagnesaemia, urinary calcium excretion is increased in Bartter syndrome but decreased in Gitelman syndrome, analogous to the effects of the loop and thiazide diuretics, respectively, on calcium transport (see Box 19.9).

If hypokalaemia occurs in the presence of a normal blood pressure and metabolic acidosis, renal tubular acidosis (proximal or 'classical' distal) should be suspected.

When hypokalaemia is due to potassium wasting through the gastrointestinal tract, the cause is usually obvious clinically. In some cases, when there is occult induction of vomiting, hypokalaemia is characteristically associated with metabolic alkalosis, due to loss of gastric acid. If, however, potassium loss has occurred through the surreptitious use of aperients, the hypokalaemia is generally associated with metabolic acidosis. In both cases, urinary potassium excretion is low unless there is significant extracellular volume depletion, which can raise urinary potassium levels by stimulating aldosterone production.

Hypokalaemia can also be caused by redistribution of potassium into cells as outlined above or as the result of K+ flux into muscle in hypokalaemic periodic paralysis, which is associated with variants in several genes that regulate transmembrane ion flow into muscle cells. Finally, reduced dietary intake of potassium can contribute to hypokalaemia but is seldom the only cause, except in extreme cases.

Clinical features

Patients with mild hypokalaemia (plasma K+ 3.0–3.5 mmol/L) are generally asymptomatic, but more profound reductions in plasma potassium often lead to muscular weakness and associated tiredness. Ventricular ectopic beats or more serious arrhythmias may occur and the arrhythmogenic effects of digoxin may be potentiated. Typical electrocardiogram (ECG) changes occur, affecting the T wave in particular. Functional bowel obstruction may occur due to paralytic ileus. Long-standing hypokalaemia may cause renal tubular damage (hypokalaemic nephropathy) and can interfere with the tubular response to vasopressin (acquired nephrogenic diabetes insipidus), resulting in polyuria and polydipsia.

Investigations

Measurement of plasma electrolytes, bicarbonate, urine potassium and sometimes of plasma calcium and magnesium is usually sufficient to establish the diagnosis. If the diagnosis remains unclear, plasma renin should be measured. Levels are low in patients with primary hyperaldosteronism and other forms of mineralocorticoid excess, but raised in other causes of hypokalaemia. Measurement of urinary potassium may also be helpful; if the kidney is the route of potassium loss, the urine potassium is high (>30 mmol/24 hrs), whereas if potassium is being lost through the gastrointestinal tract, the kidney retains potassium, resulting in a lower urinary potassium (generally <20 mmol/24 hrs). It should be noted, however, that if gastrointestinal fluid loss is also associated with hypovolaemia, activation of the renin–angiotensin–aldosterone system may occur, causing increased loss of potassium in the urine.

The cause of hypokalaemia may remain unclear despite the above investigations when urinary potassium measurements are inconclusive and the history is incomplete or unreliable. Many such cases are associated with metabolic alkalosis, and in this setting the measurement of urine chloride concentration can be helpful. A low urine chloride (<30 mmol/L) is characteristic of vomiting (spontaneous or self-induced, in which chloride is lost in HCl in the vomit), while a urine chloride >40 mmol/L suggests diuretic therapy (acute phase) or a tubular disorder such as Bartter or Gitelman syndromes. Differentiation between occult diuretic use and primary tubular disorders can be achieved by performing a screen of urine for diuretic drugs.

Management

Treatment of hypokalaemia involves first determining the cause and correcting this where possible. If the problem is mainly one of redistribution of potassium into cells, reversal of the process responsible may be sufficient to restore plasma potassium without providing supplements. In most cases, however, some form of potassium replacement will be required. This can generally be achieved with slow-release potassium chloride tablets, but in more acute circumstances intravenous potassium chloride may be necessary. The rate of administration depends on the severity of hypokalaemia and the presence of cardiac or neuromuscular complications, but should generally not exceed 10 mmol of potassium per hour. In patients with severe, life-threatening hypokalaemia, infusion rates of up to 20 mmol/hr can be used with continuous cardiac monitoring.

In the less common situation where hypokalaemia occurs in the presence of metabolic acidosis, alkaline salts of potassium, such as potassium bicarbonate, can be given by mouth. If magnesium depletion is also present, replacement of magnesium may also be required, since low cellular magnesium can promote tubular potassium secretion, causing ongoing urinary losses. In some circumstances, potassium-sparing diuretics, such as amiloride, can assist in the correction of hypokalaemia, hypomagnesaemia and metabolic alkalosis, especially when renal loss of potassium is the underlying cause.

Hyperkalaemia

Hyperkalaemia is a common electrolyte disorder, which is defined as existing when serum K^+ is >5 mmol/L. The causes of hyperkalaemia are summarised in Box 19.16.

Pathophysiology

It is important to remember that hyperkalaemia can be artefactual due to haemolysis of blood specimens during collection or in vitro, or due to release of potassium from platelets in patients with thrombocytosis.

True hyperkalaemia, however, can occur either because of redistribution of potassium between the ICF and ECF, or because potassium intake exceeds excretion. Redistribution of potassium from the ICF to the ECF may take place in the presence of systemic acidosis, or when the circulating levels of insulin, catecholamines and aldosterone are reduced, or when the effects of these hormones are blocked.

High dietary potassium intake may contribute to hyperkalaemia, but is seldom the only explanation unless renal excretion mechanisms are impaired. The mechanism of hyperkalaemia in acute kidney injury and chronic kidney disease is impaired excretion of potassium into the urine as the result of a reduced GFR. In addition, acute kidney injury can be associated with severe hyperkalaemia when there is an increased potassium load, such as in rhabdomyolysis or in sepsis, particularly when acidosis is present. In chronic kidney disease, adaptation to moderately elevated plasma potassium levels commonly occurs. However, acute rises in potassium triggered by excessive dietary intake, hypovolaemia or drugs (see below) may occur and destabilise the situation.

Hyperkalaemia can also develop when tubular potassium secretory processes are impaired, even if the GFR is normal. This can arise in association with low levels of aldosterone, as is found in Addison's disease, hyporeninaemic hypoaldosteronism or inherited disorders such as congenital isolated hypoaldosteronism, in which there is a defect in aldosterone biosynthesis, and pseudohypoaldosteronism type 2 (Gordon syndrome), caused by variants in the *WNK2* and *WNK4* genes, which causes decreased potassium secretion in the renal tubules.

Drug-induced causes include ACE inhibitors, angiotensin-receptor blockers (ARBs), non-steroidal anti-inflammatory drugs (NSAIDs) and β-adrenoceptor antagonists (β-blockers). In aldosterone deficiency or aldosterone resistance, hyperkalaemia may be associated with acid retention, giving rise to the pattern of hyperkalaemic distal ('type 4') renal tubular acidosis.

In another group of conditions, tubular potassium secretion is impaired as the result of aldosterone resistance. This can occur in a variety of diseases in which there is inflammation of the tubulointerstitium, such as systemic lupus erythematosus; following renal transplantation; during treatment with potassium-sparing diuretics; and in a number of inherited disorders of tubular transport.

Clinical features

Mild to moderate hyperkalaemia (<6.5 mmol/L) is usually asymptomatic. More severe hyperkalaemia can present with progressive muscular weakness, but sometimes there are no symptoms until cardiac arrest

i	19.16 Causes of hyperkalaemia	
Cause		**Other features and comment**
Artefactual		
Haemolysis during venepuncture		Release of intracellular K^+ during sample collection, transit or clotting
Haemolysis in vitro		
Thrombocytosis/leucocytosis		
Increased intake		
Dietary potassium		
Potassium-containing intravenous fluids		
Redistribution from cells		
Acidosis		
Insulin deficiency		
Severe hyperglycaemia		
β-blockers		Caused by flux of intracellular K^+ into plasma
Hyperkalaemic periodic paralysis		
Rhabdomyolysis		
Severe haemolysis		
Tumour lysis syndrome		
Reduced urinary excretion		
Reduced glomerular filtration:		
Acute kidney injury		Plasma creatinine typically >500 μmol/L (5.67 mg/dL)
Chronic kidney disease		
Reduced mineralocorticoid receptor activation:		
Addison's disease		
Congenital adrenal hyperplasia		
Isolated aldosterone deficiency		
ACE inhibitors		Both reduce aldosterone levels
Angiotensin-receptor blockers		
Calcineurin inhibitors		All block the mineralocorticoid receptor
Spironolactone		
Eplerenone		
Heparin		Inhibits aldosterone production
Inhibitors of renin production:		
Non-steroidal anti-inflammatory drugs		
β-blockers		
Tubulointerstitial disease:		
Interstitial nephritis		
Diabetic nephropathy		
Obstructive uropathy		
Other:		
Amiloride		Blocks K^+ exchange in distal tubule
Gordon syndrome		Direct effect on K^+ transport in renal tubule

19

occurs. The typical ECG changes are shown on page 615. Peaking of the T wave is an early ECG sign but widening of the QRS complex presages a dangerous cardiac arrhythmia. However, these characteristic ECG findings are not always present, even in severe hyperkalaemia.

Investigations

Measurement of electrolytes, creatinine and bicarbonate, when combined with clinical assessment, usually provides the explanation for hyperkalaemia. In aldosterone deficiency, plasma sodium concentration is characteristically low, although this can occur with many causes of hyperkalaemia. Addison's disease should be excluded unless there is an obvious alternative diagnosis

Management

Treatment of hyperkalaemia depends on its severity and the rate of development, but opinions vary as to what level of serum potassium constitutes severe hyperkalaemia and requires urgent treatment.

19.17 Treatment of severe hyperkalaemia

Objective	Therapy
Stabilise cell membrane potential[1]	IV calcium gluconate (10 mL of 10% solution)
Shift K⁺ into cells	Inhaled β_2-adrenoceptor agonist IV glucose (50 mL of 50% solution) and 5–10 IU rapidly acting insulin IV sodium bicarbonate[2]
Remove K⁺ from body	IV furosemide and normal saline[3] Ion-exchange resin orally or rectally Dialysis

[1]If severe hyperkalaemia (K⁺ typically > 6.5 mmol/L). [2]If acidosis present. [3]If adequate residual renal function.
(IV = intravenous)

Patients who have potassium concentrations <6.5 mmol/L in the absence of neuromuscular symptoms or ECG changes can be treated with a reduction of potassium intake and correction of predisposing factors. However, in acute and/or severe hyperkalaemia (plasma potassium >6.5–7.0 mmol/L), more urgent measures must be taken (Box 19.17). The first step should be infusion of 10 mL 10% calcium gluconate to stabilise conductive tissue membranes (calcium has the opposite effect to potassium on conduction of an action potential). Measures to shift potassium from the ECF to the ICF should also be applied, as they generally have a rapid effect and may avert arrhythmias. Ultimately, a means of removing potassium from the body is generally necessary. When renal function is reasonably preserved, loop diuretics (accompanied by intravenous saline if hypovolaemia is present) may be effective. In renal failure, dialysis may be required. Ion exchange resins, such as calcium resonium (which can be given orally or rectally) and oral sodium polystyrene sulfonate (SPS), have traditionally been used to bind and excrete gastrointestinal potassium. There are concerns, however, with regard to SPS's lack of proven efficacy and safety, with a number of reports of intestinal necrosis associated with its use. Newer cation exchange resins, which include sodium zirconium cyclosilicate and patiromer sorbitex calcium, have been developed. These are safe and effective treatments for hyperkalaemia and are preferred to SPS. However, they are not yet available in all countries for this indication.

Acid–base homeostasis

The pH of arterial plasma is normally 7.40, corresponding to an H⁺ concentration of 40 nmol/L, and under normal circumstances H⁺ concentrations do not vary outside the range of 37–45 nmol/L (pH 7.35–7.43). Abnormalities of acid–base balance can occur in a wide range of diseases. Increases in H⁺ concentration cause acidosis with a decrease in pH, whereas decreases in H⁺ concentration cause alkalosis with a rise in pH.

Functional anatomy and physiology

A variety of physiological mechanisms maintain pH of the ECF within narrow limits. The first is the action of blood and tissue buffers, of which the most important involves reaction of H⁺ ions with bicarbonate to form carbonic acid, which, under the influence of the enzyme carbonic anhydrase (CA), dissociates to form CO_2 and water:

$$CO_2 + H_2O \underset{CA}{\leftrightarrow} H_2CO_3 \rightleftharpoons H^+ + HCO_3^-$$

This buffer system is important because bicarbonate is present at a relatively high concentration in ECF (21–29 mmol/L), and two of its key components are under physiological control: CO_2 by the lungs, and bicarbonate by the kidneys. These relationships are illustrated in Figure 19.9 (a form of the Henderson–Hasselbalch equation).

Respiratory compensation for acid–base disturbances can occur quickly. In response to acid accumulation, pH changes in the brainstem stimulate ventilatory drive which reduces PCO_2 and subsequently increases pH. Conversely, systemic alkalosis leads to inhibition of ventilation, causing a rise in PCO_2 and reduction in pH, although it should be noted that this mechanism has limited capacity to change pH because hypoxia provides an alternative stimulus to drive ventilation.

The kidneys provide a third line of defence against disturbances of arterial pH. When acid accumulates due to chronic respiratory or metabolic (non-renal) causes, the kidneys have the capacity to enhance urinary excretion of acid, effectively increasing the plasma bicarbonate.

Renal control of acid–base balance

Regulation of acid–base balance occurs at several sites in the kidney. The proximal tubule reabsorbs about 85% of the filtered bicarbonate ions, through the mechanism illustrated in panel (A) in Figure 19.2. This is dependent on the enzyme carbonic anhydrase, which is present both in the cytoplasm of the proximal tubular cells and on the luminal surface of the brush border membranes. The system has a high capacity for reabsorption of filtered bicarbonate but does not lead to significant acidification of the luminal fluid.

Distal nephron segments also have an important role in bicarbonate reabsorption and acid excretion. Dissociation of H_2CO_3 occurs in the distal tubular cells, under the influence of carbonic anhydrase generating H⁺ ions and HCO_3^- ions. The H⁺ ions are secreted to the lumen by an H⁺-ATPase in the alpha intercalated cells of the cortical collecting duct and the outer medullary collecting duct cells and the HCO_3 passes across the basolateral membrane into the blood. Within the tubular lumen, H⁺ combines with hydrogen phosphate (HPO_4^{2-}) in the distal tubular lumen to form dihydrogen phosphate ($H_2PO_4^-$), which is excreted in the urine with sodium. Similarly, H⁺ combines with NH_3 in the luminal fluid to form ammonium (NH_4^+) ions, which are trapped and excreted in the urine combined with chloride ions. The NH_3 necessary for this reaction is generated in tubular cells by the enzyme glutaminase which acts on the amino acid glutamine. Both of these buffers help to prevent the urinary pH falling below 5, which would create an unfavourable gradient that would stop further secretion of H⁺ ions into the urine.

Titratable acid and ammonium excretion removes approximately 1 mmol/kg of hydrogen ions from the body per day, which equates to the non-volatile acid load arising from the metabolism of dietary protein. The slightly alkaline plasma pH of 7.4 (H⁺ 40 nmol/L) that is maintained

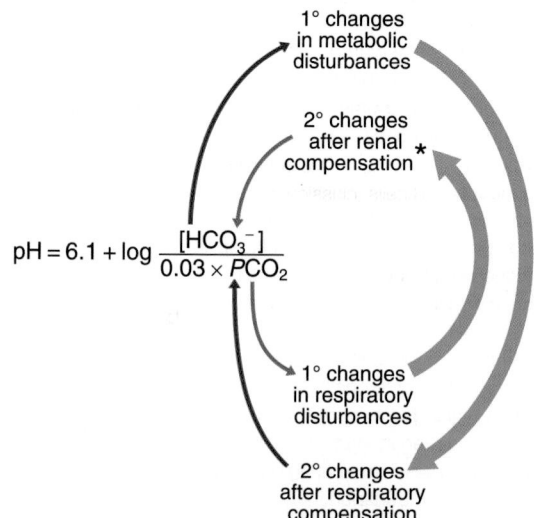

$$pH = 6.1 + \log \frac{[HCO_3^-]}{0.03 \times PCO_2}$$

Fig. 19.9 Relationship between pH, PCO_2 (in mmHg) and plasma bicarbonate concentration (in mmol/L).*Note that changes in HCO_3^- concentration are also part of the renal correction for sustained metabolic acid–base disturbances as long as the kidney itself is not the cause of the primary disturbance.

during health can be accounted for by the kidney's ability to generate an acidic urine (typically pH 5–6 (H^+ 1000–10 000 nmol/L), in which the net daily excess of metabolic acid produced by the body can be excreted.

Presenting problems in acid–base balance

Patients with disturbances of acid–base balance may present clinically either with the effects of tissue malfunction due to disturbed pH (such as altered cardiac and central nervous system function), or with secondary changes in respiration that occur as a response to the underlying metabolic change (such as Kussmaul respiration during metabolic acidosis). The clinical picture is often dominated by the underlying cause rather than the acid–base abnormality itself. Frequently, acid–base disturbances only become evident when the venous plasma bicarbonate concentration is measured and found to be abnormal, or when blood gas analysis shows abnormalities in pH, PCO_2 or bicarbonate.

The most common patterns of abnormality in blood gas parameters are shown in Box 19.18. Interpretation of arterial blood gases in respiratory failure is described in Box 17.16.

In metabolic disturbances, respiratory compensation is almost immediate, so that the predicted compensatory change in PCO_2 is achieved soon after the onset of the metabolic disturbance. In respiratory disorders, on the other hand, a small initial change in bicarbonate occurs as a result of chemical buffering of CO_2, chiefly within red blood cells, but over days and weeks the kidney achieves further compensatory changes in bicarbonate concentration as a result of chronic adjustments in acid secretory capacity. When the clinically obtained acid–base parameters do not accord with the predicted compensation shown, a mixed acid–base disturbance should be suspected.

Metabolic acidosis

Metabolic acidosis occurs when an acid other than carbonic acid (due to CO_2 retention) accumulates in the body, resulting in a fall in the plasma bicarbonate. The causes of metabolic acidosis are summarised in Box 19.19, subdivided into two categories, depending on whether the anion gap is normal or raised. When plasma bicarbonate falls, another anion needs to take its place. This is either chloride (normal anion gap) or an unmeasured anion (raised anion gap). The causes are discussed in more detail below.

Pathophysiology

Metabolic acidosis with a normal anion gap occurs when there is poisoning with or therapeutic infusion of a chloride-containing acid such as hydrochloric acid or ammonium chloride or when there is a primary loss of bicarbonate from the ECF (via the GI tract or from the kidneys). Renal tubular acidosis (RTA) can be caused by a defect in one of three processes:

- impaired bicarbonate reabsorption in the proximal tubule (proximal RTA)
- impaired acid secretion in the late distal tubule or cortical collecting duct intercalated cells (classical distal RTA)

- impaired sodium reabsorption in the late distal tubule or cortical collecting duct, which is associated with reduced secretion of both potassium and H^+ ions (hyperkalaemic distal RTA).

Various subtypes of RTA are recognised and the most common causes are shown in Box 19.20. The inherited forms of RTA are due to variants in the genes that regulate acid or bicarbonate transport in the renal tubules (see Fig. 19.2).

Acidosis with an increased anion gap is most commonly seen in ketoacidosis, lactic acidosis and late kidney failure, where there is endogenous production of anions distinct from Cl^- and HCO_3^-. Ketoacidosis is caused by insulin deficiency and is exacerbated by catecholamine and stress hormone excess, which combine to cause lipolysis and the formation of acidic ketones (acetoacetate, 3-hydroxybutyrate and acetone). The most common cause of ketoacidosis is diabetic ketoacidosis (DKA); its aetiology and management are discussed in Chapter 21. Starvation ketoacidosis occurs when there is reduced food intake in situations of high glucose demand, such as in neonates, and in pregnant or breast-feeding women. In alcoholic ketoacidosis, there is usually a background of chronic malnutrition and a recent alcohol binge. Two subtypes of lactic acidosis have been defined:

19.19 Causes of metabolic acidosis

Disorder	Mechanism
Normal anion gap	
Ingestion or infusion of inorganic acid	Therapeutic infusion of or poisoning with NH_4Cl, HCl
Gastrointestinal HCO_3^- loss	Loss of HCO_3^- in diarrhoea, small bowel fistula, urinary diversion procedure
Renal tubular acidosis (RTA)	Urinary loss of HCO_3^- in proximal RTA; impaired tubular acid secretion in distal RTA
Increased anion gap	
Endogenous acid load	
Diabetic ketoacidosis	Accumulation of ketones[1] with hyperglycaemia
Starvation ketosis	Accumulation of ketones without hyperglycaemia
Alcoholic ketoacidosis	
Lactic acidosis	Shock, liver disease, drugs
Kidney disease	Accumulation of organic acids
Exogenous acid load	
Aspirin poisoning	Accumulation of salicylate[2]
Methanol poisoning	Accumulation of formate
Ethylene glycol poisoning	Accumulation of glycolate, oxalate

[1]Ketones include acid anions acetoacetate and β-hydroxybutyrate. [2]Salicylate poisoning is also associated with respiratory alkalosis due to direct ventilatory stimulation.

19.18 Principal patterns of acid–base disturbance

Disturbance	Blood H^+	Primary change	Compensatory response	Predicted compensation
Metabolic acidosis	>40[1]	HCO_3^- <24 mmol/L	PCO_2 <5.33 kPa[2]	PCO_2 fall in kPa = 0.16 × HCO_3^- fall in mmol/L
Metabolic alkalosis	<40[1]	HCO_3^- >24 mmol/L	PCO_2 >5.33 kPa[2,3]	PCO_2 rise in kPa = 0.08 × HCO_3^- rise in mmol/L
Respiratory acidosis	>40[1]	PCO_2 >5.33 kPa[2]	HCO_3^- >24 mmol/L	Acute: HCO_3^- rise in mmol/L = 0.75 × PCO_2 rise in kPa Chronic: HCO_3^- rise in mmol/L = 2.62 × PCO_2 rise in kPa
Respiratory alkalosis	<40[1]	PCO_2 <5.33 kPa[2]	HCO_3^- <24 mmol/L	Acute: HCO_3^- fall in mmol/L = 1.50 × PCO_2 fall in kPa Chronic: HCO_3^- fall in mmol/L = 3.75 × PCO_2 fall in kPa

[1]H^+ of 40 nmol/L = pH of 7.40. [2]PCO_2 of 5.33 kPa = 40 mmHg. [3]PCO_2 does not rise above 7.33 kPa (55 mmHg) because hypoxia then intervenes to drive respiration.

19.20 Causes of renal tubular acidosis

Proximal renal tubular acidosis (type II RTA)

- Inherited:
  Fanconi syndrome
  Cystinosis
  Wilson's disease
- Paraproteinaemia:
  Myeloma
  Amyloidosis

- Heavy metal toxicity:
  Lead, cadmium and mercury
  poisoning
- Drugs:
  Carbonic anhydrase inhibitors
  Ifosfamide
- Primary hyperparathyroidism

Classical distal renal tubular acidosis (type I RTA)

- Inherited
- Autoimmune diseases:
  Systemic lupus
  erythematosus
  Sjögren syndrome

- Hyperglobulinaemia
- Primary hyperparathyroidism
- Toxins and drugs:
  Toluene
  Lithium
  Amphotericin

Hyperkalaemic distal renal tubular acidosis (type IV RTA)

- Hypoaldosteronism (primary or
  secondary)
- Obstructive nephropathy
- Renal transplant rejection

- Drugs:
  Amiloride
  Spironolactone

- *type I*, due to tissue hypoxia and peripheral generation of lactate, as in patients with circulatory failure and shock
- *type II*, due to impaired metabolism of lactate, as in liver disease or by a number of drugs and toxins, including metformin, which inhibit lactate metabolism.
  Metabolic acidosis with an increased anion gap may also be a consequence of exogenous acid loads from poisoning with aspirin, methanol or ethylene glycol. Typically, metabolic acidosis in chronic kidney disease is associated wth a normal anion gap until late in the disease process when the gap widens due to the lack of excretion of anions such as phosphate, sulphate and urate.

Clinical features

Normal anion gap metabolic acidosis is usually due either to bicarbonate loss in diarrhoea, where the clinical diagnosis is generally obvious, or to RTA. Although some forms of RTA are inherited, it may also be an acquired disorder, and in these circumstances the discovery of metabolic acidosis may serve as an early clue to the underlying diagnosis. The presentation of increased anion gap acidosis is usually dominated by clinical features of the underlying disease, such as uncontrolled diabetes mellitus, kidney failure or shock, or may be suggested by the clinical history of starvation, alcoholism or associated symptoms, such as visual complaints in methanol poisoning.

Investigations

The different types of metabolic acidosis can be distinguished by blood gas measurements, along with measurements of creatinine, electrolytes and bicarbonate. Under normal circumstances, the anion gap, defined as the numerical difference between the main measured cations (Na^+ + K^+) and the anions (Cl^- + HCO_3^-) is about 5–11 mmol/L. This gap is normally made up of various unmeasured anions, such as phosphate and sulphate, as well as albumin. RTA should be suspected when there is a hyperchloraemic acidosis with a normal anion gap in the absence of gastrointestinal disturbance. The diagnosis can be confirmed by finding an inappropriately high urine pH (>5.5) in the presence of systemic acidosis. Sometimes, distal RTA may be incomplete, such that the plasma bicarbonate concentration may be normal. In this case, an acid challenge test can be performed by administration of an acid load in the form of ammonium chloride to reduce plasma bicarbonate. The diagnosis of incomplete distal RTA can be confirmed if the urine pH fails to fall below 5.3 in the presence of a low bicarbonate.

The different subtypes of RTA can be differentiated by various biochemical features. Patients with proximal and distal RTA often present with features of profound hypokalaemia, while type IV RTA is associated with hyperkalaemia. Proximal RTA is frequently associated with urinary wasting of amino acids, phosphate and glucose (Fanconi syndrome), as well as bicarbonate and potassium. Patients with this disorder can lower the urine pH when the acidosis is severe and plasma bicarbonate levels have fallen below 16 mmol/L, since distal H^+ secretion mechanisms are intact. In the classical form of distal RTA, however, acid accumulation is relentless and progressive, resulting in mobilisation of calcium from bone and osteomalacia with hypercalciuria, renal stone formation and nephrocalcinosis. Potassium is also lost in classical distal RTA, while it is retained in hyperkalaemic distal RTA.

Investigations in patients with raised anion gap metabolic acidosis show features of the underlying cause, such as reduced GFR in kidney failure and raised urine or blood ketones in ketoacidosis. In DKA, blood glucose is raised, while in starvation and alcoholic acidosis blood glucose is not elevated and may be low. Measurement of plasma lactate is helpful in the diagnosis of lactic acidosis when values are increased over the normal maximal level of 2 mmol/L.

Management

The first step in management of metabolic acidosis is to identify and correct the underlying cause when possible (see Box 19.19). This may involve controlling diarrhoea, treating diabetes mellitus, correcting shock, stopping drugs that might cause the condition, or using dialysis to remove toxins. Since metabolic acidosis is frequently associated with sodium and water depletion, resuscitation with intravenous fluids is often needed. In alcoholism and starvation ketosis, intravenous glucose is indicated. By stimulating endogenous insulin secretion, this will reverse hepatic ketone production. Malnourished patients may also require thiamin, potassium, magnesium and phosphate supplements. Use of intravenous bicarbonate in metabolic acidosis is controversial. Because rapid correction of acidosis can induce hypokalaemia or a fall in plasma ionised calcium, the use of bicarbonate infusions is best reserved for situations where the underlying disorder cannot be readily corrected and acidosis is severe (H^+ >100 nmol/L, pH < 7.00) or associated with evidence of tissue dysfunction.

The acidosis in RTA can sometimes be controlled by treating the underlying cause (see Box 19.20), but usually supplements of sodium and potassium bicarbonate are also necessary in types I and II RTA to achieve a target plasma bicarbonate level of >18 mmol/L and normokalaemia. In type IV RTA, loop diuretics, thiazides or fludrocortisone (as appropriate to the underlying diagnosis) may be effective in correcting the acidosis and the hyperkalaemia.

Metabolic alkalosis

Metabolic alkalosis is characterised by an increase in the plasma bicarbonate concentration and the plasma pH (see Box 19.18). There is a compensatory rise in PCO_2 due to hypoventilation but this is limited by the need to avoid hypoxia. Classical causes include Conn syndrome, Cushing's syndrome and glucocorticoid therapy. Occasionally, overuse of antacid salts for treatment of dyspepsia produces a similar pattern.

Pathophysiology

Metabolic alkalosis is best classified according to the accompanying changes in ECF volume. Hypovolaemic metabolic alkalosis is the most common pattern. This can be caused by sustained vomiting, in which acid-rich fluid is lost directly from the body, or by treatment with loop diuretics or thiazides. In the case of sustained vomiting, loss of gastric acid is the immediate cause of the alkalosis, but several factors act to sustain or amplify this in the context of volume depletion (Fig. 19.10). Loss of sodium and fluid leads to hypovolaemia and secondary hyperaldosteronism, triggering proximal sodium bicarbonate reabsorption and additional acid secretion by the distal tubule. Hypokalaemia occurs due to potassium loss in the vomitus and by the kidney as the result of secondary hyperaldosteronism, and itself is a stimulus to acid secretion. Additionally, the compensatory rise in PCO_2 further enhances tubular acid secretion. The net result is sustained metabolic alkalosis with an inappropriately acid urine, which cannot be corrected until the deficit in circulating volume has been replaced.

Normovolaemic (or hypervolaemic) metabolic alkalosis occurs when bicarbonate retention and volume expansion occur simultaneously.

Clinical features

Clinically, apart from manifestations of the underlying cause, there may be few symptoms or signs related to alkalosis itself. When the rise in systemic pH is abrupt, however, plasma ionised calcium falls and signs of increased neuromuscular irritability, such as tetany, may develop.

Investigations

The diagnosis can be confirmed by measurement of electrolytes and arterial blood gases.

Management

Metabolic alkalosis with hypovolaemia can be corrected by intravenous infusions of 0.9% saline with potassium supplements. This reverses the secondary hyperaldosteronism and allows the kidney to excrete the excess alkali in the urine. Management of metabolic alkalosis in the absence of hypovolaemia should focus on management of the underlying endocrine cause such as Conn syndrome, Cushing's syndrome or corticosteroid excess.

Respiratory acidosis

Respiratory acidosis occurs when there is accumulation of CO_2 due to type II respiratory failure. This results in a rise in the PCO_2, with a compensatory increase in plasma bicarbonate concentration, particularly when the disorder is of long duration and the kidney has fully developed its capacity for increased acid excretion.

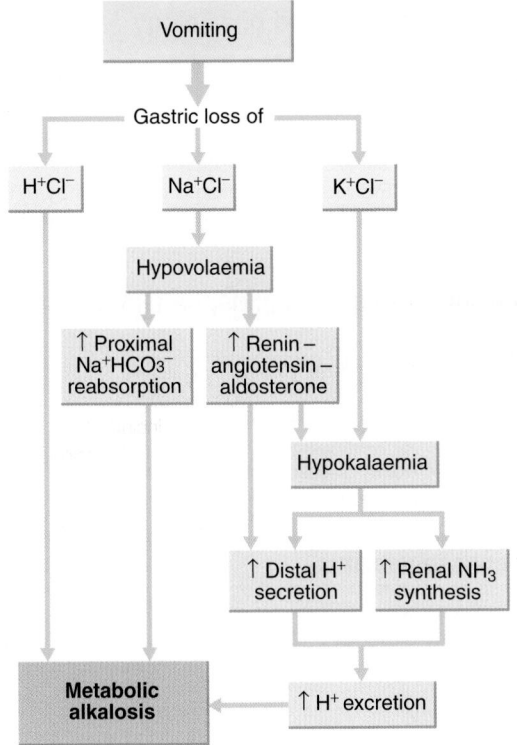

Fig. 19.10 Generation and maintenance of metabolic alkalosis during prolonged vomiting. Loss of H+Cl− generates metabolic alkalosis, which is maintained by renal changes.

This acid–base disturbance can arise from lesions anywhere along the neuromuscular pathways from the brain to the respiratory muscles that result in impaired ventilation. It can also arise during intrinsic lung disease if there is significant mismatching of ventilation and perfusion.

Clinical features are primarily those of the underlying cause of the respiratory disorder, such as paralysis, chest wall injury or chronic obstructive lung disease, but the CO_2 accumulation may itself lead to drowsiness that further depresses respiratory drive.

Management involves correction of causative factors where possible, but ultimately ventilatory support may be necessary.

Respiratory alkalosis

Respiratory alkalosis develops when there is a period of sustained hyperventilation, resulting in a reduction of PCO_2 and increase in plasma pH. If the condition is sustained, renal compensation occurs, such that tubular acid secretion is reduced and the plasma bicarbonate falls.

Respiratory alkalosis is usually of short duration, occurring in anxiety states or as the result of over-vigorous assisted ventilation. It can be prolonged in the context of pregnancy, pulmonary embolism, chronic liver disease and ingestion of certain drugs such as salicylates that directly stimulate the respiratory centre in the brainstem.

Clinical features are those of the underlying cause but agitation associated with perioral and digital tingling may also occur, as alkalosis promotes the binding of calcium to albumin, resulting in a reduction in ionised calcium concentrations. In severe cases, Trousseau's sign and Chvostek's sign may be positive, and tetany or seizures can occur.

Management involves correction of identifiable causes, reduction of anxiety, and a period of rebreathing into a closed bag to allow CO_2 levels to rise.

Mixed acid–base disorders

It is not uncommon for more than one disturbance of acid–base metabolism to be present at the same time in the same patient: for example, a respiratory acidosis due to narcotic overdose with metabolic alkalosis due to vomiting. In these situations, the arterial pH will represent the net effect of all primary and compensatory changes. Indeed, the pH may be normal, but the presence of underlying acid–base disturbances can be gauged from concomitant abnormalities in the PCO_2 and bicarbonate concentration.

In assessing these disorders, all clinical influences on the patient's acid–base status should be identified, and reference should be made to the table of predicted compensation given in Box 19.18. If the compensatory change is discrepant from the rules of thumb provided, more than one disturbance of acid–base metabolism may be suspected.

Calcium homeostasis

Disorders of calcium homeostasis are discussed in Chapter 20 and bone disease is discussed in Chapter 26.

Magnesium homeostasis

Magnesium is mainly an intracellular cation. It is important to the function of many enzymes, including the Na,K-ATPase, and can regulate both potassium and calcium channels. Its overall effect is to stabilise excitable cell membranes.

Functional anatomy and physiology

Renal handling of magnesium involves filtration of free plasma magnesium at the glomerulus (about 70% of the total), with extensive reabsorption (50%–70%) in the loop of Henle and other parts of the proximal and distal renal tubule. Magnesium reabsorption is also enhanced by parathyroid hormone (PTH).

19

Presenting problems in magnesium homeostasis

Disturbances in magnesium homeostasis usually occur because of increased loss of magnesium through the gut or kidney or inability to excrete magnesium normally in patients with renal impairment.

Hypomagnesaemia

Hypomagnesaemia is defined as existing when plasma magnesium concentrations are below the reference range of 0.75–1.0 mmol/L (1.5–2.0 mEq/L).

Pathophysiology

Hypomagnesaemia usually is a reflection of magnesium depletion (Box 19.21), which can be caused by excessive magnesium loss from the gastrointestinal tract (notably in chronic diarrhoea) or the kidney (during prolonged use of loop diuretics). Excessive alcohol ingestion can cause magnesium depletion through both gut and renal losses. Some inherited tubular transport disorders, such as Gitelman and Bartter syndromes, can also result in urinary magnesium wasting. Magnesium depletion has important effects on calcium homeostasis because magnesium is required for the normal secretion of PTH in response to a fall in serum calcium, and because hypomagnesaemia causes end-organ resistance to PTH.

Clinical features

Mild degrees of hypomagnesaemia may be asymptomatic but more severe hypomagnesaemia may be associated with symptoms of hypocalcaemia, such as tetany, cardiac arrhythmias (notably torsades de pointes), central nervous excitation and seizures, vasoconstriction and hypertension. Hypomagnesaemia and magnesium depletion are also associated (through uncertain mechanisms) with hyponatraemia and hypokalaemia, which may contribute to some of the clinical manifestations.

i	19.21 Causes of hypomagnesaemia	
Mechanism	**Examples**	
Inadequate intake	Starvation	
	Malnutrition	
	Alcoholism	
	Parenteral nutrition	
Excessive losses		
Gastrointestinal	Prolonged vomiting/nasogastric aspiration	
	Chronic diarrhoea/laxative abuse	
	Malabsorption	
	Small bowel bypass surgery	
	Fistulae	
	Proton pump inhibitors	
Urinary	Diuretic therapy	
	Alcohol	
	Tubulotoxic drugs:	
	Gentamicin	
	Cisplatin	
	Herceptin	
	Volume expansion	
	Diabetic ketoacidosis	
	Post-obstructive diuresis	
	Recovery from acute tubular necrosis	
	Inherited tubular transport defect:	
	Bartter syndrome	
	Gitelman syndrome	
	Primary renal magnesium wasting	
Miscellaneous	Acute pancreatitis	
	Foscarnet therapy	
	Proton pump inhibitor therapy	
	Hungry bone syndrome	
	Diabetes mellitus	

Management

The underlying cause should be identified and treated where possible. When symptoms are present, the treatment of choice is intravenous magnesium chloride at a rate not exceeding 0.5 mmol/kg in the first 24 hours. If intravenous access is not feasible, magnesium sulphate can be given intramuscularly. Oral magnesium salts have limited effectiveness due to poor absorption and may cause diarrhoea. If hypomagnesaemia is caused by diuretic treatment, adjunctive use of a potassium-sparing agent can also help by reducing magnesium loss into the urine.

Hypermagnesaemia

This is a much less common abnormality than hypomagnesaemia. Predisposing conditions include acute kidney injury, chronic kidney disease and adrenocortical insufficiency. The condition is generally precipitated in patients at risk from an increased intake of magnesium, or from the use of magnesium-containing medications, such as antacids, laxatives and enemas.

Clinical features include bradycardia, hypotension, reduced consciousness and respiratory depression.

Management involves ceasing all magnesium-containing drugs and reducing dietary magnesium intake, improving renal function if possible, and promoting urinary magnesium excretion using a loop diuretic with intravenous hydration, if residual renal function allows. Calcium gluconate may be given intravenously to ameliorate cardiac effects. Dialysis may be necessary in patients with poor renal function.

Phosphate homeostasis

Inorganic phosphate (mainly present as HPO_4^{2-}) is intimately involved in cell energy metabolism, intracellular signalling and bone and mineral homeostasis (Ch. 26). The normal plasma concentration is 0.8–1.4 mmol/L (2.48–4.34 mg/dL).

Functional anatomy and physiology

Phosphate is freely filtered at the glomerulus and approximately 65% is reabsorbed by the proximal tubule, through an apical sodium–phosphate co-transport carrier. A further 10%–20% is reabsorbed in the distal tubules, leaving a fractional excretion of some 10% to pass into the urine, usually as $H_2PO_4^-$. Proximal reabsorption is decreased by PTH, fibroblast growth factor 23 (FGF23), volume expansion, osmotic diuretics and glucose infusion.

Presenting problems in phosphate homeostasis

The following section deals primarily with conditions that cause acute disturbances in serum phosphate concentrations. Chronic disorders that are accompanied by phosphate depletion, such as osteomalacia and hypophosphataemic rickets, are discussed in Chapter 26. Acute kidney injury and chronic kidney disease, which are associated with hyperphosphataemia, are discussed below and also in Chapter 18.

Hypophosphataemia

Hypophosphataemia is defined as existing when serum phosphate values fall below 0.8 mmol/L (2.48 mg/dL). The causes are shown in Box 19.22, subdivided into the underlying pathogenic mechanisms.

Pathophysiology

Phosphate may redistribute into cells during periods of increased energy utilisation (such as refeeding after a period of starvation) and during systemic alkalosis. However, severe hypophosphataemia usually represents an overall body deficit due to either inadequate intake or absorption through the gut, or excessive renal losses, most notably in primary hyperparathyroidism or as the result of acute plasma volume expansion, osmotic diuresis and diuretics acting on the proximal renal tubule. Less common causes include inherited defects of proximal sodium–phosphate co-transport and tumour-induced osteomalacia due to ectopic production of the hormone FGF23.

Clinical features

The clinical features of phosphate depletion are wide-ranging, reflecting the involvement of phosphate in many aspects of metabolism. Defects appear in the blood (impaired function and survival of all cell lineages), skeletal muscle (weakness, respiratory failure), cardiac muscle (congestive cardiac failure), smooth muscle (ileus), central nervous system (decreased consciousness, seizures and coma) and bone (osteomalacia and rickets in severe prolonged hypophosphataemia).

Investigations

Measurement of creatinine, electrolytes, phosphate, albumin, calcium and alkaline phosphatase should be performed. In selected cases, measurement of PTH and 25(OH)D and FGF23 may be helpful. The combination of hypophosphataemia and hypercalcaemia suggests primary hyperparathyroidism, which should be further investigated by measurements of PTH. The combination of hypophosphataemia with raised FGF23 levels and normal levels of 25(OH)D suggests either hereditary hypophosphataemic rickets or tumour-induced osteomalacia.

Management

Management of hypophosphataemia due to decreased dietary intake or excessive losses involves administering oral phosphate supplements and high-protein/high-dairy dietary supplements that are rich in naturally occurring phosphate. Intravenous treatment with sodium or potassium phosphate salts can be used in critical situations, but there is a risk of precipitating hypocalcaemia and metastatic calcification. Management of primary hyperparathyroidism is discussed in Chapter 18 and of hypophosphataemic rickets in Chapter 26.

Hyperphosphataemia

Hyperphosphataemia is most commonly caused by acute kidney injury or chronic kidney disease. Rarely, hyperphosphataemia can occur in association with hypercalcaemia in the inherited disorder tumoral calcinosis due to loss-of-function variants in *FGF23* or *GALTN3*.

Pathophysiology

In acute kidney injury and chronic kidney disease, the primary cause is reduced phosphate excretion as the result of a low GFR. In contrast, the hyperphosphataemia in hypoparathyroidism and pseudohypoparathyroidism is due to increased tubular phosphate reabsorption.

19.22 Causes of hypophosphataemia

Mechanism	Examples
Redistribution into cells	Refeeding after starvation Respiratory alkalosis Treatment for diabetic ketoacidosis
Inadequate intake or absorption	Malnutrition Malabsorption Chronic diarrhoea Phosphate binders Antacids Vitamin D deficiency or resistance
Increased renal excretion	Hyperparathyroidism Extracellular fluid volume expansion with diuresis Osmotic diuretics Fanconi syndrome Familial hypophosphataemic rickets Tumour-induced hypophosphataemic rickets

Redistribution of phosphate from cells into the plasma can also be a contributing factor in the tumour lysis syndromes and other catabolic states. Phosphate accumulation can be aggravated in any of these conditions if the patient takes phosphate-containing preparations or inappropriate vitamin D therapy.

Clinical features

The clinical features relate to hypocalcaemia and metastatic calcification, particularly in chronic kidney disease with tertiary hyperparathyroidism (when a high calcium–phosphate product occurs). Tumoral calcinosis is characterised by musculoskeletal pain due to deposition of calcium and phosphate in the joints and soft tissues.

Management

Hyperphosphataemia in patients with kidney disease should be treated with dietary phosphate restriction and the use of oral phosphate binders. Hyperphosphataemia in hypoparathyroidism and pseudohypoparathyroidism does not usually require treatment. Hyperphosphataemia associated with tumour lysis syndromes and catabolic states can be treated with intravenous normal saline, which is given to promote phosphate excretion.

Lipids and lipoprotein metabolism

The three main biological classes of lipid are:
- cholesterol, which is composed of hydrocarbon rings
- triglycerides (TGs), which are esters composed of glycerol linked to three long-chain fatty acids
- phospholipids, which are composed of a hydrophobic 'tail' consisting of two long-chain fatty acids linked through glycerol to a hydrophilic head containing a phosphate group.

Phospholipids are present in cell membranes and are important signalling molecules.

Despite their poor water solubility, lipids need to be absorbed from the gastrointestinal tract and transported throughout the body. This is achieved by incorporating lipids within lipoproteins. Plasma cholesterol and TGs are clinically important because they are major treatable risk factors for cardiovascular disease, while severe hypertriglyceridaemia also predisposes to acute pancreatitis.

Functional anatomy and physiology

Lipids are transported and metabolised by apolipoproteins, which combine with lipids to form spherical or disc-shaped lipoproteins, consisting of a hydrophobic core and a less hydrophobic coat (Fig. 19.11). The structure of some apolipoproteins also enables them to act as enzyme co-factors or cell receptor ligands. Variations in lipid and apolipoprotein composition result in distinct classes of lipoprotein that perform specific metabolic functions.

Processing of dietary lipid

The mechanisms responsible for intestinal absorption of dietary lipid are described in Chapter 23 but the most salient features relevant to lipid metabolism are summarised in Figure 19.12. Enterocytes lining the gut extract mono and diglycerides and free fatty acids from micelles. These are re-esterified into TGs, which are combined with a truncated form of apolipoprotein B (Apo B48) as it is synthesised. Intestinal cholesterol derived from dietary and biliary sources is also absorbed through a specific intestinal membrane transporter termed NPC1L1. This produces chylomicrons containing TG and cholesterol ester that are secreted basolaterally into lymphatic lacteals and carried to the circulation through the thoracic duct. On entering the blood stream, nascent chylomicrons are modified by further exchange of apolipoproteins. Chylomicron TGs are hydrolysed by lipoprotein lipase located on the endothelium of tissue capillary beds. This releases fatty acids that are used locally for energy production or stored as TG in muscle or fat. The residual 'remnant' chylomicron particle is avidly cleared by low-density lipoprotein receptors (LDLRs) and other receptors in the liver, which recognise Apo E on the remnant lipoproteins. Complete absorption of dietary lipids takes about 6–10 hours, so chylomicrons are usually undetectable in the plasma after a 12-hour fast.

The main dietary determinants of plasma cholesterol concentrations are the intake of saturated and *trans*-unsaturated fatty acids, which reduce LDLR activity (see below), whereas dietary cholesterol has surprisingly little effect on plasma cholesterol levels. Plant sterols and drugs that inhibit cholesterol absorption are effective because they also reduce the re-utilisation of biliary cholesterol. The dietary determinants of plasma TG concentrations are complex since excessive intake of carbohydrate, fat or alcohol may all contribute to increased plasma TG by different mechanisms.

Endogenous lipid synthesis

In the fasting state, the liver is the major source of plasma lipids (see Fig. 19.12). The liver may acquire lipids by uptake, synthesis or conversion from other macronutrients. These lipids are transported to other tissues by secretion of very low-density lipoproteins (VLDLs), which are rich in

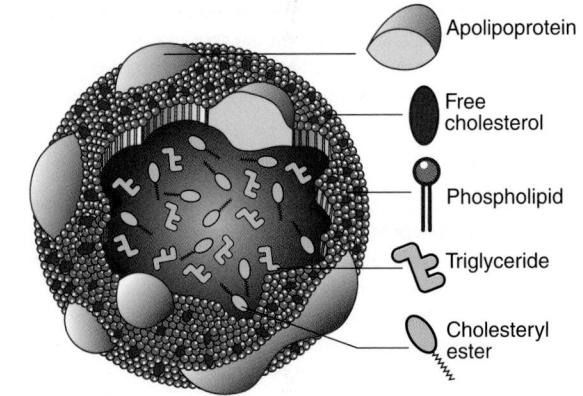

Fig. 19.11 Structure of lipoproteins.

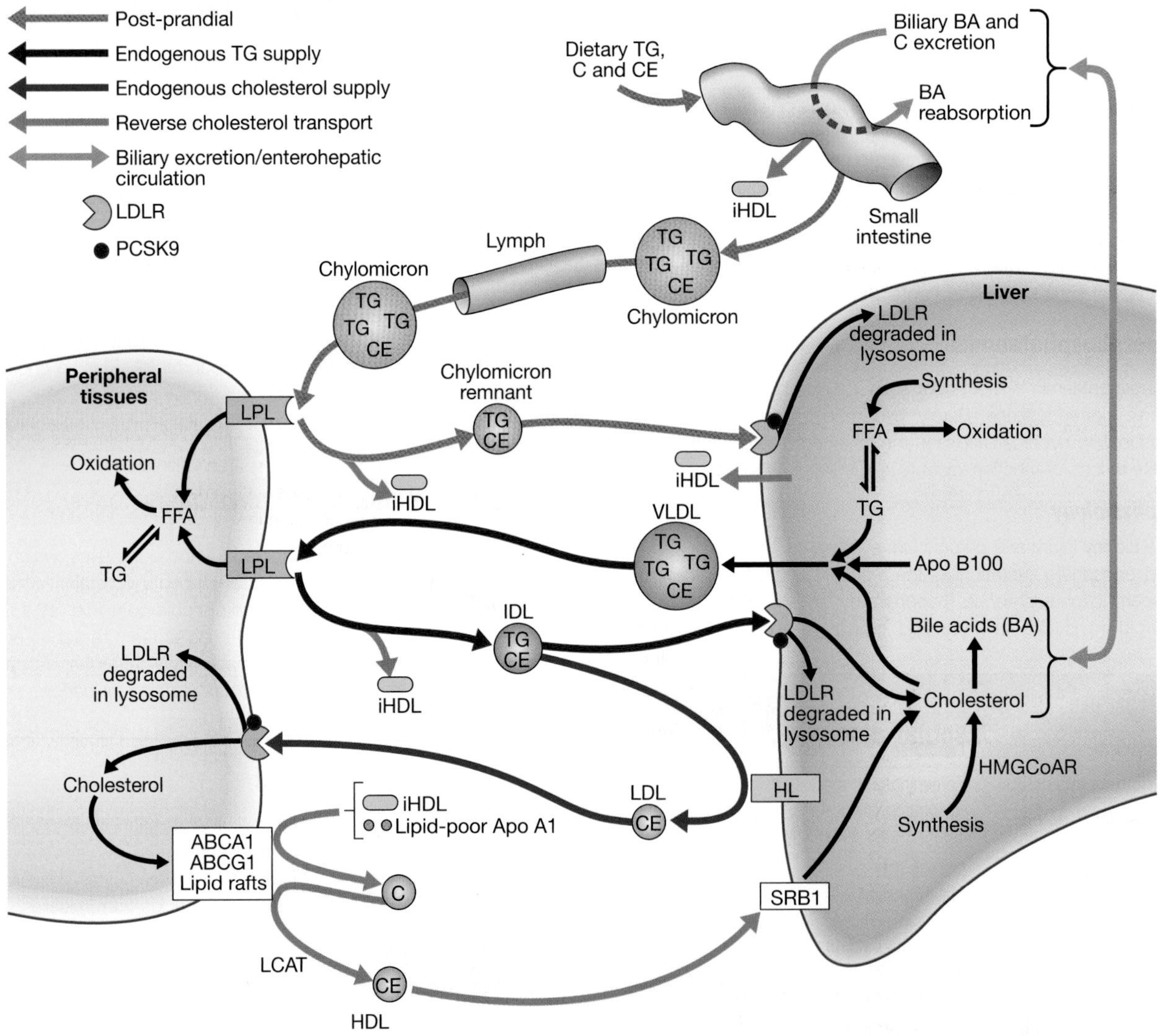

Fig. 19.12 Absorption, transport and storage of lipids. Pathways of lipid transport are shown; in addition, cholesterol ester transfer protein exchanges triglyceride and cholesterol ester between very low-density lipoprotein/chylomicrons and high-/low-density lipoprotein, and free fatty acids released from peripheral lipolysis can be taken up in the liver. (ABCA1/ABCG1 = adenosine triphosphate-binding cassette A1/G1; Apo = apolipoprotein; BA = bile acids; C = cholesterol; CE = cholesterol ester; FFA = free fatty acids; HDL = mature high-density lipoprotein; HL = hepatic lipase; HMGCoAR = hydroxy-methyl-glutaryl-co-enzyme A reductase; IDL = intermediate-density lipoprotein; iHDL = immature high-density lipoprotein; LCAT = lecithin cholesterol acyl transferase; LDL = low-density lipoprotein; LDLR = low-density lipoprotein receptor (Apo B100 receptor); LPL = lipoprotein lipase; PCSK9 = proprotein convertase subtilisin kexin 9; SRB1 = scavenger receptor B1; TG = triglyceride; VLDL = very low-density lipoprotein)

TG but differ from chylomicrons in that they are less massive and contain full-length Apo B100. Following secretion into the circulation, VLDLs undergo metabolic processing similar to that of chylomicrons. Hydrolysis of VLDL TG releases fatty acids to tissues and converts VLDLs into 'remnant' particles, referred to as intermediate-density lipoproteins (IDLs). Most IDLs are rapidly cleared by LDLRs in the liver but some are processed by hepatic lipase, which converts the particle to an LDL by removing TG and most materials other than Apo B100, and free and esterified cholesterol. The catabolism of TG-rich chylomicrons and VLDL by lipoprotein lipase is modulated by Apos C2 and C3 on the surface of these particles.

Cholesterol transport

The LDL particles act as a source of cholesterol for cells and tissues (see Fig. 19.12). LDL cholesterol is internalised by receptor-mediated endocytosis via the LDLR. Delivery of cholesterol by this mechanism contributes to the homeostatic control of intracellular cholesterol levels via sterol regulatory element binding protein (SREBP), which coordinates intracellular cholesterol metabolism via several mechanisms. Decline in SREBP down-regulates expression of LDLR and reduces the synthesis and activity of the rate-limiting enzyme for cholesterol synthesis, hydroxy-methyl-glutaryl-co-enzyme A (HMGCoA) reductase. Counterintuitively, this is accompanied by an increase in an important regulator of LDLR levels, proprotein convertase subtilisin kexin 9 (PCSK9), which targets LDLR for degradation. Intracellular free cholesterol concentrations are maintained within a narrow range by the inhibitory effects of LDL on expression of LRLR, modulation of the half-life of LDLR through PCSK9, and control of cholesterol synthesis and esterification.

Peripheral tissues are guarded against excessive cholesterol accumulation by high-density lipoproteins (HDLs; see Fig. 19.12). Lipid-poor Apo A1 (derived from the liver, intestine and the outer layer of chylomicrons and VLDL) accepts cellular cholesterol and phospholipid from a specific membrane transporter known as the ATP-binding cassette A1 (ABCA1). This produces small HDLs that are able to accept more free cholesterol from cholesterol-rich regions of the cell membrane known as 'rafts' via another membrane transporter (ABCG1). The cholesterol that has been accepted by these small HDLs is esterified by lecithin cholesterol acyl transferase (LCAT), thus maintaining an uptake gradient and remodelling the particle into a mature spherical HDL. These HDLs release their cholesterol to the liver and other cholesterol-requiring tissues via the scavenger receptor B1 (SRB1).

The cholesterol ester transfer protein (CETP) in plasma allows transfer of cholesterol from HDLs or LDLs to VLDLs or chylomicrons in exchange for TG. When TG is elevated, the action of CETP may reduce HDL cholesterol and remodel LDLs into 'small, dense' LDL particles that may be more atherogenic in the blood-vessel wall. Animal species that lack CETP seem resistant to atherosclerosis.

Lipids and cardiovascular disease

Plasma lipoprotein levels are major modifiable risk factors for cardiovascular disease. Increased levels of atherogenic lipoproteins (especially LDL, but also IDL, and possibly chylomicron remnants) contribute to the development of atherosclerosis. A sub-population of LDL particles bears an additional protein known as apolipoprotein (a), which shares homology with plasminogen. The combination of LDL and apolipoprotein (a) is known as lipoprotein (a) (Lp(a)). It transports oxidised phospholipid and is regarded as atherogenic because its plasma concentration is an independent risk factor for cardiovascular disease. Following chemical modifications such as oxidation, Apo B-containing lipoproteins are no longer cleared by the normal LDLR pathway. They trigger a self-perpetuating inflammatory response, during which they are taken up by macrophage 'scavenger receptors' to form foam cells, a hallmark of atherosclerotic lesions. These processes also have an adverse effect on endothelial function.

Conversely, HDL removes cholesterol from the tissues to the liver, where it is metabolised and excreted in bile. HDL may also counteract some components of the inflammatory response, such as the expression of vascular adhesion molecules by the endothelium. Low HDL cholesterol levels (HDL-C) are usually associated with TG elevation. This inverse relationship may confound the associations between HDL-C and/or TG with atherosclerosis.

Investigations

Lipid measurements are usually performed for the following reasons:

- screening for primary or secondary prevention of cardiovascular disease
- investigation of patients with clinical features of lipid disorders and their relatives
- monitoring of response to diet, weight control and medication.

Abnormalities of lipid metabolism most commonly come to light following these tests. Convenient non-fasting measurements of total cholesterol (TC) and HDL cholesterol (HDL-C) allow estimation of non-HDL cholesterol (non-HDLC, calculated as TC − HDL-C). A 12-hour fasting sample is required to standardise TG measurement and allow calculation of LDL cholesterol (LDL-C) according to the Friedewald formula:

$$LDL-C = TC - HDL-C - (TG/2.2)\, mmol/L$$

or

$$LDL-C = TC - HDL-C - (TG/5)\, mg/dL$$

The formula becomes unreliable when TG levels exceed 4 mmol/L (350 mg/dL). Measurements of non-HDLC or Apo B100 may assess risk of cardiovascular disease more accurately than LDL-C, particularly when TG levels are increased. Furthermore, non-fasting TG is a more sensitive marker of the risk of cardiovascular disease. A 12-hour fast is still required for formal diagnosis of hypertriglyceridaemia or use of the Friedewald equation. Consideration must be given to confounding factors, such as recent illness, after which cholesterol, LDL-C and HDL-C levels temporarily decrease in proportion to severity of the episode. Results that will affect major decisions, such as initiation of drug therapy, should be confirmed with a repeat measurement.

Elevated levels of TG are common in obesity, diabetes and insulin resistance and are frequently associated with low HDL and increased 'small, dense' LDL. Under these circumstances, LDL-C may underestimate risk. This is one situation in which measurement of non-HDLC or Apo B may provide more accurate risk assessment.

Presenting problems in lipid metabolism

Hyperlipidaemia can occur in association with various diseases and drugs, as summarised in Box 19.23. Overt or subclinical hypothyroidism may cause hypercholesterolaemia. Measurement of thyroid function is warranted in most cases, even in the absence of typical symptoms and signs.

Once secondary causes are excluded, primary lipid abnormalities may be diagnosed. Primary lipid abnormalities can be classified according to the predominant lipid problem: hypercholesterolaemia, hypertriglyceridaemia or mixed hyperlipidaemia (Box 19.24). Although single-gene disorders are encountered in all three categories, most cases are due to multiple-gene (polygenic) loci interacting with environmental factors. The clinical features and complicaions of dyslipidaemia vary somewhat between these causes.

Hypercholesterolaemia

Hypercholesterolaemia is a polygenic disorder that is the most common cause of a mild to moderate increase in LDL-C (Box 19.24). Physical signs, such as corneal arcus, xanthelasma, tendon xanthoma and eruptive xanthoma (see p. 615) may be found in this as well as other forms of hyperlipidaemia. The risk of cardiovascular disease is

19

proportional to the degree of LDL-C (or Apo B) elevation, but is modified by other major risk factors, including low HDL-C and high Lp(a).

Familial hypercholesterolaemia (FH) is a more severe disorder with a prevalence of approximately 0.3% in most populations. It is usually caused by loss-of-function variants affecting the *LDLR* gene, which results in an autosomal dominant pattern of inheritance. A similar syndrome can arise with loss-of-function variants in the ligand-binding domain of Apo B100 or gain-of-function variants in *PCSK9*, which promote LDLR degradation. Pathological variants can be detected in one of these three genes by genetic testing in about 70% of patients with FH. Most patients with FH have LDL-C levels that are approximately twice as high as in normal subjects of the same age and gender. FH may be accompanied by xanthomas of the Achilles or extensor digitorum tendons (p. 614), which are strongly suggestive of FH. The onset of corneal arcus before age 40 is also suggestive of this condition. Identification of an index case of FH (the first case of FH in a family) should trigger genetic and biochemical screening of other family members, which is a cost-effective method for case detection. Affected individuals should be managed from childhood (Box 19.25) because affected patients face the risk of a 20–40-year acceleration of the risk of premature cardiovascular disease.

Homozygous FH may occur sporadically, especially in populations in which there is a 'founder' gene effect or consanguineous marriage. Homozygosity results in more extensive xanthomas and precocious cardiovascular disease, often in childhood. Hyperalphalipoproteinaemia refers to increased levels of HDL-C. This condition rarely causes cardiovascular disease, but it may reflect HDL dysfunction, so it should not be regarded as universally benign.

Familial combined hyperlipidaemia, and dysbetalipoproteinaemia, may present with the pattern of predominant hypercholesterolaemia (see 'Mixed hyperlipidaemia' below).

Hypertriglyceridaemia

Hypertriglyceridaemia also usually involves polygenic factors (see Box 19.24). Other common causes include excess alcohol intake, medications (such as β-blockers and retinoids), type 2 diabetes, impaired glucose tolerance, central obesity or other manifestations of insulin resistance and impaired absorption of bile acids. It is often accompanied by post-prandial hyperlipidaemia and reduced HDL-C, both of which may contribute to cardiovascular risk. Excessive intake of alcohol or dietary fat, or other exacerbating factors, may precipitate a massive increase in TG levels, which, if they exceed 10 mmol/L (880 mg/dL), may pose a risk of acute pancreatitis.

Monogenic forms of hypertriglyceridaemia also occur due to loss-of-function variants in the genes encoding lipoprotein lipase and Apo C2, which coordinate the lipolytic breakdown of TG-rich lipoproteins. These cause recessively inherited severe hypertriglyceridaemia that is not readily amenable to drug treatment. It may present in childhood with episodes of acute abdominal pain or pancreatitis. In common with other causes of severe hypertriglyceridaemia, hepatomegaly, lipaemia retinalis and eruptive xanthomas may occur (p. 614). Familial hypertriglyceridaemia may also be inherited in a dominant manner due to loss-of-function variants in the *APOA5* gene, which encodes Apo A5 – a co-factor that is essential for lipoprotein lipase activity. Conversely, loss-of-function variants for genes encoding ANGPTL 3 and 4, or Apo C3, may increase lipoprotein lipase activity and reduce TG. Individuals with *APOA5* variants have an increased risk of cardiovascular disease whereas those with *ANGPTL3*, *ANGPTL4* and *APOC3* variants have a reduced risk.

Familial combined hyperlipidaemia, and dysbetalipoproteinaemia, may present with the pattern of predominant hypertriglyceridaemia (see 'Mixed hyperlipidaemia', below).

---

i 19.23 Causes of secondary hyperlipidaemia

Secondary hypercholesterolaemia

Moderately common

- Drugs:
  Diuretics
  Ciclosporin
  Glucocorticoids
  Androgens
  Antiretroviral agents
- Hypothyroidism
- Pregnancy
- Cholestatic liver disease

Less common

- Nephrotic syndrome
- Anorexia nervosa
- Porphyria
- Hyperparathyroidism

Secondary hypertriglyceridaemia

Common

- Type 2 diabetes mellitus
- Chronic renal disease
- Abdominal obesity
- Excess alcohol
- Hepatocellular disease
- Drugs:
  β-blockers
  Retinoids
  Glucocorticoids
  Antiretroviral agents

---

i 19.24 Classification of hyperlipidaemia

Disease	Elevated lipid results	Elevated lipoprotein	CHD risk	Pancreatitis risk
Predominant hypercholesterolaemia				
Polygenic (majority)	TC ± TG	LDL ± VLDL	+	−
Familial hypercholesterolaemia (LDLR defect, defective Apo B100, increased function of *PCSK9*)	TC ± TG	LDL ± VLDL	+++	−
Hyperalphalipoproteinaemia	TC ± TG	HDL	−	−
Predominant hypertriglyceridaemia				
Polygenic (majority)	TG	VLDL ± LDL	Variable	+
Lipoprotein lipase deficiency	TG ≫ TC	Chylo	?	+++
Familial hypertriglyceridaemia	TG > TC	VLDL ± chylo	?	++
Mixed hyperlipidaemia				
Polygenic (majority)	TC + TG	VLDL + LDL	Variable	+
Familial combined hyperlipidaemia*	TC and/or TG	LDL and/or VLDL	++	+
Dysbetalipoproteinaemia*	TC and/or TG	IDL	+++	+

*Familial combined hyperlipidaemia and dysbetalipoproteinaemia may also present as predominant hypercholesterolaemia or predominant hypertriglyceridaemia.
(Apo B100 = apolipoprotein B100; CHD = coronary heart disease; chylo = chylomicrons; HDL = high-density lipoprotein; IDL = intermediate-density lipoprotein; LDL = low-density lipoprotein; LDLR = low-density lipoprotein receptor; TC = total cholesterol; TG = triglycerides; VLDL = very low-density lipoprotein)
+ = slightly increased risk; ++ = increased risk; +++ = greatly increased risk; ? = risk unclear

19.25 Familial hypercholesterolaemia in adolescence

- **Statin treatment**: may be required from the age of about 10. It does not compromise normal growth and maturation.
- **Smoking**: patients should be strongly advised not to smoke.
- **Adherence to medication:** critically important to the success of treatment. Simple regimens should be used and education and support provided.

Mixed hyperlipidaemia

It is difficult to define quantitatively the distinction between predominant hyperlipidaemias and mixed hyperlipidaemia. The term 'mixed' usually implies the presence of hypertriglyceridaemia, as well as an increase in LDL-C or IDL. Treatment of massive hypertriglyceridaemia may reduce TG faster than cholesterol, thus temporarily mimicking mixed hyperlipidaemia.

Primary mixed hyperlipidaemia is usually polygenic and, like predominant hypertriglyceridaemia, often occurs in association with type 2 diabetes, impaired glucose tolerance, central obesity or other manifestations of insulin resistance. Both components of mixed hyperlipidaemia may contribute to the risk of cardiovascular disease.

Familial combined hyperlipidaemia is a term used to identify an inherited tendency towards the over-production of atherogenic Apo B-containing lipoproteins. It results in elevation of cholesterol, TG or both in different family members at different times. It is associated with an increased risk of cardiovascular disease, but it does not produce any pathognomonic physical signs. In practice, this relatively common condition is substantially modified by factors such as age and weight. It may not be a monogenic condition, but rather one end of a heterogeneous spectrum that overlaps insulin resistance.

Dysbetalipoproteinaemia (also referred to as type 3 hyperlipidaemia, broad-beta dyslipoproteinaemia or remnant hyperlipidaemia) involves accumulation of roughly equimolar levels of cholesterol and TG. It is caused by homozygous inheritance of the Apo E2 allele, which is the isoform least avidly recognised by the LDLR. In conjunction with other exacerbating factors, such as obesity or diabetes, it leads to accumulation of atherogenic IDL and chylomicron remnants. Premature cardiovascular disease is common, as is peripheral vascular disease. It may also result in the formation of palmar xanthomas, tuberous xanthomas or tendon xanthomas.

Rare dyslipidaemias

Several rare disturbances of lipid metabolism have been described (Box 19.26). They provide important insights into lipid metabolism and its impact on risk of cardiovascular disease.

Fish eye disease, Apo A1 Milano and lecithin cholesterol acyl transferase (LCAT) deficiency demonstrate that very low HDL-C levels do not necessarily cause cardiovascular disease, but Apo A1 deficiency, and possibly Tangier disease, demonstrate that low HDL-C can be atherogenic under some circumstances. PCSK9 gain-of-function and autosomal recessive *FH* variants reveal the importance of proteins that chaperone the LDLR. Sitosterolaemia and cerebrotendinous xanthomatosis demonstrate that sterols other than cholesterol can cause xanthomas and cardiovascular disease, while *PCSK9* loss-of-function variants abetalipoproteinaemia and hypobetalipoproteinaemia suggest that low levels of Apo B-containing lipoproteins reduce the risk of cardiovascular disease. Adverse health outcomes associated with extremely low plasma lipid levels in the latter two conditions are attributable to fat-soluble vitamin deficiency, or impaired transport of lipid from intestine or liver.

Principles of management

Assessment of absolute risk of cardiovascular disease, treatment of all modifiable risk factors and optimisation of lifestyle, especially diet and exercise, are central to management in all cases. Lipid-lowering therapies have a key role in the primary and secondary prevention of cardiovascular diseases. Patients with the greatest absolute risk of cardiovascular disease derive the greatest absolute benefit from treatment. Public health organisations recommend thresholds for the introduction of lipid-lowering therapy based on the identification of patients in very high-risk categories, or those calculated to be at high absolute risk according to algorithms or tables. The large epidemiological studies on which risk assessment is based should be recalibrated for the local population where possible. The decision to commence lipid-lowering therapy is usually made on the basis of the lifetime risk of cardiovascular disease which takes lipid concentrations into account along with other risk factors and age. This diminishes the pressure to treat older adults who are less likely to benefit and supports earlier intervention in patients who are not yet in old age. Recently released guidelines include ACC/AHA or ESC/EAS guidelines, which differ in some respects (see 'Further information'). Important common themes include additional clinical input for risk calculation tables, expanded lists of risk-enhancing factors, use of coronary calcium scores in intermediate-risk patients and adoption of more aggressive LDL-C treatment goals. Target levels for LDL-C are at less than 1.8 mmol/l (70 mg/dL) on one hand, or less than 1.4 mmol/l in addition to 50% reduction on the other.

Non-pharmacological management

Patients with lipid abnormalities should receive medical advice and, if necessary, dietary counselling couched in terms of practical dietary and culinary advice:

- replace sources of saturated fat and cholesterol with alternative foods, such as lean meat, low-fat dairy products, polyunsaturated spreads and low-glycaemic-index carbohydrates
- reduce energy-dense foods such as fats and soft drinks, while increasing activity and exercise to maintain or lose weight
- increase consumption of cardioprotective and nutrient-dense foods, such as vegetables, unrefined carbohydrates, fish, pulses, nuts, legumes and fruit
- adjust alcohol consumption, reducing intake if excessive or if associated with hypertension, hypertriglyceridaemia or central obesity
- achieve additional benefits with preferential intake of foods containing lipid-lowering nutrients such as n-3 fatty acids, dietary fibre and plant sterols
- reduce intake of saturated and *trans*-unsaturated fat to less than 7%–10% of total energy
- reduce intake of cholesterol to <250 mg/day.

These measures should achieve a response within 3–4 weeks but dietary adjustment may need to be introduced gradually. Although

19

i 19.26 Miscellaneous and rare forms of hyperlipidaemia		
Condition	**Lipoprotein pattern**	**CVD risk**
Tangier disease	Very low HDL, low TC	+
Apo A1 deficiency	Very low HDL	++
Apo A1 Milano	Very low HDL	−
Fish eye disease	Very low HDL, high TG	−
LCAT deficiency	Very low HDL, high TG	?
Autosomal recessive FH	Very high LDL	++
Sitosterolaemia	High plant sterols including sitosterol	+
Cerebrotendinous xanthomatosis	Bile acid defect (cholestanol accumulation)	+

+ = slightly increased risk; ++ = increased risk
(CVD = cardiovascular disease; FH = familial hypercholesterolaemia; HDL = high-density lipoprotein; LCAT = lecithin cholesterol acyl transferase; LDL = low-density lipoprotein; TC = total cholesterol; TG = triglycerides)

hyperlipidaemia in general, and hypertriglyceridaemia in particular, can be very responsive to these measures, LDL-C reductions are often only modest in routine clinical practice. Explanation, encouragement and persistence are often required to assist patient adherence. Even minor weight loss can substantially reduce cardiovascular risk, especially in centrally obese patients.

All other modifiable cardiovascular risk factors should be assessed and treated. If possible, intercurrent drug treatments that adversely affect the lipid profile should be replaced.

Pharmacological management

The main diagnostic categories provide a useful framework for management and the selection of first-line pharmacological treatment (Fig. 19.13). Depending on the response, treatment with more than one drug may be required. Advances in understanding the genetic factors that regulate lipid metabolism have led to the identification of several new lipid-lowering agents. Monoclonal antibodies and antisense mRNA therapies directed against PCSK9 are already used in clinical practice whereas antisense mRNA directed against apolipoprotein C3 (APOC3) and angiopoietin-like 3 (ANGPTL3) are under investigation for the treatment of hypercholesterolaemia and hypertriglyceridaemia.

Hypercholesterolaemia

The drugs used in the treatment of hypercholesterolaemia target the pathways responsible for cholesterol synthesis, its clearance from the circulation, or its absorption from the diet. Homeostatic mechanisms orchestrated by steroid regulatory element binding protein (SREBP) to maintain intracellular cholesterol concentrations, blunt the effectiveness of statins, ezetimibe and resins but this does not apply to PCSK9 inhibitors, which are extremely effective cholesterol-lowering agents, as summarised in (Fig. 19.14).

Statins

Statins reduce cholesterol synthesis by inhibiting the HMGCoA reductase enzyme. The reduction in cholesterol synthesis up-regulates production of the LDLR, which increases clearance of LDL and its precursor, IDL, resulting in a secondary reduction in LDL synthesis. Statins reduce LDL-C by up to 60%, reduce TG by up to 40% and increase HDL-C by

up to 10%. They also reduce the concentration of intermediate metabolites such as isoprenes, which may lead to other effects such as suppression of the inflammatory response. There is clear evidence of protection against total and coronary mortality, stroke and cardiovascular events across the spectrum of cardiovascular disease risk.

Statins are generally well tolerated and serious side-effects are infrequent. Liver function test abnormalities and muscle problems, such as myalgia, asymptomatic increase in creatine kinase (CK), myositis and, infrequently, rhabdomyolysis, are the most common. Side-effects are more likely in older adults and in patients who are debilitated or receiving other drugs that interfere with statin degradation, which usually involves cytochrome P450 3A4 or glucuronidation.

PCSK9 inhibitors

Several drugs have been developed that neutralise PCSK9, an enzyme that degrades the LDLR. This causes levels of LDLR to increase, which markedly reduces LDL-C by clearing LDL from the circulation. The PCSK9 inhibitors currently available are the monoclonal antibodies (Mab) evolocumab and alirocumab, which are administered by subcutaneous injection every 2–4 weeks, and the PCSK9 antisense mRNA inclisiran, which is administered subcutaneously every 6 months. These drugs are all highly effective. Inclisiran inhibits PCSK9 by binding to and degrading its mRNA intracellularly whereas the Mab bind and inhibit PCSK9 at the cell surface. Reductions in LDL-C of about 50%–60% have been observed with these agents in patients who have not responded adequately to standard lipid-lowering therapy and this has been accompanied by a reduction in the risk of cardiovascular events of about 15%. The reason PCSK9 inhibitors are so highly effective is that they do not lower intracellular levels of cholesterol and hence do not trigger the compensatory mechanisms that blunt the effect of other cholesterol-lowering medications (Fig. 19.14). The PCSK9 inhibitors also act synergistically with statins and ezetimibe and lower lipoprotein (a) by mechanisms that are unclear.

Ezetimibe

Ezetimibe inhibits activity of the intestinal mucosal transporter NPC1L1, which is responsible for absorption of dietary and biliary cholesterol. The resulting depletion of hepatic cholesterol up-regulates hepatic LDLR production. This mechanism of action is synergistic with the effect of statins. Monotherapy in a 10 mg/day dose reduces LDL-C by 15%–20%. Slightly

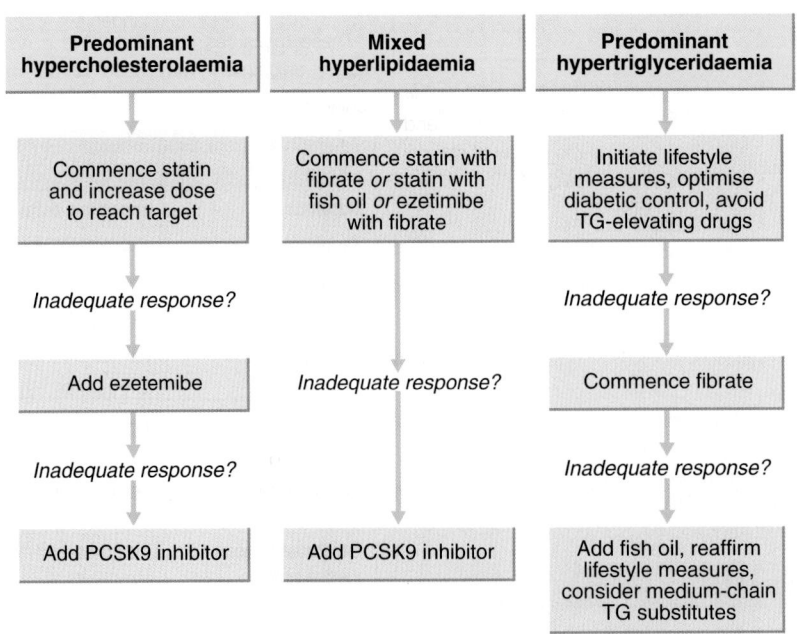

Fig. 19.13 **Flow chart for the drug treatment of hyperlipidaemia.** Triglyceride (TG) elevating drugs include glucocorticoids, antipsychotics, isotretinoin and β-blockers. See text for more details of drugs and dosages. (PCSK9 = proprotein convertase subtilisin kexin 9)

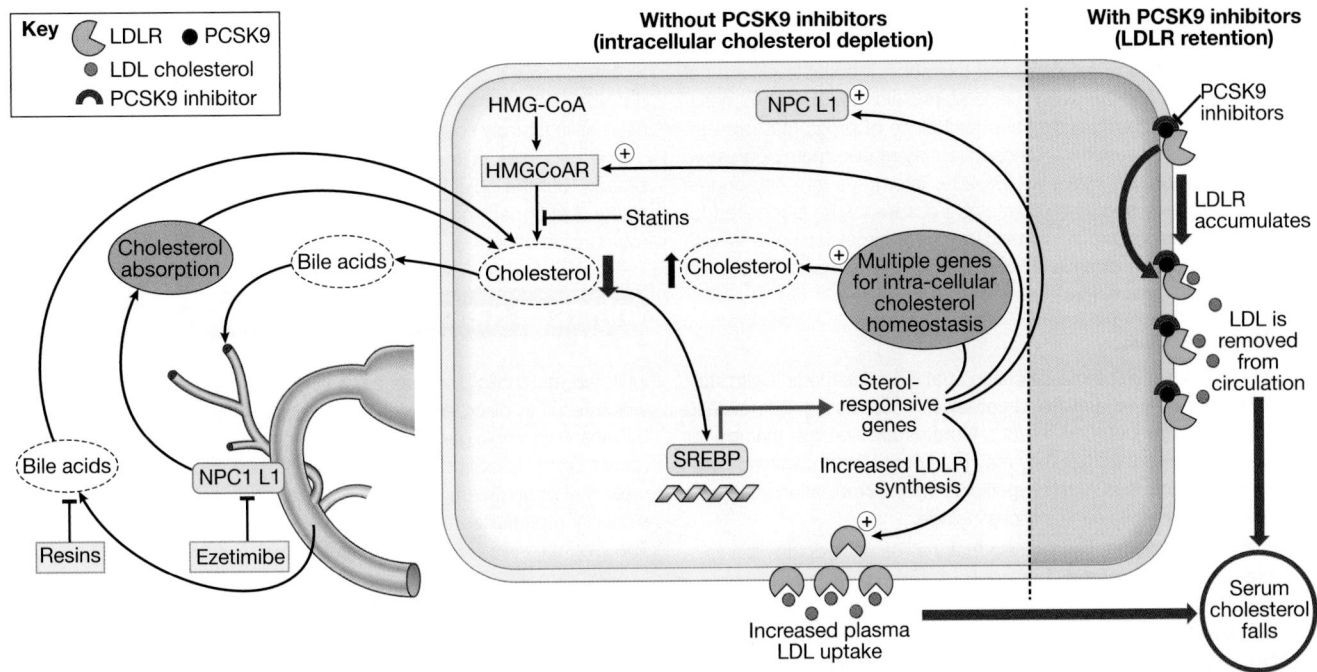

Fig. 19.14 Mechanism of action for cholesterol-lowering drugs. Traditional cholesterol-lowering drugs such as statins and ezetimibe lower intracellular cholesterol, causing activation of steroid regulatory element binding protein (SREBP) which increases expression of sterol responsive genes, particularly LDLR, leading to lower plasma LDL. Activation of SREBP also stimulates cholesterol synthesis and absorption which may blunt the therapeutic response to these drugs. SREBP also fine-tunes the restoration of intracellular cholesterol by up-regulating PCSK9 which assists degradation of LDLRs. Inhibitors of PCSK9 do not affect intracellular cholesterol but instead work by causing LDLR to accumulate at the cell surface thereby removing cholesterol bound to LDL from the circulation. (HMGCoA = hydroxy-methyl-glutaryl-co-enzyme A; HMGCoAR = hydroxy-methyl-glutaryl-co-enzyme A reductase; LDL = low-density lipoprotein; LDLR = low-density lipoprotein receptor; PCSK9 = proprotein convertase subtilisin kexin 9)

greater (17%–25%) incremental LDL-C reduction occurs when ezetimibe is added to statins. Ezetimibe is well tolerated, and evidence of a beneficial effect on cardiovascular disease endpoints is now available. Plant sterol-supplemented foods, which also reduce cholesterol absorption, lower LDL-C by 7%–15%.

Bile acid-sequestering resins

Drugs in this class include colestyramine, colestipol and colesevelam, although their use and availability is declining. They prevent the reabsorption of bile acids, thereby increasing de novo bile acid synthesis from hepatic cholesterol. The depletion of bile acids is sensed via the farnesyl X receptor and the response may also improve glucose metabolism. The resultant depletion of hepatic cholesterol up-regulates LDLR activity and reduces LDL-C in a manner that is synergistic with the action of statins. Resins may increase TG or interfere with bioavailability of other drugs. Colesevelam has fewer gastrointestinal effects than the other drugs in this class.

Combination therapy

In many patients, treatment of predominant hypercholesterolaemia can be achieved by diet plus the use of a statin in sufficient doses to achieve target LDL-C levels. Patients who do not reach LDL targets on the highest tolerated statin dose, or who are intolerant of statins, may receive plant sterols, ezetimibe, PCSK9 inhibitors, or resins. Ezetimibe and resins are safe and effective in combination with a statin because the mechanisms of action of individual therapies complement each other while blunting each other's compensatory mechanisms.

Hypertriglyceridaemia

Predominant hypertriglyceridaemia can be treated with one of the TG-lowering drugs described below, in combination with lifestyle measures such as weight reduction, reduction in alcohol consumption and optimisation of diabetic control.

Fibrates

These stimulate peroxisome proliferator-activated receptor (PPAR) alpha, which controls the expression of gene products that mediate the metabolism of TG and HDL. As a result, synthesis of fatty acids, TG and VLDL is reduced, while that of lipoprotein lipase, which catabolises TG, is enhanced. In addition, production of Apo A1 and ABC A1 is up-regulated leading to increased reverse cholesterol transport via HDL. Consequently, fibrates reduce TG by up to 50% and increase HDL-C by up to 20%, but LDL-C changes are variable.

Fewer large-scale trials have been conducted with fibrates than with statins. The results are less conclusive, but reduced rates of cardiovascular disease have been reported with fibrate therapy in the subgroup of patients with low HDL-C levels and elevated TG (TG >2.3 mmol/L (200 mg/dL)). Fibrates are usually well tolerated but share a similar side-effect profile to statins. In addition, they may increase the risk of cholelithiasis and prolong the action of anticoagulants. Accumulating evidence suggests that they may also have a protective effect against diabetic microvascular complications.

Highly polyunsaturated long-chain n-3 fatty acids

These include eicosapentaenoic acid (EPA) and docosahexaenoic acid (DHA), which comprise approximately 30% of the fatty acids in fish oil. Both are potent inhibitors of VLDL TG formation. Intakes of more than 2 g n-3 fatty acid (equivalent to 6 g of most forms of fish oil) per day lower TG in a dose-dependent fashion. Up to 50% reduction in TG may be achieved with 15 g fish oil per day. Changes in HDL-C are variable but fish oils do not usually reduce LDL-C. Fish oil fatty acids have also been shown to inhibit platelet aggregation and improve cardiac arrhythmia in animal models. Dietary and pharmacological trials suggest that n-3 fatty acids may reduce mortality from coronary heart disease. The benefit of n-3 fatty acid supplements has been confirmed in a recent trial amongst hypertriglyceridaemic patients. They appear to be safe and well tolerated. Dietary fish consumption is the preferred source for the general population.

19

Patients with predominant hypertriglyceridaemia who do not respond to lifestyle intervention can be treated with fibrates or n-3 fatty acids, depending on individual response and tolerance. If target levels are not achieved, fibrates and fish oil can be combined along with lifestyle measures, optimising diabetic control and avoidance of drugs that raise triglycerides. Massive hypertriglyceridaemia may require more aggressive limitation of dietary fat intake (<10%–20% energy as fat). Any degree of insulin deficiency should be corrected because insulin is required for optimal activity of lipoprotein lipase. The initial target for patients with massive hypertriglyceridaemia is TG <10 mmol/L (880 mg/dL), to reduce the risk of acute pancreatitis.

Mixed hyperlipidaemia

Mixed hyperlipidaemia can be difficult to treat. First-line therapy with statins alone is unlikely to achieve target levels once fasting TGs exceed approximately 4 mmol/L (350 mg/dL). Fibrates are first-line therapy for dysbetalipoproteinaemia, but they may not control the cholesterol component in other forms of mixed hyperlipidaemia. Combination therapy is often required. Effective combinations include:

- statin plus fenofibrate (recognising that the risk of myopathy is increased with gemfibrozil, but fenofibrate is relatively safe in this regard)
- statin plus fish oil when TG is not too high
- fibrate plus ezetimibe when cholesterol is not too high.

Monitoring of therapy

The effects of lipid-lowering therapy should be assessed after 6 weeks (12 weeks for fibrates). At this point, it is prudent to review side-effects, lipid response (see target levels above), CK and liver function tests. During longer-term follow-up, adherence to treatment, diet and exercise should be assessed, with monitoring of weight, blood pressure and lipid levels. The presence of cardiovascular symptoms or signs should be noted, and absolute cardiovascular risk assessed periodically. Effective statin therapy may be associated with a paradoxical and as yet unexplained increase in coronary calcium score.

It is not necessary to perform routine checks of CK and liver function unless symptoms occur, or if statins are used in combination with fibrates, or other drugs that may interfere with their clearance. If myalgia or weakness occurs in association with CK elevation over 5–10 times the upper limit of normal, or if sustained alanine aminotransferase (ALT) elevation more than 2–3 times the upper limit of normal occurs that is not accounted for by fatty liver, treatment should be discontinued and alternative therapy sought.

The principles of the management of dyslipidaemia can be applied broadly, but the objectives of treatment in old age (Box 19.27) and the safety of pharmacological therapy in pregnancy (Box 19.28) warrant special consideration.

Inherited metabolic disorders

Inherited metabolic disorders are a large group of rare genetic diseases which result in disordered cellular metabolism. The majority are caused by variants in single genes that code for enzymes, leading to defective or absent enzyme activity. This leads to: (1) the accumulation of toxic metabolites that lie upstream within the pathway or (2) an inability to synthesise essential metabolites that are required for cellular function (Fig. 19.15). The vast majority of disorders are autosomal recessive.

Newborn screening, the availability of specific therapies, increased access to genetic testing and the recognition of attenuated, later-onset forms has led to a significant increase in the incidence and prevalence of inherited metabolic disorders, many of which are treatable. Treatment options are rapidly expanding with the use of gene therapies, RNA-based therapies and precision medicine techniques.

Disorders of amino acid metabolism

Inherited disorders of amino acid metabolism usually present in the neonatal period, but some disorders, especially of amino acid transport, may not present until later in life.

Phenylketonuria

The identification and successful dietary treatment of babies with phenylketonuria (PKU) has profoundly changed the outcome of this disorder, with patients now expected to live normal lives. PKU is caused by loss-of-function variants in the *PAH* gene, which encodes phenylalanine hxdroxylase, an enzyme required for the degradation of phenylalanine, an essential amino acid. Undegraded phenylalanine accumulates, causing direct neurotoxicity and profound neurodevelopmental disability. Treatment involves lifelong adherence to a low-phenylalanine diet with additional amino acid and nutrient supplements. Early and adequate dietary treatment prevents major neurodisability, and lifelong adherence is thought to prevent psychiatric morbidity and improve cognitive function. Treatment with sapropterin, which acts as a co-factor for phenylalanine hydroxylase, has been shown to reduce blood phenylalanine concentrations and increase phenylalanine tolerance in adults and children with PKU. However, its use is limited to patients with milder variants as well as by cost.

Maternal phenylketonuria syndrome, causing microcephaly, developmental delay and cardiac defects, is caused by exposure of the developing fetus to high levels of phenylalanine. Strict dietary adherence, both preconception and during pregnancy, prevents any deleterious effects in the offspring.

Homocystinuria

Homocystinuria is usually caused by variants in the *CBS* gene, leading to defective activity of the enzyme cystathione beta-synthase. This prevents homocysteine degradation, and causes toxic accumulation of homocysteine and methionine (upstream of the metabolic block). Multiple body systems are affected, including the central nervous system (developmental delay, intellectual disability, seizures and psychiatric disturbance); skeleton (tall stature, osteoporosis); eye (ectopia lentis – lens displacement) and cardiovascular system (arterial and venous thromboembolic disease). The

19.27 Management of hyperlipidaemia in old age

- Prevalence of atherosclerotic cardiovascular disease: greatest in old age.
- Associated cardiovascular risk: lipid levels become less predictive, as do other risk factors apart from age itself.
- Benefit of statin therapy: maintained up to the age of 80 years but evidence is lacking beyond this.
- Life expectancy and statin therapy: lives saved by intervention are associated with shorter life expectancy than in younger patients, and so the impact of statins on quality-adjusted life years is smaller in old age.

19.28 Dyslipidaemia in pregnancy

- **Lipid metabolism**: lipid and lipoprotein levels increase during pregnancy. This includes an increase in low-density lipoprotein cholesterol, which resolves postpartum. Remnant dyslipidaemia and hypertriglyceridaemia may be exacerbated during pregnancy.
- **Treatment**: dyslipidaemia is rarely thought to warrant urgent treatment so pharmacological therapy is usually contraindicated when conception or pregnancy is anticipated. Teratogenicity has been reported with systemically absorbed agents, and non-absorbed agents may interfere with nutrient bioavailability.
- **Monitoring**: while still uncommon among women of child-bearing age, cardiovascular disease is increasing in prevalence. Pre-conception cardiovascular review should be considered for women at high risk to optimise medications for pregnancy and to ensure that the patient will be able to withstand the demands of pregnancy and labour.

Normal metabolic pathway

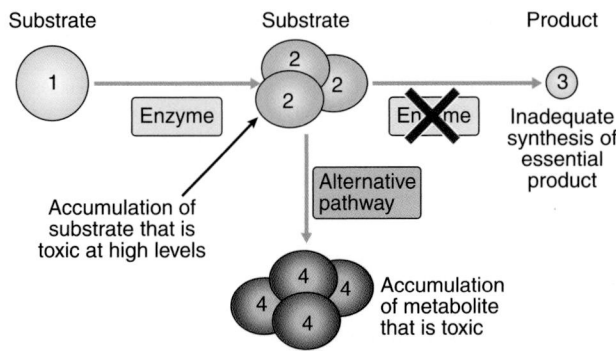

Inherited metabolic disorder

Fig. 19.15 Pathophysiology of inherited metabolic disorders. Inherited metabolic disorders cause disease either because there is lack of synthesis of an essential metabolite as the result of enzyme deficiency, or because there is accumulation of a toxic metabolite upstream of the deficient enzyme.

phenotypic spectrum is extremely variable and adults may present later in life, often with thromboembolic disease. Treatment aims to reduce homocysteine levels – through vitamin B6 (pyridoxine) – which acts as a cofactor to increase CBS enzyme activity, betaine, folate and vitamin B12 (to utilise the alternative homocysteine remethylation pathway) and consumption of a low-methionine diet. Early treatment and good compliance can prevent many of the expected complications.

Disorders of the urea cycle

Ammonia is generated by metabolism in all organs and transported to the liver for disposal by the urea cycle. Defects in any of the six urea cycle enzymes prevents normal ammonia degradation and can lead to life-threatening hyperammonaemia.

Ornithine tricarboxylase deficiency

Ornithine tricarboxylase (OTC) deficiency is the most common urea cycle disorder, and is an X-linked recessive disorder. Males often have severe neonatal disease, but the phenotypic spectrum, especially among women, is extremely wide. It may present later in life, often following a physiological stress such as trauma, surgery or post-partum. Acute hyperammonaemia may present as unexplained encephalopathy, often with respiratory alkalosis. If unrecognized, it can rapidly lead to cerebral oedema and death. Severe, neonatal onset disease can be treated by liver transplantation (the donated liver has normal enzyme activity). Later-onset disease can be managed with a protein-restricted diet, arginine supplementation and urea-scavenging medication (sodium benzoate and sodium or glycerol phenylbutyrate) to promote nitrogen excretion via alternative pathways.

Disorders of carbohydrate metabolism

Galactosaemia

Inherited variations in the *GALT* gene, causing loss of function of the enzyme galactose-1-phosphate uridyl transferase, lead to galactosaemia and an inability to metabolise galactose. In countries that do not screen for galactosaemia, patients usually present with neonatal crisis, with life-threatening liver and kidney failure, diarrhoea and cataracts,

often complicated by fulminant sepsis. Treatment is with a lactose- and galactose-free diet. This effectively prevents acute symptoms, but even with treatment there is almost always neuropsychological impairment and many patients exhibit slowly progressive neurological dysfunction over time. Premature ovarian failure occurs in almost all affected women.

Glycogen storage diseases

Glycogen storage diseases are a group of rare disorders that result from inherited defects in one of the many enzymes responsible for the formation, mobilisation or breakdown of glycogen, or of utilisation of glucose. The classification and enzyme defects responsible are summarised in Box 19.29. While glycogen storage disease type II (Pompe) is listed in this box, it is caused by deficiency in alpha glucosidase which is a lysosomal enzyme responsible for degradation of glycogen. Accordingly it is now classified as a lysosomal storage disease. The specific enzyme defect predicts symptomology and age of onset. Management is based upon avoidance of fasting, dietary modifications with frequent administration of carbohydrates and carefully managed exercise programmes to avoid hypoglycaemia. Enzyme replacement therapy with alglucosidase alfa is available for the treatment of Pompe disease.

Disorders of mitochondrial energy metabolism

During fasting or increased energy demand, fatty acid oxidation is an important source of mitochondrial energy production. Inherited variants causing loss of function in many of the enzymes involved in fatty acid oxidation and electron transfer within mitochondria have been identified. Many disorders have a catastrophic neonatal presentation, with hypoketotic hypoglycaemia, encephalopathy and liver dysfunction. Attenuated adult-onset forms are increasingly recognised, often with significant myopathy and/or acute rhabdomyolysis. Common precipitants in adulthood are endurance exercise events, such as running marathons, and alcohol. Management centres on the avoidance of fasting and provision of a regular carbohydrate energy source, with or without dietary modification of long chain or medium chain fats. Examples include carnitine palmitoyltransferase 2 (CPT2) deficiency, very long-chain acyl-CoA dehydrogenase (VLCAD) deficiency, medium-chain acyl-CoA dehydrogenase (MCAD) deficiency and multiple acyl-CoA dehydrogenase (MADD) deficiency.

Lysosomal storage disorders

The lysosome is an organelle responsible for the breakdown and resynthesis of macromolecules – essentially recycling and waste disposal – within the cell. Variants in genes encoding specific lysosomal enzymes cause loss of enzymatic function, and the accumulation of undegraded or partially degraded macromolecules within the lysosome, eventually leading to tissue damage in multiple body systems (Box 19.30). Biologic therapies with recombinant enzyme replacement therapy (ERT) have been developed to correct the metabolic defect and slow disease progression. The greatest benefit of ERT is seen with early treatment but it does does not penetrate the blood–brain barrier and is ineffective in treating neurological manifestations of disease. Some diseases appear more amenable to therapy than others. As ever, there is usually a spectrum of disease severity depending on the degree of residual enzyme function, and treating partial-loss-of-function variants with small molecule therapies to improve trafficking or support enzyme function, or as substrate reduction therapy, has shown promise as an alternative therapeutic strategy.

The porphyrias

These disorders are caused by enzymatic defects in the heme-biosynthesis pathway. Most are partial loss of function, with autosomal dominant inheritance and variable penetrance. Diagnosis relies on the detection of characteristic biochemical metabolites, as well as genetic variants and/or enzyme activity levels (Box 19.31)

19

i | **19.29 Glycogen storage diseases***

Type	Enzyme/transporter deficiency	Major phenotype	Clinical features/complications	Other names
0	Glycogen synthase	Liver	Fasting ketotic hypoglycaemia, postprandial lactic acidaemia	
I	Glucose-6-phosphatase	Liver Kidney Neutropenia	Infantile hypoglycaemia, ketosis, lactic acidosis and hepatomegaly	Von Gierke
II	Alpha-glucosidase	Muscle Heart Brain	Hypotonia, hypertrophic cardiomyopathy and developmental delay in infancy Limb girdle myopathy. Respiratory muscle weakness in adulthood	Pompe
III	Glycogen debrancher	Muscle Heart Liver	Infantile hepatomegaly and hypoglycaemia. Rhabdomyolysis, myopathy and cardiomyopathy in adulthood	Coris/Forbes
IV	Brancher	Muscle Brain Liver	Hepatomegaly, liver failure, myopathy	Anderson
V	Myophosphorylase	Muscle	Exercise intolerance and rhabdomyolysis	McArdle
VI	Glycogen phosphorylase	Liver	Hepatomegaly	Hers
VII	Muscle phosphofructokinase	Muscle	Exercise intolerance, rhabdomyolysis	Tarui
IX	Glycogen phosphorylase kinase	Liver Muscle	Hypoglycaemia Hepatomegaly	
X	Phosphoglcyerate mutase	Muscle	Exercise intolerance, rhabdomyolysis	
XI	GLUT-2	Liver Kidney	Hypoglycaemia, tubular dysfunction, hepatosplenomegaly, bone disease	Fanconi–Bickel

*Types II and IV are the most common syndromes. Some rarer causes of glycogen storage disease have not been included in this box.

i | **19.30 Lysosomal storage diseases***

Disease	Enzyme deficiency	Inheritance	Clinical features	Treatment
Fabry disease 1	Alpha-galactosidase	XLR	Acroparaesthesia, angiokeratoma, corneal verticillata Kidney disease (proteinuria and progressive CKD) Cardiomyopathy and arrhythmias Stroke and white matter changes	Enzyme replacement therapy Small molecule chaperone (amenable variants)
Gaucher disease	Glucocerebrocidase	AR	Hepatosplenomegaly Bone marrow infiltration and skeletal disease Thrombocytopenia Infantile neuronopathic form	Enzyme replacement therapy (not for neuronopathic disease) Substrate reduction therapies
Mucopolysaccharidosis	Eight different enzymes involved in the degradation of glycosaminoglycans	AR	Vary dependent on syndrome Skeletal, joint, valvular disease Characteristic facies Intellectual disability	Enzyme replacement therapy for MPSI; MPSII; MPS IV Limited by lack of efficacy in CNS disease
Gangliosidosis*	GM-1 beta-galactosidase GM-2 beta-hexosaminidase	AR	Severe progressive neurological disease	No specific treatment

*Some rare lysosomal storage diseases have been described which are not included in this box.
(AR = autosomal recessive; CKD = chronic kidney disease; CNS = central nervous system; MPS = mucopolysaccharidosis; XLR = X-linked recessive)

Acute porphyrias (the neurovisceral form) are characterised by acute attacks of abdominal pain and neuropathic symptoms, with neuropsychiatric symptoms, tachycardia, hypertension and hyponatraemia. Classically, the urine is pigmented, and darkens on exposure to light. The most common form is acute intermittent porphyria, caused by variants in *PBGD*, which encodes the enzyme porphobilinogen deaminase. Attacks are provoked by a relative depletion of heme, which removes the negative feedback regulation of the heme production pathway and stimulates heme biosynthesis. This results in the accumulation of delta-aminolaevulinic acid (ALA) and porphobilinogen (PBG) pre-cursors upstream of the metabolic block. ALA causes direct neurotoxicity. Urgent testing of urine for the presence of ALA and/or PBG will confirm the presence of an acute attack, and can be useful to differentiate between acute porphyria attacks and other causes.

Attacks can be provoked by fasting, trauma, intercurrent infection, alcohol, drugs, the menstrual cycle and hormonal contraceptives. A list of safe drugs can be found at www.drugs-porphyria.org. Cyclical attacks in menstruating women can respond to suppression of the menstrual cycle with gonadotrophin-releasing hormone analogues.

19.31 Diagnostic biochemical findings in the porphyrias

Condition	Biochemical abnormalities (protect specimens from light)		
	Urine	Blood	Faeces
Acute intermittent porphyria	↑ALA ↑ PBG		
Hereditary coproporphyria	↑ALA ↑ PBG ↑ Copro III		↑ Copro III
Variegate porphyria	↑ALA ↑PBG ↑ Copro III		↑ Proto IX
Erythropoietic protoporphyria		↑ Proto IX	↑ Proto IX
Porphyria cutanea tarda	↑ Uro I		

(ALA = delta-aminolaevulinic acid; Copro III = coproporphyrin III; PBG = porphobilinogen; Proto IX = protoporphorin IX; Uro I = uroporphyrin I)

Management centres on the avoidance of provoking factors, and the provision of an 'emergency protocol' to administer oral carbohydrates (glucose polymer) or intravenous dextrose with electrolytes in order to terminate an acute attack. In severe cases, intravenous heme arginate inhibits the heme biosynthesis pathway, thereby reducing the production of toxic metabolites. However, it is an irritant and frequently causes local phlebitis. Recently, RNA interference therapy has been shown to inhibit ALA synthesis and reduce the rate of acute porphyria attacks in severely affected patients.

Cutaneous porphyrias

The cutaneous manifestations of porphyria cutanea tarda, erythropoietic porphyria, variegate porphyria and hereditary coproporphyria are discussed in more detail in Chapter 27. It should be noted, however, that variegate porphyria and hereditary coproporphyria can have both neurovisceral and cutaneous features.

Further information

Journal articles

Lachmann RH. Treating lysosomal storage disorders: What have we learnt? J Inherit Metab Dis 2020;43(1):125–132.
Lilleker JB, Keh YS, Roncaroli F, et al. Metabolic myopathies: a practical approach. Pract Neurol 2018;18(1):14–26.
Spasovski G, Vanholder R, Allolio B, et al. Clinical practice guideline on diagnosis and treatment of hyponatraemia. Eur J Endocrinol 2014;170:G1–G47.
Stein P, Badminton M, Barth J, et al. Best practice guidelines on clinical management of acute attacks of porphyria and their complications. Ann Clin Biochem 2013;50(3):217–223.
Walsh S, Unwin R. Renal tubular disorders. Clin Med 2012;12(5):476–479.

Websites

emedicine.medscape.com The Nephrology link on this site contains a useful compendium of articles.
escardio.org/Guidelines/Clinical-Practice-Guidelines/Dyslipidaemias-Management-of European Cardiac Society guidelines on management of hyperlipidaemia.
ncbi.nlm.nih.gov The link to OMIM (Online Mendelian Inheritance in Man) provides updated information on the genetic basis of metabolic disorders.
porphyria.eu and drugs-porphyria.org Excellent resources on drug safety in porphyria.
www.BIMDG.org.uk Emergency treatment guidance for inherited metabolic disorders.

19

JDC Newell-Price
FW Gibb

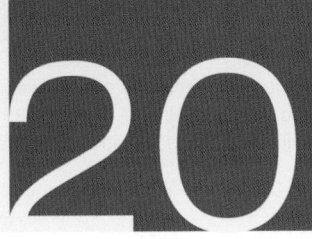

20

Endocrinology

Clinical examination in endocrine disease

Endocrine disease causes clinical syndromes with symptoms and signs involving many organ systems. The emphasis of the clinical examination depends on the gland or hormone that is thought to be abnormal.

Diabetes mellitus (described in detail in Ch. 21) and thyroid disease are the most common endocrine disorders.

5 Blood pressure
Hypertension in Cushing's and Conn syndromes, phaeochromocytoma
Hypotension in adrenal insufficiency

4 Pulse
Atrial fibrillation
Sinus tachycardia
Bradycardia

3 Skin
Hair distribution
Dry/greasy
Pigmentation/pallor
Bruising
Vitiligo
Striae
Thickness

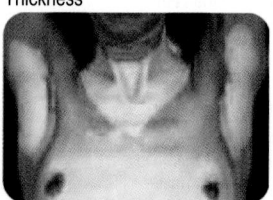

▲ Vitiligo in organ-specific autoimmune disease

2 Hands
Palmar erythema
Tremor
Acromegaly
Carpal tunnel syndrome

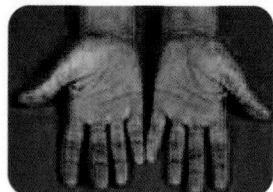

▲ Pigmentation of creases due to high ACTH levels in Addison's disease

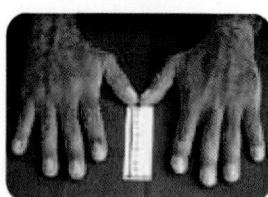

▲ Acromegalic hands. Note soft tissue enlargement causing 'spade-like' changes

1 Height and weight

6 Head

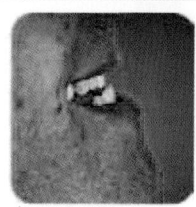

▲ Prognathism in acromegaly

Eyes
  Graves' disease (see opposite)
  Diplopia
  Visual field defect (see opposite)
Hair
  Alopecia
  Frontal balding

Facial features
  Hypothyroid
  Hirsutism
  Acromegaly
  Cushing's

Mental state
  Lethargy
  Depression
  Delirium
  Libido

7 Neck
Voice
  Hoarse, e.g. hypothyroid
  Virilised
Thyroid gland (see opposite)
  Goitre
  Nodules

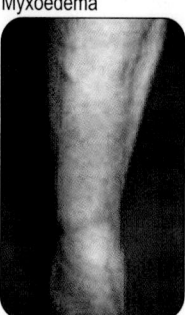

Multinodular goitre ◀

8 Breasts
Galactorrhoea
Gynaecomastia

9 Body fat
Central obesity in Cushing's syndrome and growth hormone deficiency

10 Bones
Fragility fractures (e.g. of vertebrae, neck of femur or distal radius)

11 Genitalia
Virilisation
Pubertal development
Testicular volume

12 Legs
Proximal myopathy
Myxoedema

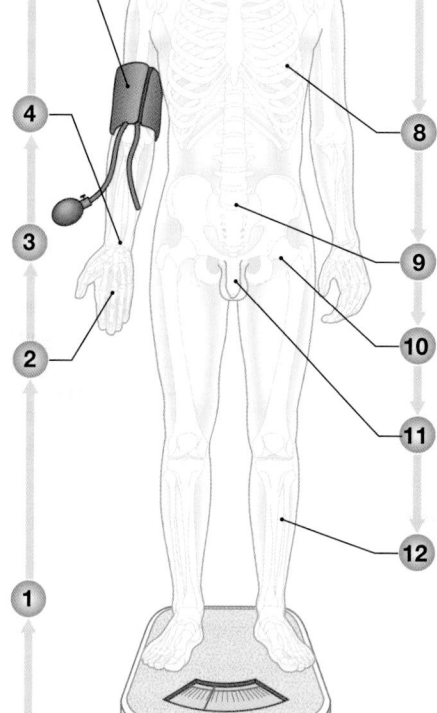

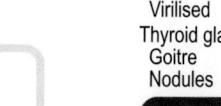
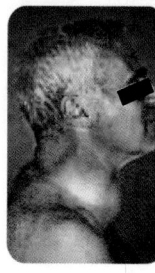

Observation
- Most examination in endocrinology is by observation
- Astute observation can often yield 'spot' diagnosis of endocrine disorders
- The emphasis of examination varies depending on which gland or hormone is thought to be involved

▲ Pretibial myxoedema in Graves' disease

(6) Examination of the visual fields by confrontation

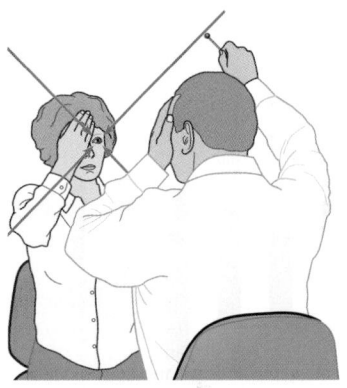

- Sit opposite patient
- You and patient cover opposite eyes
- Bring red pin (or wiggling finger) slowly into view from extreme of your vision, as shown
- Ask patient to say 'now' when it comes into view
- Continue to move pin into centre of vision and ask patient to tell you if it disappears
- Repeat in each of four quadrants
- Repeat in other eye

A bitemporal hemianopia is the classical finding in pituitary macroadenomas (p. 695)

(6) Examination in Graves' ophthalmopathy

- **Inspect** from front and side
  Periorbital oedema (Fig. 20.9)
  Conjunctival inflammation (chemosis)
  Corneal ulceration
  Proptosis (exophthalmos)*
  Lid retraction*

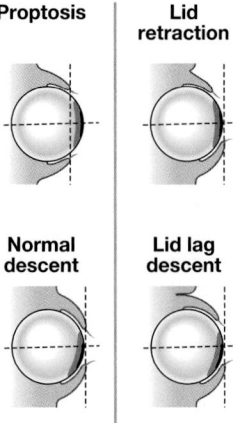

- **Range of eye movements**
  Lid lag on descending gaze*
  Diplopia on lateral gaze

- **Pupillary reflexes**
  Afferent defect (pupils constrict further on swinging light to unaffected eye, Box 28.21)

- **Vision**
  Visual acuity impaired
  Loss of colour vision
  Visual field defects

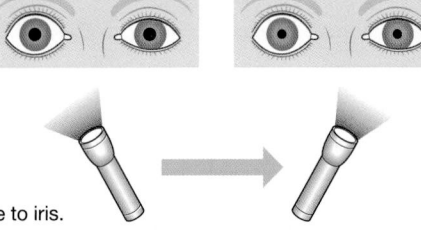

Right proptosis and afferent pupillary defect

- **Ophthalmoscopy**
  Optic disc pallor
  Papilloedema

*Note position of eyelids relative to iris.

(7) Examination of the thyroid gland

- **Inspect** from front to side

- **Palpate** from behind
  Thyroid moves on swallowing
  Check if lower margin is palpable
  Cervical lymph nodes
  Tracheal deviation

- **Auscultate** for bruit
  Ask patient to hold breath
  If present, check for radiating murmur

- **Percuss** for retrosternal thyroid

- Consider systemic signs of thyroid dysfunction (Box 20.7) incl. tremor, palmar erythema, warm peripheries, tachycardia, lid lag

- Consider signs of Graves' disease incl. ophthalmopathy, pretibial myxoedema

- Check for Pemberton's sign, i.e. facial engorgement when arms raised above head

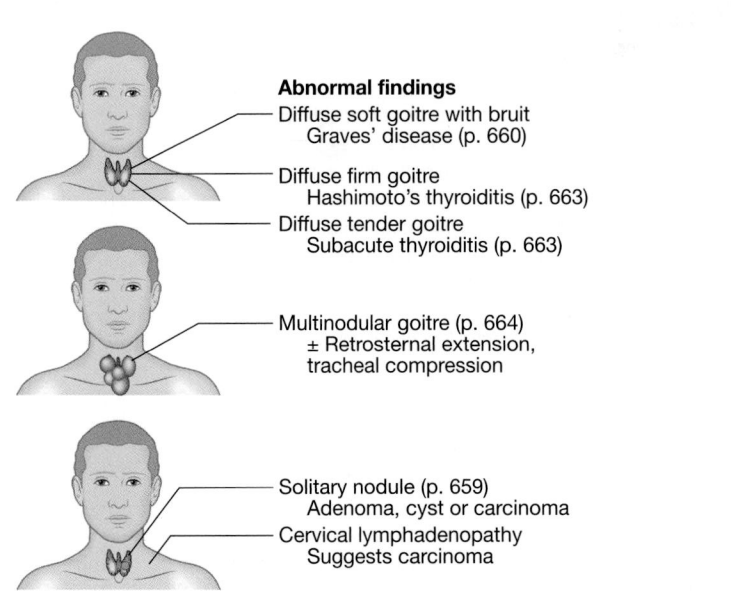

Abnormal findings
Diffuse soft goitre with bruit
  Graves' disease (p. 660)

Diffuse firm goitre
  Hashimoto's thyroiditis (p. 663)
Diffuse tender goitre
  Subacute thyroiditis (p. 663)

Multinodular goitre (p. 664)
  ± Retrosternal extension, tracheal compression

Solitary nodule (p. 659)
  Adenoma, cyst or carcinoma
Cervical lymphadenopathy
  Suggests carcinoma

20

Endocrinology concerns the synthesis, secretion and action of hormones. These are chemical messengers released from endocrine glands that coordinate the activities of many different cells. Endocrine diseases can therefore affect multiple organs and systems. This chapter describes the principles of endocrinology before dealing with the function and diseases of each gland in turn.

Some endocrine disorders are common, particularly those of the thyroid, parathyroid glands, reproductive system and β cells of the pancreas (Ch. 21). For example, thyroid dysfunction occurs in more than 10% of the population in areas with iodine deficiency, such as the Himalayas, and 4% of women aged 20–50 years in the UK. Less common endocrine syndromes are described later in the chapter.

Few endocrine therapies have been evaluated by randomised controlled trials, in part because hormone replacement therapy (e.g. with levothyroxine) has obvious clinical benefits and placebo-controlled trials would be unethical. Where trials have been performed, they relate mainly to use of therapy that is 'optional' and/or more recently available, such as oestrogen replacement in post-menopausal women, androgen therapy in older men and growth hormone replacement.

An overview of endocrinology

Functional anatomy and physiology

Some endocrine glands, such as the parathyroids and pancreas, respond directly to metabolic signals, but most are controlled by hormones released from the pituitary gland. Anterior pituitary hormone secretion is controlled in turn by substances produced in the hypothalamus and released into portal blood, which drains directly down the pituitary stalk (Fig. 20.1). Posterior pituitary hormones are synthesised in the hypothalamus and transported down nerve axons, to be released from the posterior pituitary. Hormone release in the hypothalamus and pituitary is regulated by numerous stimuli and through feedback control by hormones produced by the target glands (thyroid, adrenal cortex and gonads). These integrated endocrine systems are called 'axes' and are listed in Figure 20.2.

A wide variety of molecules can act as hormones, including peptides such as insulin and growth hormone, glycoproteins such as thyroid-stimulating hormone, and amines such as noradrenaline (norepinephrine). The biological effects of hormones are mediated by binding to receptors. Many receptors are located on the cell surface. These interact with various intracellular signalling molecules on the cytosolic side of the plasma membrane to affect cell function, usually through changes in gene expression. Some hormones, most notably steroids, bind to specific intracellular receptors. The hormone/receptor complex forms a ligand-activated transcription factor, which regulates gene expression directly.

The classical model of endocrine function involves hormones synthesised in endocrine glands, which are released into the circulation and act at sites distant from those of secretion (as in Fig. 20.1). However, additional levels of regulation are now recognised. Many other organs secrete hormones or contribute to the peripheral metabolism and activation of prohormones. A notable example is the production of oestrogens from adrenal androgens in adipose tissue by the enzyme aromatase. Some hormones, such as neurotransmitters, act in a paracrine fashion to affect adjacent cells, or act in an autocrine way to affect behaviour of the cell that produces the hormone.

Endocrine pathology

For each endocrine axis or major gland, diseases can be classified as shown in Box 20.1. Pathology arising within the gland is often called 'primary' disease (e.g. primary hypothyroidism in Hashimoto's thyroiditis), while abnormal stimulation of the gland is often called 'secondary' disease (e.g. secondary hypothyroidism in patients with a pituitary tumour

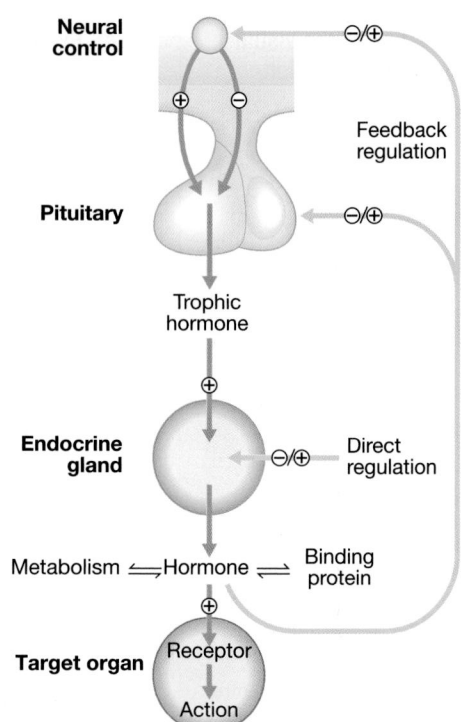

Fig. 20.1 An archetypal endocrine axis. Regulation by negative feedback and direct control is shown, along with the equilibrium between active circulating free hormone and bound or metabolised hormone.

---

i   20.1 Classification of endocrine disease

Hormone excess
- Primary gland over-production
- Secondary to excess trophic substance

Hormone deficiency
- Primary gland failure
- Secondary to deficient trophic hormone

Hormone hypersensitivity
- Failure of inactivation of hormone
- Target organ over-activity/hypersensitivity

Hormone resistance
- Failure of activation by hormone
- Target organ resistance

Non-functioning tumours
- Benign
- Malignant

---

and thyroid-stimulating hormone deficiency). Some pathological processes can affect multiple endocrine glands; these may have a genetic basis (such as organ-specific autoimmune endocrine disorders and the multiple endocrine neoplasia (MEN) syndromes) or be a consequence of therapy for another disease (e.g. following treatment of childhood cancer with chemotherapy and/or radiotherapy).

Investigation of endocrine disease

Biochemical investigations play a central role in endocrinology. Most hormones can be measured in blood but the circumstances in which the sample is taken are often crucial, especially for hormones with pulsatile secretion, such as growth hormone; those that show circadian variation,

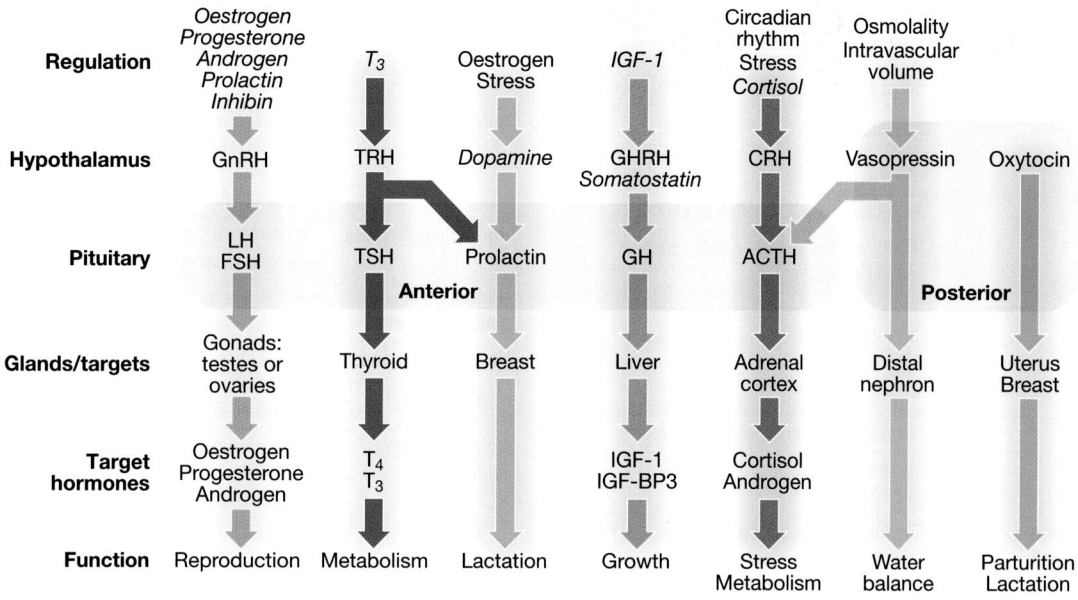

Fig. 20.2 The principal endocrine 'axes'. Some major endocrine glands are not controlled by the pituitary. These include the parathyroid glands (regulated by calcium concentrations, p. 675), the adrenal zona glomerulosa (regulated by the renin–angiotensin system, p.679) and the endocrine pancreas (p. 689). Italics show negative regulation. (ACTH = adrenocorticotrophic hormone; CRH = corticotrophin-releasing hormone; FSH = follicle-stimulating hormone; GH = growth hormone; GHRH = growth hormone-releasing hormone; GnRH = gonadotrophin-releasing hormone; IGF-1 = insulin-like growth factor-1; IGF-BP3 = IGF-binding protein-3; LH = luteinising hormone: T_3 = triiodothyronine; T_4 = thyroxine; TRH = thyrotrophin-releasing hormone; TSH = thyroid-stimulating hormone; vasopressin = antidiuretic hormone (ADH))

such as cortisol; or those that demonstrate monthly variation, such as oestrogen or progesterone. Some hormones are labile and need special collection, handling and processing requirements, e.g. collection in a special tube and/or rapid transportation to the laboratory on ice. Local protocols for hormone measurement should be carefully followed. Other investigations, such as imaging and biopsy, are more frequently reserved for patients who present with a tumour. The principles of investigation are shown in Box 20.2. The choice of test is often pragmatic, taking local access to reliable sampling facilities and laboratory measurements into account.

Presenting problems in endocrine disease

Endocrine diseases present in many different ways and to clinicians in many different disciplines. Classical syndromes are described in relation to individual glands in the following sections. Often, however, the presentation is with non-specific symptoms (Box 20.3) or with asymptomatic biochemical abnormalities. In addition, endocrine diseases are encountered in the differential diagnosis of common complaints discussed in other chapters of this book, including electrolyte abnormalities (Ch. 19, hypertension (Ch. 16), obesity (Ch. 22) and osteoporosis (Ch. 26). Although diseases of the adrenal glands, hypothalamus and pituitary are relatively rare, their diagnosis often relies on astute clinical observation in a patient with non-specific complaints, so it is important that clinicians are familiar with their key features.

The thyroid gland

Diseases of the thyroid, summarised in Box 20.4, predominantly affect females and are common, occurring in about 5% of the population. The thyroid axis is involved in the regulation of cellular differentiation and metabolism in virtually all nucleated cells, so that disorders of thyroid function have diverse manifestations. Structural diseases of the thyroid gland, such as goitre, commonly occur in patients with normal thyroid function.

 20.2 Principles of endocrine investigation

Timing of measurement
- Release of many hormones is rhythmical (pulsatile, circadian or monthly), so random measurement may be invalid and sequential or dynamic tests may be required

Choice of dynamic biochemical test
- Abnormalities are often characterised by loss of normal regulation of hormone secretion
- If hormone deficiency is suspected, choose a stimulation test
- If hormone excess is suspected, choose a suppression test
- The more tests there are to choose from, the less likely it is that any single test is infallible, so avoid interpreting one result in isolation

Imaging
- 'Functional' as well as conventional 'structural' imaging can be performed as secretory endocrine cells can also take up labelled substrates, e.g. radio-labelled iodine or octreotide
- Most endocrine glands have a high prevalence of 'incidentalomas', so do not scan unless the biochemistry confirms endocrine dysfunction or the primary problem is a tumour

Biopsy
- Many endocrine tumours are difficult to classify histologically (e.g. adrenal carcinoma and adenoma)

20

Functional anatomy, physiology and investigations

Thyroid physiology is illustrated in Figure 20.3. The parafollicular C cells secrete calcitonin, which is of no apparent physiological significance in humans. The follicular epithelial cells synthesise thyroid hormones by incorporating iodine into the amino acid tyrosine on the surface of thyroglobulin (Tg), a protein secreted into the colloid of the follicle. Iodide is a key substrate for thyroid hormone synthesis; a dietary intake in excess of 100 µg/day is required to maintain thyroid function in adults. The thyroid secretes predominantly thyroxine (T_4) and only a small amount of

i | **20.3 Examples of non-specific presentations of endocrine disease***

Symptom	Most likely endocrine disorder(s)
Lethargy and depression	Hypothyroidism, diabetes mellitus, hyperparathyroidism, hypogonadism, adrenal insufficiency, Cushing's syndrome
Weight gain	Hypothyroidism, Cushing's syndrome
Weight loss	Thyrotoxicosis, adrenal insufficiency, diabetes mellitus
Polyuria and polydipsia	Diabetes mellitus, diabetes insipidus, hyperparathyroidism, hypokalaemia (Conn syndrome)
Heat intolerance*	Thyrotoxicosis
Palpitation	Thyrotoxicosis, phaeochromocytoma
Headache	Acromegaly, pituitary tumour, phaeochromocytoma
Muscle weakness (usually proximal)	Thyrotoxicosis, Cushing's syndrome, hypokalaemia (e.g. Conn syndrome), hyperparathyroidism, hypogonadism
Coarsening of features	Acromegaly, hypothyroidism

*Heat intolerance is a common feature of menopause.

i | **20.4 Classification of thyroid disease**

	Primary	Secondary
Hormone excess	Graves' disease Multinodular goitre Adenoma Subacute thyroiditis	TSHoma
Hormone deficiency	Hashimoto's thyroiditis Atrophic hypothyroidism	Hypopituitarism
Hormone hypersensitivity	–	
Hormone resistance	Thyroid hormone resistance syndrome 5′-monodeiodinase deficiency	
Non-functioning tumours	Differentiated carcinoma Medullary carcinoma Lymphoma	

triiodothyronine (T_3); approximately 85% of T_3 in blood is produced from T_4 by a family of monodeiodinase enzymes that are active in many tissues, including liver, muscle, heart and kidney. Selenium is an integral component of these monodeiodinases. T_4 can be regarded as a pro-hormone, since it has a longer half-life in blood than T_3 (approximately 1 week compared with approximately 18 hours), and binds and activates thyroid hormone receptors less effectively than T_3. T_4 can also be converted to the inactive metabolite, reverse T_3.

T_3 and T_4 circulate in plasma almost entirely (>99%) bound to transport proteins, mainly thyroxine-binding globulin (TBG). It is the unbound or free hormones that diffuse into tissues and exert diverse metabolic actions. Some laboratories use assays that measure total T_4 and T_3 in plasma but it is increasingly common to measure free T_4 and free T_3. The theoretical advantage of the free hormone measurements is that they are not influenced by changes in the concentration of binding proteins. For example, TBG levels are increased by oestrogen (such as in the combined oral contraceptive pill) and this will result in raised total T_3 and T_4, although free thyroid hormone levels are normal.

Production of T_3 and T_4 in the thyroid is stimulated by thyrotrophin (thyroid-stimulating hormone, TSH), a glycoprotein released from the thyrotroph cells of the anterior pituitary in response to the hypothalamic tripeptide, thyrotrophin-releasing hormone (TRH). A circadian rhythm of TSH secretion can be demonstrated with a peak at 0100 hrs and trough at 1100 hrs, but the variation is small so that thyroid function can be assessed reliably from a single blood sample taken at any time of day and does not usually require any dynamic stimulation or suppression tests. There is a negative feedback of thyroid hormones on the hypothalamus and pituitary such that in thyrotoxicosis, when plasma concentrations of T_3 and T_4 are raised, TSH secretion is suppressed. Conversely, in hypothyroidism due to disease of the thyroid gland, low T_3 and T_4 are associated with high circulating TSH levels. The relationship between TSH and T_4 is classically described as inverse log-linear (Fig. 20.4). The anterior pituitary is, though, very sensitive to minor changes in thyroid hormone levels within the reference range. For example, in an individual whose free T_4 level is usually 15 pmol/L (1.17 ng/dL), a rise or fall of 5 pmol/L (0.39 ng/dL) would be associated on the one hand with undetectable TSH, and on the other hand with a raised TSH. For this reason, TSH is usually regarded as the most useful investigation of thyroid function. However, interpretation of TSH values without considering thyroid hormone levels may be misleading in patients with pituitary disease; for example, TSH is inappropriately low or 'normal' in secondary hypothyroidism (see Box 20.5 and Box 20.51). Moreover, TSH may take several weeks to 'catch up' with T_4 and T_3 levels; for example, levothyroxine therapy will raise T_4 and T_3 levels within approximately 2 weeks but it may take 4–6 weeks for the TSH to reach a steady state. Heterophilic antibodies (host antibodies with affinity to the animal antibodies used in biological assays) can also interfere with the TSH assay and cause a spurious high or low measurement. Common patterns of abnormal thyroid function test results and their interpretation are shown in Box 20.5.

Other modalities commonly employed in the investigation of thyroid disease include measurement of antibodies against the TSH receptor or other thyroid antigens (see Box 20.8), radioisotope imaging, fine needle aspiration biopsy and ultrasound. Their use is described below.

Presenting problems in thyroid disease

The most common presentations are hyperthyroidism (thyrotoxicosis), hypothyroidism and enlargement of the thyroid (goitre or thyroid nodule). Widespread availability of thyroid function tests has led to the increasingly frequent identification of patients with abnormal results who either are asymptomatic or have non-specific complaints such as tiredness and weight gain.

Thyrotoxicosis

Thyrotoxicosis describes a constellation of clinical features arising from elevated circulating levels of thyroid hormone. The most common causes are Graves' disease, multinodular goitre, autonomously functioning thyroid nodules (toxic adenoma) and thyroiditis (Box 20.6).

Clinical assessment

The clinical manifestations of thyrotoxicosis are shown in Box 20.7 and an approach to differential diagnosis is given in Figure 20.5. The most common symptoms are weight loss with a normal or increased appetite, heat intolerance, palpitations, tremor and irritability. Tachycardia, palmar erythema and lid lag are common signs. Not all patients have a palpable goitre, but experienced clinicians can discriminate the diffuse soft goitre of Graves' disease from the irregular enlargement of a multinodular goitre. All causes of thyrotoxicosis can cause lid retraction and lid lag, due to potentiation of sympathetic innervation of the levator palpebrae muscles, but only Graves' disease causes other features of ophthalmopathy, including periorbital oedema, conjunctival irritation, exophthalmos

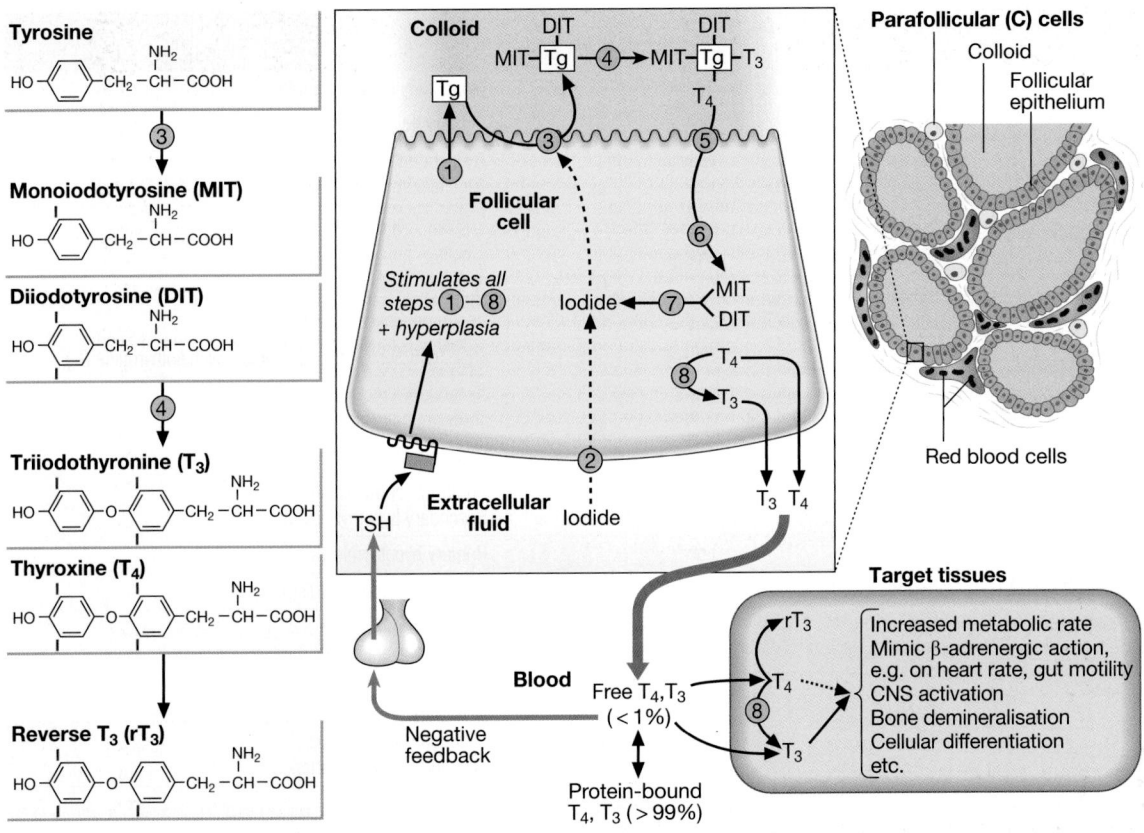

Fig. 20.3 Structure and function of the thyroid gland. (1) Thyroglobulin (Tg) is synthesised and secreted into the colloid of the follicle. (2) Inorganic iodide (I^-) is actively transported into the follicular cell ('trapping'). (3) Iodide is transported on to the colloidal surface by a transporter (pendrin, defective in Pendred syndrome, p. 667) and 'organified' by the thyroid peroxidase enzyme, which incorporates it into the amino acid tyrosine on the surface of Tg to form monoiodotyrosine (MIT) and diiodotyrosine (DIT). (4) Iodinated tyrosines couple to form triiodothyronine (T_3) and thyroxine (T_4). (5) Tg is endocytosed. (6) Tg is cleaved by proteolysis to free the iodinated tyrosine and thyroid hormones. (7) Iodinated tyrosine is dehalogenated to recycle the iodide. (8) T_4 is converted to T_3 by 5'-monodeiodinase. (CNS = central nervous system; TSH = thyroid-stimulating hormone)

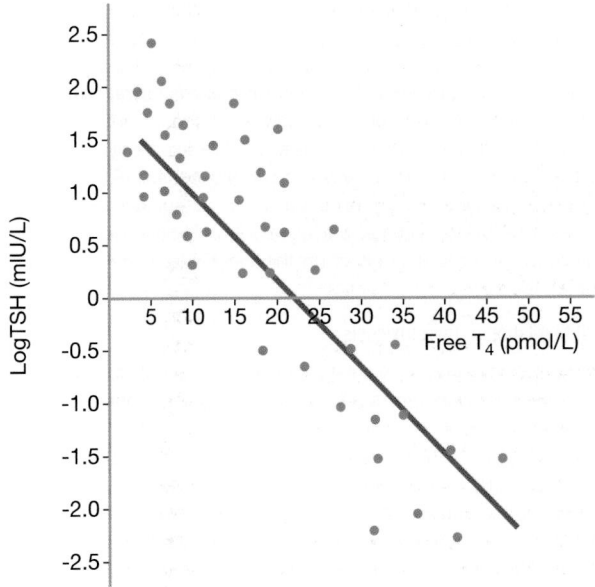

Fig. 20.4 The relationship between serum thyroid-stimulating hormone (TSH) and free T_4. Due to the classic negative feedback loop between T_4 and TSH, there is an inverse relationship between serum free T_4 and the log of serum TSH. To convert pmol/L to ng/dL, divide by 12.87.

and diplopia. Pretibial myxoedema (see p. 663) and the rare thyroid acropachy (a periosteal hypertrophy, indistinguishable from finger clubbing) are also specific to Graves' disease.

Investigations

The first-line investigations are serum T_3, T_4 and TSH. If abnormal values are found, the tests should be repeated and the abnormality confirmed in view of the likely need for prolonged medical treatment or destructive therapy. In most patients, serum T_3 and T_4 are both elevated, but T_4 is in the upper part of the reference range and T_3 is raised (T_3 toxicosis) in about 5%. Serum TSH is undetectable in primary thyrotoxicosis, but values can be raised in the very rare syndrome of secondary thyrotoxicosis caused by a TSH-producing pituitary adenoma. When biochemical thyrotoxicosis has been confirmed, measurement of TSH receptor antibodies (TRAb, elevated in Graves' disease; Box 20.8) is recommended. Where TRAb is not available, radioisotope scanning is an alternative diagnostic approach, as shown in Figure 20.5. Other non-specific abnormalities are common (Box 20.9). An electrocardiogram (ECG) may demonstrate sinus tachycardia or atrial fibrillation.

Radio-iodine uptake tests measure the proportion of isotope that is trapped in the whole gland but have been largely superseded by ^{99m}technetium scintigraphy scans, which also indicate trapping, are quicker to perform with a lower dose of radioactivity, and provide a higher-resolution image. In low-uptake thyrotoxicosis, the cause is usually a transient thyroiditis. Occasionally, patients induce 'factitious thyrotoxicosis' by consuming excessive amounts of a thyroid hormone preparation, most often levothyroxine. The exogenous levothyroxine suppresses pituitary TSH secretion and hence iodine uptake, serum thyroglobulin and release

i 20.5 How to interpret thyroid function test results

TSH	T_4	T_3	Most likely interpretation(s)
Undetectable	Raised	Raised	Primary thyrotoxicosis
Undetectable or low	Raised	Normal	Over-treatment of hypothyroidism with levothyroxine Factitious thyrotoxicosis
Undetectable	Normal[1]	Raised	Primary T_3 toxicosis
Undetectable	Normal[1]	Normal[1]	Subclinical thyrotoxicosis
Undetectable or low	Raised	Low or normal	Non-thyroidal illness Amiodarone therapy
Undetectable or low	Low	Raised	Over-treatment of hypothyroidism with liothyronine (T_3)
Undetectable	Low	Low	Secondary hypothyroidism[4] Transient thyroiditis in evolution
Normal	Low	Low[2]	Secondary hypothyroidism[4]
Mildly elevated 5–20 mIU/L	Low	Low[2]	Primary hypothyroidism Secondary hypothyroidism[4]
Elevated >20 mIU/L	Low	Low[2]	Primary hypothyroidism
Mildly elevated 5–20 mIU/L	Normal[3]	Normal[2]	Subclinical hypothyroidism
Elevated 20–500 mIU/L	Normal	Normal	Artefact Heterophilic antibodies (host antibodies with affinity to the animal antibodies used in TSH assays)
Elevated	Raised	Raised	Non-adherence to levothyroxine replacement – recent 'loading' dose Secondary thyrotoxicosis[4] Thyroid hormone resistance

[1]Usually upper part of reference range. [2]T_3 is not a sensitive indicator of hypothyroidism and should not be requested. [3]Usually lower part of reference range. [4]i.e. Secondary to pituitary or hypothalamic disease. Note that TSH assays may report detectable TSH.
(TSH = thyroid-stimulating hormone)

i 20.6 Causes of thyrotoxicosis and their relative frequencies

Cause	Frequency[1] (%)
Graves' disease	76
Multinodular goitre	14
Solitary thyroid adenoma	5
Thyroiditis Subacute (de Quervain's)[2] Post-partum[2]	 3 0.5
Iodide-induced Drugs (amiodarone)[2] Radiographic contrast media[2] Iodine supplementation programme[2]	 1 – –
Extrathyroidal source of thyroid hormone Factitious thyrotoxicosis[2] Struma ovarii[2,3]	 0.2 –
TSH-induced TSH-secreting pituitary adenoma Choriocarcinoma and hydatidiform mole[4] Follicular carcinoma±metastases	 0.2 – 0.1

[1]In a series of 2087 patients presenting to the Royal Infirmary of Edinburgh over a 10-year period. [2]Characterised by negligible radioisotope uptake. [3]i.e. Ovarian teratoma containing thyroid tissue. [4]Human chorionic gonadotrophin has thyroid-stimulating activity.
(TSH = thyroid-stimulating hormone)

of endogenous thyroid hormones. The T_4:T_3 ratio (typically 30:1 in conventional thyrotoxicosis) is increased to above 70:1 because circulating T_3 in factitious thyrotoxicosis is derived exclusively from the peripheral monodeiodination of T_4 and not from thyroid secretion. The combination of negligible iodine uptake, high T_4:T_3 ratio and a low or undetectable thyroglobulin is diagnostic.

Management

Definitive treatment of thyrotoxicosis depends on the underlying cause and may include antithyroid drugs, radioactive iodine or surgery. A non-selective β-adrenoceptor antagonist (β-blocker), such as propranolol (160 mg daily), will alleviate but not abolish symptoms in most patients within 24–48 hours. Beta-blockers should not be used for long-term treatment of thyrotoxicosis but are extremely useful in the short term, while patients are awaiting hospital consultation or following ^{131}I therapy. Verapamil may be used as an alternative to β-blockers, e.g. in patients with asthma, but usually is only effective in improving tachycardia and has little effect on the other systemic manifestations of thyrotoxicosis.

Atrial fibrillation in thyrotoxicosis

Atrial fibrillation occurs in about 10% of patients with thyrotoxicosis. The incidence is higher in men and increases with age, so that almost half of all males with thyrotoxicosis over the age of 60 are affected. Moreover, subclinical thyrotoxicosis (see p. 659) is a risk factor for atrial fibrillation. Characteristically, the ventricular rate is little influenced by digoxin but responds to the addition of a β-blocker. Thromboembolic vascular complications are particularly common in thyrotoxic atrial fibrillation so that anticoagulation is required, unless contraindicated. Once thyroid hormone and TSH concentrations have been returned to normal, atrial fibrillation will spontaneously revert to sinus rhythm in about 50% of patients but cardioversion may be required in the remainder.

Thyrotoxic crisis ('thyroid storm')

This is a rare but life-threatening complication of thyrotoxicosis. The most prominent signs are fever, agitation, delirium, tachycardia or atrial fibrillation and, in the older patient, cardiac failure. Thyrotoxic crisis is a

i | **20.7 Clinical features of thyroid dysfunction**

Thyrotoxicosis		Hypothyroidism	
Symptoms	**Signs**	**Symptoms**	**Signs**
Common			
Weight loss despite normal or increased appetite	Weight loss	Weight gain	Weight gain
Heat intolerance, sweating	Tremor	Cold intolerance	
Palpitations, tremor	Palmar erythema	Fatigue, somnolence	
Dyspnoea, fatigue	Sinus tachycardia	Dry skin	
Irritability, emotional lability	Lid retraction, lid lag	Dry hair	
		Menorrhagia	
Less common			
Osteoporosis (fracture, loss of height)	Goitre with bruit[1]	Constipation	Hoarse voice
Diarrhoea, steatorrhoea	Atrial fibrillation[2]	Hoarseness	Facial features:
Angina	Systolic hypertension/increased pulse pressure	Carpal tunnel syndrome	Purplish lips
Ankle swelling		Alopecia	Malar flush
Anxiety, psychosis	Cardiac failure[2]	Aches and pains	Periorbital oedema
Muscle weakness	Hyper-reflexia	Muscle stiffness	Loss of lateral eyebrows
Periodic paralysis (predominantly in Chinese and other Asian groups)	Ill-sustained clonus	Deafness	Anaemia
	Proximal myopathy	Depression	Carotenaemia
Pruritus, alopecia	Bulbar myopathy[2]	Infertility	Erythema ab igne
Amenorrhoea/oligomenorrhoea			Bradycardia hypertension
Infertility, spontaneous abortion			Delayed relaxation of reflexes
Loss of libido, impotence			Dermal myxoedema
Excessive lacrimation			
Rare			
Vomiting	Gynaecomastia	Psychosis (myxoedema madness)	Ileus, ascites
Apathy	Spider naevi	Galactorrhoea	Pericardial and pleural effusions
Anorexia	Onycholysis	Impotence	Cerebellar ataxia
Exacerbation of asthma	Pigmentation		Myotonia

[1]In Graves' disease only. [2]Features found particularly in older patients.

i | **20.8 Prevalence of thyroid autoantibodies (%)**

	Antibodies to:		
	Thyroid peroxidase[1]	**Thyroglobulin**	**TSH receptor[2]**
Normal population	8–27	5–20	0
Graves' disease	50–80	50–70	>95
Autoimmune hypothyroidism	90–100	80–90	10–20
Multinodular goitre	~30–40	~30–40	0
Transient thyroiditis	~30–40	~30–40	0

[1]Thyroid peroxidase (TPO) antibodies are the principal component of what was previously measured as thyroid 'microsomal' antibodies. [2]Thyroid-stimulating hormone receptor antibodies (TRAb) can be agonists (stimulatory, causing Graves' thyrotoxicosis) or antagonists ('blocking', causing hypothyroidism).

medical emergency and has a mortality of 10% despite early recognition and treatment. It is most commonly precipitated by infection in a patient with previously unrecognised or inadequately treated thyrotoxicosis. It may also develop in known thyrotoxicosis shortly after thyroidectomy in an ill-prepared patient or within a few days of ^{131}I therapy, when acute radiation damage may lead to a transient rise in serum thyroid hormone levels. Urgent specialist endocrine input should be sought in cases of suspected 'thyroid storm', both to confirm the diagnosis and provide advice on appropriate treatment.

Patients should be rehydrated and given propranolol, either orally (80 mg 4 times daily) or intravenously (1–5 mg 4 times daily). Both glucocorticoids (hydrocortisone 100 mg IV every 8 hours) and iodine are important in reducing the conversion of T_4 to active T_3. Sodium ipodate, a radiographic contrast medium (500 mg per day orally), will restore serum T_3 levels to normal in 48–72 hours. Where sodium ipodate is not available, potassium iodide or Lugol's solution are reasonable alternatives. Oral propylthiouracil (PTU) (200 mg every 4 hours) should be given to inhibit the synthesis of new thyroid hormone. PTU is preferred to carbimazole (20 mg every 6 hours) as it also inhibits the conversion of T_4 to T_3. If the patient is unconscious or uncooperative, PTU and propranolol can be administered by nasogastric tube. After 10–14 days the patient can usually be maintained on carbimazole alone.

Hyperthyroidism in old age

Some of the diagnostic and management challenges of hyperthyroidism in older people are highlighted in Box 20.12.

Hypothyroidism

Hypothyroidism is a common condition with various causes (Box 20.10), but autoimmune disease (Hashimoto's thyroiditis) and thyroid failure following ^{131}I or surgical treatment of thyrotoxicosis account for over 90% of cases, except in areas where iodine deficiency is endemic. Women are affected approximately six times more frequently than men.

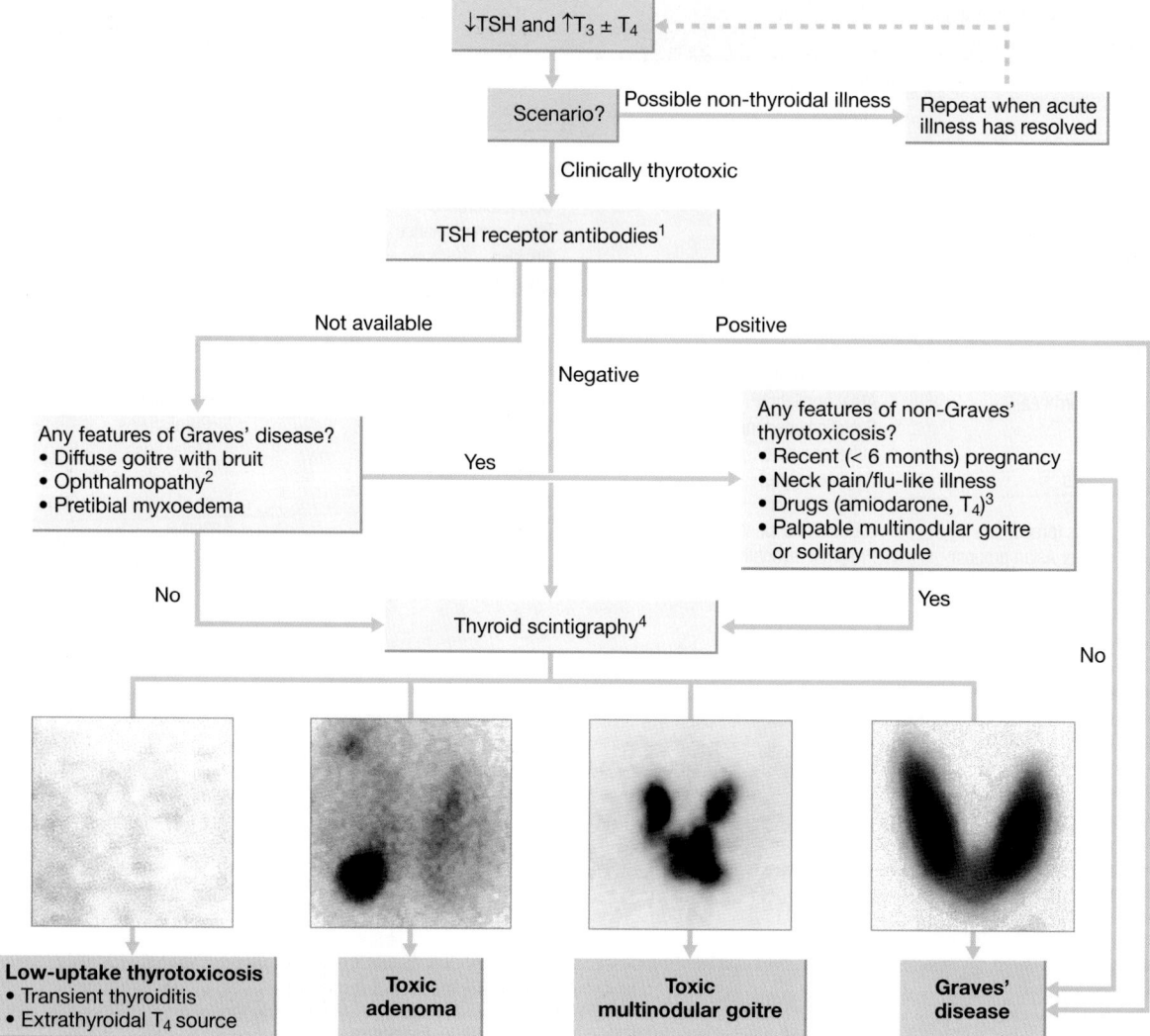

Fig. 20.5 Establishing the differential diagnosis in thyrotoxicosis. [1]Thyroid-stimulating hormone (TSH) receptor antibodies are very rare in patients without autoimmune thyroid disease but occur in only 80%–95% of patients with Graves' disease; a positive test is therefore confirmatory but a negative test does not exclude Graves' disease. Other thyroid antibodies (e.g. anti-peroxidase and anti-thyroglobulin antibodies) are unhelpful in the differential diagnosis since they occur frequently in the population and are found with several of the disorders that cause thyrotoxicosis. [2]Graves' ophthalmopathy refers to clinical features of exophthalmos and periorbital and conjunctival oedema, not simply the lid lag and lid retraction that can occur in all forms of thyrotoxicosis. [3]Scintigraphy is not necessary in most cases of drug-induced thyrotoxicosis. [4] [99m]Technetium pertechnetate scans of patients with thyrotoxicosis. In low-uptake thyrotoxicosis, most commonly due to a viral, post-partum or iodine-induced thyroiditis, there is negligible isotope detected in the region of the thyroid, although uptake is apparent in nearby salivary glands (not shown here). In a toxic adenoma there is lack of uptake of isotope by the rest of the thyroid gland due to suppression of serum TSH. In multinodular goitre there is relatively low, patchy uptake within the nodules; such an appearance is not always associated with a palpable thyroid. In Graves' disease there is diffuse uptake of isotope.

| **i** | **20.9 Non-specific laboratory abnormalities in thyroid dysfunction*** |

Thyrotoxicosis

- Serum enzymes: raised alanine aminotransferase, γ-glutamyl transferase (GGT), and alkaline phosphatase from liver and bone
- Raised bilirubin
- Mild hypercalcaemia
- Glycosuria: associated diabetes mellitus, 'lag storage' glycosuria

Hypothyroidism

- Serum enzymes: raised creatine kinase, aspartate aminotransferase, lactate dehydrogenase (LDH)
- Hypercholesterolaemia
- Anaemia: normochromic normocytic or macrocytic
- Hyponatraemia

*These abnormalities are not useful in differential diagnosis, so the tests should be avoided and any further investigation undertaken only if abnormalities persist when the patient is euthyroid.

Clinical assessment

The clinical presentation depends on the duration and severity of the hypothyroidism. Those in whom complete thyroid failure has developed insidiously over months or years may present with many of the clinical features listed in Box 20.7. A consequence of prolonged hypothyroidism is the infiltration of many body tissues by the mucopolysaccharides hyaluronic acid and chondroitin sulphate, resulting in a low-pitched voice, poor hearing, slurred speech due to a large tongue, and compression of the median nerve at the wrist (carpal tunnel syndrome). Infiltration of the dermis gives rise to non-pitting oedema (myxoedema), which is most marked in the skin of the hands, feet and eyelids. The resultant periorbital puffiness is often striking and may be combined with facial pallor due to vasoconstriction and anaemia, or a lemon-yellow tint to the skin caused by carotenaemia, along with purplish lips and malar flush. Most cases of hypothyroidism are not clinically obvious, however, and a high index of suspicion needs to be maintained so that the diagnosis is not overlooked in individuals complaining of non-specific symptoms such as tiredness, weight gain, depression or carpal tunnel syndrome.

20.10 Causes of hypothyroidism

Causes	Anti-TPO antibodies[1]	Goitre[2]
Autoimmune		
Hashimoto's thyroiditis	++	±
Spontaneous atrophic hypothyroidism	−	−
Graves' disease with TSH receptor-blocking antibodies	+	±
Iatrogenic		
Radioactive iodine ablation	+	±
Thyroidectomy	+	−
Drugs		
Carbimazole, methimazole, propylthiouracil	+	±
Amiodarone	+	±
Lithium	−	±
Transient thyroiditis		
Subacute (de Quervain's) thyroiditis	+	±
Post-partum thyroiditis	+	±
Iodine deficiency		
e.g. In mountainous regions	−	++
Congenital		
Dyshormonogenesis	−	++
Thyroid aplasia	−	−
Infiltrative		
Amyloidosis, Riedel's thyroiditis, sarcoidosis etc.	+	++
Secondary hypothyroidism		
TSH deficiency	−	−

[1]As shown in Box 20.8, thyroid autoantibodies are common in the healthy population, so might be present in anyone. ++ high titre; + more likely to be detected than in the healthy population; − not especially likely. [2]Goitre: − absent; ± may be present; ++ characteristic. (TPO = thyroid peroxidase; TSH = thyroid-stimulating hormone)

The key discriminatory features in the history and examination are highlighted in Figure 20.6. Care must be taken to identify patients with transient hypothyroidism, in whom life-long levothyroxine therapy is inappropriate. This can be observed during the first 6 months after ^{131}I treatment of Graves' disease, in the post-thyrotoxic phase of subacute thyroiditis and in post-partum thyroiditis. In these conditions, levothyroxine treatment is not always necessary, as the patient may be asymptomatic during the short period of thyroid failure.

Investigations

In the vast majority of cases, hypothyroidism results from an intrinsic disorder of the thyroid gland (primary hypothyroidism). In this situation, serum T_4 is low and TSH is elevated, usually in excess of 20 mIU/L. Measurements of serum T_3 are unhelpful since they do not discriminate reliably between euthyroidism and hypothyroidism. Measurement of thyroid peroxidase antibodies is helpful but further investigations are rarely required (Fig. 20.6). Secondary hypothyroidism is rare and is caused by failure of TSH secretion in an individual with hypothalamic or anterior pituitary disease. Other non-specific abnormalities are shown in Box 20.9. In severe, prolonged hypothyroidism, the ECG classically demonstrates sinus bradycardia with low-voltage complexes and ST-segment and T-wave abnormalities.

Management

Treatment is with levothyroxine replacement. The average replacement dose of levothyroxine is 1.6 µg/kg, which equates to around 100 µg in a 70 kg adult. In healthy younger adults it is safe to commence an estimated full dose. In older individuals, and those with a history of cardiovascular disease, it is customary to start with a low dose of 50 µg per day for 3 weeks before increasing to the estimated full dose. Levothyroxine has a half-life of 7 days so it should always be taken as a single daily dose and at least 10 weeks should pass before repeating thyroid function tests (as TSH takes several weeks to reach a steady state) and adjusting the dose. Patients feel better within 2–3 weeks. Reduction in weight and periorbital puffiness occurs quickly but the restoration of skin

20

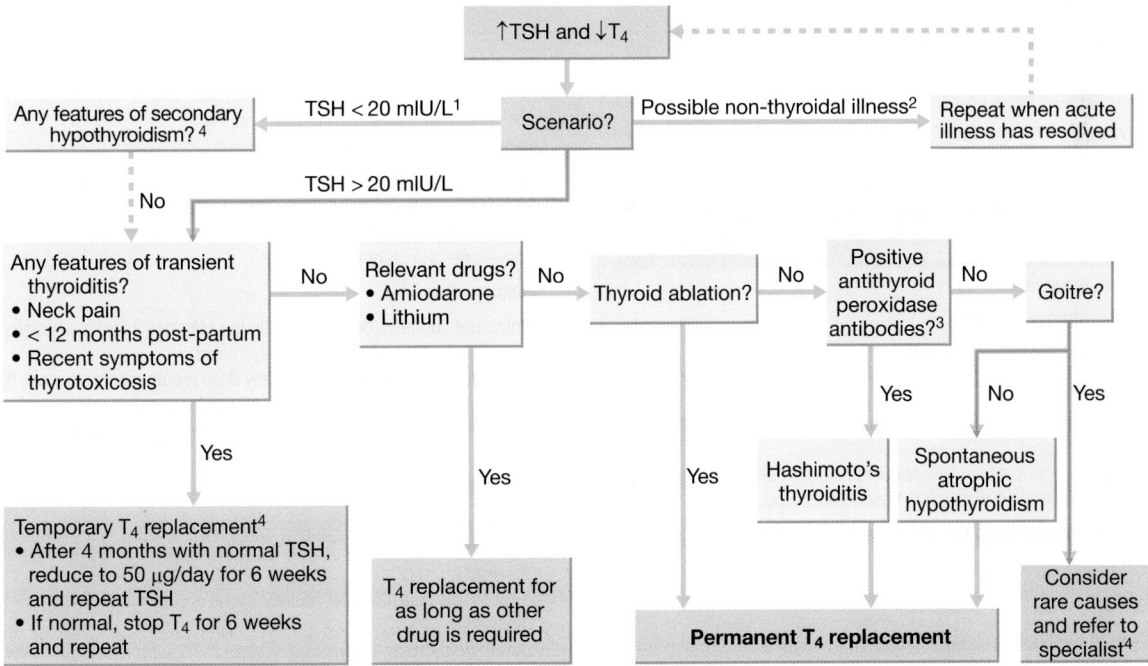

Fig. 20.6 An approach to adults with suspected primary hypothyroidism. This scheme ignores congenital causes of hypothyroidism (see Box 20.10), such as thyroid aplasia and dyshormonogenesis (associated with nerve deafness in Pendred syndrome, p. 667), which are usually diagnosed in childhood. [1]Immunoreactive thyroid-stimulating hormone (TSH) may be detected at normal or even modestly elevated levels in patients with pituitary failure; unless T_4 is only marginally low, TSH should be >20 mIU/L to confirm the diagnosis of primary hypothyroidism. [2]The usual abnormality in sick euthyroidism is a low TSH but any pattern can occur. [3]Thyroid peroxidase (TPO) antibodies are highly sensitive but not very specific for autoimmune thyroid disease (see Boxes 20.8 and 20.10). [4]Specialist advice is most appropriate where indicated. Secondary hypothyroidism is rare, but is suggested by deficiency of pituitary hormones or by clinical features of pituitary tumour such as headache or visual field defect (p. 695). Rare causes of hypothyroidism with goitre include dyshormonogenesis and infiltration of the thyroid (see Box 20.10).

and hair texture and resolution of any effusions may take 3–6 months. As illustrated in Figure 20.6, most patients do not require specialist review but will need life-long levothyroxine therapy.

The dose of levothyroxine should be adjusted to maintain serum TSH within the reference range. To achieve this, serum T_4 often needs to be in the upper part of the reference range because the T_3 required for receptor activation is derived exclusively from conversion of T_4 within the target tissues, without the usual contribution from thyroid secretion. Some physicians advocate combined replacement with T_4 (levothyroxine) and T_3 (liothyronine) or preparations of animal thyroid extract but this approach remains controversial and is not supported by robust evidence. Some patients remain symptomatic despite normalisation of TSH and may wish to take extra levothyroxine, which suppresses TSH. However, suppressed TSH is a risk factor for osteoporosis and atrial fibrillation (see below; subclinical thyrotoxicosis), so this approach cannot be recommended.

It is important to measure thyroid function every 1–2 years once the dose of levothyroxine is stabilised. This encourages adherence to therapy and allows adjustment for variable underlying thyroid activity and other changes in levothyroxine requirements (Box 20.11). Some patients have a persistent elevation of serum TSH despite an ostensibly adequate replacement dose of levothyroxine; most commonly, this is a consequence of suboptimal concordance. There may be differences in bioavailability between the numerous generic preparations of levothyroxine and so, if an individual is experiencing marked changes in serum TSH despite optimal adherence, the prescription of a branded preparation of levothyroxine could be considered. There is some limited evidence that suggests levothyroxine absorption may be better when the drug is taken before bed. In some individuals with variable concordance, levothyroxine is taken diligently or even in excess for a few days prior to a clinic visit, resulting in the seemingly anomalous combination of a high serum T_4 and high TSH (see Box 20.5).

Levothyroxine replacement in ischaemic heart disease

Hypothyroidism and ischaemic heart disease are common conditions that often occur together. Although angina may remain unchanged in severity or paradoxically disappear with restoration of metabolic rate, exacerbation of myocardial ischaemia, infarction and sudden death are recognised complications of levothyroxine replacement, even using doses as low as 25 µg per day. In patients with known ischaemic heart disease, thyroid hormone replacement should be introduced at low dose and increased very slowly under specialist supervision. Coronary intervention may be required if angina is exacerbated by levothyroxine replacement therapy.

Hypothyroidism in old age

Box 20.12 illustrates some of the diagnostic and management challenges of hypothyroidism in older people.

Hypothyroidism in pregnancy

Women with hypothyroidism usually require an increased dose of levothyroxine in pregnancy; inadequately treated hypothyroidism in pregnancy has been associated with impaired cognitive development in the fetus. This is discussed in more detail on page 1273 (see also Box 20.13).

20.12 The thyroid gland in old age

Thyrotoxicosis

- **Causes:** commonly due to multinodular goitre.
- **Clinical features:** apathy, anorexia, proximal myopathy, atrial fibrillation and cardiac failure predominate.
- **Non-thyroidal illness:** thyroid function tests are performed more frequently in older patients but interpretation may be altered by intercurrent illness.

Hypothyroidism

- **Clinical features:** non-specific features, such as physical and mental slowing, are often attributed to increasing age and the diagnosis is delayed.
- **Myxoedema coma:** more likely in older people.
- **Levothyroxine dose:** to avoid exacerbating latent or established heart disease, the starting dose should be 25–50 µg daily. Levothyroxine requirements fall with increasing age and few patients need more than 100 µg daily.
- **Other medication** (see Box 20.10): may interfere with absorption or metabolism of levothyroxine, necessitating an increase in dose.

20.13 Thyroid disease in pregnancy

Normal pregnancy

- **Trimester-specific reference ranges:** should be used to interpret thyroid function test results in pregnancy.

Iodine deficiency

- **Iodine requirements:** increased in pregnancy. The World Health Organization (WHO) recommends a minimum intake of 250 µg/day.
- **Iodine deficiency:** the major cause of preventable impaired cognitive development in children worldwide.

Hypothyroidism

- **Impaired cognitive development in the offspring:** may be associated with hypothyroidism that is not adequately treated.
- **Levothyroxine replacement therapy dose requirements:** increase by 30%–50% from early in pregnancy. Monitoring to maintain TSH results within the trimester-specific reference range is recommended in early pregnancy and at least once in each trimester.

Thyrotoxicosis

- **Gestational thyrotoxicosis:** associated with multiple pregnancies and hyperemesis gravidarum. Transient and usually does not require antithyroid drug treatment.
- **Graves' disease:** the most common cause of sustained thyrotoxicosis in pregnancy.
- **Antithyroid drugs:** propylthiouracil should be used in the first trimester, with carbimazole substituted in the second and third trimesters.

Post-partum thyroiditis

- **Screening:** not recommended for every woman, but thyroid function should be tested 4–6 weeks post partum in those with a personal history of thyroid disease, goitre or other autoimmune disease including type 1 diabetes, in those known to have positive antithyroid peroxidase antibodies, or when there is clinical suspicion of thyroid dysfunction.

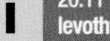

20.11 Situations in which an adjustment of the dose of levothyroxine may be necessary

Increased dose required

Pregnancy or oestrogen therapy

- Increases concentration of serum thyroxine-binding globulin

Use of other medication

- Increase T_4 clearance: phenobarbital, phenytoin, carbamazepine, rifampicin, sertraline*, chloroquine*
- Interfere with intestinal T_4 absorption: colestyramine, sucralfate, aluminium hydroxide, ferrous sulphate, dietary fibre supplements, calcium carbonate

After surgical or ¹³¹I ablation of Graves' disease

- Reduces thyroidal secretion with time

Malabsorption

Decreased dose required

Ageing

- Decreases T4 clearance

Graves' disease developing in patient with long-standing primary hypothyroidism

- Switch from production of blocking to stimulating TSH receptor antibodies

*Mechanism not fully established.

Myxoedema coma

This is a very rare presentation of hypothyroidism in which there is a depressed level of consciousness, usually in an older patient who appears myxoedematous. Body temperature may be as low as 25°C, convulsions are not uncommon, and cerebrospinal fluid (CSF) pressure and protein content are raised. The mortality rate is 50% and survival depends on early recognition and treatment of hypothyroidism and other factors contributing to the altered consciousness level, such as medication, cardiac failure, pneumonia, dilutional hyponatraemia and respiratory failure.

Myxoedema coma is a medical emergency and treatment must begin before biochemical confirmation of the diagnosis. Suspected cases should be treated with an intravenous injection of 20 μg liothyronine, followed by further injections of 20 μg 3 times daily until there is sustained clinical improvement. In survivors, there is a rise in body temperature within 24 hours and, after 48–72 hours, it is usually possible to switch patients to oral levothyroxine in a dose of 50 μg daily. Unless it is apparent that the patient has primary hypothyroidism, the thyroid failure should also be assumed to be secondary to hypothalamic or pituitary disease and treatment given with hydrocortisone 100 mg intramuscularly 3 times daily, pending the results of T_4, TSH and cortisol measurement. Other measures include slow rewarming, cautious use of intravenous fluids, broad-spectrum antibiotics and high-flow oxygen.

Symptoms of hypothyroidism with normal thyroid function tests

The classic symptoms of hypothyroidism are, by their very nature, non-specific (see Box 20.3). There is a wide differential diagnosis for symptoms such as 'fatigue', 'weight gain' and 'low mood'. As has been noted, outside the context of pituitary and hypothalamic disease, serum TSH is an excellent measure of an individual's thyroid hormone status. However, some individuals believe that they have hypothyroidism despite normal serum TSH concentrations. There are a large number of websites that claim that serum TSH is not a good measure of thyroid hormone status and suggest that other factors, such as abnormalities of T_4 to T_3 conversion, may lead to low tissue levels of active thyroid hormones. Such websites often advocate a variety of tests of thyroid function of dubious scientific validity, including measurement of serum reverse T_3, 24-hour urine T_3, basal body temperature, skin iodine absorption, and levels of selenium in blood and urine. Individuals who believe they have hypothyroidism, despite normal conventional tests of thyroid function, can be difficult to manage. They require reassurance that their symptoms are being taken seriously and that organic disease has been carefully considered; if their symptoms persist, referral to a team specialising in medically unexplained symptoms should be considered.

Asymptomatic abnormal thyroid function tests

One of the most common problems in medical practice is how to manage patients with abnormal thyroid function tests who have no obvious signs or symptoms of thyroid disease. These can be divided into three categories.

Subclinical thyrotoxicosis

Serum TSH is undetectable and serum T_3 and T_4 are at the upper end of the reference range. This combination is most often found in older patients with multinodular goitre. These patients are at increased risk of atrial fibrillation and osteoporosis, and hence the consensus view is that they have mild thyrotoxicosis and require therapy, either with ^{131}I or low dose thionamide. Otherwise, annual review is essential, as the conversion rate to overt thyrotoxicosis with elevated T_4 and/or T_3 concentrations is 5% each year.

Subclinical hypothyroidism

Serum TSH is raised and serum T_3 and T_4 concentrations are at the lower end of the reference range. This may persist for many years, although there is a risk of progression to overt thyroid failure, particularly if antibodies to thyroid peroxidase are present or if the TSH rises above 10 mIU/L. In patients with non-specific symptoms, a trial of levothyroxine therapy may be appropriate. In those with positive autoantibodies or a TSH greater than 10 mIU/L, it is better to treat the thyroid failure early rather than risk loss to follow-up and subsequent presentation with profound hypothyroidism. Levothyroxine should be given in a dose sufficient to restore the serum TSH concentration to normal.

Non-thyroidal illness ('sick euthyroidism')

This typically presents with a low serum TSH, raised T_4 and normal or low T_3 in a patient with systemic illness who does not have clinical evidence of thyroid disease. These abnormalities are caused by decreased peripheral conversion of T_4 to T_3 (with conversion instead to reverse T_3), altered levels of binding proteins and their affinity for thyroid hormones, and often reduced secretion of TSH. During convalescence, serum TSH concentrations may increase to levels found in primary hypothyroidism. As thyroid function tests are difficult to interpret in patients with non-thyroidal illness, it is wise to avoid performing thyroid function tests unless there is clinical evidence of concomitant thyroid disease. If an abnormal result is found, treatment should only be given with specialist advice and the diagnosis should be re-evaluated after recovery.

Thyroid lump or swelling

A lump or swelling in the thyroid gland can be a source of considerable anxiety for patients. There are numerous causes but, broadly speaking, a thyroid swelling is either a solitary nodule, a multinodular goitre or a diffuse goitre (Box 20.14). Nodular thyroid disease is more common in women and occurs in approximately 30% of the adult female population. The majority of thyroid nodules are impalpable but may be identified when imaging of the neck is performed for another reason, such as during Doppler ultrasonography of the carotid arteries or computed tomographic pulmonary angiography. Increasingly, thyroid nodules are identified during staging of patients with cancer with computed tomography (CT), magnetic resonance imaging (MRI) or positron emission tomography (PET) scans. Palpable thyroid nodules occur in 4%–8% of adult women and 1%–2% of adult men, and classically present when the individual (or a friend or relative) notices a lump in the neck. Multinodular goitre and solitary nodules sometimes present with acute painful enlargement due to haemorrhage into a nodule.

Patients with thyroid nodules often worry that they have cancer but the reality is that only 5%–10% of thyroid nodules are malignant. A nodule presenting in childhood or adolescence, particularly if there is a past history of head and neck irradiation, or one presenting in an older patient should heighten suspicion of a primary thyroid malignancy. The presence of cervical lymphadenopathy also increases the likelihood of malignancy.

20

i	20.14 Causes of thyroid enlargement

Diffuse goitre

• Simple goitre	• Transient thyroiditis[2]
• Hashimoto's thyroiditis[1]	• Dyshormonogenesis[1]
• Graves' disease	• Infiltrative: amyloidosis, sarcoidosis etc.
• Drugs: iodine, amiodarone, lithium	• Riedel's thyroiditis[2]
• Iodine deficiency (endemic goitre)[1]	
• Suppurative thyroiditis[2]	

Multinodular goitre

Solitary nodule

• Colloid cyst	• Medullary cell carcinoma
• Hyperplastic nodule	• Anaplastic carcinoma
• Follicular adenoma	• Lymphoma
• Papillary carcinoma	• Metastasis
• Follicular carcinoma	

[1]Goitre likely to shrink with levothyroxine therapy. [2]Usually tender.

Rarely, a secondary deposit from a renal, breast or lung carcinoma presents as a painful, rapidly growing, solitary thyroid nodule. Thyroid nodules identified on PET scanning have an approximately 33% chance of being malignant.

Clinical assessment and investigations

Swellings in the anterior part of the neck most commonly originate in the thyroid and this can be confirmed by demonstrating that the swelling moves on swallowing. It is often possible to distinguish clinically between the three main causes of thyroid swelling. There is a broad differential diagnosis of anterior neck swellings, which includes lymphadenopathy, branchial cysts, dermoid cysts and thyroglossal duct cysts (the latter are classically located in the midline and move on protrusion of the tongue). An ultrasound scan should be performed urgently, if there is any doubt as to the aetiology of an anterior neck swelling.

Serum T_3, T_4 and TSH should be measured in all patients with a goitre or solitary thyroid nodule. The finding of biochemical thyrotoxicosis or hypothyroidism (both of which may be subclinical) should lead to investigations, as already described in Box 20.5 and on page 657.

Thyroid scintigraphy

Thyroid scintigraphy with ^{99m}technetium should be performed in an individual with a low serum TSH and a nodular thyroid to confirm the presence of an autonomously functioning ('hot') nodule (see Fig. 20.5). In such circumstances, further evaluation is not necessary. 'Cold' nodules on scintigraphy have a much higher likelihood of malignancy, but the majority are benign and so scintigraphy is not routinely used in the evaluation of thyroid nodules when TSH is normal.

Thyroid ultrasound

If thyroid function tests are normal, an ultrasound scan will often determine the nature of the thyroid swelling. Ultrasound can establish whether there is generalised or localised swelling of the thyroid. Inflammatory disorders causing a diffuse goitre, such as Graves' disease and Hashimoto's thyroiditis, demonstrate a diffuse pattern of hypoechogenicity and, in the case of Graves' disease, increased thyroid blood flow may be seen on colour-flow Doppler (although ultrasound should not form part of the routine investigation of Graves' disease). The presence of thyroid autoantibodies will support the diagnosis of Graves' disease or Hashimoto's thyroiditis, while their absence in a younger patient with a diffuse goitre and normal thyroid function suggests a diagnosis of 'simple goitre'.

Ultrasound can readily determine the size and number of nodules within the thyroid and can distinguish solid nodules from those with a cystic element. Ultrasound is used increasingly as the key investigation in defining the risk of malignancy in a nodule. Size of the nodule is not a predictor of the risk of malignancy but there are other ultrasound characteristics that are associated with a higher likelihood of malignancy. These include hypoechogenicity, intranodular vascularity, the presence of microcalcification and irregular or lobulated margins. A purely cystic nodule is highly unlikely to be malignant and a 'spongiform' appearance is also highly predictive of a benign aetiology. Each individual nodule within a multinodular goitre has the same risk of malignancy as a solitary nodule. Thyroid ultrasonography is a highly specialised investigation and the accurate stratification of risk of malignancy of a thyroid nodule requires skill and expertise.

Fine needle aspiration cytology

Fine needle aspiration cytology is recommended for thyroid nodules that are suspicious for malignancy or are radiologically indeterminate. Fine needle aspiration of a thyroid nodule can be performed in the outpatient clinic, usually under ultrasound guidance. Aspiration may be therapeutic for a cyst, although recurrence on more than one occasion is an indication for surgery or alcohol ablation. Fine needle aspiration cytology cannot differentiate between a follicular adenoma and a follicular carcinoma, and in 10%–20% of cases an inadequate specimen is obtained.

Management

Nodules with a benign appearance on ultrasound may be observed in an ultrasound surveillance programme; when the suspicion of malignancy is very low, the patient may be reassured and discharged. In regions with borderline low iodine intake, there is evidence that levothyroxine therapy, in doses that suppress serum TSH, may reduce the size of some nodules. This should not be routine practice in iodine-sufficient populations.

Nodules that are suspicious for malignancy are treated by surgical excision, by either lobectomy or thyroidectomy. Nodules that are radiologically and/or cytologically indeterminate are more of a management challenge and often end up being surgically excised. Molecular techniques may, in the future, improve the diagnostic accuracy of thyroid cytology and allow a more conservative strategy for individuals with an indeterminate biopsy. Nodules in which malignancy is confirmed by formal histology are treated as described on page 665.

A diffuse or multinodular goitre may also require surgical treatment for cosmetic reasons or if there is compression of local structures (resulting in stridor or dysphagia). ^{131}I therapy may also cause some reduction in size of a multinodular goitre. Levothyroxine therapy may shrink the goitre of Hashimoto's disease, particularly if serum TSH is elevated.

Autoimmune thyroid disease

Thyroid diseases are amongst the most prevalent antibody-mediated autoimmune diseases and are associated with other organ-specific autoimmune diseases. Autoantibodies may produce inflammation and destruction of thyroid tissue, resulting in hypothyroidism, goitre (in Hashimoto's thyroiditis) or sometimes even transient thyrotoxicosis ('Hashitoxicosis'), or they may stimulate the TSH receptor to cause thyrotoxicosis (in Graves' disease). There is overlap between these conditions, since some patients have multiple autoantibodies.

Graves' disease

Graves' disease can occur at any age but is unusual before puberty and most commonly affects women aged 30–50 years. The most common manifestation is thyrotoxicosis with or without a diffuse goitre. The clinical features and differential diagnosis are described on page 652. Graves' disease also causes ophthalmopathy and, rarely, pretibial myxoedema (p. 663). These extrathyroidal features usually occur in thyrotoxic patients but can arise in the absence of thyroid dysfunction.

Graves' thyrotoxicosis
Pathophysiology

The thyrotoxicosis results from the production of IgG antibodies directed against the TSH receptor on the thyroid follicular cell, which stimulate thyroid hormone production and proliferation of follicular cells, leading to goitre in the majority of patients. These antibodies are termed thyroid-stimulating immunoglobulins or TSH receptor antibodies (TRAb) and can be detected in the serum of >95% of patients with Graves' disease. The concentration of TRAb in the serum is presumed to fluctuate to account for the natural history of Graves' thyrotoxicosis (Fig. 20.7). Thyroid failure seen in some patients may result from the presence of blocking antibodies against the TSH receptor, and from tissue destruction by cytotoxic antibodies and cell-mediated immunity.

Graves' disease has a strong genetic component. There is 20%–40% concordance for thyrotoxicosis between monozygotic twins but only 5% concordance between dizygotic twins. Genome-wide association studies have identified several genes associated with susceptibility. These include HLA-DRß-Arg74, CTLA4, PTPN22, TSHR1, CD25 and CD40. Many of these loci have been implicated in the pathogenesis of other autoimmune diseases.

A suggested trigger for the development of thyrotoxicosis in genetically susceptible individuals may be infection with viruses or bacteria.

In regions of iodine deficiency, iodine supplementation can precipitate thyrotoxicosis, but only in those with pre-existing subclinical Graves' disease. Smoking is associated with Graves' thyrotoxicosis and strongly linked with the development of ophthalmopathy.

Management

Symptoms of thyrotoxicosis respond to β-blockade but definitive treatment requires control of thyroid hormone secretion. The different options are compared in Box 20.15. Some clinicians adopt an empirical approach of prescribing a course of antithyroid drug therapy and then recommending ^{131}I or surgery if relapse occurs. In many centres, however, ^{131}I is used extensively as a first-line therapy, given the high risk of relapse following a course of antithyroid drugs (>60%). A number of observational studies have linked therapeutic ^{131}I with increased incidence of some malignancies, particularly of the thyroid and gastrointestinal tract, but the results have been inconsistent; the association may be with Graves' disease rather than its therapy, and the magnitude of the effect, if any, is small. Experience from the disaster at the Chernobyl nuclear power plant in 1986 suggests that younger people are more sensitive to radiation-induced thyroid cancer.

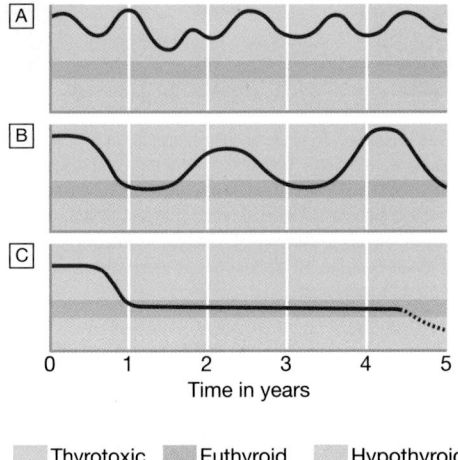

Fig. 20.7 Natural history of the thyrotoxicosis of Graves' disease. [A] and [B] The majority (60%) of patients have either prolonged periods of thyrotoxicosis of fluctuating severity, or periods of alternating relapse and remission. [C] It is the minority who experience a single short-lived episode followed by prolonged remission and, in some cases, by the eventual onset of hypothyroidism.

Antithyroid drugs The most commonly used are carbimazole and its active metabolite, methimazole (not available in the UK). Propylthiouracil is equally effective. These drugs reduce the synthesis of new thyroid hormones by inhibiting the iodination of tyrosine (see Fig. 20.3). Carbimazole may also have an immunosuppressive action, leading to a reduction in serum TRAb concentrations, but this is not enough to influence the natural history of the thyrotoxicosis significantly.

Antithyroid drugs are typically introduced at high doses (carbimazole 40–60 mg daily or propylthiouracil 400–600 mg daily), although lower doses are reasonable in individuals with only modest elevation of T_4 and T_3. Usually, this results in subjective improvement within 10–14 days and renders the patient clinically and biochemically euthyroid at 6–8 weeks. At this point, the dose can be reduced and titrated to maintain T_4 and TSH within their reference range. In most patients, carbimazole is continued at 5–20 mg per day for 12–18 months in the hope that remission will occur. Between 50% and 70% of patients with Graves' disease will subsequently relapse, usually within 2 years of stopping treatment. Risk factors for relapse include younger age, male sex, presence of a goitre and higher TRAb titres at both diagnosis and cessation of antithyroid therapy. Rarely, T_4 and TSH levels fluctuate between those of thyrotoxicosis and hypothyroidism at successive review appointments, despite good drug adherence, presumably due to rapidly changing concentrations of TRAb. In these patients, satisfactory control can be achieved by blocking thyroid hormone synthesis with carbimazole 30–40 mg daily and adding levothyroxine 100–150 μg daily as replacement therapy (a 'block and replace' regimen).

Antithyroid drugs can have adverse effects. The most common is a rash. Agranulocytosis is a rare but potentially serious complication (0.2%–0.5%) that cannot be predicted by routine measurement of white blood cell count but which is reversible on stopping treatment. Patients should be warned to stop the drug and seek medical advice immediately, should a severe sore throat or fever develop while on treatment. Propylthiouracil is associated with a small but definite risk of hepatotoxicity, which, in some instances, has resulted in liver failure requiring liver transplantation, and even in death. It should therefore be considered second-line therapy to carbimazole and be used only during pregnancy or breastfeeding, or if an adverse reaction to carbimazole has occurred.

Thyroid surgery Patients should be rendered euthyroid with antithyroid drugs before operation. Oral potassium iodide, 60 mg three times daily, is often added for 10 days before surgery to inhibit thyroid hormone release and reduce the size and vascularity of the gland, making surgery technically easier. The optimal surgical approach is a 'near-total'

20

	20.15 Comparison of treatments for the thyrotoxicosis of Graves' disease		
Management	**Common indications**	**Contraindications**	**Disadvantages/complications**
Antithyroid drugs (carbimazole, propylthiouracil)	First episode in patients <40 years	Breastfeeding (propylthiouracil suitable)	Hypersensitivity rash 2% Agranulocytosis 0.2% Hepatotoxicity (with propylthiouracil) – very rare but potentially fatal >50% relapse rate usually within 2 years of stopping drug
Thyroidectomy	Large goitre Poor drug adherence, especially in young patients Recurrent thyrotoxicosis after course of antithyroid drugs in young patients	Previous thyroid surgery Dependence on voice, e.g. singer, lecturer[1]	Hypothyroidism (~25%) Transient hypocalcaemia (10%) Permanent hypoparathyroidism (1%) Recurrent laryngeal nerve palsy[1] (1%)
Radio-iodine	Patients >40 years[2] Recurrence following surgery irrespective of age Other serious comorbidity	Pregnancy or planned pregnancy within 6 months of treatment Active Graves' ophthalmopathy[3]	Hypothyroidism: ~40% in first year, 80% after 15 years Most likely treatment to result in exacerbation of ophthalmopathy[3]

[1]It is not only vocal cord palsy due to recurrent laryngeal nerve damage that alters the voice following thyroid surgery; the superior laryngeal nerves are frequently transected and this results in minor changes in voice quality. [2]In many institutions, ^{131}I is used more liberally and is prescribed for much younger patients. [3]The extent to which radio-iodine exacerbates ophthalmopathy is controversial and practice varies; some use prednisolone to reduce this risk.

thyroidectomy, leaving behind only a small portion of gland adjacent to the recurrent laryngeal nerves. This strategy invariably results in permanent hypothyroidism and is probably associated with a higher risk of hypoparathyroidism, compared to 'subtotal' thyroidectomy, but maximises the potential for cure of thyrotoxicosis.

Radioactive iodine ^{131}I is administered orally as a single dose and is trapped and organified in the thyroid (see Fig. 20.3). [131]I emits both β and γ radiation and, although it decays within a few weeks, it has long-lasting inhibitory effects on survival and replication of follicular cells. The variable radio-iodine uptake and radiosensitivity of the gland means that the choice of dose is empirical; in most centres, approximately 400–600 MBq (approximately 10–15 mCi) is administered. This regimen is effective in 75% of patients within 4–12 weeks. During the lag period, symptoms can be controlled by a β-blocker or, in more severe cases, by carbimazole. However, carbimazole reduces the efficacy of ^{131}I therapy because it prevents organification of ^{131}I in the gland, and so should be avoided until 48 hours after radio-iodine administration. If thyrotoxicosis persists after 6 months, a further dose of ^{131}I can be given. The disadvantage of ^{131}I treatment is that the majority of patients eventually develop hypothyroidism. [131]I is usually avoided in patients with Graves' ophthalmopathy and evidence of significant active orbital inflammation. It can be administered with caution in those with mild or 'burnt-out' eye disease, when it is customary to cover the treatment with a 6-week tapering course of oral prednisolone. In women of reproductive age, pregnancy must be excluded before administration of ^{131}I and avoided for at least 6 months thereafter; men are also advised to use strict contraceptive measures for at least 4 months after receiving ^{131}I, to avoid the possibility of conceiving with sperm that have been exposed to radioactive iodine.

Thyrotoxicosis in pregnancy Thyrotoxicosis in pregnancy may be associated with significant maternal and fetal morbidity. Management is very specialised and is discussed on page 1273 (see also Box 20.13).

Thyrotoxicosis in adolescence Thyrotoxicosis can occasionally occur in adolescence and is almost always due to Graves' disease. The presentation may be atypical and management challenging, as summarised in Box 20.16.

Graves' ophthalmopathy

This condition is immunologically mediated with the TSH receptor identified as the main autoantigen. Within the orbit (and the dermis) there is cytokine-mediated proliferation of fibroblasts that secrete hydrophilic glycosaminoglycans. The resulting increase in interstitial fluid content, combined with a chronic inflammatory cell infiltrate, causes marked swelling and ultimately fibrosis of the extraocular muscles (Fig. 20.8) and a rise in retrobulbar pressure. The eye is displaced forwards (proptosis, exophthalmos) and in severe cases there is optic nerve compression.

Ophthalmopathy, like thyrotoxicosis (see Fig. 20.7), typically follows an episodic course and it is helpful to distinguish patients with active inflammation (periorbital oedema and conjunctival inflammation with changing orbital signs) from those in whom the inflammation has 'burnt out'. Eye disease is detectable in up to 50% of thyrotoxic patients at

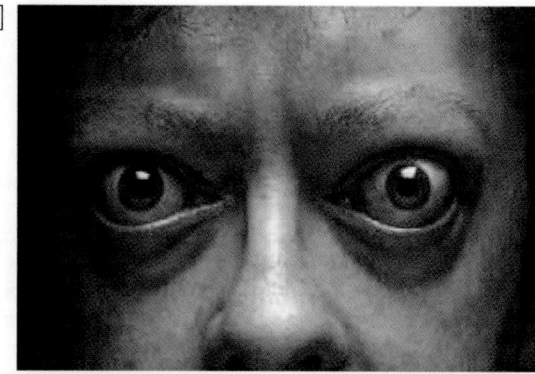
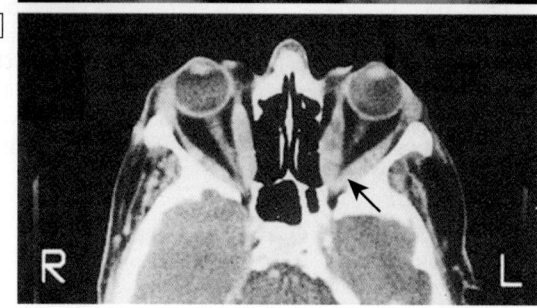

Fig. 20.8 Graves' disease. [A] Bilateral ophthalmopathy in a 42-year-old man. The main symptoms were diplopia in all directions of gaze and reduced visual acuity in the left eye. The periorbital swelling is due to retrobulbar fat prolapsing into the eyelids, and increased interstitial fluid as a result of raised intraorbital pressure. [B] Transverse CT of the orbits, showing the enlarged extraocular muscles. This is most obvious at the apex of the left orbit (arrow), where compression of the optic nerve caused reduced visual acuity.

presentation (although moderate to severe in only 5%), but active ocular inflammation may occur before or after thyrotoxic episodes (exophthalmic Graves' disease). Ophthalmopathy is more common in men and cigarette smokers. It may be exacerbated by radioiodine therapy and poor control of thyroid function, especially hypothyroidism. The most frequent presenting symptoms are related to increased exposure of the cornea, resulting from proptosis and lid retraction. There may be excessive lacrimation made worse by wind and bright light, a 'gritty' sensation in the eye and pain due to conjunctivitis or corneal ulceration. In addition, there may be reduction of visual acuity and/or visual fields as a consequence of corneal oedema or optic nerve compression. Other signs of optic nerve compression include reduced colour vision and a relative afferent pupillary defect (see page 649, Fig. 30.6 and Box 30.8). If the extraocular muscles are involved and do not act in concert, diplopia results.

The majority of patients require no treatment other than reassurance. Smoking cessation should be actively encouraged. Methylcellulose eye drops and gel counter the gritty discomfort of dry eyes, and tinted glasses or side shields attached to spectacle frames reduce the excessive lacrimation triggered by sun or wind. In patients with mild Graves' ophthalmopathy, oral selenium (100 μg twice daily for 6 months) improves quality of life, reduces ocular involvement and slows progression of disease; the mechanism of action is not known but may relate to an antioxidant effect. Moderate to severe ophthalmopathy is optimally managed by an expert multidisciplinary service. More severe inflammatory episodes are treated with glucocorticoids (e.g. pulsed intravenous methylprednisolone) and sometimes orbital radiotherapy. In recent years evidence has emerged to support the use of immunosuppressive therapies (e.g. rituximab and tocilizumab) and the IGF-1 receptor inhibitor teprotumumab in moderate to severe ophthalmopathy. Loss of visual acuity is an indication for urgent surgical decompression of the orbit. In 'burnt-out' disease, surgery to the extraocular muscles,

---

👪 20.16 Thyrotoxicosis in adolescence

- **Presentation**: may present with a deterioration in school performance or symptoms suggestive of attention deficit hyperactivity disorder.
- **Antithyroid drug therapy**: prolonged courses may be required because remission rates following an 18-month course of therapy are much lower than in adults.
- **Adherence**: adherence to antithyroid drug therapy is often suboptimal, resulting in poor disease control that may adversely affect performance at school.
- **Radio-iodine therapy**: usually avoided in adolescents because of concerns about risk of future malignancy.

and later the eyelids, may improve diplopia, conjunctival exposure and cosmetic appearance.

Pretibial myxoedema

This infiltrative dermopathy occurs in fewer than 5% of patients with Graves' disease and has similar pathological features as occur in the orbit. It takes the form of raised pink-coloured or purplish plaques on the anterior aspect of the leg, extending on to the dorsum of the foot (see p. 648). The lesions may be itchy and the skin may have a 'peau d'orange' appearance with growth of coarse hair; less commonly, the face and arms are affected. Treatment is rarely required but in severe cases topical glucocorticoids may be helpful.

Hashimoto's thyroiditis

Hashimoto's thyroiditis (or 'chronic autoimmune thyroiditis') is characterised by destructive lymphocytic infiltration of the thyroid, ultimately leading to a varying degree of fibrosis and thyroid enlargement. It has atrophic and goitrous variants.

Hashimoto's thyroiditis increases in incidence with age and affects approximately 3.5 per 1000 women and 0.8 per 1000 men each year. Many present with a small or moderately sized diffuse goitre, which is characteristically firm or rubbery in consistency. Around 25% of patients are hypothyroid at presentation. In the remainder, serum T_4 is normal and TSH normal or raised, but these patients are at risk of developing overt hypothyroidism in future years. Antithyroid peroxidase antibodies are present in the serum in more than 90% of patients with Hashimoto's thyroiditis. There is an increased risk of thyroid lymphoma, although this is exceedingly rare.

Levothyroxine therapy is indicated as treatment for hypothyroidism and also to shrink an associated goitre. In this context, the dose of levothyroxine should be sufficient to suppress serum TSH to low but detectable levels.

Transient thyroiditis

Subacute (de Quervain's) thyroiditis

In its classical painful form, subacute thyroiditis is a transient inflammation of the thyroid gland occurring after infection with Coxsackie, mumps or adenoviruses. There is pain in the region of the thyroid that may radiate to the angle of the jaw and the ears, and is made worse by swallowing, coughing and movement of the neck. The thyroid is usually palpably enlarged and tender. Systemic upset is common. Affected patients are usually females aged 20–40 years. Painless transient thyroiditis can also occur after viral infection and in patients with underlying autoimmune disease. The condition can also be precipitated by drugs, including interferon-α and lithium.

Irrespective of the clinical presentation, inflammation in the thyroid gland occurs and is associated with release of colloid and stored thyroid hormones, but also with damage to follicular cells and impaired synthesis of new thyroid hormones. As a result, T_4 and T_3 levels are raised for 4–6 weeks until the pre-formed colloid is depleted. Thereafter, there is usually a period of hypothyroidism of variable severity before the follicular cells recover and normal thyroid function is restored within 4–6 months (Fig. 20.9). In the thyrotoxic phase, the iodine uptake is low because the damaged follicular cells are unable to trap iodine and because TSH secretion is suppressed. Low-titre thyroid autoantibodies appear transiently in the serum, and the erythrocyte sedimentation rate (ESR) is usually raised. High-titre autoantibodies suggest an underlying autoimmune pathology and greater risk of recurrence and ultimate progression to hypothyroidism.

The pain and systemic upset usually respond to simple measures such as non-steroidal anti-inflammatory drugs (NSAIDs). Occasionally, however, it may be necessary to prescribe prednisolone 40 mg daily for 3–4 weeks. The thyrotoxicosis is mild and treatment with a β-blocker is

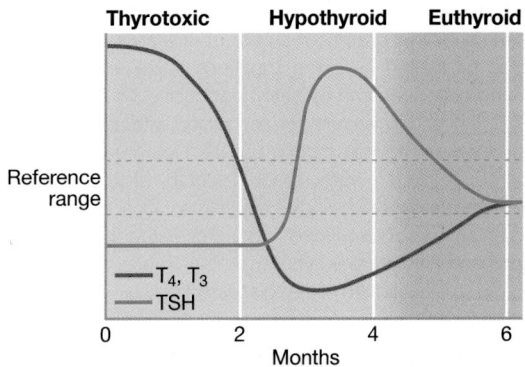

Fig. 20.9 Thyroid function tests in an episode of transient thyroiditis. This pattern might be observed in classical subacute (de Quervain's) thyroiditis, painless thyroiditis or post-partum thyroiditis. The duration of each phase varies between patients. (T_3 = triiodothyronine; T_4 = thyroxine; TSH = thyroid-stimulating hormone)

usually adequate. Antithyroid drugs are of no benefit because thyroid hormone synthesis is impaired rather than enhanced. Careful monitoring of thyroid function and symptoms is required so that levothyroxine can be prescribed temporarily in the hypothyroid phase. Care must be taken to identify patients presenting with hypothyroidism who are in the later stages of a transient thyroiditis, since they are unlikely to require life-long levothyroxine therapy (see Fig. 20.6).

Post-partum thyroiditis

The maternal immune response, which is modified during pregnancy to allow survival of the fetus, is enhanced after delivery and may unmask previously unrecognised subclinical autoimmune thyroid disease. Surveys have shown that transient biochemical disturbances of thyroid function occur in 5%–10% of women within 6 months of delivery (see Box 20.13). Those affected are likely to have antithyroid peroxidase antibodies in the serum in early pregnancy. Symptoms of thyroid dysfunction are rare and there is no association between postnatal depression and abnormal thyroid function tests. However, symptomatic thyrotoxicosis presenting for the first time within 12 months of childbirth is likely to be due to post-partum thyroiditis and the diagnosis is confirmed by a negligible radio-isotope uptake. The clinical course and treatment are similar to those of painless subacute thyroiditis (see above). Post-partum thyroiditis tends to recur after subsequent pregnancies, and eventually patients progress over a period of years to permanent hypothyroidism (see also Box 20.13).

Iodine-associated thyroid disease

Iodine deficiency

Iodine is an essential micronutrient and is a key component of T_4 and T_3. The World Health Organization (WHO) recommends a daily intake of iodine of 150 μg/day for adult men and women; higher levels are recommended for pregnant women (see p. 1273) as iodine deficiency is associated with impaired fetal brain development, and severe deficiency can cause cretinism. Dietary sources of iodine include seafood, dairy products, eggs and grains. Dietary iodine deficiency is a major worldwide public health issue, with an estimated one-third of the world population living in areas of iodine insufficiency. Iodine deficiency is particularly common in Central Africa, South-east Asia and the Western Pacific. It is associated with the development of thyroid nodules and goitre (endemic goitre); the reduced substrate available for thyroid hormone production increases thyroid activity to maximise iodine uptake and recycling, and this acts as a potent stimulus for enlargement of the thyroid and nodule formation. Most affected patients are euthyroid with normal or raised TSH levels, although hypothyroidism can occur with severe iodine

20

deficiency. Suspected iodine deficiency can be assessed by measuring iodine in urine (either a 24-hour collection or a spot sample). Endemic goitre can be treated by iodine supplementation, and a reduction in nodule and goitre size can be seen, particularly if it is commenced in childhood. Iodine deficiency is not associated with an increased risk of Graves' disease or thyroid cancer, but the high prevalence of nodular autonomy does result in an increased risk of thyrotoxicosis and this risk may be further increased by iodine supplementation. Conversely, iodine supplementation may also increase the prevalence of subclinical hypothyroidism and autoimmune hypothyroidism. These complex effects of iodine supplementation are further discussed below.

Iodine-induced thyroid dysfunction

Iodine has complex effects on thyroid function. Very high concentrations of iodine inhibit thyroid hormone synthesis and release (known as the Wolff–Chaikoff effect) and this forms the rationale for iodine treatment in thyroid crisis and prior to thyroid surgery for thyrotoxicosis. This is an autoregulatory response to protect the body from the sudden release of large amounts of thyroid hormone in response to the ingestion of a substantial load of iodine. This effect only lasts for about 10 days, after which it is followed by an 'escape phenomenon': essentially, the return to normal organification of iodine and thyroid peroxidase action (see Fig. 20.3). Therefore, if iodine is given to prepare an individual with Graves' disease for surgery, the operation must happen within 10–14 days; otherwise, a significant relapse of the thyrotoxicosis could occur.

Iodine deficiency and underlying thyroid disease can both moderate the effects of iodine on thyroid function. In iodine-deficient parts of the world, transient thyrotoxicosis may be precipitated by prophylactic iodinisation programmes. In iodine-sufficient areas, thyrotoxicosis can be precipitated by iodine-containing radiographic contrast medium or expectorants in individuals who have underlying thyroid disease predisposing to thyrotoxicosis, such as multinodular goitre or Graves' disease in remission. Induction of thyrotoxicosis by iodine is called the Jod–Basedow effect. Chronic excess iodine administration can also result in hypothyroidism; this is, in effect, a failure to escape from the Wolff–Chaikoff effect and usually occurs in the context of prior insult to the thyroid by, for example, autoimmune disease, thyroiditis, lithium, antithyroid drugs or surgery.

Amiodarone

The anti-arrhythmic agent amiodarone has a structure that is analogous to that of T_4 (Fig. 20.10) and contains huge amounts of iodine; a 200 mg dose contains 75 mg iodine. Amiodarone also has a cytotoxic effect on thyroid follicular cells and inhibits conversion of T_4 to T_3 (increasing the ratio of T_4 : T_3). Most patients receiving amiodarone have normal thyroid function but up to 20% develop hypothyroidism or thyrotoxicosis, and so thyroid function should be monitored regularly. TSH provides the best indicator of thyroid function.

The thyrotoxicosis can be classified as either:

- *type I*: iodine-induced excess thyroid hormone synthesis in patients with an underlying thyroid disorder, such as nodular goitre or latent Graves' disease (an example of the Jod–Basedow effect), or

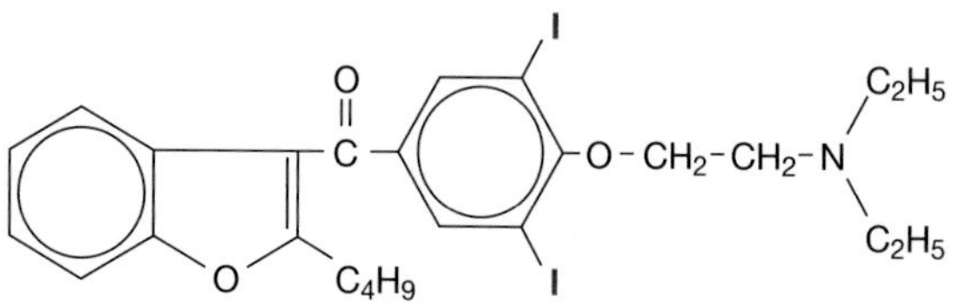

Fig. 20.10 The structure of amiodarone. Note the similarities to thyroxine (T_4) (see Fig. 20.3).

- *type II*: thyroiditis due to a direct cytotoxic effect of amiodarone administration.

These patterns can overlap and may be difficult to distinguish clinically, as iodine uptake is low in both. There is no widely accepted management algorithm, although the iodine excess renders the gland resistant to [131]I. Antithyroid drugs may be effective in patients with the type I form but are ineffective in type II thyrotoxicosis. Prednisolone is beneficial in the type II form. A pragmatic approach is to commence combination therapy with an antithyroid drug and glucocorticoid in patients with significant thyrotoxicosis. A rapid response (within 1–2 weeks) usually indicates a type II picture and permits withdrawal of the antithyroid therapy; a slower response suggests a type I picture, in which case antithyroid drugs may be continued and prednisolone withdrawn. If the cardiac state allows, amiodarone should be discontinued, but it has a long half-life (50–60 days) and so its effects are long-lasting. To minimise the risk of type I thyrotoxicosis, thyroid function should be measured in all patients prior to commencement of amiodarone therapy, and amiodarone should be avoided if TSH is suppressed.

Hypothyroidism should be treated with levothyroxine, which can be given while amiodarone is continued.

Simple and multinodular goitre

These terms describe diffuse or multinodular enlargement of the thyroid, which occurs sporadically and is of unknown aetiology.

Simple diffuse goitre

This form of goitre usually presents between the ages of 15 and 25 years, often during pregnancy, and tends to be noticed by friends and relatives rather than the patient. Occasionally, there is a tight sensation in the neck, particularly when swallowing. The goitre is soft and symmetrical, and the thyroid enlarged to two or three times normal. There is no tenderness, lymphadenopathy or overlying bruit. Concentrations of T_3, T_4 and TSH are normal and no thyroid autoantibodies are detected in the serum. No treatment is necessary and the goitre usually regresses. In some, however, the unknown stimulus to thyroid enlargement persists and, as a result of recurrent episodes of hyperplasia and involution during the following 10–20 years, the gland becomes multinodular with areas of autonomous function.

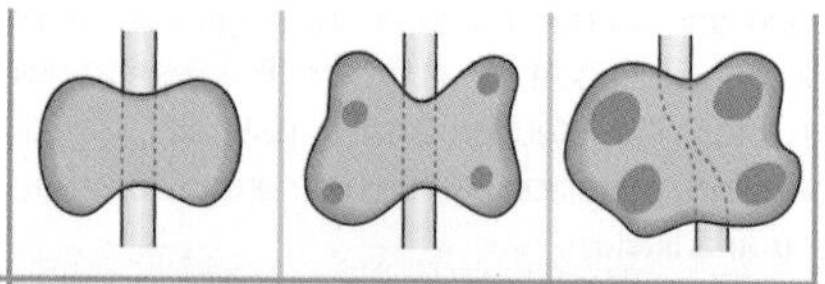

Age (in years)	15–25	26–55	> 55
Goitre	Diffuse	Nodular	Nodular
Tracheal compression/ deviation	No	Minimal	Yes
T_3, T_4	Normal	Normal	Raised
TSH	Normal	Normal or undetectable	Undetectable

Fig. 20.11 Natural history of simple goitre. (T_3 = triiodothyronine; T_4 = thyroxine; TSH = thyroid-stimulating hormone)

Multinodular goitre

The natural history is shown in Figure 20.11. Patients with thyroid enlargement in the absence of thyroid dysfunction or positive autoantibodies (i.e. with 'simple goitre'; see above) as young adults may progress to develop nodules. These nodules grow at varying rates and secrete thyroid hormone 'autonomously', thereby suppressing TSH-dependent growth and function in the rest of the gland. Ultimately, complete suppression of TSH occurs in about 25% of cases, with T_4 and T_3 levels often within the reference range (subclinical thyrotoxicosis), but sometimes elevated (toxic multinodular goitre; see Fig. 20.5).

Clinical features and investigations

Multinodular goitre is usually diagnosed in patients presenting with thyrotoxicosis, a large goitre with or without tracheal compression, or sudden painful swelling caused by haemorrhage into a nodule or cyst. The goitre is nodular or lobulated on palpation and may extend retrosternally; however, not all multinodular goitres causing thyrotoxicosis are easily palpable. Very large goitres can cause mediastinal compression with stridor (Fig. 20.12), dysphagia and obstruction of the superior vena cava. Hoarseness due to recurrent laryngeal nerve palsy can occur but is far more suggestive of thyroid carcinoma.

The diagnosis can be confirmed by ultrasonography and/or thyroid scintigraphy (see Fig. 20.5). In patients with large goitres, a flow-volume loop is a good screening test for significant tracheal compression (see Fig. 17.7). If intervention is contemplated, a CT or MRI of the thoracic inlet should be performed to quantify the degree of tracheal displacement or compression and the extent of retrosternal extension. Nodules should be evaluated for the possibility of thyroid neoplasia.

Management

If the goitre is small, no treatment is necessary but annual thyroid function testing should be arranged, as the natural history is progression to a toxic multinodular goitre. Thyroid surgery is indicated for large goitres that cause mediastinal compression or that are cosmetically unattractive. ^{131}I can result in a significant reduction in thyroid size and may be of value in older patients. Levothyroxine therapy is of no benefit in shrinking multinodular goitres in iodine-sufficient countries and may simply aggravate any associated thyrotoxicosis.

In toxic multinodular goitre, treatment is usually with ^{131}I. The iodine uptake is lower than in Graves' disease, so a higher dose may be administered (up to 800 Mbq (approximately 20 mCi)) and hypothyroidism is less common. In thyrotoxic patients with a large goitre, thyroid surgery may be indicated. Long-term treatment with antithyroid drugs is not usually employed, as relapse is invariable after drug withdrawal; drug therapy

is normally reserved for frail older patients in whom surgery or ^{131}I is not an appropriate option.

Asymptomatic patients with subclinical thyrotoxicosis are increasingly being treated with ^{131}I on the grounds that a suppressed TSH is a risk factor for atrial fibrillation and, particularly in post-menopausal women, osteoporosis.

Thyroid neoplasia

Patients with thyroid tumours usually present with a solitary nodule. Most are benign and a few of these, called 'toxic adenomas', secrete excess thyroid hormones. Primary thyroid malignancy is rare, accounting for less than 1% of all carcinomas, and has an incidence of 25 per million per annum. As shown in Box 20.17, it can be classified according to the cell type of origin. With the exception of medullary carcinoma, thyroid cancer is more common in females.

Toxic adenoma

A solitary toxic nodule is the cause of less than 5% of all cases of thyrotoxicosis. The nodule is a follicular adenoma, which autonomously secretes excess thyroid hormones and inhibits endogenous TSH secretion, with subsequent atrophy of the rest of the thyroid gland. The adenoma is usually greater than 3 cm in diameter.

Most patients are female and over 40 years of age. Although many nodules are palpable, the diagnosis can be made with certainty only by thyroid scintigraphy (see Fig. 20.5). The thyrotoxicosis is usually mild and in almost 50% of patients the plasma T_3 alone is elevated (T_3 thyrotoxicosis). ^{131}I (400–800 MBq (10–20 mCi)) is highly effective and is an ideal treatment since the atrophic cells surrounding the nodule do not take up iodine and so receive little or no radiation. For this reason, permanent hypothyroidism is unusual. Hemithyroidectomy is an alternative management option.

Differentiated carcinoma

The incidence of thyroid carcinoma has increased significantly since the early 1990s although this has not been paralleled by any significant increase in thyroid carcinoma deaths over the same period (Fig. 20.13). Increasing incidence of thyroid carcinoma is, at least in part, explained by an increased rate of incidental detection, which tracks greater use of neck imaging.

Papillary carcinoma

This is the most common of the malignant thyroid tumours and accounts for 90% of radiation-induced thyroid cancer. It may be multifocal and

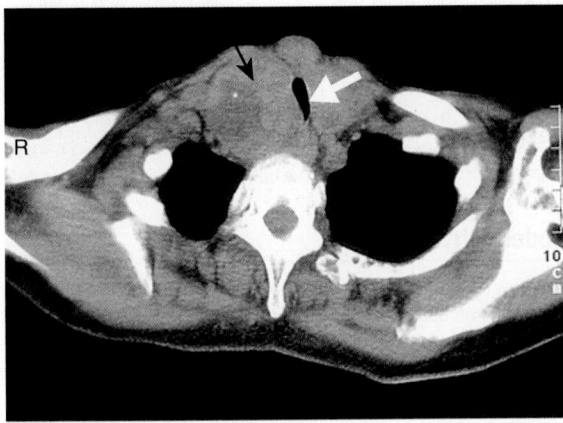

Fig. 20.12 Computed tomogram showing retrosternal multinodular goitre. The goitre (black arrow) is causing acute severe breathlessness and stridor due to tracheal compression (white arrow).

i | **20.17 Malignant thyroid tumours**

Type of tumour	Frequency (%)	Age at presentation (years)	10-year survival (%)
Follicular cells			
Differentiated carcinoma:			
Papillary	75–85	20–40	98
Follicular	10–20	40–60	94
Anaplastic	<5	>60	9
Parafollicular C cells			
Medullary carcinoma	5–8	>40*	78
Lymphocytes			
Lymphoma	<5	>60	45

*Patients with medullary carcinoma as part of multiple endocrine neoplasia (MEN) types 2a and 2b (p. 700) may present in childhood.

20

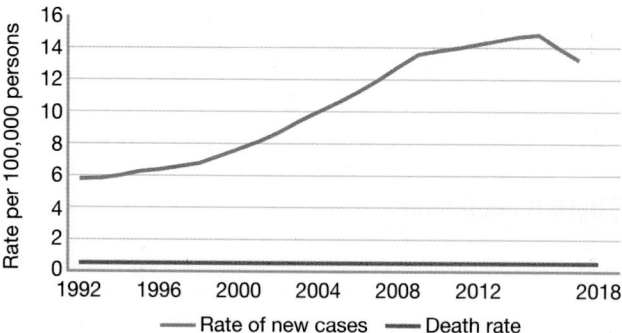

Fig. 20.13 Incidence and death rates of thyroid cancer. Although the incidence has increased from 1990 because of higher rates of discovery due to the use of more imaging, the overall death rate remains very low with an overall 5-year survival of >98%. *From National Cancer Institute https://seer.cancer.gov/statfacts/html/thyro.html.*

spread is initially to regional lymph nodes. Some patients present with cervical lymphadenopathy and no apparent thyroid enlargement; in such instances, the primary lesion may be less than 10 mm in diameter.

Follicular carcinoma

This is usually a single encapsulated lesion. Spread to cervical lymph nodes is rare. Metastases are blood-borne and are most often found in bone, lungs and brain.

Management

The management of thyroid cancers should be individualised and planned in multidisciplinary team meetings that include all specialists involved in the service; this should include thyroid surgeons, endocrinologists, oncologists, pathologists, radiologists and nurse specialists. Large tumours, those with adverse histological features and/or tumours with metastatic disease at presentation are usually managed by total thyroidectomy followed by a large dose of [131]I (1100 or 3700 MBq (approximately 30 or 100 mCi)) to ablate any remaining normal or malignant thyroid tissue. Thereafter, long-term treatment with levothyroxine in a dose sufficient to suppress TSH (usually 150–200 μg daily) is given, as there is evidence that growth of differentiated thyroid carcinomas is TSH-dependent. Smaller tumours with no adverse histological features may require only thyroid lobectomy.

Follow-up involves measurement of serum thyroglobulin, which should be undetectable in patients whose normal thyroid has been ablated and who are taking a suppressive dose of levothyroxine. Thyroglobulin antibodies may interfere with the assay and, depending on the method employed, may result in a falsely low or high result. Detectable thyroglobulin, in the absence of assay interference, is suggestive of tumour recurrence or metastases, particularly if the thyroglobulin titre is rising across serial measurements. Local recurrence or metastatic disease may be localised by ultrasound, CT, MRI and/or whole-body scanning with ^{131}I, and may be treated with further surgery and/or ^{131}I therapy. [131]I treatment in thyroid cancer and isotope scanning both require serum TSH concentrations to be elevated (>20 mIU/L). This may be achieved by levothyroxine withdrawal for 3–4 weeks, inducing symptomatic hypothyroidism, or by administering intramuscular injections of recombinant human TSH. Patients usually find the latter approach preferable but it is more expensive. Those with locally advanced or metastatic papillary and follicular carcinoma that is refractive to ^{131}I may be considered for therapy with sorafenib, lenvatinib or vandetanib. These drugs are multi-targeted tyrosine kinase inhibitors and have been shown in trials to prolong progression-free survival by between 5 and 14 months. They have multiple toxicities, however, including poor appetite, weight loss, fatigue, diarrhoea, mucositis, rashes, hypertension and blood dyscrasias. The potential benefits of therapy therefore have to be carefully weighed against side-effects that can significantly impair quality of life.

Prognosis

Most patients with papillary and follicular thyroid cancer will be cured with appropriate treatment. Adverse prognostic factors include older age at presentation, the presence of distant metastases, male sex and certain histological subtypes. However, ^{131}I therapy can be effective in treating those with distant metastases, particularly small-volume disease in the lungs, and so prolonged survival is quite common.

Anaplastic carcinoma and lymphoma

These two conditions are difficult to distinguish clinically but are distinct cytologically and histologically. Patients are usually over 60 years of age and present with rapid thyroid enlargement over 2–3 months. The goitre is hard and there may be stridor due to tracheal compression and hoarseness due to recurrent laryngeal nerve palsy. There is no effective treatment for anaplastic carcinoma, although surgery and radiotherapy may be considered in some circumstances. In older patients, median survival is only 7 months.

The prognosis for lymphoma, which may arise from pre-existing Hashimoto's thyroiditis, is better, with a median survival of 9 years. Some 98% of tumours are non-Hodgkin lymphomas, usually the diffuse large B-cell subtype. Treatment is with combination chemotherapy and external beam radiotherapy.

Medullary carcinoma

This tumour arises from the parafollicular C cells of the thyroid. In addition to calcitonin, the tumour may secrete 5-hydroxytryptamine (5-HT, serotonin), various peptides of the tachykinin family, adrenocorticotrophic hormone (ACTH) and prostaglandins. As a consequence, carcinoid syndrome (see Box 20.49) and Cushing's syndrome (see p. 679) may occur.

Patients usually present in middle age with a firm thyroid mass. Cervical lymph node involvement is common but distant metastases are rare initially. Serum calcitonin levels are raised and are useful in monitoring response to treatment. Despite the very high levels of calcitonin found in some patients, hypocalcaemia is extremely rare; however, hypercalcitoninaemia can be associated with severe, watery diarrhoea.

Treatment is by total thyroidectomy with removal of regional cervical lymph nodes. Since the C cells do not concentrate iodine and are not responsive to TSH, there is no role for ^{131}I therapy or TSH suppression with levothyroxine. External beam radiotherapy may be considered in some patients at high risk of local recurrence. Vandetanib and cabozantinib are tyrosine kinase inhibitors licensed for patients with progressive advanced medullary cancer. The prognosis is less good than for papillary and follicular carcinoma, but individuals can live for many decades with persistent disease that behaves in an indolent fashion.

Medullary carcinoma of the thyroid occurs sporadically in 70%–90% cases; in 10%–30% there is a genetic predisposition that is inherited in an autosomal dominant fashion and due to an activating mutation in the *RET* gene. This inherited tendency normally forms part of one of the MEN syndromes (MEN 2a (formerly known as MEN 2) or MEN 2b (formerly known as MEN 3), p. 700) but, occasionally, susceptibility to medullary carcinoma is the only inherited trait (familial medullary thyroid cancer and this depends on the particular codon of the *RET* gene that is mutated).

Riedel's thyroiditis

This is not a form of thyroid cancer but the presentation is similar and the differentiation can usually be made only by thyroid biopsy. It is an exceptionally rare condition of unknown aetiology, in which there is extensive infiltration of the thyroid and surrounding structures with fibrous tissue. There may be associated mediastinal and retroperitoneal fibrosis. Presentation is with a slow-growing goitre that is irregular and stony-hard. There is usually tracheal and oesophageal compression necessitating partial thyroidectomy. Other recognised complications include recurrent laryngeal nerve palsy, hypoparathyroidism and eventually hypothyroidism.

Congenital thyroid disease

Early treatment with levothyroxine is essential to prevent irreversible brain damage in children (cretinism) with congenital hypothyroidism. Routine screening of TSH levels in heel-prick blood samples obtained 5–7 days after birth (as part of the Guthrie test) has revealed an incidence of approximately 1 in 3000, resulting from thyroid agenesis, ectopic or hypoplastic glands, or dyshormonogenesis. Congenital hypothyroidism is thus six times more common than phenylketonuria. It is now possible to start levothyroxine replacement therapy within 2 weeks of birth. Developmental assessment of infants treated at this early stage has revealed no differences between cases and controls in most children.

Dyshormonogenesis

Several autosomal recessive defects in thyroid hormone synthesis have been described; the most common results from deficiency of the intrathyroidal peroxidase enzyme. Homozygous individuals present with congenital hypothyroidism; heterozygotes present in the first two decades of life with goitre, normal thyroid hormone levels and a raised TSH. The combination of dyshormonogenetic goitre and nerve deafness is known as Pendred syndrome. Most cases of Pendred syndrome are caused by mutations in the *SLC26A4* gene, which encodes pendrin, the protein that transports iodide to the luminal surface of the follicular cell (see Fig. 20.3).

Thyroid hormone resistance

This is a rare disorder in which the pituitary and hypothalamus are resistant to feedback suppression of TSH by T_3, sometimes due to mutations in the thyroid hormone receptor β gene or because of defects in monodeiodinase activity. The result is high levels of TSH, T_4 and T_3, often with a moderate goitre that may not be noted until adulthood. Thyroid hormone signalling is highly complex and involves different isozymes of both monodeiodinases and thyroid hormone receptors in different tissues. For that reason, other tissues may or may not share the resistance to thyroid hormone and there may be features of thyrotoxicosis (e.g. tachycardia). This condition can be difficult to distinguish from an equally rare TSH-producing pituitary tumour (TSHoma; see Box 20.5); administration of TRH results in elevation of TSH in thyroid hormone resistance and not in TSHoma, but an MRI scan of the pituitary may be necessary to exclude a macroadenoma.

The reproductive system

Clinical practice in reproductive medicine is shared between several specialties, including gynaecology, urology, paediatric endocrinologists, psychiatry and endocrinology. The following section is focused on disorders managed by adult endocrinologists.

Functional anatomy, physiology and investigations

The physiology of male and female reproductive function is illustrated in Figures 20.14 and 20.15, respectively. Pathways for synthesis of sex steroids are shown in Figure 20.20.

The male

In the male, the testis serves two principal functions: synthesis of testosterone by the interstitial Leydig cells under the control of luteinising hormone (LH), and spermatogenesis by Sertoli cells under the control of follicle-stimulating hormone (FSH) (but also requiring adequate testosterone). Negative feedback suppression of LH is mediated principally by testosterone, while secretion of another hormone produced by the testis, inhibin, suppresses FSH. The axis can be assessed easily by a random blood sample for testosterone, LH and FSH. Testosterone levels are higher in the morning and

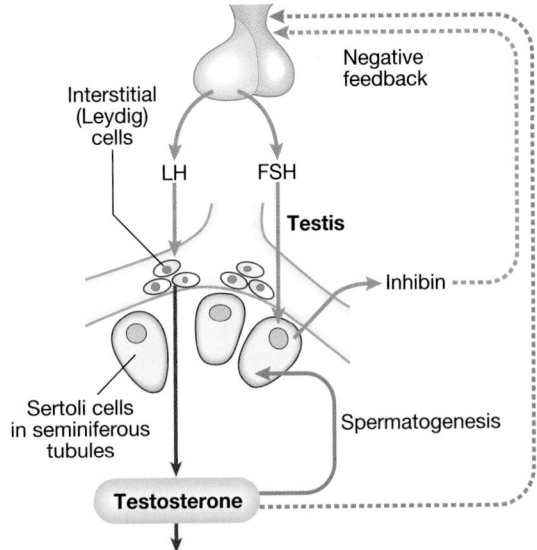

Fig. 20.14 Male reproductive physiology. (FSH = follicle-stimulating hormone; LH = luteinising hormone)

therefore, if testosterone is marginally low, sampling should be repeated with the patient fasted at 0900 hrs. Testosterone is largely bound in plasma to sex hormone-binding globulin and this can also be measured to calculate the 'free androgen index' or the 'bioavailable' testosterone. Testicular function can also be tested by semen analysis.

There is no equivalent of the menopause in men, although testosterone concentrations decline slowly from the fourth decade onwards.

The female

In the female, physiology varies during the normal menstrual cycle. FSH stimulates growth and development of ovarian follicles during the first 14 days after the menses. This leads to a gradual increase in oestradiol production from granulosa cells, which initially suppresses FSH secretion (negative feedback) but then, above a certain level, stimulates an increase in both the frequency and amplitude of gonadotrophin-releasing hormone (GnRH) pulses, resulting in a marked increase in LH secretion (positive feedback). The mid-cycle 'surge' of LH induces ovulation. After release of the ovum, the follicle differentiates into a corpus luteum, which secretes progesterone. Unless pregnancy occurs during the cycle, the corpus luteum regresses and the fall in progesterone levels results in menstrual bleeding. Circulating levels of oestrogen and progesterone in pre-menopausal women are, therefore, critically dependent on the time of the cycle. The most useful 'test' of ovarian function is a careful menstrual history: if menses are regular, measurement of gonadotrophins and oestrogen is not necessary. In addition, ovulation can be confirmed by measuring plasma progesterone levels during the luteal phase ('day 21 progesterone').

Cessation of menstruation (the menopause) occurs at an average age of approximately 50 years in high-income countries. In the 5 years before, there is a gradual increase in the number of anovulatory cycles and this is referred to as the climacteric. Oestrogen and inhibin secretion falls and negative feedback results in increased pituitary secretion of LH and FSH (both typically to levels above 30 IU/L (3.3 μg/L)).

20

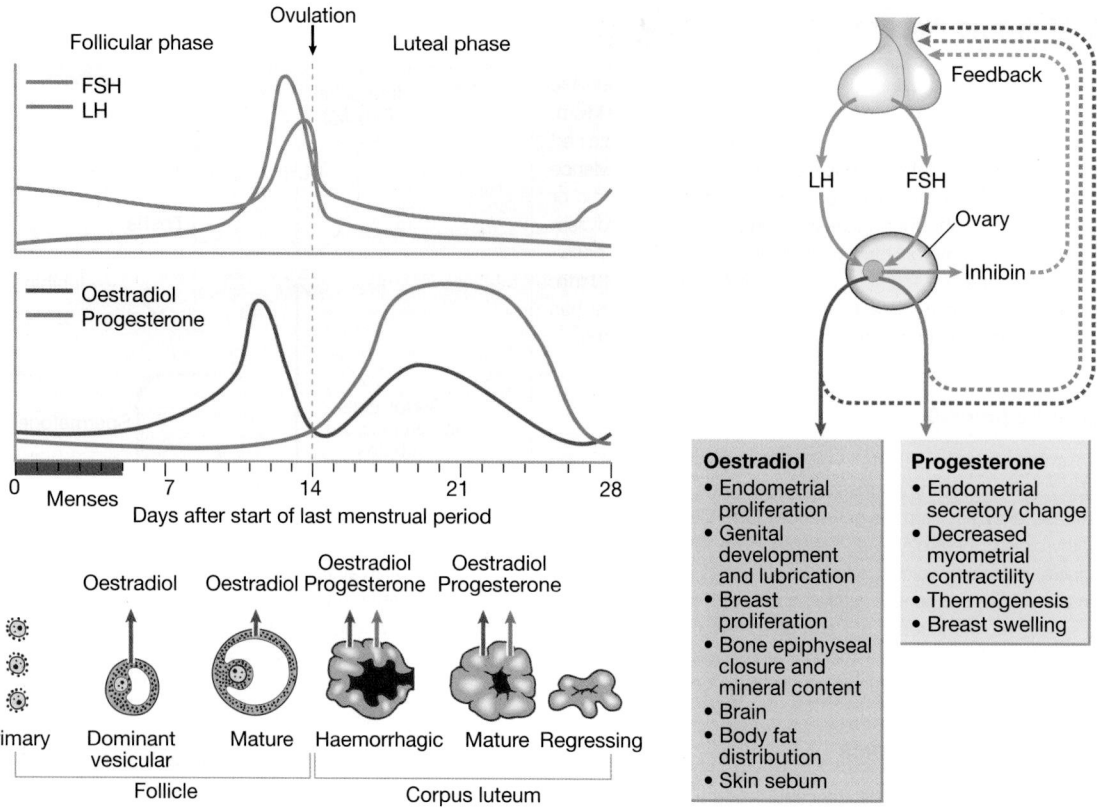

Fig. 20.15 Female reproductive physiology and the normal menstrual cycle. (FSH = follicle-stimulating hormone; LH = luteinising hormone)

The pathophysiology of male and female reproductive dysfunction is summarised in Box 20.18.

20.18 Classification of diseases of the reproductive system

	Primary	Secondary
Hormone excess	Polycystic ovary syndrome Granulosa cell tumour Leydig cell tumour Teratoma	Pituitary gonadotrophinoma
Hormone deficiency	Hypogonadism (see Box 20.19) Turner syndrome Klinefelter syndrome	Hypopituitarism Kallmann syndrome (isolated GnRH deficiency) Severe systemic illness, including anorexia nervosa
Hormone hypersensitivity	Idiopathic hirsutism	

Hormone resistance	Androgen resistance syndromes
	    Complete ('testicular feminisation')
	    Partial (Reifenstein syndrome)
	    5α-reductase type 2 deficiency	

Non-functioning tumours	Ovarian cysts Carcinoma Teratoma Seminoma	

(GnRH = gonadotrophin-releasing hormone)

Presenting problems in reproductive disease

Delayed puberty

Normal pubertal development is discussed in Chapter 33. Puberty is considered to be delayed if the onset of the physical features of sexual maturation has not occurred by a chronological age that is 2.5 standard deviations (SD) above the national average. In the UK, this is by the age of 14 in boys and 13 in girls. Genetic factors have a major influence in determining the timing of the onset of puberty, such that the age of menarche (the onset of menstruation) is often comparable within sibling and mother–daughter pairs and within ethnic groups. However, because there is also a threshold for body weight that acts as a trigger for normal puberty, the onset of puberty can be influenced by other factors, including nutritional status and chronic illness.

Clinical assessment

The differential diagnosis is shown in Box 20.19. The key issue is to determine whether the delay in puberty is simply because the 'clock is running slow' (constitutional delay of puberty) or because there is pathology in the hypothalamus/pituitary (hypogonadotrophic hypogonadism) or the gonads (hypergonadotrophic hypogonadism). A general history and physical examination should be performed with particular reference to previous or current medical disorders, social circumstances and family history. Body proportions, sense of smell and pubertal stage should be carefully documented and, in boys, the presence or absence of testes in the scrotum noted. Current weight and height may be plotted on centile charts, along with parental heights. Previous growth measurements in childhood, which can usually be obtained from health records, are extremely useful. Healthy growth usually follows a centile. Usually, children with constitutional delay have always been small but have maintained a normal growth velocity that is appropriate for bone age. Poor linear growth, with 'crossing of the height centiles', is more likely to be

i **20.19 Causes of delayed puberty and hypogonadism**

Constitutional delay

Hypogonadotrophic hypogonadism

- Structural hypothalamic/pituitary disease (see Box 20.53)
- Functional gonadotrophin deficiency:
    Chronic systemic illness (e.g. asthma, malabsorption, coeliac disease, cystic fibrosis, renal failure)
    Psychological stress
    Anorexia nervosa
    Excessive physical exercise
    Hyperprolactinaemia
    Other endocrine disease (e.g. Cushing's syndrome, primary hypothyroidism)
- Isolated gonadotrophin deficiency (Kallmann syndrome)

Hypergonadotrophic hypogonadism

- Acquired gonadal damage:
    Chemotherapy/radiotherapy to gonads
    Trauma/surgery to gonads
    Autoimmune gonadal failure
    Mumps orchitis
    Tuberculosis
    Haemochromatosis
- Developmental/congenital gonadal disorders:
    Steroid biosynthetic defects
    Anorchidism/cryptorchidism in males
    Klinefelter syndrome (47,XXY, male phenotype)
    Turner syndrome (45,X, female phenotype)

  20.20 Delayed puberty

- **Aetiology**: in boys the most common cause is constitutional delay, whereas in girls there is inevitably a structural hypothalamic/pituitary abnormality or a factor that affects their function.
- **Psychological effects**: whatever the underlying cause, delayed puberty is often associated with substantial psychological distress.
- **Investigations**: a karyotype should be performed in all adolescents with hypergonadotrophic hypogonadism, to exclude Turner and Klinefelter syndromes, unless there is an obvious precipitating cause.
- **Medical induction of puberty**: if this is being considered, it needs to be managed carefully and carried out in a controlled fashion, to avoid premature fusion of the epiphyses.

associated with acquired disease. Issues that are commonly encountered in the management of adolescents with delayed puberty are summarised in Box 20.20.

Constitutional delay of puberty

This is the most common cause of delayed puberty, but is a much more frequent explanation for lack of pubertal development in boys than in girls. Affected children are healthy and have usually been more than 2 SD below the mean height for their age throughout childhood. There is often a history of delayed puberty in siblings or parents. Since sex steroids are essential for fusion of the epiphyses, 'bone age' can be estimated by X-rays of epiphyses, usually in the wrist and hand; in constitutional delay, bone age is lower than chronological age. Constitutional delay of puberty should be considered as a normal variant, as puberty will commence spontaneously. However, affected children can experience significant psychological distress because of their lack of physical development, particularly when compared with their peers.

Hypogonadotrophic hypogonadism

This may be due to structural, inflammatory or infiltrative disorders of the pituitary and/or hypothalamus (see Box 20.53). In such circumstances, other pituitary hormones, such as growth hormone, are also likely to be deficient.

'Functional' gonadotrophin deficiency is caused by a variety of factors, including low body weight, chronic systemic illness (as a consequence

of the disease itself or secondary malnutrition), endocrine disorders and profound psychosocial stress.

Isolated gonadotrophin deficiency is usually due to a genetic abnormality that affects the synthesis of either GnRH or gonadotrophins. The most common form is Kallmann syndrome, in which there is primary GnRH deficiency and, in most affected individuals, agenesis or hypoplasia of the olfactory bulbs, resulting in anosmia or hyposmia. If isolated gonadotrophin deficiency is left untreated, the epiphyses fail to fuse, resulting in tall stature with disproportionately long arms and legs relative to trunk height (eunuchoid habitus).

Cryptorchidism (undescended testes) and gynaecomastia are commonly observed in all forms of hypogonadotrophic hypogonadism.

Hypergonadotrophic hypogonadism

Hypergonadotrophic hypogonadism associated with delayed puberty is usually due to Klinefelter syndrome in boys and Turner syndrome in girls. Other causes of primary gonadal failure are shown in Box 20.19.

Investigations

Key measurements are LH and FSH, testosterone (in boys) and oestradiol (in girls). Chromosome analysis should be performed if gonadotrophin concentrations are elevated. If gonadotrophin concentrations are low, then the differential diagnosis lies between constitutional delay and hypogonadotrophic hypogonadism. A plain X-ray of the wrist and hand may be compared with a set of standard films to obtain a bone age. Full blood count, renal function, liver function, thyroid function and coeliac disease autoantibodies (see p. 819) should be measured, but further tests may be unnecessary if the blood tests are normal and the child has all the clinical features of constitutional delay. If hypogonadotrophic hypogonadism is suspected, neuroimaging and further investigations are required (see Box 20.51).

Management

Puberty can be induced using low doses of oral oestrogen in girls (e.g. ethinylestradiol 2 μg daily) or testosterone in boys (testosterone gel or depot testosterone esters). Higher doses carry a risk of early fusion of epiphyses. This therapy should be given in a specialist clinic where the progress of puberty and growth can be carefully monitored. In children with constitutional delay, this 'priming' therapy can be discontinued when endogenous puberty is established, usually in less than a year. In children with hypogonadism, the underlying cause should be treated and reversed if possible. If hypogonadism is permanent, sex hormone doses are gradually increased during puberty and full adult replacement doses given when development is complete.

Amenorrhoea

Primary amenorrhoea may be diagnosed in a female who has never menstruated; this usually occurs as a manifestation of delayed puberty but may also be a consequence of anatomical defects of the female reproductive system, such as endometrial hypoplasia or vaginal agenesis. Secondary amenorrhoea describes the cessation of menstruation in a female who has previously had periods. The causes of this common presentation are shown in Box 20.21. In non-pregnant women, secondary amenorrhoea is almost invariably a consequence of either ovarian or hypothalamic/pituitary dysfunction. Premature ovarian failure (premature menopause) is defined, arbitrarily, as occurring before 40 years of age. Rarely, endometrial adhesions (Asherman syndrome) can form after uterine curettage, surgery or infection with tuberculosis or schistosomiasis, preventing endometrial proliferation and shedding.

Clinical assessment

The underlying cause can often be suspected from associated clinical features and the patient's age. Hypothalamic/pituitary disease and premature ovarian failure result in oestrogen deficiency, which causes a variety of symptoms usually associated with the menopause (Box 20.22). A history of galactorrhoea should be sought. Significant weight loss of

20

---

i   20.21 Causes of secondary amenorrhoea

Physiological
- Pregnancy
- Menopause

Hypogonadotrophic hypogonadism (see Box 20.19)

Ovarian dysfunction
- Hypergonadotrophic hypogonadism (see Box 20.19)
- Polycystic ovary syndrome
- Androgen-secreting tumours

Uterine dysfunction
- Asherman syndrome

---

i   20.22 Symptoms of oestrogen deficiency

Vasomotor effects
- Hot flushes
- Sweating

Psychological
- Anxiety
- Irritability
- Emotional lability

Genitourinary
- Dyspareunia
- Urgency of micturition
- Vaginal infections

---

any cause can cause amenorrhoea by suppression of gonadotrophins. Weight gain may suggest hypothyroidism, Cushing's syndrome (if other discriminatory features are present), or very rarely, a hypothalamic lesion. Hirsutism, obesity and long-standing irregular periods suggest polycystic ovary syndrome (PCOS). The presence of other autoimmune disease raises the possibility of autoimmune premature ovarian failure.

Investigations

Pregnancy should be excluded in women of reproductive age by measuring urine or serum hCG. Serum LH, FSH, oestradiol, prolactin, testosterone, T_4 and TSH should be measured and, in the absence of a menstrual cycle, can be taken at any time. Investigation of hyperprolactinaemia is described on page 697. High concentrations of LH and FSH with low or low-normal oestradiol suggest primary ovarian failure. Ovarian autoantibodies may be positive when there is an underlying autoimmune aetiology, and a karyotype should be performed in younger women to exclude mosaic Turner syndrome. Elevated LH, prolactin and testosterone levels with normal oestradiol are common in PCOS. Low levels of LH, FSH and oestradiol suggest hypothalamic or pituitary disease and a pituitary MRI is indicated.

There is some overlap in gonadotrophin and oestrogen concentrations between women with hypogonadotrophic hypogonadism and PCOS. If there is doubt as to the underlying cause of secondary amenorrhoea, then the response to 5 days of treatment with an oral progestogen (e.g. medroxyprogesterone acetate 10 mg twice daily) can be assessed. In women with PCOS, the progestogen will cause maturation of the endometrium and menstruation will occur a few days after the progestogen is stopped. In women with hypogonadotrophic hypogonadism, menstruation does not occur following progestogen withdrawal because the endometrium is atrophic as a result of oestrogen deficiency. If doubt persists in distinguishing oestrogen deficiency from a uterine abnormality, the capacity for menstruation can be tested with 1 month of treatment with cyclical oestrogen and progestogen (usually administered as a combined oral contraceptive pill).

Assessment of bone mineral density by dual X-ray absorptiometry (DXA, see Ch. 26) may be appropriate in patients with low androgen and oestrogen levels.

Management

Where possible, the underlying cause should be treated. For example, women with functional amenorrhoea due to excessive exercise and low weight should be encouraged to reduce their exercise and regain some weight. The management of structural pituitary and hypothalamic disease is described on page 693 and that of PCOS on page 673.

In oestrogen-deficient women, replacement therapy may be necessary to treat symptoms and/or to prevent osteoporosis. Women who have had a hysterectomy can be treated with oestrogen alone but those with a uterus should be treated with combined oestrogen/progestogen therapy, since unopposed oestrogen increases the risk of endometrial cancer. Cyclical hormone replacement therapy (HRT) regimens typically involve giving oestrogen on days 1–21 and progestogen on days 14–21 of the cycle, and this can be conveniently administered as the oral contraceptive pill. If oestrogenic side-effects (fluid retention, weight gain, hypertension and thrombosis) are a concern, then lower-dose oral or transdermal HRT may be more appropriate.

The timing of the discontinuation of oestrogen replacement therapy is still a matter of debate. In post-menopausal women, HRT has been shown to relieve menopausal symptoms and to prevent osteoporotic fractures but is associated with adverse effects, which are related to the duration of therapy and to the patient's age. In patients with premature menopause, HRT should be continued up to the age of around 50 years, but continued beyond this age only if there are continued symptoms of oestrogen deficiency on discontinuation.

Management of infertility in oestrogen-deficient women is described below.

Male hypogonadism

The clinical features of both hypo- and hypergonadotrophic hypogonadism include loss of libido, lethargy with muscle weakness and decreased frequency of shaving. Patients may also present with gynaecomastia, infertility, delayed puberty, osteoporosis or anaemia of chronic disease. The causes of hypogonadism are listed in Box 20.19. Mild hypogonadism may also occur in older men, particularly in the context of central adiposity and the metabolic syndrome. Postulated mechanisms are complex and include reduction in sex hormone-binding globulin by insulin resistance and reduction in GnRH and gonadotrophin secretion by cytokines or oestrogen released by adipose tissue. Testosterone levels also fall gradually with age in men (see Box 20.24) and this is associated with gonadotrophin levels that are low or inappropriately within the 'normal' range. There is an increasing trend to measure testosterone in older men, typically as part of an assessment of erectile dysfunction and lack of libido.

Investigations

Male hypogonadism is confirmed by demonstrating a low fasting 0900-hr serum testosterone level. The distinction between hypo- and hypergonadotrophic hypogonadism is by measurement of random LH and FSH. Patients with hypogonadotrophic hypogonadism should be investigated as described for pituitary disease on page 692. Patients with hypergonadotrophic hypogonadism should have the testes examined for cryptorchidism or atrophy, and a karyotype should be performed (to identify Klinefelter syndrome).

Management

Testosterone replacement is clearly indicated in younger men with significant hypogonadism to prevent osteoporosis and to restore muscle power and libido. Debate exists as to whether replacement therapy is of benefit in mild hypogonadism associated with ageing and central adiposity, particularly in the absence of structural pituitary/hypothalamic disease or other pituitary hormone deficiency. In such instances, a therapeutic trial of testosterone therapy may be considered if symptoms are present (e.g. low libido and erectile dysfunction) and the serum testosterone is consistently low, but the benefits of therapy must be carefully weighed against the potential for harm.

Routes of testosterone administration are shown in Box 20.23. First-pass hepatic metabolism of testosterone is highly efficient, so bioavailability of ingested preparations is poor. Doses of systemic testosterone can be titrated against symptoms; circulating testosterone

20.23 Options for androgen replacement therapy

Route of administration	Preparation	Dose	Frequency	Comments
Intramuscular	Testosterone undecanoate	1000 mg	Every 3 months	Smoother profile than testosterone enantate, with less frequent injections
	Testosterone enanthate	50–250 mg	Every 3–4 weeks	Produces peaks and troughs of testosterone levels that are outside the physiological range and may be symptomatic
Transdermal	Testosterone gel	50–100 mg	Daily	Stable testosterone levels; transfer of gel can occur following skin-to-skin contact with another person

20.24 Gonadal function in old age

- **Post-menopausal osteoporosis**: a major public health issue due to the high incidence of associated fragility fractures, especially of hip.
- **Hormone replacement therapy**: should be prescribed only above the age of 50 for the short-term relief of symptoms of oestrogen deficiency.
- **Sexual activity**: many older people are sexually active.
- **'Male menopause'**: does not occur, although testosterone concentrations do fall with age. Testosterone therapy in mildly hypogonadal men may be of benefit for body composition, muscle and bone. Large randomised trials are required to determine whether benefits outweigh potentially harmful effects on the prostate and cardiovascular system.
- **Androgens in older women**: hirsutism and balding occur. In those rare patients with elevated androgen levels, this may be pathological, e.g. from an ovarian tumour.

20.25 Causes of infertility

Female factors (35%–40%)

- Ovulatory dysfunction:
  Polycystic ovary syndrome
  Hypogonadotrophic hypogonadism (see Box 20.19)
  Hypergonadotrophic hypogonadism (see Box 20.19)
- Tubular dysfunction:
  Pelvic inflammatory disease (chlamydia, gonorrhoea)
  Endometriosis
  Previous sterilisation
  Previous pelvic or abdominal surgery
- Cervical and/or uterine dysfunction:
  Congenital abnormalities
  Fibroids
  Treatment for cervical carcinoma
  Asherman syndrome

Male factors (35%–40%)

- Reduced sperm quality or production:
  Y chromosome microdeletions
  Varicocele
  Hypergonadotrophic hypogonadism (see Box 20.19)
  Hypogonadotrophic hypogonadism (see Box 20.19)
- Tubular dysfunction:
  Varicocele
  Congenital abnormality of vas deferens/epididymis
  Previous sexually transmitted infection (chlamydia, gonorrhoea)
  Previous vasectomy

Unexplained or mixed factors (20%–35%)

levels may provide only a rough guide to dosage because they may be highly variable (Box 20.23). Testosterone therapy can aggravate prostatic carcinoma; prostate-specific antigen (PSA) should be measured before commencing testosterone therapy in men older than 50 years and monitored annually thereafter. Haemoglobin concentration should also be monitored, as androgen replacement can cause polycythaemia. Testosterone replacement inhibits spermatogenesis; treatment for fertility is described below.

Some important aspects of gonadal function in older women and men are summarized in Box 20.24.

Infertility

Infertility affects around 1 in 7 couples of reproductive age, often causing psychological distress. The main causes are listed in Box 20.25. In women, it may result from anovulation or abnormalities of the reproductive tract that prevent fertilisation or embryonic implantation, often damaged Fallopian tubes from previous infection. In men, infertility may result from impaired sperm quality (e.g. reduced motility) or reduced sperm number. Azoospermia or oligospermia is usually idiopathic but may be a consequence of hypogonadism (see Box 20.19). Microdeletions of the Y chromosome are increasingly recognised as a cause of severely abnormal spermatogenesis. In many couples more than one factor causing subfertility is present, and in a large proportion no cause can be identified.

Clinical assessment

A history of previous pregnancies, relevant infections and surgery is important in both men and women. A sexual history must be explored sensitively, as some couples have intercourse infrequently or only when they consider the woman to be ovulating, and psychosexual difficulties are common. Irregular and/or infrequent menstrual periods are an indicator of anovulatory cycles in the woman, in which case causes such as PCOS should be considered. In men, the testes should be examined to confirm that both are in the scrotum and to identify any structural abnormality, such as small size, absent vas deferens or the presence of a varicocele.

Investigations

Investigations should generally be performed after a couple has failed to conceive despite unprotected intercourse for 12 months, unless there is an obvious abnormality like amenorrhoea. Both partners need to be investigated. The male partner needs a semen analysis to assess sperm count and quality. Home testing for ovulation (by commercial urine dipstick kits, temperature measurement, or assessment of cervical mucus) is not recommended, as the information is often counterbalanced by increased anxiety if interpretation is inconclusive. In women with regular periods, ovulation can be confirmed by an elevated serum progesterone concentration on day 21 of the menstrual cycle. Transvaginal ultrasound can be used to assess uterine and ovarian anatomy. Tubal patency may be examined at laparoscopy or by hysterosalpingography (HSG; a radio-opaque medium is injected into the uterus and should normally outline the Fallopian tubes). In vitro assessments of sperm survival in cervical mucus may be done in cases of unexplained infertility but are rarely helpful.

Management

Couples should be advised to have regular sexual intercourse, ideally every 2–3 days throughout the menstrual cycle. It is not uncommon for 'spontaneous' pregnancies to occur in couples undergoing investigations for infertility or with identified causes of male or female subfertility.

20

In women with anovulatory cycles secondary to PCOS, clomifene, which has partial anti-oestrogen action, blocks negative feedback of oestrogen on the hypothalamus/pituitary, causing gonadotrophin secretion and thus ovulation. In women with gonadotrophin deficiency or in whom anti-oestrogen therapy is unsuccessful, ovulation may be induced by direct stimulation of the ovary by daily injection of FSH and an injection of hCG to induce follicular rupture at the appropriate time. In hypothalamic disease, pulsatile GnRH therapy with a portable infusion pump can be used to stimulate pituitary gonadotrophin secretion (note that non-pulsatile administration of GnRH or its analogues paradoxically suppresses LH and FSH secretion). Whatever method of ovulation induction is employed, monitoring of response is essential to avoid multiple ovulation. For clomifene, ultrasound monitoring is recommended for at least the first cycle. During gonadotrophin therapy, closer monitoring of follicular growth by transvaginal ultrasonography and blood oestradiol levels is mandatory. 'Ovarian hyperstimulation syndrome' is characterised by grossly enlarged ovaries and capillary leak with circulatory shock, pleural effusions and ascites. Anovulatory women who fail to respond to ovulation induction or who have primary ovarian failure may wish to consider using donated eggs or embryos, surrogacy and adoption.

Surgery to restore Fallopian tube patency can be effective but in vitro fertilisation (IVF) is normally recommended. IVF is widely used for many causes of infertility and in unexplained cases of prolonged (>3 years) infertility. The success of IVF depends on age, with low success rates in women over 40 years.

Men with hypogonadotrophic hypogonadism who wish fertility are usually given injections of hCG several times a week (recombinant FSH may also be required in men with hypogonadism of pre-pubertal origin); it may take up to 2 years to achieve satisfactory sperm counts. Surgery is rarely an option in primary testicular disease but removal of a varicocele can improve semen quality. Extraction of sperm from the epididymis for IVF, and intracytoplasmic sperm injection (ICSI, when single spermatozoa are injected into each oöcyte) are being used increasingly in men with oligospermia or poor sperm quality who have primary testicular disease. Azoospermic men may opt to use donated sperm but this may be in short supply.

Gynaecomastia

Gynaecomastia is the presence of glandular breast tissue in males. Normal breast development in women is oestrogen-dependent, while androgens oppose this effect. Gynaecomastia results from an imbalance between androgen and oestrogen activity, which may reflect androgen deficiency or oestrogen excess. Causes are listed in Box 20.26. The most common are physiological: for example, in the newborn baby (due to maternal and placental oestrogens), in pubertal boys (in whom oestradiol concentrations reach adult levels before testosterone) and in older men (due to decreasing testosterone concentrations). Prolactin excess alone does not cause gynaecomastia.

Clinical assessment

A drug history is important. Gynaecomastia is often asymmetrical and palpation may allow breast tissue to be distinguished from the prominent adipose tissue (lipomastia) around the nipple that is often observed in obesity. Features of hypogonadism should be sought (see above) and the testes examined for evidence of cryptorchidism, atrophy or a tumour.

Investigations

If a clinical distinction between gynaecomastia and adipose tissue cannot be made, then ultrasonography or mammography is required. A random blood sample should be taken for testosterone, LH, FSH, oestradiol, prolactin and hCG. Elevated oestrogen concentrations are found in testicular tumours and hCG-producing neoplasms.

Management

An adolescent with gynaecomastia who is progressing normally through puberty may be reassured that the gynaecomastia will usually resolve once development is complete. If puberty does not proceed normally, then there may be an underlying abnormality that requires investigation. Gynaecomastia may cause significant psychological distress, especially in adolescent boys, and surgical excision may be justified for cosmetic reasons. Androgen replacement will usually improve gynaecomastia in hypogonadal males and any other identifiable underlying cause should be addressed if possible. The anti-oestrogen tamoxifen may also be effective in reducing the size of the breast tissue.

Hirsutism

Hirsutism refers to the excessive growth of terminal hair (the thick, pigmented hair usually associated with the adult male chest) in an androgen-dependent distribution in women (upper lip, chin, chest, back, lower abdomen, thigh, forearm) and is one of the most common presentations of endocrine disease. It should be distinguished from hypertrichosis, which is generalised excessive growth of vellus hair (the thin, non-pigmented hair that is typically found all over the body from childhood onwards). The aetiology of androgen excess is shown in Box 20.27.

Clinical assessment

The severity of hirsutism is subjective. Some women suffer profound embarrassment from a degree of hair growth that others would not consider remarkable. Important observations are a drug and menstrual history, calculation of body mass index, measurement of blood pressure and examination for virilisation (clitoromegaly, deep voice, male-pattern balding, breast atrophy) and associated features, including acne vulgaris or Cushing's syndrome. Hirsutism of recent onset associated with virilisation is suggestive of an androgen-secreting tumour but this is rare.

Investigations

A random blood sample should be taken for testosterone, prolactin, LH and FSH. If there are clinical features of Cushing's syndrome, further investigations should be performed as detailed on page 679.

If testosterone levels are more than twice the upper limit of normal for females, idiopathic hirsutism and PCOS are less likely, especially if LH and FSH levels are low. Under these circumstances, other causes of androgen excess should be sought. Congenital adrenal hyperplasia due to 21-hydroxylase deficiency is diagnosed by a short ACTH stimulation test with measurement of 17-OH-progesterone. In post-menopausal women with significant hyperandrogenism, administration of GnRH analogue can be helpful in differentiating between an ovarian (>50% suppression of testosterone) or adrenal source (≤50% suppression) of androgen excess. The tumour should then be sought by CT or MRI of the adrenals and ovaries, as indicated by biochemical testing.

20.26 Causes of gynaecomastia

Idiopathic

Physiological

Drug-induced

- Cimetidine
- Digoxin
- Anti-androgens (cyproterone acetate, spironolactone)
- Some exogenous anabolic steroids (diethylstilbestrol)
- Cannabis

Hypogonadism (see Box 20.19)

Androgen resistance syndromes

Oestrogen excess

- Liver failure (impaired steroid metabolism)
- Oestrogen-secreting tumour (e.g. of testis)
- Human chorionic gonadotrophin-secreting tumour (e.g. of testis or lung)

i 20.27 Causes of hirsutism			
Cause	**Clinical features**	**Investigation findings**	**Treatment**
Idiopathic	Often familial Mediterranean or Asian background	Normal	Cosmetic measures Anti-androgens
Polycystic ovary syndrome	Obesity Oligomenorrhoea or secondary amenorrhoea Infertility	LH:FSH ratio >2.5:1 Minor elevation of androgens* Mild hyperprolactinaemia	Weight loss Cosmetic measures Anti-androgens (Metformin, glitazones may be useful)
Congenital adrenal hyperplasia (95% 21-hydroxylase deficiency)	Pigmentation History of salt-wasting in childhood, ambiguous genitalia, or adrenal crisis when stressed	Elevated androgens* that suppress with dexamethasone Abnormal rise in 17-OH-progesterone with ACTH	Glucocorticoid replacement administered in reverse rhythm to suppress early morning ACTH
Exogenous androgen administration	Athletes Virilisation	Low LH and FSH Analysis of urinary androgens may detect drug of misuse	Stop steroid misuse
Androgen-secreting tumour of ovary or adrenal cortex	Rapid onset Virilisation: clitoromegaly, deep voice, balding, breast atrophy	High androgens* that do not suppress with GnRH analogues Low LH and FSH CT or MRI usually demonstrates a tumour	Surgical excision
Cushing's syndrome	Clinical features of Cushing's syndrome	Normal or mild elevation of adrenal androgens* See investigations (p. 679)	Treat the cause

*e.g. Serum testosterone levels in women: <2 nmol/L (<58 ng/dL) is normal; 2–5 nmol/L (58–144 ng/dL) is minor elevation; >5 nmol/L (>144 ng/dL) is high and requires further investigation.
(ACTH = adrenocorticotrophic hormone; CT = computed tomography; FH = follicle-stimulating hormone; GnRH = gonadotrophin releasing hormone; LH = luteinising hormone; MRI = magnetic resonance imaging)

Management

This depends on the cause (Box 20.27). Options for the treatment of PCOS and idiopathic hirsutism are similar and are described below.

Polycystic ovary syndrome

Polycystic ovary syndrome (PCOS) affects up to 10% of women of reproductive age. It is a heterogeneous disorder (Box 20.28), often associated with obesity, for which the primary cause remains uncertain. Genetic factors probably play a role, since PCOS often affects several family members. The severity and clinical features of PCOS vary markedly between individual patients but diagnosis is usually made during the investigation of hirsutism or amenorrhoea/oligomenorrhoea. Infertility may also be present. There is no universally accepted definition but it has been recommended that a diagnosis of PCOS requires the presence of two of the following three features:

- menstrual irregularity
- clinical or biochemical androgen excess
- multiple cysts in the ovaries (most readily detected by transvaginal ultrasound; Fig. 20.16).

Women with PCOS are at increased risk of glucose intolerance and some authorities recommend screening for type 2 diabetes and other cardiovascular risk factors associated with the metabolic syndrome.

Management

This should be directed at the presenting complaint but all women with PCOS who are overweight should be encouraged to lose weight, as this can improve several symptoms, including menstrual irregularity, and reduces the risk of type 2 diabetes.

Menstrual irregularity and infertility

Most women with PCOS have oligomenorrhoea, with irregular, heavy menstrual periods. This may not require treatment unless fertility is

i 20.28 Features of polycystic ovary syndrome	
Mechanisms*	**Manifestations**
Pituitary dysfunction	High serum LH High serum prolactin
Anovulatory menstrual cycles	Oligomenorrhoea Secondary amenorrhoea Cystic ovaries Infertility
Androgen excess	Hirsutism Acne
Obesity	Hyperglycaemia Elevated oestrogens
Insulin resistance	Dyslipidaemia Hypertension

*These mechanisms are interrelated; it is not known which, if any, is primary. PCOS probably represents the common endpoint of several different pathologies.
(LH = luteinising hormone)

desired. Metformin may restore regular ovulatory cycles in overweight women by reducing insulin resistance, although it is less effective than clomifene at restoring fertility as measured by successful pregnancy.

In women who have very few periods each year or are amenorrhoeic, the high oestrogen concentrations associated with PCOS can cause endometrial hyperplasia. Progestogens can be administered on a cyclical basis to induce regular shedding of the endometrium and a withdrawal bleed, or a progestogen-impregnated intrauterine coil can be fitted.

Hirsutism

For hirsutism, most patients will have used cosmetic measures, such as shaving, bleaching and waxing, before consulting a doctor. Electrolysis and laser treatment are effective for small areas like the upper lip and for

20

i 20.29 Anti-androgen therapy

Mechanism of action	Drug	Dose	Hazards
Androgen receptor antagonism	Cyproterone acetate	2, 50 or 100 mg on days 1–11 of 28-day cycle with ethinylestradiol 30 μg on days 1–21	Hepatic dysfunction Feminisation of male fetus Progesterone receptor agonist Dysfunctional uterine bleeding
	Spironolactone Flutamide	100–200 mg daily Not recommended	Electrolyte disturbance Hepatic dysfunction
5α-reductase inhibition (prevent conversion of testosterone to active dihydrotestosterone)	Finasteride	5 mg daily	Limited clinical experience; possibly less efficacious than other treatments
Suppression of ovarian steroid production and elevation of sex hormone-binding globulin	Oestrogen	See combination with cyproterone acetate above or Conventional oestrogen-containing contraceptive	Venous thromboembolism Hypertension Weight gain Dyslipidaemia Increased breast and endometrial carcinoma

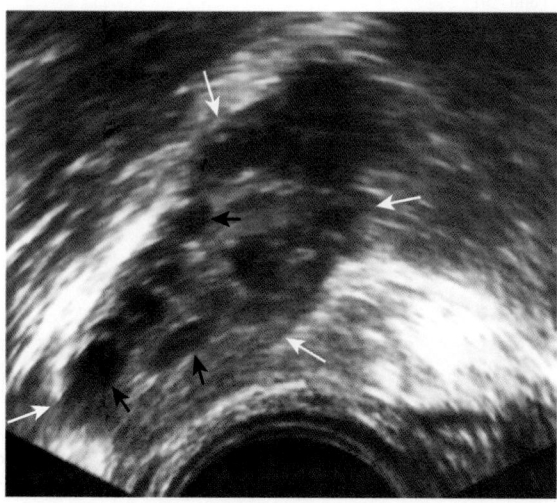

Fig. 20.16 Polycystic ovary. A transvaginal ultrasound scan showing multiple cysts (some indicated by black arrows) in the ovary (highlighted by white arrows) of a woman with polycystic ovary syndrome.

chest hair but are expensive. Eflornithine cream inhibits ornithine decarboxylase in hair follicles and may reduce hair growth when applied daily to affected areas of the face.

If conservative measures are unsuccessful, anti-androgen therapy is given (Box 20.29). The life cycle of a hair follicle is at least 3 months and no improvement is likely before this time, when follicles have shed their hair and replacement hair growth has been suppressed. Metformin and thiazolidinediones are less effective at treating hirsutism than at restoring menstrual regularity. Unless weight is lost, hirsutism will return if therapy is discontinued. The patient should know that prolonged exposure to some agents may not be desirable and they should be stopped before pregnancy.

Turner syndrome

Turner syndrome affects around 1 in 2500 females. It is classically associated with a 45,X karyotype but other cytogenetic abnormalities may be responsible, including mosaic forms (e.g. 45,X/46,XX or 45,X/46,XY) and partial deletions of an X chromosome.

Clinical features

These are shown in Figure 20.17.

Individuals with Turner syndrome invariably have short stature from an early age and this is often the initial presenting symptom. It is probably

due to haploinsufficiency of the *SHOX* gene, one copy of which is found on both the X and Y chromosomes, which encodes a protein that is predominantly found in bone fibroblasts.

The genital tract and external genitalia in Turner syndrome are female in character, since this is the default developmental outcome in the absence of testes. Ovarian tissue develops normally until the third month of gestation, but thereafter there is gonadal dysgenesis with accelerated degeneration of oöcytes and increased ovarian stromal fibrosis, resulting in 'streak ovaries'. The inability of ovarian tissue to produce oestrogen results in loss of negative feedback and elevation of FSH and LH concentrations.

There is a wide variation in the spectrum of associated somatic abnormalities. The severity of the phenotype is, in part, related to the underlying cytogenetic abnormality. Mosaic individuals may have only mild short stature and may enter puberty spontaneously before developing gonadal failure.

Diagnosis and management

The diagnosis of Turner syndrome can be confirmed by karyotype analysis. Short stature, although not directly due to growth hormone deficiency, responds to high doses of growth hormone. Prophylactic gonadectomy is recommended for individuals with 45,X/46,XY mosaicism because there is an increased risk of gonadoblastoma. Pubertal development can be induced with oestrogen therapy but causes fusion of the epiphyses and cessation of growth. The timing of pubertal induction therefore needs to be carefully planned. Adults with Turner syndrome require long-term oestrogen replacement therapy and should be monitored periodically for the development of aortic root dilatation, hearing loss and other somatic complications.

Klinefelter syndrome

Klinefelter syndrome affects approximately 1 in 1000 males and is usually associated with a 47,XXY karyotype. However, other cytogenetic variants may be responsible, especially 46,XY/47,XXY mosaicism. The principal pathological abnormality is dysgenesis of the seminiferous tubules. This is evident from infancy (and possibly even in utero) and progresses with age. By adolescence, hyalinisation and fibrosis are present within the seminiferous tubules and Leydig cell function is impaired, resulting in hypogonadism.

Clinical features

The diagnosis is typically made in adolescents who have presented with gynaecomastia and failure to progress normally through puberty. Affected individuals usually have small, firm testes. Tall stature is apparent from early childhood, reflecting characteristically long leg length associated with 47,XXY, and may be exacerbated by androgen deficiency with

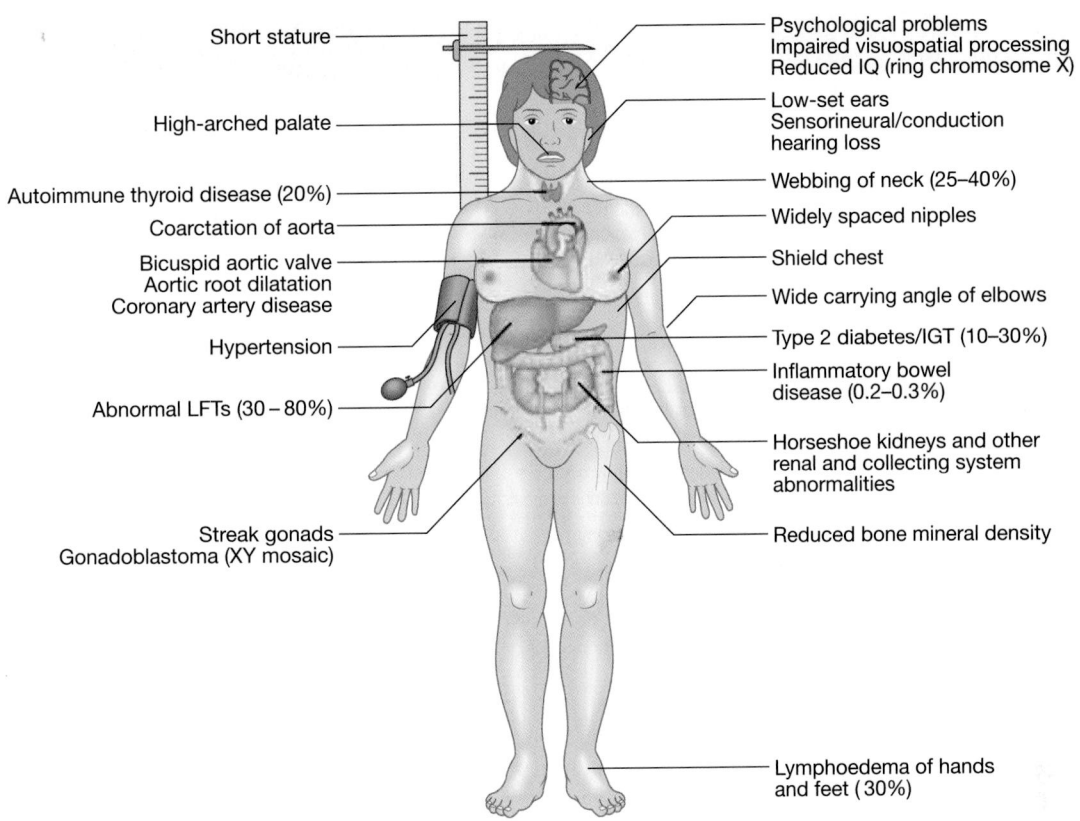

Short stature

High-arched palate

Autoimmune thyroid disease (20%)

Coarctation of aorta

Bicuspid aortic valve
Aortic root dilatation
Coronary artery disease

Hypertension

Abnormal LFTs (30 – 80%)

Streak gonads
Gonadoblastoma (XY mosaic)

Psychological problems
Impaired visuospatial processing
Reduced IQ (ring chromosome X)

Low-set ears
Sensorineural/conduction
hearing loss

Webbing of neck (25–40%)

Widely spaced nipples

Shield chest

Wide carrying angle of elbows

Type 2 diabetes/IGT (10–30%)

Inflammatory bowel
disease (0.2–0.3%)

Horseshoe kidneys and other
renal and collecting system
abnormalities

Reduced bone mineral density

Lymphoedema of hands
and feet (30%)

Fig. 20.17 Clinical features of Turner syndrome (45,X). (IGT = impaired glucose tolerance; LFTs = liver function tests).

lack of epiphyseal closure in puberty. Other clinical features may include learning difficulties and behavioural disorders, as well as an increased risk of breast cancer and type 2 diabetes in later life. The spectrum of clinical features is wide and some individuals, especially those with 46,XY/47,XXY mosaicism, may pass through puberty normally and be identified only during investigation for infertility.

Diagnosis and management

Klinefelter syndrome is suggested by the typical phenotype in a patient with hypergonadotrophic hypogonadism and can be confirmed by karyotype analysis. Individuals with clinical and biochemical evidence of androgen deficiency require androgen replacement (see Box 20.23). There are reports of successful pregnancy occurring following ICSI therapy where spermatocytes have been retrieved from the gonads of men with Klinefelter syndrome.

The parathyroid glands

Parathyroid hormone (PTH) plays a key role in the regulation of calcium and phosphate homeostasis and vitamin D metabolism, as shown in Fig. 26.62. The consequences of altered function of this axis in gut and renal disease are covered in Chapters 23 and 18, respectively. Other metabolic bone diseases are explored in Chapter 26. Here, the investigation of hypercalcaemia and hypocalcaemia and disorders of the parathyroid glands are discussed.

Functional anatomy, physiology and investigations

The four parathyroid glands lie behind the lobes of the thyroid and are approximately the size of a grain of rice. The parathyroid chief cells respond directly to changes in calcium concentrations via a

G protein-coupled cell surface receptor (the calcium-sensing receptor) located on the cell surface (see Fig. 26.62). When serum ionised calcium levels fall, PTH secretion rises. PTH is a single-chain polypeptide of 84 amino acids. It acts on the renal tubules to promote reabsorption of calcium and reduce reabsorption of phosphate, and on the skeleton to increase osteoclastic bone resorption and bone formation. PTH also promotes the conversion of 25-hydroxyvitamin D to the active metabolite, 1,25-dihydroxyvitamin D; the 1,25-dihydroxyvitamin D, in turn, enhances calcium absorption from the gut.

More than 99% of total body calcium is in bone. Prolonged exposure of bone to high levels of PTH is associated with increased osteoclastic activity and new bone formation, but the net effect is to cause bone loss with mobilisation of calcium into the extracellular fluid. In contrast, pulsatile release of PTH causes net bone gain. This effect is exploited therapeutically in the treatment of osteoporosis, as discussed in Chapter 26.

The differential diagnosis of disorders of calcium metabolism requires measurement of calcium phosphate, alkaline phosphatase, renal function, PTH and 25-hydroxyvitamin D. Although the parathyroid glands detect and respond to ionised calcium levels, most clinical laboratories measure only total serum calcium levels. About 50% of total calcium is bound to organic ions, such as citrate or phosphate, and to proteins, especially albumin. Accordingly, if the serum albumin level is reduced, total calcium concentrations should be 'corrected' by adjusting the value for calcium upwards by 0.02 mmol/L (0.08 mg/dL) for each 1 g/L reduction in albumin below 40 g/L. If albumin concentrations are significantly low, as in severe acute illness and other chronic illness such as liver cirrhosis, this correction is less accurate and measurement of ionised calcium is needed.

Calcitonin is secreted from the parafollicular C cells of the thyroid gland. Although it is a useful tumour marker in medullary carcinoma of thyroid, its release from the thyroid is of no clinical relevance to calcium homeostasis in humans.

20

i | 20.30 Classification of diseases of the parathyroid glands

	Primary	Secondary
Hormone excess	Primary hyperparathyroidism Parathyroid adenoma Parathyroid carcinoma[1] Parathyroid hyperplasia[2] Tertiary hyperparathyroidism Following prolonged secondary hyperparathyroidism	Secondary hyperparathyroidism Chronic kidney disease Malabsorption Vitamin D deficiency
Hormone deficiency	Hypoparathyroidism Post-surgical Autoimmune Inherited	
Hormone hypersensitivity	Autosomal dominant hypercalciuric hypocalcaemic (CASR-activating mutation)	
Hormone resistance	Pseudohypoparathyroidism Familial hypocalciuric hypercalcaemia	
Non-functioning tumours	Parathyroid carcinoma[1]	

[1]Parathyroid carcinomas may or may not produce parathyroid hormone. [2]In multiple endocrine neoplasia (MEN) syndromes (p. 700).
(CASR = calcium-sensing receptor)

20.31 The parathyroid glands in old age

- **Osteoporosis**: always exclude osteomalacia and hyperparathyroidism by checking vitamin D and calcium concentrations.
- **Primary hyperparathyroidism**: more common with ageing. Older people can often be observed without surgical intervention.
- **Hypercalcaemia**: may cause delirium.
- **Vitamin D deficiency**: common because of limited exposure to the sun and reduced ability of older skin to synthesise cholecalciferol.

i | 20.32 Causes of hypercalcaemia

With normal or elevated parathyroid hormone (PTH) levels

- Primary or tertiary hyperparathyroidism
- Lithium-induced hyperparathyroidism
- Familial hypocalciuric hypercalcaemia

With low PTH levels

- Malignancy (lung, breast, myeloma, renal, lymphoma, thyroid)
- Elevated 1,25-dihydroxyvitamin D (vitamin D intoxication, sarcoidosis, human immunodeficiency virus, other granulomatous disease)
- Thyrotoxicosis
- Paget's disease with immobilisation
- Milk-alkali syndrome
- Thiazide diuretics
- Glucocorticoid deficiency

Disorders of the parathyroid glands are summarised in Box 20.30. Some specific features of parathyroid disease in older people are summarised in Box 20.31.

Presenting problems in parathyroid disease

Hypercalcaemia

Hypercalcaemia is one of the most common biochemical abnormalities and is often detected during routine biochemical analysis in asymptomatic patients. However, it can present with chronic symptoms, as described below, and occasionally as an acute emergency with severe hypercalcaemia and dehydration.

Causes of hypercalcaemia are listed in Box 20.32. Of these, primary hyperparathyroidism and malignant hypercalcaemia are by far the most common. Familial hypocalciuric hypercalcaemia (FHH) is a rare but important cause that needs differentiation from primary hyperparathyroidism (HPT). Lithium may cause hyperparathyroidism by reducing the sensitivity of the calcium-sensing receptor.

Clinical assessment

Symptoms and signs of hypercalcaemia include polyuria and polydipsia, renal colic, lethargy, anorexia, nausea, dyspepsia and peptic ulceration, constipation, depression, drowsiness and impaired cognition. Patients with malignant hypercalcaemia can have a rapid onset of symptoms and may have clinical features that help to localise the tumour.

The classic symptoms of primary hyperparathyroidism are described by the adage 'bones, stones and abdominal groans', but few patients present in this way nowadays and the disorder is most often picked up as an incidental finding on biochemical testing. About 50% of patients with primary hyperparathyroidism are asymptomatic while others have non-specific symptoms such as polyuria, thirst, fatigue, depression and generalised aches and pains. Some present with renal calculi and it has been estimated that 5% of first stone formers and 15% of recurrent stone formers have primary hyperparathyroidism. Hypertension is a common feature of hyperparathyroidism. Parathyroid tumours are almost never palpable.

A family history of hypercalcaemia raises the possibility of FHH or MEN.

Investigations

The most discriminatory investigation is measurement of PTH. If PTH levels are detectable or elevated in the presence of hypercalcaemia, then primary hyperparathyroidism is the most likely diagnosis. High plasma phosphate and alkaline phosphatase accompanied by renal impairment suggest tertiary hyperparathyroidism. Hypercalcaemia may cause nephrocalcinosis and renal tubular impairment, resulting in hyperuricaemia and hyperchloraemia.

Patients with FHH can present with a similar biochemical picture to primary hyperparathyroidism but typically have low urinary calcium excretion (a ratio of urinary calcium clearance to creatinine clearance of <0.01). The diagnosis of FHH can be confirmed by screening family members for hypercalcaemia and/or identifying an inactivating mutation in the gene encoding the calcium-sensing receptor. It is important, when considering the differential diagnosis of hypercalcaemia, to recognise that FHH is at least 100 times less common than primary hyperparathyroidism.

If PTH is low and no other cause is apparent, then malignancy with or without bony metastases is likely. PTH-related peptide, which is often responsible for the hypercalcaemia associated with malignancy, is not detected by PTH assays, but can be measured by a specific assay (although this is not usually necessary). Unless the source is obvious, the patient should be screened for malignancy with a chest X-ray, myeloma screen (see p. 975) and CT as appropriate.

Management

Treatment of severe hypercalcaemia and primary hyperparathyroidism is described below and on p. 142. FHH does not require any specific intervention.

Hypocalcaemia

Aetiology

Hypocalcaemia is much less common than hypercalcaemia. The differential diagnosis is shown in Box 20.33. The most common cause of hypocalcaemia is a low serum albumin with normal ionised calcium concentration. Conversely, ionised calcium may be low in the face of normal total serum calcium in patients with alkalosis: for example, as a result of hyperventilation.

Hypocalcaemia may also develop as a result of magnesium depletion and should be considered in patients with malabsorption, those on diuretic or proton pump inhibitor therapy, and/or those with a history of alcohol excess. Magnesium deficiency causes hypocalcaemia by impairing the ability of the parathyroid glands to secrete PTH (resulting in PTH concentrations that are low or inappropriately in the reference range) and may also impair the actions of PTH on bone and kidney.

Clinical assessment

Mild hypocalcaemia is often asymptomatic but, with more profound reductions in serum calcium, tetany can occur. This is characterised by muscle spasms due to increased excitability of peripheral nerves.

Children are more liable to develop tetany than adults and present with a characteristic triad of carpopedal spasm, stridor and convulsions, although one or more of these may be found independently of the others. In carpopedal spasm, the hands adopt a characteristic position with flexion of the metacarpophalangeal joints of the fingers and adduction of the thumb ('main d'accoucheur'). Pedal spasm can also occur but is less frequent. Stridor is caused by spasm of the glottis. Adults can also develop carpopedal spasm in association with tingling of the hands and feet and around the mouth, but stridor and fits are rare.

Latent tetany may be detected by eliciting Trousseau's sign: inflation of a sphygmomanometer cuff on the upper arm to more than the systolic blood pressure is followed by carpal spasm within 3 minutes. Less specific is Chvostek's sign, in which tapping over the branches of the facial nerve as they emerge from the parotid gland produces twitching of the facial muscles.

Hypocalcaemia can cause papilloedema and prolongation of the ECG QT interval, which may predispose to ventricular arrhythmias. Prolonged hypocalcaemia and hyperphosphataemia (as in hypoparathyroidism) may cause calcification of the basal ganglia, grand mal epilepsy, psychosis and cataracts. Hypocalcaemia associated with hypophosphataemia, as in vitamin D deficiency, causes rickets in children and osteomalacia in adults.

Management

Emergency management of hypocalcaemia associated with tetany is given in Box 20.34. Treatment of chronic hypocalcaemia is described on p. 1053.

Primary hyperparathyroidism

Primary hyperparathyroidism is caused by autonomous secretion of PTH, usually by a single parathyroid adenoma, which can vary in diameter from a few millimetres to several centimetres. It should be distinguished from secondary hyperparathyroidism, in which there is a physiological increase in PTH secretion to compensate for prolonged hypocalcaemia (such as in vitamin D deficiency); and from tertiary hyperparathyroidism, in which continuous stimulation of the parathyroids over a prolonged period of time results in adenoma formation and autonomous PTH secretion (Box 20.35). This is most commonly seen in individuals with advanced chronic kidney disease.

 20.34 Management of severe hypocalcaemia

Immediate management

- 10–20 mL 10% calcium gluconate IV over 10–20 mins
- Continuous IV infusion may be required for several hours (equivalent of 10 mL 10% calcium gluconate/hr)
- Cardiac monitoring is recommended

If associated with hypomagnesaemia

- 50 mmol (1.23 g) magnesium chloride IV over 24 hrs
- Most parenteral magnesium will be excreted in the urine, so further doses may be required to replenish body stores

(IV = intravenous)

---

i 20.33 Differential diagnosis of hypocalcaemia

	Total serum calcium	Ionised serum calcium	Serum phosphate	Serum PTH	Comments
Hypoalbuminaemia	↓	↔	↔	↔	Adjust calcium upwards by 0.02 mmol/L (0.1 mg/dL) for every 1 g/L reduction in albumin below 40 g/L
Alkalosis	↔	↓	↔	↔ or ↑	p. 632
Vitamin D deficiency	↓	↓	↓	↑	p. 1053
Chronic renal failure	↓	↓	↑	↑	Due to impaired vitamin D hydroxylation. Serum creatinine ↑
Hypoparathyroidism	↓	↓	↑	↓	See text
Pseudohypoparathyroidism	↓	↓	↑	↑	Characteristic phenotype (see text)
Acute pancreatitis	↓	↓	↔ or ↓	↑	Usually clinically obvious. Serum amylase ↑
Hypomagnesaemia	↓	↓	Variable	↓ or ↔	Treatment of hypomagnesaemia may correct hypocalcaemia

(↑ = levels increased; ↓ = levels reduced; ↔ = levels normal)

i	20.35 Hyperparathyroidism		
Type		**Serum calcium**	**PTH**
Primary Single adenoma (90%) Multiple adenomas (4%) Nodular hyperplasia (5%) Carcinoma (1%)		Raised	Not suppressed
Secondary Chronic renal failure Malabsorption Osteomalacia and rickets		Low	Raised
Tertiary		Raised	Not suppressed

The prevalence of primary hyperparathyroidism is about 1 in 500 and it is 2–3 times more common in women than men; 90% of patients are over 50 years of age. It also occurs in the familial MEN syndromes, in which case hyperplasia or multiple adenomas of all four parathyroid glands are more likely than a solitary adenoma.

Clinical and radiological features

The clinical presentation of primary hyperparathyroidism is described on page 676. Parathyroid bone disease is now extremely rare due to earlier diagnosis and treatment and plain X-ray assessment is not routinely recommended. Osteitis fibrosa results from increased bone resorption by osteoclasts with fibrous replacement in the lacunae. This may present as bone pain and tenderness, fracture and deformity. Chondrocalcinosis can occur due to deposition of calcium pyrophosphate crystals within articular cartilage. It typically affects the menisci at the knees and can result in secondary degenerative arthritis or predispose to attacks of acute pseudogout. Skeletal X-rays are usually normal in mild primary hyperparathyroidism but DXA should be obtained as a matter of routine in people with primary hyperparathyroidism to exclude osteoporosis (a potential indication for surgical intervention). Renal imaging (typically ultrasound) is recommended to screen for asymptomatic nephrocalcinosis or nephrolithiasis.

Investigations

The diagnosis can be confirmed by finding a raised (or inappropriately normal) PTH level in the presence of hypercalcaemia, provided that FHH is excluded. Parathyroid scanning by ultrasound examination is often sufficient to localise an adenoma prior to surgery, although it is highly dependent on an experienced operator. Where ultrasound is equivocal, or does not identify an adenoma, a range of additional imaging modalities are available. These include 99mTc-sestamibi scintigraphy (MIBI; Fig. 20.18), 99mTc-SPECT/CT and, most recently, 18F-fluorocholine PET/CT. Negative imaging does not exclude the diagnosis, however, and four-gland exploration may be needed. Genetic testing should be considered when primary hyperparathyroidism is diagnosed before the age of 40, as the likelihood of underlying MEN syndromes is greater in this situation.

Management

The treatment of choice for primary hyperparathyroidism is surgery, with excision of a solitary parathyroid adenoma or hyperplastic glands. Experienced surgeons will identify solitary tumours in more than 90% of cases. Patients with parathyroid bone disease run a significant risk of developing hypocalcaemia post-operatively but the risk of this can be reduced by correcting vitamin D deficiency pre-operatively.

Surgery is usually indicated for individuals with clear-cut symptoms or documented complications (such as renal stones, renal impairment or osteoporosis), and (in asymptomatic patients) significant hypercalcaemia (corrected serum calcium >2.85 mmol/L (>11.4 mg/dL)). Patients who are treated conservatively without surgery should have calcium biochemistry and renal function checked annually and bone density monitored periodically. They should be encouraged to maintain a high oral fluid intake to avoid renal stones.

Occasionally, primary hyperparathyroidism presents with severe life-threatening hypercalcaemia. This is often due to dehydration and should be managed medically with intravenous fluids and bisphosphonates, as described on page 142. If this is not effective, then urgent parathyroidectomy should be considered.

Cinacalcet is a calcimimetic that enhances the sensitivity of the calcium-sensing receptor, so reducing PTH levels, and is licensed for tertiary hyperparathyroidism (page 592) and as a treatment for patients with primary hyperparathyroidism who are unwilling to have surgery or are medically unfit.

Familial hypocalciuric hypercalcaemia

This autosomal dominant disorder is caused by an inactivating mutation in one of the alleles of the calcium-sensing receptor gene, which reduces the ability of the parathyroid gland to 'sense' ionised calcium concentrations. As a result, higher than normal calcium levels are required to suppress PTH secretion. The typical presentation is with mild hypercalcaemia with PTH concentrations that are 'inappropriately' at the upper end of the reference range or are slightly elevated. Calcium-sensing receptors in the renal tubules are also affected and this leads to increased renal tubular reabsorption of calcium and hypocalciuria (as measured in the vitamin D-replete individual by a fractional calcium excretion or 24-hour calcium excretion). The hypercalcaemia of FHH is always asymptomatic and complications do not occur. The main risk of FHH is that of the patient being subjected to an unnecessary (and ineffective) parathyroidectomy if misdiagnosed as having primary hyperparathyroidism. Testing of family members for hypercalcaemia is helpful in confirming the diagnosis and it is also possible to perform genetic testing. No treatment is necessary.

Hypoparathyroidism

The most common cause of hypoparathyroidism is damage to the parathyroid glands (or their blood supply) during thyroid surgery. Rarely, hypoparathyroidism can occur as a result of infiltration of the glands with iron in haemochromatosis or copper in Wilson's disease.

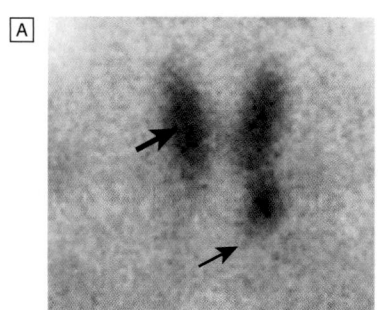
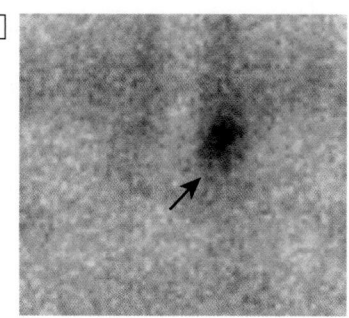

Fig. 20.18 99mTc-sestamibi scan of a patient with primary hyperparathyroidism secondary to a parathyroid adenoma. **A** After 1 hour, there is uptake in the thyroid gland (thick arrow) and the enlarged left inferior parathyroid gland (thin arrow). **B** After 3 hours, uptake is evident only in the parathyroid (thin arrow).

There are a number of rare congenital or inherited forms of hypoparathyroidism. One form is associated with autoimmune polyendocrine syndrome type 1 and another with DiGeorge syndrome. Autosomal dominant hypoparathyroidism is the mirror image of FHH (see above), in that an activating mutation in the calcium-sensing receptor reduces PTH levels, resulting in hypocalcaemia and hypercalciuria.

Pseudohypoparathyroidism

In this disorder, the individual is functionally hypoparathyroid but, instead of PTH deficiency, there is tissue resistance to the effects of PTH, such that PTH concentrations are markedly elevated. The PTH receptor itself is normal but the downstream signalling pathways are defective due to mutations that affect *GNAS1*, which encodes the Gsα protein, a molecule involved in signal transduction downstream of the PTH receptor and other G protein-coupled receptors. There are several subtypes but the most common (pseudohypoparathyroidism type 1a) is characterised by hypocalcaemia and hyperphosphataemia, in association with short stature, short fourth metacarpals and metatarsals, rounded face, obesity and subcutaneous calcification; these features are collectively referred to as Albright's hereditary osteodystrophy (AHO). Type 1a pseudohypoparathyroidism occurs only when the *GNAS1* mutation is inherited on the maternal chromosome.

The term pseudopseudohypoparathyroidism is used to describe patients who have clinical features of AHO but normal serum calcium and PTH concentrations; it occurs when the *GNAS1* mutation is inherited on the paternal chromosome. The inheritance of these disorders is an example of genetic imprinting (see Ch. 3). The difference in clinical features occurs as a result of the fact that renal cells exclusively express the maternal *GNAS1* allele, whereas both maternal and paternal alleles are expressed in other cell types; this explains why maternal inheritance is associated with hypocalcaemia and resistance to PTH (which regulates serum calcium and phosphate levels largely by an effect on the renal tubule), and why paternal inheritance is associated with skeletal and other abnormalities in the absence of hypocalcaemia and raised PTH values.

Management of hypoparathyroidism

Persistent hypoparathyroidism and pseudohypoparathyroidism are treated with oral calcium salts and vitamin D analogues, either 1α-hydroxycholecalciferol (alfacalcidol) or 1,25-dihydroxycholecalciferol (calcitriol). This therapy needs careful monitoring because of the risks of iatrogenic hypercalcaemia, hypercalciuria and nephrocalcinosis. Recombinant PTH is available as a subcutaneous injection and has been used in hypoparathyroidism (but not in pseudohypoparathyroidism). It is much more expensive than calcium and vitamin D analogues and remains a second-line therapy but has the advantage that it is less likely to cause hypercalciuria. There is no specific treatment for AHO other than to try to maintain calcium levels within the reference range using active vitamin D metabolites.

The adrenal glands

The adrenals comprise several separate endocrine glands within a single anatomical structure. The adrenal medulla is an extension of the sympathetic nervous system that secretes catecholamines into capillaries rather than synapses. Most of the adrenal cortex is made up of cells that secrete cortisol and adrenal androgens, and form part of the hypothalamic–pituitary–adrenal (HPA) axis. The small outer glomerulosa of the cortex secretes aldosterone under the control of the renin–angiotensin system. These functions are important in the integrated control of cardiovascular, metabolic and immune responses to stress.

There is increasing evidence that subtle alterations in adrenal function contribute to the pathogenesis of common diseases such as hypertension, obesity and type 2 diabetes mellitus. However, classical syndromes of adrenal hormone deficiency and excess are relatively rare.

Functional anatomy and physiology

Adrenal anatomy and function are shown in Figure 20.19. Histologically, the cortex is divided into three zones, but these function as two units (zona glomerulosa and zonae fasciculata/reticularis) that produce corticosteroids in response to humoral stimuli. Pathways for the biosynthesis of corticosteroids are shown in Figure 20.20. Investigation of adrenal function is described under specific diseases below. The different types of adrenal disease are shown in Box 20.36.

Glucocorticoids

Cortisol is the major glucocorticoid in humans. Levels are highest in the morning on waking and lowest in the middle of the night. Cortisol rises dramatically during stress, including any illness. This elevation protects key metabolic functions (such as the maintenance of cerebral glucose supply during starvation) and inhibits potentially damaging inflammatory responses to infection and injury. The clinical importance of cortisol deficiency is, therefore, most obvious at times of stress.

More than 95% of circulating cortisol is bound to protein, principally cortisol-binding globulin, which is increased by oestrogens. It is the free fraction that is biologically active. Cortisol regulates cell function by binding to glucocorticoid receptors that regulate the transcription of many genes. Cortisol can also activate mineralocorticoid receptors, but it does not normally do so because most cells containing mineralocorticoid receptors also express an enzyme called 11β-hydroxysteroid dehydrogenase type 2 (11β-HSD2), which inactivates cortisol by converting it to cortisone. Inhibitors of 11β-HSD2 (such as some liquorice) or mutations in the gene that encodes 11β-HSD2 cause cortisol to act as a mineralocorticoid, resulting in sodium retention and hypertension (see Box 20.45).

Mineralocorticoids

Aldosterone is the most important mineralocorticoid. It binds to mineralocorticoid receptors in the kidney and causes sodium retention and increased excretion of potassium and protons (see Fig. 19.2). The principal stimulus to aldosterone secretion is angiotensin II, a peptide produced by activation of the renin–angiotensin system (see Fig. 20.19). Renin activity in the juxtaglomerular apparatus of the kidney is stimulated by low perfusion pressure in the afferent arteriole, low sodium filtration leading to low sodium concentrations at the macula densa, or increased sympathetic nerve activity. As a result, renin activity is increased in hypovolaemia and renal artery stenosis, and is approximately doubled when standing up from a recumbent position.

Catecholamines

In humans, only a small proportion of circulating noradrenaline (norepinephrine) is derived from the adrenal medulla; much more is released from sympathetic nerve endings. Conversion of noradrenaline to adrenaline (epinephrine) is catalysed by catechol *O*-methyltransferase (COMT), which is induced by glucocorticoids. Blood flow in the adrenal is centripetal, so that the medulla is bathed in high concentrations of cortisol and is the major source of circulating adrenaline. However, after surgical removal of the adrenal medullae, there appear to be no clinical consequences attributable to deficiency of circulating catecholamines.

Adrenal androgens

Adrenal androgens are secreted in response to ACTH and are the most abundant steroids in the blood stream. They are probably important in the initiation of puberty (adrenarche). The adrenals are also the major source of androgens in adult females and may be important in female libido.

Presenting problems in adrenal disease

Cushing's syndrome

Cushing's syndrome is caused by excessive activation of glucocorticoid receptors. It is most commonly iatrogenic, due to prolonged administration

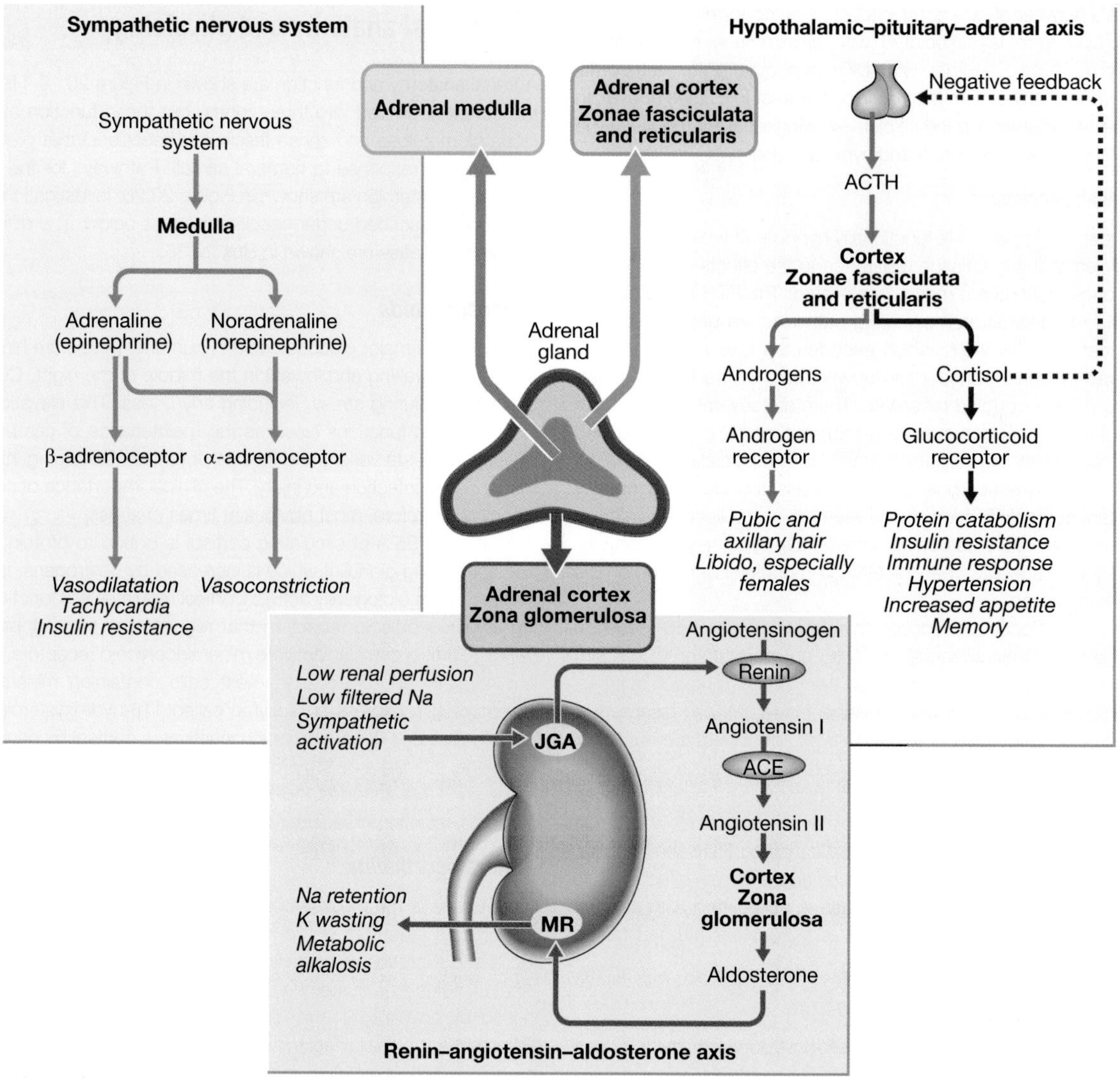

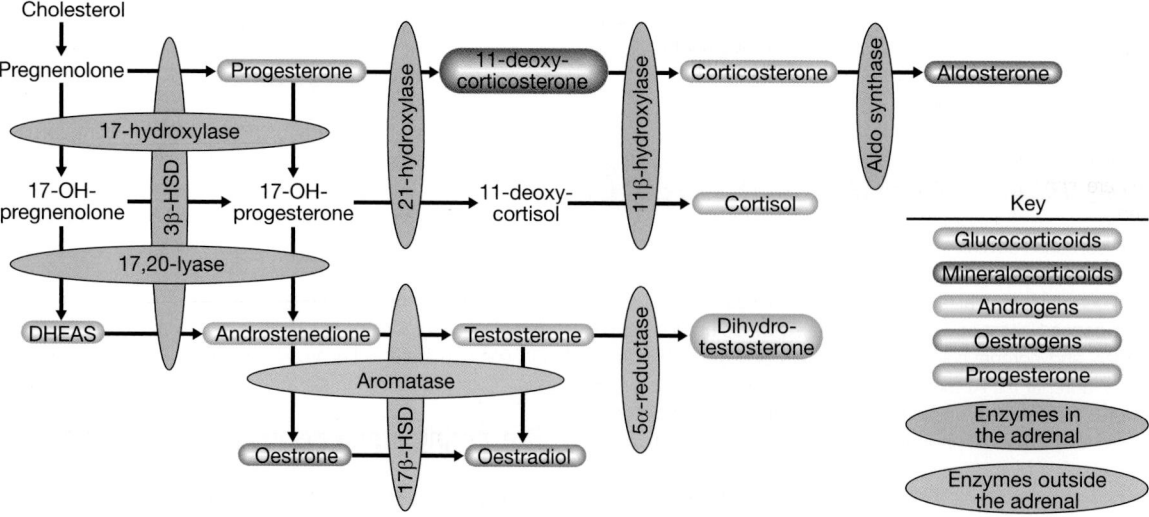

Fig. 20.19 Structure and function of the adrenal glands. (ACE = angiotensin-converting enzyme; ACTH = adrenocorticotrophic hormone; JGA = juxtaglomerular apparatus; MR = mineralocorticoid receptor)

Fig. 20.20 The major pathways of synthesis of steroid hormones. (DHEAS = dehydroepiandrosterone sulphate; HSD = hydroxysteroid dehydrogenase)

i 20.36	Classification of diseases of the adrenal glands		
	Primary		**Secondary**
Hormone excess	Non-ACTH-dependent Cushing's syndrome Primary hyperaldosteronism Phaeochromocytoma		ACTH-dependent Cushing's syndrome Secondary hyperaldosteronism
Hormone deficiency	Addison's disease Congenital adrenal hyperplasia		Hypopituitarism
Hormone hypersensitivity	11β-hydroxysteroid dehydrogenase type 2 deficiency Liddle syndrome		
Hormone resistance	Pseudohypoaldosteronism Glucocorticoid resistance syndrome		
Non-functioning tumours	Adenoma Carcinoma (usually functioning) Metastatic tumours		

(ACTH = adrenocorticotrophic hormone)

---

i 20.37	Classification of endogenous Cushing's syndrome

ACTH-dependent – 80%

- Pituitary adenoma secreting ACTH (Cushing's disease) – 70%
- Ectopic ACTH syndrome (bronchial carcinoid, small-cell lung carcinoma, other neuro-endocrine tumour) – 10%

Non-ACTH-dependent – 20%

- Adrenal adenoma – 15%
- Adrenal carcinoma – 5%
- ACTH-independent macronodular hyperplasia; primary pigmented nodular adrenal disease; McCune–Albright syndrome (together < 1%)

Hypercortisolism due to other causes (also referred to as pseudo-Cushing's syndrome)

- Alcohol excess (biochemical and clinical features)
- Major depressive illness (biochemical features only, some clinical overlap)
- Primary obesity (mild biochemical features, some clinical overlap)

(ACTH = adrenocorticotrophic hormone)

of synthetic glucocorticoids such as prednisolone. Endogenous Cushing's syndrome is uncommon but is caused by chronic over-production of cortisol by the adrenal glands, either as the result of an adrenal tumour or because of excessive production of ACTH by a pituitary tumour or ectopic ACTH production by other tumours.

Aetiology

The causes are shown in Box 20.37. Amongst endogenous causes, pituitary-dependent cortisol excess (by convention, called Cushing's disease) accounts for approximately 80% of cases. Both Cushing's disease and cortisol-secreting adrenal tumours are four times more common in women than men. In contrast, ectopic ACTH syndrome (often due to a small-cell carcinoma of the bronchus) is more common in men.

Clinical assessment

The diverse manifestations of glucocorticoid excess are shown in Figure 20.21. Many of these are not specific to Cushing's syndrome and, because spontaneous Cushing's syndrome is rare, the positive predictive value of any single clinical feature alone is low. Moreover, some common disorders can be confused with Cushing's syndrome because they are associated with alterations in cortisol secretion, e.g. obesity and

depression (Box 20.37). Features that favour Cushing's syndrome in an obese patient are those of protein-wasting, including bruising, proximal myopathy and thin skin. Any clinical suspicion of cortisol excess is best resolved by further investigation.

It is vital to exclude iatrogenic causes in all patients with Cushing's syndrome since even inhaled or topical glucocorticoids can induce the syndrome in susceptible individuals. A careful drug history must therefore be taken before embarking on complex investigations. An 0800–0900 hrs serum cortisol of <100 nmol/L (3.6 μg/dL) in a patient with a normal sleep–wake pattern and Cushingoid appearance is consistent with exogenous synthetic glucocorticoid use (common) or cyclical secretion of cortisol from endogenous Cushing's (uncommon).

Some clinical features are more common in ectopic ACTH syndrome. While ACTH-secreting pituitary tumours retain some negative feedback sensitivity to cortisol, this is absent in tumours that produce ectopic ACTH, typically resulting in higher levels of both ACTH and cortisol than are observed in pituitary-driven disease. The high ACTH levels are associated with marked pigmentation because of binding to melanocortin 1 receptors on melanocytes in the skin. The high cortisol levels also overcome the capacity of 11β-HSD2 to inactivate cortisol in the kidney, causing hypokalaemic alkalosis that aggravates myopathy and hyperglycaemia (by inhibiting insulin secretion). When the tumour that is secreting ACTH is malignant, then the onset is usually rapid and may be associated with cachexia. For these reasons, the classical features of Cushing's syndrome are less common in ectopic ACTH syndrome; if present, they suggest that a less aggressive tumour, such as a bronchial carcinoid, is responsible.

In Cushing's disease, the pituitary tumour is usually a microadenoma (<10 mm in diameter); hence other features of a pituitary macroadenoma (visual failure or disconnection hyperprolactinaemia, p. 696) are rare, but there may be secondary hypogonadism due to the inhibitory effects of excess glucocorticoids on gonadotropin secretion. If a diagnosis of Cushing's is suspected, early discussion/referral to a specialist is recommended.

Investigations

The large number of tests available for Cushing's syndrome reflects the fact that each one has limited specificity and sensitivity in isolation. Accordingly, several tests are usually combined to establish the diagnosis. Testing for Cushing's syndrome should be avoided under conditions of stress, such as an acute illness, because this activates the HPA axis, causing potentially spurious results. The diagnosis of Cushing's is a two-step process:

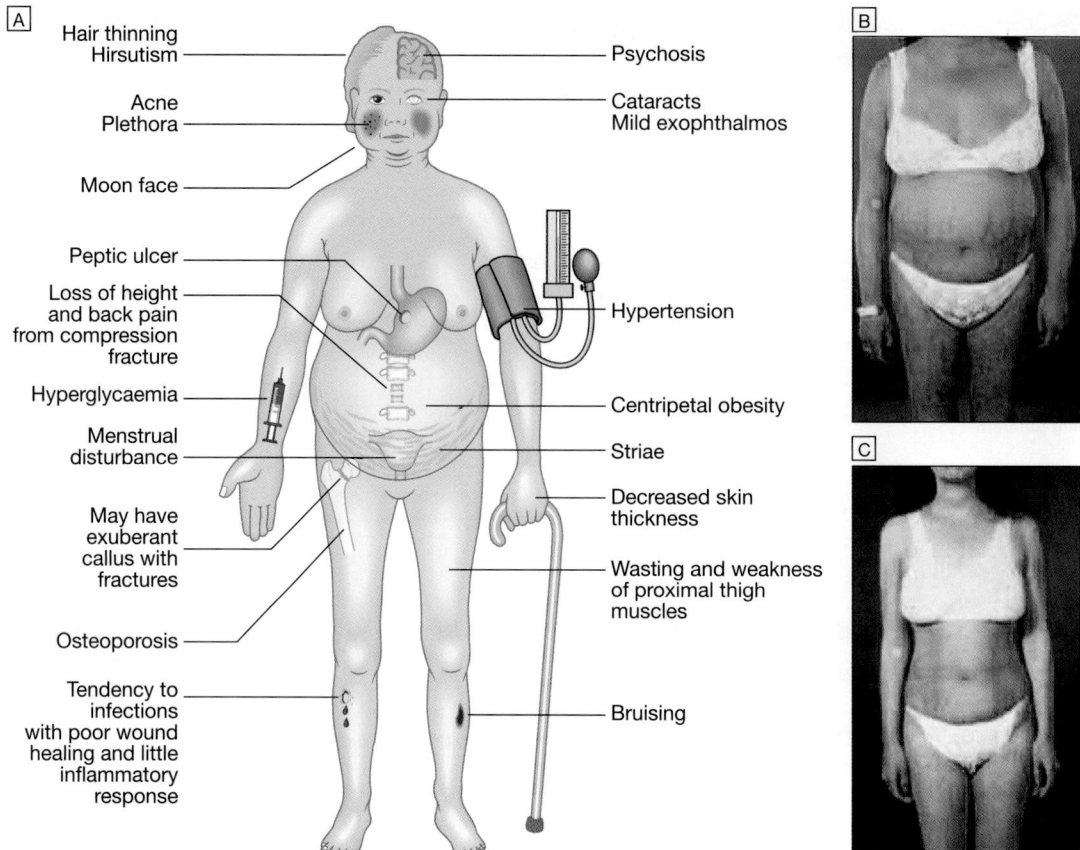

Fig. 20.21 Cushing's syndrome. A Clinical features common to all causes. B A patient with Cushing's disease before treatment. C The same patient 1 year after the successful removal of an ACTH-secreting pituitary microadenoma by trans-sphenoidal surgery.

1. to establish whether the patient has Cushing's syndrome (Fig. 20.22), and
2. to define its cause (Fig. 20.23).

Some additional tests are useful in all cases of Cushing's syndrome, including plasma electrolytes, glucose, glycosylated haemoglobin and bone mineral density measurement.

Establishing the presence of Cushing's syndrome

In patients where there is appropriate clinical suspicion, Cushing's syndrome is confirmed by using two of three main tests:

1. Failure to suppress serum cortisol with low doses of oral dexamethasone
2. Loss of the normal circadian rhythm of cortisol, with inappropriately elevated late-night serum or salivary cortisol
3. Increased 24-hour urine free cortisol (lower sensitivity than the above tests) (see Fig. 20.22).

Dexamethasone is used for suppression testing because it does not cross-react in immunoassays for cortisol. An overnight dexamethasone suppression test (ONDST) involves administration of 1 mg dexamethasone at 2300 hrs and measurement of serum cortisol at 0900 hrs the following day. In a low-dose dexamethasone suppression test (LDDST), serum cortisol is measured following administration of 0.5 mg dexamethasone 4 times daily for 48 hours. For either test, a normal response is a serum cortisol of <50 nmol/L (1.8 μg/dL). It is important for any oestrogens to be stopped for 6 weeks prior to investigation to allow corticosteroid-binding globulin (CBG) levels to return to normal and to avoid false-positive responses, as most cortisol assays measure total cortisol, including that bound to CBG. Cyclicity of cortisol

secretion is a feature of all types of Cushing's syndrome and, if very variable, can confuse diagnosis. Use of multiple salivary cortisol samples over weeks or months can be helpful in diagnosis but an elevated salivary cortisol alone should not be taken as proof of diagnosis. In iatrogenic Cushing's syndrome, cortisol levels are low unless the patient is taking a glucocorticoid (such as prednisolone) that cross-reacts in immunoassays with cortisol.

Determining the underlying cause

Once the presence of Cushing's syndrome is confirmed, measurement of plasma ACTH is the key to establishing the differential diagnosis; it is best measured in the morning around 0900 hrs. In the presence of excess cortisol secretion, an undetectable ACTH (<1.1 pmol/L (5 ng/L)) indicates an adrenal cause, while ACTH levels of >3.3 pmol/L (15 ng/L) suggest a pituitary cause or ectopic ACTH. ACTH levels between these values represent a 'grey area' and further evaluation by a specialist is required. Tests to discriminate pituitary from ectopic sources of ACTH rely on the fact that pituitary tumours, but not ectopic tumours, retain some features of normal regulation of ACTH secretion. Thus, in pituitary-dependent Cushing's disease, ACTH secretion is suppressed by high-dose dexamethasone and ACTH is stimulated by corticotrophin-releasing hormone (CRH). In a high-dose dexamethasone suppression test (HDDST), serum cortisol is measured before and after administration of 2 mg of dexamethasone 4 times daily for 48 hours.

Techniques for localisation of tumours secreting ACTH or cortisol are listed in Figure 20.23. MRI detects around 60% of pituitary microadenomas secreting ACTH. If available, bilateral inferior petrosal sinus sampling (BIPSS) with measurement of plasma ACTH near the pituitary and comparing this to peripheral levels is the best means of confirming Cushing's disease (increased gradient), unless MRI shows a tumour bigger than 6 mm, in which case it may not be needed. CT or MRI detects most

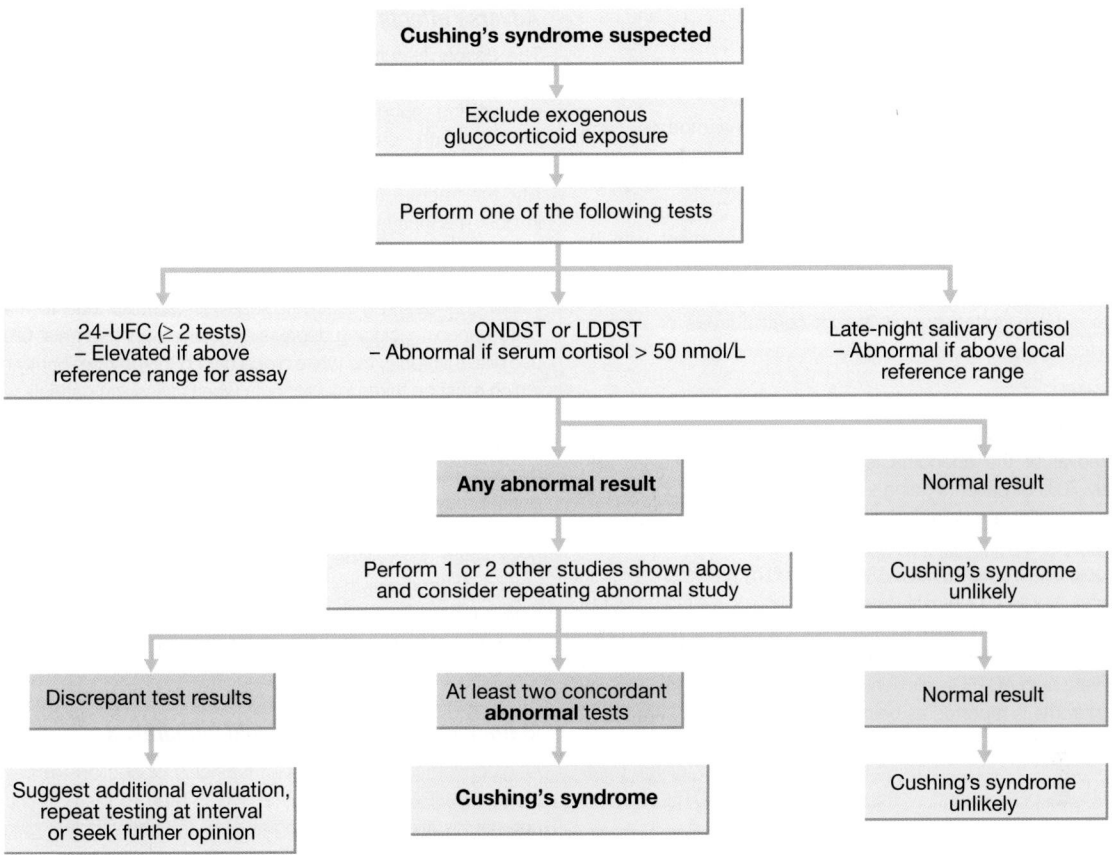

Fig. 20.22 Sequence of investigations in suspected spontaneous Cushing's syndrome. A serum cortisol of 50 nmol/L is equivalent to 1.8 μg/dL. (LDDST = low-dose dexamethasone suppression test; ONDST = overnight dexamethasone suppression test; UFC = urinary free cortisol)

20

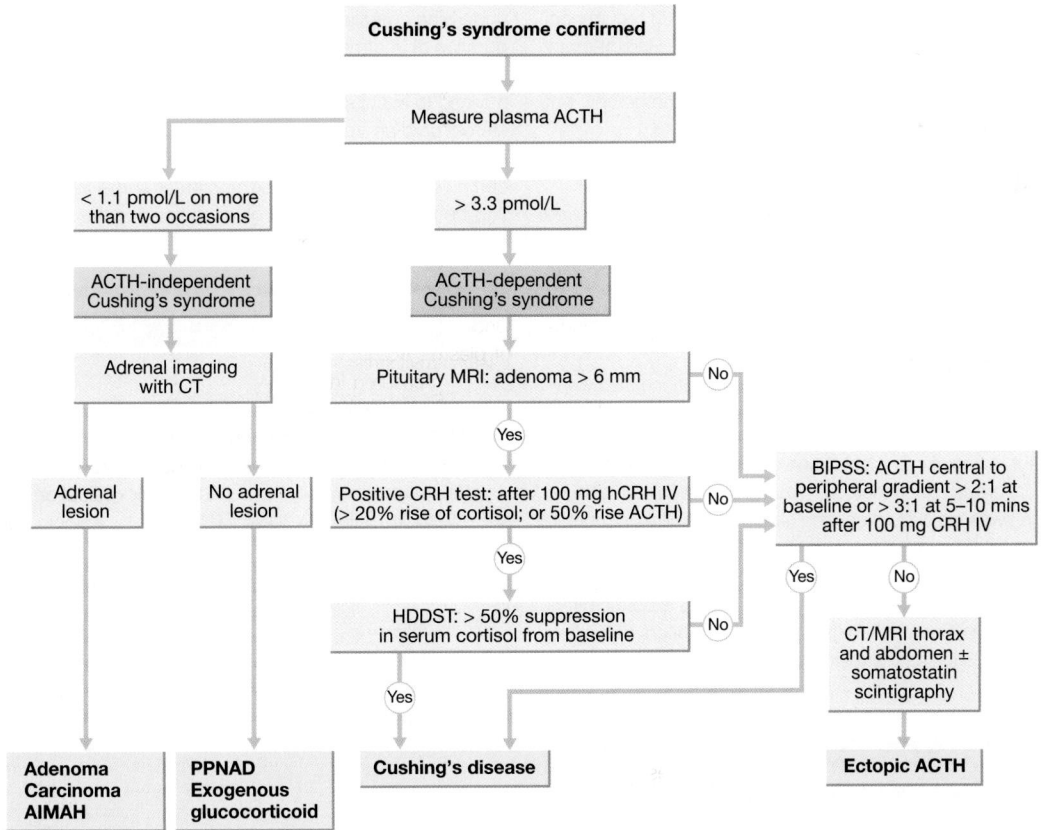

Fig. 20.23 Determining the cause of confirmed Cushing's syndrome. To convert pmol/L to ng/L, multiply by 4.541. (ACTH = adrenocorticotrophic hormone; AIMAH = ACTH-independent macronodular adrenal hyperplasia; BIPSS = bilateral inferior petrosal sinus sampling; hCRH = human corticotrophin-releasing hormone; HDDST = high-dose dexamethasone suppression test; IV = intravenous; MRI = magnetic resonance imaging; PPNAD = primary pigmented nodular adrenal disease)

adrenal tumours; adrenal carcinomas are usually large (>5 cm) and have other features of malignancy.

Management

Untreated severe Cushing's syndrome has a 50% 5-year mortality. Most patients are treated surgically, but medical therapy may be given in severe cases for a few weeks prior to operation to improve the clinical state, or where there is recurrent or incurable disease. Drugs that inhibit glucocorticoid biosynthesis form the mainstay or management, with the most widely available and established being metyrapone and ketoconazole, with osilodrostat becoming available more recently. The dose of these agents is best titrated against serum cortisol levels or 24-hour urine free cortisol.

Cushing's disease

Trans-sphenoidal surgery carried out by an experienced surgeon with selective removal of the adenoma is the treatment of choice, with approximately 70% of patients going into immediate remission. Around 20% of patients suffer a recurrence, often years later, emphasising the need for life-long follow-up.

Laparoscopic bilateral adrenalectomy performed by an expert surgeon effectively cures any type of ACTH-dependent Cushing's syndrome, but in patients with Cushing's disease (pituitary) this can result in Nelson syndrome – an invasive pituitary macroadenoma (which causes local mass effects) and very high ACTH levels (which cause pigmentation). The risk of Nelson syndrome is reported as being reduced by pituitary irradiation in some series, but not all.

The somatostatin analogue pasireotide is also licensed for the treatment of Cushing's disease and works by suppressing ACTH secretion by the tumour.

Adrenal tumours

Laparoscopic adrenal surgery is the treatment of choice for adrenal adenomas. Surgery offers the only prospect of cure for adrenocortical carcinomas but, in general, prognosis is poor with high rates of recurrence, even in patients with localised disease at presentation. Radiotherapy to the tumour bed reduces the risk of local recurrence; systemic therapy consists of the adrenolytic drug mitotane and chemotherapy, but responses are often poor.

Ectopic ACTH syndrome

Localised tumours, such as bronchial carcinoids, should be removed surgically. In patients with incurable malignancy, it is important to reduce the severity of the Cushing's syndrome using medical therapy (see above) or, if appropriate, bilateral adrenalectomy.

Therapeutic use of glucocorticoids

The remarkable anti-inflammatory properties of glucocorticoids have led to their use in a wide variety of clinical conditions but the hazards are significant. Equivalent doses of commonly used glucocorticoids are listed in Box 20.38. Topical preparations (dermal, rectal and inhaled) can also be absorbed into the systemic circulation, and although this rarely occurs to a sufficient degree to produce clinical features of Cushing's syndrome, it can result in significant suppression of endogenous ACTH and cortisol secretion. Severe Cushing's syndrome can result if there is concomitant administration of inhaled glucocorticoids and strong inhibitors of the liver enzyme CYP450 3A4, such as the antiretroviral drug ritonavir.

i	**20.38 Approximate equivalent doses of glucocorticoids**

- Hydrocortisone: 20 mg
- Cortisone acetate: 25 mg
- Prednisolone: 5 mg
- Dexamethasone: 0.5 mg

Adverse effects of glucocorticoids

The clinical features of glucocorticoid excess are illustrated in Figure 20.21. Adverse effects are related to dose, duration of therapy, and pre-existing conditions that might be worsened by glucocorticoid therapy, such as diabetes mellitus or osteoporosis. Osteoporosis is a particularly important problem because, for a given bone mineral density, the fracture risk is greater in glucocorticoid-treated patients than in post-menopausal osteoporosis. Therefore, when systemic glucocorticoids are prescribed and the anticipated duration of steroid therapy is more than 3 months, bone-protective therapy should be considered. Rapid changes in glucocorticoid levels can also lead to marked mood disturbances, including depression, mania and insomnia. Glucocorticoid use also increases the white blood cell count (predominantly neutrophils), which must be taken into account when assessing patients with possible infection.

The anti-inflammatory effect of glucocorticoids may mask signs of disease. For example, perforation of a viscus may be masked and the patient may show no febrile response to an infection. Although there is debate about whether or not glucocorticoids increase the risk of peptic ulcer when used alone, they act synergistically with NSAIDs, including aspirin, to increase the risk of serious gastrointestinal adverse effects. Latent tuberculosis may be reactivated and patients on glucocorticoids are at risk of severe varicella zoster virus infection, so should avoid contact with chickenpox or shingles if they are non-immune.

Management of glucocorticoid withdrawal

All glucocorticoid therapy, even if inhaled or applied topically, can suppress the HPA axis. In practice, this is likely to result in a crisis due to adrenal insufficiency on withdrawal of treatment only if glucocorticoids have been administered orally or systemically for longer than 3 weeks, if repeated courses have been prescribed within the previous year, or if the dose is higher than the equivalent of 7.5 mg prednisolone per day. In these circumstances, the drug, when it is no longer required for the underlying condition, must be withdrawn slowly at a rate dictated by the duration of treatment. If glucocorticoid therapy has been prolonged, then it may take many months for the HPA axis to recover. All patients must be advised to avoid sudden drug withdrawal. They should be issued with a steroid card and/or wear an engraved bracelet (Box 20.39).

Recovery of the HPA axis is aided if there is no exogenous glucocorticoid present during the nocturnal surge in ACTH secretion. This can be achieved by giving glucocorticoid in the morning. Giving ACTH

i	**20.39 Advice to patients on glucocorticoid replacement therapy**

Intercurrent stress

- Febrile illness: double dose of hydrocortisone

Surgery

- Minor operation: hydrocortisone 100 mg IM with pre-medication
- Major operation: hydrocortisone 100 mg 4 times daily for 24 hrs, then 50 mg IM 4 times daily until ready to take tablets

Vomiting

- Patients must have parenteral hydrocortisone if unable to take it by mouth

Steroid card

- Patient should carry this at all times; it should give information regarding diagnosis, steroid, dose and doctor

Bracelet and emergency pack

- Patients should be encouraged to buy a bracelet and have it engraved with the diagnosis, current treatment and a reference number for a central database
- Patients should be given a hydrocortisone emergency pack and trained in the self-administration of hydrocortisone 100 mg IM; they should be advised to take the pack on holidays/trips abroad

(IM = intramuscular)

to stimulate adrenal recovery is of no value, as the pituitary remains suppressed.

In patients who have received glucocorticoids for longer than a few weeks, especially if the period is months to years, it is often valuable to confirm that the HPA axis is recovering during glucocorticoid withdrawal. Withdrawal has to be very slow, usually by a dose reduction equivalent of prednisolone 1 mg per month or slower. Once the dose of glucocorticoid is reduced to a minimum (e.g. 5 mg prednisolone), then serum cortisol can be measured at 0900 hrs before the next dose. If this is <100 nmol/L (3.6 µg/dL), slow reduction should be continued with a repeat 0900 hrs serum cortisol when the dose of prednisolone is 3 mg per day. Once 0900 hrs serum cortisol is >150–200 nmol/L, then an ACTH stimulation test should be performed (see Box 20.42) to confirm if glucocorticoids can be withdrawn completely. Even when glucocorticoids have been successfully withdrawn, short-term replacement therapy is often advised during significant intercurrent illness occurring in subsequent months, as the HPA axis may not be able to respond fully to severe stress.

Adrenal insufficiency

Adrenal insufficiency results from inadequate secretion of cortisol and/or aldosterone. It is potentially fatal and notoriously variable in its presentation. A high index of suspicion is therefore required in patients with unexplained fatigue, hyponatraemia or hypotension. Causes are shown in Box 20.40. The most common is ACTH deficiency (secondary adrenocortical failure), usually because of inappropriate withdrawal of chronic glucocorticoid therapy or a pituitary tumour. Congenital adrenal hyperplasia and Addison's disease (primary adrenocortical failure) are rare causes.

Clinical assessment

The clinical features of adrenal insufficiency are shown in Box 20.41. In Addison's disease, either glucocorticoid or mineralocorticoid deficiency may come first, but eventually all patients fail to secrete both classes of corticosteroid.

Patients may present with chronic features and/or in acute circulatory shock. With a chronic presentation, initial symptoms are often misdiagnosed as chronic fatigue syndrome or depression. In primary adrenal insufficiency, weight loss is a uniform presenting feature. Adrenocortical insufficiency should also be considered in patients with hyponatraemia, even in the absence of symptoms.

Features of an acute adrenal crisis include circulatory shock with severe hypotension, hyponatraemia, hyperkalaemia and, in some instances, hypoglycaemia and hypercalcaemia. Muscle cramps, nausea, vomiting, diarrhoea and unexplained fever may be present. The crisis is often precipitated by intercurrent disease, surgery or infection.

Vitiligo occurs in 10%–20% of patients with autoimmune Addison's disease.

Investigations

Treatment should not be delayed to wait for results in patients with suspected acute adrenal crisis. Here, a random blood sample should be stored for subsequent measurement of serum cortisol and, if possible, plasma ACTH; if the patient's clinical condition permits, it may be appropriate to spend 30 minutes performing a short ACTH stimulation test (Box 20.42) before administering hydrocortisone, but delays must be avoided if there is circulatory compromise. Investigations should be

---

> **i** | **20.40 Causes of adrenocortical insufficiency**
>
> **Secondary (↓ACTH)**
> - Withdrawal of suppressive glucocorticoid therapy
> - Hypothalamic or pituitary disease
>
> **Primary (↑ACTH)**
>
> **Addison's disease**
>
> | *Common causes* | *Rare causes* |
> |---|---|
> | • Autoimmune:
  Sporadic
• Polyendocrine syndromes (APS types 1 and 2)
• Tuberculosis
• HIV/AIDS
• Metastatic carcinoma
• Bilateral adrenalectomy | • Lymphoma
• Intra-adrenal haemorrhage (Waterhouse–Friderichsen syndrome following meningococcal sepsis)
• Amyloidosis
• Haemochromatosis |
>
> **Corticosteroid biosynthetic enzyme defects**
> - Congenital adrenal hyperplasias
> - Drugs: metyrapone, ketoconazole, etomidate
>
> (ACTH = adrenocorticotrophic hormone; APS = autoendocrine polyendocrine syndromes; HIV/AIDS = human immunodeficiency virus/acquired immune deficiency syndrome)

> **i** | **20.41 Clinical and biochemical features of adrenal insufficiency**
>
> | | Glucocorticoid insufficiency | Mineralocorticoid insufficiency | ACTH excess | Adrenal androgen insufficiency |
> |---|---|---|---|---|
> | **Withdrawal of exogenous glucocorticoid** | + | – | – | + |
> | **Hypopituitarism** | + | – | – | + |
> | **Addison's disease** | + | + | + | + |
> | **Congenital adrenal hyperplasia (21-hydroxylase deficiency)** | + | + | + | – |
> | **Clinical features** | Weight loss, anorexia
Malaise, weakness
Nausea, vomiting
Diarrhoea or constipation
Postural hypotension
Shock
Hypoglycaemia
Hyponatraemia (dilutional)
Hypercalcaemia | Hypotension
Shock
Hyponatraemia (depletional)
Hyperkalaemia | Pigmentation of:
Sun-exposed areas
Pressure areas (e.g. elbows, knees)
Palmar creases, knuckles
Mucous membranes
Conjunctivae
Recent scars | Decreased body hair and loss of libido, especially in females |
>
> (ACTH = adrenocorticotrophic hormone)

20

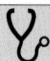

20.42 How and when to do an ACTH stimulation test

Use

- Diagnosis of primary or secondary adrenal insufficiency
- Assessment of HPA axis in patients taking suppressive glucocorticoid therapy
- Relies on ACTH-dependent adrenal atrophy in secondary adrenal insufficiency, so may not detect acute ACTH deficiency[1] (e.g. in pituitary apoplexy)

Dose

- 250 μg ACTH$_{1-24}$ (Synacthen) by IM injection at any time of day

Blood samples

- 0 and 30 mins for plasma cortisol
- 0 mins also for ACTH (on ice) if Addison's disease is being considered (patient not known to have pituitary disease or to be taking exogenous glucocorticoids)

Results

- Normal subjects: plasma cortisol >430 nmol/L (approximately 15.6 μg/dL)[2] either at baseline or at 30 mins
- Incremental change in cortisol is not a criterion

[1]In acute secondary adrenal insufficiency the adrenal cortex will still respond normally on the SST making the test unreliable in that setting. It usually takes around 6 weeks of ACTH-deficiency for the adrenal cortex to atrophy sufficiently for the response on and SST to be inadequate.[2]The exact cortisol concentration depends on the cortisol assay being used.(ACTH = adrenocorticotrophic hormone; HPA = hypothalamic–pituitary–adrenal; IM = intramuscular)

performed before treatment is given in patients who present with features suggestive of chronic adrenal insufficiency.

Assessment of glucocorticoids

Random plasma cortisol is usually low in patients with adrenal insufficiency but it may be within the reference range, yet inappropriately low, for a seriously ill patient. Random measurement of normal levels of plasma cortisol cannot therefore be used to confirm or refute the diagnosis, unless the value is above 430 nmol/L (>15.6 μg/dL), which effectively excludes adrenal insufficiency.

More useful is the short ACTH stimulation test (also called the tetracosactrin or short Synacthen test) described in Box 20.42. Cortisol levels fail to increase in response to exogenous ACTH in patients with primary or secondary adrenal insufficiency. These can be distinguished by measurement of ACTH (which is low in ACTH deficiency and high in Addison's disease).

Assessment of mineralocorticoids

Mineralocorticoid secretion in patients with suspected Addison's disease cannot be adequately assessed by electrolyte measurements since hyponatraemia occurs in both aldosterone and cortisol deficiency (see Box 20.41 and page 629). Hyperkalaemia is common, but not universal, in aldosterone deficiency. Plasma renin and aldosterone should be measured in the supine position. In mineralocorticoid deficiency, plasma renin activity is high, with plasma aldosterone being either low or in the lower part of the reference range.

Assessment of adrenal androgens

This is not necessary in men because testosterone from the testes is the principal androgen. In women, dehydroepiandrosterone sulphate (DHEAS) and androstenedione may be measured in a random specimen of blood, though levels are highest in the morning.

Other tests to establish the cause

Patients with unexplained secondary adrenocortical insufficiency should be investigated as described in Box 20.51. In patients with elevated ACTH, further tests are required to establish the cause of Addison's disease. Adrenal autoantibodies to 21-hydroxylase are frequently positive in autoimmune adrenal failure. If antibody tests are negative, imaging of the adrenal glands with CT or MRI is indicated. Tuberculosis causes adrenal calcification, visible on plain X-ray or ultrasound scan. A human immunodeficiency virus (HIV) test should be performed if relevant risk factors

are present. Adrenal metastases are a rare cause of adrenal insufficiency. Patients with evidence of autoimmune adrenal failure should be screened for other organ-specific autoimmune diseases, such as thyroid disease, pernicious anaemia and type 1 diabetes.

Management

Patients with adrenocortical insufficiency always need glucocorticoid replacement therapy and usually, but not always, mineralocorticoid therapy. There is some evidence that adrenal androgen replacement may also be beneficial in some women. Other treatments depend on the underlying cause. The emergency management of adrenal crisis is described in Box 20.43.

Glucocorticoid replacement

Adrenal replacement therapy consists of oral hydrocortisone (cortisol) 15–20 mg daily in divided doses, typically 10 mg on waking and 5 mg at around 1500 hrs. These are physiological replacement doses that should not cause Cushingoid side-effects. The dose may need to be adjusted for the individual patient but this is subjective. Excess weight gain usually indicates over-replacement, while persistent lethargy or hyperpigmentation may be due to an inadequate dose or lack of absorption. Measurement of serum cortisol levels is not usually helpful. Advice to patients dependent on glucocorticoid replacement is given in Box 20.39 and considerations in respect of glucocorticoids in old age are given in Box 20.44.

Mineralocorticoid replacement

Fludrocortisone (9α-fluoro-hydrocortisone) is administered at the usual dose of 0.05–0.15 mg daily, and adequacy of replacement may be assessed by measurement of blood pressure, plasma electrolytes and

20.43 Management of adrenal crisis

Correct volume depletion

- IV saline as required to normalise blood pressure and pulse
- In severe hyponatraemia (<125 mmol/L) avoid increases of plasma Na >10 mmol/L/day to prevent pontine demyelination
- Fludrocortisone is not required during the acute phase of treatment

Replace glucocorticoids

- IV hydrocortisone succinate 100 mg stat, and 100 mg 4 times daily for first 12–24 hrs
- Continue parenteral hydrocortisone (50–100 mg IM 4 times daily) until patient is well enough for reliable oral therapy

Correct other metabolic abnormalities

- Acute hypoglycaemia: IV 10% glucose
- Hyperkalaemia: should respond to volume replacement but occasionally requires specific therapy (see Box 19.17)

Identify and treat underlying cause

- Consider acute precipitant, such as infection
- Consider adrenal or pituitary pathology (see Box 20.40)

(IM = intramuscular; IV = intravenous)

20.44 Glucocorticoids in old age

- **Adrenocortical insufficiency**: often insidious and may present with tiredness, drowsiness, delirium, falls, immobility and orthostatic hypotension.
- **Glucocorticoid therapy**: especially hazardous in older people, who are already relatively immunocompromised and susceptible to osteoporosis, diabetes, hypertension and other complications.
- **'Physiological' glucocorticoid replacement therapy**: increased risk of adrenal crisis because adherence may be poor and there is a greater incidence of intercurrent illness. Patient and carer education, with regular reinforcement of the principles described in Box 20.39, is crucial.

plasma renin. It is indicated for virtually every patient with primary adrenal insufficiency but is not needed in secondary adrenal insufficiency.

Androgen replacement

Androgen replacement with DHEAS (50 mg/day) is occasionally given to women with primary adrenal insufficiency who have symptoms of reduced libido and fatigue, but the evidence in support of this is not robust and treatment may be associated with side-effects such as acne and hirsutism.

Incidental adrenal mass

Enlarged or hyperplastic adrenal glands are commonly found on CT or MRI scans of the abdomen that have been performed for other indications. Such lesions are known as adrenal 'incidentalomas'. The prevalence increases with age and they are present in up to 10% of adults aged 70 years and older.

Sixty per cent of adrenal incidentalomas are non-functioning adrenal adenomas. The remainder includes functional tumours of the adrenal cortex (secreting cortisol, aldosterone or androgens), phaeochromocytomas, primary and secondary carcinomas, hamartomas and other rare disorders, including granulomatous infiltrations.

Clinical assessment and investigations

There are two key questions to be resolved: is the lesion secreting hormones, and is it benign or malignant? These are best assessed by a dedicated adrenal multidisciplinary team (MDT).

Patients with an adrenal incidentaloma are usually asymptomatic. However, clinical signs and symptoms of excess glucocorticoids, mineralocorticoids, catecholamines and, in women, androgens should be sought, as discussed elsewhere in this chapter. Investigations should include a dexamethasone suppression test, urine or plasma metanephrines and, in virilised women, measurement of serum testosterone, DHEAS and androstenedione. Patients with hypertension should be investigated for mineralocorticoid excess, as described below. In bilateral masses consistent with adrenocortical lesions, 17-OH-progesterone should also be measured.

CT and MRI are equally effective in assessing the malignant potential of an adrenal mass, using the following parameters:

- *Size*. The larger the lesion, the greater the malignant potential. Around 90% of adrenocortical carcinomas are over 4 cm in diameter, but specificity is poor since only approximately 25% of such lesions are malignant.
- *Configuration*. Homogeneous and smooth lesions are more likely to be benign. The presence of metastatic lesions elsewhere increases the risk of malignancy, but as many as two-thirds of adrenal incidentalomas in patients with cancer are benign.
- *Presence of lipid*. Adenomas are usually lipid-rich, resulting in an attenuation of below 10 Hounsfield units (HU) on an unenhanced CT, and in signal dropout on chemical shift MRI.
- *Enhancement*. Benign lesions demonstrate rapid washout of contrast, whereas malignant lesions tend to retain contrast.

Histology in a sample obtained by CT-guided biopsy is rarely indicated, and is not useful in distinguishing an adrenal adenoma from an adrenocortical carcinoma. Biopsy is occasionally helpful in confirming adrenal metastases from other cancers, but should be avoided if either phaeochromocytoma or primary adrenal cancer is suspected in order to avoid precipitation of a hypertensive crisis or seeding of tumour cells, respectively. An endocrine opinion must be sought before any biopsy.

Management

In patients with radiologically benign, non-functioning lesions of less than 4 cm in diameter, surgery is not usually indicated. Functional lesions and tumours of more than 4 cm in diameter with indeterminate or concerning features, should be considered for surgery, and many centres will not

---

i | **20.45 Causes of mineralocorticoid excess**

With renin high and aldosterone high (secondary hyperaldosteronism)

- Inadequate renal perfusion (diuretic therapy, cardiac failure, liver failure, nephrotic syndrome, renal artery stenosis)
- Renin-secreting renal tumour (very rare)

With renin low and aldosterone high (primary hyperaldosteronism)

- Adrenal adenoma secreting aldosterone (Conn syndrome)
- Idiopathic bilateral adrenal hyperplasia
- Glucocorticoid-suppressible hyperaldosteronism (rare)

With renin low and aldosterone low (non-aldosterone-dependent activation of mineralocorticoid pathway)

- Ectopic ACTH syndrome
- Liquorice misuse (inhibition of 11β-HSD2)
- Liddle syndrome
- 11-deoxycorticosterone-secreting adrenal tumour
- Rare forms of congenital adrenal hyperplasia and 11β-HSD2 deficiency

(11β-HSD2 = 11β-hydroxysteroid dehydrogenase type 2; ACTH = adrenocorticotrophic hormone)

---

operate on tumours >4 cm if all other characteristics suggest benign disease. Optimal management of patients with low-grade cortisol secretion, as demonstrated by the dexamethasone suppression test, remains to be established.

Primary hyperaldosteronism

Estimates of the prevalence of primary hyperaldosteronism vary according to the screening tests employed, but it may occur in as many as 10% of people with hypertension. Indications to test for mineralocorticoid excess in hypertensive patients include hypokalaemia (including hypokalaemia induced by thiazide diuretics), poor control of blood pressure with conventional therapy, a family history of early-onset hypertension, or presentation at a young age.

Causes of excessive activation of mineralocorticoid receptors are shown in Box 20.45. It is important to differentiate primary hyperaldosteronism, caused by an intrinsic abnormality of the adrenal glands resulting in aldosterone excess, from secondary hyperaldosteronism, which is usually a consequence of enhanced activity of renin in response to inadequate renal perfusion and hypotension. Most individuals with primary hyperaldosteronism have bilateral adrenal hyperplasia (idiopathic hyperaldosteronism), while only a minority have an aldosterone-producing adenoma (APA; Conn syndrome). Glucocorticoid-suppressible hyperaldosteronism is a rare autosomal dominant condition in which aldosterone is secreted 'ectopically' from the adrenal zonae fasciculata/reticularis in response to ACTH. Rarely, the mineralocorticoid receptor pathway in the distal nephron is activated, even though aldosterone concentrations are low.

Clinical features

Individuals with primary hyperaldosteronism are usually asymptomatic but may have features of sodium retention or potassium loss. Sodium retention may cause oedema, while hypokalaemia may cause muscle weakness (or even paralysis, especially in South-east Asian populations), polyuria (secondary to renal tubular damage, which produces nephrogenic diabetes insipidus) and occasionally tetany (because of associated metabolic alkalosis and low ionised calcium). Blood pressure is elevated but accelerated phase hypertension is rare.

Investigations

Biochemical

Routine blood tests may show a hypokalaemic alkalosis. Sodium is usually at the upper end of the reference range in primary hyperaldosteronism, but is characteristically low in secondary hyperaldosteronism (because low

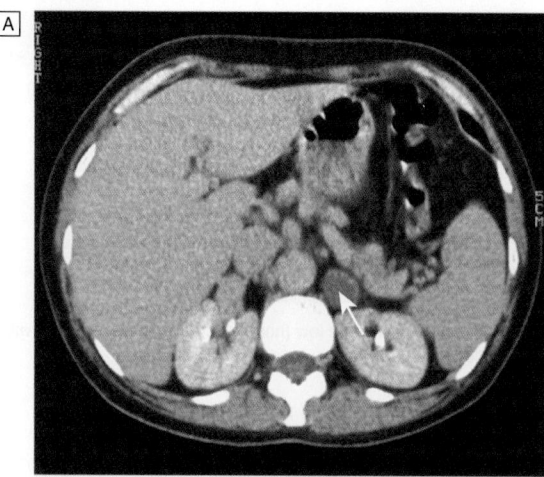

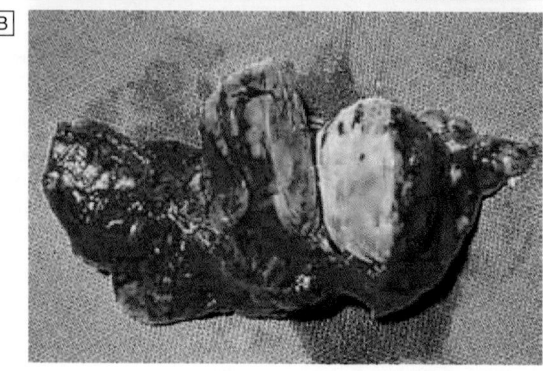

Fig. 20.24 Aldosterone-producing adenoma causing Conn syndrome. [A] CT scan of left adrenal adenoma (arrow). [B] The tumour is 'canary yellow' because of intracellular lipid accumulation.

plasma volume stimulates vasopressin (antidiuretic hormone, ADH) release and high angiotensin II levels stimulate thirst). The key measurements are plasma renin and aldosterone (Box 20.45), and in many centres the aldosterone:renin ratio (ARR) is employed as a screening test for primary hyperaldosteronism in hypertensive patients. Almost all antihypertensive drugs interfere with this ratio (β-blockers inhibit while diuretics stimulate renin secretion). Thus, individuals with an elevated ARR require further testing after stopping many antihypertensive drugs for at least 4 weeks (although if the ratio is still high despite a patient taking ACE inhibitors or angiotensin receptor-blocking drugs then this need not be done as these agents would normally cause a lowering of the ratio). If necessary, antihypertensive agents that have minimal effects on the renin–angiotensin system, such as calcium antagonists and α-blockers, may be substituted. Oral potassium supplementation may also be required, as hypokalaemia itself suppresses renin activity. If, on repeat testing, plasma renin is low and aldosterone concentrations are elevated, then further investigation under specialist supervision may include saline or fludrocortisone suppression tests.

Imaging and localisation

Imaging with CT or MRI will identify most APAs (Fig. 20.24A) but it is important to recognise the risk of false positives (non-functioning adrenal adenomas are common) and false negatives (imaging may have insufficient resolution to identify adenomas with a diameter of less than 0.5 cm). If the imaging is inconclusive and there is an intention to proceed with surgery on the basis of strong biochemical evidence of an APA, then adrenal vein catheterisation with measurement of aldosterone (and cortisol to confirm positioning of the catheters) is usually required. In some centres, this is performed even in the presence of a unilateral 'adenoma', to avoid inadvertent removal of an incidental non-functioning adenoma contralateral to a radiologically inapparent cause of aldosterone excess.

> **i** 20.46 Clinical features of phaeochromocytoma
>
> - Hypertension (usually paroxysmal; often postural drop of blood pressure)
> - Paroxysms of:
>   - Pallor (occasionally flushing)
>   - Palpitations, sweating
>   - Headache
>   - Anxiety (angor animi)
> - Abdominal pain, vomiting
> - Constipation
> - Weight loss
> - Glucose intolerance

Management

Mineralocorticoid receptor antagonists (spironolactone and eplerenone) are valuable in treating both hypokalaemia and hypertension in all forms of mineralocorticoid excess. Up to 20% of males develop gynaecomastia on spironolactone. Amiloride (10–40 mg/day), which blocks the epithelial sodium channel regulated by aldosterone, is an alternative.

In patients with an APA, medical therapy is usually given for a few weeks to normalise whole-body electrolyte balance before unilateral adrenalectomy. Laparoscopic surgery cures the biochemical abnormality but, depending on the pre-operative duration, hypertension remains in as many as 70% of cases, probably because of irreversible damage to the systemic microcirculation.

Phaeochromocytoma and paraganglioma

These are rare neuro-endocrine tumours that may secrete catecholamines (adrenaline/epinephrine, noradrenaline/norepinephrine). Approximately 80% of these tumours occur in the adrenal medulla (phaeochromocytomas), while 20% arise elsewhere in the body in sympathetic ganglia (paragangliomas). Most are benign but approximately 15% show malignant features. Around 40% are associated with inherited disorders, including neurofibromatosis, von Hippel–Lindau syndrome, MEN 2a and MEN 2b. Paragangliomas are particularly associated with mutations in the succinate dehydrogenase A, B, C and D genes. Other genetic causes include mutations in *SDHA*, *SDHAF2*, *TMEN127* and *MAX*.

Clinical features

These depend on the pattern of catecholamine secretion and are listed in Box 20.46.

Some patients present with hypertension, although it has been estimated that phaeochromocytoma accounts for less than 0.1% of cases of hypertension. The presentation may be with a complication of hypertension, such as stroke, myocardial infarction, left ventricular failure, hypertensive retinopathy or accelerated phase hypertension. The apparent paradox of postural hypotension between episodes is explained by 'pressure natriuresis' during hypertensive episodes so that intravascular volume is reduced. There may also be features of the familial syndromes associated with phaeochromocytoma. Paragangliomas are often non-functioning.

Investigations

Excessive secretion of catecholamines can be confirmed by measuring metabolites in plasma and/or urine (metanephrine and normetanephrine). There is a high 'false-positive' rate, as misleading metanephrine concentrations may be seen in stressed patients (during acute illness, following vigorous exercise or severe pain) and following ingestion of some drugs such as tricyclic antidepressants. For this reason, a repeat sample should usually be requested if elevated levels are found, although, as a rule, the higher the concentration of metanephrines, the more likely the diagnosis of phaeochromocytoma/paraganglioma. Serum chromogranin A is often elevated and may be a useful tumour marker in patients with non-secretory tumours and/or metastatic disease. Genetic testing should be considered in individuals with other features of a

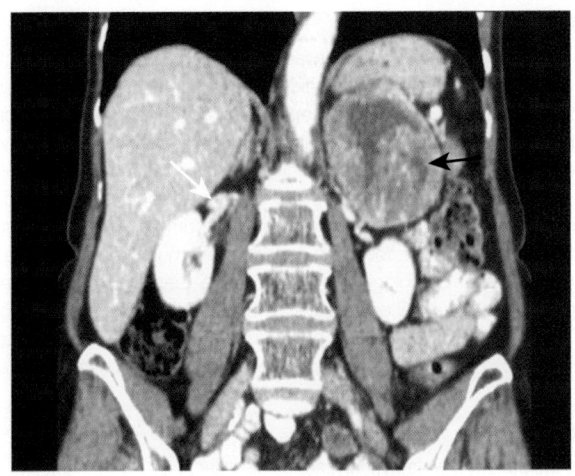

Fig. 20.25 CT scan of abdomen showing large left adrenal phaeochromocytoma. The normal right adrenal (white arrow) contrasts with the large heterogeneous phaeochromocytoma arising from the left adrenal gland (black arrow).

genetic syndrome, in those with a family history of phaeochromocytoma/paraganglioma, and in those presenting under the age of 50 years.

Localisation

Phaeochromocytomas are usually identified by abdominal CT or MRI (Fig. 20.25). Localisation of paragangliomas may be more difficult. Scintigraphy using meta-iodobenzyl guanidine (MIBG) can be useful, particularly if combined with CT, for adrenal phaeochromocytoma but is often negative in paraganglioma. ^{18}F-deoxyglucose PET or ^{68}Ga-DOTANOC or DOTATATE-PET CT are especially useful for detection of malignant disease and for confirming an imaging abnormality as a paraganglioma in an individual with underlying risk due to genetic mutation.

Management

In functioning tumours, medical therapy is required to prepare the patient for surgery, preferably for a minimum of 6 weeks, to allow restoration of normal plasma volume. The most useful drug in the face of very high circulating catecholamines is the α-blocker phenoxybenzamine (10–20 mg orally 3–4 times daily) because it is a non-competitive antagonist, unlike prazosin or doxazosin. If α-blockade produces a marked tachycardia, then a β-blocker such as propranolol can be added. On no account should a β-blocker be given before an α-blocker, as this may cause a paradoxical rise in blood pressure due to unopposed α-mediated vasoconstriction.

During surgery, sodium nitroprusside and the short-acting α-antagonist phentolamine are useful in controlling hypertensive episodes, which may result from anaesthetic induction or tumour mobilisation. Postoperative hypotension may occur and require volume expansion and, very occasionally, noradrenaline (norepinephrine) infusion, but is uncommon if the patient has been prepared with phenoxybenzamine.

Metastatic tumours may behave in an aggressive or a very indolent fashion. Management options include debulking surgery, radionuclide therapy with ^{131}I-MIBG or ^{177}Lutetium DOTATATE, chemotherapy and (chemo)embolisation of hepatic metastases; some may respond to tyrosine kinase and angiogenesis inhibitors.

Congenital adrenal hyperplasia

Pathophysiology and clinical features

Inherited defects in enzymes of the cortisol biosynthetic pathway (see Fig. 20.20) result in insufficiency of hormones downstream of the block, with impaired negative feedback and increased ACTH secretion. ACTH then stimulates the production of steroids upstream of the enzyme block. This produces adrenal hyperplasia and a combination of clinical features

that depend on the severity and site of the defect in biosynthesis. All of these enzyme abnormalities are inherited as autosomal recessive traits.

The most common enzyme defect is 21-hydroxylase deficiency. This results in impaired synthesis of cortisol and aldosterone, and accumulation of 17-OH-progesterone, which is then diverted to form adrenal androgens. In about one-third of cases, this defect is severe and presents in infancy with features of glucocorticoid and mineralocorticoid deficiency (see Box 20.41) and androgen excess, such as ambiguous genitalia in girls. In the other two-thirds, mineralocorticoid secretion is adequate but there may be features of cortisol insufficiency and/or ACTH and androgen excess, including precocious pseudo-puberty, which is distinguished from 'true' precocious puberty by low gonadotrophins. Sometimes the mildest enzyme defects are not apparent until adult life, when females may present with amenorrhoea and/or hirsutism. This is called 'non-classical' or 'late-onset' congenital adrenal hyperplasia.

Defects of all the other enzymes in Figure 20.20 are rare. Both 17-hydroxylase and 11β-hydroxylase deficiency may produce hypertension due to excess production of 11-deoxycorticosterone, which has mineralocorticoid activity.

Investigations

Circulating 17-OH-progesterone levels are raised in 21-hydroxylase deficiency but this may be demonstrated only after ACTH administration in late-onset cases. To avoid salt-wasting crises in infancy, 17-OH-progesterone can be routinely measured in heelprick blood spot samples taken from all infants in the first week of life. Assessment is otherwise as described earlier for adrenal insufficiency.

In siblings of affected children, antenatal genetic diagnosis can be made by amniocentesis or chorionic villus sampling. This allows prevention of virilisation of affected female fetuses by administration of dexamethasone to the mother to suppress ACTH levels.

Management

The aim is to replace deficient corticosteroids and to suppress ACTH-driven adrenal androgen production. A careful balance is required between adequate suppression of adrenal androgen excess and excessive glucocorticoid replacement resulting in features of Cushing's syndrome. In children, growth velocity is an important measurement, since either under- or over-replacement with glucocorticoids suppresses growth. In adults, there is no uniformly agreed adrenal replacement regimen, and clinical features (menstrual cycle, hirsutism, weight gain, blood pressure) and biochemical profiles (plasma renin, 17-OH-progesterone and testosterone levels) provide a guide.

Women with late-onset 21-hydroxylase deficiency may not require corticosteroid replacement. If hirsutism is the main problem, anti-androgen therapy may be just as effective.

The endocrine pancreas and gastrointestinal tract

A series of hormones are secreted from cells distributed throughout the gastrointestinal tract and pancreas. Functional anatomy and physiology are described in Chapter 23 and 24. Diseases associated with abnormalities of these hormones are listed in Box 20.47. Most are rare, with the exception of diabetes mellitus (Ch. 21).

Presenting problems in endocrine pancreas disease

Spontaneous hypoglycaemia

Hypoglycaemia most commonly occurs as a side-effect of treatment with insulin or sulphonylurea drugs in people with diabetes mellitus. In non-diabetic individuals, symptomatic hypoglycaemia is rare, but it is not uncommon to detect venous blood glucose concentrations below 3.0 mmol/L

20

i | **20.47 Classification of endocrine diseases of the pancreas and gastrointestinal tract**

	Primary	Secondary
Hormone excess	Insulinoma Gastrinoma (Zollinger–Ellison syndrome) Carcinoid syndrome (secretion of 5-HT) Glucagonoma VIPoma Somatostatinoma	Hypergastrinaemia of achlorhydria Hyperinsulinaemia after bariatric surgery
Hormone deficiency	Diabetes mellitus	
Hormone resistance	Insulin resistance syndromes (e.g. type 2 diabetes mellitus, lipodystrophy, Donohue syndrome)	
Non-functioning tumours	Pancreatic carcinoma Pancreatic neuro-endocrine tumour	

(5-HT = 5-hydroxytryptamine, serotonin)

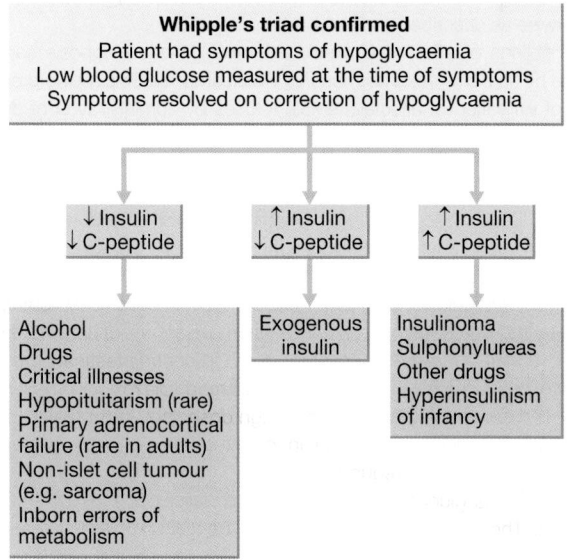

Whipple's triad confirmed
Patient had symptoms of hypoglycaemia
Low blood glucose measured at the time of symptoms
Symptoms resolved on correction of hypoglycaemia

↓ Insulin ↓ C-peptide

↑ Insulin ↓ C-peptide

↑ Insulin ↑ C-peptide

Alcohol
Drugs
Critical illnesses
Hypopituitarism (rare)
Primary adrenocortical failure (rare in adults)
Non-islet cell tumour (e.g. sarcoma)
Inborn errors of metabolism

Exogenous insulin

Insulinoma
Sulphonylureas
Other drugs
Hyperinsulinism of infancy

Fig. 20.26 Differential diagnosis of spontaneous hypoglycaemia. Measurement of insulin and C-peptide concentrations during an episode is helpful in determining the underlying cause.

(54 mg/dL) in asymptomatic patients. For this reason, and because the symptoms of hypoglycaemia are non-specific, a hypoglycaemic disorder should be diagnosed only if all three conditions of Whipple's triad are met (Fig. 20.26). There is no specific blood glucose concentration at which spontaneous hypoglycaemia can be said to occur, although the lower the blood glucose concentration, the more likely it is to have pathological significance. Investigations are unlikely to be needed unless glucose concentrations below 3.0 mmol/L are observed, many patients with true hypoglycaemia demonstrating glucose levels below 2.2 mmol/L (40 mg/dL).

With the increasing use of bariatric surgery, and more specifically gastric bypass surgery, more patients are presenting with post-prandial hypoglycaemia due to excess stimulated insulin secretion due to the rapid carbohydrate loads being delivered directly to the small intestine. Careful history-taking is needed to distinguish between post-prandial and spontaneous hypoglycaemia, and oral glucose tolerance or mixed meal testing may invoke observed hypoglycaemia in the former.

Clinical assessment

The clinical features of hypoglycaemia are described in the section on insulin-induced hypoglycaemia in Chapter 21. Individuals with chronic spontaneous hypoglycaemia often have attenuated autonomic responses and 'hypoglycaemia unawareness', and may present with a wide variety of features of neuroglycopenia, including odd behaviour and convulsions. The symptoms are usually episodic and relieved by consumption of carbohydrate. Symptoms occurring while fasting (such as before breakfast) or following exercise are much more likely to be representative of pathological hypoglycaemia than those that develop after food (post-prandial or 'reactive' symptoms). Hypoglycaemia should be considered in all comatose patients, even if there is an apparently obvious cause, such as hemiplegic stroke or alcohol intoxication.

Investigations

Does the patient have a hypoglycaemic disorder?

Patients who present acutely with delirium, coma, convulsions or stroke should be tested for hypoglycaemia at the bedside with a capillary blood sample and an automated meter. While this is sufficient to exclude hypoglycaemia, blood glucose meters are relatively inaccurate in the hypoglycaemic range and the diagnosis should always be confirmed by a laboratory-based glucose measurement. At the same time, a sample should be taken for later measurement of alcohol, insulin, C-peptide, cortisol and sulphonylurea levels, if hypoglycaemia is confirmed. Taking these samples during an acute presentation prevents subsequent unnecessary dynamic tests and is of medico-legal importance in cases where poisoning is suspected.

Patients who attend the outpatient clinic with episodic symptoms suggestive of hypoglycaemia present a more challenging problem. The main diagnostic test is the prolonged (72-hour) fast. If symptoms of hypoglycaemia develop during the fast, then blood samples should be taken to confirm hypoglycaemia and for later measurement of insulin and C-peptide. Hypoglycaemia is then corrected with oral or intravenous glucose and Whipple's triad completed by confirmation of the resolution of symptoms. The absence of clinical and biochemical evidence of hypoglycaemia during a prolonged fast effectively excludes the diagnosis of a hypoglycaemic disorder.

What is the cause of the hypoglycaemia?

In the acute setting, the underlying diagnosis is often obvious. In non-diabetic individuals, alcohol excess is the most common cause of hypoglycaemia in the UK, but other drugs – e.g. salicylates, quinine and pentamidine – may also be implicated. Hypoglycaemia is one of many metabolic derangements that occur in patients with hepatic failure, renal failure, adrenal insufficiency, sepsis or malaria.

Hypoglycaemia in the absence of insulin, or any insulin-like factor, in the blood indicates impaired gluconeogenesis and/or availability of glucose from glycogen in the liver. Hypoglycaemia associated with high insulin and low C-peptide concentrations is indicative of administration of exogenous insulin, either factitiously or feloniously. Adults with high insulin and C-peptide concentrations during an episode of hypoglycaemia are most likely to have an insulinoma but sulphonylurea ingestion should also be considered (particularly in individuals with access to such medication, such as health-care professionals or family members of someone with type 2 diabetes). Suppressed plasma β-hydroxybutyrate helps confirm inappropriate insulin secretion during fasting. Usually, insulinomas in the pancreas are small (<5 mm diameter) but can be identified by CT, MRI or ultrasound (endoscopic or laparoscopic). Imaging should include the liver since around 10% of insulinomas are malignant and may metastasise to the liver. Rarely, large non-pancreatic tumours, such as sarcomas, may cause recurrent hypoglycaemia because of their ability to produce excess pro-insulin-like growth factor-2 (pro-IGF-2), which has considerable structural homology to insulin.

Management

Treatment of acute hypoglycaemia should be initiated as soon as laboratory blood samples have been taken and should *not* be deferred until formal laboratory confirmation has been obtained. Intravenous dextrose (5% or 10%) is effective in the short term in the obtunded patient and should be followed on recovery with oral unrefined carbohydrate (starch). Continuous dextrose infusion may be necessary, especially in sulphonylurea poisoning. Intramuscular glucagon (1 mg) stimulates hepatic glucose release but is ineffective in patients with depleted glycogen reserves, such as in alcohol excess or liver disease.

Chronic recurrent hypoglycaemia in insulin-secreting tumours can be treated by regular consumption of oral carbohydrate combined with agents that inhibit insulin secretion (diazoxide or somatostatin analogues). Insulinomas are resected when benign, providing the individual is fit enough to undergo surgery. Metastatic malignant insulinomas may be incurable and are managed along the same lines as other metastatic neuro-endocrine tumours (see below).

Gastroenteropancreatic neuro-endocrine tumours

Neuro-endocrine tumours (NETs) are a heterogeneous group derived from neuro-endocrine cells in many organs, including the gastrointestinal tract, lung, adrenals (phaeochromocytoma) and thyroid (medullary carcinoma). Most NETs occur sporadically but a proportion are associated with genetic cancer syndromes, such as MEN 1, 2a and 2b, and neurofibromatosis type 1. NETs may secrete hormones into the circulation.

Gastroenteropancreatic NETs arise in organs that are derived embryologically from the gastrointestinal tract. Most commonly, they occur in the small bowel but they can also arise elsewhere in the bowel, pancreas, thymus and bronchi. The term 'carcinoid' is often used when referring to non-pancreatic gastroenteropancreatic NETs because, when initially described, they were thought to behave in an indolent fashion compared with conventional cancers. It is now recognised that there is a wide spectrum of malignant potential for all NETs; some are more usually benign (most insulinomas and appendiceal carcinoid tumours), while others have an aggressive clinical course with widespread metastases (small-cell carcinoma of the lung). The majority of gastroenteropancreatic NETs behave in an intermediate manner, with relatively slow growth but a propensity to invade and metastasise to remote organs, especially the liver.

Clinical features

Patients with gastroenteropancreatic NETs often have a history of abdominal pain over many years prior to diagnosis and usually present with local mass effects, such as small-bowel obstruction, appendicitis and pain from hepatic metastases. Thymic and bronchial carcinoids occasionally present with ectopic ACTH syndrome. Pancreatic NETs can also cause hormone excess (Box 20.48) but most are non-functional.

20.48 Pancreatic neuro-endocrine tumours		
Tumour	**Hormone**	**Effects**
Gastrinoma	Gastrin	Peptic ulcer and steatorrhoea (Zollinger–Ellison syndrome)
Insulinoma	Insulin	Recurrent hypoglycaemia (see above)
VIPoma	Vasoactive intestinal peptide (VIP)	Watery diarrhoea and hypokalaemia
Glucagonoma	Glucagon	Diabetes mellitus, necrolytic migratory erythema
Somatostatinoma	Somatostatin	Diabetes mellitus and steatorrhoea

20.49 Clinical features of the carcinoid syndrome

- Episodic flushing, wheezing and diarrhoea
- Facial telangiectasia
- Cardiac involvement (tricuspid regurgitation, pulmonary stenosis, right ventricular endocardial plaques) leading to heart failure

The classic 'carcinoid syndrome' (Box 20.49) occurs when vasoactive hormones reach the systemic circulation. In the case of gastrointestinal carcinoids, this invariably means that the tumour has metastasised to the liver or there are peritoneal deposits, which allow secreted hormones to gain access to the systemic circulation; hormones secreted by the primary tumour into the portal vein are metabolised and inactivated in the liver. The features of Zollinger–Ellison syndrome are described on page 816.

Investigations

A combination of imaging with ultrasound, CT, MRI and/or radio-labelled somatostatin analogue (Fig. 20.27) will usually identify the primary tumour and allow staging, which is crucial for determining prognosis. Biopsy of the primary tumour or a metastatic deposit is required to confirm the histological type. NETs demonstrate immunohistochemical staining for the proteins chromogranin A and synaptophysin, and the histological grade provides important prognostic information: the higher the Ki67 proliferation index, the worse the prognosis.

Carcinoid syndrome is confirmed by measuring elevated concentrations of 5-hydroxyindoleacetic acid (5-HIAA), a metabolite of serotonin, in a 24-hour urine collection. False positives can occur, particularly if the individual has been eating serotonin-rich foods, such as avocado and pineapple. Plasma chromogranin A can be measured in a fasting blood sample, along with the hormones listed in Box 20.48. All of these can be useful as tumour markers.

Management

Treatment of solitary tumours is by surgical resection. If metastatic or multifocal primary disease is present, then surgery is usually not indicated, unless there is a complication such as gastrointestinal obstruction, but debulking surgery may be performed. Diazoxide can reduce insulin secretion in insulinomas, and high doses of proton pump inhibitors suppress acid production in gastrinomas. Somatostatin analogues are effective in reducing the symptoms of carcinoid syndrome and of excess glucagon and vasoactive intestinal peptide (VIP) production. The slow-growing nature of NETs means that conventional cancer therapies, such as chemotherapy and radiotherapy, have limited efficacy, but use of somatostatin analogues is associated with improved progression-free survival, and [177]Lutetium DOTATATE is indicated for many patients with further disease progression. Other treatments, such as interferon, targeted radionuclide therapy with ^{131}I-MIBG and resection/embolisation/ablation of hepatic metastases, may have a role in the palliation of symptoms but debate exists as to whether this prolongs life. The tyrosine kinase inhibitor sunitinib and the mammalian target of rapamycin (mTOR) inhibitor everolimus have shown significant improvements in progression-free survival in patients with advanced and progressive pancreatic and lung NETS that are not poorly differentiated.

The hypothalamus and the pituitary gland

Diseases of the hypothalamus and pituitary have an annual incidence of approximately 3:100 000 and a prevalence of 30–70 per 100 000. The pituitary plays a central role in several major endocrine axes, so that investigation and treatment invariably involve several other endocrine glands.

20

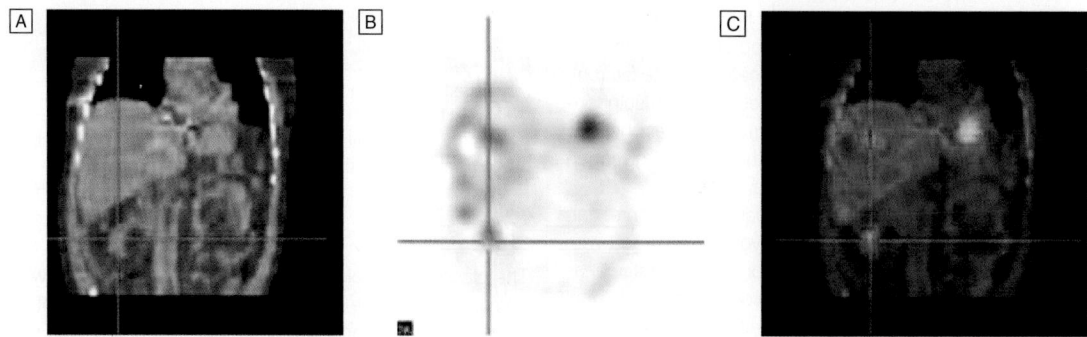

Fig. 20.27 Octreotide scintigraphy in a metastatic neuro-endocrine tumour. [A] Coronal CT scan showing hepatomegaly and a mass inferior to the liver (at the intersection of the horizontal and vertical red lines). [B] Octreotide scintogram showing patches of increased uptake in the upper abdomen. [C] When the octreotide and CT scans are superimposed, it shows that the areas of increased uptake are in hepatic metastases and in the tissue mass, which may be lymph nodes or a primary tumour.

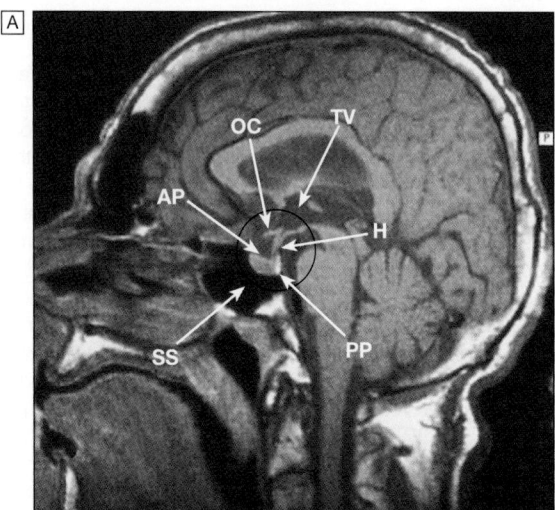

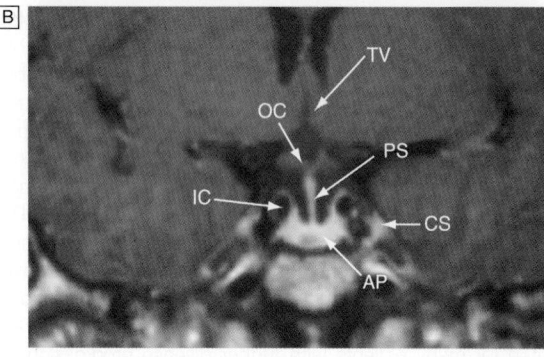

Fig. 20.28 Anatomical relationships of the normal pituitary gland and hypothalamus. See also Fig. 20.2. [A] Sagittal MRI. [B] Coronal MRI. (AP = anterior pituitary; CS = cavernous sinus; H = hypothalamus; IC = internal carotid artery; OC = optic chiasm; PP = posterior pituitary; PS = pituitary stalk; SS = sphenoid sinus; TV = third ventricle)

20.50 Classification of diseases of the pituitary and hypothalamus

	Primary	Secondary
Non-functioning tumours	Pituitary adenoma Craniopharyngioma Metastatic tumours	
Hormone excess		
Anterior pituitary Hypothalamus and posterior pituitary	Prolactinoma Acromegaly Cushing's disease Rare TSH-, LH- and FSH-secreting adenomas Syndrome of inappropriate antidiuretic hormone (SIADH, p. 624)	Disconnection hyperprolactinaemia
Hormone deficiency		
Anterior pituitary Hypothalamus and posterior pituitary	Hypopituitarism Cranial diabetes insipidus	GnRH deficiency (Kallmann syndrome)
Hormone resistance	Growth hormone resistance (Laron dwarfism) Nephrogenic diabetes insipidus	

(FSH = follicle-stimulating hormone; GnRH = gonadotrophin-releasing hormone; LH = luteinising hormone; TSH = thyroid-stimulating hormone)

Functional anatomy, physiology and investigations

The anatomical relationships of the pituitary are shown in Figure 20.28 and its numerous functions are shown in Figure 20.2. The pituitary gland is enclosed in the sella turcica and bridged over by a fold of dura mater called the diaphragma sellae, with the sphenoidal air sinuses below and the optic chiasm above. The cavernous sinuses are lateral to the pituitary fossa and contain the 3rd, 4th and 6th cranial nerves and the internal carotid arteries. The gland is composed of two lobes, anterior and posterior, and is connected to the hypothalamus by the infundibular stalk, which has portal vessels carrying blood from the median eminence of the hypothalamus to the anterior lobe and nerve fibres to the posterior lobe.

Diseases of the hypothalamus and pituitary are classified in Box 20.50. By far the most common disorder is an adenoma of the anterior pituitary gland.

Investigation of patients with pituitary disease

Although pituitary disease presents with diverse clinical manifestations (see below), the approach to investigation is similar in all cases (Box 20.51).

The approach to testing for hormone deficiency is outlined in Box 20.51. Details are given in the sections on individual glands elsewhere in this chapter. Tests for hormone excess vary according to the hormone in question. For example, prolactin is not secreted in pulsatile fashion, although it rises with significant psychological stress. Assuming that the patient was not distressed by venepuncture, a random measurement of

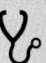

20.51 How to investigate patients with suspected pituitary hypothalamic disease

Identify pituitary hormone deficiency

ACTH deficiency
- Short ACTH stimulation test (see Box 20.42)
- Insulin tolerance test (see Box 20.55): only if there is uncertainty in interpretation of short ACTH stimulation test (e.g. acute presentation)

LH/FSH deficiency
- In the male, measure random serum testosterone, LH and FSH
- In the pre-menopausal female, ask if the menses are regular
- In the post-menopausal female, measure random serum LH and FSH (FSH normally >30 IU/L and LH >20 IU/L)

TSH deficiency
- Measure random serum T$_4$
- Note that TSH is often detectable in secondary hypothyroidism

Growth hormone deficiency
Only investigate if growth hormone replacement therapy is being contemplated
- Measure immediately after exercise
- Consider other stimulatory tests (see Box 20.54)

Cranial diabetes insipidus
Only investigate if patient complains of polyuria/polydipsia, which may be masked by ACTH or TSH deficiency
- Exclude other causes of polyuria with blood glucose, potassium and calcium measurements
- Water deprivation test (see Box 20.60) or 5% saline infusion test

Identify hormone excess
- Measure random serum prolactin
- Investigate for acromegaly (glucose tolerance test) or Cushing's syndrome if there are clinical features

Establish the anatomy and diagnosis
- Consider visual field testing
- Image the pituitary and hypothalamus by MRI or CT

(ACTH = adrenocorticotrophic hormone; CT = computed tomography; FSH = follicle-stimulating hormone; LH = luteinising hormone; MRI = magnetic resonance imaging; TSH = thyroid-stimulating hormone)

serum prolactin is sufficient to diagnose hyperprolactinaemia. In contrast, growth hormone is secreted in a pulsatile fashion. A high random level does not confirm acromegaly; the diagnosis is confirmed only by failure of growth hormone to be suppressed during an oral glucose tolerance test, and a high serum insulin-like growth factor-1 (IGF-1). Similarly, in suspected ACTH-dependent Cushing's disease, random measurement of plasma cortisol is unreliable and the diagnosis is usually made by a dexamethasone suppression, and other tests.

The most common local complication of a large pituitary tumour is compression of the optic pathway. The resulting visual field defect can be documented using a Goldmann perimetry chart or with an automated perimetry method (see p. 1222).

MRI reveals 'abnormalities' of the pituitary gland in as many as 10% of 'healthy' middle-aged people. It should therefore be performed only if there is a clear biochemical abnormality or if a patient presents with clinical features of pituitary tumour (see below). A pituitary tumour may be classified as either a macroadenoma (>10 mm diameter) or a microadenoma (<10 mm diameter).

Surgical biopsy is usually only performed as part of a therapeutic operation. Conventional histology identifies tumours as chromophobe (usually non-functioning), acidophil (typically prolactin- or growth hormone-secreting) or basophil (typically ACTH-secreting); immunohistochemistry may confirm their secretory capacity but is poorly predictive of growth potential of the tumour.

Presenting problems in hypothalamic and pituitary disease

The clinical features of pituitary disease are shown in Figure 20.29. Younger women with pituitary disease most commonly present with secondary amenorrhoea or galactorrhoea (in hyperprolactinaemia). Post-menopausal women and men of any age are less likely to report symptoms of hypogonadism and so are more likely to present late with larger tumours causing visual field defects. The presentation and management of pituitary and hypothalamic disease may be affected by old age (Box 20.52). Nowadays, many patients present with the incidental finding of a pituitary tumour on a CT or MRI scan.

20

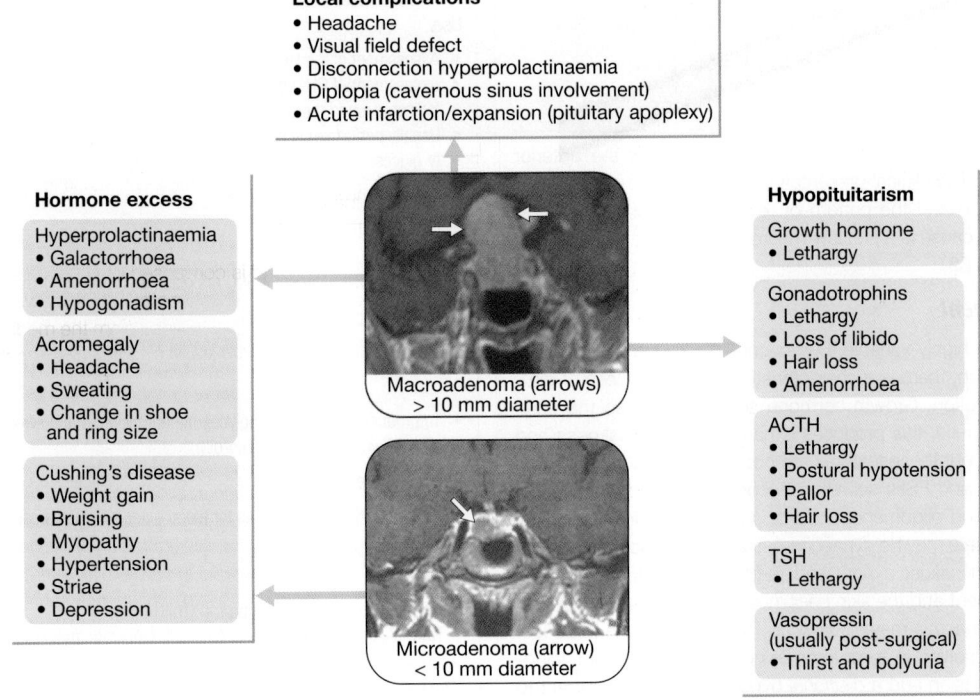

Local complications
- Headache
- Visual field defect
- Disconnection hyperprolactinaemia
- Diplopia (cavernous sinus involvement)
- Acute infarction/expansion (pituitary apoplexy)

Hormone excess

Hyperprolactinaemia
- Galactorrhoea
- Amenorrhoea
- Hypogonadism

Acromegaly
- Headache
- Sweating
- Change in shoe and ring size

Cushing's disease
- Weight gain
- Bruising
- Myopathy
- Hypertension
- Striae
- Depression

Macroadenoma (arrows) > 10 mm diameter

Microadenoma (arrow) < 10 mm diameter

Hypopituitarism

Growth hormone
- Lethargy

Gonadotrophins
- Lethargy
- Loss of libido
- Hair loss
- Amenorrhoea

ACTH
- Lethargy
- Postural hypotension
- Pallor
- Hair loss

TSH
- Lethargy

Vasopressin (usually post-surgical)
- Thirst and polyuria

Fig. 20.29 Common symptoms and signs to consider in a patient with suspected pituitary disease. (ACTH = adrenocorticotrophic hormone; TSH = thyroid-stimulating hormone)

20.52 The pituitary and hypothalamus in old age

- **Late presentation**: often with large tumours causing visual disturbance, because early symptoms such as amenorrhoea and sexual dysfunction do not occur or are not recognised.
- **Coincidentally discovered pituitary tumours**: may not require surgical intervention if the visual apparatus is not involved, because of slow growth.
- **Hyperprolactinaemia**: less impact in post-menopausal women who are already 'physiologically' hypogonadal. Macroprolactinomas, however, require treatment because of their potential to cause mass effects.

20.53 Causes of anterior pituitary hormone deficiency

Structural

- Primary pituitary tumour
- Adenoma*
- Carcinoma (exceptionally rare)
- Craniopharyngioma*
- Meningioma*
- Secondary tumour (including leukaemia and lymphoma)
- Chordoma
- Germinoma (pinealoma)
- Arachnoid cyst
- Rathke's cleft cyst
- Haemorrhage (apoplexy)

Inflammatory/infiltrative

- Sarcoidosis
- Infections, e.g. pituitary abscess, tuberculosis, syphilis, encephalitis
- Lymphocytic hypophysitis
- Haemochromatosis
- Langerhans cell histiocytosis

Congenital deficiencies

- GnRH (Kallmann syndrome)*
- GHRH*
- TRH
- CRH

Functional*

- Chronic systemic illness
- Anorexia nervosa
- Excessive exercise

Other

- Head injury*
- (Para)sellar surgery*
- (Para)sellar radiotherapy*
- Post-partum necrosis (Sheehan syndrome)
- Opiate analgesia

*The most common causes of pituitary hormone deficiency.
(CRH = corticotrophin-releasing hormone; GHRH = growth hormone-releasing hormone; GnRH = gonadotrophin-releasing hormone; TRH = thyrotrophin-releasing hormone)

Hypopituitarism

Hypopituitarism describes combined deficiency of any of the anterior pituitary hormones. The clinical presentation is variable and depends on the underlying lesion and the pattern of resulting hormone deficiency. The most common cause is a pituitary macroadenoma but other causes are listed in Box 20.53.

Clinical assessment

The presentation is highly variable. For example, following radiotherapy to the pituitary region, there is a characteristic sequence of loss of pituitary hormone secretion. Growth hormone secretion is often the earliest to be lost. In adults, this produces lethargy, muscle weakness and increased fat mass but these features are not obvious in isolation. Next, gonadotrophin (LH and FSH) secretion becomes impaired with loss of libido in the male and oligomenorrhoea or amenorrhoea in the female. Later, in the male there may be gynaecomastia and decreased frequency of shaving. In both sexes, axillary and pubic hair eventually become sparse or even absent and the skin becomes characteristically finer and wrinkled. Chronic anaemia may also occur. The next hormone to be lost is usually ACTH, resulting in symptoms of cortisol insufficiency (including postural hypotension and a *dilutional* hyponatraemia). In contrast to primary adrenal insufficiency, angiotensin II-dependent zona glomerulosa function is not lost and hence aldosterone secretion maintains normal

plasma potassium. In contrast to the pigmentation of Addison's disease due to high levels of circulating ACTH acting on the skin melanocytes, a striking degree of pallor is usually present. Finally, TSH secretion is lost with consequent secondary hypothyroidism. This contributes further to apathy and cold intolerance. In contrast to primary hypothyroidism, frank myxoedema is rare, presumably because the thyroid retains some autonomous function. The onset of all of the above symptoms is notoriously insidious. However, patients sometimes present acutely unwell with glucocorticoid deficiency. This may be precipitated by a mild infection or injury, or may occur secondary to pituitary apoplexy.

Other features of pituitary disease may be present (Fig. 20.29).

Investigations

The strategy for investigation of pituitary disease is described in Box 20.51. In acutely unwell patients, the priority is to diagnose and treat cortisol deficiency. Other tests can be undertaken later. Specific dynamic tests for diagnosing hormone deficiency are described in Box 20.42 and Box 20.54. More specialised biochemical tests, such as insulin tolerance tests (Box 20.55), GnRH and TRH tests, are rarely required. All patients with biochemical evidence of pituitary hormone deficiency should have an MRI or CT scan to identify pituitary or hypothalamic tumours. If a tumour is not identified, then further investigations are indicated to exclude infectious or infiltrative causes.

20.54 Tests of growth hormone secretion

GH levels are commonly undetectable, so a choice from the range of 'stimulation' tests is required:

- Insulin-induced hypoglycaemia
- Arginine (may be combined with GHRH)
- Glucagon
- Clonidine (in children)

(GH = growth hormone; GHRH = growth hormone-releasing hormone)

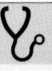

20.55 How and when to do an insulin tolerance test

Use

- Assessment of the HPA axis
- Assessment of GH deficiency
- Indicated when there is doubt after the other tests in Box 20.51
- Usually performed in specialist centres, especially in children
- IV glucose and hydrocortisone must be available for resuscitation

Contraindications

- Ischaemic heart disease
- Epilepsy
- Severe hypopituitarism (0800 hrs plasma cortisol <180 nmol/L (6.6 µg/dL))

Dose

- 0.15 U/kg body weight soluble insulin IV

Aim

- To produce adequate hypoglycaemia (tachycardia and sweating with blood glucose <2.2 mmol/L (40 mg/dL))

Blood samples

- 0, 30, 45, 60, 90, 120 mins for blood glucose, plasma cortisol and growth hormone

Results

- Normal subjects: GH >6.7 µg/L (20 mIU/L)*
- Normal subjects: cortisol >500 nmol/L (approximately 20.2 µg/dL)*

*The precise cut-off figure for a satisfactory cortisol and GH response depends on the assay used and so varies between centres.
(GH = growth hormone; HPA = hypothalamic–pituitary–adrenal; IV = intravenous)

Management

Treatment of acutely ill patients is similar to that described for adrenocortical insufficiency, except that sodium depletion is less likely to be present as there is still mineralocorticoid activity due to the renin–angiotensin–aldosterone system (which is lost in primary adrenal insufficiency). Chronic hormone replacement therapies are described below. Once the cause of hypopituitarism is established, specific treatment – of a pituitary macroadenoma, for example (see below) – may be required.

Cortisol replacement

Hydrocortisone should be given if there is ACTH deficiency. Suitable doses are described in the section on adrenal disease on page 679. Mineralocorticoid replacement is not required.

Thyroid hormone replacement

Levothyroxine 50–150 µg once daily should be given as described on page 657. Unlike in primary hypothyroidism, measuring TSH is not helpful in adjusting the replacement dose because patients with hypopituitarism often secrete glycoproteins that are measured in the TSH assays but are not bioactive. The aim is to maintain serum T_4 in the upper part of the reference range. It is dangerous to give thyroid replacement in adrenal insufficiency without first giving glucocorticoid therapy, since this may precipitate adrenal crisis.

Sex hormone replacement

This is indicated if there is gonadotrophin deficiency in women under the age of 50 and in men to restore normal sexual function and to prevent osteoporosis.

Growth hormone replacement

Growth hormone (GH) is administered by daily subcutaneous self-injection to children and adolescents with GH deficiency and, until recently, was discontinued once the epiphyses had fused. However, although hypopituitary adults receiving 'full' replacement with hydrocortisone, levothyroxine and sex steroids are usually much improved by these therapies, some individuals remain lethargic and unwell compared with a healthy population. Some of these patients feel better, and have objective improvements in their fat:muscle mass ratio and other metabolic parameters, if they are also given GH replacement. Treatment with GH may also help young adults to achieve a higher peak bone mineral density. The principal side-effect is sodium retention, manifest as peripheral oedema or carpal tunnel syndrome if given in excess. For this reason, GH replacement should be started at a low dose, with monitoring of the response by measurement of serum IGF-1.

Pituitary tumour

Pituitary tumours produce a variety of mass effects, depending on their size and location, but also present as incidental findings on CT or MRI, or with hypopituitarism, as described above. A wide variety of disorders can present as mass lesions in or around the pituitary gland (see Box 20.53). Most intrasellar tumours are pituitary macroadenomas (most commonly non-functioning adenomas; see Fig. 20.29), whereas suprasellar masses may be craniopharyngiomas (see Fig. 20.32). The most common cause of a parasellar mass is a meningioma.

Clinical assessment

Clinical features are shown in Figure 20.29. A common but non-specific presentation is with headache, which may be the consequence of stretching of the diaphragma sellae. Although the classical abnormalities associated with compression of the optic chiasm are bitemporal hemianopia (see Fig. 20.30) or upper quadrantanopia, any type of visual field defect can result from suprasellar extension of a tumour because it may compress the optic nerve (unilateral loss of acuity or scotoma) or the optic tract (homonymous hemianopia). Optic atrophy may be apparent on ophthalmoscopy. Lateral extension of a sellar mass into the

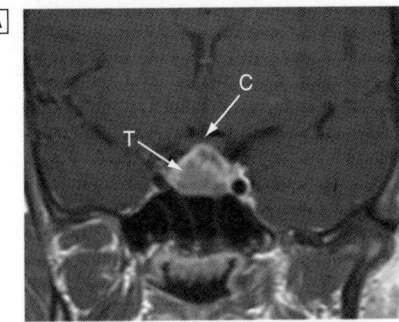
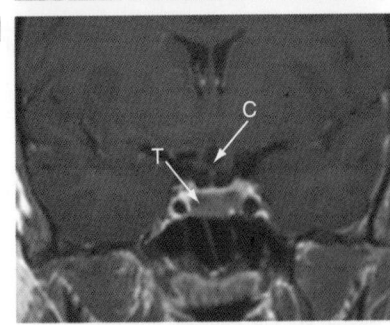

Fig. 20.30 Shrinkage of a macroprolactinoma following treatment with a dopamine agonist. [A] MRI scan showing a pituitary macroadenoma (T) compressing the optic chiasm (C). [B] MRI scan of the same tumour following treatment with a dopamine agonist. The macroadenoma, which was a prolactinoma, has decreased in size substantially and is no longer compressing the optic chiasm.

cavernous sinus with subsequent compression of the 3rd, 4th or 6th cranial nerve may cause diplopia and strabismus, but in anterior pituitary tumours this is an unusual presentation.

Occasionally, pituitary tumours infarct or there is bleeding into cystic lesions. This is termed 'pituitary apoplexy' and may result in sudden expansion with local compression symptoms and acute-onset hypopituitarism. Non-haemorrhagic infarction can also occur in a normal pituitary gland; predisposing factors include catastrophic obstetric haemorrhage (Sheehan syndrome), diabetes mellitus and raised intracranial pressure.

Investigations

Patients suspected of having a pituitary tumour should undergo MRI. If MRI is not available CT may be used but is inferior for assessment of pituitary disease and will not show the majority of small pituitary tumours. For patients intolerant of MRI this investigation may be performed under general anaesthesia if needed, or imaging performed by CT. While some lesions have distinctive neuro-radiological features, the definitive diagnosis is made on histology after surgery. All patients with (para)sellar space-occupying lesions should have pituitary function assessed as described in Box 20.51.

Management

Modalities of treatment of common pituitary and hypothalamic tumours are shown in Box 20.56. Associated hypopituitarism should be treated as described above.

Urgent treatment is required if there is evidence of pressure on visual pathways. The chances of recovery of a visual field defect are proportional to the duration of symptoms, with full recovery unlikely if the defect has been present for longer than 4 months. In the presence of a sellar mass lesion, it is crucial that serum prolactin is measured before emergency surgery is performed. If the prolactin is over 5000 mIU/L (236 ng/mL), then the lesion is likely to be a macroprolactinoma and should respond to a dopamine agonist with shrinkage of the lesion, making surgery unnecessary (see Fig. 20.30).

20

i	20.56 Therapeutic modalities for functioning and non-functioning hypothalamic and pituitary tumours				
		Surgery	Radiotherapy	Medical	Comment
Non-functioning pituitary macroadenoma		1st line	2nd line	–	
Prolactinoma		2nd line	2nd line	1st line Dopamine agonists	Dopamine agonists usually cause macroadenomas to shrink
Acromegaly		1st line	2nd line	2nd line Somatostatin analogues Dopamine agonists GH receptor antagonists	Medical therapy does not reliably cause macroadenomas to shrink Radiotherapy and medical therapy are used in combination for inoperable tumours
Cushing's disease		1st line	2nd line	2nd line Steroidogenesis inhibitors Pasireotide	Radiotherapy may take many years to reduce ACTH excess and medical therapies may be used as a bridge. Bilateral adrenalectomy may also be considered if the pituitary tumour is not completely resectable
Craniopharyngioma		1st line	2nd line	–	

(ACTH = adrenocorticotrophic hormone; GH = growth hormone)

Most operations on the pituitary are performed using the trans-sphenoidal approach via the nostrils, while transfrontal surgery via a craniotomy is occasionally needed for suprasellar tumours. It is uncommon to be able to resect lateral extensions into the cavernous sinuses, although with modern endoscopic techniques this is more feasible. All operations on the pituitary carry a risk of damaging normal endocrine function; this risk increases with the size of the primary lesion.

Pituitary function (see Box 20.51) should be retested 4–6 weeks following surgery, primarily to detect the development of any new hormone deficits. Rarely, the surgical treatment of a sellar lesion can result in recovery of hormone secretion that was deficient pre-operatively.

Following surgery, usually after 3–6 months, imaging should be repeated. If there is a significant residual mass and the histology confirms an anterior pituitary tumour, external radiotherapy may be given to reduce the risk of recurrence but the risk:benefit ratio needs careful individualised discussion. Radiotherapy is not useful in patients requiring urgent therapy because it takes many months or years to be effective and there is a risk of acute swelling of the mass. Fractionated radiotherapy carries a life-long risk of hypopituitarism (50%–100% in the first 10 years) and annual pituitary function tests are obligatory. There is also concern that radiotherapy might impair cognitive function, cause vascular changes and even induce primary brain tumours, but these side-effects have not been quantified reliably and are likely to be rare. Stereotactic radiosurgery allows specific targeting of residual disease in a more focused fashion.

Non-functioning tumours should be followed up by repeated imaging at intervals that depend on the size of the lesion and on whether or not radiotherapy has been administered. For smaller lesions that are not causing mass effects, therapeutic surgery may not be indicated and the lesion may simply be monitored by serial neuroimaging without a clear-cut diagnosis having been established.

Hyperprolactinaemia/galactorrhoea

Hyperprolactinaemia is a common abnormality that usually presents with hypogonadism and/or galactorrhoea (lactation in the absence of breastfeeding). Since prolactin stimulates milk secretion but not breast development, galactorrhoea rarely occurs in men and only does so if gynaecomastia has been induced by hypogonadism. The differential diagnosis of hyperprolactinaemia is shown in Box 20.57. Many drugs, especially dopamine antagonists, elevate prolactin concentrations. Pituitary tumours can cause hyperprolactinaemia by directly secreting prolactin (prolactinomas, see below), or by compressing the infundibular stalk and thus interrupting the tonic inhibitory effect

i	20.57 Causes of hyperprolactinaemia

Physiological

- Stress (e.g. post-seizure)
- Pregnancy
- Lactation
- Nipple stimulation
- Sleep
- Coitus
- Exercise
- Baby crying

Drug-induced

Dopamine antagonists

- Antipsychotics (phenothiazines and butyrophenones)
- Antidepressants
- Antiemetics (e.g. metoclopramide, domperidone)

Dopamine-depleting drugs

- Reserpine
- Methyldopa

Oestrogens

- Oral contraceptive pill

Pathological

Common

- Disconnection hyperprolactinaemia (e.g. non-functioning pituitary macroadenoma)
- Prolactinoma (usually microadenoma)
- Primary hypothyroidism
- Polycystic ovary syndrome

Uncommon

- Pituitary tumour secreting prolactin and growth hormone
- Hypothalamic disease
- Renal failure

Rare

- Chest wall reflex (e.g. post herpes zoster)

of hypothalamic dopamine on prolactin secretion ('disconnection' hyperprolactinaemia).

Prolactin usually circulates as a free (monomeric) hormone in plasma but, in some individuals, prolactin becomes bound to an IgG antibody. This complex is known as macroprolactin and such patients have macroprolactinaemia (not to be confused with macroprolactinoma, a prolactin-secreting pituitary tumour of more than 1 cm in diameter). Since macroprolactin cannot cross blood-vessel walls to reach prolactin receptors in target tissues, it is of no pathological significance. Some commercial prolactin assays do not distinguish prolactin from macro-prolactin and so macroprolactinaemia is a cause of spurious hyper-prolactinaemia. Identification of macroprolactin requires gel filtration chromatography or polyethylene glycol precipitation techniques, and one of these tests should be performed in all patients with hyperprolactinae-mia if the prolactin assay is known to cross-react.

Clinical assessment

In women, in addition to galactorrhoea, hypogonadism associated with hyperprolactinaemia causes secondary amenorrhoea and anovulation with infertility. Important points in the history include drug use, recent pregnancy and menstrual history. The quantity of milk produced is var-iable and it may be observed only by manual expression. In men there is decreased libido, reduced shaving frequency and lethargy. Unilateral galactorrhoea may be confused with nipple discharge, and breast exam-ination to exclude malignancy or fibrocystic disease is important. Further assessment should address the features in Figure 20.29.

Investigations

Pregnancy should first be excluded before further investigations are per-formed in women of child-bearing potential. The upper limit of normal for many assays of serum prolactin is approximately 500 mIU/L (24 ng/mL). In non-pregnant and non-lactating patients, monomeric prolac-tin concentrations of 500–1000 mIU/L (24–47 ng/mL) are likely to be induced by stress or drugs, and a repeat measurement is indicated. Levels between 1000 and 5000 mIU/L (47–236 ng/mL) are likely to be due to drugs, a microprolactinoma or 'disconnection' hyperprolactinae-mia. Levels above 5000 mIU/L (236 ng/mL) are highly suggestive of a macroprolactinoma.

Patients with prolactin excess should have tests of gonadal func-tion (p. 667), and T_4 and TSH should be measured to exclude primary

hypothyroidism causing TRH-induced prolactin excess. Unless the pro-lactin falls after withdrawal of relevant drug therapy, a serum prolactin consistently above the reference range is an indication for MRI or CT scan of the hypothalamus and pituitary. Patients with a macroadenoma also need tests for hypopituitarism (see Box 20.51).

Management

If possible, the underlying cause should be corrected (e.g. cessation of offending drugs and giving levothyroxine replacement in primary hypothyroidism). If dopamine antagonists are the cause, then dopa-mine agonist therapy is contraindicated; if gonadal dysfunction is the primary concern, sex steroid replacement therapy may be indicated. Troublesome physiological galactorrhoea can also be treated with dopamine agonists (see Box 20.58). Management of prolactinomas is described below.

Prolactinoma

Most prolactinomas in pre-menopausal women are microadenomas because the symptoms of prolactin excess usually result in early pres-entation. Prolactin-secreting cells of the anterior pituitary share a com-mon lineage with GH-secreting cells, so occasionally prolactinomas can secrete excess GH and cause acromegaly. In prolactinomas there is a relationship between prolactin concentration and tumour size: the higher the level, the bigger the tumour. Some macroprolactinomas can elevate prolactin concentrations above 100000 mIU/L (4700 ng/mL). The inves-tigation of prolactinomas is the same as for other pituitary tumours (see above).

Management

As shown in Box 20.56, several therapeutic modalities can be employed in the management of prolactinomas.

Medical

Dopamine agonist drugs are first-line therapy for the majority of patients (Box 20.58). They usually reduce serum prolactin concentrations and cause significant tumour shrinkage after several months of therapy (Fig. 20.30), but visual field defects, if present, may improve within days of first administration. It is possible to withdraw dopamine agonist therapy without recurrence of hyperprolactinaemia after a few years of treatment in some patients with a microadenoma. Also, after the menopause, sup-pression of prolactin is required in microadenomas only if galactorrhoea is troublesome, since hypogonadism is then physiological and tumour growth unlikely. In patients with macroadenomas, drugs can be withdrawn only after curative surgery or radiotherapy and under close supervision.

Ergot-derived dopamine agonists (bromocriptine and cabergoline) can bind to 5-HT_{2B} receptors in the heart and elsewhere and have been associated with fibrotic reactions, particularly tricuspid valve regurgita-tion, when used in high doses in patients with Parkinson's disease. At the relatively low doses used in prolactinomas most data suggest that systematic screening for cardiac fibrosis is unnecessary, but if dopamine agonist therapy is prolonged, periodic screening by echocardiography or use of non-ergot agents (quinagolide) may be indicated. Dopamine agonists can affect mood and behaviour, including depression, psycho-sis and risk-taking behaviour (e.g. gambling), and patients should be warned about these potential side-effects.

Surgery and radiotherapy

Surgical decompression is usually necessary only when a macropro-lactinoma has failed to shrink sufficiently with dopamine agonist therapy, and this may be because the tumour has a significant cystic component. Surgery may also be performed in patients who are intolerant of dopamine agonists. Microadenomas can be removed selectively by trans-sphenoidal surgery with a cure rate of about 80%, but recurrence is possible; the cure rate for surgery in macroadenomas is substantially lower.

External irradiation may be required for some macroadenomas to prevent regrowth if dopamine agonists are stopped.

	20.58 Dopamine agonist therapy: drugs used to treat prolactinomas		
Drug	Oral dose*	Advantages	Disadvantages
Bromocriptine	2.5–15 mg/day 2–3 times daily	Available for parenteral use Short half-life; useful in treating infertility Proven long-term efficacy	Ergotamine-like side-effects (nausea, headache, postural hypotension, constipation) Frequent dosing so poor adherence Rare reports of fibrotic reactions in various tissues
Cabergoline	250–1000 μg/week 2 doses/week	Long-acting, so missed doses less important Reported to have fewer ergotamine-like side-effects	Limited data on safety in pregnancy Associated with cardiac valvular fibrosis in Parkinson's disease
Quinagolide	50–150 μg/day Once daily	A non-ergot with few side-effects in patients intolerant of the above	Limited data on safety in pregnancy

*Tolerance develops for the side-effects. All of these agents, especially bromocriptine, must be introduced at low dose and increased slowly. If several doses of bromocriptine are missed, the process must start again.

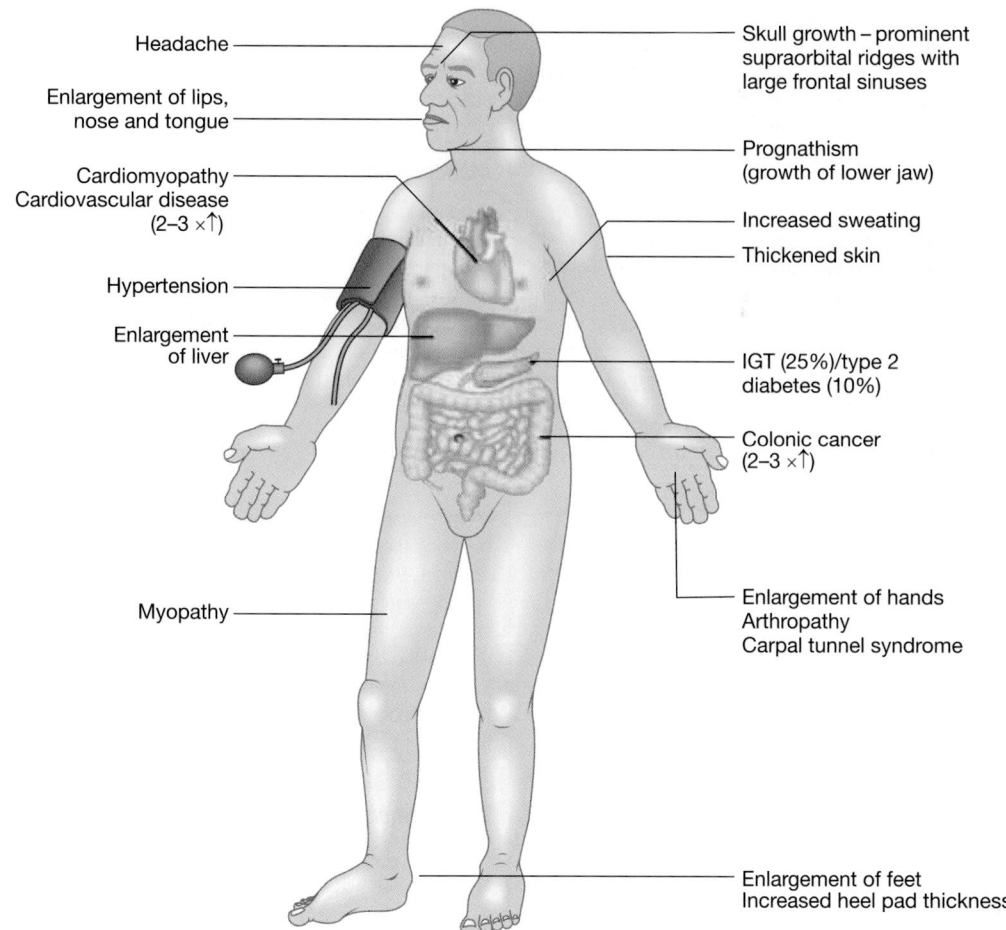

Fig. 20.31 Clinical features of acromegaly. (IGT = impaired glucose tolerance)

Labels in figure:
- Headache
- Enlargement of lips, nose and tongue
- Cardiomyopathy Cardiovascular disease (2–3 ×↑)
- Hypertension
- Enlargement of liver
- Myopathy
- Skull growth – prominent supraorbital ridges with large frontal sinuses
- Prognathism (growth of lower jaw)
- Increased sweating
- Thickened skin
- IGT (25%)/type 2 diabetes (10%)
- Colonic cancer (2–3 ×↑)
- Enlargement of hands Arthropathy Carpal tunnel syndrome
- Enlargement of feet Increased heel pad thickness

Pregnancy

Hyperprolactinaemia often presents with infertility, so dopamine agonist therapy may be followed by pregnancy. Patients with microadenomas should be advised to withdraw dopamine agonist therapy as soon as pregnancy is confirmed. In contrast, macroprolactinomas may enlarge rapidly under oestrogen stimulation and these patients should continue dopamine agonist therapy and need measurement of prolactin levels and visual fields during pregnancy. All patients should be advised to report headache or visual disturbance promptly.

Acromegaly

Acromegaly is caused by growth hormone (GH) secretion from a pituitary tumour, usually a macroadenoma, and carries an approximate twofold excess mortality when untreated.

Clinical features

If GH hypersecretion occurs before puberty, then the presentation is with gigantism. More commonly, GH excess occurs in adult life and presents with acromegaly. If hypersecretion starts in adolescence and persists into adult life, then the two conditions may be combined. The clinical features are shown in Figure 20.31. The most common complaints are headache and sweating. Additional features include those of any pituitary tumour (see Fig. 20.29).

Investigations

The clinical diagnosis must be confirmed by measuring GH levels during an oral glucose tolerance test and measuring serum IGF-1.

In normal subjects, plasma GH suppresses to below 0.5 μg/L (approximately 2 mIU/L). In acromegaly, GH does not suppress and in about 30% of patients there is a paradoxical rise; IGF-1 is also elevated. The rest of pituitary function should be investigated as described in Box 20.51. Prolactin concentrations are elevated in about 30% of patients due to co-secretion of prolactin from the tumour. Additional tests in acromegaly may include screening for colonic neoplasms with colonoscopy.

Management

The main aims are to improve symptoms and to normalise serum GH and IGF-1 to reduce morbidity and mortality. Treatment is summarised in Box 20.56.

Surgical

Trans-sphenoidal surgery is usually the first line of treatment and may result in cure of GH excess, especially in patients with microadenomas. More often, surgery serves to debulk the tumour and further second-line therapy is required, according to post-operative imaging and glucose tolerance test results.

Medical

If acromegaly persists after surgery, medical therapy is usually employed to lower GH levels to below 1.0 μg/L (approximately 3 mIU/L) and to normalise IGF-1 concentrations. Medical therapy may be discontinued after several years in patients who have received radiotherapy once the latter has been effective. Somatostatin analogues (such as octreotide, lanreotide or pasireotide) can be administered as slow-release injections every few weeks. Somatostatin

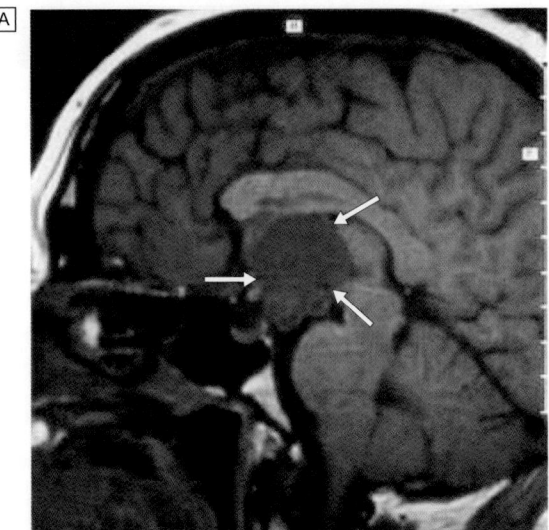

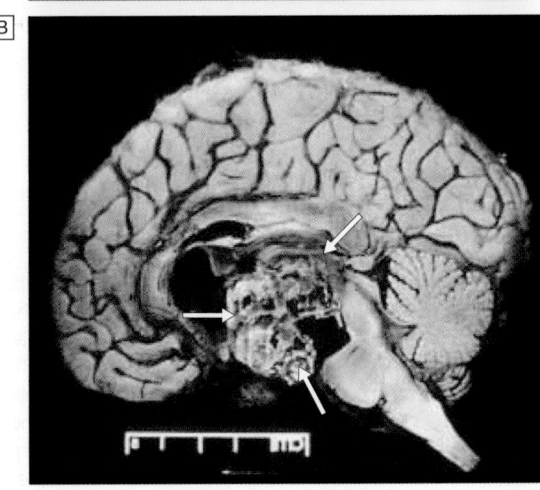

Fig. 20.32 Craniopharyngioma. [A] This developmental tumour characteristically presents in younger patients; it is often cystic and calcified, as shown in this MRI scan (arrows). [B] Pathology specimen.

analogues can also be used as primary therapy for acromegaly either as an alternative or in advance of surgery, given evidence that they can induce modest tumour shrinkage in some patients. Dopamine agonists are less effective at lowering GH but may sometimes be helpful, especially with associated prolactin excess. Pegvisomant is a peptide GH receptor antagonist administered by daily self-injection and may be indicated in some patients whose GH and IGF-1 concentrations fail to suppress sufficiently following somatostatin analogue therapy.

Radiotherapy

External radiotherapy is increasingly employed as third-line treatment if acromegaly persists after surgery, to stop tumour growth and lower GH levels. However, GH levels fall slowly (over many years) and there is a risk of hypopituitarism.

Craniopharyngioma

Craniopharyngiomas are benign tumours that develop in cell rests of Rathke's pouch, and may be located within the sella turcica, or commonly in the suprasellar space. They are often cystic, with a solid component that may or may not be calcified (Fig. 20.32). In young people, they are diagnosed more commonly than pituitary adenomas. They may present with pressure effects on adjacent structures, hypopituitarism

20.59 Causes of diabetes insipidus

Cranial

Structural hypothalamic or high stalk lesion

- See Box 20.53

Idiopathic

Genetic defect

- Dominant (*AVP* gene mutation)
- Recessive (DIDMOAD syndrome – association of diabetes insipidus with diabetes mellitus, optic atrophy, deafness)

Nephrogenic

Genetic defect

- V2 receptor mutation
- Aquaporin-2 mutation
- Cystinosis

Metabolic abnormality

- Hypokalaemia
- Hypercalcaemia

Drug therapy

- Lithium
- Demeclocycline

Poisoning

- Heavy metals

Chronic kidney disease

- Polycystic kidney disease
- Sickle-cell anaemia
- Infiltrative disease

and/or cranial diabetes insipidus. Other clinical features directly related to hypothalamic damage may also occur. These include hyperphagia and obesity, loss of the sensation of thirst and disturbance of temperature regulation, and these features can be significant clinical challenges to manage.

Craniopharyngiomas can be treated by the trans-sphenoidal route but surgery may also involve a craniotomy, with a relatively high risk of hypothalamic damage and other complications. If the tumour has a large cystic component, it may be safer to place in the cyst cavity a drain that is attached to a subcutaneous access device, rather than attempt a resection. Whatever form it takes, surgery is unlikely to be curative and radiotherapy may often be given to reduce the risk of relapse. Unfortunately, craniopharyngiomas often recur, requiring repeated surgery. They often cause considerable morbidity, usually from hypothalamic obesity, water balance problems and/or visual failure.

Diabetes insipidus

This uncommon disorder is characterised by the persistent excretion of excessive quantities of dilute urine and by thirst. It is classified into two types:

- cranial diabetes insipidus, in which there is deficient production of vasopressin by the hypothalamus
- nephrogenic diabetes insipidus, in which the renal tubules are unresponsive to vasopressin.

The underlying causes are listed in Box 20.59.

Clinical features

The most marked symptoms are polyuria (>3 L per 24 hours) and polydipsia. The patient may pass 5–20 L or more of urine in 24 hours. This

20

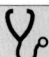

20.60 How and when to do a water deprivation test

Use

- To establish a diagnosis of diabetes insipidus and to differentiate cranial from nephrogenic causes

Protocol

- No coffee, tea or smoking on the test day
- Free fluids until 0730 hrs on the morning of the test, but discourage patients from 'stocking up' with extra fluid in anticipation of fluid deprivation
- No fluids from 0730 hrs
- Attend at 0830 hrs for measurement of body weight and plasma and urine osmolality
- Record body weight, urine volume, urine and plasma osmolality and thirst score on a visual analogue scale every 2 hrs for up to 8 hrs
- Stop the test if the patient loses 3% of body weight
- If plasma osmolality reaches >300 mOsmol/kg and urine osmolality <600 mOsmol/kg, then administer DDAVP (see text) 2 µg IM

Interpretation

- Diabetes insipidus is confirmed by a plasma osmolality >300 mOsmol/kg with a urine osmolality <600 mOsmol/kg
- Cranial diabetes insipidus is confirmed if urine osmolality rises by at least 50% after DDAVP
- Nephrogenic diabetes insipidus is confirmed if DDAVP does not concentrate the urine
- Primary polydipsia is suggested by low plasma osmolality at the start of the test

20.61 Multiple endocrine neoplasia (MEN) syndromes

MEN 1 (Wermer syndrome)

- Primary hyperparathyroidism
- Pituitary tumours
- Pancreatic neuro-endocrine tumours (e.g. non-functioning, insulinoma, gastrinoma)
- Bronchial and thymic carcinoids
- Adrenal tumours
- Cutaneous lesions (e.g. lipomas, collagenomas, angiofibromas)

MEN 2a (Sipple syndrome, and formerly known as MEN 2)

- Primary hyperparathyroidism
- Medullary carcinoma of thyroid
- Phaeochromocytoma

MEN 2b (formerly MEN 3)

- As for MEN 2a above (though medullary thyroid cancer occurs earlier, even within the first year of life)
- Marfanoid habitus
- Skeletal abnormalities (e.g. craniosynostosis)
- Abnormal dental enamel
- Multiple mucosal neuromas

MEN 4

- Primary hyperparathyroidism
- Pituitary tumours
- Possible tumours in the adrenals, reproductive organs, kidneys
- Possible pancreatic, gastric, bronchial and cervical neuro-endocrine tumours

is of low specific gravity and osmolality. If the patient has an intact thirst mechanism, is conscious and has access to oral fluids, then he or she can maintain adequate fluid intake. However, in an unconscious patient or a patient with damage to the hypothalamic thirst centre, diabetes insipidus is potentially lethal. If there is associated cortisol deficiency, then diabetes insipidus may not be manifest until glucocorticoid replacement therapy is given. The most common differential diagnosis is primary polydipsia, caused by drinking excessive amounts of fluid in the absence of a defect in vasopressin or thirst control.

Investigations

Diabetes insipidus can be confirmed if serum vasopressin is undetectable (although the assay for this is not widely available) or the urine is not maximally concentrated (i.e. <600 mOsmol/kg) in the presence of increased plasma osmolality (i.e. >300 mOsmol/kg). Sometimes, the diagnosis can be confirmed or refuted by random simultaneous samples of blood and urine, but more often a dynamic test is required. The water deprivation test described in Box 20.60 is widely used, but an alternative is to infuse hypertonic (5%) saline and measure vasopressin or better still co-peptin secretion in response to increasing plasma osmolality. Thirst can also be assessed during these tests on a visual analogue scale. Anterior pituitary function and suprasellar anatomy should be assessed in patients with cranial diabetes insipidus (see Box 20.51).

In primary polydipsia, the urine may be excessively dilute because of chronic diuresis, which 'washes out' the solute gradient across the loop of Henle, but plasma osmolality is low rather than high. DDAVP (see below) should not be administered to patients with primary polydipsia, since it will prevent excretion of water and there is a risk of severe water intoxication if the patient continues to drink fluid to excess.

In nephrogenic diabetes insipidus, appropriate further tests may include plasma electrolytes, calcium, ultrasound of the kidneys and urinalysis.

Management

Treatment of cranial diabetes insipidus is with des-amino-des-aspartate-arginine vasopressin (desmopressin, DDAVP), an analogue of vasopressin that has a longer half-life. For chronic replacement therapy

DDAVP may be administered intranasally and orally, although the latter formulation has variable bioavailability. In sick patients, DDAVP should be given by intramuscular injection. The dose of DDAVP should be adjusted on the basis of serum sodium concentrations and/or osmolality. The principal hazard is excessive treatment, resulting in water intoxication and hyponatraemia. Conversely, inadequate treatment results in thirst and polyuria. The ideal dose prevents nocturia but allows a degree of polyuria from time to time before the next dose (e.g. DDAVP nasal dose 5 µg in the morning and 10 µg at night).

The polyuria in nephrogenic diabetes insipidus is improved by thiazide diuretics (e.g. bendroflumethiazide 5–10 mg/day), amiloride (5–10 mg/day) and NSAIDs (e.g. indometacin 50 mg 3 times daily), although the last of these carries a risk of reducing glomerular filtration rate.

Disorders affecting multiple endocrine glands

Multiple endocrine neoplasia

Multiple endocrine neoplasias (MEN) are rare autosomal dominant syndromes characterised by hyperplasia and formation of adenomas or malignant tumours in multiple glands. They fall into four groups, as shown in Box 20.61. Some other genetic diseases also have an increased risk of endocrine tumours; for example, phaeochromocytoma is associated with von Hippel–Lindau syndrome and neurofibromatosis type 1.

The MEN syndromes should be considered in all patients with two or more endocrine tumours and in patients with solitary tumours who report other endocrine tumours in their family. Inactivating mutations in *MEN1* (*MENIN*), a tumour suppressor gene on chromosome 11, cause MEN 1, whereas MEN 2a and 2b are caused by gain-of-function mutations in the *RET* proto-oncogene on chromosome 10. These cause constitutive activation of the membrane-associated tyrosine kinase RET, which controls the development of cells that migrate from the neural crest. In contrast, loss-of-function mutations of the RET kinase cause Hirschsprung's disease. MEN 4 is extremely rare and is associated with loss-of-function mutations in the *CDNK1B* gene on chromosome 12;

20.62	Autoimmune polyendocrine syndromes (APS)*

Type 1 (APECED)

- Addison's disease
- Hypoparathyroidism
- Type 1 diabetes
- Primary hypothyroidism
- Chronic mucocutaneous candidiasis
- Nail dystrophy
- Dental enamel hypoplasia

Type 2 (Schmidt syndrome)

- Addison's disease
- Primary hypothyroidism
- Graves' disease
- Pernicious anaemia
- Primary hypogonadism
- Type 1 diabetes
- Vitiligo
- Coeliac disease
- Myasthenia gravis

*In both types of APS, the precise pattern of disease varies between affected individuals. (APECED = autoimmune poly-endocrinopathy-candidiasis-ectodermal dystrophy)

this gene codes for the protein p27, which has putative tumour suppressor activity. Predictive genetic testing can be performed on relatives of individuals with MEN syndromes, after appropriate counselling.

Individuals who carry mutations associated with MEN should be entered into a surveillance programme. In MEN 1, this typically involves annual history, examination and measurements of serum calcium and prolactin, and MRI of the pituitary and pancreas every 2 years; some centres also perform regular CT or MRI scans of the chest. In individuals with MEN 2a and 2b, annual history, examination and measurement of serum calcium, calcitonin and urinary or plasma catecholamine metabolites should be performed. Because the penetrance of medullary carcinoma of the thyroid approaches 100% in individuals with a *RET* mutation, prophylactic thyroidectomy should be performed in early childhood in most patients. The precise timing of surgery in childhood should be guided by the specific mutation in the *RET* gene.

Autoimmune polyendocrine syndromes

Two distinct autoimmune polyendocrine syndromes are known: APS types 1 and 2.

The most common is APS type 2 (Schmidt syndrome), which typically presents in women between the ages of 20 and 60. It is usually defined as the occurrence in the same individual of two or more autoimmune endocrine disorders, some of which are listed in Box 20.62. The mode of inheritance is autosomal dominant with incomplete penetrance and there is a strong association with HLA-DR3 and CTLA-4.

Much less common is APS type 1, which is also termed autoimmune poly-endocrinopathy-candidiasis-ectodermal dystrophy (APECED). This is inherited in an autosomal recessive fashion and is caused by loss-of-function mutations in the autoimmune regulator gene *AIRE*, which is

responsible for the presentation of self-antigens to thymocytes in utero. This is essential for the deletion of thymocyte clones that react against self-antigens and hence for the development of immune tolerance. The most common clinical features are described in Box 20.62, although the pattern of presentation is variable and other autoimmune disorders are often observed.

Endocrine effects of cancer immunotherapy

Modern cancer treatment increasingly uses immunotherapy, including immune check-point inhibitors. Whilst highly effective anti-cancer agents, these may cause endocrine dysfunction, most commonly hypopituitarism and hypothyroidism. It is crucial that these axes are monitored during therapy and that there is a high index of suspicion for potential secondary hypoadrenalism in patients presenting with fatigue and tiredness, especially in those on the anti-CTLA-4 antibody ipilumumab, and a low threshold for glucocorticoid replacement.

Late effects of childhood cancer therapy

The therapies used to treat cancers in children and adolescents, including radiotherapy and chemotherapy, may cause long-term endocrine dysfunction. These complications are discussed in detail in Chapter 33).

Opioid-induced endocrine dysfunction

Opioids may cause secondary hypoadrenalism and hypogonadism. With the increasingly widespread use of these analgesics more patients will present with vague features of lethargy that may represent secondary adrenal insufficiency, which needs to be investigated and treated as described on p. 685.

Further information

Websites

british-thyroid-association.org *British Thyroid Association: provider of guidelines, e.g. treatment of hypothyroidism and the investigation and management of thyroid cancer.*

btf-thyroid.org *British Thyroid Foundation: a resource for patient leaflets and support for patients with thyroid disorders.*

endocrinology.org *British Society for Endocrinology: useful online education resources and links to patient support group.*

endo-society.org *American Endocrine Society: provider of clinical practice guidelines.*

pituitary.org.uk *Pituitary Foundation: a resource for patient and general practitioner leaflets and further information.*

thyroid.org *American Thyroid Association: provider of clinical practice guidelines.*

20

JR Petrie
JG Boyle

21

Diabetes mellitus

Clinical examination of people with diabetes

6 Head
Xanthelasma
Cranial nerve palsy/eye
movements/ptosis

5 Neck
Carotid pulse
Bruits
Thyroid enlargement

4 Axillae

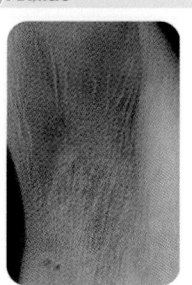

▲ Acanthosis nigricans
in insulin resistance

3 Blood pressure

2 Skin
Bullae
Granuloma annulare
Vitiligo

1 Hands
(see opposite)

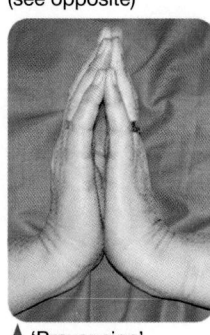

▲ 'Prayer sign'

7 Eyes (see opposite)
Visual acuity
Cataract/lens opacity
Fundoscopy

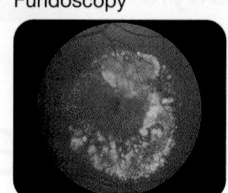

▲ Exudative maculopathy

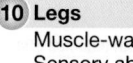
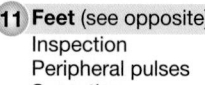

Observation
- Weight loss in insulin deficiency
- Obesity in type 2 diabetes
- Mucosal candidiasis
- Dehydration – dry mouth,
  ↓tissue turgor
- Air hunger – Kussmaul breathing
  in ketoacidosis

8 Insulin injection sites
(see opposite)

9 Abdomen
Hepatomegaly
(fatty infiltration of liver)

10 Legs
Muscle-wasting
Sensory abnormality
Hair loss
Tendon reflexes

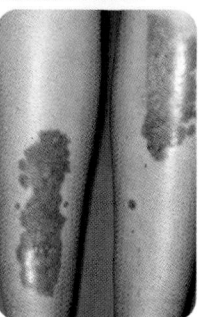

▲ Necrobiosis lipoidica

11 Feet (see opposite)
Inspection
Peripheral pulses
Sensation

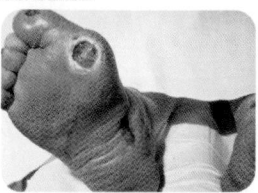

▲ Neuropathic foot ulcer

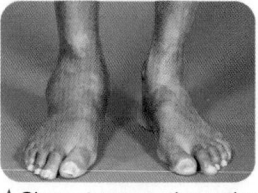

▲ Charcot neuroarthropathy

Insets (Acanthosis nigricans) From Lim E (ed.). Medicine and surgery: an integrated textbook. Edinburgh: Elsevier Ltd; 2007. (Exudative maculopathy) Courtesy of Dr A.W. Patrick and Dr I.W. Campbell.

Diabetes affects every system in the body. Clinical assessment is dominated by history and investigation rather than clinical examination. In routine clinical practice, the most important aspects of clinical examination relate to complication screening:

- Blood pressure measurement
- Foot examination (for pulses and sensation) to determine risk of (or presence of) ulceration (p. 752)
- Insulin injection sites (if applicable): inspect to check they are not over-used as this leads to impaired or unpredictable insulin absorption (lipohypertrophy, see Box 8)
- Retinal screening (see Box 7): check this has been performed according to local guidelines

Other clinically useful information:

- Technology: clinical inspection of the arm and abdomen may reveal the use of a continuous glucose monitoring (CGM) device and/or insulin pump delivering a continuous subcutaneous insulin infusion (CSII)

Other relevant clinical signs:

- Hands: there may be thickening of the skin and tendons (due to non-enzymatic glycation of collagen from long-term hyperglycaemia, see Box 1)
- Skin (uncommon):
  - Acanthosis nigricans (axilla and neck): associated with forms of diabetes involving severe insulin resistance (see Box 4)
  - Necrobiosis lipoidica diabeticorum: rash with scarred central yellow area (red margin when active) over the shins (see Box 10)

7 Examination of the eyes
Visual acuity[1]

- Check distance vision using Snellen chart at 6 m
- Check near vision using standard reading chart

Lens opacification

- Look for a normal red reflex using the ophthalmoscope held 30 cm from the eye

Fundal examination

- Use digital retinal photography (where available)[2]
- Where not available (or in an emergency), dilate pupils with mydriatic drops (unless contraindicated) and examine using direct ophthalmoscopy in a darkened room
- Note features of diabetic retinopathy (p. 1230), including photocoagulation scars from previous laser treatment

[1]Note that visual acuity can alter reversibly with acute hyperglycaemia due to osmotic changes affecting the lens. Most patients with retinopathy do not have altered visual acuity, except after a vitreous haemorrhage or in some cases of maculopathy. [2]The number of fields captured, the use of mydriatic drops (e.g. tropicamide) and how images are read depends on the setting and technology available.

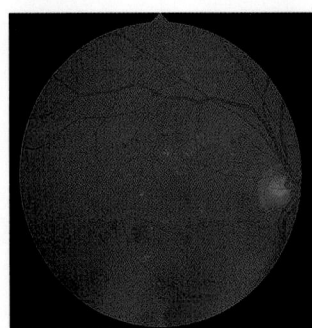

Background retinopathy. *Courtesy of Dr A.W. Patrick and Dr I.W. Campbell.*

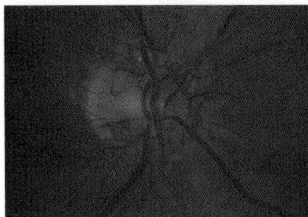

Proliferative retinopathy. *Courtesy of Dr A.W. Patrick and Dr I.W. Campbell.*

1 Examination of the hands*
Several abnormalities are more common in diabetes than in the general population:

- Limited joint mobility ('cheiroarthropathy') causes painless stiffness. The inability to extend (to 180°) the metacarpophalangeal or interphalangeal joints of at least one finger bilaterally can be demonstrated in the 'prayer sign' (see Box 1)
- Dupuytren's contracture (p. 1061) causes nodules or thickening of the skin and knuckle pads
- Carpal tunnel syndrome (p. 1193) presents with wrist pain radiating into the hand
- Trigger finger (flexor tenosynovitis) may be present
- Muscle-wasting/sensory changes may be present in peripheral sensorimotor neuropathy (more common in the lower limbs)

*Usually only examined if symptoms reported

8 Insulin injection sites*
Main areas used

- Anterior abdominal wall
- Upper thighs
- Upper outer arms

Inspection

- Bruising
- Subcutaneous fat deposition (lipohypertrophy)
- Erythema, infection (rare)

*If applicable should be checked at **all** consultations

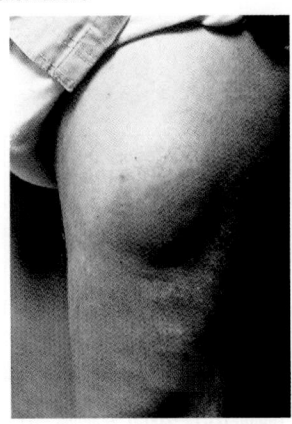

Lipohypertrophy of the upper arm.

11 Annual examination of the feet
Focus on detecting abnormal sensation and circulation to determine appropriate level of care required and prevent future ulceration/amputation.

Inspection

- Ulcers or skin breaks (require urgent referral for podiatry assessment and treatment)
- Localised bacterial or fungal infection (may require antibiotic/antifungal treatment)
- Discoloration (dusky colour) of the skin indicating critical ischaemia (if confirmed requires urgent vascular assessment)
- Callus (hard skin) formation on weight-bearing areas, ingrowing toenails (these require routine referral for podiatry to prevent ulceration)
- Fungal infection may affect skin between toes, and nails (topical or systemic antifungal treatment may be appropriate)
- Clawing of the toes/loss of the plantar arch (may reflect neuropathy)
- Severe deformity may reflect Charcot neuroarthropathy (see p. 752)

Circulation

- Peripheral pulses – dorsalis pedis and posterior tibial (**document at least annually**). If neither is palpable, the foot is at 'moderate' risk of ulceration, even if sensation is normal
- Assess capillary refill in nail-beds if pulses absent
- Skin temperature is raised in Charcot neuroarthropathy

Sensation

- 'Stocking' distribution in typical peripheral sensorimotor neuropathy
- Test light touch with a 10 gram monofilament on the dorsal surfaces of the toes and metatarsals. If absent in one or more of five places, the risk of foot ulceration is increased 5–10-fold ('moderate'), even if pulses are present (**document at least annually**)
- Testing of other sensation modalities (vibration, pain, proprioception) is not routine unless neuropathy is being fully evaluated

Reflexes (not routinely performed)

- Ankle reflexes are lost in severe sensorimotor neuropathy

  People with diabetes who have: (i) normal pulses and sensation, (ii) good footcare (nail cutting, lack of callus) and (iii) well-fitting footwear can be reassured and reviewed annually without regular podiatry.

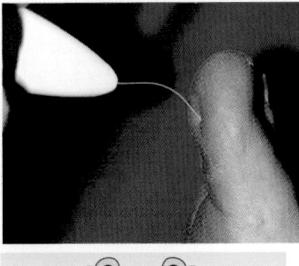

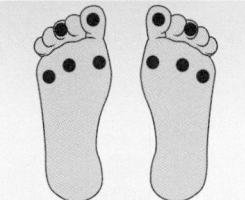

Monofilament. This is applied gently until it bends at each of five points on both feet. Areas of callus should be avoided as sensation is reduced.

Diabetes mellitus is a clinical syndrome with many causes (see Box 21.6), which is characterised by the presence of hyperglycaemia (*mellitus* being Latin for 'sweet'). Type 2 diabetes accounts for around 90% of cases, while type 1 diabetes accounts for most of the remainder. In the United States, more than 20% of adults over the age of 65 years have type 2 diabetes, while in the UK people with diabetes occupy almost 20% of acute hospital beds.

All forms of diabetes are ultimately a consequence of *absolute* or *relative* insulin deficiency. Although type 1 and type 2 diabetes share the clinical phenotype of hyperglycaemia and carry risks of similar complications, their aetiology and pathophysiology are very different. In type 1 diabetes, there is an *absolute* deficiency of insulin because of an immune-mediated destruction of insulin-producing β cells in the pancreatic islets of Langerhans. In contrast, in type 2 diabetes, concentrations of circulating insulin are typically elevated, but there is a *relative* deficiency of insulin because there is reduced sensitivity to insulin in peripheral tissues (due to obesity) and the β cells cannot make sufficient insulin to overcome this 'insulin resistance'.

Diabetes carries a heavy personal burden for those affected as well as high financial costs to health-care systems and society at large. In 2017, diabetes caused 4 million deaths globally, and health-care expenditure attributed to diabetes was estimated to be at least 727 billion US dollars, or 10% of total health-care expenditure. Acutely, high glucose results in marked symptoms of thirst, polydipsia and polyuria. If left untreated, it can lead to life-threatening metabolic decompensation requiring hospitalisation, especially in type 1 diabetes. Long-term hyperglycaemia is responsible for diabetes-specific 'microvascular' complications, particularly affecting the eyes (retinopathy), kidneys (nephropathy) and feet (neuropathy). These occur at a younger age in type 1 diabetes due to its earlier average age of onset.

Although the onset of clinical diabetes is often experienced as sudden in individual cases, there may have been a pre-clinical phase of months or even years when abnormal glucose values were not identified. Scientifically, there is no clear 'cut off' between normal and abnormal glucose levels, so international bodies have derived diagnostic criteria for diabetes (Box 21.2) based on blood glucose concentrations above which there is an appreciable risk of developing diabetic retinopathy, the most common microvascular complication (Fig. 21.1). Lower levels of hyperglycaemia (above normal) are classified as 'pre-diabetes' (Box 21.2).

The prevalence of diabetes is rising. Globally, it is estimated that 463 million people had diabetes in 2019 (9.3% of the world adult population), approximately 90% with type 2 diabetes. This figure is expected to reach 700 million by 2045. Prevalence is highest in the Middle East and lowest in parts of Africa, varying around the world (Fig. 21.2) according to

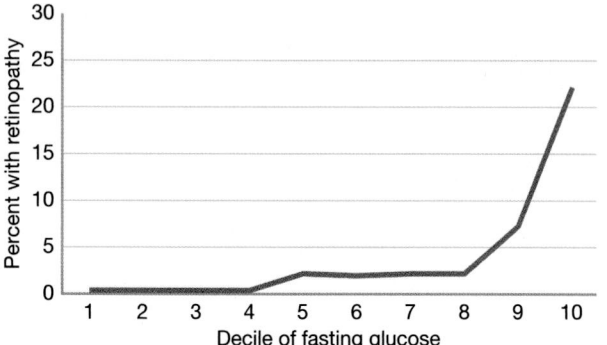

Fig. 21.1 Prevalence of retinopathy by decile of fasting glucose. There is a small inflection point at 4 mmol/L, but a major inflection at 8 mmol/L. *Adapted from World Health Organization and International Diabetes Federation. Definition and diagnosis of diabetes mellitus and intermediate hyperglycaemia: report of a WHO/ IDF consultation. Geneva: World Health Organization; 2006. https://apps.who.int/iris/handle/10665/43588*

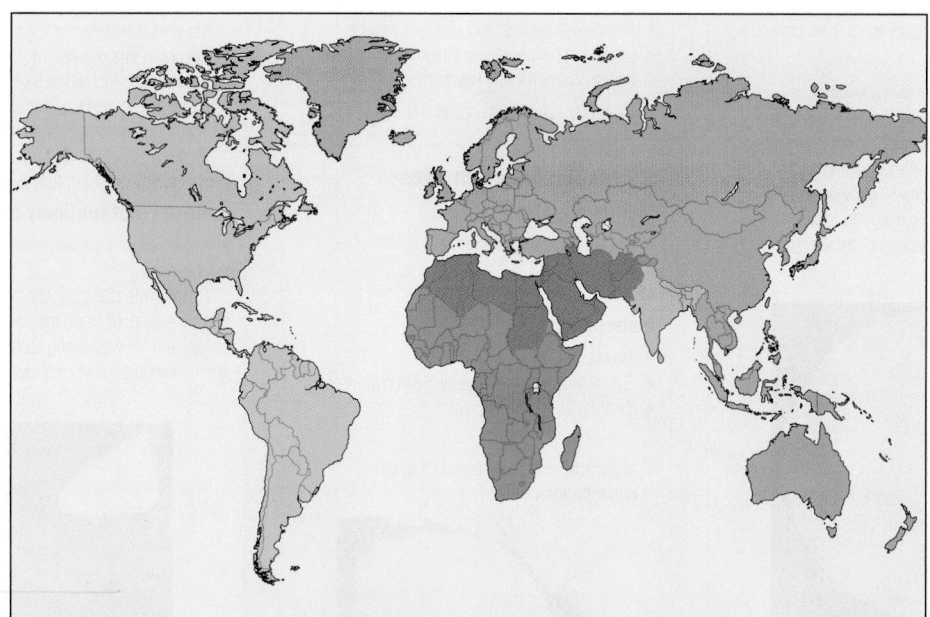

	2045	2030	2019
World	9.6%	9.2%	8.3%
Middle East and North Africa	13.9%	13.3%	12.2%
North America and Caribbean	13.0%	12.3%	11.1%
Western Pacific	12.8%	12.4%	11.4%
South Asia	12.6%	12.2%	11.3%
South and Central America	9.9%	9.5%	8.5%
Europe	7.8%	7.3%	6.3%
Africa	5.2%	5.1%	4.7%

Fig. 21.2 Current and projected diabetes prevalence in adults by region (2019–2045). *Adapted from International Diabetes Federation. IDF Diabetes Atlas, 9th edn. Brussels; 2019. Available at https://www.diabetesatlas.org.*

ethnicity as well as environmental factors (obesity, diet, habitual physical activity, urbanisation and economic development). A pronounced rise in the prevalence of type 2 diabetes occurs in migrant populations from low-income to industrialised countries. In many high-income countries, type 2 diabetes is no longer rare in children and adolescents, particularly in people of Hispanic, non-Hispanic Black and South Asian ethnicity. In some of these countries, increased survival is a factor underlying rising prevalence.

Type 1 diabetes is also subject to geographical variation and is generally more prevalent in countries closer to the polar regions. Finland, for instance, has the highest rate of type 1 diagnosis per year at >60 per 100 000 of the population, whereas in China, India and Venezuela the incidence is only 0.1 per 100 000. The incidence of type 1 diabetes is also increasing: between 1989 and 2013, 3.4 % more children were diagnosed worldwide each year. Type 1 diabetes is more common in people of European descent than in other ethnic groups and, for reasons that are not understood, more people are diagnosed in the winter months.

Functional anatomy and physiology

As a supply (and uptake) of glucose is essential for the functioning of all organs and tissues, a host of metabolic and physiological processes are involved in precise regulation of its levels in blood.

Insulin

Insulin is synthesised in the β cells of the pancreatic islets of Langerhans as a pro-hormone (pro-insulin), consisting of A- and B-chains, linked by C-peptide (see Fig. 21.23). C-peptide is cleaved by β-cell peptidases to create insulin (the A- and B-chains are joined by two disulfide bonds) and free C-peptide. In a healthy individual, around 10 days' supply of insulin is stored (~200–250 units). There are around one thousand β cells (approximately 70% of the islet cell population) in each of around one million islets scattered diffusely throughout the pancreas. The islets also contain α and δ cells, which synthesise respectively glucagon and somatostatin; F cells (also known as PP cells) synthesise pancreatic polypeptide. The islets are highly metabolically active, but each individual has a total mass of less than 1 g (see Fig. 21.3B). They are highly vascularised, to allow synthesised hormones to enter the portal circulation; despite making up only 1%–2% of total pancreatic mass, they receive 10%–15% of pancreatic blood flow.

Fig. 21.3 Pancreatic structure and endocrine function. [A] The normal adult pancreas contains about 1 million islets, which are scattered throughout the exocrine parenchyma. Histology is shown in Figure 21.8. [B] The core of each islet consists of β cells that produce insulin and is surrounded by a cortex of endocrine cells that produce other hormones, including glucagon (α cells), somatostatin (δ cells) and pancreatic polypeptide (F or PP cells). [C] Schematic representation of the pancreatic β cell. (1) Glucose enters the cell via a glucose transporter (GLUT1 or GLUT2). (2) Glucose then enters glycolysis, and subsequent oxidative phosphorylation in the mitochondria results in a rise in intracellular adenosine triphosphate (ATP). (3) This ATP acts to close the K_{ATP} channel (which consists of four KIR6.2 subunits and four SUR1 subunits). This leads to membrane depolarisation. (4) The rise in membrane potential results in calcium influx due to opening of a voltage-gated calcium channel. This rise in intracellular calcium causes insulin secretory vesicles to fuse with the cell membrane, leading to insulin secretion. (5) Other stimuli, such as glucagon-like peptide-1 (GLP-1) or gastric inhibitory polypeptide (GIP), act on G-protein-coupled receptors to increase cyclic adenosine monophosphate (cAMP) and amplify the insulin secretion. Genetic defects in the β cell result in diabetes. The primary genes are glucokinase (the initial step in glycolysis) and *HNF1α*, *HNF4α* and *HNF1β* (nuclear transcription factors). Two groups of drugs act on the β cell to promote insulin secretion. Sulphonylureas act to close the K_{ATP} channel, causing membrane depolarisation, calcium influx and insulin secretion. Incretin-acting drugs either increase the concentration of endogenous GLP-1 and GIP (the dipeptidyl peptidase 4, or DPP-4, inhibitors) or act as directly on the GLP-1 receptor (GLP-1 receptor agonists). Both of these drug groups act to augment insulin secretion, but only following an initial stimulus to insulin secretion through closure of β cell K_{ATP} channels by glucose (or sulphonylureas).

Regulation of insulin secretion

The pancreatic β cell is designed to regulate blood glucose concentrations tightly by coupling glucose and other nutrient stimuli with insulin secretion (Fig. 21.3). Entry of glucose into the pancreatic β cell is by facilitated diffusion down its concentration gradient through insulin-independent cell membrane glucose transporters (GLUT1 or GLUT2). Glucose is metabolised by glycolysis and oxidative phosphorylation. The first step of the glycolytic pathway, the conversion of glucose to glucose-6-phosphate, is catalysed by the enzyme glucokinase (GK). The generation of glucose-6-phosphate is directly proportional to the concentration of glucose, thus making GK a very effective physiological glucose sensor in the β cell. When glucose is metabolised, adenosine triphosphate (ATP) is generated, closing an ATP-sensitive potassium channel (K_{ATP}). This depolarises the cell membrane, triggering release of calcium, which in turn activates voltage-sensitive calcium channels resulting in secretion of

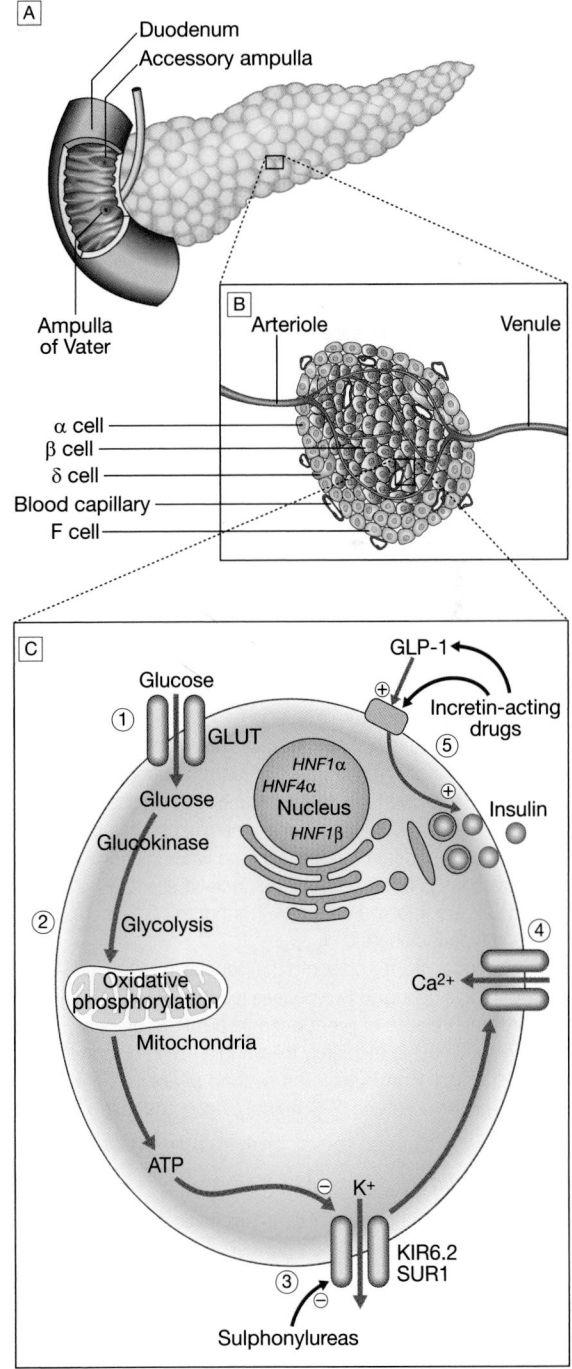

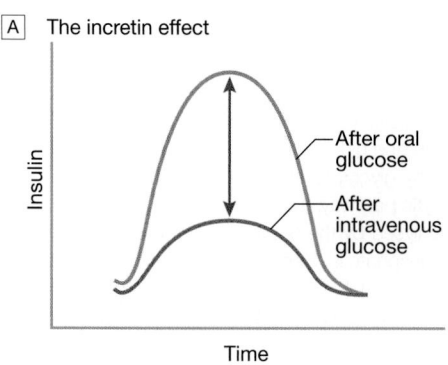

A The incretin effect

Insulin (y-axis)

After oral glucose

After intravenous glucose

Time

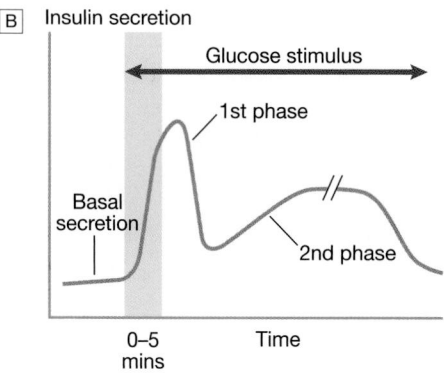

B Insulin secretion

Glucose stimulus

1st phase

Basal secretion

2nd phase

0–5 mins   Time

Fig. 21.4 Insulin secretion in response to elevated glucose. A The incretin effect describes the observation that insulin secretion is greater when glucose is given by mouth than when glucose is administered intravenously to achieve the same rise in blood glucose concentrations. The additional stimulus to insulin secretion is mediated by release of peptides from the gut and these actions are exploited in incretin-based therapies (p. 735). B An acute first phase of insulin secretion occurs in response to an elevated blood glucose, followed by a sustained second phase.

insulin. Therefore, the amount of insulin released in response to this simple pathway at any given time is intrinsically linked to the blood glucose concentration at that moment.

Insulin release can be potentiated by other nutrients and peptides and by neuronal control via the sympathetic and parasympathetic nervous system. Two peptides that potentiate insulin release from β cells following ingestion of food are glucagon-like peptide-1 (GLP-1) and gastric inhibitory polypeptide (GIP), which are released from gastrointestinal L cells and K cells respectively when nutrients reach the duodenum and upper jejunum. Thus, for a given ambient concentration of glucose sensed by the β cell, more insulin is secreted when the glucose has been ingested orally (when gut peptides are released) than when glucose was administered intravenously. This is termed the 'incretin effect' (Fig. 21.4A) and GLP-1 and GIP are known as 'incretin hormones'. The incretin effect is diminished in type 2 diabetes.

Insulin is secreted from β cells into the portal circulation (see Fig. 21.3) and classically this occurs in two phases (see Fig. 21.4B). The rapid first phase represents release of pre-formed insulin from granules within the β cells, starting almost immediately following a rise in blood glucose and is completed within 15 minutes. The second phase is more prolonged (occurring over the following 2–3 hours) and is a consequence of de novo insulin synthesis.

Actions of insulin

Insulin is an anabolic hormone (i.e. it promotes the storage of nutrients) and has pleiotropic effects on glucose, fat and protein metabolism (Box 21.1). It also stimulates cell proliferation and reduces apoptosis. The actions of insulin are mediated through the cell membrane insulin receptor. The receptor belongs to the tyrosine kinase superfamily and is coupled to an extremely complicated intracellular signalling network. A key action of

i 21.1 Metabolic actions of insulin

Increase	Decrease
Carbohydrate metabolism	
Glucose transport (muscle, adipose tissue)	Gluconeogenesis
Glycogen synthesis	Glycogenolysis
Glycolysis	
Lipid metabolism	
Triglyceride synthesis	Lipolysis
Fatty acid synthesis (liver)	Lipoprotein lipase (muscle)
Lipoprotein lipase activity (adipose tissue)	Ketogenesis
	Fatty acid oxidation (liver)
Protein metabolism	
Amino acid transport	Protein degradation
Protein synthesis	

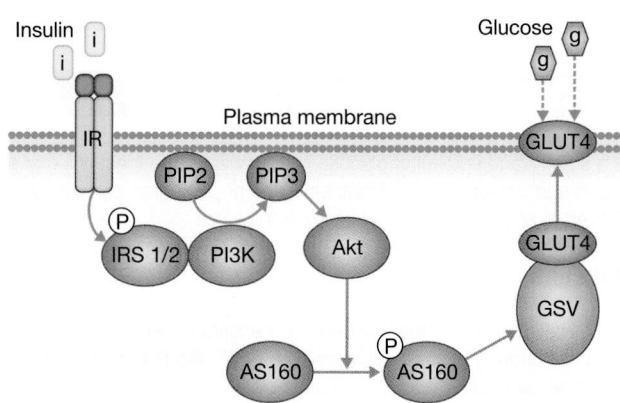

Fig. 21.5 Insulin receptor signalling. Insulin (i) binds to the insulin receptor (IR) triggering a complex signalling cascade including phosphorylation (P) of insulin receptor substrate (IRS) by tyrosine kinase. IRS associates with and activates phosphoinositide 3-kinase (PI3K). PI3K stimulates Akt, which phosphorylates and inactivates AS160. This leads ultimately to translocation of glucose transporter 4 (GLUT4) from GLUT4 storage vesicles (GSVs) to the cell surface, allowing cells to take up interstitial glucose (g). Note that there are many other elements of insulin receptor signalling (not shown) that mediate the other aspects of insulin's pleiotropic actions.

insulin is to lower blood glucose and, in part, this is mediated by promoting the uptake of glucose into muscle and adipose tissue; at a cellular level, the binding of insulin to its receptor causes cell membrane glucose transporter GLUT4 to translocate from the cytoplasm to the cell membrane, permitting the uptake of glucose into adipose and muscle cells (Fig. 21.5).

Glucagon

Alpha cells make up about 20% of the human islet cell population. Glucagon has opposite effects to insulin: for example, it acts on the liver to stimulate glycogenolysis, releasing stored glucose ('hepatic glucose production') and causing blood glucose levels to rise. Glucagon is critically important in the defence against hypoglycaemia. Its secretion by α cells is inhibited locally by β-cell insulin secretion (i.e. a 'paracrine' effect) and also by somatostatin from δ cells. Glucagon secretion is also inhibited by islet amyloid polypeptide (amylin), which is co-secreted from β cells with insulin. Thus insulin and glucagon are tightly and reciprocally regulated, such that the ratio of insulin to glucagon in the portal vein is a major determinant of hepatic glucose production and other metabolic processes, including lipolysis and ketogenesis.

Blood glucose homeostasis

Blood glucose is precisely regulated and maintained within a narrow range (between 4.0 and 5.4 mmol/L (72–99 mg/dL)) when fasting. This is essential for ensuring a physiological continuous supply of glucose to

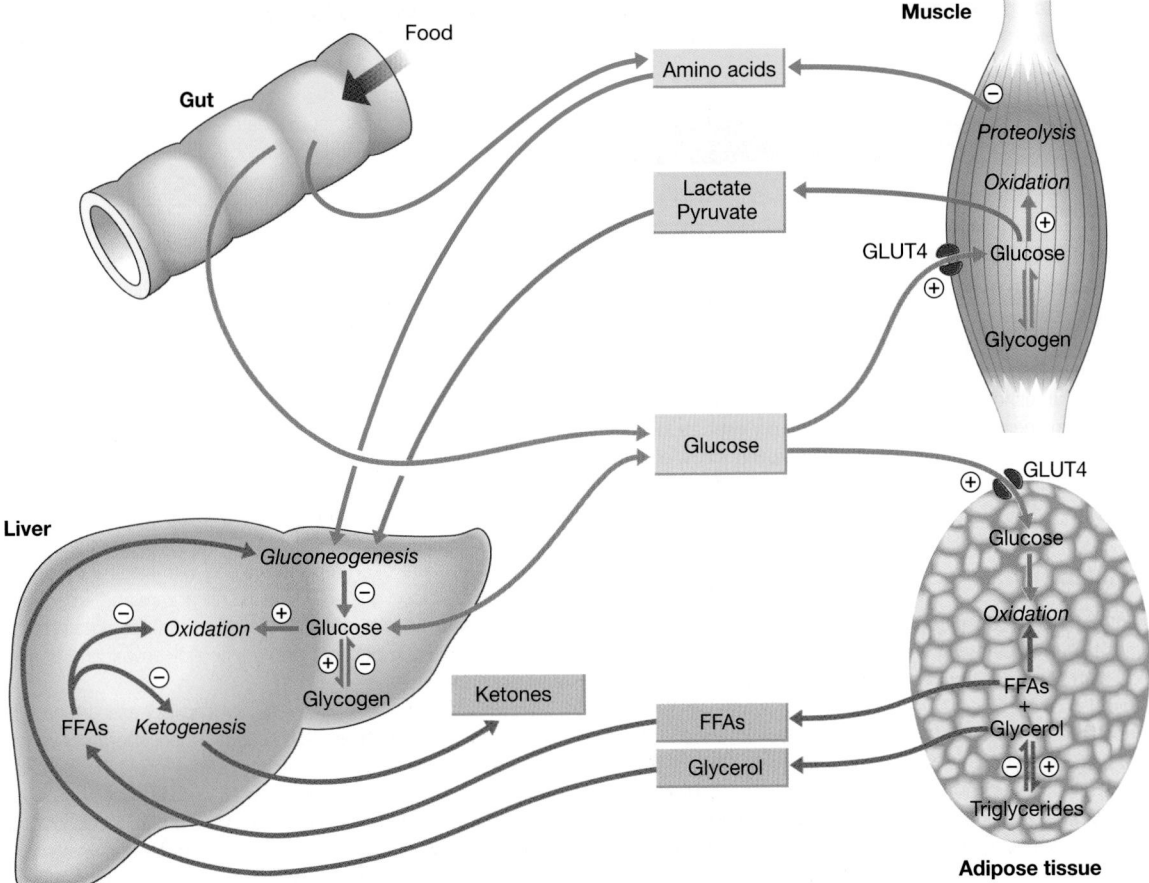

Fig. 21.6 Major metabolic pathways of fuel metabolism and the actions of insulin. ⊕ indicates stimulation and ⊖ indicates suppression by insulin. In response to a rise in blood glucose, e.g. after a meal, insulin is released, suppressing gluconeogenesis and promoting glycogen synthesis and storage. Insulin promotes the peripheral uptake of glucose, particularly in skeletal muscle, and encourages storage (as muscle glycogen). It also promotes protein synthesis and lipogenesis, and suppresses lipolysis. The release of intermediate metabolites, including amino acids (glutamine, alanine), 3-carbon intermediates in oxidation (lactate, pyruvate) and free fatty acids (FFAs), is controlled by insulin. In the absence of insulin, e.g. during fasting, these processes are reversed and favour gluconeogenesis in liver from glycogen, glycerol, amino acids and other 3-carbon precursors.

the central nervous system. The brain has little capacity to store energy in the form of glycogen or triglyceride, while the blood–brain barrier is largely impermeable to fatty acids. Therefore, the brain depends on the liver for a constant supply of glucose for oxidation and hence generation of ATP.

Glucose homeostasis is achieved through the coordinated actions of multiple organs, but mainly reflects a balance between the entry of glucose into the circulation from the liver, supplemented by intestinal absorption of glucose after meals, and the uptake of glucose by peripheral tissues, particularly skeletal muscle and brain. After ingestion of a meal containing carbohydrate, a substantial rise in blood glucose levels is prevented by:

- suppression of hepatic glucose production (by gluconeogenesis and glycogenolysis)
- stimulation of hepatic glucose uptake (and its subsequent storage as glycogen, i.e. glycogen synthesis)
- stimulation of glucose uptake by peripheral tissues (muscle and adipose) (Fig. 21.6).

These effects are mediated primarily by a post-prandial rise in portal vein insulin in response to increasing blood glucose, augmented by incretin hormones, together with a fall in portal glucagon concentrations. Depending on the size of the carbohydrate load, around one-quarter to one-third of ingested glucose is taken up in the liver.

When intestinal glucose absorption declines between meals, blood glucose levels are maintained by increased hepatic glucose output via both gluconeogenesis and glycogenolysis. This is a consequence of falling portal vein insulin concentrations and rising glucagon levels. The main substrates for gluconeogenesis are glycerol and amino acids, as shown in Figure 21.6. At times of substantially increased metabolic demand for energy, such as during exercise or other acute stress, hepatic glucose output can be further transiently increased by activation of the sympathetic nervous system and release of hormones such as adrenaline (epinephrine), noradrenaline (norepinephrine), cortisol and growth hormone, which antagonise the actions of insulin.

Fat metabolism

Adipocytes (and the liver) synthesise triglyceride from non-esterified ('free') fatty acids (FFAs) and glycerol. High circulating insulin levels after meals promote triglyceride accumulation and storage in adipose tissue. In contrast, in the fasting state, low insulin levels permit lipolysis and the release into the circulation of FFAs, which can be oxidised by many tissues. Their partial oxidation in the liver provides substrate (glycerol) and energy (in the form of ATP) to drive gluconeogenesis, but also ketones (acetoacetate, which can be reduced to 3-hydroxybutyrate or decarboxylated to acetone), which are generated in hepatocyte mitochondria. Ketones (also known as ketone bodies) are organic acids that can be oxidised and utilised as an alternative metabolic fuel for the brain when glucose is not available (e.g. during illness and prolonged fasting). Thus, when insulin levels are low (and glucagon and catecholamine levels are high), increased lipolysis and delivery of FFAs to the liver results in the production of ketones (see Fig. 21.6). However, the rate at which ketones can be utilised by peripheral tissues is 'capped': blood ketone concentrations therefore rise (hyperketonaemia) when the rate of production by the liver exceeds their removal.

Investigations

Urine glucose

While a colorimetric test for glucose is included in all standard urine 'dipsticks', it is no longer used as a screening procedure and is rarely of clinical value. If apparent glycosuria is detected, it will always require further assessment by blood testing (see below), e.g. there can be cross-reaction with β-lactam antibiotics, levodopa and salicylates. Some individuals have a high 'renal threshold' for glucose excretion, i.e. glucose is not detected in their urine despite a high blood glucose concentration. A low renal threshold for glucose (i.e. decreased reabsorption following filtration) is common during pregnancy and in healthy young adults, and is of no consequence.

Blood glucose

Measurement of blood glucose concentration is the cornerstone of diabetes diagnosis, but varies markedly according to whether taken in the fasted or fed state. Glucose concentrations are slightly lower in venous than in arterial or capillary blood, as tissues extract glucose. Whole-blood glucose concentrations are lower than separated plasma concentrations, because red blood cells contain relatively little glucose. Venous plasma measurements are the most reliable for diagnostic purposes (Boxes 21.2 and 21.3). Laboratory venous plasma glucose testing utilises a simple enzymatic reaction (glucose oxidase) and is cheap, reliable and usually automated.

21.2 Diagnostic criteria for diabetes and pre-diabetes

Diabetes is confirmed by international consensus as:

- plasma glucose in random sample or 2 hrs after a 75 g glucose load ≥ 11.1 mmol/L (200 mg/dL) *or*
- fasting plasma glucose ≥7.0 mmol/L (126 mg/dL) *or*
- HbA$_{1c}$ ≥ 48 mmol/mol

In asymptomatic patients, two diagnostic tests are required to confirm diabetes

Definitions of 'pre-diabetes' vary between expert bodies:

- impaired fasting glucose:
  - fasting plasma glucose ≥ 6.1 mmol/L (110 mg/dL) and <7.0 mmol/L (126 mg/dL) (World Health Organization) *or*
  - fasting plasma glucose ≥5.6 mmol/L (100 mg/dL) and <7.0 mmol/L (126 mg/dL) (American Diabetes Association)
- impaired glucose tolerance:
  - fasting plasma glucose <7.0 mmol/L (126 mg/dL) *and* 2-hr glucose after 75 g oral glucose drink ≥7.8 (140 mg/dL) and <11.1 mmol/L (200 mg/dL)
- HbA$_{1c}$
  - 42–47 mmol/mol (National Institute for Health and Care Excellence [NICE] guidelines, UK) *or*
  - 39–47 mmol/mol (American Diabetes Association)

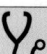

21.3 How to perform an oral glucose tolerance test (OGTT)

Preparation before the test

- Unrestricted carbohydrate diet for 3 days
- Fasted overnight for at least 8 hours
- Rest for 30 mins
- Remain seated for the duration of the test, with no smoking

Sampling

- Measure plasma glucose before and 2 hours after a 75 g oral glucose drink

Glucose can also be measured in capillary blood from a 'fingerprick' sample using test strips read with a portable electronic meter. This has been the traditional method by which people with type 1 diabetes adjust their insulin doses and detect impending hypoglycaemia. The same applies for people with insulin-treated type 2 diabetes and to a lesser extent for those treated with sulphonylureas (in whom hypoglycaemia occurs about 10 times less frequently, but is nevertheless a risk). The main limitation of capillary glucose monitoring (other than the transient pain associated with the fingerprick) is the practical limit on the number of measurements that can be performed over a 24-hour period. Blood glucose can be extremely variable, especially in people with type 1 diabetes, and so intermittent testing (such as 4–6 capillary measurements per day) may miss substantial peaks and troughs in blood glucose, especially overnight when no 'routine' measurements are usually performed.

Capillary blood glucose testing is also used as a 'near-patient test' to monitor glucose levels at the bedside in hospitalised patients with diabetes and in situations where hyperglycaemia or hypoglycaemia is a potential consequence of a medical condition or its treatment, e.g. intravenous insulin therapy (hyper- and hypoglycaemia), high-dose glucocorticoids (hyperglycaemia) and acute liver failure (hypoglycaemia). Arterial blood glucose levels are often reported, along with several other analytes, by 'near-patient' blood gas analysers in critical care and emergency departments. As with capillary testing, the blood glucose data provided can be useful in monitoring patients who are acutely unwell and at risk of hyper- and/or hypoglycaemia.

It is important to note, however, that capillary and arterial whole blood glucose measurements are *less accurate* than laboratory venous plasma glucose measurements. The capillary and arterial glucose measurement devices are designed to give patients and/or clinicians an *approximation* of the prevailing blood glucose. Where high levels of precision are required, e.g. when making a diagnosis of diabetes (which will have substantial implications for the patient) or in the evaluation of spontaneous hypoglycaemia (see Ch. 20), *laboratory* venous plasma blood glucose concentrations should be measured.

Interstitial glucose

An increasingly established approach to measure glucose in people with diabetes is continuous glucose monitoring (CGM). CGM systems use a tiny sensor inserted under the skin to measure glucose in interstitial fluid. CGM devices display both the current glucose and trend arrows, by automatically transmitting to a receiver, smartphone or smartwatch application. CGM devices can also be downloaded onto a personal computer. The use of CGM has accelerated in recent years and is becoming a standard of care in type 1 diabetes management in high-income countries. CGM can be intermittently scanned (isCGM or 'flash' CGM) or provide real-time CGM (rtCGM). The sensor can stay in place for up to 2 weeks before being replaced and provides measurements of glucose levels every 5 minutes for rtCGM or every 15 minutes for isCGM. The most recent devices do not require calibration against capillary blood glucose measurements. Less expensive (isCGM) devices require to be scanned at least once every 8 hours or the data stored in the sensor are lost (see Fig. 21.7).

Interstitial glucose correlates well with blood glucose, but has a 10- to-15-minute lag when blood glucose is rapidly changing. This can lead to discrepancies between contemporaneous CGM and capillary blood glucose measurements; these can also occur due to intrinsic inaccuracies (neither is as accurate as a laboratory measurement). Accuracy of CGM devices is constantly improving, with newer devices reporting mean absolute relative difference (MARD) of interstitial fluid and blood glucose of <11%.

Daily use of CGM improves glycaemic control in type 1 diabetes, providing useful information on daily glucose profiles and, in particular, night-time glucose patterns. It can reveal high and low glycaemic excursions that are not identified by capillary glucose testing. Alarms are incorporated into all rtCGM and some isCGM devices to warn about impending low glucose and high glucose events. Alarms are particularly important

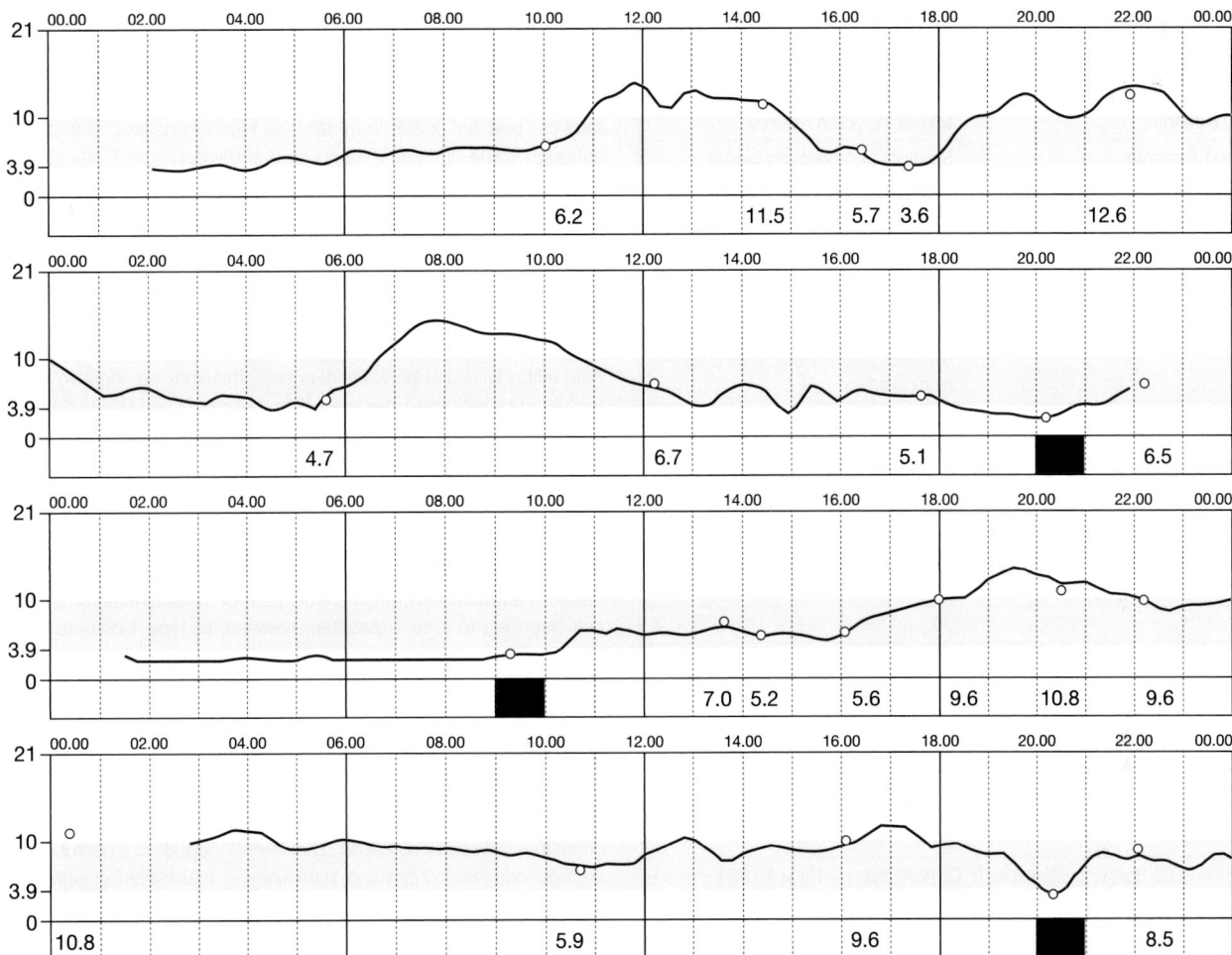

Fig. 21.7 Download from intermittently scanned ('flash') continuous glucose monitor (isCGM). Glucose data from four consecutive days are shown. Each small open circle (o) on the graph represents an occasion when the sensor has been scanned by the patient and there is a corresponding glucose level displayed at the bottom of the graph. The grey section represents the ideal target range of 3.9–10.0 mmol/L. Low glucose episodes are in red. Note the substantial variation in glucose within each 24-hour period (with frequent episodes of low and high glucose) and the variation between comparable time points on different days. Such variation could not be detected by intermittent capillary glucose testing. Each daily graph has a short period when no data are provided; this is because the time between sensor scans exceeded 8 hours.

during the night (when periods of even quite severe biochemical hypoglycaemia may go undetected) and for people with impaired awareness of hypoglycaemia (see p. 725). Early identification of low glucose (by alarm or a trend arrow showing rapidly declining glucose) allows prompt corrective action (i.e. ingesting sugar-containing foods and drinks), and thus may prevent a mild episode of hypoglycaemia becoming a severe episode. Identification of high glucose also allows self-administration, if appropriate, of additional 'correction' doses of insulin.

Initiation of CGM requires education and support to overcome potential information overload and extract meaningful from the extensive data generated. Online resources are provided by the manufacturing companies and also by user forums. The functionality that allows people with diabetes to remotely share their glucose levels with family members (e.g. a child with diabetes can share data with a parent), caregivers and their diabetes specialist team (e.g. facilitating remote consultations) is an important advance. CGM can be linked with continuous subcutaneous insulin infusion (CSII) devices ('insulin pumps') to permit the creation of 'sensor-augmented' systems; such systems can be life-transforming for people with type 1 diabetes and are discussed in detail on p. 741.

Urine and blood ketones

Ketones can be measured in either urine (using dipsticks) or blood using portable electronic meters (integrated into some capillary glucose meters). Urine tests detect acetoacetate (by the nitroprusside reaction), while blood testing strips detect beta-hydroxybutyrate (β-OHB), the major ketone found in blood during diabetic ketoacidosis (DKA). Blood testing is particularly useful to guide self-management during 'sick days' as an early warning sign of incipient DKA, but also to guide emergency in-patient management (see p. 721) e.g. monitoring resolution of DKA (Box 21.4).

Ketonuria/ketonaemia is not pathognomonic of diabetes and can be found after exercise in non-diabetic people who have been fasting or exercising strenuously, repeated vomiting, or eating a 'ketogenic' diet (with a macronutrient composition that is both high in fat and low in carbohydrate).

Glycated haemoglobin

Glycated haemoglobin is accepted as the international standard method for assessing glycaemic control in diabetes as it reflects average blood glucose over a period of weeks or months.

During hyperglycaemia, slow non-enzymatic covalent attachment of glucose to haemoglobin (glycation) increases the proportion in the HbA_1 (and specifically HbA_{1c}) fraction, relative to non-glycated adult haemoglobin (HbA_0). These fractions can be separated by chromatography although other laboratory methods can also be used. The rate of formation of HbA_{1c} is directly proportional to ambient blood glucose

i	21.4 Interpretation of capillary blood ketone measurements	
Measurement[1]	**Interpretation**	
<0.6 mmol/L	Normal; no action required	
0.6–1.5 mmol/L	Suggests metabolic control may be deteriorating; the patient should continue to monitor and seek medical advice if sustained/progressive	
1.5–3.0 mmol/L	High risk of diabetic ketoacidosis; seek medical advice	
>3.0 mmol/L	Severe ketosis suggests presence of diabetic ketoacidosis; seek urgent medical advice	

[1]To convert to mg/dL, multiply values by 18.

i	21.5 Conversion between DCCT and IFCC units for HbA$_{1c}$
DCCT units (%)	**IFCC units (mmol/mol)**
4	20
5	31
6	42
7	53
8	64
9	75
10	86
IFCC HbA$_{1c}$ (mmol/mol) = [DCCT HbA$_{1c}$(%) − 2.15] × 10.929	

(DCCT = Diabetes Control and Complications Trial; IFCC = International Federation of Clinical Chemistry and Laboratory Medicine)

concentration: a rise of 11 mmol/mol in HbA$_{1c}$ corresponds to an approximate average increase of 2 mmol/L (36 mg/dL) in blood glucose. Although HbA$_{1c}$ concentration reflects the integrated blood glucose control over the lifespan of erythrocytes (typically 120 days), HbA$_{1c}$ is most sensitive to changes in glycaemic control occurring in the month before measurement.

Since 2011, the International Federation of Clinical Chemistry and Laboratory Medicine (IFCC) has developed a standard system for reporting HbA$_{1c}$ (IFCC-standardised HbA$_{1c}$) reported in mmol/mol. However, it is important to be aware of the 'percentage' units that were previously used as many people with diabetes are more familiar with these (and many specialist publications use dual-reporting) (Box 21.5).

HbA$_{1c}$ may be erroneously low (i.e. lower than would be anticipated for the prevailing average blood glucose) in conditions associated with shorter red cell lifespan (e.g., chronic blood loss, sickle cell anaemia, thalassaemia, pregnancy) and after blood transfusion (as transfused red cell concentrate usually comes from non-diabetic donors). Conversely, HbA$_{1c}$ may be erroneously high in conditions that increase red cell lifespan (iron, vitamin B$_{12}$ or folate deficiency anaemia, splenectomy). It may be difficult to interpret with some assay methods in patients who have uraemia or a haemoglobinopathy. It is particularly important to be aware of this in pregnancy care and also in health-care settings in which red cell disorders and nutritional deficiency are prevalent, especially if HbA$_{1c}$ is used in the diagnosis of diabetes (see below).

Islet autoantibodies

As type 1 diabetes is characterised by inflammatory infiltration of pancreatic β cells, it can be useful when making a diagnosis of diabetes to identify evidence of autoimmunity. Islet antibodies include:

anti-insulin, anti-glutamic acid decarboxylase (GAD), anti-protein tyrosine phosphatase-related proteins (IA-2) and anti-zinc transporter 8 (ZnT8). They are generally measured using specific immunoassays and, as with other such assays, 'false-positive' results can occur due to assay interference. Islet antibodies may also be found in healthy individuals and although some of these may go on and develop type 1 diabetes in the future (particularly if they have first-degree relatives with type 1 diabetes), many will not develop diabetes. The significance of islet antibodies is greater when they are detected at concentrations greater than the 95th centile of the general population (i.e. in 'high titre') and if multiple antibodies are detectable. A single positive autoantibody confers a 5-year risk of type 1 diabetes of 20%–25%, rising to 50%–60% risk with two autoantibodies and 70% with three autoantibodies. Conversely, as autoantibody levels can wane over time, they may be negative in people with established type 1 diabetes. Pragmatically, if anti-GAD and anti-IA-2 antibodies are measured together, either or both will be 'positive' in approximately 85% of newly diagnosed type 1 diabetes; measurement of anti-ZnT8 antibodies at the same time increases sensitivity to over 90% (i.e. fewer than 10% of cases will be antibody negative). Islet autoantibody testing is becoming standard in some high-income countries for people commenced on insulin therapy within 3 years of diagnosis. A negative autoantibody result should prompt consideration of an alternative diagnosis to type 1 diabetes; however, as type 1 diabetes can still occur in people with negative antibodies, the clinical diagnosis of type 1 diabetes should not immediately be rejected.

C-peptide

C-peptide (see Fig. 21.23) can be readily measured in blood and urine. It is secreted by β cells in equimolar concentrations to insulin, but is not a constituent of synthetic insulin. Therefore C-peptide is a useful marker of *endogenous insulin secretion*, particularly in insulin-treated individuals (in whom a direct measurement of insulin does not distinguish exogenous from endogenous insulin).

Severe endogenous insulin deficiency (typically serum C-peptide < 200 pmol/L) is found in type 1 diabetes, diabetes secondary to other pancreatic disorders and some forms of monogenic diabetes (see p. 719). 'Undetectable' serum C-peptide was traditionally considered pathognomonic of type 1 diabetes; however, the use of modern high-sensitivity C-peptide immunoassays (e.g. with a lower limit of detection of 3 pmol/L) has demonstrated that there is a spectrum of retained endogenous insulin secretion in type 1 diabetes. Persistent endogenous insulin secretion, in any form of diabetes, even though insufficient to maintain normoglycaemia, can have a smoothing effect on blood glucose, i.e. peaks and troughs in glucose are reduced because there is a retained ability to vary insulin secretion (upwards or downwards) in response to prevailing blood glucose.

In type 2 diabetes, C-peptide concentrations are usually significantly elevated (typically > 900 pmol/L) reflecting increased insulin secretion in response to tissue insulin resistance. However, in forms of type 2 diabetes where there is a degree of endogenous insulin deficiency (such as with long diabetes duration), lower levels of C-peptide may occur.

Although there is overlap between C-peptide levels in the different forms of diabetes, a one-off measurement of random (non-fasting) serum C-peptide can be used to identify individuals who have been misclassified, e.g. labelled as type 1 diabetes, when they have type 2 diabetes or vice versa. If C-peptide is used in this way, blood glucose must be checked simultaneously to ensure it is > 4.0 mmol/L (> 72 mg/dL), as hypoglycaemia lowers endogenous insulin secretion and thus C-peptide. C-peptide measurement is also used in the diagnosis of spontaneous hypoglycaemia (p. 689).

Urine albumin ('microalbuminuria')

Standard urine dipstick testing for albumin detects urinary albumin at concentrations above 300 mg/L, but much lower concentrations can be measured using specific albumin dipsticks or quantitative biochemical laboratory tests, permitting detection of microalbuminuria (≥30 mg/L, see Box 18.11). Microalbuminuria (in the absence of urinary tract infection) has therapeutic implications as it is an important early indicator of diabetic nephropathy and a risk marker for macrovascular complications. Microalbuminuria may progress to overt (dipstick positive) proteinuria.

Establishing the diagnosis of diabetes

Glycaemia can be classified into three categories: normal, impaired (pre-diabetes) and diabetes (see Box 21.2). The glycaemia cut-off that defines diabetes is based on a level above which there is a significant risk of microvascular complications, particularly retinopathy (see Fig. 21.1). People categorised as having pre-diabetes have blood glucose levels that carry a negligible risk of microvascular complications, but are at increased risk of developing diabetes (5%–10% in this category develop diabetes each year).

Diabetes has traditionally been diagnosed using venous plasma glucose measurements (random or fasting) and (if required) a 75 g oral glucose tolerance test (OGTT; see Box 21.3). When a person has symptoms of diabetes, the diagnosis can be confirmed with either a fasting glucose of ≥7.0 mmol/L (126 mg/dL) or a random glucose of ≥11.1 mmol/L (200 mg/dL) (see Box 21.2). Asymptomatic individuals should have a second confirmatory test. Diabetes should not be diagnosed on capillary blood glucose results. In 2011, the World Health Organization (WHO) began to advocate the use of glycated haemoglobin (HbA₁c) as a diagnostic test, with an HbA₁c of ≥48 mmol/mol indicative of diabetes. This has been adopted in some countries, including the UK where it is recommended by the National Institute for Health and Care Excellence (NICE). However, in part due to the analytical issues raised by prevalent haemoglobinopathies and other factors that affect HbA₁c independent of average blood glucose (see p. 711), diagnosis by HbA1c has not been adopted by the International Diabetes Federation. As HbA₁c reflects the last 2–3 months of glycaemia, it should not be used to diagnose diabetes when the duration of onset of symptoms has been short; in this context, fasting or random glucose measurements are still required to confirm or rule out a diagnosis.

Pre-diabetes has two forms based on blood glucose criteria, namely 'impaired glucose tolerance' (IGT) and 'impaired fasting glucose' (IFG). In IGT, fasting glucose is normal, but 2-hour glucose is elevated above normal (but not high enough for diabetes). In IFG, fasting glucose is elevated above normal (not high enough for diabetes), but 2-hour glucose is normal. Pre-diabetes may also be diagnosed using HbA₁c, but criteria vary between international bodies (see Box 21.2). Pre-diabetic states are not associated with a substantial risk of microvascular disease, but with an increased risk of conversion to diabetes (particularly IFG) and an increased risk of macrovascular disease, i.e. myocardial infarction, stroke and peripheral vascular disease (particularly IGT) (see Box 21.3). Individuals in whom pre-diabetes is detected (often when screening for diabetes) should be advised of their risk of progression to diabetes, given advice about lifestyle modification to reduce this risk (as for type 2 diabetes), and be screened for treatable cardiovascular risk factors such as hypertension and dyslipidaemia.

The diagnostic criteria for diabetes in pregnancy (gestational diabetes) are more stringent (see Box 32.12). HbA₁c should not be used to diagnose diabetes in pregnancy.

Aetiology and pathogenesis of diabetes

At a fundamental level, diabetes is a consequence of *absolute* or *relative* deficiency of insulin, although the underlying genes, precipitating environmental factors and pathophysiology differ substantially between the various forms. In type 1 diabetes and diabetes secondary to pancreatic pathology there is an *absolute* insulin deficiency that requires treatment with insulin. At the other end of the spectrum, mutations in the insulin

receptor cause diabetes due to severe insulin resistance (e.g. Rabson–Mendenhall and Donohue syndromes); such individuals have extremely high levels of insulin, but have a *relative* deficiency because insulin cannot exert a functional effect via an abnormal receptor. In type 2 diabetes, there is usually a combination of both β-cell dysfunction and insulin resistance, although here the insulin resistance is usually a consequence of signalling effects downstream from the insulin receptor (see below). Although it is generally helpful to classify diabetes on an aetiological basis (Box 21.6), many individuals have diabetes due to a combination of factors, e.g. an individual with type 1 diabetes who becomes obese and insulin resistant (sometimes known as 'double diabetes'); an individual with significant obesity *and* a previous distal pancreatectomy; or an individual with a pathogenic monogenic diabetes gene mutation and strongly positive islet autoantibodies.

Pathogenesis of diabetes

Insulin resistance and the metabolic syndrome

The precise mechanisms causing insulin resistance are complicated. Abnormalities have been reported in many post-receptor intracellular signalling pathways downstream from the insulin receptor, including phosphoinositide 3-kinase (PI3K), but none of the common abnormalities are sufficient to cause type 2 diabetes in the absence of other abnormalities. A single abnormality can usually be compensated for by other pathways ('redundancy'), so 'multiple hits' may be necessary for significant insulin resistance to occur. The exact combination of abnormalities present differs between individuals (i.e. the condition is 'heterogeneous') and there is a wide range of physiological insulin sensitivity even in non-diabetic individuals. Factors associated with insulin resistance are shown in Box 21.7.

Obesity is a major cause of insulin resistance. Intra-abdominal 'central' adipose tissue is metabolically active and releases large quantities of FFAs, which may induce insulin resistance because they compete with (or inhibit use of) glucose as a fuel supply for oxidation, e.g. in muscle. In addition, adipose tissue releases a number of hormones (including a variety of peptides, called 'adipokines') that act on specific receptors to influence sensitivity to insulin in other tissues. Examples of adipokines include leptin, adiponectin, interleukin-6 and tumour necrosis factor alpha. Venous drainage of visceral adipose tissue is into the portal vein and so central obesity may have a particularly potent influence on hepatic insulin sensitivity and thereby adversely affect hepatic glucose and lipid metabolism.

---

i 21.6 Aetiological classification of diabetes mellitus

Type 1 diabetes*

Type 2 diabetes*

Other specific types
- Genetic defects of β-cell function (see Box 21.8)
- Genetic defects of insulin action (e.g., lipodystrophies)
- Pancreatic disease (e.g. pancreatitis, pancreatectomy, neoplastic disease, cystic fibrosis, haemochromatosis, fibrocalculous pancreatopathy)
- Excess endogenous production of hormonal antagonists to insulin, e.g.:
    - Growth hormone – acromegaly
    - Glucocorticoids – Cushing's syndrome
    - Glucagon – glucagonoma
    - Catecholamines – phaeochromocytoma
    - Thyroid hormones – thyrotoxicosis
- Drug-induced (e.g. glucocorticoids, thiazide diuretics, HIV drugs, immune checkpoint inhibitors)
- Associated with genetic syndromes (e.g. Down syndrome, Klinefelter syndrome, Turner syndrome, DIDMOAD (Wolfram syndrome), Friedreich's ataxia, myotonic dystrophy)
- Gestational diabetes

*The World Health Organization also recognises 'slowly evolving, immune-mediated diabetes of adults' and 'ketosis-prone type 2 diabetes' as 'hybrid' forms of diabetes. (DIDMOAD = diabetes insipidus, diabetes mellitus, optic atrophy, nerve deafness)

Some ethnic groups, e.g. South Asians and certain indigenous peoples of America and Australasia, have a very high prevalence of insulin resistance. In part this may simply relate to genetic and environmental factors associated with increased obesity in general. However, a common feature in these groups is that for a given body mass index, there is a greater degree of central rather than peripheral adiposity when compared, for example, to people of European descent.

Physical activity is another important determinant of insulin sensitivity. Inactivity is associated with down-regulation of intracellular insulin-sensitive kinases (enzymes that increase the activity of other enzymes by phosphorylation) and may promote accumulation of FFAs within skeletal muscle. Sedentary people are therefore more insulin-resistant than active people with the same degree of obesity. Moreover, physical activity allows non-insulin-dependent glucose uptake into muscle, reducing the 'demand' on pancreatic β cells to produce insulin.

Although the pathogenic mutations in single genes with a large effect (e.g. mutations in the insulin receptor that negatively impact on its function as mentioned above) are extremely rare, genetic factors nevertheless play a very important role in the pathogenesis of insulin resistance. Genome-wide association studies have shown that many common and rare gene variants are associated with increased and decreased sensitivity to insulin. Obesity has a strong genetic element (see p. 764), often relating to impaired hypothalamic mechanisms of appetite and satiety, and so many of the identified gene variants associated with obesity are also associated with insulin resistance. Ethnic differences in adipose deposition are also likely to have a genetic basis, although this has not yet been conclusively proven (many genetic studies to date have had included mainly participants of European descent). Non-obesity related genetic variants associated with insulin resistance are mostly either directly involved in glucose metabolism or in the insulin intracellular signalling cascade.

Increasing age is associated with reduced insulin sensitivity, but this may be a consequence of increased adiposity and reduced lean muscle mass rather than a direct effect of ageing. Drugs (notably glucocorticoids) and excess of hormones such as cortisol and growth hormone (see Box 21.6) can also antagonise the action of insulin.

As well as being associated with hyperglycaemia, insulin resistance is also associated with a cluster of other conditions. These include hypertension, dyslipidaemia (elevated small dense low-density lipoprotein (LDL) cholesterol, elevated triglycerides and low high-density lipoprotein (HDL) cholesterol), non-alcoholic fatty liver disease (Ch. 24) and, in women, polycystic ovarian syndrome. This cluster has been termed the 'insulin resistance syndrome' or 'metabolic syndrome' and is usually associated with central obesity, impaired glucose tolerance and an increased risk of macrovascular disease. Severe insulin resistance is also associated with acanthosis nigricans (see p. 704), i.e. dark pigmentation of body folds and creases, particularly in the axillae, groins and neck.

β-cell dysfunction

Insulin deficiency occurs across a spectrum that ranges from complete deficiency (e.g. following a total pancreatectomy), through the severe insulin deficiency of type 1 diabetes, to more minor degrees of insulin insufficiency that only become important if increased demand is placed upon the pancreas, e.g. by obesity-induced insulin resistance. In this latter situation, insulin deficiency may be more relative than absolute, i.e. the β cells may produce substantial amounts of insulin, but not in sufficient quantities to overcome an insulin-resistant state. Insulin deficiency may be the consequence of a number of different factors, some of which are listed in Box 21.7.

There is wide variation in the capacity of the pancreas to produce insulin, because of natural variation in β-cell mass and the inherent efficiency of the β cells. Single gene mutations with a large effect on β-cell mass and function are uncommon, but form the basis of most forms of monogenic diabetes (Box 21.8). Most of the variation in β-cell mass and function is mediated by multiple genes, each with a very small effect. However, where a large number of adverse genetic variants are

inherited, their cumulative effect can be significant. Individuals with genetically lower β-cell mass and function may not have abnormal blood glucose at birth, but are more susceptible to developing diabetes in later life, particularly if the individual becomes insulin resistant or acquires additional loss of β cells (e.g. through exposure to a toxin or following pancreatic surgery). Genetic variants may also code for proteins that increase susceptibility of β cells to environmental toxins or pro-inflammatory cytokines.

Autoimmune destruction and other disorders of the pancreas leading to loss of β-cell mass are discussed in subsequent sections. Increasing age is associated with a decline in β-cell mass and function and exposure to certain chemicals (notably alcohol) can also be toxic to β cells.

Elevated plasma glucose and FFAs exert toxic (and potentially reversible) effects on pancreatic β cells, respectively known as glucotoxicity and lipotoxicity. These effects are often apparent as severe hyperglycaemia (and even ketoacidosis) and may occur at the time of diagnosis of diabetes.

In type 2 diabetes, deposition of a peptide known as islet amyloid polypeptide may be observed in islets. It is not entirely clear if this contributes to the decline in β-cell function in type 2 diabetes or if it is simply a manifestation of other insults to the pancreas. Obesity is a pro-inflammatory state and cytokines released from adipose tissue (including IL-1β, IFN-γ, TNF-α, leptin and resistin) may also contribute to β-cell dysfunction in type 2 diabetes.

---

i 21.7 Factors associated with insulin resistance and insulin deficiency

Insulin resistance	Insulin deficiency
Genetic factors*	Genetic factors*
Single gene mutations	Single gene mutations
Multiple gene variants	Multiple gene variants
Central obesity	Increasing age
Ethnicity	Autoimmune destruction
Reduced physical activity	Pancreatic pathology (see Box 21.6)
Hormone excess (see Box 21.6)	Toxins, e.g. alcohol, cytokines
Drugs, e.g. glucocorticoids	Infections, e.g. SARS-CoV-2
	Glucotoxicity
	Lipotoxicity
	Deposition of islet amyloid polypeptide

*Single gene mutations generally have a large effect size, while gene variants individually have a small effect size, but collectively the effect size can be important.

---

i 21.8 Monogenic diabetes mellitus: maturity-onset diabetes of the young (MODY)

Functional defect	Main type*	Gene mutated*
β-cell glucose sensing	MODY2	GCK

The set point for basal insulin release is altered, causing a high fasting glucose, but sufficient insulin is released after meals. As a result, the HbA_{1c} is often normal and microvascular complications are rare. Treatment is rarely required.

β-cell transcriptional regulation	MODY3	HNF1α
	MODY5	HNF1β
	MODY1	HNF4α

Diabetes develops during adolescence/early adulthood and can be managed with diet and tablets for many years, but ultimately, insulin treatment is required. The HNF1α and 4α forms respond particularly well to sulphonylurea drugs. All types are associated with microvascular complications. HNF1β mutations also cause renal cysts and renal failure.

*Other gene mutations have been found in rare cases. For further information, see diabetesgenes.org.

Type 1 diabetes

Pathogenesis

Type 1 diabetes is an immune-mediated disorder involving T-cell destruction of β cells in the pancreatic islets ('insulitis'). The natural history of type 1 diabetes is classically based on a 'gene-environment interaction' model, i.e. genetically susceptible individuals develop β-cell autoimmunity following exposure to an environmental trigger. This results in a progressive loss of β cells over a period of months or years, until they have little functional capacity (Fig. 21.8). Although insulitis is a T-cell-mediated response, circulating autoantibodies to islet and/or β-cell antigens can be present long before the clinical presentation of type 1 diabetes (see p. 712).

The histological appearance of insulitis is of an inflammatory infiltrate of mononuclear cells (activated macrophages, helper cytotoxic and suppressor T lymphocytes, natural killer cells and B lymphocytes) within islets (see Fig. 21.8). The specific mechanisms inducing this process are unknown, but the hypothesis that it is triggered in susceptible individuals by viral infection has been supported by detection of enterovirus-specific mRNA in fresh pancreatic tissue samples from recently diagnosed adults. Even when type 1 diabetes is established, heavily infiltrated islets may be seen adjacent to unaffected lobules. Although the principal metabolic effect of insulitis is β cell destruction, inflammation can also be detected in adjacent exocrine (acinar) tissue.

Genetic predisposition

Type 1 diabetes is strongly influenced by genetic factors, but does not follow a simple Mendelian pattern of inheritance. Monozygotic twins have a concordance rate of 30%–50% for the condition, while dizygotic twins have a concordance of 6%–10%. In the United States, the risk of developing type 1 diabetes is 1:20 for those with a first-degree relative, compared with 1:300 in the general population. Children of mothers with type 1 diabetes have a 1%–4% risk of developing type 1 diabetes, but children of fathers with type 1 diabetes have a 10% risk. If both parents have the condition the risk is up to 30%. Notwithstanding this genetic influence, 80%–85% of new cases do not have a family history.

These observations are consistent with polygenic inheritance (see Box 21.6); over 20 different regions of the human genome have an association with type 1 diabetes risk. Most interest has focused on the human leucocyte antigen (HLA) region within the major histocompatibility complex on the short arm of chromosome 6. The HLA haplotypes DR3 and/or DR4 are associated with increased susceptibility to type 1

diabetes in people of European descent and are in 'linkage disequilibrium' (i.e. tend to be transmitted together) with the neighbouring alleles of the HLA-DQA1 and DQB1 genes. The latter may be the main determinants of genetic susceptibility, since these HLA class II genes code for proteins on the surface of cells that present foreign and self-antigens to T lymphocytes (p. 78). However, candidate gene studies and genome-wide association studies have also implicated other genes, e.g. CD25, PTPN22, SH2B3, IL2RA and IL-10. The majority of these risk loci are involved in immune responsiveness, such as recognition of pancreatic islet antigens, T cell development and immune regulation. The genes associated with type 1 diabetes overlap with those for coeliac disease and thyroid disease, consistent with clustering of these conditions in individuals or families.

Environmental predisposition

The wide geographical and seasonal variations in incidence, and the rapid acquisition of local disease incidence rates in migrants from low- to high-incidence countries, suggest that environmental factors have an important role in precipitating the development of type 1 diabetes.

Although there are many hypotheses, the nature of these environmental factors is unknown. They may trigger type 1 diabetes through direct toxicity to β cells or by stimulating an autoimmune reaction directed against β cells. Potential candidates fall into four main categories:

1. Viruses: in addition to enteroviruses (e.g. Coxsackie B4), other viruses including mumps, rubella (in utero), cytomegalovirus, Epstein–Barr virus and most recently retroviruses.
2. Toxins: various dietary nitrosamines (found in smoked and cured meats) and coffee. Bovine serum albumin (BSA), a major constituent of cow's milk, has also been implicated, since children who are given cow's milk early in infancy are more likely to develop type 1 diabetes than those who are breastfed. BSA may cross the neonatal gut wall and raise antibodies that cross-react with a heat-shock protein expressed by β cells.
3. Hygiene hypothesis: it has been proposed that reduced exposure to microorganisms in early childhood limits maturation of the immune system and increases susceptibility to autoimmune disease.
4. Vitamin D: as the highest incidences are in areas where there is less sunlight (including northern Europe), low levels of vitamin D may be important. However, no clear cause–effect relationship has been identified.

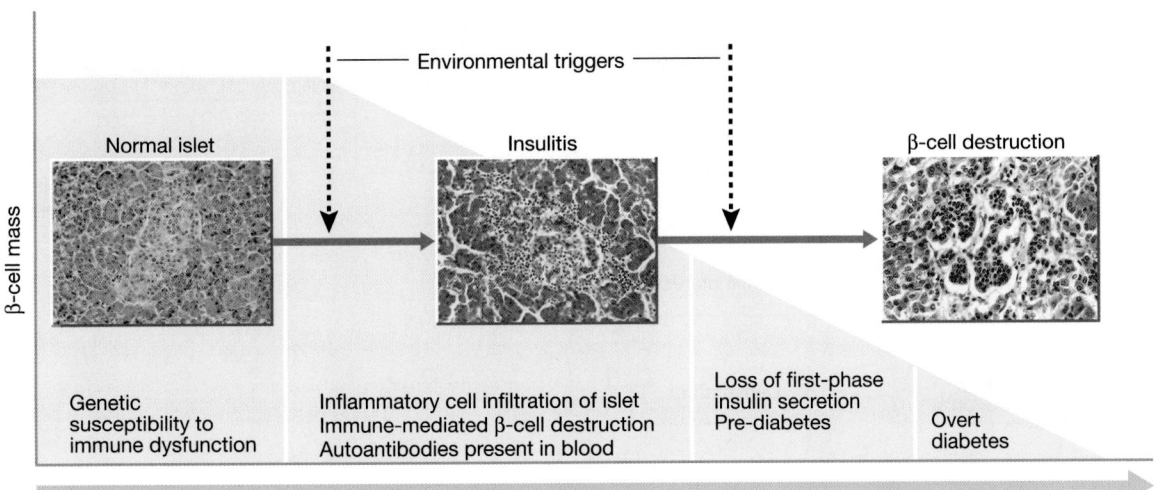

Fig. 21.8 Pathogenesis of type 1 diabetes. Proposed sequence of events in the development of type 1 diabetes. Environmental triggers are described in the text. *Insets (normal islet, β-cell destruction) Courtesy of Dr A. Foulis, Department of Pathology, University of Glasgow.*

Immune checkpoint inhibitors, increasingly used in oncology, can trigger the development of autoimmune disorders, including type 1 diabetes (see Ch. 7). The natural history of the onset of immune-mediated destruction of the pancreas seems to occur at an accelerated rate compared to the standard trajectory of type 1 diabetes, and there is often very severe insulin deficiency resulting in marked glycaemic variability.

Metabolic disturbances in type 1 diabetes

Type 1 diabetes presents when progressive β-cell destruction has crossed a threshold at which adequate insulin secretion and normal blood glucose levels can no longer be sustained. Above a certain level, high glucose levels are toxic to the remaining β cells (glucotoxicity) so that profound insulin deficiency rapidly ensues, causing the metabolic sequelae shown in Figure 21.9. Hyperglycaemia leads to glycosuria and dehydration, while glycosuria, lipolysis and proteolysis result in weight loss. Ketoacidosis occurs when generation of ketones exceeds the capacity for their metabolism. Elevated blood H+ ions drive K+ out of the intracellular compartment, while secondary hyperaldosteronism encourages urinary loss of K+. Thus, new cases of type 1 diabetes usually present with a short history (typically a few weeks) of hyperglycaemic symptoms (see Box 21.9) and weight loss, and in the most severe cases (usually when the diagnosis is delayed) DKA can develop (p. 721).

Clinical course of type 1 diabetes

The natural course of type 1 diabetes involves initially a loss of first-phase insulin secretion, followed by a period of pre-diabetes and then clinically undiagnosed diabetes, before a diagnosis of diabetes is made (Fig. 21.8). By this point, more than 80%–90% of β-cell mass has usually been destroyed. Following institution of insulin therapy, there may be a 'honeymoon period' lasting several weeks or months, during which there is a partial recovery in β-cell function as the glucotoxic effect is reversed by correction of hyperglycaemia. During the honeymoon period, the production of significant endogenous insulin means that exogenous insulin requirements may be very low and some individuals may even be able to stop insulin for a few weeks or months. Typically glycaemic control is good during this period, with modest glucose variability and a low risk of hypoglycaemia. In most patients, the immune-mediated process eventually destroys the majority of remaining β-cells, resulting in severe insulin deficiency, increased requirements for exogenous insulin and more marked glycaemic variability.

It is increasingly recognised that a proportion of individuals with type 1 diabetes retain in the long term a subset of viable β cells with a capacity to secrete small amounts of endogenous insulin. The resulting spectrum of retained endogenous insulin production can be identified by measuring C-peptide (see p. 712). A shorter duration of diabetes and a later age at onset are associated with increased likelihood of significant detectable C-peptide. As exemplified by the honeymoon period, higher C-peptide concentrations are associated with reduced glucose variability and hypoglycaemia, and increased time in range (Fig. 21.10). Higher C-peptide concentrations are also associated with reduced HbA$_{1c}$, exogenous insulin requirements, frequency of ketoacidosis and microvascular

i	21.9 Symptoms of hyperglycaemia

- Polyuria
- Nocturia
- Thirst, dry mouth
- Polydipsia
- Tiredness, fatigue, lethargy
- Change in weight (usually weight loss)
- Blurring of vision
- Pruritus vulvae, balanitis (genital candidiasis)

- Nausea
- Headache
- Hyperphagia; predilection for sweet foods
- Mood change, irritability, difficulty in concentrating, apathy

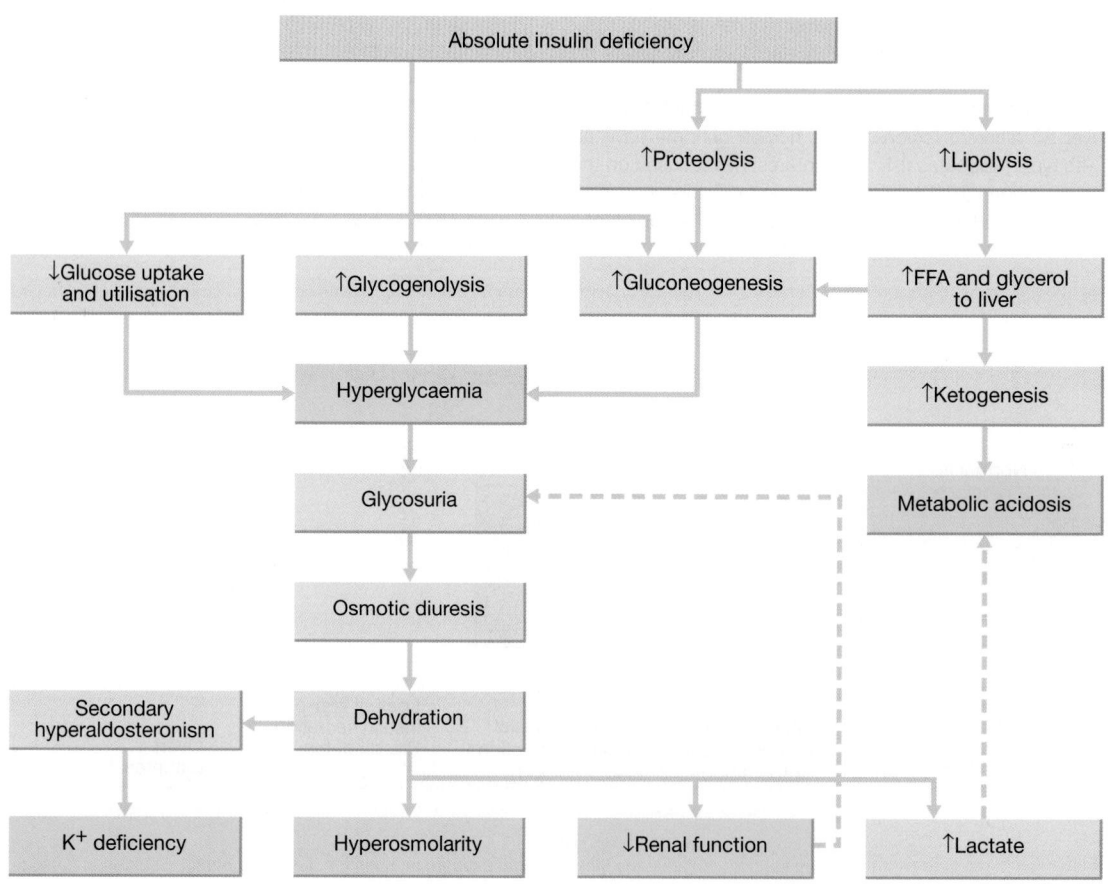

Fig. 21.9 Acute metabolic complications of insulin deficiency. (FFA = free fatty acid)

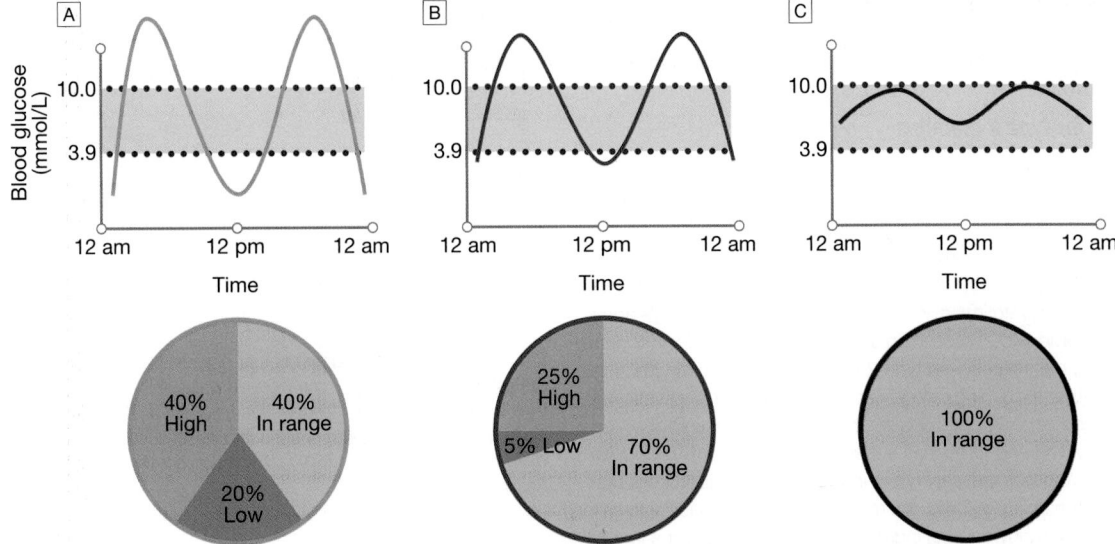

Fig. 21.10 Patterns of glycaemic variability in type 1 diabetes. Three patterns of glycaemic variability are shown, all associated with the same average blood glucose (8.6 mmol/L). **A** High variability with only 40% time in range (TIR); **B** Acceptable variability with 70% TIR. **C** Ideal profile with 100% TIR. Glycaemic variability is affected by many factors including individual behaviours (carbohydrate intake, timing and dose of insulin) and C-peptide status (high C-peptide associated with low glycaemic variability).

complications. There is currently much research activity aimed at halting or slowing the decline in endogenous insulin production early in the course of type 1 diabetes ('C-peptide preservation'), using agents such as biologic immunosuppressants.

Type 1 diabetes presenting in adults

While type 1 diabetes is classically thought of as a disease of children and young adults (most commonly presenting between 5 and 7 years of age and at or near puberty), it can manifest at any age. Over 40% of cases developing in adults over 30 years of age – although some of these diagnoses may be incorrect, with a small proportion actually having unrecognised type 2 diabetes or monogenic diabetes.

Some adults have a more insidious onset of hyperglycaemia and have 'slowly evolving immune-mediated diabetes of adults', previously known as 'latent autoimmune diabetes of adulthood' (LADA). This is essentially a subset of type 1 diabetes with usually a single islet autoantibody present in high titre (usually anti-GAD), greater retention of β-cell function and hyperglycaemia that does not require immediate commencement of insulin therapy. Affected individuals often have features of the metabolic syndrome and are initially managed with a working diagnosis of type 2 diabetes, but recognised retrospectively as having progressed more rapidly to requiring insulin treatment than is typical for type 2 diabetes.

Type 2 diabetes

Pathogenesis

Type 2 diabetes is a heterogeneous condition characterised by varying degrees of insulin resistance and β-cell dysfunction, commonly associated with obesity. Approximately 40% of overall type 2 diabetes risk is determined by genetic factors, with the rest due to environmental (acquired) factors. Insulin resistance and β-cell dysfunction have both genetic and environmental determinants (see relevant sections above). The relative contribution of insulin resistance and β-cell dysfunction varies between individuals, with most having an important contribution from both factors, but some having severe insulin resistance with less marked β-cell dysfunction, and others having significant insulin deficiency and minimal insulin resistance. For example, type 2 diabetes is increasingly seen in children and young adults, usually driven by insulin resistance due to extreme obesity (often on a background of an ethnic predisposition to diabetes). By contrast, type 2 diabetes may also occur in non-obese individuals (who have more pronounced β-cell dysfunction), particularly in the elderly. Many of the rarer types of diabetes (see Box 21.6) were

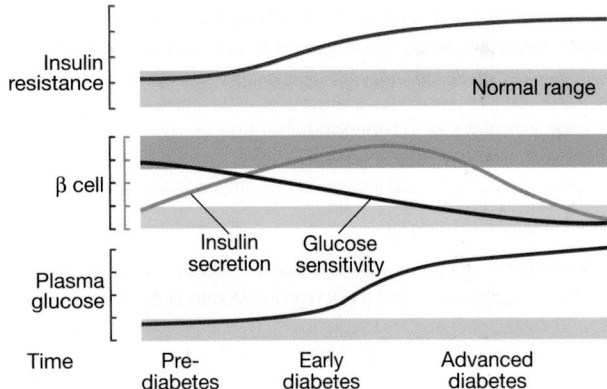

Fig. 21.11 Natural history of type 2 diabetes. Individuals predisposed to type 2 diabetes may have insulin levels at the lower end of normal and higher than normal insulin resistance (not shown in this figure), due to genetic factors. As insulin resistance increases (green) there is a compensatory increase in insulin secretion (grey), which initially maintains plasma glucose (blue) in the normal range. Eventually, the β cells are unable to compensate adequately and blood glucose rises, producing hyperglycaemia. Normal ranges are shown by horizontal bars shaded in same colours. Redrawn with permission from the original courtesy of Professor E. Ferrannini, University of Pisa.

previously categorised as type 2 diabetes, and it is likely that this list will expand in time as genetic studies provide more insights into the aetiology of diabetes. The natural history of 'typical' type 2 diabetes is shown in Figure 21.11. Individuals at high risk of type 2 diabetes usually have a degree of genetic predisposition to either pancreatic β-cell dysfunction (measured as β-cell glucose sensitivity), insulin resistance (measured as insulin-mediated glucose uptake) or both. Each of these phenotypes declines with age and the trajectory of decline is particularly determined by weight gain. The resulting rise in glucose levels over time (initially small) is compensated by an increase in insulin secretion rate, which is teleologically a homeostatic attempt to maintain normal blood glucose levels. However, unless weight gain can be reversed at an early stage, β-cell function continues to decline such that a relative state of insulin deficiency in prediabetes and early diabetes becomes absolute. This is mediated by obesity-associated factors such as glucotoxicity, lipotoxicity, pro-inflammatory cytokines and/or the deposition of amyloid polypeptide in pancreatic islets. It has been estimated that at the time of diagnosis of type 2 diabetes, around 50% of β-cell function has been lost. As β-cell function continues to decline over time, there is an escalating requirement for glucose-lowering therapy. In the most extreme form, there is pancreatic β-cell 'exhaustion' and, as in type 1 diabetes, insulin therapy is required to prevent ketoacidosis.

Risk factors for type 2 diabetes

Genetic predisposition

Genetic factors are important in type 2 diabetes, as shown by marked differences in susceptibility in different ethnic groups and by studies in monozygotic twins in whom concordance rates for type 2 diabetes approach 100%. People with an affected sibling with onset before the age of 40 have a 50% lifetime risk, declining to 30% if the sibling's age is >65 years. Genome-wide association studies have identified >400 gene variants that are associated with type 2 diabetes, each exerting a small effect and together explaining only about 10% of the overall genetic variance. Most code either for proteins involved in β-cell function or in regulation of cell cycling and turnover (i.e. β-cell mass); a smaller proportion affect control of appetite and satiety (i.e. individual susceptibility to weight gain) and insulin resistance. Thus, the major genetic susceptibility to type 2 diabetes relates to how well an individual's pancreas produces insulin. The largest population genetic effect described to date is a variation in *TCF7L2* (a transcription factor involved in glucose metabolism in pancreas and liver); 10% of the population have two copies of the risk variant for this gene and have a nearly two-fold increase in risk of developing type 2 diabetes. Other common variants explain much lower risk than this, with many explaining less than a 10% increase. However, an individual with a high genetic burden (e.g. more than 40 risk variants) compared to one with very few is more than 2.5 times more likely to develop diabetes. Rarer variants tend to have larger effects on type 2 diabetes risk than common variants: e.g. in Greenland 3% of people carry a homozygous variant in an insulin signalling gene, *TBC1D4*, that results in muscle insulin resistance and a 10-fold increased risk of type 2 diabetes.

Lifestyle factors and obesity

Epidemiological studies show that type 2 diabetes is associated with reduced physical activity and a diet high in saturated fats and refined sugars, and low in fresh fruit and vegetables. Type 2 diabetes is also strongly associated with economic deprivation, social disadvantage, excess alcohol consumption and smoking. These factors are all in turn associated with obesity, which is strongly linked with insulin resistance. The risk of developing type 2 diabetes increases with rising body mass index (BMI), such that risk is increased 10-fold in people with a BMI of more than 30 kg/m² (Ch. 22). However, although the majority of individuals with type 2 diabetes are obese, only a minority of obese people develop diabetes, as most obese people are able to increase insulin secretion to compensate for the increased demand resulting from obesity and insulin resistance. Those who develop type 2 diabetes are less able to produce sufficient insulin to overcome insulin resistance because of genetic and/or acquired factors.

Age

Type 2 diabetes is more common with increasing age (see Fig. 21.12). In the UK, it now affects approximately 25% of people aged between 60 and 80 years. In 2019, over 80% of all cases of type 2 diabetes in Scotland occurred after the age of 50 years. This association reflects declining β-cell mass and function with increasing age and the increasing tendency to insulin resistance due to greater obesity and reduced lean muscle mass.

Ethnicity

The prevalence of type 2 diabetes varies considerably according to ethnicity. For example, Figure 21.12 shows that within the United States the prevalence of diabetes is lowest in those of non-Hispanic White ethnicity and increases across the categories of non-Hispanic Black, Hispanic, Asian and finally Indigenous peoples. Genetic factors are likely to explain some of this variance, but environmental factors are also important, such as cultural practices and socio-economic status, which in turn are reflected in diet, physical activity and levels of obesity.

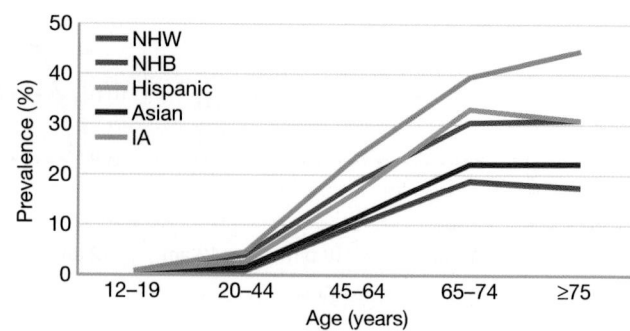

Fig. 21.12 Age-specific prevalence of diagnosed type 2 diabetes in the United States by ethnicity. NHW = non-Hispanic White; NHB = non-Hispanic Black; IA = Indigenous American. *Adapted from Golden et al. Racial/ethnic differences in the burden of type 2 diabetes over the life course: a focus on the USA and India. Diabetologia 2019; 62(10):1751–1760.* © Springer-Verlag GmbH Germany, part of Springer Nature, 2019.

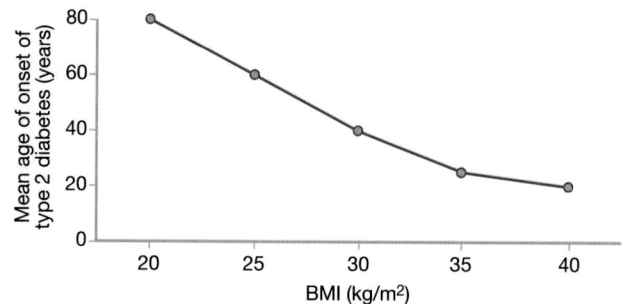

Fig. 21.13 Relationship between age of onset of type 2 diabetes and body mass index. On average, type 2 develops at a younger age in people with increased body mass index.

Interaction of risk factors for type 2 diabetes

In addition to the risk factors described above, type 2 diabetes is also more common in people with previous 'stress hyperglycaemia', in women with previous gestational diabetes and in those who had a very low birth weight. All the risk factors for type 2 diabetes are inter-related and usually have additive effects. For example, increasing BMI is associated with a younger age of onset of type 2 diabetes (Fig. 21.13), because increased insulin resistance unmasks the genetic inability of the pancreas to produce adequate amounts of insulin. Type 2 diabetes also occurs at a younger age and lower BMI in people whose father and mother are both affected, presumably because they have inherited an increased number of genetic variants associated with β-cell dysfunction and insulin resistance. The threshold of weight gain at which type 2 diabetes occurs is lower for South Asians, who develop the condition on average 5–10 years earlier than people of European descent.

Clinical course and metabolic disturbances in type 2 diabetes

In comparison with type 1 diabetes, the risk of acute metabolic decompensation is low in type 2 diabetes due to relative rather than absolute insulin deficiency. Even small amounts of insulin are sufficient to suppress lipolysis and proteolysis, so profound weight loss and DKA are much less common. Hyperglycaemia may therefore be detected incidentally on screening, or even following detection of retinal abnormalities at a routine optician appointment, i.e. before the onset of symptoms. The proportion of cases remaining undetected at any one time varies among healthcare systems, but is estimated to be as high as 20%. At diagnosis, there may be a history of fatigue and 'osmotic symptoms' (thirst, polyuria and nocturia) for many months.

However, despite the 'typical' natural history of type 2 diabetes, it is important to remember that some people with type 2 diabetes develop marked and acute osmotic symptoms and weight loss. This may be a late presentation with advanced β-cell failure (and absolute insulin deficiency), but more often acute decompensation reflects a 'vicious spiral' of decline which is at least in part reversible. In this scenario, severe hyperglycaemia is associated with a craving for sugar, with large volumes of sugary drinks consumed in an effort to quench thirst. This causes glucotoxicity leading to reduced insulin secretion and increased lipolysis with high circulating FFAs aggravating the decompensation (lipotoxicity). Education and dietary intervention can lead to rapid symptomatic improvement, but in the most severe instances, hyperglycaemic hyperosmolar state (p. 723) and even diabetic ketoacidosis (DKA) can occur.

Ketosis and DKA in type 2 diabetes is referred to as 'ketosis-prone' diabetes or 'Flatbush syndrome'. This was named after the Flatbush neighbourhood of New York, which had a large population of African American and African Carribean origin and in which presentation with DKA was noted in the 1980s to be as common with type 2 diabetes as with type 1 diabetes. It remains unclear whether ketosis-prone diabetes is a unique type or a subset of more severe type 2 diabetes, but it is now recognised to occur in sub-Saharan African, South Asian and Hispanic populations. Importantly in this scenario, insulin treatment is required initially, but as glucose and lipid levels are controlled, β cells recover and oral treatments such as metformin can be effective within 3 months, i.e. insulin treatment can be carefully discontinued.

Intercurrent illness, e.g. infection (including with COVID-19, p. 293) or acute myocardial infarction, increases the production of stress hormones that oppose insulin action. This can precipitate an acute exacerbation of insulin resistance and insulin deficiency, and result in more severe hyperglycaemia and dehydration with ketosis (p. 745). If the hyperglycaemia resolves following successful treatment of the illness, then this is retrospectively termed 'stress hyperglycaemia'. Affected individuals have a significantly increased risk of type 2 diabetes in subsequent years, presumably because they had pre-existing β-cell dysfunction and/or insulin resistance. In some individuals, hyperglycaemia persists, probably because of undiagnosed type 2 diabetes that was exacerbated by the acute illness.

Other forms of diabetes

Other causes of diabetes are shown in Box 21.6. These can broadly be classified as:

- genetic disorders, which are either monogenic (mutation in or deletion of a single gene) or part of a genetic syndrome
- secondary to endocrine disorders, e.g. excess secretion of counter-regulatory hormones (those that oppose the effects of insulin)
- secondary to more generalised diseases of the pancreas (most commonly pancreatitis and cystic fibrosis)
- drug-induced causes, e.g. glucocorticoid therapy, which may precipitate hyperglycaemia ('steroid-induced diabetes') in susceptible individuals (i.e. with pre-existing insulin-resistance and/or β-cell dysfunction). Affected individuals who recover normal glucose tolerance after cessation of the precipitating drug remain at increased risk of type 2 diabetes.

Pancreatic diabetes

Diabetes due to more generalised pancreatic disease is a common form of 'secondary diabetes', which is often not accurately distinguished from other forms of diabetes. It may be caused by acute or chronic pancreatitis, either due to alcohol excess or to gall bladder (stone) disease. While chronic pancreatitis may be associated with recurrent abdominal pain, it can also be asymptomatic in many patients. As it may go unrecognised, it is important to be aware of the possibility of pancreatic exocrine deficiency in all cases of diabetes; this can be detected by screening for low faecal enzyme elastase in a stool sample, particularly in the presence of chronic diarrhoea (see p. 850). Adequate oral pancreatic enzyme replacement can reduce abdominal pain, improve absorption of ingested nutrients and enhance well-being. This may facilitate adjustment of insulin doses and reduces risk of hypoglycaemia in affected individuals, who usually require insulin therapy.

In some geographical regions, including South Asia, a form of chronic calcific pancreatitis heralded by chronic abdominal pain can present in adolescence or early adulthood (known as fibrocalculous pancreatic diabetes). It is associated with mutations in the gene *SPINK1*, which codes for an anti-protease enzyme and is therefore now thought to result from slow pancreatic auto-digestion. It is also associated with a high risk of pancreatic cancer.

Diabetes may also be a consequence of other disorders involving the pancreas, including haemochromatosis ('bronze diabetes'), cystic fibrosis and pancreatic carcinoma.

Monogenic diabetes

Monogenic diabetes accounts for approximately 4% of diabetes in those diagnosed under the age of 30 in the UK. While there are a number of monogenic disorders of insulin action, the most common are caused by defects in insulin secretion. Monogenic disorders of the β cell cause two diabetes subtypes: maturity-onset diabetes of the young (MODY; see Box 21.8) and neonatal diabetes. The common genes involved in MODY and neonatal diabetes are shown in Figure 21.3C.

The term MODY was coined in 1974 to signify non-insulin-requiring diabetes developing under the age of 25 years in at least one family member. It is dominantly inherited, which means that many cases have a family history of diabetes spanning three generations or more. MODY has been recognised since the 1990s to be a heterogeneous condition, with multiple single gene subtypes. One form is caused by a mutation in the β-cell glucose sensor enzyme glucokinase (see Fig. 21.3B) and affected individuals have an altered set-point for glucose. Glucokinase MODY results in a high fasting glucose (usually >5.5 mmol/L (99 mg/dL)), but a normal post-prandial response and slight elevation of HbA$_{1c}$. It is important to identify these individuals as they do not develop diabetes complications and do not require glucose-lowering drug therapy and monitoring. The other forms of MODY are mostly caused by defective transcription factors that play a key role in β-cell development and function (hepatocyte nuclear factor (HNF) 1α, 1β and 4α). Patients with transcription factor MODY develop progressive diabetes in adolescence or early adulthood and the diabetes is progressive, requiring oral glucose-lowering therapy before eventually needing insulin. Patients with HNF1α and 4α MODY are extremely sensitive to sulphonylureas, so this is the treatment of choice for these individuals. Many cases have been described in which after genetic diagnosis it has been possible to discontinue long-term insulin therapy. As HNF1β is a critical transcription factor not only in pancreatic development, but also in renal and genital tract development in utero, individuals with *HNF1β* mutations often have renal cystic disease and genital tract malformation including infertility.

Neonatal diabetes is variably defined as diabetes that presents in the first 6 months of life, presenting as profound insulin deficiency with hyperglycaemia and DKA. Approximately half of patients with neonatal diabetes have a transient form that remits by about one year of age, with diabetes recurring in adolescence or early adulthood; the remainder have permanent neonatal diabetes. Approximately two-thirds of individuals with the permanent form have an activating mutation in genes encoding the KIR6.2 and SUR1 subunits of the K$_{ATP}$ channel (see Fig. 21.3C). These cause it to be insensitive to glucose-mediated increase in intracellular ATP; as a result, pancreatic β cells do not secrete insulin and insulin treatment is required from soon after birth. However, as affected individuals respond to sulphonylureas, genetic diagnosis can transform their lives, with over 90% managed with oral sulphonylurea treatment. The K$_{ATP}$ channel is found in neurons so mutations can severely affect their function causing developmental delay and epilepsy. Early sulphonylurea treatment can in some cases prevent or improve these neurological consequences.

Presenting problems in diabetes

Hyperglycaemia

Although the presence or absence of diabetes is simply based on confirmation of hyperglycaemia above the diagnostic threshold, defining

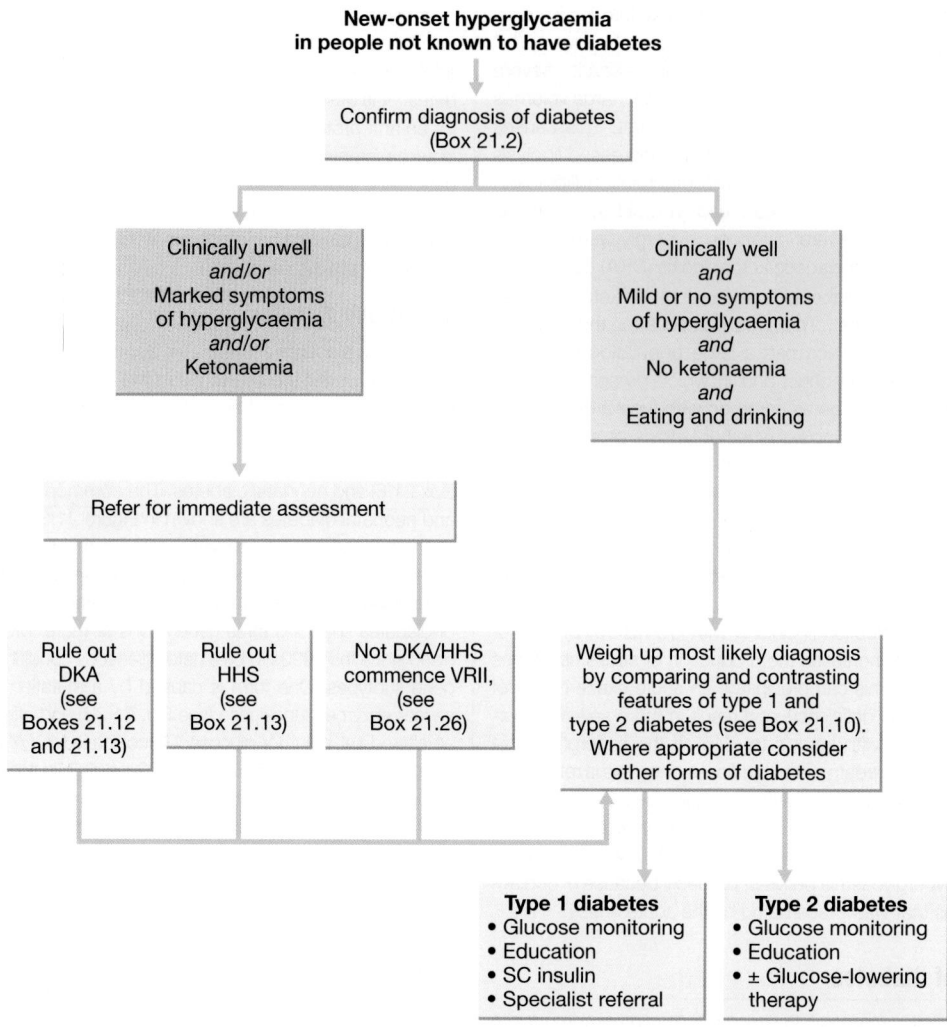

Fig. 21.14 Assessment and initial management of new-onset hyperglycaemia. (DKA = diabetic ketoacidosis; HHS = hyperosmotic hyperglycaemic state; VRII = variable rate insulin infusion)

which type of diabetes has developed can be more complex in some individuals. Initial management involves a careful clinical assessment to decide whether (and if so what type of) immediate treatment is required (Fig. 21.14). Failure to initiate insulin treatment when it is required can result in the development of DKA and even death. Therefore, when the cause of diabetes is in doubt, it may be necessary to start insulin treatment with a view to later withdrawal if it becomes apparent alternative glucose-lowering therapy is sufficient. Such decisions require careful discussion and explanation at a time of high stress.

The classical symptoms of hyperglycaemia and clinical features of type 1 and type 2 diabetes are shown respectively in Box 21.9 and Box 21.10. The classic 'osmotic symptoms' of polyuria (including nocturia), thirst and polydipsia are a consequence of the diuretic effect of significant glycosuria. Weight loss is due to dehydration and loss of calories in urine from glycosuria and, in type 1 diabetes, proteolysis and lipolysis. Severe osmotic symptoms and rapid weight loss are classically associated with the onset of type 1 diabetes, but type 2 diabetes may also present with these symptoms. Uncontrolled hyperglycaemia is associated with increased susceptibility to infection, such as skin infection (boils), genital candidiasis (with pruritus) or urine infection (see p. 748).

At the extremes of age, the distinction between type 1 and type 2 diabetes is usually obvious, but uncertainty can occur, particularly between the ages of 25 and 50 years. However, although type 2 diabetes is classically a condition of middle and old age, it is increasingly diagnosed in children and young adults. Type 1 diabetes most commonly occurs in younger people, but can occur at any age and may develop more insidiously in older individuals (p. 717). Family history of diabetes is common in type 2 diabetes and MODY and there may be a family history of autoimmune conditions in type 1 diabetes. Ethnicity and obesity may point to a diagnosis of type 2 diabetes, but type 1 diabetes can present in any race and at any weight, and it is important not to assign an incorrect diagnostic label at an early stage simply based on stereotypical features. Other causes of diabetes (see Box 21.6), such as pancreatic diabetes, should not be forgotten, particularly if there are suggestive symptoms or signs (e.g. chronic alcohol excess).

All patients presenting with hyperglycaemia should be tested for ketonuria/ketonaemia. The presence of raised ketones implies absolute insulin deficiency and indicates the need for referral to a secondary care centre for further assessment and treatment. This will usually indicate a diagnosis of type 1 diabetes but it should be remembered that 10%–15% of cases of DKA occur in people with type 2 diabetes. Islet autoantibody and C-peptide testing can be helpful in establishing the underlying cause of diabetes (p. 712), although C-peptide is most discriminatory when used at least 3 years after diagnosis (see Box 21.10). Sometimes it may be necessary for clinicians to counsel patients that their diagnosis is provisional and that a definitive diagnosis will only be possible once time has elapsed, the results of supplementary investigations are available and the responsiveness to different therapies can be assessed

i	21.10 Typical characteristics of type 1 and type 2 diabetes[1]		
		Type 1	Type 2
Age at onset		< 40 years	> 50 years
Duration of symptoms		Weeks	Months to years
Body weight		Normal or low	Obese
Ketonuria		Yes	No
Non-fasting serum C-peptide[2]		<200 pmol/L	>900 pmol/l
Rapid ketosis/ decompensation without insulin treatment		Yes	No
Autoantibodies		Positive	Negative
Family history of diabetes		Less common	Common
Other autoimmune disease		Common	Uncommon

[1]The data in this table are typical examples; however, none of these are perfect discriminators, e.g. obese people can get type 1 diabetes; young adults can get type 2 diabetes. [2]C-peptide is most discriminatory when used >3 years after diagnosis. C-peptide may be >200 pmol/L in people with type 1 diabetes in the 'honeymoon period' and may be <600 pmol/l in people with type 2 diabetes who have a marked hyperglycaemia (due to glucotoxicity).

Diabetic ketoacidosis

DKA is an acute metabolic complication of diabetes that is a consequence of *absolute* insulin deficiency. It is a medical emergency with important complications including hypoglycaemia, hypokalaemia, pulmonary oedema, acute respiratory distress syndrome and cerebral oedema. Although mortality rates have fallen in the UK over the past two decades, a single episode of DKA is associated with an approximate 5% risk of death, rising to almost 25% in those with recurrent DKA, particularly in low- and middle-income countries. Death most commonly relates to the underlying precipitating illness rather than direct metabolic complications. DKA most commonly occurs in people with type 1 diabetes and can be the first presentation of the condition (see Box 21.10). It can also occur in type 2 diabetes, particularly if it has been longstanding or in individuals who are ketosis-prone (i.e. have significant β-cell dysfunction) or who have been misclassified as type 2 rather than type 1 diabetes. In established diabetes, DKA may be precipitated by an underlying illness or physiological stress. Infection is the most common of these: pneumonia and urinary tract infection are often implicated. Acute myocardial infarction, cerebrovascular disease and pancreatitis are other common examples of a precipitating illness. Physiological stress such as surgery, trauma and pregnancy can also be implicated. The second most common cause of DKA is insulin deficiency due to discontinuation (accidental or deliberate) or inadequate delivery (error in administration, insulin pump failure, pen malfunction, out of date or inadequate storage) of insulin. Drug and social history may reveal glucocorticoid, sodium-glucose co-transporter 2 (SGLT2) inhibitors or cocaine use, all of which have been associated with DKA. In young people with recurrent episodes of DKA, psychological or personality factors are frequent causes of insulin omission and infrequent or absent monitoring of glucose levels.

Pathogenesis

A clear understanding of the biochemical basis and pathophysiology of DKA is fundamental for its efficient treatment (see Fig. 21.9). DKA is characterised by the cardinal biochemical triad of:

- hyperglycaemia (blood glucose >11.1 mmol/L (200 mg/dL)) or known diabetes* *and*

- hyperketonaemia (≥3.0 mmol/L on fingerprick testing) or ketonuria (more than 2+ on urine dipstick testing) *and*
- metabolic acidosis (venous bicarbonate <15 mmol/L and/or venous pH <7.3 (H+ >50 nmol/L)).

*DKA can occur without hyperglycaemia ('euglycaemic DKA', i.e. glucose <11 mmol/L (<198 mg/dL)), but this occurs in fewer than 5% of cases.

Severe hyperglycaemia (in some cases >100 mmol/L (1800 mg/dL)) causes a profound osmotic diuresis leading to dehydration and electrolyte loss, particularly of sodium and potassium. Ketosis is a consequence of insulin deficiency, exacerbated by elevated catecholamines and other stress hormones, leading to unrestrained lipolysis and supply of free fatty acids (FFAs) for hepatic ketogenesis. When this exceeds the capacity to metabolise acidic ketones, these accumulate in blood. The resulting metabolic acidosis forces hydrogen ions into cells, displacing potassium ions.

There are significant deficits of water and electrolytes in DKA. The average loss of water in moderately severe DKA in an adult is around 100 ml/kg. About half the deficit of total body water is derived from the intracellular compartment and occurs comparatively early in the development of acidosis with few clinical features; the remainder represents loss of extracellular fluid sustained in the later stages, when marked contraction of extracellular fluid volume occurs, with haemoconcentration, a decreased blood volume, and finally a fall in blood pressure and subsequent oliguria (<0.5 ml/kg/hr). There are also deficits in sodium (7–10 mmol/kg), chloride (3–5 mmol/kg) and potassium (3–5 mmol/kg). The plasma concentration of potassium gives very little indication of the total body deficit. Plasma potassium may even be raised initially due to disproportionate loss of water, catabolism of protein and glycogen, and displacement of potassium from the intracellular compartment by H+ ions. However, soon after treatment is started, there is likely to be a precipitous fall in the plasma potassium due to dilution of extracellular potassium by administration of intravenous fluids, the movement of potassium into cells induced by insulin, and the continuing renal loss of potassium (due to secondary hyperaldosteronism as a result of reduced renal perfusion).

The level of hyperglycaemia does not correlate with the severity of the metabolic acidosis, i.e. moderate elevation of blood glucose may be associated with life-threatening ketoacidosis. Type 1 diabetes in pregnancy and the use of sodium-glucose co-transporter 2 (SGLT2) inhibitors are two situations in which euglycaemic DKA can occur. Conversely, in other situations, hyperglycaemia predominates and acidosis is minimal, resulting in a hyperosmolar state (p. 723).

Clinical assessment

The clinical features of ketoacidosis are listed in Box 21.11. These usually progress rapidly over the course of several hours. DKA should be considered if there are the typical presenting symptoms of diabetes in association with nausea, vomiting, abdominal pain, hyperventilation, dehydration or reduced consciousness. In a severe and rapidly progressing case, the striking features are volume depletion, sunken eyes, dry mucous membranes (mouth and nose), dry axillae, decreased skin turgor (e.g. at the subclavicular area), reduced jugular venous pressure, tachycardia and hypotension. Breathing may be deep and sighing (Kussmaul's breathing) due to the compensatory hyperventilation of severe metabolic acidosis. The breath may have the sweet smell of acetone, similar to nail polish remover or pear drops. Acute confusion, a reduced conscious level, or even coma may be present. In infected patients, including those with sepsis, pyrexia may not be present initially because of vasodilatation secondary to acidosis, indeed mild hypothermia may be present. Abdominal pain and vomiting are common features of DKA and may mimic an acute abdomen (see Ch. 9). It is important to examine for signs of a precipitant; auscultation of the chest for signs of consolidation, examination of the abdomen for peritonism or obstruction and inspection of the skin for cellulitis or wounds. Careful examination of the feet for new ulceration or ischaemia is imperative.

---

i 21.11 Clinical features of diabetic ketoacidosis

Symptoms

- Polyuria, thirst
- Weight loss
- Weakness
- Nausea, vomiting

- Leg cramps
- Blurred vision
- Abdominal pain

Signs

- Dehydration
- Hypotension (postural or supine)
- Cold extremities/peripheral cyanosis
- Tachycardia

- Air hunger (Kussmaul's breathing)
- Smell of acetone
- Hypothermia
- Delirium, drowsiness, coma (10%)

---

i 21.12 Indicators of severe diabetic ketoacidosis

- Blood ketones >6 mmol/L
- Bicarbonate <5 mmol/L
- Venous/arterial pH <7.0 (H+ >100 nmol/L)

May also be:

- Persistent hypotension or oliguria
- Hypokalaemia (<3.5 mmol/L)
- Glasgow Coma Scale score <12
- O$_2$ saturation <92% on air
- Systolic blood pressure <90 mmHg
- Heart rate >100 or <60 beats per minute
- Anion gap >16 mmol/L

(pH 7.0–7.25 = moderate DKA; pH 7.26–7.30 = 'mild' DKA)

Investigations

Initial assessment should include the following:

- *Venous blood*: for urea and electrolytes, glucose, bicarbonate and acid–base status to confirm the presence of hyperglycaemia and acidosis. Hyponatraemia and hyperkalaemia are common. Serum amylase is usually elevated in DKA, but rarely indicates coexisting pancreatitis.
- *Blood (or urine if unavailable) analysis for ketones* (p. 710).
- *Electrocardiogram (ECG)* to look for evidence of acute myocardial infarction or electrolyte abnormalities.
- *Chest X-ray* to look for evidence of lung consolidation or pulmonary oedema.
- *Infection screen*: full blood count, blood and urine culture, C-reactive protein, COVID-19 swab if at risk. (N.B. leucocytosis occurs commonly in DKA, but generally represents a stress response rather than infection.)
- *Pregnancy test*: in all women of childbearing age.

Assessment of severity

The presence of one or more of the features listed in Box 21.12 is indicative of severe DKA.

Management

DKA is a medical emergency that should be treated in hospital, preferably in a high-dependency area. The aims of DKA management are to correct circulating volume and electrolyte imbalance while halting lipolysis and suppressing ketogenesis. It is important to identify and treat precipitating causes as well as to prevent complications. The central tenets of the management of DKA include intravenous insulin, intravenous fluid and potassium replacement. An agreed evidence-based protocol should be in place. A referral to the diabetes specialist team should be made as early as possible with review within 24 hours. Regular clinical and biochemical review is essential, particularly during the first 24 hours of treatment. Monitoring for complications is paramount during management. Vital signs including cardiac monitoring should be regularly assessed per protocol: low oxygen saturations may suggest the development of pulmonary oedema and acute respiratory distress syndrome (ARDS). In children and adolescents, the Glasgow Coma Scale (GCS) should be monitored hourly for cerebral oedema. Supportive measures may include nasogastric tube insertion for persistent vomiting or reduced level of consciousness and urinary catheter insertion to assess urine output and monitor treatment of oliguria (<0.5 ml urine/kg/hr). An example of the implementation of a UK guideline for the management of DKA is shown in Figure 21.15.

Fluid replacement

In adults, rapid fluid replacement should be commenced as soon as a diagnosis of DKA is confirmed (see Fig. 21.15). A rapid fluid bolus over 10–15 minutes may be required if systolic blood pressure is <90 mmHg. A more cautious approach is advised in young adults, in pregnancy, in older adults and those with a history of kidney or heart failure. Most guidelines favour correction of the extracellular fluid deficit with isotonic saline (0.9% sodium chloride). Introduction of 10% glucose is recommended when the blood glucose falls below 14 mmol/L (252 mg/dL). The 0.9% saline infusion should be continued to correct circulating volume, with glucose infusion concurrently to prevent hypoglycaemia during rapid uptake of circulating glucose into cells.

Insulin replacement

A fixed-rate intravenous insulin infusion should be commenced according to local protocols (for example a UK guideline recommends 0.1 U/kg body weight/hr (see Fig. 21.15). Blood glucose and blood ketones should be monitored hourly. Response to treatment should be assessed by a blood ketone concentration falling by at least 0.5 mmol/L/hr. Venous bicarbonate or glucose can be used if blood ketone testing is unavailable (aiming for an increase or decrease by 3.0 mmol/L/hr respectively). If blood ketones are not falling by at least 0.5 mmol/L/hr then the insulin infusion should be increased according to local protocols, after checking for malfunction of the insulin infusion. A long-acting insulin analogue in a dose equivalent to the individual's usual regimen should continue to be administered subcutaneously during the initial management of DKA. This provides basal insulin for when the intravenous insulin is discontinued and reduces the risk of rebound hyperglycaemia (or even DKA) recurring in hospital due to insulin interruption or omission – this should be a 'never event'. The fixed rate insulin infusion should be continued until DKA has resolved, defined as blood ketone <0.6 mmol/L, bicarbonate >15 mmol/L and venous pH >7.3.

Potassium replacement

Careful monitoring of potassium is essential to the management of DKA as both hypo- and hyperkalaemia can occur (see above) and are life-threatening. Potassium is not usually recommended with the initial 1 litre of 0.9% sodium chloride as the primary focus at this stage is on restoring circulating volume and renal failure may be present. Potassium should be measured urgently on a venous blood gas sample and then reassessed after 1 hour, 2 hours and then 2 hourly thereafter. Treatment with 0.9% sodium chloride with potassium chloride 40 mmol/L is recommended if the serum potassium is between 3.5 and 5.5 mmol/L and there is no evidence of oliguria (see Fig. 21.15). If potassium is >5.5 mmol/L then potassium is not added to fluid replacement. If potassium is <3.5 mmol/L at presentation then begin cardiac monitoring and involve the critical care team as additional potassium will be required. Most guidelines aim to maintain potassium between 4.0 and 5.0 mmol/L.

Intravenous bicarbonate and phosphate

Adequate fluid and insulin replacement should resolve the acidosis. The use of intravenous bicarbonate therapy is not generally recommended (due to lack of evidence of benefit), but may be considered in the context of a pH of <6.9 following discussion with a senior specialist clinician. Acidosis may reflect an adaptive response, improving oxygen delivery to the tissues, and so excessive bicarbonate may induce a paradoxical fall

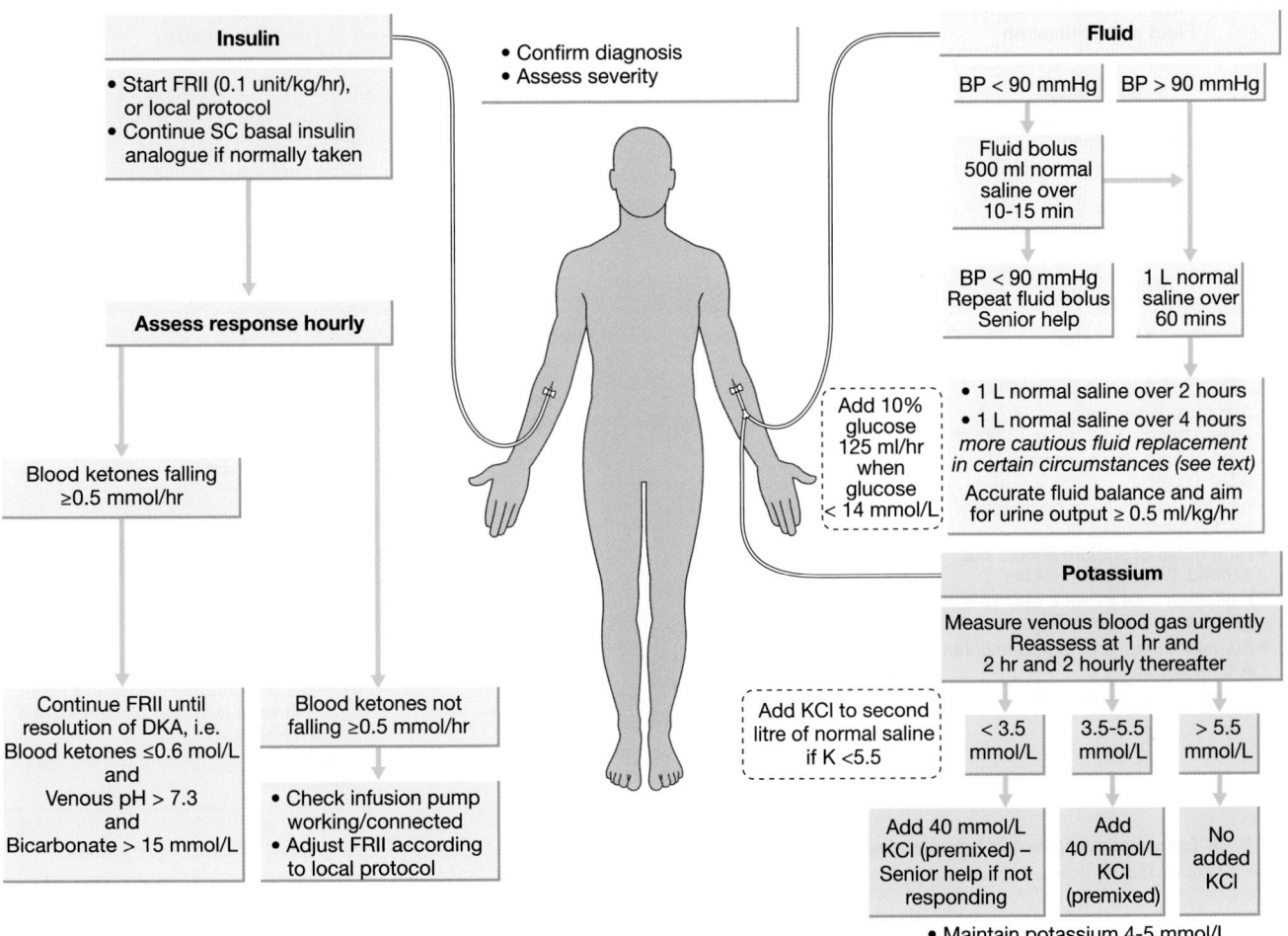

Fig. 21.15 Emergency management of diabetic ketoacidosis. (BP = blood pressure; FRII = fixed rate insulin infusion; KCl = potassium chloride; SC = subcutaneous)

in cerebrospinal fluid pH; this has been implicated in the pathogenesis of cerebral oedema in children and young adults. There is little evidence for intravenous phosphate replacement, but levels of <0.6 mmol/L are often corrected, particularly in the presence of respiratory or muscle weakness.

Ongoing management

Restoration of the usual insulin regimen, by subcutaneous injection, should not be instituted until the patient is: (i) biochemically stable and (ii) able to eat and drink normally. The fixed rate insulin infusion should be continued for 30 minutes after short-acting (or premixed) insulin is given at a mealtime. If using an insulin pump, then the infusion should be started during the daytime at the usual basal rate (commencement overnight is not recommended as ward staff may be unfamiliar with this method of insulin delivery) and the fixed insulin rate infusion should be continued until the next meal bolus is given.

It is important to review the precipitating factors that led to DKA. Glycaemic control, glucose monitoring, insulin injection technique and injection sites should all be considered. If insulin pump therapy is used then it is important to ensure that there is an adequate supply of equipment, the insulin pump is working (for example not out of warranty) and that there is access to 'back up' insulin within expiry date via pen injector devices. DKA prevention should be discussed and written guidance on 'sick day rules' provided or reinforced. A blood ketone meter should be provided. A telephone number for the diabetes specialist team should be made available at the point of discharge from hospital. Given the mortality rates associated with DKA, early educational assessment and the provision of a personalised management plan are critical. Specialist psychological support may also be necessary.

Hyperglycaemic hyperosmolar state

Hyperglycaemic hyperosmolar state (HHS) is a medical emergency that is a consequence of prolonged *relative* insulin deficiency and so requires a different management approach from DKA. There is no precise definition of HHS, but it is characterised by hypovolaemia, severe hyperglycaemia (> 30 mmol/L (>540 mg/dL)) and hyperosmolality (serum osmolality > 320 mOsmol/kg), without significant ketonaemia (<3 mmol/L) or acidosis (pH >7.3 (H+ <50 nmol/L), bicarbonate >15 mmol/L). It most often occurs in older people (often in long-term care) who may have impaired thirst perception, cognitive impairment or reduced ability to drink water. Conscious level is often impaired, particularly when osmolality is >340 mOsmol/L. Mortality rates are higher than DKA (up to 20%) reflecting the age and frailty of the population, but it is increasingly seen in younger adults particularly at the time of diagnosis of type 2 diabetes.

The pathogenesis of HHS is incompletely understood. As with DKA, there is glycosuria, leading to an osmotic diuresis, but renal loss of water is in excess to that of sodium and potassium (hypernatraemia is a common finding). In HHS, hyperglycaemia usually develops over a longer period than in DKA (a few days to weeks), causing more profound hyperglycaemia and dehydration (fluid loss may be 10–22 L in a person weighing 100 kg). The reason that people with HHS do not develop significant ketoacidosis is unclear, although it has been speculated that insulin levels, although too low to stimulate glucose uptake in insulin-sensitive tissues, are still sufficient to prevent lipolysis and subsequent ketogenesis. Differentiating HHS and DKA in individual cases can be challenging, particularly in the setting of severe intercurrent illness that can be complicated by starvation ketosis, non-ketotic acidosis (acute kidney injury, lactic acidosis) and the increased prescription of SGLT2 inhibitors.

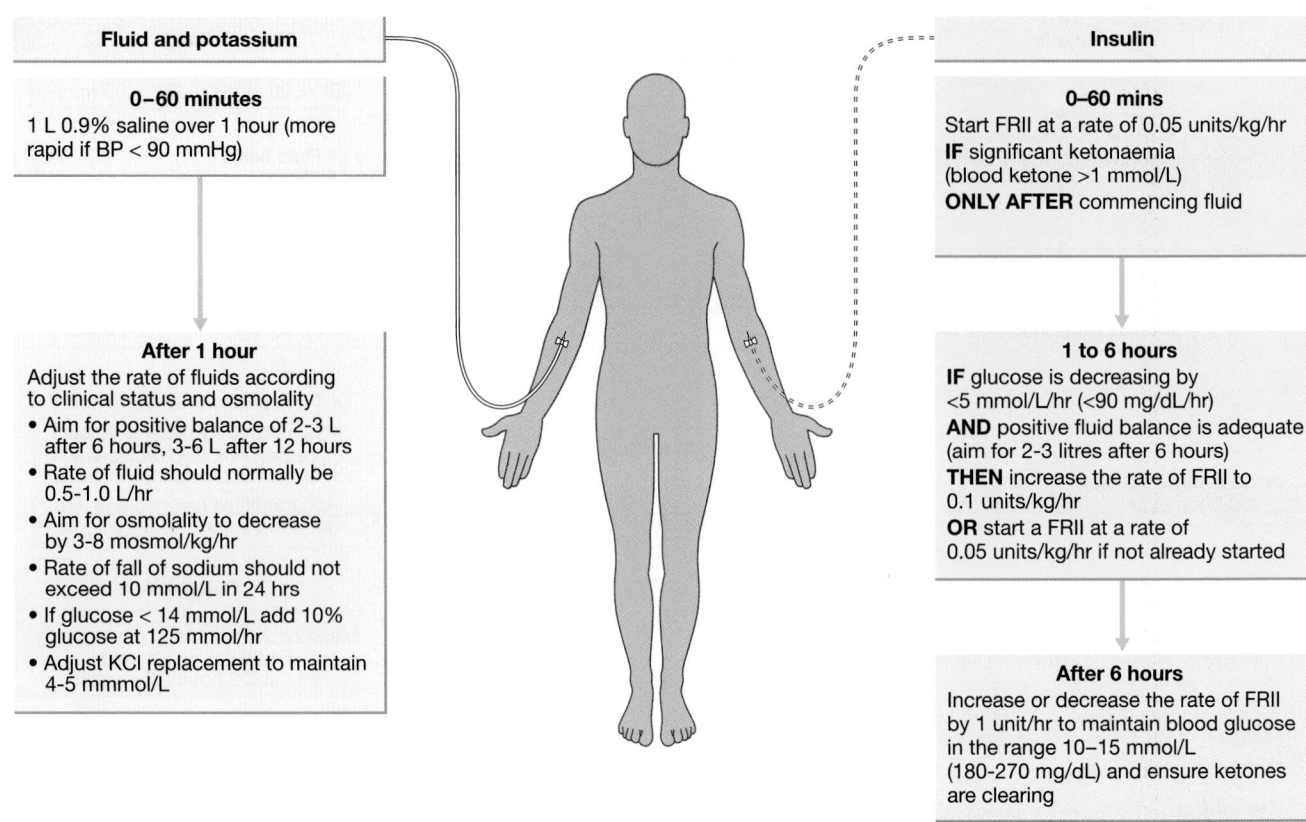

Fig. 21.16 Emergency management of hyperglycaemic hyperosmolar state. Dashed intravenous infusion line represents 'if required'. (FRII = fixed rate insulin infusion; KCl = potassium chloride)

i 21.13	Typical characteristics of HHS and DKA	
	HHS	**DKA**
Age	Older	Younger
Classification	Established pre-diabetes/type 2 diabetes or first presentation	Established type 1 diabetes or first presentation
Duration of onset	Days to weeks	Hours to days
Abdominal pain	Uncommon	Common
Volume depletion	10%–20%	5%–10%
Insulin deficiency	Relative	Absolute
Glucose	Usually >30 mmol/L	Usually >11.1 mmol/L
Ketonaemia	<3.0 mmol/L	>3.0 mmol/L
Acidosis	Bicarbonate >15 pH >7.3	Bicarbonate <15 pH 7.0–7.3

(DKA = diabetic ketoacidosis; HHS = hyperglycaemic hyperosmolar state)

The clinical features of HHS and DKA are compared and contrasted in Box 21.13. A mixed picture of HHS and DKA can occur in up to one-third of hyperglycaemic crises. If the predominant diagnosis is unclear then early specialist input is required to guide management and if necessary adjust local protocols.

HHS is more likely to occur when high glucose levels are sustained over many weeks or months. Common precipitating factors include infection (such as pneumonia or urinary tract infection) and other acute illness (such as acute myocardial infarction, cerebrovascular events), leading to an increase in counter-regulatory hormones. HHS can also occur in the context of drug therapy, such as glucocorticoids, and post-operatively in

hospital. Poor prognostic signs include hypothermia, hypotension (systolic blood pressure <90 mmHg), tachy- or bradycardia, severe hypernatraemia (sodium >160 mmol/L), serum osmolality >360 mOsmol/kg, and the presence of multiple comorbidities.

The principles of therapy are shown in Figure 21.16. The aims are to normalise osmolality and blood glucose, replace fluid and electrolyte losses, and prevent complications such as arterial or venous thrombosis (via subcutaneous thromboprophylaxis), foot ulceration (with careful protection of feet – see p. 751), cerebral oedema and central pontine myelinosis (see Ch. 19). Co-morbidities also need to be taken into account; for example, rapid fluid replacement may precipitate cardiac failure in patients with coronary artery disease, while delirium commonly occurs in older patients. Historically, management of HHS was modelled on DKA protocols, but there is increasing recognition of better outcomes using a slower approach to correction of the electrolyte and other metabolic abnormalities (in contrast to DKA there is no urgent need to correct ketoacidosis). As HHS occurs in people whose brains are at higher risk of injury, rapid shifts in osmolality should be avoided with less aggressive fluid replacement and rate of glucose lowering guided by serial calculations of serum osmolality and glucose. Key recommendations are that 0.9% sodium chloride solution alone is used for initial treatment and that insulin is introduced only when the rate of fall in blood glucose has plateaued.

If osmolality cannot be measured frequently, osmolarity can be calculated using the following equation from measurements of plasma electrolytes and glucose (in mmol/L) and used as a surrogate (the normal range is 280–296 mOsmol/L):

$$\text{Plasma osmolarity} = 2[\text{Na}^+] + [\text{glucose}] + [\text{urea}]$$

A limitation of this approach is that hyperglycaemia, by increasing serum osmolality, causes the movement of water out of cells into plasma, reducing Na^+ levels by dilution. Therefore, in the presence of hyperglycaemia, a corrected $[\text{Na}^+]$ can be calculated for use in this formula by

- Level 1 hypoglycaemia (*alert value*) as <3.9 mmol/L but ≥3.0 mmol/L (<70 mg/dL but ≥54 mg/dL)
- Level 2 hypoglycaemia (*clinically significant*) is defined as <3.0 mmol/L (<54 mg/dL). This level is unequivocally low and suggests clinically important biochemical hypoglycaemia
- Level 3 hypoglycaemia (*severe*) is defined as any low blood glucose level leading to cognitive impairment and the need for external assistance to provide glucose, glucagon or other corrective activity

adding 1.6 mmol/L to the measured [Na⁺] for every 5.55 mmol/L (100 mg/dL) increment of serum glucose above normal.

Hypoglycaemia

Hypoglycaemia has been defined by the American Diabetes Association in three distinct levels (see Box 21.14) – level 1 (alert value), level 2 (clinically significant) and level 3 (severe). When hypoglycaemia develops in people without diabetes, it is called 'spontaneous' hypoglycaemia: definition, causes and investigation are described on page 689. Hypoglycaemia seldom occurs in people without diabetes, but is very common in people with diabetes, mainly due to insulin and (to a lesser extent) sulphonylurea therapy. Unlike endogenous insulin, secretion of which is down-regulated when blood glucose falls, these therapies continue to act even when blood glucose is low.

More than 10% of people with type 1 diabetes report an episode of level 3 hypoglycaemia per year. CGM devices show more frequent episodes of level 2 hypoglycaemia – up to every 2 days in some studies. Importantly this is more frequent than hypoglycaemia measured by self-reported events or blood glucose monitoring. This finding is likely related to the improved detection by CGM. There may be an element of over-reporting at lower levels of interstitial fluid glucose, owing to lower reliability of some CGM devices, but accuracy of CGM devices is constantly improving.

The critical importance of glucose as a fuel source for the brain means that, in health, a number of mechanisms are in place to ensure that glucose homeostasis is maintained. If blood glucose falls, three primary physiological defence mechanisms operate:

- endogenous insulin release from pancreatic β cells is suppressed
- release of glucagon from pancreatic α cells is increased
- the autonomic nervous system is activated, with release of catecholamines both systemically and within tissues.

In addition, stress hormones, such as cortisol and growth hormone, are released into the blood. These actions reduce peripheral glucose uptake and increase hepatic glucose production, maintaining a glucose supply to the brain. Retained endogenous insulin secretion in people with type 1 diabetes (measured using C-peptide) has a glucose smoothing effect that reduces the frequency of hypoglycaemia, as insulin secretion is inhibited by falling blood glucose levels. However, in most individuals with type 1 diabetes endogenous insulin production falls to minimal amounts within a few years of diagnosis, increasing glucose variability and the risk of hypoglycaemia. In addition, within 5 years of diagnosis, many people with type 1 diabetes lose their ability to release glucagon during hypoglycaemia. The reasons for this are unknown and may result from loss of α-cell regulation by insulin or other products of the β cell.

Rates of hypoglycaemia are generally lower in insulin-treated type 2 diabetes than in type 1 diabetes, particularly in individuals with shorter duration of diabetes. This is likely due to preservation of significant endogenous insulin release for longer in most individuals, but also to differences in insulin regimens, i.e. more frequent use of intermediate- or longer- (rather than short-) acting insulins.

Autonomic

- Sweating
- Trembling
- Pounding heart
- Hunger
- Anxiety

Neuroglycopenic

- Delirium
- Drowsiness
- Speech difficulty
- Inability to concentrate
- Incoordination
- Irritability, anger

Non-specific

- Nausea
- Tiredness
- Headache

N.B. Symptoms differ with age; children exhibit behavioural changes (such as naughtiness or irritability), while older people experience more prominent neurological symptoms (such as visual disturbance and ataxia).

Level 3 hypoglycaemia is about 10 times less common in people with type 2 diabetes treated with sulphonylureas than in those treated with insulin therapy. As these agents were previously widely prescribed, the proportion of cases of hypoglycaemia attributable to their use was high. However, with decreasing use of sulphonylureas over the last 20 years (due to the advent of newer agents), this proportion has dramatically fallen. Nevertheless, hypoglycaemia remains a significant risk in older people who are taking these agents, particularly those with renal impairment.

Clinical assessment

Symptoms of hypoglycaemia (Box 21.15) comprise two main groups: those related to acute activation of the autonomic nervous system and those secondary to glucose deprivation of the brain (neuroglycopenia). Symptoms of hypoglycaemia are idiosyncratic, differing with age and duration of diabetes, and also depending on the circumstances in which hypoglycaemia occurs. Hypoglycaemia also affects mood, inducing a state of increased tension and low energy. Learning to recognise the early onset of hypoglycaemia is an important aspect of the education of people with diabetes managed with insulin.

Awareness of hypoglycaemia

For most individuals, the glucose level (threshold) at which they first become aware of hypoglycaemia is not constant, but varies according to the circumstances in which hypoglycaemia arises (e.g. during the night or during exercise). In addition, with longer duration of diabetes, and particularly in response to frequent hypoglycaemia, the threshold for generation of symptom responses to hypoglycaemia shifts to a lower glucose concentration. This cerebral adaptation has a similar effect on the counter-regulatory hormonal response to hypoglycaemia. Taken together, this means that individuals with type 1 diabetes may develop reduced (impaired) awareness of hypoglycaemia. Symptoms can be experienced less intensely, or even be absent, despite blood glucose concentrations below level 2 hypoglycaemia. Such individuals are at an especially high risk of level 3 hypoglycaemia. The prevalence of impaired awareness of hypoglycaemia increases with time; overall, it affects around 20%–25% of people with type 1 diabetes and under 10% with insulin-treated type 2 diabetes.

Risk factors and causes of hypoglycaemia

Risk factors and causes of hypoglycaemia in patients taking insulin or sulphonylurea drugs are listed in Box 21.16. Hypoglycaemia is the limiting factor in glycaemic management for people with type 1 diabetes: it is unpleasant and fear of the lived experience and its consequences is understandable. In some people with diabetes, fear can have a major impact on their willingness and ability to achieve target glucose levels. Level 3 hypoglycaemia can cause serious morbidity (e.g. convulsions, coma, cerebral oedema, focal neurological lesions) and has a mortality

21.16 Hypoglycaemia in diabetes: common causes and risk factors

Excess insulin

- Erroneous injection of insulin (e.g. dose miscalculation or injection of incorrect insulin type)
- Deliberate overdose
- Lipohypertrophy at injection sites (causing variable insulin absorption)
- Bariatric surgery (can cause hyperinsulinaemia)

Increased sensitivity to insulin

- Exercise
- Weight loss
- Sudden reduction in glucocorticoids
- Unrecognised Addison's disease

Reduced carbohydrate intake/increased metabolic demand

- Irregular or missed meal
- Gastroparesis due to autonomic neuropathy causing variable carbohydrate absorption
- Bariatric surgery
- Malabsorption, e.g. coeliac disease
- Eating disorder
- Early pregnancy
- Breast feeding

Reduced gluconeogenesis and/or glycogen reserves

- Alcohol
- Chronic kidney disease*
- Advanced liver disease*

Increased glucose variability

- Absent/minimal endogenous insulin secretion (reduced C-peptide)
- Long-duration type 1 diabetes/insulin-treated type 2 diabetes
- Young age of onset of type 1 diabetes

Reduced ability to detect hypoglycaemia

- Impaired awareness of hypoglycaemia
- Rapid improvement in and/or strict glycaemic control
- Previous severe hypoglycaemia
- Long-duration type 1 diabetes/duration of insulin-treated type 2 diabetes
- Older age
- Dementia
- Sleep
- No or inadequate glucose monitoring

*Also cause reduced insulin clearance.

21.17 Emergency treatment of hypoglycaemia

Biochemical or symptomatic hypoglycaemia (Levels 1 and 2)

In the UK, it is recommended that all glucose levels <4.0 mmol/L[1] are treated ('4 is the floor'). People with diabetes who recognise developing hypoglycaemia are encouraged to treat immediately. Options available include:

- Oral fast-acting carbohydrate (10–15 g) is taken as glucose drink or tablets or confectionery, e.g. 5–7 Dextrosol tablets (or 4–5 Glucotabs)
- Repeat capillary glucose measurement 10–15 mins later. If still < 4.0 mmol/L, repeat above treatment
- If blood glucose remains < 4.0 mmol/L after three cycles (30–45 mins), contact a doctor. Consider glucagon 1 mg IM or IV 10% glucose (600–800 mL/hour – caution in renal and cardiac disease)
- Once blood glucose is >4.0 mmol/L, take additional long-acting carbohydrate of choice
- Do not omit insulin injection if due but review regimen

Severe (Level 3)

This means individuals are either unconscious or unable to treat hypoglycaemia themselves. Treatment is usually by a relative or by paramedical or medical staff. Immediate treatment as below is needed.

- If patient is unconscious/fitting or very aggressive or nil by mouth, parenteral treatment is required:
  IV 75 mL 20% dextrose over 15 mins (= 15 g)[2]
  Or
  IV 150 mL 10% dextrose over 15 mins
  Or
  IM glucagon (1 mg) – may be ineffective in undernourished people, severe liver disease and in repeated hypoglycaemia. Caution in hypoglycaemia induced by oral glucose-lowering therapy.
- If patient is conscious and able to swallow, but confused, disorientated or aggressive:
  Give 2 tubes of 40% glucose gel – squeezed into mouth between teeth and gums
  Repeat blood glucose measurement after 10–15 mins and if ineffective after 3 cycles call doctor and consider IM glucagon (1 mg) or IV 10% glucose

[1]4.0 mmol/L = 72 mg/dL. [2]Use of 50% dextrose is no longer recommended.
(IM = intramuscular; IV = intravenous)
Adapted from updated JBDS Diabetes at the Front Door guideline, March 2020. Available at: abcd.care/resource/diabetes-front-door.

of up to 4% in people treated with insulin. Rarely, sudden death during sleep occurs in otherwise healthy young patients with type 1 diabetes ('dead-in-bed syndrome'); this may be a consequence of hypoglycaemia-induced cardiac arrhythmia. Hypoglycaemia is very disruptive to normal daily activities including employment, driving (see Box 21.22), travel, sport and personal relationships.

Nocturnal hypoglycaemia in people with type 1 diabetes is common, but often undetected as it may not cause waking from sleep. People with diabetes may describe poor quality of sleep, morning headaches and vivid dreams or nightmares, or a partner may observe profuse sweating, restlessness, twitching or even seizures. The only reliable way to identify this problem is to use a CGM device with a low glucose alarm.

In healthy individuals, muscle contraction during exercise causes insulin-independent glucose uptake into muscle. Suppression of endogenous insulin secretion is key to the normal physiological response to exercise as glucose derived from hepatic glucose production can be transported into muscle via other pathways; this physiological mechanism minimises any risk of 'spontaneous' exercise-induced hypoglycaemia. However, in insulin-treated diabetes, circulating insulin levels may actually increase with exercise because of improved blood flow at the site of injection, causing a significant risk of hypoglycaemia. This occurs most commonly with prolonged and/or aerobic exercise. In addition, the 'double hit' of hypoglycaemia and exercise is responsible for the additional increased risk of nocturnal hypoglycaemia that

can occur after exercise, possibly as a result of glycogen depletion. In contrast, high-intensity exercise may initially cause blood glucose to rise significantly because of stimulation of adrenaline (epinephrine) production. Close monitoring of blood glucose, education and lived experience (usually with an element of trial and error) are key in preventing exercise-induced hypoglycaemia.

Unfortunately, hypoglycaemia sometimes occurs within the hospital setting. This may result from errors in insulin dose or type of insulin prescribed or infusion of IV insulin without glucose. In addition, hypoglycaemia may occur due to changes in meal timings (e.g. fasting for procedures) or content, failure to provide usual snacks, reduced carbohydrate intake because of vomiting or reduced appetite, or factors related to the hospital admission, e.g. concurrent illness or discontinuation of long-term glucocorticoid therapy. The diabetes team has a role in continuing education of healthcare staff in all areas to prevent these situations occurring; regular review of any adverse events is also critical to prevention.

Management

Reversing hypoglycaemia

Treatment of hypoglycaemia depends on its severity and on whether the patient is conscious and able to swallow (Box 21.17). Levels 1 and 2 hypoglycaemia should be reversed with fast-acting carbohydrate, repeated measurements of glucose and, if necessary, adjustment of glucose lowering therapy. There is an understandable tendency to 'overtreat' episodes of hypoglycaemia, resulting in significant hyperglycaemia in the aftermath. Level 3 hypoglycaemia may also be treated with oral carbohydrate if the patient does not have impaired consciousness. If parenteral therapy is required, then as soon as the individual is able to swallow, oral glucose should be given. Full recovery may not occur immediately and reversal of cognitive impairment may not be complete until 60 minutes after normoglycaemia is restored. When hypoglycaemia has occurred in a patient treated with a long- or intermediate-acting insulin or a long-acting sulphonylurea, such as glibenclamide, the possibility of recurrence should be anticipated; to prevent this, infusion of 10% dextrose titrated to the patient's blood glucose, or provision of additional oral carbohydrate may be necessary.

If a person with diabetes fails to regain consciousness after blood glucose is restored to normal, then cerebral oedema and other causes of impaired consciousness – such as alcohol intoxication, a post-ictal state or cerebral haemorrhage – should be considered. Cerebral oedema is associated with a high mortality and morbidity.

Following recovery, it is important to try to identify a cause and make appropriate adjustments to therapy. Unless the reason for a hypoglycaemic episode is clear, people with diabetes should be advised to reduce the next dose of insulin by 10%–20% and seek medical advice about further adjustments in dose.

The management of self-poisoning with oral glucose-lowering agents is described on page 228.

Reducing future risk of hypoglycaemia

Every diabetes consultation should include gathering information about any low glucose levels measurements, the nature of symptoms with the measured levels of hypoglycaemia and whether there have been any episodes of level 3 hypoglycaemia. It is important to review blood glucose monitoring and CGM data with the patient to determine the details around each episode: recognition of patterns can be aided by increasing the number of measurements and triangulation with diary recordings of insulin dosing, carbohydrate intake and physical activity. The lived experience of previous hypoglycaemia and any resultant fear should be explored. Education is fundamental to the prevention of hypoglycaemia and should focus on risk factors for, and treatment of, hypoglycaemia. The importance of regular glucose monitoring, flexible insulin regimens and the need to have glucose (and glucagon) readily available should be reinforced. Relatives and friends also need to be familiar with the symptoms and signs of hypoglycaemia and should be instructed in how to help (including how to inject glucagon).

The goal is always to minimise the risk of hypoglycaemia while still reaching target glucose levels and HbA$_{1c}$. Adjustments in insulin regimen based on patterns of glucose should be agreed with the person with diabetes over time to achieve their goals. HbA$_{1c}$ targets should be individualised to balance the risk of hypoglycaemia with the risk of complications. Upgrading insulin regimens to rapid-acting and long-acting insulin analogues is associated with a lower frequency of nocturnal hypoglycaemia. The use of CGM devices (particularly those with low glucose alarms), is invaluable. CGM values and trend arrows provide important information upon which to base decisions on doses of short-acting (bolus) insulin to be administered in relation to planned carbohydrate ingestion; thus, glucose can be kept to target while hypoglycaemia is prevented. The use of sensor-augmented CSII systems, particularly those that incorporate a 'low glucose suspend' feature, can virtually abolish hypoglycaemia. Transplantation should be considered in cases of severe intractable hypoglycaemia (see p. 742).

Management of diabetes

Contemporary specialist diabetes care is delivered by a multidisciplinary team including medical staff, specialist nurses, nursing assistants, dieticians, podiatrists, pharmacists, retinal screeners, psychologists, health care assistants and administrative staff. Ideally these staff are co-located in an ambulatory care or diabetes centre, which need not necessarily be on a hospital site, and there should be close and dynamic links with primary care and community-based diabetes specialist nurses, all involved in continuing professional development.

The aims for both types 1 and 2 diabetes are initially to relieve osmotic symptoms (see p. 725) and then to minimise the risks of long-term microvascular and macrovascular complications. Microvascular complications are prevented by targeting hyperglycaemia, but control of macrovascular complications also requires management of associated risk factors, particularly hypertension, dyslipidaemia and cigarette smoking. Initial investigation and management is outlined in Figure 21.20.

Due to the risk of complications, people with all forms of diabetes should be kept under review with regular monitoring, adjustment of treatment, and screening to detect treatable complications as early as possible. Diabetes care is delivered in primary care for the majority of people with type 2 diabetes and in specialist centres for those with type 1 diabetes or complex treatment regimens and/or complications. A checklist for follow-up visits is given in Box 21.18. Frequency of appointments usually ranges from 3-monthly to annually depending on whether targets are being achieved.

Type 2 diabetes Where there are no 'red flags' of ketosis or rapid weight loss, initial management of type 2 diabetes involves dietary and lifestyle advice, which should aim at inducing remission of the condition (see p. 732). However, adding in oral glucose-lowering drugs is more likely to be required at an early stage for those who have symptomatic hyperglycaemia or a high HbA$_{1c}$. Education is key to achieving and maintaining a healthy lifestyle in type 2 diabetes. Management should be individualised, taking into account personal and cultural beliefs, individual circumstances, comorbidities and other factors.

Type 1 diabetes People with a new diagnosis of type 1 diabetes require substantial initial education and support around diet, glucose monitoring, the technicalities of insulin administration and dose adjustment, and the recognition and treatment of hypoglycaemia (Box 21.19). A diagnosis of type 1 diabetes can be profoundly life-altering not least because individuals have often previously been healthy and have now been diagnosed with a long-term condition that requires restrictions to diet and lifestyle, regular finger-pricks and multiple daily injections. Hypoglycaemia is unpleasant, can be socially embarrassing and can have significant morbidity and indeed mortality. Type 1 diabetes also has significant potential impact on employment, education, driving, overseas travel, family planning and can result in increased travel and life insurance premiums. Therefore, people living with type 1 diabetes often have higher levels of psychological and psychiatric morbidity and require substantial ongoing support and encouragement from diabetes healthcare professionals, including psychological support.

As duration of type 1 diabetes increases, maintenance of good glycaemic control can become progressively more challenging, despite the lived experience of managing insulin therapy. Hypoglycaemia tends to become more frequent, as protective counter-regulatory hormone responses and warning symptoms diminish. Maintaining strict glycaemic control, with minimal hypoglycaemia, is extremely challenging with conventional subcutaneous insulin therapy and requires motivation and meticulous attention in terms of dietary factors, glucose monitoring and decision-making around insulin dosing.

Some individuals with type 1 diabetes have long-term sub-optimal glycaemic control. The reasons for this are complex, but in many cases relate to difficulty finding time to devote the effort required to self-manage the condition in the context of other events and demands within their personal, family and work lives. Such factors vary across the lifespan with major differences between individuals. Other individuals have more serious psychological problems in accepting or adjusting to the diagnosis. These factors can lead to behaviours that have a negative impact on glycaemic control such as: omission of insulin injections (either deliberate or accidental), taking insulin injections after meals, taking fixed doses of insulin or doses based on symptoms (e.g. taking extra insulin when person feels thirsty), under-dosing with insulin to reduce risk of hypoglycaemia, consumption of foods high in unrefined carbohydrate,

21.18 How to review a patient in the diabetes clinic

Approach to the diabetes consultation

Introduction (agenda-setting)	'How are you?' 'What matters to you?' (Is translator required?)
Demographics	Age, type of diabetes, duration of diabetes
Microvascular complications	Retinopathy/maculopathy Renal function (eGFR) Microalbuminuria/proteinuria Foot examination
Macrovascular complications	Cardiovascular disease Cerebrovascular disease Peripheral vascular disease
Metabolic	BMI/weight trajectory Diet (quality/calories)/CHO counting Current glucose-lowering treatment (adherence/administration) HbA$_{1c}$ Step-wise approach to glucose monitoring (frequency, timing, representativeness or reliability of data) Hypoglycaemia (frequency, timing, symptoms, context, episodes of level 3 hypoglycaemia, consequences, driving) Hyperglycaemia (frequency, timing, symptoms, context, episodes of DKA/ HHS, consequences) Glycaemic variability if AGP available
Cardiovascular risk	BP Cholesterol Smoking cessation
Other	Pregnancy/contraception Exercise Sexual dysfunction Alcohol Driving
Summarise	Main action points Goal setting Changes to treatment Referrals within team Other referrals Accessing support prior to next appointment

Remember:
- Person-centred (lifestyle, occupation, travel, behaviour)
- Language matters
- Start with the 'Good News'
- Culturally sensitive
- Collaborative
- Empathetic
- Empowering
- Reassuring
- Non-judgemental

(AGP = Ambulatory Glucose Profile; BMI = Body Mass Index; CHO = carbohydrate; DKA = diabetic ketoacidosis; eGFR = estimated glomerular filtration rate; HHS = hyperglycaemic hyperosmolar state).

21.19 Learning outcomes on the day of type 1 diabetes diagnosis

- Explain what is type 1 diabetes
- Explore any fears and anxieties and ask questions
- Be able to check blood glucose/ketones
- Be able to administer insulin and understand the correct storage of insulin
- Understand the target blood glucose
- Understand the role of rapid-acting insulin and its relationship with food
- Understand how to safely dispose of used needles and lancets
- Appreciate that people with diabetes should follow similar dietary recommendations as appropriate for non-diabetic people and that insulin is adjusted to carbohydrate content of diet
- Understand what a 'hypo' is and how to treat it
- Be aware they can access their own diabetes health records
- Understand what to expect from the diabetes team, how to make contact and the date/time/mode of their next interaction
- Understand that notifying DVLA* about the diagnosis of type 1 diabetes is a legal requirement and the precautions to be taken before driving
- Understand that sub-optimal glycaemic control increases risks to both mother and baby
- Understand that their employer should know they have been diagnosed with type 1 diabetes

*Or equivalent in other countries.
(DVLA = United Kingdom Driver and Vehicle Licensing Agency)

Type 1 diabetes is associated with other immune-mediated disorders (see Ch. 4), including thyroid disease, coeliac disease, Addison's disease, pernicious anaemia and vitiligo. Awareness of these is important so that they can be diagnosed promptly and managed appropriately. Approximately 30% of women and 15% of men with type 1 diabetes have at least one related immune-mediated condition. The association with hypothyroidism is strongest (present in ~20% overall); coeliac disease is the second most common (present in 4%) and is particularly associated with childhood-onset diabetes. Thyroid function should be checked annually in all patients with type 1 diabetes and systematic screening for coeliac disease is recommended in many countries.

Self-assessment of glycaemic control

Type 2 diabetes People with type 2 diabetes usually only need to self-test capillary blood glucose regularly if they require insulin or sulphonylurea therapy. For those on insulin, blood glucose testing 1–4 times daily (depending on the intensity of the prescribed regimen) helps guide insulin dosing and to manage diet, exercise and illness. It also helps detect and protect against hypoglycaemia. This is also the case for sulphonylurea therapy. People with type 2 diabetes who are on neither of these therapies do not have an absolute need to test blood glucose, but it can be useful, e.g. for self-education on the effects of food and exercise on glycaemia. Fasting or pre-meal blood glucose target is usually 5.0–7.0 mmol/L (90–126 mg/dL). Those who require to test should be taught how to monitor their own blood glucose using an electronic meter and prescribed adequate supplies of blood glucose testing strips.

Type 1 diabetes People with type 1 diabetes are advised to test capillary blood glucose four or more times per day as they usually require intensive insulin regimens. Blood glucose meters with dual functionality for ketone testing are particularly useful to provide early warning of ketosis and help prevent ketoacidosis when blood glucose is high and/or during intercurrent illness.

CGM systems are increasingly becoming a standard of care in type 1 diabetes. Specific devices are funded by the NHS in the UK, as their use is associated with improved glycaemic control and is cost-effective. CGM widens the lens through which day-to-day glycaemia can be monitored

non-adherence to carbohydrate counting, over-treatment of episodes of hypoglycaemia and avoidance of glucose monitoring. Attempts to improve glycaemic control may involve enhanced input and support from diabetes specialist nurses and dietitians, more regular review in out-patient clinics, referral into structured education programmes and (increasingly) provision or recommendation of technologies like CGM and CSII therapy (where resources permit). However, even with these potentially life-transforming interventions and technologies, type 1 diabetes remains a very challenging condition.

by people with diabetes and provides a more holistic view of the lived experience of diabetes. CGM data are summarised in an Ambulatory Glucose Profile (AGP). This display provides a graphical representation of interstitial glucose over time, allowing trends to be readily identified (Fig. 21.17). Summary metrics include: mean glucose, time in range, time above range and time below range (see below). Glucose variability over time is reported as standard deviation and percentage coefficient of variation. A 'Glucose Management Indicator' is now available on some CGM devices corresponding to 'estimated HbA_{1c}' (eA_{1c}): the accuracy of this statistic increases with the volume of CGM data available (minimum 10 days and preferably >14 days).

The proportion of time spent within an optimal glycaemic range is increasingly recognised as a clinically meaningful tool. Time in range (TIR) denotes the percentage of time each day spent within agreed glucose targets (Fig. 21.18). The international consensus for 'in range' glucose values is between 3.9 and 10 mmol/L (70–180 md/dL) inclusive, with lower and higher levels termed time below range (TBR) and time above range (TAR). TIR of >70% is considered the optimum target for most people living with diabetes on the basis of extrapolation from the Diabetes Control and Complications Trial. In people at higher risk of hypoglycaemia, 50% TIR is accepted, with an understanding that this means more TAR. In pregnancy stricter glucose targets are specified (3.5–7.8 mmol/L (63–140 mg/dL)), with 70% TIR (see Ch. 32).

Therapeutic goals

HbA_{1c} targets

Type 1 diabetes The first evidence that improved glycaemic control decreases the risk of microvascular complications in diabetes came in 1993 from the Diabetes Control and Complications Trial (DCCT). The DCCT randomised adolescents and young adults with type 1 diabetes in the United States and Canada to intensive treatment (mean HbA_{1c} 53 mmol/mol) or conventional treatment (mean HbA_{1c} 75 mmol/mol) for 6.5 years. There was a 60% overall reduction in the risk of developing microvascular complications with an intensive therapy strategy, although severe hypoglycaemia was increased up to threefold in those in whom HbA_{1c} was most reduced. Thirty-year follow-up of both groups of DCCT participants demonstrated that macrovascular complications were also reduced even many years after a period of intensive control – this was termed 'metabolic memory'.

Type 2 diabetes In the UK Prospective Diabetes Study (UKPDS), published in 1998, adults with type 2 diabetes were randomised to intensive blood glucose control mainly with sulphonylureas and insulin (mean HbA_{1c} 53 mmol/mol) versus conventional glucose control mainly with dietary

treatment (mean HbA_{1c} 64 mmol/mol) for 10 years. Rates of microvascular complications were reduced in those who received intensive therapy, but a beneficial effect on macrovascular complications was observed only with metformin in overweight participants in whom there was a reduction in the rate of diabetes-related death. Follow-up of UKPDS participants over further decades reinforced the microvascular benefits of glucose lowering and the specific macrovascular benefits of metformin.

Other trials that examined whether lowering HbA_{1c} below 53 mmol/mol could further reduce rates of complications in type 2 diabetes suggested that a lower target of 48 mmol/mol may only be safe for younger people in the initial years following diagnosis due to the risks associated with hypoglycaemia (see Box 21.20).

Therefore, the usual target HbA_{1c} is 53 mmol/mol for both type 1 and type 2 diabetes. However, an individualised target is appropriate depending on the needs of the person in question. For example, in recently diagnosed individuals with type 2 diabetes not requiring any agents that cause hypoglycaemia or patients with type 1 diabetes using sensor-augmented CSII (which can substantially reduce the risks of hypoglycaemia), a target of 48 mmol/mol or less may be appropriate. Explicit setting of a higher target (e.g. 58 mmol/mol) is acceptable in some cases, for example older people with shorter duration of diabetes (i.e. at lower lifetime risk of complications), individuals with a high risk of level 3 hypoglycaemia (e.g. those with impaired awareness of hypoglycaemia or cognitive impairment) or those in whom hypoglycaemia could have a particularly adverse consequence (e.g. individuals at high fall risk; Box 21.20). In general, the benefits of lower target HbA_{1c} (primarily a lower risk of microvascular disease) need to be weighed against increased risks (primarily hypoglycaemia). The risks of hypoglycaemia are higher in individuals with absent or minimal endogenous insulin (e.g. type 1 diabetes and following total pancreatectomy), in whom there is more marked glycaemic variability (see Fig. 21.10). Achieving strict glycaemic targets in such individuals can be particularly challenging. Type 2 diabetes is associated with much lower glycaemic variability (due to retained endogenous insulin production), but unless major diet and lifestyle changes are achieved, it is usually a progressive condition and so there is usually a need to increase diabetes medication over time to achieve the individualised target HbA_{1c}.

Control of other risk factors

Type 2 diabetes Due to underlying insulin resistance, most people with type 2 diabetes have hypertension and dyslipidaemia in addition to hyperglycaemia. Targeting of these cardiovascular risk factors is crucial in reducing risk of macrovascular complications. UKPDS participants were

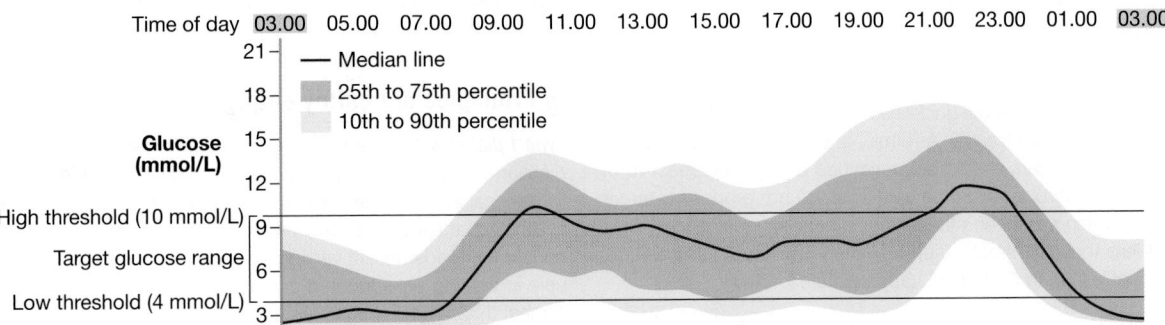

Fig. 21.17 Ambulatory blood glucose profile. The Ambulatory Glucose Profile (AGP) is generated by combining continuous glucose monitor (CGM) data over a prolonged period (usually 14 days). It provides an example of a 'typical day' allowing the person with diabetes and health-care professionals to make more rational adjustments to insulin therapy. An estimated HbA can also be derived from these data. Black/blue solid line (median line) – the average (middle) point of all glucose levels. Ideally this should be in the target glucose range with mimimal variability. Inner blue-shaded band (25th to 75th percentile) – most common glucose levels and how they vary from day to day. Outer light blue-shaded band (10th to 90th percentile) – less common glucose levels and how they vary from day to day. *Adapted from DPC Toolkits, The Ambulatory Glucose Profile (AGP) in 4 steps. https://cdn.asp.events/CLIENT_CloserSt_D86EA381_5056_B739_5482D50A1A831DDD/sites/DPC2020/media/toolkits-2018/The-Ambulatory-Glucose-Profile-AGP-in-4-steps.pdf.*

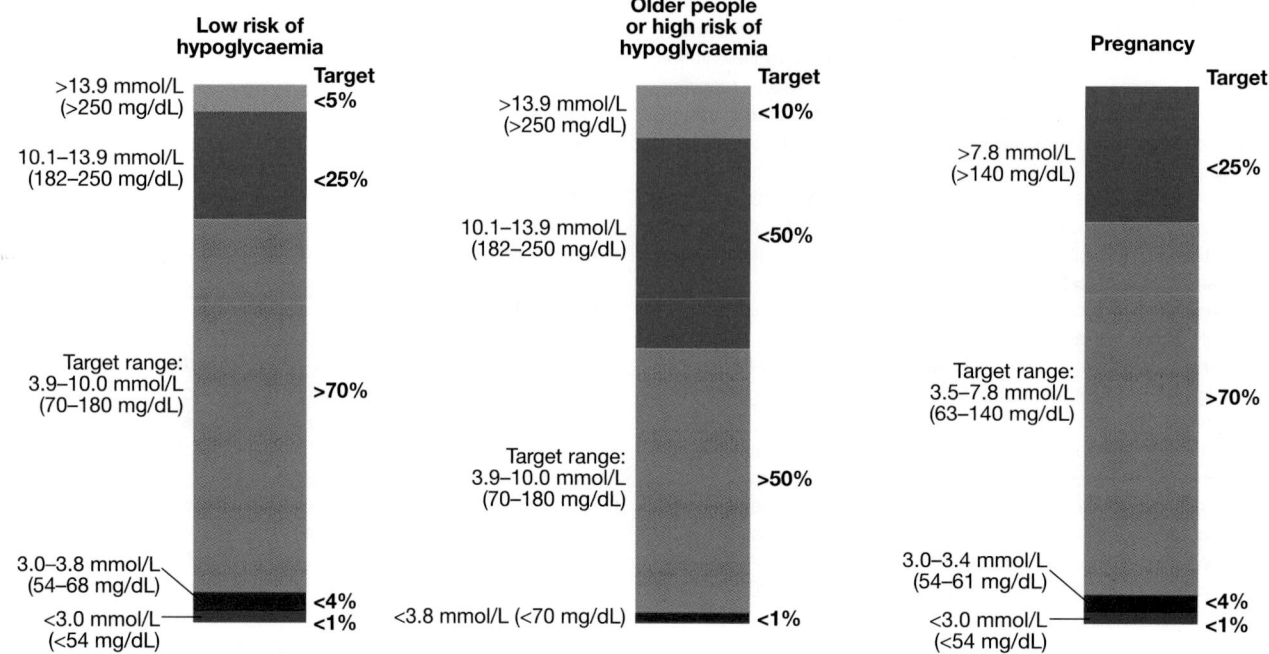

Fig. 21.18 Target time in range for different groups of people with type 1 diabetes. The different coloured sections represent the proportion of time spent within a glucose range: Green = proportion of time spent within range; yellow = time above range; orange = time significantly above range; red = time below range; brown = time significantly below range. 'In range' glucose levels are much lower for women who are pregnant. A lower 'time in range' is accepted for people at higher risk of hypoglycaemia and in older people. Note: as the percentages are targets they do not add up to 100%. *Adapted from Battelino T, et al. Clinical targets for continuous glucose monitoring data interpretation: recommendations from the international consensus on time in range. Diabetes Care 2019, dci190028.*

 21.20 Diabetes in old age

- **Incidence:** type 2 diabetes becomes more common with increasing age.
- **Aetiology:** almost any form of diabetes can present in older people; do not presume that a new diagnosis of diabetes in an older person is automatically due to type 2 diabetes.
- **Hypoglycaemia:** older people may not recognise hypoglycaemia, increasing their risk of severe hypoglycaemia.
- **Glycaemic targets:** need moderated in frail older people, especially if using agents that cause hypoglycaemia (insulin and sulphonylureas).
- **Dementia:** both Alzheimer's disease and vascular dementia are more common in people with diabetes, which can significantly affect ability to manage diabetes safely. Input from family, carers and community nurses may be essential.

also randomised to tight (<150/85 mmHg) or less tight (<180/105 mmHg) blood pressure control: the former was associated with a reduction in the risk of death as well as fewer complications overall (including retinopathy). The target for blood pressure is now usually below 140/80 mmHg, although some guidelines suggest below 130/80 mmHg (e.g. in those with renal disease). As a rule, anyone with type 2 diabetes over the age of 40 years should be prescribed a statin, irrespective of their blood cholesterol level. Some guidelines do not propose a target level once a statin has been started, but others suggest a total cholesterol of less than 4.0 mmol/L (approximately 150 mg/dL) and an LDL cholesterol of less than 2.0 mmol/L (approximately 75 mg/dL).

Type 1 diabetes Elevation of the same cardiovascular risk factors also commonly occurs over time in type 1 diabetes, but is thought at least in the early years to be of secondary importance to hyperglycaemia. Guidelines suggest targeting risk factors in those with a duration of type 1 diabetes of over 15–20 years, or aged over 35–40 years. Similar BP and cholesterol treatment targets are recommended as for people with type 2 diabetes. Caution should be exercised in prescribing for women of childbearing potential, especially drugs with teratogenic potential (including ACE inhibitors and statins).

Education, diet and lifestyle

Broadly, people with diabetes should follow similar dietary recommendations as appropriate for non-diabetic people, but if overweight or obese should seek to lose weight. However, this can be difficult as 'healthy' diet recommendations are rarely followed by the general population, particularly in countries in which cheap calorie-rich foods are widely available and heavily advertised. Labelling of foods as 'suitable for diabetics' was prohibited in the UK in 2016, but some products labelled 'diabetic' are still available. These should be avoided as they are often expensive, sweet-tasting foods (jam, biscuits, chocolate, ice-cream) that can contain synthetic sugars that raise blood glucose. People with diabetes may be misled into believing these products are essential or especially suitable. Diabetes prevention programmes are in place in many countries, essentially supporting low-fat healthy eating, weight reduction and increased physical activity (often referred to as 'non-pharmacological intervention').

Principles of healthy eating

Type 1 diabetes Soon after diagnosis patients should have access to a dietitian for education on 'carbohydrate counting', as this is essential for rational insulin dose adjustment. Books and smartphone apps are available that show carbohydrate content next to pictures of commonly consumed foodstuffs, in varying portion sizes; these can assist individuals in making an educated estimate of the carbohydrate content of a meal (Fig. 21.19). Highly accurate information on the carbohydrate content of pre-prepared foods and basic ingredients is provided on package labels; some people with type 1 diabetes weigh food portions to get as precise information as possible. Carbohydrate counting requires patience and diligence, but becomes easier with lived experience. In theory, people with type 1 diabetes with a normal weight should be able to eat unrestricted types and amounts of carbohydrate, as they can simply take an appropriate amount of insulin to 'cover' the carbohydrate content of the meal. However, in practice, because the time action profiles of available exogenous insulins do not exactly

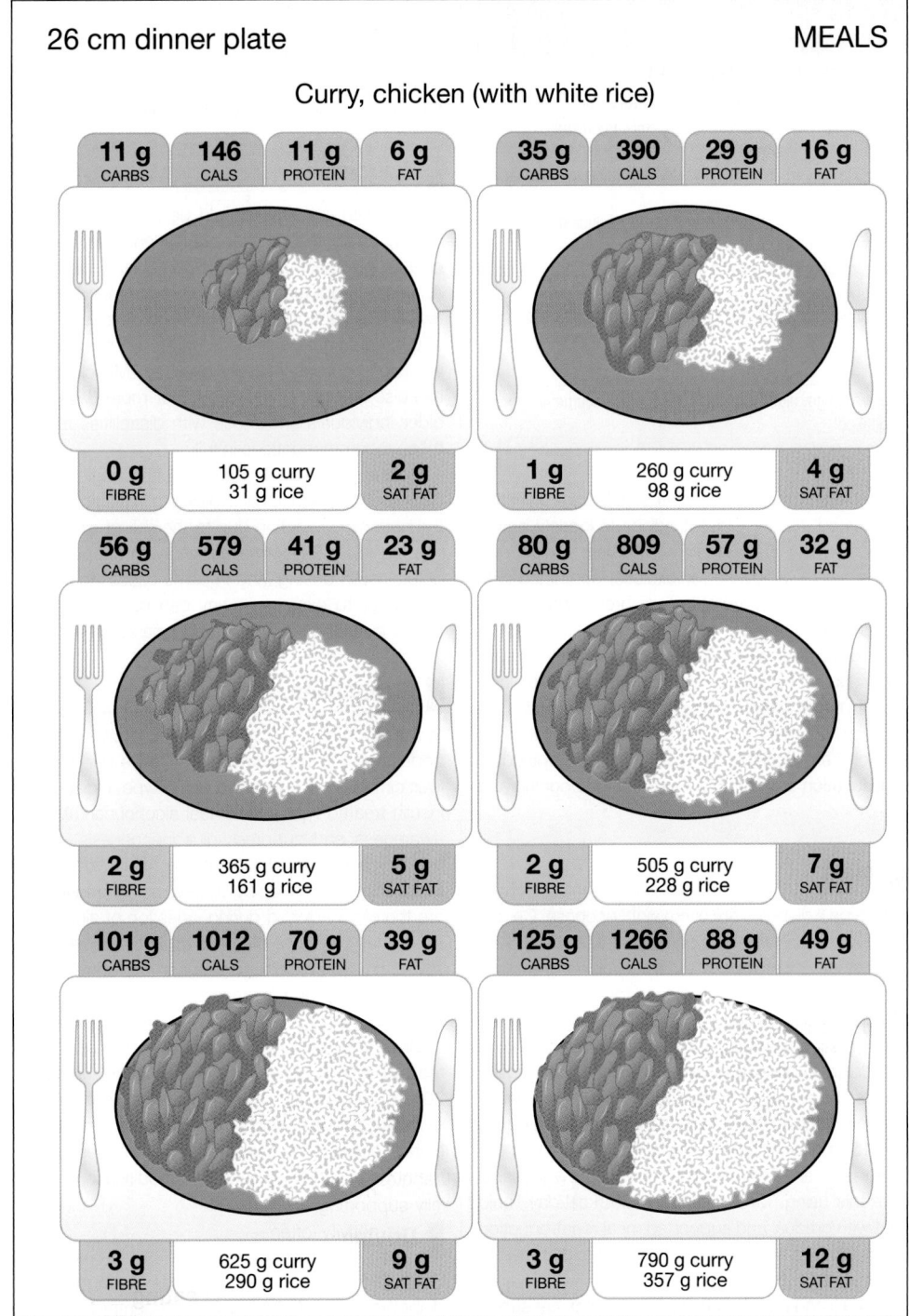

Fig. 21.19 Example of a 'carbohydrate counting' guide for people with diabetes. Books and smart phone apps are available that give illustrative examples of different foods, in different portion sizes. The macronutrient and calorie content is provided for each portion. *From Cheyette C, Balolia Y. Carbs and Cals. Carb & Calorie Counter, 6th edition; 2016. Chello Publishing Limited.*

match physiological variations in endogenous insulin, the consumption of unrefined carbohydrate (such as sweets and sugar-rich drinks) and large portions of carbohydrate (>60 g) invariably results in 'spikes' in blood glucose. Therefore, the best glycaemic control is generally seen in individuals who mostly avoid unrefined carbohydrate and limit carbohydrate portion size.

Education on advanced carbohydrate counting and how to manage diet and insulin therapy during daily life (e.g. in the context of exercise, alcohol and intercurrent illness) is provided in formal structured and cost-effective programmes, such as 'Dose Adjustment for Normal Eating' (DAFNE). This involves one week of small group learning with other individuals with the condition supported by a diabetes specialist nurse and a dietician. The COVID-19 pandemic has led to an increased use of remote 'flipped classroom' models of education supported by videotelephony platforms.

Type 2 diabetes There is no 'one size fits all' way of eating for people with type 2 diabetes, beyond making healthy choices more often and in smaller portions, as recommended by the Food Standards Agency (Box 21.21). There is no fixed formula for the balance of carbohydrate,

21.21 Dietary management of diabetes

Food Standards Agency Eatwell recommendations 2020

- Eat at least 5 portions of a variety of fruit and vegetables every day
- Base meals on potatoes, bread, rice, pasta or other starchy carbohydrates; choosing wholegrain versions where possible
- Have some dairy or dairy alternatives (such as soya drinks), choosing lower fat and lower sugar options
- Eat some beans, pulses, fish, eggs, meat and other proteins (including 2 portions of fish every week, one of which should be oily)
- Choose unsaturated oils and spreads and eat in small amounts
- Drink 6-8 cups/glasses of fluid a day
- If consuming foods and drinks high in fat, salt or sugar have these less often and in small amounts
- Eat <6.0 g salt per day

Available from: https://www.food.gov.uk/sites/default/files/media/document/eatwell-guide-master-digital.pdf.

fat and protein ('macronutrient composition'); neither is there a universal 'diet sheet' or list of 'banned' foods. Current advice is loosely based on the principles of a 'Mediterranean' diet (for which there is high level evidence of protection against cardiovascular disease) combined with a focus on choosing unrefined carbohydrates (e.g. brown rice, brown pasta, brown noodles, porridge, granary bread, and beans and lentils) rather than refined carbohydrates (fruit juices, pastries, white bread, white pasta, white rice). Nutritional advice should be tailored to individuals and take account of age, lifestyle, culture and personal circumstances. A variety of structured education programmes, which focus on dietary and lifestyle factors, are available for type 2 diabetes, including DESMOND (Diabetes Education and Self Management for Ongoing and Newly Diagnosed).

Weight management

Over 80% of people with type 2 diabetes are overweight or obese. Central obesity with increased waist circumference is particularly associated with insulin resistance and increased cardiovascular risk. Following a diagnosis of type 2 diabetes, there should be an intense focus on reversing any unhealthy habits and behaviours with the aim, where appropriate, of weight loss. It is extremely challenging for most overweight people (with or without type 2 diabetes) to lose body weight and avoid regain. However, if weight loss can be achieved, it markedly improves glycaemic control and slows diabetes progression. Substantial weight loss in obese people (usually around 15 kg or about 15% initial body weight) can put type 2 diabetes into remission and there are programmes now available to help people achieve this using, for example, an 800 kcal/day liquid 'meal replacement' diet with gradual and supported meal re-introduction at 3 months (see p. 765). Trained supervision is essential and in the UK is increasingly provided by the NHS.

Some health professionals and people with type 2 diabetes are strong advocates of low-carbohydrate, high-fat ('ketogenic' or 'Atkins') diets to promote weight loss, or alternatively intermittent fasting 2 days out of every 5 ('5:2' diet). Perhaps because they help to provide and sustain motivation, these approaches are successful in achieving and sustaining weight loss in some individuals, but to date it has not been possible to predict in advance who will respond or to demonstrate general efficacy of these diets in controlled trials. They must only be used with extreme caution in type 1 diabetes due to the risks of hypoglycaemia or ketoacidosis.

Bariatric surgery (see p. 766) induces marked weight loss in obese individuals with type 2 diabetes and this is often associated with significant improvements in HbA$_{1c}$ and withdrawal of or reduction in diabetes medications. Shared decision-making is important as surgery is not without risk of short- and long-term complications.

Over 50% of adults with type 1 diabetes are now also obese, at least in the United States and the UK. Insulin is an anabolic hormone, so if

insulin dosing is imperfectly matched to carbohydrate intake, calorie ingestion may at times be required to prevent hypoglycaemia. Some individuals appear to be more susceptible to insulin-induced weight gain than others. Increasing use of technology (CSII and CGM) may help with this problem, as may adjunct therapy with SGLT2 inhibitors.

Exercise

People with diabetes should be advised to follow advice on physical activity as for the general population. Supervised and structured exercise programmes may be of particular benefit in type 2 diabetes. The American Diabetes Association recommends that all adults with diabetes reduce sedentary time (avoiding periods >90 minutes) and do either 150 minutes per week of moderate-intensity exercise or 75 minutes per week of vigorous-intensity exercise. Muscle-strengthening (resistance) exercise is recommended on 2 or more days of the week. Of course, older individuals and those with disabilities may not be able to follow these recommendations in full.

People with type 1 diabetes (and people with insulin-treated type 2 diabetes) face additional challenges in relation to exercise compared with the general population due to the risk of exercise-induced hypoglycaemia (see p. 725). However, following support in planning reduction of bolus insulin dosing (and in some cases increased carbohydrate ingestion) prior to exercise, many can participate in high-level competitive sports including golf, rowing and marathon running.

Alcohol and smoking

In type 2 diabetes, recommendations on alcohol are as for the general population (i.e. no more than 14 units per week for adults) to prevent liver cirrhosis and weight gain. In type 1 diabetes (and for people with insulin-treated type 2 diabetes) alcohol can also reduce hypoglycaemia awareness and suppress gluconeogenesis, increasing risk of level 3 hypoglycaemia. In addition, the signs of hypoglycaemia can be mistaken for alcohol intoxication by observers. People with insulin-treated diabetes are therefore advised during ingestion of alcohol to: (i) let a companion know that they have diabetes and how to treat them if they have hypoglycaemia; (ii) continue to monitor and correct blood glucose by eating while drinking; and (iii) measure and ensure glucose is not low before retiring to bed.

Given the risk of cardiovascular complications associated with diabetes and despite increasing access to smoking cessation support, around 20% of people with type 1 diabetes and 15% of people with type 2 diabetes in most cohorts are current cigarette smokers (rates similar or higher to that in the general population). Research is required into better methods of achieving behaviour modification.

Driving

European legislation on driving has had a major impact on people with diabetes. Legislation varies from country to country and so individuals should discuss with their diabetes health-care professional if their treatment necessitates reporting to the licensing authority (Box 21.22). To drive a car or ride a motorcycle in the UK, people with diabetes who take insulin therapy must notify the Driver and Vehicle Licensing Agency (DVLA). They must have adequate awareness of hypoglycaemia, have had no more than one episode of level 3 hypoglycaemia in the preceding 12 months, meet the standards for visual acuity and visual fields, and not be regarded as a likely risk to the public while driving. In addition, blood glucose testing is required to be performed no more than 2 hours before the start of a journey and every 2 hours while driving. Blood glucose levels should be over 5.0 mmol/L (90 mg/dL) before driving; if they are below 4.0 mmol/L (72 mg/dL) or there are symptoms of hypoglycaemia, the person should not drive. CGM has been approved for monitoring glucose at times relevant for driving in the UK, provided the glucose level is above 4.0 mmol/L, there are no symptoms of hypoglycaemia and the CGM device reading is consistent with symptoms experienced. Legislative requirements in the UK for people on insulin therapy who have Group 2 licences to drive larger vehicles such as buses or lorries require, in addition, an annual examination by a diabetes specialist, along with review of 3 months of glucose readings.

Ramadan

The Quran requires Muslims to fast from sunrise to sunset during the 29 or 30 days of Ramadan, the ninth month of the Muslim calendar. While people with diabetes are a recognised exception to this and are not required to fast, many choose to do so. In this context, people with diabetes should schedule a visit with a diabetes health-care professional 6–12 weeks before Ramadan. Prior to fasting the person should be counselled on their personal risk of fasting and an individualised management plan should be developed. This should include: structured education around fluids and meal planning, when to exercise, the role of increased frequency and/or timing of glucose monitoring (which does not invalidate the fast) and adjustment to the dose time and/or frequency of glucose-lowering agents. The majority of people with type 2 diabetes can be supported to fast during Ramadan provided they are prepared to stop the fast in the case of frequent hypo- or hyperglycaemia or worsening of other related medical conditions. While people with type 1 diabetes are advised not to fast, this advice should be considered on a case-by-case basis. The highest risk of hypoglycaemia is in people who are managed with sulphonylureas and insulin (especially if they are older age, or have renal failure or advanced macrovascular complications); such individuals need careful blood glucose monitoring and, if necessary, their treatment regimens may need to be adjusted. Glucose-lowering therapies that do not cause hypoglycaemia are safest during Ramadan, if glycaemic control permits. Dipeptidyl peptidase (DPP-4) inhibitors or glucagon-like peptide-1 (GLP-1) receptor agonists provided they are initiated at least 6–8 weeks before, may be especially useful because their effect on insulin secretion is glucose-dependent. Published guidance is available to help guide dose and timing adjustments from the International Diabetes Federation and the Diabetes and Ramadan International Alliance (IDF-DAR).

Glucose-lowering agents

Type 1 diabetes is managed with insulin from the time of diagnosis. When glucose levels are above target in type 2 diabetes despite appropriate lifestyle advice, drug therapy will usually be initiated and subsequently increased ('intensified') with the aim of establishing or re-establishing adequate glucose control, abolishing osmotic symptoms and preventing microvascular complications. Some individuals require pharmacological therapy from the time of (or very soon after) diagnosis. Over the following years and decades, the majority will require to take combinations of glucose-lowering drugs, oral or injectable, and some will also require insulin.

Seven main classes of glucose-lowering drugs are generally used to manage type 2 diabetes (Box 21.23). Four are oral agents: metformin (the only available biguanide), sulphonylureas, pioglitazone (the only available thiazolidinedione), DPP-4 inhibitors and sodium glucose transporter-2 (SGLT2) inhibitors. GLP-1 receptor agonists are usually given by subcutaneous injection, but an oral preparation is available. Insulin is given by subcutaneous injection. The effects of these drugs are compared in Box 21.23. Acarbose (an intestinal disaccharidase inhibitor that prevents dietary glucose absorption) and meglitinides (oral agents that stimulate endogenous insulin) are also available, but little used due to relatively low efficacy and, in the case of acarbose, frequent (gastrointestinal) side effects. Other agents are in development.

To date, the totality of evidence confirms that any agent that reduces blood glucose will also reduce the long-term risk of microvascular complications. Factors that determine which of these drugs should be prescribed first – and then which should subsequently be added in – include:

- individual profile (severity of initial symptoms, degree of obesity)
- glucose-lowering efficacy
- protective properties in relation to cardiovascular and renal complications (see below)

---

i 21.22 Diabetes and driving

The main risk is hypoglycaemia due to insulin treatment. Health professionals should be proactive in supporting people with diabetes on insulin therapy to drive safely within the regulations while following legislation designed to protect road-users.

- Licensing regulations vary considerably between countries.
- In the UK, it is a legal requirement for people with diabetes requiring insulin therapy to notify the Driver and Vehicle Licensing Agency (DVLA)
- Group 1 licences (car, motorcycle, van) are 'period-restricted' for insulin-treated drivers, i.e. usually renewable every 3 years but with specific criteria: particularly no more than one episode of level 3 hypoglycaemia while awake in the preceding 12 months (the most recent episode more than 3 months ago)
- Group 2 licences (bus and lorry) may be granted for insulin-treated drivers: stricter criteria to be met – in particular no episode of level 3 hypoglycaemia (see Box 21.14) within the last 12 months and full awareness of hypoglycaemia regardless of whether this occurred when asleep. The licence is renewable annually.
- Blood glucose must be monitored appropriately. Those with a Group 1 licence may use continuous glucose monitoring systems, but must confirm the reading using a capillary blood glucose reading in specific circumstances (e.g. glucose ≤4.0 mmol/L)
- Insulin-treated drivers should:
  Check blood glucose before driving and 2-hourly during long journeys
  Keep an accessible supply of fast-acting carbohydrate in the vehicle
  Take regular snacks or meals during long journeys
  Stop driving if hypoglycaemia develops
  Pull over and sit in the passenger seat
  Wait 45 mins after correction of hypoglycaemia before resuming driving (delayed recovery of cognitive function)
  Carry identification in case of injury

Note: Intermittently scanned monitoring (isCGM) is now approved in the UK for Group 1 licences provided the driver has the facility to check capillary blood glucose if symptoms of hypoglycaemia or hyperglycaemia are experienced. *See: Assessing fitness to drive: a guide for medical professionals* (ch. 3). https://assets.publishing.service.gov.uk/government/uploads/system/uploads/attachment_data/file/866655/assessing-fitness-to-drive-a-guide-for-medical-professionals.pdf.

---

i 21.23 Glucose-lowering agents in type 2 diabetes: additional information (see also Fig. 21.20)

	Insulin	Sulphonylureas	Metformin	Thiazolidinediones ('glitazones')	DPP-4 inhibitors ('gliptins')	GLP-1 receptor agonists	SGLT2 inhibitors
Introduced	1922	1956	1957	1999	2006	2007	2013
Route of administration	SC injection	Oral	Oral	Oral	Oral	SC injection (oral)	Oral
Cost	High	Low	Very low	Low	Moderate	Very high	High

(DPP-4 = dipeptidyl peptidase 4; GLP-1 = glucagon-like peptide 1; SC = subcutaneous; SGLT2 = sodium and glucose transporter 2)

- adverse effect profile (hypoglycaemia, weight gain)
- renal function
- drug factors (mechanism of clearance/metabolism)
- ability or willingness to self-inject
- occupation (e.g. driving, working at heights)
- cost: important whether covered by a national health-care system, reimbursed by an insurance company, or paid for 'out-of-pocket'.

Algorithms to guide prescribing decisions are available, e.g. consensus documents from the American Diabetes Association and the European Association for the Study of Diabetes (ADA/EASD; Fig. 21.20). These are frequently updated.

Metformin is often positioned as first-line, with second-line treatment personalised for each patient according to the above factors. A third or even fourth oral agent may be added in over time, but injectable therapy (GLP-1 receptor agonists or insulin) should not be delayed while levels of glycaemia above target are sustained for months or years; this will almost inevitably result in severe complications years later.

Unlike microvascular complications, it cannot be assumed that all agents that lower glucose also reduce rates of macrovascular complications, i.e. myocardial infarction and stroke. Some newer agents clearly protect against cardiovascular disease (GLP-1 receptor agonists and SGLT2 inhibitors), but are more expensive. Others (metformin and thiazolidinediones) provide some cardiovascular protection, but are cheaper, while others do not (sulphonlyureas, DPP-4 inhibitors and insulin). SGLT2 inhibitors have additional protective properties in heart failure and diabetic kidney disease, while TZDs (thiazolidinediones) increase rates of heart failure. It is therefore likely that the protective (and adverse) effects of these different classes of glucose-lowering agents are via 'off-target' mechanisms, i.e. unrelated to glucose-lowering.

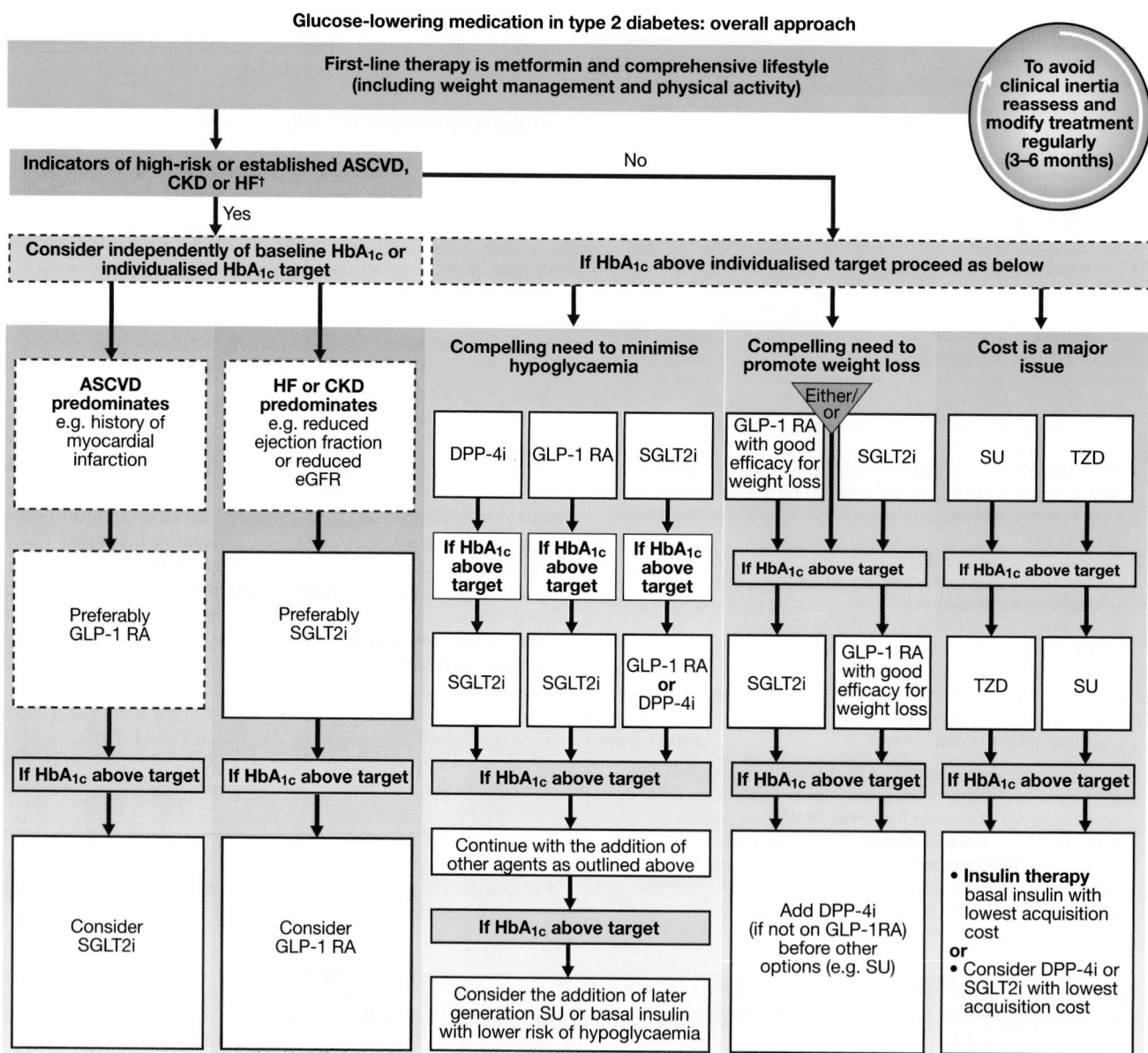

Fig. 21.20 Guidelines for glucose-lowering treatment in type 2 diabetes: adapted from ADA-EASD 2020. This pathway is illustrative – for treatment decisions please refer to the figure provided in the full guideline (https://doi.org/10.1007/s00125-019-05039-w) and region-specific drug licensing information. (DPP-4i = dipeptidyl peptidase 4 inhibitor; GLP-1 RA = glucagon-like peptide 1 receptor agonist; SGLT2i = sodium and glucose co-transporter 2 inhibitor; TZD = thiazolidinedione; SU = sulphonylurea; eGFR, estimated glomerular filtration rate; ASCVD = atherosclerotic cardiovascular disease; CKD = chronic kidney disease; HF = heart failure; LVH = left ventricular hypertrophy) Adapted from: Buse JB, Wexler DJ, Tsapas A, et al. 2019 update to: Management of hyperglycaemia in type 2 diabetes, 2018. A consensus report by the American Diabetes Association (ADA) and the European Association for the Study of Diabetes (EASD). Diabetologia 2020; 63, 221–228.

The adverse risk profile of each agent plays an important role in personalisation of second- and third-line therapy. For example, agents that cause hypoglycaemia should be avoided in those who drive for a living (particularly those holding Group 2 licences in the UK) or who work at heights.

There is little evidence to help the clinician and patient select the optimal second- or third-line treatment in advance, so a trial-and-error approach is often used, i.e. stopping a drug that does not seem to be effective (or that causes side-effects) and trying another. It is hoped that biomarkers will in the future help predict who will respond better and/or experience fewer side-effects with one drug rather than another.

Biguanides

Metformin is the only biguanide available. Its long-term benefits include not just reduction in rates of microvascular complications, but also reducing the risk of myocardial infarction, as shown in the UKPDS. It is widely used as first-line therapy for type 2 diabetes. Approximately 15% of individuals experience significant gastrointestinal side-effects, including bloating, nausea, diarrhoea and abdominal pain, such that they are unable to tolerate metformin. Metformin monotherapy may not be sufficient to provide rapid relief from symptoms in individuals with marked osmotic symptoms and weight loss at diagnosis (see sulphonylureas below).

Mechanism of action

The mechanism of action of metformin has not been precisely defined. While classically considered an 'insulin sensitiser' because it tends to lower (rather than raise) insulin levels, its main effects are on fasting glucose. Metformin reduces hepatic glucose production, may also increase insulin-mediated glucose uptake, and has effects on gut glucose uptake and utilisation. At the molecular level, metformin acts as a weak inhibitor of mitochondrial respiration, which increases intracellular adenosine monophosphate (AMP) and reduces adenosine triphosphate (ATP). This has direct effects on the flux through gluconeogenesis and activates the intracellular energy sensor, AMP-activated protein kinase (AMPK), leading to multiple beneficial effects. However, although metformin has been available for more than 60 years, it is not yet clear whether other AMPK-independent mechanisms may be just as important.

Clinical use

Metformin causes modest sustained weight loss (on average 1–2 kg), does not cause hypoglycaemia and has established benefits in microvascular disease. It is prescribed first-line therapy for the majority of people unless they do not tolerate it, and it is usually maintained when additional agents are required (see Fig. 21.20). Metformin is usually introduced at low dose (500 mg twice daily) to minimise the risk of gastrointestinal side-effects. The usual maintenance dose is 1000 mg twice daily (maximum licensed dose 1000 mg three times daily). Modified-release formulations of metformin are better tolerated by some individuals with gastrointestinal side-effects on the regular preparation.

Due to inhibition of mitochondrial respiration, metformin can cause asymptomatic hyperlactataemia, which during acute illness can present as lactic acidosis. However, this is much less common than previously thought and most instances of lactic acidosis that occur in the context of metformin prescription are due to other factors. As metformin is cleared by the kidneys, it can accumulate in renal impairment, so the dose should be halved when estimated glomerular filtration rate (eGFR) is below 45 mL/min/1.73 m^2, and it should not be used below an eGFR of 30 mL/min/1.73 m^2. It should be omitted temporarily during any acute illness potentially involving dehydration as acute kidney injury greatly increases the risk of lactic acidosis. Metformin is contraindicated in the presence of significantly impaired hepatic function and in those who drink alcohol to excess as they are more vulnerable to lactic acidosis.

Sulphonylureas

Sulphonylureas are 'insulin secretagogues', i.e. they promote pancreatic β-cell insulin secretion. Similar to metformin, the long-term benefit of sulphonylureas in reducing rates of microvascular complications was established in the UKPDS.

Mechanism of action

Sulphonylureas act by closing the pancreatic β cell ATP-sensitive potassium (K_{ATP}) channel, decreasing K$^+$ efflux, and triggering insulin secretion by a series of molecular events (see Fig. 21.3C).

Clinical use

Sulphonylureas are an effective therapy for lowering blood glucose. They may be used to relieve osmotic symptoms in individuals with newly diagnosed diabetes who have very high blood glucose, although insulin should also be considered in this context, particularly if a diagnosis of new-onset type 1 diabetes remains possible (as in this context they are dangerous because they are ineffective). They are more often used as an add-on to other glucose-lowering therapy when glycaemia is inadequately controlled (see Fig. 21.20) or in non-obese people with type 2 diabetes (who likely have significant β-cell dysfunction). Sulphonylureas are also particularly effective in some forms of monogenic and neonatal diabetes (see p. 719). The main adverse effects of sulphonylureas are weight gain and hypoglycaemia (as insulin secretion occurs irrespective of the prevailing blood glucose). A number of sulphonylureas are available: gliclazide is most commonly used in the UK and glibenclamide (known as glyburide) in the United States. Glibenclamide, however, is long-acting and prone to inducing hypoglycaemia, so should be avoided in older people. Other sulphonylureas include glimepiride and glipizide. The dose–response of all sulphonylureas is steepest at low doses, i.e. little additional benefit is obtained when the dose is increased above half-maximal doses.

Thiazolidinediones

Mechanism of action

These drugs (also called TZDs, 'glitazones' or PPARγ agonists) bind and activate peroxisome proliferator-activated receptor-γ, nuclear receptors present mainly in adipose tissue (similar to steroid and thyroid nuclear receptors), which regulate the expression of several genes involved in adipocyte differentiation. By promoting adipogenesis in subcutaneous depots, TZDs decrease circulating concentrations of free fatty acids, enhancing the actions of endogenous insulin. Therefore, they tend to increase body weight. They also alter release of 'adipokines', e.g. increasing levels of adiponectin improves insulin sensitivity in the liver. TZDs appear to be particularly effective at improving glycaemic control in women and people with a raised BMI.

Clinical use

TZDs were widely prescribed in the late 1990s and 2000s, but their use declined with the advent of other agents with fewer adverse effects and greater efficacy. One popular TZD, rosiglitazone, was withdrawn from the market in 2010 due to a subsequently disproven concern that it might increase rates of myocardial infarction. Pioglitazone, the other drug in this class, remains in use and may reduce hepatic steatosis and NASH (see Fig. 21.20) as well as providing protection from stroke. However, it exacerbates cardiac failure by causing fluid retention and increases the risk of bone fracture (and possibly bladder cancer) with long-term use.

DPP-4 inhibitors

Mechanism of action

The incretin hormones (see Fig. 21.4) GLP-1 and GIP are gut hormones that potentiate post-prandial insulin secretion (see Fig. 21.3). GLP-1 and GIP are rapidly broken down by dipeptidyl peptidase 4 (DPP-4). The 'gliptins', or DPP-4 inhibitors, prevent physiological breakdown of endogenous GLP-1 and GIP and so enhance their circulating concentrations. Incretin-based therapies (DPP-4 inhibitors and GLP-1 agonists) are 'glucose-dependent', i.e. promote insulin secretion only when glucose is high

(Fig. 21.21). Thus, insulin secretion is not augmented when blood glucose is normal, i.e. there is minimal risk of hypoglycaemia when these therapies are used as monotherapy or in combination with other drugs that do not cause hypoglycaemia.

Clinical use

DPP-4 inhibitors include sitagliptin, linagliptin, alogliptin, vildagliptin and saxagliptin. All are well tolerated and have a neutral effect on weight, but are less potent than GLP-1 receptor agonists and provide only moderate glucose-lowering activity (see Box 21.23). They are safe but do not improve cardiovascular outcomes. The DPP4 inhibitors are useful in combination with other drugs to get HbA$_{1c}$ to target when it is only modestly elevated and are commonly used in older people as they have few adverse effects. Linagliptin is the only DPP4 inhibitor that does not require dose reduction in renal impairment.

GLP-1 receptor agonists

Mechanism of action

The GLP-1 receptor agonists are peptide hormones that mimic the action of GLP-1; most require to be given by subcutaneous injection. Some have a high degree of structural homology to native GLP-1, but are modified at the sites usually cleaved by DPP-4 to prevent breakdown (liraglutide, semaglutide, dulaglutide). Others are synthetic forms of exendin-4, a 39 amino acid peptide originally isolated from the salivary secretions of the Gila monster, native to the Arizona desert (exenatide, lixisenatide). As incretin-based therapies, they potentiate release of insulin, but with greater potency than DPP-4 inhibitors. However, they also have central actions, acting centrally on receptors in specific areas of the hypothalamus (including the arcuate nucleus); in addition they delay

gastric emptying, giving a feeling of satiety after eating (see Fig. 21.21). GLP-1 receptor agonists therefore decrease appetite and feeding behaviour, resulting in weight loss of on average 3–5 kg. Modifications of either the molecule or the formulation allow some agents within the class to be injected once weekly (semaglutide, dulaglutide, extended-release exenatide), rather than once daily (liraglutide) or twice daily (exenatide). An orally administered GLP-1 receptor agonist has now been approved (encapsulated semaglutide with an advanced gastrointestinal delivery system), although it must be taken once daily on an empty stomach with a sip of water and nothing should be consumed for 30 minutes afterwards.

Clinical use

The main side-effect of GLP-1 receptor agonists is nausea (and even vomiting) in the first few days of use; this is prevented in many individuals by slowly uptitrating from a low starting dose to a therapeutic dose. Several of the GLP-1 receptor agonist class, particularly those with high structural homology to native GLP-1 (liraglutide, semaglutide and dulaglutide), have been shown in large cardiovascular outcome trials to reduce rates of major cardiovascular adverse events. These are now the most frequently prescribed drugs in the class, although as they are expensive compared with other agents, guidelines in the UK recommend that they should only be used third-line, as add-on therapy with other agents and only in those with a BMI of >30 kg/m^2 (Scottish Intercollegiate Guideline Network, SIGN) or even 35 kg/m^2 (National Institute for Health and Care Excellence NICE). However, some international guidelines (e.g. European Society for Cardiology) now recommend they should be started earlier, even before metformin, in individuals at high risk of a cardiovascular event.

Since their initial launch in 2007, GLP-1 receptor agonists have contributed to a revolution in the treatment of type 2 diabetes. For several

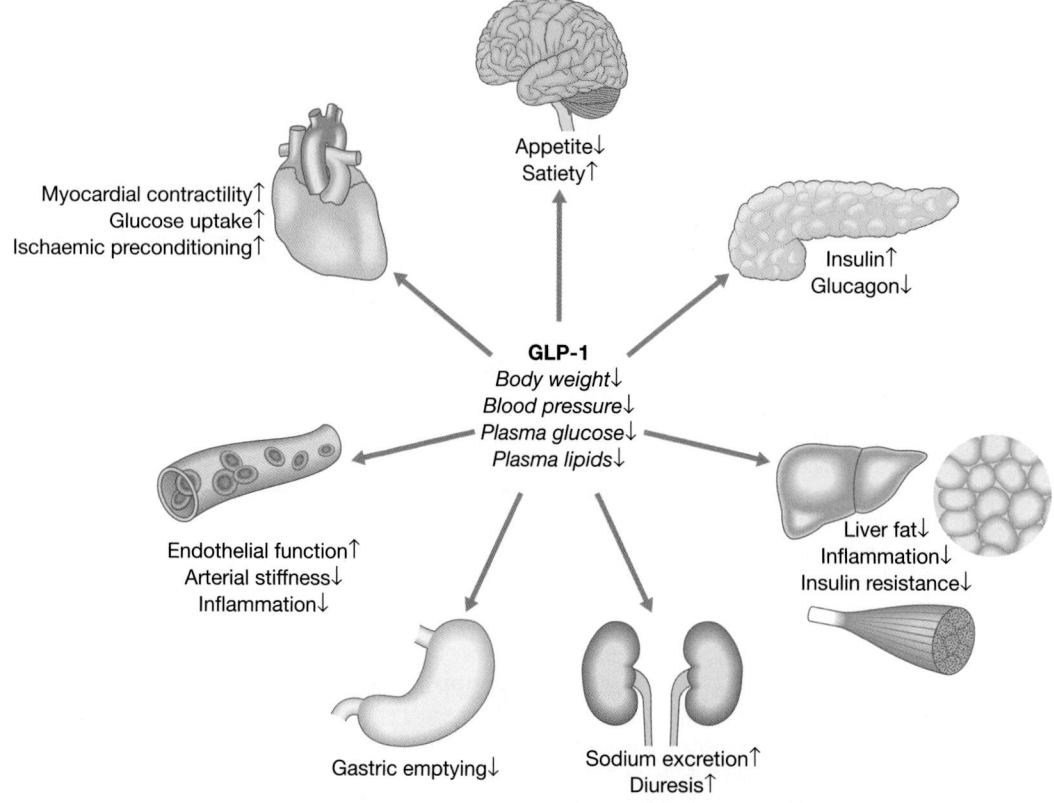

Fig. 21.21 Actions of incretin-based therapies. GLP-1 receptor agonists (GLP-RA) mediate all of the actions shown and have potent effects on blood glucose and weight. Many GLP-1 RAs are associated with a reduction in cardiovascular events. Dipeptidyl peptidase 4 inhibitors (DPP-4i) have less potent glucose-lowering ability and have a neutral effect on weight and cardiovascular disease. DPP-4is do not mediate all of the actions shown, e.g. do not reduce gastric emptying or have significant effects on appetite. (GLP-1 = glucagon-like peptide 1)

years, there was a concern that they (and DPP4-inhibitors) might increase the risk of pancreatitis or pancreatic cancer, but meta-analysis of large clinical trials has demonstrated this is not the case. Even more potent 'dual agonist' agents (with GIP agonist activity) are now in development.

SGLT2 inhibitors

Mechanism of action

Sodium-glucose co-transporter 2 (SGLT2) inhibitors are derived from apple tree bark and were first licensed for type 2 diabetes in 2013. The best-known drugs in the class are dapagliflozin, empagliflozin and canagliflozin. The mechanism by which they lower blood glucose exploits the handling of glucose in the kidneys. Glucose is filtered freely in the glomerulus and then completely reabsorbed in the proximal tubules

with sodium (mainly via SGLT2) (Fig. 21.22). During hyperglycaemia, this response reaches saturation and glucose is lost in the urine. Glycosuria is a hallmark feature of type 2 diabetes, but in many cases there is a paradoxical increase in reabsorption of glucose such that the threshold blood glucose value at which glucose is lost in the urine is higher than the usual physiological level; this may be due to increased expression of SGLT2.

SGLT2 inhibitors act by lowering the renal threshold for glucose excretion, such that typically 25% of filtered glucose is not reabsorbed. As well as lowering blood glucose, a negative energy balance is created with 200–300 kcal being lost each day (as glucose in the urine), resulting in significant weight loss. As sodium is also lost in the urine (also known as natriuresis), blood pressure is also reduced.

SGLT2 inhibitors reduce rates of major adverse cardiovascular outcomes, particularly heart failure, and also have a reno-protective effect,

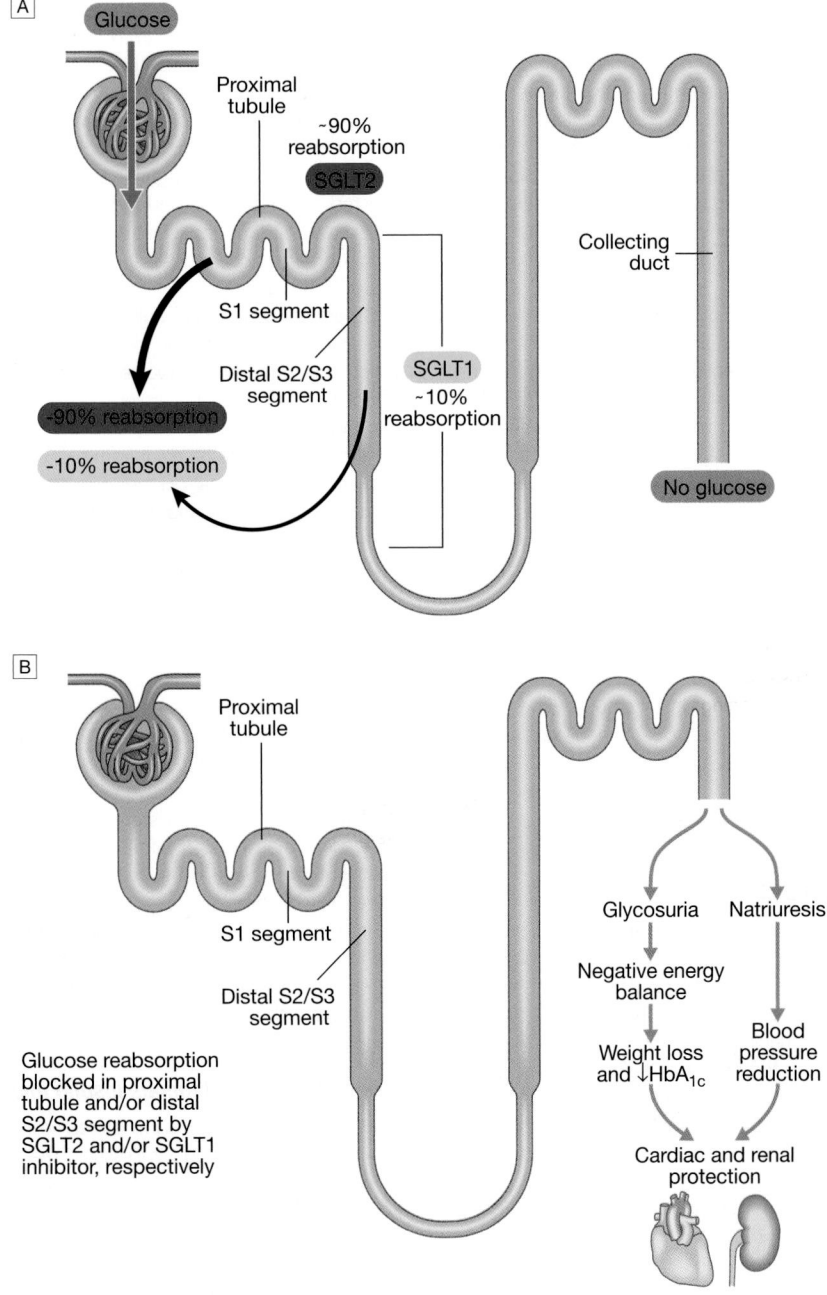

Fig. 21.22 **A** Glucose filtration and reabsorption by the nephron. Some 90% of filtered glucose is reabsorbed by sodium and glucose transporter (SGLT) 2 and 10% by SGLT1. SGLT2 inhibitors reduce net reabsorbed glucose by 25%. For a mean plasma glucose of 8 mmol/L (144 mg/dL) this results in a glucose loss of approximately 80 g per day in the urine, which in turn reduces plasma glucose. This equates to 320 kcal per day and subsequent weight loss. **B** SGLT2 inhibition leads to glycosuria and is associated with improved glycaemia, blood pressure reduction and weight loss.

i.e. reducing rates of death, dialysis and transplantation. These beneficial effects are at least in part due to blood pressure and weight lowering but other more complex mechanisms are also of clinical relevance. Compensatory glucagon release from pancreatic α cells (in response to urinary loss of glucose) decreases the circulating ratio of insulin to glucagon, promoting lipolysis and even mild ketosis; however, because of weight loss this is not sufficient to exacerbate insulin resistance. The work of the myocardium is more efficient when it utilises free fatty acids (and ketones) for fuel than it is when metabolising glucose (as it does in heart failure). Renal benefits of SGLT2 inhibitors are due to constriction of the afferent arteriole (as a reflex response to increased renal tubular loss of sodium, termed 'tubuloglomerular feedback'). This decreases intraglomerular pressure in a complementary manner to ACE inhibitors (p. 619), which cause relaxation of the efferent arteriole by opposing the action of angiotensin II.

Clinical use

SGLT2 inhibitors are effective oral glucose-lowering agents that are usually added in with other agents second-line after metformin. They help with body weight reduction and are associated with improvements in cardiovascular and renal outcomes that have substantially advanced the treatment of type 2 diabetes. They should now be prescribed for all individuals with type 2 diabetes and prior myocardial infarction, coronary artery disease, stroke, unstable angina, occlusive peripheral arterial disease or cardiac failure. Dapagliflozin is also licensed for use in type 1 diabetes, but must be used with caution due to the increased risk of ketoacidosis (see below).

The main adverse effect (in 5%–10% of those who take these agents) is genital mycotic (fungal) infections usually with *Candida albicans*, i.e. vaginal 'thrush' and balanitis. Urine infection is also more common and, very rarely, severe genital infection (Fournier's gangrene, see Ch. 13) can occur. It is essential for prescribers to mention these side-effects, to ensure that prompt measures can be taken to treat the infection; good genital hygiene is also necessary. Once blood glucose is under control, genital infections are much less likely to occur. Euglycaemic diabetic ketoacidosis (i.e. DKA not associated with marked hyperglycaemia) is a rare complication of this class of drugs, presumably driven by reduced insulin:glucagon ratio and consequent increased levels of circulating ketones. It can be minimised by education about 'sick day rules', i.e. interrupting therapy during acute illness (e.g. gastrointestinal or respiratory), avoiding dehydration and seeking medical attention. The provision of a glucose meter with additional functionality for blood ketone monitoring can also be useful as an early warning of DKA for individuals considered to be at higher risk (e.g. type 1 diabetes).

Insulin therapy

Manufacture and formulations

Insulin was first isolated in Toronto in 1921, transforming the previously short life expectancy of children and young adults with type 1 diabetes. It was obtained for therapeutic use by extraction and purification from pancreases of cows and pigs (bovine and porcine insulins), until the emergence of recombinant DNA technology enabled large-scale production of human sequence insulin from the early 1980s. From the mid-1990s, 'analogue insulins', gradually gained ground; these contain alterations to the amino acid sequence and/or additional molecules covalently added to confer desirable pharmacological profiles. They have now largely replaced human sequence insulin.

The underlying principles of insulin pharmacology are simple, but the naming of the various available insulin preparations is complicated by trade names conferred on similar or equivalent products by different manufacturers. The time-action profile of an insulin describes its pharmacodynamic properties as time to onset and peak action as well as its overall duration of action after subcutaneous injection. These properties are depicted using simplified graphs (see Fig. 21.24) as an educational tool for insulin users and health-care professionals. With only a

few exceptions, insulin concentration is standardised internationally at 100 U/mL, using a system based on the one developed by the team in Toronto. Expert advice should be sought before using more concentrated insulins and in the UK these are now provided via dedicated pen devices to avoid confusion and prevent prescribing errors.

Unmodified ('soluble' or 'regular') short-acting insulin is clear in appearance and has an onset of action within 30 minutes of injection, wearing off by 6–8 hours. Extending this duration of action was initially achieved in the 1930s by adding protamine and zinc at neutral pH to create Neutral Protamine Hagedorn insulin (known as 'isophane' or NPH insulin) – this has a cloudy appearance (and requires to be resuspended by shaking before use). It is now referred to as 'intermediate-acting' with onset of action at 60–90 minutes, peaking at 6 hours and wearing off by 12–16 hours.

When insulin is injected into subcutaneous tissues, it aggregates into hexamers; these polymers of six insulin molecules must dissociate before systemic absorption can occur. The speed of dissociation can be altered by making small changes to the amino acid sequence (insulin analogues). For example, in insulin lispro, the penultimate lysine and proline residues on the C-terminal end of the B-chain are reversed (Fig. 21.23). This prevents hexamer formation leading to a more rapid onset and shorter duration of action than soluble insulin (Box 21.24). Short-acting insulin analogues allow greater flexibility as they can be injected closer to mealtimes (ideally 15–30 minutes before). Onset of action may be further hastened by the addition of excipients to the formulation (e.g. nicotinamide and L-arginine to insulin aspart to create 'faster insulin aspart').

Other changes to the insulin molecule have been engineered to produce long-acting analogue insulins. An example is insulin glargine, in which a substitution of glycine for asparagine in the A-chain and the addition of two additional arginine residues to the C-terminal end of the B-chain serves to prolong its duration of action to nearly 24 hours by increasing its isoelectric point from pH 5.4 to 6.7, i.e. making it less soluble at a physiological pH (see Fig. 21.23). Other long-acting insulins include insulin detemir and degludec; their duration of action is extended by adding fatty acid side chains to the C-terminal end of the B-chain (Fig. 21.23). Following subcutaneous injection, insulin detemir and degludec bind to albumin in the blood, from which insulin slowly disassociates. The duration of action of insulin degludec is almost 48 hours as the fatty acid moiety also promotes subcutaneous formation of multi-hexamers of insulin (see Box 21.24). It is termed a second generation long-acting insulin. However, a comparable pharmacological profile can be achieved by using a triple concentrated form of insulin glargine ('U300 glargine'); this can also be useful to decrease injection volume for individuals who require high doses to achieve glycaemic control. Modern long-acting insulins provide more consistent basal insulin levels during the day and night and are associated with lower rates of hypoglycaemia, particularly overnight. A long-acting insulin that requires injection only once weekly is currently in development.

Pre-mixed formulations containing short-acting and isophane insulins in various proportions ('biphasic', see below) are also available and widely prescribed in some countries, particularly for individuals with type 2 diabetes with regular mealtimes who wish to avoid injecting more than twice a day (see below).

Intermittent subcutaneous insulin injection therapy

Insulin is most commonly administered several times a day as an injection into the subcutaneous adipose tissue of the anterior abdominal wall, upper arms or outer thighs with the needle sited at a right-angle to the skin. Even with careful technique, the rate of absorption of insulin is influenced by the site, depth and volume of injection, skin temperature (warming) and exercise. Accidental intramuscular injection results in more rapid absorption and hypoglycaemia; it is more likely to occur in children and slim adults (with little subcutaneous adipose tissue) and can be minimised by using shorter needles (e.g. 4 mm rather than 8 mm). A clinically important reason for delayed absorption is lipohypertrophy, which can develop at over-used injection sites (see p. 738). This is due to the local trophic (growth factor)

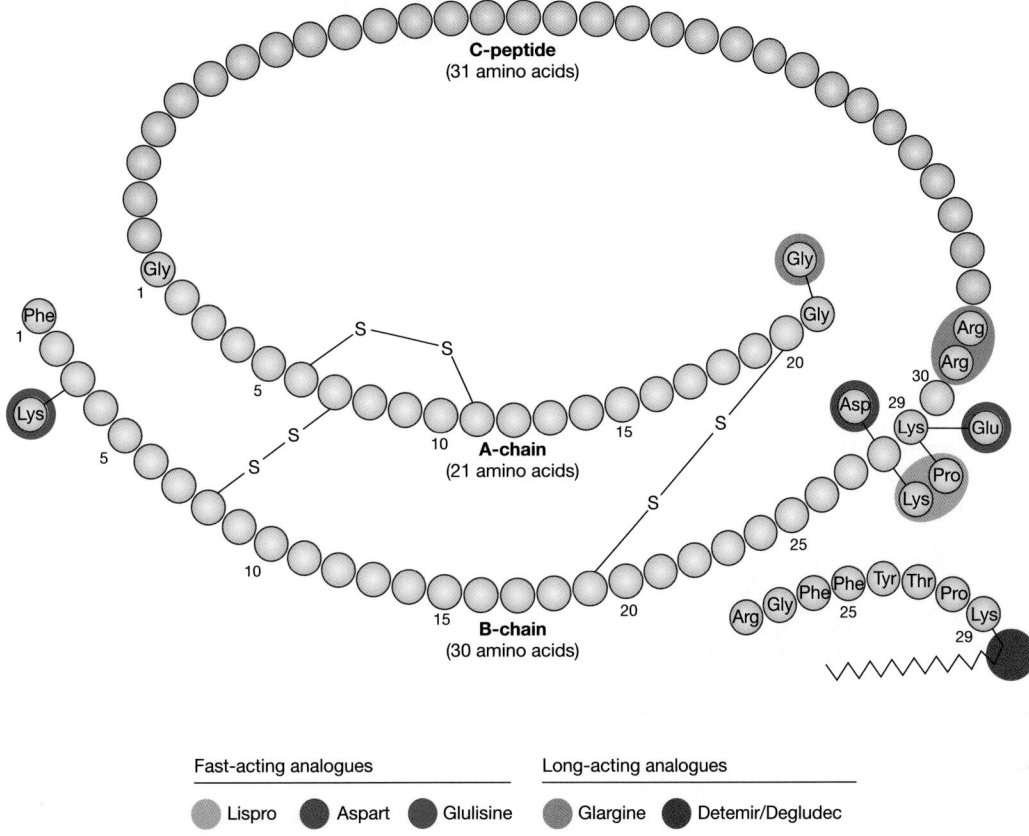

Fig. 21.23 **Schematic structure of insulin and insulin analogues.** Insulin is created when C-peptide is cleaved from the A- and B-chains of proinsulin. The areas in the shaded colours show the modifications made to the normal structure of insulin to create analogues. These are important in altering the pharmacokinetic properties of the analogues. Long-acting insulin analogues detemir and degludec are synthesised by adding specific fatty acid chains (shown) at position 29 (lysine) on the B-chain.

i	21.24 Duration of action (in hours) of insulin preparations		
Insulin	**Onset**	**Peak**	**Duration**
Rapid-acting insulin analogues: lispro, aspart, glulisine, fiasp	<0.5	0.5–2.5	3–4.5
Short-acting soluble (regular)	0.5–1	1–4	4–8
Intermediate-acting isophane (NPH), lente	1–3	3–8	7–14
Long-acting insulin analogues: glargine, detemir, degludec	1–2	None	18–26

action of insulin and results in greater variability in blood glucose. It can be avoided by not injecting into the same place and instead 'rotating' injections around (and within) the recommended sites.

Following absorption into blood, circulating insulin has a half-life of just a few minutes as it is cleared by the liver and kidneys. The total daily dose required may therefore diminish in individuals who develop liver disease or renal failure.

Traditional insulin syringes have largely been replaced by unobtrusive portable 'pen' devices, sufficient for multiple dosing and either disposable or designed to accept insulin in cartridges. Insulin users are advised to keep their stock in a refrigerator (approximately 4°C), but to keep their current pen at room temperature (as cold insulin is more painful to inject). Insulin will denature and become inactive if accidentally frozen and thawed. The complications of insulin therapy include hypoglycaemia (p. 719), weight gain, peripheral oedema, insulin antibodies, local allergy (rare) and lipohypertrophy or lipoatrophy at injection sites. Fasting hyperglycaemia (referred to as the 'Somogyi effect') has in the past been attributed to a rebound driven by counter-regulatory hormones (cortisol, growth hormone and catecholamines) following undetected overnight hypoglycaemia. However, systematic investigation in the era of CGM has detected little supporting evidence for this as high blood glucose on rising is more often due to a combination of the circadian cycle (or 'dawn phenomenon') and inadequate overnight basal insulin dosing.

Intermittent subcutaneous insulin injection regimens

The choice of insulin injection regimen depends on the agreed target for glycaemic control (set using the principle of 'shared decision-making'), need for flexibility in lifestyle and whether an individual can safely and reliably learn to adjust insulin doses in response to counting the carbohydrate content of planned meals. Time–action profiles for different insulin regimens are shown in Figure 21.24.

In general, people with type 1 diabetes should be prescribed either multiple daily insulin injections (MDI) or continuous subcutaneous insulin infusion therapy (CSII). MDI or 'basal-bolus'| therapy consists of four or five daily injections: one or two 'basal' injections (with an intermediate- or long-acting insulin, respectively) and an injection of 'bolus' insulin (usually with a rapid-acting analogue) 15–30 minutes before each of three main meals. The purpose of bolus insulin is to limit the magnitude of the rise in blood glucose following a meal. The purpose of basal ('background') insulin is to ensure there are adequate amounts of insulin to reduce hepatic glucose output, both overnight and during periods of the daytime when there is little bolus insulin activity (i.e. if there is a long time-gap between bolus injections). An MDI regimen allows greater freedom of meal timing as bolus insulin is simply administered before the meal.

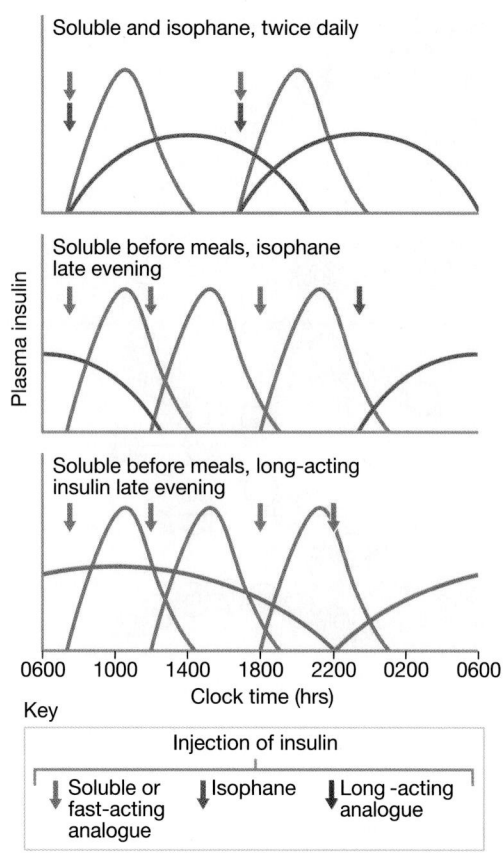

Fig. 21.24 Profiles of plasma insulin associated with different insulin regimens. These are theoretical patterns of plasma insulin and may differ considerably in magnitude and duration of action between individuals.

---

i | **21.25 Example of bolus insulin dose calculation**

You are about to eat a meal with 60 g carbohydrate

Your pre-meal blood glucose is 13.0 mmol/l

Your personalised diabetes data:

Insulin to carbohydrate ratio = 1:10

Insulin sensitivity factor = 3, i.e.1 unit of insulin lowers blood glucose by 3 mmol/L

Target blood glucose = 7 mmol/L

Bolus dose calculation

1. Bolus dose of insulin to cover meal = 60 g ÷ 10 g
   = **6 units**

2. Blood glucose correction = Actual glucose − target glucose
   = 13.0 − 7.0 mmol/L
   = **6.0 mmol/L**

3. Correction dose of insulin sensitivity factor = Blood glucose correction ÷ insulin sensitivity factor
   = 6.0 ÷ 3
   = **2 units**

4. Total bolus dose of insulin = Meal dose + correction dose
   = 6 + 2 units
   = **8 units**

The dose of bolus insulin administered at any one meal is primarily determined by the carbohydrate content of the meal, the prevailing glucose level and the target glucose for the individual. Each patient is advised by health-care professionals of their 'insulin to carbohydrate ratio', i.e. the amount of insulin to take for each carbohydrate portion. In most people, this ratio is around 1:10 (i.e. 1 unit of insulin is taken for each 10 g carbohydrate portion in the meal to be consumed), but may be higher or lower depending on the individual's insulin sensitivity. It may also vary between meals (e.g. breakfast vs evening meal). Patients are also advised of their 'insulin sensitivity factor' (or 'correction factor'), i.e. the amount that 1 unit of insulin lowers blood glucose. In most people, 1 unit of insulin lowers glucose by 3 or 4 mmol/l, although this again varies according to insulin sensitivity. Box 21.25 shows a worked example of how a person with diabetes may use this information to determine the dose of insulin to be administered with a meal. Additional adjustments to the final dose also may need to take into account other variables, including exercise and alcohol consumption. Thus, bolus insulin may need to be reduced to cover a meal taken 2 hours prior to vigorous exercise or if consuming large amounts of alcohol (see p. 732).

Basal insulin doses are determined with reference to fasting glucose levels and overnight profiles. Thus, the dose may be decreased if there is overnight or fasting hypoglycaemia and increased if there is overnight hyperglycaemia. Further refinement of daytime basal insulin can be made with reference to daytime glucose profiles following a series of carbohydrate-free meals (which do not require injection of bolus insulin) as the glucose levels in this context are mainly dependent on basal insulin.

The foregoing shows how the therapeutic use of insulin demands considerable attention to detail, with respect to a whole variety of factors, as well as significant numeracy skills. Many people understandably struggle to maintain the motivation required to monitor glucose regularly, count carbohydrate accurately, remember to take all their insulin injections and to leave an adequate gap between the bolus injection and the start of a meal.

In type 2 diabetes, insulin is usually initiated as a once-daily long-acting insulin, either alone or in combination with oral glucose-lowering agents. However, in time, more frequent insulin injections may be required. Recently, long-acting insulin analogues have been combined with GLP-1 receptor agonists, enabling co-administration of insulin and GLP-1 receptor agonists in a single daily injection.

Twice-daily administration of a short-acting and intermediate-acting insulin (usually soluble and isophane insulins), given in combination before breakfast and the evening meal, is still commonly used in many countries. Initially, two-thirds of the total daily requirement of insulin is given in the morning in a fixed ratio of short-acting to intermediate-acting preparation and the remaining third is given in the evening. Pre-mixed formulations are available that contain different proportions of soluble and isophane insulins (e.g. 30:70 and 50:50). These offer convenience in that only two injections per day are required (before breakfast and before the evening meal), but are inflexible as the individual components cannot be adjusted independently, i.e. a late meal or unexpected physical exercise can result in hypoglycaemia. Such regimens usually only provide optimal glycaemic control in individuals who prefer set meal-times with little dietary flexibility and who take part in little moderate or vigorous physical exercise.

Continuous subcutaneous insulin infusion therapy (insulin pump)

Continuous subcutaneous insulin infusion (CSII), commonly known as insulin pump therapy, is a system of insulin delivery that uses a battery-operated medical device to deliver insulin continuously to people with type 1 diabetes. A variety of insulin pumps are available and the choice is often framed by cost, compatibility with CGM systems and the personal preference or circumstances of the person with diabetes. When using a traditional pump, rapid-acting insulin is infused from a disposable insulin cartridge/reservoir within the pump (which has controls, a processing module and batteries). The disposable insulin cartridge/reservoir is attached to a tubing system that connects to a cannula, which is inserted subcutaneously (disposable infusion set) and secured by an adhesive dressing. The insulin infusion set and site should be changed every 3 days to avoid superficial infection of the site and compromise to the subcutaneous infusion of insulin. Patch pumps eliminate tubing from insulin infusion set as the cannula, cartridge/reservoir and batteries are located in a wearable disposable 'pod'. The controls and processing module are located in a handheld 'personal diabetes manager' that communicates wirelessly to the pod, which is changed every 3 days, as with the traditional pump. Examples of a traditional pump and patch pump are shown in Figure 21.25.

Basal insulin is delivered in the form of continuous infusion of rapid-acting insulin, usually 40%–50% of total daily dose (TDD). The proportion of basal insulin to TDD can vary, particularly in people who consume low or high carbohydrate diets. The number of units per hour can be calculated simply by dividing the TDD by 24. The basal rate is adjusted by fasting for periods of at least 4 hours while periodically evaluating the blood glucose levels and adjusting the pump infusion rate to maintain glucose in the normal range. Adjustments are made by approximately 10% at a time, 2 hours before a change in blood glucose is required, because of the kinetics of insulin absorption and time to reach steady state. One of the key advantages of CSII is that basal rates can be varied *within* a 24-hour period (this is in contrast to basal insulin in an MDI regimen, for which the dose can be altered, but the basal levels then remain relatively constant for the duration of action of that injection). This flexibility to pre-program adjustments is especially useful overnight, e.g. when basal rates can be reduced to prevent low glucose and then increased pre-dawn to prevent high morning (fasting) glucose. In addition, temporary basal rates can be used to lessen the risk of hypoglycaemia with daily activity (e.g. commuting, grocery shopping) or aerobic exercise (e.g. running, cycling).

Pre-meal boluses are administered 15–30 minutes before food via the insulin pump to limit post-prandial glucose excursions. As with MDI, bolus dosing is determined by the carbohydrate content of the meal, a personalised insulin to carbohydrate ratio and pre-meal glucose levels. Insulin pumps allow more flexibility with bolus insulin infusions in both timing and shape (e.g. using an extended or dual-wave bolus when covering high-fat/protein meals such as pizza or steak, or when diabetes is complicated by gastroparesis). Additionally, insulin pumps have calculators or 'bolus wizards' that calculate the 'active insulin on board', for precise calculation of pre-meal boluses and to allow safer 'correction' doses during periods of hyperglycaemia. This helps reduce the risk of hypoglycaemia from boluses given close together in time, an effect known as 'insulin stacking'.

Overall, CSII reduces blood glucose variability in type 1 diabetes and in some people can help improve HbA$_{1c}$. However, the benefits of insulin pump therapy can only be fully realised with meticulous and attentive carbohydrate counting and glucose monitoring, and pro-active adjustment of bolus and basal insulin in response to glucose levels. There are also risks to pump therapy that limit its suitability for some people. Pump failure leading to an interruption of the subcutaneous insulin infusion can occur for a variety of reasons. Causes include detachment or kinking of the insulin infusion set cannula or malfunction due to expiry of the battery. As the pump delivers rapid-acting insulin and there is no depot of intermediate or long-acting insulin, pump failure can very quickly (within a matter of hours) lead to insulin deficiency and DKA. Therefore, insulin pump users must regularly monitor glucose and promptly check for ketones and change the infusion set and cannula site if they have concerns about pump failure. 'Back-up' unexpired insulin pens should always be available. Individuals who are not prepared or able to monitor glucose regularly are not suitable for CSII because of the risks of DKA. Cannula site infection is another recognised complication of pump therapy; this risk can be reduced by good hygiene and by ensuring the cannula is changed every three days.

Sensor-augmented CSII therapy

A further iteration in insulin pump therapy in recent years is communication with certain CGM devices via computerised algorithms (Fig. 21.26). Senor-augmented insulin pumps can use data from CGM and, with knowledge of the amount of 'active insulin on board', can adjust basal rates towards a target glucose. Rather than preset basal rate infusions, such 'hybrid closed-loop' systems (also known as an 'artificial pancreas') automatically decide whether to infuse a small amount of basal insulin every 5 minutes, with decisions about pre-meal boluses still determined by the person with diabetes (Fig. 21.27). Features also include 'low-glucose suspend' or 'suspend before low' functions, such that detection of hypoglycaemia or a glucose level falling below a pre-set threshold (e.g. 5.0 mmol/L (90 mg/dL)) respectively, signal the pump to stop infusing insulin temporarily, leading to a substantial reduction in hypoglycaemia without rebound hyperglycaemia. Finally, bi-hormonal fully automated closed-loop systems (containing separate syringe drivers with insulin and glucagon), also known as the 'bionic pancreas', are now in clinical trials but not yet commercially available. The current systems are not perfect (e.g. recurrent low glucose sensor alarms can be irritating), but sensor-augmented CSII technologies are rapidly improving and offer the real prospect of a 'technological cure' for type 1 diabetes, i.e. delivering near normal blood glucose, with little or no hypoglycaemia and with minimal input

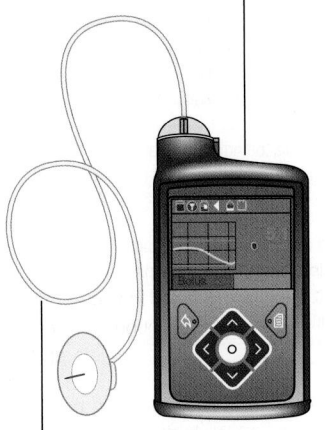

A
Electronic device containing a plastic cartridge of insulin, battery and internal computer to program insulin delivery

B
Integrated (tubeless) pump and infusion device

1,35u
10B

LAST BOLUS 3u LAST BG 5.1 mmol/L

Insulin infusion set containing flexible tubing and cannula for insertion

Control system which can communicate wirelessly with the pump

Fig. 21.25 Insulin pumps. An insulin pump is an alternative means of delivering insulin in type 1 diabetes. **A** Different types are available and include the pump device itself (with controls, processing module and batteries), a disposable reservoir for insulin (inside the pump) and a disposable infusion set (with tubing and a cannula for subcutaneous insertion). **B** Alternative configurations include disposable or semi-disposable pumps without infusion tubing. Insulin pumps deliver rapid-acting insulin continuously and can be adjusted by the user, based on regular glucose monitoring and carbohydrate counting.

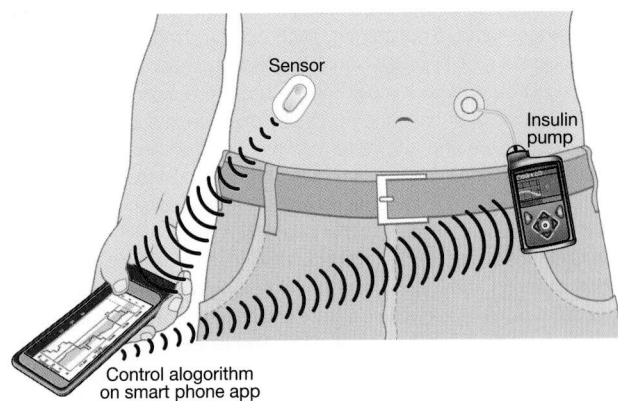

Sensor

Insulin pump

Control algorithm on smart phone app

Fig. 21.26 Sensor-augmented insulin pump system. The artificial pancreas (AP) can vary in its set up but, core to an AP system are: (1) a continuous glucose monitor (CGM) measuring interstitial glucose levels every 5–15 minutes; (2) a smartphone (or personal diabetes manager) with an app that uses the glucose information from the CGM, along with modifications inserted by the user, to calculate how much insulin should be delivered. This is communicated wirelessly to (3) the insulin pump that delivers insulin subcutaneously as directed.

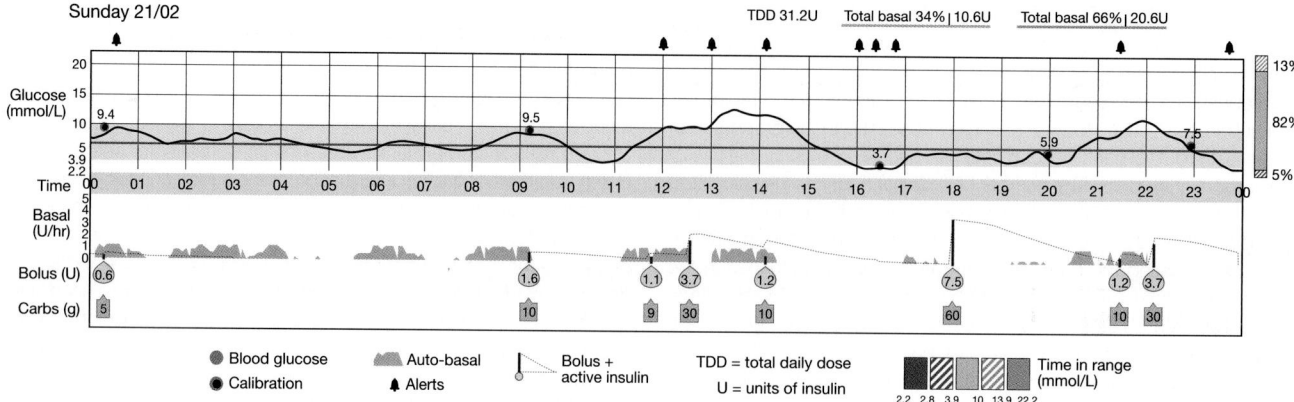

Fig. 21.27 Download from a sensor-augmented insulin pump system. The user is required to enter the carbohydrate content of meals and snacks. Bolus doses of insulin are determined in part on this information (purple). Basal insulin administration is determined by an algorithm using glucose data and 'active insulin'. Note how the basal insulin infused (pink) varies substantially with time, such that basal insulin ceases when glucose levels are falling (especially if there is still active insulin present from a previous bolus dose). The user is also alerted when there are impending low or high glucose events. These functions facilitate excellent glycaemic control (especially overnight when there is no impact on glucose from food ingestion and exercise) and prevent or minimise low glucose events.

required from the user. However, these technologies are expensive and widespread use may be limited by cost for some time to come. The use of do-it-yourself artificial pancreas systems (DIY-APS), also known as 'looping', is increasing, particularly in high-income countries. DIY-APS are by definition not approved by regulatory bodies, but use existing insulin pumps and CGM devices with free open resource software to link the systems and provide much of the functionality described above.

Intravenous insulin therapy

Circulating insulin has a half-life of approximately 2.5 minutes (the longer duration of action of subcutaneous insulin is because of the time taken for insulin to be absorbed from subcutaneous sites to the blood). Therefore, direct infusion of insulin via the intravenous route gives maximum flexibility in regulating blood glucose concentrations: an increase in the infusion rate will rapidly correct hyperglycaemia, while cessation of intravenous insulin will arrest a rapidly declining blood glucose. This inherent flexibility makes intravenous insulin a powerful tool in the management of hyperglycaemic emergencies and in stabilising blood glucose in a perioperative situation or in individuals who are unwell, e.g. with poor oral intake or delayed gastric emptying. Subcutaneous insulin does not lower blood glucose quickly enough for hyperglycaemic emergencies, particularly if skin perfusion is reduced during sepsis, while its duration of action may also be too long (i.e. result in hypoglycaemia) if given to an unwell patient who subsequently cannot eat or vomits. Intravenous insulin is, however, a dangerous therapy if not properly supervised and monitored. There are substantial risks of hypoglycaema, hypokalaemia and hyperglycaemia (including DKA) and so it must only be used in a setting where medical and nursing staff have the necessary experience and time to safely prescribe, prepare and administer the therapy. Standardised ward-level documentation and protocols are essential to support the clinical team.

Intravenous insulin is most commonly given via an electronic syringe driver (insulin injected directly into a bag of intravenous glucose and potassium is now rarely used). Usually, 50 units of soluble insulin (Actrapid® or Humulin S®) is diluted in 50 mL 0.9% sodium chloride, to provide an infusion of 1 unit insulin/mL. In hyperglycaemic emergencies (especially DKA), it is usually given as a fixed rate insulin infusion (FRII). This avoids the possibility of the infusion rate reducing to zero, as can occur with a variable rate insulin infusion (VRII), which might cause a worsening of acidosis and ketosis.

In perioperative and medically unwell patients insulin is usually given as a VRII (formerly called an 'insulin sliding scale'). Indications and principles of using VRII in the hospital setting are outlined in Box 21.26. An example of a VRII prescription chart is shown in Figure 21.28. Bedside capillary blood glucose monitoring should be performed on an hourly basis. Due to the short half-life of intravenous insulin, the insulin infusion must be monitored regularly to ensure it is continuously running;

21.26 Variable rate insulin infusion (VRII)

Principles

- Desired glucose targets are achieved and maintained
- Avoidance of hypoglycaemia
- Avoidance of ketonaemia by providing adequate carbohydrate and insulin
- Maintenance of fluid and electrolyte balance

Indications

- People with diabetes undergoing operations, e.g. fasting >24 hours, emergency surgery
- People with diabetes who have uncontrolled hyperglycaemia or who are unable to eat and drink due to prolonged fasting, nausea, vomiting or reduced consciousness

Do not use

- Diabetic ketoacidosis (DKA)
- Hyperglycaemic hyperosmolar state (HHS)

Additional requirements

- Capillary blood glucose should be checked at least hourly
- The standard regimen for intravenous fluid prescription is 0.45% sodium chloride + 5% glucose + 0.15% potassium chloride (pre-prepared infusion bags) run at 100 mL/hr through a volumetric pump only
- Potassium monitoring is required to maintain serum level between 4 and 5 mmol/L
- Specialty input is required to guide fluid replacement in special situations, such as cardiac failure, renal failure, following head injury and after neurosurgery

Considerations when stopping

- Continue long-acting insulin at usual time while on VRII to allow stopping at any time
- Pre-mixed insulin should not be administered on VRII – if stopping VRII give usual dose at breakfast/dinner and stop VRII after 2 hours (due to short half-life of intravenous insulin and risk of rebound hyperglycaemia)

if there is interruption to the infusion even for a relatively short period of time (e.g. a 'tissued' intravenous cannula, a kink in the infusion tube, a mechanical failure in the pump or the syringe simply running-out), significant hyperglycaemia can quickly ensue. With a VRII, intravenous glucose (e.g. 0.45% sodium chloride + 5% glucose + 0.15% potassium chloride infused at 100 mL/hr) should be prescribed to provide some energy substrate and to reduce the risk of hypoglycaemia and hypokalaemia. Where possible, the glucose and insulin infusions should be given through a volumetric infusion device via the same intravenous catheter with a Y-connector, so that if the cannula blocks or 'tissues', then both infusions simultaneously cease, reducing the risk of hypoglycaemia from unopposed insulin. If additional fluids or potassium replacement

Variable Rate Insulin Infusion (VRII): prescription, administration and monitoring record (adults)						
1. Prescription: insulin infusion details						
Medicine	**Total amount of insulin in syringe**	**Name of diluent**	**Total volume in syringe**	**Insulin concentration**	**Route**	**Comments**
SOLUBLE INSULIN (Actrapid® or Humulin S®)	50 units	Sodium chloride 0.9%	50 ml	1 unit /ml	IV	

2. Prescription: insulin dose variable rate

Capillary blood glucose (CBG)- mmol/L	Insulin infusion rate (units/hour)		
	Recommended initial rate	**Alternative rate**	**Alternative rate**
< 4	**Prescriber: tick below as appropriate** **0** (if long-acting insulin given) ☐ **0.5** (if long-acting insulin not given) ☐ Date ┆ Time ┆ Initial		
4–7	1		
7.1–9	2		
9.1–11	3		
11.1–14	4		
14.1–17	5 (check ketones if type 1 diabetes)		
17.1–20	6 (check ketones if type 1 diabetes)		
>20	**Seek senior medical advice** (check ketones)		
Signature of prescriber			
Date			

Fig. 21.28 Example of a prescription document for a variable rate insulin infusion (VRII). The insulin infusion has a standard concentration of 1 unit/mL. The rate of insulin infusion is adjusted according to the prevailing blood glucose level. Adjustments are made to the infusion rates as capillary blood glucose falls and rises.

are required, depending on the volume and potassium status of the individual, they should be given via a separate infusion. Unused insulin should be discarded every 24 hours and a new infusion prepared. VRIIs should be reviewed at least every 24 hours to ensure that the infusion rates prescribed for a given blood sugar level have resulted in stable glucose levels. If blood sugar levels have been very variable, with frequent adjustments to the infusion rate, this is usually a sign that the prescription needs to be modified (or that it is time for the VRII to be discontinued as the patient has begun to eat).

Transplantation

The goal of transplantation is to facilitate independence from insulin, reduce complications and improve quality of life.

The American Diabetes Association (ADA) criteria for transplantation include three main types of pancreas transplantation:

- Simultaneous pancreas–kidney (SPK) transplant, when pancreas and kidney are transplanted simultaneously from the same deceased donor, or pancreas-after-kidney (PAK) transplant, when a cadaveric donor pancreas transplant is performed after a previous, and different, living or deceased donor kidney transplant
- Pancreas transplant alone (PTA)
- Islet transplantation

Whole pancreas transplantation is carried out in a relatively small number of people each year. SPK is the most commonly performed procedure. Most SPK and PAK are undertaken in people with diabetes and end-stage kidney disease, in whom successful transplantation will improve glycaemia and may improve kidney survival. PTA is generally considered for people with progressive complications leading to significant loss of quality of life (for example recurrent level 3 hypoglycaemia). The principal complications occurring immediately after surgery include thrombosis, pancreatitis, infection, bleeding and rejection. Prognosis is improving: 1 year after transplantation >95% of all patients are still alive and 80%–85% of all pancreases are still functional. After transplantation, people will need life-long immunosuppression, which carries with it an increased risk of infection and skin cancer.

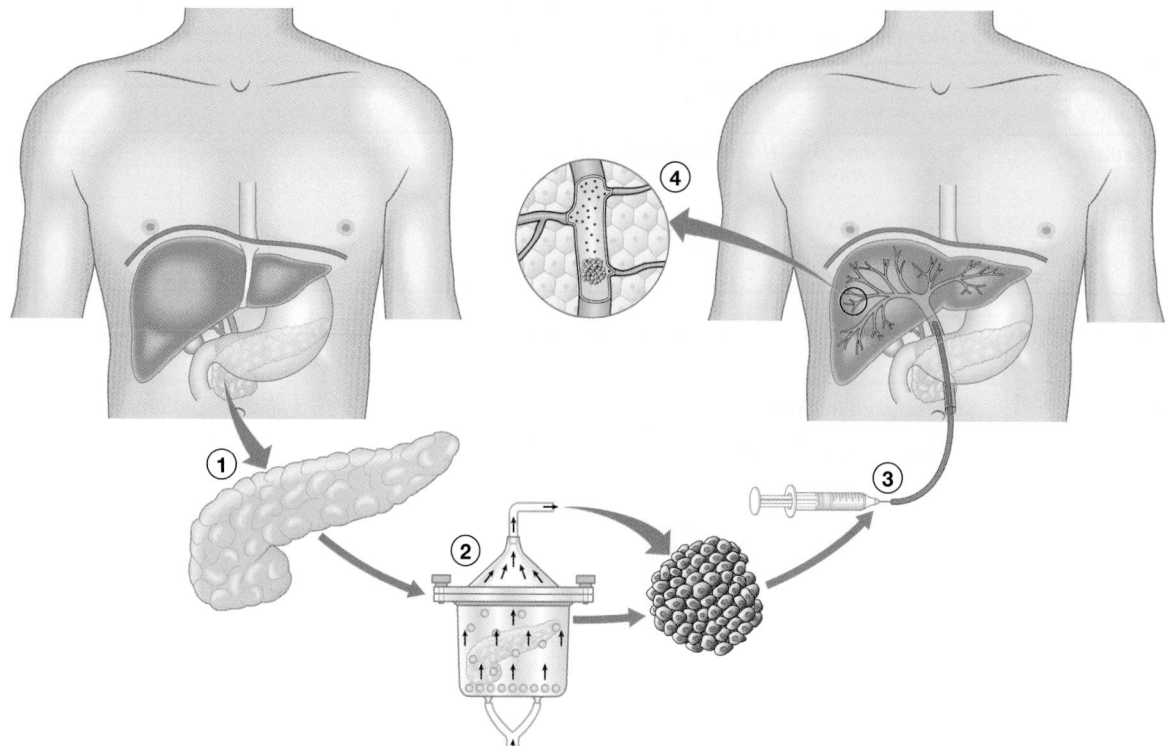

Fig. 21.29 Transplanting islet cells. (1) Pancreas obtained from suitable human donor. (2) Pancreatic islets containing insulin-producing β cells are isolated first in a Ricordi chamber. (3) Islets, once separated and purified, are infused into the hepatic portal vein. (4) Once embedded in the liver, pancreatic islets secrete insulin in response to changes in portal vein glucose.

Islet transplantation involves the transplantation of islets from a donor pancreas into a person with type 1 diabetes. The isolated pancreatic islets are usually infused into the patient's liver via the portal vein. This approach has now been successfully adopted in a number of centres around the world (Fig. 21.29). At present, islet transplantation is usually suitable only for people with unstable glycaemic control characterised by severe intractable hypoglycaemia that cannot be corrected by structured education, modern insulin regimens and technology. Progress is being made towards meeting the needs of supply, purification and storage of islets, but problems remain relating to transplant rejection and destruction by the immune-mediated process against β cells that caused type 1 diabetes in the first place. Nevertheless, the development of methods of inducing tolerance to transplanted islets and the potential use of stem cells mean that this may still prove a promising approach in the long term. Adoption of newer immunosuppressive protocols has resulted in far better outcomes and now nearly 50% of people with diabetes transplanted will be insulin-independent at 3 years post transplantation. This is an evolving therapy area with many new experimental techniques under development. There are no direct comparisons between whole pancreas and islet transplantation, but it appears that whole pancreas transplantation results in higher rates of insulin independence albeit with the greater morbidity of surgery.

Management of diabetes in special situations

Diabetes in pregnancy

The management of women with diabetes who are pregnant or who have developed diabetes during pregnancy (gestational diabetes) is discussed in detail in Chapter 32. This is a highly specialised area and requires careful management, as elevated maternal blood glucose in pregnancy is associated with significant maternal and fetal morbidity.

 21.27 Diabetes in adolescence

- **Type of diabetes**: type 1 diabetes is predominant in children and adolescents, but type 2 diabetes is now presenting in unprecedented numbers of obese, inactive teenagers. Monogenic diabetes (MODY) should also be considered (see Box 21.8).
- **Physiological changes**: hormonal, physical and lifestyle changes in puberty affect dietary intake, exercise patterns and sensitivity to insulin, necessitating alterations in insulin regimen.
- **Emotional changes**: adolescence is a phase of transition into independence (principally from parental care). Periods of rebellion against parental control, experimentation (e.g. with alcohol and recreational drugs) and a more chaotic lifestyle are common, and often impact adversely on control of diabetes.
- **Glycaemic control**: a temporary deterioration in control is common, although not universal. It is sometimes more important to maintain contact and engagement with a young person than to insist on tight glycaemic control.
- **Diabetic ketoacidosis**: a few adolescents and young adults present with frequent episodes of DKA, often because of suboptimal adherence to insulin therapy. This is more common in females. Precipitating factors include desire for weight loss, personality and even manipulation of family or schooling circumstances.
- **Adolescent diabetes clinics**: these challenges are best tackled with support from a specialised multidisciplinary team, including paediatricians, physicians, nurses and psychologists. Support is required for the patient and parents.

Children, adolescents and young adults with diabetes

Most type 1 diabetes is diagnosed in children below 18 years of age, with peak incidence rates between 5 and 7 years of age and at puberty. The management of diabetes in children and adolescents has important differences to adults, which should be addressed in specialised clinics with multidisciplinary input (Box 21.27). Some of the unique aspects of childhood type 1 diabetes management include changing insulin sensitivity related to sexual maturity and physical growth, unique vulnerability to hypoglycaemia (especially in children below 6 years of age) and DKA. Family dynamics, child-care and schooling, developmental stages and ability to self-care all have to be considered in the personalised management plan. In older children and adolescents, there may be issues of body image, eating disorders and recreational drug and alcohol use. Innovative models of education such as digital comics and gamification are emerging. It is also notable that there is very limited clinical research in children with diabetes and so most recommendations are based on expert opinion. The prevalence of type 2 diabetes in those below 20 years of age is increasing and is estimated to increase 4-fold in the next 40 years.

Diabetes in hospital

People with diabetes account for around 20% of all hospital in-patients in the UK. The vast majority (around 9 out of 10) are admitted to hospital for a cause unrelated to diabetes or for a condition where diabetes may be a contributory factor (e.g. an acute cardiovascular event or elective surgery for cataract). Common causes for diabetes-specific admission include foot ulceration, DKA, HHS, newly diagnosed diabetes and hyperglycaemia. Any person with diabetes presenting to hospital acutely unwell should have a blood glucose measurement.

People with diabetes often report unhappiness with how their diabetes was managed during a hospital admission. Clearly admission to hospital disturbs an individual's usual daily routine, including the timings and types of meal being offered, and the amount of physical activity. Acute illness and surgery can cause blood glucose levels to rise and the

individual may not be able to eat or drink for extended periods. Insulin and other glucose-lowering medication may be prescribed by relatively inexperienced trainees or non-specialists and some people with diabetes report a feeling of 'loss of control' in the management of their condition. When the prescribed dose of insulin is different from what is considered appropriate by the person with diabetes this should be discussed and handled sensitively with clear explanations for the rationale behind prescribing decisions. Through lived experience, the person with diabetes may well know more about their condition than the doctor.

Errors in prescriptions of glucose-lowering therapies (especially insulin) are extremely common and may be due to lack of knowledge on the part of medical staff, inadvertent error due to time pressures or other human or system factors (see Chapter 1). It is important that medical staff are proactive in adjusting glucose-lowering therapy to avoid extreme glucose excursions. Hyperglycaemia and hypoglycaemia are unpleasant and potentially harmful; they are also associated with increased length of stay.

Hyperglycaemia in acute admissions to hospital

Hyperglycaemia is often found in patients who are admitted to hospital as an emergency. In most instances, this occurs in people with known diabetes, but it may also be due to undiagnosed diabetes or stress hyperglycaemia (see p. 719). An example of decision-making support around the management of hyperglycaemia on admission to hospital can be found in Figure 21.30.

Acute intercurrent illness causes catabolic stress and secretion of counter-regulatory hormones (including catecholamines and cortisol) in both normal and diabetic individuals. This results in increased

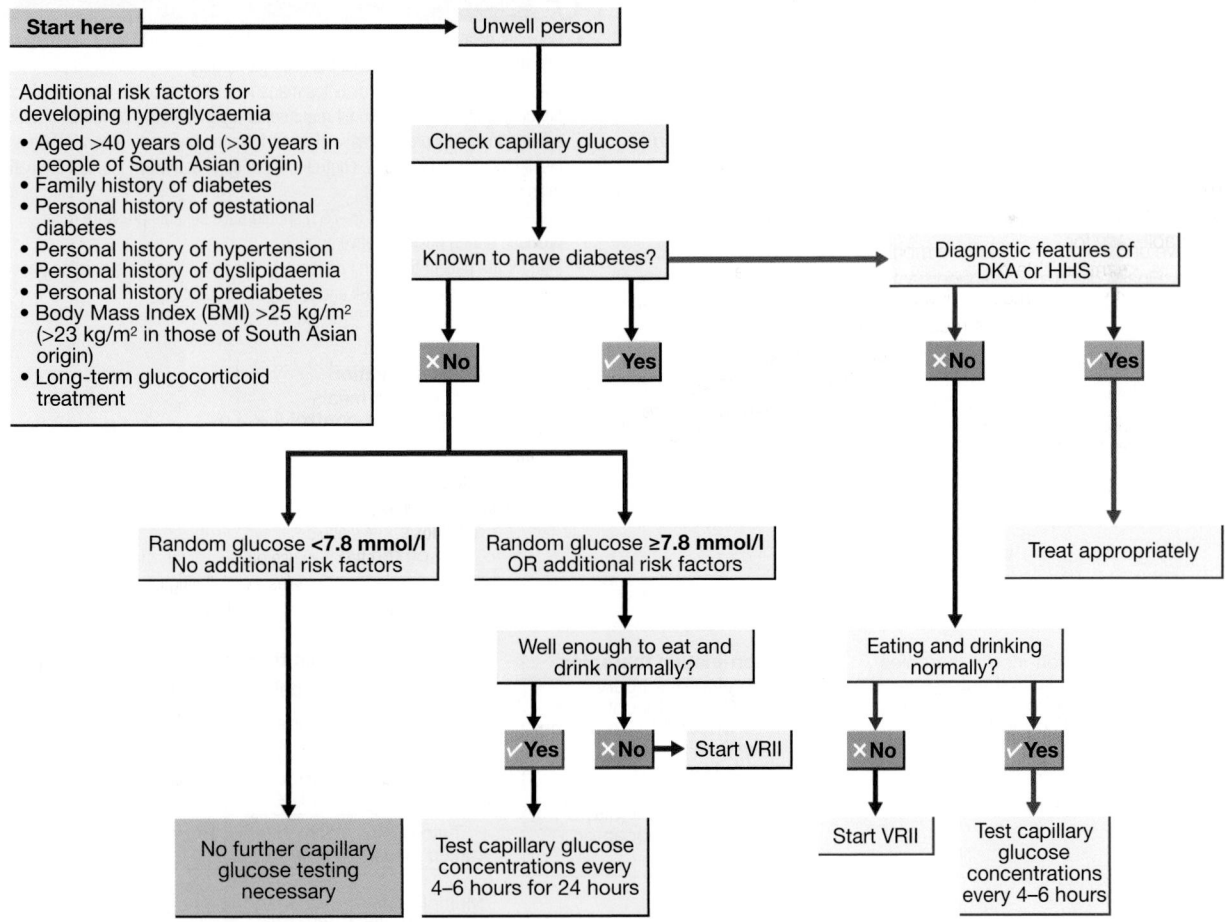

Fig. 21.30 Decision-making algorithm for an individual presenting to hospital with hyperglycaemia. The target glucose of individuals with established diabetes is 6–10 mmol/L, but a range of 4–12 mmol/L is acceptable. (DKA = diabetic ketoacidosis; HHS = hyperglycaemic hyperosmolar state; VRII = variable rate insulin infusion)
Adapted from Joint British Diabetes Societies for Inpatient Care, Diabetes at the Front Door; 2021. https://abcd.care/joint-british-diabetes-societies-jbds-inpatient-care-group.

glycogenolysis, gluconeogenesis, lipolysis, proteolysis and insulin resistance. Starvation exacerbates this process by increasing lipolysis. In a person without diabetes, these metabolic effects lead to a secondary increase in the secretion of insulin, which exerts a controlling influence. In people with untreated or poorly controlled diabetes, the uptake of metabolic substrate into tissues is significantly reduced because of insulin deficiency (relative or absolute), catabolism is increased and, ultimately, metabolic decompensation in the form of DKA or HHS may develop.

Hyperglycaemia on admission to hospital is associated with increased length of stay and increased mortality in a wide variety of acute medical emergencies, including acute myocardial infarction and acute stroke. This may be a direct consequence of hyperglycaemia (perhaps through volume depletion from osmotic diuresis, electrolye imbalance, a secondary pro-coagulant state, and/or negative effects on the immune system) or simply a consequence that more severe illness (with a worse prognosis) causes greater degrees of hyperglycaemia. Intuitively, intensive glycaemic control with intravenous insulin should improve outcomes during acute illness. However, studies to date have shown that strategies aiming for near-normal blood glucose levels in acutely ill patients are associated with either increased mortality or no overall benefit. The reasons for the adverse outcomes are not established, but intensive glycaemic control is inevitably associated with an increased risk of hypoglycaemia, because of the inherent limitations of modern insulins, the limited frequency of glucose monitoring in a ward environment and the relative imprecision of near-patient blood glucose meters. Activation of the sympathetic nervous system and release of counter-regulatory hormones during acute hypoglycaemia likely has deleterious consequences for the acutely ill patient. Therefore, a target blood glucose of between 6 and 10 mmol/L (105 and 180 mg/dL) with an acceptable range of 4–12 mmol/L (72–220 mg/dL) is recommended for in-patients with diabetes. VRII is sometimes used for uncontrolled hyperglycaemia in hospital.

Surgery and diabetes

People with diabetes are reported to have up to 50% higher perioperative mortality than people without diabetes. Surgery has the same metabolic consequences, described above, as acute intercurrent illness. In addition, hyperglycaemia impairs wound healing and innate immunity, leading to increased risk of infection. People with diabetes are also more likely to have underlying pre-operative morbidity, especially cardiovascular disease. Finally, glycaemic management errors may cause dangerous hyperglycaemia or hypoglycaemia. Careful pre-operative assessment and perioperative management are therefore essential, ideally with support from the diabetes specialist team.

Pre-operative assessment

Unless a surgical intervention is an emergency, people with diabetes should be assessed well in advance of surgery so that glycaemic control can be achieved and other risk factors can be addressed (Box 21.28). There is good evidence that a higher HbA$_{1c}$ is associated with adverse perioperative outcome. In general, the upper limit for an acceptable HbA$_{1c}$ in this context is 69 mmol/mol (8.5%). However, since optimisation of care may take weeks or months to achieve, the potential benefits of improved glycaemia need to be weighed against the potential benefits for early surgical intervention.

Perioperative management

Figure 21.31 outlines a general approach to perioperative management of diabetes, although this may need to be adapted according to the individual, the surgical procedure and local guidelines, i.e. there is no 'one size fits all' approach. People with diabetes who are considered low-risk can attend as day cases or be admitted on the day of surgery. Occasionally, they may be admitted the night before surgery to ensure optimal management.

Postoperative management

People with diabetes who need to continue fasting after surgery should be maintained on a VRII until they are able to eat and drink. During this time, care must be taken with fluid balance and electrolyte levels; the ideal glucose range is 6–10 mmol/L (105–180 mg/dL), with an acceptable range

21.28 Pre-operative assessment

- Consider delaying surgery and refer to the diabetes team if HbA$_{1c}$ >69 mmol/mol; this should be weighed against the need for surgery
- Establish an individualized diabetes management plan for the pre-admission period (including optimization if required) and perioperative period (this will be determined by pre-operative glucose-lowering regimens – non-insulin and insulin therapies, glycaemic control and period of starvation (i.e. will the patient miss more than one meal)
- Patients with high-risk feet (p. 751) should have suitable pressure relief provided during post-operative nursing
- Plan for the patient to be first on the list. This minimises the starvation period and thereby the need for VRII and length of inpatient stay

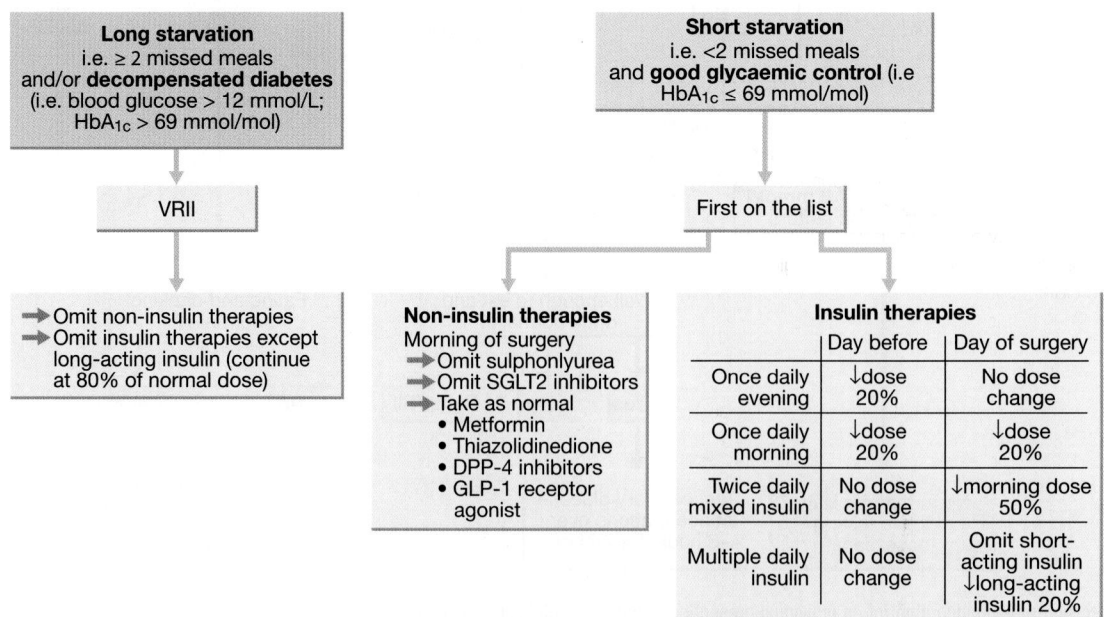

Fig. 21.31 A suggested approach to the perioperative management of diabetes. *Adapted from Joint British Diabetes Societies for Inpatient Care, Management of adults with diabetes undergoing surgery and elective procedures: Improving standards. March 2016.*

of 4–12 mmol/L (72–220 mg/dL). Once usual glucose-lowering treatment has been reinstated, good blood glucose control should be maintained to optimise wound healing and recovery.

Diabetes footcare in hospital

Diabetes foot disease is discussed in detail on p. 751. Between 2% and 3% of people with diabetes admitted to hospital develop a foot ulcer during the admission. Pressure ulceration (due to prolonged contact between part of the foot, such as the heel, and a firm surface, such as a mattress) can occur due to prolonged immobility in a hospital bed and is associated with peripheral vascular disease, poor glycaemic control, malnourishment and dehydration. Delirium, dementia and peripheral neuropathy all increase the risk of developing pressure ulceration, because the individual does not recognise the sensation of abnormal heel pressure. The feet of all people with diabetes should be examined on admission to hospital. Those with feet 'vulnerable' for ulceration must be given protection for their feet. Individuals who are bedbound should wear special 'foot protectors' – moulded plastic boots with padding that specifically redistribute pressure and off-load the heel areas as these are particularly susceptible to pressure ulceration. Pressure relief pads are also available that can be fitted to the end of a bed and are indicated for people with 'at risk' feet who are ambulant. If ulceration is identified on the initial foot assessment or occurs during admission (something that should be a 'never event'), then the patient should be immediately referred to the multidisciplinary diabetes foot team.

Complications of diabetes

Chronic hyperglycaemia causes irreversible damage over time to a number of tissues: particularly the small blood vessels of the retina (retinopathy), the glomerulus (nephropathy) and peripheral nerves (peripheral neuropathy) (Box 21.29). These so-called microvascular complications are amongst the commonest causes of visual loss, end-stage renal failure (dialysis) and foot ulceration (amputation) in most global populations and have a major adverse impact on quality of life. They are strongly linked to hyperglycaemia and increased duration of diabetes. Hyperglycaemia causes tissue damage via four main biochemical pathways: the polyol pathway, the hexosamine pathway, accumulation of advanced glycation end products and activation of protein kinase C. Each of these leads to overproduction of reactive oxygen species by the mitochondrial electron transport chain, giving rise to oxidative stress. The histopathological hallmark of diabetic microangiopathy is thickening of the capillary basement membrane, with associated increased vascular permeability. This occurs throughout the body resulting in the characteristic microvascular complications and accelerated atherosclerosis.

In the 1990s over 20% of people with type 2 diabetes in the UK had evidence of microvascular complications at the time of diagnosis, but this rate has fallen dramatically in many countries (e.g. to as low as 1% in parts of Germany) with better awareness and screening in the community and consequently earlier diagnosis. Microvascular complications are strongly linked to long-term elevated blood glucose (usually manifest as an elevated HbA_{1c}) and individuals with strict glycaemic control have a much lower risk of developing these complications.

Macrovascular complications are less closely linked to blood glucose, particularly in type 2 diabetes. In type 2 diabetes, insulin resistance is also directly and pathophysiologically linked with hypertension and dyslipidaemia (as part of the metabolic syndrome, each of which is also a risk factor for atherosclerosis). Thus, even individuals with impaired glucose tolerance (i.e. who do not have high enough blood glucose to be diagnosed with diabetes) already have an elevated risk of cardiovascular disease. Management of blood pressure and dyslipidaemia in diabetes are discussed briefly on p. 729), while the investigation and management of cardiovascular disease are discussed in detail in Chapters 16 and 29.

In addition to vascular complications, diabetes is associated with an increased susceptibility to infection and increased severity of infection.

> ### 🛈 21.29 Complications of diabetes
>
> **Microvascular/neuropathic**
>
> **Retinopathy, cataract**
> - Common cause of visual loss
>
> **Nephropathy**
> - Renal failure, requirement for dialysis
>
> **Peripheral neuropathy (foot disease)**
> - Sensory loss
> - Pain
> - Ulceration
> - Charcot neuroarthropathy
>
> **Autonomic neuropathy**
> - Postural hypotension
> - Gastroparesis
> - Sexual dysfunction
>
> **Macrovascular**
>
> **Coronary circulation**
> - Angina
> - Acute coronary syndrome/ myocardial infarction
>
> **Cerebral circulation**
> - Transient ischaemic attack
> - Stroke
>
> **Peripheral circulation (foot disease)**
> - Claudication
> - Ischaemia
> - Ulceration
>
> **Infection**
> - Increased risk of certain infections, e.g. *Candida* spp., urine infection, fungal nail disease
> - Increased risk of severe forms of infection, e.g. COVID-19, influenza, tuberculosis
> - Increased risk of opportunistic infections, e.g. emphysematous pyelonephritis
>
> **Rheumatological complications**
> - Cheiroarthropathy, limited joint movement
> - Dupuytren's contracture
> - Adhesive capsulitis
> - Trigger finger
>
> **Skin complications**
> - Diabetic dermopathy
> - Necrobiosis lipoidica
> - Xerosis

Glycation of soft tissues and periarticular structures can cause a variety of rheumatological disorders, including diabetic cheiroarthropathy and adhesive capsulitis. Glycation and subsequent osmotic changes in the lens of the eye can cause reversibly reduced visual acuity at presentation of diabetes and can predispose to cataracts. Type 2 diabetes is associated with a 2-fold increased risk of dementia with increased risk of both Alzheimer's disease and vascular dementia. The mechanisms underpinning this association are complex and may involve factors such as micro- and macrovascular disease, abnormalities in insulin action in the brain and glycosylation of neuronal tissue.

Life expectancy/mortality

The life expectancy of people with type 2 diabetes in the UK is similar to that of the general population for those of higher socioeconomic status. However, those who are subject to social deprivation lose on average 4–5 years of life, even in countries where there is universal access to health care and free prescriptions. This gradient of life expectancy according to factors that are not classically 'biomedical' is more difficult to measure in countries that do not have universal health-care coverage, but is likely even steeper in those countries with an 'uninsured' section of the population.

Excess mortality in type 2 diabetes is caused mainly by cardiovascular disease, particularly myocardial infarction and stroke. There is also substantial morbidity from myocardial infarction, stroke, angina, cardiac failure and intermittent claudication. The pathological changes of atherosclerosis in type 2 diabetes are similar to those in non-diabetic individuals, but occur earlier in life and are more extensive and severe with the effects of associated major cardiovascular risk factors (smoking, hypertension and dyslipidaemia) amplified. Rates of mortality adjusted for age and socio-economic status are 38% higher in men and 49% higher in women with type 2 diabetes, mainly driven by cardiovascular disease. In the United States, hospitalisation rates for stroke are 1.5 times higher in adults with type 2 diabetes while 60% of non-traumatic amputations are in people with diabetes.

In type 1 diabetes, life expectancy is reduced on average by 11 years in men and 13 years in women. Under the age of 30 years, most deaths occur due to severe acute metabolic complications (DKA and hypoglycaemia). Cardiovascular disease accounts for almost as many deaths aged 30–39 years and predominates after the age of 40 years. Death may also be a consequence of renal failure caused by diabetic nephropathy. In addition, microvascular complications are responsible for substantial morbidity and disability: for example, blindness from diabetic retinopathy, lifestyle restrictions associated with renal dialysis, difficulty in walking and chronic ulceration of the feet from peripheral neuropathy, and bowel and bladder dysfunction from autonomic neuropathy.

Infections and diabetes

People with diabetes are at increased risk of infection and when such infections occur they may be more severe. Hyperglycaemia affects the function of key aspects of the cellular innate immune system, notably the function of neutrophils and monocytes/macrophages, with reduced chemotaxis, phagocytosis and killing of pathogens. Abnormalities in humoral immunity are also seen, such as reduced levels of complement proteins and cytokines, but the significance of this is less clear. Therefore, diabetes is in effect an immunocompromised state and, as a consequence, infections are more common and more likely to be caused by opportunistic pathogens, such as anaerobic organisms and fungi. In addition, microbes grow better in a high glucose environment and this may contribute to increased virulence. Finally, peripheral vascular disease and neuropathy, especially in the feet, predispose to skin ulceration. Breaks in the skin act as a portal for bacteria to enter the body and, if there is associated vascular disease, the reduced blood supply to the injured tissue impairs wound healing so there is reduced access for neutrophils and other components of the immune system to the damaged tissues. Individuals with glycaemic control above target (raised HbA_{1c}) are at higher risk of infection and its consequences, including COVID-19 (see below), although risk remains increased in all people with diabetes.

Urogenital, skin and soft tissue infections

As already noted, one of the commonest sites of infection in people with diabetes is the urogenital system. Genital infections, especially from yeasts such as *Candida* species, causing balanitis in men and vulvovaginitis in women are common at diagnosis of diabetes, in those taking SGLT2 inhibitors and in individuals with poor glycaemic control. Urine infections, including pyelonephritis, are also more common in people with diabetes and may progress to sepsis and acute kidney injury; rarely, even more serious forms of pyelonephritis can occur in which gas is formed in the renal parenchyma (emphysematous pyelonephritis).

Fungal nail infections and infections of skin and soft tissues are also more prevalent in people with diabetes. Skin and soft tissue infections, e.g. cellulitis, abscesses and boils, are usually caused by *Staphylococcus aureus* or β-haemolytic streptococci, as in non-diabetic patients. However, people with diabetes are more likely to experience polymicrobial and anaerobic infections, such as necrotising fasciitis, gas gangrene and synergistic gangrene (including Fournier gangrene of genital and perineal skin), presumably because of the combination of relative immunosuppression and poor tissue perfusion (p. 271).

Bone and joint infection

Approximately 30% of all cases of osteomyelitis are associated with diabetes (see Ch. 26). The most commonly affected sites are the bones of the feet, because of the strong association with peripheral neuropathy, peripheral vascular disease and foot ulceration. Osteomyelitis may occur as a primary consequence of a puncture injury (which has introduced microbes into the wound) or secondary to a long-term skin ulcer or other breach in the skin. Approximately 90% of cases of diabetic foot osteomyelitis occur in the forefoot, with approximately 5% of cases in the mid- and hindfoot, respectively. Osteomyelitis results in destruction of the bone and potentially adjacent joints. It can present as an acute infection, but more commonly is a chronic, insidious infection that progressively worsens.

The clinical features of osteomyelitis in people with diabetes often appear non-severe and may be more suggestive of a soft tissue infection than bone infection. The diagnosis may, therefore, be delayed unless clinicians have a low threshold for suspecting osteomyelitis and carrying out appropriate investigations. Larger ulcers (>2 cm) and deeper ulcers (>3 mm) are associated with an increased risk of osteomyelitis, as is the presence of visible bone in the wound or bone that can be probed. However, none of these signs are diagnostic for osteomyelitis. Plain X-rays are insensitive, especially in milder infections, only showing features of osteomyelitis if more than 30%–50% of bone is lost. MRI and bone scintigraphy have higher sensitivity. Although *Staphylococcus aureus* is most commonly involved, Gram-negative and anaerobic organisms can also be detected. Wound swabs are usually unhelpful, because of contamination from organisms on the skin that are not involved in the bone infection; the most useful microbiological data comes if a bone fragment can be obtained for culture. Osteomyelitis is particularly difficult to treat because many antibiotics do not reach adequate concentrations in bone. Primary antibiotic therapy can be used in milder infections, though often a prolonged course of antibiotics (of many weeks and months) is required. Surgical débridement of infected soft tissue and bone is often required and can reduce the need for amputation. However, osteomyelitis, particularly in the hindfoot, is associated with a poor prognosis and a very high risk of below-knee amputation (~50%).

Septic arthritis and discitis are also more common in people with diabetes, either as a consequence of a direct puncture injury, haematogenous spread from an infection elsewhere or direct spread from an adjacent area of osteomyelitis. *Staphylococcus aureus* is the most commonly implicated organism in both instances: investigation and management are discussed on pages 1025 and 1026.

COVID-19

Severe infection with SARS-CoV-2, i.e. that resulting in death and/or admission to a critical care unit, is much more common in people with diabetes. Precise estimates of the increased risk vary, but people with type 1 diabetes are at approximately 2.5–3.5 times increased risk, while people with type 2 diabetes are at 1.5–2.0 times increased risk. There is a strong association with glycaemic control, such that those individuals with chronically elevated blood glucose are at the highest risk.

SARS-CoV-2 infection, in turn, appears to have an adverse impact on diabetes itself. There are many reports of people with COVID-19, with or without a previous diagnosis of diabetes, presenting with severe hyperglycaemia and DKA. The mechanisms underlying this remain unclear. It may in part be a consequence of worsening insulin resistance precipitated by severe intercurrent illness (see p. 745). However, SARS-CoV-2 gains entry to cells via the angiotensin-converting enzyme 2 (ACE2) receptor; this is highly expressed in β cells in the pancreas. Thus, tropism of SARS-CoV-2 for β cells could trigger damage that impairs insulin secretion, resulting in hyperglycaemia and DKA. It has been suggested that SARS-Co-V-2 may act as a trigger for type 1 diabetes, as some paediatric diabetes centres reported increased incidence during the pandemic; however, this association has not consistently been demonstrated.

Diabetic eye disease

Diabetic retinopathy and diabetic maculopathy are together the most common causes of visual impairment and loss in many countries. The pathogenesis, clinical features and management of diabetic retinopathy and other eye conditions (including cataract) relevant to diabetes are described in Chapter 30.

Diabetic kidney disease

Diabetes is the most common cause of end-stage renal disease globally, and approximately 40% of people requiring renal replacement therapy (i.e. dialysis or transplantation) have diabetes. In people with type 1 diabetes, kidney disease is most often caused by *diabetic nephropathy* (see below), but in people with type 2 diabetes it may also be caused by other conditions to which people with hyperglycaemia are predisposed (e.g. recurrent sepsis and acute kidney injury as a result of urinary tract infection, hypertension and renal vascular disease). Forty per cent of people with type 2 diabetes have chronic kidney disease (CKD) and usually it is multifactorial in aetiology.

About 30% of individuals with type 1 diabetes develop diabetic nephropathy from 10–20 years after diagnosis, but the incidence after this time falls to less than 1% per year. The risk of nephropathy in populations of European descent with type 2 diabetes is similar to that with type 1 diabetes, but the rate of progression may be exacerbated by concomitant obesity and other risk factors. It is much higher in some ethnic groups (e.g. African Caribbeans, South Asians and Japanese), with epigenetic and genetic factors thought to influence this increased risk. It should be noted that some individuals with long-standing hyperglycaemia do not develop nephropathy, suggesting the presence of as-yet-undiscovered protective (potentially genetic) factors. With improved standards of care focusing on glycaemic control and more widespread use of blood pressure-lowering medication targeting the renin-angiotensin system, the proportion of people with diabetes and CKD is reducing. However, due to the global rise in the incidence of type 2 diabetes, the absolute number of people with diabetes and end-stage renal failure continues to rise.

The pathophysiology underlying diabetic nephropathy is not fully understood. A key molecule is transforming growth factor β, which upregulates flux of glucose into renal cells and activates the renin–angiotensin system leading to renal inflammation and fibrosis. The classical pattern of progression of renal abnormalities in diabetes is shown schematically in Figure 21.32. Initially there is hyperfiltration in the glomeruli, then onset of microalbuminuria due to damage (and thickening) of the glomerular basement membrane causing leaking of protein, which can then progress to frank (dipstick-positive) proteinuria. Matrix material also accumulates in the mesangium and, as disease advances, nodular deposits form in the glomeruli ('focal' glomerulosclerosis; Fig. 21.33). As glomeruli are progressively lost, renal function deteriorates, which manifests as a declining glomerular filtration rate.

Diagnosis and screening

Urine should be tested for microalbuminuria and a blood test sent for estimated glomerular filtration rate (eGFR) on an annual basis in all adults with diabetes. CKD in diabetes is defined using criteria listed in Box 18.3. Microalbuminuria is the presence in the urine of small amounts of albumin at a concentration below that detectable using a standard urine dipstick. As the measurement is physiologically variable, a single measurement is not considered informative: it should be confirmed as present in at least two of three 'first-morning' specimens taken on separate days (Box 21.30). Microalbuminuria is usually reported as a proportion of the concentration or weight of creatinine present in the sample (mg/mmol

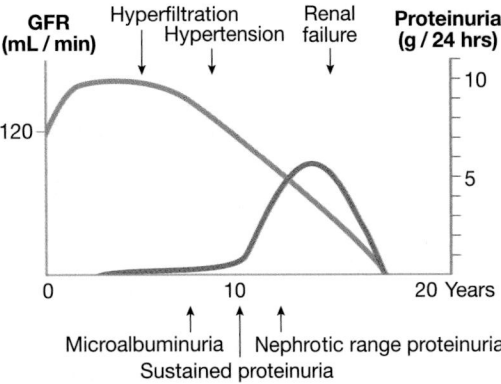

Fig. 21.32 Natural history of diabetic nephropathy. In the first few years of type 1 diabetes mellitus, there is hyperfiltration; thereafter glomerular filtration rate declines fairly steadily to return to a normal value at approximately 10 years (blue line). In susceptible patients (about 30%), there is sustained proteinuria after about 10 years and by approximately 14 years this has reached the nephrotic range (red line).

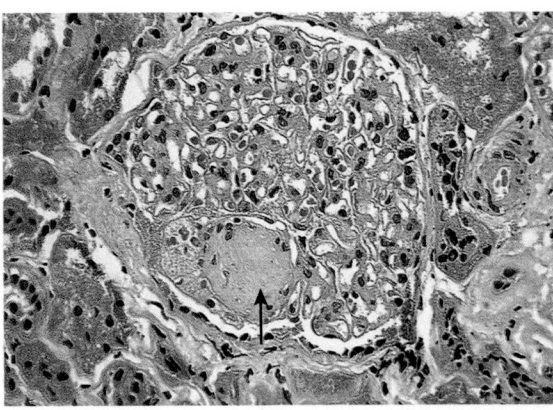

Fig. 21.33 Nodular diabetic glomerulosclerosis. There is thickening of basement membranes, mesangial expansion and a Kimmelstiel–Wilson nodule (arrow), which is pathognomonic of diabetic kidney disease.

---

i 21.30 Screening for microalbuminuria

- Early morning urine is measured for the albumin:creatinine ratio (ACR)
- Microalbuminuria is present if:
  Male: ACR 2.5–30 mg/mmol creatinine or 25–300 mg/g
  Female: ACR 3.5–30 mg/mmol creatinine or 35–300 mg/g
- An elevated ACR should be followed by a repeat test:
  There is established microalbuminuria if 2 out of 3 tests are positive
- Proteinuria (overt or dipstick-postive nephropathy) is likely to be present if ACR > 30 mg/mmol
- This is confirmed by a protein: creatinine ratio (PCR) of >45 mg/mmol
- Nephrotic range proteinuria is present when PCR >300 mg/mmol

---

or mg/g) to reduce variability, with the threshold for diagnosis higher in women (see Box 18.9). Overt nephropathy is the presence of macroalbuminuria equivalent to the level of protein detectable on a standard urine dipstick. Microalbuminuria is a good predictor of progression to nephropathy in type 1 diabetes and an indication for ACE inhibitor or angiotensin II receptor blocker therapy to protect the kidneys. It is also a risk marker for macrovascular disease, especially in type 2 diabetes.

Management

Establishing the presence of microalbuminuria should prompt vigorous efforts to reduce the risk of progression to nephropathy (and to protect against cardiovascular disease) by:

- control of blood pressure
- reduction of cardiovascular risk factors
- optimisation of glycaemic control.

Blockade of the renin–angiotensin system using either ACE inhibitors or angiotensin 2 receptor blockers (ARBs) has been shown to have an additional benefit over similar levels of blood pressure control achieved with other antihypertensive agents and is recommended as first-line therapy. This relieves angiotensin II-mediated vasoconstriction of efferent arterioles downstream from the glomerular capillary tuft (see Fig. 18.1D), decreasing glomerular filtration pressure and, therefore, hyperfiltration and protein leak. Electrolytes and renal function should be checked after initiation or dose increase of these agents as they can cause a marked deterioration in renal function if there is occult stenosis of the main renal artery, i.e. when adequate intraglomerular pressure is critically dependent on efferent arteriolar tone. There is no additional benefit of combining agents from these two classes. However, addition of other antihypertensive agents is required to achieve target BP control in many cases, e.g. calcium channel blockers, diuretics and α-adrenoceptor antagonists (α-blockers).

Halving the amount of albuminuria with an ACE inhibitor or ARB results in a nearly 50% reduction in long-term risk of progression to end-stage renal disease and requirement for renal replacement therapy, often in the form of haemodialysis (p. 593). SGLT2 inhibitor therapy in people with type 2 diabetes, overt proteinuria (>300 mg/day) and eGFR >30 ml/min/1.73m^2 reduces the risk of progression to end-stage kidney disease by approximately 30%. SGLT2 inhibitor therapy also reduces cardiovascular events in people with CKD and is rapidly becoming a standard of care as an add-on to ACE inhibitor or ARB therapy.

Individuals with CKD stages 3–5, but no proteinuria, may have CKD due to other factors, e.g. hypertension rather than diabetic nephropathy, and it is not yet clear if SGLT2 inhibitors slow progression of CKD in this group.

Renal transplantation is indicated for people with end-stage kidney disease, who are fit enough to undergo the procedure; it dramatically improves lives of organ recipients (see Ch. 18). Simultaneous pancreas transplantation should be performed, where possible, in people with type 1 diabetes. Anti-rejection immunosuppression carries risks and requires careful monitoring. Recurrence of diabetic nephropathy in the transplanted organ (allograft) is usually too slow to be a serious problem, although other complications may continue to progress.

Diabetic neuropathy

Diabetic neuropathy causes substantial morbidity, particularly due to foot ulceration. It is diagnosed on the basis of symptoms and signs after the exclusion of other causes of neuropathy (see Ch. 28). It is more common with increased duration of either type 1 or 2 diabetes. The most common type is a 'polyneuropathy' (i.e. evidence that more than one type of nerve fibre is affected). About 25%–30% of adults have evidence of neuropathy 10–15 years on from diagnosis and about half of these have painful diabetic neuropathy (PDN). Like retinopathy, neuropathy occurs secondary to hyperglycaemia and is related to duration of diabetes. Motor, sensory and autonomic nerves may be involved in varying combinations.

Pathological features can occur in any peripheral nerves. They include axonal degeneration of both myelinated and unmyelinated fibres, with thickening of the Schwann cell basal lamina, patchy segmental demyelination and abnormal intraneural capillaries (with basement membrane thickening and microthrombi).

Clinical features

Symmetrical sensory polyneuropathy

This is the commonest type of diabetic neuropathy and is a diffuse, small-fibre neuropathy that is, at least initially, frequently asymptomatic. There is impairment, in a 'glove and stocking' distribution, of all modalities of sensation including diminished vibration sensation (Fig. 21.34). Symptoms may include paraesthesiae in the feet, sharp pain in the lower limbs (worse at night and felt mainly on the anterior aspect of the legs), burning sensations in the soles of the feet and cutaneous hyperaesthesia. As the condition advances, weakness and atrophy of the interosseous muscles may develop leading to structural changes in the foot with loss of lateral and transverse arches, clawing of the toes and exposure of the metatarsal heads. This results in increased pressure on the plantar aspects of the metatarsal heads, with hard 'callus' skin at these and other pressure points, leading to ulceration and even Charcot neuroarthropathy (see below).

In practice, loss of sensation to a 10 g monofilament provides evidence of increased risk and requirement for increased foot care (e.g. regular foot inspection, care from podiatry, attention to appropriate footwear). When diagnosis is uncertain, formal electrophysiological tests (p. 1132) may be performed demonstrating slowing of both motor and sensory conduction as well as abnormal vibration sensitivity and thermal thresholds.

Asymmetrical motor diabetic neuropathy (diabetic amyotrophy)

This is much less common; it presents as severe, progressive weakness and wasting of the proximal muscles of the lower limbs. It is accompanied by severe pain, felt mainly on the anterior aspect of the leg, hyperaesthesia and paraesthesiae. This condition is thought to involve acute infarction of the lower motor neurons of the lumbosacral plexus. Partial recovery usually occurs within 12 months; management is supportive.

Mononeuropathy

Mononeuropathies of a single sensory or motor, peripheral or cranial nerve are rare, but more often affect people with diabetes. The nerves most likely to be affected are the 6th and 3rd cranial nerves (resulting in diplopia), the 7th cranial nerve (resulting in Bell's palsy) and the femoral and sciatic nerves. The mononeuropathy is usually severe and of rapid onset, but eventually recovers. Nerve compression palsies are more common in diabetes, e.g. the median nerve, resulting in carpal tunnel syndrome, and less commonly, the ulnar nerve. Compression palsies may be a consequence of glycation and thickening of connective tissue and/or diabetic microangiopathy.

Autonomic neuropathy

This may occur independently of other types of neuropathy. It is less clearly associated with glycaemic control and improving control does not usually relieve the symptoms. Parasympathetic or sympathetic nerves may be predominantly affected. Common symptoms include dizziness, nausea and vomiting, post-gustatory sweating, difficulty with micturition, and diarrhoea/faecal incontinence. A postural drop may be detected on lying and standing BP measurement with a resting tachycardia. Pupils may be pinpoint.

Formal testing is rarely performed but involves the 'Ewing tests', which screen for evidence of lack of heart rate variability in response to manoeuvres designed to alter the activity of the autonomic nerve system (Valsalva manoeuvre, deep breathing, sustained handgrip).

Support stockings and fludrocortisone therapy may be helpful for symptoms of postural hypotension. Due to the risk of sudden cardiorespiratory arrest, there is only 50%–70% survival within 10 years of developing overt autonomic neuropathy. Fortunately, severe cases are infrequent.

Gastroparesis This is one of the most disabling complications of diabetes. It usually affects people with type 1 diabetes. Following exclusion of mechanical forms of obstruction (by upper gastrointestinal endoscopy), delayed gastric emptying is demonstrated using scintigraphy following a ^{99m}-technetium-labelled standard meal. Gastroparesis is a prominent feature of severe autonomic neuropathy, but can also occur secondary to a co-existent primary eating disorder. The main symptoms (the severity of which tend to wax and wane) are nausea and vomiting (especially of undigested food), abdominal pain and a feeling of fullness/early satiety. It can contribute to increased variability in blood glucose, as there can be

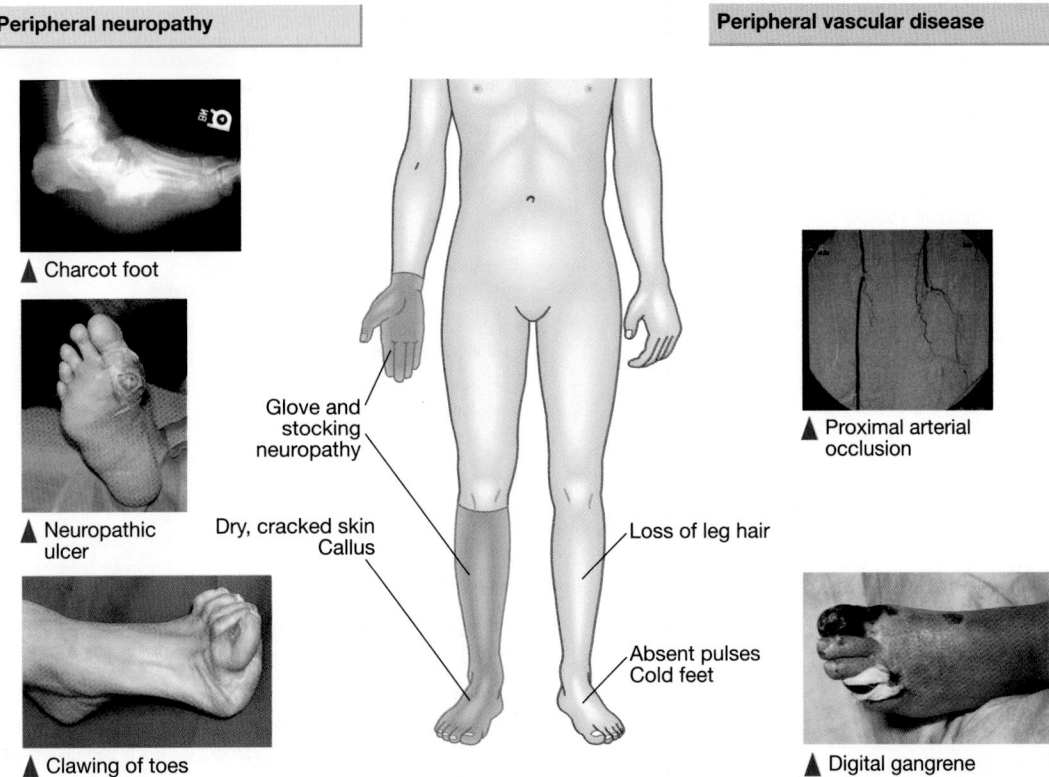

Peripheral neuropathy

▲ Charcot foot

▲ Neuropathic ulcer

▲ Clawing of toes

Glove and stocking neuropathy

Dry, cracked skin
Callus

Peripheral vascular disease

▲ Proximal arterial occlusion

Loss of leg hair

Absent pulses
Cold feet

▲ Digital gangrene

Fig. 21.34 Diabetic foot disease. Patients with diabetes can have neuropathy, peripheral vascular disease or both. Clawing of the toes is thought to be caused by intrinsic muscle atrophy and subsequent imbalance of muscle function, and causes greater pressure on the metatarsal heads and pressure on flexed toes, leading to increased callus and risk of ulceration. A Charcot foot occurs only in the presence of neuropathy, and results in bony destruction and ultimately deformity (this X-ray shows a resulting 'rocker bottom foot'). The angiogram reveals disease of the superficial femoral arteries (occlusion of the left and stenosis of the right). *Insets (Proximal arterial occlusion) From http:// emedicine.medscape.com/article/460178-overview#a0104; (Toe clawing) Bowker JH, Pfeifer MA. Levin and O'Neal's The diabetic foot, 7th edn. Philadelphia: Mosby, Elsevier Inc.; 2008; (Neuropathic foot ulcer) Levy MJ, Valabhji J. Vascular II: The diabetic foot. Surgery 2008; 26:25–28; (Digital gangrene) Swartz MH. Textbook of physical diagnosis, 5th edn. Philadelphia: WB Saunders, Elsevier Inc.; 2006.*

a mismatch between the delayed rise in post-prandial glucose and the time-action profile of injected insulin.

Improving quality of life and achieving glycaemic control is difficult. Low-fibre and low-residue diets may be tried, as well as eating smaller amounts more frequently. Prokinetic dopamine antagonist anti-emetics (metoclopramide, domperidone) are often prescribed in an effort to accelerate gastric emptying, but are not recommended for long-term use due to adverse effects. For individuals on MDI, rapid-acting insulin may be better taken after rather than before a meal and CSII is beneficial for some. There may be frequent hospital admissions during 'flare-ups.' A 'gastric pacemaker' device is of benefit in some cases; others may benefit from endoscopic injection of botulinum toxin into the gastric pylorus (to increase gastric emptying). Enteral nutrition is rarely required unless gastroparesis is very severe.

Sexual dysfunction Men with type 2 diabetes are 30% more likely than non-diabetic men to have erectile dysfunction, rising to 70% with more than 20 years' duration of diabetes. In type 1 diabetes, the risk of erectile dysfunction is elevated threefold. This is mainly due to autonomic neuropathy and vascular disease (cavernosal microangiopathy). The approach to treatment options is as for non-diabetic men (for further information, see page 612). Women with diabetes also have higher rates of sexual dysfunction, including vaginal dryness, dyspareunia and increased susceptibility to urinary tract infections.

Management

Tricyclic antidepressants (low dose amitryptiline, duloxetine) and anticonvulsants (pregabalin, gabapentin) – combined if necessary with opiate

analgesia (tramadol, oxycodone) – can improve quality of life in PDN. Management of other forms of neuropathy is shown in Box 21.31

Diabetic foot disease

The feet are especially vulnerable in diabetes as there may be loss of protective sensation (due to neuropathy), inadequate blood supply (due to small and large blood vessel disease) or both. For this reason foot care is particularly important. Foot ulceration and associated complications are the most common reasons for prolonged hospital admission for people with diabetes.

Aetiology

In a vulnerable foot, ulceration is initiated by (often minor) trauma (p. 340 and Fig. 21.34). Disruption of the protective epidermis then permits infection, particularly in the presence of hyperglycaemia. Most ulcers develop at the site of a plaque of callus skin, which has developed on a 'pressure point' typically on the plantar aspect of the foot, on the metatarsal heads or the tips of clawed toes. The majority of foot ulcers are neuropathic or neuroischaemic. Neuroischaemic ulcers classically occur on the margins of the foot as they are often precipitated by compression of the foot by ill-fitting shoes. Hence, they are seen over the medial aspect of the first metatarsophalangeal joint, the styloid process of the 5th metatarsal and the tips of the toes.

Management

Systematic annual screening to estimate and record risk of foot ulceration in order to ensure appropriate access to podiatry has been shown to reduce rates of ulceration and amputation. Two simple tests are

ℹ 21.31 Management options for peripheral sensorimotor and autonomic neuropathies

Pain and paraesthesiae from peripheral somatic neuropathies

- Insulin therapy (intensive glycaemic control)
- Anticonvulsants (gabapentin, pregabalin)
- Tricyclic antidepressants (low-dose amitriptyline, imipramine)
- Other antidepressants (duloxetine)
- Substance P depleter (capsaicin – topical)
- Opiates (tramadol, oxycodone)
- Antioxidant α-lipoic acid

Postural hypotension

- Support stockings
- Fludrocortisone
- Midodrine

Gastroparesis

- Dopamine antagonists (metoclopramide, domperidone)*
- Erythromycin
- Botulinum toxin (endoscopic injection into pylorus)
- Gastric pacemaker; percutaneous enteral (jejunal) feeding (see Fig. 22.11)

Diarrhoea (p. Ch. 23)

- Loperamide
- Rifaxamin (for suspected bacterial overgrowth)

Constipation

- Stimulant laxatives (senna)

Excessive sweating

- Anticholinergic drugs (propantheline, poldine, oxybutinin)
- Clonidine
- Topical antimuscarinic agent (glycopyrrolate cream)

Erectile dysfunction (p. Ch. 18)

- Phosphodiesterase type 5 inhibitors (sildenafil, vardenafil, tadalafil) – oral
- Dopamine agonist (apomorphine) – sublingual
- Prostaglandin E₁ (alprostadil) – injected into corpus cavernosum or intra-urethral administration of pellets
- Vacuum tumescence devices
- Implanted penile prosthesis
- Psychological counselling; psychosexual therapy

*Not licensed for long-term use due to risk of dystonia.

ℹ 21.32 Care of the feet in diabetes

Advice aimed at prevention of ulceration

Low risk (as per general population)

- Wash feet every day
- Cut or file toenails regularly
- Change socks or stockings every day
- Moisturise skin if dry
- Cover minor cuts with sterile dressings
- Treat fungal skin and nail infections promptly
- Do not burst blisters

Moderate and high risk

- Inspect feet every day
- Avoid walking barefoot
- Wear well-fitting shoes (e.g. trainers)
- Avoid over-the-counter corn/callus remedies
- Do not attempt corn removal
- Check footwear for foreign bodies
- Avoid high and low temperatures

Podiatry

- Access should be available appropriate to level of risk (see Fig. 21.35)
- Access to a multidisciplinary foot team including a specialised podiatrist should be available for urgent referrals and care of active foot ulcers

Orthotic footwear

- Specially manufactured and fitted orthotic footwear is required to prevent recurrence of ulceration and to protect the feet of patients with Charcot neuroarthropathy

required to grade risk according to a 'traffic light' system (Fig. 21.35): a 10 g monofilament should be used to assess sensation at five points on each foot and foot pulses should be palpated (dorsalis pedis and/or posterior tibial).

- Green: People with normal protective sensation and palpable pulses are at 'low risk' and can be educated and reassured regarding foot care until next screening (Box 21.32).
- Amber: Those who have reduction or loss of sensation to monofilament, or in whom no pulse can be palpated in at least one foot, are at 'moderate' risk. A assessment and development of a care plan by a trained podiatrist is recommended when first identified and annual screening thereafter. Regular support with foot care may be offered. Well-fitting footwear is essential.
- Red: As for amber, but there is both reduced sensation and absent pulses in at least one foot or callus/structural foot deformity in the presence of either reduced sensation or absent pulses. Assessment and treatment by a specialist podiatrist is required. Orthotic footwear may be recommended.

People with diabetes and their relatives or carers can easily learn to use the Ipswich Touch Test to screen for neuropathy: this involves lightly and briefly (for 1–2 seconds) touching the tips of the first, third and fifth toes of both feet with the index finger: an abnormal result is when touch cannot be felt on two or more toes.

Foot ulceration

People with a foot ulcer require urgent assessment by a multidisciplinary foot team, involving a diabetes specialist, a podiatrist, a vascular surgeon and an orthotist.

Management involves:

- Débridement of necrotic tissue
- Antibiotic therapy (may be prolonged as infection can accelerate tissue necrosis and lead to gangrene)
- Pressure relief (depending on site, severity and stage of healing): customised insoles, specialised orthotic footwear, total contact plaster cast, irremovable aircast boot.

Ulcers that do not heal promptly may progress to osteomyelitis (infection of the underlying bone). If an ulcer is neuroischaemic, a vascular assessment is often carried out by ultrasound or angiography, as revascularisation by angioplasty or surgery may be required to allow the ulcer to heal. In cases of severe secondary infection or gangrene, amputation of the affected toe or of the limb (below or above knee) may be required depending on the severity.

Charcot neuroarthropathy

This is a rare but severe complication of neuropathy affecting the bones and joints of the foot characterised by early inflammation and then joint dislocation, subluxation and pathological fractures of the foot. It was originally described as a complication of neurosyphilis, but now that this is near eradicated it is almost exclusively seen in diabetes. The pathophysiological mechanisms remain poorly understood.

Charcot neuroarthropathy presents in a structurally abnormal foot with localised swelling, erythema and increased temperature (>2°C compared with the contralateral foot). Early diagnosis can prevent progressive and debilitating deformity (see Fig. 21.34) and sepsis. The initial X-ray may show bony destruction but is often normal. As about 40% of patients with a Charcot joint also have a foot ulcer, it can be difficult to differentiate from osteomyelitis. Magnetic resonance imaging (MRI) of the foot is a sensitive diagnostic test. Management

Diabetic foot risk stratification and triage

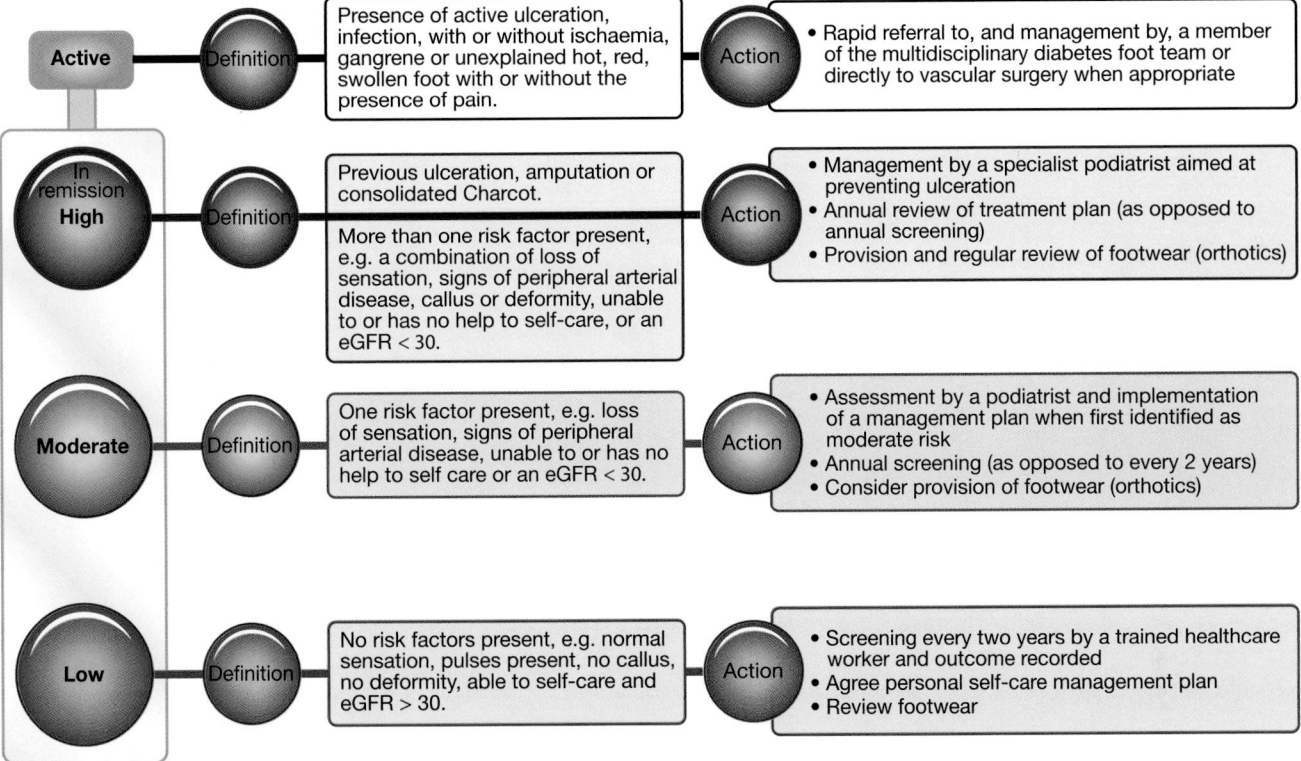

All people with diabetes should have written information on how to access podiatry (urgent or otherwise), cardiovascular risk reduction and access to a smoking cessation programme

Fig. 21.35 Risk assessment and management of foot problems in diabetes. *Reproduced with permission of the Scottish Diabetes Foot Action Group.*

involves pressure relief and immobilisation (with a plaster cast or inflatable 'aircast' boot) and treating infection. This may take 3–6 months and sometimes longer.

Skin and rheumatological complications of diabetes

Glycation of collagen in skin, subcutaneous and periarticular tissues, perhaps supplemented by an effect of tissue ischaemia from micro-angiopathy, can cause thickening of the skin, leading to a painless limited mobility of the joints of the hands and feet (cheiroarthropathy or 'diabetic stiff hand syndrome') and a waxy, tight feel to the skin. In the most severe cases it can resemble scleroderma. The inability to extend to 180° the metacarpophalangeal or interphalangeal joints of at least one finger bilaterally can be demonstrated in the 'prayer sign'. Adhesive capsulitis (e.g. causing frozen shoulder), Dupuytren's contracture and trigger finger are all more common in people with diabetes.

Diabetic dermopathy manifests as rounded red papules in the pre-tibial area that become pigmented with time. It is commoner in men and is associated with other complications of diabetes. Necrobiosis lipoidica is a rare granulomatous disorder that occurs predominantly in women with type 1 diabetes and is characterised by reddened plaques, with a yellowish central area that has atrophic skin and telangiectasia (see pages 704 and 1113). Xerosis (or abnormal dryness of the skin) may be a cutaneous manifestation of autonomic neuropathy and can lead to cracks in the skin that act as a portal for infection.

Further information

Journal articles
Holman RR, Paul SK, Bethel MA, et al. 10-year follow-up of intensive glucose control in type 2 diabetes. N Engl J Med 2008;359(15):1577–1589.
Nathan DM, for the DCCT/EDIC Research Group The Diabetes Control and Complications Trial/Epidemiology of Diabetes Interventions and Complications Study at 30 Years: Overview. Diabetes Care 2014;37(1):9–16.

Books
Jörgens V, Porta M (eds). Unveiling diabetes - historical milestones in diabetology. Frontiers in Diabetes, vol. 29. Basle: Karger; 2020. *Insights into the history of diabetes and its treatment.*

Websites
sign.ac.uk/media/1090/sign154.pdf *Scottish Intercollegiate Guideline Network (SIGN) evidence-based guideline (2017) on 'Pharmacological management of glycaemia' in type 2 diabetes.*
care.diabetesjournals.org/content/diacare/suppl/2019/12/20/43.Supplement_1. DC1/Standards_of_Care_2020.pdf *American Diabetes Association (ADA) Standards of Medical Care in Diabetes (2020) – updated at least annually.*
diabetes.org.uk/ *Diabetes UK. Includes information for healthcare professionals and for people with diabetes.*
idf.org/ *International Diabetes Federation. 'E-library' contains consensus statements and guidelines.*
elearning.mydiabetesmyway.scot.nhs.uk/ *An interactive diabetes website including practical learning modules for people living with diabetes.*
diabetes.org.uk/resources-s3/2018-09/language-matters_language%20and%20 diabetes.pdf *An NHS England document about why language matters in diabetes care.*
revolvecomics.com/read-diabetes-type-1-comics/ *Open access digital comics for people and families with type 1 diabetes.*

AG Shand
MEJ Lean

22

Nutritional factors in disease

Clinical examination in nutritional disorders

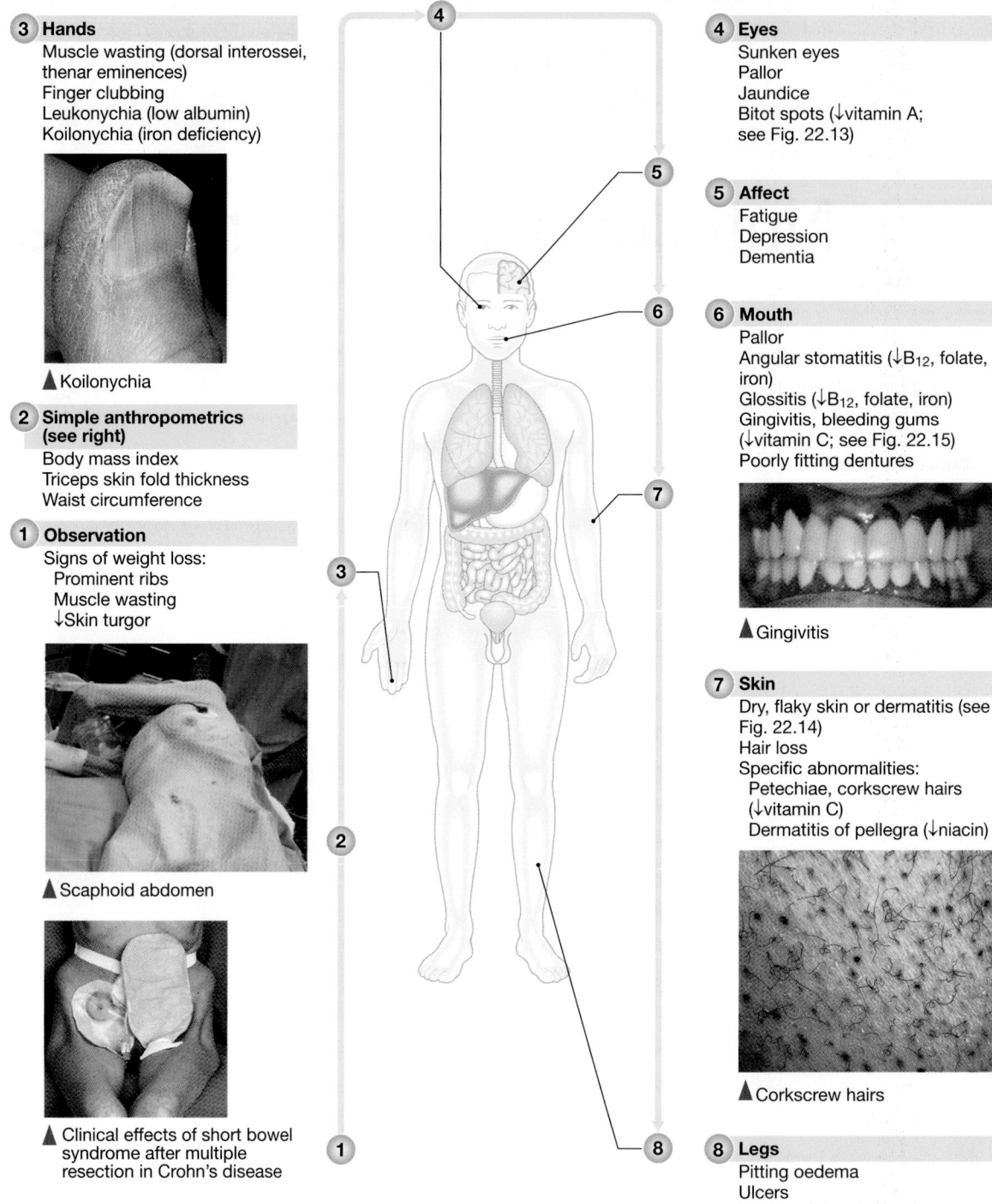

3 Hands
Muscle wasting (dorsal interossei, thenar eminences)
Finger clubbing
Leukonychia (low albumin)
Koilonychia (iron deficiency)

▲ Koilonychia

2 Simple anthropometrics (see right)
Body mass index
Triceps skin fold thickness
Waist circumference

1 Observation
Signs of weight loss:
  Prominent ribs
  Muscle wasting
  ↓Skin turgor

▲ Scaphoid abdomen

▲ Clinical effects of short bowel syndrome after multiple resection in Crohn's disease

4 Eyes
Sunken eyes
Pallor
Jaundice
Bitot spots (↓vitamin A; see Fig. 22.13)

5 Affect
Fatigue
Depression
Dementia

6 Mouth
Pallor
Angular stomatitis (↓B_{12}, folate, iron)
Glossitis (↓B_{12}, folate, iron)
Gingivitis, bleeding gums (↓vitamin C; see Fig. 22.15)
Poorly fitting dentures

▲ Gingivitis

7 Skin
Dry, flaky skin or dermatitis (see Fig. 22.14)
Hair loss
Specific abnormalities:
  Petechiae, corkscrew hairs (↓vitamin C)
  Dermatitis of pellegra (↓niacin)

▲ Corkscrew hairs

8 Legs
Pitting oedema
Ulcers
Bruising (vitamin K)

Insets (Scaphoid abdomen) From Chandra A, Quinones-Baldrich WJ. Chronic mesenteric ischemia: How to select patients for invasive treatment. Sem Vasc Surg 2010;23: 21–28; (Koilonychia) Habif TP. Clinical dermatology, 6th edn. Philadelphia: Saunders, Elsevier Inc.; 2016; (Gingivitis) Newman MG, Takei H, Klokkevold PR, et al. Carranza's Clinical periodontology, 12th edn. Philadelphia: Saunders, Elsevier Inc.; 2015; (Corkscrew hairs) Bolognia JL, Jorizzo JL, Schaffer JV, et al. Dermatology, 3rd edn. Philadelphia: Saunders, Elsevier Inc.; 2012.

Clinical assessment and investigation of nutritional status

Nutritional status is a conceptual term, with no simple measurement test. It incorporates three interrelated components (see Box below), all needed to perform all the functions required in health and to respond to stresses. (1) 'What we eat' – diet composition, reflecting both availability and supply of nutrients; (2) 'What we are' – body composition, overall size and amounts of components (e.g. body fat, muscle mass, micronutrients, haemoglobin, etc); (3) 'What we can do' – our functional capacity, for physical, mental, metabolic and social functions.

Grasping the circular complexity of nutritional status is important for understanding any disease and to optimise management. It is not sufficient to consider just one or two of the three components in isolation. While certain elements within each of the three components can be measured, and they may point towards a nutritional problem, it is not possible to 'measure' nutritional status with any simple test. Its assessment requires clinical skills and experience.

While body compositional measures are valuable, biochemistry has limited value in assessing nutritional status. Many micronutrient assays are heavily affected by acute-phase responses during illness, so do not reflect whole body status. Moreover, functional micronutrient deficiencies can occur despite body stores being adequate; for example, vitamin A deficiency can occur during illness if its transport to tissues is frustrated by a decline in retinol-binding protein.

Under-nutrition can go unnoticed in patients with multiple comorbidities. Simple, validated tools (e.g. MUST) are available to screen patients for nutritional problems. It is vital to be aware of under-nutrition as a possible contributor to any acute medical presentation. Early nutritional assessment is crucial: past medical and surgical history (e.g. intestinal surgery), drug history and specific diet history about eating habits and food preferences (ideally by a trained dietitian). Evidence of recent weight loss and muscle wasting should be sought. Body composition can be assessed by clinical anthropomorphic measurements, or more sophisticated methods if required.

 The inter-related components that define nutritional status

What we eat – diet composition

- Self-reported intake (retrospective)
- Objectively observed food consumption
- Estimated or measured nutrient consumption

What we are – body composition

- Water content, chemical composition
- 2-compartment (fat/lean tissue), imaging
- Bone mass/specific tissue composition

What we (can) do – functions

- Metabolic, cellular
- Organ/whole-body function
- Physical, mental and social activities

 Important elements of the diet history

Ask about weight

- Current weight
- Weight 2 weeks, 1 month and 6 months ago
- Assessment of degree of change: clothes, loose skin, muscle, stretch marks

Ask about current food intake

- Quantity of food and if any change
- Quality of food taken
- Whether normal food is being eaten
- Avoidance of specific food types (e.g. solids)
- Any nutritional supplements
- Reliance on supplements/tube feeding
- Any change in appetite or interest in food
- Any taste disturbance

Ask about symptoms that interfere with eating

- Oral ulcers or oral pain
- Difficulties swallowing
- Nausea/vomiting
- Early satiety
- Alteration in bowel habit
- Abdominal (or other) pain

Ask about activity levels/performance status

- Normal activity
- Slightly reduced activity
- Inactive < 50% of the time
- Inactive most of the time

---

2 Body mass index (BMI)

$$BMI = \frac{wt(kg)}{ht(m)^2}$$

Example: an adult of 70 kg with a height of 1.75 m has a BMI of $70/1.75^2 = 22.9$ kg/m²

- BMI is a useful way of identifying under- or over-nutrition but cannot discriminate between high lean body or muscle mass and fat mass (e.g. boxers have low fat mass but high BMI)
- Fat mass is also subject to ethnic variation; for the same BMI, South Asians tend to have more body fat than Europeans
- If height cannot be determined (e.g. in older people or those unable to stand), measurement of the femoral length or 'knee height' is a good surrogate

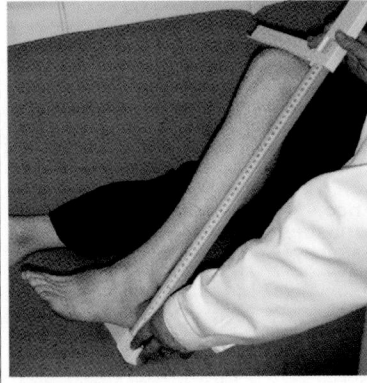

Measurement of knee height.

---

2 Measures of body composition and nutritional status

Body composition

- Anthropometry (see below)
- Bioelectrical impedance
- Dual X-ray absorptiometry (DXA)
- Magnetic resonance imaging (MRI)

Muscle function and global nutritional status

- Hand grip strength (dynamometer test) – poor grip associated with increased mortality

Obesity and fat distribution (android vs gynoid)

- Waist circumference (useful up to BMI 35 kg/m²) measured midway between superior iliac crest and lower border of rib cage

Body fat content and muscle mass

- Triceps skinfold thickness (when combined with mid-/upper arm circumference estimates muscle mass)

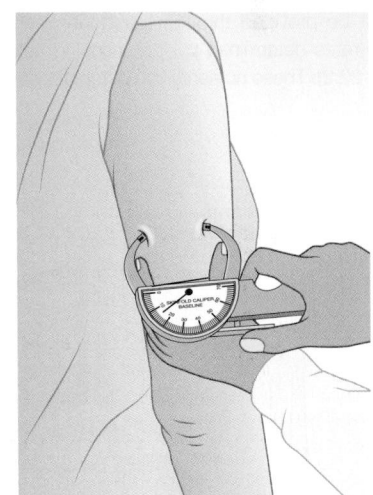

Triceps skinfold thickness. Lean patients 6–12 mm; obese patients 40–50 mm.

22

Nutritional factors and disease

Obtaining adequate nutrition is a fundamental requirement for optimal growth, function and health of every cell, and every organ, determining the health, and ultimately survival, of every individual and even species.

Nutritional adequacy can be threatened by natural supply, by competition, and by ignorance or trickery. The politics of human food provision constitute a prominent factor in wars, natural disasters and the profit-driven global economy. In recent decades, stable plentiful nutrition unknown to previous generations has led to a pandemic of obesity and its health consequences in post-industrial countries. However, shockingly, famine and under-nutrition still dominate ill-health in lower-income countries until they transition suddenly into Westernised overnutrition. Quality, or nutritional balance, of food consumption, and thus the food supply, also influences health (Fig. 22.1). Nutrients are classified into 'macronutrients', which contribute energy (measured as calories or kilojoules), and are eaten in relatively large amounts, and 'micronutrients' (vitamins and minerals), which do not contribute to energy balance but are required in small amounts because they are not synthesised in the body. The fact that we cannot synthesise them tells us that they were plentiful in traditional human diets. When they are lacking, or poorly absorbed, classical deficiency diseases develop, such as anaemia from folate or iron deficiency, or blindness from vitamin A deficiency, which still occur in current medical practice, even with obesity. Foods may contain bioactive compounds, such as caffeine, and toxins, but modern diets cause much more ill-heath by contributing to chronic diseases – type 2 diabetes, coronary heart disease and some major cancers.

All doctors must be alert to the three roles of nutrition. In every case, consider if nutrition (1) might contribute to the cause of disease, thus a means of prevention; (2) might be impaired as a result of disease; and (3) might contribute to recovery. A clear understanding of nutrition is thus essential to deal with the needs of individual patients and inform public policy.

Physiology of nutrition

There are some 27 essential nutrients required by every cell, which must be provided through the bloodstream continuously but at variable rates determined by the changing activities of different cell types (Fig. 22.2). These nutrients come from foods, of different types which are

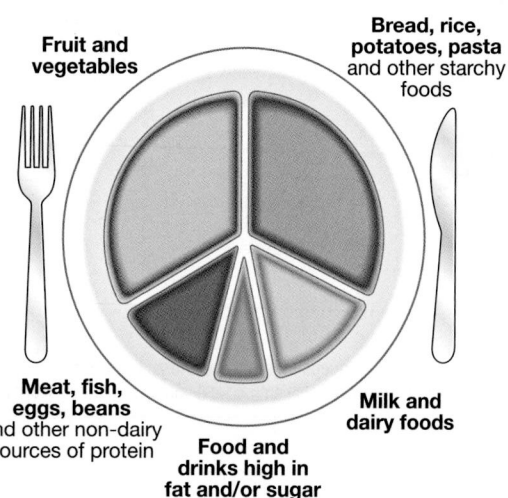

Fig. 22.1 Proportion of key food groups recommended for a healthy, well-balanced diet. *Crown copyright. Department of Health in association with the Welsh Government, the Scottish Government and the Food Standards Agency in Northern Ireland.*

consumed intermittently and sometimes only occasionally. The physiology and language of nutrition is therefore similar to economics, involving intermittent supply, losses at different rates, storage, obligatory costs, impacts on function, and mitigation of impacts by alterations in the internal economy.

Energy balance

The laws of thermodynamics dictate that *energy intake = energy expenditure ± changes in energy storage* (Fig. 22.3). The largest component of 24 hour energy expenditure is basal metabolic rate (BMR) – obligatory energy expenditure required to maintain metabolic functions of tissues at rest. It is closely predicted by body weight, and lower in females and older or inactive people (Fig. 22.3B). Extra energy is needed for growth, pregnancy and lactation and for physical activity, which varies considerably with occupation and lifestyle. Physical activity levels are usually defined as multiples of BMR (Fig. 22.3C). The energy required to digest food (generating heat as 'diet-induced thermogenesis' Fig. 22.3D) accounts for approximately 10% of total energy expenditure, protein requiring more energy than other macronutrients.

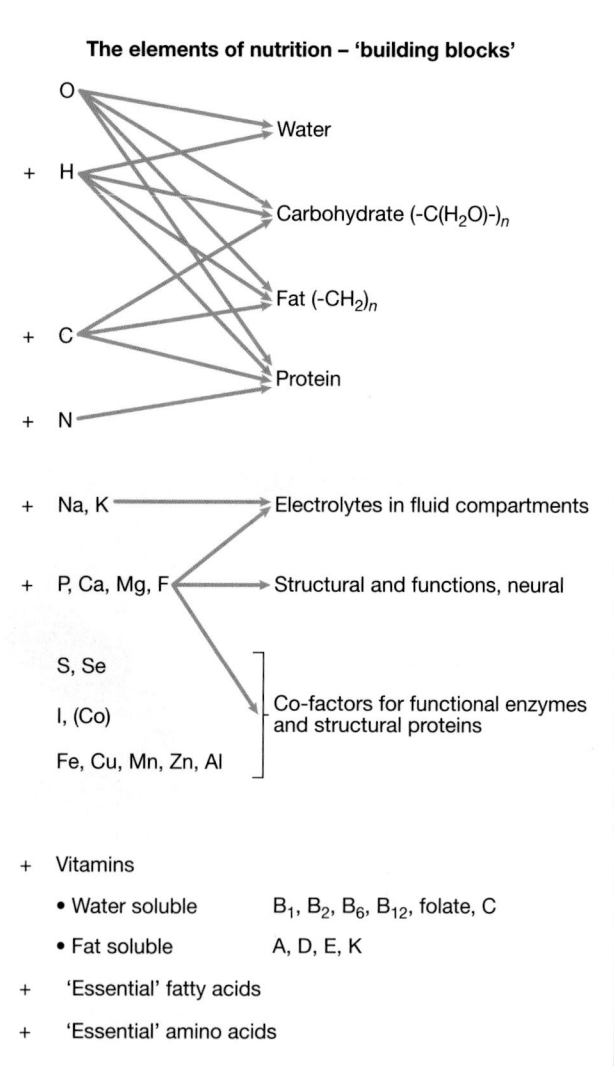

Fig. 22.2 The 18 essential chemical elements in our bodies, required to be absorbed after digestion of our foods, are used in a variety of ways by human metabolism to build the compounds needed to grow, function in health and respond to stresses. The essential vitamins, aminoacids and fatty acids must be consumed 'ready-made' in foods.

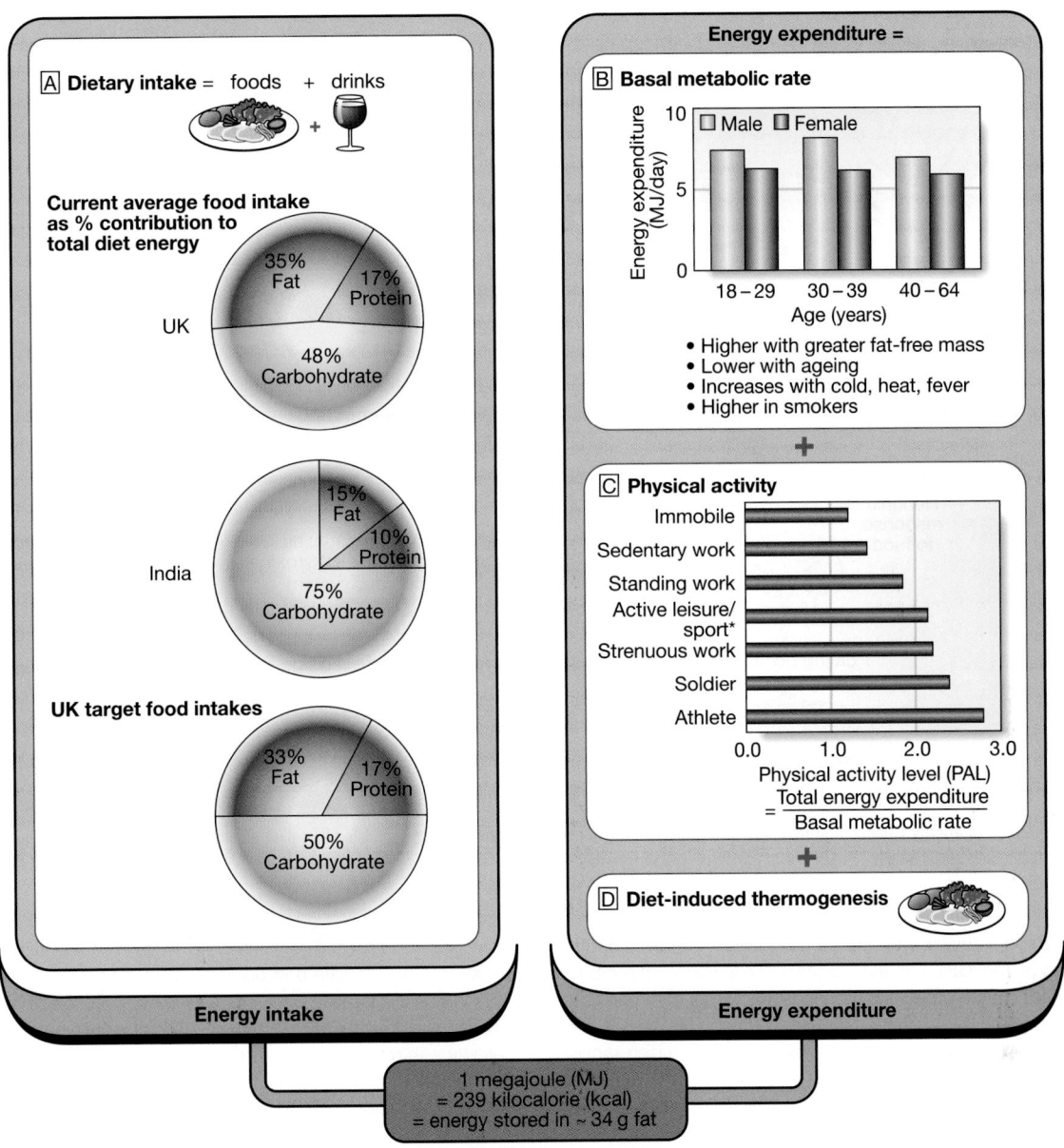

Fig. 22.3 Determinants of energy balance. [A] Energy intake is shown as national averages, highlighting the differences in sources of energy in different countries (but obscuring substantial regional variations). The targets are recommendations as a percentage of food energy only. (For WHO targets, see Box 22.4.) In the UK, it is assumed that 5% of energy intake will be derived from alcohol. [B] Data for normal basal metabolic rate (BMR) were obtained from healthy men and women in various countries. BMR declines from middle age and is lower in women, even after adjustment for body size because of differences in fat-free mass. [C] Energy is required for movement and activity. Physical activity level (PAL) is the multiple of BMR by which total energy expenditure is increased by activity. [D] Energy is consumed in order to digest food. *Leisure or sport activity increases PAL by ~0.3 for each 30–60 minutes of moderate exercise performed 4–5 times per week. The UK population median for PAL is 1.6, with estimates of 1.5 for the 'less active' and 1.8 for the 'more active'. *(A) Source: Department of Health.*

Energy intake is determined by the '*macronutrients*'. Carbohydrate, fat, protein and alcohol provide fuel for mitochondrial oxidation to generate energy (as adenosine triphosphate (ATP)). The energy provided, and the amounts that can be stored in the body, differs:

- fat — 37 kJ/g (9 kcal/g) Stored as body fat, usually sufficient for >40 days
- alcohol — 29 kJ/g (7 kcal/g) Not stored: toxic, must be metabolised immediately
- protein — 17 kJ/g (4 kcal/g) Not stored, but can be oxidised in extreme starvation
- carbohydrate — 16 kJ/g (3.75 kcal/g) Stored as glycogen in liver and muscle, sufficient for 12–24 hours

Regulation of energy balance

Energy intake and expenditure are highly regulated (Fig. 22.4). In general, appetite matches requirement very closely: even when body weight is doubled by obesity, the mismatch between intake and expenditure is usually under 1%. Food shortage, with loss of weight, is the main threat to survival faced by any organism, and negative energy balance immediately signals a range of physiological messages. Energy is conserved by dropping core temperature, and by reducing BMR and physical activity acutely. Chronic food shortage, or micronutrient deficiency, prevents growth and blocks reproductive function, delaying maturation and halting ovulation. Thus pregnancy is most likely to occur during times of nutritional plenty, when both mother and baby have a better chance of survival. Anorexia nervosa and excessive exercise, as well as

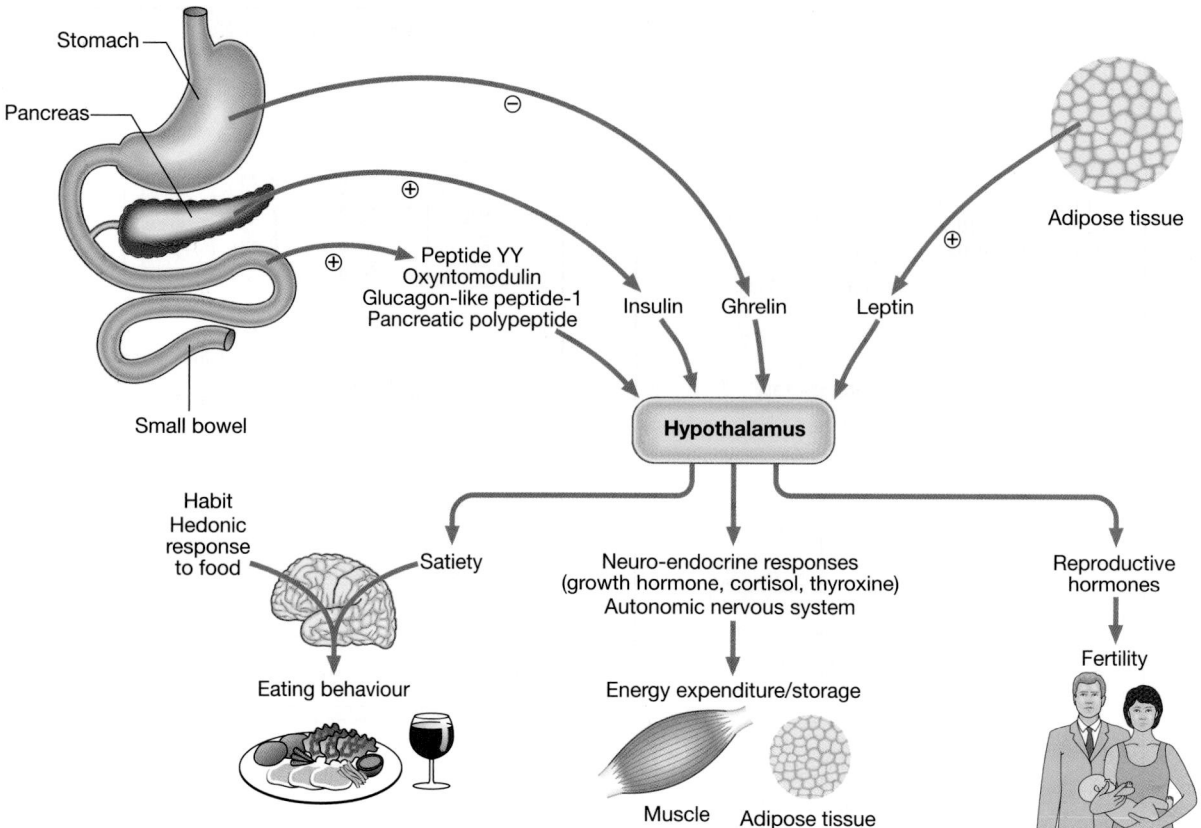

Fig. 22.4 Regulation of energy balance and its link with reproduction. ⊕ indicates factors that are stimulated by eating and induce satiety. ⊖ indicates factors that are suppressed by eating and inhibit satiety.

weight loss through illness, can cause amenorrhoea. Improved nutrition is thought to be the reason for the increasingly early onset of puberty in many societies. At the other extreme, obesity is also a common cause of amenorrhoea.

Energy balance is coordinated in the hypothalamus, which receives afferent signals that indicate nutritional status in the short term (e.g. the stomach hormone ghrelin, which falls immediately after eating and rises gradually thereafter, to suppress satiety and signal that it is time for the next meal) and the long term (e.g. the adipose hormone leptin, which increases with growing fat mass and also links fat mass to reproductive function). The hypothalamus responds with changes in many local neurotransmitters that alter activity in pathways that influence energy balance (see Fig. 22.3), including hormones acting on the pituitary gland (see Fig. 20.2), and neural control circuits that connect with the cerebral cortex and autonomic nervous system.

Responses to under- and over-nutrition

These complex regulatory pathways allow adaptation to variations in nutrition. In response to starvation, reproductive function is suppressed, BMR is reduced, and there are profound psychological effects, including energy conservation through lethargy. These adjustments can 'defend' body weight within certain limits. In the low-insulin state of starvation (see Fig. 21.6), however, fuels are liberated from stores, initially from glycogen (in liver and muscle), then from triglyceride (lipolysis in adipose tissue, with excess free fatty acid supply to the liver leading to ketosis) and finally in protein (proteolysis in muscle). In neonates and in women who are pregnant or breastfeeding, with high glucose requirements, starvation can result in ketoacidosis with normal or low blood glucose.

In response to over-nutrition, BMR rises, and extra energy is required to carry increased body weight, so the original body weight is again 'defended' within certain limits. In the high-insulin state of over-nutrition, excess energy is stored principally as fat in adipose tissue but in

individuals predisposed to 'metabolic syndrome' and type 2 diabetes it may also accumulate and damage organ function in liver (non-alcoholic fatty liver disease), pancreas and skeletal muscle. If hypothalamic function is abnormal (e.g. in those with craniopharyngioma) or in rare patients with mutations (e.g. in leptin or melanocortin-4 receptors), loss of response to satiety signals, together with loss of adaptive changes in energy expenditure, result in relentless weight gain.

Macronutrients (energy-yielding nutrients)

Carbohydrates

Types of carbohydrate and their dietary sources are listed in Box 22.1. The 'available' carbohydrates (starches and sugars) are broken down to monosaccharides for absorption from the gut and supply about half the energy in a well-balanced healthful diet (see Fig. 22.3A). Carbohydrates can be synthesised de novo in small amounts from glycerol or protein. If the available carbohydrate intake is less than 100 g per day, increased lipolysis and fat oxidation leads to dietary ketosis (see Fig. 21.9).

There is much public and media confusion arising from equating carbohydrates with sugars, and a belief that sugars (the product of photosynthesis, on which all life depends) are hazardous. Dietary guidelines do correctly restrict the intake of 'non-milk extrinsic', added, sugars (sucrose, maltose, fructose), which promote dental caries when there is fluoride insufficiency, and may lead to greater energy consumption by children. However, sugars in fruits and milk, or generated by starch hydrolysis in the gut, present no hazard in their natural whole-food matrix. Starches in cereal foods, root foods and legumes provide the largest proportion of energy in most diets around the world, and a high carbohydrate intake in traditional diets is associated with freedom from non-communicable diseases. Starches are polymers of glucose, linked by the same 1–4 glycosidic linkages. Some starches are digested promptly by

22.1 Dietary carbohydrates			
Class	**Components**	**Examples**	**Source**
Free sugars	Monosaccharides Disaccharides	Glucose, fructose Sucrose, lactose, maltose, galactose	Intrinsic: fruits, milks, vegetables Extrinsic (extracted, refined): beet or cane sucrose, high-fructose corn syrup
Short-chain carbohydrates	Oligosaccharides	Maltodextrins, fructo-oligosaccharides	
Starch polysaccharides	Rapidly digestible Slowly digestible		Cereals (wheat, rice), root vegetables (potato), legumes (lentils, beans, peas)
Resistant starch	Not digested	Starch altered by cooking	Cooked and cooled potato, pasta Some lactose from milk in infancy
Non-starch polysaccharides **(NSPs; dietary fibre)**	Fibrous Viscous	Cellulose Hemicellulose Pectins Gums	Many plant foods Pulses
Sugar alcohols		Sorbitol, xylitol	Sorbitol: stone fruits (apples, peaches, prunes) Xylitol: maize, berry fruits Both used as low-calorie sugar alternatives

salivary and then pancreatic amylase, however, producing rapid delivery of glucose to the blood. Other starches are digested more slowly, either because they are protected in the structure of the food, or because the molecule is unbranched (amylose). The area under the curve of blood glucose concentration over 2 hours after eating 50 g carbohydrate in a food, expressed as a percentage of the response to 50 g carbohydrate as glucose or white bread, is termed the 'glycaemic index' of that food. High consumption of high-glycaemic-index foods is weakly associated with type 2 diabetes, but it should be noted that table sugar (sucrose) has a relatively low glycaemic index, being only 50% glucose. Sugar alcohols (e.g. sorbitol), sweeteners that are not absorbed from the gut cause diarrhoea if eaten in large amounts. The main sugar in milk is lactose, a vital energy source for infants, hydrolysed by intestinal lactase for absorption. Some older people, especially East and South East Asians, produce much less lactase, so must limit unfermented milk products. Temporary lactose intolerance is common after any gastroenteritis, but lactase production can be restored by cautious lactose reintroduction.

Dietary fibre

Dietary fibre is carbohydrate that is not digested and absorbed in the small intestine, so passes into the large bowel as the main nutrient for the gut microbiota. Most dietary fibre is 'non-starch polysaccharides' (NSPs) (see Box 22.1), plus some 'resistant' dietary starch, altered by cooking to escape hydrolysis in the small intestine. The many bacterial species which make up the colonic microbiota digest fibre to produce short-chain fatty acids, which are absorbed as fuel for the colonic epithelium and contribute to bowel health and also bioactive, stimulating hormones like glucagon-like peptide (GLP-1) from colon 'H' cells. In infancy, some lactose in milk is not absorbed, and serves the same functions.

Some types of NSP, notably the hemicellulose of wheat, increase the water-holding capacity of the colonic contents and the bulk of faeces. They relieve simple constipation, appear to prevent diverticulosis and may reduce the risk of colon cancer. Viscous dietary fibres, like pectin and guar gum, delay glucose absorption and thus reduce glycaemic index, and reduce bile salt absorption hence plasma cholesterol concentration.

Fats

Fat is the highest-energy density macronutrient, and incurs minimal energy costs for absorption and storage. Highly prized in ancient times, it is now cheap and carries flavours, so is commercially important by providing 'added-value' for manufactured foods. Quite minor excess consumption is an insidious cause of obesity (see Fig. 22.3A).

Free fatty acids are absorbed, reassembled in chylomicrons (see Fig. 23.5), to enter the circulation directly or via the lymph. Fatty acid

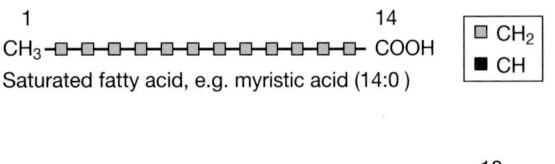

Fig. 22.5 Schematic representation of fatty acids. Standard nomenclature specifies the number of carbon atoms and indicates the number and position of the double bond(s) relative to the methyl ($-CH_3$, ω) end of the molecule after a colon.

structures are shown in Figure 22.5. The principal polyunsaturated fatty acids (PUFA) in plant seed oils, linoleic acid (18:2 ω6) and α-linolenic acid (18:3 ω3) are the 'essential' fatty acids, which humans cannot synthesise de novo. They undergo further desaturation and elongation, to produce, for example, γ-linolenic acid (18:3 ω6) and arachidonic acid (20:4 ω6). These are precursors of prostaglandins and eicosanoids, and form part of the structure of lipid membranes in all cells. Pellagic (shoaling) fish and fish oils are rich in ω3 PUFA (e.g. eicosapentaenoic (20:5 ω3) and docosahexaenoic (22:6 ω3), which promote the anti-inflammatory cascade of prostaglandin production and occur in the lipids of the human brain and retina. They also reduce blood pressure, improve glucose tolerance and inhibit thrombosis by competitively antagonising thromboxane A_2 formation. Saturated fats have high melting points, mostly coming from warm-blooded animal sources: those with shorter chain lengths, from dairy foods, appear relatively safe, but those with long chain lengths, found particularly in animal fat and manufactured meat products, elevate LDL cholesterol and promote cardiovascular disease. Replacing them with PUFAs may help prevent coronary heart disease, provided the PUFAs are protected by their natural antioxidants. High intakes of *trans* fatty acids (TFAs; isomers of the natural *cis* fatty acids) reflect the use of oils that have been partially hydrogenated in the food industry to raise their melting point for use in manufactured foods. They behave like the long-chain saturated fats to promote cardiovascular disease, so it is recommended that TFAs are limited to <2% of dietary fat intake. Changes in industrial practice in the UK and United States have brought most people's TFA intakes below 1%, with the residual amount coming from ruminant digestion in milk.

22

i 22.2 Amino acids

Essential amino acids

- Tryptophan
- Histidine
- Methionine
- Threonine
- Isoleucine
- Valine
- Phenylalanine
- Lysine
- Leucine

Conditionally essential amino acids and their precursors

- Cysteine: methionine, serine
- Tyrosine: phenylalanine
- Arginine: glutamine/glutamate, aspartate
- Proline: glutamate
- Glycine: serine, choline

i 22.3 Daily adult energy requirements in health

Circumstances	Daily requirements*	
	Females	Males
At rest (basal metabolic rate)	5.4 MJ (1300 kcal)	6.7 MJ (1600 kcal)
Less active	8.0 MJ (1900 kcal)	9.9 MJ (2400 kcal)
Population median	8.8 MJ (2100 kcal)	10.8 MJ (2600 kcal)
More active	9.6 MJ (2300 kcal)	11.8 MJ (2800 kcal)

*These are based on a healthy target body mass index (BMI) of 22.5 kg/m². For a female, height is 162 cm and weight 59.0 kg; for a male, height is 175 cm and weight 68.8 kg. Previous average recommendations of 8.1 MJ (1950 kcal, usually rounded up to 2000 kcal) for females and 10.7 MJ (2500 kcal) for males should continue to be used, as these fall within experimental error.

i 22.4 WHO recommended population macronutrient goals

Nutrient	Target limits for population average intakes (% of total energy unless indicated)	
	Lower	Upper
Protein	10	
Total fat	15	30
Saturated fatty acids	0	10
Polyunsaturated fatty acids	6	10
Trans fatty acids	0	1
Dietary cholesterol (mg/day)	0	300
Total carbohydrate	55	75
Free (added) sugars	0	10
Complex carbohydrate	50	70
Dietary fibre (g/day)		
As non-starch polysaccharides	>20	
As total dietary fibre	>25	
Total fruit and vegetables	>400	

Cholesterol is also absorbed from food in chylomicrons and is an important substrate for steroid and sterol synthesis, but not an important source of energy, nor a major contributor to plasma cholesterol concentration as it is also synthesised in the liver.

Proteins

Proteins, with all their complexity for structural and metabolic/enzymic functions, are made up of some 20 different amino acids. Nine are 'essential' (Box 22.2), i.e. they cannot be synthesised by healthy humans, but are required for synthesis of important proteins, so must always be provided by the diet. While amino acids are well preserved by recycling, there are no stores, so a regular supply is needed to replace losses. Five other amino acids are 'conditionally essential': they can usually be synthesised from other amino acids, but synthesis may be insufficient, demanding a greater dietary supply under certain conditions (e.g. poor diet, pregnancy, growth, illness). The remaining necessary amino acids can be synthesised in the body by transamination, provided there is a sufficient supply of amino groups.

Dietary proteins of animal origin contain a mix of amino acids well matched to human needs, so have greater biological value than proteins of vegetable origin, which are low in one or more of the essential amino acids. However, when different vegetable proteins are eaten together, classically a cereal and a legume, their amino acid contents are complementary and produce an adequate mix, a key feature of most surviving traditional diets, and an important principle for vegan diets.

Dietary recommendations for macronutrients

Recommendations for energy intake (Box 22.3) and proportions of macronutrients (Box 22.4) in the general population have been developed from detailed analyses, and quality assessment, of the totality of the scientific evidence and have changed little over the last 50 years. Recommended ranges or limits aim to provide sufficient essential nutrients for the great majority of healthy people at different life-stages, and also to minimise the risks of chronic non-communicable diseases (obesity, type 2 diabetes, coronary heart disease, diverticulosis, cancers). The requirements during and after illness may be different, and pre-term infants have particular needs.

Disorders of altered energy balance

Obesity

Obesity is regarded as a global pandemic, or 'syndemic' as it entails potentially disastrous consequences for human health. In 2020, almost 30% of adults in the UK were obese (i.e. BMI ≥30 kg/m²) compared with 7% in 1980 and 16% in 1995. Moreover, almost 66% of the total UK adult population is overweight (BMI ≥25 kg/m²). The proportion with a normal weight (BMI 18.5–25 kg/m²) falls to only about 11% by age 65, presenting a problem for interpreting disease associations because those 11% include very fit people, but also a relatively high proportion who have remained or become thinner through illness.

In low- and middle-income countries, average obesity rates are lower, but these figures may disguise high rates of obesity and non-communicable diseases emerging in urban communities.

Complications

Obesity affects both mortality and morbidity (Fig. 22.6). Changes in mortality are difficult to analyse due to the confounding effects of lower body weight in cigarette smokers and those with other illnesses (such as cancer). The lowest mortality rates in Europeans are still in the BMI range 18.5–25 kg/m² (and at lower BMI in South-east Asians), but there is only a minor rise until BMI is above 30 kg/m². A BMI above 35 kg/m² at age 40 years reduces life expectancy by up to 7 years for non-smokers and by 13 years for smokers, and if type 2 diabetes develops, almost always with moderate overweight, life expectancy is reduced by about 7 years at any BMI. Coronary heart disease (Fig. 22.7) is the major cause of death but cancer rates are also increased in the overweight, especially colorectal cancer in males and cancer of the gallbladder, biliary tract, breast, endometrium and cervix in females. Obesity has little effect on life expectancy above 70 years of age, but the severely obese often spend much of their life disabled, physically, mentally and socially. Although an increased body weight results in greater bone density through increased mechanical stress, this does not translate into a lower incidence of osteoporotic fractures. Obesity may have profound psychological consequences, compounded by stigmatisation and victim blaming, rather than offering sympathetic support for effective treatment.

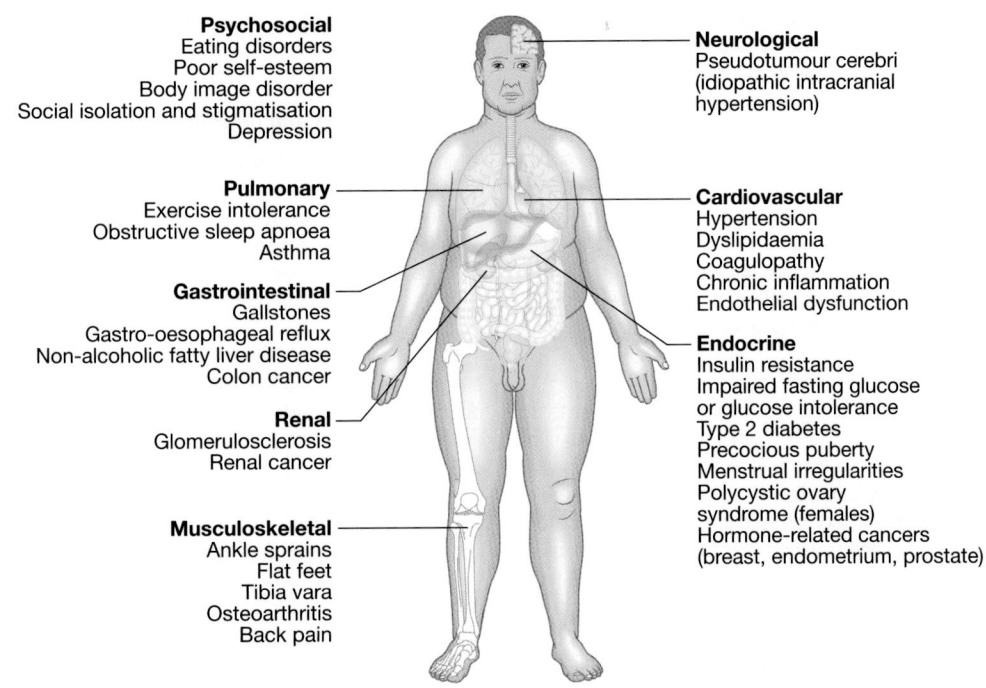

Psychosocial
Eating disorders
Poor self-esteem
Body image disorder
Social isolation and stigmatisation
Depression

Neurological
Pseudotumour cerebri
(idiopathic intracranial
hypertension)

Pulmonary
Exercise intolerance
Obstructive sleep apnoea
Asthma

Cardiovascular
Hypertension
Dyslipidaemia
Coagulopathy
Chronic inflammation
Endothelial dysfunction

Gastrointestinal
Gallstones
Gastro-oesophageal reflux
Non-alcoholic fatty liver disease
Colon cancer

Endocrine
Insulin resistance
Impaired fasting glucose
or glucose intolerance
Type 2 diabetes
Precocious puberty
Menstrual irregularities
Polycystic ovary
syndrome (females)
Hormone-related cancers
(breast, endometrium, prostate)

Renal
Glomerulosclerosis
Renal cancer

Musculoskeletal
Ankle sprains
Flat feet
Tibia vara
Osteoarthritis
Back pain

Fig. 22.6 Complications of obesity.

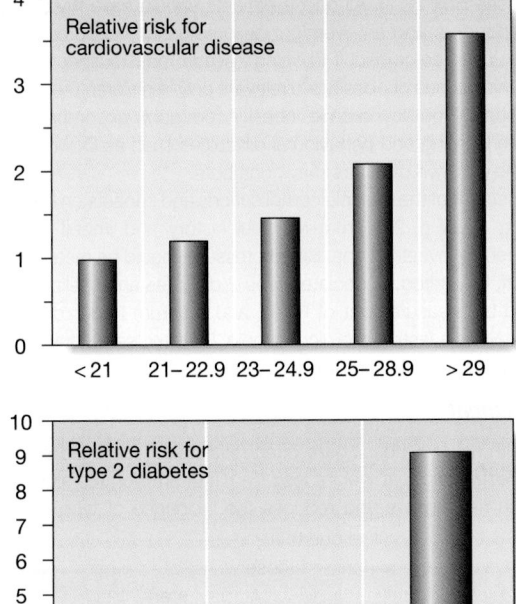

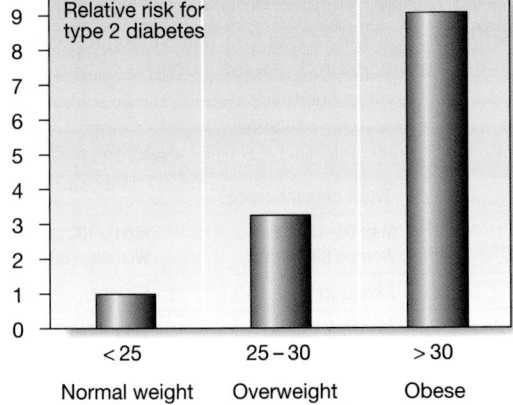

Body mass index (kg/m²)

Fig. 22.7 Risks of diabetes and cardiovascular disease in overweight and obese women. Data are from the Nurses' Health Study in the United States and mostly relate to women of predominantly European descent. In some ethnic groups (e.g. South Asians, Indigenous Americans) and in people with higher waist circumference, the metabolic complications are even more severe at a given level of body mass index.

Body fat distribution

For some complications of obesity, the distribution rather than the absolute amount of excess adipose tissue appears to be important. Increased intra-abdominal fat causes a 'central' ('abdominal', 'visceral', 'android' or 'apple-shaped') shape, which contrasts with subcutaneous fat accumulation causing 'generalised' ('gynoid' or 'pear-shaped') obesity. The former, more common in men, incurs ectopic fat accumulation with impaired functions in liver, pancreas, skeletal and cardiac muscle, promoting type 2 diabetes, metabolic syndrome and cardiovascular disease (see Fig. 22.6). The intra-abdominal fat drains into the portal vein and thence directly to the liver, thus many factors released from adipose tissue (including free fatty acids; 'adipokines', such as tumour necrosis factor alpha, adiponectin and resistin) are at higher concentration in the liver and muscle, inducing insulin resistance and promoting type 2 diabetes. The key to remission of type 2 diabetes, with restoration of the first-phase insulin response to glucose appears to be loss of ectopic fat in liver and pancreas.

Aetiology

Accumulation of fat results from a discrepancy between energy consumption and energy expenditure that is too large to be defended by the hypothalamic regulation of BMR. A continued small daily positive energy balance of only 0.1 MJ (50 kcal; ~2% of intake) would lead to weight gain of ~25 kg over 10 years. With habituation to a subtle energy excess, body fat content shows 'tracking' with age within obesogenic environments, such that children of obese families usually become obese adults. If physical activity decreases with age, which is now common, but food consumption is more driven by habit and marketing than physiology, BMR tends to fall and weight increases throughout adult life (see Fig. 22.3).

The obesity pandemic reflects dramatic changes over the last 40–50 years in both energy intake and expenditure (Box 22.5), although both are difficult to measure reliably. The estimated average global daily supply of food energy per person increased from approximately 9.8 MJ (2350 kcal) in the 1960s to approximately 11.7 MJ (2800 kcal) in the 1990s, but its delivery is unequal. For example, in India it is estimated that 5% of the population receives 40% of the available food energy, leading to obesity in the urban population in parallel with under-nutrition in some rural

22

communities. In affluent societies, a significant proportion of this food supply is discarded. In the United States, men's average daily energy intake reportedly rose from 10.2 MJ (2450 kcal) in 1971 to 11.0 MJ (2618 kcal) in 2000. Portion sizes, particularly of energy-dense foods such as drinks with highly refined sugar content and salty snacks, have increased, and the 'food disappearance' rate (i.e. production and sales) has increased for all food groups, with greater consumption of catered meals and less food waste. Obesity is correlated positively with the number of hours spent watching screens, inversely with sleep time, and inversely with levels of physical activity. Labour-saving devices play a part and minor activities such as fidgeting, termed non-exercise activity thermogenesis (NEAT), may contribute to energy expenditure and protect against obesity.

Susceptibility to obesity

Susceptibility to obesity varies between individuals. Obese subjects do not have a 'slow metabolism': their BMR is higher than that of lean subjects. Twin and adoption studies confirm a familial influence on obesity, but both environment and genes contribute to 'heritability'. The pattern of inheritance suggests a polygenic disorder, with small contributions from a number of different genes, together accounting for 25%–70% of variation in weight. Genome-wide association studies of polymorphisms have identified a handful of genes, some of which encode proteins known to be involved in the control of appetite or metabolism function. However, these account for less than 5% of variation in body weight. Genes also influence fat distribution and therefore risk of metabolic consequences of obesity.

A few rare single-gene disorders have been identified that lead to severe childhood obesity. These include mutations of the melanocortin-4 receptor (*MC4R*), which account for approximately 5% of severe early-onset obesity; defects in the enzymes processing propiomelanocortin (*POMC*, the precursor for adrenocorticotrophic hormone (ACTH)) in the hypothalamus; and mutations in the leptin gene (see Fig. 22.4). The latter can be treated by leptin injections. Additional genetic conditions in which obesity is a feature include Prader–Willi and Lawrence–Moon–Biedl syndromes.

Clinical features and investigations

- In assessing an individual presenting with obesity, the aims are to: exclude an underlying cause,
- identify complications,
- quantify the current and potential problems and
- agree a management plan with the individual, based on evidence, proportionate to the problem and optimally supported.

Measuring waist circumference is useful with BMI under 35 kg/m²: above this level, it is unnecessary and becomes unreliable as the waist descends under gravity. Risks of metabolic and cardiovascular complications are worse with a high waist circumference; lower cut-offs of BMI and waist circumference indicate higher risk in South Asians (Box 22.6).

A very general history of dietary patterns and preferences may be helpful in guiding dietary advice but substantial under-reporting of food consumption is almost universal among overweight people. Pathological eating behaviours such as binge eating, nocturnal eating or bulimia demand specific management. Alcohol is rarely a major source of energy intake but should be considered as a possible obstacle to effective treatment. Many commonly prescribed drugs cause weight gain, and impede effective weight loss (Box 22.7). If possible these should be withdrawn or doses minimised.

In a small minority of patients presenting with a short history of marked change in adult weight gain trajectory, specific causal factors such as hypothyroidism or Cushing's syndrome can be identified and treated (see Box 22.7). All obese patients should have thyroid function tests performed, and an overnight dexamethasone suppression test or 24-hour urine free cortisol if Cushing's syndrome is suspected clinically. Monogenic causes of obesity are relevant only in children presenting with severe obesity, but 'syndromic' obesity commonly accompanies conditions with learning and behavioural difficulties such as Down syndrome, where the goodwill of carers may contribute.

Assessment of the multiple complications and impacts on life and work of obesity (see Fig. 22.6) requires a full history, and limited examination and screening investigations. Blood pressure should be measured with a large cuff, if required. Associated type 2 diabetes and dyslipidaemia are detected by measurement of HbA$_{1c}$ and a serum lipid profile, respectively, ideally in a fasting morning sample. Elevated serum transaminases occur in patients with non-alcoholic fatty liver disease.

Management

The health risks of obesity are often reversible if identified and treated early. Effective modest weight loss (5–10 kg) ameliorates all the cardiometabolic risk factors and reduces the incidence of type 2 diabetes.

---

i 22.5 Some reasons for the increasing prevalence of obesity – the 'obesogenic' environment

Increasing energy intake

- ↑ Portion sizes
- ↑ Snacking, grazing and loss of regular meals
- ↑ Energy-dense 'added-value' food (fat and sugars)
- ↑ Affluence
- Effective marketing

Decreasing energy expenditure

- ↑ Car ownership
- ↓ Walking to school/work
- ↑ Automation/domestic labour-saving
- ↓ Manual labour in occupations
- ↓ Sports in schools
- ↑ Time spent on computer games and watching TV
- ↑ Central heating, washing machines

---

i 22.6 Quantifying obesity with BMI and waist circumference for risk of type 2 diabetes and cardiovascular disease[1]

BMI (weight in kg/height in m²)	Classification[2]	Waist circumference[3]		
		Men < 94 cm / Women < 80 cm	Men 94–102 cm / Women 80–88 cm	Men > 102 cm / Women > 88 cm
18.5–24.9	Reference range	Low	*Increased*	**Severe**
25.0–29.9	Overweight	Low	*Moderate*	**Very severe**
>30.0	**Obese**			
30.0–34.9	Class I	*Moderate*	**Severe**	**Very severe**
35.0–39.9	Class II	(not possible)	**Very severe**	**Very severe**
>40.0	Class III	(not possible)	**Very severe**	**Very severe**

[1]Lower cut-offs apply for people of South Asian ancestry, see note 2. High waist circumference is the more potent risk indicator, reflecting increase intra-abdominal and ectopic fat accumulation in vital organs. [2]Classification of the World Health Organization (WHO) and International Obesity Task Force. The Western Pacific Region Office of WHO recommends that, among South Asians, BMI > 23.0 is overweight and > 25.0 is obese. Lower cut-offs for waist circumference have also been proposed for South Asians but have not been validated. [3]When BMI is > 35 kg/m², waist circumference is difficult to measure because the waist descends under gravity, so does not add to the increased risk.

i 22.7 Secondary causes of weight gain

Endocrine factors

- Hypothyroidism
- Cushing's syndrome
- Insulinoma
- Hypothalamic tumours or injury

Drug treatments (worse in combination)

- Atypical antipsychotics (e.g. olanzapine)
- Antidepressants (e.g. amitryptyline, mirtazepine)
- Gabapentin, pregabalin
- Sulphonylureas, thiazolidinediones, insulin
- Pizotifen
- Glucocorticoids
- Sodium valproate
- β-blockers

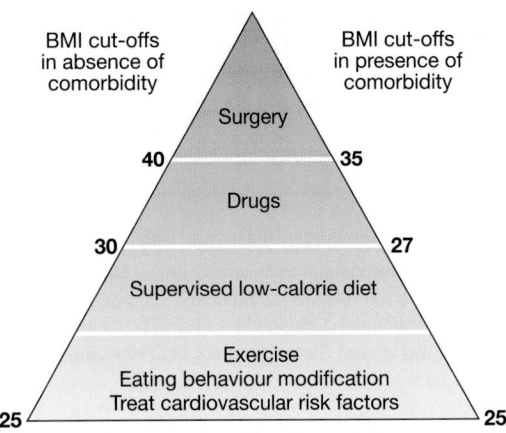

Fig. 22.8 Therapeutic options for obesity. Relevant comorbidities include type 2 diabetes, hypertension, cardiovascular disease, sleep apnoea, and waist circumference of >102 cm in men or 88 cm in women. This is an approximate consensus of the numerous national guidelines, which vary slightly in their recommendations and are revised every few years. (BMI = body masss index).

More substantial weight loss (10–15 kg or more) is needed to gain remission of established type diabetes, or of sleep apnoea. Sustaining substantial weight loss is notoriously hard, so population strategies to prevent and reverse obesity are high on public health priority agendas. Many initiatives have evidence for limited success while the initiative is in place, including promoting 'healthy eating' in schools, enhancing walking and cycling options for commuters, and liaising with the food industry to reduce energy, sugar and fat content and to label foods appropriately. Unfortunately these measures tend most to benefit those better educated who already suffer less from overweight and obesity. Taxes on high-sugar drinks have been introduced in some countries, with some evidence for short-term changes in consumption but not in effect on body weights, probably because artificially sweetened alternatives still stimulate an appetite for more energy-dense foods. Unfortunately, many heavily promoted 'low-fat' foods are often still energy-dense.

Most patients seeking assistance with obesity appear motivated to lose weight and have often done so previously, without long-term success. These patients may hold inaccurate perceptions of their energy intake and expenditure, and an unrealistic view of the target weight that they would regard as a 'success'. An empathetic explanation of energy balance, which recognises that some individuals are more susceptible to obesity than others, and find it more difficult to lose body weight and sustain this loss, is important. Reassurance that there is no underlying endocrine or metabolic problem can be helpful, especially for family members or carers. Appropriate goals for weight loss should be agreed, recognising that a given amount of weight loss achieves greater risk reduction at higher levels of BMI, but accommodating the perceptions of the patient. An initial reasonable goal for most patients with BMI up to 30 kg/m^2 is to lose 5%–10% of body weight using conventional diet and lifestyle modifications. With BMI above 30 kg/m^2, or if type 2 diabetes or other serious complications are present, greater weight loss of over 10–15 kg is recommended, and more intensive intervention is indicated, with separate strategies for inducing and for maintaining weight loss of this order (Fig. 22.8). Modern adjunctive drug treatment can be very effective (e.g. GLP-1 agonists), but mainly to sustain major weight losses for those who alter their diet substantially.

Lifestyle advice

Behavioural modification to avoid or mitigate some effects of the 'obesogenic' environment (see Box 22.5) is the cornerstone of long-term control of weight. Adopting more disciplined eating patterns, and preplanned meals, is advised. Advising modest extra activity to increase physical activity level (PAL) ratios (see Fig. 22.3C), may be successful for younger people, but this must be sustainable and regular as a daily routine (e.g. walking rather than driving to work): older patients, and those with arthritis or type 2 diabetes find increasing physical activity very hard. Regular support, and positive strategic encouragement when problems arise, from a dietitian or weight loss group is very valuable.

Weight loss diets

The general lifestyle advice above, with medical encouragement, may gradually induce weight loss and a grateful patient. However, regain is a huge problem, as people slip back to their 'normal' diets and lifestyles, especially when life-events step in. Contrary to much previous teaching, the evidence is now consistent that more rapid and greater early weight loss tends to result in better quality of life, and to better long-term maintenance. More rapid weight loss may also be required to prepare for surgery.

Very-low-energy diets (VLEDs, under 800 kcal/day) or low energy diets of 800–1000 kcal/day are similarly effective for rapid weight loss of 1.5–2.5 kg/week, compared to 0.5 kg/week on conventional regimens. Both are safe if provided as a nutritionally complete formula diet, and most successful with encouragement from an experienced and supportive physician or nutritionist. A minimum content of 40–50 g protein daily minimises muscle degradation, over 20 g of fat helps to avoid gallstone formation, with sufficient magnesium to avoid constipation, and fluid intake of at least 2.5 L/day to avoid dehydration which can cause orthostatic hypotension, headache, constipation and nausea. Medical supervision is needed for patients whose glucose-lowering and antihypertensive medications need withdrawal or reduction with rapid weight loss.

Drugs

The obesity pandemic has stimulated huge investment by the pharmaceutical industry in finding drugs for obesity, unfortunately hitherto directed and licensed only for 'weight loss' although the greater problem for patients is in fact long-term maintenance of a lower weight. There is no role for diuretics, or for thyroxine. Metformin does generate an average weight loss of about 2 kg, but is not licensed or effective for weight management. Drug therapy should only be used as an adjunct to optimal, evidence-based, lifestyle advice and support, which should be continued throughout treatment.

Orlistat inhibits pancreatic and gastric lipases. The standard dose of 120 mg taken with each of the three main meals reduces dietary fat absorption by about 30%. It is not absorbed, and adverse effects relate to fat malabsorption if the diet still contains too much fat: loose oily stools, faecal urgency, flatus and malabsorption of fat-soluble vitamins. Its efficacy is partly explained because patients taking orlistat adhere better to low-fat diets in order to avoid unpleasant gastrointestinal side-effects, but it is favoured by few patients. The combination of low-dose phentermine and topiramate extended release, approved in the United States, results in weight loss of ~6% greater than placebo. Concerns over teratogenicity of topiramate and cardiovascular effects of

22

both phentermine and topiramate (albeit at higher doses) have blocked its approval in Europe. The combination of the opioid antagonist naltrexone and the noradrenaline (norepinephrine)/dopamine re-uptake inhibitor bupropion is similarly effective, and approved in both the United States and Europe. Its main adverse effects are dry mouth and constipation.

The most effective medications for obesity treatment are the glucagon-like peptide-1 (GLP-1) receptor agonists, usually at higher doses than are used to treat type diabetes. These drugs are remarkably safe, their main drawback being high cost. Their main side-effects are gastrointestinal and avoided if the dose is very low to start, and then slowly increased. Patients are very willing to accept subcutaneous administration for effective treatment. Liraglutide is approved for obesity treatment in Europe and the United States, and for high-risk obese patients, at a daily subcutaneous dose up to 3 mg. The mean weight loss in randomised trials was about 10 kg, including trials of people with type 2 diabetes. Even better results can be achieved in routine practice if it is stopped early when it proves ineffective. It is recommended to stop liraglutide if 3 mg/day for 3 months fails to generate >5% weight loss (usually indicating poor dietary compliance). Another GLP-1 agonist, semaglutide, also already licensed for type 2 diabetes, is under consideration in both the United States and Europe for approval at a dose of 2.4 mg/day subcutaneously. It generates even greater weight losses than liraglutide, with similar safety, and weekly injection and an oral form are in trials.

Drug therapy is usually reserved for patients with high risk of complications from obesity (see Fig. 22.8). All licensed drugs do reduce the cardiovascular and diabetes risks and weight loss of >10% is associated with reduced cardiac events. However, approvals are currently for weight loss, not maintenance, so duration of drug treatment is controversial. Withdrawing an effective drug means it no longer works, so weight regain is usual. Although life-long therapy is advocated on the basis of short-term research trials for many drugs that reduce risks (e.g. drugs for hypertension and osteoporosis), this is not yet widely accepted for obesity treatment. Weight regain despite continued drug treatment generally reflects reduction in professional support and relaxation of dietary control, for which reinforcement and new lifestyle measures are needed. Patients who demonstrate early weight loss (e.g. >5% after 12 weeks on the optimum dose) achieve greater and longer-term weight loss. Treatment can be stopped in non-responders at this point and alternative treatments considered.

Surgery

'Bariatric' surgery is the most effective treatment for obesity, in terms of amount and duration of weight loss (see Fig. 22.8 and Box 22.8), and associated with improvements in all obesity-related risk factors and reduced mortality. Bariatric surgery should be contemplated in motivated patients who have very high risks of complications of obesity, when optimal dietary and drug therapy has been insufficiently effective. It is usually reserved for those with severe obesity (BMI >40 kg/m²), or those with a BMI >35 kg/m² and significant complications, such as type 2 diabetes or obstructive sleep apnoea, although some evidence-based guidelines now suggest surgery can be considered at a lower weight with recent-onset diabetes and a BMI >30 kg/m². Only experienced specialist surgeons should undertake these procedures, in collaboration with a multidisciplinary team and plans for lifelong follow-up. Several approaches are used (Fig. 22.9) and all can be performed laparoscopically. The mechanism of weight loss, and its maintenance, after bariatric surgery is controversial. It may not simply relate to limiting the stomach size, or absorptive capacity, but also in disrupting release of ghrelin from the stomach or promoting release of other peptides from the small bowel, thereby enhancing satiety signalling in the hypothalamus. Diabetes usually improves rapidly after surgery, particularly after gastric bypass, but this is mainly attributable to severe energy restriction in the perioperative period. Increased release of incretin hormones such as GLP-1 may contribute to improved glucose control.

Bariatric surgery has taught us a lot about the pathogenesis of obesity and the health improvements possible with substantial weight loss, but it

i | **22.8 Effectiveness and adverse effects of laparoscopic bariatric surgical procedures***

Procedure	Expected 2-year weight loss (kg)	Adverse effects
Gastric banding	19–25	Band slippage, erosion, stricture Port site infection Mortality <0.2% in experienced centres
Sleeve gastrectomy	20–30	Iron deficiency Vitamin B_{12} deficiency Mortality <0.2% in experienced centres
Roux-en-Y gastric bypass	20–40	Internal hernia Stomal ulcer Dumping syndrome Hypoglycaemia Iron deficiency Vitamin B_{12} deficiency Vitamin D deficiency Mortality 0.5%

*Weight regain is a frequent problem beyond 5 years after all bariatric surgery, particularly banding and sleeve gastrectomy.

is not a 'one-step solution'. Complications of one kind or another, often multiple and some serious, affect almost all patients after bariatric surgery, depending on the approach. Perioperative mortality is now under 1% in experienced centres, but post-operative respiratory problems, wound infection and dehiscence, staple leaks, stomal stenosis, marginal ulcers and venous thrombosis may occur. Additional problems may arise at a later stage, such as pouch and distal oesophageal dilatation with loss of effectiveness, persistent vomiting, hypoglycaemic or hypotensive 'dumping' syndromes, hypoglycaemia and micronutrient deficiencies, particularly of folate, vitamin B_{12} and iron, which are of special concern to women contemplating pregnancy; this should be delayed for at least 2 years following surgery.

Cosmetic surgical procedures may be needed for a full physical and mental recovery after major weight loss. Apronectomy is a major operation to remove an overhang of unsightly, infected or ulcerated abdominal skin, a common problem in obese women after the menopause. This operation is not without risks, and of no value for long-term weight reduction if food intake remains unrestricted.

Treatment of additional risk factors

Obesity must not be treated in isolation. Other risk factors must be addressed, including smoking, excess alcohol consumption, diabetes, hyperlipidaemia, hypertension and obstructive sleep apnoea.

Under-nutrition

Starvation and famine

There remain regions of the world, particularly rural Africa, where under-nutrition due to famine is endemic, where up to 20% of adults have BMI <18.5 kg/m² (Box 22.9), and stunting due to under-nutrition affects 50% of children. The World Health Organization (WHO) reports that chronic under-nutrition is responsible for more than half of all childhood deaths worldwide. Starvation is manifest as marasmus (malnutrition with marked muscle wasting) or, when added complications such multiple infections and oxidative stress come into play, kwashiorkor (malnutrition with oedema). Growth retardation is due to deficiencies of key nutrients (protein, zinc, potassium, phosphate and sulphur). Treatment of these childhood conditions is not discussed in this adult medical textbook. In adults, starvation is the result of chronic sustained negative energy (calorie) balance, commonly with coexisting micronutrient deficiencies and many possible causes (Box 22.10).

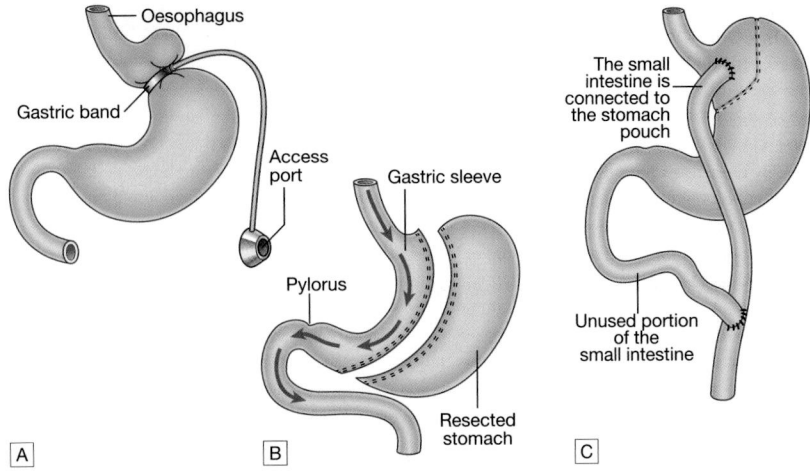

Fig. 22.9 Bariatric surgical procedures. [A] Laparoscopic banding, with the option of a reservoir band and subcutaneous access to restrict the stomach further after compensatory expansion has occurred. [B] Sleeve gastrectomy. [C] Roux-en-Y gastric bypass.

22.9 Classification of under-nutrition in adults by body mass index (weight/height²)

BMI (kg/m²)	Classification
>20	Adequate nutrition
18.5–20	Marginal
<18.5	**Under-nutrition**
17–18.4	Mild
16–17	Moderate
<16	Severe

22.10 Causes of under-nutrition and weight loss in adults

Decreased energy intake

- Famine
- Persistent regurgitation or vomiting
- True anorexia from depression
- True anorexia from drug side-effects
- Eating disorders (e.g. anorexia nervosa https://we.tl/t-KFTRESkTDA)
- Malabsorption (e.g. small intestinal disease)
- Maldigestion (e.g. pancreatic exocrine insufficiency)

Increased energy expenditure

- Increased basal metabolic rate (thyrotoxicosis, trauma, fever, cancer cachexia, anxiety)
- Excessive physical activity (e.g. marathon runners)
- Energy loss (e.g. glycosuria in diabetes)
- Impaired energy storage (e.g. Addison disease, phaeochromocytoma)

22.11 Clinical features of severe under-nutrition in adults

- Weight loss
- Thirst, craving for food, weakness and feeling cold
- Nocturia, amenorrhoea or impotence
- Lax, pale, dry skin with loss of turgor and, occasionally, pigmented patches
- Cold and cyanosed extremities, pressure sores
- Hair thinning or loss (except in adolescents)
- Muscle-wasting, best demonstrated by the loss of the temporalis and periscapular muscles and reduced mid-arm circumference
- Loss of subcutaneous fat, reflected in reduced skinfold thickness and mid-arm circumference
- Hypothermia, bradycardia, hypotension and small heart
- Oedema, which may be present without hypoalbuminaemia ('famine oedema')
- Distended abdomen with diarrhoea
- Diminished tendon jerks
- Apathy, loss of initiative, depression, introversion, aggression if food is nearby
- Susceptibility to infections (see Box 22.12)

22.12 Infections associated with starvation

- Gastroenteritis and Gram-negative sepsis
- Respiratory infections, especially bronchopneumonia
- Certain viral diseases, especially measles and herpes simplex
- Tuberculosis
- Streptococcal and staphylococcal skin infections
- Helminthic infestations

Clinical features

In starvation, the severity of malnutrition can be assessed by anthropometric measurements, such as BMI (see p. 757 and Box 22.9). Demispan and mid-arm circumference measurements are most useful in monitoring progress during treatment. The clinical features of severe under-nutrition in adults are listed in Box 22.11.

Under-nutrition often includes vitamin deficiencies, especially of thiamin, folate and vitamin C (see below). Diarrhoea can lead to depletion of sodium, potassium and magnesium. The high mortality rate in famine situations is often due to outbreaks of infection, such as gastroenteritis, typhus or cholera (Box 22.12), but the usual signs of infection (e.g. fever, tachycardia) may not be apparent. In advanced starvation, patients shut down non-essential metabolism, with hypothermia and bradycardia, and become physically inactive in a flexed, fetal position, minimising heat loss. In the last stage of starvation, death comes quietly and often quite suddenly, commonly through asymptomatic pneumonia or primary arrhythmia. The very old are most vulnerable: younger people may be able to adapt to prolonged undernutrition. At necropsy all organs are atrophied, except the brain, which tends to maintain its weight.

Investigations

In a famine, laboratory investigations may be impractical but will show that plasma free fatty acids are increased and there is ketosis and a mild metabolic acidosis. Plasma glucose is low but albumin concentration is often maintained because the liver still functions reasonably normally. Insulin secretion is diminished, glucagon and cortisol tend to increase, and reverse T_3 replaces normal triiodothyronine. The resting metabolic rate falls, partly because of falling lean body mass, and partly because of hypothalamic compensation (see Fig. 22.3). The urine has a fixed specific gravity and creatinine excretion becomes low. There may be

22

mild pancytopenia. The erythrocyte sedimentation rate (ESR) is normal unless there is infection. Tests of delayed skin hypersensitivity, e.g. to tuberculin, become falsely negative. The electrocardiogram shows sinus bradycardia and low voltage.

Management

Undernutrition in a famine, or with anorexia nervosa, tends to preserve muscle mass, while with prolonged infections and inflammation, muscle tends to be lost more rapidly, reflected in lower mid upper arm circumference (MUAC). Undernutrition represents the only emergency in clinical nutrition. Starvation kills, but usually slowly: an average man or woman has enough body fat to live on for about 40 days, provided fluids are still consumed but ill-guided attempts at treating undernutrition can rapidly kill an otherwise healthy patient.

The severity of under-nutrition is graded according to BMI (see Box 22.9). People with mild starvation are not in great danger; those with moderate starvation need extra feeding; and those who are severely underweight need hospital care, particularly to avoid death from 'refeeding syndrome' (Box 22.13). Correcting fluids and electrolytes first, and their careful monitoring for at least 7 days of refeeding, is vital as there is often marked depletion of potassium, phosphate and magnesium after starvation. If insulin is stimulated by food without correcting these, their sudden movement into cells can cause a sudden arrhythmic death.

It is also essential to give thiamine to all severely undernourished patients (initially parenterally to be sure of absorption) to correct possible deficiency before food is administered, in order to avoid precipitating beri beri. Thiamine should be given on suspicion, without waiting for confirmatory blood tests, and without waiting for clinical signs of beri beri to emerge: a delay could be catastrophic, with permanent sequelae.

When food becomes available, and can be taken, it should be given by mouth in small, frequent amounts at first, using a suitable formula preparation (Box 22.14). Gastrointestinal involution often causes a degree of malabsorption, and diarrhoea, initially. Secondary lactose intolerance is common so milk-based foods are inappropriate. Individual energy requirements can vary by 30%, but minor over-feeding is more hazardous, causing fatty liver, than modest under-feeding, so rapid refeeding should be avoided. During rehabilitation, more concentrated formula can be given with additional more palatable foods similar to the usual staple meal. Salt should be restricted and micronutrient supplements (e.g. potassium, magnesium, zinc and multivitamins) may be essential. Between 6.3 and 8.4 MJ/day (1500–2000 kcal/day) will arrest progressive under-nutrition but additional energy may be required for regain of weight. During refeeding, a weight gain of 5% body weight per month indicates satisfactory progress. Other care is supportive and includes attention to the skin, adequate hydration, treatment of infections and careful monitoring of body temperature, since thermoregulation may be impaired.

Circumstances and resources are different in every famine but many problems are non-medical and concern organisation, infrastructure, liaison, politics, procurement, security and ensuring that food is distributed on the basis of need. Lastly, plans must be made for the future for prevention and/or earlier intervention if similar circumstances prevail.

Under-nutrition in hospital

It is a worry that under-nutrition remains a serious issue in many sectors of high-income countries, particularly for older people and those who are less independent. In the UK, 30% of people requiring acute admission to hospital show evidence of under-nutrition and 65% of those admitted will lose an average of 5% of their total body weight during that admission. In the older population, levels of under-nutrition and vitamin deficiencies parallel levels of independent living. In Scotland, 33% of those aged over 65 who are living in their own home are deficient in folic acid and 10% are deficient in vitamin C. The prevalence of vitamin deficiencies rises further in less independent groups in residential homes.

Under-nutrition is poorly recognised and poorly documented in hospital admissions and discharges, with potentially serious medical and medico-legal consequences. Physical effects include impaired immunity,

22.13 Recognition and management of refeeding syndrome

- Refeeding after undernutrition is essential, but:
  - Refeeding without correcting K/Mg/PO₄ is a common cause of death
  - Refeeding without correcting subclinical thiamine deficiency causes permanent brain injury (Korsakoff psychosis). Always give IV thiamine before commencing refeeding – do not wait for biochemical confirmation of deficiency
- Classical patients at risk: kwashiorkor/marasmus, chronic malnutrition, alcoholism
- Others risk factors: BMI <16 kg/m²; unintentional weight loss >15% in 3–6 months; little/no oral intake for >10 days; low K+, Mg++, PO₄ before feeding
- Can occur with lesser degrees of weight loss and higher BMI levels; also in 'sarcopoenic obesity'
- Refeeding leads to: uptake of glucose, K+, Mg++ and PO₄ into cells, and reduced plasma levels; thiamine utilisation and depletion; and retention of Na+ and water
- General treatment measures: careful monitoring, daily weights, cautious rehydration, cardiac monitoring if ECG changes, e.g. prolonged QTc interval
- Give repeated IV infusions of small doses of PO₄ (10–20 mmol)
- IV correction of hypokalaemia and hypomagnesaemia
- Energy: start at 10–20 kcal/kg daily increasing to meet energy needs over 5–7 days

(BMI – body mass index; ECG = electrocardiogram; IV = intravenous)

22.14 WHO recommended diets for refeeding

Nutrient (per 100 mL)	F-75 diet[1]	F-100 diet[2]
Energy	315 kJ (75 kcal)	420 kJ (100 kcal)
Protein (g)	0.9	2.9
Lactose (g)	1.3	4.2
Potassium (mmol)	3.6	5.9
Sodium (mmol)	0.9	1.9
Magnesium (mmol)	0.43	0.73
Zinc (mg)	2.0	2.3
Copper (mg)	0.25	0.25
Percentage of energy from:		
Protein	5	12
Fat	32	53
Osmolality (mOsmol/kg)	333	419
Dose	170 kJ/kg (40 kcal/kg)	630–920 kJ/kg (150–220 kcal/kg)
Rate of feeding by mouth	2.2 (mL/kg/hr)	Gradual increase in volume, 6 times daily

[1]F-75 is prepared from milk powder (25 g), sugar (70 g), cereal flour (35 g), vegetable oil (27 g) and vitamin and mineral supplements, made up to 1 L with water. [2]F-100 (1 L) contains milk powder (80 g), sugar (50 g), vegetable oil (60 g) and vitamin and mineral supplements (no cereal).

muscle weakness, which in turn affects cardiac and respiratory function, osteomalacia, and delayed wound healing with increased risks of secondary infection. The under-nourished patient is often withdrawn and this may be mistaken for depressive illness. Engagement with treatment and rehabilitation can be adversely affected. Much of this can be avoided through better awareness of under-nutrition, prompt nutritional assessment and monitoring with appropriate intervention. Screening systems, such as the Malnutrition Universal Screening Tool (MUST) (Fig. 22.10), raise awareness across multidisciplinary teams, and encourage staff to assess and monitor food intake and weigh patients regularly.

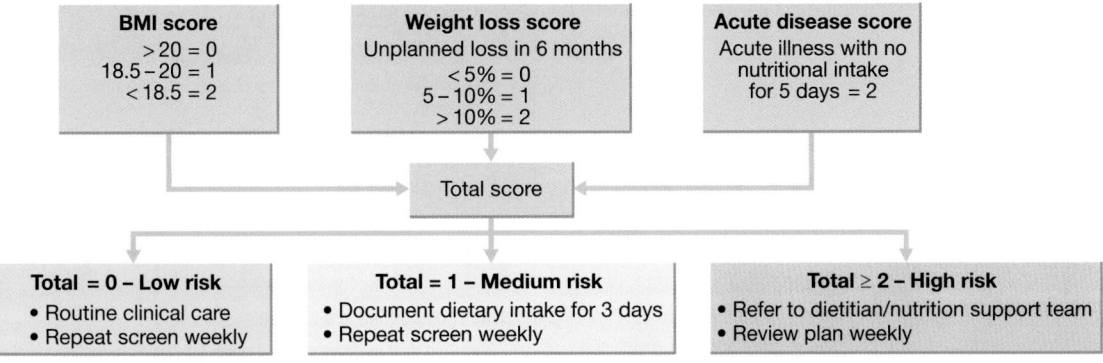

Fig. 22.10 Screening hospitalised patients for risk of malnutrition. Acute illnesses include decompensated liver disease, cancer cachexia or being kept 'nil by mouth'. *Adapted from the British Association of Parenteral and Enteral Nutrition Malnutrition Universal Screening Tool (www.bapen.org.uk).*

Causes are often complex (see Box 22.10). Social issues impact on food choices and may cause or exacerbate disease. Social isolation, low levels of disposable income and a lack of knowledge or interest in healthy eating may increase reliance on calorie-dense convenience foods of poor nutritional quality. The non-specific effects of chronic inflammation, infection or malignancy, as well as specific gastrointestinal disorders, may adversely affect appetite, reducing food intake.

Loss of appetite is common with gastrointestinal diseases, but occurs as a non-specific response to myriad other conditions or their treatments. The most frequent side-effects of many prescription drugs are nausea and gastrointestinal disturbance. Surgical resection of the gastrointestinal tract can have major nutritional sequelae in the years following, ranging from intolerance of normal volumes of food, or specific nutrient malabsorption, to intestinal failure (where there is partial or complete failure of the intestine to perform its vital functions). This is especially so after partial or total gastrectomy, extensive small bowel surgery or pancreatic (Whipple's) resection. It helps to consider systematically where the problem(s) might lie (Box 22.15).

An approach to assisted nutrition in hospital patients

All patients in hospital or a care home should be screened periodically for possible malnutrition using the MUST tool (Fig. 22.10), and formally assessed if indicated. Poor appetite, immobility, poor dentition or even being kept 'nil by mouth' for hospital procedures all contribute to weight loss. A decision to intervene to tackle and reverse nutritional difficulties may involve simply ensuring that adequate supplies of suitable food are delivered accessibly (it is difficult to eat lying down) or that dentures fit properly, but may require an assessment of a patient's swallow or of the intestine's ability to digest foods. Whenever possible, it is best to use the most physiological means of feeding, i.e. by mouth, reserving more invasive interventions for when swallowing and digestion are impaired or absent. Enteral feeding is always preferred to parenteral, with its multiple hazards, provided the intestine is accessible and functioning.

Oral nutritional supplements

Where swallow and intestinal function remain intact, the simplest form of assisted nutrition is the use of oral nutritional supplements, starting with attractive foods. Most branded supplement products are nutritionally complete (fortified with the daily requirements of vitamins, minerals and trace elements) and come in various formulations and textures, including 'shakes' and 'puddings' with a thicker consistency. They are expensive, but can be cost-effective and useful for people who may require just a small number of additional calories each day to maintain or gain weight in the short or longer term. However, they should not be used to replace normal meals or snacks. And their use and effect must be monitored. In spite of their nutritional value, small volume and range of flavours, many people find them unpalatable or difficult to tolerate, in which case they will be ineffective, but patients may not volunteer this information.

> **i** **22.15 Factors affecting adequacy of nutritional intake in hospitalised patients**
>
> **Factors affecting appetite**
> - Unfamiliar or ill-prepared food
> - Altered taste or smell
> - Anxiety (social, cultural, financial, general and mental health issues may all be relevant, individually or in combination)
> - Nausea and/or vomiting
> - Non-specific effects of illness and/or drugs
>
> **Issues of quantity**
> - Insufficient food on the plate?
> - Reliance on 3 meals a day without the normal 4th meal or snacks
>
> **Getting the food from the plate to the mouth**
> - Generalised reduced mobility
> - Reduced manual dexterity
> - Horizontal posture, bedrest
> - Loss of upper limb or hand function
>
> **Difficulties chewing food and initiating swallow**
> - Tooth loss
> - Poorly fitting dentures
> - Pain in the mouth, tongue or jaws
> - Respiratory failure
>
> **Specific problems with the oesophagus and gastrointestinal tract**
> - Obstruction (intrinsic or extrinsic)
> - Ischaemia
> - Inflammation
> - Malabsorption
>
> **Cultural issues**
> - Is the food provided appropriate to the patient's beliefs?
>
> **More general evidence of self-neglect**
> - Evidence of chronic coexisting illness
> - Evidence of mental health problems – low mood may be 'cause' or 'effect' in under-nutrition

Enteral feeding

Where swallowing or food ingestion is impaired but intestinal function remains intact enteral tube feeding is the next choice (naso-enteral, gastrostomy or jejunostomy feeding). There are a number of theoretical advantages to enteral feeding, as opposed to parenteral, with uncertain evidence. These include:

- preservation of intestinal mucosal architecture, gut-associated lymphoid tissue and hepatic and pulmonary immune function
- reduced levels of systemic inflammation and hyperglycaemia
- interference with pathogenicity of gut micro-organisms.

However, the areas in which advantage has been consistently *proven* are:

- fewer episodes of infection
- lower cost
- earlier return to intestinal function
- shorter length of hospital stay.

The risks of enteral feeding are those related to tube insertion (Box 22.16) and diarrhoea (Box 22.17).

Nasogastric tube feeding

This is simple, readily available, comparatively low-cost and most suitable for short-term feeding (up to 4 weeks). Insertion of a nasogastric tube requires care and training (see Box 23.40 and Box 22.16). Patients with reduced conscious level may pull at tubes and displace them: a nasal 'bridle' device can help by fixing the tube around the nasal septum, unless forcible tugging is likely.

Gastrostomy feeding

Gastrostomy is a more invasive insertion technique, but easier to manage when longer-term feeding (>4 weeks) is required. Gastrostomies are less liable to displacement than nasogastric tubes and allow for fewer feed interruptions, so more of the prescribed feeds can be administered. An endoscopic, minimally invasive, technique is usual. Both endoscopic and radiological gastrostomy insertion involve inflating the stomach, thus opposing it to the anterior abdominal wall. The stomach is then punctured percutaneously and a suitable tube placed (Fig. 22.11) with an internal retainer device (plastic 'bumper' or balloon) that sits snugly against the gastric mucosa, and an external retainer to limit movement. These retainers hold the gastric wall against the abdominal wall, effectively creating a controlled gastrocutaneous ('Eck') fistula that matures over 2–4 weeks. Patient assessment and selection prior to gastrostomy placement should be done by a multidisciplinary nutrition support team, to weigh benefits against risks, recognising the need for stoma care (Box 22.18 and see Box 22.26).

Post-pyloric feeding

In patients with a high risk of pulmonary aspiration or gastroparesis, it may be preferable to feed into the jejunum (via a nasojejunal tube,

i · 22.16 Complications of nasogastric tube feeding

- Tube misplacement, e.g. tracheal or bronchial placement (*rarely*, intracranial placement)
- Reflux of gastric contents and pulmonary aspiration
- Interrupted feeding or inadequate feed volumes
- Refeeding syndrome

i · 22.17 Diarrhoea related to enteral feeding

Factors contributing to diarrhoea

- Fibre-free feed may reduce short-chain fatty acid production in colon
- Fat malabsorption
- Inappropriate osmotic load
- Pre-existing primary gut problem (e.g. lactose intolerance)
- Infection

Management

- Often responds well to a fibre-containing feed or a switch to an alternative feed
- Simple antidiarrhoeal agents (e.g. loperamide) can be very effective

i · 22.18 Complications of gastrostomy tube feeding

- Reflux of gastric contents and pulmonary aspiration (same as nasogastric tube)
- Risks of insertion (pain, damage to intra-abdominal structures, intestinal perforation, pulmonary aspiration, infection, death)
- Risk of tumour 'seeding' if an endoscopic 'pull-through' technique is used in head and neck or oesophageal cancer patients
- Refeeding syndrome

gastrostomy with jejunal extension or direct placement into jejunum by radiological, endoscopic or surgical means).

Parenteral nutrition

This is strictly reserved for clinical situations where the absorptive functioning of the intestine is severely impaired, usually by resection, and will remain so indefinitely. Nutrition is delivered directly into a large-diameter systemic vein, completely bypassing the intestine and portal

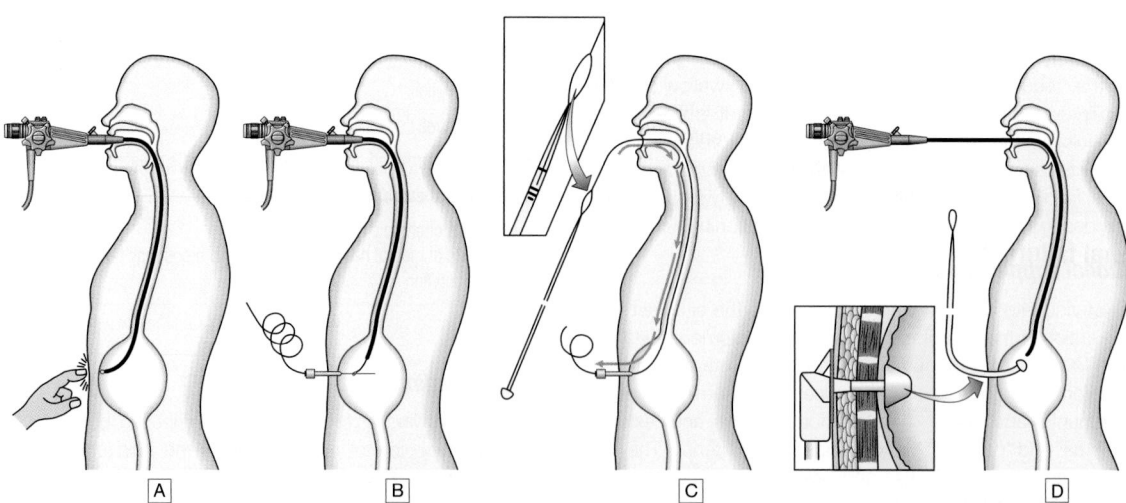

Fig. 22.11 Percutaneous endoscopic gastrostomy (PEG) placement. **A** Finger pressure on the anterior abdominal wall is noted by the endoscopist. **B** Following insertion of a cannula through the anterior abdominal wall into the stomach, a guidewire is threaded through the cannula and grasped by the endoscopic forceps or snare. **C** The endoscope is withdrawn with the guidewire. The gastrostomy tube is then attached to the guidewire. **D** The guidewire and tube are pulled back through the mouth, oesophagus and stomach to exit on the anterior abdominal wall, and the endoscope is repassed to confirm the site of placement of the retention device. The latter closely abuts the gastric mucosa; its position is maintained by an external fixation device (see inset). It is also possible to place PEG tubes using fluoroscopic guidance when endoscopy is difficult (radiologically inserted gastrostomy).

22.19 Complications of parenteral nutrition

Intravenous catheter complications

- Insertion (pneumothorax, haemothorax, arterial puncture)
- Catheter infection (sepsis, discitis, pulmonary or cerebral abscess)
- Central venous thrombosis

Metabolic complications

- Refeeding syndrome
- Electrolyte imbalance
- Hyperglycaemia
- Hyperalimentation
- Fluid overload
- Hepatic steatosis/fibrosis/cirrhosis

22.20 Parameters for monitoring parenteral nutrition in hospital

Parameter	Monitoring requirement
Electrolytes (sodium, potassium, magnesium) **Bone profile** (calcium, phosphate) **Liver function tests** (bilirubin, alanine aminotransferase, alkaline phosphatase, γ-glutamyl transferase) **Markers of inflammation** (C-reactive protein, leucocyte count)	Daily until stable and then 2–3 times per week
Blood glucose	At least twice daily until stable and then daily
Cholesterol and triglycerides	Weekly initially, reducing to every 3 months when stable

22.21 Causes of short bowel syndrome in adults

- Mesenteric ischaemia
- Post-operative complications
- Crohn's disease
- Trauma
- Neoplasia
- Radiation enteritis

22.22 Likely requirements for support according to length of intact residual small bowel

Residual length of jejunum (cm)	Oral fluid restriction	Oral glucose/ electrolyte solution	Intravenous fluids	Parenteral nutrition
<200	Yes	Yes	May avoid	May avoid
<100	Yes	Yes	Yes	May avoid
<75	Yes	Yes	Yes	Yes

venous system. As well as being more invasive, more expensive and less physiological than the enteral route, parenteral nutrition has many more complications (Box 22.19), mainly infective and metabolic (disturbances of electrolytes, hyperglycaemia). Strict adherence to aseptic practice in handling catheters and careful monitoring of clinical (pulse, blood pressure and temperature) and biochemical (urea, electrolytes, glucose and liver function tests) parameters are necessary to minimise risk (Box 22.20). Overfeeding is a particular hazard, causing fatty liver and potentially liver failure and death: accurate estimation of energy requirement is needed, preferably measurement using a metabolic cart.

The parenteral route is most often required in acutely ill patients with multi-organ failure, in severely under-nourished patients undergoing surgery which cannot be delayed, and with short bowel syndrome following resection. One by one, previous indications for parenteral feeding, e.g. thoracic duct rupture, have been found responsive to enteral feeding. There are major ethical issues around starting, and stopping, parenteral feeding, particularly if the patient lacks capacity.

Intestinal failure ('short bowel syndrome')

Intestinal failure (IF) is defined as a reduction in gut function to below the minimum necessary for both adequate absorption of macronutrients and/or water and electrolytes. Intravenous supplementation is then required to support health and/or growth.

IF can be classified according to its onset, metabolic consequences and expected outcome.

- *Type 1 IF*: a common acute-onset, usually self-limiting condition with few long-term sequelae. It is most often seen following abdominal surgery or in the context of critical illness. Intravenous fluid and electrolyte support may be required for a few days to weeks.
- *Type 2 IF*: far less common, following an acute intra-abdominal event (ischaemia, volvulus, trauma or perioperative complication) often with septic and metabolic problems, creating complex

nutritional issues, requiring support for weeks to months with multidisciplinary input (nursing, dietetic, medical, biochemical, surgical, radiological and microbiological).
- *Type 3 IF*: a chronic condition in which patients are metabolically stable but require full intravenous nutrition support over months to years. It may or may not be reversible.

Management

IF is a complex clinical problem with profound and wide-ranging physiological and psychological effects, which is best cared for by a dedicated multidisciplinary team. Most IF results from short bowel syndrome (Box 22.21), with chronic intestinal dysmotility and chronic intestinal pseudo-obstruction accounting for most of the remainder. The severity of the physiological upset correlates well with how much functioning intestine remains (rather than how much has been removed). Measuring the remaining small bowel (from the duodeno-jejunal flexure) at the time of surgery is essential to plan future therapy (Box 22.22). The aims of treatment are to:

- provide nutrition, water and electrolytes to maintain health with normal body weight (and allow normal growth in affected children)
- utilise the enteral or oral routes as much as possible
- minimise the burden of complications of the underlying disease, as well as the IF and its treatment
- allow a good quality of life.

If the ileum and especially the ileum and colon remain intact, long-term nutritional support can usually be avoided. Unlike the jejunum, the ileum can adapt to increase absorption of water and electrolytes over time. The presence of the colon (part or wholly intact) further improves fluid absorption, and can contribute energy from absorption of bacterially produced short-chain fatty acids.

Jejunum–colon patients

Those with an anastomosis between jejunum and residual colon (jejunum–colon patients) may look well in the days or initial weeks following the acute insult but develop protein-energy malnutrition and significant weight loss, becoming seriously under-nourished over weeks to months.

Stool volume is determined by oral intake, with higher intakes causing more diarrhoea and the potential for dehydration, sodium and magnesium depletion and acute renal failure. The absence of the ileum leads to deficiencies of vitamin B_{12} and fat-soluble vitamins. The absorption of various drugs, including thyroxine, digoxin and warfarin, can be reduced. Approximately 45% of patients will develop gallstones due to disruption of the enterohepatic circulation of bile acids, and 25% develop calcium oxalate renal stones due to increased colonic absorption of oxalate (see Fig. 23.44).

22

22.23 Management of short bowel patients (and 'high-output' stoma)

Accurate charting of fluid intake and losses

- Vital: oral intake determines stool volume and should be *restricted* rather than encouraged

Dehydration and hyponatraemia

- Must first be corrected intravenously to restore circulating volume and reduce thirst
- Stool volume should be minimised and any ongoing fluid imbalance between oral intake and stool losses replenished intravenously

Measures to reduce stool volume losses

- *Restrict* oral fluid intake to ≤500 mL/24 hrs
- Give a further 1000 mL oral fluid as oral rehydration solution containing 90–120 mmol Na/L
- Slow intestinal transit (to maximise opportunities for absorption):
  - Loperamide, codeine phosphate
- Reduce volume of intestinal secretions:
  - Gastric acid: omeprazole 20 mg/day orally
  - Other secretions: octreotide 50–100 μg 3 times daily by subcutaneous injection

Measures to increase absorption

- Teduglutide (a recombinant glucagon-like peptide 2) significantly reduces requirements for intravenous fluid and nutritional support by promoting growth and integrity of small bowel mucosa

22.24 Potential indications for small bowel transplantation

Complications of central venous catheters

- Central venous thrombosis leading to loss of two or more intravenous access points
- Severe or recurrent line sepsis
- Recurrent severe acute kidney injury related to dehydration

Metabolic complications of parenteral nutrition

- Parenteral nutrition-related liver fibrosis, cirrhosis and liver failure

22.25 Complications of small bowel/multivisceral transplantation

- Sepsis:
  Enteric bacterial species
  Staphylococci
  Fungal species
- Cytomegalovirus infection
- Post-transplantation lymphoproliferative disease (PTLD)
- Graft-versus-host disease
- Acute and chronic rejection
- Chronic renal impairment

Jejunostomy patients

Patients left with a stoma (usually a jejunostomy) behave very differently, although stool volumes are again determined by oral intake. The jejunum is intrinsically highly permeable, and in the absence of the ileum and its net absorptive role, high losses of fluid, sodium and magnesium dominate the clinical picture from the outset. Dehydration, hyponatraemia, hypomagnesaemia and acute renal failure are the most immediate problems but protein-energy malnutrition will also develop. The jejunum has no real potential for adaptation in terms of absorption, so it is essential to recognise and address dehydration and electrolyte disturbance early as it is likely to be permanent (Box 22.23).

Small bowel and multivisceral transplantation

Long-term intravenous nutritional support is the mainstay of therapy for chronic IF but has its own morbidity and mortality. The 10-year survival for patients on long-term home parenteral nutrition is approximately 90%. Most deaths are due to the underlying disease process but 5%–11% will die from direct complications of parenteral nutrition itself (especially catheter-related sepsvis). A minority of patients with chronic IF, for whom the safe administration of parenteral nutrition has become difficult or impossible, may benefit from small bowel transplantation (Box 22.24). The first successful small bowel transplant was carried out in 1988. The introduction of tacrolimus allowed a satisfactory balance of immunosuppression, avoiding rejection while minimising sepsis. Since then, over 2000 transplants have been performed worldwide. Survival rates continue to improve, for both isolated small bowel and multivisceral transplantation (small bowel along with a combination of liver and/or kidney and/or pancreas), although major complications are still frequent (Box 22.25). Current 5-year survival rates are 50%–80%, with better outcomes for younger patients and those receiving isolated small bowel procedures.

Further developments in treatment of intestinal failure

Long-acting recombinant human GLP-2 analogues, such as teduglutide and apraglutide, enhance intestinal absorption by:

- increasing intestinal blood flow to the intestine
- increasing portal blood flow away from the intestine
- slowing intestinal transit times
- reducing gastric acid secretion.

In patients with short bowel syndrome and IF, the increased intestinal absorptive function induced by teduglutide can significantly reduce the volumes of parenteral fluids and nutrition required, and may allow some patients to regain independence from parenteral support. Side-effects include abdominal cramps and distension (seen in 50%), peristomal swelling, pain, nausea, vomiting and local injection site reactions. Since teduglutide stimulates proliferation of the intestinal epithelium, it should be avoided in those with history of gastrointestinal malignancy. In patients with a colon, a pre-treatment screening colonoscopy should be undertaken to detect and remove any polyps. Use of teduglutide is currently limited by high costs.

Artificial nutrition at the end of life

In some situations, assisted nutrition may not reverse weight loss or improve quality and duration of life. Such scenarios may present when approaching the end of life, or with weight loss due to progressive incurable disease, such as advanced respiratory or cardiac failure, malignancy or dementia. A decision not to intervene may then be appropriate. An intervention that merely prolongs life without preserving or adding to its quality is seldom justified as in the patient's best interest, particularly if the intervention is not without risk itself. A thoughtful and sensitive discussion explaining what artificial nutrition can and cannot achieve is vital, involving the multidisciplinary team looking after the patient, along with carers, next of kin and, in some cases, legal representatives (Box 22.26).

Nutrition and dementia

Weight loss is seen commonly in older people (Box 22.27) or in those with dementia, and nutritional and eating problems are a significant source of concern for those caring for them. It is appropriate to:

- screen for malnutrition
- assess specific eating difficulties (e.g. Edinburgh Feeding Evaluation in Dementia questionnaire)
- monitor and document body weight
- encourage adequate intake of food
- therapeutic trial of oral nutritional supplements.

Undernutrition can be distressing and there may be specific circumstances where a trial of enteral feeding can be justified (see Box 22.26).

22.26 Ethical and legal considerations in the management of artificial nutritional support	

- Care of the sick involves the duty of providing adequate fluid and nutrients
- Food and fluid should not be withheld from a patient who expresses a desire to eat and drink, unless there is a medical contraindication (e.g. risk of aspiration)
- A treatment plan should include consideration of nutritional issues and should be agreed by all members of the health-care team
- In the situation of palliative care, tube feeding should be instituted only if it is needed to relieve symptoms
- Tube feeding is usually regarded in law as a medical treatment. Like other treatments, the need for such support should be reviewed on a regular basis and changes made in the light of clinical circumstances
- A competent adult patient must give consent for any invasive procedures, including passage of a nasogastric tube or insertion of a central venous cannula
- If a patient is unable to give consent, the health-care team should act in that person's best interests, taking into account any wishes previously expressed by the patient and the views of family
- Under certain specified circumstances (e.g. anorexia nervosa), it is appropriate to provide artificial nutritional support to the unwilling patient

Adapted from British Association for Parenteral and Enteral Nutrition guidelines, www.bapen.org.uk.

22.27 Energy balance in old age	

- **Body composition**: muscle mass falls with inactivity, and percentage of body fat increases.
- **Energy expenditure**: with lower lean body mass, basal metabolic rate is decreased and energy requirements are reduced.
- **Weight loss**: after weight gain throughout adult life, weight often falls beyond the age of 75–80 years. This may reflect decreased appetite, loss of smell and taste, and decreased interest in and financial resources for food preparation, especially after loss of a partner.
- **BMI**: less reliable in old age as height is lost (due to kyphosis, osteoporotic crush fractures, loss of intervertebral disc spaces). Alternative measurements include arm demispan and knee height, which can be extrapolated to estimate height.

Success is more likely in those with mild to moderate dementia, after a reversible crisis precipitated by some acute event. In dementia, tube feeding rarely improves quality of life (Fig. 22.12), but PEG is better tolerated than the nasal route.

Micronutrients, minerals and their diseases

Vitamins

Vitamins are organic compounds with vital roles as cofactors in certain metabolic pathways. They are categorised into the fat-soluble (vitamins A, D, E and K) and water-soluble (vitamins of the B complex group and vitamin C).

Recommended daily intakes of micronutrients (Box 22.28) vary between countries. In the UK, the 'reference nutrient intake' (RNI) has been calculated as the mean plus two standard deviations (SD) of daily intake in the population, which therefore describes intake that satisfies 97.5% of the population. The lower reference nutrient intake (LRNI) is the mean minus 2 SD, below which may be insufficient for 2.5% of the population. These dietary reference values (DRV) have superseded the terms RDI (recommended daily intake) and RDA (recommended daily amount) still used in other countries. Additional amounts of some micronutrients may be required in pregnancy and lactation (Box 22.29).

Vitamin deficiency diseases are most prevalent in lower-income countries, but still occur in high-income countries. Older people (Box 22.30) and alcohol misusers are at risk of deficiencies in B vitamins and in vitamins D

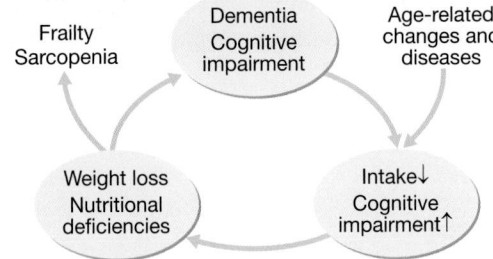

Fig. 22.12 Malnutrition in dementia – a vicious circle. *From Volkert D, Chourdakis M, Faxen-Irving G, et al. ESPEN guidelines on nutrition in dementia. Clin Nutr 2015; 34:1052–1073.*

and C. Nutritional deficiencies in pregnancy can affect either the mother or the developing fetus, and extra increments of vitamins are recommended in the UK (see Box 22.29). Darker-skinned individuals living at higher latitude, and those who cover up or do not go outside are at increased risk of vitamin D deficiency due to inadequate sunlight exposure. Fat-soluble deficiencies, notably and catastrophically vitamin E, can result from rare abetalipoproteinaemia. Deficiencies of vitamins occur with intestinal malabsorption, both primary gastrointestinal problems and secondary to hepatic or pancreatic diseases or to autoimmune conditions (e.g. coeliac, pernicious anaemia) (Box 22.31). Routine dietary supplements are recommended for these 'at-risk' groups. Doctors must also be alert to micronutrient deficiencies induced by some drugs, and from extreme diets. Severe carbohydrate restriction limits thiamine consumption and beri beri can develop. Some extreme, non-evidence-based, diets can jeopardise vitamin A status.

There is a great deal of unscrupulous marketing and claims about vitamins. Some vitamins may have pharmacological actions when given at supraphysiological doses, such vitamin A for acne. Taking vitamin supplements is highly promoted for commercial reasons, and fashionable in many population sectors, although there is no evidence of benefit. Serious toxic effects are met with high dosages of vitamins A, B$_6$ and D. Cocktails of micronutrients referred to as 'antioxidant' (vitamin C, beta-carotene and often selenium or zinc) are still marketed as remedies to prevent heart disease, although large clinical trials have shown more, not less, heart disease in supplemented groups.

Investigation of suspected vitamin deficiency or excess may involve biochemical assessment of body stores (Box 22.32). Measurements in blood should be interpreted carefully, however, in conjunction with the clinical presentation.

Fat-soluble vitamins

Vitamin A (retinol)

Pre-formed retinol is found only in foods of animal origin. Vitamin A can also be derived from carotenes, which are present in green and coloured vegetables and some fruits. Carotenes provide most of the total vitamin A in the UK and constitute the only supply in vegans. Retinol is converted to several other important molecules:

- *11-cis-retinaldehyde* is part of the photoreceptor complex in rods of the retina.
- *Retinoic acid* induces differentiation of epithelial cells by binding to specific nuclear receptors, which induce responsive genes. In vitamin A deficiency, mucus-secreting cells are replaced by keratin-producing cells.
- *Retinoids* are necessary for normal growth, fetal development, fertility, haematopoiesis and immune function.

The most important consequence of vitamin A deficiency is irreversible blindness in young children, and it also contributes to worse outcomes from many infections, such as measles. Asia is most notably affected and the problem is being addressed through widespread vitamin A

22

22.28 Summary of clinically important vitamins and WHO recommended daily intakes[1]

Vitamin	Sources[2] Rich	Important	Reference nutrient intake (RNI)[3]
Fat-soluble			
A (retinol)	Liver	Milk and milk products, eggs, fish oils	700 µg men 600 µg women
D (cholecalciferol)	Fish oils	Ultraviolet exposure to skin Egg yolks, margarine, fortified cereals	10 µg if >65 years or no sunlight exposure
E (tocopherol)	Sunflower oil	Vegetables, nuts, seed oils	No RNI. Safe intake: 4 mg men 3 mg women
K (phylloquinone, menaquinone)	Soya oil, menaquinones produced by intestinal bacteria	Green vegetables	No RNI. Safe intake: 1 µg/kg
Water-soluble			
B$_1$ (thiamin)	Pork	Cereals, grains, beans	0.8 mg per 9.68 MJ (2000 kcal) energy intake
B$_2$ (riboflavin)	Milk	Milk and milk products, breakfast cereals, bread	1.3 mg men 1.1 mg women
B$_3$ (niacin, nicotinic acid, nicotinamide)	Meat, cereals		17 mg men 13 mg women
B$_6$ (pyridoxine)	Meat, fish, potatoes, bananas	Vegetables, intestinal microflora synthesis	1.4 mg men 1.2 mg women
Folate	Liver	Green leafy vegetables, fortified breakfast cereals	200 µg
B$_{12}$ (cobalamin)	Animal products	Bacterial colonisation	1.5 µg
Biotin	Egg yolk	Intestinal flora	No RNI. Safe intake: 10–200 µg
C (ascorbic acid)	Citrus fruit	Fresh fruit, fresh and frozen vegetables	40 mg

[1]See WHO document: https://apps.who.int/iris/bitstream/handle/10665/42716/9241546123.pdf?ua = 1. [2]Rich sources contain the nutrient in high concentration but are not generally eaten in large amounts; important sources contain less but contribute most because larger amounts are eaten. [3]Requirements vary by age, and recommendations differ between countries. These figures are mostly generous: deficiency is unlikely unless intakes are well below them.

22.29 Nutrition in pregnancy and lactation

- **Weight gain** to reach BMI = 30 kg/m^2 in the third trimester is desirable. Heavier women need not gain so much.
- **Obesity:** promotes gestational diabetes and fetal abnormalities, but weight loss is undesirable during pregnancy. Overweight women should reach a healthier weight before pregnancy.
- **Energy requirements:** increased in both mother and fetus but can be met through reduced maternal energy expenditure.
- **Micronutrient requirements:** adaptive mechanisms ensure increased uptake of minerals in pregnancy, but extra increments of some are required during lactation (see Box 22.32). Additional increments of some vitamins are recommended during pregnancy and lactation:
  Vitamin A: for growth and maintenance of the fetus, and to provide some reserve (important in some countries to prevent blindness associated with vitamin A deficiency). Teratogenic in excessive amounts.
  Vitamin D: to ensure bone and dental development in the infant. Higher incidences of hypocalcaemia, hypoparathyroidisim and defective dental enamel have been seen in infants of women not taking vitamin D supplements at >50° latitude.
  Folate: taken pre-conceptually and during the first trimester, reduces the incidence of neural tube defects by 70%.
  Vitamin B$_{12}$: in lactation only.
  Thiamin: to meet increased fetal energy demands.
  Riboflavin: to meet extra demands.
  Niacin: in lactation only.
  Vitamin C: for the last trimester to maintain maternal stores as fetal demands increase.
  Iodine: in countries with high consumption of staple foods (e.g. brassicas, maize, bamboo shoots) that contain goitrogens (thiocyanates or perchlorates) that interfere with iodine uptake, supplements prevent infants being born with cretinism.

22.30 Vitamin deficiency in old age

- **Requirements:** although requirements for energy fall with age, those for micronutrients do not. If dietary energy intake falls, a vitamin-rich diet is required to compensate.
- **Vitamin D:** levels are commonly low due to low total dietary intake, low sun exposure and less efficient skin conversion. This leads to bone loss and fractures. Supplements have modest effectiveness for preventing fractures, so should be given to those at risk of falls in institutional care, but other measures to prevent falls are vital.
- **Vitamin B$_{12}$ deficiency:** a causal relationship with dementia has not been identified, but it does produce neuropsychiatric effects and should be checked in all those with declining cognitive function.

22.31 Common gastrointestinal disorders that may be associated with malabsorption of fat-soluble vitamins

- Biliary obstruction
- Pancreatic exocrine insufficiency
- Coeliac disease
- Ileal inflammation or resection

supplementation programmes. Adults are not usually at risk because liver stores can supply vitamin A when foods containing vitamin A are unavailable.

Early deficiency causes impaired adaptation to the dark (night blindness), but this is rarely recognised. Keratinisation of the cornea (xerophthalmia) gives rise to characteristic Bitot's spots and progresses to keratomalacia, with corneal ulceration, scarring and irreversible blindness

22.32 Biochemical assessment of vitamin status

Nutrient	Biochemical assessments of deficiency or excess
Vitamin A	Serum retinol may be low in deficiency Serum retinyl esters: when vitamin A toxicity is suspected
Vitamin D	Plasma/serum 25-hydroxyvitamin D (25(OH)D): reflects body stores (liver and adipose tissue) Plasma/serum 1,25(OH)$_2$D: difficult to interpret
Vitamin E	Serum tocopherol:cholesterol ratio
Vitamin K	Coagulation assays (e.g. prothrombin time) Plasma vitamin K
Vitamin B$_1$ (thiamin)	Whole-blood vitamin B$_1$ or red blood cell transketolase activity (Treat suspected deficiency without waiting for results)
Vitamin B$_2$ (riboflavin)	Red blood cell glutathione reductase activity or whole-blood vitamin B$_2$
Vitamin B$_3$ (niacin)	Urinary metabolites: 1-methyl-2-pyridone-5-carboxamide, 1-methylnicotinamide
Vitamin B$_6$	Plasma pyridoxal phosphate or erythrocyte transaminase activation coefficient
Vitamin B$_{12}$	Plasma B$_{12}$: poor measure of overall vitamin B$_{12}$ status but will detect severe deficiency Alternatives (methylmalonic acid and holotranscobalamin) are not used routinely
Folate	Red blood cell folate Plasma folate: reflects recent intake but also detects unmetabolised folic acid from foods and supplements
Vitamin C	Leucocyte ascorbic acid: assesses vitamin C tissue stores Plasma ascorbic acid: reflects recent (daily) intake

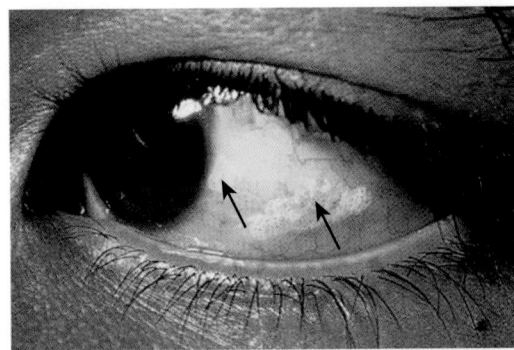
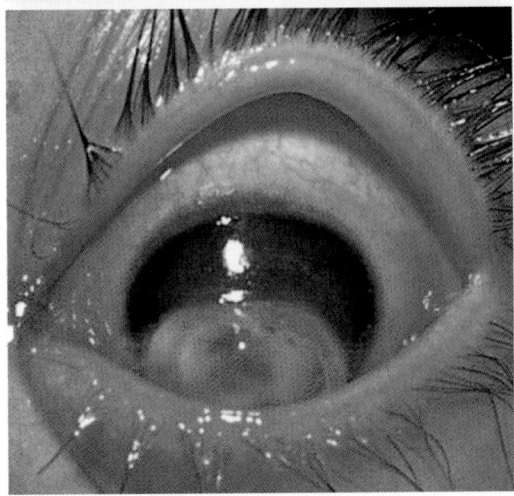

Fig. 22.13 Eye signs of vitamin A deficiency. A Bitot spots in xerophthalmia, showing the white triangular plaques (arrows). B Keratomalacia in a 14-month-old child. There is liquefactive necrosis affecting the greater part of the cornea, with typical sparing of the superior aspect. *(A) Courtesy of Institute of Ophthalmology, Moorfields Eye Hospital, London. (B) From WHO. Report of a joint WHO/USAID meeting, vitamin A deficiency and xerophthalmia (WHO technical report series no. 5W); 1976.*

(Fig. 22.13). In countries where vitamin A deficiency is endemic, pregnant women should be advised to eat dark green, leafy vegetables and yellow fruits (to build up stores of retinol in the fetal liver), and infants should be fed the same. The WHO is according high priority to prevention in communities where xerophthalmia occurs, giving single prophylactic oral doses of 60 mg retinyl palmitate (providing 200 000 U retinol) to pre-school children. This also reduces mortality from gastroenteritis and respiratory infections.

Repeated moderate or high doses of retinol can cause liver damage, hyperostosis and teratogenicity. Women in countries where deficiency is not endemic are therefore advised not to take vitamin A supplements in pregnancy. Acute overdose leads to nausea and headache, increased intracranial pressure and skin desquamation. Excessive intake of carotene causes harmless orange pigmentation of the skin (hypercarotenosis).

Vitamin D

Vitamin D is required for musculoskeletal health, specifically preventing rickets and osteomalacia. Adequate levels of vitamin D may also be important in some other conditions and may improve immune function. The natural form of vitamin D, cholecalciferol, is formed in the skin by the action of ultraviolet (UV) light on 7-dehydrocholesterol, a metabolite of cholesterol. Vitamin D is converted in the liver to 25-hydroxyvitamin D (25(OH)D), which is further hydroxylated in the kidneys to 1,25-dihydroxyvitamin D (1,25(OH)$_2$D), the most active form of the vitamin (see Fig. 26.62). This 1,25(OH)$_2$D activates specific intracellular receptors that influence calcium metabolism, bone mineralisation and tissue differentiation. The synthetic form, ergocalciferol or vitamin D$_2$, is considered to be less potent than endogenous D$_3$.

In much of the world, skin exposure to sunlight is the main source. Moving away from the equator, the intensity of UV light decreases, so

that at a latitude above 50° (including northern Europe) vitamin D is not synthesised in winter, and even above 30° there is seasonal variation. The large body store, in the liver, normally accumulated during the summer, is consumed during the winter. The limited sunlight exposure in the UK has led to recommendations that everyone over the age of 1 should be given 10 μg vitamin D supplement daily, with a lower dose of 8.5–10 μg in breastfed babies under 1 year of age. Formula milk is fortified with vitamin D so further supplements are only necessary when <500 mL of formula milk is consumed daily. Supplementation at these doses is appropriate for babies and people in old age who are confined indoors, and those who habitually cover up their skin when outdoors. The richest food sources are oily fish such as salmon, sardines, herring and mackerel, red meat, liver and eggs. Breakfast cereals, margarines and milk products are widely fortified with vitamin D in some parts of Europe and in North America.

The effects of vitamin D deficiency (calcium deficiency, rickets and osteomalacia) are described on page 1053. An analogue of vitamin D (calcipotriol) is used for treatment of skin conditions such as psoriasis.

Excessive doses of cholecalciferol, ergocalciferol or the hydroxylated metabolites cause hypercalcaemia. Partly because redundant receptors for vitamin D are present in most tissues, commercial agencies have proposed a role for vitamin D in nearly every human disease, and market it in large doses. Randomised trials are required to refute each claim, and they have nearly all been refuted.

22

Vitamin E

There are eight related fat-soluble substances with vitamin E activity. The most important dietary form is α-tocopherol. Vitamin E has many direct metabolic actions:

- It prevents oxidation of polyunsaturated fatty acids in cell membranes by free radicals.
- It helps maintain cell membrane structure.
- It affects DNA synthesis and cell signalling.
- It is involved in the anti-inflammatory and immune systems.

Human deficiency is rare and has been described only in premature infants and in malabsorption, notably with abetalipoproteinaemia. It can cause a mild haemolytic anaemia, ataxia and visual scotomas. Vitamin E intakes of up to 3200 mg/day (1000-fold greater than recommended intakes) are considered safe. Diets rich in vitamin E (e.g. vegetable oils, nuts and seeds) are consumed in countries with lower rates of coronary heart disease, but randomised controlled trials have not demonstrated cardioprotective effects of vitamin E or other antioxidants.

Vitamin K

Vitamin K is supplied in the diet mainly as vitamin K$_1$ (phylloquinone) in the UK, or as vitamin K$_2$ (menaquinone) from fermented products in parts of Asia. Vitamin K$_2$ is also synthesised by bacteria in the colon. Vitamin K is a co-factor for carboxylation reactions: in particular, the production of γ-carboxyglutamate (gla). Gla residues are found in four of the coagulation factor proteins (II, VII, IX and X; p. 927), conferring their capacity to bind to phospholipid surfaces in the presence of calcium. Other important gla proteins are osteocalcin and matrix gla protein, which are important in bone mineralisation.

Vitamin K deficiency leads to delayed coagulation and bleeding. In obstructive jaundice, dietary vitamin K is not absorbed and it is essential to administer the vitamin in parenteral form before surgery. Warfarin and related anticoagulants act by antagonising vitamin K. Vitamin K is given routinely to newborn babies to prevent haemorrhagic disease. Symptoms of excess have been reported only in infants, with synthetic preparations linked to haemolysis and liver damage.

Water-soluble vitamins

Thiamin (vitamin B$_1$)

Thiamin is mainly supplied by nuts and seeds, including legumes and whole-grain cereals. Thiamin pyrophosphate (TPP) is a co-factor for enzyme reactions involved in the metabolism of macronutrients (carbohydrate, fat and alcohol), including:

- decarboxylation of pyruvate to acetyl-co-enzyme A, which bridges between glycolysis and the tricarboxylic acid (Krebs) cycle
- transketolase activity in the hexose monophosphate shunt pathway
- decarboxylation of α-ketoglutarate to succinate in the Krebs cycle.

In thiamin deficiency, cells cannot metabolise glucose aerobically to generate energy as ATP. Neuronal cells are most vulnerable because they depend almost exclusively on glucose for energy requirements. Impaired glucose oxidation also causes an accumulation of pyruvic and lactic acids, which produce vasodilatation and increased cardiac output.

Deficiency – beri-beri

Thiamin deficiency constitutes a clinical emergency, causing sudden catastrophic and often permanent damage if treatment is delayed. It occurs when sufficient whole-grain cereals or other seeds and nuts are not consumed, classically in the developing world, from diets based on polished rice. It also occurs among people who follow extreme low-carbohydrate diets, for example for weight loss. It is especially encountered in chronic alcohol misusers, among whom poor diet, impaired absorption, storage and phosphorylation of thiamin in the liver, and the increased requirements for thiamin to metabolise ethanol, all contribute to deficiency.

The body has very limited stores of thiamin, so deficiency can develop after only 1 month on a thiamin-free diet. There are two forms of the disease in adults, which may coexist:

- Dry (or neurological) beri-beri may manifest with chronic peripheral neuropathy and with wrist and/or foot drop. However its most dramatic presentation is with Wernicke encephalopathy, the triad of ophthalmoplegia, ataxia and confusion, which may progress to permanent Korsakoff psychosis.
- Wet (or cardiac) beri-beri causes generalised oedema due to biventricular heart failure with pulmonary congestion and ECG changes.

Wet beri-beri usually recovers full and swiftly with thiamin replacement. However, with dry beri-beri, response to thiamin administration is not uniformly good. Multivitamin and mineral therapy seems to produce some improvement, however, suggesting that other dietary deficiencies may be involved, with zinc particularly incriminated.

Possible thiamin deficiency, and any clinical suggestions of Wernicke encephalopathy or wet beri-beri, should be treated on suspicion, immediately, without waiting for biochemical confirmation of the diagnosis, with intravenous vitamin B and C mixture. Korsakoff psychosis, brain damage with failure to create memory, can develop rapidly, and is irreversible and does not respond to thiamin treatment.

Riboflavin (vitamin B$_2$)

Riboflavin is required for the flavin co-factors involved in oxidation–reduction reactions. It is widely distributed in animal and vegetable foods. Levels are low in staple cereals but germination, e.g. as bean sprouts, increases its content. It is destroyed under alkaline conditions by heat and by exposure to sunlight. Deficiency is rare in developed countries. It mainly affects the tongue and lips and manifests as glossitis, angular stomatitis and cheilosis. The genitals may be involved, as well as the skin areas rich in sebaceous glands, causing nasolabial or facial dyssebacea. Rapid recovery usually follows administration of riboflavin 10 mg daily by mouth.

Niacin (vitamin B$_3$)

Niacin encompasses nicotinic acid and nicotinamide. Nicotinamide is an essential part of the two pyridine nucleotides, nicotinamide adenine dinucleotide (NAD) and nicotinamide adenine dinucleotide phosphate (NADP), which play a key role as hydrogen acceptors and donors for many enzymes. Niacin can be synthesised in the body in limited amounts from the amino acid tryptophan.

Deficiency – pellagra

Pellagra was formerly endemic among poor people who subsisted chiefly on maize, which contains niacytin, a form of niacin that the body is unable to utilise. Pellagra can develop in only 8 weeks in individuals eating diets that are very deficient in niacin and tryptophan. It remains a problem in parts of Africa, and is occasionally seen in alcohol misusers and in patients with chronic small intestinal disease in developed countries. Pellagra can occur in Hartnup disease, a genetic disorder characterised by impaired absorption of several amino acids, including tryptophan. It is also seen occasionally in carcinoid syndrome, when tryptophan is consumed in the excessive production of 5-hydroxytryptamine (5-HT, serotonin). Pellagra is the 'Disease of the three Ds':

- Dermatitis. Characteristic erythema resembling severe sunburn, appearing symmetrically over the parts of the body exposed to sunlight, particularly the limbs (Fig. 22.14) and especially on the neck but not the face (Casal's necklace). The skin lesions may progress to vesiculation, cracking, exudation and secondary infection.
- Diarrhoea. Often associated with anorexia, nausea, glossitis and dysphagia, reflecting the presence of a non-infective inflammation that extends throughout the gastrointestinal tract.
- Dementia. In severe deficiency, delirium occurs acutely and dementia develops if untreated.

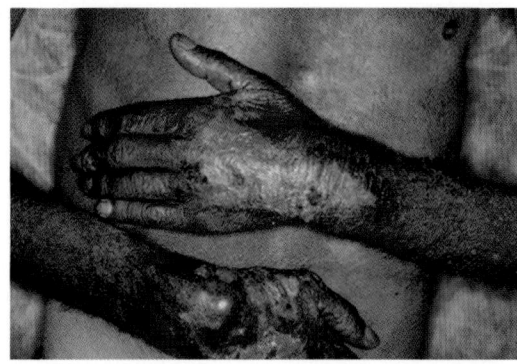

Fig. 22.14 Dermatitis in niacin deficiency (pellagra). There are red, scaly, cracked areas with sharply demarcated borders and surrounding pigmented skin. *From Piqué-Duran E, Pérez-Cejudo JA, Cameselle D, et al. Pellagra: A clinical, histopathological, and epidemiological study of 7 cases. Actas Dermosifiliogr 2012; 103(1):51–58.*

Treatment is with nicotinamide, 100 mg 3 times daily orally or parenterally. The response is usually rapid. Within 24 hours the erythema diminishes, the diarrhoea ceases and a striking improvement occurs in the patient's mental state.

Toxicity

Excessive intakes of niacin may lead to reversible hepatotoxicity. Nicotinic acid is a lipid-lowering agent but doses above 200 mg a day cause vasodilatory symptoms ('flushing' and/or hypotension).

Pyridoxine (vitamin B₆)

Pyridoxine, pyridoxal and pyridoxamine are different forms of vitamin B_6 that undergo phosphorylation to produce pyridoxal 5-phosphate (PLP). PLP is the co-factor for a large number of enzymes involved in the metabolism of amino acids. Vitamin B_6 is available in most foods.

Deficiency is rare, although certain drugs, such as isoniazid and penicillamine, act as chemical antagonists to pyridoxine. Pyridoxine administration is effective in isoniazid-induced peripheral neuropathy and some cases of sideroblastic anaemia. Large doses of vitamin B_6 have an antiemetic effect in radiotherapy-induced nausea. Although vitamin B_6 supplements have become popular in the treatment of nausea in pregnancy, carpal tunnel syndrome and pre-menstrual syndrome, there is no convincing evidence of benefit. Very high doses of vitamin B_6 taken for several months can cause unpleasant sensory polyneuropathy, which may become permanent.

Biotin

Biotin is a co-enzyme in the synthesis of fatty acids, isoleucine and valine, and is also involved in gluconeogenesis. Deficiency results from consuming very large quantities of raw egg whites (> 30% energy intake) because the avidin they contain binds to and inactivates biotin in the intestine. It may also be seen after long periods of total parenteral nutrition. The clinical features of deficiency include scaly dermatitis, alopecia and paraesthesia.

Folate (folic acid)

Folates exist in many forms. The main circulating form is 5-methyltetrahydrofolate. The natural forms, in plant foods, are prone to oxidation. Folic acid is the stable synthetic form. Folate works as a methyl donor for cellular methylation and protein synthesis, particularly for haematopoiesis. It is also directly involved in DNA and RNA synthesis, and requirements increase during embryonic development. Deficiency states include dietary insufficiency and also altered folate metabolism, which may be genetic.

The commonest clinical presentation of folate deficiency is as macrocytic anaemia, which may extend to pancytopenia, in people with poor consumption of fruit and green vegetables. It is particularly frequent among alcohol misusers. Folate deficiency in early pregnancy may cause three major birth defects (spina bifida, anencephaly and encephalocele) resulting from imperfect closure of the neural tube, which takes place 3–4 weeks after conception. Women who have experienced a pregnancy affected by a neural tube defect should take 5 mg of folic acid daily from before conception and throughout the first trimester; this reduces the incidence of these defects by 70%. All women planning a pregnancy are advised to include good sources of folate in their diet, and to take folate supplements throughout the first trimester. Liver is the richest source of folate but an alternative source (e.g. leafy vegetables) is advised in early pregnancy because of the high vitamin A content of liver. Folate deficiency has also been associated with heart disease, dementia and cancer. There is mandatory fortification of flour with folic acid in the United States and voluntary fortification of many foods across Europe. Neural tube defects have declined dramatically, but there are some concerns about increased incidence of colon cancer, through accelerating the growth of polyps.

Hydroxycobalamin (vitamin B₁₂)

Vitamin B_{12} is a co-factor in folate co-enzyme recycling and nerve myelination. Vitamin B_{12} and folate are particularly important in DNA synthesis in red blood cells. The haematological disorders (macrocytic or megaloblastic anaemias) caused by their deficiency are discussed in Chapter 25. Vitamin B_{12}, but not folate, is needed for the integrity of myelin, so that vitamin B_{12} deficiency is also associated with neurological disease (see Box 25.33).

In older people and chronic alcohol misusers, or after bowel surgery, vitamin B_{12} deficiency arises from insufficient intake and/or from malabsorption, but purely dietary deficiency is rare, as it is synthesised by colonic bacteria. The classic cause is malabsorption through pernicious anaemia. Several drugs, including neomycin, can render vitamin B_{12} inactive. Adequate intake of folate maintains erythropoiesis and there is a concern that fortification of foods with folate may delay recognition of underlying vitamin B_{12} deficiency.

In severe deficiency there is insidious, diffuse and uneven demyelination. It may be clinically manifest as peripheral neuropathy or spinal cord degeneration affecting both posterior and lateral columns ('subacute combined degeneration of the spinal cord'), or there may be cerebral manifestations (resembling dementia) or optic atrophy. Vitamin B_{12} therapy improves symptoms in most cases.

Vitamin C (ascorbic acid)

Ascorbic acid is a natural antioxidant in fruit and vegetables. It serves as an essential cofactor in the hydroxylation of proline and lysine in protocollagen, to hydroxyproline and hydroxylysine in mature collagen. It is also an active reducing agent in the aqueous phase of living tissues, and is involved in intracellular electron transfer. It is very easily destroyed by heat, increased pH and light, and is very soluble in water; hence many traditional cooking methods reduce it. Claims that high-dose vitamin C improves immune function (including resistance to the common cold), prevents cancers or heart disease and cholesterol turnover are unsubstantiated.

Deficiency – scurvy

Vitamin C deficiency causes defective formation of collagen with impaired healing of wounds, capillary haemorrhage and reduced platelet adhesiveness (normal platelets are rich in ascorbate) (Fig. 22.15). Precipitants and clinical features of scurvy are shown in Box 22.33. A dose of 250 mg vitamin C 3 times daily by mouth should saturate the tissues quickly. The deficiencies in the patient's food choices also need to be corrected, and other vitamin supplements given if necessary, for example for alcohol misusers. Daily intakes above 1 g/day can cause diarrhoea and the formation of renal oxalate stones.

Other bioactive dietary compounds

There are a number of non-essential organic compounds found in vegetable foods with purported health benefits, such as reducing risk of heart disease or cancers. Groups of compounds such as the flavonoids and phytoestrogens do show bioactivity through their respective antioxidant and oestrogenic or anti-oestrogenic activities. Flavonoids (of which there are many different classes) are potent antioxidants found

22

22.33 Scurvy – vitamin C deficiency

Precipitants

Increased requirement

- Trauma, surgery, burns, infections
- Smoking
- Drugs (glucocorticoids, aspirin, indometacin, tetracycline)

Dietary deficiency

- Lack of dietary fruit and vegetables for > 2 months
- Infants fed exclusively on boiled milk

Clinical features

- Swollen gums that bleed easily
- Perifollicular and petechial haemorrhages
- Ecchymoses
- Haemarthrosis
- Gastrointestinal bleeding
- Anaemia
- Poor wound healing

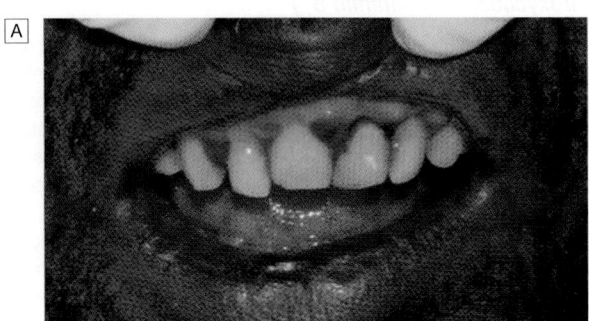

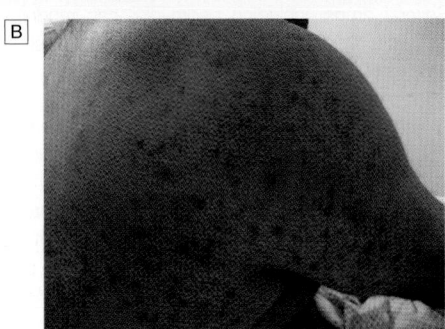

Fig. 22.15 Scurvy. A Gingival swelling and bleeding. B Perifollicular hyperkeratosis. *(A,B) From Ho V, Prinsloo P, Ombiga J. Persistent anaemia due to scurvy. J NZ Med Assoc 2007; 120:62. Reproduced with permission.*

in fruit and vegetables, tea and wine; phytoestrogens are found in soy products (with higher intakes in parts of Asia compared to Europe and the United States) and other pulses. Caffeine and related compounds in tea and coffee, can with habituation improve mental performance in the short term, with adverse effects including agitation and tachycardia at higher intakes. Acute withdrawal of usual caffeine intake (e.g. in a hospital admission) can provoke headaches, indicating its addictive quality. It is added to carbonated beverages and 'tonic wines', ostensibly as a flavouring, but increases their consumption.

Inorganic micronutrients

A number of inorganic elements are necessary for structure and growth, as electrolytes, or as cofactors in enzymes and are thus essential dietary constituents for humans (Box 22.34). Deficiency is seen when there is inadequate dietary intake or excessive loss from the body. Toxic effects have also been observed from self-medication and disordered absorption or excretion. Examples of clinical toxicity include excess of iron (haemochromatosis or haemosiderosis), fluoride (fluorosis), copper (Wilson's disease) and selenium (selenosis, seen in parts of China). For most minerals, the available biochemical plasma markers do not accurately reflect whole-body status or dietary intake, and dietary assessment is required.

Calcium and phosphorus

Calcium is the most abundant cation in the body and powerful homeostatic mechanisms control circulating ionised calcium levels. WHO dietary guidelines for calcium differ between countries, with higher intakes usually recommended in places with higher fracture prevalence. Between 20% and 30% of calcium in the diet is absorbed, depending on vitamin D status and food source. Calcium requirements depend on phosphorus intakes, with an optimum molar ratio (Ca:P) of 1:1. Excessive phosphorus intakes (e.g. 1–1.5 g/day) with a Ca:P of 1:3 have been shown to cause hypocalcaemia and secondary hyperparathyroidism.

Calcium absorption may be impaired in vitamin D deficiency and in malabsorption secondary to small intestinal disease. Calcium deficiency causes impaired bone mineralisation and can lead to osteomalacia in adults. The potential benefits of high calcium intake in osteoporosis are discussed on p. 1052. Too much calcium can lead to constipation, and toxicity has been observed in 'milk-alkali syndrome'.

Dietary insufficiency of phosphorus is rare as a cause of deficiency (except in older people with limited diets, and importantly in severe starvation) because it is present in nearly all foods and phosphates are added to a number of processed foods. Phosphate deficiency in adults occurs:

- in patients with renal tubular phosphate loss
- in patients with diabetic ketoacidosis
- in patients receiving a prolonged high dosage of aluminium hydroxide
- in alcohol misusers, sometimes when they are fed with high-carbohydrate foods
- in patients receiving parenteral nutrition if inadequate phosphate is provided.

Deficiency causes hypophosphataemia and muscle weakness secondary to ATP deficiency.

Iron

Iron is involved in the synthesis of haemoglobin and is required for the transport of electrons within cells and for a number of enzyme reactions. Non-haem iron in cereals and vegetables is poorly absorbed but makes the greater contribution to overall intake, compared to the well-absorbed haem iron from animal products. Fruits and vegetables containing vitamin C enhance iron absorption, while the tannins in tea reduce it. Dietary calcium reduces iron uptake from the same meal, which may precipitate iron deficiency in those with borderline iron stores. There is no physiological mechanism for excretion of iron, so homeostasis depends on the regulation of iron absorption (see Fig. 25.20). This is regulated at the level of duodenal enterocytes by hepcidin (a peptide secreted by hepatocytes in the duodenum). The normal daily loss of iron is 1 mg, arising from desquamated surface cells and intestinal losses. A regular loss of only 2 mL of blood per day doubles the iron requirement. On average, an additional 20 mg of iron is lost during menstruation, so pre-menopausal women require about twice as much iron as men (and more if menstrual losses are heavy).

The major consequence of iron deficiency is anaemia. This is one of the most important nutritional causes of ill health in all parts of the world. In the UK, it is estimated that 10% women are iron-deficient. Dietary iron overload is occasionally observed and results in iron accumulation in the liver and, rarely, cirrhosis. Haemochromatosis results from an inherited increase in iron absorption.

Normally, only a small proportion of dietary iron is absorbed. Iron absorption mechanisms are up-regulated, to absorb a greater proportion if dietary provision is low. Iron shares and competes for a pathway for absorption with zinc. Indiscriminate iron supplementation can therefore impair zinc status. In overdosage, iron supplements are highly toxic and can be fatal for children.

22.34 Summary of clinically important minerals

Mineral	Sources[1] Rich	Important	Reference nutrient intake (RNI)
Calcium	Milk and milk products, tofu	Milk, boned fish, green vegetables, beans	700 mg[2]
Phosphorus	Most foods contain phosphorus		550 mg[2]
	Marmite and dry-roasted peanuts	Milk, cereal products, bread and meat	
Magnesium	Whole grains, nuts	Unprocessed and wholegrain foods	300 mg men 270 mg women[2]
Iron	Liver, red meat (haem iron)	Non-haem iron from vegetables, wholemeal bread	8.7 mg 14.8 mg women <50 years
Zinc	Red meat, seafood	Dairy produce, wholemeal bread	9.5 mg men 7 mg women[2]
Iodine	Edible seaweeds Sea fish	Milk and dairy products Sea food products	140 µg
Selenium	Fish, food crops grown in selenium-rich soils	Fish	75 µg men 60 µg women[2]
Copper	Shellfish, liver	Bread, cereal products, vegetables	1.2 mg[2]
Fluoride	Tea	Drinking water, tea	No RNI. Safe intake: 0.5 mg/kg
Potassium	Dried fruit, potatoes, coffee	Fresh fruit, vegetables, meat and dairy foods	3500 mg
Sodium	Table salt, anchovies	Processed foods, bread, bacon	1600 mg

[1]Rich sources contain the nutrient in high concentration but are not generally eaten in large amounts; important sources contain less but contribute most because larger amounts are eaten. [2]Increased amounts are required in women during lactation.

Iodine

Iodine is required, in very small amounts, for synthesis of thyroid hormones and thus for neurodevelopment. It is present in sea fish, seaweed and most plant foods grown near the sea. The amount of iodine in soil and water influences the iodine content of plant foods, and of animals grazing on them. Iodine is lacking, giving rise in older times to endemic goitre and cretinism, in the highest mountainous areas of the world (e.g. the Alps and the Himalayas) and in the soil of frequently flooded plains (e.g. Bangladesh). In the UK, most dietary iodine in human diets until recently came from disinfectant used to wash cows' udders before milking. Milk and sea fish are now the main sources, but many people have inadequate intakes.

About a billion people in the world are estimated to have an inadequate iodine intake and hence are at risk of iodine deficiency disorder. Goitre is the most common manifestation, affecting about 200 million people.

In areas where women have endemic goitre, 1% or more of babies are born with cretinism (characterised by impaired growth and neurological development and physical deformities). There is a higher than usual prevalence of deafness, slowed reflexes and poor learning in the remaining population. The best way of preventing neonatal cretinism is to ensure adequate levels of iodine during pregnancy. This can be achieved by intramuscular injections with 1–2 mL of iodised poppy seed oil (475–950 mg iodine) to women of child-bearing age every 3–5 years, by administration of iodised oil orally at 6-monthly or yearly intervals to adults and children.

In many countries foods are fortified with iodine to avoid iodine deficiency, especially reported among young people who avoid fish and/or dairy products. Iodised salt is most common, but with health advice to minimise sodium consumption, other common foods such as milk and breads can be fortified, provided their cumulative consumption does not become excessive.

Zinc

Zinc is present in most foods of vegetable and animal origin, and is stored in the liver. It is an essential component of many enzymes, including carbonic anhydrase, alcohol dehydrogenase and alkaline phosphatase.

Acute zinc deficiency has been reported in patients receiving prolonged zinc-free parenteral nutrition and causes diarrhoea, mental apathy, a moist, eczematoid dermatitis, especially around the mouth, and loss of hair. Chronic zinc deficiency occurs in dietary deficiency, malabsorption syndromes, when there are chronic losses (e.g. of exudates from leg ulcers), in alcoholism and in cirrhosis. It causes the clinical features seen in the very rare congenital disorder known as acrodermatitis enteropathica (growth retardation, hair loss and chronic diarrhoea). Zinc deficiency is thought to be responsible for one-third of the world's population not reaching their optimal height. In the Middle East, chronic deficiency has been associated with dwarfism and hypogonadism. In starvation, zinc deficiency causes thymic atrophy; zinc supplements may accelerate the healing of skin lesions, promote general well-being, improve appetite and reduce the morbidity associated with the under-nourished state, and lower the mortality associated with diarrhoea and pneumonia in children.

Selenium

The family of seleno-enzymes includes glutathione peroxidase, which helps prevent free radical damage to cells, and monodeiodinase, which converts thyroxine to triiodothyronine. North American soil has a higher selenium content than European and Asian soil, and the decreasing reliance of Europe on imported American food in recent decades has resulted in a decline in dietary selenium intake.

Selenium deficiency can cause hypothyroidism, cardiomyopathy in children (Keshan disease) and myopathy in adults. Excess selenium can cause heart disease, and has been linked to industrial pollution.

Fluoride

Fluoride is an essential nutrient necessary for normal dental enamel, and also incorporated as a component of bone mineral. Fluoride is most important for young children, before the permanent teeth erupt, while their enamel is being laid down, but also for healthy enamel recycling and repair after damage. Fluoride deficiency results in weakened dental enamel, vulnerable to attack by acid produced from sugars by oral bacteria, and thus to dental caries and tooth loss. Fluoride in normal amounts may help strengthen bone and protect against fractures. Excessive intakes cause a brown mottling of dental enamel, and may compromise bone structure, making them more brittle.

Fluoride is an unusual micronutrient in being supplied almost entirely from drinking water, including local water and that consumed from other areas as bottled or canned drinks. If the water supply contains more than 1 part per million (ppm) of fluoride, the incidence of dental caries is low. Very hard waters may contain over 10 ppm, presenting no problem other than some discoloration of teeth. However, soft waters contain little or no fluoride, so dental caries and loss is very frequent without supplementation. Almost no foods provide significant amounts of fluoride, an exception being tea, permitting strong teeth in areas where both tea and sugar cane are grown and consumed by children.

Adding of traces of fluoride to public water supplies, to maintain a normal healthful concentration of 1 ppm, is now a widespread practice but, where this is not policy, dental health must depend on education, supplementation to children, and provision of fluoride-containing toothpaste.

Chronic fluoride poisoning is occasionally seen where the water supply contains >10 ppm fluoride. It can also occur in workers handling cryolite (aluminium sodium fluoride), used in smelting aluminium. Pitting of teeth is a result of excess fluoride intake as a child.

Sodium, potassium and magnesium

Most animal and plant foods are low in natural sodium, and rich in potassium and magnesium. Western diets are high in sodium due to the sodium chloride (salt) that is added to processed food. In the UK, it is recommended that daily salt intakes are kept well below 6 g, and potassium and magnesium intakes maintained at levels a little greater than currently, principally to prevent the common gradual rise in blood pressure which occurs if children are weaned onto a lifelong higher sodium diet. The pathophysiological roles of sodium, potassium and magnesium are discussed in Chapter 14.

Other essential inorganic nutrients

These include chloride (a counter-ion to sodium and potassium), cobalt (required for vitamin B_{12}), sulphur (a constituent of methionine and cysteine), manganese (needed for or activates many enzymes) and chromium (necessary for insulin action). Deficiency of chromium presents as hyperglycaemia and has been reported in adults as a rare complication of prolonged parenteral nutrition.

Copper metabolism is abnormal in Wilson's disease. Deficiency occasionally occurs but only in young children, causing microcytic hypochromic anaemia, neutropenia, retarded growth, skeletal rarefaction and dermatosis.

Further information

Websites

gov.uk/government/groups/scientific-advisory-committee-on-nutrition *Scientific Advisory Committee on Nutrition (SACN): UK recommended dietary consumptions.*

diabetes.org.uk/professionals/position-statements-reports/food-nutrition-lifestyle/evidence-based-nutrition-guidelines-for-the-prevention-and-management-of-diabetes *Diabetes UK dietary guidelines for diabetes.*

bapen.org.uk *British Society for Parenteral and Enteral Nutrition; includes the MUST tool.*

bsg.org.uk *British Society of Gastroenterology: guidelines on management of patients with a short bowel, enteral feeding for adult hospital patients and the provision of a percutaneously placed enteral tube feeding service.*

espen.org *European Society for Parenteral and Enteral Nutrition: guidelines for adult parenteral nutrition; perioperative care in elective colonic and rectal/pelvic surgery; nutrition in dementia; acute and chronic intestinal failure in adults; and nutrition in cancer patients.*

nice.org.uk *National Institute for Health and Care Excellence: guidance for nutritional support in adults.*

A Rej
TS Chew
DS Sanders

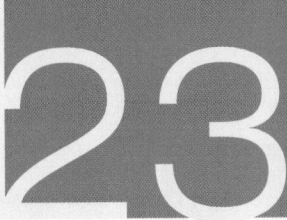

23

Gastroenterology

Clinical examination of the gastrointestinal tract

3 Head and neck
Pallor
Jaundice
Angular stomatitis
Glossitis
Parotid enlargement
Mouth ulcers
Dentition
Lymphadenopathy

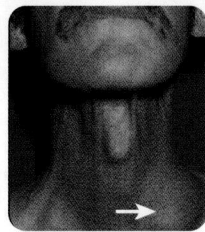
▲ Virchow's gland in gastric cancer

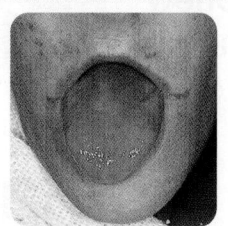
▲ Atrophic glossitis and angular stomatitis in vitamin B$_{12}$ deficiency

2 Hands
Clubbing
Koilonychia
Signs of liver disease (Ch. 24)

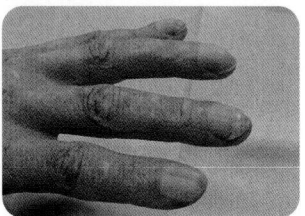
▲ Clubbing in patient with malabsorption

1 Skin and nutritional status
Muscle bulk
Subcutaneous fat
Signs of weight loss
Erythema nodosum

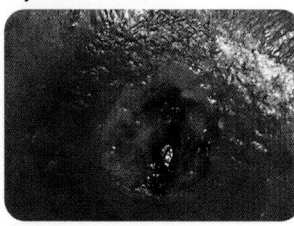
▲ Pyoderma gangrenosum in ulcerative colitis

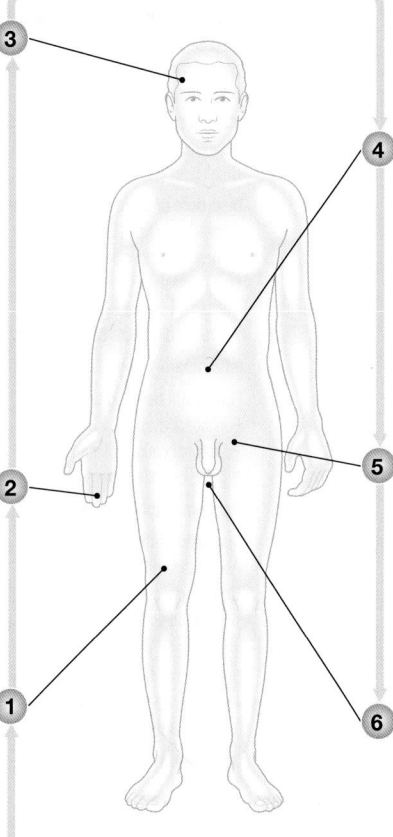

Observation
• Distressed/in pain?
• Fever?
• Dehydrated?
• Habitus
• Skin

4 Abdominal examination
(see opposite)
Observe
Distension
Respiratory movements
Scars
Colour

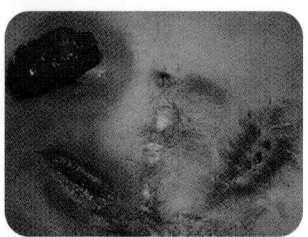
▲ Multiple surgical scars, a prolapsing ileostomy and enterocutaneous fistulae in a patient with Crohn's disease

Palpate
Tender/guarding
Masses
Viscera
  Liver (Ch. 24)
  Kidneys (Ch. 18)
  Spleen

Percuss
Ascites
Viscera

Auscultate
Bowel sounds
Bruits

5 Groin
Herniae
Lymph nodes

6 Perineum/rectal
(see opposite)
Fistulae
Skin tags
Haemorrhoids
Masses

4 **Abdominal examination: possible findings**

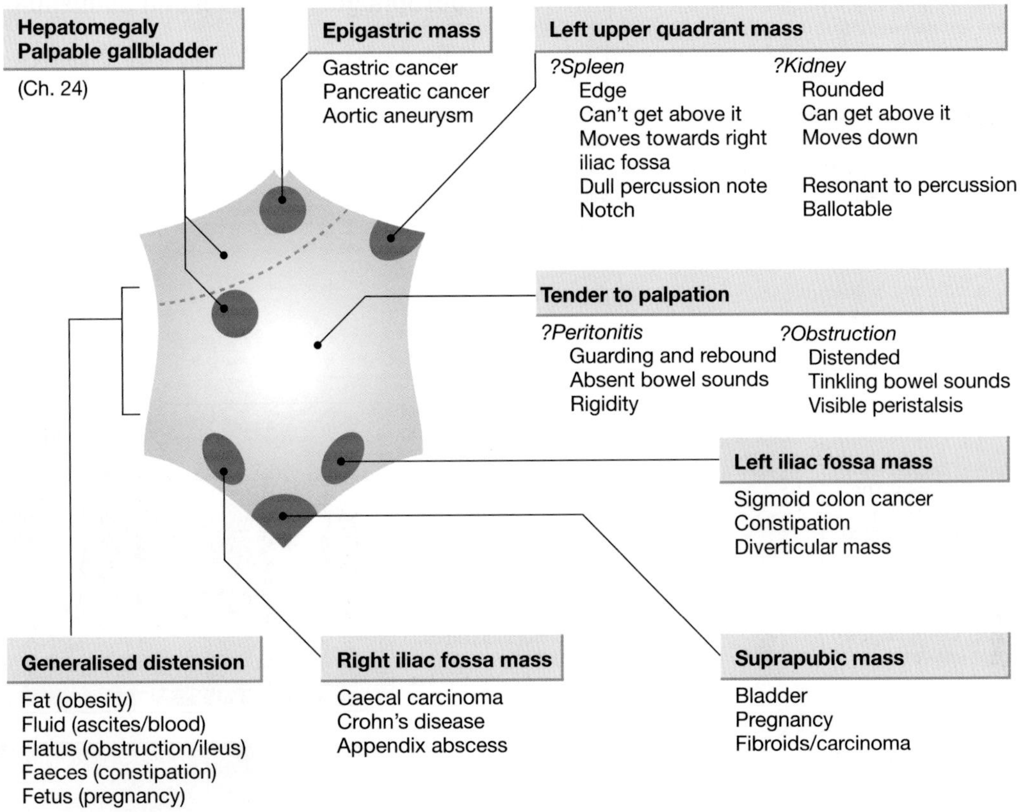

Hepatomegaly
Palpable gallbladder

(Ch. 24)

Epigastric mass

Gastric cancer
Pancreatic cancer
Aortic aneurysm

Left upper quadrant mass

?Spleen
  Edge
  Can't get above it
  Moves towards right
  iliac fossa
  Dull percussion note
  Notch

?Kidney
  Rounded
  Can get above it
  Moves down

  Resonant to percussion
  Ballotable

Tender to palpation

?Peritonitis
  Guarding and rebound
  Absent bowel sounds
  Rigidity

?Obstruction
  Distended
  Tinkling bowel sounds
  Visible peristalsis

Left iliac fossa mass

Sigmoid colon cancer
Constipation
Diverticular mass

Generalised distension

Fat (obesity)
Fluid (ascites/blood)
Flatus (obstruction/ileus)
Faeces (constipation)
Fetus (pregnancy)

Right iliac fossa mass

Caecal carcinoma
Crohn's disease
Appendix abscess

Suprapubic mass

Bladder
Pregnancy
Fibroids/carcinoma

6 **Rectal examination: common findings**

23

Anal disease

Tags
Haemorrhoids
Polyps
Crohn's disease

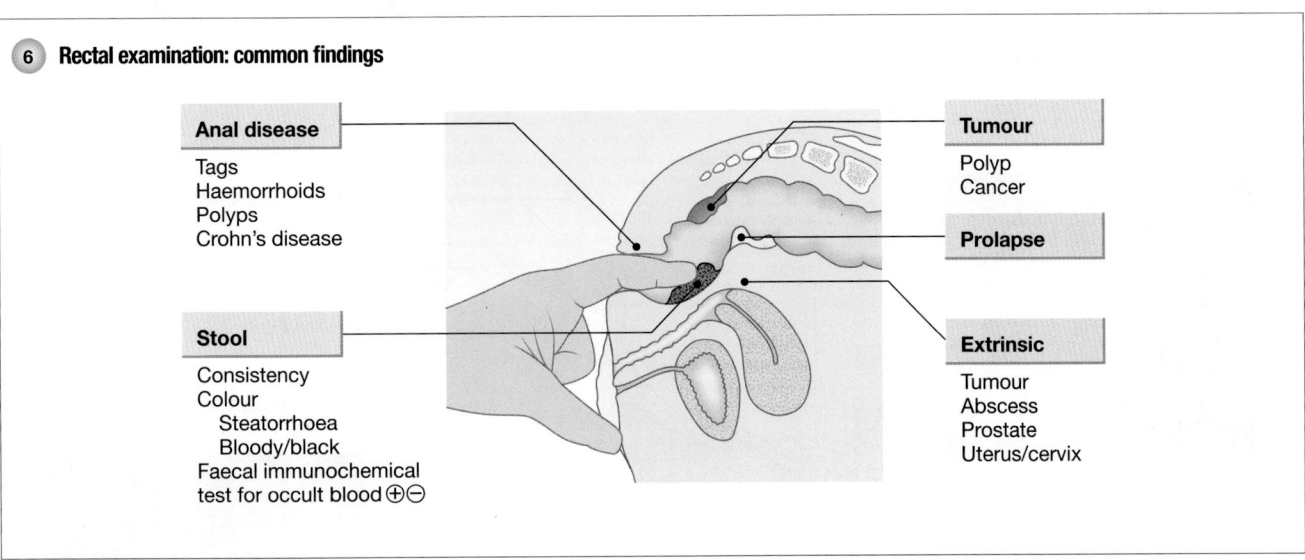

Tumour

Polyp
Cancer

Prolapse

Stool

Consistency
Colour
  Steatorrhoea
  Bloody/black
Faecal immunochemical
test for occult blood ⊕⊖

Extrinsic

Tumour
Abscess
Prostate
Uterus/cervix

Diseases of the gastrointestinal tract are a major cause of morbidity and mortality. Around 10% of all consultations in primary care are for gastroenterological problems, split equally between the upper and lower gastrointestinal tract. Infective diarrhoea and malabsorption are responsible for much ill health and many deaths in low- and middle-income countries. The gastrointestinal tract is the most common site for cancer development. Colorectal cancer is the third most common cancer in men and second most common in women, with population-based screening programmes existing in many countries. Functional gastrointestinal disorders account for at least 40% of all referrals to gastroenterology services and consume considerable health-care resources. The inflammatory bowel diseases, Crohn's disease and ulcerative colitis, together affect 1 in 250 people in the Western world, with substantial associated morbidity.

Functional anatomy and physiology

Oesophagus, stomach and duodenum

The oesophagus is a muscular tube that extends 25 cm from the cricoid cartilage to the cardiac orifice of the stomach, with the gastroesophageal junction being 40 cm from the incisors. The oesophagus has both an upper and a lower sphincter. A peristaltic swallowing wave propels the food bolus into the stomach (Fig. 23.1).

The stomach acts as a 'hopper', retaining and grinding food, and then actively propelling it into the upper small bowel (Fig. 23.2).

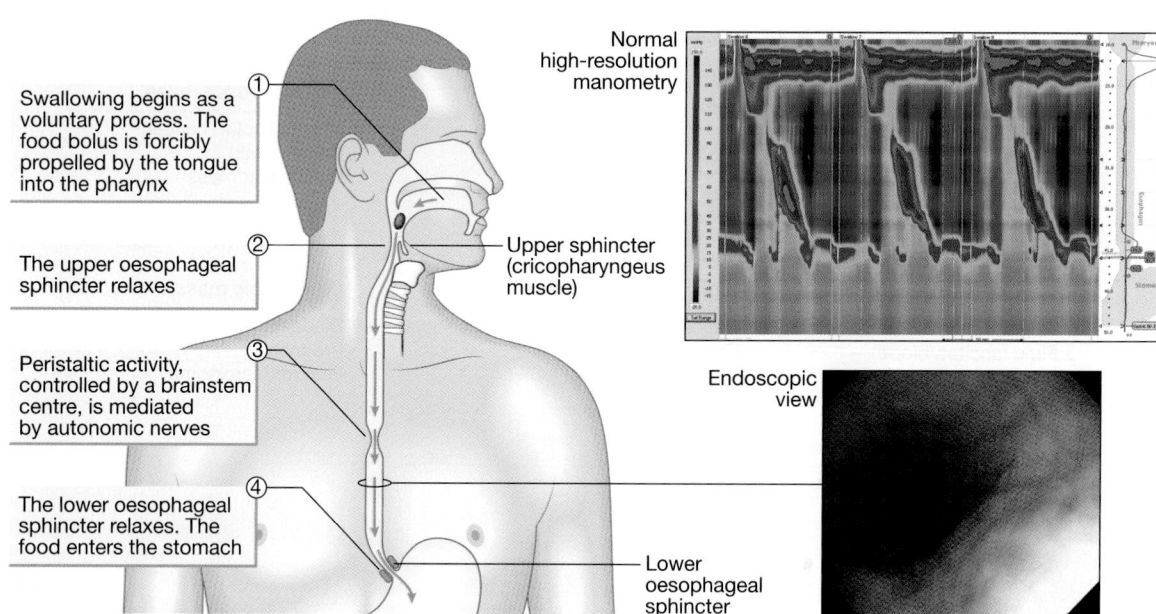

① Swallowing begins as a voluntary process. The food bolus is forcibly propelled by the tongue into the pharynx

② The upper oesophageal sphincter relaxes

③ Peristaltic activity, controlled by a brainstem centre, is mediated by autonomic nerves

④ The lower oesophageal sphincter relaxes. The food enters the stomach

Upper sphincter (cricopharyngeus muscle)

Lower oesophageal sphincter

Normal high-resolution manometry

Endoscopic view

Fig. 23.1 The oesophagus: anatomy and function. The swallowing wave.

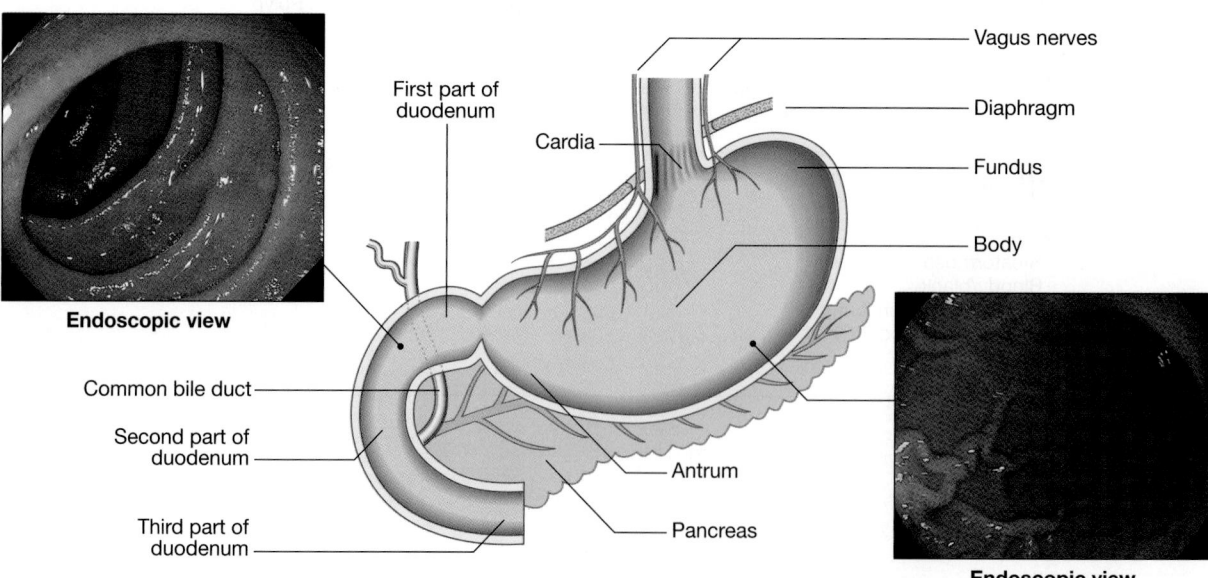

Endoscopic view

First part of duodenum

Cardia

Common bile duct

Second part of duodenum

Third part of duodenum

Vagus nerves

Diaphragm

Fundus

Body

Antrum

Pancreas

Endoscopic view

Fig. 23.2 Normal gastric and duodenal anatomy.

Gastric secretion

Gastrin, histamine and acetylcholine are the key stimulants of acid secretion. Hydrogen and chloride ions are secreted from the apical membrane of gastric parietal cells into the lumen of the stomach by a hydrogen–potassium adenosine triphosphatase (ATPase) ('proton pump') (Fig. 23.3). The hydrochloric acid sterilises the upper gastrointestinal tract and converts the zymogen pepsinogen, which is secreted by chief cells, to pepsin, which digests proteins to polypeptides. The glycoprotein intrinsic factor, secreted in parallel with acid, is necessary for vitamin B_{12} absorption in the terminal ileum.

Gastrin, somatostatin and ghrelin

The hormone gastrin is produced by G cells mainly in the gastric antrum, with somatostatin being secreted from D cells throughout the gastrointestinal tract. Gastrin stimulates acid secretion and mucosal growth while somatostatin suppresses it. Ghrelin, secreted from oxyntic glands, stimulates acid secretion, as well as appetite and gastric emptying.

Protective factors

Bicarbonate ions, stimulated by prostaglandins, mucins and trefoil factor family (TFF) peptides, together protect the gastroduodenal mucosa from the ulcerative properties of acid and pepsin.

Small intestine

The jejunum extends from the ligament of Treitz to the ileocaecal valve (Fig. 23.4). During fasting, a wave of peristaltic activity passes down the small bowel every 1–2 hours. Entry of food into the gastrointestinal tract stimulates small bowel peristaltic activity. Functions of the small intestine are:

- digestion (mechanical, enzymatic and peristaltic)
- absorption – the products of digestion, water, electrolytes and vitamins
- protection against ingested toxins
- immune regulation.

Digestion and absorption

Fat

Dietary lipids comprise long-chain triglycerides, cholesterol esters and lecithin. Lipids are insoluble in water and undergo lipolysis and incorporation into mixed micelles before they can be absorbed into enterocytes

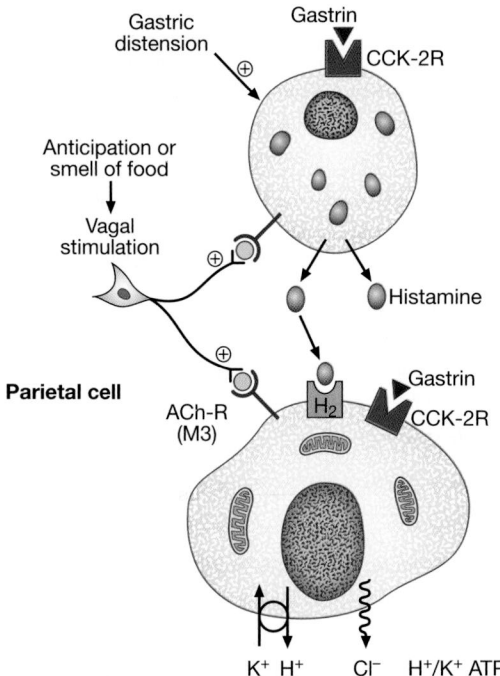

Fig. 23.3 Control of acid secretion. Gastrin released from antral G cells in response to food (protein) binds to cholecystokinin receptors (CCK-2R) on the surface of enterochromaffin-like (ECL) cells, which in turn release histamine. The histamine binds to H_2 receptors on parietal cells and this leads to secretion of hydrogen ions in exchange for potassium ions at the apical membrane. Parietal cells also express CCK-2R and it is thought that activation of these receptors by gastrin is involved in regulatory proliferation of parietal cells. Cholinergic (vagal) activity and gastric distension also stimulate acid secretion; somatostatin, vasoactive intestinal polypeptide (VIP) and gastric inhibitory polypeptide (GIP) may inhibit it. (ACh-R = acetylcholine receptor; ATPase = adenosine triphosphatase)

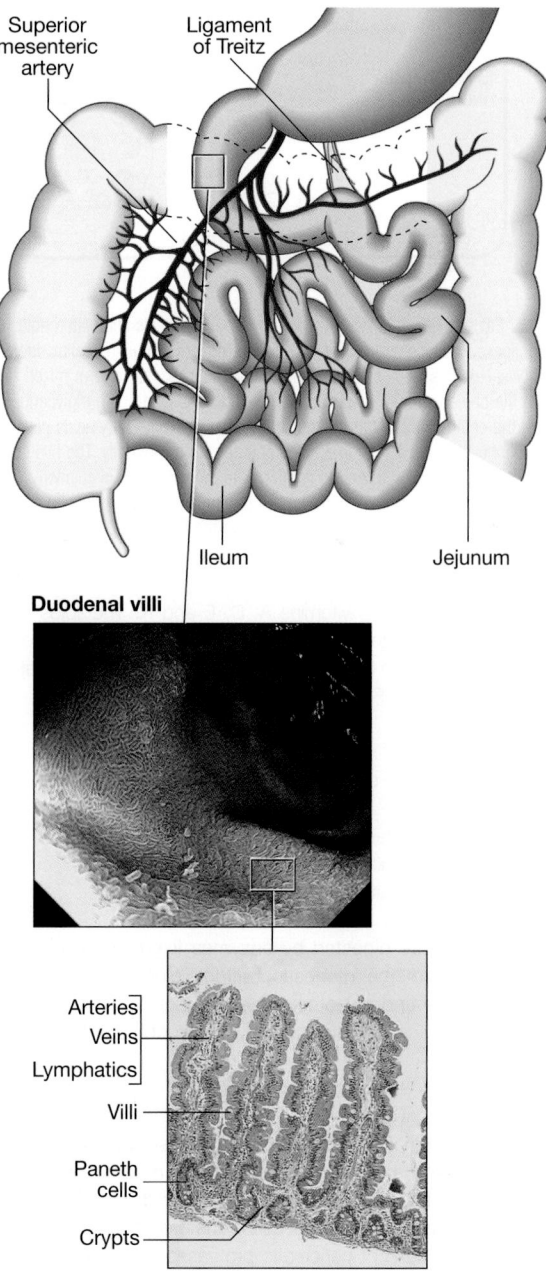

Fig. 23.4 Small intestine: anatomy. Epithelial cells are formed in crypts and differentiate as they migrate to the tip of the villi to form enterocytes (absorptive cells) and goblet cells.

23

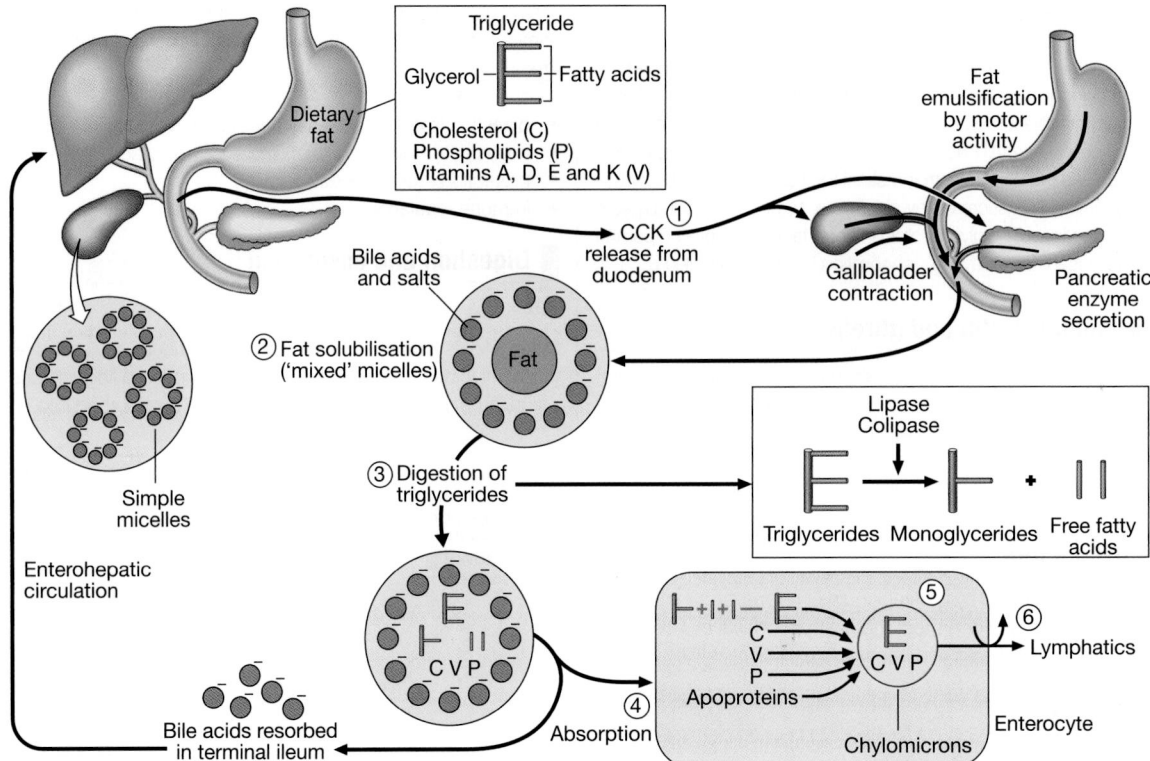

Fig. 23.5 Fat digestion. *Step 1: Luminal phase.* Fatty acids stimulate cholecystokinin (CCK) release from the duodenum and upper jejunum. The CCK stimulates release of amylase, lipase, colipase and proteases from the pancreas, causes gallbladder contraction and relaxes the sphincter of Oddi, allowing bile to flow into the intestine. *Step 2: Fat solubilisation.* Bile acids and salts combine with dietary fat to form mixed micelles, which also contain cholesterol and fat-soluble vitamins. *Step 3: Digestion.* Pancreatic lipase, in the presence of its co-factor, colipase, cleaves long-chain triglycerides, yielding fatty acids and monoglycerides. *Step 4: Absorption.* Mixed micelles diffuse to the brush border of the enterocytes. Within the brush border, long-chain fatty acids bind to proteins, which transport the fatty acids into the cell, whereas cholesterol, short-chain fatty acids, phospholipids and fat-soluble vitamins enter the cell directly. The bile salts remain in the small intestinal lumen and are actively transported from the terminal ileum into the portal circulation and returned to the liver (the enterohepatic circulation). *Step 5: Re-esterification.* Within the enterocyte, fatty acids are re-esterified to form triglycerides. Triglycerides combine with cholesterol ester, fat-soluble vitamins, phospholipids and apoproteins to form chylomicrons. *Step 6: Transport.* Chylomicrons leave the enterocytes by exocytosis, enter mesenteric lymphatics, pass into the thoracic duct and eventually reach the systemic circulation.

along with the fat-soluble vitamins A, D, E and K. The lipids are processed within enterocytes and pass via lymphatics into the systemic circulation. Fat absorption and digestion can be considered as a stepwise process, as outlined in Figure 23.5.

Carbohydrates

Starch is hydrolysed by salivary and pancreatic amylases to:

- α-limit dextrins containing 4–8 glucose molecules
- the disaccharide maltose
- the trisaccharide maltotriose.

Disaccharides are digested by enzymes fixed to the microvillous membrane to form the monosaccharides glucose, galactose and fructose. Glucose and galactose enter the cell by an energy-requiring process involving a carrier protein, and fructose enters by simple diffusion.

Protein

The steps involved in protein digestion are shown in Figure 23.6. Intragastric digestion by pepsin is quantitatively modest, but important, because the resulting polypeptides and amino acids stimulate cholecystokinin (CCK) release from the mucosa of the proximal jejunum, which in turn stimulates release of pancreatic proteases, including trypsinogen, chymotrypsinogen, pro-elastases and procarboxypeptidases, from the pancreas. On exposure to brush border enterokinase, inert trypsinogen is converted to the active proteolytic enzyme trypsin, which activates

the other pancreatic pro-enzymes. Trypsin digests proteins to produce oligopeptides, peptides and amino acids. Oligopeptides are further hydrolysed by brush border enzymes to yield dipeptides, tripeptides and amino acids. These small peptides and the amino acids are actively transported into the enterocytes, where intracellular peptidases further digest peptides to amino acids. Amino acids are then actively transported across the basal cell membrane of the enterocyte into the portal circulation and the liver.

Water and electrolytes

Absorption and secretion of electrolytes and water occur throughout the intestine. Electrolytes and water are transported by two pathways:

- *the paracellular route*, in which passive flow through tight junctions between cells is a consequence of osmotic, electrical or hydrostatic gradients
- *the transcellular route* across apical and basolateral membranes by energy-requiring specific active transport carriers (pumps).

In healthy individuals, fluid balance is tightly controlled, such that only 100 mL of the 8 litres of fluid entering the gastrointestinal tract daily is excreted in stools (Fig. 23.7).

Vitamins and trace elements

Water-soluble vitamins are absorbed throughout the intestine. The absorption of folic acid, vitamin B$_{12}$, calcium and iron is described in Chapter 25.

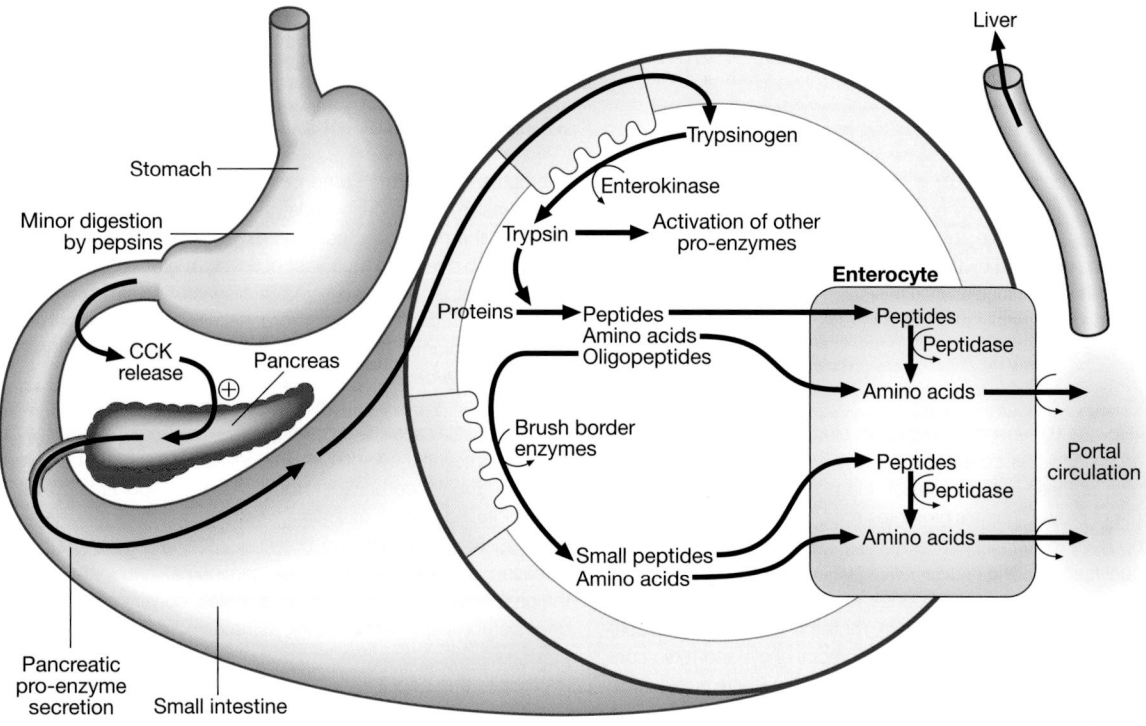

Fig. 23.6 Protein digestion. (CCK = cholecystokinin)

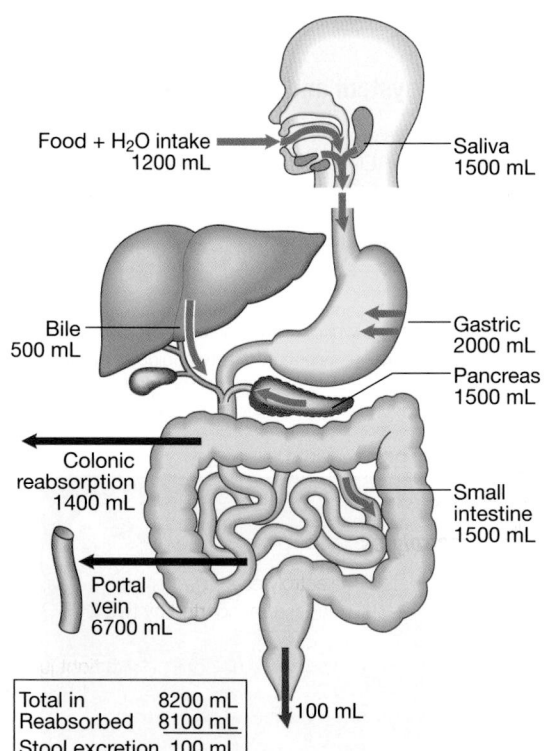

Fig. 23.7 Fluid homeostasis in the gastrointestinal tract.

Total in	8200 mL
Reabsorbed	8100 mL
Stool excretion	100 mL

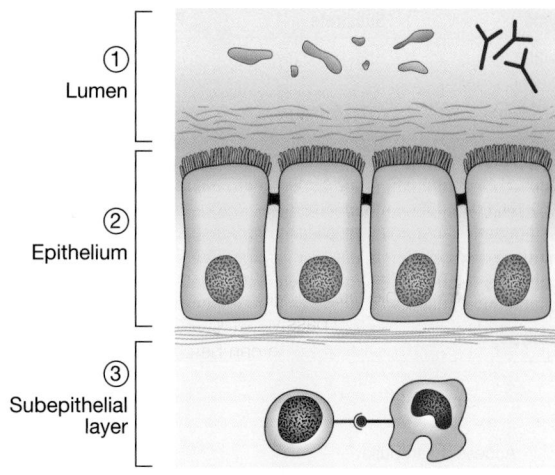

Fig. 23.8 Intestinal defence mechanisms. See text for details.

impermeable brush border membranes and passage between cells is prevented by tight and adherens junctions. These cells can react to foreign peptides ('innate immunity') using pattern recognition receptors found on cell surfaces (Toll receptors) or intracellularly. Lastly, in the sub-epithelial layer, immune responses occur under control of the adaptive immune system in response to pathogenic compounds.

Immunological defence mechanisms

Gastrointestinal mucosa-associated lymphoid tissue (MALT) constitutes 25% of the total lymphatic tissue of the body and is at the heart of adaptive immunity. Within Peyer's patches, B lymphocytes differentiate to plasma cells following exposure to antigens and these migrate to mesenteric lymph nodes to enter the blood stream via the thoracic duct. The plasma cells return to the lamina propria of the gut through the circulation and release immunoglobulin A (IgA), which is transported into the lumen of the intestine. Intestinal T lymphocytes help localise plasma cells to the site of antigen exposure, as well as producing inflammatory mediators. Macrophages in the gut phagocytose foreign materials and secrete a

Protective function of the small intestine

Physical defence mechanisms

There are several levels of defence in the small bowel (Fig. 23.8). Firstly, the gut lumen contains host bacteria, mucins and secreted antibacterial products, including defensins and immunoglobulins that help combat pathogenic infections. Secondly, epithelial cells have relatively

range of cytokines, which mediate inflammation. Similarly, activation of mast-cell surface IgE receptors leads to degranulation and release of other molecules involved in inflammation.

Pancreas

The exocrine pancreas (Box 23.1) is necessary for the digestion of fat, protein and carbohydrate. Pro-enzymes are secreted from pancreatic acinar cells in response to circulating gastrointestinal hormones (Fig. 23.9) and are activated by trypsin. Bicarbonate-rich fluid is secreted from ductular cells to produce an optimum alkaline pH for enzyme activity. The endocrine pancreas is discussed in Chapters 20 and 21.

Colon

The colon (Fig. 23.10) absorbs water and electrolytes. It also acts as a storage organ and has contractile activity. Two types of contraction occur. The first of these is segmentation (ring contraction), which leads to mixing but not propulsion; this promotes absorption of water and electrolytes. Propulsive (peristaltic contraction) waves occur several times a day and propel faeces to the rectum. All activity is stimulated after meals through the gastrocolic reflex in response to release of hormones such as 5-hydroxytryptamine (5-HT, serotonin), motilin and CCK. Faecal continence depends on maintenance of the anorectal angle and tonic contraction of the external anal sphincters. On defecation, there is relaxation of the anorectal muscles, increased intra-abdominal pressure from the Valsalva manoeuvre and contraction of abdominal muscles, and relaxation of the anal sphincters.

Intestinal microbiota

The human microbiota comprises 10^{14} microbial residents in the human body, vastly outnumbering host cells. Indeed, the number of bacterial genes in the microbiota genome exceeds that of the host by 100-fold or more. This represents a vast ecosystem that is central to health and homeostasis, and is disordered in disease. In terms of nomenclature, 'microbiota' refers to the microorganisms that live in a particular niche, while 'microbiome' refers to the collective genomes of these microbiota. There is a degree of heritability of this microbiota, but it is clear that there are many environmental factors that can affect it, including diet, drugs, physical activity, smoking, stress and natural ageing. Generally, the adult intestinal microbiota is acquired by the age of 2 years. A dysbiosis or imbalance between the different components of the intestinal microbiota has been associated with diseases of the gastrointestinal tract, such as inflammatory bowel disease and colorectal cancer; liver disease, including hepatocellular carcinoma; and pathologies outside the gastrointestinal tract, such as diabetes, obesity, cardiovascular disorders, cerebrovascular disorders, asthma and psychiatric disorders, such as depression. Many challenges remain in understanding the intestinal microbiota and how it impacts on health and disease.

Control of gastrointestinal function

Secretion, absorption, motor activity, growth and differentiation of the gut are all modulated by a combination of neuronal and hormonal factors.

The nervous system and gastrointestinal function

The central nervous system (CNS), the autonomic system (ANS) and the enteric nervous system (ENS) interact to regulate gut function. The ANS comprises:

- *parasympathetic pathways* (vagal and sacral efferent), which are cholinergic, and increase smooth muscle tone and promote sphincter relaxation
- *sympathetic pathways*, which release noradrenaline (norepinephrine), reduce smooth muscle tone and stimulate sphincter contraction.

i 23.1	Pancreatic enzymes	
Enzyme	**Substrate**	**Product**
Amylase	Starch and glycogen	Limit dextrans Maltose Maltriose
Lipase **Colipase**	Triglycerides	Monoglycerides and free fatty acids
Proteolytic enzymes **Trypsinogen** **Chymotrypsinogen** **Pro-elastase** **Pro-carboxypeptidases**	Proteins and polypeptides	Short polypeptides

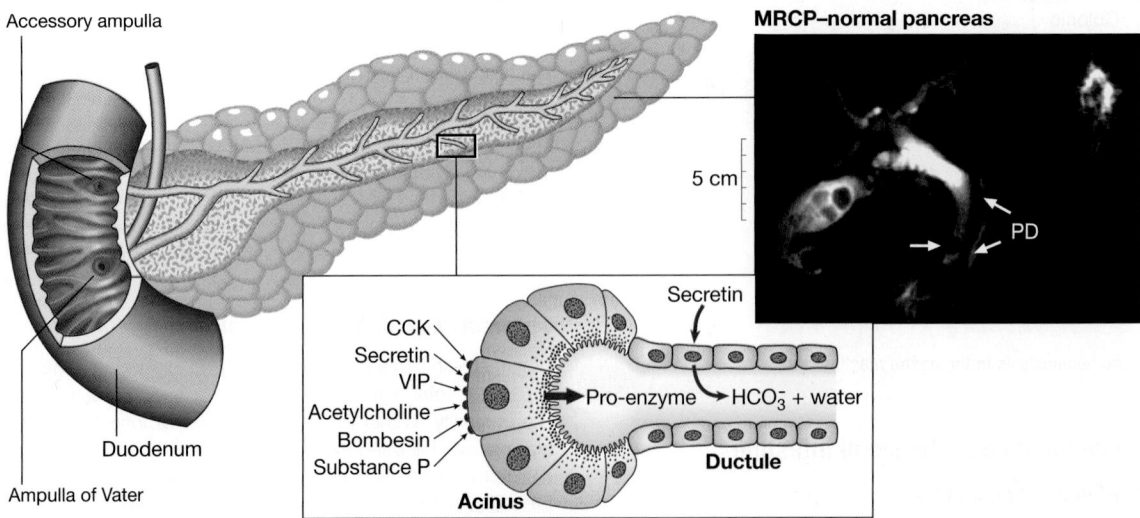

Fig. 23.9 Pancreatic structure and function. Ductular cells secrete alkaline fluid in response to secretin. Acinar cells secrete digestive enzymes from zymogen granules in response to a range of secretagogues. The photograph shows a normal pancreatic duct (PD) and side branches, as defined at magnetic resonance cholangiopancreatography (MRCP). Note the incidental calculi in the gallbladder and common bile duct (arrow). (CCK = cholecystokinin; VIP = vasoactive intestinal polypeptide)

The enteric nervous system

In conjunction with the ANS, the ENS senses gut contents and conditions, and regulates motility, fluid exchange, secretion, blood flow and other key gut functions. It comprises two major networks intrinsic to the gut wall. The myenteric (Auerbach's) plexus in the smooth muscle layer regulates motor control; and the submucosal (Meissner's) plexus exerts secretory control over the epithelium, entero-endocrine cells and submucosal vessels. Together, these plexuses form a two-layered neuronal mesh along the length of the gut. Although connected centrally via the ANS, the ENS can function autonomously using a variety of transmitters, including acetylcholine, noradrenaline (norepinephrine), 5-HT, nitric oxide, substance P and calcitonin gene-related peptide (CGRP). There are local reflex loops within the ENS but also loops involving the coeliac and mesenteric ganglia and the paravertebral ganglia. The parasympathetic system generally stimulates motility and secretion, while the sympathetic system generally acts in an inhibitory manner.

Peristalsis

Peristalsis is a reflex triggered by gut wall distension, which consists of a wave of circular muscle contraction to propel contents from the oesophagus to the rectum. It can be influenced by innervation but functions independently. It results from a basic electrical rhythm originating from the interstitial cells of Cajal in the circular layer of intestinal smooth muscle. These are stellate cells of mesenchymal origin with smooth muscle features, which act as the 'pacemaker' of the gut.

Migrating motor complexes

Migrating motor complexes (MMCs) are waves of contraction spreading from the stomach to the ileum, occurring at a frequency of about 5 per minute every 90 minutes or so, between meals and during fasting. They may serve to sweep intestinal contents distally in preparation for the next meal and are inhibited by eating.

Gut hormones

The origin, action and control of the major gut hormones, peptides and non-peptide signalling transmitters are summarised in Box 23.2.

Investigation of gastrointestinal disease

A wide range of tests is available for the investigation of patients with gastrointestinal symptoms. These can be classified broadly into tests of structure, tests for infection and tests of function.

Imaging

Plain X-rays

Plain X-rays of the abdomen are useful in the diagnosis of intestinal obstruction or paralytic ileus, where dilated loops of bowel and (in the erect position) fluid levels may be seen (Fig. 23.11). Calcified lymph nodes, gallstones and renal stones can also be detected. Chest X-ray (performed with the patient in erect position) is useful in the diagnosis of suspected perforation, as it shows subdiaphragmatic free air (see Fig. 23.11).

Contrast studies

X-rays with contrast medium are usually performed to assess not only anatomical abnormalities but also motility. Barium sulphate provides good mucosal coating and excellent opacification but can precipitate impaction proximal to an obstructive lesion. Water-soluble contrast is used to opacify bowel prior to abdominal computed tomography and in cases of suspected perforation. The double contrast technique improves mucosal visualisation by using gas to distend the barium-coated

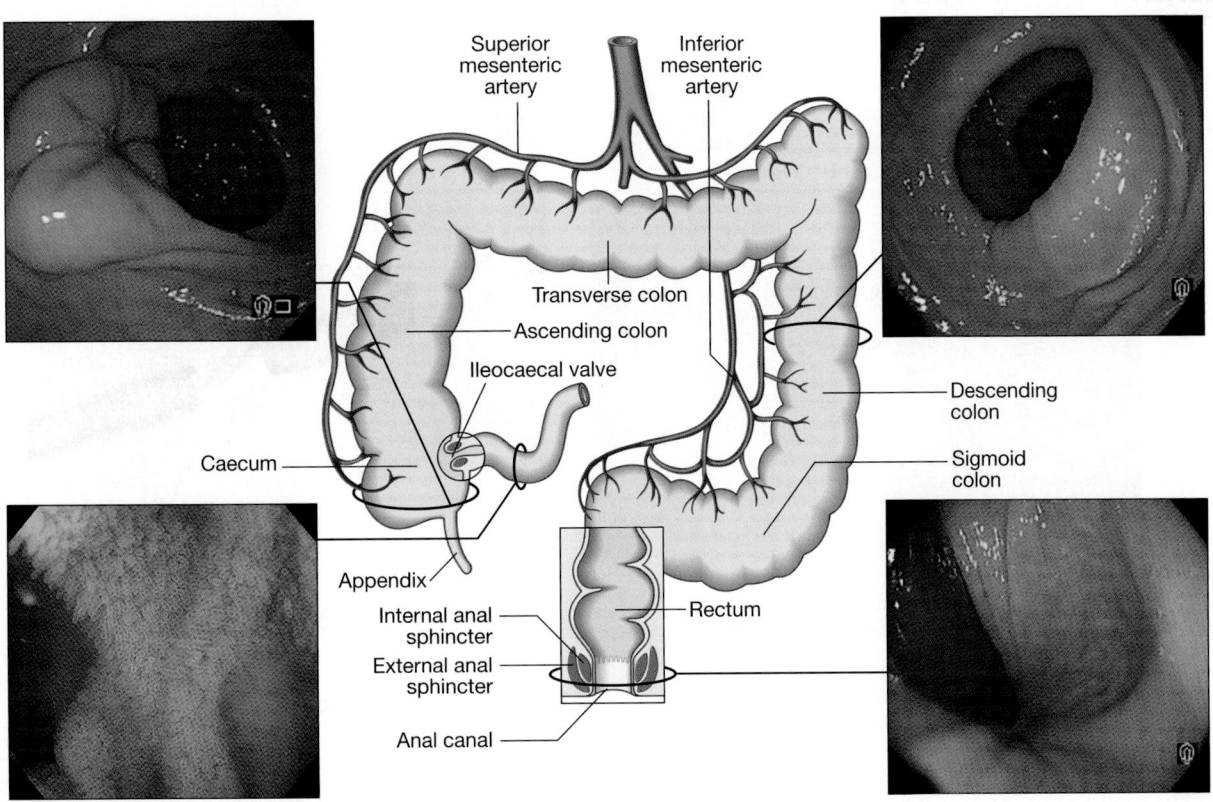

Fig. 23.10 The normal colon, rectum and anal canal.

i 23.2 Gut hormones and peptides

Hormone	Origin	Stimulus	Action
Gastrin	Predominantly stomach (G cell)	Products of protein digestion Suppressed by acid and somatostatin	Stimulates gastric acid secretion Stimulates growth of gastrointestinal mucosa
Somatostatin	Throughout gastrointestinal tract (D cell)	Fat ingestion	Inhibits gastrin and insulin secretion Decreases acid secretion Decreases absorption Inhibits pancreatic secretion
Cholecystokinin (CCK)	Duodenum and jejunum (I cells); also ileal and colonic nerve endings	Products of protein digestion Fat and fatty acids Suppressed by trypsin	Stimulates pancreatic enzyme secretion Stimulates gallbladder contraction Relaxes sphincter of Oddi Modulates satiety Decreases gastric acid secretion Reduces gastric emptying Regulates pancreatic growth
Secretin	Duodenum and jejunum (S cells)	Duodenal acid Fatty acids	Stimulates pancreatic fluid and bicarbonate secretion Decreases acid secretion Reduces gastric emptying
Motilin	Duodenum, small intestine and colon (Mo cells)	Fasting Dietary fat	Regulates peristaltic activity, including migrating motor complexes (MMCs)
Gastric inhibitory polypeptide (GIP)	Duodenum (K cells) and jejunum	Glucose and fat	Stimulates insulin release (also known as glucose-dependent insulinotrophic polypeptide) Inhibits acid secretion Enhances satiety
Glucagon-like peptide-1 (GLP-1)	Ileum and colon (L cells)	Carbohydrates, protein and fat	Stimulates insulin release Inhibits acid secretion and gastric emptying Enhances satiety
Vasoactive intestinal peptide (VIP)	Nerve fibres throughout gastrointestinal tract	Unknown	Has vasodilator action Relaxes smooth muscle Stimulates water and electrolyte secretion
Ghrelin	Stomach	Fasting Inhibited by eating	Stimulates appetite, acid secretion and gastric emptying
Peptide YY	Ileum and colon	Feeding	Modulates satiety

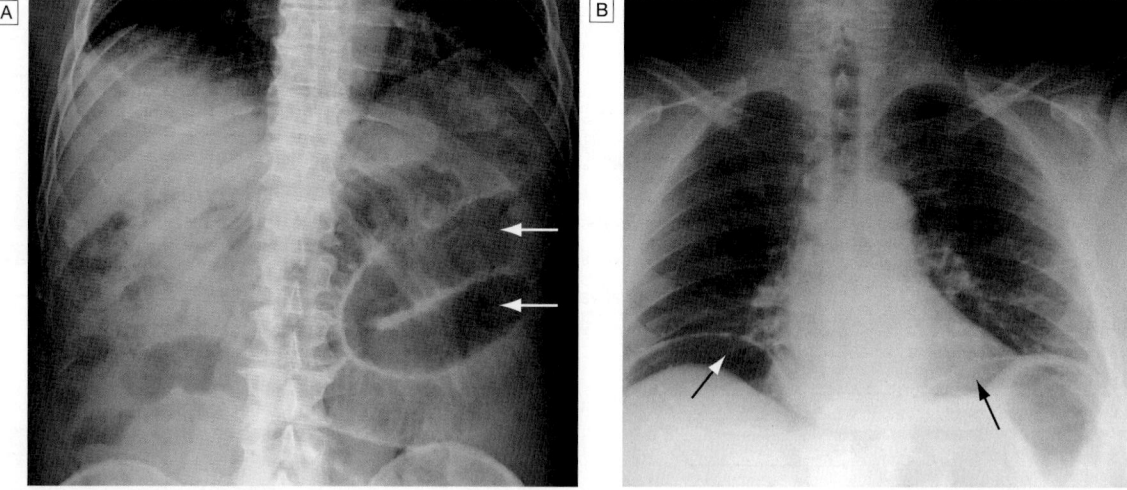

Fig. 23.11 Examples of plain X-rays. [A] Abdominal X-ray showing dilatation of loops of small bowel (arrows), which are indicative of obstruction (in this case due to adhesions from previous surgery). [B] Chest X-ray showing free air under both hemi-diaphragms (arrows), which is indicative of acute perforation of an abdominal viscus.

intestinal surface. Contrast studies are useful for detecting filling defects, such as tumours, strictures, ulcers and motility disorders, but are inferior to endoscopic procedures and more sophisticated cross-sectional imaging techniques, such as computed tomography and magnetic resonance imaging. The major uses and limitations of various contrast studies are shown in Box 23.3 and Figure 23.12.

Ultrasound, computed tomography and magnetic resonance imaging

Ultrasound, computed tomography (CT) and magnetic resonance imaging (MRI) are key tests in the evaluation of intra-abdominal disease. They are non-invasive and offer detailed images of the abdominal contents; portable ultrasound devices are increasingly used at the bedside to provide rapid diagnostic information, e.g. in acute abdominal pain and to assist with investigations such as paracentesis. Fluorodeoxyglucose-positron emission tomography (FDG-PET) is used in the staging of malignancies and images may be fused with CT to enhance localisation. Their main applications are summarised in Box 23.4 and Figure 23.13.

i	**23.3**	**Contrast radiology in the investigation of gastrointestinal disease**	
	Barium swallow/meal	Barium follow-through	Barium enema
Indications and major uses	Motility disorders (achalasia and gastroparesis) Perforation or fistula (non-ionic contrast)	Diarrhoea and abdominal pain of small bowel origin Possible obstruction by strictures Suspected malabsorption Assessment of Crohn's disease	Altered bowel habit Evaluation of strictures or diverticular disease Megacolon
Limitations	Risk of aspiration Poor mucosal detail Low sensitivity for early cancer Inability to biopsy	Time-consuming nature Radiation exposure Relative insensitivity	Difficulty in frail or incontinent patients Sigmoidoscopy needed to see rectum Low sensitivity for lesions < 1 cm

Endoanal ultrasound and anorectal manometry

Endoanal ultrasound is primarily used in the evaluation of anal fistula and anal sphincter pathology, in individuals presenting with faecal incontinence. In conjunction with this, anorectal manometry is commonly performed to detect abnormalities of sphincter function and recto-anal coordination. Anorectal manometry is also commonly used to assess constipation, particularly when thought due to obstructive defecation.

Endoscopy

Videoendoscopes provide high-definition imaging and accessories can be passed down the endoscope to allow both diagnostic and therapeutic procedures, some of which are illustrated in Figure 23.14. Endoscopes with magnifying lenses allow almost microscopic detail to be observed, and imaging modalities, such as confocal endomicroscopy, autofluorescence and 'narrow-band imaging', are increasingly used to detect subtle abnormalities not visible by standard 'white light' endoscopy. The implications of endoscopic procedures in older people are shown in Box 23.5.

Upper gastrointestinal endoscopy

This is performed under light sedation, or using only local anaesthetic throat spray after the patient has fasted for at least 4 hours. With the patient in the left lateral position, the entire oesophagus (excluding pharynx), stomach and first two parts of duodenum can be seen. Indications, contraindications and complications are given in Box 23.6. While upper gastrointestinal endoscopy is mainly performed via the transoral route, transnasal endoscopy is becoming an emerging alternative in some units.

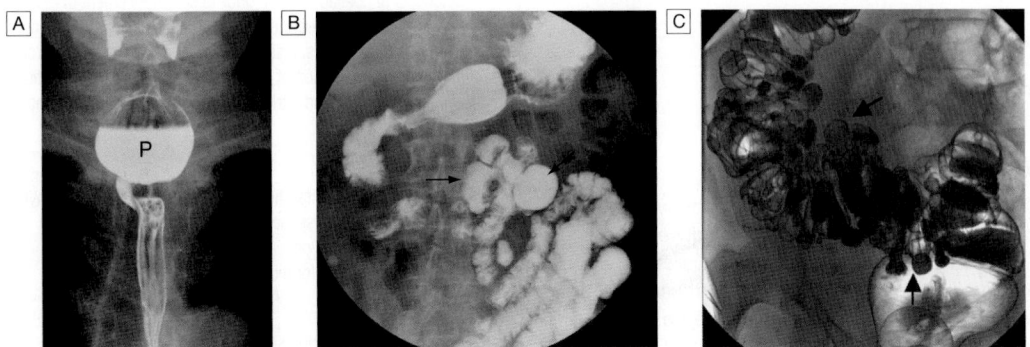

Fig. 23.12 Examples of contrast radiology. [A] Barium swallow showing a large pharyngeal pouch (P) with retained contrast creating an air–fluid level. [B] Barium follow-through. There are multiple diverticula (arrows) in this patient with jejunal diverticulosis. [C] Barium enema showing severe diverticular disease. There is tortuosity and narrowing of the sigmoid colon with multiple diverticula (arrows).

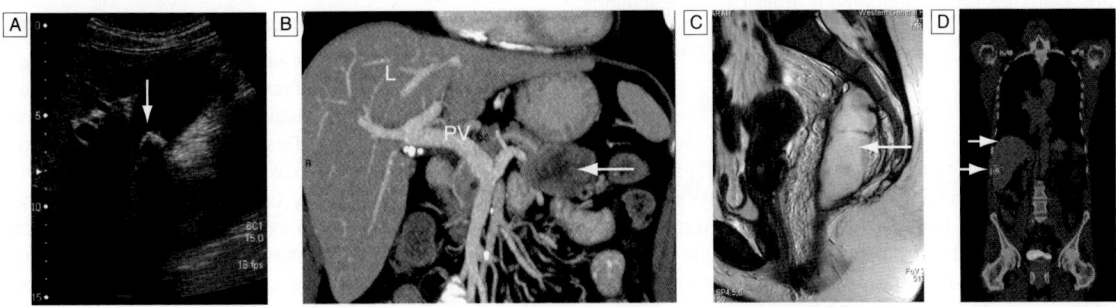

Fig. 23.13 Examples of ultrasound, CT and MRI. [A] Ultrasound showing large gallstone (arrow) with acoustic shadowing. [B] Multidetector coronal CT showing large solid and cystic malignant tumour in the pancreatic tail (arrow). (PV = portal vein; L = liver) [C] Pelvic MRI showing large pelvic abscess (arrow) posterior to the rectum in a patient with Crohn's disease. [D] Fused CT-PET image showing two liver metastases (arrows).

23

23.4 Imaging in gastroenterology				
	Ultrasound	Computed tomography (CT)	Magnetic resonance imaging (MRI)	Positron emission tomography-CT (PET-CT)
Indications and major uses	Abdominal masses Organomegaly Ascites Biliary tract dilatation Gallstones Guided biopsy of lesions Small bowel imaging	Assessment of pancreatic disease Hepatic tumour deposits CT colonography ('virtual colonoscopy') Tumour staging Assessment of lesion vascularity Abscesses and collections	Hepatic tumour staging MRCP Pelvic/perianal disease Crohn's fistulae Small bowel visualisation	Detection of metastases not seen on ultrasound or CT Images can be fused with CT to form composite image
Limitations	Low sensitivity for small lesions Little functional information Operator-dependent Gas and obesity may obscure view	Cost Radiation dose	Claustrophobic patients Contraindicated in presence of metallic prostheses, cardiac pacemaker, cochlear implants	Signal detection depends on metabolic activity within tumour – not all are metabolically active

(MRCP = magnetic resonance cholangiopancreatography)

23.5 Endoscopy in old age

- **Tolerance**: endoscopic procedures are generally well tolerated, even in very old people.
- **Side-effects from sedation**: older people are more sensitive, and respiratory depression, hypotension and prolonged recovery times are more common.
- **Bowel preparation for colonoscopy**: can be difficult in frail, immobile people. Sodium phosphate-based preparations can cause dehydration or hypotension and should be avoided in those with underlying cardiac or renal failure. Minimal-preparation CT colonograms provide an excellent alternative in these individuals.
- **Antiperistaltic agents**: hyoscine should be avoided in those with glaucoma and can also cause tachyarrhythmias. Glucagon is preferred if an antiperistaltic agent is needed.

(CT = computed tomography)

Endoscopic ultrasound

Endoscopic ultrasound (EUS) combines endoscopy with intraluminal ultrasonography using a high-frequency transducer to produce high-resolution ultrasound images. This allows visualisation through the wall of the gastrointestinal tract and into surrounding tissues, e.g. the pancreas or lymph nodes. It can therefore be used to perform fine needle aspiration or biopsy of mass lesions. EUS is helpful in the diagnosis of pancreatic tumours, chronic pancreatitis, pancreatic cysts, cholangiocarcinoma, common bile duct stones, ampullary lesions and submucosal tumours. It also plays an important role in the staging of certain cancers, e.g. those of oesophagus and pancreas. The role of EUS as a therapeutic modality has increased, and can be used in the drainage of pancreatic fluid collections and coeliac plexus block for pain management. Possible complications of EUS include bleeding, infection, cardiopulmonary events and perforation.

Capsule endoscopy

Capsule endoscopy (Fig. 23.15) uses a capsule containing an imaging device, battery, transmitter and antenna; as it traverses the small intestine, it transmits images to a battery-powered recorder worn on a belt round the patient's waist. After approximately 8 hours, the capsule is excreted. Images from the capsule are analysed as a video sequence and it is usually possible to localise the segment of small bowel where lesions are seen. Abnormalities detected usually require enteroscopy for confirmation and therapy. Indications, contraindications and complications are listed in Box 23.7.

23.6 Upper gastrointestinal endoscopy

Indications

- Dyspepsia in patients > 55 years of age or with alarm symptoms
- Atypical chest pain
- Dysphagia
- Vomiting
- Weight loss
- Acute or chronic gastrointestinal bleeding
- Screening for oesophageal varices in chronic liver disease
- Abnormal CT scan or barium meal
- Duodenal biopsies in the investigation of malabsorption and confirmation of a diagnosis of coeliac disease prior to commencement of gluten-free diet
- Therapy, including treatment of bleeding lesions, banding/injection of varices, dilatation of strictures, insertion of stents, placement of percutaneous gastrostomies, ablation of Barrett's oesophagus and resection of high-grade dysplastic lesions and early neoplasia in the upper gastrointestinal tract

Contraindications

- Severe shock
- Recent myocardial infarction, unstable angina, cardiac arrhythmia
- Severe respiratory disease*
- Atlantoaxial subluxation*
- Possible visceral perforation

Complications

- Cardiorespiratory depression due to sedation
- Aspiration pneumonia
- Perforation

*These are 'relative' contraindications; in experienced hands, endoscopy can be safely performed.
(CT = computed tomography)

Enteroscopy – push enteroscopy/double balloon enteroscopy

While upper gastrointestinal endoscopy can reach the proximal small intestine in most patients, enteroscopy is an endoscopic technique that allows more extensive evaluation of the small intestine, extending into the jejunum and/or ileum. Push enteroscopy uses a long endoscope to examine up to the proximal jejunum. Deeper evaluation of the small bowel can be assessed by using a technique called double balloon enteroscopy, which uses a long endoscope with a flexible overtube. Sequential and repeated inflation and deflation of balloons on the tip of the overtube and enteroscope allow the operator to push and pull along the entire length of the small intestine to the terminal ileum, to diagnose or treat small bowel lesions detected by capsule endoscopy or other imaging modalities. This technique can be performed via an antegrade approach (via the mouth) or retrograde approach (via the anus),

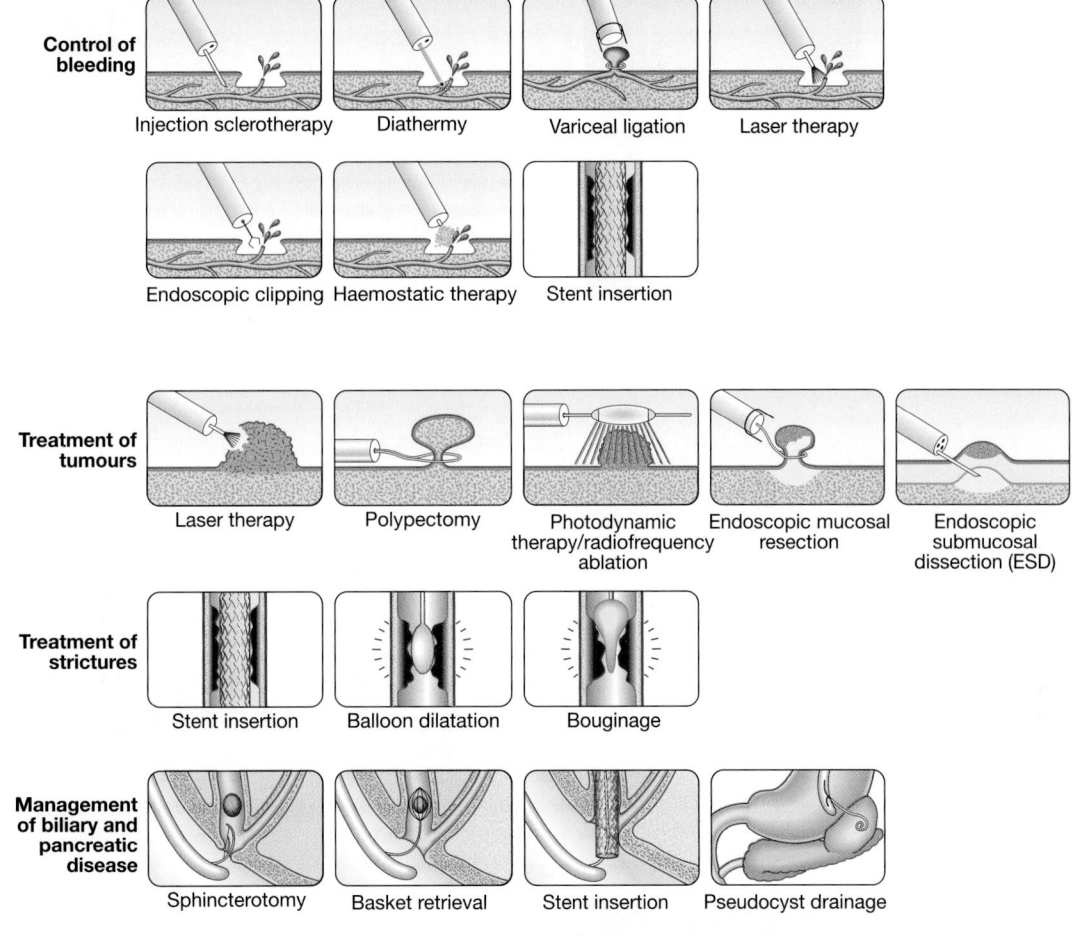

Fig. 23.14 Examples of therapeutic techniques in endoscopy.

dependent upon the site of the lesion. Indications, contraindications and complications are listed in Box 23.8.

Sigmoidoscopy and colonoscopy

Sigmoidoscopy can be carried out either in the outpatient clinic using a rigid plastic sigmoidoscope or in the endoscopy suite using a colonoscope following bowel preparation. When sigmoidoscopy is combined with proctoscopy, accurate detection of haemorrhoids, ulcerative colitis and distal colorectal neoplasia is possible. After full bowel cleansing, it is possible to examine the entire colon and the terminal ileum using a colonoscope. Indications, contraindications and complications of colonoscopy are listed in Box 23.9.

Magnetic resonance cholangiopancreatography

Magnetic resonance cholangiopancreatography (MRCP) has largely replaced endoscopic retrograde cholangiopancreatography (ERCP) in the evaluation of obstructive jaundice since it produces comparable images of the biliary tree and pancreas, providing information that complements that obtained from CT and EUS.

Endoscopic retrograde cholangiopancreatography

Using a side-viewing duodenoscope, it is possible to cannulate the main pancreatic duct and common bile duct. ERCP is used mainly in the treatment of a range of biliary and pancreatic diseases that have been identified by other imaging techniques such as MRCP, EUS and CT. Indications for and risks of ERCP are listed in Box 23.10.

▍ Histology

Biopsy material obtained endoscopically or percutaneously can provide useful information (Box 23.11).

Tests of infection

▍ Bacterial cultures

Stool cultures are essential in the investigation of diarrhoea, especially when it is acute or bloody, in order to identify pathogenic organisms (see Ch. 13).

▍ Serology

Detection of antibodies plays a limited role in the diagnosis of gastrointestinal infection caused by organisms such as *Helicobacter pylori*, *Salmonella* species and *Entamoeba histolytica*.

▍ Breath tests

Non-invasive breath tests for *H. pylori* infection are discussed on page 814 and breath tests for suspected small intestinal bacterial overgrowth on page 822.

Tests of function

A number of dynamic tests can be used to investigate aspects of gut function, including digestion, absorption, inflammation and epithelial permeability. Some of the more common ones are listed in Box 23.12. In the assessment of suspected malabsorption, blood tests (full blood count, erythrocyte sedimentation rate (ESR)), and measurement of C-reactive protein (CRP), folate, vitamin B$_{12}$, iron status, albumin, calcium and phosphate) are essential, and endoscopy is undertaken to obtain mucosal biopsies. Faecal calprotectin is very sensitive at detecting mucosal inflammation.

23

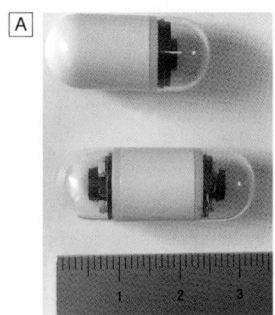
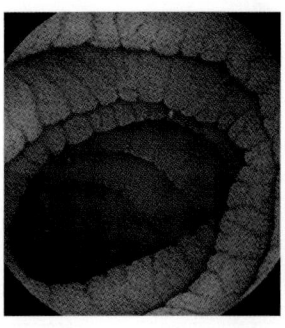

Fig. 23.15 Wireless capsule endoscopy. A Examples of capsules. B Capsule endoscopy image of scalloping of the small bowel suggestive of coeliac disease.

 23.7 Wireless capsule endoscopy

Indications

- Obscure gastrointestinal bleeding
- Small bowel Crohn's disease
- Assessment of coeliac disease and its complications
- Screening and surveillance in familial polyposis syndromes

Contraindications

- Known or suspected small bowel stricture (risk of capsule retention)
- Caution in people with pacemakers or implantable defibrillators

Complications

- Capsule retention (< 1%)

 23.8 Double balloon enteroscopy

Indications

Diagnostic
- Obscure gastrointestinal bleeding
- Malabsorption or unexplained diarrhoea
- Suspicious radiological findings
- Suspected small bowel tumour
- Surveillance of polyposis syndromes

Therapeutic
- Coagulation/diathermy of bleeding lesions
- Jejunostomy placement

Contraindications
- As for upper gastrointestinal endoscopy

Complications

- As for upper gastrointestinal endoscopy
- Post-procedure abdominal pain (≤ 20%)
- Pancreatitis (1%–3%)
- Perforation (especially after resection of large polyps)

Oesophageal motility

A barium swallow can give useful information about oesophageal motility. Videofluoroscopy, with joint assessment by a speech and language therapist and a radiologist, may be necessary in difficult cases. High resolution oesophageal manometry (see Fig. 23.1), often in conjunction with 24-hour pH measurements, is of value in diagnosing cases of refractory gastro-oesophageal reflux, achalasia and non-cardiac chest pain. Oesophageal impedance testing is useful for detecting non-acid or gas reflux events, especially in patients with atypical symptoms or those who respond poorly to acid suppression.

 23.9 Colonoscopy

Indications*

- Suspected inflammatory bowel disease
- Chronic diarrhoea
- Altered bowel habit
- Rectal bleeding or iron deficiency anaemia
- Assessment of abnormal CT colonogram or barium enema
- Colorectal cancer screening
- Colorectal adenoma and carcinoma follow-up
- Therapeutic procedures, including endoscopic resection, dilatation of strictures, laser, stent insertion and argon plasma coagulation

Contraindications

- Acute severe ulcerative colitis (unprepared flexible sigmoidoscopy is preferred)
- As for upper gastrointestinal endoscopy

Complications

- Cardiorespiratory depression due to sedation
- Perforation
- Bleeding following polypectomy

*Colonoscopy is not useful in the investigation of constipation.
(CT = computed tomography)

 23.10 Endoscopic retrograde cholangiopancreatography (ERCP)

Indications

Diagnostic
- Biliary or pancreatic disease where other imaging is equivocal or contraindicated
- Ampullary biopsy or biliary cytology

Therapeutic
- Biliary disease:
  Removal of common bile duct calculi*
  Palliation of malignant biliary obstruction
  Management of biliary leaks/damage complicating surgery
  Dilatation of benign strictures
  Primary sclerosing cholangitis
- Pancreatic disease:
  Drainage of pancreatic pseudocysts and fistulae
  Removal of pancreatic calculi (selected cases)

Contraindications

- Severe cardiopulmonary comorbidity
- Coagulopathy

Complications

- Occur in 5%–10% with a 30-day mortality of 0.5%–1%

General
- As for upper endoscopy

Specific
- Biliary disease:
  Bleeding following sphincterotomy
  Cholangitis (if biliary obstruction is not relieved by ERCP)
  Gallstone impaction
- Pancreatic disease:
  Acute pancreatitis
  Infection of pseudocyst

*Laparoscopic surgery is preferred in fit individuals who also require cholecystectomy.

 23.11 Reasons for biopsy or cytological examination

- Suspected malignant lesions
- Assessment of mucosal abnormalities
- Diagnosis of infection (*Candida, Helicobacter pylori, Giardia lamblia*)
- Analysis of genetic mutations

i	23.12	Tests of gastrointestinal function		
Process	Test	Principle		Comments
Absorption Lactose	Lactose H_2 breath test	Measurement of breath H_2 content after 50 g oral lactose. Undigested sugar is metabolised by colonic bacteria in hypolactasia and expired hydrogen is measured		Non-invasive and accurate. May provoke pain and diarrhoea in sufferers
Fructose	Fructose H_2 breath test	Measurement of breath H_2 content after 25–50 g oral fructose. Unabsorbed fructose is fermented by colonic bacteria with expired hydrogen measured		Results can be difficult to interpret as breath testing does not reflect fructose ingestion in everyday life
Bile acids	^{75}SeHCAT test Serum 7α-hydroxycholestenone	Isotopic quantification of 7-day whole-body retention of oral dose ^{75}Se-labelled homocholyltaurine (>15% = normal, 5%–15% borderline, < 5% = abnormal) Intermediate metabolite of the bile acid synthetic pathway. Serum levels indicate activity of the pathway and are elevated in bile acid diarrhoea		Accurate and specific but requires two visits and involves radiation. Results can be equivocal. Serum 7α-hydroxycholestenone is almost as sensitive and specific Simple test to perform and only marginally less sensitive and specific than ^{75}SeHCAT test
Pancreatic exocrine function	Faecal elastase	Immunoassay of pancreatic enzymes on stool sample		Simple, quick and avoids urine collection. Does not detect mild disease
Mucosal inflammation/ permeability	Faecal calprotectin or lactoferrin	Proteins secreted non-specifically by neutrophils into the colon in response to inflammation or neoplasia		Useful screening test for gastrointestinal inflammation and for monitoring patients with Crohn's disease and ulcerative colitis. Poor sensitivity for cancer

(^{75}SeHCAT = ^{75}Se-homocholic acid taurine)

Gastric emptying

This involves administering a test meal containing solids and liquids labelled with different radioisotopes and measuring the amount retained in the stomach afterwards (Box 23.13). It is useful in the investigation of suspected delayed gastric emptying (gastroparesis), when other studies are normal.

Colonic and anorectal motility

A plain abdominal X-ray taken on day 5 after ingestion of different-shaped inert plastic pellets on days 1–3 gives an estimate of whole-gut transit time. The test is useful in the evaluation of chronic constipation, when the position of any retained pellets can be observed, and helps to differentiate cases of slow transit from those due to dyssynergic defecation. The mechanism of defecation and anorectal function can be assessed by anorectal manometry, electrophysiological tests and defecating proctography.

Radioisotope tests

Many different radioisotope tests are used (Boxes 23.12 and 23.13). In some, structural information is obtained, such as the localisation of a Meckel's diverticulum. Others provide functional information, such as the rate of gastric emptying or ability to reabsorb bile acids. Others are tests of infection and rely on the presence of bacteria to hydrolyse a radio-labelled test substance followed by detection of the radioisotope in expired air, such as the urea breath test for *H. pylori*.

Gut hormone testing

Excess gut hormone secretion by some gastrointestinal and pancreatic neuro-endocrine tumours can be assessed by measuring levels in blood. Commonly measured hormones include gastrin, somatostatin, vasoactive intestinal polypeptide (VIP) and pancreatic polypeptide.

Presenting problems in gastrointestinal disease

Dysphagia

Dysphagia is defined as difficulty in swallowing. It may coexist with heartburn or vomiting but should be distinguished from both globus sensation

i	23.13	Tests involving radioisotopes	
Test	Isotope		Major uses and principle of test
Gastric emptying study	^{99m}Tc-sulphur ^{111}In-DTPA		Assessment of gastric emptying, particularly for possible gastroparesis
Urea breath test	^{13}C-urea		Non-invasive diagnosis of *Helicobacter pylori*. Bacterial urease enzyme splits urea to ammonia and CO_2, which is detected in expired air
Meckel's scan	^{99m}Tc-pertechnetate		Diagnosis of Meckel's diverticulum in cases of obscure gastrointestinal bleeding. Isotope is injected intravenously and localises in ectopic parietal mucosa within diverticulum
Somatostatin receptor scintigraphy (SRS)	^{111}In-DTPA-octreotide ^{99m}Tc-tektrotyd		Staging neuro-endocrine tumours. Labelled somatostatin analogues bind to cell surface somatostatin receptors on neuro-endocrine cancer cells
Positron emission tomography-CT (PET-CT)	^{18}F-FDG ^{68}Ga-labelled somatostatin analogue		Staging high-grade cancers More sensitive and specific than SRS for staging neuro-endocrine tumours

(C = carbon; DTPA = diethylenetriaminepentaacetic acid; FDG = fluorodeoxyglucose; In = indium; Tc = technetium)

(in which anxious people feel a lump in the throat without organic cause) and odynophagia (pain during swallowing, usually from gastro-oesophageal reflux or candidiasis).

Dysphagia can occur due to problems in the oropharynx or oesophagus (Fig. 23.16). Oropharyngeal disorders affect the initiation of swallowing at the pharynx and upper oesophageal sphincter. The patient has difficulty initiating swallowing and complains of choking, nasal regurgitation or tracheal aspiration. Drooling, dysarthria, hoarseness and cranial nerve or other neurological signs may be present. Oesophageal disorders cause dysphagia by obstructing the lumen or by affecting motility. Patients with oesophageal disease complain of food 'sticking' after

23

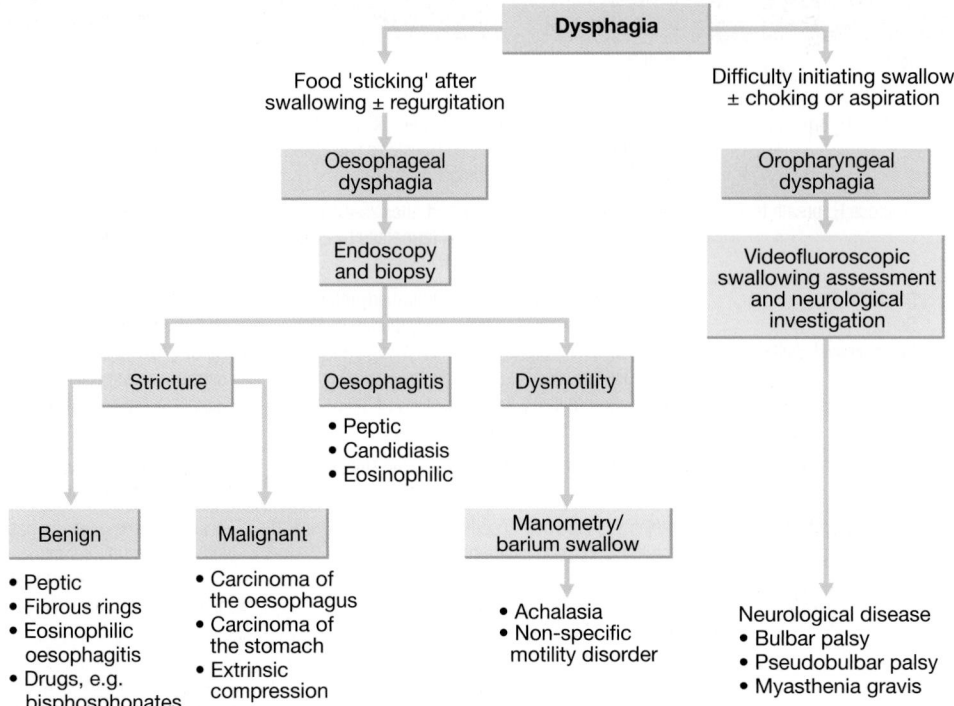

Fig. 23.16 Investigation of dysphagia.

swallowing, although the level at which this is felt correlates poorly with the true site of obstruction. Swallowing of liquids is normal until strictures become extreme.

Investigations

Dysphagia should always be investigated urgently. Endoscopy is the investigation of choice because it allows biopsy and dilatation of strictures. Even if the appearances are normal, biopsies should be taken to look for eosinophilic oesophagitis. If no abnormality is found, then barium swallow with videofluoroscopic swallowing assessment can be used to detect major motility disorders. In some cases, high-resolution oesophageal manometry is required, allowing accurate classification of abnormalities. Figure 23.16 summarises a diagnostic approach to dysphagia and lists the major causes.

Dyspepsia

Dyspepsia describes symptoms such as discomfort, bloating and nausea, which are thought to originate from the upper gastrointestinal tract. There are many causes (Box 23.14), including some arising outside the digestive system. Heartburn and other 'reflux' symptoms are separate entities and are considered elsewhere. Although symptoms often correlate poorly with the underlying diagnosis, a careful history is important to detect 'alarm' features requiring urgent investigation (Box 23.15) and to detect atypical symptoms that might be due to problems outside the gastrointestinal tract.

Dyspepsia affects up to 80% of the population at some time in life and most patients have no serious underlying disease. People who present with new dyspepsia at an age of more than 55 years and younger patients unresponsive to empirical treatment require investigation to exclude serious disease. An algorithm for the investigation of dyspepsia is outlined in Figure 23.17.

Heartburn and regurgitation

Heartburn describes retrosternal, burning discomfort, often rising up into the chest and sometimes accompanied by regurgitation of acidic or bitter fluid into the throat. These symptoms often occur after meals, on lying down or with bending, straining or heavy lifting. They are classical

i	**23.14 Causes of dyspepsia**

Upper gastrointestinal disorders

- Peptic ulcer disease
- Acute gastritis
- Gallstones
- Oesophageal spasm
- Non-ulcer dyspepsia
- Irritable bowel syndrome

Other gastrointestinal disorders

- Pancreatic disease (cancer, chronic pancreatitis)
- Colonic carcinoma
- Hepatic disease (hepatitis, metastases)

Systemic disease

- Renal failure
- Hypercalcaemia

Drugs

- Non-steroidal anti-inflammatory drugs (NSAIDs)
- Glucocorticoids
- Iron and potassium supplements
- Digoxin

Others

- Psychological (anxiety, depression)
- Alcohol

i	**23.15 Alarm features in dyspepsia**

- Unintentional weight loss
- Anaemia
- Persistent vomiting
- Haematemesis and/or melaena
- Dysphagia
- Palpable abdominal mass

symptoms of gastro-oesophageal reflux but up to 50% of patients present with other symptoms, such as chest pain, belching, halitosis, chronic cough or sore throats. In young patients with typical symptoms and a good response to dietary changes, antacids or acid suppression investigation is not required, but patients aged over 55 years and those with alarm symptoms or atypical features need urgent endoscopy.

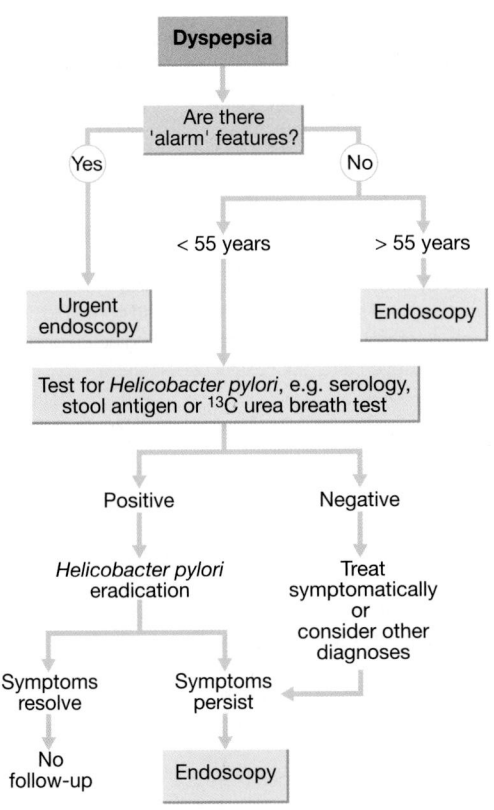

Fig. 23.17 **Investigation of dyspepsia.**

Vomiting

Vomiting is a complex reflex involving both autonomic and somatic neural pathways. Synchronous contraction of the diaphragm, intercostal muscles and abdominal muscles raises intra-abdominal pressure and, combined with relaxation of the lower oesophageal sphincter, results in forcible ejection of gastric contents. It is important to distinguish true vomiting from regurgitation and to elicit whether the vomiting is acute or chronic (recurrent), as the underlying causes may differ. The major causes are shown in Figure 23.18.

Gastrointestinal bleeding

Acute upper gastrointestinal bleeding

This is the most common gastrointestinal emergency, with an estimated incidence of 134 per 100 000 of the population in the UK; the mortality of patients admitted to hospital is around 10%. Risk scoring systems have been developed to stratify the risk of needing endoscopic therapy or of having a poor outcome (Box 23.16). The advantage of the Blatchford score is that it may be used before endoscopy to predict the need for intervention to treat bleeding. Low scores (2 or less) are associated with a very low risk of adverse outcome. The common causes are shown in Figure 23.19.

Clinical assessment

Haematemesis is red with clots when bleeding is rapid and profuse, or black ('coffee grounds') when less severe. Syncope may occur and is caused by hypotension from intravascular volume depletion. Symptoms of anaemia suggest chronic bleeding. Melaena is the passage of black, tarry stools containing altered blood; it is usually caused by bleeding from the upper gastrointestinal tract, although haemorrhage from the right side of the colon is occasionally responsible. The characteristic colour and smell are the result of the action of digestive enzymes and of bacteria on haemoglobin. Severe acute upper gastrointestinal bleeding can sometimes cause maroon or bright red stool.

Management

The principles of emergency management of non-variceal bleeding are discussed in detail below. Management of variceal bleeding is discussed on page 882.

1. Intravenous access

The first step is to gain intravenous access, ideally using two large-bore cannulae.

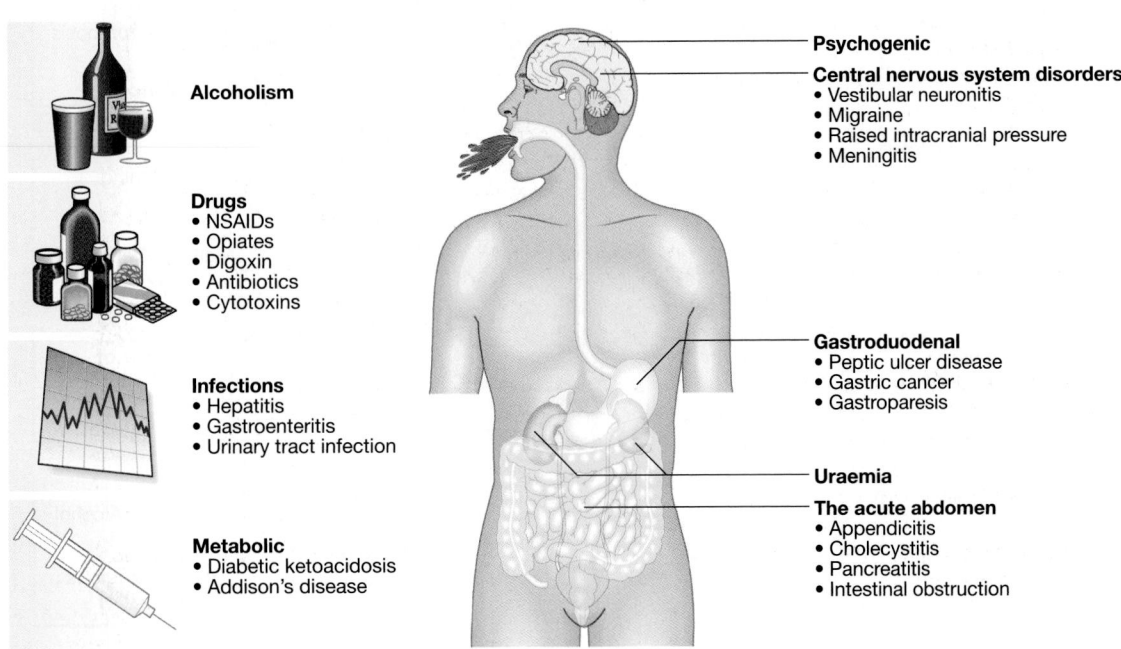

Fig. 23.18 **Causes of vomiting.** (NSAIDs = non-steroidal anti-inflammatory drugs)

i 23.16 Modified Blatchford score: risk stratification in acute upper gastrointestinal bleeding

Admission risk marker	Score component value
Blood urea	
≥ 25 mmol/L (70 mg/dL)	6
10–25 mmol/L (28–70 mg/dL)	4
8–10 mmol/L (22.4–28 mg/dL)	3
6.5–8 mmol/L (18.2–22.4 mg/dL)	2
< 6.5 mmol/L (18.2 mg/dL)	0
Haemoglobin for men	
< 100 g/L (10 g/dL)	6
100–119 g/L (10–11.9 g/dL)	3
120–129 g/L (12–12.9 g/dL)	1
≥ 130 g/L (13 g/dL)	0
Haemoglobin for women	
< 100 g/L (10 g/dL)	6
100–119 g/L (10–11.9 g/dL)	1
≥ 120 g/L (12 g/dL)	0
Systolic blood pressure	
< 90 mmHg	3
90–99 mmHg	2
100–109 mmHg	1
> 109 mmHg	0
Other markers	
Presentation with syncope	2
Hepatic disease	2
Cardiac failure	2
Pulse ≥ 100 beats/min	1
Presentation with melaena	1
None of the above	0

2. Initial clinical assessment

- *Define circulatory status.* Severe bleeding causes tachycardia, hypotension and oliguria. The patient is cold and sweating, and may be agitated.
- *Seek evidence of liver disease* (p. 860). Jaundice, cutaneous stigmata, hepatosplenomegaly and ascites may be present in decompensated cirrhosis.
- *Identify comorbidity.* The presence of cardiorespiratory, cerebrovascular or renal disease is important, both because these may be worsened by acute bleeding and because they increase the hazards of endoscopy and surgical operations. These comorbidities are, therefore, a common cause of death following acute gastrointestinal haemorrhage, even after successful haemostasis.

3. Basic investigations

- *Full blood count.* Chronic or subacute bleeding leads to anaemia, but the haemoglobin concentration may be normal after sudden, major bleeding until haemodilution occurs. Thrombocytopenia may be a clue to the presence of hypersplenism in chronic liver disease.
- *Urea and electrolytes.* This test may show evidence of renal failure. The blood urea rises as the absorbed products of luminal blood are metabolised by the liver; an elevated blood urea with normal creatinine concentration implies severe bleeding.
- *Liver function tests.* These may show evidence of chronic liver disease.
- *Prothrombin time.* Check when there is a clinical suggestion of liver disease or patients are anticoagulated.
- *Cross-matching.* At least 2 units of blood should be cross-matched if a significant bleed is suspected.

4. Resuscitation

Intravenous crystalloid fluids should be given to raise the blood pressure, with a 500 ml bolus recommended over less than 15 minutes in haemodynamically unstable patients. In most patients, blood should be transfused when haemoglobin is less than 70 g/L, although transfusion should be considered at higher levels in those with haemodynamic instability or ischaemic heart disease.

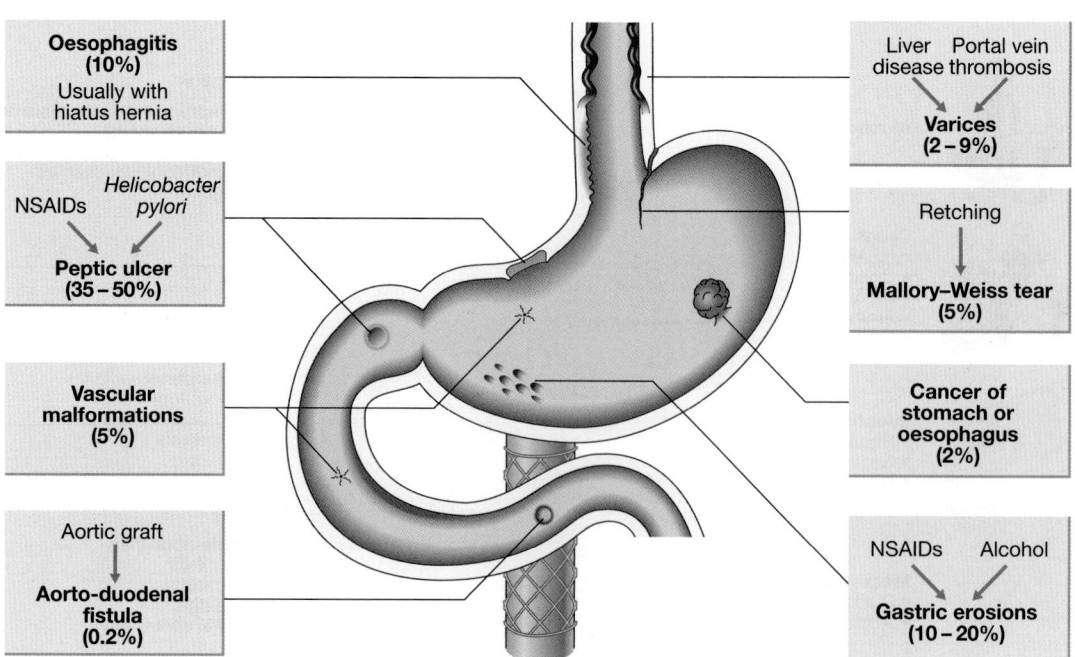

Fig. 23.19 Causes of acute upper gastrointestinal haemorrhage. Frequency is given in parentheses. (NSAIDs = non-steroidal anti-inflammatory drugs)

5. Oxygen

Oxygen saturations should be monitored with pulse oximetry, with a target saturation of 94%–98% and oxygen prescribed as required.

6. Antithrombotic drugs

An increasing number of individuals present with an upper gastrointestinal bleed while using antithrombotic medication. Aspirin can be continued during an upper gastrointestinal bleed. P2Y12-receptor antagonists (e.g. clopidogrel) should be temporarily stopped (unless prescribed following coronary artery stenting), as well as warfarin and direct oral anticoagulant therapy. However, early reintroduction of these medications should occur after haemostasis has been achieved to reduce thrombotic events and death.

7. Proton pump inhibitor (PPI) therapy

Intravenous PPI infusion should be given in non-variceal bleeding, in individuals who have a high-risk ulcer post endoscopy (e.g. ulcers with a clot and/or requiring endoscopic haemostasis). PPIs work by reducing gastric acid secretion, neutralising intragastric pH, promoting clot stability by reducing pepsin-induced clot lysis and increasing platelet aggregation. While intravenous PPI infusion is most frequently used, intermittent intravenous PPI and oral high-dose PPI can be considered as alternatives. Box 23.17 outlines some common PPIs used.

i 23.17 Common proton pump inhibitors (PPIs) and dosage for peptic ulcer disease		
Oral administration		
	Standard dose	High dose
Lansoprazole	30 mg OD	30 mg BD
Omeprazole	20 mg OD	40 mg OD
Pantoprazole	40 mg OD	40 mg BD
Rabeprazole	20 mg OD	20 mg BD
Esomeprazole	20 mg OD	40 mg OD
Intravenous infusion		
	Dose	
Omeprazole Pantoprazole Esomeprazole	80 mg IV bolus, followed by 8 mg/hr for 72 hrs	
(BD = twice daily; IV = intravenous; OD = once daily)		

8. Endoscopy

This should be carried out after adequate resuscitation, ideally within 24 hours; it yields a diagnosis in approximately 80% of cases. Patients with major endoscopic stigmata of recent haemorrhage (Fig. 23.20) can be treated endoscopically using a thermal or mechanical modality, such as a 'heater probe' or endoscopic clips, combined with injection of dilute adrenaline (epinephrine) into the bleeding point ('dual therapy'). A biologically inert haemostatic mineral powder (TC325, 'haemospray') can be used as rescue therapy when standard therapy fails. This may stop active bleeding and combined with PPI therapy may prevent rebleeding, thus avoiding the need for surgery. Newer techniques, such as 'over-the-scope clips', may also be used as a rescue therapy when standard therapy fails, treating large vessels or fibrotic lesions. Patients found to have bled from varices should be treated by band ligation (p. 883); balloon tamponade is another option if this fails, while arrangements are made for a transjugular intrahepatic portosystemic shunt (TIPSS). Balloon tamponade can be associated with serious complications, and newer techniques, such as removable, self-expanding, covered metal oesophageal stents may be used as an alternative option.

9. Monitoring

Patients should be closely observed, with hourly measurements of pulse, blood pressure, oxygen saturations and urine output.

10. Radiology and surgery

Patients who have recurrent bleeding, where endoscopic attempts at haemostasis have failed, should be considered for radiological or surgical intervention. If available, angiographic control of bleeding is generally preferred to surgery in older, frail patients. If surgery is required, the choice of operation depends on the site and diagnosis of the bleeding lesion. Duodenal ulcers are treated by under-running, with or without pyloroplasty. Under-running for gastric ulcers can also be carried out (a biopsy must be taken to exclude carcinoma). Local excision may be performed, but when neither is possible, partial gastrectomy is required.

11. Eradication

Following treatment for ulcer bleeding, all patients should avoid non-steroidal anti-inflammatory drugs (NSAIDs) and those who test positive for *H. pylori* infection should receive eradication therapy (p. 814). Successful eradication should be confirmed by urea breath or faecal antigen testing.

23

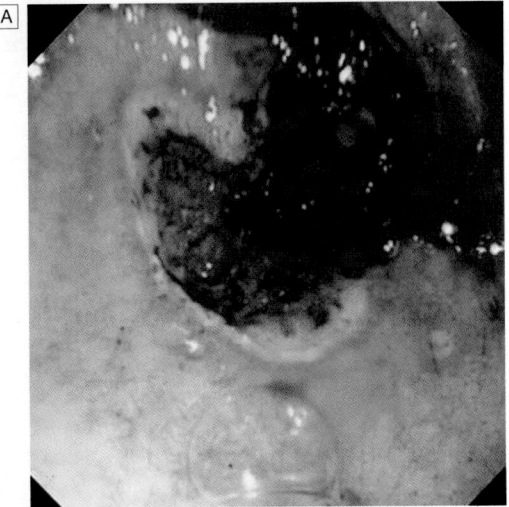 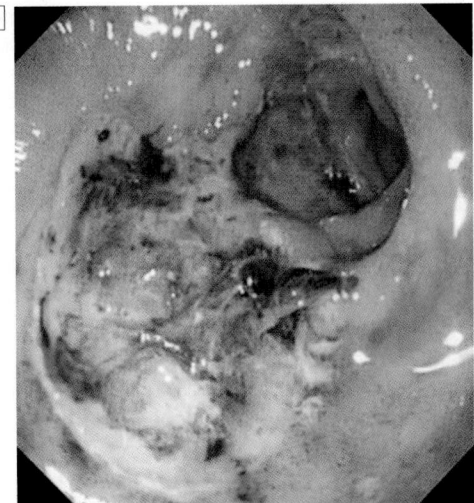

Fig. 23.20 Major stigmata of recent haemorrhage and endoscopic treatment. [A] Active bleeding from a duodenal ulcer. [B] Haemostasis is achieved after endoscopic injection of adrenaline (epinephrine) and application of a heater probe.

Lower gastrointestinal bleeding

The incidence of lower gastrointestinal bleeding is around 30–90 per 100 000 of the population in the UK, with an in-hospital mortality of around 4%. This may be caused by haemorrhage from the colon, anal canal or small bowel. It is useful to distinguish those patients who present with profuse, acute bleeding from those who present with chronic or subacute bleeding of lesser severity (see Box 23.18).

Severe acute lower gastrointestinal bleeding

This presents with profuse red or maroon diarrhoea and with hypovolaemic shock. If available, CT angiography should be performed initially to localise the site of blood loss. If the bleeding source is identified, then catheter angiography with embolisation should be performed. If no source of bleeding is found then a colonoscopy should be performed. Some patients presenting with an apparent severe lower GI bleed are ultimately found to have a significant upper GI bleed.

The commonest cause of lower GI bleeding is diverticular disease, with up to two-thirds of cases being classified as severe. Bleeding from diverticular disease is often due to erosion of an artery within the mouth of a diverticulum. Multiple endoscopic options are available, with endoscopic clipping either alone or after the injection of dilute adrenaline (epinephrine) considered as first-line treatment in the UK. Angiodysplasia is a disease of older adults, in which vascular malformations develop within the GI tract, commonly in the caecum. Bleeding can be acute and profuse; it usually stops spontaneously, but commonly recurs. Diagnosis is often difficult. Colonoscopy may reveal characteristic vascular spots and, in the acute phase, angiography can show bleeding into the intestinal lumen and an abnormal large, draining vein. The treatment of choice is endoscopic thermal ablation, but resection of the affected bowel may be required if bleeding continues. Bowel ischaemia due to occlusion of the inferior mesenteric artery can present with abdominal colic and rectal bleeding. It should be considered in patients (particularly older patients) who have evidence of generalised atherosclerosis. The diagnosis is made at colonoscopy. Resection is required only in the presence of peritonitis. Meckel's diverticulum with ectopic gastric epithelium may ulcerate and erode into a major artery. The diagnosis should be considered in children or adolescents who present with profuse or recurrent lower gastrointestinal bleeding. A Meckel's ^{99m}Tc-pertechnetate scan is sometimes positive, but the diagnosis is commonly made only by laparotomy, at which time the diverticulum is excised.

Subacute or chronic lower gastrointestinal bleeding

This can occur at all ages and is usually due to haemorrhoids or anal fissure. Haemorrhoidal bleeding is bright red and occurs during or after defecation. Proctoscopy can be used to make the diagnosis, but individuals who have altered bowel habit and those who present over the age of 40 years should undergo colonoscopy to exclude coexisting colorectal cancer. Anal fissure should be suspected when fresh rectal bleeding and anal pain occur during defecation.

i	23.18 Causes of lower gastrointestinal bleeding
Severe acute	
• Diverticular disease	• Meckel's diverticulum
• Angiodysplasia	• Inflammatory bowel disease (rarely)
• Ischaemia	
Moderate, chronic/subacute	
• Fissure	• Large polyps
• Haemorrhoids	• Angiodysplasia
• Inflammatory bowel disease	• Radiation enteritis
• Carcinoma	• Solitary rectal ulcer

Major gastrointestinal bleeding of unknown cause

In some patients who present with major gastrointestinal bleeding, upper endoscopy, colonoscopy and CT angiography may fail to reveal a diagnosis. Wireless capsule endoscopy is increasingly used in such patients. The diagnostic yield is highest when performed as close as possible to the bleeding episode, particularly within the first 48 hours of presenting with bleeding. Wireless capsule endoscopy is often used to define a source of bleeding prior to enteroscopy (Fig. 23.21), with push or double balloon enteroscopy being used to visualise the small intestine and treat the bleeding source. When all else fails, laparotomy with on-table endoscopy is indicated.

Chronic occult gastrointestinal bleeding

In this context, occult means that blood or its breakdown products are present in the stool but cannot be seen by the naked eye. Occult bleeding may reach 200 mL per day and cause iron deficiency anaemia. Any cause of gastrointestinal bleeding may be responsible, but the most important is colorectal cancer, particularly carcinoma of the caecum, which may produce no gastrointestinal symptoms. In clinical practice, investigation of the upper and lower gastrointestinal tract should be considered whenever a patient presents with unexplained iron deficiency anaemia.

Diarrhoea

Diarrhoea is defined as the passage of three or more loose or liquid stools per day. Stool weight was previously used to define diarrhoea (> 200 g stool per day), but is no longer recommended as normal stool volumes can exceed this value. The most severe symptom in many patients is urgency of defecation, while faecal incontinence can occur in acute and chronic diarrhoeal illnesses.

Acute diarrhoea

This is extremely common and is usually caused by faecal–oral transmission of bacteria or their toxins, viruses or parasites (see Ch. 13). Infective diarrhoea is usually short-lived and patients who present with a history of diarrhoea lasting more than 10 days rarely have an infective cause. A variety of drugs, including antibiotics, cytotoxic drugs, PPIs and NSAIDs, may be responsible.

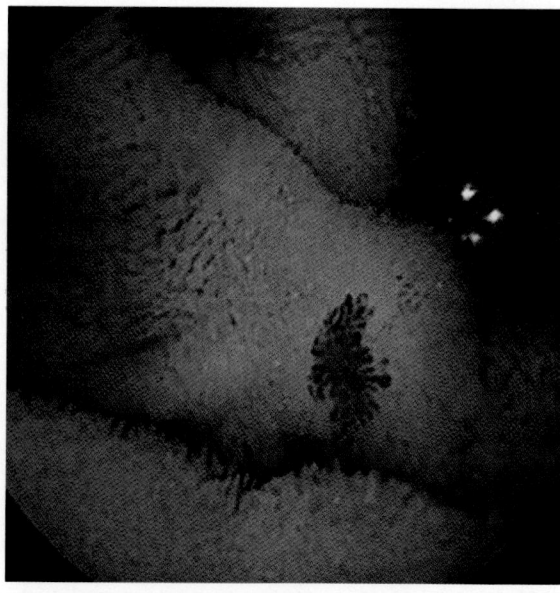

Fig. 23.21 Angiodysplastic lesion noted on capsule endoscopy.

	23.19 Chronic or relapsing diarrhoea		
	Colonic	**Malabsorption**	**Small bowel**
Clinical features	Blood and mucus in stool Cramping lower abdominal pain	Steatorrhoea Undigested food in the stool Weight loss and nutritional disturbances	Large-volume, watery stool Abdominal bloating Cramping mid-abdominal pain

Some causes	Inflammatory bowel disease
	Microscopic colitis
	Neoplasia
	Ischaemia
	Irritable bowel syndrome
		Pancreatic:
		  Chronic pancreatitis
		  Cancer of pancreas
		  Cystic fibrosis
		Enteropathy:
		  Coeliac disease
		  Tropical sprue
		  Lymphoma
		  Lymphangiectasia
			Crohn's disease
			Neuro-endocrine tumour
			Small bowel carcinoid
			VIPoma
			Drug-induced:
			  NSAIDs
			  Aminosalicylates
			  SSRIs

Investigations	Faecal calprotectin Ileocolonoscopy with biopsies	Faecal elastase Ultrasound, CT and MRCP Small bowel biopsy Barium follow-through or small bowel MRI	Faecal calprotectin Stool volume Serum gut hormone profile and 24 hr urine 5HIAA Barium follow-through or small bowel MRI

(CT = computed tomography; 5HIAA = 5-hydroxyindoleacetic acid; MRCP = magnetic resonance cholangiopancreatography; MRI = magnetic resonance imaging; NSAIDs = non-steroidal anti-inflammatory drugs; SSRIs = selective serotonin re-uptake inhibitors; VIP = vasoactive intestinal polypeptide)

Chronic or relapsing diarrhoea

Chronic diarrhoea can be categorised as being caused by disease of the colon or small bowel, or due to malabsorption (Box 23.19). Clinical presentation, examination of the stool, routine blood tests and imaging reveal a diagnosis in many cases. Young patients (< 40 years) with typical symptoms of a functional bowel disorder, with negative initial investigations, may have a diagnosis of irritable bowel syndrome (p. 847).

Malabsorption

Diarrhoea and weight loss in patients with a normal diet are likely to be caused by malabsorption. The symptoms are diverse in nature and variable in severity. A few patients have apparently normal bowel habit, but diarrhoea usually occurs and may be watery and voluminous. Bulky, pale and offensive stools that float in the toilet (steatorrhoea) signify fat malabsorption. Abdominal distension, borborygmi, cramps, weight loss and undigested food in the stool may be present. Some patients complain only of malaise and lethargy. In others, symptoms related to deficiencies of specific vitamins, trace elements and minerals may occur (Fig. 23.22).

Pathophysiology

Malabsorption results from abnormalities of the three processes that are essential to normal digestion:

- *Intraluminal maldigestion* occurs when deficiency of bile or pancreatic enzymes results in inadequate solubilisation and hydrolysis of nutrients. Fat and protein malabsorption results. This may also occur with small bowel bacterial overgrowth.
- *Mucosal malabsorption* results from small bowel resection or conditions that damage the small intestinal epithelium, thereby diminishing the surface area for absorption and depleting brush border enzyme activity.
- *'Post-mucosal' lymphatic obstruction* prevents the uptake and transport of absorbed lipids into lymphatic vessels. Increased pressure in these vessels results in leakage into the intestinal lumen, leading to protein-losing enteropathy.

Investigations

Investigations should be performed both to confirm the presence of malabsorption and to determine the underlying cause. Routine blood tests may show one or more of the abnormalities listed in Box 23.20. Tests to confirm fat and protein malabsorption should be performed (see Box 23.12). An approach to the investigation of malabsorption is shown in Figure 23.23.

Weight loss

Weight loss may be physiological, due to dieting, exercise, starvation, or the decreased nutritional intake that accompanies old age. Weight loss of more than 5% of usual body weight over 6–12 months is clinically important and can indicate the presence of an underlying disease. Hospital and general practice weight records may be valuable in confirming that weight loss has occurred, as may reweighing patients at intervals; sometimes weight is regained or stabilises in those with no obvious cause. Pathological weight loss can be due to psychiatric illness, systemic disease, gastrointestinal causes or advanced disease of many organ systems (Fig. 23.24).

Physiological causes

Weight loss can occur in the absence of serious disease in healthy individuals who have changes in physical activity or social circumstances. It may be difficult to be sure of this diagnosis in older patients, when the dietary history may be unreliable, and professional help from a dietitian may be required.

Psychiatric illness

Features of anorexia nervosa, bulimia and affective disorders (see Ch. 31) may be apparent only after formal psychiatric input. Patients with alcohol dependence lose weight as a consequence of self-neglect and poor dietary intake. Depression may cause weight loss.

Systemic disease

Chronic infections, including tuberculosis (Ch. 17), recurrent urine or chest infections, and a range of parasitic and protozoan infections (Ch. 13), should be considered. A history of foreign travel, high-risk activities and specific features, such as fever, night sweats, rigors, productive cough and dysuria, must be sought. High-risk sexual activity and recreational drug misuse may suggest human immunodeficiency virus (HIV)-related illness (Ch. 14). Weight loss is a late feature of disseminated malignancy, but by the time the patient presents, other features of cancer are often present. Chronic inflammatory diseases, such as rheumatoid arthritis and polymyalgia rheumatica (Ch. 26), are often associated with weight loss.

Gastrointestinal disease

Almost any disease of the gastrointestinal tract can cause weight loss. Dysphagia and gastric outflow obstruction (p. 816) cause weight loss by

23

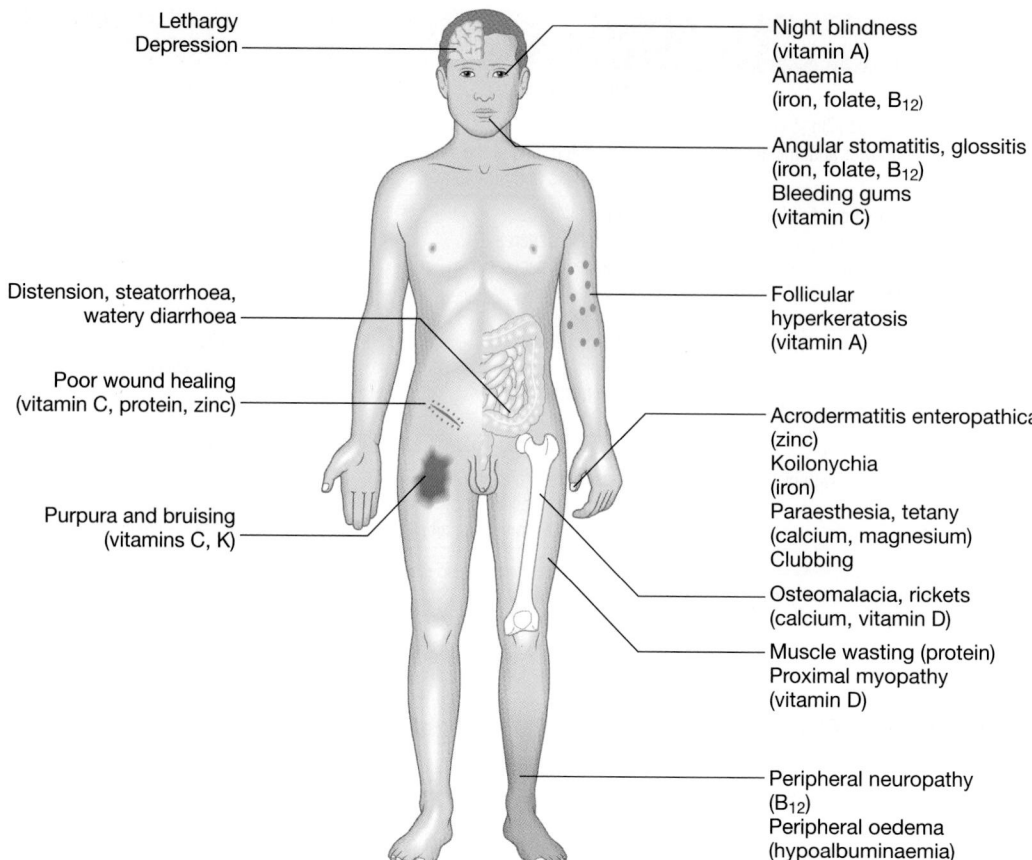

Lethargy
Depression

Distension, steatorrhoea,
watery diarrhoea

Poor wound healing
(vitamin C, protein, zinc)

Purpura and bruising
(vitamins C, K)

Night blindness
(vitamin A)
Anaemia
(iron, folate, B$_{12}$)

Angular stomatitis, glossitis
(iron, folate, B$_{12}$)
Bleeding gums
(vitamin C)

Follicular
hyperkeratosis
(vitamin A)

Acrodermatitis enteropathica
(zinc)
Koilonychia
(iron)
Paraesthesia, tetany
(calcium, magnesium)
Clubbing

Osteomalacia, rickets
(calcium, vitamin D)

Muscle wasting (protein)
Proximal myopathy
(vitamin D)

Peripheral neuropathy
(B$_{12}$)
Peripheral oedema
(hypoalbuminaemia)

Fig. 23.22 Possible physical consequences of malabsorption.

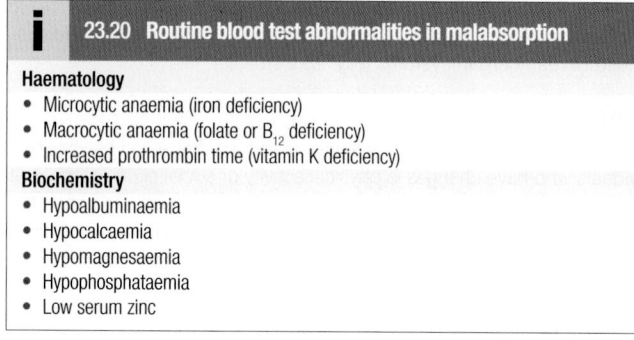

23.20 Routine blood test abnormalities in malabsorption

Haematology
- Microcytic anaemia (iron deficiency)
- Macrocytic anaemia (folate or B$_{12}$ deficiency)
- Increased prothrombin time (vitamin K deficiency)

Biochemistry
- Hypoalbuminaemia
- Hypocalcaemia
- Hypomagnesaemia
- Hypophosphataemia
- Low serum zinc

reducing food intake. Malignancy at any site may cause weight loss by mechanical obstruction, anorexia or cytokine-mediated systemic effects. Malabsorption from pancreatic diseases (p. 850) or small bowel causes may lead to profound weight loss with specific nutritional deficiencies (p. 766). Inflammatory diseases, such as Crohn's disease or ulcerative colitis (p. 835), cause anorexia, fear of eating and loss of protein, blood and nutrients from the gut.

Metabolic disorders and miscellaneous causes

Weight loss may occur in association with metabolic disorders, such as a new presentation of type 1 diabetes or thyrotoxicosis, as well as end-stage respiratory and cardiac disease.

Investigations

In cases where the cause of weight loss is not obvious after thorough history-taking and physical examination, or where an existing condition is considered unlikely, the following investigations are indicated: urinalysis for glucose, protein and blood; blood tests, including liver

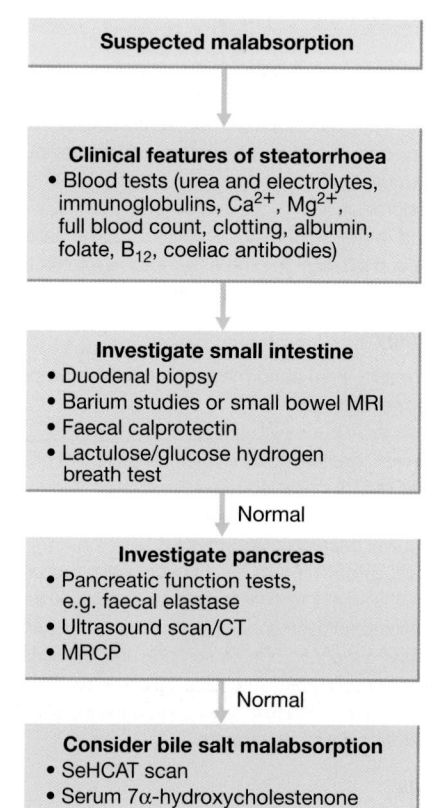

Suspected malabsorption

↓

Clinical features of steatorrhoea
- Blood tests (urea and electrolytes, immunoglobulins, Ca^{2+}, Mg^{2+}, full blood count, clotting, albumin, folate, B$_{12}$, coeliac antibodies)

↓

Investigate small intestine
- Duodenal biopsy
- Barium studies or small bowel MRI
- Faecal calprotectin
- Lactulose/glucose hydrogen breath test

↓ Normal

Investigate pancreas
- Pancreatic function tests, e.g. faecal elastase
- Ultrasound scan/CT
- MRCP

↓ Normal

Consider bile salt malabsorption
- SeHCAT scan
- Serum 7α-hydroxycholestenone

Fig. 23.23 Investigation for suspected malabsorption. (CT = computed tomography; MRCP = magnetic resonance cholangiopancreatography; MRI = magnetic resonance imaging; ^{75}SeHCAT = ^{75}Se-homocholic acid taurine)

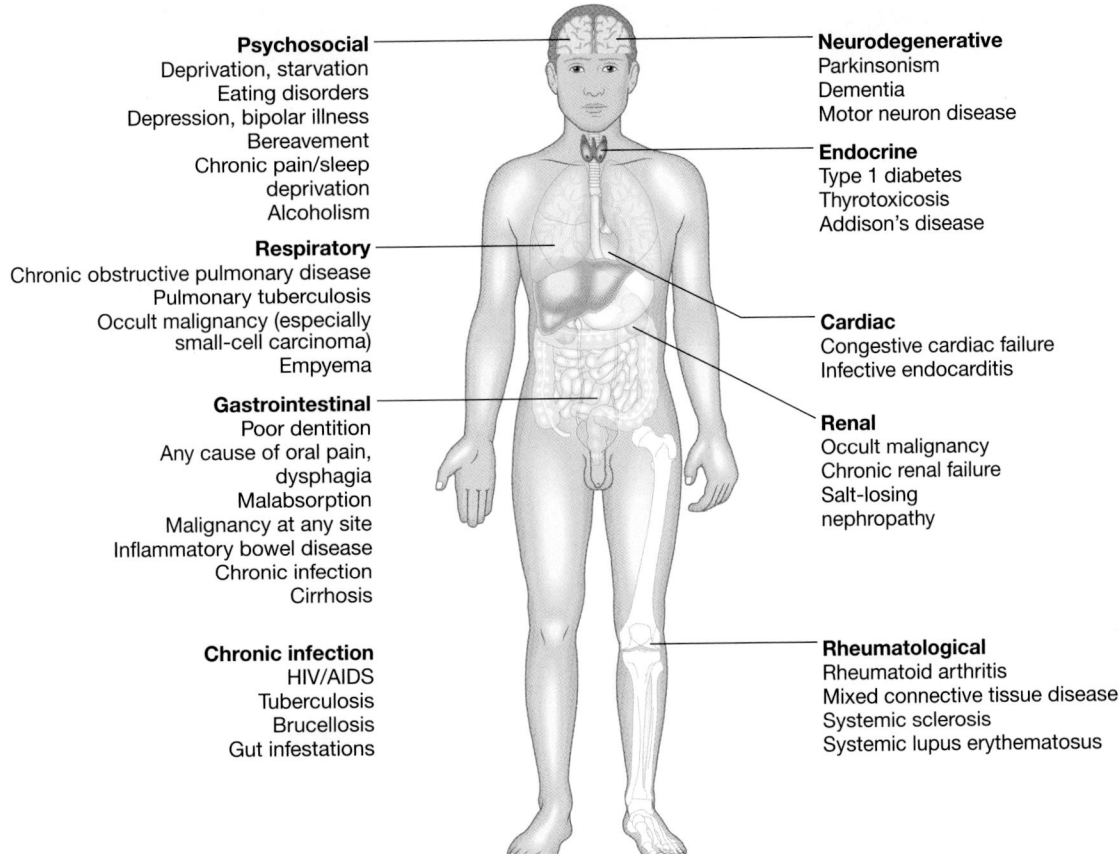

Psychosocial
Deprivation, starvation
Eating disorders
Depression, bipolar illness
Bereavement
Chronic pain/sleep
deprivation
Alcoholism

Respiratory
Chronic obstructive pulmonary disease
Pulmonary tuberculosis
Occult malignancy (especially
small-cell carcinoma)
Empyema

Gastrointestinal
Poor dentition
Any cause of oral pain,
dysphagia
Malabsorption
Malignancy at any site
Inflammatory bowel disease
Chronic infection
Cirrhosis

Chronic infection
HIV/AIDS
Tuberculosis
Brucellosis
Gut infestations

Neurodegenerative
Parkinsonism
Dementia
Motor neuron disease

Endocrine
Type 1 diabetes
Thyrotoxicosis
Addison's disease

Cardiac
Congestive cardiac failure
Infective endocarditis

Renal
Occult malignancy
Chronic renal failure
Salt-losing
nephropathy

Rheumatological
Rheumatoid arthritis
Mixed connective tissue disease
Systemic sclerosis
Systemic lupus erythematosus

Fig. 23.24 Some important causes of weight loss.

function tests, random blood glucose and thyroid function tests; CRP and ESR (may be raised in unsuspected infections, such as tuberculosis, connective tissue disorders and malignancy); and faecal calprotectin. Where the cause of weight loss is still unclear, chest X-ray, whole-body CT imaging and/or endoscopic investigation may be required. Rarely, tests such as bone marrow aspiration or liver biopsy may be necessary to identify conditions like cryptic miliary tuberculosis (Ch. 17). Before embarking on invasive or very costly investigations, it is always worth revisiting the patient's history and reweighing at intervals.

Constipation

Constipation is defined as infrequent passage of hard stools. Patients may also complain of straining, a sensation of incomplete evacuation and either perianal or abdominal discomfort. Constipation can be acute, typically lasting less than 1 week, or chronic, lasting greater than 4 weeks. Chronic constipation is normally due to a primary cause, such as dietary intake (e.g. insufficient fibre), lifestyle factors (e.g. sedentary lifestyle) or disorders of rectal evacuation.

Secondary causes of chronic constipation are numerous, including drugs such as opiates. Box 23.21 outlines causes of constipation.

Clinical assessment and management

The onset, duration and characteristics are important; for example, a neonatal onset suggests Hirschsprung's disease, while a recent change in bowel activity in middle age should raise the suspicion of an organic disorder, such as colonic carcinoma. The presence of rectal bleeding, pain and weight loss is important, as are excessive straining, symptoms suggestive of irritable bowel syndrome, a history of childhood constipation and emotional distress.

Careful examination contributes more to the diagnosis than extensive investigation. A search should be made for general medical disorders, as well as signs of intestinal obstruction. Neurological disorders, especially spinal cord lesions, should be sought. Perineal inspection and rectal examination are essential and may reveal abnormalities of the pelvic floor (abnormal descent, impaired sensation), anal canal or rectum (masses, faecal impaction, prolapse).

It is neither possible nor appropriate to investigate every person with constipation. For those with chronic constipation, investigation will usually proceed along the lines described below.

Initial investigations

A thorough history and physical examination should be performed. Careful digital rectal examination and inspection of the perineum is essential, and useful in the assessment of pelvic floor abnormalities. A full blood count, routine biochemistry, including serum calcium and thyroid function tests, should be carried out. If these are normal, then dietary and lifestyle modifications should be advised, such as increased fluid intake, dietary fibre supplementation and exercise. Laxatives should be commenced if individuals fail to respond. Organic causes should be explored using colonoscopy in individuals with concerning symptoms (e.g. rectal bleeding, pain or weight loss).

Further investigations

If no cause is found and disabling symptoms are present, then specialist referral for investigation of possible dysmotility may be necessary. The problem may be due to delayed transit of stool in the colon (slow transit constipation) or from functional abnormalities in the pelvic floor and anal sphincter muscles (dyssynergic defecation). Intestinal marker studies, anorectal manometry, electrophysiological studies and magnetic resonance proctography can all be used to define the problem.

23

i 23.21 Causes of constipation

Gastrointestinal causes

Dietary

• Lack of fibre and/or fluid intake

Motility

• Slow-transit constipation
• Irritable bowel syndrome
• Drugs (see below)

• Chronic intestinal pseudo-obstruction

Structural

• Colonic carcinoma
• Diverticular disease

• Hirschsprung's disease

Defecation

• Anorectal disease (Crohn's, fissures, haemorrhoids)

• Dyssynergic defecation

Non-gastrointestinal causes

Drugs

• Opiates
• Anticholinergics
• Calcium antagonists

• Iron supplements
• Aluminium-containing antacids

Neurological

• Multiple sclerosis
• Spinal cord lesions

• Cerebrovascular accidents
• Parkinsonism

Metabolic/endocrine

• Diabetes mellitus
• Hypercalcaemia

• Hypothyroidism
• Pregnancy

Others

• Any serious illness with immobility, especially in old age

• Depression

i 23.22 Extra-intestinal causes of chronic or recurrent abdominal pain

Retroperitoneal

• Aortic aneurysm
• Malignancy

• Lymphadenopathy
• Abscess

Psychogenic

• Depression
• Anxiety

• Hypochondriasis
• Somatisation

Locomotor

• Vertebral compression/fracture

• Abdominal muscle strain

Metabolic/endocrine

• Diabetes mellitus
• Acute intermittent porphyria

• Hypercalcaemia

Drugs/toxins

• Glucocorticoids
• Azathioprine

• Lead
• Alcohol

Haematological

• Sickle-cell disease

• Haemolytic disorders

Neurological

• Spinal cord lesions
• Tabes dorsalis

• Radiculopathy

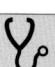 23.23 How to assess abdominal pain

• Duration
• Site and radiation
• Severity
• Precipitating and relieving factors (food, drugs, alcohol, posture, movement, defecation)
• Nature (colicky, constant, sharp or dull, wakes patient at night)
• Pattern (intermittent or continuous)
• Associated features (vomiting, dyspepsia, altered bowel habit)

Abdominal pain

There are four types of abdominal pain:

• *Visceral*. Gut organs are insensitive to stimuli such as burning and cutting but are sensitive to distension, contraction, twisting and stretching. Pain from unpaired structures is usually, but not always, felt in the midline.
• *Parietal*. The parietal peritoneum is innervated by somatic nerves and its involvement by inflammation, infection or neoplasia causes sharp, well-localised and lateralised pain.
• *Referred pain*. Gallbladder pain, for example, may be referred to the back or shoulder tip.
• *Psychogenic*. Cultural, emotional and psychosocial factors influence everyone's experience of pain. In some patients, no organic cause can be found despite investigation, and psychogenic causes (depression or somatisation disorder) may be responsible (see Ch. 31).

The causes, assessment and management of acute abdominal pain are discussed in Chapter 9.

Chronic or recurrent abdominal pain

It is essential to take a detailed history, paying particular attention to features of the pain and any associated symptoms (Boxes 23.22 and 23.23). Note should be made of the patient's general demeanour, mood and emotional state, signs of weight loss, fever, jaundice or anaemia. If a thorough abdominal and rectal examination is normal, a careful search should be made for evidence of disease affecting other structures, particularly the vertebral column, spinal cord, lungs and cardiovascular system.

Investigations will depend on the clinical features elicited during the history and examination:

• Endoscopy and ultrasound are indicated for epigastric pain, and for dyspepsia and symptoms suggestive of gallbladder disease.
• Colonoscopy is indicated for patients with altered bowel habit, rectal bleeding or features of obstruction suggesting colonic disease.
• CT or MR angiography should be considered when pain is provoked by food in a patient with widespread atherosclerosis, as this may indicate mesenteric ischaemia.
• Persistent symptoms require exclusion of colonic or small bowel disease. However, young patients with pain related to defecation, bloating and alternating bowel habit are more likely to have irritable bowel syndrome (p. 847). Simple investigations (blood tests, faecal calprotectin and sigmoidoscopy) are sufficient in the absence of rectal bleeding, weight loss and abnormal physical findings.
• Ultrasound, CT and faecal elastase are required for patients with upper abdominal pain radiating to the back. A history of alcohol misuse, weight loss and diarrhoea suggests chronic pancreatitis or pancreatic cancer.
• Recurrent attacks of pain in the loins radiating to the flanks with urinary symptoms should prompt investigation for renal or ureteric stones by abdominal X-ray, ultrasound and computed tomography of the kidneys, ureters and bladder (CT KUB).
• Chronic abdominal wall pain (CAWP) should be considered when pain is clearly related to movement, with the commonest cause being anterior cutaneous nerve entrapment syndrome. A positive Carnett's sign (abdominal pain is unchanged or worsened when abdominal muscles are tensed, e.g. by asking the patient to lift their head and shoulders from the examination couch) may point towards

the diagnosis. CAWP is frequently overlooked and patients are often mis-diagnosed as having a functional disorder.

- A past history of psychiatric disturbance, repeated negative investigations or vague symptoms that do not fit any disease or organ pattern suggest a psychological origin for the pain. Careful review of case notes and previous investigations, along with open and honest discussion with the patient, reduces the need for further cycles of unnecessary and invasive tests. Care must always be taken, however, not to miss rare pathology, such as acute intermittent porphyria (p. 644) or atypical presentations of common diseases.

Constant abdominal pain

Patients with chronic pain that is constant or nearly always present usually have features to suggest the underlying diagnosis. No cause will be found in a minority, despite thorough investigation, leading to consideration of functional causes of abdominal pain. Centrally mediated abdominal pain syndrome is characterised by severe constant or frequent abdominal pain that is rarely related to gut function, thought to result from abnormal CNS processing of normal visceral afferent sensory input and psychosocial factors are often operative (see Ch. 31). The management is reliant on establishing an effective patient–physician relationship, psychological support and the appropriate use of drugs such as tricyclic antidepressants to minimise the effects of the pain on social, personal and occupational life. Narcotic bowel syndrome may also present with constant abdominal pain, and is associated with increased or continuous use of opioids, with opioid-induced hyperalgesia thought to be the cause for symptoms. Patients tend to have an improvement in pain on withdrawal of opiates.

Disorders of the mouth and salivary glands

Aphthous ulceration

Aphthous ulcers are superficial and painful; they occur in any part of the mouth. Recurrent ulcers occur in around 20% of the population and are particularly common in women prior to menstruation. The cause is unknown, but in severe cases other causes of oral ulceration must be considered (Box 23.24). Biopsy is occasionally necessary for diagnosis.

Treatment is generally not required. Acute episodes may be treated with topical glucocorticoids (such as 0.1% triamcinolone in Orabase) or choline salicylate (8.7%) gel. Symptomatic relief is achieved using local anaesthetic mouthwashes. Rarely, patients with very severe, recurrent aphthous ulcers may need oral glucocorticoids.

Oral cancer

Squamous carcinoma of the oral cavity is common worldwide and is more common in males. Five-year survival is around 50%, largely as a result of late diagnosis. Poor diet, alcohol excess and smoking or tobacco chewing are the traditional risk factors but high-risk, oncogenic strains of human papillomavirus (HPV-16 and HPV-18) have been identified as being responsible for much of the recent increase in incidence, especially in cases affecting the base of tongue, soft palate and tonsils. In parts of Asia, the disease is common among people who chew areca nuts wrapped in leaves of the betel plant ('betel nuts').

Oral cancer may present in many ways (Box 23.25) and a high index of suspicion is required. All possible sources of local trauma or infection should be treated in patients with suspicious lesions and they should be reviewed after 2 weeks, with biopsy if the lesion persists. Small cancers can be resected but extensive surgery, with neck dissection to remove involved lymph nodes, may be necessary. Some patients can be treated with radical radiotherapy alone, and sometimes chemoradiotherapy is also given after surgery to treat microscopic residual disease. Some tumours may be amenable to photodynamic therapy (PDT), avoiding the need for surgery. Recurrent or metastatic disease may require treatment with the monoclonal antibody cetuximab

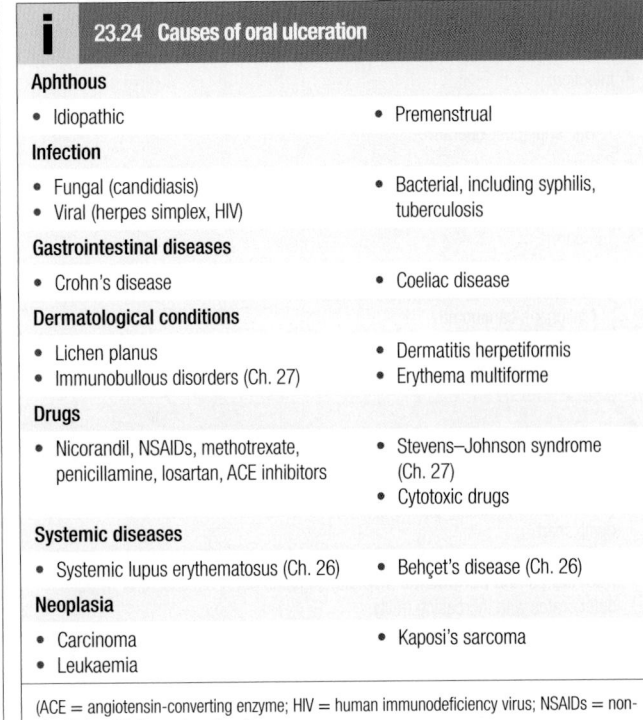

i | **23.24 Causes of oral ulceration**

Aphthous
- Idiopathic
- Premenstrual

Infection
- Fungal (candidiasis)
- Viral (herpes simplex, HIV)
- Bacterial, including syphilis, tuberculosis

Gastrointestinal diseases
- Crohn's disease
- Coeliac disease

Dermatological conditions
- Lichen planus
- Immunobullous disorders (Ch. 27)
- Dermatitis herpetiformis
- Erythema multiforme

Drugs
- Nicorandil, NSAIDs, methotrexate, penicillamine, losartan, ACE inhibitors
- Stevens–Johnson syndrome (Ch. 27)
- Cytotoxic drugs

Systemic diseases
- Systemic lupus erythematosus (Ch. 26)
- Behçet's disease (Ch. 26)

Neoplasia
- Carcinoma
- Leukaemia
- Kaposi's sarcoma

(ACE = angiotensin-converting enzyme; HIV = human immunodeficiency virus; NSAIDs = non-steroidal anti-inflammatory drugs)

i | **23.25 Symptoms and signs of oral cancer**

- Solitary ulcer without precipitant, e.g. local trauma
- Solitary white patch ('leukoplakia') that fails to wipe off
- Solitary red patch
- Fixed lump
- Lip numbness in absence of trauma or infection
- Trismus (pain/difficulty in opening the mouth)
- Cervical lymphadenopathy

(an epidermal growth factor receptor inhibitor), in combination with chemotherapy.

Candidiasis

The yeast *Candida albicans* is a normal mouth commensal, but it may proliferate to cause thrush. This occurs in babies, debilitated patients, people receiving glucocorticoid or antibiotic therapy, individuals with diabetes and immunosuppressed patients, especially those receiving cytotoxic therapy and those with HIV infection. White patches are seen on the tongue and buccal mucosa. Odynophagia or dysphagia suggests pharyngeal and oesophageal candidiasis. A clinical diagnosis is sufficient to instigate therapy, although brushings or biopsies can be obtained for mycological examination. Oral thrush can be treated using topical treatments such as miconazole or nystatin. Resistant cases or immunosuppressed patients may require oral fluconazole.

Parotitis

Parotitis is caused by viral or bacterial infection. Mumps causes a self-limiting acute parotitis (p. 284). Bacterial parotitis usually occurs as a complication of major surgery. It is a consequence of dehydration and poor oral hygiene, and can be avoided by good post-operative care. Patients present with painful parotid swelling and this can be complicated by abscess formation. Broad-spectrum antibiotics are required, while surgical drainage is necessary for abscesses. Other causes of salivary gland enlargement are listed in Box 23.26 and implications of oral health in older people are discussed in Box 23.27.

23

- Infection:
  - Mumps
  - Bacterial (post-operative)
- Calculi
- Sjögren syndrome (Ch. 26)
- Sarcoidosis
- Tumours:
  - Benign: pleomorphic adenoma (95% of cases)
  - Intermediate: mucoepidermoid tumour
  - Malignant: carcinoma

23.27 Oral health in old age

- **Dry mouth**: affects around 40% of healthy older people.
- **Gustatory and olfactory sensation**: declines and chewing power is diminished.
- **Salivation**: baseline salivary flow falls, but stimulated salivation is unchanged.
- **Root caries and periodontal disease**: common partly because oral hygiene deteriorates with increasing frailty.
- **Bacteraemia and sepsis**: may complicate Gram-negative anaerobic infection in the periodontal pockets of the very frail.

Disorders of the oesophagus

Gastro-oesophageal reflux disease

Gastro-oesophageal reflux resulting in heartburn affects approximately 15% of the general population.

Pathophysiology

Occasional episodes of gastro-oesophageal reflux are common in healthy individuals. Reflux is normally followed by oesophageal peristaltic waves that efficiently clear the gullet, alkaline saliva neutralises residual acid and symptoms do not occur. Gastro-oesophageal reflux disease develops when the oesophageal mucosa is exposed to gastroduodenal contents for prolonged periods of time, resulting in symptoms and, in a proportion of cases, oesophagitis. Several factors are known to be involved in the development of gastro-oesophageal reflux disease and these are shown in Figure 23.25.

Abnormalities of the lower oesophageal sphincter

The lower oesophageal sphincter is tonically contracted under normal circumstances, relaxing only during swallowing (see Fig. 23.1).

Some patients with gastro-oesophageal reflux disease have reduced lower oesophageal sphincter tone, permitting reflux when intra-abdominal pressure rises. In others, basal sphincter tone is normal, but reflux occurs in response to frequent episodes of inappropriate sphincter relaxation.

Hiatus hernia

Hiatus hernia (Box 23.28 and Fig. 23.26) causes reflux because the pressure gradient is lost between the abdominal and thoracic cavities, which normally pinches the hiatus. In addition, the oblique angle between the cardia and oesophagus disappears. Many patients who have large hiatus hernias develop reflux symptoms but the relationship between the presence of a hernia and symptoms is poor. Nevertheless, almost all patients who develop oesophagitis, Barrett's oesophagus or peptic strictures are found to have a hiatus hernia.

Delayed oesophageal clearance

Defective oesophageal peristaltic activity is commonly found in patients who have oesophagitis. It is a primary abnormality, since it persists after

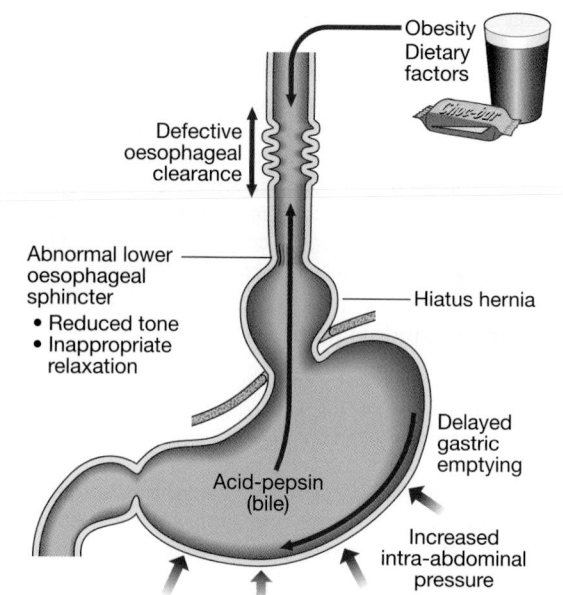

Fig. 23.25 Factors associated with the development of gastro-oesophageal reflux disease.

- Herniation of the stomach through the diaphragm into the chest
- Occurs in 30% of the population over the age of 50 years
- Often asymptomatic
- Heartburn and regurgitation can occur
- Gastric volvulus may complicate large hernias

oesophagitis has been healed by acid-suppressing drug therapy. Poor oesophageal clearance leads to increased acid exposure time.

Gastric contents

Gastric acid is the most important oesophageal irritant and there is a close relationship between acid exposure time and symptoms. Pepsin and bile also contribute to mucosal injury.

Defective gastric emptying

Gastric emptying is delayed in patients with gastro-oesophageal reflux disease. The reason is unknown.

Increased intra-abdominal pressure

Pregnancy and obesity are established predisposing causes. Weight loss may improve symptoms.

Dietary and environmental factors

Dietary fat, chocolate, alcohol, tea and coffee relax the lower oesophageal sphincter and may provoke symptoms. The foods that trigger symptoms vary widely between affected individuals.

Patient factors

Visceral sensitivity and patient vigilance play a role in determining symptom severity and consulting behaviour in individual patients.

Clinical features

The major symptoms are heartburn and regurgitation, often provoked by bending, straining or lying down. 'Waterbrash', which is salivation due to reflex salivary gland stimulation as acid enters the gullet, is often present. Gastro-oesophageal reflux is commoner in older people (Box 23.29) and in those who are overweight. Some patients are woken at night by

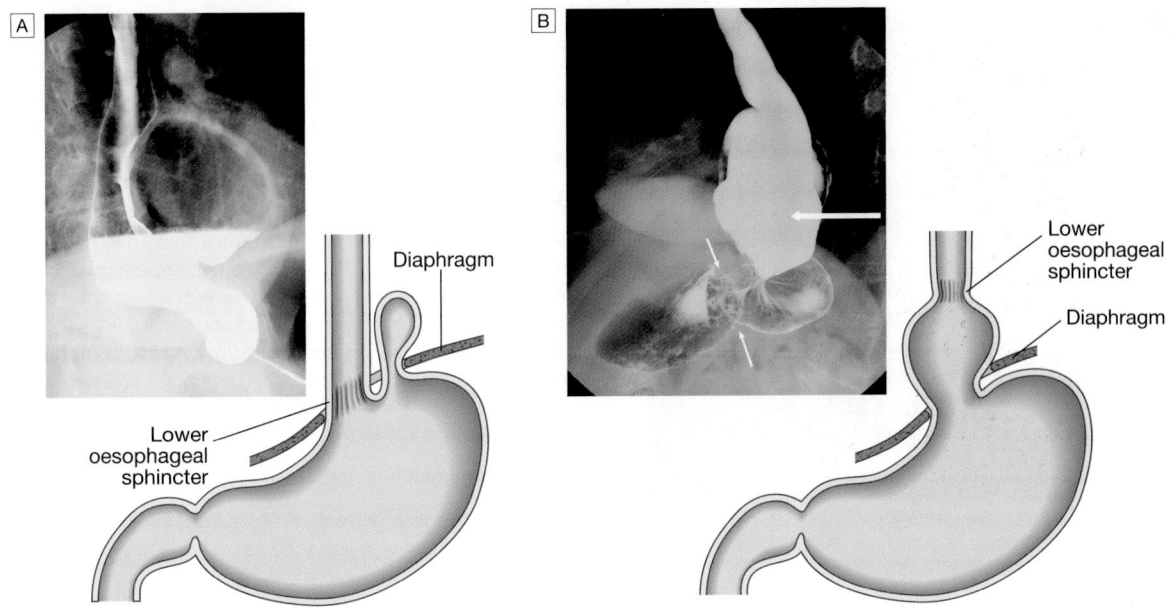

Fig. 23.26 **Types of hiatus hernia.** A Rolling or para-oesophageal. *Inset:* Barium meal showing a large para-oesophageal hernia with intrathoracic stomach. B Sliding. *Inset:* Barium meal showing a gastric volvulus (small arrows) complicating a sliding hiatus hernia (large arrow).

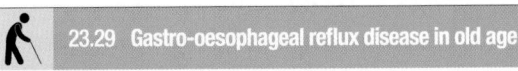

| 23.29 | **Gastro-oesophageal reflux disease in old age** |

- **Prevalence**: higher.
- **Severity of symptoms**: does not correlate with the degree of mucosal inflammation.
- **Complications**: late complications, such as peptic strictures or bleeding from oesophagitis, are more common.
- **Recurrent pneumonia**: consider aspiration from occult gastro-oesophageal reflux disease.

choking as refluxed fluid irritates the larynx. Others develop odynophagia or dysphagia. A variety of other features have been described, such as atypical chest pain that may be severe and can mimic angina; it may be due to reflux-induced oesophageal spasm. Others include hoarseness ('acid laryngitis'), recurrent chest infections, chronic cough and asthma. The true relationship of these features to gastro-oesophageal reflux disease remains unclear.

Complications

Oesophagitis

A range of endoscopic findings is recognised, from mild redness to severe bleeding ulceration with stricture formation, although appearances may be completely normal (Fig. 23.27). There is a poor correlation between symptoms and histological and endoscopic findings.

Barrett's oesophagus

Barrett's oesophagus is a pre-malignant condition, in which the normal squamous lining of the lower oesophagus is replaced by columnar mucosa (columnar lined oesophagus; CLO) that may contain areas of intestinal metaplasia (Fig. 23.28). Patients are often asymptomatic until discovered, and can present with oesophageal cancer. Barrett's oesophagus is an adaptive response to chronic gastro-oesophageal reflux and is found in 10% of patients undergoing gastroscopy for reflux symptoms. The estimated prevalence in Western countries is 1%–2% of the population. The relative risk of oesophageal cancer is increased 40–120-fold, but the absolute risk is low (0.1%–0.5% per year). The epidemiology and aetiology of Barrett's oesophagus are poorly understood. The prevalence

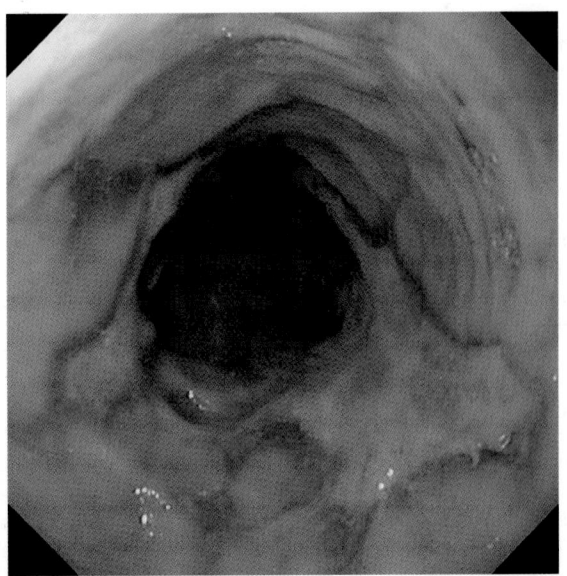

Fig. 23.27 **Severe reflux oesophagitis.** There is near-circumferential superficial ulceration and inflammation extending up the gullet.

is increasing, and it is more common in men (especially of European ancestry), the obese (central obesity in particular) and those over 50 years of age. Cigarette smoking is a moderate risk factor, while there is a less clear association with alcohol. The risk of cancer seems to relate to the severity and duration of reflux rather than the presence of Barrett's oesophagus per se, and it has been suggested that duodenogastro-oesophageal reflux of bile, pancreatic enzymes and pepsin, as well as gastric acid, may be important in the pathogenesis. The molecular events underlying progression of Barrett's oesophagus to dysplasia and cancer are incompletely understood, but inactivation of the tumour suppression protein p16 by loss of heterozygosity or promoter hypermethylation is a key event, followed by somatic inactivation of *TP53*, which promotes aneuploidy and tumour progression. Studies are in progress to develop biomarkers that will allow detection of those at higher cancer risk, but are currently not used in clinical practice.

23

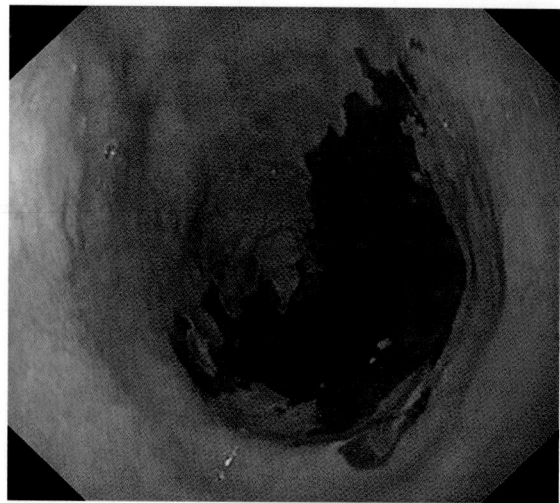

Fig. 23.28 Barrett's oesophagus. Tongues of pink columnar mucosa are seen extending upwards above the oesophago-gastric junction.

Diagnosis

Endoscopy is the gold standard for diagnosis. Multiple systematic biopsies are taken, in addition to sampling any visible lesions, to maximise the chance of detecting intestinal metaplasia and/or dysplasia.

Management

Neither potent acid suppression nor anti-reflux surgery stops progression or induces regression of Barrett's oesophagus, and treatment is indicated only for symptoms of reflux or complications, such as stricture. Endoscopic therapies can induce regression and at present may be used for those with dysplasia and mucosal oesophageal adenocarcinoma. Regular endoscopic surveillance can detect dysplasia at an early stage and may improve survival but, because most Barrett's oesophagus is undetected until cancer develops, surveillance strategies are unlikely to influence the overall mortality rate of oesophageal cancer. Surveillance is expensive and the cost-effectiveness of this approach is debatable. Currently, surveillance intervals for Barrett's oesophagus are risk stratified by the length of the Barrett's oesophagus segment, and by the presence and grade of dysplasia.

For those with high-grade dysplasia or intramucosal carcinoma, the treatment options are either oesophagectomy or endoscopic therapy, with a combination of endoscopic resection of any visibly abnormal areas and radiofrequency ablation (RFA) of the remaining Barrett's mucosa, as an 'organ-preserving' alternative to surgery. Promising alternative ablative therapies to RFA are in development, such as cryoablation, but further studies are required before recommending these as a second-line option for patients who fail to respond to RFA.

Anaemia

Iron deficiency anaemia can occur as a consequence of occult blood loss from long-standing oesophagitis. Most patients have a large hiatus hernia and bleeding can stem from subtle erosions in the neck of the sac ('Cameron lesions'). Nevertheless, hiatus hernia is very common and other causes of blood loss, particularly colorectal cancer, must be considered in anaemic patients, even when endoscopy reveals oesophagitis.

Benign oesophageal stricture

Fibrous strictures can develop as a consequence of long-standing oesophagitis, especially in older people and those with poor oesophageal peristaltic activity. The typical presentation is with dysphagia that is worse for solids than for liquids. Bolus obstruction following ingestion of meat causes absolute dysphagia. A history of heartburn is common but not invariable; many patients presenting in old age with strictures have no preceding heartburn.

Diagnosis is by endoscopy, when biopsies of the stricture can be taken to exclude malignancy. Endoscopic balloon dilatation or bouginage is helpful. Subsequently, long-term therapy with a PPI at full dose should be started to reduce the risk of recurrent oesophagitis and stricture formation. The patient should be advised to chew food thoroughly and it is important to ensure adequate dentition.

Gastric volvulus

Occasionally, a massive intrathoracic hiatus hernia may twist on itself, leading to a gastric volvulus. This gives rise to complete oesophageal or gastric obstruction and the patient presents with severe chest pain, vomiting and dysphagia. The diagnosis is made by chest X-ray (air bubble in the chest) and barium swallow (see Fig. 23.26B). A nasogastric tube is normally inserted in the acute phase to facilitate decompression, with surgery usually advised after the acute episode. Endoscopic decompression may be an alternative option in selected patients in old age.

Investigations

Young patients who present with typical symptoms of gastro-oesophageal reflux, without worrying features such as dysphagia, weight loss or anaemia, can be treated empirically without investigation. Investigation is advisable if patients present over the age of 50–55 years, if symptoms are atypical or if a complication is suspected. Endoscopy is the investigation of choice. This is performed to exclude other upper gastrointestinal diseases that can mimic gastro-oesophageal reflux and to identify complications. A normal endoscopy in a patient with compatible symptoms should not preclude treatment for gastro-oesophageal reflux disease.

Oesophageal pH monitoring is indicated if the diagnosis is unclear or surgical intervention is under consideration. This involves tethering a slim catheter with a terminal radiotelemetry pH-sensitive probe above the gastro-oesophageal junction; wireless oesophageal pH monitoring is available in some centres for those intolerant of catheter-based monitoring. Intraluminal pH is recorded while the patient undergoes normal activities, and episodes of symptoms are noted and related to pH. An oesophageal pH of less than 4 for more than 6% of the study time is considered diagnostic for reflux disease. In patients with difficult reflux, impedance testing can detect weakly acidic or alkaline reflux that is not revealed by standard pH testing.

Management

A treatment algorithm for gastro-oesophageal reflux is outlined in Figure 23.29. Lifestyle advice should be given, including weight loss, avoidance of dietary items that worsen symptoms, elevation of the bed head in those who experience nocturnal symptoms, avoidance of late meals and cessation of smoking. Patients who fail to respond to these measures should be offered PPIs, which are usually effective in resolving symptoms and healing oesophagitis. Recurrence of symptoms is common when therapy is stopped and some patients require life-long treatment at the lowest acceptable dose. When dysmotility features are prominent, prokinetics such as domperidone (not available in the United States) or metoclopramide can be helpful. There is no evidence that *H. pylori* eradication has any therapeutic value. Proprietary antacids and alginates can also provide symptomatic benefit. H_2-receptor antagonist drugs relieve symptoms without healing oesophagitis.

Long-term PPI therapy can lead to the development of parietal cell hyperplasia and hypertrophy, leading to acid rebound on withdrawal of PPIs after long-term usage. PPI therapy is also associated with reduced absorption of iron, B_{12} and magnesium. The drugs may also predispose to enteric infections with *Salmonella*, *Campylobacter* and possibly *Clostridioides difficile*. They may have an undesirable impact on the composition of the gut microbiota, although the clinical importance of this is unclear. An association between microscopic colitis and PPIs has also been suggested, as well as with acute interstitial nephritis. Long-term therapy increases the risk of *Helicobacter*-associated progression of gastric mucosal atrophy (see below) and *H. pylori* eradication is advised in patients requiring PPIs for more than 1 year. The risks described with PPIs are relatively modest, but patients should receive the lowest dose of PPIs to manage their symptoms.

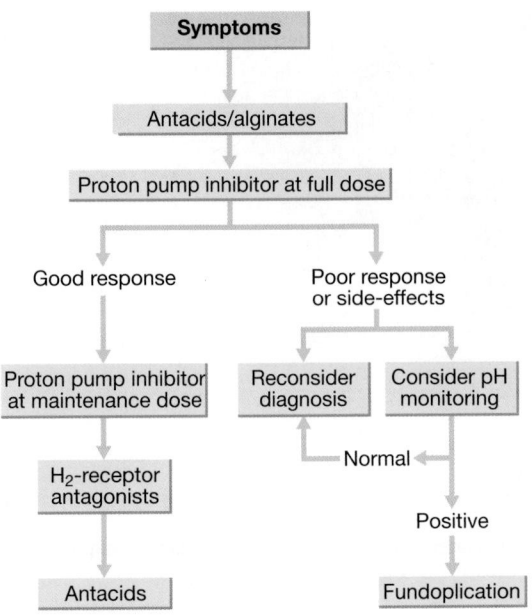

Fig. 23.29 **Treatment of gastro-oesophageal reflux disease: a 'step-down' approach.**

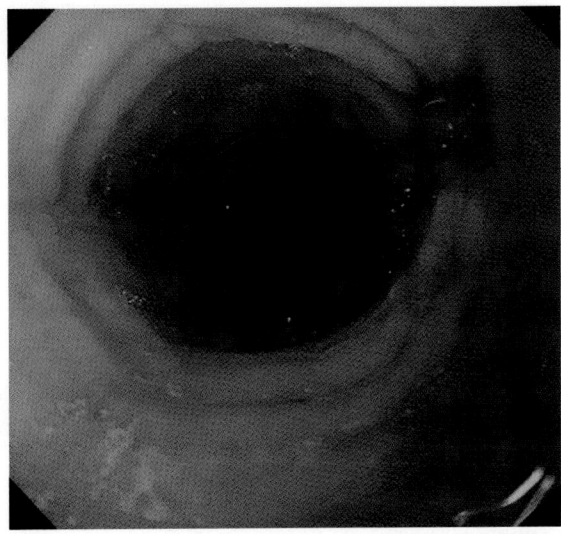

Fig. 23.30 **Endoscopic features suggestive of eosinophilic oesophagitis.**

Patients who fail to respond to medical therapy, those who are unwilling to take long-term PPIs and those whose major symptom is severe regurgitation should be considered for laparoscopic fundoplication (see this book's companion text, *Principles and Practice of Surgery*); endoscopic anti-reflux procedures are currently in development.

Other causes of oesophagitis

Infection

Oesophageal candidiasis occurs in debilitated patients and those taking broad-spectrum antibiotics or cytotoxic drugs. It is a particular problem in patients with HIV/AIDS, who are also susceptible to a spectrum of other oesophageal infections (p. 359).

Corrosives

Suicide attempt by ingestion of caustic acid (e.g. vinegar) or alkaline agents (e.g. bleach) is followed by painful burns of the mouth and pharynx and by extensive erosive oesophagitis (p. 234). Late complications include oesophageal strictures, which may require endoscopic dilatation or stent insertion, or surgery in severe cases.

Drugs

Potassium supplements and NSAIDs may cause oesophageal ulcers when the tablets are trapped above an oesophageal stricture. Liquid preparations of these drugs should be used in such patients. Bisphosphonates cause oesophageal ulceration and should be used with caution in patients with known oesophageal disorders. Tetracyclines, such as doxycycline, can also cause oesophagitis.

Eosinophilic oesophagitis

This is an increasingly recognised condition, that affects both children and adults, and is more common in males.. It occurs more often in atopic individuals and is characterised by eosinophilic infiltration of the oesophageal mucosa. Children commonly present with vomiting, difficulty feeding or failure to thrive. In contrast, adults present with dysphagia or food bolus obstruction more often than heartburn, while other symptoms, such as chest pain may be present. Endoscopy is usually normal, but mucosal rings, longitudinal furrows, exudates, oedema, strictures or a narrow-calibre oesophagus can occur (Fig. 23.30). To obtain a diagnosis, multiple biopsies should be taken from different levels of the oesophagus.

One of the features noted on histology is an increase in eosinophil density (≥ 15 eosinophils per high-powered field (HPF)).

Dietary modifications are an effective first-line treatment for this condition, and include elemental and elimination diets. Adherence to these diets can be challenging, particularly in adults. In terms of pharmacological management, an empiric 8-week trial of high-dose PPI can be used in the first instance. Around one-third of patients will respond to this, known as PPI-responsive oesophageal eosinophilia. In patients who do not respond, 8–12 weeks of therapy with topical glucocorticoids can be used, such as fluticasone and budesonide. Fluticasone is delivered by spraying into the mouth via a metered-dose inhaler, and swallowed rather than inhaled. Budesonide is administered as an oral viscous solution. There are few pharmacological options beyond this, with biologic agents currently experimental. Endoscopic oesophageal dilatation may be considered in individuals with strictures or mucosal rings that have failed to respond to medical therapy.

Benign oesophageal stricture

Benign oesophageal stricture is usually a consequence of gastro-oesophageal reflux disease (Box 23.30) and occurs most often in older adults who have poor oesophageal clearance. Rings, caused by submucosal fibrosis, are found at the oesophago-gastric junction ('Schatzki ring') and cause intermittent dysphagia, often starting in middle age. A post-cricoid web is a rare complication of iron deficiency anaemia (Paterson–Kelly or Plummer–Vinson syndrome), and may be complicated by the development of squamous carcinoma. Benign strictures can be treated by endoscopic dilatation, in which wire-guided bougies or balloons are used to disrupt the fibrous tissue of the stricture.

Tumours of the oesophagus

Benign tumours

The most common is a leiomyoma. This is usually asymptomatic, but may cause bleeding or dysphagia.

Carcinoma of the oesophagus

Squamous oesophageal cancer (Box 23.31) accounts for 90% of oesophageal cancers globally, being more common in Iran, areas of Africa and China. Squamous cancer can occur in any part of the oesophagus, although almost all tumours in the upper oesophagus are squamous cancers. Adenocarcinomas typically arise in the lower third

23

23.30 Causes of oesophageal stricture

- Gastro-oesophageal reflux disease
- Webs and rings
- Carcinoma of the oesophagus or cardia
- Eosinophilic oesophagitis
- Extrinsic compression from bronchial carcinoma
- Corrosive ingestion
- Post-operative scarring following oesophageal resection
- Following radiotherapy
- Following long-term nasogastric intubation
- Bisphosphonates

23.31 Squamous carcinoma: aetiological factors

- Smoking
- Alcohol excess
- Chewing betel nuts or tobacco
- Achalasia of the oesophagus
- Coeliac disease
- Post-cricoid web
- Post-caustic stricture
- Tylosis (familial hyperkeratosis of palms and soles)

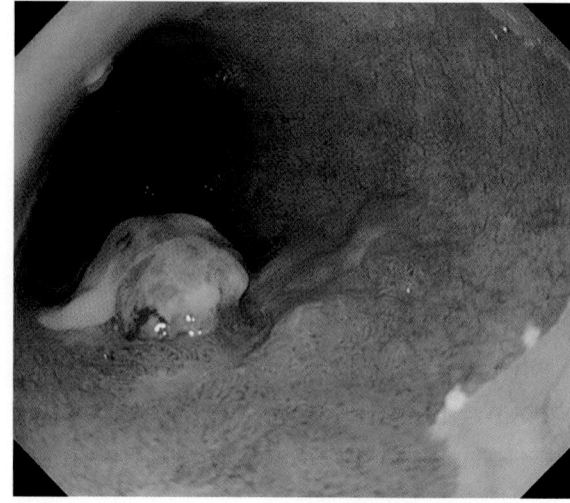

Fig. 23.31 Adenocarcinoma of the lower oesophagus. A polypoidal adenocarcinoma in association with Barrett's oesophagus.

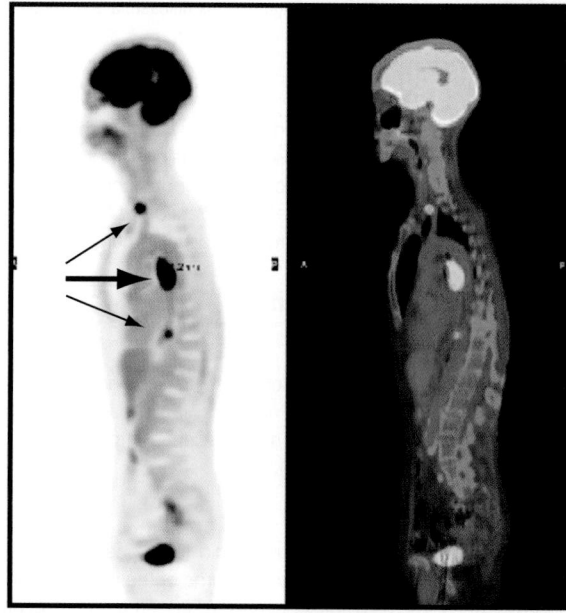

Fig. 23.32 Positron emission tomography–computed tomography (PET-CT) staging of oesophageal carcinoma. Whole-body PET scan showing avid uptake in the primary tumour (thick arrow) but also in distant paratracheal (superior thin arrow) and gastro-oesophageal (inferior thin arrow) lymph nodes.

of the oesophagus from Barrett's oesophagus or from the cardia of the stomach, and are more common in America, Australia and Europe. The incidence is increasing possibly as a result of the high prevalence of gastro-oesophageal reflux and Barrett's oesophagus in Western populations. Despite modern treatment, the overall 5-year survival of patients presenting with oesophageal cancer is less than 20%.

Clinical features

Most patients have a history of progressive, painless dysphagia for solid foods. Others present acutely because of food bolus obstruction. In the late stages, weight loss is often extreme; chest pain or hoarseness suggests mediastinal invasion. Fistulation between the oesophagus and the trachea or bronchial tree leads to coughing after swallowing, pneumonia and pleural effusion. Physical signs may be absent but, even at initial presentation, cachexia, cervical lymphadenopathy or other evidence of metastatic spread is common.

Investigations

The investigation of choice is upper gastrointestinal endoscopy (Fig. 23.31) with biopsy. Once a diagnosis has been made, investigations should be performed to stage the tumour and define operability. Thoracic and abdominal CT, often combined with positron emission tomography (PET-CT), should be carried out to identify metastatic spread and local invasion (Fig. 23.32). Invasion of the aorta, major airways or coeliac axis usually precludes surgery, but patients with resectable disease on imaging should undergo EUS to determine the depth of penetration of the tumour into the oesophageal wall and to detect locoregional lymph node involvement (Fig. 23.33). These investigations will define the TNM (tumour, node, metastases) stage of the disease (Box 7.3).

Management

Endoscopic management is an option in specialist centres for very early superficial tumours. Techniques such as endoscopic mucosal resection or endoscopic submucosal dissection with or without radiofrequency ablation, have become established for Barrett's oesophagus and, in particular, adenocarcinoma. Oesophagectomy is the treatment of choice for limited and locally advanced tumours where resection is possible. For locally advanced tumours, neoadjuvant and perioperative chemotherapy or chemoradiotherapy (e.g. cisplatin and capecitabine) can reduce the tumour bulk and increase the chances of complete (R0) surgical resection. Neoadjuvant therapy can also relieve dysphagia and improve nutritional status. Some patients with squamous carcinoma can have a complete response following definitive chemoradiotherapy, with a subset not requiring surgery initially but close surveillance. All cases should be discussed within a multidisciplinary oesophageal cancer team (MDT).

Approximately 70% of patients have extensive disease at presentation; in these, treatment is palliative and should focus on relief of dysphagia and pain. Palliative radiotherapy or stent placement can be used for symptom control. Palliative chemotherapy can be used for selected patients, particularly for those with adenocarcinoma. Quality of life can be improved by nutritional support and appropriate analgesia.

Perforation of the oesophagus

Oesophageal perforation is a rare but potentially life-threatening clinical condition. The most common cause is iatrogenic endoscopic perforation complicating dilatation or intubation. Malignant, corrosive or post-radiotherapy strictures are more likely to be perforated than peptic strictures.

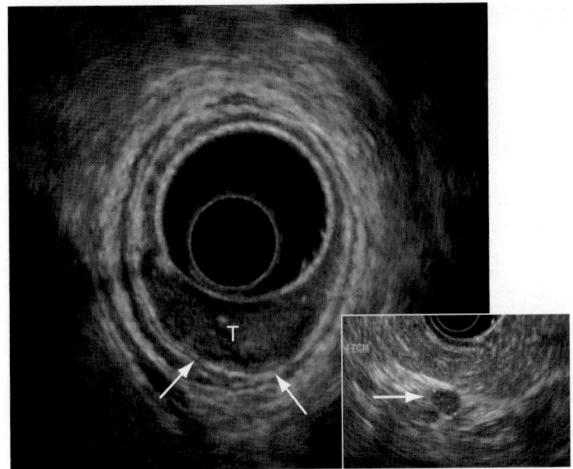

Fig. 23.33 Endoscopic ultrasound staging of oesophageal carcinoma. There is a superficial adenocarcinoma of the oesophagus (T). The submucosa (white band, white arrows) is not involved but there is a small involved local lymph node (white arrow, inset). The tumour is therefore staged T1a, N1.

Spontaneous oesophageal perforation ('Boerhaave syndrome') results from forceful vomiting and retching, accounting for around 15% of cases. Severe chest pain and shock occur as oesophago-gastric contents enter the mediastinum and thoracic cavity. Subcutaneous emphysema, pleural effusions and pneumothorax develop. The diagnosis can be made using a water-soluble contrast swallow but, in difficult cases, both CT and careful endoscopy (usually in an intubated patient) may be required. Delay in diagnosis is a key factor in the high mortality associated with this condition.

Surgery remains the mainstay of treatment for oesophageal perforation. However, an increasing subgroup of patients are being managed via non-operative measures, such as individuals with small well-defined tears. Non-operative options include conservative management involving broad spectrum antibiotics and parental nutrition, and endoscopic management such as clip placement.

Oesophageal motility disorders

Pharyngeal pouch

This occurs because of incoordination of swallowing within the pharynx, which leads to herniation through the cricopharyngeus muscle and formation of a pouch. It is rare, affecting 1 in 100 000 people; it occurs predominantly in men, and is most common in the seventh and eighth decades of life. Many patients have no symptoms, but regurgitation, halitosis and dysphagia can be present. Some notice gurgling in the throat after swallowing. The investigation of choice is a barium swallow (see Fig. 23.12A), which demonstrates the pouch and reveals incoordination of swallowing, often with pulmonary aspiration. Treatment is indicated in symptomatic patients, and can be via a surgical approach, such as cricopharyngeus myotomy (diverticulotomy), with or without resection of the pouch. Recently, there has been the development of minimally invasive endoscopic approaches, such as endoscopic diverticulectomy.

Achalasia of the oesophagus

Pathophysiology

Achalasia is characterised by:

- a hypertonic lower oesophageal sphincter, which fails to relax in response to the swallowing wave
- failure of propagated oesophageal contraction, leading to progressive dilatation of the gullet.

The cause is unknown. It is associated with autoimmune diseases, such as type 1 diabetes mellitus, systemic lupus erythematosus, rheumatoid arthritis and Sjögren syndrome. Defective release of nitric oxide by inhibitory neurons in the lower oesophageal sphincter has been reported, and there is degeneration of ganglion cells within the sphincter and the body of the oesophagus. Loss of the dorsal vagal nuclei within the brainstem can be demonstrated in later stages. Infection with *Trypanosoma cruzi* in Chagas' disease (Ch. 13) causes a syndrome that is clinically indistinguishable from achalasia.

Clinical features

The presentation is with dysphagia, typically to solids and liquids. Regurgitation to saliva and food can also occur, as well as some patients experiencing episodes of chest pain due to oesophageal spasm. Around one-third of patients can experience weight loss. As the disease progresses, dysphagia worsens, the oesophagus empties poorly and nocturnal pulmonary aspiration develops. Achalasia predisposes to squamous carcinoma of the oesophagus.

Investigations

Endoscopy should always be carried out because carcinoma of the cardia can mimic the presentation and radiological and manometric features of achalasia ('pseudo-achalasia'). A barium swallow shows tapered narrowing of the lower oesophagus and, in late disease, the oesophageal body is dilated, aperistaltic and food-filled (Fig. 23.34A). Manometry confirms the high-pressure, non-relaxing lower oesophageal sphincter with poor contractility of the oesophageal body (Fig. 23.34B).

Management

Endoscopic

Forceful pneumatic dilatation using a 30–35 mm-diameter, fluoroscopically positioned balloon disrupts the oesophageal sphincter and improves symptoms in 80% of patients. Some patients require more than one dilatation, but those needing frequent dilatation are best treated surgically. Endoscopically directed injection of botulinum toxin into the lower oesophageal sphincter induces clinical remission, but relapse is common, with worsening response on repeated treatments. It tends to be reserved for frail individuals in old age where other treatments are too risky. Peroral endoscopic myotomy (POEM) is a newer advanced endoscopic technique for the management of achalasia, but is currently only performed in specialist centres (Fig. 23.35).

Surgical

Surgical myotomy (Heller's operation), commonly performed laparoscopically or as an open operation, is effective but is more invasive than endoscopic dilatation. Both pneumatic dilatation and myotomy may be complicated by gastro-oesophageal reflux, and this can lead to severe oesophagitis because oesophageal clearance is so poor. For this reason, Heller's myotomy is accompanied by a partial fundoplication anti-reflux procedure. PPI therapy is often necessary after surgery.

Other oesophageal motility disorders

Distal oesophageal spasm presents in late middle age with episodic chest pain that may mimic angina, but is sometimes accompanied by transient dysphagia. Some cases occur in response to gastro-oesophageal reflux. Treatment is based on the use of PPIs when gastro-oesophageal reflux is present. Oral or sublingual nitrates or nifedipine may relieve attacks of pain. The results of drug therapy are often disappointing, as are the alternatives such as pneumatic dilatation and surgical myotomy. 'Nutcracker' oesophagus is a condition in which extremely forceful peristaltic activity leads to episodic chest pain and dysphagia. Treatment is with nitrates or nifedipine. Some patients present with oesophageal motility disorders that do not fit into a specific disease entity. The patients usually present in old age and with dysphagia and chest pain. Manometric abnormalities occur, ranging from poor peristalsis to spasm. Treatment is with dilatation and/or vasodilators for chest pain.

23

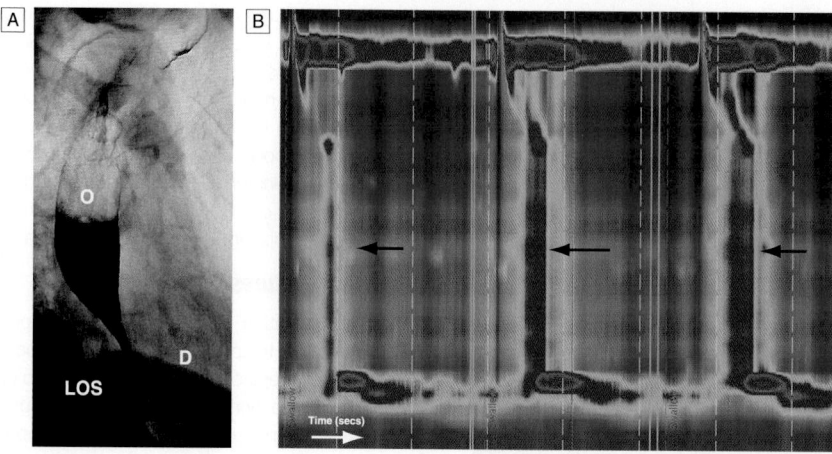

Fig. 23.34 Achalasia. $\boxed{A}$ X-ray showing a dilated, barium-filled oesophagus (O) with fluid level and distal tapering, and a closed lower oesophageal sphincter (LOS). (D = diaphragm) $\boxed{B}$ High-resolution manometry in achalasia showing absence of peristaltic swallowing wave in oesophageal body (black arrows) and raised LOS pressure with failure of relaxation on swallowing (white arrow). Compare with normal appearances in Figure 23.1.

Secondary causes of oesophageal dysmotility

In systemic sclerosis or CREST syndrome (p. 1040) the muscle of the oesophagus is replaced by fibrous tissue, which causes failure of peristalsis leading to heartburn and dysphagia. Oesophagitis is often severe and benign fibrous strictures occur. These patients require long-term therapy with PPIs. If patients remain symptomatic, endoscopic dilatation may be considered. Dermatomyositis, rheumatoid arthritis and myasthenia gravis may also cause dysphagia.

Disorders of the stomach and duodenum

Gastritis

Gastritis is a histological diagnosis, although it can also be recognised at endoscopy.

Acute gastritis

Acute gastritis is often erosive and haemorrhagic. Neutrophils are the predominant inflammatory cell in the superficial epithelium. Many cases result from alcohol, aspirin or NSAID ingestion (Box 23.32). Acute gastritis often produces no symptoms, but may cause dyspepsia, anorexia, nausea or vomiting, and haematemesis or melaena. Many cases resolve quickly and do not merit investigation; in others, endoscopy and biopsy may be necessary to exclude peptic ulcer or cancer. Treatment should be directed at the underlying cause. Short-term symptomatic therapy with antacids, and acid suppression using PPIs, prokinetics (domperidone) or antiemetics (metoclopramide) may be necessary.

Chronic gastritis due to *Helicobacter pylori* infection

This is the most common cause of chronic gastritis (see Box 23.32). The predominant inflammatory cells are lymphocytes and plasma cells. Correlation between symptoms and endoscopic or pathological findings is poor. Most patients are asymptomatic and do not require treatment, but patients with dyspepsia may benefit from *H. pylori* eradication.

Autoimmune chronic gastritis

This involves the body of the stomach but spares the antrum; it results from autoimmune damage to parietal cells. The histological features are diffuse chronic inflammation, atrophy and loss of fundic glands, intestinal metaplasia and sometimes hyperplasia of enterochromaffin-like (ECL)

cells. Circulating antibodies to parietal cell and intrinsic factor may be present. In some patients, the degree of gastric atrophy is severe and loss of intrinsic factor secretion leads to pernicious anaemia (p. 954). The gastritis itself is usually asymptomatic. Some patients have evidence of other organ-specific autoimmunity, particularly thyroid disease. In the long-term, there is a two- to threefold increase in the risk of gastric cancer (see below).

Ménétrier's disease

In this rare condition, the gastric pits are elongated and tortuous, with replacement of the parietal and chief cells by mucus-secreting cells. The cause is unknown but there is excessive production of transforming growth factor alpha (TGF-α). As a result, the mucosal folds of the body and fundus are greatly enlarged. Most patients are hypochlorhydric. While some patients have upper gastrointestinal symptoms, the majority present in middle or old age with protein-losing enteropathy (p. 824) due to exudation from the gastric mucosa. Endoscopy shows enlarged, nodular and coarse folds, although biopsies may not be deep enough to show all the histological features. Treatment with antisecretory drugs, such as PPIs with or without octreotide, may reduce protein loss and *H. pylori* eradication may be effective, but unresponsive patients require partial gastrectomy.

Peptic ulcer disease

Peptic ulcers are most commonly located in the stomach or duodenum, but can also occur in the lower oesophagus, in the jejunum after surgical anastomosis to the stomach or, rarely, in the ileum adjacent to a Meckel's diverticulum. Ulcers in the stomach or duodenum may be acute or chronic; both penetrate the muscularis mucosae, but the acute ulcer shows no evidence of fibrosis. Erosions do not penetrate the muscularis mucosae.

Gastric and duodenal ulcer

The lifetime prevalence of peptic ulcer is around 5%–10%. The incidence is decreasing in many high-income societies as a result of widespread use of *Helicobacter pylori* eradication therapy. The male-to-female ratio for duodenal ulcer varies from 5:1 to 2:1, while that for gastric ulcer is 2:1 or less. Chronic gastric ulcer is usually single; 90% are situated on the lesser curve within the antrum or at the junction between body and antral mucosa. Chronic duodenal ulcer usually occurs in the first part of the duodenum and 50% are on the anterior wall. Gastric and duodenal ulcers coexist in 10% of patients and more than one peptic ulcer is found in 10%–15% of patients.

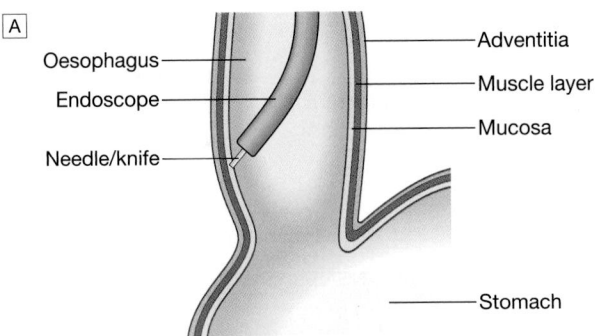

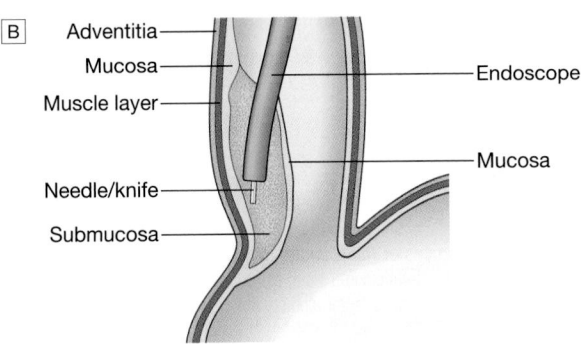

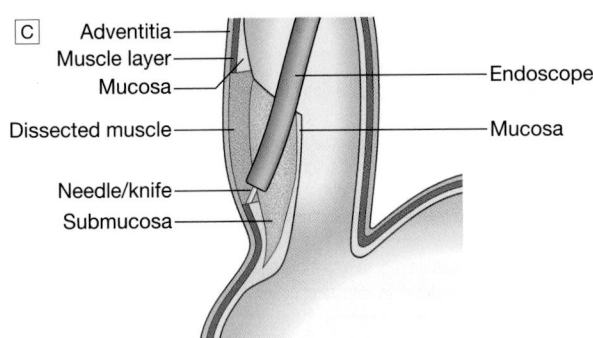

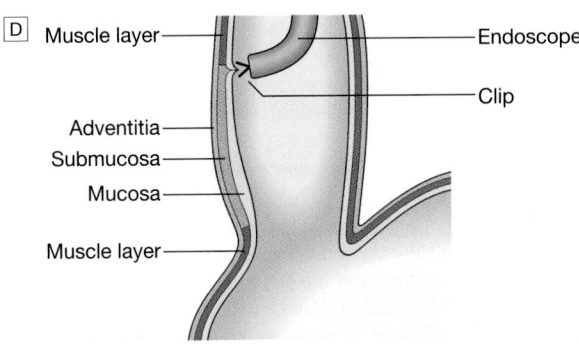

Fig. 23.35 Per-oral endoscopic myotomy. [A] Mucosal surface opened to access submucosal space. [B] A submucosal tunnel is created. [C] Circular muscle is dissected – endoscopic myotomy. [D] The entry site is closed with clips.

Pathophysiology

Helicobacter pylori

Peptic ulceration is strongly associated with *H. pylori* infection. The prevalence of the infection in high-income societies rises with age and in the UK approximately 50% of people over the age of 50 years are infected. In low- and middle-income countries, infection is more common, affecting up to 90% of adults. These infections are probably acquired in childhood by person-to-person contact. The vast majority of colonised people

---

i 23.32 Common causes of gastritis

Acute gastritis (often erosive and haemorrhagic)

- Aspirin, NSAIDs
- *Helicobacter pylori* (initial infection)
- Alcohol
- Other drugs, e.g. iron preparations
- Severe physiological stress, e.g. burns, multi-organ failure, central nervous system trauma
- Bile reflux, e.g. following gastric surgery
- Viral infections, e.g. CMV, herpes simplex virus in HIV/AIDS (Ch. 14)

Chronic non-specific gastritis

- *H. pylori* infection
- Autoimmune (pernicious anaemia)
- Post-gastrectomy

Chronic 'specific' forms (rare)

- Infections, e.g. CMV, tuberculosis
- Gastrointestinal diseases, e.g. Crohn's disease
- Systemic diseases, e.g. sarcoidosis, graft-versus-host disease
- Idiopathic, e.g. granulomatous gastritis

(CMV = cytomegalovirus; HIV/AIDS = human immunodeficiency virus/acquired immunodeficiency syndrome; NSAIDs = non-steroidal anti-inflammatory drugs)

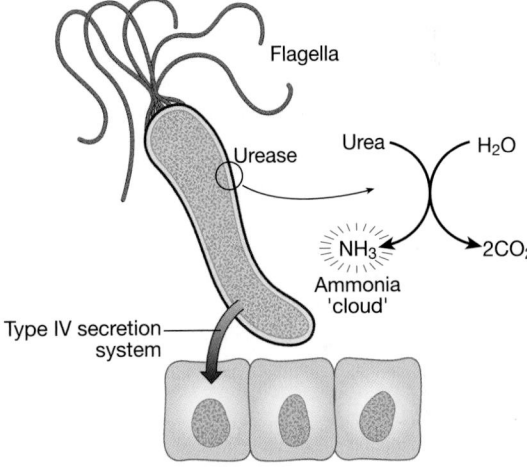

Other factors
- Vacuolating cytotoxin (vacA)
- Cytotoxin-associated gene (cagA)
- Adhesins (babA)
- Outer inflammatory protein A (oipA)

Fig. 23.36 Factors that influence the virulence of *Helicobacter pylori*.

remain healthy and asymptomatic, and only a minority develop clinical disease. Around 90% of duodenal ulcer patients and 70% of gastric ulcer patients are infected with *H. pylori*.

H. pylori is Gram-negative and spiral, and has multiple flagella at one end, which make it motile, allowing it to burrow and live beneath the mucus layer adherent to the epithelial surface. It uses an adhesin molecule (BabA) to bind to the Lewis b antigen on epithelial cells. Here the surface pH is close to neutral and any acidity is buffered by the organism's production of the enzyme urease. This produces ammonia from urea and raises the pH around the bacterium and between its two cell membrane layers. *H. pylori* exclusively colonises gastric-type epithelium and is found in the duodenum only in association with patches of gastric metaplasia. It causes chronic gastritis by provoking a local inflammatory response in the underlying epithelium (Fig. 23.36). This depends on numerous factors, notably expression of bacterial *CagA* and *VacA* genes. The CagA gene product is injected into epithelial cells, interacting with numerous cell-signalling pathways involved in cell replication and apoptosis. *H. pylori* strains expressing

23

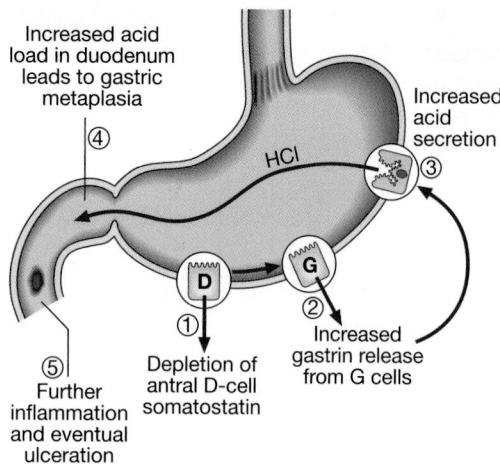

Fig. 23.37 **Sequence of events in the pathophysiology of duodenal ulceration.**

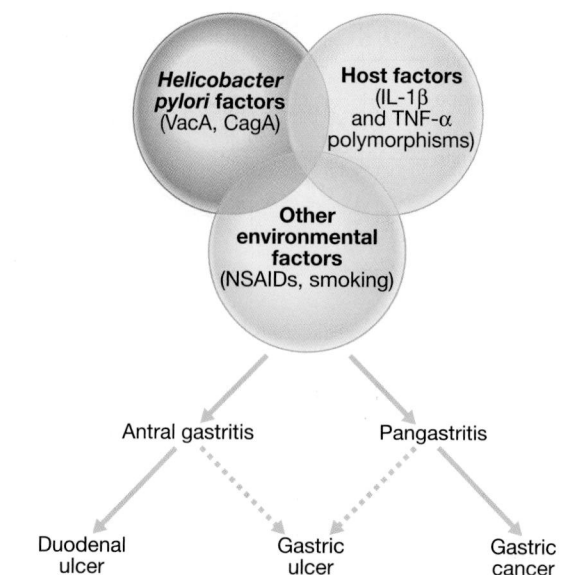

Fig. 23.38 **Consequences of *Helicobacter pylori* infection.** (CagA = cytotoxin-associated gene; IL-1β = interleukin-1 beta; NSAIDs = non-steroidal anti-inflammatory drugs; TNF-α = tumour necrosis factor alpha; VacA = vacuolating cytotoxin)

CagA (CagA⁺) are more often associated with disease than CagA⁻ strains. Most strains also secrete a large pore-forming protein called VacA, which causes increased cell permeability, efflux of micronutrients from the epithelium, induction of apoptosis and suppression of local immune cell activity. Several forms of VacA exist and pathology is most strongly associated with the s1/ml form of the toxin.

The distribution and severity of *H. pylori*-induced gastritis determine the clinical outcome. In most people, *H. pylori* causes a mild pangastritis with little effect on acid secretion and the majority develop no significant clinical outcomes. In a minority (up to 10% in the West), the infection causes an antral-predominant pattern of gastritis characterised by hypergastrinaemia and a very exaggerated acid production by parietal cells, which could lead to duodenal ulceration (Fig. 23.37). In a much smaller number of infected people, *H. pylori* causes a corpus-predominant pattern of gastritis leading to gastric atrophy and hypochlorhydria. This phenotype is much more common in Asian countries, particularly Japan, China and Korea. The hypochlorhydria allows other bacteria to proliferate within the stomach; these other bacteria continue to drive the chronic inflammation and produce mutagenic nitrites from dietary nitrates, predisposing to the development of gastric cancer (Fig. 23.38). The effects of *H. pylori* are more complex in gastric ulcer patients compared to those with duodenal ulcers. The ulcer probably arises because of impaired mucosal defence resulting from a combination of *H. pylori* infection, NSAIDs and smoking, rather than excess acid.

NSAIDs

There has been an increase in the use of NSAIDs and aspirin; these drugs account for 10% of peptic ulcers. NSAIDs increase the risk of complication of peptic ulcer disease four-fold, due to impairment of mucosal defences, as discussed on page 1009.

Smoking

Smoking confers an increased risk of gastric ulcer and, to a lesser extent, duodenal ulcer. Once the ulcer has formed, it is more likely to cause complications and less likely to heal if the patient continues to smoke.

Clinical features

Peptic ulcer disease is a chronic condition with spontaneous relapses and remissions lasting for decades, if not for life. The most common presentation is with recurrent abdominal pain that has three notable characteristics: localisation to the epigastrium, relationship to food and episodic occurrence. Occasional vomiting occurs in about 40% of ulcer subjects; persistent daily vomiting suggests gastric outlet obstruction. In one-third, the history is less characteristic, especially in older people or those taking NSAIDs (Box 23.33). In this situation, pain may be absent or so slight that it is experienced only as a vague sense of epigastric unease. Occasionally, the only symptoms are

23.33 Peptic ulcer disease in old age

- **Gastroduodenal ulcers**: have a greater incidence, admission rate and mortality.
- **Causes**: high prevalence of *Helicobacter pylori*, use of non-steroidal anti-inflammatory drugs and impaired defence mechanisms.
- **Atypical presentations**: pain and dyspepsia are frequently absent or atypical. Older people often develop complications, such as bleeding or perforation, without a dyspeptic history.
- **Bleeding**: older patients require more intensive management because they have more limited reserve to withstand hypovolaemia.

anorexia and nausea, or early satiety after meals. In some patients, the ulcer is completely 'silent', presenting for the first time with anaemia from chronic undetected blood loss, as abrupt haematemesis or as acute perforation; in others, there is recurrent acute bleeding without ulcer pain. The diagnostic value of individual symptoms for peptic ulcer disease is poor; the history is therefore a poor predictor of the presence of an ulcer.

Investigations

Endoscopy is the preferred investigation (Fig. 23.39). Gastric ulcers may occasionally be malignant and therefore must always be biopsied and followed up to ensure healing. Patients should be tested for *H. pylori* infection. The current options available are listed in Box 23.34. Some are invasive and require endoscopy; others are non-invasive. They vary in sensitivity and specificity. Breath tests or faecal antigen tests are best because of accuracy, simplicity and non-invasiveness.

Management

The aims of management are to relieve symptoms, induce healing and prevent recurrence. *H. pylori* eradication is the cornerstone of therapy for peptic ulcers, as this will successfully prevent relapse and eliminate the need for long-term therapy in the majority of patients.

H. pylori eradication

All patients with proven ulcers who are *H. pylori*-positive should be offered eradication as primary therapy. Treatment is based on a PPI taken simultaneously with two antibiotics (from amoxicillin, clarithromycin and metronidazole) for at least 7 days. High-dose, twice-daily PPI therapy

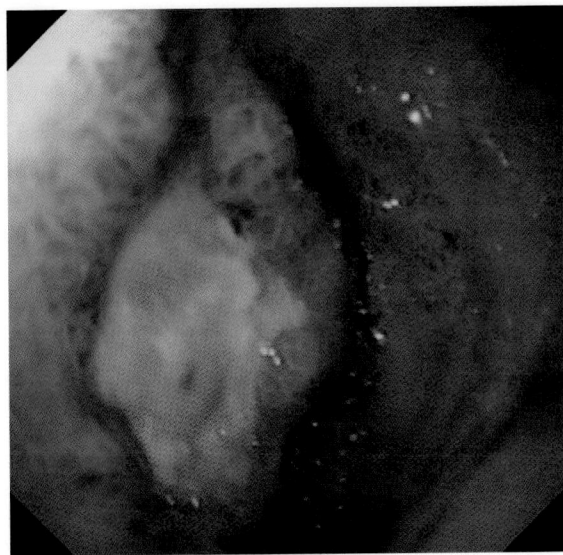

Fig. 23.39 Endoscopic identification of a duodenal ulcer. The ulcer has a clean base and there are no stigmata of recent haemorrhage.

23.34 Methods for the diagnosis of *Helicobacter pylori* infection		
Test	**Advantages**	**Disadvantages**
Non-invasive		
Serology	Rapid office kits available Good for population studies	Lacks specificity Cannot differentiate current from past infection
^{13}C-urea breath test	High sensitivity and specificity	Requires expensive mass spectrometer
Faecal antigen test	Cheap, specific (> 95%)	Acceptability
Invasive (antral biopsy)		
Histology	Specificity	False negatives Takes several days to process
Rapid urease test	Cheap, quick, specific (> 95%)	Sensitivity 85%
Microbiological culture	'Gold standard' Defines antibiotic sensitivity	Slow and laborious Lacks sensitivity

23.35 Common side-effects of *Helicobacter pylori* eradication therapy

- Diarrhoea: 30%–50% of patients; usually mild, but *Clostridioides difficile*-associated diarrhoea can occur
- Flushing and vomiting when taken with alcohol (metronidazole)
- Nausea, vomiting
- Abdominal cramps
- Headache
- Rash

23.36 Indications for *Helicobacter pylori* testing

Definite

- Active or past history of peptic ulcer disease
- Extranodal marginal-zone lymphomas of MALT type
- Previous endoscopic resection for early gastric cancer
- Dyspepsia
- Long-term NSAID or low-dose aspirin users
- Extragastric disorders:
  - Idiopathic thrombocytopenic purpura
  - Unexplained iron deficiency anaemia
- Unexplained Vitamin B_{12} deficiency

Not indicated

- Gastro-oesophageal reflux disease
- Asymptomatic people

(MALT = mucosa-associated lymphoid tissue; NSAID = non-steroidal anti-inflammatory drug)

23.37 Indications for surgery in peptic ulcer

Emergency

- Perforation
- Haemorrhage

Elective

- Gastric outflow obstruction
- Persistent ulceration despite adequate medical therapy
- Recurrent ulcer following gastric surgery

General measures

Cigarette smoking, aspirin and NSAIDs should be avoided. Alcohol in moderation is not harmful and no special dietary advice is required.

Maintenance treatment

Continuous maintenance treatment should not be necessary after successful *H. pylori* eradication. For the minority who do require it, the lowest effective dose of PPI should be used.

Surgical treatment

Surgery is now rarely required for peptic ulcer disease, but it is needed in some cases (Box 23.37).

Complications of gastric resection or vagotomy

Up to 50% of patients who undergo gastric surgery for peptic ulcer experience long-term adverse effects. In most cases these are minor, but in 10% they significantly impair quality of life.

Dumping

Symptoms of dumping syndrome can be either early or late. Early dumping is more common, and occurs within 30 minutes following a meal. Rapid gastric emptying leads to distension of the proximal small intestine as the hypertonic contents draw fluid into the lumen. This leads to

increases efficacy of treatment, as does extending treatment to 10–14 days. Success used to be achieved in greater than 90% of patients, but this has now fallen to below 70% in many countries as a result of antibiotic resistance. In addition, adherence and side effects (Box 23.35) may influence success of eradication.

H. pylori and NSAIDs are independent risk factors for ulcer disease and patients requiring long-term NSAID therapy should first undergo eradication therapy to reduce ulcer risk. Subsequent co-prescription of a PPI along with the NSAID is advised, but is not always necessary for patients being given low-dose aspirin, in whom the risk of ulcer complications is lower.

Other indications for *H. pylori* testing are shown in Box 23.36. Eradication of the infection has proven benefits in several extragastric disorders, including unexplained B_{12} deficiency and iron deficiency anaemia, once sources of gastrointestinal bleeding have been looked for and excluded. Platelet counts improve and may normalise after eradication therapy in patients with idiopathic thrombocytopenic purpura (p. 981); the mechanism for this is unclear.

23

abdominal discomfort and diarrhoea after eating. Autonomic reflexes release a range of gastrointestinal hormones that provoke vasomotor features, such as flushing, palpitations, sweating, tachycardia and hypotension. Patients should therefore avoid large meals with high carbohydrate content. Late dumping occurs 1–3 hours following a meal, with symptoms related to reactive hypoglycaemia, such as nausea, tremor and sweating, which are relieved by eating more food.

Chemical (bile reflux) gastropathy

Duodenogastric bile reflux leads to chronic gastropathy. Treatment with ursodeoxycholic acid may be effective. A few patients require revisional surgery with creation of a Roux en Y loop to prevent bile reflux.

Diarrhoea and maldigestion

Diarrhoea may develop after any peptic ulcer operation and usually occurs 1–2 hours after eating. Poor mixing of food in the stomach, with rapid emptying, inadequate mixing with pancreaticobiliary secretions, rapid transit and bacterial overgrowth, may lead to malabsorption. Diarrhoea often responds to small, dry meals with a reduced intake of refined carbohydrates. Antidiarrhoeal drugs, such as codeine phosphate (15–30 mg 4–6 times daily) or loperamide (2 mg after each loose stool), are helpful.

Weight loss

Most patients lose weight shortly after surgery and 30%–40% are unable to regain all the weight that is lost. The usual cause is reduced intake because of a small gastric remnant, but diarrhoea and mild steatorrhoea also contribute.

Anaemia

Anaemia is common many years after subtotal gastrectomy. Iron deficiency is the most common cause; folic acid and B_{12} deficiency are much less frequent. Inadequate dietary intake of iron and folate, lack of acid and intrinsic factor secretion, mild chronic low-grade blood loss from the gastric remnant and recurrent ulceration are responsible.

Metabolic bone disease

Both osteoporosis and osteomalacia can occur as a consequence of calcium and vitamin D malabsorption.

Gastric cancer

An increased risk of gastric cancer has been reported from several epidemiological studies. Surgery itself is an independent risk factor for late development of malignancy in the gastric remnant, but the risk is higher in those with hypochlorhydria, duodenogastric reflux of bile, smoking and *H. pylori* infection. Although the relative risk is increased, the absolute risk of cancer remains low and endoscopic surveillance is not indicated following gastric surgery.

Complications of peptic ulcer disease

Perforation

When perforation occurs, the contents of the stomach escape into the peritoneal cavity, leading to peritonitis. This is more common in duodenal than in gastric ulcers and is usually found with ulcers on the anterior wall. About one-quarter of all perforations occur in acute ulcers and NSAIDs are often incriminated. Perforation can be the first sign of ulcer and a history of recurrent epigastric pain is uncommon. The most striking symptom is sudden, severe pain; its distribution follows the spread of the gastric contents over the peritoneum. The pain initially develops in the upper abdomen and rapidly becomes generalised; shoulder tip pain is caused by irritation of the diaphragm. The pain is accompanied by shallow respiration, due to limitation of diaphragmatic movements, and by shock. The abdomen is held immobile and there is generalised 'board-like' rigidity. Bowel sounds are absent and liver dullness to percussion decreases due to the presence of gas under the diaphragm. After some hours, symptoms may improve, although abdominal rigidity remains.

i	23.38 Differential diagnosis and management of gastric outlet obstruction	
Cause		**Management**
Fibrotic stricture from duodenal ulcer (pyloric stenosis)		Balloon dilatation or surgery
Oedema from pyloric channel or duodenal ulcer		Proton pump inhibitor therapy
Carcinoma of antrum		Surgery
Adult hypertrophic pyloric stenosis		Surgery

Later, the patient's condition deteriorates as general peritonitis develops. In at least 50% of cases, an erect chest X-ray shows free air beneath the diaphragm (see Fig. 23.11B). If not, a water-soluble contrast swallow will confirm leakage of gastroduodenal contents. After resuscitation, the acute perforation should be treated surgically, either by simple closure or by conversion of the perforation into a pyloroplasty if it is large. On rare occasions, a 'Polya' partial gastrectomy is required. Following surgery, *H. pylori* should be treated (if present) and NSAIDs avoided. Perforation carries a mortality of around 25%, reflecting the advanced age and significant comorbidity of the population that are affected.

Gastric outlet obstruction

The causes are shown in Box 23.38. The most common is an ulcer in the region of the pylorus. The presentation is with nausea, vomiting and abdominal distension. Large quantities of gastric content are often vomited and food eaten 24 hours or more previously may be recognised. Physical examination may show evidence of wasting and dehydration. A succussion splash may be elicited 4 hours or more after the last meal or drink. Visible gastric peristalsis is diagnostic of gastric outlet obstruction. Endoscopy should be performed after the stomach has been emptied using a wide-bore nasogastric tube. Intravenous correction of dehydration is undertaken and, in severe cases, at least 4 L of isotonic saline and 80 mmol of potassium may be necessary during the first 24 hours. In some patients, PPIs heal ulcers, relieve pyloric oedema and overcome the need for surgery. Endoscopic balloon dilatation of benign stenoses may be possible in some patients, but in others partial gastrectomy is necessary; this is best done after a 7-day period of nasogastric aspiration, which enables the stomach to return to normal size. A gastroenterostomy is an alternative operation but, unless this is accompanied by vagotomy, patients will require long-term PPI therapy to prevent stomal ulceration.

Bleeding

See page 797.

Zollinger–Ellison syndrome

This is a rare disorder characterised by gastric acid hypersecretion and severe peptic ulceration, caused by a gastrin-secreting neuro-endocrine tumour ('gastrinoma') (Ch. 21). It probably accounts for about 0.1% of all cases of duodenal ulceration. The syndrome occurs in either sex at any age, although it is most common between 30 and 50 years of age.

Pathophysiology

Elevated gastrin stimulates acid secretion to its maximal capacity and increases the parietal cell mass three- to sixfold. The acid output may be so great that it reaches the upper small intestine, reducing the luminal pH to 2 or less. Pancreatic lipase is inactivated and bile acids are precipitated. Diarrhoea and steatorrhoea result. Around 90% of tumours occur in the pancreatic head or proximal duodenal wall. Between 20% and 60% of patients have multiple endocrine neoplasia (MEN) type 1 (p. 700). In sporadic disease, the tumours are usually unifocal, but in MEN 1 there are invariably multifocal tumours. Individual tumour size can vary from 1 mm to 20 cm; approximately one-half to two-thirds are malignant, but like many neuro-endocrine tumours they are often slow-growing.

Clinical features

The presentation is with severe and often multiple peptic ulcers in unusual sites, such as the post-bulbar duodenum, jejunum or oesophagus. There is a poor response to standard ulcer therapy. The history is usually short, and bleeding and perforations are common. Diarrhoea is seen in one-third or more of patients and can be the presenting feature.

Investigations

Serum gastrin levels are normally grossly elevated (10- to 1000-fold). Injection of the hormone secretin normally causes no change or a slight decrease in circulating gastrin concentrations, but in Zollinger–Ellison syndrome it produces a paradoxical and dramatic increase in gastrin. Tumour localisation (and staging) is best achieved by a combination of CT and EUS; radio-labelled somatostatin receptor scintigraphy and [68]gallium DOTATATE PET scanning may also be used for tumour detection and staging.

Management

Unifocal tumours may be resected, but surgery may not be appropriate when there are multi-focal tumours or if there is metastatic disease. In this situation, continuous therapy with a PPI in high dose can be successful in healing ulcers and alleviating diarrhoea. Somatostatin analogue therapy may reduce gastrin secretion and have an anti-tumour effect; other treatment options for pancreatic neuro-endocrine tumours are discussed on page 700). Overall 5-year survival is 60%–75% and all patients should undergo genetic screening for MEN 1.

Tumours of the stomach

Gastric carcinoma

Around 90% of gastric cancers are adenocarcinomas. Gastric cancer is the fifth most common cancer, with marked geographical variation in incidence. It is most common in China, Japan, South Korea, Eastern Europe and parts of South America. In most countries the incidence is 50% lower in women. In both sexes it rises sharply after 50 years of age. Studies of Japanese migrants to the United States have revealed a much lower incidence in the second generation, confirming the importance of environmental factors. The overall prognosis is poor, with less than 30% surviving 5 years, except in Japan where there are much higher survival rates. The best hope for improved survival lies in more efficient detection of tumours at an earlier stage, with screening for early gastric cancers performed in Japan and South Korea.

Pathophysiology

Infection with *H. pylori* plays a key pathogenic role and the infection has been classified by the International Agency for Research on Cancer (IARC) as a definite human carcinogen. It is associated with chronic atrophic gastritis, gastric mucosal atrophy and gastric cancer (Fig. 23.40). It has been estimated that *H. pylori* infection may contribute to the occurrence of gastric cancer in 70% of cases. Although the majority of *H. pylori*-infected individuals have normal or increased acid secretion, a few become hypo- or achlorhydric and these people are thought to be at greatest risk. *H. pylori*-induced chronic inflammation with generation of reactive oxygen species and depletion of the normally abundant antioxidant ascorbic acid are also important. There is strong evidence that *H. pylori* eradication, especially if achieved before irreversible pre-neoplastic changes (atrophy and intestinal metaplasia) have developed, reduces the risk of cancer development in high-risk populations and is cost-effective.

Diets rich in salted, smoked or pickled foods and the consumption of nitrites and nitrates may increase cancer risk. Carcinogenic *N*-nitroso-compounds are formed from nitrates by the action of nitrite-reducing bacteria that colonise the achlorhydric stomach. Diets lacking in fresh fruit and vegetables, as well as vitamins C and A, may also contribute. Other risk factors are listed in Box 23.39. Genetic risk factors also play

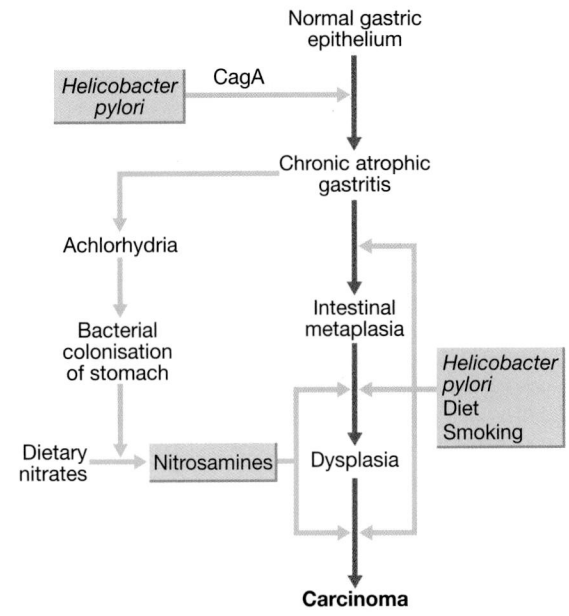

Fig. 23.40 Gastric carcinogenesis: a possible mechanism. (CagA = cytotoxin-associated gene)

---

i | **23.39 Risk factors for gastric cancer**

- *Helicobacter pylori*
- Smoking
- Alcohol
- Dietary associations (see text)
- Autoimmune gastritis (pernicious anaemia)
- Adenomatous gastric polyps
- Previous partial gastrectomy (> 20 years)
- Ménétrier's disease
- Hereditary diffuse gastric cancer families (*CDH1* mutations)
- Familial adenomatous polyposis (p. 831)

---

a role, with 10%-20% of gastric cancers showing familial history of the disease. Rarely, gastric cancer may be inherited in an autosomal dominant manner in association with mutations of the *E-cadherin* (*CDH1*) gene. There are eight genomic regions associated with an increased risk of gastric cancer.

Virtually all tumours are adenocarcinomas arising from mucus-secreting cells in the base of the gastric crypts. Most develop on a background of chronic atrophic gastritis with intestinal metaplasia and dysplasia. Cancers are either 'intestinal', arising from areas of intestinal metaplasia with histological features reminiscent of intestinal epithelium, or 'diffuse', arising from normal gastric mucosa. Intestinal-type carcinomas are more common and arise against a background of chronic mucosal injury. Diffuse cancers tend to be poorly differentiated and occur in younger patients. In low- and middle-income countries, 50% of gastric cancers develop in the antrum; 20%–30% occur in the gastric body, often on the greater curve; and 20% are found in the cardia. In Western populations, however, proximal gastric tumours are more common than those arising in the body and distal stomach. This change in disease pattern may be a reflection of changes in lifestyle or the decreasing prevalence of *H. pylori* in high-income countries. Diffuse submucosal infiltration by a scirrhous cancer (linitis plastica) is uncommon. Early gastric cancer is defined as cancer confined to the mucosa or submucosa. It is more often recognised in Japan, where widespread screening is practised. Some cases can be cured by endoscopic mucosal or submucosal resection. The majority of patients (> 80%) in the West, however, present with advanced gastric cancer.

23

Clinical features

Early gastric cancer is usually asymptomatic, but may be discovered during endoscopy for investigation of dyspepsia. Two-thirds of patients with advanced cancers have weight loss and 50% have ulcer-like pain. Anorexia and nausea occur in one-third, while early satiety, haematemesis, melaena and dyspepsia alone are less common. Dysphagia occurs in tumours of the gastric cardia that obstruct the gastro-oesophageal junction. Anaemia from occult bleeding is also common. Examination may reveal no abnormalities, but signs of weight loss, anaemia and a palpable epigastric mass may be present. Jaundice or ascites signifies metastatic spread. Occasionally, tumour spread occurs to the supraclavicular lymph nodes (Virchow's node), umbilicus (Sister Joseph's nodule) or ovaries (Krukenberg tumour). Paraneoplastic phenomena, such as acanthosis nigricans, thrombophlebitis (Trousseau's sign) and dermatomyositis may rarely occur. Metastases arise most commonly in the liver, lungs, peritoneum and bone marrow.

Investigations

Upper gastrointestinal endoscopy is the investigation of choice (Fig. 23.41) and should be performed promptly in any dyspeptic patient with 'alarm features' (see Box 23.15). Multiple biopsies from the edge and base of a gastric ulcer are required. Once the diagnosis is made, further imaging is necessary for staging and assessment of resectability. EUS and CT can be used to stage locally advanced gastric cancer; laparoscopy may be required to assess for peritoneal metastatic disease if resection is being contemplated.

Management

Surgery

Resection offers the only hope of cure and this can be achieved in about 90% of patients with early gastric cancer. While surgery is the gold standard, endoscopic mucosal resection or endoscopic submucosal dissection can be considered for very early tumours. For the majority of patients with locally advanced disease, total gastrectomy with lymphadenectomy is the operation of choice, preserving the spleen if possible. Proximal tumours involving the oesophago-gastric junction also require a distal oesophagectomy. Small tumours sited distally can be managed by a partial gastrectomy with lymphadenectomy and either a Billroth I or a Roux-en-Y reconstruction. More extensive lymph node resection may increase survival rates, but carries greater morbidity. Even for those who cannot be cured, palliative resection may be necessary when patients present with bleeding or gastric outflow obstruction. Perioperative chemotherapy is recommended for patients with locally advanced disease (e.g. epirubicin, cisplatin and 5-fluorouracil). For individuals who did not receive pre-operative chemotherapy, post-operative chemoradiotherapy (e.g. 5-flurouracil and leucovorin with radiotherapy) or adjuvant chemotherapy (e.g. 5-fluorouracil) is recommended.

Palliative treatment

Metastatic gastric cancer has a poor outlook, with survival around 4 months with best supportive care. Patients with inoperable locally advanced disease, or metastatic disease should be considered for palliative chemotherapy depending upon fitness, which may extend survival to 12 months. The biologic agent trastuzumab is recommended in conjunction with chemotherapy for patients whose tumours overexpress HER2 (p. 137). Endoscopic laser ablation for control of dysphagia or recurrent bleeding benefits some patients. Carcinomas at the cardia or pylorus may require endoscopic dilatation or insertion of expandable metallic stents for relief of dysphagia or vomiting. A nasogastric tube may offer temporary relief of vomiting due to gastric outlet obstruction (Box 23.40).

Gastric lymphoma

This is a rare tumour, accounting for less than 5% of all gastric malignancies. The stomach is, however, the most common site for extranodal non-Hodgkin lymphoma and 60% of all primary gastrointestinal lymphomas occur at this site. Gastric lymphoma is 2 to 3 times more common in males than females. Lymphoid tissue is not found in the normal stomach, but lymphoid aggregates develop in the presence of *H. pylori* infection. Indeed, *H. pylori* infection is closely associated with the development of a low-grade lymphoma (classified as extranodal marginal-zone lymphomas of MALT type). EUS plays an important role in staging these lesions by accurately defining the depth of invasion into the gastric wall.

The clinical presentation is similar to that of gastric cancer and endoscopically the tumour appears as a polypoid or ulcerating mass. While initial treatment of low-grade lesions confined to the superficial layers

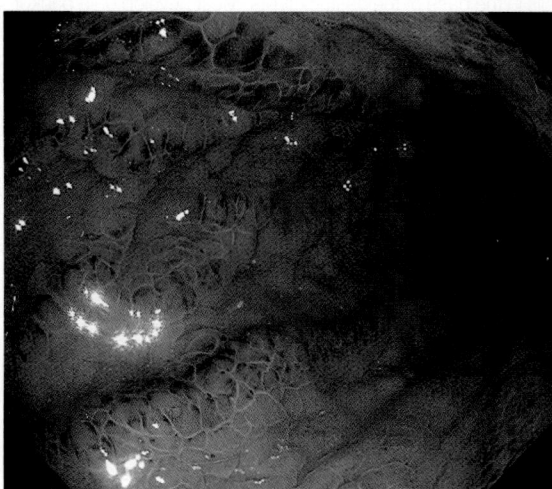

Fig. 23.41 Gastric carcinoma. Endoscopic finding of an early gastric cancer.

23.40 How to insert a nasogastric tube

Equipment

- 8–9 F 'fine-bore' tube for feeding or 16–18 F 'wide-bore' tube for drainage
- Lubricant jelly
- Cup of water and straw for sipping
- Adhesive tape
- pH (not litmus) paper
- Sickness bowl and tissues
- Catheter drainage bag and clamp (for drainage)

Technique

- A clear explanation and a calm patient are essential
- Establish a 'stop signal' for the patient to use, if needed
- Ask the patient to sit semi-upright
- Examine the nose for deformity or blockage to determine which side to use
- Measure the distance from ear to xiphoid process via the nose and mark the position on the tube
- Advance the lubricated tube tip slowly along the floor of the nasal passage to the oropharynx
- Ask the patient to sip water and advance the tube 2–3 cm with each swallow
- Stop, withdraw and retry if the patient is distressed or coughing, as the tube may have entered the larynx
- Advance until the mark on the tube reaches the tip of the nose and secure with tape
- Aspirate the contents and check pH (gastric acid confirmed if pH < 5). If in doubt, perform a chest X-ray to confirm tube position (usually necessary with feeding tubes)
- Attach the catheter drainage bag, if necessary, and clamp

Aftercare

- Flush the tube daily after feeding or drug dosing
- Check position regularly and look for signs of displacement
- Check with the pharmacist what drugs, if any, can be safely given via the tube

of the gastric wall consists of *H. pylori* eradication and close observation, 25% contain t(11:18) chromosomal translocations. In these cases, additional radiotherapy or chemotherapy is usually necessary. High-grade B-cell lymphomas should be treated by a combination of rituximab, chemotherapy (p. 971), surgery and radiotherapy. The choice depends on the site and extent of tumour, the presence of comorbid illnesses, and other factors, such as symptoms of bleeding and gastric outflow obstruction. The prognosis depends on the stage at diagnosis. Features predicting a favourable prognosis are stage I or II disease, small resectable tumours, tumours with low-grade histology and age below 60 years.

Other tumours of the stomach

Gastrointestinal stromal cell tumours (GISTs), arising from the interstitial cells of Cajal, are occasionally found incidentally at endoscopy and account for 1%–2% of gastrointestinal neoplasms. They are differentiated from other mesenchymal tumours by expression of the *c-kit* proto-oncogene, which encodes a tyrosine kinase receptor. These tumours, particularly the smaller lesions of less than 2 cm, are usually benign and asymptomatic, but larger ones may have malignant potential and may occasionally be responsible for dyspepsia, ulceration and gastrointestinal bleeding. Small lesions (< 2 cm) are usually monitored by endoscopy, while larger ones require surgical resection. Very large lesions should be treated pre-operatively with imatinib (a tyrosine kinase inhibitor) to reduce their size and make surgery easier. Imatinib can also provide prolonged control of metastatic GISTs. Sunitinib and regorafenib are used as second-line agents.

A variety of different types of gastric polyps occur. Fundic gland polyps are common and usually not associated with an increased risk of malignancy, other than in the context of familial adenomatous polyposis (FAP) (see p. 834). Hyperplastic polyps are also common, with regression generally occurring after *H. pylori* eradication. Adenomatous polyps are rare but have malignant potential and should be removed endoscopically with subsequent surveillance by periodic endoscopy.

Occasionally, gastric neuro-endocrine (carcinoid) tumours are seen in the fundus and body in patients with long-standing pernicious anaemia. These benign tumours arise from ECL or other endocrine cells, and are often multiple, but rarely invasive. Unlike carcinoid tumours arising elsewhere in the gastrointestinal tract, they usually run a benign and favourable course. Large (> 2 cm) carcinoids may, however, metastasise and should be removed. Rarely, small nodules of ectopic pancreatic exocrine tissue are found. These 'pancreatic rests' may be mistaken for gastric neoplasms and usually cause no symptoms. EUS is the most useful investigation.

Gastric motility disorders

Gastroparesis

Defective gastric emptying without mechanical obstruction of the stomach or duodenum can occur as a primary event, due to inherited or acquired disorders of the gastric pacemaker, or can be secondary to disorders of autonomic nerves (particularly diabetic neuropathy) or the gastroduodenal musculature (systemic sclerosis, myotonic dystrophies and amyloidosis). Drugs such as opiates, calcium channel antagonists and those with anticholinergic activity (tricyclics, phenothiazines) can also cause gastroparesis. Early satiety and recurrent vomiting are the major symptoms; abdominal fullness and a succussion splash may be present on examination. Symptoms may overlap with functional dyspepsia (postprandial distress syndrome). Treatment is based on small, frequent, low-fat meals and the use of metoclopramide and domperidone. In severe cases, nutritional failure can occur and long-term jejunostomy feeding or total parenteral nutrition is required. Surgical insertion of a gastric neurostimulator may be considered in refractory cases, especially those complicating diabetic autonomic neuropathy.

Disorders of the small intestine

Disorders causing malabsorption

Coeliac disease

Coeliac disease is an inflammatory disorder of the small bowel occurring in genetically susceptible individuals, which results from intolerance to wheat gluten and similar proteins found in rye, barley and, to a lesser extent, oats. It can result in malabsorption and responds to a gluten-free diet. The condition occurs worldwide, but is more common in northern Europe. The prevalence in the UK is approximately 1%, although 50% of these people are asymptomatic. These include both undiagnosed 'silent' cases of the disease and cases of 'latent' coeliac disease – genetically susceptible people who may later develop clinical coeliac disease.

Pathophysiology

The precise mechanism of mucosal damage is unclear, but immunological responses to gluten play a key role (Fig. 23.42). There is a strong genetic component, with around 8% of first-degree relatives of an index case affected, and there is strong (approximately 80%) concordance in monozygotic twins. There is a strong association with human leukocyte antigen (HLA)-DQ2/DQ8. Dysbiosis of the intestinal microbiota has been identified, but it is unclear if this is pathological or a response to the underlying mucosal changes.

Clinical features

Coeliac disease can present at any age. In infancy, it occurs after weaning on to cereals and typically presents with diarrhoea, malabsorption and failure to thrive. In older children, it may present with non-specific features, such as delayed growth. Features of malnutrition are found on examination and mild abdominal distension may be present. Affected children have growth and pubertal delay, leading to short stature in adulthood.

In adults, the disease usually presents during the third or fourth decade and females are affected twice as often as males. The presentation is highly variable, depending on the severity and extent of small bowel involvement. Some have florid malabsorption, while others develop non-specific symptoms, such as tiredness, weight loss, folate deficiency or iron deficiency anaemia. Other symptoms include oral ulceration, dyspepsia and bloating; such non-specific symptomatology is more common in older people (see Box 23.41). Unrecognised coeliac disease is associated with mild under-nutrition and osteoporosis.

Coeliac disease is associated with other HLA-linked autoimmune disorders and with certain other diseases (Box 23.42). In some centres, individuals at higher risk of developing coeliac disease, e.g. people with type 1 diabetes, undergo periodic antibody screening. This may identify people with asymptomatic or minimally symptomatic disease.

Investigations

These are performed to confirm the diagnosis and to look for consequences of malabsorption.

Duodenal biopsy

Endoscopic small bowel biopsy is the gold standard. Endoscopic appearances should not preclude biopsy, as the mucosa usually looks normal. As the histological changes can be patchy, an adequate number of biopsies (four biopsies from the second part of the duodenum plus one from the duodenal bulb) should be taken. The histological features are usually characteristic, but other causes of villous atrophy should be considered (Box 23.43 and Fig. 23.43).

Antibodies

Antibody tests constitute a valuable screening tool in patients with diarrhoea or other suggestive symptoms, but are not a diagnostic substitute for small bowel biopsy at present. Tissue transglutaminase (tTG) is now recognised

23

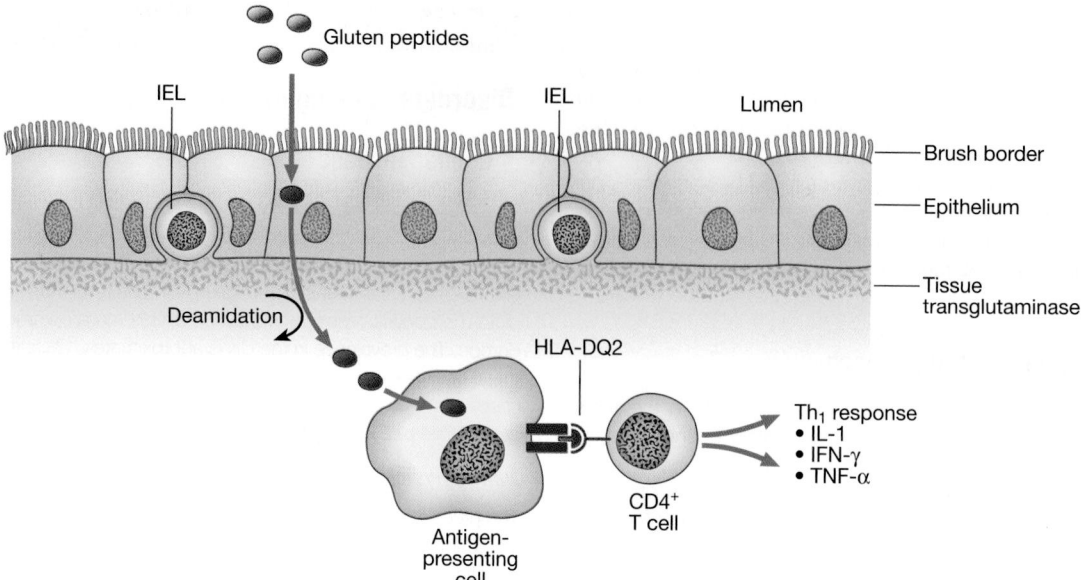

Fig. 23.42 Pathophysiology of coeliac disease. After being taken up by epithelial cells, gluten peptides are deamidated by the enzyme tissue transglutaminase in the subepithelial layer. They are then able to fit the antigen-binding motif on human leucocyte antigen (HLA)-DQ2-positive antigen-presenting cells. Recognition by CD4+ T cells triggers a Th$_1$ immune response with generation of pro-inflammatory cytokines: interleukin-1 (IL-1), interferon gamma (IFN-γ) and tumour necrosis factor alpha (TNF-α). Lymphocytes infiltrate the lamina propria and an increase in intra-epithelial lymphocytes (IELs), crypt hyperplasia and villous atrophy ensue.

23.41 Malabsorption in old age

- **Coeliac disease**: symptoms such as dyspepsia tend to be vague; only 25% present classically with diarrhoea and weight loss. Metabolic bone disease, folate or iron deficiency, coagulopathy and small bowel lymphoma are more common.
- **Small bowel bacterial overgrowth**: more common due to atrophic gastritis, resulting in hypo- or achlorhydria, increased prevalence of jejunal diverticulosis and long-term adverse effects of gastric surgery for ulcer disease.

23.42 Disease associations of coeliac disease

- Type 1 diabetes mellitus (2%–8%)
- Thyroid disease (5%)
- Primary biliary cholangitis (3%)
- Sjögren syndrome (3%)
- Immunoglobulin A deficiency (2%)
- Pernicious anaemia
- Sarcoidosis
- Neurological complications:
  Encephalopathy
  Cerebellar atrophy
  Peripheral neuropathy
  Epilepsy
- Myasthenia gravis
- Dermatitis herpetiformis
- Down syndrome
- Enteropathy-associated T-cell lymphoma
- Small bowel carcinoma
- Squamous carcinoma of oesophagus
- Ulcerative jejunitis
- Pancreatic insufficiency
- Microscopic colitis
- Splenic atrophy

23.43 Important causes of subtotal villous atrophy

- Coeliac disease
- Tropical sprue
- Dermatitis herpetiformis
- Lymphoma
- HIV-related enteropathy
- Giardiasis
- Hypogammaglobulinaemia
- Radiation
- Whipple's disease
- Zollinger–Ellison syndrome

(HIV = human immunodeficiency virus)

as the autoantigen for anti-endomysial antibodies. If the antibody screen is positive, adult patients should remain on a gluten-containing diet until duodenal biopsies are taken. High-titre serology in symptomatic children can be considered diagnostic without the need for endoscopy and biopsy. The use of this approach for diagnosis in adults is currently being explored.

Anti-endomysial antibodies of the IgA class are detectable by immunofluorescence in most untreated cases. They are sensitive (85%–95%) and specific (approximately 99%) for the diagnosis, except in very young infants. IgG antibodies, however, must be measured in patients with coexisting IgA deficiency. Measurement of the concentration of tTG antibodies has become the serological test of choice in many countries, as it is easier to perform, is semi-quantitative, has more than 95% sensitivity and specificity, and is more accurate in patients with IgA deficiency.

Haematology and biochemistry

A full blood count may show microcytic or macrocytic anaemia from iron or folate deficiency and features of hyposplenism (target cells, spherocytes and Howell–Jolly bodies). Biochemical tests may reveal reduced concentrations of calcium, magnesium, total protein, albumin or vitamin D. Serum IgA measurement is required to ensure an appropriate IgA response and to allow accurate analysis of serological testing.

Other investigations

Measurement of bone density should be considered to look for osteopenia or osteoporosis, especially in older patients and post-menopausal women.

Management

The aims are to correct existing deficiencies of micronutrients, such as iron, folate, calcium and/or vitamin D, and to achieve mucosal healing through a life-long gluten-free diet. This requires the exclusion of wheat, rye, barley and initially oats, although oats may be re-introduced safely in most patients after 6–12 months. Initially, frequent dietary counselling is required to make sure the diet is being observed, as the most common reason for failure to improve with dietary treatment is accidental or unrecognised gluten ingestion. Mineral and vitamin supplements are also given when indicated, but are seldom necessary when a strict gluten-free diet is adhered to. Booklets

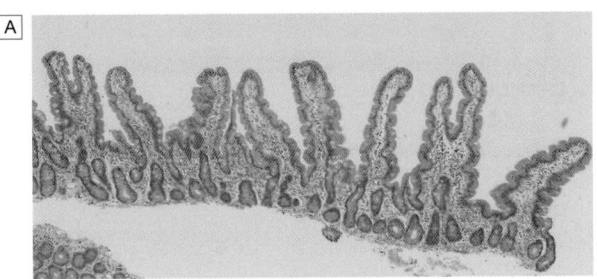 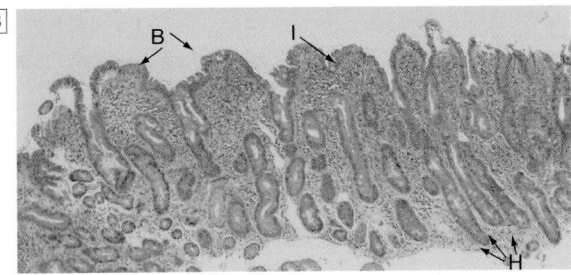

Fig. 23.43 Jejunal mucosa. [A] Normal. [B] Subtotal villous atrophy in coeliac disease. There is blunting of villi (B), crypt hyperplasia (H) and inflammatory infiltration of the lamina propria (I).

produced by 'coeliac societies' in many countries contain diet sheets and recipes using gluten-free flour, and are of great value. Dietetic follow-up is key to management. Patients should be followed up after initiation of a gluten-free diet, with assessment of symptoms, weight and nutritional status, and blood should be taken for measurement of tTG or anti-endomysial antibodies. There are currently no effective non-invasive tests to assess small bowel mucosal healing. Repeat small bowel biopsies should be considered in patients whose symptoms fail to improve and those in whom antibody levels remain high. In these circumstances, if the diet is satisfactory, then other conditions, such as pancreatic insufficiency or microscopic colitis, should be sought, as should complications of coeliac disease, such as ulcerative jejunitis or enteropathy-associated T-cell lymphoma. Some patients who fail to respond adequately to a gluten-free diet may require therapy with glucocorticoids or immunosuppressive drugs, and may be classified as refractory coeliac disease (RCD). RCD can be classified as type 1, characterised as a normal intraepithelial lymphocyte phenotype, or type 2, characterised by an abnormal expansion of a subset of small intestinal intraepithelial lymphocytes. Type 2 RCD has a 5-year survival of around 50%, compared to 90% in type 1 RCD.

Complications

A twofold-increased risk of malignancy, particularly of enteropathy-associated T-cell lymphoma, small bowel carcinoma and squamous carcinoma of the oesophagus, has been reported.

A few patients develop ulcerative jejuno-ileitis. This may present with fever, pain, obstruction or perforation. This diagnosis can be made by barium studies or enteroscopy but laparotomy and full-thickness biopsy may be required. Treatment is difficult. Glucocorticoids are used with mixed success and some patients require surgical resection and parenteral nutrition. The course is often progressive.

Osteoporosis and osteomalacia may occur in patients with long-standing, poorly controlled coeliac disease. These complications are less common in those who adhere strictly to a gluten-free diet.

Dermatitis herpetiformis

This is characterised by crops of intensely itchy blisters over the elbows, knees, back and buttocks (Ch. 27). Immunofluorescence shows granular or linear IgA deposition at the dermo-epidermal junction. Almost all patients have partial villous atrophy on duodenal biopsy, identical to that seen in coeliac disease, even though they usually have no gastrointestinal symptoms. In contrast, fewer than 10% of coeliac patients have evidence of dermatitis herpetiformis, although both disorders are associated with the same histocompatibility antigen groups. The rash usually responds to a gluten-free diet, but some patients require additional treatment with dapsone (100–150 mg daily).

Tropical sprue

Tropical sprue is defined as chronic, progressive malabsorption in a patient in or from a tropical country, associated with abnormalities of small intestinal structure and function. The disease occurs mainly in the West Indies and in southern India, Malaysia and Indonesia.

Pathophysiology

The epidemiological pattern and occasional epidemics suggest that an infective agent may be involved. Although no single bacterium has been isolated, the condition often begins after an acute diarrhoeal illness. Small bowel bacterial overgrowth with *Escherichia coli*, *Enterobacter* and *Klebsiella* is frequently seen. The changes closely resemble those of coeliac disease.

Clinical features

There is diarrhoea, abdominal distension, anorexia, fatigue and weight loss. In visitors to the tropics, the onset of severe diarrhoea may be sudden and accompanied by fever. When the disorder becomes chronic, the features of megaloblastic anaemia (vitamin B_{12} and folic acid malabsorption) and other deficiencies, including ankle oedema, glossitis and stomatitis, are common. Remissions and relapses may occur. The differential diagnosis in the indigenous tropical population is an infective cause of diarrhoea. The important differential diagnosis in visitors to the tropics is giardiasis (Ch. 13).

Management

Tetracycline (250 mg 4 times daily for 28 days) is the treatment of choice and brings about long-term remission or cure. In most patients, pharmacological doses of folic acid (5 mg daily) improve symptoms and jejunal morphology. In some cases, treatment must be prolonged before improvement occurs and occasionally patients must leave the tropics.

Small intestinal bacterial overgrowth

The normal duodenum and jejunum contain fewer than 10^4/mL organisms and these are usually derived from saliva. The count of coliform organisms never exceeds 10^3/mL. In bacterial overgrowth, there may be 10^8–10^{10}/mL organisms, most of which are normally found only in the colon. Disorders that impair the normal physiological mechanisms controlling bacterial proliferation in the intestine predispose to bacterial overgrowth (Box 23.44). The most important are loss of gastric acidity, impaired intestinal motility and structural abnormalities that allow colonic bacteria to gain access to the small intestine or provide a secluded haven from the peristaltic stream.

Pathophysiology

Bacterial overgrowth can occur in patients with small bowel diverticuli or following surgery that creates 'blind loops' of bowel, e.g. Billroth II or Roux-en-Y reconstructions. Diabetic autonomic neuropathy reduces small bowel motility and affects enterocyte secretion. In systemic sclerosis, bacterial overgrowth arises because the circular and longitudinal layers of the intestinal muscle are fibrosed and motility is abnormal. In idiopathic hypogammaglobulinaemia, bacterial overgrowth occurs because the IgA and IgM levels in serum and jejunal secretions are reduced. Chronic diarrhoea and malabsorption occur because of

23

i	23.44 Causes of small intestinal bacterial overgrowth	
Mechanism	**Examples**	
Hypo- or achlorhydria	Pernicious anaemia Partial gastrectomy Long-term proton pump inhibitor therapy	
Impaired intestinal motility	Systemic sclerosis Diabetic autonomic neuropathy	
Structural abnormalities	Gastric surgery (e.g. blind loop after Billroth II operation) Jejunal diverticulosis Enterocolic fistulae* Extensive small bowel resection Strictures*	
Impaired immune function	Hypogammaglobulinaemia	

*Most commonly caused by Crohn's disease.

bacterial overgrowth and recurrent gastrointestinal infections (particularly giardiasis, Ch. 13).

Clinical features

Patients commonly present with bloating, abdominal pain, distension and diarrhoea. Nutritional deficiencies can occur in severe cases, e.g. vitamin B_{12} deficiency can arise as the bacteria utilise vitamin B_{12}. Nutritional deficiencies are more commonly seen in patients with structural abnormalities, such as 'blind loop syndrome' or systemic sclerosis. Symptoms can commonly overlap with other diagnoses such as IBS and functional dyspepsia. There may also be symptoms from any underlying intestinal cause.

Investigations

Culture of small bowel aspirate, obtained at endoscopy, is the gold standard for diagnosis. However, this is a time-consuming, invasive and expensive technique. Bacterial overgrowth can also be diagnosed non-invasively using hydrogen breath tests, although they lack sensitivity. These simple, non-radioactive tests involve serial measurement of breath samples for hydrogen after oral ingestion of 75 g glucose or 10 g lactulose. If bacteria are present within the small bowel, they rapidly metabolise the glucose/lactulose, causing an early rise in exhaled hydrogen, in advance of that normally resulting from metabolism by colonic flora. Lactulose breath tests have a higher sensitivity than glucose, although may be less specific, as a rise in hydrogen can coincide with the arrival of lactulose in the caecum, leading to a false-positive result.

Management

The underlying cause of small intestinal bacterial overgrowth should be addressed, where possible. A course of broad-spectrum antibiotic for 2 weeks is the first-line treatment, although there is no consensus on agent or dose. Examples include rifaximin (which is not absorbed from the gut after oral administration), as well as systemic antibiotics such as ciprofloxacin, metronidazole and amoxicillin. Around 30%–40% of patients do not respond adequately and relapse rates are high. Some patients require up to 4 weeks of treatment and, in a few, continuous rotating courses of antibiotics are necessary. Consideration needs to be given to the risk of emerging antimicrobial resistance. Intramuscular vitamin B_{12} supplementation may be needed in chronic cases. Patients with motility disorders, such as diabetes and systemic sclerosis, can sometimes benefit from antidiarrhoeal drugs (diphenoxylate or loperamide orally). Giardiasis should be controlled in patients with hypogammaglobulinaemia, using metronidazole or tinidazole, but if symptoms fail to respond adequately, immunoglobulin infusions may be required.

i	23.45 Clinical features of Whipple's disease	
Gastrointestinal (> 70%)		
• Diarrhoea (75%) • Steatorrhoea • Weight loss (90%)	• Protein-losing enteropathy • Ascites • Hepatosplenomegaly (< 5%)	
Musculoskeletal (65%)		
• Seronegative large joint arthropathy	• Sacroiliitis	
Cardiac (10%)		
• Pericarditis • Myocarditis	• Endocarditis • Coronary arteritis	
Neurological (10%–40%)		
• Apathy • Fits • Dementia	• Myoclonus • Meningitis • Cranial nerve lesions	
Pulmonary (10%–20%)		
• Chronic cough • Pleurisy	• Pulmonary infiltrates	
Haematological (60%)		
• Anaemia	• Lymphadenopathy	
Other (40%)		
• Fever	• Pigmentation	

Whipple's disease

This rare condition is characterised by infiltration of small intestinal mucosa by 'foamy' macrophages, which stain positive with periodic acid–Schiff (PAS) reagent. The disease is a multisystem one and almost any organ can be affected, sometimes long before gastrointestinal involvement becomes apparent (Box 23.45).

Pathophysiology

Whipple's disease is caused by infection with the Gram-positive bacillus *Tropheryma whipplei*, which becomes resident within macrophages in the bowel mucosa. Villi are widened and flattened, containing densely packed macrophages in the lamina propria, which obstruct lymphatic drainage and cause fat malabsorption. Between 50% and 70% of the individuals have antibodies against *Tropheryma whipplei* worldwide, indicating prior environmental exposure, and yet Whipple's disease only occurs in a minority. This is presumably because host, bacterial and environmental factors are contributory in its pathogenesis.

Clinical features

Middle-aged men of European descent are most frequently affected and presentation depends on the pattern of organ involvement. Low-grade fever is common and most patients have joint symptoms to some degree, often as the first manifestation. Occasionally, neurological manifestations may predominate, due to CNS infection. Endocarditis can also occur, but usually only in a late phase.

Investigations

Diagnosis is made by the characteristic features on small bowel biopsy, with characterisation of the bacillus by polymerase chain reaction (PCR).

Management

Whipple's disease is often fatal if untreated but responds well, at least initially, to intravenous ceftriaxone (2 g daily for 2 weeks), followed by oral co-trimoxazole for at least 1 year. Symptoms usually resolve quickly and biopsy changes revert to normal in a few weeks. Long-term follow-up is essential, as clinical relapse occurs in up to one-third of patients, often within the CNS; in this case, the same therapy is repeated or else treatment with doxycycline and hydroxychloroquine is necessary.

Bile acid diarrhoea

Causes of bile acid diarrhoea are shown in Box 23.46. The population prevalence is estimated at around 1% and it is often under-diagnosed. It is now appreciated that up to a third of patients diagnosed with diarrhoea-predominant irritable bowel syndrome have evidence of bile acid diarrhoea. A common scenario is in patients with Crohn's disease who have undergone ileal resection, which can also lead to other malabsorptive manifestations (Fig. 23.44). Unabsorbed bile salts pass into the colon, stimulating water and electrolyte secretion and causing diarrhoea. If hepatic synthesis of new bile acids cannot keep pace with faecal losses, fat malabsorption occurs. Another consequence is the formation of lithogenic bile, leading to gallstones. Renal calculi, rich in oxalate, develop. Normally, oxalate in the colon is bound to and precipitated by calcium. Unabsorbed bile salts preferentially bind calcium, leaving oxalate to be absorbed, with development of urinary oxalate calculi.

Patients have urgent watery diarrhoea or mild steatorrhoea. Contrast studies and tests of B_{12} and bile acid absorption, such as the ^{75}Se-homocholic acid taurine (SeHCAT) test (see Box 23.12), are useful investigations but are not available throughout the world due to use of synthetic radio-labelled compound. An elevated serum 7α-hydroxycholestenone is a useful non-invasive marker of bile acid diarrhoea. Diarrhoea usually responds well to bile acid sequestrants, such as colestyramine or colesevelam, which bind bile salts in the intestinal lumen. Bile acid sequestrants can also be used as a diagnostic trial, where investigations are unavailable.

Short bowel syndrome

This is discussed in detail in Chapter 22.

i	23.46 Classification of bile acid diarrhoea	
Type	**Cause**	
Type 1	Terminal ileal disease leading to malabsorption of bile acids from terminal ileum, e.g. Crohn's disease, terminal ileal resection	
Type 2	Primary or idiopathic – no anatomical abnormalities or risk factors present	
Type 3	Other conditions that affect GI absorption, e.g. chronic pancreatitis, coeliac disease, small intestinal bacterial overgrowth	

Radiation enteropathy

Intestinal damage occurs in 10%–15% of patients undergoing radiotherapy for abdominal or pelvic malignancy. The risk varies with total dose, dosing schedule and the use of concomitant chemotherapy.

Pathophysiology

The rectum, sigmoid colon and terminal ileum are most frequently involved. Radiation causes acute inflammation, shortening of villi, oedema and crypt abscess formation. These usually resolve completely, but some patients develop an obliterative endarteritis affecting the endothelium of submucosal arterioles over 2–12 months. In the longer term, this can provoke a fibrotic reaction, leading to adhesions, ulceration, strictures, obstruction or fistula to adjacent organs.

Clinical features

In the acute phase, there is nausea, vomiting, cramping abdominal pain and diarrhoea. When the rectum and colon are involved, rectal mucus, bleeding and tenesmus occur. The chronic phase develops after 3 or more months in some patients and produces one or more of the problems listed in Box 23.47.

Investigations

In the acute phase, the rectal changes at sigmoidoscopy resemble ulcerative proctitis (see Fig. 23.64). The extent of the lesion can be assessed by colonoscopy. Barium follow-through or MRI enterography can be of diagnostic value in showing small bowel strictures, ulcers and fistulae.

Management

Diarrhoea in the acute phase should be treated with codeine phosphate, diphenoxylate or loperamide. Antibiotics may be required for bacterial

i	23.47 Chronic complications of intestinal irradiation
• Proctocolitis
• Bleeding from telangiectasia
• Small bowel strictures
• Fistulae: rectovaginal, colovesical, enterocolic
• Adhesions
• Malabsorption: bacterial overgrowth, bile acid diarrhoea (ileal damage)

23

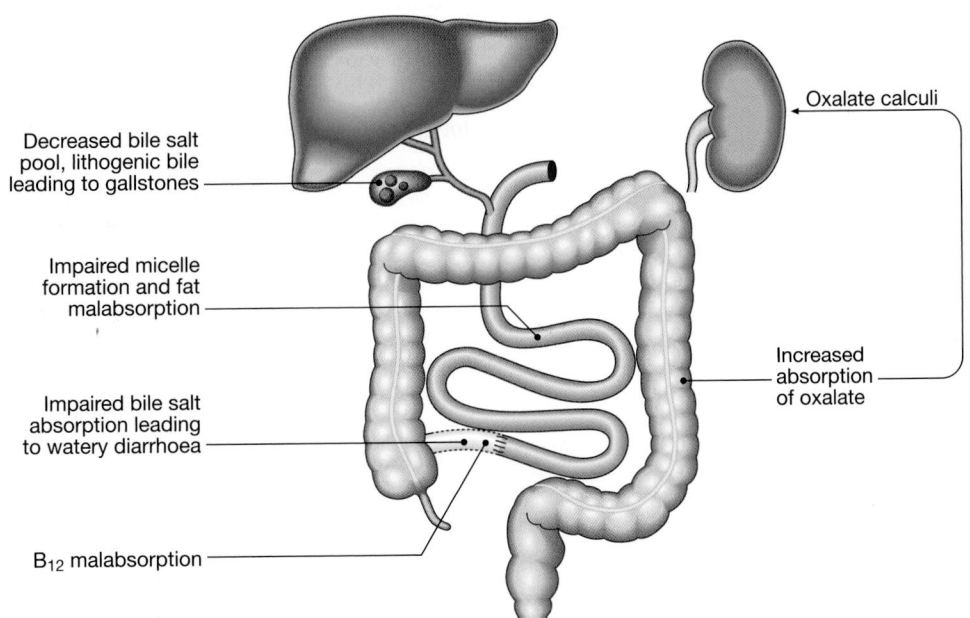

Decreased bile salt pool, lithogenic bile leading to gallstones

Impaired micelle formation and fat malabsorption

Impaired bile salt absorption leading to watery diarrhoea

B_{12} malabsorption

Oxalate calculi

Increased absorption of oxalate

Fig. 23.44 Consequences of ileal resection.

overgrowth. Nutritional supplements are necessary when malabsorption is present. Colestyramine or colesevelam is useful for associated bile acid diarrhoea. In radiation enteropathy, the underlying pathophysiology is tissue ischaemia rather than inflammation; glucocorticoid enemas are therefore not effective. Treatments include sucralfate enema and hyperbaric oxygen. Different endoscopic techniques may also be used, including argon plasma coagulation, radiofrequency ablation and heater probe thermocoagulation. Surgery should be avoided, if possible, because the injured intestine is difficult to resect and anastomose, but may be necessary if there is obstruction, perforation or fistula.

Abetalipoproteinaemia

This rare autosomal recessive disorder is caused by deficiency of apolipoprotein B, which results in failure of chylomicron formation. It leads to fat malabsorption and deficiency of fat-soluble vitamins. Jejunal biopsy reveals enterocytes distended with resynthesised triglyceride and normal villous morphology. Serum cholesterol and triglyceride levels are low. A number of other abnormalities occur in this syndrome, including acanthocytosis, retinitis pigmentosa and a progressive neurological disorder with cerebellar and dorsal column signs. Symptoms may be improved by a low-fat diet supplemented with medium-chain triglycerides and vitamins A, D, E and K.

Miscellaneous disorders of the small intestine

Protein-losing enteropathy

This term is used when there is excessive loss of protein into the gut lumen, sufficient to cause hypoproteinaemia. Protein-losing enteropathy occurs in many gut disorders but is most common in those where ulceration occurs (Box 23.48). In other disorders, protein loss can result from increased mucosal permeability or obstruction of intestinal lymphatic vessels. Patients present with peripheral oedema and hypoproteinaemia (reduced serum albumin and immunoglobulins), in the context of normal liver function and absent proteinuria.. The diagnosis can be confirmed by measurement of faecal clearance of α_1-antitrypsin or ^{51}Cr-labelled albumin after intravenous injection. Other investigations should be performed to determine the underlying cause. Treatment is that of the underlying disorder, with nutritional support and measures to control peripheral oedema.

Intestinal lymphangiectasia

This may be primary, resulting from congenital malunion of lymphatics, or secondary to lymphatic obstruction due to lymphoma, filariasis or constrictive pericarditis. Impaired drainage of intestinal lymphatic vessels leads to discharge of protein and fat-rich lymph into the gastrointestinal lumen. The condition presents with peripheral lymphoedema, pleural effusions or chylous ascites, and steatorrhoea. Investigations reveal hypoalbuminaemia, lymphopenia and reduced serum immunoglobulin concentrations. The diagnosis can be made by CT or MRI scanning and by enteroscopy with jejunal biopsy, which shows greatly dilated lacteals. Treatment consists of a low-fat diet with medium-chain triglyceride supplements.

Ulceration of the small intestine

Small bowel ulcers are uncommon and are either idiopathic or secondary to underlying intestinal disorders (Box 23.49). Ulcers are more common in the ileum and cause bleeding, perforation, stricture formation or obstruction. Capsule endoscopyand enteroscopy confirm the diagnosis.

NSAID-associated small intestinal toxicity

NSAIDs cause a spectrum of small intestinal lesions, ranging from erosions and ulcers to mucosal webs, strictures and, rarely, a condition known as 'diaphragm disease', in which intense submucosal fibrosis results in circumferential stricturing. The condition can present with pain,

---

i | **23.48 Causes of protein-losing enteropathy**

With mucosal erosions or ulceration

- Crohn's disease
- Ulcerative colitis
- Radiation damage
- Oesophageal, gastric or colonic cancer
- Lymphoma

Without mucosal erosions or ulceration

- Ménétrier's disease
- Bacterial overgrowth
- Coeliac disease
- Tropical sprue
- Eosinophilic gastroenteritis
- Systemic lupus erythematosus

With lymphatic obstruction

- Intestinal lymphangiectasia
- Constrictive pericarditis
- Lymphoma
- Whipple's disease

---

i | **23.49 Causes of small intestinal ulcers**

- Idiopathic
- Inflammatory bowel disease
- Non-steroidal anti-inflammatory drugs
- Ulcerative jejuno-ileitis
- Lymphoma and carcinoma
- Infections (tuberculosis, typhoid, *Yersinia enterocolitica*)
- Others (radiation, vasculitis)

---

obstruction, bleeding or anaemia, and may mimic Crohn's disease, carcinoma or lymphoma. Enteroscopy or capsule endoscopy can reveal the diagnosis but sometimes this is discovered only at laparotomy.

Eosinophilic gastroenteritis

This disorder of unknown aetiology can affect any part of the gastrointestinal tract, with the stomach and small intestine being the areas most commonly affected; it is characterised by eosinophil infiltration involving the gut wall, in the absence of parasitic infection or eosinophilia of other tissues. It may be mucosal, muscular or subserosal. Peripheral blood eosinophilia is present in around 70% of cases.

Clinical features

There are features of obstruction and inflammation, such as colicky pain, nausea and vomiting, diarrhoea and weight loss. Protein-losing enteropathy occurs and up to 50% of patients have a history of other allergic disorders. Steatorrhoea may be present in around 30% of patients. Serosal involvement may produce eosinophilic ascites.

Investigations and management

The diagnosis is made by histological assessment of multiple endoscopic biopsies, although full-thickness biopsies are occasionally required. Other investigations should be performed to exclude parasitic infection and other causes of eosinophilia. Serum IgE concentration is raised in around two-thirds of cases. Dietary manipulations can be considered as an initial strategy, but are rarely effective, although elimination diets (especially of milk) may benefit a few patients. Severe symptoms are treated with prednisolone (20–40 mg daily) and/or sodium cromoglicate, which stabilises mast cell membranes. The prognosis is good in the majority of patients.

Meckel's diverticulum

This is the most common congenital anomaly of the gastrointestinal tract and occurs in 0.3%–3% of people, but the vast majority of affected individuals are asymptomatic throughout life. The diverticulum results from failure of closure of the vitelline duct, with persistence of a blind-ending sac arising from the anti-mesenteric border of the ileum; it usually occurs within 100 cm of the ileocaecal valve and is up to 5 cm long. Approximately 50% contain ectopic gastric mucosa; rarely, colonic, pancreatic or endometrial tissue is present. Complications most commonly occur in the first 2 years of life, but are occasionally seen in young adults. Bleeding can result from ulceration of ileal mucosa adjacent to the ectopic parietal cells and presents as recurrent melaena or altered blood per rectum. The diagnosis can be made by scanning the abdomen using a gamma camera following an intravenous injection of ^{99m}Tc-pertechnetate, which is concentrated by ectopic parietal cells. Other complications include intestinal obstruction, diverticulitis, intussusception and perforation. Intervention is unnecessary unless complications occur.

Adverse food reactions

Adverse food reactions are common and are subdivided into food intolerance and food allergy, the former being much more common. In food intolerance, there is an adverse reaction to food that is not immune-mediated and results from pharmacological (histamine, tyramine or monosodium glutamate), metabolic (lactase deficiency) or other mechanisms (toxins or chemical contaminants in food). Food allergies (discussed in the section on 'Allergy' in Chapter 4) are immune-mediated disorders, most commonly due to type I hypersensitivity reactions with production of IgE antibodies, although type IV delayed hypersensitivity reactions are also seen.

Lactose intolerance

Human milk contains around 200 mmol/L (68 g/L) of lactose, which is normally digested to glucose and galactose by the brush border enzyme lactase prior to absorption. In most populations, enterocyte lactase activity declines throughout childhood. The enzyme is deficient in up to 90% of adult Africans, Asians and South Americans, but only 5% of northern Europeans.

In cases of genetically determined (primary) lactase deficiency, jejunal morphology is normal. 'Secondary' lactase deficiency occurs as a consequence of disorders that damage the jejunal mucosa, such as coeliac disease and viral gastroenteritis. Unhydrolysed lactose enters the colon, where bacterial fermentation produces volatile short-chain fatty acids, hydrogen and carbon dioxide.

Clinical features

In most people, lactase deficiency is completely asymptomatic. However, some complain of colicky pain, abdominal distension, increased flatus, borborygmi and diarrhoea after ingesting milk or milk products. Irritable bowel syndrome may be suspected, but the correct diagnosis is suggested by clinical improvement on lactose withdrawal. The lactose hydrogen breath test is a useful non-invasive investigation.

Dietary exclusion of lactose is recommended, although most sufferers are able to tolerate small amounts of milk (up to 250 mL milk, 12 g lactose) without symptoms. Addition of commercial lactase preparations to milk may be effective, but is costly.

Infections of the small intestine

Infections of the small intestine are discussed in other chapters. For travellers' diarrhoea, giardiasis and amoebiasis, see Chapter 13. Abdominal tuberculosis is discussed on page 520. Cryptosporidiosis and other protozoal infections, including cystoisosporiasis (Cystoisospora belli) and microsporidiosis, are covered Chapters 13 and 14.

Tumours of the small intestine

The small intestine is rarely affected by neoplasia and fewer than 5% of all gastrointestinal tumours occur at this site.

Benign tumours

The most common are adenomas, GISTs, lipomas and hamartomas. Adenomas are most often found in the periampullary region and are usually asymptomatic, although occult bleeding or obstruction due to intussusception may occur. Transformation to adenocarcinoma is rare.

Multiple adenomas are common in the duodenum of patients with familial adenomatous polyposis (FAP), who require regular endoscopic surveillance. Hamartomatous polyps with almost no malignant potential occur in Peutz–Jeghers syndrome (p. 832).

Malignant tumours

These are rare and include, in decreasing order of frequency, neuro-endocrine tumours, adenocarcinoma, malignant GIST and lymphoma. The majority occur in middle age or later. Kaposi's sarcoma of the small bowel may arise in patients with HIV/AIDS.

Adenocarcinomas

Adenocarcinomas occur with increased frequency in patients with FAP, coeliac disease, small bowel Crohn's disease and Peutz–Jeghers syndrome. This rare cancer accounts for fewer than 5% of all gastrointestinal malignancies. The non-specific presentation and rarity of these lesions often lead to a delay in diagnosis. Most are noted during assessment of anaemia or obscure GI bleeding. Capsule endoscopy or device-assisted enteroscopy, and small bowel enterography studies (CT or MRI) can be used to identify lesions. Treatment is by surgical resection.

Neuro-endocrine tumours

These are discussed in detail on page 691.

Lymphoma

Non-Hodgkin lymphoma (Ch. 25) may involve the gastrointestinal tract as part of more generalised disease or may rarely arise in the gut, the small intestine being most commonly affected. Lymphomas occur with increased frequency in patients with coeliac disease, HIV/AIDS and other immunodeficiency states. Most are of B-cell origin, although lymphoma associated with coeliac disease is derived from T cells (enteropathy-associated T-cell lymphoma).

Colicky abdominal pain, obstruction and weight loss are the presenting features and perforation is also seen occasionally. Malabsorption is a feature of diffuse bowel involvement and hepatosplenomegaly is rare.

The diagnosis is made by small bowel biopsy, radiological contrast studies and CT. Staging investigations should be performed as for lymphomas occurring elsewhere (p. 133). Surgical resection, where possible, is the treatment of choice, with radiotherapy and combination chemotherapy reserved for those with advanced disease. The prognosis depends largely on the stage at diagnosis, cell type, patient age and the presence of 'B' symptoms (fever, weight loss, night sweats).

Immunoproliferative small intestinal disease

Immunoproliferative small intestinal disease (IPSID), also known as alpha heavy chain disease, is a rare condition occurring mainly in Mediterranean countries, the Middle East, India, Pakistan and North America. It is a variant of B-cell lymphoma of MALT type and often associated with Campylobacter jejuni infection. The condition varies in severity from relatively benign to frankly malignant.

The small intestinal mucosa is diffusely affected, especially proximally, by a dense lymphoplasmacytic infiltrate. Enlarged mesenteric lymph nodes are also common. Most patients are young adults who present with malabsorption, anorexia and fever. Serum electrophoresis confirms the presence of alpha heavy chains (from the F_c portion of IgA). Prolonged remissions can be obtained with long-term antibiotic therapy, but chemotherapy is required for those who fail to respond or who have aggressive disease.

Small intestine motility disorders

Chronic small intestine pseudo-obstruction

Small intestinal motility is disordered in conditions that affect the smooth muscle or nerves of the intestine. Many cases are 'primary' (idiopathic), while others are 'secondary' to a variety of disorders or drugs (Box 23.50).

23

i 23.50 Causes of chronic intestinal pseudo-obstruction

Primary or idiopathic

- Rare familial visceral myopathies or neuropathies
- Congenital aganglionosis

Secondary

- Drugs (opiates, tricyclic antidepressants, phenothiazines)
- Smooth muscle disorders (systemic sclerosis, amyloidosis, mitochondrial myopathies)
- Myenteric plexus disorders, e.g. paraneoplastic syndrome in small-cell lung cancer
- Central nervous system disorders (Parkinson's disease, autonomic neuropathy)
- Endocrine and metabolic disorders (hypothyroidism, diabetic autonomic neuropathy, phaeochromocytoma, acute intermittent porphyria)

Clinical features

There are recurrent episodes of nausea, vomiting, abdominal discomfort and distension, often worse after food. Alternating constipation and diarrhoea occur and weight loss results from malabsorption (due to bacterial overgrowth) and fear of eating. There may also be symptoms of dysmotility affecting other parts of the gastrointestinal tract, such as dysphagia, and features of bladder dysfunction in primary cases. Some patients develop severe abdominal pain for reasons that are poorly understood and this can be difficult to manage.

Investigations

The diagnosis is often delayed and a high index of suspicion is needed. Plain X-rays show distended loops of bowel and air–fluid levels, with abdominal CT and small bowel MRI used to exclude mechanical obstruction. Laparotomy is sometimes required to exclude obstruction and to obtain full-thickness biopsies of the intestine. Examination of biopsy material using specialised techniques, such as electron microscopy and immunohistochemistry can diagnose the many rare diseases of enteric smooth muscle and nerves that can cause this syndrome.

Management

This is often difficult. Underlying causes should be addressed and further surgery avoided. Metoclopramide or domperidone may enhance motility and antibiotics are given for bacterial overgrowth. Nutritional and psychological support is also necessary.

Disorders of the colon and rectum

Colorectal polyps

Types of colorectal polyps

In the colon, polyps usually arise from the mucosal layer. These can vary in number and size, from a few millimetres to several centimetres. They are commonly described based on their appearance as sessile, pedunculated, flat, elevated or depressed (Fig. 23.45). In addition, they are classified histologically, as neoplastic or non-neoplastic polyps (Box 23.51). This is important to help predict their malignant potential.

Non-neoplastic polyps include hamartomas, inflammatory polyps and hyperplastic polyps, which harbour no malignant potential. Hyperplastic polyps are the commonest type of colorectal polyp, and are a subgroup of so-called serrated polyps, often small in size, and frequently found in the distal colon. Hamartomas can occur sporadically, or as part of a polyposis syndrome. Inflammatory polyps are commonly seen in the context of IBD and are due to inflammation within the colon with distorted mucosa.

The most well-known neoplastic polyps are conventional adenomas, which harbour malignant potential and are extremely common in the

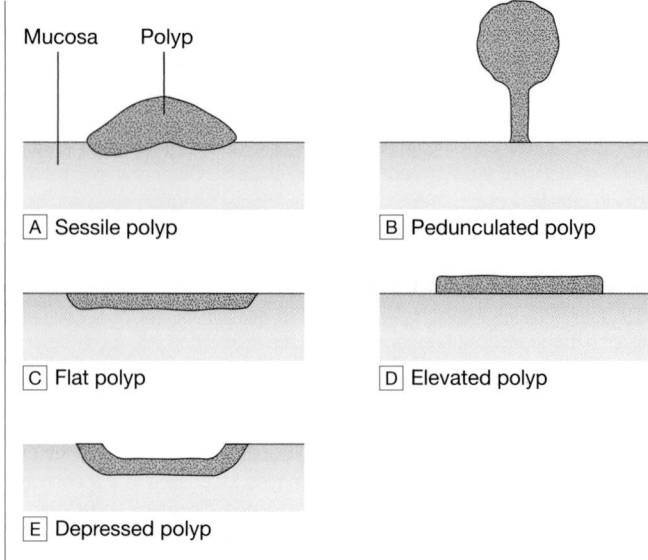

Fig. 23.45 Polyp morphology.

A Sessile polyp
B Pedunculated polyp
C Flat polyp
D Elevated polyp
E Depressed polyp

i 23.51 Neoplastic and non-neoplastic polyps

Neoplastic polyps	Non-neoplastic polyps
• Conventional adenoma	• Hamartoma
• Sessile serrated lesion	• Inflammatory
• Traditional serrated adenoma	• Hyperplastic

Western world. The prevalence of adenomas increases with age; 50% of people over 60 years of age have colorectal adenomas and in half of these the polyps are multiple. Adenomas can be found throughout the colon, although larger polyps, harbouring a higher risk of malignancy, tend to be more common in the rectum and distal colon. They can be further sub-classified histologically, as either tubular, villous or tubulovillous, according to the glandular architecture. Features associated with a higher risk of subsequent malignancy are listed in Box 23.52. Adenomas are usually asymptomatic and discovered incidentally. Larger adenomas can occasionally cause bleeding and anaemia. Rarely, large villous adenomas can secrete significant amounts of mucus, causing diarrhoea and hypokalaemia (McKittrick-Wheelock syndrome).

Traditionally, it was thought that adenomas were the only type of neoplastic polyp. However, it is now known that sessile serrated lesions and traditional serrated adenomas, further subgroups of serrated polyps, bear malignant potential. Sessile serrated lesions are more common in the right colon, tend to be flatter than conventional adenomas and are often covered with a mucus cap, making them hard to detect. They are now thought to account for between 15%–30% of colorectal cancers. Traditional serrated adenomas are relatively rare, accounting for <1% of all polyps, commonly found in the distal colon and can also harbour malignant potential.

Assessment and treatment of colorectal polyps

Colonic polyps are commonly found incidentally during endoscopy. If a polyp is found during sigmoidoscopy, a colonoscopy should be subsequently performed, as up to 40%–50% of affected individuals have further polyps more proximally in the colon. As neoplastic colonic polyps have malignant potential, these should be removed via colonoscopic polypectomy, as this considerably reduces subsequent colorectal cancer risk (Fig. 23.46). When cancer cells are found within 2 mm of the resection margin of the polyp, when the polyp cancer is poorly differentiated or when lymphatic invasion is present, segmental colonic resection is recommended because residual tumour or lymphatic spread (in up to 10%) may be present. Malignant polyps without these features can be followed up by surveillance colonoscopy.

Very large sessile polyps can sometimes be removed safely by endoscopic mucosal resection (EMR), but many require surgery. Endoscopic submucosal dissection (ESD) can be used for some lesions with a high suspicion of limited submucosal invasion, although this is a technically challenging procedure that is not routinely performed. Once all polyps have been removed, surveillance colonoscopy should be undertaken in individuals with high-risk findings, as new polyps develop in 50% of patients. Patients over 75 years of age tend not to require repeated colonoscopies, as their subsequent lifetime cancer risk is low.

Colorectal cancer

Globally, colorectal cancer is the third most commonly diagnosed cancer in males and second in females. High-income countries have the highest incidence of colorectal cancer, while Africa and South Asia have the lowest incidence. Worldwide incidence is continuing to increase, although incidence rates have stabilised in high-income countries. In the UK, the incidence is around 70 per 100000 of the population. The condition becomes increasingly common over the age of 50 years.

Pathophysiology

Both environmental and genetic factors are important in colorectal carcinogenesis. The majority (75%) of colorectal cancers are sporadic, with 20% of patients having genetic predisposition and a small minority (5%) being hereditary. Figure 23.47 outlines the key pathophysiological factors.

Genetics

Colorectal cancer development results from the accumulation of multiple genetic mutations. There are also associated epigenetic influences, such as microRNA expression signature, and potential influences from non-coding genetic variation. Currently, there are three main pathways

> **i** | **23.52 Risk factors for malignant change in colonic polyps**
>
> • Large size (> 2 cm)
> • Multiple polyps
> • Serrated polyps (excluding small rectal hyperplastic polyps)
> • Villous architecture
> • High-grade dysplasia

of genetic instability and each is associated with histological, clinical and prognostic parameters:

• *Chromosomal instability*. Mutations or deletions of portions of chromosomes arise, with loss of heterozygosity (LOH) and inactivation of specific tumour suppressor genes. In LOH, one allele of a gene is deleted, but gene inactivation occurs only when a subsequent unrelated mutation affects the other allele. Chromosomal instability (CIN) occurs in around 85% of colorectal cancers.
• *Microsatellite instability*. This involves germline mutations in one of six genes encoding enzymes involved in repairing errors that occur normally during DNA replication (DNA mismatch repair); these genes are designated *hMSH2*, *hMSH6*, *hMLH1*, *hMLH3*, *hPMS1* and *hPMS2*. Replication errors accumulate and can be detected in 'microsatellites' of repetitive DNA sequences. They also occur in important regulatory genes, resulting in a genetically unstable phenotype and accumulation of multiple somatic mutations throughout the genome that eventually lead to cancer. Around 15% of sporadic cancers develop this way, as do most cases of hereditary non-polyposis colon cancer (HNPCC).
• *CpG island methylator phenotype (CIMP)*. This phenotype is found in approximately 20%–30% of colorectal cancers and results in widespread gene hypermethylation. The result is functional loss of tumour suppressor genes.

There are two distinct pathways of carcinogenesis: the classical adenoma–carcinoma pathway and the more recently discovered alternate serrated neoplasia pathway. The classical adenoma–carcinoma pathway is characterised by an adenoma as the precursor lesion. Adenomas tend to result in carcinoma through the sequential acquisition of mutations, through chromosomal and microsatellite instability (Fig. 23.48). The time period for an adenoma to develop into a carcinoma is thought to take between 5 and 10 years. The serrated neoplasia pathway is characterised by a serrated polyp as a precursor lesion. Serrated polyps (hyperplastic, sessile serrated lesions, traditional serrated adenomas) were all thought to be non-neoplastic previously. However, it is now thought that sessile serrated lesions and traditional serrated adenomas are precursor lesions for malignancy. While hyperplastic polyps are generally still viewed as non-neoplastic, some subtypes are thought to be precursors of sessile serrated lesions. There are two pathways of carcinoma formation via the serrated neoplasia pathway, through the traditional serrated and sessile routes, with genetic instability through microsatellite instability and CIMP (Fig. 23.49), although molecular pathways are still not well understood. The serrated neoplasia pathway is associated with faster carcinoma development in comparison to the classical adenoma–carcinoma pathway.

23

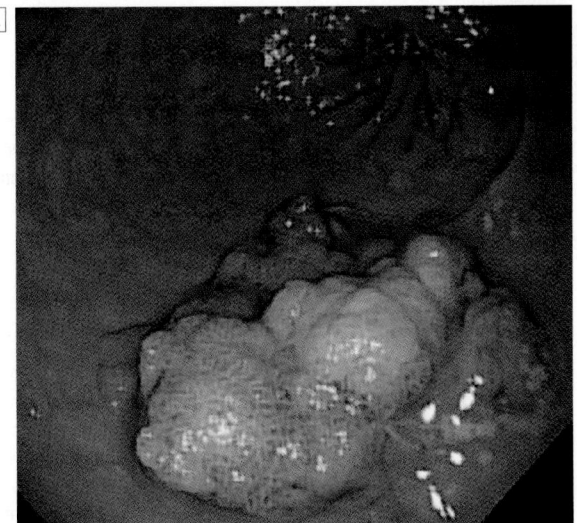
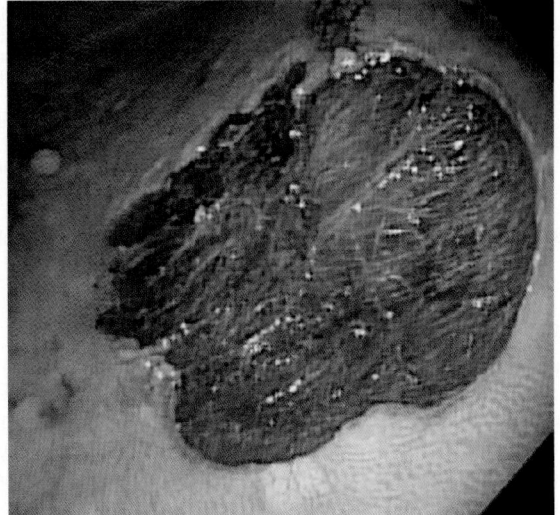

Fig. 23.46 Large rectal adenomatous polyp. A Before colonoscopic polypectomy. B After polypectomy.

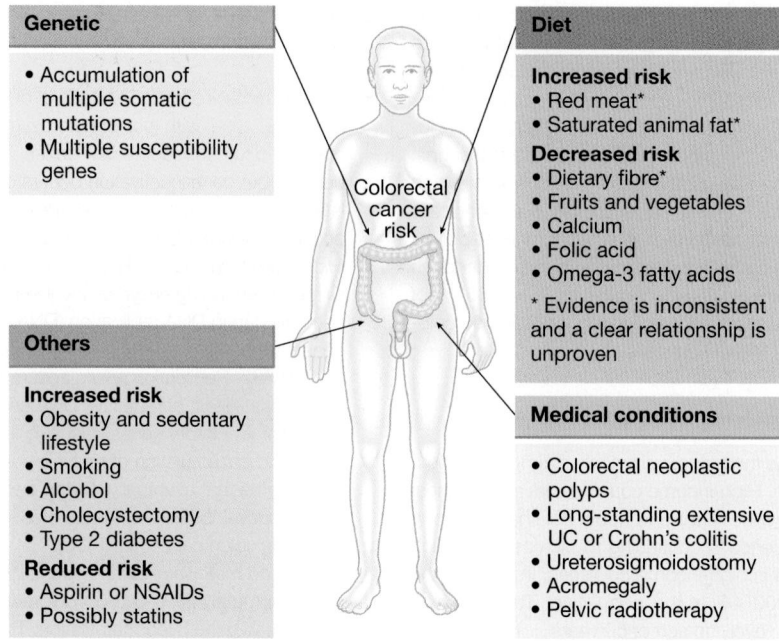

Fig. 23.47 Risk factors for colorectal cancer. (NSAIDs = non-steroidal anti-inflammatory drigs; UC = ulcerative colitis)

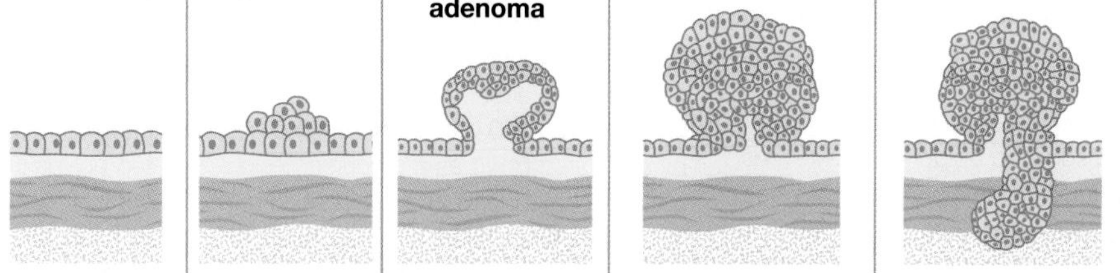

	Normal	Early adenoma	Intermediate adenoma	Late adenoma	Carcinoma
Key gene(s)		*APC* (adenomatous polyposis coli)	*KRAS*	*DCC* (deleted in colon cancer) *SMAD4*	*TP53*
Chromosome		5q	12p	18q	17p
Normal function		Inhibits translocation of β-catenin to nucleus and suppresses cell growth	Transmembrane GTP-binding protein mediating mitogenic signals (p21)	*DCC* regulates apoptosis and has a tumour suppressor function *SMAD4* regulates cell growth	Up-regulated during cell damage to arrest cell cycle and allow DNA repair or apoptosis to occur
Alteration		Truncating mutations	Gain-of-function mutations	Allelic deletion or silencing (*DCC*) Gain-of-function mutations (*SMAD4*)	Allelic deletion; gain-of-function mutations
Effect		Progression to early adenoma development	Cell proliferation	Enhanced tumour growth, invasion and metastasis	Cell proliferation; impaired apoptosis

Further mutations
- Anchorage independence
- Protease synthesis
- Telomerase synthesis
- Multidrug resistance
- Evasion of immune system

Fig. 23.48 The multistep origin of cancer: molecular events implicated in colorectal carcinogenesis. (GTP = guanine triphosphate)

Environment

The majority of colorectal cancers are sporadic, with the development of carcinoma being dependent upon the penetrance of a genetic predisposition and the severity of environmental insult. It is thought that up to 50% of cases of colorectal cancer may potentially be preventable by lifestyle modifications. Several risks factors increase the risk of colorectal cancer, such as smoking, alcohol and type 2 diabetes. In addition, dietary factors are also key in the pathophysiology of colorectal cancer, such as fruit and vegetable intake (see Fig. 23.47).

Clinical features

Symptoms vary, depending on the site of the carcinoma. However, the disease is largely asymptomatic until at an advanced stage. In tumours of the left colon, fresh rectal bleeding is common and obstruction occurs early. Tumours of the right colon present with anaemia from occult bleeding or with altered bowel habit, but obstruction is a late feature. Colicky lower abdominal pain is present in two-thirds of patients and rectal bleeding occurs in 50%. A minority present with features of either obstruction or perforation, leading to peritonitis, localised abscess or

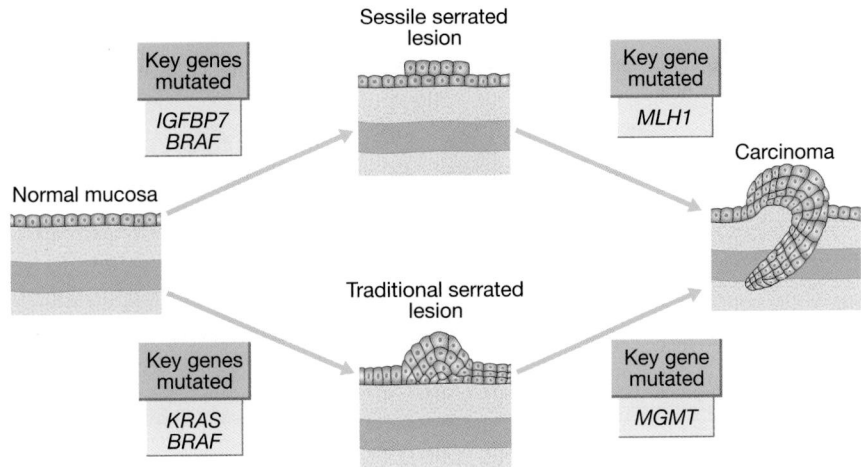

Gene	IGFBP7	BRAF	KRAS	MLH1	MGMT
Chromosome	4q	7q	12p	3p	10q
Normal function	Interacts with insulin-like growth factors that are involved in preventing apoptosis	Regulates cell proliferation, differentiation, migration and apoptosis	Transmembrane GTP-binding protein mediating mitogenic signals (p 21)	Mismatch repair gene that repairs errors made during DNA replication	DNA-repair protein involved in defence against mutagenesis and toxicity

Fig. 23.49 The serrated neoplasia pathway.

fistula formation. Carcinoma of the rectum usually causes early bleeding, mucus discharge or a feeling of incomplete emptying. Between 10% and 20% of patients present with iron deficiency anaemia or weight loss. On examination, there may be a palpable mass, signs of anaemia or hepatomegaly from metastases. Low rectal tumours may be palpable on digital examination.

Investigations

Colonoscopy is the investigation of choice because it is more sensitive and specific than barium enema. Furthermore, lesions can be biopsied and polyps removed. Patients in whom colonoscopy is incomplete and those who are at high risk of complications can be investigated by CT colonography (virtual colonoscopy). This is a sensitive and non-invasive technique for diagnosing tumours and polyps of more than 6 mm diameter. When the diagnosis of colon cancer has been made, CT of the chest, abdomen and pelvis should be performed as a staging investigation, particularly to detect hepatic metastases, with an increasing role of MRI for further characterisation of liver lesions. Pelvic MRI or endoanal ultrasound should be used for local staging of rectal cancer. Measurement of serum carcinoembryonic antigen (CEA) levels is of limited value in diagnosis, since values are normal in many patients, but CEA testing can be helpful during follow-up to monitor for recurrence. FDG PET-CT is being increasingly used, although its exact role is still debated. Tumour stage (TNM) at diagnosis is the most important determinant of prognosis (Fig. 23.50).

Management

Endoscopy

Early colorectal cancers may be amenable to endoscopic treatment, using techniques such as endoscopic mucosal resection, endoscopic submucosal dissection and endoscopic full-thickness resection. Endoscopic submucosal dissection and endoscopic full-thickness resection tend to be used when there is suspicion of superficial submucosal invasion and

needs a highly skilled endoscopist. In addition to such a procedure, surgical mesenteric lymphadenectomy may be required.

Surgery

Surgery for colorectal cancer remains the cornerstone of treatment with curative intent. Rectal cancers can be complex to operate on due to the anatomy of the pelvis. Neoadjuvant radiotherapy or chemoradiotherapy should be offered to individuals with high-risk rectal cancers to increase the subsequent chance of a complete (R0) subsequent surgical resection. Colorectal cancer may present as an emergency with obstruction or perforation. Obstruction can be treated by either a decompressing colostomy or endoscopic stenting. Metastatic disease confined to liver or lung should be considered for resection, as this can be potentially curative if there is truly no disease at other sites. Metastatic disease confined to the peritoneum can be considered for cytoreductive surgery and hyperthermic intraperitoneal chemotherapy, which shows benefit in survival in a subset of patients. Postoperatively, patients should undergo colonoscopy after 1 year and then 3 years later to search for local recurrence or development of new lesions.

Adjuvant therapy

About 30%–40% of patients have lymph node involvement at presentation and are therefore at risk of recurrence. Most recurrences are within 3 years of diagnosis and affect the liver, lung, distant lymph nodes and peritoneum. Adjuvant chemotherapy with 5-fluorouracil/folinic acid or capecitabine, preferably in combination with oxaliplatin, can reduce the risk of recurrence.

Palliation of advanced disease

Surgical resection of the primary tumour is appropriate for some patients with metastases to treat obstruction, bleeding or pain. *RAS* and *BRAF* V600E mutations are tested for in metastatic colorectal cancer in individuals being considered for systemic anti-cancer treatment, with outcomes worse if these mutations are present. Palliative chemotherapy with

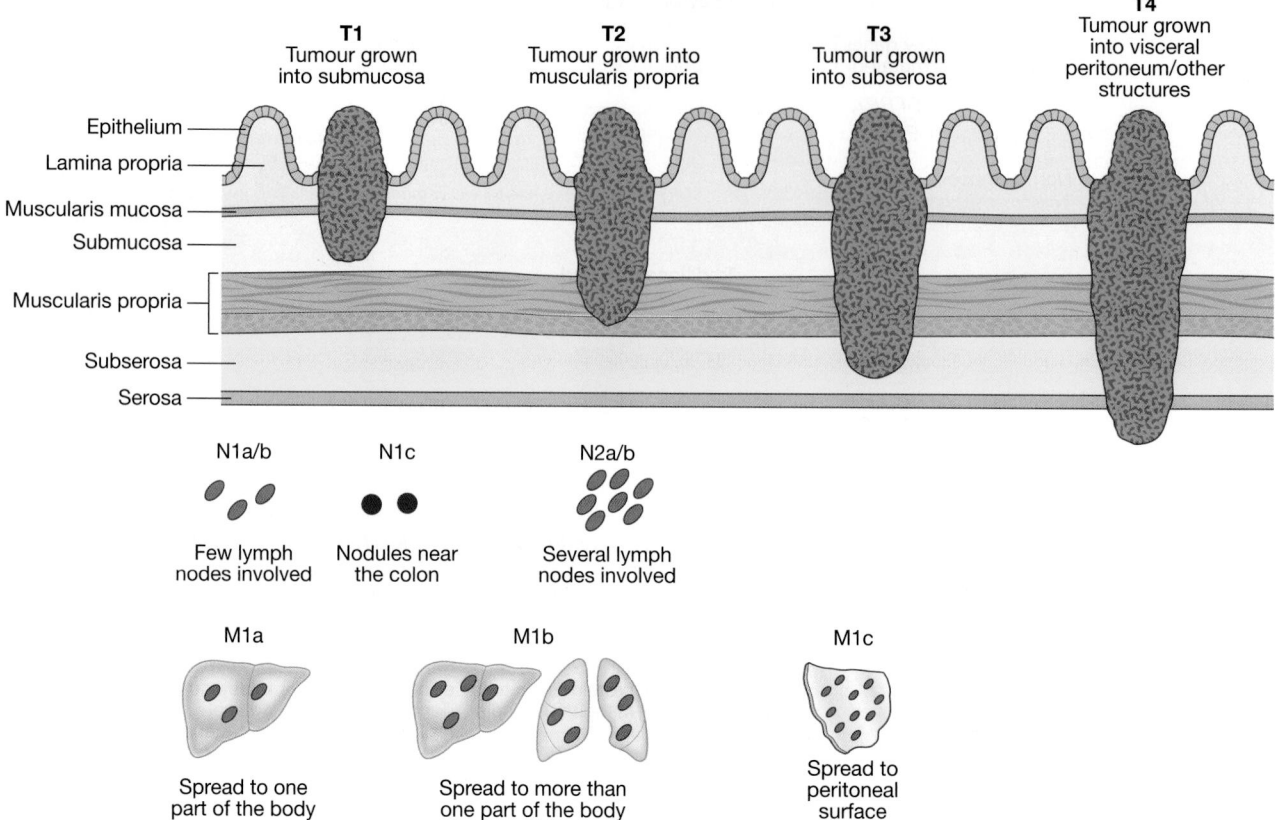

Fig. 23.50 TNM classification in colorectal cancer.

5-fluorouracil/folinic acid, capecitabine, oxaliplatin or irinotecan improves survival. Patients with advanced metastatic disease may be treated with monoclonal antibodies such as panitumumab or cetuximab, which bind to and inhibit the epidermal growth factor receptor. They are often given together with chemotherapy. Pelvic radiotherapy is sometimes useful for distressing rectal symptoms, such as pain, bleeding or severe tenesmus. Endoscopic laser therapy or insertion of an expandable metal stent can be used to relieve obstruction.

Prevention and screening

Secondary prevention aims to detect and remove lesions at an early or pre-malignant stage by screening the asymptomatic general population. Several potential methods exist:

- Population-based screening of people between the age of 50 to 74 years by regular *faecal immunochemical testing (FIT)* reduces colorectal cancer mortality and increases the proportion of early cancers detected. Serial stool testing with or without subsequent colonoscopy is the screening method of choice in the UK.
- *Colonoscopy* remains the gold standard and allows preventative polypectomy, but is expensive, requires bowel preparation and carries risks (perforation approximately 1:1000). Many countries lack the resources to offer this form of screening.
- *Flexible sigmoidoscopy* is an alternative option and has been shown to reduce overall colorectal cancer mortality by approximately 35% (70% for cases arising in the rectosigmoid). It is recommended in England, where available, as a one-off test in individuals aged 55 years, with subsequent FIT from age 60 years.
- *CT colonography* is fast and low-risk, and offers equivalent sensitivity to colonoscopy. Disadvantages include reduced sensitivity to detect polyps of less than 6mm, the requirement for bowel preparation, exposure to ionising radiation and its inability to offer therapeutic intent.

Hereditary syndromes predisposing to colorectal cancer

Whilst hereditary syndromes are rare, collectively accounting for 3%–5% of colorectal carcinomas, they are important to identify, as the risk of colorectal carcinoma is high in these individuals.

Non-polyposis syndromes

Hereditary non-polyposis colorectal cancer (HNPCC), also known as Lynch syndrome, has an autosomal dominant mode of inheritance, with a positive family history of colon cancer occurring at a young age. It is the commonest hereditary cancer syndrome, accounting for 1%–3% of all colorectal cancer cases. The lifetime risk in affected individuals is 80%, with a mean age at cancer development of 45 years. In contrast to sporadic colon cancer, two-thirds of tumours occur proximally. The clinical diagnostic criteria are listed in Box 23.53, with diagnosis now shifting from such criteria to testing of tumour material by microsatellite instability polymerase chain reaction and immunohistochemistry for mismatch repair proteins. In a subset of patients, there is also an increased incidence of cancers of the endometrium, ovary, urinary tract, stomach, pancreas, small intestine and CNS, related to inheritance of different mismatch repair gene mutations. Those who fulfil the criteria for HNPCC should be referred for pedigree assessment, genetic testing (see above) and colonoscopy. These should begin at either 25 years or 35 years (dependent upon the specific genetic abnormalities detected). Colonoscopy needs to be repeated every 2 years, but despite this, interval cancers can still occur. Regular daily use of aspirin is thought to reduce colorectal cancer risk.

Polyposis syndromes

Polyposis syndromes are classified by histopathology (Box 23.54). It is important to note that, while the hamartomatous polyps in Peutz–Jeghers syndrome and juvenile polyposis are not themselves neoplastic, these disorders are associated with an increased risk of malignancy of the breast, colon, ovary and thyroid.

Familial adenomatous polyposis

Familial adenomatous polyposis (FAP) is an uncommon autosomal dominant disorder affecting 1 in 14000 of the population and accounting for 0.07% of colorectal cancers. It results from germline mutation of the tumour suppressor *APC* gene, followed by acquired mutation of the remaining allele (Ch. 3). The *APC* gene is large and over 1400 different mutations have been reported, but most are loss-of-function mutations resulting in a truncated APC protein. This protein normally binds to and sequesters β-catenin, but is unable to do so when mutated, allowing β-catenin to translocate to the nucleus, where it up-regulates the expression of many genes. Gene mutations are detected in around 95% of FAP cases. Around 25% of cases arise as new mutations and have no family history.

Hundreds to thousands of adenomatous colonic polyps develop in 80% of patients by age 15 (Fig. 23.51), with symptoms such as rectal bleeding beginning a few years later. In those affected, cancer will develop within 10–15 years of the appearance of adenomas and 90% of patients will develop colorectal cancer by the age of 50 years. Despite surveillance, approximately 1 in 4 patients with FAP have cancer by the time they undergo colectomy. There appears to be phenotypic variability in FAP, with an attenuated form resulting in fewer than 100 adenomatous polyps and later onset of polyposis and cancer.

A second gene involved in base excision repair (MutY homolog, *MUTYH*) has been identified and may give rise to colonic polyposis. *MUTYH* displays autosomal recessive inheritance and leads to tens to hundreds of polyps and proximal colon cancer. This variant is referred to as MUTYH-associated polyposis (MAP).

In FAP, non-neoplastic cystic fundic gland polyps occur in the stomach, but adenomatous polyps also arise uncommonly. Duodenal adenomas are found in over 90% and are most common around the ampulla of Vater. Malignant transformation to adenocarcinoma takes place in 10% and is the leading cause of death in those who have had prophylactic colectomy. Many extra-intestinal features are also seen (Box 23.55).

Desmoid tumours occur in up to one-third of patients and usually arise in the mesentery or abdominal wall. Although benign, they may become very large, causing compression of adjacent organs, intestinal obstruction or vascular compromise and are difficult to remove. They sometimes respond to hormonal therapy with tamoxifen, and the NSAID sulindac may bring about regression in some, by unknown mechanisms. Congenital hypertrophy of the retinal pigment epithelium (CHRPE) occurs in some cases and is seen as dark, round, pigmented retinal lesions. When present in an at-risk individual, these are 100% predictive of the presence of FAP. A variant, Turcot syndrome, is characterised by FAP with primary CNS tumours (astrocytoma or medulloblastoma).

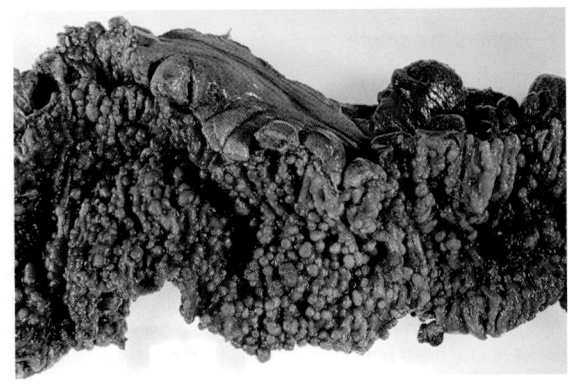

Fig. 23.51 Familial adenomatous polyposis. There are hundreds of adenomatous polyps throughout the colon.

ℹ 23.53 Modified Amsterdam criteria* for hereditary non-polyposis colon cancer

- Three or more relatives with colon cancer (at least one first-degree)
- Colorectal cancer in two or more generations
- At least one member affected under 50 years of age
- Familial adenomatous polyposis excluded

*These criteria are strict and may miss some families with mutations. Hereditary non-polyposis colon cancer should also be considered in individuals with colorectal or endometrial cancer under 45 years of age.

ℹ 23.55 Extra-intestinal features of familial adenomatous polyposis

- Congenital hypertrophy of the retinal pigment epithelium (CHRPE, 70%–80%)
- Epidermoid cysts (extremities, face, scalp)* (50%)
- Benign osteomas, especially skull and angle of mandible* (50%–90%)
- Dental abnormalities (15%–25%)*
- Desmoid tumours (10%–15%)
- Other malignancies (brain, thyroid, liver, adrenal, 1%–3%)

*Gardner syndrome.

23

ℹ 23.54 Gastrointestinal polyposis syndromes

	Neoplastic		Non-neoplastic[1]		
	Familial adenomatous polyposis	**Peutz–Jeghers syndrome**	**Juvenile polyposis**	**Cronkhite–Canada syndrome**	**Cowden disease**
Inheritance	Autosomal dominant[2]	Autosomal dominant	Autosomal dominant in one-third	None	Autosomal dominant
Oesophageal polyps	–	–	–	+	+
Gastric polyps	+	+	+	+++	+++
Small bowel polyps	++	+++	++	++	++
Colonic polyps	+++	++	++	+++	+
Other features	Colorectal cancer, bleeding, extra-intestinal features (see Box 23.55)	Pigmentation, bleeding, intussusception, bowel and other cancers	Colorectal cancer	Hair loss, pigmentation, nail dystrophy, malabsorption	Many congenital anomalies, oral and cutaneous hamartomas, thyroid and breast tumours

[1]The polyps themselves are not neoplastic but cancer risk is increased in several syndromes. [2]Rare autosomal recessive variant *MUTYH* (see text).
(– = absent; + = may occur; ++ = common; +++ = very common)

Early identification of affected individuals before symptoms develop is essential. The diagnosis can be excluded if sigmoidoscopy is normal. In newly diagnosed cases, genetic testing should be carried out to confirm the diagnosis and identify the causal mutation. Subsequently, all first-degree relatives should undergo genetic testing (Ch. 3). In families with known FAP, adolescents should undergo mutation testing at 13–14 years of age and patients who are found to have the mutation should be offered colectomy after school or college education has been completed. The operation of choice is total proctocolectomy with ileal pouch–anal anastomosis. Ileoanal pouch construction may be associated with reduced fertility in women, which may be due to fallopian tube scarring post surgery. Therefore, colectomy with ileorectal anastomosis can be used, but is associated with a risk of cancer in the retained rectum. Periodic upper gastrointestinal endoscopy every 1–3 years is recommended to detect and monitor duodenal and periampullary adenomas. If large, these may be amenable to endoscopic resection.

Peutz–Jeghers syndrome

Puetz-Jeghers syndrome occurs in around 1 in 120 000 of the population, accounting for less than 0.01% of colorectal cancer cases. Multiple hamartomatous polyps occur in the small intestine and colon, as well as melanin pigmentation of the lips, mouth and digits (Fig. 23.52). Most cases are asymptomatic, although chronic bleeding, anaemia or intussusception can occur. There is a significant risk of small bowel or colonic adenocarcinoma and of cancer of the pancreas, lung, testis, ovary, breast and endometrium. Peutz–Jeghers syndrome is an autosomal dominant disorder with high penetrance, most commonly resulting from truncating mutations in a serine–threonine kinase gene on chromosome 19p (*STK11*). Diagnosis requires two of the three following features:

- small bowel polyposis
- mucocutaneous pigmentation
- a family history suggesting autosomal dominant inheritance.

The diagnosis can be made by genetic testing, but this may be inconclusive, since mutations in genes other than *STK11* can cause the disorder. Affected people should undergo regular upper endoscopy, colonoscopy and small bowel and pancreatic imaging. Polyps greater than 1 cm in size should be removed. Testicular examination is essential for men, while women should undergo pelvic examination, cervical smears and regular mammography (lifetime risk of breast cancer of 50%). Asymptomatic relatives of affected patients should also undergo screening.

Juvenile polyposis

In juvenile polyposis, tens to hundreds of mucus-filled hamartomatous polyps are found in the colorectum. One-third of cases are inherited in an autosomal dominant manner and up to one-fifth develop colorectal cancer before the age of 40. The criteria for diagnosis are:

- ten or more colonic juvenile polyps
- juvenile polyps elsewhere in the gut, *or*
- any polyps in those with a family history.

Germline mutations in the *SMAD4* gene are often found, as well as mutations in the *BMPR1A* gene. *SMAD4* mutations may have a more aggressive clinical phenotype, while *BMPR1A* is particularly implicated in European populations. Colonoscopy with polypectomy should be performed every 1–2 years and colectomy considered for extensive involvement. Periodic upper gastrointestinal endoscopy should be performed every 1–2 years, in view of the risk of gastric and duodenal cancer.

Diverticulosis

Diverticula are acquired and are most common in the sigmoid and descending colon of middle-aged people. Asymptomatic diverticula (diverticulosis) are present in over 50% of people above the age of

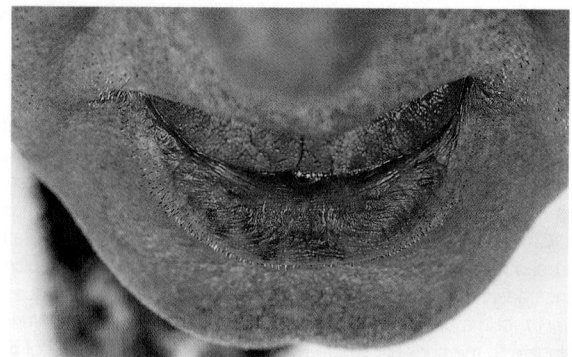

Fig. 23.52 Peutz–Jeghers syndrome. Typical lip pigmentation.

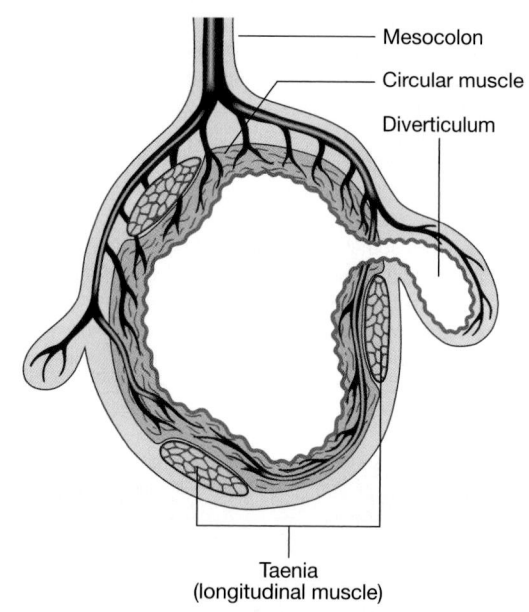

Mesocolon
Circular muscle
Diverticulum
Taenia (longitudinal muscle)

Fig. 23.53 The human colon in diverticulosis. The colonic wall is weak between the taeniae. The blood vessels that supply the colon pierce the circular muscle and weaken it further by forming tunnels. Diverticula usually emerge through these points of least resistance.

70 years. Symptomatic diverticular disease supervenes in 10%–25% of cases, while complicated diverticulosis (acute diverticulitis, pericolic abscess, bleeding, perforation or stricture) is uncommon.

Pathophysiology

A life-long refined diet with a relative deficiency of fibre is thought to be responsible and the condition is rare in populations with a high dietary fibre intake, such as in Asia, where it more often affects the right side of the colon. It is postulated that small-volume stools require high intracolonic pressures for propulsion and this leads to herniation of mucosa between the taeniae coli (Fig. 23.53). Whilst the pathophysiology of diverticular disease is thought to be mainly due to environmental risk factors, recent evidence suggests the involvement of predisposing genetic factors. Diverticula consist of protrusions of mucosa covered by peritoneum. There is commonly hypertrophy of the circular muscle coat. Inflammation is thought to result from impaction of diverticula with faecoliths. This may resolve spontaneously or progress to cause haemorrhage, perforation, local abscess formation, fistula and peritonitis. Repeated attacks of inflammation lead to thickening of the bowel wall, narrowing of the lumen and eventual obstruction.

Clinical features

Symptoms are usually the result of associated constipation or spasm. Colicky pain is suprapubic or felt in the left iliac fossa. The sigmoid colon may be palpable and, in attacks of diverticulitis, there is local tenderness, guarding, rigidity ('left-sided appendicitis') and sometimes a palpable mass. During these episodes, there may be diarrhoea, rectal bleeding or fever. The differential diagnosis includes colorectal cancer, ischaemic colitis, IBD and infection. Diverticular disease may be complicated by perforation, pericolic abscess, fistula formation (usually colovesical), acute lower gastrointestinal bleeding and obstruction. These complications are more common in patients who take NSAIDs or aspirin. After one attack of diverticulitis, the recurrence rate is around 3% per year. Over 10–30 years, perforation, obstruction or bleeding may occur, each affecting 5% of patients.

Investigations

Investigations are usually performed to exclude colorectal neoplasia. Diverticula can be seen during colonoscopy or on imaging modalities such as CT scan, CT colonography or barium enema (see Fig. 23.12C). In severe diverticulosis, colonoscopy requires expertise and carries a risk of perforation. CT is used to assess complications, such as perforation or pericolic abscess.

Management

Diverticular disease that is asymptomatic and discovered coincidentally requires no treatment. Constipation can be relieved by a high-fibre diet, with or without a bulking laxative (ispaghula husk, 1–2 sachets daily), taken with plenty of fluids. Stimulant laxatives (see Box 23.56) should be avoided. Antispasmodics may sometimes help. Acute attacks of diverticulitis can be treated with antibiotics active against Gram-negative and anaerobic organisms. Severe cases require intravenous fluids, intravenous antibiotics, analgesia and nasogastric suction, but randomised trials show no benefit from acute resection compared to conservative management. Emergency surgery is reserved for severe haemorrhage or perforation. Percutaneous drainage of acute paracolic abscesses can be effective and avoids the need for emergency surgery. Patients who have repeated attacks of obstruction should undergo elective surgery once the acute episode has settled, in order to resect the affected segment of bowel with restoration of continuity by primary anastomosis.

Colonic motility disorders

The clinical approach to patients with constipation and its aetiology have been described on page 803.

Simple constipation

Simple constipation is extremely common and does not signify underlying organic disease. It usually responds to increased dietary fibre or the use of bulking agents; an adequate fluid intake is also essential. Many types of laxative are available, and these are listed in Box 23.56.

Severe idiopathic constipation

This occurs almost exclusively in young women and often begins in childhood or adolescence. The cause is unknown, but some have 'slow transit' with reduced motor activity in the colon. Others have 'dyssynergic defecation', resulting from inappropriate contraction of the external anal sphincter and puborectalis muscle (anismus). The condition is often resistant to treatment. Bulking agents may exacerbate symptoms, but prokinetic agents or balanced solutions of polyethylene glycol '3350' benefit some patients with slow transit. Glycerol suppositories and biofeedback techniques are used for those with dyssynergic defecation. Others benefit from agents such as prucalopride or linaclotide. Rarely, subtotal colectomy may be necessary as a last resort.

Faecal impaction

In faecal impaction, a large, hard mass of stool fills the rectum. This tends to occur in disabled, immobile or institutionalised patients, especially frail older adults or those with dementia (see Box 23.57). Constipating drugs, autonomic neuropathy and painful anal conditions also contribute. Megacolon, intestinal obstruction and urinary tract infections may supervene. Perforation and bleeding from pressure-induced ulceration are occasionally seen. Overflow diarrhoea may also be a presenting feature, sometimes leading to worsening of symptoms with the incorrect use of antidiarrhoeal medication. Treatment should involve adequate hydration and careful digital disimpaction after softening the impacted stool with arachis oil enemas. Stimulants should be avoided.

Melanosis coli and laxative misuse syndromes

Long-term consumption of stimulant laxatives leads to accumulation of lipofuscin pigment in macrophages in the lamina propria. This imparts a brown discoloration to the colonic mucosa, often described as resembling 'tiger skin'. The condition is benign and resolves when the laxatives are stopped. Prolonged laxative use may rarely result in megacolon or 'cathartic colon', in which barium enema demonstrates a featureless mucosa, loss of haustra and shortening of the bowel. Surreptitious laxative misuse is a psychiatric condition seen in young women, some of whom have a history of bulimia or anorexia nervosa (Ch. 31). They complain of refractory watery diarrhoea. Laxative use is usually denied and may continue, even when patients are undergoing investigation. Screening of urine for laxatives may reveal the diagnosis.

Hirschsprung's disease

This disease is characterised by constipation and colonic dilatation (megacolon) due to congenital absence of ganglion cells in the large intestine. Incidence is approximately 1:5000. About one-third of patients have a positive family history and, in these families, the disease is inherited in

23

Class	Examples
i 23.56 Laxatives	
Bulk-forming laxatives	Ispaghula husk, methylcellulose
Stimulants	Bisacodyl, dantron (only for terminally ill patients), docusate, senna
Faecal softeners	Docusate, arachis oil enema
Osmotic laxatives	Lactulose, lactitol, magnesium salts
Serotonergic agents	Prucalopride
Prosecretory agents	Linaclotide, lubiprostone, plecanatide
Others	Polyethylene glycol (PEG)*, phosphate enema*

*Also used for bowel preparation prior to investigation or surgery.

23.57 Constipation in old age

- **Evaluation**: particular attention should be paid to immobility, dietary fluid and fibre intake, drugs and depression.
- **Immobility**: predisposes to constipation by increasing the colonic transit time; the longer this is, the greater the fluid absorption and the harder the stool.
- **Bulking agents**: can make matters worse in patients with slow transit times and should be avoided.
- **Overflow diarrhoea**: if faecal impaction develops, paradoxical overflow diarrhoea may occur. If antidiarrhoeal agents are given, the underlying impaction may worsen and result in serious complications, such as stercoral ulceration and bleeding.

an autosomal dominant manner with incomplete penetrance. About 50% of familial cases and 15% of sporadic cases have mutations affecting the RET proto-oncogene, which is also implicated in multiple endocrine neoplasia (MEN) types 2a and 2b (p. 700). Unlike MEN 2a and 2b, which are caused by activating RET mutations, Hirschsprung's disease is caused by loss-of-function mutations. In some kindreds, Hirschsprung's disease and MEN can actually co-segregate and this presumably represents both 'switch off' and 'switch on' of RET in different tissues. Although RET is the most important susceptibility gene, some patients with RET mutations do not develop clinical Hirschsprung's disease and mutations in other genes have been identified that interact to cause the disease. All of the genes implicated in Hirschsprung's disease are involved in the regulation of enteric neurogenesis and the mutations cause failure of migration of neuroblasts into the gut wall during embryogenesis. Ganglion cells are absent from nerve plexuses, most commonly in a short segment of the rectum and/or sigmoid colon. As a result, the internal anal sphincter fails to relax. Constipation, abdominal distension and vomiting usually develop immediately after birth but a few cases do not present until childhood or adolescence. The rectum is empty on digital examination.

A plain abdominal X-ray or barium enema shows a small rectum and colonic dilatation above the narrowed segment. Full-thickness biopsies are required to demonstrate nerve plexuses and confirm the absence of ganglion cells. Histochemical stains for acetylcholinesterase are also used. Anorectal manometry demonstrates failure of the internal sphincter to relax with balloon distension. Treatment involves resection of the affected segment.

Acquired megacolon

This may develop in childhood as a result of voluntary withholding of stool during toilet training and can present with faecal impaction and soiling. In such cases, it presents after the first year of life and is distinguished from Hirschsprung's disease by the urge to defecate and the presence of stool in the rectum. It usually responds to osmotic laxatives.

In adults, acquired megacolon has several causes. It is seen in patients with depression or dementia, either as part of the condition or as a side-effect of antidepressant drugs. Prolonged misuse of stimulant laxatives may cause degeneration of the myenteric plexus, while interruption of sensory or motor innervation may be responsible in a number of neurological disorders. Patients taking large doses of opioid analgesics can develop a megacolon: so-called 'narcotic bowel syndrome'. Systemic sclerosis and hypothyroidism are other recognised causes.

Most patients can be managed conservatively by treatment of the underlying cause, high-residue diets, laxatives and the judicious use of enemas. Prokinetics are helpful in a minority of patients. Opioid-induced constipation can be treated with the specific peripheral opioid receptor antagonists, such as naloxegol, methylnaltrexone and naldemedine. Subtotal colectomy is a last resort for the most severely affected patients.

Acute colonic pseudo-obstruction

Acute colonic pseudo-obstruction (Ogilvie syndrome) has many causes (Box 23.58) and is characterised by sudden onset of painless, massive enlargement of the proximal colon; there are no features of mechanical obstruction. Bowel sounds are normal or high-pitched, rather than absent. Left untreated, it may progress to perforation, peritonitis and death.

i	**23.58** Causes of acute colonic pseudo-obstruction

- Trauma, burns
- Recent surgery
- Drugs (opiates, phenothiazines)
- Respiratory failure
- Electrolyte and acid–base disorders (e.g. hypokalaemia, hypomagnesaemia)
- Diabetes mellitus – autonomic dysfunction
- Uraemia

Abdominal X-rays show colonic dilatation with air extending to the rectum. Caecal diameter greater than 10 cm is associated with a high risk of perforation. CT with contrast demonstrates the absence of mechanical obstruction.

Management consists of treating the underlying disorder and correcting any biochemical abnormalities. The anticholinesterase neostigmine is effective in enhancing parasympathetic activity and gut motility. Decompression, with either a rectal tube or colonoscope, may be effective but needs to be repeated until the condition resolves. In severe cases, surgical or fluoroscopic defunctioning caecostomy is necessary.

Anorectal disorders

Haemorrhoids

Haemorrhoids (commonly known as piles) arise from congestion of the internal and/or external venous plexuses around the anal canal. They are extremely common in adults. The aetiology is unknown, although they are associated with constipation and straining, and may develop for the first time during pregnancy. First-degree piles bleed, while second-degree piles prolapse but retract spontaneously. Third-degree piles are those that require manual replacement after prolapsing. Bright red rectal bleeding occurs after defecation. Other symptoms include pain, pruritus ani and mucus discharge; thrombosis can occur in prolapsed piles, which can be very painful (Fig. 23.54). Treatment involves measures to prevent constipation and straining. Band ligation is effective for many, but a minority of patients require haemorrhoidectomy, which is usually curative. Haemorrhoidal artery ligation operation (HALO) procedures have been developed and may replace surgery. HALO involves using Doppler ultrasound to identify all the arteries feeding the haemorrhoids and subsequent ligation.

Pruritus ani

This is common and can stem from many causes (Box 23.59), most of which result in contamination of the perianal skin with faecal contents.

Itching may be severe and results in an itch–scratch–itch cycle that exacerbates the problem. When no underlying cause is found, all local barrier ointments and creams must be stopped. Good personal hygiene is essential, with careful washing after defecation. The perineal area must be kept dry and clean. Bulk-forming laxatives may reduce faecal soiling.

Solitary rectal ulcer syndrome

This is most common in young adults and occurs on the anterior rectal wall. It is thought to result from localised chronic trauma and/or ischaemia

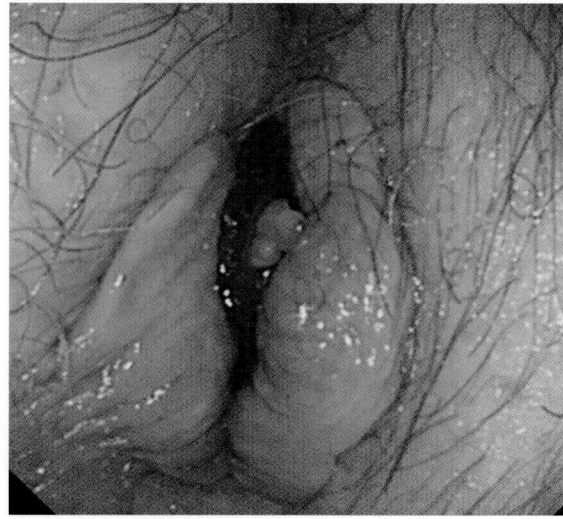

Fig. 23.54 Thrombosed prolapsed haemorrhoids.

i 23.59 Causes of pruritus ani

Local anorectal conditions

- Haemorrhoids
- Fistula, fissures
- Poor hygiene

Infections

- Threadworms
- Candidiasis

Skin disorders

- Contact dermatitis
- Psoriasis
- Lichen planus

Other

- Diarrhoea or incontinence of any cause
- Irritable bowel syndrome
- Anxiety

i 23.60 Causes of faecal incontinence

- Obstetric trauma: childbirth, hysterectomy
- Severe diarrhoea
- Faecal impaction
- Congenital anorectal anomalies
- Anorectal disease: haemorrhoids, rectal prolapse, Crohn's disease
- Neurological disorders: spinal cord or cauda equina lesions, dementia

associated with disordered puborectalis function and mucosal prolapse. The ulcer is seen at sigmoidoscopy and biopsies show a characteristic accumulation of collagen.

Symptoms include minor bleeding and mucus per rectum, tenesmus and perineal pain. Treatment is often difficult, but avoidance of straining at defecation is important and treatment of constipation may help. Marked mucosal prolapse is treated surgically.

Anal fissure

In this common problem, traumatic or ischaemic damage to the anal mucosa results in a superficial mucosal tear, most commonly in the midline posteriorly. Spasm of the internal anal sphincter exacerbates the condition. Severe pain occurs on defecation and there may be minor bleeding, mucus discharge and pruritus. The skin may be indurated and an oedematous skin tag, or 'sentinel pile', adjacent to the fissure is common.

Avoidance of constipation with bulk-forming laxatives and increased fluid intake is important. Relaxation of the internal sphincter is normally mediated by nitric oxid and 0.2% glyceryl trinitrate, which donates nitric oxide and improves mucosal blood flow, is effective in 60%–80% of patients. Diltiazem cream (2%) can be used as an alternative. Resistant cases may respond to injection of botulinum toxin into the internal anal sphincter to induce relaxation. Manual dilatation under anaesthesia leads to long-term incontinence and should not be considered. The majority of cases can be treated without surgery, but where these measures fail, healing can be achieved surgically by lateral internal anal sphincterotomy or advancement anoplasty.

Anorectal abscesses and fistulae

Perianal abscesses develop between the internal and external anal sphincters and may point at the perianal skin. Ischiorectal abscesses occur lateral to the sphincters in the ischiorectal fossa. They usually result from infection of anal glands by normal intestinal bacteria. Crohn's disease (see below) is sometimes responsible.

Patients complain of extreme perianal pain, fever and/or discharge of pus. Spontaneous rupture may lead to the development of fistulae. These may be superficial or track through the anal sphincters to reach the rectum. Abscesses are drained surgically and superficial fistulae are laid open with care to avoid sphincter damage.

Faecal incontinence

The normal control of anal continence is described on page 788. Common causes of incontinence are listed in Box 23.60. High-risk patients include frail older people, women after childbirth and those with severe neurological/spinal disorders, learning disabilities or cognitive impairment.

Patients are often embarrassed to admit to incontinence and may complain only of 'diarrhoea'. A careful history and examination, especially

of the anorectum and perineum, may help to establish the underlying cause. Endoanal ultrasound is valuable for defining the integrity of the anal sphincters, while anorectal physiology and MR proctography are also useful investigations.

Management

This is often very difficult. Underlying disorders should be treated and diarrhoea managed with loperamide, diphenoxylate or codeine phosphate. Attention must be paid to a proper diet and adequate fluid intake. Pelvic floor exercises, biofeedback and bowel retraining techniques help some patients, and those with confirmed anal sphincter defects may benefit from sphincter repair operations. Where sphincter repair is not appropriate, a trial of sacral nerve stimulation is undertaken with a view to insertion of a permanent stimulator but, if unsuccessful, creation of a neo-sphincter may be possible, by graciloplasty or by an artificial anal sphincter.

Inflammatory bowel disease

Ulcerative colitis and Crohn's disease are chronic inflammatory bowel diseases that pursue a protracted relapsing and remitting course, usually extending over years. The diseases have many similarities and it is sometimes impossible to differentiate between them. One crucial distinction is that ulcerative colitis involves only the colonic mucosa, while Crohn's disease can involve any part of the gastrointestinal tract from mouth to anus. A summary of the main features of ulcerative colitis and Crohn's disease is provided in Box 23.61.

The incidence of inflammatory bowel disease (IBD) varies widely between populations. The highest incidence is in North America, Europe and Oceania. A rapid increase in incidence in the 21st century has been seen in newly industrialised countries in Asia, Africa and South America, with the adoption of an increasingly Westernised lifestyle.

Both diseases most commonly start in the second and third decades of life, with a second smaller incidence peak in the seventh decade. The number of people with IBD over the age of 65 years, however, is increasing, and it is becoming more common in younger children. Approximately 620 000 people are affected by IBD in the UK, with a prevalence of 0.5%–1%. Life expectancy in patients with IBD is similar to that of the general population. Although many patients require surgery and admission to hospital for other reasons, with substantial associated morbidity, the majority have an excellent work record and pursue a normal life.

Pathophysiology

IBD has both environmental and genetic components, and evidence from genome-wide association studies suggests that genetic variants that predispose to Crohn's disease may have undergone positive selection by protecting against infectious diseases, including tuberculosis (Box 23.62). It is thought that IBD develops because these genetically susceptible individuals mount an abnormal inflammatory response to environmental triggers, such as intestinal bacteria. This leads to inflammation of the intestine with involvement of a wide array of innate and adaptive immune cell responses, with release of inflammatory mediators, including tumour necrosis factor alpha (TNF-α), interleukin (IL)-12 and IL-23, which cause tissue damage (Fig. 23.55). There appears to be an association between microbial dysbiosis and IBD. For example, there is a reduced diversity, primarily of *Firmicutes* and *Bacteroides*,

i 23.61 Comparison of ulcerative colitis and Crohn's disease

	Ulcerative colitis	Crohn's disease
Age group	Any	Any
Gender	M = F	Slight female preponderance
Incidence	Stable	Increasing
Ethnic group	Any	Any; more common in Ashkenazi Jews
Genetic factors	HLA-DR*103; colonic epithelial barrier function (HNF4α, LAMB1, CDH1)	Defective innate immunity and autophagy (NOD2, ATG16L1, IRGM)
Risk factors	More common in non-/ex-smokers Appendicectomy protects	More common in smokers
Anatomical distribution	Colon only; begins at anorectal margin with variable proximal extension	Any part of gastrointestinal tract; perianal disease common; patchy distribution, skip lesions
Extra-intestinal manifestations	Common	Common
Presentation	Bloody diarrhoea	Variable; pain, diarrhoea, weight loss all common
Histology	Inflammation limited to mucosa; crypt distortion, cryptitis, crypt abscesses, loss of goblet cells	Submucosal or transmural inflammation common; deep fissuring ulcers, fistulae; patchy changes; granulomas
Management	5-ASA; glucocorticoids; azathioprine; biologic therapy (anti-TNF, anti-α4β7 integrin, anti-p40, Janus kinase inhibitor); colectomy is curative	Glucocorticoids; azathioprine; methotrexate; biologic therapy (anti-TNF, anti-α4β7 integrin, anti-p40); nutritional therapy; smoking cessation; surgery for complications is not curative; 5-ASA is not effective

(5-ASA = 5-aminosalicylic acid; TNF = tumour necrosis factor)

i 23.62 Factors associated with the development of inflammatory bowel disease

Genetic

- Both CD and UC are common in Ashkenazi Jews
- 10% have first-degree relative/one or more close relative with IBD
- High concordance in identical twins (40%–50% CD; 20%–25% UC)
- 163 susceptibility loci identified at genome-wide levels of significance; most confer susceptibility to both CD and UC; many are also susceptibility loci for other inflammatory conditions (especially ankylosing spondylosis and psoriasis)
- UC and CD are both associated with genetic variants at HLA locus, and with multiple genes involved with immune signalling (especially IL-23 and IL-10 pathways)
- CD is associated with genetic defects in innate immunity and autophagy (NOD2, ATG16L1 and IRGM genes)
- UC is associated with genetic defects in barrier function
- NOD2 is associated with ileal and stricturing disease, and hence a need for resectional surgery
- HLA-DR*103 is associated with severe UC

Environmental

- UC is more common in non-smokers and ex-smokers
- CD is more common in smokers (relative risk = 3)
- CD is associated with a low-residue, high-refined-sugar diet
- Commensal gut microbiota are altered (dysbiosis) in CD and UC
- Appendicectomy protects against UC

(CD = Crohn's disease; HLA = human leucocyte antigen; IBD = inflammatory bowel disease; IL = interleukin; UC = ulcerative colitis)

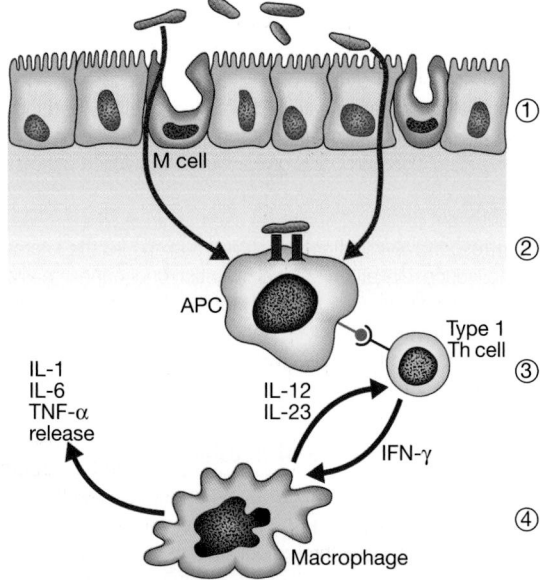

Fig. 23.55 Pathogenesis of inflammatory bowel disease. (1) Bacterial antigens are taken up by specialised M cells, pass between leaky epithelial cells or enter the lamina propria through ulcerated mucosa. (2) After processing, they are presented to type 1 T-helper cells by antigen-presenting cells (APCs) in the lamina propria. (3) T-cell activation and differentiation results in a Th₁ T cell-mediated cytokine response (4) with secretion of cytokines, including interferon gamma (IFN-γ). Further amplification of T cells perpetuates the inflammatory process with activation of non-immune cells and release of other important cytokines, including interleukin (IL)-12, IL-23, IL-1, IL-6 and tumour necrosis factor alpha (TNF-α). These pathways occur in all normal individuals exposed to an inflammatory insult and this is self-limiting in healthy subjects. In genetically predisposed persons, dysregulation of innate immunity may trigger inflammatory bowel disease.

Ulcerative colitis

Inflammation invariably involves the rectum (proctitis) and spreads proximally in a continuous manner to involve the entire colon in some cases (pancolitis). In long-standing pancolitis, the bowel can become

and a relative increase in Enterobacteriaceae. Functional changes in the bacteria are important and include a reduction of anti-inflammatory metabolites, such as butyrate and other short-chain fatty acids. While microbial dysbiosis has been recognised in IBD, a causal role has yet to be established. There is emerging evidence that the virome and mycobiome (fungal species) may be important in the development of IBD. In both diseases, the intestinal wall is infiltrated with acute and chronic inflammatory cells, but there are important differences between the conditions in the distribution of lesions and in histological features (Fig. 23.56).

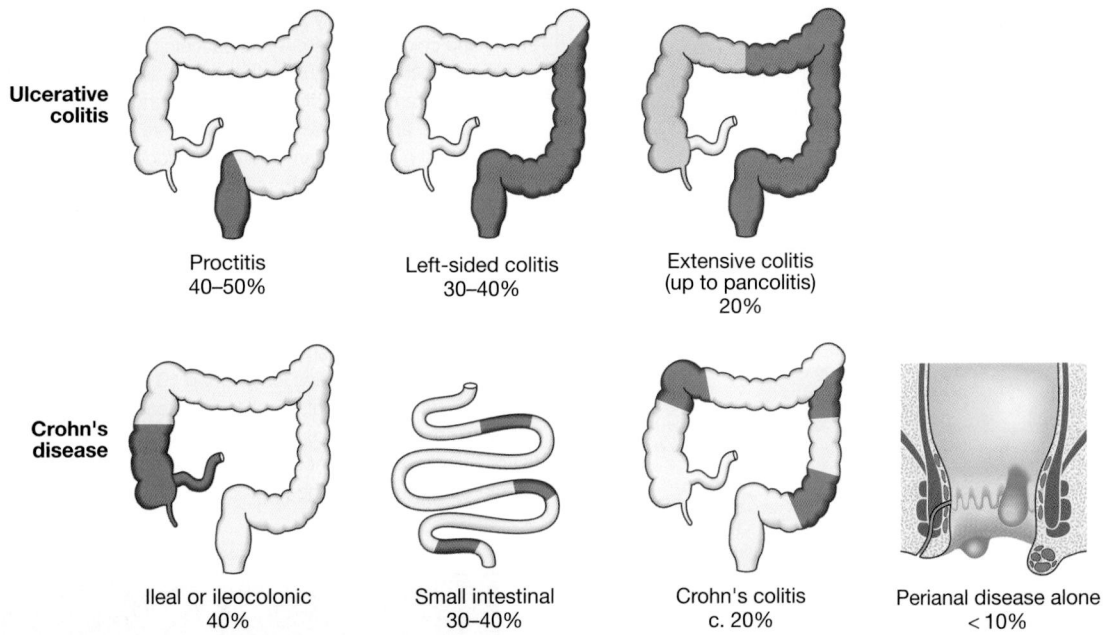

Ulcerative colitis

Proctitis
40–50%

Left-sided colitis
30–40%

Extensive colitis
(up to pancolitis)
20%

Crohn's disease

Ileal or ileocolonic
40%

Small intestinal
30–40%

Crohn's colitis
c. 20%

Perianal disease alone
< 10%

Fig. 23.56 Common patterns of disease distribution in inflammatory bowel disease.

shortened and post-inflammatory 'pseudopolyps' develop; these are normal or hypertrophied residual mucosa within areas of atrophy (Fig. 23.57). The inflammatory process is limited to the mucosa and spares the deeper layers of the bowel wall (Fig. 23.58). Both acute and chronic inflammatory cells infiltrate the lamina propria and the crypts ('cryptitis'). Crypt abscesses are typical. Goblet cells lose their mucus and, in long-standing cases, glands become distorted. Dysplasia, characterised by heaping of cells within crypts, nuclear atypia and increased mitotic rate, may herald the development of colon cancer.

Crohn's disease

The sites most commonly involved, in order of frequency, are the terminal ileum and right side of the colon, the small intestine, the colon alone, and the perianal region (Fig. 23.56). The entire wall of the bowel is oedematous and thickened, and there are deep ulcers that often appear as linear fissures; thus the mucosa between them is described as 'cobblestone'. These may penetrate through the bowel wall to initiate abscesses or fistulae involving the bowel, bladder, uterus, vagina and skin of the perineum. The mesenteric lymph nodes are enlarged and the mesentery is thickened. Crohn's disease has a patchy distribution and the inflammatory process is interrupted by islands of normal mucosa, resulting in 'skip lesions'. On histological examination, the bowel wall is thickened with a chronic inflammatory infiltrate throughout all layers (Fig. 23.59).

Clinical features

Ulcerative colitis

The cardinal symptoms are rectal bleeding with passage of mucus and bloody diarrhoea. The presentation varies, depending on the site and severity of the disease (see Fig. 23.56), as well as the presence of extra-intestinal manifestations. The first attack is usually the most severe and is followed by relapses and remissions. Emotional stress, intercurrent infection, gastroenteritis, antibiotics or NSAID therapy may all provoke a relapse. Proctitis causes rectal bleeding and mucus discharge, accompanied by tenesmus. Some patients pass frequent, small-volume fluid stools, while others pass pellety stools due to constipation upstream of the inflamed rectum. Constitutional symptoms rarely occur. Left-sided and extensive colitis causes bloody diarrhoea with mucus, often with abdominal cramps. In severe cases, anorexia, malaise, weight loss and abdominal pain occur and the patient is toxic, with fever, tachycardia and signs of peritoneal inflammation (Box 23.63).

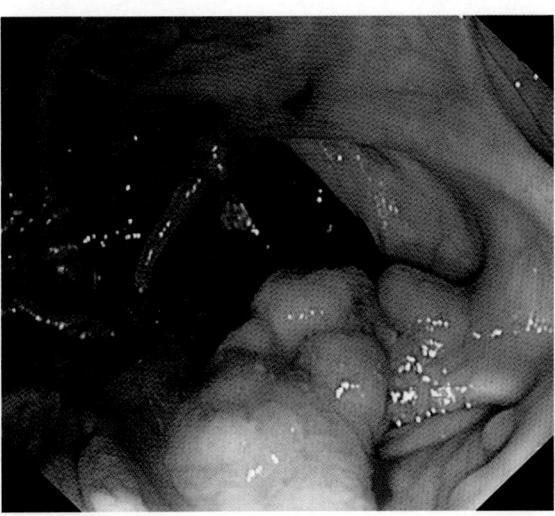

Fig. 23.57 Pseudopolyposis in ulcerative colitis.

23

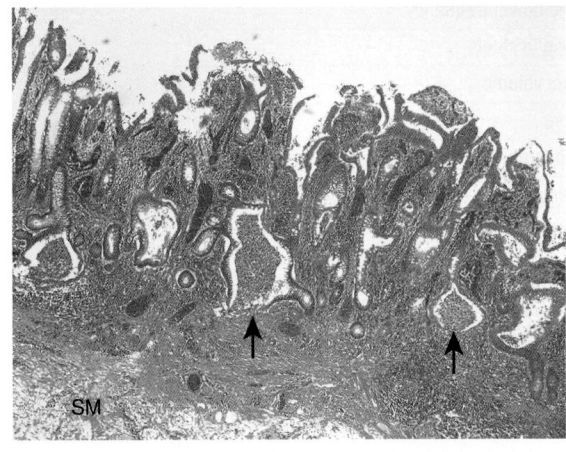

Fig. 23.58 Histology of ulcerative colitis. There is surface ulceration and inflammation is confined to the mucosa with excess inflammatory cells in the lamina propria, loss of goblet cells and crypt abscesses (arrows). (SM = submucosa)

Crohn's disease

The major symptoms are abdominal pain, diarrhoea and weight loss. Ileal Crohn's disease (Figs. 23.60 and 23.61) may cause subacute or even acute intestinal obstruction. Patients can occasionally present with a perforated abscess. Abdominal pain is often associated with diarrhoea, which is usually watery and does not contain blood or mucus. Patients may lose weight because they avoid food, since eating provokes pain. Weight loss may also be due to malabsorption and some patients present with features of fat, protein or vitamin deficiencies. Crohn's colitis presents in an identical manner to ulcerative colitis, but rectal sparing and the presence of perianal disease are features that favour a diagnosis of Crohn's disease. Many patients present with symptoms of both small bowel and colonic disease. A few patients present with isolated perianal disease, vomiting from jejunal strictures or severe oral ulceration.

Physical examination often reveals evidence of weight loss, anaemia with glossitis and angular stomatitis. There is abdominal tenderness, most marked over the inflamed area. An abdominal mass may be palpable and is due to matted loops of thickened bowel or an intra-abdominal abscess. Perianal skin tags, fissures or fistulae are found in at least 50% of patients.

Differential diagnosis

The differential diagnosis is summarised in Box 23.64. The most important issue is to distinguish the first attack of acute colitis from infection. In general, diarrhoea lasting longer than 10 days in Western countries is unlikely to be the result of infection, whereas a history of foreign travel, antibiotic exposure (*Clostridioides difficile*/pseudomembranous colitis) or homosexual contact increases the possibility of infection, which should be excluded by the appropriate investigations (see below). The

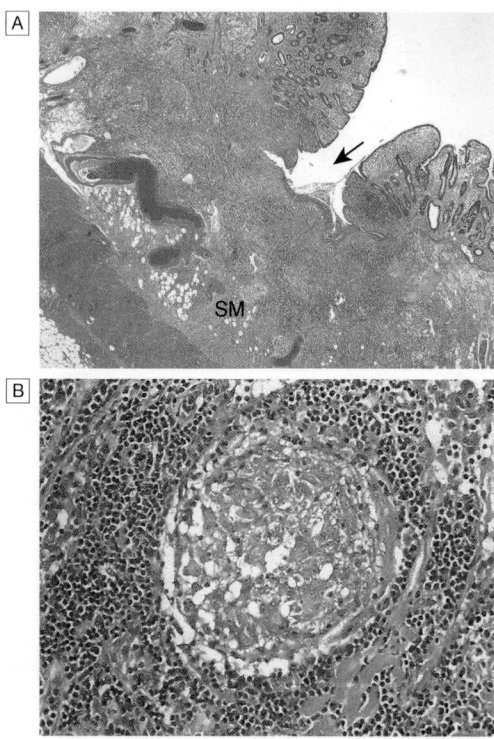

Fig. 23.59 Histology of Crohn's disease. [A] Inflammation is 'transmural'; there is fissuring ulceration (arrow), with inflammation extending into the submucosa (SM). [B] At higher power, a characteristic non-caseating granuloma is seen.

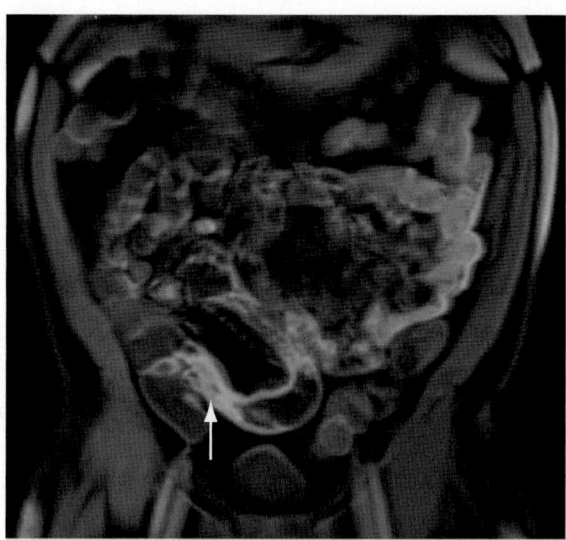

Fig. 23.60 Ileal Crohn's disease. Small bowel magnetic resonance image showing a terminal ileum that is thickened, narrowed and enhancing (arrow), with dilatation immediately proximal to this.

23.63 Assessment of disease severity in ulcerative colitis			
	Mild	**Moderate**	**Severe**
Daily bowel frequency	< 4	4–6	≥ 6*
Blood in stools	+/−	+/++	+++
Stool volume	< 200 g/24 hrs	200–400 g/24 hrs	> 400 g/24 hrs
Pulse	< 90 beats/min	< 90 beats/min	≥ 90 beats/min*
Temperature	Normal	Normal	≥ 37.8°C*
Haemoglobin	Normal	Normal	< 100 g/L (< 10 g/dL)*
Erythrocyte sedimentation rate	Normal	Normal	> 30 mm/hr* (or equivalent C-reactive protein)
Serum albumin	> 35 g/L (> 3.5 g/dL)		< 30 g/L (< 3 g/dL)
Abdominal X-ray	Normal	Normal	Dilated bowel, mucosal islands, thumb-printing of mucosa, or absence of features
Sigmoidoscopy	Normal or erythema/granular mucosa		Severe mucosal inflammatory changes; ulceration; blood in lumen

*The Truelove–Witts criteria for acute severe ulcerative colitis are ≥ 6 bloody stools/24 hrs plus one or more of: anaemia, fever, tachycardia and high inflammatory markers.

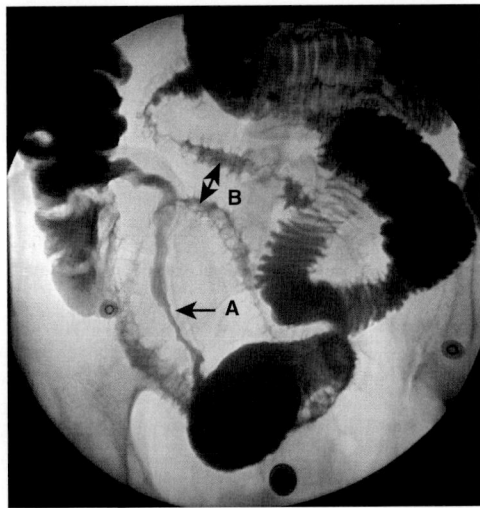

Fig. 23.61 Barium follow-through showing terminal ileal Crohn's disease. A long stricture is present (arrow A), and more proximally there is ulceration with characteristic 'rose thorn' ulcers (arrow B).

i	**23.64 Conditions that can mimic ulcerative or Crohn's colitis**

Infective

Bacterial

- Salmonella
- Shigella
- Campylobacter jejuni
- Escherichia coli O157

- Gonococcal proctitis
- Pseudomembranous colitis
- Chlamydia proctitis

Viral

- Herpes simplex proctitis
- Cytomegalovirus

Protozoal

- Amoebiasis

Non-infective

- Ischaemic colitis
- Collagenous colitis
- Non-steroidal anti-inflammatory drugs

- Diverticulitis
- Radiation proctitis
- Behçet's disease
- Colonic carcinoma

i	**23.65 Differential diagnosis of small bowel Crohn's disease**

- Other causes of right iliac fossa mass:
  - Caecal carcinoma
  - Appendix abscess*
- Infection (tuberculosis, *Yersinia*, actinomycosis)
- Mesenteric adenitis
- Pelvic inflammatory disease
- Lymphoma

*Common; other causes are rare.

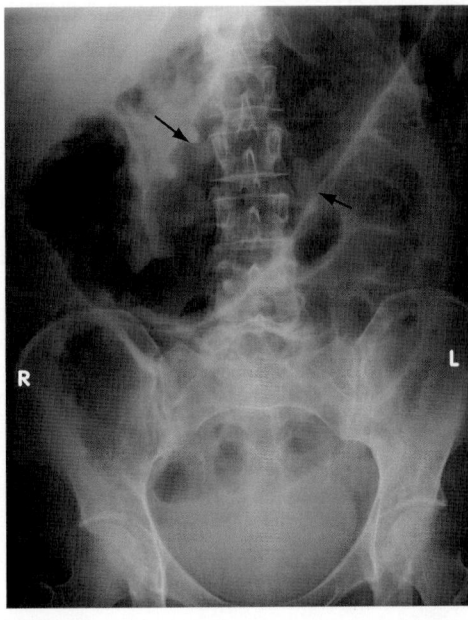

Fig. 23.62 Plain abdominal X-ray showing a grossly dilated colon due to severe ulcerative colitis. There is also marked mucosal oedema and 'thumb-printing' (arrows).

diagnosis of Crohn's disease is usually more straightforward and is made on the basis of imaging and clinical presentation, but in atypical cases biopsy or surgical resection is necessary to exclude other diseases (Box 23.65).

Complications

Life-threatening colonic inflammation

This can occur in both ulcerative colitis and Crohn's colitis. In the most extreme cases, the colon dilates (toxic megacolon) and bacterial toxins pass freely across the diseased mucosa into the portal and then systemic circulation. This complication arises most commonly during the first attack of colitis and is recognised by the features described in Box 23.63. An abdominal X-ray should be taken daily because, when the transverse colon is dilated to more than 6 cm (Fig. 23.62), there is a high risk of colonic perforation, although this complication can also occur in the absence of toxic megacolon. Severe colonic inflammation with toxic dilatation is a surgical emergency and often requires colectomy.

Haemorrhage

Haemorrhage due to erosion of a major artery is rare, but can occur in both conditions. This is more common in Crohn's disease, where deep ulceration erodes larger vessels.

Fistulae

These are specific to Crohn's disease. Enteroenteric fistulae can cause diarrhoea and malabsorption due to blind loop syndrome. Enterovesical fistulation causes recurrent urinary infections and pneumaturia. An enterovaginal fistula causes a faeculent vaginal discharge. Fistulation from the bowel may also cause perianal or ischiorectal abscesses, fissures and fistulae.

Cancer

Colorectal cancer accounts for one in six deaths in ulcerative colitis. The risk of dysplasia and cancer increases with the duration and extent of uncontrolled colonic inflammation. Thus patients who have long-standing, extensive colitis are at highest risk. 5-ASA therapy may reduce the risk of dysplasia and neoplasia in ulcerative colitis. Thiopurines also seem to reduce the risk of colorectal cancer in ulcerative colitis, but not Crohn's disease. However, these benefits must be weighed against the very small increase in lymphoma, especially in older patients. The cumulative incidence for IBD-associated colorectal cancer has been reported at 1% at 10 years after diagnosis, which increases to 7% after 30 years. For unknown reasons, the risk is particularly high in patients who have concomitant primary sclerosing cholangitis. Tumours develop in areas of dysplasia and may be multiple. Patients with long-standing colitis are therefore entered into surveillance programmes beginning 8 years after diagnosis, with patients with primary sclerosing cholangitis having annual surveillance colonoscopy from diagnosis. Targeted biopsies of areas that show abnormalities on

23

staining with indigo carmine or methylene blue increase the chance of detecting dysplasia and this technique (termed pancolonic chromo-endoscopy) has replaced colonoscopy with random biopsies taken every 10 cm in screening for malignancy. The procedure allows patients to be stratified into high-, medium- or low-risk groups to determine the interval between surveillance procedures. Family history of colon cancer is also an important factor to consider. If high-grade dysplasia is found, panproctocolectomy is usually recommended because of the high risk of colon cancer.

Extra-intestinal complications

Extra-intestinal complications are common in IBD and may dominate the clinical picture. Some of these occur during relapse of intestinal disease; others appear to be unrelated to intestinal disease activity (Fig. 23.63).

Investigations

Investigations are necessary to confirm the diagnosis, define disease distribution and activity, and identify complications. Full blood count may show anaemia resulting from bleeding or malabsorption of iron, folic acid or vitamin B_{12}. Platelet count can also be high as a marker of chronic inflammation. Serum albumin concentration falls as a consequence of protein-losing enteropathy, inflammatory disease or poor nutrition. ESR and CRP are elevated in exacerbations and in response to abscess formation. Faecal calprotectin has a high sensitivity for detecting gastrointestinal inflammation and may be elevated, even when the CRP is normal. It is particularly useful for distinguishing inflammatory bowel disease from irritable bowel syndrome at diagnosis, and for subsequent monitoring of disease activity.

Bacteriology

At initial presentation, stool microscopy, culture and examination for *Clostridiodes difficile* toxin or for ova and cysts, blood cultures and serological tests should be performed. These investigations should be repeated in established disease to exclude superimposed enteric infection in patients who present with exacerbations of IBD. During acute flares necessitating hospital admission, three separate stool samples should be sent for bacteriology to maximise sensitivity.

Endoscopy

Patients who present with diarrhoea plus raised inflammatory markers or alarm features, such as weight loss, rectal bleeding and anaemia, should undergo ileocolonoscopy. Flexible sigmoidoscopy is occasionally performed to make a diagnosis, especially during acute severe presentations when ileocolonoscopy may confer an unacceptable risk; ileocolonoscopy should still be performed at a later date, however, in order to evaluate disease extent. In ulcerative colitis, there is loss of vascular pattern, granularity, friability and contact bleeding, with or without ulceration (Fig. 23.64). In Crohn's disease, patchy inflammation, with discrete, deep ulcers, strictures and perianal disease (fissures, fistulae and skin tags), is typically observed, often with rectal sparing. In established disease, colonoscopy may show active inflammation with pseudo-polyps or a complicating carcinoma. Biopsies should be taken from each anatomical segment (terminal ileum, right colon, transverse colon, left colon and rectum) to confirm the diagnosis and define disease extent, and also to seek dysplasia in patients with long-standing colitis guided by pancolonic chromo-endoscopy. In Crohn's disease, wireless capsule

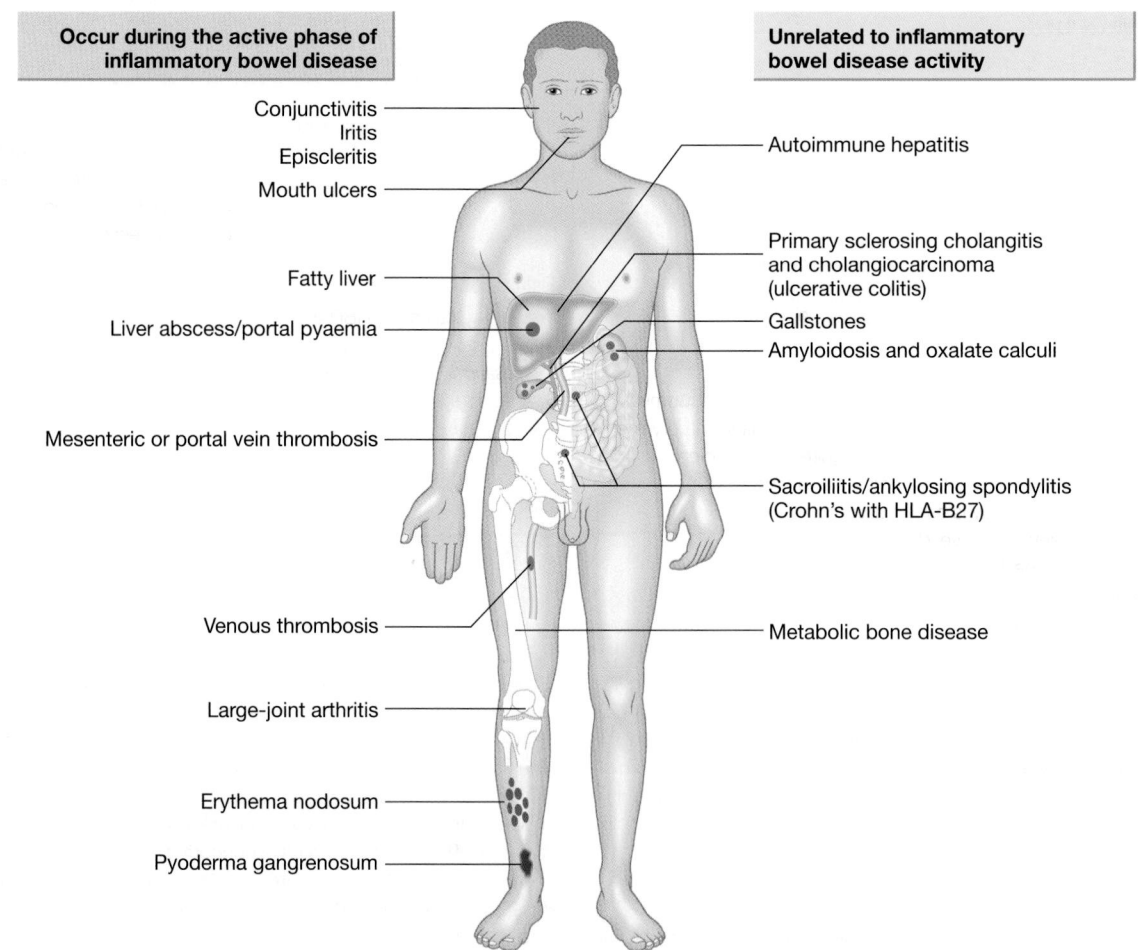

Fig. 23.63 Systemic complications of inflammatory bowel disease. See also Chapters 24 and 26. (HLA = human leucocyte antigen)

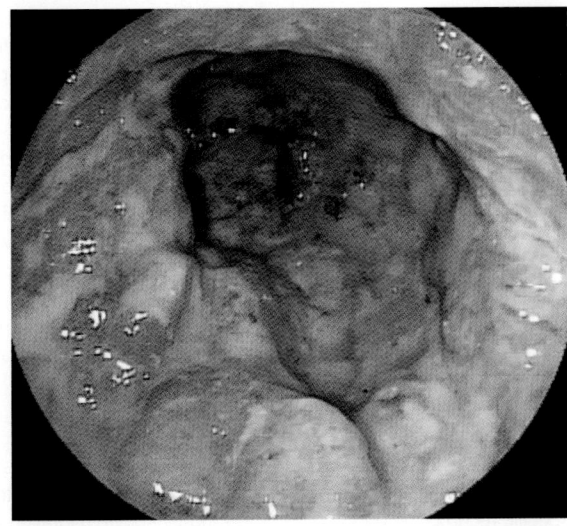

Fig. 23.64 Sigmoidoscopic view of moderately active ulcerative colitis.
Mucosa is erythematous and friable with contact bleeding. Submucosal blood vessels are no longer visible.

i	23.66 Non-biologic agents used in the treatment of inflammatory bowel disease		
Class	**Drug**	**Indication**	
Aminosalicylates	Mesalazine Olsalazine Sulfasalazine Balsalazide	Induce remission or maintenance in mild/ moderate ulcerative colitis	
Glucocorticoids	Prednisolone Hydrocortisone Budesonide Beclomethasone Methylprednisolone	Induce remission in acute ulcerative colitis or Crohn's disease	
Anti-metabolites	Azathioprine Mercaptopurine	Maintenance therapy in ulcerative colitis or Crohn's disease	
	Methotrexate	Maintenance therapy in Crohn's disease	
Calcineurin inhibitors	Ciclosporin	Severe ulcerative colitis refractory to glucocorticoids	
Antibiotics	Ciprofloxacin Metronidazole	Peri-anal Crohn's disease and pouchitis	

endoscopy has a greater sensitivity for detecting small bowel disease in comparison to radiological techniques and is useful when there is a high suspicion of Crohn's despite normal imaging. Enteroscopy may be required to make a histological diagnosis of small bowel Crohn's disease, when the inflamed segment is out of reach of standard endoscopes, or for a therapeutic indication, such as dilatation of strictures. In individuals with upper gastrointestinal symptoms, an upper gastrointestinal endoscopy may be useful. However, this is not routinely used in adults with suspected or proven Crohn's disease.

Radiology

Where colonoscopy is incomplete, a CT colonogram is preferred. Small bowel imaging is essential to complete staging of Crohn's disease. Traditional contrast imaging by barium follow-through demonstrates affected areas of the bowel as narrowed and ulcerated, often with multiple strictures (see Fig. 23.61). This has largely been replaced by MRI enterography, which does not involve exposure to radiation and is a sensitive way of detecting extra-intestinal manifestations and of assessing pelvic and perineal involvement. These studies use an orally administered small bowel-distending agent and intravenous contrast to provide transmural imaging that can usefully distinguish between predominantly inflammatory strictures (that should respond to anti-inflammatory medical strategies) and fibrotic strictures (that require a mechanical solution, such as surgical resection, stricturoplasty or endoscopic balloon dilatation). A plain abdominal X-ray is essential in the management of patients who present with severe active disease. Dilatation of the colon (see Fig. 23.62), mucosal oedema (thumb-printing) or evidence of perforation may be found. Patients with proctitis may have features of proximal faecal loading. In small bowel Crohn's disease, there may be evidence of intestinal obstruction or displacement of bowel loops by a mass. Ultrasound is a very powerful tool to detect small bowel inflammation and stricture formation, but it is operator-dependent. The role of CT is limited to screening for complications, such as perforation or abscess formation, in the acutely unwell.

Management

Medical therapy plays an important role in the management of IBD. However, optimal management depends on establishing a multidisciplinary team-based approach involving physicians, surgeons, radiologists, nurse specialists and dietitians. Both ulcerative colitis and Crohn's disease are life-long conditions and have important psychosocial implications; specialist nurses, counsellors and patient support groups have key

roles in education, reassurance and coping. The key aims of medical therapy are to:

- treat acute attacks (induce remission)
- prevent relapses (maintain remission)
- prevent bowel damage
- detect dysplasia and prevent carcinoma
- select appropriate patients for surgery.

Medical therapy

Several medical treatment options exist in the management for IBD. Whilst traditional management for IBD has been through the use of non-biologic treatments, there has been a rapid expansion in the use of biologics, with common treatments described below.

Non-biologic therapies

Non-biologics used in IBD are summarised in Box 23.66.

Aminosalicylates (5-ASA)

5-ASAs are more commonly used in ulcerative colitis than in Crohn's disease. 5-ASAs are thought to have multiple anti-inflammatory effects, including inhibition of mediatiors of lipoxygenase and cyclooxygenase, modulating cytokine release from the mucosa. Several types are available, with different means of delivery to the colon; pH-dependent (Asacol, Salofalk), time-dependent (Pentasa) or bacterial breakdown by colonic bacteria from a carrier molecule (sulfasalazine, balsalazide). While sulfasalazine was the first 5-ASA to be used in IBD, side-effects are common, such as headache, nausea, diarrhoea and blood dyscrasias. Other 5-ASAs are better tolerated. 5-ASAs can be administered orally or topically (suppositories or enema). Patients commencing a 5-ASA should have their urea and electrolytes checked at baseline, after 2–3 months and then annually, as nephrotoxicity can occur rarely (1 in 4000 patient years).

Glucocorticoids

Glucocorticoids such as prednisolone, hydrocortisone, budesonide and beclomethasone can be used to induce clinical remission in both ulcerative colitis and Crohn's disease, but have no role in preventing relapse. They can be administered orally, topically (suppositories or enema) or intravenously and have powerful anti-inflammatory effects. When administered, it is important to have high vigilance for complications, such as osteoporosis, diabetes and weight gain. Simultaneous calcium and vitamin D supplementation should be given for bone protection. Budesonide is a potent glucocorticoid, which is efficiently cleared from circulation by the liver, thereby minimising adrenocortical suppression and side-effects. It is commonly considered for active ileitis and ileocolitis.

Thiopurines

Thiopurines used in IBD are azathioprine and mercaptopurine. They are immunmodulators that induce T-cell apoptosis. Azathioprine and mercaptopurine are administered orally and metabolised to thioguanine nucleotides (TGNs). Thiopurine methyltransferase (TPMT) methylates thiopurine metabolites away from TGNs and affects drug levels. Leucopenia can occur in 3%, particularly in inherited TPMT deficiency. TPMT levels are checked prior to starting treatment and thiopurines are avoided if deficient/very low due to risk of toxicity. Thiopurines take around 6 weeks after starting treatment to be effective. Around 20% of patients will have complications leading to drug withdrawal. Complications include influenza-like syndrome with myalgia, nausea and vomiting. Genetic variation of NUDT15 has been described in association with myelosuppression and testing is performed if available. Other adverse effects include hepatotoxicity and pancreatitis. Patients are counselled on the increase lymphoma (approximately 2–3-fold) and non-melanoma skin cancer (life-long sun protection advised) risk. Caution is taken in prescribing thiopurines in patients presenting over the age of 60 years due to risk of malignancy.

Methotrexate

Methotrexate can be used for maintanence therapy in Crohn's disease, with no role in ulcerative colitis. It is commonly used in individuals who have failed to respond with thiopurines. It is a folic acid antagonist, which inhibits dihydrofolate reductase, preventing DNA synthesis. The bioavailability of oral methotrexate is variable when compared to parental administration, with the subcutaneous injection being generally preferred to intramuscular due to ease of administration. Nausea, stomatitis, diarrhoea, hepatotoxicity and pneumonitis can occur with methotrexate. Folic acid should be given concurrently to reduce gastrointestinal and liver toxicity. Women of child-bearing potential must use a robust contraceptive method and should be counselled to plan pregnancy with a 6-month methotrexate-free period prior to conception as it is teratogenic.

Ciclosporin

Ciclosporin is a calcineurin inhibitor, inhibiting in particular the transcription of interleukin-2. It is used in ulcerative colitis that has responded poorly to glucocorticoids and has no role in Crohn's disease. Major side-effects include nephrotoxicity, infections and neurotoxicity (including fits). Minor complications include tremor, paraesthesiae, abnormal liver function tests and hirsutism. Acutely, ciclosporin is usually administered intravenously, with responders to treatment converted to oral administration, which is continued for several months as a bridging therapy. Thiopurine manintence therapy is commonly given as maintenance subsequently, as ciclosporin has no benefit as maintenance therapy.

Antibiotics

Antibiotics are useful in perianal Crohn's disease and pouchitis. There is little evidence comparing different antibiotics for acute pouchitis, although ciprofloxacin is better tolerated with fewer adverse effects than metronidazole. The major concern is peripheral neuropathy with long-term metronidazole, with tendon inflammation and damage potentially occurring with ciprofloxacin. Combination antibiotics may be needed for chronic pouchitis. Antibiotics tend to be used in combination with thiopurines and anti-TNF therapy in perianal disease.

Biologic agents

Several classes of biologic agents are used in the management of IBD, with their indication shown in Box 23.67 and site of action shown in Fig. 23.65. The majority of biologics are administered either intravenously or subcutaneously, with the exception of tofacitinib, which is administered orally.

Anti-TNF antibodies

These include infliximab, adalimumab, golimumab and certolizumab. They are monoclonal antibodies that bind to TNF-α, preventing proinflammatory and pathological cytokine release by TNF-α. Acute (anaphylactic) and delayed (serum sickness) infusion reactions can occur after multiple infusions. Anti-drug antibody titres and drug levels can be also measured to assess efficacy. Anti-TNF antibodies are contraindicated in infection; reactivation of latent tuberculosis and moderate to severe cardiac failure can occur. In view of this, assessment for latent tuberculosis and hepatitis B and C prior to commencement is required. There is a possible increased risk of malignancy and, rarely, neurological adverse events. Treatment should occur until treatment failure, or should be reassessed after 12 months.

Anti-α4β7 integrin

Vedolizumab is a monoclonal antibody that blocks α4β7 integrin expressed on leukocytes and inhibits leukocyte interaction with a gut-specific receptor on endothelium, reducing leukocyte migration into gut mucosa. It is a gut-selective biologic used in both ulcerative colitis and Crohn's disease. Side-effects include nasopharyngitis, arthralgia and headache. Treatment is discontinued if there is no improvement after 14 weeks. Treatment should occur until treatment failure, or should be reassessed after 12 months.

Janus kinase inhibitor

Tofacitinib is a Janus kinase inhibitor that selectively inhibits the Janus-associated tyrosine kinases JAK1 and JAK3, blocking proinflammatory cytokine signalling via the STAT pathway. It has the advantage of oral administration in comparison to other biologics being used in ulcerative colits. High doses should be avoided in patients at risk of pulmonary embolism and it is contraindicated in pregnancy. Herpes zoster has been noted to occur more often on active treatment; zoster vaccination is therefore recommended in those over age of 70 years or high-risk individuals (recurrent shingles) over 50 years.

Anti-p40 antibodies

Ustekinumab is a monoclonal antibody that binds to p-40 subunit of both IL-12 and IL-23 to prevent T-cell activation; it is used in both ulcerative colitis and Crohn's disease. Side-effects include nasopharyngitis, headache and arthralgia. Treatment should occur until treatment failure or should be reassessed after 12 months.

Therapeutic drug monitoring

Up to one-third of patients do not respond to biologic therapy (primary non-response), with up to a half discontinuing biologic therapy after initial response due to secondary loss of response or adverse effects. This can be due to pharmokinetic or pharmodynamic issues of the drug. Favourable outcomes have been associated with good drug concentrations, with low levels leading to immunogenicity and drug failure. Therapeutic drug monitoring can be performed with biologic therapy, ensuring patients have adequate drug levels, pre-emptively preventing flares due to low drug levels. Combination treatment of biologics with thiopurines or methotrexate can be used to prevent and reduce anti-drug antibodies. Drug monitoring can also be performed with thiopurines, with thiopurine metabolites measured to tailor therapy.

Ulcerative colitis

Active ulcerative colitis

Patients with active ulcerative colitis are initially treated with topical or oral 5-aminosalicylate (5-ASA) therapy. Patients with left-sided or extensive ulcerative colitis should continue oral 5-ASA in the long term to prevent relapse and minimise the risk of dysplasia. Individuals with an incomplete response to 5-ASA treatment may require treatment with systemic glucocorticoids, immunomodulator or biologic therapy. Glucocorticoids

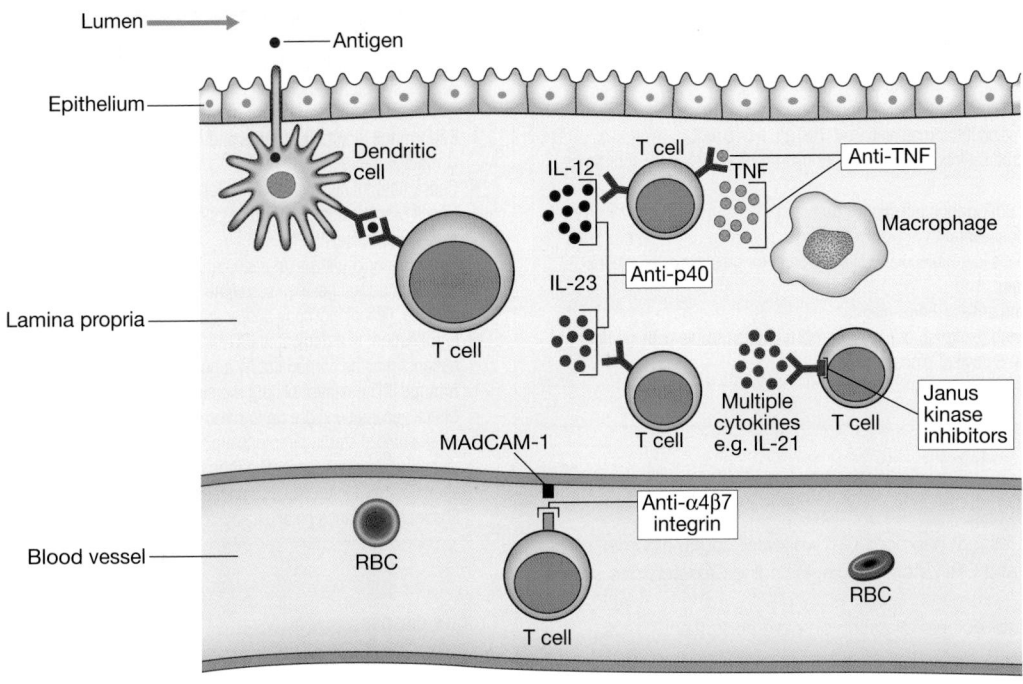

Fig. 23.65 Site of action of biologics. (TNF = tumour necrosis factor; IL = interleukin; RBC = red blood cell)

i	**23.67 Biologic agents used in the treatment of inflammatory bowel disease**		
Class	**Drug**	**Indication**	
Anti-TNF antibodies	Infliximab	Moderate to severe Crohn's disease and ulcerative colitis	
		Acute severe ulcerative colitis as rescue therapy	
	Adalimumab	Moderate to severe Crohn's disease and ulcerative colitis	
	Golimumab	Moderate to severe ulcerative colitis	
	Certolizumab	Moderate to severe Crohn's disease	
Anti-α4β7 integrin	Vedolizumab	Moderate to severe Crohn's disease and ulcerative colitis	
Janus kinase inhibitor	Tofacitinib	Moderate to severe ulcerative colitis	
Anti-p40 antibodies	Ustekinumab	Moderate to severe Crohn's disease and ulcerative colitis	

should never be used for maintenance therapy. An algorithm for the management of active ulcerative colitis is shown in Fig. 23.66.

Severe ulcerative colitis

Patients who fail to respond to maximal oral therapy and those who present with acute severe colitis (meeting the Truelove–Witts criteria; see Box 23.63) are best managed in hospital and should be monitored jointly by a physician and surgeon:

- *clinically*: for the presence of abdominal pain, temperature, pulse rate, stool blood and frequency

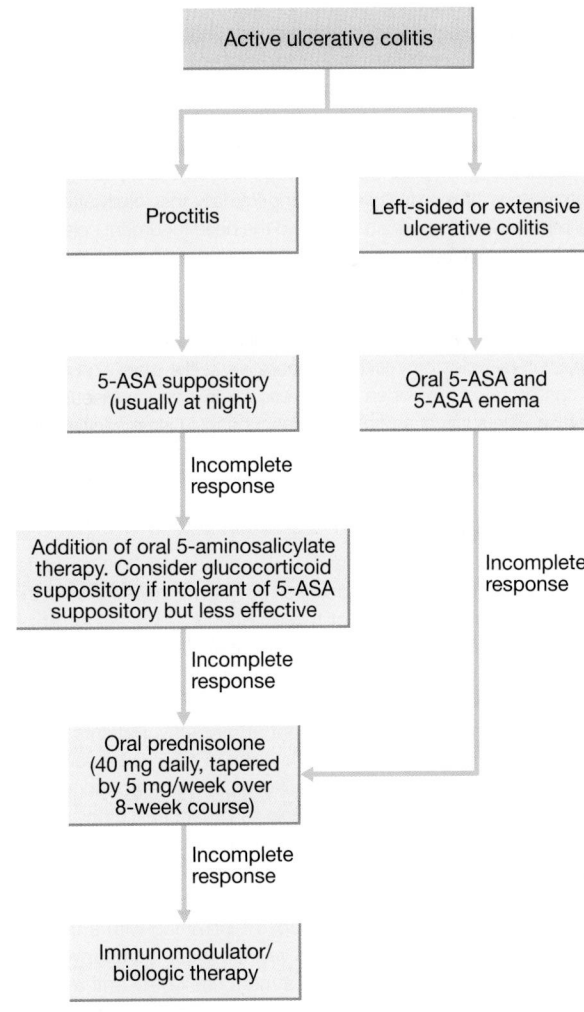

Fig. 23.66 Medical management of active ulcerative colitis.

23

23.68 Medical management of fulminant ulcerative colitis

- Admit to hospital for intensive therapy and monitoring
- Give IV fluids and correct electrolyte imbalance
- Consider transfusion if haemoglobin is < 100 g/L (< 10 g/dL)
- Give IV methylprednisolone (60 mg daily) or hydrocortisone (100 mg four times daily)
- Give antibiotics until enteric infection is excluded
- Arrange nutritional support
- Give subcutaneous low-molecular-weight heparin for prophylaxis of venous thromboembolism
- Avoid opiates and antidiarrhoeal agents
- Consider infliximab (5 mg/kg) or ciclosporin (2 mg/kg) in stable patients not responding to 3–5 days of glucocorticoids

(IV = intravenous)

23.69 Monitoring of inflammatory bowel disease (IBD)

- Assess symptoms, including extra-intestinal manifestations
- Examine for abdominal mass or perianal disease
- Perform full blood count, urea and electrolytes, liver function tests, albumin, C-reactive protein (CRP)
- Check haematinics (vitamin B_{12}, folate, iron studies) at least annually
- Check faecal calprotectin (to monitor each disease flare/change in therapy and assess response)
- Perform stool cultures (at each flare to exclude infection)
- Assess mucosal healing: surrogate markers (CRP/calprotectin), small bowel capsule, ileocolonoscopy and/or small bowel magnetic resonance imaging
- Enrol patient in a dedicated IBD clinic (monitoring of stable, uncomplicated patients may be carried out by a nurse or phone clinic)
- Arrange IBD multidisciplinary meeting for acutely ill or complex patients
- Check vaccinations are up to date; live vaccinations may be given at least 4 weeks before starting immunosuppressive therapy and at least 3 months after stopping immunosuppressive therapy. Patients on immunosuppressive therapy should receive influenza and pneumococcal vaccination
- Ensure surveillance colonoscopy is scheduled where appropriate

- *by laboratory testing*: haemoglobin, white cell count, albumin, electrolytes, ESR and CRP, stool culture, including *Clostridioides difficile* toxin assay
- *radiologically*: for colonic dilatation on plain abdominal X-rays.

All patients should be given supportive treatment with intravenous fluids to correct dehydration and enteral nutritional support should be provided for malnourished patients (Box 23.68). Intravenous glucocorticoids (methylprednisolone 60 mg every 24 hours or hydrocortisone 100 mg four times daily) should be given by infusion or bolus injection. Patients should receive prophylactic low-molecular weight heparin, as the risk of venous thromboembolism is 2–3-fold higher compared to inpatients without IBD. Topical and oral aminosalicylates have no role to play in the acute severe attack. Response to therapy is judged over the first 3 days. Patients who do not respond promptly to glucocorticoids should be considered for medical rescue therapy with ciclosporin (2 mg/kg daily by intravenous infusion followed by 5 mg/kg daily, then orally after 7 days) or infliximab (5 mg/kg), which can avoid the need for urgent colectomy in approximately 60% of cases.

Patients who develop colonic dilatation (> 6 cm), those whose clinical and laboratory measurements deteriorate and those who do not respond after 7–10 days' maximal medical treatment usually require urgent surgery. Subtotal colectomy with end ileostomy is the operation of choice and can be performed open or laparoscopically, dependent upon local expertise. The surgical and medical teams should liaise early in the disease course and, if possible, the patient should have the opportunity to speak with the stoma nurse prior to colectomy.

Maintenance of remission

Life-long maintenance therapy is recommended for all patients with left-sided or extensive disease, but is not necessary in those with proctitis (although 20% of these patients will develop proximal 'extension' over the lifetime of their disease). Once-daily oral 5-aminosalicylates are the preferred first-line agents. Sulfasalazine has a higher incidence of side-effects, but is equally effective and can be considered in patients with coexistent arthropathy. Patients who frequently relapse despite aminosalicylate drugs have in the past always been offered thiopurines (azathioprine or 6-mercaptopurine). While thiopurines still have an important role for treatment, other immunosuppressive drugs may also be used. Biologic therapy with anti-TNF antibodies (infliximab, adalimumab or golimumab) can be considered for maintenance treatment in patients with moderate to severe ulcerative colitis. Combination therapy of infliximab with a thiopurine should be used, as it is more effective than monotherapy with infliximab. In patients where anti-TNF treatment has failed, anti-α4β7 integrin antibodies (vedolizumab), Janus kinase inhibitors (tofacitinib) and anti-p40 antibodies (ustekinumab), can be considered to maintain remission.

Crohn's disease

Principles of management

Crohn's disease is a progressive condition that may result in stricture or fistula formation if suboptimally treated. It is therefore important to agree long-term treatment goals with the patient; these are to induce remission and then maintain glucocorticoid-free remission with a normal quality of life. Treatment should focus on monitoring the patient carefully for evidence of disease activity and complications (Box 23.69), and ensuring that mucosal healing is achieved.

Induction of remission in mild to moderate disease

Glucocorticoids remain the mainstay of treatment for active Crohn's disease. The drug of first choice in patents with ileal disease is budesonide, since it undergoes 90% first-pass metabolism in the liver and has very little systemic toxicity. A typical regimen is 9 mg once daily for 4 weeks, with a stepwise reduction of 3 mg every 4 weeks until therapy is stopped. If there is no response to budesonide within 2 weeks, the patient should be switched to prednisolone, which has greater potency. This is typically given in a dose of 40 mg daily, reducing by 5 mg/week over 8 weeks, at which point treatment is stopped. Oral prednisolone in the dose regimen described above is the treatment of choice for inducing remission in colonic Crohn's disease.

As an alternative to glucocorticoid therapy, enteral nutrition with either an elemental (constituent amino acids) or polymeric (liquid protein) diet may induce remission. Both types of diet are equally effective, but the polymeric one is more palatable when taken by mouth, and this improves adherence. It is particularly effective in children, in whom equal efficacy to glucocorticoids has been demonstrated, and in extensive ileal disease in adults. As well as resting the gut and providing excellent nutritional support, it also has a direct anti-inflammatory effect. It is an effective bridge to urgent staging investigations at first presentation and can be given by mouth or by nasogastric tube. With sufficient explanation, encouragement and motivation, most patients will tolerate it well.

Induction of remission in severe disease

Patients with severe disease can be treated with systemic glucocorticoids. The early introduction of biologics can also be considered, providing that acute perforating complications, such as abscess, have not arisen. Anti-TNF (infliximab or adalimumab), anti-α4β7 integrin (vedolizumab) and anti-p40 (ustekinumab) therapy can be considered as first-line biologics. Patients with evidence of persistently active disease require further maintenance treatment (see below).

Maintenance therapy

Glucocorticoids are not effective at maintaining remission in Crohn's disease. Immunosuppressive treatment with thiopurines (azathioprine and

23.70 How to give anti-tumour necrosis factor (TNF) therapy in inflammatory bowel disease

- Infliximab (5 mg/kg IV infusion) is given as three loading doses (at 0, 2 and 6 weeks), with 8-weekly maintenance thereafter. Some patients may require dose escalation to 10 mg/kg up to 4 weekly
- Adalimumab is given as SC injections, which patients can be trained to give themselves. Loading dose is 160 mg, followed by 80 mg 2 weeks later and 40 mg every second week thereafter; some patients require dose escalation to 40 mg once weekly
- Concomitant immunosuppression with a thiopurine or methotrexate may be more efficacious than monotherapy but has more side-effects
- Anti-TNF therapy is contraindicated in the presence of active infection and latent tuberculosis without appropriate prophylaxis; it carries an increased risk of opportunistic infections and a possible increased risk of malignancy; rarely, multiple sclerosis may be unmasked in susceptible individuals. Counselling about the balance of risk and benefit for each patient is important
- Prior to therapy, latent tuberculosis must be excluded, as well as checking immunisation status, as well as hepatitis B, hepatitis C, HIV and VZV status
- Live vaccines should not be given
- Golimumab is effective for ulcerative colitis
- Certolizumab is effective for luminal Crohn's disease, but is not licensed in Europe

(HIV = human immunodeficiency virus; IV = intravenous; SC = subcutabeous; TNF = tumour necrosis factor; VZV = varicella zoster virus)

mercaptopurine) may be used as maintenance therapy, but methotrexate is also effective and can be given once weekly, either orally or by subcutaneous injection; subcutaneous administration has better bioavailability. Patients refractory to immunomodulator therapy should be considered for biologic therapy with anti-TNF (infliximab or adalimumab) (Box 23.70), anti-α4β7 integrin (vedolizumab) or anti-p40 (ustekinumab) therapies). Combination therapy of infliximab with a thiopurine should be used, as it is more effective than monotherapy with infliximab. Combination therapy of infliximab with methotrexate may also be used to reduce immunogenicity. In patients who still require glucocorticoids despite optimal treatment with biologics, other options must be considered including surgery.

Cigarette smokers with Crohn's disease should be strongly counselled to stop smoking at every possible opportunity. Those that do not manage to stop smoking fare much worse, with increased rates of relapse and surgical intervention, with adverse effects of smoking being more pronounced in women than in men. Careful monitoring of disease activity (see Box 23.69) is the key to maintaining sustained remission and preventing the accumulation of bowel damage in Crohn's disease.

Fistulae and perianal disease

Fistulae may develop in relation to active Crohn's disease and are often associated with sepsis. The first step is to define the site by imaging (usually MRI of the pelvis). Endoanal ultrasound is another option for assessment, but is limited in patients with luminal stenoses, as well as by local expertise. Surgical exploration by examination under anaesthetic is usually then required, to delineate the anatomy and drain abscesses. Seton sutures can be inserted through fistula tracts to ensure adequate drainage and to prevent future sepsis. Glucocorticoids are ineffective. Use of antibiotics, such as metronidazole and/or ciprofloxacin, can aid healing as an adjunctive treatment. Thiopurines can be used in chronic disease, but do not usually result in fistula healing. Anti TNF therapy can heal fistulae and perianal disease in many patients and are indicated when the measures described above have been ineffective. Higher trough infliximab drug levels are aimed for in perianal Crohn's disease. The evidence of benefit in perianal fistulating disease for the newer biologics is presently unclear. Other options for refractory perianal disease are proctectomy or faecal diversion with an upstream stoma.

23.71 Indications for surgery in ulcerative colitis

Impaired quality of life
- Loss of occupation or education
- Disruption of family life

Failure of medical therapy
- Dependence on oral glucocorticoids
- Resistant to drug therapy
- Intolerable side-effects of drug therapy

Fulminant colitis
- Life-threatening bleeding

Toxic megacolon
- Perforation

Colon cancer or severe dysplasia

Surgical management

Ulcerative colitis

Up to 60% of patients with extensive ulcerative colitis eventually require surgery. The indications are listed in Box 23.71. Impaired quality of life, with its impact on occupation and social and family life, is the most important of these. Surgery involves removal of the entire colon and rectum, and cures the patient. One-third of those with pancolitis undergo colectomy within 5 years of diagnosis. Before surgery, patients should be counselled by doctors, stoma nurses and patients who have undergone similar surgery. The procedure of choice is usually an initial subtotal colectomy with ileostomy and a subsequent ileorectal anastomosis, or a proctocolectomy and ileal pouch–anal anastomosis. The companion text to this book, *Principles and Practice of Surgery*, should be consulted for further details.

Crohn's disease

Operations are often necessary to deal with fistulae, abscesses and perianal disease, and may also be required to relieve small or large bowel obstruction. In contrast to ulcerative colitis, surgery is not curative and disease recurrence is the rule. The only method that has consistently been shown to reduce post-operative recurrence is smoking cessation. Antibiotics are effective in the short term only. Use of thiopurines post surgery is suggested if there are indicators of a high chance of recurrence, i.e. more than one resection or evidence of penetrating disease, such as fistulae or abscess. Otherwise, it is common to undertake colonoscopy 6 months after surgery to inspect and biopsy the anastomosis and neo-terminal ileum. Patients with endoscopic recurrence are then prescribed immunomodulators or biologics to prevent further complications.

Surgery should be as conservative as possible in order to minimise the loss of viable intestine and to avoid the creation of a short bowel syndrome (p. 771). Obstructing or fistulating small bowel disease may require resection of affected tissue. Patients who have localised segments of Crohn's colitis may be managed by segmental resection and/or multiple strictureplasties, in which the stricture is not resected but instead incised in its longitudinal axis and sutured transversely. Others who have extensive colitis require total colectomy but ileal pouch formation should be avoided because of the high risk of recurrence within the pouch and subsequent fistulae, abscess formation and pouch failure.

Historical datasets show that around 80% of Crohn's patients undergo surgery at some stage and 70% of these require more than one operation during their lifetime. Clinical recurrence following resectional surgery is present in 50% of all cases at 10 years. Emerging data demonstrate that aggressive medical therapy, coupled with intense monitoring, probably reduces the requirement for surgery substantially.

23

IBD in special circumstances

Childhood

Children developing IBD tend to have more extensive disease than adults. Chronic ill health in childhood or adolescence may result in impaired growth, metabolic bone disease and delayed puberty. Loss of schooling and social contact, as well as frequent hospitalisation, can have important psychosocial consequences. Treatment is similar to that described for adults and may involve glucocorticoids, immunosuppressive drugs, biologic agents and surgery. However, exclusive enteral nutrition can also be used to induce disease remission in Crohn's disease, as well as aiding with growth and nutritional status. Monitoring of height, weight and sexual development is crucial. Children with IBD should be managed by specialised paediatric gastroenterologists and transitioned to adult care in dedicated clinics (Box 23.72).

Pregnancy

Pregnant women with IBD are best managed in an MDT approach involving an IBD physician and an obstetrician. A woman's ability to become pregnant is adversely affected by active IBD. Pre-conceptual counselling should focus on optimising disease control. During pregnancy, roughly one-third of women improve, one-third get worse and one-third remain stable with active disease. In the post-partum period, these changes sometimes reverse spontaneously, e.g. improvement during pregnancy is followed by post-partum relapse. Drug therapy, including aminosalicylates, glucocorticoids, thiopurines and biologics can be safely continued throughout pregnancy, but methotrexate and tofacitinib must be avoided, both during pregnancy and pre-conception (Box 23.73). Biologics such as infliximab, adalimumab, vedolizumab and ustekinumab may pass across the placenta and concentrate in the fetus, especially in the last trimester. Some women who are in deep remission may therefore choose to omit their biologics in the last trimester. However, biologics can be safely continued throughout the pregnancy, especially in women with ongoing active disease, at high risk of relapse or when limited treatment options. Breast feeding is recommended in all women and the use of thiopurines and biologics does not preclude women from breastfeeding. Thiopurine drug levels in breast milk are very low, with negligible levels measured in breast-fed infants of mothers on thiopurines. Levels of biologics are also very low in breastmilk and lead to negligible levels in the breast-fed infant due to normal gut digestion. Mode of delivery should be discussed with pregnant women and in the absence of active rectal or perianal fistulating disease, where a caesarean section is recommended, a vaginal delivery is safe.

Metabolic bone disease

Patients with IBD are prone to developing osteoporosis due to the effects of chronic inflammation, glucocorticoids, weight loss, malnutrition and malabsorption. Osteomalacia can also occur in Crohn's disease that is complicated by malabsorption, but is less common than osteoporosis. The risk of osteoporosis increases with age and with the dose and duration of glucocorticoid therapy. Patients should have their fracture risk assessed prior to glucocorticoid therapy. Individuals who receive prolonged (> 3 months) or repeated courses of oral glucocorticoid therapy should have bone densitometry assessed. Oral bisphosphonates, in the form of alendronate and risedronate, are commonly used for treatment if required. Denosumab and high dose intravenous bisphosphonates should be avoided in women of childbearing age, due to their unknown effects on the fetus.

Microscopic colitis

Microscopic colitis, which comprises two related conditions called lymphocytic colitis and collagenous colitis, has no known cause. Both forms are commoner in women with a mean age of presentation of around 60 years. The presentation is with chronic non-bloody watery diarrhoea. The colonoscopic appearances are normal, but histological examination of

23.72 Inflammatory bowel disease in adolescence

- **Delayed growth and pubertal development**: chronic active inflammation, malabsorption, malnutrition and long-term glucocorticoids contribute to short stature and delayed development, with physical and psychological consequences.
- **Metabolic bone disease**: more common with chronic disease beginning in childhood, resulting from chronic inflammation, dietary deficiency and malabsorption of calcium and vitamin D.
- **Drug side-effects and adherence issues**: young people are more likely to require azathioprine or biologic therapy than adults. Poor adherence to therapy is more common than with adults, as younger patients may feel well, lack self-motivation to adhere and believe that drugs are ineffective or cause side-effects.
- **Loss of time from education**: physical illness, surgery, fatigue in chronic inflammatory bowel disease, privacy and dignity issues, and social isolation may all contribute.
- **Emotional difficulties**: may result from challenges in coping with illness, problems with forming interpersonal relationships, and issues relating to body image or sexual function.

23.73 Pregnancy and inflammatory bowel disease (IBD)

Pre-conception

- Outcomes are best when pregnancy is carefully planned and disease is in remission
- Methotrexate must be stopped 6 months prior to conception; other IBD drugs should be continued until discussed with a specialist
- Aminosalicylates and azathioprine are safe in pregnancy
- Glucocorticoids are probably safe
- Biologic therapy (infliximab, adalimumab, vedolizumab, ustekinumab) in pregnancy can continue if established pre-pregnancy
- Tofacitinib should be avoided in pregnancy
- Folic acid (5 mg/day) is recommended pre-conception. Consider high-dose supplements in small bowel Crohn's disease with low levels despite 5 mg dose

Pregnancy

- Two-thirds of patients in remission will remain so in pregnancy
- Active disease is likely to remain active
- Severe active disease carries an increased risk of premature delivery and low birth weight
- Perform endoscopy only when absolutely essential for clinical decision-making (ideally in second trimester)
- X-rays can be performed if clinically indicated, but discuss with the radiologist first. Ultrasound is preferable but is operator-dependent. MRI small bowel can be performed without intravenous gadolinium and oral contrast

Labour

- This needs careful discussion between patient, gastroenterologist and obstetrician
- Normal labour and vaginal delivery are possible for most
- Caesarean section may be preferred for patients with perianal Crohn's or an ileo-anal pouch to reduce risks of pelvic floor damage, fistulation and late incontinence
- Venous thromboembolism prophylaxis is important if in hospital

Breastfeeding

- This is safe and does not exacerbate IBD
- Data on the risk to babies from drugs excreted in breast milk are limited; most of these drugs are probably safe
- Patients should discuss breastfeeding and drug therapy with their doctor

biopsies shows a range of abnormalities. It is therefore recommended that biopsies of the right and left colon plus the terminal ileum should be undertaken in all patients undergoing colonoscopy for diarrhoea. An increased number of intraepithelial and lamina propria lymphocytes is noted in both forms of microscopic colitis, with a thickened subepithelial collagen band also noted in collagenous colitis. Microscopic colitis may be associated with autoimmune diseases such as coeliac disease, rheumatoid arthritis and thyroid disease, and some drug therapies, such as NSAIDs and PPIs. Bile acid diarrhoea has also been reported to be more prevalent in this group. Treatment with budesonide is usually effective for inducing remission. Up to 70% of individuals can relapse and require further treatment, but others can remain symptom free.

Functional bowel disorders

Functional gastrointestinal disorders are a common diagnosis in gastroenterology, accounting for around 40% of all referrals to gastroenterology. They are thought to be disorders of brain–gut interaction, with alterations in motility, visceral hypersensitivity, gut microbiota, immune and mucosal function, as well as alterations in central nervous system processing.

Functional dyspepsia

Functional dyspepsia can be diagnosed in patients presenting with dyspepsia where organic disease has been excluded. Patients are usually young (< 40 years) and women are affected twice as commonly as men. There are subtypes of this condition, with individuals being classified as having postprandial distress syndrome, epigastric pain syndrome or a mixture of both.

Pathophysiology

The cause is poorly understood, but probably covers a spectrum of mucosal, motility and psychological factors.

Clinical features

Symptoms such as bloating, early satiety, loss of appetite, nausea, vomiting or retching may suggest a diagnosis of postprandial distress syndrome, whereas symptoms of epigastric pain or epigastric burning may suggest a diagnosis of epigastric pain syndrome. Symptoms seen in functional dyspepsia can significantly overlap with symptoms of an organic disease, and alarm features should be sought (see Box 23.15). While patients with functional dyspepsia can experience vomiting, persistent vomiting may suggest an underlying organic disorder. Peptic ulcer disease must be considered, while in older people intra-abdominal malignancy is a prime concern. There are no diagnostic signs, although there may be inappropriate tenderness on abdominal palpation. A drug history should be taken and the possibility of a depressive illness should be considered. Pregnancy should be ruled out in young women before radiological studies are undertaken. Alcohol misuse should be suspected when early-morning nausea and retching are prominent.

Investigations

The history will often suggest the diagnosis. All patients should be checked for *H. pylori* infection and patients with alarm features should undergo endoscopy to exclude mucosal disease. While an ultrasound scan may detect gallstones, these are rarely responsible for dyspeptic symptoms, unless the patient has features to suggest biliary pathology.

Management

Up to 10% of patients benefit from *H. pylori* eradication therapy and this should be offered to infected individuals. Eradication also removes a major risk factor for peptic ulcers and gastric cancer, but at the cost of a small risk of side-effects and worsening symptoms of underlying gastro-oesophageal reflux disease. Idiosyncratic and restrictive diets are of little benefit but smaller portions and fat restriction may help.

Drug treatment is targeted on the subtype of functional dyspepsia. Prokinetic drugs (e.g. metoclopramide), fundus-relaxing drugs (e.g. buspirone) or centrally acting neuromodulators (e.g. mirtazapine) can be used in postprandial distress syndrome. Acid suppression medication (e.g. PPI) and tricyclic antidepressants (e.g. amitriptyline) may be used in epigastric pain syndrome. Patients with major psychological disorders

that result in persistent or recurrent symptoms may require behavioural or other formal psychotherapy (Ch. 31).

Functional causes of vomiting

Cyclical vomiting syndrome (CVS) is an increasingly recognised cause of functional vomiting. It is characterised by distinct phases. There tends to be a prodrome phase, where symptoms of nausea, pallor and sweating are noted. This is then followed by an intense vomiting phase, with other associated symptoms such as abdominal pain, which can last up to a week. After this, patients enter a recovery phase, with improvement and resolution of symptoms. There will then be a period of time without symptoms. Triggers can include stress, fatigue and menstruation. The cause of CVS is unknown, although an association with migraine headaches is recognised. A subset of adults with CVS have symptoms triggered by chronic cannabis use, known as cannabinoid hyperemesis syndrome. Patients with CVS are managed with general lifestyle advice, with avoidance of triggers such as cannabis. Acute episodes can be managed with medications, such as anxiolytics (e.g. lorazepam) and antiemetics (e.g. ondansetron). Prophylactic treatment includes the use of tricyclic antidepressants (e.g. amitryptiline) and antiepileptic medication (e.g. levetiracetam).

In all patients it is essential to exclude other common causes of vomiting (see; Fig. 23.18). Patients who do not have characteristic symptoms seen in CVS, with nausea or vomiting occurring weekly, in the absence of organic disease may be diagnosed as having chronic nausea and vomiting syndrome (CNVS). These patients may respond to treatments including antiemetics (e.g. ondansetron) and tricyclic antidepressants (e.g. amitriptyline).

Irritable bowel syndrome

Irritable bowel syndrome (IBS) has an estimated worldwide prevalence of around 5%. It is characterised by recurrent abdominal pain in association with abnormal defecation in the absence of a structural abnormality of the gut. IBS accounts for frequent absenteeism from work and impaired quality of life. Young women are affected more often than men.

Pathophysiology

The cause of IBS is incompletely understood but biopsychosocial factors are thought to play an important role, along with luminal factors, such as diet and the gut microbiota, as discussed below.

Behavioural and psychosocial factors

Early learning difficulties or emotionally challenging interactions during childhood may contribute to IBS in later life. Most patients seen in general practice do not have psychological problems but about 50% of patients referred to hospital have a psychiatric illness, such as anxiety, depression, somatisation and neurosis. Panic attacks are also common. Acute psychological stress and overt psychiatric disease are known to alter visceral perception and gastrointestinal motility. There is an increased prevalence of abnormal illness behaviour, with frequent consultations for minor symptoms and reduced coping ability (Ch. 31). These factors contribute to but do not cause IBS.

Physiological factors

The pathophysiology of IBS is still not fully understood. IBS is thought to be a disorder of the brain–gut axis, with alterations in visceral hypersensitivity. There is some evidence that IBS may be a serotoninergic (5-HT) disorder, as evidenced by relatively excessive release of 5-HT in diarrhoea-predominant IBS (IBS-D) and relative deficiency with constipation-predominant IBS (IBS-C). Accordingly, 5-HT_3 receptor antagonists are effective in IBS-D, while 5-HT_4 agonists improve bowel function in IBS-C. There is some evidence that IBS may represent a state of low-grade gut inflammation or immune activation, not detectable by tests, with raised numbers of mucosal mast cells that sensitise enteric neurons by releasing histamine and tryptase. Some patients respond positively to mast cell stabilisers,

23

such as ketotifen, which supports a pathogenic role of mast cells in at least some patients. Immune activation may be associated with altered CNS processing of visceral pain signals. This is more common in women and in IBS-D, and may be triggered by a prior episode of gastroenteritis with *Salmonella* or *Campylobacter* species.

Luminal factors

Both quantitative and qualitative alterations in intestinal bacterial microbiota have been reported. Small intestinal bacterial overgrowth (SIBO) may be present in some patients and lead to symptoms. This 'gut dysbiosis' may explain the response to probiotics or the non-absorbable antibiotic rifaximin.

Dietary factors are also important. Some patients have chemical food intolerances (not allergy) to poorly absorbed, short-chain carbohydrates (lactose, fructose and sorbitol, among others), collectively known as FODMAPs (fermentable oligo-, di- and monosaccharides, and polyols). Whilst their fermentation in the colon is normal physiology, this leads to bloating, pain, wind and altered bowel habit in patients with IBS, thought to be due to visceral hypersensitivity. Gluten exposure seems to cause symptoms in some IBS patients and there is an overlap with the diagnosis of non-coeliac gluten sensitivity (negative coeliac serology and normal duodenal biopsies).

Clinical features

The key symptoms of IBS include recurrent abdominal pain and altered bowel habit (Box 23.74). Abdominal pain is usually colicky or cramping in nature, felt in the lower abdomen and related to defecation. The bowel habit is variable, with IBS stratified by predominant bowel habit; those with mainly constipation (IBS-C), mainly diarrhoea (IBS-D), mixed bowel habit (IBS-M) or unsubtyped (IBS-U). Those with constipation tend to pass infrequent pellety stools, usually in association with abdominal pain or proctalgia. Those with diarrhoea have frequent defecation but produce low-volume stools and rarely have nocturnal symptoms. Passage of mucus is common but rectal bleeding does not occur. Patients do not lose weight and are constitutionally well. Diagnosis is made through a careful history, exploring diet, medical, surgical and psychological history. The presence of other functional gastrointestinal disorders may also support the diagnosis, in addition to non-gastrointestinal symptoms such as migraine headaches, dyspareunia and interstitial cystitis. Onset after gastroenteritis may point towards a diagnosis of post-infectious IBS. Physical examination is generally unremarkable, with the exception of variable tenderness to palpation.

Investigations

The diagnosis is clinical in nature and can be made confidently in most patients using the Rome IV criteria, combined with the absence of alarm symptoms and without resorting to complicated tests (Box 23.75). Limited laboratory tests are normally performed prior to making a diagnosis of IBS, including full blood count, faecal calprotectin and C-reactive protein, which are all normal. Colonoscopy should be undertaken when patients present with alarm features, to exclude other diagnoses such as colorectal cancer and inflammatory bowel disease. Those who present atypically require investigations to exclude other gastrointestinal diseases. Diarrhoea-predominant patients justify investigations to exclude coeliac disease, microscopic, lactose intolerance, bile acid diarrhoea (see earlier in this chapter), thyrotoxicosis (Ch. 20) and, in relevant countries, parasitic infection.

Management

The most important steps are to make a positive diagnosis, as well as educating and reassuring the patient. Communicating diagnostic certainty is crucial, to prevent further unwarranted testing. Many people are concerned that they have developed cancer. A cycle of anxiety leading to colonic symptoms, which further heighten anxiety, can be broken by explaining that symptoms are not due to a serious underlying disease, but instead are the result of behavioural, psychosocial, physiological and luminal factors. In individuals who fail to respond to reassurance, treatment is traditionally tailored to the predominant symptoms (Fig. 23.67).

23.74 Rome IV criteria for diagnosis of irritable bowel syndrome

Recurrent abdominal pain at least 1 day per week on average in the last 3 months (onset at least 6 months before diagnosis), associated with *two or more* of the following:
- Related to defecation
- Onset associated with a change in frequency of stool
- Onset associated with a change in form (appearance) of stool

23.75 Alarm features in suspected irritable bowel syndrome

- Age >50 years
- Unintentional weight loss
- Nocturnal symptoms
- Recent change in bowel habit
- Palpable abdominal mass or lymphadenopathy
- Family history of colon cancer or inflammatory bowel disease
- Anaemia
- Evidence of overt gastrointestinal bleeding (i.e. melaena or fresh blood in stools (haematochezia))

A large proportion of IBS patients report symptoms triggered by food, with diet being shown to be an effective management option for many patients (Box 23.76). Dietary advice should be implemented under the expert guidance of a dietitian, to prevent potential nutritional deficiencies of restrictive diets. General dietary advice is the first-line option recommended in the UK, with advice on regular meals, adjustment of fibre intake, adequate fluid intake, assessment of alcohol and caffeine intake, decreasing fat intake and assessing components of spicy meals which may be contributing to symptoms. If these measures fail, a low FODMAP diet may help some patients, as may a trial of a gluten-free diet. Up to 30% may benefit from a wheat-free diet, some may respond to lactose exclusion and excess intake of artificial sweeteners, such as sorbitol, should be addressed. Probiotics, in capsule form, may be effective if taken for several months, although the optimum combination of bacterial strains and dose have yet to be clarified.

Patients with intractable symptoms sometimes benefit from several months of therapy with a tricyclic antidepressant, such as amitriptyline or imipramine. Side-effects include dry mouth and drowsiness, but these are usually mild and the drug is generally well tolerated, although patients with features of somatisation tolerate the drug poorly and lower doses should be used. It may act by reducing visceral sensation and by altering gastrointestinal motility. Anxiety and affective disorders may also require specific treatment (Ch. 31). The 5-HT$_4$ agonist prucalopride, the guanylate cyclase-C receptor agonist linaclotide and chloride channel activators, such as lubiprostone, can be effective in IBS-C.

Systemic and nonabsorbable antibiotics, such as rifaximin, that act strictly on the gut lumen are sometimes used to manage symptoms, although the mechanism of action remains uncertain.

Psychological interventions, such as cognitive behavioural therapy, relaxation and gut-directed hypnotherapy, should be reserved for the most difficult cases. Cognitive behavioural therapy is the most widely studied psychotherapy treatment for IBS and may improve bowel symptoms, quality of life and psychological distress. A range of complementary and alternative therapies exist; most lack a good evidence base but are popular and help some patients (Box 23.77).

Most patients have a relapsing and remitting course. Exacerbations often follow stressful life events, occupational dissatisfaction and difficulties with interpersonal relationships.

Ischaemic gut injury

Ischaemic gut injury is usually the result of arterial occlusion. Severe hypotension and venous insufficiency are less frequent causes. The presentation is variable, depending on the different vessels involved and the acuteness of the event. Diagnosis is often difficult.

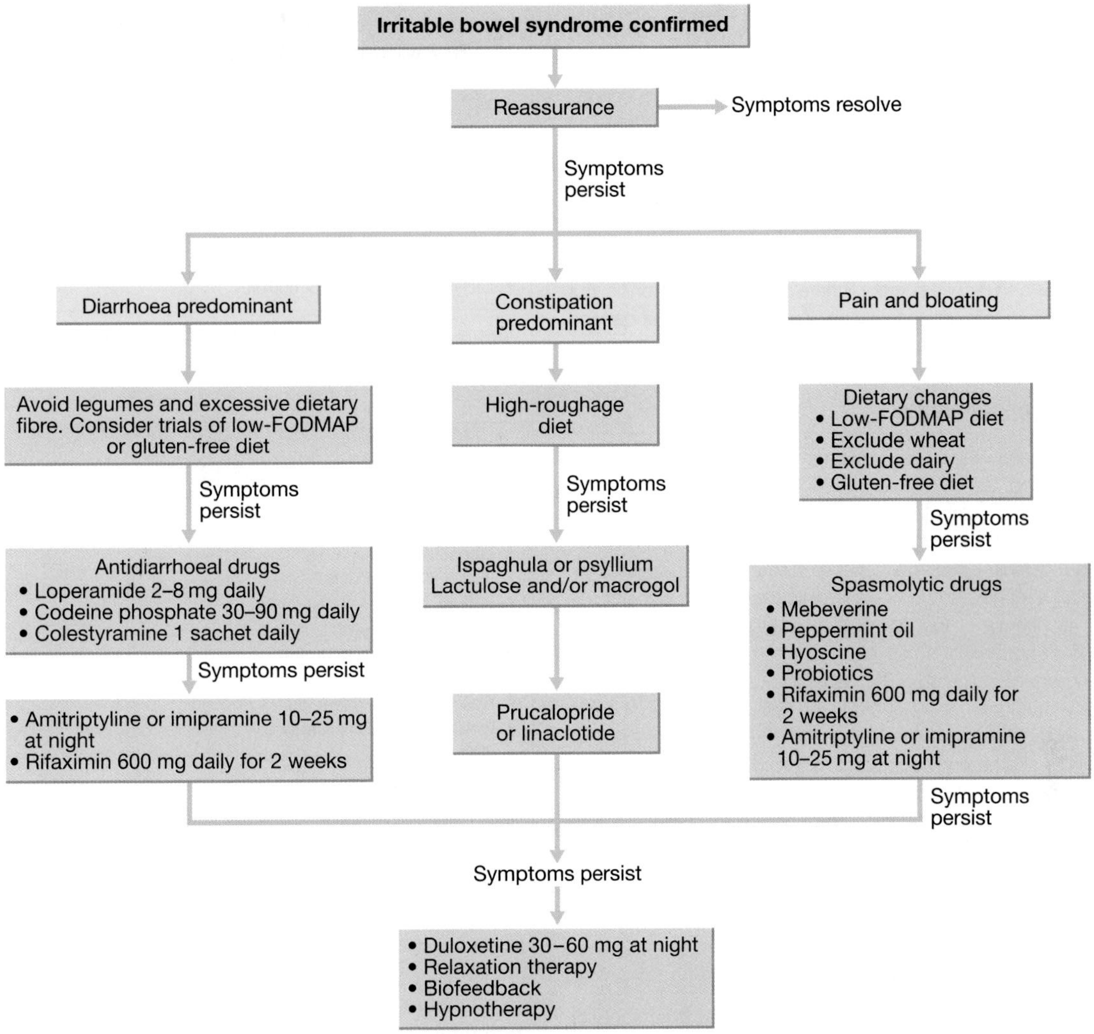

Irritable bowel syndrome confirmed

Reassurance → Symptoms resolve

Symptoms persist

| Diarrhoea predominant | Constipation predominant | Pain and bloating |

Diarrhoea predominant

Avoid legumes and excessive dietary fibre. Consider trials of low-FODMAP or gluten-free diet

Symptoms persist

Antidiarrhoeal drugs
• Loperamide 2–8 mg daily
• Codeine phosphate 30–90 mg daily
• Colestyramine 1 sachet daily

Symptoms persist

• Amitriptyline or imipramine 10–25 mg at night
• Rifaximin 600 mg daily for 2 weeks

Constipation predominant

High-roughage diet

Symptoms persist

Ispaghula or psyllium
Lactulose and/or macrogol

Prucalopride or linaclotide

Pain and bloating

Dietary changes
• Low-FODMAP diet
• Exclude wheat
• Exclude dairy
• Gluten-free diet

Symptoms persist

Spasmolytic drugs
• Mebeverine
• Peppermint oil
• Hyoscine
• Probiotics
• Rifaximin 600 mg daily for 2 weeks
• Amitriptyline or imipramine 10–25 mg at night

Symptoms persist

Symptoms persist

• Duloxetine 30–60 mg at night
• Relaxation therapy
• Biofeedback
• Hypnotherapy

Fig. 23.67 Management of irritable bowel syndrome. (FODMAP = fermentable oligo-, di- and monosaccharides, and polyols)

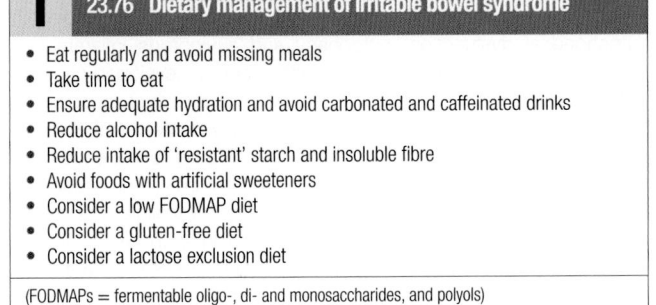

i 23.76 Dietary management of irritable bowel syndrome

• Eat regularly and avoid missing meals
• Take time to eat
• Ensure adequate hydration and avoid carbonated and caffeinated drinks
• Reduce alcohol intake
• Reduce intake of 'resistant' starch and insoluble fibre
• Avoid foods with artificial sweeteners
• Consider a low FODMAP diet
• Consider a gluten-free diet
• Consider a lactose exclusion diet

(FODMAPs = fermentable oligo-, di- and monosaccharides, and polyols)

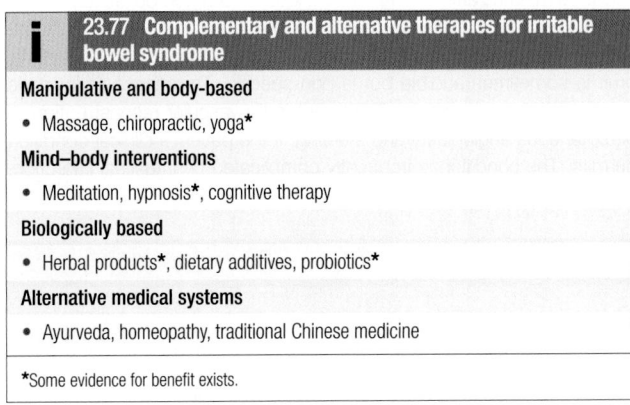

i 23.77 Complementary and alternative therapies for irritable bowel syndrome

Manipulative and body-based

• Massage, chiropractic, yoga*

Mind–body interventions

• Meditation, hypnosis*, cognitive therapy

Biologically based

• Herbal products*, dietary additives, probiotics*

Alternative medical systems

• Ayurveda, homeopathy, traditional Chinese medicine

*Some evidence for benefit exists.

23

Acute small bowel ischaemia

An embolus from the heart or aorta to the superior mesenteric artery is responsible for 40%–50% of cases, thrombosis of underlying atheromatous disease for approximately 25% and non-occlusive ischaemia due to hypotension complicating myocardial infarction, heart failure, arrhythmias or sudden blood loss for approximately 25%. Vasculitis and venous occlusion are rare causes. The clinical spectrum ranges from transient alteration of bowel function to transmural haemorrhagic necrosis and gangrene. Patients usually have evidence of cardiac disease and arrhythmia. Almost all develop abdominal pain that is more impressive than the physical findings. In the early stages, the only physical signs may be a silent, distended abdomen or diminished bowel sounds, with peritonitis developing only later.

Leucocytosis, lactic acidosis, hyperphosphataemia and hyperamylasaemia are typical. Plain abdominal X-rays show 'thumb-printing' due to mucosal oedema. CT with contrast has replaced percutaneous angiography as the gold standard for diagnosis and may demonstrate features such as occlusion of the mesenteric vessels and bowel wall thickening. Laparoscopy may also be used for diagnosis. Resuscitation, management of cardiac disease and intravenous broad-spectrum antibiotic therapy, followed by laparotomy, are key steps. If treatment is instituted early, embolectomy and vascular reconstruction may salvage some small bowel. In these rare cases, a 'second look' laparotomy should be undertaken 24 hours later and further necrotic bowel resected. While laparotomy is the established approach, endovascular techniques may be considered, such as thrombolysis or percutaneous transluminal angioplasty. The results of therapy depend on early intervention; patients treated late have a 75% mortality rate. Survivors often have nutritional failure from short bowel syndrome (Ch. 22) and require intensive nutritional support, including home parenteral nutrition and anticoagulation. Small bowel transplantation can be considered in selected patients. Patients with mesenteric venous thrombosis also require surgery if there are signs of peritonitis, but are otherwise treated with anticoagulation. Investigations for underlying prothrombotic disorders should be performed (p. 988).

Acute colonic ischaemia

The splenic flexure and descending colon have little collateral circulation and lie in 'watershed' areas of arterial supply. The spectrum of injury ranges from reversible colopathy to transient colitis, colonic stricture, gangrene and fulminant pancolitis. Arterial thromboembolism is usually responsible, but colonic ischaemia can also follow severe hypotension, colonic volvulus, strangulated hernia, systemic vasculitis or hypercoagulable states. Ischaemia of the descending and sigmoid colon is also a complication of abdominal aortic aneurysm surgery (where the inferior mesenteric artery is ligated). The patient is usually an older adult who presents with sudden onset of cramping, left-sided, lower abdominal pain and rectal bleeding. Symptoms usually resolve spontaneously over 24–48 hours and healing occurs in 2 weeks. Some may develop a fibrous stricture or segment of colitis. A minority develop gangrene and peritonitis. CT with contrast is the imaging of choice for diagnosis, with early colonoscopy within 48 hours of presentation recommended; otherwise, mucosal ulceration may have resolved. Resection is required for peritonitis; colonoscopy should not be performed in this circumstance.

Chronic mesenteric ischaemia

This results from atherosclerotic stenosis of the coeliac axis, superior mesenteric artery and inferior mesenteric artery. At least two of the three vessels must be affected for symptoms to develop. The typical presentation is with dull but severe mid- or upper abdominal pain developing about 30 minutes after eating. Weight loss is common because patients are reluctant to eat and some experience diarrhoea. Physical examination shows evidence of generalised arterial disease. An abdominal bruit is sometimes audible but is non-specific. The diagnosis is made by mesenteric angiography. Treatment is by vascular reconstruction or percutaneous angioplasty and stenting, if the patient's clinical condition permits. The condition is frequently complicated by intestinal infarction, if left untreated.

Diseases of the pancreas

Acute pancreatitis

Acute pancreatitis accounts for 3% of all cases of abdominal pain admitted to hospital. It affects 2–28 per 100000 of the population and is increasing in incidence. It is a potentially serious condition with an overall mortality of 10%. About 80% of all cases are mild and have a favourable outcome. Approximately 98% of deaths from pancreatitis occur in the 20% of patients with severe disease and about one-third of these arise within the first week, usually from multi-organ failure. After this time, the majority of deaths result from sepsis, especially that complicating infected necrosis. At admission, it is possible to predict patients at risk of these complications (Box 23.78). Individuals who are predicted to have severe pancreatitis (Box 23.79) and those with necrosis or other complications should be managed in a specialist centre with an intensive care unit and multidisciplinary hepatobiliary specialists.

23.78 Glasgow criteria for prognosis in acute pancreatitis*

- Age > 55 years
- PO_2 < 8 kPa (60 mmHg)
- White blood cell count > 15×10^9/L
- Albumin < 32 g/L (3.2 g/dL)
- Serum calcium <2 mmol/L (8 mg/dL) (corrected)
- Glucose > 10 mmol/L (180 mg/dL)
- Urea > 16 mmol/L (45 mg/dL) (after rehydration)
- Alanine aminotransferase > 200 U/L
- Lactate dehydrogenase > 600 U/L

*Severity and prognosis worsen as the number of these factors increases. More than three implies severe disease.

23.79 Features that predict severe pancreatitis

Initial assessment
- Clinical impression of severity
- Body mass index > 30 kg/m²
- Pleural effusion on chest X-ray
- APACHE II score > 8 (see Box 9.55)

24 hours after admission
- Clinical impression of severity
- APACHE II score > 8
- Glasgow score > 3 (see Box 23.78)
- Persisting organ failure, especially if multiple
- CRP > 150 mg/L

48 hours after admission
- Clinical impression of severity
- Glasgow score > 3
- CRP > 150 mg/L
- Persisting organ failure for 48 hours
- Multiple or progressive organ failure

(CRP = C-reactive protein)

Pathophysiology

Acute pancreatitis occurs as a consequence of premature intracellular trypsinogen activation, releasing proteases that digest the pancreas and surrounding tissue. Triggers for this are many, including alcohol, gallstones and pancreatic duct obstruction (Fig. 23.68). There is simultaneous activation of nuclear factor kappa B (NFκB), leading to mitochondrial dysfunction, autophagy and a vigorous inflammatory response. The normal pancreas has only a poorly developed capsule, and adjacent structures, including the common bile duct, duodenum, splenic vein and transverse colon, are commonly involved in the inflammatory process. The severity of acute pancreatitis is dependent on the balance between the activity of released proteolytic enzymes and antiproteolytic factors. The latter comprise an intracellular pancreatic trypsin inhibitor protein and circulating β_2-macroglobulin, α_1-antitrypsin and C1-esterase inhibitors. The causes of acute pancreatitis are listed in Box 23.80. Acute pancreatitis is often self-limiting, but in some patients with severe disease, local complications, such as necrosis, pseudocyst or abscess, occur, as well as systemic complications that lead to multi-organ failure.

Clinical features

The typical presentation is with severe, constant upper abdominal pain, of increasing intensity over 15–60 minutes, which radiates to the back. Nausea and vomiting are common. There is marked epigastric tenderness, but in the early stages (and in contrast to a perforated peptic ulcer), guarding and rebound tenderness are absent because the inflammation is principally retroperitoneal. Bowel sounds become quiet or absent as paralytic ileus develops. In severe cases, the patient becomes hypoxic and develops hypovolaemic shock with oliguria. Discoloration of the flanks (Grey Turner's sign) or the periumbilical region

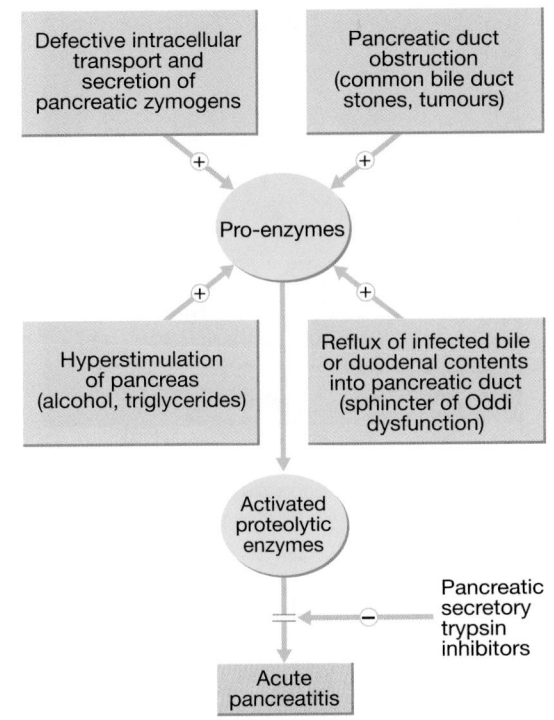

Fig. 23.68 Pathophysiology of acute pancreatitis.

i	23.81	Complications of acute pancreatitis
Complication		**Cause**
Systemic		
Systemic inflammatory response syndrome (SIRS)		Increased vascular permeability from cytokine, platelet-aggregating factor and kinin release
Hypoxia		Acute respiratory distress syndrome (ARDS) due to microthrombi in pulmonary vessels
Hyperglycaemia		Disruption of islets of Langerhans with altered insulin/glucagon release
Hypocalcaemia		Sequestration of calcium in fat necrosis, fall in ionised calcium
Reduced serum albumin concentration		Increased capillary permeability
Pancreatic		
Necrosis		Non-viable pancreatic tissue and peripancreatic tissue death; frequently infected
Abscess		Circumscribed collection of pus close to the pancreas and containing little or no pancreatic necrotic tissue
Pseudocyst		Disruption of pancreatic ducts
Pancreatic ascites or pleural effusion		Disruption of pancreatic ducts
Gastrointestinal		
Upper gastrointestinal bleeding		Gastric or duodenal erosions
Variceal haemorrhage		Splenic or portal vein thrombosis
Erosion into colon		Erosion by pancreatic pseudocyst
Duodenal obstruction		Compression by pancreatic mass
Obstructive jaundice		Compression of common bile duct

i	23.80	Causes of acute pancreatitis

Common (90% of cases)

- Gallstones
- Alcohol
- Idiopathic causes
- Post-ERCP

Rare

- Post-surgical (abdominal, cardiopulmonary bypass)
- Trauma
- Drugs (azathioprine/mercaptopurine, thiazide diuretics, sodium valproate)
- Metabolic (hypercalcaemia, hypertriglyceridaemia)
- Pancreas divisum (p. 854)
- Sphincter of Oddi dysfunction
- Infection (mumps, Coxsackie virus)
- Hereditary factors
- Renal failure
- Organ transplantation (kidney, liver)
- Severe hypothermia
- Petrochemical exposure
- Scorpion sting

(ERCP = endoscopic retrograde cholangiopancreatography)

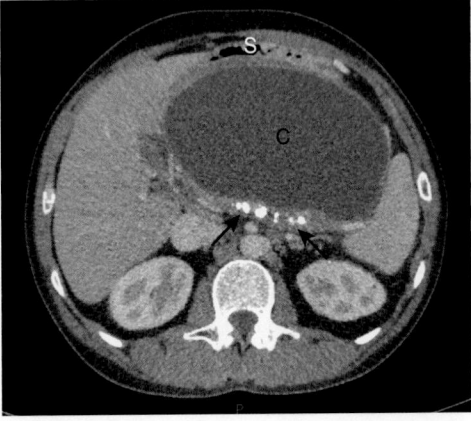

Fig. 23.69 Computed tomogram showing large pancreatic pseudocyst (C) compressing the stomach (S). The pancreas is atrophic and calcified (arrows).

(Cullen's sign) is a feature of severe pancreatitis with haemorrhage. The differential diagnosis includes a perforated viscus, acute cholecystitis and myocardial infarction. Various complications may occur and these are listed in Box 23.81.

A collection of fluid and debris may develop in the lesser sac, following inflammatory rupture of the pancreatic duct; this is known as a pancreatic fluid collection. It is initially contained within a poorly defined, fragile wall of granulation tissue, which matures over a 6-week period to form a fibrous capsule (Fig. 23.69). Such 'pseudocysts' are common and usually asymptomatic, resolving as the pancreatitis recovers. Pseudocysts greater than 6 cm in diameter seldom disappear spontaneously and can cause constant abdominal pain and compress or erode surrounding

structures, including blood vessels, to form pseudoaneurysms. Large pseudocysts can be detected clinically as a palpable abdominal mass.

Pancreatic ascites occurs when fluid leaks from a disrupted pancreatic duct into the peritoneal cavity. Leakage into the thoracic cavity can result in a pleural effusion or a pleuro-pancreatic fistula.

Investigations

The diagnosis is based on raised serum amylase or lipase concentrations and ultrasound or CT evidence of pancreatic swelling. Plain X-rays should be taken to exclude other diagnoses, such as perforation or

23

obstruction and to identify pulmonary complications. Amylase is efficiently excreted by the kidneys and concentrations may have returned to normal if measured 24–48 hours after the onset of pancreatitis. A persistently elevated serum amylase concentration suggests pseudocyst formation. Peritoneal amylase concentrations are massively elevated in pancreatic ascites. Serum amylase concentrations are also elevated (but less so) in intestinal ischaemia, perforated peptic ulcer and ruptured ovarian cyst, while the salivary isoenzyme of amylase is elevated in parotitis. If available, serum lipase measurements are preferable to amylase, as they have greater diagnostic accuracy for acute pancreatitis.

Ultrasound scanning can confirm the diagnosis, although in the earlier stages the gland may not be grossly swollen. An ultrasound scan is also useful because it may show gallstones, biliary obstruction or pseudocyst formation.

Contrast-enhanced pancreatic CT performed at least 3 days after admission can be useful in assessing viability of the pancreas if persisting organ failure, sepsis or clinical deterioration is present, since these features may indicate that pancreatic necrosis has occurred. Necrotising pancreatitis is associated with decreased pancreatic enhancement on CT, following intravenous injection of contrast material. The presence of gas within necrotic material (Fig. 23.70) suggests infection and impending abscess formation, in which case percutaneous aspiration of material for bacterial culture should be carried out and appropriate antibiotics prescribed. Involvement of the colon, blood vessels and other adjacent structures by the inflammatory process is best seen on CT.

Certain investigations stratify the severity of acute pancreatitis and have important prognostic value at the time of presentation (see Boxes 23.78 and 23.79). In addition, serial assessment of CRP is a useful indicator of progress. A peak CRP of > 210mg/L in the first 4 days predicts severe acute pancreatitis with 80% accuracy. It is worth noting that the serum amylase concentration has no prognostic value.

Management

Management comprises several related steps:

- establishing the diagnosis and disease severity
- early resuscitation, according to whether the disease is mild or severe
- detection and treatment of complications
- treatment of the underlying cause.

Opiate analgesics should be given to treat pain and hypovolaemia should be corrected using normal saline or other crystalloids. All severe cases should be managed in a high-dependency or intensive care unit. A urinary catheter should be inserted in patients with shock, with a central venous line inserted if required. Oxygen should be given to hypoxic patients and those who develop systemic inflammatory response syndrome (SIRS) may require ventilatory support. Hyperglycaemia should be corrected using insulin and hypocalcaemia by intravenous calcium injection.

Nasogastric aspiration is required only if paralytic ileus is present. Enteral feeding, if tolerated, should be started at an early stage in patients with severe pancreatitis because they are in a severely catabolic state and need nutritional support. Enteral feeding decreases endotoxaemia and so may reduce systemic complications. Nasogastric feeding is just as effective as feeding by the nasojejunal route. Prophylaxis of thromboembolism with subcutaneous low-molecular-weight heparin is also advisable. The use of prophylactic, broad-spectrum intravenous antibiotics to prevent infection of pancreatic necrosis is not indicated, but infected necrosis is treated with antibiotics that penetrate necrotic tissue, e.g. carbapenems or quinolones, and metronidazole.

Patients who present with cholangitis in association with severe acute pancreatitis should undergo urgent ERCP to diagnose and treat choledocholithiasis. In less severe cases of gallstone pancreatitis, biliary imaging (using MRCP or EUS) can be carried out after the acute phase has resolved. If the liver function tests return to normal and ultrasound has not demonstrated a dilated biliary tree, laparoscopic cholecystectomy with an on-table cholangiogram is appropriate because any common bile

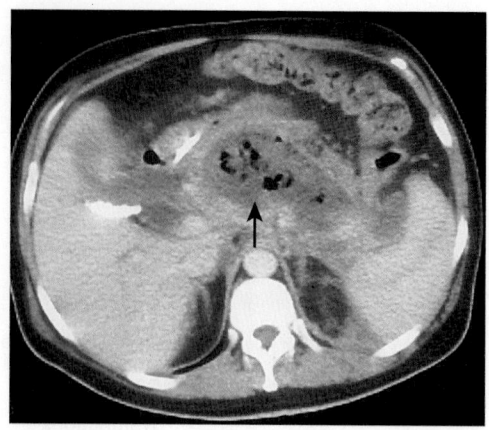

Fig. 23.70 Pancreatic necrosis. Lack of vascular enhancement of the pancreas during contrast-enhanced computed tomography indicates necrosis (arrow). The presence of gas suggests that infection has occurred.

duct stones have probably passed. When the operative cholangiogram detects residual common bile duct stones, these should be removed by laparoscopic exploration of the duct or by post-operative ERCP. Cholecystectomy should be undertaken within 2 weeks of resolution of pancreatitis – and preferably during the same admission – to prevent further potentially fatal attacks of pancreatitis. Patients with infected pancreatic necrosis or pancreatic abscess require urgent endoscopic drainage or minimally invasive retroperitoneal pancreatic (MIRP) necrosectomy to debride all cavities of necrotic material. Pancreatic pseudocysts can be treated by drainage into the stomach or duodenum. This is usually performed after an interval of at least 6 weeks, once a pseudocapsule has matured, by surgical or endoscopic cystogastrostomy.

Chronic pancreatitis

Chronic pancreatitis is a chronic inflammatory disease characterised by fibrosis and destruction of exocrine pancreatic tissue. Diabetes mellitus occurs in advanced cases because the islets of Langerhans are involved (Ch. 21).

Pathophysiology

Around 80% of cases in Western countries result from alcohol misuse, with idiopathic chronic pancreatitis being the second most common cause. In southern India, severe chronic fibrocalcific pancreatitis occurs in non-alcoholics, possibly as a result of malnutrition, deficiency of trace elements and micronutrients, and cassava consumption. Other causes are listed in Box 23.82. The pathophysiology of chronic pancreatitis is shown in Figure 23.71.

Clinical features

Chronic pancreatitis predominantly affects middle-aged men with alcohol dependence. More than 80% present with abdominal pain. In 50%, this occurs as episodes of 'acute pancreatitis', although each attack results in a degree of permanent pancreatic damage. Relentless, slowly progressive chronic pain without acute exacerbations affects 35% of patients, while the remainder have no pain but present with diarrhoea. Pain is due to a combination of increased pressure within the pancreatic ducts and direct involvement of peripancreatic nerves by the inflammatory process. Pain may be relieved by leaning forwards or by drinking alcohol. Approximately one-fifth of patients chronically consume opiate analgesics. Weight loss is common and results from a combination of anorexia, avoidance of food because of post-prandial pain, malabsorption and/or diabetes. Steatorrhoea occurs when more than 90% of the exocrine tissue has been destroyed; protein malabsorption develops only in the most advanced cases. Overall, 30% of patients have (secondary) diabetes, but this figure rises to 70% in those with chronic fibrocalcific pancreatitis. Physical examination reveals a thin, malnourished patient with epigastric tenderness. Skin pigmentation over the abdomen and back is common and results from chronic use of a hot water bottle (erythema ab igne). Many patients have features of other alcohol- and smoking-related diseases. Complications are listed in Box 23.83.

Investigations

Investigations (Box 23.84 and Fig. 23.72) are carried out to:

- make a diagnosis of chronic pancreatitis
- define pancreatic function
- demonstrate anatomical abnormalities prior to surgical intervention.

---

i | 23.82 Causes of chronic pancreatitis*

Toxic–metabolic

- Alcohol
- Tobacco
- Hypercalcaemia
- Chronic kidney disease

Idiopathic

- Tropical
- Early-/late-onset types

Genetic

- Hereditary pancreatitis (cationic trypsinogen mutation)
- *SPINK-1* mutation
- Cystic fibrosis

Autoimmune

- In isolation or as part of multi-organ problem

Recurrent and severe acute pancreatitis

- Recurrent acute pancreatitis
- Post-necrotic

Obstructive

- Ductal adenocarcinoma
- Intraductal papillary mucinous neoplasia
- Pancreas divisum
- Sphincter of Oddi stenosis

*These can be memorised by the mnemonic 'TIGARO'. Gallstones do not cause chronic pancreatitis but may be observed as an incidental finding.

Management

Alcohol misuse

Alcohol avoidance is crucial in halting progression of the disease and reducing pain.

---

i | 23.83 Complications of chronic pancreatitis

- Pseudocysts and pancreatic ascites, which occur in both acute and chronic pancreatitis
- Obstructive jaundice due to benign stricture of the common bile duct as it passes through the diseased pancreas
- Duodenal stenosis
- Portal or splenic vein thrombosis leading to segmental portal hypertension and gastric varices
- Peptic ulcer
- Secondary diabetes mellitus
- Pancreatic cancer
- Pancreatic exocrine insufficiency
- Osteopenia or osteoporosis

---

i | 23.84 Investigations in chronic pancreatitis

Tests to establish the diagnosis

- Ultrasound
- Computed tomography (may show atrophy, calcification or ductal dilatation)
- Abdominal X-ray (may show calcification)
- Magnetic resonance cholangiopancreatography
- Endoscopic ultrasound

Tests to define pancreatic function

- Collection of pure pancreatic juice after secretin injection (gold standard but invasive and seldom used)
- Faecal pancreatic elastase (see Box 23.12)

Tests to demonstrate anatomy prior to surgery

- Magnetic resonance cholangiopancreatography

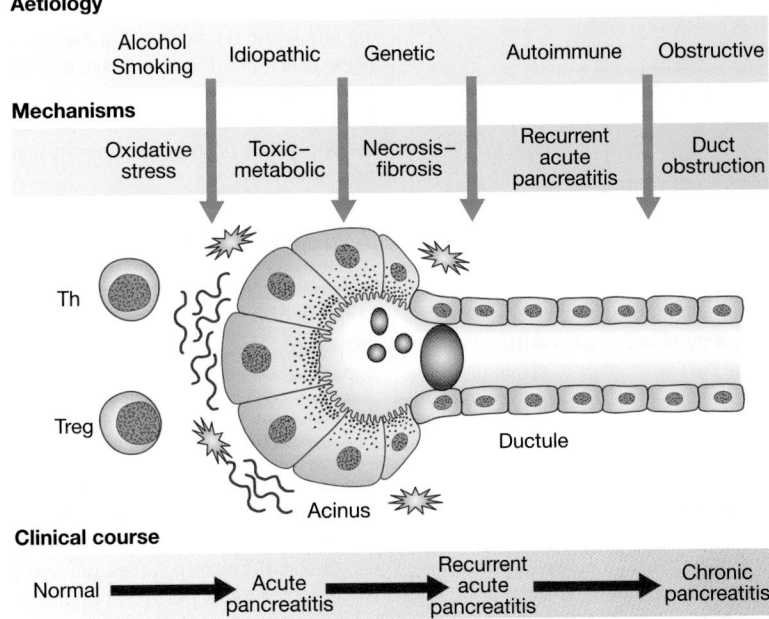

Fig. 23.71 Pathophysiology of chronic pancreatitis. Alcohol and other risk factors may trigger acute pancreatitis through multiple mechanisms. The first (or 'sentinel') episode of acute pancreatitis initiates an inflammatory response involving T-helper (Th) cells. Ongoing exposure to alcohol drives further inflammation but this is modified by regulatory T cells (Treg) with subsequent fibrosis, via activation of pancreatic stellate cells. A cycle of inflammation and fibrosis ensues, with development of chronic pancreatitis. Alcohol is the most relevant risk factor, as it is involved at multiple steps.

23

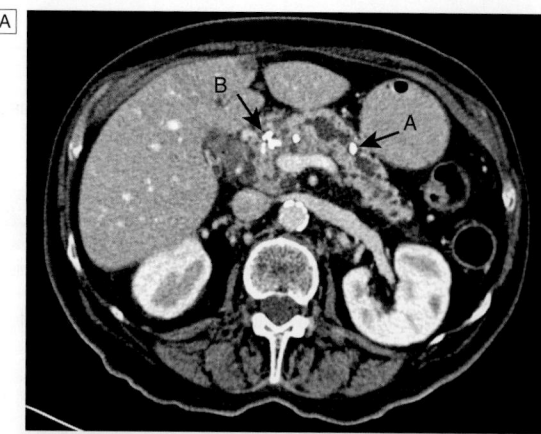

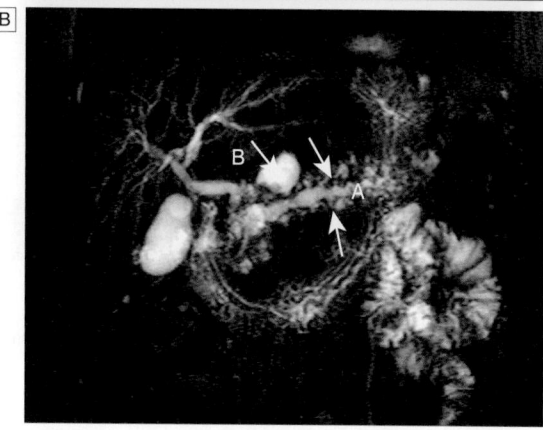

Fig. 23.72 Imaging in chronic pancreatitis. A Computed tomogram showing a grossly dilated and irregular duct with a calcified stone (arrow A). Note the calcification in the head of the gland (arrow B). B Magnetic resonance cholangiopancreatogram of the same patient showing marked ductal dilatation with abnormal dilated side branches (arrows A). A small cyst is also present (arrow B).

---

i   23.85 Intervention in chronic pancreatitis

Endoscopic therapy

- Dilatation or stenting of pancreatic duct strictures
- Removal of calculi (mechanical or shock-wave lithotripsy)
- Drainage of pseudocysts

Surgical methods

- Partial pancreatic resection, preserving the duodenum
- Pancreatico-jejunostomy

Pain relief

A range of analgesic drugs, particularly NSAIDs, are valuable but the severe and unremitting nature of the pain often leads to opiate use with the risk of addiction. Analgesics, such as pregabalin and tricyclic antidepressants at a low dose, may be effective. Oral pancreatic enzyme supplements suppress pancreatic secretion and their regular use reduces analgesic consumption in some patients. Patients who are abstinent from alcohol and who have severe chronic pain that is resistant to conservative measures should be considered for surgical or endoscopic pancreatic therapy (Box 23.85). Coeliac plexus neurolysis sometimes produces long-lasting pain relief, although relapse occurs in the majority of cases. In some patients, MRCP does not show a surgically or endoscopically correctable abnormality and, in these individuals, the only surgical approach is total pancreatectomy. Unfortunately, even after this operation, some continue to experience pain. Moreover, the procedure causes diabetes, which may be difficult to control, with a high risk of

hypoglycaemia (since both insulin and glucagon are absent) and significant morbidity and mortality.

Malabsorption

This is treated by dietary fat restriction (with supplementary medium-chain triglyceride therapy in malnourished patients) and oral pancreatic enzyme supplements. A PPI is added to optimise duodenal pH for pancreatic enzyme activity.

Management of complications

Surgical or endoscopic therapy may be necessary for the management of pseudocysts, pancreatic ascites, common bile duct or duodenal stricture and the consequences of portal hypertension. Many patients with chronic pancreatitis also require treatment for other alcohol- and smoking-related diseases and for the consequences of self-neglect and malnutrition.

Autoimmune pancreatitis

Autoimmune pancreatitis (AIP) is a chronic fibroinflammatory disease of the pancreas that can mimic cancer, but which responds to glucocorticoids. There are two different subtypes, type 1 and type 2 AIP. Type 1 AIP belongs to IgG4-related disorders, which can include various organs such as bile ducts, salivary glands, kidneys, lungs and thyroid glands. Type 2 AIP affects the pancreas only, but is strongly associated with inflammatory bowel disease, particularly ulcerative colitis. AIP can present with obstructive jaundice, weight loss and abdominal pain. Blood tests may reveal increased serum IgG4 in type 1 AIP, with no reliable serological markers for type 2 AIP. Imaging in type 1 AIP may show a diffusely enlarged pancreas, narrowing of the pancreatic duct and stricturing of the lower bile duct. Focal mass-like pancreatic lesions may be seen in type 2 AIP. The symptom response to glucocorticoids is usually good in AIP, but recurrence can occur after initial response, particularly in type 1 AIP, with some patients requiring immunomodulators (e.g. azathioprine) or rituximab.

Congenital abnormalities affecting the pancreas

Pancreas divisum

This is due to failure of the primitive dorsal and ventral ducts to fuse during embryonic development of the pancreas. As a consequence, most of the pancreatic drainage occurs through the smaller accessory ampulla rather than through the major ampulla. The condition occurs in 7%–10% of the normal population and is usually asymptomatic, but some patients develop acute pancreatitis, chronic pancreatitis or atypical abdominal pain.

Annular pancreas

In this congenital anomaly, the pancreas encircles the second/third part of the duodenum, leading to gastric outlet obstruction. Annular pancreas is associated with malrotation of the intestine, atresias and cardiac anomalies.

Cystic fibrosis

This disease is considered in detail on page 510. The major gastrointestinal manifestations are pancreatic insufficiency and meconium ileus. Peptic ulcer and hepatobiliary disease may also occur. In cystic fibrosis, pancreatic secretions are protein- and mucus-rich. The resultant viscous juice forms plugs that obstruct the pancreatic ductules, leading to progressive destruction of acinar cells. Steatorrhoea is universal and the large-volume bulky stools predispose to rectal prolapse. Malnutrition is compounded by the metabolic demands of respiratory failure and by diabetes, which develops in 40% of patients by adolescence.

Nutritional counselling and supervision are important to ensure intake of high-energy foods, providing 120%–150% of the recommended intake for normal subjects. Fats are an important calorie source and, despite the presence of steatorrhoea, fat intake should not be restricted. Supplementary fat-soluble vitamins are also necessary. High-dose oral pancreatic enzymes are required, in doses sufficient to control steatorrhoea and stool frequency. A PPI aids fat digestion by producing an optimal duodenal pH.

Meconium ileus

Mucus-rich plugs within intestinal contents can obstruct the small or large intestine of a newborn child. Meconium ileus is treated by the mucolytic agent N-acetylcysteine, given orally, by Gastrografin enema or by gut lavage using polyethylene glycol. In resistant cases of meconium ileus, surgical resection may be necessary.

Tumours of the pancreas

Adenocarcinoma of the pancreas

Some 90% of pancreatic neoplasms are adenocarcinomas that arise from the pancreatic ducts. These tumours involve local structures and metastasise to regional lymph nodes at an early stage. Most patients have advanced disease at the time of presentation. Neuro-endocrine tumours also arise in the pancreas, but tend to grow more slowly and have a better prognosis; these are discussed in detail on page 691. The incidence of pancreatic adenocarcinoma is higher in high-income countries, affecting 10–15 per 100 000 in Western populations, rising to 100 per 100 000 in those over the age of 70. Men are affected more often than women. The disease is associated with increasing age, smoking, diabetes and chronic pancreatitis. Between 5% and 10% of patients have a genetic predisposition: hereditary pancreatitis, HNPCC and familial atypical mole multiple melanoma syndrome (FAMMM). Overall survival is only 3%–5%, with a median survival of 6–10 months for those with locally advanced disease and 3–5 months if metastases are present.

Clinical features

Many patients are asymptomatic until an advanced stage, when they present with central abdominal pain, weight loss and obstructive jaundice (Fig. 23.73). The pain results from invasion of the coeliac plexus and is characteristically incessant and gnawing. It often radiates from the upper abdomen through to the back and may be eased a little by bending forwards. Almost all patients lose weight and many are cachectic. Around 60%–70% of tumours arise from the head of the pancreas, and involvement of the common bile duct results in the development of obstructive jaundice, often with severe pruritus. Some patients present with diarrhoea, vomiting from duodenal obstruction, diabetes mellitus, recurrent venous thrombosis, acute pancreatitis or depression. Physical examination reveals clear evidence of weight loss. An abdominal mass due to the tumour, a palpable gallbladder or hepatic metastases is commonly found. A palpable gallbladder in a jaundiced patient is usually the consequence of distal biliary obstruction by a pancreatic cancer (Courvoisier's sign).

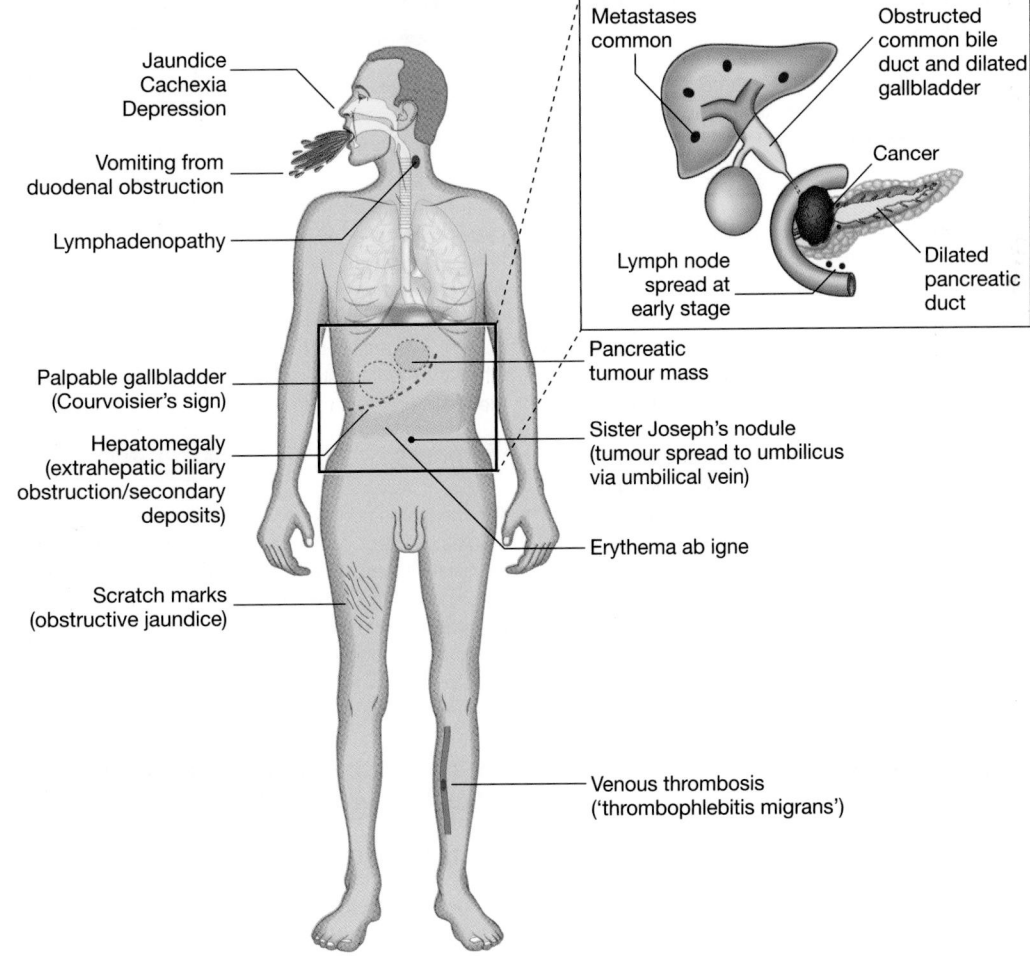

Fig. 23.73 Features of pancreatic cancer.

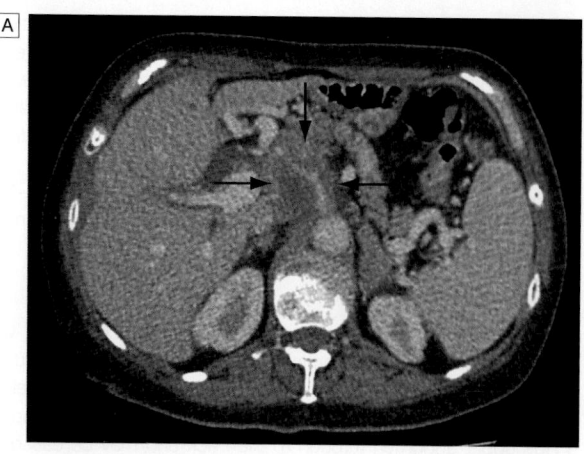
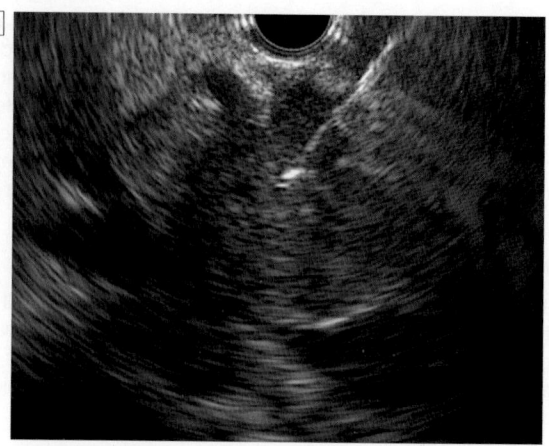

Fig. 23.74 Carcinoma of the pancreas. [A] A computed tomogram showing a large, necrotic mass encasing the coeliac axis (arrows). [B] Endoscopic ultrasound was subsequently performed to enhance staging and to obtain a fine needle aspiration biopsy, which confirmed pancreatic ductal adenocarcinoma.

Investigations

The diagnosis is usually made by ultrasound and contrast-enhanced CT (Fig. 23.74). Diagnosis in non-jaundiced patients is often delayed because presenting symptoms are relatively non-specific. Fit patients with small, localised tumours should undergo staging to define operability. EUS or laparoscopy with laparoscopic ultrasound will define tumour size, involvement of blood vessels and metastatic spread. In patients unsuitable for surgery because of advanced disease, frailty or comorbidity, EUS- or CT-guided cytology or biopsy can be used to confirm the diagnosis (see Fig. 23.74). MRCP and ERCP are sensitive methods of diagnosing pancreatic cancer and are valuable when the diagnosis is in doubt, although differentiation between cancer and localised chronic pancreatitis can be difficult. The main role of ERCP is to insert a stent into the common bile duct to relieve obstructive jaundice in inoperable patients. Serum cancer antigen 19-9 (CA 19-9) can be used to monitor response to treatment and as a marker of recurrent disease. It has a poor predictive value for diagnosis.

Management

Surgical resection is the only method of effecting cure and 5-year survival in patients undergoing a complete resection is around 12%. Adjuvant chemotherapy can also be used in these patients, using gemcitabine and capecitabine. Only 10%–15% of tumours are resectable with potential curative intent, since most are locally advanced at the time of diagnosis. For the great majority of patients, treatment is palliative. Chemotherapy with FOLFIRINOX (5-fluorouracil, leucovorin, irinotecan and oxaliplatin) improves median survival to 11 months. Pain relief can be achieved using analgesics, but in some patients coeliac plexus neurolysis may be required. Jaundice can be relieved by choledochojejunostomy in fit patients, whereas percutaneous or endoscopic stenting is preferable in older patients and those with very advanced disease. Ampullary or periampullary adenocarcinomas are rare neoplasms that arise from the ampulla of Vater or adjacent duodenum. They are often polypoid and may ulcerate; they frequently infiltrate the duodenum, but behave less aggressively than pancreatic adenocarcinoma. Around 25% of patients undergoing resection of ampullary or periampullary tumours survive for 5 years, in contrast to patients with pancreatic ductal cancer.

Incidental pancreatic mass

Cystic neoplasms of the pancreas are increasingly being seen with widespread use of CT. These are a heterogeneous group; serous cystadenomas rarely, if ever, become malignant and do not require surgery. Mucinous cysts occur more often in women, are usually in the pancreatic tail and display a spectrum of behaviour from benign to frankly malignant. Aspiration of the cyst contents for cytology and measurement of CEA and amylase concentrations in fluid obtained at EUS can help determine

whether a lesion is mucinous or not. In fit patients, all mucinous lesions should be resected. A variant, called intraductal papillary mucinous neoplasia (IPMN), is often discovered coincidentally on CT, frequently in men in old age. This may affect the main pancreatic duct with marked dilatation and plugs of mucus, or may involve a side branch. The histology varies from villous adenomatous change to dysplasia or carcinoma. Since IPMN is a pre-malignant, but indolent, condition, the decision to resect or to monitor depends on age and fitness of the patient and location, size and evolution of lesions.

Diseases of the peritoneal cavity

Peritonitis

Surgical peritonitis occurs as the result of a ruptured viscus (for details see this book's companion text, *Principles and Practice of Surgery*). Peritonitis may also complicate ascites in chronic liver disease (spontaneous bacterial peritonitis, p. 877) or may occur in children in the absence of ascites, due to infection with *Streptococcus pneumoniae* or β-haemolytic streptococci (p. 301).

Chlamydial peritonitis is a complication of pelvic inflammatory disease (p. 375). The patient presents with right upper quadrant pain, pyrexia and a hepatic rub (the Fitz-Hugh–Curtis syndrome). Tuberculosis may cause peritonitis and ascites (p. 518).

Tumours

The most common is secondary adenocarcinoma from the ovary or gastrointestinal tract. Mesothelioma is a rare tumour complicating asbestos exposure. It presents as a diffuse abdominal mass, due to omental infiltration, and with ascites. The prognosis is extremely poor. Pseudomyxoma peritonei is a rare tumour of the appendix that spreads into the peritoneal cavity and is often found incidentally. Diagnosis can be confirmed by abdominal CT or MRI, with cytoreductive surgery and hyperthermic intraperitoneal chemotherapy being used for curative treatment.

Other disorders

Endometriosis

Ectopic endometrial tissue can become embedded on the serosal aspect of the intestine, most frequently in the sigmoid and rectum. The overlying mucosa is usually intact. Cyclical engorgement and inflammation result in pain, bleeding, diarrhoea, constipation and adhesions or obstruction. Low backache is frequent. The onset is usually between 20 and 45 years and the condition is more common in nulliparous women. Bimanual examination may reveal tender nodules in the pouch of Douglas. Endoscopic studies reveal the diagnosis only if carried out during menstruation, when a bluish mass with intact overlying mucosa is apparent. In some patients, laparoscopy is required. Treatment options include laparoscopic diathermy and hormonal therapy with progestogens (e.g. norethisterone), gonadotrophin-releasing hormone analogues or danazol.

Pneumatosis cystoides intestinalis

In this rare condition, multiple gas-filled submucosal cysts line the colonic and small bowel walls. The cause is unknown but the condition may be seen in patients with chronic cardiac or pulmonary disease, pyloric obstruction, systemic sclerosis or dermatomyositis. Most patients are asymptomatic, although there may be abdominal cramp, diarrhoea, tenesmus, rectal bleeding and mucus discharge. The cysts are recognised on sigmoidoscopy, plain abdominal X-rays, CT or MRI. Therapies reported to be effective include prolonged high-flow oxygen, elemental diets and antibiotics.

HIV/AIDS and the gastrointestinal tract

Patients with human immunodeficiency virus/acquired immunodeficiency syndrome (HIV/AIDS) may develop several symptoms referable to the gastrointestinal tract, as discussed in detail on page 359. HIV testing should be considered in all patients with atypical or unexplained gastrointestinal symptoms and in those resident in areas of high prevalence.

Further information

Books and journal articles

Feldman M, Friedman LS, Brandt LJ. Sleisenger and Fordtran's Gastrointestinal and liver disease, 11th edn. Elsevier; 2020.
Podolsky DK, Camilleri M, Gregory Fitz J, et al. Yamada's Textbook of gastroenterology, 6th edn. Wiley–Blackwell; 2015.

Websites

bsg.org.uk *British Society of Gastroenterology*.
crohnsandcolitis.org.uk *Crohn's and Colitis UK*.
coeliac.org.uk *Coeliac UK*.
ecco-ibd.eu *European Crohn's and Colitis Organisation*.
esge.com *European Society of Gastrointestinal Endoscopy*.
gastro.org *American Gastroenterological Association and American Digestive Health Foundation*.
isg.org.in *Indian Society of Gastroenterology*.

23

MJ Williams
TT Gordon-Walker

24

Hepatology

Clinical examination of the abdomen for liver and biliary disease

2 Face
Jaundice
Spider naevi
Parotid swelling

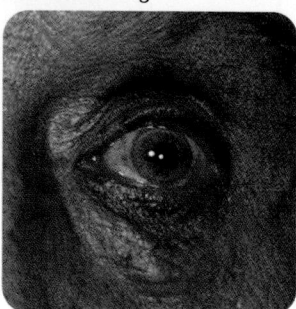

▲ Xanthelasma and jaundiced sclera in a patient with chronic cholestasis

1 Hands
Clubbing
Dupuytren's contracture
Leuconychia
Bruising
Flapping tremor (hepatic encephalopathy)

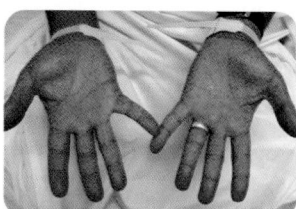

▲ Palmar erythema

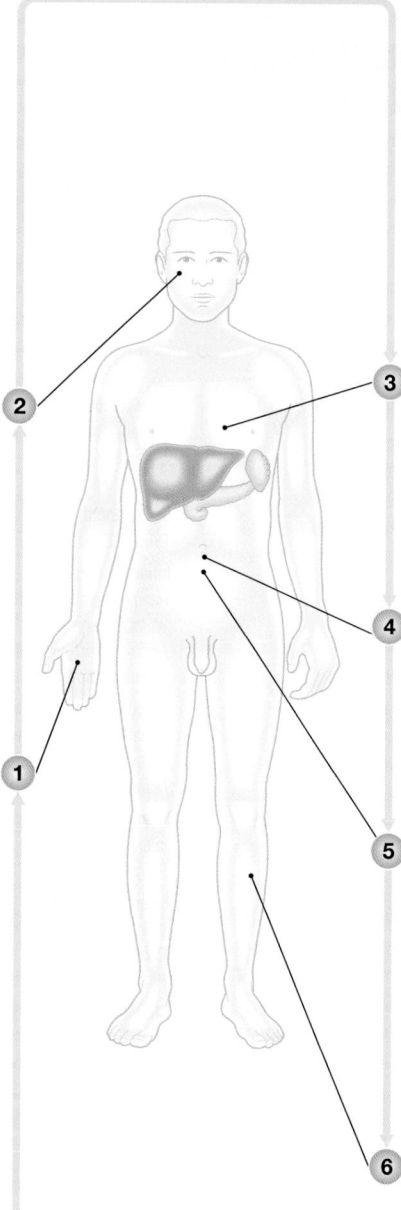

Observation
• Smell of alcohol or fetor hepaticus
• Encephalopathy
• Weight loss
• Scratch marks from itching

3 Chest
Loss of body hair

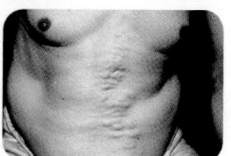

▲ Gynaecomastia

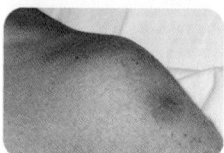

▲ Spider naevi

4 Abdomen: inspection
Scars
Distension
Veins
Testicular atrophy

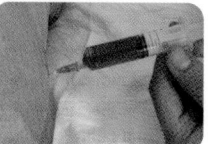

▲ Aspiration of ascitic fluid

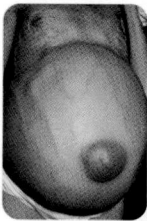

▲ Dilated abdominal wall veins (caput medusae)

5 Abdomen: palpation/ percussion/auscultation
Hepatomegaly
Splenomegaly
Ascites
Palpable gallbladder
Hepatic bruit (rare)
Tumour

6 Legs
Bruising
Oedema

Insets (Spider naevi) From Hayes P, Simpson K. Gastroenterology and liver disease. Edinburgh: Churchill Livingstone, Elsevier Ltd; 1995; (Aspiration) Strachan M. Davidson's Clinical cases. Edinburgh: Churchill Livingstone, Elsevier Ltd; 2008; (Palmar erythema) Goldman L, Schafter AI. Goldman's Cecil medicine, 24th edn. Philadelphia: WB Saunders, Elsevier Inc.; 2012.

History and significance of abdominal signs

 Interpretation of physical signs in cirrhosis

Signs of cirrhosis

- Spider naevi
- Palmar erythema
- Leuconychia
- Bruising (low platelets)
- Loss of body hair (increased oestrogens)
- Gynaecomastia (increased oestrogens)

Signs of portal hypertension

- Splenomegaly
- Dilated abdominal wall veins

Signs of decompensation

- Jaundice
- Ascites/peripheral oedema
- Flapping tremor (encephalopathy)

Signs related to specific aetiologies

- Dupuytren's contracture (alcohol)
- Parotid swelling (alcohol)
- Intoxication/withdrawal (alcohol)
- Xanthelasma (PBC, NAFLD)
- Scratch marks (cholestatic liver disease)
- Clubbing (hepatopulmonary syndrome)

(NAFLD = non-alcoholic fatty liver disease; PBC = primary biliary cholangitis)

 Silent presentation of liver disease

It is important to note that patients with liver disease can present silently following detection of abnormality on screening investigation. This occurs frequently in practice in three settings:

Biochemical abnormality

- Liver enzyme abnormality detected during health screening or drug monitoring

Radiological abnormality

- Observation of an unexpected structural abnormality such as an altered liver texture or contour, or a mass lesion on ultrasound, computed tomography or other imaging undertaken for reasons unrelated to the liver

Serological abnormality

- Detection of a liver-related autoantibody

 Ascites

Causes	Associated clinical findings
Exudative (high protein)	
Carcinoma	Weight loss
	Abdominal mass
	'Craggy' hepatomegaly
Tuberculosis	Weight loss ± fever
Transudative (low protein)	
Cirrhosis	Stigmata of cirrhosis (see above)
Renal failure (including nephrotic syndrome)	Severe generalised oedema
Congestive heart failure	Elevated jugular venous pressure
	Peripheral oedema

5 **Assessment of liver size**

Clinical assessment of hepatomegaly is important in diagnosing liver disease.

- Start in the right iliac fossa.
- Press hand gently up towards ribcage as patient breathes in.
- Progress up the abdomen 2 cm with each breath.
- Detect if smooth or irregular, tender or non-tender; ascertain the shape.
- Confirm the lower border of the liver by percussion.
- Identify the upper border by percussion.

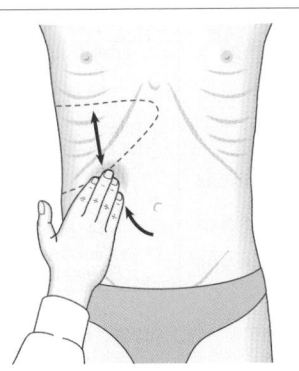

1 **Assessment of encephalopathy**

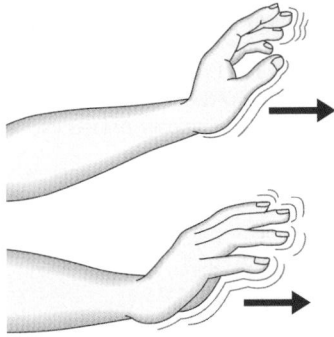

Flapping tremor. Jerky forward movements every 5–10 secs, when arms are outstretched and hands are dorsiflexed, suggest hepatic encephalopathy. The movements are coarser than those seen in tremor.

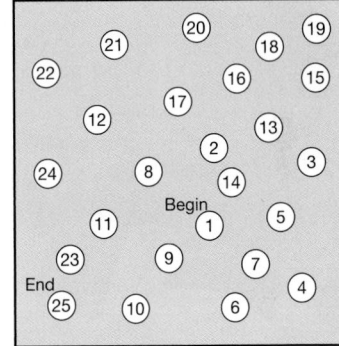

Number connection test. These 25 numbered circles can normally be joined together within 30 secs. Serial observations may provide useful information, as long as the position of the numbers is varied to avoid the patient learning their pattern.

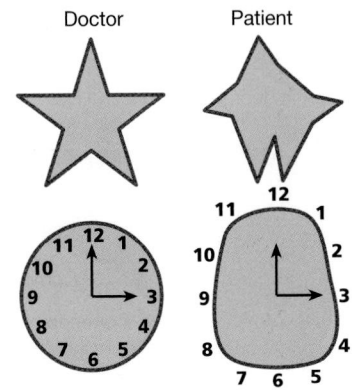

Constructional apraxia. Drawing stars and clocks may reveal marked abnormality.

24

Functional anatomy and physiology

Applied anatomy

Normal liver structure and blood supply

The liver weighs 1.2–1.5 kg and has multiple functions, including roles in metabolism, control of infection, and elimination of toxins and by-products of metabolism. It is classically divided into left and right lobes by the

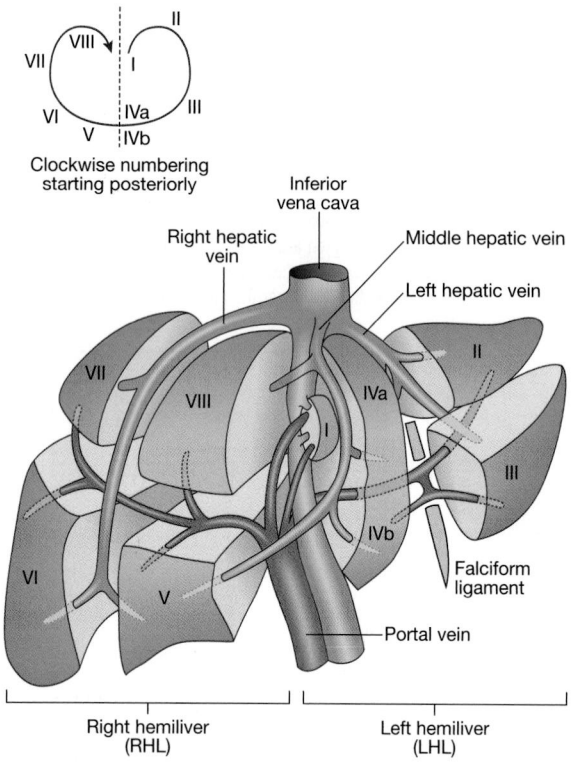

Fig. 24.1 Liver blood supply.

falciform ligament, but a more useful functional division is into the right and left hemilivers, based on blood supply (Fig. 24.1). These are further divided into eight segments, according to subdivisions of the hepatic and portal veins. Each segment has its own branch of the hepatic artery and biliary tree. The segmental anatomy of the liver has an important influence on imaging and treatment of liver tumours, given the increasing use of surgical resection. A liver segment is made up of multiple smaller units known as lobules, comprised of a central vein, radiating sinusoids separated from each other by single liver cell (hepatocyte) plates, and peripheral portal tracts containing terminal branches of the hepatic artery, portal vein and bile duct. The functional unit of the liver is the hepatic acinus (Fig. 24.2).

Blood flows into the acinus via a single branch of the portal vein and hepatic artery situated centrally in the portal tract. Blood flows outwards along the hepatic sinusoids into one of several tributaries of the hepatic vein at the periphery of the acinus. Bile is excreted by hepatocytes into channels called cholangioles, which lie between them, and flows in the opposite direction from the periphery of the acinus back to the interlobular bile duct in the portal tract. The hepatocytes in each acinus lie in three zones, depending on their position relative to the portal tract. Those in zone 1 are closest to the terminal branches of the portal vein and hepatic artery, and are richly supplied with oxygenated blood, and with blood containing the highest concentration of nutrients and toxins. Conversely, hepatocytes in zone 3 are furthest from the portal tracts and closest to the hepatic veins, and are therefore relatively hypoxic and exposed to lower concentrations of nutrients and toxins compared to zone 1. The different perfusion and toxin exposure patterns, and thus vulnerability, of hepatocytes in the different zones contribute to the often patchy nature of liver injury.

Liver cells

Hepatocytes comprise 80% of liver cells. The remaining 20% are the endothelial cells lining the sinusoids, cholangiocytes lining the intrahepatic bile ducts, cells of the immune system including macrophages (Kupffer cells) and key populations of non-parenchymal cells, including hepatic stellate cells (Ito cells) and other myofibroblast precursors.

Endothelial cells line the sinusoids (Fig. 24.3), a network of capillary vessels that differ from other capillary beds in the body, in that there is no basement membrane. The endothelial cells have gaps between them

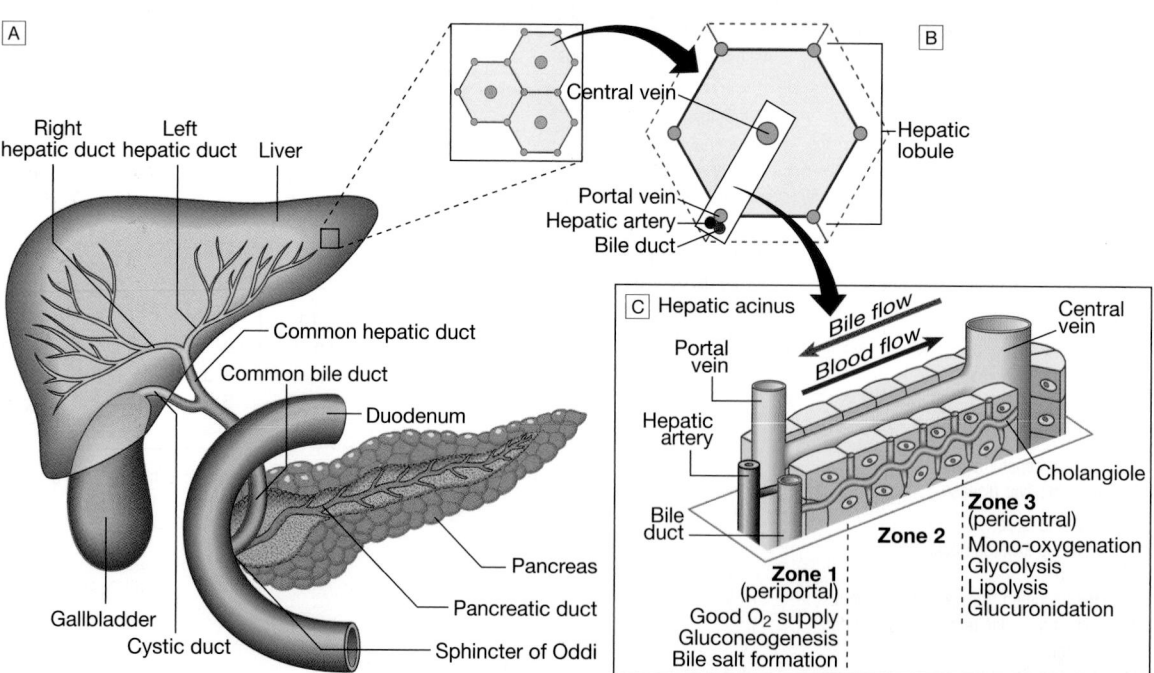

Fig. 24.2 Liver structure and microstructure. A Liver anatomy showing relationship with pancreas, bile duct and duodenum. B Hepatic lobule. C Hepatic acinus.

(fenestrae) of about 0.1 μm in diameter, allowing free flow of fluid and particulate matter to the hepatocytes. Individual hepatocytes are separated from the leaky sinusoids by the space of Disse, which contains stellate cells that store vitamin A and play an important part in regulating liver blood flow. They may also be immunologically active and play a role in the liver's contribution to defence against pathogens. The key role of stellate cells in terms of pathology is in the development of hepatic fibrosis, the precursor of cirrhosis. They undergo activation in response to cytokines produced following liver injury, differentiating into myofibroblasts, which are the major producers of the collagen-rich matrix that forms fibrous tissue (Fig. 24.4).

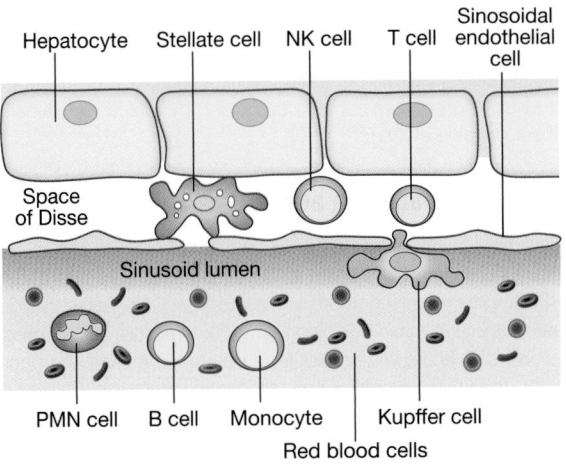

Fig. 24.3 Non-parenchymal liver cells. (B cell = B lymphocyte; NK cell = natural killer cell; PMN cell = polymorphonuclear leucocyte; T cell = T lymphocyte).

Blood supply

The liver is unique as an organ, as it has dual perfusion. The majority of its blood supply (50%–90%) is via the portal vein, which drains blood from the gut via the superior mesenteric vein and from the spleen, and is the principal route for nutrient trafficking to the liver. A minority of inflow is oxygenated blood from the hepatic artery. The dual perfusion system, and the variable contribution from portal vein and hepatic artery, can have important effects on the clinical expression of liver ischaemia (which typically exhibits a less dramatic pattern than ischaemia in other organs, a fact that can sometimes lead to it being missed clinically), and can raise practical challenges in liver surgery.

Biliary system and gallbladder

Hepatocytes provide the driving force for bile flow by creating osmotic gradients of bile acids, which form micelles in bile (bile acid-dependent bile flow), and of sodium (bile acid-independent bile flow). Hepatocytes secrete bile into the biliary canaliculi that then progressively merge into a system of interlobular, septal and major ducts. The right and left hepatic ducts join as they emerge from the liver to form the common hepatic duct, which becomes the common bile duct after joining the cystic duct (see Fig. 24.2). The common bile duct is approximately 5 cm long and 4–6 mm wide. The distal portion of the duct passes through the head of the pancreas and usually joins the pancreatic duct before entering the duodenum through the ampullary sphincter (sphincter of Oddi). It should be noted, though, that the anatomy of the lower common bile duct can vary widely. Common bile duct pressure is maintained by rhythmic contraction and relaxation of the sphincter of Oddi; this pressure exceeds gallbladder pressure in the fasting state, so that bile normally flows into the gallbladder, where it is concentrated 10-fold by resorption of water and electrolytes.

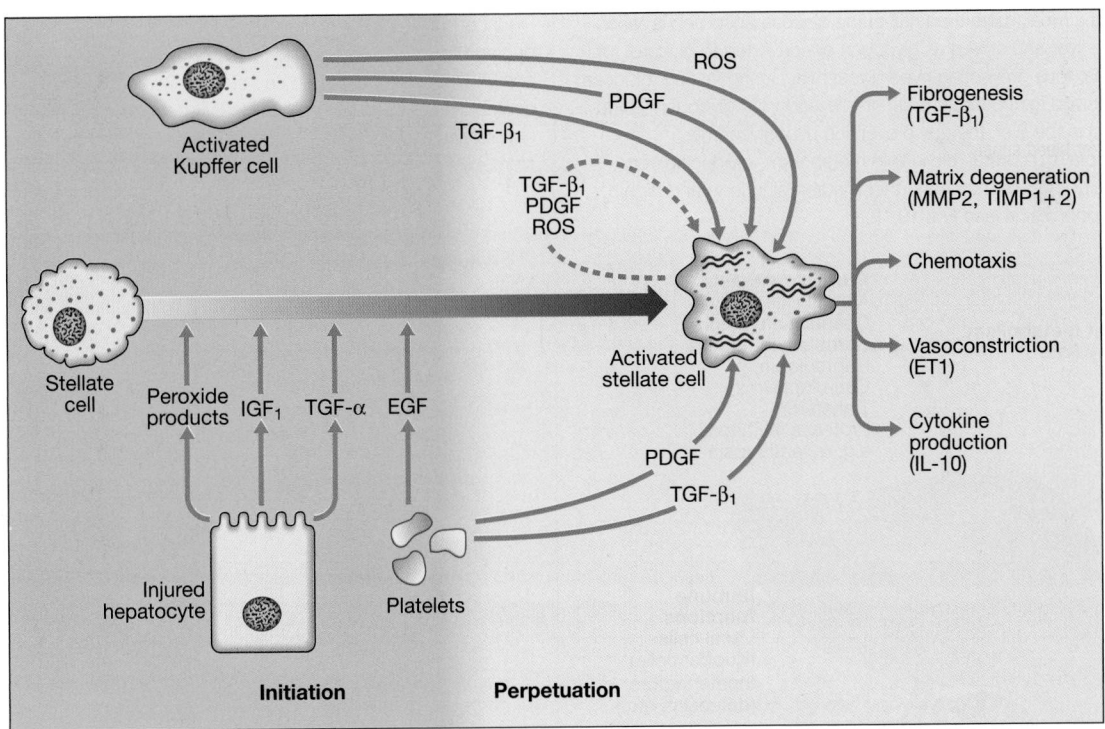

Fig. 24.4 Pathogenic mechanisms in hepatic fibrosis. Stellate cell activation occurs under the influence of cytokines released by other cell types in the liver, including hepatocytes, Kupffer cells (tissue macrophages), platelets and lymphocytes. Once stellate cells become activated, they can perpetuate their own activation by synthesis of transforming growth factor beta (TGF-β_1), and platelet-derived growth factor (PDGF) through autocrine loops. Activated stellate cells produce TGF-β_1, stimulating the production of collagen matrix, as well as inhibitors of collagen breakdown. The inhibitors of collagen breakdown, matrix metalloproteinase 2 and 9 (MMP2 and MMP9), are inactivated in turn by tissue inhibitors TIMP1 and TIMP2, which are increased in fibrosis. Inflammation also contributes to fibrosis, with the cytokine profile produced by Th2 lymphocytes, such as interleukin-6 and 13 (IL-6 and IL-13). Activated stellate cells also produce endothelin 1 (ET1), which may contribute to portal hypertension. (EGF = epidermal growth factor; IGF$_1$ = insulin-like growth factor 1; ROS = reactive oxygen species)

24

The gallbladder is a pear-shaped sac typically lying under the right hemiliver, with its fundus located anteriorly behind the tip of the 9th costal cartilage. Anatomical variation is common. The function of the gallbladder is to concentrate, and provide a reservoir for, bile. Gallbladder tone is maintained by vagal activity, and cholecystokinin released from the duodenal mucosa during feeding causes gallbladder contraction and reduces sphincter pressure, so that bile flows into the duodenum. The body and neck of the gallbladder pass posteromedially towards the porta hepatis, and the cystic duct then joins it to the common hepatic duct. The cystic duct mucosa has prominent crescentic folds (valves of Heister), giving it a beaded appearance on cholangiography.

Hepatic function

Carbohydrate, amino acid and lipid metabolism

The liver plays a central role in carbohydrate, lipid and amino acid metabolism, and is also involved in metabolising drugs and environmental toxins (Fig. 24.5). An important and increasingly recognised role for the liver is in the integration of metabolic pathways, regulating the response of the body to feeding and starvation. Abnormality in metabolic pathways and their regulation can play an important role both in liver disease (e.g. non-alcoholic fatty liver disease, NAFLD) and in diseases that are not conventionally regarded as diseases of the liver (such as type 2 diabetes and inborn errors of metabolism). Hepatocytes have specific pathways to handle each of the nutrients absorbed from the gut and carried to the liver via the portal vein:

- Amino acids from dietary proteins are used for synthesis of plasma proteins, including albumin. The liver produces 8–14 g of albumin per day, and this plays a critical role in maintaining oncotic pressure in the vascular space and in the transport of small molecules like bilirubin, hormones and drugs throughout the body. Amino acids that are not required for the production of new proteins are broken down, with the amino group being converted ultimately to urea.
- Following a meal, more than half of the glucose absorbed is taken up by the liver and stored as glycogen or converted to glycerol and fatty acids, thus preventing hyperglycaemia. During fasting, glucose is synthesised (gluconeogenesis) or released from glycogen (glycogenolysis) in the liver, thereby preventing hypoglycaemia.
- The liver plays a central role in lipid metabolism, producing very low-density lipoproteins and further metabolising low- and high-density lipoproteins (see Fig. 19.12).

Clotting factors

The liver produces key proteins that are involved in the coagulation cascade. Many of these coagulation factors (II, VII, IX and X) are post-translationally modified by vitamin K-dependent enzymes, and their synthesis is impaired in vitamin K deficiency. Reduced clotting factor synthesis is an important and easily accessible biomarker of liver function in the setting of liver injury. The short half-life of clotting factors makes the prothrombin time (PT; or the International Normalised Ratio, INR) a rapidly responsive measure of hepatocyte function. However, the deranged PT or INR seen in liver disease does not directly equate to increased bleeding risk, as these tests do not capture the concurrent reduced synthesis of *anticoagulant* factors, including protein C and protein S. In stable patients with liver disease the coagulation is rebalanced by these offsetting factors that restore a neutral or marginally pro-thrombotic state (balanced coagulopathy). Correction of PT using blood products before minor invasive procedures should be guided by clinical risk rather than the absolute value of the PT.

Bilirubin metabolism and bile

The liver plays a central role in the metabolism of bilirubin and is responsible for the production of bile (Fig. 24.6). Between 425 and 510 mmol (250–300 mg) of unconjugated bilirubin is produced from the catabolism of haem daily. Bilirubin in the blood is normally almost all unconjugated and, because it is not water-soluble, is bound to albumin and does not pass into the urine. Unconjugated bilirubin is taken up by hepatocytes at the sinusoidal membrane, where it is conjugated in the endoplasmic reticulum by UDP-glucuronyl transferase, producing bilirubin mono- and diglucuronide. Impaired conjugation by this enzyme is a cause of inherited hyperbilirubinaemias (see Box 24.18). These bilirubin conjugates are water-soluble and are exported into the bile canaliculi by specific carriers on the hepatocyte membranes. The conjugated bilirubin is excreted in the bile and passes into the duodenal lumen.

Once in the intestine, conjugated bilirubin is metabolised by colonic bacteria to form stercobilinogen, which may be further oxidised to stercobilin. Both stercobilinogen and stercobilin are then excreted in the stool, contributing to its brown colour. Biliary obstruction results in reduced stercobilinogen in the stool, and the stools become pale. A small amount of stercobilinogen (4 mg/day) is absorbed from the bowel, passes through

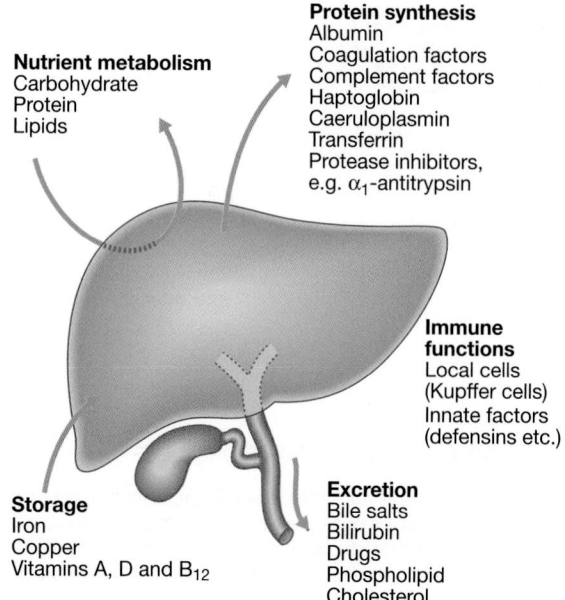

Nutrient metabolism
Carbohydrate
Protein
Lipids

Protein synthesis
Albumin
Coagulation factors
Complement factors
Haptoglobin
Caeruloplasmin
Transferrin
Protease inhibitors,
e.g. α₁-antitrypsin

Immune functions
Local cells
(Kupffer cells)
Innate factors
(defensins etc.)

Storage
Iron
Copper
Vitamins A, D and B$_{12}$

Excretion
Bile salts
Bilirubin
Drugs
Phospholipid
Cholesterol

Fig. 24.5 Important liver functions.

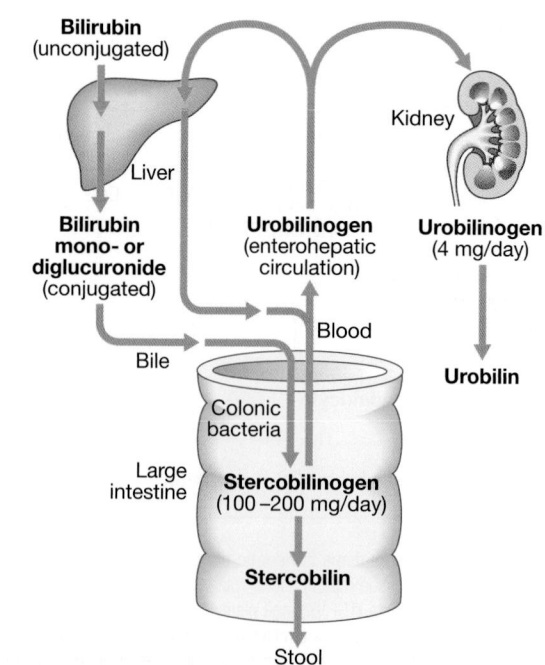

Fig. 24.6 Pathway of bilirubin excretion.

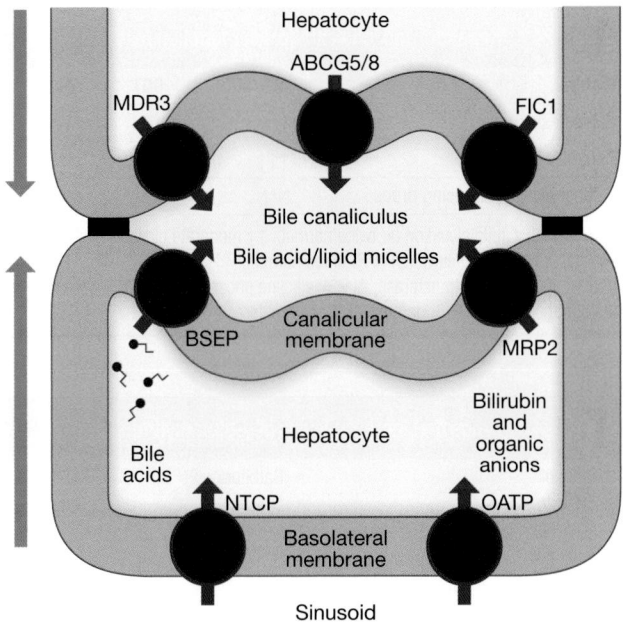

Fig. 24.7 Biliary transporter proteins. On the hepatocyte basolateral membrane, sodium taurocholate co-transporting polypeptide (NTCP) mediates uptake of conjugated bile acids from portal blood. At the canalicular membrane, bile salts are secreted via the bile salt export pump (BSEP) into bile. Multidrug resistance protein 3 (MDR3) transports (flips) phospholipid onto the outer side of the canalicular membrane. The ATP-binding cassette subgroup G 5 and 8 transporters (ABCG5/8) transport sterols including cholesterol into bile. These lipids form mixed micelles with bile salts and protect the membranes lining the biliary tree against the detergent action of bile salts. Familial intrahepatic cholestasis 1 (FIC1), now known as ATP8B1, transports phosphatidylserine to the outer side of the canalicular membrane and is essential for normal bile flow. Mutations in FIC1 can result in either progressive familial intrahepatic cholestasis (PFIC) in children or benign recurrent intrahepatic cholestasis (BRIC). Organic anion transporter protein (OATP) transports bilirubin and organic anions from portal blood into hepatocytes. Multidrug resistance protein 2 (MRP2) transports bilirubin, a range of organic anions and conjugates into bile.

the liver and is excreted in the urine, where it is known as urobilinogen or, following further oxidisation, urobilin. The liver secretes 1–2 L of bile daily. Bile contains bile acids (formed from cholesterol), phospholipids, bilirubin and cholesterol. Several biliary transporter proteins have been identified (Fig. 24.7). Mutations in genes encoding these proteins have been identified in inherited intrahepatic biliary diseases presenting in childhood, and in adult-onset disease such as intrahepatic cholestasis of pregnancy and gallstone formation.

Storage of vitamins and minerals

Vitamins A, D and B$_{12}$ are stored by the liver in large amounts, while others, such as vitamin K and folate, are stored in smaller amounts and disappear rapidly if dietary intake is reduced. The liver is also able to metabolise vitamins to more active compounds, e.g. 7-dehydrocholesterol to 25(OH) vitamin D. Vitamin K is a fat-soluble vitamin and so the inability to absorb fat-soluble vitamins, as occurs in biliary obstruction, results in a coagulopathy. The liver also stores minerals such as iron, in ferritin and haemosiderin, and copper, which is excreted in bile.

Immune regulation

Approximately 9% of the normal liver is composed of immune cells (see Fig. 24.3). Cells of the innate immune system include Kupffer cells derived from blood monocytes, the liver macrophages and natural killer (NK) cells, as well as 'classical' B and T cells of the adaptive immune response. Additional populations of atypical lymphocytes, with phenotypic features of both T cells and NK cells, are thought to play an

important role in host defence through linking of innate and adaptive immunity. The enrichment of such cells in the liver reflects the unique importance of the liver in preventing microorganisms from the gut from entering the systemic circulation.

Kupffer cells constitute the largest single mass of tissue-resident macrophages in the body and account for 80% of the phagocytic capacity of this system. They remove aged and damaged red blood cells, bacteria, viruses, antigen–antibody complexes and endotoxin. They also produce a wide variety of inflammatory mediators that can act locally or may be released into the systemic circulation.

The immunological environment of the liver is unique in that antigens presented within it tend to induce immunological tolerance. This is of importance in liver transplantation, where classical major histocompatibility (MHC) barriers may be crossed, and also in chronic viral infections, when immune responses may be attenuated. The mechanisms that underlie this phenomenon have not been fully defined.

Investigation of liver and hepatobiliary disease

Investigations play an important role in the management of liver disease in three settings:

- identifying the presence of liver disease in those with risk factors
- establishing the aetiology in those with incidentally found liver disease
- understanding disease severity (in particular, identification of fibrosis which leads to cirrhosis with its complications).

When planning investigations, it is important to be clear as to which of these goals is being addressed.

Suspicion of the presence of liver disease is normally based on blood biochemistry abnormality ('liver function tests', or 'LFTs').

Aetiology is typically established through a combination of history, specific blood tests and, where appropriate, imaging and liver biopsy.

Staging of disease involves the assessment of fibrosis and identification of cirrhosis and its complications. Although histology remains the gold standard for staging liver fibrosis, it has been largely replaced by non-invasive approaches, including novel imaging modalities, elastography, serum markers of fibrosis and predictive scoring systems.

The aims of investigation in patients with suspected liver disease are shown in Box 24.1.

Liver blood biochemistry

Liver blood biochemistry (LFTs) includes the measurement of serum bilirubin, aminotransferases, alkaline phosphatase, γ-glutamyl transferase and albumin. Most analytes measured by LFTs are not truly 'function' tests but enzymes that are released by injured hepatocytes and provide biochemical evidence of liver cell damage. The pattern of liver enzyme abnormalities can help to distinguish the likely cause of injury (hepatitic or cholestatic). Liver function per se is best assessed by the serum bilirubin, albumin and prothrombin time because of the role played by the liver in clearance of bilirubin and in synthesis of albumin and clotting factors. These measures reflect the severity of liver disease

---

i **24.1 Aims of investigations in patients with suspected liver disease**

- Detect hepatic abnormality
- Measure the severity of liver damage
- Detect the pattern of liver function test abnormality: hepatitis, cholestatic or mixed
- Identify the specific cause
- Investigate possible complications

24

and are related to clinical outcomes, reflected by their use in several prognostic scores: the Child–Pugh and MELD (Model for End-stage Liver Disease) scores in cirrhosis (see Boxes 24.31 and 24.32), the Glasgow score in alcoholic hepatitis (see Box 24.49) and the King's College Hospital criteria for liver transplantation in acute liver failure (see Box 24.18).

Bilirubin

The degree of elevation of bilirubin can reflect the degree of liver damage. A raised bilirubin often occurs earlier in the natural history of biliary disease (e.g. primary sclerosing cholangitis) than in disease of the liver parenchyma (e.g. cirrhosis), where the hepatocytes are primarily involved. Swelling of the liver within its capsule in inflammation can, however, sometimes impair bile flow and cause an elevation of bilirubin level that is disproportionate to the degree of liver injury. Caution is therefore needed in interpreting the level of liver injury purely on the basis of bilirubin elevation. Bilirubin may also be elevated in the absence of liver injury as a result of haemolysis (resulting in increased bilirubin production) or inherited disorders of bilirubin metabolism (see Box 24.12).

Albumin

Serum albumin levels are often low in patients with cirrhosis. This is due to a change in the volume of distribution of albumin, and to reduced synthesis. Since the plasma half-life of albumin is about 2 weeks, albumin levels may be normal in acute liver failure but are almost always reduced in chronic liver failure. Albumin is not a specific marker of liver disease and is reduced in a range of conditions, including sepsis, malnutrition, nephrotic syndrome and protein-losing enteropathy.

Alanine aminotransferase and aspartate aminotransferase

Alanine aminotransferase (ALT) and aspartate aminotransferase (AST) are intracellular enzymes that are released during damage to hepatocytes. Although AST may also be released from heart or skeletal muscle, expression of ALT outside the liver is relatively low and this enzyme is therefore considered more specific for hepatocellular damage. Large increases of aminotransferase activity favour hepatocellular damage, and this pattern of enzyme abnormality is known as 'hepatitic'.

The AST level is usually lower than the ALT, resulting in an AST/ALT ratio of less than 0.8. This ratio reverses in two situations: in alcohol-related liver disease (particularly in alcoholic hepatitis where the ratio can be > 2), or as an indicator of advanced fibrosis in non-alcohol-related liver disease such as hepatitis C or NAFLD.

Alkaline phosphatase and γ-glutamyl transferase

Alkaline phosphatase (ALP) is the collective name given to several different enzymes that hydrolyse phosphate esters at alkaline pH. These enzymes are widely distributed in the body but the main sites of production are the liver, bone and placenta. ALPs are post-translationally modified, resulting in the production of several different isoenzymes, which differ in abundance in different tissues. ALP enzymes in the liver are located in cell membranes of the hepatic sinusoids and the biliary canaliculi. Accordingly, levels rise with biliary injury and with sinusoidal obstruction, as occurs in infiltrative liver disease.

Gamma-glutamyl transferase (GGT) is a microsomal enzyme found in many cells and tissues of the body. The highest concentrations are located in the liver, where it is produced by hepatocytes and biliary epithelium.

The pattern of a modest increase in aminotransferase activity and large increases in ALP and GGT activity suggests impaired bile flow and is commonly described as 'cholestatic' (Box 24.2). Isolated elevation of the serum GGT is relatively common and may occur during ingestion of

24.2 'Hepatitic' and 'cholestatic' liver function tests			
Pattern	AST/ALT	GGT	ALP
Cholestasis	↑	↑↑	↑↑↑
Hepatitis	↑↑↑	↑	↑
Alcohol/enzyme-inducing drugs	N/↑	↑↑	N

N = normal; ↑ mild elevation (< twice normal); ↑↑ moderate elevation (2–5 times normal); ↑↑↑ marked elevation (> 5 times normal).
(ALT = alanine aminotransferase; ALP = alkaline phosphatase; AST = aspartate aminotransferase; GGT = gamma-glutamyltransferase)

24.3 Drugs that increase levels of γ-glutamyltransferase	
• Ethanol	• Barbiturates
• Phenytoin	• Oral contraceptive pill
• Carbamazepine	• Griseofulvin
• Valproate	• Isotretinoin

microsomal enzyme-inducing drugs, including alcohol (Box 24.3), but also in NAFLD. Elevated ALP with normal GGT is suggestive of non-hepatic origin, e.g. bone disease or pregnancy.

Other biochemical tests

Other widely available biochemical tests may become altered in patients with liver disease:

• Hyponatraemia occurs in severe liver disease despite a high total body sodium content due to increased production of vasopressin (antidiuretic hormone, ADH; see Fig. 19.7), and may be exacerbated by diuretic use. A low sodium level predicts a poor prognosis in cirrhosis.
• Serum urea may be reduced in hepatic failure or due to loss of muscle mass, whereas levels of urea may be increased following gastrointestinal haemorrhage.
• Ferritin is elevated in patients with haemochromatosis, systemic inflammatory disease and a range of conditions causing significant parenchymal inflammation, including alcohol excess and NAFLD.

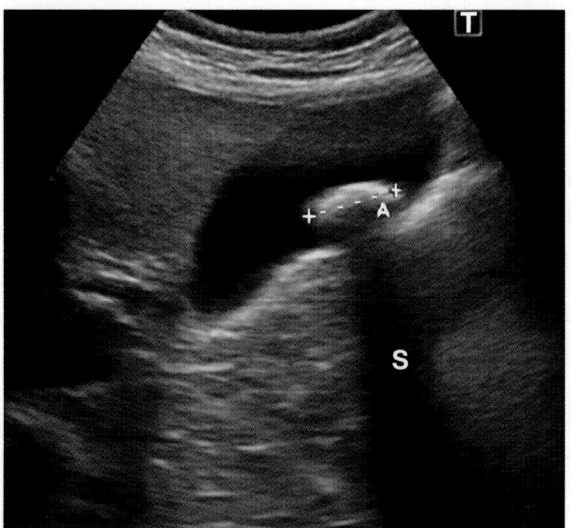

Fig. 24.8 Ultrasound showing a stone in the gallbladder (A) with acoustic shadow (S).

Haematological tests

Blood count

The peripheral blood count is often abnormal and can give a clue to the underlying diagnosis:

- *A normochromic normocytic anaemia* may reflect anaemia of chronic disease or recent gastrointestinal haemorrhage, whereas chronic blood loss is characterised by a hypochromic microcytic anaemia secondary to iron deficiency. A high erythrocyte mean cell volume (macrocytosis) is associated with alcohol misuse or haemolysis, but target cells in any jaundiced patient also result in a macrocytosis.
- *Leucopenia* may complicate portal hypertension and hypersplenism, whereas leucocytosis may occur with cholangitis, alcoholic hepatitis and hepatic abscesses. Atypical lymphocytes are seen in infectious mononucleosis, which may be complicated by an acute hepatitis.
- *Thrombocytopenia* is common in cirrhosis and is due to reduced platelet production and increased breakdown because of hypersplenism. Thrombopoietin, required for platelet production, is produced in the liver and levels fall with worsening liver function. Thus platelet levels are usually more depressed than white cells and haemoglobin in the presence of hypersplenism in patients with cirrhosis. Thrombocytosis is unusual in patients with liver disease but may occur in those with active gastrointestinal haemorrhage and, rarely, in hepatocellular carcinoma.

Coagulation tests

These are often abnormal in patients with liver disease. An increased PT is an indicator of impaired liver function. The normal half-lives of the vitamin K-dependent coagulation factors in the blood are short (5–72 hours), and so changes in the PT occur relatively quickly following liver damage; these changes provide valuable prognostic information in patients with both acute and chronic liver failure. Vitamin K does not reverse this deficiency if it is due to liver disease, but will correct the PT if the cause is vitamin K deficiency, as may occur with cholestasis due to malabsorption of fat-soluble vitamins, or poor diet.

24.4 Chronic liver disease screen

- Hepatitis B surface antigen
- Hepatitis C antibody
- Liver autoantibodies (antinuclear antibody, smooth muscle antibody, antimitochondrial antibody, anti-liver–kidney microsomal antibody)
- Immunoglobulins
- Ferritin
- α_1-antitrypsin
- Caeruloplasmin

Immunological tests

A variety of tests are available to evaluate the aetiology of hepatic disease (Boxes 24.4 and 24.5). The presence of liver-related autoantibodies can be suggestive of autoimmune liver disease (although false-positive results can occur in other inflammatory diseases such as NAFLD). Elevation in overall serum immunoglobulin levels (either IgG or IgM) can also indicate autoimmunity. In contrast, elevated serum IgA may be seen in alcohol-related liver disease and NAFLD.

Imaging

Several imaging techniques can be used to determine the site and nature of structural lesions in the liver and biliary tree. In general, however, imaging techniques are unable to identify hepatic inflammation and have poor sensitivity for liver fibrosis unless advanced cirrhosis with portal hypertension is present.

Ultrasound

Ultrasound is non-invasive and most commonly used as a 'first-line' test to identify gallstones, biliary obstruction (Fig. 24.8) or thrombosis in the hepatic vasculature. Ultrasound may show changes of cirrhosis (nodular liver contour, coarse echotexture, right lobe atrophy and left lobe hypertrophy) or portal hypertension (splenomegaly, ascites) but has a relatively low sensitivity for diagnosing compensated cirrhosis. Focal lesions, such as tumours, may not be detected if they are less than 2 cm in diameter

24.5 How to identify the cause of liver function test (LFT) abnormality

Diagnosis	Clinical clue	Initial test	Additional tests
Alcohol-related liver disease	History	LFTs AST > ALT; high MCV	Random blood alcohol
Non-alcoholic fatty liver disease (NAFLD)	Metabolic syndrome (central obesity, diabetes, hypertension)	LFTs Ultrasound showing fatty liver	
Chronic hepatitis B	Born in high-prevalence area; injection drug use; blood transfusion	HBsAg	HBeAg, HBeAb HBV-DNA
Chronic hepatitis C	Injection drug use; blood transfusion	HCV antibody	HCV-RNA
Primary biliary cholangitis	Itch; raised ALP	AMA Raised IgM	
Primary sclerosing cholangitis	Inflammatory bowel disease	MRCP	
Autoimmune hepatitis	Other autoimmune diseases	ASMA, ANA, LKM, raised IgG	Liver biopsy
Haemochromatosis	Diabetes/joint pain	Transferrin saturation, ferritin	HFE gene test
Wilson's disease	Neurological signs; haemolysis	Caeruloplasmin	24-hour urinary copper
Alpha-1-antitrypsin deficiency	Lung disease	α_1-antitrypsin level	α_1-antitrypsin genotype
Drug-induced liver disease	Drug/herbal remedy history	LFTs	Liver biopsy

(ALP = alkaline phosphatase; ALT = alanine aminotransferase; AMA = antimitochondrial antibody; ANA = antinuclear antibody; ASMA = anti-smooth muscle antibody; AST = aspartate aminotransferase; HBeAb = antibody to hepatitis B e antigen; HBeAg = hepatitis B e antigen; HBsAg = hepatitis B surface antigen; HBV = hepatitis B virus; HCV = hepatitis C virus; HFE = haemochromatosis (high iron/Fe); IgM = immunoglobulin M; IgG = immunoglobulin G; LKM = liver–kidney microsomal antibody; MCV = mean cell volume; MRCP = magnetic resonance cholangiopancreatography)

24

and have similar echogenicity to normal liver tissue. Bubble-based contrast media can enhance discriminant capability. Doppler ultrasound allows blood flow in the hepatic artery, portal vein and hepatic veins to be investigated. Endoscopic ultrasound provides high-resolution images of the pancreas, biliary tree and liver (see below and Fig. 24.46).

Computed tomography and magnetic resonance imaging

Computed tomography (CT) detects smaller focal lesions in the liver, especially when combined with contrast injection (Fig. 24.9). Magnetic resonance imaging (MRI) can also be used to localise and confirm the aetiology of focal liver lesions, particularly primary and secondary tumours.

Hepatic angiography is seldom used nowadays as a diagnostic tool, since CT and MRI are both able to provide images of hepatic vasculature, but it still has a therapeutic role in the embolisation of vascular tumours, such as hepatocellular carcinoma. Hepatic venography is now rarely performed.

Cholangiography

Cholangiography can be undertaken by magnetic resonance cholangiopancreatography (MRCP; Fig. 24.10), endoscopy (endoscopic retrograde cholangiopancreatography, ERCP) or the percutaneous approach (percutaneous transhepatic cholangiography, PTC). The latter does not allow the ampulla of Vater or pancreatic duct to be visualised. Endoscopic ultrasound can also provide high-quality biliary imaging safely (see below). MRCP is as good as ERCP at providing images of the biliary tree but is safer, and there is now little, if any, role for diagnostic ERCP. Both endoscopic and percutaneous approaches allow therapeutic interventions, such as the insertion of biliary stents across bile duct strictures. The percutaneous approach is used only if it is not possible to access the bile duct endoscopically.

Endoscopic ultrasound

Endoscopic ultrasound (EUS) is complementary to MRCP in the diagnostic evaluation of the extrahepatic biliary tree, ampulla of Vater and pancreas. With the ultrasonic probe in the duodenum, high-quality images are obtained, tissue sampling can be performed and, increasingly, therapeutic drainage of biliary obstruction can be performed. EUS has the advantage over ERCP of not exposing patients to the risk of pancreatitis, among other complications of bile duct cannulation.

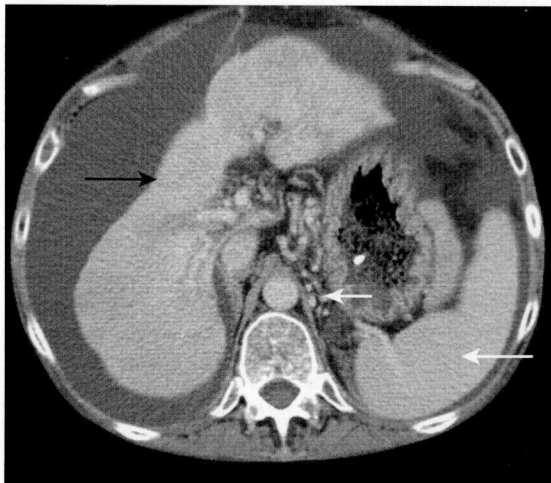

Fig. 24.9 Computed tomography in a patient with cirrhosis. The liver is small and has an irregular outline (black arrow), the spleen is enlarged (long white arrow), fluid (ascites) is seen around the liver, and collateral vessels are present around the proximal stomach (short white arrow).

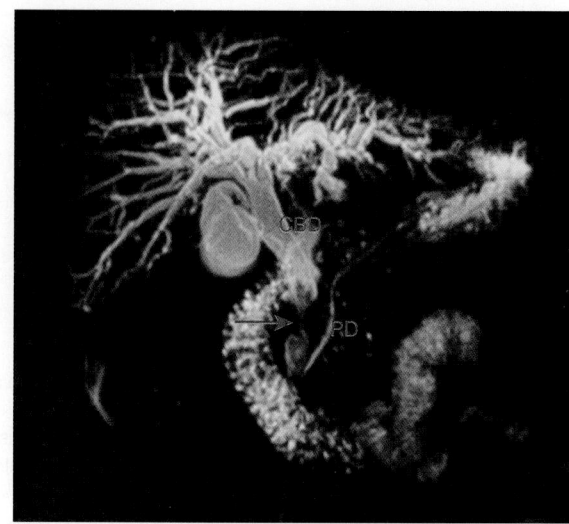

Fig. 24.10 Magnetic resonance cholangiopancreatography showing a biliary stricture due to cholangiocarcinoma in the distal common bile duct (arrow). The proximal common bile duct (CBD) is dilated but the pancreatic duct (PD) is normal.

Non-invasive markers of hepatic fibrosis

Fibrosis is a key predictor of prognosis in chronic liver disease, and can help to guide monitoring and treatment decisions. This is now largely assessed by non-invasive markers of liver fibrosis. A number of indirect fibrosis markers have been described, including bilirubin, AST/ALT ratio and platelet count. Simple scoring systems such as the FIB-4 score and NAFLD fibrosis score combine routinely available blood tests and clinical risk factors, and are often used as screening tests for fibrosis risk. These tests have a high negative predictive value, with a normal value making advanced fibrosis very unlikely, but a relatively low positive predictive value. Whilst these have been validated across a range of aetiologies, the cut-off values used (e.g. for FIB-4) may differ according to aetiology, and serum-based tests are less reliable in alcohol-related liver disease.

Fibrosis can also be assessed using more specific serum tests. Fibrotest® combines five serum markers including α_2-macroglobulin, haptoglobin and apolipoprotein A1. The Enhanced Liver Fibrosis (ELF®) serological assay provides direct assessment of fibrogenesis and fibrolysis using a combination of hyaluronic acid, procollagen peptide III (PIIINP) and tissue inhibitor of metalloproteinase 1 (TIMP1).

An alternative to serological markers is transient elastography (Fibroscan®), in which ultrasound-based shock waves are sent through the liver to measure stiffness as a surrogate for hepatic fibrosis. This is quick, non-invasive and provides immediate results. Depending on the threshold used, this can exclude significant fibrosis or diagnose cirrhosis. However, results can be influenced by the presence of severe inflammation and become less reliable with increasing obesity. Magnetic resonance elastography appears more reliable and is not influenced by obesity, but is costly and not widely available.

Histological examination

A liver biopsy can confirm the severity of liver damage and provide aetiological information. It is performed percutaneously with a Trucut or Menghini needle, usually through an intercostal space under local anaesthesia, or radiologically using a transjugular approach.

Percutaneous liver biopsy is a relatively safe procedure if the conditions detailed in Box 24.6 are met, but carries a mortality of about 0.01%. The main complications are abdominal and/or shoulder pain, bleeding and biliary peritonitis. Liver biopsies can be carried out in patients with defective haemostasis if:

- the defect is corrected with fresh frozen plasma and platelet transfusion,
- the biopsy is obtained by the transjugular route, *or*

- Cooperative patient
- It is recommended that for non-lesional liver biopsy in patients with chronic liver disease a transvenous route should be used if INR > 1.4
- For percutaneous lesional biopsies the INR should be < 2
- Platelet count > 50 × 10⁹/L
- Exclusion of bile duct obstruction, localised skin infection, advanced chronic obstructive pulmonary disease, marked ascites and severe anaemia
- Liver biopsy should be avoided in unstable patients with uncontrolled bleeding, bacterial infection and significant renal impairment.

(INR = International Normalised Ratio)

- the procedure is conducted percutaneously under ultrasound control and the needle track is then plugged with procoagulant material.

In patients with potentially resectable malignancy, biopsy should be avoided due to the potential risk of tumour dissemination (biopsy track seeding). Operative or laparoscopic liver biopsy may sometimes be valuable.

Liver biopsy is used where there is uncertainty as to the cause of liver disease, or to quantify the degree of inflammation ('grade') or fibrosis ('stage'). Semi-quantitative scoring systems may be used to describe the degree of inflammation or fibrosis. Although often regarded as the 'gold standard' investigation for liver disease, liver biopsies are limited by sampling error, with studies showing significant variation in both grade and stage between simultaneous paired biopsies. The use of special histological stains can help in determining aetiology. The clinical features and prognosis of these changes are dependent on the underlying aetiology and are discussed in the relevant sections below.

Presenting problems in liver disease

Liver injury may be either acute or chronic. The main causes are listed in Fig. 24.11 and discussed in detail later in the chapter. In the UK, liver disease is the only one of the top causes of mortality that is steadily increasing (Fig. 24.12). Mortality rates have risen substantially over the last 30 years, with a near-fivefold increase in liver-related mortality in

people younger than 65 years. The rate of increase is substantially higher in the UK than in other countries in Western Europe.

- *Acute liver injury* may present with non-specific symptoms of fatigue and abnormal LFTs, or with jaundice and acute liver failure.
- *Chronic liver injury* is defined as hepatic injury, inflammation and/or fibrosis occurring in the liver for more than 6 months. In the early stages, patients can be asymptomatic with fluctuating abnormal LFTs. With more severe liver damage, however, the presentation can be with jaundice, portal hypertension or other signs of cirrhosis and hepatic decompensation (Box 24.7). Patients with clinically silent chronic liver disease frequently present when abnormalities in liver function are observed on routine blood testing, or when clinical events, such as an intercurrent infection or surgical intervention, cause the liver to decompensate. Patients with compensated cirrhosis can undergo most forms of surgery without significantly increased risk. Surgical complications are more common in patients with decompensated cirrhosis and the presence of portal hypertension with intra-abdominal varices can make abdominal surgery more hazardous. The possibility of undiagnosed liver disease should be borne

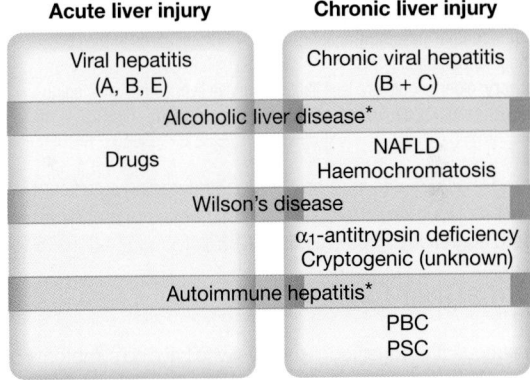

Fig. 24.11 Causes of acute and chronic liver injury. *Although there is often evidence of chronic liver disease at presentation, may present acutely with jaundice. In alcoholic liver disease this is due to superimposed alcoholic hepatitis. (NAFLD = non-alcoholic fatty liver disease; PBC = primary biliary cholangitis; PSC = primary sclerosing cholangitis)

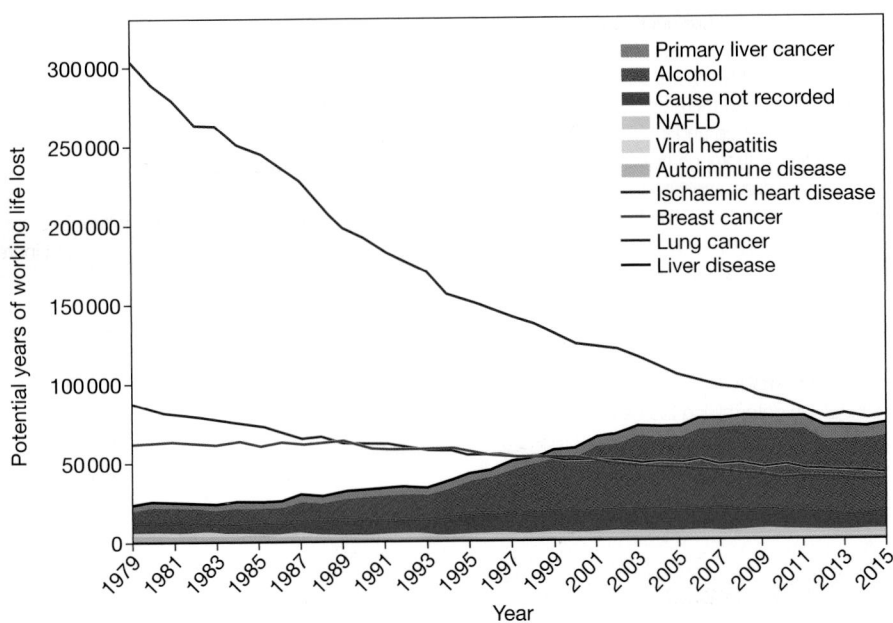

Fig. 24.12 Potential years of working life lost (before 65 years of age) estimated with Office for National Statistics mortality data for 1979–2015. *From Williams R, Alexander G, Armstrong I, et al. Disease burden and costs from excess alcohol consumption, obesity, and viral hepatitis: fourth report of the Lancet Standing Commission on Liver Disease in the UK. Reprinted with permission from Elsevier (The Lancet 2018; 391:1097–1107).*

i	**24.7 Presentation of liver disease**	
Severity	**Acute liver injury**	**Chronic liver injury**
Mild/moderate	Abnormal liver function tests	Abnormal liver function tests
Severe	Jaundice	Signs of cirrhosis ± portal hypertension
Very severe	Acute liver failure	Chronic liver failure* Jaundice Ascites Hepatic encephalopathy Portal hypertension with variceal bleeding

*May not occur until several years after cirrhosis has presented.

24.8 Liver disease in old age

- **Alcoholic liver disease**: 10% of cases present over the age of 70 years, when disease is more likely to be severe and has a worse prognosis.
- **Hepatitis A**: causes more severe illness and runs a more protracted course.
- **Primary biliary cholangitis**: one-third of cases are over 65 years.
- **Liver abscess**: more than 50% of all cases in the UK are over 60 years.
- **Hepatocellular carcinoma**: approximately 50% of cases in the UK present over the age of 65 years.
- **Surgery**: older people are less likely to survive liver surgery (including transplantation) because comorbidity is more prevalent.

in mind in all patients in at-risk groups undergoing significant surgery. Many liver disorders are more common in older age and can pursue a more aggressive course (Box 24.8).

Abnormal liver function tests

LFTs are frequently requested in patients who have no symptoms or signs of liver disease, as part of routine health checks, insurance medicals or drug monitoring. The prevalence of abnormal LFTs has been reported to be as high as 10%–20% in some studies. In the majority of cases, these will not reflect significant underlying liver disease. However, many patients with chronic liver disease are asymptomatic or have vague, non-specific symptoms. The most common abnormalities are alcohol-related or non-alcoholic fatty liver disease. Since effective medical treatments are now available for many types of chronic liver disease, further evaluation is usually warranted to make sure the patient does not have a treatable condition. Biochemical abnormalities in chronic liver disease often fluctuate over time; even mild abnormalities can therefore indicate significant underlying disease and so warrant follow-up and investigation.

When abnormal LFTs are detected, a thorough history should be compiled to determine the patient's alcohol consumption, drug use (prescribed, over-the-counter or recreational), risk factors for viral hepatitis (e.g. blood transfusion, injection drug use, tattoos), the presence of autoimmune diseases, family history, neurological symptoms and the presence of features of the metabolic syndrome, including diabetes and/or obesity (see Box 24.5 and Fig. 22.6). Stigmata of chronic liver disease should be looked for but further investigations are indicated even in the absence of these signs.

Both the pattern of enzyme abnormality (hepatitic or cholestatic) and the degree of elevation are helpful in determining the cause of underlying liver disease (Boxes 24.9 and 24.10). The investigations that make up a standard liver screen and additional or confirmatory tests are shown in Boxes 24.4 and 24.5. An algorithm for investigating abnormal LFTs is provided in Fig. 24.13.

Jaundice

Jaundice is usually detectable clinically when the plasma bilirubin exceeds 40 μmol/L (~2.5 mg/dL). The causes of jaundice overlap with the causes of abnormal LFTs discussed above. In a patient with jaundice it is useful to consider whether the cause might be pre-hepatic, hepatic or post-hepatic, and there are often important clues in the history (Box 24.11).

Pre-hepatic jaundice

This is caused either by haemolysis or by congenital hyperbilirubinaemia, and is characterised by an isolated raised bilirubin level.

In haemolysis, destruction of red blood cells or their marrow precursors causes increased bilirubin production. Jaundice due to haemolysis is usually mild because a healthy liver can excrete a bilirubin load six-times greater than normal before unconjugated bilirubin accumulates in the plasma. This does not apply to newborns, who have less capacity to metabolise bilirubin.

The most common form of non-haemolytic hyperbilirubinaemia is Gilbert syndrome, an inherited disorder of bilirubin metabolism (Box 24.12). Other inherited disorders of bilirubin metabolism are very rare.

Hepatic jaundice

This is characterised by jaundice due to hepatic dysfunction (usually indicated by abnormal liver enzymes) but normal biliary imaging. This can be due to acute hepatocellular injury (see Box 24.9), intrahepatic cholestasis (see Box 24.10) or decompensation of cirrhosis. 'Hepatic' jaundice can be a manifestation of extrahepatic disease such as sepsis or right heart failure. In all of these, jaundice results from an inability of the liver to transport bilirubin into the bile, occurring at any point between uptake of unconjugated bilirubin into the cells and transport of conjugated bilirubin into the canaliculi. In addition, swelling of cells and oedema resulting

---

24.9 Common causes of elevated serum transaminases

Minor elevation (< 100 U/L*)
- Chronic hepatitis C
- Chronic hepatitis B
- Fatty liver disease
- Alcoholic hepatitis
- Haemochromatosis

Moderate elevation (100–300 U/L*)
As above plus:
- Non-alcoholic steatohepatitis
- Autoimmune hepatitis
- Wilson's disease

Major elevation (> 300 U/L*)
- Drugs (e.g. paracetamol)
- Acute viral hepatitis
- Autoimmune hepatitis
- Ischaemic hepatitis
- Toxins (e.g. *Amanita phalloides* poisoning)
- Flare of chronic hepatitis B

*These ranges are indicative but do not rigidly discriminate between different aetiologies.

24.10 Causes of cholestatic jaundice

Hepatic
- Primary biliary cholangitis
- Primary sclerosing cholangitis
- Alcohol
- Drugs
- Hepatic infiltrations (lymphoma, granuloma, amyloid, metastases)
- Cystic fibrosis
- Sepsis
- Pregnancy
- Inherited cholestatic liver disease (e.g. benign recurrent intrahepatic cholestasis)
- Right heart failure

Post-hepatic
- Carcinoma:
  - Ampullary
  - Pancreatic
  - Bile duct (cholangiocarcinoma)
  - Liver metastases
- Choledocholithiasis
- Primary sclerosing cholangitis
- Parasitic infection
- Traumatic biliary strictures
- Chronic pancreatitis
- IgG4 cholangitis

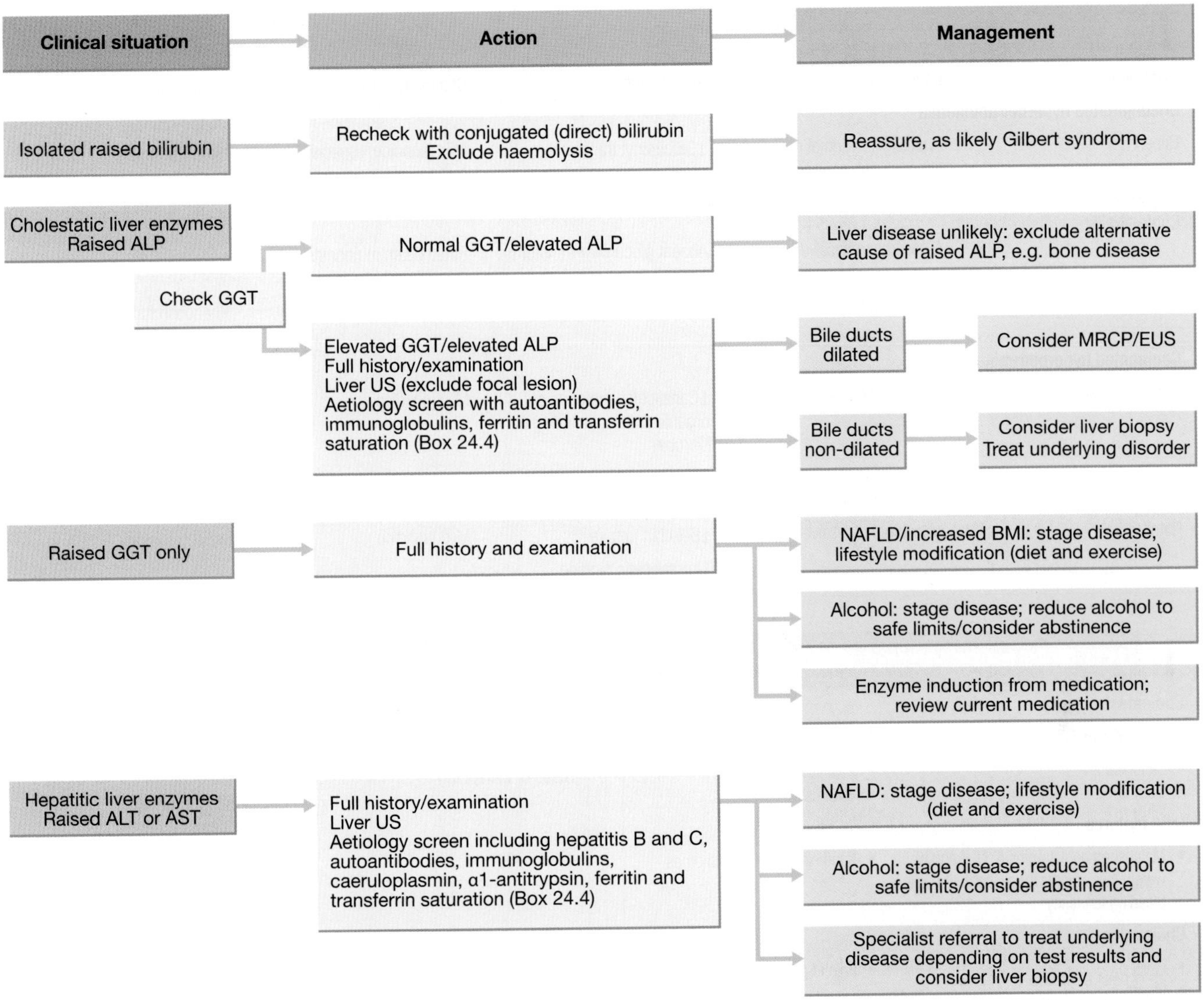

Clinical situation	Action	Management

Isolated raised bilirubin → Recheck with conjugated (direct) bilirubin / Exclude haemolysis → Reassure, as likely Gilbert syndrome

Cholestatic liver enzymes Raised ALP → Check GGT

Normal GGT/elevated ALP → Liver disease unlikely: exclude alternative cause of raised ALP, e.g. bone disease

Elevated GGT/elevated ALP
Full history/examination
Liver US (exclude focal lesion)
Aetiology screen with autoantibodies, immunoglobulins, ferritin and transferrin saturation (Box 24.4)

→ Bile ducts dilated → Consider MRCP/EUS

→ Bile ducts non-dilated → Consider liver biopsy / Treat underlying disorder

Raised GGT only → Full history and examination →

- NAFLD/increased BMI: stage disease; lifestyle modification (diet and exercise)
- Alcohol: stage disease; reduce alcohol to safe limits/consider abstinence
- Enzyme induction from medication; review current medication

Hepatitic liver enzymes Raised ALT or AST → Full history/examination
Liver US
Aetiology screen including hepatitis B and C, autoantibodies, immunoglobulins, caeruloplasmin, α1-antitrypsin, ferritin and transferrin saturation (Box 24.4)

- NAFLD: stage disease; lifestyle modification (diet and exercise)
- Alcohol: stage disease; reduce alcohol to safe limits/consider abstinence
- Specialist referral to treat underlying disease depending on test results and consider liver biopsy

Fig. 24.13 Suggested management of abnormal liver function tests in asymptomatic patients. (ALP = alkaline phosphatase; ASP = aspartate aminotransferase; BMI = body mass index; EUS = endoscopic ultrasound; GGT = γ-glutamyl transferase; MRCP = magnetic resonance cholangiopancreatography; NAFLD = non-alcoholic fatty liver disease; US = ultrasound)

24

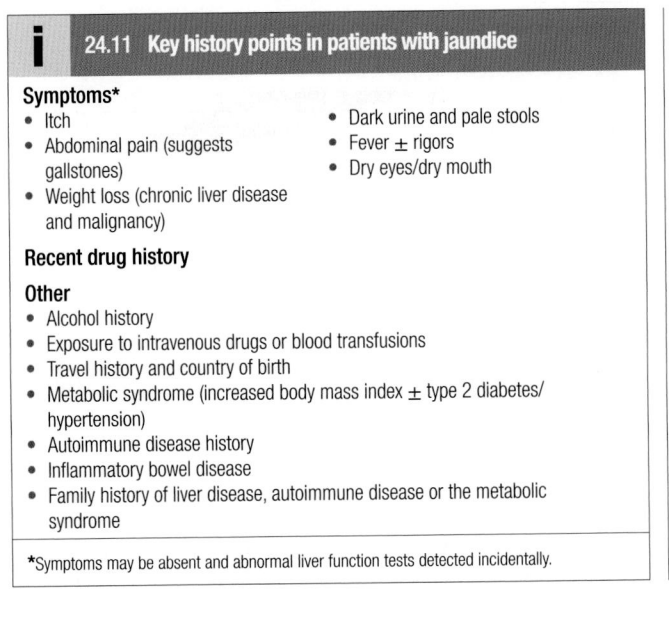

i 24.11 Key history points in patients with jaundice

Symptoms*
- Itch
- Abdominal pain (suggests gallstones)
- Weight loss (chronic liver disease and malignancy)
- Dark urine and pale stools
- Fever ± rigors
- Dry eyes/dry mouth

Recent drug history

Other
- Alcohol history
- Exposure to intravenous drugs or blood transfusions
- Travel history and country of birth
- Metabolic syndrome (increased body mass index ± type 2 diabetes/ hypertension)
- Autoimmune disease history
- Inflammatory bowel disease
- Family history of liver disease, autoimmune disease or the metabolic syndrome

*Symptoms may be absent and abnormal liver function tests detected incidentally.

from parenchymal damage may cause obstruction of the biliary canaliculi. Consequently, the concentrations of both unconjugated and conjugated bilirubin in the blood increase. Jaundice due to acute parenchymal liver disease is associated with increases in transaminases (AST/ALT), but increases in cholestatic enzymes (GGT/ALP) may occur and suggest specific aetiologies (see below). Acute jaundice in the presence of an ALT of > 1000 U/L is highly suggestive of an infectious cause (e.g. hepatitis A, B or E), drugs (e.g. paracetamol) or hepatic ischaemia. Imaging is essential, not only to exclude a post-hepatic cause but to identify features suggestive of cirrhosis or portal hypertension, and to define the patency of the hepatic vasculature. Liver biopsy has an important role in defining the aetiology of unexplained hepatocellular jaundice and the extent of liver injury.

Post-hepatic jaundice

Post-hepatic jaundice may be caused by obstruction of the larger bile ducts, usually between the hilum and the ampulla of Vater, resulting in biliary dilatation on imaging.

The causes of post-hepatic jaundice are listed in Box 24.10. Post-hepatic jaundice is most commonly due to diseases affecting the

i 24.12 Congenital non-haemolytic hyperbilirubinaemia

Syndrome	Inheritance	Abnormality	Clinical features	Treatment
Unconjugated hyperbilirubinaemia				
Gilbert	Typically autosomal recessive, although autosomal dominant forms are also described	↓Glucuronyl transferase ↓Bilirubin uptake	Mild jaundice, especially with fasting	None necessary
Crigler–Najjar:				
Type I	Autosomal recessive	Absent glucuronyl transferase	Rapid death in neonate (kernicterus)	
Type II	Autosomal recessive	↓↓Glucuronyl transferase	Presents in neonate	Phenobarbital, phototherapy or liver transplant
Conjugated hyperbilirubinaemia				
Dubin–Johnson	Autosomal recessive	↓Canalicular excretion of organic anions, including bilirubin Pigmentation of liver biopsy tissue	Mild jaundice	None necessary
Rotor	Autosomal recessive	↓Bilirubin uptake ↓Intrahepatic binding	Mild jaundice	None necessary

i 24.13 Clinical features and complications of cholestatic jaundice

Cholestasis

Early features

- Jaundice
- Dark urine
- Pale stools
- Pruritus

Late features

- Malabsorption (vitamins A, D, E and K): weight loss, steatorrhoea, osteomalacia, bleeding tendency
- Xanthelasma and xanthomas

Cholangitis

- Fever
- Rigors
- Pain (if gallstones present)

i 24.14 Clinical features suggesting an underlying cause of cholestatic jaundice*

Clinical feature	Causes
Jaundice	
Static or increasing	Carcinoma Primary biliary cholangitis Primary sclerosing cholangitis
Fluctuating	Choledocholithiasis Stricture Pancreatitis Choledochal cyst Primary sclerosing cholangitis
Abdominal pain	Choledocholithiasis Pancreatitis Choledochal cyst
Cholangitis	Choledocholithiasis Stricture Choledochal cyst
Abdominal scar	Stone Stricture
Irregular hepatomegaly	Hepatic carcinoma
Palpable gallbladder	Carcinoma below cystic duct (usually pancreas)
Abdominal mass	Carcinoma Pancreatitis (cyst) Choledochal cyst
Occult blood in stools	Ampullary tumour

*Each of these diseases can give rise to almost any of the clinical features shown but the box indicates the most likely cause of the clinical features listed.

extrahepatic bile ducts, which are often amenable to surgical or endoscopic correction.

Clinical features (Box 24.13) comprise those due to cholestasis itself, those due to secondary infection (cholangitis) and those of the underlying condition (Box 24.14). Post-hepatic jaundice is characteristically associated with pale stools, dark urine and itch, although these features also occur with intrahepatic cholestasis. If the gallbladder is palpable, the jaundice is unlikely to be caused by biliary obstruction due to gallstones, probably because a chronically inflamed, stone-containing gallbladder cannot readily dilate. This is Courvoisier's Law, and suggests that jaundice is due to a malignant biliary obstruction (e.g. pancreatic cancer). Cholangitis is characterised by 'Charcot's triad' of jaundice, right upper quadrant pain and fever.

Cholestatic jaundice is characterised by a relatively greater elevation of ALP and GGT than ALT, although a high ALT is often seen with ductal gallstones presumably due to a cholangitic element. Ultrasound is usually the first-line imaging to determine whether there is dilatation of the biliary tree (Fig. 24.14). MRCP provides a more detailed assessment of the biliary tree, especially where ductal stones are suspected, whereas CT is preferred for assessing malignant lesions. EUS provides an additional modality for investigation of lower common bile duct obstruction.

Management of post-hepatic jaundice depends on the underlying cause and is discussed in the relevant sections below.

Acute liver failure

Acute liver failure is a rare but life-threatening condition characterised by a rapid progressive deterioration in liver function. A variety of insults can lead to marked elevation of transaminases, or acute liver injury. This is considered severe if it results in jaundice and coagulopathy. A small number of such patients will go on to develop encephalopathy, which is the cardinal feature of acute liver failure. The absence of evidence of

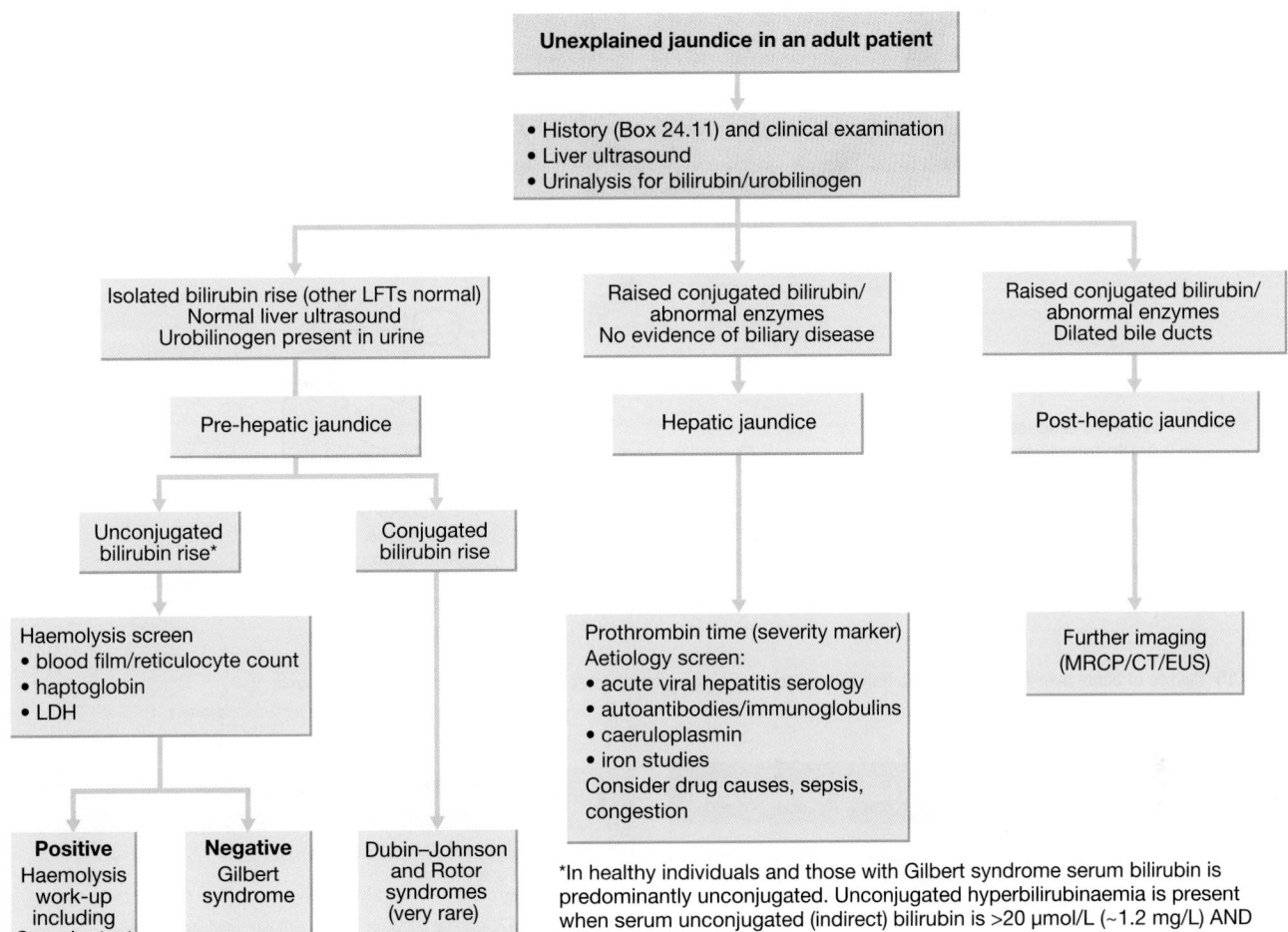

Fig. 24.14 Investigation of jaundice. (CT = computed tomography; ERCP = endoscopic retrograde cholangiopancreatography; EUS = endoscopic ultrasound; LDH = lactate dehydrogenase; LFTs = liver function tests; MRCP = magnetic resonance cholangiopancreatography)

pre-existing liver disease distinguishes it from encephalopathy due to decompensated cirrhosis or acute-on-chronic liver failure. It is critical, therefore, to understand whether liver failure is a truly acute event or an acute deterioration on a background of pre-existing injury (which may itself not have been diagnosed). Although liver biopsy may ultimately be necessary, it is the presence or absence of the clinical features suggesting chronicity that guides the clinician.

Acute liver failure may be subclassified into hyperacute, acute and subacute, according to the interval between onset of jaundice and encephalopathy (Box 24.15). This can help to identify likely cause and predict prognosis. Patients with subacute liver failure are more likely to be drug-induced or of indeterminate cause, and have a worse outcome with medical care alone than those with a hyperacute course.

Pathophysiology

Any cause of hepatocyte damage can produce acute liver failure, provided it is sufficiently severe (Fig. 24.15). Acute viral hepatitis is the most common cause worldwide, whereas paracetamol toxicity is the most frequent cause in the UK. Acute liver failure occurs occasionally with other drugs (prescription, recreational or herbal), or from *Amanita phalloides* (mushroom) poisoning, in autoimmune hepatitis, in acute fatty liver of pregnancy, in Wilson's disease, following shock and, rarely, in extensive malignant disease of the liver. In 10% of cases, the cause of acute liver failure remains unknown and these patients are often labelled as having 'non-A–E viral hepatitis' or 'cryptogenic' acute liver failure.

Clinical assessment

Cerebral disturbance (hepatic encephalopathy and/or cerebral oedema) is the cardinal manifestation of acute liver failure. The initial clinical features

i	24.15	**Classification of acute liver failure**		
Type		**Time: jaundice to encephalopathy**	**Cerebral oedema**	**Common causes**
Hyperacute		< 7 days	Common	Viral, paracetamol
Acute		8–28 days	Common	Cryptogenic, drugs
Subacute		29 days to 12 weeks	Uncommon	Cryptogenic, drugs, autoimmune hepatitis

24

are often subtle and include reduced alertness and poor concentration, progressing through behavioural abnormalities, such as restlessness and aggressive outbursts, to drowsiness and coma (Box 24.16). Cerebral oedema may occur due to increased intracranial pressure, causing unequal or abnormally reacting pupils, fixed pupils, hypertensive episodes, bradycardia, hyperventilation, profuse sweating, local or general myoclonus, focal fits or decerebrate posturing. Papilloedema occurs rarely and is a late sign.

More general symptoms include weakness, nausea and vomiting. The patient may be jaundiced but jaundice may not be present at the outset (e.g. in paracetamol overdose), and there are a number of exceptions, including Reye syndrome, in which jaundice is rare. Occasionally, death may occur in hyperacute liver failure before jaundice develops. Fetor hepaticus can be present. The liver is usually of normal size but later

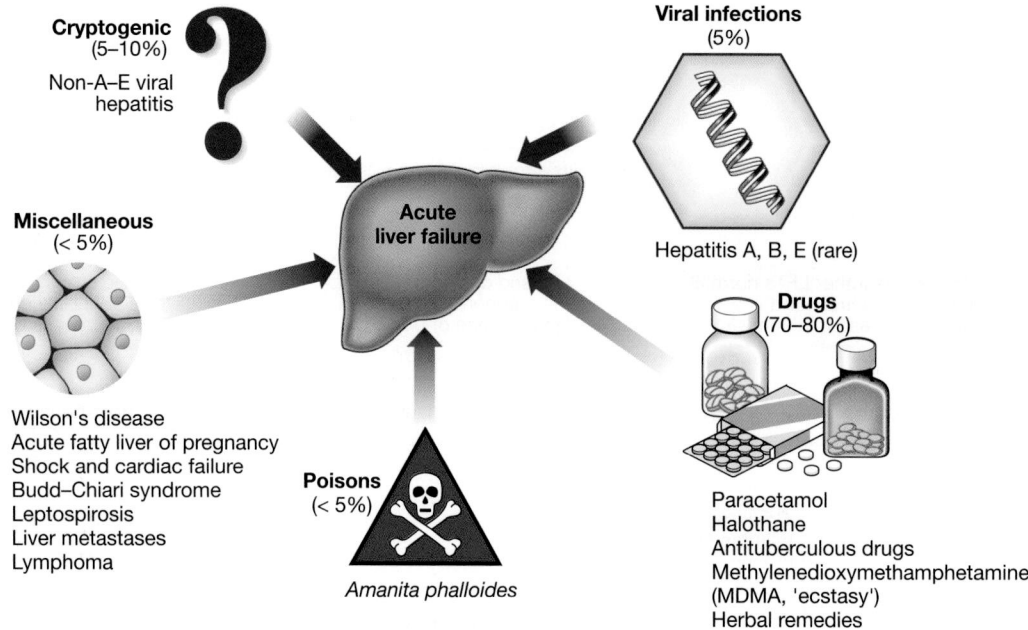

Fig. 24.15 Causes of acute liver failure in the UK. The relative frequency of the different causes varies according to geographical area.

24.16 How to assess clinical grade of hepatic encephalopathy	
Clinical grade	**Clinical signs**
Grade 1	Poor concentration, slurred speech, slow mentation, disordered sleep rhythm
Grade 2	Drowsy but easily rousable, occasional aggressive behaviour, lethargic
Grade 3	Marked delirium, drowsy, sleepy but responds to pain and voice, gross disorientation
Grade 4	Unresponsive to voice, may or may not respond to painful stimuli, unconscious

24.17 Investigations to determine the cause of acute liver failure

- Toxicology screen of blood and urine
- HBsAg, IgM anti-HBc
- IgM anti-HAV
- Anti-HEV, HCV, cytomegalovirus, herpes simplex, Epstein–Barr virus
- Caeruloplasmin, serum copper, urinary copper, slit-lamp eye examination
- Autoantibodies: ANA, ASMA, LKM, SLA
- Immunoglobulins
- Ultrasound of liver and Doppler of hepatic veins

(ANA = antinuclear antibody; anti-HBc = antibody to hepatitis B core antigen; ASMA = anti-smooth muscle antibody; HAV = hepatitis A virus; HBsAg = hepatitis B surface antigen; HCV = hepatitis C virus; HEV = hepatitis E virus; IgM = immunoglobulin M; LKM = liver–kidney microsomal antibody; SLA = soluble liver antigen)

24.18 Adverse prognostic criteria in acute liver failure[1]

Paracetamol overdose

- pH < 7.25 at or beyond 24 hours following the overdose and after fluid resuscitation
  Or
- Prothrombin time > 100 secs *plus* encephalopathy grade 3 or 4 *plus* serum creatinine > 300 μmol/L (≅ 3.38 mg/dL) or anuria
  Or
- Arterial lactate > 5 mmol/L at presentation and > 4 mmol/L 24 hours later after fluid resuscitation

Non-paracetamol cases

- Prothrombin time > 100 secs (or INR > 6.5) with any grade of encephalopathy
  Or
- Any three of the following[2]:
  Jaundice to encephalopathy time > 7 days
  Age < 10 or > 40 years
  Bilirubin > 300 μmol/L (≅ 17.6 mg/dL)
  Prothrombin time > 50 secs (or INR > 3.5)
  Unfavourable aetiology, e.g. seronegative hepatitis or idiosyncratic drug reaction

[1]Predict a mortality rate of ≥ 90% and are an indication for possible liver transplantation. [2]In the absence of encephalopathy INR > 2 after vitamin K repletion is mandatory.
(INR = International Normalised Ratio)

becomes smaller. Hepatomegaly is unusual and, in the presence of a sudden onset of ascites, suggests venous outflow obstruction as the cause (Budd–Chiari syndrome, p. 909). Splenomegaly is uncommon and never prominent. Ascites and oedema are late developments and may be a consequence of fluid therapy.

Investigations

The patient should be investigated to determine the cause of the liver failure and the prognosis (Boxes 24.17 and 24.18). Hepatitis B core IgM antibody is the best screening test for acute hepatitis B infection, as liver damage is due to the immunological response to the virus, which has often been eliminated, and the test for hepatitis B surface antigen (HBsAg) may be negative by the time liver failure develops. The PT rapidly becomes prolonged as coagulation factor synthesis fails; this is the laboratory test of greatest prognostic value and should be carried out at least twice daily. Vitamin K should be given to ensure that the PT is not prolonged as a result of underlying vitamin K deficiency, but fresh frozen plasma should be avoided except in major bleeding as it will interfere with the use of PT for monitoring. Factor V levels can be used instead of the PT to assess the degree of liver impairment. Plasma bilirubin also predicts outcome in non-paracetamol causes of acute liver failure. Plasma aminotransferase activity is particularly high after paracetamol overdose, reaching 100–500 times normal, but falls as liver damage progresses and is not helpful in determining prognosis. Plasma albumin remains normal unless the course is prolonged. Percutaneous liver biopsy is contraindicated because of the severe coagulopathy, but biopsy can be undertaken using the transjugular route if appropriate.

Management

Patients with acute liver failure should be treated in a high-dependency or intensive care unit as soon as progressive prolongation of the PT occurs or hepatic encephalopathy is identified (Box 24.19), so that prompt treatment of complications can be initiated (Box 24.20). Conservative treatment aims to support other organ systems in the hope that hepatic regeneration will occur. *N*-acetylcysteine therapy should be given early to all patients in whom paracetamol toxicity is suspected, although the benefits are less clear in non-paracetamol-induced acute liver failure. Liver transplantation is an increasingly important treatment option for acute liver failure, and criteria have been developed to identify patients unlikely to survive without a transplant (see Box 24.18). Patients should, wherever possible, be transferred to a transplant centre before these criteria are met to allow time for assessment and to maximise the time for a donor liver to become available. Survival following liver transplantation for acute liver failure is improving and 1-year survival rates of 80%–90% can be expected. A number of artificial liver support systems have been developed and evaluated for use as a bridge to either transplantation or recovery. None, however, has entered routine clinical use.

Hepatomegaly

Hepatomegaly may occur as the result of a general enlargement of the liver or because of primary or secondary liver tumour (Box 24.21). The most common liver tumours in Western countries are liver metastases, whereas primary liver cancer complicating chronic viral hepatitis is more common in the Far East. Unlike carcinoma metastases, those from neuro-endocrine tumours typically cause massive hepatomegaly but without significant weight loss. Cirrhosis can be associated with either hepatomegaly or reduced liver size in advanced disease.

Ascites

Ascites is present when there is accumulation of free fluid in the peritoneal cavity. Small amounts of ascites are asymptomatic, but with larger accumulations of fluid (> 1 L) there is abdominal distension, fullness in the flanks, shifting dullness on percussion and, when the ascites is marked, a fluid thrill/fluid wave. Other features include eversion of the umbilicus, herniae, abdominal striae, divarication of the recti and scrotal oedema. Dilated superficial abdominal veins may be seen if the ascites is due to portal hypertension.

Pathophysiology

The most common causes of ascites are cirrhosis, intra-abdominal malignancy and heart failure. Many primary disorders of the peritoneum and visceral organs can also cause ascites, and these need to be considered even in a patient with chronic liver disease (Box 24.22). Splanchnic arterial vasodilatation is thought to be the main factor leading to ascites in cirrhosis. This is mediated by vasodilators (mainly nitric oxide) that are released when portal hypertension causes shunting of blood into the systemic circulation. Systemic arterial pressure falls due to pronounced splanchnic

24.19 Monitoring in acute liver failure

Cardiorespiratory
- Pulse
- Blood pressure
- Central venous pressure
- Respiratory rate

Neurological
- Signs of intracranial hypertension including pupillary responses. Invasive intracranial pressure monitor is now less commonly used
- Conscious level

Fluid balance
- Hourly output (urine, vomiting, diarrhoea)
- Input: oral, intravenous

Blood analyses
- Arterial blood gases
- Peripheral blood count (including platelets)
- Sodium, potassium, HCO_3^-, calcium, magnesium
- Creatinine, urea
- Glucose (2-hourly in acute phase)
- Prothrombin time

Infection surveillance
- Cultures: blood, urine, throat, sputum, cannula sites
- Chest X-ray
- Temperature

24.20 Complications of acute liver failure
- Encephalopathy and cerebral oedema
- Hypoglycaemia
- Metabolic acidosis
- Infection (bacterial, fungal)
- Renal failure
- Multi-organ failure (hypotension and respiratory failure)

24.21 Causes of change in liver size

Large liver (hepatomegaly)
- Liver metastases
- Cirrhosis (early): non-alcoholic fatty liver disease, alcohol, haemochromatosis
- Right heart failure
- Multiple or large hepatic cysts
- Hepatic vein outflow obstruction
- Infiltration: amyloid

Small liver
- Cirrhosis (late)

24.22 Causes of ascites

Low SAAG	High SAAG
Common causes	

Malignant disease:
  Hepatic
  Peritoneal
	Cirrhosis
	Cardiac failure

Other causes	

Acute pancreatitis
Lymphatic obstruction
Infection:
  Tuberculosis
Nephrotic syndrome
Protein-losing enteropathy
Severe malnutrition
	Hepatic venous occlusion:
	  Budd–Chiari syndrome[1]
	  Sinusoidal obstruction syndrome
	  (Veno-occlusive disease)

Rare causes	
Hypothyroidism Meigs syndrome[2]	Constrictive pericarditis

[1]Early Budd–Chiari syndrome presents with ascites with high protein content (> 25 g/L) and elevated SAAG. In chronic Budd–Chiari syndrome the protein concentration may fall but SAAG remains elevated. [2]Meigs syndrome is the association of a right pleural effusion with or without ascites and a benign ovarian tumour. The ascites resolves on removal of the tumour. Although usually reported as being associated with a low SAAG, it can also be seen with a high SAAG.

(SAAG = serum–ascites albumin gradient; see text)

24

vasodilatation as cirrhosis advances. This leads to activation of the renin–angiotensin system with secondary aldosteronism, increased sympathetic nervous activity, increased atrial natriuretic hormone secretion and altered activity of the kallikrein–kinin system (Fig. 24.16). These systems tend to normalise arterial pressure initially but produce salt and water retention. In this setting, the combination of splanchnic arterial vasodilatation and portal hypertension alters intestinal capillary permeability, promoting accumulation of fluid within the peritoneum.

Investigations

Ultrasonography is the best means of detecting ascites, particularly in the obese and those with small volumes of fluid. Paracentesis (if necessary under ultrasonic guidance) can be used to obtain ascitic fluid for analysis. The

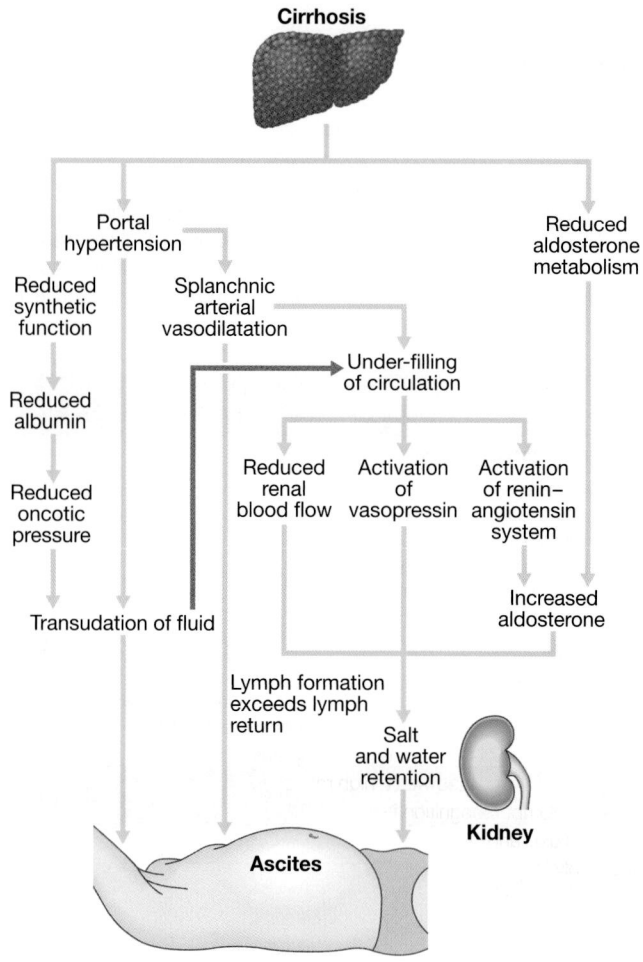

Fig. 24.16 Pathogenesis of ascites.

i 24.23 Ascitic fluid: appearance and analysis

Cause/appearance

- Cirrhosis: clear, straw-coloured or light green
- Malignant disease: bloody
- Infection: cloudy
- Biliary communication: heavy bile staining
- Lymphatic obstruction: milky-white (chylous)

Useful investigations

- Total albumin (plus serum albumin) and protein*
- Amylase
- Neutrophil count
- Cytology
- Microscopy and culture

*To calculate the serum–ascites albumin gradient (SAAG).

appearance of ascitic fluid may point to the underlying cause (Box 24.23). Pleural effusions are found in about 10% of patients, usually on the right side (hepatic hydrothorax); most are small and identified only on chest X-ray, but occasionally a massive hydrothorax occurs. Pleural effusions, particularly those on the left side, should not be assumed to be due to the ascites.

Measurement of the protein concentration and the serum–ascites albumin gradient (SAAG) can be a useful tool to distinguish ascites of different aetiologies. Cirrhotic patients typically develop ascites with a low protein concentration ('transudate'; protein concentration <25 g/L (2.5 g/dL)) and relatively few cells. In up to 30% of patients, however, the total protein concentration is > 30 g/L (3.0 g/dL). In these cases, it is useful to calculate the SAAG by subtracting the concentration of the ascites fluid albumin from the serum albumin. A gradient of > 11 g/L (1.1 g/dL) is 96% predictive that ascites is due to portal hypertension. Venous outflow obstruction due to cardiac failure or hepatic venous outflow obstruction can also cause a SAAG of > 11 g/L (1.1 g/dL) but, unlike in cirrhosis, the total protein content is usually > 25 g/L (2.5 g/dL). Conversely, conditions including nephrotic syndrome, protein-losing enteropathy and severe malnutrition result in ascites with low protein concentration and a SAAG of < 11 g/L (1.1 g/dL) due to diminished serum oncotic pressure.

High protein ascites ('exudate'; protein concentration > 25 g/L (2.5 g/dL) or a SAAG of < 11 g/L (1.1 g/dL) raises the possibility of infection (especially tuberculosis), malignancy, pancreatic ascites or, rarely, hypothyroidism). Ascitic amylase activity of > 1000 U/L identifies pancreatic ascites, whereas low ascites glucose concentrations suggest malignant disease or tuberculosis. Cytological examination may reveal malignant cells but has a low sensitivity unless large volumes are sent. Polymorphonuclear leucocyte counts of > 250×10^6/L strongly suggest infection (spontaneous bacterial peritonitis; see below). Laparoscopy can be valuable in detecting peritoneal disease.

The presence of triglyceride at a level > 1.1 g/L (110 mg/dL) is diagnostic of chylous ascites and suggests anatomical or functional abnormality of lymphatic drainage from the abdomen. Chylous ascites has a characteristic milky-white appearance.

Management

Successful treatment relieves discomfort but does not prolong life; if over-vigorous, it can produce serious disorders of fluid/electrolyte balance, and precipitate hepatic encephalopathy (see below). Treatment of transudative ascites is based on restricting sodium intake, promoting urine output with diuretics and, if necessary, removing ascites directly by paracentesis. Exudative ascites due to malignancy is treated with paracentesis but fluid replacement is generally not required. During management of ascites, the patient should be weighed regularly. Diuretics should be titrated to remove no more than 1 L of fluid (or 1 kg body weight) daily to avoid excessive fluid depletion.

Sodium restriction

Restriction of dietary sodium intake is essential to achieve negative sodium balance and a few patients can be managed satisfactorily by this alone. Restriction of sodium intake to 100 mmol/24 hrs ('no added salt diet') is usually adequate. Drugs containing relatively large amounts of sodium, and those promoting sodium retention, such as non-steroidal anti-inflammatory drugs (NSAIDs), must be avoided (Box 24.24). Restriction of water intake to 1.0–1.5 L/24 hrs is rarely needed unless the plasma sodium falls below 125 mmol/L.

Diuretics

Most patients require diuretics in addition to sodium restriction. Spironolactone (100–400 mg/day) is the first-line drug because it is a powerful aldosterone antagonist; it can, however, cause painful gynaecomastia and hyperkalaemia, in which case amiloride (5–10 mg/day) can be substituted. This is often combined with a loop diuretic, such as furosemide (40–160 mg/day). Patients must be monitored for electrolyte imbalance and renal dysfunction. Diuresis may be improved if patients are rested in bed, perhaps because renal blood flow increases in the horizontal position. Patients who do not respond to maximal doses of

i | **24.24 Some drugs containing relatively large amounts of sodium or causing sodium retention**

High sodium content

- Alginates
- Antacids
- Antibiotics
- Phenytoin

- Effervescent preparations (e.g. aspirin, calcium, paracetamol)
- Sodium valproate

Sodium retention

- Carbenoxolone
- Glucocorticoids
- Metoclopramide

- Non-steroidal anti-inflammatory drugs
- Oestrogens

i | **24.25 Diagnostic criteria for HRS-AKI**

- Diagnosis of cirrhosis, acute liver failure, acute on chronic liver failure
- Increase in serum creatinine $\geq 26.5\,\mu mol/L$ ($\geq 0.3\,mg/dl$) within 48 hours or $\geq 50\%$ from baseline according to IAC-AKI criteria
  and/or
- Urinary output $\leq 0.5\,ml/kg$ per hr for $\geq 6\,hrs$
- No response after 2 consecutive days of diuretic withdrawal and volume expansion with albumin. The recommended dose of albumin is 1 g/kg body weight to a maximum of 100 g
- Absence of shock
- No current or recent treatment with nephrotoxic drugs
- Absence of parenchymal kidney disease, as defined as
  1 Absence of proteinuria (> 500 mg/day)
  2 Absence of microhaematuria (> 50 RBC per high power field)
  3 Normal findings on renal ultrasound

(AKI = acute kidney injury; HRS = hepatorenal syndrome; IAC = International Aascites Club; RBC = red blood cells)

spironolactone and furosemide (diuretic-resistant), or who are unable to tolerate these doses due to hyponatraemia or renal impairment (diuretic-intolerant), are considered to have refractory ascites and should be treated by other measures.

Paracentesis

First-line treatment of refractory ascites is large-volume paracentesis. Paracentesis to dryness is safe, provided the circulation is supported with an intravenous colloid such as human albumin (6–8 g per litre of ascites removed, usually as 100 mL of 20% or 25% human albumin solution (HAS) for every 2–3 L of ascites drained). Paracentesis can be used as an initial therapy or when other treatments fail. Drains should be removed after 6–12 hours to reduce risk of infection.

Transjugular intrahepatic portosystemic stent shunt

A transjugular intrahepatic portosystemic stent shunt (TIPSS; p. 883) can relieve resistant ascites but does not prolong life; it may be an option where the only alternative is frequent, large-volume paracentesis. TIPSS can be used in patients awaiting liver transplantation or in those with reasonable liver function, but can aggravate encephalopathy in those with poor function.

Complications

Renal failure

Renal dysfunction is commonly seen in patients with liver cirrhosis, related to pre-renal, intrinsic and post-renal causes. It is most frequently related to dehydration, diuretic therapy and/or sepsis. However, patients with cirrhosis and ascites may develop a distinct type of renal dysfunction termed hepatorenal syndrome (HRS).

Hepatorenal syndrome

HRS is renal dysfunction that occurs due to reduced renal perfusion, resulting from both haemodynamic alterations in the arterial circulation (splanchnic vasodilatation/renal vasoconstriction) and overactivity of endogenous vasoactive systems. HRS has traditionally been classified into two subtypes but the terminology has recently changed to reflect changes in the understanding and definition of both acute kidney injury (AKI) and chronic kidney disease (CKD).

Type-1 HRS (now termed HRS-AKI) involves a rapid reduction in renal function (AKI) that is usually precipitated by an acute event, including bacterial infection, GI haemorrhage, alcoholic hepatitis or acute liver failure, which disturbs the abnormal renal haemodynamics and has a poor prognosis.

Traditionally HRS was diagnosed with a serum creatinine cutoff of > 1.5 g/dL (> 133 µmol/L) but this has been modified to use a change in renal function from baseline and removing the cutoff threshold. This was necessary to avoid delay in diagnosis and initiation of treatment for HRS. The diagnostic criteria from HRS AKI are shown in Box 24.25.

Type II HRS (now termed HRS non-acute kidney injury or HRS-NAKI) is a stable or slowly progressive form of renal dysfunction developing over weeks to months, in the absence of an obvious precipitant. It is characterised clinically by diuretic-resistant ascites.

Management of HRS-AKI involves identifying and treating precipitating factors. Diuretics and beta-blockers should be discontinued. Nephrotoxic drugs including vasodilators and non-steroidal anti-inflammatories should be stopped. Infections should be sought and treated. Volume replacement should be used to treat fluid loss/deficits. Intravenous albumin infusions in combination with terlipressin (1–2 mg every 4–6 hours) have been shown to improve short-term survival. In countries where terlipressin is not available, a combination of midodrine, octreotide and albumin may be used. TIPSS may be effective for treatment of HRS in highly selected patients. Haemodialysis may be considered in patients who fail to respond to treatment as either a bridge to transplant (in suitable patients) or as a bridge to recovery in patients with a reversible liver injury (typically acute liver failure).

Spontaneous bacterial peritonitis

Spontaneous bacterial peritonitis (SBP) is the most common bacterial infection in patients with cirrhosis, and results from translocation of bacteria from the intestine into ascites. It may present with abdominal pain or fever in a patient with obvious features of cirrhosis and ascites. However, abdominal signs are mild or absent in about one-third of patients, and it may present with hepatic encephalopathy or a non-specific deterioration. SBP is associated with a high rate of acute kidney injury and mortality, and prompt recognition is critical. Diagnostic paracentesis may show cloudy fluid, and an ascites neutrophil count of $> 250 \times 10^6/L$ almost invariably indicates infection. Most organisms isolated are of enteric origin and *Escherichia coli* is the most frequently found. Ascitic culture in blood culture bottles gives the highest yield of organisms. SBP needs to be differentiated from other intra-abdominal emergencies, and the finding of multiple organisms on culture should arouse suspicion of a perforated viscus.

Treatment should be started immediately with broad-spectrum antibiotics, such as cefotaxime or piperacillin/tazobactam). Patients with jaundice or renal impairment also benefit from intravenous albumin (1.5 g/kg on day 1 and 1.0 g/kg on day 3). Recurrence of SBP is common, but is reduced by prophylactic antibiotics such as norfloxacin (400 mg/day), ciprofloxacin (750 mg/week) or cotrimoxazole (960 mg/day). Primary antibiotic prophylaxis also reduces the incidence of SBP in patients with low ascitic protein < 15 g/L.

Prognosis

Only 10%–20% of patients survive for 5 years from the first appearance of ascites due to cirrhosis. The outlook is not universally poor, however, and is best in those with well-maintained liver function and a good response to therapy. The prognosis is also better when a treatable cause for the underlying cirrhosis is present or when a precipitating cause for ascites, such as excess salt intake, is found. The mortality at 1 year is 50% following the first episode of bacterial peritonitis.

24

Hepatic encephalopathy

Hepatic encephalopathy is a neuropsychiatric syndrome caused by liver disease that occurs in 30%–40% of patients with cirrhosis. It causes a spectrum of symptoms ranging from mild fluctuating cognitive impairment to coma. The degree of encephalopathy can be graded from 1 to 4, and this is useful in assessing progression or response to therapy (see Box 24.10). The earliest features are very mild and easily overlooked, but as the condition becomes more severe, inability to concentrate, delirium, disorientation, drowsiness, slurring of speech and eventually coma develop. Seizures are rare. Examination usually shows a flapping tremor (asterixis), inability to perform simple mental arithmetic tasks or to draw objects such as a star (constructional apraxia, p. 861) and, as the condition progresses, hyper-reflexia and bilateral extensor plantar responses. Hepatic encephalopathy rarely causes focal neurological signs; if these are present, other causes must be sought. Fetor hepaticus, a sweet musty odour to the breath, is usually present but is more a sign of liver failure and portosystemic shunting than of hepatic encephalopathy. Rarely, chronic hepatic encephalopathy (hepatocerebral degeneration) gives rise to variable combinations of cerebellar dysfunction, Parkinsonian syndromes, spastic paraplegia and dementia.

Many conditions can cause similar presentations to encephalopathy. Simple delirium needs to be differentiated from infection, alcohol withdrawal and Wernicke's encephalopathy, and coma from subdural haematoma, which can occur after a fall, especially in alcohol misuse (Box 24.26). When an episode develops acutely, a precipitating factor may be found (Box 24.27).

Pathophysiology

Hepatic encephalopathy is thought to be due to a disturbance of brain function provoked by circulating gut-derived neurotoxins that are normally metabolised by the liver and excluded from the systemic circulation. Affected patients usually have evidence of both liver failure and portosystemic shunting of blood, but the balance between these varies between individuals. Some degree of liver failure is a key factor, as portosystemic shunting of blood alone hardly ever causes encephalopathy. The 'neurotoxins' causing encephalopathy are unknown but are thought to be mainly nitrogenous substances produced in the gut, at least in part by bacterial action. Ammonia has traditionally been considered an important factor, but the correlation between serum ammonia levels and encephalopathy is poor. Recent interest has focused on γ-aminobutyric acid (GABA) as a mediator, along with octopamine, amino acids, mercaptans and fatty acids that can act as neurotransmitters. The brain in cirrhosis may also be sensitised to other factors, such as drugs that can precipitate hepatic encephalopathy (see Box 24.27). Disruption of the function of the blood–brain barrier is a feature of acute hepatic failure and may lead to cerebral oedema.

---

i | **24.26 Differential diagnosis of hepatic encephalopathy**

- Intracranial bleed (subdural/extradural haematoma)
- Drug or alcohol intoxication
- Delirium tremens/alcohol withdrawal
- Wernicke's encephalopathy
- Primary psychiatric disorders
- Hypoglycaemia
- Neurological Wilson's disease
- Post-ictal state

---

i | **24.27 Factors precipitating hepatic encephalopathy**

- Drugs (especially sedatives, antidepressants)
- Dehydration (including diuretics, paracentesis)
- Portosystemic shunting
- Infection
- Hypokalaemia
- Hyponatraemia
- Constipation
- ↑Protein load (including gastrointestinal bleeding)

Investigations

The diagnosis can usually be made clinically; when doubt exists, an electroencephalogram shows diffuse slowing of the normal alpha waves with eventual development of delta waves. The arterial ammonia is usually increased in patients with hepatic encephalopathy. Increased concentrations can, however, occur in the absence of clinical encephalopathy, rendering this investigation of little diagnostic value.

Management

The principles are to treat or remove precipitating causes (Box 24.27) and to suppress the production of neurotoxins by bacteria in the bowel. Lactulose (15–30 mL 3 times daily) is increased gradually until the bowels are moving twice daily. It produces an osmotic laxative effect, reduces the pH of the colonic content, thereby limiting colonic ammonia absorption, and promotes the incorporation of nitrogen into bacteria. Phosphate enemas may be required in patients where the oral route is compromised or in patients with refractory constipation. Rifaximin (550 mg twice daily) is a well-tolerated, non-absorbed antibiotic that acts by reducing the bacterial content of the bowel and is effective in reducing episodes of recurrent hepatic encephalopathy. There is some evidence to support the amino acid combination l-ornithine l-arginine (LOLA) in lowering ammonia levels and improving encephalopathy. In cases of reduced conscious level, endotracheal intubation may be required for airway protection. Dietary protein restriction is no longer recommended because it can

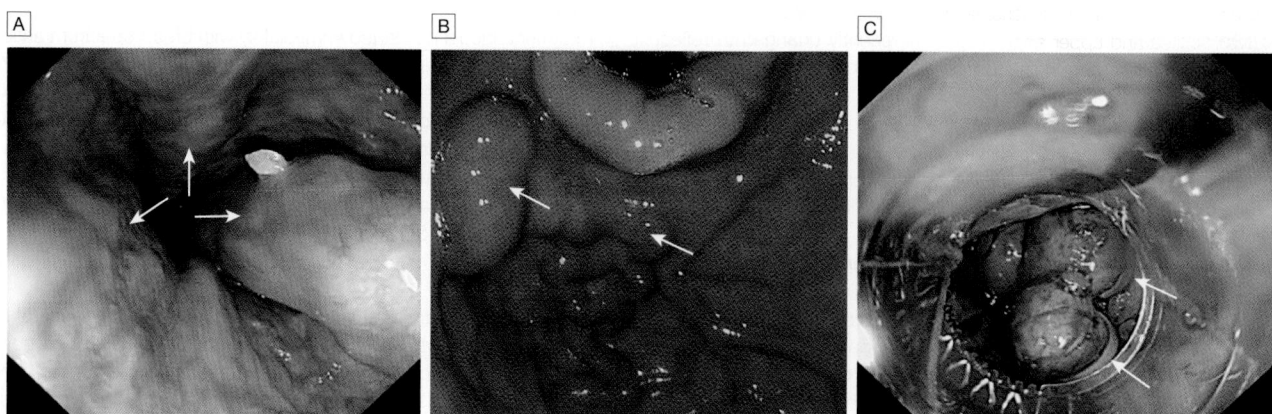

Fig. 24.17 Varices: endoscopic views. [A] Oesophageal varices (arrows) at the lower end of the oesophagus with a prominent white fibrin plug at the site of recent haemorrhage. [B] Gastric varices (arrows). [C] Appearance of oesophageal varices following application of strangulating bands (band ligation, arrows).

lead to a worsening nutritional state in already malnourished patients. Chronic or refractory encephalopathy is one of the main indications for liver transplantation.

Variceal bleeding

Acute upper gastrointestinal haemorrhage from gastro-oesophageal varices (Fig. 24.17) is common in chronic liver disease. Investigation and management are discussed on page 797 and the specific management of variceal bleeding on page 882.

Cirrhosis

Cirrhosis is characterised by diffuse hepatic fibrosis and nodule formation. It can occur at any age, has significant morbidity and is an important cause of premature death. It is the most common cause of portal hypertension. Worldwide, the most common causes are chronic viral hepatitis, prolonged excessive alcohol consumption and NAFLD, but any condition leading to persistent or recurrent hepatocyte injury may lead to cirrhosis. The causes of cirrhosis are listed in Box 24.28.

Cirrhosis may also occur in prolonged biliary injury, as is found in primary biliary cholangitis (PBC), primary sclerosing cholangitis (PSC) and post-surgical biliary strictures. Persistent impairment of venous return from the liver, such as is found in sinusoidal obstruction syndrome (SOS; veno-occlusive disease), Budd–Chiari syndrome and cardiac hepatopathy, can also result in cirrhosis.

Pathophysiology

Following liver injury, stellate cells in the space of Disse (see Fig. 24.3) are activated by cytokines produced by Kupffer cells and hepatocytes. This transforms the stellate cell into a myofibroblast-like cell, capable of producing collagen, pro-inflammatory cytokines and other mediators that promote hepatocyte damage and tissue fibrosis (see Fig. 24.4).

Cirrhosis is technically a histological diagnosis (Fig. 24.18), although most cases will be diagnosed on a combination of imaging, clinical signs and fibrosis markers. Fibrosis evolves over years, and the progression can be described semi-quantitatively (Fig. 24.19). Fibrosis and widespread hepatocyte loss lead to distortion of the normal liver architecture that disrupts the hepatic vasculature, causing portosystemic shunts. These changes usually affect the whole liver, but in biliary cirrhosis (e.g. PBC) they can be patchy.

Clinical features

The clinical presentation is highly variable. Some patients are asymptomatic and the diagnosis is made incidentally at ultrasound or at surgery. Others present with isolated hepatomegaly, splenomegaly, signs of portal hypertension or hepatic insufficiency. When symptoms are present, they are often non-specific and include weakness, fatigue, muscle cramps, weight loss, anorexia, nausea and upper abdominal discomfort (Box 24.29). Cirrhosis will occasionally present because of shortness of breath due to a large right pleural effusion, or with hepatopulmonary syndrome (p. 909).

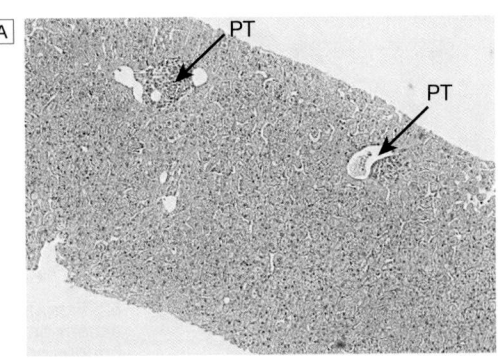

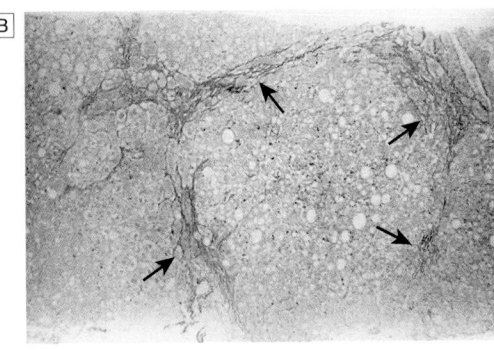

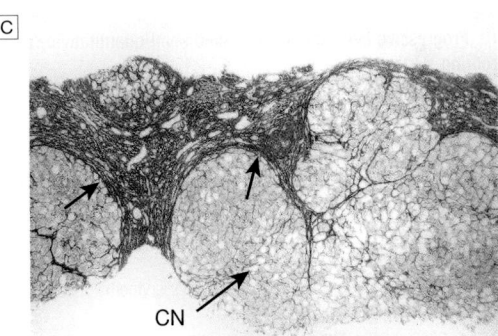

Fig. 24.18 Histological features in normal liver, hepatic fibrosis and cirrhosis. **A** Normal liver. Columns of hepatocytes 1–2 cells thick radiate from the portal tracts (PT) to the central veins. The portal tract contains a normal intralobular bile duct branch of the hepatic artery and portal venous radical. **B** Bridging fibrosis (stained pink, arrows) spreading out around the hepatic vein and single liver cells (pericellular) and linking adjacent portal tracts and hepatic veins. **C** A cirrhotic liver. The liver architecture is disrupted. The normal arrangement of portal tracts and hepatic veins is now lost and nodules of proliferating hepatocytes are broken up by strands of pink-/orange-staining fibrous tissue (arrows) forming cirrhotic nodules (CN).

24

Hepatomegaly is common when the cirrhosis is due to alcoholic liver disease or haemochromatosis. Progressive hepatocyte destruction and fibrosis gradually reduce liver size as the disease progresses in other causes of cirrhosis. The liver is often hard, irregular and non-tender. Jaundice is mild when it first appears and is due primarily to a failure to excrete bilirubin. Palmar erythema (redness over the thenar and hypothenar eminences) can be seen early in the disease but is of limited diagnostic value, as it occurs in many other conditions associated with a hyper-dynamic circulation, including pregnancy, as well as being found in some healthy people. Spider telangiectasias (or spider naevi) occur and comprise a central arteriole (that occasionally raises the skin surface), from which small vessels radiate. They blanch with pressure and refill from the centre outwards, are usually found on the hands, face and upper chest. One or two small spider telangiectasias may be present in up to 15% of young healthy adults and may occur transiently in greater numbers in the third trimester of pregnancy, but otherwise multiple spider telangiectasias are a strong

---

24.28 Causes of cirrhosis

- Alcohol
- Chronic viral hepatitis (B or C)
- Non-alcoholic fatty liver disease
- Immune:
  - Primary sclerosing cholangitis
  - Autoimmune liver disease
- Biliary:
  - Primary biliary cholangitis
  - Secondary biliary cirrhosis
  - Cystic fibrosis
- Genetic:
  - Haemochromatosis
  - Wilson's disease
  - Alpha-1-antitrypsin deficiency
- Cryptogenic (unknown – 15%)
- Chronic venous outflow obstruction
- Cardiac hepatopathy with chronic hepatic congestion
- Any chronic liver disease

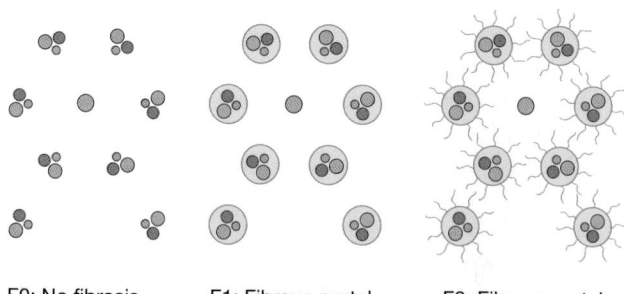

F0: No fibrosis
F1: Fibrous portal expansion
F2: Fibrous portal expansion with few bridges or septa

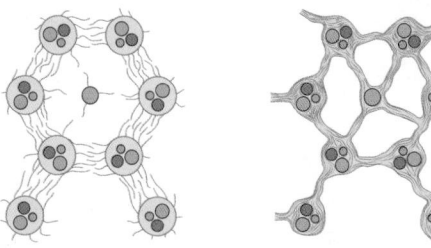

F3: Severe fibrosis with numerous bridges or septa
F4: Cirrhosis

Fig. 24.19 Progressive liver fibrosis assessed semi-quantitatively using Metavir scoring system.

---

i   24.29 Clinical features of hepatic cirrhosis

- Hepatomegaly (although liver may also be small)
- Jaundice
- Ascites
- Circulatory changes: spider telangiectasia, palmar erythema
- Endocrine changes: loss of libido, hair loss
    Men: gynaecomastia, testicular atrophy, impotence
    Women: breast atrophy, irregular menses, amenorrhoea
- Haemorrhagic tendency: bruises, purpura, epistaxis
- Portal hypertension: splenomegaly, collateral vessels, variceal bleeding
- Hepatic encephalopathy
- Other features: pigmentation (haemochromatosis), Dupuytren's contracture (alcohol excess)

---

indicator of liver disease. Florid spider telangiectasia and gynaecomastia are most common in alcohol-related cirrhosis, possibly related to phyto-oestrogens in alcoholic drinks. Pigmentation is most striking in haemochromatosis and in any cirrhosis associated with prolonged cholestasis. Clubbing of the fingers and toes is not a sign of cirrhosis but is seen in combination with hypoxia in hepatopulmonary syndrome.

Endocrine changes are noticed more readily in men, who show loss of male hair distribution and testicular atrophy. Gynaecomastia is common and can be due to drugs such as spironolactone. Easy bruising becomes more frequent as cirrhosis advances.

Splenomegaly and collateral vessel formation are features of portal hypertension, which occurs in more advanced disease (see below).

Jaundice, ascites, encephalopathy and variceal bleeding signify advanced disease, and are associated with a worse prognosis. The term 'hepatic decompensation' or 'decompensated liver disease' is often used when any of these are present.

Other clinical and laboratory features may be present (Box 24.30); these include peripheral oedema, renal failure, and hypoalbuminaemia and coagulation abnormalities due to defective protein synthesis.

---

i   24.30 Features of chronic liver failure

- Worsening synthetic liver function:
    Prolonged prothrombin time
    Low albumin
- Jaundice
- Variceal bleeding
- Hepatic encephalopathy
- Ascites:
    Spontaneous bacterial peritonitis
    Hepatorenal failure

Anaemia is common and often multifactorial, due to a combination of chronic inflammation, bone marrow suppression, haemolysis or chronic blood loss.

Management

This includes treatment of the underlying cause, maintenance of nutrition and treatment of complications, including ascites, hepatic encephalopathy, portal hypertension and varices.

Nutrition in cirrhosis

Malnutrition is a frequent complication, affecting up to 50% of patients with decompensated cirrhosis. Loss of muscle mass (sarcopenia) is associated with a higher rate of complications including infections, encephalopathy and ascites. Although BMI is the most widely used measure of nutritional status, sarcopenia can coexist with obesity especially in patients with NAFLD. Handgrip strength is a simple and inexpensive way to assess muscle function, and predicts morbidity and mortality in cirrhosis. Daily calorie intake should be no lower than 35 kcal/kg body weight with a daily protein intake of 1.2–1.5 g/kg. A late evening snack will help to minimise overnight fasting which could otherwise trigger a catabolic state in cirrhosis. If patients are unable to achieve adequate oral intake, enteral feeding should be considered.

Screening for complications

Once the diagnosis of cirrhosis is made, endoscopy should be considered to screen for oesophageal varices. As cirrhosis is associated with an increased risk of hepatocellular carcinoma, patients should be placed under regular surveillance for it. Cirrhosis is associated with an increased risk of osteoporosis and associated fractures, and bone mineral density measurement is recommended.

Chronic liver failure due to cirrhosis can also be treated by liver transplantation. This currently accounts for about three-quarters of all liver transplants.

Prognosis

Most chronic liver diseases run a gradually progressive course, although many patients present with advanced disease and/or serious complications that carry a high mortality. Prognosis is more favourable when the underlying cause can be corrected. Cirrhosis can be categorised into two prognostic groups: compensated and decompensated. Decompensated cirrhosis is defined by the presence of complications, including ascites, variceal bleeding, jaundice and encephalopathy, which are the main determinants of patient survival. Compensated patients have a relatively good prognosis with median survival >12 years. However, in decompensated cirrhosis median survival is around 2 years, albeit with significant patient-to-patient variability.

Raised bilirubin, low albumin and prolonged PT reflect impaired liver function. Along with renal dysfunction and hyponatraemia, these are all bad prognostic features (Box 24.31 and Fig. 24.20). Prognostic scores including Child–Pugh and MELD (Model for End-stage Liver Disease) scores can be used to assess prognosis in chronic liver disease. MELD is a complex algorithm including serum creatinine, serum bilirubin and INR (Box 24.32). The MELD-Na score incorporates serum sodium into this calculation and provides better prognostic accuracy in predicting mortality in patients awaiting liver transplantation. The UKELD (United Kingdom Model of End-stage Liver Disease) score is based on the same variables as MELD-Na and is used in the United Kingdom to determine the need for liver transplantation. A score ≥49 indicates a 9% 1-year risk of death and is the minimum score required for listing for liver transplantation for liver failure. Although these scores give a guide to prognosis, the course of cirrhosis is unpredictable, being heavily influenced by the incidence of sporadic decompensating events (e.g. sepsis, variceal bleeding, etc.).

24.31 Child–Pugh classification of prognosis in cirrhosis

Score	1	2	3
Encephalopathy	None	Mild	Marked
Bilirubin (μmol/L (*mg/dL*))*			
Primary biliary cholangitis/sclerosing cholangitis	< 68 (*4*)	68–170 (*4–10*)	>170 (*10*)
Other causes of cirrhosis	<34 (*2*)	34–50 (*2–3*)	>50 (*3*)
Albumin (g/L (*g/dL*))	>35 (*3.5*)	28–35 (*2.8–3.5*)	<28 (*2.8*)
Prothrombin time (secs prolonged)	< 4	4–6	> 6
Ascites	None	Mild	Marked
Add the individual scores: <7 = Child's A, 7–9 = Child's B, >9 = Child's C			

*To convert bilirubin in μmol/L to mg/dL, divide by 17.

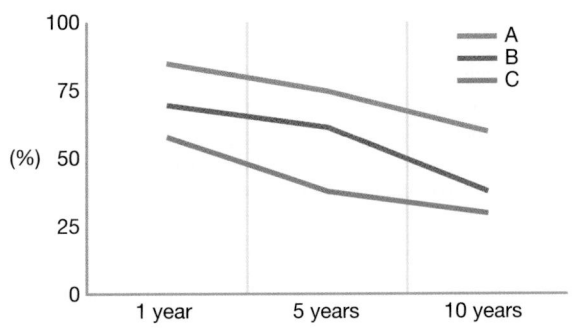

Fig. 24.20 Survival in cirrhosis by Child–Pugh score.

24.32 One-year survival rate depending on MELD score

MELD score	1-year survival (%)	
	No complications	Complications*
< 9	97	90
10–19	90	85
20–29	70	65
30–39	70	50
MELD from SI units		
10×(0.378 [ln serum bilirubin (μmol/L)] + 1.12 [ln INR] + 0.957 [ln serum creatinine (μmol/L)] + 0.643)		
MELD from non-SI units		
3.8 [ln serum bilirubin (mg/dL)] + 11.2 [ln INR] + 9.3 [ln serum creatinine (mg/dL)] + 6.4		
ln = natural log. To calculate online, go to https://optn.transplant.hrsa.gov/resources/allocation-calculators/meld-calculator/		

*'Complications' means the presence of ascites, encephalopathy or variceal bleeding.
(INR = International Normalised Ratio; MELD = Model for End-stage Liver Disease)

Acute on chronic liver failure

Acute on chronic liver failure (ACLF) is a term used to describe acute decompensation of chronic liver disease with features of liver failure (jaundice and coagulopathy) and other extra-hepatic organ failures. It is associated with a high short-term mortality. Common triggering events include alcoholic hepatitis, systemic infection or viral hepatitis. However up to 40% of patients have no identifiable precipitant. Persistent inflammation and immune dysfunction results in a systemic inflammatory response syndrome leading to extra-hepatic organ failure. The number of extra-hepatic organs involved determines prognosis. The 28-day mortality with single organ failure (typically renal failure or hepatic encephalopathy) is 23%, increasing to 32% in patients with two organ failures and >75% in patients with three or more organ failures. Management involves identification and treatment of the precipitating event and organ support as required.

Portal hypertension

Portal hypertension frequently complicates cirrhosis but has other causes. The normal hepatic venous pressure gradient (HVPG – difference between the wedged hepatic venous pressure (WHVP) and free hepatic venous pressure (FHVP); see below) is 5–6 mmHg. Clinically significant portal hypertension is present when the gradient exceeds 10 mmHg and risk of variceal bleeding increases beyond a gradient of 12 mmHg. Causes are classified in accordance with the main sites of obstruction to blood flow in the portal venous system (Fig. 24.21). Extrahepatic portal vein obstruction is the usual source of portal hypertension in childhood and adolescence, while cirrhosis causes at least 90% of cases of portal hypertension in adults in developed countries. Schistosomiasis is the most common cause of portal hypertension worldwide but is infrequent outside endemic areas, such as Egypt.

Clinical features

The clinical features result principally from portal venous congestion and collateral vessel formation (Box 24.33). Splenomegaly is a cardinal finding and a diagnosis of portal hypertension is unusual when splenomegaly cannot be detected clinically or by ultrasonography. The spleen is rarely enlarged more than 5 cm below the left costal margin in adults but more marked splenomegaly can occur in childhood and adolescence. Collateral vessels may be visible on the anterior abdominal wall and occasionally several radiate from the umbilicus to form a 'caput medusae' (p. 860). Rarely, a large umbilical collateral vessel has a blood flow sufficient to give a venous hum on auscultation (Cruveilhier–Baumgarten syndrome). The most important collateral vessel formation occurs in the oesophagus and stomach, as this can be a source of severe bleeding. Rectal varices also cause bleeding and are often mistaken for haemorrhoids (which are no more common in portal hypertension than in the general population). Fetor hepaticus results from portosystemic shunting of blood, which allows mercaptans to pass directly to the lungs.

Ascites occurs as a result of renal sodium retention and portal hypertension that may be due, for example, to post-hepatic causes (hepatic outflow obstruction, p. 875) or cirrhosis.

The most important consequence of portal hypertension is variceal bleeding, which commonly arises from oesophageal varices located within 3–5 cm of the gastro-oesophageal junction, or from gastric varices. The size of the varices, endoscopic variceal features such as red spots and stripes, high portal pressure and liver failure are all factors that predispose to bleeding. Drugs capable of causing mucosal erosion, such as salicylates and NSAIDs, can also precipitate bleeding. Variceal bleeding is often severe, and recurrent if preventative treatment is not given.

24

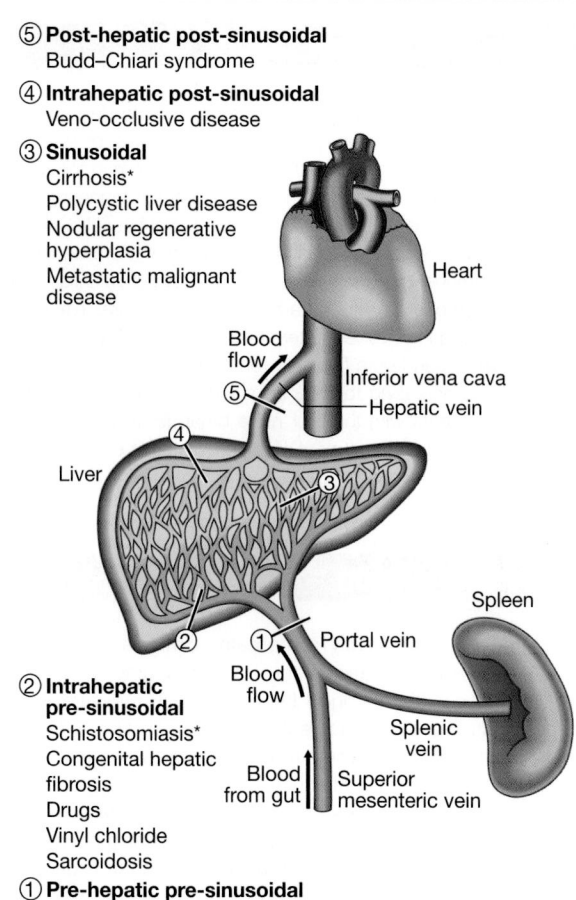

⑤ **Post-hepatic post-sinusoidal**
Budd–Chiari syndrome

④ **Intrahepatic post-sinusoidal**
Veno-occlusive disease

③ **Sinusoidal**
Cirrhosis*
Polycystic liver disease
Nodular regenerative
hyperplasia
Metastatic malignant
disease

② **Intrahepatic
pre-sinusoidal**
Schistosomiasis*
Congenital hepatic
fibrosis
Drugs
Vinyl chloride
Sarcoidosis

① **Pre-hepatic pre-sinusoidal**
Portal vein thrombosis due to sepsis (umbilical,
portal pyaemia) or procoagulopathy or secondary
to cirrhosis
Abdominal trauma including surgery

Fig. 24.21 Classification of portal hypertension according to site of vascular obstruction. *Most common cause. Note that splenic vein occlusion can also follow pancreatitis, leading to gastric varices.

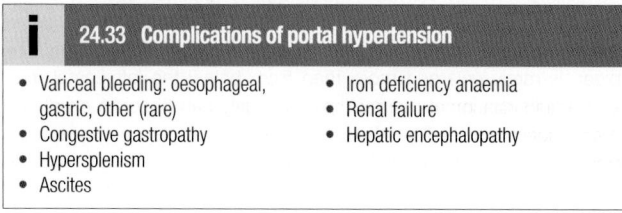

i 24.33 Complications of portal hypertension

- Variceal bleeding: oesophageal, gastric, other (rare)
- Congestive gastropathy
- Hypersplenism
- Ascites
- Iron deficiency anaemia
- Renal failure
- Hepatic encephalopathy

Pathophysiology

Increased portal vascular resistance leads to a gradual reduction in the flow of portal blood to the liver and simultaneously to the development of collateral vessels, allowing portal blood to bypass the liver and enter the systemic circulation directly. Portosystemic shunting occurs, particularly in the gastrointestinal tract and especially the distal oesophagus, stomach and rectum, in the anterior abdominal wall, and in the renal, lumbar, ovarian and testicular vasculature. Stomal varices can also occur at the site of an ileostomy. As collateral vessel formation progresses, more than half of the portal blood flow may be shunted directly to the systemic circulation. Increased portal flow contributes to portal hypertension but is not the dominant factor.

Investigations

The diagnosis is often made clinically. Portal venous pressure measurements are rarely needed for clinical assessment or routine management but can be used to confirm portal hypertension and to differentiate sinusoidal and pre-sinusoidal forms. Pressure measurements are made by using a balloon catheter inserted using the transjugular route (via the inferior vena cava into a hepatic vein and then hepatic venule) to measure the WHVP. This is an indirect measurement of portal vein pressure. Thrombocytopenia is common due to hypersplenism, and platelet counts are usually in the region of 100×10^9/L; values below 50×10^9/L are uncommon. Leucopenia occurs occasionally but anaemia is seldom attributed directly to hypersplenism.

Endoscopy is the most useful investigation to determine whether gastro-oesophageal varices are present (see Fig. 24.17). When cirrhosis is diagnosed, endoscopy should be performed to screen for oesophageal varices (and repeated every 2–3 years if initially absent). However, this may not be needed in patients with a normal platelet count and low liver stiffness (<20 kPa) who are at low risk of significant varices. Ultrasonography often shows features of portal hypertension, such as splenomegaly and collateral vessels, and can sometimes indicate the cause, such as cirrhosis or portal vein thrombosis. CT and magnetic resonance angiography can identify the extent of portal vein clot and check hepatic vein patency.

Management

Acute upper gastrointestinal haemorrhage from gastro-oesophageal varices is a common manifestation of chronic liver disease. In the presence of portal hypertension, the risk of a variceal bleed occurring within 2 years varies from 7% for small varices up to 30% for large varices. The mortality following a variceal bleed has improved to around 15% overall but is still about 45% in those with poor liver function (i.e. Child–Pugh C).

The management of portal hypertension is largely focused on the prevention and/or control of variceal haemorrhage. It is important to remember, though, that bleeding can also result from peptic ulceration, which is more common in patients with liver disease than in the general population. The investigation and management of gastrointestinal bleeding are dealt with in more detail on page 797.

Primary prevention of variceal bleeding

If non-bleeding varices are identified at endoscopy, non-selective β-adrenoceptor antagonist (β-blocker) therapy with propranolol (80–160 mg/day) or nadolol (40–240 mg/day) is effective in reducing portal venous pressure. Administration of these drugs at doses that reduce the heart rate by 25% has been shown to be effective in the primary prevention of variceal bleeding. In patients with cirrhosis, treatment with propranolol reduces variceal bleeding by 47% (number needed to treat for benefit (NNT$_B$) 10), death from bleeding by 45% (NNT$_B$ 25) and overall mortality by 22% (NNT$_B$ 16). The efficacy of β-blockers in primary prevention is similar to that of prophylactic banding, which may also be considered, particularly in patients who are unable to tolerate or adhere to β-blocker therapy. Carvedilol, a non-cardioselective vasodilating β-blocker, is also effective and may be better tolerated at doses of 6.25–12.5 mg/day.

Management of acute variceal bleeding

The priority in acute bleeding is to restore the circulation, not least because shock reduces liver blood flow and causes further deterioration of liver function. However, restrictive transfusion (aiming for a haemoglobin level >70 g/L) is associated with better outcomes than liberal transfusion. The source of bleeding should always be confirmed by endoscopy because about 20% of patients are bleeding from non-variceal lesions. Management of acute variceal bleeding is described in Box 24.34 and illustrated in Fig. 24.22. All patients with cirrhosis and gastrointestinal bleeding should receive prophylactic broad-spectrum antibiotics, such as intravenous cephalosporin or piperacillin/tazobactam, because sepsis is common and treatment with antibiotics improves survival. The measures used to control acute variceal bleeding include vasoactive medications (e.g. terlipressin), endoscopic therapy (banding), balloon tamponade and TIPSS.

Pharmacological reduction of portal venous pressure Terlipressin is a synthetic vasopressin analogue that, in contrast to vasopressin, can be given by intermittent injection rather than continuous infusion. It reduces

24.34 Emergency management of bleeding	
Management	**Reason**
Intravenous fluids	To replace extracellular volume
Vasopressor (terlipressin)*	To reduce portal pressure, acute bleeding and risk of early rebleeding
Prophylactic antibiotics (cephalosporin IV)	To reduce incidence of spontaneous bacterial peritonitis
Emergency endoscopy	To confirm variceal rather than ulcer bleed
Variceal band ligation	To stop bleeding
Proton pump inhibitor	To prevent peptic ulcers
Phosphate enema and/or lactulose	To prevent hepatic encephalopathy

*Caution in patients with significant coronary artery, peripheral or other vascular disease.

portal blood flow and/or intrahepatic resistance and hence brings down portal pressure. It lowers mortality in the setting of acute variceal bleeding. The dose of terlipressin is 2 mg intravenously 4 times daily until bleeding stops, and then 1 mg 4 times daily for up to 72 hours. Caution is needed in patients with severe ischaemic heart disease or peripheral vascular disease because of the drug's vasoconstrictor properties. In countries where terlipressin is not available, octreotide is a frequently used alternative.

Variceal ligation ('banding') This is the most widely used initial treatment and is undertaken, if possible, at the time of diagnostic endoscopy (see Fig. 24.17C). It stops variceal bleeding in over 90% of patients and can be repeated if bleeding recurs. Band ligation involves the varices being sucked into a cap placed on the end of the endoscope, allowing them to be occluded with a tight rubber band. The occluded varix subsequently sloughs with variceal obliteration. Banding is repeated every 2–4 weeks until all varices are obliterated. Regular follow-up endoscopy is required to identify and treat any recurrence of varices. Band ligation has fewer side-effects than sclerotherapy, a technique in which varices were injected with a sclerosing agent, and has largely replaced it. Prophylactic acid suppression with proton pump inhibitors may reduce the risk of secondary bleeding from banding-induced ulceration.

In the case of gastric varices, banding is less effective and so endoscopic therapy relies on injection of agents such as thrombin or cyanoacrylate glue directly into the varix to induce thrombosis. Although highly effective, cyanoacrylate injection treatment may be complicated by 'glue embolism' to the lungs.

Active bleeding may make endoscopic therapy difficult. Protection of the patient's airway with endotracheal intubation aids the endoscopist, facilitating therapy and significantly reducing the risk of pulmonary aspiration.

Balloon tamponade This technique employs a Minnesota tube, which consists of two balloons that can be positioned in the fundus of the stomach and in the lower oesophagus, respectively (Fig. 24.23). Additional lumens allow contents to be aspirated from the stomach and from the oesophagus. This technique may be used in the event of life-threatening haemorrhage if early endoscopic therapy is not available or is unsuccessful.

Endotracheal intubation prior to tube insertion reduces the risk of pulmonary aspiration. The tube should be passed through the mouth into the stomach. The gastric balloon should be inflated with 200–250 mL of air, and gentle traction applied to compress the gastro-oesophageal junction. Inadvertent inflation in the oesophagus can result in oesophageal rupture so, ideally, the gastric balloon should be inflated under direct endoscopic vision. Tamponade of the gastro-oesophageal junction with the gastric balloon will almost always control bleeding from oesophageal

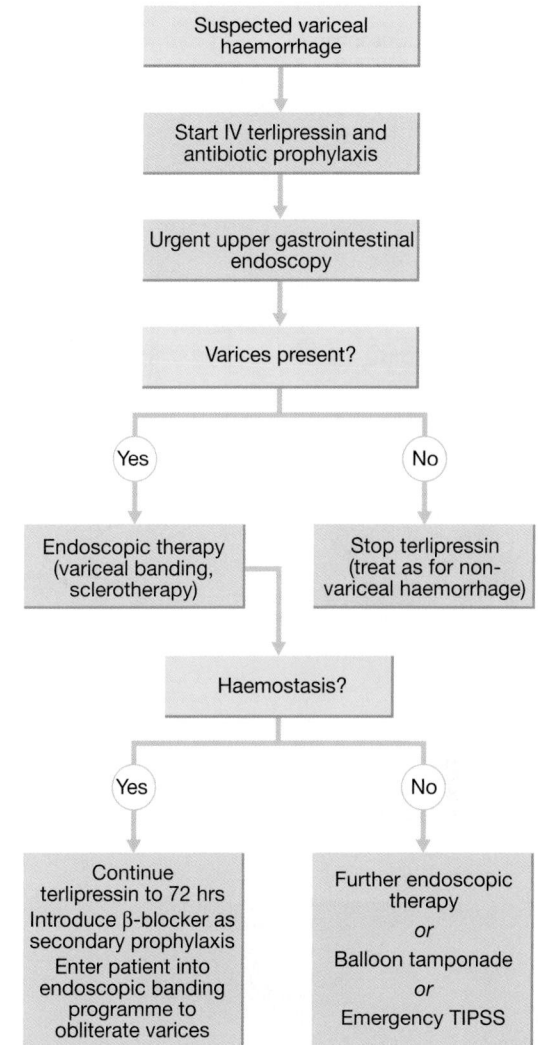

Fig. 24.22 Management of acute bleeding from oesophageal varices. (TIPSS = transjugular intrahepatic portosystemic stent shunt)

varices and inflation of the oesophageal balloon is rarely required. If the oesophageal balloon needs to be used because of continued bleeding, pressure should be monitored with a sphygmomanometer (to maintain < 40 mmHg) and it should be deflated for about 10 minutes every 3 hours to avoid oesophageal mucosal damage. Balloon tamponade is only a bridge to more definitive therapy. Novel endoscopic therapies such as self-expanding removable oesophageal stents and haemostatic powder spray also appear to be effective short-term alternatives in small case series.

TIPSS This technique uses a stent placed between the portal vein and the hepatic vein within the liver to provide a portosystemic shunt and reduce portal pressure (Fig. 24.24). It is carried out under radiological control via the internal jugular vein; prior patency of the portal vein must be determined angiographically, coagulation deficiencies may require correction with fresh frozen plasma, and antibiotic cover is provided. Successful shunt placement stops and prevents further variceal bleeding, and is an effective treatment for both oesophageal and gastric varices. Further bleeding necessitates investigation and treatment (e.g. angioplasty) because it is usually associated with shunt narrowing or occlusion. Hepatic encephalopathy occurs in up to a third of patients following TIPSS and may require reducing the shunt diameter. Although TIPSS is associated with less rebleeding than endoscopic therapy, survival is not improved.

24

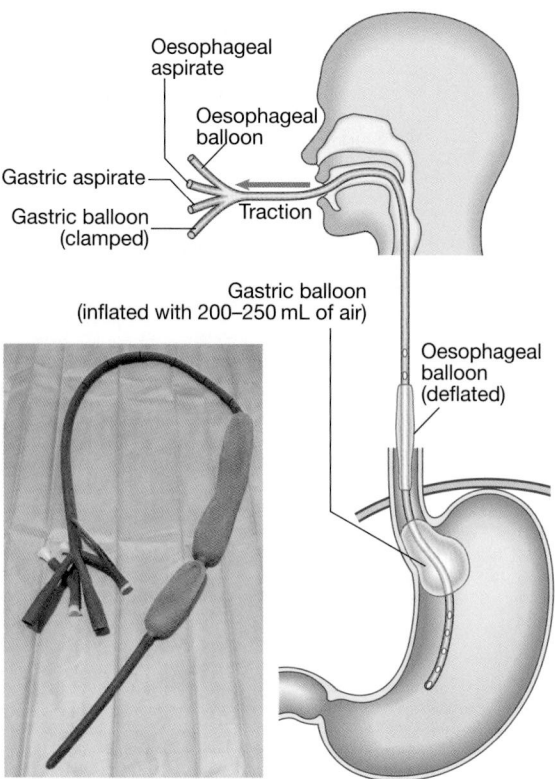

Fig. 24.23 **Minnesota tube.**

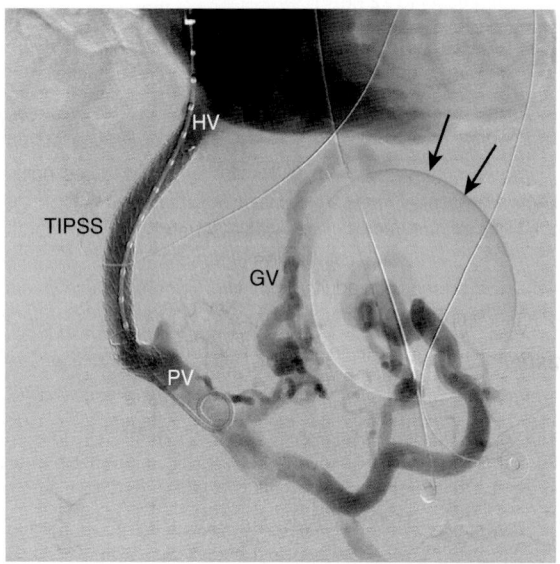

Fig. 24.24 **Transjugular intrahepatic portosystemic stent shunt (TIPSS).** X-ray showing placement of a TIPSS, allowing blood to flow from the portal vein (PV) into the hepatic vein (HV). Contrast can be also be seen in gastric varices (GV). Arrows show the outline of the gastric balloon of a Sengstaken tube.

Portosystemic shunt surgery Surgery prevents recurrent bleeding but carries a high mortality and often leads to encephalopathy. In practice, portosystemic shunts are now reserved for when other treatments have not been successful and are offered only to patients with good liver function.

Oesophageal transection Rarely, surgical transection of the varices may be performed as a last resort when bleeding cannot be controlled by other means but operative mortality is high.

Secondary prevention of variceal bleeding

Beta-blockers are used as a secondary measure to prevent recurrent variceal bleeding. Following successful endoscopic therapy, patients should be entered into an oesophageal banding programme with repeated sessions of therapy at 2–4-week intervals until the varices are obliterated. There is some evidence that early TIPSS after successful endoscopic therapy may improve survival in selected patients with advanced liver disease.

Congestive 'portal hypertensive' gastropathy

Long-standing portal hypertension causes chronic gastric congestion, which is recognisable at endoscopy as multiple areas of punctate erythema ('portal hypertensive gastropathy' or 'snakeskin gastropathy') in the proximal stomach. Similar lesions may also occur more distally in the gastrointestinal tract (enteropathy and colopathy). These areas may become eroded, causing oozing from multiple sites. Acute bleeding can occur but repeated minor bleeding causing iron deficiency anaemia is more common. Anaemia may be prevented by oral iron supplements but repeated blood transfusions can become necessary. Reduction of the portal pressure using propranolol (80–160 mg/day) is the best initial treatment. In selected cases TIPSS procedure can be considered.

Gastric antral vascular ectasia (GAVE) is an alternative cause of mucosal oozing in patients with cirrhosis. This is characterised by red spots in the distal stomach, often arranged in stripes around the pylorus ('watermelon stomach'). Therapy for GAVE is focused on endoscopic ablation using argon plasma coagulation (APC) or radiofrequency ablation (RFA).

Infections and the liver

The liver may be subject to a number of different infections. These include hepatotropic viral infections and bacterial and protozoal infections. Each has specific clinical features and requires targeted therapies.

Viral hepatitis

This must be considered in anyone presenting with hepatitic liver blood tests (high transaminases). The causes are listed in Box 24.35.

All these viruses cause illnesses that have similar clinical and pathological features and are frequently anicteric or even asymptomatic. They differ in their tendency to cause acute and chronic infections. The features of the major hepatitis viruses are shown in Box 24.36.

Clinical features of acute infection

A non-specific prodromal illness characterised by headache, myalgia, arthralgia, nausea and anorexia usually precedes the development of jaundice by a few days to 2 weeks. Vomiting and diarrhoea may follow and abdominal discomfort is common. Dark urine and pale stools may precede jaundice. There are usually few physical signs. The liver is often tender but only minimally enlarged. Occasionally, mild splenomegaly and

ⓘ	24.35 **Causes of viral hepatitis**
Common	
• Hepatitis A	• Hepatitis C
• Hepatitis B ± hepatitis D	• Hepatitis E
Less common	
• Cytomegalovirus	• Epstein–Barr virus
Rare	
• Herpes simplex	• Yellow fever

24.36 Features of the main hepatitis viruses

	Hepatitis A	Hepatitis B	Hepatitis C	Hepatitis D	Hepatitis E
Virus					
Group	Enterovirus	Hepadnavirus	Flavivirus	Incomplete virus	Calicivirus
Nucleic acid	RNA	DNA	RNA	RNA	RNA
Size (diameter)	27 nm	42 nm	30–38 nm	35 nm	27 nm
Incubation (weeks)	2–4	4–20	2–26	6–9	3–8
Spread*					
Faeces	Yes	No	No	No	Yes (1–2)
Ingestion of infected meat	No	No	No	No	Yes (3–4)
Blood	Uncommon	Yes	Yes	Yes	No
Saliva	Yes	Yes	Yes	Unknown	Unknown
Sexual	Uncommon	Yes	Uncommon	Yes	Unknown
Vertical	No	Yes	Uncommon	Yes	No
Chronic infection	No	Yes	Yes	Yes	No (except immune-compromised)
Prevention					
Active	Vaccine	Vaccine	No	Prevented by hepatitis B vaccination	No
Passive	Immune serum globulin	Hyperimmune serum globulin	No		No

*All body fluids are potentially infectious, although some (e.g. urine) are less infectious than others.

24.37 Complications of acute viral hepatitis

- Acute liver failure
- Cholestatic hepatitis (hepatitis A)
- Aplastic anaemia
- Chronic liver disease and cirrhosis (hepatitis B and C)
- Relapsing hepatitis

cervical lymphadenopathy are seen. These features are more frequent in children or those with Epstein–Barr virus (EBV) infection. Symptoms rarely last longer than 3–6 weeks. Complications may occur but are rare (Box 24.37).

Investigations

A hepatitic pattern of LFTs develops, with serum transaminases typically between 200 and 2000 U/L in an acute infection (usually lower and fluctuating in chronic infections). The ALP rarely exceeds twice the upper limit of normal. The plasma bilirubin and prothrombin time (PT) reflect the degree of liver damage. Prolongation of the PT rarely exceeds 25 seconds, except in rare cases of acute liver failure. The white cell count is usually normal with a relative lymphocytosis. Serological tests confirm the aetiology of the infection.

Management

Most individuals do not need hospital care. Drugs such as sedatives and narcotics, which are metabolised in the liver, should be avoided. Alcohol should not be taken during the acute illness. Elective surgery should be avoided in cases of acute viral hepatitis, as there is a risk of post-operative liver failure.

Liver transplantation is very rarely indicated for acute viral hepatitis complicated by liver failure.

Hepatitis A

The hepatitis A virus (HAV) belongs to the picornavirus group of enteroviruses. HAV is highly infectious and is spread by the faecal–oral route. Risk of infection is associated with a lack of safe water and poor sanitation. In occasional outbreaks, water and shellfish have been the vehicles of transmission. Infection may be asymptomatic or produce symptoms after an average incubation period of 28 days. The likelihood of symptoms relates to age, with most children under 6 years of age having no symptoms but most adults developing jaundice. Up to 30% of adults will have serological evidence of past infection but give no history of jaundice. Infected individuals excrete the virus in faeces for about 2–3 weeks before the onset of symptoms and then for a further 2 weeks or so.

In contrast to hepatitis B and C, chronic infection does not occur. Almost all cases will recover fully with lifelong immunity, but a very small proportion develop acute liver failure (0.1%) and may die. Infection in patients with pre-existing chronic liver disease may cause serious or life-threatening disease. In adults, a cholestatic phase with elevated ALP levels may complicate infection.

Investigations

Diagnosis of HAV infection is based on antibody testing. Only one HAV antigen has been found and infected people make an antibody to this antigen (anti-HAV). Anti-HAV immunoglobulin (Ig) M antibody is detectable in the blood 5–10 days before the onset of symptoms and falls to low levels within about 3 months of recovery, so is diagnostic of acute HAV infection. Anti-HAV IgG antibody persists for years after infection, and is a marker of previous HAV infection with resulting immunity.

Management

Infection in the community is best prevented by improving social conditions, especially overcrowding and poor sanitation. Individuals can be given substantial protection from infection by active immunisation with an inactivated virus vaccine. Immunisation should be considered for those at particular risk, such as people travelling to endemic areas, close contacts of HAV-infected patients, older individuals, those with other major disease (including chronic liver disease) and perhaps pregnant women.

Immediate protection can also be provided by immune serum globulin if this is given soon after exposure to the virus. The protective effect of immune serum globulin is attributed to its anti-HAV content. Intramuscular injection of immune serum globulin is recommended for close contacts of infected individuals who are less able to respond to

24

vaccination, such as those aged 60 years or over, immunocompromised individuals or those with chronic liver disease. It may also be effective in an outbreak of hepatitis, in a school or nursery, as injection of those at risk prevents secondary spread to families.

There is no role for antiviral drugs in the therapy of HAV infection.

Hepatitis B

The hepatitis B virus (HBV) consists of a core containing DNA and a DNA polymerase enzyme needed for virus replication, surrounded by surface protein (Fig. 24.25). The virus and an excess of its surface protein (known as hepatitis B surface antigen, HBsAg) circulate in the blood. The virus replicates and assembles within hepatocytes but is not directly cytotoxic; hepatocyte damage occurs during immune-mediated clearance of infected hepatocytes.

Hepatitis B is one of the most common causes of chronic liver disease and hepatocellular carcinoma worldwide. Approximately 250 million people have chronic HBV infection. There is large regional variation, with the highest rates seen in the Western Pacific and African regions.

Hepatitis B can cause acute or chronic infection. The risk of developing chronic HBV infection depends on the source and timing of exposure. Infections may occur via a number of routes (Box 24.38). In endemic areas, vertical transmission from mother to child in the perinatal period is the most common cause of infection and carries the highest risk of ongoing chronic infection (90%–95%). In contrast, exposure to HBV at an older age is much more likely to result in an acute hepatitis, with chronic infection developing in less than 5% of adult-acquired HBV.

In perinatal infection, adaptive immune responses to HBV may be absent initially, with apparent immunological tolerance. Although HBV-specific T-cells are detectable in this setting, they are weak and functionally impaired. The mechanisms underlying this are incompletely understood.

Chronic hepatitis can lead to cirrhosis or hepatocellular carcinoma, usually after decades of infection (Fig. 24.26). Chronic HBV infection is a dynamic process that can be divided into five phases (Box 24.39); these are not necessarily strictly sequential, however, and not all patients will go through all phases. Phases are considered as either 'infection' where circulating HBsAg is detectable but is not resulting in any current liver injury, or 'hepatitis' where this is accompanied by liver inflammation and fibrosis.

Investigations

Assessment of hepatitis B infection relies on looking at a combination of viral markers (surface antigen, e-antigen and viral load) and liver markers (ALT and fibrosis markers) to determine the stage of disease.

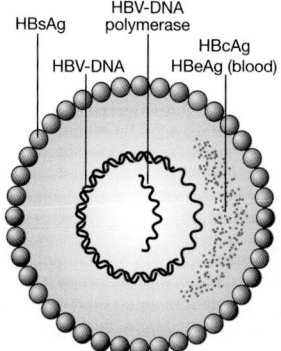

Fig. 24.25 Schematic diagram of the hepatitis B virus. Hepatitis B surface antigen (HBsAg) is a protein that makes up part of the viral envelope. Hepatitis B core antigen (HBcAg) is a protein that makes up the capsid or core part of the virus (found in the liver but not in blood). Hepatitis B e antigen (HBeAg) is part of the HBcAg that can be found in the blood and indicates infectivity. (HBV = hepatitis B virus)

24.38 Risk factors for the acquisition of hepatitis B infection

Vertical transmission
- Hepatitis B surface antigen (HBsAg)-positive mother (especially if e-antigen-positive)

Horizontal transmission
- Sexual transmission
- Intravenous drug use
- Infected unscreened blood products
- Tattoos/acupuncture needles
- Needlestick injury
- Sharing toothbrush/razor
- Close living quarters/playground play as a toddler (may contribute to high rate of horizontal transmission in Africa)

Serology

HBV contains several antigens to which infected persons can make immune responses (Fig. 24.27); these antigens and their antibodies are important in identifying the stage of HBV infection (see Box 24.39 and Box 24.40), in addition to direct assessment of viral load by polymerase chain reaction (PCR) for HBV DNA.

Hepatitis B surface antigen Hepatitis B surface antigen (HBsAg) is the main indicator of active infection, and a negative test for HBsAg makes HBV infection very unlikely. The exception is in acute liver failure from hepatitis B, where the liver damage is mediated by viral clearance and so HBsAg may be negative at presentation, with evidence of recent infection provided by the presence of hepatitis B core (anti-HBc) IgM (see below). In resolving acute HBV infection, antibody to HBsAg (anti-HBs) usually appears after about 3–6 months and persists for many years or perhaps permanently. Anti-HBs implies either a previous infection, in which case anti-HBc (see below) is usually also present, or previous vaccination, in which case anti-HBc is not present.

Hepatitis B core antigen Hepatitis B core antigen (HBcAg) is not found in the blood, but antibody to it (anti-HBc) appears early in the illness and rapidly reaches a high titre, which subsides gradually but then persists. Anti-HBc is initially of IgM type, with IgG antibody appearing later (see Fig. 24.27 and Box 24.40).

Hepatitis B e antigen Hepatitis B e antigen (HBeAg) is part of the core antigen that is detectable in the blood and can be used as an indicator of viral replication. Seroconversion to e antigen (i.e. loss of HBeAg and development of anti-HBe antibody) indicates a partial immune control of the virus and is associated with a significant drop in viral load. This typically occurs after 10–30 years in perinatally acquired infection, but within 3–6 months in adult-acquired acute infections.

Viral load and genotype

HBV-DNA can be measured by PCR in the blood. Viral loads are usually highest (in excess of 10^7 copies/mL) in HBeAg-positive infection, making this the most infectious phase. Once patients undergo HBeAg seroconversion, viral loads drop to less than 10^5 copies/mL in HBeAg-negative infection. Around 15%–20% of patients will subsequently develop further rises in viral load, due to mutations in the pre-core or core promoter region (Fig. 24.28). Such patients are classified as having HBeAg-negative chronic hepatitis.

Measurement of viral load is important in detecting flares of HBeAg-negative hepatitis and in monitoring response to antiviral therapy. Ten HBV genotypes (A–J) can also be identified using PCR. These affect the likelihood of response to pegylated interferon.

Management of acute hepatitis B

Full spontaneous recovery occurs in more than 95% of adults following acute HBV infection. Fulminant liver failure due to acute hepatitis B

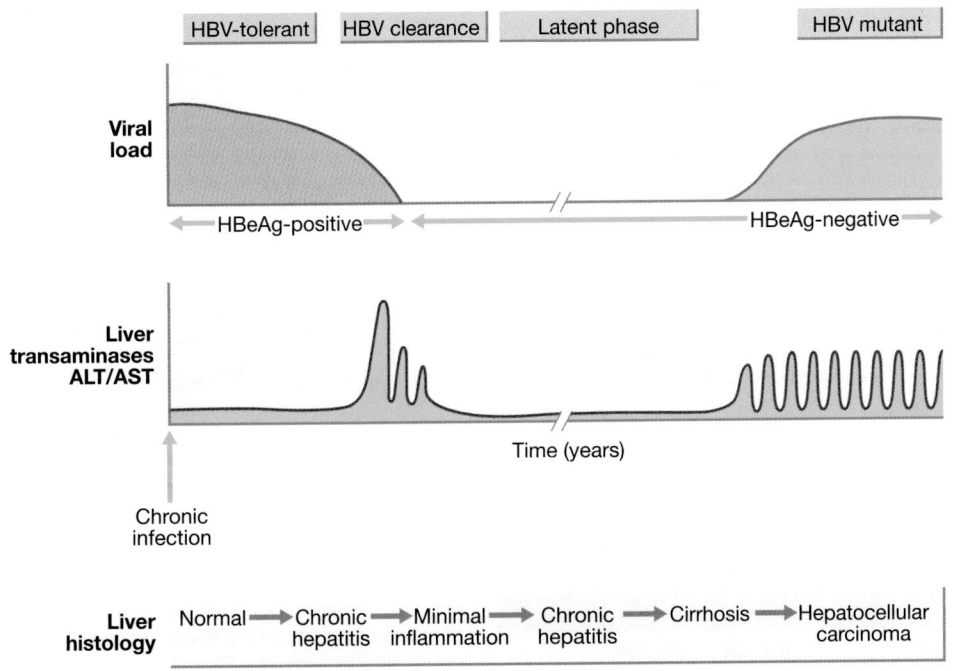

Fig. 24.26 Natural history of chronic hepatitis B virus (HBV) infection. There is an initial immunotolerant phase with high levels of virus and normal liver biochemistry. An immunological response to the virus then occurs, with elevation in serum transaminases, which causes liver damage: chronic hepatitis. If this response is sustained over many years and viral clearance does not occur promptly, chronic hepatitis may result in cirrhosis. In individuals with a successful immunological response, viral load falls, HBe antibody (HBeAg) develops and there is no further liver damage. Some individuals may subsequently develop HBV-DNA mutants that escape from immune regulation, and viral load again rises with further chronic hepatitis. Mutations in the core protein result in the virus's inability to secrete HBe antigen despite high levels of viral replication; such individuals have HBeAg-negative chronic hepatitis. (ALT = alanine aminotransferase; AST = aspartate aminotransferase)

i | 24.39 The five phases of chronic hepatitis B virus (HBV) infection

Phase	HBsAg	HBeAg	Viral load	ALT	Histology	Notes
HBeAg positive chronic infection	+	+	+++ ($>10^7$ IU/ml)	Normal	Normal/minimal necroinflammation	Prolonged in perinatally infected individuals; may be short or absent if infected as an adult. High viral load and so very infectious. Previously known as 'immune-tolerant'
HBeAg-positive chronic hepatitis	+	+	++ (10^4–10^7 IU/ml)	Raised	Moderate/severe necroinflammation	May last weeks or years. Risk of cirrhosis or HCC if prolonged. Previously known as 'immune-reactive'
HBeAg-negative chronic infection	+	−	+/− (<2000 IU/ml)	Normal	Normal/minimal necroinflammation	Low risk of cirrhosis or HCC in majority. Previously known as 'inactive carrier'.
HBeAg-negative chronic hepatitis	+	−	Fluctuating +/++ (>2000 IU/ml)	Raised/ fluctuating	Moderate/severe necroinflammation	May represent late immune reactivation or presence of 'pre-core mutant' HBV. High risk of cirrhosis or HCC
HBsAg-negative phase	−	−	−/±	Normal	Normal	Ultrasensitive techniques may detect low-level HBV DNA even after HBsAg loss

(HBeAg = hepatitis B e antigen; HBsAg = hepatitis B surface antigen; HCC = hepatocellular carcinoma)

24

occurs in fewer than 1% of cases but can be life-threatening and require liver transplantation. The remaining <5% develop chronic infection.

Treatment of acute HBV infection is supportive, with monitoring for acute liver failure. Antiviral therapy is usually only considered in those with evidence of severe liver injury with coagulopathy (INR > 1.5) or a protracted course with persistent symptoms for >4 weeks.

Recovery from acute HBV infection occurs within 6 months and is characterised by the appearance of antibody to viral antigens. Persistence of Persistence of HBeAg or HBsAg indicates chronic infection.

Management of chronic hepatitis B

Once hepatitis B infection has been present for more than 6 months, spontaneous clearance is uncommon. Most patients with chronic hepatitis B are asymptomatic and develop complications, such as cirrhosis

and hepatocellular carcinoma, only after many years (see Fig. 24.26). Fibrosis accumulates during periods of liver injury (the 'hepatitis' phases) and results in cirrhosis in 15%–20% of patients with chronic HBV over 5–20 years. The rate of progression to cirrhosis is higher in HBeAg-negative hepatitis (8%–10% incidence per annum) than HBeAg-positive hepatitis (2%–5% per annum).

The ideal goal of treatment would be to achieve long-term viral clearance with loss of HBsAg, but this is rarely achieved with current therapies. Instead, treatment is aimed at suppressing viral replication to prevent disease progression to cirrhosis or hepatocellular carcinoma. The goals of treatment are therefore HBeAg seroconversion, reduction in HBV-DNA and normalisation of the LFTs. Only a proportion (10%–40%) of patients with chronic hepatitis B will require treatment. This is usually targeted at those in the 'hepatitis' phases with high viral load and

Relative amount of product detectable

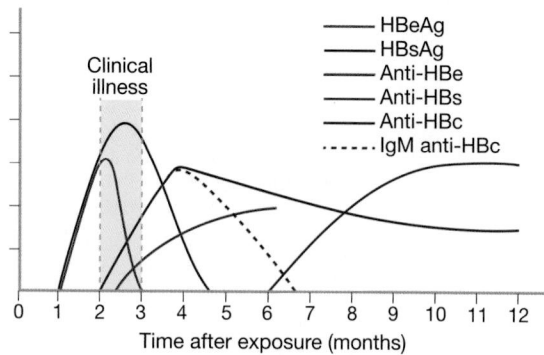

Fig. 24.27 Serological responses to hepatitis B virus infection. (anti-HBc = antibody to hepatitis B core antigen; anti-HBe = antibody to HBeAg; anti-HBs = antibody to HBsAg; HBeAg = hepatitis B e antigen; HBsAg = hepatitis B surface antigen; IgM = immunoglobulin M)

i	24.40 How to interpret the serological tests of acute hepatitis B virus infection				
Interpretation	**HBsAg**	**Anti-HBc IgM**	**Anti-HBc IgG**	**Anti-HBs**	
Incubation period	+	+	–	–	
Acute hepatitis					
Early	+	+	–	–	
Established	+	+	+	–	
Convalescence					
(3–6 months)	–	±	+	±	
(6–9 months)	–	–	+	+	
Post-infection	–	–	+	±	
Immunisation without infection	–	–	–	+	

+ = positive; – = negative; ± = present at low titre or absent.
(anti-HBc IgM/IgG = antibody to hepatitis B core antigen of immunoglobulin M/G type; anti-HBs = antibody to HBsAg; HBsAg = hepatitis B surface antigen)

accompanying liver injury, either in terms of necroinflammation (raised ALT) or established fibrosis (on biopsy or raised liver stiffness on transient elastography). All patients with cirrhosis should be treated to prevent decompensation. Treatment may also be initiated during pregnancy in the absence of liver injury to prevent mother-to-child transmission.

Two different types of drug are used to treat hepatitis B: direct-acting nucleoside/nucleotide analogues and pegylated interferon-alfa.

Direct-acting nucleoside/nucleotide antiviral agents

Orally administered nucleoside/nucleotide antiviral agents are the mainstay of therapy. These act by inhibiting the reverse transcription of pregenomic RNA to HBV-DNA by HBV-DNA polymerase but do not directly affect the covalently closed circular DNA (cccDNA) template for viral replication, and so relapse is common if treatment is withdrawn. One major concern is the selection of antiviral-resistant mutations with long-term treatment. This is particularly important with some of the older agents, such as lamivudine, as mutations induced by previous antiviral exposure may also induce resistance to newer agents. Entecavir and tenofovir (see below) are potent antivirals with a high barrier to genetic resistance and so are the most appropriate first-line agents.

Lamivudine Although initially effective, long-term therapy is often complicated by the development of HBV-DNA polymerase mutants (e.g. the 'YMDD variant'), which lead to viral resistance. These occur in around half of patients after 3 years and are characterised by a rise in viral load

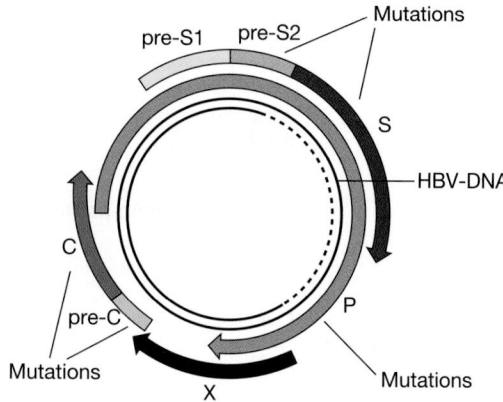

Fig. 24.28 The site of hepatitis B virus (HBV)-DNA mutations. HBV-DNA encodes four proteins: a DNA polymerase needed for viral replication (P), a surface protein (S), a core protein (C) and an X protein. The pre-C and C regions encode a core protein and an e antigen. Although mutations in the hepatitis B virus are frequent, certain mutations have important clinical consequences. Pre-C encodes a signal sequence needed for the C protein to be secreted from the liver cell into serum as e antigen. A mutation in the pre-core region leads to a failure of secretion of e antigen into serum, and so individuals have high levels of viral production but no detectable e antigen in the serum. Mutations can also occur in the surface protein and may lead to the failure of vaccination to prevent infection, since surface antibodies are produced against the native S protein. Mutations also occur in the DNA polymerase during antiviral treatment with lamivudine.

during treatment. Outside resource-limited settings, this agent is now seldom used for the treatment of HBV but may be used to prevent reactivation in patients with past HBV infection (HBsAg-negative but HBcAb-positive) if they are undergoing treatment with rituximab or chemotherapy.

Entecavir and tenofovir Monotherapy with entecavir or tenofovir is substantially more effective than lamivudine in reducing viral load in HBeAg-positive and HBeAg-negative chronic hepatitis. Antiviral resistance mutations occur very rarely, in <1% after 5 years of entecavir and with no evidence of resistance after 8 years of tenofovir. Both drugs have action against human immunodeficiency virus (HIV) and so their use as monotherapy is contraindicated in HIV-positive patients, as it may lead to HIV antiviral drug resistance. Current European guidelines advise that the other nucleoside/nucleotide antivirals should not be used as first-line monotherapy due to the induction of viral mutations, unless entecavir or tenofovir are not available or appropriate.

Pegylated interferon-alfa

Pegylated interferon-alfa (PEG-IFN) acts by augmenting the host immune response. This is most effective in patients with a pre-treatment low viral load and serum transaminases greater than twice the upper limit of normal. Treatment is for a finite period (typically around 1 year), and is associated with higher rates of HBsAg and HBeAg seroconversion than nucleoside/nucleotide agents but with greater side-effects. Interferon is contraindicated in the presence of cirrhosis, as it may cause a rise in serum transaminases and precipitate liver failure. In HBeAg-positive chronic hepatitis, PEG-IFN results in sustained HBeAG seroconversion in around 30%, and HBsAg seroconversion in 3%–5%. Response rates are higher in those with genotype A or B virus, and those with low viral load and high ALT. Sustained response rates are lower in HBeAg-negative chronic hepatitis.

Liver transplantation

Patients with advanced liver disease or hepatocellular carcinoma (HCC) may require liver transplantation. The use of nucleoside/nucleotide analogues post-transplant (with hepatitis B immunoglobulin in high-risk individuals) has made recurrent disease due to graft re-infection very uncommon, and outcomes are comparable with other indications.

Hepatocellular carcinoma risk

Chronic HBV infection is associated with an increased risk of hepatocellular carcinoma, even in the absence of cirrhosis. This risk increases with age, male sex, smoking, diabetes, family history of HCC and high viral loads. A number of scoring systems (such as REACH-B and PAGE-B) have been developed to identify high-risk non-cirrhotic patients who may benefit from HCC screening.

Prevention

Individuals are most infectious when high levels of HBV-DNA are present in the blood, typically in the HBeAg-positive infection phase. HBV-DNA can be found in saliva, urine, semen and vaginal secretions (although urine is not usually considered to be capable of transmitting infection). The virus is about ten times more infectious than hepatitis C.

A recombinant hepatitis B vaccine containing HBsAg is available (Engerix) and is capable of producing active immunisation in 95% of normal individuals. The vaccine should be offered to those at increased risk of infection who are not already immune, as evidenced by anti-HBs in the blood (Box 24.41). The vaccine is ineffective in those already infected by HBV. Following known exposure, infection can also be prevented or minimised by the intramuscular injection of specific hepatitis B immunoglobulin (HBIg) prepared from blood containing anti-HBs. This should be given within 48 hours, or at most a week, of exposure to infected blood (e.g. needlestick injury, contamination of cuts or mucous membranes). Vaccine can be given together with HBIg (active–passive immunisation).

Neonates born to hepatitis B-infected mothers should be immunised at birth and given immunoglobulin. Hepatitis B serology should then be checked at 12 months of age.

Co-infection with HIV

Around 10% of the HIV-infected population has concurrent HBV and this figure may be as high as 25% in areas where both viruses are prevalent. Up to half of injection drug users with HIV are co-infected with HBV. Co-infection increases the morbidity and mortality compared to either infection alone: there are greater levels of HBV viraemia, faster progression to chronic infection and greater risk of cirrhosis and hepatocellular carcinoma than with HBV infection alone. The immunosuppression that is seen in HIV infection can lead to loss of anti-HBs antibodies, reactivation of infection and a poorer antibody response to HBV vaccination. Pregnancy poses particular problems in co-infected patients, with increased risk of perinatal transmission of HBV to the child.

Treatment can also be problematic. Several nucleoside analogues have dual antiviral activity and some regimens have been associated with emergence of drug resistance. Co-infection is also associated with diminished response to interferons and increased resistance to lamivudine in some patients. Co-infection should be managed by specialists with expertise in this area and combinations of antiviral agents need to be thought through carefully. Antiviral therapy should be considered for co-infected pregnant women, using drugs with dual activity, e.g. tenofovir with emtricitabine or lamivudine.

Globally, there is a need to identify co-infected patients earlier, especially in endemic areas, as well as a need for early effective interventions, particularly in pregnant women, to reduce perinatal transmission.

i	24.41 At-risk groups meriting hepatitis B vaccination in low-endemic areas

- Parenteral drug users
- Men who have sex with men
- Close contacts of infected individuals:
     Newborn of infected mothers
     Regular sexual partners
- Patients on chronic haemodialysis
- Patients with chronic liver disease
- Medical, nursing and laboratory personnel

Hepatitis D (Delta virus)

The hepatitis D virus (HDV) is an RNA-defective virus that has no independent existence; it requires HBV for replication and has the same sources and modes of spread. It can infect individuals simultaneously with HBV or can superinfect those who already have chronic HBV. Simultaneous infections give rise to acute hepatitis, which is often severe but is limited by recovery from the HBV infection. Infections in individuals with chronic HBV can cause acute hepatitis with spontaneous recovery, and occasionally there is simultaneous cessation of the chronic HBV infection. Chronic infection with HBV and HDV can also occur, and this frequently causes rapidly progressive chronic hepatitis and eventually cirrhosis.

HDV has a worldwide distribution. It is endemic in parts of the Mediterranean basin, Africa and South America, where transmission is mainly by close personal contact and occasionally by vertical transmission from mothers with HBV. In non-endemic areas, transmission is mainly a consequence of parenteral drug misuse.

Investigations

HDV contains a single antigen to which infected individuals make an antibody (anti-HDV). Delta antigen appears in the blood only transiently, and in practice diagnosis depends on detecting anti-HDV. Simultaneous infection with HBV and HDV, followed by full recovery, is associated with the appearance of low titres of anti-HDV IgM within a few days of the onset of the illness. This antibody generally disappears within 2 months but persists in a few patients. Super-infection of patients with chronic HBV infection leads to the production of high titres of anti-HDV, initially IgM and later IgG. Such patients may then develop chronic infection with both viruses, in which case anti-HDV titres plateau at high levels.

Management

Effective management of hepatitis B prevents hepatitis D.

Hepatitis C

This is caused by an RNA flavivirus. Acute symptomatic infection with hepatitis C is rare. Most individuals are unaware of when they became infected and are identified only when they develop chronic liver disease. Around 70% of individuals exposed to the virus become chronically infected and late spontaneous viral clearance is rare. It is estimated that around 70 million individuals have chronic hepatitis C worldwide, with the highest prevalence in the Eastern Mediterranean region. There is no active or passive protection against hepatitis C virus (HCV).

Hepatitis C infection is usually identified in asymptomatic individuals screened because they have risk factors for infection, such as previous injecting drug use (Box 24.42), or have incidentally been found to have abnormal liver blood tests. Although most people remain asymptomatic until progression to cirrhosis occurs, fatigue can complicate chronic infection and is unrelated to the degree of liver damage.

If hepatitis C infection is left untreated, progression from chronic hepatitis to cirrhosis may occur, with 20% developing cirrhosis over 20 years. Risk factors for progression include male gender, immunosuppression (such as co-infection with HIV), prothrombotic states and heavy alcohol misuse. Once cirrhosis is present, 2%–5% per year will develop primary hepatocellular carcinoma, although this rate falls by around 75% following successful antiviral therapy.

Investigations
Serology and virology

The HCV genome encodes a large polypeptide precursor that is modified post-translationally to at least 10 proteins, including several antigens that give rise to antibodies in an infected person; these are used in diagnosis. Following an acute infection (such as a needlestick injury), HCV RNA can be detected in the blood within 2–4 weeks but it may take 6–12 weeks for antibodies to appear. Anti-HCV antibodies persist in serum even after

24

- Intravenous drug use (95% of new cases in the UK)
- Unscreened infected blood products
- Vertical transmission (3% risk)
- Needlestick injury (3% risk)
- Iatrogenic parenteral transmission (e.g. contaminated vaccination needles)
- Sharing toothbrushes/razors
- Sexual transmission (uncommon)

viral clearance, whether spontaneous or post-treatment. Anti-HCV antibodies are used as the initial screening test for chronic infection but if positive, the presence of serum HCV RNA or hepatitis C core antigen is required to confirm active infection. In cases of suspected acute infection, negative testing should be repeated after 4 weeks.

Molecular analysis

There are six common viral genotypes, the distribution of which varies worldwide. The most common genotypes are 1 (45%) and 3 (25%). Genotype has no effect on progression of liver disease but historically had a major effect on response to treatment: genotype 1 was less easy to eradicate than genotypes 2 and 3 with traditional pegylated interferon alfa-/ribavirin-based treatments. All genotypes now have highly successful treatment options, although genotype may still be used to guide the choice of direct-acting antiviral drugs.

Liver function tests

LFTs may be normal or show fluctuating serum transaminases between 50 and 200 U/L. Jaundice can occasionally occur during acute infection and confers an increased likelihood of spontaneous viral clearance, but otherwise only appears in end-stage cirrhosis.

Fibrosis assessment

Serum transaminase levels in hepatitis C are a poor predictor of the degree of liver fibrosis. This should be assessed at diagnosis using transient elastography, blood biomarkers or non-invasive fibrosis scoring systems such as the Fibrosis-4 (FIB4) score or aspartate aminotransferase to platelet ratio index (APRI). Where there is diagnostic uncertainty, a liver biopsy may be required to stage the extent of liver damage.

Management

The aim of treatment is to eradicate infection and all patients with chronic HCV infection should be treated where possible. Sustained virological response (SVR) refers to undetectable HCV RNA at least 12 weeks after treatment completion, and carries a very low chance (< 1%) of subsequent relapse. In recent years, there have been substantial advances in treatment, with rates of SVR rising from less than 40% a decade ago to levels approaching 100% with newer direct-acting antivirals (DAAs). Whilst the cost of these new treatments initially posed a significant financial challenge, the price of DAAs has fallen significantly in recent years and the challenges now include identification and engagement of patients with infection.

Until 2013, the treatment of choice was combination therapy with pegylated interferon and ribavirin for up to 48 weeks. Treatment had many side-effects and a low SVR rate of 40%–70% depending on genotype.

Since 2013, new classes of DAAs have allowed interferon-free regimens with substantially shorter treatment duration, minimal side-effects and high cure rates. There are four main classes of DAA, which are defined according to their mechanism of action and therapeutic target (Box 24.43). These compounds are targeted to specific steps in the hepatitis C viral life cycle to disrupt viral replication (Fig. 24.29). These drugs are now frequently combined into single pill combinations that can be taken once daily for 8–12 weeks with SVR rates of over 95%. Whilst some DAA combinations are only licensed for specific viral genotypes, several pan-genotypic treatments are now available.

Liver transplantation should be considered when complications of cirrhosis occur. However, DAAs can be safely used even in patients with

i	24.43 Direct-acting antiviral agents for hepatitis C		
Drug class	**Therapeutic target**	**Selected drugs**	
Protease inhibitors (PIs)	Non-structural viral protein NS3/4 A (protease that cleaves the HCV polyprotein)	Paritaprevir Grazoprevir Voxilaprevir Glecaprevir	
Nucleoside polymerase inhibitors (NPIs)	Non-structural viral protein NS5B (RNA-dependent RNA polymerase needed for viral replication)	Sofosbuvir	
Non-nucleoside polymerase inhibitors (NNPIs)	Non-structural viral protein NS5B (RNA-dependent RNA polymerase needed for viral replication)	Dasabuvir	
NS5A replication complex inhibitors	Non-structural viral protein NS5A (assembly of viral replication complex)	Velpatasvir Ledipasvir Ombitasvir Elbasvir Pibrentasvir	
Host-targeting antiviral drugs (HTAs)	Cyclophilin (pharmacological inhibitor targets host cell functions involved in the HCV life cycle)	Alisporivir	

(HCV = hepatitis C virus)

decompensated cirrhosis, and successful treatment can be associated with an improvement in liver function. It is therefore becoming less common to require liver transplantation for liver failure secondary to hepatitis C, although it may still be required for hepatocellular carcinoma. Whilst most patients will now be able to have successful anti-viral treatment before transplantation, DAAs can also be used post-transplant and recurrent hepatitis C in the transplanted liver is now very rare.

Hepatitis E

Hepatitis E virus (HEV) is an RNA virus that is now thought to be the most common cause of acute viral hepatitis worldwide. Four major genotypes are described. Genotypes 1 and 2 exclusively infect humans via the faecal–oral route and cause waterborne epidemics, mainly in Asia. Genotypes 3 and 4 are mostly zoonotic (in pigs, wild boars and deer) and are transmitted to humans through undercooked meat. HEV can rarely be transmitted by blood transfusion, and blood donations in the United Kingdom are now routinely screened for hepatitis E.

HEV causes a self-limiting acute hepatitis that does not require any specific treatment. However, it can cause chronic hepatitis, progressing to cirrhosis, in immunocompromised patients, especially organ-transplant recipients. This may require a reduction in the level of immunosuppression and/or treatment with ribavirin.

Infection with genotype 1 or 2 virus during pregnancy carries a high risk of acute liver failure, which has a high mortality. Hepatitis E also causes more severe disease in those with underlying cirrhosis, resulting in decompensation or acute-on-chronic liver failure. Extrahepatic manifestations are increasingly recognised and include neurological problems such as Guillain-Barré syndrome and neuralgic amyotrophy.

Diagnosis of acute infection is usually based on detection of anti-HEV IgM antibodies but it is possible to measure HEV RNA or capsid antigen in the blood and stool (especially in immunocompromised patients).

Other forms of viral hepatitis

Non-A–E hepatitis is the term used to describe hepatitis thought to be due to a virus that is not HAV, HBV, HCV or HEV. Although the viruses

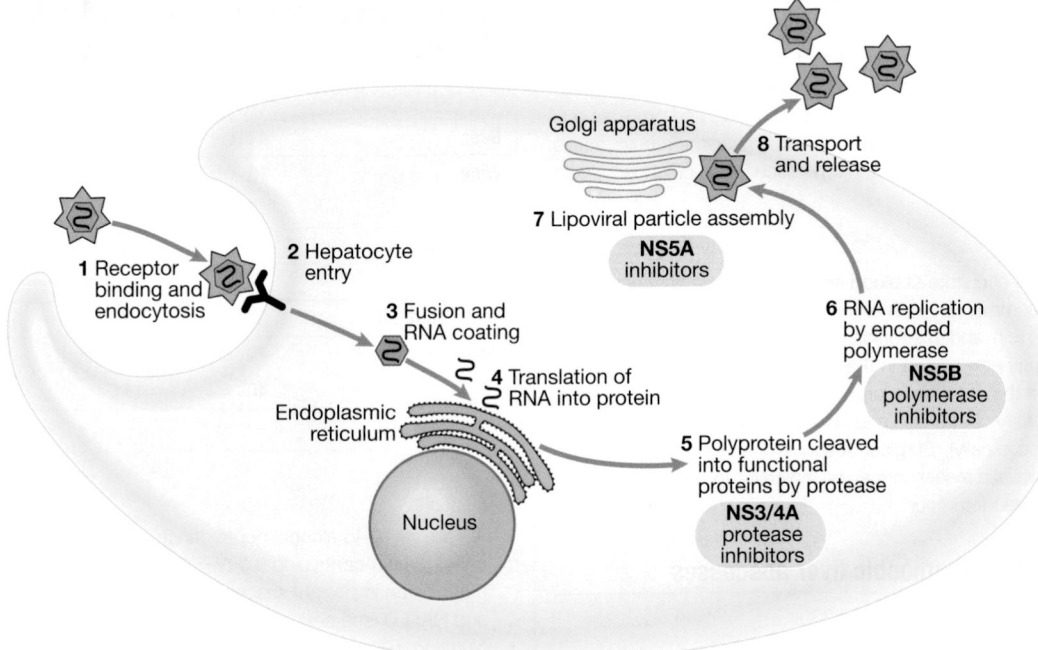

Fig. 24.29 Direct-acting antiviral agents. These compounds are targeted to specific steps in the hepatitis C viral life cycle to disrupt replication. (NS = non-structural viral protein)

above account for the majority of clinically significant hepatitis infections, other viruses can affect the liver. Cytomegalovirus and EBV infection causes abnormal LFTs in most patients and occasionally jaundice occurs. Herpes simplex is a rare cause of hepatitis in adults, most of whom are immunocompromised but can be very severe in pregnancy. Abnormal LFTs are also common in chickenpox, measles, rubella, acute HIV and COVID-19 infection.

HIV infection and the liver

Several causes of abnormal LFTs occur in HIV infection, as shown in Box 24.44. This topic is discussed in more detail in Chapter 14. Co-infection with HIV and HBV is discussed on page 889.

Liver abscess

Liver abscesses are classified as pyogenic (bacterial), hydatid (protozoal) or amoebic.

Pyogenic liver abscess

Pyogenic liver abscesses are uncommon but important because they are potentially curable but carry significant morbidity and mortality if untreated. The mortality of liver abscesses is 5%–25%. Mortality is higher in those with multiple abscesses, underlying malignancy or other comorbidities, and delayed diagnosis.

Pathophysiology

Infection can reach the liver in several ways (Box 24.45). Pyogenic abscesses are most common in older patients and usually result from ascending infection due to biliary obstruction (cholangitis) or contiguous spread from an empyema of the gallbladder. They can also complicate dental sepsis or colonic pathology, e.g. cancer, diverticulitis or inflammatory bowel disease causing portal pyaemia. Abscesses complicating suppurative appendicitis used to be common in young adults but are now rare. Immunocompromised or diabetic patients are particularly likely to develop liver abscesses. Multiple abscesses are usually due to biliary obstruction and may be polymicrobial. *Escherichia coli*, *Klebsiella pneumonia* and *Streptococcus milleri* are the most common organisms;

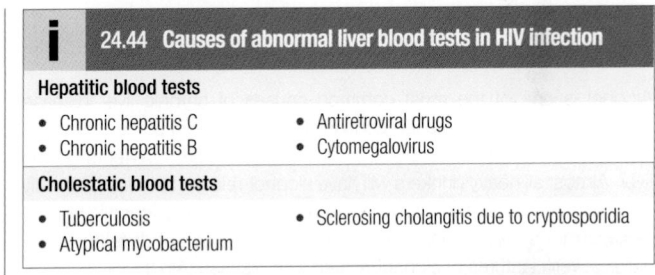

i 24.44 Causes of abnormal liver blood tests in HIV infection

Hepatitic blood tests

- Chronic hepatitis C
- Chronic hepatitis B
- Antiretroviral drugs
- Cytomegalovirus

Cholestatic blood tests

- Tuberculosis
- Atypical mycobacterium
- Sclerosing cholangitis due to cryptosporidia

i 24.45 Causes of pyogenic liver abscesses

- Biliary obstruction (cholangitis)
- Haematogenous:
    Portal vein (intra-abdominal infections)
    Hepatic artery (bacteraemia)
- Direct extension (cholecystitis)
- Trauma:
    Penetrating or non-penetrating
- Infection of liver tumour or cyst

anaerobes such as *Bacteroides* can often be found when infection has been transmitted from large bowel pathology.

Clinical features

Patients are generally ill with fever and sometimes rigors and weight loss. Right upper quadrant abdominal pain is common, sometimes with radiation to the right shoulder. The pain may be pleuritic in nature. Tender hepatomegaly is found in more than 50% of patients. Mild jaundice may be present, becoming severe if large abscesses cause biliary obstruction. Atypical presentations are common and include anorexia, diarrhoea, dyspnoea and pyrexia of unknown origin. Necrotic colorectal metastases can be misdiagnosed as hepatic abscess.

Investigations

A raised white cell count and neutrophilia is common. Alkaline phosphatase is often raised and albumin levels are low. Blood cultures are

24

positive in 50%–80%. The chest X-ray may show a raised right diaphragm and lung collapse, or an effusion at the base of the right lung. Liver imaging is key; ultrasound will detect at least 80% of pyogenic abscesses and CT with contrast will detect over 95%. Needle aspiration under ultrasound guidance confirms the diagnosis and provides pus for culture. Abscesses caused by gut-derived organisms require active exclusion of significant colonic pathology, such as a colonoscopy to exclude colorectal carcinoma.

Management

Pending the results of culture of blood and pus from the abscess, treatment should be commenced with a combination of antibiotics, such as ampicillin, gentamicin and metronidazole. Percutaneous aspiration or drainage with a catheter placed in the abscess under ultrasound guidance is required if the abscess is large or not responding to antibiotics. Any associated biliary obstruction and cholangitis require biliary drainage (preferably endoscopically). Surgical abscess drainage is rarely undertaken, although hepatic resection may be indicated for a chronic persistent abscess or 'pseudotumour'.

Hydatid cysts and amoebic liver abscesses

These are described on pages 342 and 330.

Leptospirosis

This is described on page 305.

Alcohol-related liver disease

Alcohol is one of the most common causes of chronic liver disease worldwide, with consumption continuing to increase in some countries. Excessive alcohol consumption produces a spectrum of effects on the liver. Almost all heavy drinkers will have alcohol-related fatty liver, but only a minority will develop clinically significant liver disease (alcoholic hepatitis or cirrhosis). A number of factors influence the risk of developing the more severe features of alcohol-related liver disease (ALD):

- *Amount of alcohol consumed*. In the UK, a 'unit' of alcohol contains 8 g of ethanol (Box 24.46). There is significant variability between countries in advice with regard to alcohol consumption but current UK guidelines recommend drinking less than 14 units of alcohol per week. This threshold is based on a wide range of health issues, including cancer risk. The threshold of alcohol consumption required to develop liver disease varies considerably between individuals but begins at around 30 g/day (25–30 units/week) of ethanol. However, there is not a linear relationship between dose and liver damage. For many, consumption of more than 80 g/day, for more than 5 years, is required to confer significant risk of advanced liver disease. The average alcohol consumption of a man with cirrhosis is 160 g/day for over 8 years. However, even at this level of consumption, many patients will not develop advanced liver disease.
- *Drinking pattern*. There are conflicting data with regard to drinking pattern but it is generally thought that liver damage is more likely to occur in continuous rather than intermittent or 'binge' drinkers, as this pattern gives the liver a chance to recover. It is therefore recommended that people should have at least two alcohol-free days each week. The type of beverage does not affect risk.
- *Sex*. Women who drink heavily are at higher risk of developing cirrhosis than men. This may relate to the higher blood ethanol levels seen in women compared to men after consuming the same amount of alcohol.
- *Genetics*. Genetic factors predispose to both alcohol use disorders and risk of disease progression. Polymorphisms in genes involved in alcohol metabolism (alcohol dehydrogenase and acetaldehyde dehydrogenase) and in neurotransmitter pathways (GABA receptor

i	24.46 Amount of alcohol in an average drink			
Alcohol type	% Alcohol by volume	Amount	Units*	
Beer	4	568 mL (1 pint)	2.3	
Wine	13	175 mL	2.3	
	13	750 mL	10	
'Alcopops'	6	330 mL	2	
Sherry	17.5	750 mL	13	
Vodka/rum/gin	37.5	25 mL	1	
Whisky/brandy	40	700 mL	28	
	40	1 L	40	

*1 unit = 8 g.

A2) are linked to alcohol dependence. The patatin-like phospholipase domain-containing 3 (*PNPLA3*) gene, also known as adiponutrin, is an important susceptibility gene for cirrhosis in both ALD and NAFLD (see next section).
- *Nutrition*. Being either obese or underweight increases mortality in alcohol-related liver disease. Ethanol itself produces 7 kcal/g (29.3 kJ/g) and many alcoholic drinks also contain sugar, which further increases the calorific value and may contribute to weight gain. Excess alcohol consumption is also frequently associated with nutritional deficiencies such as thiamine and folate deficiency.
- *Coexistent liver disease*. Patients with coexistent chronic hepatitis C or NAFLD who drink heavily have accelerated disease progression compared with non-drinkers.

Pathophysiology

Alcohol reaches peak blood concentrations after about 20 minutes, although this may be influenced by stomach contents. It is metabolised almost exclusively by the liver via one of two pathways (Fig. 24.30).

Approximately 80% of alcohol is metabolised by alcohol dehydrogenase to acetaldehyde, and then by aldehyde dehydrogenase to acetate. This process converts NAD (nicotinamide adenine dinucleotide) to NADH, altering the redox potential of the cell. Up to 20% of alcohol is metabolised by the microsomal ethanol-oxidising system (MEOS), predominantly through the inducible cytochrome p450 2E1, also generating acetaldehyde along with oxygen free radicals. The CYP2E1 enzyme also metabolises acetaminophen, and hence chronic alcoholics are more susceptible to hepatotoxicity from low doses of paracetamol. Acetaldehyde from either pathway is toxic and causes structural alterations of cellular proteins. This results in altered mitochondrial function and generation of reactive oxygen species, leading to oxidative stress. The altered ratio of reduced/oxidised NAD interrupts beta-oxidation of fatty acids and causes upregulation of sterol regulatory element-binding protein 1 (SREBP1), promoting fatty acid synthesis.

Damage to hepatocytes leads to stimulation of immune cells via damage-associated molecular patterns (DAMPs) such as mitochondrial DNA or necrotic debris. Alcohol also affects the gut leading to dysbiosis and increased gut permeability, delivering pathogen-associated molecular patterns (PAMPs) such as lipopolysaccharide and bacterial DNA via the portal vein which stimulate immune cells, leading to release of tumour necrosis factor alpha (TNF-α) and interleukin (IL)-1, IL-2 and IL-8. All of these cytokines have been implicated in the pathogenesis of liver fibrosis (see Fig. 24.4).

The pathological features of ALD are shown in Box 24.47. The most common manifestation is accumulation of triglycerides within hepatocytes (hepatic steatosis), or alcohol-related fatty liver. This progresses in some patients to cause hepatocyte injury and inflammation, or steatohepatitis. This can present acutely with a clinical syndrome of rapid onset jaundice (alcoholic hepatitis) or can result in progressive fibrosis leading

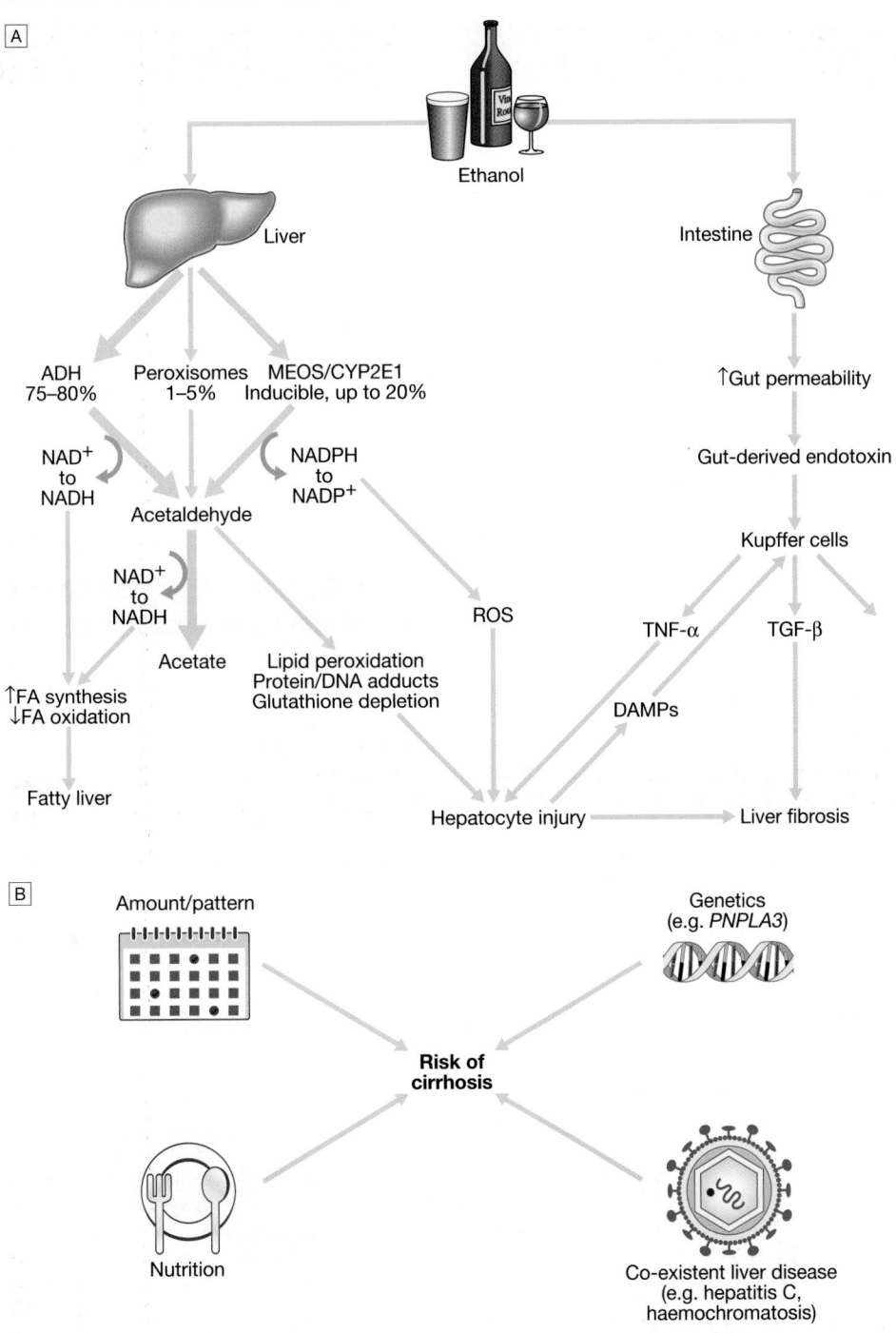

Fig. 24.30 Factors involved in the pathogenesis of alcohol-related liver disease. [A] Main biochemical pathways in alcohol-related liver disease. [B] Modulating factors in pathogenesis of alcohol-related liver disease. (ADH = alcohol dehydrogenase; DAMPs = damage-associated molecular patterns; FA = fatty acid; MEOS = microsomal ethanol oxidising system; NAD = nicotinamide adenine dinucleotide; NADH = NAD-hydrogen; NADP = nicotinamide adenine dinucleotide phosphate; NADPH = NADP-hydrogen; ROS = reactive oxygen species; TGF-β = transforming growth factor beta; TNF-α = tumour necrosis factor alpha)

to cirrhosis; these two presentations can coexist. Iron deposition is common and does not necessarily indicate haemochromatosis. Fig. 24.31 shows the histological features of alcohol-related liver disease, which are identical to those of non-alcoholic steatohepatitis.

Clinical features

Three types of ALD are recognised (Box 24.48) but these may overlap. Alcohol misuse may also cause damage of other organs and this should be specifically looked for (see Box 31.24). Dupuytren's contracture (thickening of the palmar fascia) is associated with chronic alcohol excess, but is not predictive of underlying liver disease.

Alcohol-related fatty liver disease

Alcohol-related fatty liver disease (AFLD) usually presents with an incidental finding of elevated transaminases or an echogenic liver on ultrasound. It is generally asymptomatic, has a good prognosis and steatosis usually disappears within 3 months of abstinence.

Alcoholic hepatitis

Alcoholic hepatitis (AH) presents with rapid onset jaundice in the context of recent heavy alcohol use. This is commonly associated with tender hepatomegaly and features of the systemic inflammatory response syndrome. Unlike other types of hepatitis, the ALT level is only mildly raised

24.47 Pathological features of alcohol-related liver disease

- Macrovesicular steatosis
- Alcoholic hepatitis:
  - Ballooning degeneration of hepatocytes
  - Neutrophil infiltration
  - Mallory's hyaline
  - Pericellular fibrosis
- Fibrous septa, leading to cirrhosis
- Lipogranuloma
- Central hyaline sclerosis
- Mega-mitochondria

(<300) and may even be normal, but the AST/ALT ratio is often greater than 1.5–2. It carries a significant short-term risk of death, often due to sepsis or renal failure. Severe AH is associated with a 15% 1-month mortality and 50% 1-year mortality. Cirrhosis may coexist in patients with acute alcoholic hepatitis. Patients often deteriorate during the first 1–3 weeks in hospital. Even if they abstain, it may take up to 6 months for jaundice to resolve. In patients presenting with jaundice who subsequently abstain, the 3- and 5-year survival is 70%. In contrast, those who continue to drink have 3- and 5-year survival rates of 60% and 34%, respectively.

Alcoholic cirrhosis

Palmar erythema, spider naevi and gynaecomastia are more common in alcoholic cirrhosis than in cirrhosis of other aetiologies. Alcoholic cirrhosis often presents with a serious complication, such as variceal haemorrhage or ascites, and only half of such patients will survive for 5 years from presentation. However, most who survive the initial illness and who become abstinent will survive beyond 5 years.

Investigations

Investigations aim to establish alcohol misuse, exclude alternative or additional coexistent causes of liver disease, and assess the severity of liver damage. The clinical history from patient, relatives and friends is important to establish alcohol misuse duration and severity. Biological markers, particularly macrocytosis in the absence of anaemia, may suggest and support a history of alcohol misuse. A raised GGT is commonly seen in alcohol-related fatty liver and generally falls within 2–6 weeks of abstinence but is not specific and may also be elevated in the presence of other conditions, including NAFLD. Carbohydrate-deficient transferrin (CDT) is also a serum biomarker of recent alcohol excess.

The extent of fibrosis can be assessed using either serum fibrosis markers or transient elastography. A liver biopsy is occasionally required if there is diagnostic uncertainty.

In alcoholic hepatitis, a number of prognostic scoring systems are available. The prothrombin time (PT) and bilirubin are used to calculate a 'modified discriminant function' (mDF), also known as the Maddrey score, which enables the clinician to assess prognosis (serum bilirubin in μmol/L is divided by 17 to convert to mg/dL):

$$DF = [4.6 \times \text{Increase in PT (sec)}] + \text{Bilirubin (mg/dL)}$$

24.48 Clinical syndromes of alcohol-related liver disease

Fatty liver (>90%)	
• Asymptomatic abnormal liver enzymes	• Bright (echogenic) liver on ultrasound
Alcoholic hepatitis (10%–35%)	
• Rapid onset jaundice • Coagulopathy • Tender hepatomegaly	• High short-term mortality
Cirrhosis (10%–20%)	
• Stigmata of chronic liver disease • Ascites/varices/encephalopathy	• Nodular liver (large, normal or small) • Risk of hepatocellular carcinoma

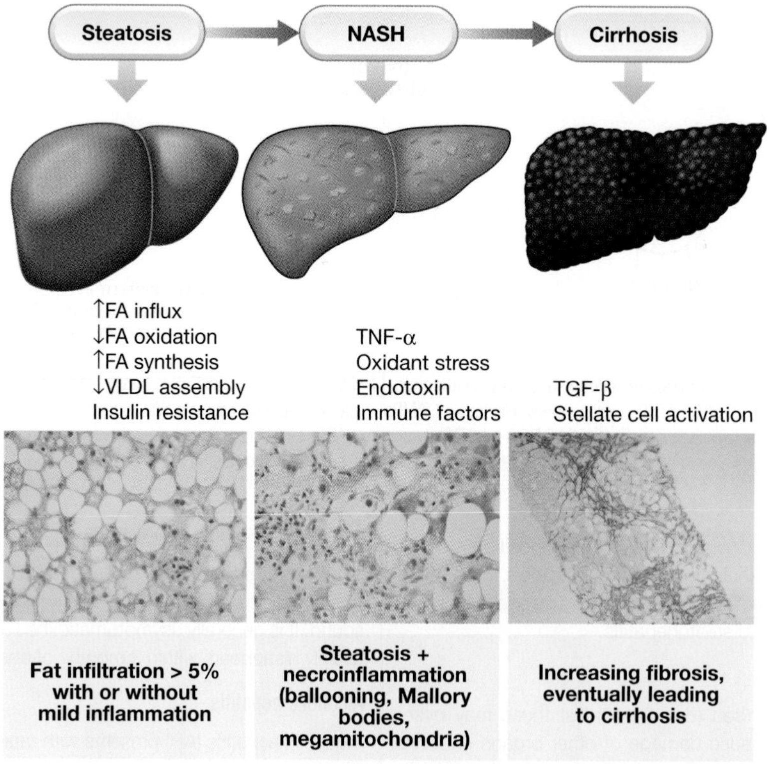
Steatosis
NASH
Cirrhosis
↑FA influx
↓FA oxidation
↑FA synthesis
↓VLDL assembly
Insulin resistance
TNF-α
Oxidant stress
Endotoxin
Immune factors
TGF-β
Stellate cell activation
Fat infiltration > 5% with or without mild inflammation
Steatosis + necroinflammation (ballooning, Mallory bodies, megamitochondria)
Increasing fibrosis, eventually leading to cirrhosis

Fig. 24.31 Non-alcoholic fatty liver disease (NAFLD) and non-alcoholic steatohepatitis (NASH). Rate of progression is determined by environmental (dietary) and genetic factors. (FA = fatty acid; TGF-β = transforming growth factor beta; TNF-α = tumour necrosis factor alpha; VLDL = very low-density lipoprotein)

A value over 32 implies severe disease. Historically, this group had a 40%–50% 1 month mortality but this has dropped to 15% in a recent large study, reflecting improved medical management. A second scoring system, the Glasgow Alcoholic Hepatitis Score, uses the age, white cell count and renal function, in addition to PT and bilirubin, to assess prognosis (Box 24.49). A score of 9 or more identifies an even higher risk group with a 60% 1-month mortality.

Management

Cessation of alcohol consumption is the single most important treatment and prognostic factor. Life-long abstinence is the best advice. General health and life expectancy are improved when this occurs, irrespective of the stage of liver disease. Abstinence is even effective at preventing progression, hepatic decompensation and death once cirrhosis is present. Treatment of alcohol dependency is discussed Chapter 31. In the acute presentation of ALD it is important to identify and anticipate alcohol withdrawal and Wernicke's encephalopathy, in parallel with the liver disease.

Nutrition

Nutrition is very important, and calorie intake correlates with survival in severe alcoholic hepatitis. Enteral feeding via a fine-bore nasogastric tube may be needed in patients unable to meet their requirements.

Drug therapy

The optimal treatment of severe alcoholic hepatitis (Maddrey's discriminative score >32) has been widely debated. The STOPAH study was a large, multicentre, double-blind, randomised trial in patients with a clinical diagnosis of severe alcoholic hepatitis. This showed no effect of pentoxifylline (a weak anti-TNF agent) on survival. There was a borderline reduction in 28-day mortality with prednisolone, but no benefit by 3 months or 1 year. Prednisolone was associated with increased rates of sepsis and gastrointestinal bleeding. N-acetyl cysteine (NAC) may also limit oxidative stress but initial trials failed to show any benefit. A single trial has suggested a benefit of intravenous NAC in patients also treated with prednisolone. If the bilirubin has not fallen 7 days after starting glucocorticoids, the drugs are unlikely to reduce mortality and should be stopped.

Liver transplantation

ALD is a common indication for liver transplantation in Europe and the United States. The outcome of transplantation for ALD is good, with survival rates similar to other indications and if the patient remains abstinent there is no risk of disease recurrence. The challenge is to identify patients with an unacceptable risk of returning to harmful alcohol consumption. Many programmes require a 6-month period of abstinence from alcohol before a patient is considered for transplantation. Although duration of abstinence is only one factor in predicting risk of relapse and the length

required is debatable, a period of abstinence will allow recovery of liver function sufficient to avoid transplantation in some, as well as identify those at highest risk of early recidivism. Transplantation for alcoholic hepatitis has been described in highly selected individuals with acceptable short-term outcomes but it is seldom performed due to concerns about longer-term risk of recidivism.

Non-alcoholic fatty liver disease

Increasingly sedentary lifestyles and changing dietary patterns mean that the prevalence of obesity and insulin resistance has increased worldwide, and so fat accumulation in the liver is a common finding during abdominal imaging studies and on liver biopsy. This results in a similar spectrum of liver disease to alcohol excess, so when these changes were observed in the absence of high alcohol consumption, this was called non-alcoholic fatty liver disease (NAFLD).

NAFLD includes a spectrum of progressive liver disease. The majority will have fatty infiltration alone (steatosis) but a minority (10%–20%) will develop accompanying inflammation (non-alcoholic steatohepatitis, NASH) and/or fibrosis, and may progress to cirrhosis and primary liver cancer. NAFLD is considered by many to be the hepatic manifestation of the 'metabolic syndrome' as it is strongly associated with obesity, type 2 diabetes, dyslipidaemia and hypertension. Initial definitions used a threshold of alcohol consumption (typically 28 units per week for men or 21 units for women) for diagnosis. However, an alternative nomenclature of metabolic (dysfunction)-associated fatty liver disease, or MAFLD, has recently been proposed to reflect our better understanding of the risk factors and to describe those patients in whom this coexists with alcohol excess.

Overall, NAFLD is estimated to have a global prevalence of 24%. A large European study found NAFLD to be present in 94% of obese patients (body mass index (BMI) >30kg/m²), 67% of overweight patients (BMI >25kg/m²) and 25% of normal-weight patients. The overall prevalence of NAFLD in patients with type 2 diabetes ranges from 40% to 70%. The frequency of steatosis varies with ethnicity (45% in patients of Hispanic origin, 33% in those of European ancestry and 24% in those of African ancestry) and gender (in those of European descent, 42% males vs 24% females).

Fibrosis is the main determinant of outcome. Patients with cirrhosis have a high risk of liver-related adverse outcomes, whereas those with less advanced fibrosis are more likely to have extra-hepatic cancers and vascular events. Patients with NASH have significantly higher rates of fibrosis progression than those with simple steatosis. Due to its increasing prevalence, NAFLD cirrhosis is predicted to become the main aetiology in patients undergoing liver transplantation during the next 5 years.

Pathophysiology

The initiating events in NAFLD are typically based on the development of obesity and insulin resistance, leading to increased hepatic free fatty acid flux. This imbalance between the rate of import/synthesis and the rate of export/catabolism of fatty acids in the liver leads to the development of steatosis. This may be an adaptive response through which hepatocytes store potentially toxic lipids as relatively inert triglyceride. A 'two-hit' hypothesis has been proposed to describe the pathogenesis of NAFLD, the 'first hit' causing steatosis that then progresses to NASH or fibrosis if a 'second hit' occurs. In reality, progression probably follows hepatocellular injury caused by a combination of several different 'hits', including:

- oxidative stress due to free radicals produced during fatty acid oxidation
- direct lipotoxicity from fatty acids and other metabolites in the liver
- endoplasmic reticulum stress
- gut-derived endotoxin
- cytokine release (TNF-α etc.) and immune-mediated hepatocellular injury.

24.49 How to assess prognosis using the Glasgow Alcoholic Hepatitis Score			
Score	1	2	3
Age	<50	>50	
White cell count (×10⁹/L)	<15	>15	
Urea (mmol/L (BUN mg/dl))	<5 (14)	>5 (14)	
PT ratio	<1.5	1.5–2.0	>2.0
Bilirubin (μmol/L (mg/dL))	<125 (7.4)	125–250 (7.4–14.8)	>250 (14.8)

A score of ≥9 is associated with a 40% 28-day survival, compared to 80% for patients with a score of <9.

(BUN = blood urea nitrogen; PT = prothrombin time)

24

Cellular damage triggers cell death and inflammation, which leads to stellate cell activation and development of hepatic fibrosis that culminates in cirrhosis (see Fig. 24.31).

As with many other liver diseases, genetic and environmental factors interact to determine disease progression:

- *Genetics*. Several genetic modifiers of disease severity have been identified, with *PNPLA3* and its product, adiponutrin, being the best validated.
- *Demographics*. Cirrhosis is more common with increasing age, although possibly just reflecting longer duration of disease. Higher rates of fibrosis progression are observed in men and post-menopausal women.
- *Diet*. Excessive alcohol consumption leads to increased fibrosis progression, whereas coffee consumption appears to be protective against fibrosis and HCC in NAFLD.
- *Intestinal microbiota*. Obesity, diabetes and NAFLD are all linked with gut dysbiosis, with several microbial signatures associated with advanced fibrosis. The gut microbiome may influence intestinal permeability and delivery of pathogen-associated molecular patterns (PAMPs) through the portal circulation that trigger liver inflammation.
- *Comorbidity*. The presence of type 2 diabetes and severe obesity are associated with higher rates of cirrhosis in NAFLD.

NAFLD should not be confused with acute fatty liver, which can occur in hepatic mitochondrial cytopathies, e.g. acute fatty liver of pregnancy or drug toxicity (sodium valproate, tetracyclines), or with bacterial toxins (e.g. *Bacillus cereus*). In these, defective mitochondrial beta-oxidation of lipids leads to fat droplet accumulation in hepatocytes and microvesicular steatosis.

Clinical features

NAFLD is frequently asymptomatic, although it may be associated with fatigue and mild right upper quadrant discomfort. It is commonly identified as an incidental biochemical abnormality during routine blood tests or as a fatty liver on abdominal imaging. Alternatively, patients may present late in the natural history of the disease with complications of cirrhosis and portal hypertension, such as variceal haemorrhage, or with hepatocellular carcinoma.

The average age of NAFLD cirrhosis patients is currently 50–60 years; however, the emerging epidemic of childhood obesity means that NAFLD is present in increasing numbers of younger patients. NAFLD is also associated with polycystic ovary syndrome and obstructive sleep apnoea.

Investigations

Investigation of patients with suspected NAFLD should aim to confirm the presence of fat in the liver and determine the extent of fibrosis. It is important to assess alcohol consumption as a contributory factor and check for medications that cause fatty liver, such as tamoxifen, amiodarone and corticosteroids. Investigations should exclude other coexistent liver diseases (including viral, autoimmune and inherited causes).

Biochemical tests

There is no single diagnostic blood test for NAFLD. Serum GGT is often raised. ALT and AST may be normal or modestly raised, usually less than twice the upper limit of normal. ALT levels fall as hepatic fibrosis increases and the normal AST:ALT ratio of < 1 reverses as advanced fibrosis develops. Other laboratory abnormalities that may be present include low-titre antinuclear antibody (ANA) in 20%–30% of patients and elevated ferritin levels.

Although routine blood tests are unable to determine the degree of liver fibrosis accurately, several calculated scores, such as the NAFLD Fibrosis Score and FIB-4 Score, which are based on the results of routinely available blood tests and anthropometrics, have a high negative predictive value for advanced fibrosis/cirrhosis (Box 24.50). A low score can therefore be used to rule out advanced fibrosis in many NAFLD patients, allowing care to focus on those most likely to have advanced disease. Specific serum fibrosis markers such as the Enhanced Liver Fibrosis panel may also be used.

Imaging

Ultrasound is most often used and provides a qualitative assessment of hepatic fat content, as the liver appears 'bright' due to increased echogenicity; however, sensitivity is limited when fewer than 33% of hepatocytes are steatotic. CT, MRI or MR spectroscopy offer greater sensitivity for detecting lesser degrees of steatosis, but these are resource-intensive and not widely used. No routine imaging modality can distinguish simple steatosis from steatohepatitis or accurately quantify hepatic fibrosis short of cirrhosis.

Transient elastography

Transient elastography (TE) is often used to assess those with indeterminate fibrosis scores. Liver stiffness can predict the likelihood of advanced fibrosis and is well validated in NAFLD, although readings may get less reliable with BMI over 40. Controlled Attenuation Parameter (CAP) is an ultrasound-based technique which can be performed simultaneously with TE to quantify steatosis non-invasively.

Liver biopsy

Although it is frequently not required for either diagnosis or staging, liver biopsy remains the 'gold standard' investigation for diagnosis and assessment of degree of inflammation and extent of liver fibrosis. The histological changes seen in NAFLD are identical to those described in ALD (see previous section). The definition of NASH is based on a combination of three lesions (steatosis, hepatocellular injury and inflammation; see Fig. 24.31) with a mainly centrilobular, acinar zone 3 distribution. Perisinusoidal fibrosis is a characteristic feature of NAFLD. Histological scoring systems are widely used to assess both necroinflammation and fibrosis severity semi-quantitatively.

It is important to note that hepatic fat content tends to diminish as cirrhosis develops and so NAFLD is likely to be under-diagnosed in the setting of advanced liver disease, where it is thought to be the underlying cause of 30%–75% of cases in which no specific aetiology is readily identified (so-called 'cryptogenic cirrhosis').

i	**24.50 Simple non-invasive scores for NAFLD/fibrosis[1]**		
		Thresholds	
Test	**Key variables**	**Age <65 yr**	**Age >65 yr**
NAFLD Fibrosis Score (NFS)[2]	Age BMI Diabetes/IFG AST ALT Platelets Albumin	**High risk** >0.676 **Indeterminate risk** −1.455–0.676 **Low risk** <−1.455	**High risk** >0.676 **Indeterminate risk** 0.12–0.676 **Low risk** <0.12
FIB-4 Score[3]	Age AST Platelets ALT	**High risk** >2.67 **Indeterminate risk** 1.30–2.67 **Low risk** <1.30	**High risk** >2.67 **Indeterminate risk** 2.00–2.67 **Low risk** <2.00

[1]Predict advanced fibrosis and cirrhosis (F3–4). Simple scores like NFS and FIB-4 are based on the results of routinely available blood tests and anthropometrics. [2]www.nafldscore.com. [3]http://gihep.com/calculators/hepatology/fibrosis-4-score/.
(ALT = alanine aminotransferase; AST = aspartate aminotransferase; BMI = body mass index; IFG = impaired fasting glucose)
NFS from Angulo P, Hui JM, Marchesini G, et al. The NAFLD Fibrosis Score. A noninvasive system that identifies liver fibrosis in patients with NAFLD. Hepatology 2007;45(4):846–854; FIB-4 from Vallet-Pichard A, Mallet V, Nalpas B, et al. FIB-4: an inexpensive and accurate marker of fibrosis in HCV infection. comparison with liver biopsy and fibrotest. Hepatology 2007; 46(1):32–36.

Management

As it is a marker of the metabolic syndrome, identification of NAFLD should prompt screening for and treatment of cardiovascular risk factors in all patients. It is also necessary to assess whether patients have advanced fibrosis so that liver-targeted treatment can be focused particularly on those patients. An example of an algorithm for the assessment and risk stratification of patients with NAFLD is provided in Fig. 24.32.

Non-pharmacological treatment

Current treatment comprises lifestyle interventions to promote weight loss and improve insulin sensitivity through dietary changes and physical exercise. Sustained weight reduction of 7%–10% is associated with significant improvement in histological and biochemical NASH severity. However, this is only achieved by a small proportion of patients, focusing attention on other strategies. A Mediterranean diet pattern and reduced fructose consumption may also be helpful.

Pharmacological treatment

No pharmacological agents are currently licensed specifically for NAFLD therapy. Treatment directed at coexisting metabolic disorders, such as dyslipidaemia and hypertension, should be given. Although HMG-CoA reductase inhibitors (statins) do not ameliorate NAFLD, there does not appear to be any increased risk of hepatotoxicity or other side-effects, and so they may be used safely to treat dyslipidaemia. Specific insulin-sensitising agents, in particular glitazones, may help selected patients. Positive results with high-dose vitamin E (800 U/day) have been tempered by evidence that high doses may be associated with an increased risk of prostate cancer and all-cause mortality, which has limited its use. Obeticholic acid, a farnesoid X receptor agonist, appears to improve fibrosis in non-cirrhotic NASH in an interim analysis but the trial is ongoing. Several other new medicines are currently in late-phase clinical trials and so liver-targeted pharmacological treatments are likely to be available within the next few years.

Autoimmune liver and biliary disease

The liver is an important target for autoimmune injury. The clinical picture is dictated by the nature of the autoimmune process and, in particular, the target cell for immune injury. The disease patterns are quite distinctive for primary hepatocellular injury (autoimmune hepatitis) and biliary epithelial cell injury (primary biliary cholangitis and primary sclerosing cholangitis).

Autoimmune hepatitis

Autoimmune hepatitis (AIH) is a disease of immune-mediated injury targeting hepatocytes, which can present either as an acute severe hepatitis or chronic hepatitis leading to cirrhosis. It is a lifelong disease which often runs a relapsing and remitting course. It can develop at any age, with peaks around the second and sixth decades. It is more common in women with a 5:1 predominance. It has a strong association with other autoimmune diseases (Box 24.51).

Pathophysiology

It is characterised by the presence of serum antibodies and peripheral blood T lymphocytes reactive with self-proteins, and high levels of serum immunoglobulins – in particular, IgG. The reasons for the breakdown in immune tolerance in autoimmune hepatitis remain unclear. There are strong HLA associations (typically DR3 and DR4), indicating an underlying genetic predisposition, with a presumed environmental trigger. Exposure to the antibiotic nitrofurantoin can induce autoimmune hepatitis in a small number of cases, and cross-reactivity to viruses such as HAV and EBV has been proposed as an alternative trigger.

Clinical features

Some patients may be asymptomatic, with a raised ALT detected on blood tests. The onset of symptoms is usually insidious, with fatigue, anorexia and arthralgia. The non-specific nature of the early features can lead to the diagnosis being missed in the early disease stages. In about one-quarter of patients the onset is acute, resembling viral hepatitis, but

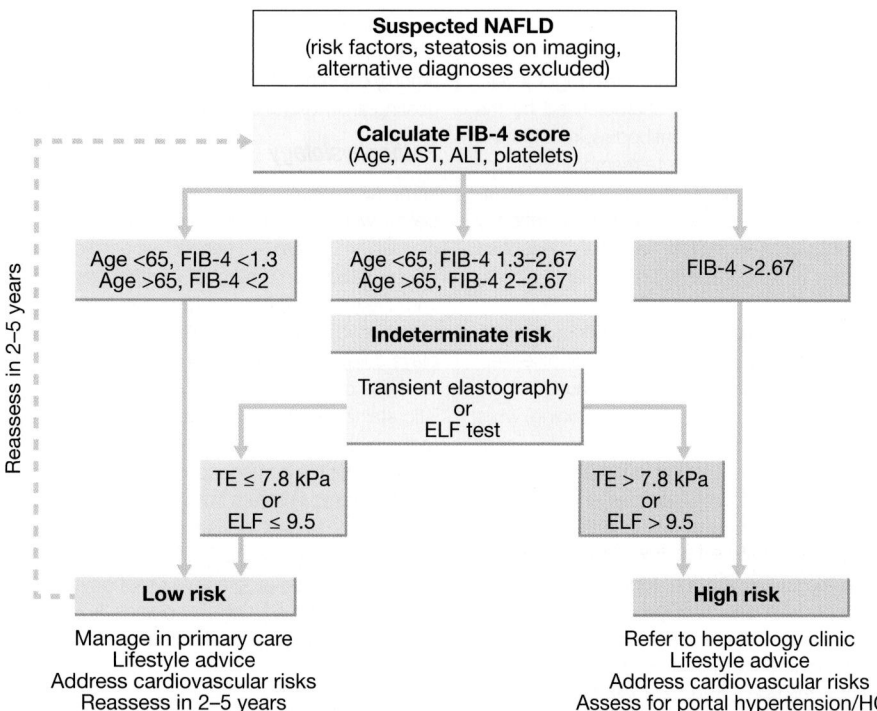

Fig. 24.32 Assessment and risk stratification of patients with non-alcoholic fatty liver disease (NAFLD). (ALT = alanine aminotransferase; AST = aspartate aminotransferase; ELF = enhanced liver fibrosis; FIB-4 = fibrosis-4; HCC = hepatocellular carcinoma; TE = transient elastography)

24.51 Conditions associated with autoimmune hepatitis

- Autoimmune thyroiditis
- Systemic lupus erythematosus
- Rheumatoid arthritis
- Primary sclerosing cholangitis
- Coeliac disease
- Type 1 diabetes
- Dermatomyositis
- Coombs-positive haemolytic anaemia
- Ulcerative colitis

24.52 Frequency of autoantibodies in chronic non-viral liver diseases and in healthy people

Disease	Antinuclear antibody (%)	Anti-smooth muscle antibody (%)	Antimitochondrial antibody*
Healthy controls	5	1.5	0.01
Autoimmune hepatitis	80	70	15
Primary biliary cholangitis	25	35	95
Cryptogenic cirrhosis	40	30	15

*Patients with antimitochondrial antibody frequently have cholestatic liver function tests and may have primary biliary cholangitis (see text).

resolution does not occur. This acute presentation can lead to extensive liver necrosis and liver failure. Signs of chronic liver disease, especially spider naevi and hepatosplenomegaly, can be present. Approximately 25% of patients will have cirrhosis at diagnosis, and some will progress to cirrhosis despite treatment.

Investigations

There is no single diagnostic test for autoimmune hepatitis. Liver enzymes typically show raised ALT and AST, although these fluctuate. Serological tests for autoantibodies are often positive (Box 24.52). The most frequently seen autoantibody pattern is high titre of antinuclear and/or anti-smooth muscle antibodies, typically associated with raised IgG levels, frequently seen in young adult females. Disease characterised by the presence of anti-liver–kidney microsomal (LKM) antibodies, recognising cytochrome P450-IID6 expressed on the hepatocyte membrane, is typically seen in paediatric populations and can be more resistant to treatment than ANA-positive disease. More recently, a pattern of antibody reactivity with anti-soluble liver antigen (anti-SLA) has been described typically in adult patients, often with aggressive disease and lacking autoantibodies of other specificities.

It should be noted that low titres of these antibodies occur in some healthy people and in patients with other inflammatory liver diseases. ANA also occur in connective tissue diseases and other autoimmune diseases (with an identical pattern of homogenous nuclear staining) while anti-smooth muscle antibody has been reported in infectious mononucleosis, chronic hepatitis C infection and a variety of malignant diseases.

Elevated serum IgG levels are an important diagnostic and treatment response feature if present, but the diagnosis is still possible in the presence of normal IgG levels. If the diagnosis of autoimmune hepatitis is suspected, liver biopsy should be performed both to confirm the diagnosis before commencing long-term immunosuppression and to stage any liver fibrosis. It typically shows an abundance of lymphocytes and plasma cells around the portal tracts (portal lymphoplasmacytic hepatitis) with inflammation extending out from the edge of the portal tracts into the lobule (interface hepatitis). Scoring systems, such as the International Autoimmune Hepatitis Group (IAIHG) criteria, are useful for epidemiological study and for assessing trial eligibility but are complex for normal clinical practice.

Management

Treatment with glucocorticoids is life-saving in autoimmune hepatitis, particularly during exacerbations of active and symptomatic disease. Initially, prednisolone (30–40mg/day) is given orally; the dose is then gradually reduced as the patient and LFTs improve. Budesonide may be used in non-cirrhotic patients if steroid side-effects are problematic. Maintenance therapy is usually with azathioprine (1–2mg/kg daily), although introduction of this is often delayed by around a month to allow the liver enzymes to settle in case it causes drug-induced hepatotoxicity. Maintenance azathioprine can be used as monotherapy, or may be combined with low-dose prednisolone (ideally, below 5mg/day). Second-line therapies are unlicensed with little long-term outcome data. However, in case series, mycophenolate mofetil (MMF) appears effective in patients who are azathioprine-intolerant, but less so in azathioprine non-responders. Similarly, tacrolimus appears helpful in refractory disease.

The aims of treatment are to achieve resolution of symptoms and to completely control inflammatory activity to prevent progressive fibrosis, especially in younger patients or those with cirrhosis. As flares may be asymptomatic but increase the risk of cirrhosis or decompensation, disease activity (indicated by rising ALT and IgG levels) should be monitored regularly. Maintenance treatment is required for at least 3 years and is often continued long term, as relapse rates are high if immunosuppression is withdrawn.

Primary biliary cholangitis

Primary biliary cholangitis (PBC, formerly known as primary biliary cirrhosis until 2015, when the name was changed to reflect the large proportion of non-cirrhotic patients) is a chronic, progressive cholestatic liver disease that predominantly affects women aged 30 and over. It is strongly associated with the presence of antimitochondrial antibodies (AMA), which in combination with cholestatic liver enzymes are diagnostic of PBC. It is characterised by granulomatous inflammation of the portal tracts, leading to progressive damage and eventually loss of the small and middle-sized bile ducts. This, in turn, leads to fibrosis and cirrhosis of the liver.

Epidemiology

The prevalence of PBC varies across the world. It is relatively common in northern Europe and North America but is rare in Africa and Asia. There is a strong female-to-male predominance of 9:1; it is also more common among cigarette smokers. Clustering of cases has been reported, suggesting an environmental trigger in susceptible individuals.

Pathophysiology

Immune mechanisms are clearly involved. The condition is closely associated with other autoimmune non-hepatic diseases, such as thyroid disease, and there is a genetic association with HLA-DR8, together with polymorphisms in a number of other genes regulating the nature of the immune response (e.g. IL-12 and its receptor). AMA is directed at pyruvate dehydrogenase complex, a mitochondrial enzyme complex that plays a key role in cellular energy generation. PBC-specific ANAs (such as those directed at the nuclear pore antigen gp210) have a characteristic staining pattern in immunofluorescence assays (selectively binding to the nuclear rim or nuclear dots), which means that they should not be mistaken for the homogenously staining ANA seen in autoimmune hepatitis. Increases in serum immunoglobulin levels are frequent but, unlike in autoimmune hepatitis, it is typically IgM that is elevated.

Pathologically, chronic granulomatous inflammation destroys the interlobular bile ducts; progressive lymphocyte-mediated inflammatory damage causes fibrosis, which spreads from the portal tracts to the liver parenchyma and eventually leads to cirrhosis.

Clinical features

PBC may be detected incidentally on routine blood tests, but systemic symptoms such as fatigue and generalised itch are common. The severity of these symptoms does not correlate with the severity of the liver disease. Although there may be right upper abdominal discomfort, the typical biliary-type pain, fever and rigors seen with bacterial cholangitis do not occur in PBC. Bone pain or fractures can rarely result from osteomalacia (fat-soluble vitamin malabsorption) or, more commonly, from osteoporosis. Xanthomatous deposits occur in a minority, especially around the eyes. Scratch marks may be found in patients with severe pruritus.

Associated diseases

Autoimmune and connective tissue diseases occur with increased frequency in PBC, particularly the sicca syndrome, systemic sclerosis, coeliac disease and thyroid diseases. Hypothyroidism should always be considered in patients with fatigue.

Diagnosis and investigations

The LFTs show a pattern of cholestasis (see Box 24.2). Hypercholesterolaemia is common and worsens as disease progresses but appears not to be associated with increased cardiovascular risk. AMA is present in over 95% of patients; when it is absent, the diagnosis should not be made without obtaining histological evidence and considering cholangiography (typically MRCP) to exclude other biliary disease. Due to the peripheral nature of the ducts affected by PBC, the biliary tree should appear normal on imaging. ANA and anti-smooth muscle antibodies are present in around 15% of patients (see Box 24.52); autoantibodies found in associated diseases may also be present. Fibrosis stage should be assessed, usually using transient elastography. Liver biopsy is necessary only if there is diagnostic uncertainty. The histological features of PBC correlate poorly with the clinical features; portal hypertension can develop before the histological onset of cirrhosis.

Management

The hydrophilic bile acid ursodeoxycholic acid (UDCA), at a dose of 13–15 mg/kg daily, improves bile flow, replaces toxic hydrophobic bile acids in the bile acid pool and reduces apoptosis of the biliary epithelium. Clinically, UDCA improves LFTs, may slow down histological progression and has few side-effects; it is therefore widely used in the treatment of PBC and should be regarded as the optimal first-line treatment. Eighty percent of patients will have a good biochemical response to UDCA with a reduction in serum alkaline phosphatase to normal or near-normal levels, and this corresponds to very good long-term outcomes. However, a significant minority of patients, especially those presenting under the age of 50 years, show an inadequate response to UDCA, and have an increased risk of developing end-stage liver disease. Obeticholic acid (OCA) is a second-generation bile acid therapeutic that acts as an agonist for the nuclear farnesoid X receptor. It improves alkaline phosphatase in more than half of patients who did not respond to or tolerate UDCA, and is licensed for second-line therapy in PBC. Bezafibrate, a peroxisome proliferator-activated receptor-alpha (PPARα) agonist used predominantly to treat hyperlipidaemia, has also been shown to improve alkaline phosphatase in the majority of UDCA non-responders, although it is not licensed for this use. Due to the short-term nature of the studies, neither drug has yet been shown to alter clinically significant outcomes. Despite the autoimmune aetiology, immunosuppressants, such as glucocorticoids, azathioprine, penicillamine and ciclosporin, have all failed to show any overall benefit when given to unselected PBC patients.

Liver transplantation should be considered once liver failure has developed and may also be indicated in patients with intractable pruritus. Serum bilirubin remains the most reliable marker of declining liver function. Transplantation is associated with an excellent 5-year survival of over 80%, although the disease will recur in over one-third of patients at 10 years.

Pruritus

This is the main symptom requiring treatment. The cause is unknown, but up-regulation of opioid receptors and increased levels of endogenous opioids may play a role. First-line treatment is with the anion-binding resin colestyramine, which probably acts by binding potential pruritogens in the intestine and increasing their excretion in the stool. A dose of 4–16 g/day orally is used. The powder is mixed in orange juice and the main dose (8 g) taken before and after breakfast, when maximal duodenal bile acid concentrations occur. Colestyramine may bind other drugs in the gut (most obviously UDCA) and adequate spacing should be used between drugs. Colestyramine is sometimes ineffective and can be difficult for some patients to tolerate. Alternative treatments include rifampicin (150 mg/day, titrated up to a maximum of 600 mg/day as required with close monitoring of LFTs), naltrexone (an opioid antagonist; 25 mg/day initially, increasing up to 300 mg/day), plasmapheresis and a liver support device (e.g. a molecular adsorbent recirculating system, MARS).

Fatigue

Fatigue affects about one-third of patients with PBC. The cause is unknown but it may reflect intracerebral changes due to cholestasis. Unfortunately, once depression, hypothyroidism and coeliac disease have been excluded, there is currently no specific treatment. The impact on patients' lives can be substantial.

Malabsorption

Prolonged cholestasis is associated with steatorrhoea and malabsorption of fat-soluble vitamins, which should be replaced as necessary. Coeliac disease should be excluded since its incidence is increased in PBC.

Bone disease

Osteopenia and osteoporosis are common and normal post-menopausal bone loss is accelerated. Baseline bone density should be measured and treatment started with replacement calcium and vitamin D_3. Bisphosphonates should be used if there is evidence of osteoporosis. Osteomalacia is rare.

Overlap syndromes

AMA-negative PBC ('autoimmune cholangitis')

A few patients demonstrate the clinical, biochemical and histological features of PBC but do not have detectable AMA in the serum. Serum transaminases, serum immunoglobulin levels and titres of ANA tend to be higher than in AMA-positive PBC. The clinical course mirrors classical PBC, however, and these patients should be considered as having a variant of PBC.

PBC/autoimmune hepatitis overlap

A few patients with AMA and cholestatic LFTs have elevated transaminases, high serum immunoglobulin IgG levels and interface hepatitis on liver histology. In such individuals, a trial of glucocorticoid therapy may be beneficial.

Primary sclerosing cholangitis

Primary sclerosing cholangitis (PSC) is an immune-mediated cholestatic liver disease characterised by multifocal stricturing of the larger bile ducts of the extra- and/or intrahepatic biliary tree, often in association with inflammatory bowel disease. This is also associated with progressive hepatic fibrosis which can lead to cirrhosis and portal hypertension, along with an increased risk of various cancers (cholangiocarcinoma, gallbladder, colon).

The incidence is about 6.3/100 000 in people of European ancestry. Unlike most other autoimmune diseases, PSC is twice as common in men as women. Most patients present at age 25–40 years, although the condition may be diagnosed at any age and is an important cause of chronic liver disease in children. The generally accepted diagnostic criteria are:

- generalised beading and stenosis of the biliary system on cholangiography (Fig. 24.33)
- absence of choledocholithiasis (or history of bile duct surgery)
- exclusion of bile duct cancer, by prolonged follow-up.

24

The term 'secondary sclerosing cholangitis' is used to describe the typical changes described above when a clear predisposing factor for duct fibrosis can be identified. The causes of secondary sclerosing cholangitis are shown in Box 24.53.

Pathophysiology

The cause of PSC is unknown but there is a close association with inflammatory bowel disease, particularly ulcerative colitis (Box 24.54). About 70%–80% of PSC patients have coexisting ulcerative colitis, and PSC is the most common form of chronic liver disease in ulcerative colitis. Between 3% and 10% of patients with ulcerative colitis develop PSC, particularly those with extensive colitis or pancolitis. The distribution of PSC-associated colitis is often predominantly right-sided with relative distal sparing, and may be less symptomatic that non-PSC IBD. The prevalence of PSC is lower in patients with Crohn's colitis (about 1%). Patients with PSC and ulcerative colitis are at greater risk of colorectal neoplasia than those with ulcerative colitis alone, and individuals who develop colorectal neoplasia are at greater risk of cholangiocarcinoma.

PSC is thought to be an immunologically mediated disease, triggered in genetically susceptible individuals by toxic or infectious agents, which may gain access to the biliary tract through a leaky, diseased colon. A close link has been identified with HLA haplotype A1-B8-DR3-DRW52A, which is commonly found in association with other organ-specific autoimmune diseases (e.g. autoimmune hepatitis).

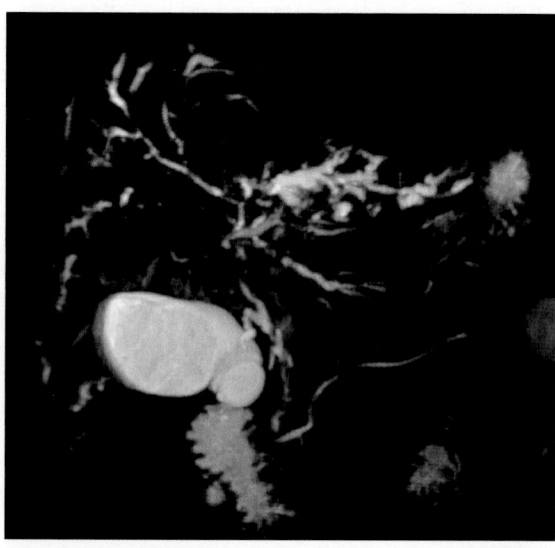

Fig. 24.33 Magnetic resonance cholangiopancreatogram showing typical changes of primary sclerosing cholangitis. There is intrahepatic bile duct beading, stricturing and dilatation. The extrahepatic bile duct is also diffusely strictured. *Courtesy of Dr Dilip Patel, Royal Infirmary of Edinburgh.*

Perinuclear antineutrophil cytoplasmic antibodies (ANCA) have been detected in the sera of 60%–80% of patients with PSC with or without ulcerative colitis, and in 30%–40% of patients with ulcerative colitis alone. The antibody is not specific for PSC and is found in other chronic liver diseases (e.g. 50% of patients with autoimmune hepatitis), so is of little diagnostic use on its own.

Clinical features

The diagnosis is often made incidentally when persistently raised serum ALP is discovered in an individual with ulcerative colitis. Patients may present with episodes of biliary obstruction, or with symptoms of cirrhosis or portal hypertension. Common symptoms include fatigue, intermittent jaundice, weight loss, right upper quadrant abdominal pain and pruritus. Attacks of acute cholangitis are uncommon and usually follow biliary instrumentation.

Investigations

Biochemical screening usually reveals a cholestatic pattern of LFTs but ALP and bilirubin levels may vary widely in individual patients during the course of the disease. For example, ALP and bilirubin values increase during acute cholangitis, decrease after therapy and sometimes fluctuate for no apparent reason. Modest elevations in serum transaminases are usually seen, whereas hypoalbuminaemia and clotting abnormalities are found at a late stage only. In addition to ANCA, low titres of serum ANA and anti-smooth muscle antibodies may be found in PSC but have no diagnostic significance; serum AMA is absent.

The key investigation is MRCP, which is usually diagnostic and reveals multiple irregular stricturing and dilatation (see Fig. 24.33). ERCP should be reserved for therapeutic interventions.

On liver biopsy, the characteristic early features of PSC are periductal 'onion skin' fibrosis and inflammation, with portal oedema and bile ductular proliferation resulting in expansion of the portal tracts (Fig. 24.34). Later, fibrosis spreads, progressing inevitably to biliary cirrhosis; obliterative cholangitis leads to the so-called 'vanishing bile duct syndrome'.

The link with IBD and associated colon cancer risk is sufficiently strong that all patients diagnosed with PSC should undergo an initial colonoscopy, even in the absence of bowel symptoms.

Management

There is no cure for PSC but management of cholestasis and its complications and specific treatment of the disease process are indicated. UDCA is widely used, although the evidence to support this is limited. UDCA may have benefit in terms of reducing colon carcinoma risk.

The course of PSC is variable. Overall, the median time from diagnosis to death or transplant is around 20 years. Prognosis is worse in

---

i 24.53 Causes of secondary sclerosing cholangitis

- Previous bile duct surgery with stricturing and cholangitis
- Bile duct stones causing cholangitis
- Traumatic or ischaemic bile duct injury
- Critical illness ischaemic cholangiopathy
- Intrahepatic infusion of 5-fluorodeoxyuridine
- Insertion of formalin into hepatic hydatid cysts
- Insertion of alcohol into hepatic tumours
- Parasitic infections (e.g. *Clonorchis*)
- Autoimmune pancreatitis/immunoglobulin G4-associated cholangitis
- Acquired immunodeficiency syndrome (AIDS; probably infective as a result of cytomegalovirus or *Cryptosporidium*)

---

i 24.54 Comparison of primary biliary cholangitis (PBC) and primary sclerosing cholangitis (PSC)

	PBC	PSC
Gender (F:M)	9:1	1:3
Age	Older: median age 50–55 years	Younger: median age 20–40 years
Disease associations	Non-organ-specific autoimmune disease (e.g. Sjögren syndrome) and autoimmune thyroid disease	Ulcerative colitis
Autoantibody profile	90% AMA +ve	65%–85% pANCA +ve (but this is non-specific and not diagnostic)
Predominant bile-duct injury	Intrahepatic	Extrahepatic > intrahepatic

(AMA = antimitochondrial antibody; pANCA = perinuclear antineutrophil cytoplasmic antibody)

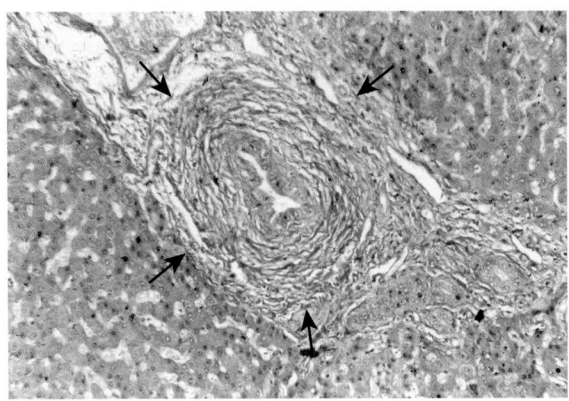

Fig. 24.34 Primary sclerosing cholangitis. Note onion skin scarring (arrows) surrounding a bile duct.

symptomatic patients, possibly reflecting a later disease stage at diagnosis. In recent series, the leading cause of death in PSC is cholangiocarcinoma (58% of deaths), with lower rates attributable to liver failure (30%) and variceal bleeding (9%). Immunosuppressive agents, including prednisolone, azathioprine, methotrexate and ciclosporin, have been tried; results have generally been disappointing.

Symptomatic patients often have pruritus. Management is as for PBC. Fatigue appears to be less prominent than in PBC, although it is still present in some patients.

Cancer screening

Patients with PSC should have annual ultrasound scans to assess for gallbladder polyps, to aid early detection of gallbladder cancer. Patients with PSC and colitis should undergo annual colonoscopy to screen for colorectal cancer. There is not an established role for routine screening for cholangiocarcinoma with either imaging or serum CA19-9 levels, due to both the low specificity and the low likelihood of successful intervention, even with earlier diagnosis.

Management of complications

Broad-spectrum antibiotics (e.g. ciprofloxacin) should be given for acute attacks of cholangitis. If new symptoms or worsening liver tests, non-invasive imaging such as MRCP and/or contrast CT should be performed to assess for a dominant stricture (which may be either inflammatory or malignant). If a dominant stricture is associated with either jaundice or infection, ERCP may be performed for sampling (via brush cytology) to exclude cholangiocarcinoma and to relieve the obstruction, usually through balloon dilatation rather than stenting. Fat-soluble vitamin replacement is necessary in jaundiced patients. Metabolic bone disease (usually osteoporosis) is a common complication that requires treatment.

Surgical treatment

Surgical resection of the extrahepatic bile duct and biliary reconstruction have a limited role in the management of non-cirrhotic patients with dominant extrahepatic disease. Orthotopic transplantation is the only surgical option in patients with advanced liver disease; 5-year survival is 80%–90% in most centres. Unfortunately, the condition may recur in the graft in around 20% of patients and there are no identified therapies able to prevent this. Cholangiocarcinoma is a contraindication to transplantation. Colon carcinoma risk persists following transplantation (and may be increased because of immunosuppression) so colonoscopic surveillance should continue.

A comparison of PBC and PSC is shown in Box 24.53.

IgG4-associated cholangitis

This disease (as well as its nomenclature) is closely related to autoimmune pancreatitis (which is present in more than 90% of the patients).

 24.55 Manifestations of IgG4-related disease

- Autoimmune pancreatitis
- Sialadenitis (especially submandibular gland)
- Dacryoadenitis (lacrimal gland)
- Retroperitoneal fibrosis
- Riedel's thyroiditis
- Retro-orbital tumours
- Periaortitis and periarteritis

IgG4-associated cholangitis (IAC) often presents in middle-aged to older men with obstructive jaundice (due to either hilar stricturing/intrahepatic sclerosing cholangitis or a low bile duct stricture). Cholangiographic appearances can resemble PSC or hilar cholangiocarcinoma. Patients may have past or concurrent evidence of IgG4 disease in other organs (Box 24.55).The serum IgG4 is often raised and liver biopsy shows a lymphoplasmacytic infiltrate, with IgG4-positive plasma cells. It is important not to miss the diagnosis as it responds well to glucocorticoid therapy, often with complete normalisation of liver enzymes and resolution of strictures on serial imaging.

Liver tumours and other focal liver lesions

Identification of a hepatic mass lesion is common, both in patients with known pre-existing liver disease and as a primary presentation. Although primary and secondary malignant tumours are important potential diagnoses, benign disease is frequent. The critical steps to be taken in diagnosing hepatic mass lesions are:

- determining the presence, nature and severity of any underlying chronic liver disease, as the differential diagnosis is very different in patients with and those without chronic liver disease
- using optimal (usually multiple) imaging modalities.

Primary malignant tumours

Hepatocellular carcinoma

Hepatocellular carcinoma (HCC) is the most common primary liver tumour, and the sixth most frequent cause of cancer worldwide. Cirrhosis is present in 75%–90% of individuals with HCC and is an important risk factor for the disease. The risk is between 1% and 5% in cirrhosis caused by hepatitis B and C. There is also an increased risk in cirrhosis due to haemochromatosis, alcohol, NAFLD and alpha-1-antitrypsin deficiency. In northern Europe, 90% of those with HCC have underlying cirrhosis, compared with 30% in Taiwan, where hepatitis B is the main risk factor. The age-adjusted incidence rates vary from 28 per 100000 in Southeast Asia (reflecting the prevalence of hepatitis B) to 10 per 100000 in southern Europe and 5 per 100000 in northern Europe. Chronic hepatitis B infection increases the risk of HCC 100-fold and is the major risk factor worldwide. The risk of HCC is 0.4% per year in the absence of cirrhosis and 2%–6% in cirrhosis. The risk is four times higher in HBeAg-positive individuals than in those who are HBeAg-negative. Hepatitis B vaccination has led to a fall in HCC in countries with a high prevalence of hepatitis B. The incidence in Europe and North America has risen recently, probably related to the increased prevalence of hepatitis C and NAFLD cirrhosis. The risk is higher in men and rises with age.

Macroscopically, the tumour usually appears as a single mass in the absence of cirrhosis, or as a single nodule or multiple nodules in the presence of cirrhosis. It takes its blood supply from the hepatic artery and tends to spread by invasion into the portal vein and its radicals. Lymph node metastases are common, while lung and bone metastases are rare. Well-differentiated tumours can resemble normal hepatocytes and can be difficult to distinguish from normal liver.

24

Clinical features

HCC may present with symptoms or through screening of high-risk patients. Commonly, liver function deteriorates in those with underlying cirrhosis, with worsening ascites, jaundice or variceal haemorrhage. Other symptoms can include weight loss, anorexia and abdominal pain. This often rapid deterioration may be the first presentation of previously undiagnosed cirrhosis. Examination may reveal hepatomegaly or a right hypochondrial mass. Tumour vascularity can lead to an abdominal bruit, and hepatic rupture with intra-abdominal bleeding may occur. The advanced nature of disease that presents in this way makes curative therapy unlikely.

HCC found through screening is typically detected much earlier in its natural history, significantly increasing the treatment options.

Investigations

Serum markers

Alpha-fetoprotein (AFP) is produced by 60% of HCCs. Levels increase with the size of the tumour and are often normal or only minimally elevated in small tumours detected by ultrasound screening. Serum AFP can also rise in the presence of active hepatitis B and C viral replication; very high levels are seen following acute hepatic necrosis, such as that following paracetamol toxicity. AFP is used in conjunction with ultrasound in screening but, in view of low sensitivity and specificity, levels need to be interpreted with caution. Nevertheless, in the absence of active liver inflammation, a significantly elevated or progressively rising AFP warrants an aggressive search for HCC (normal range is < 10 ng/ml [8 IU/ml]). In HCC patients with elevated AFP levels, serial measurements can be a useful biomarker of disease progression or response to treatment.

Imaging

Ultrasound will detect focal liver lesions as small as 1 cm. The use of ultrasound contrast agents has increased sensitivity and specificity but is highly user-dependent. Ultrasound may also show evidence of portal vein involvement and features of coexistent cirrhosis. The diagnosis is usually confirmed on either multi-phase contrast-enhanced CT or MRI, which demonstrate the typical hallmarks of HCC: arterial enhancement with washout on the portal venous phase (Fig. 24.35). Small lesions of less than 2 cm can be difficult to differentiate from hyperplastic nodules in cirrhosis. A combination of imaging modalities (CT and MRI) may be required for indeterminate or probable HCC when the typical radiological features are absent (Fig. 24.36).

Liver biopsy

Histological confirmation is advisable in patients with large tumours who do not have cirrhosis or hepatitis B, in order to confirm the diagnosis and exclude metastatic tumour. Biopsy should be avoided in patients who may be eligible for transplantation or surgical resection because there is a small (1.8%–4%) risk of tumour seeding along the needle tract. In all cases of potential HCC where biopsy is being considered, the impact that a confirmed diagnosis will have on therapy must be weighed against the risks of bleeding.

Role of screening

Screening for HCC, by ultrasound scanning, with or without AFP measurements, every 6 months is indicated in high-risk patients who would be suitable for therapy if diagnosed with HCC. The risk is highest in patients with chronic hepatitis B and cirrhosis due to viral hepatitis and haemochromatosis, and lower in patients with cirrhosis due to Wilson's disease and autoimmune hepatitis. Cost-effectiveness studies suggest that HCC surveillance is warranted in cirrhotic patients where there is an annual incidence of HCC of ≥ 1.5% per year. Screening may also be indicated in those with chronic hepatitis B (who carry an increased risk of HCC, even in the absence of cirrhosis). Although many studies investigating the efficacy of HCC surveillance are affected by lead-time and length-time bias, the current evidence base supports the continued use of HCC surveillance. Screening identifies smaller tumours, often less than 3 cm in size, which are more likely to be cured by surgical resection, local ablative therapy or transplantation.

Management

This is different for patients with cirrhosis and those without. In the presence of cirrhosis, treatment options depend on tumour size and number, severity of liver disease (Child–Pugh score) and performance status. An algorithm for managing those with cirrhosis is shown in Fig. 24.36.

Hepatic resection

This is the treatment of choice for non-cirrhotic patients. The 5-year survival in this group is about 50%. There is a 50% recurrence rate at 5 years, however, which may be due to a second de novo tumour or recurrence of the original tumour. Few patients with cirrhosis are suitable for hepatic resection because of the high risk of hepatic failure. Nevertheless, surgery can be safely performed in cirrhotic patients with small tumours, good liver function (Child–Pugh A) and the absence of clinically relevant portal hypertension (HVPG ≤ 10 mmHg). In experienced centres, advances in surgical technique and pre-operative assessment have permitted liver resection to be performed safely in selected patients with more advanced liver disease and tumour burden.

Liver transplantation

Transplantation has the benefit of curing underlying cirrhosis and removing the risk of a second, de novo tumour in an at-risk patient. The requirement for immunosuppression creates its own risks of reactivation,

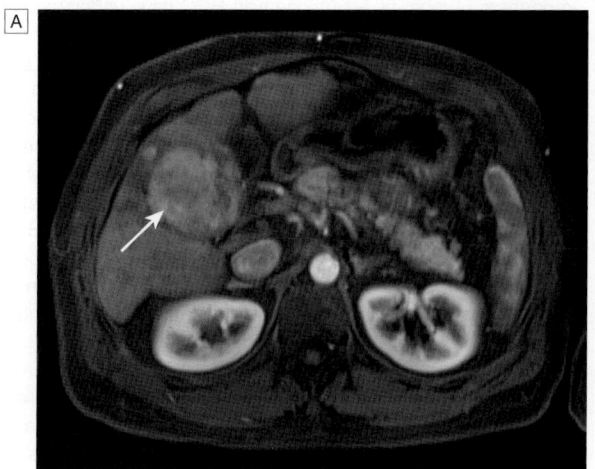
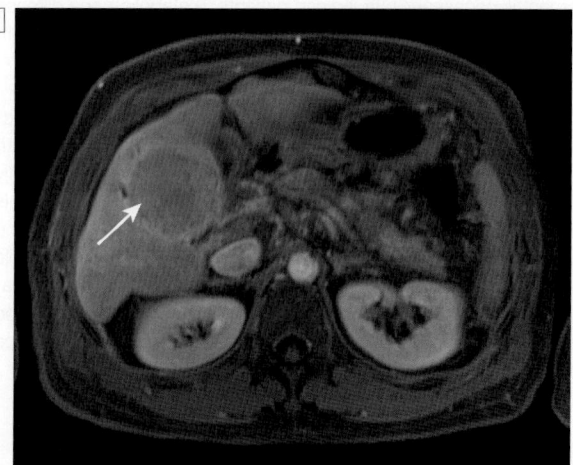

Fig. 24.35 Contrast-enhanced MRI liver showing a large hepatocellular carcinoma. The tumour (marked by the arrows) demonstrates contrast uptake (enhancement) in the arterial phase (A) and washout in the portal venous phase (B). *Courtesy of Dr Hamish Ireland, Royal Infirmary of Edinburgh.*

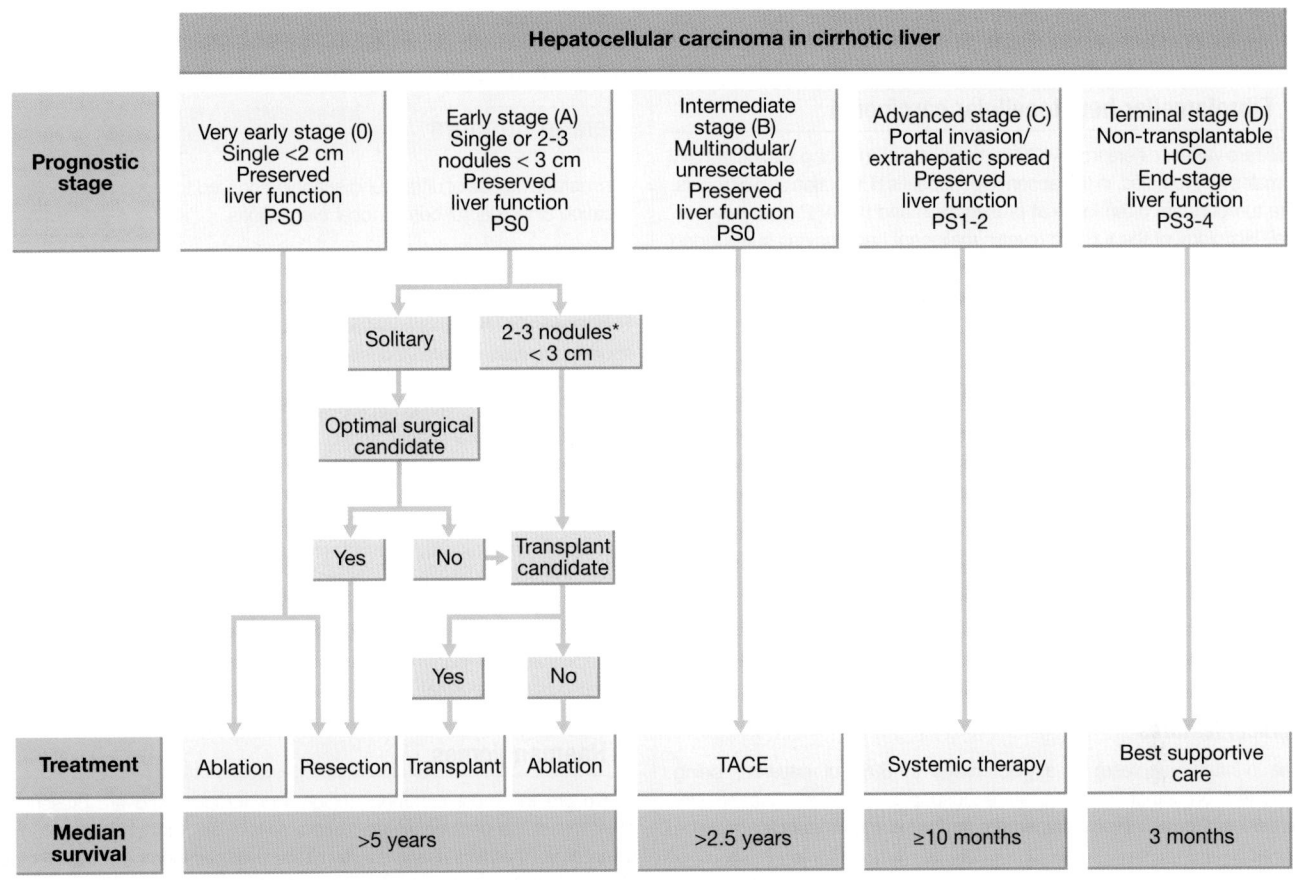

Fig. 24.36 Management of hepatocellular carcinoma complicating cirrhosis. Modified Barcelona Clinic Liver Cancer (BCLC) staging system. Patient management is determined by the size and number of tumours, evidence of portal invasion or extrahepatic spread, severity of underlying liver cirrhosis and performance status. Preserved liver function refers to Childs–Pugh A cirrhosis without ascites. Performance status (PS): 0 = fully active, no symptoms, >2 = limited self-care, confined to bed or chair for more than 50% of waking hours. Optimal surgical candidate refers to a global assessment of a patient's suitability based on compensated liver disease (Child–Pugh A), acceptable grade of portal hypertension, acceptable amount of remaining parenchyma and possibility of using a laparoscopic or minimally invasive approach.
*In some countries, including the United Kingdom, transplant may be considered in patients with up to five tumours, each less than 3 cm. (HCC = hepatocellular carcinoma; TACE = transarterial chemoembolisation) *Adapted from European Association for the Study of the Liver (EASL) Clinical Practice Guidelines: Management of Hepatocellular Carcinoma. Journal of Hepatology. 2018: 69;182–236.*

however, if residual or metastatic disease is present, and assessment of patients for suitability for liver transplantation focuses on the exclusion of extrahepatic disease and vascular invasion. The 5-year survival following liver transplantation is 75% for patients with single tumours of less than 5 cm in size or three tumours smaller than 3 cm (the Milan criteria). Extended criteria have been developed in a number of countries, including the UK, allowing patients to be transplanted with a greater number of small tumours (≤5) or larger single tumours (5–7 cm) that have demonstrated stability after a period of observation (6 months), either with or without locoregional therapy.

Ablative therapy

Ablative therapies use a number of different techniques to achieve localised destruction of tumour tissue. US or CT-guided thermal ablative techniques, including radiofrequency ablation (RFA) and microwave ablation, have largely replaced percutaneous ethanol injection in the treatment of HCC. Alternative techniques include cryoablation and irreversible electroporation. Loco-regional ablative therapies may be curative for patients with early HCC. Thermal ablation in single tumours <3 cm in size is an alternative to surgery based on technical factors (position of the tumour), severity of underlying liver disease and comorbidity.

Transarterial chemoembolisation

Transarterial chemoembolisation (TACE) is the most widely used palliative treatment for patients with HCC not amenable to surgery or potentially curative ablative techniques. TACE involves the selective intra-arterial infusion of chemotherapeutic agents followed by embolisation of the tumour feeding vessels with absorbable gelatin powder (Gelfoam) to achieve localised tumour necrosis and devascularisation. Conventional TACE achieves response rates of 52% with 1-year and 3-year survival rates of 70% and 40%, respectively. Modifications of this technique include the use of drug-eluting beads. TACE should not be used in patients with advanced liver or renal dysfunction, vascular invasion or extra-hepatic spread. TACE is widely used as a bridging therapy for patients awaiting liver transplant and increasingly has found a role in down-staging therapy in patients being considered for liver transplant. Selective internal radiation therapy (SIRT) involves intra-arterial infusion of radioactive substances or microspheres into the hepatic artery. Its use is being investigated as an alternative to TACE or systemic therapy and as a bridging therapy to liver transplant.

Systemic therapy

Sorafenib improves survival from 8 to 11 months in cirrhotic patients, but often with significant side-effects. The drug is a multikinase inhibitor with activity against Raf, vascular endothelial growth factor (VEGF) and platelet-derived growth factor (PDGF) signalling, and is the first systemic therapy to prolong survival in HCC. Levantinib is an alternative oral multi-kinase inhibitor that has demonstrated non-inferiority to sorafinib but with a different side-effect profile. Second-line therapies include regorafenib and cabozantinib. Trials of immune therapy are

24

ongoing. Pre-treatment with sorafenib 2–3 weeks before TACE appears to improve progression-free survival, as reported in the TACTICS trial.

Fibrolamellar hepatocellular carcinoma

This rare variant differs from HCC in that it occurs in young adults, equally in males and females, in the absence of hepatitis B infection and cirrhosis. The tumours are often large at presentation and the AFP is usually normal. Histology of the tumour reveals malignant hepatocytes surrounded by a dense fibrous stroma. The treatment of choice is surgical resection. This variant of HCC has a better prognosis following surgery than an equivalent-sized HCC, two-thirds of patients surviving beyond 5 years.

Other primary malignant tumours

These are rare but include haemangio-endothelial sarcomas. Cholangiocarcinoma (bile duct cancer) typically presents with bile duct obstruction rather than as a hepatic mass lesion, although intra-hepatic cholangiocarcinoma can present as a focal liver tumour.

Secondary malignant tumours

These are common and usually originate from carcinomas in the lung, breast, abdomen or pelvis. They may be single or multiple. Peritoneal dissemination frequently results in ascites.

Clinical features

The primary neoplasm is asymptomatic in 50% of patients, being detected on either radiological, endoscopic or blood biochemistry screening. There is liver enlargement and weight loss; jaundice may be present.

Investigations

A raised ALP activity is the most common biochemical abnormality but LFTs may be normal. Ascitic fluid, if present, has a high protein content and may be blood-stained; cytology sometimes reveals malignant cells. Imaging shows filling defects (Fig. 24.37); laparoscopy may reveal the tumour and facilitates liver biopsy.

Management

Hepatic resection can improve survival for slow-growing colonic carcinoma metastases, and is an approach that should be actively explored in patients who are fit for liver resection and have had the primary tumour resected, once extrahepatic disease has been excluded. Patients with neuro-endocrine tumours (NETs), such as gastrinomas, insulinomas and glucagonomas, and those with lymphomas may benefit from surgery, hormonal treatment or chemotherapy. Unfortunately, palliative treatment to relieve pain is all that is available for most patients.

Benign tumours

The increasing use of ultrasound scanning has led to more frequent identification of incidental benign focal liver lesions.

Hepatic adenomas

These are rare benign hepatocellular tumours that may present as an abdominal mass or with abdominal pain but now more typically present as an incidental finding on imaging.

They are more common in women (female : male ratio 10:1) and are associated with oral contraceptive, androgen and anabolic steroid use. Hepatic adenomas can increase in size during pregnancy. Large or rapidly growing adenomas can rarely rupture, causing intraperitoneal bleeding. In women, resection is indicated for hepatic adenomas ≥5 cm in diameter or with exophytic protrusion, as this is associated with higher rates of bleeding. Hepatic adenomas <5 cm rarely bleed and there is a low rate of malignant transformation. Management involves avoidance of the oral contraceptive pill and weight loss. Resection is recommended for hepatic adenoma in men, irrespective of size because of a higher rate of malignant transformation.

Haemangiomas

These are the most common benign liver tumours and are present in 1%–20% of the population. Most are smaller than 3 cm and rarely cause symptoms. The diagnosis is usually made by ultrasound but CT/MRI may show a low-density lesion with delayed arterial filling. Surgery is needed only for very large symptomatic lesions or where the diagnosis is in doubt.

Focal nodular hyperplasia

Focal nodular hyperplasia (FNH) is a benign polyclonal hepatocellular proliferation resulting from an arterial malformation. FNH is more common in women (female : male ratio 9:1) and typically present between 35 and 50 years. Most are solitary and <5 cm but 20%–30% are multiple. The lesions are usually asymptomatic. They can be differentiated from adenoma by a focal central scar seen on CT or MRI (Fig. 24.38). Histologically, they consist of nodular regeneration of hepatocytes without fibrosis. In the absence of symptoms, surgical resection is not required. If a confident diagnosis of FNH can be made then follow-up imaging is not required. There is no need to discontinue the oral contraceptive pill or monitor in pregnancy.

Cystic liver disease and liver abscess

Isolated or multiple simple cysts are common in the liver and are a relatively frequent finding on ultrasound screening. They can be associated with polycystic renal disease (Fig. 24.39). They are intrinsically benign and require no therapy, other than in rare cases where the mass effect of very large or multiple cysts causes abdominal discomfort. In such cases, percutaneous or surgical debulking can be attempted but recurrence is typical. Liver transplant may rarely be required in severe cases. Liver abscesses are discussed on page 891.

Drugs and the liver

The liver is the primary site of drug metabolism and an important target for drug-induced injury. Pre-existing liver disease may affect the capacity of the liver to metabolise drugs and unexpected toxicity may occur when patients with liver disease are given drugs in normal doses. Box 24.56

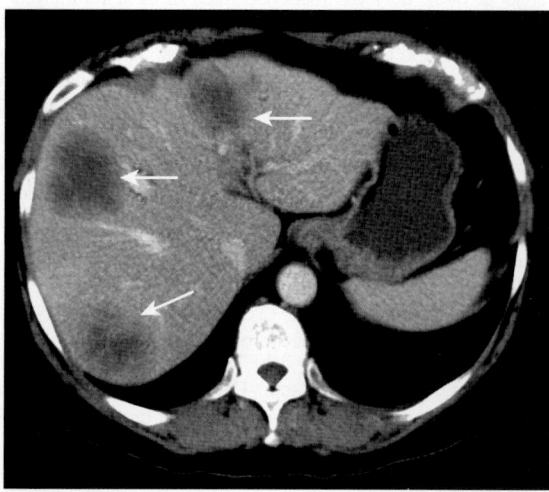

Fig. 24.37 CT liver showing multiple hypo-attenuating liver metastases (arrows). *Courtesy of Dr Hamish Ireland, Royal Infirmary of Edinburgh.*

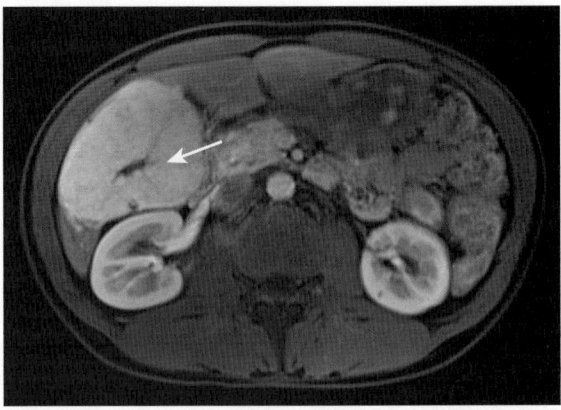

Fig. 24.38 MRI liver showing a large focal nodular hyperplasia with central scar (arrow). *Courtesy of Dr Hamish Ireland, Royal Infirmary of Edinburgh.*

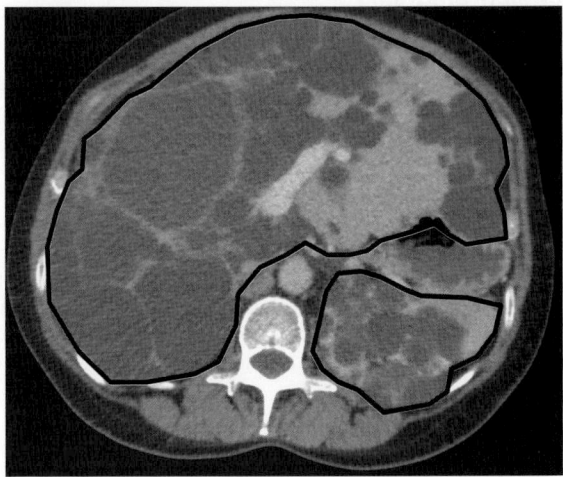

Fig. 24.39 CT abdomen from a patient with polycystic liver and kidney disease. Multiple low attenuation cysts are seen within the liver (highlighted in blue) and left kidney (red). *Courtesy of Dr Hamish Ireland, Royal Infirmary of Edinburgh.*

i	**24.56 Drugs to be avoided in cirrhosis**		
Drug		**Problem**	**Toxicity**
Non-steroidal anti-inflammatory drugs		Reduced renal blood flow Mucosal ulceration	Hepatorenal failure Bleeding varices
Angiotensin-converting enzyme inhibitors		Reduced renal blood flow	Hepatorenal failure
Codeine		Constipation	Hepatic encephalopathy
Narcotics		Constipation, drug accumulation	Hepatic encephalopathy
Anxiolytics		Drug accumulation	Hepatic encephalopathy

i	**24.57 Examples of common causes of drug-induced hepatotoxicity**	
Pattern		**Drug**
Cholestasis		Chlorpromazine High-dose oestrogens
Cholestatic hepatitis		Non-steroidal anti-inflammatory drugs Co-amoxiclav Statins
Acute hepatitis		Rifampicin Isoniazid
Non-alcoholic steatohepatitis		Amiodarone
Venous outflow obstruction		Busulfan Azathioprine
Fibrosis		Methotrexate
Autoimmune hepatitis-like		Nitrofurantoin Checkpoint inhibitors (nivolumab/pembrolizumab)

i	**24.58 Diagnosing acute drug-induced liver disease**

- Tabulate the drugs taken:
  Prescribed and self-administered
- Establish whether hepatotoxicity is reported in the literature
- Relate the time the drugs were taken to the onset of illness: 4 days to 8 weeks (usual)
- Establish the effect of stopping the drugs on normalisation of liver biochemistry:
  Hepatitic liver function tests (2 months)
  Cholestatic/mixed liver function tests (6 months)
  N.B. *Challenge tests with drugs should be avoided*
- Exclude other causes:
  Viral hepatitis
  Biliary disease
- Consider liver biopsy

also shows drugs that should be avoided in patients with cirrhosis, as they can exacerbate known complications of cirrhosis. The possibility of undiagnosed underlying liver injury should always be considered in patients exhibiting unexpected effects following drug exposure.

Drug-induced liver injury

Drug toxicity should always be considered in the differential diagnosis of patients presenting with acute liver failure, jaundice or abnormal liver biochemistry. Drug-induced liver injury (DILI) can be classified as either intrinsic (predictable dose-related toxicity occurring in a large proportion of individuals exposed to a drug) or idiosyncratic (occurring unpredictably in a small proportion of patients exposed to a drug). Typical patterns of drug toxicity are listed in Box 24.57; the most common picture is a mixed cholestatic hepatitis. The presence of jaundice indicates more severe liver damage. Although acute liver failure can occur, most drug reactions are self-limiting and chronic liver damage is rare. Abnormal LFTs often take weeks to normalise following a drug-induced hepatitis, and it may be months before they normalise after a cholestatic hepatitis. Occasionally, permanent bile duct loss (ductopenia) follows a cholestatic drug reaction, such as that due to co-amoxiclav, resulting in chronic cholestasis with persistent symptoms such as itching.

The key to diagnosis is a detailed drug history (Box 24.58), looking for temporal relationships between drug exposure and onset of liver abnormality (bearing in mind the fact that liver injury can frequently take weeks or even months to develop following exposure). A liver biopsy should be considered if there is suspicion of pre-existing liver disease or if blood tests fail to improve when the suspect drug is withdrawn.

Where drug-induced liver injury is suspected or cannot be excluded, the potential culprit drug should be discontinued unless it is impossible to do so safely.

Types of liver injury

Different histological patterns of liver injury may occur with drug injury.

Cholestasis

Pure cholestasis (selective interference with bile flow in the absence of liver injury) can occur with oestrogens; this was common when high concentrations of oestrogens (50 μg/day) were used as contraceptives. Both the current oral contraceptive pill and hormone replacement therapy can be safely used in chronic liver disease.

Chlorpromazine and antibiotics such as flucloxacillin are examples of drugs that cause cholestatic hepatitis, which is characterised by inflammation and canalicular injury. Co-amoxiclav is the most common antibiotic to cause abnormal LFTs but, unlike other antibiotics, it may not produce symptoms until 10–42 days after it is stopped. Anabolic steroids used by body-builders may also cause a cholestatic hepatitis. In some cases (e.g. NSAIDs and cyclo-oxygenase 2 (COX-2) inhibitors), there is overlap with acute hepatocellular injury.

Hepatocyte necrosis

Many drugs cause an acute hepatocellular necrosis with high serum transaminase concentrations; paracetamol is the best known. Inflammation is not always present but does accompany necrosis in liver injury due to diclofenac (an NSAID) and isoniazid (an anti-tuberculous drug). Granulomas may be seen in liver injury following the use of allopurinol. Acute hepatocellular necrosis has also been described following the use of several herbal remedies, including germander, comfrey and jin bu huan. Recreational drugs, including cocaine and ecstasy, can also cause severe acute hepatitis.

Steatosis

Microvesicular hepatocyte fat deposition, due to direct effects on mitochondrial beta-oxidation, can follow exposure to tetracyclines and sodium valproate. Macrovesicular hepatocyte fat deposition has been described with tamoxifen, and amiodarone toxicity can produce a similar histological picture to NASH.

Vascular/sinusoidal lesions

Drugs such as the alkylating agents used in oncology can damage the vascular endothelium and lead to hepatic venous outflow obstruction. Chronic overdose of vitamin A can damage the sinusoids and trigger local fibrosis that can result in portal hypertension.

Hepatic fibrosis

Most drugs cause reversible liver injury and hepatic fibrosis is very uncommon. Methotrexate, however, as well as causing acute liver injury when it is started, can lead to cirrhosis when used in high doses over a long period of time. Risk factors for drug-induced hepatic fibrosis include pre-existing liver disease and a high alcohol intake.

Autoimmune hepatitis-like

Nitrofurantoin is a commonly used antibiotic for urinary tract infections which can cause a liver injury with the features of autoimmune hepatitis, with raised ALT and IgG levels and anti-nuclear or anti-smooth muscle antibodies. Immune checkpoint inhibitors (such as nivolumab and pembrolizumab) are increasingly used as immunotherapy in cancer treatments. A well-recognised side-effect is the development of florid organ-specific autoimmune disease, including an autoimmune hepatitis which can require high-dose steroids to control it.

Inherited liver diseases

The inherited diseases are an important and probably under-diagnosed group of liver diseases. In addition to the 'classical' conditions, such as haemochromatosis and Wilson's disease, the important role played by the liver in the expression of the inborn errors of metabolism should be remembered, as should the potential for genetic underpinning for intrahepatic cholestasis.

 24.59 Causes of haemochromatosis

Primary haemochromatosis

- HFE-associated haemochromatosis (AR)
- Juvenile haemochromatosis (hemojuvelin/hepcidin mutation, AR)
- Transferrin receptor 2 deficiency (*TFR2* mutation, AR)
- Ferroportin disease (*SLC40A1* mutation, AD)

Secondary iron overload

- Transfusional or dietary iron overload
- Iron-loading anaemia (thalassaemia, sideroblastic anaemia, chronic haemolytic anaemias)
- Liver disease (ALD, NAFLD, hepatitis C)

(AD = autosomal dominant, AR = autosomal recessive)

Haemochromatosis

Haemochromatosis is a condition in which the amount of total body iron is increased; the excess iron is deposited in, and causes damage to, several organs, including the liver. It may be primary or secondary to other diseases (Box 24.59).

Genetic haemochromatosis

In genetic haemochromatosis (GH), iron is deposited throughout the body and total body iron may reach 20–60 g (normally 4 g). The important organs involved are the liver, pancreatic islets, endocrine glands, joints and heart. In the liver, iron deposition occurs first in the periportal hepatocytes, extending later to all hepatocytes, with associated fibrosis and eventually cirrhosis.

Pathophysiology

Body iron content is controlled by regulation of iron absorption from diet and its storage in the reticuloendothelial system. The hormone hepcidin inhibits iron transport by binding to ferroportin on enterocytes and macrophages (see Fig. 25.20). Approximately 90% of GH patients are homozygous for a single point mutation resulting in a cysteine to tyrosine substitution at position 282 (C282Y) in the HFE protein, which leads to reduced hepcidin levels and ultimately, uncontrolled increased iron absorption. This is one of the most frequent genetic disorders in Northern European populations. However, penetrance is variable and fewer than 50% of C282Y homozygotes will develop clinical features of haemochromatosis. Iron loss in menstruation and pregnancy can delay the onset of GH in females. A single copy of the C2828Y mutation can also cause GH if also accompanied by a histidine-to-aspartic acid mutation at position 63 (H63D), referred to as compound heterozygosity. This genotype has a lower risk of iron overload and typically causes a less severe form of haemochromatosis. A number of other rare autosomal recessive mutations leading to GH are described. The second most common form of inherited iron disorder is *ferroportin disease*, an autosomal dominant disorder which typically has a milder clinical phenotype than HFE-associated haemochromatosis.

Clinical features

Symptomatic disease usually presents in men over 40 years of age with features of liver disease (often with hepatomegaly), diabetes or heart failure. Fatigue and arthropathy are early symptoms but are frequently absent. Leaden-grey skin pigmentation can sometimes occur due to excess melanin, especially in exposed parts, axillae, groins and genitalia: hence the term 'bronzed diabetes'. Impotence, loss of libido and testicular atrophy are recognised complications, as are early-onset osteoarthritis targeting unusual sites such as the metacarpophalangeal joints, chondrocalcinosis and pseudogout. Cardiac failure or cardiac dysrhythmia may occur due to iron deposition in the heart.

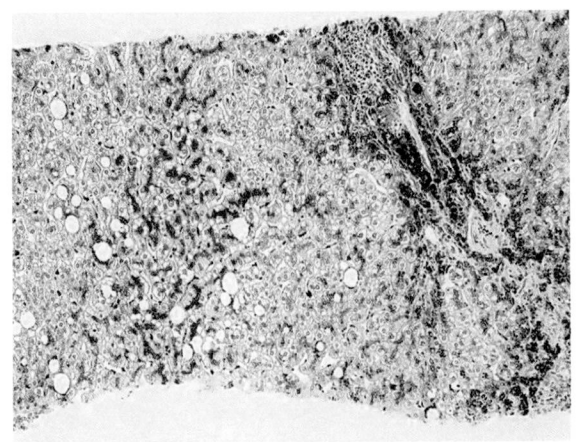

Fig. 24.40 Liver histology: haemochromatosis. This Perls stain shows accumulating iron within hepatocytes, which is stained blue. There is also accumulation of large fat globules in some hepatocytes (macrovesicular steatosis). Iron also accumulates in Kupffer cells and biliary epithelial cells.

Investigations

In the absence of inflammation, serum ferritin is proportional to iron stores and is used as a screening test for iron overload. Patients with GH have raised ferritin and raised transferrin saturations (> 40% in women, > 50% in men), and this pattern should prompt molecular testing for HFE mutations. If HFE-associated GH is confirmed, those with raised transaminases or a ferritin over 1000 μg/L (100 μg/dL) are at highest risk for liver disease and should also undergo fibrosis assessment (usually with transient elastography). If GH is suspected but HFE genotyping is normal, MRI liver or liver biopsy can be used to assess for significant iron overload to identify patients requiring extended genetic testing. Liver biopsy allows assessment of the distribution of iron, with deposition predominantly within hepatocytes being characteristic of haemochromatosis, while accumulation within reticuloendothelial cells is more suggestive of secondary iron overload. The Hepatic Iron Index (HII) provides quantification of liver iron (μmol of iron per gram dry weight of liver/age in years). An HII of more than 1.9 suggests genetic haemochromatosis (Fig. 24.40). The differential diagnoses for elevated ferritin are systemic inflammatory diseases, alcohol-related liver disease and NAFLD. Very significant ferritin elevation can be seen in adult Still's disease.

Management

Treatment consists of weekly venesection of 500 mL blood (250 mg iron) to reduce ferritin to under 50 μg/L (5 μg/dL) and transferrin saturations to under 50%. Thereafter, venesection is continued as required to maintain these parameters. Liver and cardiac problems improve after iron removal, but joint pain is less predictable and can improve or worsen after iron removal. Diabetes does not resolve. First-degree family members should be investigated, preferably by genetic screening, to identify and treat other cases early.

Pre-cirrhotic patients with GH have a normal life expectancy, and even cirrhotic patients have a good prognosis compared with other forms of cirrhosis (three-quarters of patients are alive 5 years after diagnosis). This is probably because liver function is often well preserved at diagnosis and improves with therapy. Screening for hepatocellular carcinoma (p. 901) is mandatory because this is the main cause of death, affecting one-third of patients with cirrhosis. Venesection reduces but does not abolish the risk of hepatocellular carcinoma in the presence of cirrhosis.

Secondary haemochromatosis

Many conditions, including chronic haemolytic disorders, sideroblastic anaemia, other conditions requiring multiple blood transfusion (generally over 50 L), porphyria cutanea tarda, dietary iron overload and occasionally alcohol-related cirrhosis, are associated with widespread secondary iron overload. The features are similar to those of primary haemochromatosis but the history and clinical findings point to the true diagnosis. Some patients are heterozygotes for *HFE* mutations and this may contribute to the development of iron overload.

Wilson's disease

Wilson's disease (hepatolenticular degeneration) is a rare but important autosomal recessive disorder of copper metabolism caused by a variety of mutations in the *ATP7B* gene. Pathological copper accumulation leads to damage to liver, brain and other organs.

Pathophysiology

Copper acts as a cofactor for a number of essential enzymes. Dietary absorption is usually balanced by excretion into bile. The *ATP7B* gene encodes a transmembrane copper-transporting ATPase which excretes copper into bile, and loss of function causes excessive copper accumulation. This transporter is also required for synthesis of functional caeruloplasmin, the circulating copper-binding protein. The amount of copper in the body at birth is normal but thereafter it increases steadily; the organs most affected are the liver, basal ganglia of the brain, eyes, kidneys and skeleton.

At least 700 different mutations have been described. Most cases are compound heterozygotes with two different mutations in *ATP7B*. Attempts to correlate the genotype with the mode of presentation and clinical course have not shown any consistent patterns. The large number of culprit mutations means that, in contrast to haemochromatosis, genetic diagnosis is not routine in Wilson's disease, although it may have a role in screening families following identification of the genotype in an index patient.

Clinical features

Symptoms usually arise between the ages of 5 and 45 years. Hepatic disease occurs predominantly in childhood and early adolescence. Neurological damage causes movement disorders and dementia, which tends to present in later adolescence. These features can occur alone or simultaneously. Other manifestations include renal tubular damage and osteoporosis, but these are rarely presenting features.

Liver disease

There is a wide spectrum of acute and chronic presentations of liver disease, including asymptomatic elevated liver enzymes, acute hepatitis, recurrent jaundice and silent progression to cirrhosis. Fulminant liver failure can occur, especially in young women. This causes the liberation of free copper into the blood stream, causing massive haemolysis and renal tubulopathy. The possibility of Wilson's disease should be considered in any patient under the age of 40 presenting with recurrent acute hepatitis or chronic liver disease of unknown cause, especially when this is accompanied by haemolytic anaemia.

Neurological disease

Clinical features include a variety of extrapyramidal features, particularly tremor, choreoathetosis, dystonia, parkinsonism and dementia. Neurological disease typically develops after the onset of liver disease and can be prevented by effective treatment. This increases the importance of diagnosis in the liver phase beyond just allowing effective management of liver disease.

Kayser–Fleischer rings

These constitute the most important single clinical clue to the diagnosis and can be seen in 60% of adults with Wilson's disease (less often in children but almost always in neurological Wilson's disease), but require slit-lamp examination for correct identification. Kayser–Fleischer rings are characterised by greenish-brown discoloration of the corneal margin appearing first at the upper periphery. They disappear with treatment.

24

Investigations

Diagnosis of Wilson's disease is based on algorithms incorporating symptoms and signs, measures of copper metabolism and DNA analysis. A low serum caeruloplasmin is the best single laboratory clue to the diagnosis. However, advanced liver failure from any cause can also reduce the serum caeruloplasmin, and conversely a normal value does not exclude the diagnosis if there is a high index of suspicion. Other features of disordered copper metabolism should therefore be sought; these include a high free serum copper concentration, a high urine copper excretion of greater than 0.6 μmol/24 hrs (38 μg/24 hrs) and a very high hepatic copper content. Measuring 24-hour urinary copper excretion while giving D-penicillamine is a useful confirmatory test; more than 25 μmol/24 hrs is considered diagnostic of Wilson's disease.

Management

Pharmacological treatment is with either chelating-agents (D-penicillamine or trientene) that increase urinary copper excretion, or zinc salts, which reduce absorption of dietary copper. The copper-binding agent penicillamine is the drug of choice. The dose given must be sufficient to produce cupriuresis and most patients require 1.5 μg/day (range 1–4 μg). The dose can be reduced once the disease is in remission but treatment must continue for life, even through pregnancy. Care must be taken to ensure that re-accumulation of copper does not occur. Abrupt discontinuation of treatment must be avoided because this may precipitate acute liver failure. Toxic effects occur in one-third of patients and include rashes, protein-losing nephropathy, lupus-like syndrome and bone marrow depression. If these arise, trientine dihydrochloride (1.2–2.4 μg/day) and zinc (50 mg 3 times daily) are potential alternatives.

Prognosis is excellent with early treatment, and presymptomatic patients compliant with treatment have comparable survival to the general population. Liver transplantation is indicated for fulminant liver failure or for advanced cirrhosis with liver failure. The value of liver transplantation in severe neurological Wilson's disease is unclear. Siblings and children must be investigated and treatment should be given to all affected individuals, even if they are asymptomatic.

Alpha-1-antitrypsin deficiency

Alpha-1-antitrypsin (α_1-AT) is a serine protease inhibitor (Serpin, or Pi) produced by the liver and secreted into the circulation. One of its main functions is the breakdown of neutrophil elastase. Circulating levels of α1-AT can double during the acute phase response and play a key anti-inflammatory role, preventing damage to normal tissue. Numerous variants of the *SERPINA1* gene have been described but there are two common mutations. The wild type is known as the M allele. Ninety-five percent of cases of severe deficiency are due to homozygosity of the Z allele. Mild deficiency can result from the less-severe S allele. The mutated α_1-AT forms polymers within the endoplasmic reticulum of hepatocytes, with reduced secretion into the blood. The accumulation of polymers within hepatocytes causes the liver toxicity, whereas the unopposed neutrophil elastase activity causes damage to structural proteins in the lungs. Homozygous individuals (PiZZ) have low plasma α_1-AT concentrations, although globules containing α_1-AT are found in the liver, and these people may develop hepatic and pulmonary disease. Liver manifestations include cholestatic jaundice in the neonatal period (neonatal hepatitis), which can resolve spontaneously; and chronic hepatitis leading to cirrhosis in adults. Alpha$_1$-AT deficiency is an exacerbating factor for liver disease of other aetiologies, and the possibility of dual pathology should be considered when severity of disease, such as ALD, appears disproportionate to the level of underlying insult.

There are no clinical features that distinguish liver disease due to α_1-AT deficiency from liver disease due to other causes, and the diagnosis is made from the low plasma α_1-AT concentration and genotyping for the presence of the mutation. Alpha$_1$-AT-containing globules can be demonstrated in the liver (Fig. 24.41) but this is not necessary to make the diagnosis.

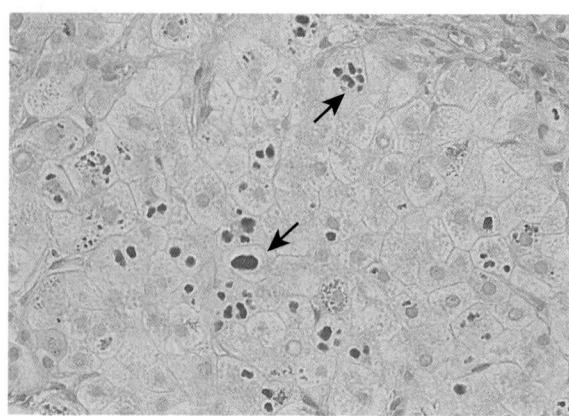

Fig. 24.41 Liver histology in alpha-1-antitrypsin deficiency. Accumulation of periodic acid–Schiff-positive granules (arrows) within individual hepatocytes is shown in this section from a patient with α_1-AT deficiency.

There is no specific treatment. The risk of severe and early-onset emphysema means that all patients should be advised to stop smoking.

Gilbert syndrome

Gilbert syndrome is by far the most common inherited disorder of bilirubin metabolism (see Box 24.12). It is an autosomal recessive trait when caused by a mutation in the promoter region of the gene for UDP-glucuronyl transferase enzyme (*UGT1A1*), which leads to reduced enzyme expression. It can be inherited in a dominant fashion when there is a missense mutation in the gene. This results in decreased conjugation of bilirubin, which accumulates as unconjugated bilirubin in the blood. The levels of unconjugated bilirubin increase during fasting, as fasting reduces levels of UDP-glucuronyl transferase.

Clinical features

The typical presentation is with isolated elevation of bilirubin, typically, although not exclusively, in the setting of physical stress or illness. There are no stigmata of chronic liver disease other than jaundice. Increased excretion of bilirubin and hence stercobilinogen leads to normal-coloured or dark stools, and increased urobilinogen excretion causes the urine to turn dark on standing as urobilin is formed. In the presence of haemolysis, pallor due to anaemia and splenomegaly due to excessive reticuloendothelial activity are usually present.

Investigations

The plasma bilirubin is usually less than 100 μmol/L (~6 mg/dL) and the LFTs are otherwise normal. There is no bilirubinuria because the hyperbilirubinaemia is predominantly unconjugated. Hepatic histology is normal and liver biopsy is not recommended for the investigation of patients with possible Gilbert syndrome. The condition is not associated with liver injury and thus has an excellent prognosis, needs no treatment, and is clinically important only because it may be mistaken for more serious liver disease.

Vascular liver disease

Metabolically, the liver is highly active and has large oxygen requirements. This places it at risk of ischaemic injury in settings of impaired perfusion. The risk is mitigated, however, by the dual perfusion of the liver (via the portal vein as well as hepatic artery), with the former representing a low-pressure perfusion system that offers protection against the potential effects of arterial hypotension. The single outflow through the hepatic vein and the low-pressure perfusion system of the portal vein make the liver vulnerable to venous thrombotic ischaemia in the context of Budd–Chiari syndrome and portal vein thrombosis, respectively.

Hepatic arterial disease

Liver ischaemia

Liver ischaemic injury (ischaemic hepatitis) is relatively common during hypotensive or hypoxic events and is under-diagnosed. The characteristic pattern is one of rising transaminase values in the days following such an event (e.g. prolonged seizures). Ischaemic hepatitis is more common in patients with pre-existing hepatic congestion (e.g. congestive cardiac failure) or underlying liver disease. Liver synthetic dysfunction and encephalopathy are uncommon but can occur. Liver failure is very rare. Diagnosis typically rests on clinical suspicion and exclusion of other potential aetiologies. Treatment is aimed at optimising liver perfusion and oxygen delivery. Outcome is dictated by the morbidity and mortality associated with the underlying disease, given that liver ischaemia frequently occurs in the context of other organ ischaemia in high-risk patients.

Liver arterial disease

Hepatic arterial disease is rare outside the setting of liver transplantation and is difficult to diagnose. It can cause significant liver damage. Hepatic artery occlusion may result from inadvertent injury during biliary surgery or may be caused by emboli, neoplasms, polyarteritis nodosa, blunt trauma or radiation. It usually causes severe upper abdominal pain with or without signs of circulatory shock. LFTs show raised transaminases (AST or ALT usually > 1000 U/L), as in other causes of acute liver damage. Patients usually survive if the liver and portal blood supply are otherwise normal.

Hepatic artery aneurysms are extrahepatic in three-quarters of cases and intrahepatic in one-quarter. Atheroma, vasculitis, bacterial endocarditis and surgical or biopsy trauma are the main causes. They usually lead to bleeding into the biliary tree, peritoneum or intestine. CT scans are helpful in identifying the location of the aneurysm, adjacent structures and evidence of rupture. Angiography remains the gold standard for diagnosis. Treatment is radiological or surgical. Any of the vasculitides can affect the hepatic artery but this rarely causes symptoms.

Hepatic artery thrombosis (HAT) is a recognised complication of liver transplantation and typically occurs in the early post-transplant period. Clinical features are often related to bile duct rather than liver ischaemia because of the dominant role of the hepatic artery in extrahepatic bile duct perfusion. Manifestations can include bile duct anastomotic failure with bile leak or the development of late bile duct strictures (ischaemic cholangiopathy). Diagnosis and initial intervention are radiological in the first instance, with ERCP and biliary stenting being the principal approaches to the treatment of biliary strictures causing significant cholestasis.

Portal venous disease

Portal hypertension

See page 881.

Portal vein thrombosis

Portal venous thrombosis as a primary event is rare but can occur in any condition predisposing to thrombosis. It may also complicate intra-abdominal inflammatory or neoplastic disease and is a recognised cause of portal hypertension. Acute portal venous thrombosis causes abdominal pain and diarrhoea, and may rarely lead to bowel infarction, requiring surgery. Underlying thrombophilia needs to be excluded. Treatment is based on anticoagulation, which is associated with increased recanalisation rates following acute portal vein thrombosis. Subacute thrombosis can be asymptomatic but may subsequently lead to extrahepatic portal hypertension. Ascites is unusual in non-cirrhotic portal hypertension, unless the albumin is particularly low.

Portal vein thrombosis can arise as a secondary event in patients with cirrhosis and portal hypertension, and is a recognised cause of decompensation in patients with previously stable cirrhosis. In individuals showing such decompensation, portal vein patency should be assessed by ultrasound with Doppler flow studies. The role of anticoagulation in patients with chronic portal vein thrombosis is unclear, but it is recommended in potential transplant candidates to reduce the risk of clot propagation. Chronic portal vein thrombosis can be a cause of portal hypertension.

Hepatopulmonary syndrome

This condition is characterised by resistant hypoxaemia (PaO_2 < 9.3 kPa (70 mmHg)), intrapulmonary vascular dilatation in patients with cirrhosis, and portal hypertension. Clinical features include finger clubbing, cyanosis and a characteristic reduction in arterial oxygen saturation on standing (orthodeoxia). The hypoxia is due to intrapulmonary shunting through direct arteriovenous communications. Nitric oxide (NO) over-production may be important in pathogenesis. The hepatopulmonary syndrome can be treated by liver transplantation but, if severe (PaO_2 < 6.7 kPa (50 mmHg)), is associated with an increased operative risk.

Portopulmonary hypertension

This unusual complication of portal hypertension is similar to 'primary pulmonary hypertension' (p. 549). It is defined as pulmonary hypertension with increased pulmonary vascular resistance and a normal pulmonary artery wedge pressure in a patient with portal hypertension. The condition is caused by vasoconstriction and obliteration of the pulmonary arterial system and leads to breathlessness and fatigue.

Hepatic venous disease

Obstruction to hepatic venous blood flow can occur in the small central hepatic veins, the large hepatic veins, the inferior vena cava or the heart. The clinical features depend on the cause and on the speed with which obstruction develops, and can mimic many other forms of chronic liver disease, sometimes leading to delayed diagnosis. Congestive hepatomegaly and ascites are the most consistent features. The possibility of hepatic venous obstruction should always be considered in patients with an atypical liver presentation.

Budd–Chiari syndrome

This uncommon condition is caused by thrombosis of the larger hepatic veins and sometimes the inferior vena cava. Many patients have haematological disorders such as myelofibrosis, primary proliferative polycythaemia, paroxysmal nocturnal haemoglobinuria, or antithrombin III, protein C or protein S deficiencies (Ch. 25). Pregnancy and oral contraceptive use, obstruction due to tumours (particularly carcinomas of the liver, kidneys or adrenals), congenital venous webs and occasionally inferior vena caval stenosis are the other main causes. The underlying cause cannot be found in about 30% of patients, although this percentage is falling as molecular diagnostic tools (e.g. for the *JAK2* mutation in myelofibrosis) increase the capacity to diagnose underlying haematological disorders. Hepatic congestion affecting the centrilobular areas is followed by centrilobular fibrosis, and eventually cirrhosis supervenes in those who survive long enough.

Clinical features

Acute venous occlusion causes rapid development of upper abdominal pain, marked ascites and occasionally acute liver failure. More gradual occlusion causes gross ascites and, often, upper abdominal discomfort. Hepatomegaly, frequently with tenderness over the liver, is almost always present. Peripheral oedema occurs only when there is inferior vena cava obstruction. Features of cirrhosis and portal hypertension develop in those who survive the acute event.

24

Investigations

The LFTs vary considerably, depending on the presentation, and can show the features of acute hepatitis. Ascitic fluid analysis shows a protein concentration above 25 g/L (2.5 g/dL) (exudate) in the early stages; however, this often falls later in the disease. Doppler ultrasound may reveal obliteration of the hepatic veins and reversed flow or associated thrombosis in the portal vein. CT may show enlargement of the caudate lobe, as this often has a separate venous drainage system that is not involved in the disease. CT and MRI may also demonstrate occlusion of the hepatic veins and inferior vena cava. Liver biopsy demonstrates centrilobular congestion with fibrosis, depending on the duration of the illness. Venography is needed only if CT and MRI are unable to demonstrate the hepatic venous anatomy clearly.

Management

Predisposing causes should be treated as far as possible; where recent thrombosis is suspected, thrombolysis with recombinant tissue plasminogen activator or streptokinase, followed by heparin and oral anticoagulation, should be considered. Long-term anticoagulation is required. Ascites is initially treated medically but often with only limited success. Short hepatic venous strictures can be treated with angioplasty. In the case of more extensive hepatic vein occlusion, many patients can be managed successfully by insertion of a covered TIPSS, followed by anticoagulation. Surgical shunts, such as portacaval shunts, are rarely performed now that TIPSS is available. Approximately 40% of patients will require TIPSS following failure of medical management. Survival at 1 year and 5 years following TIPSS is 88% and 78%, respectively. Occasionally, a web can be resected or an inferior vena caval stenosis dilated. Progressive liver failure is an indication for liver transplantation and life-long anticoagulation.

Sinusoidal obstruction syndrome (veno-occlusive disease)

Sinusoidal obstruction syndrome (SOS; previously known as veno-occlusive disease) is a rare condition characterised by widespread occlusion of the small central hepatic veins. Pyrrolizidine alkaloids in *Senecio* and *Heliotropium* plants used to make teas, as well as cytotoxic drugs and hepatic irradiation, are all recognised causes. SOS may develop in 10%–20% of patients following haematopoietic stem cell transplantation (usually within the first 20 days) and carries a 90% mortality in severe cases. Pathogenesis involves obliteration and fibrosis of terminal hepatic venules due to deposition of red cells, haemosiderin-laden macrophages and coagulation factors. In this setting, SOS is thought to relate to pre-conditioning therapy with irradiation and cytotoxic chemotherapy. The clinical features are similar to those of the Budd–Chiari syndrome (see above). Investigations show evidence of venous outflow obstruction histologically but, in contrast to Budd–Chiari, the large hepatic veins appear patent radiologically. Transjugular liver biopsy (with portal pressure measurements) may facilitate the diagnosis. Treatment involves close supportive care/fluid management to maintain intravascular filling, and in severe cases, defibrotide, a drug that binds to vascular endothelial cells, promoting fibrinolysis and suppressing coagulation, is recommended.

Cardiac disease

Hepatic damage, due primarily to congestion, may develop in all forms of right heart failure; usually, the clinical features are predominantly cardiac. Very rarely, long-standing cardiac failure and hepatic congestion give rise to liver cirrhosis. Liver cirrhosis is a recognised complication of some forms of congenital heart disease. Fontan-associated liver disease develops in patients with diverse forms of congenital cardiac disease resulting in a single functioning ventricle, treated with the Fontan procedure. Chronic hepatic congestion resulting from passive filling of the pulmonary arterial circulation results in progressive liver fibrosis and cirrhosis. Severe left ventricular dysfunction is a cause of ischaemic hepatitis. Cardiac causes of acute and chronic liver disease are typically under-diagnosed. Treatment is principally that of the underlying heart disease with supportive treatment for the liver component.

Nodular regenerative hyperplasia of the liver

This is the most common cause of non-cirrhotic portal hypertension in developed countries; it is characterised by small hepatocyte nodules throughout the liver without fibrosis, which can result in sinusoidal compression. It is believed to be due to damage to small hepatic arterioles and portal venules. It occurs in older people and is associated with many conditions, including connective tissue disease, haematological diseases and immunosuppressive drugs, such as azathioprine. The condition is usually asymptomatic but occasionally presents with portal hypertension or with an abdominal mass. The diagnosis is made by liver biopsy, which, in contrast to cirrhosis, shows nodule formation in the absence of fibrous septa. Liver function is good and the prognosis is very favourable. Management is based on treatment of the portal hypertension.

Pregnancy and the liver

The inter-relationship between liver disease and pregnancy can be a complex one and a source of real anxiety for both patient and clinician. Three possibilities need to be borne in mind when treating a pregnant woman with a liver abnormality:

- This represents a worsening of pre-existing chronic liver or biliary disease (although pregnancy may be the first time a woman's liver biochemistry has been tested, so this may not have previously been diagnosed).
- This represents a genuine first presentation of liver disease that is not intrinsically related to pregnancy.
- This represents a genuine pregnancy-associated liver injury process.

It is critical to obtain information relating to liver disease risk factors and pre-pregnancy liver status to establish whether any abnormality was present before pregnancy. In general, the earlier in pregnancy that liver abnormality presents, the more likely it is to represent either pre-existing liver disease or non-pregnancy-related acute liver disease. Equally, the best outcome for both mother and baby results from optimising the physical condition of the mother, and in situations of deteriorating liver function (which can be steep in late pregnancy) consideration should always be given to early delivery if the fetus is viable. Joint management between hepatologists and obstetricians is essential.

Intercurrent and pre-existing liver disease

Acute hepatitis A can occur during pregnancy but has no effect on the fetus. Chronic hepatitis B requires identification in pregnancy because of long-term health implications for the mother and the effectiveness of perinatal vaccination (with or without pre-delivery maternal antiviral therapy) in reducing neonatal acquisition of chronic hepatitis B. Maternal transmission of hepatitis C occurs in 1% of cases and there is no convincing evidence that the mode of delivery affects this. Hepatitis E (genotypes 1 and 2) is reported to progress to acute liver failure much more commonly in pregnancy, with a 20% maternal mortality. Pregnancy may be associated with either worsening or improvement of autoimmune hepatitis, although improvement during pregnancy and rebound post-partum is the most common pattern seen. Complications of portal hypertension may be a particular issue in the second and third trimesters.

Gallstones are more common during pregnancy and may present with cholecystitis or biliary obstruction. The diagnosis can usually be made

Box 24.60 Abnormal liver function tests in pregnancy

- **Liver function tests**: alkaline phosphatase (ALP) levels and albumin normally fall in pregnancy. ALP levels can rise due to the contribution of placental ALP.
- **Pre-existing liver disease**: pregnancy is uncommon in cirrhosis because cirrhosis causes relative infertility. Varices can enlarge in pregnancy, and ascites should be treated with amiloride rather than spironolactone. Penicillamine for Wilson's disease and azathioprine for autoimmune liver disease should be continued during pregnancy. Autoimmune liver disease can flare up post partum.
- **Incidental**: viral, autoimmune and drug-induced hepatitis must be excluded in the presence of an elevated alanine aminotransferase (ALT). Immunoglobulin/vaccination given to the fetus at birth prevents transmission of hepatitis B to the fetus if the mother is infected. Gallstones are more common in pregnancy and post partum, and are a cause of a raised ALP level. Biliary imaging with ultrasound and magnetic resonance cholangiopancreatography is safe. Endoscopic retrograde cholangiopancreatography to remove stones can be performed safely with shielding of the fetus from radiation.
- **Pregnancy-related liver diseases**: occur predominantly in the third trimester and resolve post partum. Maternal and fetal mortality and morbidity are reduced by expediting delivery.

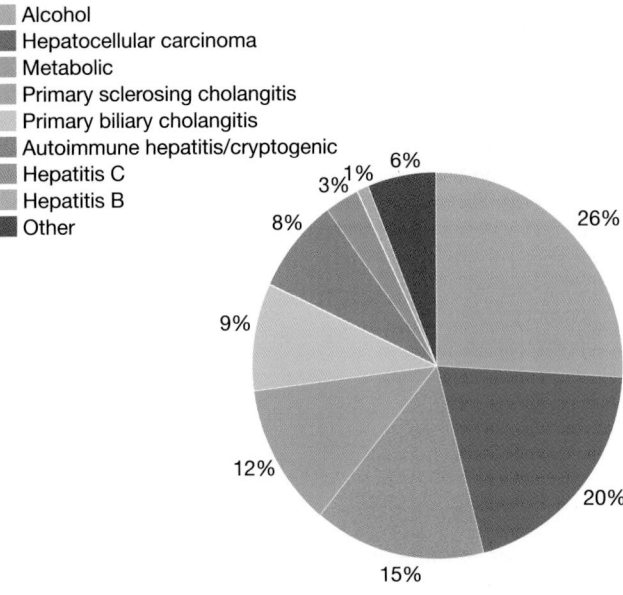

Fig. 24.42 Indications for elective adult liver transplantation in the UK, 2019–2020.

with ultrasound. In biliary obstruction due to gallstones, therapeutic ERCP can be safely performed but lead protection for the fetus is essential and X-ray screening must be kept to a minimum.

Pregnancy-associated liver disease

Several conditions occur only during pregnancy, may recur in subsequent pregnancies and resolve after delivery of the baby, and these are discussed in Chapter 32. The causes of abnormal LFTs in pregnancy, which include pregnancy-associated liver disease, are shown in Box 24.60.

Liver transplantation

Liver transplantation is an effective treatment for end-stage liver disease. However, the number of procedures is limited by cadaveric donor availability and 5%–15% of those listed for liver transplantation will die while awaiting a donor liver. The main complications of liver transplantation relate to long-term immunosuppression, rejection or disease recurrence in the liver graft.

Indications and contraindications

More than 30000 liver transplants are performed worldwide each year. The main indications vary between regions. In Europe, the majority of liver transplants are for decompensated cirrhosis (56%), most frequently due to alcohol, hepatitis C or NAFLD, followed by hepatocellular carcinoma (17%), with 8% for acute liver failure. Fig. 24.42 shows indications for transplantation in the UK. In Asia, the most common indication is hepatocellular carcinoma related to hepatitis B. Patterns are changing over time, with reducing need for transplant in hepatitis C as a result of improved antiviral therapy, but increasing prevalence of NAFLD. Liver transplantation is increasingly being undertaken in older patients, with 30% of liver transplants in Europe now in patients aged over 60 years, but only a very small number aged over 70 years.

Transplant may be undertaken to improve survival in advanced liver disease or to alleviate symptoms. Common indications for elective transplant assessment are listed in Box 24.61. There are various criteria for HCC based on the size and number of lesions and level of serum alpha-fetoprotein (as these factors predict risk of recurrence post-transplant). Current UK guidelines allow transplant for a single lesion below

 24.61 Indications for liver transplant assessment for cirrhosis

Complications

- First episode of bacterial peritonitis
- Diuretic-resistant ascites
- Recurrent variceal haemorrhage
- Hepatocellular carcinoma
- Persistent hepatic encephalopathy

Poor liver function

- Bilirubin > 100 μmol/L (5.8 mg/dL) in primary biliary cholangitis
- MELD score > 12 (Box 24.32)
- UKELD score ≥ 49
- Child–Pugh grade C (Box 24.31)

(MELD = Model for End-stage Liver Disease; UKELD United Kingdom Model for End-stage Liver Disease)

5 cm, or up to five lesions all below 3 cm, provided there is no macrovascular invasion or extrahepatic spread. Larger lesions may be suitable if stable following treatment. Specific criteria exist for patients with acute liver failure, depending on aetiology.

The main contraindications to transplantation are extrahepatic sepsis or malignancy, active alcohol or other substance misuse, and significant cardiorespiratory disease.

Patients are matched for ABO blood group and size but do not require HLA matching with donors, as the liver is a relatively immune-privileged organ compared with the heart or kidneys.

Organ allocation is often based on greatest need, estimating short-term mortality using the MELD or UKELD scores (see Box 24.32). The United Kingdom has recently moved to a national allocation system based on Transplant Benefit Score, which uses donor and recipient variables to calculate the difference between the mortality without transplant (need) and the predicted 5-year survival with transplant (utility), to identify those with the greatest net benefit.

Approaches to increase the availability of donor organs include:

- *Split liver transplantation*. Due to the liver's regenerative capacity, a cadaveric donor liver can be split into two, with the larger right lobe used in an adult and the smaller left lobe used in a child.

24

- *Living donor transplantation*. This is normally performed using the left lateral segment or the right lobe from a healthy donor. The donor mortality is significant, at 0.5%–1%. Pre-operative assessment includes looking at donor liver size and psychological status.
- *Use of marginal grafts*. Higher-risk livers (older donors, steatotic livers, non-heart-beating donors) are being used in selected patients. Novel organ perfusion technologies may help to improve graft selection and outcomes in this group.
- *Increased donation*. Improved infrastructure to support organ donation, increased public awareness of transplantation and changes to consent process ('opt-out', or presumed consent) may all increase donation rates.

Complications

Early complications

Primary graft non-function

This is due to a severe ischaemia--reperfusion injury, resulting in irreversible graft failure and requiring early re-transplantation in around 4%–6% of recipients. Factors that increase the likelihood of primary non-function include increasing donor age, degree of steatosis in the liver and the length of ischaemia.

Technical complications

These include hepatic artery thrombosis, which may necessitate re-transplantation. Anastomotic biliary strictures can also occur; these may respond to endoscopic stenting, or require surgical reconstruction. Portal vein thrombosis following transplant is rare.

Rejection

Lifelong immunosuppression is required in most liver transplant recipients, although at lower levels than with kidney or heart/lung transplants. Immunosuppression is maximal in the early post-operative period, with reducing levels over time. A number of different regimens are used but the majority include a calcineurin inhibitor (usually tacrolimus) with or without an antimetabolite (azathioprine or mycophenolate) or tapering steroids. Some patients can eventually be maintained on a single agent. Acute cellular rejection occurs in 15%–25% of patients, commonly presenting as raised liver enzymes at 5–30 days post-transplant, but can arise later. This normally responds to 3 days of high-dose intravenous methylprednisolone.

Infections

Bacterial infections, such as pneumonia and wound infections, can occur in the first few weeks after transplantation. Opportunistic infections are also seen, and prophylaxis against fungal infections and *Pneumocystis jirovecii* may be given during the first few months. Cytomegalovirus (primary infection or reactivation) is common in the 3 months after transplantation and can cause fevers, bone marrow suppression and hepatitis. Patients who have never had cytomegalovirus infection but who receive a liver from a donor who has been exposed are at greatest risk and are usually given prophylactic antiviral therapy, such as valganciclovir. Patients with latent tuberculosis should receive prophylaxis against reactivation.

Late complications

Late complications are mostly consequences of long-term immunosuppression. These include malignancy (especially skin cancers and lymphoma), renal failure and cardiovascular disease. Weight gain is common following liver transplantation, leading to obesity and diabetes. Chronic rejection is rare, occurring in only 5% of cases. Recurrence of the initial disease can occur, especially with autoimmune liver diseases or hepatocellular carcinoma.

Prognosis

Current UK data show 1-year survival for patients transplanted for cirrhosis of 94%, with 5-year survival of 84%. Outcomes are worse in patients transplanted for acute liver failure as they often have multi-organ failure at the time of transplantation, and in patients transplanted for hepatocellular carcinoma, due to disease recurrence.

Cholestatic and biliary disease

The concepts of biliary and cholestatic disease, and the important distinctions between them, can be a source of confusion. 'Cholestasis' relates to impaired bile flow, usually detected as a biochemical abnormality (typically, elevation of ALP and elevation in serum bile acid levels and bilirubin). This can be due to failure of bile acid transport across the hepatocyte membrane, or physical obstruction of the bile duct. 'Biliary disease' relates to pathology at any level from the small intrahepatic bile ducts to the sphincter of Oddi. Although there is very significant overlap between cholestatic and biliary disease, there are scenarios where cholestasis can exist without biliary disease (transporter disease or pure drug-induced cholestasis) and where biliary disease can exist without cholestasis (when disease of the bile duct does not impact on bile flow).

Chemical cholestasis

Pure cholestasis can occur as an inherited condition (p. 906), as a consequence of cholestatic drug reactions (p. 906) or as acute cholestasis of pregnancy. A more frequent, but less recognised, acquired biochemical cholestasis occurs in sepsis ('cholangitis lenta'). This biochemical phenomenon is one of the causes of LFT abnormality in sepsis. Also termed subacute non-suppurative cholangitis, it is characterised by inspissated bile plugs in dilated bile ductules in the absence of mechanical obstruction. It does not require specific treatment and has a prognostic significance conferred by the underlying septic process.

Mutations in the biliary transporter proteins on the hepatocyte canalicular membrane (familial intrahepatic cholestasis 1, FIC1), illustrated in Fig. 24.7, have been shown to cause an inherited intrahepatic biliary disease in childhood, characterised by raised ALP levels and progression to a biliary cirrhosis. It is also becoming increasingly clear that these proteins contribute to intrahepatic biliary disease in adulthood.

Benign recurrent intrahepatic cholestasis

Benign recurrent intrahepatic cholestasis (BRIC) is a rare autosomal recessive genetic disorder characterised by recurrent episodes of cholestatic jaundice lasting weeks to months. It usually presents in adolescence. Prodromal symptoms include pruritus, nausea, vomiting and weight loss. Patients are asymptomatic between episodes. Blood tests typically show conjugated hyperbilirubinaemia with elevated alkaline phosphatase. Cholangiography shows no evidence of biliary obstruction. Liver biopsy shows cholestasis during episodes but is normal between episodes.

BRIC is associated with mutations in the genes for two bile acid transporters: ATP8B1 (BRIC1) encoding FIC1 and ABCB11 (BRIC2) encoding the bile salt export pump (BSEP). Treatment is required to relieve symptoms and the long-term prognosis is good.

Intrahepatic biliary disease

Inflammatory and immune disease

The small intrahepatic bile ducts appear to be specifically vulnerable to immune injury, and ductopenic injury ('vanishing bile duct syndrome') can be a feature of a number of chronic conditions, including graft-versus-host disease (GVHD), sarcoidosis and, in the setting of liver transplantation, ductopenic rejection. Intrahepatic small bile duct injury occurs most frequently in primary biliary cholangitis, an autoimmune cholestatic disease, and less frequently in primary sclerosing cholangitis (see Box 24.54).

Caroli's disease

Caroli's disease and Caroli's syndrome are rare congenital disorders characterised by multifocal saccular dilatation of the intrahepatic bile ducts. Bile duct ectasia may involve the entire liver, a lobe or a single segment. In Caroli's disease, biliary ectasia occurs in isolation. However, in the more common variant, Caroli's syndrome, the bile duct dilatation is associated with congenital hepatic fibrosis. The molecular pathogenesis is incompletely understood. Most cases are transmitted in an autosomal recessive manner and are associated with autosomal recessive polycystic kidney disease (ARPKD). In both conditions, focal dilatation of bile ducts leads to cholestasis with formation of biliary sludge and intraductal calculi. Recurrent attacks of cholangitis require antibiotic therapy and predispose to hepatic abscess formation. There is an increased risk of cholangiocarcinoma affecting 2.5%–16% of patients. Prognosis is generally poor. Localised disease may be treated by segmental liver resection. Patients with diffuse disease complicated by recurrent biliary sepsis or portal hypertension may require liver transplantation.

Congenital hepatic fibrosis

Congenital hepatic fibrosis (CHF) is a rare developmental disorder characterised by broad bands of fibrous tissue linking portal tracts and irregular-shaped proliferating bile ducts, resulting from ductal plate malformation. CHF may be inherited in an autosomal recessive manner and is associated with a range of disorders with multisystem involvement, including: Caroli's syndrome, polycystic kidney disease, Joubert syndrome and Bardet–Biedl syndrome. The renal tubules may show cystic dilatation (medullary sponge kidney) and renal cysts/renal failure may develop. The condition typically present in childhood or early adulthood, although late presentation is described. Patients may present with symptoms of portal hypertension, including painful splenomegaly and variceal bleeding with preserved hepatic function, or with symptoms of cholestasis and recurrent cholangitis (Caroli's syndrome). However, patients frequently present with symptoms related to other organ systems (e.g. kidney, central nervous system).

Cystic fibrosis

The term cystic fibrosis-associated liver disease (CFLD) encompasses the range of liver disease seen in patients with cystic fibrosis. Liver function test abnormalities are common, with persistent abnormalities affecting 40% of patients with cystic fibrosis. Biliary cirrhosis develops in 5%–10% of individuals by adolescence/early adulthood when complications such as variceal haemorrhage may occur. Non-cirrhotic portal hypertension may develop as a consequence of pre-sinusoidal obliterative portal venopathy. UDCA improves liver biochemistry but it is unclear whether the drug can prevent progression of liver disease. Deficiency of fat-soluble vitamins (A, D, E and K) may need to be treated in view of biliary and pancreatic disease.

Extrahepatic biliary disease

Diseases of the extrahepatic biliary tree typically present with the clinical features of impaired bile flow (jaundice, itch and fat malabsorption). Obstructive disease is frequently a consequence of ductal gallstones, sometimes with associated infection or inflammatory strictures, or post-surgical strictures. Malignant diseases (cholangiocarcinoma or carcinoma of the head of pancreas) should be considered in all patients with extrahepatic biliary obstruction. PSC frequently involves the extrahepatic biliary tree and its differential, IgG4 disease, is an important and potentially treatable cause of disease.

Choledochal cysts

Choledochal cysts are uncommon congenital cysts of the biliary tree (Fig. 24.43). They are usually diagnosed in the first decade of life. The majority cause diffuse dilatation of the common bile duct (type I). Others represent true diverticulae of the common bile duct (type II), dilatation of the intra-duodenal bile duct at the pancreatico-biliary junction (type III) or dilatation of the intrahepatic and/or the extrahepatic biliary ducts (type IV). Type IV choledochal cysts are subdivided into those affecting the intrahepatic and extrahepatic ducts (type IVA) or multiple cysts affecting extrahepatic ducts with normal intrahepatic ducts (type IVB). Type V choledochal cysts refer to one or more cystic dilatations of intrahepatic ducts with normal extrahepatic ducts, with multiple cystic dilatations of intrahepatic ducts referred to as Caroli's disease. Children may present with abdominal mass, jaundice or biliary peritonitis from cyst rupture. Adults more commonly present with jaundice, abdominal pain and cholangitis. Liver abscess and biliary cirrhosis may develop. There is an increased incidence of cholangiocarcinoma. Cyst excision with hepaticojejunostomy is the treatment of choice.

Secondary biliary cirrhosis

Secondary biliary cirrhosis develops after prolonged large duct biliary obstruction due to gallstones, benign bile duct strictures or sclerosing cholangitis (see below). Carcinomas rarely cause secondary biliary cirrhosis because few patients survive long enough. The clinical features are those of chronic cholestasis with episodes of ascending cholangitis or even liver abscess. Cirrhosis, ascites and portal hypertension are late features. Relief of biliary obstruction may require endoscopic or surgical intervention. Cholangitis dictates treatment with antibiotics, which can be given continuously if attacks recur frequently.

Gallstones

Gallstone formation is the most common disorder of the biliary tree and it is unusual for the gallbladder to be diseased in the absence of gallstones. In high-income countries, gallstones occur in 7% of males and 15% of females aged 18–65 years, with an overall prevalence of 11%. In individuals under 40 years there is a 3:1 female preponderance, whereas in older people the sex ratio is about equal. Gallstones are less frequent in Asia and Africa. There has been much debate over the role of diet

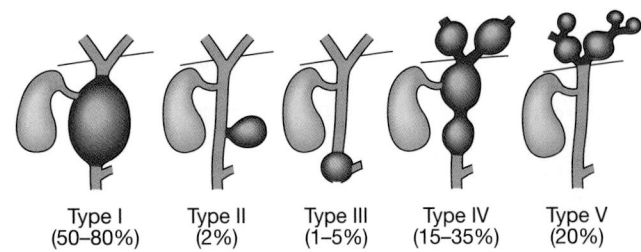

| Type I (50–80%) | Type II (2%) | Type III (1–5%) | Type IV (15–35%) | Type V (20%) |

Fig. 24.43 Classification and frequency of choledochal cysts. *Adapted from the Todani Classification of Choledochal Cysts (1977).*

24

in cholesterol gallstone disease; an increase in dietary cholesterol, fat, total calories and refined carbohydrate or lack of dietary fibre has been implicated.

Pathophysiology

Gallstones are conventionally classified into cholesterol or pigment stones, although the majority are of mixed composition. Gallstones contain varying quantities of calcium salts, including calcium bilirubinate, carbonate, phosphate and palmitate, which are radio-opaque. Gallstone formation is multifactorial and the factors involved are related to the type of gallstone (Boxes 24.62 and 24.63).

Cholesterol gallstones

Cholesterol is held in solution in bile by its association with bile acids and phospholipids in the form of micelles and vesicles. Biliary lipoproteins may also have a role in solubilising cholesterol. In gallstone disease, the liver produces bile that contains an excess of cholesterol because there is either a relative deficiency of bile salts or a relative excess of cholesterol ('lithogenic' bile). Abnormalities of bile salt synthesis and circulation, cholesterol secretion and gallbladder function may make production of lithogenic bile more likely.

Pigment stones

Brown, crumbly pigment stones are almost always the consequence of bacterial or parasitic biliary infection. They are common in the Far East, where infection allows bacterial β-glucuronidase to hydrolyse conjugated bilirubin to its free form, which then precipitates as calcium bilirubinate. The mechanism of black pigment gallstone formation in high-income countries is not satisfactorily explained. Haemolysis is important as a contributing factor for the development of black pigment stones that occur in chronic haemolytic disease.

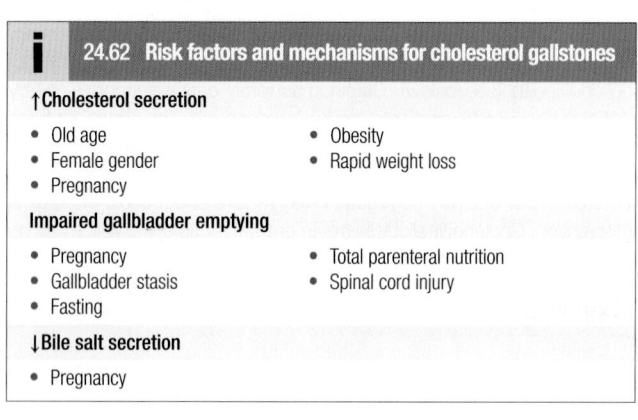

i 24.62 Risk factors and mechanisms for cholesterol gallstones

↑Cholesterol secretion

- Old age
- Female gender
- Pregnancy
- Obesity
- Rapid weight loss

Impaired gallbladder emptying

- Pregnancy
- Gallbladder stasis
- Fasting
- Total parenteral nutrition
- Spinal cord injury

↓Bile salt secretion

- Pregnancy

i 24.63 Composition of and risk factors for pigment stones

Black	Brown
Composition	
Polymerised calcium bilirubinates*	Calcium bilirubinate crystals*
Mucin glycoprotein	Mucin glycoprotein
Calcium phosphate	Cholesterol
Calcium carbonate	Calcium palmitate/stearate
Cholesterol	
Risk factors	
Haemolysis	Infected bile
Age	Stasis
Hepatic cirrhosis	
Ileal resection/disease	

*Major component.

Biliary sludge

This describes gelatinous bile that contains numerous microspheroliths of calcium bilirubinate granules and cholesterol crystals, as well as glycoproteins; it is an important precursor to the formation of gallstones in the majority of patients. Biliary sludge is frequently formed under normal conditions but then either dissolves or is cleared by the gallbladder; only in about 15% of patients does it persist to form cholesterol stones. Fasting, parenteral nutrition and pregnancy are also associated with sludge formation.

Clinical features

Only 10% of individuals with gallstones develop clinical evidence of gallstone disease. However, once symptoms occur they are likely to recur. Symptomatic stones within the gallbladder (Box 24.64) manifest as either biliary pain ('biliary colic') or cholecystitis (see below). If a gallstone becomes acutely impacted in the cystic duct, the patient will experience pain. The term 'biliary colic' is a misnomer because the pain does not rhythmically increase and decrease in intensity like other forms of colic. Typically, the pain occurs suddenly and persists for several hours; if it continues for more than 6 hours, a complication such as cholecystitis or pancreatitis may be present. Pain is usually felt in the epigastrium (70% of patients) or right upper quadrant (20%) and radiates to the interscapular region or the tip of the right scapula, but other sites include the left upper quadrant and the lower chest. The pain can mimic intrathoracic disease, oesophagitis, myocardial infarction or aortic dissection.

Combinations of fatty food intolerance, dyspepsia and flatulence not attributable to other causes have been referred to as 'gallstone dyspepsia'. These symptoms are not now recognised as being caused by gallstones and are best regarded as functional dyspepsia. Acute and chronic cholecystitis is described below.

A mucocele may develop if there is slow distension of the gallbladder from continuous secretion of mucus; if this material becomes infected, an empyema supervenes. Calcium may be secreted into the lumen of the hydropic gallbladder, causing 'limey' bile, and if calcium salts are precipitated in the gallbladder wall, the radiological appearance of 'porcelain' gallbladder results.

Gallstones in the gallbladder (cholecystolithiasis) migrate to the common bile duct (choledocholithiasis; p. 916) in approximately 10%–20% of patients and can cause biliary colic. Rarely, stones can fistulate between the gallbladder and the gastric outlet or duodenum (causing obstruction, known as Bouveret syndrome) or colon. If this occurs, air will be seen in the biliary tree on plain abdominal X-rays. If a stone larger than 2.5 cm in diameter has migrated into the gut, it may then impact either at the terminal ileum or sigmoid colon. The resultant intestinal obstruction may be followed by 'gallstone ileus'. Gallstones impacted in the cystic duct may cause obstruction to the common hepatic duct and the clinical picture of extrahepatic biliary diseases ('Mirizzi syndrome', with its important differential of malignant bile duct stricture). The more common cause of jaundice due to gallstones is a stone passing from the cystic duct into the common bile duct (choledocholithiasis), which may also result in cholangitis or acute pancreatitis. It is usually very small stones that precipitate acute pancreatitis, due to oedema at the ampulla as the stone

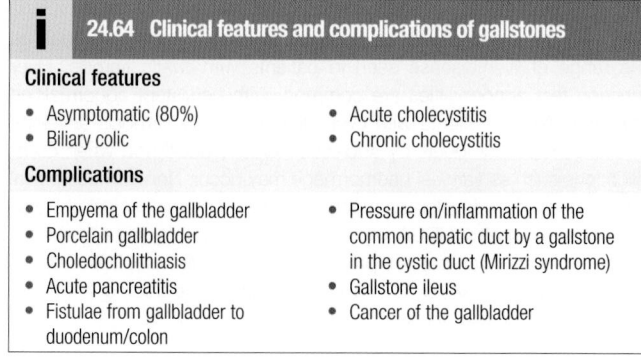

i 24.64 Clinical features and complications of gallstones

Clinical features

- Asymptomatic (80%)
- Biliary colic
- Acute cholecystitis
- Chronic cholecystitis

Complications

- Empyema of the gallbladder
- Porcelain gallbladder
- Choledocholithiasis
- Acute pancreatitis
- Fistulae from gallbladder to duodenum/colon
- Pressure on/inflammation of the common hepatic duct by a gallstone in the cystic duct (Mirizzi syndrome)
- Gallstone ileus
- Cancer of the gallbladder

24.65 Gallbladder disease in old age

- **Gallstones**: by the age of 70 years, prevalence is around 30% in women and 19% in men.
- **Acute cholecystitis**: tends to be severe, may have few localising signs and is associated with a high frequency of empyema and perforation. If such complications supervene, mortality may reach 20%.
- **Cholecystectomy**: mortality after urgent cholecystectomy for acute uncomplicated cholecystitis is not significantly higher than in younger patients.
- **Endoscopic sphincterotomy and removal of common duct stones**: well tolerated by older patients, with lower mortality than surgical common bile duct exploration.
- **Cancer of the gallbladder**: a disease of old age, with a 1-year survival of 10%.

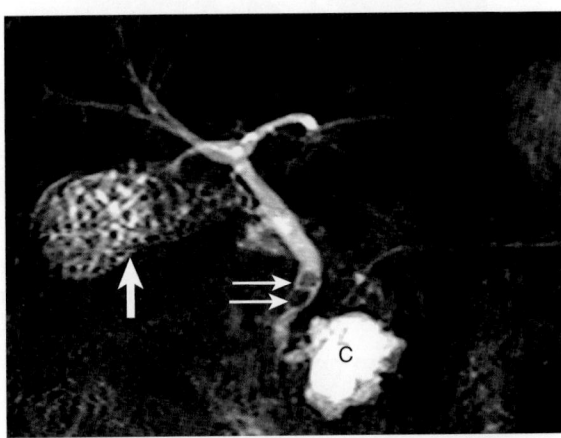

Fig. 24.44 Magnetic resonance cholangiopancreatogram showing multiple small stones in the gallbladder (large arrow), two larger stones in the distal common bile duct (smaller arrows) and also a cystic lesion in the head of pancreas (C).

passes into the duodenum. No stone is seen within the bile duct in 80% of cases of presumed gallstone pancreatitis, suggesting stone passage. Previous stone passage is also the likely cause of most cases of benign papillary fibrosis, which is most commonly seen in patients with previous or present gallstone disease. It presents with biliary pain (often following cholecystectomy) with cholestatic LFTs and biliary dilatation, or acute pancreatitis, and is treated by ERCP and sphincterotomy.

Cancer of the gallbladder is increasing in frequency but in over 85% of cases is associated with the presence of gallstones. Previously, the diagnosis was typically made as an incidental histological finding following cholecystectomy for gallstone disease. Increasing awareness of the risk of gallbladder carcinoma and of the role played by polyps in the natural history has led to an increase in screening activity and prospective diagnosis. Biliary disease is common in the elderly and can be challenging to manage in frail patients (Box 24.65).

Investigations

Ultrasound is the investigation of choice for diagnosing gallstones. Most stones are diagnosed by transabdominal ultrasound, which has more than 84% sensitivity and 99% specificity for gallbladder stones (see Fig. 24.8). CT, MRCP (Fig. 24.44) and, increasingly, EUS are excellent modalities for detecting complications of gallstones (distal bile duct stone or gallbladder empyema) but are inferior to ultrasound in defining their presence in the gallbladder. When recurrent attacks of otherwise unexplained acute pancreatitis occur, they may result from 'microlithiasis' in the gallbladder or common bile duct and are best assessed by EUS.

Management

Asymptomatic gallstones found incidentally in the gallbladder should not be treated because the majority will never cause symptoms.

24.66 Treatment of gallstones

Gallbladder stones
- Cholecystectomy: laparoscopic or open
- Oral bile acids: chenodeoxycholic or ursodeoxycholic (low rate of stone dissolution)

Bile duct stones
- Endoscopic sphincterotomy and stone extraction
- Surgical bile duct exploration
- Lithotripsy (endoscopic or extracorporeal shock wave, ESWL)

Symptomatic gallstones are best treated surgically by laparoscopic cholecystectomy; the severity of symptoms should be balanced against the individual patient surgical risk in order to decide whether surgery is warranted. Asymptomatic common bile duct stones should also be removed due to the high risk of complications (Box 24.66).

Cholecystitis

Acute cholecystitis

Pathophysiology

Acute cholecystitis is almost always associated with obstruction of the gallbladder neck or cystic duct by a gallstone. Occasionally, obstruction may be by mucus, parasitic worms or a biliary tumour, or may follow endoscopic bile duct stenting. The pathogenesis is unclear but the initial inflammation is possibly chemically induced. This leads to gallbladder mucosal damage, which releases phospholipase, converting biliary lecithin to lysolecithin, a recognised mucosal toxin. At the time of surgery, approximately 50% of cultures of the gallbladder contents are sterile. Infection occurs eventually, and in older patients or those with diabetes mellitus a severe infection with gas-forming organisms can cause emphysematous cholecystitis. Acalculous cholecystitis can occur in the intensive care setting and in association with parenteral nutrition, sickle cell disease and diabetes mellitus.

Clinical features

The cardinal feature is pain in the right upper quadrant but also in the epigastrium, the right shoulder tip or the interscapular region. Differentiation between biliary colic and acute cholecystitis may be difficult; features suggesting cholecystitis include severe and prolonged pain, fever and leucocytosis.

Examination shows right hypochondrial tenderness with guarding, worse on inspiration (Murphy's sign) and occasionally a gallbladder mass (30% of cases). Fever is present but rigors are unusual and suggest cholangitis. Jaundice occurs in less than 10% of patients and is usually due to passage of stones into the common bile duct, or to compression or even stricturing of the common bile duct following stone impaction in the cystic duct (Mirizzi syndrome). Gallbladder perforation occurs in 10%–15% of cases and gallbladder empyema may arise.

Investigations

Peripheral blood leucocytosis is common, except in older patients, in whom the signs of inflammation may be minimal. Minor increases of transaminases and amylase may be encountered. Amylase should be measured to detect acute pancreatitis, which may be a potentially serious complication of gallstones. Only when the amylase is higher than 1000 U/L can pain be confidently attributed to acute pancreatitis, since moderately elevated levels of amylase can occur with many other causes of abdominal pain. Plain X-rays of the abdomen and chest may show radio-opaque gallstones, and rarely intrabiliary gas due to fistulation of a gallstone into the intestine; they are important in excluding lower lobe pneumonia and a perforated viscus. Ultrasonography detects gallstones and gallbladder thickening due to cholecystitis but gallbladder empyema or perforation is best assessed by CT.

24

Management

Medical

Medical management consists of bed rest, pain relief, antibiotics and intravenous fluids. Moderate pain can be treated with NSAIDs but more severe pain should be managed with opiates. A cephalosporin (such as cefuroxime) or piperacillin/tazobactam is the usual antibiotic of choice, but metronidazole is normally added in severely ill patients and local prescribing practice may vary. Cholecystitis usually resolves with medical treatment but the inflammation may progress to an empyema or perforation and peritonitis.

Surgical

Urgent surgery is the optimal treatment when cholecystitis progresses in spite of medical therapy and when complications such as empyema or perforation develop. The operation should be carried out within 5 days of the onset of symptoms. Delayed surgery after 2–3 months is no longer favoured. When cholecystectomy may be difficult due to extensive inflammatory change, percutaneous gallbladder drainage can be performed, with subsequent cholecystectomy 4–6 weeks later. Recurrent biliary colic or cholecystitis is frequent if the gallbladder is not removed.

Chronic cholecystitis

Chronic inflammation of the gallbladder is almost invariably associated with gallstones. The usual symptoms are those of recurrent attacks of upper abdominal pain, often at night and following a heavy meal. The clinical features are similar to those of acute calculous cholecystitis but milder. Patients may recover spontaneously or following analgesia and antibiotics. They are usually advised to undergo elective laparoscopic cholecystectomy.

Acute cholangitis

Acute cholangitis is caused by bacterial infection of bile ducts and occurs in patients with other biliary problems, such as choledocholithiasis (see below), biliary strictures or tumours, or after ERCP. Jaundice, fever (with or without rigors) and right upper quadrant pain are the main presenting features ('Charcot's triad'). Treatment is with antibiotics, relief of biliary obstruction and removal (if possible) of the underlying cause.

Choledocholithiasis

Stones in the common bile duct (choledocholithiasis) occur in 10%–15% of patients with gallstones (Fig. 24.45), which have usually migrated from the gallbladder. Primary bile duct stones are rare but can develop within the common bile duct many years after a cholecystectomy, and are sometimes related to biliary sludge arising from dysfunction of the sphincter of Oddi. In Far Eastern countries, primary common bile duct stones are thought to follow bacterial infection secondary to parasitic infections with *Clonorchis sinensis*, *Ascaris lumbricoides* or *Fasciola hepatica*. Common bile duct stones can cause bile duct obstruction and may be complicated by cholangitis due to secondary bacterial infection, sepsis, liver abscess and biliary stricture.

Clinical features

Choledocholithiasis may be asymptomatic, may be found incidentally by operative cholangiography at cholecystectomy or on abdominal imaging, or may manifest as biliary colic, jaundice, cholangitis or pancreatitis. If the gallbladder is still present, it is usually small, fibrotic and impalpable.

Investigations

The LFTs show a cholestatic pattern. If cholangitis is present, the patient usually has a leucocytosis. Initial imaging is with transabdominal ultrasound which often show dilated extrahepatic and intrahepatic bile ducts, together with gallbladder stones (Fig. 24.46), but does not always reveal the cause of the obstruction in the common bile duct; 50% of bile duct stones are missed on ultrasound, particularly those in the distal common bile duct. MRCP and EUS both have a high sensitivity for ductal stones,

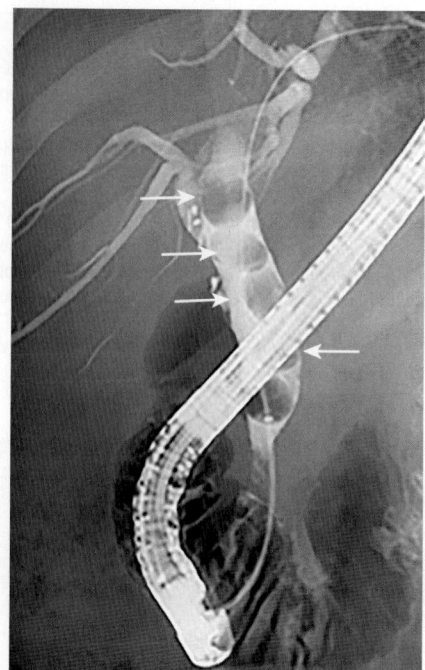

Fig. 24.45 Endoscopic retrograde cholangiopancreatogram showing common duct stones (arrows).

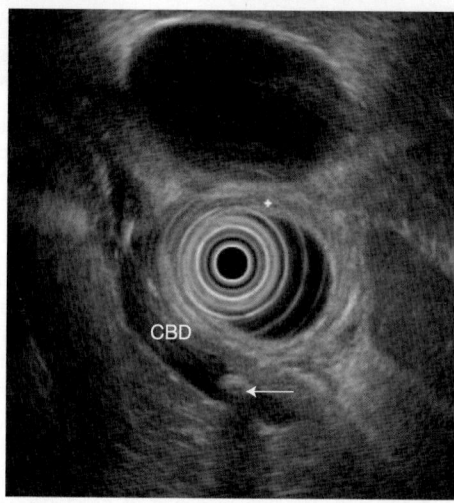

Fig. 24.46 Endoscopic ultrasonography (EUS) image showing a prominent common bile duct (CBD) containing a small stone (arrow) causing acoustic shadowing.

and can also help to define biliary anatomy prior to intervention. MRCP is often preferred as it is non-invasive.

Management

Cholangitis should be treated with analgesia, intravenous fluids and broad-spectrum antibiotics, such as cefuroxime and metronidazole (local prescribing practice may vary). Blood cultures should be taken before the antibiotics are administered. Patients also require urgent decompression of the biliary tree and stone removal. ERCP with biliary sphincterotomy and stone extraction is the treatment of choice and is successful in about 90% of patients. In some complex cases cholangioscopy ('SpyGlass'™) with electrohydraulic lithotripsy may be required. If ERCP fails, other approaches include percutaneous transhepatic drainage and combined ('rendezvous') endoscopic procedures, extracorporeal shock wave lithotripsy (ESWL) and surgery.

Surgical treatment of choledocholithiasis is performed less frequently than ERCP. The CBD may be explored laparoscopically, either transcystic (via the gallbladder) or trans-ductal, or at laparotomy.

Recurrent pyogenic cholangitis

This disease occurs predominantly in South-east Asia. Biliary sludge, calcium bilirubinate concretions and stones accumulate in the intrahepatic bile ducts, with secondary bacterial infection. Patients present with recurrent attacks of upper abdominal pain, fever and cholestatic jaundice. Investigation of the biliary tree demonstrates that both the intrahepatic and the extrahepatic portions are filled with soft biliary mud. Eventually, the liver becomes scarred and liver abscesses and secondary biliary cirrhosis develop. The condition is difficult to manage and requires drainage of the biliary tract with extraction of stones, antibiotics and, in certain patients, partial resection of damaged areas of the liver.

Tumours of the gallbladder and bile duct

Carcinoma of the gallbladder

This is an uncommon tumour, occurring more often in females and usually in those over the age of 70 years. More than 90% are adenocarcinomas; the remainder are anaplastic or, rarely, squamous tumours. Gallstones are present in 70%–80% of cases and are thought to be important in the aetiology of the tumour. Individuals with a calcified gallbladder ('porcelain gallbladder') are at high risk of malignant change, and gallbladder polyps greater than 1 cm in size are associated with increased risk of malignancy; preventative cholecystectomy should be considered in such patients. Chronic infection with *Salmonella*, especially in areas where typhoid is endemic, is also a risk factor.

Carcinoma of the gallbladder may be diagnosed incidentally and is found in 0.2%–3% of gallbladders removed at cholecystectomy for gallstone disease. It may manifest as repeated attacks of biliary pain and, later, persistent jaundice and weight loss. A gallbladder mass may be palpable in the right hypochondrium. LFTs show cholestasis, and calcification of the gallbladder wall ('porcelain gallbladder') may be found on X-ray. The tumour can be diagnosed by ultrasonography and staged by CT. The treatment is surgical excision but local extension of the tumour beyond the wall of the gallbladder into the liver, lymph nodes and surrounding tissues is common at diagnosis. Only a minority of pre-operatively diagnosed gallbladder cancers are suitable for resection. Palliative management is usually all that can be offered. Survival is generally short, death typically occurring within 1 year in patients presenting with symptoms.

Cholangiocarcinoma

Cholangiocarcinoma (CCA) is an uncommon tumour that can arise anywhere in the biliary tree, from the intrahepatic bile ducts (20%–25% of cases) and the confluence of the right and left hepatic ducts at the liver hilum (50%–60%) to the distal common bile duct (20%). It accounts for only 1.5% of all cancers but the incidence is increasing. The cause is unknown but the tumour is associated with gallstones, primary and secondary sclerosing cholangitis, Caroli's disease and choledochal cysts (see Fig. 24.43). In the Far East, particularly northern Thailand, chronic liver fluke infection (*Clonorchis sinensis*) is a major risk factor for the development of CCA in men. Primary sclerosing cholangitis carries a lifetime risk of CCA of 5%–20%, although only 5% of CCAs relate to primary sclerosing cholangitis. Cirrhosis is a risk factor for intrahepatic cholangiocarcinoma. Chronic biliary inflammation appears to be a common factor in the development of biliary dysplasia and cancer that is shared by all the predisposing causes.

Tumours typically invade the lymphatics and adjacent vessels, with a predilection for spread within perineural sheaths. The presentation is usually with obstructive jaundice. About 50% of patients also have upper abdominal pain and weight loss. The diagnosis is made using a combination of CT and MRI (see Fig. 24.10) but can be difficult to confirm in patients with sclerosing cholangitis. Serum levels of the tumour marker CA19-9 are elevated in up to 80% of cases, although this may occur in biliary obstruction of any cause. In the setting of biliary obstruction, ERCP may result in positive biliary cytology. The sensitivity of biliary brushing cytology is low (20%–43%) but can be improved with analysis for chromosomal aneuploidy using fluorescent in situ hybridisation (FISH). Endoscopic ultrasound–fine needle aspiration (EUS–FNA) of bile duct masses or lymph nodes is sometimes possible, and in specialist centres cholangioscopy with biopsy is now established. CCAs can be treated surgically in about 20% of patients, which improves 5-year survival from less than 5% to 20%–40%. Surgery involves excision of the extrahepatic biliary tree with or without a liver resection and a Roux loop reconstruction. Liver transplant is generally not recommended as a treatment for CCA due to high recurrence rate and poor long-term survival. Neoadjuvant chemotherapy followed by liver transplant is effective in highly selected patients with perihilar CCA, but is not a widely accepted or available treatment.

Most patients with CCA are treated with stent insertion across the malignant biliary stricture, using endoscopic or percutaneous transhepatic techniques to achieve relief of jaundice (Fig. 24.47). Patients with unresectable disease may receive chemotherapy and selected

24

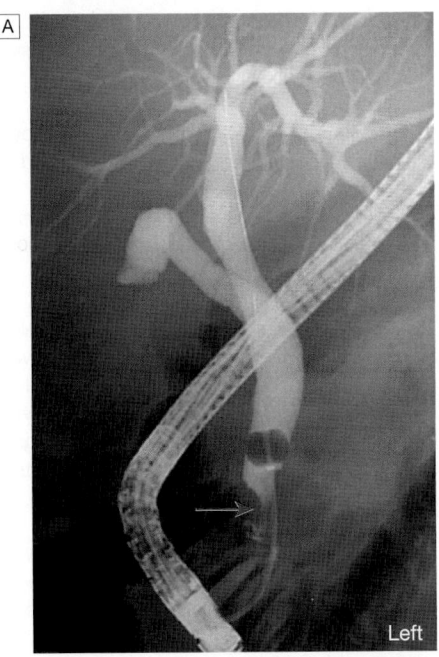
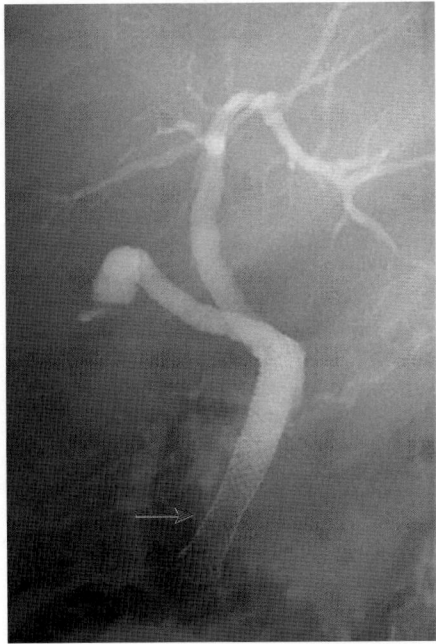

Left

Fig. 24.47 Cholangiocarcinoma. A Endoscopic retrograde cholangiopancreatogram showing a malignant distal biliary stricture (arrow) and dilated duct above this. B A self-expanding metallic stent (SEMS) has been placed across the stricture to relieve jaundice (arrow).

patients may benefit from combined chemotherapy and radiotherapy. Loco-regional therapies with chemotherapy may be effective for locally advanced unresectable tumours, but particularly intrahepatic CCA. Palliation with endoscopic photodynamic therapy has provided encouraging results for extrahepatic CCA.

Carcinoma at the ampulla of Vater

Nearly 40% of all adenocarcinomas of the small intestine arise in relationship to the ampulla of Vater and present with pain, anaemia, vomiting and weight loss. Jaundice may be intermittent or persistent. The diagnosis is made by duodenal endoscopy and biopsy of the tumour but staging by CT/MRI and EUS is essential. Ampullary carcinoma must be differentiated from carcinoma of the head of the pancreas and a CCA because these last two conditions both have a worse prognosis. Imaging may show a 'double duct sign' with dilatation of both the common bile duct and pancreatic duct due to obstruction at the ampulla. EUS is the most sensitive method of assessing and staging ampullary or periampullary tumours.

Curative surgical treatment can be undertaken by pancreaticoduodenectomy and the 5-year survival may be as high as 50%. If resection is impossible, palliative surgical bypass or stenting may be necessary.

Benign gallbladder tumours

These are uncommon, often asymptomatic and usually found incidentally at operation or postmortem. Cholesterol polyps, sometimes associated with cholesterolosis, papillomas and adenomas, are the main types.

Miscellaneous biliary disorders

Functional gallbladder disorder

Functional gallbladder disorder refers to symptoms of biliary-type pain in the absence of gallstones, sludge or microlithiasis. Gallstone disease needs to be excluded by means of abdominal US ± EUS to exclude microlithiasis. Other diagnostic tests may be required to exclude peptic ulcer disease, pancreatitis or musculoskeletal syndromes. Cholecystokinin-stimulated hepatobiliary scintigraphy can be used to evaluate gallbladder ejection fraction.

Symptoms suggestive of functional gallbladder disorder often improve spontaneously so urgent surgical intervention is not required. Management involves patient education and reassurance. Pharmacological therapy with analgesia, neuromodulators and antispasmodics may be beneficial. Cholecystectomy can improve symptoms in many patients with recurrent functional biliary pain. It is suggested that a low gallbladder ejection fraction (<40%) may identify a subset of patients likely to benefit from surgery but evidence is contradictory.

Post-cholecystectomy syndrome

Post-cholecystectomy syndrome refers to a complex of heterogeneous symptoms including abdominal pain and dyspepsia that recur and/or persist following cholecystectomy. It occurs in 10%–30% of patients depending on how the condition is defined, how actively symptoms are sought and what the original indication for cholecystectomy was. The syndrome occurs most frequently in women, in patients who have had symptoms for more than 5 years before cholecystectomy, and in cases when the operation was undertaken for non-calculous gallbladder disease. An increase in bowel frequency resulting from bile acid diarrhoea occurs in about 5%–10% of patients after cholecystectomy and often responds to colestyramine (4–8 g daily). Severe post-cholecystectomy syndrome occurs in only 2%–5% of patients. The main causes are listed in Box 24.67.

The usual symptoms include right upper quadrant pain, flatulence, fatty food intolerance and occasionally jaundice and cholangitis. The LFTs may be abnormal and sometimes show cholestasis. Ultrasonography is used to detect biliary obstruction, and EUS or MRCP to seek common

i	**24.67 Causes of post-cholecystectomy symptoms**

Immediate post-surgical
- Bleeding
- Biliary peritonitis
- Abscess
- Bile duct trauma/transection
- Fistula

Biliary
- Common bile duct stones
- Benign stricture
- Tumour
- Cystic duct stump syndrome
- Disorders of the ampulla of Vater (e.g. benign papillary fibrosis; sphincter of Oddi dysfunction)

Extrabiliary
- Functional dyspepsia
- Peptic ulcer
- Pancreatic disease
- Gastro-oesophageal reflux
- Irritable bowel syndrome
- Functional abdominal pain

bile duct stones. If retained bile duct stones are excluded, sphincter of Oddi dysfunction should be considered (see below). Other investigations that may be required include upper gastrointestinal endoscopy, small bowel radiology and pancreatic function tests. The possibility of a functional illness should also be considered.

Functional biliary sphincter disorders ('sphincter of Oddi dysfunction')

The sphincter of Oddi is a small smooth-muscle sphincter situated at the junction of the bile duct and pancreatic duct in the duodenum. It has been believed that sphincter of Oddi dysfunction (SOD) was characterised by an increase in contractility that produces a benign non-calculous obstruction to the flow of bile or pancreatic juice. This may cause pancreaticobiliary pain, deranged LFTs or recurrent pancreatitis. Classification systems, based on clinical history, laboratory results, findings on investigation and response to interventions, are difficult because of the fluctuating nature of symptoms and the well-recognised placebo effect of interventions. SOD was previously classified into types I–III but these have been replaced by newer terminology (Boxes 24.68 and 24.69).

Clinical features

Patients with functional biliary sphincter disorders, who are predominantly female, present with symptoms and signs suggestive of either biliary or pancreatic disease:

- *Patients with biliary sphincter disorders* experience recurrent, episodic biliary-type pain. They have often had a cholecystectomy but the gallbladder may be intact.
- *Patients with pancreatic sphincter disorders* usually present with unexplained recurrent attacks of pancreatitis.

Investigations

The diagnosis is established by excluding gallstones, including microlithiasis, and by demonstrating a dilated or slowly draining bile duct. The gold standard for diagnosis is sphincter of Oddi manometry. This is not widely available, however, and is associated with a high rate of procedure-related pancreatitis. Hepatobiliary scintigraphy may have value in the second-line investigation of post-cholecystectomy syndrome.

Management

All patients with organic stenosis are treated with endoscopic sphincterotomy. The results are good but patients should be warned that there is a high risk of complications, particularly acute pancreatitis (10%–15%). Manometry should ideally be performed in all suspected functional sphincter of Oddi disorder patients, and results of sphincterotomy in those with high pressures are good, but this should be avoided in

24.68 Classification of biliary sphincter of Oddi dysfunction (SOD)

Organic stenosis (formerly SOD type I)

- Biliary-type pain
- Abnormal liver enzymes (ALP or ALT/AST > twice normal on two or more occasions)
- Dilated common bile duct (> 12 mm diameter on US or > 10 mm on cholangiography)
- Delayed drainage of ERCP contrast beyond 45 mins

Functional sphincter of Oddi disorder (formerly SOD type II)

- Biliary-type pain
- Absence of bile duct stones or other structural abnormalities
- Elevated liver enzymes or dilated bile duct (but not both)

Functional biliary-type pain (formerly SOD type III)

- Biliary-type pain with no other abnormalities

(ALT = alanine aminotransferase; ALP = alkaline phosphatase; AST = aspartate aminotransferase; ERCP = endoscopic retrograde cholangiopancreatography; US = ultrasound)

24.69 Criteria for pancreatic sphincter of Oddi dysfunction

- Recurrent attacks of acute pancreatitis – pancreatic-type pain with amylase or lipase 3 times normal and/or imaging evidence of acute pancreatitis
- Other aetiologies of acute pancreatitis excluded
- Normal pancreas at endoscopic ultrasound
- Abnormal sphincter manometry

---

patients with functional biliary-type pain as it is of no benefit. Medical therapy with nifedipine and/or low-dose amitriptyline may be tried. Pancreatic SOD can be treated with biliary sphincterotomy, carried out in specialist centres, but this should be undertaken with caution and careful consideration.

Routine prophylactic pancreatic duct stenting in patients undergoing ERCP for sphincter of Oddi disorders is no longer encouraged. Prophylactic administration of rectal NSAIDs (e.g. diclofenac 100 mg) is recommended instead because this significantly reduces the risk of procedure-related acute pancreatitis.

Cholesterolosis of the gallbladder

In this condition, lipid deposits in the submucosa and epithelium appear as multiple yellow spots on the pink mucosa, giving rise to the description 'strawberry gallbladder'. Cholesterolosis of the gallbladder is usually asymptomatic. Larger polypoid deposits occur in a third of cases leading to the formation of cholesterol polyps that can detach resulting in complications similar to small gallstones, including right upper quadrant pain. Small,

fixed filling defects may be visible on ultrasonography; the radiologist can usually differentiate between gallstones and cholesterolosis. The condition is usually diagnosed at cholecystectomy; if the diagnosis is made radiologically, cholecystectomy may be indicated, depending on symptoms.

Adenomyomatosis of the gallbladder

In this condition, there is hyperplasia of the muscle and mucosa of the gallbladder. The projection of pouches of mucous membrane through weak points in the muscle coat produces Rokitansky–Aschoff sinuses. There is much disagreement over whether adenomyomatosis is a cause of right upper quadrant pain or other gastrointestinal symptoms. It may be diagnosed by oral cholecystography, when a halo or ring of opacified diverticula can be seen around the gallbladder. Other appearances include deformity of the body of the gallbladder or marked irregularity of the outline. Localised adenomyomatosis in the region of the gallbladder fundus causes the appearance of a 'Phrygian cap'. Most patients are treated by cholecystectomy but only after other diseases in the upper gastrointestinal tract have been excluded.

IgG4-associated cholangitis

This often presents with obstructive jaundice and is described on page 901.

Further information

Books and journal articles

EASL Clinical practice guidelines: Autoimmune hepatitis. J Hepatol 2015; 63:971–1004.

EASL Clinical practice guidelines: The diagnosis and treatment of primary biliary cholangitis. J Hepatol 2017; 67(1):145–172.

EASL Clinical practice guidelines: Liver transplantation. J Hepatol 2016; 64:433–485.

EASL Recommendations on the treatment of hepatitis C. J Hepatol 2018; 69(2):461–511.

EASL 2017 Clinical practice guidelines on the management of hepatitis B infection. J Hepatol 2017; 67(2):370–398.

EASL Clinical practice guidelines: Management of hepatocellular carcinoma. J Hepatol 2018; 69(1):182–236.

EASL–EASD–EASO Clinical practice guidelines for the management of non-alcoholic fatty liver disease. J Hepatol 2016; 64:1388–1402.

Williams R, Aithal G, Alexander GJ, et al. Unacceptable failures: the final report of the Lancet Commission into liver disease in the UK. Lancet 2020; 395:226-239.

Websites

aasld.org *American Association for the Study of Liver Diseases (guidelines available).*

bsg.org.uk *British Society of Gastroenterology (guidelines available).*

easl.eu *European Association for the Study of the Liver (guidelines available).*

eltr.org *European Liver Transplant Registry.*

unos.org *United Network for Organ Sharing: US transplant register.*

24

HG Watson
DJ Culligan
LM Manson

25

Haematology and transfusion medicine

Clinical examination in blood disease

4 Conjunctivae
Pallor
Jaundice

3 Mouth
Lips: angular stomatitis, telangiectasia
Gum hypertrophy
Tongue: colour, smoothness
Buccal mucosa: petechiae
Tonsils: size

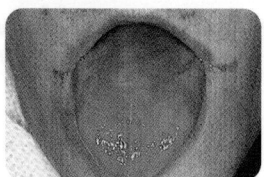

▲ Glossitis and angular stomatitis in iron deficiency

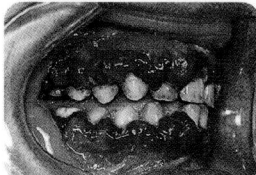

▲ Gum hypertrophy in acute myeloid leukaemia

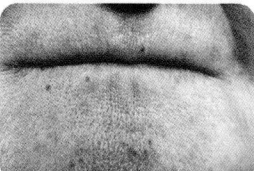

▲ Hereditary haemorrhagic telangiectasia

2 Pulse
Rate

1 Hands
Perfusion
Telangiectasia
Skin crease pallor
Koilonychia

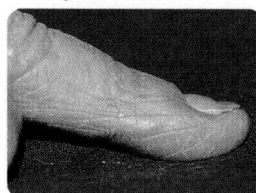

▲ Koilonychia in iron deficiency

5 Fundi
Hyperviscosity
Engorged veins
Papilloedema
Haemorrhage

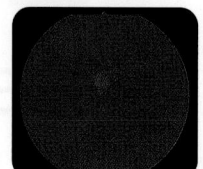

▲ Fundal haemorrhage in thrombocytopenia

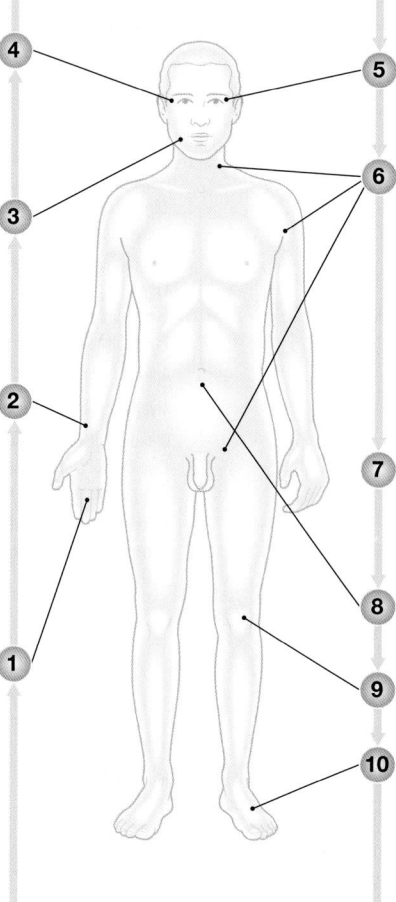

Observation
• General well-being
• Colour: pallor, plethora
• Breathlessness

6 Lymph nodes
(see opposite)

7 Skin
Purpura
Bruising

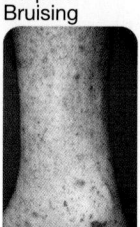

▲ Purpura/petechiae in thrombocytopenia

8 Abdomen
Masses
Ascites
Hepatomegaly
Splenomegaly
Inguinal and femoral lymph nodes

9 Joints
Deformity
Swelling
Restricted movement

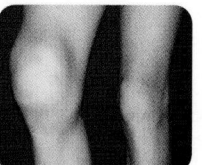

▲ Swollen joint in haemophilia

10 Feet
Peripheral circulation
Toes: gangrene

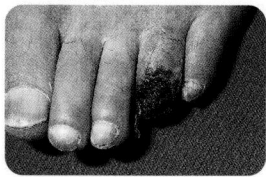

▲ Gangrenous toe in thrombocytosis

11 Urinalysis
Blood
Urobilinogen

Insets (Glossitis) From Hoffbrand VA, John E, Pettit JE, Vyas P. Color atlas of clinical hematology, 4th edn. Philadelphia: Mosby, Elsevier Inc.; 2010; (Petechiae) From Young NS, Gerson SL, High KA (eds). Clinical hematology. St Louis: Mosby, Elsevier Inc.; 2006.

Abnormalities detected in the blood are caused not only by primary diseases of the blood and lymphoreticular systems, but also by diseases affecting other systems of the body. The clinical assessment of patients with haematological abnormalities must include a general history and examination, as well as a search for symptoms and signs of specific primary haematological and other disorders that result in abnormalities of red cells, white cells, platelets, coagulation, lymph nodes and lymphoreticular tissues.

Anaemia

Symptoms and signs help to indicate the clinical severity of anaemia. A full history and examination is needed to identify the underlying cause.

6 Lymphadenopathy

Lymphadenopathy can be caused by benign or malignant disease. The clinical points to clarify are shown in the box.

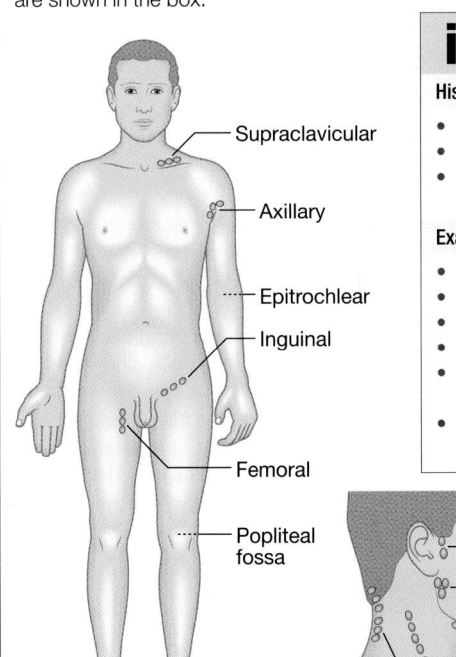

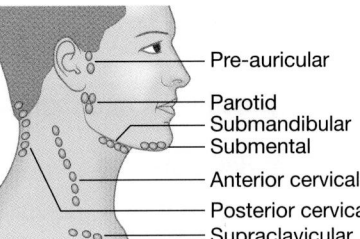

i	**Lymphadenopathy**

History

- Speed of onset, rate of enlargement
- Painful or painless
- Associated symptoms: weight loss, night sweats, itch

Examination

- Sites: localised, generalised
- Size (cm)
- Character: hard, soft, rubbery
- Fixed, mobile
- Search area that node drains for abnormalities (e.g. dental abscess)
- Other general examination (e.g. joints, rashes, finger clubbing)

Supraclavicular
Axillary
Epitrochlear
Inguinal
Femoral
Popliteal fossa

Pre-auricular
Parotid
Submandibular
Submental
Anterior cervical
Posterior cervical
Supraclavicular

i	**Anaemia**

Non-specific symptoms

- Tiredness
- Lightheadedness
- Breathlessness
- Development/worsening of ischaemic symptoms, e.g. angina or claudication

Non-specific signs

- Mucous membrane pallor
- Tachypnoea
- Raised jugular venous pressure
- Tachycardia
- Flow murmurs
- Ankle oedema
- Postural hypotension

Bleeding

Bleeding can be due to congenital or acquired abnormalities in the coagulation system. History and examination help to clarify the severity and the underlying cause of the bleeding problem.

8 Examination of the spleen

- Move your hand up from the right iliac fossa, towards the left upper quadrant on expiration.
- Keep your hand still and ask the patient to take a deep breath through the mouth to feel the spleen edge being displaced downwards.

- Place your left hand around the patient's lower ribs and approach the costal margin to pull the spleen forwards.
- To help palpate a spleen that is only slightly enlarged, roll the patient on to the right side and examine as before.

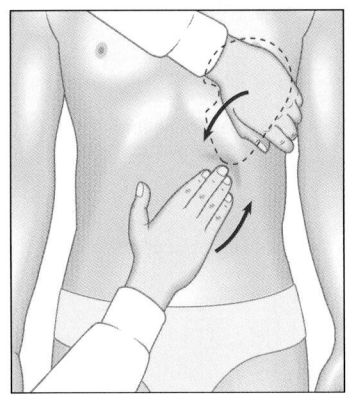

i	**Characteristics of the spleen**

- Notch
- Superficial
- Dull to percussion
- Cannot get examining hand between ribs and spleen
- Moves well with respiration

i	**Bleeding**

History

- Site of bleed
- Duration of bleed
- Precipitating causes, including previous surgery or trauma
- Family history
- Drug history
- Age at presentation
- Other medical conditions, e.g. liver disease

Examination

There are two main patterns of bleeding:

1. Mucosal bleeding
   Reduced number or function of platelets (e.g. bone marrow failure or aspirin) or von Willebrand factor (e.g. von Willebrand disease)
       Skin: petechiae, bruises
       Gum and mucous membrane bleeding
       Fundal haemorrhage
       Post-surgical bleeding
2. Coagulation factor deficiency (e.g. haemophilia or warfarin/anticoagulant)
       Bleeding into joints (haemarthrosis) or muscles
       Bleeding into soft tissues
       Retroperitoneal haemorrhage
       Intracranial haemorrhage
       Post-surgical bleeding

Disorders of the blood cover a wide spectrum of illnesses, ranging from some of the most common disorders affecting humans (anaemias) to relatively rare conditions such as leukaemias and congenital coagulation disorders. Although the latter are uncommon, advances in cellular and molecular biology have had major impacts on their diagnosis, treatment and prognosis. Haematological changes occur as a consequence of diseases affecting any system and give important information in the diagnosis and monitoring of many conditions.

Functional anatomy and physiology

Blood flows throughout the body in the vascular system, and consists of:

- red cells, which transport oxygen from the lungs to the tissues
- white cells, which defend against infection
- platelets, which interact with blood vessels and clotting factors to maintain vascular integrity and prevent bleeding
- plasma, which contains proteins with many functions, including antibodies and coagulation factors.

Haematopoiesis

Haematopoiesis describes the formation of blood cells, an active process that must maintain normal numbers of circulating cells and be able to respond rapidly to increased demands such as bleeding or infection. During development, haematopoiesis occurs in the yolk sac, liver and spleen, and subsequently in red bone marrow in the medullary cavity of all bones. In childhood, red marrow is progressively replaced by fat (yellow marrow) so that, in adults, normal haematopoiesis is restricted to the vertebrae, pelvis, sternum, ribs, clavicles, skull, upper humeri and proximal femora. However, red marrow can expand in response to increased demands for blood cells.

Bone marrow contains a range of immature haematopoietic precursor cells and a storage pool of mature cells for release at times of increased demand. Haematopoietic cells interact closely with surrounding connective tissue stroma, made up of reticular cells, macrophages, fat cells, blood vessels and nerve fibres (Fig. 25.1). In normal marrow, nests of red cell precursors cluster around a central macrophage, which provides iron and also phagocytoses nuclei from red cells prior to their release into the circulation. Megakaryocytes are large cells that produce and release platelets into vascular sinuses. White cell precursors are clustered next to the bone trabeculae; maturing cells migrate into the marrow spaces towards the vascular sinuses. Plasma cells are antibody-secreting mature B cells that normally represent less than 5% of the marrow population and are scattered throughout the intertrabecular spaces.

Stem cells

All blood cells are derived from pluripotent haematopoietic stem cells. These comprise only 0.01% of the total marrow cells, but they can self-renew (i.e. make more stem cells) or differentiate to produce a hierarchy of lineage-committed progenitor cells. The resulting primitive progenitor cells cannot be identified morphologically, so they are named according to the types of cell (or colony) they form during cell culture experiments. CFU–GM (colony-forming unit – granulocyte, monocyte) is a progenitor cell that produces granulocytic and monocytic lines, CFU–E produce erythroid cells, and CFU–Meg produce megakaryocytes and ultimately platelets (Fig. 25.2).

Growth factors, produced in bone marrow stromal cells and elsewhere, control the survival, proliferation, differentiation and function of stem cells and their progeny. Some, such as interleukin-3 (IL-3), stem cell factor (SCF) and granulocyte, macrophage–colony-stimulating factor (GM–CSF), act on a wide number of cell types at various stages of differentiation. Others, such as erythropoietin, granulocyte–colony-stimulating factor (G–CSF) and thrombopoietin (Tpo), are lineage-specific. Many of these growth factors are now synthesised by recombinant DNA technology and used as treatments: for example, erythropoietin to correct renal anaemia and G–CSF to hasten neutrophil recovery after chemotherapy.

The bone marrow also contains stem cells that can differentiate into non-haematological cells. Mesenchymal stem cells differentiate into skeletal muscle, cartilage, cardiac muscle and fat cells while others differentiate into nerves, liver and blood vessel endothelium. This is termed stem cell plasticity and may have exciting clinical applications in the future (Ch. 3).

Blood cells and their functions

Red cells

Red cell precursors formed in the bone marrow from the erythroid (CFU–E) progenitor cells are called erythroblasts or normoblasts (Fig. 25.3). These divide and acquire haemoglobin, which turns the cytoplasm pink; the nucleus condenses and is extruded from the cell. The first non-nucleated red cell is a reticulocyte, which still contains ribosomal material in the cytoplasm, giving these large cells a faint blue tinge ('polychromasia').

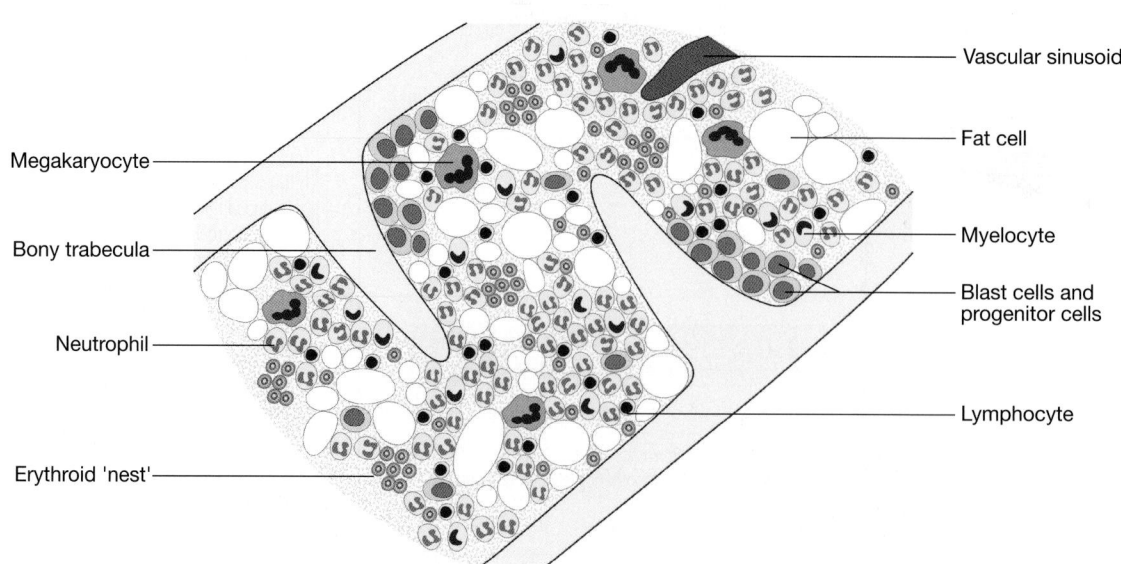

Fig. 25.1 Structural organisation of normal bone marrow.

Megakaryocyte

Bony trabecula

Neutrophil

Erythroid 'nest'

Vascular sinusoid

Fat cell

Myelocyte

Blast cells and progenitor cells

Lymphocyte

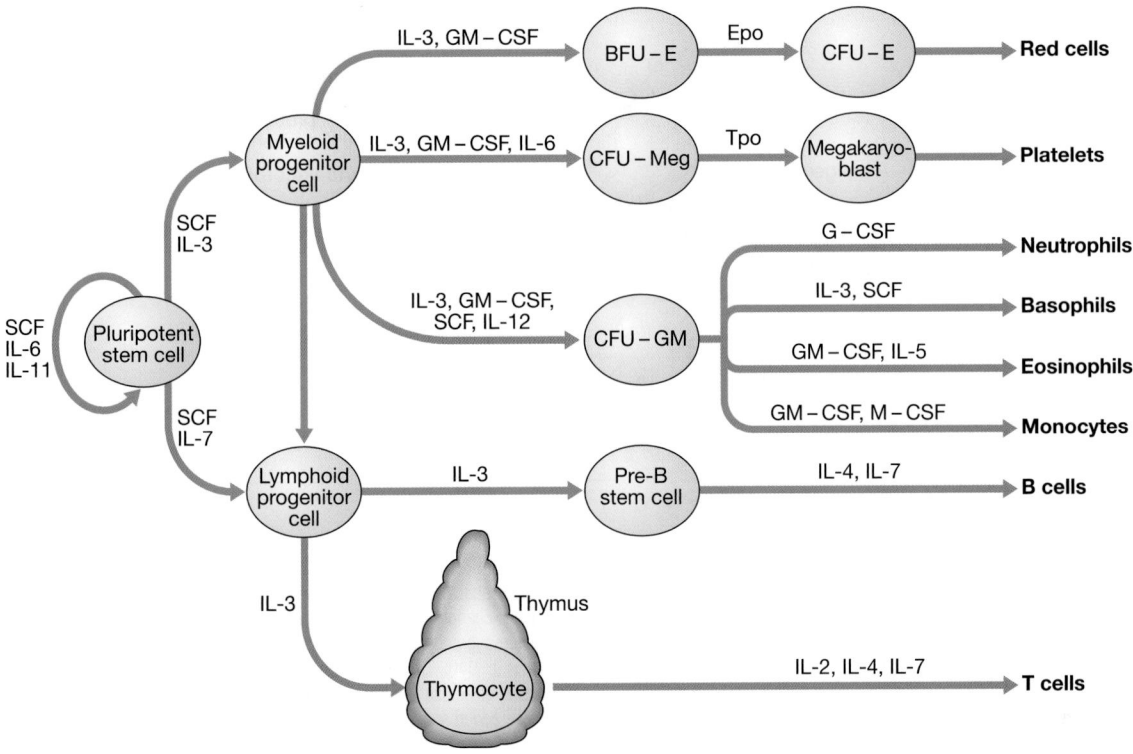

Fig. 25.2 Stem cells and growth factors in haematopoietic cell development. (BFU–E = burst-forming unit – erythroid; CFU–E = colony-forming unit – erythroid; CFU–GM = colony-forming unit – granulocyte, monocyte; CFU–Meg = colony-forming unit – megakaryocyte; Epo = erythropoietin; G–CSF = granulocyte–colony-stimulating factor; GM–CSF = granulocyte, macrophage – colony-stimulating factor; IL = interleukin; M–CSF = macrophage–colony-stimulating factor; SCF = stem cell factor; Tpo = thrombopoietin)

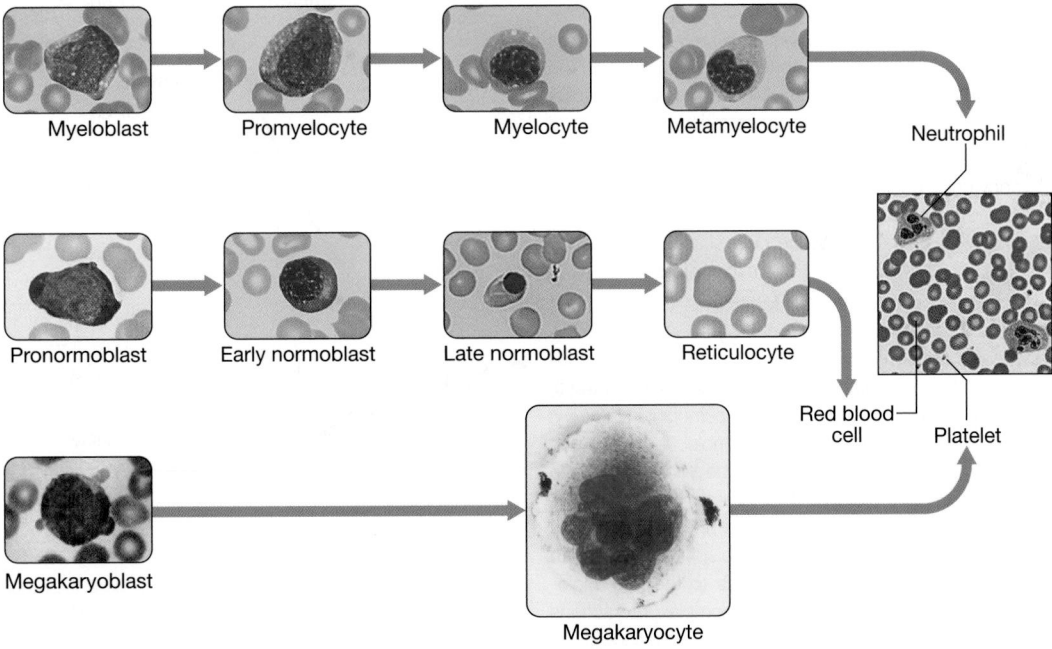

Fig. 25.3 Maturation pathway of red cells, granulocytes and platelets. The image on the right is a normal blood film.

Reticulocytes lose their ribosomal material and mature over 3 days, during which time they are released into the circulation. Increased numbers of circulating reticulocytes (reticulocytosis) reflect increased erythropoiesis. Proliferation and differentiation of red cell precursors is stimulated by erythropoietin, a polypeptide hormone produced by renal interstitial peritubular cells in response to hypoxia. Failure of erythropoietin production in patients with renal failure causes anaemia, which can be treated with exogenous recombinant erythropoietin or similar pharmacological agents called erythropoiesis-stimulating agents, e.g. darbepoetin.

Normal mature red cells circulate for about 120 days. They are 8 μm biconcave discs lacking a nucleus, but filled with haemoglobin, which delivers oxygen to the tissues. In order to pass through the smallest capillaries, the red cell membrane is deformable, with a lipid bilayer to which a 'skeleton' of filamentous proteins is attached via special linkage

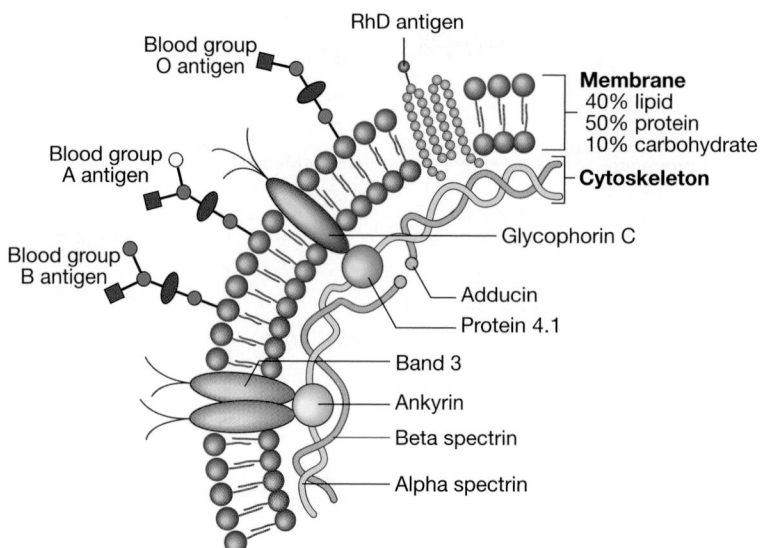

Fig. 25.4 Normal structure of red cell membrane. Red cell membrane flexibility is conferred by attachment of cytoskeletal proteins. Important transmembrane proteins include band 3 (an ion transport channel) and glycophorin C (involved in cytoskeletal attachment and gas exchange, and a receptor for *Plasmodium falciparum* in malaria). Antigens on the red blood cell determine an individual's blood group. There are currently 39 blood group systems (groups of carbohydrate or protein antigens controlled by a single gene or by multiple closely linked loci); the most important clinically are the ABO and Rhesus (Rh) systems (p. 940). The ABO genetic locus has three main allelic forms: A, B and O. The A and B alleles encode glycosyltransferases that introduce *N*-acetylgalactosamine (open circle) and *D*-galactose (blue circle), respectively, on to antigenic carbohydrate molecules on the membrane surface. People with the O allele produce an O antigen, which lacks either of these added sugar groups. Rh antigens are transmembrane proteins.

proteins (Fig. 25.4). Inherited abnormalities of any of these proteins result in loss of membrane as cells pass through the spleen, and the formation of abnormally shaped red cells called spherocytes or elliptocytes (see Fig. 25.8D). Red cells are exposed to osmotic stress in the pulmonary and renal circulation; in order to maintain homeostasis, the membrane contains ion pumps, which control intracellular levels of sodium, potassium, chloride and bicarbonate. In the absence of mitochondria, the energy for these functions is provided by anaerobic glycolysis and the pentose phosphate pathway in the cytosol. Membrane glycoproteins inserted into the lipid bilayer also form the antigens recognised by blood grouping (see Fig. 25.4). The ABO and Rhesus systems are the most commonly recognised, but over 400 blood group antigens have been described.

Haemoglobin

Haemoglobin is a protein specially adapted for oxygen transport. It is composed of four globin chains, each surrounding an iron-containing porphyrin pigment molecule termed haem. Globin chains are a combination of two alpha and two non-alpha chains; haemoglobin A ($\alpha\alpha/\beta\beta$) represents over 90% of adult haemoglobin, whereas haemoglobin F ($\alpha\alpha/\gamma\gamma$) is the predominant type in the fetus. Each haem molecule contains a ferrous ion (Fe^{2+}), to which oxygen reversibly binds; the affinity for oxygen increases as successive oxygen molecules bind. When oxygen is bound, the beta chains 'swing' closer together; they move apart as oxygen is lost. In the 'open' deoxygenated state, 2,3-bisphosphoglycerate (2,3-BPG), a product of red cell metabolism, binds to the haemoglobin molecule and lowers its oxygen affinity. These complex interactions produce the sigmoid shape of the oxygen dissociation curve (Fig. 25.5). The position of this curve depends on the concentrations of 2,3-BPG, H^+ ions and CO_2; increased levels shift the curve to the right and cause oxygen to be released more readily, e.g. when red cells reach hypoxic tissues. Haemoglobin F is unable to bind 2,3-BPG and has a left-shifted oxygen dissociation curve, which, together with the low pH of fetal blood, ensures fetal oxygenation. Strong oxidising agents, such as dapsone, can convert the ferrous iron in haemoglobin to its ferric state (Fe^{3+}). The resultant methaemoglobin also has a left-shifted oxygen dissociation curve, which can result in tissue hypoxia (see Fig. 10.1).

Genetic mutations affecting the haem-binding pockets of globin chains or the 'hinge' interactions between globin chains result in

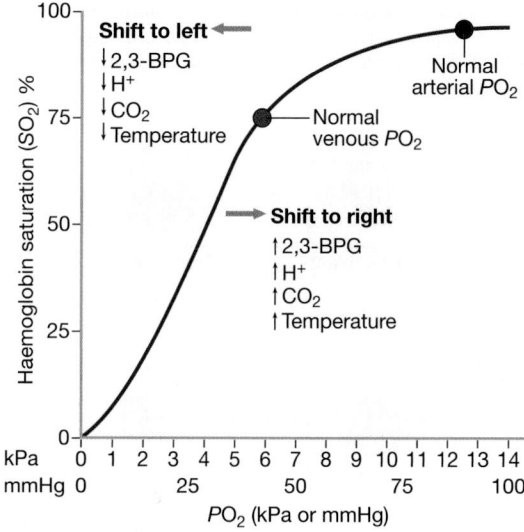

Fig. 25.5 The haemoglobin–oxygen dissociation curve. Factors are listed that shift the curve to the right (more oxygen released from blood) and to the left (less oxygen released) at given PO_2. To convert kPa to mmHg, multiply by 7.5. (2,3-BPG = 2,3-bisphosphoglycerate).

haemoglobinopathies or unstable haemoglobins. Alpha globin chains are produced by two genes on chromosome 16, and beta globin chains by a single gene on chromosome 11; imbalance in the production of globin chains results in the thalassaemias (p. 962). Defects in haem synthesis cause the porphyrias (Ch. 19).

Destruction

Red cells at the end of their lifespan of approximately 120 days are phagocytosed by the reticulo-endothelial system. Amino acids from globin chains are recycled and iron is removed from haem for reuse in haemoglobin synthesis. The remnant haem structure is degraded to bilirubin and conjugated with glucuronic acid before being excreted in bile. In the small bowel, bilirubin is converted to stercobilin; most of this is excreted, but a small amount is reabsorbed and excreted by the kidney as urobilinogen. Increased red cell destruction due to haemolysis or ineffective haematopoiesis results in jaundice and increased urinary urobilinogen. Free intravascular haemoglobin is toxic and is normally bound by haptoglobins, which are plasma proteins produced by the liver.

White cells

White cells or leucocytes in the blood consist of granulocytes (neutrophils, eosinophils and basophils), monocytes and lymphocytes (see Fig. 25.12). Granulocytes and monocytes are formed from bone marrow CFU–GM progenitor cells during myelopoiesis. The first recognisable granulocyte in the marrow is the myeloblast, a large cell with a small amount of basophilic cytoplasm and a primitive nucleus with open chromatin and nucleoli. As the cells divide and mature, the nucleus segments and the cytoplasm acquires specific neutrophilic, eosinophilic or basophilic granules (see Fig. 25.3). This takes about 14 days. The cytokines G–CSF, GM–CSF and M–CSF are involved in the production of myeloid cells, and recombinant G–CSF can be used clinically to hasten recovery of blood neutrophil counts after chemotherapy.

Myelocytes or metamyelocytes are normally found only in the marrow, but may appear in the circulation in response to infection or toxic states. The appearance of more primitive myeloid precursors in the blood is often associated with the presence of nucleated red cells and is termed a 'leucoerythroblastic' picture; this indicates a serious disturbance of marrow function.

Neutrophils

Neutrophils, the most common white blood cells in the blood of adults, are 10–14 µm in diameter, with a multilobular nucleus containing 2–5 segments and granules in their cytoplasm. Their main function is to recognise, ingest and destroy foreign particles and microorganisms see Ch. 4). A large storage pool of mature neutrophils exists in the bone marrow. Every day, some 10^{11} neutrophils enter the circulation, where cells may be circulating freely or attached to endothelium in the marginating pool. These two pools are equal in size; factors such as exercise or catecholamines increase the number of cells flowing in the blood. Neutrophils spend 6–10 hours in the circulation before being removed, principally by the spleen. Alternatively, they pass into the tissues and either are consumed in the inflammatory process or undergo apoptotic cell death and phagocytosis by macrophages.

Eosinophils

Eosinophils represent 1%–6% of the circulating white cells. They are a similar size to neutrophils, but have a bilobed nucleus and prominent orange granules on Romanowsky staining. Eosinophils are phagocytic and their granules contain a peroxidase capable of generating reactive oxygen species and proteins involved in the intracellular killing of protozoa and helminths (Ch. 13). They are also involved in allergic reactions (e.g. atopic asthma, Ch. 17; see also Ch. 4).

Basophils

These cells are less common than eosinophils, representing less than 1% of circulating white cells. They contain dense black granules that obscure the nucleus. Mast cells resemble basophils, but are found only in the tissues. These cells are involved in hypersensitivity reactions (Ch. 4).

Monocytes

Monocytes are the largest of the white cells, with a diameter of 12–20 µm and an irregular nucleus in abundant pale blue cytoplasm containing occasional cytoplasmic vacuoles. These cells circulate for a few hours and then migrate into tissue, where they become macrophages, Kupffer cells or antigen-presenting dendritic cells. The former phagocytose debris, apoptotic cells and microorganisms (see Box 4.1).

Lymphocytes

Lymphocytes are derived from pluripotent haematopoietic stem cells in the bone marrow. There are two main types: T cells (which mediate cellular immunity) and B cells (which mediate humoral immunity) (Ch. 4). Lymphoid cells that migrate to the thymus develop into T cells, whereas B cells develop in the bone marrow.

The majority (about 80%) of lymphocytes in the circulation are T cells. Lymphocytes are heterogeneous, the smallest being the size of red cells and the largest the size of neutrophils. Small lymphocytes are circular with scanty cytoplasm but the larger cells are more irregular with abundant blue cytoplasm. Lymphocyte subpopulations have specific functions and lifespan can vary from a few days to many years. Cell surface antigens ('cluster of differentiation' (CD) antigens), which appear at different points of lymphocyte maturation and indicate the lineage and maturity of the cell, are used to classify lymphomas and lymphoid leukaemias.

Haemostasis

Blood must be maintained in a fluid state in order to function as a transport system, but must be able to solidify to form a clot following vascular injury in order to prevent excessive bleeding, a process known as haemostasis. Successful haemostasis is localised to the area of tissue damage and is followed by removal of the clot and tissue repair. This is achieved by complex interactions between the vascular endothelium, platelets, von Willebrand factor, coagulation factors, natural anticoagulants and fibrinolytic enzymes (Fig. 25.6 and see Fig. 25.18). Dysfunction of any of these components may result in haemorrhage or thrombosis.

Platelets

Platelets are formed in the bone marrow from megakaryocytes. Megakaryocytic progenitor cells (CFU–Meg) divide to form megakaryoblasts, which undergo a process called 'endomitotic reduplication', in which there is division of the nucleus but not the cell. This creates mature megakaryocytes, large cells with several nuclei and cytoplasm containing platelet granules. Large numbers of platelets then fragment off from each megakaryocyte into the circulation. The formation and maturation of megakaryocytes is stimulated by thrombopoietin produced in the liver. Platelets circulate for 8–10 days before they are destroyed in the reticulo-endothelial system. Some 30% of peripheral platelets are normally pooled in the spleen and do not circulate.

Under normal conditions, platelets are discoid, with a diameter of 2–4 µm (Fig. 25.7). The surface membrane invaginates to form a tubular network, the canalicular system, which provides a conduit for the discharge of the granule content following platelet activation. Drugs that inhibit platelet function and thrombosis include aspirin (cyclo-oxygenase inhibitor), clopidogrel, prasugrel and ticagrelor (adenosine diphosphate (ADP)-mediated activation inhibitors), dipyridamole (phosphodiesterase inhibitor), and abciximab, tirofiban and eptifibatide (which prevent fibrinogen binding to glycoprotein IIb/IIIa (αiib beta3 integrin); see Fig. 25.18).

Clotting factors

The coagulation system consists of a cascade of soluble inactive zymogen proteins designated by Roman numerals. When proteolytically cleaved and activated, each is capable of activating one or more components of the cascade. Activated factors are designated by the suffix 'a'. Some of these reactions require phospholipid and calcium. Coagulation occurs by two pathways: it is initiated by the extrinsic (or tissue factor) pathway and amplified by the 'intrinsic pathway' (see Fig. 25.6D).

Clotting factors are synthesised by the liver, although factor V is also produced by platelets and endothelial cells. Factors II, VII, IX and X require post-translational carboxylation to allow them to participate in coagulation. The carboxylase enzyme responsible for this in the liver is vitamin K-dependent. Vitamin K is converted to an epoxide in this reaction and must be reduced to its active form by a reductase enzyme. This reductase is inhibited by warfarin, and this is the basis of the anticoagulant effect of coumarins (p. 947). Inherited (e.g. haemophilia) and acquired (e.g. liver failure) causes of coagulation factor deficiency are associated with bleeding.

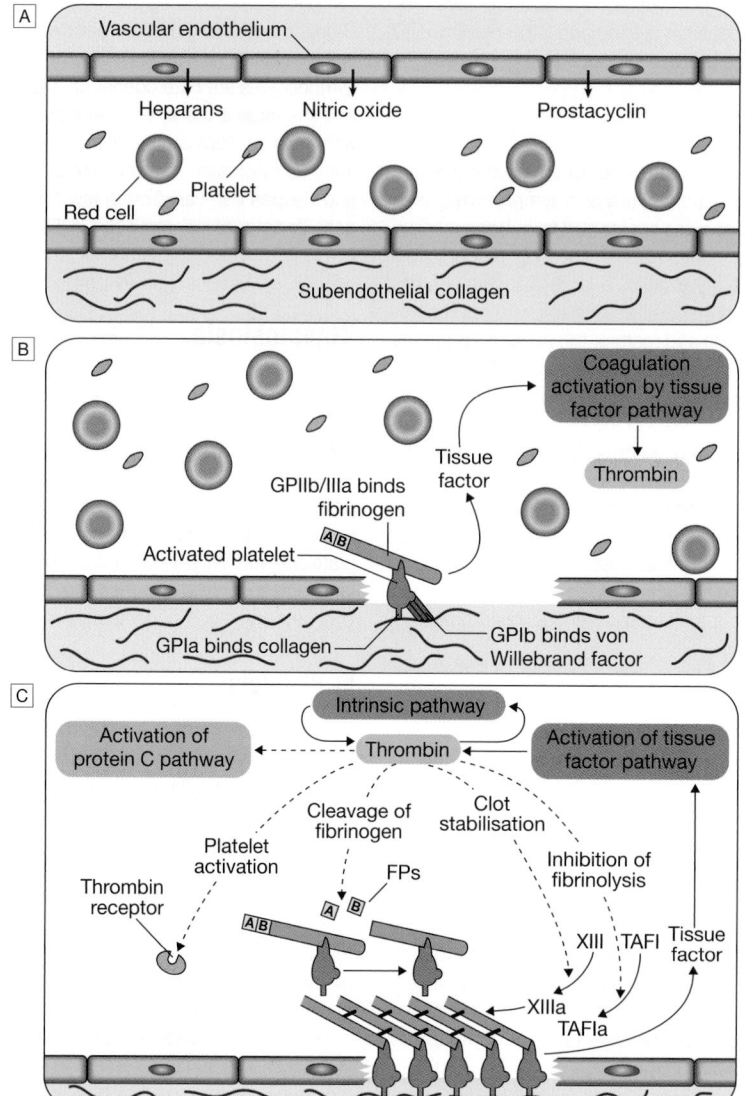

Fig. 25.6 The stages of normal haemostasis. **A** *Stage 1. Pre-injury conditions encourage flow.* The vascular endothelium produces substances (including nitric oxide, prostacyclin and heparans) to prevent adhesion of platelets and white cells to the vessel wall. Platelets and coagulation factors circulate in a non-activated state. **B** *Stage 2. Early haemostatic response: platelets adhere; coagulation is activated.* At the site of injury, the endothelium is breached, exposing subendothelial collagen. Small amounts of tissue factor (TF) are released. Platelets bind to collagen via a specific receptor, glycoprotein la (GPIa), causing a change in platelet shape and its adhesion to the area of damage by the binding of other receptors (GPIb and GPIIb/IIIa) to von Willebrand factor and fibrinogen, respectively. Coagulation is activated by the tissue factor (extrinsic) pathway, generating small amounts of thrombin. **C** and **D** *Stage 3. Fibrin clot formation: platelets become activated and aggregate; fibrin formation is supported by the platelet membrane; stable fibrin clot forms.* The adherent platelets are activated by many pathways, including binding of adenosine diphosphate (ADP), collagen, thrombin and adrenaline (epinephrine) to surface receptors. The cyclo-oxygenase pathway converts arachidonic acid from the platelet membrane into thromboxane A_2, which causes aggregation of platelets. Activation of the platelets results in release of the platelet granule contents, enhancing coagulation further (see Fig. 25.7). Thrombin plays a key role in the control of coagulation: the small amount generated via the TF pathway massively amplifies its own production; the 'intrinsic' pathway becomes activated and large amounts of thrombin are generated. Thrombin directly causes clot formation by cleaving fibrinopeptides (FPs) from fibrinogen to produce fibrin. Fibrin monomers are cross-linked by factor XIII, which is also activated by thrombin. Having had a key role in clot formation and stabilisation, thrombin then starts to regulate clot formation in two main ways: (a) activation of the protein C (PC) pathway (a natural anticoagulant), which reduces further coagulation; (b) activation of thrombin-activatable fibrinolysis inhibitor (TAFI), which inhibits fibrinolysis (see E and F). **E** *Stage 4. Limiting clot formation: natural anticoagulants reverse activation of coagulation factors.* Once haemostasis has been secured, the propagation of clot is curtailed by anticoagulants. Antithrombin is a serine protease inhibitor synthesised by the liver, which destroys activated factors such as XIa, Xa and thrombin (IIa). Its major activity against thrombin and Xa is enhanced by heparin and fondaparinux, explaining their anticoagulant effect. Tissue factor pathway inhibitor (TFPI) binds to and inactivates VIIa and Xa. Activation of PC occurs following binding of thrombin to membrane-bound thrombomodulin; activated protein C (aPC) binds to its co-factor, protein S (PS), and cleaves Va and VIIIa. PC and PS are vitamin K-dependent and are depleted by coumarin anticoagulants such as warfarin. **F** *Stage 5. Fibrinolysis: plasmin degrades fibrin to allow vessel recanalisation and tissue repair.* The insoluble clot needs to be broken down for vessel recanalisation. Plasmin, the main fibrinolytic enzyme, is produced when plasminogen is activated, e.g. by tissue plasminogen activator (t-PA) or urokinase in the clot. Plasmin hydrolyses the fibrin clot, producing fibrin degradation products, including the D-dimer. This process is highly regulated; the plasminogen activators are controlled by an inhibitor called plasminogen activator inhibitor (PAI), the activity of plasmin is inhibited by α_2-antiplasmin and α_2-macroglobulin, and fibrinolysis is further inhibited by the thrombin-activated TAFI.

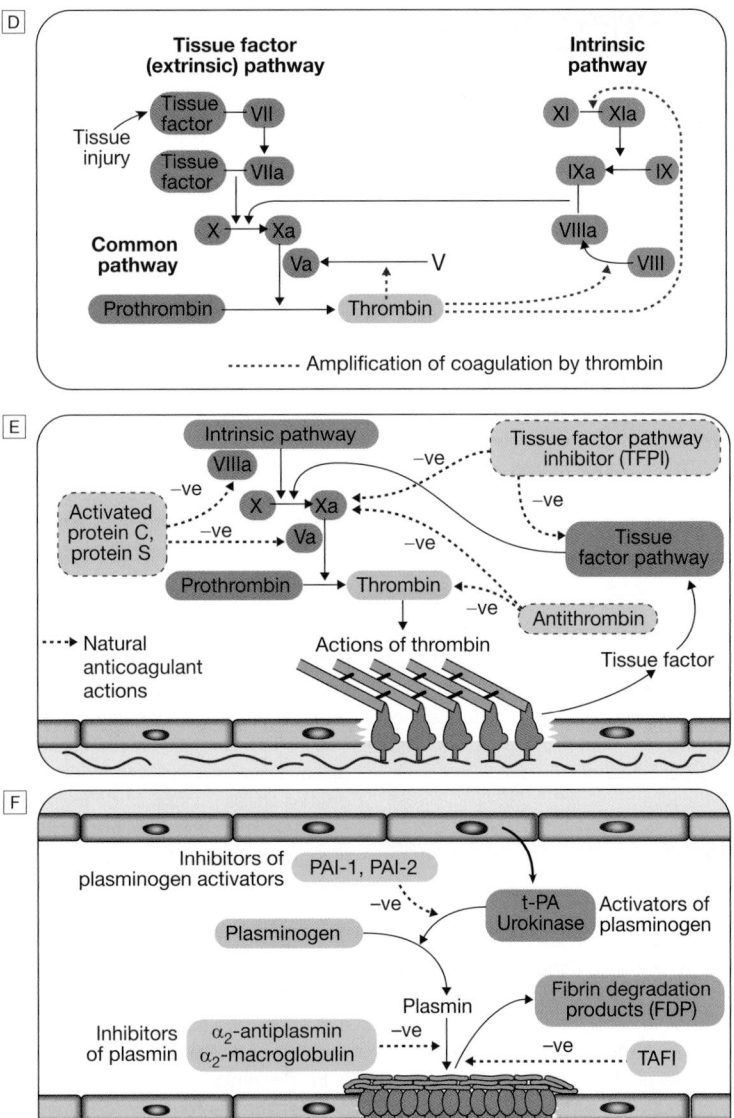

Fig. 25.6, cont'd

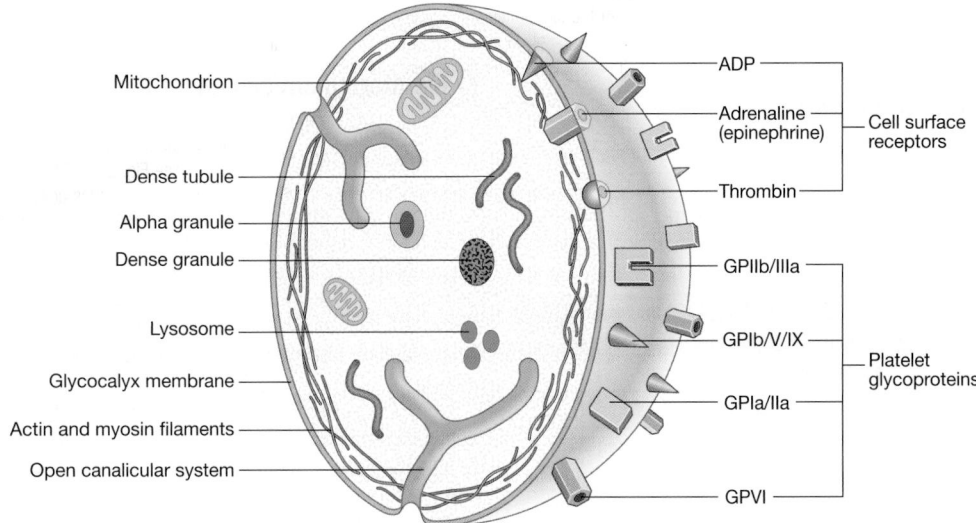

Fig. 25.7 Normal platelet structure. The platelet surface is populated by glycoproteins, which bind to key structures including fibrinogen, collagen and von Willebrand factor and cell surface receptors for thrombin, ADP and adrenaline (epinephrine). Through internal signalling pathways, platelet activation causes degranulation of alpha and dense granules, which ultimately results in platelet aggregation. Blockade of these pathways by drugs such as aspirin, clopidogrel, ticagrelor, tirofiban and abciximab forms the basis of antiplatelet therapy. (ADP = adenosine diphosphate; GP = glycoprotein)

Investigation of diseases of the blood

The full blood count

To obtain a full blood count (FBC), anticoagulated blood is processed through automated blood analysers that use a variety of technologies (particle-sizing, radiofrequency and laser instrumentation) to measure the haematological parameters. These include numbers of circulating cells, the proportion of whole blood volume occupied by red cells (the haematocrit, Hct), and the red cell indices that give information about the size of red cells (mean cell volume, MCV) and the amount of haemoglobin present in the red cells (mean cell haemoglobin, MCH). Blood analysers can differentiate types of white blood cell and give automated counts of neutrophils, lymphocytes, monocytes, eosinophils and basophils. It is important to appreciate, however, that a number of conditions can lead to spurious results (Box 25.1). The reference ranges for a number of common haematological parameters in adults are given in Chapter 35 and the effects of age are shown in Box 25.6.

Blood film examination

Although technical advances in full blood count analysers have resulted in fewer blood samples requiring manual examination, scrutiny of blood components prepared on a microscope slide (the 'blood film') can often yield valuable information (Box 25.2 and Fig. 25.8). Analysers cannot identify abnormalities of red cell shape and content (e.g. Howell–Jolly bodies, basophilic stippling, malaria parasites) or fully define abnormal white cells such as blasts.

Bone marrow examination

In adults, bone marrow for examination is usually obtained from the posterior iliac crest. After a local anaesthetic, marrow can be sucked out from the medullary space, stained and examined under the microscope (bone marrow aspirate). In addition, a core of bone may be removed (trephine biopsy), fixed and decalcified before sections are cut for staining (Fig. 25.9). A bone marrow aspirate is used to assess the composition and morphology of haematopoietic cells or abnormal infiltrates. Further investigations may be performed, such as cell surface marker analysis (immunophenotyping), chromosome (karyotyping) and molecular studies, including next generation sequencing (NGS) to identify mutated genes as part of the assessment of malignant diseases and bone marrow failure syndromes. Marrow can be cultured for suspected tuberculosis. A trephine biopsy is superior for assessing marrow cellularity, marrow fibrosis, and infiltration by abnormal cells such as metastatic carcinoma.

Investigation of coagulation

Bleeding disorders

In patients with clinical evidence of a bleeding disorder (p. 923), there are recommended screening tests (Box 25.3). Physiological activation of coagulation is predominantly by tissue factor, with amplification of the process by the small amounts of thrombin formed as a result. For ease of description, the terms extrinsic, intrinsic and common pathways are still used (see Fig. 25.6D).

Coagulation tests measure the time to clot formation in vitro in a platelet poor plasma sample after the clotting process is initiated by activators and calcium. The result of the test sample is compared with normal controls. The tissue factor ('extrinsic') pathway (see Fig. 25.6D) is assessed by the prothrombin time (PT), and the 'intrinsic' pathway by the activated partial thromboplastin time (APTT), sometimes known as the partial thromboplastin time with kaolin (PTTK). Coagulation is delayed by deficiencies of coagulation factors and by the presence of inhibitors of coagulation, such as heparin and lupus anticoagulants. The approximate reference ranges and causes of abnormalities are shown in Box 25.3. If both the PT and APTT are prolonged, this indicates either deficiency or inhibition of the final common pathway (which includes factors X, V, prothrombin and fibrinogen) or global coagulation factor deficiency involving more than one factor, as occurs in disseminated intravascular coagulation (DIC; pp. 199 and 988). Further specific tests may be performed based on interpretation of the clinical scenario and results of these screening tests. A mixing test with normal plasma allows differentiation between a coagulation factor deficiency (the prolonged time corrects) and the presence of an inhibitor of coagulation (the prolonged time does not correct); the latter may be a chemical (heparins) or an antibody (most often a lupus anticoagulant, but occasionally a specific inhibitor of one of the coagulation factors, typically factor VIII). Von Willebrand disease may present with a normal APTT; further investigation of suspected cases is detailed on page 984.

Platelet function has historically been assessed by the bleeding time, measured as the time to stop bleeding after a standardised incision. However, most centres have abandoned the use of this test. Platelet function can be assessed in vitro by measuring aggregation in response to various agonists, such as adrenaline (epinephrine), collagen, thrombin, arachidonic acid and ADP, agglutination in response to ristocetin or by measuring the constituents of the intracellular granules, e.g. adenosine triphosphate, adenosine diphosphate and their ratio to each other (ATP/ADP).

In disseminated intravascular coagulation (DIC), platelets and coagulation factors are consumed, resulting in thrombocytopenia and prolonged PT and APTT. In addition, there is evidence of active coagulation with consumption of fibrinogen and generation of fibrin degradation products (D-dimers). Note, however, that fibrinogen is an acute phase protein that may also be elevated in inflammatory disease (p. 67).

Monitoring anticoagulant therapy

The International Normalised Ratio (INR) is validated only to assess the therapeutic effect of coumarin anticoagulants, including warfarin. INR is the ratio of the patient's PT to that of a normal control, raised to the power of the international sensitivity index of the thromboplastin used in the test (ISI, derived by comparison with an international reference standard material). Concentrations of the direct oral anticoagulants (DOACs) cannot be accurately assessed from the PT or the APTT, with which they have a variable and generally poor correlation, but can be measured using appropriately calibrated specific assays.

Monitoring of heparin therapy is, on the whole, required only with unfractionated heparins (UFH). Therapeutic anticoagulation prolongs the APTT relative to a control sample by a ratio of approximately 1.5–2.5. Many laboratories now prefer to measure UFH activity by an appropriately calibrated anti-Xa assay. Low-molecular-weight heparins have such a predictable dose response that monitoring of the anticoagulant effect is not required, except in patients with renal impairment (glomerular filtration rate less than 30 mL/min). When monitoring is indicated, an anti-Xa assay is used.

25.1 Spurious full blood count results from autoanalysers

Result	Explanation
Increased haemoglobin	Lipaemia, jaundice, very high white cell count
Reduced haemoglobin	Improper sample mixing, blood taken from vein into which an infusion is flowing
Increased red cell volume (mean cell volume, MCV)	Cold agglutinins, non-ketotic hyperosmolarity
Increased white cell count	Nucleated red cells present
Reduced platelet count	Clot in sample, platelet clumping

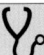

25.2 How to interpret red cell appearances

Microcytosis (reduced average cell size, MCV < 76 fL) [A]

- Iron deficiency
- Thalassaemia
- Sideroblastic anaemia

Macrocytosis (increased average cell size, MCV > 100 fL) [B]

- Vitamin B₁₂ or folate deficiency
- Liver disease, alcohol
- Hypothyroidism
- Myelodysplastic syndromes
- Drugs (e.g. zidovudine, trimethoprim, phenytoin, methotrexate, hydroxycarbamide)

Target cells (central area of haemoglobinisation) [C]

- Liver disease
- Thalassaemia
- Post-splenectomy
- Haemoglobin C disease

Spherocytes (dense cells, no area of central pallor) [D]

- Autoimmune haemolytic anaemia
- Post-splenectomy
- Hereditary spherocytosis

Red cell fragments (intravascular haemolysis) [E]

- Microangiopathic haemolysis, e.g. haemolytic urea syndrome (HUS), thrombotic thrombocytopenic purpura (TTP)
- Disseminated intravascular coagulation (DIC)

Nucleated red blood cells (normoblasts) [F]

- Marrow infiltration
- Severe haemolysis
- Myelofibrosis
- Acute haemorrhage

Howell–Jolly bodies (small round nuclear remnants) [G]

- Hyposplenism
- Post-splenectomy
- Dyshaematopoiesis

Basophilic stippling (abnormal ribosomal RNA appears as blue dots) [H]

- Dyshaematopoiesis
- Lead poisoning

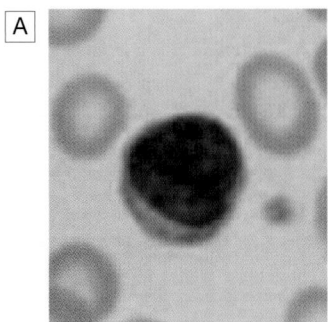
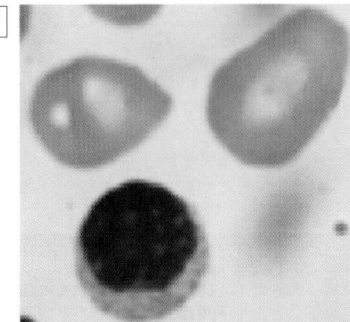
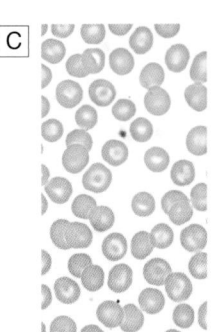
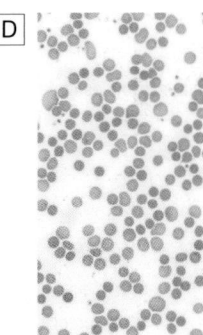
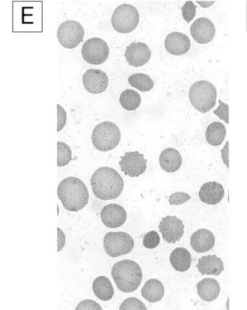
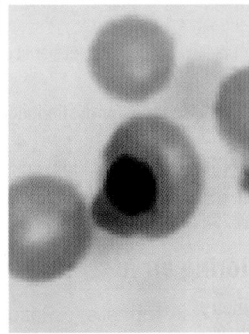
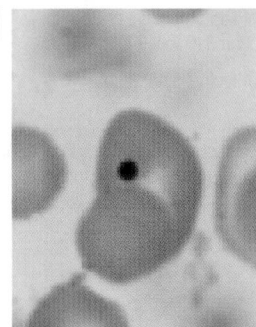
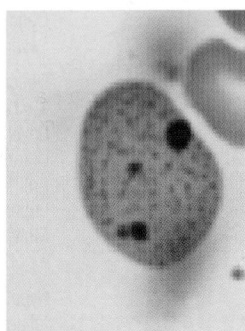

Fig. 25.8 Appearance of red blood cells. [A] Microcytosis. [B] Macrocytosis. [C] Target cells. [D] Spherocytes and polychromasia. [E] Red cell fragments. [F] Nucleated red blood cells. [G] Howell–Jolly bodies. [H] Basophilic stippling.

(MCV = mean cell volume)

Thrombotic disorders

Measurement of plasma levels of D-dimers derived from fibrin degradation is useful in excluding the diagnosis of active venous thrombosis in some patients (see Fig. 9.6).

A variety of tests exist that may help to explain an underlying propensity to thrombosis, especially venous thromboembolism (thrombophilia) (Box 25.4). Examples of possible indications for testing are given in Box 25.5. In most patients, the results of these tests do not affect clinical management (p. 984) but they may influence the duration of anticoagulation (e.g. antiphospholipid antibodies, p. XXX), justify family screening in inherited thrombophilias (p. 986), or suggest additional management strategies to reduce thrombosis risk (e.g. in myeloproliferative disease and paroxysmal nocturnal haemoglobinuria; p. 959). Anticoagulants can interfere with some of these assays. For example, warfarin reduces protein C and S levels and affects measurement of lupus anticoagulant. Heparin interferes with antithrombin and lupus anticoagulant assays and the DOACs all affect the measurement of lupus anticoagulant as well as other specific

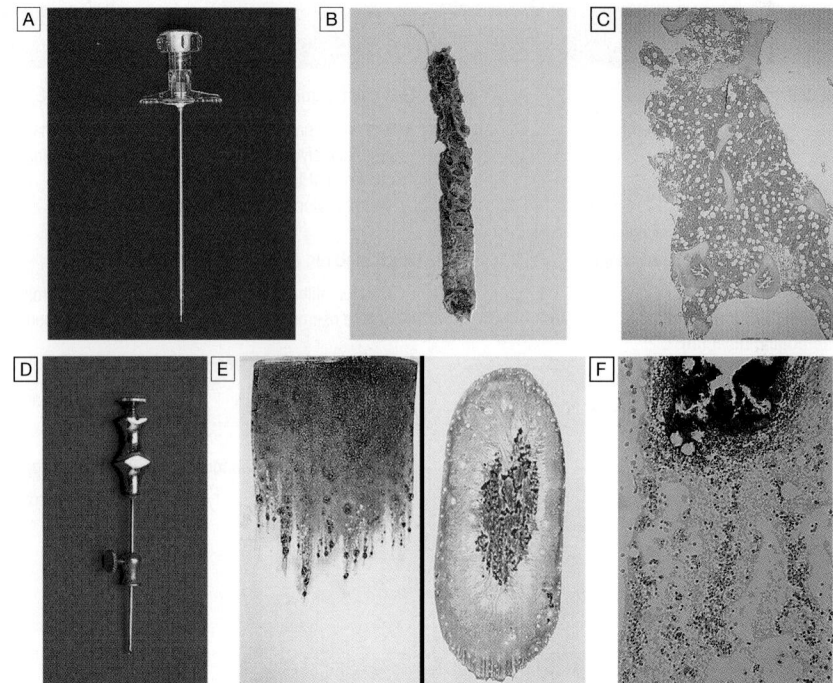

Fig. 25.9 Bone marrow aspirate and trephine. A Trephine biopsy needle. B Macroscopic appearance of a trephine biopsy. C Microscopic appearance of stained section of trephine. D Bone marrow aspirate needle. E Stained macroscopic appearance of marrow aspirate: smear (left) and squash (right). F Microscopic appearance of stained marrow particles and trails of haematopoietic cells.

i 25.3 Coagulation screening tests[1]

Investigation	Reference range[2]	Situations in which tests may be abnormal
Platelet count	150–400 × 10⁹/L	Thrombocytopenia
Prothrombin time (PT)	9–12 secs	Deficiencies of factors II, V, VII or X Severe fibrinogen deficiency, DIC
Activated partial thromboplastin time (APTT)	26–36 secs	Deficiencies of factors II, V, VIII, IX, X, XI, XII Severe fibrinogen deficiency Unfractionated heparin therapy Antibodies against clotting factors Lupus anticoagulant Multiple factor deficiency, e.g. DIC
Fibrinogen concentration	1.5–4.0 g/L	Hypofibrinogenaemia, e.g. liver failure, DIC

[1]N.B. International Normalised Ratio (INR) is used only to monitor coumarin therapy and is not a coagulation screening test. [2]Ranges are approximate and may vary between laboratories. (DIC = disseminated intravascular coagulation)

i 25.4 Investigation of possible thrombophilia

Full blood count

Plasma levels
- Antithrombin
- Protein C
- Protein S (free)
- Antiphospholipid antibodies, lupus anticoagulant, anticardiolipin antibody/anti-β_2GP1

Thrombin/reptilase time (for dysfibrinogenaemia)

Genetic testing
- Factor V Leiden
- Prothrombin G20210A
- *JAK-2 V617F* mutation
- *CALR* mutations
- *MPL 515* mutation

Flow cytometry
- Screen for GPI-linked cell surface proteins (CD14, 16, 55, 59), deficient in paroxysmal nocturnal haemoglobinuria

(CD = cluster of differentiation; GP1 = glycoprotein 1; GPI = glycerol phosphatidyl inositol)

coagulation assays. Therefore these tests, when required, should be performed when the patient is not taking anticoagulants or, if required, during temporary discontinuation to facilitate accurate measurement

Box 25.6 lists some considerations specific to all haematological investigations in old age.

Presenting problems in blood disease

Anaemia

Anaemia refers to a state in which the level of haemoglobin in the blood is below the reference range appropriate for age and sex. Other factors, including pregnancy and altitude, also affect haemoglobin levels and must

i 25.5 Possible indications for thrombophilia testing*

- Venous thrombosis <45 years
- Recurrent venous thrombosis
- Family history of unprovoked or recurrent thrombosis
- Combined arterial and venous thrombosis
- Venous thrombosis at an unusual site:
  Cerebral venous thrombosis
  Hepatic vein (Budd–Chiari syndrome)
  Portal vein, mesenteric vein, splenic vein

*Antiphospholipid antibodies should be sought where clinical criteria for antiphospholipid syndrome (APS) are fulfilled (p. 986). Thrombophilia testing may explain the diagnosis without necessarily affecting management and this limits the clinical value of such an approach.

25.6 Haematological investigations in old age

- **Blood cell counts and film components**: not altered in general by ageing alone, although haemoglobin concentrations fall with increasing age.
- **Ratio of bone marrow cells to marrow fat**: falls.
- **Neutrophils**: maintained throughout life, although leucocytes may be less readily mobilised by bacterial invasion in old age.
- **Lymphocytes**: functionally compromised by age due to a T-cell-related defect in cell-mediated immunity.
- **Clotting factors**: no major changes, although mild congenital deficiencies may be first noticed in old age.
- **Erythrocyte sedimentation rate (ESR)**: raised above the reference range, but usually in association with chronic or subacute disease. In truly healthy older people, the ESR range is very similar to that in younger people (see Ch. 4).
- **Clonal haematopoiesis.** Myeloid gene panels are more likely to demonstrate clonal haematopoiesis of indeterminate potential (CHIP) based on acquired gene mutations in the blood cells of older patients. This may occur as frequently as 20% of people aged over 80 years despite having normal blood counts.

25.7 Causes of anaemia

Decreased or ineffective marrow production

- Lack of iron, vitamin B$_{12}$ or folate
- Hypoplasia/myelodysplasia
- Invasion by malignant cells
- Renal failure
- Anaemia of chronic disease

Normal marrow production but increased removal of cells

- Blood loss
- Haemolysis
- Hypersplenism

be taken into account when considering whether an individual is anaemic. The clinical features of anaemia reflect diminished oxygen supply to the tissues (p. 922). A rapid onset of anaemia (e.g. due to blood loss) causes more profound symptoms than a gradually developing anaemia. Individuals with cardiorespiratory disease are more susceptible to symptoms of anaemia.

The clinical assessment and investigation of anaemia should gauge its severity and define the underlying cause (Box 25.7).

Clinical assessment

- *Iron deficiency anaemia* (p. 950) is the most common type of anaemia worldwide. A thorough gastrointestinal history is important, looking in particular for symptoms of blood loss. Menorrhagia is a common cause of anaemia in pre-menopausal females, so women should always be asked about menstrual periods.
- *A dietary history* should assess the intake of iron, B12 and folate, which may become deficient in comparison to needs (e.g. in pregnancy or during periods of rapid growth; see also Chs 22 and 33).
- *Past medical history* may reveal a disease that is known to be associated with anaemia, such as rheumatoid arthritis (anaemia of inflammation (AI)), or previous surgery (e.g. resection of the stomach or small bowel, which may lead to malabsorption of iron and/or vitamin B$_{12}$).
- *Family history and ethnic background* may raise suspicion of haemolytic anaemias, such as the haemoglobinopathies, oxidative enzymopathies and membranopathies. Pernicious anaemia, an autoimmune disorder, may also run in families, but is not associated with a clear Mendelian pattern of inheritance.
- *A drug history* may reveal the ingestion of drugs that cause or worsen blood loss (e.g. anticoagulants, anti-platelet drugs and anti-inflammatory drugs), haemolysis (e.g. sulphonamides and anti-malarial drugs) or aplasia (e.g. chloramphenicol, mercaptopurine).

On examination, as well as the general physical findings of anaemia shown on page, there may be specific findings related to the aetiology of the anaemia; for example, a right iliac fossa mass due to an underlying caecal carcinoma. Haemolytic anaemias can cause jaundice. Vitamin B$_{12}$ deficiency may be associated with neurological signs, including peripheral neuropathy, dementia and signs of subacute combined degeneration of the cord (Box 28.82). Sickle-cell anaemia (p. 960) may result in leg ulcers, stroke or features of pulmonary hypertension. Anaemia may be multifactorial and the lack of specific symptoms and signs does not rule out silent pathology.

Investigations

Schemes for the investigation of anaemias are often based on the size of the red cells, which is most accurately indicated by the MCV in the FBC. Commonly, in the presence of anaemia:

- A normal MCV (normocytic anaemia) suggests either acute blood loss or the anaemia of chronic disease, also known as the anaemia of inflammation (ACD/AI) (Fig. 25.10).
- A low MCV (microcytic anaemia) suggests iron deficiency or thalassaemia or sometimes ACD/AI (Fig. 25.10).
- A high MCV (macrocytic anaemia) suggests vitamin B$_{12}$ or folate deficiency or myelodysplasia (Fig. 25.11).

Specific types of anaemia and their management are described later in this chapter.

High haemoglobin

Patients with a persistently raised haematocrit (Hct) (> 0.52 males, > 0.48 females) for more than 2 months should be investigated. 'True' polycythaemia (or absolute erythrocytosis) indicates an excess of red cells, while 'relative', 'apparent' or 'low-volume' polycythaemia is due to a decreased plasma volume. Causes of polycythaemia are shown in Box 25.8. These involve increased erythropoiesis in the bone marrow, either due to a primary increase in marrow activity, or in response to increased erythropoietin (Epo) levels in chronic hypoxaemia, or due to inappropriate secretion of Epo. Some athletes improperly use Epo to increase oxygen-carrying capacity and thus enhance their physical performance.

Apparent erythrocytosis with a raised Hct, normal red cell mass (RCM) and reduced plasma volume may be associated with hypertension, smoking, alcohol and diuretic use (Gaisböck syndrome).

Clinical assessment and investigations

Males and females with Hct values of over 0.60 and over 0.56, respectively, can be assumed to have an absolute erythrocytosis. A clinical history and examination including measurement of oxygen saturation will identify most patients with polycythaemia secondary to hypoxia. The presence of hypertension, smoking, excess alcohol consumption and/or diuretic use is consistent with low-volume polycythaemia (Gaisböck syndrome). In polycythaemia rubra vera (PRV), the acquired *V617F* mutation is found in the *JAK-2* gene (a kinase) in over 90% of cases; in the remainder, mutations in exon 12 of the same gene may be identified. Patients with PRV have an increased risk of arterial thromboses, particularly stroke, and venous thromboembolism. They may also have aquagenic pruritus (itching after exposure to water), hepatosplenomegaly and gout (due to high red cell turnover).

If *JAK-2* mutations are absent and there is no obvious secondary cause, a measurement of red cell mass is required to confirm an absolute erythrocytosis, followed by further investigations to exclude hypoxia, and causes of inappropriate erythropoietin secretion.

Leucopenia (low white cell count)

A reduction in the total numbers of circulating white cells is called leucopenia. This may be due to a reduction in all types of white cell or in individual cell types (usually neutrophils or lymphocytes). Leucopenia may occur in isolation or as part of a reduction in all three haematological lineages (pancytopenia; p. 939).

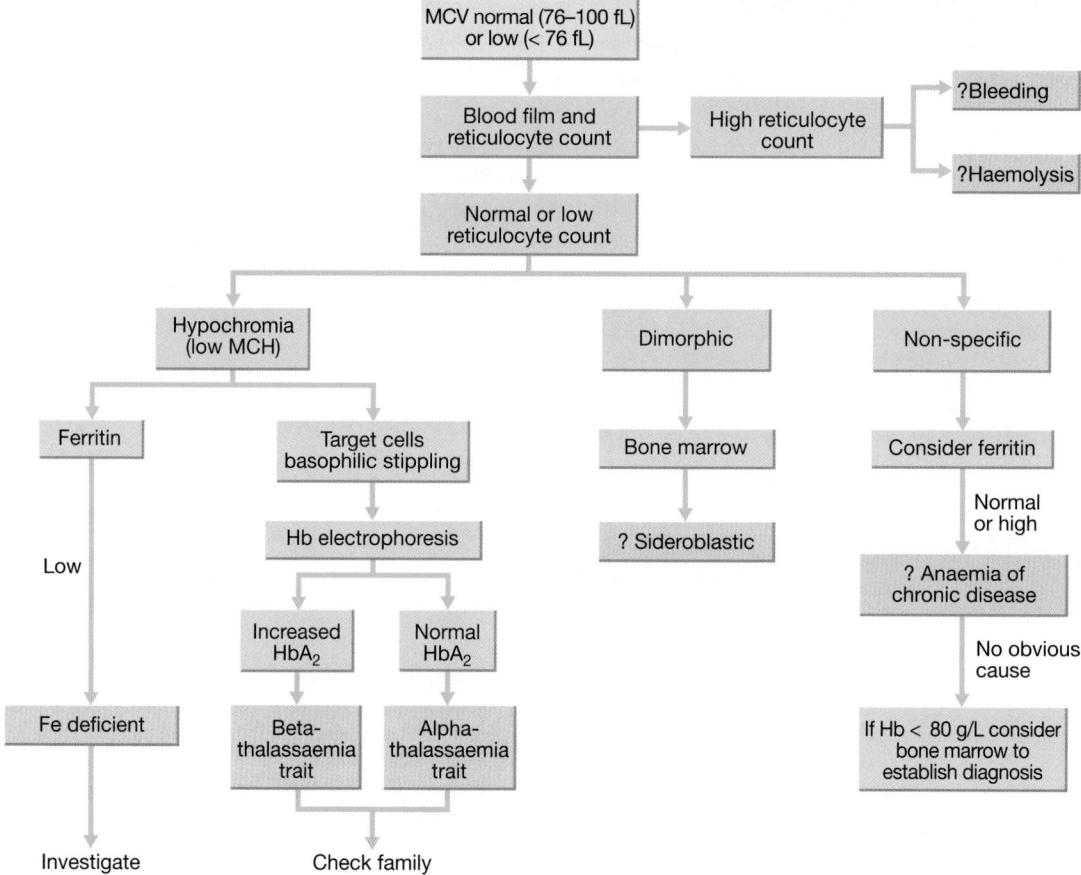

Fig. 25.10 Investigation of anaemia with normal or low mean cell volume (MCV). (Hb = haemoglobin; MCH = mean cell haemoglobin)

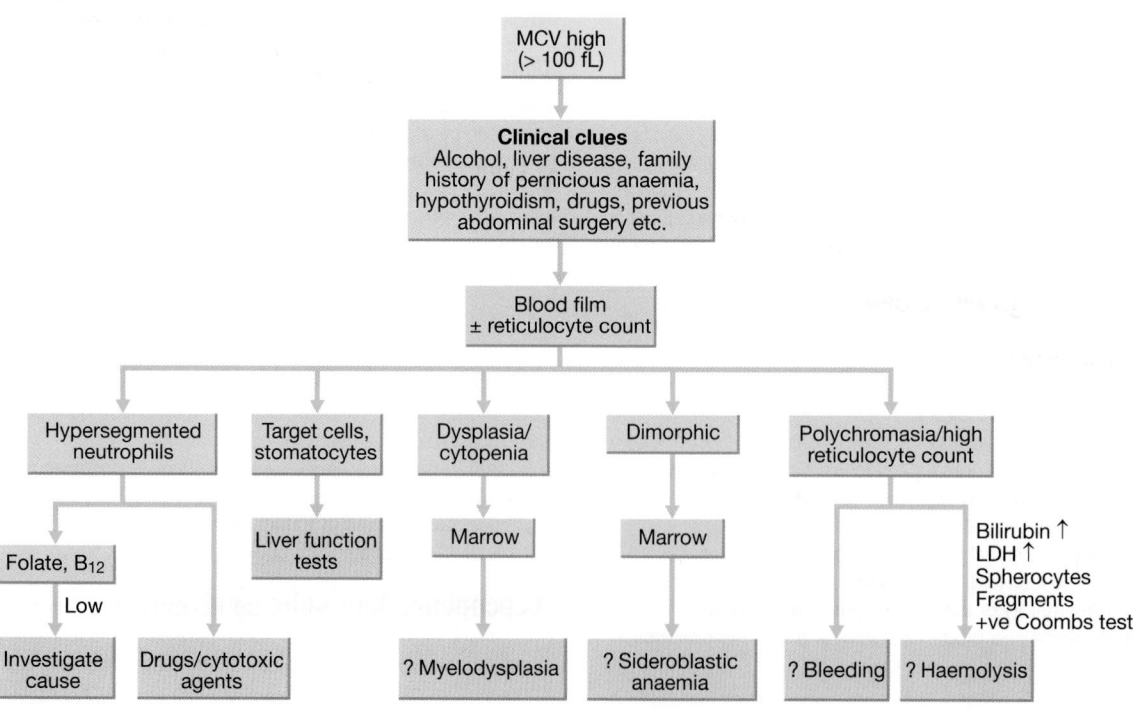

Fig. 25.11 Investigation of anaemia with high mean cell volume (MCV). (LDH = lactate dehydrogenase)

i	**25.8 Classification and causes of erythrocytosis**		
	Absolute erythrocytosis		**Relative (low-volume) erythrocytosis**
Haematocrit	High		High
Red cell mass	High		Normal
Plasma volume	Normal		Low

Causes	*Primary*
	 Myeloproliferative disorder
	 Polycythaemia rubra vera (primary proliferative polycythaemia)
	 Secondary
	 High erythropoietin due to tissue hypoxia:
	    High altitude
	    Cardiorespiratory disease
	    High-affinity haemoglobins
	 Inappropriately increased erythropoietin:
	    Renal disease (hydronephrosis, cysts, carcinoma)
	    Other tumours (hepatoma, bronchogenic carcinoma, uterine fibroids,
	    phaeochromocytoma, cerebellar haemangioblastoma)
	    Exogenous testosterone therapy
	 Exogenous erythropoietin administration:
	    Performance-enhancing drug-taking in athletes
			Diuretics
			 Smoking
			 Obesity
			 Alcohol excess
			 Gaisböck syndrome

Neutropenia

A reduction in neutrophil count (usually $<1.5 \times 10^9$/L but dependent on age and race) is called neutropenia. The main causes are listed in Box 25.9 and Fig. 25.12. Drug-induced neutropenia is not uncommon (Box 25.10). Clinical manifestations range from no symptoms to overwhelming sepsis. The risk of bacterial infection is related to the degree of neutropenia, with counts lower than 0.5×10^9/L considered to be critically low. Fever is the first and often only manifestation of infection. A sore throat, perianal pain or skin inflammation may be present. The lack of neutrophils allows the patient to become septicaemic and shocked within hours if immediate antibiotic therapy is not commenced. Management is discussed on page 269.

Lymphopenia

This is an absolute lymphocyte count of less than 1×10^9/L. The causes are shown in Box 25.9. Although minor reductions may be asymptomatic, deficiencies in cell-mediated immunity may result in infections (with organisms such as fungi, viruses and mycobacteria) and a propensity to lymphoid and other malignancies (particularly those associated with viral infections such as Epstein–Barr virus (EBV), human papillomavirus (HPV) and human herpesvirus 8 (HHV-8)). Lymphopenia without any obvious cause is common with advancing age.

Leucocytosis (high white cell count)

An increase in the total numbers of circulating white cells is called leucocytosis. This is usually due to an increase in a specific type of cell (see Box 25.9). It is important to realise that an increase in a single type of white cell (e.g. eosinophils or monocytes) may not increase the total white cell count (WCC) above the upper limit of normal and will be apparent only if the 'differential' of the white count is examined.

Neutrophilia

An increase in the number of circulating neutrophils is called a neutrophilia or a neutrophil leucocytosis. It can result from an increased production of cells from the bone marrow or redistribution from the marginated pool. The normal neutrophil count depends on age, race and certain physiological parameters. During pregnancy, not only is there an increase in neutrophils, but also earlier forms, such as metamyelocytes, can be found in the blood. The causes of a neutrophilia are shown in Box 25.9.

Eosinophilia

A high eosinophil count of more than 0.5×10^9/L is usually secondary to infection (especially parasites; Ch. 13), allergy (e.g. eczema, asthma, reactions to drugs; (Ch. 4), immunological disorders (e.g. polyarteritis, sarcoidosis) or malignancy (e.g. lymphomas) (see Box 25.9). Usually, such eosinophilia is short-lived.

In the rarer primary disorders, there is a persistently raised, often clonal, eosinophilia, e.g. in myeloproliferative disorders, subtypes of acute myeloid leukaemia and idiopathic hypereosinophilic syndrome (HES). Specific mutations in receptor tyrosine kinase genes have been found in some primary eosinophilias (e.g. causing rearrangements of platelet-derived growth factor receptors α and β or c-kit), which allow diagnosis and, in some cases, specific therapy with tyrosine kinase inhibitors such as imatinib.

Eosinophil infiltration can damage many organs (e.g. heart, lungs, gastrointestinal tract, skin, musculoskeletal system); evaluation of eosinophilia therefore includes not only the identification of any underlying cause and its appropriate treatment, but also assessment of any related organ damage.

Lymphocytosis

A lymphocytosis is an increase in circulating lymphocytes above that expected for the patient's age. In adults, this is greater than 3.5×10^9/L. Infants and children have higher counts; age-related reference ranges should be consulted. Causes are shown in Box 25.9; the most common is viral infection.

Lymphadenopathy

Enlarged lymph glands may be an important indicator of haematological disease, but they are not uncommon in reaction to infection or inflammation (Box 25.11). The sites of lymph node groups, and symptoms and signs that may help elucidate the underlying cause are shown on page 921. Nodes that enlarge in response to local infection or inflammation ('reactive nodes') usually expand rapidly and are painful, whereas those due to haematological disease are more frequently painless. Localised lymphadenopathy should elicit a search for a source of inflammation or primary malignancy in the appropriate drainage area:

- the scalp, ear, mouth and throat, face, teeth or thyroid for neck nodes
- the breast for axillary nodes
- the perineum or external genitalia for inguinal nodes.

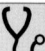

25.9 How to interpret white blood cell results

Neutrophils A

Neutrophilia

- Infection: bacterial, fungal
- Trauma: surgery, burns
- Infarction: myocardial infarct, pulmonary embolus, sickle-cell crisis
- Inflammation: gout, rheumatoid arthritis, ulcerative colitis, Crohn's disease
- Malignancy: solid tumours, Hodgkin lymphoma
- Myeloproliferative disease: polycythaemia, chronic myeloid leukaemia
- Physiological: exercise, pregnancy

Neutropenia

- Infection: viral, bacterial (e.g. *Salmonella*), protozoal (e.g. malaria)
- Drugs: see Box 25.10
- Autoimmune: connective tissue disease
- Alcohol
- Bone marrow infiltration: leukaemia, myelodysplasia
- Congenital: Kostmann syndrome
- Constitutional: African Caribbean and Middle Eastern descent

Eosinophils B

Eosinophilia

- Allergy: hay fever, asthma, eczema
- Infection: parasitic
- Drug hypersensitivity: e.g. gold, sulphonamides
- Vasculitis: e.g. eosinophilic granulomatosis with polyangiitis (Churg–Strauss), granulomatosis with polyangiitis (Wegener's)
- Connective tissue disease: polyarteritis nodosa
- Malignancy: solid tumours, lymphomas
- Primary bone marrow disorders: myeloproliferative disorders, hypereosinophilic syndrome (HES), acute myeloid leukaemia

Basophils C

Basophilia

- Myeloproliferative disease: polycythaemia vera, chronic myeloid leukaemia
- Inflammation: acute hypersensitivity, ulcerative colitis, Crohn's disease

Monocytes D

Monocytosis

- Infection: bacterial (e.g. tuberculosis)
- Inflammation: connective tissue disease, ulcerative colitis, Crohn's disease
- Malignancy: solid tumours, chronic myelomonocytic leukaemia

Lymphocytes E

Lymphocytosis

- Infection: viral, bacterial (e.g. *Bordetella pertussis*)
- Lymphoproliferative disease: chronic lymphocytic leukaemia, lymphoma
- Post-splenectomy

Lymphopenia

- Inflammation: connective tissue disease
- Lymphoma
- Renal failure
- Sarcoidosis
- Drugs: glucocorticoids, cytotoxics
- Congenital: severe combined immunodeficiency
- Human immunodeficiency virus (HIV) infection

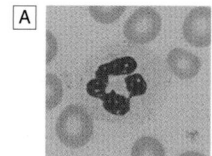 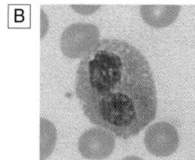 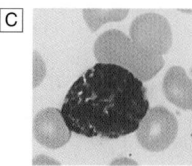 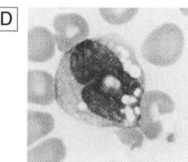 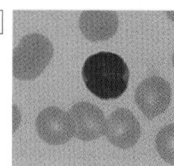

Fig. 25.12 Appearance of white blood cells. A Neutrophil. B Eosinophil. C Basophil. D Monocyte. E Lymphocyte.

25.10 Drugs that can induce neutropenia*

Group	Examples
Analgesics/anti-inflammatory agents	Gold, penicillamine, naproxen
Antithyroid drugs	Carbimazole, propylthiouracil
Anti-arrhythmics	Quinidine, procainamide
Antihypertensives	Captopril, enalapril, nifedipine
Antidepressants/psychotropics	Amitriptyline, dosulepin, mianserin
Antimalarials	Pyrimethamine, dapsone, sulfadoxine, chloroquine
Anticonvulsants	Phenytoin, sodium valproate, carbamazepine
Antibiotics	Sulphonamides, penicillins, cephalosporins
Miscellaneous	Cimetidine, ranitidine, chlorpropamide, zidovudine

*Many drugs can induce cytopenias. Many chemotherapy drugs and immunosuppressant drugs predictably cause neutropenia. In suspected cases check drug summary of product characteristics.

25.11 Causes of lymphadenopathy

Infective
- Bacterial: streptococcal, tuberculosis, brucellosis
- Viral: Epstein–Barr virus (EBV), human immunodeficiency virus (HIV)
- Protozoal: toxoplasmosis
- Fungal: histoplasmosis, coccidioidomycosis

Neoplastic
- Primary: lymphomas, leukaemias
- Secondary: lung, breast, thyroid, stomach, melanoma

Connective tissue disorders
- Rheumatoid arthritis
- Systemic lupus erythematosus (SLE)

Sarcoidosis

Amyloidosis

Drugs
- Phenytoin

Generalised lymphadenopathy may be secondary to infection, often viral, connective tissue disease or extensive skin disease (dermatopathic lymphadenopathy), but is more likely to signify underlying haematological malignancy. Weight loss and drenching night sweats that may require a change of nightclothes are associated with haematological malignancies, particularly lymphoma.

Initial investigations in lymphadenopathy include an FBC (to detect evidence of infection, inflammation or haematological disease such as leucocytosis, thrombocytosis or lymphopenia), measurement of erythrocyte sedimentation rate (ESR) and a chest X-ray (to detect mediastinal lymphadenopathy). If the findings suggest malignancy, a formal cutting needle or excision biopsy of a representative node is indicated to obtain a histological diagnosis. Increasingly, such lymph node biopsies are carried out under image guidance using ultrasound or CT scanning, rather than formal surgical excision biopsy. However, the quality of such specimens is variable and can be difficult to interpret, especially if they are small.

Splenomegaly

The spleen may be enlarged due to involvement by lymphoproliferative disease, the resumption of extramedullary haematopoiesis in myeloproliferative disease, enhanced reticulo-endothelial activity in autoimmune haemolysis, expansion of the lymphoid tissue in response to infections, or vascular congestion as a result of portal hypertension (Box 25.12).

25.12 Causes of splenomegaly

Congestive

Portal hypertension
- Cirrhosis
- Hepatic vein occlusion
- Portal vein thrombosis
- Stenosis or malformation of portal or splenic vein

Cardiac
- Chronic congestive cardiac failure
- Constrictive pericarditis

Infective

Bacterial
- Endocarditis
- Sepsis
- Tuberculosis
- Brucellosis
- *Salmonella*

Viral
- Hepatitis
- Epstein–Barr
- Cytomegalovirus

Protozoal
- Malaria*
- Leishmaniasis (kala-azar)*
- Trypanosomiasis

Fungal
- Histoplasmosis

Inflammatory/granulomatous disorders
- Felty syndrome in rheumatoid arthritis
- Systemic lupus erythematosus
- Sarcoidosis

Haematological

Red cell disorders
- Megaloblastic anaemia
- Haemoglobinopathies
- Hereditary spherocytosis

Autoimmune haemolytic anaemias

Myeloproliferative disorders
- Chronic myeloid leukaemia*
- Myelofibrosis*
- Polycythaemia rubra vera
- Essential thrombocythaemia

Neoplastic
- Leukaemias, including chronic myeloid leukaemia*
- Lymphomas

Other malignancies
- Metastatic cancer – rare

Lysosomal storage diseases
- Gaucher's disease
- Niemann–Pick disease

Miscellaneous
- Cysts, amyloid, thyrotoxicosis, haemophagocytic syndromes and other histiocytic disorders

*Causes of massive splenomegaly.

Hepatosplenomegaly is suggestive of lympho- or myeloproliferative disease, liver disease or infiltration (e.g. with amyloid). Associated lymphadenopathy is suggestive of lymphoproliferative disease. An enlarged spleen may cause abdominal discomfort, accompanied by back pain and abdominal bloating and early satiety due to stomach compression. Splenic infarction produces severe abdominal pain radiating to the left shoulder tip, associated with a splenic rub on auscultation. Rarely, spontaneous or traumatic rupture and bleeding may occur.

Investigation should focus on the suspected cause. Imaging of the spleen by ultrasound or computed tomography (CT) will detect variations in density in the spleen, which may be a feature of lymphoproliferative disease; it also allows imaging of the liver and abdominal lymph nodes. Biopsy of enlarged abdominal or superficial lymph nodes may provide the diagnosis, as might a bone marrow biopsy in splenic lymphomas. A chest X-ray or CT of the thorax will detect mediastinal lymphadenopathy. An FBC may show pancytopenia secondary to hypersplenism, when the enlarged spleen has become overactive, pooling and destroying blood cells prematurely. If other abnormalities are present, such as abnormal lymphocytes or a leucoerythroblastic blood film, a bone marrow examination is indicated. Screening for infectious or liver disease (p. 8665) may be appropriate. If all investigations are unhelpful, splenectomy may be diagnostic, but is rarely carried out in these circumstances.

Bleeding

Normal bleeding is seen following surgery and trauma. Pathological bleeding occurs when structurally abnormal vessels rupture or when a vessel is breached in the presence of a defect in haemostasis. This may be due to a deficiency or dysfunction of platelets, the coagulation factors or von Willebrand factor, or occasionally to excessive fibrinolysis, which is most commonly observed following therapeutic thrombolysis (Ch. 16).

Clinical assessment

'Screening' blood tests (see Box 25.3) do not reliably detect all causes of pathological bleeding (e.g. von Willebrand disease, scurvy, certain anticoagulant and anti-platelet drugs and the causes of purpura listed in Box 25.13) and should not be used indiscriminately. A careful clinical evaluation is the key to diagnosis of bleeding disorders (p. 980). It is important to consider the following:

- *Site of bleeding.* Bleeding into muscle and joints, along with retroperitoneal and intracranial haemorrhage, indicates a likely defect in coagulation factors. Purpura, prolonged bleeding from superficial cuts, epistaxis, gastrointestinal haemorrhage or menorrhagia is more likely to be due to thrombocytopenia, a platelet function disorder or von Willebrand disease. Recurrent bleeds at a single site suggest a local structural abnormality rather than coagulopathic bleeding.
- *Duration of history.* It may be possible to assess whether the disorder is congenital or acquired.
- *Precipitating causes.* Bleeding arising spontaneously indicates a more severe defect than bleeding that occurs only after trauma.
- *Surgery.* Ask about operations. Dental extractions, tonsillectomy and circumcision are stressful tests of the haemostatic system. Immediate post-surgical bleeding suggests defective platelet plug formation and primary haemostasis; delayed haemorrhage is more suggestive of a coagulation defect. However, in post-surgical

25.13 Causes of non-thrombocytopenic purpura

- Senile purpura
- Factitious purpura
- Henoch–Schönlein purpura (Ch. 26)
- Vasculitis (Ch. 26)
- Paraproteinaemias
- Purpura fulminans, e.g. in disseminated intravascular coagulation secondary to sepsis

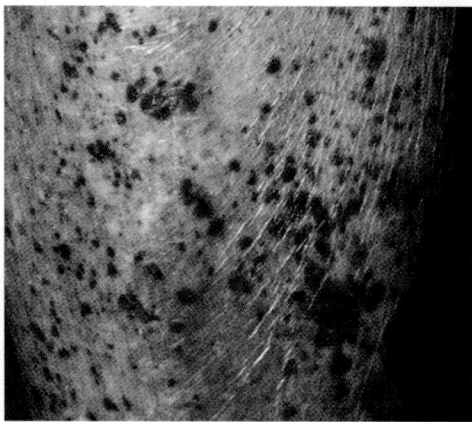

Fig. 25.13 Petechial purpura.

patients, persistent bleeding from a single site is more likely to indicate surgical bleeding than coagulopathic bleeding.

- *Family history*. While a positive family history may be present in patients with inherited disorders, the absence of affected relatives does not exclude a hereditary bleeding diathesis; about one-third of cases of haemophilia arise in individuals without a family history, and deficiencies of factor VII, X and XIII are recessively inherited. Recessive disorders are more common in cultures where there is consanguineous marriage.
- *Drugs*. Use of antithrombotic, anticoagulant and fibrinolytic drugs must be elicited. Drug interactions with warfarin and drug-induced thrombocytopenia should be considered. Some 'herbal' remedies may result in a bleeding diathesis.

Clinical examination may reveal different patterns of skin bleeding. Petechial purpura is minor bleeding into the dermis that is flat and non-blanching (Fig. 25.13). Petechiae are typically found in patients with thrombocytopenia or platelet dysfunction. Palpable purpura occurs in vasculitis. Ecchymosis, or bruising, is more extensive bleeding into deeper layers of the skin. The lesions are initially dark red or purple, but become yellow as haemoglobin is degraded. Retroperitoneal bleeding presents with a flank or peri-umbilical haematoma. Telangiectasia of lips and tongue points to hereditary haemorrhagic telangiectasia (p. 970). Joints should be examined for evidence of haemarthroses. A full examination is important, as it may give clues to an underlying associated systemic illness such as a haematological or other malignancy, liver disease, renal failure, connective tissue disease and possible causes of splenomegaly.

Investigations

Screening investigations and their interpretation are described on page 930. If the patient has a history that is strongly suggestive of a bleeding disorder and all the preliminary screening tests give normal results, further investigations, such as measurement of von Willebrand factor and assessment of platelet function, should be performed.

Thrombocytopenia (low platelet count)

A reduced platelet count may arise by one of two mechanisms:

- decreased or abnormal production (bone marrow failure and hereditary thrombocytopathies)
- increased consumption following release into the circulation (immune-mediated, DIC or sequestration).

Spontaneous bleeding does not usually occur until the platelet count falls below $20 \times 10^9/L$, unless their function is also compromised. Purpura and spontaneous bruising are characteristic, but there may also be oral,

---

> ### i 25.14 Causes of thrombocytopenia
>
> **Decreased production**
>
> **Marrow hypoplasia**
> - Childhood bone marrow failure syndromes, e.g. Fanconi's anaemia, dyskeratosis congenita, amegakaryocytic thrombocytopenia
> - Idiopathic aplastic anaemia
> - Drug-induced: cytotoxics, antimetabolites
> - Transfusion-associated graft-versus-host disease
>
> **Marrow infiltration**
> - Leukaemia
> - Myeloma
> - Carcinoma (rare)
> - Myelofibrosis
> - Osteopetrosis
> - Lysosomal storage disorders, e.g. Gaucher's disease
>
> **Haematinic deficiency**
> - Vitamin B_{12} and/or folate deficiency
>
> **Familial (macro-)thrombocytopathies**
> - Myosin heavy chain abnormalities, e.g. Alport syndrome, Fechtner syndrome, May–Hegglin anomaly
> - Bernard–Soulier syndrome
> - Montreal platelet syndrome
> - Wiskott–Aldrich syndrome (small platelets)
> - Mediterranean macrothrombocytopathy
>
> **Increased consumption**
>
> **Immune mechanisms**
> - Idiopathic thrombocytopenic purpura*
> - Neonatal alloimmune thrombocytopenia
> - Post-transfusion purpura
> - Drug-associated, especially quinine, vancomycin and heparin
>
> **Coagulation activation**
> - Disseminated intravascular coagulation (DIC) (see Box 25.70)
>
> **Mechanical pooling**
> - Hypersplenism
>
> **Thrombotic microangiopathies**
> - Haemolytic uraemic syndrome (HUS) and atypical HUS
> - Liver disease
> - Thrombotic thrombocytopenic purpura
> - Pre-eclampsia/HELLP
>
> **Others**
> - Gestational thrombocytopenia
> - Type 2B von Willebrand disease
> - Pseudo von Willebrand disease
>
> *Associated conditions include collagen vascular diseases (particularly systemic lupus erythematosus), B-cell malignancy, HIV infection and antiphospholipid syndrome.

nasal, gastrointestinal or genitourinary bleeding. Severe thrombocytopenia ($<10 \times 10^9/L$) may result in retinal haemorrhage and potentially fatal intracranial bleeding, but this is rare.

Investigations are directed at the possible causes listed in Box 25.14. A blood film is the single most useful initial investigation. Examination of the bone marrow may reveal increased megakaryocytes in consumptive causes of thrombocytopenia, or the underlying cause of bone marrow failure in leukaemia, hypoplastic anaemia or myelodysplasia.

Treatment (if required) depends on the underlying cause. Platelet transfusion is rarely required and is usually confined to patients with bone marrow failure and platelet counts below $10 \times 10^9/L$, or to clinical situations with actual or predicted serious haemorrhage.

Thrombocytosis (high platelet count)

The most common reason for a raised platelet count is that it is reactive to another process, such as infection, inflammation, connective tissue disease, malignancy, iron deficiency, acute haemolysis or gastrointestinal bleeding (Box 25.15). The presenting clinical features are usually those

25.15 Causes of a raised platelet count

Reactive thrombocytosis

- Acute and chronic inflammatory disorders
- Infection
- Malignant disease

- Tissue damage
- Haemolytic anaemias
- Post-splenectomy
- Post-haemorrhage

Clonal thrombocytosis

- Primary thrombocythaemia
- Polycythaemia rubra vera
- Chronic myeloid leukaemia
- Myelofibrosis

- Myelodysplastic syndromes (MDSs)
- MDS with ring sideroblasts and thrombocytosis
- MDS with isolated deletion of 5q

25.16 Causes of pancytopenia

Bone marrow failure

- Hypoplastic/aplastic anaemia (p. 978): inherited, idiopathic, viral, drugs

Bone marrow infiltration

- Acute leukaemia
- Myeloma
- Lymphoma
- Carcinoma
- Haemophagocytic syndrome
- Myelodysplastic syndromes

Ineffective haematopoiesis

- Megaloblastic anaemia
- Acquired immunodeficiency syndrome (AIDS)

Peripheral pooling/destruction

- Hypersplenism: portal hypertension, Felty syndrome, malaria, myelofibrosis
- Systemic lupus erythematosus

of the underlying disorder and haemostasis is rarely affected. Reactive thrombocytosis is distinguished from the myeloproliferative disorders by the presence of uniform small platelets, lack of splenomegaly and the presence of an associated underlying disorder. The key to diagnosis is the clinical history and examination, combined with observation of the platelet count over time (reactive thrombocytosis gets better with resolution of the underlying cause).

The platelets are a product of an abnormally expanding clone of cells in the myeloproliferative disorders, chronic myeloid leukaemia and some forms of myelodysplasia. As with PRV, patients with essential thrombocythaemia may present with thrombosis or, rarely, bleeding. Stroke, transient ischaemic attacks, amaurosis fugax, digital ischaemia or gangrene, aquagenic pruritus, splenomegaly and systemic upset are also features. Patients with myeloproliferative disorders may also present with features such as aquagenic pruritus, splenomegaly and systemic upset.

Pancytopenia

Pancytopenia refers to the combination of anaemia, leucopenia and thrombocytopenia. It may be due to reduced production of blood cells as a consequence of bone marrow suppression or infiltration, or there may be peripheral destruction or splenic pooling of mature cells. Causes are shown in Box 25.16. A bone marrow aspirate and trephine are usually required to establish the diagnosis.

Infection

Infection is a major complication of haematological disorders. It relates to the immunological deficit caused by the disease itself, or its treatment with chemotherapy and/or immunotherapy (pp. 268 and 933).

Principles of management of haematological disease

Blood components and transfusion

Blood transfusion from an unrelated donor to a recipient inevitably carries some risk, including adverse immunological interactions between the host and infused blood (see below), and transmission of infectious agents. Although there are many compelling clinical indications for blood component transfusion, there are also many clinical circumstances where transfusion is conventional, but the evidence for its effectiveness is limited. In these settings, allogeneic transfusion may be avoided by following protocols that recommend the use of low haemoglobin thresholds for red cell transfusion, perioperative blood salvage and antifibrinolytic drugs.

Blood components

Blood components are prepared from whole blood or specific blood constituents collected from individual donors and include red cells, platelets, plasma and cryoprecipitate (Box 25.17).

Plasma derivatives are licensed pharmaceutical products produced on a factory scale from large volumes of human plasma obtained from many people and treated to reduce the risk of transmissible infection. Examples include:

- *Coagulation factors.* Concentrates of factors VIII and IX are used for the treatment of conditions such as haemophilia A, haemophilia B and von Willebrand disease. Coagulation factors made by recombinant DNA technology are now preferred due to perceived lack of infection risk but plasma-derived products are still used in many countries.
- *Immunoglobulins.* Intravenous immunoglobulin G (IVIgG) is administered as regular replacement therapy to reduce infective complications in patients with primary and secondary immunodeficiency. A short, high-dose course of IVIgG may also be effective in some immunological disorders, including immune thrombocytopenia (p. 981) and Guillain–Barré syndrome (Ch. 28). IVIgG can cause acute reactions and must be infused strictly according to the manufacturer's product information. There is a risk of renal dysfunction in susceptible patients and in these circumstances immunoglobulin products containing low or no sucrose are preferred. Anti-zoster immunoglobulin has a role in the prophylaxis of varicella zoster (Ch. 13). Anti-Rhesus D immunoglobulin is used in pregnancy to prevent haemolytic disease of the newborn (see Box 25.19).
- *Human albumin.* This is available in two strengths. The 5% solution can be used as a colloid resuscitation fluid, but it is no more effective and is more expensive than crystalloid solutions. Human albumin 20% solution may be used in the management of hypoproteinaemic oedema in nephrotic syndrome (Ch. 18) and refractory ascites in chronic liver disease (Ch. 24). It is hyperoncotic and expands plasma volume by more than the amount infused.

Blood components and their uses are summarised in Box 25.17.

Blood donation

A safe supply of blood components depends on a well-organised system with regular donation by healthy individuals who have no excess risk of infections transmissible in blood (Fig. 25.14). Blood donations are obtained by either venesection of a unit of whole blood or collection of a specific component, such as platelets, by apheresis. During apheresis, the donor's blood is drawn via a closed system into a machine that separates the components by centrifugation and collects the desired fraction into a bag, returning the rest of the blood to the donor. Each donation must be tested for hepatitis B virus (HBV), hepatitis C virus (HCV), HIV and human T-cell lymphotropic virus (HTLV) nucleic acid

i 25.17 Blood components and their use

Component	Major haemorrhage	Other indications
Red cell concentrate[1]		
Most of the plasma is removed and replaced with a solution of glucose and adenine in saline to maintain viability of red cells ABO compatibility with recipient essential	Replace acute blood loss: increase circulating red cell mass to relieve clinical features caused by insufficient oxygen delivery. Order 4–6U initially to allow high red cell to FFP transfusion ratios of (at least) 2:1	*Severe anaemia* If no cardiovascular disease, transfuse to maintain Hb at 70 g/L If known or likely to have cardiovascular disease, maintain Hb at 90 g/L
Platelet concentrate		
One adult dose is made from four donations of whole blood, or from a single platelet apheresis donation ABO compatibility with recipient preferable	Maintain platelet count $>50 \times 10^9$/L, or in multiple or central nervous system trauma $>100 \times 10^9$/L If ongoing bleeding, order when platelets $<100 \times 10^9$/L to allow for delivery time Each adult dose has a minimum of 2.4×10^{11} platelets, which raises platelet count by 40×10^9/L unless there is consumptive coagulopathy, e.g. disseminated intravascular coagulation	*Thrombocytopenia*, e.g. in acute leukaemia Maintain platelet count $>10 \times 10^9$/L if not bleeding Maintain platelet count $>20 \times 10^9$/L if minor bleeding or at risk (sepsis, concurrent use of antibiotics, abnormal coagulation) Increase platelet count $>50 \times 10^9$/L for minor invasive procedure (e.g. lumbar puncture, gastroscopy and biopsy, insertion of indwelling lines, liver biopsy, laparotomy) or in acute, major blood loss Increase platelet count $>100 \times 10^9$/L for operations in critical sites such as brain or eyes
Fresh frozen plasma[2]		
150–300 mL plasma from one donation of whole blood ABO compatibility with recipient recommended	Dilutional coagulopathy with a PT prolonged $>50\%$ is likely after replacement of 1–1.5 blood volumes with red cell concentrate Give initially in (at least) a ratio of 1 FFP:2 red cell concentrate; order 15–20 mL/kg and allow for thawing time. Further doses only if bleeding continues and guided by PT and APTT	*Replacement of coagulation factor deficiency* If no virally inactivated or recombinant product is available *Thrombotic thrombocytopenic purpura* Plasma exchange (using virus-inactivated plasma if available) is frequently effective
Cryoprecipitate[2]		

Fibrinogen and coagulation factor concentrated from plasma by controlled thawing
10–20 mL pack contains:
  Fibrinogen 150–300 mg
  Factor VIII 80–120 U
  von Willebrand factor 80–120 U
In UK supplied as pools of 5 U
	Aim to keep fibrinogen >1.5 g/L. Pooled units (of 10 donations) will raise fibrinogen by 1 g/L	*von Willebrand disease and haemophilia*
		If virus-inactivated or recombinant products are not available

[1]Whole blood is an alternative to red cell concentrate. ABO compatibility with recipient essential. [2]Pooled plasma can be treated with solvent and detergent or single units treated with methylene blue as an additional viral inactivation step. Virus-inactivated plasma is indicated for large-volume exposure, as in treatment of thrombotic thrombocytopenic purpura.
(APTT = activated partial thromboplastin time; FFP = fresh frozen plasma; Hb = haemoglobin; PT = prothrombin time)

and/or antibodies. Platelet concentrates may be tested for bacterial contamination. The need for other microbiological tests depends on local epidemiology. For example, testing for *Trypanosoma cruzi* (Chagas' disease; Ch. 13) is necessary in areas of South America and the United States where infection is prevalent. Tests for West Nile virus have been required in the United States and UK since this agent became more prevalent. Components for use in specific patient groups are prepared from hepatitis E virus-negative donors in the UK, and plasma donated in the UK is not used at present for producing pooled plasma derivatives in view of concerns about transmission of variant Creutzfeldt–Jakob disease (vCJD; Ch. 28).

Adverse effects of transfusion

Death attributable to transfusion is rare, at 0.99 per 100 000 transfusions; this includes death where a delay in timely supply of components was contributory. Moderate or severe febrile, allergic and hypotensive reactions occur in around 12 per 100 000 transfusions and are usually seen in patients who have had repeated transfusions. Any symptoms or signs that arise during a transfusion must be taken seriously, as they may be the first warnings of a serious reaction. Fig. 25.16 outlines the symptoms and signs, management and investigation of acute reactions to blood components.

Red cell incompatibility

Red blood cell membranes contain numerous cell surface molecules that are potentially antigenic (see Fig. 25.4). The ABO and Rhesus D antigens are the most important in routine transfusion and antenatal practice.

ABO blood groups

The frequency of the ABO antigens varies among different populations. The ABO blood group antigens are oligosaccharide chains that project from the red cell surface. These chains are attached to proteins and lipids that lie in the red cell membrane. The *ABO* gene encodes a glycosyltransferase that catalyses the final step in the synthesis of the chain, which has three common alleles: A, B and O. The O allele encodes an inactive enzyme, leaving the ABO antigen precursor (called the H antigen) unmodified. The A and B alleles encode enzymes that differ by four amino acids and hence attach different sugars to the end of the chain. Individuals are tolerant to their own ABO antigens, but do not suppress B-cell clones producing antibodies against ABO antigens that they do not carry themselves (Box 25.18). They are, therefore, capable of mounting a humoral immune response to these 'foreign' antigens.

ABO-incompatible red cell transfusion

If red cells of an incompatible ABO group are transfused (especially if a group O recipient is transfused with group A, B or AB red cells), the

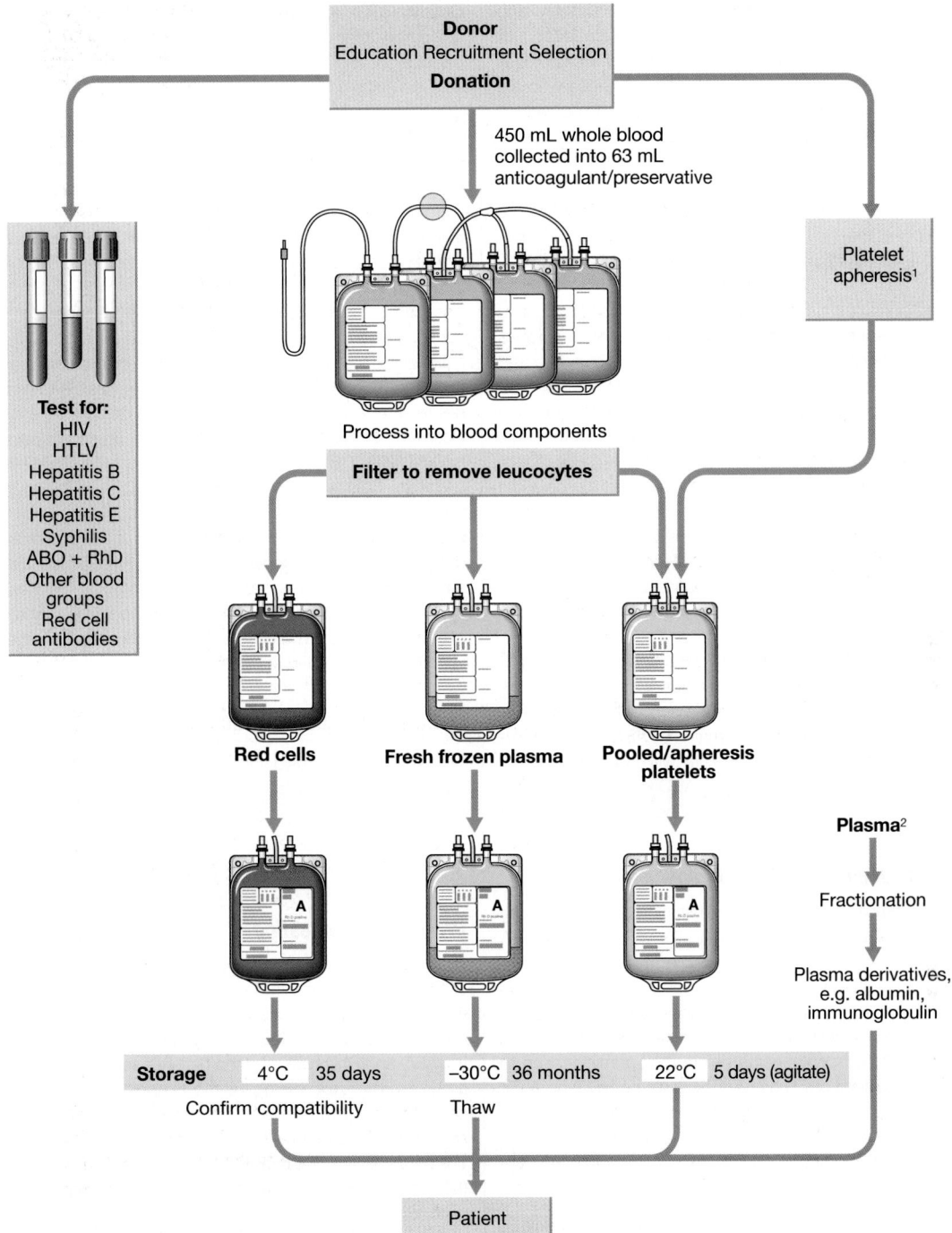

Fig. 25.14 **Blood donation, processing and storage.** [1]Platelet apheresis involves circulating the donor's blood through a cell separator to remove platelets before returning other blood components to the donor. [2]In the UK, plasma for fractionation is imported as a precautionary measure against variant Creutzfeldt–Jakob disease (vCJD). (HIV = human immunodeficiency virus; HTLV = human T-cell lymphotropic virus)

i 25.18 ABO blood group antigens and antibodies			
ABO blood group	**Red cell A or B antigens**	**Antibodies in plasma**	**UK frequency (%)**
O	None	Anti-A and anti-B	46
A	A	Anti-B	42
B	B	Anti-A	9
AB	A and B	None	3

recipient's IgM anti-A, anti-B or anti-AB binds to the *transfused* red cells. This activates the full complement pathway (Ch. 4), creating pores in the red cell membrane and destroying the transfused red cells in the circulation (intravascular haemolysis). The anaphylatoxins C3a and C5a, released by complement activation, liberate cytokines such as tumour necrosis factor (TNF), interleukin (IL)-1 and IL-8, and stimulate degranulation of mast cells with release of vasoactive mediators. All these substances may lead to inflammation, increased vascular permeability and hypotension, which may, in turn, cause shock and renal failure. Inflammatory mediators can also cause platelet aggregation, lung peribronchial oedema and smooth muscle contraction. About 20%–30% of

ABO-incompatible transfusions cause some degree of morbidity, and 5%–10% cause or contribute to a patient's death. The main reason for this relatively low morbidity is the lack of potency of ABO antibodies in group A or B subjects; even if the recipient is group O, those who are very young or very old usually have weaker antibodies that do not lead to the activation of large amounts of complement.

The Rhesus D blood group and haemolytic disease of the newborn

About 15% of populations of predominantly European descent are Rhesus-negative: that is, they lack the Rhesus D (RhD) red cell surface antigen (see Fig. 25.4). In other populations (e.g. in Chinese and Bengalis), only 1%–5% are Rhesus-negative. RhD-negative individuals do not normally produce substantial amounts of anti-RhD antibodies. However, if RhD-positive red cells enter the circulation of an RhD-negative individual, IgG antibodies are produced. This can occur during pregnancy if the mother is exposed to fetal cells via fetomaternal haemorrhage, or following transfusion. If a woman is sensitised, during a subsequent pregnancy anti-RhD antibodies can cross the placenta; if the fetus is RhD-positive, haemolysis with severe fetal anaemia and hyperbilirubinaemia can result. This can cause severe neurological damage or death due to haemolytic disease of the newborn (HDN). Therefore, an RhD-negative female who may subsequently become pregnant should never be transfused with RhD-positive blood.

In RhD-negative women, administration of anti-RhD immunoglobulin (anti-D) perinatally can block the immune response to RhD antigen on fetal cells and is the only effective product for preventing the development of Rhesus antibodies (Box 25.19).

HDN can also be caused by other alloantibodies against red cell antigens, usually after previous pregnancies or transfusions. These antigens include Rhc, RhC, RhE, Rhe, and the Kell, Kidd and Duffy antigen systems. HDN can also occur if there is fetomaternal ABO incompatibility, most commonly seen in a group O mother with a group A fetus. The fetus is generally less severely affected by ABO incompatibility than by RhD, Rhc or Kell antigen mismatch and the incompatibility is often picked up coincidentally after birth.

Other immunological complications of transfusion

Rare but serious complications include transfusion-associated lung injury (TRALI) and transfusion-associated graft-versus-host disease (TA GVHD). The latter occurs when there is sharing of a human leucocyte antigen (HLA) haplotype between donor and recipient, which allows transfused lymphocytes to engraft, proliferate and recognise the recipient as foreign, resulting in acute GVHD (p. 945). Prevention is by gamma- or X-ray irradiation of blood components before their administration to prevent lymphocyte proliferation. Those at risk of TA GVHD who must receive irradiated blood components include patients with congenital T-cell immunodeficiencies or Hodgkin lymphoma, patients with aplastic anaemia receiving immunosuppressive therapy with antithymocyte

---

globulin (ATG), recipients of haematopoietic stem cell transplants or of blood from a family member, neonates who have received an intrauterine transfusion, and patients taking T-lymphocyte-suppressing drugs, such as fludarabine and other purine analogues.

Transfusion-transmitted infection

Over the past 30 years, HBV, HIV-1 and HCV have been identified and effective tests introduced to detect and exclude infected donations. Where blood is from 'safe' donors and correctly tested, the current risk of a donated unit being infectious is very small. In the UK, the estimated chance that a unit of blood from a 'safe' donor might be infected with one of the viruses for which blood is tested is approximately 1 in 25 million units for HIV-1, less than 1 in 100 million for HCV and 1 in 1.2 million for HBV. However, some patients who received transfusions before these tests were available suffered serious consequences from infection; this serves as a reminder to avoid non-essential transfusion since it is impossible to exclude the emergence of new or currently unrecognised transfusion-transmissible infection. Licensed plasma derivatives that have been virus-inactivated do not transmit HIV, HTLV, HBV, HCV, cytomegalovirus or other lipid-enveloped viruses.

Variant CJD is a human prion disease linked to bovine spongiform encephalitis (BSE; Ch. 28). The risk of a recipient acquiring the agent of vCJD from a transfusion is uncertain, but of 16 recipients of blood from donors who later developed the disease, 3 have died with clinical vCJD and 1 other had postmortem immunohistological features of infection.

Bacterial contamination of a blood component – usually platelets – is extremely rare (there have been no proven cases in the UK in recent years) but can result in severe bacteraemia/sepsis in the recipient.

Safe transfusion procedures

The proposed transfusion and any alternatives should be discussed with the patient or, if that is not possible, with a relative. Their consent to proceed with transfusion should be obtained and the discussion documented. Some patients, e.g. Jehovah's Witnesses, may refuse transfusion and require specialised management to survive profound anaemia following blood loss.

Pre-transfusion testing

To ensure that red cells supplied for transfusion are compatible with the intended recipient, the transfusion laboratory will perform either a 'group and screen' procedure or a 'cross-match'. In the group and screen procedure, the red cells from the patient's blood sample are tested to determine the ABO and RhD type, and the patient's serum is also tested against an array of red cells expressing the most important antigens to detect any red cell antibodies. Any antibody detected can be identified by further testing, so that red cell units that lack the corresponding antigen can be selected. The patient's sample can be held in the laboratory for up to a week, so that the hospital blood bank can quickly prepare compatible blood without the need for a further patient sample. Conventional cross-matching consists of the group and antibody screen, followed by direct confirmation of the compatibility of individual units of red cells with the patient's serum. Full cross-matching takes about 45 minutes, if no red cell antibodies are present, but may require hours if a patient has multiple antibodies.

Blood can be supplied by 'electronic issue', without the need for compatibility cross-matching, if the laboratory's computer system shows that the patient's ABO and RhD groups have been identified and confirmed on two separate occasions and their antibody screen is negative. This allows group-specific units to be issued quickly and safely, for elective and emergency transfusion.

Bedside procedures for safe transfusion

Errors leading to patients receiving the wrong blood are an important avoidable cause of mortality and morbidity. Most incompatible transfusions result from failure to adhere to standard procedures for taking correctly labelled blood samples from the patient and ensuring that the correct pack of blood component is transfused into the intended patient. In the UK in 2019, the annual incidence of transfusion of an incorrect

---

25.19 Rhesus D blood groups in pregnancy

- **Haemolytic disease of the newborn (HDN)**: occurs when the mother has anti-red cell immunoglobulin G (IgG) antibodies that cross the placenta and haemolyse fetal red cells.
- **Screening for HDN in pregnancy**: at the time of booking (12–16 weeks) and again at 28–34 weeks' gestation, every pregnant woman should have a blood sample sent for determination of ABO and Rhesus D (RhD) group and testing for red cell alloantibodies that may be directed against paternal blood group antigens present on fetal red cells.
- **Anti-D immunoglobulin prophylaxis in a pregnant woman who is RhD-negative**: antenatal anti-D prophylaxis is offered at 28–34 weeks to RhD-negative pregnant women who have no evidence of immune anti-D. This prevents the formation of antibodies that could cause HDN. Following delivery of an RhD-positive baby, the mother is given further anti-D within 72 hours; a maternal sample is checked for remaining fetal red cells and additional anti-D is given if indicated. Additional anti-D is also given after potential sensitising events antenatally (e.g. early bleeding). Doses vary according to national recommendations.

blood component is approximately 15 per 100000 units transfused. Every hospital where blood is transfused should have a written transfusion policy used by all staff who order, check or administer blood products (Fig. 25.15). Management of suspected transfusion reactions is shown in Fig. 25.16.

Transfusion in major haemorrhage

The successful management of a patient with major haemorrhage requires frontline clinical staff to be trained to recognise significant blood loss early and to intervene before shock is established. Hospitals should have local major haemorrhage protocols and all clinical staff must be familiar with their content. Good team working and communication are essential to prevent poor clinical outcome, suboptimal or inappropriate transfusion practice and component wastage. Fresh frozen plasma (FFP) should be given as part of initial resuscitation in (at least) a 1:2 ratio with red cell concentrate (RCC) until coagulation results are available. If the patient is bleeding, a ratio of FFP to RCC of 1:1 should be given

until laboratory results are available and use of cryoprecipitate should be considered. Once the bleeding is under control, further FFP transfusion should be guided by laboratory results with transfusion triggers of PT and/or APTT above 1·5 times normal for a standard dose of FFP (15–20 mL/kg). Cryoprecipitate should be given if the fibrinogen level falls below 1.5 g/L. Platelets should be kept above 50 × 10⁹/L; to allow for delivery time, platelets should be requested if there is ongoing bleeding and the platelet count has fallen below 100 × 10⁹/L. Blood component use in major haemorrhage is summarised in Box 25.17 and key points in transfusion medicine in Box 25.20.

Anti-cancer drugs

Cytotoxic chemotherapy

Many haematological malignancies are sensitive to the effects of cytotoxic chemotherapy drugs and, as such, they remain the mainstay of treatment for most haematological cancers (Box 25.21; see also Fig. 7.2). There is a wide range of drugs available that work by damaging DNA or disrupting cellular metabolism, in such a way that natural apoptosis mechanisms, such as *TP53*, are activated and the cell dies. Despite cancer cells being more sensitive, chemotherapy is largely non-specific and kills some normal cells as well as cancer cells. This leads to common side-effects of treatment, such as transient bone marrow failure, hair loss, mucositis and infertility. The supportive care of patients undergoing chemotherapy is critical in overcoming these side-effects. It is this supportive care, including blood product support, antibiotics, antifungal drugs, growth factors and antiemetics, that has allowed specialist haematology units to achieve the best possible results from intensive chemotherapy: for example, when treating acute leukaemia.

The basic principles of chemotherapy include combining several non-cross-reacting drugs in a regimen that kills a fixed proportion of cancer cells with a given dose. Several cycles of the combination are given to achieve gradual reduction of the tumour burden, to induce remission and, in some instances, to produce a cure (Ch. 7).

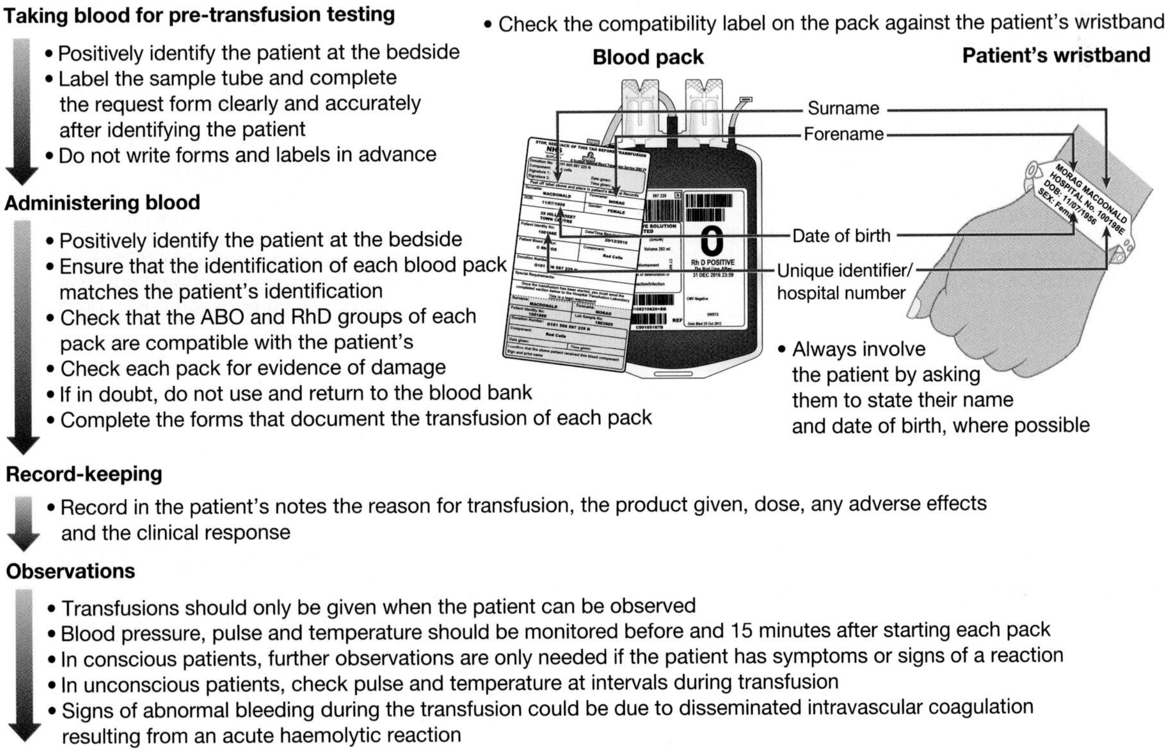

 25.20 Key points in transfusion medicine

- A restrictive strategy for red cell transfusion (Hb <70 g/L) is at least as effective as a liberal strategy (<100 g/L).
- The majority of reports in haemovigilance schemes such as SHOT relate to errors in the process of transfusion.
- Although transfusion-transmitted infection is a major concern for patients receiving transfusion, it is rare.
- In patients with trauma or burns or those who have had surgery, there is no evidence that resuscitation with albumin or other colloid solutions reduces the risk of death compared to resuscitation with crystalloid solutions.
- It is recommended that transfusion should be carried out overnight only in unavoidable circumstances.

(SHOT = Serious Hazards of Transfusion)

Taking blood for pre-transfusion testing
- Positively identify the patient at the bedside
- Label the sample tube and complete the request form clearly and accurately after identifying the patient
- Do not write forms and labels in advance

Administering blood
- Positively identify the patient at the bedside
- Ensure that the identification of each blood pack matches the patient's identification
- Check that the ABO and RhD groups of each pack are compatible with the patient's
- Check each pack for evidence of damage
- If in doubt, do not use and return to the blood bank
- Complete the forms that document the transfusion of each pack

Record-keeping
- Record in the patient's notes the reason for transfusion, the product given, dose, any adverse effects and the clinical response

Observations
- Transfusions should only be given when the patient can be observed
- Blood pressure, pulse and temperature should be monitored before and 15 minutes after starting each pack
- In conscious patients, further observations are only needed if the patient has symptoms or signs of a reaction
- In unconscious patients, check pulse and temperature at intervals during transfusion
- Signs of abnormal bleeding during the transfusion could be due to disseminated intravascular coagulation resulting from an acute haemolytic reaction

• Check the compatibility label on the pack against the patient's wristband

Blood pack   **Patient's wristband**

— Surname —
— Forename —
— Date of birth —
— Unique identifier/ hospital number —

- Always involve the patient by asking them to state their name and date of birth, where possible

Fig. 25.15 Bedside procedures for safe blood transfusion. The patient's safety depends on adherence to standard procedures for taking samples for compatibility testing, administering blood, record-keeping and observations.

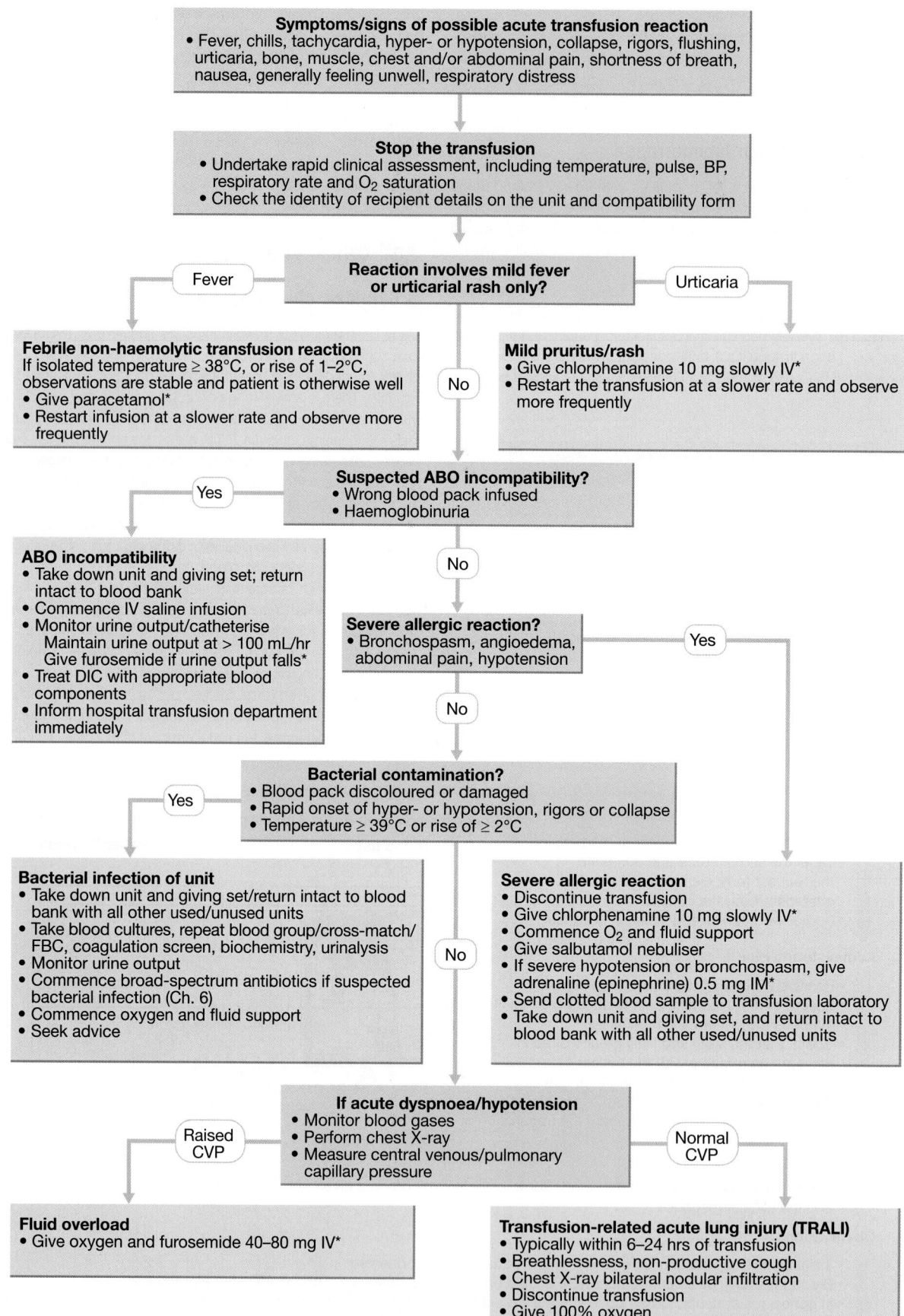

Fig. 25.16 Investigation and management of acute transfusion reactions. *Use size-appropriate dose in children. (ARDS = acute respiratory distress syndrome; BP = blood pressure; CVP = central venous pressure; DIC = disseminated intravascular coagulation; FBC = full blood count; IV = intravenous)

Monocolonal antibodies

In recent years, chemotherapy has been improved by the addition of treatments that are more targeted to the cancer cell, particularly monoclonal antibodies; for example, rituximab (anti-CD20) has been added to CHOP (cyclophosphamide doxorubicin, vincristine, prednisolone) and other regimens. This has significantly improved the outcome in a range of CD20-positive B-cell lymphomas, including diffuse large B-cell lymphoma, follicular lymphoma and mantle cell lymphoma. As well as 'naked' monoclonal antibodies that kill malignant cells by engaging antibody-dependent cytotoxic T cells or complement, chemotherapy drugs can also be linked to a monoclonal antibody to allow targeting of the chemotherapy drug to the specific cancer cell. Examples of such antibody–drug conjugates (ADCs) or 'payload' antibodies include the linking of the intercalating antibiotic calicheamicin to anti-CD33 (gemtuzumab ozogamicin) in the treatment of acute myeloid leukaemia (see Fig. 25.27) and to anti-CD22 (inotuzumab ozogamicin) in the treatment of acute lymphoblastic leukaemia (see Fig. 25.28).

Small molecule targeted therapies

Small molecules targeted at the mechanisms causing cancer are replacing cytotoxic chemotherapy in some disease situations. The most successful of these to date are tyrosine kinase inhibitors targeting BCR-ABL in chronic myeloid leukaemia, which have transformed the treatment of this disease over the last 20 years (see Fig. 25.29). This is a rapidly growing area of medicine and now includes inhibitors of B-cell signalling in chronic lymphocytic leukaemia and lymphomas (see Fig. 25.30) and drugs that target mutated gene products, such as FMS-like tyrosine kinase 3-internal tandem duplication (*FLT3-ITD*) in acute myeloid leukaemia. More details of specific therapies are given later in the chapter.

Immunotherapy

This includes cellular immunotherapy (see below) and non-cellular immunotherapy such as antibody and antibody-conjugate mediated cytotoxicity as outlined above and checkpoint inhibitor therapy as described in Chapter 7. Checkpoint inhibitor therapy has, to date, proved less useful in haematological malignancies than in solid tumours. This might be because haematological malignancies tend to have less acquired mutations to stimulate T-cell attack than do solid tumours.

Haematopoietic stem cell transplantation

Transplantation of haematopoietic stem cells (HSCT) has offered the only hope of 'cure' in a variety of haematological and non-haematological disorders (Box 25.22). As standard treatment improves, the indications for HSCT are being refined and extended, although its use remains most common in haematological malignancies. The type of HSCT is defined according to the donor and source of stem cells:

• In *allogeneic* HSCT, the stem cells come from a *donor* – either a related donor (usually an HLA-identical sibling) or a closely HLA-matched volunteer unrelated donor (VUD).
• In an *autologous* transplant, the stem cells are harvested from the *patient* and stored in the vapour phase of liquid nitrogen until required. Stem cells can be harvested from the bone marrow or, most commonly nowadays, from the blood.

Allogeneic HSCT

Healthy bone marrow or blood stem cells from a donor are infused intravenously into the recipient, who has been suitably 'conditioned'. The conditioning treatment (chemotherapy with or without radiotherapy) is 'myeloablative' or, increasingly, 'non-myeloablative'. Myeloablative conditioning destroys malignant cells and immunosuppresses the recipient, as well as ablating the recipient's haematopoietic tissues. Reduced intensity conditioning (non-myeloablative) relies on intense immunosuppression to

provide 'immunological space' for transplanted stem cells. The infused donor cells 'home' to the marrow, engraft and produce enough erythrocytes, granulocytes and platelets for the patient's needs after about 2–4 weeks. During this period of aplasia, patients are at risk of infection and bleeding, and require intensive supportive care as described on page 966. It may take several years to regain normal immunological function and patients remain at risk from opportunistic infections, particularly in the first year.

An advantage of receiving allogeneic donor stem cells is that the donor's immune system can recognise residual recipient malignant cells and destroy them. This immunological 'graft-versus-disease' effect is a powerful tool against many haematological tumours and can be boosted post-transplantation by the infusion of T cells taken from the donor: so-called donor lymphocyte infusion (DLI).

Considerable morbidity and mortality are associated with HSCT. The best results are obtained in younger patients (<40 years) with minimal residual disease, who have an HLA-identical sibling donor. However, reduced-intensity conditioning (RIC) has enabled treatment of older or less fit patients, in whom the majority of haematological malignancies occur. In this form of transplantation, rather than using very intensive myeloablative conditioning, which causes morbidity from organ damage, relatively low doses of chemotherapy drugs, such as fludarabine and cyclophosphamide or busulfan, are used in combination with antibodies such as alemtuzumab (which targets CD52 on mature lymphoid cells) or anti-thymocyte globulin (ATG) to immunosuppress the recipient and allow donor stem cells to engraft. The emerging donor immune system then eliminates malignant cells via the 'graft-versus-disease' effect, which may be boosted by the elective use of donor T-cell infusions post-transplant. Such transplants have produced long-term remissions in some patients with acute leukaemia and myelodysplastic syndromes aged 40–70 years, who would not previously have been considered for a myeloablative allograft.

Complications

These are outlined in Boxes 25.23 and 25.24. The risks and outcomes of transplantation depend upon several patient- and disease-related factors. In general, 25% die from procedure-related complications, such as infection and GVHD, and there remains a significant risk of the haematological malignancy relapsing. The long-term survival for patients undergoing allogeneic HSCT in acute leukaemia is around 50%.

Graft-versus-host disease

GVHD is caused by the cytotoxic activity of donor T lymphocytes that become sensitised to their new host, regarding it as foreign. This may cause either an acute or a chronic form of GVHD.

Acute GVHD occurs in the first 100 days after transplant in about one-third of patients. It can affect the skin, causing rashes, the liver, causing jaundice, and the gut, causing diarrhoea, and may vary from mild to lethal. Prevention includes HLA-matching of the donor, immunosuppressant drugs, including methotrexate, ciclosporin, alemtuzumab or ATG. Severe presentations are very difficult to control and, despite high-dose glucocorticoids, may result in death.

Chronic GVHD may follow acute GVHD or arise independently; it occurs later than acute GVHD. It often resembles a connective tissue disorder, although in mild cases a rash may be the only manifestation. Chronic GVHD is usually treated with glucocorticoids and prolonged immunosuppression with, for example, ciclosporin. Chronic GVHD results in an increased infection risk. However, associated with chronic GVHD is the 'graft-versus-disease' effect and a lower relapse rate of the underlying malignancy.

Autologous HSCT

This procedure can also be used in haematological malignancies. The patient's stem cells from blood or marrow are first harvested and frozen when their disease is in remission. After conditioning myeloablative therapy, the autologous stem cells are reinfused into the blood stream in order to rescue the patient from the marrow damage and aplasia caused by chemotherapy. This is an effective way of safely delivering high-dose chemotherapy to chemosensitive cancers. Autologous

25.21 Examples of commonly used cytotoxic chemotherapy drugs in haematology*

Alkylating agents (cross-link double-stranded DNA by adding an alkyl group)

- Cyclophosphamide
- Melphalan
- Chlorambucil

Anthracyclines (intercalate between base pairs in the DNA molecule)

- Daunorubicin
- Doxorubicin
- Idarubicin

Antimetabolites (inhibit DNA and RNA synthesis)

- Cytosine arabinoside
- Fludarabine
- Methotrexate

Vinca alkaloids (cause disruption of tubulin)

- Vincristine
- Vinblastine

Topoisomerase II inhibitors (prevent DNA repair)

- Etoposide
- Daunorubicin
- Mitoxantrone

Monoclonal antibodies

Naked antibodies engaging antibody-dependent cytotoxic T cell or complement
Anti-CD20

- Rituximab,
- Obinotuzumab

Anti-CD19

- Blinatumumab – bi-specific T-cell engager (BITE)

Antibody-delivered cytotoxicity (ADC or 'payload antibodies')
Anti-CD33 linked to calicheamicin

- Gemtuzumab ozogomicin

Anti-CD22 linked to calicheamicin

- Inotuzumab ozogamicin

Anti-CD30 linked to monomethyl auristatin E

- Brentuximab vedotin

Targeted small molecules

Inhibitors of tyrosine kinases (TKIs)
- Imatinib, dasatinib, nilotinib, ponatinib and bosutinib in CML
- Midostaurin and gilteritinib in *FLT-3*-positive AML

Inhibitors of B-cell signalling in lymphoid malignancies
- Inhibitors of Bruton's tyrosine kinase in CLL, ibrutinib and acalabrutinib
- Inhibitors of PI3 kinase in CLL and follicular lymphoma, idelalisib

*For sites of action of these agents in the cell cycle, see Fig. 7.2.
(AML = acute myeloid leukaemia; CD = cluster of differentiation; CLL = chronic lymphocytic leukaemia; CML = chronic myeloid leukaemia; FLT-3 = FMS-like tyrosine kinase 3; PI3 = phosphatidylinositol-3)

25.22 Indications for allogeneic haematopoietic stem cell transplantation

- Neoplastic disorders affecting stem cell compartments (e.g. leukaemias, MDSs)
- Failure of haematopoiesis (e.g. aplastic anaemia)
- Major inherited defects in blood cell production (e.g. thalassaemia, immunodeficiency diseases)
- Inborn errors of metabolism with missing enzymes or cell lines

(MDSs = myelodysplastic syndromes)

25.23 Complications of allogeneic haematopoietic stem cell transplantation

Early

- Anaemia
- Infections
- Bleeding
- Acute GVHD
- Mucositis – pain, nausea, diarrhoea
- Liver veno-occlusive disease

Late

- Chronic GVHD
- Infertility
- Cataracts
- Second malignancy

(GVHD = graft-versus-host disease)

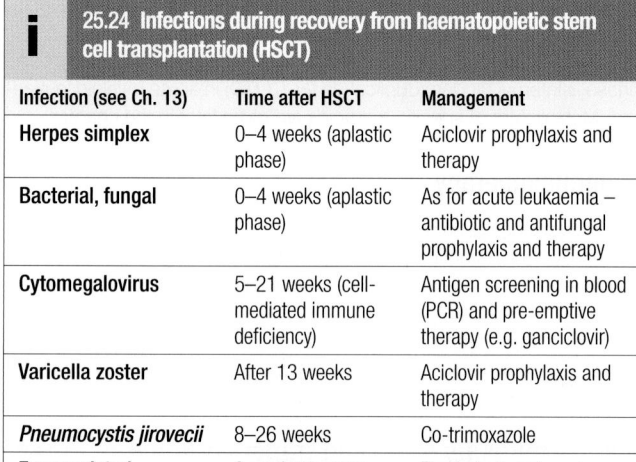

25.24 Infections during recovery from haematopoietic stem cell transplantation (HSCT)

Infection (see Ch. 13)	Time after HSCT	Management
Herpes simplex	0–4 weeks (aplastic phase)	Aciclovir prophylaxis and therapy
Bacterial, fungal	0–4 weeks (aplastic phase)	As for acute leukaemia – antibiotic and antifungal prophylaxis and therapy
Cytomegalovirus	5–21 weeks (cell-mediated immune deficiency)	Antigen screening in blood (PCR) and pre-emptive therapy (e.g. ganciclovir)
Varicella zoster	After 13 weeks	Aciclovir prophylaxis and therapy
Pneumocystis jirovecii	8–26 weeks	Co-trimoxazole
Encapsulated bacteria	8 weeks to years (immunoglobulin deficiency, prolonged with GVHD)	Prophylaxis and revaccination

(GVHD = graft-versus-host disease; PCR = polymerase chain reaction)

HSCT may be used as consolidation chemotherapy for disorders that do not primarily involve the haematopoietic tissues, or for patients in whom very good remissions have been achieved. The most common indications are lymphomas and myeloma. The preferred source of stem cells for autologous transplants is peripheral blood (PBSCT). These stem cells engraft more quickly, marrow recovery occurring within 2–3 weeks. There is no risk of GVHD and no immunosuppression is required. Thus autologous HSCT carries a lower procedure-related mortality rate than allogeneic HSCT at aroun 1%–5%, but there is a higher rate of recurrence of malignancy because the anti-malignancy effect is solely dependent on the conditioning chemotherapy with no 'graft-versus-disease' effect. There is ongoing interest in using autologous HSCT to treat severe autoimmune diseases. The theory is that the patient's immune system is 'reset' to not attack host tissues. Early success in multiple sclerosis has led to current randomised controlled trials in this area.

Alternative cellular therapies

While HSCT remains a major cellular therapy for a range of malignant and some non-malignant haematological conditions, newer cell-based treatments have been recently introduced into practice. These include donor T cells primed to respond to specific viruses, including cytomegalovirus (CMV) and Epstein–Barr Virus (EBV). Immunocompromised patients, such as those post solid organ or haematopoietic transplantation, can suffer from reactivation of latent CMV or EBV infection and develop life-threatening complications, e.g. pneumonitis (CMV) and post-transplant lymphoproliferative disease (EBV). Primed donor T cells can be used to treat these

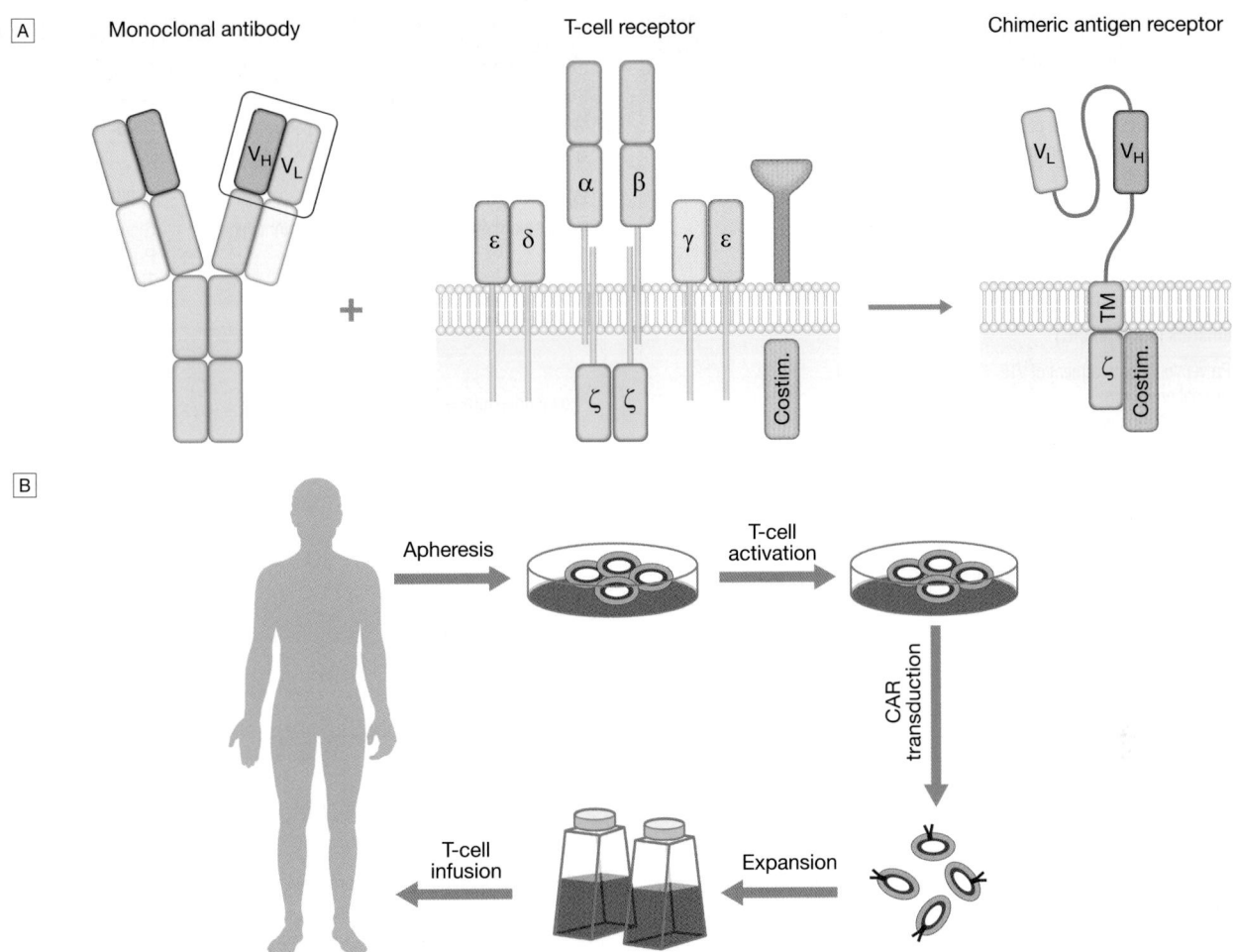

Fig. 25.17 The manufacturing process for CAR-T cells. [A] The chimeric antigen receptor (CAR) is genetically engineered by combining the extracellular antigen receptor binding domain from a monoclonal antibody (V_H and V_L are the heavy and light chain variable regions) with the intracellular activation domain from a T-cell receptor (ζ) and a costimulatory subunit (Costim.); they are linked by a transmembrane (TM) component. During the process the extracellular domain of the T-cell receptor is cleaved and removed ($\alpha-\epsilon$). The new CAR uses the monoclonal antibody binding domain, e.g. anti-CD19, to bind to the target CD19 on the lymphoma cell surface and this can now activate the T-cell effector killing mechanisms via the activation domain, allowing the CAR-T cell to kill the lymphoma cell. [B] The CAR-T cells are manufactured by transducing the new gene for CAR into the patient's T cells. T cells are harvested from the patient by apheresis and then genetically altered in a laboratory process that takes about 4 weeks. The manufactured CAR-T cells are expanded in numbers during this time in tissue culture before being reinfused into the patient. *(Modified from Fesnak A O'Doherty U. Clinical development and manufacture of chimeric antigen receptor T cells and the role of leukapheresis. Eur Oncol Haematol 2017; 13(1):28–34 and Majzner RG, Mackall CL. Clinical lessons learned from the first leg of the CAR T cell journey. Nat Med 2019; 25:1341–1355 with permission.)*

conditions, especially when alternative approaches such as reduction in immunosuppression or anti-viral drugs have failed.

Another exciting new cellular therapy, called chimeric antigen receptor T-cell (CAR-T) therapy, has been developed for patients with some B-cell malignancies where alternative treatments have failed. This technology is based on genetic engineering where a patient's own T cells are harvested and have a new chimeric receptor gene introduced into the cell. This produces a cell surface receptor that uses the antigen binding domain of an antibody molecule to recognise a target on the malignant B cell (CD19) coupled to a T-cell receptor-activating domain (Fig. 25.17). This chimeric B/T receptor can effectively bind to the malignant B cell and activate the T cell to kill it. This treatment is licensed and available for children and young adults with relapsed acute lymphoblastic leukaemia and patients with multiply relapsed diffuse large B-cell lymphoma. This novel therapy has cured some patients who were in a desparate situation, with some data suggesting 60%–70% alive after one year.

Anticoagulant and antithrombotic therapy

There are numerous indications for anticoagulant and antithrombotic medications (Box 25.25). The guiding principles are outlined here, but management in specific indications is discussed elsewhere in the book. Broadly speaking, antiplatelet medications are of greater efficacy in the

prevention of arterial thrombosis and of less value in the prevention of venous thromboembolism (VTE). Thus, antiplatelet agents, such as aspirin, clopidogrel and, increasingly, ticagrelor, are the drugs of choice in acute coronary events (Ch. 16) and in ischaemic cerebrovascular disease, while warfarin and other anticoagulants are favoured in VTE (p. 985) and management of atrial fibrillation (Ch. 16). In some extremely prothrombotic situations, such as coronary artery stenting, a combination of anticoagulant and antiplatelet drugs is used.

A wide range of anticoagulant and antithrombotic drugs is used in clinical practice. These drugs and their modes of action are given in Box 25.26 and Fig. 25.18. Newer agents allow predictable anticoagulation without the need for frequent monitoring and dose titration. Although warfarin remains an option for oral anticoagulation, newer oral anticoagulants (dabigatran, rivaroxaban, edoxaban and apixaban), which can be given at fixed doses with predictable effects and no need for monitoring, have now been approved for the prevention of perioperative VTE, the treatment of established VTE and the prevention of cardioembolic stroke in patients with atrial fibrillation.

Heparins

Unfractionated heparin (UFH) and low-molecular-weight heparins (LMWHs) act as anticoagulants by binding a specific pentasaccharide

i | **25.25 Indications for anticoagulation**

Heparin/LMWH/fondaparinux

- Prevention and treatment of VTE
- Percutaneous coronary intervention
- Post-thrombolysis for MI
- Unstable angina pectoris
- Non-Q wave MI
- Acute peripheral arterial occlusion
- Cardiopulmonary bypass
- Haemodialysis and haemofiltration

Coumarins (warfarin etc.)

- Prevention and treatment of VTE
- Arterial embolism
- Atrial fibrillation with specific risk factors for stroke (p. 414)
- Mobile mural thrombus post-MI
- Extensive anterior MI   Therapeutic INR 2.5
- Dilated cardiomyopathy
- Cardioversion
- Ischaemic stroke in antiphospholipid syndrome
- Mitral stenosis and mitral regurgitation with atrial fibrillation

- Recurrent venous thrombosis while on warfarin   INR 3.5
- Mechanical prosthetic cardiac valves}

Rivaroxaban

- Prevention and treatment of VTE
- Atrial fibrillation with risk factors for stroke
- Post acute coronary syndrome
- Symptomatic coronary artery disease and peripheral vascular disease

Dabigatran etexilate

- Prevention and treatment of VTE
- Atrial fibrillation with risk factors for stroke

Apixaban

- Prevention and treatment of VTE
- Atrial fibrillation with risk factors for stroke

Edoxaban

- Treatment of VTE
- Atrial fibrillation with risk factors for stroke

(INR = international normalised ratio; LMWH = low-molecular-weight heparin; MI = myocardial infarction; VTE = venous thromboembolism)

i | **25.26 Modes of action of anticoagulant and antithrombotic drugs**

Mode of action	Drug
Antiplatelet drugs	
Cyclo-oxygenase (COX) inhibition	Aspirin
Adenosine diphosphate (ADP) receptor inhibition	Clopidogrel Prasugrel Ticagrelor
Glycoprotein IIb/IIIa inhibition	Abciximab Tirofiban Eptifibatide
Phosphodiesterase inhibition	Dipyridamole
Oral anticoagulants	
Vitamin K antagonism	Warfarin/coumarins
Direct thrombin inhibition	Dabigatran
Direct Xa inhibition	Rivaroxaban Apixaban Edoxaban
Injectable anticoagulants	
Antithrombin-dependent inhibition of thrombin and Xa	Heparin LMWH
Antithrombin-dependent inhibition of Xa	Fondaparinux Danaparoid
Direct thrombin inhibition	Argatroban Bivalirudin

UFH is, however, more completely reversed by protamine sulphate in the event of bleeding and at the end of cardiopulmonary bypass, for which UFH remains the drug of choice (Box 25.27).

LMWHs are widely used for the prevention and treatment of VTE, the management of acute coronary syndromes and for most other scenarios listed in Box 25.25. In some situations, UFH is still favoured by some clinicians, though there is little evidence that it is advantageous, except when rapid reversibility is required. UFH is useful in patients with a high risk of bleeding, e.g. those who have peptic ulceration or who may require urgent surgery. It is also favoured in the treatment of life-threatening thromboembolism, e.g. major pulmonary embolism with significant hypoxaemia, hypotension and right-sided heart strain. In this situation, UFH is started with a loading intravenous dose of 80U/kg, followed by a continuous infusion of 18U/kg/hr initially. The level of anticoagulation should be assessed by the APTT after 6 hours and, if satisfactory, twice daily thereafter. It is usual to aim for a patient APTT that is 1.5–2.5 times the control time of the test. Monitoring of UFH treatment by APTT is not without difficulties and other assays, such as the specific anti-Xa assay calibrated for measurement of UFH, provides more accurate guidance.

Heparin-induced thrombocytopenia

Heparin-induced thrombocytopenia (HIT) is a rare complication of heparin therapy, caused by induction of anti-heparin/PF4 antibodies that bind to and activate platelets via an Fc receptor. This results in platelet activation and a prothrombotic state, with a paradoxical thrombocytopenia. HIT is more common in surgical than medical patients (especially cardiac and orthopaedic patients), with use of UFH rather than LMWH, and with higher doses of heparin. Some adenovirus vector-based SARS-CoV-2 RNA vaccines have been associated with a similar condition characterised by venous thrombosis (often cerebral) and paradoxical thrombocytopenia.

Clinical features

Patients present, typically 5–14 days after starting heparin treatment, with a fall in platelet count of more than 30% from baseline. The count may still be in the reference range. The patient may be asymptomatic, or develop venous or arterial thrombosis and skin lesions, including overt skin

sequence to antithrombin. This enhances the avidity of anti-thrombin for its substrates, which are the activated proteases of the coagulation pathway such as Xa and thrombin (see Fig. 25.6E and Fig. 25.18). Fondaparinux is a synthetic pentasaccharide, which also binds antithrombin and has similar properties to LMWH. LMWHs preferentially augment antithrombin activity against factor Xa. For the licensed indications, LMWHs are at least as efficacious as UFH, but have several advantages:

- LMWHs are nearly 100% bioavailable and so produce reliable dose-dependent anticoagulation.
- LMWHs do not require monitoring of their anticoagulant effect (except possibly in patients with very low body weight and with a glomerular filtration rate below 30mL/min).
- LMWHs have a half-life of around 4 hours when given subcutaneously, compared with 1 hour for UFH. This permits once-daily dosing by the subcutaneous route, rather than the therapeutic continuous intravenous infusion or twice-daily subcutaneous administration required for UFH.
- While rates of bleeding are similar between products, the risk of osteoporosis and heparin-induced thrombocytopenia is much lower for LMWH.

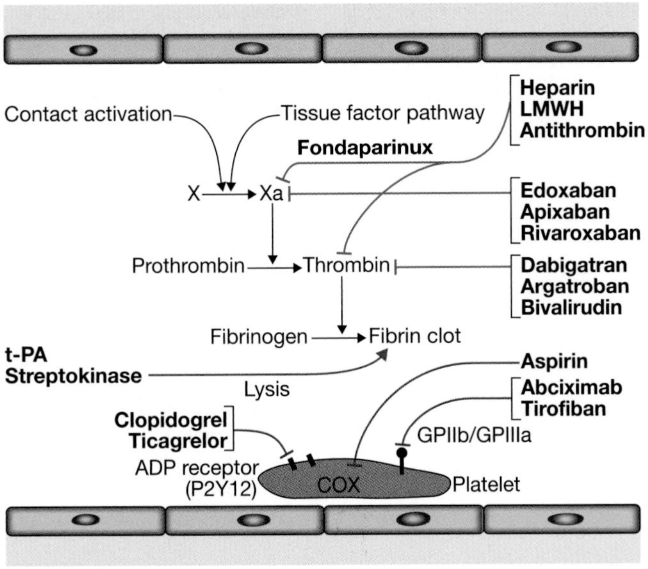

Fig. 25.18 Sites of action of antithrombotic and fibrinolytic medicines. Heparin and low molecular weight heparin (LMWH) enhance the avidity of antithrombin for Factor Xa and thrombin (Factor IIa). Fondaparinux also binds antithrombin, but only inhibits Factor Xa. The direct oral anticoagulants (DOACs) rivaroxaban, apixaban, edoxaban and dabigatran directly inhibit specific proteases in the common pathway. Glycoprotein (GP) IIb/IIIa is a receptor for fibrinogen and von Willebrand factor and aids platelet activation and aggregation. P2Y12 is the receptor for adenosine diphosphate (ADP) and its activation also triggers platelet aggregation. Aspirin is an inhibitor of cyclo-oxygenase (COX) in platelets. (t-PA = tissue plasminogen activator)

25.27 Treatments for emergencies in haematological practice

- Reversal of life- and limb-threatening haemorrhage in anticoagulated patients:
  Warfarin: prothrombin complex concentrate and IV vitamin K$_1$
  Unfractionated heparin: protamine sulphate
  Dabigatran: idarucizumab
  Rivaroxaban and apixaban: andexanet alfa
- Recognition of thrombotic thrombocytopenic purpura and treatment with plasma exchange
- Recognition of coagulopathy associated with acute promyelocytic leukaemia and treatment with all-trans-retinoic acid and fibrinogen replacement
- Recognition of chest syndrome and stroke in patients with sickle-cell anaemia and red cell transfusion or exchange transfusion
- Recognition of neutropenic sepsis in patients receiving chemotherapy and early treatment with empirical broad-spectrum antibiotics

(IV = intravenous)

---

necrosis. Affected patients may complain of pain or itch at injection sites and of systemic symptoms, such as shivering, following heparin injections. Patients who have received heparin in the preceding 100 days and who have preformed antibodies may develop acute systemic symptoms and an abrupt fall in platelet count in the first 24 hours after re-exposure.

Investigations

The pre-test probability of the diagnosis is assessed using the 4Ts scoring system. This assigns a score based on:

- the **T**hrombocytopenia
- the **T**iming of the fall in platelet count
- the presence of new **T**hrombosis
- the likelihood of ano**T**her cause for the thrombocytopenia.

Individuals at low risk need no further test. Those with intermediate and high likelihood scores should have the diagnosis confirmed or refuted using an anti-PF4 enzyme-linked immunosorbent assay (ELISA).

Management

Heparin should be discontinued as soon as HIT is diagnosed and an alternative anticoagulant that does not cross-react with the antibody should be substituted. Argatroban (a direct thrombin inhibitor) and danaparoid

(a heparin analogue) are licensed for use in the UK. Fonaparinux is not licensed for this indication but can also be used. In asymptomatic patients with HIT who do not receive an alternative anticoagulant, around 50% will sustain a thrombosis in the subsequent 30 days. Patients with established thrombosis have a poorer prognosis.

Coumarins

Although several coumarin anticoagulants are used around the world, warfarin is the most common.

Coumarins inhibit the vitamin K-dependent post-translational carboxylation of factors II (prothrombin), VII, IX and X in the liver (see Fig. 25.6D). This results in anticoagulation due to an effective deficiency of these factors. This is monitored by the INR, a standardised test based on measurement of the prothrombin time (see Box 25.3). Recommended target INR values for specific indications are given in Box 25.25.

Warfarin anticoagulation typically takes more than 3–5 days to become established, even using loading doses. Patients who require rapid initiation of therapy may receive higher initiation doses of warfarin. A typical regimen in this situation is to give 10 mg warfarin on the first and second days, with 5 mg on the third day; subsequent doses are titrated against the INR. Patients without an urgent need for anticoagulation (e.g. atrial fibrillation) can have warfarin introduced slowly using lower doses. Low-dose regimens are associated with a lower risk of the patient developing a supratherapeutic INR, and hence a lower bleeding risk. The duration of warfarin therapy depends on the clinical indication and while treatment of deep vein thrombosis (DVT) or preparation for cardioversion may require a finite duration, anticoagulation to prevent cardioembolic stroke in atrial fibrillation or from heart valve disease is long-term.

The major problems with warfarin are:

- a narrow therapeutic window
- metabolism that is affected by many factors
- numerous drug interactions.

Drug interactions are common through protein binding and metabolism by the cytochrome P450 system. Inter-individual differences in warfarin doses required to achieve a therapeutic INR are mostly accounted for by naturally occurring polymorphisms in the *CYP2C9* and the *VKORC1* genes (which predict the metabolism and function of warfarin, respectively) and dietary intake of vitamin K.

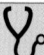

25.28 How to assess risks of anticoagulation

Contraindications

- Recent surgery, especially to eye or central nervous system
- Pre-existing haemorrhagic state, e.g. advanced liver disease, haemophilia, thrombocytopenia
- Pre-existing structural lesions, e.g. peptic ulcer
- Recent cerebral or gastrointestinal haemorrhage
- Uncontrolled hypertension
- Cognitive impairment
- Frequent falls

Bleeding risk score

- Several bleeding risk scores exist for different indications for anticoagulation
- The validation of most bleeding risk scores has been poor
- Many risk factors for thrombosis are also risk factors for bleeding
- HAS BLED is the best validated score for patients with atrial fibrillation. Following anticoagulant-related bleeding, reassessment of bleeding and thrombosis risk is indicated
- In many cases, patients benefit from recommencing anticoagulants after bleeding

Major bleeding is the most common serious side-effect of warfarin and occurs in 1%–2% of patients each year. Fatal haemorrhage, which is most commonly intracranial, occurs in about 0.25% per annum. There are scoring systems that predict the annual bleeding risk and these can be used to help compare the risks and benefits of warfarin for an individual patient (Box 25.28). There are also some specific contraindications to anticoagulation (Box 25.28). Management of warfarin includes strategies for over-anticoagulation and for bleeding:

- If the INR is above the therapeutic level, warfarin should be withheld or the dose reduced. If the patient is not bleeding, it may be appropriate to give a small dose of vitamin K either orally or intravenously (1–2.5 mg), especially if the INR is greater than 8.
- In the event of bleeding, withhold further warfarin. Minor bleeding can be treated with 1–2.5 mg of vitamin K intravenously (IV). Major haemorrhage should be treated as an emergency with vitamin K 5–10 mg slowly IV, combined with coagulation factor replacement (see Box 25.27). This should optimally be a prothrombin complex concentrate (30–50 U/kg) that contains factors II, VII, IX and X; if that is not available, fresh frozen plasma (15–30 mL/kg) should be given.

Direct oral anticoagulants

The direct oral anticoagulants (DOACs) are specific inhibitors of key proteases in the common pathway and offer an alternative to coumarins in the management of VTE and the prevention of stroke and systemic embolism in patients with atrial fibrillation. Dabigatran inhibits thrombin while rivaroxaban, apixaban and edoxaban inhibit Xa (see Fig. 25.18). The key features of these drugs include the fact that they are efficacious in fixed oral doses, have a short half-life of around 10 hours, achieve peak plasma levels 2–4 hours after oral intake, have very few drug interactions and are all moderately dependent on renal function for their excretion. An initial perceived drawback was the lack of specific reversal agents for these drugs, but the monoclonal antibody idarucizumab is now available for the reversal of dabigatran and andexanet alfa, a site-inactivated Xa molecule, has recently been licensed for the reversal of apixaban and rivaroxaban (see Box 25.27).

DOACs are now licensed for the prevention of VTE following high-risk orthopaedic surgery (except edoxaban), the acute management and prevention of recurrence of VTE and the prevention of stroke and systemic embolism in patients with atrial fibrillation with risk factors. Dosing is standard across a range of conditions, but is affected by extremes (low and high) of body weight and impaired renal function. The general perception is that in these indications they are at least as efficacious as dose-adjusted coumarin and probably associated with less clinically significant bleeding.

Anaemias

Around 30% of the total world population is anaemic and half of these, some 600 million people, have iron deficiency. The classification of anaemia by the size of the red cells (MCV) indicates the likely cause (see Figs. 25.10 and 25.11).

Red cells in the bone marrow must acquire a minimum level of haemoglobin before being released into the blood stream (Fig. 25.19). While in the marrow compartment, red cell precursors undergo cell division driven by erythropoietin. If red cells cannot acquire haemoglobin at a normal rate, they will undergo more divisions than normal and will have a low MCV when released into the blood. The MCV is low because component parts of the haemoglobin molecule are not fully available: that is, iron in iron deficiency, globin chains in thalassaemia, haem ring in congenital sideroblastic anaemia and, occasionally, poor iron utilisation in the anaemia of chronic disease/anaemia of inflammation.

In megaloblastic anaemia, the biochemical consequence of vitamin B_{12} or folate deficiency is an inability to synthesise new bases to make DNA. A similar defect of cell division is seen in the presence of cytotoxic drugs or haematological disease in the marrow, such as myelodysplasia. In these states, cells haemoglobinise normally, but undergo fewer cell divisions, resulting in circulating red cells with a raised MCV. The red cell membrane is composed of a lipid bilayer that will freely exchange with the plasma pool of lipid. Conditions such as liver disease, hypothyroidism, hyperlipidaemia and pregnancy are associated with raised lipids and may also cause a raised MCV. Reticulocytes are larger than mature red cells, so when the reticulocyte count is raised – e.g. in haemolysis – this may also increase the MCV.

Iron deficiency anaemia

This occurs when iron losses or physiological requirements exceed absorption.

Blood loss

The most common explanation in men and post-menopausal women is gastrointestinal blood loss (Ch. 23). This may result from occult gastric or colorectal malignancy, gastritis, peptic ulceration, inflammatory bowel disease, diverticulitis, polyps and angiodysplastic lesions. Worldwide, hookworm and schistosomiasis are the most common causes of gut blood loss (Ch. 13). Gastrointestinal blood loss may be exacerbated by the chronic use of aspirin or non-steroidal anti-inflammatory drugs (NSAIDs), which cause intestinal erosions and impair platelet function. In women of child-bearing age, menstrual blood loss, pregnancy and breastfeeding contribute to iron deficiency by depleting iron stores; in developed countries, one-third of pre-menopausal women have low iron stores, but only 3% display iron-deficient haematopoiesis. Very rarely, chronic haemoptysis or haematuria may cause iron deficiency.

Malabsorption

A dietary assessment should be made in all patients to ascertain their iron intake (Ch. 22). Gastric acid is required to release iron from food and helps to keep iron in the soluble ferrous state (Fig. 25.20). Achlorhydria in older people or that due to drugs such as proton pump inhibitors may contribute to the lack of iron availability from the diet, as may previous gastric surgery. Iron is absorbed actively in the upper small intestine and hence can be affected by coeliac disease (p. 819).

Physiological demands

At times of rapid growth, such as infancy and puberty, iron requirements increase and may outstrip absorption. In pregnancy, iron is diverted to the fetus, the placenta and the increased maternal red cell mass, and is lost with bleeding at parturition (Box 25.29).

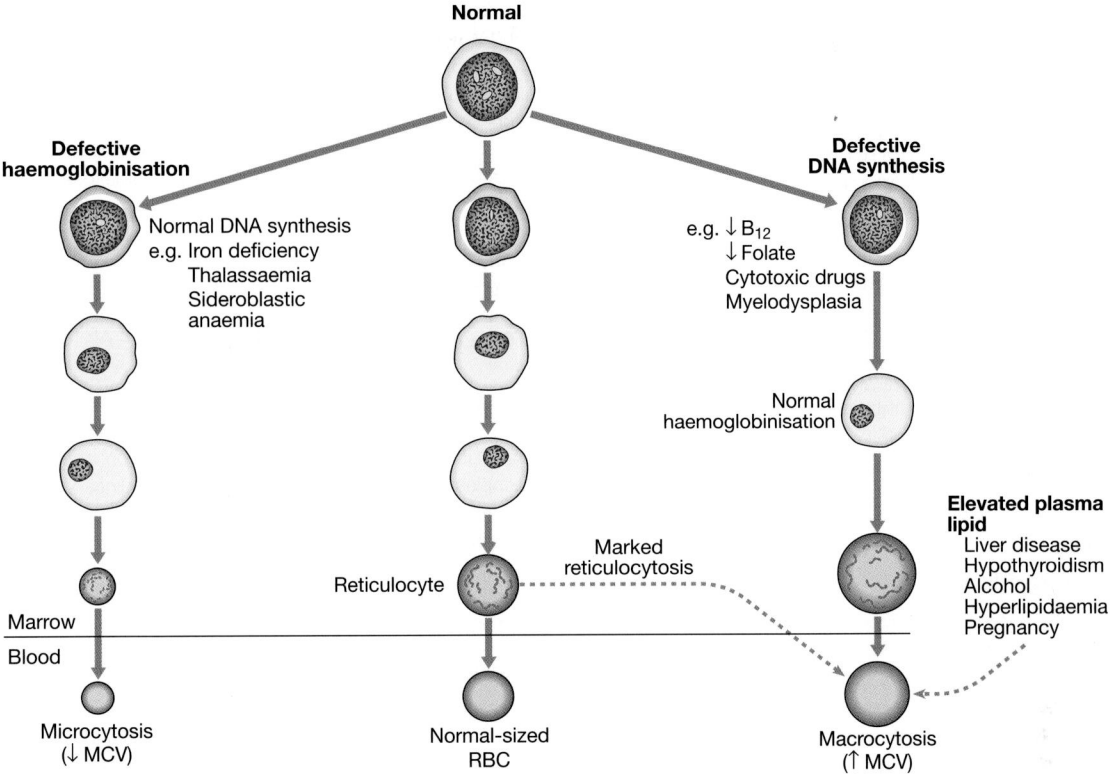

Fig. 25.19 Factors that influence the size of red cells in anaemia. In microcytosis, the MCV is <76 fL. In macrocytosis, the MCV is >100 fL. (MCV = mean cell volume; RBC = red blood cell)

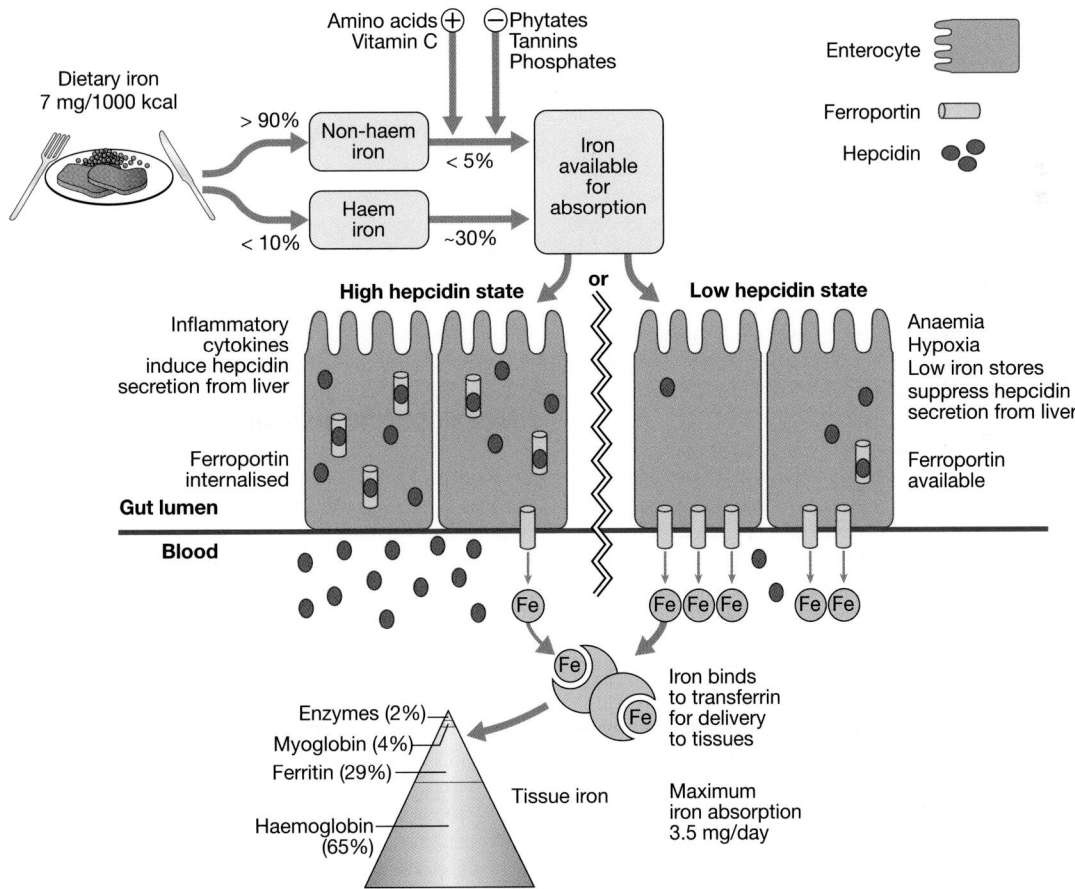

Fig. 25.20 The regulation of iron absorption, uptake and distribution in the body. The transport of iron is regulated in a similar fashion to enterocytes in other iron-transporting cells such as macrophages.

25.29 Haematological physiology in pregnancy

- **Full blood count**: increased plasma volume (40%) lowers normal haemoglobin (reference range reduced to > 105 g/L at 28 weeks). The mean cell volume (MCV) may increase by 5 fL. A progressive neutrophilia occurs. Gestational thrombocytopenia (rarely <60 × 10⁹/L) is a benign phenomenon.
- **Depletion of iron stores**: iron deficiency is a common cause of anaemia in pregnancy and, if present, should be treated with oral iron supplement.
- **Vitamin B₁₂**: serum levels are physiologically low in pregnancy but deficiency is uncommon.
- **Folate**: tissue stores may become depleted, and folate supplementation is recommended in all pregnancies (see Box 22.29).
- **Coagulation factors**: from the second trimester, procoagulant factors increase approximately threefold, particularly fibrinogen, von Willebrand factor and factor VIII. This causes activated protein C resistance and a shortened activated partial thromboplastin time (APTT), and contributes to a prothrombotic state.
- **Anticoagulants**: levels of protein C increase from the second trimester, while levels of free protein S fall as C4b binding protein increases.

Investigations

Confirmation of iron deficiency

Serum ferritin is a measure of iron stores in tissues and is the best single test to confirm iron deficiency (Box 25.30). A subnormal level is most often due to iron deficiency or, very rarely, hypothyroidism or vitamin C deficiency. Ferritin levels can be raised in liver disease and in the acute phase response; in these conditions, a ferritin level of up to 100 μg/L may still be compatible with low bone marrow iron stores.

Plasma iron and total iron binding capacity (TIBC) are measures of iron availability; hence they are affected by many factors besides iron stores. Plasma iron has a marked diurnal and day-to-day variation and becomes very low during an acute phase response, but is raised in liver disease and haemolysis. Levels of transferrin, the binding protein for iron, are lowered by malnutrition, liver disease, the acute phase response and nephrotic syndrome, but raised by pregnancy and the oral contraceptive pill. A transferrin saturation (i.e. iron/TIBC×100) of less than 16% is consistent with iron deficiency, but is less specific than a low ferritin measurement.

All proliferating cells express membrane transferrin receptors to acquire iron; a small amount of this receptor is shed into blood, where it can be detected in a free soluble form. When iron stores are low, cells up-regulate transferrin receptor expression and the levels of soluble plasma transferrin receptor increase. This can be measured by immunoassay and used to distinguish storage iron depletion in the presence of an acute phase response or liver disease, when a raised level indicates iron deficiency. In difficult cases, it may still be necessary to examine a bone marrow aspirate for iron stores.

Investigation of the cause

This will depend on the age and sex of the patient, as well as the history and clinical findings. In men and in post-menopausal women with a normal diet, the upper and lower gastrointestinal tract should be investigated by endoscopy or radiological studies. Current guidelines suggest exclusion of coeliac disease by antibody testing at an early stage of investigation of iron deficiency. In the tropics, stool and urine should be examined for parasites (Box 13.19).

Management

Unless the patient has angina, heart failure or evidence of cerebral hypoxia, transfusion is not indicated and oral iron replacement is appropriate. Ferrous sulphate 200 mg 3 times daily (195 mg of elemental iron per day) is adequate and should be continued for 3–6 months to replete iron stores. Many patients suffer gastrointestinal side-effects with ferrous sulphate, including dyspepsia and altered bowel habit. When this occurs, reduction in dose or another alternative oral preparation should be tried. Delayed-release preparations are not useful, since they release iron beyond the upper small intestine, where it cannot be absorbed.

The haemoglobin should rise by around 10 g/L every 7–10 days and a reticulocyte response will be evident within a week. A failure to respond adequately may be due to non-adherence, continued blood loss, malabsorption or an incorrect diagnosis. Patients with malabsorption, chronic gut disease or inability to tolerate any oral preparation may need parenteral iron therapy. Previously, iron dextran or iron sucrose was used, but new preparations of ferric isomaltose and ferric carboxymaltose have fewer allergic effects and are preferred. Doses required can be calculated based on the patient's starting haemoglobin and body weight. Observation for anaphylaxis following an initial test dose is recommended.

Anaemia of chronic disease

Anaemia of chronic disease (ACD), also known as anaemia of inflammation (AI), is a common type of anaemia, particularly in hospital populations. It occurs in the setting of chronic infection, chronic inflammation or neoplasia. The anaemia is not related to bleeding, haemolysis or marrow infiltration, is mild, with haemoglobin in the range of 85–115 g/L, and is usually associated with a normal MCV (normocytic, normochromic), though this may be reduced in long-standing inflammation. The serum iron is low, but iron stores are normal or increased, as indicated by the ferritin or stainable marrow iron.

Pathogenesis

It has become clear that the key regulatory protein that accounts for the findings characteristic of ACD/AI is hepcidin, which is produced by the liver (see Fig. 25.20). Hepcidin production is induced by pro-inflammatory cytokines, especially IL-6. Hepcidin binds to ferroportin on the membrane of iron-exporting cells, such as small intestinal enterocytes and macrophages, internalising the ferroportin and thereby inhibiting the export of iron from these cells into the blood. The iron remains trapped inside the cells in the form of ferritin, levels of which are therefore normal or high in the face of significant anaemia. Inhibition or blockade of hepcidin is a potential target for treatment of this form of anaemia.

Diagnosis and management

It is often difficult to distinguish ACD associated with a low MCV from iron deficiency. Box 25.30 summarises the investigations and results. Examination of the marrow may ultimately be required to assess iron stores directly. A trial of oral iron can be given in difficult situations. A positive response occurs in true iron deficiency, but not in ACD. Measures that reduce the severity of the underlying disorder generally help to improve the ACD. Trials of higher-dose intravenous iron are under way to try to bypass the hepcidin-induced blockade.

Megaloblastic anaemia

This results from a deficiency of vitamin B₁₂ or folic acid, or from disturbances in folic acid metabolism. Folate is an important substrate of, and vitamin B₁₂ a co-factor for, the generation of the essential amino acid methionine from homocysteine. This reaction produces tetrahydrofolate, which is converted to thymidine monophosphate for incorporation into DNA. Deficiency of either vitamin B₁₂ or folate will therefore produce high plasma levels of homocysteine and impaired DNA synthesis.

The end result is cells with arrested nuclear maturation, but normal cytoplasmic development: so-called nucleocytoplasmic asynchrony. All proliferating cells will exhibit megaloblastosis; hence changes are evident in the buccal mucosa, tongue, small intestine, cervix, vagina and uterus. The high proliferation rate of bone marrow results in striking changes in the haematopoietic system in megaloblastic anaemia. Cells become arrested in development and die within the marrow; this ineffective erythropoiesis results in an expanded hypercellular marrow. The megaloblastic changes are most evident in the early-nucleated red cell precursors and haemolysis within the marrow results in a raised bilirubin and lactate dehydrogenase (LDH), but without the reticulocytosis

i 25.30 Investigations to differentiate anaemia of chronic disease from iron deficiency anaemia

	Ferritin	Iron	TIBC	Transferrin saturation	Soluble transferrin receptor
Iron deficiency anaemia	↓	↓	↑	↓	↑
Anaemia of chronic disease	↑/Normal	↓	↓	↓	↓/Normal

(TIBC = total iron binding capacity)

i 25.31 Clinical features of megaloblastic anaemia

Symptoms

- Malaise (90%)
- Breathlessness (50%)
- Paraesthesiae (80%)
- Sore mouth (20%)
- Weight loss
- Impotence
- Poor memory
- Depression
- Personality change
- Hallucinations
- Visual disturbance

Signs

- Smooth tongue
- Angular cheilosis
- Vitiligo
- Skin pigmentation
- Heart failure
- Pyrexia

i 25.32 Investigations in megaloblastic anaemia

Investigation	Result
Haemoglobin	Often reduced, may be very low
Mean cell volume	Usually raised, commonly >120 fL
Erythrocyte count	Low for degree of anaemia
Blood film	Oval macrocytosis, poikilocytosis, red cell fragmentation, neutrophil hypersegmentation
Reticulocyte count	Low for degree of anaemia
Leucocyte count	Low or normal
Platelet count	Low or normal
Bone marrow	Increased cellularity, megaloblastic changes in erythroid series, giant metamyelocytes, dysplastic megakaryocytes, increased iron in stores, pathological non-ring sideroblasts
Serum ferritin	Elevated
Plasma lactate dehydrogenase	Elevated, often markedly

characteristic of other forms of haemolysis (see Box 25.31). Iron stores are usually raised. The mature red cells are large and oval, and sometimes contain nuclear remnants. Nuclear changes are seen in the immature granulocyte precursors and a characteristic appearance is that of 'giant' metamyelocytes with a large 'sausage-shaped' nucleus. The mature neutrophils show hypersegmentation of their nuclei, with cells having six or more nuclear lobes. If severe, a pancytopenia may be present in the peripheral blood.

Vitamin B$_{12}$ deficiency, but not folate deficiency, is associated with neurological disease in up to 40% of cases, although advanced neurological disease due to B$_{12}$ deficiency is now uncommon in the developed world. The main pathological finding is focal demyelination affecting the spinal cord, peripheral nerves, optic nerves and cerebrum. The most common manifestations are sensory, with peripheral paraesthesiae and ataxia of gait. The clinical and diagnostic features of megaloblastic anaemia are summarised in Boxes 25.31 and 25.32, and the neurological features of B$_{12}$ deficiency in Box 25.33.

Vitamin B$_{12}$

Vitamin B$_{12}$ absorption

The average daily diet contains 5–30 µg of vitamin B$_{12}$, mainly in meat, fish, eggs and milk – well in excess of the 1 µg daily requirement. In the stomach, gastric enzymes release vitamin B$_{12}$ from food and at gastric pH it binds to a carrier protein termed R protein. The gastric parietal cells produce intrinsic factor, a vitamin B$_{12}$-binding protein that optimally binds vitamin B$_{12}$ at pH 8. As gastric emptying occurs, pancreatic secretion raises the pH and vitamin B$_{12}$ released from the diet switches from the R protein to intrinsic factor. Bile also contains vitamin B$_{12}$ that is available for reabsorption in the intestine. The vitamin B$_{12}$–intrinsic factor complex binds to specific receptors in the terminal ileum, and vitamin B$_{12}$ is actively transported by the enterocytes to plasma, where it binds to transcobalamin II, a transport protein produced by the liver, which carries it to the tissues for utilisation. The liver stores enough vitamin B$_{12}$ to last for approximately 3 years and this, together with the enterohepatic circulation, means that vitamin B$_{12}$ deficiency takes years to become manifest, even if all dietary intake is stopped or severe B$_{12}$ malabsorption supervenes.

Blood levels of vitamin B$_{12}$ (cobalamin) provide a reasonable indication of tissue stores, are usually diagnostic of deficiency and remain the first-line tests for most laboratories. Additional tests have been evaluated,

i 25.33 Neurological findings in B$_{12}$ deficiency

Peripheral nerves

- Glove and stocking paraesthesiae
- Loss of ankle reflexes

Spinal cord

- Subacute combined degeneration of the cord
  Posterior columns – diminished vibration sensation and proprioception
  Corticospinal tracts – upper motor neuron signs

Cerebrum

- Dementia
- Optic atrophy
- Autonomic neuropathy

including measurement of methylmalonic acid, holotranscobalamin and plasma homocysteine levels, but do not add much in most clinical situations. Levels of cobalamins fall in normal pregnancy. Reference ranges vary between laboratories, but levels below 150 ng/L are common and, in the last trimester, 5%–10% of women have levels below 100 ng/L. Spuriously low B$_{12}$ values occur in women using the oral contraceptive pill and in patients with myeloma, in whom paraproteins can interfere with vitamin B$_{12}$ assays.

Causes of vitamin B$_{12}$ deficiency

Dietary deficiency

This occurs only in strict vegans, but the onset of clinical features can occur at any age between 10 and 80 years. Less strict vegetarians often have slightly low vitamin B$_{12}$ levels, but are not tissue vitamin B$_{12}$-deficient.

Gastric pathology

Release of vitamin B$_{12}$ from food requires normal gastric acid and enzyme secretion and this is impaired by hypochlorhydria in older patients or following gastric surgery. Total gastrectomy invariably results in vitamin B_{12} deficiency within 5 years, often combined with iron deficiency; these patients need life-long 3-monthly vitamin B_{12} injections. After partial gastrectomy, vitamin B_{12} deficiency only develops in 10%–20% of patients by 5 years; an annual injection of vitamin B_{12} should prevent deficiency in this group. Patients may develop B_{12} deficiency after certain types of bariatric surgery (see Ch. 22).

Pernicious anaemia

This is an organ-specific autoimmune disorder in which the gastric mucosa is atrophic, with loss of parietal cells causing intrinsic factor deficiency. In the absence of intrinsic factor, less than 1% of dietary vitamin B_{12} is absorbed. Pernicious anaemia has an incidence of 25/100000 population over the age of 40 years in developed countries, but an average age of onset of 60 years. It is more common in individuals with other autoimmune disease (Hashimoto's thyroiditis, Graves' disease, vitiligo or Addison's disease; Ch. 20) or a family history of these or pernicious anaemia. The finding of anti-intrinsic factor antibodies in the context of B_{12} deficiency is diagnostic of pernicious anaemia without further investigation. Antiparietal cell antibodies are present in over 90% of cases, but are also present in 20% of normal females over the age of 60 years; a negative result makes pernicious anaemia less likely, but a positive result is not diagnostic. The Schilling test, involving measurement of absorption of radio-labelled B_{12} after oral administration before and after replacement of intrinsic factor, has fallen out of favour with the availability of autoantibody tests, greater caution in the use of radioactive tracers and limited availability of intrinsic factor.

Small bowel pathology

One-third of patients with pancreatic exocrine insufficiency fail to transfer dietary vitamin B_{12} from R protein to intrinsic factor. This usually results in slightly low vitamin B_{12} values, but no tissue evidence of vitamin B_{12} deficiency. Inflammatory disease of the terminal ileum, such as Crohn's disease, may impair the absorption of vitamin B_{12}–intrinsic factor complex, as may surgery on that part of the bowel. Motility disorders or hypogammaglobulinaemia can result in bacterial overgrowth and the ensuing competition for free vitamin B_{12} can lead to deficiency. A small number of people heavily infected with the fish tapeworm (Ch. 13) develop vitamin B_{12} deficiency.

Folate

Folate absorption

Folates are produced by plants and bacteria; hence dietary leafy vegetables (spinach, broccoli, lettuce), fruits (bananas, melons) and animal protein (liver, kidney) are a rich source. An average Western diet contains more than the minimum daily intake of 50 μg, but excess cooking destroys folates. Most dietary folate is present as polyglutamates; these are converted to monoglutamate in the upper small bowel and actively transported into plasma. Plasma folate is loosely bound to plasma proteins such as albumin and there is an enterohepatic circulation. Total body stores of folate are small and deficiency can occur in a matter of weeks.

Folate deficiency

The causes and diagnostic features of folate deficiency are shown in Boxes 25.34 and 25.35. Edentulous older people or psychiatric patients are particularly susceptible to dietary deficiency and this is exacerbated in the presence of gut disease or malignancy. Pregnancy-induced folate deficiency is the most common cause of megaloblastosis worldwide and is more likely in the context of twin pregnancies, multiparity and hyperemesis gravidarum. Serum folate measurement is very sensitive to dietary intake; a single folate-rich meal can normalise it in a patient with true folate deficiency, whereas anorexia, alcohol and anticonvulsant therapy can reduce it in the absence of megaloblastosis. For this reason, red cell folate levels are a more accurate indicator of folate stores and tissue folate deficiency.

25.34 Causes of folate deficiency

Diet
- Poor intake of vegetables

Malabsorption
- e.g. Coeliac disease, small bowel surgery including some forms of bariatric surgery

Increased demand
- Cell proliferation, e.g. haemolysis
- Pregnancy

Drugs*
- Certain anticonvulsants (e.g. phenytoin)
- Contraceptive pill
- Certain cytotoxic drugs (e.g. methotrexate)

*Usually only a problem in patients deficient in folate from another cause.

25.35 Investigation of folic acid deficiency

Diagnostic findings
- Serum folate levels may be low but are difficult to interpret
- Low red cell folate levels indicate prolonged folate deficiency and are probably the most relevant measure

Corroborative findings
- Macrocytic dysplastic blood picture
- Megaloblastic marrow

Management of megaloblastic anaemia

If a patient with a severe megaloblastic anaemia is very ill and treatment must be started before vitamin B_{12} and red cell folate results are available, that treatment should always include both folic acid and vitamin B_{12}. The use of folic acid alone in the presence of vitamin B_{12} deficiency may result in worsening of neurological features.

Rarely, if severe angina or heart failure is present, transfusion can be used. The cardiovascular system is adapted to the chronic anaemia present in megaloblastosis and the volume load imposed by transfusion may result in decompensation and severe cardiac failure. In such circumstances, exchange transfusion or slow administration of 1 U of red cells with diuretic cover may be given.

Vitamin B₁₂ deficiency

Vitamin B_{12} deficiency is treated with hydroxycobalamin. In cases of malabsorption, 1000 μg IM for 6 doses 2 or 3 days apart, followed by maintenance therapy of 1000 μg every 3 months for life, is recommended. In the presence of neurological involvement, a dose of 1000 μg on alternate days until there is no further improvement, followed by maintenance as above, is recommended. In dietary deficiency oral B_{12} replacement will suffice. The reticulocyte count will peak by the 5th–10th day after starting replacement therapy. The haemoglobin will rise by 10 g/L every week until normalised. The response of the marrow is associated with a fall in plasma potassium levels and rapid depletion of iron stores. If an initial response is not maintained and the blood film is dimorphic (i.e. shows a mixture of microcytic and macrocytic cells), the patient may need additional iron therapy. A sensory neuropathy may take 6–12 months to correct; long-standing neurological damage may not improve.

Folate deficiency

Oral folic acid (5 mg daily for 3 weeks) will treat acute deficiency and 5 mg once weekly is adequate maintenance therapy. Prophylactic folic acid in pregnancy prevents megaloblastosis in women at

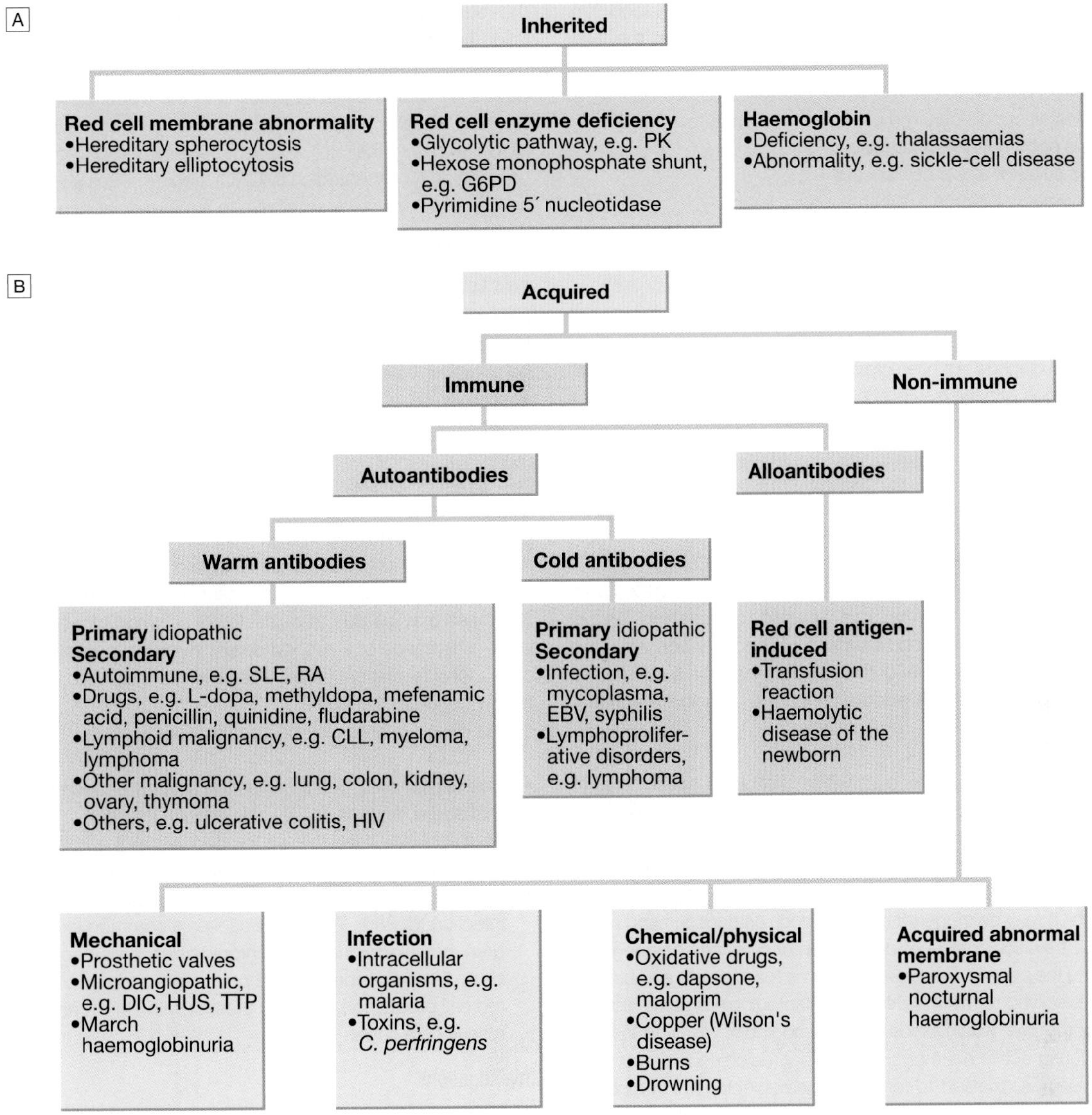

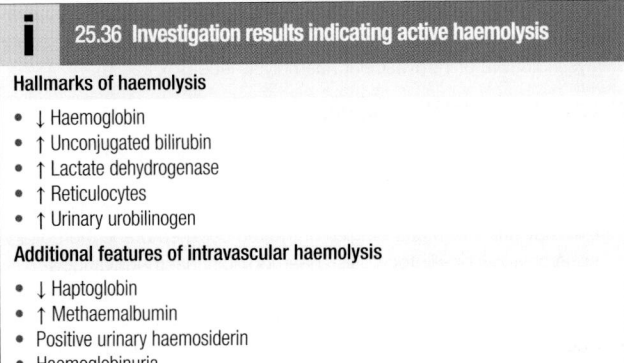

A Inherited

Red cell membrane abnormality
•Hereditary spherocytosis
•Hereditary elliptocytosis

Red cell enzyme deficiency
•Glycolytic pathway, e.g. PK
•Hexose monophosphate shunt, e.g. G6PD
•Pyrimidine 5′ nucleotidase

Haemoglobin
•Deficiency, e.g. thalassaemias
•Abnormality, e.g. sickle-cell disease

B

Acquired

Immune

Non-immune

Autoantibodies

Alloantibodies

Warm antibodies

Cold antibodies

Primary idiopathic
Secondary
•Autoimmune, e.g. SLE, RA
•Drugs, e.g. L-dopa, methyldopa, mefenamic acid, penicillin, quinidine, fludarabine
•Lymphoid malignancy, e.g. CLL, myeloma, lymphoma
•Other malignancy, e.g. lung, colon, kidney, ovary, thymoma
•Others, e.g. ulcerative colitis, HIV

Primary idiopathic
Secondary
•Infection, e.g. mycoplasma, EBV, syphilis
•Lymphoprolifer-ative disorders, e.g. lymphoma

Red cell antigen-induced
•Transfusion reaction
•Haemolytic disease of the newborn

Mechanical
•Prosthetic valves
•Microangiopathic, e.g. DIC, HUS, TTP
•March haemoglobinuria

Infection
•Intracellular organisms, e.g. malaria
•Toxins, e.g. *C. perfringens*

Chemical/physical
•Oxidative drugs, e.g. dapsone, maloprim
•Copper (Wilson's disease)
•Burns
•Drowning

Acquired abnormal membrane
•Paroxysmal nocturnal haemoglobinuria

Fig. 25.21 Causes and classification of haemolysis. A Inherited causes. B Acquired causes. (CLL = chronic lymphocytic leukaemia; DIC = disseminated intravascular coagulation; EBV = Epstein–Barr virus; G6PD = glucose-6-phosphate dehydrogenase; HUS = haemolytic uraemic syndrome; PK = pyruvate kinase; RA = rheumatoid arthritis; SLE = systemic lupus erythematosus; TTP = thrombotic thrombocytopenic purpura)

risk and reduces the risk of fetal neural tube defects (Box 22.29). Prophylactic supplementation is also given in chronic haematological disease associated with reduced red cell lifespan (e.g. haemolytic anaemias).

Haemolytic anaemia

Haemolysis indicates that there is shortening of the normal red cell lifespan of 120 days. There are many causes, as shown in Fig. 25.21. To compensate, the bone marrow may increase its output of red cells six- to eightfold by increasing the proportion of red cells produced, expanding the volume of active marrow, and releasing reticulocytes prematurely. Anaemia occurs only if the rate of destruction exceeds this increased production rate.

There are some general features of haemolysis and other specific features that help to identify the reason for haemolysis. Results of investigations that establish the presence of haemolysis are shown in Box 25.36. Red cell destruction overloads pathways for haemoglobin breakdown in the liver (p. 864), causing a modest rise in unconjugated bilirubin in the blood and mild jaundice. Increased reabsorption of urobilinogen from the

i	**25.36 Investigation results indicating active haemolysis**

Hallmarks of haemolysis

- ↓ Haemoglobin
- ↑ Unconjugated bilirubin
- ↑ Lactate dehydrogenase
- ↑ Reticulocytes
- ↑ Urinary urobilinogen

Additional features of intravascular haemolysis

- ↓ Haptoglobin
- ↑ Methaemalbumin
- Positive urinary haemosiderin
- Haemoglobinuria

gut results in an increase in urinary urobilinogen (pp. 870 and 924). Red cell destruction releases LDH into the serum. The bone marrow compensation results in a reticulocytosis and sometimes nucleated red cell precursors appear in the blood. Increased proliferation of the bone marrow can result in a thrombocytosis, neutrophilia and, if marked, immature granulocytes in the blood, producing a leucoerythroblastic blood film. The appearances of the red cells may give an indication of the likely cause of the haemolysis:

- spherocytes are small, dark red cells that suggest autoimmune haemolysis or hereditary spherocytosis
- sickle cells suggest sickle-cell disease
- red cell fragments indicate microangiopathic haemolysis
- bite cells (normal-sized red cells that look as if they have been partially eaten) suggest oxidative haemolysis.

The compensatory erythroid hyperplasia may give rise to folate deficiency, with megaloblastic blood features.

The differential diagnosis of haemolysis is determined by the clinical scenario in combination with the results of blood film examination and Coombs testing for antibodies directed against red cells (see below and Fig. 25.21).

Extravascular haemolysis

Physiological red cell destruction occurs in the reticulo-endothelial cells in the liver or spleen, so avoiding free haemoglobin in the plasma. In most haemolytic states, haemolysis is predominantly extravascular.

To confirm the haemolysis, patients' red cells can be labelled with ^{51}chromium. When re-injected, they can be used to determine red cell survival; when combined with body surface radioactivity counting, this test may indicate whether the liver or the spleen is the main source of red cell destruction. However, this is seldom performed in clinical practice.

Intravascular haemolysis

Less commonly, red cell lysis occurs within the blood stream due to membrane damage by complement (ABO transfusion reactions, paroxysmal nocturnal haemoglobinuria), infections (malaria, *Clostridium perfringens*), mechanical trauma (heart valves, DIC) or oxidative damage (e.g. enzymopathies such as glucose-6-phosphate dehydrogenase deficiency, which may be triggered by drugs such as dapsone and maloprim). When intravascular red cell destruction occurs, free haemoglobin is released into the plasma. Free haemoglobin is toxic to cells and binding proteins have evolved to minimise this risk. Haptoglobin is an α_2-globulin produced by the liver which binds free haemoglobin, resulting in a fall in its levels during active haemolysis. Once haptoglobins are saturated, free haemoglobin is oxidised to form methaemoglobin, which binds to albumin in turn forming methaemalbumin, which can be detected spectrophotometrically in Schumm's test. Methaemoglobin is degraded and any free haem is bound to a second binding protein called haemopexin. If all the protective mechanisms are saturated, free haemoglobin may appear in the urine (haemoglobinuria). When fulminant, this gives rise to black urine, as in severe *falciparum* malaria infection (Ch. 13). In smaller amounts, renal tubular cells absorb the haemoglobin, degrade it and store the iron as haemosiderin. When the tubular cells are subsequently sloughed into the urine, they give rise to haemosiderinuria, which is always indicative of intravascular haemolysis (see Box 25.36).

Causes of haemolytic anaemia

These can be classified as inherited or acquired (see Fig. 25.21).

- *Inherited* red cell abnormalities resulting in chronic haemolytic anaemia may arise from pathologies of the red cell membrane (hereditary spherocytosis or elliptocytosis), haemoglobin (haemoglobinopathies), or protective enzymes that prevent cellular oxidative damage, such as glucose-6-phosphate dehydrogenase (G6PD).
- *Acquired* causes include auto- and alloantibody-mediated destruction of red blood cells and other mechanical, toxic and infective causes.

Red cell membrane defects

The structure of the red cell membrane is shown in Fig. 25.4. The basic structure is a cytoskeleton 'stapled' on to the lipid bilayer by special protein complexes. This structure ensures great deformability and elasticity;

the red cell diameter is 8 μm, but the narrowest capillaries in the circulation are in the spleen, measuring just 2 μm in diameter. When the normal red cell structure is disturbed, usually by a quantitative or functional deficiency of one or more proteins in the cytoskeleton, cells lose their elasticity. Each time such cells pass through the spleen, they lose membrane relative to their cell volume. This results in an increase in mean cell haemoglobin concentration (MCHC), abnormal cell shape (see Box 25.2) and reduced red cell survival due to extravascular haemolysis.

Hereditary spherocytosis

This is usually inherited as an autosomal dominant condition, although 25% of cases have no family history and represent new mutations. The incidence is approximately 1:5000 in high-income countries, but this may be an under-estimate since the disease may present de novo in patients aged over 65 years and is often discovered as a chance finding on a blood count. The most common abnormalities are deficiencies of beta spectrin or ankyrin (see Fig. 25.4). The severity of spontaneous haemolysis varies. Most cases are associated with an asymptomatic compensated chronic haemolytic state with spherocytes present on the blood film, a reticulocytosis and mild hyperbilirubinaemia. Pigment gallstones are present in up to 50% of patients and may cause symptomatic cholecystitis. Occasional cases are associated with more severe haemolysis; these may be due to coincidental polymorphisms in alpha spectrin or co-inheritance of a second defect involving a different protein. These cases tend to present earlier in life with symptomatic, sometimes transfusion-dependent anaemia.

The clinical course may be complicated by crises:

- *Haemolytic crisis* occurs when the severity of haemolysis increases; this is rare, and usually associated with infection.
- *Megaloblastic crisis* follows the development of folate deficiency; this may occur as a first presentation of the disease in pregnancy.
- *Aplastic crisis* occurs in association with parvovirus (erythrovirus) infection (p. 280). Parvovirus causes a common exanthem in children, but if individuals with chronic haemolysis become infected, the virus directly invades red cell precursors and temporarily switches off red cell production. Patients present with severe anaemia and a low reticulocyte count.

Investigations

The patient and other family members should be screened for features of compensated haemolysis (see Box 25.36). This may be all that is required to confirm the diagnosis. Haemoglobin levels are variable, depending on the degree of compensation. The blood film will show spherocytes, but the direct Coombs test (Fig. 25.22) is negative, excluding immune haemolysis. An osmotic fragility test may show increased sensitivity to lysis in hypotonic saline solutions, but is limited by lack of sensitivity and specificity. More specific flow cytometric tests detecting binding of eosin-5-maleimide to red cells are recommended in borderline cases.

Management

Folic acid prophylaxis (5 mg daily) should be given for life. In severe cases, consideration may be given to splenectomy, which improves but does not normalise red cell survival. Potential indications for splenectomy include moderate to severe haemolysis with complications (anaemia and gallstones), although splenectomy should be delayed where possible until after 6 years of age in view of the subsequent risk of sepsis. Guidelines for the management of patients after splenectomy are presented in Box 25.37.

Acute, severe haemolytic crises require transfusion support, but cross-matched blood must be transfused slowly as haemolytic transfusion reactions may occur (see Fig. 25.16).

Hereditary elliptocytosis

This term refers to a heterogeneous group of disorders that produce an increase in elliptocytic red cells on the blood film and a variable degree of haemolysis. This is due to a functional abnormality of one or more anchor proteins in the red cell membrane, e.g. alpha spectrin or protein 4.1

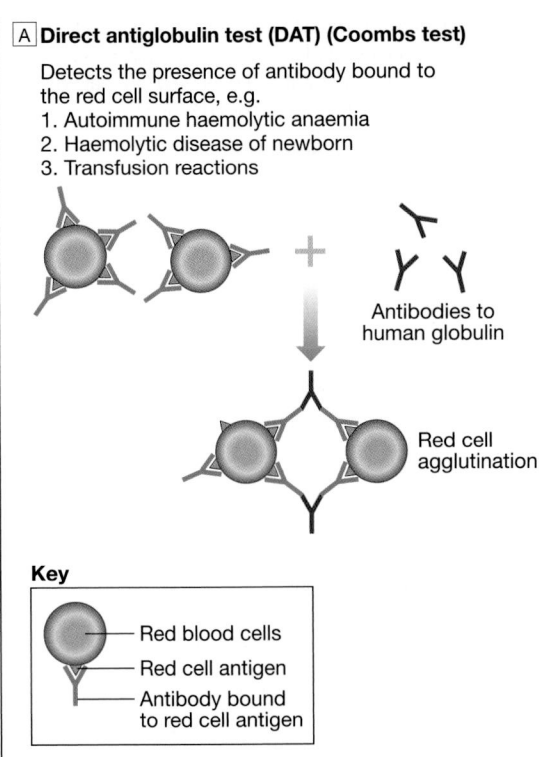

A | **Direct antiglobulin test (DAT) (Coombs test)**

Detects the presence of antibody bound to the red cell surface, e.g.
1. Autoimmune haemolytic anaemia
2. Haemolytic disease of newborn
3. Transfusion reactions

Antibodies to human globulin

Red cell agglutination

Key

Red blood cells

Red cell antigen

Antibody bound to red cell antigen

B | **Indirect antiglobulin test (IAT) (indirect Coombs test)**

Detects antibodies in the plasma, e.g.
1. Antibody screen in pre-transfusion testing
2. Screening in pregnancy for antibodies that may cause haemolytic disease of newborn

Patient's plasma

Stage 1

Red cells with known antigen expression

Red cells with Ag – Ab complex on cell surface

Stage 2

Antibodies to human globulin

Red cell agglutination

Fig. 25.22 Direct and indirect antiglobulin tests.

> **i** | **25.37 Management of the splenectomised patient**
>
> - Vaccinate with pneumococcal, *Haemophilus influenzae* type B, meningococcal group C and influenza vaccines at least 2–3 weeks before elective splenectomy. Vaccination should be given after emergency surgery but may be less effective
> - Pneumococcal re-immunisation should be given at least 5-yearly and influenza annually. Vaccination status must be documented
> - Life-long prophylactic penicillin V (500 mg twice daily) is recommended. In penicillin-allergic patients, consider a macrolide
> - Patients should be educated regarding the risks of infection and methods of prophylaxis
> - A card or bracelet should be carried to alert health professionals to the risk of overwhelming sepsis
> - In sepsis, patients should be resuscitated and given intravenous antibiotics to cover pneumococcus, *Haemophilus* and meningococcus, according to local resistance patterns
> - The risk of cerebral malaria is increased in the event of infection
> - Animal bites should be promptly treated with local disinfection and antibiotics to prevent serious soft tissue infection and sepsis

(see Fig. 25.4). Inheritance may be autosomal dominant or recessive. Hereditary elliptocytosis is less common than hereditary spherocytosis in Western countries, with an incidence of 1/10000, but is more common in equatorial Africa and parts of South-east Asia. The clinical course is variable and depends on the degree of membrane dysfunction caused by the inherited molecular defect(s); most cases present as an asymptomatic blood film abnormality, but occasional cases result in neonatal haemolysis or a chronic compensated haemolytic state. Management of the latter is the same as for hereditary spherocytosis.

A characteristic variant of hereditary elliptocytosis occurs in South-East Asia, particularly Malaysia and Papua New Guinea, with stomatocytes and ovalocytes in the blood. This has a prevalence of up to 30% in some communities because it offers relative protection from malaria and thus has sustained a high gene frequency. The blood film is often very abnormal and immediate differential diagnosis is broad.

Red cell enzymopathies

The mature red cell must produce energy via ATP to maintain a normal internal environment and cell volume while protecting itself from the oxidative stress presented by oxygen carriage. ATP is generated by glycolysis, while the hexose monophosphate shunt produces nicotinamide adenine dinucleotide phosphate (NADPH) and glutathione to protect against oxidative stress. The impact of functional or quantitative defects in the enzymes in these pathways depends on the importance of the steps affected and the presence of alternative pathways. In general, defects in the hexose monophosphate shunt pathway result in periodic haemolysis precipitated by episodic oxidative stress, while those in the glycolysis pathway result in shortened red cell survival and chronic haemolysis.

Glucose-6-phosphate dehydrogenase deficiency

The enzyme glucose-6-phosphate dehydrogenase (G6PD) is pivotal in the hexose monophosphate shunt pathway. Deficiencies result in the most common human enzymopathy, affecting 10% of the world's population, with a geographical distribution that parallels the malaria belt because heterozygotes are protected from malarial parasitisation. The enzyme is a heteromeric structure made of catalytic subunits that are encoded by a gene on the X chromosome. The deficiency therefore affects males and rare homozygous females (Ch. 3), but it is carried by females. Carrier heterozygous females are usually only affected in the neonatal period or in the presence of skewed X-inactivation.

Over 400 subtypes of G6PD are described. The most common types associated with normal activity are the B+ enzyme present in most populations of European descent and 70% of those of African Caribbean origin, and the A+ variant present in 20% of African Caribbeans. The two common variants associated with reduced activity are the A− variety in approximately 10% of African Caribbeans, and the Mediterranean or B− variety in those of European origin. In East and West Africa, up to 20% of males and 4% of females (homozygotes) are affected and have enzyme levels of about 15% of normal. The deficiency in European and East Asian populations is more severe, with enzyme levels as low as 1%.

25.38 Glucose-6-phosphate dehydrogenase deficiency

Clinical features

- Acute drug-induced haemolysis to (e.g.):
   Analgesics: aspirin, phenacetin
   Antimalarials: primaquine, quinine, chloroquine, pyrimethamine
   Antibiotics: sulphonamides, nitrofurantoin, ciprofloxacin
   Miscellaneous: quinidine, probenecid, vitamin K, dapsone
- Chronic compensated haemolysis
- Infection or acute illness
- Neonatal jaundice: may be a feature of the B⁻ enzyme
- Favism, i.e. acute haemolysis after ingestion of broad beans (*Vicia fava*)

Laboratory features

Non-spherocytic intravascular haemolysis during an attack
The blood film will show:
- Bite cells (red cells with a 'bite' of membrane missing)
- Blister cells (red cells with surface blistering of the membrane)
- Irregularly shaped small cells
- Polychromasia reflecting the reticulocytosis
- Denatured haemoglobin visible as Heinz bodies within the red cell cytoplasm with a supravital stain such as methyl violet

G6PD level
- Can be indirectly assessed by screening methods that usually depend on the decreased ability to reduce dyes
- Direct assessment of G6PD is made in those with low screening values
- Care must be taken close to an acute haemolytic episode because reticulocytes may have higher enzyme levels and give rise to a false normal result

Clinical features and investigation findings are shown in Box 25.38.

Management aims to stop the intake of any precipitant drugs or foods and treat any underlying infection. Favism due to the consumption of fava beans is the classically described precipitant of haemolysis in patients with G6PD deficiency. Acute transfusion support may be life-saving.

Pyruvate kinase deficiency

This is the second most common red cell enzyme defect. It results in deficiency of ATP production and a chronic haemolytic anaemia. It is inherited as an autosomal recessive trait. The extent of anaemia is variable; the blood film shows characteristic 'prickle cells' that resemble holly leaves. Enzyme activity is only 5%–20% of normal. Transfusion support may be necessary during periods of haemolysis.

Pyrimidine 5' nucleotidase deficiency

The pyrimidine 5' nucleotidase enzyme catalyses the dephosphorylation of nucleoside monophosphates and is important during the degradation of RNA in reticulocytes. It is inherited as an autosomal recessive trait and is as common as pyruvate kinase deficiency in Mediterranean, African and Jewish populations. The accumulation of excess ribonucleoprotein results in coarse basophilic stippling (see Box 25.2), associated with a chronic haemolytic state. The enzyme is very sensitive to inhibition by lead and this is the reason why basophilic stippling is a feature of lead poisoning.

Autoimmune haemolytic anaemia

This results from increased red cell destruction due to red cell autoantibodies. The antibodies may be IgG or IgM, or more rarely IgE or IgA. If an antibody avidly fixes complement, it will cause intravascular haemolysis, but if complement activation is weak, the haemolysis will be extravascular (in the reticulo-endothelial system). Antibody-coated red cells lose membrane to macrophages in the spleen and hence spherocytes are present in the blood. The optimum temperature at which the antibody is active (thermal specificity) is used to classify immune haemolysis:

- *Warm antibodies* bind best at 37°C and account for 80% of cases. The majority are IgG and often react against Rhesus antigens.

- *Cold antibodies* bind best at 4°C but can bind up to 37°C in some cases. They are usually IgM and bind complement. To be clinically relevant, they must act within the range of normal body temperatures. They account for the other 20% of cases.

Warm autoimmune haemolysis

The incidence of warm autoimmune haemolysis is approximately 1/100 000 population per annum; it occurs at all ages, but is more common in middle age and in females. No underlying cause is identified in up to 50% of cases. The remainder are secondary to a wide variety of other conditions (see Fig. 25.21B).

Investigations

There is evidence of haemolysis, spherocytes and polychromasia on the blood film. The diagnosis is confirmed by the direct Coombs or antiglobulin test (see Fig. 25.22). The patient's red cells are mixed with Coombs reagent, which contains antibodies against human IgG/IgM/complement. If the red cells have been coated by antibody in vivo, the Coombs reagent will induce their agglutination and this can be detected visually. The relevant antibody can be eluted from the red cell surface and tested against a panel of typed red cells to determine against which red cell antigen it is directed. The most common specificity is for Rhesus antigens and most often anti-e; this is helpful when choosing blood to cross-match. The direct Coombs test can be negative in the presence of brisk haemolysis. A positive test requires about 200 antibody molecules to attach to each red cell; with a very avid complement-fixing antibody, haemolysis may occur at lower levels of antibody-binding. The standard Coombs reagent will miss IgA or IgE antibodies. Around 10% of all warm autoimmune haemolytic anaemias are Coombs test-negative.

Management

If the haemolysis is secondary to an underlying cause, this must be treated and any implicated drugs stopped.

It is usual to treat patients initially with prednisolone (1 mg/kg orally). A response is seen in 70%–80% of cases, but may take up to 3 weeks; a rise in haemoglobin will be matched by a fall in bilirubin, LDH and reticulocyte levels. Once the haemoglobin has normalised and the reticulocytosis resolved, the glucocorticoid dose can be reduced slowly over several weeks. Glucocorticoids probably work by decreasing macrophage destruction of antibody-coated red cells and reducing antibody production.

Transfusion support may be required for life-threatening problems, such as the development of heart failure or rapid unabated falls in haemoglobin. The least incompatible blood should be used, but this may still give rise to transfusion reactions or the development of alloantibodies.

If the haemolysis fails to respond to glucocorticoids or can only be stabilised by large doses, then second-line therapy with the anti-CD20 monoclonal antibody rituximab should be considered. Failure to respond to rituximab can be followed by consideration of treatment with a range of immunomodulatory/ immunosuppressive agents or splenectomy. Pharmacological agents include azathioprine, ciclosporin, danazol and mycophenolate mofetil. Splenectomy is associated with a good response in 50%–60% of cases. The operation can be performed laparoscopically with reduced morbidity. There are concerns about all modes of third-line therapy as long-term immunosuppression carries a risk of malignancy, while splenectomy is associated with an excess of severe infection due to the capsulate organisms pneumococcus and meningococcus (see Box 25.40).

Cold agglutinin disease

This is mediated by antibodies, usually IgM, which bind to the red cells at low temperatures and cause them to agglutinate. It may cause intravascular haemolysis if complement fixation occurs. This can be chronic when the antibody is monoclonal, or acute or transient when the antibody is polyclonal.

Chronic cold agglutinin disease

This typically affects older adult patients and may be associated with an underlying low-grade B-cell lymphoma. It causes a low-grade intravascular haemolysis with cold, painful and often blue fingers, toes, ears or nose (so-called acrocyanosis). The latter is due to red cell agglutination in the small vessels in these colder, exposed areas. The blood film shows red cell agglutination and the MCV may be spuriously high because the automated analysers detect red cell aggregates as single cells. Monoclonal IgM usually has anti-I or, less often, anti-i specificity. Treatment is primarily by transfusion support, but may also be directed at any underlying lymphoma. Patients must keep extremities warm, especially in winter. Some patients respond to rituximab. Fludarabine can be added in if a clonal abnormality is detected. For patients requiring blood transfusion, the cross-match sample must be placed in a transport flask at a temperature of 37°C and blood must be administered via a bloodwarmer. All patients should receive folic acid supplementation.

Other causes of cold agglutination

Cold agglutination can occur in association with *Mycoplasma pneumoniae* or with infectious mononucleosis. Paroxysmal cold haemoglobinuria is a very rare cause seen in children, in association with viral or bacterial infection. An IgG antibody binds to red cells in the peripheral circulation, but lysis occurs in the central circulation when complement fixation takes place. This antibody is termed the Donath–Landsteiner antibody and has specificity against the P antigen on the red cells.

Alloimmune haemolytic anaemia

Alloimmune haemolytic anaemia is caused by antibodies against non-self red cells. It has two main causes, occurring after:

- unmatched blood transfusion (see Fig. 25.16)
- maternal sensitisation to paternal antigens on fetal cells (haemolytic disease of the newborn, see Box 25.19).

Non-immune haemolytic anaemia

Endothelial damage

Disruption of red cell membrane may occur in a number of conditions and is characterised by the presence of red cell fragments on the blood film and markers of intravascular haemolysis:

- *Mechanical heart valves*. High flow through incompetent valves or periprosthetic leaks through the suture ring holding a valve in place result in shear stress damage.
- *March haemoglobinuria*. Vigorous exercise, such as prolonged marching or marathon running, can cause red cell damage in the capillaries in the feet.
- *Thermal injury*. Severe burns cause thermal damage to red cells, characterised by fragmentation and the presence of microspherocytes in the blood.
- *Microangiopathic haemolytic anaemia*. Fibrin deposition in capillaries can cause severe red cell disruption. It may occur in a wide variety of conditions: disseminated carcinomatosis, malignant or pregnancy-induced hypertension, haemolytic uraemic syndrome (Ch. 18), thrombotic thrombocytopenic purpura and disseminated intravascular coagulation (p. 988).

Infection

Plasmodium falciparum malaria (p. 319) may be associated with intravascular haemolysis; when severe, this is termed blackwater fever because of the associated haemoglobinuria. *Clostridium perfringens* sepsis (p. 271), usually in the context of ascending cholangitis or necrotising fasciitis, may cause severe intravascular haemolysis with marked spherocytosis due to bacterial production of a lecithinase that destroys the red cell membrane.

Chemicals or drugs

Dapsone and sulfasalazine cause haemolysis by oxidative denaturation of haemoglobin. Denatured haemoglobin forms Heinz bodies in the red cells, visible on supravital staining with brilliant cresyl blue. Arsenic gas, copper, chlorates, nitrites and nitrobenzene derivatives may all cause haemolysis.

Paroxysmal nocturnal haemoglobinuria

Paroxysmal nocturnal haemoglobinuria (PNH) is a rare acquired, non-malignant clonal expansion of haematopoietic stem cells deficient in glycosylphosphatidylinositol (GPI) anchor protein. GPI anchors several key molecules to cells and its absence results in clinical outcomes that reflect this, causing intravascular haemolysis and anaemia because of increased sensitivity of red cells to lysis by complement. This happens because key defence mechanisms that protect cells from complement-mediated lysis (CD55 and CD59) are GPI-anchored to red cells under normal circumstances. Episodes of intravascular haemolysis result in haemoglobinuria, most noticeable in early morning urine, which has a characteristic red–brown colour. The disease is associated with an increased risk of venous and arterial thrombosis in unusual sites, such as the liver or abdomen. PNH clones are also associated with hypoplastic bone marrow failure, aplastic anaemia and myelodysplastic syndrome (see later). Management is supportive with transfusion and folate supplements and prophylaxis or treatment of thrombosis. Standard care now includes the anti-complement C5 monoclonal antibodies eculizimab and ravulizumab. This has been shown to be effective in reducing haemolysis, transfusion requirements and thrombotic risk. The C5 inhibitory antibodies both carry a risk of infection, particularly for *Neisseria meningitidis*, and all treated patients must be vaccinated against this organism.

Haemoglobinopathies

These disorders are caused by mutations affecting the genes encoding the globin chains of haemoglobin. Normal haemoglobin is composed of two alpha and two non-alpha globin chains. Alpha globin chains are produced throughout life, including in the fetus, so severe mutations in these may cause intrauterine death. Production of non-alpha chains varies with age; fetal haemoglobin (HbF-$\alpha\alpha/\gamma\gamma$) has two gamma chains, while the predominant adult haemoglobin (HbA-$\alpha\alpha/\beta\beta$) has two beta chains. Thus, disorders affecting the beta chains do not present until after 6 months of age. A constant small amount of haemoglobin A_2 (HbA$_2$-$\alpha\alpha/\delta\delta$, usually less than 2%) is made from birth.

The geographical distribution of the common haemoglobinopathies is shown in Fig. 25.23. The haemoglobinopathies can be classified into qualitative or quantitative abnormalities.

Qualitative abnormalities – abnormal haemoglobins

In qualitative abnormalities (called the abnormal haemoglobins) there is a functionally important alteration in the amino acid structure of the polypeptide chains of the globin chains. Several hundred such variants are known; they were originally designated by letters of the alphabet, e.g. S, C, D or E, but the more recently described ones are known by names that are usually taken from the town or district in which they were first described. The best-known example is haemoglobin S, found in sickle-cell anaemia. Mutations around the haem-binding pocket cause the haem ring to fall out of the structure and produce an unstable haemoglobin. These substitutions often change the charge of the globin chains, producing different electrophoretic mobility, and this forms the basis for the diagnostic use of haemoglobin electrophoresis to identify haemoglobinopathies.

Quantitative abnormalities – thalassaemias

In quantitative abnormalities (the thalassaemias), there are mutations causing a reduced rate of production of one or other of the globin chains,

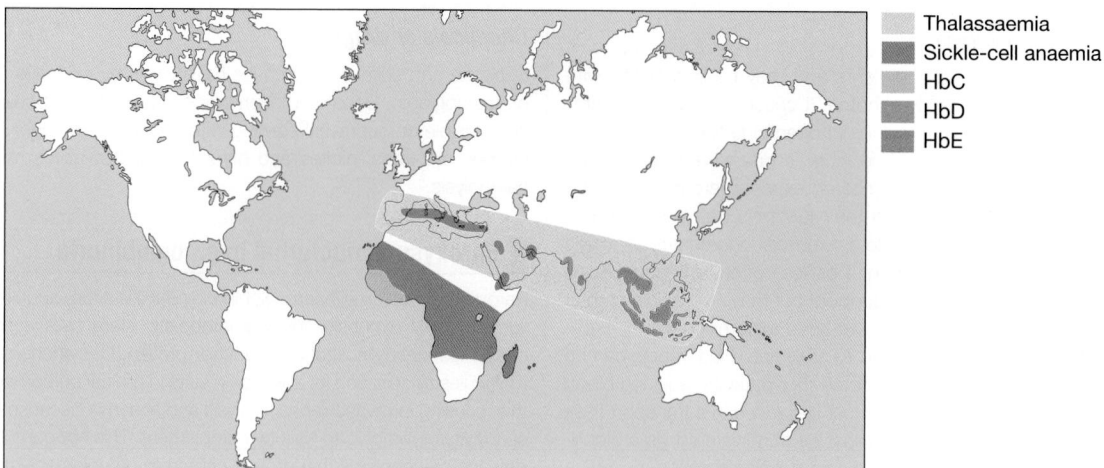

Fig. 25.23 **The geographical distribution of the haemoglobinopathies.** *From Hoffbrand AV, Pettit JE. Essential haematology, 3rd edn. Edinburgh: Blackwell Science; 1992.*

altering the ratio of alpha to non-alpha chains. In alpha-thalassaemia excess beta chains are present, while in beta-thalassaemia excess alpha chains are present. The excess chains precipitate, causing red cell membrane damage and reduced red cell survival due to haemolysis.

Sickle-cell anaemia

Sickle-cell disease results from a single glutamic acid to valine substitution at position 6 of the beta globin polypeptide chain. It is inherited as an autosomal recessive trait (Ch. 3). Homozygotes only produce abnormal beta chains that make haemoglobin S (HbS, termed SS), and this results in the clinical syndrome of sickle-cell disease. Heterozygotes produce a mixture of normal and abnormal beta chains that make normal HbA and HbS (termed AS), and this results in sickle-cell trait; although this was previously thought of as asymptomatic, it may be associated with an increased risk of sudden and cardiovascular death in young adults.

Epidemiology

The heterozygote frequency is over 20% in tropical Africa (see Fig. 25.23). In African American populations, sickle-cell trait has a frequency of 8%. Individuals with sickle-cell trait are relatively resistant to the effects of *falciparum* malaria in early childhood; the high prevalence in equatorial Africa can thus be explained by the survival advantage it confers in areas where *falciparum* malaria is endemic. However, homozygous patients with sickle-cell anaemia do not have correspondingly greater resistance to *falciparum* malaria.

Pathogenesis

When haemoglobin S is deoxygenated, the molecules of haemoglobin polymerise to form pseudocrystalline structures known as 'tactoids'. These distort the red cell membrane and produce characteristic sickle-shaped cells (Fig. 25.24). The polymerisation is reversible when re-oxygenation occurs. The distortion of the red cell membrane, however, may become permanent and the red cell 'irreversibly sickled'. The greater the concentration of sickle-cell haemoglobin in the individual cell, the more easily tactoids are formed, but this process may be enhanced or retarded by the presence of other haemoglobins. Thus the abnormal haemoglobin C variant participates in polymerisation more readily than haemoglobin A, whereas haemoglobin F strongly inhibits polymerisation.

Clinical features

Sickling is precipitated by hypoxia, acidosis, dehydration and infection. Irreversibly sickled cells have a shortened survival and plug vessels in the microcirculation. This results in a number of acute syndromes, termed 'crises', and chronic organ damage (see Fig. 25.24):

- *Painful vaso-occlusive crisis*. Plugging of small vessels in the bone produces acute severe bone pain. This affects areas of active marrow: the hands and feet in children (so-called dactylitis) or the femora, humeri, ribs, pelvis and vertebrae in adults. Patients usually have a systemic response with tachycardia, and fever. This is the most common form of crisis.
- *Stroke*. The single most devastating consequence of sickle-cell disease is stroke. Stroke or silent stroke occurs in 10%–15% of children with sickle-cell disease. Children at risk of stroke can be identified by screening with transcranial Doppler ultrasound, with fast flow associated with increased stroke risk. These children may be offered strategies such as transfusion or treatment with hydroxycarbamide to reduce the risk of stroke.
- *Sickle chest syndrome*. This may follow a vaso-occlusive crisis and is the most common cause of death in adult sickle-cell disease. Bone marrow infarction results in fat emboli to the lungs, which cause further sickling and infarction, leading to ventilatory failure if not treated.
- *Sequestration crisis*. Thrombosis of the venous outflow from an organ causes loss of function and acute painful enlargement. In children, the spleen is the most common site. Massive splenic enlargement may result in severe anaemia, circulatory collapse and death. Recurrent sickling in the spleen in childhood results in infarction and adults may have no functional spleen. In adults, the liver may undergo sequestration with severe pain due to capsular stretching. Priapism may occur in affected individuals.
- *Aplastic crisis*. Infection of adult sicklers with human parvovirus B19 (erythrovirus) may result in a severe but self-limiting red cell aplasia. This results in profound anaemia, which may cause heart failure. Unlike in all other sickle crises, the reticulocyte count is low.
- *Pregnancy*. Pregnancy in sickle-cell disease requires planning and multidisciplinary management. Women with sickle-cell disease have increased pregnancy-related morbidity, which includes painful crisis, placental failure and thrombosis (Box 25.39).

Investigations

Patients with sickle-cell disease have a compensated anaemia, usually around 60–80 g/L. The blood film shows sickle cells, target cells and features of hyposplenism from a young age. A reticulocytosis is present. The presence of HbS can be demonstrated by exposing red cells to a reducing agent such as sodium dithionite; HbA gives a clear solution, whereas HbS polymerises to produce a turbid solution. This forms the basis of

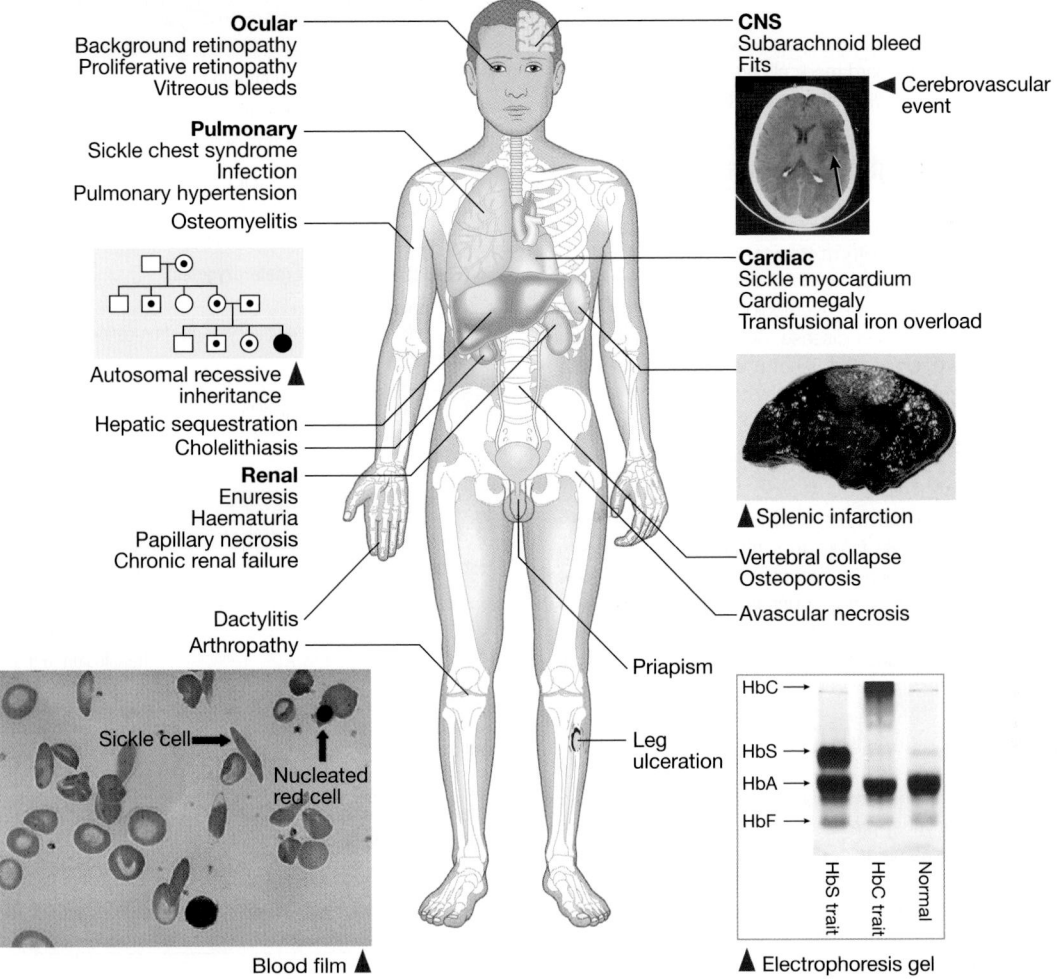

Ocular
Background retinopathy
Proliferative retinopathy
Vitreous bleeds

Pulmonary
Sickle chest syndrome
Infection
Pulmonary hypertension
Osteomyelitis

Autosomal recessive ▲
inheritance

Hepatic sequestration
Cholelithiasis

Renal
Enuresis
Haematuria
Papillary necrosis
Chronic renal failure

Dactylitis
Arthropathy

Sickle cell ➡
Nucleated
red cell

Blood film ▲

CNS
Subarachnoid bleed
Fits
◀ Cerebrovascular
event

Cardiac
Sickle myocardium
Cardiomegaly
Transfusional iron overload

▲ Splenic infarction

Vertebral collapse
Osteoporosis

Avascular necrosis

Priapism

Leg
ulceration

HbC ➡
HbS ➡
HbA ➡
HbF ➡

HbS trait
HbC trait
Normal

▲ Electrophoresis gel

Fig. 25.24 Clinical and laboratory features of sickle-cell disease.

 25.39 Sickle-cell disease in pregnancy

- **Pre-conceptual counselling**: advice on the effect of sickle-cell disease on pregnancy, and vice versa, should be offered.
- **Vaccination status**: should be updated before conception.
- **Testing of partner**: testing for haemoglobinopathy status is advised.
- **Folic acid**: should be taken in high dose (5 mg daily) prior to and throughout pregnancy.
- **Hydroxycarbamide**: should be discontinued 3 months prior to conception.
- **Angiotensin-converting enzyme (ACE) inhibitors**: should be discontinued prior to conception.
- **Pulmonary hypertension**: should be excluded prior to conception.
- **Placental failure**: women with sickle-cell disease have increased rates, resulting in pre-eclampsia and intrauterine growth retardation.
- **Aspirin 75 mg**: should be given throughout pregnancy.
- **Thromboprophylaxis after delivery**: all women with sickle-cell disease should receive thromboprophylaxis with low-molecular-weight heparin for at least 10 days post vaginal delivery and for 6 weeks post caesarean section. Antenatal thromboprophylaxis should be considered for women with additional risk factors for venous thromboembolism (see Box 25.67).
- **Transfusion**: extended cross-matched blood for Rhesus and Kell status should be provided. Blood should be cytomegalovirus-negative.

emergency screening tests before surgery in appropriate ethnic groups, but cannot distinguish between sickle-cell trait and disease. The definitive diagnosis requires haemoglobin electrophoresis to demonstrate the absence of HbA, 2%–20% HbF and the predominance of HbS. Both parents of the affected individual will have sickle-cell trait.

Management

All patients with sickle-cell disease should receive prophylaxis with daily folic acid, and appropriate management of the hyposplenic state that is uniformly found in these patients from an early age (see Box 25.37). Seasonal vaccination against influenza is also advised.

Vaso-occlusive crises are managed by aggressive rehydration, oxygen therapy, adequate analgesia (which often requires opiates) and antibiotics. Transfusion should be with fully genotyped blood wherever possible. Simple top-up transfusion may be used in a sequestration or aplastic crisis. A regular transfusion programme to suppress HbS production and maintain the HbS level below 30% may be indicated in patients with recurrent severe complications, such as cerebrovascular accidents in children or chest syndromes in adults. Exchange transfusion, in which a patient is simultaneously venesected and transfused to replace HbS with HbA, may be used in life-threatening crises or to prepare patients for surgery.

A high HbF level inhibits polymerisation of HbS and reduces sickling. Patients with sickle-cell disease and high HbF levels have a mild clinical course with few crises. Some agents are able to increase synthesis of HbF and this has been used to reduce the frequency of severe crises. The oral cytotoxic agent hydroxycarbamide has been shown to have clinical benefit with acceptable side-effects in children and adults who have recurrent severe crises. The P-selectin inhibitor, crizanlizumab, is currently under review as an agent to reduce vasoocclusive crisis.

Relatively few allogeneic stem cell transplants from HLA-matched siblings have been performed, but this procedure appears to be potentially curative (p. 945).

Prognosis

In Africa, few children with sickle-cell anaemia survive to adult life without medical attention. Even with standard medical care, approximately 15% die by the age of 20 years and 50% by the age of 40 years.

Other abnormal haemoglobins

Haemoglobin C (HbC) disease, another beta-chain haemoglobinopathy, is clinically silent but associated with microcytosis and target cells on the blood film. Compound heterozygotes inheriting one *HbS* gene and one *HbC* gene from their parents have haemoglobin SC disease, which behaves like a mild form of sickle-cell disease. SC disease is associated with a reduced frequency of crises, but is not uncommonly associated with complications in pregnancy and retinopathy.

Thalassaemias

Thalassaemia is an inherited impairment of haemoglobin production, in which there is partial or complete failure to synthesise a specific type of globin chain. In alpha-thalassaemia, disruption of one or both alleles on chromosome 16 may occur, with production of some or no alpha globin chains. In beta-thalassaemia, defective production usually results from disabling point mutations causing no (β^0) or reduced (β^-) beta chain production.

Beta-thalassaemia

Failure to synthesise beta chains (beta-thalassaemia) is the most common type of thalassaemia, most prevalent in the Mediterranean area. Heterozygotes have thalassaemia minor, a condition in which there is usually mild microcytic anaemia and little or no clinical disability, which may be detected only when iron therapy for a mild microcytic anaemia fails. Homozygotes (thalassaemia major) either are unable to synthesise haemoglobin A or, at best, produce very little; after the first 4–6 months of life, they develop profound transfusion-dependent hypochromic anaemia. The diagnostic features are summarised in Box 25.40. Intermediate grades of severity occur.

Management and prevention

See Box 25.41. Cure is now a possibility for selected children, with allogeneic HSCT (p. 945).

It is possible to identify a fetus with homozygous beta-thalassaemia by obtaining chorionic villous material for DNA analysis sufficiently early in pregnancy to allow termination. This examination is appropriate only if both parents are known to be carriers (beta-thalassaemia minor) and will accept a termination.

Alpha-thalassaemia

Reduced or absent alpha-chain synthesis is common in South-east Asia. There are two alpha gene loci on chromosome 16 and therefore each individual carries four alpha gene alleles.

- If one is deleted, there is no clinical effect.
- If two are deleted, there may be a mild hypochromic anaemia.
- If three are deleted, the patient has haemoglobin H disease.
- If all four are deleted, the baby is stillborn (hydrops fetalis).

Haemoglobin H is a beta-chain tetramer, formed from the excess of beta chains, which is functionally useless, so that patients rely on their low levels of HbA for oxygen transport. Treatment of haemoglobin H disease is similar to that of beta-thalassaemia of intermediate severity, involving folic acid supplementation, transfusion if required and avoidance of iron therapy.

Some considerations specific to anaemia in old age are listed in Box 25.42.

---

i 25.40 Diagnostic features of beta-thalassaemia

Beta-thalassaemia major (homozygotes)

- Profound hypochromic anaemia
- Evidence of severe red cell dysplasia
- Erythroblastosis
- Absence or gross reduction of the amount of haemoglobin A
- Raised levels of haemoglobin F
- Evidence that both parents have thalassaemia minor

Beta-thalassaemia minor (heterozygotes)

- Mild anaemia
- Microcytic hypochromic erythrocytes (not iron-deficient)
- Some target cells
- Punctate basophilia
- Raised haemoglobin A_2 fraction

---

i 25.41 Treatment of beta-thalassaemia major

Problem	Management
Erythropoietic failure	Allogeneic HSCT from HLA-compatible sibling Transfusion to maintain Hb >100 g/L Folic acid 5 mg daily
Iron overload	Iron therapy contraindicated Iron chelation therapy
Splenomegaly causing mechanical problems, excessive transfusion needs	Splenectomy; see Box 25.37

(Hb = haemoglobin; HLA = human leucocyte antigen; HSCT = haematopoietic stem cell transplantation)

25.42 Anaemia in old age

- **Mean haemoglobin**: falls with age in both sexes but remains well within the reference range. When a low haemoglobin does occur, it is generally due to disease.
- **Anaemia can never be considered 'normal' in old age**.
- **Symptoms**: may be subtle and insidious. Cardiovascular features such as dyspnoea and oedema, and cerebral features such as dizziness and apathy, tend to predominate.
- **Ferritin**: if lower than 45 µg/L in older people, is highly predictive of iron deficiency. Conversely, ferritin may be raised by chronic disease and so a normal ferritin does not exclude iron deficiency.
- **Serum iron and transferrin**: fall with age because of the prevalence of other disorders, and are not reliable indicators of deficiency.
- **Most common cause of iron deficiency**: gastrointestinal blood loss.
- **Most common cause of vitamin B$_{12}$ deficiency**: pernicious anaemia, as the prevalence of chronic atrophic gastritis rises in old age.
- **Neuropsychiatric symptoms associated with vitamin B$_{12}$ deficiency**: well-established association but a causal relationship has not been clearly shown. Dementia associated with vitamin B$_{12}$ deficiency in the absence of haematological abnormalities is rare.
- **Anaemia of chronic disease**: frequent in old age because of the rising prevalence of diseases that inhibit iron transport.

Haematological malignancies

Haematological malignancies arise when the processes controlling proliferation or apoptosis are corrupted in blood cells because of acquired mutations in key regulatory genes. If mature differentiated cells are involved, the cells will have a low growth fraction and produce indolent

25.43 Consequences of haematological malignancy in adolescence

- **Tailored management protocols**: the most effective treatment schedules for leukaemia and lymphoma differ between children and adults. Adolescent patients may be most appropriately managed in specialist centres.
- **Psychosocial effects**: adolescents undergoing treatment for haematological malignancy may suffer significant consequences for their schooling and social development, and require support from a multidisciplinary team.
- **'Late effects'**: adolescents who have been treated with chemotherapy and/or radiotherapy in childhood may be at risk of a wide range of complications, depending on the region irradiated, radiation dose and the drugs used. Particularly relevant complications in this age group include short stature, growth hormone deficiency, delayed puberty and cognitive dysfunction affecting schooling (after cranial irradiation). Life-long follow-up is often undertaken to detect and manage these late effects and to deal with consequences such as infertility and second malignancy.

neoplasms, such as the low-grade lymphomas or chronic leukaemias, when patients have an expected survival of many years. In contrast, if more primitive stem or progenitor cells are involved, the cells can have the highest growth fractions of all human neoplasms, producing rapidly progressive, life-threatening illnesses such as the acute leukaemias or high-grade lymphomas. Involvement of pluripotent stem cells produces the most aggressive acute leukaemias. In general, haematological neoplasms are diseases of older patients, the exceptions being acute lymphoblastic leukaemia, which predominantly affects children, and Hodgkin lymphoma, which affects people aged 20–40 years. Management of young patients with haematological malignancy is particularly challenging (Box 25.43).

Leukaemias

Leukaemias are malignant disorders of the white cell compartment, characteristically associated with increased numbers of white cells in the bone marrow and/or peripheral blood. The course of leukaemia may vary from a few days or weeks to many years, depending on the type.

Terminology and classification

Leukaemias are traditionally classified into four main groups:

- acute lymphoblastic leukaemia (ALL)
- acute myeloid leukaemia (AML)
- chronic lymphocytic leukaemia (CLL)
- chronic myeloid leukaemia (CML).

In acute leukaemia, there is proliferation of mutated haematopoietic stem and progenitor cells, with limited accompanying differentiation, leading to an accumulation of blasts, predominantly in the bone marrow, which causes bone marrow failure. In chronic leukaemia, the malignant clone is able to differentiate, resulting in an accumulation of more mature cells. Lymphocytic and lymphoblastic cells are those derived from the lymphoid progenitor cells (B cells and T cells). Myeloid refers to the other lineages: that is, precursors of red cells, granulocytes, monocytes and platelets (see Fig. 25.2).

The diagnosis of leukaemia is usually suspected from an abnormal blood count, often including a raised white count, and is confirmed by examination of the bone marrow. This includes the morphology of the abnormal cells, analysis of cell surface markers (immunophenotyping), clone-specific chromosome abnormalities and molecular changes. These results are incorporated in the World Health Organization (WHO) classification of tumours of haematopoietic and lymphoid tissues; the subclassification of acute leukaemias is shown in Box 25.44. The features in the bone marrow not only provide an accurate diagnosis, but also give valuable prognostic information, increasingly allowing therapy to be tailored to the patient's disease.

25.44 WHO classification of acute leukaemia

Acute myeloid leukaemia (AML) with recurrent genetic abnormalities
- AML with t(8;21)(q22;q22.1), gene product *RUNX1-RUNX1T1*
- AML with inv(16)(p13.1;q22), gene product *CBFB-MYHL1*
- Acute promyelocytic leukaemia t(15;17), gene product *PML-RARA*
- AML with t(9;11)(p21.3;q23.3), gene product *MLLT3-KMT2A*
- AML with t(6;9)(p23;q34), gene product *DEK-NUP214*
- AML with inv(3)(q21.3;q26.2) or t(3;3)(q21.3;q26.2), gene products *GATA2, MECOM*
- AML (megakaryoblastic) with t(1;22)(p13.3;q13.3), gene product *RBM15-MKL1*
- AML with mutated *NPM1*
- AML with biallelic mutations of *CEBPA*

Acute myeloid leukaemia with myelodysplasia-related changes
- e.g. Following a myelodysplastic syndrome

Therapy-related myeloid neoplasms
- e.g. Alkylating agent or topoisomerase II inhibitor

Myeloid sarcoma
Myeloid proliferations related to Down syndrome
Acute myeloid leukaemia not otherwise specified
- e.g. AML with or without differentiation, acute myelomonocytic leukaemia, erythroleukaemia, megakaryoblastic leukaemia

Acute lymphoblastic leukaemia (ALL)
- B-lymphoblastic leukaemia/lymphoma
- T-lymphoblastic leukaemia/lymphoma

25.45 Risk factors for leukaemia

Ionising radiation
- After atomic bombing of Japanese cities (myeloid leukaemia)
- Radiotherapy
- Diagnostic X-rays of the fetus in pregnancy

Cytotoxic drugs
- Especially alkylating agents and topoisomerase II inhibitors (therapy-related myeloid malignancies), usually after a latent period of several years with alkylating agents and a few months to 2 years with topoisomerase II inhibitors
- Industrial exposure to benzene

Retroviruses
- Adult T-cell leukaemia/lymphoma (ATLL) caused by human T-cell lymphotropic virus 1(HTLV-1), most prevalent in Japan, the Caribbean and some areas of Central and South America and Africa

Genetic
- Identical twin of patients with leukaemia
- Down syndrome and certain other genetic disorders

Immunological
- Immune deficiency states (e.g. hypogammaglobulinaemia)

Epidemiology and aetiology

The incidence of leukaemia of all types in the population is approximately 10/10 000 per annum, of which just under half are cases of acute leukaemia. Males are affected more frequently than females, the ratio being about 3:2 in acute leukaemia, 2:1 in chronic lymphocytic leukaemia and 1.3:1 in chronic myeloid leukaemia. Geographical variation in incidence does occur, the most striking being the rarity of chronic lymphocytic leukaemia in Chinese and related races. Acute leukaemia occurs at all ages. Acute lymphoblastic leukaemia shows a peak of incidence in children aged 1–5 years. All forms of acute myeloid leukaemia have their lowest incidence in children and young adult life and there is a striking rise over the age of 50. Chronic leukaemias occur mainly in middle and old age.

The cause of the leukaemia is unknown in the majority of patients. Several risk factors have been identified (Box 25.45).

Acute leukaemia

Mutations in haematopoietic stem cells produce leukaemic stem cells. Proliferation of these cells that do not mature leads to an accumulation of primitive cells that take up more and more marrow space at the expense of the normal haematopoietic cells. Eventually, this proliferation spills into the blood. Acute myeloid leukaemia (AML) is about four times more common than acute lymphoblastic leukaemia (ALL) in adults. In children, the proportions are reversed, the lymphoblastic variety being more common. The clinical features are usually those of bone marrow failure (anaemia, bleeding or infection; pp. 932, 937 and 939).

Investigations

Blood examination usually shows anaemia with a normal or raised MCV. The leucocyte count may vary from as low as 1×10^9/L to as high as 500×10^9/L or more. In the majority of patients, the count is below 100×10^9/L. Severe thrombocytopenia is usual but not invariable. Frequently, blast cells are seen in the blood film, but sometimes the blast cells may be infrequent or absent. A bone marrow examination will confirm the diagnosis. The bone marrow is usually hypercellular, with replacement of normal elements by leukaemic blast cells in varying degrees (but more than 20% of the cells) (Fig. 25.25). The presence of Auer rods in the cytoplasm of blast cells indicates a myeloblastic type of leukaemia. Classification and prognosis are determined by immunophenotyping and chromosome and molecular analysis, as shown in Fig. 25.26.

Management

Ideally, whenever possible, patients with acute leukaemia should be treated within a clinical trial. If a decision to embark on specific therapy has been taken, the patient should be prepared as recommended in Box 25.46. It is unwise to attempt aggressive management of acute leukaemia unless adequate supportive therapy can be provided.

The aim of treatment is to destroy the leukaemic clone of cells without destroying the residual normal stem cell compartment from which repopulation of the haematopoietic tissues will occur. The detail of the schedules for treatments can be found in specialist texts. The drugs most commonly employed are listed in Box 25.47. Generally, if a patient fails to go into remission with induction treatment, alternative drug combinations may be tried, but the outlook is poor unless remission can be achieved. Disease that relapses during treatment or soon after the end of treatment, including after HSCT, carries a poor prognosis and is difficult to treat. The longer after the end of treatment that relapse occurs, the more likely it is that further treatment will be effective. In some patients, alternative palliative chemotherapy, not designed to achieve remission, may be used to curb excessive leucocyte proliferation. Drugs used for this purpose include hydroxycarbamide and mercaptopurine. The aim is to reduce the blast count without inducing bone marrow failure.

Specific therapy

Acute myeloid leukaemia (AML) AML is predominantly a disease of those in old age and many patients are frail. Treatment has become more complex in the recent years and is increasingly tailor-made for AML subgroups defined by genetic abnormalities or persistence of measurable residual disease (MRD). The first decision must be whether or not to give specific treatment to attempt to achieve remission. The most effective remission induction therapy is based around intensive combination chemotherapy. This is generally aggressive, has numerous side-effects and may not be appropriate for the very old or patients with serious comorbidities. In these patients, supportive treatment can effect considerable improvement in well-being, but there remains considerable unmet need. Low-intensity chemotherapy, such as low-dose cytosine arabinoside or azacitidine, is frequently used in older and frailer patients, but this induces remission in less than 20% of patients. Recently, the addition of the BCL-2 inhibitor venetoclax to cytosine and azacitdine has shown improved overall survival, especially the combination with azacitidine (Fig. 25.27).

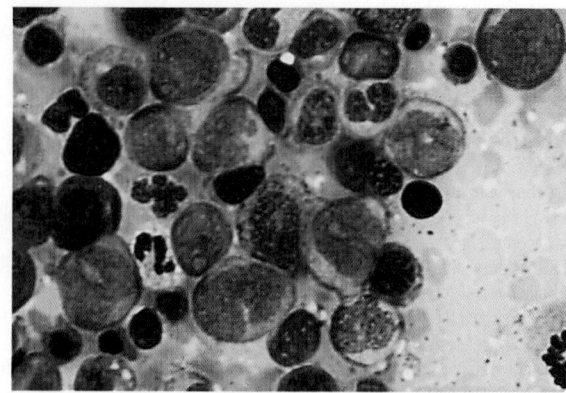

Fig. 25.25 Acute myeloid leukaemia. Bone marrow aspirate showing infiltration with large blast cells, which display nuclear folding and prominent nucleoli.

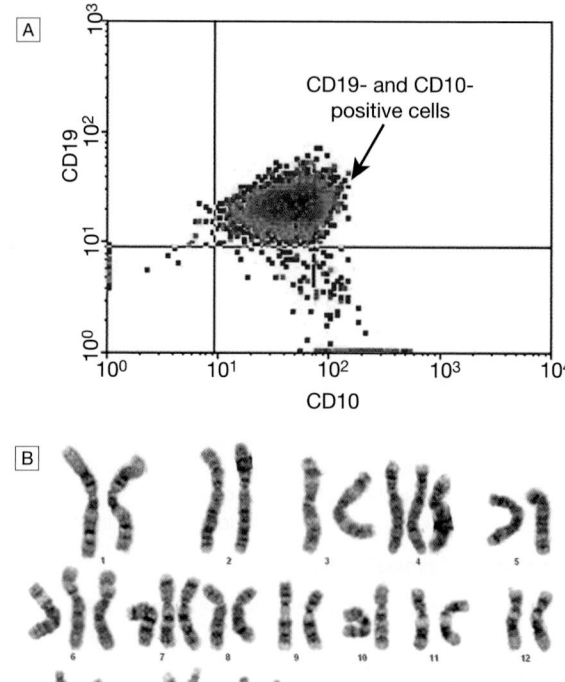

Fig. 25.26 Investigation of acute lymphoblastic leukaemia (ALL). $\boxed{A}$ Flow cytometric analysis of blasts labelled with the fluorescent antibodies anti-CD19 (*y* axis) and anti-CD10 (*x* axis). ALL blasts are positive for both CD19 and CD10 (arrow). $\boxed{B}$ Chromosome analysis (karyotype) of blasts showing additional chromosomes X, 4, 6, 7, 14, 18 and 21.

There are currently three phases of specific treatment for AML:

- *Remission induction*. In this phase, a fraction of the tumour is killed by combinations of chemotherapy drugs. The standard of care for remission induction in AML is daunorubicin with cytosine arabinoside given for 7–10 days in two cycles. Patients with a good or standard risk karyotype, including normal karyotype, benefit from the addition of the antibody-drug conjugate gemtuzumab ozagomicin which targets CD33 on the AML cell and delivers the DNA damaging drug calicheamicin directly into the cell (see Fig. 25.27), while AML with the *FLT3-ITD* mutation benefits from the addition of the

25.46 Preparation for specific therapy in acute leukaemia

- Existing infections identified and treated (e.g. urinary tract infection, oral candidiasis, dental, gingival and skin infections)
- Screen for COVID-19
- Anaemia corrected by red cell concentrate transfusion
- Thrombocytopenic bleeding controlled by platelet transfusions
- If possible, central venous catheter (e.g. Hickman line) inserted to facilitate access to the circulation for delivery of chemotherapy, fluids, blood products and other supportive drugs
- Tumour lysis risk assessed and prevention started: fluids with allopurinol or rasburicase
- Therapeutic regimen carefully explained to the patient and informed consent obtained
- Consideration of entry into clinical trial

i **25.47 Drugs commonly used in the treatment of acute leukaemia**

Phase	Acute lymphoblastic leukaemia	Acute myeloid leukaemia
Induction	Vincristine (IV) Prednisolone (oral) L-Asparaginase (IM) Daunorubicin (IV) Methotrexate (intrathecal) Imatinib (oral)*	Daunorubicin (IV) Cytarabine (IV) Etoposide (IV and oral) Gentuzumab ozogamicin (IV) All-*trans* retinoic acid (ATRA) (oral) Arsenic trioxide (ATO) (IV)
Consolidation	Daunorubicin (IV) Cytarabine (IV) Etoposide (IV) Methotrexate (IV) Imatinib (oral)*	Cytarabine (IV) Amsacrine (IV) Mitoxantrone (IV)
Maintenance	Prednisolone (oral) Vincristine (IV) Mercaptopurine (oral) Methotrexate (oral) Imatinib (oral)*	
Relapse	Fludarabine (IV) Cytarabine (IV) Idarubicin (IV)	Fludarabine (IV) Cytarabine (IV) Arsenic trioxide (ATO) (IV) Idarubicin (IV)

*If Philadelphia chromosome-positive.
(IM = intramuscular; IV = intravenous)

FLT3 inhibitor midostaurin (see Fig. 25.27). The patient goes through a period of severe bone marrow hypoplasia lasting 3–4 weeks and requires intensive support and inpatient care from a specially trained multidisciplinary team. The aim is to achieve remission, a state in which the blood counts return to normal and the marrow blast count is less than 5%. Quality of life is highly dependent on achieving remission, hence remission induction is the preferred therapy for all patients who are considered fit enough to undergo such treatment.

- *Remission consolidation*. If remission has been achieved, residual disease is attacked by therapy during the consolidation phase. This consists of a number of courses of chemotherapy, most commonly 1–2 courses of high-dose cytosine arabinoside, again resulting in periods of marrow hypoplasia. In poor-prognosis AML, defined by poor risk cytogenetic/molecular genetic abnormalities or persistent MRD, this may include allogeneic HSCT.
- *Remission maintenance*. Maintenance therapy has only recently become an effective tool for some patients with AML compared to its long-established role in ALL. Patients not undergoing allogeneic HSCT with *FLT3* mutated AML receive one year of maintenance with midostaurin and other patients may benefit from azacitidine.

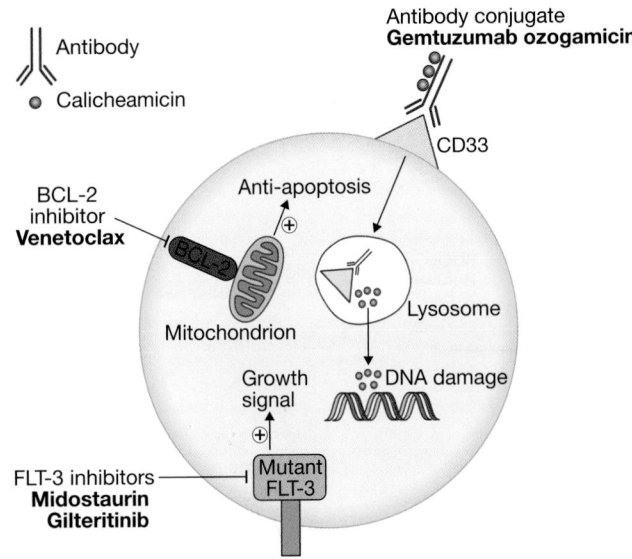

Fig. 25.27 Targeted therapies for acute myeloid leukaemia (AML). Small molecule midostaurin inhibits mutant FLT3 molecules and is used in combination with chemotherapy. Gilteritinib inhibits mutant FLT3 and is used on its own for relapsed patients. Venetoclax inhibits BCL-2 and so induces apoptosis; it is used with the drug azacitidine in older, frailer patients. Gemtuzumab ozogamicin is a conjugate of an antibody and a chemotherapy agent. The antibody binds to CD33 on the cell surface; antibody and CD33 are internalised and the chemotherapy agent calicheamicin causes DNA damage. (BCL-2 = B-cell lymphoma 2; FLT-3 = FMS-like tyrosine kinase)

Relapsed AML carries a poor prognosis. Increasingly, this is pre-empted by monitoring MRD and intervening before haematological relapse occurs. However, the aim is to attempt to achieve further remission and deliver an allogeneic HSCT, if possible.

Acute promyelocytic leukaemia (APML) A subtype of AML, called acute promyelocytic leukaemia (APML), is characterised by a block in differentiation of malignant promyelocytes. These cells accumulate and lead to bone marrow failure and a tendency to severe bleeding, including into the CNS, because of enhanced fibrinolysis and DIC induced by the procoagulant proteins in the malignant cells, e.g. tPA and uPA. This leukaemia is caused by a translocation of genes on chromosomes 15 (*PML*) and 17 (*RARA*) producing the *PML-RARA* rearrangement which drives the leukaemia. APML carries the best prognosis of all AML if the patient survives the initial bleeding risk. Furthermore, low risk cases can be treated with a non-chemotherapy regimen of differentiation therapy with all-trans-retinoic acid (ATRA) and arsenic trioxide (ATO). Higher-risk patients are treated with ATRA and anthracycline-based chemotherapy. The prognosis is excellent with 90% cure rate for patients receiving treatment. However, the early death rate from bleeding remains problematic and intensive supportive care and immediate introduction of ATRA therapy is vital to prevent this.

Acute lymphoblastic leukaemia (ALL) This is predominantly a disease of childhood with a mean age of 2–4 years. However, it also occurs in adulthood where it is more difficult to treat and carries a poorer prognosis. Once again there are three phases of therapy with treatment tailor-made to risk groups based on genetic abnormaliites and levels of MRD:

- *Remission induction* – As with AML the aim is to achieve remission using a combination of chemotherapy drugs given over a 4-week period. The drugs commonly used are dexamethasone, vincristine, anthracyclines, methotrexate, mercaptopurine and asparaginase. Induction therapy in ALL is often less damaging and better tolerated than AML, however, the high dosage of steroids coupled with neutropenia carries a high risk of infections, including fungal

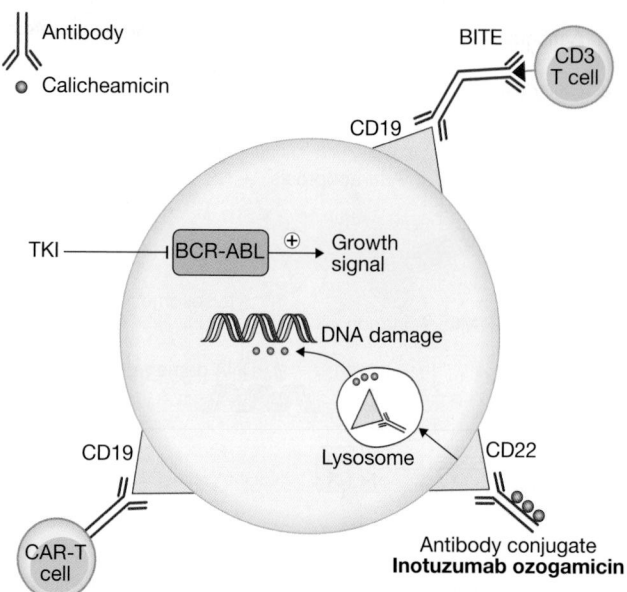

Fig. 25.28 Targeted therapies for acute lymphoblastic leukaemia (ALL). Chimeric antigen receptor T (CAR-T) cells and bi-specific T-cell engager (BITE) both promote T-cell killing of the ALL cell. CAR-T as described in Fig. 25.17 and BITE by using an antibody that can simultaneously bind to a leukaemia cell and a T cell to bring them together. TKIs include imatinib, dasatinib and ponatinib. Inotuzumab–ozogamicin is a conjugate of an antibody and a chemotherapy agent. The antibody binds to CD22 on the cell surface; antibody and CD22 are internalised and the chemotherapy agent calicheamicin causes DNA damage. (TKI = tyrosine kinase inhibitor)

infections. Adult patients are more likely to have a poor-risk genetic abnormality. A *BCR-ABL* rearrangement occurs in about 25% of adult patients and TKI therapy, e.g. dasatinib, is included with the chemotherapy (Fig. 25.28). Once again, old and frail patients tolerate treatment much less well and treatment is modified accordingly. Adolescent and young adult patients require special support and have been shown to do better with children's protocols than adult protocols.

- *Remission consolidation* – The consolidation phase builds on the remission by further decreasing the leukaemic burden. The intensity of consolidation depends on the level of MRD at the end of remission induction and includes blocks of chemotherapy drugs. Allogeneic HSCT is used as consolidation for fit adults with ALL and a suitable donor, but rarely in children unless they relapse.
- Remission maintenance – If the patient is still in remission after the consolidation phase for ALL, a period of maintenance therapy is given, with the individual as an outpatient and treatment consisting of a repeating cycle of drug administration. This may extend for up to 3 years if relapse does not occur. In ALL prophylactic treatment to the central nervous system is required, as this is a sanctuary site where standard therapy does not penetrate. This usually consists of a combination of cranial irradiation, intrathecal chemotherapy and high-dose methotrexate, which crosses the blood–brain barrier. Such therapy is integrated into the induction, remission and consolidation phases of therapy

Relapsed ALL is a complex area and ranges from positive MRD, isolated CNS or testicular relapse to full blown haematological relapse. The aim is once again to achieve further remission and frequently to deliver allogeneic HSCT. Newer therapies for relapse include blinatumomab, a bi-specific antibody against CD19 and CD3 to promote T-cell killing (BITE – bi-specific antibody T-cell engager), inotuzumab ozogamicin (which targets CD22 and delivers calicheamicin directly into the cell; see Fig. 25.28), nelarabine in T-cell ALL and CAR-T-cell therapy (see Fig. 25.17). Some long-term cures have been achieved with these therapies.

Supportive therapy

Aggressive and potentially curative therapy, which involves periods of severe bone marrow failure, would not be possible without appropriate supportive care. The following problems commonly arise.

Anaemia Anaemia is treated with red cell concentrate transfusions.

Bleeding Thrombocytopenic bleeding requires platelet transfusions, unless the bleeding is trivial. Recent trials have confirmed that in acute leukaemia prophylactic platelet transfusion should be given to maintain the platelet count above 10×10^9/L. Coagulation abnormalities occur and need accurate diagnosis and treatment, especially in APML (see above).

Infection So-called neutropenic sepsis is a major complication of acute leukaemia and its treatment. Every leukaemia centre will have a written definition and management policy for this common event. UK NICE guidelines define neutropenic sepsis as fever (>38°C) lasting over 1 hour in a neutropenic patient (neutrophils <0.5×10^9/l) or with other signs or symptoms of significant sepsis (see also p. 198). Parenteral broad-spectrum antibiotic therapy is essential. Empirical therapy is given according to the perceived severity of the sepsis illness and local bacteriological resistance patterns. Increasingly, low-risk cases of neutropenic sepsis are treated with single antibiotics, e.g. piperacillin/tazobactam. Higher-risk cases are managed with regimens such as a combination of an aminoglycoside (e.g. gentamicin) and a broad-spectrum penicillin (e.g. piperacillin/tazobactam) or a single-agent beta-lactam (e.g. meropenem). The organisms most commonly associated with severe neutropenic sepsis are Gram-positive bacteria, such as *Staphylococcus aureus* and *Staphylococcus epidermidis*, which are present on the skin and gain entry via cannulae and central lines. Gram-negative infections often originate from the gastro-intestinal tract, which is affected by chemotherapy-induced mucositis; organisms such as *Escherichia coli*, *Pseudomonas* and *Klebsiella* spp. are likely to cause rapid clinical deterioration and must be covered with initially empirical antibiotic therapy. Gram-positive infection may require vancomycin or teicoplanin therapy. If fever has not resolved after 3–5 days and there is evidence for a disseminated fungal infection on CT scans or sensitive blood tests, empirical antifungal therapy (e.g. a liposomal amphotericin B preparation, voriconazole or caspofungin) is added.

Patients with ALL are susceptible to infection with *Pneumocystis jirovecii* (Ch. 14), which causes a severe pneumonia. Prophylaxis with co-trimoxazole is given during chemotherapy. Diagnosis may require either induced sputum, bronchoalveolar lavage or open lung biopsy. Treatment is with high-dose co-trimoxazole, initially intravenously, changing to oral treatment as soon as possible.

Oral and pharyngeal *Candida* infection is common. Fluconazole is effective for the treatment of established local infection and for prophylaxis against systemic candidaemia. Prophylaxis against other systemic fungal infections including *Aspergillus*, for example itraconazole or posaconazole, is usual practice during high-risk intensive chemotherapy. This is often used along with sensitive markers of early fungal infection to guide treatment initiation (a 'pre-emptive approach').

For systemic fungal infection with *Candida* or aspergillosis, intravenous liposomal amphotericin, caspofungin or voriconazole is required for up to 3 weeks. In systemic *Candida* infection intravenous catheters should be removed.

Reactivation of herpes simplex infection (Ch. 13) occurs frequently around the lips and nose during ablative therapy for acute leukaemia, and is treated with aciclovir. This may also be prescribed prophylactically to patients with a history of cold sores or elevated antibody titres to herpes simplex. Herpes zoster manifesting as chickenpox or, after reactivation, as shingles (Ch. 13) should be treated in the early stage with high-dose aciclovir, as it can be fatal in immunocompromised patients.

The value of isolation facilities, such as laminar flow rooms, is debatable but may contribute to staff awareness of careful reverse barrier nursing practice. The isolation can be psychologically stressful for the patient.

Metabolic problems Frequent monitoring of fluid balance and renal, hepatic and haemostatic function is necessary. Patients are often severely anorexic and diarrhoea is common as a consequence of the side-effects of therapy; they may find drinking difficult and hence require intravenous fluids and electrolytes. Renal toxicity occurs with some antibiotics (e.g. aminoglycosides) and antifungal agents (amphotericin). Cellular breakdown during induction therapy (tumour lysis syndrome; p. 142) releases intracellular ions and nucleic acid breakdown products, causing hyperkalaemia, hyperuricaemia, hyperphosphataemia and hypocalcaemia. This may lead to renal failure. Allopurinol and intravenous hydration are given to try to prevent this. In patients at high risk of tumour lysis syndrome, e.g. acute leukaemia with a white cell count of more than 100×10^9/L, prophylactic rasburicase (a recombinant urate oxidase enzyme) is used. Occasionally, dialysis may be required.

Psychological problems Psychological support is a key aspect of care. Patients should be kept informed, and their questions answered and fears allayed as far as possible. A multidisciplinary approach to patient care involves input from many services, including psychology. Key members of the team include haematology specialist nurses, who are often the central point of contact for patients and families throughout the illness.

Haematopoietic stem cell transplantation (HSCT)

This is described on page 945. In patients with high-risk acute leukaemia, allogeneic HSCT can improve 5-year survival from 20% to around 50%. Reduced-intensity conditioning has allowed HSCT to be delivered to a higher proportion of patients with acute leukaemias, up to the age of about 65 years. Improved knowledge of the biology of leukaemia alters the definition of high risk. For example, patients with AML with a normal karyotype and isolated *NPM1* gene mutations are considered good risk and are not routinely transplanted in first remission. However, otherwise similar patients with isolated *FLT3-ITD* mutations are poor risk and considered for transplant in first remission.

Prognosis

Without treatment, the median survival of patients with acute leukaemia is about 5 weeks. This may be extended to a number of months with supportive treatment. Patients who achieve remission with specific therapy have a better outlook. Around 80% of adult patients under 60 years of age with ALL or AML achieve remission, although remission rates are lower for older patients. However, the relapse rate continues to be high. Box 25.48 shows the survival in ALL and AML and the influence of prognostic features. The level of detectable leukaemia cells after induction therapy, called measurable residual disease (MRD), can be a powerful prognostic tool and is now used routinely in some forms of acute leukaemia (e.g. ALL and AML with NPM1 mutation) to determine subsequent consolidation therapy.

Advances in treatment have led to steady improvement in survival from acute leukaemia. Some 90% of children with ALL are cured and about 50% of adults aged less than 60 years are cured from AML. As discussed above, APML has a 90% cure rate. Prognosis remains poor in most other groups of patients with acute leukaemias, especially in old age. Current trials aim to improve survival, especially in standard and poor-risk disease, with strategies that include better use of allogeneic HSCT, better ability to predict relapse using MRD and new targeted therapies (see Figs. 25.27 and 25.28).

Chronic myeloid leukaemia

Chronic myeloid leukaemia (CML) is a myeloproliferative stem cell disorder resulting in proliferation of all haematopoietic lineages, but manifesting predominantly in the granulocytic series. Maturation of cells proceeds fairly normally. The disease occurs chiefly between the ages of 30 and 80 years, with a peak incidence at 55 years. It is rare, with an annual incidence in the UK of 1.8/100 000, and accounts for 15% of all leukaemias. It is found in all races.

	25.48 Outcome in adult acute leukaemia	
Disease/risk	**Risk factors**	**5-year overall survival**
Acute myeloid leukaemia (AML)		
Good risk	Promyelocytic leukaemia t(15;17)	90%
	t(8;21)	65%
	inv(16) or t(16;16)	70%
Poor risk	Cytogenetic abnormalities −5, −7, del 5q, abn(3q), complex (>5)	21%
Intermediate risk	AML with none of the above	48%
Acute lymphoblastic leukaemia (ALL)		
Poor risk	Philadelphia chromosome High white count >100 × 10⁹/L Abnormal short arm of chromosome 11 t(1;19)	20%
Standard	ALL with none of the above	37%

The defining characteristic of CML is the chromosome abnormality known as the Philadelphia (Ph) chromosome. This is a shortened chromosome 22 resulting from a reciprocal translocation of material with chromosome 9. The break on chromosome 22 occurs in the breakpoint cluster region (BCR). The fragment from chromosome 9 that joins the BCR carries the *abl* oncogene, which forms a fusion gene with the remains of the BCR. This *BCR-ABL* fusion gene codes for a 210 kDa protein with tyrosine kinase activity, which plays a causative role in the disease as an oncogene (p. 132), influencing cellular proliferation, differentiation and survival and is a target for very effective tyrosine kinase inhibitor (TKI) therapy (Fig. 25.29 and see Box 25.21). In some patients in whom conventional chromosomal analysis does not detect a Ph chromosome, the BCR-ABL gene product is detectable by molecular techniques.

Natural history

The disease has three phases:

- *A chronic phase*, in which the disease is responsive to treatment and is easily controlled, which used to last 3–5 years. With the introduction of the tyrosine kinase inhibitors (TKI) (Box 25.49), this phase has been prolonged to encompass a normal life expectancy in many patients.
- *An accelerated phase* (not always seen), in which disease control becomes more difficult.
- *Blast crisis*, in which the disease transforms into an acute leukaemia, either myeloblastic (70%) or lymphoblastic (30%), which is relatively refractory to treatment. This is the cause of death in the majority of patients; survival is therefore dictated by the timing of blast crisis, which cannot be predicted. Prior to TKI therapy (see below), approximately 10% of patients per year would transform; the transformation rate has been reduced to 0.5%–2.5% per year with TKI therapy.

Clinical features

Symptoms at presentation may include lethargy, weight loss, abdominal discomfort, gout and sweating, but about 25% of patients are asymptomatic at diagnosis. Splenomegaly is present in 90%; in about 10% the enlargement is massive, extending to over 15 cm below the costal margin. A friction rub may be heard in cases of splenic infarction. Hepatomegaly occurs in about 50%. Lymphadenopathy is unusual.

Investigations

FBC results are variable between patients. There is usually a normocytic, normochromic anaemia. The leucocyte count can vary from 10 to 600 × 10⁹/L. In about one-third of patients, there is a very high platelet

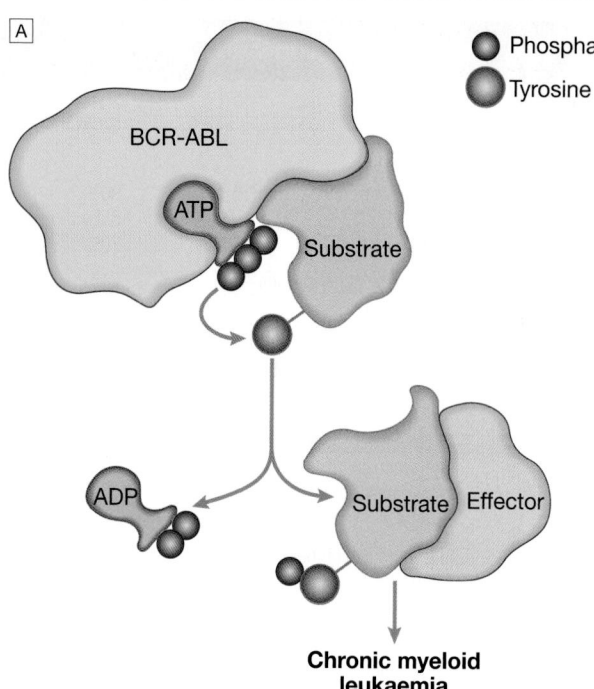

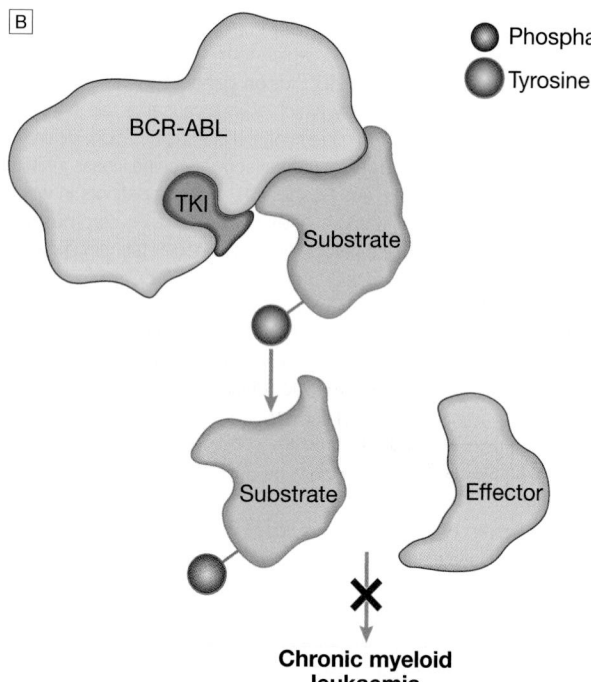

Fig. 25.29 Mode of action in tyrosine kinase inhibition of BCR-ABL.
[A] Untreated CML. The BCR-ABL protein acts as 'rogue' tyrosine kinase. It phosphorylates tyrosine residues on substrate molecules, and hence activates these molecules, by transferring phosphate groups from ATP. In turn these molecules activate down-stream effector molecules that cause CML. [B] Tyrosine kinase inhibitor (TKI) treatment (imatinib, dasatinib, nilotinib, posatinib, bosutanib). These molecules bind to the tyrosine kinase domain of BCR-ABL and block the phosphorylation process and hence inhibit the downstream effector pathways, so reversing the process causing CML. (CML = chronic myeloid leukaemia)

count, sometimes as high as 2000×10^9/L. In the blood film, the full range of granulocyte precursors, from myeloblasts to mature neutrophils, is seen but the predominant cells are neutrophils and myelocytes (see Fig. 25.3). Myeloblasts usually constitute less than 10% of all white cells. There is often an absolute increase in eosinophils and basophils,

	25.49 Tyrosine kinase inhibition in chronic myeloid leukaemia
Agents	

First-line
- Imatinib
- Nilotinib
- Dasatinib

Second-line
- Imatinib
- Nilotinib
- Dasatinib
- Bosutinib
- Ponatinib*

Outcomes
- 90% achieve complete cytogenetic response
- Responses faster with nilotinib and dasatinib
- Median survival comparable to normal population

*For patients with T315I kinase domain mutations use ponatinib.

and nucleated red cells are common. If the disease progresses through an accelerated phase, the percentage of more primitive cells increases. Blast transformation is characterised by a dramatic increase in the number of circulating blasts. In patients with thrombocytosis, very high platelet counts may persist during treatment, in both chronic and accelerated phases, but usually drop dramatically at blast transformation. Basophilia tends to increase as the disease progresses.

Bone marrow should be obtained to confirm the diagnosis and phase of disease by morphology, chromosome analysis to demonstrate the presence of the Ph chromosome, and RNA analysis to demonstrate the presence of the BCR-ABL gene product. Blood LDH is elevated and uric acid may be high due to increased cell breakdown.

Management

Chronic phase

There are now five available tyrosine kinase inhibitors (TKIs) for the treatment of CML (see Box 25.49). These specifically inhibit BCR-ABL tyrosine kinase activity. Imatinib, nilotinib and dasatinib are recommended as first-line therapy in chronic phase CML; they usually normalise the blood count within a month and within 3–6 months produce complete cytogenetic response (disappearance of the Ph chromosome) in some 90% of patients. Patients are monitored by 3-monthly real-time quantitative polymerase chain reaction (PCR) for BCR-ABL mRNA transcripts in blood. The aim is to reduce the BCR-ABL transcript levels by 3–5 logs from baseline and this is called major molecular response (MR3–MR5). A proportion of patients achieve a complete molecular response where the transcripts are not detectable by PCR. Up to 50% of patients with a complete or major molecular response may be able to discontinue TKI therapy. For those failing to respond or who lose their response and progress on first-line therapy, options include switching to a different TKI (see Box 25.49). Some patients develop detectable mutations in the BCR-ABL gene, which causes resistance to one or more of the TKIs. The *T315I* mutation is particularly problematic as this causes wide-ranging resistance, but the third-generation TKI ponatinib can be effective. Allogeneic HSCT (p. 945) is now reserved for patients who fail TKI therapy. Hydroxycarbamide and interferon were previously used for control of disease. Hydroxycarbamide is still useful in palliative situations and interferon is used in women planning pregnancy.

Accelerated phase and blast crisis

Management is more difficult. For patients in accelerated phase, TKI therapy is indicated, most commonly with nilotinib or dasatinib. When blast transformation occurs, the type of blast cell should be determined. Response to appropriate acute leukaemia treatment (see Box 25.49) is better if disease is lymphoblastic rather than myeloblastic. Second- or third-generation TKIs such as dasatinib are used in combination with chemotherapy to try to achieve remission. In younger and fitter patients

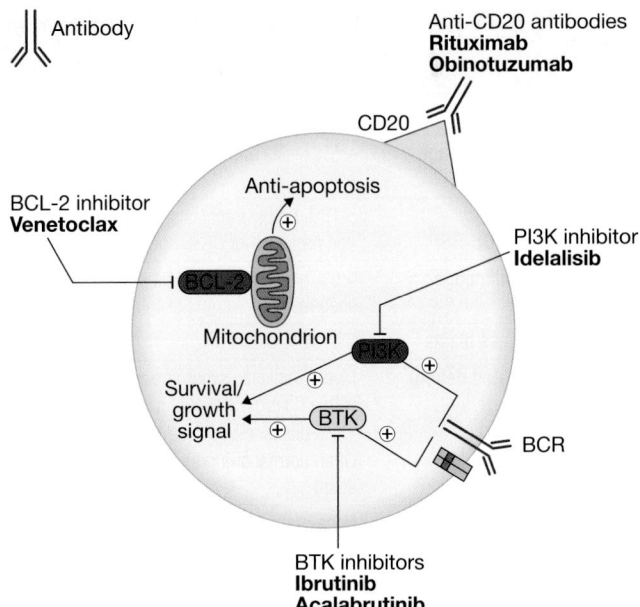

Fig. 25.30 Targeted therapies for chronic lymphocytic leukaemia (CLL). CLL cells are 'addicted' to stimulation of the B-cell receptor (BCR), which is surface immunoglobulin. This pathway can now be inhibited by drugs that block the downstream effector pathways of BCR involving BTK and PI3K molecules. CLL cells also depend on anti-apoptosis signals, especially increased BCL-2. Venetoclax inhibits BCL-2 and induces apoptosis. The anti-CD20 'naked' antibodies are used with chemotherapy to enhance CLL cell killing. (BCR = B-cell receptor; BTK = Bruton's tyrosine kinase; PI3K = phosphatidylinositol-3-kinase)

an allogeneic HSCT is appropriate therapy if a return to chronic phase is achieved. Hydroxycarbamide can be an effective single agent and low-dose cytarabine can also be used palliatively in older patients.

Chronic lymphocytic leukaemia

Chronic lymphocytic leukaemia (CLL) is the most common variety of leukaemia, accounting for 30% of cases. The male-to-female ratio is 2:1 and the median age at presentation is 65–70 years. CLL is characterised by the clonal expansion of small mature-looking B cells. Failure to apoptose because of overexpression of BCL-2 and in some cases mutations in *TP53* leads to an ever-increasing accumulation of immuno-incompetent leukaemic B cells. This is to the detriment of immune function and normal bone marrow haematopoiesis. CLL cells are dependent on abnormal and persistent signalling through the B-cell receptor (BCR) pathway. Drugs that can inhibit these pathways are now available and show great promise (Fig. 25.30).

Clinical features

The onset is usually insidious. Indeed, in around 70% of patients the diagnosis is made incidentally on a routine FBC. Presenting problems may be anaemia, infections, painless lymphadenopathy, and systemic symptoms such as night sweats or weight loss; these more often occur later in the course of the disease or in disease that is advanced at presentation.

Investigations

The diagnosis is based on the peripheral blood findings of a mature lymphocytosis (>5 × 10⁹/L) with characteristic morphology and cell surface markers. Immunophenotyping reveals the lymphocytes to be monoclonal B cells expressing the B-cell antigens CD19 and CD23, with either kappa or lambda immunoglobulin light chains and, characteristically, an aberrant T-cell antigen CD5. On flow cytometry, some people are shown to have circulating CLL cells at a level less than 5 × 10⁹/L. This is known

as monoclonal B lymphocytosis of uncertain significance (MBL). Such patients progress to CLL at a rate of 1% per year.

Other useful investigations in CLL include a reticulocyte count and a direct Coombs test, as autoimmune haemolytic anaemia may occur (p. 958). Serum immunoglobulin levels should be estimated to establish the degree of hypogammaglobulinaemia, which is common and progressive. Bone marrow examination by aspirate and trephine is not essential for the diagnosis of CLL, but may be helpful in difficult cases, for prognosis (patients with diffuse marrow involvement have a poorer prognosis) and to monitor response to therapy. The main prognostic factor is stage of disease (Box 25.50); however, loss of chromosome 17p or mutation in the *TP53* gene, which resides at this genetic locus, is a powerful prognostic marker of poor outcome and predictor of response to therapy. A mutation in *TP53* is present in <10% of patients at presentation, but rises to 30% of cases at relapse. This test should be performed in all patients prior to the initiation of therapy.

Management

No specific treatment is required for most clinical stage A patients, unless progression occurs. The patient should be offered clear information about CLL and be reassured about the indolent nature of the disease, as the diagnosis of leukaemia inevitably causes anxiety.

Treatment is required only if there is evidence of bone marrow failure, massive or progressive lymphadenopathy or splenomegaly, systemic symptoms such as weight loss or night sweats, a rapidly increasing lymphocyte count, autoimmune haemolytic anaemia or thrombocytopenia. Initial therapy for those requiring treatment (progressive stage A and stages B and C) is based on the age and fitness of the patient and the *TP53* mutation status. For patients who are under 70 years, fit and *TP53* mutation-negative, fludarabine in combination with the alkylating agent cyclophosphamide and the anti-CD20 monoclonal antibody rituximab (FCR) is standard care. For older, less fit patients, rituximab is combined with gentler chemotherapy: bendamustine or oral chlorambucil. A more potent anti-CD20 antibody, obinutuzumab, produces better responses in combination with chlorambucil than rituximab.

Ibrutinib inhibits Bruton's tyrosine kinase and idelalisib inhibits PI3 kinase, both components of the BCR pathway (see Fig. 25.30). Ibrutinib and idelalisib are licensed for relapsed CLL, but are effective in *TP53*-mutated disease at all stages. Ibrutinib is first-line standard of care in *TP53*-mutated CLL. CLL cells are resistant to apoptosis and express increased levels of anti-apoptotic proteins, including BCL-2. Venetoclax is an inhibitor of BCL-2 and is so effective at killing CLL cells that it frequently causes tumour lysis syndrome when first administered. Venetoclax is licensed in combination with obinutuzumab for the treatment of adult patients with previously untreated CLL and is attractive as it is given for a fixed period of two years. Venetoclax can also be used for patients with *TP53* mutation or who have failed previous therapy. Bone marrow failure or autoimmune cytopenias may respond to glucocorticoid treatment or rituximab.

Supportive care is increasingly required in progressive disease, such as transfusions for symptomatic anaemia or thrombocytopenia, prompt treatment of infections and, for some patients with hypogammaglobulinaemia, immunoglobulin replacement. Radiotherapy may be used for lymphadenopathy that is causing discomfort or local obstruction and for symptomatic splenomegaly. Splenectomy may be required to improve low blood counts due to autoimmune destruction or to hypersplenism and can relieve massive splenomegaly.

Prognosis

The majority of clinical stage A patients have a normal life expectancy, but patients with advanced CLL are more likely to die from their disease or infectious complications. Survival is influenced by other prognostic features of the leukaemia, particularly *TP53* mutation status, and traditionally whether patients can tolerate and respond to fludarabine-based treatment. In those able to be treated with chemotherapy and rituximab, 90% are alive 4 years later. The newer agents may replace and surpass immunochemotherapy as first-line therapy. As in other haematological malignancies the presence of MRD is prognostically important. Ibrutinib and especially venetoclax are more likely to produce an MRD negative state. Rarely, CLL transforms to an aggressive high-grade lymphoma, called Richter's transformation.

Prolymphocytic leukaemia

Prolymphocytic leukaemia (PLL) is a form of chronic leukaemia found mainly in males over the age of 60 years; 25% of cases are of T cell origin. There is typically massive splenomegaly with little lymphadenopathy and a very high leucocyte count, often in excess of 400×10^9/L. Effusions and involvement of skin are well recognized. The characteristic cell is a large lymphocyte with a prominent nucleolus. Treatment is generally unsuccessful and the prognosis very poor. Leukapharesis, splenectomy and chemotherapy may be tried. The anti-CD52 antibody alemtuzumab, when given intravenously, has produced responses in some 90% of patients with T-PLL. Younger patients who respond to treatment may be considered for allogeneic HSCT.

Hairy cell leukaemia

This is a rare chronic B-cell lymphoproliferative disorder. The male-to-female ratio is 6:1 and the median age at diagnosis is 50 years. Presenting symptoms are general ill health and recurrent infections. Splenomegaly occurs in 90% but lymph node enlargement is unusual.

Severe neutropenia, monocytopenia and the characteristic hairy cells in the blood and bone marrow are typical. These cells usually have a B-lymphocyte immunotype, but they also characteristically express CD25 and CD103. Recently, all patients with hairy cell leukaemia have been found to have a mutation in the *BRAF* gene and this may become a therapeutic target. Chemotherapy treatments such as cladribine and deoxycoformycin can produce long-lasting remissions.

Myelodysplastic syndromes

Myelodysplastic syndromes (MDSs) constitute a group of clonal haematopoietic disorders with the common features of ineffective blood cell production and a tendency to progress to AML. As such, they are pre-leukaemic and represent genetic steps in the development of leukaemia. These genetic abnormalities have been identified and are increasingly present with age as a manifestation of clonal haematopoiesis, occurring in about 20% of patients over the age of 80. Blood counts are normal (clonal haematopoiesis of indeterminate potential, CHIP), but there is an increased risk of developing MDS, AML or non-haematological disease such as coronary artery disease. The common CHIP gene mutations include *DNMT3a*, *TET2* and *ASXL1*.

Some 80% of patients with MDS have one or more acquired mutations in specific genes and these are now routinely identified by multi-gene next generation sequencing (NGS) using a so-called 'myeloid gene panel'. Some are associated with specific phenotypes of MDS, e.g. 80% of cases with ring sideroblasts have a mutation in the splice factor gene *SF3B1*. Others have prognostic significance, e.g. *TP53* or two or

i	25.51 WHO classification of myelodysplastic syndromes (MDS)	
Disease		**Bone marrow findings**
MDS with single-lineage dysplasia		<5% blasts and single-lineage dysplasia only
MDS with ring sideroblasts (MDS-RS)		>15% ring sideroblasts, or 6%–14% and presence of *SF3B1* gene mutation
MDS with multilineage dysplasia		<5% blasts and dysplasia in two or more lineages
MDS with excess blasts		5%–19% blasts
MDS with isolated del(5q)		Myelodysplastic syndrome associated with a del(5q) cytogenetic abnormality <5% blasts Often normal or increased blood platelet count
MDS, unclassifiable		None of the above or inadequate material

more mutations carry a poor prognosis. Chromosome analysis frequently reveals abnormalities, particularly of chromosome 5 or 7.

MDS presents with consequences of bone marrow failure (anaemia, recurrent infections or bleeding), usually in older people (median age at diagnosis is 73 years). The overall incidence is 4/100000 in the population, rising to more than 30/100000 in the over-seventies. The blood film is characterised by cytopenias and abnormal-looking (dysplastic) blood cells, including macrocytic red cells and hypogranular neutrophils with nuclear hyper- or hyposegmentation. The bone marrow is hypercellular, with dysplastic changes in at least 10% of cells of one or more cell lines. Blast cells may be increased but do not reach the 20% level that indicates acute leukaemia. The WHO classification of MDS is shown in Box 25.51.

Prognosis

The natural history of MDS is progressive worsening of dysplasia leading to fatal bone marrow failure or progression to AML in 30% of cases. The time to progression varies (from months to years) with the subtype of MDS, being slowest in MDS with ring sideroblasts and single-lineage dysplasia and most rapid in MDS with excess blasts. The revised International Prognostic Scoring System (IPSS-R) predicts clinical outcome based on karyotype and cytopenias in blood, as well as percentage of bone marrow blasts (Box 25.52). There are five prognostic groups. The median survival for low-risk patients (IPSS-R very low and low) is 5–9 years, that for the intermediate group is 3 years and that for high-risk patients (IPSS-R high and very high) is 1–1.5 years.

Management

For the vast majority of patients who are in old age, the disease is incurable, and supportive care with red cell and platelet transfusions is the mainstay of treatment. A trial of erythropoiesis stimulating agents (ESA) is recommended in some patients with low-risk MDS (IPSS-R very low, low and intermediate) to improve haemoglobin. Responders have better quality of life, lower risk of progression to AML and possibly better overall survival. Granulocyte colony stimulating factor (G-CSF) is recommended for short-term use in neutropenic patients with active infection. A rare subtype called MDS with isolated del(5q) responds well to the immunomodulatory drug lenalidomide, with two-thirds of anaemic patients becoming transfusion-independent for up to 2 years. Allogeneic stem cell transplantation may afford a cure in patients with a good performance status and is considered in high-risk patients (IPSS-R high and very high) and some low-risk patients. The hypomethylating agent azacitidine has improved survival by a median of 9 months compared to supportive care or low intensity chemotherapy for high-risk patients, and is a recommended standard of care for those not eligible for transplantation.

25.52 Revised International Prognostic Scoring System and outcomes in myelodysplasia*

Risk category	Overall score	Median survival (years)	25% progression to acute myeloid leukaemia (years)
Very low	≤1.5	8.8	Not reached
Low	>1.5–3	5.3	10.8
Intermediate	>3–4.5	3.0	3.2
High	>4.5–6	1.6	1.4
Very high	>6	0.8	0.73

*The IPSS-R is based on three prognostic factors: the blast percentage in bone marrow; karyotype; and number and degree of blood cytopenias. A score is derived from which patients can be stratified into five risk categories for survival and leukaemic transformation.

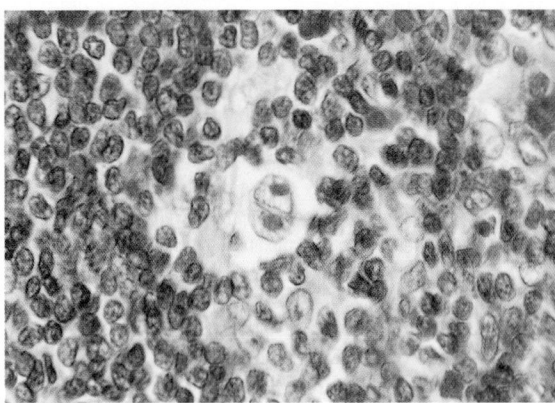

Fig. 25.32 Hodgkin lymphoma. In the centre of this lymph node biopsy is a large typical Reed–Sternberg cell with two nuclei containing a prominent eosinophilic nucleolus.

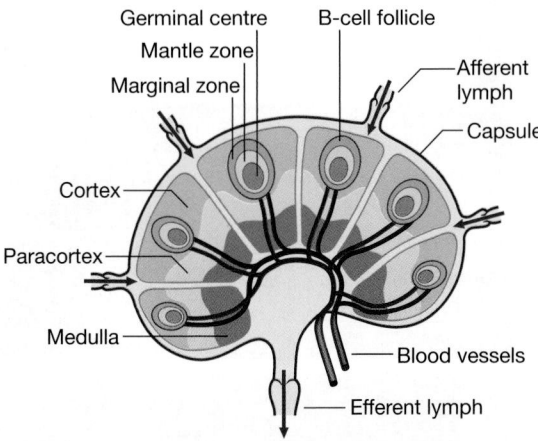

Fig. 25.31 Schema of lymph node architecture. Different lymphocyte populations reside in different areas of the node: B cells in the follicles, T cells in the paracortex and plasma cells in the medulla. B cells are selected for antigen in the follicle centre. Errors during this process result in B-cell lymphomas, which are by far the most common type.

Lymphomas

These neoplasms arise from lymphoid tissues and are diagnosed from the pathological findings on biopsy as Hodgkin or non-Hodgkin lymphoma. The majority are of B-cell origin. Non-Hodgkin lymphomas are classified as low- or high-grade tumours on the basis of their proliferation rate. The normal architecture of the lymph node is outlined in Fig. 25.31.

- *High-grade tumours* divide rapidly, are typically present for a matter of weeks before diagnosis, and may be life-threatening with high risk of extranodal involvement.
- *Low-grade tumours* divide slowly, may be present for many months before diagnosis, and typically behave in an indolent fashion.

Hodgkin lymphoma

The histological hallmark of Hodgkin lymphoma (HL) is the presence of Reed–Sternberg cells: large, malignant lymphoid cells of B-cell origin (Fig. 25.32). They are often present only in small numbers, but are surrounded by large numbers of reactive non-malignant T cells, plasma cells and granulocytes, including eosinophils.

The epidemiology of HL is shown in Box 25.53 and its histological WHO classification in Box 25.54.

25.53 Epidemiology and aetiology of Hodgkin lymphoma

Incidence
- Approximately 4 new cases/100 000 population/year

Sex ratio
- Slight male excess (1.5:1)

Age
- Median age 31 years; first peak at 20–35 years and second at 50–70 years

Aetiology
- Unknown
- More common in patients from well-educated backgrounds and small families
- Three times more likely with a past history of infectious mononucleosis but no definitive causal link to Epstein–Barr virus infection proven

25.54 WHO pathological classification of Hodgkin lymphoma (HL)

Type	Histology classification	Proportion of HL
Nodular lymphocyte-predominant HL		5%
Classical HL	Nodular sclerosing	70%
	Mixed cellularity	20%
	Lymphocyte-rich	5%
	Lymphocyte-depleted	Rare

Nodular lymphocyte-predominant HL is slow-growing, localised and rarely fatal. It has biological features, such as CD20-positive Hodgkin cells, and clinical features that make it more akin to a low-grade B-cell non-Hodgkin lymphoma. Classical HL is divided into four histological subtypes from the appearance of the Reed–Sternberg cells and surrounding reactive cells. The nodular sclerosing type is more common in young patients and in women. Mixed cellularity is more common in older patients. Lymphocyte-rich HL usually presents in men. Lymphocyte-depleted HL is rare and probably represents large-cell or anaplastic non-Hodgkin lymphoma.

Clinical features

There is painless, rubbery lymphadenopathy, usually in the neck or supraclavicular fossae; the lymph nodes may fluctuate in size. Young patients with nodular sclerosing disease may have large mediastinal masses that are surprisingly asymptomatic, but may cause dry cough and some

	25.55 Clinical stages of Hodgkin lymphoma (Ann Arbor classification)	
Stage	**Definition**	
I	Involvement of a single lymph node region (I) or extralymphatic* site (I$_E$)	
II	Involvement of two or more lymph node regions (II) or an extralymphatic site and lymph node regions on the same side of (above or below) the diaphragm (II$_E$)	
III	Involvement of lymph node regions on both sides of the diaphragm with (III$_E$) or without (III) localised extralymphatic involvement or involvement of the spleen (III$_S$), or both (III$_{SE}$)	
IV	Diffuse involvement of one or more extralymphatic tissues, e.g. liver or bone marrow	
Each stage is subclassified		
A	No systemic symptoms	
B	Weight loss >10%, drenching sweats, fever	

*The lymphatic structures are defined as the lymph nodes, spleen, thymus, Waldeyer's ring, appendix and Peyer's patches.

breathlessness. Isolated subdiaphragmatic nodes occur in fewer than 10% at diagnosis. Hepatosplenomegaly may be present, but does not always indicate disease in those organs. Spread is contiguous from one node to the next, and extranodal disease, such as bone, brain or skin involvement, is rare. Systemic symptoms include so-called 'B symptoms' of drenching night sweats, fever and loss of 10% body weight. Other symptoms can include pruritis and rarely, but dramtically, alcohol-induced pain within lymph nodes.

Investigations

Treatment of HL depends on the stage at presentation; investigations therefore aim not only to diagnose lymphoma, but also to determine the extent of disease (Box 25.55).

- *FBC* may be normal. If a normochromic, normocytic anaemia or lymphopenia is present, this is a poor prognostic factor, particularly in advanced disease. An eosinophilia, neutrophilia or thrombocytosis may be present.
- *ESR* may be raised and is an adverse prognostic factor.
- *Renal function tests* are required to ensure function is normal prior to treatment.
- *Liver function* may be abnormal in the absence of disease or may reflect hepatic infiltration. An obstructive pattern may be caused by nodes at the porta hepatis.
- *LDH* may be raised and is an adverse prognostic factor.
- *Chest X-ray* may show a mediastinal mass.
- *CT scan* of chest, abdomen and pelvis permits staging. Bulky disease (>10 cm in a single node mass) is an adverse prognostic feature.
- *Positron emission tomography-CT (PET-CT) scanning* identifies nodes involved with HL that are [18]fluorodeoxyglucose (FDG)-avid and this allows more accurate staging and monitoring of response (Fig. 25.33).
- *Lymph node biopsy* may be undertaken surgically or by percutaneous needle biopsy under radiological guidance (Fig. 25.34).

Management

Given the high cure rate and excellent prognosis of a majority of young and middle-aged patients with HL, the aim is to maximize cure rates while minimising long-term treatment-related toxicity. Treatment approaches involve defining patients as early-stage disease (stages IA and IIA) or advanced stage disease (IB, IIB, III and IV). The ABVD regimen (doxorubicin (adriamycin), bleomycin, vinblastine and dacarbazine) is widely

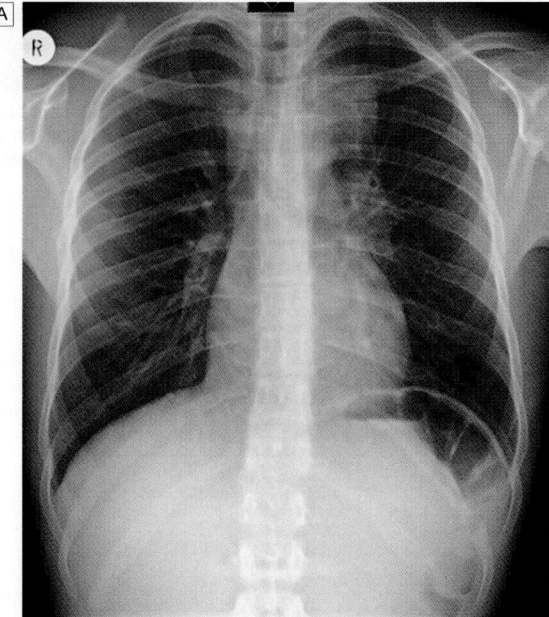
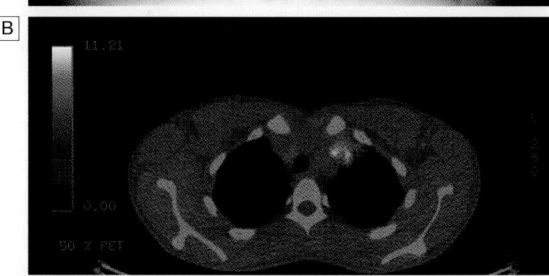
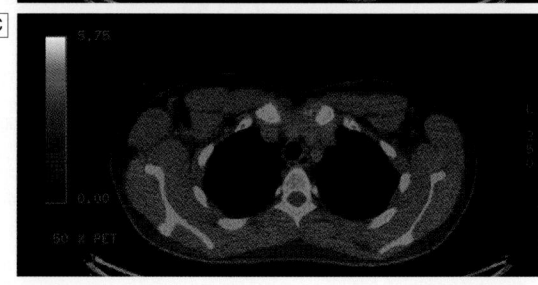

Fig. 25.33 Positron emission tomography (PET) scans in Hodgkin lymphoma, demonstrating response to treatment. A Chest X-ray from a young man with Hodgkin lymphoma at presentation, showing a left-sided anterior–superior mediastinal mass with tracheal deviation to the right. B Fused PET-CT image showing intense fluorodeoxyglucose (FDG) uptake (avidity) in the mass at presentation. C Fused PET-CT image showing no FDG uptake (PET negativity), representing complete response at the end of treatment.

used in the UK, while the more intensive BEACOPP regimen (bleomycin, etoposide, doxorubicin (adriamycin), cyclophosphamide, vincristine (oncovin), procarbazine, prednisolone) is a more effective alternative, though with a greater risk of side-effects including infertility and treatment-related MDS and AML.

Standard therapy for early-stage patients without additional risk factors, such as bulk disease or high ESR, is two cycles of ABVD combined with 20 Gy radiotherapy to the involved sites of disease. Standard therapy for early-stage patients with additional risk factors is four cycles of ABVD combined with 30 Gy radiotherapy. Careful planning of radiotherapy is required to limit the doses delivered to normal tissues and new planning techniques continue to improve targeting of radiotherapy. Nevertheless, the long-term risks of second cancers and heart and lung disease within the radiation fields remain a concern, especially for young people with a high cure rate and potentially decades of life ahead of them. Early-stage patients who have a negative FDG PET-CT scan after

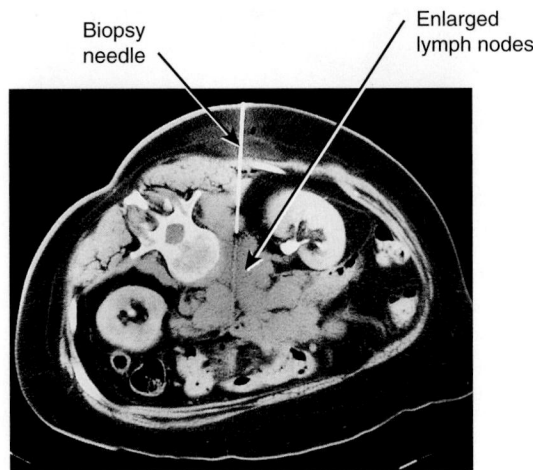

Fig. 25.34 **CT-guided percutaneous needle biopsy of retroperitoneal nodes involved by lymphoma.**

25.56 The Hasenclever prognostic index for advanced Hodgkin lymphoma

Score 1 for each of the following risk factors present at diagnosis:
- Age >45 years
- Male gender
- Serum albumin <40 g/L
- Hb <105 g/L
- Stage IV disease
- White blood cell count >15 × 10⁹/L
- Lymphopenia <0.6 × 10⁹/L

Score	5-year rate of freedom from progression (%)	5-year rate of overall survival (%)
0–1	79	90
>2	60	74
>3	55	70
>4	47	59

three or four cycles of combination chemotherapy can safely omit radiotherapy. Young women receiving breast irradiation during the treatment of chest disease have an increased risk of breast cancer and should participate in a breast screening programme. Patients continuing to smoke after lung irradiation are at particular risk of future lung cancer.

ABVD chemotherapy can cause cardiac and pulmonary toxicity, due to doxorubicin and bleomycin, respectively. The incidence of infertility and secondary myelodysplasia/AML is low with this regimen but higher with BEACOPP.

Patients with advanced-stage disease are most commonly managed with chemotherapy alone. Standard treatment in the UK is 6–8 cycles of ABVD, followed by an assessment of response. A negative FDG PET-CT after two cycles of ABVD (interim PET-2 response) predicts a very good outcome from continuing with up to six cycles of ABVD. Indeed, the same outcome can be achieved by omitting the bleomycin from the last four cycles and using just AVD, thus reducing the risk of lung toxicity. Even more impressive results of >90% 5-year progression-free survival can be achieved with just four cycles of BEACOPP if the interim PET-2 scan is negative. Patients who have a positive FDGPET-CT after two cycles, however, have a very high relapse risk if they continue with ABVD, with only 13% being relapse-free at 2 years. Switching to BEACOPP from ABVD or continuing with BEACOPP for six cycles in these patients improves the relapse-free survival to approximately 65%–90%.

Patients with relapsed disease that responds to salvage chemotherapy and ideally becomes FDG PET-CT-negative should be considered for autologous stem cell transplantation (p. 945). Those with resistant disease might benefit from an allogeneic stem cell transplant. Brentuximab vedotin is an antibody–drug conjugate directed against CD30 on the Reed–Sternberg cell surface. This antibody delivers the antimitotic toxin monomethyl auristatin E to the Hodgkin cells and, as a single agent, can produce good responses in patients who have failed, or are not suitable for, an autologous transplant and can be a 'bridge' to an allogeneic transplant. Reed–Sternberg cells over-express the cell surface protein Programme Death Ligand 1 (PDL-1). This engages with Programmed Death Protein 1 (PD-1) on T cells and leads to T-cell 'exhaustion' (see Fig. 7.12). This 'immune checkpoint' is an important survival mechanism for Reed–Sternberg cells. The immunotherapy drugs pembrolizumab and nivolumab can inhibit this 'checkpoint' in the immune response and allow T-cell killing of Reed–Sternberg cells. Both drugs are available for patients who have failed multiple lines of treatment and can produce further remissions.

Prognosis

Over 90% of patients with early-stage HL achieve complete remission when treated with chemotherapy, followed by involved field radiotherapy,

and the great majority are cured. The major challenge is how to reduce treatment intensity, and hence long-term toxicity, without reducing the excellent cure rates in this group. Omitting radiotherapy in the majority of FDG PET-CT-negative patients is one major step forward in this regard.

Historically, between 50% and 70% of those with advanced-stage HL were cured. The Hasenclever index (Box 25.56) can be helpful in assigning approximate chances of cure when discussing treatment plans with patients. More recent data using FDG PET-CT to direct therapy suggests that long-term survival is improving to beyond 80%. Patients who fail to respond to initial chemotherapy or relapse within a year of initial therapy have a poor prognosis, but some may achieve long-term survival after autologous HSCT. Patients relapsing after 1 year may obtain long-term survival with further chemotherapy alone, but fit patients frequently proceed to autologous HSCT.

Non-Hodgkin lymphoma

Non-Hodgkin lymphoma (NHL) represents a monoclonal proliferation of lymphoid cells of B-cell (90%) or T-cell (10%) origin. The incidence of these tumours increases with age, to 62.8/million population per annum at age 75 years, and the overall rate is increasing at about 3% per year.

The epidemiology of NHL is shown in Box 25.57. Previous classifications were based principally on histological appearances. The current WHO classification stratifies according to cell lineage (T or B cells) and incorporates clinical features, histology, genetic abnormalities and concepts related to the biology of the lymphoma. Clinically, the most important factor is grade, which is a reflection of proliferation rate. High-grade NHL has high proliferation rates, rapidly produces symptoms, is fatal if untreated, but is potentially curable. Low-grade NHL has low proliferation rates, may be asymptomatic for many months or even years before presentation, runs an indolent course, but is frequently disseminated at diagnosis and not curable by conventional therapy. Of all cases of NHL in the developed world, over 50% are either diffuse large B-cell NHL (high-grade) or follicular NHL (low-grade) (Fig. 25.35). Other forms of NHL, including Burkitt lymphoma, mantle cell lymphoma, mucosa-associated lymphoid tissue (MALT) lymphomas and T-cell lymphomas, are individually less common.

Clinical features

Unlike Hodgkin lymphoma, NHL is often widely disseminated at presentation, including in extranodal sites. Patients present with lymph node enlargement (Fig. 25.36), which may be associated with systemic upset: weight loss, sweats, fever and itching. Hepatosplenomegaly may be present. Sites of extranodal involvement include the bone marrow, gut, thyroid, lung, skin, testis, brain and, more rarely, bone. Bone marrow involvement is more common in low-grade (50%–60%) than high-grade

25.57 Epidemiology and aetiology of non-Hodgkin lymphoma

Incidence

- 12 new cases/100 000 people/year

Sex ratio

- Slight male excess

Age

- Median age 65–70 years

Aetiology

- No single causative abnormality described
- Lymphoma is a late manifestation of HIV infection (Ch. 14)
- Specific lymphoma types are associated with viruses: e.g. Epstein–Barr virus (EBV) with post-transplant NHL, human herpesvirus 8 (HHV8) with a primary effusion lymphoma, and human T-cell lymphotropic virus (HTLV-1) with adult T-cell leukaemia lymphoma
- Gastric lymphoma can be associated with *Helicobacter pylori* infection
- Some lymphomas are associated with specific chromosomal translocations:
  The t(14;18) in follicular lymphoma results in the dysregulated expression of the *BCL-2* gene product, which inhibits apoptotic cell death
  The t(8;14) found in Burkitt lymphoma and the t(11;14) in mantle cell lymphoma alter function of *c-myc* and *cyclin D1*, respectively, resulting in malignant proliferation
  Large B-cell lymphomas with rearrangements of *c-myc* with *BCL-2* and/or *BCL-6* (double and triple hit lymphomas)
- Lymphoma occurs in congenital immunodeficiency states and in immunosuppressed patients after organ transplantation

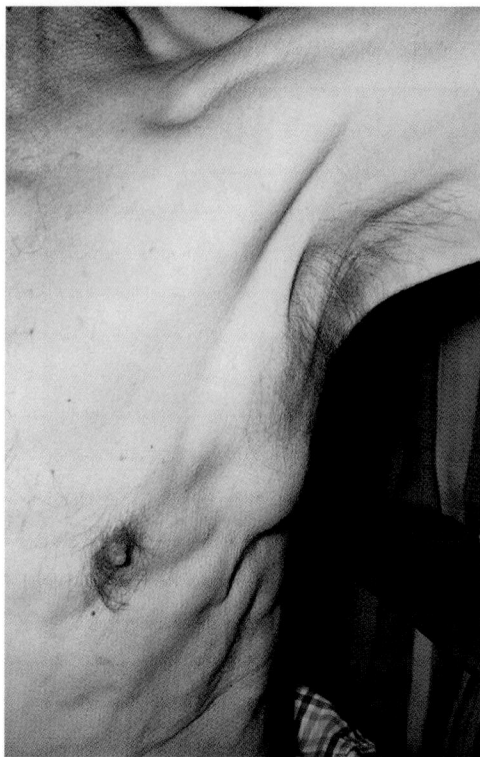

Fig. 25.36 Bulky axillary lymphadenopathy with distended superficial veins in a patient presenting with high-grade lymphoma. *From Howard MR, Hamilton PJ. Haematology: An illustrated colour text, 4th edn. Edinburgh: Elsevier Ltd; 2013.*

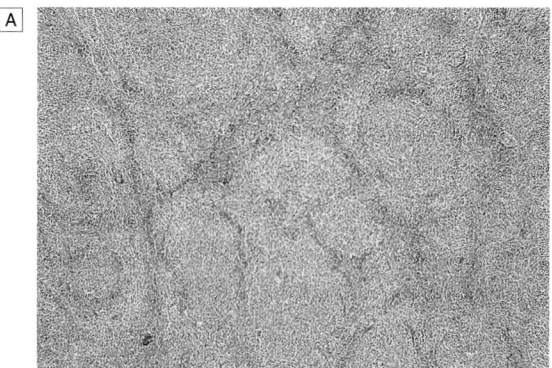

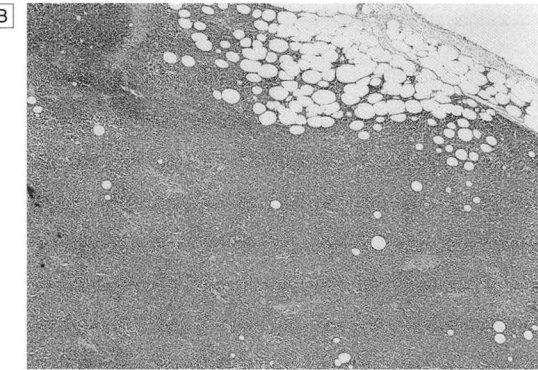

Fig. 25.35 Histology of non-Hodgkin lymphoma. A (Low-grade) follicular or nodular pattern. B (High-grade) diffuse pattern.

Investigations

These are as for HL, but in addition the following should be performed:

- *Bone marrow aspiration and trephine* to identify bone marrow involvement.
- *Immunophenotyping of surface antigens to distinguish T-cell from B-cell tumours*. This may be done on blood, marrow or nodal material.
- *Cytogenetic analysis to detect chromosomal translocations*, particularly rearrangements of the oncogene *c-MYC* and molecular testing for T-cell receptor or immunoglobulin gene rearrangements.
- *Immunoglobulin determination*. Some lymphomas are associated with IgG or IgM paraproteins, which serve as markers for treatment response.
- *Measurement of urate levels*. Some very aggressive high-grade NHLs are associated with very high urate levels, which can precipitate renal failure when treatment is started as a consequence of tumour lysis syndrome.
- *HIV testing*. HIV is a risk factor for some lymphomas and affects treatment decisions.
- *Hepatitis B and C testing*. This should be done prior to therapy with rituximab.

Management

Low-grade NHL

The majority of patients (80%) present with advanced stage disease and will run a relapsing and remitting course over several years. Overall survival has improved in recent years with more treatment options. Asymptomatic patients may not require therapy and are managed by 'watching and waiting'. Indications for treatment include marked systemic symptoms, lymphadenopathy causing discomfort or disfigurement,

(10%) disease. Other extranodal sites tend to be more common in high-grade disease, particularly CNS involvement. Compression syndromes may occur, including gut obstruction, ascites, superior vena cava obstruction and spinal cord compression.

The same staging system (see Box 25.55) is used for both HL and NHL, but NHL is more likely to be stage III or IV at presentation.

bone marrow failure or compression syndromes. In follicular lymphoma, the options are:

- *Radiotherapy*. This can be used for localised stage I disease, which is rare. FDG PET-CT-confirmed stage I disease has a 70% cure rate with radiotherapy.
- *Chemotherapy*. Most patients will respond to oral therapy with chlorambucil, which is well tolerated, but not curative and is reserved nowadays for older/frail patients. More intensive intravenous chemotherapy in younger patients produces better quality of life through long periods of remission.
- *Monoclonal antibody therapy*. Humanised monoclonal antibodies ('biologic therapy'; p. 945) can be used to target surface antigens on tumour cells and to induce tumour cell apoptosis directly. The anti-CD20 antibody rituximab has been shown to induce durable clinical responses in up to 60% of patients when given alone, and acts synergistically when given with chemotherapy. Rituximab (R) in combination with cyclophosphamide, vincristine and prednisolone (R-CVP), cyclophosphamide, doxorubicin (hydroxydaunorubicin), vincristine (oncovin), prednisolone (R-CHOP) or bendamustine (R-bendamustine) is commonly used as first-line therapy. Two years of maintenance therapy with single-agent rituximab, following achievement of first or second response, especially if this is only a partial response, delays the time to next treatment. As yet, however, rituximab maintenance has not shown a survival benefit. New and more potent monoclonal antibodies are in development; a recent trial of obinutuzumab combined with chemotherapy showed longer progression-free survival compared to similar chemotherapy with rituximab.
- *Targeted therapy*. The PI3 kinase inhibitor idelalisib is approved for relapsed follicular lymphoma and ibrutinib (Fig. 25.30) is approved for relapsed mantle cell lymphoma (a poor-prognosis lymphoma with low-grade histology, but aggressive clinical behaviour) and for relapsed Waldenstrom's macroglobulinaemia (also known as lymphoplasmacytic lymphoma, see below. Newer targeted therapies are likely to become more widely used in low-grade lymphomas in the near future.
- *Transplantation*. High-dose chemotherapy and autologous HSCT can produce long remissions in patients with relapsed disease. Decisions on the timing of such treatment are complex in the context of rituximab maintenance and newer targeted therapies. However, younger patients with short first or second remissions or who relapse during rituximab maintenance should be considered.

High-grade NHL

Patients with diffuse large B-cell NHL need treatment at initial presentation:

- *Chemotherapy*. The majority (>90%) are treated with intravenous combination chemotherapy, typically with the CHOP regimen (cyclophosphamide, doxorubicin (hydroxydaunorubicin), vincristine (oncovin) and prednisolone).
- *Monoclonal antibody therapy*. When combined with CHOP chemotherapy, rituximab (R) increases the complete response rates and improves overall survival. R-CHOP, 4–6 cycles, is currently recommended as first-line therapy for all relatively fit patients. Dose reduction (R-mini CHOP) is preferable in those over 80 years of age and replacement of doxorubicin with gemcitibine (R-GCVP) is considered in those with impaired cardiac function.
- *Radiotherapy*. Stage I patients without bulky disease are treated with four cycles of CHOP or R-CHOP, followed by involved site radiotherapy. Radiotherapy is also indicated for a residual localised site of bulk disease after chemotherapy and for spinal cord and other compression syndromes.
- *HSCT*. Autologous HSCT (p. 945) benefits patients with relapsed disease that is sensitive to salvage immunochemotherapy. As with HL, achieving a negative FDG PTC-CT negativity to autologous transplantation is desirable.
- *CAR-T-cell therapy* (Fig. 25.17) is licensed for certain patients with multiply relapsed DLBL or high-grade transformation of follicular lymphoma and can salvage patients from a desparate situation.

Prognosis

Low-grade NHL runs an indolent remitting and relapsing course, with an overall median survival of 12 years. Transformation to a high-grade NHL occurs in 3% per annum and is associated with poor survival.

In diffuse large B-cell NHL treated with R-CHOP, some 75% of patients overall respond initially to therapy and 50% will have disease-free survival at 5 years. The prognosis for patients with high grade NHL is further refined according to the international prognostic index (IPI). For high-grade NHL, 5-year survival ranges from over 75% in those with low-risk scores (age <60 years, stage I or II, one or fewer extranodal sites, normal LDH and good performance status) to 25% in those with high-risk scores (increasing age, advanced stage, concomitant disease and a raised LDH).

Rearrangements of the *c-MYC* oncogene, either alone (more commonly Burkitt lymphoma) or with rearrangements of *BCL-2* and/or *BCL-6* (double or triple hit high-grade lymphomas) are recognised entities in WHO classification with poor prognoses and are increasingly treated more aggressively.

Relapse is associated with a poor response to further chemotherapy (<10% 5-year survival), but in patients under 65 years HSCT improves survival.

Paraproteinaemias

A gammopathy refers to over-production of one or more classes of immunoglobulin. It may be polyclonal in association with acute or chronic inflammation, such as infection including HIV, sarcoidosis, autoimmune disorders or some malignancies. Alternatively, a monoclonal increase in a single immunoglobulin class may occur in association with normal or reduced levels of the other immunoglobulins. Such monoclonal proteins (also called M-proteins, paraproteins or monoclonal gammopathies) occur as a feature of myeloma, solitary plasmacytomas, lymphoma and amyloidosis, in connective tissue disease such as rheumatoid arthritis or polymyalgia rheumatica, in infection such as HIV and in solid tumours. In addition, they may be present with no underlying disease. Gammopathies are detected by plasma immunoelectrophoresis.

Monoclonal gammopathy of uncertain significance

In monoclonal gammopathy of uncertain significance (MGUS, also known as benign monoclonal gammopathy), a paraprotein is present in the blood but there are no other features of myeloma, Waldenström macroglobulinaemia (see below), lymphoma or related disease. It is a common condition associated with increasing age; a paraprotein can be found in 1% of the population aged over 50 years, increasing to 5% over 80 years.

Clinical features and investigations

Patients are usually asymptomatic and the paraprotein is found on blood testing for other reasons. The routine blood count and biochemistry are normal, the paraprotein is usually present in small amounts with no associated immune paresis and there are no lytic bone lesions. The bone marrow may have increased plasma cells, but these usually constitute less than 10% of nucleated cells.

Prognosis

After follow-up of 20 years, only one-quarter of cases will progress to myeloma or a related disorder (i.e. around 1% per annum). There is no certain way of predicting progression in an individual patient. However, an abnormal ratio of kappa to lambda light chains (serum free light chain ratio, SFLR) increases the risk of progression. Patients with an abnormal ratio should be monitored for progression on an annual basis.

Waldenström macroglobulinaemia

This is a low-grade lymphoplasmacytic lymphoma associated with an IgM paraprotein, causing clinical features of hyperviscosity syndrome. It is a rare tumour occurring in old age and more commonly affects males.

Patients classically present with features of hyperviscosity, such as nosebleeds, bruising, delirium and visual disturbance. However, presentation is more commonly with anaemia, systemic symptoms, splenomegaly or lymphadenopathy, or may be asymptomatic with an IgM paraprotein detected on routine screening. Patients are found on investigation to have an IgM paraprotein associated with a raised plasma viscosity. The bone marrow has a characteristic appearance, with infiltration of lymphoid cells, plasma cells and sometimes prominent mast cells. A high proportion of patients have a mutation in the *MYD88* gene.

Management

If patients show symptoms of hyperviscosity and anaemia, plasmapheresis is required to remove IgM and make blood transfusion possible. Chemotherapy with alkylating agents, such as chlorambucil, has historically been the mainstay of treatment, controlling disease in over 50%. Fludarabine may be more effective in this disease, but has more side-effects. Rituximab in combination with chemotherapy, e.g bendamustine, is now most commonly used; ibrutinib is very effective and has recently been licensed for use. Rituximab alone can cause a rapid release of IgM and increase in viscosity. The median survival is 5 years.

Multiple myeloma

This is a malignant proliferation of plasma cells. Normal plasma cells are derived from B cells and produce immunoglobulins that contain heavy and light chains. Normal immunoglobulins are polyclonal, which means that a variety of heavy chains are produced and each may be of kappa or lambda light chain type (Ch. 4). In myeloma, plasma cells produce immunoglobulin of a single heavy and light chain, a monoclonal protein commonly referred to as a paraprotein. In most cases an excess of light chain is produced and in some cases only light chain is produced; this appears in the urine as Bence Jones proteinuria and can be measured in the urine or serum as free light chain. The frequency of different isotypes of monoclonal protein in myeloma is shown in Box 25.58.

Although a small number of malignant plasma cells are present in the circulation, the majority are present in the bone marrow. The malignant plasma cells produce cytokines, which stimulate osteoclasts and result in net bone reabsorption. The resulting lytic lesions cause bone pain, fractures and hypercalcaemia. Marrow involvement can result in anaemia or pancytopenia.

Clinical features and investigations

The incidence of myeloma is 4/100 000 new cases per annum, with a male-to-female ratio of 2:1. The median age at diagnosis is 60–70 years and the disease is more common in people of African Caribbean origin. The clinical features are demonstrated in Fig. 25.37.

Diagnosis of myeloma requires two of the following criteria to be fulfilled:

- increased malignant plasma cells in the bone marrow
- serum and/or urinary M-protein
- skeletal lytic lesions.

Bone marrow aspiration, plasma and urine electrophoresis, and a skeletal survey are thus required; the latter is classically a series of plain X-rays, but more often now low-dose CT scan or whole-body MRI is performed. Normal immunoglobulin levels, i.e. the absence of immunoparesis, should cast doubt on the diagnosis. Paraproteinaemia can cause an elevated ESR, but this is a non-specific test; only approximately 5% of patients with a persistently elevated ESR above 100 mm/hr have underlying myeloma. Serum albumin and β_2-microglobulin are measured for prognostic purposes, along with a cytogenetic analysis of the tumour cells.

25.58 Classification of multiple myeloma

Type of monoclonal (M)-protein	Relative frequency (%)
IgG	55
IgA	21
Light chain only	22
Others (D, E, non-secretory)	2

Management

If patients are asymptomatic with no evidence of end-organ damage (e.g. to kidneys, bone marrow or bone), treatment may not be required. So-called asymptomatic myeloma should be monitored closely for the development of end-organ damage.

Immediate support

- High fluid intake to treat renal impairment and hypercalcaemia (p. 676)
- Analgesia for bone pain
- Bisphosphonates for hypercalcaemia and to delay other skeletal-related events (p. 1051)
- Allopurinol to prevent urate nephropathy
- Plasmapheresis, if necessary, for hyperviscosity
- Antibiotic prophylaxis with levofloxacin during the first 3 months of therapy.

Chemotherapy with or without HSCT

Patients are initially assessed for their fitness and eligibility for autologous HSCT and treatment pathways vary accordingly. Myeloma therapy has improved with the addition of novel agents, initially the immunomodulatory drug thalidomide and more recently the proteasome inhibitors bortezomib and carfilzomib, the second- and third-generation immunomodulatory drugs lenalidomide and pomalidomide and the anti-myeloma antibodies daratumumab and isatuximab, which binds to CD 38 on the malignant plasma cell (Fig. 25.38).

For first-line therapy in older patients who are unsuitable for transplant, thalidomide combined with the alkylating agent melphalan and prednisolone (MPT) has increased the median overall survival to more than 4 years. Lenalidomide is approved first-line treatment for patients not eligible for transplantation and who are intolerant of, or unsuitable for, thalidomide. Thalidomide and lenalidomide both have anti-angiogenic effects against tumour blood vessels and immunomodulatory effects. Both can cause somnolence, constipation, peripheral neuropathy and thrombosis, though lenalidomide has a better side-effect profile. It is vital that females of child-bearing age use adequate contraception, as thalidomide and lenalidomide are teratogenic. Treatment is administered until paraprotein levels have stopped falling. This is termed 'plateau phase' and can last for weeks or years.

In younger, fitter patients considered eligible for transplant, standard treatment includes first-line therapies, such as cyclophosphamide, thalidomide and dexamethasone (CTD) or bortezomib (Velcade), thalidomide and dexamethasone (VTD) to maximum response, and then autologous HSCT. This improves quality of life and prolongs survival, but does not cure myeloma. In all patients who have achieved maximal response, lenalidomide maintenance has been shown to prolong the response.

When myeloma progresses, treatment is given to induce a further plateau phase. In the UK, the proteosome inhibitor bortezomib and lenalidomide have been used as second- and third-line therapy, as appropriate. However, as they have been used more frequently in the first or second line with prognostic benefit, subsequent relapses are more difficult to treat. Pomalidomide, carfilzomib and daratumumab show promise in relapsed/refractory disease and are increasingly used. Patients who respond may benefit from a second autologous HSCT.

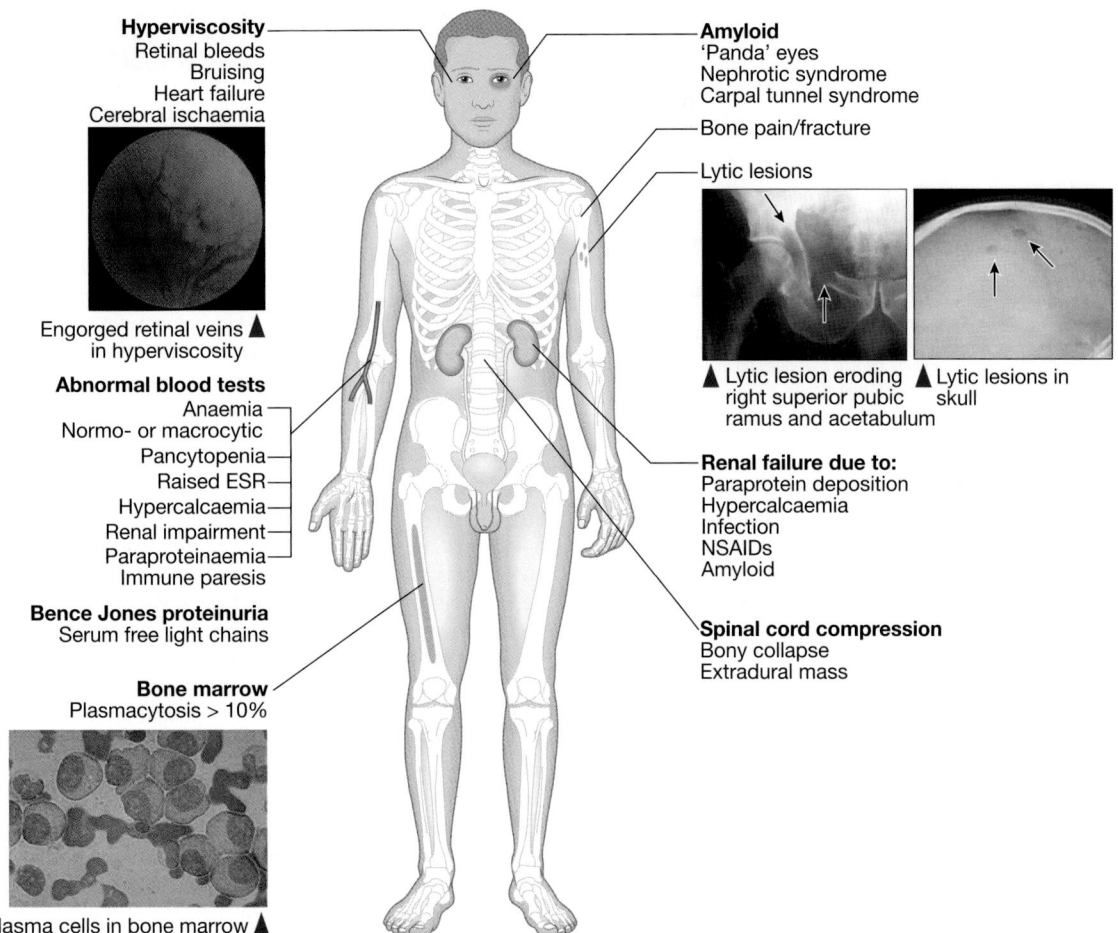

Hyperviscosity
Retinal bleeds
Bruising
Heart failure
Cerebral ischaemia

Engorged retinal veins ▲
in hyperviscosity

Abnormal blood tests
Anaemia
Normo- or macrocytic
Pancytopenia
Raised ESR
Hypercalcaemia
Renal impairment
Paraproteinaemia
Immune paresis

Bence Jones proteinuria
Serum free light chains

Bone marrow
Plasmacytosis > 10%

Plasma cells in bone marrow ▲

Amyloid
'Panda' eyes
Nephrotic syndrome
Carpal tunnel syndrome

Bone pain/fracture

Lytic lesions

▲ Lytic lesion eroding   ▲ Lytic lesions in
right superior pubic   skull
ramus and acetabulum

Renal failure due to:
Paraprotein deposition
Hypercalcaemia
Infection
NSAIDs
Amyloid

Spinal cord compression
Bony collapse
Extradural mass

Fig. 25.37 Clinical and laboratory features of multiple myeloma. (ESR = erythrocyte sedimentation rate; NSAIDs = non-steroidal anti-inflammatory drugs)

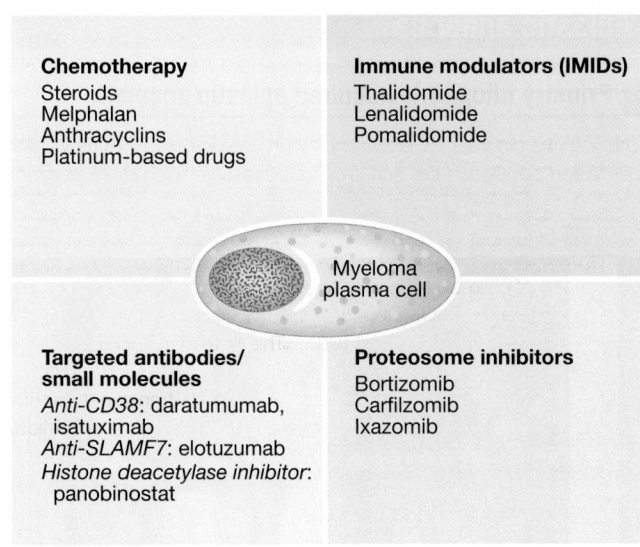

Chemotherapy
Steroids
Melphalan
Anthracyclins
Platinum-based drugs

Immune modulators (IMIDs)
Thalidomide
Lenalidomide
Pomalidomide

Myeloma
plasma cell

**Targeted antibodies/
small molecules**
Anti-CD38: daratumumab,
isatuximab
Anti-SLAMF7: elotuzumab
Histone deacetylase inhibitor:
panobinostat

Proteosome inhibitors
Bortizomib
Carfilzomib
Ixazomib

Fig. 25.38 Myeloma therapy. The four main groups of drugs that may be used in the management of myeloma. (IMIDs = immunomodulatory imide drugs)

Radiotherapy

This is effective for localised bone pain not responding to simple analgesia and for pathological fractures. It is also useful for the emergency treatment of spinal cord compression complicating extradural plasmacytomas.

Bisphosphonates

Long-term bisphosphonate therapy reduces bone pain and skeletal events. These drugs protect bone and may cause apoptosis of malignant plasma cells. There is evidence that intravenous zoledronate in combination with anti-myeloma therapy confers a survival advantage over oral bisphosphonates. Osteonecrosis of the jaw may be associated with long-term use or poor oral hygiene and gum sepsis; regular dental review, including a check before starting therapy, is therefore important.

Prognosis

The international staging system (ISS) identifies poor prognostic features, including a high β_2-microglobulin and low albumin at diagnosis (ISS stage 3, median survival 29 months). Those with a normal albumin and a low β_2-microglobulin (ISS stage 1) have a median survival of 62 months. Increasingly, cytogenetic analysis is used to identify poor-risk patients, e.g. t(4;14), del(17/17p), t(14;16), t(14;20), non-hyperdiploidy and gain(1q). Use of autologous HSCT and advances in drug therapy with the newer agents have increased survival. Over one-third of patients are now surviving for 5 years, compared with only one-quarter 10 years ago. The outlook may improve further with new drugs and combinations of treatments.

Some general considerations regarding haematological malignancy in old age are summarised in Box 25.59.

Solitary plasmacytomas

These are rare presentations of plasma cell malignancy in which an isolated tumour occurs in soft tissues or bone. Two-thirds of cases occur in soft tissues and are commoly centred around the upper aero-digestive tract, but can occur anywhere. Others present as bone tumours,

25.59 Haematological malignancy in old age

- **Median age**: approximately 70 years for most haematological malignancies.
- **Poor-risk biological features**: adverse cytogenetics or the presence of a multidrug resistance phenotype are more frequent.
- **Prognosis**: increasing age is an independent adverse variable in acute leukaemia and aggressive lymphoma.
- **Chemotherapy**: may be less well tolerated. Older people are more likely to have antecedent cardiac, pulmonary or metabolic problems, tolerate systemic infection less well and metabolise cytotoxic drugs differently.
- **Cure rates**: similar to those in younger patients, in those who do tolerate treatment.
- **Decision to treat**: should be based on the individual's biological status, the level of social support available, and the patient's wishes and those of the immediate family, but not on chronological age alone.

25.60 Histiocytic disorders

- Langerhans cell histiocytosis (LCH)
- Cutaneous and mucocutaneous histiocytosis (C)
- Malignant histiocytosis (M)
- Rosai–Dorfman disease (RD)
- Haemophagocytic lymphohistiocytosis (HLH)

commonly in long bones and vertebrae. Patients present with pain, palpable lumps or compression symptoms, such as difficulty swallowing, shortness of breath or cord compression.

Diagnosis involves tissue biopsy, which demonstrates a solid tumour of monoclonal plasma cells, and staging to exclude disseminated multiple myeloma. Some cases are associated with a low-level paraprotein, but other features of myeloma are absent.

Primary treatment is usually with radiotherapy. This can be curative, especially in soft tissue plasmacytomas, which less frequently progress to myeloma. Plasmacytomas of bone have a high rate of progression to myeloma and must be monitored carefully or treated as myeloma from the outset. Rarely myeloma presents as multiple plasmacytomas of bone.

Histiocytic disorders

These are a group of rare tissue infiltrating conditions affecting children and less commonly adults. Histiocytes are immune cells found in various tissues throughout the body whose functions include phagocytosis (tissue macrophages), activation of the immune system and promoting immune tolerance via antigen presentation to T cells (Fig. 25.39). Disorders resulting from pathological infiltration of tissues by histocytes are shown in Box 25.60.

LCH is the commonest type and is caused by mutations in cell signalling known as the MAPKinase pathway. Key genes mutated in this pathway include *BRAF* (65%–70%) and *MAP2K* (20%). LCH can present with isolated painless lumps, e.g. of bone (eosinophilic granuloma) or with symptoms of disseminated tissue involvement including bone, lung, skin

(e.g. persistent nappy rash), lymphadenopathy, splenomegaly and periodontal disease. Diagnosis can be difficult because of the rarity and multiple symptoms at presentation. Management includes surgical excision or radiotherapy of an isolated lesion or topical or systemic chemotherapy drugs, including methotrexate, etoposide and cladribine in disseminated LCH. The *BRAF* inhibitors, e.g. vemurafenib, have shown promising activity in relapsed LCH.

HLH results from mutations in immune genes, e.g. perforin. Presentation is predominantly in children with tissue infiltration by histiocytes and macrophages. Abnormal cytokine production, e.g. interferon-gamma and activation of complement, leads to hyperinflammation and associated haemophagocytosis of blood cells producing pancytopenia. Treatment is based around immunosuppression with glucocorticoids, chemotherapy or ciclosporin, all with the aim of proceeding to allogeneic stem cell transplantation. Newer treatments aimed at inhibiting cytokines or complement activation are being studied.

An acquired form of reactive haemophagocytosis called macrophage activation syndrome (MAS) or secondary HLH is associated with a range of conditions including rheumatological conditions, e.g. juvenile idiopathic arthritis, SLE and Kawasaki disease, acute viral infections, e.g. EBV, CMV and HHV6 and T-cell lymphomas. These diverse conditions generate a cytokine storm, which drives the MAS. Patients present very unwell with fever, severe pancytopenia, deranged coagulation tests, hepatomegaly and a very high ferritin level (often measured in the tens of thousands μg/L). Management includes supportive care, glucocorticoids or other immunosuppression, inhibition of IL-1 with anakinra and, if possible, treatment of the underlying condition.

Aplastic anaemia

Primary idiopathic acquired aplastic anaemia

This is a rare disorder in Europe and North America, with 2–4 new cases per million population per annum. The disease is much more common

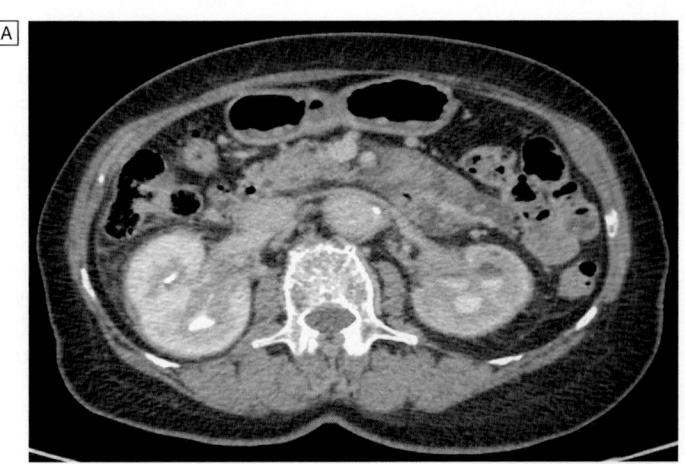
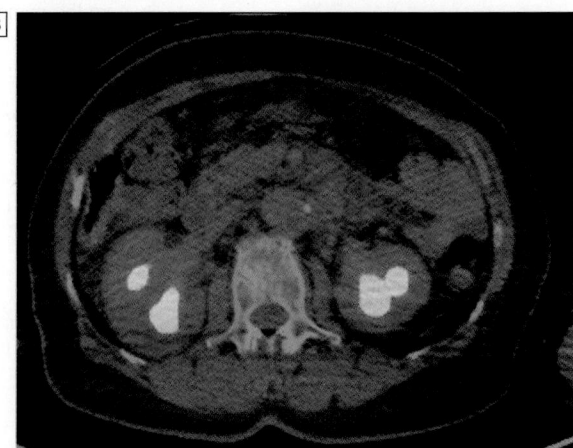

Fig. 25.39 Histiocytic disorder. A CT scan demonstrating bilateral histiocytic infiltration of the kidneys with typical 'hair on end' appearance of the renal cortex. The patient is an older woman with Langerhan cell histiocytosis involving kidneys, lymph nodes and skin. B PET scan of the same patient showing PET positivity in the renal cortex, most noticeable on the right. The intense PET signal relates to excretion of radioactive glucose in urine into the renal pelvis. *Courtesy of Dr Mark Gandhi, Radiology Department, Aberdeen Royal Infirmary.*

in certain other parts of the world, e.g. east Asia. The basic problem is failure of the pluripotent stem cells because of an autoimmune attack, producing hypoplasia of the bone marrow with a pancytopenia in the blood. The diagnosis rests on exclusion of other causes of secondary aplastic anaemia (see below) and rare congenital causes, such as Fanconi's anaemia.

Clinical features and investigations

Patients present with symptoms of bone marrow failure, usually anaemia or bleeding, and less commonly, infections. An FBC demonstrates pancytopenia, low reticulocytes and often macrocytosis. Bone marrow aspiration and trephine reveal hypocellularity. The severity of aplastic anaemia is graded according to the Camitta criteria (Box 25.61).

Management

All patients will require blood product support and aggressive management of infection. The prognosis of severe aplastic anaemia managed with supportive therapy only is poor and more than 50% of patients die, usually in the first year. The curative treatment for patients under 35 years of age with severe idiopathic aplastic anaemia is allogeneic HSCT if there is an available sibling donor (p. 945). Patients aged 35–50 may be candidates if they have no comorbidities. Those with a compatible sibling donor should proceed to transplantation as soon as possible; they have a 75%–90% chance of long-term cure. In older patients and those without a suitable donor, immunosuppressive therapy (IST) with anti-thymocyte globulin (ATG) and ciclosporin is the treatment of choice and gives 5-year survival rates of 75%. Unrelated donor allografts are considered for suitable patients who fail IST. The thrombopoietin receptor agonist eltrombopag has produced trilineage responses in patients who fail IST and is licensed for this indication. Non-transplanted patients may relapse or other clonal disorders of haematopoiesis may evolve, such as paroxysmal nocturnal haemoglobinuria (p. 959), myelodysplastic syndrome (p. 970) and AML (p. 964). Patients with aplastic anaemia must be followed up long-term.

Secondary aplastic anaemia

Causes of this condition are listed in Box 25.62. It is not practical to list all the drugs that have been suspected of causing aplasia. It is important to check the reported side-effects of all drugs taken over the preceding months. In some instances, the cytopenia is more selective and affects only one cell line, most often the neutrophils. Frequently, this is an incidental finding, with no ill health. It probably has an immune basis, but this is difficult to prove.

The clinical features and methods of diagnosis are the same as for primary idiopathic aplastic anaemia. An underlying cause should be treated or removed, but otherwise management is as for the idiopathic form.

 25.61 Camitta criteria

Severe AA (SAA)

- Marrow cellularity <25% (or 25%–50% with <30% residual haematopoietic cells), plus at least two of:
    Neutrophils <0.5 × 10⁹/L
    Platelets <20 × 10⁹/L
    Reticulocyte count <20 × 10⁹/L

Very severe AA (VSAA)

- As for SAA but neutrophils <0.2 × 10⁹/L

Non-severe AA (NSAA)

- AA not fulfilling the criteria for SAA or VSAA

 25.62 Causes of secondary aplastic anaemia

- Drugs:
    Cytotoxic drugs
    Antibiotics – chloramphenicol, sulphonamides
    Antirheumatic agents – penicillamine, gold, phenylbutazone, indometacin
    Antithyroid drugs – carbimazole, propylthiouracil
    Anticonvulsants
    Immunosuppressants – azathioprine
- Chemicals:
    Benzene, toluene solvent misuse – glue-sniffing
    Insecticides – chlorinated hydrocarbons (DDT), organophosphates and carbamates (Ch. 10)
- Radiation
- Viral hepatitis
- Pregnancy
- Paroxysmal nocturnal haemoglobinuria

Myeloproliferative neoplasms

These make up a group of chronic conditions characterised by clonal proliferation of marrow stem/precursor cells. Polycythaemia rubra vera (PRV), essential thrombocythaemia and myelofibrosis are the non-leukaemic myeloproliferative neoplasms. Although the majority of patients are classifiable as having one of these disorders, some have overlapping features and there is often progression from one to another, e.g. PRV to myelofibrosis. A mutation in the gene on chromosome 9 encoding the signal transduction molecule *JAK-2* (*JAK-2 V617F*) has been found in more than 90% of PRV cases and 50% of those with essential thrombocythaemia and myelofibrosis; less frequently, mutations may be identified in exon 12 of *JAK-2*. Mutations in the calreticulin gene (*CALR*), which produces a chaperone protein that protects proteins moving from the endoplasmic reticulin to the cytoplasm, have been found in a further 25% of patients with essential thrombocythaemia. Less commonly, mutations can be detected in the thrombopoietin receptor gene *MPL*.

Myelofibrosis

In myelofibrosis, the marrow is initially hypercellular, with an excess of abnormal megakaryocytes that release growth factors, such as platelet-derived growth factor, to the marrow microenvironment, resulting in a reactive proliferation of fibroblasts. As the disease progresses, the marrow becomes fibrosed.

Most patients present over the age of 50 years, with lassitude, weight loss and night sweats. The spleen can be massively enlarged due to extramedullary haematopoiesis (blood cell formation outside the bone marrow), and painful splenic infarcts may occur.

The characteristic blood picture is leucoerythroblastic anaemia, with circulating immature red blood cells (increased reticulocytes and nucleated red blood cells) and granulocyte precursors (myelocytes). The red cells are shaped like teardrops (teardrop poikilocytes), and giant platelets may be seen in the blood. The white count varies from low to moderately high and the platelet count may be high, normal or low. Urate levels may be high due to increased cell breakdown, and folate deficiency is common. The marrow is often difficult to aspirate and a trephine biopsy shows an excess of megakaryocytes, increased reticulin and fibrous tissue replacement. The presence of a pathological *JAK-2* mutation supports the diagnosis.

Management and prognosis

Median survival is 4 years from diagnosis, but ranges from 1 year to over 20 years. Treatment is directed at control of symptoms, e.g. red cell transfusions for anaemia. Folic acid should be given to prevent deficiency. Cytotoxic therapy with hydroxycarbamide may help control spleen size, the white cell count or systemic symptoms. Splenectomy may be required for a grossly enlarged spleen or symptomatic pancytopenia secondary to splenic pooling of cells and hypersplenism. Allogeneic HSCT may be considered for younger patients. Ruxolitinib, an inhibitor of *JAK-2*, is effective at reducing systemic symptoms and splenomegaly and may improve life expectancy with longer-term use.

Essential thrombocythaemia

Uncontrolled proliferation of megakaryocytes results in a raised level of circulating platelets that are often dysfunctional. Prior to a diagnosis of essential thrombocythaemia being made, reactive causes of thrombo- cytosis must be excluded (see Box 25.15). The presence of pathogenic *JAK-2 V617F, CALR* or, rarely, *MPL* mutations supports the diagnosis, but is not universal. Patients present at a median age of 60 years with vascular occlusion, acrocyanosis (painful discoloured finger tips) or bleeding, or with an asymptomatic isolated raised platelet count. A small percentage (around 5%) will transform to acute leukaemia and others to myelofibrosis.

It is likely that most patients with essential thrombocythaemia benefit from low-dose aspirin to reduce the risk of occlusive vascular events. Low-risk patients (age <40 years, platelet count <1500 × 10^9/L and no bleeding or thrombosis) may not require treatment to reduce the platelet count. For those with a platelet count above 1500 × 10^9/L, with symptoms, or with other risk factors for thrombosis such as diabetes or hypertension, treatment to control platelet counts should be given. Agents include oral hydroxycarbamide or anagrelide, an inhibitor of megakaryocyte matura- tion. Intravenous radioactive phosphorus (^{32}P) may be useful in old age, but is rarely available nowadays, and interferon-alfa has a role in younger patients, including pregnant women and women planning to conceive.

Polycythaemia rubra vera

PRV occurs mainly in patients over the age of 40 years and presents either as an incidental finding of a high haemoglobin, or with symptoms of hyperviscosity, such as lassitude, loss of concentration, headaches, dizziness, blackouts, pruritus and epistaxis. Some patients present with manifestations of peripheral arterial or cerebrovascular disease. Venous thromboembolism may also occur. Peptic ulceration is common, some- times complicated by bleeding. Patients are often plethoric and many have a palpable spleen at diagnosis.

Investigation of polycythaemia is discussed on page 933. The diag- nosis of PRV now rests on the demonstration of a high haematocrit and the presence of a pathogenic *JAK-2* mutation (positive in 95% of cases). In the occasional *JAK-2*-negative cases, a raised red cell mass and absence of causes of a secondary erythrocytosis must be established. The spleen may be enlarged and neutrophil and platelet counts are fre- quently raised, an abnormal karyotype may be found in the marrow and in vitro culture of the marrow can be used to demonstrate autonomous growth in the absence of added growth factors.

Management and prognosis

Aspirin reduces the risk of thrombosis. Venesection gives prompt relief of hyperviscosity symptoms. Between 400 and 500 mL of blood (less if the patient is in old age) are removed and the venesection is repeated every 5–7 days until the haematocrit is reduced to below 45%. Less frequent, regular venesection will maintain this level until the haemoglobin remains reduced because of iron deficiency.

Suppression of marrow proliferation with hydroxycarbamide or interferon-alfa may reduce the risk of vascular occlusion, control spleen size and reduce transformation to myelofibrosis. The JAK-2 inhibitor ruxolitinib is licensed for patients whose disease is not controlled by hydroxycarbamide. Median survival after diagnosis in treated patients exceeds 10 years. Some patients survive more than 20 years; however, cerebrovascular or coronary events occur in up to 60% of patients. The disease may convert to another myelopro- liferative disorder, with about 15% developing acute leukaemia or myelofibrosis.

Bleeding disorders

Disorders of primary haemostasis

The initial formation of the platelet plug (see Fig. 25.6A; also known as 'primary haemostasis') may fail in thrombocytopenia (p. 938), von Willebrand disease (p. 984), and also in platelet function disorders and diseases affecting the vessel wall.

Vessel wall abnormalities

Vessel wall abnormalities may be:

• congenital, such as hereditary haemorrhagic telangiectasia
• acquired, as in a vasculitis (Ch. 26) or scurvy.

Hereditary haemorrhagic telangiectasia

Hereditary haemorrhagic telangiectasia (HHT) is a dominantly inher- ited condition caused by mutations in the genes encoding endoglin and activin receptor-like kinase, which are endothelial cell receptors for transforming growth factor-beta (TGF-β), a potent angiogenic cytokine. Telangiectasia and small aneurysms are found on the fingertips, face and tongue, and in the nasal passages, lung and gastrointestinal tract. A sig- nificant proportion of these patients develop larger pulmonary arterio- venous malformations (PAVMs) that cause arterial hypoxaemia due to a right-to-left shunt. These predispose to paradoxical embolism, resulting in stroke or cerebral abscess. All patients with HHT should be screened for PAVMs and cerebral AVMs; if these are found, ablation by embolisa- tion should be considered.

Patients present either with recurrent bleeds, particularly epistaxis, or with iron deficiency due to occult gastrointestinal bleeding. Treatment can be difficult because of the multiple bleeding points, but regular iron therapy often allows the marrow to compensate for blood loss. Local cautery or laser therapy may prevent single lesions from bleeding. A vari- ety of medical therapies have been tried but none has been found to be universally effective.

Ehlers–Danlos disease

Vascular Ehlers–Danlos syndrome (type 4) is a rare autosomal dominant disorder (1/100 000) caused by a defect in type 3 collagen that results in fragile blood vessels and organ membranes, leading to bleeding and organ rupture. Classical joint hypermobility (Ch. 26) is often limited in this form of the disease, but skin changes and facial appearance are typical. The diagnosis should be considered when there is a history of bleeding with normal laboratory tests.

Scurvy

Vitamin C deficiency affects the normal synthesis of collagen and results in a bleeding disorder characterised by perifollicular and petechial haem- orrhage, bruising and subperiosteal bleeding. The key to diagnosis is the dietary history (Ch. 22).

Platelet function disorders

Bleeding may result from thrombocytopenia (see Box 25.14) or from congenital or acquired abnormalities of platelet function. The most com- mon acquired disorders are iatrogenic, resulting from the use of aspirin, clopidogrel, ticagrelor, dipyridamole and the glycoprotein IIb/IIIa inhibitors to prevent arterial thrombosis (see Box 25.26). Inherited platelet function abnormalities are relatively rare. Congenital abnormalities may be due to deficiency of the membrane glycoproteins, e.g. Glanzmann's thrombas- thenia (IIb/IIIa) or Bernard–Soulier syndrome (Ib), or due to the presence of defective platelet granules, e.g. a deficiency of dense (delta) gran- ules (see Fig. 25.7) giving rise to storage pool disorders. The congenital macrothrombocytopathies that are due to mutations in the myosin heavy chain gene *MYH-9* are characterised by large platelets, inclusion bodies in the neutrophils (Döhle bodies) and a variety of other features, including sensorineural deafness and renal abnormalities. Other familial thrombocytopathies are important, as they can be associated with somatic features (TAR; thrombocytopenia with absent radii (TAR)), and some are associated with a propensity for development of bone marrow failure or dysplasia (e.g. mutations in *RUNX-1* and *ANKRD 26*).

Apart from Glanzmann's thrombasthenia, these conditions are mild disorders, with bleeding typically occurring after trauma or surgery, but rarely spontaneous. Glanzmann's thrombasthenia is an autosomal recessive condition associated with a variable, but often severe bleeding disorder. These conditions are usually managed by local mechanical measures, but antifibrinolytics, such as tranexamic acid, may be useful and, in severe bleeding, platelet transfusion may be required. Recombinant VIIa is licensed for the treatment of resistant bleeding in Glanzmann's thrombasthenia.

Thrombocytopenia

Thrombocytopenia occurs in many disease processes, as listed in Box 25.14, many of which are discussed elsewhere in this chapter.

Idiopathic thrombocytopenic purpura

Idiopathic thrombocytopenic purpura (ITP) is immune-mediated with involvement of autoantibodies, most often directed against the platelet membrane glycoprotein IIb/IIIa, which sensitise the platelet, resulting in premature removal from the circulation by cells of the reticulo-endothelial system. It is not a single disorder; some cases occur in isolation while others are associated with underlying immune dysregulation in conditions such as connective tissue diseases, HIV infection, B-cell malignancies, pregnancy and certain drug therapies. The clinical presentation and pathogenesis are similar, whatever the cause of ITP.

Clinical features and investigations

The presentation depends on the degree of thrombocytopenia. Spontaneous bleeding typically occurs only when the platelet count is below 20 × 10⁹/L. At higher counts, the patient may complain of easy bruising or sometimes epistaxis or menorrhagia. Many cases with counts of more than 50 × 10⁹/L are discovered by chance.

In adults, ITP more commonly affects females and may have an insidious onset. Unlike ITP in children, it is unusual for there to be a history of a preceding viral infection. The development of ITP in the context of COVID-19 infection has been documented. Symptoms or signs of a connective tissue disease may be apparent at presentation or emerge several years later. Patients aged over 65 years should be considered for a bone marrow examination to look for an accompanying B-cell malignancy and appropriate autoantibody testing performed if a diagnosis of connective tissue disease is suspected. HIV testing should be considered because a positive result will have major implications for appropriate therapy. The peripheral blood film is normal, apart from a greatly reduced platelet number, while the bone marrow reveals an obvious increase in megakaryocytes.

Management

Many patients with stable compensated ITP and a platelet count of more than 30 × 10⁹/L do not require treatment to raise the platelet count, except at times of increased bleeding risk, such as surgery and biopsy. First-line therapy for patients with spontaneous bleeding is with high doses of glucocorticoids, either prednisolone (1 mg/kg daily) or dexamethasone (40 mg daily for 4 days), to suppress antibody production and inhibit phagocytosis of sensitised platelets by reticulo-endothelial cells. Administration of intravenous immunoglobulin can raise the platelet count by blocking antibody receptors on reticulo-endothelial cells and is combined with glucocorticoid therapy if there is severe haemostatic failure, especially with evidence of significant mucosal bleeding or a slow response to glucocorticoids alone. Persistent or potentially life-threatening bleeding should be treated with platelet transfusion in addition to the other therapies.

The condition may become chronic, with remissions and relapses. Relapses should be treated by re-introducing glucocorticoids. If a patient has two relapses or primary refractory disease, second-line therapies are considered. The options for second-line therapy include the thrombopoietin receptor agonists (TPO-RA) eltrombopag and romiplostim (which stimulate new platelet formation), the splenic tyrosine kinase inhibitor fostamatinib, splenectomy and immunosuppression. Where splenectomy is considered, the precautions shown in Box 25.37 need to be in place. Splenectomy produces complete remission in about 70% of patients and improvement in a further 20%–25% in favourable cases. The TPO-RAs induce response in around 75% of cases, usually within 10–14 days. Low-dose glucocorticoid therapy and immunosuppressants such as rituximab, ciclosporin, mycophenolate and tacrolimus may also produce remissions. The order in which therapies should be used is not entirely clear, although the TPO-RAs and fostamatinib are licensed for this indication, while the immunosuppressive agents are not.

Coagulation disorders

Normal coagulation is explained in Figure 25.6 and the effects of age are discussed in Box 25.63. Coagulation factor deficiency may be congenital or acquired and may affect one or several of the coagulation factors (Box 25.64). Inherited disorders are almost uniformly related to decreased synthesis, as a result of mutation in the gene encoding a key protein in coagulation. Von Willebrand disease is the most common inherited bleeding disorder. Haemophilia A and B are the most common single coagulation factor deficiencies, but inherited deficiencies of all the other coagulation factors are seen. Acquired disorders may be due to under-production (e.g. in liver failure), increased consumption (e.g. in DIC) or inhibition of function of coagulation factors (such as heparin therapy or immune inhibitors of coagulation, e.g. acquired haemophilia A).

Haemophilia A

Factor VIII deficiency resulting in haemophilia A affects 1/10 000 individuals. It is the most common congenital coagulation factor deficiency. Factor VIII is primarily synthesised by the liver and endothelial cells and has a half-life of about 12 hours. It is protected from proteolysis in the circulation by binding to von Willebrand factor (vWF).

Genetics

The factor VIII gene is located on the X chromosome. Haemophilia is associated with a range of mutations in the factor VIII gene; these include major inversions, large deletions and missense, nonsense and splice site abnormalities. As the factor VIII gene is on the X chromosome, haemophilia A is a sex-linked disorder (Ch. 3). Thus all daughters of a patient with haemophilia are obligate carriers and they, in turn, have a 1 in 4 chance of each pregnancy resulting in the birth of an affected male baby, a normal male baby, a carrier female or a normal female. Antenatal diagnosis by chorionic villous sampling is possible in families with a known mutation.

Haemophilia 'breeds true' within a family; all members have the same factor VIII gene mutation and a similarly severe or mild phenotype. Female carriers of haemophilia may have reduced factor VIII levels because of random inactivation of their normal X chromosome in the developing fetus. This can result in a mild bleeding disorder; thus all known or suspected carriers of haemophilia A should have their factor VIII level measured.

Clinical features

The extent and patterns of bleeding are closely related to residual factor VIII levels (Box 25.65). Patients with severe haemophilia (factor VIII levels <0.01 U/mL) present with spontaneous bleeding into skin, muscle and joints. Retroperitoneal and intracranial bleeding is also a feature. Babies with severe haemophilia have an increased risk of intracranial haemorrhage and, although there is insufficient evidence to recommend routine

25.63 Haemostasis and thrombosis in old age

- **Thrombocytopenia**: reasonably common because of the rising prevalence of disorders in which it may be a secondary feature and also because of the greater use of drugs that can cause it.
- **'Senile' purpura**: presumed to be due to an age-associated loss of subcutaneous fat and the collagenous support of small blood vessels, making them more prone to damage from minor trauma.
- **Thrombosis**: incidence of thromboembolic disease rises with increasing age. This may be due to stasis and concurrent illness, to which older people are prone. Some studies show increased platelet aggregation with age and others age-associated hyperactivity of the haemostatic system, which could contribute to a prothrombotic state.
- **Thromboprophylaxis**: should be considered in all older patients who are immobile as a result of acute illness. Prophylaxis is not required in chronic immobility without a medical cause, as there is no associated increase in thromboembolism.
- **Anticoagulation**: older patients are more sensitive to the anticoagulant effects of warfarin, partly due to the concurrent use of other drugs and the presence of other pathology. Life-threatening or fatal bleeds on warfarin are significantly more common in those over 80 years.

25.64 Causes of coagulopathy

Congenital

X-linked
- Haemophilia A and B

Autosomal
- Von Willebrand disease
- Factor II, V, VII, X, XI and XIII deficiencies
- Combined II, VII, IX and X deficiency
- Combined V and VIII deficiency
- Hypofibrinogenaemia
- Dysfibrinogenaemia

Acquired

Under-production
- Liver failure
- Vitamin K deficiency

Increased consumption
- Coagulation activation:
  Disseminated intravascular coagulation (DIC)
- Immune-mediated:
  Acquired haemophilia and von Willebrand syndrome
- Others:
  Acquired factor X deficiency (in amyloid)
  Acquired von Willebrand syndrome in Wilms' tumour
  Acquired factor VII deficiency in sepsis

Drug-induced
- Inhibition of function:
  Heparins
  Argatroban
  Bivalirudin
  Fondaparinux
  Rivaroxaban
  Apixaban
  Dabigatran
  Edoxaban
- Inhibition of post-translational modification:
  Warfarin

caesarean section for these births, it is appropriate to avoid head trauma and to perform cranial imaging of the newborn within the first 24 hours of life. Individuals with moderate and mild haemophilia (factor VIII levels 0.01–0.4 U/mL) present with the same pattern of bleeding, but usually after trauma or surgery when bleeding is disproportionate to the severity of the insult.

25.65 Severity of haemophilia (ISTH criteria)

Severity	Factor VIII or IX level	Clinical presentation
Severe	<0.01 U/mL	Spontaneous haemarthroses and muscle haematomas
Moderate	0.01–0.05 U/mL	Mild trauma or surgery causes bleeding
Mild	>0.05–0.4 U/mL	Major injury or surgery results in excess bleeding

(ISTH = International Society on Thrombosis and Haemostasis)

The major morbidity of recurrent bleeding in severe haemophilia is musculoskeletal. Bleeding is typically into large joints, especially knees, elbows, ankles and hips. Muscle haematomas are also characteristic, most commonly in the calf and psoas muscles. If early treatment is not given to arrest bleeding, a hot, swollen and very painful joint or muscle haematoma develops. Recurrent bleeding into joints leads to synovial hypertrophy, destruction of the cartilage and chronic haemophilic arthropathy (Fig. 25.40). Complications of muscle haematomas depend on their location. A large psoas bleed may extend to compress the femoral nerve; calf haematomas may increase pressure within the inflexible fascial sheath, causing a compartment syndrome with ischaemia, necrosis, fibrosis, and subsequent contraction and shortening of the Achilles tendon.

Management

The aim of management of severe haemophilia A (and B; see below) in high-income countries is to render patients 'bleed free'. This can be achieved by prophylaxis using coagulation factor concentrates or, in haemophilia A, by a bispecific monoclonal antibody called emicizumab that mimics factor VIII activity. Emicizumab binds to both activated factor IX and factor X to allow the formation of the tenase complex that results in thrombin and clot formation (Fig. 25.41). Prophylaxis using concentrates aims to achieve trough levels of factor VIII or IX that protect the patient against spontaneous bleeding. There is debate about optimal trough values needed to achieve this aim. Prophylaxis can be provided in many different ways: daily, on alternate days, or on information from pharmacokinetic studies that inform on the best way of scheduling prophylaxis. Practice in haemophilia A and B is also changing due to the introduction of recombinant factor concentrates that have been manipulated to alter their half-life. In addition to standard half-life recombinant factor VIII and IX, there are new products produced by Fc fusion and pegylation/glycopegylation that extend the half-life of the coagulation factor to the degree that it can be used to alter dosing schedules for prophylaxis.

The alternative approach, which still needs to be used in low- and middle-income countries, is to treat on demand. In severe haemophilia A, bleeding episodes should be treated by raising the factor VIII level, usually by intravenous infusion of factor VIII concentrate. Factor VIII concentrates are freeze-dried and stable at 4°C and can therefore be stored in domestic refrigerators, allowing patients to treat themselves at home at the earliest indication of bleeding. Coagulation factor concentrates prepared from blood donor plasma are now screened for many blood-borne pathogens including HBV, HCV and HIV, and undergo two separate virus inactivation or removal processes during manufacture; these preparations have a good safety record. However, factor concentrates prepared by recombinant technology are now widely available and, although more expensive, are perceived as being safer than those derived from human plasma in relation to infection risk. In addition to raising factor VIII or IX concentrations, resting of the bleeding site with either bed rest or a splint reduces continuing haemorrhage. Once bleeding has settled, the patient should be mobilised and physiotherapy used to restore strength to the surrounding muscles. All non-immune potential recipients of pooled blood products should be offered hepatitis A and B immunisation.

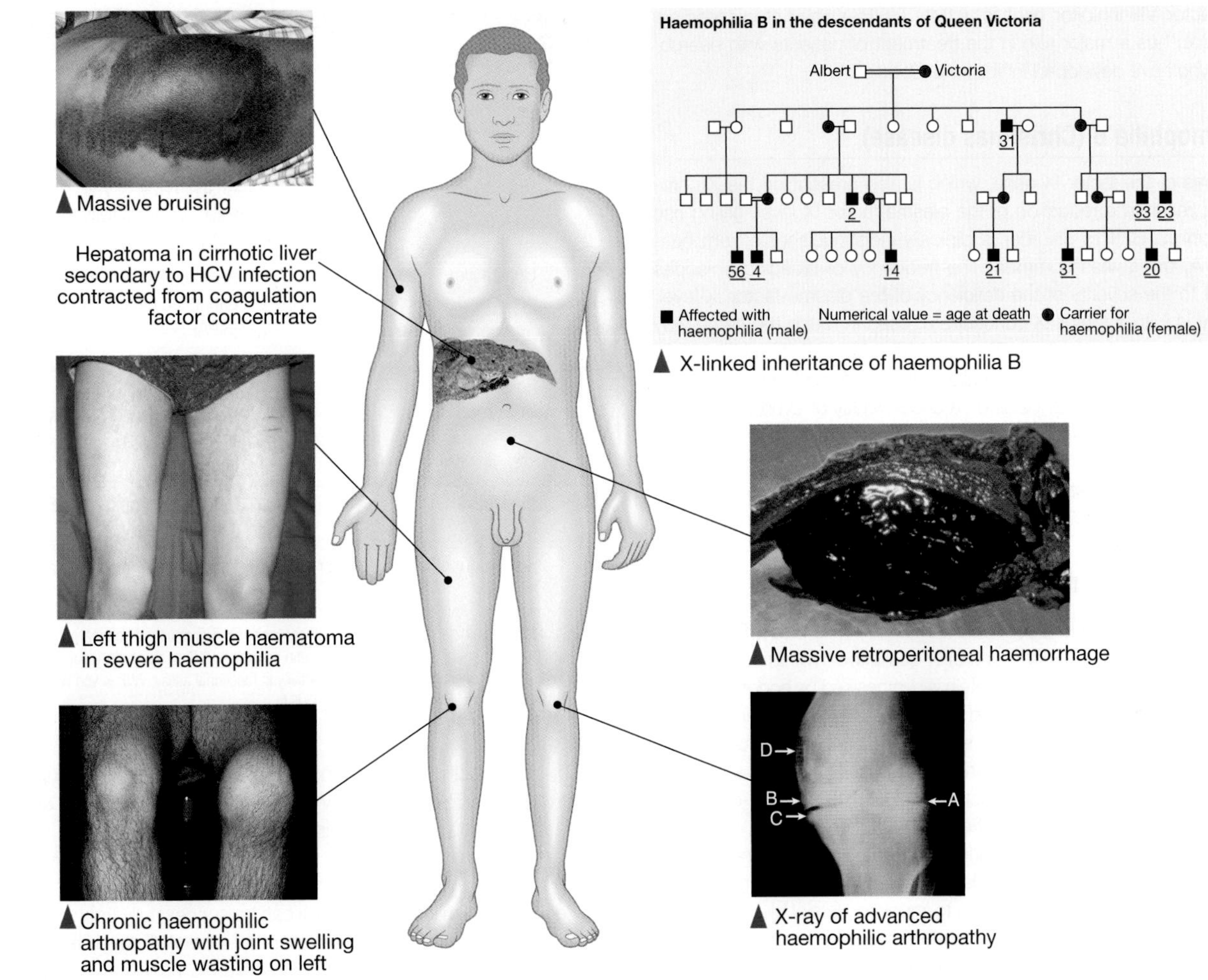

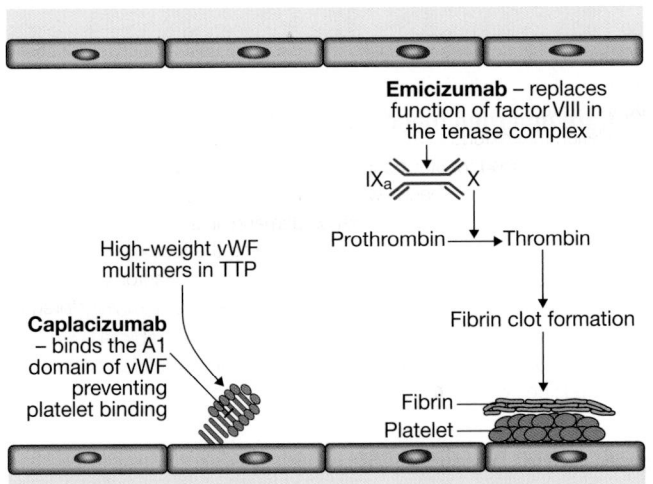

Massive bruising

Hepatoma in cirrhotic liver secondary to HCV infection contracted from coagulation factor concentrate

Left thigh muscle haematoma in severe haemophilia

Chronic haemophilic arthropathy with joint swelling and muscle wasting on left

Haemophilia B in the descendants of Queen Victoria

Albert ☐━━━● Victoria

■ Affected with haemophilia (male)   Numerical value = age at death   ● Carrier for haemophilia (female)

X-linked inheritance of haemophilia B

Massive retroperitoneal haemorrhage

D→ B→ C→ ←A

X-ray of advanced haemophilic arthropathy

Fig. 25.40 Clinical manifestations of haemophilia. On the knee X-ray, repeated bleeds have led to broadening of the femoral epicondyles, and there is no cartilage present, as evidenced by the close proximity of the femur and tibia (A); sclerosis (B), osteophyte (C) and bony cysts (D) are present. (HCV = hepatitis C virus) *Inset (Massive bruising) From Hoffbrand VA. Color atlas of clinical hematology, 3rd edn. Philadelphia: Mosby, Elsevier Inc.; 2000.*

Emicizumab – replaces function of factor VIII in the tenase complex

IXₐ ⟩⟨ X

Prothrombin ──→ Thrombin

High-weight vWF multimers in TTP

Caplacizumab – binds the A1 domain of vWF preventing platelet binding

Fibrin clot formation

Fibrin
Platelet

Fig. 25.41 Mechanism of action of novel agents in haemostasis and thrombosis. Emicizumab is a bispecific antibody that acts in a similar manner to Factor VIIIa by binding to factor IXa and factor X and so can be used in haemophilia A. Capalacizumab inhibits the A1 domain on von Willebrand factor (vWF), preventing binding to platelets and subsequent platelet aggregation. It is increasingly used in the treatment of thrombotic thrombocytopenic purpura (TTP).

The vasopressin receptor agonist desmopressin raises the vWF and factor VIII levels 3–4-fold, which is useful in arresting bleeding in patients with mild or moderate haemophilia A. The dose required for this purpose is higher than that used in diabetes insipidus, usually 0.3 µg/kg, and is given intravenously or subcutaneously. Alternatively, the same effect can be achieved by intranasal administration of a 300 µg dose. Following repeated administration of desmopressin, patients need to be monitored for evidence of water retention, which can result in significant hyponatraemia. Desmopressin is contraindicated in patients with a history of severe arterial disease, because of a propensity to provoke a thrombotic event, and in young children where hyponatraemia can result in fits.

Complications of coagulation factor therapy

Before 1986, coagulation factor concentrates from human plasma were not fully virus-inactivated and many patients became infected with HIV and HBV/HCV. Concern that the infectious agent that causes variant Creutzfeldt–Jakob disease (vCJD) (Ch. 28) might be transmissible by blood and blood products has been confirmed in recipients of red cell transfusion (p. 940), and in one recipient of factor VIII. Another serious complication of factor VIII treatment is the development of anti-factor VIII antibodies, which arise in about 25% of those with severe haemophilia. These antibodies rapidly neutralise therapeutic infusions, making treatment relatively ineffective. Infusions of activated clotting factors, e.g.

VIIa or factor VIII inhibitor bypass activity (FEIBA), may stop bleeding. Emicizumab has a major role in the treatment of patients with haemophilia A who have developed inhibitory antibodies.

Haemophilia B (Christmas disease)

Aberrations of the factor IX gene, which is also present on the X chromosome, result in a reduction of the plasma factor IX level, giving rise to haemophilia B. This disorder is clinically indistinguishable from haemophilia A, but is less common. The frequency of bleeding episodes is related to the severity of the deficiency of the plasma factor IX level. Treatment is with a factor IX concentrate, used in much the same way as factor VIII for haemophilia A. The new extended half-life recombinant factor IX products made by Fc fusion, albumin fusion and pegylation offer the possibility of prophylaxis on a once-weekly or even two-weekly schedule. Although factor IX concentrates shared the problems of virus transmission seen with factor VIII, they do not commonly induce inhibitory antibodies (<1% patients); when this does occur, however, it may be heralded by the development of a severe allergic-type reaction.

Von Willebrand disease

Von Willebrand disease is a common and usually mild bleeding disorder caused by a quantitative (types 1 and 3) or qualitative (type 2) deficiency of von Willebrand factor (vWF). This protein is synthesised by endothelial cells and megakaryocytes, and is involved in both platelet function and coagulation. It normally forms a multimeric structure that is essential for its interaction with subendothelial collagen and platelets (see Figs. 25.6 and 25.7). vWF acts as a carrier protein for factor VIII, to which it is non-covalently bound; deficiency of vWF lowers the plasma factor VIII level. vWF also forms bridges between platelets and subendothelial components (e.g. collagen; see Fig. 25.6B), allowing platelets to adhere to damaged vessel walls; deficiency of vWF therefore leads to impaired platelet plug formation. Blood group antigens (A and B) are expressed on vWF, reducing its susceptibility to proteolysis; as a result, people with blood group O have lower circulating vWF levels than individuals with non-O groups.

Most patients with von Willebrand disease have a type 1 disorder, characterised by a quantitative decrease in a normal functional protein. This usually arises through reduced synthesis or increased clearance of vWF. Patients with type 2 disorders inherit vWF molecules that are functionally abnormal. The type of abnormality depends on the site of the mutation in the vWF gene and how it affects binding to platelets, collagen and factor VIII. Patients with type 2A disease have abnormalities in vWF-dependent platelet adhesion; those with mutations in the platelet glycoprotein Ib binding site, resulting in increased affinity for glycoprotein 1b, have type 2B disease; those with mutations in the factor VIII binding site have type 2N disease; and those with other abnormalities in platelet binding, but with normal vWF multimeric structure, have type 2M disease. The patterns of laboratory abnormality accompanying these types are described in Box 25.66. The gene for vWF is located on chromosome 12 and the disease is usually autosomal dominantly inherited, except in type 2N and type 3, where inheritance is autosomal recessive.

Clinical features

Patients present with haemorrhagic manifestations similar to those in individuals with reduced platelet function. Superficial bruising, epistaxis, menorrhagia and gastrointestinal haemorrhage are common. Bleeding episodes are usually much less frequent than in severe haemophilia, and excessive haemorrhage may be observed only after trauma or surgery. Within a single family, the disease has variable penetrance, so that some members may have quite severe and frequent bleeds, whereas others are relatively asymptomatic.

Investigations

The disorder is characterised by reduced activity of vWF and factor VIII. The disease can be classified using a combination of assays that include functional and antigenic measures of vWF, multimeric analysis of the

i	25.66 Classification of von Willebrand disease			
Type	Defect	Inheritance	Investigations/patterns
1	Partial quantitative	AD	Parallel decrease in vWF:Ag, RiCoF and VIII:c
2A	Qualitative	AD	Absent HWM of vWF Ratio of vWF activity to antigen <0.7
2B	Qualitative	AD	Reduced HWM of vWF Enhanced platelet agglutination (RIPA)
2M	Qualitative	AD	Ratio of vWF activity to antigen <0.7 Normal multimers of vWF Abnormal vWF/platelet interactions
2N	Qualitative	AR	Defective binding of vWF to VIII Low VIII
3	Severe quantitative	AR or CH	Very low vWF and VIII:c activity Absent multimers

(AD = autosomal dominant; AR = autosomal recessive; CH = compound heterozygote; HWM = high-weight multimers of vWF; RiCoF = ristocetin co-factor; RIPA = ristocetin-induced platelet agglutination; VIII:c = coagulation factor VIII activity in functional assay; vWF = von Willebrand factor; vWF:Ag = vWF antigen measured by ELISA)

protein, and specific tests of function to determine binding to platelet glycoprotein Ib (RIPA) and factor VIII (see Box 25.66). In addition, analysis for mutations in the vWF gene can be informative.

Management

Many episodes of mild haemorrhage can be successfully treated by local means or with desmopressin, which raises the vWF level, resulting in a secondary increase in factor VIII. Tranexamic acid may be useful in mucosal bleeding. For more serious or persistent bleeds, haemostasis can be achieved with selected factor VIII concentrates, which contain considerable quantities of vWF in addition to factor VIII. Pure plasma-derived and recombinant vWF concentrates are now available, improving the options and the perceived safety of treatment. Young children and patients with severe arterial disease should not receive desmopressin, and patients with type 2B disease develop thrombocytopenia that may be troublesome following desmopressin. Bleeding in type 3 patients responds only to factor VIII/vWF concentrate.

Rare inherited bleeding disorders

Severe deficiencies of factor VII, X and XIII occur as autosomal recessive disorders. They are rare, but are associated with severe bleeding. Typical features include haemorrhage from the umbilical stump and intracranial haemorrhage. Factor XIII deficiency in women is typically associated with recurrent fetal loss.

Factor XI deficiency may occur in heterozygous or homozygous individuals. Bleeding is very variable and is not accurately predicted by coagulation factor levels. In general, severe bleeding is confined to patients with levels below 15% of normal.

Acquired bleeding disorders

DIC is an important cause of bleeding that begins with exaggerated and inappropriate intravascular coagulation. It is discussed later under thrombotic disorders.

Liver disease

Although, traditionally, severe parenchymal liver disease is associated with an excess of bleeding, it is now clear that these patients also have an increased risk of venous thrombosis. The description of end-stage liver disease as a state of auto-anticoagulation is misleading. Although there is reduced hepatic synthesis of procoagulant factors, this is balanced to a degree by the reduced production of natural anticoagulant proteins and reduced fibrinolytic activity in patients with advanced liver disease. In severe parenchymal liver disease, bleeding may arise from many different causes. Major bleeding, is often from structural abnormalities such as oesophageal varices or peptic ulcer, and sepsis and volume overload are common precipitants of bleeding. There is reduced hepatic synthesis, for example, of factors V, VII, VIII, IX, X, XI, prothrombin and fibrinogen. Clearance of plasminogen activator is reduced. Thrombocytopenia may occur secondary to hypersplenism in the presence of portal hypertension and due to reduced production and activity of thrombopoietin in advanced liver disease. In cholestatic jaundice, there is reduced vitamin K absorption, leading to deficiency of factors II, VII, IX and X, but also of proteins C and S. Treatment with plasma products or platelet transfusion should be reserved for acute bleeds or to cover interventional procedures such as liver biopsy. Vitamin K deficiency can be readily corrected with parenteral administration of vitamin K.

Renal failure

The severity of the haemorrhagic state in renal failure is proportional to the plasma urea concentration. Bleeding manifestations are those of platelet dysfunction, with gastrointestinal haemorrhage being particularly common. The causes are multifactorial and include anaemia, mild thrombocytopenia and the accumulation of low-molecular-weight waste products, normally excreted by the kidney, that inhibit platelet function. Treatment is by dialysis to reduce the urea concentration. Rarely, in severe or persistent bleeding, platelet concentrate infusions and red cell transfusions are indicated. Increasing the concentration of vWF, either by cryoprecipitate or by desmopressin, may promote haemostasis. Patients with significant renal impairment have an increased risk of anticoagulant-related bleeding, particularly with drugs that are at least partially renally excreted.

Thrombotic disorders

Venous thromboembolic disease (venous thromboembolism)

While the most common presentations of venous thromboembolism (VTE) are deep vein thrombosis (DVT) of the leg (p. 188) and/or pulmonary embolism (PE; see also p. 546), similar management principles apply to rarer manifestations such as jugular vein thrombosis, upper limb DVT, cerebral sinus thrombosis (p. 1186) and intra-abdominal venous thrombosis (e.g. Budd–Chiari syndrome; p. 909).

VTE has an annual incidence of approximately 1:1000 in Western populations. The relative incidence of DVT:PE is approximately 2:1. Mortality 30 days after DVT is approximately 10%, compared to 15% for PE. All forms of VTE are increasingly common with age and many of the deaths are related to coexisting medical conditions, such as active cancer or inflammatory disease, which predispose the patient to thrombosis in the first place. Risk factors for VTE are often present (Box 25.67) and it is appropriate to seek evidence of these risk factors in determining the long-term management strategy. Figure 25.42 illustrates some of the causes and consequences of VTE. The diagnosis of DVT and PE are discussed on pages 188 and 546, respectively.

Management of VTE

The mainstay of treatment for all forms of VTE is anticoagulation. This can be achieved in several ways. One option is to use LMWH followed by a coumarin anticoagulant, such as warfarin. Treatment of acute VTE with LMWH should continue for a minimum of 5 days. Patients treated with warfarin should achieve a target INR of 2.5 (range 2–3; pp. 930 and Box 25.25) with LMWH continuing until the INR is above 2. Alternatively, patients may be treated with a DOAC. Rivaroxaban and apixaban may be used immediately from diagnosis without the need for LMWH, while

i	**25.67 Factors predisposing to venous thrombosis**

Patient factors
- Increasing age
- Obesity
- Varicose veins
- Previous deep vein thrombosis
- Family history, especially of unprovoked venous thromboembolism when young
- Transient additional risk factors:
  - Pregnancy/puerperium
  - Oestrogen-containing oral contraceptives and hormone replacement therapy
  - Immobility, e.g. long-distance travel (>4 hrs)
  - Intravenous drug use involving the femoral vein
  - Surgery (see below)
  - Medical illnesses (see below)

Surgical conditions
- Major surgery, especially if >30 mins' duration
- Abdominal or pelvic surgery, especially for cancer
- Major lower limb orthopaedic surgery, e.g. joint replacement and hip fracture surgery

Medical conditions
- Myocardial infarction/heart failure
- Inflammatory conditions: inflammatory bowel disease, connective tissue disorders and vasculitis
- Malignancy (anti-cancer chemotherapy increases the risk of venous thromboembolism compared with cancer alone)
- Nephrotic syndrome
- Chronic obstructive pulmonary disease
- Severe infection, bacterial or viral
- Neurological conditions associated with immobility, e.g. stroke, paraplegia, Guillain–Barré syndrome
- Any high-dependency admission

Haematological disorders
- Polycythaemia rubra vera
- Essential thrombocythaemia
- Deficiency of natural anticoagulants: antithrombin, protein C, protein S
- Paroxysmal nocturnal haemoglobinuria
- Gain-of-function prothrombotic mutations: factor V Leiden, prothrombin gene G20210A
- Myelofibrosis

Antiphospholipid syndrome

the licences for dabigatran and edoxaban include initial treatment with LMWH for a minimum of 5 days before commencing the DOAC (see Fig. 25.41). In patients with active cancer and VTE, maintenance anticoagulation with LMWH is associated with a lower recurrence rate than warfarin. The use of DOACs in cancer-associated thrombosis is under study. Small studies suggest a possible role for apixaban and rivaroxaban in this context. Patients who have had VTE and have a strong contraindication to anticoagulation and those who continue to have new pulmonary emboli despite therapeutic anticoagulation should have an inferior vena cava (IVC) filter inserted to prevent life-threatening PE.

The optimal *initial* period of anticoagulation is between 6 weeks and 6 months. Patients with a provoked VTE in the presence of a temporary risk factor, which is then removed, can usually be treated for short periods (e.g. 3 months), and indeed anticoagulation for more than 6 months does not alter the rate of recurrence following discontinuation of therapy. If there are ongoing risk factors that cannot be alleviated, such as active cancer, long-term anticoagulation is usually recommended, provided that the risk of bleeding is not deemed excessive.

For patients with unprovoked VTE, the optimum duration of anticoagulation can be difficult to establish. Recurrence of VTE is about 2%–3% per annum in patients who have a temporary medical risk factor at presentation and about 7%–10% per annum in those with apparently unprovoked VTE. This plateaus at around 30%–40% recurrence at 5 years. As such, many patients who have had unprovoked episodes of VTE will benefit from long-term anticoagulation. Several factors predict risk of recurrence following an episode of unprovoked VTE. The strongest

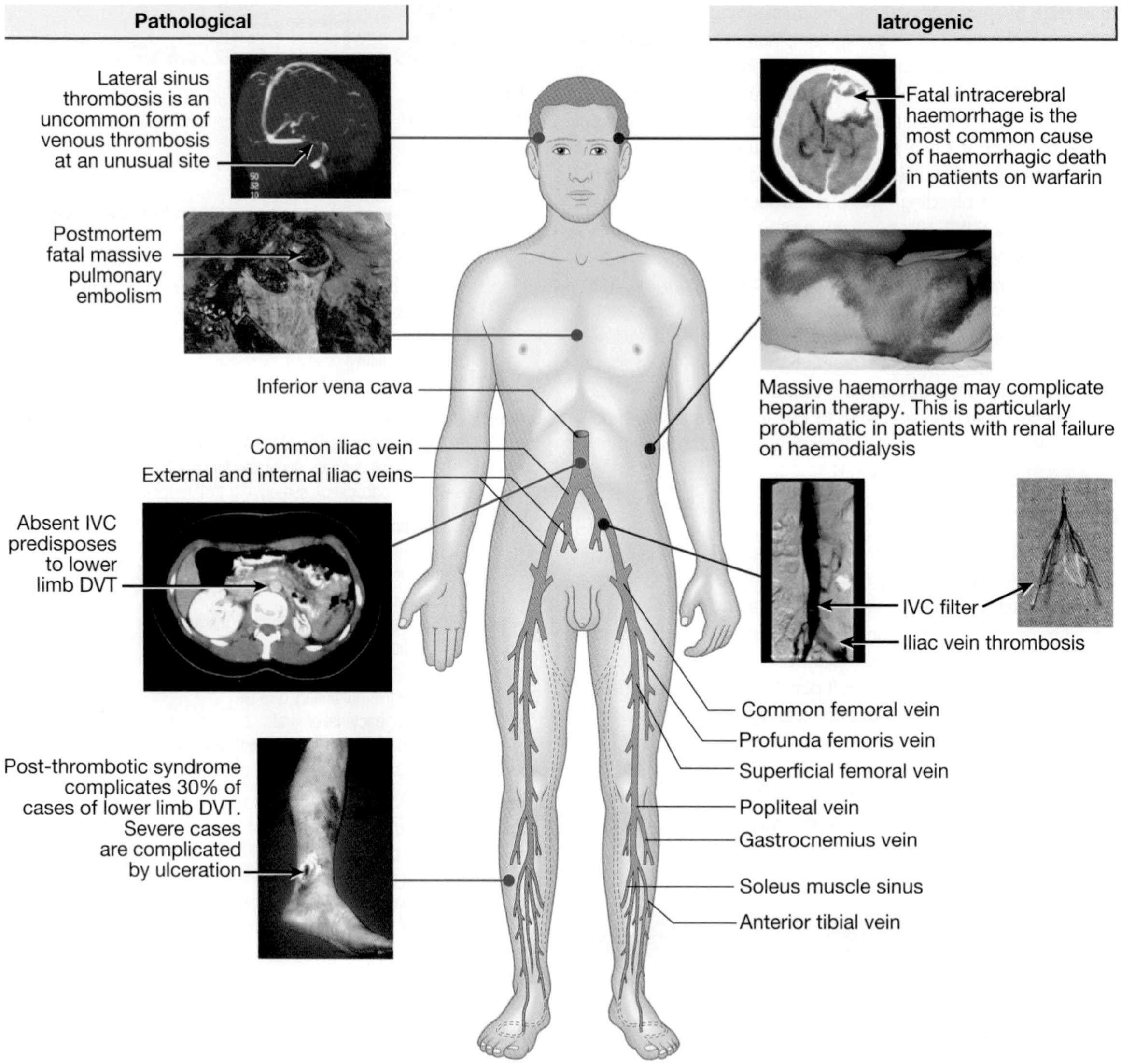

Pathological	Iatrogenic

Lateral sinus thrombosis is an uncommon form of venous thrombosis at an unusual site

Fatal intracerebral haemorrhage is the most common cause of haemorrhagic death in patients on warfarin

Postmortem fatal massive pulmonary embolism

Massive haemorrhage may complicate heparin therapy. This is particularly problematic in patients with renal failure on haemodialysis

Inferior vena cava

Common iliac vein

External and internal iliac veins

Absent IVC predisposes to lower limb DVT

IVC filter

Iliac vein thrombosis

Common femoral vein

Profunda femoris vein

Superficial femoral vein

Popliteal vein

Gastrocnemius vein

Post-thrombotic syndrome complicates 30% of cases of lower limb DVT. Severe cases are complicated by ulceration

Soleus muscle sinus

Anterior tibial vein

Fig. 25.42 Causes and consequences of venous thromboembolic disease and its treatment. (DVT = deep vein thrombosis; IVC = inferior vena cava)

predictors of recurrence are male sex and a positive D-dimer assay measured 1 month after stopping anticoagulant therapy. These factors are incorporated into scoring systems to predict recurrence such as the DASH score, HERDOO2 score and the Vienna prediction model.

The management of DVT of the leg should also include elevation and analgesia; in limb-threatening DVT, thrombolysis may also be considered. Thrombolysis for PE is discussed in Chapter 17. Post-thrombotic syndrome is due to damage of venous valves by the thrombus. It occurs in around 30% of patients who sustain a proximal lower limb DVT and results in persistent leg swelling, heaviness and discoloration. The most severe complication of this syndrome is ulceration around the medial malleolus (see Fig. 25.42). Use of elastic compression stockings following a DVT does not reduce the incidence of post-thrombotic syndrome.

Prophylaxis of VTE

All patients admitted to hospital should be assessed for their risk of developing VTE and appropriate prophylactic measures should be put in place. Both medical and surgical patients are at increased risk. A summary of the risk categories is given in Box 25.68. Early mobilisation of patients is important to prevent DVT and those at medium or high risk require additional antithrombotic measures; these may be pharmacological or mechanical. There is increasing evidence in high-risk groups, such as patients who have had major lower limb orthopaedic surgery and abdominal or pelvic cancer surgery, for protracted thromboprophylaxis

for as long as 30 days or so after the procedure. Particular care should be taken with the use of pharmacological prophylaxis in patients with a high risk of bleeding or with specific risks of haemorrhage related to the site of surgery or the use of spinal or epidural anaesthesia.

Inherited and acquired thrombophilia and prothrombotic states

Several inherited conditions predispose to VTE (see Box 25.67), and have several points in common that are worth noting:

- None of them is strongly associated with arterial thrombosis.
- All are associated with a slightly increased incidence of adverse outcome of pregnancy, including recurrent early fetal loss, but there are no data to indicate that any specific intervention changes that outcome.
- Apart from in antithrombin deficiency and homozygous factor V Leiden, most carriers of these genes will never have an episode of VTE; if they do, it will be associated with the presence of an additional temporary risk factor.
- There is little evidence that detection of these abnormalities predicts recurrence of VTE over and above the validated scoring systems mentioned above.

25.68 Antithrombotic prophylaxis

Indications

Patients in the following categories should be considered for specific antithrombotic prophylaxis:

Moderate risk of DVT
- Major surgery:
  In patients >40 years or with other risk factor for VTE
- Major medical illness, e.g.:
  Heart failure
  Myocardial infarction with complications
  Sepsis
  Inflammatory conditions, including inflammatory bowel disease
  Active malignancy
  Nephrotic syndrome
  Stroke and other conditions leading to lower limb paralysis

High risk of DVT
- Major abdominal or pelvic surgery for malignancy or with history of DVT or known thrombophilia (see Box 25.4)
- Major hip or knee surgery
- Neurosurgery

Methods of VTE prophylaxis

Mechanical
- Intermittent pneumatic compression
- Mechanical foot pumps
- Graduated compression stockings

Pharmacological
- LMWHs
- Unfractionated heparin
- Fondaparinux
- Dabigatran
- Rivaroxaban
- Apixaban
- Warfarin

(DVT = deep vein thrombosis; VTE = venous thromboembolism)

- None of these conditions per se requires treatment with anticoagulants. Patients with thrombosis should receive anticoagulation, as discussed earlier. Patients who are deemed to be at high risk of thrombosis, e.g. those with antithrombin deficiency in pregnancy, should receive treatment or prophylactic doses of unfractionated or LMW heparin to cover the period of risk only.

Antithrombin deficiency

Antithrombin (AT) is a serine protease inhibitor (SERPIN) that inactivates the activated coagulation factors IIa, IXa, Xa and XIa. Heparins and fondaparinux achieve their therapeutic effect by potentiating the activity of AT. Familial deficiency of AT is inherited in an autosomal dominant manner; homozygosity for mutant alleles is not compatible with life. Around 70% of affected individuals will have an episode of VTE before the age of 60 years and the relative risk for thrombosis compared with the background population is 10–20-fold. Pregnancy is a high-risk period for VTE and this requires fairly aggressive management with doses of LMWH that are greater than the usual prophylactic doses (≥100 U/kg/day). AT concentrate (either plasma-derived or recombinant) is available; this is required for cardiopulmonary bypass and may be used as an adjunct to heparin in surgical prophylaxis and in the peripartum period.

Protein C and S deficiencies

Protein C and its co-factor protein S are vitamin K-dependent natural anticoagulants involved in switching off coagulation factor activation (factors Va and VIIIa) and so thrombin generation (see Fig. 25.6F). Inherited deficiency of either protein C or S results in a prothrombotic state with a 5-fold relative risk of VTE compared with the background population.

Factor V Leiden

Factor V Leiden results from a gain-of-function, single-base-pair mutation, which prevents the cleavage and hence inactivation of activated

factor V. This results in a relative risk of venous thrombosis of 5 in heterozygotes and 50 or more in rare homozygotes. The mutation is found in about 5% of Northern Europeans, 2% of Hispanics, 1.2% of African Americans, 0.5% of Asian Americans and 1.25% of Indigenous Americans, and is rare in Chinese and Malay people.

Prothrombin G20210A

This gain-of-function mutation in the non-coding 3′ end of the prothrombin gene is associated with an increased plasma level of prothrombin. It is present in about 2% of Northern Europeans, but is rare in native populations of Korea, China, India and Africa. In the heterozygous state, it is associated with a 2–3-fold increase in risk of VTE compared with the background population.

Antiphospholipid syndrome

Antiphospholipid syndrome (APS) is a clinicopathological entity in which a constellation of clinical conditions, alone or in combination, is found in association with a persistently positive test for an antiphospholipid antibody. The antiphospholipid antibodies are heterogeneous and typically are directed against proteins that bind to phospholipids (Box 25.69). Although causal roles for these antibodies have been proposed, the mechanisms underlying the clinical features of APS are not clear. In clinical practice, two types of test are used, which detect:

- antibodies that bind to negatively charged phospholipid on an ELISA plate (called an anticardiolipin antibody test); these assays usually contain β_2-glycoprotein 1 (β_2-GP1)
- those that interfere with phospholipid-dependent coagulation tests like the APTT or the dilute Russell viper venom time (DRVVT; called a lupus anticoagulant test).

The term antiphospholipid antibody encompasses both a lupus anticoagulant and an anticardiolipin antibody/anti-β_2-GP1; individuals may be positive for one, two or all three of these activities. It has been shown that patients who are 'triple positive' have an increased likelihood of thrombotic events compared with single or double positives.

Clinical features and management

APS may present in isolation (primary APS) or in association with one of the conditions shown in Box 25.69, most typically systemic lupus erythematosus (secondary APS). Most patients present with a single manifestation and APS is now most frequently diagnosed in women with

 25.69 Antiphospholipid syndrome (APS)

Clinical manifestations

- Adverse pregnancy outcome
  Recurrent first trimester abortion (≥3)
  Unexplained death of morphologically normal fetus after 10 weeks' gestation
  Severe early pre-eclampsia
- Venous thromboembolism
- Arterial thromboembolism
- Livedo reticularis, catastrophic APS, transverse myelitis, skin necrosis, chorea

Conditions associated with secondary APS

- Systemic lupus erythematosus
- Rheumatoid arthritis
- Systemic sclerosis
- Behçet's disease
- Temporal arteritis
- Sjögren syndrome

Targets for antiphospholipid antibodies

- β_2-glycoprotein 1
- Protein C
- Annexin V
- Prothrombin (may result in haemorrhagic presentation)

adverse outcomes of pregnancy. It is extremely important to make the diagnosis in patients with APS, whatever the manifestation, because it affects the prognosis and management of arterial thrombosis, VTE and pregnancy.

Arterial thrombosis, typically stroke, associated with APS should probably be treated with anti-coagulation, as opposed to anti-platelet therapy. APS-associated VTE is one of the situations in which the predicted recurrence rate is high enough to indicate long-term anti-coagulation after a first event. Recent evidence suggests that patients with APS presenting with thrombotic events should receive warfarin as opposed to a DOAC as anticoagulant of choice. In women with obstetric presentations of APS, intervention with heparin and aspirin is almost routinely prescribed, although there is little evidence from clinical trials that it is an effective therapy in increasing the chance of a successful pregnancy outcome.

Disseminated intravascular coagulation

Disseminated intravascular coagulation (DIC) may complicate a range of illnesses (Box 25.70). It is characterised by systemic activation of the pathways involved in coagulation and its regulation. This may result in the generation of intravascular fibrin clots causing multi-organ failure, with simultaneous coagulation factor and platelet consumption, causing bleeding. The systemic coagulation activation is induced either through cytokine pathways, which are activated as part of a systemic inflammatory response, or by the release of procoagulant substances such as tissue factor. In addition, suboptimal function of the natural anticoagulant pathways and dysregulated fibrinolysis contribute to DIC. There is consumption of platelets, coagulation factors (notably factors V and VIII) and fibrinogen. The lysis of fibrin clot results in production of fibrin degradation products (FDPs), including D-dimers.

25.70 Disseminated intravascular coagulation (DIC)	
Underlying conditions	
• Infection/sepsis	
• Trauma	
• Obstetric, e.g. amniotic fluid embolism, placental abruption, pre-eclampsia	
• Severe liver failure	
• Malignancy, e.g. solid tumours and leukaemias	
• Tissue destruction, e.g. pancreatitis, burns	
• Vascular abnormalities, e.g. vascular aneurysms, liver haemangiomas	
• Toxic/immunological, e.g. ABO incompatibility, snake bites, recreational drugs	
ISTH scoring system for diagnosis of DIC	
Presence of an associated disorder	Essential
Platelets (× 10⁹/L)	>100 = 0
	<100 = 1
	<50 = 2
Elevated fibrin degradation products	No increase = 0
	Moderate = 2
	Strong = 3
Prolonged prothrombin time	<3 secs = 0
	>3 secs but <6 secs = 1
	>6 secs = 2
Fibrinogen	>1 g/L = 0
	<1 g/L = 1
Total score	
≥5 = Compatible with overt DIC	
<5 = Repeat monitoring over 1–2 days	
(ISTH = International Society for Thrombosis and Haemostasis)	

Investigations

DIC should be suspected when any of the conditions listed in Box 25.70 are met. Measurement of coagulation times (APTT and PT; see Box 25.3) along with fibrinogen, platelet count and FDPs, helps in the assessment of prognosis and aids clinical decision-making with regard to both bleeding and thrombotic complications.

Management

Therapy is primarily aimed at the underlying cause. These patients will often require intensive care to deal with concomitant issues, such as acidosis, dehydration, renal failure and hypoxia. Blood component therapy, such as fresh frozen plasma, cryoprecipitate and platelets, should be given if the patient is bleeding or to cover interventions with a high bleeding risk, but should not be prescribed routinely based on coagulation tests and platelet counts alone. Prophylactic doses of heparin should be given, unless there is a clear contraindication. Established thrombosis should be treated cautiously with therapeutic doses of unfractionated heparin, unless clearly contraindicated. Patients with DIC should not, in general, be treated with antifibrinolytic therapy, e.g. tranexamic acid.

Thrombotic thrombocytopenic purpura

Like DIC and also heparin-induced thrombocytopenia (p. 937), thrombotic thrombocytopenic purpura (TTP) is a disorder in which thrombosis is accompanied by paradoxical thrombocytopenia. TTP is characterised by a pentad of findings, although few patients have all five components:

• thrombocytopenia
• microangiopathic haemolytic anaemia
• neurological sequelae
• fever
• renal impairment.

It is an acute autoimmune disorder mediated by antibodies against ADAMTS-13 (a disintegrin and metalloproteinase with a thrombospondin type 1 motif).

This enzyme normally cleaves vWF multimers to produce normal functional units, and its deficiency results in large vWF multimers that cross-link platelets. The features are of microvascular occlusion by platelet thrombi affecting key organs, principally brain and kidneys. It is a rare disorder (1 in 750 000 per annum), which may occur alone or in association with drugs (ticlopidine, ciclosporin), HIV, shiga toxins (Ch. 13) and malignancy. It should be treated by emergency plasma exchange. Glucocorticoids, aspirin and rituximab also have a role in management. Caplacizumab, a monoclonal antibody directed against the A domain of vWF, is associated with improved outcomes, less relapse and faster time to recovery in patients with acquired TTP. Untreated mortality rates are 90% in the first 10 days, and even with appropriate therapy, the mortality rate is 20%–30% at 6 months.

Further information

Websites

b-s-h.org.uk/guidelines *Guidelines from the British Society for Haematology.*
cibmtr.org *Center for International Blood & Marrow Transplant Research.*
transfusionguidelines.org.uk *Contains the UK Transfusion Services' Handbook of Transfusion Medicine and links to other relevant sites.*
ukhcdo.org *UK Haemophilia Centre Doctors' Organisation.*

GPR Clunie
SH Ralston

26

Rheumatology and bone disease

Clinical examination of the musculoskeletal system

2 Extensor surfaces
Rheumatoid nodules
Swollen bursa
Psoriasis rash

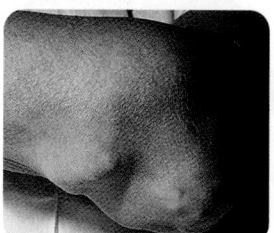

▲ Rheumatoid nodules

1 Hands
Swelling
Deformity
Nail changes
Tophi
Raynaud's

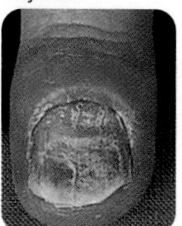

▲ Nail dystrophy in psoriatic arthritis

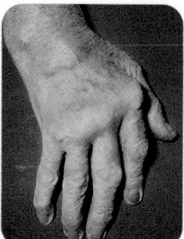

▲ Synovitis and deformity in rheumatoid arthritis

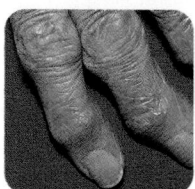

▲ Heberdens and Bouchard's nodes in osteoarthritis

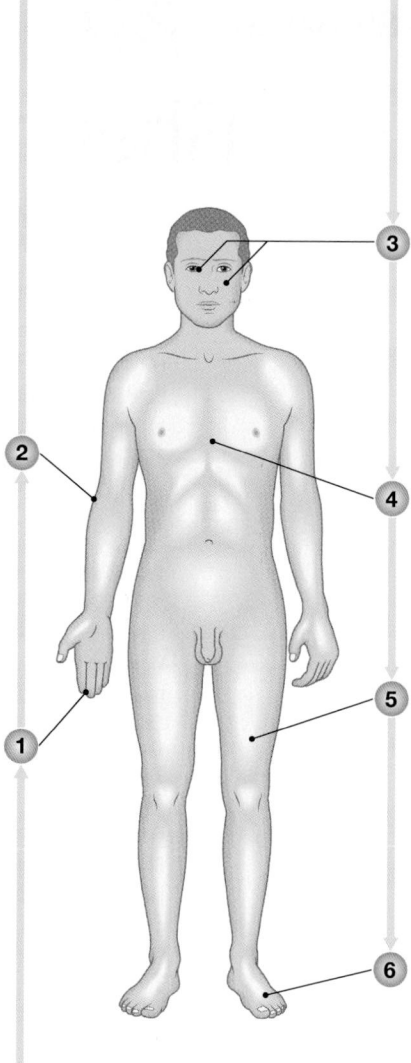

Observation
• General appearance
• Gait
• Deformity
• Swelling
• Redness
• Rash

3 Face
Rash
Alopecia
Mouth ulcers
Eyes

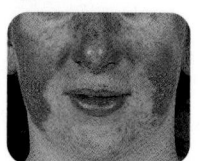

▲ Butterfly rash in systemic lupus erythematosus

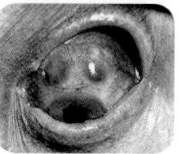

▲ Scleritis in rheumatoid arthritis

4 Trunk
Kyphosis
Scoliosis
Tender spots (fibromyalgia, enthesitis)

5 Legs
Deformity
Swelling
Restricted movement

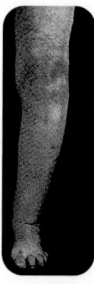

▲ Bone deformity in Paget's disease

6 Feet
Deformity
Swelling (gout, dactylitis)
Redness

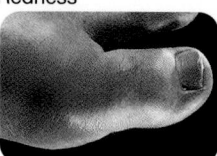

▲ Acute gout

General Assessment of Locomotor System (GALS) and Schöber's test

1 Gait

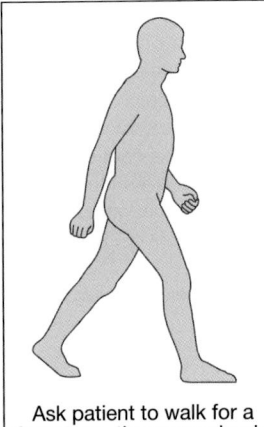

Ask patient to walk for a few steps, then come back. Look for pain or limp

2 Arms

Inspect hands for swelling or deformity

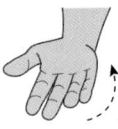

Ask patient to make a fist and open and close fingers (tests hand function)

Squeeze metacarpals (tests for inflammation)

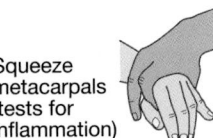

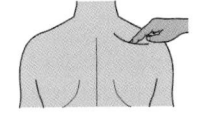

Press over supraspinatus (tests for hyperalgesia)

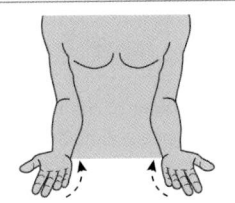

Patient turns palms up and down with elbows at side (tests supination and pronation of wrists and elbow)

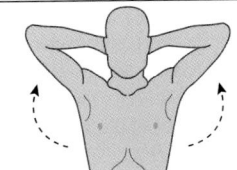

Ask patient to put hands behind head (tests shoulder movements)

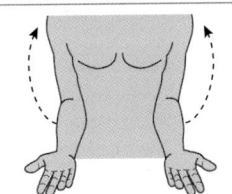

Patient flexes elbows to touch shoulder (tests elbow flexion)

3 Legs

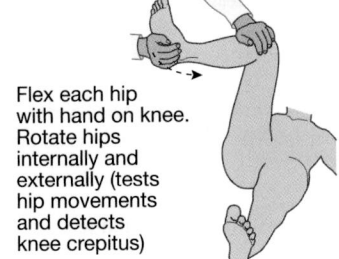

Flex each hip with hand on knee. Rotate hips internally and externally (tests hip movements and detects knee crepitus)

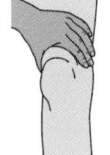 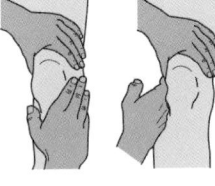

Palpate each knee for warmth and swelling (tests for synovitis and effusion)

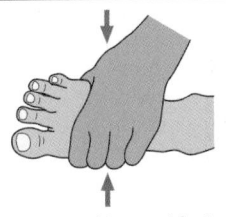

Inspect ankles and feet. Squeeze forefoot (tests for metatarsophalangeal synovitis)

4 Spine

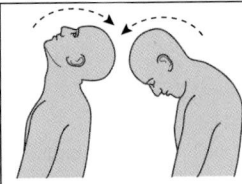

Patient looks at ceiling and then puts chin on chest (tests flexion and extension cervical spine)

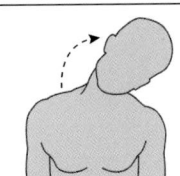

Ask patient to try to put ear on shoulder (tests lateral flexion cervical spine)

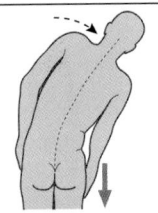

Patient slides hand down leg to knee (tests lateral spine flexion)

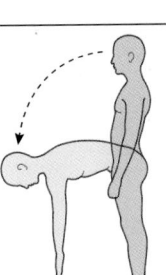

Inspect spine from behind and side, looking for scoliosis, kyphosis or localised deformity. Ask patient to touch toes

5 Schöber's test

Mark skin with pen in midline about 4 cm below superior iliac crest. Make another mark in midline 10 cm above first. Ask patient to bend forwards. Normally, distance between marks should increase to 15 cm

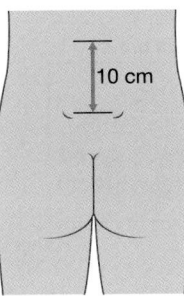

10 cm

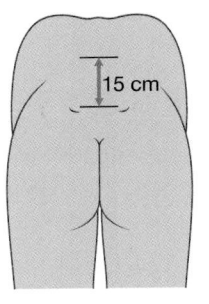

15 cm

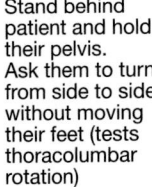
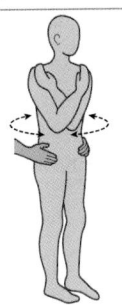

Stand behind patient and hold their pelvis. Ask them to turn from side to side without moving their feet (tests thoracolumbar rotation)

26

Disorders of the musculoskeletal system affect all ages and ethnic groups. In the UK, about 25% of new consultations in general practice are for musculoskeletal symptoms. Musculoskeletal diseases may arise from processes affecting bones, joints, muscles, or connective tissues such as skin and tendon. The principal manifestations are pain and impairment of locomotor function.

Diseases of the musculoskeletal system tend to be more common in women and most increase in frequency with increasing age. They are the most common cause of physical disability in older people and account for one-third of physical disability at all ages.

Functional anatomy and physiology

The musculoskeletal system is responsible for movement of the body, provides a structural framework to protect internal organs and acts as a reservoir for storage of calcium and phosphate in the regulation of mineral homeostasis. The main components of the musculoskeletal system are depicted in Figure 26.1.

Bone

Bones fall into two main types, based on their embryonic development. Flat bones, such as the skull, develop by intramembranous ossification, in which embryonic fibroblasts differentiate directly into bone within condensations of mesenchymal tissue during early fetal life. Long bones, such as the femur and radius, develop by endochondral ossification from a cartilage template. During development, the cartilage is invaded by vascular tissue containing osteoprogenitor cells and is gradually replaced by bone from centres of ossification situated in the middle and at the ends of the bone. A thin remnant of cartilage called the growth plate or epiphysis remains at each end of long bones and chondrocyte proliferation here is responsible for skeletal growth during childhood and adolescence. At the end of puberty, the increased levels of sex hormones halt cell division in the growth plate. The cartilage remnant then disappears as the epiphysis fuses and longitudinal bone growth ceases.

Two types of bone tissue are present in the normal skeleton (Fig. 26.1). Cortical bone is formed from Haversian systems, comprising concentric lamellae of bone tissue surrounding a central canal that contains blood vessels. Cortical bone is dense and forms a hard envelope around the long bones. Trabecular or cancellous bone fills the centre of the bone and consists of an interconnecting meshwork of trabeculae, separated by spaces filled with bone marrow. Important cell types in bone are:

- *Osteoclasts*: multinucleated cells of haematopoietic origin, responsible for bone resorption.
- *Osteoblasts*: mononuclear cells derived from marrow stromal cells responsible for bone formation.
- *Osteocytes*: cells that differentiate from osteoblasts that become embedded in bone matrix during bone formation. They are responsible for sensing and responding to mechanical stimuli and for coordinating osteoclast and osteoblast activity by producing receptor activator of nuclear factor kappa B ligand (RANKL) and sclerostin (SOST).
- *Bone marrow stromal cells*: cells that produce RANKL and macrophage colony-stimulating factor (M-CSF), which act together to stimulate osteoclast formation, and other cytokines that support haematopoiesis.
- *Bone lining cells*: flattened cells lining the bone surface that differentiate from osteoblasts when bone formation is complete.

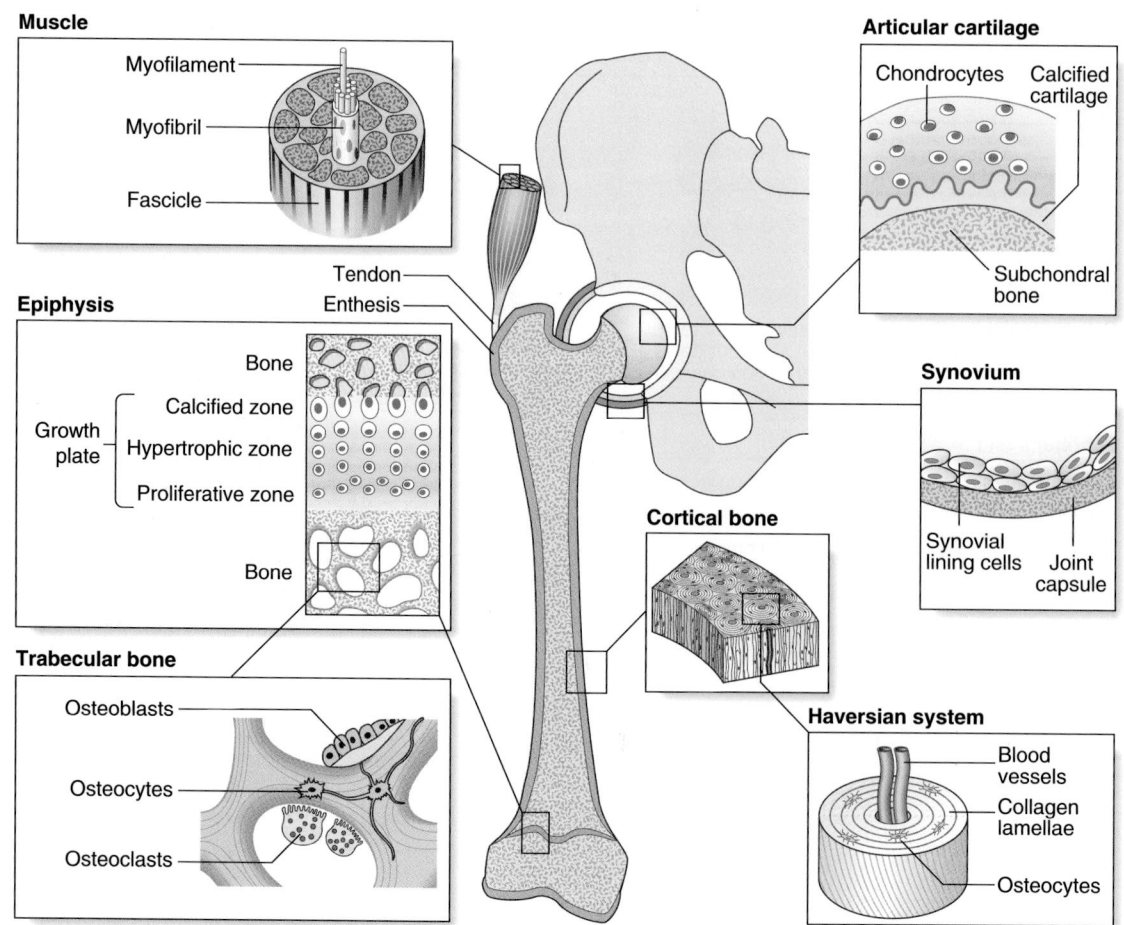

Fig. 26.1 Structure of the major musculoskeletal tissues.

Bone matrix and mineral

The most abundant protein of bone is type I collagen, which is formed from two α1 peptide chains and one α2 chain wound together in a triple helix. Type I collagen is proteolytically processed inside the cell before being laid down in the extracellular space, releasing propeptide fragments that can be used as biochemical markers of bone formation. Subsequently, the collagen fibrils become 'cross-linked' to one another

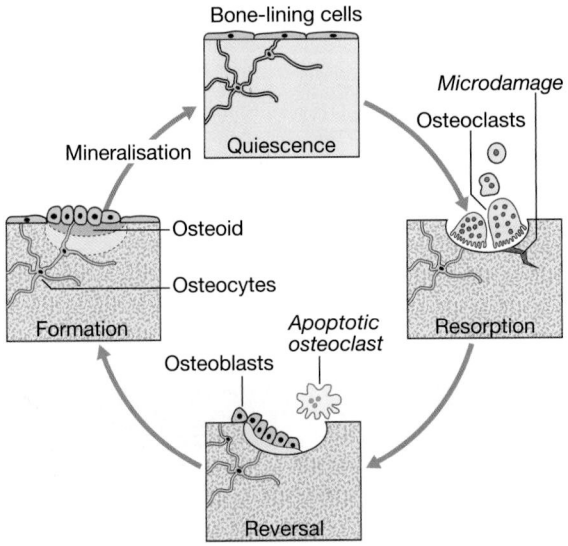

Fig. 26.2 The bone remodelling cycle. Bone is renewed and repaired by the process of bone remodelling. This begins by removal of old and damaged bone by osteoclasts during the phase of bone resorption. After about 10 days, the osteoclasts undergo programmed cell death (apoptosis) and during the reversal phase are replaced by osteoblasts, which begin to fill in the resorbed area with new bone matrix, heralding the start of bone formation. The bone matrix is initially uncalcified (osteoid) but then becomes mineralised to form mature bone.

by pyridinium molecules, a process that enhances bone strength. When bone is broken down by osteoclasts, the cross-links are released into the circulation. These can be measured biochemically and are sometimes used clinically to assess levels of bone resorption. Bone is normally laid down in an orderly fashion, but when bone turnover is high, as in Paget's disease or severe hyperparathyroidism, it is laid down in a chaotic pattern, giving rise to 'woven bone' that is mechanically weak. Bone matrix also contains growth factors, other structural proteins and proteoglycans, thought to be involved in helping bone cells attach to bone matrix and in regulating bone cell activity. The other major component of bone is mineral, comprised of calcium and phosphate crystals deposited between the collagen fibrils in the form of hydroxyapatite $[Ca_{10}(PO_4)_6(OH)_2]$. Mineralisation is essential for bone rigidity and strength, but over-mineralisation causes bone to become brittle. In clinical practice, increased mineralisation can occur in some types of osteogenesis imperfecta and in response to long-term bisphosphonate therapy.

Bone remodelling

Bone remodelling is required for renewal and repair of the skeleton throughout life. This is a cyclical process that has four phases: quiescence, resorption, reversal and formation, as illustrated in Figure 26.2. Remodelling starts with the attraction of osteoclast precursors in peripheral blood to the target site, probably by local release of chemotactic factors from areas of microdamage. The osteoclasts resorb bone and, after about 10 days, undergo programmed cell death (apoptosis), heralding the start of the reversal phase when osteoblast precursors are recruited to the resorption site. The osteoblast precursors differentiate into mature osteoblasts and form new bone during the formation phase. Initially, the matrix is unmineralised (osteoid) but eventually becomes mineralised to form mature bone. Some osteoblasts become trapped in bone matrix and differentiate into osteocytes, which play a key regulatory role in coordinating bone formation and resorption, whereas others differentiate into bone-lining cells.

The cellular and molecular mediators of this bone remodelling are shown in more detail in Figure 26.3. Osteoclast precursors are derived from haematopoietic stem cells and differentiate into mature osteoclasts

26

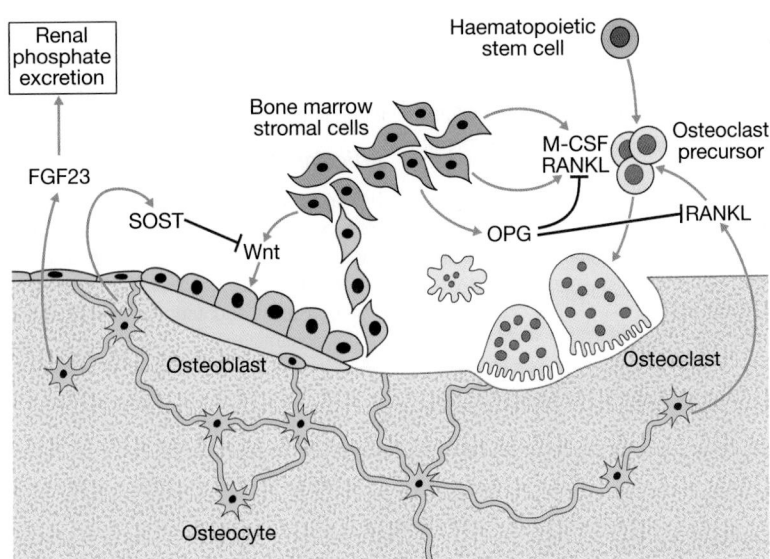

Fig. 26.3 Cellular and molecular regulators of bone remodelling. Osteoclast precursors are derived from haematopoietic stem cells. They differentiate into mature osteoclasts in response to the receptor activator of nuclear factor kappa B ligand (RANKL), which is produced by osteocytes, bone marrow stromal cells and activated T cells (not shown), and macrophage colony-stimulating factor (M-CSF), which is produced by bone marrow stromal cells. Osteoprotegerin (OPG) is also produced in the bone microenvironment, where it inhibits osteoclastic bone resorption by blocking the effect of RANKL. Osteoblasts, which are derived from bone marrow stromal cells, are responsible for bone formation. Osteoblast activity is stimulated by signalling molecules in the Wnt family but inhibited by sclerostin (SOST), which is produced by osteocytes. In addition to their role in regulating osteoclast and osteoblast activity, osteocytes have an endocrine function in regulating phosphate homeostasis by producing fibroblast growth factor 23 (FGF23), which acts on the kidney to promote phosphate excretion.

i | **26.1 Key regulators of bone remodelling**

Mediator	Source	Main effects	Comment
RANKL	Osteocytes Stromal cells Activated T cells	Stimulates bone resorption	Activates RANK
Osteoprotegerin	Stromal cells Lymphocytes	Inhibits bone resorption	Acts as decoy receptor for RANKL
Wnt	Stromal cells	Stimulates bone formation	Activates LRP receptors
Sclerostin	Osteocytes	Inhibits bone formation	Blocks effect of Wnt on LRP receptors
Parathyroid hormone	Parathyroid glands	Increases bone resorption and formation	
Thyroid hormone	Thyroid gland	Increases bone resorption and formation	
Oestrogen	Ovary	Inhibits bone resorption	
Glucocorticoid	Adrenal gland Exogenous	Inhibits bone formation	

(LRP = lipoprotein receptor-related protein; RANKL = receptor activator of nuclear factor kappa B ligand)

in response to M-CSF, produced by bone marrow stromal cells, and RANKL, produced by both osteocytes and bone marrow stromal cells. The RANKL binds to and activates a receptor called RANK (receptor activator of nuclear factor kappa B) on osteoclast precursors, promoting osteoclast differentiation and bone resorption. This effect is blocked by osteoprotegerin (OPG), which is a decoy receptor for RANKL that inhibits osteoclast formation. Once formed, mature osteoclasts attach to the bone surface by a tight sealing zone and secrete hydrochloric acid and proteolytic enzymes, including cathepsin K, into the space underneath, which is known as the Howship's lacuna. The acid dissolves the mineral and cathepsin K degrades collagen. Osteocytes also produce sclerostin (SOST), which is a potent inhibitor of bone formation. Under conditions of mechanical loading, sclerostin production by osteocytes is inhibited, allowing bone formation to proceed, stimulated by members of the Wnt family of signalling proteins. The Wnt molecules stimulate bone formation by activating members of the lipoprotein receptor-related protein (LRP) family, the most important of which are LRP4, LRP5 and LRP6. Sclerostin antagonises the effects of Wnt family members by blocking their interaction with LRP family members. Finally, osteocytes play a critical role in phosphate homeostasis by producing the hormone FGF23, which regulates renal tubular phosphate reabsorption. Key regulators of bone remodelling are summarised in Box 26.1.

Mineralisation of bone is critically dependent on the enzyme alkaline phosphatase (ALP), which is produced by osteoblasts and degrades pyrophosphate, an inhibitor of mineralisation. Bone remodelling is predominantly regulated at a local level but can be influenced by circulating hormones or mechanical loading, which can up-regulate or down-regulate remodelling across the whole skeleton (Box 26.1).

Joints

There are three main types of joint: fibrous, fibrocartilaginous and synovial (Box 26.2).

Fibrous and fibrocartilaginous joints

These comprise a simple bridge of fibrous or fibrocartilaginous tissue joining two bones together where there is little requirement for movement such as the symphysis pubis. The intervertebral disc is a special type of fibrocartilaginous joint in which an amorphous area, called the nucleus pulposus, lies in the centre of the fibrocartilaginous bridge. The nucleus has a high water content and acts as a cushion to improve the disc's shock-absorbing properties.

i | **26.2 Types of joint**

Type	Range of movement	Examples
Fibrous	Minimal	Skull sutures
Fibrocartilaginous	Limited	Symphysis pubis Costochondral junctions Intervertebral discs Sacroiliac joints
Synovial	Large	Most limb joints Temporomandibular Costovertebral

Synovial joints

These are complex structures containing several cell types. They are found where a wide range of movement is needed (Fig. 26.4).

Articular cartilage

This avascular tissue covers the bone ends in synovial joints. Cartilage cells (chondrocytes) are responsible for synthesis and turnover of cartilage, which consists of a mesh of type II collagen fibrils that extend through a hydrated 'gel' of proteoglycan molecules. The most important proteoglycan is aggrecan, which consists of a core protein to which several glycosaminoglycan (GAG) side chains are attached (Fig. 26.5). The GAGs are polysaccharides that consist of long chains of disaccharide repeats comprising one normal sugar and an amino sugar. The most abundant GAGs in aggrecan are chondroitin sulphate and keratan sulphate. Hyaluronan is another important GAG that binds to aggrecan molecules to form very large complexes with a total molecular weight of more than 100 million. Aggrecan has a strong negative charge and avidly binds water molecules to assume a shape that occupies the maximum possible volume available. The expansive force of the hydrated aggrecan, combined with the restrictive strength of the collagen mesh, gives articular cartilage excellent shock-absorbing properties.

With ageing, the concentration of chondroitin sulphate decreases, whereas that of keratan sulphate increases, resulting in reduced water content and shock-absorbing properties. These changes differ from those found in osteoarthritis, where there is abnormal chondrocyte division, loss of proteoglycan from matrix and an increase in water content.

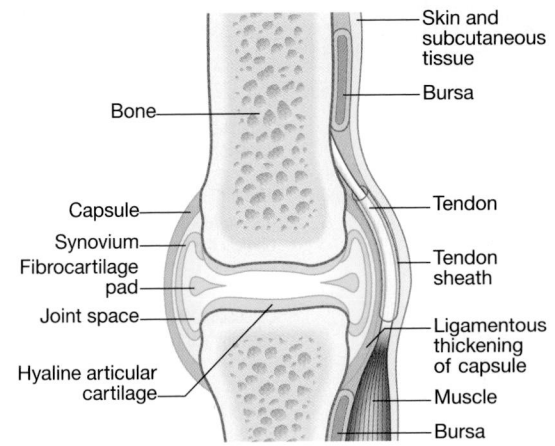

Fig. 26.4 Structure of a synovial joint.

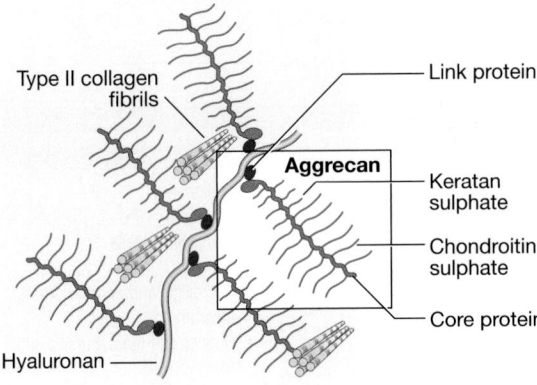

Fig. 26.5 Ultrastructure of articular cartilage.

Cartilage matrix is constantly turning over and in health there is a perfect balance between synthesis and degradation. Degradation of cartilage matrix is carried out by aggrecanases and matrix metalloproteinases, responsible for the breakdown of proteins and proteoglycans, and by glycosidases, responsible for the breakdown of GAGs. Pro-inflammatory cytokines, such as interleukin (IL)-1 and tumour necrosis factor (TNF), which are released during inflammation, stimulate production of aggrecanase and metalloproteinases, causing cartilage degradation.

Synovial fluid

The surfaces of articular cartilage are separated by a space filled with synovial fluid (SF), a viscous liquid that lubricates the joint. It is an ultrafiltrate of plasma, into which synovial cells secrete hyaluronan and proteoglycans.

Intra-articular discs

Some joints contain fibrocartilaginous discs within the joint space that act as shock absorbers. The most clinically important are the menisci of the knee. These are avascular structures that remain viable because of diffusion of oxygen and nutrients from the SF.

Synovial membrane, joint capsule and bursae

The bones of synovial joints are connected by the joint capsule, a fibrous structure richly supplied with blood vessels, nerves and lymphatics which encases the joint. Ligaments are discrete, regional thickenings of the capsule that act to stabilise joints (see Fig. 26.4). The inner surface of the joint capsule is the synovial membrane, comprising an outer layer of blood vessels and loose connective tissue that is rich in type I collagen,

and an inner layer 1–4 cells thick consisting of two main cell types. Type A synoviocytes are phagocytic cells derived from the monocyte/macrophage lineage and are responsible for removing particulate matter from the joint cavity; type B synoviocytes are fibroblast-like cells that secrete SF. Most inflammatory and degenerative joint diseases are associated with thickening of the synovial membrane and infiltration by lymphocytes, polymorphs and macrophages.

Bursae are hollow sacs lined with synovium and contain a small amount of SF. They help tendons and muscles move smoothly in relation to bones and other articular structures.

Skeletal muscle

Skeletal muscles are responsible for body movements and respiration. Muscle consists of bundles of cells (myocytes) embedded in fine connective tissue containing nerves and blood vessels. Myocytes are large, elongated, multinucleated cells formed by fusion of mononuclear precursors (myoblasts) in early embryonic life. The nuclei lie peripherally and the centre of the cell contains actin and myosin molecules, which interdigitate with one another to form the myofibrils that are responsible for muscle contraction. The molecular mechanisms of skeletal muscle contraction are the same as for cardiac muscle (p. 389). Myocytes contain many mitochondria that provide the large amounts of adenosine triphosphate (ATP) necessary for muscle contraction and are rich in the protein myoglobin, which acts as a reservoir for oxygen during contraction.

Individual myofibrils are organised into bundles (fasciculi) that are bound together by a thin layer of connective tissue (the perimysium). The surface of the muscle is surrounded by a thicker layer of connective tissue, the epimysium, which merges with the perimysium to form the muscle tendon. Tendons are tough, fibrous structures that attach muscles to a point of insertion on the bone surface called the enthesis. Entheses transmit tensile load from soft tissues to bone and are composed of either fibrous tissue or fibrocartilage, depending on the local needs of the tissue in adapting to physical stress. The entheses are particularly affected by inflammation in patients with spondyloarthritis, as discussed later in this chapter.

Investigation of musculoskeletal disease

Clinical history and examination usually provide sufficient information for the diagnosis and management of many musculoskeletal diseases. Investigations are helpful in confirming the diagnosis, assessing disease activity and indicating prognosis. Investigations that are commonly used in musculoskeletal disease are discussed in more detail below

Joint aspiration

Joint aspiration with examination of SF is pivotal in patients with suspected septic arthritis, crystal arthritis or intra-articular bleeding. It should be carried out in all individuals with acute monoarthritis and samples should be sent for microbiology and clinical chemistry.

It is possible to obtain SF by aspiration from most peripheral joints and only a small amount is required for diagnostic purposes. Normal SF is present in small volume, is clear and either colourless or pale yellow, and has a high viscosity. It contains few cells. With joint inflammation, the volume increases, the cell count and the proportion of neutrophils rise (causing turbidity), and the viscosity reduces (due to enzymatic degradation of hyaluronan and aggrecan). Turbid fluid with a high neutrophil count occurs in septic arthritis, crystal arthritis and reactive arthritis. High concentrations of urate crystals or cholesterol can make SF appear white. Non-uniform blood-staining usually reflects needle trauma to the synovium. Uniform blood-staining is most commonly due to a bleeding diathesis, trauma or pigmented villonodular synovitis, but can also occur in severe inflammatory synovitis. A lipid layer floating above blood-stained

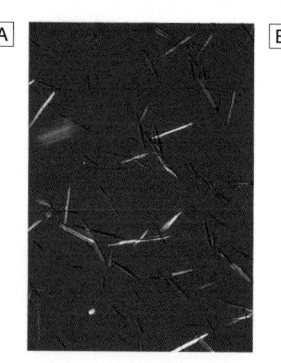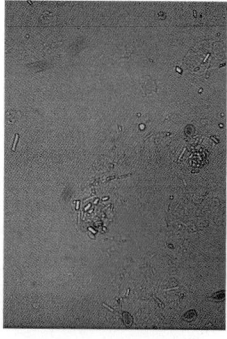

Fig. 26.6 Compensated polarised light microscopy of synovial fluids (× 400). [A] Monosodium urate crystals show bright negative birefringence under polarised light and needle-shaped morphology. [B] Calcium pyrophosphate crystals show weak positive birefringence under polarised light and are few in number. They are more difficult to detect than urate crystals.

fluid is diagnostic of intra-articular fracture and is caused by release of bone marrow fat into the joint.

Crystals can be identified by compensated polarised light microscopy of fresh SF (to avoid crystal dissolution and post-aspiration crystallisation). Urate crystals are long and needle-shaped, and show a strong light intensity and negative birefringence (Fig. 26.6A). Calcium pyrophosphate crystals are smaller, rhomboid in shape and usually less numerous than urate crystals; they have weak intensity and positive birefringence (Fig. 26.6B).

Imaging

Plain X-rays

X-rays show structural changes that are of value in the differential diagnosis and monitoring of many bone and joint diseases (Box 26.3).

They are of diagnostic value in osteoarthritis (OA), where they demonstrate joint space narrowing that tends to be focal rather than widespread (as seen in inflammatory arthritis). Other features of OA detected on X-rays include osteophytes, subchondral sclerosis, bone cysts and calcified loose bodies within the synovium (see Fig. 26.18). Erosions and sclerosis of the sacroiliac joints and syndesmophytes in the spine may be observed in spondyloarthritis (SpA; see Fig. 26.41). Erosions, associated with new bone formation and periosteal reaction, also occur in peripheral joints and at entheses in SpA. In tophaceous gout, well-defined punched-out erosions may occur (see Fig. 26.27). Calcification of cartilage, tendons and soft tissues or muscle occurs mainly in chondrocalcinosis (see Fig. 26.28), calcium-containing crystal diseases, tumoral calcinosis and autoimmune connective tissue diseases.

X-rays are of limited value in the diagnosis of rheumatoid arthritis (RA) because features such as erosions, joint space narrowing and periarticular osteoporosis may be detectable only after several months or even years. The main indication for X-rays in RA is in the assessment of disease over time when structural damage to the joints is suspected.

Radionuclide bone scintigraphy

Radionuclide bone scintigraphy is mainly used in the diagnosis of metastatic bone disease and Paget's disease of bone. Abnormalities may also be observed in primary bone tumours, complex regional pain syndrome, OA and different types of inflammatory arthritis, but the changes are non-specific and other imaging modalities are more commonly used. Bone scintigraphy involves gamma-camera imaging following an intravenous injection of ^{99m}Tc-labelled bisphosphonate. Early post-injection images reflect blood flow and can show increased perfusion of inflamed synovium, Pagetic bone or primary or secondary bone tumours. Delayed images taken a few hours later reflect bone remodelling as the

---

26.3 Radiographic abnormalities in selected rheumatic diseases

Rheumatoid arthritis
- Periarticular osteoporosis
- Marginal joint erosions
- Joint subluxation
- Joint space narrowing

Osteoporosis
- Osteopenia
- Vertebral fractures
- Non-vertebral fractures
- Cortical thinning

Paget's disease
- Bone expansion
- Abnormal trabecular pattern
- Osteosclerosis and lysis
- Pseudofractures

Psoriatic arthritis
- Sacroiliitis
- Syndesmophytes
- Bone sclerosis
- Proliferative enthesis erosions
- Enthesophytes
- Juxta-articular new bone

Osteoarthritis
- Joint space narrowing
- Osteophytes
- Subchondral sclerosis
- Joint deformity
- Subchondral cysts

26.4 Conditions detected by magnetic resonance imaging

- Osteonecrosis
- Intervertebral disc disease
- Nerve root entrapment
- Spinal cord compression
- Spinal stenosis
- Infection
- Complex regional pain syndrome
- Malignancy
- Fractures
- Meniscal disease
- Synovitis
- Sacroiliitis and enthesitides
- Inflammatory myositis
- Rotator cuff tears, bursitis and tenosynovitis

---

^{99m}Tc-labelled bisphosphonate localises to sites of active bone turnover. Single photon emission computed tomography (SPECT) combines radionuclide imaging with computed tomography. Bone radionuclide SPECT can provide accurate anatomical localisation of abnormalities within bone and is of particular value in the assessment of patients with chronic low back and pelvic pain where standard scintigraphy has yielded inconclusive results.

Magnetic resonance imaging

Magnetic resonance imaging (MRI) gives detailed information on anatomy, allowing three-dimensional visualisation of bone and soft tissues that cannot be adequately assessed by plain X-rays. The technique is valuable in the assessment and diagnosis of many musculoskeletal diseases (Box 26.4). T1-weighted sequences are useful for defining anatomy, whereas T2-weighted sequences are useful for assessing tissue water content, which is often increased in synovitis and other inflammatory disorders (Fig. 26.7). MRI sequences that suppress signal from fat, such as short TI inversion recovery (STIR), are helpful when evaluating inflammatory disease. Contrast agents, such as gadolinium, can be administered to increase sensitivity in detecting erosions and synovitis.

Ultrasonography

Ultrasonography is a useful investigation for confirmation of small joint synovitis and erosions, for anatomical location of periarticular lesions, for characterisation of tendon lesions and for guided injection of joints and bursae. Ultrasonography is more sensitive than clinical examination for the detection of early synovitis and can be helpful in the diagnosis and assessment of patients with suspected inflammatory arthritis. In addition to locating synovial thickening and effusions, ultrasound can detect

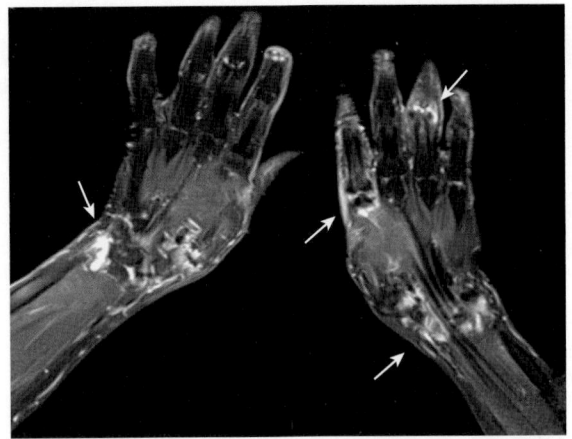

Fig. 26.7 Magnetic resonance image showing joint synovitis. Coronal post-contrast T1-weighted image shows extensive enhancement consistent with synovitis (white areas, arrowed) in both wrists, at the second metacarpophalangeal joint and proximal interphalangeal joints of the right hand. *Courtesy of Dr I. Beggs.*

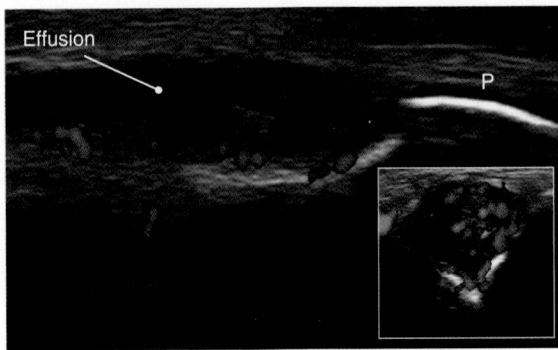

Fig. 26.8 Ultrasound image showing synovitis. Lateral image of a metacarpophalangeal joint in inflammatory arthritis. The periosteum (P) of the phalanx shows as a white line. The dark, hypo-echoic area indicates an effusion. The coloured areas demonstrated by power Doppler indicate increased vascularity. The inset shows a transverse image of the same joint. *Courtesy of Dr N. McKay.*

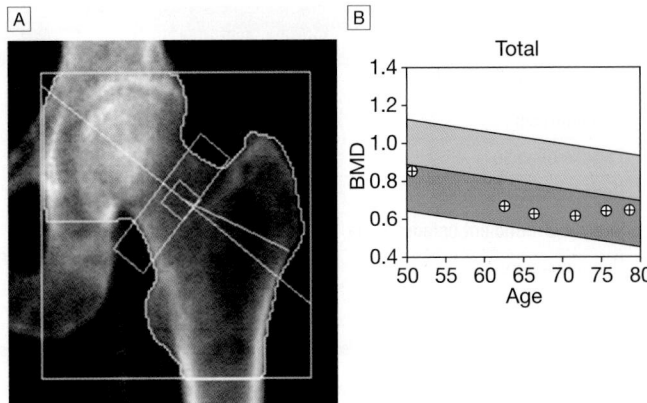

Scan date	Age	BMD	T-score	BMD change vs baseline	BMD change vs previous
11.01.2021	78	0.648	-2.4	-24.5%#	0.5%
03.01.2018	75	0.645	-2.4	-24.8%#	3.9%
21.01.2014	71	0.620	-2.6	-27.7%#	-1.6%
05.09.2008	66	0.630	-2.6	-26.5%#	-5.7%*
13.12.2004	62	0.668	-2.2	-22.1%#	-22.1%#
21.01.1993	50	0.857	-0.7		

*Statistically significant change since the previous scan results.
#Statistically significant change since baseline data in 1993.

Fig. 26.9 Left hip dual X-ray absorptiometry (DXA) scan. [A] The regions of interest (ROI) of the hip that are scanned. [B] Graph showing the changes in bone mineral density (BMD) of the total hip ROI over time. The extent of the blue panels above and below the central line represents ±2 standard deviations from the average BMD of the reference population for age. Data panel: BMD estimates, corresponding T-scores (see text for explanation) and changes in BMD over time (and with ageing) are shown. By 2008 this patient had become osteoporotic (T-score < −2.5). Since 2014 (age 71 years) the patient has been benefitting from effective osteoporosis treatment and BMD has increased.

increased blood flow within synovium using power Doppler imaging, an option that is available on most modern ultrasound machines (Fig. 26.8). Ultrasound is also used in the differential diagnosis of giant cell arteritis (GCA) to look for evidence of thickening of the vessel wall in the temporal or axillary arteries.

Computed tomography

Computed tomography (CT) is used selectively for assessing patients with bone and joint disease. CT may be used when skeletal anatomy needs defining, when calcific lesions are being assessed, when MRI is contraindicated, or when articular regions are being evaluated in which an adjacent joint replacement creates signal artefacts on MRI (using specific metal artefact reduction algorithms).

Dual X-ray absorptiometry

Dual X-ray absorptiometry (DXA) is used to measure bone mineral density (BMD) and has a key role in the diagnosis and management of osteoporosis. Measurements at lumbar spine, hip and sometimes forearm are obtained. DXA works on the principle that calcium in bone attenuates passage of X-rays through the tissue in proportion to the amount of mineral present: the more bone mineral present, the higher the BMD value. The results are presented in terms of BMD (in grams of hydroxyapatite per cm^2)

and as the T-score, which reflect the number of standard deviations by which the patient's BMD value differs from that in a young healthy control (Fig. 26.9). Osteoporosis is defined to be present when the T-score is −2.5 or below; osteopenia is defined to be present when the T-score lies between −1.0 and −2.5; and normal BMD is defined to be present when the T-score lies between −1.0 and below +2.5. T score values above +2.5 indicate high bone density. It is important to recognize that T-score values fall with age in the whole population as bone density falls, meaning that many people aged 60 and above have osteopenia or osteoporosis based on T-score, even though the BMD results are in the 'normal range' for that age group. Bone density needs to be interpreted carefully taking into account coexisting conditions, such as aortic calcification, vertebral fractures, degenerative disc disease and OA, all of which can cause high BMD results even in the presence of osteoporosis. Radiographic correlation is helpful in these circumstances.

Blood tests

Haematology

Abnormalities in the full blood count (FBC) often occur in inflammatory rheumatic diseases, but changes are usually non-specific. Examples include neutrophilia in crystal arthritides and septic arthritis neutropenia in systemic lupus erythematosus (SLE) and lymphopenia in autoimmune rheumatic and connective tissue diseases. Reduced levels of

26

i | **26.5 Typical biochemical features in various bone diseases**

	Calcium	Phosphate	ALP	PTH	FGF23	25(OH)D
Osteoporosis	N	N	N (↑ after fracture)	N or ↑	N	N or ↓
Paget's disease	N	N	↑↑	N or ↑	N	N or ↓
Renal osteodystrophy	N or ↓	↑	↑	↑↑	↑↑	N or ↓
Vitamin D-deficient osteomalacia	N or ↓	N or ↓	↑	↑↑	N or ↓	↓↓
Hypophosphataemic rickets	N	↓↓	↑	N or ↑	↑↑	N or ↓
Primary hyperparathyroidism	↑/↑↑	N or ↓	N or ↑	↑/↑↑	N or ↑	N or ↓

(N = normal; single arrow = increased or decreased; double arrow = greatly increased or decreased; ALP = alkaline phosphatase; FGF23 = fibroblast growth factor 23; 25(OH)D = 25 hydroxy-vitamin D; PTH = parathyroid hormone)

i | **26.6 Causes of an elevated serum creatinine phosphokinase (CPK)**

- Inflammatory myositis ± vasculitis
- Muscular dystrophy
- Motor neuron disease
- Alcohol, drugs (especially statins)
- Myocardial infarction*
- Trauma, strenuous exercise, prolonged immobilisation after a fall
- Hypothyroidism, metabolic myopathy
- Viral myositis

*The CK-MB cardiac-specific isoform is disproportionately elevated compared with total CPK.

i | **26.7 Conditions associated with a positive rheumatoid factor***

Condition	Approximate frequency (%)
Rheumatoid arthritis with nodules and extra-articular manifestations	100
Rheumatoid arthritis (overall)	70
Primary Sjögren syndrome	90
Mixed essential cryoglobulinaemia	90
Primary biliary cholangitis	50
Infective endocarditis	40
Systemic lupus erythematosus	30
Tuberculosis	15
Age > 65 years	20

*Normal healthy people can be positive for rheumatoid factor.

haemoglobin and raised platelets are a common and important finding in active inflammatory diseases. Some disease-modifying anti-rheumatic drugs (DMARDs) and biologics can cause marrow toxicity and require regular monitoring of the FBC. Additional tests that are useful in assessing rheumatic diseases include the direct antiglobulin test (which can indicate intravascular haemolysis in SLE).

Biochemistry

Routine biochemistry is useful for assessing metabolic bone disease, muscle diseases and gout, and is essential in monitoring DMARDs and biologic drugs (renal and hepatic function). Several bone diseases, including Paget's disease, renal bone disease and osteomalacia, give a characteristic pattern that can be helpful diagnostically (Box 26.5). Serum levels of uric acid are usually raised in gout, but a normal level does not exclude it, especially during an acute attack when uric acid levels temporarily fall. Equally, an elevated serum uric acid does not confirm the diagnosis, since most hyperuricaemic people never develop gout. Levels of C-reactive protein (CRP) are a useful marker of infection and inflammation, and are more specific than the erythrocyte sedimentation rate (ESR). An exception is in autoimmune connective tissue diseases, such as SLE and systemic sclerosis, where CRP may be normal but the ESR raised in active disease. Accordingly, an elevated CRP in a patient with SLE or systemic sclerosis suggests an intercurrent illness, such as sepsis, rather than active disease. Serum creatine phosphokinase (CK) levels are useful in the diagnosis of myopathy or myositis, but specificity and sensitivity are poor and raised levels may occur in other conditions (Box 26.6).

Immunology

Autoantibody tests are widely used in the diagnosis of rheumatic diseases. Whatever test is used, the results must be interpreted in light of the clinical picture and the different detection and assay systems used in different hospitals.

Rheumatoid factor

Rheumatoid factor (RF) is an antibody directed against the Fc fragment of human immunoglobulin. In routine clinical practice, immunoglobulin M

(IgM) RF is usually measured. About 70% of patients with RA test positive for RF, but the specificity for RA is poor (Box 26.7). High RF titres in RA are associated with more severe disease and extra-articular features.

Anti-citrullinated peptide antibodies

Anti-citrullinated peptide antibodies (ACPA) recognise peptides in which the amino acid arginine has been converted to citrulline by peptidylarginine deiminase, an enzyme abundant in inflamed synovium and in a variety of mucosal structures. Like RF, ACPA is positive in around 70% of people with RA, but specificity is higher (> 95%) and consequently ACPA has largely superseded RF in the diagnosis of RA. Like RF, ACPA positivity is associated with more severe disease and extra-articular features. It is important to emphasise that ACPA positivity does not equate to a diagnosis of RA since a proportion of people in the normal population are ACPA positive. These individuals are at increased risk of developing RA at some point in life, but may never do so. The pathogenic role of ACPAs is still debated but they may amplify the synovial response to an inflammatory stimulus.

Antinuclear antibodies

Antinuclear antibodies (ANAs) are directed against one or more components of the cell nucleus, including nucleic acids and the proteins that process DNA or RNA. They occur in many inflammatory rheumatic diseases, but are also found at low titre in normal individuals and in other diseases (Box 26.8). ANAs are not associated with disease severity or activity. The most common indication for ANA testing is in patients suspected of having SLE or other autoimmune connective tissue diseases. ANA has high sensitivity for SLE (100%), but low specificity (10%–40%). A negative ANA virtually excludes SLE but a positive result does not confirm it.

i	**26.8 Conditions associated with a positive antinuclear antibody***

Condition	Approximate frequency (%)
Systemic lupus erythematosus	100
Systemic sclerosis	90–95
Sjögren syndrome	40–70
Dermatomyositis or polymyositis	30–80
Mixed connective tissue disease	100
Autoimmune hepatitis	100
Rheumatoid arthritis	30–50
Autoimmune thyroid disease	30–50
Malignancy	Varies widely
Infectious diseases	Varies widely

*Low-titre positive antinuclear antibody can occur in people without autoimmune disease, without obvious clinical consequences, particularly in older adults.

i	**26.9 Conditions associated with antibodies to extractable nuclear antigens**

Antibody (target/other name)	Disease association
Anti-centromere antibody	Localised cutaneous systemic sclerosis (sensitivity 60%, specificity 98%)
Anti-histone antibody	Drug-induced lupus (80%)
Anti-Jo-1 (anti-histidyl-tRNA synthetase)	Polymyositis, dermatomyositis or polymyositis–systemic sclerosis overlap (20%–30%) Particularly associated with interstitial lung disease
Anti-La antibody (anti-SS-B)	Sjögren syndrome (60%) SLE (20%–60%)
Anti-ribonucleoprotein antibody (anti-RNP)	Mixed connective tissue disease (100%) SLE (25%–50%), usually in conjunction with anti-Sm antibodies
Anti-Ro antibody (anti-SS-A)	SLE (35%–60%): associated with photosensitivity, thrombocytopenia and subacute cutaneous lupus Maternal anti-Ro antibodies associated with neonatal lupus and congenital heart block Sjögren syndrome (40%–80%)
Anti-RNA polymerase	Diffuse systemic sclerosis (15%)
Anti Sm (anti-Smith antibody)	SLE (15%–30%); associated with renal disease
Anti-Scl-70 (anti-topoisomerase I antibody)	Diffuse systemic sclerosis (15%); associated with more severe organ involvement, including pulmonary fibrosis

(SLE = systemic lupus erythematosus)

Anti-DNA antibodies bind to double-stranded DNA (dsDNA). They are useful in SLE monitoring as high titres are associated with more severe disease and an increase in antibody titre may precede relapse. Most commonly, testing for anti-DNA antibodies is performed by enzyme-linked immunosorbent assay (ELISA) but immunofluorescent staining of DNA from the microorganism *Crithidia luciliae* is also used and has a much higher specificity than dsDNA ELISA for the diagnosis of SLE. It is primarily used in patients where the clinical suspicion of SLE is high but where standard dsDNA tests have yielded equivocal results.

It is also possible to screen for antibodies to various extractable nuclear antigens (ENA). These act as biomarkers for certain subtypes of autoimmune connective tissue diseases and some complications of SLE, but for most disorders their sensitivity and specificity are poor (Box 26.9).

Antiphospholipid antibodies

These antibodies can be detected in patients with SLE and in the antiphospholipid syndrome (see Box 25.69). In clinical practice the most commonly used tests are for antibodies to cardiolipin/beta$_2$-glycoprotein 1 (β_2GP1) and the dilute Russell viper venom test, which is a functional assay for antibodies that interfere with the clotting mechanism in vitro.

Antineutrophil cytoplasmic antibodies

Antineutrophil cytoplasmic antibodies (ANCA) are IgG antibodies directed against the cytoplasmic constituents of neutrophils and are useful in the diagnosis and monitoring of systemic vasculitis. Two common patterns are described by immunofluorescence: cytoplasmic fluorescence (c-ANCA), which is caused by antibodies to proteinase-3 (PR3); and perinuclear fluorescence (p-ANCA), which is caused by antibodies to myeloperoxidase (MPO) and other proteins, such as lactoferrin and elastase. These antibodies are not specific for vasculitis and positive results may be found in autoimmune liver disease, malignancy, infection (bacterial and human immunodeficiency virus, HIV), inflammatory bowel disease (IBD), RA, SLE and pulmonary fibrosis.

Complement and complement component antibodies

Low complement C3 is an indicator of active SLE and some forms of vasculitis owing to consumption of complement by immune complexes (see Fig. 4.4). Low C4 is less specific for SLE activity. High C3 and functional measures of complement activation are non-specific features of inflammation. It is possible to screen for autoantibodies directed against a variety of other complement components. Some have clinical utility. For example, anti-C1q antibodies are associated with SLE, but also occur in hypocomplementemic urticarial vasculitis syndrome (HUVS).

Approach to autoantibody testing and interpretation

Testing for autoantibodies should only be performed to gain support for the diagnosis when clinical assessment suggests there may be an underlying autoimmune disease. They are not screening tests for the presence of autoimmune disease since they have limited sensitivity and specificity (see Box 26.9). Routine re-testing of autoantibody profiles is seldom helpful unless the clinical features of the disease change or evolve with time.

Tissue biopsy

Tissue biopsy is useful in confirming the diagnosis in certain musculoskeletal diseases.

Synovial biopsy can be useful in selected patients with chronic inflammatory monoarthritis or tenosynovitis to rule out chronic infectious causes, especially mycobacterial infections. Synovial biopsy can be obtained arthroscopically or by using ultrasound guidance under local anaesthetic.

Temporal artery biopsy can be of value in patients suspected of having giant cell arteritis.

Biopsies of affected tissues, such as skin, lung, nasopharynx, gut, kidney and muscle, are of value in confirming a diagnosis of systemic vasculitis.

Muscle biopsy is important in the investigation of myopathy and inflammatory myositis. It is usually taken from the quadriceps or deltoid through a small skin incision under local anaesthetic. Since myositis can be patchy in nature, MRI is sometimes used to localise the best site for biopsy. Immunohistochemical staining, together with plain histology, gives information on primary and secondary muscle and neuromuscular

26

disease. Repeat biopsies are sometimes used to monitor the response to treatment.

Bone biopsy is occasionally required in patients with infiltrative disorders of bone, renal bone disease, suspected chronic infection or malignancy and rarely to confirm or exclude the presence of osteomalacia. For focal lesions, the biopsy should be taken under X-ray guidance or at open surgery, from an affected site. If a systemic bone disease or disorder of mineralisation is suspected, biopsies are usually taken from the iliac crest using a large-diameter (8 mm) trephine needle under local anaesthetic and processed without demineralisation.

Electromyography

Electromyography is of value in the investigation of suspected myopathy and inflammatory myositis, when it shows the diagnostic triad of:

- spontaneous fibrillation
- short-duration action potentials in a polyphasic disorganised outline
- repetitive bouts of high-voltage oscillations on needle contact with diseased muscle.

Presenting problems in musculoskeletal disease

The pattern of joint involvement and time-course can often provide valuable clues to the underlying diagnosis. The most common clinical presentations of musculoskeletal disease are discussed in this section.

Monoarthritis

This refers to pain and swelling affecting a single joint. The most common causes are crystal arthritis, sepsis, reactive arthritis and oligoarticular juvenile idiopathic arthritis. Other potential causes are shown in Box 26.10.

Clinical assessment

The clinical history, pattern of joint involvement, speed of onset, and age and gender of the patient all give clues to the most likely diagnosis. A very rapid onset (6–12 hours) is suggestive of either gout or acute calcium pyrophosphate arthritis (CPPA), which is also known as pseudogout. Both may be triggered by an intercurrent illness, dehydration or surgery. Gout classically affects younger men and particularly targets the first metatarsophalangeal (MTP) joint, whereas CPPA tends to affect older women, often with pre-existing OA or calcium pyrophosphate deposition (CPPD) disease. Reactive arthritis can also develop acutely and may be preceded by a diarrhoeal illness or genital infection. Septic arthritis develops more slowly and continues to progress until treated. Haemarthrosis usually follows an injury and may be associated with a large effusion,

in the absence of periarticular swelling or skin change. Pigmented villonodular synovitis also presents with synovial swelling and a large effusion, affecting a single joint but with a gradual onset. Rheumatoid arthritis seldom presents with monoarthritis, but psoriatic arthritis (PsA) can present this way, although the onset is usually more gradual in both conditions. Osteoarthritis can present with pain affecting a single joint, but the onset is gradual. Although there may be bony swelling of joints affected by OA, synovitis and effusions are uncommon.

Investigations

Aspiration of the affected joint is mandatory in patients with sudden onset of a hot swollen joint. The fluid should be sent for culture and Gram stain to seek the presence of organisms and should be checked by polarised light microscopy for crystals. Blood cultures should also be taken in patients suspected of having septic arthritis. CRP and ESR should be measured. While values are raised with both infection and inflammation, serial measurements can be useful in assessing the response to treatment. Serum uric acid measurements are of limited value since urate is a negative acute phase reactant and values can fall to within the normal range in acute gout. If investigations suggest CPPA, an elevated serum calcium may suggest underlying primary hyperparathyroidism.

Management

If there is any suspicion of septic arthritis, intravenous antibiotics should be given promptly, pending the results of cultures (see Box 26.50). Patients with suspected crystal-induced arthritis or reactive arthritis may be given intra-articular glucocorticoid injections to help the pain and swelling, but only if Gram stain is negative and synovial fluid culture has been negative for 48 hours. Longer-term management should be directed towards the underlying cause.

Polyarthritis

This term is used to describe pain and swelling affecting five or more joints or joint groups. The possible causes are listed in Box 26.11 and extra-articular features are listed in Box 26.12.

Clinical assessment

The hallmarks of an inflammatory polyarthritis are early-morning stiffness and worsening of symptoms with inactivity, along with synovial swelling and tenderness on examination.

The pattern of involvement can be helpful in reaching a diagnosis (Fig. 26.10). In RA there is typically symmetrical involvement targeting the metacarpophalangeal (MCP) and proximal interphalangeal (PIP) joints of the hands and wrists as well as the ankles and metatarsophalangeal (MTP) and PIP joints of the feet. Other large joints may also be affected. In psoriatic arthritis (PsA), the PIP and distal interphalangeal (DIP) joints of the hands are usually affected, often in an asymmetrical pattern and accompanied by nail pitting or early onycholysis. Large joints may also be affected, and psoriasis may or may not be present. In SLE there may be a polyarthritis, but this more usually causes polyarthralgia and tenosynovitis, mainly of distal limb joints and tendons. OA has a similar pattern of involvement to PsA in the hands, but can usually be distinguished by the presence of Heberden's and Bouchard's nodes and lack of synovitis and other features of PsA.

Investigations

Blood samples should be taken for routine haematology, biochemistry, ESR, CRP, viral serology and an immunological screen, including ANA and ACPA (or RF). If there is clinical suspicion of an inflammatory arthritis, but clinical signs of synovitis are absent, ultrasound examination or MRI may be helpful in confirming the diagnosis.

Management

Management should be tailored to the underlying diagnosis. While investigations are in progress non-steroidal anti-inflammatory drugs (NSAIDs) and analgesics may be considered for symptom control. While

i	**26.10 Causes of monoarthritis**

Common

• Gout	• Spondyloarthritis
• Pseudogout	• Psoriatic arthritis
• Trauma	• Reactive arthritis
• Haemarthrosis	• Enteropathic arthritis

Less common

• Rheumatoid arthritis	• Tuberculosis
• Juvenile idiopathic arthritis	• Leukaemia*
• Pigmented villonodular synovitis	• Gonococcal infection
• Foreign body reaction	• Osteomyelitis*

*In children, both leukaemia and osteomyelitis may present with monoarthritis.

i | 26.11 Common causes of polyarthritis

Cause	Characteristics
Rheumatoid arthritis	Symmetrical, small and large joints, upper and lower limbs
Viral arthritis	Symmetrical, small joints; may be associated with rash and prodromal illness; self-limiting
Osteoarthritis	Symmetrical, targets PIP, DIP and first CMC joints in hands, knees, hips, back and neck; associated with Heberden's and Bouchard's nodes
Psoriatic arthritis	Tends to be asymmetrical, affecting PIP and DIP joints in the hands but large joints may also be affected; often associated with nail pitting/onycholysis, dactylitis and enthesitis
Axial spondyloarthritis and enteropathic arthritis	Tends to affect mid-size and large joints and entheses, lower more than upper limbs; history of inflammatory back pain
Systemic lupus erythematosus	Symmetrical, typically affecting small joints; clinical evidence of synovitis unusual
Juvenile idiopathic arthritis	Various patterns including: polyarticular, oligoarticular and systemic but also enthesitis-predominant
Chronic gout	Affects distal more than proximal joints; history of acute attacks
Chronic sarcoidosis	Small and large joints, often involves ankles
Poncet's disease	A reactive arthritis often affecting large joints associated with tuberculosis
Calcium pyrophosphate arthritis	Chronic polyarthritis with involvement of wrists, ankles, knees and oligoarticular small hand joints

(CMC = carpometacarpal; DIP = distal interphalangeal; PIP = proximal interphalangeal)

i | 26.12 Extra-articular features of inflammatory arthritis

Clinical feature	Disease association
Skin, nails and mucous membranes	
Psoriasis, nail pitting and dystrophy	Psoriatic arthritis
Raynaud's phenomenon	Systemic sclerosis, antiphospholipid syndrome, SLE
Photosensitivity	SLE
Livedo reticularis	SLE, antiphospholipid syndrome
Splinter haemorrhages, nail-fold infarcts, purpuric lesions	Vasculitis
Urticaria and erythemas	SLE, adult-onset Still's disease, systemic JIA, rheumatic fever
Oral ulcers	SLE, reactive arthritis, Behçet's disease
Nodules	RA (mainly extensor surfaces), gout (tophi; eccentric, white deposits within), rheumatic fever
Xerostomia, dry skin, various rashes	Primary Sjögren syndrome
Eyes	
Uveitis	SpA, sarcoid, JIA, Behçet's disease
Conjunctivitis	Reactive arthritis
Episcleritis, scleritis	RA, vasculitis
Heart, lungs	
Pleuro-pericarditis	SLE, RA, rheumatic fever
Aortic valve/root disease	HLA-B27-related SpA
Interstitial lung disease	RA, SLE, primary Sjögren syndrome
Abdominal organs	
Hepatosplenomegaly	RA, SLE
Haematuria, proteinuria	SLE, vasculitis, systemic sclerosis
Urethritis	Reactive arthritis and SpA (sterile)
Fever, lymphadenopathy	Infection, systemic JIA, rheumatic fever

(HLA = human leucocyte antigen; JIA = juvenile idiopathic arthritis; RA = rheumatoid arthritis; SLE = systemic lupus erythematosus; SpA = spondyloarthritis)

glucocorticoids can be helpful in treating symptoms of inflammatory arthritis they should generally be avoided until a definitive diagnosis has been made.

Fracture

Fractures are a common presenting symptom of osteoporosis, but they also occur in other bone diseases, in osteopenia and in some people with a normal skeleton where there has been a high trauma injury.

Clinical assessment

The presentation is with localised bone pain, which is worsened by movement of the affected limb or region. There is usually a history of trauma, but spontaneous fractures can occur in the absence of trauma in severe osteoporosis. Fractures can be divided into several subtypes, based on the precipitating event and presence or absence of an underlying disease (Box 26.13). The main differential diagnosis is soft tissue injury, but fracture should be suspected when there is marked pain and swelling, abnormal movement of the affected limb, crepitus or deformity. Femoral neck fractures typically produce a shortened, externally rotated leg that is painful to move. The pain from vertebral fracture is variable and a high index of suspicion is key to making the diagnosis by imaging, as discussed below.

Investigations

X-rays of the affected site should be taken in at least two planes and examined for discontinuity of the cortical outline (Box 26.14). In addition to demonstrating the fracture, X-rays may also show evidence of an underlying disorder, such as osteoporosis, Paget's disease or osteomalacia. If the X-ray fails to show evidence of a fracture, but clinical suspicion remains high, MRI should be obtained. In many countries patients with low trauma fractures above the age of 50 are referred for a DXA scan to screen for osteoporosis. DXA is also indicated in those under 50 with very strong clinical risk factors for osteoporosis.

Management

Management of fracture in the acute stage requires adequate pain relief, with opiates if necessary, reduction of the fracture to restore normal anatomy and immobilisation of the affected limb to promote healing. This can be achieved either by the use of an external cast or splint, or by internal fixation. Femoral neck fractures present a special management problem since non-union and osteonecrosis are common. This is especially true with intracapsular hip fractures, which should be treated by joint replacement surgery. Following the fracture, rehabilitation is required with physiotherapy and a supervised exercise programme. If the DXA scan shows evidence of osteoporosis or other metabolic bone disease, this should be treated appropriately as described later in this chapter.

Generalised musculoskeletal pain

Clinical assessment

There are a variety of causes of generalised pain, as summarised in Box 26.15. Relentlessly progressive pain occurring in association with weight loss suggests malignant disease with bone metastases. Generalised bone pain may also arise in osteomalacia, primary

26

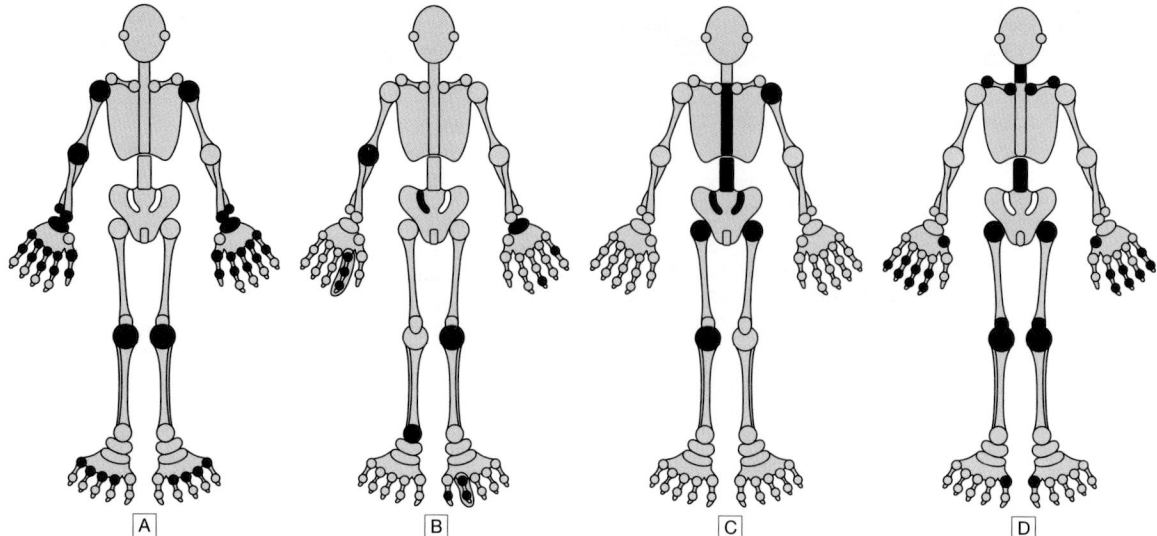

Fig. 26.10 Patterns of joint involvement in different forms of polyarthritis. [A] Rheumatoid arthritis typically targets the metacarpophalangeal and proximal interphalangeal joints of the hands and metatarsophalangeal joints of the feet, as well as other joints, in a symmetrical pattern. [B] Psoriatic arthritis targets proximal and distal interphalangeal joints of the hands, entheses and larger joints in an asymmetrical pattern. Sacroiliitis (often asymmetrical) may occur. [C] Axial spondyloarthritis/ankylosing spondylitis targets the spine, sacroiliac joints, entheses and large peripheral joints in an asymmetrical pattern. [D] Osteoarthritis targets the proximal and distal interphalangeal joints of the hands, first carpometacarpal joint at the base of the thumb, knees, hips, lumbar and cervical spine.

---

i **26.13 Characteristics of different fracture types**

Fracture type	Precipitation factor	Disease
Fragility fracture	Fall from standing height or less	Osteoporosis Osteopenia
Vertebral fracture	Bending, lifting, falling	Osteoporosis
Stress fracture	Running, excessive training	Normal
High-energy fracture	Major trauma	Normal
Pathological fracture	Spontaneous, minimal trauma	Malignancy Paget's disease Osteomalacia

---

26.14 How to investigate a suspected fracture

- Order X-rays in two projections at right-angles to one another
- Include the whole bone and the joints at either end (this may reveal an additional unsuspected fracture)
- Check for evidence of displacement
- Check for a break in the cortex
- In suspected vertebral fracture, check for depression of the end plate
- If clinical suspicion is high but no fracture is seen, request magnetic resonance imaging

---

hyperparathyroidism and polyostotic Paget's disease. An important common cause is fibromyalgia (FM) syndrome, which presents with generalised pain that particularly affects the trunk, back and neck. Accompanying features include fatigue, poor concentration and focal areas of hyperalgesia. Widespread pain may also occur in association with Ehlers–Danlos syndrome hypermobility subtype (hEDS). Pain is a prominent feature in patients with polymyalgia rheumatica and GCA, but this tends to be localised to the pelvic and shoulder girdle. Similarly, pain is also a common feature of inflammatory arthritis and OA but tends to be localised to affected joints. Widespread pain can occur in PsA if there is extensive enthesitis.

---

i **26.15 Some common causes of generalised pain**

- Myositis
- Psoriatic arthritis (enthesopathic)
- Fibromyalgia
- Ehlers–Danlos syndrome, hypermobility type
- Parvovirus arthromyalgia
- Rheumatic fever/post-streptococcal infection
- Metastatic cancer
- Severe osteomalacia

Investigations

Bone scintigraphy is of value in patients with suspected bone metastases or Paget's disease and can also reveal evidence of stress fractures in osteomalacia. FBC, ESR and CRP may be abnormal in the presence of inflammatory disease and myeloma. Plasma and urine protein electrophoresis should be performed to screen for myeloma, and if abnormalities are detected further imaging should be considered with X-ray, low-dose CT or MRI. Routine biochemistry, vitamin D and parathyroid hormone (PTH) should be measured if osteomalacia is suspected. In Paget's disease, the typical picture is of an elevation in ALP with otherwise normal biochemistry. Investigations are unremarkable in patients with FM and hEDS.

Management

Management should be directed towards the underlying cause. Chronic pain of unknown cause and that associated with FM respond poorly to analgesics and NSAIDs, but may respond partially to antineuropathic agents, such as amitriptyline, duloxetine, gabapentin and pregabalin.

Muscle weakness

Muscle weakness can arise from a variety of causes, as shown in Box 26.16. It is important to distinguish between a subjective feeling of generalised weakness occurring with fatigue, and an objective weakness with loss of muscle power and function. The former is a non-specific manifestation of many systemic conditions.

> **i 26.16 Causes of proximal muscle weakness**
>
> **Inflammatory**
>
> - Polymyositis
> - Dermatomyositis
> - Other autoimmune connective tissue disease
> - Inclusion body myositis
> - Sarcoid
> - Myasthenia gravis
>
> **Endocrine** (Ch. 20)
>
> - Hypothyroidism
> - Hyperthyroidism
> - Cushing's syndrome
> - Addison's disease
>
> **Metabolic** (Ch. 19)
>
> - Myophosphorylase deficiency
> - Phosphofructokinase deficiency
> - Hypokalaemia
> - Carnitine deficiency
> - Osteomalacia
> - Hypercalcaemia
>
> **Genetic**
>
> - Muscular dystrophy
> - Mitochondrial disease
>
> **Drugs/toxins**
>
> - Alcohol
> - Cocaine
> - Glucocorticoids
> - Statins and fibrates
> - Tumour necrosis factor inhibitors
> - Zidovudine
>
> **Infections** (Ch. 13)
>
> - Viral (HIV, cytomegalovirus, rubella, Epstein–Barr, echovirus)
> - Parasitic (schistosomiasis, cysticercosis, toxoplasmosis)
> - Bacterial (*Clostridium perfringens*, staphylococci, tuberculosis, *Mycoplasma*)

Clinical assessment

Clinical examination should document the presence, pattern and severity of muscle weakness assessed using the Medical Research Council (MRC) scale (no power (0) to full power (5)). Proximal muscle weakness suggests the presence of a myopathy or myositis, which typically causes difficulty in standing from a seated position, walking up steps, squatting and lifting overhead. Worsening of symptoms on exercise and post-exertional cramps suggest a metabolic myopathy, such as glycogen storage disease. A strong family history and onset in childhood or early adulthood suggest muscular dystrophy. Alcohol excess can cause an inflammatory myositis and atrophy of type 2 muscle fibres. Proximal myopathy may be a complication of Cushing's syndrome, glucocorticoid therapy and osteomalacia. Myopathy and myositis can also occur in association with many drugs (see Box 26.78) and viral infections, including HIV; in the latter case, it may be due to HIV itself or to treatment with zidovudine. Polymyositis and dermatomyositis in adults are frequently associated with an occult malignancy, emphasising the importance of a thorough general examination of patients with this presentation.

Investigations

Investigations should include routine biochemistry and haematology, ESR, CRP, creatine kinase, serum 25(OH)-vitamin D, PTH, parvovirus, hepatitis B/C, HIV and streptococcus serology, serum and urine protein electrophoresis, serum ACE, ANAs/ENAs, RF, complement and myositis-specific autoantibodies such as Jo-1. Open muscle biopsy (site-guided by MRI detection of abnormal muscle) and electromyography (EMG) are usually required to make the diagnosis. Genetic testing may be of value in patients where an inherited disorder is suspected. Patients suspected to have myositis should be screened for malignancy. Initially this involves a CT scan of the chest, abdomen and pelvis followed by upper gastrointestinal endoscopy and colonoscopy if necessary.

Management

Management is determined by the underlying cause, but all patients with muscle disease should be referred for physiotherapy and graded exercises to maximise muscle function while specific treatment is introduced.

> **i 26.17 Causes of low back pain**
>
> - Mechanical (soft-tissue lesion) back pain
> - Intervertebral disc disease (degenerative or annulus tear and prolapse)
> - Facet joint disease (osteoarthritis, psoriatic arthritis)
> - Vertebral fracture
> - Paget's disease
> - Axial spondyloarthritis
> - Discitis (infective or inflammatory ['spondylodiscitis'])
> - Bone metastases
> - Spondylolisthesis

Regional musculoskeletal pain

Regional musculoskeletal pain is a common presenting complaint, usually occurring as the result of age-related degenerative disease of tendons and ligaments, OA and trauma.

Back pain

Back pain is a common symptom that affects 60%–80% of people at some time in their lives. Although the prevalence has not increased, reported disability from back pain has risen significantly in the last 30 years. In Western countries, back pain is the most common cause of sickness-related work absence. In the UK, 7% of adults consult their GP each year with back pain. Globally, low back pain is thought to affect about 9% of the population. The most important causes of low back pain are summarised in Box 26.17.

Clinical assessment

The main purpose of clinical assessment is to differentiate the self-limiting disorder of acute mechanical back pain from serious spinal pathology, as summarised in Figure 26.11. Mechanical back pain is the most common cause of acute back pain in people aged 20–55. This accounts for more than 90% of episodes, is usually acute and associated with lifting or bending. It is exacerbated by activity and is generally relieved by rest (Box 26.18). It is usually confined to the lumbar–sacral region, buttock or thigh, is asymmetrical and does not radiate beyond the knee (which would imply nerve root irritation). On examination, there may be asymmetric local paraspinal muscle spasm and tenderness, with painful restriction of some, but not all, movements. Low back pain is more common in manual workers, particularly those in occupations that involve heavy lifting and twisting. The prognosis is generally good. After 2 days, 30% are better and 90% have recovered by 6 weeks. Recurrences of pain may occur and about 10%–15% of patients go on to develop chronic back pain that may be difficult to treat. Psychological elements, such as job dissatisfaction, depression and anxiety, are important risk factors for the transition to chronic pain and disability.

Back pain secondary to serious spinal pathology has different characteristics (Box 26.19). If there is clinical evidence of spinal cord or nerve root compression, or a cauda equina lesion, then urgent investigation is needed. Spinal stenosis presents insidiously with leg discomfort on walking that is relieved by rest, bending forwards or walking uphill. Patients may adopt a characteristic simian posture, with a forward stoop and slight flexion at hips and knees. The most common cause is the gradual development of coexisting contributing lesions such as facet joint arthritis, ligament flavum thickening or degenerative spondylolisthesis.

Degenerative disc disease and osteoarthritis is a common cause of chronic low back pain in middle-aged and older adults. Prolapse of an intervertebral disc presents when discs are still well hydrated (in young and early middle age) with nerve root pain, which can be accompanied by characteristic features such as sensory deficit, motor weakness and asymmetrical reflexes (Box 26.20). Examination may reveal a positive sciatic or femoral stretch test. About 70% of patients improve by 4 weeks. Inflammatory back pain (IBP) due to axial spondyloarthritis (axSpA) or

26

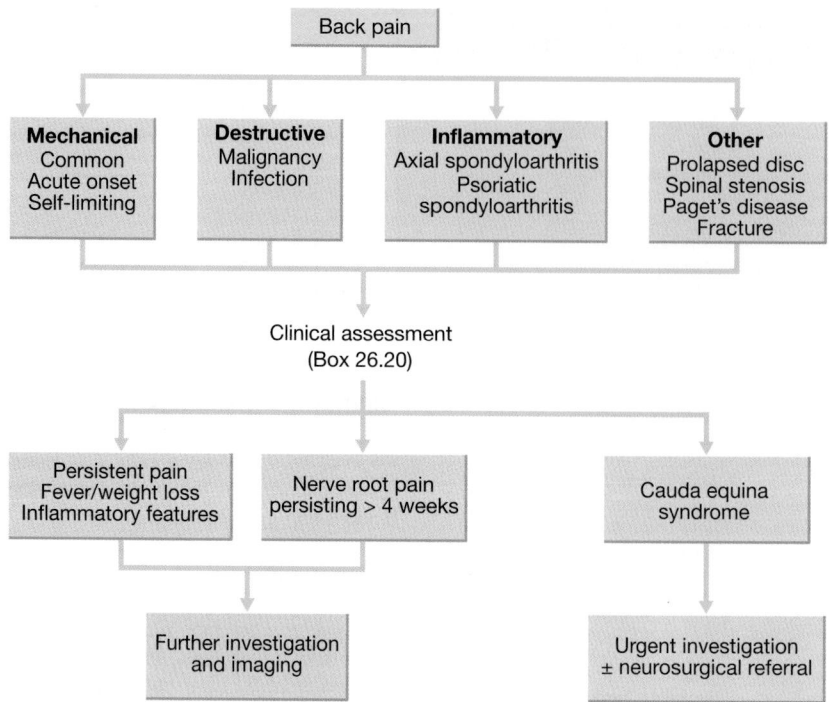

Fig. 26.11 Initial triage assessment of back pain.

---

i 26.18 Features of mechanical low back pain

- Pain varies with physical activity (improved with rest)
- Onset often sudden and precipitated by lifting or bending
- Recurrent episodes
- Pain limited to back or upper leg
- No clear-cut nerve root distribution
- No systemic features
- Self-limiting with recovery at 6 weeks in 90%

---

i 26.19 Red flags for possible spinal pathology

History

- Age < 20 years or > 55 years at presentation
- Character: constant, progressive pain unrelieved by rest
- Location: thoracic pain
- Past medical history: carcinoma, tuberculosis, HIV, systemic glucocorticoid use, osteoporosis
- Constitutional: systemic upset, sweats, weight loss
- Major trauma

Examination

- Painful spinal deformity
- Severe/symmetrical spinal deformity
- Saddle anaesthesia
- Progressive neurological signs/muscle-wasting
- Multiple levels of root signs

---

i 26.20 Clinical features of radicular pain

Nerve root pain

- Unilateral leg pain worse than low back pain
- Pain radiates beyond knee
- Paraesthesia in same distribution
- Nerve irritation signs (reduced straight leg raising that reproduces leg pain)
- Motor, sensory or reflex signs (limited to one or adjacent nerve roots)
- Often self-limiting, with 50% recovery at 6 weeks

Cauda equina syndrome

- Difficulty with micturition
- Loss of anal sphincter tone or faecal incontinence
- Saddle anaesthesia
- Gait disturbance
- Pain, numbness or weakness affecting one or both legs

Investigations

Investigations are not required in patients with acute mechanical back pain. Those with persistent pain (> 6 weeks) or red flags (see Box 26.19) should undergo further investigation. MRI is the investigation of choice because it can demonstrate spinal stenosis, cord compression or nerve root compression, as well as inflammatory changes in axSpA, malignancy and sepsis. Plain X-rays can be of value in patients suspected of having vertebral compression fractures, OA and degenerative disc disease. If metastatic disease is suspected, bone scintigraphy or CT should be considered. Additional investigations that may be required include routine biochemistry and haematology, ESR and CRP (to screen for infection and inflammatory disease), protein and urine electrophoresis (for myeloma), human leucocyte antigen (HLA)-B27 for axSpA and prostate-specific antigen for prostate carcinoma.

Management

Education is important in patients with mechanical back pain. It should emphasise the self-limiting nature of the condition and the fact that exercise is helpful rather than damaging. Regular analgesia and/or NSAIDs may be required to improve mobility and facilitate exercise. Return to

---

PsA has a gradual onset and almost always occurs before the age of 40. It is associated with morning stiffness and improves with movement. Spondylolisthesis may cause back pain that is typically aggravated by standing and walking. Occasionally, diffuse idiopathic skeletal hyperostosis (DISH) can cause back pain, but this is not a prominent feature. Arachnoiditis is a rare cause of chronic severe low back pain. It is caused by chronic inflammation of the nerve root sheaths in the spinal canal and can complicate meningitis, spinal surgery or myelography with oil-based contrast agents.

26.21 Causes of neck pain

Mechanical

- Postural
- Whiplash injury
- Cervical spondylosis

Inflammatory

- Infections
- Axial spondyloarthritis
- Psoriatic arthritis
- Rheumatoid arthritis
- Polymyalgia rheumatica
- Discitis

Metabolic

- Axial CPPD disease
- Fibrous dysplasia
- Paget's disease

Neoplastic

- Metastases
- Myeloma
- Lymphoma
- Intrathecal tumours

Other

- Fibromyalgia
- Torticollis

Referred

- Pharynx
- Cervical lymph nodes
- Dental disease
- Angina pectoris
- Aortic aneurysm
- Pancoast tumour
- Diaphragm

(CPPD = calcium pyrophosphate deposition)

26.22 Clinical findings in shoulder pain

Rotator cuff and subacromial lesions

- Pain reproduced by resisted active movement:
  Abduction: supraspinatus
  External rotation: infraspinatus, teres minor
  Internal rotation: subscapularis

Acromioclavicular joint

- Pain on full abduction and adduction (at 90° of forward elevation)

Bicipital (long head) tendinitis

- Tenderness over bicipital groove
- Pain reproduced by resisted active wrist supination or elbow flexion

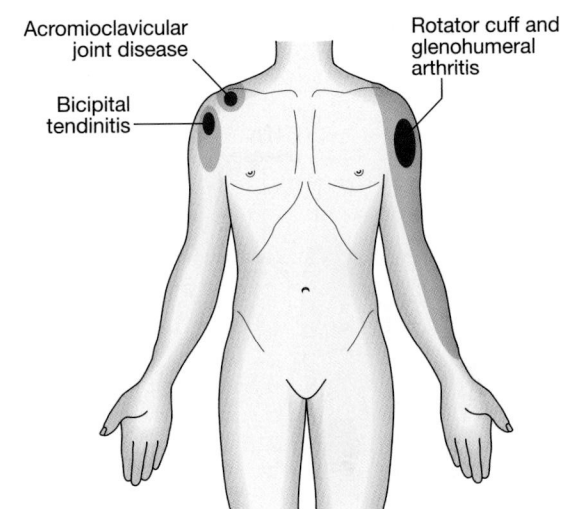

Fig. 26.12 Pain patterns around the shoulder. The dark shading indicates sites of maximum pain.

work and normal activity should take place as soon as possible. Bed rest is not helpful and may increase the risk of chronic disability. Referral for physiotherapy should be considered if a return to normal activities has not been achieved by 6 weeks. Low-dose tricyclic antidepressant drugs may help pain, sleep and mood.

Other treatment modalities that are occasionally used include epidural and facet joint injection, traction and lumbar supports, though there is limited randomised controlled trial evidence to support their use. Malignant disease, osteoporosis, Paget's disease and SpAs require specific treatment of the underlying condition.

Surgery is required in less than 1% of patients with low back pain, but may be needed in progressive spinal stenosis, in spinal cord compression and in some patients with nerve root compression.

Neck pain

Neck pain is a common symptom that can occur following an injury or falling asleep in an awkward position, as a result of stress or in association with OA of the spine. The causes are shown in Box 26.21. Most cases resolve spontaneously or with a short course of NSAIDs or analgesics and some exercise therapy. Patients with persistent pain that follows a nerve root distribution and those with upper or lower limb neurological signs should be investigated by MRI and, if necessary, referred for a neurosurgical opinion.

Shoulder pain

Shoulder pain is a common complaint over the age of 40 (Box 26.22). Varying pain patterns associated with common lesions are shown in Figure 26.12. For most shoulder lesions, general management is with analgesics, NSAIDs, local glucocorticoid injections and physiotherapy aimed at restoring normal movement and function. Surgery may be required in patients who have debilitating or persistent symptoms in association with rotator cuff lesions or severe acromioclavicular joint arthritis. If there is subacromial impingement, without evidence of a rotator cuff tear on MRI, subacromial glucocorticoid injection and physiotherapy constitute a reasonable first step. Calcific supraspinatus tendonitis unresponsive to glucocorticoid injection can be treated with barbotage (needle disruption of deposit under ultrasound guidance).

Complete rotator cuff tears in people under 40 years of age may respond well to full surgical repair, but results are less good in older people. Adhesive capsulitis (frozen shoulder) presents with pain associated with marked restriction of elevation and external rotation. Adhesive capsulitis is commonly associated with diabetes mellitus and neck/radicular lesions. Treatment in the early stage is with analgesia, intra- and extracapsular glucocorticoid injection, and regular 'pendulum' exercises of the arm to mobilise. Complete recovery sometimes takes up to 2 years. For severe or persistent symptoms, joint distension and manipulation under anaesthesia are surgical options.

Elbow pain

The most common causes are repetitive trauma causing lateral epicondylitis (tennis elbow) and medial epicondylitis (golfer's elbow) (Box 26.23). SpAs, including psoriatic disease, can present with the same symptoms (tendon insertion enthesitis). Management is by rest, analgesics and topical or systemic NSAIDs. Local glucocorticoid injections may be required in resistant cases. Olecranon bursitis can also follow local repetitive trauma, but other causes include infections and gout.

Hand and wrist pain

Pain from hand or wrist joints is well localised to the affected joint, except for pain from the first carpometacarpal (CMC) joint, commonly targeted by OA or PsA; although maximal at the thumb base, the pain often radiates down the thumb and to the radial aspect of the wrist. Non-articular causes of hand pain include:

26

26.23 Common local causes of elbow pain

Lesion	Pain	Examination findings
Lateral humeral epicondylitis (traumatic 'tennis elbow' or SpA-related enthesitis)	Lateral epicondyle Radiation to extensor forearm	Tenderness over epicondyle Pain reproduced by resisted active wrist extension
Medial humeral epicondylitis (traumatic 'golfer's elbow' or SpA-related enthesitis)	Medial epicondyle Radiation to flexor forearm	Tenderness over epicondyle Pain reproduced by resisted active wrist flexion
Olecranon bursitis (gout, rheumatoid arthritis or infection)	Olecranon	Tender swelling

(SpA = spondyloarthritis)

- *Tenosynovitis*: affects flexor or extensor digital tendons. Pain and tenderness are well localised to the tendon lesions. There is often early-morning 'claw-like' digit stiffness. De Quervain's tenosynovitis involves the tendon sheaths of abductor pollicis longus and extensor pollicis brevis. It produces pain maximal over the radial aspect of the distal forearm and wrist and marked pain on forced ulnar deviation of the wrist with the thumb held across the patient's palm (Finkelstein's sign). This test is not specific for this lesion alone.
- *Raynaud's phenomenon*: digital vasospasm triggered mostly by cold.
- *C6, C7 or C8 radiculopathy*.
- *Carpal tunnel syndrome*: hand position-dependent and/or nocturnal pain, numbness and paraesthesia of thumb and second to fourth digits.

Hip pain

Pain from the hip joint is usually felt deep in the groin, with variable radiation to the buttock, anterolateral thigh or knee (Fig. 26.13). A lay person's description of their 'hip pain' will often locate the pain to the greater trochanter area. A common cause in older people is OA, which should be suspected if the pain is worse on weight bearing. Paget's disease can also enter into the differential diagnosis. Occasionally, inflammatory disease secondary to axSpA or PsA can present with groin, greater trochanter area or hip pain. Greater trochanter pain syndrome is usually due to either gluteus medius insertional tendonitis/enthesitis, trochanteric bursitis or referred pain (Box 26.24). Pain at this site may also be referred from the lumbosacral spine. Other less common causes of pain in the hip/groin area include inguinal hernia, adductor tendonitis and enthesitis of anterior superior/inferior iliac spines.

Knee pain

In middle and older age, the most common cause of knee pain is OA, the features of which are described later in this chapter. Pain that is associated with locking of the knee (sudden painful inability to extend fully) is usually due to a meniscal tear or osteochondritis dissecans. Referred pain from the hip may present at the knee and is reproduced by hip, not knee, movement. Pain from periarticular lesions is well localised to the involved structure (Box 26.25). Anterior knee pain may be due to patellar ligament or retinacular lesions (enthesitis, tendonitis, fat-pad syndrome) occurring typically from overuse and/or axSpA. Anterior knee pain is relatively common in adolescents and may be the result of patellar articular cartilage or ligament insertion osteochondritis.

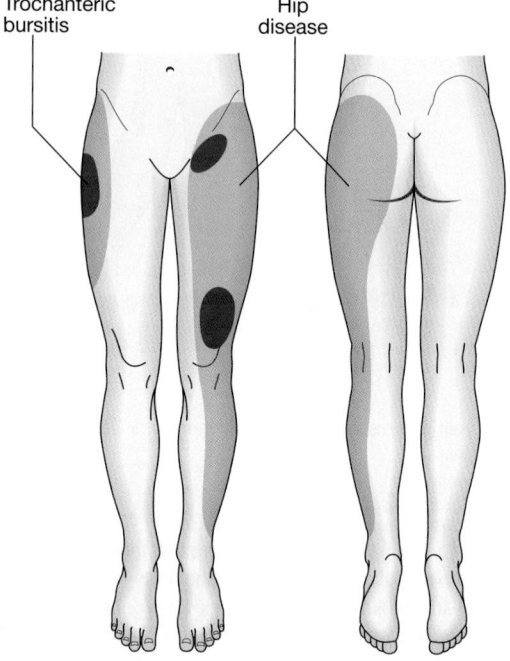

Trochanteric bursitis

Hip disease

Fig. 26.13 Pain patterns of hip disease and trochanteric pain syndrome. The dark shading indicates sites of maximum pain.

26.24 Local causes of hip pain

Lesion	Pain	Examination findings
Osteoarthritis	Groin pain, worse on weight bearing	Limited range of movement and/or pain on examination of hip
Gluteus medius enthesitis	Upper lateral thigh, worse on lying on that side at night	Tenderness over greater trochanter
Trochanteric bursitis	As above	As above
Adductor tendinitis (SpA-related enthesitis or sports-related trauma)	Upper inner thigh	Tenderness over adductor origin/tendon/muscle Pain reproduced by resisted active hip adduction
Ischiogluteal enthesitis/bursitis	Buttock, worse on sitting	Tenderness over ischial prominence
Pubic symphysitis (can mimic intra-articular hip lesions)	Medial groin pain, can radiate to inner or even outer upper thighs	Tenderness over symphysis joint If pain is worse on trunk curl/rectus activation under symphysis-resting hand, it may be insertional rectus enthesitis (SpAs)

(SpA = spondyloarthritis)

i	26.25	Local causes of knee pain

Lesion	Pain	Examination findings
Osteoarthritis	Weight bearing or on ascending and descending starts	Enlargement of knee joint, tenderness at joint margins, crepitus on flexion, small effusions, quadriceps wasting
Pre-patellar bursitis	Over patella	Tender fluctuant swelling in front of patella
Superficial and deep infrapatellar bursitis and fat-pad syndrome	Anterior knee, inferior to patella	Tenderness in front of (superficial) or behind (deep) patellar tendon Pain on full flexion
Anserine bursitis/ enthesitis	Upper medial tibia	Tenderness (± swelling) over upper medial tibia
Medial collateral ligament lesions (injury or enthesitis)	Upper medial tibia	Localised tenderness of upper medial tibia Pain reproduced by valgus stress on partly flexed knee
Popliteal cyst (Baker's cyst)	Popliteal fossa	Tender swelling of popliteal fossa
Patellar ligament enthesopathy	Anterior upper tibia	Tenderness over tibial tubercle
Osteochondritis of patellar ligament (Osgood–Schlatter disease)	Anterior upper tibia	Pain on resisted active knee extension

Ankle and foot pain

Pain from the ankle (tibiotalar) joint due to OA or osteochondral defect is felt between the malleoli and is worse on weight-bearing. Pain from the subtalar joint (from the same lesions) is also worse on weight-bearing. Inflammatory arthritis of either of these joints (RA, PsA, CPPD arthritis or gout) often worsens and swells with rest. These diagnoses can be associated with hindfoot tenosynovitis (peroneal or posterior tibial). Pain under the heel is typically due to plantar fasciitis. This can occur as the result of overuse, in which case it may respond to rest, padded footwear and local glucocorticoid injections, but can also arise in SpA as a manifestation of enthesitis. Pain affecting the back of the heel may be due to Achilles tendinitis or enthesitis. The MTP joints of the feet are commonly involved symmetrically in RA. The presentation is with pain on walking felt below the metatarsal heads, often described as 'walking on marbles'. Patients with active inflammation of the MTP joints have pain when the forefoot is squeezed. Involvement of the first MTP joint is common in OA or PsA and is associated, respectively, with hallux valgus and dactylitis. The hallux is also a classical target in acute gout. Morton's neuroma is a neuropathy of an interdigital nerve and is usually located between the third and fourth metatarsal heads. Women are most commonly affected (tight shoes can be to blame). Local sensory loss and a palpable tender swelling between the metatarsal heads may be detected. Footwear adjustment often helps, with or without a local glucocorticoid injection, but surgical decompression may be required if symptoms persist.

Principles of management

The management of rheumatological disorders should be tailored to the underlying diagnosis. Certain aspects are common to many disorders,

i	26.26	Interventions for patients with rheumatic diseases

Core interventions

- Education
- Aerobic conditioning
- Muscle strengthening
- Simple analgesics
- Disease-modifying therapy

- Reduction of adverse mechanical factors
- Pacing of activities
- Appropriate footwear
- Weight reduction if obese

Other options

- Other analgesic drugs:
  Oral non-steroidal anti-inflammatory drugs
  Topical agents
  Opioid analgesics
  Amitriptyline
  Gabapentin/pregabalin

- Local glucocorticoid injections
- Physical treatments:
  Heat, cold, aids, appliances
- Surgery
- Coping strategies (see Box 26.27)

however, and the general principles are discussed here. The therapeutic aims are:

- to educate patients about their disease so as to enhance self-management
- to control pain, if it is present
- to optimise function
- to modify the disease process where this is possible
- to identify and treat comorbidity.

These aims are interrelated and success in one area often benefits others. Successful management requires careful assessment of the person as a whole. The management plan should be individualised and patient-centred, should involve relevant members of the multidisciplinary team, and should be agreed and understood by both the patient and all the practitioners that are involved. It must also take into account:

- the patient's activity requirements and occupational and recreational aspirations
- risk factors that may influence the disease
- the patient's perceptions and knowledge of the condition
- medications and coping strategies that have already been tried
- comorbid disease and its therapy
- the availability, costs and logistics of appropriate evidence-based interventions.

Generally, the simplest and safest interventions should be tried first. Symptoms and signs may change with time, so the management plan for most patients requires regular review and re-adjustment.

Core interventions that should be considered for everyone with a painful musculoskeletal condition are listed in Box 26.26. There are also other non-pharmacological and drug options, the choice of which depends on the nature and severity of the diagnosis.

Education and lifestyle interventions

Education

Patients must always be informed about the nature of their condition and its investigation, treatment and prognosis, since education can improve outcome. Information and therapist contact can reduce pain and disability, improve self-efficacy and reduce the health-care costs of many musculoskeletal conditions, including OA and RA. The mechanisms are unclear, but in part may result from improved adherence. Benefits are modest, but potentially long-lasting, safe and cost-effective. Education can be provided through one-to-one discussion, written literature, patient-led group education classes and interactive computer programs. Inclusion of the patient's partner or carer is often appropriate;

26

this is essential for childhood conditions but also helps in many chronic adult conditions.

For children and adolescents with chronic diseases such as JIA, education and support of the whole family, schooling and psychological support is essential and best delivered through a multidisciplinary team.

Patient-run charitable organisations provide a wealth of information and support to patients (see 'Further information'). The detail of the educational materials and services that organisations can provide should be known to the multidisciplinary team and organisation contact details should be made available to patients.

Exercise

Several types of exercise can be prescribed:

- *Aerobic fitness training* can produce long-term reduction in pain and disability. It improves well-being, encourages restorative sleep and benefits common comorbidity, such as obesity, diabetes, chronic heart failure and hypertension.
- *Local strengthening exercise* for muscles that act over compromised joints also reduces pain and disability, with improvements in the reduced muscle strength, proprioception, coordination and balance that associate with chronic arthritis. 'Small amounts often' of strengthening exercise are better than protracted sessions performed infrequently.
- *Weight-bearing exercise* is of value in osteoporosis, where it can result in modest increases in bone density and slow bone loss.

Joint protection

Excessive impact-loading and adverse repetitive use of a compromised joint or periarticular tissue can worsen symptoms in patients with arthritis. This can be mitigated by cessation of contact sports and by pacing of activities by dividing physical tasks into shorter segments with brief breaks in between. Other strategies include adaptations to machinery or tools at the workplace; the use of shock-absorbing footwear with thick soft soles, which can reduce impact-loading through feet, knees, hips and back; and the use of a walking stick on the contralateral side to a painful hip, knee or foot.

Non-pharmacological interventions

Physical and occupational therapy

Local heat, ice packs, wax baths and other local external applications can induce muscle relaxation and provide temporary relief of symptoms in a range of rheumatic diseases.

Hydrotherapy and balneotherapy (immersion in a bath) induce muscle relaxation and facilitate movement in a warm, pain-relieving environment without the restraints of gravity and normal load-bearing. Various manipulative techniques may also help improve restricted movement.

Splints can give temporary rest and support for painful joints and periarticular tissues, and can prevent harmful involuntary postures during sleep. Prolonged rest must be avoided. Orthoses are more permanent appliances used to reduce instability and excessive abnormal movement and provide support and comfort. They include working wrist splints, knee braces, iron and T-straps to control ankle instability and a multitude of (often custom made) foot insole supports to offload painful or deformed foot structures. Orthoses are particularly suited to severely disabled patients in whom a surgical option is inappropriate and often need to be custom-made for the individual.

Aids and appliances can provide dignity and independence for patients with respect to activities of daily living. Common examples are a raised toilet seat, raised chair height, extended handles on taps, a shower instead of a bath, thick-handled cutlery and extended 'hands' to pull on tights and socks. Full assessment and advice from an occupational therapist maximise the benefits of these aids.

> **i** 26.27 Self-help and coping strategies
>
> - Yoga, Pilates and relaxation techniques to reduce stress
> - Avoidance of negative situations or activities that produce stress and increase in pleasant activities that give satisfaction
> - Information and discussion to alter beliefs about and perspectives on disease
> - Reduction or avoidance of catastrophising and maladaptive pain behaviour
> - Imagery and distraction techniques for pain
> - Expansion of social contact and better use of social services

Self-help and coping strategies

These plans help patients to cope better with, and adjust to, chronic pain and disability. They may be useful at any stage but are particularly beneficial for patients with incurable problems who have tried all available treatment options. The aim is to increase self-management through self-assessment and problem-solving, so that patients can recognise negative, but potentially remediable, aspects of their mood (stress, frustration, anger or low self-esteem) and their situation (physical, social, financial). These may then be addressed by changes in attitude and behaviour, as shown in Box 26.27.

Involvement of the spouse or partner in mutual goal-setting can improve partnership adjustment. Such approaches are often an element of group education classes and pain clinics, but may require more formal clinical psychological input.

Tailored multidisciplinary approaches are required for patients with juvenile idiopathic arthritis (JIA) and other chronic childhood diseases, dependent on age and maturity. Adolescents and young adults have specific demands, different to those of young children and adults, which are influenced by many issues in their lives impinging on the disease process, its impact and their ability to cope with it.

Weight control

Obesity aggravates pain at most sites through increased mechanical strain and is a risk factor for progression of joint damage in patients with OA and other types of arthritis. Obesity may contribute, through its metabolic and inflammatory effects, to amplifying symptoms of rheumatic disease and in certain scenarios has been linked with poorer immunotherapy responses (e.g. anti-TNF-α in PsA). This should be explained to obese patients and strategies offered on how to lose and maintain an appropriate weight. By contrast, excessive weight loss is also detrimental and low weight (body mass index (BMI) < 20 kg/m^2) is associated with an increased risk of fractures. Patients should therefore be advised to maintain BMI within the 20–25 kg/m^2 range.

Surgery

A variety of surgical interventions can relieve pain and conserve or restore function in patients with bone, joint and periarticular disease (Box 26.28). Soft tissue release and tenosynovectomy can reduce inflammatory symptoms, improve function and prevent or retard tendon damage for variable periods, sometimes indefinitely. Synovectomy does not prevent disease progression, but may be indicated for pain relief when drugs, physical therapy and intra-articular injections have provided insufficient relief. The main approaches for damaged joints are osteotomy (cutting bone to alter joint mechanics and load transmission), excision arthroplasty (removing part or all of the joint), joint replacement (insertion of prosthesis in place of the excised joint) and arthrodesis (joint fusion). Surgical fixation of fractures is frequently required in patients with osteoporosis and other bone diseases.

The main aims of surgery are to provide pain relief and improve function and quality of life. If surgery is to be successful, the aims and consequences of each operation should be considered as part of an integrated programme of management and rehabilitation by multidisciplinary teams of surgeons, allied health professionals and physicians, and carefully explained to the patient. Assessment of motivation, social support and

26.28 Surgical procedures in rheumatological and bone diseases

Procedure	Indication
Soft tissue release	
Carpal tunnel	Median nerve compression
Tarsal tunnel	Posterior tibial nerve entrapment
Flexor tenosynovectomy	Relief of 'trigger' fingers
Ulnar nerve transposition	Ulnar nerve entrapment at elbow
Fasciotomy	Severe Dupuytren's contracture
Tendon repairs and transfers	
Hand extensor tendons	Extensor tendon rupture
Thumb and finger flexor tendons	Flexor tendon rupture
Synovectomy	
Wrist and extensor tendon sheath (+ excision of radial head)	Pain relief and prevention of extensor tendon rupture in RA, resistant inflammatory synovitis
Knee synovectomy	Resistant inflammatory synovitis
Osteotomy	
Femoral osteotomy	Early OA of hip
Tibial osteotomy	Uni-compartmental knee OA Deformed tibia in OA or Paget's disease
Excision arthroplasty	
First metatarsophalangeal joint (Keller's procedure)	Painful hallux valgus
Radial head	Painful distal radio-ulnar joint
Lateral end of clavicle	Painful acromioclavicular joint
Metatarsal head	Painful subluxed metatarsophalangeal joints
Joint replacement arthroplasty	
Knee, hip, shoulder, elbow	Painful damaged joints in OA and RA
Arthrodesis	
Wrist	Damaged joint: pain relief, improvement of grip
Ankle/subtalar joints	Damaged joint: pain relief, stabilisation of hindfoot
Fracture repair	
Hip arthroplasty	Fractured neck of femur
External fixation	Multiple fractures, open fractures
Intramedullary nailing	Tibial and femur fractures
Screw, plating and wiring	Wrist and other fractures
Other procedures	
Nerve root decompression	Spinal stenosis, nerve entrapment
Vertebroplasty and kyphoplasty	Painful vertebral fracture (evidence base for efficacy poor)

(OA = osteoarthritis; RA = rheumatoid arthritis)

environment is no less important than careful consideration of patients' general health, their risks for major surgery, the extent of disease in other joints, and their ability to mobilise following surgery. For some severely compromised people, pain relief and functional independence are better served by provision of a suitable wheelchair, home adjustments and social services than by surgery that is technically successful, but following which the patient cannot mobilise.

Pharmacological treatment

Analgesics

Paracetamol (1 g up to 4 times daily) is the oral analgesic of first choice for mild to moderate pain. It is thought to work by inhibiting prostaglandin synthesis in the brain while having little effect on peripheral prostaglandin production. It is well tolerated and has few adverse effects and drug interactions. An increased risk of gastrointestinal events and cardiovascular disease has been reported with chronic usage in observational studies, but this may be due to channelling of patients at higher risk of these events for treatment with paracetamol rather than an NSAID. Paracetamol can be combined with codeine (co-codamol) or dihydrocodeine (co-dydramol). These compound analgesics are more effective than paracetamol, but have more side-effects, including constipation, headache and delirium (especially in older adults). The centrally acting opioid analgesics tramadol and meptazinol may be useful for temporary control of severe pain unresponsive to other measures, but can cause nausea, bowel upset, dizziness and somnolence, and withdrawal symptoms after chronic use. The non-opioid analgesic nefopam (30–90 mg three times daily) can help moderate pain, though side-effects (nausea, anxiety, dry mouth) often limit its use. Patients with severe or intractable pain may require strong opioid analgesics, such as oxycodone or morphine.

Non-steroidal anti-inflammatory drugs (NSAIDs)

These are among the most widely prescribed drugs, but their use has declined over recent years because long-term prescription is associated with an increased risk of cardiovascular disease. Oral NSAIDs are useful in the treatment of a range of rheumatic diseases with an inflammatory component. They inhibit the cyclo-oxygenase (COX) and prostaglandin H synthase enzymes, which convert arachidonic acid, derived from membrane phospholipids, to prostaglandins and leukotrienes by the COX and 5-lipoxygenase pathways, respectively (Fig. 26.14). There are two COX isoforms; COX-1 is constitutively expressed in gastric mucosa, platelets and kidneys, and production of prostaglandins at these sites protects against mucosal damage and regulates platelet aggregation and renal blood flow. The COX-2 enzyme is induced at sites of inflammation, producing prostaglandins that cause local pain and swelling. Inflammation also up-regulates COX-2 in the spinal cord, where it modulates pain perception. Ibuprofen, diclofenac and naproxen are non-selective drugs that inhibit both COX enzymes, whereas celecoxib and etoricoxib are

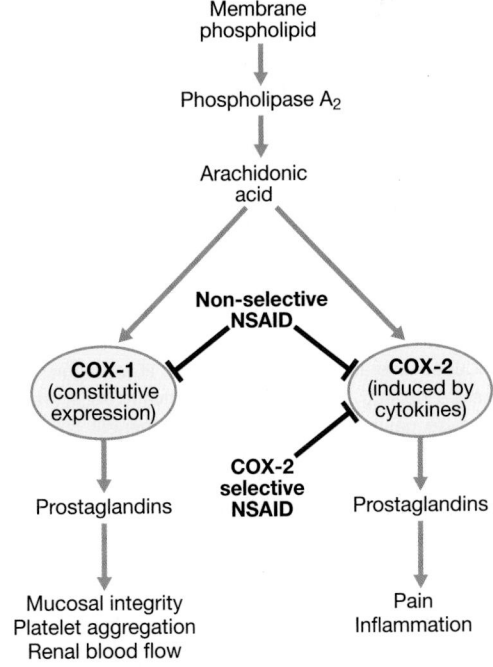

Fig. 26.14 Mechanism of action of non-steroidal anti-inflammatory drugs (NSAIDs). (COX = cyclo-oxygenase)

26.29 Commonly used NSAIDs and their risk of gastrointestinal bleeding and perforation

Drug	Daily adult dose	Doses/day	Idiosyncratic side-effects, comments
Low risk			
Celecoxib	100–200 mg	1–2	Selective COX-2 inhibitor
Etoricoxib	60–120 mg	1	Selective COX-2 inhibitor
Medium risk			
Ibuprofen	1600–2400 mg	3–4	Gastrointestinal adverse effects more likely than with COX-2 inhibitors, even with PPI therapy
Naproxen	500–1000 mg	1–2	
Diclofenac	75–150 mg	2–3	
High risk			
Indometacin	50–200 mg	3–4	High incidence of dyspepsia and CNS side-effects

(CNS = central nervous system; COX = cyclo-oxygenase; PPI = proton pump inhibitor)

26.30 Risk factors for NSAID-induced peptic ulcers

- Age > 60 years*
- Past history of peptic ulcer*
- Past history of adverse event with NSAID
- Concomitant glucocorticoid use
- High-dose or multiple NSAIDs
- High-risk NSAIDs (see Box 26.29)

*The most important risk factors.

26.31 Recommendations for the use of NSAIDs

- Use the lowest dose for the shortest time possible to control symptoms
- Avoid NSAIDs in patients on warfarin
- Allow 2–3 weeks to assess efficacy. If response is inadequate, consider a trial of another NSAID
- Never prescribe more than one NSAID at a time
- Co-prescribe a proton pump inhibitor for patients with risk factors for gastrointestinal adverse effects (see Box 26.30)
- Avoid in patients with cardiovascular disease

26.32 Use of oral NSAIDs in old age

- **Gastrointestinal complications:** age is a strong risk factor for enteral bleeding and perforation, and for peptic ulceration. Older adults are more likely to die if they suffer NSAID-associated enteral bleeding or perforation.
- **Cardiovascular disease:** use NSAIDs with caution in patients with cardiovascular disease. Therapy with NSAIDs may exacerbate hypertension and heart failure.
- **Renal disease:** use of NSAIDs may cause or worsen renal impairment.

Recommendations for NSAID prescribing are summarised in Box 26.31. Because of the risk of adverse effects, NSAIDs should be used with great care in older patients (Box 26.32).

Topical agents

Topical NSAID creams and gels and capsaicin cream can help in the treatment of OA and superficial periarticular lesions affecting hands, elbows and knees. They may be used as monotherapy or as an adjunct to oral analgesics. Topical NSAIDs can penetrate superficial tissues and even reach the joint capsule, though intrasynovial levels mainly reflect blood-borne drug delivery. Capsaicin selectively binds to the protein transient receptor potential vanilloid type 1 (TRPV1), which is a heat-activated calcium channel on the surface of peripheral type C nociceptor fibres. Initial application causes a burning sensation, but continued use depletes presynaptic substance P, with subsequent pain reduction that is optimal after a period of 1–2 weeks. Lidocaine 5% medicated patches are licensed for the treatment of post-herpetic neuropathic pain, but are also used off label for a variety of painful conditions including painful vertebral fractures, sometimes with good effects.

Disease-modifying anti-rheumatic drugs

Disease-modifying anti-rheumatic drugs (DMARDs) comprise small-molecule inhibitors of the immune response, glucocorticoids and biologic DMARDs. DMARDs not only improve symptoms but also favourably modify disease progression in a variety of inflammatory rheumatic diseases. Small-molecule inhibitors are either classical DMARDs (cDMARDs), which have relatively non-specific inhibitory effects on the immune response (Box 26.33), or targeted synthetic DMARDs (tsD-MARDs), which are designed to inhibit the effects of a specific target molecule (Box 26.34). Biologic DMARDs ('biologics') are monoclonal antibodies, fusion proteins or decoy receptors targeted towards specific cytokines, receptors and other cell-surface molecules regulating the immune response (Fig. 26.15). Most cDMARDs have the potential to cause bone marrow suppression or liver dysfunction and require regular blood monitoring, as summarised in Box 26.33. If toxicity occurs, treatment may need to be stopped temporarily and resumed at a lower dose or withdrawn completely if toxicity is severe.

Classical DMARDs (cDMARDs)

Methotrexate (MTX) is the core cDMARD in RA, JIA and PsA. It inhibits folic acid reductase, preventing formation of tetrahydrofolate, which is necessary for DNA synthesis in leucocytes and other cells. It is given

selective inhibitors of COX-2. While NSAIDs have anti-inflammatory activity, they are not thought to have a disease-modifying effect in either OA or inflammatory rheumatic diseases.

Non-selective NSAIDs can damage the gastric and duodenal mucosal barrier and are associated with an increased risk of upper gastrointestinal ulceration, bleeding and perforation. The adjusted increased risk (odds ratio) of bleeding or perforation from non-selective NSAIDs is 4–5, though differences exist between NSAIDs (Box 26.29). Dyspepsia is a poor guide to the presence of NSAID-associated ulceration and bleeding, and the principal risk factors are shown in Box 26.30. Co-prescription of a proton pump inhibitor (PPI) or misoprostol (200 µg twice or 3 times daily) reduces the risk of NSAID-induced ulceration and bleeding, but H₂-antagonists in standard doses are ineffective. The COX-2 selective NSAIDs are much less likely to cause gastrointestinal toxicity, but benefit is attenuated in patients on low-dose aspirin. The UK National Institute for Health and Care Excellence (NICE) guidelines advise that a PPI should be co-prescribed with all NSAIDs, including COX-2-selective NSAIDs, even though the risk of gastrointestinal events with these is low. Since chronic PPI therapy is associated with an increased risk of hip fracture, the merits of giving PPI therapy with a COX-2-selective drug need to be carefully considered.

Other side-effects of NSAIDs include fluid retention and renal impairment due to inhibition of renal prostaglandin production, non-ulcer-associated dyspepsia, abdominal pain, altered bowel habit and rashes. Interstitial nephritis, asthma and anaphylaxis can also occur but are rare.

i 26.33 Classical disease-modifying anti-rheumatic drugs (DMARDs)

Drug	Maintenance dose	Monitoring*			Indications
		FBC	LFTs	Other	
Methotrexate (MTX)	15–25 mg weekly orally or s/c	✓	✓		RA, PsA, JIA, axSpA, CPP disease
Sulfasalazine (SSZ)	2–4 g daily orally	✓	✓		RA, PsA, axSpA,
Hydroxychloroquine (HCQ)	200–400 mg daily orally	–	–	Visual function	RA, SLE, CPP disease
Leflunomide (LEF)	10–20 mg daily orally	✓	✓	BP	RA, PsA
Azathioprine (AZA)	1–2.5 mg/kg daily orally	✓	✓		SLE, SV
Cyclophosphamide	2 mg/kg daily orally or 15 mg/kg IV	✓	✓	eGFR	SLE, SV
Mycophenolate mofetil (MMF)	2–4 g daily orally	✓	✓	–	SLE, SV
Ciclosporin A	3–5 mg/kg daily orally	–	–	BP, eGFR	RA, PsA

*Monitoring tests are usually done every 2 weeks on initiation of treatment for 6 weeks, then monthly for 3 months, then 3-monthly.
(axSpA = axial spondyloarthritis; BP = blood pressure; CPP = calcium pyrophosphate; eGFR = estimated glomerular filtration rate; FBC = full blood count; IM = intramuscular; IV = intravenous; JIA = juvenile idiopathic arthritis; LFTs = liver function tests; PsA = psoriatic arthritis; RA = rheumatoid arthritis; SLE = systemic lupus erythematosus; SV = systemic vasculitis)

i 26.34 Targeted synthetic disease-modifying anti-rheumatic drugs

Drug	Maintenance dose	Regular monitoring			Indications
		FBC	LFT	Other	
Apremilast	30 mg twice daily orally	–	–	–	PsA
Tofacitinib	5 mg twice daily orally	✓	✓	Infection	RA. PsA
Baricitinib	2–4 mg daily orally	–	–	Infection	RA
Upadacitinib	15–30 mg daily orally	–	–	Infection	RA, PsA, axSpA
Filgotinib	200 mg daily orally	–	–	Infection	RA

orally or subcutaneously using a variety of dose increment schedules, to a maximum of 25 mg weekly (in adults) and 15 mg/m²/week in JIA, until benefit or toxicity occurs. Folic acid (5 mg/week) should be co-prescribed to be taken the day after MTX since it reduces adverse effects without impairing efficacy. Benefit is usually observed after 4–8 weeks, but treatment should continue for 3 months before reaching the conclusion that MTX has been ineffective. The most common adverse effects are nausea, vomiting and malaise, which usually occur one 1–2 days after the weekly dose. Patients should be warned of drug interaction with sulphonamides and the importance of avoiding excess alcohol, which enhances MTX hepatotoxicity. Acute pulmonary toxicity (pneumonitis) is rare, but can occur at any time during treatment and patients should be warned to stop therapy and seek advice if they develop any new respiratory symptoms. If pneumonitis occurs, treatment should be withdrawn and high-dose glucocorticoids given. MTX must be co-prescribed with robust contraception in women of child-bearing potential and treatment must be stopped for 3 months in advance of planning a pregnancy.

Sulfasalazine (SSZ) can be used alone or in combination with other drugs in the treatment of RA and PsA. Its mechanism of action is incompletely understood. Nausea and gastrointestinal intolerance are the main adverse effects but leucopenia, abnormal liver function tests (LFTs) and rashes may occur. The usual starting dose is 500 mg daily, escalating in 500 mg increments every 2 weeks to a maintenance dose of 2–4 g daily until benefit or toxicity occurs. Benefit may be observed after 4–8 weeks, but treatment should be continued for 3 months before concluding that it has been ineffective. Orange staining of urine and contact lenses may occur. SSZ is generally considered to be safe during pregnancy.

Hydroxychloroquine (HCQ) can be used alone or in combination with other drugs in the treatment of RA and SLE in a dose of 200–400 mg daily. It acts by modulating lysosomal activity and autophagy causing inhibition of inflammatory responses. While a wide range of side-effects can theoretically occur, it is generally well tolerated in practice. With long-term use (> 5 years) there is a risk of ocular toxicity due to accumulation in the retina, although this is uncommon. It is usual to check visual function before starting treatment and to repeat this periodically while treatment is continued. HCQ is generally considered to be safe during pregnancy

Leflunomide (LEF) can be used alone or in combination with other drugs for the treatment of RA and PsA in a dose of 10–20 mg/day. It works by inhibiting dihydro-orotate dehydrogenase, an enzyme used by activated lymphocytes to synthesise pyrimidines necessary for DNA synthesis. It has low marrow toxicity, but may cause liver dysfunction, hypertension and hirsutism. It must be co-prescribed with robust contraception in women of child-bearing potential. Treatment must be stopped for a period of 2 years in advance of planning a pregnancy or undergo a washout procedure with cholestyramine to remove the drug from the system.

Azathioprine (AZA) is most commonly used in vasculitis and SLE, often in combination with other drugs. It is metabolised to 6-mercaptopurine (6-MP), which blocks lymphocyte proliferation by inhibiting DNA synthesis. The typical starting dose is 1 mg/kg body weight per day, increasing to 2.5 mg/kg until a response is observed or toxicity occurs. Bone marrow suppression is the most important side-effect, but nausea may also occur. Genetic polymorphisms in the enzyme thiopurine S-methyltransferase (TPMT) influence catabolism of 6-MP and sometimes genetic testing for TPMT variants is done to guide dosages. Allopurinol inhibits catabolism of azathioprine, necessitating a 75% reduction in azathioprine dose.

Cyclophosphamide is a cytotoxic alkylating agent that cross-links DNA and halts cell division, causing immunosuppression. It is mainly used to induce remission in life-threatening systemic vasculitis and SLE. It can be given orally in a dose of 2 mg/kg/day for 3–6 months or intravenously in a dose of 15 mg/kg every 3–4 weeks on 6–8 occasions. Adverse effects include nausea, anorexia, vomiting, bone marrow suppression, cardiac toxicity, alopecia and haemorrhagic cystitis. The risk of cystitis can be mitigated by co-administration of mesna (2-mercaptoethane sulfonate, which binds its urotoxic metabolites) and a high fluid intake.

26

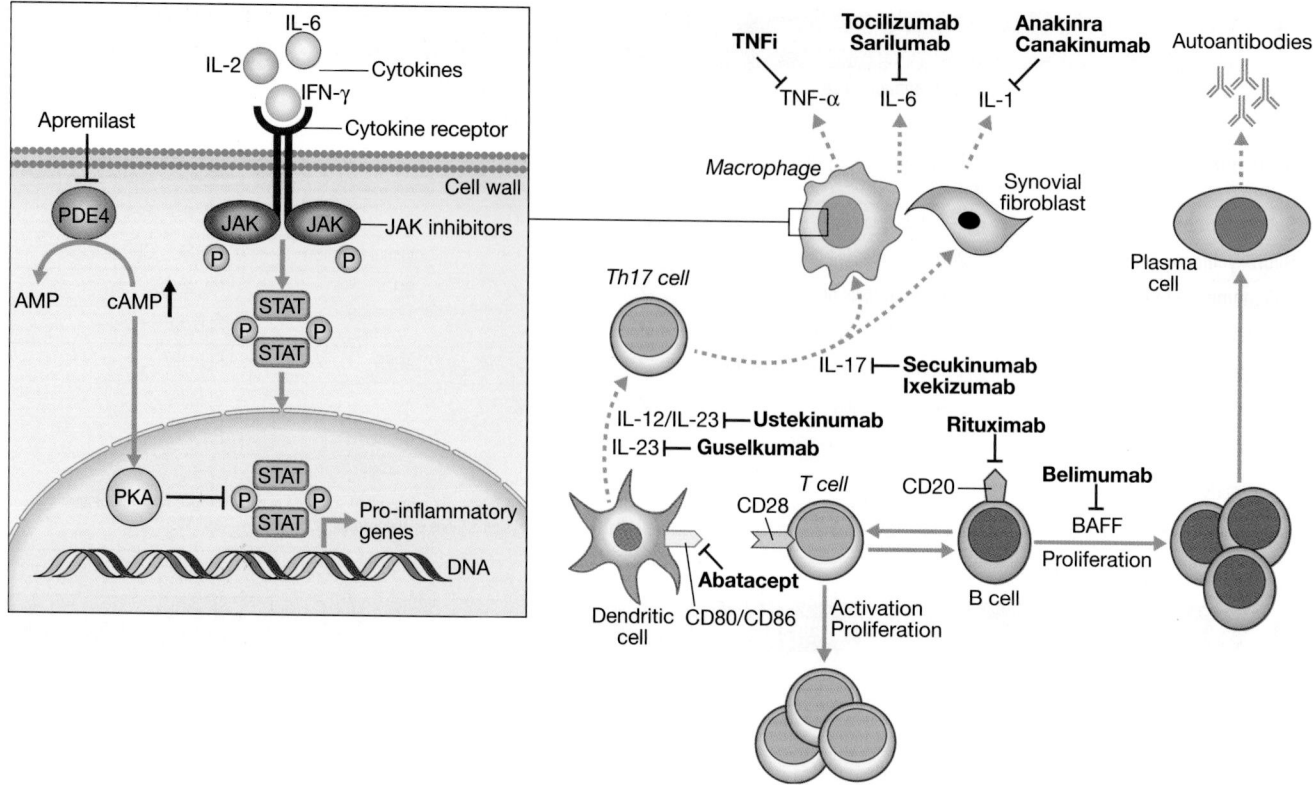

Fig. 26.15 Targets for biologic therapies in inflammatory rheumatic diseases. Biologic treatments for inflammatory rheumatic diseases work by targeting key cytokines and other molecules involved in regulating the immune response. (BAFF = B-cell-activating factor of the TNF family; AMP = adenosine monophosphate; cAMP = cyclic AMP; CD = cluster of differentiation; IL = interleukin; JAK = Janus activated kinase; P = phosphate; PDE = phosphodiesterase; PKA = protein kinase A; STAT = signal transducers and activators of transcription; TNF-α = tumour necrosis factor alpha; TNFi = inhibitor of tumour necrosis factor)

Mycophenolate mofetil (MMF) works by inhibiting inosine monophosphate dehydrogenase, a rate-limiting enzyme in the synthesis of guanosine nucleotides in lymphocytes. MMF is used in SLE and vasculitis in doses of 2–4 g daily orally. Haematological toxicity is the main adverse effect.

Ciclosporin A is a calcineurin inhibitor that inhibits lymphocyte activation. It is occasionally used in the treatment of RA and PsA at a dose of 2.5–4 mg/kg/day orally.

Glucocorticoids have powerful anti-inflammatory and immunosuppressive effects and have been shown to have disease-modifying effects in various inflammatory rheumatic diseases. They promote apoptosis of many immune cells and activation of a wide range of pro-inflammatory signalling pathways. They are used orally, intravenously, intramuscularly and by intra-articular injection in the treatment of a wide range of inflammatory rheumatic diseases, as well as by local injection in patients with soft tissue rheumatism.

Systemic glucocorticoids are widely used in moderate to high doses to induce remission in early RA, systemic and polyarticular JIA, giant cell arteritis, polymyalgia rheumatica, vasculitis and SLE. Many patients with SLE require low dose maintenance therapy with glucocorticoids and this is sometimes also required in RA when other options are unsuitable. They are widely used in the short-term treatment of flares in many inflammatory rheumatic diseases. Glucocorticoids should be used with caution in PsA because of a rebound increase in activity of psoriasis when the effects wear off.

Intra-articular glucocorticoids are employed in the treatment of a wide range of inflammatory arthritides and are primarily indicated when there are one or two problem joints with persistent synovitis despite good general control of the disease. Methylprednisolone is one of the most widely used, typically in doses of 40–80 mg.

Intramuscular methylprednisolone (80–120 mg) is a useful way of controlling inflammatory arthritis while waiting for the effects of newly introduced drugs to take effect. It can also be helpful in patients with stable disease who have a disease flare where a major change in DMARD strategy is not thought to be necessary.

Targeted synthetic DMARDs (tsDMARDs)

These are small molecules targeted at specific intracellular targets involved in regulating the immune response. Treatment costs are high and these drugs are generally used as second-line agents in patients who have responded inadequately to cDMARDs.

Janus-activated kinase (JAK) inhibitors work by inhibiting JAK enzymes, which are a family of intracellular signalling molecules that play a key role in transducing the effects of several pro-inflammatory cytokines. The main adverse effects of JAK inhibitors are an increased risk of infections, and because of this, it is customary to screen patients for evidence of occult infection with HIV, hepatitis C, hepatitis B and previous TB before commencing therapy. Currently there are four drugs in this class. Tofacitinib (5 mg twice daily or 10 mg daily) is indicated for adults with RA and PsA. It is usually prescribed in combination with MTX, but can be used as monotherapy in patients where MTX is poorly tolerated or contraindicated. Baricitinib (2–4 mg once daily) and filgotinib (200 mg daily) are both indicated for RA. Upadacitinib (15 mg daily) is also indicated as monotherapy or in combination with MTX, for RA, PsA and AxSpA. Tofacitinib requires long-term blood monitoring for marrow and liver toxicity, but this is not required with the other JAK inhibitors once the first 3 months of therapy have been completed.

Apremilast is used in the treatment of PsA. It is a small molecule inhibitor of phosphodiesterase 4, an enzyme that breaks down cyclic adenosine monophosphate (cAMP). This suppresses production of pro-inflammatory cytokines, thereby reducing inflammation. Apremilast is given orally in a dose of 30 mg twice daily. The main adverse effects are gastrointestinal upset, weight loss and an increased risk of depression.

| | 26.35 Biologic therapies for inflammatory rheumatic disease |

Drug	Maintenance dose	Mechanism of action	Indications
Etanercept	50 mg weekly SC	Decoy receptor for TNF-α	RA, PsA, AxSpA, JIA
Infliximab	3–5 mg/kg 8-weekly IV	Antibody to TNF-α	RA, PsA, AxSpA, JIA
Adalimumab	40 mg 2-weekly SC		
Certolizumab	200 mg 2-weekly SC		
Golimumab	50 mg 4-weekly SC		
Rituximab	2×1 g 2 weeks apart IV	Antibody to CD20; destroys B cells	RA, vasculitis
Belimumab	200 mg weekly SC or 10 mg/kg 4-weekly IV	Antibody to BAFF; inhibits B-cell activation	SLE
Abatacept	125 mg weekly SC or 10 mg/kg 4-weekly IV	Inhibits T-cell activation	RA, PsA, JIA
Tocilizumab	162 mg weekly SC or 8 mg/kg 8-weekly IV	Antibody to IL-6 receptor	RA, JIA, GCA
Sarilumab	200 mg 2-weekly SC	Antibody to IL-6 receptor	RA
Ustekinumab	45 mg 12-weekly SC	Antibody to IL-12 and IL-23	PsA
Secukinumab	150 mg 4-weekly SC	Antibody to IL-17A	PsA, axSpA
Ixekizumab	80 mg 4-weekly SC.	Antibody to IL-17A/F	PsA and AxSpA
Anakinra	100 mg daily SC	Decoy receptor for IL-1	RA, CAPS, AOSD, gout
Canakinumab	150 mg or 2 mg/kg 8-weekly SC	Antibody to IL-1β	CAPS, sJIA, AOSD, gout
Guselkumab	100 mg 8-weekly SC	Antibody to IL-23	PsA

(AOSD = adult-onset Still's disease; axSpA = axial spondyloarthritis; BAFF = B cell-activating factor of the TNF family; CAPS = cryopyrin-associated periodic syndromes; CD = cluster of differentiation; GCA = giant cell arteritis; IL = interleukin; IV = intravenous; JIA = juvenile idiopathic arthritis; PsA = psoriatic arthritis; RA = rheumatoid arthritis; SC = subcutaneous; sJIA = systemic juvenile idiopathic arthritis; SLE = systemic lupus erythematosus; TNF-α = tumour necrosis factor alpha)

Biologic DMARDs

'Biologics' (monoclonal antibodies, fusion proteins or decoy receptors) are given either as self-administered subcutaneous injections every 1–4 weeks or as infusions every few weeks. The main adverse effect of biologics as a class is an increased risk of infections, and screening for occult infections is generally performed before commencing therapy as described for JAK inhibitors. Biologics are not carcinogenic, but patients who develop cancer while on treatment may exhibit accelerated progression of the tumour due to suppression of the immune response. Treatment costs are higher than with cDMARDs and tsDMARDs and many countries have set guidelines and funding restrictions that limit their use. Their mechanisms of action, dosages and indications are summarised in Box 26.35.

TNF-α inhibitors. Most drugs in this class are monoclonal antibodies that bind to and neutralise TNF-α, but etanercept is a decoy receptor that prevents TNF-α binding to its receptor. Anti-TNF-α therapy is frequently used as the first-line biologic in RA, JIA and PsA when cDMARD therapy has been incompletely effective and as first line biologic in axSpA/AS in patients who have failed to respond adequately to NSAID therapy. Anti-TNF-α is contraindicated in patients with active infections and those with indwelling catheters, due to the high risk of infection. Other contraindications are heart failure (New York Heart Association grade 3 or 4) and multiple sclerosis, both of which may be worsened by treatment. Anti-TNF-α therapies can be used during pregnancy, but should be stopped in the third trimester since most cross the placenta and can cause immunosuppression in the neonate. An exception is certolizumab, which does not cross the placenta and can be used safely throughout pregnancy.

Rituximab is an antibody directed against the CD20 receptor, which is expressed on B lymphocytes and immature plasma cells. Rituximab causes profound B cell lymphopenia for several months due to complement-mediated lysis of cells that express CD20. Rituximab is indicated in RA patients where response to cDMARDs has been inadequate and to induce remission in adults and children with ANCA-associated vasculitis. In RA, treatment can be repeated when signs of improvement are wearing off (6 months to 1 year or longer). In ANCA-positive vasculitis, a single cycle of treatment may last for up to 18 months. Adverse effects include hypogammaglobulinaemia, infusion reactions, an increased risk of infections and, rarely, progressive multifocal leucoencephalopathy

(PML), a serious and potentially fatal infection of the central nervous system caused by reactivation of JC virus.

Belimumab is a monoclonal antibody that blocks the effects of the cytokine B cell-activating factor of the TNF family (BAFF), which is required for B cell survival and function. It is indicated in juvenile and adult patients with SLE who have had an inadequate response to cDMARDs. The main adverse effects are an increased risk of infection, leucopenia and hypersensitivity reactions following infusion.

Abatacept is a fusion protein in which the Fc domain of IgG has been combined with the extracellular domain of CTLA4, which blocks T-cell activation by acting as a decoy for CD28, a co-stimulatory molecule necessary for T-cell activation. It is indicated for RA and PsA and polyarticular onset JIA where the response to cDMARDs is inadequate. The main adverse effect is an increased risk of infections.

IL-6 inhibitors. There are two drugs in this class. Tocilizumab is a monoclonal antibody that competes with IL-6 for binding to the IL-6 receptor, thereby inhibiting IL-6 signalling. It is indicated in RA with or without MTX after inadequate response to cDMARDs and in patients 12 years of age and older with systemic JIA, who have responded inadequately to therapy with NSAIDs and systemic glucocorticoids. It is also indicated as a steroid-sparing agent in GCA. Sarilumab is a monoclonal antibody (IgG1) that works in a similar way to tocilizumab, which is licensed for treating adult RA (with concomitant MTX), where there has been an inadequate response to cDMARDs. Adverse effects of both agents include leucopenia, abnormal LFTs, hypercholesterolaemia and hypersensitivity reactions. Both drugs should be avoided during pregnancy if possible.

Ustekinumab is an antibody to p40, which is a subunit shared by the cytokines IL-23 and IL-12. It acts as an inhibitor of both IL-12 and IL-23 signalling and is indicated in adults with PsA who have not responded adequately to cDMARDs. It can be used as monotherapy or in combination with MTX. Adverse effects include an increased risk of infections, hypersensitivity reactions and an exfoliative dermatitis. Guselkumab is an antibody directed against the p19 protein of IL-23, which acts as a specific inhibitor of IL-23 signalling. It is effective in the treatment of PsA and can be used alone or in combination with MTX.

IL-17 inhibitors. There are two drugs in this class; secukinumab is a monoclonal antibody to IL-17A and ixekizumab, which binds both

IL-17A and IL-17A/F. These drugs are indicated in adults with PsA and axSpA who have not responded adequately to cDMARDs and/or anti-TNF-α. Adverse effects include an increased risk of triggering bouts of IBD, infections, nasopharyngitis and headache. Adverse effects include infections and exacerbation of IBD. Clinical experience indicates that these drugs are probably safe during pregnancy, but information is limited.

Interleukin-1 inhibitors. There are two drugs in this class. Anakinra is a human IL-1 receptor antagonist, which neutralises the effects of interleukin-1α (IL-1α) and interleukin-1β (IL-1β) by inhibiting binding to interleukin-1 type I receptor (IL-1RI). Its most frequent use is for the treatment of adult-onset Still's disease and for periodic fever syndromes (p. 76). It has some efficacy in RA, but is seldom used since other drugs are more effective. Other indications include acute gout, although it is not licensed for this condition, and chronic non-infectious osteomyelitis (see p. 1062). Adverse effects include an increased risk of infections, hypersensitivity reactions and neutropenia. Canakinumab is a monoclonal antibody directed against IL-1β, which is indicated for the treatment of systemic JIA (Still's disease), adult-onset Still's disease and acute flares of gout resistant to other treatments. The usual maintenance dose in adults is 150–300 mg every 8 weeks. Adverse effects include an increased risk of infections, hypersensitivity reactions and neutropenia.

Osteoarthritis

Osteoarthritis (OA) is by far the most common form of arthritis and is a major cause of pain and disability in older people. It is characterised by focal loss of articular cartilage, subchondral osteosclerosis, osteophyte formation at the joint margin and remodelling of joint contour with enlargement of affected joints.

Epidemiology

The prevalence rises progressively with age and it has been estimated that 45% of all people develop knee OA and 25% hip OA at some point during life. Although some are asymptomatic, the lifetime risk of having a total hip or knee replacement for OA in someone aged 50 is about 11% for women and 8% for men in the UK. There are major ethnic differences in susceptibility: the prevalence of hip OA is lower in Africa, China, Japan and South Asia than in European countries, while that of knee OA is higher.

Pathophysiology

OA is a complex disorder, with both genetic and environmental components (Box 26.36). Family-based studies have estimated that the heritability of OA ranges from about 43% at the knee to between 60% and 65% at the hip and hand, respectively. In most cases, the inheritance is polygenic and mediated by several genetic variants of small effect. OA can be a component of multiple epiphyseal dysplasias, which are caused by single gene mutations affecting components of cartilage matrix. Structural abnormalities, such as slipped femoral epiphysis and developmental dysplasia of the hip, are also associated with a high risk of OA, presumably due to abnormal load distribution across the joint. Similar mechanisms probably explain the increased risk of OA in patients with limb deformity secondary to Paget's disease of bone. Biomechanical factors play an important role in OA related to certain occupations, such as farmers (hip OA), miners (knee OA) and elite or professional athletes (knee and ankle OA). It has been speculated that the higher prevalence of knee OA in South and East Asia might be accounted for by squatting. There is also a high risk of knee OA in people who have had destabilising injuries, such as cruciate ligament rupture, and those who have had meniscectomy. For most individuals, however, participation in recreational sport does not appear to increase the risk significantly. There is a strong association between obesity and OA, particularly of the hip knee. This is thought to be due partly to biomechanical factors, but it has also been speculated that cytokines released from adipose tissue may play a role. Oestrogen appears important; lower rates of OA have been

Genetics
- Skeletal dysplasias
- Polygenic inheritance

Developmental abnormalities
- Developmental dysplasia of the hip
- Slipped femoral epiphysis

Repetitive loading
- Farmers
- Miners
- Elite athletes

Adverse biomechanics
- Meniscectomy
- Ligament rupture
- Paget's disease

Obesity

Trauma

Hormonal
- Oestrogen deficiency
- Aromatase inhibitors

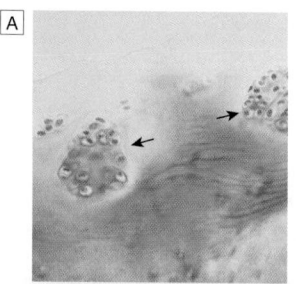
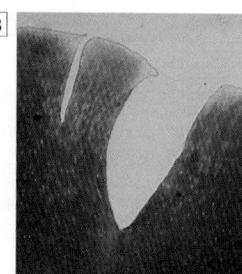
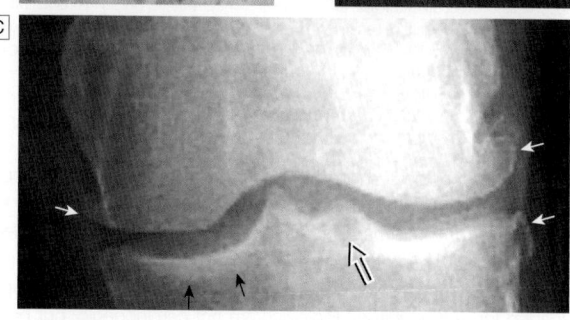

Fig. 26.16 Pathological changes in osteoarthritis. A Abnormal nests of proliferating chondrocytes (arrows) interspersed with matrix devoid of normal chondrocytes. B Fibrillation of cartilage in osteoarthritis (OA). C X-ray of knee joint affected by OA, showing osteophytes at joint margin (white arrows), subchondral sclerosis (black arrows) and a subchondral cyst (open arrow).

observed in women who use hormone replacement therapy (HRT), while women who receive aromatase inhibitor therapy for breast cancer often experience a flare in symptoms of OA.

Degeneration of articular cartilage is the defining feature of OA. Under normal circumstances, chondrocytes are terminally differentiated cells, but in OA they start dividing to produce nests of metabolically active cells (Fig. 26.16A). Initially, matrix components are produced by these cells at an increased rate, but at the same time there is accelerated degradation of the major structural components of cartilage matrix, including aggrecan and type II collagen (see Fig. 26.5). Eventually, the concentration of aggrecan in cartilage matrix falls and makes the cartilage vulnerable to load-bearing injury. Fissuring of the cartilage surface ('fibrillation') then occurs, leading to the development of deep vertical clefts (Fig. 26.16B), localised chondrocyte death and decreased cartilage thickness. This is initially focal, mainly targeting the maximum load-bearing part of the joint, but eventually large parts of the cartilage surface are damaged. CPP and basic calcium phosphate crystals often become deposited in the abnormal cartilage.

OA is also accompanied by abnormalities in subchondral bone, which becomes sclerotic and the site of subchondral cysts (Fig. 26.16C). Fibrocartilage is produced at the joint margin, which undergoes endochondral ossification to form osteophytes. Bone remodelling and cartilage thinning slowly alter the shape of the OA joint, increasing its surface area. It is almost as though there is a homeostatic mechanism operative in

OA that causes enlargement of the failing joint to spread the mechanical load over a greater surface area.

Patients with OA also have higher BMD values at sites distant from the joint and this is particularly associated with osteophyte formation. This is in keeping with observations made in epidemiological studies that show that patients with OA are partially protected from developing osteoporosis and vice versa. This is likely to be due to the fact that the genetic factors that predispose to osteoporosis might be protective for OA.

The synovium in OA is often hyperplastic and may be the site of inflammatory change, but to a much lesser extent than in RA and other inflammatory arthropathies. Osteochondral bodies commonly occur within the synovium, reflecting chondroid metaplasia or secondary uptake and growth of damaged cartilage fragments. The outer capsule also thickens and contracts, usually retaining the stability of the remodelling joint. The muscles surrounding affected joints commonly show evidence of wasting and non-specific type II fibre atrophy.

Clinical features

Osteoarthritis has a characteristic distribution, mainly targeting the hips, knees, PIP and DIP joints of the hands, neck and lumbar spine (see Fig. 26.10). The main presenting symptoms are pain and functional restriction. The causes of pain in OA are not completely understood, but may relate to increased pressure in subchondral bone (mainly causing night pain), trabecular microfractures, capsular distension and low-grade synovitis. Pain may also result from bursitis and enthesopathy secondary to altered joint mechanics. Typical OA pain has the characteristics listed in Box 26.37. For many people, functional restriction of the hands, knees or hips is an equal, if not greater, problem than pain. The clinical findings vary according to severity, but are principally those of joint damage.

The correlation between the presence of structural change, as assessed by imaging, and symptoms such as pain and disability varies markedly according to site. It is stronger at the hip than at the knee and weak at most small joints. This suggests that the risk factors for pain and disability may differ from those for structural change. At the knee, for example, reduced quadriceps muscle strength and adverse psychosocial factors (anxiety, depression) correlate more strongly with pain and disability than the degree of radiographic change.

Radiological evidence of OA is very common in middle-aged and older people, and the disease may coexist with other conditions, so it is important to remember that pain in a patient with OA may be due to another cause.

Generalised nodal OA

Characteristics of this common form of OA are shown in Box 26.38. Some patients are asymptomatic whereas others develop pain, stiffness and swelling of one or more PIP and DIP joints of the hands from the age of about 40 years onwards. Gradually, these develop posterolateral swellings on each side of the extensor tendon, which slowly enlarge and harden to become Heberden's (DIP) and Bouchard's (PIP) nodes (Fig. 26.17). Typically, each joint goes through a phase of episodic symptoms (1–5 years) while the node evolves and OA develops. Once OA is fully established, symptoms may subside and hand function often remains good. Affected joints are enlarged as a result of osteophyte formation and often show characteristic lateral deviation, reflecting the asymmetric focal cartilage loss of OA (Fig. 26.18). Involvement of the first carpometacarpal (CMC) joint is also common, leading to pain on trying to open bottles and jars, and functional impairment. Clinically, it may be detected by the presence of crepitus on joint movement and squaring of the thumb base.

Generalised nodal OA has a very strong genetic component: the daughter of an affected mother has a 1 in 3 chance of developing nodal OA herself. People with nodal OA are also at increased risk of OA at other sites, especially the knee.

Knee OA

At the knee, OA principally targets the patello-femoral and medial tibio-femoral compartments, but eventually spreads to affect the whole of the

26.37 Symptoms and signs of osteoarthritis

Pain
- Insidious onset over months or years
- Variable or intermittent nature over time ('good days, bad days')
- Mainly related to movement and weight-bearing, relieved by rest
- Mild morning stiffness (< 15 mins) and inactivity gelling (< 5 mins) after rest
- Usually only one or a few joints painful

Clinical signs
- Restricted movement due to capsular thickening or blocking by osteophyte
- Palpable, sometimes audible, coarse crepitus due to rough articular surfaces
- Bony swelling around joint margins
- Deformity, usually without instability
- Joint-line or periarticular tenderness
- Muscle weakness and wasting
- Mild or absent synovitis

26.38 Characteristics of generalised nodal osteoarthritis

- Polyarticular finger interphalangeal joint osteoarthritis
- Heberden's (± Bouchard's) nodes
- Marked female preponderance
- Peak onset in middle age
- Good functional outcome for hands
- Predisposition to osteoarthritis at other joints, especially knees
- Strong genetic predisposition

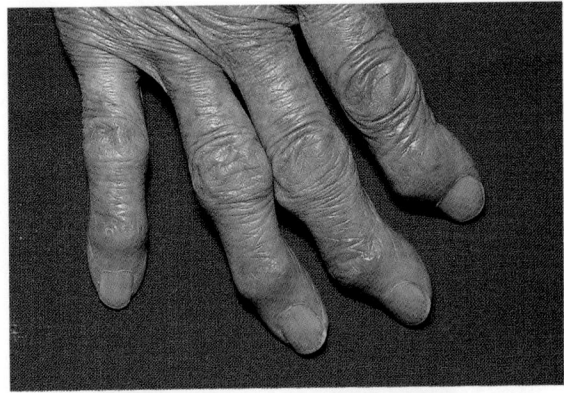

Fig. 26.17 Nodal osteoarthritis. Heberden's nodes and lateral (radial to ulnar) deviation of distal interphalangeal joints, with mild Bouchard's nodes at the proximal interphalangeal joints.

joint (Fig. 26.19). It may be isolated or occur as part of generalised nodal OA. Most patients have bilateral and symmetrical involvement. In men, trauma is often a more important risk factor and may result in unilateral OA.

The pain is usually localised to the anterior or medial aspect of the knee and upper tibia. Patello-femoral pain is usually worse going up and down stairs or inclines. Posterior knee pain suggests the presence of a complicating popliteal cyst (Baker's cyst). Prolonged walking, rising from a chair, getting in or out of a car, or bending to put on shoes and socks may be difficult. Local examination findings may include:

- a jerky, asymmetric (antalgic) gait with less time weight-bearing on the painful side
- a varus (Fig. 26.20) or, less commonly, valgus and/or a fixed flexion deformity
- joint-line and/or periarticular tenderness (secondary anserine bursitis and medial ligament enthesopathy (see Box 26.25), causing tenderness of the upper medial tibia)

26

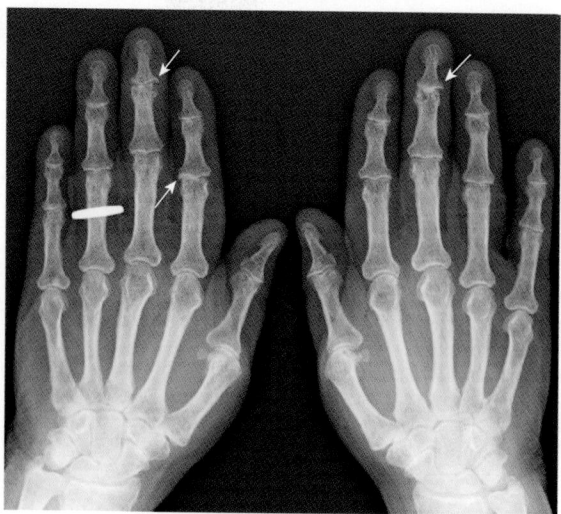

Fig. 26.18 X-ray appearances in hand osteoarthritis. There is joint space narrowing affecting the proximal interphalangeal (PIP) and distal interphalangeal (DIP) joints in both hands. There are typical articular subchondral and 'gull wing' appearances to some osteoarthritis-affected joints, as well as osteophyte formation that is most marked at the second DIP joints bilaterally and the first PIP joint on the right hand (arrows).

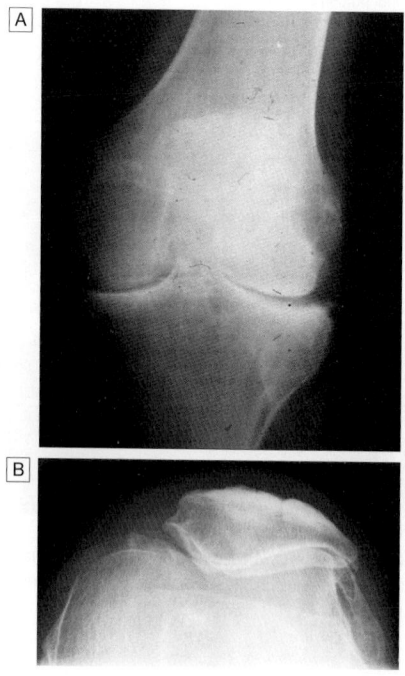

Fig. 26.19 X-ray appearances in knee osteoarthritis. **A** Advanced osteoarthritis showing almost complete loss of joint space affecting both compartments and sclerosis of subchondral bone. **B** Skyline view of the patella femoral joint in a patient with severe patello-femoral osteoarthritis. There is almost complete loss of joint space and lateral displacement of the patella.

- weakness and wasting of the quadriceps muscle
- restricted flexion and extension with crepitus
- bony swelling around the joint line.

CPP crystal deposition in association with OA is common at the knee. This may result in a more overt inflammatory component (stiffness, effusions) and super-added acute attacks of synovitis (acute CPP crystal arthritis), which may be associated with more rapid radiographic and clinical progression.

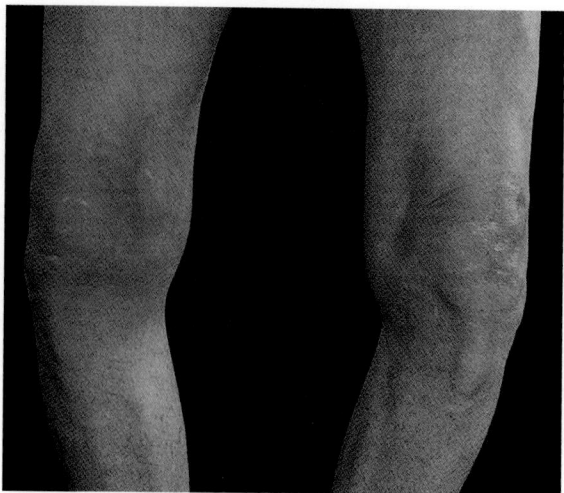

Fig. 26.20 Typical varus knee deformity resulting from marked medial tibio-femoral osteoarthritis.

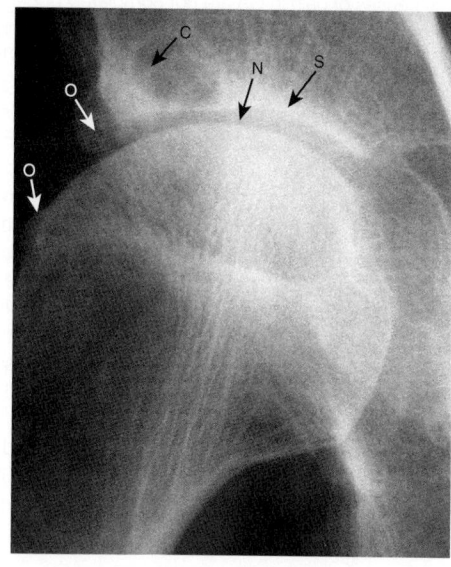

Fig. 26.21 X-ray of hip showing changes of osteoarthritis. Note the superior joint space narrowing (N), subchondral sclerosis (S), marginal osteophytes (O) and cysts (C).

Hip OA

Hip OA most commonly targets the superior aspect of the joint (Fig. 26.21). It is often unilateral at presentation, frequently progresses with superolateral migration of the femoral head and has a poor prognosis. The less common central (medial) OA shows more central cartilage loss and is largely confined to women. It is often bilateral at presentation and can be associated with generalised nodal OA. It has a better prognosis than superior hip OA and progression to axial migration of the femoral head is uncommon.

The hip shows the best correlation between symptoms and radiographic change. Hip pain is usually maximal deep in the anterior groin, with variable radiation to the buttock, anterolateral thigh, knee or shin. Lateral hip pain, worse on lying on that side with tenderness over the greater trochanter, suggests secondary trochanteric bursitis. Common functional difficulties are the same as for knee OA; in addition, restricted hip abduction in women may cause pain during sexual intercourse. Examination may reveal:

- an antalgic gait
- weakness and wasting of quadriceps and gluteal muscles

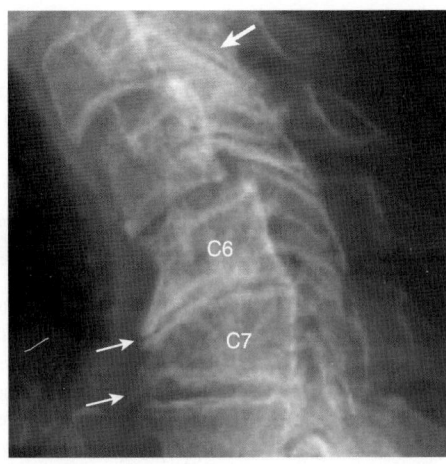

Fig. 26.22 X-ray of spine showing typical changes of osteoarthritis. Cervical spondylosis showing disc space narrowing between C6 and C7, osteophytes at the anterior vertebral body margins (thin arrows) and osteosclerosis at the apophyseal joints (thick arrow).

26.39 Causes of early-onset osteoarthritis

Monoarticular

- Previous trauma, localised instability

Pauciarticular or polyarticular

- Juvenile idiopathic arthritis
- Metabolic or endocrine disease:
  Haemochromatosis
  Ochronosis
  Acromegaly
  Alkaptonuria
- Spondylo-epiphyseal dysplasia
- Late osteonecrosis
- Neuropathic joint
- Kashin–Beck disease

- pain and restriction of internal rotation with the hip flexed – the earliest and most sensitive sign of hip OA; other movements may subsequently be restricted and painful
- anterior groin tenderness just lateral to the femoral pulse
- fixed flexion, external rotation deformity of the hip
- ipsilateral leg shortening with severe joint attrition and superior femoral migration.

Obesity is associated with more rapid progression of hip OA.

Spine OA

The cervical and lumbar spine are the sites most often targeted by OA, where it is referred to as cervical spondylosis and lumbar spondylosis, respectively (Fig. 26.22). Spine OA may occur in isolation or as part of generalised OA. The typical presentation is with pain localised to the low back region or the neck, although radiation of pain to the arms, buttocks and legs may also occur due to nerve root compression. The pain is typically relieved by rest and worse on movement. On physical examination, the range of movement may be limited and loss of lumbar lordosis is typical. The straight leg-raising test or femoral stretch test may be positive and neurological signs may be seen in the legs where there is complicating spinal stenosis or nerve root compression.

Early-onset OA

Rarely, OA may present before the age of 45. In most cases, a single joint is affected and there is a clear history of previous trauma. However, specific causes of OA need to be considered in people with early-onset disease affecting several joints, especially those not normally targeted by OA, in which case rare causes need to be considered (Box 26.39).

26.40 Osteoarthritis in old age

- **Pain and disability**: osteoarthritis is the principal cause in old age.
- **Calcium phosphate deposition disease**: may cause acute attacks of synovitis (pseudogout) on a background of chronic osteoarthritis.
- **Falls**: reduced muscle strength and pain associated with lower limb osteoarthritis increase the risk.
- **Muscle-strengthening exercises**: safely reduce the pain and disability of knee osteoarthritis with accompanying improvements in balance and reduced tendency to fall.
- **Oral paracetamol and topical non-steroidal anti-inflammatory drugs**: safe in older people, with no important drug interactions or contraindications.
- **Intra-articular injection of glucocorticoid**: a very safe and often effective treatment, particularly useful for tiding a patient over a special event.
- **Total joint replacement**: an excellent cost-effective treatment for severe disabling knee or hip osteoarthritis in older people. There is no age limit for joint replacement surgery.

Kashin–Beck disease is a rare form of OA that occurs in children, typically between the ages of 7 and 13, in some regions of China. The cause is unknown, but suggested predisposing factors are selenium deficiency and contamination of cereals with mycotoxin-producing fungi.

Erosive OA

This term is used to describe an unusual group of patients with hand OA who have a more prolonged symptom phase, more overt inflammation, more disability and worse outcome than those with nodal OA. Distinguishing features include preferential targeting of PIP joints, subchondral erosions on X-rays, occasional ankylosis of affected joints and lack of association with OA elsewhere. It is unclear whether erosive OA is part of the spectrum of hand OA or a discrete subset.

Investigations

A plain X-ray of the affected joints should be performed and often will show one or more of the typical features of OA (see Fig. 26.16 and Figs. 26.18–26.22). In addition to providing diagnostic information, X-rays are of value in assessing the severity of structural change, which is helpful if joint replacement surgery is being considered. Non-weight-bearing postero-anterior views of the pelvis are adequate for assessing hip OA. Patients with suspected knee OA should have standing anteroposterior X-rays taken to assess tibio-femoral cartilage loss and a flexed skyline view to assess patello-femoral involvement. Spine OA can often be diagnosed on a plain X-ray, which typically shows evidence of disc space narrowing and osteophytes. If nerve root compression or spinal stenosis is suspected, MRI should be performed.

Routine biochemistry, haematology and autoantibody tests are usually normal, though inflammatory OA can be associated with a mild acute phase response. Synovial fluid aspirated from an affected joint is viscous, with a low cell count.

Unexplained early-onset OA requires additional investigation, guided by the suspected underlying condition. X-rays may show typical features of dysplasia or osteonecrosis, widening of joint spaces in acromegaly, multiple cysts, chondrocalcinosis and MCP joint involvement in haemochromatosis or disorganised architecture in neuropathic joints.

Management

Treatment follows the general principles outlined earlier this chapter. Measures that are pertinent in older people are summarised in Box 26.40.

Education

It is important to explain the nature of the condition fully, outlining the role of relevant risk factors such as obesity, heredity and trauma. The patient should be informed that established structural changes are permanent and that, although a cure is not possible, pain and function can often be improved. The prognosis should also be discussed, mentioning that it is generally good for nodal hand OA and better for knee than hip OA.

26

Lifestyle advice

Weight loss has a substantial beneficial effect on symptoms if the patient is obese and is probably one of the most effective treatments available for OA of the lower limbs. Strengthening and aerobic exercises also have beneficial effects in OA and should be advised, preferably with reinforcement by a physiotherapist. Quadriceps strengthening exercises are particularly beneficial in knee OA. Shock-absorbing footwear, pacing of activities, use of a walking stick for painful knee or hip OA, and provision of built-up shoes to equalise leg lengths can all improve symptoms.

Non-pharmacological therapy

Acupuncture and transcutaneous electrical nerve stimulation (TENS) can be effective in knee OA. Local physical therapies, such as heat or cold, can sometimes give temporary relief.

Pharmacological therapy

If symptoms do not respond to non-pharmacological measures, paracetamol should be tried. Addition of a topical NSAID and then capsaicin for knee and hand OA can also be helpful. Oral NSAIDs should be considered in patients who remain symptomatic. These drugs are significantly more effective than paracetamol and can be successfully combined with paracetamol or compound analgesics if the pain is severe. Strong opiates may occasionally be required. Antineuropathic drugs, such as amitriptyline, gabapentin and pregabalin, are sometimes used in patients with symptoms that are difficult to control, but the evidence base for their use is poor. Neutralising antibodies to nerve growth factor have been developed and are effective treatment for pain in OA, but they are not yet licensed for routine clinical use.

Intra-articular injections

Intra-articular glucocorticoid injections are effective in the treatment of knee OA and are also used for symptomatic relief in the treatment of OA at the first CMC joint. The duration of effect is usually short, but trials of serial glucocorticoid injections every 3 months in knee OA have shown efficacy for up to 1 year. Intra-articular injections of hyaluronic acid can help to an extent in knee OA, but the treatment is expensive and the effect short-lived. In the UK they have not been considered to be cost-effective by NICE.

Neutraceuticals

Chondroitin sulphate and glucosamine sulphate have been used alone and in combination for the treatment of knee OA. There is evidence from randomised controlled trials that these agents can improve knee pain to a small extent (3%–5%) compared with placebo.

Surgery

Surgery should be considered for patients with OA whose symptoms and functional impairment impact significantly on their quality of life despite optimal medical therapy and lifestyle advice. Total joint replacement surgery is by far the most common surgical procedure for patients with OA. It can transform the quality of life for people with severe knee or hip OA and is indicated when there is significant structural damage on X-ray. Although surgery should not be undertaken at an early stage during the development of OA, it is important to consider it before functional limitation has become advanced since this may compromise outcome. Patient-specific factors, such as age, gender, smoking and presence of obesity, should not be barriers to referral for joint replacement.

Only a small proportion of patients with OA progress to the extent that total joint replacement is required, but OA is by far the most frequent indication for this. Over 95% of joint replacements continue to function well into the second decade after surgery and most provide life-long, pain-free function. Up to 20% of patients are not satisfied with the outcome, however, and a few experience little or no improvement in pain. Other surgical procedures are performed much less frequently. Resurfacing of the femoral head can be considered for younger patients with hip OA (age <60) as an alternative to total joint replacement. Tibial osteotomy represents an alternative to total joint replacement in younger patients with knee OA and can be effective at improving pain by altering alignment of the lower leg. Cartilage repair is sometimes performed to treat focal cartilage defects resulting from joint injury.

Crystal-induced arthritis

A variety of crystals can deposit in and around joints and structures in the spine and cause an acute inflammatory or even chronic inflammatory arthritis or disease (Box 26.41). Several factors influence crystal formation (Fig. 26.23). There must be sufficient concentration of the chemical components (ionic product), but whether a crystal then forms depends on the balance of tissue factors that promote and inhibit crystal nucleation and growth. The inflammatory potential of crystals resides in their physical irregularity and high negative surface charge, which can induce inflammation and damage cell membranes. Crystals may also cause mechanical damage to tissues and act as wear particles at the joint surface. They can reside in cartilage or tendon for years without causing inflammation or symptoms and it is only when they are released that they trigger inflammation. This may occur spontaneously but can also result from local trauma, rapid changes in the concentration of the components that form crystals, or in association with an acute phase response triggered by intercurrent illness or surgery. In the longer term, a reduction in concentrations of the solutes that form crystals causes dissolution of crystals and remission of the arthritis.

Gout

Gout is the most common inflammatory arthritis in men and in older women though robust epidemiological data on the prevalence of CPPD are lacking. Gout is caused by deposition of monosodium urate monohydrate crystals in and around synovial joints.

Epidemiology

The prevalence of gout is approximately 1%–2%, with a greater than 5:1 male preponderance. Gout has become progressively more common over recent years in affluent societies due to the increased prevalence of obesity and metabolic syndrome, of which hyperuricaemia is

i	26.41 Crystal-associated arthritis and deposition in connective tissue	
Crystal		**Disease**
Common		
Monosodium urate monohydrate		Acute gout
		Chronic tophaceous gout
Calcium pyrophosphate (CPP)		Acute CPP crystal arthritis
		Chronic CPP crystal arthritis
		Chondrocalcinosis
		Axial disease (e.g. crowned dens syndrome)
Basic calcium phosphate (BCP)		Calcific periarthritis
		Calcinosis
Uncommon		
Cholesterol		Chronic effusions in rheumatoid arthritis
Calcium oxalate		Acute arthritis in dialysis patients
Extrinsic crystals/semi-crystalline particles:		
Synthetic crystals		Acute synovitis
Plant thorns/sea urchin spines		Chronic monoarthritis, tenosynovitis

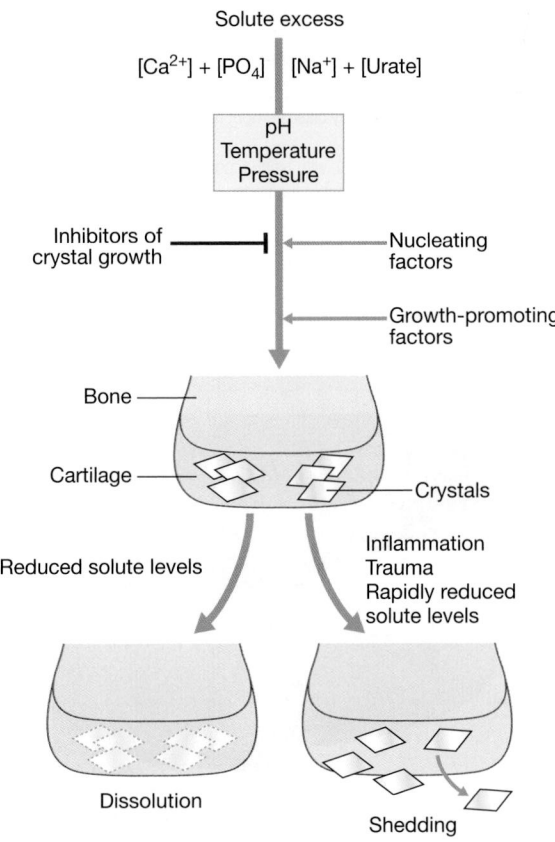

Fig. 26.23 Mechanisms of crystal formation.

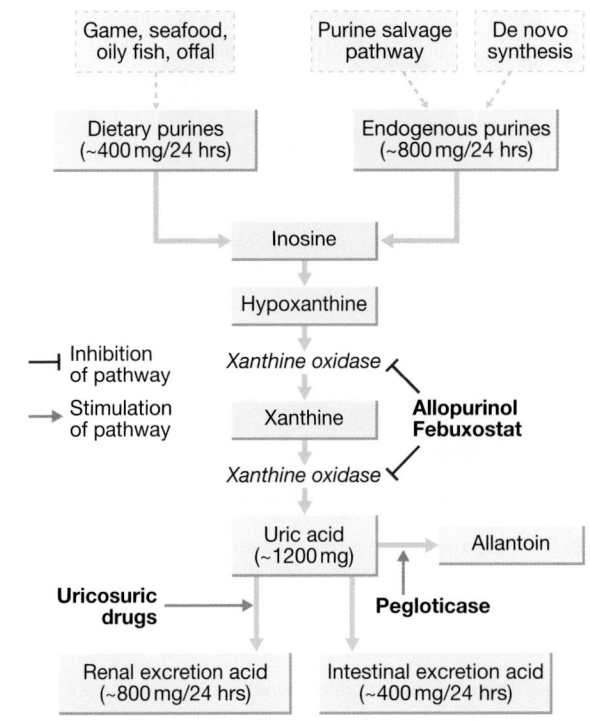

Fig. 26.24 Uric acid metabolism. The main pathways for uric acid production and elimination are shown, along with the site of action for urate-lowering therapies.

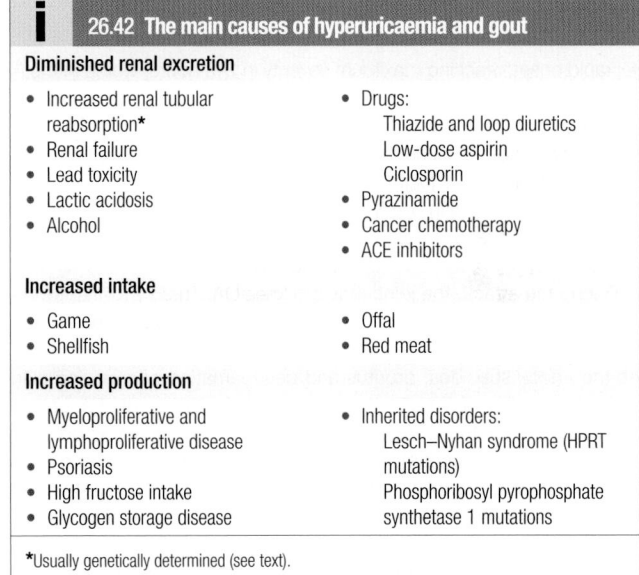

i 26.42 The main causes of hyperuricaemia and gout

Diminished renal excretion

- Increased renal tubular reabsorption*
- Renal failure
- Lead toxicity
- Lactic acidosis
- Alcohol

- Drugs:
  Thiazide and loop diuretics
  Low-dose aspirin
  Ciclosporin
- Pyrazinamide
- Cancer chemotherapy
- ACE inhibitors

Increased intake

- Game
- Shellfish

- Offal
- Red meat

Increased production

- Myeloproliferative and lymphoproliferative disease
- Psoriasis
- High fructose intake
- Glycogen storage disease

- Inherited disorders:
  Lesch–Nyhan syndrome (HPRT mutations)
  Phosphoribosyl pyrophosphate synthetase 1 mutations

*Usually genetically determined (see text).
(ACE = angiotensin-converting enzyme; HPRT = hypoxanthine guanine phosphoribosyl transferase)

an integral component. The risk of developing gout increases with age and with serum uric acid (SUA) levels. These are normally distributed in the general population and hyperuricaemia is defined as an SUA of more than 2 standard deviations above the mean for the population. SUA levels are higher in men, increase with age and are positively associated with body weight. Levels are higher in some ethnic groups (such as Maoris and Pacific islanders). Although hyperuricaemia is a strong risk factor for gout, only a minority of hyperuricaemic individuals actually develop gout.

Pathophysiology

About one-third of the body uric acid pool is derived from dietary sources and two-thirds from endogenous purine metabolism (Fig. 26.24). The concentration of uric acid in body fluids depends on the balance between endogenous synthesis and elimination by the kidneys (two-thirds) and gut (one-third). Purine nucleotide synthesis and degradation are regulated by a network of enzyme pathways, but xanthine oxidase plays a pivotal role in catalysing the conversion of hypoxanthine to xanthine and xanthine to uric acid.

The causes of hyperuricaemia are shown in Box 26.42. In over 90% of patients, the main abnormality is reduced uric acid excretion by the kidney, which is genetically determined. Impaired renal excretion of urate also accounts for the occurrence of hyperuricaemia in chronic renal failure and for hyperuricaemia associated with thiazide diuretic therapy.

Other risk factors for gout include metabolic syndrome, high alcohol intake (predominantly beer, which contains guanosine), generalised OA and a diet relatively high in game, offal, seafood, red meat and fructose, or low in vitamin C. Lead poisoning may cause gout (saturnine gout). The association between OA and gout is thought to be due to a reduction in levels of proteoglycan and other inhibitors of crystal formation in osteoarthritic cartilage, predisposing to crystal formation.

Some patients develop gout because they over-produce uric acid. The mechanisms are poorly understood, except in the case of a few single gene disorders where there are mutations in genes that regulate purine metabolism (see Box 26.42). Lesch–Nyhan syndrome is an X-linked recessive form of gout that is also associated with mental retardation, self-mutilation and choreoathetosis. An inherited cause should be suspected if other clinical features are present or there is an early age at onset with a positive family history. Severe hyperuricaemia can also occur in patients with haematological and other cancers who are undergoing chemotherapy due to increased purine turnover (tumour lysis

26

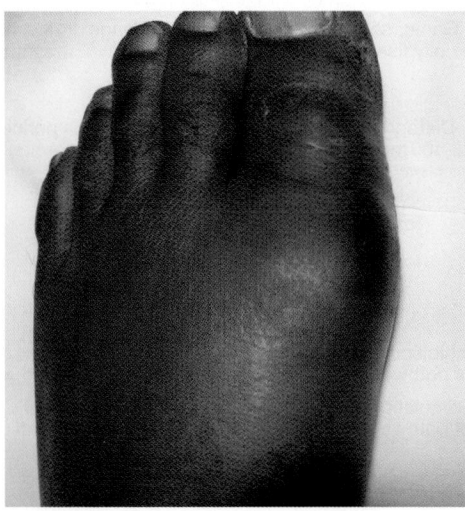

Fig. 26.25 Podagra. Acute gout causing swelling, erythema, and extreme pain and tenderness of the first metatarsophalangeal joint. *From Goldman L, Shafer AI. Goldman-Cecil medicine, 26th edn. Philadelphia: Elsevier; 2020.*

syndrome). This acute rise in urate seldom, if ever, causes gout but can cause acute kidney injury.

Clinical features

The classical presentation is with an acute monoarthritis, which affects the first MTP joint in over 50% of cases (Fig. 26.25). Other common sites are the ankle, midfoot, knee, small joints of hands, wrist and elbow. The axial skeleton and large proximal joints are rarely involved. Typical features include:

- rapid onset, reaching maximum severity in 2–6 hours, worse in the early morning
- severe pain, often described as the 'worst pain ever'
- extreme tenderness, so the patient is unable to wear a sock or to let bedding rest on the joint
- marked swelling with overlying red, shiny skin
- self-limiting over 5–14 days, with complete resolution.

During the attack, the joint shows signs of marked synovitis, swelling and erythema. There may be accompanying fever, malaise and even delirium, especially if a large joint such as the knee is involved. As the attack subsides, pruritus and desquamation of overlying skin are common. The main differential diagnosis is septic arthritis, cellulitis and reactive arthritis. Acute attacks may also manifest as bursitis, or tenosynovitis. Sometimes an acute attack will be followed by further attacks in other joints a few days later (cluster attacks), the first possibly acting as a trigger. Simultaneous polyarticular attacks are unusual.

Some people never have a second episode and in others several years may elapse before a second attack occurs. Patients with repeated attacks may progress to chronic gout, with chronic pain, joint damage, deformity and functional impairment. Patients with uncontrolled hyperuricaemia who suffer multiple attacks of acute gout may also progress to chronic gout.

The presentation of gout in old age may be atypical, with chronic symptoms rather than acute attacks (Box 26.43).

Crystals may be deposited in the joints and soft tissues to produce irregular firm nodules called tophi. These have a predilection for the extensor surfaces of fingers, hands, forearm, elbows, Achilles tendons and sometimes the helix of the ear. Tophi have a white colour (Fig. 26.26), differentiating them from rheumatoid nodules. Tophi can ulcerate, discharging white gritty material, become infected or induce a local inflammatory response, with erythema and pus in the absence of secondary infection. They are

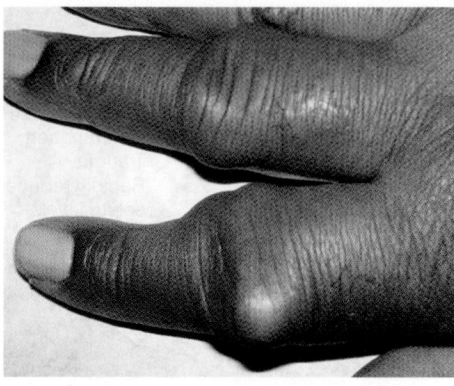

Fig. 26.26 Tophi over the proximal interphalangeal joints of the hands. *From Goldman L, Shafer AI. Goldman-Cecil medicine, 25th edn. Elsevier; 2016.*

usually a feature of long-standing gout, but can sometimes develop within 12 months in patients with chronic renal failure. Occasionally, tophi may develop in the absence of previous acute attacks, especially in patients on thiazide therapy who have coexisting OA.

In addition to causing musculoskeletal disease, chronic hyperuricaemia may be complicated by renal stone formation and, if severe, renal impairment due to the development of interstitial nephritis as a result of urate deposition in the kidney. This is particularly common in patients with chronic tophaceous gout who are on diuretic therapy.

Investigations

The diagnosis of gout can be confirmed by the identification of urate crystals in the aspirate from a joint, bursa or tophus (see Fig. 26.6A). In acute gout, the synovial fluid may be turbid due to an elevated neutrophil count. In chronic gout, the appearance is more variable, but occasionally the fluid appears white due to the presence of urate crystals. Between attacks, aspiration of an asymptomatic first MTP joint or knee may still reveal crystals.

A biochemical screen, including renal function, uric acid, glucose and lipid profile, should be performed because of the association with metabolic syndrome. Hyperuricaemia is usually present in gout, but levels may be normal during an attack because serum urate falls during inflammation. Acute gout is characterised by an elevated ESR and CRP and with a neutrophilia, all of which return to normal as the attack subsides. Tophaceous gout may be accompanied by a modest but chronic elevation in ESR and CRP.

X-rays are usually normal in acute gout, but well-demarcated erosions may be seen in patients with chronic or tophaceous gout (Fig. 26.27). Tophi may also be visible on X-rays as soft tissue swellings. In late disease, destructive changes may occur that are similar to those in other forms of advanced inflammatory arthritis.

Management

Management should focus on first dealing with the acute attack and then giving prophylaxis to lower SUA and prevent further attacks.

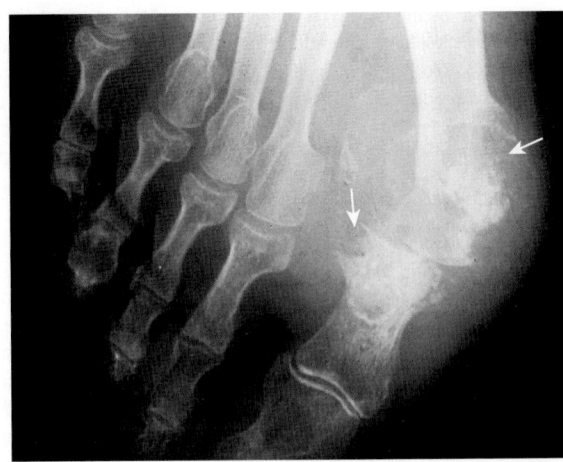

Fig. 26.27 Erosive arthritis in chronic gout. Punched-out ('Lulworth Cove') erosions (arrows) in association with a destructive arthritis affecting the first metatarsophalangeal joint.

> **i** | **26.44 Indications for urate-lowering drugs**
>
> - Recurrent attacks of acute gout
> - Evidence of bone or joint damage
> - Tophi
> - Renal impairment
> - Nephrolithiasis
> - Chemotherapy-related hyperuricemia

Acute gout

Oral colchicine given in doses of 0.5 mg 2–4 times daily is the treatment of first choice in acute gout. It works by inhibiting the inflammasome (see Fig. 4.2), which reduces IL-1β production by macrophages. The most common adverse effects are nausea, vomiting and diarrhoea. Oral NSAIDs are also effective, but are used less commonly since many patients affected by acute gout have coexisting cardiovascular, cerebrovascular or chronic kidney disease. Oral prednisolone (15–20 mg daily for 2–3 days) or intramuscular methylprednisolone (80–120 mg daily) are highly effective and are a good choice in older patients where there is an increased risk of toxicity with colchicine and NSAID (see Box 26.43). IL-1 inhibition with anakinra or canakinumab (see Box 26.35) is effective but both treatments are expensive and so are seldom given. Local ice packs can also be used for symptomatic relief. Patients with recurrent episodes can keep a supply of an NSAID, colchicine or prednisolone and take it as soon as the first symptoms occur, continuing until the attack resolves. Joint aspiration can give pain relief, particularly if a large joint is affected, and may be combined with an intra-articular glucocorticoid injection if the diagnosis is clear and infection can be excluded.

Prophylaxis

Patients who have had a single attack of gout do not necessarily need to be given urate-lowering therapy, but it should be offered to individuals who have more than one acute attack within 12 months and those with complications such as tophi or erosions (Box 26.44). The long-term therapeutic aim is to prevent attacks occurring by bringing SUA below the level at which monosodium urate monohydrate crystals form. A therapeutic target of <300 μmol/L (5 mg/dL) is recommended in the British Society of Rheumatology guidelines, whereas the European League Against Rheumatism guidelines recommend a threshold of <360 μmol/L (6 mg/dL) or <300 μmol/L (5 mg/dL) in those with severe gout.

Allopurinol is the drug of first choice. It inhibits xanthine oxidase, which reduces the conversion of hypoxanthine and xanthine to uric acid. The recommended starting dose is 100 mg daily, or 50 mg in older patients and in renal impairment. The dose of allopurinol should be increased by 100 mg every 4 weeks (50 mg in older patients and those with renal impairment) until the target uric acid level is achieved, side-effects occur or the maximum recommended dose is reached (900 mg/day). Acute flares of gout often follow initiation of urate-lowering therapy. The patient should be warned about this and told to continue therapy, even if an attack occurs. The risk of flares can be reduced by prophylaxis with oral colchicine (0.5–1 mg daily) or an NSAID for the first few months. Alternatively, patients can be given a supply of colchicine, an NSAID or prednisolone to be taken at the first sign of an acute attack. In the longer term, annual monitoring of uric acid levels is recommended. In most patients, urate-lowering therapy needs to be continued indefinitely.

Febuxostat also inhibits xanthine oxidase. It is typically used in patients with an inadequate response to allopurinol and when allopurinol is contraindicated or causes adverse effects. Febuxostat undergoes hepatic metabolism and no dose adjustment is required for renal impairment. It is more effective than allopurinol, but commonly provokes acute attacks when therapy is initiated. The usual starting dose is 40–80 mg daily, increasing to 120 mg daily in patients with an inadequate response. Prophylaxis against acute attacks should be given on initiating therapy, as described for allopurinol.

Uricosuric drugs, such as probenecid, sulfinpyrazone and benzbromarone, lower urate levels but are seldom used in routine clinical practice. They are contraindicated in urate over-producers and those with renal impairment or urolithiasis and require patients to maintain a high fluid intake to avoid uric acid crystallisation in the renal tubules.

Pegloticase is a biologic treatment comprised of the enzyme uricase conjugated to monomethoxypolyethylene glycol. It breaks down uric acid and is indicated for the treatment of tophaceous gout resistant to standard therapy and is administered as an intravenous infusion every 2 weeks for up to 6 months. It is highly effective at controlling hyperuricaemia and can cause regression of tophi. The main adverse effects are infusion reactions (which can be treated with antihistamines or glucocorticoids) and flares of gout during the first 3 months of therapy. A limiting factor for longer-term treatment is the development of antibodies to pegloticase, which occur in a high proportion of cases and are associated with an impaired therapeutic response.

Lifestyle measures are as important as drug therapy in treatment of gout. Patients should be advised to lose weight if appropriate and reduce excessive alcohol intake, especially beer. Several antihypertensive drugs, including thiazides, β-adrenoceptor antagonists (β-blockers) and angiotensin converting enzyme (ACE) inhibitors, increase uric acid levels, whereas losartan has a uricosuric effect and should be substituted for other drugs if possible. Patients should avoid large amounts of seafood and offal, which have a high purine content, but a highly restrictive diet is not necessary.

Calcium pyrophosphate deposition (CPPD) disease

Calcium pyrophosphate deposition (CPPD) disease encompasses a range of clinical presentations. Crystals can deposit in articular cartilage, synovium, entheses, tendons and ligaments – both axial and peripheral skeletal sites. The acute form of CPPD disease is acute calcium pyrophosphate (CPP) crystal arthritis ('pseudogout'). Acute CPP crystal arthritis is rare under the age of 55 years, but occurs in 10%–15% of people between 65 and 75 years and 30%–60% of those over 85 years old. It typically involves the knee, wrist, ankle, shoulder and hip. Acute CPP inflammation can also affect axial skeletal structures. Risk factors for CPPD disease are shown in Box 26.45. Frequently, patients with CPPD disease have multiple joint chondrocalcinosis and a proportion present with *chronic* CPP crystal arthritis without a history of previous *acute* CPP crystal arthritis. The picture is typically an inflammatory polyarthritis superimposed on a background of OA – typically of the wrist, shoulder or knee (Fig. 26.28). Chronic CPP crystal arthritis can be mistaken for RA by the unwary, as MCP joints can be affected (usually just 2nd and 3rd, sparing the 4th and 5th) and low titre RF is a common incidental finding in old age. The prevalence of CPPD disease affecting the axial skeletal is unknown.

26

26.45 The main risk factors for calcium pyrophosphate deposition disease

Common

- Older age
- Osteoarthritis*
- Hyperparathyroidism (both primary and secondary)
- Hypovitaminosis-D (by causing secondary hyperparathyroidism)

Rare

- Familial factors*
- Haemochromatosis*
- Hypophosphatasia
- Hypomagnesaemia
- Hypoparathyroidism
- Wilson's disease

*May be associated with structural damage to affected joints.

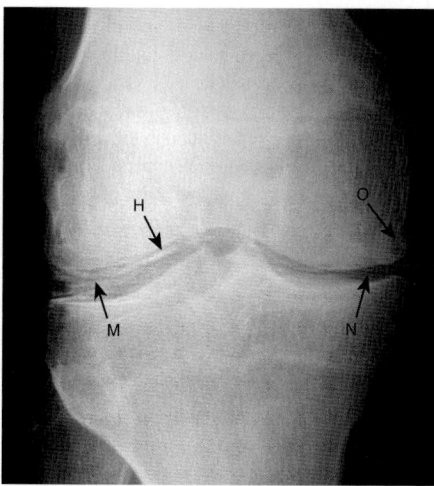

Fig. 26.28 Chondrocalcinosis of the knee. The X-ray shows calcification of the fibrocartilaginous menisci (M) and articular hyaline cartilage (H). There is also narrowing (N) of the medial tibio-femoral compartment and osteophyte (O) formation.

Pathophysiology

The underlying mechanisms of crystal deposition are poorly understood. Clinical studies have shown that CPP levels are raised in patients with CPPD disease, possibly due to over-production, but why this happens is unclear. In hypophosphatasia (see Box 26.75), the predisposing factor is thought to be impaired degradation of CPP due to deficiency of ALP. In OA, it is thought that a reduction in the amounts of proteoglycan and other natural inhibitors of crystal formation in the abnormal cartilage also predispose to crystal deposition (see Fig. 26.23).

Clinical features

The typical acute CPP crystal arthritis presentation is with a swollen tender joint that is warm and erythematous with a large effusion. Fever is common and the patient may appear confused and ill. The knee is most commonly affected, followed by the wrist, shoulder, ankle and elbow. Trigger factors include trauma, intercurrent illness, dehydration and surgery. Septic arthritis and gout are the main differential diagnoses.

Chronic CPP crystal arthritis can mimic RA, though joint involvement patterns are generally different (in chronic CPP crystal arthritis: wrists, MCP joints 2 and 3, ankles, shoulders). Affected joints usually show features of OA, with varying degrees of synovitis. Effusion and synovial thickening are usually most apparent at knees and wrists. Wrist involvement may result in carpal tunnel syndrome. Inflammatory changes can occur

at entheses such as the gluteal tendon insertions at the greater trochanters and may involve tendons and the ligamentum flavum. Inflammation around the odontoid may occur secondary to CPP crystal deposition, leading to crowned dens syndrome; this presents clinically with neck and occipital neck pain (with neck rotation being the most severely affected movement). Severe damage and instability of knees, hips or shoulders can mimic a neuropathic joint.

Investigations

The pivotal investigation in diagnosing acute CPP crystal arthritis is joint aspiration, followed by examination of synovial fluid using compensated polarised microscopy to demonstrate CPP crystals (see Fig. 26.6B). The aspirated fluid is often turbid and may be uniformly blood-stained, reflecting the severity of inflammation. Since sepsis and acute CPP crystal arthritis can coexist, Gram stain and culture of the fluid should be performed to exclude sepsis, even if CPP crystals are identified in synovial fluid.

For diagnosing chronic CPP crystal arthritis and CPP axial skeletal disease, X-rays of the affected joints, carefully reviewed, may show evidence of calcification in hyaline cartilage and/or fibrocartilage or at periarticular entheses. Reviewing CT images if available (and windowed for bone), are often helpful in revealing CPP deposition in pelvic and spine structures. Screening for secondary causes (see Box 26.45) and metabolic risk factors should be undertaken in all cases of CPPD disease and abnormalities treated.

Management

In acute CPP crystal arthritis, ice packs, joint elevation and joint aspiration provides symptomatic relief. Once infection is excluded, intra-articular glucocorticoid can be injected. NSAIDs and colchicine (0.5–2 mg daily) are helpful, but must be used with caution in older patients. Chronic CPP crystal arthritis can respond to low-dose oral glucocorticoids, methotrexate and hydroxychloroquine. Colchicine long-term (0.5–1 mg daily) may play a role in preventing acute CPP inflammatory flare-ups. Little is known about the optimum drug management of chronic CPPD disease in the axial skeletal.

Basic calcium phosphate deposition disease

Basic calcium phosphate (BCP) deposition disease is caused by the deposition of hydroxyapatite or apatite crystals and other basic calcium phosphate salts (octacalcium phosphate, tricalcium phosphate) in soft tissues. The main affected sites are tendons, ligaments and hyaline cartilage in patients with degenerative disease, and skeletal muscle and subcutaneous tissues in connective tissue diseases.

Pathophysiology

Under normal circumstances, inhibitors of mineralisation, such as pyrophosphate and proteoglycans, prevent calcification of soft tissues. When these protective mechanisms break down, abnormal calcification occurs. There are many causes (Box 26.46). In most situations, calcification is of no consequence, but when the crystals are released an inflammatory reaction may be initiated, causing local pain and inflammation.

Calcific periarthritis

This occurs as the result of deposition of BCP in tendons, which provokes an acute inflammatory response. Commonly the supraspinatus tendon is affected (Fig. 26.29), but other sites may also be involved, including the tendons around the hip, feet and hands. The presentation is with acute pain, swelling and local tenderness that develops rapidly over 4–6 hours. The overlying skin may be hot and red, raising the possibility of infection. Attacks sometimes occur spontaneously, but can also be triggered by trauma. Modest systemic upset and fever are common. Tendon calcification may be seen on X-ray. If the affected joint or bursa is aspirated, inflammatory fluid containing many calcium-staining (alizarin red S) aggregates may be obtained. During an acute attack, there may be a neutrophilia with an elevation in ESR and CRP. Routine biochemistry is normal. Treatment is with analgesics and NSAIDs. Attacks may also respond to a local injection of glucocorticoid. The condition usually resolves spontaneously over 1–3 weeks and this is often accompanied by dispersal and disappearance of calcific deposits on X-ray. Large deposits sometimes accumulate, causing limitation of joint movement, and may require surgical removal.

Acute inflammatory arthritis

Deposition of BCP occurs commonly in OA, both alone and in combination with CPP crystals, in which case it is referred to as mixed crystal deposition disease. An acute crystal-induced arthritis can occur, identical to pure acute CPP crystal arthritis.

Milwaukee shoulder syndrome

This is a rare syndrome, in which extensive deposition of BCP crystals in large joints is associated with progressive joint destruction. It is more common in women than in men. The onset is gradual, with joint pain, sometimes precipitated by injury or overuse. The disease progresses over a few months to cause severe pain and disability, associated with joint destruction. X-rays show joint space narrowing, osteophytes and calcification. Aspiration yields large volumes of relatively non-inflammatory fluid containing abundant BCP aggregates and often cartilage fragments. The differential diagnosis is end-stage osteonecrosis, chronic sepsis or neuropathic joint. There is no acute phase response and synovial fluid cultures are negative.

Treatment is with analgesics, intra-articular injection of glucocorticoids, local physical treatments and physiotherapy. The clinical outcome is poor, however, and most patients require joint replacement. The cause is incompletely understood, but it has been speculated that deposition of BCP crystals activates collagenase and other proteases in articular cells, which are responsible for the tissue damage.

Autoimmune connective tissue disease

Deposition of BCP may occur in the subcutaneous tissues and muscle of patients with systemic sclerosis and other autoimmune connective tissue diseases. Usually, the deposits are asymptomatic, but they may be associated with pain and local ulceration. The mechanism by which this occurs is unclear and there is no specific treatment.

Fibromyalgia

Fibromyalgia (FM) is a condition of generalised pain and consequent disability. It is frequently associated with medically unexplained symptoms in other systems. The prevalence in the UK and United States is about 2%–3%. Although FM can occur at any age, including adolescence, it increases in prevalence with age, to reach a peak of 7% in women aged over 70. There is a strong female predominance of around 10:1. Risk factors include life events that cause (unresolved) psychosocial distress relating to previous abuse, marital disharmony, alcoholism or illness in the family, poor sleep health, previous injury or assault and low income. FM arises in a variety of races and cultures. FM may co-exist with other inflammatory rheumatic diseases, including axSpA and SLE.

Pathophysiology

The cause of FM is poorly understood, but two abnormalities that may be interrelated (Fig. 26.30), and have been consistently reported in affected patients, are disturbed, non-restorative sleep and pain sensitisation, probably caused by abnormal central pain processing.

Clinical features

The main presenting feature is widespread pain, which is often worst in the neck and back (Box 26.47). It is characteristically diffuse and unresponsive to analgesics and NSAIDs. Physiotherapy often makes FM pain worse. Fatiguability, most prominent in the morning, is another major problem and disability is often marked. Although people can usually undertake self-care (such as eating, washing and dressing), they may be unable to perform tasks such as shopping or housework. They may

𝒊	26.46 Rheumatic diseases associated with basic calcium phosphate deposition	
Disease		**Site of calcification**
Calcific periarthritis		Tendons and ligaments
Dermatomyositis and polymyositis		Subcutaneous tissue
Systemic sclerosis (lcSScl)		Subcutaneous tissue
Mixed connective tissue disease		Subcutaneous tissue
Paget's disease of bone		Blood vessels
Ankylosing spondylitis		Ligaments
Fibrodysplasia ossificans progressiva		Subcutaneous tissues and muscle
Milwaukee shoulder syndrome		Tendons and ligaments
Albright's hereditary osteodystrophy		Muscle

(lcSScl = localised cutaneous systemic sclerosis)

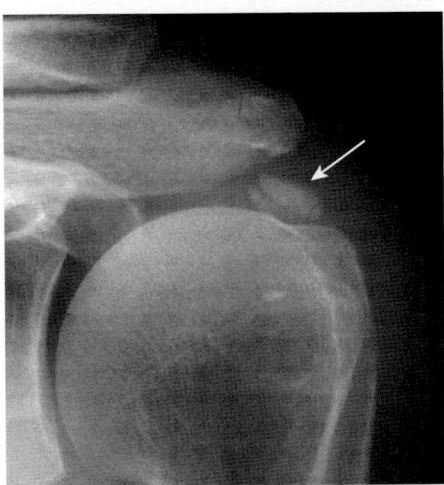

Fig. 26.29 Shoulder X-ray showing supraspinatus tendon calcification (arrow).

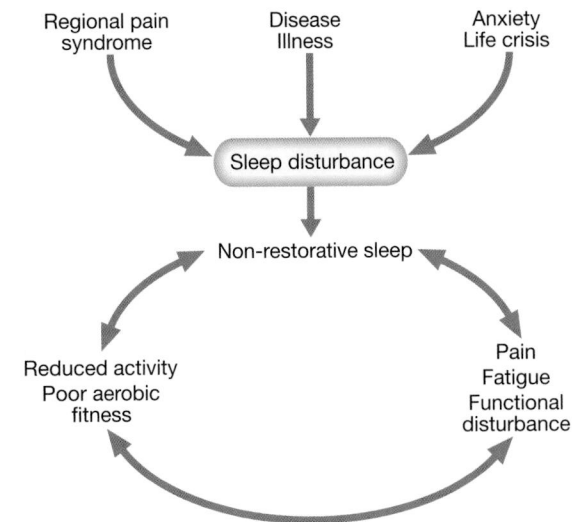

Fig. 26.30 Possible causative mechanisms in fibromyalgia.

26

experience major performance difficulties at work, and may even stop working, because of pain and fatigue.

Examination is unremarkable, apart from the presence of hyperalgesia on moderate digital pressure (enough just to whiten the nail of the examiner) over multiple sites (Fig. 26.31).

Investigations and management

There are no abnormalities on routine blood tests or imaging, but it is important to screen for other conditions that could account for all or some of the patient's symptoms (Box 26.48). Imaging is not generally recommended except to exclude other causes of pain if these are suspected clinically.

The aims of management are to educate the patient about the condition, address unresolved psychological issues, achieve pain control and improve sleep. Wherever possible, education should include the spouse, family or carer. It is conventional to acknowledge that the cause of FM is not fully understood, but the widespread pain does not reflect inflammation, tissue damage or disease. The model of a self-perpetuating cycle of poor sleep and pain (see Fig. 26.30) is a useful framework for problem-based management. Understanding the diagnosis can often help the patient come to terms with the symptoms. Repeat or drawn-out investigation may reinforce beliefs in occult serious pathology and should be avoided.

Low-dose amitriptyline (10–75 mg at night), with or without fluoxetine, may help by encouraging delta sleep and reducing spinal cord wind-up. Many people with FM, however, are intolerant of even small doses of amitriptyline. There is limited evidence for the use of tramadol, serotonin–noradrenaline (norepinephrine) re-uptake inhibitors (SNRIs) such as duloxetine, and the anticonvulsants pregabalin and gabapentin. A graded increase in aerobic exercise can improve well-being and sleep quality.

---

i | **26.47 The spectrum of symptoms in fibromyalgia**

Usual symptoms

- Widespread pain
- Fatiguability
- Disability
- Broken, non-restorative sleep
- Low affect, irritability, poor concentration

Variable locomotor symptoms

- Early-morning stiffness
- Feeling of swelling in hands
- Distal finger tingling

Additional, variable, non-locomotor symptoms

- Non-throbbing bifrontal headache (tension headache)
- Colicky abdominal pain, bloating, variable bowel habit (irritable bowel syndrome)
- Bladder fullness, nocturnal frequency (irritable bladder)
- Hyperacusis, dyspareunia, discomfort when touched (allodynia)
- Frequent side-effects with drugs (chemical sensitivity)

---

i | **26.48 Laboratory investigations recommended before finalising a diagnosis of fibromyalgia**

Test	Condition screened for
Full blood count, liver and renal function tests	General disease indicators
Erythrocyte sedimentation rate, C-reactive protein, serum amyloid A, immunoglobulins, faecal calprotectin	Inflammatory disease, Inflammatory bowel disease
Thyroid function	Hypo-/hyperthyroidism
Calcium, albumin, phosphate, alkaline phosphatase, parathyroid hormone, 25 hydroxy-vitamin D, serum angiotensin-converting enzyme	Hyperparathyroidism, osteomalacia, sarcoid
Antinuclear antibodies, extractable nuclear antigens, rheumatoid factor, anti-cyclic citrullinated peptide antibodies, complement C3 and C4, lupus anticoagulant, anti-cardiolipin antibodies	Autoinflammatory and autoimmune diseases

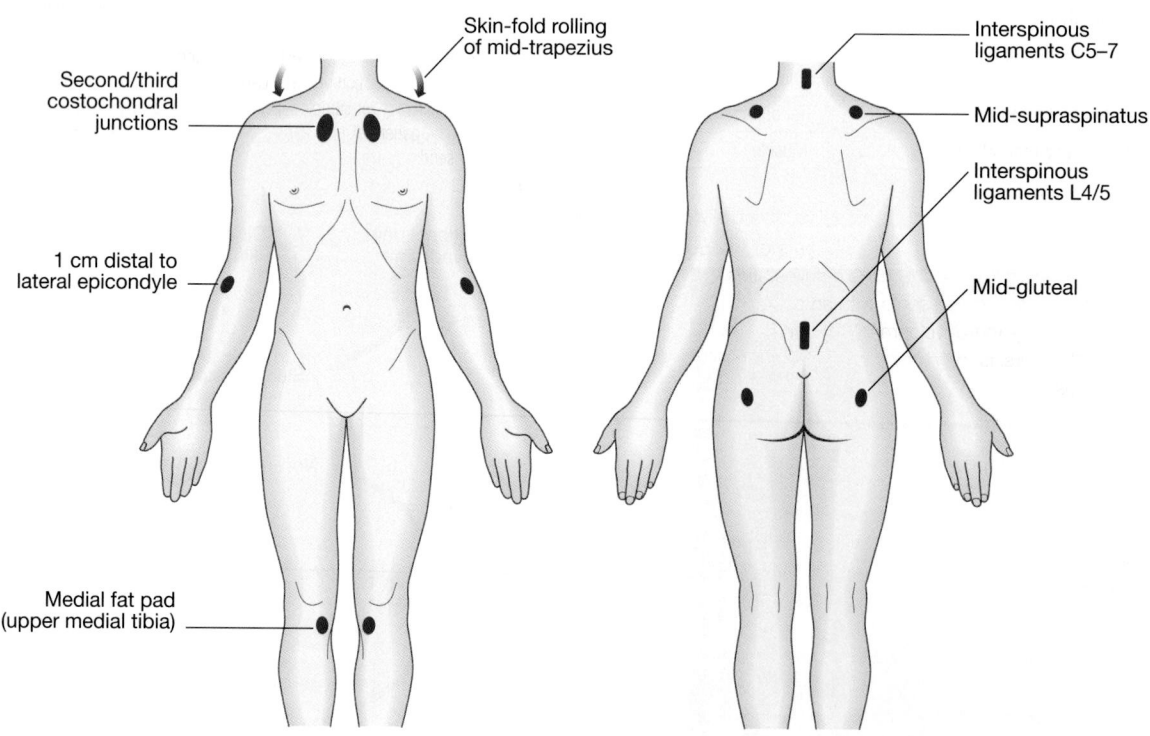

Fig. 26.31 Typical tender points in fibromyalgia.

The use of self-help strategies and a cognitive behavioural approach with relaxation techniques should be encouraged. Sublimated anxiety relating to distressing life events should be specifically explored with appropriate counselling. There are patient organisations that provide additional information and support. Although treatment may improve quality of life and ability to cope, most people remain symptomatic for many years.

Bone and joint infections

Septic arthritis

Septic arthritis is the most rapid and destructive joint disease. The incidence is 2–10 per 100 000 in the general population and 30–70 per 100 000 in those with pre-existing joint disease or joint replacement. Septic arthritis is associated with significant morbidity and still has a mortality of about 10% despite advances in antimicrobial therapy. The most important risk factor for mortality is increasing age.

Pathogenesis

Septic arthritis usually occurs as a result of haematogenous spread from infections of the skin or upper respiratory tract; infection from direct puncture wounds or secondary to joint aspiration is uncommon. Risk factors include increasing age, pre-existing joint disease (principally RA), diabetes mellitus, advanced renal disease, immunosuppression (by drugs or disease) and intravenous drug misuse. In RA, the skin is a frequent portal of entry because of maceration of skin between the toes due to joint deformity and difficulties with foot hygiene caused by hand deformity. Box 26.49 describes the particular considerations in old age.

Clinical features

The usual presentation is with acute or subacute monoarthritis and fever. The joint is usually swollen, hot and red, with pain at rest and on movement. Although any joint can be affected, lower limb joints, such as the knee and hip, are most commonly targeted. Patients with pre-existing arthritis may present with multiple joint involvement.

The most common organism in adults is *Staphylococcus aureus*, particularly in patients with RA and diabetes, but infections with ß-haemolytic streptococci and Gram-negative bacilli are also frequent. Tuberculosis should always be considered where local population infection prevalence is high. Gonococcal infection can present with a migratory arthralgia, low-grade fever and tenosynovitis, which may precede the development of an oligo- or monoarthritis. Painful pustular skin lesions may also be present. Gram-negative bacilli or group B, C and G streptococci are important causes among older adults and intravenous drug users. Less commonly, septic arthritis may be caused by group A streptococci, pneumococci, meningococci and *Haemophilus influenzae*. Arthritis may be a feature of Lyme disease caused by members of the *Borrelia* species of microorganisms. It is generally a late manifestation, which usually affects large joints. Brucellosis presents with an acute febrile illness, followed in some cases by the development of localised infection, which can result in arthritis, bursitis, osteomyelitis, sacroiliitis and paravertebral or psoas abscesses.

26.49 Joint and bone infection in old age

- **Vertebral infection**: more common. Recognition may be delayed, as symptoms may be attributed to compression fractures caused by osteoporosis.
- **Peripheral vascular disease**: leads to more frequent involvement of the bones of the feet, and diabetic foot ulcers are also commonly complicated by osteomyelitis.
- **Prosthetic joint infections**: now more common because of the increased frequency of prosthetic joint insertion in older people.
- **Gram-negative bacilli**: more frequent pathogens than in younger people.
- **Cephalosporins**: contraindicated due to the high risk of *Clostridioides difficile.*
- **Septic arthritis**: mortality is high in older patients.

Investigations

The pivotal investigation is joint aspiration, but blood cultures should also be taken. The synovial fluid is usually turbid or blood-stained but may appear normal. If the joint is not readily accessible, aspiration should be performed under imaging guidance or in theatre. Prosthetic joints should only be aspirated in theatre to minimise the risk of introducing infection.

Synovial fluid should be sent for Gram stain and culture; cultures are positive in around 90% of cases, but the Gram stain is positive in only 50%. In contrast, synovial fluid culture is positive in only 30% of gonococcal infections, making it important to obtain concurrent cultures from the genital tract (positive in 70%–90% of cases).

There is a leucocytosis with raised CRP in most patients, but these features may be absent in older or immunocompromised patients, or early in the disease course. Serial measurements of CRP are useful in following the response to treatment.

Management

The principles of management are summarised in Box 26.50. The patient should be admitted to hospital for pain relief and administration of parenteral antibiotics. Flucloxacillin (2 g IV 4 times daily) is the antibiotic of first choice pending the results of cultures, since it will cover most staphylococcal and streptococcal infections. If there is reason to suspect meticillin-resistant *Staphylococcus aureus* (such as a known carrier), vancomycin should be used instead while awaiting cultures. If a Gram-negative infection is suspected, initial antibiotic treatment should cover Gram-negative bacilli as well as staphylococci and streptococci. Cephalosporins are a reasonable choice in this situation, but carry a high risk of *Clostridioides difficile* infection in those aged over 65; gentamicin is a good alternative.

26.50 Emergency management of suspected septic arthritis

Admit patient to hospital

Perform urgent investigations
- Aspirate joint (use imaging guidance as needed). Send synovial fluid for Gram stain and culture
- Send blood for culture, routine biochemistry and haematology, including erythrocyte sedimentation rate and C-reactive protein
- Consider sending other samples (sputum, urine, wound swab) for culture, depending on patient history, to determine primary source of infection
- Consider sending serum sample (and later a paired sample) for *Neisseria* and *Brucella* serology

Commence intravenous antibiotic*
- Flucloxacillin (2 g four times daily) to cover *Staph. aureus*
- If penicillin-allergic:
    Clindamycin (450–600 mg four times daily in younger patients)
    Intravenous vancomycin (1 g twice daily if age > 65 years)
- If high risk of Gram-negative infection, in the immunocompromised and in IV drug users, add a 3rd generation cephalosporin
- When treating empirically before culture results are available, always seek local microbiology advice

Relieve pain
- Oral and/or intravenous analgesics or NSAID (caution in older patients)
- Consider local ice-packs

Aspirate joint
- Perform serial needle aspiration to dryness (1–3 times daily or as required)
- Consider arthroscopic drainage if needle aspiration difficult
- Consider synovial biopsy at arthroscopy for tissue for PCR analysis for TB

Arrange physiotherapy
- Early regular passive movement, progressing to active movements once pain controlled and effusion not re-accumulating

*Antibiotic choice should take local epidemiology and patient risk factors into account and be supported by local guidelines where available.

26

26.51 Musculoskeletal manifestations of HIV	
Condition	**Comment**
Non-specific arthralgia and mechanical low back pain	Most common
Reactive arthritis Psoriatic arthritis Idiopathic inflammatory arthritis	Especially in men who have sex with men. Idiopathic arthritis is usually of lower limb joints and may be of SpA aetiology
Osteonecrosis Myositis or vasculitis Osteoporosis Sjögren-like disease	May be either related to HIV, to its treatment or intercurrent disease

Whatever antimicrobial regimen is chosen; changes may be required depending on the organism that is isolated. Microbiology advice should always be sought in complicated situations, such as when treating intravenous drug users, patients in intensive care and those who might be colonised by resistant organisms. It is traditional to continue intravenous antibiotics for 2 weeks and to follow this with oral treatment for another 4 weeks, but there is no evidence to support the optimal duration of treatment. Joint aspiration should be performed using a large-bore needle once or twice daily. If this is not possible, arthroscopic or open surgical drainage may be needed. Regular passive movement should be undertaken from the outset and active movements encouraged once the condition has stabilised. Infected prosthetic joints require management by the orthopaedic team, but prolonged antibiotic treatment on its own is often ineffective and removal of the prosthesis may be required for eradication of the infection.

Viral arthritis

The usual presentation is with acute polyarthritis following a febrile illness, which may be accompanied by a rash. Most cases of viral arthritis are self-limiting and settle down within 4–6 weeks. Human parvovirus arthropathy (mainly B19) is the most common in Europe; adults may not have the characteristic 'slapped cheek' facial rash seen in children. The diagnosis can be confirmed by a rise in specific IgM. Polyarthritis may also occur rarely with hepatitis B and C, rubella (including rubella vaccination) and HIV infection. A variety of mosquito-borne viruses may cause epidemics of acute polyarthritis, including Ross River (Australia, Pacific), Chikungunya and O'nyong-nyong (Asia, Africa) and Mayaro viruses (South America). A wide variety of articular symptoms have been associated with HIV, mainly in the later stages of infection (Box 26.51). Management is symptomatic, with NSAIDs and analgesics.

Osteomyelitis

In osteomyelitis, the primary sites of infection are bone and bone marrow. Any part of a bone may be involved, but there is preferential targeting of the juxta-epiphyseal regions of long bones adjacent to joints. The risk of osteomyelitis increases with age; the incidence is about 9 cases per 100 000 person-years in those under 18, rising to 41 cases in those aged 60–69 and 88 cases in those above the age of 80.

Pathogenesis

Haematogenous spread is the most common cause in children. In adults, contiguous spread of infection from adjacent soft tissues is more common, usually in patients with infected skin ulcers (pressure sores, neuropathic or ischaemic ulcers) or following surgery. Diabetes is a particularly important risk factor, accounting for about 30% of cases in recent series. Other risk factors include immunosuppressive therapy, HIV infection and sickle-cell disease, which particularly increases the risk of *Salmonella* infection. The organisms most frequently implicated are *Staph. aureus* and ß-haemolytic streptococci. Tuberculosis also needs

to be considered as a cause in high prevalence areas. Osteomyelitis secondary to pyogenic organisms often results in a florid inflammatory response, with a greatly increased intraosseous pressure. If untreated, the condition may cause localised areas of osteonecrosis, leading to the development of a fragment of necrotic bone that is called a sequestrum. Eventual perforation of the cortex by pus stimulates local new bone formation (involucrum) in the periosteum, often leading to the development of sinuses that discharge through the skin.

Clinical features

The presentation is usually with localised bone pain and tenderness, often accompanied by malaise, night sweats and pyrexia. The adjacent joint may be painful to move and may develop a sterile effusion or secondary septic arthritis. Where the osteomyelitis is due to contiguous spread, there will be an overlying skin ulcer or wound, which often has necrotic tissue, purulent discharge and an offensive smell. In diabetic foot osteomyelitis, there may be no pain due to co-existent peripheral neuropathy.

Investigations

Patients suspected of having osteomyelitis should have an MRI, which is more sensitive than X-ray for detecting early changes. Where possible, cultures should be obtained by open or imaging-guided biopsy of the lesion. If tuberculosis is suspected, PCR-based analysis of synovial fluid or biopsy material should be considered. Evidence of osteopenia, localised osteolysis and osteonecrosis may be seen on X-ray. Blood cultures should be taken, which may also reveal the causative organism. Routine bloods typically show evidence of an acute phase response with a neutrophilia and raised ESR and CRP.

Management

Early recognition is critical as once osteomyelitis becomes established and chronic, it may prove very hard to eradicate with antibiotics alone. Ideally, antibiotics should not be started until the microbiological cause has been established. The principles are those followed for septic arthritis. An exception is in localised osteomyelitis of the toes and fingers, which can often be treated successfully with a prolonged course of oral antibiotics. Resection of the infected bone and subsequent reconstruction may be required. Complications of chronic osteomyelitis include secondary amyloidosis and skin malignancy at the margin of a discharging sinus (Marjolin's ulcer).

Discitis

Discitis is an unusual condition in which there is infection of the intervertebral disc, often extending into the epidural space or paravertebral soft tissues. *Staph. aureus* is the most common pathogen. Risk factors include diabetes mellitus, immunodeficiency or immunosuppressive therapy, and intravenous drug use. The presentation is with back pain accompanied by fever, and an acute phase response with high ESR and CRP and a neutrophilia. If the diagnosis is suspected, an MRI should be performed and blood cultures taken. If blood cultures are negative, open or imaging-guided biopsy of the lesion should be performed to try to identify the organism responsible. Management is with supportive care and parenteral antibiotics followed by oral antibiotics, as described for osteomyelitis.

Tuberculosis

Tuberculosis (TB) of the musculoskeletal system is now rare in Europe and the United States, but remains common in sub-Saharan Africa and South Asia. It has been estimated to occur in about 1%–3% of patients with TB overall. In about 50% of cases, the spine is affected (Pott's disease). Tuberculous osteomyelitis can also occur. Osteoarticular TB is thought to occur as the result of haematogenous spread from the site of primary infection, but a reactive arthritis (Poncet's disease) can also occur in TB in the absence of direct infection. Peripheral arthritis tends

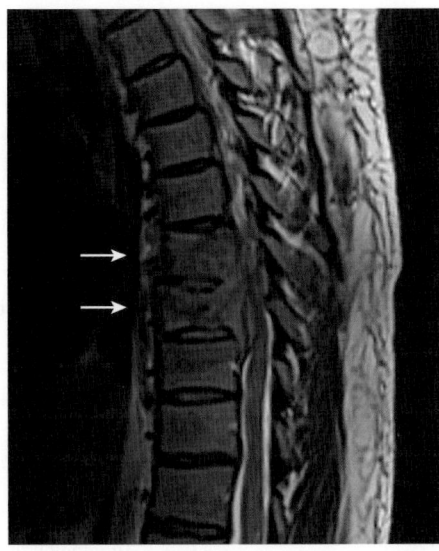

Fig. 26.32 Tuberculosis of the spine. MRI scan of a patient with tuberculosis of the spine, showing destruction of vertebrae T7 and T8 (arrows) with a soft tissue mass encroaching on the spinal cord posteriorly. A plain X-ray of the thoracic spine taken at the same time (not shown) was normal.

to affect weight-bearing joints such as the hip, knee and ankle, and presents with pain, swelling and restriction of movement on examination. The initial presentation of spinal TB is with back pain, progressing to cause deformity and spinal cord compression if untreated. Systemic symptoms such as fever and weight loss may or may not be present. Radiological changes develop slowly and are relatively non-specific, consisting of periarticular osteoporosis, bone erosions and joint space narrowing. In the spine, X-rays may show evidence of bone destruction and disc narrowing but appearances may be normal in early disease. Imaging with MRI is more sensitive than X-rays at detecting the features of osteoarticular TB and is the imaging investigation of first choice, although the appearances are non-specific (Fig. 26.32). The gold standard for diagnosis is synovial or tissue biopsy, which yields positive results in about 80% of cases in showing the characteristic histological features of TB. Culture of synovial fluid is positive in between 20% and 40% of cases, but examination of synovial fluid or synovial tissue by PCR can yield the diagnosis more rapidly, with positive results in more than 95% of culture-positive cases and 50%–60% of culture-negative cases. The key to treatment is to initiate appropriate anti-tuberculous therapy. According to WHO guidelines, quadruple therapy with isoniazid, rifampicin, pyrazinamide and ethambutol should be given as first-line therapy for 2 months and followed by 4 months of isoniazid and rifampicin. Treatment may be required for extended periods of 12–18 months in some cases depending on the extent of disease and clinical response. Alternative agents may be required in patients with resistant organisms, as discussed in Chapter 17. In some cases, surgical débridement may be required for extensive peripheral joint disease and surgical decompression and stabilisation for patients with severe spinal disease.

Rheumatoid arthritis

Rheumatoid arthritis (RA) is a common form of inflammatory arthritis, occurring throughout the world and in all ethnic groups. The prevalence of RA is approximately 0.8%–1.0% in Europe and South Asia, with a female-to-male ratio of 3:1. The prevalence is lower in South-east Asia (0.4%). The highest prevalence in the world is in Pima Indians (5%). It is a chronic disease characterised by a clinical course of exacerbations and remissions.

Pathophysiology

RA is a complex disease with both genetic and environmental components. The importance of genetic factors is demonstrated by higher concordance of RA in monozygotic (12%–15%) compared with dizygotic twins (3%) and an increased frequency of disease in first-degree relatives of patients. Genome-wide association studies have detected nearly 100 loci that are associated with the risk of developing RA. The strongest association is with variants in the HLA region and is determined by variations in three amino acids in the HLA-DRβ1 molecule (positions 11, 71 and 74) and single variants in HLA-B (at position 9) and HLA-DPβ1 (at position 9). The non-HLA loci generally lie within or close to genes involved in regulating the immune response. It is believed that RA occurs when an environmental stimulus, such as infection, triggers autoimmunity in a genetically susceptible host by modifying host proteins, through processes like citrullination, so that they become immunogenic. However, no single specific pathogen has been identified as a cause. An important environmental risk factor is cigarette smoking, which is also associated with more severe disease and reduced responsiveness to treatment. Remission may occur during pregnancy and sometimes RA first presents post partum. This is likely to be due to suppression of the immune response during pregnancy, but hormonal changes may also play a role.

The disease is characterised by infiltration of synovium with lymphocytes, plasma cells, dendritic cells and macrophages. There is evidence that CD4+ T and B cells play important roles in the pathogenesis of RA by interacting with other cells in the synovium, as illustrated in Figure 26.33. Lymphoid follicles form within the synovium in which T- and B-cell interactions occur, causing activation of T cells to produce cytokines and activation of B cells to produce autoantibodies, including RF and ACPA. Synovial macrophages are activated by TNF-α and interferon-gamma (IFN-γ), produced by T cells. The macrophages produce several pro-inflammatory cytokines, including TNF-α, IL-1 and IL-6, which act on synovial fibroblasts to produce further cytokines, setting up a positive feedback loop. The synovial fibroblasts proliferate, causing synovial hypertrophy and producing matrix metalloproteinases and the proteinase ADAMTS-5, which degrade soft tissues and cartilage. Prostaglandins and nitric oxide produced within inflamed synovium cause vasodilatation, resulting in swelling and pain. Systemic release of IL-6 triggers production of acute phase proteins by the liver. At the joint margin, the inflamed synovium (pannus) directly invades bone and cartilage to cause joint erosions. A key pathogenic factor in bone erosions and periarticular osteoporosis is osteoclast activation, stimulated by the production of M-CSF by synovial cells and RANKL by activated T cells (see Fig. 26.33). New blood-vessel formation (angiogenesis) occurs, causing the inflamed synovium to become highly vascular. Within these blood vessels, pro-inflammatory cytokines activate endothelial cells, which support recruitment of yet more leucocytes to perpetuate the inflammatory process.

Later, fibrous or bony ankylosis may occur. Muscles adjacent to inflamed joints atrophy and may be infiltrated with lymphocytes. This leads to progressive biomechanical joint dysfunction, which may further amplify joint destruction.

Rheumatoid nodules occur in patients who are RF- or ACPA-positive and primarily affect extensor tendons. They consist of a central area of fibrinoid material surrounded by a palisade of proliferating mononuclear cells. Granulomatous lesions may occur in the pleura, lung, pericardium and sclera.

Clinical features

The typical presentation is with pain, joint swelling and stiffness affecting the small joints of the hands, feet and wrists in a symmetrical fashion. Large joint involvement, systemic symptoms and extra-articular features may also occur. Clinical criteria for the diagnosis of RA are shown in Box 26.52.

Sometimes RA has an acute onset, with severe early morning stiffness, polyarthritis and pitting oedema. This occurs more commonly in old age. Another presentation is with proximal muscle stiffness mimicking polymyalgia rheumatica. Occasionally, the onset is palindromic, with relapsing and remitting episodes of pain, stiffness and swelling that last for only a few hours or days.

26

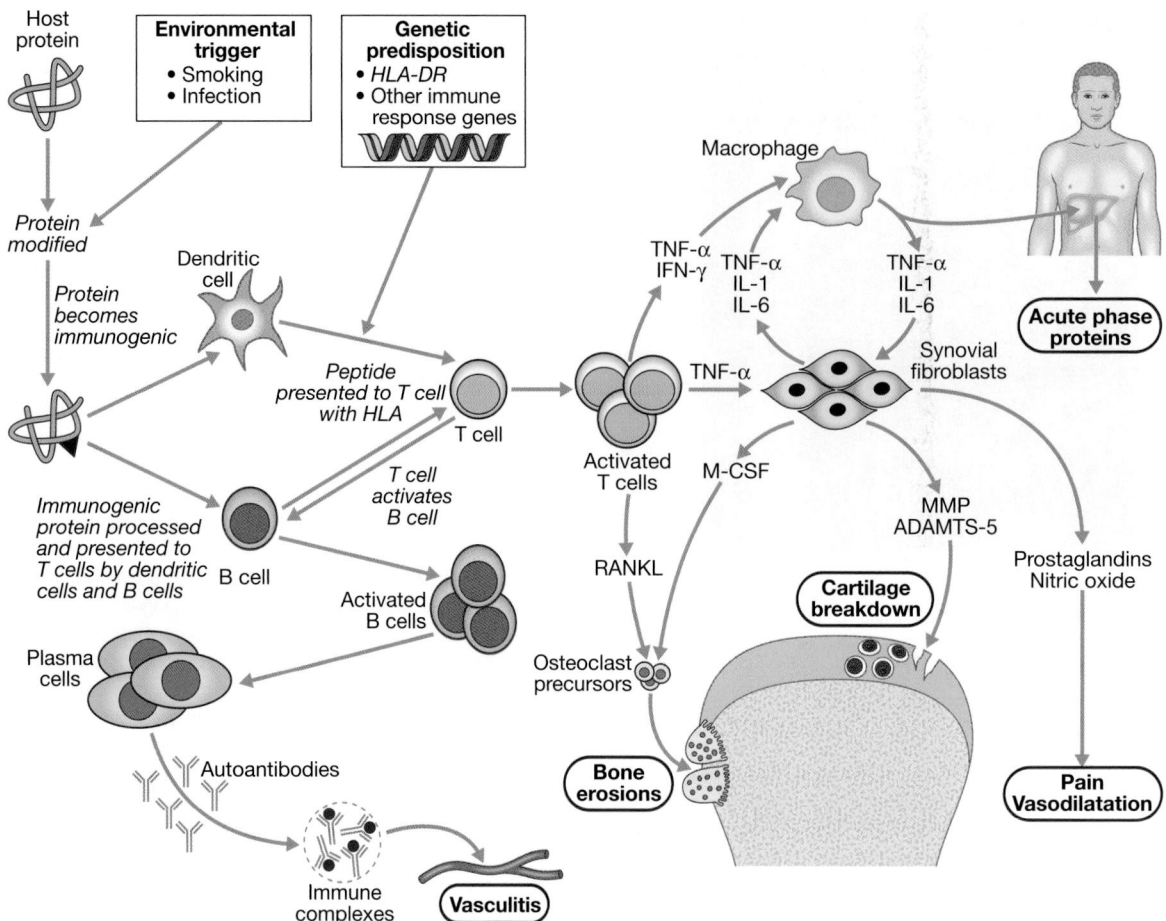

Fig. 26.33 Pathophysiology of rheumatoid arthritis. Some of the cytokines and cellular interactions that are important in rheumatoid arthritis are shown. (ADAMTS5 = aggrecanase; HLA = human leucocyte antigen; IFN = interferon; IL = interleukin; M-CSF = macrophage colony-stimulating factor; MMP = matrix metalloproteinase; RANKL = receptor activator of nuclear factor kappa B ligand; TNF = tumour necrosis factor)

i	26.52 Criteria for diagnosis of rheumatoid arthritis*	
Criterion		**Score**
Joints affected		
1 large joint		0
2–10 large joints		1
1–3 small joints		2
4–10 small joints		3
> 10 joints (at least 1 small joint)		5
Serology		
Negative RF and ACPA		0
Low positive RF or ACPA		2
High positive RF or ACPA		3
Duration of symptoms		
< 6 weeks		0
> 6 weeks		1
Acute phase reactants		
Normal CRP and ESR		0
Abnormal CRP or ESR		1
Patients with a score ≥ 6 are considered to have definite RA.		

*European League Against Rheumatism/American College of Rheumatology 2010 criteria. (ACPA = anti-citrullinated peptide antibody; CRP = C-reactive protein; ESR = erythrocyte sedimentation rate; RF = rheumatoid factor)

Examination typically reveals swelling and tenderness of the affected joints. Erythema is unusual and its presence suggests coexistent infection. Characteristic deformities may develop with long-standing uncontrolled disease, although these have become less common over recent years with more aggressive management. They include ulnar deviation of the fingers, 'swan neck' deformity, the boutonnière or 'button hole' deformity and a Z deformity of the thumb (Fig. 26.34). Dorsal subluxation of the ulna at the distal radio-ulnar joint may occur and contribute to rupture of the fourth and fifth extensor tendons. Triggering of fingers may occur because of nodules in the flexor tendon sheaths. Subluxation of the MTP joints of the feet may result in 'cock-up' toe deformities, causing pain on weight-bearing on the exposed MTP heads and the development of secondary adventitious bursae and callosities. In the hindfoot, a valgus deformity of the calcaneus may be observed as the result of damage to the posterior tibial tendon, then ankle and subtalar joints. This is often associated with loss of the longitudinal arch (flat foot) due to rupture of the tibialis posterior tendon. Popliteal (Baker's) cysts may occur in patients with knee synovitis, in which synovial fluid communicates with the cyst, but is prevented from returning to the joint by a valve-like mechanism; this is not specific to RA. Rupture may be induced by knee flexion, leading to calf pain and swelling that may mimic a deep venous thrombosis (DVT).

Systemic features

Anorexia, weight loss and fatigue may occur throughout the disease course. Osteoporosis is a common complication and muscle-wasting may occur as the result of systemic inflammation and reduced activity. Extra-articular features are most common in patients with long-standing seropositive erosive disease, but may occasionally occur at presentation,

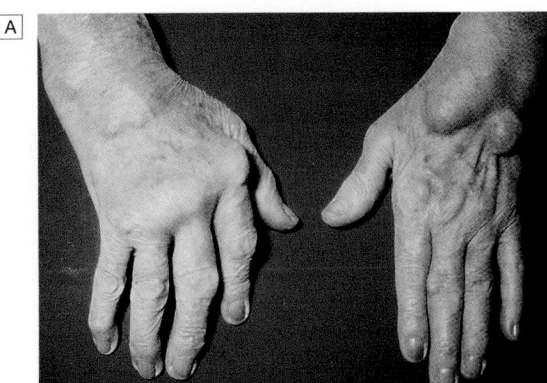

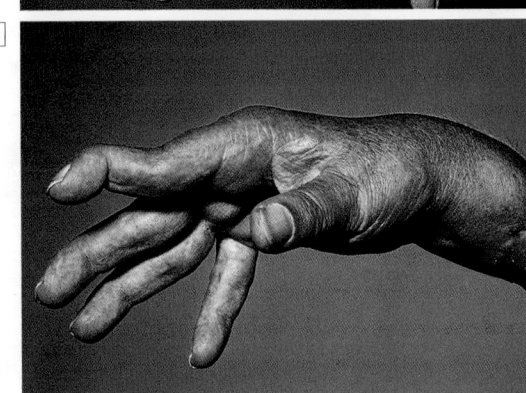

Fig. 26.34 The hand in rheumatoid arthritis. A Ulnar deviation of the fingers with wasting of the small muscles of the hands and synovial swelling at the wrists, the extensor tendon sheaths, the metacarpophalangeal and proximal interphalangeal joints. B 'Swan neck' deformity of the fingers.

especially in men. Most are due to serositis, granuloma and nodule formation or vasculitis (Box 26.53).

Nodules

Rheumatoid nodules occur almost exclusively in RF or ACPA-positive patients, usually in extensor tendons (Fig. 26.35). They are frequently asymptomatic, but some may be complicated by ulceration and secondary infection. Nodules are more common in smokers.

Vasculitis

This is uncommon, but may occur in seropositive patients. The presentation is with systemic symptoms, such as fatigue and fever and nail-fold infarcts. Rarely, cutaneous ulceration, skin necrosis and mesenteric, renal or coronary artery occlusion may occur.

Ocular involvement

The most common symptom is dry eyes (keratoconjunctivitis sicca) due to secondary Sjögren syndrome. Scleritis and peripheral ulcerative keratitis are uncommon, but are more serious and potentially sight-threatening complications that usually present with pain and redness. Clinical features and management are discussed in more detail in Chapter 30.

Serositis

Serositis is usually asymptomatic, but may present with pleural or pericardial pain and breathlessness. Pericardial effusion and constrictive pericarditis may rarely occur.

Cardiac involvement

Heart block, cardiomyopathy, coronary artery occlusion and aortic regurgitation have all been reported, but are rare. The risk of cardiovascular disease is increased due to a combination of conventional risk factors, such as high cholesterol, smoking, hypertension, reduced

---

i | 26.53 Extra-articular manifestations of rheumatoid disease

Systemic
- Fever
- Weight loss
- Fatigue
- Susceptibility to infection

Musculoskeletal
- Muscle-wasting
- Tenosynovitis
- Bursitis
- Osteoporosis

Haematological
- Anaemia
- Thrombocytosis
- Eosinophilia

Lymphatic
- Felty syndrome (Box 26.54)
- Splenomegaly

Nodules
- Sinuses
- Fistulae

Ocular
- Episcleritis
- Scleritis
- Scleromalacia
- Keratoconjunctivitis sicca

Vasculitis
- Digital arteritis
- Ulcers
- Pyoderma gangrenosum
- Mononeuritis multiplex
- Visceral arteritis

Cardiac
- Pericarditis
- Myocarditis
- Endocarditis
- Conduction defects
- Coronary vasculitis
- Granulomatous aortitis

Pulmonary
- Nodules
- Pleural effusions
- Pulmonary fibrosis
- Obliterative bronchiolitis
- Caplan syndrome
- Bronchiectasis
- Pneumothorax

Neurological
- Cervical cord compression
- Compression neuropathies
- Peripheral neuropathy
- Mononeuritis multiplex

Amyloidosis

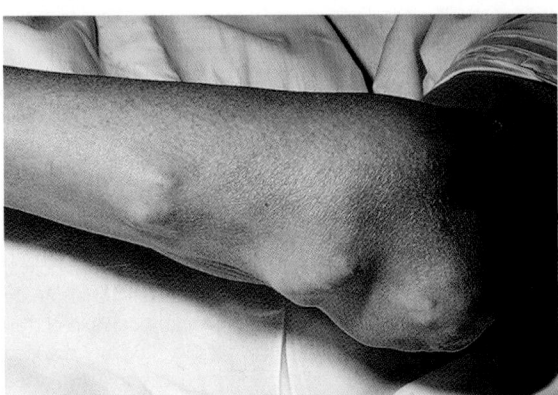

Fig. 26.35 Rheumatoid nodules and olecranon bursitis. Nodules were palpable within, as well as outside, the bursa.

physical activity, NSAIDs, glucocorticoids and the effects of inflammatory cytokines on vascular endothelium.

Pulmonary involvement

Pulmonary fibrosis may occur, but is often asymptomatic. There is some evidence that the risk of pulmonary fibrosis is increased by anti-TNF-α therapy, although it is uncertain whether this is causal or a marker of more severe disease in patients who require anti-TNF-α treatment.

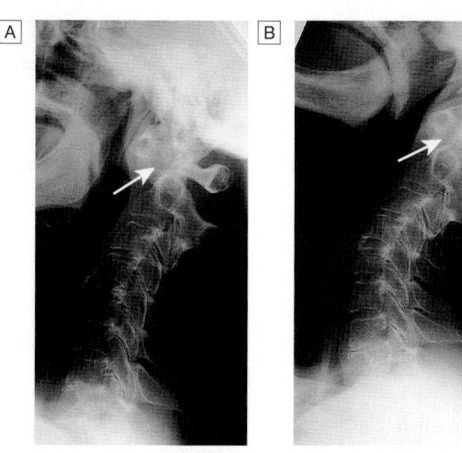

Fig. 26.36 Subluxation of cervical spine. [A] Flexion, showing widening of the space (arrow) between the odontoid peg of the axis (behind) and the anterior arch of the atlas (in front). [B] Extension, showing reduction in this space (arrow).

Peripheral neuropathy

Entrapment neuropathies may result from compression by hypertrophied synovium or by joint subluxation. Median nerve compression is the most common and bilateral carpal tunnel syndrome can occur as a presenting feature of RA. Other syndromes include ulnar nerve compression at the elbow or wrist, compression of the lateral popliteal nerve at the head of the fibula, and tarsal tunnel syndrome (entrapment of the posterior tibial nerve in the flexor retinaculum), which causes burning, tingling and numbness in the distal sole and toes. Diffuse symmetrical peripheral neuropathy and mononeuritis multiplex may occur in patients with rheumatoid vasculitis.

Spinal cord compression

This rare complication is caused by compression of the spinal cord from subluxation of the cervical spine at the atlanto-axial joint or at a subaxial level (Fig. 26.36). Atlanto-axial subluxation is due to erosion of the transverse ligament posterior to the odontoid peg. It can lead to cord compression or sudden death following minor trauma or manipulation. It should be suspected in any RA patient who describes new onset of occipital headache, particularly if symptoms of paraesthesia or electric shock are present in the arms. The onset is often insidious, with subtle loss of function that may initially be attributed to active disease. Reflexes and power can be difficult to assess in patients with extensive joint disease and therefore sensory or upper motor signs are most important. Patients with evidence of spinal cord compression require urgent neurosurgical referral for stabilisation and fixation.

Other complications

Amyloidosis is a rare complication of long-standing disease that usually presents with nephrotic syndrome. Microcytic anaemia can occur due to iron deficiency resulting from NSAID-induced gastrointestinal blood loss, whereas normochromic, normocytic anaemia with thrombocytosis occurs in patients with active disease. Felty syndrome is a rare complication of seropositive RA in which splenomegaly occurs in combination with neutropenia and thrombocytopenia (Box 26.54). Localised or generalised lymphadenopathy can occur in patients with active disease, but persistent lymphadenopathy may indicate the development of lymphoma, which is more common in patients with long-standing RA.

Investigations

The diagnosis of RA is essentially clinical, but investigations are useful in confirming the diagnosis and assessing disease activity (Box 26.55). The ESR and CRP are usually raised, but normal results do not exclude the diagnosis, especially if only a few joints are involved. Tests for ACPA are positive in about 70% of cases and are highly specific for RA, occurring in many patients before clinical onset of the disease. Similarly, RF is also positive in about 70% of cases, most of whom also test positive for ACPA. RF is less specific than ACPA, however, and positive tests can occur in other diseases (see Box 26.7).

---

i | 26.54 Felty syndrome

Risk factors

- Age of onset 50–70 years
- Female > male
- European > African ancestry
- Long-standing rheumatoid arthritis
- Deforming, but inactive disease
- Seropositive for rheumatoid factor

Common clinical features

- Splenomegaly
- Lymphadenopathy
- Weight loss
- Skin pigmentation
- Keratoconjunctivitis sicca
- Vasculitis, leg ulcers
- Recurrent infections
- Nodules

Laboratory findings

- Normochromic, normocytic anaemia
- Neutropenia
- Abnormal liver function
- Thrombocytopenia
- Impaired T- and B-cell immunity

---

i | 26.55 Investigations and monitoring of rheumatoid arthritis

To establish diagnosis

- Clinical criteria
- Erythrocyte sedimentation rate and C-reactive protein
- Ultrasound or magnetic resonance imaging
- Rheumatoid factor and anti-citrullinated peptide antibodies

To monitor disease activity and drug efficacy

- Pain (visual analogue scale)
- Early morning stiffness (minutes)
- Joint tenderness
- Joint swelling
- DAS28 (Fig. 26.37)
- Erythrocyte sedimentation rate and C-reactive protein

To monitor disease damage

- X-rays
- Functional assessment

To monitor drug safety

- Urinalysis
- Full blood count
- Chest X-ray
- Urea and creatinine
- Liver function tests

Ultrasound examination and MRI are not routinely required, but can be of value in patients with symptoms suggestive of RA where there is clinical uncertainty about the presence of synovitis. Plain X-rays of the hands, wrist and feet are usually normal in early RA, but periarticular osteoporosis and marginal joint erosions may be observed with more advanced disease. The main indication for an X-ray is in the assessment of patients with painful joints to determine whether significant structural damage has occurred. Patients who are suspected of having atlanto-axial disease should have lateral X-rays taken in flexion and extension, and an MRI. In those with suspected Baker's cyst, ultrasound may be required to establish the diagnosis.

The Disease Activity Score in 28 joints (DAS28) is widely used to assess disease activity, response to treatment and need for biologic therapy. It involves counting the number of swollen and tender joints in the upper limbs and knees, and combining this with the ESR and the patient's assessment of the activity of their arthritis on a visual analogue scale, where 0 indicates no symptoms and 100 the worst symptoms possible. Data are entered into a calculator to generate a numerical score. The higher the value, the more active the disease (Fig. 26.37).

Management

The treatment goal is to suppress inflammation, control symptoms, prevent joint damage and maintain function. This involves a combination of pharmacological and non-pharmacological therapies. When RA occurs in women of child-bearing age, additional considerations need to be taken into account and these are summarised in Box 26.56.

Pharmacological therapy

Prompt initiation of cDMARD therapy is indicated in all patients as this improves outcome. A variety of therapeutic regimens exist. A typical

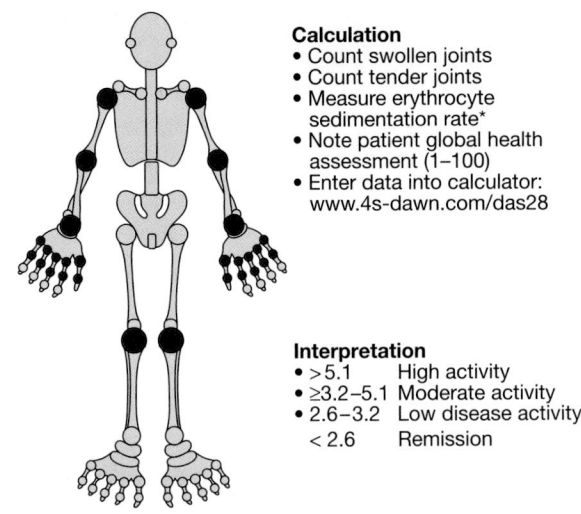

Calculation
- Count swollen joints
- Count tender joints
- Measure erythrocyte sedimentation rate*
- Note patient global health assessment (1–100)
- Enter data into calculator: www.4s-dawn.com/das28

Interpretation
- >5.1   High activity
- ≥3.2–5.1   Moderate activity
- 2.6–3.2   Low disease activity
- < 2.6   Remission

Fig. 26.37 Calculation of the Disease Activity Score 28 (DAS28).
*Erythrocyte sedimentation rate or C-reactive protein can be used for the calculation.

26.56 Rheumatoid arthritis in pregnancy

- **Immunological changes in pregnancy**: many patients with rheumatoid arthritis go into remission during pregnancy.
- **Conception**: methotrexate should be discontinued for ≥ 3 months and leflunomide discontinued for ≥ 24 months before trying to conceive.
- **Paracetamol**: the oral analgesic of choice during pregnancy.
- **Oral non-steroidal anti-inflammatory drugs and selective cyclo-oxygenase 2 (COX-2) inhibitors**: can be used from implantation to 20 weeks' gestation.
- **Glucocorticoids**: may be used to control disease flares; the main maternal risks are hypertension, glucose intolerance and infection.
- **DMARDs that may be used**: sulfasalazine, azathioprine and hydroxychloroquine if required to control inflammation.
- **DMARDs that must be avoided**: methotrexate, leflunomide, cyclophosphamide and mycophenolate.
- **Biologic** therapy experience is limited but anti-TNF-α therapy appears to be safe during pregnancy. The main risk is immunosuppression in the neonate, except for certolizumab, which does not cross the placenta in appreciable amounts.
- **Breastfeeding**: methotrexate, leflunomide and cyclophosphamide are contraindicated.

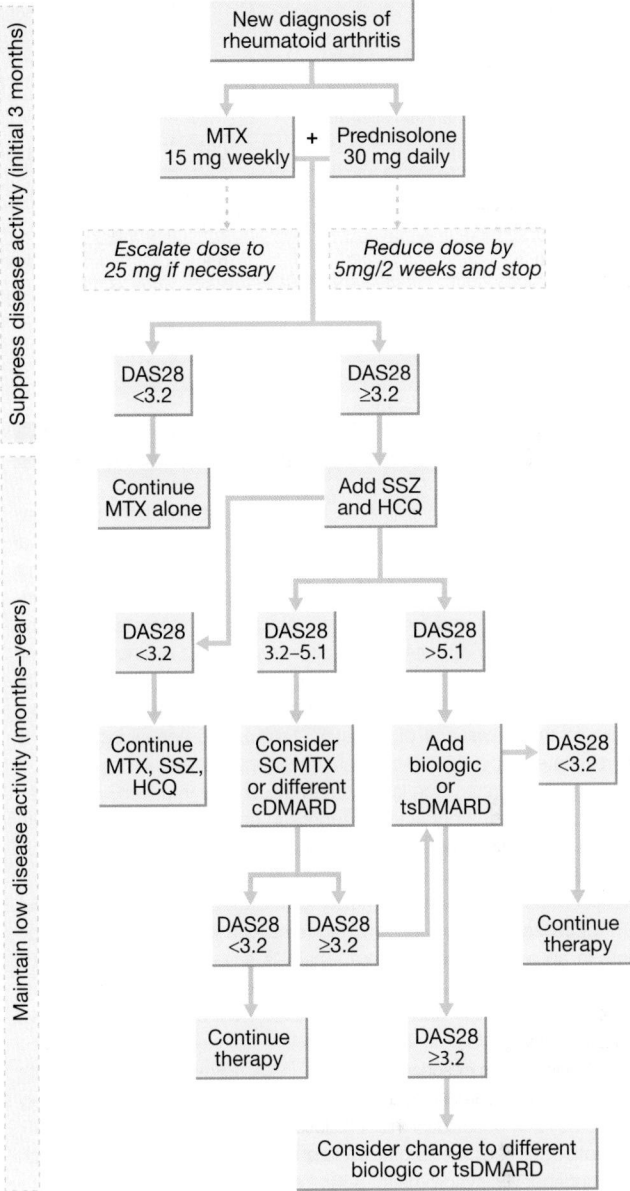

Fig. 26.38 Algorithm for the management of rheumatoid arthritis.
(DAS28 = Disease Activity Score 28; DMARD = disease-modifying antirheumatic drug; HCQ = hydroxychloroquine; MTX = methotrexate; SSZ = sulfasalazine; ts = targeted synthetic; SC = subcutaneous)

---

algorithm is shown in Figure 26.38. For example: on first diagnosis, prednisolone can be started in a dose of 30 mg daily gradually reducing in 5 mg increments every 2 weeks until therapy is withdrawn after about 12 weeks. At the same time, methotrexate (MTX) should be started in an initial dose of 15 mg weekly, along with folic acid 5 mg weekly, and escalated up to a maximum of 25 mg weekly, depending on the response. If the patient fails to respond adequately or dose-limiting toxicity occurs, then an additional cDMARD should be commenced in combination with MTX. A common combination is triple therapy, in which MTX, SSZ and HCQ are combined (see Fig. 26.38). Other cDMARD can be substituted or added, or subcutaneous MTX substituted for oral therapy, if the patient fails to respond fully. If disease activity remains high despite these measures, it is usual to progress to biologic or tsDMARD therapy. The most commonly used first-line biologic in RA is anti-TNF-α therapy, although several other options are available both in terms of tsDMARD (see Box 26.34) and other biologics (see Box 26.35). A reduction in biologic dose can be considered in patients who have been stable for 12 months or more on therapy, since it is possible to reduce the dose in up to 50% of patients without loss of therapeutic effect. Studies show that efficacy and durability of response to biologics is enhanced by co-treatment with MTX.

Disease flares can occur from time to time even in patients who are established on DMARD and biologic therapy. Transient flares can be dealt with by local joint or deep IM 'depot' steroid injections or a short course of oral prednisolone, but if a sustained flare occurs, a change in DMARD and/or biologic should be considered.

Non-pharmacological therapy

Physiotherapy, occupational therapy and psychologist support are all important for RA patients. Liaison with social services may be appropriate and enhance the holistic support of patients whose lives are changed by the chronic disease. Patient-run charitable organisations can offer a wealth of education and support to RA patients and their families.

Surgery

Synovectomy can be helpful in joints that have failed to respond adequately to systemic therapy and intra-articular injections. Joint arthroplasty may be required where secondary OA evolves, but the need for this has diminished as the result of more aggressive medical management. Other surgical procedures that can be helpful are metatarsal osteotomies, ulna head excision with wrist synovectomy (and to prevent overlying extensor tendon rupture) and upper cervical spine fixation where there is progressive atlanto-axial subluxation. Joint fusion (wrist or triple hindfoot) can reduce pain where joint changes are severe/advanced (see Box 26.28).

26

i	26.57	The main clinical features of juvenile idiopathic arthritis		
Subtype	Frequency	Clinical features		Immunology
Systemic juvenile idiopathic arthritis	5%	Fever, rash, arthralgia, hepatosplenomegaly		Autoantibody-negative
Oligoarthritis (≤ 4 joints)	60%	Large-joint arthritis, uveitis		ANA-positive
Polyarthritis (≥ 5 joints)	20%	Polyarthritis; may be extended form of oligoarthritis		ANA-positive
Enthesis-related	5%	Sacroiliitis, enthesopathy		HLA-B27-positive
RF-positive	5%	Polyarthritis, similar to RA		RF-positive, ACPA-positive
Psoriatic arthritis	5%	Same as adult disease		Autoantibody-negative

(ACPA = anti-citrullinated peptide antibody; ANA = antinuclear antibody; HLA = human leucocyte antigen; RA = rheumatoid arthritis; RF = rheumatoid factor)

Juvenile idiopathic arthritis

Juvenile idiopathic arthritis (JIA) is the term accepted by the international community for several forms of arthritis defined by the International League of Associations for Rheumatology 2001 criteria (Box 26.57). This includes juvenile forms of psoriatic arthritis (JPsA), rheumatoid arthritis (JRA) and more undifferentiated forms of inflammatory arthritis. The majority of patients with JIA have a phenotype that is distinct from adult inflammatory arthritis and includes a strong association with uveitis. JIA affects about 1:1000 children and young people up to 16 years of age – similar to the prevalence of diabetes (1:700). The annual incidence is approximately 1 per 10 000 children and young people.

Whereas joint restriction is attributed to damage in adults, in children it indicates inflammatory activity. Arthritis in children affects limb growth and has a negative effect on height and weight attainment. In young children, effective disease control can repair joint damage before puberty.

Oligoarthritis is the most common form of JIA, accounting for about 60% of cases. It is more common in females and tends to affect large joints in an asymmetrical pattern. There is an association with uveitis and many patients are ANA-positive. Polyarticular JIA is heterogeneous: some patients are RF and/or ACPA-positive, while others are negative for autoantibodies.

Systemic juvenile idiopathic arthritis (sJIA, formerly known as Still's disease) is characterised by fever, rash, arthritis, hepatosplenomegaly and serositis in association with anaemia and a raised ESR and CRP. Autoantibody tests are negative. This form of JIA is associated with haemophagocytic syndrome (p. 939).

Many cases of enthesitis-related arthritis (ERA) are likely to be self-limiting forms of SpA. ERA can progress over time into a more obviously defined SpA.

Investigations

The ESR and CRP do not correlate well with the extent or severity of inflammation and may be normal. A very high ESR may indicate the presence of inflammatory bowel disease or (very rarely) leukaemia. Low haemoglobin is likely to be due to anaemia of chronic disease rather than iron deficiency. A positive ANA occurs in 40%–75% of cases of JIA and indicates an increased risk of eye disease. Ultrasound is the radiological investigation of choice to confirm synovitis or tenosynovitis. The false-negative rate is higher in foot and ankle disease than in other joints. Arthroscopy should be avoided unless a biopsy is required. Synovial fluid aspiration is essential if there is suspicion of infection.

Management

The key approach is to gain early rapid control of inflammation, minimise the adverse effects of treatment and support the general physical and mental health of the patient, and family, which requires full multidisciplinary team input. Standard therapy is MTX (subcutaneous MTX is typically used in the young child). Alternative treatment includes LEF, SSZ and HCQ. AZA and ciclosporin can be used to treat JIA with uveitis. MMF and tacrolimus are considered to have a specific role in treating uveitis alone. Drug

	26.58	Juvenile idiopathic arthritis in adolescence

- **Uveitis**: may be clinically silent and persist into adulthood. All (not just those who are ANA-positive) need ophthalmic screening for eye involvement.
- **Persistence into adulthood**: occurs in 50% of cases, especially in systemic disease. Specific supportive management through transition from adolescence to adulthood should be planned.
- **Reduced peak bone mass**: common in polyarthritis and systemic juvenile idiopathic arthritis but there are few data on fracture risk and the evidence base for treatment is poor.
- **Therapy**: methotrexate is standard treatment, used after NSAIDs alone are insufficient. Anti-TNF therapy is effective in all forms of juvenile idiopathic arthritis, but long-term safety remains unclear.

(ANA = antinuclear antibody; NSAIDs = non-steroidal anti-inflammatory drugs; TNF-α = tumour necrosis factor alpha)

combinations are not well studied in JIA. Where DMARDs fail, biologics (see Box 26.35), including anti-TNF-α, abatacept and tocilizumab, are effective in JIA, though precise indications and licensed use alone or with MTX do vary in parts of the world and according to local protocols and guidelines. Anakinra and canakinumab can be used to treat sJIA.

Prognosis

Suboptimal outcomes are associated with delayed diagnosis and referral to the specialist multidisciplinary team, inadequate disease control, presentation with uveitis, sJIA in males and poor engagement with services. Psychological support of affected children and their families is associated with improved outcome. Oligo-JIA often resolves at puberty. Polyarticular disease and sJIA remain active into adulthood in about 50% of cases. Common issues around the transition of adolescent patients into adulthood are shown in Box 26.58.

Spondyloarthritides

The spondyloarthritides comprise a group of related inflammatory diseases that show overlap in their clinical features and have a shared immunogenetic association with HLA-B27 (Box 26.59). The spectrum of spondyloarthritis (SpA) includes:

- axial spondyloarthritis (axSpA) comprising:
  - non-radiographic SpA (nr-axSpA)
  - radiographic axSpA (ankylosing spondylitis [AS])
- reactive SpA
- psoriatic arthritis
- arthritis with inflammatory bowel disease (enteropathic SpA).

In axSpA the axial skeleton is predominantly affected. In contrast to RA, in SpAs there are frequent and notable non-synovial musculoskeletal lesions – mainly inflammatory in nature – of ligaments, tendons,

26.59 Features common to all spondyloarthritides

- Asymmetrical inflammatory oligoarthritis (lower > upper limb)
- History of inflammatory back pain
- Sacroiliitis
- Osteitis (bone marrow oedema on MRI)
- Enthesitis (Achilles' tendonitis, plantar fasciitis)
- Dactylitis
- Family history common
- HLA-B27 association
- Psoriasis (of skin and/or nails)
- Uveitis
- Sterile urethritis and/or prostatitis
- Inflammatory bowel disease
- Aortic root lesions (aortic incompetence, conduction defects)

(HLA = human leucocyte antigen; MRI = magnetic resonance imaging)

26.60 Classification criteria for axial spondyloarthritis (ASAS)

In patients with > 3 months' back pain and age at onset < 45 years, either A or B is present:

A: Sacroiliitis on imaging* plus ≥ 1 SpA feature

B: HLA-B27 plus ≥ 2 SpA features

SpA features are:
- Inflammatory back pain
- Arthritis
- Enthesitis (heel)
- Uveitis
- Dactylitis
- Psoriasis
- Crohn's/colitis
- Good response to NSAIDs
- SpA family history
- HLA-B27
- Elevated CRP

*'Sacroiliitis on imaging' here is defined as *either* active (acute) inflammation on MRI highly suggestive of sacroiliitis associated with SpA, *or* definite radiographic sacroiliitis according to the modified New York criteria.
(ASAS = Assessment of Spondylitis International Society; CRP = C-reactive protein; HLA = human leucocyte antigen; MRI = magnetic resonance imaging; NSAID = non-steroidal anti-inflammatory drug)

periosteum and other bone lesions. A hallmark lesion of SpAs is enthesitis, which is inflammation at the site of a ligament or tendon insertion into bone. Dactylitis, inflammation of a whole finger or toe, may also occur (see Fig. 26.44).

It has been estimated that about 1% of the adult population in the United States may have a SpA (about 2.7 million). There is a striking association with HLA-B27, particularly for AS (> 95%). For AS there is a male-to-female ratio of about 3:1. In Europe, more than 90% of those affected are HLA-B27-positive (HLA-B27 population prevalence in those of European origin is 9%). The overall prevalence of AS is below 0.5% in most populations. Additionally, SpAs are thought to arise as the result of an aberrant host response to infection and abnormal mucosal immunity primarily mediated through increased production of IL-23, which in turn causes activation of Th17 lymphocytes that produce IL-17, TNF-α and other inflammatory cytokines. In some situations, a triggering organism can be identified, as in reactive arthritis following bacterial dysentery or chlamydial urethritis, but in others the environmental trigger remains obscure. Familial clustering not only is common to the specific condition occurring in the proband, but also may extend to other diseases in the SpA group.

Axial spondyloarthritis

Axial spondyloarthritis (axSpA) is the diagnostic term that includes patients with non-radiographic axial SpA (nr-axSpA) and ankylosing spondylitis (AS; also termed radiographic axSpA, Box 26.60). Inflammatory changes in the axial skeleton (such as sacroiliitis, see Fig. 26.40) are characteristic of axSpA and are visualised by MRI. Radiographic alterations, such as new bone formation with syndesmophytes and ankylosis, develop later in the course of the disease and, by definition, are not present in patients with nr-axSpA. A diagnosis of AS (radiographic axSpA), which requires evidence of these radiographic changes on X-ray, may only be applied many years after a patient's symptoms started. It is important to recognise that not all patients with nr-axSpA will go on to develop AS.

Pathophysiology

Axial SpA arises from an interaction between environmental pathogens and the host immune system in genetically susceptible individuals. Increased faecal carriage of *Klebsiella aerogenes* has been reported in patients with AS and may relate to exacerbation of both joint and eye disease. There is increasing evidence that axSpA is due to an abnormal host response to the intestinal microbiota with involvement of Th17 cells, which have a key role in mucosal immunity. This leads to production of various inflammatory cytokines, including IL-23, IL-17 and TNF-α, which play vital roles in the pathogenesis of enthesitis and other inflammatory lesions (Fig. 26.39).

There a strong association between axSpA and carriage of the major histocompatibility complex (MHC) class I molecule HLA-B27. This is

particularly striking in patients defined as having AS, more than 95% of whom are positive for HLA-B27. Other susceptibility genes also implicated in susceptibility to AS include *ERAP-1* (an endoplasmic reticulum protein with a role facilitating intracellular antigen processing and binding with its presenting MHC molecule HLA-B27), the IL-23 receptor and downstream signalling molecules involved in directing Th17 cell responses, such as *STAT3* (see Fig. 4.3). The HLA-B27 molecule itself is implicated through its antigen-presenting function or because of its propensity to form homodimers that activate leucocytes. HLA-B27 molecules may also misfold, causing increased endoplasmic reticulum stress. This could lead to inflammatory cytokine release by macrophages and dendritic cells, thus triggering inflammatory disease.

Clinical features

The cardinal feature of axSpA is inflammatory back pain and early morning stiffness, with low back pain radiating to the buttocks or posterior thighs if the sacroiliac joints are involved. Symptoms are exacerbated by inactivity and relieved by movement. Musculoskeletal symptoms may be prominent at entheses, may be episodic and, if persistent, can present as widespread pain and be mistaken for fibromyalgia. Fatigue is common. A history of psoriasis (current, previous or in a first-degree relative) and inflammatory bowel symptoms (current or previous) are important clues. Physical signs include a reduced range of lumbar spine movements in all directions, pain on sacroiliac stressing and a high enthesitis index. Entheses that are typically affected include Achilles' insertion, plantar fascia origin, patellar ligament entheses, gluteus medius insertion at the greater trochanter and tendon attachments at humeral epicondyles. Acute anterior uveitis is the most common extra-articular feature, which occasionally precedes joint disease. The extent of extra-articular features are shown in Box 26.61.

A number of validated clinical questionnaires, such as the Bath Ankylosing Spondylitis Disease Activity Index (BASDAI), Bath Ankylosing Spondylitis Functional Index (BASFI) and Ankylosing Spondylitis Disease Activity Score (ASDAS-CRP), can be used to assess disease activity and functional status.

Spinal fusion can develop as AS progresses, but it does so over many years, varies in its extent and in most cases does not cause a gross flexion deformity. However, a few patients develop marked kyphosis of the dorsal and cervical spine that may interfere with forward vision. This may prove incapacitating, especially when associated with fixed flexion contractures of hips or knees. Osteoporosis is a common complication, particularly of the spine, leading to an increased risk of vertebral fracture.

Investigations

The diagnosis of axSpA is aided by ultrasound or MRI of entheses, or by MRI of the sacroiliac joints and spine (Fig. 26.40). Other findings may include raised ESR and CRP (although these can be normal), anaemia

26

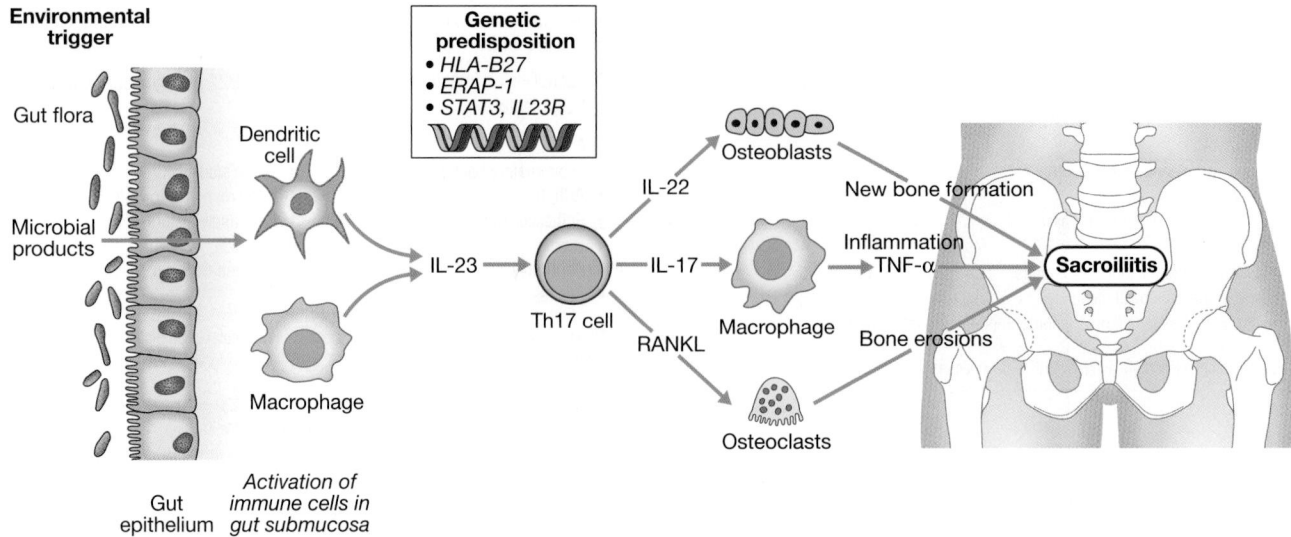

Fig. 26.39 Pathophysiology of axial spondyloarthropathy. In genetically susceptible individuals, it is thought that bacterial components penetrate the mucosal barrier to activate macrophages and dendritic cells in the intestinal submucosa. These cells produce increased amounts of interleukin (IL)-23, which activate Th17 cells resulting in production of IL-17, tumour necrosis factor (TNF)-α and other inflammatory mediators. IL-17 has a pivotal role in driving inflammation, causing sacroiliitis and enthesitis. Production of IL-22 by T cells is thought to be involved in causing the new bone formation that occurs in of axial spondyloarthropathy. (RANKL = receptor activator of nuclear factor kappa B ligand)

	26.61 Extra-articular features of axial spondyloarthritis

- Fatigue, anaemia
- Anterior uveitis (25%)
- Prostatitis (80% of men) and sterile urethritis
- Inflammatory bowel disease (in up to 50%)
- Osteoporosis
- Osteoproliferation and osteosclerosis
- Cardiovascular disease (aortic valve disease 20%)
- Amyloidosis (rare)
- Atypical upper lobe pulmonary fibrosis (very rare)

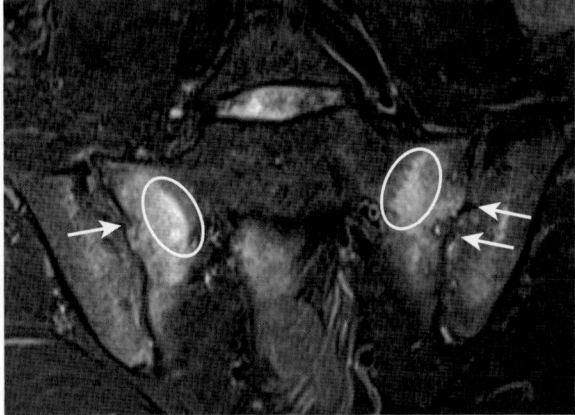

Fig. 26.40 Magnetic resonance imaging appearances in sacroiliitis. Coronal MRI short T1 inversion recovery (STIR) sequence showing bilateral sacroiliitis in axial spondyloarthritis. Bone marrow oedema (circles) is present around both sacroiliac joints, which show irregularities due to erosions (arrows).

and positive HLA-B27. Faecal calprotectin is a useful screening test for associated inflammatory bowel disease.

By definition, abnormalities are not seen in X-rays in nr-axSpA. In AS, X-rays of the sacroiliac joint show irregularity and loss of cortical margins, widening of the joint space and subsequently sclerosis, joint space narrowing and fusion. Lateral thoracolumbar spine X-rays may show anterior 'squaring' of vertebrae due to erosion and sclerosis of the anterior corners and periostitis of the waist. Bridging syndesmophytes may also be seen. These are areas of calcification that follow the outermost fibres of the annulus (Fig. 26.41). In advanced disease, ossification of the anterior longitudinal ligament and facet joint fusion may also be visible. The combination of these features may result in the typical 'bamboo' spine (Fig. 26.42). Erosive changes may be seen in the symphysis pubis, ischial tuberosities and peripheral joints. Osteoporosis is common and vertebral fractures may occur. Atlanto-axial dislocation can arise as a late feature. MRI is more sensitive for detection of early sacroiliitis than X-rays (see Fig. 26.40) and can also detect inflammatory changes in the lumbar spine. DXA scanning or vertebral quantitative CT is important as part of a fragility fracture assessment.

Management

Patient education, NSAID use (optimally, once daily or slow release taken at bedtime) and physical therapy are key interventions at the outset. For severe and/or persistent peripheral joint involvement, both SSZ and MTX are reasonable therapy choices. These medications have no impact on spinal symptoms or disease progression. In patients who fail to respond adequately or who cannot tolerate NSAIDs, progression to biologic therapy with either TNF-α, or IL-17A inhibitors should be considered. Anti-TNFα therapy is effective for both the axial and peripheral lesions of axSpA, but it is as yet unclear whether anti-TNF-α therapy modifies the natural history of the disease.

Local glucocorticoid injections can be useful for persistent plantar fasciitis, other enthesopathies and peripheral arthritis. Oral glucocorticoids may be required for acute uveitis, but do not help spinal disease. Severe hip, knee or shoulder arthritis with secondary OA may require

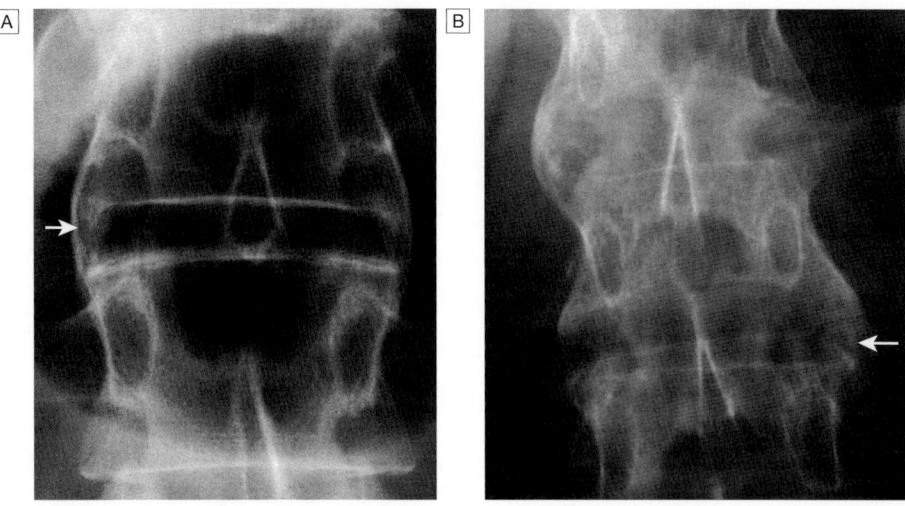

Fig. 26.41 Radiographic changes in spondyloarthritis. [A] Fine symmetrical marginal syndesmophytes typical of ankylosing spondylitis (arrow). [B] Coarse, asymmetrical non-marginal syndesmophytes typical of psoriatic spondylitis (arrow).

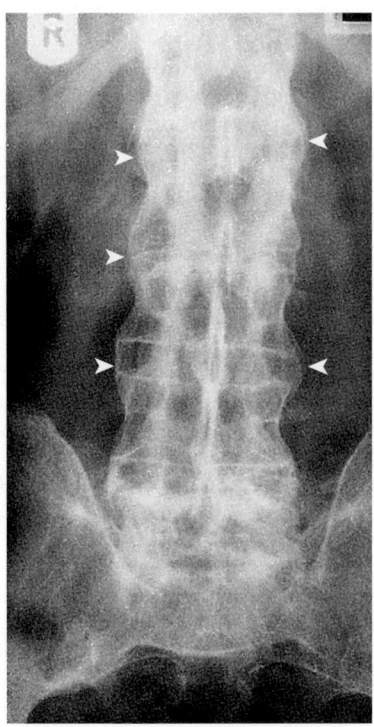

Fig. 26.42 'Bamboo' spine of advanced ankylosing spondylitis. Note the symmetrical marginal syndesmophytes (arrows), sacroiliac joint fusion and generalised osteopenia.

arthroplasty. In AS, spinal osteotomy, to correct stoop and make eyeline/posture 'more normal', can make a significant difference to patients with severe ankylosed kyphotic spines.

Prognosis

With such a recent definition of disease, the markers of prognosis in patients diagnosed with nr-axSpA are not fully understood. It is clear that axSpA can remain mild and/or episodic in many patients for many years but persistently high inflammatory markers and functional incapacity are markers of a poor outcome. Nonetheless, over 75% of patients with AS are able to remain in employment and enjoy a good quality of life. Even if severe ankylosis develops, functional limitation may not be marked, as long as the spine is fused in an erect posture.

Reactive arthritis

Reactive (spondylo)arthritis (ReA) is a 'reaction' to a number of bacterial triggers with clinical features in keeping with all SpA conditions. The known triggers are *Chlamydia*, *Campylobacter*, *Salmonella*, *Shigella* and *Yersinia*. Notably, non-SpA-related reactive arthritis can occur following infection with many viruses, *Mycoplasma*, *Borrelia*, streptococci and mycobacteria, including *M. leprae*, which causes leprosy (Hansen's disease); however, the 'reaction' in these instances consists typically of myoarthralgias, is not associated with HLA-B27 and is generally not chronic. The arthritis associated with rheumatic fever is also an example of a reactive arthritis that is not associated with HLA-B27.

Sexually acquired reactive arthritis (SARA) is predominantly a disease of young men, with a male preponderance of 15:1. This may reflect a difficulty in diagnosing the condition in young women, in whom *Chlamydia* infection is often asymptomatic and hard to detect in practical terms. Between 1% and 2% of patients with non-specific urethritis seen at genitourinary medicine clinics have SARA. The syndrome of chlamydial urethritis, conjunctivitis and reactive arthritis was formerly known as Reiter's disease.

With enteric triggering infections (enteropathic ReA), HLA-B27 may predict the reactive arthritis and its severity, though the condition occurs in HLA-B27-negative people. The incidence of specific triggering infections causing ReA around the world varies, depending on the epidemiology of the infection and prevalence of HLA-B27 in the local population.

Clinical features

The onset is typically acute, with an inflammatory enthesitis, oligoarthritis, sacroiliitis and/or spinal inflammation. Lower limb joints and entheses are predominantly affected. In all types of ReA, there may be considerable systemic disturbance, with fever and weight loss. Achilles insertional enthesitis/tendonitis or plantar fasciitis may also be present. The first attack of arthritis is usually self-limiting, but recurrent or chronic arthritis can develop and about 10% of patients will still have active disease 20 years after the initial presentation. Low back pain and stiffness due to enthesitis and osteitis are common and 15%–20% of patients develop sacroiliitis. Many extra-articular features in ReA involve the skin, especially in SARA:

- circinate balanitis, which starts as vesicles on the coronal margin of the prepuce and glans penis, later rupturing to form superficial erosions with minimal surrounding erythema, some coalescing to give a circular pattern

26

- keratoderma blennorrhagica, which begins as discrete waxy, yellow–brown vesico-papules with desquamating margins, occasionally coalescing to form large crusty plaques on the palms and soles of the feet
- pustular psoriasis
- nail dystrophy with subungual hyperkeratosis
- mouth ulcers
- conjunctivitis
- uveitis, which is rare with the first attack, but arises in 30% of patients with recurring or chronic arthritis.

Other complications in ReA are very rare but include aortic incompetence, conduction defects, pleuro-pericarditis, peripheral neuropathy, seizures and meningoencephalitis.

Investigations

The diagnosis is usually made clinically, but joint aspiration may be required to exclude crystal arthritis and articular infection. ESR and CRP are raised. High vaginal swabs may reveal *Chlamydia* on culture. Except for post-*Salmonella* arthritis, stool cultures are usually negative by the time the arthritis presents, but serology may help confirm previous dysentery. RF, ACPA and ANA are negative.

In chronic or recurrent disease, X-rays show periarticular osteoporosis; proliferative erosions, notably at entheses; periostitis, especially of metatarsals, phalanges and pelvis; and large, 'fluffy' calcaneal spurs. In contrast to AS, radiographic sacroiliitis is often asymmetrical and sometimes unilateral, and syndesmophytes are predominantly coarse and asymmetrical, often extending beyond the contours of the annulus ('non-marginal') (see Fig. 26.41B). Radiographic changes in the peripheral joints and spine are identical to those seen in psoriasis.

Management

Acute ReA should be treated with rest, NSAIDs and analgesics. Intra-articular or systemic glucocorticoids may be required in patients with severe monarticular synovitis or polyarticular disease, respectively. There is no convincing evidence for the use of antibiotics unless a triggering infection is identified. If chlamydial urethritis is diagnosed, it should be treated empirically with a short course of doxycycline or a single dose of azithromycin. Treatment with DMARDs (usually SSZ or MTX) should be considered for patients with persistent marked symptoms, recurrent arthritis or severe keratoderma blennorrhagica. Anterior uveitis is a medical emergency requiring topical, subconjunctival or systemic glucocorticoids. For DMARD-recalcitrant cases, anti-TNF-α therapy should be considered.

Psoriatic arthritis

Based on data from the UK and Denmark, the estimated population prevalence of psoriatic arthritis (PsA) from registry and coding data is approximately 0.2%. It is likely the true prevalence is considerably higher, but this has not been extensively studied. The prevalence of PsA in psoriasis patients is variable, based on clinical assessment, but may be up to 40%. Early PsA may present as axSpA. The onset is usually between 25 and 40 years of age, but juvenile forms exist. Occasionally, the arthritis and psoriasis develop synchronously, but the onset of musculoskeletal and skin disease is frequently separated by many years. Classification of PsA requires key assessments of family history and screening for enthesitis (Box 26.62).

Pathophysiology

Genetic factors have an important role in PsA and family studies have suggested that heritability may exceed 80%. Variants in the *HLA-B* and *HLA-C* genes are the strongest genetic risk factors, but more than 30 other variants also play a part. Carriage of the HLA B27 allele in those with PsA of European descent is about 20% as compared with the background rate of 9%. Many of these variants overlap with those implicated in psoriasis, where there are more than 40 susceptibility loci. These lie

26.62 The CASPAR criteria for psoriatic arthritis

Inflammatory articular disease (joint, spine or enthesis) with ≥ 3 points from the following (1 point each unless stated):
- Current psoriasis (scores 2 points)
- History of psoriasis in first- or second-degree relative
- Psoriatic nail dystrophy
- Negative IgM rheumatoid factor[1]
- Current dactylitis
- History of dactylitis
- Juxta-articular new bone[2]

[1]Established by any method except latex. [2]Ill-defined ossification near joint margins (excluding osteophytes) on X-rays of hands or feet.
(CASPAR = ClASsification for Psoriatic ARthritis)

within or close to genes in the IL-12, IL-23 and nuclear factor kappa B (NFκB) signalling pathways. It is thought that an environmental factor, probably infectious in nature, triggers the disease in genetically susceptible individuals, leading to immune activation involving dendritic cells and T cells. CD8+ T cells (which recognise antigen presented in the context of HLA class I) are more abundant than CD4+ T cells within the joint, which is in keeping with the genetic association between PsA and HLA-C and B variants. There is increasing evidence that the IL-23/IL-17 pathway plays a pivotal role in PsA. It is thought that the triggering stimulus causes over-production of IL-23 by dendritic cells, which in turn promotes differentiation and activation of Th17 cells that produce the pro-inflammatory cytokine IL-17. This, along with Th1 cytokines like IFN-γ and TNF-α, acts on macrophages and tissue-resident stromal cells at entheses, in bone and within the joint to produce additional pro-inflammatory cytokines and other mediators, which contribute to inflammation and tissue damage, as shown in Figure 26.43.

Clinical features

The presentation is with pain and stiffness affecting joints, tendons, spine and entheses. Joints are typically not swollen; however, several patterns of joint involvement are recognised (see below), including an oligoarticular form. These patterns are not mutually exclusive. Marked variation in disease patterns exists, including a disease course of intermittent exacerbation and remission. Destructive arthritis and disability are uncommon, except in the case of arthritis mutilans. Though both psoriasis and PsA are associated with obesity, it is not clear if the latter plays a role in aetiopathogenesis.

Asymmetrical inflammatory mono-/oligoarthritis

This often presents abruptly with a combination of synovitis and adjacent periarticular inflammation. It occurs most characteristically in the hands and feet, when synovitis of a finger or toe is coupled with tenosynovitis, enthesitis and inflammation of intervening tissue to give a 'sausage digit' or dactylitis (Fig. 26.44A). Large joints, such as the knee and ankle, may also be involved, sometimes with very large effusions.

Symmetrical polyarthritis

This accounts for about 25% of cases. It predominates in women and may resemble RA, with symmetrical involvement of small and large joints in both upper and lower limbs. Nodules and other extra-articular features of RA are absent and arthritis is generally less extensive and more benign.

Distal interphalangeal joint arthritis

This is quite a common pattern. It can be difficult to distinguish from inflammatory generalised OA, but in PsA psoriatic nail disease is usually present (Fig. 26.44B).

Psoriatic spondylitis

This type presents with inflammatory back or neck pain and stiffness. Any structure in the spine can be involved, including intervertebral discs, entheses and facet joints. It may occur alone or with any of the other clinical patterns and is typically unilateral or asymmetric in severity.

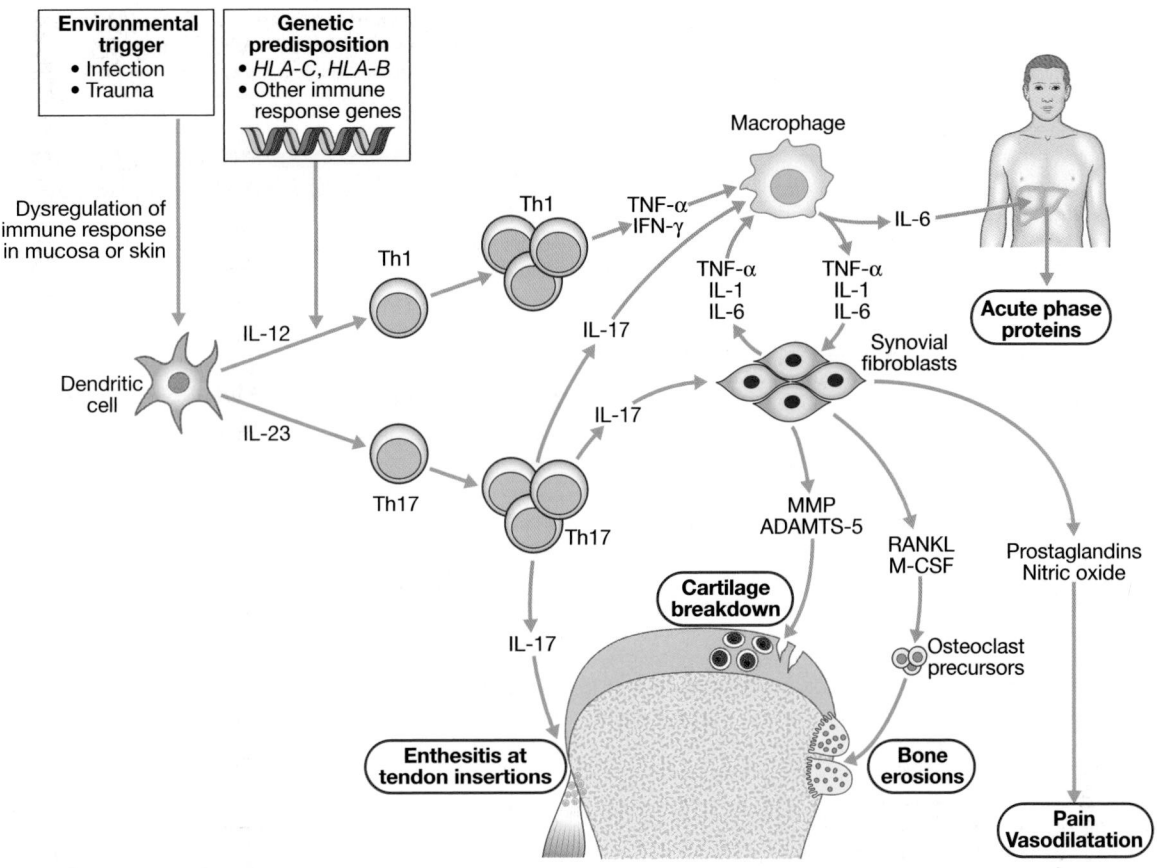

Fig. 26.43 Pathogenesis of psoriatic arthritis. As in the case of axSpA, the IL-23/IL-17 axis is thought to play a key role in PsA. Some of the cytokines and cellular interactions important in psoriatic arthritis are also shown. (ADAMTS-5 = aggrecanase; IFN = interferon; IL = interleukin; M-CSF = macrophage colony-stimulating factor; MMP = matrix metalloproteinase; TNF = tumour necrosis factor; RANKL = receptor activator of nuclear factor kappa B ligand)

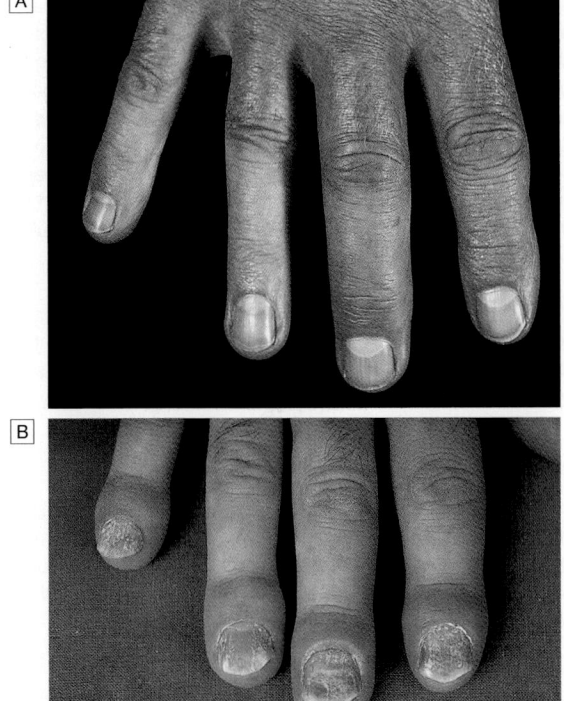

Fig. 26.44 Psoriatic arthropathy. [A] Dactylitis. [B] Distal interphalangeal joint pattern with accompanying nail dystrophy (pitting and onycholysis).

Arthritis mutilans

This is a deforming erosive arthritis targeting the fingers and toes; it occurs in 5% of cases of PsA. Prominent cartilage and bone destruction results in marked digital instability. The encasing skin appears invaginated and 'telescoped' ('main en lorgnette') and the finger can be pulled back to its original length.

Enthesitis-predominant

This form of disease presents with pain and stiffness at the insertion sites of tendons and ligaments into bone (enthesitis). Symptoms can be extensive or localised. Patients often report muscle stiffness or aches. Typically affected entheses include Achilles tendon insertions, plantar fascia origins, patellar ligament attachments, hip abductor complex insertion at lateral femoral condyle, gluteus medius insertion at greater trochanter, humeral epicondyle tendon attachments, deltoid origin at acromial edge, intercostal muscle attachments at ribs, and pelvic ligament attachments. This form of PsA can be mistaken for fibromyalgia by the unwary.

Nail changes

Nail changes include pitting, onycholysis, subungual hyperkeratosis and horizontal ridging, which are found in 85% of patients with PsA and can occur in the absence of skin disease. The characteristic rash of psoriasis may be widespread, or confined to the scalp, natal cleft, umbilicus and genitals, or in areas where there are frictional skin effects (e.g. from clothing) where it is easily overlooked. Obtaining a history of psoriasis in a first-degree relative can be tricky but is important, given that a positive response contributes to making a diagnosis. Psoriasis and PsA may be discordant in the same individual, with onset of features sometimes years apart. The absence of psoriasis, or history of it, does not preclude a diagnosis of PsA (see Box 26.62).

26

Investigations

The diagnosis is made on clinical grounds. Autoantibodies are usually negative, though low-dose RF, ACPA and ANA can be detected, and acute phase reactants, such as ESR and CRP, are raised in only a proportion of patients with active disease. X-rays may be normal or show juxta-articular osteoproliferation or erosive change with joint space narrowing. Features that favour PsA over RA include the characteristic distribution (see Fig. 26.10) of erosions with osteoproliferation, absence of periarticular osteoporosis and osteosclerosis. Imaging of the axial skeleton, in advanced disease, can show coarse, asymmetrical, non-marginal syndesmophytes, juxta-facet joint osteoproliferation and sacroiliitis. MRI and ultrasound with power Doppler are increasingly employed to detect synovial inflammation and inflammation at the entheses.

Management

Patient education to understand the breadth, episodic nature and variability of disease is important. Weight loss may play a therapeutic role to limit clinical impact. Therapy with NSAIDs and analgesics may be sufficient to manage symptoms in mild disease. Intra-articular glucocorticoid injections can control isolated synovitis or enthesitis. Splints and prolonged rest should be avoided because of the tendency to fibrous and bony ankylosis. Patients with spondylitis should be prescribed the same exercise and posture regime as in axSpA. Therapy with cDMARDs should be considered for polyenthesitis or synovitis unresponsive to conservative treatment. MTX is the drug of first choice and is also effective for skin disease. Other cDMARDs may also be helpful, including SSZ, ciclosporin and LEF. Particular attention should be paid to monitoring liver function in patients treated with cDMARDs, since abnormalities are common in PsA. HCQ is not generally used in PsA, but can be tried if other options are unsuitable. Anti-TNF-α should be considered for individuals with active synovitis who respond inadequately to cDMARDs, and treatment is effective for both PsA and psoriasis. Ustekinumab, a monoclonal antibody that binds to and neutralises the p40 subunit of IL-12 and IL-23, improves joint, dactylitis and enthesitis lesions in PsA, as does guselkumab which is a specific inhibitor of IL-23. Secukinumab and ixekizumab, monoclonal antibodies that target IL-17, have similar or even greater efficacy than TNF-α inhibitors in PsA. Apremilast is effective in PsA when cDMARD therapy fails, but is less efficacious than biologic treatments.

Enteropathic (spondylo)arthritis

The overall prevalence of inflammatory musculoskeletal disease in inflammatory bowel diseases (IBDs: Crohn's disease and ulcerative colitis) is not well known, as studies have not adequately assessed enthesitis and osteitis lesions, but the musculoskeletal manifestations are in keeping with a SpA phenotype. Involvement of the peripheral joints is seen in about 20% of IBD patients. Oligoarticular disease predominantly affects the large lower limb joints (knees, ankles and hips). Evidence of sacroiliitis can also be detected by imaging in a proportion of patients with IBD. Imaging evidence of sacroiliitis is present in about 15%–20% of IBD patients. Osteitis pubis is also a typical lesion. In Crohn's disease, more than in colitis, the arthritis usually coincides with exacerbations of the underlying bowel disease and the arthritis improves with effective treatment of the bowel disease. There is some suggestion that the severity and onset of inflammatory musculoskeletal symptoms can vary in association with changes in the integrity of the ileocaecal valve, raising the possibility that changes in gut flora may act as triggers for the associated SpA.

NSAIDs are best avoided, since they can exacerbate IBD. Instead, judicious use of glucocorticoids, SSZ and MTX may be considered. Liaison is necessary between gastroenterologist and rheumatologist with regard to choice of therapy. Anti-TNF-α therapy is effective in enteropathic arthritis, but etanercept should be avoided as it has no efficacy in IBD. Anti-IL-17A therapy should be avoided as it can trigger flares of IBD. Tofacitinib, while not specifically licensed for enteropathic arthritis,

is efficacious in ulcerative colitis and might be a further treatment option. When musculoskeletal symptoms worsen despite anti-TNF-α therapy, it is wise to exclude small intestinal bacterial overgrowth as a triggering cause.

Autoimmune connective tissue diseases

Autoimmune connective tissue diseases (AICTDs) share many clinical features and are characterised by dysregulation of immune responses, with autoantibody production that is often directed at components of the cell nucleus, and tissue damage.

Systemic lupus erythematosus

Systemic lupus erythematosus (SLE) is a rare disease with a prevalence that ranges from about 0.03% in people of European descent to 0.2% in people of African Caribbean origin. Some 90% of affected patients are female and the peak age at onset is between 20 and 30 years. SLE is associated with considerable morbidity and a fivefold increase in mortality compared to age- and gender-matched controls, mainly because of an increased risk of premature cardiovascular disease.

Pathophysiology

The cause of SLE is incompletely understood. Genetic factors play a role and the strongest region of association lies with alleles in the HLA-DR and DQ regions. However, approximately 100 other susceptibility loci, which lie within or close to genes involved in the immune response, have also been identified by genome-wide association studies. The overall heritability of SLE has been estimated to be about 40%–60%, illustrating the importance of environmental influences, although the nature of these are unclear. In a few instances, SLE is associated with inherited mutations in complement components C1q, C2 and C4, in the immunoglobulin receptor FcγRIIIb and in the DNA exonuclease *TREX*. From an immunological standpoint, the characteristic feature of SLE is autoantibody production. These autoantibodies have specificity for a wide range of targets, but many are directed against antigens present within the cell or within the nucleus. This has led to the hypothesis that SLE may occur because of defects in apoptosis or in the clearance of apoptotic cells, which causes inappropriate exposure of intracellular antigens on the cell surface, leading to polyclonal B- and T-cell activation, and autoantibody production. In support of this, environmental factors that cause flares of SLE, such as ultraviolet light and infections, increase oxidative stress and cause cell damage. Whatever the underlying cause, autoantibody production and immune complex formation are thought to be important mechanisms of tissue damage in active SLE, leading to vasculitis and organ damage.

Clinical features

Symptoms such as fever, weight loss and mild lymphadenopathy may occur during flares of disease activity, whereas others such as fatigue and low-grade joint pains can be constant and not particularly associated with active inflammatory disease.

Arthritis

Arthralgia is a common symptom, occurring in 90% of patients, and is often associated with early morning stiffness. Tenosynovitis may also occur, but clinically apparent synovitis with joint swelling is unusual. Joint deformities may arise (Jaccoud's arthropathy) as the result of tendon damage, but joint erosions are not a feature.

Raynaud's phenomenon

Raynaud's phenomenon (RP) is characterised by vasoconstriction of the small vessels of the hand and feet in response to cold, leading to pallor followed by cyanosis of the affected digits followed by vasodilatation causing the affected digits to turn red. This is a common feature of SLE and may antedate other symptoms by months or years. Raynaud's

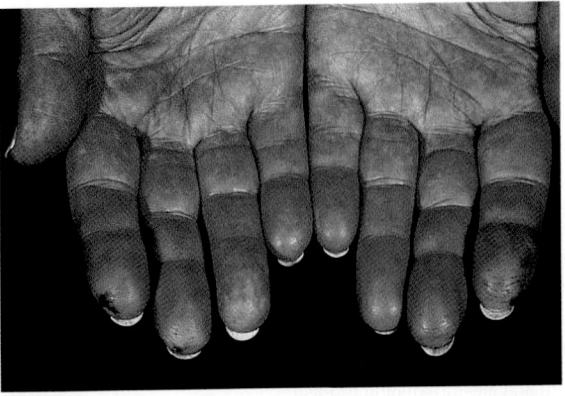

Fig. 26.45 Severe secondary Raynaud's phenomenon leading to ischaemic digital ulceration.

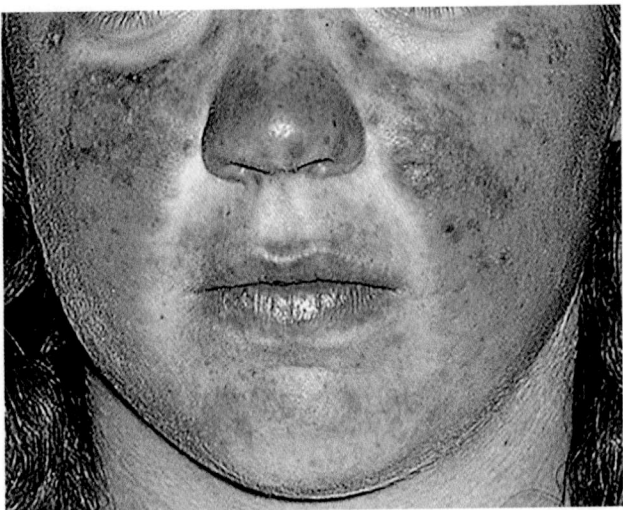

Fig. 26.46 Malar rash of systemic lupus erythematosus, sparing the nasolabial folds. The rash, when mild, can be notably similar to rosacea, which may itself be associated with inflammatory joint diseases that are associated with enteral diseases.

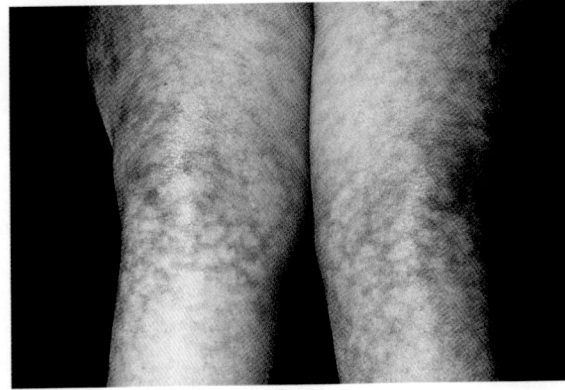

Fig. 26.47 Livedo reticularis (as typically occurs in systemic lupus erythematosus and antiphospholipid syndrome).

phenomenon associated with SLE and other AICTDs (secondary RP) needs to be differentiated from primary RP, which is a benign disorder that is common in the general population (up to 5%). Features of secondary RP include age at onset of over 25 years, other features of AICTD, absence of a family history of RP, severity of symptoms, presence of digital ulceration (Fig. 26.45) and male gender. Examination of capillary nail-fold loops using an ophthalmoscope (with oil placed on the skin) can show loss of the normal loop pattern, with capillary 'fallout' and dilatation and branching of loops; these features support a diagnosis of secondary RP, but can be observed in severe primary RP.

Skin

The skin is commonly involved in SLE and many eruptions are precipitated by exposure to ultraviolet light. The main types of skin involvement are:

- The classic malar facial rash (up to 20% of patients). This is erythematous, raised and painful or itchy, and occurs over the cheeks with sparing of the nasolabial folds (Fig. 26.46). Rosacea may mimic this rash.
- A discoid rash characterised by hyperkeratosis and follicular plugging, with scarring alopecia if it occurs on the scalp.
- Diffuse, usually non-scarring alopecia, which may also occur with active disease.
- Urticarial eruptions.

- Livedo reticularis (Fig. 26.47), which is also a feature of antiphospholipid syndrome and can become frankly vasculitic, if severe.

Kidney

Renal involvement is one of the main determinants of prognosis and regular monitoring of urinalysis and blood pressure is essential. The typical renal lesion is a proliferative glomerulonephritis, characterised by heavy haematuria, proteinuria and casts on urine microscopy.

Cardiovascular

The most common manifestation is pericarditis. Myocarditis and Libman–Sacks endocarditis can also occur. The endocarditis is due to accumulation on the heart valves of sterile fibrin-containing vegetations, which is thought to be a manifestation of hypercoagulability associated with antiphospholipid antibodies. The risk of atherosclerosis is greatly increased, as is the risk of stroke and myocardial infarction. This is thought to be multifactorial due to the adverse effects of inflammation on the endothelium, chronic glucocorticoid therapy and the procoagulant effects of antiphospholipid antibodies.

Lung

Lung involvement is common and most frequently manifests as pleuritic pain (serositis) or pleural effusion. Other features include pneumonitis, atelectasis, reduced lung volume and pulmonary fibrosis. The risk of thromboembolism is increased, especially in patients with antiphospholipid antibodies.

Neurological

Fatigue, headache and poor concentration are common and often occur in the absence of laboratory evidence of active disease. More specific features of cerebral SLE include visual hallucinations, chorea, organic psychosis, transverse myelitis and lymphocytic meningitis.

Haematological

Neutropenia, lymphopenia, thrombocytopenia and haemolytic anaemia may occur, due to antibody-mediated destruction of peripheral blood cells. The degree of lymphopenia can be a guide to disease activity.

Gastrointestinal

Mouth ulcers may occur and can be painful. Peritoneal serositis can cause acute pain. Mesenteric vasculitis is a serious complication, which can present with abdominal pain, bowel infarction or perforation. Hepatitis is a recognised, though rare, feature.

Paediatric disease

Renal disease and cutaneous manifestations are more frequent in juvenile-onset SLE compared to disease in adults. Similarly, there is

26

<table>
<tr><td colspan="2">i   26.63 Criteria for the classification of systemic lupus erythematosus</td></tr>
</table>

Features	Characteristics
Malar rash	Fixed erythema, flat or raised, sparing the nasolabial folds
Discoid rash	Erythematous raised patches with adherent keratotic scarring and follicular plugging
Photosensitivity	Rash due to unusual reaction to sunlight
Oral ulcers	Oral or nasopharyngeal ulceration, which may be painless
Arthritis	Non-erosive, involving two or more peripheral joints
Serositis	Pleuritis (history of pleuritic pain or rub, or pleural effusion) *or* pericarditis (rub, electrocardiogram evidence or effusion)
Renal disorder	Persistent proteinuria > 0.5 g/24 hrs *or* cellular casts (red cell, granular or tubular)
Neurological disorder	Seizures or psychosis, in the absence of provoking drugs or metabolic derangement
Haematological disorder	Haemolytic anaemia *or* leucopenia* ($<4 \times 10^9$/L) *or* lymphopenia* ($<1 \times 10^9$/L) *or* thrombocytopenia* ($<100 \times 10^9$/L) in the absence of offending drugs
Immunological	Anti-DNA antibodies in abnormal titre *or* presence of antibody to Sm antigen *or* positive antiphospholipid antibodies
Antinuclear antibody (ANA)	Abnormal titre of ANA by immunofluorescence
An adult has SLE if any 4 of 11 features are present serially or simultaneously	

*On two separate occasions.

subsequently a higher incidence of renal disease, malar rash, Raynaud's phenomenon, cutaneous vasculitis and neuropsychiatric manifestations than in adults.

Investigations

The diagnosis is based on a combination of clinical features and laboratory abnormalities. To fulfil the classification criteria for SLE, at least 4 of the 11 factors shown in Box 26.63 must be present or have occurred in the past. Checking of ANAs, antibodies to ENAs and complement, routine haematology, biochemistry and urinalysis are mandatory. Patients with active SLE are almost always positive for ANA. ANA-negative SLE can occur, but this is rare and in such cases antibodies to the ENA Ro or antiphospholipid antibodies are present. Anti-dsDNA antibodies are positive in most patients and are quite specific for SLE. Serum levels of C3 may be low in active SLE due to complement consumption, but in some people low C3 and C4 can also be caused by inherited deficiencies in C1, C2 or C4, all of which predispose to SLE. Studies of other family members can help to differentiate inherited deficiencies from complement consumption. A raised ESR, leucopenia and lymphopenia are typical of active SLE, and this may be accompanied by anaemia, haemolytic anaemia and thrombocytopenia. CRP is often normal in active SLE and presence of an elevated CRP in SLE raises the possibility of either serositis, or co-existing infection.

Management

The therapeutic goals are to educate the patient about the nature of the illness, to control symptoms and to prevent organ damage and maintain normal function. Patients should be advised to avoid sun and ultraviolet light exposure and to employ sun blocks (sun protection factor 25–50).

Mild to moderate disease

Patients with mild disease restricted to skin and joints can sometimes be managed with analgesics, NSAIDs and HCQ. Frequently, however, glucocorticoids are also necessary (prednisolone 5–20 mg/day), often in combination with immunosuppressants such as MTX, azathioprine or mycophenolate mofetil (MMF). Increased doses of glucocorticoids may be required for flares in activity or complications such as pleurisy or pericarditis. The monoclonal antibody belimumab has been shown to be effective in patients with active SLE who have responded inadequately to standard therapy. Fatigue may be problematic, but there is some evidence that low intensity regular aerobic exercise can be helpful. Poor sleep hygiene should be addressed to try to combat this symptom.

Severe and life-threatening disease

High-dose glucocorticoids and immunosuppressants are required for the treatment of renal, CNS and cardiac involvement. A commonly used regimen is pulsed methylprednisolone (10 mg/kg IV) plus cyclophosphamide (15 mg/kg IV), repeated at 2–3-weekly intervals for six cycles. Cyclophosphamide may cause haemorrhagic cystitis, but the risk can be minimised by good hydration and co-prescription of mesna (2-mercaptoethane sulfonate), which binds its urotoxic metabolites. Because of the risk of azoospermia and premature menopause, sperm or oocyte collection and storage need to be considered prior to treatment with cyclophosphamide.

MMF has been used successfully with high-dose glucocorticoids for renal involvement with results similar to those of pulsed cyclophosphamide, but fewer adverse effects. Belimumab in combination with standard therapy significantly decreases disease activity in SLE patients and is safe and well tolerated. Its role in patients with renal and neurological disease is still under investigation.

Rituximab has been reported as being effective in case reports and case series, but randomised placebo-controlled trials have not shown benefit.

Maintenance therapy

Following control of acute disease, oral prednisolone can be commenced in a dose of 40–60 mg daily, gradually reducing to 10–15 mg/day or less by 3 months. Azathioprine (2–2.5 mg/kg/day), MTX (10–25 mg/week) or MMF (2–3 g/day) may also be prescribed as steroid-sparing agents. The long-term aim is to try to maintain remission with the lowest dose of glucocorticoid and immunosuppressant possible. Cardiovascular risk factors, such as obesity, hypertension and hyperlipidaemia, should be controlled and patients should be advised to stop smoking and reduce excess alcohol intake.

Patients with SLE and the antiphospholipid antibody syndrome, who have had previous thrombosis, require life-long warfarin therapy. Patients with SLE are at risk of osteoporosis and hypovitaminosis D, and accordingly should be screened with biochemistry and DXA scanning.

Systemic sclerosis

Systemic sclerosis (SScl) is an autoimmune disorder of connective tissue, which results in fibrosis affecting the skin, internal organs and vasculature. It is characterised by severe Raynaud's phenomenon, digital ischaemia (Fig. 26.48), sclerodactyly, cardiac, lung, gut and renal disease. The peak age of onset is in the fourth and fifth decades. It is a rare condition with a prevalence of 10–20 per 100 000, with a 4:1 female-to-male ratio. It is subdivided into limited cutaneous systemic sclerosis (lcSScl: 70% of cases) and diffuse cutaneous systemic sclerosis (dcSScl: 30% of cases) depending on the extent of skin involvement and presence of major organ involvement. Some patients with lcSScl have calcinosis and telangiectasia and when combined with Raynaud's phenomenon, oesophageal involvement and sclerodactyly this is referred to as the CREST syndrome (Calcinosis, Raynaud's, oEsophageal involvement, Sclerodactyly and Telangiectasia), which has a good prognosis. The prognosis in dcSScl is poor (5-year survival about 70%). Features that associate with a poor prognosis include older age, diffuse skin disease, proteinuria, high ESR, a low gas transfer factor for carbon monoxide (TLCO) and pulmonary hypertension.

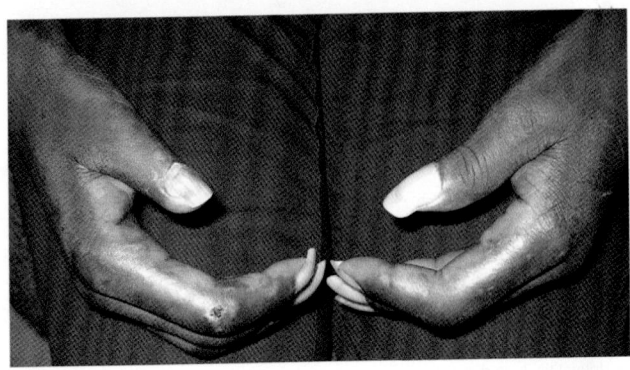

Fig. 26.48 Systemic sclerosis. Hands showing tight, shiny skin, sclerodactyly and flexion contractures of the fingers. *From Callen J, Jorizzo J, Zone J, Piette W, Rosenbach M, Vleugels RA. Dermatological signs of systemic disease, 5th edn. Elsevier; 2017.*

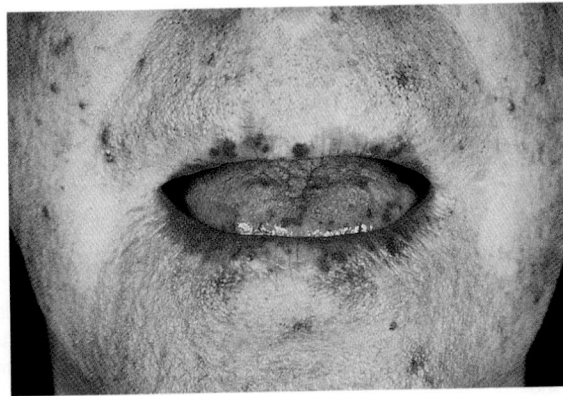

Fig. 26.49 Typical facial appearance showing telangiectasias in localised cutaneous systemic sclerosis.

Pathophysiology

The cause of SScl is not completely understood. There is evidence for a genetic component and associations with alleles at the HLA locus have been found. The disease occurs in all ethnic groups and race may influence severity. Isolated cases have been reported in which an SScl-like disease has been triggered by exposure to silica dust, vinyl chloride, epoxy resins and trichloroethylene. There is clear evidence of immunological dysfunction: T lymphocytes, especially those of the Th17 subtype, infiltrate the skin and there is abnormal fibroblast activation, leading to increased production of extracellular matrix in the dermis, primarily type I collagen. This results in symmetrical thickening, tightening and induration of the skin (scleroderma). Arterial and arteriolar narrowing occurs due to intimal proliferation and vessel wall inflammation. Endothelial injury causes release of vasoconstrictors and platelet activation, resulting in further ischaemia, which is thought to exacerbate the fibrotic process.

Clinical features

Skin

Initially, there is non-pitting oedema of fingers and flexor tendon sheaths. Subsequently, the skin becomes shiny and taut, and distal skin creases disappear. There can be capillary loss. The face and neck are often involved, with thinning of the lips and radial furrowing. In some patients, skin thickening stops at this stage. Skin involvement restricted to sites distal to the elbow or knee (apart from the face) is thus classified as lcSScl (Fig. 26.49). Involvement proximal to the knee and elbow and on the trunk is classified as 'diffuse disease' (dcSScl).

Raynaud's phenomenon

This is a universal feature and can precede other features by many years. Involvement of small blood vessels in the extremities may cause critical tissue ischaemia, leading to localised distal skin infarction and necrosis.

Musculoskeletal features

Arthralgia and flexor tenosynovitis are common. Restricted hand function is due to skin involvement rather than joint disease and erosive arthropathy is uncommon. Muscle weakness and wasting can result from myositis.

Gastrointestinal involvement

Smooth muscle atrophy and fibrosis in the lower two-thirds of the oesophagus lead to reflux with erosive oesophagitis. Dysphagia and odynophagia may also occur. Involvement of the stomach causes early satiety and occasionally outlet obstruction. Recurrent occult upper gastrointestinal bleeding may indicate a 'watermelon' stomach (antral vascular ectasia; up to 20% of patients). Small intestine involvement may lead to malabsorption due to bacterial overgrowth and intermittent bloating, pain or constipation. Dilatation of bowel due to autonomic neuropathy may cause pseudo-obstruction with nausea, vomiting, abdominal discomfort and distension, often worse after food (symptoms can mimic those of an acute abdomen and can lead to erroneous laparotomy).

Pulmonary involvement

Pulmonary hypertension complicates long-standing disease and is six times more prevalent in lcSScl than in dcSScl. It usually presents with insidiously evolving exertional dyspnoea and signs of right heart failure. Interstitial lung disease is common in patients with dcSScl who have topoisomerase 1 antibodies (Scl70). Dyspnoea can evolve slowly over time or rapidly in occasional cases.

Renal involvement

One of the main causes of death is hypertensive renal crisis, characterised by rapidly developing accelerated phase hypertension and renal failure. Hypertensive renal crisis is much more likely to occur in dcSScl than in lcSScl, and in patients with topoisomerase 1 and RNP antibodies.

Investigations

As SScl can affect multiple organs, routine haematology, renal, liver and bone function tests and urinalysis are essential. ANA is positive in about 95%. About 30% of patients with dcSScl have antibodies to topoisomerase 1 (Scl70). About 60% of patients have anticentromere antibodies and this is a biomarker for lcSScl and CREST syndrome. Chest X-ray, transthoracic echocardiography and lung function tests are recommended to assess for interstitial lung disease and pulmonary hypertension (low corrected transfer factor may indicate early pulmonary hypertension). High-resolution lung CT is recommended if interstitial lung disease is suspected. If pulmonary hypertension is suspected, right heart catheter measurements should be arranged at a specialist cardiac centre. A barium swallow can assess oesophageal involvement. A hydrogen breath test can indicate small intestinal bacterial overgrowth.

Management

For most patients, the focus of management is to ameliorate symptoms and combat the effects of the disease on target organs. In patients with severe dcSScl, encouraging results have been obtained with autologous stem cell transplantation following myeloablative therapy with cyclophosphamide.

- *Raynaud's phenomenon and digital ulcers*. Avoidance of cold exposure, use of thermal insulating gloves/socks and maintenance of a high core temperature all help. If symptoms are persistent, calcium channel blockers, losartan, fluoxetine, sildenafil and tadalafil can be effective. Courses of intravenous prostacyclin are used for severe disease and critical ischemia. The endothelin-1 antagonist bosentan is

26

licensed for treating ischaemic digital ulcers and digital tip tissue health can be maintained with regular use of fucidin–hydrocortisone cream.

- *Gastrointestinal complications*. Oesophageal reflux should be treated with proton pump inhibitors and anti-reflux agents. Rotating courses of antibiotics may be required for small intestinal bacterial overgrowth (p. 848), while metoclopramide or domperidone may help patients with symptoms of dysmotility/pseudo-obstruction.
- *Hypertension*. Aggressive treatment with ACE inhibitors is needed, even if renal impairment is present.
- *Joint involvement*. This may be treated with analgesics and/or NSAIDs. If synovitis is present then therapy with MTX or other cDMARD can be of value.
- *Progressive pulmonary hypertension*. Early treatment with bosentan is required. In severe or progressive disease, heart–lung transplant may be considered.
- *Interstitial lung disease*. Cyclophosphamide is effective in slowing progression of interstitial lung disease and similar results have been observed with MMF. More recently the tyrosine kinase inhibitor nintedanib (150 mg twice daily) has shown efficacy in slowing decline of lung function in dcSScl.

Mixed connective tissue disease

Mixed connective tissue disease (MCTD) is a condition in which some clinical features of SScl, myositis and SLE all occur in the same patient. It commonly presents with indolent puffiness of the fingers (the appearance is between that of SpA-type dactylitis and sclerodactyly) with Raynaud's phenomenon and myalgias. Most patients have anti-RNP antibodies. Management focuses on treating the individual components of the disease (see other sections).

Sjögren syndrome

Sjögren syndrome (SS) is characterised by grittiness of the eyes and dryness of the mouth due to lymphocytic infiltration of salivary and lacrimal glands, leading to glandular fibrosis and exocrine failure. The typical age of onset is between 40 and 50 years, with a 9:1 female-to-male ratio. It is subdivided into primary Sjögren syndrome (PSS), which occurs in the absence of other autoimmune disease, and secondary Sjögren syndrome, where it occurs in association with other conditions like RA and SLE.

Clinical features

The eye symptoms, termed keratoconjunctivitis sicca, are due to a lack of lubricating tears, which reflects inflammatory infiltration of the lacrimal glands. Conjunctivitis and blepharitis are frequent and may lead to filamentary keratitis due to binding of tenacious mucous filaments to the cornea and conjunctiva. Oral involvement manifests as a dry mouth (xerostomia). There is a high incidence of dental caries, gingivitis, periodontitis and other dental problems. Lymphadenopathy is present in about two-thirds of patients and other sites of extraglandular involvement are listed in Box 26.64. Often the most disabling symptom is fatigue. There may be an association with inflammatory small-joint OA, although formal studies have not been done to determine if this is a chance association. Sialadenitis, osteoarthritis and xerostomia (SOX) syndrome has been described; this may occur independently of PSS or, more likely, constitutes a mild form. Both interstitial lung disease (presenting with dry cough, dyspnoea and course crackles on lung auscultation) and interstitial nephritis (presenting with polyuria and sometimes complicated by renal tubular acidosis) may occur and both require proactive screening. PSS is associated with a 40-fold increased lifetime risk of lymphoma, though the complication is still very rare. This should be suspected if there is progressive worsening of lymphadenopathy.

Investigations

Support for the diagnosis can be obtained by the Schirmer tear test, which measures tear flow over 5 minutes using absorbent paper strips placed

i	**26.64 Features of primary Sjögren syndrome**

Risk factors

• Age of onset 40–60	• HLA-B8/DR3
• Female > male	

Common clinical features

• Keratoconjunctivitis sicca	• Non-erosive arthralgia
• Xerostomia	• Generalised osteoarthritis
• Salivary gland enlargement	• Raynaud's phenomenon
• Rashes/skin irritation	• Fatigue

Less common features

• Low-grade fever	• Peripheral neuropathy
• Interstitial lung disease	• Lymphadenopathy
• Anaemia, leucopenia	• Lymphoreticular lymphoma
• Thrombocytopenia	• Glomerulonephritis
• Cryoglobulinaemia	• Interstitial nephritis
• Vasculitis	• Renal tubular acidosis

Autoantibodies frequently detected

• Rheumatoid factor	• SS-B (anti-La)
• Antinuclear antibody	• Gastric parietal cell
• SS-A (anti-Ro)	• Thyroid

Associated autoimmune disorders

• Systemic lupus erythematosus	• Primary biliary cholangitis
• Systemic sclerosis	• Chronic active hepatitis
• Coeliac disease	• Myasthenia gravis

(HLA = human leucocyte antigen)

on the lower eyelid; a normal result is more than 5 mm of wetting. Corneal staining with rose bengal may show punctate epithelial abnormalities over the area not covered by the open eyelid. If the diagnosis remains in doubt, it can be confirmed by demonstrating focal lymphocytic infiltrate in a minor salivary gland biopsy. Most patients have an elevated ESR and hypergammaglobulinaemia, and one or more autoantibodies, including ANA and RF are usually present. ANA-negative disease does exist, but in this case anti-Ro and anti-La antibodies are usually detectable (see Box 26.9). A chest X-ray, high resolution CT and lung function tests should be performed if symptoms suggestive of lung disease are present. Routine biochemistry and tests of urinary concentrating ability may be required if interstitial nephritis is suspected. Lymph node biopsy should be performed to exclude lymphoma in patients with progressive lymphadenopathy.

Management

No treatments can significantly modify the course of SS and so management is essentially symptomatic. Lacrimal substitutes, such as hypromellose, should be used during the day in combination with more viscous lubricating application at night. Soft contact lenses can be useful for corneal protection in patients with filamentary keratitis and occlusion of the lacrimal ducts is occasionally needed. Artificial saliva sprays, saliva-stimulating tablets, pastilles and oral gels can be tried for xerostomia, but often chewing gum is most effective. Adequate post-prandial oral hygiene and prompt treatment of oral candidiasis are essential. Vaginal dryness is treated with lubricants. A trial of systemic pilocarpine (5–30 mg daily in divided doses) is worthwhile in early disease to increase salivary and lacrimal secretions. HCQ (200 mg twice daily) is sometimes used in the treatment of SS, but clinical trials have not shown convincing evidence of benefit. Immunosuppression does not improve sicca symptoms, but is often used in the treatment of interstitial lung disease and interstitial nephritis although the evidence base for benefit is limited.

Polymyositis and dermatomyositis

Polymyositis (PM) and dermatomyositis (DM) are characterised by an inflammatory infiltrate of both skeletal and smooth muscle. In DM,

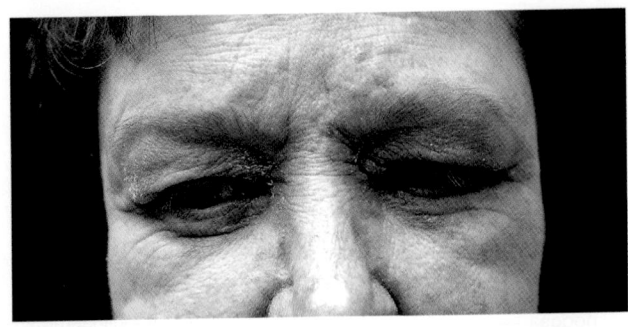

Fig. 26.50 Heliotrope rash and eyelid oedema in dermatomyositis. *From Callen JP, Jorisso JL, Bolognia JL, Piette WW, Zone JZ. Dermatological signs of internal disease, 4th edn. Elsevier; 2009.*

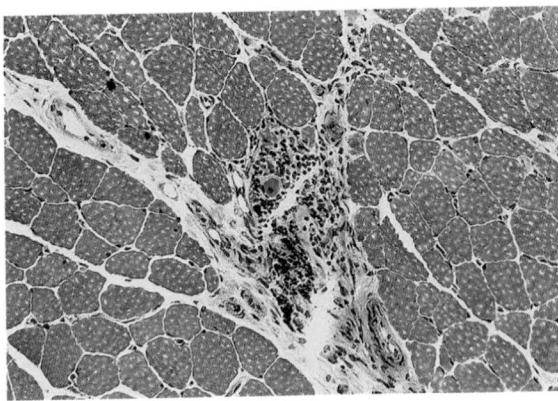

Fig. 26.51 Muscle biopsy from a patient with polymyositis. The sample shows an intense inflammatory cell infiltrate in an area of degenerating and regenerating muscle fibres.

characteristic skin changes also occur. Both diseases are rare, with an incidence of 2–10 cases per million/year. They can occur in isolation or in association with other autoimmune diseases and both may be the presenting features of a previously undiagnosed malignancy.

Clinical features

The typical presentation of PM and DM is with symmetrical proximal muscle weakness over a few weeks, usually affecting the lower limbs more than the upper, in adults between 40 and 60 years of age. Patients report difficulty rising from a chair, climbing stairs and lifting. Muscle pain is not a prominent feature but may be present in up to one-third of patients. Systemic features of fever, weight loss and fatigue are common. Subcutaneous calcification associated with skin ulceration may occur in both DM and PM. Respiratory or pharyngeal muscle involvement can lead to ventilatory failure or aspiration that requires urgent treatment. Interstitial lung disease occurs in up to 30% of patients and is associated with the presence of antisynthetase (Jo-1) antibodies.

The skin lesions in DM include Gottron's papules, which are scaly, erythematous or violaceous, psoriasiform plaques occurring over the extensor surfaces of PIP and DIP joints, and a heliotrope rash that is a violaceous discoloration of the eyelid in combination with periorbital oedema (Fig. 26.50). Similar rashes occur on the upper back, chest and shoulders over a 'shawl' distribution. Periungual nail-fold capillaries are often enlarged and tortuous.

Investigations

Muscle biopsy is the pivotal investigation and shows the typical features of fibre necrosis, regeneration and inflammatory cell infiltrate (Fig. 26.51). Since muscle involvement may be patchy, it is common to perform an MRI scan prior to biopsy, which often shows features of increased signal intensity in STIR sequence images. This not only provides support for the diagnosis, but also can help choose the optimal site for a biopsy. Serum levels of creatine kinase are typically raised and are a useful measure of disease activity, although a normal creatine kinase does not exclude the diagnosis, particularly in juvenile myositis. Electromyography is very useful for highlighting non-autoimmune/non-inflammatory myopathies. Screening for underlying malignancy should be undertaken routinely (full examination, chest X-ray, serum urine and protein electrophoresis, CT of chest/abdomen/pelvis; prostate-specific antigen in men and mammography in women).

Management

Oral glucocorticoids (prednisolone 1 mg/kg daily) are the first-line treatment of PM and DM, but high-dose intravenous methylprednisolone (1 g/day for 3 days) may be required in patients with respiratory or pharyngeal weakness. If there is a good response, glucocorticoids should be reduced by approximately 25% per month aiming for a maintenance dose of 5–7.5 mg daily. Glucocorticoid-induced myopathy should be considered in patients who initially respond but then relapse. A second muscle biopsy can be of diagnostic value to guide further treatment in this situation since in the case of glucocorticoid myopathy type II fibre atrophy is observed as compared with fibre necrosis and regeneration in active myositis. Treatment should be adjusted accordingly. Although most patients respond well to glucocorticoids, additional immunosuppressive therapy may be required as steroid-sparing agents in the form of MTX, azathioprine, MMF or ciclosporin. Rituximab is sometimes used in refractory cases, but the only randomised trial of this agent did not show benefit over placebo. Intravenous immunoglobulin (IVIg) has been shown to be effective in the treatment of DM and is often used in the treatment of refractory PM and DM. Antimalarials such as HCQ and mepacrine have been used for skin-predominant disease, but the evidence for benefit is limited and based on case reports.

Juvenile dermatomyositis

Juvenile dermatomyositis (JDM) is by far the most common inflammatory myopathy in children and adolescents, and typically does not require a search for malignancy. The incidence is 2–4 per million (United States and UK), with a median age of onset of 7 years (25% are below 4 years at diagnosis). Many clinical features are similar to those in the adult disease. JDM can be monocyclic, lasting up to 3 years (25%–40%), or polycyclic with periods of remission and relapse (60%–75%). In some cases, polycyclic JDM can be chronic and life-long. Skin ulceration occurs in 10%–20% of cases and calcinosis in about 30%.

Intravenous methylprednisolone, then oral glucocorticoids and MTX produce a rapid response in many cases. Cyclophosphamide may be used for resistant disease with skin ulceration. IVIg is given in resistant cases.

Undifferentiated autoimmune connective tissue disease

The term undifferentiated autoimmune connective tissue disease is used to describe the situation where patients present with individual clinical features of AICTD, either simultaneously or sequentially, but do not meet the criteria for diagnosis of a specific disease. Some of these individuals may progress to develop a specific AICTD with time; others continue to have an undifferentiated disease that remains the same for many years, and in others the symptoms will recede. These patients should be kept under review with management directed at treating individual symptoms as they arise.

26

Adult-onset Still's disease

Adult-onset Still's disease is a rare systemic inflammatory disorder of unknown cause with features that are in some respects similar to sJIA and familial fever syndromes (p. 71). The presentation is with intermittent fever, rash and polyarthritis or polyarthralgia. There is evidence that increased production of the pro-inflammatory cytokine interleukin-1 may play a pathogenic role. Splenomegaly, hepatomegaly and lymphadenopathy may be present. Investigations typically provide evidence of an acute phase response with raised ESR and CRP and a markedly elevated serum ferritin. Tests for RF and ANA are negative. Treatment with NSAIDs can be effective in mild cases, but in more severe disease, glucocorticoids with or without DMARD such as azathioprine, MTX or MMF, are indicated. In resistant disease, the interleukin-1 inhibitors canakinumab or anakinra can be highly effective.

Vasculitis

Vasculitis is characterised by inflammation and necrosis of blood vessel walls, with associated damage to skin, kidney, lung, heart, brain and gastrointestinal tract. There is a wide spectrum of involvement and severity, ranging from mild and transient disease affecting only the skin, to life-threatening fulminant disease with multiple organ failure. Principal sites of involvement for the main types of vasculitis are summarised in Figure 26.52. The clinical features result from a combination of local tissue ischaemia (due to vessel inflammation and narrowing) and the systemic effects of widespread inflammation. Systemic vasculitis should be considered in any patient with fever, weight loss, fatigue, evidence of multisystem involvement, rashes, raised inflammatory markers and abnormal urinalysis (Box 26.65).

Antineutrophil cytoplasmic antibody-associated vasculitis

Antineutrophil cytoplasmic antibody (ANCA)-associated vasculitis (AAV) is a life-threatening disorder characterised by inflammatory infiltration of small blood vessels, fibrinoid necrosis and the presence of circulating antibodies to antineutrophil cytoplasmic antibody (ANCA). The combined incidence is about 10–15/1 000 000. There are three main subtypes with differing clinical features:

Microscopic polyangiitis

Microscopic polyangiitis (MPA) is a necrotising small-vessel vasculitis found with rapidly progressive glomerulonephritis, often in association with alveolar haemorrhage. Cutaneous and gastrointestinal involvement is common and other features include neuropathy (15%) and pleural effusions (15%). Patients are usually myeloperoxidase (MPO) antibody-positive.

Granulomatosis with polyangiitis

Granulomatosis with polyangiitis (GPA), also known as Wegener's granulomatosis, is characterised by granuloma formation, mainly affecting the nasal passages, airways and kidney. A minority of patients present with glomerulonephritis. The most common presentation of GPA is with epistaxis, nasal crusting and sinusitis, but haemoptysis and mucosal ulceration may also occur. Deafness may be a feature due to inner ear involvement and proptosis may occur because of inflammation of the retro-orbital tissue (Fig. 26.53). This causes diplopia due to entrapment of the extra-ocular muscles, or loss of vision due to optic nerve compression. Disturbance of colour vision is an early feature of optic nerve compression. Untreated nasal disease ultimately leads to destruction of bone and cartilage. Migratory pulmonary infiltrates and nodules occur in 50% of patients (as seen on high-resolution CT of lungs). Patients with GPA are usually proteinase-3 (PR3) antibody-positive.

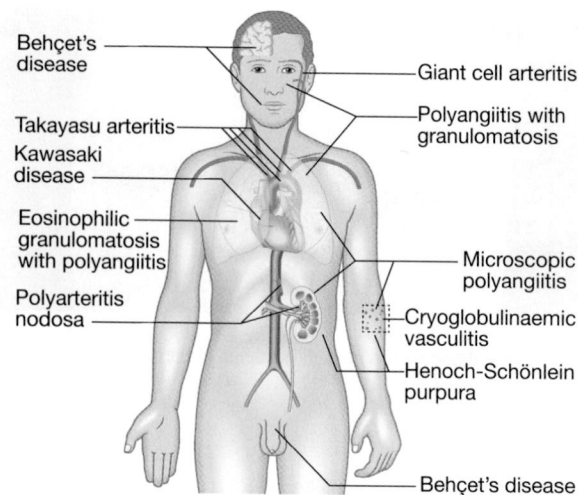

Fig. 26.52 Types of vasculitis. The anatomical targets of different forms of vasculitis are shown.

---

i | 26.65 Clinical features of systemic vasculitis

Systemic
- Malaise
- Fever
- Night sweats
- Weight loss
- Myoarthralgias

Rashes
- Palpable purpura
- Pulp infarcts
- Ulceration
- Livedo reticularis

Ear, nose and throat
- Epistaxis
- Recurrent sinusitis
- Deafness

Respiratory
- Haemoptysis
- Cough
- Poorly controlled asthma

Gastrointestinal
- Abdominal pain (due to mucosal inflammation or enteric ischaemia)
- Mouth ulcers
- Diarrhoea

Neurological
- Sensory or motor neuropathy

Eosinophilic granulomatosis with polyangiitis

Eosinophilic granulomatosis with polyangiitis (EGPA), also known as Churg–Strauss syndrome, is a small-vessel vasculitis with an incidence of about 1–3 per 1 000 000. Antibodies to MPO or PR3 can be detected in up to 60% of cases. It is somewhat distinct from MPA and GPA in that eosinophilia is a prominent feature. Some patients have a prodromal period for many years, characterised by allergic rhinitis, nasal polyposis and late-onset asthma that is often difficult to control. The typical acute presentation is with a triad of skin lesions (purpura or nodules), asymmetric mononeuritis multiplex and eosinophilia. Pulmonary infiltrates and pleural or pericardial effusions due to serositis may be present. Up to 50% of patients have abdominal symptoms provoked by mesenteric vasculitis.

Investigation of AAV

Patients with active disease usually have a leucocytosis with elevated CRP and ESR. Complement levels are usually normal or slightly elevated. Eosinophilia is common in EGPA. Imaging of the upper airways, chest and nasal passages with MRI can be useful in localising abnormalities in

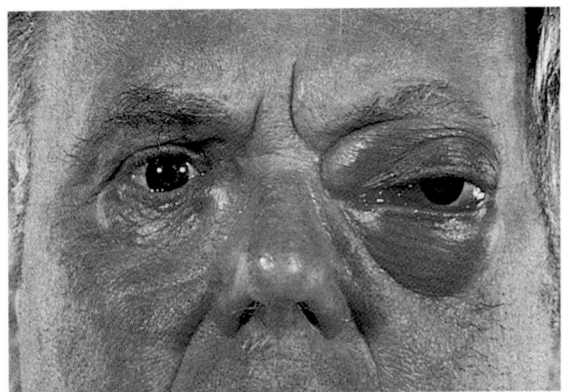

Fig. 26.53 Eye involvement in antineutrophil cytoplasmic antibody-associated vasculitis.

GPA. Often, the diagnosis of AAV can be made on clinical and serological grounds in combination with the laboratory abnormalities described above, but if there is any doubt the diagnosis should be confirmed by biopsy of the kidney, skin or lesions in the sinuses and upper airways.

Management

Management of organ-threatening AAV is with high-dose glucocorticoids and immunosuppressive therapy. A commonly used regimen is pulse intravenous methylprednisolone 0.5–1 g for 3 days coupled with intravenous cyclophosphamide 15 mg/kg every 2 weeks for 3 months. This is followed by maintenance therapy with lower-dose glucocorticoids and azathioprine, MTX or MMF. Rituximab in combination with high-dose glucocorticoids has been shown to be equally effective as oral cyclophosphamide and glucocorticoids at inducing remission in AAV. Plasmapheresis should be considered for fulminant lung disease. High dose glucocorticoids and MTX are an effective combination for treating limited AAV where there is indolent sinus, lung or skin disease. Recently mepolizumab, an inhibitor of IL-5, has been shown to reduce the risk of relapse when combined with glucocorticoids in EGPA. Patients with AAV must be followed on a regular and long-term basis since the condition has a tendency to relapse, monitoring urinalysis for blood and protein, plasma creatinine, FBC, ESR, CRP, lung function and PR3 or MPO antibody titres.

Takayasu arteritis

Takayasu arteritis affects the aorta, its major branches and occasionally the pulmonary arteries. The typical age at onset is 25–30 years, with an 8:1 female-to-male ratio. It has a worldwide distribution, but is most common in Asia. It is characterised by granulomatous inflammation of the vessel wall, leading to its occlusion or weakening. It presents with claudication, fever, arthralgia and weight loss. Clinical examination may reveal loss of pulses, bruits, hypertension and aortic incompetence. Investigation typically shows a raised ESR and CRP and a normocytic, normochromic anaemia. The pivotal investigation is CT or MRI angiography, which reveals thickening of the vessel wall and narrowing of the lumen. Aortic coarctation, and aneurysmal dilatation may also occur. The diagnosis can also be made by ^{18}fluorodeoxyglucose PET-CT imaging, where there is increased tracer uptake in affected vessels. Treatment is with high-dose glucocorticoids and immunosuppressants, as described for ANCA-associated vasculitis. With successful treatment, the 5-year survival is 83%.

Kawasaki disease

Kawasaki disease is a vasculitis that mostly involves the coronary vessels. It presents as an acute systemic disorder, usually affecting children under 5 years. It occurs mainly in Japan and other Asian countries,

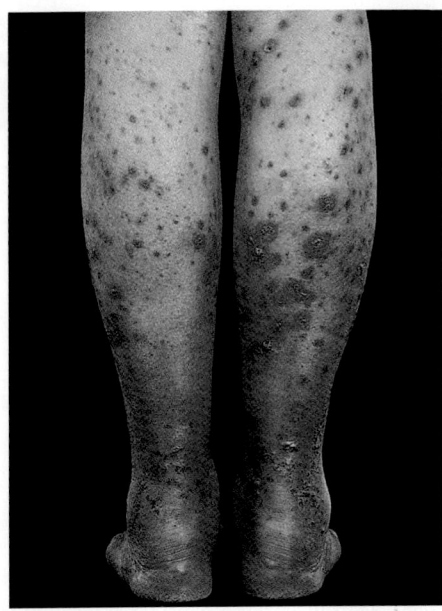

Fig. 26.54 Rash of systemic vasculitis (palpable purpura).

such as China and Korea, but other ethnic groups may also be affected. Presentation is with fever, generalised rash (including palms and soles), inflamed oral mucosa and conjunctival injection resembling a viral exanthem. The cause is unknown, but is thought to be an abnormal immune response to an infectious trigger. A syndrome with some similarities to Kawasaki disease has recently been reported to be a complication of COVID-19 infection in children. Cardiovascular complications include coronary arteritis, leading to myocardial infarction, transient coronary dilatation, myocarditis, pericarditis, peripheral vascular insufficiency and gangrene. Treatment is with aspirin (5 mg/kg daily for 14 days) and IVIg (400 mg/kg daily for 5 days). Ciclosporin (5 mg/kg/day) in combination with IVIg can be effective in patients with resistant disease.

Polyarteritis nodosa

Polyarteritis nodosa has a peak incidence between the ages of 40 and 50, with a male-to-female ratio of 2:1. The annual incidence is about 2/1 000 000. Hepatitis B is an important risk factor and the incidence is 10 times higher in the Inuit of Alaska, in whom hepatitis B infection is endemic. Presentation is with fever, myalgia, arthralgia and weight loss, in combination with manifestations of multisystem disease. The most common skin lesions are palpable purpura (Fig. 26.54), ulceration, infarction and livedo reticularis (see Fig. 26.47). Pathological changes comprise necrotising inflammation and vessel occlusion, and in 70% of patients, arteritis of the vasa nervorum leads to neuropathy, which is typically symmetrical and affects both sensory and motor function. Severe hypertension and/or renal impairment may occur due to multiple renal infarctions, but glomerulonephritis is rare (in contrast to MPA). The diagnosis is confirmed by conventional or MR angiography, which shows multiple aneurysms and smooth narrowing of mesenteric, hepatic or renal systems, or by muscle or sural nerve biopsy, which reveals the histological changes described above. Treatment is with high-dose glucocorticoids and cyclophosphamide, as described for ANCA-associated vasculitis.

Giant cell arteritis and polymyalgia rheumatica

Giant cell arteritis (GCA) is a granulomatous arteritis that affects medium- and large-sized arteries. It is commonly associated with polymyalgia rheumatica (PMR), which presents with symmetrical pain and stiffness affecting the shoulder and pelvic girdle. There is evidence that these symptoms are due to an inflammatory infiltrate of the synovium and

26

> **26.66 Conditions that can cause 'polymyalgic' axial and proximal limb inflammatory symptoms or mimic polymyalgia rheumatica**
>
> - Calcium pyrophosphate disease
> - Spondyloarthritis
> - Rheumatoid arthritis
> - Hyper-/hypothyroidism
> - Psoriatic arthritis (enthesopathic)
> - Systemic vasculitis
> - Myeloma
> - Inflammatory myopathy (particularly inclusion body myositis)
> - Lambert–Eaton syndrome
> - Multiple separate lesions (cervical spondylosis, cervical radiculopathy, bilateral subacromial impingement, facet joint arthritis, osteoarthritis of the acromioclavicular joint)

> **26.67 Emergency management of giant cell arteritis**
>
> - Take blood for CRP, ESR and FBC
> - Commence prednisolone (40–60 mg daily)
> - Consider urgent ophthalmology examination in patients with visual symptoms
> - Consider temporal artery biopsy or ultrasound
> - Review within 1 week and adjust glucocorticoid doses according to clinical response and results of investigations
>
> (ACPA = anti-citrullinated peptide antibody; ANA = antinuclear antibody; ANCA = antineutrophil cytoplasmic antibody; CPK = creatine phosphokinase; CRP = C-reactive protein; ESR = erythrocyte sedimentation rate; FBC = full blood count)

tendon sheaths in the affected regions. Since many patients with GCA have symptoms of PMR, and some patients with PMR go on to develop GCA if untreated, many rheumatologists consider them to be different manifestations of the same underlying disorder. Both diseases are rare under the age of 60 years. The average age at onset is 70, with a female-to-male ratio of about 3:1. The prevalence of GCA in people of European descent is about 20 per 100 000 in those over the age of 50 years, while PMR affect abouts 60 per 100 000. Both conditions are much less common (1 in 100 000) in African and Asian populations. The cause is unknown, but there is a strong genetic component such that GCA is strongly associated with genetic variation at the HLA-DRB1 locus.

Clinical features

The cardinal symptom of GCA is headache, which is often localised to the temporal or occipital region and may be accompanied by scalp tenderness. Jaw pain develops in some patients, brought on by chewing or talking and is referred to as jaw claudication. Visual disturbance can occur (most specifically amaurosis) and a catastrophic presentation is with blindness in one eye due to occlusion of the posterior ciliary artery. In such cases the optic disc may appear pale and swollen with haemorrhages, but these changes may take 24–36 hours to develop and the fundi may initially appear normal. Rarely, neurological involvement may occur, with transient ischaemic attacks, brainstem infarcts and hemiparesis.

In GCA, constitutional symptoms, such as weight loss, fatigue, malaise and night sweats, are common. With PMR, there may be stiffness and painful restriction of active shoulder movements on waking. Sometimes patients can present with symptoms that are similar to RA. The affected muscles are not tender and there is no weakness or muscle-wasting. Other conditions that cause PMR-like symptoms are shown in Box 26.66.

Investigations

The typical laboratory abnormality is an elevated ESR and CRP, often with a normochromic, normocytic anaemia. Abnormal liver function tests may also occur. Very rarely, PMR and GCA can present with a normal ESR in the early stages of disease evolution. More objective evidence for GCA should be obtained whenever possible. The two most commonly used investigations are temporal artery biopsy and ultrasound of the temporal arteries. Characteristic biopsy findings are fragmentation of the internal elastic lamina with necrosis of the media in combination with a mixed inflammatory cell infiltrate. The sensitivity is about 70% with multiple biopsies and multiple section analysis (to detect 'skip' lesions), but a negative biopsy does not exclude the diagnosis. The characteristic finding on Doppler ultrasound examination is the 'halo' sign, where the thickened vessel wall shows as a dark area surrounding a positive Doppler signal within the vessel. The overall sensitivity is about 55% and specificity about 70% in routine clinical practice. A negative result does not exclude the diagnosis.

Management

Prednisolone should be commenced urgently in suspected GCA because of the risk of visual loss (Box 26.67). Response is dramatic, such that symptoms largely resolve within 48–72 hours of starting therapy in virtually all patients. It is customary to use higher doses in GCA (40–60 mg prednisolone) than in PMR (15–20 mg). In both conditions, the glucocorticoid dose should be progressively reduced, guided by symptoms and ESR, with the aim of reaching a dose of 10–15 mg by about 8 weeks. The rate of reduction should then be slowed by 1 mg per month. The IL-6 inhibitor tocilizumab has been shown to reduce the risk of relapse following glucocorticoid dose reductions in GCA and is of value in patients at high risk of glucocorticoid side effects. The long-term efficacy of tocilizumab in GCA remains under investigation. If symptoms recur, the dose should be increased to that which previously controlled the symptoms and reduction attempted again in another few weeks. Immunosuppressive therapy with MTX or azathioprine may be required as steroid-sparing agents in patients where it is not possible to reduce the prednisolone dose below 10 mg daily. Most patients need glucocorticoids for an average of 12–24 months and in view of this bisphosphonate therapy is often required to protect against osteoporosis.

Henoch–Schönlein purpura

Henoch–Schönlein purpura is a small-vessel vasculitis caused by immune complex deposition following an infectious trigger. It is predominantly a disease of children and young adults. The usual presentation is with purpura over the buttocks and lower legs, accompanied by abdominal pain, gastrointestinal bleeding and arthralgia. Nephritis can also occur and may present up to 4 weeks after the onset of other symptoms. Biopsy of affected tissue shows a vasculitis with IgA deposits in the vessel wall. Henoch–Schönlein purpura is usually a self-limiting disorder that settles spontaneously without specific treatment. Glucocorticoids and immunosuppressive therapy may be required in patients with more severe disease, particularly in the presence of nephritis.

Cryoglobulinaemic vasculitis

This is a small-vessel vasculitis that occurs when immunoglobulins precipitate out in the cold. Cryoglobulins are classified into three types (see Box 4.16). Types II and III are associated with vasculitis. The typical presentation is with a vasculitic rash over the lower limbs, arthralgia, Raynaud's phenomenon and neuropathy. The ESR and CRP are elevated in active disease and C3 levels may be reduced. Some cases are secondary to hepatitis C infection and others are associated with other autoimmune diseases. Affected patients should be screened and, if positive, treated for hepatitis C. There is no consensus as to how best to treat cryoglobulinaemic vasculitis in the absence of an obvious trigger. Glucocorticoids and immunosuppressive therapy are often used empirically, but their efficacy is uncertain. In severe cases, plasmapheresis can be considered.

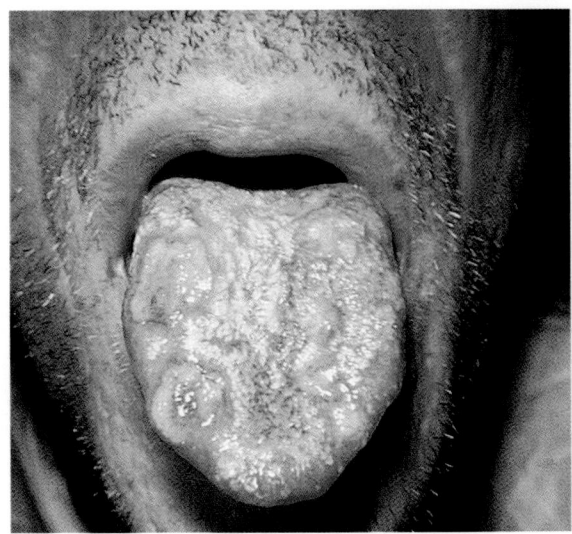

Fig. 26.55 Oral ulceration in Behçet's disease.

---

i	26.68 Criteria for the diagnosis of Behçet's disease

Recurrent oral ulceration: minor aphthous, major aphthous or herpetiform ulceration at least three times in 12 months *plus* two of the following:
- Recurrent genital ulceration
- Eye lesions: anterior uveitis, posterior uveitis, cells in vitreous on slit-lamp examination, retinal vasculitis
- Skin lesions: erythema nodosum, pseudofolliculitis, papulopustular lesions, acneiform nodules
- Positive pathergy test

Behçet's disease

This is a vasculitis of unknown aetiology that characteristically targets small arteries and venules. It is rare in Western Europe but more common in 'Silk Route' countries, around the Mediterranean and in Japan, where there is a strong genetic association with HLA-B51.

Oral ulcers are invariably present (Fig. 26.55). Unlike aphthous ulcers, they are usually deep and multiple, and last for 10–30 days. Genital ulcers are also a common problem, occurring in 60%–80% of cases. The usual skin lesions are erythema nodosum or acneiform lesions, but migratory thrombophlebitis and vasculitis also occur. Ocular involvement is common and may include anterior or posterior uveitis or retinal vasculitis. Neurological involvement occurs in 5% and mainly involves the brainstem, although the meninges, hemispheres and cord can also be affected, causing pyramidal signs, cranial nerve lesions, brainstem symptoms or hemiparesis. Recurrent thromboses also occur. Renal involvement is extremely rare.

The diagnosis is primarily made on clinical grounds (Box 26.68), but one characteristic feature that can be of diagnostic value is the pathergy test, which involves pricking the skin with a needle and looking for evidence of pustule development within 48 hours.

Oral and genital ulceration can be managed with a combination of colchicine and topical glucocorticoid preparations. Colchicine can be effective for erythema nodosum and arthralgia. Glucocorticoids and immunosuppressants such as azathioprine are indicated for uveitis, recurrent venous thrombosis and neurological disease. Anti-TNF-α therapy and/or thalidomide may be required in refractory patients.

Relapsing polychondritis

Relapsing polychondritis is a rare inflammatory disease of cartilage that classically presents with acute pain and swelling of one or both ear pinnae, sparing the lower non-cartilaginous portion. Around 30% of patients have coexisting autoimmune or connective tissue disease. Involvement of tracheobronchial cartilage may lead to a hoarseness, cough, stridor or expiratory wheeze. Other manifestations include collapse of the bridge of the nose, scleritis, hearing loss and cardiac valve dysfunction. Cartilage biopsy shows an inflammatory infiltrate in the perichondrium. Both ESR and CRP are raised in active disease. Pulmonary function tests, including flow–volume loops, should be performed to assess the degree of laryngotracheal disease, since this is an important cause of mortality. Mild disease usually responds to low-dose glucocorticoids or NSAIDs, whereas major tracheobronchial involvement requires high-dose glucocorticoids and immunosuppressants, as described for SLE.

IgG4 disease

This is a rare condition (1–3/100 000) characterised by an inflammatory infiltrate of affected tissues in the early stages followed by fibrotic damage as the disease progresses. The disease may present in many ways, including with swelling of the lacrimal and salivary glands (mimicking Sjögren syndrome) and proptosis, sinusitis, hearing loss, interstitial lung disease and cranial nerve lesions (mimicking GPA). Inflammatory disease of the great vessels may occur while abdominal pain may result from infiltration of the pancreas or retroperitoneum. Thyroid involvement may manifest as Hashimoto's thyroiditis and Reidel's thyroiditis. The diagnosis may be suspected by the presence of an lymphocytic infiltrate on tissue biopsy, which is rich in IgG4-secreting plasma cells, and raised serum IgG4. Management is with glucocorticoids (prednisolone 30–40 mg/day with progressive dose reduction guided by symptoms, inflammatory markers and IgG4 levels) and an immunosuppressive such as MTX, azathioprine or MMF. Intravenous rituximab has also been used successfully using a similar regimen as in RA.

Diseases of bone

Osteoporosis

Osteoporosis is the most common bone disease. It has been estimated that more than 8.9 million fractures occur annually worldwide and most of these occur in patients with osteopenia or osteoporosis. About one-third of all women and one-fifth of men aged 50 and above suffer fractures at some point in life. The burden of osteoporosis-related fractures is predicted to increase by two- to threefold by 2050 on a worldwide basis, due to ageing of the population. Osteoporosis is under-diagnosed and under-treated throughout Asia, particularly in rural areas, due to low provision of technologies like DXA, which are required to make the diagnosis. Osteoporosis-related fractures can affect any bone, but common sites are the forearm (Colles' fracture), spine (vertebral fractures), humerus and hip. All of these fractures become more common with increasing age (Fig. 26.56). Since only about one-third of vertebral fractures come to medical attention (clinical vertebral fractures), the true number of patients with vertebral fracture is likely to be much greater than that shown in Figure 26.56. Hip fractures are the most serious complication of osteoporosis and have an immediate mortality of about 12% and a continued increase in mortality of about 20% when compared with age-matched controls. Treatment of hip fracture accounts for the majority of the health-care costs associated with osteoporosis.

Pathophysiology

The defining feature of osteoporosis is reduced bone density, which causes micro-architectural deterioration of bone tissue and leads to an increased risk of fracture, in response to minor trauma. The risk of fracture increases markedly with age in both genders (see Fig. 26.56). This is mostly attributable to an increased risk of falling with age, but is also due in part to an age-related decline in bone density, especially in

26

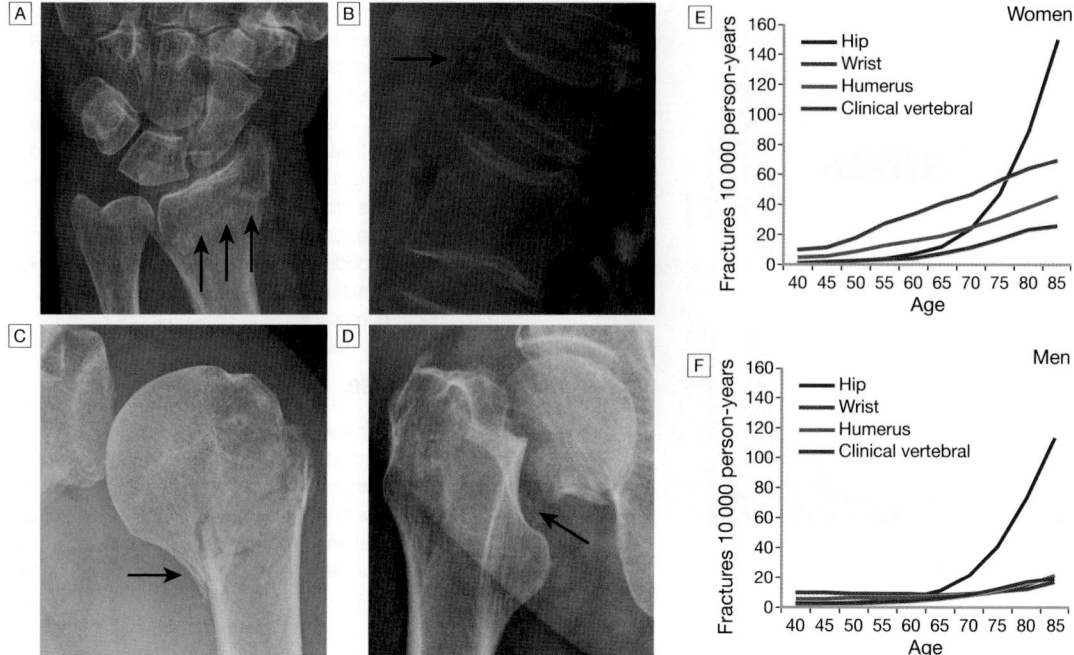

Fig. 26.56 Fractures associated with osteoporosis. [A] Wrist. [B] Vertebrae. [C] Humerus. [D] Hip. The fracture sites are indicated by black arrows. [E] and [F] The changing incidence of each of these fractures with age in women and men, respectively. *From Curtis EM, van der Velde R, Moon RJ, et al. Epidemiology of fractures in the United Kingdom, 1988–2012: variation with age, sex, geography, ethnicity and socioeconomic status. Bone 2016; 87:19–26.*

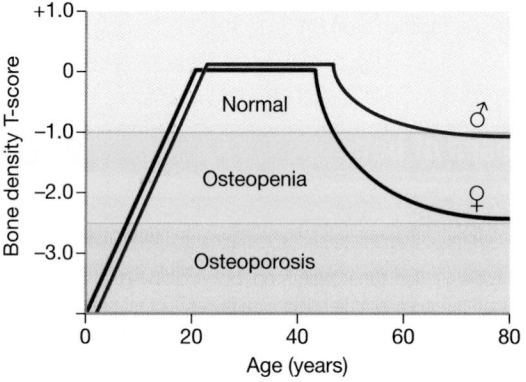

Fig. 26.57 Changes in bone mass with age. Changes in men (blue line) and women (red line).

women (Fig. 26.57). Bone mass increases during growth to reach a peak between the ages of 20 and about 45 years, but falls thereafter in both genders with an accelerated phase of bone loss after the menopause in women due to oestrogen deficiency. The loss of bone with ageing is caused by an imbalance in the bone remodelling cycle, whereby the amount of new bone formed by osteoblasts cannot keep pace with the amount that is removed by osteoclasts (see Fig. 26.2). The reduction in bone formation is thought to be partly due to differentiation of bone marrow stem cells to adipocytes, as opposed to osteoblasts. Osteoporosis sometimes occurs because of failure to attain adequate levels of peak bone mass, but is more commonly due to age-related bone loss.

Osteoporosis is a complex disease that can occur in association with a wide variety of risk factors, as summarised in Box 26.69. Genetic factors account for up to 80% of variation in bone density and genome-wide association studies have shown that susceptibility is determined in part by a large number of common variants, some of which are involved in the RANK and Wnt signalling pathways (see Fig. 26.3). Rarely, osteoporosis may be caused by mutations in single genes. Environmental factors, such as exercise and calcium intake during growth and adolescence,

i	**26.69 Risk factors for osteoporosis**

Genetics

- Single-gene disorders:
- *LRP5* mutations
- Oestrogen receptor mutations
- Polygenic inheritance:
- Common variants in many pathways

Endocrine disease

- Hypogonadism
- Hyperthyroidism
- Hyperparathyroidism
- Cushing's syndrome

Inflammatory disease

- Inflammatory bowel disease
- Ankylosing spondylitis
- Rheumatoid arthritis

Drugs

- Glucocorticoids
- Gonadotrophin-releasing hormone (GnRH) agonists
- Levothyroxine over-replacement
- Aromatase inhibitors
- Thiazolidinediones
- Anticonvulsants
- Alcohol intake > 3 U/day
- Heparin

Gastrointestinal disease

- Malabsorption
- Chronic liver disease

Lung disease

- Chronic obstructive pulmonary disease
- Cystic fibrosis

Miscellaneous

- Myeloma
- Homocystinuria
- Anorexia nervosa*
- Highly trained athletes*
- HIV infection
- Gaucher's disease
- Systemic mastocytosis
- Immobilisation
- Low body mass index
- Heavy smoking
- Autoantibodies to osteoprotegerin (OPG)

*Hypogonadism also plays a role in osteoporosis associated with these conditions.

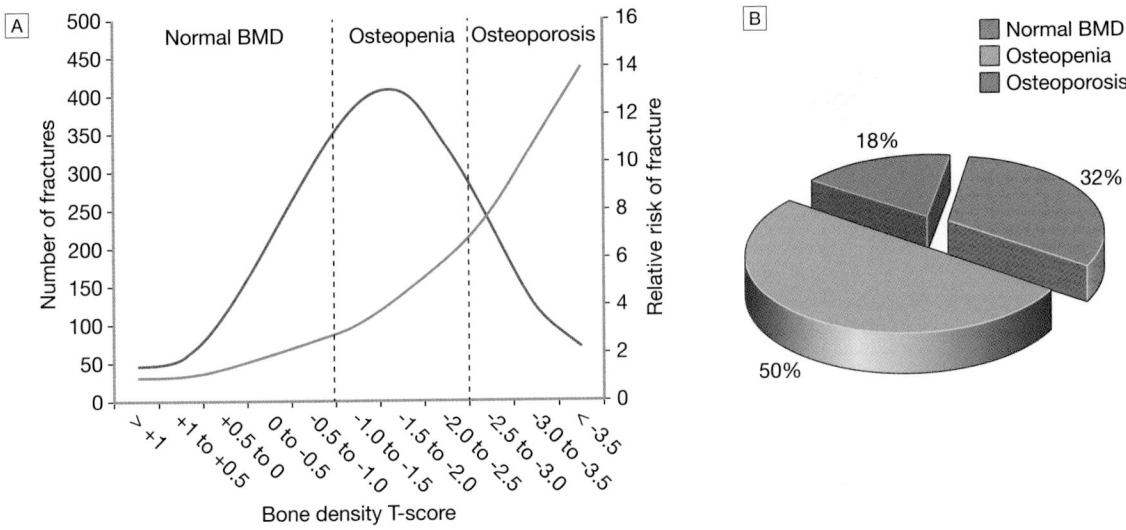

Fig. 26.58 Relation between bone mineral density (BMD) and fractures. [A] The relative risk of fracture increases exponentially as BMD falls (blue line), and is 14-fold higher in people with a T-score of <−3.5 compared with those with normal BMD. In absolute terms, however, more fractures occur in people with normal BMD or osteopenia (red line). [B] The number of fractures that occur in people with normal BMD, osteopenia and osteoporosis.

are important in maximising peak bone mass and in regulating rates of post-menopausal bone loss. Smoking has a detrimental effect on BMD and is associated with an increased fracture risk, partly because female smokers have an earlier menopause than non-smokers. Heavy alcohol intake is a recognised cause of osteoporosis and fractures, but moderate intake does not substantially alter risk.

Idiopathic osteoporosis

The term idiopathic osteoporosis is frequently used to describe the occurrence of osteoporosis in patients with no specific underlying cause. It is slightly misleading, since most, if not all, patients in this category have age-related osteoporosis or osteoporosis associated with inheritance of genetic variants that regulate bone density.

Secondary osteoporosis

Osteoporosis can occur in association with a variety of diseases and drug treatments, and in many cases more than one disease or risk factor is operative. The most important causes are summarised in Box 26.69. Secondary causes of osteoporosis are particularly common in men, occurring in up to 50% of patients. Hypogonadism, glucocorticoid use (see below) and alcohol excess are the most important predisposing factors.

Glucocorticoid-induced osteoporosis

Glucocorticoid-induced osteoporosis is a common problem in patients with systemic inflammatory and chronic pulmonary diseases. The risk of osteoporosis is related to dose and duration of glucocorticoid therapy and increases substantially in patients who have taken more than 7.5 mg of prednisolone daily for more than 3 months (or an equivalent dose of another glucocorticoid). Inhaled glucocorticoids can reduce bone density, but the risk of osteoporosis is much lower than with systemic therapy. Glucocorticoids mainly cause osteoporosis by inhibiting bone formation and causing apoptosis of osteoblasts and osteocytes. Other contributory mechanisms include inhibition of intestinal calcium absorption, increased renal excretion of calcium and secondary hyperparathyroidism, which stimulates osteoclastic bone resorption.

Pregnancy-associated osteoporosis

This is a rare form of osteoporosis that typically presents with back pain and multiple vertebral fractures usually during the third trimester or puerperium. It is discussed in more detail in Chapter 32.

i	26.70 Indications for dual X-ray absorptiometry (DXA)

- Low-trauma fracture, age > 50 years
- Clinical risk factors and 10-year fracture risk > 10%
- Glucocorticoid therapy (> 7.5 mg prednisolone daily for > 3 months)
- Baseline and follow-up assessment of response of osteoporosis to treatment
- Assessment of progression of osteopenia to osteoporosis
- Age < 50 years and strong risk factors for osteoporosis

Clinical features

Osteoporosis does not cause symptoms until a fracture occurs. Non-vertebral fractures are almost always caused by a traumatic event, most usually a simple fall. The term 'fragility fracture' is used to describe a fracture that occurs as the result of a fall from standing height or less. These are typical of osteoporosis. It is important to remember that the majority of people who suffer a fragility fracture do not have osteoporosis; some have normal BMD, but most have osteopenia (Fig. 26.58). The clinical signs of fracture are pain, local tenderness and deformity. In hip fracture, the patient is (with rare exceptions) unable to weight-bear and has a shortened and externally rotated limb on the affected side. The presentation of vertebral fractures is variable. Some patients present with acute severe back pain. This may radiate to the anterior chest or abdominal wall and be mistaken for a myocardial infarction, aortic dissection or intra-abdominal pathology. In others the presentation is with height loss and kyphosis in the absence of pain or with chronic back pain. Osteoporosis may be suspected by the finding of radiological osteopenia or vertebral deformities on imaging that has been performed for other reasons.

Investigations

The most important investigation is DXA (see Fig. 26.9). This should be considered in patients aged over 50 who have already suffered a fragility fracture, and in those with clinical risk factors (Box 26.70) when a fracture risk assessment tool has returned an elevated value. The risk at which DXA should be performed remains a subject of debate, but a 10-year risk of over 10% has been suggested, since there is evidence of benefit from treatment at this level. Other indications for DXA are in patients under 50 years who have very strong risk factors, such as premature menopause or high-dose glucocorticoids. Figure 26.59 provides a suggested algorithm for the investigation of patients with suspected osteoporosis.

26

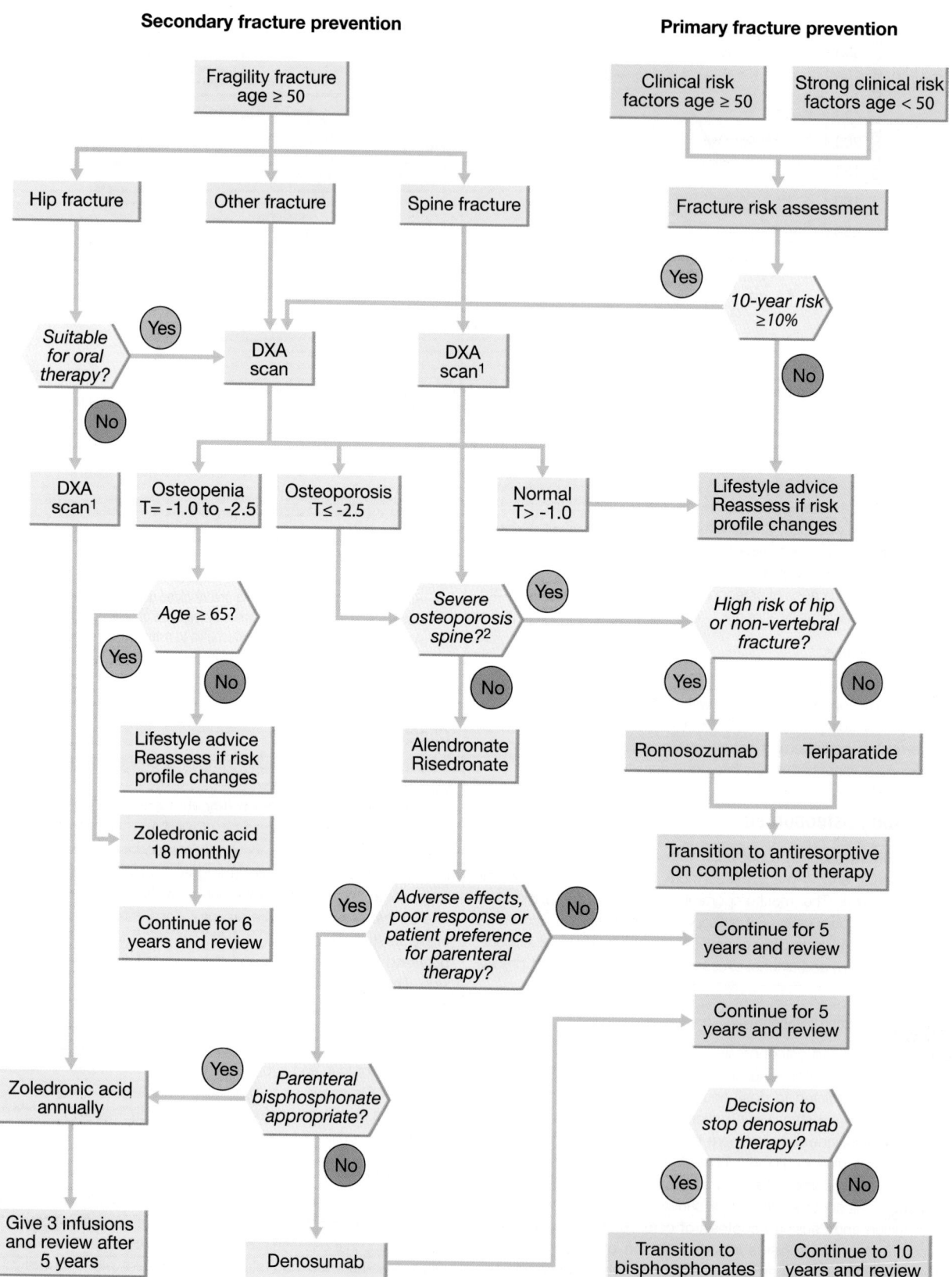

Fig. 26.59 Algorithm for the diagnosis and management of osteoporosis. [1]DXA scan advisable to obtain baseline BMD but not necessary to initiate treatment. [2]One severe or two or more moderate vertebral fractures on X-ray, and T-score < −1.5 at any site or spine T score < −4.0. *Adapted from SIGN 142. www.sign/ac/uk*

A history should be taken to identify any predisposing causes, such as early menopause, excessive alcohol intake, smoking and glucocorticoid therapy. Signs of endocrine disease, neoplasia and inflammatory disease should be sought on clinical examination. A falls history should be taken and screening tests performed to assess the risk of falls (p. 1297). Screening for secondary causes of osteoporosis should be performed, as summarised in Box 26.71.

Management

The aim of treatment is to reduce the risk of fracture and this can be achieved by a combination of approaches.

Non-pharmacological interventions

Advice on smoking cessation, moderation of alcohol intake, adequate dietary calcium intake and exercise should be given. Those with recurrent falls or unsteadiness on a 'get up and go' test (p. 1297) should be referred to a multidisciplinary falls-prevention team. Hip protectors can reduce the risk of hip fracture in selected patients, but adherence is often poor.

Pharmacological interventions

Several drug treatments are now available to reduce the risk of fracture in osteoporosis. The dosages, mode of administration and indications are summarised in Box 26.72. More detail on the individual drugs is provided below.

Bisphosphonates Bisphosphonates are the first-line treatment for osteoporosis. These are a class of drugs with a central core of P-C-P atoms, to which various side-chains are attached. Following administration, they target bone surfaces and are ingested by osteoclasts during the process of bone resorption. The bisphosphonate is released within the osteoclast, causing cell death and thereby bone resorption. This in turn causes an increase in bone density, but this is principally due to increased mineralisation of bone, rather than an increase in bone mass (Fig. 26.60). Bisphosphonates reduce the risk of fractures in osteoporosis, but do not completely prevent the occurrence of fractures.

Oral bisphosphonates are typically given for a period of 5 years, at which point the need for continued therapy should be evaluated, with a repeat DXA if possible. If patients have remained free of fractures after 5 years and if BMD levels have increased and no longer remain in the osteoporotic range, it is usual to instigate a 5-year spell off therapy. Treatment may be continued for up to 10 years in patients whose BMD levels remain in the osteoporotic range after 5 years and in those with pre-existing vertebral fractures. A change in treatment should be considered in patients who have lost BMD despite oral bisphosphonates (more than 4% at any site). Most commonly, this will be a switch to parenteral zoledronic acid which is often given by annual infusion of 5 mg for 3 consecutive years followed by a spell of 2 years without treatment. Infusions every 18 months over a spell of 6 years have also been found to be effective for fracture prevention.

Oral bisphosphonates are poorly absorbed from the gastrointestinal tract and should be taken on an empty stomach with plain water; no

26.71 Investigations to consider in suspected osteoporosis

Investigation	Secondary cause of osteoporosis
Urea, creatinine and electrolytes	Chronic kidney disease
Liver function tests and albumin	Chronic liver disease
Full blood count, erythrocyte sedimentation rate	Inflammatory disease Myeloma
Tissue transglutaminase antibodies	Coeliac disease
Serum calcium and phosphate, 25(OH)D, PTH	Primary and secondary hyperparathyroidism, vitamin D deficiency. Normocalcaemic PHPT exists with reference range calcium
Thyroid function tests	Hyperthyroidism
Serum protein electrophoresis	Myeloma Monoclonal gammopathy of uncertain significance
Urine Bence Jones protein	Myeloma
Testosterone and gonadotrophins	Male hypogonadism
Oestrogen and gonadotrophins	Female hypogonadism[1]
Bone biopsy	Unexplained early-onset osteoporosis[2]

[1]Only required for unexplained osteoporosis in young women who are amenorrhoeic. [2]Seldom required.
(25(OH)D = 25 hydroxy-vitamin D; PTH = parathyroid hormone)

26.72 Drug treatments for osteoporosis

Drug	Regimen	Postmenopausal osteoporosis	Glucocorticoid osteoporosis	Male osteoporosis
Alendronic acid	70 mg/week orally	✓	✓	✓
Risedronate	35 mg/week orally	✓	✓	✓
Ibandronate	150 mg/monthly orally 3 mg/3-monthly IV	✓	✓	✓
Zoledronic acid	5 mg annually IV	✓	✓	✓
Denosumab	60 mg 6-monthly SC	✓	✓	✓
Calcium/vitamin D	Calcium 500–1000 mg daily Vitamin D 400–800 IU orally	✓	✓	✓
Teriparatide	20 µg/day SC	✓	✓	✓
Abaloparatide	80 µg/day SC	✓	–	–
Romosozumab	210 mg/month SC	✓		
Hormone replacement therapy	Various preparations	✓	–	–
Raloxifene	60 mg/day orally	✓	–	–
Tibolone	1.25 mg/day orally	✓	–	–

(IV = intravenous; SC = subcutaneous)

26

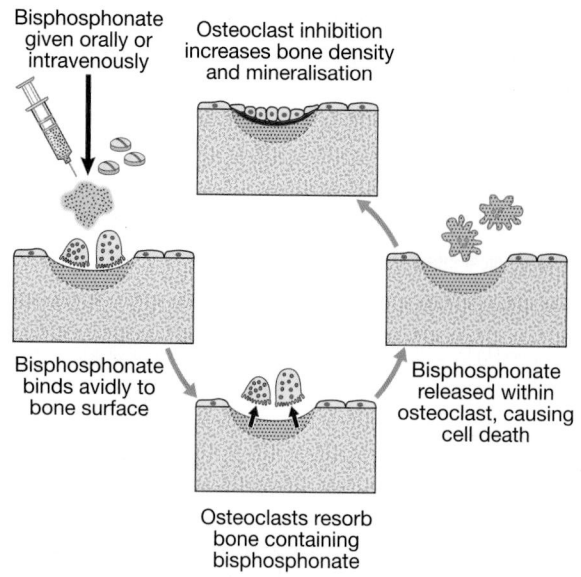

Fig. 26.60 Mechanism of action of bisphosphonates.

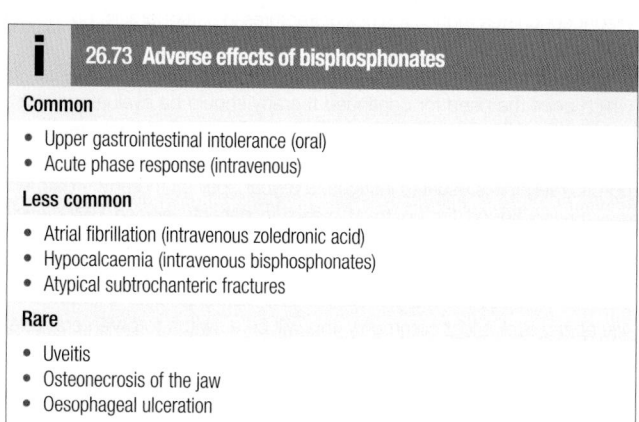

i · 26.73 Adverse effects of bisphosphonates

Common

• Upper gastrointestinal intolerance (oral)
• Acute phase response (intravenous)

Less common

• Atrial fibrillation (intravenous zoledronic acid)
• Hypocalcaemia (intravenous bisphosphonates)
• Atypical subtrochanteric fractures

Rare

• Uveitis
• Osteonecrosis of the jaw
• Oesophageal ulceration

food should be eaten for 30–45 minutes after administration. They are contraindicated in patients with oesophageal stricture or achalasia, since tablets may stick in the oesophagus, causing ulceration and perforation. Upper gastrointestinal upset occurs in about 5% of cases. Oral bisphosphonates can be used in patients with gastro-oesophageal reflux disease, but may cause worsening of symptoms. The most common adverse effect with intravenous bisphosphonates is a transient influenza-like illness with fever, malaise, anorexia and generalised aches, which occurs 24–48 hours after administration. This is self-limiting, but can be treated with paracetamol or NSAIDs if necessary. It predominantly occurs after the first exposure and tolerance develops thereafter. Other adverse effects are shown in Box 26.73. Osteonecrosis of the jaw is characterised by the presence of necrotic bone in the mandible or maxilla, typically occurring after tooth extraction when the socket fails to heal. This complication is very rare in osteoporosis, but patients receiving bisphosphonates should be advised to pay attention to good oral hygiene. There is no evidence that temporarily stopping bisphosphonates for tooth extraction alters the risk of osteonecrosis of the jaw. Atypical subtrochanteric fractures have been described in patients who have received long-term bisphosphonates and appear to be the result of over-suppression of normal bone remodelling. In the vast majority, the benefits of bisphosphonate therapy far outweigh the risks, but it is important for treatment to be targeted to patients with low BMD who are most likely to benefit.

Denosumab Denosumab is a monoclonal antibody that inhibits bone resorption by neutralising the effects of RANKL (see Fig. 26.2). It is administered by subcutaneous injection of 60 mg every 6 months in the

👤 26.74 Osteoporosis in old age

• **Bone loss:** due to increased bone turnover, with an age-related defect switch in differentiation of bone marrow stromal cells to form adipocytes as opposed to osteoblasts.
• **Fractures due to osteoporosis:** common cause of morbidity and mortality, although fracture healing is not delayed by age.
• **Recurrent fractures:** those who suffer a fragility fracture are at increased risk of further fracture, so should be investigated for osteoporosis and treated if this is confirmed.
• **Falls:** risk factors for falls (such as visual and neuromuscular impairments) are independent risk factors for hip fracture in older people, so intervention to prevent falls is as important as treatment of osteoporosis.
• **Intravenous zoledronic acid:** reduces mortality and subsequent fracture in selected older patients with hip fractures.
• **Calcium and vitamin D:** reduce the risk of fractures in those who are housebound or living in care homes.

treatment of osteoporosis and has similar efficacy to zoledronic acid. One potential adverse effect is hypocalcaemia, but this can be mitigated by calcium and vitamin D supplements. Denosumab may rarely cause osteonecrosis of the jaw and atypical subtrochanteric fractures. When denosumab is stopped, there is a rebound increase in bone turnover that can be associated with an increased risk of vertebral fracture and even hypercalcaemia. Because of this denosumab needs to be continued on a long-term basis; if it has to be stopped for any reason, bisphosphonate therapy should be given to inhibit the rebound increase in bone turnover.

Calcium and vitamin D Combined calcium and vitamin D supplements have limited efficacy in the prevention of osteoporotic fractures when given alone, but are widely used as an adjunct to other treatments. A typical daily dosage is 1000 mg calcium and 800 IU vitamin D. Calcium and vitamin D supplements have efficacy in preventing fragility fractures in old age or in institutionalised patients, who are at high risk of deficiency (Box 26.74). Vitamin D supplements alone do not prevent fractures in osteoporosis, but there is evidence that the response to bisphosphonates is blunted in patients with vitamin D deficiency. If the patient's dietary calcium is sufficient, stand-alone vitamin D supplements (800 IU daily) can be prescribed as an adjunct to anti-osteoporosis therapies. Calcitriol ($1,25(OH)_2D_3$), the active metabolite of vitamin D, is licensed for treatment of osteoporosis but it is seldom used because the data on fracture prevention are less robust than for other agents.

Teriparatide Teriparatide (TPTD) is the 1-34 fragment of human PTH. It is an effective treatment for osteoporosis, which works by stimulating new bone formation. Although TPTD also stimulates bone resorption, the increase in bone formation is greater, resulting in increased bone density, particularly at sites rich in trabecular bone such as the spine. It is given by a self-administered subcutaneous injection in a dose of 20 μg daily for 2 years. At the end of this period, bisphosphonate therapy or another inhibitor of bone resorption should be administered to maintain the increase in BMD. Oral bisphosphonates and TPTD should not be given in combination, however, since the bisphosphonate blunts the anabolic effect. The efficacy of TPTD for prevention of non-vertebral fractures is similar to that of bisphosphonates, but it is superior to oral bisphosphonates in preventing vertebral fractures. The most common adverse effects are headache, muscle cramps and dizziness. Mild hypercalcaemia may occur, but it is usually asymptomatic and does not require discontinuation of treatment. Monitoring of serum calcium is not required during TPTD treatment.

Abaloparatide Abaloparatide is the 1-34 fragment of PTH-related protein which has effects similar to those of TPTD. It is given as a self-administered injection of 80 μg daily for 18 months. At the end of this period an inhibitor of bone resorption should be given to maintain the increase in bone mass. Efficacy has been demonstrated for the prevention of vertebral fractures.

i | **26.75 Causes of osteomalacia and rickets**

Cause	Predisposing factor	Mechanism
Vitamin D deficiency		
Classical	Lack of sunlight exposure and poor diet	Reduced cholecalciferol synthesis in the skin/low levels of vitamin D in the diet
Gastrointestinal disease	Malabsorption	Malabsorption of dietary vitamin D and calcium
Failure of 1,25 vitamin D synthesis		
Chronic renal failure	Hyperphosphataemia and kidney damage	Impaired conversion of $25(OH)D_3$ to $1,25(OH)_2D_3$
Vitamin D-resistant rickets type I (autosomal recessive)	Loss-of-function mutations in renal 25(OH)D 1α-hydroxylase enzyme	Impaired conversion of $25(OH)D_3$ to $1,25(OH)_2D_3$
Vitamin D receptor defects		
Vitamin D-resistant rickets type II (autosomal recessive)	Loss-of-function mutations in vitamin D receptor	Impaired response to $1,25(OH)_2D_3$
Defects in phosphate and pyrophosphate metabolism		
Hypophosphataemic rickets (X-linked dominant)	Mutations in *PHEX*	Increased FGF23 production (mechanism unclear)
Autosomal dominant hypophosphataemic rickets	Mutation in *FGF23*	Mutant FGF23 is resistant to degradation
Autosomal recessive hypophosphataemic rickets	Mutations in *DMP1*	Increased production of FGF23. Local deficiency of DMP1 inhibits mineralisation
Tumour-induced hypophosphataemic osteomalacia	Ectopic production of FGF23 by tumour	Over-production of FGF23
Hypophosphatasia	Mutations in *ALPL*, which encodes alkaline phosphatase	Inhibition of bone mineralisation due to accumulation of pyrophosphate in bone
Iatrogenic and other causes		
Bisphosphonate therapy	High-dose etidronate/pamidronate	Drug-induced impairment of mineralisation
Aluminium	Use of aluminium-containing phosphate binders or aluminium in dialysis fluid	Aluminium-induced impairment of mineralisation
Fluoride	High fluoride in water	Inhibition of mineralisation by fluoride

(FGF23 = fibroblast growth factor 23)

Romosozumab This is a neutralising antibody to sclerostin, which is produced by osteocytes and acts to inhibit bone formation (see Fig. 26.3). Romosozumab is a highly effective treatment for osteoporosis and works by inhibiting bone resorption and stimulating bone formation. It is indicated for the treatment of severe osteoporosis, where it is given by self-administered subcutaneous injection 210 mg once a month for 12 months. Following completion of treatment, an inhibitor of bone resorption should be given to maintain the increase in bone density. Romosozumab is significantly more effective than oral alendronic acid at preventing fractures of all types and it is one of the most effective treatments for osteoporosis currently available. Adverse effects are uncommon, although a slight excess of cardiovascular events was observed in some clinical trials and because of that it is contraindicated in patients with a previous history of myocardial infarction or stroke.

Hormone replacement therapy Cyclical HRT with oestrogen and progestogen prevents post-menopausal bone loss and reduces the risk of vertebral and non-vertebral fractures in post-menopausal women. It is primarily indicated for the prevention of osteoporosis in women with an early menopause and for treatment of women with osteoporosis in their early fifties who have troublesome menopausal symptoms. It is not recommended above the age of 60 because of an increased risk of breast cancer, cardiovascular disease and venous thromboembolism.

Raloxifene Raloxifene is a selective oestrogen receptor modulator (SERM) that acts as a partial agonist at oestrogen receptors in bone and liver, but as an antagonist in breast and endometrium. It is effective in reducing the risk of vertebral fractures, but does not influence the risk of non-vertebral fracture and is seldom used. Adverse effects include muscle cramps, worsening of hot flushes and an increased risk of venous thromboembolism. Bazedoxifene is a related SERM that has similar effects to raloxifene.

Tibolone

Tibolone has partial agonist activity at oestrogen, progestogen and androgen receptors. It has been shown to prevent vertebral and non-vertebral fractures in post-menopausal osteoporosis. Treatment is associated with a slightly increased risk of stroke, but a reduced risk of breast cancer.

Surgery

Orthopaedic surgery with internal fixation is frequently required to reduce and stabilise osteoporotic fractures. Patients with intracapsular fracture of the femoral neck generally need hemi-arthroplasty or total hip replacement in view of the high risk of osteonecrosis.

Vertebroplasty is sometimes used in the treatment of painful vertebral compression fractures. It involves injecting methyl methacrylate (MMA) into the affected vertebral body under sedation and local anaesthesia. Randomised trials have not shown convincing evidence of benefit as compared with a sham procedure. Kyphoplasty is used under similar circumstances, but in this case a needle is introduced into the affected vertebral body and a balloon is inflated, which is then filled with MMA. It has similar efficacy to vertebroplasty. Serious adverse effects may occur with both procedures, including spinal cord compression due to leakage of MMA and fat embolism.

Osteomalacia, rickets and vitamin D deficiency

Osteomalacia and rickets are characterised by defective mineralisation of bone. The most common cause is vitamin D deficiency, but both conditions can also occur as the result of inherited defects in renal phosphate excretion, inherited defects in the vitamin D receptor and in the pathways responsible for vitamin D activation. Other causes are summarised in Box 26.75 and are discussed in more detail below. The term osteomalacia refers to the syndrome when it occurs in adults; rickets is the equivalent in children.

26

Vitamin D deficiency

Vitamin D deficiency is a biochemical diagnosis, which is defined to be present when serum 25(OH)D concentrations are below 25 nmol/L (10 ng/mL). People with vitamin D levels in the range 25–50 nmol/L (10–20 ng/mL) are said to have vitamin D insufficiency, whereas those with 25(OH)D levels above 50 nmol/L (20 ng/mL) are classified as having normal vitamin D status. The likelihood of developing vitamin D deficiency is strongly related to sunlight exposure. It is common in northern latitudes (or southern latitudes in the southern hemisphere) and shows seasonal variation. Vitamin D deficiency is more common in the winter and spring and less common in summer and autumn (for a UK example, see Fig. 26.61). People with dark skin and those who wear facial coverings are more prone to developing vitamin D deficiency.

Pathogenesis

The source of vitamin D and pathways involved in regulating its metabolism are shown in Figure 26.62. In normal individuals, vitamin D (also known as cholecalciferol) comes from two sources: about 70% is made in the skin, where 7-dehydrocholesterol is converted to cholecalciferol under the influence of ultraviolet light, whereas the remaining 30% is derived from the diet. The main dietary sources are oily fish and meat, although bread and dairy products are fortified with vitamin D in some countries. On entering the circulation, vitamin D is hydroxylated in the liver to form 25(OH)-vitamin D and this is further hydroxylated in the kidney to form 1,25(OH)$_2$D, the biologically active metabolite. The 1,25(OH)$_2$D primarily acts on the gut to increase intestinal calcium absorption, but also acts on the skeleton to stimulate bone remodelling. Synthesis of 1,25(OH)$_2$D is regulated by a negative feedback loop orchestrated by the parathyroid glands. When vitamin D levels fall – as the result of lower sunlight exposure or dietary lack – production of 1,25(OH)$_2$D is reduced, causing a reduction in calcium absorption from the gut. This causes a transient fall in serum calcium, which is detected by calcium-sensing receptors on the parathyroid chief cells; this increases PTH secretion, which restores calcium levels to normal. Vitamin D deficiency is, therefore, usually characterised by a low level of 25(OH)D and a raised level of PTH. Sometimes, low 25(OH)D levels may be observed in the presence of a normal PTH concentration. This is of uncertain clinical significance and can be due to variations in levels of vitamin D-binding protein. Serum concentrations of vitamin D are under genetic control and are associated with variants close to the *GC* gene, which encodes vitamin D-binding

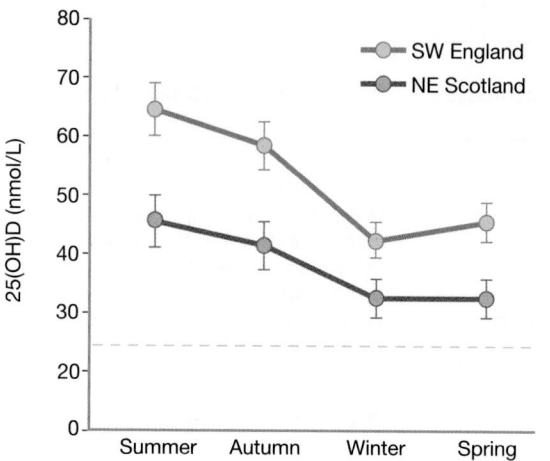

Fig. 26.61 Seasonal changes in vitamin D concentrations. (To convert nmol/L to ng/mL, multiply by 2.5.) *Adapted from McDonald HM, Mavroeidi A, Fraser WD, et al. Sunlight and dietary contributions to the seasonal vitamin D status of cohorts of healthy postmenopausal women living at northerly latitudes: a major cause for concern? Osteoporosis Int 2011; 22:2461–2472.*

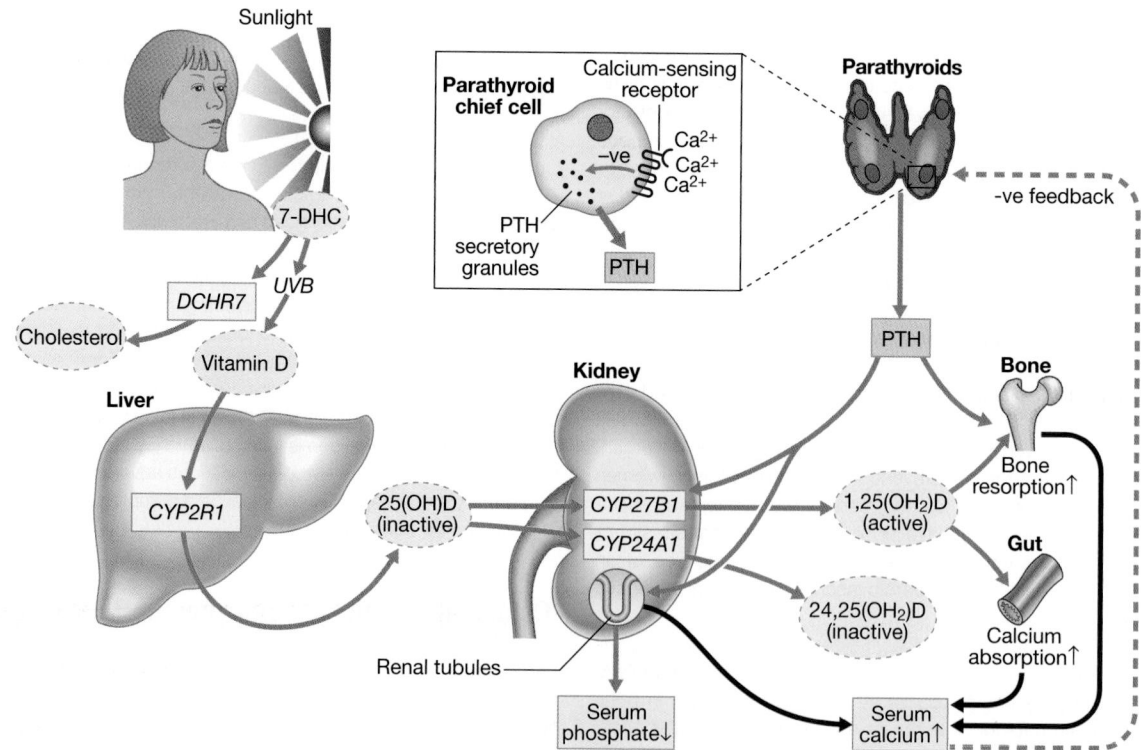

Fig. 26.62 Vitamin D metabolism. Vitamin D is produced in the skin from 7-dehydrocholesterol (7-DHC) by ultraviolet B (UVB) light. The 7-dehydrocholesterol reductase enzyme, which is encoded by the *DHCR7* gene, opposes the effect of UVB by converting 7-DHC to cholesterol. The vitamin D then undergoes hydroxylation steps in the liver and kidney to form the active metabolite 1,25(OH)$_2$D, which regulates calcium homeostasis by stimulating calcium absorption from the diet and bone resorption. See text for details. (PTH = parathyroid hormone)

protein; the *DHCR7* gene, which encodes 7-dehydrocholesterol reductase, responsible for catalysing conversion of 7-DHC to cholesterol; the *CYP2R1* gene, which encodes vitamin D-25-hydroxylase, responsible for hydroxylation of vitamin D in the liver; and the *CYP24A1* gene, which encodes vitamin D-24-hydroxylase, responsible for converting 25(OH)D to the inactive metabolite 24,25(OH)$_2$D.

Clinical features

Low circulating levels of vitamin D do not cause symptoms unless the vitamin D deficiency is severe, so the diagnosis of vitamin D deficiency is primarily made as the result of biochemical testing. A wide range of diseases, including most types of cancer, diabetes, multiple sclerosis and chronic inflammatory diseases have been associated with vitamin D deficiency. Current evidence suggests that these are not causal associations, but explained by confounding whereby people who are unwell have reduced sunlight exposure and poor diet. If vitamin D deficiency is prolonged and severe, then osteomalacia and rickets may occur, as discussed below.

Investigations

The diagnosis can be made by measurement of serum 25(OH)D. In patients with low 25(OH)D, measurements of PTH, serum calcium, phosphate and ALP should also be considered. Low levels of 25(OH)D in the absence of other abnormalities is unlikely to be of any clinical significance and in many cases is likely to be due to low levels of vitamin D-binding protein, the levels of which are genetically determined. If low 25(OH)D levels are combined with raised levels of PTH, this is of more significance since it indicates secondary hyperparathyroidism, which if untreated and prolonged, may impair bone health and eventually lead to osteomalacia or rickets.

Management

Vitamin D supplements should be considered in patients who have low 25(OH)D levels and raised levels of PTH. In most young adults, greater exposure to UV light and cholecalciferol in a dose of 800 IU daily should be sufficient to correct the deficiency. Short courses of high-strength vitamin D can also be used, such as 20000 IU once weekly for 4–6 weeks. The benefit of treating low 25(OH)D values in the absence of other abnormalities of calcium biochemistry is uncertain. There is some evidence that response to bisphosphonate treatment of osteoporosis is impaired in patients with vitamin D deficiency and this is an indication for supplements. Similarly, patients who are receiving intravenous bisphosphonates and denosumab for osteoporosis should have vitamin D deficiency corrected by supplementation to reduce the risk of hypocalcaemia.

Osteomalacia and rickets

Severe and prolonged vitamin D deficiency can result in the occurrence of osteomalacia in adults and rickets in children. Improvements in nutrition mean that these are now relatively uncommon conditions in high-income countries, but they remain prevalent in older housebound individuals, who may have a poor diet and limited sunlight exposure, in women who wear facial coverings such as the niqab or burka, and in people with malabsorption.

Pathogenesis

Osteomalacia and rickets occur as the result of chronic secondary hyperparathyroidism, which invariably accompanies severe and long-standing vitamin D deficiency. The sustained elevation in PTH levels maintains normal levels of serum calcium by increasing bone resorption, which eventually causes progressive demineralisation of the skeleton. Phosphate released during the process of bone resorption is lost through increased renal excretion, resulting in hypophosphataemia. The raised levels of PTH stimulate osteoblast activity and cause new bone formation, but the matrix is not mineralised properly because of deficiency of calcium and phosphate. The under-mineralised bone is soft, mechanically weak and subject to fractures, particularly stress fractures. Normal levels of serum calcium tend to be maintained until a very advanced stage, when hypocalcaemia may occur.

Clinical features

Vitamin D deficiency in children causes delayed development, muscle hypotonia, craniotabes (small unossified areas in membranous bones of the skull that yield to finger pressure with a cracking feeling), bossing of the frontal and parietal bones and delayed anterior fontanelle closure, enlargement of epiphyses at the lower end of the radius and swelling of the rib costochondral junctions ('rickety rosary'). Osteomalacia in adults can present with fractures and low BMD, mimicking osteoporosis. Other symptoms include bone pain and general malaise. Proximal muscle weakness is prominent and the patient may walk with a waddling gait and struggle to climb stairs or stand up from a chair. There may be bone and muscle tenderness on pressure and focal bone pain can be due to fissure fractures of the ribs and pelvis.

Investigations

The diagnosis can usually be made by measurement of serum 25(OH)D, PTH, calcium, phosphate and ALP. Typically, serum ALP levels are raised, 25(OH)D levels are undetectable and PTH is markedly elevated. Serum phosphate levels tend to be low, but serum calcium is usually normal, unless the disease is advanced. X-rays often show osteopenia or vertebral crush fractures and, with more advanced disease, focal radiolucent areas (pseudofractures or Looser zones) may be seen in ribs, pelvis and long bones (Fig. 26.63). In children, there is thickening and widening of the epiphyseal plate. A radionuclide bone scan may show multiple hot spots in the ribs and pelvis at the site of fractures and the appearance may be mistaken for metastases. Where there is doubt, the diagnosis can be confirmed by bone biopsy, which shows the pathognomonic increased thickness and extent of osteoid seams (see Fig. 26.63).

Management

Osteomalacia and rickets respond promptly to treatment with vitamin D. A wide variety of doses can be used. Treatment with between 10000 and 25000 IU daily for 2–4 weeks is associated with rapid clinical improvement, an elevation in serum 25(OH)D and a reduction in PTH. Serum ALP levels sometimes rise initially as mineralisation of bone increases, but eventually fall to within the reference range as the bone disease heals. Subsequently, the dose of vitamin D can usually be reduced to a maintenance level of 800–1600 IU daily (10–20 µg), except in patients with malabsorption, who may require higher maintenance doses.

Vitamin D-resistant rickets

This is a genetically determined condition that presents in childhood with rickets that is resistant to therapy with vitamin D in standard dosages.

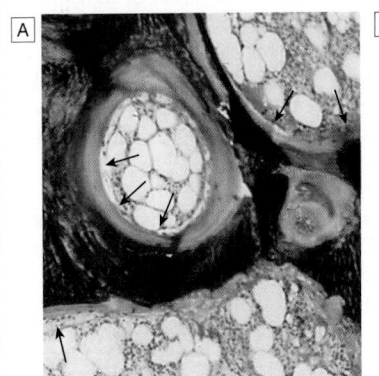
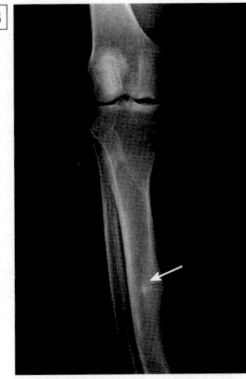

Fig. 26.63 Osteomalacia. **A** Photomicrograph of a toluidine blue-stained bone biopsy from a patient with osteomalacia showing thickened osteoid seams, stained light blue (arrows) covering most of the bone surface (left). Calcified bone is stained purple. **B** X-ray of a patient with osteomalacia showing a stress fracture of the tibia (arrow).

26

Pathogenesis

Type I vitamin D-resistant rickets (VDRR) is caused by inactivating mutations in the 25(OH)D-1α-hydroxylase (*CYP27B1*) enzyme, which converts 25(OH)D to the active metabolite $1,25(OH)_2D_3$. Type II VDRR is caused by inactivating mutations in the vitamin D receptor, which impair its ability to activate gene transcription. Both are recessive disorders and consanguinity is common.

Clinical features

These are as described above for infantile rickets. The diagnosis is usually first suspected when the patient fails to respond to vitamin D supplementation.

Investigations

The biochemical features of type I VDRR are similar to those of ordinary vitamin D deficiency, except that levels of 25(OH)D are normal, but $1,25(OH)_2D$ is low. In type II VDRR, 25(OH)D is normal, but PTH and $1,25(OH)_2D_3$ values are raised. The diagnosis can be confirmed by genetic testing.

Management

Type I VDRR responds fully to treatment with the active vitamin D metabolites 1α-hydroxy-vitamin D (1–2 μg daily, orally) or 1,25-dihydroxy-vitamin D (0.25–1.5 μg daily, orally). Calcium supplements are not necessary unless there is dietary deficiency. Type II VDRR sometimes responds partially to very high doses of active vitamin D metabolites, which can activate the mutant receptor, although additional calcium and phosphate supplements are also necessary.

Hereditary hypophosphataemic rickets

This group of disorders are caused by inherited defects in renal tubular phosphate reabsorption. The most common is X-linked hypophosphataemic rickets (XLH), but autosomal dominant and autosomal recessive forms also occur (see Box 26.75).

Pathophysiology

Most forms of hereditary hypophosphataemic rickets are associated with raised circulating concentrations of the phosphate-regulating hormone fibroblast growth factor 23 (FGF23). This hormone is produced by osteocytes (see Fig. 26.3) and enters the circulation, where it is normally inactivated by proteolytic cleavage. Production of FGF23 by osteocytes is under tonic inhibition by DMP1 and PHEX. In XLH, the inhibitory effect on FGF23 production is lost due to mutations in *PHEX* and a similar situation occurs in autosomal recessive hypophosphataemic rickets (ARHR1) due to loss-of-function mutations in *DMP1*. In autosomal dominant hypophosphataemic rickets (ADHR), the FGF23 protein carries mutations that prevent FGF23 being degraded, thereby causing accumulation of intact FGF23 hormone in the circulation. In all three diseases, the elevation in FGF23 results in osteomalacia and rickets by causing phosphaturia by up-regulation of sodium-dependent phosphate transporters in the renal tubules, and also by inhibiting conversion of 25(OH)D to $1,25(OH)_2D$ by the kidney, which in turn causes reduced calcium and phosphate absorption from the gut.

Clinical features

The presentation is with symptoms and signs of rickets during childhood that do not respond to vitamin D supplementation. In adults, hypophosphataemic rickets may be accompanied by dental abscesses, and by bone and joint pain due to the development of an enthesopathy.

Investigations

The diagnosis can be confirmed by the finding of low serum phosphate levels and a reduction in tubular reabsorption of phosphate. Serum levels of vitamin D are normal and PTH is normal or elevated. Serum concentrations of FGF23 are markedly elevated. The causal mutations can be identified by genetic testing.

Management

The aim of treatment is to ameliorate symptoms, restore normal growth and maintain serum phosphate levels within the reference range. Traditionally, treatment has been with phosphate supplements (1–4 g daily) and alfacalcidol (1–2 μg daily) or calcitriol (0.5–1.5 μg daily), with the aim of promoting intestinal calcium and phosphate absorption. Levels of calcium and phosphate, as well as renal function, should be monitored regularly and the doses of phosphate and vitamin D metabolites carefully titrated to maintain serum phosphate within the normal range, but avoid hypercalcaemia. Burosumab is a neutralising antibody to FGF23 which can reverse the biochemical abnormalities in hereditary hypophosphataemic rickets. It is currently licensed for the treatment of XLH in children where it has been shown to be superior to standard therapy with phosphate supplements and active vitamin D metabolites at healing rickets. It is also effective at reversing hypophosphataemia in adults, and trials are currently in progress to examine the effects on clinical outcome of the disease in adults.

Tumour-induced osteomalacia

This is a rare syndrome caused by over-production of FGF23 by mesenchymal tumours. The presentation is with severe osteomalacia and hypophosphataemia in an adult patient with no obvious predisposing risk factor for vitamin D deficiency. Biochemical findings are as described for hereditary hypophosphataemic rickets. The underlying tumour can be difficult to find and multiple modality imaging with whole-body MRI, CT and somatostatin or gallium-68 DOTATATE scintigraphy is often needed. Options for medical management include phosphate supplements and active vitamin D metabolites or burosumab, but the treatment of choice is surgical resection of the primary tumour, which is curative.

Hypophosphatasia

Hypophosphatasia is an autosomal recessive disorder caused by loss-of-function mutations in the *TNALP* gene, which results in accumulation of pyrophosphate and inhibition of bone mineralisation. The typical presentation is with severe intractable rickets during infancy, sometimes in association with seizures. Investigations show low or undetectable levels of serum ALP, but normal levels of calcium, phosphate, PTH and vitamin D metabolites. Urine excretion of pyridoxal 5′ phosphate and phosphoethanolamine (substrates for ALP) is increased. In severely affected patients, remarkable therapeutic responses have been obtained with recombinant ALP therapy (asfotase alfa), which is curative. Heterozygous carriers of mutation in *TNALP* may present in adulthood with osteoporosis, fractures and low ALP values. The best mode of treatment for these patients remains to be determined.

Other causes of osteomalacia

These are summarised in Box 26.75. Osteomalacia may occur as a component of renal osteodystrophy in patients with chronic kidney disease. The mechanism is reduced conversion of 25(OH)D into the active metabolite $1,25(OH)_2D$ by the failing kidney. Aluminium intoxication is now rare due to reduced use of aluminium-containing phosphate binders and removal of aluminium from the water supplies used in dialysis. If aluminium intoxication is suspected, the diagnosis can be confirmed by demonstration of aluminium at the calcification front in a bone biopsy. Osteomalacia due to bisphosphonates has mostly been described in patients with Paget's disease who are receiving etidronate and high-dose pamidronate. It is usually asymptomatic and healing occurs when treatment is stopped. Excessive fluoride intake causes osteomalacia due to direct inhibition of mineralisation and is common in parts of the world where there is a high fluoride content in drinking water. The condition reverses when fluoride intake is reduced.

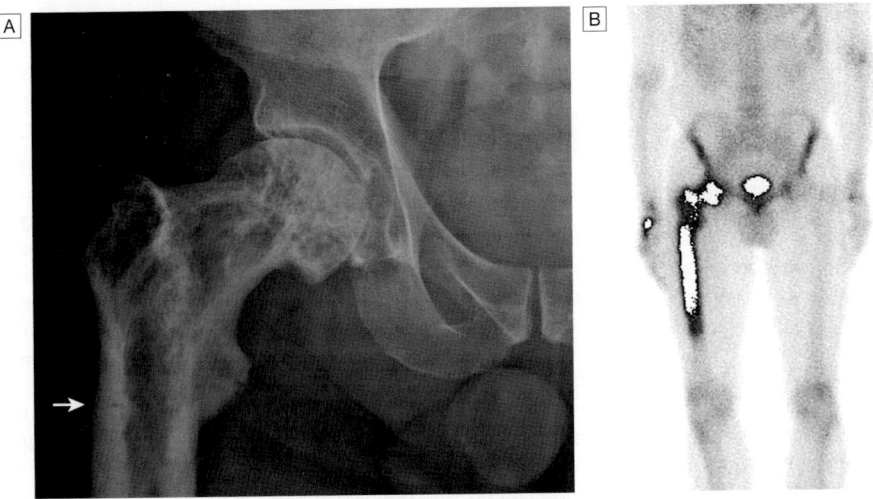

Fig. 26.64 Paget's disease of bone. **A** X-ray showing Paget's disease of the upper right femur illustrating osteolytic and osteosclerotic bone, a coarsened trabecular pattern and bone expansion with a stress fracture (arrow) visible on the lateral aspect of the femur. **B** Bone scintigraphy from the same patient showing intense tracer uptake in the affected bone.

Paget's disease of bone

Paget's disease of bone (PDB) is characterised by focal areas of increased and disorganised bone remodelling involving one or more skeletal sites. The disease is common in the UK, affecting about 1% of those aged above 55, and in other countries in Europe. It is rare in Scandinavia and Asia. The prevalence doubles each decade from the age of 50 onwards and affects up to 8% of the UK population by the age of 85.

Pathophysiology

The primary abnormality is increased osteoclastic bone resorption, accompanied by marrow fibrosis, increased vascularity of bone and increased, but disorganised, bone formation. Osteoclasts in PDB are greater in number and unusually large, containing characteristic nuclear inclusion bodies. Genetic factors are important and mutations in the *SQSTM1* gene are a common cause of classical PDB. The presence of nuclear inclusion bodies in osteoclasts has fuelled speculation that PDB might be caused by a slow virus infection, but this remains unproven. Biomechanical factors may influence which bones are affected, as PDB often starts at sites of muscle insertions into bone and, in some cases, localises to bones or limbs that have been subjected to repetitive trauma or overuse. Involvement of subchondral bone can compromise the joint and predispose to OA. The prevalence of PDB has fallen in many countries over recent decades, suggesting that environmental factors play a role, but their identity remains unclear.

Clinical features

The axial skeleton is predominantly affected and common sites of involvement are the pelvis, femur, tibia, lumbar spine, skull and scapula. The most common presentation is with bone pain localised to an affected site, but bone deformity, deafness and pathological fractures may also be presenting features. Many patients are asymptomatic and in about 20% of cases the diagnosis is made on the basis of an X-ray or blood test performed for another reason. Clinical signs include bone deformity and expansion, and increased warmth over an affected bone. Neurological problems, such as deafness, cranial nerve defects, nerve root pain, spinal cord compression and spinal stenosis, may occur due to enlargement of affected bones and encroachment on the spinal cord and nerve foramina. Surprisingly, deafness is seldom due to compression of the auditory nerve, but instead is conductive in nature due to osteosclerosis of the temporal bone. The increased vascularity of pagetic bone can very rarely precipitate high-output cardiac failure in older patients with limited cardiac

reserve. Osteosarcoma is an unusual but serious complication that presents with increasing pain and swelling of an affected site.

Investigations

The characteristic features are an isolated elevation in ALP and bone expansion on X-rays, with alternating areas of radiolucency and osteosclerosis (Fig. 26.64A). Levels of ALP can be normal if only a single bone is affected. The best way of identifying affected sites is a radionuclide bone scan, which shows increased uptake in affected bones (Fig. 26.64B). If the bone scan is positive, X-rays should be taken to confirm the diagnosis. Bone biopsy is not usually required, but may help to exclude osteosclerotic metastases in cases of diagnostic uncertainty.

Management

The main indication for treatment with inhibitors of bone resorption is bone pain, which is thought to be due to increased metabolic activity (Box 26.76). Patients should be carefully assessed to determine the cause of the pain since it can be difficult to differentiate the pain caused by increased metabolic activity of PDB from that caused by complications such as bone deformity, nerve compression symptoms and OA. Zoledronic acid is considered the treatment of choice since it is highly effective at suppressing elevated bone turnover in PDB and is most likely to give a favourable pain response. Intravenous pamidronate and oral risedronate can also be effective. If there is doubt about whether the pain is due to PDB, it can be worthwhile giving a therapeutic trial of bisphosphonate to determine whether the symptoms improve. Although there is always the possibility of a 'placebo effect', a positive response usually indicates that the pain was due to increased metabolic activity. Repeated courses of bisphosphonates can be given if symptoms recur. There is not any firm evidence as yet to suggest

i	**26.76 Medical management of Paget's disease**	
Drug	**Route of administration**	**Dose**
Risedronate	Oral	30 mg daily for 2 months
Pamidronate	IV	1–3 × 60 mg infusions
Zoledronic acid	IV	1 × 5 mg infusion
Calcitonin	SC	100–200 IU 3 times weekly for 2–3 months

(IV = intravenous; SC = subcutaneous)

26

that prophylactic bisphosphonates prevent the development of complications in PDB, but this issue is under investigation.

Other bone diseases

Complex regional pain syndrome type 1

Complex regional pain syndrome (CRPS) type 1 is characterised by gradual onset of pain, swelling and local tenderness, usually affecting a limb extremity. It may be triggered by fracture, but can also occur in association with soft tissue injury, pregnancy and intercurrent illness or can develop spontaneously. The cause is unknown, but abnormalities of the sympathetic nervous system are thought to play a pathogenic role. The affected limb is swollen and tender, and there may be evidence of regional autonomic dysfunction with abnormal sweating and changes in skin colour and temperature. The diagnosis is primarily clinical, based on the features shown in Box 8.12. Support for the diagnosis can be obtained with MRI, which shows bone marrow oedema, or radionuclide bone scan, which shows a local increase in tracer uptake. X-rays typically show localised patchy osteoporosis. Haematology, biochemistry and immunology are normal.

The aims of treatment are to control pain and encourage mobilisation. Analgesics, NSAIDs, antineuropathic agents, calcitonin, glucocorticoids, β-adrenoceptor antagonists (β-blockers), sympathectomy and bisphosphonates have all been tried, but none is particularly effective. Although some cases resolve with time, many individuals have persistent symptoms and fail to regain normal function.

Osteonecrosis

Osteonecrosis is the term used to describe death of bone due to impairment of its blood supply. The most commonly affected sites are the femoral head, humeral head navicular and scaphoid. In some cases, the condition occurs as the result of direct trauma that interrupts the blood supply to the affected bone. This is the reason for osteonecrosis of the femoral head following fractures of the femoral neck and in patients with thrombophilia, antiphospholipid syndrome, Gaucher's disease and haemoglobinopathies, such as sickle cell disease. Other important predisposing factors include high-dose glucocorticoid treatment, alcohol excess, SLE, HIV and radiotherapy, but in many of these conditions the pathophysiology is poorly understood. The presentation is with pain localised to the affected site, which is exacerbated by weight-bearing. The diagnosis can be confirmed by MRI, which shows evidence of subchondral necrotic bone and bone marrow oedema. X-rays are normal in the early stages, but later may show evidence of osteosclerosis and deformity of the affected bone. There is no specific treatment. Management should focus on controlling pain and encouraging mobilisation. Symptoms often improve spontaneously with time, but joint replacement may be required in patients who have persisting pain in association with significant structural damage to the affected joint.

Scheuermann's osteochondritis

This disorder predominantly affects adolescent boys, who develop a dorsal kyphosis in association with irregular radiographic ossification of the vertebral end plates. It has a strong genetic component and may sometimes be inherited in an autosomal dominant manner. Most patients are asymptomatic, but back pain aggravated by exercise and relieved by rest may occur. Excessive exercise and heavy manual labour before epiphyseal fusion has occurred may aggravate symptoms. Management consists of advice to avoid excessive activity and provision of protective postural exercises. Rarely, corrective surgery may be required if there is severe deformity. Scheuermann's disease can sometimes present for the first time in adulthood, when it can be confused with osteoporotic vertebral fractures. It can be differentiated from osteoporosis by the characteristic X-ray changes, which show mild wedge deformity of 3–4

adjacent vertebrae, irregularity of the vertebral end plates, and normal BMD on DXA examination.

Fibrous dysplasia

This is an acquired systemic disorder that mainly affects the skeleton and is caused by somatic mutations in the GNAS1 gene. The characteristic presentation is with bone pain and pathological fractures. Associated features include endocrine dysfunction, especially precocious puberty, and café-au-lait skin pigmentation (McCune–Albright syndrome). The diagnosis can usually be made by imaging, which shows focal, predominantly osteolytic lesions with bone expansion on X-rays (Fig. 26.65), and focal increased uptake on bone scan. The condition may cause a single (monostotic) or multiple (polyostotic) lesions. The condition can superficially resemble Paget's disease of bone, but the earlier age of onset and pattern of involvement are usually distinctive. Very rarely, malignant change can occur and should be suspected if there is a sudden increase in pain and swelling. Management is symptomatic. Intravenous bisphosphonates are often used in an attempt to control pain, but the evidence base for their efficacy is weak. Orthopaedic surgery may be required for treatment of fracture and deformity or to prevent a pathological fracture in a weight-bearing bone. Endocrine manifestations, such as precocious puberty, may require specific treatment.

Osteogenesis imperfecta

Osteogenesis imperfecta (OI) is the name given to a group of disorders characterised by severe osteoporosis and multiple fractures in infancy and childhood. Most cases are caused by mutations in the COL1A1 and COL1A2 genes, which encode the proteins that make type I collagen. These result in reduced collagen production (in mild OI) or in formation of abnormal collagen chains that are rapidly degraded (in severe OI). Mutations in several other genes have been described that can cause OI, some of which affect post-translational modification of collagen and

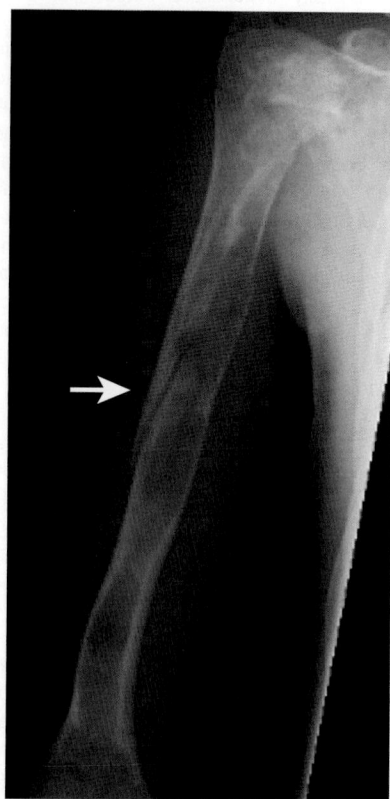

Fig. 26.65 Fibrous dysplasia. X-ray of the right humerus in a patient with polyostotic fibrous dysplasia showing multiple expansile osteolytic lesions and a pathological fracture in the humeral mid-shaft (arrowed).

others that affect bone formation. Many patients have no family history. Some of these have new mutations whereas others may have recessive forms of the disease. The Sillence classification is commonly used to grade severity. This varies from neonatal lethal OI (type II), through very severe OI with multiple fractures in infancy and childhood (types III and IV), to mild (type I), in which affected patients typically have blue sclerae. The diagnosis of OI is usually obvious clinically, based on the presentation with multiple low-trauma fractures during infancy. The disease can be mistaken for non-accidental injury in childhood and for osteoporosis in adulthood; in such cases, genetic testing can be of diagnostic value. Treatment is multidisciplinary, involving surgical reduction and fixation of fractures and correction of limb deformities, with physiotherapy and occupational therapy for rehabilitation of patients with bone deformity. Bisphosphonates are widely used in the treatment of OI, especially intravenous pamidronate and zoledronic acid in children, but there is limited evidence for efficacy in fracture prevention.

Osteopetrosis

Osteopetrosis is the collective name given to a rare group of inherited diseases caused by failure of osteoclast function. Presentation is highly variable, ranging from a lethal disorder that presents with bone marrow failure in infancy to a milder and sometimes asymptomatic form that presents in adulthood. Severe osteopetrosis is inherited in an autosomal recessive manner and presents with failure to thrive, delayed dentition, cranial nerve palsies (due to absent cranial foramina), blindness, anaemia and recurrent infections due to bone marrow failure. The adult-onset type (Albers–Schönberg disease) shows autosomal dominant inheritance and presents with bone pain, cranial nerve palsies, osteomyelitis, OA or fracture; it is sometimes detected as an incidental radiographic finding. The responsible mutations affect either the genes that regulate osteoclast differentiation (*RANK*, *RANKL*), causing 'osteoclast-poor' osteopetrosis, or the genes involved in bone resorption, causing 'osteoclast-rich' osteopetrosis. These include mutations in the *TCIRG1* gene, which encodes a component of the osteoclast proton pump, and mutations in the *CLCN7* gene, which encodes the osteoclast chloride pump. The most effective treatment is bone marrow transplantation that can provide a source of osteoclasts that resorb bone normally, but this is not effective in patients with *RANKL* mutations. Medical management has generally limited efficacy, but IFNγ treatment may improve blood counts and reduce the frequency of infections.

Sclerosing bone dysplasias

These are rare diseases characterised by osteosclerosis and increased bone formation. Van Buchem disease and sclerosteosis are recessive disorders caused by loss-of-function mutations in the *SOST* gene, which normally suppresses bone formation (see Fig. 26.3). The resulting lack of functional sclerostin causes increased bone formation and bone overgrowth, leading to enlargement of the cranium and jaw, tall stature and cranial nerve palsies. There is no effective treatment. High bone mass syndrome is a benign disorder caused by mutations in the *LRP4* or *LRP5* gene, which is characterised by unusually high bone density. The mutations render the LRP receptors resistant to the inhibitory effects of SOST. Most patients are asymptomatic, but bone overgrowth in the palate (torus palatinus) and enlargement of the mandible can occur in later life. Treatment is not usually required. Camurati–Engelmann disease is an autosomal dominant condition caused by gain of function in the *TGFB1* gene. It presents with bone pain, muscle weakness and osteosclerosis mainly affecting the diaphysis of long bones. Glucocorticoids can help the bone pain, although usually analgesics are also required.

Bone and joint tumours

Primary tumours of bones and joints are rare, have a peak incidence in childhood and adolescence, and can be benign or malignant

i	**26.77 Primary tumours of the musculoskeletal system**	
Cell type	**Benign**	**Malignant**
Osteoblast	Osteoid osteoma	Osteosarcoma
Chondrocyte	Chondroma Osteochondroma	Chondrosarcoma
Fibroblast	Fibroma	Fibrosarcoma
Bone marrow cell	Eosinophilic granuloma	Ewing's sarcoma
Endothelial cell	Haemangioma	Angiosarcoma
Osteoclast precursor	Giant cell tumour	Malignant giant cell tumour

(Box 26.77). Paget's disease of bone accounts for most cases of osteosarcoma occurring above the age of 40.

Osteosarcoma

This is a rare tumour with an incidence of 0.6–0.85 per 100 000 population. It is the most common primary bone tumour. Most patients present under the age of 30, but osteosarcoma also occurs in old age in association with Paget's disease. The presentation is with local pain and swelling. X-rays show expansion of the bone with a surrounding soft tissue mass, often containing islands of calcification. If the diagnosis is being considered, MRI or CT should be performed to determine the extent of tumour. Patients suspected of having osteosarcoma should be referred to a specialist team for biopsy. Treatment depends on histological type, but generally involves surgical removal of the tumour, followed by chemotherapy and radiotherapy. The prognosis is normally good in cases that present in childhood and adolescence, but poor in older patients.

Chondrosarcoma

This is the second most common primary bone tumour. Presentation is as described for osteosarcoma. The treatment of choice is surgical resection since chondrosarcomas are relatively resistant to chemotherapy and radiotherapy. The prognosis is good for low-grade tumours, but poor for anaplastic tumours.

Ewing's sarcoma

This is the third most common sarcoma, which presents almost exclusively under the age of 40. Presentation is as described for osteosarcoma. Treatment is by local excision and surgical resection. The prognosis is excellent for patients who present before metastasis has occurred.

Metastatic bone disease

Metastatic bone disease may present in a variety of ways: with localised or generalised progressive bone pain, generalised regional pain, symptoms of spinal cord compression, or acute pain due to pathological fracture. Systemic features, such as weight loss and anorexia, and symptoms referable to the primary tumour are often present. The tumours that most commonly metastasise to bone are myeloma and those of bronchus, breast, prostate, kidney and thyroid. Management is discussed in Chapter 7.

Rheumatological involvement in other diseases

Many systemic diseases can affect the locomotor system and many drugs may cause adverse musculoskeletal effects (Box 26.78). The most

26

common examples are described here. Bone disease may also occur in sarcoidosis, haemophilia and sickle-cell anaemia.

Malignant disease

Malignant disease can cause a variety of non-metastatic musculoskeletal problems (Box 26.79). One of the most striking is hypertrophic pulmonary osteoarthropathy (HPOA), characterised by clubbing and painful swelling of the limbs, periosteal new bone formation and arthralgia/arthritis. The most common causes are bronchial carcinoma and mesothelioma. Bone scans show increased periosteal uptake before new bone is apparent on X-ray. The course follows that of the underlying malignancy and HPOA resolves if this is cured.

Endocrine disease

Hypothyroidism may present with carpal tunnel syndrome or, rarely, with painful, symmetrical proximal myopathy and muscle hypertrophy. Both resolve with levothyroxine replacement. Primary hyperparathyroidism is associated with osteoporosis and also predisposes to CPPD disease and to calcific periarthritis, especially in patients with renal disease.

Diabetes mellitus commonly causes diabetic cheirarthropathy, characterised by tightening of skin and periarticular structures, causing flexion deformities of the fingers that may be painful. Diabetic osteopathy presents as forefoot pain with radiographic progression from osteopenia to complete osteolysis of the phalanges and metatarsals. Diabetes also predisposes to osteoporosis, fragility fractures, adhesive capsulitis, Dupuytren's contracture, osteomyelitis, septic arthritis and Charcot's joints.

Acromegaly can be associated with mechanical back pain, with normal or excessive movement; carpal tunnel syndrome; Raynaud's syndrome and an arthropathy (50%). This arthropathy mainly affects the large joints and has clinical similarities to OA, but with a normal or increased range of movement. X-rays may show widening of joint spaces, squaring of bone ends, generalised osteopenia and tufting of terminal phalanges. It does not improve with treatment of the acromegaly and is an important cause of reduced quality of life in affected individuals.

Haematological disease

Haemochromatosis is complicated by an arthropathy in about 50% of cases. It typically presents between the ages of 40 and 50 and may predate other features of the disease. The small joints of the hands and wrists are typically affected but the hips, shoulders and knees may also be involved. The X-ray changes resemble OA, but cysts are often multiple and prominent with little osteophyte formation. Involvement of the radiocarpal and MCP joints may occur, which is unusual in primary OA, and about 30% have CPPD. Treatment of the haemochromatosis does not influence the arthropathy and management is as described for OA. Haemophilia can be complicated by haemarthrosis, which, if recurrent, can result in the development of secondary OA. Sickle-cell disease may be associated with bone pain, osteonecrosis and osteomyelitis. Thalassaemia may be complicated by bone deformity, especially affecting the craniofacial bones, and by osteoporosis.

Neurological disease

Neurological disease may result in rapidly destructive arthritis of joints, first described by Charcot in association with syphilis. The cause is incompletely understood, but may involve repetitive trauma as the result of sensory loss and altered blood flow secondary to impaired sympathetic nervous system control. The main predisposing diseases and sites of involvement are:

- diabetic neuropathy (hindfoot)
- syringomyelia (shoulder, elbow, wrist)
- leprosy (hands, feet)
- tabes dorsalis (knees, spine).

i	26.78 Drug-induced effects on the musculoskeletal system	
Musculoskeletal problem	**Principal drug**	
Secondary gout	Thiazides, furosemide, alcohol	
Osteoporosis	Glucocorticoids, heparin, glitazones, aromatase inhibitors, GnRH agonists	
Osteomalacia	Anticonvulsants, etidronate and pamidronate (high-dose)	
Osteonecrosis	Glucocorticoids, alcohol	
Drug-induced lupus syndrome	Procainamide, hydralazine, isoniazid, chlorpromazine, minocycline, anti-TNF-α biologics	
Arthralgias	Glucocorticoid withdrawal, glibenclamide, methyldopa, ciclosporin, isoniazid, barbiturates, bisphosphonates, aromatase inhibitors	
Myalgia	Glucocorticoid withdrawal, L-tryptophan, fibrates, statins	
Myopathy/myositis	Glucocorticoids, chloroquines, penicillamine, statins, zidovudine, colchicine, fibrates, alcohol	
Arthritis	Immune checkpoint inhibitors (ICIs)	
Vasculitis	Penicillins, cephalosporins, sulphonamides, thiazides, phenytoin, allopurinol	

(ACTH = adrenocorticotrophic hormone; GnRH = gonadotrophin-releasing hormone)

---

i	26.79 Rheumatological manifestations of malignancy

- Polyarthritis
- Dermatomyositis and polymyositis
- Hypophosphataemic osteomalacia
- Hypertrophic osteoarthropathy
- Vasculitis, connective tissue disease
- Raynaud's syndrome
- Polymyalgia rheumatica-like syndrome

The presentation is with subacute or chronic monoarthritis. Pain can occur, especially at the onset, but once the joint is severely deranged, pain is often minimal and signs become disproportionately greater than symptoms. The joint is often grossly swollen, with effusion, crepitus, marked instability and deformity, but usually no increased warmth. X-rays show disorganisation of normal joint architecture and often multiple loose bodies (Fig. 26.66), and either no (atrophic) or gross (hypertrophic) new bone formation. Management principally involves orthoses and occasionally arthrodesis.

Miscellaneous conditions

Anterior tibial compartment syndrome

This is characterised by severe pain in the front of the lower leg, aggravated by exercise and relieved by rest. Symptoms result from fascial compression of the muscles in the anterior tibial compartment and may be associated with foot drop. Treatment is by surgical decompression.

Carpal tunnel syndrome

This is a common nerve entrapment syndrome caused by compression of the median nerve at the wrist. It presents with numbness, tingling

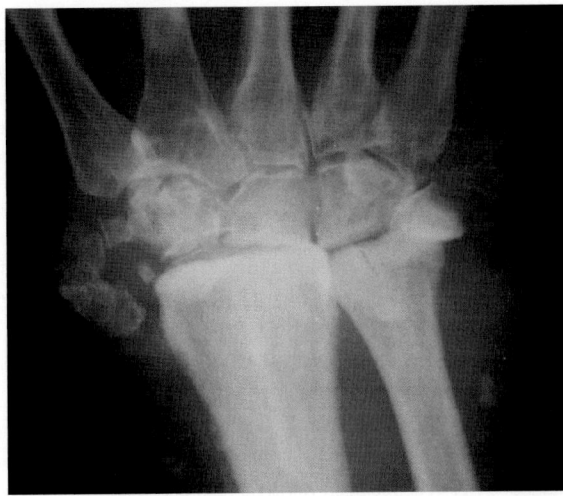

Fig. 26.66 Wrist X-ray showing a neuropathic (Charcot) joint in a patient with syringomyelia. Note the disorganised architecture with complete loss of the proximal carpal row, bony fragments and soft tissue swelling.

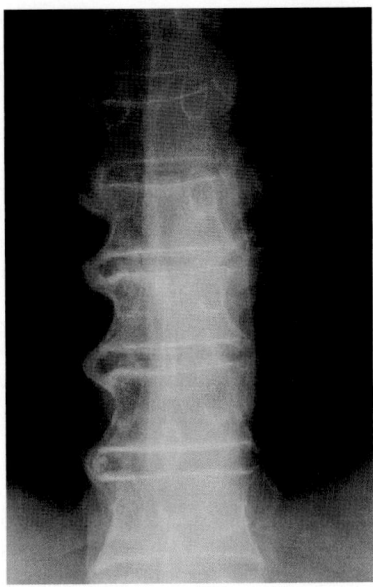

Fig. 26.67 Diffuse idiopathic skeletal hyperostosis (DISH). Anteroposterior X-ray of the thoracic spine showing right-sided, flowing new bone joining contiguous thoracic vertebrae. The disc spaces are preserved.

and pain in a median nerve distribution. The most common causes are hypothyroidism, diabetes mellitus, rheumatoid arthritis, obesity and pregnancy (especially in the third trimester). In some patients, no underlying cause may be identified. Carpal tunnel syndrome often responds to treatment of the underlying condition, but other options include local glucocorticoid injections and surgical decompression.

Diffuse idiopathic skeletal hyperostosis

Diffuse idiopathic skeletal hyperostosis (DISH) is a common disorder, affecting 10% of men and 8% of women over the age of 65, but its prevalence increases further with age and is associated with obesity, hypertension and type 2 diabetes mellitus. It is characterised by syndesmophytes and florid new bone formation along the anterolateral aspect of contiguous vertebral bodies (Fig. 26.67). DISH is distinguished from lumbar spondylosis by the absence of disc space narrowing and marginal vertebral body sclerosis, and from ankylosing spondylitis by the absence of sacroiliitis or apophyseal joint fusion. It is usually an asymptomatic radiographic finding, but can cause back pain or pain at peripheral sites, such as the heel, in association with enthesophyte formation.

Dupuytren's contracture

Dupuytren's contracture is characterised by fibrosis and contracture of the superficial palmar fascia of the hands. The patient is unable to extend the fingers fully and there is puckering of the skin with palpable nodules. The ring and little fingers are usually the first and worst affected. Dupuytren's contracture is usually painless, but causes problems due to limitation of hand function and snagging of the curled fingers in pockets. It is age-related, usually bilateral and more common in men. There is a strong genetic component and sometimes may be familial, with dominant inheritance. The condition can be associated with plantar fibromatosis, Peyronie's disease, alcohol misuse and chronic vibration injury. It is very slowly progressive. Often no treatment is required, but it can be treated medically by local injections of collagenase or surgically by fasciotomy if symptoms are troublesome.

Joint hypermobility

Joint hypermobility is caused by increased laxity of connective tissues. It is commonly observed in a number of hereditary conditions including: Marfan syndrome, which arises from mutations in the *FBN1* gene; osteogenesis imperfecta and Ehlers–Danlos syndrome types I, II and IV, caused by mutations in the *COL3A1*, *COL5A1* and *COL5A2* genes.

i 26.80 Modified Beighton score for joint hypermobility	
Clinical test	**Score**
Extend little finger > 90°	1 point each side
Bring thumb back parallel to/touching forearm	1 point each side
Extend elbow > 10°	1 point each side
Extend knee > 10°	1 point each side
Touch floor with flat of hands, legs straight	1 point
Hypermobile = a score of 6 or more points out of a possible 9 for epidemiological studies, or 4 or more points (with arthralgia in four or more joints) for a clinical diagnosis of the benign joint hypermobility syndrome	

The term hypermobile Ehlers–Danlos syndrome (hEDS), which is also known as EDS type III, is used to describe a polygenic form of joint hypermobility. Patients with this condition have hypermobile joints in combination with a range of symptoms such as chronic joint and ligamentous pain, fibromyalgia-like symptoms, recurrent dislocations, easy bruising, abdominal symptoms, insensitivity to local anaesthetic, mitral valve prolapse and postural orthostatic tachycardia syndrome (POTS), in which there is dizziness, hypotension and an increased heart rate on standing. The diagnosis of hEDS can be made if the modified Beighton score is 4 or above (Box 26.80) in the presence of one or more of the above clinical features. It is useful to distinguish hEDS from the milder hypermobility spectrum disorder (HSD), which is the name given to the syndrome where joint hypermobility is accompanied by some, but not all, features of hEDS.

Inclusion body myositis

Inclusion body myositis (IBM) is the most frequent primary myopathy in middle age and after. It is characterised by slowly progressive muscle weakness and atrophy, with pathological changes of inflammation, degeneration and mitochondrial abnormality in affected muscle fibres. IBM typically presents with distal muscle weakness. In time, muscles atrophy. Investigation is the same as for polymyositis. There is typically a slightly elevated creatine kinase and myopathic changes on EMG.

26

Muscle biopsy shows abnormal fibres containing rimmed vacuoles and filamentous inclusions in the nucleus and cytoplasm. Therapeutic response to glucocorticoids and immunosuppressants is poor. There is anecdotal report of efficacy with IVIg, but trial evidence is lacking.

Pigmented villonodular synovitis

Pigmented villonodular synovitis is an uncommon proliferative disorder of synovium, which typically affects young adults. It is caused by a somatic chromosomal translocation in synovial cells that places the *CSF1* gene downstream of the *COL6A3* gene promoter. The result is local over-production of M-CSF, which causes accumulation of macrophages in the joint. The presentation is with joint swelling, limitation of movement and local discomfort. The diagnosis can be confirmed by MRI or synovial biopsy. Treatment is by surgical or radiation synovectomy.

Scoliosis

Scoliosis is characterised by an abnormal lateral curvature of the spine of greater than 10 degrees. Scoliosis may be secondary to known disorders or idiopathic. In about 20% of cases, scoliosis is secondary to a neuromuscular disorder, such as muscular dystrophy, cerebral palsy or neurofibromatosis. It may also occur in association with hereditary connective tissue diseases, such as Marfan syndrome. Scoliosis may also develop in later life, usually as a result of structural changes in the spine from degenerative change. The term idiopathic scoliosis is used to described the remaining cases where there is no obvious cause. In fact, there is strong evidence from twin studies that idiopathic scoliosis is genetically mediated, in keeping with the finding that it is evident during childhood or adolescence. It is often asymptomatic, but it can persist into adulthood and may become symptomatic, associated with evolving degenerative changes.

The diagnosis of scoliosis can be made clinically by physical examination and confirmed by X-ray. External bracing and/or surgical intervention are considered in adolescents with severe deformities to correct deformity or prevent progression, but the evidence base is poor. In adulthood, treatment is symptomatic in nature with analgesics, NSAIDs or antineuropathic medications.

Spondylolysis

Spondylolysis describes a break in the integrity of the vertebral neural arch. The principal cause is an acquired defect in the pars interarticularis due to a fracture, mainly seen in gymnasts, dancers and runners, in whom it is an important cause of back pain. Spondylolisthesis describes the condition in which a defect causes slippage of a vertebra on the one below. This may be congenital, post-traumatic or degenerative. Rarely, it can result from metastatic destruction of the posterior elements. Uncomplicated spondylolysis does not cause symptoms, but spondylolisthesis can lead to low back pain aggravated by standing and walking. Occasionally, symptoms of nerve root or spinal compression may occur. The diagnosis can be made on oblique X-rays of the lumbar spine, but MRI may be required if there is neurological involvement. Advice on posture and muscle-strengthening exercises is required in mild cases. Surgical fusion is indicated for severe and recurrent low back pain. Surgical decompression is mandatory prior to fusion in patients with significant lumbar stenosis or symptoms of cauda equina compression.

Chronic non-infectious osteomyelitis

Chronic non-infectious osteomyelitis (CNO) is characterised by pain, swelling and osteosclerosis of affected bones. It may target a single bone or multiple bones when it is called chronic recurrent multifocal osteomyelitis (CRMO). The conditions can occur in the absence of other features or be part of the synovitis–acne–pustulosis–hyperostosis–osteitis (SAPHO) syndrome. These disorders often target the clavicles and bones of the anterior chest wall but other bones may be affected, including the mandible and lower limb bones. SAPHO syndrome may be part of a spectrum of autoinflammatory bone disease that includes chronic recurrent (sterile) multifocal osteomyelitis in children and adolescents. Other features of SAPHO include a pustular rash affecting the palms and soles of the feet, enthesitis, spondylodiscitis, sacroiliitis and synovitis of peripheral joints. These disorders tend to present in children or young adults. Radionuclide bone scans show increased uptake in affected bones with osteosclerosis and bone expansion on X-rays and CT scans. Various treatments have been used, including glucocorticoids, DMARDs, bisphosphonates, anakinra and anti-TNF-α, with most success arising from biologic use. The cause is unknown, but has been suggested to be an autoinflammatory process triggered by a micro-organism.

Trigger finger

This occurs as the result of stenosing tenosynovitis in the flexor tendon sheath, with intermittent locking of the finger in flexion. It can arise spontaneously or in association with inflammatory diseases such as RA. Symptoms usually respond to local glucocorticoid injections, but surgical decompression is occasionally required.

Further information

Journal articles

Campion EW. Calcium pyrophosphate deposition disease. N Engl J Med 2016;374:2575–2578.

Gossec L, Smolen JS, Ramiro S, et al. European League Against Rheumatism (EULAR) recommendations for the management of psoriatic arthritis with pharmacological therapies: 2015 update. Ann Rheum Dis 2016;75:499–510.

Guo Q, Wang Y, Xu D, et al. Rheumatoid arthritis: pathological mechanisms and modern pharmacological therapies. Bone Res 2018;6:15.

Hellmich B, Agueda A, Monti S, et al. 2018 Update of the EULAR recommendations for the management of large vessel vasculitis. Ann Rheum Dis 2020;79:19–30.

Hui M, Carr A, Cameron S, et al. The British Society for Rheumatology Guideline for the Management of Gout. Rheumatology 2017;56:e1–e20. https://doi.org/10.1093/rheumatology/kex156.

Ralston SH, Corral-Gudino L, Cooper C, et al. Diagnosis and management of Paget's disease of bone in adults: a clinical guideline. J Bone Miner Res 2019;34(4):579–604.

Smolen JS, Landewé RBM, Bijlsma JWJ, et al. EULAR recommendations for the management of rheumatoid arthritis with synthetic and biological disease-modifying antirheumatic drugs: 2019 update. Ann Rheum Dis 2020;79: 685–699.

Taurog JD, Avneesh C, Colbert RA. Ankylosing spondylitis and axial spondyloarthritis. N Engl J Med 2016;374:2563–2567.

Zhang W, Doherty M, Pascuale E, et al. EULAR recommendations for calcium pyrophosphate deposition. Part II Management. Ann Rheum Dis 2011;70: 571–575.

Websites

4s-dawn.com/DAS28 *Calculator for this measure of activity in rheumatoid arthritis.*

asas-group.org *Repository of resources to aid assessment of spondyloarthritis.*
basdai.com/BASDAI.php *BASDAI calculator for assessing ankylosing spondylitis.*
omim.org *Online Mendelian Inheritance in Man (OMIM): genetic diseases.*
shef.ac.uk/FRAX/tool.jsp and qfracture.org/ *Fracture risk assessment tools.*
sign.ac.uk *Scottish Intercollegiate Guidelines Network 142 – Management of osteoporosis and the prevention of fragility fractures (2020 update).*
thefreelibrary.com *Information on drug-induced myopathies.*
vasculitis.org/ *Vasculitis resources from the European Vasculitis Society.*

Patient organisations

ARMA arma.uk.net/membership/ *A UK-based umbrella organisation for numerous patient-advocacy groups covering a wide area of musculoskeletal disease. Extensive weblinks.*

NRAS nras.org.uk/useful-links/category/international-links *A UK-based patient-run, patient-advocacy organisation for people with RA. There are weblinks to many international RA groups including in India, the United States, Canada and South Africa.*

IOF iofbonehealth.org/ *US-based globally active organisation promoting the detection, management and education of osteoporosis.*

SH Ibbotson

27

Dermatology

Clinical examination in skin disease

8 Detailed morphology of individual lesions
Use a magnifying lens in good lighting to assist
Use correct terminology (see definitions throughout text)

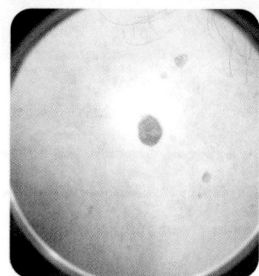

▲ Magnifying lens image of benign naevus

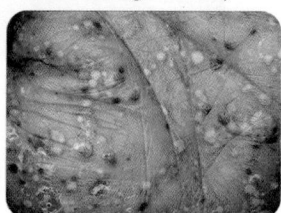

▲ Palmoplantar pustulosis

7 Overall description of individual lesions
Discrete, grouped, confluent, reticulate (lace-like), linear

6 Morphology of rash
Monomorphic or polymorphic

5 Involvement of axillae/groins
e.g. hidradenitis suppurativa

4 Nail involvement

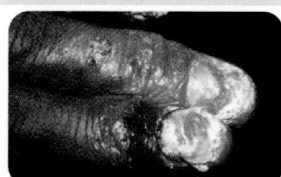

▲ Psoriatic changes in nails and peri-ungual involvement

3 Involvement of hands, including nail folds and finger webs

2 If symmetrical

■ Extensor, e.g. psoriasis

□ Flexor, e.g. eczema

1 Distribution of rash
Symmetrical vs asymmetrical
Proximal vs distal vs facial
Localised vs widespread

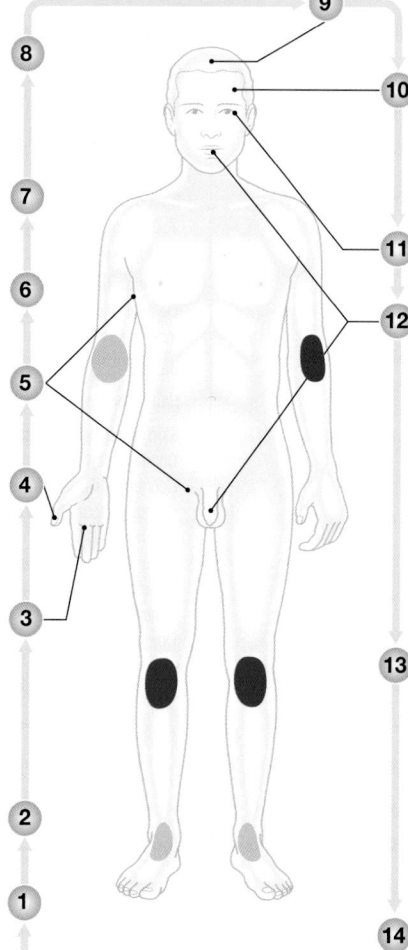

Observation
The patient must be undressed, with make-up and dressings removed, and examined in good lighting. Consider the following:
• Age
• General health
• Distress
• Scratching

9 Examination of scalp
Hair loss
Scalp changes

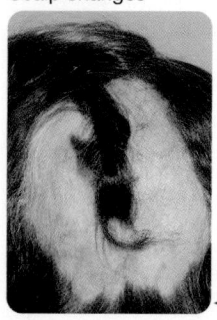

▲ Alopecia areata

10 Involvement of face
Central
Hairline
Cheeks and nasal bridge: 'butterfly' distribution
Sparing of light-protected sites, e.g. behind ears, under chin

11 Eye involvement
e.g. Conjunctivitis/blepharitis in rosacea or eyelash loss in alopecia areata

12 Oral and genital involvement

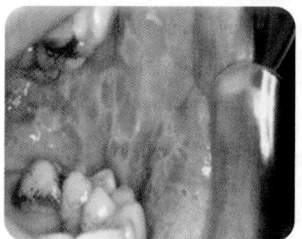

▲ Reticulate (lacy) network on buccal mucosa in lichen planus. May also be genital involvement

13 Joint involvement
e.g. Psoriatic arthritis

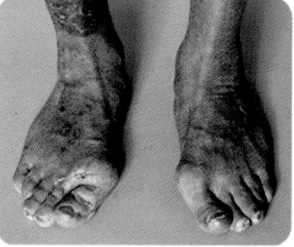

▲ Arthritis, plaque psoriasis and psoriatic nail dystrophy

14 General medical examination
Including lymph nodes and other systems as indicated

It is tempting to examine the skin first. This is a mistake; take a history, then examine the skin and the rest of the patient.

1. History-taking	2. Drug/allergy history	3. Examination of skin	4. Closer inspection	5. General examination
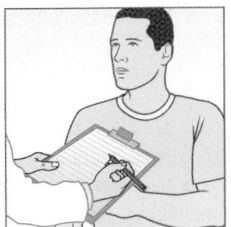	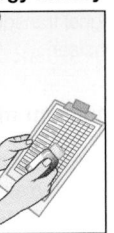	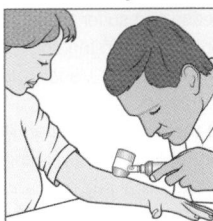	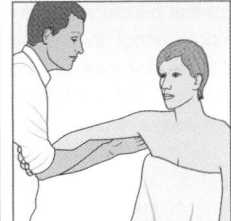	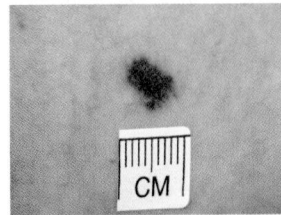

Include:
- Onset and course
- Exacerbating/relieving factors
- Past history of skin disease, atopy or autoimmune disease
- Social history, occupation, recreation
- Psychological impact, gauged by health-related life quality indices

- Always take a detailed drug and allergy history
- Include all systemic and topical drugs, and over-the-counter preparations

- Examine skin, hair, nails and mucous membranes
- Is it a rash or a lesion?
- Distribution and morphology important for rash

- Use of a magnifying lens and/or dermatoscope may be invaluable
- Site, size and detailed morphology of a lesion are essential factors to elicit

- General examination, incl. peripheral lymph nodes, may be indicated/important
- Skin diseases may have systemic features (e.g. cardiovascular disease in psoriasis); many systemic diseases have dermatological features (e.g. diabetes)

6. Define type of lesion using correct terminology

Helps in differential diagnosis and allows colleagues to visualise the process. Other definitions are provided in the chapter.

Macule/patch

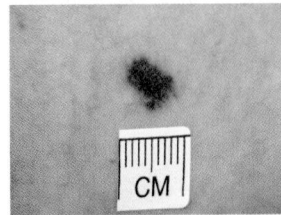

Macule: circumscribed flat area of colour change ≤ 1 cm diameter; patch: > 1 cm

Papule

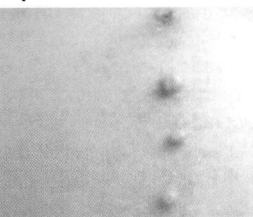

Discrete elevation ≤ 1 cm diameter

Nodule

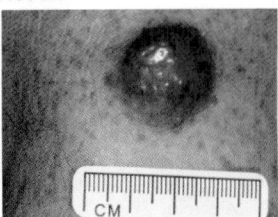

Like papule but deeper (into dermis or subcutaneous layer), > 1 cm diameter

Plaque

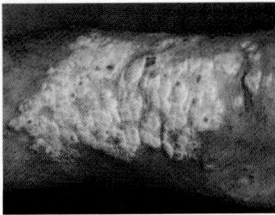

Raised area > 1 cm diameter with flat top

Vesicle

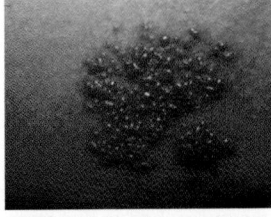

Small (≤ 1 cm diameter) fluid-filled blister

Blisters/bullae

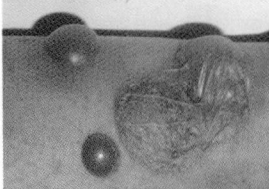

Large (> 1 cm diameter) fluid-filled blister

Pustule

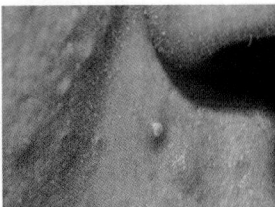

Visible accumulation of pus in blister

Petechiae/purpura

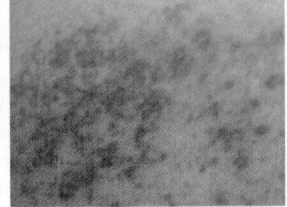

Petechiae: tiny macules due to extravascular blood in dermis; purpura: larger, may be palpable

7. Score activity

Tools for objective assessment of disease severity, such as the Psoriasis Area and Severity Index (PASI), are important in assessing severity and treatment responses.

■ Four body parts are each scored individually

(A) Each of the four body parts is scored:

Redness (erythema)	0–4
Thickness (induration)	0–4
Scaling (desquamation)	0–4

(B) The area of each involved body part is scored:

0	0%
1	< 10%
2	10–29%
3	30–49%
4	50–69%
5	70–89%
6	90–100%

(C) 10%   20%   30%   40%

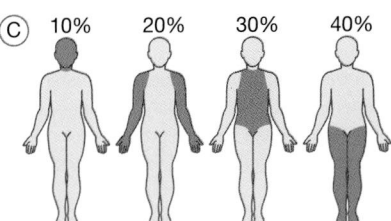

To find the PASI score, add together: (A) Sum for each part × (B) % of that part involved × (C) % weighting of that body part

Minimum = 0; maximum = 72

27

Diseases affecting the skin are common, and important because the absence of normal skin function, as well as sometimes being life-threatening, can severely impair quality of life. This may be exacerbated by the fact that people with skin disease can suffer the effects of stigma, often brought about by the ill-informed understanding of others with respect to skin diseases, particularly as regards visually disfiguring skin changes or the belief that they are contagious.

Skin diseases affect all ages and there are more than 2000 different types and presentations. Assessment of the skin is valuable in the management of anyone presenting with a medical problem and, conversely, assessment of the other body systems is important when managing primary skin diseases. This chapter concentrates on common skin diseases and those that are important components of general medical conditions. Skin infections, including those related to the human immunodeficiency virus (HIV), tuberculosis, leprosy (Hansen's disease) and syphilis, are also discussed in Chapters 14, 17, 13 and 15, respectively.

Functional anatomy and physiology

The skin covers just under $2\,m^2$ in the average adult. The outer layer is the epidermis, a stratified squamous epithelium consisting mainly of keratinocytes. The epidermis is attached to, but separated from, the underlying dermis by the basement membrane. The dermis is less cellular and supports blood vessels, nerves and epidermal-derived appendages (hair follicles and sweat glands). Below it is the subcutis, consisting of adipose tissue.

Epidermis

In most sites, the epidermis is only 0.1–0.2 mm thick, except on the palms or soles, where it can extend to several millimetres. Keratinocytes make up approximately 90% of epidermal cells (Fig. 27.1). The main proliferative compartment is the basal layer. Keratinocytes synthesise a range of structural proteins, such as keratins, loricrin and filaggrin (filament aggregating protein), which play key roles in maintaining the skin's barrier function. Keratinocytes are also responsible for synthesis of vitamin D under the influence of ultraviolet B (UVB) light. There are more than 50 types of keratin and their expression varies by body site, site within the epidermis and disease state. Mutations of certain keratin genes can result in blistering disorders and ichthyosis (characterised by scale without major inflammation). As keratinocytes migrate from the basal layer, they differentiate, producing a variety of protein and lipid products. Keratinocytes undergo apoptosis in the granular layer before losing their nuclei and becoming the flattened corneocytes of the stratum corneum (keratin layer). The epidermis is a site of lipid production, and the ability of the stratum corneum to act as a hydrophobic barrier is the result of its 'bricks and mortar' design; dead corneocytes with highly cross-linked protein membranes ('bricks') lie within a metabolically active lipid layer synthesised by keratinocytes ('mortar'). Terminal differentiation of keratinocytes relies on the keratin filaments being aggregated and this is, in part, mediated by filaggrin. Mutations of the filaggrin gene are found in icthyosis vulgaris and in some patients with atopic eczema.

The skin is a barrier against physical stresses and infections. Cell-to-cell attachments must be able to transmit and dissipate stress, a function performed by desmosomes. Diseases that affect desmosomes, such as pemphigus, result in blistering due to keratinocyte separation.

The remaining 10% of epidermal cells are:

- *Langerhans' cells*: these are dendritic, bone marrow-derived cells that circulate between the epidermis and local lymph nodes. Their prime function is antigen presentation to lymphocytes. Other dermal antigen-presenting dendritic cells are also present.
- *Melanocytes*: these occur predominantly in the basal layer and are of neural crest origin. They synthesise the pigment melanin from tyrosine, package it in melanosomes and transfer it to surrounding keratinocytes via their dendritic processes.
- *Merkel cells*: these occur in the basal layer and are thought to play a role in signal transduction of fine touch. Their embryological derivation is unclear.

Basement membrane

The basement membrane (see Fig. 27.1) is an anchor for the epidermis and allows movement of cells and nutrients between dermis and epidermis. The cell membrane of the epidermal basal cell is attached to the basement membrane via hemi-desmosomes. The lamina lucida lies immediately below the basal cell membrane and is composed predominantly of laminin. Anchoring filaments extend through the lamina lucida to attach to the lamina densa. This electron-dense layer consists mostly of type IV collagen; from it extend loops of type VII collagen, forming anchoring fibrils that fasten the basement membrane to the dermis.

Dermis

The dermis is vascular and supports the epidermis structurally and nutritionally. It varies in thickness from just over 1 mm on the inner forearm to 4 mm on the back. Fibroblasts are the predominant cells but others include mast cells, mononuclear phagocytes, T lymphocytes, dendritic cells, neurons and endothelial cells. The acellular part of the dermis consists mainly of collagen I and III, elastin and reticulin, synthesised by fibroblasts. Support is provided by an amorphous ground substance (mostly glycosaminoglycans, hyaluronic acid and dermatan sulphate), whose production and catabolism are altered by hormonal changes and ultraviolet radiation (UVR). Based on the pattern of collagen fibrils, the superficial dermis is termed the 'papillary dermis', and the deeper, coarser part is the 'reticular dermis'.

Epidermal appendages

Hair follicles

There are 3–5 million hair follicles, epidermal invaginations that develop during the second trimester. They occur throughout the skin, with the exception of palms, soles and parts of the genitalia (glabrous skin). The highest density of hair follicles is on the scalp ($500-1000/cm^2$). Newborns are covered with fine 'lanugo' hairs, which are usually non-pigmented and lack a central medulla; these are subsequently replaced by vellus hair, which is similar but more likely to be pigmented. By contrast, scalp hair becomes terminal hair, which is thicker with a central medulla, is usually pigmented and grows longer. At puberty, vellus hairs in hormonally sensitive regions, such as the axillary and genital areas, become terminal hairs.

Human hairs grow in a cycle with three phases: anagen (active hair growth), catagen (transitional phase) and telogen (resting phase). The duration of each phase varies by site. On the scalp, anagen lasts several years, catagen a few days and telogen around 3 months. The length of hair at different sites reflects the differing lengths of anagen.

Sebaceous glands

Sebaceous glands are epidermal downgrowths, usually associated with hair follicles and composed of modified keratinocytes. The cells of the sebaceous gland (sebocytes) produce a range of lipids, discharging the contents into the duct around the hair follicle. Sebum excretion is under hormonal control, with androgens increasing it (as do progesterones, to a lesser degree) and oestrogens reducing it. In animals, sebum is important for hair waterproofing but its role in humans is unclear.

Sweat glands

Eccrine sweat glands develop in the second trimester and are also epidermal invaginations found all over the body. Their coiled ducts open directly on to the skin surface. They play a major role in

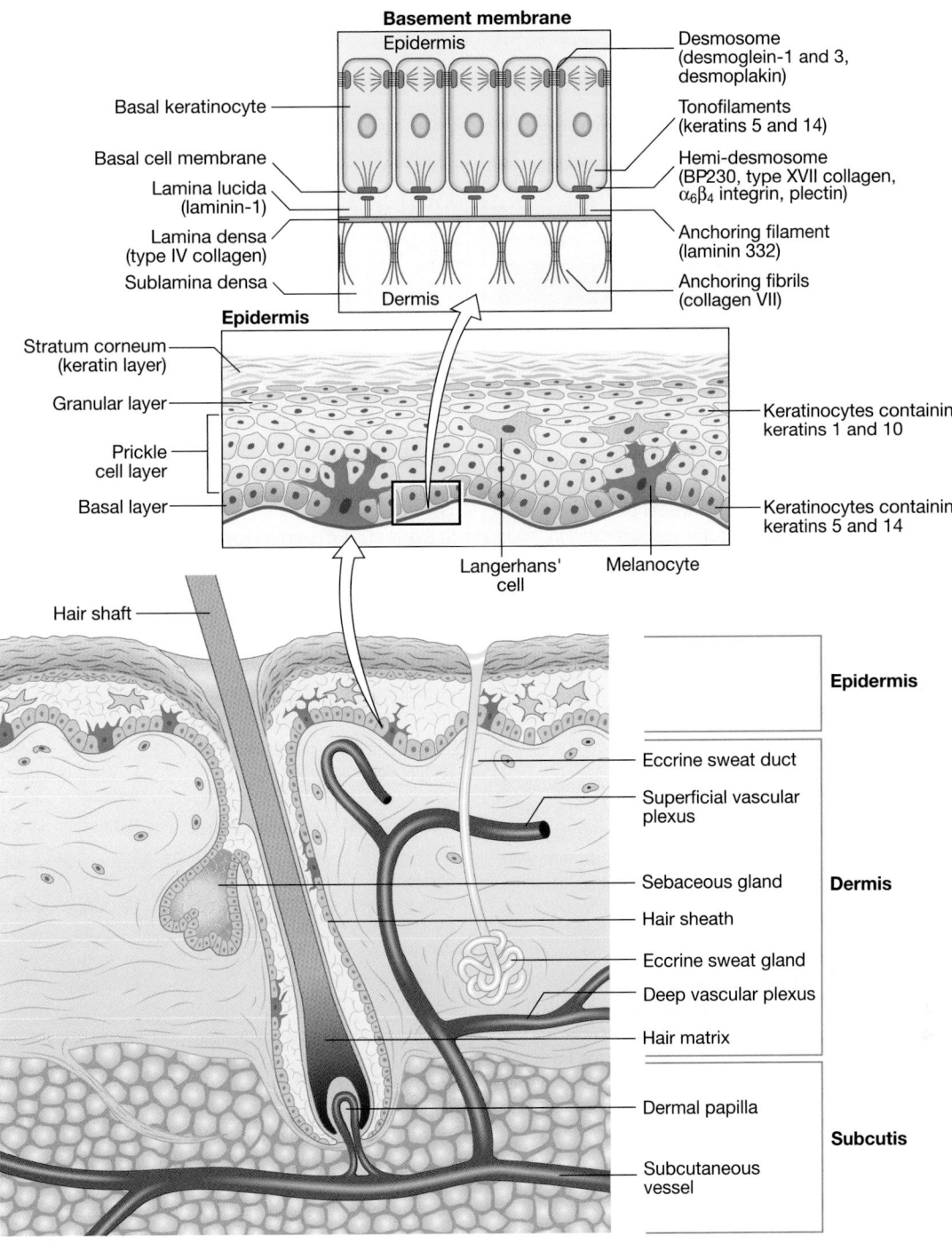

Basement membrane

Epidermis

Basal keratinocyte

Basal cell membrane
Lamina lucida
(laminin-1)
Lamina densa
(type IV collagen)
Sublamina densa

Dermis

Desmosome
(desmoglein-1 and 3,
desmoplakin)
Tonofilaments
(keratins 5 and 14)
Hemi-desmosome
(BP230, type XVII collagen,
$\alpha_6\beta_4$ integrin, plectin)
Anchoring filament
(laminin 332)
Anchoring fibrils
(collagen VII)

Epidermis

Stratum corneum
(keratin layer)
Granular layer
Prickle
cell layer
Basal layer

Keratinocytes containing
keratins 1 and 10

Keratinocytes containing
keratins 5 and 14

Langerhans'
cell

Melanocyte

Hair shaft

Epidermis

Eccrine sweat duct
Superficial vascular
plexus

Sebaceous gland

Hair sheath

Eccrine sweat gland

Deep vascular plexus

Hair matrix

Dermis

Dermal papilla

Subcutaneous
vessel

Subcutis

Fig. 27.1 Structure of normal skin.

27

thermoregulation and, unusually, are innervated by cholinergic fibres of the sympathetic nervous system. Eccrine glands of the palms and soles are innervated differently and are activated in the 'fight or flight' response. Apocrine sweat glands are restricted to the axillae and the mammary and genital areas, are connected to hair follicles and are not involved in thermoregulation.

Nails

Fingernail growth commences at approximately 8 weeks of gestation and is complete by 32 weeks. Toenails develop slightly later. The anatomy of the nail apparatus is described later in the chapter.

Blood vessels and nerves

Human skin has a plentiful blood supply, arranged in superficial and deep plexuses consisting of arterioles, arterial and venous capillaries, and venules. The upper plexus in the papillary dermis communicates with the lower plexus at the junction between the dermis and the subcutis. Capillary loops arise from terminal arterioles in the horizontal papillary plexus. Blood vessels are supplied by sympathetic and parasympathetic nerves, with the relative contributions of the pathways differing by site. Sympathetic signals are important in mediating autonomic-induced vasoconstriction. The blood supply of skin is far greater than that required for normal skin physiology and reflects the importance of skin in thermoregulation.

Functions of the skin

The skin has many functions, all of which can be affected by disease (Box 27.1). Skin changes associated with ageing are shown in Box 27.2.

Investigation of skin disease

Magnifying glass

A hand-held or freestanding magnifying lens used under good lighting conditions (ideally daylight) is valuable for examination of the skin.

Wood's light

Wood's light is a long-wavelength UVA/short-wavelength visible (violet) light source that can be used in various ways. In hypopigmentation, such as in vitiligo, it can help in appreciating the extent of disease. In pigmented conditions, such as melasma, it can determine whether pigmentation is mainly epidermal (sharp cut-off under Wood's lamp) or mixed epidermal and dermal (ill-defined cut-off). Wood's lamp can also be used to help with the diagnosis of some fungal infections because of their characteristic fluorescence.

Dermatoscopy and diascopy

Dermatoscopy (also known as dermoscopy and epiluminescence microscopy) is increasingly performed with hand-held dermatoscopes. What makes dermatoscopy unique is the fact that it allows visualisation through contact of a glass plate on the instrument with a liquid film applied to the skin, or through special optics to allow non-contact dermatoscopy, enabling deeper structures to be seen without interference from reflection and refraction of light in the epidermis.

Diascopy is simply pressing on the lesion with a glass slide. This provides some of the effect of dermatoscopy, but is mainly used to remove blood from vascular lesions to make the appearance of the lesion clearer. Granulomatous skin diseases may have a characteristic appearance under diascopy, such as in lupus vulgaris (cutaneous tuberculosis), in which 'apple jelly nodules' are typically seen on diascopy.

Skin biopsy

Skin biopsy is a pivotal investigation in dermatology and can be used in a range of dermatological presentations. In the most common scenario, a skin biopsy is undertaken in order to obtain tissue on which to perform standard histopathology. However, tissue may also be subjected to a variety of staining and culture techniques, including immunostaining. Histopathological examination of skin biopsies is especially useful for tumour diagnosis. When a dermatologist or pathologist with dermatopathology expertise is involved, it can also assist in the diagnosis of inflammatory skin diseases. It is rare for histopathology of a previously undiagnosed inflammatory skin disease to provide a diagnosis on its own; clinico-pathological correlation is critical. Most biopsies are stained with haematoxylin and eosin but other stains may be useful in special situations, such as for fungal hyphae, iron or mucin. Direct immunofluorescence can also be undertaken on a fresh skin biopsy, allowing antigen visualisation using fluorescein-labelled antibodies; this is especially important in the diagnosis of autoimmune bullous disorders or connective tissue disease, such as cutaneous lupus.

---

i | 27.1 Functions of the skin

Function	Structure/cell involved
Protection against:	
Chemicals, particles, desiccation	Stratum corneum
Ultraviolet radiation	Melanin produced by melanocytes and transferred to keratinocytes
	Stratum corneum hyperproliferation
Antigens, haptens	Langerhans' cells, lymphocytes, mononuclear phagocytes, mast cells, dermal dendritic cells
Microorganisms	Stratum corneum, Langerhans' cells, mononuclear phagocytes, mast cells, dermal dendritic cells
Maintenance of fluid balance Prevents loss of water, electrolytes and macromolecules	Stratum corneum
Shock absorber Strong, elastic and compliant covering	Dermis and subcutaneous fat
Sensation	Specialised nerve endings mediating pain and withdrawal Itch leading to scratch and removal of a parasite
Metabolism Detoxification of xenobiotics, retinoid metabolism, isomerisation of urocanic acid	Predominantly keratinocytes
Temperature regulation	Eccrine sweat glands and blood vessels
Protection, and fine manipulation of small objects	Nails
Hormonal Steroidogenesis, testosterone synthesis and conversion to other androgenic steroids	Hair follicles, sebaceous glands
Conversion of thyroxine (T_4) to triiodothyronine (T_3)	Keratinocytes
Conversion of 7-dehydrocholesterol to vitamin D	Keratinocytes
Pheromonal Importance unknown in humans	Apocrine sweat glands, possibly sebaceous glands
Psychosocial, grooming and sexual behaviour	Appearance, tactile quality of skin, hair, nails

---

 ### 27.2 Skin changes in old age

- **Chronological ageing**: due to the intrinsic ageing process.
- **Photo-ageing**: due to cumulative ultraviolet radiation (UVR) exposure and superimposed on intrinsic ageing.
- **Typical changes**: include atrophy, laxity, yellow discoloration, wrinkling, dryness, irregular pigmentation, and thinning and greying of hair.
- **Causes**: age-related alterations in structure and function of the skin, cumulative effects of environmental insults, especially UVR and smoking, cutaneous consequences of disease in other organ systems.
- **Consequences**: reduction in immune and inflammatory responses, reduction in absorption and clearance of topical medications, reduced healing, increased susceptibility to irritants, dermatitis, adverse drug effects (including topical glucocorticoid-induced atrophy and purpura) and diseases such as skin cancer.

Microbiology

Bacteriology

Bacterial swabs may identify a causative infective agent. However, organisms identified from the skin surface may not be the cause of the skin disease but instead may simply reflect colonisation of skin that has already been damaged by a primary skin disease.

Virology

A number of techniques, including immunofluorescence and polymerase chain reaction (PCR), are available to diagnose herpes simplex or herpes zoster viruses from vesicle fluid.

Mycology

Scale, nail clippings (or scrapings of crumbly subungual hyperkeratosis) and plucked hairs can be examined by light microscopy. If potassium hydroxide and a simple light microscope are available, this can be performed in any outpatient clinic. Microbiology laboratories will also routinely undertake microscopy and culture for fungi and yeasts.

Patch testing

Patch testing is the investigation of choice for delayed, cell-mediated, type IV hypersensitivity reactions to topical agents, which clinically manifest as dermatitis. Potential allergens (see Box 27.23) are applied as patches to the back under occlusion for 48 hours, in vehicles and at concentrations that minimise false-positive and false-negative reactions. After 48 hours the patches are removed and patch-test readings are undertaken at time points of up to 7 days after patch-test application, with the most typical time point being at 96 hours. When interpreting patch test readings, it is important to determine the clinical relevance of any allergic reactions before giving avoidance advice.

Photopatch testing is similar to patch testing but investigates delayed hypersensitivity reactions to a topically applied agent (usually a sunscreen or topical non-steroidal anti-inflammatory drug (NSAID)) after the absorption of UVR. It involves applying substances in duplicate and irradiating one set with UVR (typically UVA, 5 J/cm^2), readings then being conducted in a similar manner to patch testing.

Prick tests and specific immunoglobulin E testing

Prick tests are used to investigate cutaneous type I (immediate) hypersensitivity reactions to various antigens such as pollen, house dust mite or dander. The skin is pricked with commercially available stylets through a dilution of the appropriate antigen solution. Alternatively, specific immunoglobulin E (IgE) levels to antigens can be measured in serum. If challenge tests are undertaken for patients with suspected allergy, these must be performed under controlled conditions due to the potential risk of triggering a severe reaction. More details of IgE testing are provided in Chapter 4.

Phototesting

Phototesting is extremely valuable in the assessment of suspected photosensitivity. The mainstay investigation is monochromator phototesting, which involves exposing the patient's back to increasing doses of irradiation using narrow wavebands across the solar spectrum and then assessing responses at each waveband, using the minimal erythema dose (MED) as the endpoint. This is the dose required to cause just perceptible skin reddening (erythema) and is compared with values for the normal population. If a patient has reduced MEDs (develops erythema at lower doses than healthy subjects), this indicates abnormal photosensitivity. Thus, monochromator phototesting can be used to determine whether a patient is abnormally photosensitive, which wavebands are involved and how sensitive the patient is. Provocation testing can be performed with a broadband (usually UVA) source to induce rash at a test site (most useful for polymorphic light eruption) and is a helpful diagnostic

test. Provocation testing to a variety of light sources, including artificial compact fluorescent lamps, may also be indicated, the latter being most relevant in patients with severe photosensitivity.

Patients who are referred for phototherapy will also commonly undergo an MED test, in which they are exposed to a series of test doses of the light source that will be used therapeutically (often narrowband UVB); the MED is determined 24 hours later (or 72–96 hours for the psoralen–ultraviolet A (PUVA) minimal phototoxic dose. This allows treatment regimens to be individualised, based on a patient's erythemal responses. The MED can also detect abnormal photosensitivity, and represents a safety measure prior to starting a course of phototherapy.

Blood tests

Although most patients presenting with a skin problem do not need blood tests as part of their investigations, there are many systemic diseases that can present with skin features and, indeed, blood tests may also be indicated in the investigation of primary skin disease. A wide range of possible investigations may be required and some examples include haemoglobin, iron studies and thyroid function tests in pruritus or hair loss; autoantibody screening if lupus is suspected; measurement of porphyrins for skin fragility and hypertrichosis; and hepatitis screening in lichen planus. These diverse examples emphasise the importance of considering an underlying systemic disease when assessing a patient with a dermatological presentation.

Imaging

Imaging techniques are not typically required but X-rays, ultrasound, magnetic resonance imaging (MRI) or computed tomography (CT) may occasionally be indicated in specific situations, such as in metastatic melanoma or in a patient presenting with a diagnosis of cutaneous sarcoid.

Presenting problems in skin disease

The major presentations in dermatology are outlined below. Detail of the underlying disorders is mostly provided in the disease-specific sections further on in the chapter.

Lumps and lesions

The term lump or lesion is typically used to describe a papule or nodule, although sometimes may refer to a macule or plaque. A new or changing lump is one of the key dermatology presentations.

Clinical assessment

Detailed history-taking and examination are essential:

- *Change*: Is the lump new or has there been a change in a pre-existing lesion? What is the nature of the change – size, colour, shape or surface change? Has change been rapid or slow? Are there other features – pain, itch, inflammation, bleeding or ulceration (**definition** of 'ulcer': an area from which the epidermis and at least the upper part of the dermis have been lost – see Fig. 27.9)?
- *Patient*: What is the patient's age? Are they fair-skinned and freckled? Have they got multiple naevi? Has there been much sun exposure? Have they used sunbeds or lived and worked in sunny climates? Have they used photoprotection? Have they had skin cancer before or is there a family history of skin cancer? What medications are they taking? Are they immunosuppressed?
- *Site*: Is it on a sun-exposed or covered site? The scalp, face, upper limbs and back in men, and face, hands and lower legs in women, are the most chronically sun-exposed sites.
- *Are there other similar lesions?* These might include actinic keratoses (see Fig. 27.14) or basal cell papillomas (see Fig. 27.18).

27

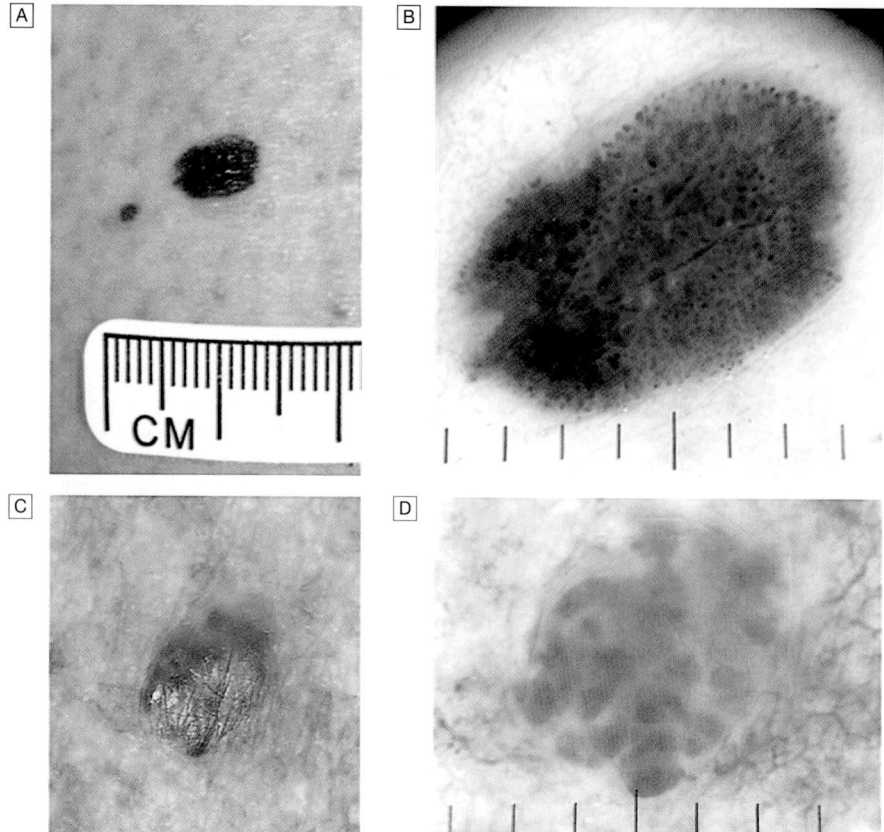

Fig. 27.2 Dermatoscopy. [A] A changing lesion. [B] Dermatoscopy highlights the abnormal pigment network and other features suggestive of melanoma. Excision biopsy confirmed the diagnosis of superficial spreading malignant melanoma (Breslow thickness 0.8 mm). [C] Another changing lesion. [D] Dermatoscopy highlights the vascular lacunae of this benign angioma and the patient was reassured.

- *Morphology*: Tenderness, size, symmetry, regularity of border, colour, surface characteristics and the presence of features such as crust (**definition**: dried exudate of blood or serous fluid – see Fig. 27.20), scale (**definition**: a flake arising from the stratum corneum; any condition with a thickened stratum corneum can cause scaling – see Fig. 27.14) and ulceration must be assessed. Stretching the skin and using a magnifying lens can be helpful, such as for detecting the raised, pearled edge of a basal cell carcinoma (see Fig. 27.12).
- *Dermatoscopy*: This can be used to detect the presence of abnormal vessels, such as in basal cell carcinoma or the characteristic keratin cysts in basal cell papillomas. It is invaluable for assessing pigmented and vascular lesions (Fig. 27.2).

Is it a melanocytic naevus or a malignant melanoma?

This is a common clinical scenario and one that it is critical to resolve correctly.

- The precise nature of the change should be determined (as above). Listen to the patient and pay attention to subtle changes, as people know their skin well.
- If the patient has other pigmented lesions, then these should be examined too, as they may be informative. For example, if the presenting lesion looks different from the others, then suspicion of melanoma is increased; conversely, if the patient has multiple basal cell papillomas, this may be reassuring – although do not be falsely reassured.
- Is there a positive family history of melanoma? A suspicious naevus in a patient with a first-degree relative with melanoma probably warrants excision.

> **i**   **27.3 ABCDE features of malignant melanoma**
>
> - **A**symmetry
> - **B**order irregular
> - **C**olour irregular
> - **D**iameter >0.5 cm
> - **E**levation irregular
> - (+ Loss of skin markings)

The ABCDE 'rule' is a guide to the characteristic features of melanoma (Box 27.3 and see Figs. 27.2 and 27.16), although melanomas should ideally be diagnosed before the diameter is greater than 0.5 cm. Loss of normal skin markings in a pigmented lesion may be suggestive of melanoma. Conversely, normal skin markings and fine hairs dispersed evenly over a lesion are reassuring but do not exclude melanoma. The Glasgow seven-point checklist is another useful guide:

- *major features*: change in size, shape and colour
- *minor features*: diameter >0.5 cm, inflammation, oozing, bleeding, itch or altered sensation.

Patients with one major or one minor feature should be referred for further evaluation.

Investigations and management

If a benign diagnosis, such as basal cell papilloma, is made on clinical grounds, then the patient can be reassured and the lesion either left or treated: for example, with cryotherapy. If there are concerns about the diagnosis or malignancy is suspected, then skin biopsy in order to obtain a tissue diagnosis is the usual approach. An incisional biopsy may be indicated, although if the lesion is small, excision may be most appropriate. If significant concern exists about the possibility of malignant melanoma, initial excision with a 2 mm margin would usually be undertaken prior to more definitive management once histology was confirmed. Further management of a changed lesion would, of course, depend on histological analysis of the diagnostic biopsy.

Rash

A rash is the other common presentation in dermatology. The main categories of scaly rashes are listed in Box 27.4. The most common type of rash presentation is maculopapular. Diagnosis can often be made on clinical grounds, although a biopsy may be required.

Clinical assessment

Important aspects of the history include:

- *Age at onset and duration of rash*. Atopic eczema often starts in early childhood and psoriasis between 15 and 40 years, and both may be chronic. Infective or drug-induced rashes are more likely to be of short duration and the latter to occur in relation to drug ingestion. Duration of individual lesions is also important, as in urticaria, for example, where lesions will come and go over short periods of time and do not persist beyond 24 hours.
- *Body site at onset and distribution*. Flexural sites are more typically involved in atopic eczema, and extensor surfaces and scalp in psoriasis. Symmetry is often indicative of an endogenous disease, such as psoriasis, whereas asymmetry is more common with exogenous causes, such as contact dermatitis or infections like herpes zoster.
- *Itch*. Eczema is usually extremely itchy and psoriasis may be less so.
- *Preceding illness and systemic symptoms*. Guttate psoriasis may be precipitated by a β-haemolytic streptococcal throat infection; almost

all patients with infectious mononucleosis treated with amoxicillin will develop an erythematous maculopapular eruption; a history of chancre at the site of inoculation may be elicited in a presentation of secondary syphilis; malaise and arthralgia are common in drug eruptions and vasculitis.

The morphology of the rash and the characteristics of individual lesions are important (see Box 27.4).

Investigations and management

It is important to have a short differential diagnosis based on clinical assessment in order to direct investigations. For example, in psoriasis, no investigations may be needed and initial management with patient counselling and topical therapies may suffice. If the diagnosis is unclear, then a diagnostic skin biopsy and other targeted investigations based on the clinical picture may be required. An initial management plan should also be implemented. For example, in a child presenting with a rash that has features suggestive of impetigo, skin and nasal swabs should be performed and, once these have been taken, topical or systemic antibiotics should be introduced, depending on clinical extent of disease, and management should be adjusted accordingly, dependent on investigation findings and clinical course. In contrast, if a patient presents with a maculopapular rash shortly after introduction of a new drug, then drug withdrawal, diagnostic biopsy, full blood count, including eosinophil count, and liver and renal function tests, in parallel with topical emollients and glucocorticoids, may be indicated.

Blisters

A blister is a fluid-filled collection in the skin. The term vesicle is used for small lesions and bulla for larger lesions. Blistering occurs due to loss of cell adhesion within the epidermis or subepidermal region (see Fig. 27.1). The clinical presentation depends on the site or level of blistering within the skin, which in turn reflects the underlying cause. There are a limited number of conditions that present with blisters (Box 27.5):

i 27.4	Causes and clinical features of common scaly rashes		
Diagnosis	**Distribution**	**Morphology**	**Associated signs**
Atopic eczema (p.1096)	Face and flexures	Poorly defined erythema, scaling Vesicles Lichenification if chronic	Shiny nails Infra-orbital crease 'Dirty neck' (grey–brown discoloration)
Psoriasis (p. 1099)	Extensor surfaces Lower back	Well-defined Erythematous plaques Silvery scale	Nail pitting, onycholysis Scalp involvement Axillae and genital areas often affected Joint involvement Köbner phenomenon (p. 1103)
Pityriasis rosea (p. 1102)	'Fir tree' pattern on trunk	Well-defined Small, erythematous plaques Collarette of scale	Herald patch
Drug eruption (p. 1115)	Widespread	Macules and papules Erythema and scale Exfoliation	Possible mucosal involvement or erythroderma
Pityriasis versicolor (p. 1093)	Upper trunk and shoulders	Hypo- and hyper-pigmented scaly patches	
Lichen planus (p. 1103)	Distal limbs Flexural aspect of wrists Lower back	Shiny, flat-topped, violaceous papules Wickham's striae	White, lacy network on buccal mucosa Nail changes Scarring alopecia Köbner phenomenon
Tinea corporis (p. 1092)	Asymmetrical Often isolated lesions	Erythematous, often annular plaques Peripheral scale (sometimes pustules) Expansion with central clearing	Possible nail, scalp, groin involvement
Secondary syphilis (p. 377)	Trunk and proximal limbs Palms and soles	Red macules and papules, which become 'gun-metal' grey	History of chancre Systemic symptoms, e.g. malaise and fever

27

i	**27.5 Causes of acquired blisters**	
	Localised	**Generalised**
Vesicular	Herpes simplex Herpes zoster Impetigo Pompholyx	Eczema herpeticum* Dermatitis herpetiformis Acute eczema
Bullous	Impetigo Cellulitis Stasis oedema Acute eczema Insect bites Fixed drug eruption	Toxic epidermal necrolysis* Erythema multiforme Stevens–Johnson syndrome* Bullous pemphigoid Pemphigus* Epidermolysis bullosa acquisita Lupus erythematosus Porphyria cutanea tarda Pseudoporphyria Drug eruptions

*Usually with mucosal involvement too.

- Intact blisters are not often seen if the split is high in the epidermis (below the stratum corneum), as the blister roof is so fragile that it ruptures easily, leaving erosions (**definition**: an area of skin denuded by complete or partial loss of the epidermis). This occurs in pemphigus foliaceus, staphylococcal scalded skin syndrome (see Fig. 27.21) and bullous impetigo.
- If the split is lower in the epidermis, then intact flaccid blisters and erosions may be seen, as occurs in pemphigus vulgaris and toxic epidermal necrolysis (see Fig. 27.41).
- If the split is subepidermal, then tense-roofed blisters are seen. This occurs in bullous pemphigoid (see Fig. 27.42), epidermolysis bullosa acquisita and porphyria cutanea tarda (see Fig. 27.53).
- If there are foci of separation at different levels of the epidermis, such as may occur in eczema, then multilocular bullae made up of coalescing vesicles can occur.

Clinical assessment

Detailed history-taking and examination are critical. A history of onset, progression, mucosal involvement, drugs and systemic symptoms should be sought. Clinical assessment of the distribution, extent and morphology of the rash should be made. The Nikolsky sign is useful: sliding lateral pressure from a finger on normal-looking epidermis can dislodge and detach the epidermis in conditions with intra-epidermal defects, such as pemphigus and toxic epidermal necrolysis. A systematic approach to diagnosis is required (Fig. 27.3).

Investigations and management

Investigations and initial management will be guided by the clinical presentation and differential diagnosis, and are described in more detail under the specific diseases. For example, an initial approach may include

directed investigations, such as incisional diagnostic skin biopsy for histology and direct immunofluorescence, indirect immunofluorescence and other targeted blood tests or skin swabs. Management should be based on the likely diagnosis and begin in parallel with investigations, until the diagnosis is confirmed.

Itch

Itch describes the unpleasant sensation that leads to scratching or rubbing. The terms 'itch' and 'pruritus' are synonymous; however, 'pruritus' is often used when itch is generalised. Itch can arise from primary cutaneous disease or be secondary to systemic disease, which may cause itch by central or peripheral mechanisms. Even when the mechanism is peripheral, there are not always signs of primary skin disease.

The nerve endings that signal itch are in the epidermis or near the dermo-epidermal junction. The underlying mechanisms of itch are not fully understood. Transmission is by unmyelinated slow-conducting C fibres through the spinothalamic tract to the thalamus and then the cortex. Aδ fibres also seem to be involved in transmitting signals to the spinal cord, and the heat-sensitive transient receptor potential (TRP) channels 1–4 are important. There is an inhibitory relationship between pain and itch. Scratching may relieve the symptom of itch after the sensation has ceased and this is either by stimulation of ascending sensory pathways that inhibit itch-transmitting neurons at the spinal cord (Wall's 'gate' mechanism), or by direct damage to cutaneous sensory nerves.

The mechanisms of itch in most systemic diseases remain unclear. The itch of kidney disease, for example, may be mediated by circulating endogenous opioids. The clinical observation that peritoneal dialysis helps reduce itch more frequently than haemodialysis is consistent with this, with smaller molecules generally being dialysed more readily if the peritoneal membrane is used rather than a dialysis machine membrane.

Clinical assessment

It is important to determine whether skin changes are primary (a process in the skin causing itch) or secondary (skin changes caused by rubbing and scratching because of itch). This requires a thorough history and examination, sometimes with investigations, to exclude systemic disease. Many common primary skin disorders are associated with itch (Box 27.6). If itch is not connected with primary skin disease, other causes

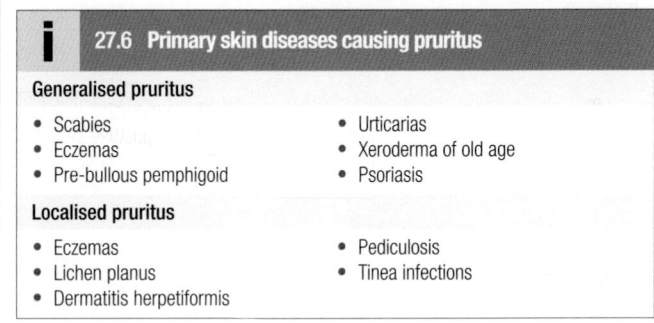

i	**27.6 Primary skin diseases causing pruritus**

Generalised pruritus

- Scabies
- Eczemas
- Pre-bullous pemphigoid
- Urticarias
- Xeroderma of old age
- Psoriasis

Localised pruritus

- Eczemas
- Lichen planus
- Dermatitis herpetiformis
- Pediculosis
- Tinea infections

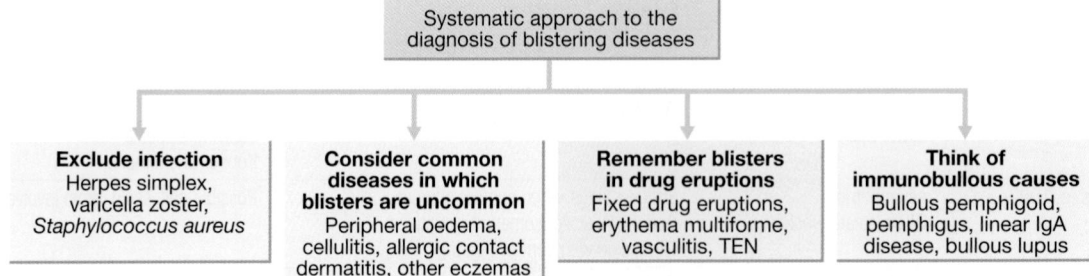

Fig. 27.3 A systematic approach to the diagnosis of blistering diseases. (TEN = toxic epidermal necrolysis)

i   27.7 Secondary causes of pruritus

Medical condition	Cause of pruritus	Treatment*	Medical condition	Cause of pruritus	Treatment*
Liver disease	Central opioid effect Elevation in bile salts may contribute	Naltrexone Colestyramine Rifampicin Sedative antihistamines UVB	**Thyrotoxicosis** **Hypothyroidism** **Carcinoid syndrome**	Unknown Unknown 5-HT-mediated	
Renal failure	Unknown; uraemia contributes	UVB Oral activated charcoal	**HIV infection**	Infection, infestation Eosinophilic folliculitis Seborrhoeic dermatitis Unknown	Treatment of infection Local corticosteroids, UVB Anti-pityrosporal treatment UVB
Haematological disease			**Malignancy**	Unknown	
Anaemia Polycythaemia rubra vera Lymphoma Leukaemia Myeloma	Iron deficiency Unknown (often aquagenic pruritus) } Unknown	Iron replacement	**Psychogenic**	Unknown	Psychotherapy, anxiolytics, antidepressants
Endocrine disease Diabetes mellitus	Infections such as candidiasis and tinea	Treatment of infection			

*In addition to specific treatment of the primary condition and symptomatic treatments, such as emollients. (5-HT = 5-hydroxytryptamine, serotonin; HIV = human immunodeficiency virus; UVB = ultraviolet B)

27.8 Causes of pruritus in pregnancy

Diagnosis	Pregnancy, gestation and features	Treatment
Polymorphic eruption of pregnancy (pruritic urticarial papules and plaques, PUPP)	Typically first pregnancy and uncommonly recurs during third trimester and after delivery Polymorphic urticated papules and plaques, start in striae	Chlorphenamine, emollients Topical glucocorticoids
Acute cholestasis of pregnancy	Third trimester and commonly recurs in subsequent pregnancies Abnormal liver function tests Increased fetal and maternal risk	Emollients Chlorphenamine Colestyramine UVB Early delivery
Pemphigoid gestationis	Any stage, often second trimester and commonly recurs in subsequent pregnancies Urticated erythema, blistering initially periumbilical Characteristic histology and immunofluorescence	Topical or oral glucocorticoids
Prurigo gestationis	Second trimester Excoriated papules	Emollients Topical glucocorticoids Chlorphenamine UVB
Pruritic folliculitis	Third trimester Sterile pustules on trunk	Topical glucocorticoids UVB

(UVB = ultraviolet B)

should be considered (Box 27.7). These include liver diseases (mainly cholestatic diseases, such as primary biliary cholangitis), malignancies (generalised itch may be the presenting feature of lymphoma), haematological conditions (generalised itch in chronic iron deficiency or water contact-provoked (aquagenic) intense itch in polycythaemia), endocrine diseases (including hypo- and hyperthyroidism), chronic kidney disease (in which severity of itch is not always clearly associated with plasma creatinine concentration) and psychogenic causes (such as in 'delusions of infestation'). Itch is common in pregnancy and may be due to one of the pregnancy-specific dermatoses. Making a correct diagnosis is particularly important in pregnancy, as some disorders can be associated with increased fetal risk (Box 27.8).

Investigations and management

Investigations should be directed towards finding an underlying cause and there will be a different approach for itch with rash, as opposed to itch with no signs of primary skin disease (Fig. 27.4). If there are no signs of primary skin disease, investigations should be undertaken to exclude systemic disease or iatrogenic causes. Psychogenic itch should be considered only if organic disease has been ruled out. There are no consistently effective therapies to suppress itch, and so establishing the underlying cause is critical. If a clear-cut diagnosis cannot be made, non-specific approaches can be used for symptom relief. These include sedation, often with H_1-receptor antihistamines, along with emollients and counter-irritants (such as topical menthol-containing preparations). UVB phototherapy is useful for generalised itch due to a variety of causes but the only randomised controlled study of efficacy is in chronic kidney disease. Other treatments include low-dose tricyclic antidepressants (probably through similar mechanisms to those involved when these drugs are used for chronic pain) and opiate antagonists. If a psychogenic itch is considered likely, antidepressants and/or cognitive behavioural therapy may be effective. Itch of any cause can be severe and its potentially major adverse effects on quality of life are not always fully appreciated. Assessments of impact on quality of life, such as Dermatology Life Quality Index (DLQI) scores, are essential.

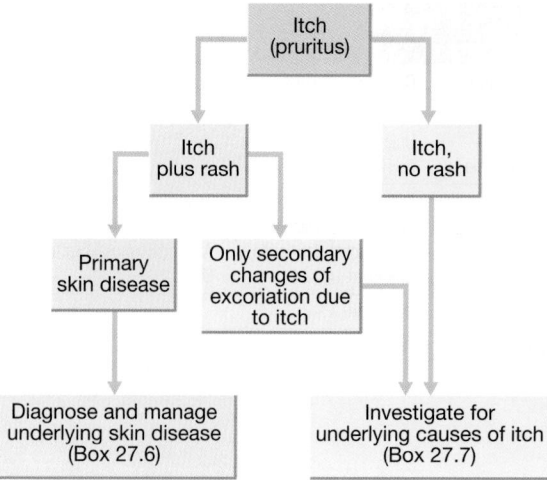

Fig. 27.4 **An overall approach to the investigation and management of itch (pruritus).**

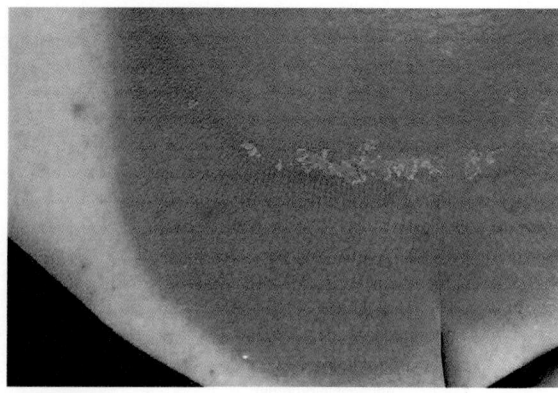

Fig. 27.5 **Sunburn.** Acute exposure to ultraviolet radiation results in an erythemal response that peaks 12–24 hours later. Sensitivity depends on the individual's constitutive skin phototype.

Photosensitivity

Cutaneous photosensitivity is an abnormal response of the skin to UVR or visible radiation. The sun is the natural source but patients may also be exposed to artificial sources of UVR through the use of sunbeds and/or phototherapy. Chronic UVR exposure increases skin cancer risk and photo-ageing. Acute exposure can induce erythema (redness) as a normal response (Fig. 27.5). However, abnormal photosensitivity occurs when a patient reacts to lower doses than would normally cause a response, either with a heightened erythemal reaction or the development of a rash. Photo-aggravated skin diseases are exacerbated by sunlight but not caused by it. The main photosensitive and photo-aggravated diseases are listed in Box 27.9.

Sunlight consists mainly of visible light, and the UVR component is divided into three wavebands (Fig. 27.6), according to the Commission Internationale de l'Eclairage (CIE):

- *UVC* (200–280 nm), which is absorbed by ozone and does not reach the Earth's surface.
- *UVB* (280–315 nm), which constitutes less than 10% of UVR exposure but is around 1000-fold more potent than UVA and so accounts for the erythemal 'sunburning' effects of sunlight.
- *UVA* (315–400 nm), which is the most abundant UVR component reaching the Earth's surface.

The arbitrary division between UVB and UVA regions is more often considered to be at 320 nm by photobiologists, and the UVA region can be further subdivided into UVA2 (320–340 nm) and UVA1 (340–400 nm). UVA2 behaves biologically more like UVB, and UVA1 can be used therapeutically for several skin conditions, such as morphoea and eczema.

Patients with photosensitivity diseases can be abnormally sensitive to UVB, UVA, visible light (over 400 nm) or, commonly, a combination of wavebands. UVB is absorbed by window glass, whereas UVA and visible light are transmitted through glass.

i	27.9 The photosensitivity and photo-aggravated diseases	
Cause	**Condition**	**Clinical features**
Immunological (previously known as idiopathic)	Polymorphic light eruption (PLE)	Seasonal, itchy, papulovesicular rash on photo-exposed sites; face and back of hands often spared. Often hours of UVR exposure needed to provoke; lasts a few days; affects about 20% in Northern Europe, more common in young women
	Chronic actinic dermatitis (CAD)	Chronic dermatitis on sun-exposed sites. Most common in older adult males. Predominantly UVB, but also often UVA and visible light photosensitivity. Most also have contact allergies
	Solar urticaria	Immediate-onset urticaria on photo-exposed sites. Usually UVA and visible light photosensitivity. Can occur at any age
	Actinic prurigo	Uncommon, presents in childhood. Often familial, with strong HLA association. Some similarities to PLE, although scarring occurs
	Hydroa vacciniforme	Rare childhood photodermatosis. Varioliform scarring
Drugs (variety of mechanisms)	Phototoxicity	Usually UVA (and visible light) photosensitivity
		Most common. Exaggerated sunburn and exfoliation. Many drugs such as thiazides, tetracyclines, fluoroquinolones, quinine, NSAIDs
	Pseudoporphyria	NSAIDs, retinoids, tetracyclines, furosemide are examples
	Photoallergy	Usually to topical agents, particularly sunscreens and NSAIDs
Metabolic	Porphyrias	Mainly porphyria cutanea tarda and erythropoietic protoporphyria
	Pellagra	Photo-exposed site dermatitis due to tryptophan deficiency (see Fig. 22.14)
Photogenodermatoses	Xeroderma pigmentosum	Rare. Defect in DNA excision repair, abnormal photosensitivity, photo-ageing and skin cancer. There may be neurological features
Photo-aggravation of pre-existing conditions	Lupus erythematosus Erythema multiforme Rosacea	Can also be drug-induced (see Box 27.36)

(HLA = human leucocyte antigen; NSAIDs = non-steroidal anti-inflammatory drugs; UVA/UVB = ultraviolet A/B; UVR = ultraviolet radiation)

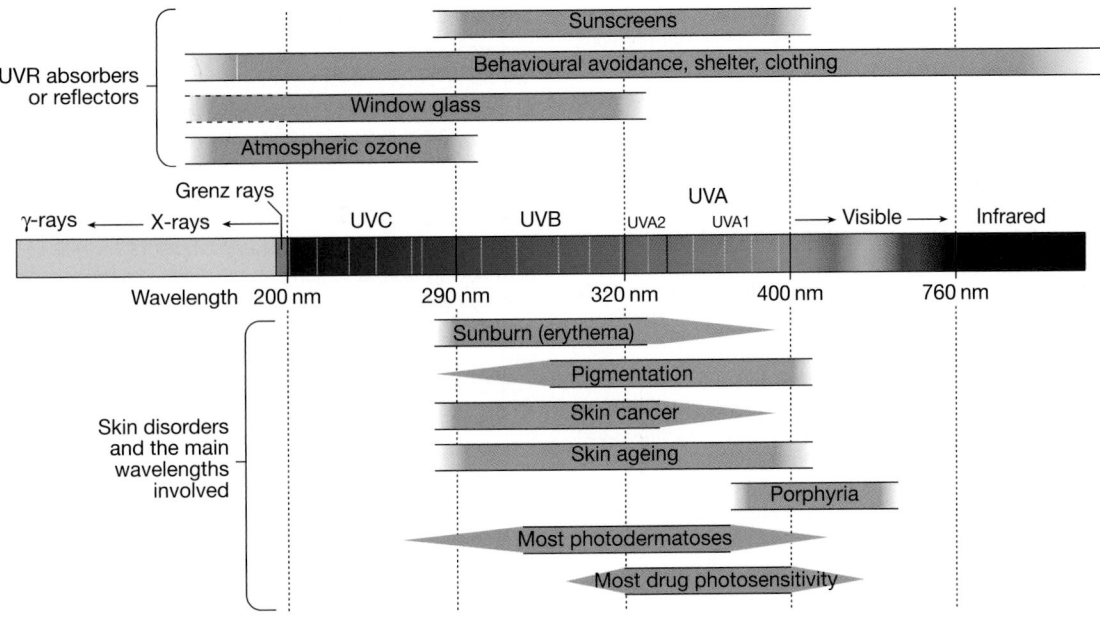

Fig. 27.6 The electromagnetic spectrum. The action spectrum is not well defined for many conditions and, for some, is approximate and may vary between patients. The action spectrum for non-melanoma skin cancer mirrors that for erythema. The action spectrum for melanoma is not known but includes UVA and UVB. Photoprotection measures vary, depending on condition, although the mainstay always includes behavioural modification, clothing cover and appropriate sunscreen choices. (UV = ultraviolet; UVR = ultraviolet radiation)

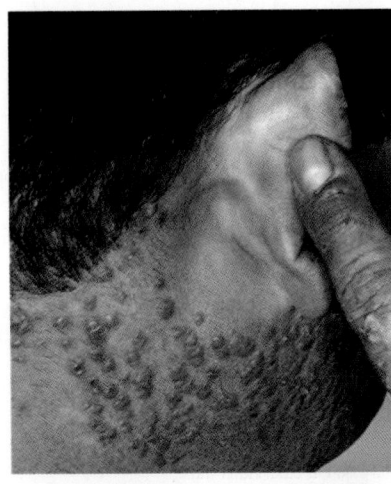

Fig. 27.7 Chronic actinic dermatitis. Note the sharp cut-off and sparing behind the ear in the shadow cast by the earlobe (Wilkinson's triangle).

Clinical assessment

Taking a careful history is essential, as the patient may not have the rash when assessed. Seasonal pattern and distribution of rash are important. Key sites are the face (particularly nose, cheeks and forehead), top of ears, neck (Fig. 27.7), bald scalp, back of hands and forearms. Sparing is often seen under the chin and nose, behind the ears, on the upper eyelids and the distal digits – as we normally walk about with our eyes open and fingers flexed! It can be misleading if there is covered site involvement. Patients who are sensitive to UVA and visible light may be affected through clothing. These patients commonly experience perennial symptoms and may not be aware of the association with daylight exposure. Other photosensitivity diseases, such as actinic prurigo or chronic actinic dermatitis, may also involve covered sites. Sparing of habitually exposed sites, such as the face and back of hands, occurs most commonly in polymorphic light eruption (PLE) and is called the

'hardening phenomenon'. Importantly, some conditions, such as solar urticaria, develop rapidly after sunlight exposure, whereas others, such as cutaneous lupus, can take several days to evolve.

Investigations and management

If photosensitivity is suspected, the patient should be referred to a specialist centre for assessment and investigation, usually involving monochromator phototesting. Other investigations will often include provocation, patch or photopatch testing and screening for lupus and the porphyrias. Rarely, investigations such as human leucocyte antigen (HLA) typing in suspected actinic prurigo, or DNA excision repair functional activity or genotyping in suspected xeroderma pigmentosum, may be required.

Management depends on the cause. If there is a phototoxic drug or chemical cause, this must be identified and addressed: for instance, by stopping the drug or treating the porphyria. Counselling in regard to sun avoidance is essential: keeping out of direct sun in the middle of the day, covering up with clothing, wearing hats with a wide brim and careful use of high-factor sunscreens. Paradoxically, in some conditions, particularly PLE and solar urticaria, phototherapy can be used to induce 'hardening', which is a term used to describe the process by which phototherapy cross-links structures in the skin; in these circumstances the mechanism of desensitisation is unclear. Other approaches may be necessary, depending on disease and severity, and may include antihistamines (useful in two-thirds of patients with solar urticaria) and systemic immunosuppression (sometimes required in the immunological photodermatoses, such as chronic actinic dermatitis). Patients with photosensitivity are at risk of vitamin D deficiency due to reduced vitamin D synthesis by the skin and often require vitamin D supplements.

Sunscreens

Sunscreens can be divided into two categories: chemical sunscreens, which absorb specific wavelengths of UVR, and physical sunscreens, which reflect UVR and the shorter visible wavelengths (see Fig. 27.6). Sunscreens are now highly sophisticated and most offer protection against UVB and most UVA wavelengths. If a patient is abnormally photosensitive to the longer wavelengths of UVA and the visible part of the spectrum (for example, in cutaneous porphyrias and solar urticaria), then conventional sunscreens are not beneficial and specific reflectant

27

sunscreens are required. Historically, these agents were less cosmetically acceptable due to visible light reflection, but current formulations, some of which are tinted, have reduced this problem.

Sunscreen protection levels are described by sun protection factor (SPF). This is the ratio of the dose of UVR required to produce skin erythema in the presence and absence of the sunscreen. A sunscreen of SPF20 means that it would take 20 times as long for a person to develop sunburn in the presence of the sunscreen, as compared to not using it. Therefore, SPF is really a sunburn protection factor and is not a good guide to how well a sunscreen will perform in protecting against other reactions (such as skin pain in erythropoietic protoporphyria or UVR-induced immunosuppression). SPF values are determined under experimental conditions whereas, in practice, people tend to use 25%–33% of the amount of sunscreen required to achieve the stated SPF and it is easy to be lulled into a false sense of security of believing that higher levels of sun protection will be achieved than in reality will be the case. Patient counselling is therefore important with regard to adequate application of sunscreen. Importantly, there is no such thing as a complete 'sunblock' as sunscreens offer, at best, partial protection and are no substitute for modifying behaviour and covering up.

Leg ulcers

Leg ulcer is not a diagnosis, but a symptom of an underlying disease in which there is complete loss of the epidermis, leaving dermal layers exposed. Ulcers on the lower leg are frequently caused by vascular disease but there are other causes, as summarised in Box 27.10.

Clinical assessment

A detailed history of the onset and course of leg ulceration and predisposing conditions should be elicited. The site and surrounding skin should be assessed. Varicose veins are often present, although not inevitably. Assessment of the venous and arterial vasculature and neurological examination are critical. The site of ulceration may also help to indicate the underlying primary cause (Fig. 27.8). Full clinical examination is essential as the ulcer may be arising in the context of systemic disease, such as vasculitis.

i | 27.10 Causes of leg ulceration

Venous hypertension

- Sometimes following deep vein thrombosis

Arterial disease

- Atherosclerosis
- Vasculitis
- Buerger's disease

Small-vessel disease

- Diabetes mellitus
- Vasculitis

Haematological disorders

- Sickle-cell disease
- Cryoglobulinaemia
- Spherocytosis
- Polycythaemia
- Myeloma
- Waldenström's macroglobulinaemia
- Immune complex disease

Neuropathy

- Diabetes mellitus
- Leprosy (Hansen's disease)
- Syphilis

Tumour

- Squamous cell carcinoma
- Basal cell carcinoma
- Malignant melanoma
- Kaposi's sarcoma

Trauma

- Injury
- Factitious

Leg ulceration due to venous disease

Varicose veins, a history of deep venous thrombosis and obesity are predisposing factors. Incompetent valves in the deep and perforating veins of the lower leg result in retrograde flow of blood to the superficial system, and a rise in capillary pressure ('venous hypertension'). Pericapillary fibrin cuffing occurs, leading to impairment of local tissue oxygenation and homeostasis.

The first symptom in venous ulceration is often heaviness of the legs, followed by oedema. Haemosiderin pigmentation, pallor and firmness of surrounding skin, and sometimes venous/gravitational eczema subsequently develop. This progresses to lipodermatosclerosis – firm induration due to fibrosis of the dermis and subcutis, which may produce the well-known 'inverted champagne bottle' appearance. Ulceration, often precipitated by trauma or infection, follows. Venous ulcers typically occur on the medial lower leg (Fig. 27.9).

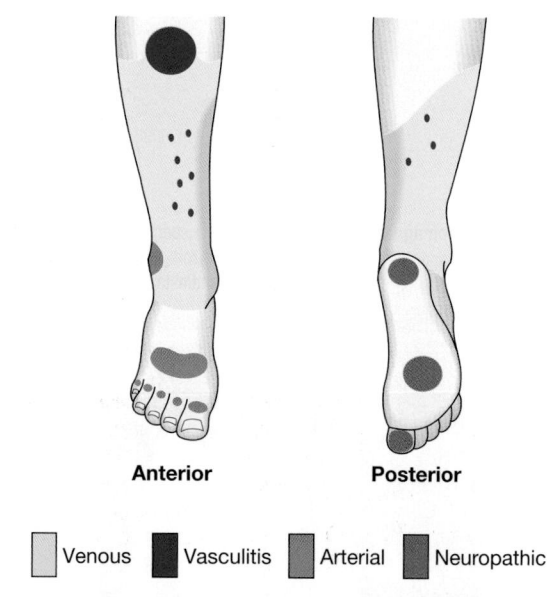

Anterior   **Posterior**

☐ Venous   ■ Vasculitis   ■ Arterial   ■ Neuropathic

Fig. 27.8 Causes of lower limb ulceration. The main types of leg ulcer tend to affect particular sites.

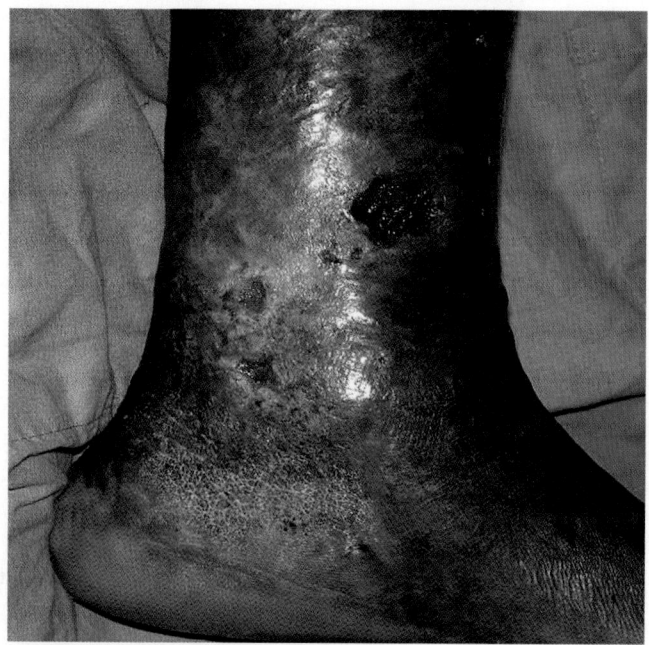

Fig. 27.9 Patient with chronic venous insufficiency who has chronic venous stasis skin changes and venous ulceration. *From Braddom RL, Chan L, Harrast MA. Physical medicine and rehabilitation, 4th edn. Elsevier; 2011.*

Complications of venous leg ulceration include bacterial colonisation and infection, and contact allergic dermatitis to topical medicaments, dressings and bandages. Lipodermatosclerosis may cause lymphoedema and hyperkeratosis; rarely, a squamous cell carcinoma (SCC) may develop in a long-standing venous ulcer (Marjolin's ulcer).

Leg ulceration due to arterial disease

Deep, painful, punched-out ulcers on the lower leg, especially the shin and foot and in the context of intermittent claudication, are likely to be due to arterial disease. Risk factors include smoking, hypertension, diabetes and hyperlipidaemia. The foot is cold and dusky, and the skin atrophic and hairless. Peripheral pulses are absent or reduced. In these circumstances a vascular surgical assessment should be sought urgently.

Leg ulceration due to vasculitis

Vasculitis can cause leg ulceration either directly through epidermal necrosis due to damage to the underlying vasculature, or indirectly due to neuropathy.

Leg ulceration due to neuropathy

The most common causes of neuropathic ulcers are diabetes and leprosy. Microangiopathy also contributes to ulceration in diabetes. The ulcers occur over weight-bearing areas, such as the heel. In the presence of neuropathy, protection of skin from trauma is essential to prevent ulceration.

Investigations

Appropriate investigations include:

- *Full blood count* to detect anaemia and blood dyscrasias.
- *Urea and electrolytes* to assess renal function.
- *Urinalysis* for glycosuria.
- *Bacterial swab* if there is a purulent discharge, rapid extension, cellulitis, lymphangitis or sepsis. This can guide antibiotic therapy for secondary infection but pathogenic bacteria are not always the same as those identified from the ulcer surface.
- *Doppler ultrasound* to assess arterial circulation. An ankle systolic pressure to brachial systolic pressure index (ABPI) of below 0.8 suggests significant arterial disease and a vascular surgery opinion should be sought. However, arterial calcification, such as in diabetes, can produce a spuriously high ABPI. Pulse oximetry may also be useful, although ABPI is the preferred investigation if feasible.

Management

General advice on exercise, weight loss and smoking cessation is important in all cases. Specific management depends on making the correct diagnosis to identify the cause(s) of ulceration. Underlying factors, such as diabetes or anaemia, must be treated. Oedema must be reduced by leg elevation and, if there is no arterial compromise, graduated compression bandaging from toes to knees to enhance venous return and improve healing. Compression bandaging is effective for individuals with an ABPI of more than 0.8 but should be avoided if the ABPI is less than 0.8.

If the ulcer is purulent, weak potassium permanganate soaks may help, and exudate and slough can be removed with normal saline or clean water. Dressings do not themselves heal leg ulcers, but can reduce discomfort and odour and, by reducing colonisation by potential pathogens, may reduce the frequency of secondary infection. A variety of dressings may be used, including non-adherent and absorbent (alginates, hydrogels, hydrocolloids) types. The frequency of dressing changes varies; heavily exudative ulcers may need daily dressings, whereas changes once weekly may suffice for drier ulcers. Occasionally, leeches may be used topically for ulcers with heavy adherent exudate.

Surrounding eczema should be suppressed with a topical glucocorticoid. Commonly, this is venous eczema, but there should be a low threshold for referral for patch testing, as contact allergy to topical applications is common. Systemic antibiotics are indicated only if there is evidence of infection, as opposed to colonisation. Various techniques of split-thickness grafting (such as pinch and mince grafts) may hasten healing of clean ulcers but do not reduce recurrence risk. Leg ulcers can be very persistent but with accurate diagnosis and optimal management, healing is usually achievable. Symptomatic relief, including oral analgesics and sometimes chronic pain management, is important. Once the ulcer has healed, ongoing use of compression hosiery is advised to limit the risk of recurrence.

Abnormal pigmentation

Loss of skin pigmentation (depigmentation), reduction in pigmentation (hypopigmentation) and increased pigment (hyperpigmentation) are features of a variety of disorders. A detailed history and examination, including use of a Wood's light, are required to establish the diagnosis. Investigations will depend on the presentation. For example, microscopy of skin scrapings should be undertaken if hypopigmentation is associated with inflammation and scaling; screening for autoimmune disease may be required if vitiligo is suspected; and investigation for endocrine disease or the porphyrias may be appropriate in hyperpigmentation. Further details of the specific conditions are discussed later in this chapter.

Hair and nail abnormalities

Many conditions affect the skin appendages, particularly hair and nails. Conditions causing hair loss (alopecia) are listed in Box 27.31. Nail changes may be a marker for systemic disease, such as iron deficiency, or be a feature of certain skin conditions, such as psoriasis.

Acute skin failure

Acute skin failure is a medical emergency. Several conditions can cause widespread and acute failure of many skin functions (see Box 27.1), including thermoregulation, fluid balance control and barrier to infection. Many of these conditions involve widespread dilatation of the dermal vasculature and can provoke high-output cardiac failure; they are also associated with increased protein loss from the skin and often from the gut. Many lead to acute skin failure by causing erythroderma (erythema affecting at least 90% of the body surface area), although severe autoimmune blistering diseases and the spectrum of Stevens–Johnson syndrome/toxic epidermal necrolysis (TEN) disease can produce acute skin failure without erythroderma.

Clinical assessment

Detailed history-taking and full examination are required. Particular attention should be paid to drug history, chronology and history of any preceding skin disease. Eczema, psoriasis, drug eruptions and cutaneous T-cell lymphoma (Sézary syndrome) are among the diseases that can either present with, or progress to, erythroderma. Other causes include the psoriasis-like condition pityriasis rubra pilaris, and rare types of ichthyosis. Erythroderma may occur at any age and is associated with severe morbidity and significant mortality (see Fig. 27.36D). Older people are at greatest risk, especially if they have comorbidities. Erythroderma may appear suddenly or evolve slowly. In dark skin, the presence of pigmentation may mask erythema, giving a purplish hue.

Erythrodermic patients are usually systemically unwell with shivering and hypothermia, secondary to excess heat loss. However, they may also be pyrexial and unable to lose heat due to damage to sweat gland function and sweat duct occlusion. Tachycardia and hypotension may be present because of volume depletion. Peripheral oedema is common in erythroderma, owing to low albumin and high-output cardiac failure. Lymph nodes may be enlarged, either as a reaction to skin inflammation or, rarely, due to lymphomatous infiltration.

Investigations and management

Investigations are required to establish the underlying cause and to identify systemic involvement, such as hypoalbuminaemia, deranged liver and renal function and electrolyte imbalance. Skin biopsy may be necessary if the cause is unclear. Regardless of the cause, important aspects of the management of erythroderma include supportive measures to ensure adequate hydration, maintenance of core temperature and adequate nutrition. Insensible fluid loss can be many litres above normal losses. Protein may be lost directly from the skin and through the gut because of the protein-losing enteropathy that often accompanies conditions such as erythrodermic psoriasis. To reduce the risks of infection, any intravenous cannulae should be sited in peripheral veins, if possible. In the initial management of acute erythroderma, urinary catheterisation is often required (for patient comfort and accurate fluid balance monitoring) but catheters should be removed as soon as possible. Frequent application of a simple ointment emollient (such as white soft paraffin/liquid paraffin mix) is usually appropriate.

Principles of management of skin disease

General measures

General measures that apply in all skin diseases include establishment of the correct diagnosis, removal of precipitating or aggravating factors, use of safe, effective treatments and consideration of the patient holistically, taking into account the impact of the disease on quality of life and the person's support network. The psychological impact of chronic skin diseases should not be under-estimated and it is important to remember that psychiatric illness can also manifest as a skin disease, such as in delusions of infestation or trichotillomania. Careful clinical assessment is essential and any management strategy must also include approaches to address the psychological well-being of the patient.

Topical treatments

Topical treatments are first-line therapy for most skin diseases, many of which can be treated effectively by topical agents alone. Selection of the appropriate active drug/ingredient and vehicle is essential. Ointments are preferred to creams for dry skin conditions, such as chronic eczemas, as they are more hydrating and contain fewer preservatives than creams, and so allergy risk is reduced. However, patients find creams easier to apply and so adherence may be better. Gels and lotions can be easier to use on hair-bearing sites. The molecular weight and lipid–water coefficient of a drug determine its skin penetration, with larger, water-soluble, polar molecules penetrating poorly. In skin disease, if the stratum corneum is impaired – as in eczema – increased drug absorption occurs. Occlusion under dressings also increases absorption. Drugs can be used in different potencies or concentrations, or in combination with other active ingredients, and many are available in more than one formulation. The properties of different vehicles are listed in Box 27.11. Overall, adherence to topical treatments can be problematic, so it is essential for patients to know exactly what is required of them and for regimens to be kept as simple as possible. Emollients, topical glucocorticoids and other selected key topical therapies that are widely used in a diverse range of skin conditions are detailed below. For the more disease-specific therapies, detailed descriptions are included in the disease sections.

Emollients

These are mainstays in the treatment of eczema, psoriasis and many other conditions, and are used to moisturise, lubricate, protect and 'soften' skin. They are essentially vehicles without active drug and are available in many formulations: creams, ointments, gels and bath, shower and soap substitutes. White soft paraffin is the most effective and is widely used.

Topical glucocorticoids

Glucocorticoids are available in a variety of formulations, potencies and strengths, most commonly as creams and ointments (Box 27.12). Selection of the correct product depends on the condition being treated, body site and duration of expected use. Mild topical glucocorticoids are used in delicate areas, such as the face or genitals, and close supervision of glucocorticoid use at these sites is required. In contrast, very potent glucocorticoids may be required under occlusion for chronic resistant disease such as nodular prurigo.

Adverse cutaneous effects of chronic glucocorticoid use include atrophy (**definition**: an area of thin, translucent skin caused by loss of

i	27.11 Characteristics of vehicles used in topical treatments				
Vehicle	**Definition**	**Use**	**Site**	**Cosmetic acceptability**	**Risk of contact sensitisation**
Creams	Emulsions of oil and water (aqueous cream)	Acute presentations Cooling, soothing Well absorbed Mild emollients	All sites, including mucous membranes and flexures, but not hair-bearing areas	Very good Helps adherence	Significant, due to preservatives, antimicrobials and often lanolin
Ointments	Greasy preparations Insoluble in water (white soft paraffin) Soluble (emulsifying ointment)	Chronic dry skin conditions Occlusive and emollient Hydrating Mildly anti-inflammatory	Avoid hair-bearing areas and flexures	Moderate	Low
Lotions	Water-based Liquid formulation Often antiseptic and astringent (potassium permanganate)	Cooling effect Cleans the skin and removes exudates	Large areas of the skin and the scalp	Good, but can sting if in an alcoholic base	Rare
Gels	Thickened lotions Hydrophilic and hydrophobic bases	For specific sites	Hair-bearing areas and the face	Good	Low
Pastes	Semi-solid preparations consisting of finely powdered solids suspended in an ointment	Occlusive, protective Hydrating Circumscribed skin lesions, (psoriasis, lichen simplex chronicus)	Any area of skin Often used in medicated bandages	Moderate	Moderate

glucocorticoids can be used in a variety of indications, including nodular prurigo, keloid scar (**definition** of 'scar': replacement of normal structures by fibrous tissue at the site of an injury, although keloid scar describes a pathological process extending beyond the site of injury), acne cysts and alopecia areata.

Anti-infective agents

Antiseptics should be considered before antibiotics, as they cover a wide range of organisms and help to reduce the risk of antibiotic resistance. Antibiotics can be used either for their anti-infective properties or for their anti-inflammatory properties. Topical antiviral and antifungal agents are also widely used for a range of mild skin infections.

Calcineurin inhibitors

The topical calcineurin inhibitors tacrolimus and pimecrolimus can be used to treat eczema and a variety of other conditions, through local cutaneous immunosuppression.

Immune response modifiers

Topical imiquimod was introduced for the treatment of anogenital warts but can be used for a diverse range of other skin diseases, including actinic keratosis, Bowen's disease, basal cell carcinoma, lentigo maligna, cutaneous lupus and common and planar warts. Its mechanism of action is via stimulation of endogenous Th2 immune responses and release of cytokines, including interferon-gamma (IFN-γ). It can cause significant inflammation, requiring dose adjustments, but subclinical disease may respond to treatment.

Dressings

A 'wound' covering is called a dressing. Box 27.13 shows the indications for their use. The active agent, vehicle and 'wound' type should be considered. Wet lesions should be treated with wet dressings. Paste bandages can be used in conjunction with topical emollients and glucocorticoids to soothe and cool, ease pruritus and scratching, and reduce inflammation. Dressings for venous leg ulcers are described later in this chapter.

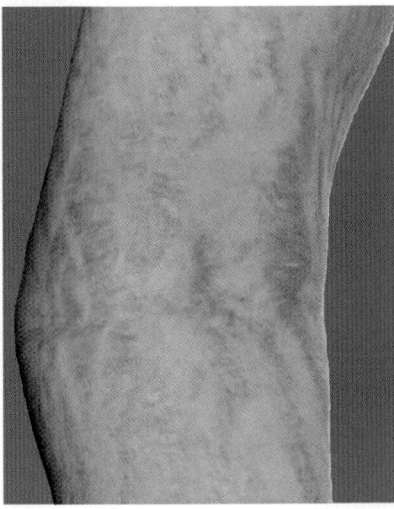

Fig. 27.10 Striae and atrophy induced by excess prolonged potent topical glucocorticoid use.

epidermis, dermis or subcutaneous fat – Fig. 27.10), striae (**definition**: linear, atrophic, pink, purple or white bands caused by connective tissue changes – Fig. 27.10), petechiae and purpura (**definition**: haemorrhagic macules or papules caused by extravasated blood) and telangiectasiae (**definition**: visible dilatations of small cutaneous blood vessels – see Fig. 27.12A), increased risk of infection and systemic absorption, causing Cushingoid features and suppression of the hypothalamic–pituitary–adrenal axis. However, under-treatment with glucocorticoids is more common than over-treatment in routine clinical practice. In general, the lowest potency of glucocorticoid should be used for the shortest period to gain control of the disease; this can be achieved by initial use of a more potent glucocorticoid, with reduction in potency or frequency of application as control is gained. Tolerance or tachyphylaxis can develop with chronic use, so intermittent courses of treatment are advised. Caution is required with glucocorticoids in psoriasis, as rebound, unstable or pustular psoriasis can occur with sudden cessation of use. Nevertheless, glucocorticoids are invaluable for many sites, particularly the flexures. Topical glucocorticoids are often formulated in combination with antiseptics, antibiotics or antifungals, and their controlled use may be appropriate in infected eczema or flexural psoriasis. Intralesional injections of

Phototherapy and photochemotherapy

Ultraviolet radiation (UVR) treatments (most commonly, narrowband ultraviolet B and psoralen–ultraviolet A (PUVA)) are used in the management of many different diseases. The best evidence for their efficacy is in psoriasis, atopic eczema, vitiligo and chronic urticaria, although there is also evidence that UVB is helpful in treating generalised itch associated with chronic kidney disease and a range of other diverse skin conditions.

Psoralens are natural photosensitisers found in a number of plants. They intercalate between the strands of DNA and, on excitation with UVA, cross-link the DNA strands. Psoralens are therefore prodrugs that are activated only in skin that is exposed to UVA. Psoralens can also be applied topically in a bath before irradiation with UVA (bath PUVA) or can

27

be applied in creams or gels for localised topical PUVA. PUVA is a more complex treatment than UVB and has more adverse effects; in particular, cumulative exposure to PUVA increases the risk of skin cancer, particularly squamous cell carcinoma. Therefore, PUVA is generally used for poor responders to UVB, or in diseases such as plaque-stage cutaneous T-cell lymphoma or pityriasis rubra pilaris, where it is the phototherapy of first choice. Phototherapy or PUVA may be offered as a whole-body or localised treatment.

Longer-wavelength UVA1 (340–400 nm) is also used for several conditions, particularly the fibrosing skin diseases such as morphoea, where efficacy has been shown and there is a lack of other well-proven therapies. The evidence base for its place in the management of several diseases, such as eczema, is not fully proven and availability of UVA1 is mainly through tertiary referral centres with expertise in photodermatology and phototherapy.

Systemic therapies

General information is provided here for drugs used in a range of skin diseases; details of other drugs are provided in disease-specific sections.

Antibiotics

Antibiotics are widely used for their anti-infective properties, particularly for staphylococcal and streptococcal skin infections. In these indications, the correct antibiotic should be selected, based on bacterial sensitivity and patient factors. As examples, oral flucloxacillin may be indicated for clinically infected eczema, intravenous flucloxacillin for cellulitis, and clarithromycin for a patient with a staphylococcal carbuncle who is penicillin-allergic. Optimal therapeutic doses and courses must be chosen, based on local antimicrobial prescribing guidelines. Several antibiotics, such as tetracyclines, erythromycin and co-trimoxazole are used predominantly for their anti-inflammatory effects in indications such as acne vulgaris, bullous pemphigoid and pyoderma gangrenosum.

Antihistamines

A range of H_1- and H_2-receptor antagonists are used in dermatology. For diseases in which histamine in the skin is relevant (such as urticaria), non-sedating antihistamines should be given: for example, fexofenadine or cetirizine. For pruritic conditions such as eczema, the sedating effect of antihistamines like hydroxyzine or chlorphenamine is important. However, antihistamines are widely used in older patients for the symptom of pruritus due to a variety of causes such as xeroderma, metabolic impairment, malignancy or concomitant drugs. Sedating antihistamines should be used with caution in older patients, as they may increase the risk of falls and accidents in the home, with disastrous consequences. Careful choice of drug and dose is therefore essential. Leukotriene receptor antagonists, such as montelukast, may be added to antihistamine regimens, for additional mast cell stabilising effects.

Retinoids

Oral retinoids are used in a range of conditions, including acne, psoriasis and other keratinisation disorders. They promote differentiation of skin cells and have anti-inflammatory effects. Isotretinoin (13-*cis*-retinoic acid) is widely used for moderate to severe acne. Acitretin can be effective in psoriasis and other keratinisation disorders, such as ichthyosis, as can alitretinoin (9-*cis*-retinoic acid) in hand and foot eczema and bexarotene in cutaneous T-cell lymphoma.

Adverse effects of retinoids include dryness of the skin and mucous membranes, abnormalities in liver function or hepatitis, increase in serum triglycerides (levels should be checked before and during therapy) and mood disturbances. Alitretinoin and bexarotene can cause hypothyroidism. Systemic retinoids are teratogenic and must be prescribed along with a robust form of contraception. Females must have a negative pregnancy test before, during and after therapy, and pregnancy must be avoided for 2 months after stopping isotretinoin and 2 years after stopping acitretin.

Immunosuppressants

Systemic glucocorticoids, particularly prednisolone, are widely used in inflammatory skin diseases, such as eczema, immunobullous disease and connective tissue disorders. Methotrexate, azathioprine and mycophenolate mofetil are effective in eczema and psoriasis either alone or as glucocorticoid-sparing agents. Further details on the mechanism of action, adverse effects and monitoring requirements for these agents are provided in Chapter 26 (see Box 26.33). Hydroxycarbamide is an alternative immunosuppressant to methotrexate in psoriasis, but is not licensed for this indication and appears to be less effective than methotrexate. The risk of myelosuppression is greater. Dimethyl fumarate is also used off label in the treatment of psoriasis. Ciclosporin has a rapid onset of action and is effective in inducing clearance of psoriasis and eczema. Monitoring of blood pressure and renal function is required. Ciclosporin should be used only with caution after phototherapy, particularly PUVA, because of the increased risk of skin cancer. Long-term use of ciclosporin is not advised. Dapsone is an immunomodulator and may be used in diseases in which neutrophils are implicated, such as dermatitis herpetiformis. Haemolysis, methaemoglobinaemia and hypersensitivity can occur, and monitoring is required. Hydroxychloroquine is of particular value in cutaneous lupus.

Biologic and other advanced therapies

Major advances in the treatment of inflammatory skin diseases have been made in recent years through increased understanding of pathophysiology, the identification of new molecular targets for drug design and the introduction of biological treatments and small molecules that target specific signalling pathways involved in the inflammatory response. Biologic treatments work by binding to and neutralising pro-inflammatory cytokines or components of their receptors whereas small molecule inhibitors target intracellular signalling pathways situated downstream of cytokine receptors.

Multiple biologics are available for the treatment of severe or treatment-resistant psoriasis. These include multiple inhibitors of tumour necrosis factor alpha (TNF-α) (adalimumab, certolizumab, etanercept and infliximab), ustekinumab, which inhibits interleukin (IL)-12 and IL-23 by binding to the p40 component of both cytokines; guselkumab, which is a specific inhibitor of IL-23; ixekizumab and secukinumab, which are inhibitors of IL-17; and brodalumab, which inhibits the IL-17 receptor (Fig. 27.11).

Dupilumab is an antibody that targets the IL-4 receptor alpha chain subunit, which is common to both IL-4 and IL-13 receptors. It has been shown to be efficacious in the treatment of severe atopic dermatitis resistant to standard therapies. Tralokinumab and lebrikizumab are specific inhibitors of IL-13 which are also showing promise in the treatment of severe atopic dermatitis but these are not yet licensed for clinical use (Box 27.14). Omalizumab, a monoclonal antibody directed against immunoglobulin E (IgE), which is used in severe asthma, also has a role in the treatment of urticaria and some patients with atopic dermatitis. Small molecule targeted synthetic immunosuppressives have also been developed. Apremilast inhibits phosphodiesterase-E4 (PDE-4) reducing cytokine production by immune cells and is used in psoriasis. Crisaborole, another PDE-4 inhibitor, is under development for the treatment of psoriasis. Baricitinib and upadacitinib, which inhibit Janus activated kinase (JAK) enzymes that are involved in signalling downstream of several cytokine receptors, are also used in psoriasis and atopic dermatitis. Rituximab, which binds to CD20 causing depletion of B cells, is used in pemphigus vulgaris. Intravenous immunoglobulin, pooled from donor plasma, may be used in the treatment of dermatomyositis and occasionally may be indicated in other dermatological diseases. More detail on the dosages, mechanism of action and adverse effects of these agents

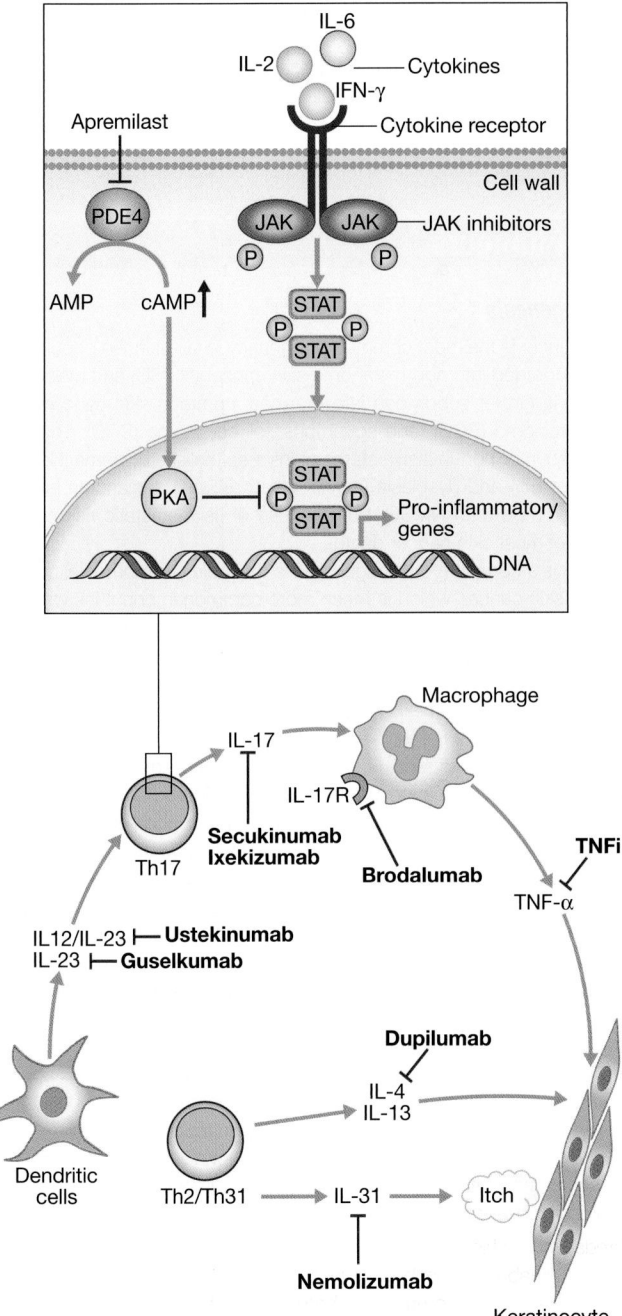

Fig. 27.11 Biologic and targeted therapies in inflammatory skin diseases.
Biologic treatments for inflammatory rheumatic diseases work by targeting key cytokines or their receptors involved in regulating the immune response. (IL = interleukin; Th = T-helper cell subtype; TNFα = tumour necrosis factor alpha; TNFi = inhibitor of tumour necrosis factor alpha; PDE4 = phosphodiesterase E4; JAK = Janus activated kinase; PKA = protein kinase A; STAT = signal transducers and activators of transcription; cAMP = cyclic adenosine monophosphate)

Drug	Class and type of drug	Molecular target	Function of target	Indication
27.14	**New and emerging therapies for inflammatory skin disease**			
Tralokinumab	Mab inhibitor	IL-13	Pro-inflammatory cytokine	Atopic dermatitis
Lebrikizumab	Mab inhibitor	IL-13	Pro-inflammatory cytokine	Atopic dermatitis
Fezakinumab	Mab inhibitor	IL-22	Pro-inflammatory cytokine	Atopic dermatitis
Nemolizumab	Mab inhibitor	IL-31	Mediator of itch	Atopic dermatitis
Crisabrole	Small molecule inhibitor	PDE4	Regulates cytokine production by immune cells	Atopic dermatitis Psoriasis
Fingolomod	Small molecule inhibitor	S1PR	Trafficking of immune cells to the skin	Atopic dermatitis
Ponesimid	Small molecule inhibitor	S1PR	Trafficking of immune cells to the skin	Atopic dermatitis
Tapinarof	Small molecule agonist	Aryl hydrocarbon receptor	Inhibits production of inflammatory cytokines	Atopic dermatitis Psoriasis

(Mab = monoclonal antibody)

involved in regulating production of IL-17 and other cytokines in the skin. Tumour targeted kinase inhibitors and biologics directed against CTLA-4 and the programmed cell death (PD1) pathways which are used in the treatment of melanoma are discussed later in this chapter.

Dermatological surgery

Most dermatological surgical procedures are performed under local anaesthetic. Knowledge of local anatomy is essential, particularly the locations of vessels and nerves. In certain sites, such as the fingers, soles of the feet and the nose, local cutaneous nerve blocks are useful. Some sites are associated with particular risks, such as keloidal scarring on the upper trunk of young patients, unsightly scars over the scapulae, and poor healing and risk of ulceration following procedures on the lower legs.

Excision biopsy

This involves surgical removal of the lesion followed by histological examination. The most common indication is suspicion of malignancy. The lesion and line of excision should be marked out and the margin of excision decided before the procedure. It is important to excise down to the appropriate anatomical plane. Depending on body site, a range of procedures can minimise the resulting defect. Healing by secondary intention may also achieve good cosmetic results.

Curettage

Curettage involves using a small, spoon-shaped implement (curette), not only as a definitive treatment but also to obtain histology. Curettage does not preserve tissue architecture very well, however, and it may be difficult to distinguish between dysplasia and invasive malignancy. It can be an effective treatment for basal cell papilloma, actinic keratosis, intra-epidermal carcinoma and superficial basal cell carcinoma.

are provided in Chapter 26 (see Box 26.35). Other new treatments that are under development include: nemolizumab, which targets the IL-31 receptor and improves itching in atopic dermatitis; ponesomid and fingolimod, which target the sphingosine-1-phosphate pathway, which is involved in trafficking immune cells into the skin; fezakinumab, which inhibits IL-22, a proinflammatory cytokine implicated in the pathogenesis of psoriasis and atopic dermatitis; and tapinarof, a small molecule modulator of the aryl hydrocarbon receptor which is a transcription factor

27

Shave excision

Shave excision using local anaesthetic may be used for simple and effective treatment of raised superficial benign skin lesions affecting epidermis and upper dermis, such as benign naevi and skin tags.

Mohs' micrographic surgery

Mohs' micrographic surgery is employed to ensure adequate tumour excision margins, while conserving unaffected tissue. It is most commonly used for basal cell carcinoma.

Non-surgical treatments

Cryotherapy

Cryotherapy is a destructive treatment using liquid nitrogen to cause cellwall and membrane destruction and cell death. Liquid nitrogen can be applied either with a cotton bud or, more effectively, with a spray gun. A wide variety of conditions can be treated but it is essential for the correct diagnosis to be made first, if necessary by diagnostic biopsy. Cryotherapy should not be used to treat melanocytic naevi. Benign lesions, such as viral warts and basal cell papilloma, respond well, and cryotherapy can also be effective for actinic keratosis, Bowen's disease or superficial non-melanoma skin cancer. Malignant indications require more vigorous treatment, usually with two cycles, and this is normally carried out in secondary care. Considerable inflammation, blistering and pigmentary change, particularly hypopigmentation, can occur. Caution is required to avoid damage to tendons and nerves, especially when using cryotherapy on digits.

Laser therapy

Laser therapy involves treatment with monochromatic light. Skin components (chromophores), such as haemoglobin and melanin, absorb specific wavelengths of electromagnetic radiation, and these wavelengths can therefore be used to destroy these targets selectively and to treat certain skin disorders. Lasers targeting haemoglobin are employed for vascular abnormalities, such as spider naevi, telangiectasiae and portwine stains, and lasers targeting melanin can treat benign pigmentary disorders or pigment in tattoos or drug-induced hyperpigmentation (for example, secondary to minocycline). Melanin-targeted lasers can also be used for hair removal if the hair is pigmented. Light delivery in short pulses restricts damage to the treated site.

The carbon dioxide laser emits infrared light that is absorbed by water in tissues and can therefore be used for destructive purposes. The depth of effect can be controlled, such that the carbon dioxide laser is widely employed for resurfacing in photorejuvenation or acne scarring. Significant morbidity is associated with this destructive laser, although this may be minimised with fractionated regimens, and general anaesthesia may be required.

Photodynamic therapy

Photodynamic therapy (PDT) is widely used in dermatology, predominantly for actinic keratoses, Bowen's disease and superficial basal cell carcinoma.

Radiotherapy and grenz (Bucky) ray therapy

Radiotherapy can be employed for several skin conditions, including non-melanoma skin cancer or lentigo maligna that is not suitable for surgical treatment, but its use in dermatology has declined. Scarring and poikiloderma can occur at treated sites, although these are minimised if fractionated regimens are chosen. Superficial radiotherapy is now rarely employed to treat benign dermatoses. Even more superficial ionising radiation (grenz (Bucky) rays) can be useful for localised dermatoses that are having severe effects on quality of life, if conventional treatments have been inadequate; for example, it may avoid the need for systemic immunosuppression in a patient with severe recalcitrant localised scalp psoriasis.

Skin tumours

Pathogenesis

Skin cancer is the most common malignancy in fair-skinned populations. It is subdivided into non-melanoma skin cancer (NMSC) and melanoma. NMSC is further subdivided into the most common skin cancer, basal cell carcinoma (BCC), and squamous cell carcinoma (SCC). The latter has precursor non-invasive states of intra-epithelial carcinoma (Bowen's disease, BD) and dysplasia (actinic keratosis, AK). Melanoma is much less common than NMSC, but because of its metastatic risk it is the cause of most skin cancer deaths.

UVR is a complete carcinogen and is the main environmental risk factor for skin cancer, which is much more common in countries with high ambient sun exposure, such as Australia. Skin cancer risk also increases if an individual migrates to such a country when young, particularly if less than 10 years of age. Epidemiological evidence supports a close link between chronic UVR exposure and risk of SCC and AK, and a modest link between sun exposure and BCC risk. Melanoma usually arises on sites that are intermittently exposed to UVR, and episodes of sunburn and recreational sun exposure have been implicated as risk factors for melanoma. There is good evidence to show that sunbed exposure is also a risk for both melanoma and NMSC, particularly when exposure starts in adolescence and early adult life. Strategies to reduce sun exposure are therefore important for skin cancer prevention, with reliance mainly on behavioural modification, covering up and judicious sunscreen use. Indeed, there is evidence to show that sunscreen use reduces naevi development in children, and in adults regular sunscreen use reduces the risk of AK and SCC and is likely also to have preventative roles in melanoma and BCC development.

There are identifiable genetic predispositions for some skin cancers, such as in xeroderma pigmentosum, an autosomal recessive condition caused by an inherited defect in DNA excision repair, and basal cell naevus (Gorlin) syndrome, an autosomal dominant disorder caused by loss-of-function mutations affecting the PTCH1 tumour suppressor genes, with consequent activation of the Hedgehog pathway. Interestingly, the Hedgehog pathway is also almost invariably activated in sporadic BCC, which usually contain somatic mutations in PTCH1 and less commonly in the SMO gene, which lies in the same signalling pathway. The genetics of SCC are heterogeneous and less clearly defined, with several mutations and pathways implicated, including TP53, CDKN2A/p16, NOTCH, EGFR and the MAPK signalling pathways. Interestingly, many of the mutations seen in SCC also occur in the pre-cancers AK and BD. The genetics of melanoma are discussed later in this chapter.

Cutaneous immune surveillance is also critical and immunosuppressed organ transplant recipients have a greatly increased risk of skin cancer, particularly SCC. Interestingly, patients who have received high treatment numbers of PUVA (more than 150), which is immunosuppressive, are also at increased risk of skin cancer, particularly SCC.

Although UVB can increase the risk of skin cancer, there is no evidence to date that UVB phototherapy significantly increases skin cancer risk. Likewise, there is no evidence that UVA1 phototherapy increases skin cancer risk, although ongoing vigilance is required. Ionising radiation, notably radiotherapy, thermal radiation and chemical carcinogens, such as arsenic or coal tar, can increase NMSC risk, particularly SCC. A role for oncogenic human papillomaviruses in SCC development is also implicated, particularly in immunosuppressed patients, where viral DNA is detected in more than 80% of tumours. Chronic inflammation is a risk factor for SCC, which may arise in chronic skin ulcers, discoid lupus erythematosus or vulgaris, and the scarring genetic skin disease dystrophic epidermolysis bullosa (see Box 27.26), in which up to 50% of patients develop SCC.

Malignant tumours

Basal cell carcinoma

The incidence of NMSC has increased dramatically in recent decades and basal cell carcinoma (BCC) accounts for more than 70% of cases. In Europe, the ratio of BCC to SCC is 4–5:1 in immunocompetent patients. It is a malignant tumour that rarely metastasises; it is thought to derive from immature pluripotent epidermal cells and is composed of cells with similarities to basal layer epidermis and appendages. Lesions typically occur at sites of moderate sun exposure, particularly the face, and are slow-growing. The incidence increases with age and males are more commonly affected. Lesions may ulcerate and invade locally; hence the term 'rodent ulcer'.

Clinical features

Early BCCs usually present as pale, translucent papules or nodules, with overlying superficial telangiectatic vessels (nodular BCC). If untreated, they increase in size and ulcerate, to form a crater with a rolled, pearled edge and telangiectatic vessels (Fig. 27.12). There may be some pigmentation or a cystic component. A superficial multifocal type can occur, frequently on the trunk, and may be large (up to 10 cm in diameter); often there are multiple lesions. Superficial BCC usually presents as a red/brown plaque or patch with a raised, thread-like edge, which is often best seen by stretching the skin; this helps to distinguish it from Bowen's disease. Less commonly, a morphoeic, infiltrative BCC presents as a poorly defined, slowly enlarging, sclerotic yellow/grey plaque.

Diagnosis and management

The diagnosis is often obvious clinically, based on the features mentioned above, although a diagnostic confirmatory biopsy may be required prior to definitive treatment. Management depends on the characteristics of the tumour and on patient factors, including comorbidities and patient wishes. Essentially, treatment will be either surgical or, in some cases, medical (Box 27.15). Surgical excision, ideally with a 4–5 mm margin, is the treatment of choice, with a cure rate of approximately 95%. Curettage and cautery may also be effective for selected lesions. Management of infiltrative morphoeic BCC and/or lesions at difficult sites, such as around

the eye, may require more complex techniques, such as Mohs' micrographic surgery, to ensure adequate tumour excision margins, while conserving unaffected tissue. This involves processing of frozen sections of all margins in stages (usually on the same day) until all the tumour is removed. The procedure is time-consuming (so can be difficult for older, frail patients) and requires particular surgical and pathology skills, but is associated with the highest long-term cure rates, with 98%–99% clear at 5-year follow-up.

If a surgical approach is used for management of BCC and the primary tumour is not completely excised, re-excision may be required, although follow-up may be appropriate as not all tumours that are incompletely excised recur. However, this is not recommended for tumours at high-risk sites or for infiltrative morphoeic BCC, where complete excision is advisable. Cryotherapy may be effective for BCC but can cause blistering and scarring, so is best suited to small, superficial lesions at low-risk sites.

Radiotherapy can be invaluable for large BCC lesions in frail patients but is less commonly used because of the risk of scarring.

Medical therapies can be used to treat low-risk BCC, particularly when surgery is not appropriate for a patient. Topical immunomodulators, such as imiquimod, are effective for low-risk BCC and may be particularly useful for patients who are not able to attend a hospital clinic setting but are able to apply a topical preparation at home over a 6-week period. Imiquimod usually induces a prominent inflammatory reaction and patients should be advised that dose adjustments may be required. Topical 5-fluorouracil can also be effective for low-risk small lesions of superficial BCC, although this usually provokes an intense inflammatory reaction. Intralesional interferon-alfa2b has been used for BCC but multiple treatments and high cost preclude its regular use.

PDT is an effective treatment for low-risk, predominantly superficial BCC, as well as AK and BD. Usually, topical porphyrin PDT is employed, which involves application of a porphyrin prodrug to the lesion to be treated. The prodrug is taken up and converted by the cell's haem cycle to protoporphyrin IX, a photosensitiser. This is

---

> **ℹ 27.15 Management of non-melanoma skin cancer and pre-cancer**
>
> **Basal cell carcinoma**
> - Excision results in the lowest recurrence rates
> - Mohs' micrographic surgery is effective for high-risk BCC
> - Medical treatments are often appropriate for low-risk superficial tumours in patients with comorbidities
> - Cryotherapy and topical 5-fluorouracil can be used for superficial BCC
> - Topical photodynamic therapy and topical imiquimod are both effective in superficial BCC
> - BCC in patients with Gorlin syndrome should not be treated with radiotherapy
> - Hedgehog pathway inhibitors can induce clinical response in patients with advanced inoperable BCC
>
> **Squamous cell carcinoma**
> - Excision is the treatment of choice for invasive SCC
> - Most recurrences or metastases occur within 5 years
> - Medical management is not usually considered for invasive SCC
>
> **Carcinoma in situ (Bowen's disease)**
> - For single/few lesions on good healing sites, cryotherapy, curettage, photodynamic therapy, topical imiquimod and 5-fluorouracil are options
> - For multiple lesions and/or poor healing sites such as the lower leg, photodynamic therapy, where feasible, is the treatment of choice, although topical 5-fluorouracil or imiquimod are alternative treatments
>
> **Actinic keratosis**
> - For single/few lesions on good healing sites, cryotherapy, curettage and 5-fluorouracil + salicylic acid are options. especially if hyperkeratotic
> - For multiple lesions/field change, topical 5-fluorouracil, conventional or daylight photodynamic therapy, imiquimod or diclofenac in hyaluronic acid gel may be effective

27

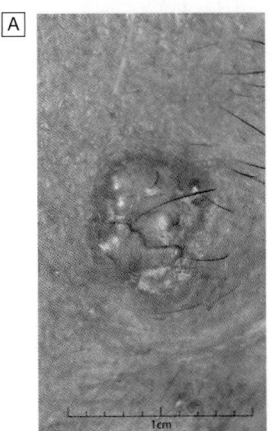
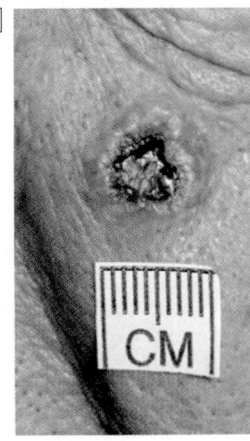

Fig. 27.12 Basal cell carcinoma. **A** A nodular BCC showing the translucent nature of the tumour and the abnormal arborising vessels. **B** An ulcerated BCC showing the raised, rolled edge.

photochemically activated by visible (normally red) light, usually delivered by a light-emitting diode (LED), in the presence of oxygen, causing the production of reactive oxygen species, which cause destruction of treated tissue. The photosensitiser is taken up preferentially by diseased skin, and adverse effects in normal skin are minimised. PDT is at least as effective as cryotherapy and surgery for superficial BCC and may be preferred at sites of poor healing, such as the lower leg, or where cosmetic outcome is important. PDT is not as effective as surgery for long-term clearance of nodular BCC but can be considered if surgery is not appropriate. Pain during irradiation may occur during PDT, although adjustments to the irradiation regime can reduce discomfort and treatment is usually well tolerated. PDT is typically undertaken in the outpatient clinic setting and is well suited to frail patients and those unable to undertake treatment with topical agents at home.

Rarely, advanced BCC may be locally invasive or even metastasise. Major advances have been made in targeted drug development, and Hedgehog pathway inhibitors, such as vismodegib and sonidegib, can be used effectively for disease control and palliation in this setting, although there may be significant associated drug-induced toxicity.

Squamous cell carcinoma

Squamous cell carcinoma (SCC) is a malignancy that arises from epidermal keratinocytes and is the second most common skin cancer, occurring most frequently in older adult males and smokers. There is a close association between cumulative UVR exposure and SCC risk, with most SCC lesions occurring on chronically sun-exposed sites in light-skinned populations and often arising at sites of field-change carcinogenesis, with coexistent precursors of AK and BD commonly evident. In the immunosuppressed patient population, such as organ transplant recipients, SCC is the most common skin cancer and its incidence is dramatically increased, particularly in association with the duration of immunosuppression and the degree of sun exposure and damage accrued pre-transplant. The risk of SCC is also increased in HIV infection. Furthermore, SCC arising in the immunosuppressed is more likely to behave aggressively or to metastasise.

Clinical features

The tumours usually occur on chronically sun-exposed sites, such as bald scalp, tops of ears, face and back of hands. The clinical presentation may be diverse, ranging from rapid development of a painful keratotic nodule in a pre-existing area of dysplasia (Fig. 27.13) to the de novo presentation of an erythematous, infiltrated, often-warty nodule or plaque that may ulcerate. The clinical appearance depends on histological grading; well-differentiated tumours more often present as defined keratotic nodules (Fig. 27.13A), whereas poorly differentiated tumours tend to be ill defined and infiltrative, and may ulcerate. SCC has metastatic potential; some tumours, such as those on lips and ears and in immunosuppressed patients, behave more aggressively and are more likely to metastasise to draining lymph nodes.

Management

Early diagnosis is important and complete surgical excision is the usual treatment of choice (see Box 27.15). Standard excision with a 4–6mm margin is advised and the cure rate is approximately 90%–95%. Mohs' surgery is an option but is used less frequently for SCC than for BCC. High-risk SCC should be treated aggressively, with a wider margin of excision of at least 6mm where feasible. This may include larger, thicker lesions, tumours at sites where metastases are more likely, such as the ear, lip or non-sun-exposed sites, and those occurring in the immunosuppressed and/or with histology showing the tumour to be poorly differentiated, with evidence of lymphatic, vascular or perineural involvement or a high mitotic index. Such patients and those with metastatic disease require management via a multidisciplinary team. In patients who are at high risk for further SCC, systemic retinoids may have a role in reducing the rate of SCC development, but rapid appearance of tumours occurs on drug cessation. Occasionally, curettage and cautery may be appropriate if the tumour is small and low-risk and either surgical excision is contraindicated or the patient is unwilling to proceed with excision. Radiotherapy may be indicated if surgical excision is not feasible. Cryotherapy and topical non-surgical therapies are not usually used in invasive SCC because of risk of recurrence and metastasis.

Actinic keratosis

Actinic keratoses (AK) are scaly, erythematous lesions arising on chronically sun-exposed sites. Histology shows dysplasia, although the diagnosis of typical AK is usually made on clinical grounds (Fig. 27.14). They are common in fair-skinned people who have had significant sun exposure, are often multiple and increase with age. The prevalence is much higher in Australia than in the UK and some surveys have shown a prevalence of more than 50% in those over 40 years old. The rate of progression to SCC is less than 0.1% and spontaneous resolution is possible. However, SCC can also arise de novo and without progression from AK. Increase in size, ulceration, bleeding, pain or tenderness can be indicative of transformation into SCC.

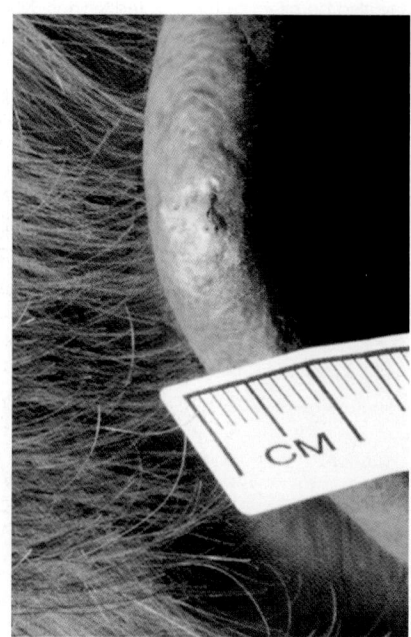

Fig. 27.14 Actinic keratosis. Close-up of a hyperkeratotic AK on the ear.

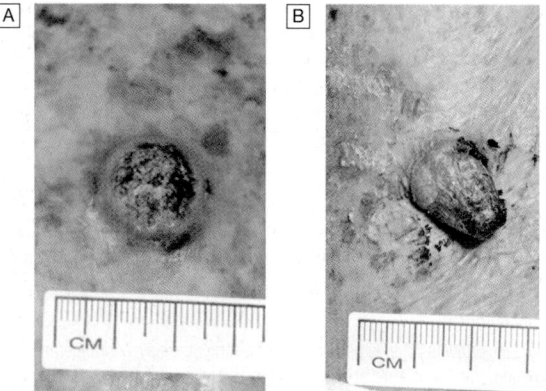

Fig. 27.13 Squamous cell carcinoma. [A] A centrally keratinous, symmetrical, well-differentiated SCC. Clinically, this could be confused with keratoacanthoma. [B] An SCC arising from an area of epidermal dysplasia.

Management

Several treatments are available for AK (see Box 27.15). Emollients and photoprotection, including high-factor sunscreens, may suffice for mild disease. Single or low numbers of lesions of AK can be effectively treated with cryotherapy. Hyperkeratotic lesions may be treated with the antimetabolite 5-fluorouracil, combined with salicylic acid, or may require curettage and cautery.

Multiple lesions require field-directed therapy; 5-fluorouracil is widely used in this setting as an effective initial therapeutic approach and topical imiquimod is an alternative. Diclofenac in a hyaluronic acid gel base can also be used topically for low-grade maintenance control of AK, the rationale for its use being the over-expression of cyclo-oxygenase (COX)-2 in AK lesions. PDT is widely used for field-change multiple AK, with high efficacy rates; it is at least as effective as cryotherapy or 5-fluorouracil. The relative selectivity of treatment allows subclinical disease to be treated, while sparing normal skin. A regimen using daylight to activate the photosensitiser is increasingly and widely used for extensive mild AK, with high efficacy rates, comparable to hospital-based PDT but without the need for specialised equipment and allowing patients to be treated at home.

Bowen's disease

Clinical features

Bowen's disease (BD) is the name given to an intra-epidermal carcinoma that usually presents as a slowly enlarging, erythematous, scaly plaque on the lower legs of fair-skinned older women (Fig. 27.15) but other sites can also be involved. It can be confused with eczema or psoriasis, but is usually asymptomatic and does not respond to topical glucocorticoids. It may also be hard to distinguish from superficial BCC. Transformation into SCC occurs in 3% or less.

Diagnosis

Incisional biopsy is usually undertaken to confirm the diagnosis. This shows an intra-epidermal carcinoma with no invasion through the basement membrane. Histology may also be obtained by curettage but this does not allow distinction from invasive SCC to be made, due to loss of tissue orientation and architecture.

Management

While curettage or excision may be appropriate in some settings, non-surgical therapies are generally preferred (see Box 27.15), especially on the lower legs. PDT, in particular, may be advantageous for BD on the lower leg because of relative selectivity of treatment and sparing of normal tissue, thus reducing the risk of poor healing and ulceration at this vulnerable site. Given the low risk of malignant transformation, the option of no active treatment may also be appropriate for some frail patients with multiple co-morbidities.

Cutaneous lymphomas

The most common form of cutaneous T-cell lymphoma is mycosis fungoides (MF). This can persist for years in patch and plaque stages,

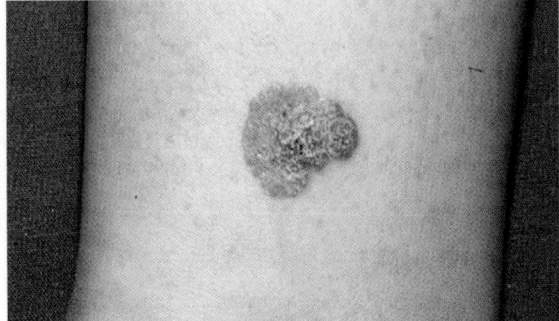

Fig. 27.15 Intra-epidermal carcinoma (Bowen's disease). The lower leg is a common site and lesions are often treated non-surgically.

often resembling eczema or psoriasis. Only sometimes does it progress through to nodules and finally a systemic stage, Sézary syndrome. B-cell lymphomas, on the other hand, usually present as nodules or plaque-like tumours. The diagnosis of cutaneous T-cell lymphoma requires a high index of suspicion, particularly in patients thought to have unusual recalcitrant forms of eczema or psoriasis.

Treatment is symptomatic and there is no evidence that it alters prognosis. In the early stages of cutaneous T-cell lymphoma, systemic or local glucocorticoids may be indicated; alternatively, narrowband UVB phototherapy (for patch-stage MF) or PUVA (for plaque-stage MF) may be used. Once lesions have moved beyond plaque stage, localised radiotherapy, electron beam radiation, the synthetic retinoid bexarotene, interferon-alfa, extracorporeal photopheresis and systemic anti-lymphoma chemotherapy regimens may be needed. Management of advanced disease invariably requires a multidisciplinary team approach, with collaboration between dermatologists, pathologists and haematological oncologists.

Melanoma

Melanoma is a malignant tumour of epidermal melanocytes. While only 4% of skin cancers are melanomas, they account for 80% of skin cancer deaths. There has been a steady rise in the incidence of melanoma in fair-skinned populations over recent decades, with the highest incidence in Australasia. Primary prevention and early detection are essential, as therapy for advanced and metastatic disease, whilst being a rapidly evolving field, remains challenging and unsatisfactory.

Pathophysiology

Risk factors for melanoma include fair skin, freckles, red hair, number of naevi and sunlight exposure. The type of sunlight exposure is under debate but intermittent exposure, such as recreational time in the sun, sunburn and sunbed use, is implicated. Patients with multiple atypical naevi (dysplastic naevus syndrome) and fair-skinned people, often with variant alleles in the melanocortin-1 gene, are at increased risk of melanoma. A family history of melanoma increases the risk but a strong family history is unusual. Rarely, autosomal dominant inheritance of melanoma with incomplete penetrance can occur due to mutations in *CDKN2A*, which encodes the p16 tumour suppressor protein. In these patients, the lifetime risk of melanoma is more than 50%. Several other susceptibility genes and potential genetic targets for therapeutic intervention in advanced disease have also been identified.

Clinical features

Melanoma can occur at any age and site and in either sex, but typically affects the leg in females and back in males. It is rare before puberty. The classification of invasive malignant melanoma is shown in Box 27.16. Early lesions may be in situ and pre-invasive before becoming invasive melanoma with metastatic potential. Any change in naevi or development of new lesions should be assessed to exclude malignancy and, for this, the dermatoscope is invaluable (see Fig. 27.2). Real-time non-invasive imaging techniques are being investigated as tools to assist in diagnosis but are largely experimental. If there is any doubt, excision is advised.

Superficial spreading melanoma

Superficial spreading melanoma (SSM) is the most common type in light-skinned populations. It usually presents as a slowly enlarging, macular, pigmented lesion, with increasing irregularity in shape and pigment; this superficial, radial growth phase can last for approximately 2 years. Subsequently, the lesion may become palpable and this is indicative of a vertical growth phase, with dermal invasion; when this occurs, the tumour has the potential to invade lymphatics and vessels and to become metastatic (Fig. 27.16A). Approximately 50% of melanomas arise from a pre-existing naevus.

Nodular melanoma

Nodular melanoma is most common in the fifth and sixth decades, particularly in men and on the trunk (Fig. 27.16B). This may account in part

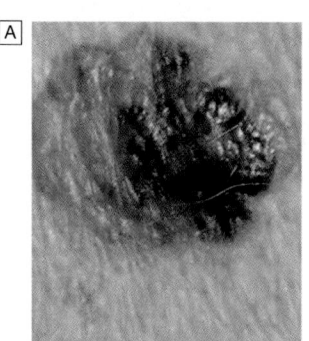 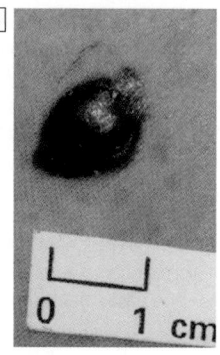

Fig. 27.16 Superficial spreading melanoma. [A] A superficial spreading malignant melanoma with a palpable area indicative of vertical growth phase (Breslow thickness 1.3 mm). [B] A nodular malignant melanoma arising de novo and with Breslow thickness of 3.5 mm.

for the increased mortality rates from melanoma in men, as these are tumours with greater metastatic risk. They often present as a rapidly growing nodule that may bleed and ulcerate. Nodular melanomas may be heavily pigmented, or relatively amelanotic and erythematous, and be confused with benign vascular lesions. A rim of pigmentation may, however, be seen under the dermatoscope. Lesions may develop de novo or from a pre-existing naevus or SSM.

Lentigo maligna melanoma

This arises from a prolonged pre-invasive phase termed lentigo maligna. It occurs as a very slowly expanding, pigmented, macular lesion, usually on photo-exposed head and neck sites of older patients; histology shows in situ changes only. This phase may last for several years before a nodule of invasive melanoma develops in a proportion of cases (lentigo maligna melanoma).

Acral lentiginous or palmoplantar melanoma

This accounts for only approximately 10% of melanomas in light-skinned races and is more common in dark-skinned people, in whom it is responsible for 50% of cases. This indicates that UVR exposure may not be implicated in acral melanoma risk.

Subungual melanoma

This form of melanoma is rare. It may present as a painless, proximally expanding streak of pigmentation arising from the nail matrix, and progresses to nail dystrophy and involvement of the adjacent nail fold (Hutchinson's sign).

Diagnosis and management

The diagnosis is made by excision biopsy of a suspicious lesion. The initial biopsy should include a 2 mm margin, followed up where possible by wider excision if the diagnosis is confirmed. Occasionally, radiotherapy or imiquimod may be used for lentigo maligna, if surgery is not feasible. The Breslow thickness of the tumour (the maximal depth from epidermal granular cell layer to deepest tumour cells) is critical for management and prognosis. The presence of ulceration may lead to under-estimation of the Breslow thickness and may also adversely affect prognosis. The mitotic rate and the presence or absence of any evidence

of lymphovascular or perineural involvement should also be ascertained. The clinical staging of melanoma extent is essential, in order to establish whether disease is primary and localised, or if there is nodal or metastatic spread.

Wide excision of melanoma with a low risk of metastasis (stage 1 disease, Breslow thickness <1 mm) with a 1 cm clear margin is accepted practice. The margin of excision for more advanced disease is controversial, although a 2–3 cm margin for thicker tumours is generally advised as an attempt to reduce risk of local recurrence. There is no evidence that more radical surgery with 4–6 cm margins is beneficial. The majority of tumours can be excised without the need for grafting. For tumours with a Breslow thickness of 0.8–1 mm or more, a sentinel lymph node biopsy is indicated and should be considered on a case-by-case basis as, in addition to provision of prognostic information, a positive sentinel node biopsy facilitates access to adjuvant treatment with either targeted therapy and/or immune checkpoint inhibitors and is often required before entry to clinical trials of new treatments. Patients must be counselled about the sentinel node biopsy procedure, which is usually performed at the time of wider excision. It involves injection of radio-labelled blue dye at the site of the primary melanoma, allowing identification of the draining 'sentinel' node by radioscintigraphy; this sentinel node is then removed and examined in detail by histology, immunohistochemistry and/or PCR of melanocyte gene products to look for tumour deposits.

If the biopsy is positive, adjuvant therapy should be considered as described below and has largely replaced the need for complete local lymphadenectomy, which is a procedure that is associated with high morbidity in terms of lymphoedema and has no proven survival benefit. Nowadays it is only undertaken if there is a high risk of bulky locoregional recurrence.

Localised cutaneous or nodal recurrence may be treated surgically and cutaneous metastases or in transit disease may be amenable to palliation with electrochemotherapy if there is no evidence of widespread metastatic disease.

There have been major advances in treatment options for advanced melanoma, such that patients are often now able to have extended survival, sometimes for many years. However, ultimately the overall prognosis for metastatic disease remains poor and treatment options remain palliative, with disease control as opposed to cure. Genetic developments have facilitated the introduction of tumour-targeted treatments for advanced, unresectable and/or metastatic disease, such as the *B-Raf* and *c-Kit* kinase inhibitors for patients expressing these gene mutations, notably dabrafenib and vemurafenib, with demonstrable clinical responses. Combined BRAF and MEK targeted inhibition, with drugs such as trametinib, may also be used. Immune checkpoint inhibition with ipilimumab, which causes T-cell activation by inhibiting CTLA-4, alone or in combination with the programmed cell death (PD1) pathway blockers nivolumab or pembrolizumab, provides clinically meaningful improvements in quality of life and survival to patients with advanced disease. Standard chemotherapy may also be used in some cases of metastatic disease, although outcomes are poor. Other biologic and gene therapies and vaccines are also being investigated. It is important for patients with advanced melanoma to be managed through a multidisciplinary team in order to optimise care, provide access to adjuvant therapy and facilitate their inclusion in clinical trials.

All patients should be advised regarding ongoing photoprotection, with sensible behaviour in the sun, covering up, wearing hats and high-factor sunscreen use. However, evidence has shown that despite patients with melanoma being advised to photoprotect, many follow this advice only for the first year following diagnosis, thus emphasising the need for ongoing reinforcement of guidance with regard to photoprotection. It is also prudent to advise patients who are photoprotecting to optimise oral vitamin D through diet and/or supplements.

Prognosis

Prognosis is influenced by several factors, including tumour characteristics and thickness (Breslow thickness) and the presence or absence of regional, nodal or metastatic disease. Patients with in situ melanoma do not have risk of metastasis and those with an invasive primary tumour of less than 1 mm Breslow thickness have more than a 90% chance of 5-year disease-free survival, but this figure drops to approximately 50% for a tumour of greater than 3.5 mm thickness. Survival rates fall to less than 10% for those with advanced nodal or metastatic disease.

Benign skin lesions

In practice, it is often difficult to distinguish between skin cancer and a benign lesion on clinical grounds; if there is any doubt, biopsy and histology are required. Benign melanocytic naevi and basal cell papilloma, in particular, can often be mistaken for melanoma, even by dermatologists. Keratoacanthoma, while benign, is also commonly considered to be invasive SCC on clinical grounds.

Keratoacanthoma

This benign tumour has a striking clinical presentation of rapid growth over weeks to months and subsequent spontaneous resolution. It is thought to be associated with chronic sun exposure and most commonly occurs on the central face. The classical appearance is of an isolated dome-shaped nodule often of 5 cm or more in diameter, with a central keratin plug (Fig. 27.17). Clinically and histologically, the lesion often resembles SCC (see Fig. 27.13A). Most are treated surgically, either by curettage and cautery or by excision, to rule out SCC and to avoid the unsightly scar after spontaneous resolution.

Freckle

Histologically, a freckle (ephelis) consists of normal numbers of melanocytes, but with focal increases in melanin in keratinocytes. They are most common on sun-exposed sites in fair-skinned individuals, particularly children and those with red hair, and on the face. There is a familial tendency. Clinically, freckles are brown macules that darken following UVR exposure.

Lentigo

A lentigo (plural lentigines) consists of increased numbers of melanocytes along the basement membrane, but without formation of the nests that occur in melanocytic naevi. These lesions usually occur at sites of chronic sun exposure (see the background skin changes in Fig. 27.13A), become more common with age, and are often referred to as 'liver spots' or 'age spots'. They can vary in colour from light to very dark brown. Distinction from melanoma is essential and histology may be required.

Haemangiomas

Benign vascular tumours or hamartomas are common and include Campbell de Morgan spots (see Fig. 27.18), which present as pink/red papules on the upper half of the body. They can sometimes be difficult to distinguish from melanocytic lesions, particularly if they are thrombosed or occur on particular sites, such as the lip or genitalia. The dermatoscope is helpful for this (see Fig. 27.2).

Basal cell papilloma

Basal cell papillomas (also known as seborrhoeic warts or keratoses) are common, benign epidermal tumours (Fig. 27.18). They may be flat, raised, pedunculated or warty-surfaced, and can appear to be 'stuck on'. They occur in both sexes and with increasing age, and are most common on the face and trunk. The colour may vary from yellow to almost black and the surface may seem 'greasy', with pinpoint keratin plugs visible, particularly with a magnifying lens. If there is no doubt about the diagnosis, they can be left alone or treated by cryotherapy or curettage if they are cosmetically troublesome. If there is a suspicion of melanoma, excision or diagnostic biopsy should be undertaken.

Melanocytic naevi

Melanocytic naevi (moles) are localised benign clonal proliferations of melanocytes. It is thought that they may arise as the result of abnormalities in the normal migration of melanocytes during development. It is quite normal to have 20–50, although, interestingly, individuals with red hair have fewer. Genetic and environmental factors are implicated. Monozygotic twins have higher concordance in naevi numbers than dizygotic twins. Individuals who have had greater sun exposure have higher numbers of naevi. Most melanocytic naevi appear in childhood and early adult life, or during pregnancy or oestrogen therapy. The onset of a new mole is less common after the age of 25 years. Congenital melanocytic naevi occur at or shortly after birth.

Clinical features

Acquired melanocytic naevi are classified according to the microscopic location of the melanocyte nests (Fig. 27.19). Junctional naevi are usually macular, circular or oval, and mid- to dark brown. Compound and intradermal naevi are nodules because of the dermal component, and may be hair-bearing. Intradermal naevi are usually less pigmented than compound naevi. Their surface may be smooth, cerebriform, hyperkeratotic or papillomatous.

Some individuals have large numbers of naevi, often at unusual sites, such as the scalp, palms or soles, and these may frequently appear 'atypical' in terms of variability in pigmentation, size and shape. Some may be very dark or pink and may show a depigmented or inflamed halo.

27

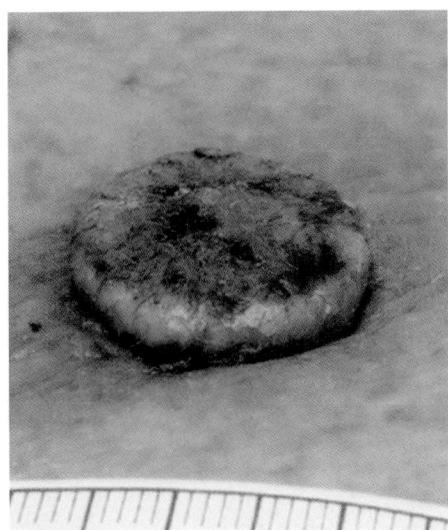

Fig. 27.17 Keratoacanthoma.

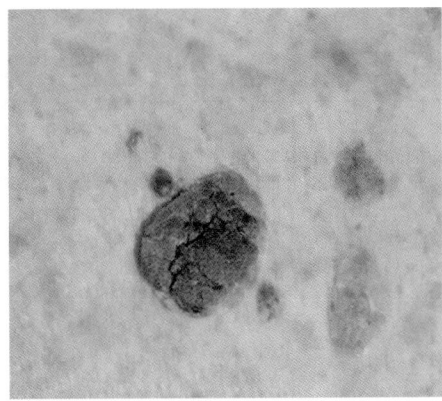

Fig. 27.18 A typical basal cell papilloma. Note the neighbouring basal cell papillomas and the coincidental benign angiomas (Campbell de Morgan spots).

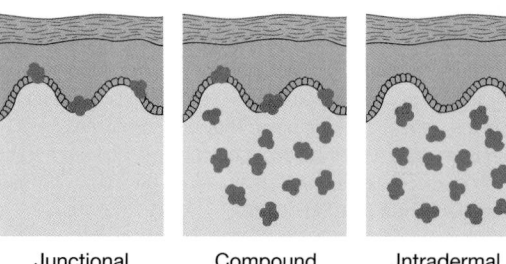

Junctional   Compound   Intradermal

Fig. 27.19 Classification of melanocytic naevi. Classification is based on microscopic location of the nests of naevus cells.

If these naevi are removed, then 'dysplastic changes' are often seen. Such naevi are known to occur in some rare families with an inherited melanoma predisposition. However, the significance of such changes in non-familial cases is unclear and there is no consensus on management and follow-up.

Although approximately 50% of melanomas arise in pre-existing naevi, most naevi do not become malignant; although a changing naevus must be taken seriously, most will not be melanomas. Malignant change is most likely in large congenital melanocytic naevi (risk may correlate with size of lesion) and possibly in families where there is a history of large numbers of atypical naevi and/or a history of melanoma.

Diagnosis and management

Melanocytic naevi are normal and do not require excision, unless malignancy is suspected or they become repeatedly inflamed or traumatised. Advice on photoprotection is important for fair-skinned individuals with multiple naevi.

Blue naevi

These are melanocytic naevi in which there is a proliferation of spindled melanocytes relatively deep within the dermis. Light scattering means that the pigment appears blue rather than brown. They may be difficult to distinguish from nodular melanoma and are therefore often excised.

Dermatofibroma

A dermatofibroma is a characteristically firm, often pigmented, raised lesion, most commonly found on the lower legs. Its aetiology is unclear, although a reactive process secondary to insect bites or trauma is one hypothesis. There is frequently a ring of pigment around the lesion and dimpling when the skin is pinched, reflecting epidermal tethering.

Acrochordon

Acrochordons, or skin tags, are benign pedunculated lesions; they are most common in skin flexures and usually have a very characteristic clinical appearance. However, they may sometimes be confused with melanocytic naevi. Treatment is not required unless there is diagnostic doubt or they are causing symptoms, such as irritation, or for cosmetic reasons. Cryotherapy or snip or shave excision may be appropriate in that situation.

Lipoma

Lipomas are benign tumours of adipocytes that are characteristically soft and lie more deeply in the skin than epidermal tumours; they are usually diagnosed easily on clinical grounds. A variant, angiolipoma, is typically

painful. Treatment is not required unless there is diagnostic doubt or they are symptomatic or cosmetically troublesome, in which case a diagnostic biopsy or surgical excision may be required.

Common skin infections and infestations

Bacterial infections

Impetigo

Impetigo is a common and highly contagious superficial bacterial skin infection. There are two main presentations: bullous impetigo, caused by a staphylococcal epidermolytic toxin, and non-bullous impetigo (Fig. 27.20), which can be caused by either *Staphylococcus aureus* or streptococci, or both together. *Staphylococcus* spp. are the most common agents in temperate climates, whereas streptococcal impetigo is more often seen in hot, humid areas. All ages can be affected but non-bullous disease particularly affects young children, often in late summer. Outbreaks can arise in conditions of overcrowding and poor hygiene or in institutions. A widespread form can occur in neonates. Predisposing factors are minor skin abrasions and the existence of other skin conditions, such as infestations or eczema.

In non-bullous impetigo, a thin-walled vesicle develops; it rapidly ruptures and is rarely seen intact. Dried exudate, forming golden crusting, arises on an erythematous base. In bullous disease, the toxins cleave desmoglein-1, causing a superficial epidermal split and the occurrence of intact blisters with clear to cloudy fluid, which last for 2–3 days. The face, scalp and limbs are commonly affected but other sites can also be involved, particularly if there are predisposing factors such as eczema. Lesions may be single or multiple and coalesce. Constitutional symptoms are uncommon. A bacterial swab should be taken from blister fluid or an active lesion before treatment commences. Around one-third of the population is a nasal carrier of *Staphylococcus*, so swabs from the nostrils should also be obtained.

In mild, localised disease, topical treatment with mupirocin or fusidic acid is usually effective and limits the spread of infection. The use of topical antiseptics and soap and water to remove infected crusts is also helpful. Staphylococcal carriage should be treated, with mupirocin topically to the nostrils, if swabs are positive. In severe cases, an oral antibiotic, such as flucloxacillin or clarithromycin, is indicated. If nephritogenic streptococci are isolated then systemic antibiotics should be considered to reduce the risk of streptococcal glomerulonephritis. Underlying disease, such as infestations, must be treated and cross-infection minimised. Scarring does not occur but there may be temporary dyspigmentation.

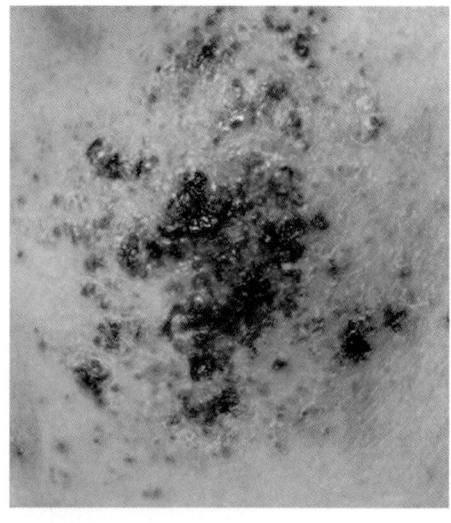

Fig. 27.20 Non-bullous impetigo.

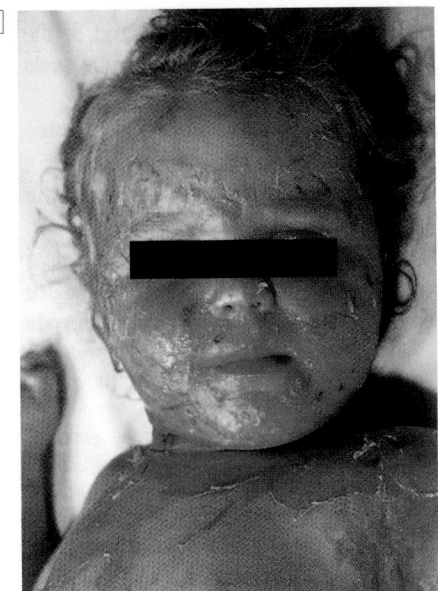

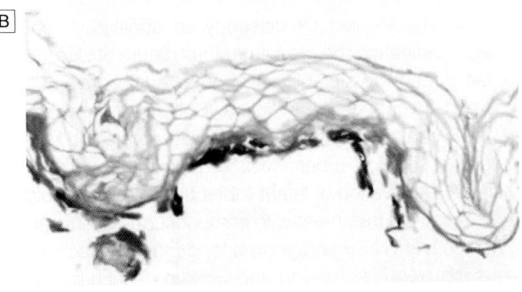

Fig. 27.21 Staphylococcal scalded skin syndrome. [A] Extensive erythema and superficial peeling of the skin. [B] The condition was rapidly diagnosed by examination of a frozen section of skin snip. *(A) From Savin JA, Dahl M, Hunter JAA. Clinical dermatology, 3rd edn. Oxford: Blackwell; 2002.*

Staphylococcal scalded skin syndrome

Staphylococcal scalded skin syndrome (SSSS) is a potentially serious exfoliating condition occurring predominantly in children, particularly neonates (Fig. 27.21). It is caused by systemic circulation of epidermolytic toxins from a *Staph. aureus* infection. The same toxins are implicated in bullous impetigo, which is a localised form of SSSS. The focus of infection may be minor skin trauma, the umbilicus, urinary tract or nasopharynx. The child presents with fever, irritability and skin tenderness. Erythema usually begins in the groin and axillae, and around the mouth. Blisters and superficial erosions develop over 1–2 days and can rapidly involve large areas, with severe systemic upset. Bacterial swabs should be obtained from possible primary sites of infection. A skin snip should also be taken for urgent histology. This is a sample of the superficial peeling skin removed by 'snipping with scissors', without the need for local anaesthetic. It shows a split beneath the stratum corneum, and differentiates SSSS from toxic epidermal necrolysis, in which the whole epidermis is affected (see Fig. 27.41). Systemic antibiotics and intensive supportive measures should be commenced immediately. Bacterial swabs from nostrils, axillae and groins should be taken from family members to exclude staphylococcal carriage. Although the acute presentation of SSSS is often severe, rapid recovery and absence of scarring are usual, as the epidermal split is superficial.

Toxic shock syndrome

This condition is characterised by fever, desquamating rash, circulatory collapse and multi-organ involvement. It is caused by staphylococcal

toxins and early cases were thought to arise with tampon use. Intensive supportive care and systemic antibiotics are required.

Ecthyma

Ecthyma is caused by either staphylococci or streptococci, or both together, and is characterised by adherent crusts overlying ulceration. It occurs worldwide but is more common in the tropics. In Europe, it occurs more frequently in children. Predisposing factors include poor hygiene, malnutrition and underlying skin disease, such as scabies. It is commonly seen in drug abusers, and minor trauma can predispose to lesion development. Management approaches are similar to impetigo as ecthyma can be considered as a deeper version of impetigo. Crust removal, antiseptics and systemic antibiotics may be required.

Folliculitis, furuncles and carbuncles

Hair follicle inflammation can be superficial, involving just the ostium of the follicle (folliculitis), or deep (furuncles and carbuncles).

Superficial folliculitis

The primary lesions are follicular pustules and erythema. Superficial folliculitis is often infective, caused by *Staph. aureus*, but can also be sterile and caused by physical (for example, traumatic epilation) or chemical (for example, mineral oil) injury. Staphylococcal folliculitis is most common in children and often occurs on the scalp or limbs. Pustules usually resolve without scarring in 7–10 days but can become chronic. In older children and adults, they may progress to a deeper form of folliculitis. The condition is often self-limiting and may respond to irritant removal and antiseptics. More severe cases may require topical or systemic antibiotics and treatment of *Staph. aureus* carrier sites.

Deep folliculitis (furuncles and carbuncles)

A furuncle (boil) is an acute *Staph. aureus* infection of the hair follicle, usually with necrosis. It is most common in young adults and males. It is usually sporadic but epidemics occasionally occur. Malnutrition, diabetes and HIV predispose, although most cases arise in otherwise healthy people. All body sites can be involved but neck, buttocks and anogenital areas are commonly affected areas. Infection is often associated with chronic *Staph. aureus* carriage in the nostrils and perineum, and may be due to resistant strains, such as methicillin-resistant organisms (MRSA). Friction caused by tight clothing may be contributory. Initially, an inflammatory follicular nodule develops and becomes pustular, fluctuant and tender. Crops of lesions sometimes occur. There may be fever and mild constitutional upset. Lesions rupture over days to weeks, discharge pus, become necrotic and leave a scar.

If a deep *Staph. aureus* infection of a group of contiguous hair follicles occurs, this is termed a carbuncle and is associated with intense deep inflammation (Fig. 27.22). This usually occurs in middle-aged men, often

27

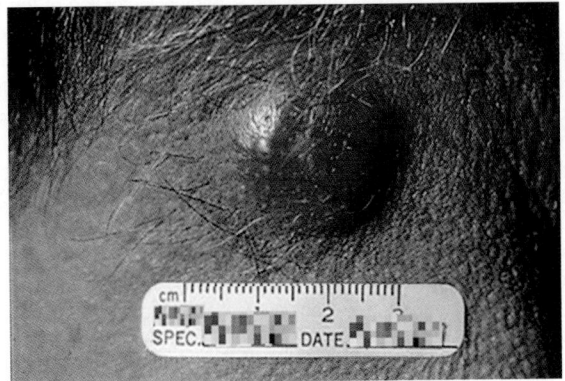

Fig. 27.22 Staphylococcal carbuncle.

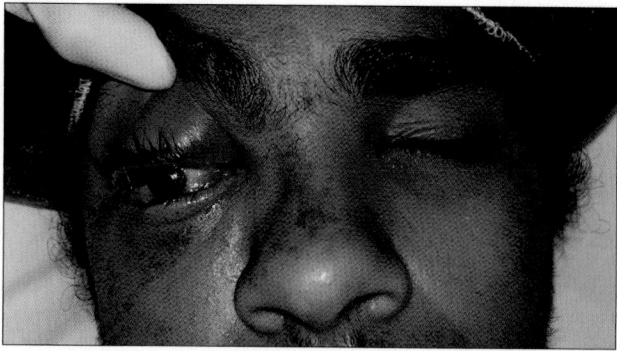

Fig. 27.23 Severe right orbital cellulitis. There is proptosis, chemosis, reduced ocular motility and reduced vision. From Yanoff M, Duker JS. Ophthalmology, 5th edn. Elsevier; 2019.

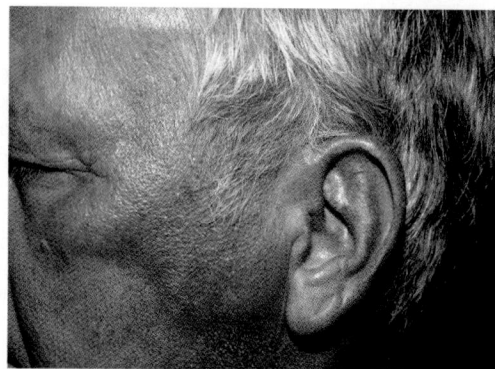

Fig. 27.24 Erysipelas. *From Schwarzenberger K, Werchniak A, Ko C. General dermatology. Elsevier; 2009.*

with predisposing conditions such as diabetes or immunosuppression. A carbuncle is an exquisitely tender nodule, usually on the neck, shoulders or hips, associated with severe constitutional symptoms. Discharge, necrosis and scarring are usual. Bacterial swabs must be taken and treatment is with anti-staphylococcal antibiotics, e.g. flucloxacillin, and sometimes incision and drainage.

Other staphylococcal toxins may also be pathogenic. For example, Panton–Valentine Leukocidin (PVL)-producing *Staph. aureus* can cause recurrent abscesses (**definition**: localised collections of pus in cavities) and may be difficult to eradicate.

Cellulitis and erysipelas

Cellulitis is inflammation of subcutaneous tissue, due to bacterial infection (Fig. 27.23). In contrast, erysipelas is bacterial infection of the dermis and upper subcutaneous tissue (Fig. 27.24), although in practice it may be difficult to distinguish between them. These conditions are most commonly caused by group A streptococci but culture of swabs from affected sites is often negative. There is frequently a source of organism entry, such as an ear infection, varicose eczema/ulcer or tinea pedis, and swabs should also be taken from these sites. Diabetes and immunosuppression are predisposing factors. The patient usually has malaise, fever and leucocytosis, and streptococcal serology will often be positive. The face (erysipelas) and legs (cellulitis) are most often affected and the site is hot, painful, erythematous and oedematous. Blistering often occurs and may be haemorrhagic. Regional lymphadenopathy is common. Erysipelas typically has a well-defined edge due to its more superficial level of involvement, whereas cellulitis is typically ill defined. Treatment is usually with intravenous flucloxacillin, with clarithromycin, clindamycin and vancomycin as alternatives for penicillin-allergic patients. Milder

cases may be treated with oral antibiotics. If cases are untreated, sequelae include lymphoedema, cavernous sinus thrombosis, sepsis and glomerulonephritis.

Mycobacterial infections

Mycobacterium leprae infection may involve the skin and its manifestations will be influenced by host immunity, patients with high levels of immunity presenting with paucibacillary tuberculoid leprosy and those with low immune resistance developing multibacillary lepromatous leprosy. Hypopigmented or erythematous patches, with associated altered or lost sensation, or skin thickening, nodules and infiltration should raise suspicion of a diagnosis of leprosy. The skin may also be an extrapulmonary site of involvement in tuberculosis, usually due to infection with *Mycobacterium tuberculosis*. Skin manifestations depend on the route of infection, previous sensitisation and host immunity. There may be a variety of cutaneous features, including the red–brown scarring inflammatory plaques seen in lupus vulgaris due to direct skin inoculation; scrofuloderma, which describes the skin changes overlying lymph nodes or joints infected with tuberculosis; and the reactive nodular and ulcerated changes seen in patients with high levels of immune response, notably the tuberculids and erythema induratum (Bazin's disease). On diascopy, an 'apple jelly' appearance is typically seen, indicating the granulomatous nature of skin involvement. Granulomas evident on skin biopsy should certainly raise suspicion of a diagnosis of mycobacterial infection. Culture of organisms may be tricky but PCR can assist with diagnosis. Patients should be thoroughly investigated for signs of tuberculosis at pulmonary or other extrapulmonary sites. Reactivation of latent tuberculosis is a particular concern for patients receiving treatment with immunosuppressants and biologic agents, particularly TNF-α antagonists for conditions such as psoriasis. Vigilance is required in screening and workup of such patients prior to consideration of these therapeutic agents. Management of tuberculosis is discussed in Chapter 17.

Other mycobacterial skin infections may occur, such as *Mycobacterium marinum*, typically seen in those who clean tropical fish tanks. Sporotrichoid spread of granulomatous nodules from the site of inoculation along lymphatics is typical; granulomatous changes are seen on histology and resolution usually occurs with a prolonged course of antibiotics such as doxycycline or minocycline. Resolution may also take place spontaneously or after destructive therapies, such as cryotherapy.

Leishmaniasis

This protozoan infection may be restricted to the skin or there may be systemic features depending on the species, which occur in different geographical areas. The clinical features and management of this condition are discussed in Chapter 13.

Necrotising soft tissue infections and anthrax

These conditions are discussed in more detail in Chapter 13.

Erythrasma

Erythrasma is a mild, chronic, localised, superficial skin infection caused by *Corynebacterium minutissimum*, which is part of the normal skin flora. Warmth and humidity predispose to this infection, which usually occurs in flexures and toe clefts. It is asymptomatic or mildly itchy and lesions are well defined, red–brown and scaly. *C. minutissimum* has characteristic coral-pink fluorescence under Wood's light. Microscopy and culture of skin scrapings can confirm the diagnosis but are not usually needed if Wood's light examination is positive. A topical azole (clotrimazole or miconazole) or fusidic acid is usually effective. Oral erythromycin can be used for extensive or resistant disease. Antiseptics can be used to prevent disease recurrence.

Pitted keratolysis

This is another superficial skin infection caused by *Corynebacterium* and *Streptomyces* spp., and possibly other organisms, producing characteristic circular erosions ('pits') on the soles. It is usually asymptomatic. The bacterium can be identified in skin scrapings and typically occurs in association with hyperhidrosis, which must be treated to prevent recurrence. Treatment is as for erythrasma.

Other bacterial skin infections

Syphilis and the non-venereal treponematoses are discussed in Chapter 15. There has been a marked increase in incidence of syphilis. Skin signs may be subtle; for example, secondary syphilis may be misdiagnosed as pityriasis rosea. Lesions on palms, soles and mucosae should raise suspicion. Microscopic identification of the spirochaete may be possible and syphilitic serology should be undertaken using enzyme immunoassay or PCR-based techniques, depending on availability. Lyme disease can also cause a skin rash; the clinical features and management are described in Chapter 13.

Viral infections

Herpesvirus infections

The cutaneous manifestations of the human herpesviruses are described in more detail in Chapter 13. Topical antivirals may suffice for prophylaxis or treatment of mild viral disease, such as herpes simplex cold sore virus infection. Systemic antivirals are indicated for significant viral skin disease. For example, systemic aciclovir should be prescribed for eczema herpeticum (see Fig. 13.15C).

Papillomaviruses and viral warts

Viral warts are extremely common and are caused by the DNA human papillomavirus (HPV). There are over 90 subtypes, based on DNA sequence analysis, causing different clinical presentations. Transmission is by direct virus contact, in living or shed skin, and is encouraged by trauma and moisture, such as in swimming pools. Genital warts are spread by sexual activity and show a clear relationship with cervical and intra-epithelial cancers of the genital area. HPV-16 and 18 appear to inactivate tumour suppressor gene pathways and lead to squamous cell carcinoma of the cervix or intra-epithelial carcinoma of the genital skin. Vaccinations are available against HPV-16 and 18 and are recommended for females and males aged 12–13 years, before they become sexually active, with the objective of offering protective effects against cervical, genital, anal and some head and neck malignancies. The relationship between skin HPV and skin cancer is unclear. Individuals who are systemically immunosuppressed – after organ transplantation, for example – have greatly increased risks of skin cancer and HPV infection but a causal link is not certain.

Clinical features

Common warts are initially smooth, skin-coloured papules, which become hyperkeratotic and 'warty'. They are most common on the hands (Fig. 27.25) but can occur on the face, genitalia and limbs, and are often multiple. Plantar warts (verrucae) have a slightly protruding rough surface and horny rim, and are often painful on walking. Paring reveals capillary loops that distinguish plantar warts from corns. Other varieties of wart include:

- *mosaic warts*: mosaic-like sheets of warts
- *plane warts*: smooth, flat-topped papules, usually on the face and backs of hands, which may be pigmented and therefore misdiagnosed
- *facial warts*: often filiform
- *genital warts*: may be papillomatous and exuberant.

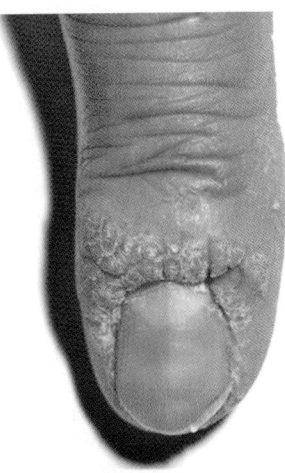

Fig. 27.25 Viral wart on the finger. The capillary loops are evident within the warty hyperkeratosis. Periungual sites are common and more difficult to treat.

Management

Most viral warts resolve spontaneously, although this may take years and active treatment is therefore often sought. However, asymptomatic warts generally should not be treated. Viral warts are particularly problematic and more recalcitrant to treatment in immunosuppressed patients following organ transplantation.

Treatments are destructive. Salicylic acid or salicylic/lactic acid combinations and regular wart paring for several months are the most consistently effective treatments. For certain types of warts, such as filiform facial warts, cryotherapy is generally the treatment of choice, but for common hand and foot warts salicylic acid wart paint should be used first. Cryotherapy is usually the next step and is repeated 2–4-weekly. However, caution is required, particularly on the hands, as over-vigorous cryotherapy can lead to scarring, nail dystrophy and even tendon rupture. Periungual and subungual warts can be problematic and nail cutting and subsequent electrodessication may help. Several other therapies have been used for recalcitrant warts, including topical formaldehyde, glutaraldehyde, podophyllotoxin, trichloroacetic acid, cantharidin, topical or systemic retinoids, intralesional bleomycin or interferon injections, and contact sensitisation with, for example, diphencyprone. Imiquimod and PDT may also be beneficial, particularly for multiple warts in immunosuppressed patients, and laser therapy can have a role in some cases.

Molluscum contagiosum

Molluscum contagiosum is caused by a DNA poxvirus skin infection. It is most common in children over the age of 1 year, particularly those with atopic dermatitis. It also occurs frequently in immunosuppressed patients, including those with HIV. Lesions are dome-shaped, 'umbilicated', skin-coloured papules with central punctum (Fig. 27.26). They

27

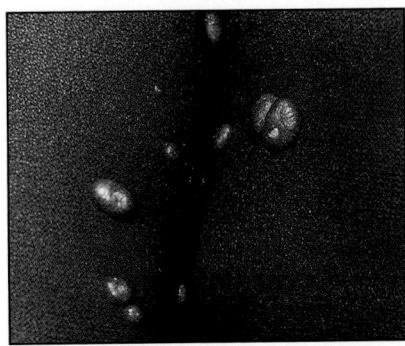

Fig. 27.26 Molluscum contagiosum. Some of the pearly lesions show characteristic umbilication. *From Lissauer T, Carroll W. Illustrated textbook of paediatrics, 6th edn. Elsevier; 2022.*

are often multiple and found at sites of apposition, such as the side of the chest and the inner arm. Spontaneous resolution occurs but can take months. Prior to resolution, they often become inflamed and may leave small, atrophic scars. Destructive therapies may be painful and risk scarring, and the decision not to treat is often sensible. Gentle squeezing with forceps after bathing can hasten resolution. If active treatment is needed, topical salicylic acid, potassium hydroxide, podophyllin, cantharidin, trichloroacetic acid, imiquimod, cryotherapy, diathermy, curettage or laser treatment are therapeutic approaches that can be considered.

Orf

Orf is a parapoxvirus skin infection and is an occupational risk for those who work with sheep and goats. Inoculation of virus, usually into finger skin, causes significant inflammation and necrosis, which typically resolves within 2–6 weeks. No specific treatment is required, unless there is secondary infection. Erythema multiforme can be provoked by orf.

Other viral exanthems

Skin rash can be a feature of various other virus infections and these are discussed in more detail in Chapter 13.

Fungal infections

Fungal skin infections can be superficial (dermatophytes and yeasts) or, less commonly, deep (chromomycosis or sporotrichosis); the latter are seen more often in tropical climates or in the immunocompromised. Dermatophyte infections (ringworm) are extremely common and usually caused by fungi of the *Microsporum*, *Trichophyton* and *Epidermophyton* species. The fungi can originate from soil (geophilic) or animals (zoophilic), or be confined to human skin (anthropophilic). Dermatophyte infections usually present with skin (tinea corporis), scalp (tinea capitis), groin (tinea cruris), foot (tinea pedis) and/or nail (onychomycosis) involvement (Fig. 27.27).

Diagnosis

Skin scrapings, hair pluckings or nail clippings must be taken from areas of disease activity – typically, the advancing lesion edge for skin involvement, the crumbling dystrophic nail and subungual hyperkeratosis for nail involvement, and plucked hair from scalp or other affected hair-bearing sites – in order to confirm the diagnosis by microscopy and culture.

Management

The azoles (ketoconazole, miconazole), triazoles (itraconazole, fluconazole) and triallylamines (terbinafine) are used most widely in fungal skin disease. Topical antifungals such as terbinafine or miconazole may suffice, although systemic treatment (terbinafine, itraconazole or griseofulvin) may be required for stubborn or extensive disease and scalp or nail involvement. Indeed, prolonged courses of systemic treatment may be needed for nail involvement. The fungistatic agent griseofulvin, given orally, is usually used for fungal infection of scalp or nails in children in the UK, as it is the only drug licensed in children for this indication; outside the UK, and in adults, terbinafine is usually the treatment of choice as it has broader range of activity and shorter treatment duration. Itraconazole is also an effective alternative. In addition to systemic antifungals, short courses of systemic or topical glucocorticoid are often used in kerion on the basis of reducing inflammation and possible hair loss. However, glucocorticoid use is controversial, with no good evidence of benefit.

Tinea corporis

Tinea corporis should feature in the differential diagnosis of a red, scaly rash. Typically, lesions are erythematous, annular and scaly, with a well-defined edge and central clearing. There may also be pustules at the active edge. Lesions are usually asymmetrical and may be single or multiple. The degree of inflammation is dependent on the organism involved and the host immune response. *Microsporum canis* (from dogs) and *T. verrucosum* (from cats) are common culprits. Ill-advised use of topical glucocorticoids can modify the clinical presentation and increase disease extension (tinea incognito).

Tinea cruris

This is extremely common worldwide and is usually caused by *T. rubrum*. Itchy, erythematous plaques develop in the groins and extend on to the thighs, with a raised active edge (see Fig. 27.27A).

Tinea pedis

Tinea pedis or 'athlete's foot' is the most common fungal infection in the UK and USA, and is usually caused by anthropophilic fungi, such as *T. rubrum*, *T. interdigitale* and *E. floccosum*. It typically presents as an itchy rash between the toes, with peeling, fissuring and maceration. Involvement of one sole or palm (tinea manuum) with fine scaling is characteristic of *T. rubrum* infection. Vesiculation or blistering is more often seen with *T. mentagrophytes*.

Tinea capitis

This is a dermatophyte infection of scalp hair shafts and is most common in children. It typically presents as an area of scalp inflammation and scaling, often with pustules and partial hair loss (Fig. 27.27B). Infection may be within the shaft (endothrix, most commonly caused by *T. tonsurans*), causing patchy hair loss with broken hairs at the surface ('black dot'), little inflammation and no fluorescence with Wood's light. Infection

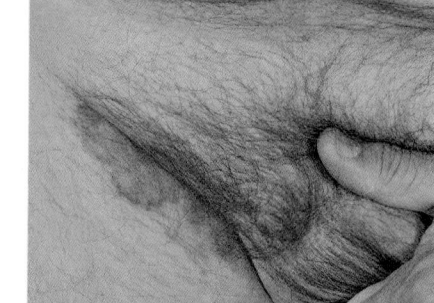
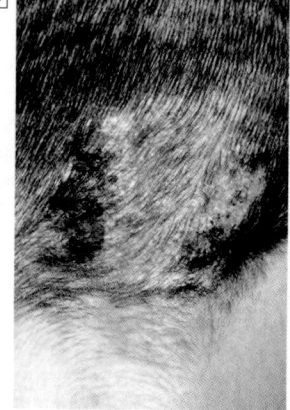

Fig. 27.27 Dermatophyte infections. A *Trichophyton rubrum* infection of the groin (tinea cruris). B *Microsporum canis* infection of the scalp (tinea capitis).

outside the hair shaft (ectothrix, most commonly caused by *M. audouinii* (anthropophilic)) shows minimal inflammation; *M. canis* (from dogs and cats) infections are more inflammatory and can be identified by green fluorescence with Wood's light. Kerion is a boggy, inflammatory area of tinea capitis, usually caused by zoophilic fungi such as cattle ringworm (*T. verrucosum*).

Onychomycosis

This is a fungal infection of the nail plate and the species involved are generally those that cause tinea capitis or tinea pedis. Onychomycosis usually presents with yellow/brown nail discoloration, crumbling, thickening and subungual hyperkeratosis. Usually, some nails are spared, there is asymmetry and toenails are more commonly involved.

Candidiasis

This is a superficial skin or mucosal infection caused by a yeast-like fungus, *Candida albicans*. Infections are usually not serious, unless the patient is immunocompromised, in which case deeper tissues can be involved. The organism has a predilection for warm, moist environments and typical presentations are napkin candidiasis in babies, genital and perineal candidiasis, intertrigo and oral candidiasis. The diagnosis can be confirmed by microscopy and culture of skin swabs, and treatment is with topical or systemic antifungals, such as azoles.

Pityriasis versicolor

Pityriasis versicolor is a persistent, superficial skin condition caused by various species of the commensal yeast *Malassezia*, most commonly *Malassezia globosa*, but sometimes *M. sympadialis* or *M. furfur*, It occurs in men and women and in different races. It is found more frequently in warmer, humid climates, and is usually more severe and persistent in the immunocompromised. It is characterised by scaly, oval macules on the upper trunk, usually hypopigmented but occasionally hyperpigmented. Hypopigmentation is more obvious after sun exposure and tanning. The diagnosis can be confirmed by microscopy of skin scrapings, showing 'spaghetti and meatballs' hyphae. Treatment with selenium sulphide or ketoconazole shampoos and topical or systemic azole antifungal agents is usually effective, although recurrence is common because these yeasts are skin commensals, and maintenance topical therapy may be required. Altered pigmentation can persist for months after treatment.

Infestations

Scabies

Scabies is caused by the mite *Sarcoptes scabiei*. It spreads in households and environments where there is intimate personal contact. The diagnosis is made by identifying the scabietic burrow (**definition**: a linear or curvilinear papule, caused by a burrowing scabies mite – Fig. 27.28) and visualising the mite (by extracting with a needle or using a dermatoscope). In small children, the palms and soles can be involved, with pustules. Pruritus is prominent. The clinical features include secondary eczematisation elsewhere on the body; the face and scalp are rarely affected, except in infants. Involvement of the genitals in males and of the nipples commonly occurs. Even after successful treatment, itch can continue and occasionally nodular lesions persist.

Topical treatment of the affected individual and all asymptomatic family members/physical contacts is required to ensure eradication. Two applications 1 week apart of an aqueous solution of permethrin or malathion to the whole body, excluding the head, are usually successful. If there is poor adherence, immunosuppression or heavy infestation (crusted 'Norwegian' scabies), systemic treatment with a single oral dose of ivermectin is sometimes appropriate.

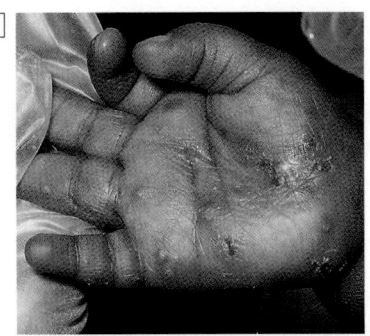
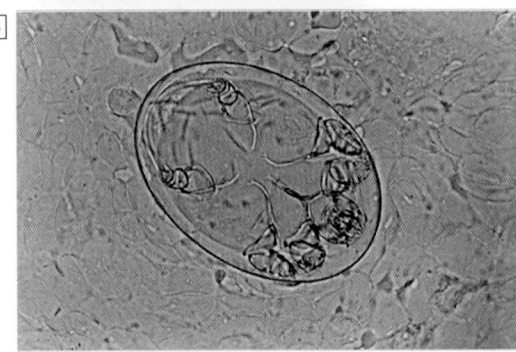

Fig. 27.28 **Scabies.** A Scabies in a young child affecting the palm. B A mite still in its egg, seen on light microscopy of scrapings over a burrow. Note that the mite has only six legs, unlike adult mites, which have eight. (A) *From Lissauer T, Carroll W. Illustrated textbook of paediatrics, 5th edn. Elsevier; 2018.*

Head lice

Infestation with the head louse, *Pediculus humanus capitis*, is common. It is highly contagious and spread by direct head-to-head contact. Scalp itch leads to scratching, secondary infection and cervical lymphadenopathy. The diagnosis is confirmed by identifying the living louse or nymph on the scalp or on a black sheet of paper after careful fine-toothed combing of wet hair following conditioner application. The empty egg cases ('nits') are easily seen on the hair shaft and are hard to dislodge.

Treatment is recommended for the affected individual and any infected household/school contacts. Eradication in school populations is difficult because of poor adherence and treatment resistance. Topical treatment with dimeticone, permethrin, carbaryl or, less often, malathion in lotion or aqueous formulations may be effective and should be applied twice at an interval of 7–10 days. Rotational treatments within a community may avoid resistance. 'Wet-combing' (physical removal of live lice by regular combing of conditioned wet hair – 'bug busting') can suffice but may be less effective than pharmacological treatments. Vaseline should be applied to eyelashes/brows twice daily for at least a fortnight. High-temperature washing of clothing and bedding is required. Treatment resistance and recurrence can be problematic.

Body lice

These are similar to head lice but live on clothing, particularly in seams, and feed on the skin. Poor hygiene and overcrowded conditions predispose. Itch, excoriation (**definition**: a linear ulcer or erosion resulting from scratching) and secondary infection occur. Dry-cleaning and high-temperature washing or insecticide treatment of clothes are required. Treatment options are as for head lice. For heavy infestation, oral ivermectin may be indicated.

Pubic (crab) lice

Usually, these are sexually acquired and very itchy. Management is as for head and body lice and whole-body treatment should be undertaken. Pubic hair may need to be shaved. Sexual and other close contacts

27

should also be treated and patients should also be screened for sexually transmitted diseases.

Acne and rosacea

Acne vulgaris

Acne is chronic inflammation of the pilosebaceous units. It is extremely common, generally starts during puberty and has been estimated to affect over 90% of adolescents. It is usually most severe in later adolescence but can persist into the thirties and forties, particularly in females (Box 27.17).

Pathogenesis

The key components are increased sebum production; colonisation of pilosebaceous ducts by *Propionibacterium acnes*, which in turn causes inflammation; and hypercornification and occlusion of pilosebaceous ducts (Fig. 27.29). Severity of acne is associated with sebum excretion rate, which increases at puberty. Both androgens and progestogens increase sebum excretion and oestrogens reduce it, but most patients with acne have normal hormone profiles. There may be a positive family history and there is high concordance in monozygotic twins, indicating that genetic factors are important, but the candidate genes are poorly defined.

Clinical features

Acne usually affects the face and often the trunk. Greasiness of the skin may be obvious (seborrhoea). The hallmark is the comedone (**definition**:

> **27.17 Acne in adolescence**
>
> **Epidemiology**: acne vulgaris is most common between the ages of 12 and 20. It often begins around 10–13 years of age, lasts 5–10 years and usually resolves by age 20–25.
> **Emotional effects**: at all ages acne can have negative effects on self-esteem, but it is especially important to assess how it affects an adolescent. Depression and suicidal ideation may occur. The consequences (whether acne is objectively severe or not) can be devastating, leading to embarrassment, school avoidance, and life-long effects on ability to form friendships, attract partners, and acquire and keep employment.
> **Treatment**: effective treatments aim to improve the condition, prevent worsening (including later scarring) and restore emotional well-being and self-esteem.

open comedones (blackheads) are dilated keratin-filled follicles, which appear as black papules due to the keratin debris; closed comedones (whiteheads) usually have no visible follicular opening and are caused by accumulation of sebum and keratin deeper in the pilosebaceous ducts – see Fig. 27.29). Inflammatory papules, nodules and cysts occur and may arise from comedones (Fig. 27.30). Scarring may follow deep-seated or superficial acne and may be keloidal.

There are also distinct clinical variants:

- *Acne conglobata*: characterised by comedones, nodules, abscesses, sinuses (**definition**: cavities or channels that permit the escape of pus or fluid) and cysts, usually with marked scarring. It is rare, usually affecting adult males, and most commonly occurs on trunk and upper limbs. It may be associated with *hidradenitis suppurativa (acne inversa)* (an occlusive follicular chronic inflammatory condition affecting apocrine glands; this predominantly affects axillae, groins, perineal and perianal sites and follows a relapsing and remitting course and often requires complex medical and surgical management approaches), scalp folliculitis and pilonidal sinus.
- *Acne fulminans*: a rare but severe presentation of acne, associated with fever, arthralgias and systemic inflammation, with raised neutrophil count and plasma viscosity. It is usually found on the trunk in adolescent males. Costochondritis can occur.
- *Acne excoriée*: self-inflicted excoriations due to compulsive picking of pre-existing or imagined acne lesions. It usually affects adolescent girls, and underlying psychological problems are common.
- *Secondary acne*: comedonal acne can be caused by greasy cosmetics or occupational exposure to oils, tars or chlorinated aromatic hydrocarbons. Predominantly pustular acne can occur in patients using systemic or topical glucocorticoids, oral contraceptives, anticonvulsants, lithium or antineoplastic drugs, such as the epidermal growth factor receptor (EGFR) inhibitors. Most patients with acne do not have an underlying endocrine disorder but acne is a common feature of polycystic ovary syndrome which should be suspected if acne is moderate to severe and associated with hirsutism and menstrual irregularities. Virilisation should also raise suspicion of an androgen-secreting tumour.

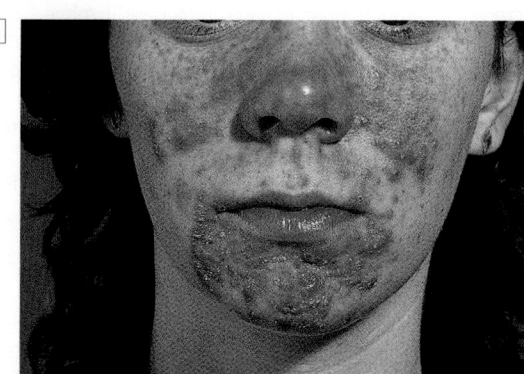

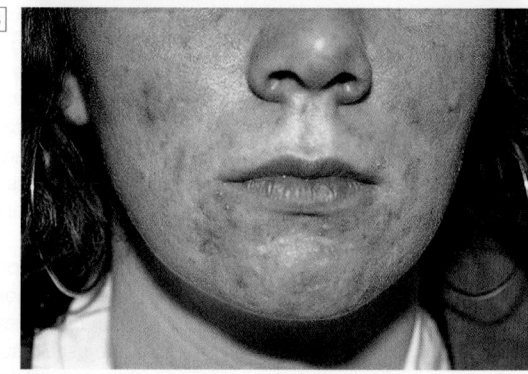

Fig. 27.30 Cystic acne in an adolescent girl. A Before treatment. B After prolonged systemic antibiotic treatment.

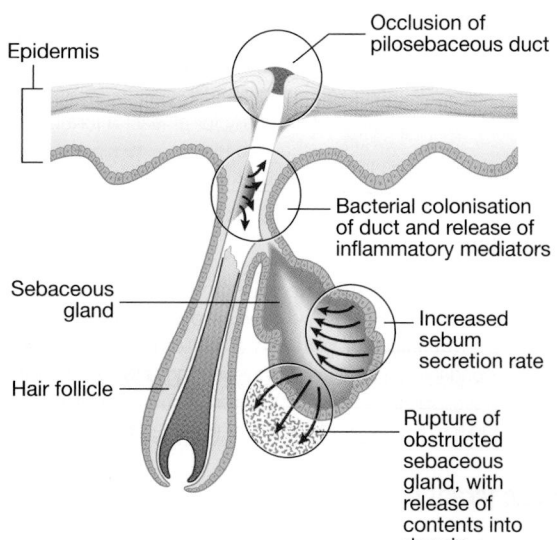

Epidermis

Occlusion of pilosebaceous duct

Bacterial colonisation of duct and release of inflammatory mediators

Sebaceous gland

Increased sebum secretion rate

Hair follicle

Rupture of obstructed sebaceous gland, with release of contents into dermis

Fig. 27.29 Pathogenesis of acne.

Investigations

Investigations are not required in typical acne vulgaris. Secondary causes and suspected underlying endocrine disease or virilisation should be investigated.

Management

Mild to moderate disease

Mild disease is usually managed with topical therapy. If comedones predominate, then topical benzoyl peroxide or retinoids should be used. Benzoyl peroxide has both anti-comedogenic and antiseptic effects. It is an irritant, which may contribute to the therapeutic response, but this can be minimised by adjusting treatment regimens. Azelaic acid may also be used for mild acne and has both antimicrobial and anti-comedogenic action. Topical retinoids, in particular *all-trans* retinoic acid and adapalene, are widely employed for mild to moderate comedonal acne vulgaris. Treatment should be initially applied at low concentrations for short duration and increased as tolerated. Patients with mild inflammatory acne should respond to topical antibiotics, such as erythromycin or clindamycin, which can be used in combination with other treatments.

For moderate inflammatory acne, a systemic tetracycline should be used at adequate dose for 3–6 months in the first instance (Fig. 27.30B). Oxytetracycline must be taken on an empty stomach, in a dose of up to 1.5 g a day. It has a good safety profile, even with long-term use, but adherence may be a challenge. Lymecycline is an alternative and is taken once daily, with or without food, thereby improving adherence. Doxycycline is another option but commonly causes photosensitivity. Minocycline is used less frequently, as it can cause hyperpigmentation, autoimmune hepatitis and drug-induced lupus, and monitoring is required. If the patient fails to respond, then alternatives include erythromycin or trimethoprim.

In women with acne, oestrogen-containing oral contraceptives can be a useful adjunct, as they are associated with a small reduction in sebum production. Combined oestrogen and anti-androgen (such as cyproterone acetate) contraceptives may provide additional efficacy, particularly in women with acne and hirsutism, as seen in polycystic ovary syndrome.

Patients should be referred for consideration of isotretinoin (13-*cis*-retinoic acid) if there is a failure to respond adequately to 6 months of therapy with these combined systemic and topical approaches.

Moderate to severe disease

Isotretinoin (13-*cis*-retinoic acid) has revolutionised the treatment of moderate to severe acne that has not responded adequately to other therapies. It has multifactorial mechanisms of action, with reduction in sebum excretion by over 90%, follicular hypercornification, *P. acnes* colonisation and inflammation. Oral isotretinoin is usually used at a dose of 0.5–1 mg/kg over 4 months. Sebum excretion typically returns to baseline within a year after treatment cessation, although clinical benefit is usually longer-lasting. Many patients will not require further treatment, although a second or third course of isotretinoin may be needed. A low-dose continuous or intermittent-dose regimen may occasionally be considered for a longer duration in patients who relapse after a higher-dose regimen, and may also be beneficial for older females with persistent acne. Combination with systemic glucocorticoid may be required in the short term for severe acne, in order to minimise the risk of disease flare early in the treatment course. Thorough screening and monitoring are required, given the side-effect profile of isotretinoin, particularly with respect to teratogenicity and possible mood disturbance. Pregnancy must be avoided during treatment and for a minimum of 2 months after drug cessation, and a strict pregnancy prevention programme and regular pregnancy testing are required. Depression and suicide have been reported in association with isotretinoin, although a causal role has not been established. However, pre-drug screening for depressive symptoms should be undertaken and mood monitored during therapy.

Other treatments and physical measures

Intralesional injections of triamcinolone acetonide may be required for inflamed acne nodules or cysts, which can also be incised and drained, or excised under local anaesthetic. Scarring may be prevented by adequate treatment of active acne. Keloid scars may respond to intralesional glucocorticoid and/or silicone dressings. Carbon dioxide laser, microdermabrasion, chemical peeling or localised excision can also be considered for scarring. UVB phototherapy or PDT can occasionally be used in patients with inflammatory acne who are unable to use conventional therapy, such as isotretinoin. There is no convincing evidence to support a causal association between diet and acne. The psychological impact of acne must not be under-estimated and should be considered in management decisions (see Box 27.17).

Rosacea

This chronic inflammatory condition affects the central face and consists of flushing, erythema, papules, pustules and telangiectasiae. The cause is unknown. Rosacea is distinct from acne vulgaris; sebum excretion is normal and comedones are absent. The relative contribution of *Demodex* mite and cutaneous vasomotor instability to the pathogenesis of rosacea remains poorly defined.

Clinical features

Rosacea most commonly affects fair-skinned, middle-aged females and can be exacerbated by heat, sunlight and alcohol. The convexities of nose, forehead, cheeks and chin are typically involved (Fig. 27.31). The condition is heterogeneous and intermittent flushing, followed by fixed erythema and telangiectasiae, predominates in some; in others, papules and pustules are prominent. Sebaceous gland hyperplasia and soft tissue overgrowth of the nose (rhinophyma) can occur, particularly in males. Conjunctivitis and blepharitis may also occur. Facial lymphoedema can be an added complication.

Investigations

Usually, no investigations are required and the diagnosis is obvious clinically. However, rosacea must be distinguished from acne vulgaris, systemic lupus erythematosus, photosensitivity disorders and seborrhoeic dermatitis (the latter may coexist with rosacea).

Management

Mild disease may respond to topical antimicrobials, such as metronidazole or azelaic acid. Topical ivermectin may be beneficial in some cases, supporting a contributory role of *Demodex* in pathogenesis. Tetracycline or erythromycin for 3–6 months is usually effective in inflammatory

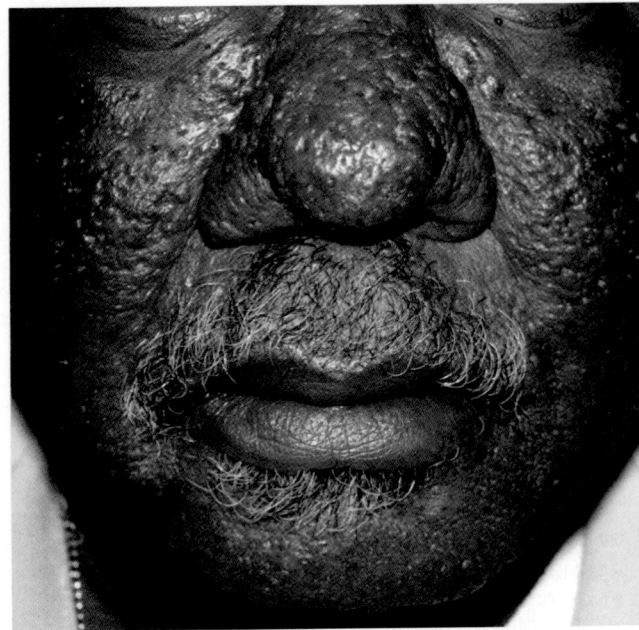

Fig. 27.31 Glandular rosacea. Showing prominent rhinophyma. *From James W, Elston D, McMahon PJ. Andrews' diseases of the skin clinical atlas. Elsevier; 2018.*

pustular disease resistant to topical therapy. Relapse may require intermittent or chronic antibiotic use. Erythema and telangiectasiae do not usually respond well to antibiotics but vascular laser therapy may be effective. Topical vasoconstrictors, such as the α_2-adrenoceptor agonist brimonidine, may be of benefit in some cases where erythema and telangiectasiae predominate. Systemic isotretinoin may be helpful in severe resistant disease and rhinophyma may require laser therapy or surgery.

Eczemas

The term 'eczema' derives from the Greek word 'to boil' and is synonymous with the other descriptive term, 'dermatitis'. Eczema describes a clinical and histological pattern, which can be acute or chronic and has several causes. Acutely, epidermal oedema (spongiosis) and intra-epidermal vesiculation (producing multilocular blisters) predominate, whereas with chronicity there is more epidermal thickening (acanthosis). Vasodilatation and T-cell lymphocytic infiltration of the upper dermis also occur.

Clinical features

There are several patterns of eczema (Box 27.18) but the clinical features are similar, irrespective of the cause (Box 27.19). Some subtypes of eczema have specific distinguishing features and these are discussed in more detail below.

Investigations

Bacterial and viral swabs for microscopy and culture are important in suspected secondary infection. Bacterial swabs are commonly positive, particularly for staphylococci, although clinical assessment is required in order to ascertain whether swab results are of clinical significance and whether antibiotic treatment is required. Individuals with atopic eczema have an increased susceptibility to herpes simplex virus (HSV) and are at risk of developing a widespread infection, eczema herpeticum. The presence of small, punched-out lesions on a background of worsening eczema suggests the possibility of secondary HSV infection. Skin scrapings to rule out secondary fungal infection should also be considered. Total IgE and specific IgE tests and skin prick tests are not routinely undertaken in atopic eczema as they are not usually helpful, although they may occasionally be indicated in some cases as directed by the history. Patch tests should be performed if contact allergic dermatitis is suspected (see Box 27.23 below). Skin biopsy is not usually required unless there is diagnostic doubt.

27.18 Classification of eczema

Endogenous

• Atopic, seborrhoeic

Exogenous

• Irritant, allergic, photo-allergic, chronic actinic dermatitis

Characteristic patterns and morphology

• Asteatotic, discoid, gravitational, lichen simplex, pompholyx

27.19 The clinical morphology of eczema

Acute

• Erythema, oedema, usually typically ill defined
• Papules, vesicles and occasionally bullae
• Exudation, fissuring
• Scaling

Chronic

• May be as above but less oedema, vesiculation and exudate
• Lichenification: skin thickening with pronounced skin markings, secondary to chronic rubbing and scratching
• Fissures (**definition**: slit-shaped deep ulcers), excoriations
• Dyspigmentation: hyper- and hypopigmentation can occur

Management

A general approach to the management of eczema includes advice, education and support, required for patients with eczema of any type (Fig. 27.32). Input from patient support groups, such as the National Eczema Society in the UK, can be very helpful. Intensive and prolonged treatments are often required and chronic eczema can have a major and devastating adverse impact on personal and family lives. Emollients and topical glucocorticoids are mainstays of treatment for all eczema types, in order to improve skin barrier function, limit transepidermal water loss and reduce inflammation. Emollients can be used as bath additives and soap substitutes, and applied directly to the skin, often combined with antiseptics. Sedative antihistamines are useful if sleep is interrupted but non-sedating antihistamines are ineffective, as the itch of eczema is not primarily mediated by histamine.

Ointments are preferred for chronic eczema, whereas cream- or lotion-based treatment may be more appropriate for acute eczema (see Box 27.11). Treatment is once to twice daily. Hydrocortisone (1%) or clobetasone butyrate is generally used on the face, with more potent glucocorticoids restricted to trunk and limbs (see Box 27.12). A good strategy is to employ an intensive regimen with more potent glucocorticoids initially and then taper use according to response. A key principle is to use the least potent glucocorticoid that is effective for the shortest possible time. The patient should be given instructions on how much to apply, using the fingertip unit for guidance (a strip of glucocorticoid cream on distal phalanx pulp should cover two palm-size areas). It is also important to monitor glucocorticoid use and the easiest way to do this is ask the patient how long it takes them to use a specific size of glucocorticoid tube. The side-effects of topical glucocorticoid therapy need to be considered but glucocorticoid phobia and under-treatment of eczema are often more of a problem than over-treatment. Particular care should be taken on certain sites, such as the face and flexures, and in children and older adults (see Box 27.2 and Fig. 27.10).

The clinical features of eczema influence the choice of topical treatment. For example, appropriate treatment of acute exudative eczema could be with potassium permanganate soaks, emollients and topical glucocorticoids under wet wraps. Chronic eczema may be best treated with a potent topical glucocorticoid in an ointment formulation and occlusion with a paste bandage to ease itching and scratching.

The topical calcineurin inhibitors tacrolimus and pimecrolimus may be useful glucocorticoid-sparing agents for eczema, particularly on the face; they cause local cutaneous immunosuppression. Initial burning and stinging may limit use but are usually transient side-effects. Bacterial and viral skin infection risk may be increased due to immunosuppression. Caution should be employed with sun exposure and these agents should not be used in combination with phototherapy because of their immunosuppressive effects.

Atopic eczema

This is the most common subtype of eczema. The prevalence has increased dramatically since the early 1980s, and the disease now affects at least 20% of schoolchildren and 5%–10% of adults in the UK.

Pathogenesis

Generalised prolonged hypersensitivity to common environmental antigens, such as pollen and house-dust mite, is the hallmark of atopy, in which there is a genetic predisposition to produce excess IgE. Atopic individuals manifest one or more of a group of diseases that includes asthma, hay fever, food and other allergies, and atopic eczema. Genetic factors play an important role in all of these conditions, supported by higher concordance of atopic disease in monozygotic twins compared with dizygotic twins. Filaggrin gene mutations increase the risk of developing atopic eczema by more than threefold, emphasising the importance of epidermal barrier impairment in this disease. Other genes are also likely to be implicated, with many other susceptibility loci identified, although these studies require further replication. Decreased skin barrier

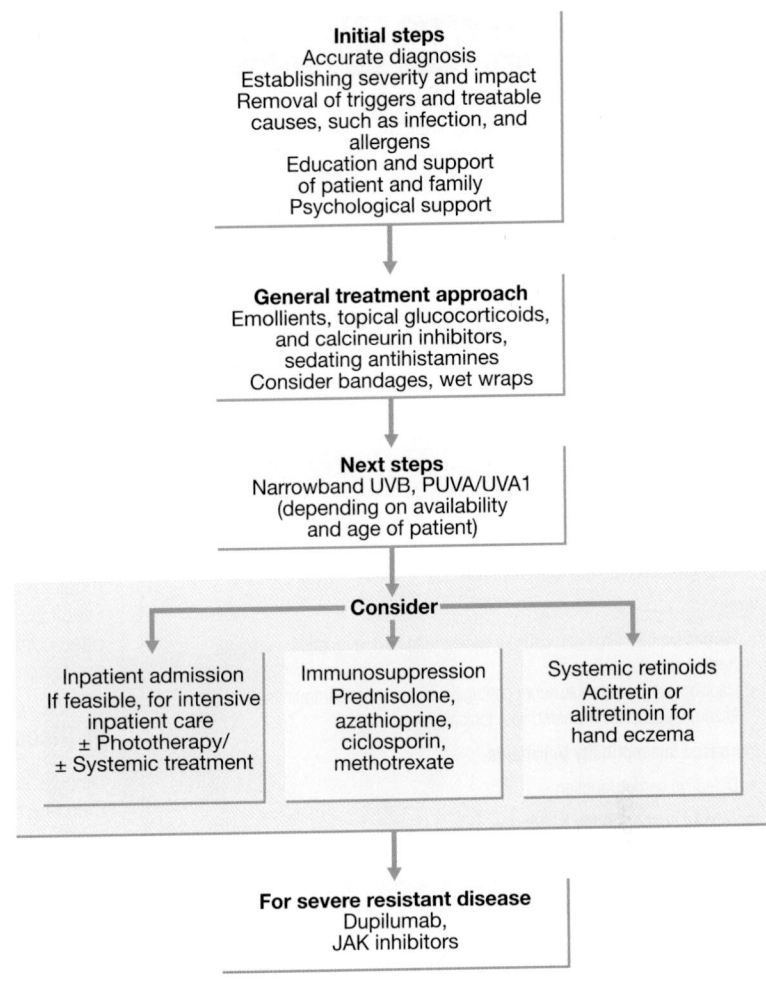

Initial steps
Accurate diagnosis
Establishing severity and impact
Removal of triggers and treatable
causes, such as infection, and
allergens
Education and support
of patient and family
Psychological support

General treatment approach
Emollients, topical glucocorticoids,
and calcineurin inhibitors,
sedating antihistamines
Consider bandages, wet wraps

Next steps
Narrowband UVB, PUVA/UVA1
(depending on availability
and age of patient)

Consider

| Inpatient admission If feasible, for intensive inpatient care ± Phototherapy/ ± Systemic treatment | Immunosuppression Prednisolone, azathioprine, ciclosporin, methotrexate | Systemic retinoids Acitretin or alitretinoin for hand eczema |

For severe resistant disease
Dupilumab,
JAK inhibitors

Fig. 27.32 General management approaches: atopic eczema.
(JAK = Janus kinase; PDE = phosphodiesterase; PUVA = psoralen-ultraviolet A; UVA1 = ultraviolet A1; UVB = narrowband ultraviolet B)

function may also allow greater penetration of allergens through the epidermis, and thus cause immune stimulation and subsequent inflammation. The interaction between genes and environment is important; it has been estimated that 60%–80% of individuals are genetically susceptible to the induction of IgE-mediated sensitisation to environmental allergens such as food and animal hair. Eczema is characterised by infiltration of Th2 cells, which are known to play a role in activating mast cells and eosinophils, as well as stimulating IgE production by IgE-producing B cells. The therapeutic inhibition of IL-4 and IL-13 and promising trials of phosphodiesterase-4 and JAK inhibitors, highlights the involvement of these targets in atopic dermatitis pathogenesis. Emerging therapeutic targets for atopic eczema both in terms of targeting Th2-driven inflammation and skin barrier dysfunction is a rapidly evolving field and further informs our understanding at a mechanistic level (see Fig. 27.34). The contributing roles of the microbiome are also being explored. Thus, the pathogenesis of atopic eczema is complex and multifactorial, involving an interplay of contributing factors.

Clinical features

Atopic eczema is extremely itchy and scratching accounts for many of the signs (Fig. 27.33). Widespread cutaneous dryness (also known as xeroderma or xerosis) is another feature. The distribution and character of the rash vary with age (Box 27.20). Complications are listed in Box 27.21.

Investigations

The diagnosis of atopic eczema is made using clinical criteria (Box 27.22). Interestingly, while most patients with atopic eczema have raised total IgE levels and IgE-specific antibodies, this is not a prerequisite for the diagnosis, as a significant minority have normal levels of IgE.

Management

The general principles of management are as described in Figure 27.32. Emollients and topical glucocorticoids, tar and ichthammol paste bandages, or wet wraps in children, are often required and are mainstays in improving barrier function and reducing inflammation, although have not been shown to have a preventative effect against

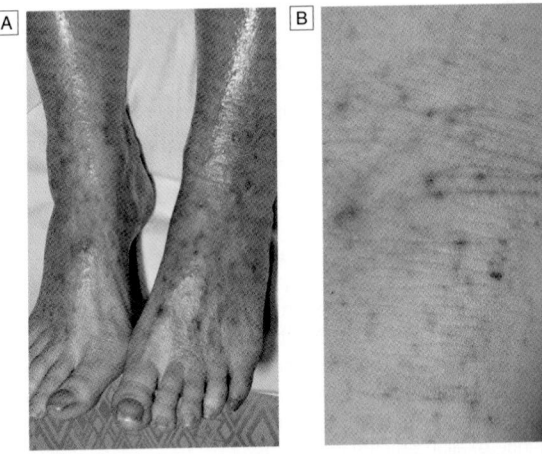

Fig. 27.33 Atopic eczema. A This patient had life-long chronic atopic eczema and experienced a generalised flare of disease triggered by infection. B Lichenification of chronic flexural eczema secondary to rubbing and scratching.

27

27.20 Atopic eczema: distribution and character of rash

Babies and infants

- Often acute and facial involvement prominent
- Trunk involved but nappy area usually spared

Children

- Flexures: behind knees, antecubital fossae, wrists and ankles

Adults

- Face and trunk usually involved, limb involvement not restricted to flexures
- Lichenification common

 27.21 Complications of atopic eczema

Secondary infection

Bacterial

- *Staphylococcus aureus* most common

Viral

- Herpes simplex virus can cause a widespread severe eruption – eczema herpeticum
- Papillomavirus and molluscum contagiosum are more common in atopic eczema, especially if treated with topical glucocorticoids

Increased susceptibility to irritants

- Defective barrier function

Increased susceptibility to allergy

- Food allergy – mainly relevant in infants; eggs, cow's milk protein, nuts, fish, wheat and soya may cause an immediate reaction with angioedema and/or urticaria rather than exacerbation of eczema
- Anaphylaxis in severe allergy
- Increased risk of sensitisation to type IV allergens because of impaired barrier function

Impact on life and health

- Poor sleep, loss of schooling, behavioural difficulties, failure to thrive in children
- Impact on sleep, work, relationships, hobbies, psychology and quality of life in adults

 27.22 Diagnostic criteria for atopic eczema

Itchy skin rash (or history of itch or rubbing from parent) and at least three of the following:

- History of involvement of skin creases (or cheeks if <4 years)
- History of atopic disease (asthma, hay fever) (or in a first-degree relative if <4 years)
- Dry skin (xeroderma)
- Visible flexural eczema (cheeks, forehead, outer limbs if <4 years)
- Onset in first 2 years of life

the subsequent development of atopic eczema when used in babies. Topical calcineurin inhibitors may be used as glucocorticoid-sparing agents but should not be used in infected eczema. Secondary infection should be treated but positive skin swabs in isolation, without clinical evidence of infection, do not necessarily require treatment with antibiotics, although antiseptics would be appropriate. Sedating antihistamines may help to break the itch/scratch cycle. Identification and avoidance of allergens are important.

Phototherapy is generally the next step, if topical therapies are insufficient (see Fig. 27.32). Narrowband UVB is usually the initial phototherapy of choice and can also be used in children. PUVA or UVA1 can also be used if UVB is ineffective, although mainly in adults as PUVA is generally avoided in children. Localised phototherapy may be used for eczema on hands and feet and PUVA may be more effective in that situation. Systemic immunosuppression with, for example, oral glucocorticoids, intermittent ciclosporin, azathioprine or methotrexate may be needed if the response to topical therapies and phototherapy is inadequate. Systemic retinoids, such as acitretin or alitretinoin, may be indicated: for example, in hand and foot eczema.

Dupilumab, which blocks the IL-4 receptor alpha chain subunit common to both IL-4 and IL-13 receptors, is now licensed for clinical use in patients with severe disease, as are the JAK inhibitors baricitinib and upadacitinib. The anti-IL-13 agents tralokinumab and lebrikizumab are also showing promise in clinical trials, as are phosphodiesterase-4 inhibitors and other therapeutic targets (see Fig. 27.11 and Box 27.14).

Seborrhoeic eczema

This is an erythematous scaly rash affecting the scalp (dandruff), central face, nasolabial folds, eyebrows, central chest and upper back. It is associated with, and may be due to, overgrowth of *Malassezia* yeasts. When severe, it may resemble psoriasis. Severe or recalcitrant seborrhoeic eczema can be a marker of immunodeficiency, including HIV infection. Topical azoles, such as ketoconazole shampoo and cream, often combined with mild glucocorticoid, are mainstays. Treatment often needs to be repeated due to disease recurrence.

Discoid eczema

Discoid eczema, which is also known as nummular eczema, is common and characteristically consists of discrete, coin-shaped eczematous lesions, which are often impetiginised and most commonly occur on the limbs of men. It is an eczema type that can be due to any chronic itchy condition, whether primarily of the skin or secondary to an underlying disease. Initial management should include topical antiseptics, in addition to emollients and topical glucocorticoids. Judicious antibiotic use may also be required for acute flares.

Irritant eczema

Detergents, alkalis, acids, solvents and abrasives are common irritants. Strong irritants have acute effects, whereas weaker irritants commonly cause chronic eczema, especially of the hands, after prolonged exposure. Individual susceptibility varies and older adults, atopic and fair-skinned individuals are predisposed. Irritant eczema accounts for most occupational cases of eczema and is a significant cause of time off work. Irritant avoidance, including protective clothing (such as gloves), is essential. Emollients and topical glucocorticoids are indicated.

Allergic contact eczema

This occurs due to a delayed hypersensitivity reaction following contact with antigens or haptens. Previous allergen exposure is required for sensitisation and the reaction is specific to the allergen or closely related chemicals. Common allergens are listed in Box 27.23.

Allergy persists indefinitely and eczema occurs at sites of allergen contact and can secondarily spread beyond this. The distribution of eczema can be very informative with regard to possible culprits. There are many recognisable patterns of sites of eczema involvement, such as earlobes, wrists and umbilicus due to contact with nickel in earrings, watches and jeans studs; hands and wrists due to rubber gloves; and upper eyelids due to colophony from rubbing of the eyes in nail varnish wearers. Oedema may also be a feature (Fig. 27.34). Allergen avoidance is key and may involve a change of occupation, recreational activities or hobbies. It is important to ensure that patients are fully informed as to the nature and likely occurrence of allergens and good detective work is required to scrutinise lifestyle and daily activities. Treatment with emollients and topical glucocorticoids helps but will not suffice if there is continued allergen exposure.

27.23 Common type IV delayed hypersensitivity allergens

Allergen	Source
Nickel	Jewellery, jean studs, bra clips, watches
Dichromate	Cement, leather, matches
Rubber chemicals	Clothing, shoes, rubber gloves, tyres
Colophony	Sticking plaster, collodion, nail varnish
Paraphenylenediamine	Hair dye, clothing, tattoos
Balsam of Peru	Perfumes, citrus fruits, shower/bath products
Neomycin, benzocaine	Topical medications
Parabens	Preservative in cosmetics and creams
Wool alcohols	Lanolin, cosmetics, creams
Epoxy resin	Resin adhesives, glues
Methyl- and chloromethyl-isothiazolinone	Preservatives, with increasing numbers of cases of allergy reported

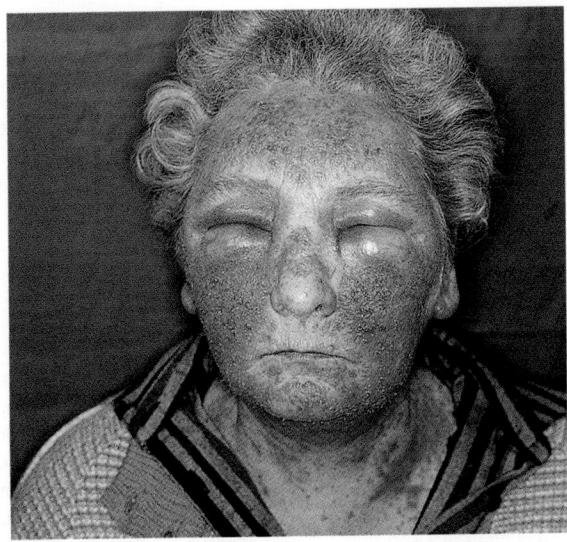

Fig. 27.34 Allergic contact eczema. This was caused by the application of an antihistamine cream. The acute eczematous reaction and bilateral periorbital oedema are typical.

Asteatotic eczema

This occurs in dry skin and is common in older adults. Low humidity caused by central heating, over-washing, diuretics and cholesterol-lowering drugs predispose. The most common site is the lower legs, and a 'crazy paving' pattern of fine fissuring on an erythematous background is seen. Emollients are a mainstay, in combination with topical glucocorticoids. Patients must be advised to use caution with flammable emollients and to avoid bathroom slippages related to emollients on floor and feet, and this is particularly relevant for older individuals.

Gravitational eczema

Gravitational or stasis eczema occurs on the lower legs and is often associated with signs of venous insufficiency: oedema, loss of hair, induration, lipodermatosclerosis and ulceration. Emollients should be used and topical glucocorticoids should be applied to eczematous areas but not to ulcers. There is a high risk of sensitisation to topical preservatives (such as chlorocresol), antibiotics (such as neomycin) and bandages

(such as rubber additives). Oedema and ulceration are treated by leg elevation and compression bandages.

Lichen simplex

Lichenification of eczema occurs secondary to chronic rubbing and scratching, and lichen simplex is a localised form. Common sites include the neck, lower legs and anogenital region. Treatment with emollients and very potent topical glucocorticoids may be required, often impregnated in tape or with occlusion.

Pompholyx

Intensely itchy vesicles and bullae occur on the palms, palmar surface and sides of the fingers and soles. Pompholyx may have several causes, which include atopic eczema, irritant and contact allergic dermatitis and fungal infection. The underlying cause must be treated or removed.

Psoriasis and other erythematous scaly eruptions

Psoriasis

Psoriasis is a chronic inflammatory, hyperproliferative skin disease. It is characterised by well-defined, erythematous scaly plaques, particularly affecting extensor surfaces, scalp and nails, and usually follows a relapsing and remitting course. Psoriasis affects approximately 1.5%–3% of populations of European ancestry but is less common in Asian, South American and African populations. It occurs equally in both sexes and at any age; although it is uncommon under the age of 5 years, more than 50% of patients present before the age of 30 years. The age of onset follows a bimodal distribution, with an early-onset type in the teenage or early adult years, often with a family history of psoriasis, a more severe disease course and strong HLA association. The later-onset type is typically seen between 50 and 60 years, usually without a family history and with a less severe disease course.

Pathogenesis

Both genetic and environmental factors are important. Twin studies show concordance rates of 60%–75% and 15%–20% for psoriasis arising in monozygotic and dizygotic twins, respectively. The age at onset and severity of disease are often similar in familial cases. If one parent has psoriasis, the chance of a child being affected is about 15%–20%; if both parents have the disease, this rises to 50% and the risk is increased further if a sibling also has the disease.

Variants of the HLA-C region within the major histocompatibility complex (MHC) on chromosome 6 account for almost half of the heritability of psoriasis. However, at least 70 other loci are implicated, with susceptibility variants that lie within or close to genes involved in regulating epidermal barrier function, antigen presentation, cytokine production, notably IL-13 and IL-23, T-cell differentiation (especially Th-1 and Th-17 subsets) and nuclear factor kappa B (NFκB) signalling. Some of the loci that predispose to psoriasis overlap with those implicated in Crohn's disease, ankylosing spondylitis and psoriatic arthritis.

Environmental triggers for psoriasis are shown in (Box 27.24). Although the theory is controversial, stress may exacerbate psoriasis in susceptible individuals and psoriasis is itself a cause of psychological stress. Likewise, there is a higher incidence of smoking and heavy alcohol consumption in patients with psoriasis but it is unclear whether this is cause or effect. There is also an association between psoriasis and metabolic syndrome.

The histological changes of psoriasis are shown in Figure 27.35. The main features are:

- keratinocyte hyperproliferation and abnormal differentiation, leading to retention of nuclei in the stratum corneum

27

- inflammation, with a T-cell (mainly activated Th-1 and Th-17) lymphocytic infiltrate and release of cytokines and adhesion molecules, such as interleukins (including IL-17, IL-23 and IL-12), TNF-α, IFN-γ and intercellular adhesion molecule (ICAM)-1
- vascular changes, with tortuosity of dermal capillary loop vessels and release of mediators, such as vascular endothelial growth factor (VEGF).

The initiating event for psoriasis is unknown. Disordered cell proliferation is a key feature; this was previously thought to be the primary event but is now considered to be secondary to inflammatory change. The transit time for keratinocyte migration, from basal layer to shedding from stratum corneum, is shortened from approximately 28 to 5 days, so that immature cells reach the stratum corneum prematurely. Proliferation rate is also increased in non-lesional skin but to a lesser extent. Similarly, even the clinically unaffected nails of patients with psoriasis grow more quickly than those of controls.

While immunological factors clearly play a key role in psoriasis, the precise mechanisms of disease initiation and the sequence of events that lead to psoriasis are not fully defined. Therapeutic efficacy through targeted biological inhibition of the effects of key cytokines, notably TNF-α, IL-17, IL-23 and IL-12, continues to provide major insight into the pathogenesis of psoriasis and the pathways and mechanisms involved.

Clinical features

Psoriasis has several different presentations (Fig. 27.36).

Plaque psoriasis

This is the most common presentation and usually represents more stable disease. The typical lesion is a raised, well-demarcated erythematous plaque of variable size (see Fig. 27.36A). In untreated disease, silver/white scale is evident and more obvious on scraping the surface, which reveals bleeding points (Auspitz sign). The most common sites are the extensor surfaces, notably elbows and knees, and the lower back. Others include:

- *Scalp*: involvement is seen in approximately 60% of patients. Typically, easily palpable, erythematous scaly plaques are evident within hair-bearing scalp and there is clear demarcation at or beyond the hair margin. Occipital involvement is common and difficult to treat. Less often, fine diffuse scaling may be present and difficult to distinguish from seborrhoeic dermatitis. Involvement of other 'seborrhoeic sites', such as eyebrows, nasolabial folds and the pre-sternal area, is not uncommon and again may be confused with seborrhoeic dermatitis. Temporary hair loss can occur but permanent loss is unusual.
- *Nails*: involvement is common, with 'thimble pitting', onycholysis (separation of the nail from the nail bed, see Fig. 27.36B), subungual hyperkeratosis and periungual involvement.
- *Flexures*: psoriasis of the natal cleft and submammary and axillary folds is usually symmetrical, erythematous and smooth, without scale.
- *Palms*: psoriasis of the palms can be difficult to distinguish from eczema.

Guttate psoriasis

This is most common in children and adolescents and is often the initial presentation (see Fig. 27.36C). It may present shortly after a streptococcal throat infection and evolves rapidly. Individual lesions are droplet-shaped, small (usually less than 1 cm in diameter), erythematous, scaly and numerous. An episode of guttate psoriasis may clear spontaneously or with topical treatment within a few months, but UVB phototherapy is often required and is highly effective. Guttate psoriasis often heralds the onset of plaque psoriasis in adulthood.

Erythrodermic psoriasis

Generalised erythrodermic psoriasis is a medical emergency (see Fig. 27.36D).

 27.24 Exacerbating factors in psoriasis

Trauma

- Lesions can appear at sites of skin trauma, such as scratches or surgical wounds (Köbner isomorphic phenomenon)

Infection

- β-haemolytic streptococcal throat infections often precede guttate psoriasis (see Fig. 27.36C)
- Severe psoriasis may be the initial presentation of HIV infection

Sunlight

- Psoriasis may occur or worsen after sun exposure, mainly due to Köbnerisation at sites of sunburn or polymorphic light eruption

Drugs

- Antimalarials, β-adrenoceptor antagonists (β-blockers), lithium, NSAIDs and TNF-α inhibitors can exacerbate psoriasis
- 'Rebound' flare of psoriasis may occur after withdrawal of systemic glucocorticoids or potent topical glucocorticoids. Rebound psoriasis is often unstable and may be pustular

Psychological factors

- Anxiety and stress may exacerbate psoriasis in predisposed individuals

(HIV = human immunodeficiency virus; NSAIDs = non-steroidal anti-inflammatory drugs; TNF-α = tumour necrosis factor alpha)

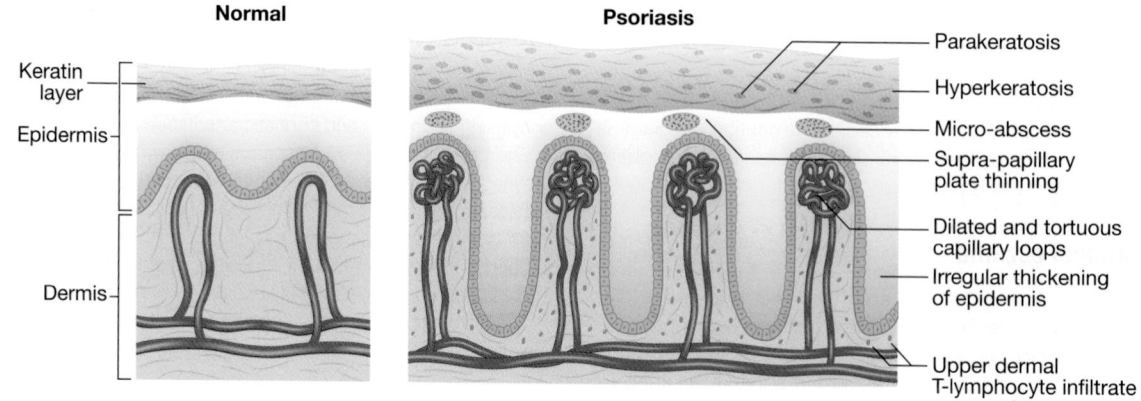

Fig. 27.35 **The histology of psoriasis.**

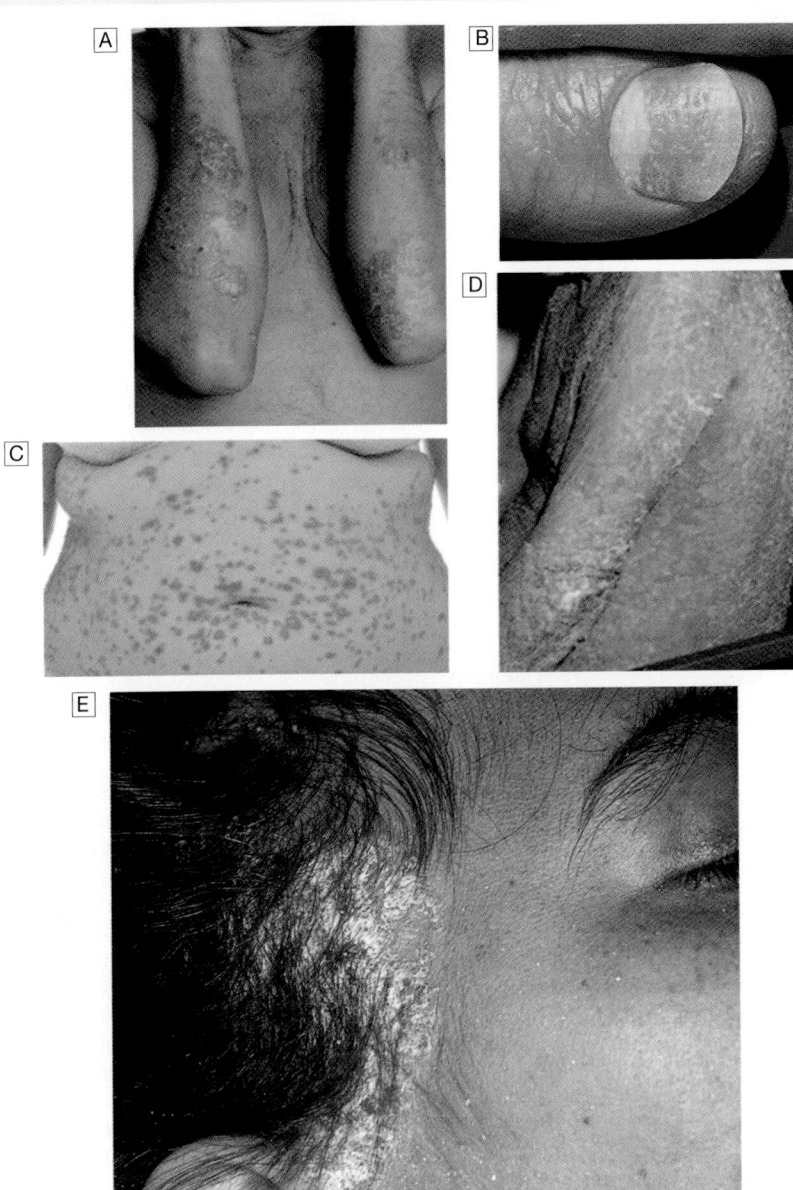

Fig. 27.36 Psoriasis. A Chronic plaque psoriasis, most prominent on extensor surfaces. B Nail involvement, with coarse pitting and separation from the nail plate (onycholysis). C Guttate psoriasis following a streptococcal throat infection. D Erythrodermic psoriasis. E Psoriasis on the scalp. (E) *From Wilson SF, Giddens JF. Health Assessment for Nursing Practice, 7th edn. Elsevier; 2022.*

Pustular psoriasis

Pustular psoriasis may be generalised or localised. Generalised pustular psoriasis is uncommon, unstable and life-threatening. It will often emerge in the context of plaque disease and the onset is usually sudden, with large numbers of small, sterile pustules on an erythematous background, often merging into sheets, with waves of new pustules in subsequent days. The patient is usually febrile and systemically unwell, and this must be dealt with as a medical emergency. Unstable pustular psoriasis may be precipitated as a rebound phenomenon following either topical or systemic glucocorticoid use in a patient with psoriasis. Localised pustular psoriasis of the palms and soles (palmoplantar pustulosis) is more common, chronic and closely associated with smoking; small, sterile pustules and erythema develop and resolve with pigmentation and scaling. A localised form of sterile pustulosis of a few digits (acropustulosis) can also occur. It is unclear whether these localised forms of pustulosis are truly psoriatic.

Arthropathy

Between 5% and 10% of individuals with psoriasis develop an inflammatory arthropathy, which can take on a number of patterns. Joint involvement is more likely in patients with psoriatic nail disease. Psoriatic arthritis is discussed in more detail in Chapter 26.

Investigations

Skin biopsy is not usually required but may be performed if there is diagnostic doubt. An infection screen, particularly throat swab and/or serology for recent streptococcal infection, may be informative in guttate psoriasis. Assessment of impact on life using the DLQI and disease extent using PASI (Psoriasis Area and Severity Index) is essential. Due to the association of psoriasis with metabolic syndrome, comorbidities and cardiovascular risk factors should be assessed and managed along usual lines. HIV testing should be considered in severe or recalcitrant psoriasis.

Management

Counselling about diagnosis and management of skin involvement and other comorbidities is paramount. Information and services must be available for patients. Psoriasis can have a major impact on all aspects of life and this must not be under-estimated. Reassurance is also needed, as the condition is generally not life-threatening. Advice regarding reduction in risk factors for cardiovascular disease should be given (smoking cessation, reduction of alcohol intake, adequate exercise and a normal body mass index). Associated diseases, such as hypertension and diabetes, should be treated.

Patients need to be involved in their own management, as the disease is usually chronic and the benefit/risk profile of treatments must be

27

discussed and tailored to individuals. The endpoint for treatment also needs to be discussed because complete disease clearance may not be practical or appropriate and patients vary considerably in their treatment requirements. Extent of disease and impact on quality of life must be taken into account. Patient adherence to topical and systemic therapies is essential and dependent on the treatment practicalities.

The treatment approach generally follows a stepwise progression, with treatment categories broadly summarised (Fig. 27.37).

Topical treatments, including emollients, are the first-line approach. Vitamin D receptor agonists, such as calcipotriol, calcitriol and tacalcitol, are often used as first-line topical treatment. The mechanism of action includes increased differentiation and reduction of proliferation, reducing plaque scale and thickness. Calcipotriol is most widely used and can be applied once to twice daily; if less than 100 g of ointment is used each week, there is no risk of hypercalcaemia. Vitamin D analogues can cause irritation but this is often temporary. Topical glucocorticoids may be required in the management of psoriasis, particularly at flexural or facial sites, and may be alternated or combined with vitamin D analogues. However, safe, appropriately supervised and judicious use is necessary, with awareness of the potential risk of rebound unstable or pustular psoriasis with glucocorticoid

over-use or sudden cessation. Dithranol and coal tar are effective and, like vitamin D analogues, work by increasing differentiation and inhibiting proliferation. Although often effective, they are messy and time-consuming. Modified versions of Goeckerman's regimen (the combination of coal tar and UVB) are still used, but coal tar has a characteristic odour and can be irritant. Short-contact dithranol therapy at relatively high concentrations applied for 15–30 minutes can be used but causes brown staining of skin and purple discoloration of light hair. In recent years, efforts have been made to improve the tolerance of tar and dithranol preparations, but at reduced efficacy. Overall, the use of tar and dithranol has reduced in recent years but they can be highly effective in selected patients.

If topical treatment is insufficient, then UVB phototherapy or PUVA should usually be the next step. If the patient continues to have active disease or early recurrence, then the addition of systemic retinoid such as acitretin to UVB or PUVA can be effective. Alternatively, immunosuppressants, such as methotrexate or ciclosporin, may be required. For difficult treatment-resistant disease, fumaric acid esters, apremilast and biologics should be considered and biologic therapies are now widely used in routine dermatology practice and have had a major impact on the management of patients with severe or poorly responsive psoriasis (see Fig. 27.11 and Box 27.14).

The active component of fumaric acid ester therapy is dimethyl fumarate and efficacy in psoriasis is established. Common adverse effects are flushing and diarrhoea. Lymphopenia is also expected at effective doses. Apremilast (a phosphodiesterase-4 inhibitor) is indicated for moderate to severe psoriasis resistant to standard measures (such as light-based therapies, methotrexate or ciclosporin). Of the biologic agents, the anti-TNF-α agents (adalimumab, etanercept, infliximab, certolizumab), ustekinumab (an inhibitor of IL-12 and IL-23), guselkumab (IL-23 inhibitor) and secukinumab, brodalumab, ixekizumab or bimekizumab (IL-17 inhibitors) may all offer high levels of efficacy.

Irrespective of the treatment chosen, individualised management is essential. For example, a patient with localised plaque psoriasis on elbows, knees and sacrum should respond to topical treatment only, whereas someone with guttate psoriasis is likely to need phototherapy as a first-line approach because of difficulties in topical drug application in extensive disease. A patient with extensive chronic plaque psoriasis and significant arthropathy would be better suited to a systemic drug, such as methotrexate, than phototherapy, which would be unlikely to improve joint symptoms. Thus, whilst a stepwise general approach to management (see Fig. 27.37) may offer guidance, the correct choice for any given patient must be determined on an individual basis.

Pityriasis rosea

This is an acute, self-limiting exanthem that particularly affects young adults and occurs worldwide, with a slight female predominance. It usually presents in spring and summer, although no infective agent has been identified and its aetiology is unknown. It is characterised by the appearance of a 'herald patch', an oval lesion (1–2 cm) with a pinkish (salmon-coloured) centre, a darker periphery and a characteristic collarette of scale. It is followed 1–2 weeks later by a widespread papulosquamous eruption, which is typically arranged in a symmetrical 'fir tree' pattern on the trunk. Individual lesions also have a collarette of scale. An inverse variant with flexural involvement can occur. Mucosal involvement is rare. There is a small risk of recurrence. Symptomatic relief can be achieved with emollients and mild topical glucocorticoids. Post-inflammatory hyperpigmentation can supervene, particularly in darker skin types.

Pityriasis lichenoides chronica

This is rare but typically presents within the first three decades of life. The aetiology is unclear but the condition is part of a spectrum and remits spontaneously. The more acute variety (pityriasis lichenoides et varioliformis acuta, PLEVA) presents as crops of papules that rapidly evolve with central necrosis, each attack lasting up to 3 months. The more chronic variety presents as a persistent, widespread, scaly

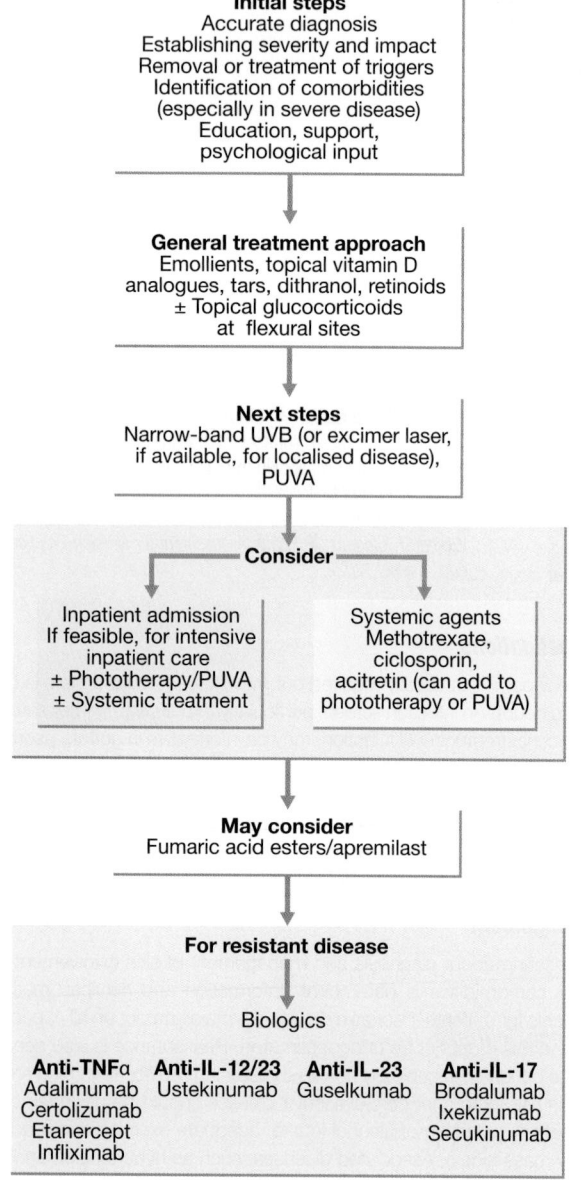

Fig. 27.37 General management approaches: psoriasis. (IL = interleukin; PUVA = psoralen–ultraviolet A; TNF-α = tumour necrosis factor alpha; UVB = ultraviolet B)

eruption. Characteristically, lesions are brown papules with a mica-like scale ('cornflake'). The condition fluctuates but can persist for months or years. Emollients, topical glucocorticoids and long-term oral erythromycin can occasionally be helpful. UVB phototherapy or PUVA is usually effective, although recurrences are high.

Drug eruptions

It is essential to consider a drug cause in anyone presenting with an erythematous maculopapular or papulosquamous eruption, and a careful drug history is critical. Exfoliation ('peeling') and post-inflammatory hyper- or, less commonly, hypopigmentation can occur.

Other causes

Secondary syphilis, pityriasis versicolor and tinea corporis fungal infection can all cause an erythematous papulosquamous rash and must be considered in the differential diagnosis of erythematous papulosquamous rashes.

Lichenoid eruptions

Lichen planus

Lichen planus occurs worldwide. It typically presents as a pruritic rash; the mucosae, hair and nails may also be involved.

Pathogenesis

The disease probably has an autoimmune basis since there is an association with inflammatory bowel disease, primary biliary cholangitis, autoimmune hepatitis, hepatitis B and C, alopecia areata, myasthenia gravis and thymoma. There are also similarities with graft-versus-host disease (GVHD). Lichen planus can occasionally occur in families and possible HLA associations have been reported but there is no clear inheritance pattern. On skin biopsy, characteristic histological changes include hyperkeratosis, basal cell degeneration and a heavy, band-like T-lymphocyte infiltrate in the papillary dermis, with affinity for the epidermis (epidermotropism). The dermo-epidermal junction has a 'sawtooth' appearance.

Clinical features

Lichen planus occurs in both sexes and at any age, although usually between 30 and 60 years. It generally presents on the distal limbs, most commonly on the flexural aspects of the wrists and forearms (Fig. 27.38), and on the lower back. It is intensely itchy and lesions are violaceous, shiny, flat-topped, polygonal papules, with a characteristic fine lacy, white network on the surface (Wickham's striae). New lesions may appear at sites of skin trauma (Köbner phenomenon) and the rash may become generalised. Individual lesions may last for many months and can become hypertrophic and modified by scratching, particularly on the lower legs.

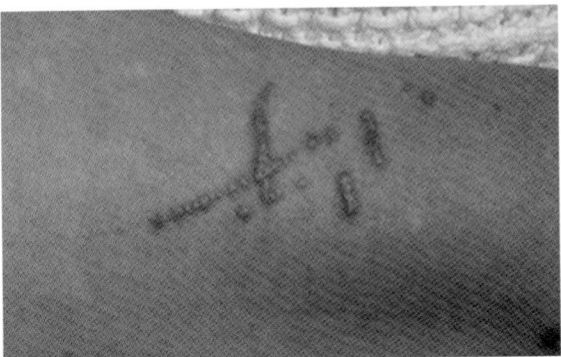

Fig. 27.38 Lichen planus. Violaceous papules on the flexural aspect of the forearm, arising at a site of minor linear trauma (Köbner phenomenon).

The eruption usually remits over months but can become chronic, particularly with hypertrophic disease. Post-inflammatory pigmentary change is common, particularly in darker skin types. Mucous membrane involvement occurs in 30%–70% of patients, usually as a network of white, lacy striae on the buccal mucosae and tongue. These oral changes are often asymptomatic and should be sought on examination. Genital and other mucosal surfaces can also be affected. Nail involvement occurs in about 10% and can range from longitudinal ridging to a destructive nail dystrophy, scarring (pterygium) and nail loss. Scalp involvement usually presents as an inflammatory scarring alopecia, often with tufting of residual hairs. The classical presentation of lichen planus is unmistakable, but less common atypical variants, which include annular, atrophic, actinic, linear, bullous, follicular, pigmented and ulcerative types, can be a diagnostic challenge.

Investigations

A skin biopsy should be performed if there is diagnostic doubt. A careful drug history must be taken, as, although the classical presentation of lichen planus is usually 'idiopathic', the main differential is a drug-induced lichenoid reaction (see below). Other differential diagnoses include psoriasis, pityriasis rosea, pityriasis lichenoides chronica and secondary syphilis. Screening for underlying disease, such as hepatitis, must be considered.

Management

The condition is usually self-limiting, although rarely it may persist for years, particularly oral lichen planus. Treatment is symptomatic and potent local glucocorticoids (topical, with occlusion or by injection for hypertrophic disease, or as oral rinse for oral involvement) may help the intense itch; short courses of systemic glucocorticoids are sometimes required for extensive disease. UVB, PUVA or UVA1 can be beneficial and, for recalcitrant disease, retinoids or immunosuppressants, such as ciclosporin or methotrexate, may be needed. A low but significant risk of malignant transformation exists with persistent oral and genital disease, so active treatment, surveillance and smoking cessation are important.

Drug-induced lichenoid eruptions

Drug-induced lichenoid reactions that are clinically and histologically difficult to distinguish from idiopathic lichen planus are important to identify. The likely culprits are gold, quinine, proton pump inhibitors, sulphonamides, penicillamine, antimalarials, antituberculous drugs, thiazide diuretics, β-adrenoceptor antagonists (β-blockers), angiotensin-converting enzyme (ACE) inhibitors, NSAIDs, sulphonylureas, lithium and dyes in colour developers (see Box 27.36).

Graft-versus-host disease

In the acute stage of graft-versus-host disease (GVHD), there is a distinctive dermatitis associated with hepatitis. After about 3 months, chronic GVHD can present with a lichenoid eruption on the palms, soles, face and upper trunk. Progressive sclerodermatous skin thickening, associated with pigmentary changes, may lead to contractures and limited mobility.

Urticaria

Urticaria ('hives') is caused by localised dermal oedema secondary to a temporary increase in capillary permeability. If oedema involves subcutaneous or submucosal layers, the term angioedema is used.

Clinical features

Acute urticaria may be associated with angioedema of the lips, face, tongue, throat and, rarely, wheezing, abdominal pain, headaches and even anaphylaxis. Urticaria present for less than 6 weeks is considered to be acute, and chronic if it continues for more than 6 weeks. Individual weals (**definition**: evanescent discrete areas of dermal oedema, often centrally white due to masking of local blood supply by fluid; weals can be papules, macules, patches and plaques – Fig. 27.39) last for less than 24 hours; if

27

they persist, urticarial vasculitis needs to be considered. Clarification of the duration of urticaria can be achieved by drawing around the weal and re-assessing 24 hours later. History-taking should probe for possible causes, including medications (Box 27.25). Physical triggers can also be assessed

Fig. 27.39 Urticaria. Erythema, reflecting dilated dermal vessels, and oedema (with upper dermal oedema obscuring the erythema centrally) are evident. Note the absence of epidermal changes.

---

i | **27.25 Causes of urticaria**

Acute and chronic urticaria

- Autoimmune: due to antibodies that cross-link the IgE receptor on mast cells
- Allergens in foods and inhalants
- Contact allergens: latex, animal saliva
- Drugs: see Box 27.36
- Physical stimuli: heat, cold, pressure, sun, sweat, water
- Infections: intestinal parasites, hepatitis
- Others: SLE, pregnancy, thyroid disease
- Idiopathic: chronic spontaneous urticaria and angioedema

Urticarial vasculitis

- Hepatitis B, SLE, idiopathic

(IgE = immunoglobulin E; SLE = systemic lupus erythematosus)

---

in challenge testing, such as eliciting dermographism or pressure testing. Enquiry about family history and medication, particularly ACE inhibitors, is important in angioedema. Examination may be unremarkable or weals may be evident (see Fig. 27.39). The skin should be stroked firmly with an orange stick in order to ascertain whether dermographism is present or not.

Mast cell degranulation and release of histamine and other vasoactive mediators is the basis of urticaria (Fig. 27.40). Chronic spontaneous urticaria (previously called 'chronic idiopathic' or 'chronic ordinary' urticaria) is the most common chronic urticaria and has an autoimmune pathogenesis in some cases.

Investigations

Investigations should be guided by the history and possible causes, but are often negative, particularly in acute urticaria. Some or all of the following may be appropriate:

- *Full blood count*: eosinophilia in parasitic infection or drug cause.
- *Erythrocyte sedimentation rate (ESR) or plasma viscosity*: elevated in vasculitis.
- *Urea and electrolytes, thyroid and liver function tests, iron studies*: may reveal an underlying systemic disorder.
- *Total IgE and specific IgE to possible allergens*: shellfish, peanut, house-dust mite. Particularly relevant if there is angioedema.
- *Autoantibodies, particularly antinuclear factor*: positive in systemic lupus erythematosus (SLE) and often positive in urticarial vasculitis. Other autoimmune diseases, such as rheumatoid arthritis and auto-immune hepatitis or thyroid disease, may be associated.
- *Complement C_3 and C_4 levels*: if these are low due to complement consumption, C_1 esterase inhibitor activity should be measured.
- *Infection screen*: hepatitis screen and HIV may be indicated.
- *Skin biopsy*: if urticarial vasculitis is suspected.
- *Challenge tests*: to confirm physical urticarias, such as dermographism, pressure, heat, cold.

Management

Removal or treatment of any trigger is essential, although this may not be identified in the majority of cases. Urticaria may be precipitated by aspirin, NSAIDs, codeine and opioids, and it is advisable to suggest alternatives such as paracetamol. In chronic urticaria, non-sedating

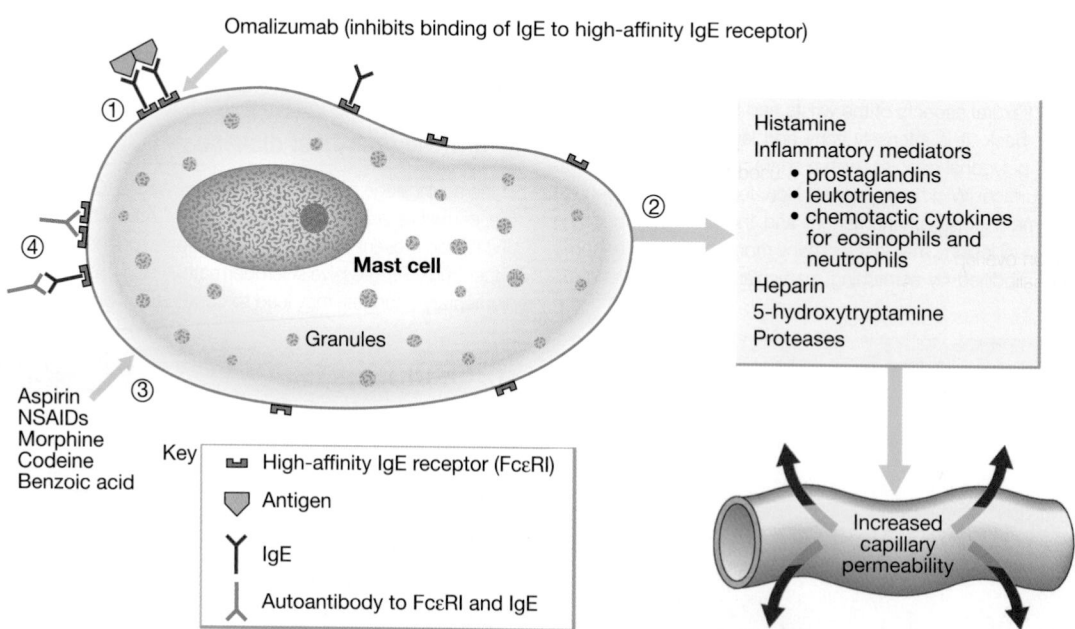

Omalizumab (inhibits binding of IgE to high-affinity IgE receptor)

Histamine
Inflammatory mediators
- prostaglandins
- leukotrienes
- chemotactic cytokines for eosinophils and neutrophils

Heparin
5-hydroxytryptamine
Proteases

Mast cell

Granules

Aspirin
NSAIDs
Morphine
Codeine
Benzoic acid

Key

- ▥ High-affinity IgE receptor (FcɛRI)
- ▽ Antigen
- Y IgE
- ⅄ Autoantibody to FcɛRI and IgE

Increased capillary permeability

Fig. 27.40 Pathogenesis of urticaria. Mast cell degranulation occurs in a variety of ways. (1) Type I hypersensitivity causes degranulation. (2) Spontaneous mast cell degranulation in chronic urticaria. (3) Chemical mast cell degranulation. (4) Autoimmunity, with IgE antibodies directed against IgE receptors or IgE itself. Histamine and the leukotrienes are especially relevant mediators in urticaria. Heparin release is probably not a major factor in urticaria but plays a role in the osteoporosis that can occur in systemic mastocytosis. (IgE = immunoglobulin E; NSAIDs = non-steroidal anti-inflammatory drugs)

antihistamines, such as fexofenadine, loratadine or cetirizine, are usually beneficial. If there is lack of response after 2 weeks, an alternative non-sedating antihistamine should be used and an H_2-blocker, such as cimetidine or ranitidine, can be added. Mast cell stabilisers or leukotriene receptor antagonists, such as montelukast, can be used for more recalcitrant disease. For chronic urticaria, narrowband UVB phototherapy is valuable and has proven efficacy. Systemic glucocorticoids are widely prescribed for urticaria but are not indicated in the majority of cases. If systemic glucocorticoids are used, efficacy may be seen only at relatively high doses and they are appropriate only for occasional short courses in the acute setting, usually in association with angioedema. Patients with a history of life-threatening anaphylaxis, as in peanut or wasp sting allergy, should carry a self-administered adrenaline (epinephrine) injection kit. The management of anaphylaxis is discussed in Chapter 9 and the management of hereditary angioedema is discussed in Chapter 4. The anti-IgE monoclonal antibody omalizumab may be effective in patients with severe recalcitrant urticaria (Fig. 27.40).

Bullous diseases

Blistering can occur at any level in the skin and there are a variety of different presentations, depending on the underlying defect and level of involvement. Knowledge of the molecular basis of many blistering disorders has advanced considerably through understanding of the basic processes of cell adhesion and studies of rare genetic blistering disorders, particularly epidermolysis bullosa (Box 27.26). This section concentrates on primary blistering skin diseases.

Toxic epidermal necrolysis

Toxic epidermal necrolysis (TEN) is a medical emergency, as the extensive mucocutaneous blistering is associated with a high mortality rate. It is usually drug-induced (see Box 27.36), with anticonvulsants, sulphonamides, sulphonylureas, NSAIDs, allopurinol and antiretroviral therapy often implicated. Usually 1–4 weeks after drug commencement, the patient becomes systemically unwell and often pyrexial. Erythema and blistering develop, initially on the trunk but rapidly involving all skin; an early warning sign is cutaneous pain. Sheets of blisters coalesce and denude, and the underlying skin is painful and erythematous (Fig. 27.41). Gentle lateral pressure on stroking the skin results in epidermal detachment (Nikolsky sign), demonstrating the severity of skin fragility. Mucous membrane involvement and blistering are usual. Blistering of skin and mucosae may be haemorrhagic. A disease severity score (Box 27.27) is used to predict outcome. The main differential diagnosis is staphylococcal scalded skin syndrome, although the diagnosis is usually obvious in an adult patient with a culprit drug. There is often overlap with Stevens–Johnson syndrome and targetoid lesions, especially on palms and soles, may be evident. Skin snip may allow early diagnosis. If there is diagnostic doubt, then full-thickness skin biopsy should be undertaken for histology and direct immunofluorescence in order to exclude immunobullous or other diagnoses.

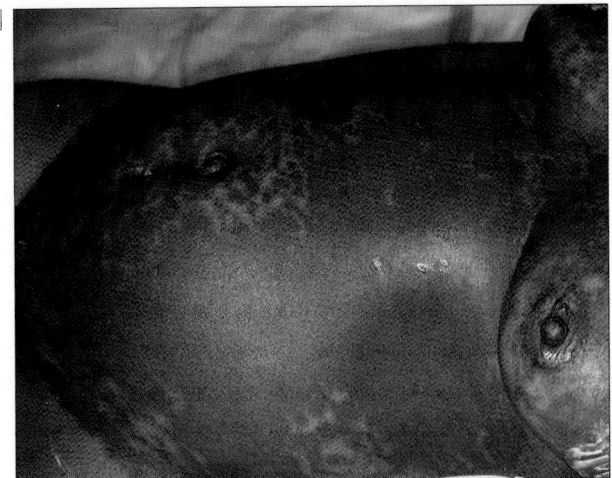

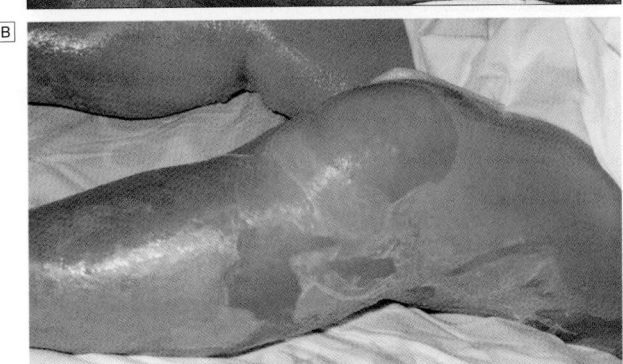

Fig. 27.41 Toxic epidermal necrolysis. A Characteristic dusky red colour of the early macular eruption in TEN. B Full-blown necrolytic lesions, note the extensive erythema, oedema and epidermal loss secondary to carbamazepine. *(A) From Bolognia JL, Schaffer JV, Jorizzo J. Dermatology, 3rd edn. Elsevier; 2012.*

i	27.27 The SCORTEN disease severity score for toxic epidermal necrolysis

Factor

- Age >40 years
- Heart rate >120 beats/min
- Cancer or haematological malignancy
- Involved body surface area >10%
- Blood urea >10 mmol/L (28 mg/dL)
- Serum bicarbonate <20 mmol/L
- Blood glucose ≥14 mmol/L (252 mg/dL)

Mortality rates

- 0–1 factor present = 3%
- 2 factors = 12%
- 3 factors = 35%
- 4 factors = 58%
- ≥5 factors = 90%

From Bastuji-Garin S, Fouchard N, Bertocchi M, et al. SCORTEN: a severity-of-illness score for toxic epidermal necrolysis. J Invest Dermatol 2000; 115:149–153.

Identification and discontinuation of the causative drug are essential. Sepsis and multi-organ failure are major risks. Intensive care in a dedicated dermatology ward or intensive care or burns unit is of paramount importance. Treatment is supportive, with regular sterile dressings and emollients, careful attention to fluid balance and treatment of infection if it develops. Urethral and ocular involvement is common and must be looked for and treated symptomatically. Chronic sequelae, including ocular and urethral scarring and adverse psychological impact can be problematic in survivors. There is no conclusive evidence that intravenous immunoglobulins, systemic glucocorticoids or ciclosporin improve outcomes and survival.

i	27.26 Classification of epidermolysis bullosa		
Type	**Mode of inheritance**	**Level of blister***	**Abnormality**
Simple	Autosomal dominant	Epidermal basal cell	Keratins 5 and 14
Junctional	Autosomal recessive	Lamina lucida	Laminin-5 and $\alpha_6\beta_4$ integrin
Dystrophic	Autosomal dominant and recessive	Dermis below lamina densa	Collagen VII

*See Figure 27.1.

27

Immunobullous diseases

There are various subtypes of immunobullous disease that affect patients of different ages and have clinical characteristics (Box 27.28). The key investigation is an elliptical biopsy taken from the edge of a recent blister (Box 27.29). The sample is halved: one half is put in formalin for subsequent histology, while the other is sent fresh for direct immunofluorescence. Serum should also be sent for indirect immunofluorescence in suspected immunobullous disease.

Bullous pemphigoid

Bullous pemphigoid (BP) is the most common immunobullous disease and occurs worldwide. It is a disease of older people, with an average age of onset of 65 years; males and females are equally affected.

Pathogenesis

The disease is caused by autoantibodies (BP-230 and BP-180) directed against the hemi-desmosomal BP antigens BPAg-1 (intracellular) and BPAg-2 (transmembranous type XVII collagen), respectively. Antibody–antigen binding initiates complement activation and inflammation, with hemi-desmosomal damage and subepidermal blistering.

Clinical features

There is often a lengthy prodrome of an itchy, urticated, erythematous rash prior to the development of tense bullae (Fig. 27.42A). Milia (definition: small epidermal keratin cysts) may develop due to basement membrane disruption. Mucosal involvement is uncommon.

Investigations

The diagnosis can be made by skin biopsy, which shows subepidermal blistering with an eosinophil-rich inflammatory infiltrate. Direct immunofluorescence demonstrates the presence of IgG and C3 at the basement membrane (Fig. 27.42B). Indirect immunofluorescence may show positive titres of circulating anti-epidermal antibodies. Distinction from epidermolysis bullosa acquisita requires immunofluorescence studies using the patient's serum on salt-split skin. In BP, the immunoreactants localise to the epidermal side (hemi-desmosome) of split skin, whereas in epidermolysis bullosa acquisita they localise to the base of the split (type VII collagen/anchoring fibrils).

Management

Very potent topical glucocorticoids are effective and may be sufficient in frail older patients; they need to be applied to all sites, however, and not just lesional skin. Tetracyclines, such as doxycycline, have important anti-inflammatory effects and may limit the use of systemic glucocorticoids. Doxycycline has been shown to be non-inferior to prednisolone for initial control of bullous pemphigoid and to have fewer long-term adverse effects, although most patients with extensive disease will go on to require systemic glucocorticoids (0.75 mg/kg/day or less), often combined with immunosuppressants as glucocorticoid-sparing agents. In severe refractory disease, other therapies, such as intravenous immunoglobulin or rituximab, are sometimes used but are of unproven efficacy. The condition does, however, often burn out spontaneously over a few years.

---

i 27.28 Age of onset in immunobullous skin disorders

Disease	Age
Pemphigus vulgaris	40–60 years
Pemphigus foliaceus	Any age (endemic form in parts of Brazil and South Africa, from adolescence on)
Bullous pemphigoid	Sixties and over
Dermatitis herpetiformis	Young, associated with coeliac disease
Linear IgA disease	Any age
Pemphigoid gestationis	Pregnant females
Epidermolysis bullosa acquisita	Any age
Bullous lupus erythematosus	Young females of African ancestry

---

i 27.29 Clinical and investigation findings in the immunobullous disorders

Disease	Site of blisters	Nature of blisters	Mucous membrane involvement	Antigen	Circulating antibody (indirect IF)	Fixed antibody (direct IF)
Pemphigus vulgaris	Trunk, head	Flaccid, fragile, many erosions	100%	Desmoglein-1 and 3 (120 kD)	IgG	IgG, C_3 intercellular (epidermal)
Pemphigus foliaceus	Trunk	Often not present, multiple erosions, may mimic dermatitis	No	Desmoglein-1	IgG	IgG, C_3 intercellular (epidermal)
Bullous pemphigoid	Trunk, flexures and limbs	Tense, milia as blisters resolve	Occasional	BP-230 and 180	IgG (70%)	IgG, C_3 at BMZ
Dermatitis herpetiformis	Elbows, lower back, buttocks	Excoriated and often not present	No	Unknown	Anti-endomysial and tissue transglutaminase	Granular IgA in papillary dermis
Linear IgA disease	Widespread	Tense, often annular configuration, 'string of beads'	Frequent	Unknown	50% have low titres of circulating antibody	Linear IgA at BMZ
Pemphigoid gestationis	Periumbilical and limbs	Tense, milia as blisters resolve	Rare	Collagen XVII (part of hemi-desmosome, BP-180)	Circulating antibodies to BP-180 (type XVII collagen) (and BP-230)	C_3 at BMZ
Epidermolysis bullosa acquisita	Widespread	Tense, scarring, milia	Common (50%)	Type VII collagen	IgG (anti-type VII collagen)	IgG at BMZ
Bullous lupus erythematosus	Widespread	Tense	Rare	Type VII collagen	Anti-type VII collagen	IgG, IgA, IgM at BMZ

(BMZ = basement membrane zone; IF = immunofluorescence; Ig = immunoglobulin)

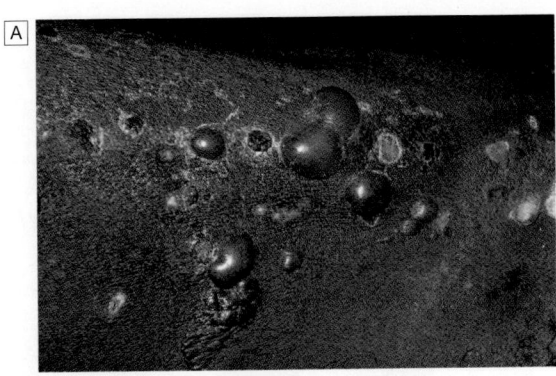 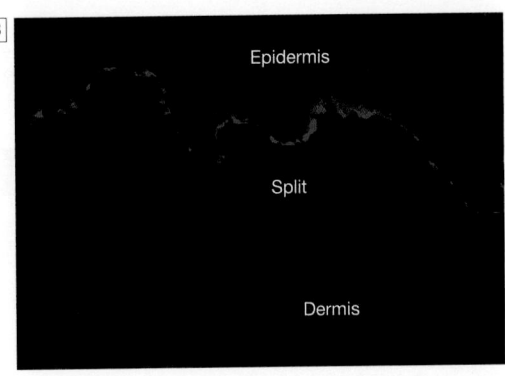

Fig. 27.42 Bullous pemphigoid. A Large, tense, unilocular blisters. B Immunofluorescence on salt-split skin, showing a subepidermal blister and linear IgG and C3 deposition at the basement membrane zone. *(A) From James W, Elston D, Treat J, Rosenbach M, Micheletti R. Andrews' Diseases of the skin, 13th edn. Elsevier: 2020.*

Pemphigus

Pemphigus is less common than BP and patients tend to be younger.

Pathogenesis

The cause is IgG1 and IgG4 autoantibodies, directed against desmogleins-1 and 3, resulting in intra-epidermal blistering. The syndrome may occur spontaneously or be secondary to drugs such as penicillamine or captopril and underlying malignancy (paraneoplastic pemphigus). Pemphigus folliaceus is a very superficial form, in which antibodies are directed against desmoglein-1 only and affect just the most superficial epidermis.

Clinical features

Skin and mucosae are usually involved, although disease may be restricted to mucosae only, which may be severely affected. Due to the higher level of split within the epidermis, the blisters are flaccid, easily ruptured and often not seen intact. Erosions are common and the Nikolsky sign is positive. The trunk is usually affected. The condition is associated with significant morbidity and mortality.

Investigations

The diagnosis can be made by skin biopsy, which shows intra-epidermal blistering and acantholysis, with positive direct immunofluorescence for IgG (usually IgG1 or IgG4) and C3 at the periphery of keratinocytes, giving a 'chicken wire' appearance within the epidermis. The titres of circulating epidermal autoantibodies can also be used to monitor disease activity. Investigations should screen for associated autoimmune disease or malignancy if paraneoplastic pemphigus is suspected.

Management

Pemphigus is more difficult to treat than BP and high-dose systemic glucocorticoids such as prednisolone (0.5–1.0 mg/kg/day) are usually required. Azathioprine and cyclophosphamide are most often used as glucocorticoid-sparing agents but a range of other immunosuppressants may be considered for severe recalcitrant disease, including methotrexate, ciclosporin, mycophenolate mofetil, intravenous immunoglobulins, plasma exchange, extracorporeal photopheresis and rituximab. Often, long-term treatment is required to prevent relapse.

Dermatitis herpetiformis

Dermatitis herpetiformis (DH) is an autoimmune blistering disorder that is strongly associated with coeliac disease (CD). While fewer than 10% of individuals with CD develop DH, almost all patients with DH have evidence of partial villous atrophy on intestinal biopsy, even if they have no gastrointestinal symptoms. It is unclear why some CD patients develop DH and others do not. Although DH is a bullous disease, intact vesicles and blisters are seldom seen, as the condition is so pruritic that excoriations on extensor surfaces of arms, knees, buttocks, shoulders and scalp may be the only signs.

The diagnosis can be made by skin biopsy, which shows subepidermal vesiculation in the dermal papillae and a neutrophil- and eosinophil-rich infiltrate. Direct immunofluorescence shows granular IgA in the papillary dermis. Anti-endomysial antibodies and tissue transglutaminase should be assessed and jejunal biopsy undertaken if indicated. The condition usually responds to a gluten-free diet but, if not, dapsone can also be used.

Linear IgA disease

This occurs in children (chronic bullous disease of childhood) and adults, and is usually self-limiting, although it can be active for a few years. Drugs, notably vancomycin, can be a secondary cause. Blisters can arise on erythematous, urticated or otherwise normal-looking skin and often form an annular configuration at the edge of the lesion: 'clusters of jewels' (herpetiform) and 'string of beads' (annular/polycyclic). Mucosal involvement is common and ophthalmology input important, as corneal scarring is a risk with longstanding disease. Linear IgA is seen at the basement membrane on direct immunofluorescence and localises to either roof or floor of salt-split skin. Dapsone, sulfapyridine, prednisolone, colchicine or intravenous immunoglobulin may be effective.

Epidermolysis bullosa acquisita

This chronic blistering disease affects skin and mucosae, and scarring, hair loss and nail dystrophy may be problematic. Blisters often follow trauma and milia develop. It can be very difficult to distinguish from other immunobullous diseases, such as bullous pemphigoid. It is caused by an IgG antibody to type VII collagen, which provokes subepidermal blistering and a mixed inflammatory infiltrate, although the latter may not be prominent. Direct immunofluorescence on perilesional skin shows IgG and C3 at the dermo-epidermal junction and pattern analysis may be helpful in distinction from bullous pemphigoid. Indirect immunofluorescence microscopy on salt-split normal human skin typically shows IgG and IgA in the floor of the artificially induced blister, whereas in BP antibody localisation would be to the roof of the blister. Epidermolysis bullosa acquisita is very difficult to treat, as it often does not respond well to immunosuppressants. Mainstays of treatment include systemic glucocorticoids in combination with dapsone or colchicine. Other immunosuppressive approaches may be required and include ciclosporin, azathioprine, immunoglobulins, plasmapheresis and rituximab. The condition may be associated with inflammatory bowel disease, rheumatoid arthritis, multiple myeloma and lymphoma, and thus associated comorbidities should be sought.

27

Porphyria cutanea tarda and pseudoporphyria

These conditions may also cause blistering (see Boxes 27.9 and 27.35). Porphyria is discussed in more detail in Chapter 19.

Pigmentation disorders

Decreased pigmentation

Disorders causing hypopigmentation and/or depigmentation include:

- vitiligo
- albinism
- pityriasis alba: depigmented areas on the face, particularly in children, with or without scale and usually considered to be eczematous
- pityriasis versicolor: hypopigmentation or, less commonly, hyperpigmentation can occur
- idiopathic guttate hypomelanosis: multiple small areas of depigmentation arising in chronically sun-exposed skin
- rarely, phenylketonuria and hypopituitarism.

Vitiligo

Vitiligo is an acquired condition affecting 1% of the population worldwide. Focal loss of melanocytes results in the development of patches of hypopigmentation. A positive family history of vitiligo is relatively common in those with extensive disease, and this type is also associated with other autoimmune diseases. Trauma and sunburn may (through the Köbner phenomenon) precipitate the appearance of vitiligo. It is thought to be the result of cell-mediated autoimmune destruction of melanocytes but why some areas are targeted and others are spared is unclear.

Clinical features

Generalised vitiligo is often symmetrical and involves hands, wrists, feet, knees and neck, as well as areas around body orifices (Fig. 27.43). The hair of the scalp, beard, eyebrows and lashes may also depigment. Segmental vitiligo is restricted to one part of the body but not necessarily a dermatome. The patches of depigmentation are sharply defined, and in light-skinned individuals may be surrounded by hyperpigmentation. Spotty perifollicular pigment may be seen within the depigmentation and is often the first sign of repigmentation. There is no history or evidence of inflammation within the patches, which may be helpful in distinguishing vitiligo from post-inflammatory hypopigmentation. Sensation in the depigmented patches is normal, unlike tuberculoid leprosy. Wood's light examination enhances the contrast between pigmented and non-pigmented skin. The course is unpredictable; most patches remain static or enlarge but a few undergo re-pigmentation spontaneously.

Management

Protecting the patches from excessive sun exposure with clothing or sunscreen may be helpful to avoid sunburn. Camouflage cosmetics may be beneficial, particularly in those with dark skin. In fair skin, photoprotection and cosmetic cover may be all that is required. Very potent or potent topical glucocorticoids have limited efficacy with respect to repigmentation. Topical pimecrolimus or tacrolimus may also have a role as a glucocorticoid-sparing agent. Phototherapy with narrowband UVB or PUVA can also be used. Narrowband UVB is the most effective repigmentary treatment available for generalised vitiligo, but even very prolonged courses often do not produce a satisfactory outcome. The absence of leucotrichia (white hairs in the area of vitiligo) and the presence of a trichrome pattern (three colours – normal skin colour, hypopigmentation and depigmentation) are good prognostic features. Vitiligo on the face, trunk and proximal limbs is more likely to respond than that on hands and feet. Exceptionally, depigmentation of normal non-lesional skin or a surgical approach with autologous melanocyte transfer, using a range of techniques including split-skin grafts and blister roof grafts, is sometimes used on dermabraded recipient skin in specific severe cases.

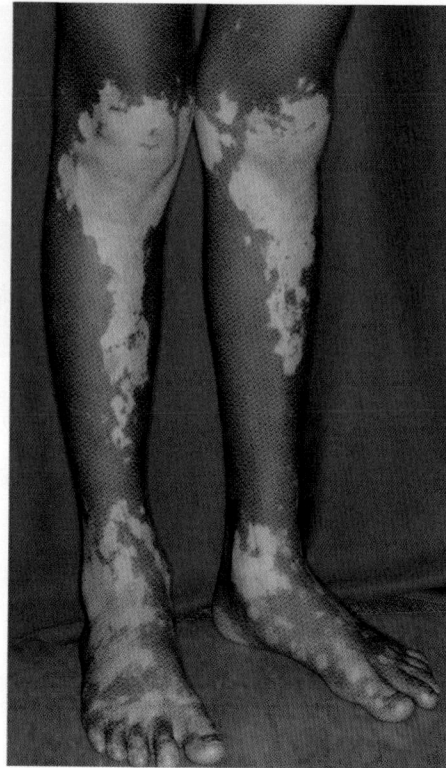

Fig. 27.43 Vitiligo. Symmetrical depigmentation of the knees and lower extremities. The dorsal aspect of the feet and hands are particularly hard to repigment. *From Mancini AJ, Paller AS. Hurwitz clinical pediatric dermatology, 5th edn. Elsevier; 2016.*

The impact of vitiligo differs markedly between populations. In South Asia the effects are more readily discernible than in light-skinned individuals in northern Europe. Depigmentation is also seen in leprosy, which means that individuals with vitiligo are often stigmatised. The emotional impact of vitiligo may be immense; psychological support is essential and is important in conveying realistic expectations of possible treatment approaches.

Oculocutaneous albinism

Albinism results from a range of genetic abnormalities that lead to reduced melanin biosynthesis in the skin and eyes; the number of melanocytes is normal (in contrast to vitiligo). Albinism is usually inherited as an autosomal recessive trait and there are several different types and presentations.

Type 1 albinism is due to a defect in the tyrosinase gene, whose product is rate-limiting in the production of melanin. Affected individuals have an almost complete absence of pigment in the skin and hair at birth, with consequent pale skin and white hair, and failure of melanin production in the iris and retina. Patients have photophobia, poor vision not correctable with refraction, rotatory nystagmus, and an alternating strabismus associated with abnormalities in the decussation of nerve fibres in the optic tract.

A second form of albinism is due to a defect in the *P* gene, which encodes an ion channel protein in the melanosome. Patients may have gross reduction of melanin in the skin and in the eyes, but may be more mildly affected than type 1 albinos. Establishing the subtype of albinism requires genetic analysis, as there is considerable phenotypic heterogeneity.

Oculocutaneous albinos are at grossly increased risk of sunburn and skin cancer. In equatorial regions, many die from squamous cell carcinoma or, more rarely, melanoma in early adult life. Interestingly, they may develop pigmented melanocytic naevi and freckles in response to sun exposure.

Management

Strict photoprotection, with sun avoidance (including occupational exposure), clothing, hats and sunscreens, is important. Early diagnosis and treatment of skin tumours is essential.

Increased pigmentation

- *Diffuse hyperpigmentation*: most commonly due to hypermelanosis but other pigments may be deposited in the skin, such as orange discoloration with carotenaemia and bronze with haemochromatosis.
- *Endocrine pigmentation*: may occur in several conditions. Melasma (chloasma) describes discrete patches of facial pigmentation that occur in pregnancy and in some women taking oral contraceptives. The mechanism for this localised increased hormonal sensitivity is unknown. Diffuse pigmentation, sometimes worse in the skin creases and mucosae, may be a feature of Addison's disease, Cushing's syndrome, Nelson syndrome and chronic renal failure due to increased levels of pituitary melanotrophic peptides, including adrenocorticotrophic hormone (ACTH)
- *Photo-exposed site hyperpigmentation*: occurs in some of the porphyrias but can also be drug-induced with amiodarone and chlorpromazine.
- *Drug-induced pigmentation* (Box 27.30): may be diffuse or localised. It is not always due to hypermelanosis but sometimes is caused by deposition of the drug or a metabolite.
- *Focal hypermelanosis*: seen in lesions such as freckles and lentigines, characterised by focal areas of increased pigmentation.

Establishing the cause is important. Photoprotection may minimise the risk of increasing pigmentation. Topical hydroquinone preparations can be used for skin lightening in some types of hyperpigmentation, although caution is required, particularly in darker skin types.

Hair disorders

These can be subdivided into disorders that cause loss of hair (alopecia) or excessive hair growth (hypertrichosis and hirsutism).

Alopecia

Alopecia is characterised by loss of hair. It can be further subdivided into localised and diffuse, and into scarring and non-scarring subtypes (Box 27.31).

Pathogenesis

Alopecia can be observed in association with inflammatory disorders that cause scarring (lichen planus, discoid lupus) and others that do not cause scarring (tinea capitis, psoriasis, seborrhoeic eczema). These conditions are discussed elsewhere. Alopecia areata has an autoimmune basis and there is a strong genetic component, with a family history in approximately 20% of cases. In addition to atopy, it is associated with other autoimmune diseases, particularly thyroid disease, and with Down syndrome. The cause of androgenetic alopecia is unclear but likely to be multifactorial, with genetic, hormonal and end-organ receptor sensitivity to the factors implicated. Developments in therapeutic approaches, such as JAK inhibition, will continue to provide evidence to inform our understanding of the pathogenesis of alopecia areata and the pathways involved.

Clinical features

Alopecia areata

This usually presents with well-defined, localised, non-inflammatory, non-scarring patches of alopecia, usually on the scalp (Fig. 27.44). Pathognomonic 'exclamation mark' hairs are seen (broken hairs, tapering towards the scalp) during active hair loss. A diffuse pattern can uncommonly occur on the scalp. Eyebrows, eyelashes, beard and body hair can be affected. Alopecia totalis describes complete loss of scalp hair, and alopecia universalis is complete loss of all hair. Nail pitting may occur. Spontaneous regrowth is usual for small patches of alopecia but the prognosis is less good for larger patches, more extensive involvement, early onset and an association with atopy.

Androgenetic alopecia

Male-pattern baldness is physiological in men over 20 years old, although it can also occur in adolescent. It is also found in women, particularly after the menopause. Characteristically, this involves bitemporal recession initially and subsequent involvement of the crown ('male pattern'), although it is often diffuse in women.

Investigations

Important investigations include full blood count, renal and liver function tests, iron studies, thyroid function, autoantibody screen and syphilis serology, as several systemic diseases, particularly iron deficiency and hypothyroidism, can cause diffuse non-scarring alopecia. Hair pull tests may help to establish the ratio of anagen to telogen hairs but require expertise for interpretation. Scrapings and pluckings should be sent for mycology if there is localised inflammation. Scalp biopsy and direct immunofluorescence of scarring alopecia may confirm a diagnosis of lichen planus or discoid lupus erythematosus but expert interpretation is needed.

i 27.30 Drug-induced pigmentation	
Drug	**Appearance**
Amiodarone	Photo-exposed sites, slate-grey
Arsenic	Diffuse bronze pigmentation Raindrop depigmentation
Bleomycin	Usually flexural, brown
Busulfan	Diffuse brown
Chloroquine	Photo-exposed sites, blue-grey
Clofazimine	Red
Mepacrine	Yellow
Minocycline	Temples, shins, gingiva, sclera, scar sites, slate-grey
Phenothiazines	Photo-exposed sites, slate-grey
Psoralens	Photo-exposed sites, brown

i 27.31 Classification and causes of alopecia	
Localised	**Diffuse**
Non-scarring	
Tinea capitis	Androgenetic alopecia
Alopecia areata	Telogen effluvium
Androgenetic alopecia	Hypothyroidism
Traumatic (trichotillomania, traction, cosmetic)	Hyperthyroidism
Syphilis	Hypopituitarism
	Diabetes mellitus
	HIV disease
	Nutritional (especially iron) deficiency
	Liver disease
	Post-partum
	Alopecia areata
	Syphilis
	Drug-induced: chemotherapy, retinoids
Scarring	
Discoid lupus erythematosus	Systemic lupus erythematosus
Lichen planopilaris	Radiotherapy
Herpes zoster	Folliculitis decalvans
Pseudopelade	Lichen planopilaris
Tinea capitis/kerion	
Morphoea (en coup de sabre)	
Idiopathic	
Developmental defects	

27

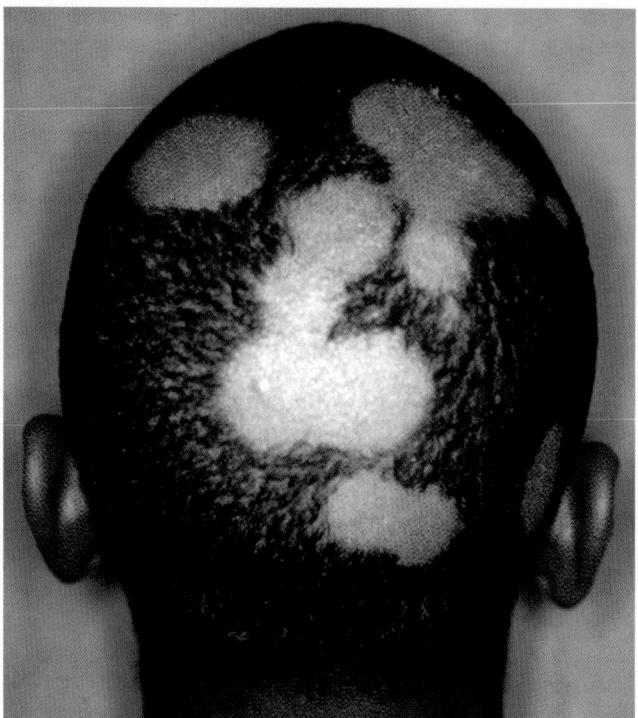

Fig. 27.44 Alopecia areata.

Management

Any underlying condition, such as iron deficiency, should be treated and may result in clinical improvement. Alopecia can have a major impact on quality of life and psychological support is usually required. It is particularly important to establish realistic expectations.

Hair may spontaneously regrow in alopecia areata and it may be appropriate to offer no active intervention as, while some treatments may induce some hair regrowth, there is no evidence that any treatment fundamentally alters the course of the disease. There may be some response to topical or intralesional glucocorticoids. PUVA or immunotherapy with diphencyprone may be effective, with evidence of hair regrowth, but there is a risk of relapse on discontinuation of treatment. Short courses of systemic glucocorticoids are occasionally used in an attempt to limit acutely progressive extensive alopecia areata but should not be used in the long term; the risk of relapse on discontinuation is high. Ongoing trials of JAK inhibitors may provide future hope for patients with this difficult disease.

Some males with androgenetic alopecia may be helped by systemic finasteride. Topical minoxidil can be used in males and females with androgenetic alopecia but, if an effect is obtained, treatment must be continued and is expensive. In females, anti-androgen therapy, such as cyproterone acetate, can be used. Wigs are often appropriate for extensive alopecia. Scalp surgery and autologous hair transplants are expensive but can be used for androgenetic alopecia.

Hypertrichosis

Hypertrichosis is a generalised or localised increase in hair and may be congenital or acquired. It can be primary or secondary: for example, to drugs such as ciclosporin, minoxidil or diazoxide, malignancy or eating disorders. Laser therapy or eflornithine, which inhibits ornithine decarboxylase and arrests hair growth while it is being used, may be helpful. When the hypertrichosis follows a male pattern, it is called hirsutism.

Hirsutism

Hirsutism is the growth of terminal hair in a male pattern in a female. The cause of most cases is unknown and, while it may occur in hyperandrogenism, Cushing's syndrome and polycystic ovary syndrome, only a small minority of patients have a demonstrable hormonal abnormality. Psychological distress is often significant and oral contraceptives containing an anti-androgen such as cyproterone acetate, laser therapy or topical eflornithine may be beneficial.

Nail disorders

The nails can be affected by both local and systemic disease. The nail apparatus consists of the nail matrix and the nail plate, which arises from the matrix and lies on the nail bed (Fig. 27.45). The cells of the matrix and, to a lesser extent the bed, produce the keratinous plate.

Important information may be obtained from nail-fold examination, including dilated capillaries and ragged cuticles in connective tissue disease (Fig. 27.46) and the boggy inflammation of paronychia. The latter commonly occurs chronically in individuals undertaking wet work, in those with diabetes or poor peripheral circulation, and subsequent to increased cosmetic nail procedures and vigorous manicuring.

Normal variants

Longitudinal ridging and beading of the nail plate occur with age. White transverse patches (striate leuconychia) are often caused by airspaces within the plate.

Nail trauma

- *Nail biting/picking* is a very common habit. Repetitive proximal nail-fold trauma (often involving the thumb nail) results in transverse ridging and central furrowing of the nail.

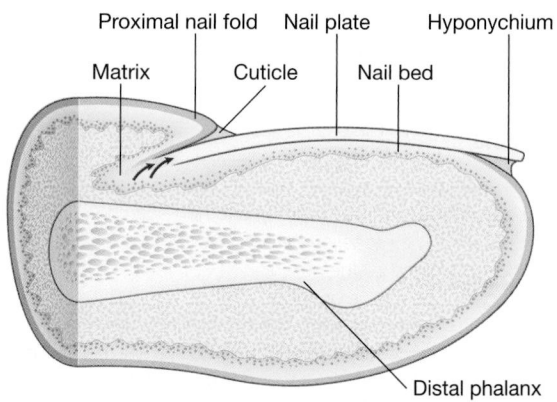

Fig. 27.45 The nail plate and bed. Arrows indicate the direction of nail growth.

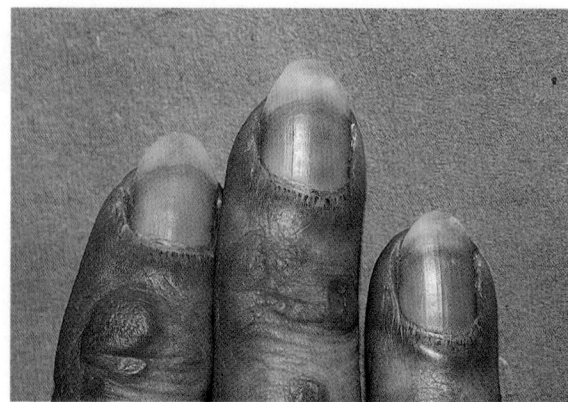

Fig. 27.46 Dermatomyositis Note the prominent periungual involvement. Erythema, dilated and tortuous capillaries in the proximal nail fold, and ragged cuticles are features of connective tissue disease.

- *Chronic trauma* from poorly fitting shoes and sport can cause thickening and disordered growth of the nail (onychogryphosis) and subsequent ingrowing toenails.
- *Splinter haemorrhages* are fine, linear, dark brown longitudinal streaks in the plate (see Fig. 16.87). They are usually caused by trauma, especially if distal. Uncommonly, they can occur in nail psoriasis and are also a hallmark of infective endocarditis.
- *Subungual haematoma* is red, purple or grey–brown discoloration of the nail plate, usually of the big toe (Fig. 27.47). These haematomas are usually due to trauma, although a history of this may not be clear. The main differential is subungual melanoma, although rapid onset, lack of nail-fold involvement and proximal clearing as the nail grows are clues to the diagnosis of haematoma. If there is diagnostic doubt, a biopsy may be needed.

Nail involvement in skin diseases

- *Dermatophyte infection/onychomycosis*: features are described earlier in the chapter in the section on skin infection.
- *Psoriasis*: nail involvement is common (see Fig. 27.36B).
- *Eczema*: nails may be shiny due to rubbing skin. Fine pitting can occur. If there is periungual eczema, the nail may become dystrophic, with thickening and transverse ridging. Paronychia is common.
- *Lichen planus*: there may be longitudinal ridging and thinning of the nail, giving a sandpaper texture (trachyonychia), erythematous streaks (erythronychia), subungual hyperkeratosis, pigmentation and, in severe cases, pterygium (splitting of nail due to central fibrosis and scarring, giving a winged appearance) and a destructive nail dystrophy.
- *Alopecia areata*: nail-plate pitting and trachyonychia can occur.

Nail involvement in systemic disease

The nails may be affected in many systemic diseases and important examples are detailed below:

- *Beau's lines*: horizontal ridges/indentations in the nail plate occur simultaneously in all nails (Fig. 27.48B). They typically follow a systemic illness and are thought to be due to temporary growth arrest of cells in the nail matrix; they subsequently migrate out as the nail grows. Normal nail growth is approximately 0.1 mm/day for fingers and 0.05 mm/day for toes, so the timing of the systemic upset can usually be estimated by the position of the Beau's lines.
- *Koilonychia*: this concave or spoon-shaped nail-plate deformity is caused by iron deficiency (Fig. 27.48C).
- *Clubbing*: in the early stages, the angle between the proximal nail and nail fold is lost. In its more established form, there may be swelling of the distal digits (Figs. 27.48D and E) or toes. Causes include bronchogenic carcinoma, asbestosis (especially with mesothelioma), suppurative or fibrosing lung disease, cyanotic congenital heart disease, infective endocarditis, inflammatory bowel disease, biliary cirrhosis and thyrotoxicosis; rarely, clubbing can be familial or idiopathic.
- *Nail discoloration*: whitening may occur in hypoalbuminaemia. 'Half-and-half' nails (white proximally and red/brown distally) may be found in renal failure. Antimalarials and some other drugs occasionally discolour nails.

Nail involvement in congenital disease

Nails can be affected in congenital diseases, such as pachyonychia congenita, a rare, usually autosomal dominant, condition caused by mutations in differentiation-specific keratin genes 6A, 6B, 16 and 17. This results in palmoplantar keratoderma and gross nail discoloration and thickening, due to subungual hyperkeratosis, from birth.

Skin disease in general medicine

Many skin conditions present to other medical specialties. These are listed in Box 27.32 and the most common ones that are not discussed elsewhere are detailed below.

Conditions involving cutaneous vasculature

Vasculitis

Vasculitic involvement of the skin usually presents as palpable purpura (see Fig. 26.54). The diagnosis is confirmed by skin biopsy, along with histology and immunofluorescence examination. Vasculitis is discussed in more detail in Chapter 26.

Pyoderma gangrenosum

The initial lesion of pyoderma gangrenosum (PG) is usually a painful, tender, inflamed nodule or pustule, which breaks down centrally and rapidly progresses to an ulcer with an indurated, undermined purplish or pustular edge (Fig. 27.49). Lesions may be single or multiple and are classified as ulcerative, pustular, bullous or vegetative. PG usually occurs in adults and, although it may occur in isolation, is usually associated with underlying disease, particularly inflammatory bowel disease, inflammatory arthritis, blood dyscrasias, immunodeficiencies and HIV infection. Investigation should be made with these associations in mind. The diagnosis is largely clinical, as histology is not specific. Analgesia, treatment of secondary bacterial infection and supportive dressings are important. Systemic treatment with glucocorticoids, dapsone, ciclosporin or other immunosuppressants is often required. Prednisolone and ciclosporin have been shown in a randomised controlled trial to be of similar efficacy and can thus both be considered in the management of pyoderma gangrenosum, allowing individual patient comorbidities and risk factors to be taken into account. Tetracyclines may be added for their anti-inflammatory effects. There are reports of efficacy with TNF-α (infliximab, adalimumab), IL-12/23 (ustekinumab) and IL-17 (brodalumab and secukinumab) inhibitors for severe recalcitrant PG, although as this is a rare orphan disease, evidence is relatively limited. Once healing has taken place, recurrences are typically only intermittent.

27

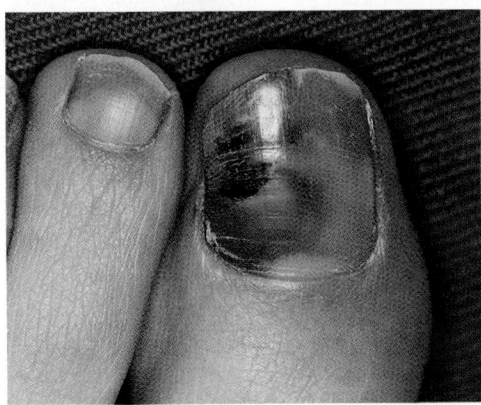

Fig. 27.47 Subungual haematoma.

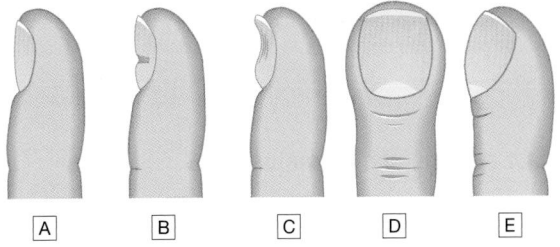

Fig. 27.48 The nail in systemic disease. [A] Normal nail. [B] Beau's line. [C] Koilonychia. [D] and [E] Digital clubbing.

Primary skin problems

- Cellulitis
- Vasculitis
- Leg ulcers
- Pressure sores

Skin involvement in multisystem disease

- Genetic: neurofibromatosis, tuberous sclerosis
- Xanthomas
- Amyloidosis
- Porphyria
- Sarcoidosis
- Systemic lupus erythematosus
- Systemic sclerosis

Non-specific and variable skin reactions to systemic disease

- Urticaria
- Erythema multiforme
- Annular erythemas
- Erythema nodosum
- Pyoderma gangrenosum
- Sweet syndrome
- Generalised pruritus

Skin conditions associated with malignancy

- Dermatomyositis
- Generalised pruritus
- Acanthosis nigricans
- Superficial thrombophlebitis

Skin problems associated with specific medical disorders

- Liver: generalised pruritus, pigmentation, spider naevi, palmar erythema, nail clubbing
- Kidney: generalised pruritus, uraemic frost, pigmentation
- Diabetes mellitus: necrobiosis lipoidica, diabetic dermopathy
- Cutaneous Crohn's disease

Skin problems secondary to treatment of systemic disease

- Drug eruptions

Miscellaneous

- Granuloma annulare
- Morphoea

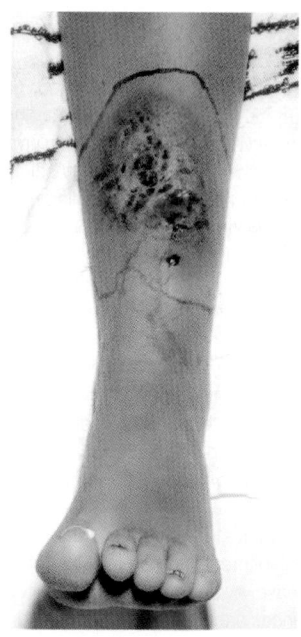

Fig. 27.49 Pyoderma gangrenosum. This young patient had Crohn's disease. Note the cribriform pattern of re-epithelialisation, which is characteristic of this condition.

Other neutrophilic dermatoses

These include Sweet's acute febrile neutrophilic dermatosis and the neutrophilic dermatosis of rheumatoid disease, which are characterised by intense inflammation, mainly consisting of neutrophils, around dermal blood vessels. There can be damage to vessels ('vasculopathy') but usually no frank vasculitis.

Pressure sores

Localised, prolonged, pressure-induced ischaemia can lead to the development of pressure sores, which can occur in up to 30% of hospitalised older adults. They are associated with considerable morbidity, mortality and expense to health services. The main risk factors are immobility, poor nutrition, local tissue hypoxia – for example, with anaemia, peripheral vascular disease, diabetes, sepsis and skin atrophy – or barrier impairment, such as in eczema.

A localised area of erythema develops at sites of bony prominences (particularly sacrum, greater trochanter, ischial and calcaneal tuberosities, and lateral malleolus). This progresses to a blister and then erosion, which will develop into a deep necrotic ulcer, usually colonised by *Pseudomonas aeruginosa* if pressure is not alleviated.

Prevention is key and involves identification of at-risk patients and regular repositioning and use of pressure-relieving mattresses. Predisposing factors, such as anaemia and poor nutrition, should be corrected. Once established, significant infection must be treated and necrotic tissue debrided. Dressings encourage granulation, although surgical intervention may sometimes be needed.

Connective tissue disease

Lupus erythematosus

This autoimmune disorder can be subdivided into systemic lupus erythematosus (SLE) and cutaneous lupus, which includes discoid lupus erythematosus (DLE) and subacute cutaneous lupus erythematosus (SCLE). The features of SLE are discussed in Chapter 26 (see Box 26.63, and Boxes 27.35 and 27.36 below). DLE typically presents as scaly red plaques with follicular plugging, usually on photo-exposed sites of the face, head and neck, which resolve with scarring and pigmentary change. If the scalp is involved, scarring alopecia usually occurs (Fig. 27.51). Most patients with DLE do not develop SLE. Patients with SCLE may have extensive cutaneous involvement, usually aggravated by sun exposure, with an annular, polycyclic or papulosquamous eruption. Systemic involvement is uncommon and the prognosis usually good. There is a strong association with antibodies to Ro/SS-A antigen. A diagnosis of cutaneous lupus is confirmed by histopathology and direct immunofluorescence. Cutaneous lupus may respond to topical glucocorticoids, antimalarials or immunosuppressants. Antimalarials and photoprotection are important mainstays in the management of cutaneous lupus, and systemic immunosuppression may be required for resistant disease. Paradoxically, low-dose UVA1 phototherapy can be effective for lupus.

Systemic sclerosis

This autoimmune multisystem disease presents with severe Raynaud's syndrome, digital ulcers and skin fibrosis. Dilated nail-fold capillaries and ragged cuticles are frequent. The clinical features and management are described in Chapter 26.

Morphoea

Morphoea is a localised cutaneous form of scleroderma that can affect any site at any age. It usually presents as a thickened violaceous plaque, which may become hyper- or hypopigmented. Plaques can become generalised. Linear forms exist and, if in the scalp, are associated with scarring hair loss (en coup de sabre). There is usually no systemic involvement. Topical glucocorticoids or immunosuppressants or phototherapy, particularly PUVA or UVA1, can be effective, and systemic immunosuppression may be used for resistant extensive disease.

Dermatomyositis

Dermatomyositis is a multisystem disease, predominantly affecting skin, muscles and blood vessels. Typical cutaneous features include a violaceous 'heliotrope' erythema periorbitally and involving the upper eyelids, but this can sometimes affect the upper trunk, shoulders ('shawl sign') and limbs. Linear erythematous streaks may also be observed on the back of hands and fingers, and papules over the knuckles (Gottron's papules). Tortuous dilated nail-fold capillaries, often best seen with a dermatoscope, and ragged cuticles are usually evident (Fig. 27.46). Photo-aggravation of the cutaneous features is often prominent (Fig. 27.50). The clinical features and management are described in Chapter 26.

Granulomatous disease

Granuloma annulare

This is common and may be reactive, although a trigger is usually not apparent. The hallmark is the presence of dermal granulomas, which are usually palisading and associated with alteration of dermal collagen (necrobiosis). The condition is generally asymptomatic and may present as an isolated dermal lesion with a raised papular annular edge, or may be more generalised. An association between generalised disease and diabetes has been proposed but not confirmed. Lesions often resolve spontaneously. Intralesional glucocorticoids or cryotherapy can be used for localised disease, and UVB or UVA1 phototherapy or PUVA for generalised disease.

Necrobiosis lipoidica

This condition has some histological features in common with granuloma annulare, although necrobiosis predominates. The lesion has a characteristic yellow, waxy, atrophic appearance, often with violaceous

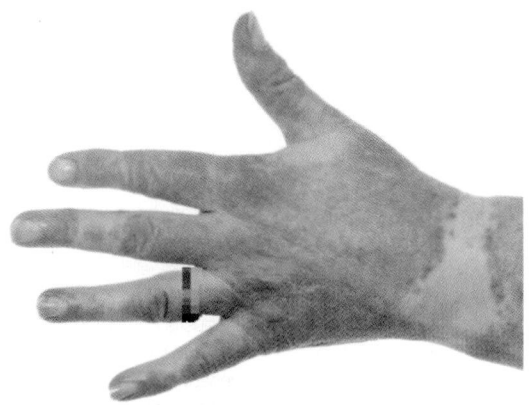

Fig. 27.50 Dermatomyositis. Photo-aggravation in dermatomyositis.

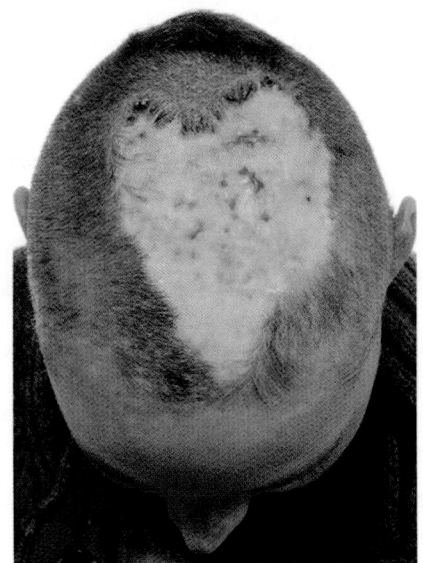

Fig. 27.51 Scarring inflammatory alopecia. This patient had systemic lupus erythematosus and additional cutaneous features of scarring inflammatory discoid lupus erythematosus.

edge (Fig. 27.52). Underlying blood vessels are easily seen because of tissue atrophy. Necrobiosis lipoidica typically appears on the shins and is prone to ulceration after trauma. There is a strong association with diabetes: most patients with necrobiosis lipoidica have or develop diabetes, although less than 1% of diabetic patients develop necrobiosis lipoidica. Treatment is difficult and includes very potent topical or intralesional glucocorticoids, topical calcineurin inhibitors, PUVA or UVA1 phototherapy and systemic immunosuppression.

Sarcoidosis

This condition is characterised by the presence of non-caseating granulomas. The cause is unknown, although infectious and genetic factors have been proposed. It is usually a multisystem disease, with skin lesions in about one-third of patients. Cutaneous features can occur in isolation and include violaceous infiltrated dermal plaques and nodules, which can affect any site but particularly digits and nose (lupus pernio), more generalised hyper- or hypopigmented or annular papules and plaques, infiltrative changes in scars and erythema nodosum (see Fig. 17.57). It has been reported more commonly and may be more severe in those of African, African American or South Asian ancestry. Cutaneous disease may respond to topical or intralesional glucocorticoids, cryotherapy, UVA1, laser or PDT. Clinical features, investigation and management of systemic disease are discussed in Chapter 17.

Cutaneous Crohn's disease

Cutaneous Crohn's disease is rare but may present as perianal and peristomal infiltrative plaques, lymphoedema, sinuses or fistulae, and oral granulomatous disease. These changes are termed 'metastatic' Crohn's and histology shows non-caseating granulomas. Reactive skin changes can also occur in the form of erythema nodosum and pyoderma gangrenosum. Treatment is of the underlying disease.

Porphyrias

The porphyrias are a diverse group of diseases, caused by reduced or absent activity of specific enzymes in the porphyrin–haem biosynthetic pathway. Due to this loss of enzyme activity, porphyrin precursors proximal to the implicated enzyme step accumulate. If the accumulated porphyrins absorb visible light, then there will be skin features and photosensitivity, which explains why some porphyrias have skin features (porphyria cutanea tarda) and others do not (acute intermittent porphyria). The most common skin presentations are photo-exposed site blistering, skin fragility and pain on daylight exposure.

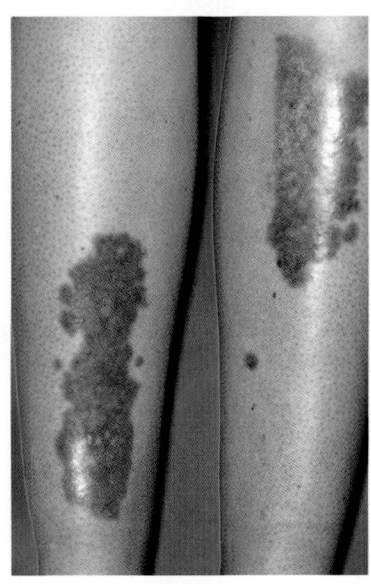

Fig. 27.52 Necrobiosis lipoidica. Atrophic yellow plaques with violaceous edges, on the shins of a patient with diabetes mellitus.

Cutaneous porphyrias: fragility and blisters

Although porphyria cutanea tarda (PCT) may be genetically inherited, this is uncommon and acquired PCT is the most common porphyria worldwide. It is caused by an underlying chronic liver disease, in association with hepatic iron overload. The liver disease is often only diagnosed through investigation of the skin presentation and it is thus an important diagnosis not to miss. Typical features are increased skin fragility, blistering, erosions, hypertrichosis, scarring and milia occurring on light-exposed areas, particularly the backs of the hands (Fig. 27.53). Less common features include facial hypertrichosis, hyperpigmentation and morphoea-like changes. Variegate porphyria (VP) and hereditary coproporphyria (HCP) may be indistinguishable on skin features and it is important to make the correct diagnosis, as acute neurovisceral attacks, which may be drug-induced, can occur in VP and HCP but not in PCT. Pseudoporphyria may also be impossible to distinguish from PCT on clinical grounds but is most frequently caused by a drug (commonly naproxen; see Box 27.36) or by sunbed use; on investigation, porphyrins are normal. A PCT-like presentation may also be seen in uraemia due to renal failure, but is caused by raised porphyrins due to impaired elimination rather than an enzyme defect.

Management of PCT requires removal or treatment of any underlying cause, which may involve venesection, iron chelation, very low-dose hydroxychloroquine once or twice per week and photoprotection.

Cutaneous porphyria: pain on sun exposure

Erythropoietic protoporphyria is caused by a genetic defect in the ferrochelatase gene that leads to ferrochelatase enzyme deficiency. It is an important diagnosis to consider. The presentation is usually in early childhood, although the diagnosis is often delayed. In part this is because, although the baby or child cries due to immediate pain on sunlight exposure, physical signs are often absent or minimal and thus a link with sunlight may not always be considered. The deficient ferrochelatase activity leads to accumulation of lipid-soluble protoporphyrins in the skin, explaining the photosensitivity manifest as pain on daylight exposure. Multiple pigment gallstones, anaemia (usually only problematic if considered to be due to iron deficiency) and, rarely, severe liver disease can occur, which may be fatal and requires liver transplantation. In addition to photoprotection, UVB phototherapy may be effective for the symptoms of photosensitivity and, more recently, the use of alpha-melanocyte-stimulating hormone (α-MSH) analogues has been explored.

Abnormal deposition disorders

Xanthomas

Deposits of fatty material in the skin, subcutaneous fat and tendons may be the first clue to primary or secondary hyperlipidaemia.

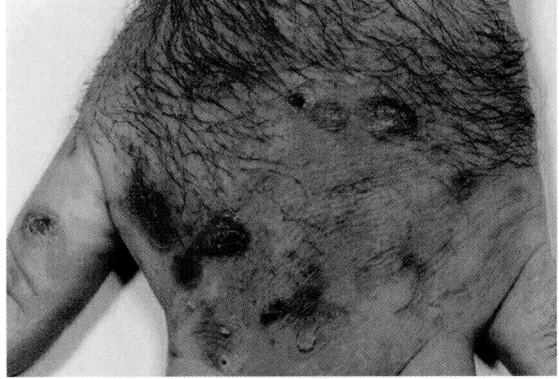

Fig. 27.53 Porphyria cutanea tarda. Skin fragility, blistering, scarring, milia and hypertrichosis on the back of hands and fingers in hepatitis C.

Amyloidosis

Cutaneous amyloid may present as periocular plaques in primary systemic amyloidosis and amyloid associated with multiple myeloma, but is uncommon in systemic amyloidosis secondary to rheumatoid arthritis or other chronic inflammatory diseases. Amyloid infiltration of blood vessels may manifest as 'pinch purpura' following skin trauma. Macular amyloid is more common in darker skin types and appears as pruritic grey/brown macules or patches, usually on the back. Potent topical glucocorticoids can be beneficial, although it is often treatment-resistant.

Genetic disorders

Neurofibromatosis

This condition can present with skin lesions. More details are provided in Chapter 28.

Tuberous sclerosis

This is an autosomal dominant condition and two genetic loci have been identified: *TSC1* (chromosome 9) encoding hamartin, and *TSC2* (chromosome 16) encoding tuberin. The hallmark is hamartomas in many systems. The classic triad of clinical features comprises learning disability, epilepsy and skin lesions but there is marked heterogeneity in clinical features. Skin changes include pale oval (ash leaf) macules that occur in early childhood; yellowish/pink papules in the mid-face (angiofibromas, 'adenoma sebaceum'), occurring in adolescence; periungual and subungual fibromas; and connective tissue naevi (shagreen patches, often on lower back). Gum hyperplasia, retinal phakomas (fibrous overgrowths), renal, lung and heart tumours, cerebral gliomas and calcified basal ganglia may also occur.

Reactive disorders

Erythema multiforme

Erythema multiforme has characteristic clinical and histological features and can be triggered by a variety of factors (Box 27.33) but a cause is not always identified. The disease is likely to have an immunological basis. Lesions are multiple, erythematous, annular, targetoid 'bull's eyes' (Fig. 27.54) and may blister. Stevens–Johnson syndrome is a severe form of erythema multiforme with marked blistering, mucosal involvement (mouth, eyes and genitals) and systemic upset.

Identification and removal/treatment of any trigger are essential. Analgesia and topical glucocorticoids may provide symptomatic relief. Supportive care is required in Stevens–Johnson syndrome, including ophthalmology input.

Erythema nodosum

This is characterised histologically by a septal panniculitis of subcutaneous fat (see Fig. 17.59). An identified trigger is often present

i	**27.33 Provoking factors in erythema multiforme**

Infections
- Viral: herpes simplex, orf, infectious mononucleosis, hepatitis B, HIV
- *Mycoplasma* and other bacterial infections

Drugs
- Sulphonamides, penicillins, barbiturates and carbamazepine

Systemic disease
- Sarcoidosis, malignancy, systemic lupus erythematosus

Other
- Radiotherapy, pregnancy

(Box 27.34). Lesions are typically painful, indurated violaceous nodules on the shins and lower legs. Systemic upset, arthralgias and fever are common. Spontaneous resolution occurs over a month or so, leaving bruise-like marks. Any underlying cause should be identified and removed or treated. Bed rest, leg elevation and an oral NSAID frequently offer symptomatic relief. Systemic glucocorticoids are effective but seldom required, and must be avoided when there is a possibility of infection. Potassium iodide, dapsone or hydroxychloroquine may be effective for resistant disease but these are rarely required.

Acquired reactive perforating dermatosis

The hallmark of this condition is transepidermal elimination of dermal material, particularly collagen and elastic tissue. It presents as keratotic papules, particularly in patients with diabetes and chronic renal disease. Treatment with topical glucocorticoids, retinoids, PUVA or UVA1 therapy may help. There are other related perforating dermopathies, with characteristic histology.

Annular erythemas

This group of chronic, poorly defined, annular, erythematous and often scaly eruptions can be further subdivided and may be secondary to an identifiable cause. Erythema chronicum migrans can be associated with Lyme disease (*Borrelia burgdorferi*). Erythema marginatum can occur in rheumatic fever or Still's disease. Erythema gyratum repens typically presents as concentric circles of erythema and scale with an advancing edge and is usually associated with underlying malignancy. Erythema annulare centrifugum presents with expanding, scaly, erythematous rings, with central fading. A trigger may not be apparent but possible associations include fungal infection, drugs, autoimmune or endocrine diseases, such as lupus or thyroid disease, and malignancy, particularly haematological. An underlying trigger must be sought and removed or treated. Topical glucocorticoids or phototherapy may be helpful for chronic disease.

Acanthosis nigricans

Hyperkeratosis and pigmentation are typical and affected sites have a velvety texture. The flexures, especially axillae and, in dark-skinned people, sides of neck, are involved. There are several types, mainly associated with insulin resistance. Most often, acanthosis nigricans is found in conjunction with obesity and regresses with weight loss. It can be associated with malignancy, usually adenocarcinoma (particularly gastric), when it is usually more extensive and pruritic, and can involve mucous membranes.

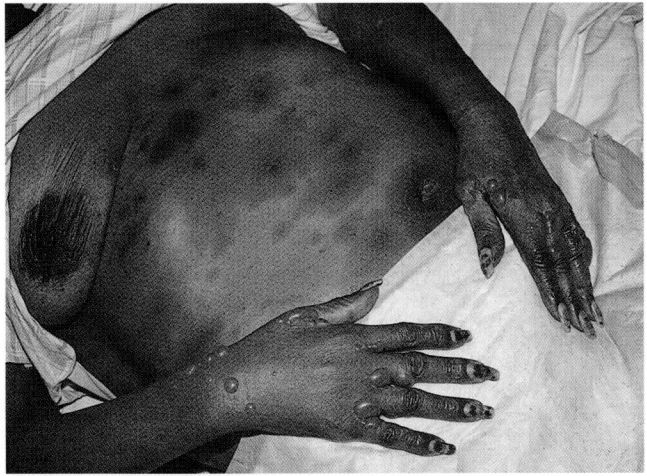

Fig. 27.54 Severe bullous erythema multiforme. *From Swartz MH. Textbook of physical diagnosis, 8th edn. Elsevier; 2021.*

Drug eruptions

Virtually all drugs may have cutaneous adverse effects (Fig. 27.55) and this should be considered in the differential diagnosis of most presentations of skin disease. Drugs can exert their adverse effects via several mechanisms, which can be broadly subdivided into non-immunological and immunological (Box 27.35).

i **27.34 Provoking factors in erythema nodosum**

Infections
- Bacteria: streptococci, mycobacteria, *Brucella*, *Mycoplasma*, *Rickettsia*, *Chlamydia*
- Viruses: hepatitis B and infectious mononucleosis
- Fungi

Drugs
- Sulphonamides, sulphonylureas, oral contraceptives

Systemic disease
- Sarcoidosis, inflammatory bowel disease, malignancy

Other
- Pregnancy

i **27.35 Types of drug eruption**

Non-immunological

Predictable
- Striae due to glucocorticoids (see Fig. 27.10)
- Asteatosis with statins
- Candidal infections with antibiotics
- Worsening of psoriasis with lithium, β-blockers, antimalarials, NSAIDs
- Urticaria with aspirin due to mast cell degranulation
- Bradykinin-mediated angioedema due to ACE inhibitors
- Doxycycline photosensitivity
- Dapsone haemolysis

Immunological

Unpredictable
- Immediate IgE-mediated hypersensitivity (type I): penicillin-induced urticaria and anaphylaxis
- Antibody-mediated (type II): penicillin-induced haemolysis
- Immune complex-mediated (type III): drug-induced serum sickness or vasculitis
- Delayed hypersensitivity (type IV): drug-induced erythema multiforme, lichenoid or pemphigus-like reaction; drug-induced lupus

(ACE = angiotensin-converting enzyme; IgE = immunoglobulin E; NSAIDs = non-steroidal anti-inflammatory drugs)

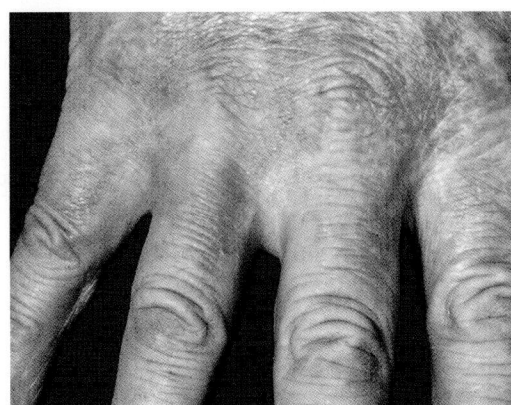

Fig. 27.55 Drug eruption. Possible drug causes of rash should always be considered. This was doxycycline-induced photosensitivity in a farmer.

27

ℹ 27.36 Clinical patterns of drug eruptions

Reaction pattern	Clinical features	Examples of causative drugs
Exanthematous	Erythema, maculopapular	Antibiotics (especially ampicillin), anticonvulsants, gold, penicillamine, NSAIDs, carbimazole, anti-TNF drugs and other biologic therapies
Urticaria and angioedema	Sometimes accompanied by angioedema Angioedema alone	Salicylates, opiates, NSAIDs, antibiotics, dextran, ACE inhibitors
Lichenoid	Violaceous, lichen planus-like, dyspigmentation	Gold, penicillamine, antimalarials, thiazides, NSAIDs, β-blockers, ACE inhibitors, sulphonamides, lithium, sulphonylureas, proton pump inhibitors, quinine, antituberculous, dyes in colour developers
Purpura and vasculitis	Palpable purpura and necrosis	Allopurinol, antibiotics, ACE inhibitors, NSAIDs, aspirin, anticonvulsants, diuretics, oral contraceptives
Erythema multiforme	Target-like lesions and bullae on extensor aspects of limbs	See Box 27.33
Erythema nodosum	Tender, painful, dusky, erythematous nodules on shins	See Box 27.34
Exfoliative dermatitis	There may be erythroderma	Allopurinol, carbamazepine, barbiturates, penicillins, PAS, isoniazid, gold, lithium, penicillamine, ACE inhibitors
Toxic epidermal necrolysis	Rapid evolution, extensive blistering, erythema, necrolysis, mucosal involvement	Anticonvulsants, antibiotics, especially sulphonamides, NSAIDs, terbinafine, sulphonylureas, antiretrovirals, allopurinol
Photosensitivity	Photo-exposed site rash, may be sunburn-like, exfoliation, lichenoid	Thiazides, amiodarone, quinine, NSAIDs, tetracyclines, fluoroquinolones, phenothiazines, sulphonamides, retinoids, psoralens
Drug-induced lupus	Photosensitivity, discoid lesions, urticarial or erythema multiforme-like. May have positive lupus serology and anti-histone antibodies	Allopurinol, thiazides, ACE inhibitors, PAS, anticonvulsants, β-blockers, gold, hydralazine, minocycline, penicillamine, lithium, proton pump inhibitors
Psoriasiform rash	Rash resembles psoriasis	See Box 27.24
DRESS	Facial oedema, fever, extensive rash, lymphadenopathy, eosinophilia and systemic involvement	Anticonvulsants, trimethoprim, minocycline, allopurinol, dapsone, terbinafine
AGEP/toxic pustuloderma	Rapid onset of sterile, non-follicular pustules on erythematous base	Ampicillin/amoxicillin, erythromycin, quinolones, sulphonamides, terbinafine, diltiazem, hydroxychloroquine
Acneiform eruptions	Rash resembles acne	Lithium, anticonvulsants, oral contraceptives, androgens, glucocorticoids, antituberculous drugs, EGFR antagonists (cetuximab and erlotinib)
Pigmentation		See Box 27.30
Bullous eruptions	Often at pressure sites and there may be other features, such as purpura, milia	Barbiturates, penicillamine, furosemide
Pseudoporphyria	May be indistinguishable from porphyria cutanea tarda clinically	NSAIDs, tetracyclines, retinoids, furosemide, nalidixic acid
Exacerbation of acute hepatic porphyrias		See page 1113 Always check all drugs for safety of use in porphyrias against standard guidelines
Drug-induced immunobullous disease	May resemble pemphigoid, pemphigus, dermatomyositis, scleroderma, epidermolysis bullosa acquisita	Penicillamine, ACE inhibitors, vancomycin
Fixed drug eruptions	Round/oval, erythema, oedema±bullae Same site every time drug is given Pigmentation on resolution	Tetracyclines, sulphonamides, penicillins, quinine, NSAIDs, barbiturates, anticonvulsants
Hair loss	Diffuse	Cytotoxic agents, oral retinoids, anticoagulants, anticonvulsants, antithyroid drugs, lithium, oral contraceptives, infliximab
Hypertrichosis	Excessive hair growth in non-androgenic distribution	Diazoxide, minoxidil, ciclosporin

(ACE = angiotensin-converting enzyme; AGEP = acute generalised exanthematous pustulosis; DRESS = drug rash with eosinophilia and systemic symptoms; EGFR = epidermal growth factor receptor; NSAIDs = non-steroidal anti-inflammatory drugs; PAS = para-aminosalicylic acid; TNF = tumour necrosis factor)

27.37 Diagnostic clues to drug eruptions

- Past history of reaction to suspected drug
- Introduction of suspected drug a few days to weeks before onset of rash
- Recent prescription of a drug commonly associated with rashes (penicillin, sulphonamide, thiazide, allopurinol)
- Symmetrical eruption that fits with a well-recognised pattern, caused by a current drug
- Resolution of rash following drug cessation

Clinical features

Cutaneous drug reactions typically present in specific patterns (Box 27.36). Non-immunologically mediated reactions can theoretically occur in anyone, given sufficient exposure to the drug, although idiosyncratic factors, such as genetic predisposition, may render some more susceptible. There is limited information on genetic determinants of drug responses and adverse effects, although advances have been made providing opportunities for personalised medicine. Immunologically mediated cutaneous drug eruptions typically commence within days to weeks of starting the drug. Detailed history-taking relating to prescribed and non-prescribed medications is essential and there may be other clues (Box 27.37).

Investigations and management

The suspected drug must be stopped. If drug-induced photosensitivity is considered, the patient should be phototested while on the drug to confirm the diagnosis, and again after drug withdrawal to confirm resolution of photosensitivity. An eosinophilia and abnormalities in liver function tests may occur in adverse drug reactions and, for example, specific IgE to penicillin may be raised in penicillin-induced rash but, otherwise, specific investigations are not available. Rechallenge with drug is not usually undertaken unless the reaction is mild, as this can be risky. Drug withdrawal may not be straightforward and substitute drugs may be required. Antihistamines and/or topical or systemic glucocorticoids may provide supportive management, depending on the type of cutaneous reaction. The management of anaphylaxis is described in Chapter 9.

Further information

Websites

bad.org.uk *British Association of Dermatologists: guidelines and patient information for many skin diseases.*

cochrane.org/cochrane-reviews *Many relevant skin reviews, including sun protection (CD011161), psoriasis (CD001213, CD001433, CD001976, CD005028, CD007633, CD009481, CD009687, CD010017, CD010497, CD0131535, CD011541, CD011571, CD011628, CD011941, CD011972), eczema (CD003871, CD004054, CD004055, CD004414, CD004416, CD005203, CD005205, CD005500, CD006135, CD007346, CD007770, CD008138, CD008426, CD008642, CD009864, CD011224, CD011380, CD012119, CD012167, CD013206), skin cancer (CD003412, CD005413, CD004415, CD004835, CD005414, CD007041, CD007281, CD007869, CD008946, CD008955, CD010307, CD010308, CD011123, CD011161, CD011901, CD011902, CD012352, CD012806, CD013186, CD013187, CD013189, CD013191, CD013192, CD013194), leg ulcers (CD000265, CD001177, CD001273, CD001733, CD001737, CD001836, CD002303, CD003557, CD008394, CD008599, CD009432, CD010182, CD012093, CD011354, CD011378, CD011979, CD012583 and others), acne, rosacea, hidradenitis suppurativa (CD000194, CD002086, CD003262, CD004425, CD007917, CD009435, CD009436, CD010081, CD011154, CD011368, CD011946), urticaria (CD007770, CD006137, CD008596), hair disorders (CD007628, CD004413, CD010334), skin infections (CD003261, CD003584, CD004685, CD004767, CD004834, CD005067, CD005068, CD007937, CD009758, CD009992, CD010031, CD010095, CD011680, CD012235), bullous pemphigoid (CD002292), autoimmune (CD002954, CD003263, CD005027), relating to skin in older adults (CD006471, CD009362, CD010891, CD011377, CD013128) and many other useful reviews.*

nice.org.uk *National Institute for Health and Care Excellence: guidance for skin cancer (NG14, NG34, PH32, CSG8, TA473, TA321, TA268, TA319, TA384, TA400, TA366, TA357, TA396, TA269, IPG446, IPG478, DG19, melanoma 2020), atopic eczema (QS44, CG57, TA81, TA82, TA177, TA534, 2020), psoriasis (CG153, TA146, TA372, TA103, TA134, TA350, TA180, TA419, TA442, TA475, TA511, TA521, TA574, TA575, QS40), sun exposure (NG34, PH32, 2020), vitamin D (PH56, ES28), urticaria (TA339, ESUOM31), rosacea (ESNM43, ESNM68), scabies (ESUOM29), photodynamic therapy (IPG155, MTG6); Grenz rays (IPG236) and COVID-19: Immunosuppression (NG169).*

sign.ac.uk *Scottish Intercollegiate Guidelines Network: 121 – Diagnosis and management of psoriasis TA81and psoriatic arthritis in adults; 125 – Management of atopic eczema in primary care; 140 – Management of primary cutaneous squamous cell carcinoma; 146 – Cutaneous melanoma skin.*

27

DPJ Hunt
MD Connor

28

Neurology

Clinical examination of the nervous system

4 **Cranial nerves**

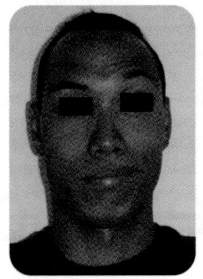 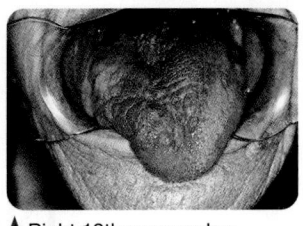

▲ Right 12th nerve palsy: wasting of right side of tongue

▲ 7th nerve palsy: drooping mouth and flattening of nasolabial skin fold

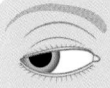 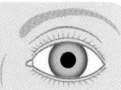

▲ 3rd nerve palsy: one eye points 'down and out'

3 **Neck and skull**

Skull size and shape
Neck stiffness and Kernig's test
Carotid bruit

2 **Back**

Scoliosis
Operative scars
Evidence of spina bifida occulta
Winging of scapula

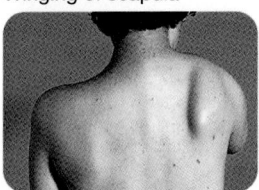

▲ Winging of right scapula (muscular dystrophy)

1 **Stance and gait**

Posture
Romberg's test
Arm swing
Pattern of gait
Tandem (heel-toe) gait

Observation/general
• General appearance
• Mood (e.g. anxious, depressed)
• Facial expression (or lack thereof)
• Handedness
• Nutritional status
• Blood pressure

5 **Optic fundi**

Papilloedema
Optic atrophy
Cupping of disc (glaucoma)
Hypertensive changes
Signs of diabetes

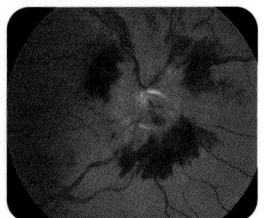

▲ Haemorrhagic papilloedema

6 **Motor**

Wasting, fasciculation
Abnormal posture
Abnormal movements
Tone (including clonus)
Strength
Coordination
Tendon reflexes
Abdominal reflexes
Plantar reflexes

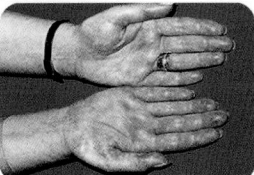

▲ Wasting of right thenar eminence due to cervical rib

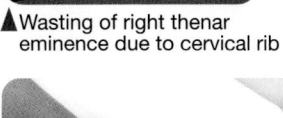

▲ Pes cavus

7 **Sensory**

Pin-prick, temperature
Joint position, vibration
Two-point discrimination

8 **Higher cerebral function**

Orientation
Memory
Speech and language
Localised cortical functions

Insets (winging of scapula, 12th nerve palsy, wasting of thenar eminence) Courtesy of Dr R.E. Cull, Western General Hospital, Edinburgh.

1 Examination of gait and posture

Procedure	Abnormality	Disease
Rising from chair	Difficulty rising	Proximal muscle weakness or joint disorders
Gait initiation	Difficulty starting to walk, frozen	Cerebrovascular disease or parkinsonism
Posture	Stooped	Parkinsonism
Retropulsion/ anteropulsion	Postural instability	Parkinsonism
Arms during walking	Reduced arm swing	Parkinsonism or upper motor neuron lesion
	Enhanced tremor	Parkinsonism
	Dystonic posturing	Dystonia
Gait pattern	Circumduction (stiff leg moves outwards in 'circular' manner)	Hemiparesis, typically after stroke
	'Slapping', high-stepping due to foot drop	L5 radiculopathy or common peroneal nerve lesion
	Narrow-based, short strides, freezing in doorways	Parkinsonism
	Stiff-legged, scissors gait	Spastic paraparesis (multiple sclerosis, vascular disease, spinal cord lesions)
	Wide-based, unsteady, unable to perform tandem gait	Cerebellar lesion
	Waddling gait	Myopathies with proximal weakness

4 Examination of cranial nerves

Nerve	Name	Tests
I	Olfactory	Ask patient about sense of smell (examine only if change is reported)
II	Optic	Visual acuity and colour vision Visual fields Pupillary responses Ophthalmoscopy
III	Oculomotor	Eyelids (ptosis) Pupil size, symmetry, reactions Eye movements
IV	Trochlear	Eye movements (superior oblique muscle)
V	Trigeminal	Facial sensation Corneal reflex Muscles of mastication
VI	Abducens	Eye movements (lateral rectus muscle)
VII	Facial	Facial symmetry and movements
VIII	Vestibulocochlear	Otoscopy Hearing Tuning fork tests (Rinne and Weber)
IX	Glossopharyngeal	Swallowing
X	Vagus	Palatal elevation (uvula deviates to side opposite lesion) Swallowing Cough (bovine) Speech
XI	Accessory	Look for wasting of trapezius/ sternocleidomastoid Elevation of shoulders Turning head to right and left
XII	Hypoglossal	Look for wasting/fasciculation Tongue protrusion (deviates to side of lesion)

6 Root values of tendon reflexes

Reflex	Root value
Arm	
Biceps jerk	C5
Supinator jerk	C6
Triceps jerk	C7
Finger jerk	C8
Leg	
Knee jerk	L3/L4
Ankle jerk	S1

Motor

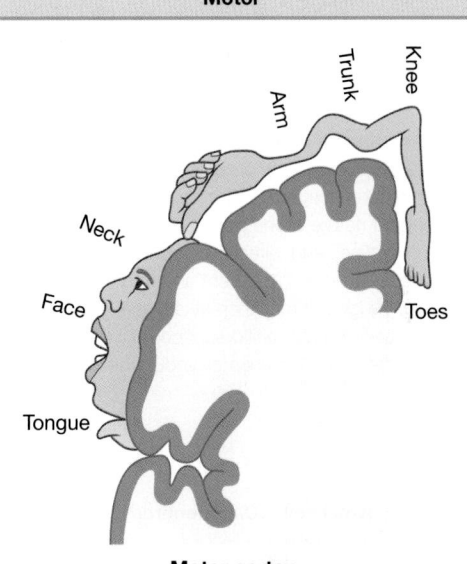

Motor cortex
(pre-central gyrus)

Sensory

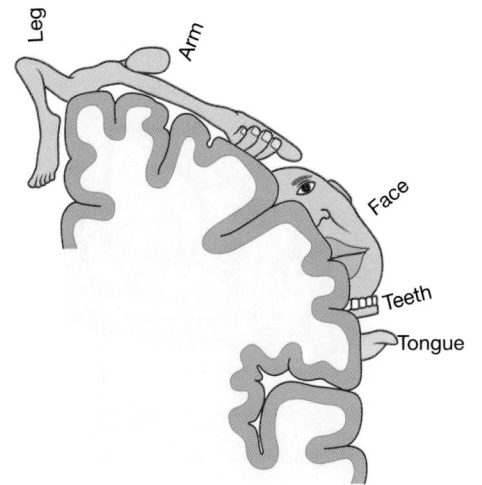

Somatic cortex
(post-central gyrus)

Motor and sensory homunculi. The motor and sensory homunculi illustrate the cortical areas serving each anatomical area within the pre-central (motor) and post-central (sensory) gyri.

28

The complexity of the brain differentiates us from other species, and its interactions with the spinal cord and peripheral nerves combine to allow us to perceive and react to the external world while maintaining a stable internal environment. The cerebral cortex provides a platform for processing information and forming a response, and in doing so, both forms and is affected by our personality and mental state.

Neurology has for too long been misperceived as a specialty in which intricate clinical examination and numerous investigations are required to diagnose obscure and untreatable conditions. In fact, nervous system disorders are common, accounting for 10% of the UK's general practice consultations, 20% of acute medical admissions and most chronic physical disability. The development of specific, effective treatments has made accurate diagnosis essential. Neurological management requires knowledge of a range of common conditions, which can be applied to individual patients after careful history-taking, with lesser contributions arising from targeted examination and considered investigation.

Pathological and anatomical localisation of symptoms and signs is important, but skill can be required to identify those *not* associated with neurological disease, differentiating patients requiring investigation and treatment from those who need reassurance.

Initially, it is important to exclude conditions that constitute neurological emergencies (Box 28.1). If the presentation is not an emergency, time can be taken to reach a diagnosis. The history should provide a hypothesis for the site and nature of the potential pathology, which a focused examination may refine, and direct appropriate further investigations. An informed discussion with the patient and family regarding diagnosis, management and prognosis may then take place.

As stroke has become a specific subspecialty in many centres, it is described in Chapter 29. This chapter should be read with it, to help clarify how the presentation, diagnosis and management of stroke present their own challenges.

Functional anatomy and physiology

Cells of the nervous system

The nervous system comprises billions of specialised cells, forming a spectacular network of connections. In addition to neurons, there are many types of glial cells. Astrocytes form the structural framework for neurons and control their biochemical environment, their foot processes adjoining small blood vessels and forming the blood–brain barrier (Fig. 28.1). Oligodendrocytes are responsible for the formation and maintenance of the myelin sheath, which surrounds axons and is essential for maintaining the speed and consistency of action potential propagation along axons. Peripheral nerves have axons invested in myelin made by oligodendrocytes (Schwann cells). Microglial cells derive

28.1 Neurological emergencies

- Status epilepticus (p. 1137)
- Stroke (if thrombolysis or mechanical thrombectomy available) (p. 1211)
- Guillain–Barré syndrome (p. 1192)
- Myasthenia gravis (if bulbar and/or respiratory) (p. 1194)
- Spinal cord compression (p. 1189)
- Subarachnoid haemorrhage (p. 1214)
- Neuroleptic malignant syndrome (p. 1252)

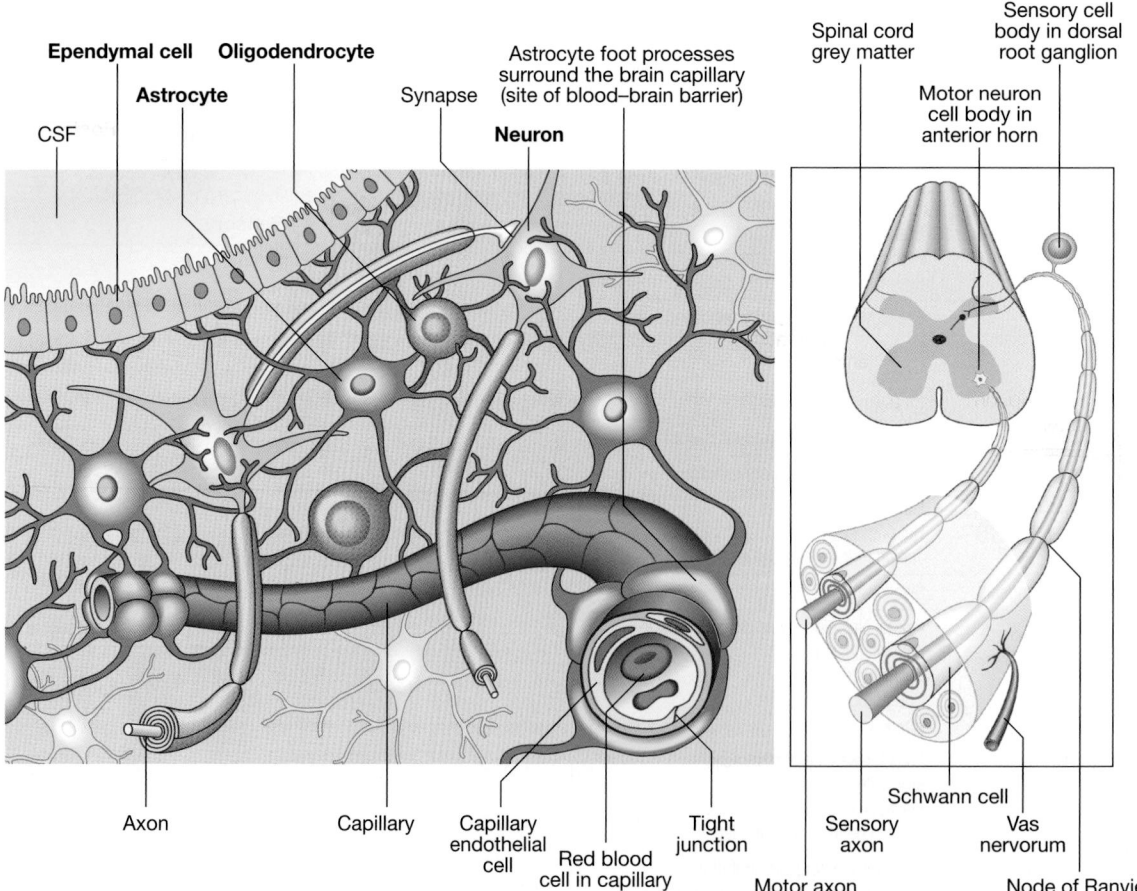

Fig. 28.1 Cells of the nervous system. (CSF = cerebrospinal fluid)

from monocytes/macrophages and play a role in fighting infection and removing damaged cells. Ependymal cells line the cerebral ventricles.

Generation and transmission of the nervous impulse

The role of the central nervous system (CNS) is to generate outputs in response to external stimuli and changes in internal conditions. The CNS has to maintain a delicate balance between responsivity to external stimuli and remaining stoic enough to remain stable in a rapidly changing environment. Each neuron receives input by synaptic transmission from dendrites (branched projections of other neurons), which sum to produce output in the form of an action potential that is then conducted along the axon, resulting in synaptic transmission to other neurons or, in the motor system, to muscle cells. Summation of the inputs causes net changes in the target neuron's electrochemical gradient, which, if large enough, will trigger an action potential. Communication between cells is by synaptic transmission that involves the release of neurotransmitters to interact with structures on the target cell's surface, including ion channels and other receptors (Fig. 28.2).

At least 20 different neurotransmitters act at different sites in the nervous system, most of which are potentially amenable to pharmacological manipulation.

Each neuronal cell body may receive synaptic input from thousands of other neurons. The synapsing neuron terminals are also subject to feedback regulation via receptor sites on the pre-synaptic membrane, modifying the release of transmitter across the synaptic cleft. In addition to such acute effects, some neurotransmitters produce long-term modulation of metabolic function or gene expression. This effect probably underlies more complex processes such as long-term memory.

Functional anatomy of the nervous system

Major components of the nervous system and their inter-relationships are depicted in Figure 28.3.

Cerebral hemispheres

The cerebral hemispheres coordinate the highest level of nervous function, the anterior half dealing with executive ('doing') functions and the posterior half constructing a perception of the environment. Each cerebral hemisphere has four functionally specialised lobes (Box 28.2 and Fig. 28.4), with some functions being distributed asymmetrically ('lateralised'), to produce cerebral dominance for functions such as motor control, speech or memory. Cerebral dominance aligns limb dominance with language function: in right-handed individuals the left hemisphere is almost always dominant, while around half of left-handers have a dominant right hemisphere.

Frontal lobes are concerned with executive function, movement, behaviour and planning. As well as the primary and supplementary motor cortex, there are specialised areas for control of eye movements, speech (Broca's area) and micturition.

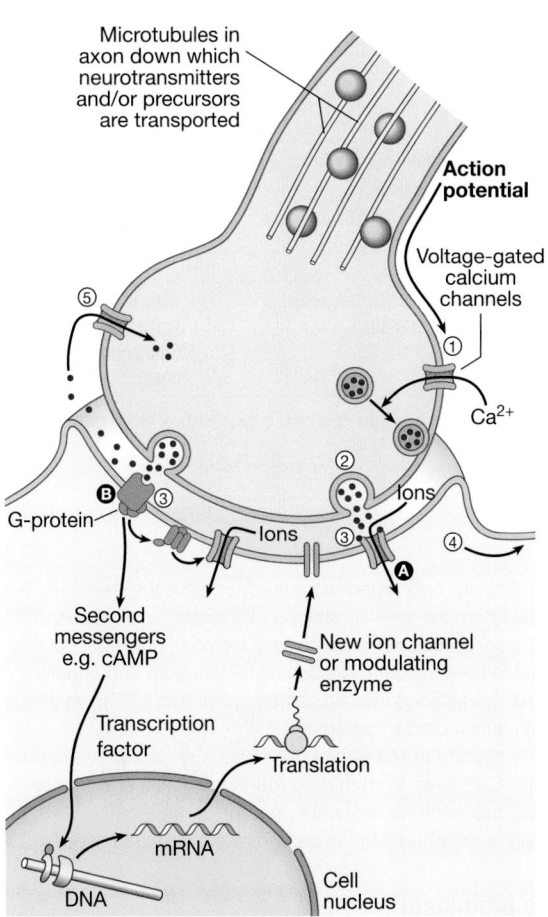

Fig. 28.2 Neurotransmission and neurotransmitters. (1) An action potential arriving at the nerve terminal depolarises the membrane and this opens voltage-gated calcium channels. (2) Entry of calcium causes the fusion of synaptic vesicles containing neurotransmitters with the pre-synaptic membrane and release of the neurotransmitter across the synaptic cleft. (3) The neurotransmitter binds to receptors on the post-synaptic membrane either (A) to open ligand-gated ion channels that, by allowing ion entry, depolarise the membrane and initiate an action potential (4), or (B) to bind to metabotropic receptors that activate an effector enzyme (e.g. adenylyl cyclase) and thus modulate gene transcription via the intracellular second messenger system, leading to changes in synthesis of ion channels or modulating enzymes. (5) Neurotransmitters are taken up at the pre-synaptic membrane and/or metabolised. (cAMP = cyclic adenosine monophosphate; DNA = deoxyribonucleic acid; mRNA = messenger ribonucleic acid)

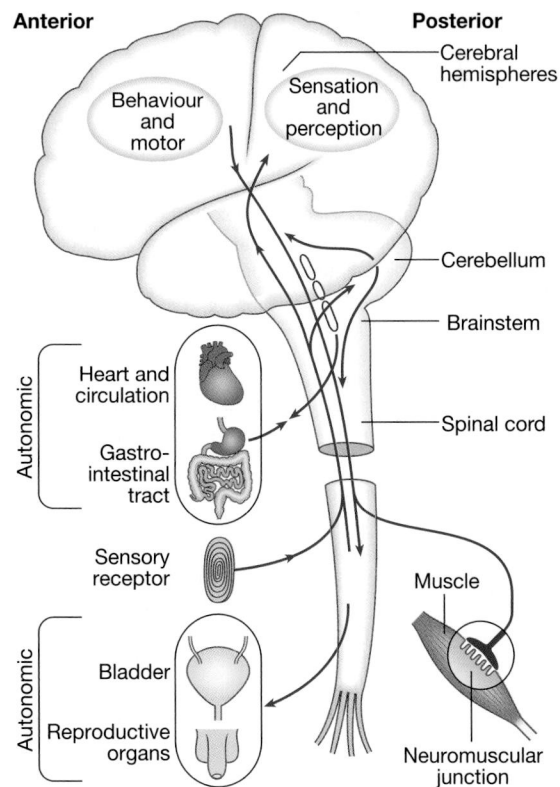

Fig. 28.3 The major anatomical components of the nervous system.

i | **28.2 Cortical lobar functions**

Lobe	Function	Effects of damage		
		Cognitive/behavioural	Associated physical signs	Positive phenomena
Frontal	Personality	Disinhibition	Impaired smell	Seizures – often nocturnal with motor activity
	Emotional control	Lack of initiation	Contralateral hemiparesis	Versive head movements
	Social behaviour	Antisocial behaviour	Frontal release signs[1]	
	Contralateral motor control	Impaired memory		
	Language	Expressive dysphasia		
	Micturition	Incontinence		
Parietal: dominant	Language	Dysphasia	Contralateral hemisensory loss	Focal sensory seizures
	Calculation	Acalculia	Astereognosis[2]	
		Dyslexia	Agraphaesthesia[4]	
		Apraxia[3]	Contralateral homonymous lower quadrantanopia	
		Agnosia[5]		
Parietal: non-dominant	Spatial orientation	Neglect of contralateral side	Contralateral hemisensory loss	Focal sensory seizures
	Constructional skills	Spatial disorientation	Astereognosis[2]	
		Constructional apraxia	Agraphaesthesia[4]	
		Dressing apraxia	Contralateral homonymous lower quadrantanopia	
Temporal: dominant	Auditory perception	Receptive aphasia	Contralateral homonymous upper quadrantanopia	Complex hallucinations (smell, sound, vision, memory)
	Language	Dyslexia		
	Verbal memory	Impaired verbal memory		
	Smell			
	Balance			
Temporal: non-dominant	Auditory perception	Impaired non-verbal memory	Contralateral homonymous upper quadrantanopia	Complex hallucinations (smell, sound, vision, memory)
	Melody/pitch perception	Impaired musical skills (tonal perception)		
	Non-verbal memory			
	Smell			
	Balance			
Occipital	Visual processing	Visual inattention	Homonymous hemianopia (macular sparing)	Simple visual hallucinations (e.g. phosphenes, zigzag lines)
		Visual loss		
		Visual agnosia		

[1]Grasp reflex, palmomental response, pout response. [2]Inability to determine three-dimensional shape by touch. [3]Inability to perform complex movements in the presence of normal motor, sensory and cerebellar function. [4]Inability to 'read' numbers or letters drawn on hand, with the eyes shut. [5]Inability to recognise familiar objects, e.g. faces.

The parietal lobes integrate sensory perception. The primary sensory cortex lies in the post-central gyrus of the parietal lobe. Much of the remainder is devoted to 'association' cortex, which processes and interprets input from the various sensory modalities. The supramarginal and angular gyri of the dominant parietal lobe form part of the language area (p. 1144). Close to these are regions dealing with numerical function. The non-dominant parietal lobe is concerned with spatial awareness and orientation.

The temporal lobes contain the primary auditory cortex and primary vestibular cortex. On the inner medial sides lie the olfactory and parahippocampal cortices, which are involved in memory function. The temporal lobes also link intimately to the limbic system, including the hippocampus and the amygdala, which are involved in memory and emotional processing. The dominant temporal lobe also participates in language functions, particularly verbal comprehension (Wernicke's area). Musical processing occurs across both temporal lobes, rhythm on the dominant side and melody/pitch on the non-dominant.

The occipital lobes are responsible for visual interpretation. The contralateral visual hemifield is represented in each primary visual cortex, with surrounding areas processing specific visual submodalities such as colour, movement or depth, and the analysis of more complex visual patterns such as faces.

Deep to the grey matter in the cortices, and the white matter (composed of neuronal axons), are collections of cells known as the basal ganglia that are concerned with motor control; the thalamus, which is responsible for the level of attention to sensory perception; the limbic system, concerned with emotion and memory; and the hypothalamus, responsible for homeostasis, such as temperature and appetite control. The cerebral ventricles contain cerebrospinal fluid (CSF), which cushions the brain during cranial movement.

CSF is formed in the lateral ventricles and protects and nourishes the CNS. CSF flows from third to fourth ventricles and through foramina in the brainstem to dissipate over the surface of the CNS, eventually being reabsorbed into the cerebral venous system (see Fig. 28.42).

The brainstem

In addition to containing all the sensory and motor pathways entering and leaving the hemispheres, the brainstem houses the nuclei and projections of most cranial nerves, as well as other important collections of neurons in the reticular formation (Fig. 28.5). Cranial nerve nuclei provide motor control to muscles of the head (including face and eyes) and coordinate sensory input from the special sense organs and the face, nose, mouth, larynx and pharynx. They also relay autonomic messages, including pupillary, salivary and lacrimal functions. The reticular formation is mainly involved in control of conjugate eye movements, the maintenance of balance and arousal, and cardiorespiratory control.

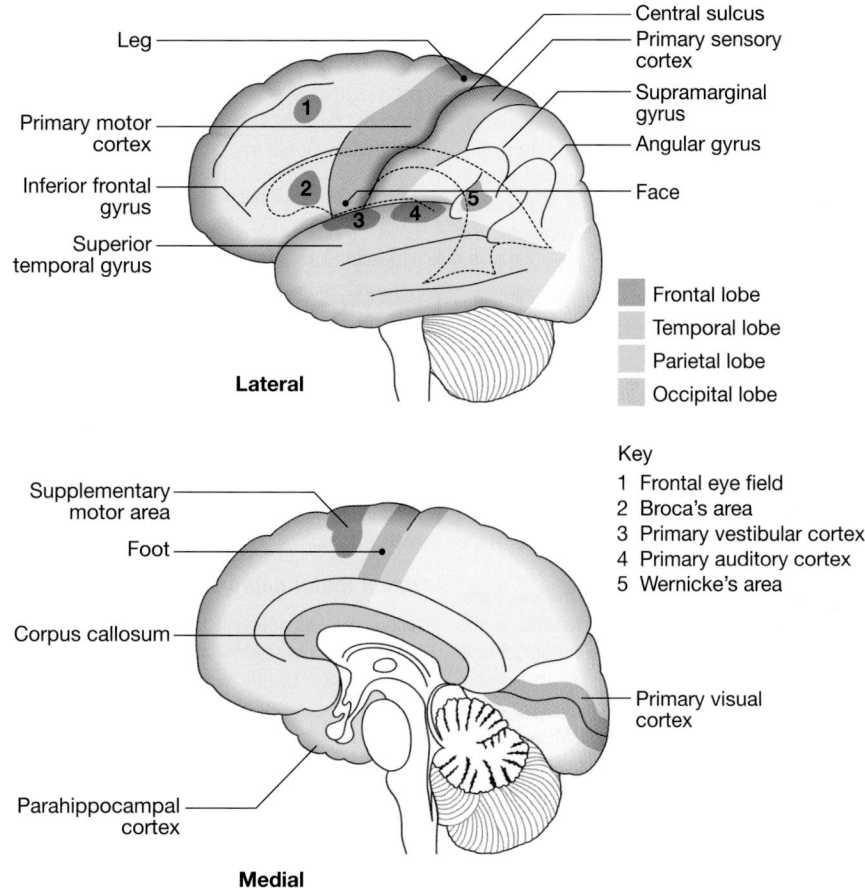

Lateral

Frontal lobe
Temporal lobe
Parietal lobe
Occipital lobe

Key
1 Frontal eye field
2 Broca's area
3 Primary vestibular cortex
4 Primary auditory cortex
5 Wernicke's area

Medial

Fig. 28.4 Anatomy of the cerebral cortex.

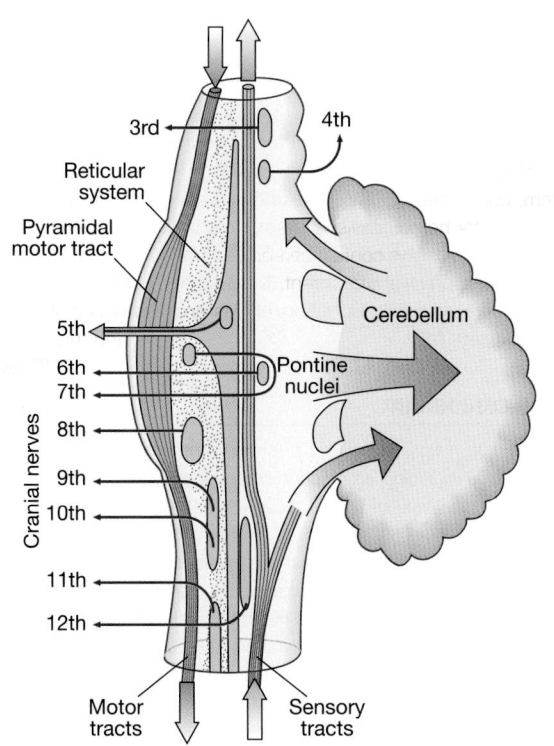

Fig. 28.5 Anatomy of the brainstem.

The spinal cord

The spinal cord is the route for virtually all communication between the extracranial structures and the CNS. Afferent and efferent fibres are grouped in discrete bundles but collections of cells in the grey matter are responsible for lower-order motor reflexes and the primary processing of sensory information.

Sensory peripheral nervous system

The sensory cell bodies of peripheral nerves are situated just outside the spinal cord, in the dorsal root ganglia in the spinal exit foramina, while the distal ends of their neurons utilise various specialised endings for the conversion of external stimuli into action potentials. Sensory nerves consist of a combination of large, fast, myelinated axons (which carry information about joint position sense and commands to muscles) and smaller, slower, unmyelinated axons (which carry information about pain and temperature, as well as autonomic function).

Motor peripheral nervous system

The anterior horns of the spinal cord comprise cell bodies of the lower motor neurons. To increase conduction speed, peripheral motor nerve axons are wrapped in myelin produced by Schwann cells. Motor neurons release acetylcholine across the neuromuscular junction, which changes the muscle end-plate potential and initiates muscle contraction.

28

The autonomic system

The autonomic system regulates the cardiovascular and respiratory systems, the smooth muscle of the gastrointestinal tract, and many exocrine and endocrine glands throughout the body. The autonomic system is controlled centrally by diffuse modulatory systems in the brainstem, limbic system, hypothalamus and frontal lobes, which are concerned with arousal and background behavioural responses to threat. Autonomic output divides functionally and pharmacologically into two divisions: the parasympathetic and sympathetic systems.

The motor system

A programme of movement formulated by the pre-motor cortex is converted into a series of excitatory and inhibitory signals in the motor cortex that are transmitted to the spinal cord in the pyramidal tract (Fig. 28.6). This passes through the internal capsule and the ventral brainstem before crossing (decussating) in the medulla to enter the lateral columns of the spinal cord. The pyramidal tract 'upper motor neurons' synapse with the anterior horn cells of the spinal cord grey matter, which form the lower motor neurons.

Any movement necessitates changes in posture and muscle tone, sometimes in quite separate muscle groups to those involved in the actual movement. The motor system consists of a hierarchy of controls that maintain body posture and muscle tone, on which any movement is superimposed. In the grey matter of the spinal cord, the lowest order of the motor hierarchy controls reflex responses to stretch. Muscle spindles sense lengthening of the muscle; they provide the afferent side of

the stretch reflex and initiate a monosynaptic reflex leading to protective or reactive muscle contraction. Inputs from the brainstem are largely inhibitory. Polysynaptic connections in the spinal cord grey matter control more complex reflex actions of flexion and extension of the limbs that form the basic building blocks of coordinated actions, but complete control requires input from the extrapyramidal system and the cerebellum.

Lower motor neurons

Lower motor neurons in the anterior horn of the spinal cord innervate a group of muscle fibres termed a 'motor unit'. Loss of lower motor neurons causes loss of contraction within this unit, resulting in weakness and reduced muscle tone. Subsequently, denervated muscle fibres atrophy, causing muscle wasting, and depolarise spontaneously, causing 'fibrillations'. Except in the tongue, these are usually perceptible only on electromyography (EMG; p. 1132). With the passage of time, neighbouring intact neurons sprout to provide re-innervation, but the neuromuscular junctions of the enlarged motor units are unstable and depolarise spontaneously, causing fasciculations (large enough to be visible). Fasciculations therefore imply chronic denervation with partial re-innervation.

Upper motor neurons

Upper motor neurons have both inhibitory and excitatory influence on the function of lower motor neurons in the anterior horn. Lesions affecting the upper motor neuron result in increased tone, most evident in the strongest muscle groups (i.e. the extensors of the lower limbs and the flexors of the upper limbs). The weakness of upper motor neuron lesions is conversely more pronounced in the opposing muscle groups. Loss of inhibition will also lead to brisk reflexes and enhanced reflex patterns of movement, such as flexion withdrawal to noxious stimuli and spasms of extension. The increased tone is more apparent during rapid stretching ('spastic catch') but may quickly give way with sustained tension (the 'clasp-knife' phenomenon). More primitive reflexes are also released, manifest as extensor plantar responses. Spasticity may not be present until some weeks after the onset of an upper motor neuron lesion.

The extrapyramidal system

Circuits between the basal ganglia and the motor cortex constitute the extrapyramidal system, which controls muscle tone, body posture and the initiation of movement (see Fig. 28.6). Lesions of the extrapyramidal system produce an increase in tone that, unlike spasticity, is continuous throughout the range of movement at any speed of stretch ('lead pipe' rigidity). Involuntary movements are also a feature of extrapyramidal lesions, and tremor in combination with rigidity produces typical 'cogwheel' rigidity. Extrapyramidal lesions also cause slowed and clumsy movements (bradykinesia), which characteristically reduce in size with repetition, as well as postural instability, which can precipitate falls.

The cerebellum

The cerebellum fine-tunes and coordinates movement initiated by the motor cortex, including articulation of speech. It also participates in the planning and learning of skilled movements through reciprocal connections with the thalamus and cortex. A lesion in a cerebellar hemisphere causes lack of coordination on the same side of the body. Cerebellar dysfunction impairs the smoothness of eye movements, causing nystagmus, and renders speech dysarthric. In the limbs, the initial movement is normal, but as the target is approached, the accuracy of the movement deteriorates, producing an 'intention tremor'. The distances of targets are misjudged (dysmetria), resulting in 'past-pointing'. The ability to produce rapid, accurate, regularly alternating movements is also impaired (dysdiadochokinesis). The central vermis of the cerebellum is concerned with the coordination of gait and posture. Disorders of this area therefore produce a characteristic ataxic gait (see below).

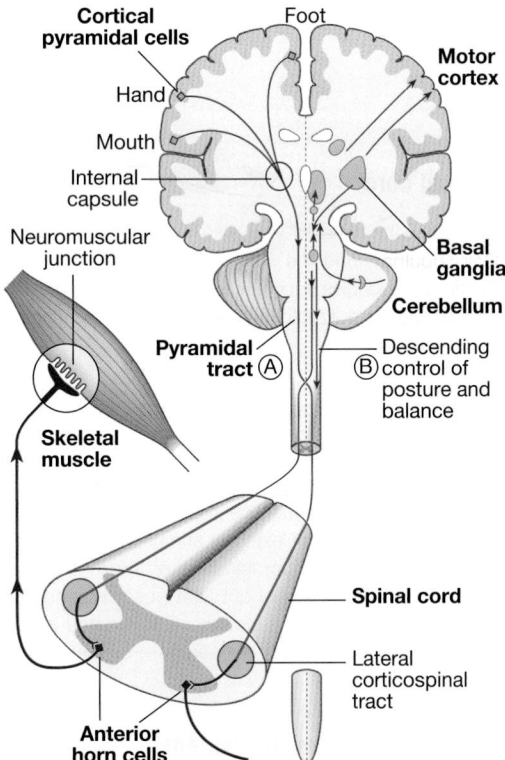

Fig. 28.6 The motor system. Neurons from the motor cortex descend as the pyramidal tract in the internal capsule and cerebral peduncle to the ventral brainstem, where most cross low in the medulla (A). In the spinal cord the upper motor neurons form the corticospinal tract in the lateral column before synapsing with the lower motor neurons in the anterior horns. The activity in the motor cortex is modulated by influences from the basal ganglia and cerebellum. Pathways descending from these structures control posture and balance (B).

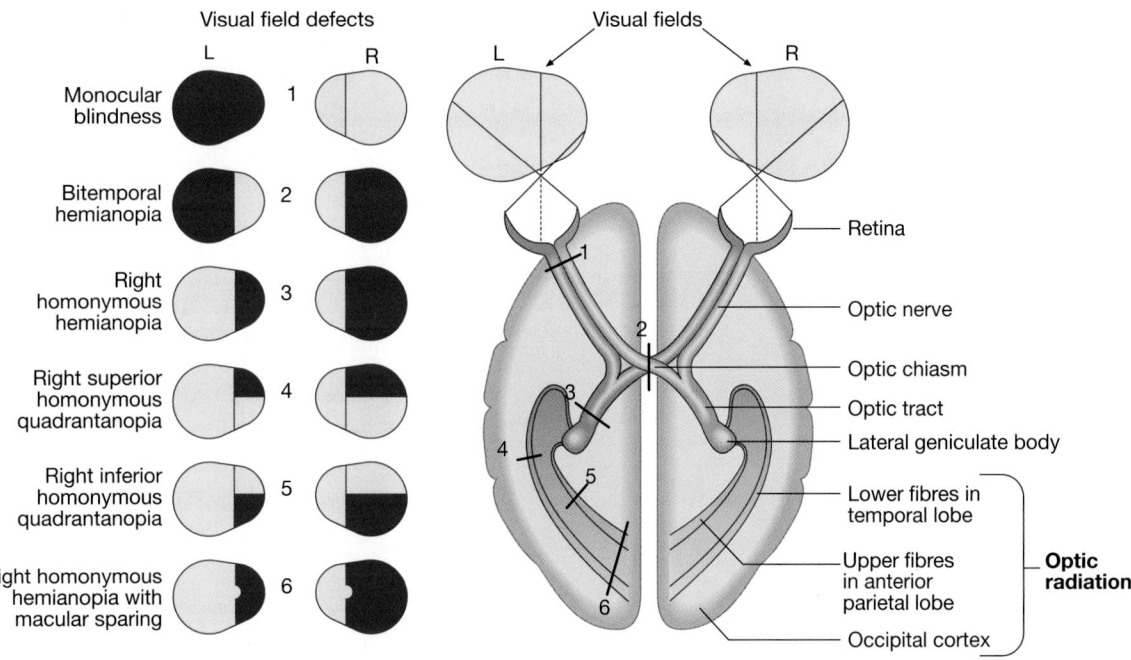

Fig. 28.7 Visual pathways and visual field defects. Schematic representation of eyes and brain in transverse section.

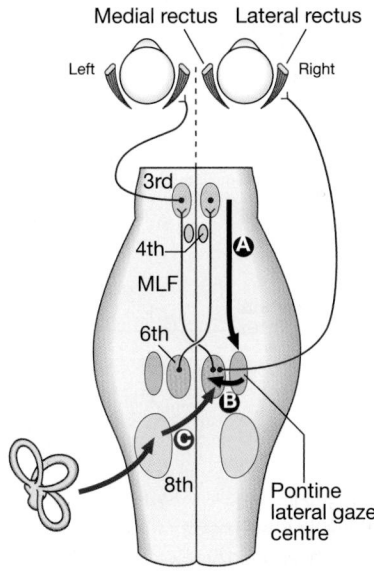

Fig. 28.8 Control of conjugate eye movements. Downward projections pass from the cortex to the pontine lateral gaze centre (A). The pontine gaze centre projects to the 6th cranial nerve nucleus (B), which innervates the ipsilateral lateral rectus and projects to the contralateral 3rd nerve nucleus (and hence medial rectus) via the medial longitudinal fasciculus (MLF). Tonic inputs from the vestibular apparatus (C) project to the contralateral 6th nerve nucleus via the vestibular nuclei.

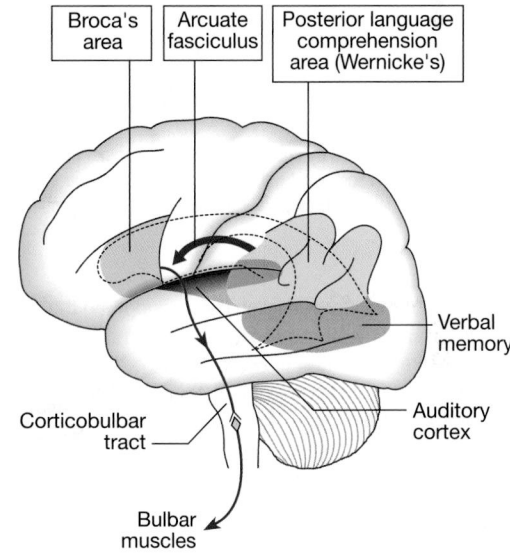

Fig. 28.9 Areas of the cerebral cortex involved in the generation of spoken language.

Vision

The neurological organisation of visual pathways is shown in Figure 28.7. Fibres from ganglion cells in the retina pass to the optic disc and then backwards through the lamina cribrosa to the optic nerve. Nasal optic nerve fibres (subserving the temporal visual field) cross at the chiasm but temporal fibres do not. Hence, fibres in each optic tract and further posteriorly carry representation of contralateral visual space. From the lateral geniculate nucleus, lower fibres pass through the temporal lobes on their way to the primary visual area in the occipital cortex, while the upper fibres pass through the parietal lobe.

Normally, the eyes move conjugately (in the same direction at the same speed), though horizontal convergence allows fusion of images at different distances. The control of eye movements begins in the cerebral hemispheres, particularly within the frontal eye fields, and the pathway then descends to the brainstem with input from the visual cortex, superior colliculus and cerebellum. Horizontal and vertical gaze centres in the pons and mid-brain, respectively, coordinate output to the ocular motor nerve nuclei (3, 4 and 6), which are connected to each other by the medial longitudinal fasciculus (MLF) (Fig. 28.8). The MLF is particularly important in coordinating horizontal movements of the eyes. The resulting signals to extraocular muscles are supplied by the oculomotor (3rd), trochlear (4th) and abducens (6th) cranial nerves.

The pupillary size is determined by a combination of parasympathetic and sympathetic activity. Parasympathetic fibres originate in the Edinger–Westphal subnucleus of the 3rd nerve, and pass with the 3rd

28

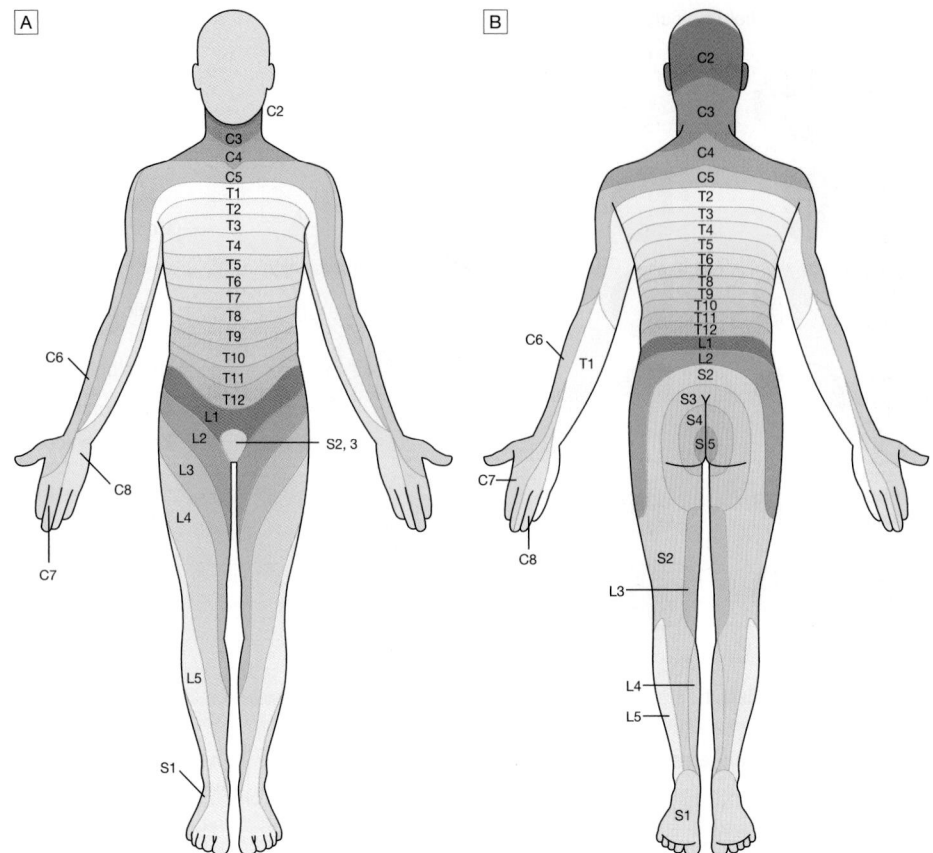

Fig. 28.10 The areas supplied by specific levels of the spinal cord. These are approximations and in practice there is much overlap. The clinical utility of these dermatomes has diminished somewhat with the advent of good magnetic resonance imaging of the spinal cord but it remains important to ascertain the presence of a 'spinal level' of sensation, to remember the supply of the saddle area, and to note the cervical descent of some facial spinothalamic pathways. **A** Anterior. **B** Posterior.

nerve to synapse in the ciliary ganglion before supplying the constrictor pupillae of the iris. Sympathetic fibres originate in the hypothalamus, pass down the brainstem and cervical spinal cord to emerge at T1, return up to the eye in association with the internal carotid artery, and supply the dilator pupillae.

Speech

Much of the cerebral cortex is involved in the process of forming and interpreting communicating sounds, especially in the dominant hemisphere (see Box 28.2). Decoding of speech sounds (phonemes) is carried out in the upper part of the posterior temporal lobe. The attribution of meaning, as well as the formulation of the language required for the expression of ideas and concepts, occurs predominantly in the lower parts of the anterior parietal lobe (the angular and supramarginal gyri). The temporal speech comprehension region is called Wernicke's area (Fig. 28.9). Other parts of the temporal lobe contribute to verbal memory, where lexicons of meaningful words are 'stored'. Parts of the non-dominant parietal lobe appear to contribute to non-verbal aspects of language in recognising meaningful intonation patterns (prosody).

The frontal language area is in the posterior end of the dominant inferior frontal gyrus known as Broca's area. This receives input from the temporal and parietal lobes via the arcuate fasciculus. The motor commands generated in Broca's area pass to the cranial nerve nuclei in the pons and medulla, as well as to the anterior horn cells in the spinal cord. Nerve impulses to the lips, tongue, palate, pharynx, larynx and respiratory muscles result in the series of ordered sounds comprising speech. The cerebellum also plays an important role in coordinating speech, and lesions of the cerebellum lead to dysarthria, where the problem lies in motor articulation of speech.

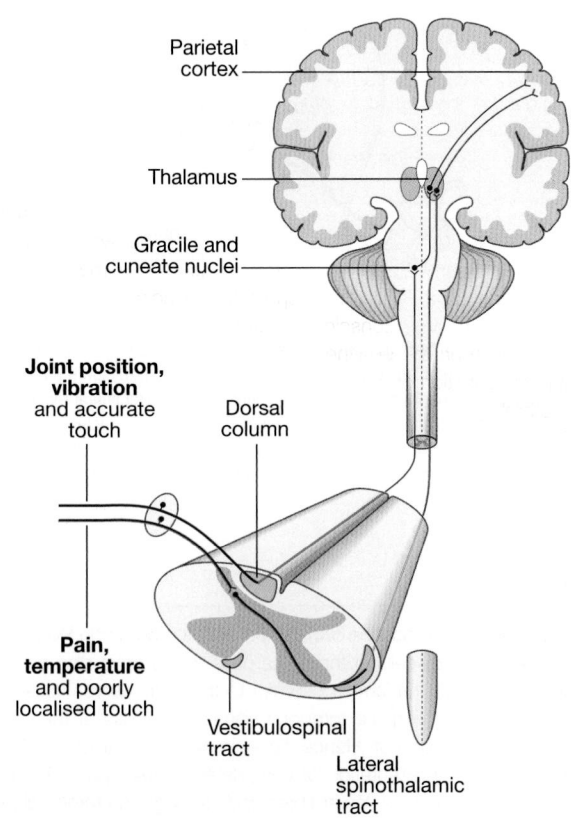

Fig. 28.11 The main somatic sensory pathways.

The somatosensory system

The body surface can be described by dermatomes, each dermatome being an area of skin in which sensory nerves derive from a single spinal nerve root (Fig. 28.10). Sensory information ascends in two anatomically discrete systems (Fig. 28.11). Fibres from proprioceptive organs and those mediating specific sensation (including vibration) enter the spinal cord at the posterior horn and pass without synapsing into the ipsilateral posterior columns. In contrast, fibres conveying pain and temperature sensory information (nociceptive neurons) synapse with second-order neurons that cross the midline in the spinal cord before ascending in the contralateral anterolateral spinothalamic tract to the brainstem.

The second-order neurons of the dorsal column sensory system cross the midline in the upper medulla to ascend through the brainstem. Here they lie just medial to the (already crossed) spinothalamic pathway. Brainstem lesions can therefore cause sensory loss affecting all modalities on the contralateral side of the body. Distribution of facial sensory loss due to brainstem lesions arises from the anatomy of the trigeminal fibres within the brainstem. Fibres from the back of the face (near the ears) descend within the brainstem to the upper part of the spinal cord before synapsing, the second-order neurons crossing the midline and then ascending with the spinothalamic fibres. Fibres conveying sensation from more anterior areas of the face descend a shorter distance in the brainstem. Thus, sensory loss in the face from low brainstem lesions is in a 'balaclava helmet' distribution, as the longer descending trigeminal fibres are affected. Both dorsal column and spinothalamic tracts end in the thalamus, relaying from there to the parietal cortex.

Pain

Pain is a complex perception that is only partly related to activity in nociceptor neurons (Fig. 8.2). Higher up, chronic and severe pain interacts extensively with mood and can exacerbate or be exacerbated by mood disorder, including depression and anxiety. Modification of psychological and psychiatric sequelae is a vital part of pain management (see Ch. 8).

Sphincter control

The sympathetic supply to the bladder arises from roots T11–L2 to synapse in the inferior hypogastric plexus, while the parasympathetic supply leaves from S2–4. In addition, a somatic supply to the external (voluntary) sphincter arises from S2–4, travelling via the pudendal nerves.

Storage of urine is maintained by inhibiting parasympathetic activity and thus relaxing the detrusor muscle of the bladder wall. Continence is also helped by simultaneous sympathetic- and somatic-mediated tonic contraction of the urethral sphincters. Voiding in adults is usually carried out under conscious control, which triggers relaxation of tonic inhibition on the pontine micturition centre from higher centres, leading to relaxation of the pelvic floor muscles and external and internal urethral sphincters, along with parasympathetic-mediated detrusor contraction.

Personality and mood

The physiology and pathology of mood disorders are discussed elsewhere (Ch. 31) but it is important to remember that any process affecting brain function may influence mood and affect. Conversely, mood disorder may have a significant effect on perception and function. It can be difficult to disentangle whether psychological and psychiatric changes are the cause or the effect of any neurological symptoms.

Sleep

The function of sleep is unknown but it is required for health. Sleep is controlled by the reticular activating system in the upper brainstem and diencephalon. It is composed of different stages that can be visualised

28.3 Major focal brainstem lesions

Site of lesions	Clinical features
Midbrain	Ipsilateral 3rd palsy Contralateral upper motor neuron 7th palsy Contralateral hemiplegia
Dorsal mid-brain (tectum)	Vertical gaze palsy Convergence disorders Convergence retraction nystagmus Pupillary and lid disorders
Pons	Ipsilateral 6th palsy Ipsilateral lower motor neuron 7th palsy Contralateral hemiplegia
Medulla (Lateral medullary syndrome)	Ipsilateral 5th, 9th, 10th, 11th palsy Ipsilateral Horner syndrome Ipsilateral cerebellar signs Contralateral spinothalamic sensory loss Vestibular disturbance

on electroencephalography (EEG). As drowsiness occurs, normal EEG background alpha rhythm disappears and activity becomes dominated by deepening slow-wave activity. As sleep deepens and dreaming begins, the limbs become flaccid, movements are 'blocked' and EEG signs of rapid eye movements (REM) are superimposed on the slow wave. REM sleep persists for a short spell before another slow-wave spell starts, the cycle repeating several times throughout the night. REM phases lengthen as sleep progresses. REM sleep seems to be the most important part of the sleep cycle for refreshing cognitive processes, and REM sleep deprivation causes tiredness, irritability and impaired judgement.

Localising lesions in the central nervous system

After taking a history and examining the patient, the clinician should have an idea of the nature and site of any pathology (see Box 28.10). Given the intricate anatomy of the brainstem, this section will dwell on the possible localisation in more detail (see Fig. 28.5).

Brainstem lesions typically present with symptoms due to cranial nerve, cerebellar and upper motor neuron dysfunction and are most commonly caused by vascular disease. Since the anatomy of the brainstem is very precisely organised, it is usually possible to localise the site of a lesion on the basis of careful history and examination in order to determine exactly which tracts/nuclei are affected, usually invoking the fewest number of lesions.

For example, in a patient presenting with sudden onset of upper motor neuron features affecting the right face, arm and leg in association with a left 3rd nerve palsy, the lesion will be in the left cerebral peduncle in the brainstem and the pathology is likely to have been a discrete stroke, as the onset was sudden. Examples of brainstem lesions are listed in Box 28.3. The effects of individual cranial nerve deficits are discussed elsewhere in this chapter in the sections on eye movements, and on facial weakness, sensory loss in brainstem lesions, dysphonia and dysarthria, and bulbar symptoms.

Investigation of neurological disease

Experienced clinicians make most neurological diagnoses on history alone, with a lesser contribution from examination and investigation. As investigations become more complex and more easily available, it is tempting to adopt a 'scan first, think later' approach to neurological symptoms. The frequency of 'false-positive' results, the wide range of normality and the negative implications for patients (unnecessary expense, inconvenience, discomfort and worry) necessitate a more thoughtful approach. Investigation may include assessment of structure

28

i 28.4 Imaging techniques for the nervous system

Technique	Applications	Advantages	Disadvantages	Comments
X-ray/CT	Plain X-rays, CT, CTA	Widely available	Ionising radiation	X-rays: used for fractures or foreign bodies
	Radiculography	Relatively cheap	Contrast reactions	CT: first line for stroke
	Myelography	Relatively quick	Invasive (myelography and angiography)	Intra-arterial angiography: gold standard for vascular lesions
	Intra-arterial angiography			
MRI	Structural imaging	High-quality soft tissue images, useful for posterior fossa and temporal lobes	Expensive	Functional MR and spectroscopy: mainly research tools
	MRA		Less widely available	
	Functional MRI			
	MR spectroscopy	No ionising radiation	MRA images blood flow, not vessel anatomy	
			Claustrophobic	
		Non-invasive	Pacemakers are a contraindication	
			Contrast (gadolinium) reactions	
Ultrasound	Doppler	Cheap	Operator-dependent	Screening tool to assess need for carotid endarterectomy
	Duplex scans	Quick	Poor anatomical definition	
		Non-invasive		
Radioisotope	Isotope brain scan	In vivo imaging of functional anatomy (ligand binding, blood flow)	Poor spatial resolution	Isotope scans: obsolete
	SPECT		Ionising radiation	SPECT: useful in movement disorders, epilepsy and dementias
	PET		Expensive	
			Not widely available	PET: mainly research tool

(CT = computed tomography; CTA = computed tomographic angiography; MRA = magnetic resonance angiography; MRI = magnetic resonance imaging; PET = positron emission tomography; SPECT = single photon emission computed tomography)

i 28.5 Different magnetic resonance imaging (MRI) sequences

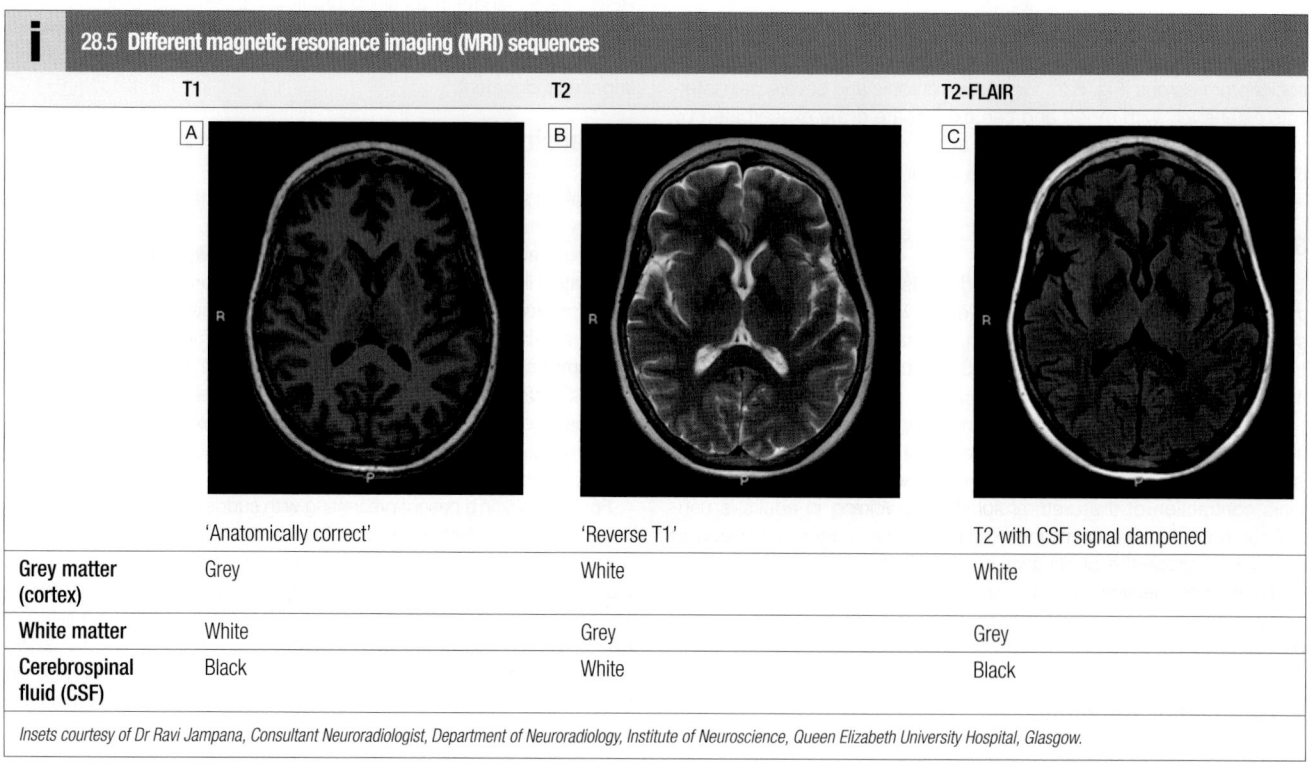

	T1	T2	T2-FLAIR
	'Anatomically correct'	'Reverse T1'	T2 with CSF signal dampened
Grey matter (cortex)	Grey	White	White
White matter	White	Grey	Grey
Cerebrospinal fluid (CSF)	Black	White	Black

Insets courtesy of Dr Ravi Jampana, Consultant Neuroradiologist, Department of Neuroradiology, Institute of Neuroscience, Queen Elizabeth University Hospital, Glasgow.

(imaging) and function (neurophysiology). Neurophysiological testing has become so complex that in some countries it constitutes a separate specialty focusing on electroencephalography, evoked potentials, nerve conduction studies and electromyography.

Neuroimaging

Neurological imaging has traditionally allowed only assessment of structure but advances are allowing much more sophistication.

Imaging modalities can use X-rays (plain X-rays, computed tomography (CT), CT angiography, myelography and angiography), magnetic resonance (MR imaging (MRI), MR angiography (MRA)), ultrasound (Doppler imaging of blood vessels) and nuclear medicine techniques (single photon emission computed tomography (SPECT) and positron emission tomography (PET)). The uses and limitations of each of these are shown in Box 28.4. Different sequences for analysing MRI signals can provide helpful information for characterising tissues and pathologies (Box 28.5).

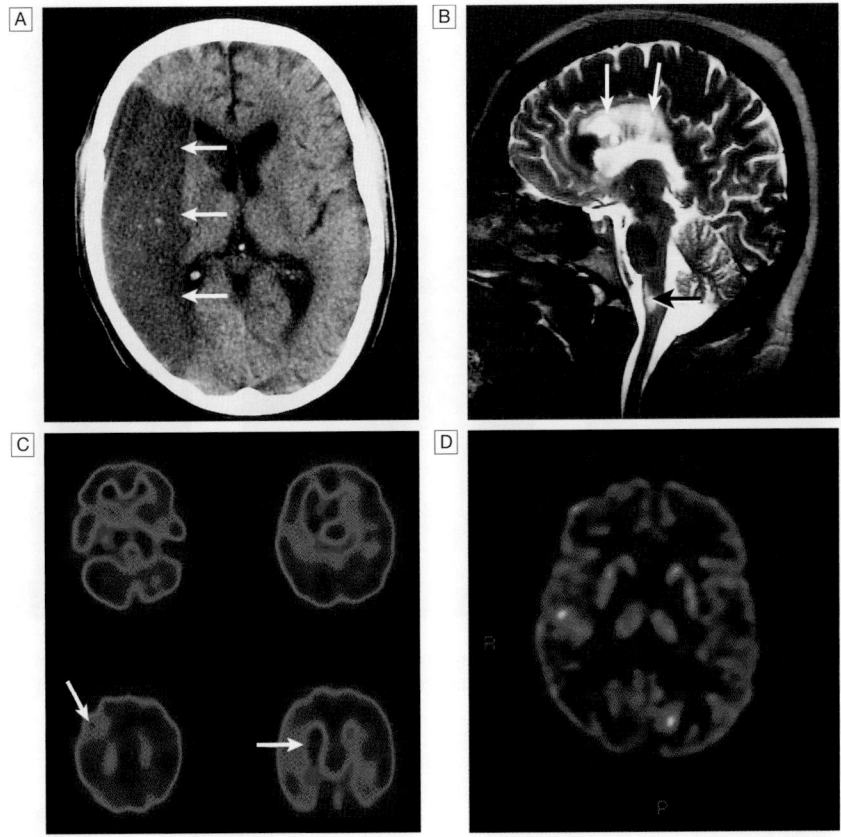

Fig. 28.12 Different techniques of imaging the head and brain. [A] Computed tomogram showing complete middle cerebral artery infarct (arrows). [B] Magnetic resonance image showing widespread areas of high signal in multiple sclerosis (arrows). [C] Single photon emission computed tomography scan after caudate infarct showing relative hypoperfusion of overlying right cerebral cortex (arrows). [D] Normal positron emission tomogram (PET scan) of brain. *(A–C) Courtesy of Dr D. Collie. (D) Courtesy of Dr Ravi Jampana, Consultant Neuroradiologist, Department of Neuroradiology, Institute of Neuroscience, Queen Elizabeth University Hospital, Glasgow.*

Advanced MR techniques, such as functional MRI (fMRI), MR spectroscopy or diffusion tensor imaging (DTI), can be used to assess brain metabolism and chemical compositions. This may be dynamic and can provide 'maps' of cortical function to help plan lesionectomy and epilepsy surgery. Similarly, MR spectroscopy can outline the chemical composition of specific regions, providing notions of whether lesions are ischaemic, neoplastic or inflammatory.

Some degenerative neurological conditions cause functional rather than structural abnormalities that make metabolic and neurochemical assessment increasingly useful. PET scanning can display glucose metabolism in dementia and epilepsy. SPECT scanning uses the lipid-soluble properties of radioactive tracers to mark cerebral blood flow at the time of injection to help in investigating seizures. Dopaminergic pathway tracers can assess the integrity of the nigrostriatal pathway in patients with possible parkinsonism.

Head and orbit

Plain skull X-rays now have a very limited role in neurological disease. CT or MRI is needed for intracranial imaging. CT is good for demonstrating bone and calcification well. It will also detect abnormalities of the brain and ventricles, such as atrophy, tumours, cysts, abscesses, vascular lesions and hydrocephalus. Diagnostic yield may be improved by the use of intravenous contrast and thinner slicing but CT is not optimal for lesions of meninges, cranial nerves or subtle parenchymal changes.

MRI resolution is unaffected by bone and so is more useful in posterior fossa disease. Its sensitivity for cortical and white matter changes makes it the modality of choice in inflammatory conditions

such as multiple sclerosis and in the investigation of epilepsy. Different MRI techniques can selectively suppress signal from fluid or fat, for example, and so increase sensitivity for more subtle pathologies.

Examples of brain imaged by the various techniques are shown in Figure 28.12.

Cervical, thoracic and lumbar spine

X-rays are useful for imaging bony structures and can show destruction or damage to vertebrae, for example, but will provide no information about non-bony tissues, such as intervertebral discs, spinal cord and nerve roots. They have some usefulness in dynamic imaging, e.g. flexion/extension of the spine, in the assessment of instability. MRI has transformed spinal investigation, as it can give information not only about vertebrae and intervertebral discs but also about their effects on the spinal cord and nerve roots. Myelography (usually with CT) is a rarely used invasive technique requiring injection of contrast into the lumbar theca. While outlining the nerve roots and spinal cord provides some detail about abnormal structure, the accuracy and availability of MRI have reduced the need for it. Myelography may still be used where MRI is unavailable, contraindicated, or precluded by a patient's claustrophobia. Examples of the cervical spine imaged by plain X-rays, myelography and MRI are shown in Figure 28.13.

Blood vessels

Imaging of the extra- and intracranial blood vessels and disturbance of arterial or venous blood flow is described on page 1214.

28

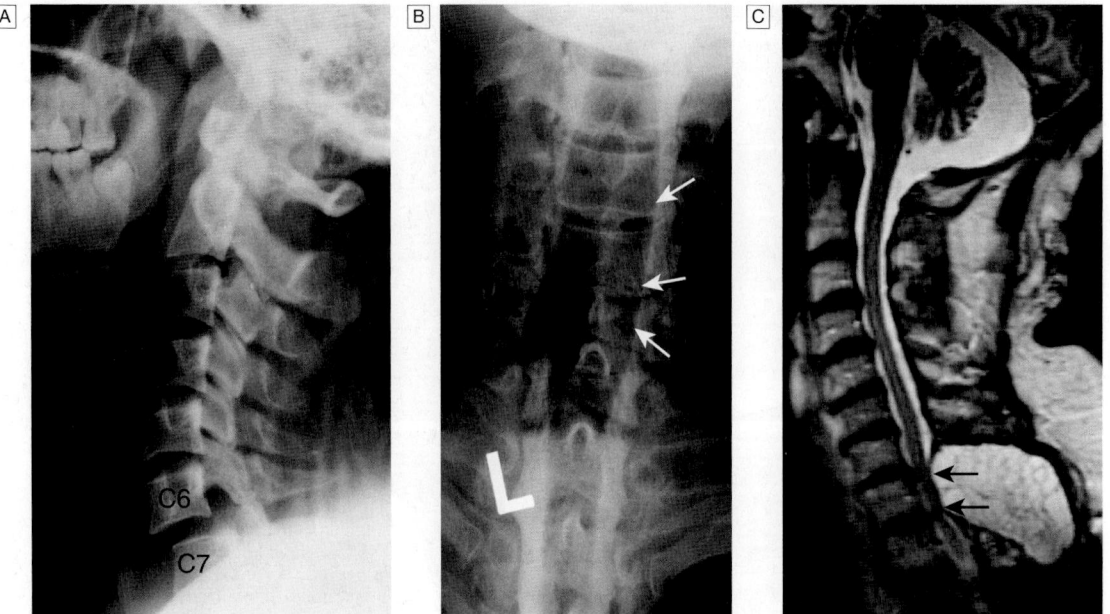

Fig. 28.13 Different techniques of imaging the cervical spine. [A] Lateral X-ray showing bilateral C6/7 facet dislocation. [B] Myelogram showing widening of cervical cord due to astrocytoma (arrows). [C] Magnetic resonance image showing posterior epidural compression from adenocarcinomatous metastasis to the posterior arch of T1 (arrows). *(A–C) Courtesy of Dr D. Collie.*

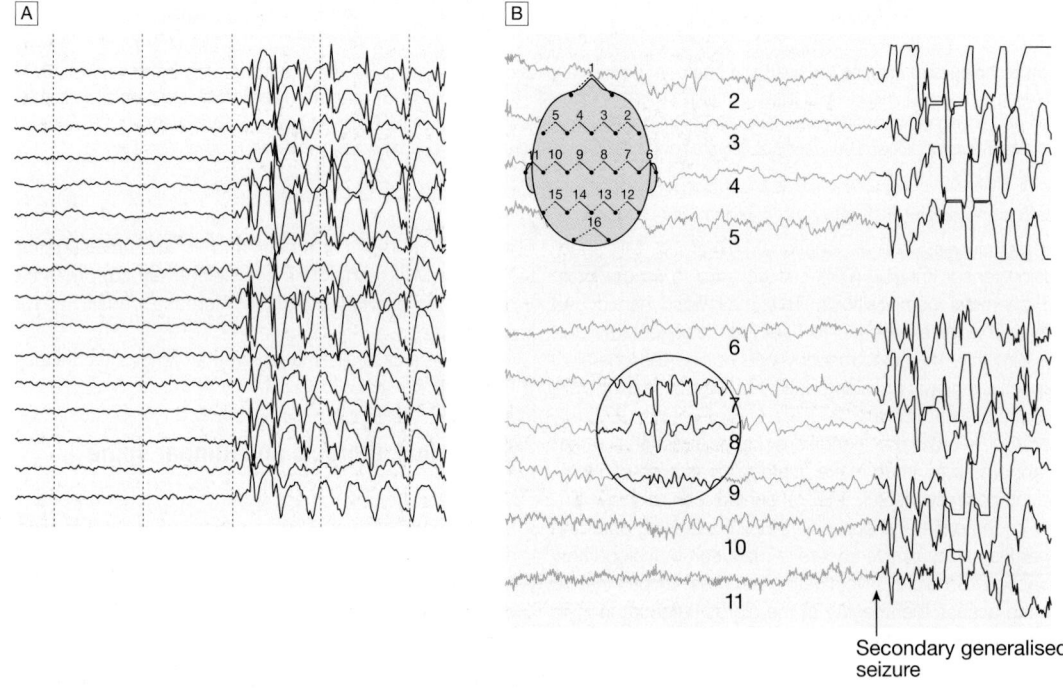

Fig. 28.14 Electroencephalograms in epilepsy. [A] Generalised epileptic discharge, as seen in epilepsy syndromes such as childhood absence or juvenile myoclonic epilepsy. [B] Focal sharp waves over the right parietal region (circled), with spread of discharge to cause a generalised tonic–clonic seizure.

Neurophysiological testing

Electroencephalography

The electroencephalogram (EEG) detects electrical activity arising in the cerebral cortex via electrodes placed on the scalp to record the amplitude and frequency of the resulting waveforms. With closed eyes, the normal background activity is 8–13 Hz (known as alpha rhythm), most prominent occipitally and suppressed on eye opening. Other frequency bands seen over different parts of the brain in different circumstances are beta (faster than 13/sec), theta (4–8/sec) and delta (slower than 4/sec). Normal EEG patterns evolve with age and alertness; lower frequencies predominate in the very young and during sleep.

In recent years digital technology has allowed longer, cleaner EEG recordings that can be analysed in a number of ways and recorded alongside contemporaneous video of any clinical 'event'. Meanwhile,

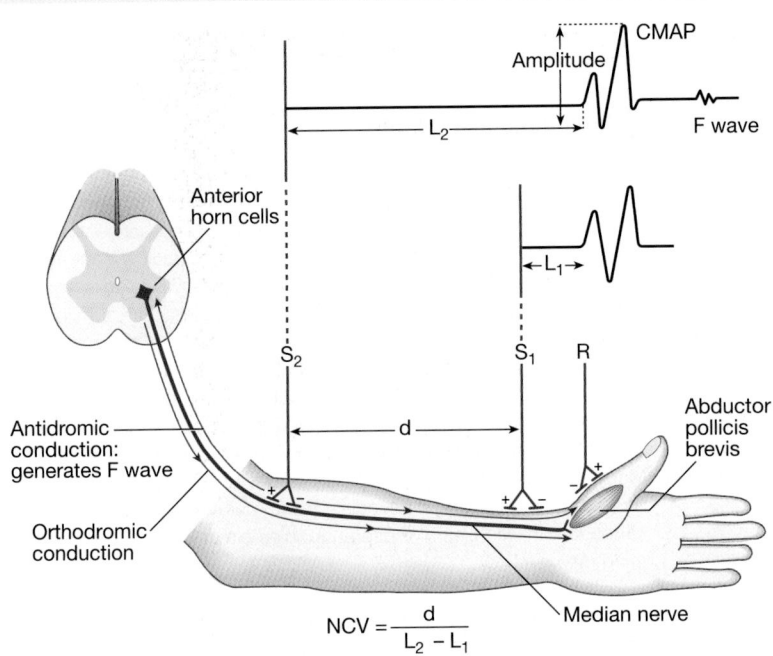

Fig. 28.15 Motor nerve conduction tests. Electrodes (R) on the muscle (abductor pollicis here) record the compound muscle action potential (CMAP) after stimulation at the median nerve at the wrist (S₁) and from the elbow (S₂). The velocity from elbow to wrist can be determined if the distance between the two stimulating electrodes (d) is known. A prolonged L₁ (L = latency) would be caused by dysfunction distally in the median nerve (e.g. in carpal tunnel syndrome). A prolonged L₂ is caused by slow nerve conduction (as in demyelinating neuropathy). The F wave is a small delayed response that appears when the electrical signal travels backwards to the anterior horn cell, sparking a second action potential in a minority of fibres (see text). (NCV = nerve conduction velocity)

the development of intracranial recording allows more sensitive monitoring via surgically placed electrodes in and around lesions to help increase the efficacy and safety of epilepsy surgery.

Abnormal EEGs result from a number of conditions. Examples include an increase in fast frequencies (beta) seen with sedating drugs such as benzodiazepines, or marked focal slowing noted over a structural lesion such as a tumour or an infarct. Improved quality and accessibility of imaging have made EEG redundant in lesion localisation, except in the specialist investigation of epilepsy (p. 1155). EEG remains useful in progressive and continuous disorders such as reduced consciousness, encephalitis, and certain dementias, such as Creutzfeldt–Jakob disease.

Since sleep induces marked changes in cerebral activity, EEG can be useful in diagnosis of sleep disturbances. In paroxysmal disorders such as epilepsy, EEG is at its most useful when it captures activity during one of the events in question. Over 50% of patients with epilepsy have a normal 'routine' EEG but, conversely, the presence of epileptiform features does not of itself make a diagnosis. Up to 5% of some normal populations may demonstrate epileptiform discharges on EEG, preventing its use as a screening test for epilepsy, most notably in younger patients with a family history of epilepsy. In view of this, the EEG should not be used where epilepsy is merely 'possible'.

Therefore the EEG in epilepsy is predominantly used for classification and prognostication, but in some patients can help localise the seat of epileptiform discharges when surgery is being considered. During a seizure, high-voltage disturbances of background activity ('discharges') are often noted. These may be generalised, as in the 3 Hz 'spike and wave' of childhood absence epilepsy, or more focal, as in localisation-related epilepsies (Fig. 28.14). Techniques such as hyperventilation or photic stimulation can be used to increase the yield of epileptiform changes, particularly in the generalised epilepsy syndromes. While some argue that it is possible to detect 'spikes' and 'sharp waves' to lend support to a clinical diagnosis, these are non-specific and therefore not diagnostic, and can lead an unwary clinician to err in ascribing other symptoms to epilepsy.

Nerve conduction studies

Electrical stimulation of a nerve causes an impulse to travel both efferently and afferently along the underlying axons. Nerve conduction studies (NCS) make use of this, recording action potentials as they pass along peripheral nerves and (with motor nerves) as they pass into the muscle belly. Digital recording has enhanced sensitivity and reproducibility of these tiny potentials. By measuring the time taken to traverse a known distance, it is possible to calculate nerve conduction velocities (NCVs). Healthy nerves at room temperature will conduct at a speed of 40–50 m/sec. If the recorded potential is smaller than expected, this provides evidence of a reduction in the overall number of functioning axons. Significant slowing of conduction velocity, in contrast, suggests impaired conduction due to peripheral nerve demyelination. Such changes in NCS may be diffuse (as in a hereditary demyelinating peripheral neuropathy), focal (as in pressure palsies) or multifocal (e.g. Guillain–Barré syndrome, mononeuritis multiplex). The information gained can allow the disease responsible for peripheral nerve dysfunction to be better deduced (see Box 28.86).

Stimulation of motor nerves allows for the recording of compound muscle action potentials (CMAPs) over muscles (Fig. 28.15). These are around 500 times larger than sensory nerve potentials, typically around 1–20 millivolts. Since a proportion of stimulated impulses in motor nerves will 'reflect' back from the anterior horn cell body (forming the 'F' wave), it is also possible to obtain some information about the condition of nerve roots.

Repetitive nerve stimulation (RNS) at 3–15/sec provides consistent CMAPs in healthy muscle. In myasthenia gravis (p. 1194), however, where there is partial blockage of acetylcholine receptors, there is a diagnostic fall (decrement) in CMAP amplitude. In contrast, an increasing CMAP with high-frequency RNS is seen in Lambert–Eaton myasthenic syndrome (p. 1195).

Electromyography

Electromyography (EMG) is usually performed alongside NCS and involves needle recording of muscle electrical potential during rest and contraction. At rest, muscle is electrically silent but loss of nerve supply causes muscle membrane to become unstable, manifest as fibrillations, positive sharp waves ('spontaneous activity') or fasciculations. Motor unit action potentials are recorded during muscle contraction. Axonal loss or destruction will result in fewer motor units. Resultant sprouting of remaining units will lead to increasing size of each individual unit on EMG. Myopathy, in contrast, causes muscle fibre splitting, which results

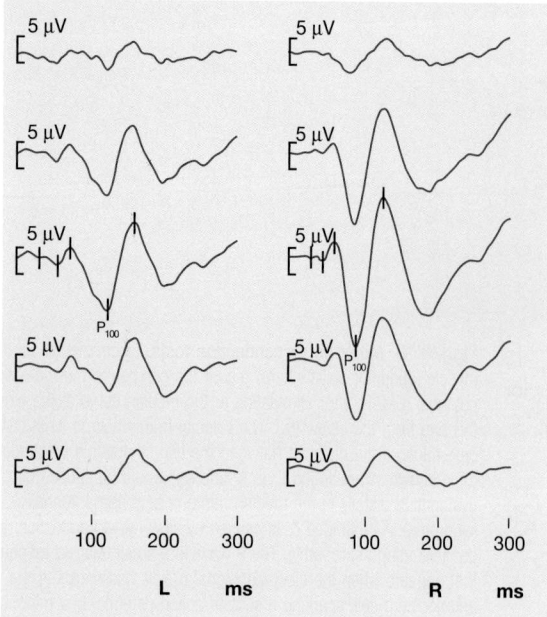

Fig. 28.16 Visual evoked potential (VEP) recording. The abnormality is in the left hemisphere, with delay in latency and a reduction in signal of the P_{100}.

in a large number of smaller units on EMG. Other abnormal activity, such as myotonic discharges, may signify abnormal ion channel conduction, as in myotonic dystrophy or myotonia congenita.

Specialised single-fibre electromyography (SFEMG) can be used to investigate neuromuscular junction transmission. Measuring 'jitter' and 'blocking' can identify the effect of antibodies in reducing the action of acetylcholine on the receptor.

Evoked potentials

The cortical response to visual, auditory or electrical stimulation can be measured on an EEG as an evoked potential (EP). If a stimulus is provided – e.g. to the eye – the tiny EEG response can be discerned when averaging 100–1000 repeated stimuli. Assessing the latency (the time delay) and amplitude can give information about the integrity of the relevant pathway. MRI now provides more information about CNS pathways, thus reducing reliance on EPs. In practice, visual evoked potentials (VEPs) are most commonly used to help differentiate CNS demyelination from small-vessel white-matter changes (Fig. 28.16).

Magnetic stimulation

Central conduction times can also be measured using electromagnetic induction of action potentials in the cortex or spinal cord by the local application of specialised coils. Again, MRI has made this technique largely redundant, other than for research.

Routine blood tests

Many systemic conditions that can affect the nervous system can be identified by simple blood tests. Nutritional deficiencies, metabolic disturbances, inflammatory conditions or infections may all present or be associated with neurological symptoms, and basic blood tests (full blood count, erythrocyte sedimentation rate, C-reactive protein, biochemical screening) may provide clues. Specific blood tests will be highlighted in the relevant subsections of this chapter. Human immunodeficiency

virus (HIV) infection is an important cause of neurological disease and the clinician should have a low threshold for checking this.

Immunological tests

Recent developments have seen a host of new immune-mediated conditions emerge in clinical neurology, with antibody targets ranging from muscle and neuromuscular junction disturbance (causing weakness and muscle pain) to specific neuroglial cell surface molecules such as ion channels (causing cognitive decline, epilepsy and psychiatric changes). Examples of autoantibodies that aid diagnosis and may play a disease-causing role include AChR antibodies (myasthenia gravis), Aquaporin 4 and MOG antibodies (neuromyelitis optica), NMDAR, Lgi1 and CASPR2 antibodies (autoimmune encephalitis). Many of these antibodies to neural/glial cell surface antigens are specifically associated with individual neurological syndromes. Many other antibodies against intracellular antigens have also been described, in particular in association with paraneoplastic syndromes, although it is less clear if these antibodies play a causal role in mediating disease.

Genetic testing

Relevant subsections will detail the increasing numbers of inherited neurological conditions that can now be diagnosed by DNA analysis (p. 52). These include diseases caused by increased numbers of trinucleotide repeats, such as Huntington's disease myotonic dystrophy; and some types of spinocerebellar ataxia. Mitochondrial DNA can also be sequenced to diagnose relevant disorders. Next-generation sequencing technologies including exome sequencing and whole genome sequencing are increasingly employed to identify undiagnosed genetic disease, but expertise is required in their interpretation (see Ch. 3).

Lumbar puncture

Lumbar puncture (LP) is the technique used to obtain both a CSF sample and an indirect measure of intracranial pressure. After local anaesthetic injection, a needle is inserted between lumbar spinous processes (usually between L3 and L4) through the dura and into the spinal canal. Intracranial pressure can be deduced (if patients are lying on their side) and CSF removed for analysis. CSF pressure measurement is important in the diagnosis and monitoring of idiopathic intracranial hypertension. In this condition, the LP itself is therapeutic.

CSF is normally clear and colourless, and the tests that are usually performed include a naked eye examination of the CSF and centrifugation to determine the colour of the supernatant (yellow, or xanthochromic, some hours after subarachnoid haemorrhage; p. 1214). Measurement of absorption of specific light wavelengths helps quantify the amount of haem metabolites in CSF. Routine analysis involves a cell count, as well as glucose and protein concentrations.

CSF assessment is important in investigating infections (meningitis or encephalitis), subarachnoid haemorrhage and inflammatory conditions. Normal values and abnormalities found in specific conditions are shown in Box 28.6. More sophisticated analysis allows measurement of antibody formation solely within the CNS (oligoclonal bands), genetic analysis (e.g. polymerase chain reaction (PCR) for herpes simplex or tuberculosis), immunological tests (NMDAR, paraneoplastic antibodies), immunophenotyping by fluorescence-activated cell sorting (FACS) and cytology (to detect malignant cells).

If there is a cranial space-occupying lesion causing raised intracranial pressure, LP presents a theoretical risk of downward shift of intracerebral contents, a potentially fatal process known as coning. Consequently, LP is contraindicated if there is any clinical suggestion of raised intracranial pressure (papilloedema), depressed level of consciousness, or focal neurological signs suggesting a cerebral lesion,

i 28.6 How to interpret cerebrospinal fluid results

	Normal	Subarachnoid haemorrhage	Multiple sclerosis	Carcinomatous/ lymphomatous meningitis	AIDP[1]
Pressure	50–250 mmH$_2$O	Increased	Normal	Normal /increased	Normal
Colour	Clear	Blood-stained Xanthochromic	Clear	Clear/xanthochromic	Clear
Red cell count (×10[6]/L)	0–4	Raised	Normal	Normal/elevated	Normal
White cell count (×10[6]/L)	0–4	Normal/slightly raised	0–50 lymphocytes	0-400 lymphocyte	0-50 (<5 in 85%)
Glucose	>50%–60% of blood level	Normal	Normal	Normal/decreased	Normal
Protein	<0.45 g/L	Increased	Normal/increased	Normal/increased	Increased[2]
Microbiology	Sterile	Sterile	Sterile	Sterile/cytology may be helpful	Sterile
Oligoclonal bands	Negative	Negative	Often positive	Uncertain	Matched bands (serum and CSF)

	Acute bacterial meningitis	Partially treated bacterial meningitis[2]	Viral meningitis[2]	Cryptococcal meningitis in HIV[1]	Tuberculous meningitis
Pressure	Normal/increased	Normal/increased	Normal	Elevated often very high	Normal/increased
Colour	Cloudy	Clear /cloudy	Clear	Clear /cloudy	Clear/cloudy
Red cell count (×10[6]/L)	Normal	Normal	Normal	Normal	Normal
White cell count (×10[6]/L)	1000–5000 polymorphs	Normal to raised; mixed cells	10–2000 lymphocytes	20-200 mainly lymphocytes	50–5000 lymphocytes
Glucose	Decreased	Normal/decreased	Normal	Normal/decreased	Decreased
Protein	Increased	Normal/increased	Normal/increased	Normal/increased	Increased
Microbiology	Organisms on Gram stain and/or culture	Greater chance of no growth	Sterile/virus detected	India ink positive (around 50%); cryptococcal antigen/culture	Ziehl–Neelsen/ auramine stain or tuberculosis culture positive
Oligoclonal bands	Can be positive	Can be positive	Can be positive	Uncertain	Can be positive

(AIDP=acute inflammatory demyelinating polyneuropathy; HIV=human immunodeficiency virus)
[1]See Chapter 14 for more detail on findings in HIV infection. [2]Cerebrospinal fluid findings in bacterial and viral meningitis are variable, and this table shows only the most common patterns.

until imaging (by CT or MRI) has excluded a space-occupying lesion or hydrocephalus. When there is a risk of local haemorrhage (thrombocytopenia, disseminated intravascular coagulation or anticoagulant treatment), then caution should be exercised or specific measures should be taken. LP can be safely performed in patients on low-dose aspirin or low-dose heparin. UK guidelines advise considering pausing other antiplatelet agents for a period before elective LP (e.g. 7 days for clopidogrel). LP may be unsafe in patients who are fully anticoagulated due to the increased risk of epidural haematoma and haematology advice should be sought.

About 30% of LPs are followed by a postural headache, due to reduced CSF pressure. The frequency of headache can be reduced by using smaller or atraumatic needles. Rarer complications involve transient radicular pain, and pain over the lumbar region during the procedure. Aseptic technique renders secondary infections such as meningitis extremely rare.

Biopsy

Biopsies of nervous tissue (peripheral nerve, muscle, meninges or brain) are occasionally required for diagnosis.

Nerve biopsy can help in the investigation of peripheral neuropathy. Usually, a distal sensory nerve (sural or radial) is targeted. Histological examination can help identify underlying causes, such as vasculitides or infiltrative disorders like amyloid. Nerve biopsy should not be undertaken lightly since there is an appreciable morbidity; it should be reserved for cases where the diagnosis is in doubt after routine investigations and where it will influence management.

Muscle biopsy is performed more frequently and is indicated for the differentiation of myositis and myopathies. These conditions can usually be distinguished by histological examination, and enzyme histochemistry can be useful when mitochondrial diseases and storage diseases are suspected. The quadriceps muscle is most commonly biopsied but other muscles may also be sampled if they are involved clinically. Although pain and infection can follow the procedure, these are less of a problem than after nerve biopsy. Imaging and clinical examination may help guide and determine biopsy site.

Brain biopsy is required when imaging fails to clarify the nature of intracerebral lesions, e.g. in unexplained degenerative diseases such as unusual cases of dementia and in patients with brain tumours. Some biopsies are performed stereotactically through a burr hole in the skull. Nevertheless, haemorrhage, infection and death still occur and brain biopsy should be considered only if a diagnosis is otherwise elusive. Discussion between neurologist, neuroradiologist, neurosurgeon and neuropathologist is important to ensure maximal diagnostic yield of these samples.

28

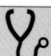

28.7 How to take a neurological history

Introduction

- Age and sex
- Handedness

Presenting complaint

- Symptoms (clarify: see text)
- Overall pattern: intermittent or persistent?
- If intermittent, how often do symptoms occur and how long do they last?
- Speed of onset: seconds, minutes, hours, days, weeks, months, years, decades?
- Better, worse or the same over time?
- Associated symptoms (including non-neurological)
- Disability caused by symptoms
- Change in walking
- Difficulty with fine hand movements, e.g. writing, fastening buttons, using cutlery
- Effect on work, family life and leisure

Background

- Previous neurological symptoms and whether similar to current symptoms
- Previous medical history
- Domestic situation
- Driving licence status
- Medications (current and at time of symptom onset)
- Alcohol/smoking habits
- Recreational drug and other toxin exposure
- Family history and developmental history
- What are patient's thoughts/fears/concerns?

28.8 The key diagnostic questions

Where is the lesion?

- Is it neurological?
- If so, to which part of the nervous system does it localise?
  Central versus peripheral

What is the lesion?

- Hereditary or congenital
- Acquired:
  Traumatic
  Infective
  Neoplastic
  Degenerative
  Inflammatory or immune-mediated
  Vascular
  Functional

28.9 Neurological examination in old age

- **Pupils**: tend to be smaller, making fundoscopy more difficult.
- **Limb tone**: more difficult to assess because of poor relaxation and concomitant joint disease.
- **Ankle reflexes**: may be absent.
- **Gait assessment**: more difficult because of concurrent musculoskeletal disease and pre-existing neurological deficits.
- **Sensory testing**: especially difficult when there is cognitive impairment.
- **Vibration sense**: may be reduced distally in the legs.

Biopsy of other organs can be useful in the diagnosis of systemic disorders presenting as neurological problems, such as tonsillar biopsy (prion diseases), or rectal or fat biopsy (for assessment of amyloid).

Presenting problems in neurological disease

While history is important in all medical specialties, it is especially key in neurology, where many neurological diagnoses have no confirmatory test. History-taking allows doctor and patient to get to know one another; many neurological diseases follow chronic paths and this may be the first of many such consultations. It also allows the clinician to obtain information about the patient's affect, cognition and psychiatric state.

History-taking is a highly active process. While there are generic templates (Box 28.7), each individual story will follow its own course, and diagnostic considerations during the history will guide further questioning.

It is important to be clear about what patients mean by certain words. They may find it difficult to describe symptoms: for instance, weakness may be called 'numbness', while there are many possible interpretations of 'dizziness'. These must be clarified; even in emergency situations, a clear, accurate history is the foundation of any management plan. While the story should come primarily from the patient, input from eye-witnesses and family members is crucial if the patient is unable to provide details or if there has been loss of consciousness. This need for corroboration and clarification means the telephone is as important as any investigation.

The aim of the history is to address two key issues: (1) *where is the lesion;* and (2) *what is the lesion?* (Box 28.8). These should remain uppermost in the doctor's mind while the history is being elicited, especially in older people (Box 28.9). Some common combinations of symptoms may suggest particular locations for a lesion (Box 28.10). Enquiry about handedness is important; lateralisation of the dominant hand helps designate the dominant hemisphere, which in turn may help to localise

any pathologies, or to plan rehabilitation or treatment strategies in asymmetrical disorders such as stroke or Parkinson's disease.

Epidemiology must be borne in mind. How likely is it that this particular patient has any specific condition under consideration? For example, a 20-year-old with right-sided headache and tenderness will not have temporal arteritis, but this is an important possibility if such symptoms present in a 78-year-old female. Global epidemiology is important and endemic infectious agents and travel history should always be considered.

Determining the evolution, speed of onset and progression of a disease is important (Box 28.11). For example, if right-hand weakness occurred overnight, it would suggest a stroke in an older person or an acute entrapment neuropathy in a younger one. Evolution over several days, however, might make demyelination (multiple sclerosis) a possible diagnosis, or perhaps a subdural haematoma if the weakness was preceded by a head injury in an older person taking warfarin. Progression over weeks might bring an intracranial mass lesion or motor neuron disease into the differential. Slow progression over a year or so, with difficulty in using the hand, could suggest a degenerative process such as Parkinson's disease. The impact on day-to-day activities, such as walking, climbing stairs and carrying out fine hand movements, should also be established in order to gauge the level of associated disability.

Estimates of the frequency and duration of specific events are essential when taking details of a paroxysmal disorder such as migraine and epilepsy. Vague terms such as 'a lot' or 'sometimes' are unhelpful, and it can assist the patient if choices are given to estimate numbers, such as once a day, week or month.

Many neurological symptoms are not explained by typical neurological disease. Describing these as 'functional' is less pejorative, more acceptable to patients and more in keeping with modern understanding of these symptoms than 'psychogenic' or 'hysterical'. Functional symptoms require considerable experience in diagnosis and are frequently missed.

28.10 How to 'localise' neurological disease

Combination of symptoms/signs	Probable site	Possible pathology	Other important information
Painless loss of hemilateral function	Cerebral cortex	Usually vascular, inflammatory or neoplastic	Associated systemic symptoms Tempo of evolution
Pyramidal weakness of all four limbs or both legs, bladder signs, sensory loss	Spinal cord	Usually vascular, inflammatory, infective, or neoplastic	Associated systemic symptoms Tempo of evolution Travel history Endemic infections
Cranial nerve lesions, with limb pyramidal signs or sensory loss ± sphincter disturbance	Brainstem Mid-brain Pons Medulla	Usually vascular or inflammatory Rarely neoplastic or infective	Associated systemic symptoms Tempo of evolution Travel history Endemic infections
Visual loss + pyramidal signs and/or cerebellar signs	Widespread cerebral lesions	Usually inflammatory	Tempo of evolution
Weakness and/or sensory loss in a combination of individual peripheral nerves	Several peripheral nerves ('mononeuritis multiplex')	Usually inflammatory or diabetic, rarely infective, such as human immunodeficiency virus	Associated systemic symptoms
Weakness with widespread LMN and UMN signs	Upper and lower motor neurons	Motor neuron disease Cervical myeloradiculopathy	Associated localised cervical symptoms
Distal loss of sensation and/or weakness	Generalised peripheral nerves	See causes of neuropathy (p. 1191)	Associated systemic symptoms

(LMN/UMN = lower/upper motor neuron)

28.11 The evolution of symptoms

Onset	Evolution	Possible causes
Sudden (minutes to hours)	Stable/improvement	Vascular (stroke/transient ischaemic attack (TIA)) Nerve entrapment syndromes Functional
Gradual	Progressive over days	Inflammation Infection
Gradual	Progressive over weeks to months	Neoplastic/paraneoplastic
Gradual	Progressive over months to years	Genetic Degenerative

Headache and facial pain

Most headaches are chronic disorders but acute presentation of headaches is an important aspect of emergency medical care. Headache may be divided into primary (benign) or secondary, and most patients, whether presenting in clinic or as emergencies, have primary syndromes (see Box 9.13). The emergency clinical assessment of headaches is dealt with on page 186.

Ocular pain

Assuming that ocular disease (such as acute glaucoma) has been excluded, ocular pain may be due to trigeminal autonomic cephalalgias (TACs) or, rarely, inflammatory or infiltrative lesions at the apex of the orbit or the cavernous sinus, when 3rd, 4th, 5th or 6th cranial nerve involvement is usually evident. Ocular pain and headache are also discussed on page 1223.

Facial pain

Pain in the face can be due to dental or temporomandibular joint problems. Acute sinusitis is usually apparent from other features of sinus congestion/infection and may cause localised pain over the affected sinus, but is almost never the explanation for persistent facial pain or headache.

Facial pain is not uncommon in migraine but some syndromes can present solely with facial pain. The most common neurological causes of facial pain are trigeminal neuralgia, herpes zoster (shingles) and post-herpetic neuralgia, all characterised by their extreme severity. In trigeminal neuralgia, the patient describes bouts of brief (seconds), lancinating pain ('electric shocks'), most frequently felt in the second and third divisions of the nerve and often triggered by talking or chewing. Facial shingles most commonly affects the first (ophthalmic) division of the trigeminal nerve, and pain usually precedes the rash. Post-herpetic neuralgia may follow, typically a continuous burning pain throughout the affected territory, with marked sensitivity to light touch (allodynia) and resistance to treatment. Destructive lesions of the trigeminal nerve usually cause numbness rather than pain.

Dizziness, blackouts and 'funny turns'

Acute onset of dizziness or blackouts will present to the acute medical department. In neurological practice, it is common to deal with patients presenting with a history of multiple events. While detailed questioning will be dealt with in the relevant section (see p. 185), the neurologist will have to tease out the pattern of each of the different attack types experienced by the patient to be able to form a treatment and investigation plan, one of the challenges of clinical neurology.

Status epilepticus

Status epilepticus is seizure activity not resolving spontaneously, or recurrent seizure with no recovery of consciousness in between. Persisting seizure activity has a recognised mortality and is a medical emergency.

Diagnosis is usually clinical and can be made on the basis of the description of prolonged rigidity and/or clonic movements with loss of awareness. As seizure activity becomes prolonged, movements may

28

become more subtle. Cyanosis, pyrexia, acidosis and sweating may occur, and complications include aspiration, hypotension, cardiac arrhythmias and renal or hepatic failure.

In patients with pre-existing epilepsy, the most likely cause is a fall in antiepileptic drug levels. In de novo status epilepticus, it is essential to exclude precipitants such as infection (meningitis, encephalitis), neoplasia and metabolic derangement (hypoglycaemia, hyponatraemia or hypocalcaemia). Treatment and investigation are outlined in Box 28.12.

Coma

Coma and loss of consciousness usually present to the acute medical admissions department (p. 197). Clarification of cause and prognosis may require specialist neurological input.

Delirium

Delirium describes cortical dysfunction and replaces the older term 'acute confusional state'. It has a range of primary causes, and given its role in precipitating acute admission, it is covered in detail on page 213.

Amnesia

Memory disturbance is a common symptom. In the absence of significant functional impairment (e.g. inability to work, dyspraxias, loss of daily function), many patients will prove to have benign memory dysfunction related to age, mood or psychiatric disorders. Investigation and treatment of the dementias are discussed elsewhere (p. 1246).

Temporary loss of memory may be due to a transient delirium related to infection, the post-ictal period after seizure, or transient global amnesia. These are usually distinguished on the basis of the history. Transient amnesia resulting directly from a seizure (transient epileptic amnesia) is a rare result of temporal lobe epilepsy.

Transient global amnesia

Transient global amnesia (TGA) predominantly affects middle-aged people, with an abrupt, discrete loss of anterograde memory function lasting up to a few hours. During the episode, patients are unable to record new memories, resulting in repetitive questioning, the hallmark of this condition. Consciousness is preserved and patients may perform even complex motor acts normally. During the attack there is retrograde amnesia for the events of the past few days, weeks or years. After 4–6 hours, memory function and behaviour return to normal but the patient has persistent, complete amnesia for the duration of the attack itself. There are no seizure markers and, unlike epileptic amnesia, transient global amnesia recurs in only around 10%–20% of cases. A vascular aetiology is unlikely (TGA is not a risk factor for subsequent vascular disease) and amnesia may be due to a benign process similar to migraine, occurring in the hippocampus. TGA causes no physical signs and, provided there is a typical history (which requires a witness), no investigation is necessary and patients may be reassured.

Persistent amnesia

Serious neurological disease must be excluded in patients with persistent memory disturbance, although many will prove to have benign symptoms. Symptoms corroborated by relatives or colleagues are likely to be more significant than those noted by the patient only. Where poor concentration is at the heart of cognitive deterioration, it is more likely to be due to an underlying mood disorder.

It is important to assess the timing of onset and to establish which aspects of memory are affected. Complaints of getting lost or of losing complex abilities are more pathological than word-finding difficulties. Disturbance of episodic or working memory (previously called 'short-term memory') must be distinguished from semantic memory (memory for concept-based knowledge unrelated to specific experiences). Episodic

28.12 Management of status epilepticus

Initial

- Ensure airway is patent; give oxygen to prevent cerebral hypoxia
- Check pulse, blood pressure, BM Stix and respiratory rate
- Secure intravenous access and initiate ECG monitoring
- Send blood for:
   Glucose, urea and electrolytes, calcium and magnesium, liver function, antiepileptic drug levels
   Full blood count and coagulation screen
   Storing a sample for future analysis (e.g. drug misuse)
- If seizures continue for > 5 mins: give midazolam 10 mg bucally or nasally or lorazepam 4 mg IV if access available or diazepam 10 mg rectally or IV if necessary; repeat *once only* after 15 mins
- Correct any metabolic trigger, e.g. hypoglycaemia, thiamine deficiency (give thiamine before glucose if suspected)

Ongoing

If seizures continue after 30 mins
- IV infusion with one of:
   Levetiracetam: 60mg/kg (max dose 4500mg) over 10 minutes
   Phenytoin: 15 mg/kg at 50 mg/min (with cardiac monitoring, risk of hypotension and bradycardia)
   Sodium valproate: 20–30 mg/kg IV at 40 mg/min
   Phenobarbital: 10 mg/kg at 100 mg/min
- Cardiac monitor and pulse oximetry:
   Monitor neurological condition, blood pressure, respiration; check blood gases
- If severe renal dysfunction with eGFR less than 30 mL/min/1.73m² avoid levetiracetam; sodium valproate is then drug of first choice

If seizures still continue after 30–60 mins
- Transfer to intensive care:
   Start treatment for refractory status with intubation, ventilation and general anaesthesia using propofol or thiopental
   EEG monitor

Once status controlled

- Commence longer-term antiepileptic medication with one of:
   Levetiracetam 1000–1500 mg IV, oral/nasogastric tube twice daily (adjust for renal impairment and start 10–12 hours after loading dose)
   Sodium valproate 10 mg/kg IV over 3–5 mins, then 800–2000 mg/day
   Phenytoin: give loading dose (if not already used as above) of 15 mg/kg, infuse at < 50 mg/min, then 300 mg/day
   Carbamazepine 400 mg by nasogastric tube, then 400–1200 mg/day
- Investigate cause

(ECG = electrocardiogram; EEG = electroencephalogram; eGFR = estimated glomerular filtration rate; IV = intravenous)

memory is selectively impaired in Korsakoff syndrome (often secondary to alcohol) or bilateral temporal lobe damage. It can also be seen in conjunction with other types of dementia. Progressive deterioration over months suggests an underlying dementia, and a full medical assessment must be performed to detect any underlying medical problem.

It is important to identify and treat depression in patients with memory loss. Depression may present as a 'pseudo-dementia', with concentration and memory impairment as dominant features, and this is often reversible with antidepressant medication. Any patient with dementia (particularly of Alzheimer type) may develop depression in the early stages of their illness, however. Specific causes of progressive dementia, with their investigation and treatment, are described elsewhere (p. 1246).

Weakness

The assessment of weakness requires the application of basic anatomy, physiology and some pathology to the interpretation of the history and clinical findings. Points to consider are shown on Figure 28.17 and in Boxes 28.13 and 28.14. The pattern and evolution of weakness and the clinical signs provide clues to the site and nature of the lesion.

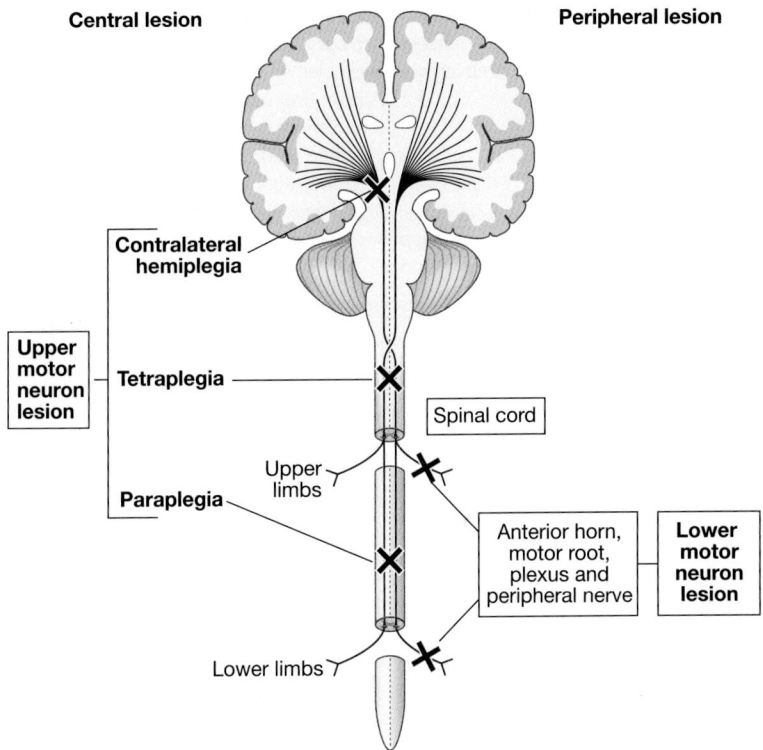

Fig. 28.17 Patterns of motor loss according to the anatomical site of the lesion.

i	28.13 Distinguishing signs in upper versus lower motor neuron syndromes	
	Upper motor neuron lesion	Lower motor neuron lesion
Inspection	Normal (may be wasting in chronic lesions)	Wasting, fasciculation
Tone	Increased with clonus	Normal or decreased, no clonus
Pattern of weakness	Preferentially affects extensors in arms, flexors in leg Hemiparesis, paraparesis or tetraparesis	Typically focal, in distribution of nerve root or peripheral nerve, with associated sensory changes
Deep tendon reflexes	Increased	Decreased/absent
Plantar response	Extensor (Babinski sign)	Flexor

28.14 How to assess weakness	
Clinical finding	Likely level of lesion/diagnosis
Pattern and distribution	
Isolated muscles	Radiculopathy or mononeuropathy
Both limbs on one side (hemiparesis)	Cerebral hemisphere, less likely cord or brainstem
One limb	Neuronopathy, plexopathy, cord/brain
Both lower limbs (paraparesis)	Spinal cord; look for a sensory level
Fatigability	Myasthenia gravis
Bizarre, fluctuating, not following anatomical rules	Functional
Signs	
Upper motor neuron	Brain/spinal cord
Lower motor neuron	Peripheral nervous system
Evolution of the weakness	
Sudden and improving	Stroke/mononeuropathy
Evolving over months or years	Meningioma, cervical spondylotic myelopathy
Gradually worsening over days or weeks	Cerebral mass, demyelination, infection
Associated symptoms	
Absence of sensory involvement	Motor neuron disease, myopathy, myasthenia

It is important to establish whether the patient has loss of power rather than reduced sensation or generalised fatigue. Pain may restrict movement and thus mimic weakness. Paradoxically, sensory neglect may leave patients unaware of severe weakness.

Patients with parkinsonism may complain of weakness; extrapyramidal signs of rigidity (cogwheel or lead pipe) and bradykinesia should be evident, and a resting tremor (usually asymmetrical) may provide a further clue. Simple observation of the patient walking into the consulting room may be diagnostic and is as important as formal strength testing. Movement restricted by pain should be apparent, and other features (contractures, wasting, fasciculations, abnormal movements/postures) all provide diagnostic clues.

Weakness is a common symptom arising without an underlying degenerative or destructive cause (functional symptom). Functional weakness does not conform to typical patterns, and the signs in Box 28.13 are absent. Clinical examination is often variable (e.g. the patient can walk but appears to have no leg movement when assessed on the couch), and strength may appear to 'give way', with the patient able to achieve full power for brief bursts, which does not occur in disease. Hoover's sign is useful to confirm functional weakness and relies on eliciting the normal phenomenon of simultaneous hip extension when the contralateral hip flexes. In functional weakness, hip extension

28

weakness may be seen; this then returns to full strength when contralateral hip flexion is tested. This sign may be demonstrated to the patient in a non-confrontational manner, to show that potential limb power is intact.

Facial weakness

Facial nerve palsy (Bell's palsy)

One of the most common causes of facial weakness is Bell's palsy, a lower motor neuron lesion of the 7th (facial) nerve, affecting all ages and both sexes. It is more common following upper respiratory tract infections, during pregnancy and in patients with diabetes, immunosuppression and hypertension. It is common in human immunodeficiency virus at the time of seroconversion.

The lesion is within the facial canal. Symptoms usually develop subacutely over a few hours, with pain around the ear preceding the unilateral facial weakness. Patients often describe the face as 'numb' but there is no objective sensory loss (except to taste, if the chorda tympani is involved). Hyperacusis may occur if the nerve to stapedius is involved and impairment of parasympathetic fibres may cause diminished salivation and tear secretion. Examination reveals an ipsilateral lower motor neuron facial nerve palsy (no sparing of forehead muscles). Vesicles in the ear or on the palate may indicate primary herpes zoster infection. A clinical search for signs of other causes of lower motor neuron facial nerve weakness, such as parotid or scalp lesions, trauma or skull base lesions, is justified.

Glucocorticoids improve recovery rates if started within 72 hours of onset but antiviral drugs are not effective. Artificial tears applied regularly prevent corneal drying, and taping the eye shut overnight helps prevent exposure keratitis and corneal abrasion. Patients unable to close the eye should be referred urgently to an ophthalmologist. About 80% of patients recover spontaneously within 12 weeks. Plastic surgery may be considered for the minority left with facial disfigurement after 12 months. Recurrence is unusual and should prompt further investigation. Aberrant re-innervation may occur during recovery, producing unwanted facial movements, such as eye closure when the mouth is moved (synkinesis) or 'crocodile tears' (tearing during salivation).

Unlike Bell's palsy, lesions with an upper motor neuron origin may spare the upper face. Cortical lesions may cause a facial weakness either in isolation or with associated hemiparesis and speech difficulties.

Sensory disturbance

Sensory symptoms are common and frequently benign. Patients often find sensory symptoms difficult to describe and sensory examination is difficult for both doctor and patient. While neurological disease can cause sensory symptoms, systemic disorders can also be responsible. Tingling in both hands and around the mouth can occur as the result of hyperventilation or hypocalcaemia. When there is dysfunction of the relevant cerebral cortex, the patient's perception of the wholeness or actual presence of the relevant part of the body may be distorted.

Numbness and paraesthesia

The history may give the best clues to localisation and pathology. Certain common patterns are recognised: in migraine, the aura may consist of spreading tingling or paraesthesia, followed by numbness evolving over 20–30 minutes over one half of the body, often splitting the tongue. Sensory loss caused by a stroke or transient ischaemic attack (TIA) occurs much more rapidly and is typically negative (numbness) rather than positive (tingling). Rarely, unpleasant paraesthesia of sensory epilepsy spreads within seconds. The sensory alteration of inflammatory spinal cord lesions often ascends from one or both lower limbs to a distinct level on the trunk over hours to days, and can give rise to a feeling of constriction, sometimes described as 'being hugged'. Sensory change can occur as a manifestation of anxiety or as part of a functional neurological disorder. In such cases, the distribution usually neither conforms to a known anatomical pattern nor fits with any typical neurological disease. Care must be taken in diagnosing functional sensory problems; a careful history and examination will ensure there is no other objective neurological deficit.

Sensory neurological examination needs to be undertaken and interpreted with care because the findings depend, by definition, on subjective reports. The reported distribution of sensory loss can be useful, however, when combined with the coexisting deficits of motor and/or cranial nerve function (Fig. 28.18).

Sensory loss in peripheral nerve lesions

Here the symptoms are usually of sensory loss and paraesthesia. Single nerve lesions cause disturbance in the sensory distribution of the nerve, whereas in diffuse neuropathies the longest neurons are affected first, giving a characteristic 'glove and stocking' distribution. If smaller nerve fibres are preferentially affected (e.g. in diabetic neuropathy), temperature and pin-prick (pain) are reduced, whilst vibration sense and proprioception (modalities served by the larger, well-myelinated, sensory nerves) may be relatively spared. In contrast, vibration and proprioception are particularly affected if the neuropathy is demyelinating in character, producing symptoms of tightness and swelling with impairment of proprioception and vibration sensation.

Sensory loss in nerve root lesions

These typically present with pain as a prominent feature, either within the spine or in the limb plexuses. Pain is often felt in the myotome rather than the dermatome. The nerve root involved may be deduced from the dermatomal pattern of sensory loss, although overlap may lead to this being smaller than expected.

Sensory loss in spinal cord lesions

Transverse lesions of the spinal cord produce loss of all sensory modalities below that segmental level, although the clinical level may only be manifest 2–3 segments lower than the anatomical site of the lesion. Very often, there is a band of paraesthesia or hyperaesthesia at the top of the area of sensory loss. Clinical examination may reveal dissociated sensory loss, i.e. different patterns in the spinothalamic and dorsal columnar pathways. If the transverse lesion is vascular due to anterior spinal artery thrombosis, the spinothalamic pathways may be affected while the posterior one-third of the spinal cord (the dorsal column modalities) may be spared.

Lesions damaging one side of the spinal cord will produce loss of spinothalamic modalities (pain and temperature) on the opposite side, and of dorsal column modalities (joint position and vibration sense) on the same side of the body – the Brown–Séquard syndrome (see Fig. 28.18E).

Lesions in the centre of the spinal cord (such as syringomyelia: see Box 28.82 and Fig. 28.49) spare the dorsal columns but involve the spinothalamic fibres crossing the cord from both sides over the length of the lesion. There is no sensory loss in segments above and below the lesion; this is described as 'suspended' sensory loss. There is sometimes reflex loss at the level of the lesion if afferent fibres of the reflex arc are affected.

An isolated lesion of the dorsal columns is not uncommon in multiple sclerosis. This produces a characteristic unpleasant, tight feeling over the limb(s) involved and, while there is no loss of pin-prick or temperature sensation, the associated loss of proprioception may severely limit function of the affected limb(s).

Sensory loss in brainstem lesions

Lesions in the brainstem can be associated with sensory loss but the distribution depends on the site of the lesion. A lesion limited to the trigeminal nucleus or its sensory projections will cause ipsilateral facial sensory disturbance. For example, pain resembling trigeminal neuralgia can be seen in patients with multiple sclerosis. The anatomy of the trigeminal connections means that lesions in the medulla or spinal cord can give rise to 'balaclava helmet' patterns of sensory loss. Sensory pathways running up from the spinal cord can also be damaged in the brainstem, resulting in simultaneous sensory loss in arm(s) and/or leg(s).

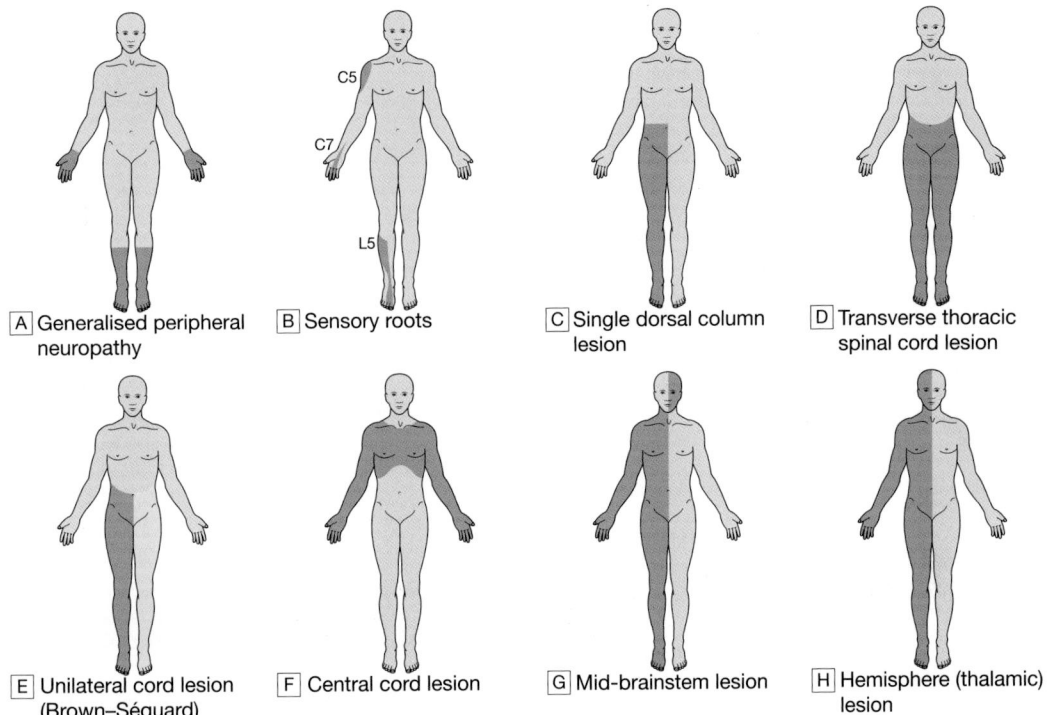

Fig. 28.18 Patterns of sensory loss. **A** Generalised peripheral neuropathy. **B** Sensory roots: some common examples. **C** Single dorsal column lesion (proprioception and some touch loss). **D** Transverse thoracic spinal cord lesion. **E** Unilateral cord lesion (Brown–Séquard): ipsilateral dorsal column (and motor) deficit and contralateral spinothalamic deficit. **F** Central cord lesion: 'cape' distribution of spinothalamic loss. **G** Mid-brainstem lesion: ipsilateral facial sensory loss and contralateral loss on body below the vertex. **H** Hemisphere (thalamic) lesion: contralateral loss on one side of face and body.

Sensory loss in hemispheric lesions

The temporal, parietal and occipital lobes receive sensory information regarding the various modalities of touch, vision, hearing and balance (see Box 28.2). The initial points of entry into the cortex are the respective primary cortical areas (see Fig. 28.4). Damage to any of these primary areas will result in reduction or loss of the ability to perceive that particular modality: 'negative' symptomatology. Abnormal excitation of these areas can result in a false perception ('positive' symptoms), the most common of which is migrainous visual aura (flashing lights or teichopsia).

Cortical lesions are more likely to cause a mixed motor and sensory loss. Substantial lesions of the parietal cortex (as in large strokes) can cause severe loss of proprioception and may even abolish conscious awareness of the existence of the affected limb(s), known as neglect; this can be difficult to distinguish from paralysis. Pathways are so tightly packed in the thalamus that even small lacunar strokes can cause isolated contralateral hemisensory loss.

Neuropathic pain

Neuropathic pain is a positive neurological symptom caused by dysfunction of the pain perception apparatus, in contrast to nociceptive pain, which is secondary to pathological processes such as inflammation. Neuropathic pain has distinctive features and typically provokes a very unpleasant, persistent, burning sensation. There is often increased sensitivity to touch, so that light brushing of the affected area causes exquisite pain (allodynia). Painful stimuli are felt as though they arise from a larger area than that touched, and spontaneous bursts of pain may also occur. Pain may be elicited by other modalities (allodynia) and is considerably affected by emotional influences. The most common causes of neuropathic pain are diabetic neuropathies, trigeminal and post-herpetic neuralgias, and trauma to a peripheral nerve. Treatment of these syndromes can be difficult. Drugs that modulate various parts of the nociceptive system, such as gabapentin, carbamazepine or tricyclic antidepressants,

may help. Localised treatment (topical treatment or nerve blocks) sometimes succeeds but may increase the sensory deficit and worsen the situation. Electrical stimulation has occasionally proved successful.

Abnormal movements

Disorders of movement lead to either extra, unwanted movement (hyperkinetic disorders) or too little movement (hypokinetic disorders) (Box 28.15). In either case, the lesion often localises to the basal ganglia, although some tremors are related to cerebellar or brainstem disturbance. Functional movement disorders are common and may mimic all of the organic syndromes below. The most important hypokinetic disorder is Parkinson's disease. Parkinsonism is a clinical description of a collection of symptoms, including tremor, bradykinesia and rigidity. While the history is always important, observation is clearly vital; much of the skill in diagnosing movement disorders lies in pattern recognition. Once it is established whether the problem is hypo- or hyperkinetic, the next task is to categorise the movements further, accepting that there is often overlap. Videoing the movements (with the patient's consent), so that they can be shown to a movement disorder expert, may provide a quick diagnosis in cases of uncertainty.

Tremor

Tremor is caused by alternating agonist/antagonist muscle contractions and produces a rhythmical oscillation of the body part affected. In the assessment of tremor, the position, body part affected, frequency and amplitude should be considered, as these provide diagnostic clues (Box 28.16).

Other hyperkinetic syndromes

Non-rhythmic involuntary movements include chorea, athetosis, ballism, dystonia, myoclonus and tics. They are categorised by clinical appearance, and coexistence and overlap are common, such as in choreoathetosis.

28

Chorea

Chorea (from the Greek word 'dance') refers to abrupt, brief, irregular, purposeless involuntary movements, appearing fidgety and clumsy and affecting different areas. They suggest disease in the caudate nucleus (as in Huntington's disease) and are a common complication of levodopa treatment for Parkinson's disease. Other causes are shown in Box 28.17.

Athetosis

Slower, writhing movements of the limbs are often combined with chorea and have similar causes.

Ballism

This more dramatic form of chorea causes often violent flinging movements of one limb (monoballism) or one side of the body (hemiballism). The lesion localises to the contralateral subthalamic nucleus and the most common cause is stroke.

Dystonia

Sustained involuntary muscle contraction causes abnormal postures or movement. It may be generalised (usually in childhood-onset genetic syndromes) or, more commonly, focal/segmental (such as in torticollis, when the head is twisted repeatedly to one side). Some dystonias occur only with specific tasks, such as writer's cramp or other occupational 'cramps'. Dystonic tremor is associated, is asymmetrical and of large amplitude.

i 28.15 Movement disorders

Description	Features	Examples
Hypokinetic disorders		
Parkinsonism	Akinesia	Idiopathic Parkinson's disease
	Rigidity	Other degenerative syndromes
	Tremor	Drug-induced
	Loss of postural reflexes	(See Box 28.51)
	Other features depending on cause	
Catatonia	Mutism	Usually psychiatric; if neurological, is most commonly of vascular origin
	Sustained posturing and waxy flexibility	
Hyperkinetic disorders		
Tremor	Rhythmical oscillation of body part (see Box 28.16)	Essential tremor
		Parkinson's disease
		Drug-induced
Chorea	Abrupt, brief, irregular, involuntary movements	Huntington's disease
		Drug-induced
Tics	Stereotyped, repetitive movements, briefly suppressible	Tourette syndrome
Myoclonus	Shock-like muscle jerks	Epilepsy
		Hypnic jerks
		Focal cortical disease
Dystonia	Sustained muscle contraction causing abnormal postures ± tremor	Genetic
		Generalised dystonic syndromes
		Focal dystonias in adults (e.g. torticollis)
Others	Various	Paroxysmal hyperkinetic dyskinesias
		Hemifacial spasm
		Tardive syndromes

i 28.17 Causes of chorea

Hereditary

- Huntington's disease (HD) and HD-like syndromes
- Wilson's disease
- Neuroacanthocytosis
- Dentato-rubro-pallidoluysian atrophy
- Benign hereditary chorea
- Paroxysmal dyskinesias

Cerebral birth injury (including kernicterus)

Cerebral trauma

Drugs

- Levodopa (long-term with Parkinson's disease)
- Antipsychotics
- Antiepileptics
- Oral contraceptive

Metabolic

- Disorders affecting thyroid, parathyroid, glucose, sodium, calcium and magnesium balance
- Pregnancy

Autoimmune

- Post-streptococcal (Sydenham's chorea)
- Antiphospholipid antibody syndrome
- Autoimmune encephalitis
- Systemic lupus erythematosus

Structural lesions of basal ganglia (usually caudate)

- Vascular
- Demyelination
- Brain tumour
- Infection

i 28.16 Causes and characteristics of tremors

	Body part affected	Position	Frequency	Amplitude	Character
Physiological	Both arms > legs	Posture, movement	High	Small (fine)	Enhanced by anxiety, emotion, drugs, toxins
Parkinsonism	Unilateral or asymmetrical Arm > leg, chin, never head	Rest Postural and re-emergent may occur	Low (3–4 Hz)	Moderate	Typically pill-rolling, thumb and index finger, other features of parkinsonism
Essential tremor	Bilateral arms, head	Movement	High (8–10 Hz)	Low to moderate	Family history; 50% respond to alcohol
Dystonic	Head, arms, legs	Posture	Variable	Variable	Other features of dystonia, often jerky tremors
Functional	Any	Any	Variable	Variable	Distractible

Myoclonus

Myoclonus consists of brief, isolated, random jerks of muscle groups. This is physiological at the onset of sleep (hypnic jerks). Similarly, a myoclonic jerk is a component of the normal startle response, which may be exaggerated in some rare (mostly genetic) disorders. Myoclonus may occur in disorders of the cerebral cortex, such as some forms of epilepsy. Alternatively, myoclonus can arise from subcortical structures or, more rarely, from segments of the spinal cord.

Tics

Tics are stereotyped repetitive movements, such as blinking, winking, head shaking or shoulder shrugging. Unlike dyskinesias, the patient may be able to suppress them, although only for a short time. Isolated tics are common in childhood and usually disappear. Tourette syndrome is defined by the presence of multiple motor and vocal tics that may evolve over time; it is frequently associated with psychiatric disease, including obsessive compulsions, depression, self-harm or attention deficit disorder. Tics may also occur in Huntington's and Wilson's diseases, or after streptococcal infection.

Abnormal perception

The parietal lobes are involved in the higher processing and integration of primary sensory information. This takes place in areas referred to as 'association' cortex, damage to which gives rise to sensory (including visual) inattention, disorders of spatial perception and disruption of spatially orientated behaviour, leading to apraxia's. Apraxia is the inability to perform complex, organised activity in the presence of normal basic motor, sensory and cerebellar function (after weakness, numbness and ataxia have been excluded as causes). Examples of complex motor activities include dressing, using cutlery and geographical orientation. Other abnormalities that can result from damage to the association cortex involve difficulty reading (dyslexia) or writing (dysgraphia), or the inability to recognise familiar objects (agnosia). The results of damage to particular lobes of the brain are given in Box 28.2.

Altered balance and vertigo

Balance is a complicated dynamic process that requires ongoing modification of both axial and limb muscles to compensate for the effects of gravity and alterations in body position and load (and hence centre of gravity) in order to prevent a person from falling. This requires input from a variety of sensory modalities (visual, vestibular and proprioceptive), processing by the cerebellum and brainstem, and output via a number of descending pathways (e.g. vestibulospinal, rubrospinal and reticulospinal tracts).

Disorders of balance can therefore arise from any part of this process. Disordered input (loss of vision, vestibular disorders or lack of joint position sense), processing (damage to vestibular nuclei or cerebellum) or motor function (spinal cord lesions, leg weakness of any cause) can all impair balance. The patient may complain of different symptoms, depending on the location of the lesion. For example, loss of joint position sense or cerebellar function may result in a sensation of unsteadiness, while damage to the vestibular nuclei or labyrinth may result in an illusion of movement, such as vertigo (see below). A careful history is vital. Since vision can often compensate for lack of joint position sense, patients with peripheral neuropathies or dorsal column loss will often find their problem more noticeable in the dark.

Examination of such patients may yield physical signs that again depend on the site of the lesion. Sensory abnormalities may be manifest as altered visual acuities or visual fields, possibly with abnormalities on fundoscopy, altered eye movements (including nystagmus, impaired vestibular function or lack of joint position sense. Disturbance of cerebellar function may be manifest as nystagmus, dysarthria or ataxia, or difficulty with gait (unsteadiness or inability to perform tandem gait; see

below). Leg weakness, if present, will be detectable on examination of the limbs.

Vertigo

Vertigo is defined as an abnormal perception of movement of the environment or self, and occurs because of conflicting visual, proprioceptive and vestibular information about a person's position in space. Vertigo commonly arises from imbalance of vestibular input and is within the experience of most people, since this is the 'dizziness' that occurs after someone has spun round vigorously and then stops. Bilateral labyrinthine dysfunction often causes some unsteadiness. Labyrinthine vertigo usually lasts days at a time, though it may recur, while vertigo arising from central (brainstem) disorders is often persistent and accompanied by other brainstem signs. Benign paroxysmal positional vertigo lasts a few seconds on head movement. A careful history will reveal the likely cause in most patients.

Abnormal gait

Many neurological disorders can affect gait. Observing patients as they walk into the consulting room can be very informative, although formal examination is also important. Neurogenic gait disorders need to be distinguished from those due to skeletal abnormalities, usually characterised by pain producing an antalgic gait, or limp. Gait alteration incompatible with any anatomical or physiological deficit may be due to functional disorders.

Pyramidal gait

Upper motor neuron lesions cause characteristic extension of the affected leg. The resultant tendency for the toes to strike the ground on walking requires the leg to swing outwards at the hip (circumduction). Nevertheless, a shoe on the affected side worn down at the toes may provide evidence of this type of gait. In hemiplegia, the asymmetry between affected and normal sides is obvious on walking, but in paraparesis both lower limbs swing slowly from the hips in extension and are dragged stiffly over the ground – described as 'walking in mud'.

Foot drop

In normal walking, the heel is the first part of the foot to hit the ground. A lower motor neuron lesion affecting the leg will cause weakness of ankle dorsiflexion, resulting in a less controlled descent of the foot, which makes a slapping noise as it hits the ground. In severe cases, the foot will have to be lifted higher at the knee to allow room for the inadequately dorsiflexed foot to swing through, resulting in a high-stepping gait.

Myopathic gait

During walking, alternating transfer of the body's weight through each leg requires adequate hip abduction. In proximal muscle weakness, usually caused by muscle disease, the hips are not properly fixed by these muscles and trunk movements are exaggerated, producing a rolling or waddling gait.

Ataxic gait

An ataxic gait can result from lesions in the cerebellum, vestibular apparatus or peripheral nerves. Patients with lesions of the central portion of the cerebellum (the vermis) walk with a characteristic broad-based gait 'as if drunk' (cerebellar function is particularly sensitive to alcohol). Patients with acute vestibular disturbances walk similarly but the accompanying vertigo is characteristic. Inability to walk heel to toe may be the only sign of less severe cerebellar dysfunction.

Proprioceptive defects can also cause an ataxic gait. The impairment of joint position sense makes walking unreliable, especially in poor light. The feet tend to be placed on the ground with greater emphasis, presumably to enhance proprioceptive input, resulting in a 'stamping' gait.

28

Apraxic gait

In an apraxic gait, power, cerebellar function and proprioception are normal on examination of the legs. The patient may be able to carry out complex motor tasks (e.g. bicycling motion) while recumbent and yet cannot formulate the motor act of walking. In this higher cerebral dysfunction, the feet appear stuck to the floor and the patient cannot walk. Gait apraxia is a sign of diffuse bilateral hemisphere disease (such as normal pressure hydrocephalus) or diffuse frontal lobe disease.

Marche à petits pas

This gait is characterised by small, slow steps and marked instability. It differs from the festination found in Parkinson's disease (see below), in that it lacks increasing pace and freezing. The usual cause is small-vessel cerebrovascular disease and there may be accompanying bilateral upper motor neuron signs.

Extrapyramidal gait

The rigidity and bradykinesia of basal ganglia dysfunction lead to a stooped posture and characteristic gait difficulties, with problems initiating walking and controlling the pace of the gait. Patients may become stuck while trying to start walking or when walking through doorways ('freezing'). The centre of gravity will be moved forwards to aid propulsion, which, with poor axial control, can lead to an accelerating pace of shuffling and difficulty stopping. This produces the festinant gait: initial stuttering steps that quickly increase in frequency while decreasing in length.

Abnormal speech and language

Speech disturbance may be isolated to disruption of sound output (dysarthria) or may involve language disturbance (dysphasia). Dysphonia (reduction in the sound/volume) is usually due to mechanical laryngeal disruption, whereas dysarthria is more typically neurological in origin. Dysphasia is always neurological and localises to the dominant cerebral hemisphere (usually left, regardless of handedness). Combinations of speech and swallowing problems are explained below.

Dysphonia

Dysphonia describes hoarse or whispered speech. The most common cause is laryngitis, but dysphonia can also result from a lesion of the 10th cranial nerve or disease of the vocal cords, including laryngeal dystonia. Parkinsonism may cause hypophonia with marked reduction in speech volume, often in association with dysarthria, making speech difficult to understand.

Dysarthria

Dysarthria is characterised by poorly articulated or slurred speech and can occur in association with lesions of the cerebellum, brainstem and lower cranial nerves, as well as in myasthenia or myopathic disease. Language function is not affected. The quality of the speech tends to differ, depending on the cause, but it can be very difficult to distinguish the different types clinically (Box 28.18). Dysarthria is discussed further in the section on bulbar symptoms below.

Dysphasia

Dysphasia (or aphasia) is a disorder of the language content of speech. It can occur with lesions over a wide area of the dominant hemisphere (Fig. 28.19). Dysphasia may be categorised according to whether the speech output is fluent or non-fluent. Fluent aphasias, also called receptive aphasias, are impairments related mostly to the input or reception of language, with difficulties either in auditory verbal comprehension or in the repetition of words, phrases or sentences spoken by others. Speech is easy and fluent but there are difficulties related to the output of language as well, such as paraphasia (either substitution of similar-sounding non-words, or incorrect words) and neologisms (non-existent words).

Non-fluent aphasias, also called expressive aphasias, are difficulties in articulating, but in most cases there is relatively good auditory verbal comprehension. Examples include Broca aphasia (associated with pathologies in the inferior frontal region), transcortical motor aphasia and global aphasia.

'Pure' aphasias are selective impairments in reading, writing or the recognition of words. These disorders may be quite selective. For example, a person is able to read but not write, or is able to write but not read. Examples include pure alexia, agraphia and pure word deafness.

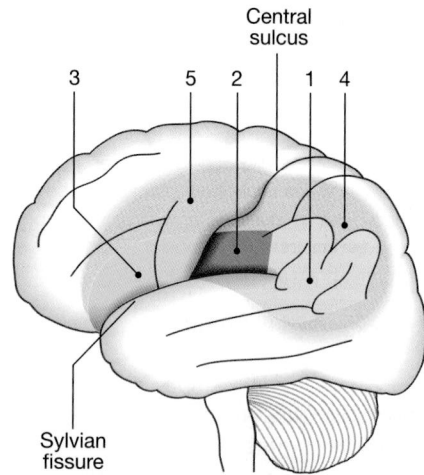

Fig. 28.19 Classification of cortical speech problems. (1) Wernicke's aphasia: fluent dysphasia with poor comprehension and poor repetition. (2) Conduction aphasia: fluent aphasia with good comprehension and poor repetition. (3) Broca's aphasia: non-fluent aphasia with good comprehension and poor repetition. (4) Transcortical sensory aphasia: fluent aphasia with poor comprehension and good repetition. (5) Transcortical motor aphasia: non-fluent aphasia with good comprehension and good repetition. Large lesions affecting all of regions 1–5 cause global aphasia.

28.18 Causes of dysarthria			
Type	Site	Characteristics	Associated features
Myopathic	Muscles of speech	Indistinct, poor articulation	Weakness of face, tongue and neck
Myasthenic	Motor end plate	Indistinct with fatigue and dysphonia Fluctuating severity	Ptosis, diplopia, facial and neck weakness
Bulbar	Brainstem	Indistinct, slurred, often nasal	Dysphagia, diplopia, ataxia
'Scanning'	Cerebellum	Slurred, impaired timing and cadence, 'sing-song'	Ataxia of limbs and gait, tremor of head/limbs Nystagmus
Spastic ('pseudo-bulbar')	Pyramidal tracts	Indistinct, nasal tone, mumbling	Poor rapid tongue movements, increased reflexes and jaw jerk
Parkinsonian	Basal ganglia	Indistinct, rapid, stammering, quiet	Tremor, rigidity, slow shuffling gait
Dystonic	Basal ganglia	Strained, slow, high-pitched	Dystonia, athetosis

Dysphasia (a focal symptom) is frequently misinterpreted as disorientation (which is non-focal) and it is important always to consider dysphasia as an alternative explanation for the apparently 'confused' patient. Dysphasia can be misheard/misspelt as dysphagia, and for this reason some prefer to use 'aphasia' to avoid confusion.

Disturbance of smell

Symptomatic olfactory loss is most commonly due to local causes (nasal obstruction) but may follow head injury. Hyposmia may predate motor symptoms in Parkinson's disease by many years, although it is rarely noticed by the patient. Frontal lobe lesions are a rare cause. Positive olfactory symptoms may arise in Alzheimer's disease or epilepsy.

Visual disturbance and ocular abnormalities

Disturbances of vision may be due to primary ocular disease or to disorders of the central connections and visual cortex. Visual symptoms are usually negative (loss of vision) but sometimes positive, most commonly in migraine. Eye movements may be disturbed, giving rise to double vision (diplopia) or blurred vision. Loss of vision is also discussed on page 1224.

Visual loss

Visual loss can occur as the result of lesions in any areas between the retina and the visual cortex. Patterns of visual field loss are explained by the anatomy of the visual pathways (see Fig. 28.7). Associated clinical manifestations are described in Box 30.8. Visual symptoms affecting one eye only are due to lesions anterior to the optic chiasm.

Transient visual loss is quite common and sudden-onset visual loss lasting less than 15 minutes is likely to have a vascular origin. It may be difficult to know whether the visual loss was monocular (carotid circulation) or binocular (vertebrobasilar circulation), and it is important to ask if the patient tried closing each eye in turn to see whether the symptom affected one eye or both. Visual field testing is an important part of the examination, either at the bedside or formally with perimetry. Field defects become more symmetrical (congruous), the closer the lesion comes to the visual cortex.

Migrainous visual symptoms are very common and, when associated with typical headache and other migraine features, rarely pose a diagnostic challenge. They may occur in isolation, however, making distinction from TIA difficult, but TIAs typically cause negative (blindness) symptoms, whereas migraine causes positive phenomena (see below). TIAs often last for a shorter time (a few minutes), compared to the 10–60-minute duration of migraine aura, and have an abrupt onset and end, unlike the gradual evolution of a migraine aura.

Positive visual phenomena

The most common cause is migraine; patients may describe silvery zigzag lines (fortification spectra) or flashing coloured lights (teichopsia), usually preceding the headache. Simple flashes of light (phosphenes) may indicate damage to the retina (e.g. detachment) or to the primary visual cortex. Formed visual hallucinations may be caused by drugs or may be due to epilepsy or 'release phenomena' in a blind visual field (Charles Bonnet syndrome).

Double vision

Diplopia arises from misalignment of the eyes, meaning that the image is not projected to the same points on the two retinas. At its most subtle it may be reported as blurred rather than double vision. Monocular diplopia indicates ocular disease, while binocular diplopia suggests a neurological cause. Closing either eye in turn will abort binocular diplopia. Once the presence of binocular diplopia is confirmed, it should be established whether the diplopia is maximal in any particular direction of gaze, whether the images are separated horizontally or vertically, and whether there are any associated symptoms or signs, such as ptosis or pupillary disturbance.

Binocular diplopia may result from central disorders or from disturbance of the ocular motor nerves, muscles or the neuromuscular junction (see Fig. 28.8). The pattern of double vision, along with any associated features, usually allows the clinician to infer which nerves/muscles are affected, while the mode of onset and other features (e.g. fatigability in myasthenia) provide further clues to the cause.

The causes of ocular motor nerve palsies are listed in Box 28.19. Examination findings are illustrated in Figure 28.20.

i 28.19 Common causes of damage to cranial nerves 3, 4 and 6			
Site	Common pathology	Nerve(s) involved	Associated features
Brainstem	Infarction	3 (mid-brain)	Contralateral pyramidal signs
	Haemorrhage	6 (ponto-medullary junction)	Ipsilateral lower motor neuron facial palsy
	Demyelination		Other brainstem/cerebellar signs
	Intrinsic tumour		
Intrameningeal	Meningitis (infective/malignant)	3, 4 and/or 6	Meningism, features of primary disease course
	Raised intracranial pressure	6	Papilloedema
		3 (uncal herniation)	Features of space-occupying lesion
	Aneurysms	3 (posterior communicating artery)	Pain
		6 (basilar artery)	Features of subarachnoid haemorrhage
	Cerebello-pontine angle tumour	6	8, 7, 5 nerve lesions (order of likelihood)
			Ipsilateral cerebellar signs
	Trauma	3, 4 and/or 6	Other features of trauma
Cavernous sinus	Infection/thrombosis	3, 4 and/or 6	May be 5th nerve involvement also
	Carotid artery aneurysm		Pupil may be fixed, mid-position
	Caroticocavernous fistula		(Sympathetic plexus on carotid may also be affected)
Superior orbital fissure	Tumour (e.g. sphenoid wing meningioma)	3, 4 and/or 6	May be proptosis, chemosis
	Granuloma		
Orbit	Vascular (e.g. diabetes, vasculitis)	3, 4 and/or 6	Pain
	Infections		Pupil often spared in vascular 3rd nerve palsy
	Tumour		
	Granuloma		
	Trauma		

28

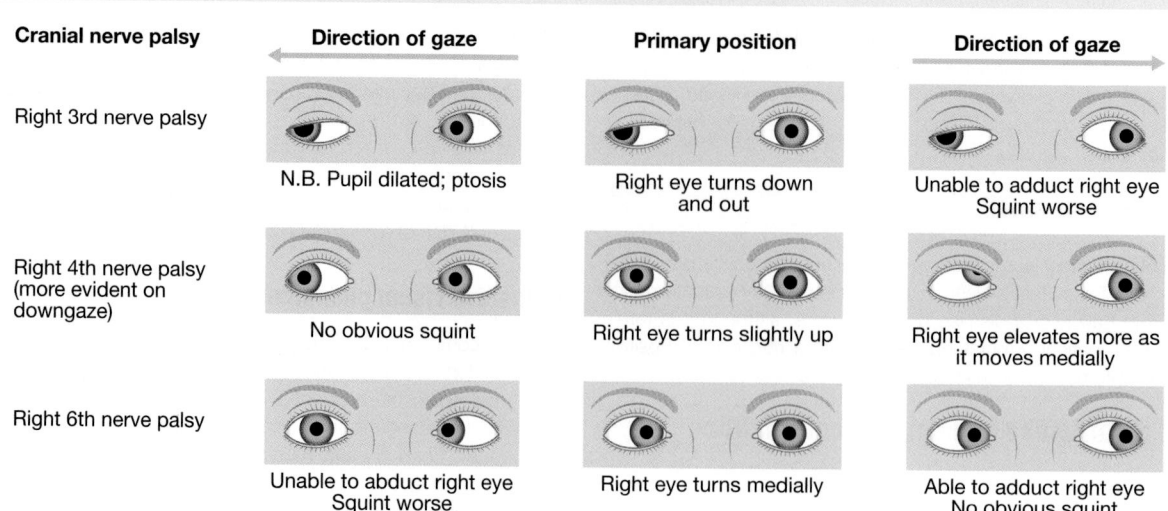

Fig. 28.20 Examination findings in 3rd, 4th and 6th nerve palsy. Diplopia tends to be more obvious on lateral gaze compared to primary position.

Nystagmus

Nystagmus describes a repetitive to-and-fro movement of the eyes. In central lesions, the slow drifts are the primary abnormal movement, each followed by fast (corrective) phases. Nystagmus occurs because the control systems of the eyes are defective, causing them to drift off target; corrections then become necessary to return fixation to the object of interest, causing nystagmus. The direction of the fast phase is usually designated as the direction of the nystagmus because it is easier to see. Nystagmus may be horizontal, vertical or torsional, and usually involves both eyes synchronously. It may be a physiological phenomenon in response to sustained vestibular stimulation or movement of the visual world (optokinetic nystagmus). There are many causes of pathological nystagmus, the most common sites of lesions being the vestibular system, brainstem and cerebellum.

The brainstem and the cerebellum are involved in maintaining eccentric positions of gaze. Lesions will therefore allow the eyes to drift back in towards primary position, producing nystagmus with fast component beats in the direction of gaze (gaze-evoked nystagmus). This is the most common type of 'central' nystagmus; it is most commonly bidirectional and not usually accompanied by vertigo. Other signs of brainstem dysfunction may be evident. Brainstem disease may also cause vertical nystagmus.

Unilateral cerebellar lesions may result in gaze-evoked nystagmus when looking in the direction of the lesion, where the fast phases are directed towards the side of the lesion. Cerebellar hemisphere lesions also cause 'ocular dysmetria', an overshoot of target-directed, fast eye movements (saccades) resembling 'past-pointing' in limbs.

In vestibular lesions, damage to one of the horizontal canals or its connections will allow the tonic output from the healthy contralateral side to cause the eyes to drift towards the side of the lesion. This elicits recurrent compensatory fast movements away from the side of the lesion, manifest as unidirectional horizontal nystagmus. Vertical and torsional components can be seen with damage to other parts of the vestibular apparatus. The nystagmus of peripheral labyrinthine lesions is accompanied by vertigo and usually by nausea, vomiting and unsteadiness, but as the CNS habituates, the nystagmus disappears (fatigues) quite quickly. Central vestibular nystagmus is more persistent.

Nystagmus also occurs as a consequence of drug toxicity and nutritional deficiency (e.g. thiamin). The severity is variable, and it may or may not result in visual degradation, though it may be associated with a sensation of movement of the visual world (oscillopsia). Nystagmus may occur as a congenital phenomenon, in which case both phases are equal and 'pendular', rather than having alternating fast and slow components.

Ptosis

Various disorders may cause drooping of the eyelids (ptosis) and these are listed in Box 28.20 and shown on Figure 28.21.

Abnormal pupillary responses

Abnormal pupillary responses may arise from lesions at several points between the retina and brainstem. Lesions of the oculomotor nerve, ciliary ganglion and sympathetic supply produce characteristic ipsilateral disorders of pupillary function. 'Afferent' defects result from damage to an optic nerve, impairing the direct response of a pupil to light, although leaving the consensual response from stimulation of the normal eye intact. Structural damage to the iris itself can also result in pupillary abnormalities. Causes are given in Box 28.21. An example is shown in Figure 28.22.

Papilloedema

There are several causes of swelling of the optic disc but the term 'papilloedema' is reserved for swelling secondary to raised intracranial pressure, when obstructed axoplasmic flow from retinal ganglion cells in swollen nerve fibres, which in turn cause capillary and venous congestion, producing papilloedema. Lack of papilloedema never excludes raised intracranial pressure. Optic disc swelling and papilloedema are also discussed on page 1226.

Optic atrophy

See Chapter 30.

Hearing disturbance

Each cochlear organ has bilateral cortical representation, so unilateral hearing loss is a result of peripheral organ damage. Bilateral hearing dysfunction is usual and is most commonly due to age-related degeneration or noise damage, although infection and drugs (particularly diuretics and aminoglycoside antibiotics) can be a primary cause. Prominent deafness may suggest a mitochondrial disorder (see Box 28.92).

Bulbar symptoms – dysphagia and dysarthria

Swallowing is a complex activity involving the coordinated action of lips, tongue, soft palate, pharynx and larynx, which are innervated by cranial nerves 7, 9, 10, 11 and 12. Structural causes of dysphagia are considered on page 795. Neurological mechanisms are vulnerable to damage

i 28.20 Common causes of ptosis

Mechanism	Causes	Associated clinical features
3rd nerve palsy	Isolated palsy (see Box 28.19) Central/supranuclear lesion	Ptosis is usually complete Extraocular muscle palsy (eye 'down and out') Depending on site of lesion, other cranial nerve palsies (e.g. 4, 5 and 6) or contralateral upper motor neuron signs
Sympathetic lesion (Horner syndrome: see Fig. 28.22)	Central (hypothalamus/brainstem) Peripheral (lung apex, carotid artery pathology) Idiopathic	Ptosis is partial Lack of sweating on affected side Depending on site of lesion, brainstem signs, signs of apical lung/brachial plexus disease, or ipsilateral carotid artery stroke
Myopathic	Myasthenia gravis Dystrophia myotonica	Extraocular muscle palsies Usually bilateral More widespread muscle weakness, with fatigability in myasthenia Progressive external ophthalmoplegia Other characteristic features of individual causes
Other	Functional ptosis Pseudo-ptosis (e.g. blepharospasm) Local orbital/lid disease Age-related levator dehiscence	Resistance to eye opening Eyebrows depressed rather than raised May be local orbital abnormality

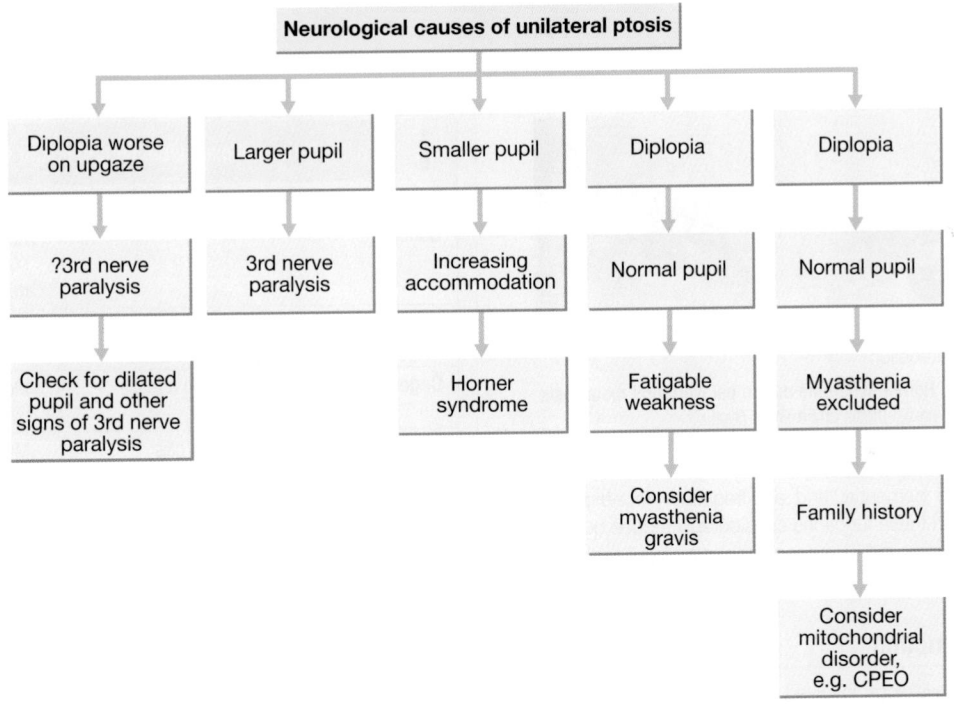

Fig. 28.21 Differential diagnosis of unilateral ptosis. (CPEO = chronic progressive external ophthalmoplegia)

28

at different points, resulting in dysphagia that is usually accompanied by dysarthria. Tempo is again crucial: acute onset of dysphagia may occur as a result of brainstem stroke or a rapidly developing neuropathy, such as Guillain–Barré syndrome or diphtheria. Intermittent fatigable muscle weakness (including dysphagia) would suggest myasthenia gravis. Dysphagia developing over weeks or months may be seen in motor neuron disease, basal meningitis and inflammatory brainstem disease. More slowly developing dysphagia suggests a myopathy or possibly a brainstem or skull-base tumour.

Pathologies affecting lower cranial nerves (9, 10, 11 and 12) frequently manifest bilaterally, producing dysphagia and dysarthria. The term 'bulbar palsy' is used to describe lower motor neuron lesions, either within the medulla or outside the brainstem. The tongue may be wasted and fasciculating, and palatal movement is reduced.

Upper motor neuron innervation of swallowing is bilateral, so persistent dysphagia is unusual with a unilateral upper motor lesion (the exception being in the acute stages of, for example, a hemispheric stroke). Widespread lesions above the medulla will cause upper motor neuron bulbar paralysis, known as 'pseudobulbar palsy'. Here the tongue is small and contracted, and moves slowly; the jaw jerk is brisk, and there may be associated emotional variability. Causes of these are shown in Box 28.22.

Bladder, bowel and sexual disturbance

While isolated disturbances of bladder, bowel and sexual function are rarely the sole presenting features of neurological disease, they are common complications of many chronic disorders such as multiple

i **28.21 Pupillary disorders**

Disorder	Cause	Ophthalmological features	Associated features
3rd nerve palsy	See Box 28.20	Dilated pupil (especially with external compression) Extraocular muscle palsy (eye is typically 'down and out') Complete ptosis	Other features of 3rd nerve palsy (see Box 28.20)
Horner syndrome (see Fig. 28.22)	Lesion to sympathetic supply	Small pupil Partial ptosis Iris heterochromia (if congenital)	Ipsilateral failure of sweating (anhidrosis)
Holmes–Adie syndrome (tonic pupil)	Lesion of ciliary ganglion (usually idiopathic)	Dilated pupil Light–near dissociation (accommodate but do not react to light) Vermiform movement of iris during contraction Disturbance of accommodation	Generalised areflexia
Argyll Robertson pupil	Dorsal mid-brain lesion (syphilis or diabetes)	Small, irregular pupils Light–near dissociation	Other features of tabes dorsalis (Box 28.69)
Local pupillary damage	Trauma/inflammatory disease	Irregular pupils, often with adhesions to lens (synechiae) Variable degree of reactivity	Other features of trauma/underlying inflammatory disease (e.g. cataract, blindness etc.)
Relative afferent pupillary defect (Marcus Gunn pupil)	Damage to optic nerve	Pupils symmetrical – swinging torch test reveals dilatation in abnormal eye	Decreased visual acuity/colour vision Central scotoma Optic disc swelling or pallor

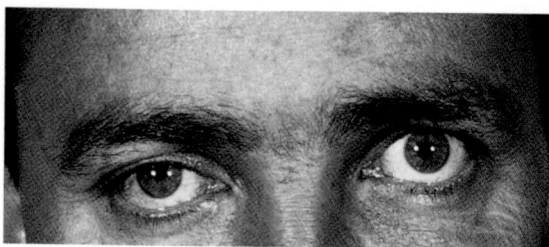

Fig. 28.22 Right-sided Horner syndrome due to paravertebral metastasis at T1. There is ipsilateral partial ptosis and a small pupil.

i **28.22 Causes of pseudobulbar and bulbar palsy**

Type	Pseudobulbar	Bulbar
Genetic	–	Kennedy's disease (X-linked bulbospinal neuronopathy)
Vascular	Bilateral hemisphere (lacunar) infarction	Medullary infarction (see Box 28.3)
Degenerative	Motor neuron disease	Motor neuron disease Syringobulbia
Inflammatory/ infective	Multiple sclerosis Cerebral vasculitis	Myasthenia Guillain–Barré syndrome Poliomyelitis Lyme disease Vasculitis
Neoplastic	High brainstem tumours	Brainstem glioma Malignant meningitis

sclerosis, stroke and dementia, and are frequently found post head injury. Abnormalities in these functions considerably reduce quality of life for patients. Incontinence and its management are discussed elsewhere (pp. 567, 833 and 1305).

Bladder dysfunction

The anatomy and physiology involved in controlling bladder functions are discussed in Chapter 18, but it is worth emphasising the role of the pontine micturition centre, which is itself under higher control via inputs from the pre-frontal cortex, mid-brain and hypothalamus.

In the absence of conscious control (e.g. in coma or dementia), distension of the bladder to near capacity evokes reflex detrusor contraction (analogous to the muscle stretch reflex), and reciprocal changes in sympathetic activation and relaxation of the distal sphincter result in coordinated bladder emptying.

Damage to the lower motor neuron pathways (the pelvic and pudendal nerves) produces a flaccid bladder and sphincter with overflow incontinence, often accompanied by loss of pudendal sensation. Such damage may be due to disease of the conus medullaris or sacral nerve roots, either within the dura (as in inflammatory or carcinomatous meningitis) or as they pass through the sacrum (trauma or malignancy), or due to damage to the nerves themselves in the pelvis (infection, haematoma, trauma or malignancy).

Damage to the pons or spinal cord results in an 'upper motor neuron' pattern of bladder dysfunction due to uncontrolled over-activity of

the parasympathetic supply. The bladder is small and highly sensitive to being stretched. This results in frequency, urgency and urge incontinence. Loss of the coordinating control of the pontine micturition centre will also result in the phenomenon of detrusor–sphincter dyssynergia, in which detrusor contraction and sphincter relaxation are not coordinated; the spastic bladder will often try to empty against a closed sphincter. This manifests as both urgency and an inability to pass urine, which is distressing and painful. The resultant incomplete bladder emptying predisposes to urinary infection, and the prolonged high intravesical pressure may result in obstructive uropathy and renal failure; post-micturition bladder ultrasound may confirm incomplete bladder emptying. More severe lesions of the spinal cord, as in spinal cord compression or trauma, can result in painless urinary retention as bladder sensation, normally carried in the lateral spinothalamic tracts, will be disrupted.

Damage to the frontal lobes gives rise to loss of awareness of bladder fullness and consequent incontinence. Coexisting cognitive impairment may result in inappropriate micturition. These features may be seen in hydrocephalus, frontal tumours, dementia and bifrontal subdural haematomas.

i	28.23 Neurogenic bladder: clinical features and treatment			
Type	Site of lesion	Result	Treatment
Atonic (lower motor neuron)	Sacral segments of cord (conus medullaris)	Loss of detrusor contraction	Intermittent self-catheterisation
	Sacral roots and nerves	Difficulty initiating micturition Bladder distension with overflow	In-dwelling catheterisation
Hypertonic (upper motor neuron)	Pyramidal tract in spinal cord or brainstem	Urgency with urge incontinence Bladder sphincter incoordination (dyssynergia)	Anticholinergics: Solifenacin Tolterodine Imipramine
		Incomplete bladder emptying	Intermittent self-catheterisation
Cortical	Post-central Pre-central Frontal	Loss of awareness of bladder fullness Difficulty initiating micturition Inappropriate micturition Loss of social control	Intermittent or in-dwelling catheterisation

When a patient presents with bladder symptoms, it is important to localise the lesion on the basis of history and examination, remembering that most bladder problems are not neurological unless there are overt neurological signs. Clinical features and management are summarised in Box 28.23.

Rectal dysfunction

The rectum has an excitatory cholinergic input from the parasympathetic sacral outflow, and inhibitory sympathetic supply similar to the bladder. Continence depends largely on skeletal muscle contraction in the puborectalis and pelvic floor muscles supplied by the pudendal nerves, as well as the internal and external anal sphincters. Damage to the autonomic components usually causes constipation (a common early symptom in Parkinson's disease) but diabetic neuropathy can be associated with diarrhoea. Lesions affecting the conus medullaris, the somatic S2–4 roots and the pudendal nerves may cause faecal incontinence.

Erectile failure and ejaculatory failure

These related functions are under autonomic control via the pelvic nerves (parasympathetic, S2–4) and hypogastric nerves (sympathetic, L1–2). Descending influences from the cerebrum are important for erection but it can occur as a reflex phenomenon in response to genital stimulation. Erection is largely parasympathetic and may be impaired by a number of drugs, including anticholinergic, antihypertensive and antidepressant agents. Sympathetic activity is important for ejaculation and may be inhibited by α-adrenoceptor antagonists (α-blockers).

Personality change

While this is often due to psychiatric illness, neurological conditions that alter the function of the frontal lobes can cause personality change and mood disorder (see Box 28.2). Personality change due to a frontal lobe disorder may occur as the result of structural damage due to stroke, trauma, tumour or hydrocephalus. The nature of any change may help localise the lesion.

Patients with mesial frontal lesions become increasingly withdrawn, unresponsive and mute (abulic), often in association with urinary incontinence, gait apraxia and an increase in tone known as 'gegenhalten' or paratonia, in which the patient varies the resistance to movement in proportion to the force exerted by the examiner.

Patients with lesions of the dorsolateral pre-frontal cortex develop a dysexecutive syndrome, which involves difficulties with speech, motor planning and organisation. Those with orbitofrontal lesions of the frontal lobes, in contrast, become disinhibited, displaying grandiosity or irresponsible behaviour. Memory is substantially intact but frontal release signs may emerge, such as a grasp reflex, palmomental response or

pout. Proximity to the olfactory bulb and tracts means that inferior frontal lobe tumours may be associated with anosmia.

Disturbance to the cortical areas responsible for speech or memory can result in changes that may be interpreted as changes in personality.

Sleep disturbance

Disturbances of sleep are common and are not usually due to neurological disease. Patients may complain of insomnia (difficulty sleeping), excessive daytime sleepiness, disturbed behaviour during night-time sleep, parasomnia (sleep walking and talking, or night terrors) or disturbing subjective experiences during sleep and/or its onset (nightmares, hypnagogic hallucinations, sleep paralysis). A careful history (from bed partner as well as patient) usually allows specific causes of sleep disturbance to be identified and these are discussed in more detail on page 1159.

Psychiatric disorders

Psychiatric disorders may cause or result from neurological problems. Care is needed in their identification, as effective management will help the underlying neurological illness.

Mood and sleep disturbance will exacerbate neurological symptoms, thus increasing disability. The best practitioners have the skill to carry the patient with them when describing the patterns of behaviour contributing to worsening symptoms.

Assessment to detect an underlying or exacerbating mood disorder is vital in all patients, ensuring that depression and anxiety are managed to minimise their secondary effects on neurological symptoms.

Headache syndromes

Acute management of headache is dealt with on page 186, but management of chronic, complex, or refractory headaches may require specialist input. Headaches may be classified as primary or secondary, depending on the underlying cause (see Box 9.13). Secondary headache may be due to structural, infective, inflammatory or vascular conditions, discussed later in this chapter. Primary headache syndromes are described here.

Tension-type headache

This is the most common type of headache and is experienced to some degree by the majority of the population.

Pathophysiology

Tension-type headache is incompletely understood, and some consider that it is simply a milder version of migraine; certainly, the original notion

28

that it is due primarily to muscle tension (hence the unsatisfactory name) has long since been dismissed. Anxiety about the headache itself may lead to continuation of symptoms, and patients may become convinced of a serious underlying condition.

Clinical features

The pain of tension headache is characterised as 'dull', 'tight' or like a 'pressure', and there may be a sensation of a band round the head or pressure at the vertex. It is of constant character and generalised, but often radiates forwards from the occipital region. It may be episodic or persistent, although the severity may vary, and there is no associated vomiting or photophobia. Tension-type headache is rarely disabling and patients appear well. The pain often progresses throughout the day. Tenderness may be present over the skull vault or in the occiput but is easily distinguished from the triggered pains of trigeminal neuralgia and the exquisite tenderness of temporal arteritis. Analgesics may be taken with chronic regularity, despite little effect, and may perpetuate the symptoms (see 'Medication overuse headache' below).

Management

Most benefit is derived from a careful assessment, followed by discussion of likely precipitants and reassurance that the prognosis is good. The concept of medication overuse headache needs careful explanation. An important therapeutic step is to allow patients to realise that their problem has been taken seriously and rigorously assessed. Physiotherapy (with muscle relaxation and stress management) may help and low-dose amitriptyline can provide benefit. Investigation is rarely required. The reassurance value of brain imaging needs careful assessment: the pick-up rate of structural abnormalities is exceedingly low, and significantly outweighed by the likelihood of identifying an incidental and irrelevant finding (e.g. an arachnoid cyst, Chiari I malformation or vascular abnormality). The value of such 'reassurance' is usually over-estimated by doctors and patients alike.

Migraine

Migraine usually appears before middle age, or occasionally in later life; it affects about 20% of females and 6% of males at some point in life. Migraine is usually readily identifiable from the history, although unusual variants can cause uncertainty.

Pathophysiology

The cause of migraine is unknown but there is increasing evidence that the aura (see below) is due to dysfunction of ion channels causing a spreading front of cortical depolarisation (excitation) followed by hyperpolarisation (depression of activity). This process (the 'spreading depression of Leão') spreads over the cortex at a rate of about 3 mm/min, corresponding to the aura's symptomatic spread. The headache phase is associated with vasodilatation of extracranial vessels and may be relayed by hypothalamic activity. Activation of the trigeminovascular system is probably important. A genetic contribution is implied by the frequently positive family history, and similar phenomena occurring in disorders such as CADASIL (cerebral autosomal dominant arteriopathy with subcortical infarcts and leukoencephalopathy) or mitochondrial disease (p. 1197). The female preponderance and the frequency of migraine attacks at certain points in the menstrual cycle also suggest hormonal influences. Oestrogen-containing oral contraception sometimes exacerbates migraine and increases the very small risk of stroke in patients who suffer from migraine with aura. Doctors and patients often over-estimate the role of dietary precipitants such as cheese, chocolate or red wine. When psychological factors contribute, the migraine attack often occurs after a period of stress, being more likely on Friday evening at the end of the working week or at the beginning of a holiday.

Clinical features

Some patients report a prodrome of malaise, irritability or behavioural change for some hours or days. Around 20% of patients experience

an aura and are said to have migraine with aura (previously known as classical migraine). The aura may manifest as almost any neurological symptom but is most often visual, consisting of fortification spectra, which are usually positive phenomena such as shimmering, silvery zigzag lines marching across the visual fields for up to 40 minutes, sometimes leaving a trail of temporary visual field loss (scotoma). Sensory symptoms characteristically spreading over 20–30 minutes, from one part of the body to another, are more common than motor ones, and language function can be affected, leading to similarities with TIA/stroke. Isolated aura may occur (i.e. the neurological symptoms are not followed by headache).

The 80% of patients with characteristic headache but no 'aura' are said to have migraine without aura (previously called 'common' migraine).

Migraine headache is usually severe and throbbing, with photophobia, phonophobia and vomiting lasting from 4 to 72 hours. Movement makes the pain worse and patients prefer to lie in a quiet, dark room.

In a small number of patients, the aura may persist, leaving more permanent neurological disturbance. This persistent migrainous aura may occur with or without evidence of brain infarction.

Management

Avoidance of identified triggers or exacerbating factors (such as the combined contraceptive pill) may prevent attacks. Treatment of an acute attack consists of simple analgesia with aspirin, paracetamol or non-steroidal anti-inflammatory agents. Nausea may require an antiemetic such as metoclopramide or domperidone. Severe attacks can be aborted by one of the 'triptans' (e.g. sumatriptan), which are potent 5-hydroxytryptamine (5-HT, serotonin) agonists. These can be administered via the oral, subcutaneous or nasal route. Caution is needed with ergotamine preparations because they may lead to dependence. Overuse of any analgesia, including triptans, may contribute to medication overuse headache.

If attacks are frequent (more than two per month), prophylaxis should be considered. Many drugs can be chosen but the most frequently used are vasoactive drugs (β-adrenoceptor antagonists (β-blockers), candesartan, lisinopril), antidepressants (amitriptyline, dosulepin) and antiepileptic drugs (topiramate). Consideration needs to be given to the teratogenicity of antiepileptic drugs in women of childbearing potential. Monoclonal antibodies to calcitonin gene-related peptide receptor are available for refractory migraine. Women with aura should avoid oestrogen treatment for either oral contraception or hormone replacement, although the increased risk of ischaemic stroke is minimal.

Medication overuse headache

With increasing availability of over-the-counter medication, headache syndromes perpetuated by analgesia intake are becoming much more common. Medication overuse headache (MOH) can complicate any headache syndrome but is especially common with migraine and chronic tension-type headache. The most frequent culprits are compound analgesics (particularly codeine and other opiate-containing preparations) and triptans, and MOH is usually associated with use on more than 10–15 days per month.

Management is by withdrawal of the responsible analgesics. Patients should be warned that the initial effect will be to exacerbate the headache, and migraine prophylactics may be helpful in reducing the rebound headaches. Relapse rates are high, and patients often need help and support in withdrawing from analgesia; a careful explanation of this paradoxical concept is vital.

Cluster headache

Cluster headaches (also known as migrainous neuralgia) are much less common than migraine. Unusually for headache syndromes, there is a significant male predominance and onset is usually in the third decade.

Pathophysiology

The cause is unknown but this type of headache differs from migraine in many ways, suggesting a different pathophysiological basis. Although uncommon, it is the most common of the trigeminal autonomic cephalalgia syndromes. Functional imaging studies have suggested abnormal hypothalamic activity. Patients are more often smokers with a higher than average alcohol consumption.

Clinical features

Cluster headache is strikingly periodic, featuring runs of identical headaches beginning at the same time for weeks at a stretch (the 'cluster'). Patients may experience either one or several attacks within a 24-hour period, and typically are awoken from sleep by symptoms ('alarm clock headache'). Cluster headache causes severe, unilateral periorbital pain with autonomic features, such as ipsilateral tearing, nasal congestion and conjunctival injection (occasionally with the other features of a Horner syndrome). The pain, though severe, is characteristically brief (30–90 minutes). In contrast to the behaviour of those with migraine, patients are highly agitated during the headache phase. The cluster period is typically a few weeks, followed by remission for months to years, but a small proportion do not experience remission.

Management

Acute attacks can usually be halted by subcutaneous injections of sumatriptan or inhalation of 100% oxygen. The brevity of the attack probably prevents other migraine therapies from being effective. Migraine prophylaxis is often ineffective too but attacks can be prevented in some patients by verapamil, sodium valproate, or short courses of oral glucocorticoids. Patients with severe debilitating clusters can be helped with lithium therapy, although this requires monitoring.

Trigeminal neuralgia

This is characterised by unilateral lancinating facial pain, most commonly involving the second and/or third divisions of the trigeminal nerve territory, usually in patients over the age of 50 years.

Pathophysiology

For most, trigeminal neuralgia remains an idiopathic condition but there is a suggestion that it may be due to an irritative lesion involving the trigeminal root zone, in some cases an aberrant loop of artery. Other compressive lesions, usually benign, are occasionally found. Trigeminal neuralgia associated with multiple sclerosis may result from a plaque of demyelination in the brainstem.

Clinical features

The pain is repetitive, severe and very brief (seconds or less). It may be triggered by touch, a cold wind or eating. Physical signs are usually absent, although the spasms may make the patient wince and sit silently (tic douloureux). There is a tendency for the condition to remit and relapse over many years. Rarely, there may be combined features of trigeminal neuralgia and cluster headache ('cluster–tic').

Management

The pain often responds to carbamazepine. It is wise to start with a low dose and increase gradually, according to effect. In patients who cannot tolerate carbamazepine, oxcarbazepine, gabapentin, pregabalin, amitriptyline or glucocorticoids may be effective alternatives, but if medication is ineffective or poorly tolerated, surgical treatment should be considered. Decompression of the vascular loop encroaching on the trigeminal root is often performed and may lead to pain relief in some cases. Otherwise, localised injection of alcohol or phenol into a peripheral branch of the nerve may be effective.

Headaches associated with specific activities

These usually affect men in their thirties and forties. Patients develop a sudden, severe headache with exertion, including sexual activity. There is usually no vomiting or neck stiffness, and the headache lasts less than 10–15 minutes, though a less severe dullness may persist for some hours. Subarachnoid haemorrhage needs to be excluded by CT and/or CSF examination (see Fig. 29.13) after a first event. The pathogenesis of these headaches is unknown. Although frightening, attacks are usually brief and patients may need only reassurance and simple analgesia for the residual headache. The syndrome may recur, and prevention may be necessary with propranolol or indometacin.

Other headache syndromes

A number of rare headache syndromes produce pains about the eye similar to cluster headaches (Box 28.24). These include chronic paroxysmal hemicrania and SUNCT (short-lasting unilateral neuralgiform headaches with conjunctival injection and tearing). The recognition of these syndromes is useful because they often respond to specific treatments such as indometacin.

28.24 Paroxysmal headaches				
Type	Character of pain	Duration	Location	Comment
Ice pick	Stabbing	Very brief (split-second)	Variable, usually temporoparietal	Benign, more common in migraine
Ice cream	Sharp, severe	30–120 secs	Bitemporal/occipital	Obvious trigger by cold stimuli
Exertional/sexual activity	Bursting, thunderclap	Severe for mins, then less severe for hours	Generalised	Subarachnoid haemorrhage needs to be excluded
Cough	Bursting	Secs to mins	Occipital or generalised	Intracranial pathology needs to be excluded (especially craniocervical junction)
Cluster headache (migrainous neuralgia)	Severe unilateral, with ptosis, tearing, conjunctival injection, unilateral nasal congestion	30–90 mins 1–3 times per day	Periorbital	Usually in men, occurring in clusters over weeks/months
Chronic paroxysmal hemicrania	Severe unilateral with cluster headache-like autonomic features (see above)	5–20 mins, frequently through day	Periorbital/temporal	Usually in women, responds to indometacin
SUNCT*	Severe, sharp, triggered by touch or neck movements	15–120 secs, repetitive through day	Periorbital	May respond to carbamazepine

*Short-lasting, unilateral, neuralgiform headache with conjunctival injection, tearing, rhinorrhoea and forehead sweating.

28

Functional neurological disorder

Many patients present with functional symptoms and some may have a functional neurological disorder (FND). FND (also known as functional neurological symptom disorder, dissociative neurological symptom disorder, or conversion disorder) is a disorder at the interface of neurology and psychiatry, reflecting function or dysfunction in the shared organ, the brain. The symptoms are involuntary and cause considerable disability. Core to the assessment and management of most patients is a diagnosis made on positive grounds, communicated to patients in a manner that contributes constructively to management.

Functional symptoms are not consistent with any other recognised neurological disease or disorder. The diagnosis depends on demonstrating internal inconsistency. The inconsistency will depend on the specific functional symptom. Functional symptoms include functional weakness, sensory disturbance, pain, movement disorders, dissociative attacks (also called non-epileptic attacks), visual symptoms, speech and cognitive symptoms. Examples of internal inconsistency include: weakness of hip extension when the patient tries to extend the hip, which is overcome when the opposite hip is flexed against resistance (Hoover's sign); marked weakness of the legs on examination in a patient able to stand and walk; a detailed description of specific events of memory loss; and expressive dysphasia with retained written language. Other findings may include: non-anatomical sensory loss, abnormal movements that are distractable, and dissociative or non-epileptic attacks occurring in the absence of concomitant EEG abnormality. Tiredness, poor concentration and sleep disturbance are also common.

Many but not all patients with FND have predisposing and perpetuating factors (Box 28.25) that may include anxiety, depression, post-traumatic stress disorder, a history of abuse or aversive events. There may be a precipitating event, which may at times appear minor in comparison to the range and severity of the patient's symptoms.

The approach to the patient with FND or functional symptoms should ideally include:

- a detailed history exploring all symptoms
- examination looking for positive findings, e.g. Hoover's sign
- review of past medical records, which often contain functional symptoms in other organ systems, e.g. irritable bowel syndrome, globus, non-cardiac chest pain
- rapid investigation to exclude a structural cause
- and a clear, constructive explanation of the diagnosis based on positive findings rather than the rather unhelpful 'medically unexplained symptom' approach of the past.

There are several useful websites that provide patients with additional information and advice (p. XXX). For many patients understanding their symptoms and the condition will be sufficient, others may require additional multidisciplinary support and treatment from a range of professionals including: physiotherapy, occupational and speech therapy, neurology and neuropsychiatry/psychiatry. Treatment may include neurophysiotherapy, use of antidepressant medication (although not all patients are depressed) and cognitive behavioural therapy. The diagnosis should not be made simply because the patient's presentation is unusual. A diagnosis of FND should be based on an appropriate history, examination and normal relevant findings on investigation.

Factitious disorders and malingering are not the same as FND. In the absence of clear objective evidence, e.g. witnessing a patient tampering with tests, diagnosis of these disorders should best be left to psychiatrists

Epilepsy

A seizure can be defined as the occurrence of signs and/or symptoms due to abnormal, excessive or synchronous neuronal activity in the brain. The lifetime risk of an isolated seizure is about 5%, although incidence is highest at the extremes of age. Epilepsy is the tendency to have unprovoked seizures. While the prevalence of active epilepsy in European countries is about 0.5%, this figure varies globally and can be influenced by the prevalence of parasitic illnesses such as cysticercosis. A recent change in definition allows the diagnosis of epilepsy to be made after a single seizure with a high risk of recurrence (e.g. a single seizure in the presence of a cortical lesion). Such changes may lead to an observed increase in epilepsy incidence.

Historical terms such as 'grand mal' (implying tonic–clonic seizures) and 'petit mal' (intended originally to mean 'absence seizures' but commonly misused to describe 'anything other than grand mal') have been superseded. Subsequent revisions, including terms such as 'complex partial' and 'simple partial', have been imprecise and carry little information about underlying pathology, treatment or prognosis. The modern equivalents for these terms will be given below, but it is preferable to adhere to the 2017 iteration of the International League Against Epilepsy's classification (Box 28.26).

Pathophysiology

To function normally, the brain must maintain a continual balance between excitation and inhibition, remaining responsive to the environment while avoiding continued unrestrained spontaneous activity. The inhibitory transmitter gamma-aminobutyric acid (GABA) is particularly important, acting on ion channels to enhance chloride inflow and reducing the chances of action potential formation. Excitatory amino acids (glutamate and aspartate) allow influx of sodium and calcium, producing the opposite effect. It is likely that many seizures result from an imbalance between this excitation and inhibition. Intracellular recordings during seizures demonstrate a paroxysmal depolarisation shift in neuronal membrane potential, an upshift in internal potential predisposing to recurrent action potentials. In vivo, epileptic cortex shows repetitive discharges involving large groups of neurons.

Focal epilepsy

Seizures may be related to a localised disturbance in the cortex, becoming manifest in the first instance as focal seizures. Any disturbance of cortical architecture and function can precipitate this, whether focal infection, tumour, hamartoma or trauma-related scarring. If focal seizures remain localised, the symptoms experienced depend on which cortical area is affected. If areas in the temporal lobes become involved, then awareness of the environment becomes impaired but without associated tonic–clonic movements. When both hemispheres become involved, the seizure becomes generalised (Fig. 28.23).

Generalised epilepsies

The new terminology is genetic generalised epilepsies (GGEs) (previously idiopathic generalised epilepsies, and many prefer to still use this term) to reflect their likely cause. These seizures are generalised at onset, abnormal activity probably originating in the central mechanisms controlling cortical activation (see Fig. 28.23) and spreading rapidly. This group constitutes around 30% of all epilepsy and is likely to reflect widespread

---

i 28.25 Clinical features suggestive of functional disorder

- Inconsistent examination findings (e.g. Hoover's sign)
- Situational provocation of events (e.g. in medical settings)
- Associated mental health disorders:
    - Anxiety
    - Depression
- Lack of anatomical coherence to neurological symptoms
- Florid or bizarre descriptions of individual symptoms
- History of multiple other systemic symptoms inadequately explained by disease (asthma/breathlessness, fatigue, pain, gastrointestinal symptoms)

28.26 Classification of seizures (2017 International League Against Epilepsy classification)

Generalised onset

Motor

- Tonic–clonic (in any combination)
- Clonic
- Tonic
- Myoclonic
- Myoclonic–tonic–clonic
- Myotonic–atonic
- Atonic
- Epileptic spasms

Non-motor (absence):

- Typical
- Atypical
- Myoclonic
- Eyelid myoclonia

Focal onset

(Can occur with retained awareness or impaired awareness)

Motor onset

- Automatisms
- Atonic
- Clonic
- Epileptic spasms
- Hyperkinetic
- Myoclonic
- Tonic

Nonmotor onset

- Autonomic
- Behaviour arrest
- Cognitive
- Emotional
- Sensory

Focal to bilateral tonic–clonic

Unknown onset

Motor

- Tonic–clonic
- Epileptic spasms

Non-motor

- Behavioural arrest

28.27 Trigger factors for seizures

- Sleep deprivation
- Missed doses of antiepileptic drugs in treated patients
- Alcohol (particularly withdrawal)
- Recreational drug misuse
- Physical and mental exhaustion
- Flickering lights, including TV and computer screens (generalised epilepsy syndromes only)
- Intercurrent infections and metabolic disturbances
- Uncommon: loud noises, music, reading, hot baths

disturbance of structure or function. GGEs almost always become apparent before the age of 35.

Seizure activity is usually apparent on EEG as spike and wave discharges (see Fig. 28.14). Other generalised seizures may involve merely brief loss of awareness (absence seizures), single jerks (myoclonus) or loss of tone (atonic seizures), as detailed in Box 28.26.

Clinical features

Seizure type and epilepsy type

Patients can experience more than one type of seizure attack, and it is important to document each attack type and the patient's age at its onset, along with its frequency, duration and typical features. Any triggers should be identified (Box 28.27). The type of seizure, other clinical features and investigations can then be used to determine the epilepsy syndrome, as discussed below. Where there is doubt about the type, this is best stated and a full classification should be deferred until the evolution of the clinical features clarifies the picture.

To classify seizure type, the clinician should ask firstly whether there is a focal onset, and secondly whether the seizures conform to one of the recognised patterns (see Box 28.26). Epilepsy that starts in patients beyond their mid-thirties will almost invariably reflect a focal cerebral event. Where activity remains focal, the classification will be obvious. With generalised tonic–clonic seizures, a focal onset will be heralded by positive neurological symptoms and signs corresponding to the normal function of that area. Occipital onset causes visual changes (lights and blobs of colour), temporal lobe onset causes false recognition (déjà vu), sensory strip involvement causes sensory alteration (burning, tingling) and motor strip involvement causes jerking.

Alternatively, patients report a previous local cortical insult, and it may be reasonably (but not invariably) inferred that this is the seat of epileptogenesis.

Focal seizures

The classification of focal seizures is shown in Box 28.26. They are caused by localised cortical activity. The localisation of such symptoms is described above. A spreading pattern of seizure may occur, the abnormal sensation spreading much faster (in seconds) than a migrainous focal sensory attack.

Awareness may become impaired if spread occurs to the temporal lobes (previously 'complex partial seizure'). Patients stop and stare blankly, often blinking repetitively, making smacking movements of their lips or displaying other automatisms, such as picking at their clothes. After a few minutes consciousness returns but the patient may be muddled and feel drowsy for a period of up to an hour. The age of onset, preceding aura, longer duration and post-ictal symptoms usually make these easy to differentiate from childhood absence seizures (see below).

Seizures arising from the anterior parts of the frontal lobe may produce bizarre behaviour patterns, including limb posturing, sleep walking or even frenetic, ill-directed motor activity with incoherent screaming. Video EEG may be necessary to differentiate these from psychogenic attacks (which are more common) but abruptness of onset, stereotyped nature, relative brevity and nocturnal preponderance may indicate a frontal origin. Causes of focal seizures are given in Box 28.28.

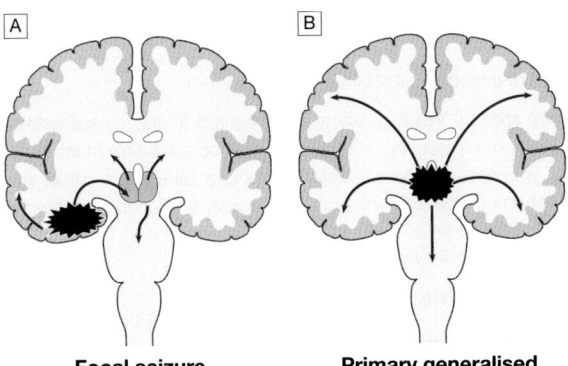

Focal seizure
± secondary generalisation

Primary generalised seizure

Fig. 28.23 The pathophysiological classification of seizures. [A] A focal seizure originates from a paroxysmal discharge in a focal area of the cerebral cortex (often the temporal lobe); the seizure may subsequently spread to the rest of the brain (secondary generalisation) via diencephalic activating pathways. [B] In genetic generalised epilepsies (GGEs) the abnormal electrical discharges originate from the diencephalic activating system and spread simultaneously to all areas of the cortex.

28

28.28 Causes of focal seizures

Idiopathic

- Benign Rolandic epilepsy of childhood
- Benign occipital epilepsy of childhood

Focal structural lesions

Genetic

- Tuberous sclerosis
- Autosomal dominant nocturnal frontal lobe epilepsy
- Autosomal dominant partial epilepsy with auditory features (ADPEAF)
- von Hippel–Lindau disease
- Neurofibromatosis
- Cerebral migration abnormalities

Infantile hemiplegia

Dysembryonic

- Cortical dysgenesis
- Sturge–Weber syndrome

Mesial temporal sclerosis (associated with febrile convulsions)

Cerebrovascular disease (see Ch. 29)

- Intracerebral haemorrhage
- Cerebral infarction
- Arteriovenous malformation
- Cavernous haemangioma

Tumours (primary and secondary)

Trauma (including neurosurgery)

Infective

- Cerebral abscess (pyogenic)
- Toxoplasmosis
- Cysticercosis
- Tuberculoma
- Subdural empyema
- Encephalitis
- Human immunodeficiency virus (HIV)

Inflammatory

- Autoimmune encephalopathies (e.g. anti-voltage-gated potassium channel antibodies, anti-NMDA receptor antibodies)
- Sarcoidosis
- Vasculitis

28.29 Causes of generalised tonic–clonic seizures

Generalisation from focal seizures

- See Box 28.28

Genetic

- Inborn errors of metabolism
- Storage diseases
- Phakomatoses (e.g. tuberous sclerosis)

Cerebral birth injury

Hydrocephalus

Cerebral anoxia

Drugs

- Antibiotics: penicillin, isoniazid, metronidazole
- Antimalarials: chloroquine, mefloquine
- Ciclosporin
- Amphetamines (withdrawal)
- Cardiac anti-arrhythmics: lidocaine, disopyramide
- Psychotropic agents: phenothiazines, tricyclic antidepressants, lithium

Alcohol (especially withdrawal)

Toxins

- Organophosphates (sarin)
- Heavy metals (lead, tin)

Metabolic disease

- Hypocalcaemia
- Hyponatraemia
- Hypomagnesaemia
- Hypoglycaemia
- Renal failure
- Liver failure

Infective

- Post-infectious encephalopathy
- Meningitis

Inflammatory

- Multiple sclerosis (uncommon)
- Systemic lupus erythematosus

Diffuse degenerative diseases

- Alzheimer's disease (uncommonly)
- Creutzfeldt–Jakob disease (rarely)

Generalised seizures

Tonic–clonic seizures An initial 'aura' may be experienced by the patient, depending on the cortical area from which the seizure originates (as above). The patient then becomes rigid (tonic) and unconscious, falling heavily if standing ('like a log') and risking facial injury. During this phase, breathing stops and central cyanosis may occur. As cortical discharges reduce in frequency, jerking (clonic) movements emerge for 2 minutes at most. Afterwards, there is a flaccid state of deep coma, which can persist for some minutes, and on regaining awareness the patient may be confused, disorientated and/or amnesic. During the attack, urinary incontinence and tongue-biting may occur. A severely bitten, bleeding tongue after an attack of loss of consciousness is pathognomonic of a generalised seizure but less marked lingual injury can occur in syncope. Subsequently, the patient usually feels unwell and sleepy, with headache and myalgia. Witnesses are usually frightened by the event, often believe the person to be dying, and may struggle to give a clear account of the episode. Some may not describe the tonic or clonic phase and may not mention cyanosis or tongue-biting. In less typical episodes, post-ictal delirium, or sequelae such as headache or myalgia, may be the main pointers to the diagnosis. Causes of generalised tonic–clonic seizures are listed in Box 28.29.

Absence seizures Absence seizures (previously 'petit mal') always start in childhood. The attacks are rarely mistaken for focal seizures because of their brevity. They can occur so frequently (20–30 times a day) that they are mistaken for daydreaming or poor concentration in school.

Myoclonic seizures These are typically brief, jerking movements, predominating in the arms. In epilepsy, they are more marked in the morning or on awakening from sleep, and tend to be provoked by fatigue, alcohol, or sleep deprivation.

Atonic seizures These are seizures involving brief loss of muscle tone, usually resulting in heavy falls with or without loss of consciousness. They occur only in the context of epilepsy syndromes that involve other forms of seizure.

Tonic seizures These are associated with a generalised increase in tone and an associated loss of awareness. They are usually seen as part of an epilepsy syndrome and are unlikely to be isolated.

Clonic seizures Clonic seizures are similar to tonic–clonic seizures. The clinical manifestations are similar but there is no preceding tonic phase.

Seizures of uncertain generalised or focal nature

Epileptic spasms While these are highlighted in the classification system, they are unusual in adult practice and occur mainly in infancy. They signify widespread cortical disturbance and take the form of marked contractions of the axial musculature, lasting a fraction of a second but recurring in clusters of 5–50, often on awakening.

Epilepsy syndromes

Many patients with epilepsy fall into specific patterns, depending on seizure type(s), age of onset and treatment responsiveness: the so-called electroclinical syndromes (Box 28.30). It is anticipated that genetic testing will ultimately demonstrate similarities in molecular pathophysiology.

Box 28.31 highlights the more common epilepsy syndromes, which are largely of early onset and are sensitive to sleep deprivation, hyperventilation, alcohol and photic stimulation. Epilepsies that do not fit into any of these diagnostic categories can be delineated firstly on the basis of the presence or absence of a known structural or metabolic condition (presumed cause), and then on the basis of the primary mode of seizure onset (generalised versus focal).

Investigations

Single seizure

All patients with transient loss of consciousness should have a 12-lead ECG. Where seizure is suspected or definite, patients should have cranial imaging with either MRI or CT, although the yield is low unless focal signs are present. EEG may help to assess prognosis once a firm diagnosis has been made. The recurrence rate after a first seizure is approximately 40% and most recurrent attacks occur within a month or two of the first. Further seizures are less likely if an identified trigger can be avoided (see Box 28.27).

Other investigations for infective, toxic and metabolic causes (Box 28.32) may be appropriate. An EEG performed immediately after a seizure may be more helpful in showing focal features than if performed after a delay.

Epilepsy

The same investigations are required in a patient with epilepsy (Box 28.32). The EEG may help to establish the type of epilepsy and guide therapy. Investigations should be revisited if the epilepsy is intractable to treatment.

Inter-ictal EEG is abnormal in only about 50% of patients with recurrent seizures, so it cannot be used to exclude epilepsy. The sensitivity can be increased to about 85% by prolonging recording time and including a period of natural or drug-induced sleep, but this does not replace a well-taken history. Ambulatory EEG recording or video EEG monitoring may help with differentiation of epilepsy from other disorders if attacks are sufficiently frequent.

 28.30 Electroclinical epilepsy syndromes

Adolescence to adulthood

- Juvenile absence epilepsy (JAE)
- Juvenile myoclonic epilepsy (JME)
- Epilepsy with generalised tonic–clonic seizures alone
- Progressive myoclonus epilepsies (PMEs)
- Autosomal dominant epilepsy with auditory features (ADEAF)
- Other familial temporal lobe epilepsies

Less specific age relationship

- Familial focal epilepsy with variable foci (childhood to adult)
- Reflex epilepsies

Distinctive constellations

- Mesial temporal lobe epilepsy with hippocampal sclerosis (MTLE with HS)
- Rasmussen syndrome
- Gelastic (from the Greek word for laughter) seizures with hypothalamic hamartoma
- Hemiconvulsion–hemiplegia–epilepsy

Epilepsies with structural–metabolic causes

- Malformations of cortical development (hemimegalencephaly, heterotopias etc.)
- Neurocutaneous syndromes (tuberous sclerosis complex, Sturge–Weber etc.)
- Tumour
- Infection
- Trauma
- Angioma
- Perinatal insults
- Stroke

Epilepsies of unknown cause

Conditions with epileptic seizures not needing long-term treatment

- Benign neonatal seizures (BNS)
- Febrile seizures (FS)

28.32 Investigation of epilepsy

From where is the epilepsy arising?

- Standard EEG
- Sleep EEG
- EEG with special electrodes (foramen ovale, subdural)

What is the cause of the epilepsy?

Structural lesion?

- CT
- MRI

Metabolic disorder?

- Urea and electrolytes
- Liver function tests
- Blood glucose
- Serum calcium, magnesium

Inflammatory or infective disorder?

- Full blood count, erythrocyte sedimentation rate, C-reactive protein
- Chest X-ray
- Serology for syphilis, HIV, collagen disease
- CSF examination

Are the attacks truly epileptic?

- Ambulatory EEG
- Videotelemetry

(CSF = cerebrospinal fluid; CT = computed tomography; EEG = electroencephalography; HIV = human immunodeficiency virus; MRI = magnetic resonance imaging)

28.31 Common generalised epilepsy syndromes

Syndrome	Age of onset	Type of seizure	EEG features	Treatment	Prognosis
Childhood absence epilepsy	4–8 years	Frequent brief absences	3/sec spike and wave	Ethosuximide Sodium valproate Levetiracetam	40% develop GTCS, 80% remit in adulthood
Juvenile absence epilepsy	10–15 years	Less frequent absences than childhood absence	Poly-spike and wave	Sodium valproate Levetiracetam	80% develop GTCS, 80% seizure-free in adulthood
Juvenile myoclonic epilepsy	15–20 years	GTCS, absences, morning myoclonus	Poly-spike and wave, photosensitivity	Sodium valproate Levetiracetam	90% remit with AEDs but relapse if AED withdrawn
GTCS on awakening	10–25 years	GTCS, sometimes myoclonus	Spike and wave on waking and sleep onset	Sodium valproate Levetiracetam	65% controlled with AEDs but relapse off treatment

(AED = antiepileptic drug; GTCS = generalised tonic–clonic seizure)

28

28.33 Indications for brain imaging in epilepsy

- Epilepsy starting after the age of 16 years
- Seizures having focal features clinically
- Electroencephalogram showing a focal seizure source
- Control of seizures difficult or deteriorating

28.34 How to administer first aid for seizures

- Move the person away from danger (fire, water, machinery, furniture)
- After convulsions cease, turn the person into the 'recovery' position (semi-prone)
- Ensure the airway is clear but do **NOT** insert anything in the mouth (tongue-biting occurs at seizure onset and cannot be prevented by observers)
- If convulsions continue for more than 5 mins or recur without the person regaining consciousness, summon urgent medical attention
- Do not leave the person alone until fully recovered (drowsiness and delirium can persist for up to 1 hr)

28.35 Epilepsy: outcome after 20 years

- 50% are seizure-free, without drugs, for the previous 5 years
- 20% are seizure-free for the previous 5 years but continue to take medication
- 30% continue to have seizures in spite of antiepileptic therapy

Indications for imaging are summarised in Box 28.33. Imaging cannot establish a diagnosis of epilepsy but identifies any structural cause. It is not required if a confident diagnosis of a recognised GGE syndrome (e.g. juvenile myoclonic epilepsy) is made. While CT excludes a major structural cause of epilepsy, MRI is required to demonstrate subtle changes such as hippocampal sclerosis, which may direct or inform surgical intervention.

Management

It is important to explain the nature and cause of seizures to patients and their relatives, and to instruct relatives in the first aid management of seizures (Box 28.34). Many people with epilepsy feel stigmatised and may become unnecessarily isolated from work and social life. It is important to emphasise that epilepsy is a common disorder that affects 0.5%–1% of the population, and that full control of seizures can be expected in approximately 70% of patients (Box 28.35).

Immediate care

Little can or needs to be done for a person during a convulsive seizure except for first aid and common-sense manoeuvres to limit damage or secondary complications (see Box 28.34). Advice should be given that on no account should anything be inserted into the patient's mouth. The management of status epilepticus is described on page 1137.

Lifestyle advice

Patients should be advised to avoid activities where they might place themselves or others at risk if they have a seizure. This applies at work, at home and at leisure. At home, only shallow baths (or showers) should be taken. Prolonged cycle journeys should be discouraged until reasonable freedom from seizures has been achieved. Activities involving prolonged proximity to water (swimming, fishing or boating) should always be carried out in the company of someone who is aware of the risks and the potential need for rescue measures. Driving regulations vary between countries and the patient should be made aware of these (Box 28.36). Certain occupations, such as firefighter or airline pilot, are not open to

28.36 UK driving regulations

The physician's prime duty is to ensure the patient is aware of the legal obligation to inform the driving authority

Private use

Single seizure
- Cease driving for 6 months; a longer period may be required if risk of recurrence is high

Epilepsy (i.e. more than one seizure over the age of 5 years)
- Cease driving immediately
- Licence restored when patient is seizure-free for 1 year, *or* an initial sleep seizure is followed by exclusively sleep seizures for 1 year, *or* mixed awake and sleep seizures are followed by 3 years of exclusively sleep seizures
- Licence will require renewal every 3 years thereafter until patient is seizure-free for 10 years

Withdrawal of antiepileptic drugs
- Cease driving during withdrawal period and for 6 months thereafter

Vocational drivers (heavy goods and public service vehicles)
- No licence permitted if any seizure has occurred after the age of 5 years until patient is off medication and seizure-free for more than 10 years, and has no potentially epileptogenic brain lesion

those with a previous or active diagnosis of epilepsy; further information is available from epilepsy support organisations.

The risk of harm from epilepsy should be discussed around the time of diagnosis. In particular epilepsy is associated with a very small, but potentially modifiable, risk of sudden death (sudden unexpected death in epilepsy, SUDEP). Explaining risks of epilepsy, including SUDEP, should be done with care and sensitivity, and with the aim of motivating the patient to adapt habits and lifestyle to optimise epilepsy control and minimise risks of serious complications.

Antiepileptic drugs

Antiepileptic drugs (AEDs) should be considered where risk of seizure recurrence is high. A diagnosis of two or more seizures is justification enough but a prolonged inter-seizure interval may deter some patients and physicians. Treatment decisions should always be shared with the patient, to enhance adherence. A wide range of drugs is available. These agents either increase inhibitory neurotransmission in the brain or alter neuronal sodium channels to prevent abnormally rapid transmission of impulses. In the majority of patients, full control is achieved with a single drug. Dose regimens should be kept as simple as possible. Guidelines are listed in Box 28.37. For focal epilepsies, one large study suggests that lamotrigine is the best-tolerated monotherapy, which, alongside its favourable adverse-effect profile and relative lack of pharmacokinetic interactions, makes it a good first-line drug, although caution must be exercised with oral contraceptive use. Unclassified or genetic generalised epilepsies respond best to valproate, although pregnancy-related problems mean that valproate should not be used in women of reproductive age unless the benefits outweigh the risks. The initial choice should be an established first-line drug (Box 28.38), with more recently introduced drugs as second choice.

Monitoring therapy

Some practitioners confuse epilepsy care with serum level monitoring. The newer drugs have much more predictable pharmacokinetics than the older ones and the only indication for measuring serum levels is if there is doubt about adherence. Blood levels need to be interpreted carefully and dose changes made to treat the patient rather than to bring a serum level into the 'therapeutic range'. Some centres advocate serum level monitoring during pregnancy (notably with lamotrigine) but the evidence of benefit for this is not strong.

28.37 Guidelines for antiepileptic drug therapy*

- Start with one first-line drug (see Box 28.38)
- Start at a low dose; gradually increase dose until effective control of seizures is achieved or side-effects develop
- Optimise adherence (use minimum number of doses per day)
- If first drug fails (seizures continue or side-effects develop), start second first-line drug, followed if possible by gradual withdrawal of first
- If second drug fails (seizures continue or side-effects develop), start second-line drug in combination with the preferred baseline drug at maximum tolerated dose (beware interactions)
- If this combination fails (seizures continue or side-effects develop), replace second-line drug with alternative second-line drug
- If this combination fails, check adherence and reconsider diagnosis. (Are events seizures? Occult lesion? Treatment adherence/alcohol/drugs confounding response?)
- Consider alternative, non-drug treatments (e.g. epilepsy surgery, vagal nerve stimulation)
- Use minimum number of drugs in combination at any one time

*See Scottish Intercollegiate Guidelines Network SIGN 143 – Diagnosis and management of epilepsy in adults (May 2015).

28.38 Guidelines for choice of antiepileptic drug[1]

Epilepsy type	First-line	Second-line	Third-line
Focal onset and/or secondary GTCS	Lamotrigine	Carbamazepine Levetiracetam Sodium valproate Topiramate Perampanel Zonisamide Lacosamide	Gabapentin Oxcarbazepine Phenytoin Pregabalin Tiagabine
GTCS[2]	Sodium valproate Levetiracetam	Lamotrigine Topiramate Zonisamide Ethosuximide	Phenytoin Primidone Acetazolamide
Absence[2]	Ethosuximide	Sodium valproate	Lamotrigine Clonazepam
Myoclonic[2]	Sodium valproate	Levetiracetam Clonazepam	Lamotrigine Phenobarbital

[1]See Scottish Intercollegiate Guidelines Network SIGN 143 – Diagnosis and management of epilepsy in adults (May 2015). [2]Genetic generalised epilepsies.
N.B. Use as few drugs as possible at the lowest possible dose. Avoid sodium valproate in women of childbearing age/potential unless benefit outweighs risk.
(GTCS = generalised tonic–clonic seizure)

Epilepsy surgery

Some patients with drug-resistant epilepsy benefit from surgical resection of epileptogenic brain tissue. Less invasive treatments, including vagal nerve stimulation or deep brain stimulation, may also be helpful in some patients. All those who continue to experience seizures despite appropriate drug treatment should be considered for surgical treatment. Planning such interventions requires intensive specialist assessment and investigation to identify the site of seizure onset and the dispensability of any target areas for resection, i.e. whether the area of brain involved is necessary for a critical function such as vision or motor function.

Withdrawing antiepileptic therapy

Withdrawal of medication may be considered after a patient has been seizure-free for more than 2 years. Childhood-onset epilepsy, particularly classical absence seizures, carries the best prognosis for successful drug withdrawal. Other epilepsy syndromes, such as juvenile myoclonic epilepsy, have a marked tendency to recur after drug withdrawal.

Focal epilepsies that begin in adult life are also likely to recur, especially if there is an identified structural lesion. Overall, the recurrence rate after drug withdrawal depends on the individual's epilepsy history. An individualised estimate may be gained from the SIGN guideline tables (see 'Further information').

Patients should be advised of the risks of recurrence, to allow them to decide whether or not they wish to withdraw. If undertaken, withdrawal should be done slowly, reducing the drug dose gradually over weeks or months. Withdrawal may necessitate precautions around driving or occupation (see Box 28.36).

Contraception

Some AEDs induce hepatic enzymes that metabolise synthetic hormones, increasing the risk of contraceptive failure. This is most marked with carbamazepine, phenytoin and barbiturates, but clinically significant effects can be seen with lamotrigine and topiramate. If the AED cannot be changed, this can be overcome by giving higher-dose preparations of the oral contraceptive. Sodium valproate and levetiracetam have no interaction with hormonal contraception.

Pregnancy and reproduction

Epilepsy presents specific management problems during pregnancy (Box 28.39). There is usually concern about the risks of teratogenesis associated with AEDs which must be balanced against the benefits of these drugs. It is important to recognise proportionate risks: background risk of severe fetal malformation in the general population is around 2%–3%, while the AED most associated with teratogenesis is sodium valproate, which, at high dose, increases the risk to up to 10%. Long-term observational studies show that most of the commonly used AEDs can be given safely in pregnancy, although the risk of congenital abnormalities in the fetus is dependent on the type, number and dose of AEDs.

Over the past few years medicines regulatory agencies have strengthened their warnings surrounding the risk of birth defects and developmental disorders in children born to women who take valproate during pregnancy. In the UK it has been emphasised that if valproate is taken during pregnancy, up to 4 in 10 babies are at risk of developmental disorders, in addition to the 1 in 10 who are at risk of birth defects. Consequently, in the UK, valproate must no longer be used in any woman or girl able to have children, unless she has a pregnancy prevention programme in place.

Pre-conception treatment with folic acid (5 mg daily), along with use of the smallest effective doses of as few AEDs as possible, may reduce the risk of fetal abnormalities. The risks of abrupt AED withdrawal to the mother should be stressed.

Seizures may become more frequent during pregnancy, particularly if pharmacokinetic changes decrease serum levels of AEDs (see Box 28.39).

Menstrual irregularities and reduced fertility are more common in women with epilepsy, and are also increased by sodium valproate. Patients with epilepsy are at greater risk of osteoporosis, apparently independently of the drug used. Some centres advocate vitamin D supplementation in any patient with epilepsy but the higher female risk of osteoporosis makes this most important in women. Oral contraception can interact with individual AEDs (see Box 28.39).

Prognosis

The outcome of newly diagnosed epilepsy is generally good. Overall, generalised epilepsies and generalised seizures are more readily controlled than focal seizures. The presence of a structural lesion reduces the chances of freedom from seizures. The overall prognosis for

28

28.39 Epilepsy in pregnancy

- **Provision of pre-conception counselling is best practice**: start folic acid (5 mg daily for 2 months) before conception to reduce the risk of fetal malformations.
- **Fetal malformation**: risk is minimised if a single drug is used.
    Carbamazepine and lamotrigine have the lowest incidence of major fetal malformations.
    The risk with sodium valproate is particularly high (see text) and should be carefully balanced against its benefits.
    Levetiracetam may be safe but avoid other newer drugs if possible.
- **Learning difficulties in children**: IQ may be lower when children are exposed to valproate in utero, so its use should always be considered carefully.
- **Haemorrhagic disease of the newborn**: enzyme-inducing antiepileptic drugs increase risk. Give IM vitamin K (1 mg) to the infant at birth.
- **Increased frequency of seizures**: where breakthrough seizures occur, monitor antiepileptic drug levels and adjust the dose regimen accordingly.
- **Pharmacokinetic effects of pregnancy**: carbamazepine levels may fall in the third trimester. Lamotrigine and levetiracetam levels may fall early in pregnancy. Some advocate monitoring of levels.

28.40 Epilepsy in old age

- **Incidence and prevalence**: late-onset epilepsy is very common and the annual incidence in those over 60 years is rising.
- **Fits and faints**: the features that usually differentiate these may be less definitive than in younger patients.
- **Non-convulsive status epilepticus**: can present as delirium in old age.
- **Cerebrovascular disease**: the underlying cause of seizures in 30%–50% of patients over the age of 50 years. A seizure may occur with an overt stroke or with occult vascular disease.
- **Neurogenerative disease** or **dementia**: should be considered when epilepsy presents in old age.
- **Antiepileptic drug regimens**: keep as simple as possible and take care to avoid interactions with other drugs being prescribed.
- **Carbamazepine-induced hyponatraemia**: increases significantly with age; this is particularly important in patients on diuretics or those with heart failure.
- **Withdrawal of antiepileptic therapy**: drug withdrawal should be attempted only where benefits exceed risk of harm from seizures.

28.41 Epilepsy in adolescence

- **Effect on school/education**: seizures, antiepileptic drugs (AEDs) and psychological complications of epilepsy may hamper education. Fear may make some educational institutions unduly restrictive.
- **Effect on family relationships**: parents may adopt a protective role, which can lead to epilepsy (and AEDs) becoming a point of assertion and rebellion.
- **Effect on career choice**: epilepsy may exclude or restrict employment in the emergency services and armed forces.
- **Alcohol**: may affect sleep pattern; excess may be associated with poor AED adherence.
- **Illicit drugs**: may affect seizure threshold and be associated with poor AED adherence.
- **Sleep disturbance**: may be worsened by social activities and computer games.
- **Oral contraception**: interactions with AED can occur. Use may not always be disclosed to parents.

epilepsy is shown in Box 28.35. Problems that epilepsy poses in older adults and in adolescents are summarised in Boxes 28.40 and 28.41, respectively.

Status epilepticus

Presentation and management are described on page 1137. While generalised status epilepticus is most easily recognised, non-convulsive status may be less dramatic and less easily diagnosed. It may cause only altered awareness, delirium or wandering with automatisms. In an intensive care unit setting, EEG monitoring is essential to ensure that diagnosis and treatment are optimised.

Non-epileptic attack disorder ('dissociative attacks')

The difficulty with nomenclature is discussed on page 1152. Patients may present with attacks that resemble epileptic seizures but are caused by psychological phenomena and have no abnormal EEG discharges. Such attacks may be very prolonged, sometimes mimicking status epilepticus. Epileptic and non-epileptic attacks may coexist and time and effort are needed to clarify the relative contribution of each, allowing more accurate and comprehensive treatment.

Non-epileptic attack disorder (NEAD) may be accompanied by dramatic flailing of the limbs and arching of the back, with side-to-side head movements and vocalising. Cyanosis and severe biting of the tongue are rare but incontinence can occur. Distress and crying are common following non-epileptic attacks. The distinction between epileptic attacks originating in the frontal lobes and non-epileptic attacks may be especially difficult, and may require videotelemetry with prolonged EEG recordings. Non-epileptic attacks are three times more common in women than in men. They are not necessarily associated with formal psychiatric illness. Patients and carers may need reassurance that hospital admission is not required for every attack. Prevention requires psychotherapeutic interventions rather than drug therapy.

Vestibular disorders

Vertigo is the typical symptom caused by vestibular dysfunction, and most patients with vertigo have acute vestibular failure, benign paroxysmal positional vertigo or Ménière's disease. Central (brain) causes of vertigo are rare by comparison, with the exception of migraine.

Acute vestibular failure

Although commonly called 'labyrinthitis' or 'vestibular neuronitis', acute vestibular failure is a more accurate term, as most cases are idiopathic. It usually presents as isolated severe vertigo with vomiting and unsteadiness. It begins abruptly, often on waking, and many patients are initially bed-bound. The vertigo settles within a few days, though head movement may continue to provoke transient symptoms (positional vertigo) for some time. During the acute attack, nystagmus will be present for a few days.

Cinnarizine, prochlorperazine or betahistine provide symptomatic relief but should not be used long term, as this may delay recovery. A small proportion of patients fail to recover fully and complain of ongoing imbalance and dysequilibrium rather than vertigo; vestibular rehabilitation by a physiotherapist may help.

Benign paroxysmal positional vertigo

Benign paroxysmal positional vertigo (BPPV) is due to the presence of otolithic debris from the saccule or utricle affecting the free flow of endolymph in the semicircular canals (cupulolithiasis). It may follow minor head injury but typically is spontaneous. The history is diagnostic, with transient (seconds) vertigo precipitated by movement (typically, rolling over in bed or getting into or out of bed). Although it is benign, and usually self-limiting after weeks or months, patients are often alarmed by the symptoms. The diagnosis can be confirmed by the 'Hallpike manoeuvre' to demonstrate positional nystagmus (Fig. 28.24). Treatment comprises explanation and reassurance, along with positioning procedures designed to return otolithic debris from the semicircular canal to saccule or utricle (such as the Epley manoeuvre) and/or to re-educate the brain to cope with the inappropriate signals from the labyrinth (such as Cawthorne–Cooksey exercises: see 'Further information').

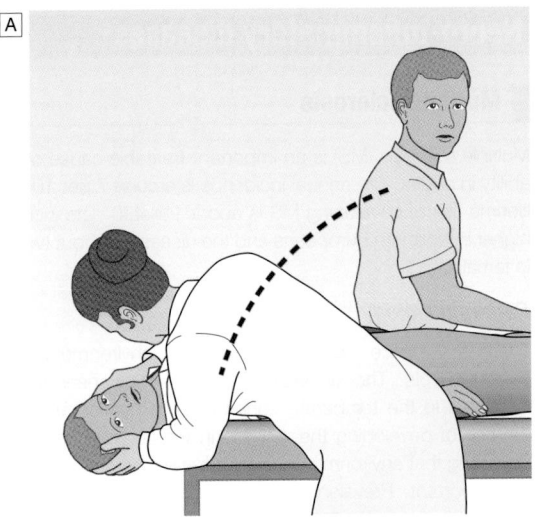
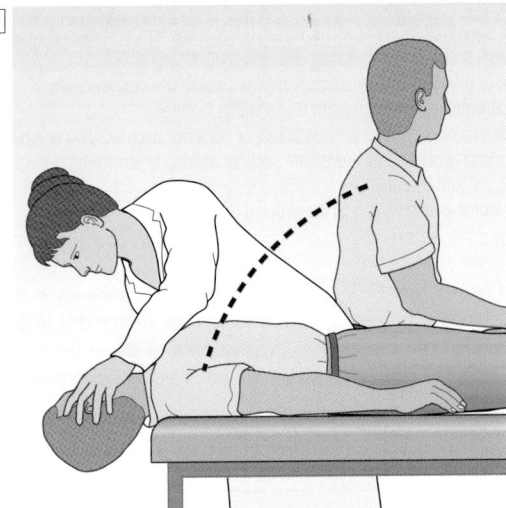

Fig. 28.24 The Hallpike manoeuvre for diagnosis of benign paroxysmal positional vertigo (BPPV). Patients are asked to keep their eyes open and look at the examiner as their head is swung briskly backwards through 120° to overhang the edge of the couch. **A** Perform first with the right ear down. **B** Perform next with the left ear down. The examiner looks for nystagmus (usually accompanied by vertigo). In BPPV, the nystagmus typically occurs in A or B only and is torsional, the fast phase beating towards the lower ear. Its onset is usually delayed a few seconds and it lasts 10–20 seconds. As the patient is returned to the upright position, transient nystagmus may occur in the opposite direction. Both nystagmus and vertigo typically decrease (fatigue) on repeat testing.

Ménière disease

This is due to an abnormality of the endolymph that causes episodes of vertigo accompanied by tinnitus and fullness in the ear, each attack typically lasting a few hours. Over the years, patients may develop progressive deafness (typically low-tone on audiometry). Examination is typically normal in between attacks. The diagnosis is clinical, supported by abnormal audiometry. Ménière disease is idiopathic but a similar syndrome may be caused by middle ear trauma or infection. Imaging may be indicated to exclude other focal brainstem or cerebellopontine angle pathology but will be normal in Ménière disease. Management includes a low-salt diet, vestibular sedatives for acute attacks (e.g. cinnarizine or prochlorperazine), and occasionally surgery to increase endolymphatic drainage from the vestibular system. Migraine may also cause episodic vertigo, and can be confused with Ménière disease, although usually other migrainous features will appear in the history.

Disorders of sleep

Sleep disturbances include too much sleep (hypersomnolence or excessive daytime sleepiness), insufficient or poor-quality sleep (insomnia) and abnormal behaviour during sleep (parasomnias). Insomnia is usually caused by psychological or psychiatric disorders, shift work and other environmental causes, pain and so on, and will not be discussed further. Many symptoms and disorders may affect sleep and sleep quality (e.g. pain, depression/anxiety, parkinsonism).

Excessive daytime sleepiness (hypersomnolence)

There are primary and secondary causes (Box 28.42). The most common causes are impaired sleep due to lifestyle issues or sleep-disordered breathing. Sleepiness may be measured using the Epworth sleepiness scale (see Box 17.86). Most causes will be identified by a detailed history from the patient and their bed partner, and a 2-week sleep diary.

Narcolepsy

This has a prevalence of about 1 in 2000, with peak onset in adolescence and early middle age. The key symptom is sudden, irresistible 'sleep attacks', often in inappropriate circumstances such as while

---

i | **28.42 Causes of hypersomnolence**

Primary causes

- Narcolepsy
- Idiopathic hypersomnolence
- Brain injury

Secondary causes (due to poor-quality sleep)

- Obstructive sleep apnoea
- Pain
- Restless legs/periodic limb movements of sleep
- Parkinsonism and other neurodegenerative diseases
- Depression/anxiety
- Medication
- Environmental factors (noise, temperature etc.)

---

i | **28.43 Narcolepsy symptoms**

Sleep attacks

- Brief, frequent and unlike normal somnolence

Cataplexy

- Sudden loss of muscle tone triggered by surprise, laughter, strong emotion etc.

Hypnagogic or hypnopompic hallucinations

- Frightening hallucinations experienced during sleep onset or waking due to intrusion of REM sleep during wakefulness (can occur in normal people)

Sleep paralysis

- Brief paralysis on waking (can occur in normal people)

---

eating or talking. Other characteristic features help distinguish this from excessive daytime sleepiness (Box 28.43). Symptoms may be due to loss of hypocretin-secreting hypothalamic neurons. Diagnosis requires sleep study with sleep latency testing (demonstrating rapid onset of REM sleep). Narcolepsy may respond to stimulants such as modafinil but more severe cases may require sodium oxybate, dexamfetamine, methylphenidate or a selective serotonin reuptake inhibitor (SSRI). Cataplexy can be debilitating and can respond to sodium oxybate or to antidepressants, such as clomipramine or venlafaxine.

Parasomnias

Parasomnias are abnormal motor behaviours that occur around sleep. They may arise in either REM or non-REM sleep, with characteristic

28.44 Diagnostic criteria for restless legs syndrome

A need to move the legs, usually accompanied or caused by uncomfortable, unpleasant sensations in the legs, with the following features:
- only present or worse during periods of rest or inactivity, such as lying or sitting
- partially or totally relieved by movement such as walking or stretching, at least as long as the activity continues
- generally worse or occurs only in the evening or night.

features and timing. Non-REM parasomnias tend to occur early in sleep. Parasomnias should be distinguished from other motor disturbances (such as periodic limb movements, hypnic jerks or sleep talking) and sleep-onset epileptic seizures. History from a sleeping partner or other witness is essential.

Non-REM parasomnias

These are due to incomplete arousal from non-REM sleep and manifest as night terrors, sleep walking and confusional arousals (sleep drunkenness). They typically occur within an hour or two of sleep onset, are common in children and usually of no pathological significance. Rarely, they persist into adulthood and may become increasingly complex, including dressing, moving objects, eating, drinking or even acts of violence. Patients have little or no recollection of the episodes, even though they appear 'awake'. The episodes may be triggered by alcohol or unfamiliar sleeping situations and can be familial. Treatment is usually not required but clonazepam can be used.

REM sleep behaviour disorder

In REM sleep behaviour disorder (RBD), patients 'act out' their dreams during REM sleep, due to failure of the usual muscle atonia. Sleep partners provide typical histories of patients 'fighting' or 'struggling' in their sleep, sometimes causing injury to themselves or to their partner. They are easily roused from this state, with recollection of their dream, unlike in non-REM states. RBD is more common in men and may be an early symptom of neurodegenerative diseases such as alpha synucleinopathies, perhaps preceding more typical symptoms of these conditions by years. Polysomnography will confirm absence of atonia during REM sleep. Clonazepam is the most successful treatment.

Restless legs syndrome

Restless legs syndrome (RLS) is common, with a prevalence of up to 10%, but many patients never seek medical attention. It is characterised by unpleasant leg (rarely, arm) sensations that are eased by movement (motor restlessness); the diagnosis is clinical (Box 28.44). It has a strong familial tendency and can present with daytime somnolence due to poor sleep. It is usually idiopathic but may be associated with iron deficiency, pregnancy, peripheral neuropathy, Parkinson's disease or uraemia. It should be distinguished from akathisia, the daytime motor restlessness that is an adverse effect of antipsychotic drugs. Treatment, if required, is with gabapentanoids, dopaminergic drugs (dopamine agonists or levodopa) or benzodiazepines. Serum ferritin should be maintained above 75 µg/L.

Periodic limb movements in sleep

Unlike RLS, periodic limb movements in sleep (PLMS) only occur during sleep and cause repetitive flexion movements of the limbs, usually in the early (non-REM) stages of sleep. Although patients are unaware of the symptoms, they may disrupt sleep quality and often disturb partners. The pathological significance of PLMS is uncertain and it often occurs in normal health. There is an overlap with RLS. Treatment is most successful with clonazepam or dopaminergic drugs.

Neuro-inflammatory diseases

Multiple sclerosis

Multiple sclerosis (MS) is an important treatable cause of long-term disability in adults. The annual incidence is around 7 per 100000, while the lifetime risk of developing MS is about 1 in 400. The incidence of MS is higher in Northern Europeans and the disease is about twice as common in females.

Pathophysiology

There is evidence that both genetic and environmental factors play a causative role. The prevalence of MS is low near the equator and increases in the temperate zones of both hemispheres. People retain the risk of developing the disease in the zone in which they grew up, indicating that environmental exposures during growth and development are important. Prevalence also correlates with environmental factors, such as sunlight exposure, vitamin D and exposure to Epstein–Barr virus (EBV), although causative mechanisms remain unclear. Genetic factors are also relevant; the risk of familial occurrence in MS is 15%, with highest risk in first-degree relatives (age-adjusted risk 4%–5% for siblings and 2%–3% for parents or offspring). Large genome-wide association studies (GWAS) of MS implicate the modest influence of hundreds of genes, in particular those with an immunological function, and there is overlap with other immune diseases. An autoimmune cause of multiple sclerosis is therefore supported by genetic studies, a prominent role of immune cells in disease pathogenesis and efficacy of multiple immune therapies.

Initial CNS inflammation in MS involves entry of lymphocytes across the blood–brain barrier, which can be inhibited by monoclonal antibodies like natalizumab which bind α4ß1-integrin. These cells proliferate in perivascular lesions and the resulting inflammatory cascade releases cytokines and initiates destruction of the oligodendrocyte–myelin unit. Histologically, the resultant lesion is a plaque of inflammatory demyelination, most commonly in the periventricular regions of the brain, the optic nerves and the spinal cord (Fig. 28.25), and also found in the cortex. After the acute attack, gliosis and repair by oligodendrocyte precursor cells follows, leaving a shrunken scar.

Much of the initial acute clinical deficit is caused by the effect of inflammation on transmission of the nervous impulse rather than structural disruption of myelin, and may explain the rapid recovery of some deficits. In the long term, accumulating myelin loss reduces the efficiency of impulse propagation or causes complete conduction block, contributing to sustained impairment of CNS functions. Inflammatory mediators released during the acute attack, and loss of structural and trophic support from myelinating cells, contribute to axonal damage, which is a feature of the latter stages of the disease and is an important substrate of disability in the later, progressive phase of MS (Fig. 28.26).

Clinical features

The diagnosis of MS requires the demonstration of otherwise unexplained CNS lesions separated in time and space (Box 28.45); traditionally, this meant two or more clinical relapses affecting different parts of the nervous system, and the first ever episode is often referred to as a 'clinically isolated syndrome' (CIS). However recent changes to diagnostic criteria mean that MS may be diagnosed after an isolated episode because MRI can identify clinically silent lesions of different ages, and the presence of unpaired oligoclonal bands in the CSF can strongly suggest the development of future events (Box 28.45). As such MS can be proactively diagnosed and treated compared to a decade ago. The peak age of onset of MS is the fourth decade; onset in childhood or after the age of 70 years is less common but can occur.

Symptoms and signs of MS usually evolve over days or weeks, resolving over weeks or months. About 85%–90% of patients have an initial relapsing and remitting clinical course with variable intervening recovery, although the majority will eventually enter a secondary progressive phase. Most of the rest follow a slowly progressive clinical course (so-called

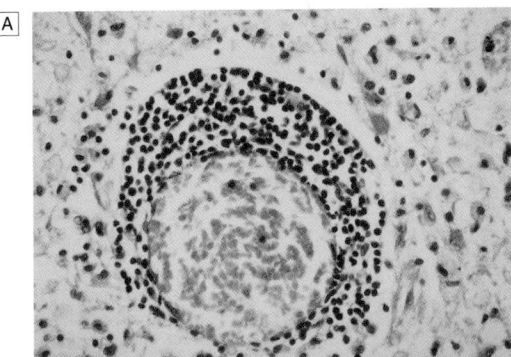

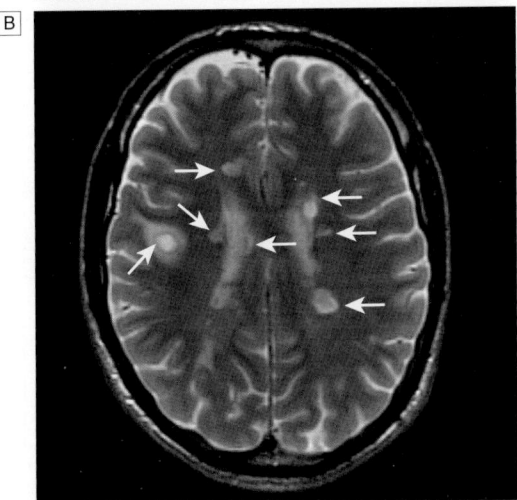

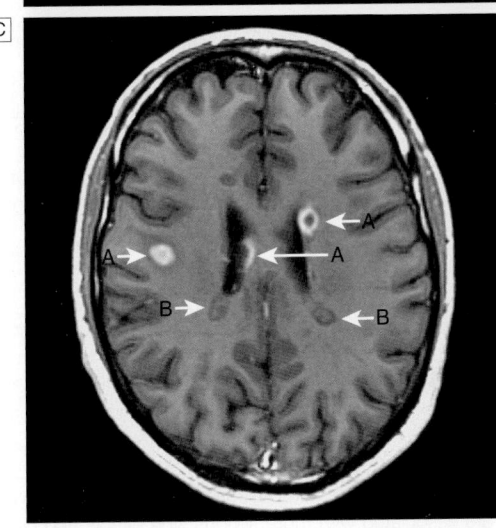

Fig. 28.25 Multiple sclerosis. **A** Photomicrograph from demyelinating plaque, showing perivascular cuffing of blood vessel by lymphocytes. **B** Brain magnetic resonance imaging in multiple sclerosis. Multiple high-signal lesions (arrows) seen particularly in the paraventricular region on T2 image. **C** In T1 image with gadolinium enhancement, recent lesions (A arrows) show enhancement, suggesting active inflammation (enhancement persists for 4 weeks); older lesions (B arrows) show no enhancement but low signal, suggesting gliosis.

<table>
<tr><td colspan="3">i   28.45 The McDonald criteria for the diagnosis of multiple sclerosis (MS) (2017)*</td></tr>
<tr><td>Number of clinical attacks</td><td>Number of lesions with objective clinical evidence</td><td>Additional evidence required to diagnose MS</td></tr>
<tr><td>≥2</td><td>≥2</td><td>None</td></tr>
<tr><td>≥2</td><td>1 (with reasonable historical evidence of a previous relapse)</td><td>None</td></tr>
<tr><td>≥2</td><td>1</td><td>Dissemination in space demonstrated by an additional clinical attack implicating a different CNS site or by MRI</td></tr>
<tr><td>1</td><td>≥2</td><td>Dissemination in time demonstrated by an additional clinical attack or by MRI or demonstration of CSF-specific oligoclonal bands</td></tr>
<tr><td>1</td><td>1</td><td>Dissemination in space demonstrated by an additional clinical attack implicating a different CNS site or by MRI *and*

Dissemination in time demonstrated by an additional clinical attack or by MRI, or demonstration of CSF-specific oligoclonal bands</td></tr>
</table>

*The diagnostic criteria require reasonable exclusion of other possible causes for central nervous system inflammation.
From Thompson A et al. Diagnosis of multiple sclerosis: 2017 revisions of the McDonald criteria. Lancet Neurology 2018;17(2):162–173.
(CSF = cerebrospinal fluid; CNS = central nervous system; MRI = magnetic resonance imaging)

i   28.46 Clinical features of multiple sclerosis

Common presentations of multiple sclerosis

- Optic neuritis
- Transverse myelitis
- Brainstem syndrome
- Cerebellar syndrome

Other symptoms and syndromes seen in MS

- Afferent pupillary defect and optic atrophy (previous optic neuritis)
- Lhermitte's symptom (tingling in spine or limbs on neck flexion)
- Progressive paraparesis
- Partial Brown–Séquard syndrome (Fig. 28.18)
- Internuclear ophthalmoplegia with ataxia
- Tremor
- Cognitive dysfunction
- Trigeminal neuralgia under the age of 50

There are a number of typical clinical symptoms and syndromes suggestive of MS, occurring either at presentation or during the course of the illness (Box 28.46). The physical signs observed in MS are determined by the anatomical site of inflammation. Combined spinal cord and brainstem signs are common, although evidence of previous optic neuritis may be found in the form of an afferent pupillary deficit. Cognitive symptoms of MS are underappreciated and can be significant, particularly in the later stages of the disease.

The prognosis for patients with MS is difficult to predict with confidence, especially early in the disease. Those with untreated relapsing and remitting MS experience, on average, 1–2 relapses every 2 years, although this may decline with time. Prognosis is better for patients with optic neuritis and only sensory relapses. Overall, about one-third of patients are disabled to the point of needing help with walking after 10 years, and this proportion rises to about half after 15 years. It would appear likely (though this is as yet unproven) that disease-modifying drugs will have an effect on long-term disability.

primary progressive MS). Aggressive variants of multiple sclerosis can occur, and this can include presentation with tumour-like lesions which may require biopsy for confirmation (see Fig. 28.26). The clinical course of multiple sclerosis is highly variable and difficult to predict. Frequent relapses with incomplete recovery indicate a poorer prognosis and the need for high efficacy therapy. Some milder cases have an interval of years or even decades between attacks.

28

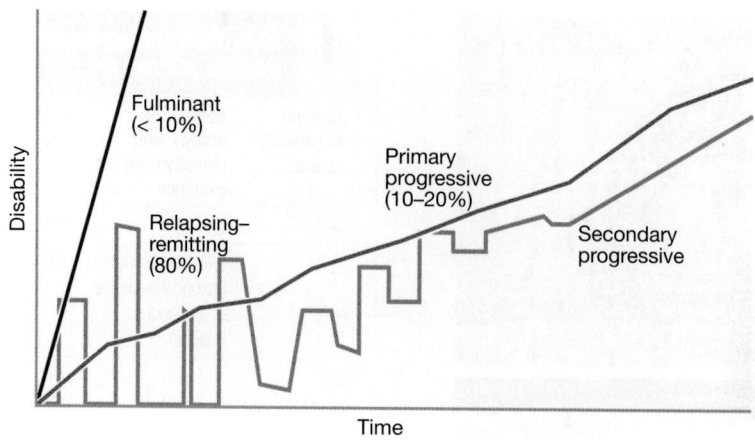

Fig. 28.26 The progression of disability in fulminant, relapsing–remitting and progressive multiple sclerosis. *Courtesy of Professor D.A.S. Compston.*

Investigations

There is no single diagnostic test that is definitive for MS and the results of investigation need to be combined with the clinical picture in order to make a diagnosis; MRI is the most important investigation (Fig. 28.27). MS mimics should be excluded (see below). Following the first clinical event, investigations help confirm the disseminated nature of the disease. MRI is the most sensitive technique for imaging lesions in brain and spinal cord (Fig. 28.28) and for excluding other causes that have provoked the neurological deficit. MS lesions often have an oval appearance and lesions which have developed in the past couple of months usually take up contrast around the lesion rim. Typical MRI lesion locations include the periventricular region, juxtacortical, infratentorial regions and spinal cord. Spinal cord lesions in MS are typically short and are asymmetric (Fig. 28.28). Longer spinal cord lesions, over 3 vertebral bodies in length, should raise the possibility of neuromyelitis optica, an antibody-mediated neuroinflammatory disease. In older age groups, MRI appearances in MS may be confused with those of small-vessel disease and non-specific white matter lesions can be seen in common conditions such as migraine. Therefore careful and experienced evaluation of brain and spinal cord imaging is important for accurate diagnosis.

In MS, the CSF typically has a normal white cell count and protein, although may show a small lymphocytic pleocytosis in active disease. CSF can be used to identify intrathecal synthesis of immunoglobulins in MS. Oligoclonal bands are found in the CSF but not the blood in about 90% of patients. The presence of these bands can help facilitate a more rapid diagnosis of MS in individuals who have had a single clinical event, since they suggest a more chronic neuroinflammatory process. Oligoclonal bands are not specific for MS and denote only intrathecal inflammation, provided they are unique for the CSF. These can appear in other disorders, which should be excluded by examination and investigation. It is important to exclude other potentially treatable conditions, such as infection, vitamin B_{12} deficiency and spinal cord compression.

Management

The management of MS involves (i) disease modifying therapies and (ii) symptomatic approaches.

Disease-modifying treatment (DMT)

The past two decades have seen enormous progress in the treatment of multiple sclerosis, in particular the treatment of early MS. There is a broad spectrum of immunotherapies for the treatment of MS, with > 10 drugs approved in Europe and the United States. These drugs are most efficacious in the relapsing–remitting phase of disease, and early diagnosis and treatment is increasingly viewed as important in improving long-term outcomes. All DMTs reduce relapse frequency and higher efficacy drugs, for example B-cell depleting monoclonal antibodies, reduce the development of disability. Recently, immunotherapies have also been approved to prevent disability in progressive forms of MS, although only where

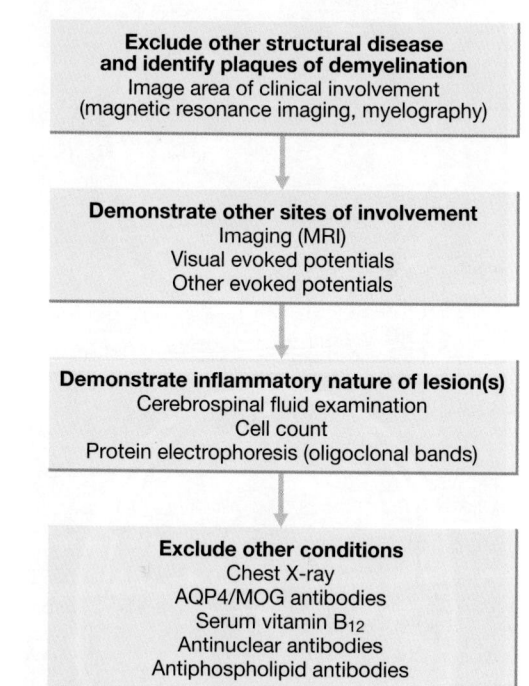

Exclude other structural disease and identify plaques of demyelination
Image area of clinical involvement
(magnetic resonance imaging, myelography)

Demonstrate other sites of involvement
Imaging (MRI)
Visual evoked potentials
Other evoked potentials

Demonstrate inflammatory nature of lesion(s)
Cerebrospinal fluid examination
Cell count
Protein electrophoresis (oligoclonal bands)

Exclude other conditions
Chest X-ray
AQP4/MOG antibodies
Serum vitamin B_{12}
Antinuclear antibodies
Antiphospholipid antibodies

Fig. 28.27 Investigations in a patient suspected of having multiple sclerosis.

active inflammation can be demonstrated. In general, drugs with higher efficacy are associated with more serious side-effects and clinical trials are under way to determine the optimum level of immune treatment early in the course of MS (Box 28.47). Careful selection and counselling of patients are necessary and these drugs should be supervised by teams experienced in their use, as recommended in national guidelines. Some DMTs can be used during pregnancy, but MS specialist advice should be sought.

Smoking, poor diet and obesity are risk factors for disease progression in MS, and should be addressed as early as possible.

The acute relapse

In a disabling relapse of MS, pulses of high-dose glucocorticoid, given either intravenously or orally over 3–5 days, will shorten the duration of the acute episode, but will not affect long-term recovery. If a patient develops a new neurological deficit whilst on a DMT, consideration should also be given to possible neurological side-effects of the drug (e.g. visual loss due to fingolimod-associated macular oedema, cognitive symptoms caused by natalizumab-associated PML)

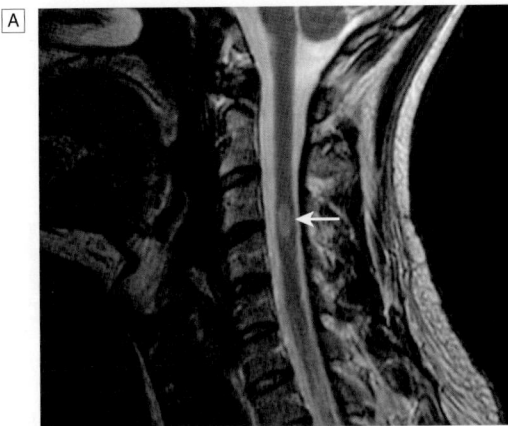
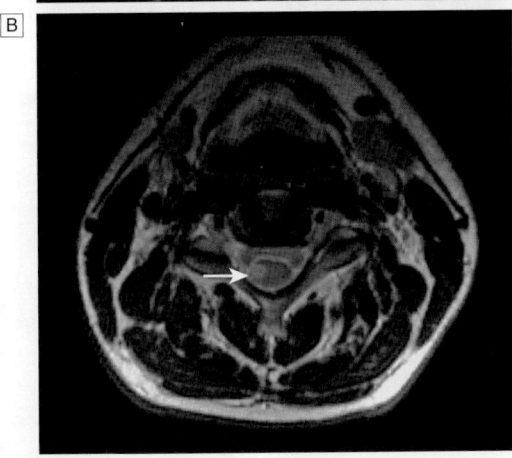

Fig. 28.28 Multiple sclerosis. Demyelinating lesion in cervical spinal cord, high-signal T2 images (arrows). [A] Sagittal plane. [B] Axial plane.

Treatment of symptoms, complications and disability

Treatments for the complications of MS are summarised in Box 28.48. It is important to provide patients with a careful explanation of the nature of the disease and its outcome. Specialist nurses working in a multidisciplinary team of health-care professionals are of great value in managing the chronic phase of the disease. Periods of physiotherapy and occupational therapy may improve functional capacity in those who become disabled, and guidance can be provided on the provision of aids at home. Bladder care is particularly important. Urgency and frequency can be treated pharmacologically (see Box 28.23) but this may lead to a degree of retention with an attendant risk of infection. Urinary retention can be managed initially by intermittent urinary catheterisation but an in-dwelling catheter may become necessary. It is important to address sexual dysfunction, which can occur and is a frequent source of distress. Pregnancy does not increase the risk of progression of MS but relapses may occur post-partum (Box 28.49).

Acute disseminated encephalomyelitis

This is an acute, often severe monophasic demyelinating condition in which areas of perivenous demyelination are widely disseminated throughout the brain and spinal cord. The illness may arise spontaneously but often occurs a week or so after a viral infection, especially measles or chickenpox, or following vaccination, suggesting that it is immunologically mediated.

Clinical features

Headache, vomiting, pyrexia, delirium and meningism may be presenting features, often with focal or multifocal brain and spinal cord signs. Seizures or coma may occur. A minority of patients who recover have further episodes.

---

i 28.47 Disease-modifying treatments in multiple sclerosis

Treatment	Route of administration/ dosing	Comment
High-efficacy biologic therapy: average relapse rate reduction > 50%		
Ocrelizumab	Intravenous infusion every 6 months	Associated with infusion reactions, increased infection risk and hypogammaglobulinaemia. Rituximab is also widely used in some countries with strong RCT evidence
Natalizumab	4-weekly intravenous infusion	Risk of PML in individuals who have evidence of JC virus infection
Alemtuzumab	Intravenous infusion over two courses separated by 12 months; 5-day infusion initially, second course 3 days	Cytokine release syndrome and infusion reactions. 30% develop secondary autoimmunity, mainly affecting thyroid
Moderate efficacy immunotherapy: average relapse rate reduction 30%–50%		
Fingolimod	Daily oral	More effective than interferon. First dose bradycardia, increased susceptibility to infections, macular oedema
Cladribine	Pulsed oral treatment	Risk of lymphopenia and infections. Some concern about longer-term cancer risk
Dimethyl fumarate	Daily oral	May cause flushing and gastrointestinal disturbance. Small risk of PML
Lower efficacy immunotherapy: average relapse rate reduction 30%		
Glatiramer acetate	Alternate-day subcutaneous injection	Similar efficacy to interferon-beta
Teriflunomide	Daily oral	May cause diarrhoea, alopecia, hepatotoxicity and teratogenicity
Interferon-beta	Alternate-day or weekly intramuscular or subcutaneous injection	In widespread use for reducing relapse rate

(JC virus = human polyoma virus 2; PML = progressive multifocal leukoencephalopathy; RCT = randomised controlled trial)

Investigations

MRI shows multiple high-signal areas in a pattern similar to that of MS, although often with large confluent areas of abnormality. CSF may be normal or show an increase in protein and lymphocytes (occasionally > 100 × 10⁶ cells/L). Oligoclonal bands may be found in the acute episode but, in contrast to MS, do not persist beyond clinical recovery. The clinical picture may be very similar to a first relapse of MS.

Management

The prognosis for acute disseminated encephalomyelitis is generally good, although occasionally it may be fatal. Treatment with high-dose intravenous methylprednisolone, using the same regimen as for a relapse of MS, is recommended.

28

i **28.48 Treatment of complications in multiple sclerosis**

i | **28.48 Treatment of complications in multiple sclerosis**

Dysaesthesia and pain

- Carbamazepine
- Gabapentin
- Duloxetine
- Amitriptyline

Walking speed

- Fampridine

Bladder symptoms

- See Box 28.23

Erectile dysfunction

- Sildenafil 50–100 mg/day
- Tadalafil

Spasticity

- Physiotherapy
- Baclofen (usually oral)
- Dantrolene
- Gabapentin
- Cannabinoids
- Tizanidine
- Intrathecal baclofen
- Local (intramuscular) injection of botulinum toxin
- Chemical neuronectomy

28.49 Multiple sclerosis in pregnancy

- **Counselling**: provision of pre-conception counselling is best practice.
- **Relapse risk**: slight reduction in relapse rate during pregnancy, but increased risk of postpartum relapse
- **Disease-modifying drugs**: some DMTs can be continued during pregnancy following assessment of risk–benefit. Specialist advice is recommended in all cases.

(DMT = disease-modifying treatment)

Transverse myelitis

Transverse myelitis is an acute, usually monophasic, demyelinating disorder affecting the spinal cord. It is sometimes thought to be post-infectious in origin. It occurs at any age and presents with a subacute paraparesis with a sensory level, accompanied by severe pain in the neck or back at the onset. MRI should distinguish this from an external lesion affecting the spinal cord. CSF examination shows cellular pleocytosis. Oligoclonal bands are usually absent. Treatment is with high-dose intravenous methylprednisolone. The outcome is variable: one-third have static deficit, one-third go on to develop MS and one-third recover with no subsequent relapse. Some clinical features may suggest a higher risk of MS after transverse myelitis.

Neuromyelitis optica

Neuromyelitis optica spectrum disorder (NMOSD, previously Devic disease) typically presents with severe optic neuritis or longitudinally extensive transverse myelitis. NMO can also cause severe vomiting or hiccups due to brainstem dysfunction. With cord presentations, spinal MRI scans show lesions that are typically longer than three spinal segments. The majority of cases are associated with an antibody against an astrocytic water channel, aquaporin 4. It is likely that this is a pathogenic antibody. The presence of aquaporin 4 antibodies is a strong predictor of future relapse. More recently it is recognised that some cases of NMOSD can be associated with myelin oligodendrocyte glycoprotein-associated MOG antibodies, although these patients might be less prone to relapse. A proportion of NMOSD are not associated with known antibodies. Brain lesions can be seen on MRI, but are less prominent than in MS and can develop in aquaporin 4-rich areas around the base of the fourth ventricle. Clinical deficits tend to recover less well than in MS, and the disease may be more aggressive with more frequent relapses. Treatment with glucocorticoids, oral immunosuppression and rituximab is often used. Recent clinical trials have suggested efficacy of B-cell depletion, IL-6 blockade and complement inhibition (Fig. 28.29).

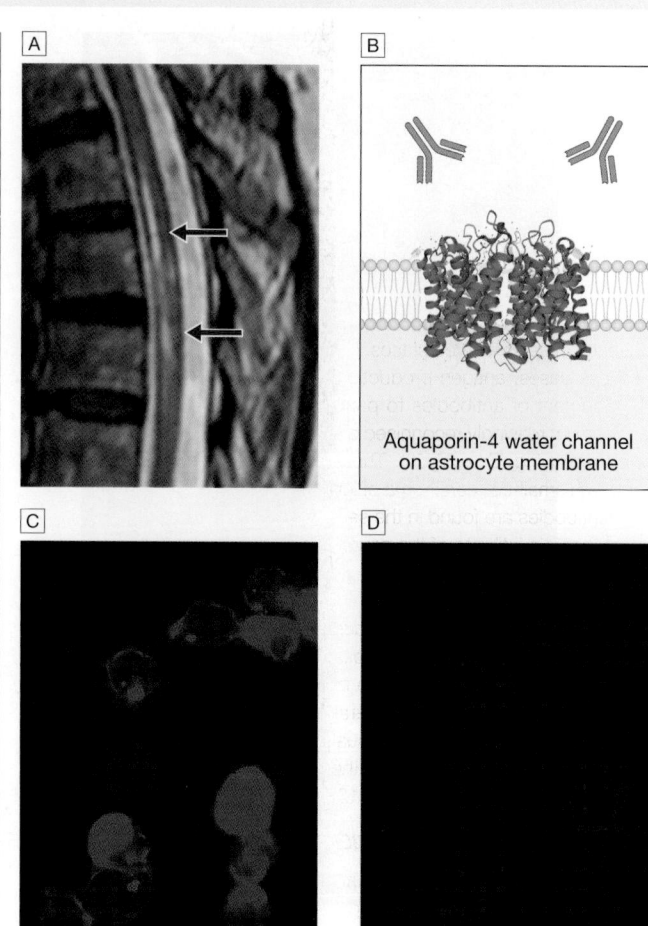

AQP4   + Patient serum

Fig. 28.29 Neuromyelitis optica. NMOSD typically causes longitudinally extensive transverse myelitis, extending over three or more vertebral segments. [A] MRI scan of spinal cord (T2-weighted) shows long hyperintense lesion within the thoracic spinal cord (red arrows). [B] NMOSD is typically associated with antibodies against the astrocytic water channel aquaporin 4. [C] These antibodies can be detected by cell-based assays, where serum is added to cells transfected with AQP4 (green). [D] If antibodies are present in serum, these bind to the surface of the transfected cells (red). *(A) From Williams J, McGlasson S, Irani S, et al. Neuromyelitis optica in patients with increased interferon alpha concentrations. Lancet Neurol 2020; 19(1):31–33. (D) Courtesy of Professor Sarosh Irani, University of Oxford.*

Autoimmune encephalitis

Autoimmune encephalitis (AE) is an immune-mediated brain disease which can occur at any age and presents with cognitive symptoms, behavioural change and seizures. AE can occasionally develop following a preceding infection and should be considered if there is an inflammatory deterioration following recovery from an initial brain infection. AE can present with distinct clinical syndromes and these are associated with specific autoantibodies directed against neuronal cell surface antigens. Limbic encephalitis presents with memory disturbance (and can mimic neurodegenerative dementia in older persons), emotional and behavioural disturbance and seizures, which can cause brief dystonic movements of the face and arm (facio-brachial dystonic seizures). MRI may show enhancement and inflammation in hippocampus and associated limbic structures, and there are often mild inflammatory changes in the CSF. There is a strong association with Lgi1 and CASPR2 antibodies.

AE can also be associated with NMDAR antibodies, and this syndrome typically presents with neuropsychiatric symptoms, movement disorders, autonomic dysfunction and seizures and often causes serious illness requiring intensive care admission. A subset of NMDAR encephalitis is associated with ovarian teratoma. Corticosteroids, immune globulin and plasma exchange are often used acutely. AE can relapse or follow a chronic course and long-term immunosuppression with oral immunosuppressants, cyclophosphamide or rituximab may be needed.

Paraneoplastic neurological disorders

Neurological disease may occur with systemic malignant tumours in the absence of cerebral metastases. It is now recognised that, in the majority of these cases, antigen production in the body of the tumour leads to development of antibodies to parts of the CNS. Paraneoplastic conditions are increasingly recognised and the number of antibodies identified is also growing (Box 28.50). These syndromes are particularly associated with small-cell carcinoma of lung, ovarian tumours and lymphomas. Autoantibodies are found in the serum and/or CSF, and biopsy will show a lymphocytic infiltrate of the neural tissue affected.

Clinical features

Clinical presentations are summarised in Box 28.50. In most instances, the neurological condition progresses quite rapidly over a few months, preceding the malignant disease in around half of cases. The range of clinical patterns is so wide that paraneoplastic disease should be considered in the diagnosis of any unusual progressive neurological syndrome. The paraneoplastic disorders of the peripheral nervous system particularly affect the synaptic cleft (p. 1122).

Investigations and management

The presence of characteristic autoantibodies in the context of a suspicious clinical picture may be diagnostic. The causative tumour may be very small and therefore CT of the chest or abdomen or PET scanning may be necessary to find it. These investigations should be pursued only when paraneoplastic disease has been proven, rather than when it is suspected. The CSF often shows an increased protein and lymphocyte count with oligoclonal bands.

Treatment is directed at the primary tumour. Occasionally, successful therapy of the tumour is associated with improvement of the paraneoplastic syndrome. Some improvement may occur following administration of intravenous immunoglobulin.

Neurodegenerative diseases

While MS is the most common cause of disability in young people in the UK, vascular and neurodegenerative diseases are increasingly important in later life. The neurodegenerative diseases are united in having a pathological process that leads to specific neuronal death, causing relentlessly progressive symptoms, with incidence rising with age. The causes are not yet known, although genetic influences are important. Alzheimer's disease and Parkinson's disease are the most common.

Movement disorders

Movement disorders present with a wide range of symptoms. They may be genetic or acquired, and the most important is Parkinson's disease. Most movement disorders are categorised clinically, with few confirmatory investigations available other than for those with a known gene abnormality.

Idiopathic Parkinson's disease

Parkinsonism is a clinical syndrome characterised primarily by bradykinesia, with associated increased tone (rigidity), tremor and loss of postural reflexes. There are many causes (Box 28.51) but the most

i	**28.50 Paraneoplastic disorders of the nervous system**
Clinical presentation	**Associated tumour**
Central nervous system	
Limbic encephalitis	SCLC, testicular, breast, thymoma, teratoma
Myelopathy	SCLC, thymoma, others
Stiff person syndrome	Breast, SCLC, thymoma, others
Cerebellar degeneration	Breast, ovarian, SCLC, lymphoma
Encephalomyelitis	SCLC, thymoma
Opsoclonus–myoclonus	Breast, ovarian, SCLC, neuroblastoma, testicular
Optic neuritis	SCLC
Peripheral nervous system	
Neuromyotonia	Thymoma, SCLC, others
Myasthenia gravis	Thymoma
Sensorimotor polyneuropathy	Lymphoma, SCLC, others
Lambert–Eaton syndrome	SCLC
Motor neuropathy	Lymphoma, SCLC, others
Sensory neuropathy	Lymphoma, SCLC, others
Polymyositis/dermatomyositis	Lung, breast

(SCLC = small cell lung cancer)

i 28.51 Causes of parkinsonism

Idiopathic Parkinson's disease (at least 80% of parkinsonism)

Cerebrovascular disease

Drugs and toxins

- Antipsychotic drugs (older and 'atypical')
- Metoclopramide, prochlorperazine
- Tetrabenazine
- Sodium valproate
- Lithium
- Manganese
- MPTP

Other degenerative diseases

- Dementia with Lewy bodies
- Progressive supranuclear palsy
- Multiple system atrophy
- Corticobasal degeneration
- Alzheimer's disease

Genetic

- Huntington's disease
- Fragile X tremor ataxia syndrome
- Dopa-responsive dystonia
- Spinocerebellar ataxias (particularly SCA 3)
- Wilson's disease

Anoxic brain injury

(MPTP = methyl-phenyl-tetrahydropyridine)

common is Parkinson's disease (PD). PD has an annual incidence of about 18/100 000 in the UK and a prevalence of about 180/100 000. Age has a critical influence on incidence and prevalence, the latter rising to 300–500/100 000 after 80 years of age. The global prevalence of PD (over 6 million in 2016) more than doubled between 1990 and 2016 with increases across all socio-demographic regions of the world, related mainly to increasing age and longer disease duration. Average age of onset is about 60 years and fewer than 5% of patients present under the age of 40. Genetic factors are increasingly recognised and several single genes causing parkinsonism have been identified. Monogenic Parkinson's disease can be caused by mutations in *SNCA* (which encode alpha-synuclein), as well as *Parkin*, *PINK1*, *DJ-1* and many more, although overall monogenic disease accounts for a very small proportion of cases overall. Mutations in the *LRRK2* gene are the most frequent genetic cause of late-onset PD. Having a first-degree relative with PD confers a 2–3 times

28

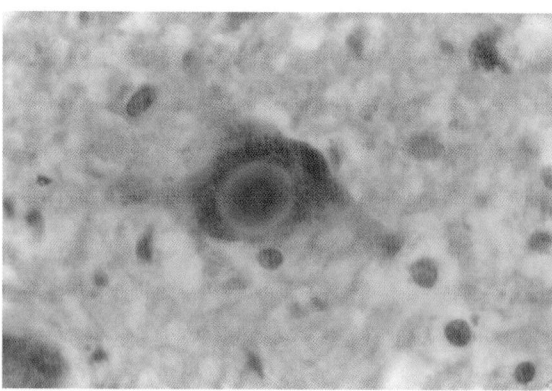

Fig. 28.30 Parkinson's disease. High power (× 400) view of substantia nigra of a patient with Parkinson's disease showing classical Lewy body (haematoxylin and eosin). *Courtesy of Dr J. Xuereb.*

General

- Expressionless face (hypomimia)
- Soft, rapid, indistinct speech (dysphonia)
- Flexed (stooped) posture
- Impaired postural reflexes

Gait

- Slow to start walking (failure of gait ignition)
- Rapid, short stride length, tendency to shorten (festination)
- Reduction of arm swing
- Impaired balance on turning

Tremor

Resting (3–4 Hz, moderate amplitude): most common

- Asymmetric, usually first in arm/hand ('pill rolling')
- May affect legs, jaw and chin but not head
- Intermittent, present at rest, often briefly abolished by movement of limb, exacerbated by walking

Postural (6–8 Hz, moderate amplitude)

- Present immediately on stretching out arms

Re-emergent tremor (3–4 Hz, moderate amplitude)

- Initially no tremor on stretching arms out, rest tremor re-emerges after a few seconds

Rigidity

- Cogwheel type, mostly upper limbs (due to tremor superimposed on rigidity)
- Lead pipe type

Akinesia (fundamental feature)

- Slowness of movement
- Fatiguing and decrease in size of repetitive movements

Normal findings (if abnormal, consider other causes)

- Power, deep tendon reflexes, plantar responses
- Eye movements
- Sensory and cerebellar examination

---

increased risk of developing the disorder. It is progressive and incurable, with a variable prognosis. While motor symptoms are the most common presenting features, non-motor symptoms (particularly cognitive impairment, depression and anxiety) become increasingly prominent as the disease progresses, and significantly reduce quality of life.

Pathophysiology

Although mutations in several genes have been identified in a few cases, in most patients the cause remains unknown. The discovery that methyl-phenyl-tetrahydropyridine (MPTP) caused severe parkinsonism in young drug users suggested that PD might be due to an environmental toxin but none has been convincingly identified. The pathological hallmarks of PD are depletion of the pigmented dopaminergic neurons in the substantia nigra and the presence of α-synuclein and other protein inclusions in nigral cells (Lewy bodies; Fig. 28.30). It is thought that environmental or genetic factors alter the α-synuclein protein, rendering it toxic and leading to Lewy body formation within the nigral cells. Lewy bodies are also found in the basal ganglia, brainstem and cortex, and increase with disease progression. PD is recognised as a synucleinopathy alongside multiple system atrophy and dementia with Lewy bodies. The loss of dopaminergic neurotransmission is responsible for many of the clinical features.

Clinical features

Non-motor symptoms, including reduction in sense of smell (hyposmia), anxiety/depression, constipation and REM sleep behavioural disturbance (RBD), may precede the development of typical motor features by many years but patients rarely present at this stage. The motor symptoms are almost always initially asymmetrical. The hallmark is bradykinesia, leading to classic symptoms such as increasingly small handwriting ('micrographia'), difficulty tying shoelaces or buttoning clothes, and difficulty rolling over in bed. Tremor is an early feature but may not be present in at least 20% of people with PD. It is typically a unilateral rest tremor affecting limbs, jaw and chin but not the head. In some patients tremor remains the dominant symptom for many years. Rigidity causes stiffness and a flexed posture. Although postural righting reflexes are impaired early on in the disease, falls tend not to occur until later. As the disease advances, speech becomes softer and indistinct. There are a number of abnormalities on neurological examination (Box 28.52).

Although features are initially unilateral, gradual bilateral involvement evolves with time. Cognition is spared in early disease; if impaired, it should trigger consideration of alternative diagnoses, such as dementia with Lewy bodies.

Non-motor symptoms

While non-motor symptoms may precede the onset of more typical symptoms by many years, for most patients these features become increasingly common and disabling as PD progresses. Cognitive impairment, including dementia, is the symptom most likely to impair quality of life for patients and their carers. Estimates of dementia frequency range from 30% to 80%, depending on definitions and length of follow-up. Other distressing non-motor symptoms include neuropsychiatric features (anxiety, depression, apathy, hallucinosis/psychosis), sleep disturbance and hypersomnolence, fatigue, pain, sphincter disturbance and constipation, sexual problems (erectile failure, loss of libido or hypersexuality), drooling and weight loss.

Investigations

The diagnosis is clinical. Structural imaging (CT or MRI) is usually normal for age and thus rarely helpful, although it may support a suspected vascular cause of parkinsonism. Functional dopaminergic imaging (SPECT or PET) is abnormal, even in the early stages (Fig. 28.31), but does not differentiate between the different forms of degenerative parkinsonism (see Box 28.51) and so is not specific for PD. In younger patients, specific investigations may be appropriate (e.g. exclusion of Huntington's or Wilson's diseases). Some patients with family histories may wish to consider genetic testing, although the role of genetic counselling is uncertain at present.

Management

Drug therapy

Drug treatment for PD remains symptomatic rather than curative, and there is no evidence that any of the currently available drugs are neuroprotective. Levodopa (LD) remains the most effective treatment

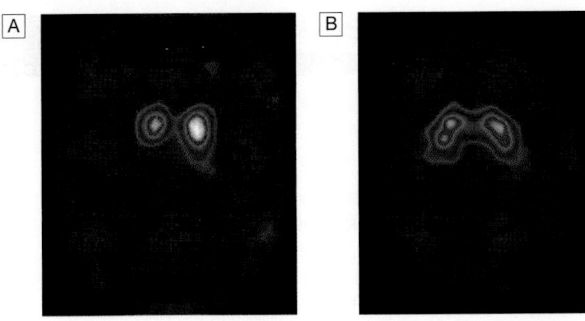

Fig. 28.31 Imaging in Parkinson's disease. A Single photon emission computed tomography (SPECT) in Parkinson's disease showing reduced dopamine activity in the basal ganglia. B Normal.

i	28.53 Dopamine agonists*

Ergot-derived

- Bromocriptine
- Lisuride
- Pergolide
- Cabergoline

Non-ergot-derived

- Ropinirole
- Pramipexole
- Rotigotine (transdermal patch)
- Apomorphine (subcutaneous, nasal, sublingual)

*Oral unless otherwise stated.

available but other agents include dopamine agonists, anticholinergics, inhibitors of monoamine oxidase (MAOI)-B and catechol-O-methyl-transferase (COMT), and amantadine. Debate continues about when and what treatment should be started. In general, most specialists recommend initiating treatment when symptoms are impacting on everyday life, although some favour treatment as soon as the diagnosis is made. Whether it is best to start with LD, a dopamine agonist or MAOI-B remains unclear but most accept that the most effective, best-tolerated and cheapest drug is LD. Many motor symptoms, such as tremor, freezing, falling, head-drop and abnormal flexion, are quite resistant to treatment. Some non-motor symptoms, such as anxiety or depression, may respond to drug or non-drug treatments. In the UK, rivastigmine is licensed for use in PD-associated dementia, although its effect is modest. Many other non-motor symptoms are resistant to treatment. Drugs for PD should not be stopped abruptly, as this can precipitate malignant hyperthermia.

Levodopa Levodopa is the precursor to dopamine. When administered orally, more than 90% is decarboxylated to dopamine peripherally in the gastrointestinal tract and blood vessels, and only a small proportion reaches the brain. This peripheral conversion is responsible for the high frequency of adverse effects. To avoid this, LD is combined with a dopa decarboxylase inhibitor (DDI); the inhibitor does not cross the blood–brain barrier, thus avoiding unwanted decarboxylation-blocking in the brain. Two DDIs, carbidopa and benserazide, are available as combination preparations with LD (Sinemet and Madopar, respectively).

LD is most effective for relieving akinesia and rigidity; tremor response is often less satisfactory and it has no effect on many motor (posture, freezing) and non-motor symptoms. Failure of akinesia/rigidity to respond to LD (1000 mg/day) should prompt reconsideration of the diagnosis. Although controlled-release versions of LD exist, these are usually best reserved for use overnight, as their variable bioavailability makes them difficult to use throughout the day. Madopar is also available as a dispersible tablet for more rapid-onset effect.

Adverse effects include postural hypotension, nausea and vomiting, which may be offset by domperidone, though this is only prescribed for brief periods, if essential, given the risk of prolonged QTc interval and arrhythmia. LD may exacerbate or trigger hallucinations, and abnormal LD-seeking behaviour (dopamine dysregulation syndrome), in which the patient takes excessive doses of LD, may occur uncommonly.

As PD progresses, the response to LD becomes less predictable in many patients, leading to motor fluctuations. This end-of-dose deterioration is due to progressive loss of dopamine storage capacity by dwindling numbers of striatonigral neurons. LD-induced involuntary movements (dyskinesia) may occur as a peak-dose phenomenon or as a biphasic phenomenon (occurring during both the build-up and wearing-off phases). More complex fluctuations present as sudden, unpredictable changes in response, in which periods of parkinsonism ('off' phases) alternate with improved mobility but with dyskinesias ('on' phases). Motor complication management is difficult; wearing-off effects may respond to increased dose or frequency of LD or the addition of a COMT inhibitor (see below). More complex fluctuations may be improved by the addition of dopamine agonists (including continuous infusion of apomorphine), use of intraintestinal LD via a percutaneous endoscopic jejunostomy, or deep brain stimulator implantation.

Dopamine receptor agonists Originally introduced in the hope of delaying the initiation of LD and thus delaying motor complications, several dopamine agonists are available, and may be delivered orally, transdermally, sublingually, intranasally or subcutaneously (Box 28.53).

The ergot-derived agonists are no longer recommended because of rare but serious fibrotic side-effects. With the exception of apomorphine, all the agonists are considerably less effective than LD in relieving parkinsonism, have more adverse effects (nausea, vomiting, disorientation and hallucinations, impulse control disorders) and are more expensive. Their role in the management of PD (monotherapy or adjunctive) remains uncertain, and evidence suggests that their usefulness as initial monotherapy is short-lasting.

MAOI-B inhibitors Monoamine oxidase type B facilitates breakdown of excess dopamine in the synapse. Two inhibitors are used in PD: selegiline and rasagiline. The effects of both are modest, although usually well tolerated. Neither is neuroprotective, despite initial hopes.

COMT inhibitors Catechol-O-methyl-transferase (along with dopa decarboxylase) is involved in peripheral breakdown of LD. Three inhibitors are available: entacapone, opicapone and tolcapone (which also inhibits central COMT). Entacapone has a modest effect and is most useful for early wearing-off. It is available either as a single tablet taken with each LD/DDI dose, or as a combination tablet with LD and DDI. The more potent tolcapone is less used because of rare but serious hepatotoxicity. Opicapone, the newest of the three, is available as a once-daily drug.

Amantadine This has a mild, usually short-lived effect on bradykinesia and is rarely used unless patients are unable to tolerate other drugs. It is more commonly employed as a treatment for LD-induced dyskinesias, although again benefit is modest and short-lived. Adverse effects include livedo reticularis, peripheral oedema, delirium and other anticholinergic effects.

Anticholinergic drugs These were the main treatment for PD prior to the introduction of LD. Their role now is limited by lack of efficacy (apart from an effect on tremor sometimes) and adverse effects, including dry mouth, blurred vision, constipation, urinary retention, delirium and hallucinosis, as well as long-term concerns regarding cognitive impairment. Several anticholinergics are available, including trihexyphenidyl (benzhexol) and orphenadrine.

28

Surgery

Destructive neurosurgery was commonly used before the introduction of LD. In the last 20 years, stereotactic surgery has emerged and most commonly involves deep brain stimulation (DBS), rather than the destructive approach of previous eras. Various targets have been identified, including the thalamus (only effective for tremor), globus pallidus and subthalamic nucleus. DBS is usually reserved for individuals with medically refractory tremor or motor fluctuations, and careful patient selection is vital to success. Intracranial delivery of fetal grafts or specific growth factors remains experimental. MRI-guided ultrasound-induced thalamotomy is a relatively new treatment for tremor; long-term outcomes are not well established.

Physiotherapy, occupational therapy and speech therapy

Patients at all stages of PD benefit from physiotherapy, which helps reduce rigidity and corrects abnormal posture. Occupational therapists can provide equipment to help overcome functional limitations, such as rails for stairs and the toilet, and bathing equipment. Speech therapy can help where dysarthria and dysphonia interfere with communication, and advice may also be provided to those with dysphagia. As with many complex neurological disorders, patients with PD should ideally be managed by a multidisciplinary team, including PD specialist nurses.

Other Parkinsonian syndromes

Cerebrovascular disease and drug-induced parkinsonism are the most common alternative causes of parkinsonism (see Box 28.51). There are several degenerative conditions that cause parkinsonism, including multiple system atrophy, progressive supranuclear palsy and corticobasal degeneration. They typically have a more rapid progression than PD and tend to be resistant to treatment with LD. They are defined pathologically and identification during life is difficult. There are other conditions that may rarely manifest as parkinsonism, including Huntington's and Wilson's diseases.

Multiple system atrophy

Multiple system atrophy (MSA) is characterised by parkinsonism, autonomic failure and cerebellar symptoms, with either parkinsonism (MSA-P) or cerebellar features (MSA-C) predominating. It is much less common than PD, with a prevalence of about 4/100000. Although early distinction between PD and MSA-P may be difficult, early falls, postural instability and lack of response to LD are clues. The pathological hallmark is α-synuclein-containing glial cytoplasmic inclusions found in the basal ganglia, cerebellum and motor cortex. Management is symptomatic and the prognosis is less good than for PD, with mean survival from symptom onset of fewer than 10 years and early disability. Cognition is usually unaffected.

Progressive supranuclear palsy

Progressive supranuclear palsy (PSP) presents with symmetrical parkinsonism, cognitive impairment, early falls and bulbar symptoms. The characteristic eye movement disorder, with slowed vertical saccades leading to impairment of up- and down-gaze, may take years to emerge. PSP has different pathological features, being associated with abnormal accumulation of tau (τ) proteins and degeneration of the substantia nigra, subthalamic nucleus and mid-brain. It is therefore considered a tauopathy rather than synucleinopathy. The prevalence is about 5/100000, with average survival similar to that in MSA. There is no treatment, and the parkinsonism usually does not respond to LD.

Corticobasal degeneration

Corticobasal degeneration (CBD) is less common than MSA or PSP, and the clinical manifestations are variable, including parkinsonism,

ℹ	28.54 Causes of acquired ataxia

Structural

- Brain tumour
- Brain abscess

Toxic

- Drugs: lithium, several antiepileptics (including phenytoin, carbamazepine, lamotrigine and valproate), amiodarone, toluene, 5-fluorouracil, cytosine arabinoside
- Alcohol
- Heavy metals/chemicals: mercury, lead, thallium

Infection/post-infectious

- HIV
- Varicella zoster
- Whipple's disease
- Miller Fisher syndrome (p. 1192)

Degenerative

- Multiple system atrophy
- Sporadic Creutzfeldt–Jakob disease
- Idiopathic (or sporadic) late-onset cerebellar ataxia

Inflammatory/immune-mediated

- Multiple sclerosis
- Gluten ataxia (coeliac disease)
- Paraneoplastic ataxia
- Hashimoto encephalopathy

Metabolic

- Vitamin B$_1$ or E deficiency
- Hypothyroidism
- Hypoparathyroidism

Vascular

- Stroke (ischaemic or haemorrhagic)
- Vascular malformations
- Superficial siderosis

dystonia, myoclonus and 'alien limb' phenomenon, whereby a limb (usually upper) moves about or interferes with the other limb without apparent conscious control. Cortical symptoms, including dementia and especially apraxia, are common and may be the only features in some cases. A number of other diseases may present with a corticobasal *syndrome*, including other dementias. CBD is a tauopathy with widespread deposition throughout the brain and has similar survival rates to MSA and PSP.

Wilson's disease

This is an autosomal recessive disorder resulting from mutation in the *ATP7B* gene, causing a defect of copper metabolism (p. 907). It is a treatable cause of various movement disorders, including tremor, dystonia, parkinsonism and ataxia; psychiatric symptoms may also occur. Wilson's disease should always be excluded in patients under the age of 50 presenting with any movement disorder.

Huntington's disease

Huntington's disease (HD) is an autosomal dominant disorder, presenting in adults usually but occasionally in children. It is due to expansion of a trinucleotide CAG repeat in the *Huntingtin* gene on chromosome 4 (see Box 3.2). The disease frequently demonstrates the phenomenon of anticipation, in which there is a younger age at onset as the disease is passed through generations, due to progressive expansion of the repeat. The prevalence is about 4–8/100000.

Clinical features

HD typically presents with a progressive behavioural disturbance, abnormal movements (usually chorea) and cognitive impairment leading to dementia. Onset under 18 years is rare but patients may then present with parkinsonism rather than chorea (the 'Westphal variant'). There is always a family history, although this may not always be apparent and can sometimes be concealed.

28.55 Inherited ataxias

Inheritance pattern	Age of onset	Clinical features
Autosomal dominant		
Episodic ataxias	Childhood and early adulthood	Brief episodes of ataxia, sometimes induced by stress or startle. May develop progressive ataxia
Spinocerebellar ataxias (SCAs)	Childhood to middle age	Over 35 subtypes identified. Progressive ataxia, sometimes associated with other features, e.g. retinitis pigmentosa, pyramidal tract abnormalities, peripheral neuropathy and cognitive deficits
Dentato-rubro-pallidoluysian atrophy (DRPLA)	Childhood to middle age	Children present with myoclonic epilepsy and progressive ataxia. Adults have progressive ataxia with psychiatric features, dementia and choreoathetosis
Autosomal recessive		
Friedreich's ataxia	Childhood/adolescence (late onset possible)	Ataxia, nystagmus, dysarthria, spasticity, areflexia, proprioceptive impairment, diabetes mellitus, optic atrophy, cardiac abnormalities. Usually chair-bound
Ataxia telangiectasia	Childhood	Progressive ataxia, athetosis, telangiectasia on conjunctivae, impaired DNA repair, immune deficiency, tendency to malignancies
Abetalipoproteinaemia	Childhood	Steatorrhoea, sensorimotor neuropathy, retinitis pigmentosa, malabsorption of vitamins A, D, E and K
Hereditary ataxia with vitamin E deficiency	< 20 years	Similar to Friedreich's ataxia, visual loss or retinitis pigmentosa, chorea
Others	Usually young onset	Numerous, with genes identified only in some
X-linked		
Fragile X tremor ataxia syndrome	> 50 years	Tremor, ataxia, parkinsonism, autonomic failure, cognitive impairment and dementia
Adrenoleukodystrophy	Childhood to adult	Impaired adrenal and cognitive function, sometimes spastic paraparesis
Mitochondrial disease	Various	Ataxia features in several mitochondrial diseases, including Kearns–Sayre syndrome, MELAS, MERRF, Leigh syndrome

(MELAS = mitochondrial myopathy, encephalopathy, lactic acidosis and stroke-like episodes; MERRF = myoclonic epilepsy with ragged red fibres)

Investigations and management

The diagnosis is confirmed by genetic testing; pre-symptomatic testing for other family members is available but must be preceded by appropriate counselling. Brain imaging may show caudate atrophy but is not a reliable test. There are a number of HD mimics.

Management is symptomatic, though antisense oligonucleotide therapy to reduce the Huntingtin gene (*HTT*) product is currently being trialled. The chorea may respond to neuroleptics such as risperidone or sulpiride, or tetrabenazine. Depression and anxiety are common and may be helped by medication.

Ataxias

The ataxias are a heterogeneous group of inherited and acquired disorders, presenting either with pure ataxia or in association with other neurological and non-neurological features. The differential is wide (Boxes 28.54 and 28.55), and diagnosis is guided by age of onset, evolution and clinical features. A significant proportion of cases remain idiopathic despite investigation.

The hereditary ataxias are a group of inherited disorders in which degenerative changes occur to varying extents in the cerebellum, brainstem, pyramidal tracts, spinocerebellar tracts and optic and peripheral nerves, and influence the clinical manifestations. Onset ranges from infancy to adulthood, with recessive, sex-linked or dominant inheritance (see Box 28.55). While the genetic abnormality has been identified for some, allowing diagnostic testing, this is not currently the case for many of the hereditary ataxias.

28.56 Drug-induced tremor (usually postural)*

- β-agonists (e.g. salbutamol)
- Theophylline
- Sodium valproate
- Thyroxine
- Lithium
- Tricyclic antidepressants
- Recreational drugs (e.g. amphetamines)
- Alcohol
- Caffeine

*Drugs causing parkinsonism and associated tremor are listed in Box 28.51.

Tremor disorders

Tremor is a feature of many disorders but the most important clinical syndromes are PD, essential tremor, drug-induced tremors (Box 28.56) and functional (psychogenic) tremors.

Essential tremor

This has a prevalence of about 300/100 000 and may display a dominant pattern of inheritance, although no genes have thus far been identified. It may present at any age with a bilateral arm tremor (8–10 Hz), rarely at rest but typical with movement. The head and voice may be involved. The tremor improves in about 50% of patients with small amounts of alcohol. There are no specific tests and essential tremor should be distinguished from other tremor syndromes, including dystonic tremor. Beta-blockers and primidone are sometimes helpful, and DBS of the thalamus is an effective treatment for severe cases.

28

Dystonia

Dystonia is characterised by a focal increase in tone affecting muscles in the limbs or trunk. It may be a feature of a number of neurological conditions (PD, Wilson's disease), or occur secondary to brain damage (trauma, stroke) or drugs (tardive syndromes). Dystonia also occurs as a primary disorder. With childhood onset the cause is usually genetic and dystonia is generalised, but adult onset is usually focal; examples include a twisted neck (torticollis), repetitive blinking (blepharospasm) or tremor. Task-specific symptoms (e.g. writer's cramp, musician's dystonia) are often dystonic. Treatment is difficult but botulinum toxin injections or DBS may be useful.

Hemifacial spasm

This usually presents after middle age with intermittent twitching around one eye, spreading ipsilaterally to other facial muscles. The spasms are exacerbated by talking, eating and stress. Hemifacial spasm is usually idiopathic, similar to trigeminal neuralgia; it has been suggested that it may be due to an aberrant arterial loop irritating the 7th nerve just outside the pons. It may, however, be symptomatic and secondary to structural lesions. Drug treatment is not effective but injections of botulinum toxin into affected muscles help, although these usually have to be repeated every 3 months or so. In refractory cases, microvascular decompression may be considered.

Motor neuron disease

Motor neuron disease (MND) is a neurodegenerative condition caused by loss of upper and lower motor neurons in the spinal cord, cranial nerve nuclei and motor cortex. Annual incidence is about 2/100000, with a prevalence of about 7/100000. Most cases are sporadic but 10% of cases are familial and mutations in *C9orf72* (repeat expansion), *SOD1*, *VCP*, *FUS* and *TARDBP/TDP43* are found in many of these monogenic cases and may influence clinical phenotype and course, in particular overlap with frontotemporal dementia. The most common form of MND (Fig. 28.32) is amyotrophic lateral sclerosis (ALS), and many use the terms MND and ALS interchangeably. ALS is characterised by a combination of upper and lower motor neuron signs; there are rarer, pure lower (progressive muscular atrophy) or upper (progressive lateral sclerosis) motor neuron variants of MND. The average age of onset is 65, with 10% presenting before 45 years.

Clinical features

Diagnosis can be difficult and is often delayed. MND typically presents focally, either with limb onset (e.g. foot drop or loss of manual dexterity) or with bulbar symptoms (dysarthria, swallowing difficulty); respiratory onset is rare but type II respiratory failure is a common cause of death. Sensory, autonomic and visual symptoms do not occur, although cramp is common (Box 28.57). Examination reveals a combination of lower and upper motor neuron signs (e.g. brisk reflexes in wasted, fasciculating muscles) without sensory involvement (see Fig. 28.32). Cognitive impairment is under-recognised in MND: up to 50% will have a mainly executive impairment on formal testing, and around 10% develop a frontotemporal dementia (FTD). About 10% of patients presenting with FTD will develop ALS within a few years of dementia onset. Even with treatment, MND is relentlessly progressive, but median survival is improved with specialist follow-up offering non-invasive ventilation, feeding measures and access to pharmacological treatment.

Investigations

Clinical features are often typical but alternative diagnoses should be excluded. Exclusion of treatable causes, such as immune-mediated

---

i   28.57 Clinical features of motor neuron disease

Onset

- Usually after the age of 50 years
- Very uncommon before the age of 30 years
- Affects males more commonly than females

Symptoms

- Limb muscle weakness, cramps, occasionally fasciculation
- Disturbance of speech/swallowing (dysarthria/dysphagia)
- Cognitive and behavioural features common (similar to frontotemporal dementia)

Signs

- Wasting and fasciculation of muscles
- Weakness of muscles of limbs, tongue, face and palate
- Pyramidal tract involvement, causing spasticity, exaggerated tendon reflexes, extensor plantar responses
- External ocular muscles and sphincters usually remain intact
- No objective sensory deficit
- Evidence of cognitive impairment with frontotemporal dominance

Course

- Symptoms often begin focally in one part and spread gradually but relentlessly to become widespread

---

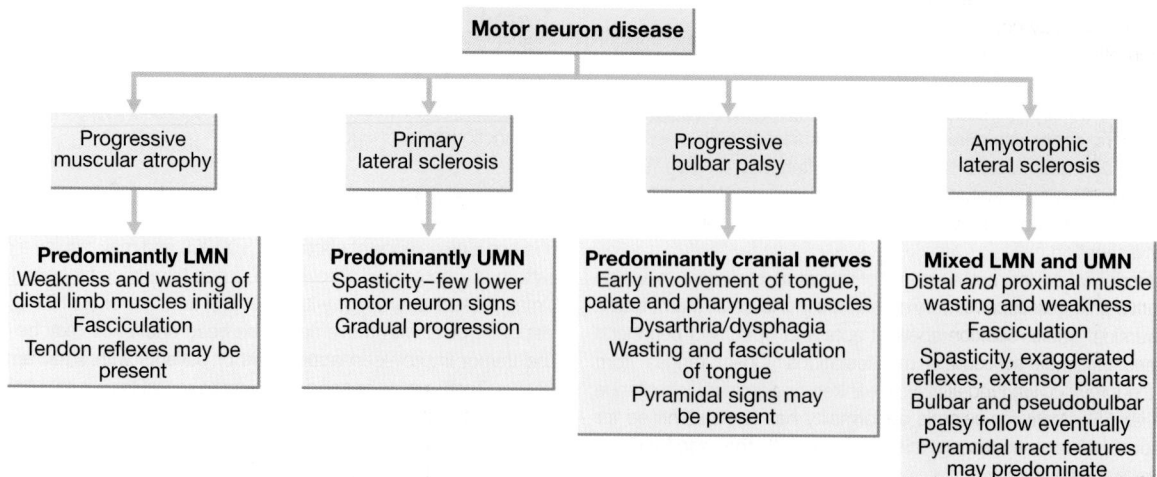

Fig. 28.32 Patterns of involvement in motor neuron disease. (LMN = lower motor neuron; UMN = upper motor neuron)

multifocal motor neuropathy with conduction block (p. 1192) and cervical myeloradiculopathy, is essential. Blood tests are usually normal, other than a mildly raised creatine kinase. Sensory and motor nerve conduction studies are normal but there may be reduction in amplitude of motor action potentials due to axonal loss. EMG will usually confirm the typical features of widespread denervation and re-innervation. Spinal fluid analysis is not usually necessary. Genetic testing is increasing in importance, with mutations found in *SOD1*, *FUS*, *TARDBP* and *C9orf72* that may help predict risk of disease in those with a family history of MND.

Management

Patients should be managed within a multidisciplinary service, including physiotherapists, speech and occupational therapists, dietitians, ventilatory and feeding support, and palliative care teams, with neurological and respiratory input. Riluzole, a glutamate release antagonist, is licensed for ALS but has only a modest effect, prolonging median survival by about 2–3 months.

Non-invasive ventilation significantly prolongs survival and improves or maintains quality of life in people with ALS. Survival and some measures of quality of life are significantly improved in the subgroup of people with better baseline bulbar function but not in those with severe bulbar impairment. Feeding by percutaneous gastrostomy may improve quality of life and prolong survival, even when done at a late stage. Rapid access to palliative care teams is essential for patients as they enter the terminal stages of MND.

Spinal muscular atrophy

This is a group of genetically determined recessive disorders affecting spinal and cranial lower motor neurons, characterised by proximal and distal wasting, fasciculation and weakness of muscles. Most SMA cases are caused by a defective *SMN1* gene. Involvement is usually symmetrical but occasional localised forms occur. With the exception of the infantile form, progression is slow and the prognosis better than for MND. Sophisticated nucleic acid-based therapies for the treatment of SMA have shown significant promise. Intrathecally delivered antisense oligonucleotide therapies can partially correct this *SMN1* genetic defect and show clinical efficacy in severe forms of the disease.

Infections of the nervous system

The clinical features of nervous system infections depend on the location of the infection (the meninges or the parenchyma of the brain and spinal cord), the causative organism (virus, bacterium, fungus or parasite), and whether the infection is acute or chronic. The major infections of the nervous system are listed in Box 28.58. The frequency of these varies geographically and in relation to socio-economic level. While certain infections, e.g. tuberculosis and cysticercosis, may not be prevalent in the United Kingdom, they are common in other regions and, therefore, occur in returning travellers or immigrants. Protozoal infections are described in Chapter 13.

Meningitis

The characteristic clinical features of acute infection of the meninges are pyrexia, headache and meningism. Meningism consists of headache, photophobia and stiffness of the neck, sometimes accompanied by other signs of meningeal irritation, including Kernig's sign (extension at the knee with the hip joint flexed causes spasm in the hamstring muscles) and Brudzinski's sign (passive flexion of the neck causes flexion of the hips and knees). However, as discussed in Chapter 1, meningitis frequently presents without meningism, and although Kernig's and Brudinski's signs are specific, their sensitivity can be as low as 5%. Therefore, meningitis should be considered in anyone who presents with fever and headache. Altered level of consciousness may occur and is more common in older people. Abnormalities in the CSF (see Box 28.6) are important in distinguishing the cause of meningitis. Causes of meningitis are listed in Box 28.59.

28.58 Infections of the nervous system

Bacterial infections
- Meningitis
- Suppurative encephalitis
- Brain abscess
- Paravertebral (epidural) abscess
- Tuberculosis
- Neurosyphilis
- Leprosy (Hansen's disease) (peripheral nerves)*
- Diphtheria (peripheral nerves)*
- Tetanus (motor cells)

Viral infections
- Meningitis
- Encephalitis
- Transverse myelitis
- Progressive multifocal leucoencephalopathy
- Poliomyelitis
- Subacute sclerosing panencephalitis (late sequel)
- Rabies
- HIV infection (Ch. 14)
- COVID-19 (SARS-CoV-2)

Prion diseases
- Creutzfeldt–Jakob disease
- Kuru

Protozoal infections (Ch. 13)
- Malaria*
- Toxoplasmosis (in immune-suppressed)*
- Trypanosomiasis*
- Amoebic abscess*

Helminthic infections
- Schistosomiasis (spinal cord)*
- Cysticercosis*
- Hydatid disease*
- Strongyloidiasis*

Fungal infections
- *Candida* meningitis or brain abscess
- Cryptococcal meningitis

*These infections are discussed in Chapter 13.

Viral meningitis

Viruses are the most common cause of meningitis, usually resulting in a benign and self-limiting illness requiring no specific therapy. It is much less serious than bacterial meningitis unless there is associated encephalitis. A number of viruses can cause meningitis (see Box 28.59), the most common being enteroviruses. Where specific immunisation is not employed, the mumps virus is a common cause.

Clinical features

Viral meningitis occurs mainly in children or young adults, with acute onset of headache and irritability and the rapid development of meningism. The headache is usually the most severe feature. There may be a high pyrexia but focal neurological signs are rare.

Investigations

The diagnosis is made by lumbar puncture, with the specific viral cause identified by a nucleic acid amplification test (NAAT). CSF usually contains an excess of lymphocytes. While glucose and protein levels are commonly normal, the latter may be raised. It is important to verify that the patient has not received antibiotics (for whatever cause) prior to the lumbar puncture, as CSF lymphocytosis can also be found in partially treated bacterial meningitis (see Box 28.6).

Management

There is no specific treatment and the condition is usually benign and self-limiting. The patient should be treated symptomatically in a quiet environment. Recovery usually occurs within days, although a lymphocytic pleocytosis may persist in the CSF. Meningitis may also occur as a complication of a systemic viral infection such as mumps, measles, infectious mononucleosis, varicella zoster and hepatitis. Whatever the virus, complete recovery without specific therapy is the rule.

28

i **28.59 Causes of meningitis**

Infective

Bacteria

- *Streptococcus pneumoniae*
- *Neisseria meningitidis* (serogroups A, B, C, Y, W135)
- *Mycobacterium tuberculosis*
- *Haemophilus influenzae*
- *Listeria monocytogenes*
- Other streptococci including *Strep. suis*
- *Staphylococcus aureus* (skull fracture)

Viruses

- Enteroviruses (echo, Coxsackie, polio)
- Herpes simplex virus type 2 (Mollaret's meningitis)
- Varicella zoster virus
- Herpes simplex type 1
- Epstein–Barr virus
- Cytomegalovirus
- Measles
- Mumps
- Other viruses that cause
  Lymphocytic choriomeningitis virus
  West Nile virus
  Human immunodeficiency virus

Fungi

- *Cryptococcus neoformans*
- *Candida*
- *Histoplasma*
- *Blastomyces*
- *Coccidioides*
- *Sporothrix*

Non-infective ('sterile')

Malignant disease

- Breast cancer
- Bronchogenic cancer
- Leukaemia
- Lymphoma

Inflammatory disease (may be recurrent)

- Sarcoidosis
- Systemic lupus erythematosus
- Behçet's disease

Bacterial meningitis

Many bacteria can cause meningitis but geographical patterns vary, as does age-related sensitivity (Box 28.60). In the 'meningitis belt' of sub-Saharan Africa, drought and dust storms are often associated with meningococcal outbreaks (Harmattan meningitis). Bacterial meningitis is usually part of a bacteraemic illness, although direct spread from an adjacent focus of infection in the ear, skull fracture or sinus can be causative. Antibiotics have rendered this less common but mortality and morbidity remain significant. An important factor in determining prognosis is early diagnosis and the prompt initiation of appropriate therapy. Most bacterial causes of meningitis are normal commensals of the upper respiratory tract. New and potentially pathogenic strains are acquired by droplet spread but close contact is necessary. Epidemics of meningococcal meningitis occur, particularly in cramped living conditions or where the climate is hot and dry. The organism invades through the nasopharynx, producing sepsis and leading to meningitis.

Pathophysiology

Streptococcus pneumoniae (pneumococcus) and *Neisseria meningitidis* (meningococcus) are the commonest cause of bacterial meningitis globally, including in the United Kingdom. *Streptococcus suis* is a rare zoonotic cause of meningitis associated with porcine contact. It is an important cause of meningitis in some parts of Asia, including Vietnam and Thailand. Some degree of hearing loss occurs in more than half of survivors. Infection stimulates an immune response, causing the pia–arachnoid membrane to become congested and infiltrated with inflammatory cells. The pro-inflammatory immune mediators released are particularly prominent in *Streptococcus pneumoniae* infection and may account for the poor prognosis associated with pneumococcal meningitis. Pus then forms in layers, which may later organise to form adhesions. These may obstruct the free flow of CSF, leading to hydrocephalus, or they may damage the cranial nerves at the base of the brain. Hearing loss is a frequent complication. The CSF pressure rises rapidly, the

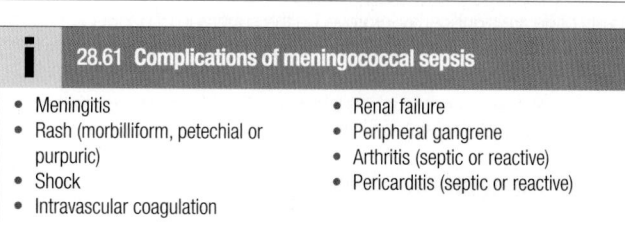

i **28.60 Bacterial causes of meningitis at different ages**

Age of onset	Common	Less common
Neonate	Gram-negative bacilli (*Escherichia coli*) Group B streptococci	*Listeria monocytogenes*
Pre-school child	*Haemophilus influenzae* *Neisseria meningitidis* (serogroups A, B, C, Y, W) *Streptococcus pneumoniae*	*Mycobacterium tuberculosis*
Older child and adult	*Strep. pneumoniae* *N. meningitidis* (serogroups A, B, C, Y, W) *M. tuberculosis* *H. influenzae*	*L. monocytogenes* Other streptococci *Staphylococcus aureus* (skull fracture)

i **28.61 Complications of meningococcal sepsis**

- Meningitis
- Rash (morbilliform, petechial or purpuric)
- Shock
- Intravascular coagulation
- Renal failure
- Peripheral gangrene
- Arthritis (septic or reactive)
- Pericarditis (septic or reactive)

protein content increases, and there is a cellular reaction that varies in type and severity according to the nature of the inflammation and the causative organism. An obliterative endarteritis of the leptomeningeal arteries passing through the meningeal exudate may produce secondary cerebral infarction. Pneumococcal meningitis is often associated with a very purulent CSF and a high mortality, especially in older adults.

Clinical features

The most common presenting features are fever and headache, which may also be associated with drowsiness and meningism. More than 90% of patients have any two of: headache, pyrexia, meningism and altered consciousness. Rash may occur in meningococcal meningitis. In severe bacterial meningitis the patient may be comatose, later developing focal neurological signs. Seizures may occur in around a quarter of patients. When accompanied by sepsis, presenting signs may evolve rapidly, with abrupt onset of obtundation due to cerebral oedema. Complications of meningococcal sepsis are listed in Box 28.61. Chronic meningococcaemia is a rare condition in which the patient can be unwell for weeks or even months with recurrent fever, sweating, joint pains and transient rash. In pneumococcal and *Haemophilus* infections there may be an accompanying otitis media. Pneumococcal meningitis may be associated with pneumonia and occurs especially in older patients and alcoholics, as well as those with hyposplenism. *Listeria monocytogenes* causes meningitis and rhombencephalitis (brainstem encephalitis) in the immunosuppressed, people at the extremes of age (neonates and older adults), with diabetes, alcoholics and pregnant women.

Investigations

Lumbar puncture is mandatory unless there are contraindications. If the patient is drowsy and has focal neurological signs or seizures, is immunosuppressed, has undergone recent neurosurgery or has suffered a head injury, it is wise to obtain a CT to exclude a mass lesion (such as a cerebral abscess) before lumbar puncture because of the risk of coning. This should not, however, delay treatment of presumed meningitis. If lumbar puncture is deferred or omitted, it is essential to take blood cultures and to start empirical treatment (Fig. 28.33). Lumbar puncture will help differentiate the causative organism but the characteristic findings in bacterial meningitis listed in Box 28.6 are far from universal. If the CSF is abnormal, the safest

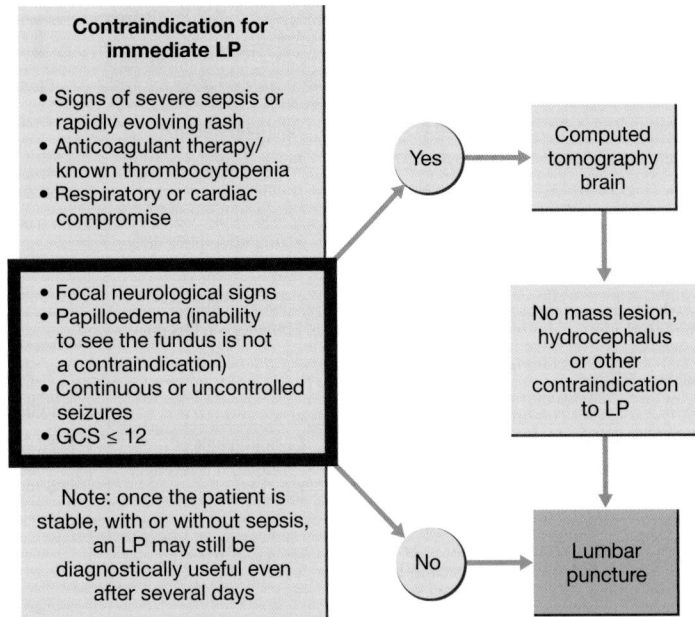

Fig. 28.33 The investigation of meningitis based on the British Infection Association acute meningitis guideline. (CRP = C-reactive protein; GCS = Glasgow Coma Scale; LP = lumbar puncture, PCR = polymerase chain reaction) *(Adapted from the UK joint specialist societies guideline on the diagnosis and management of acute meningitis and meningococcal sepsis in immunocompetent adults. Journal of Infection 2016; 72: 405–438.)*

course is to treat for bacterial meningitis. A bloody tap may complicate CSF findings. The safest approach is to treat for bacterial meningitis if the white cell count is above normal and disregard the red cell count. Gram film and culture may allow identification of the organism. Blood cultures may be positive. PCR techniques can be used on both blood and CSF to identify bacterial DNA for several days after antibiotic treatment has started.

Management

There is an untreated mortality rate of around 80%, so action must be swift. Antibiotics should ideally be given after CSF and blood cultures have been obtained, but if there is any delay obtaining these samples, antibiotic therapy should be started immediately. Recommended empirical therapies are outlined in Box 28.62, and the preferred antibiotic when the organism is known after CSF examination is stipulated in Box 28.63. Some regions of the world have a high prevalence of penicillin resistance and local guidelines or microbiologist advice should be sought. There is remarkably little evidence to guide duration of antibiotic treatment. As a guide, pneumococcal meningitis should be treated for 10–14 days, meningococcal meningitis slightly less (around 7 days) and *Listeria* meningitis for 21 days. Adjunctive glucocorticoid therapy is useful in reducing hearing loss and neurological sequelae in both children and adults in high-income countries, but evidence does not support the use of dexamethasone in lower-income countries or where there are high rates of untreated HIV.

In meningococcal disease, mortality is doubled if the patient presents with features of sepsis rather than meningitis. Individuals likely to require intensive care facilities and expertise include those with cardiac, respiratory or renal involvement, and those with CNS depression prejudicing the airway. Early endotracheal intubation and mechanical ventilation protect the airway and may prevent the development of the acute respiratory distress syndrome (ARDS). Adverse prognostic features include hypotensive shock, a rapidly developing rash, a haemorrhagic diathesis, multisystem failure and age over 60 years.

Prevention of meningococcal infection

Close contacts of patients with meningococcal infection (Box 28.64) should be given a single dose of ciprofloxacin. Rifampicin for two days is an alternative for those unable to take ciprofloxacin. If not treated with ceftriaxone or cefotaxime, the index case should be given similar treatment to clear infection from the nasopharynx before hospital discharge. Vaccines are available for most meningococcal subgroups.

 28.62 Treatment of bacterial meningitis of unknown cause (based on the British Infection Association Guideline 2016)*

1. Adults aged less than 60 years

- Cefotaxime 2 g IV 4 times daily *or*
- Ceftriaxone 2 g IV twice daily

2. Patients in whom penicillin-resistant pneumococcal infection is suspected, or in areas with a significant incidence of penicillin resistance in the community

As for (1) but add:
- Vancomycin 15–20 mg/kg IV twice daily *or*
- Rifampicin 600 mg IV or orally twice daily

3. Adults aged >60 years and those in whom *Listeria monocytogenes* infection is suspected (brainstem signs, immunosuppression, diabetic, alcohol misuser)

As for (1) but add:
- Ampicillin 2 g IV 6 times daily *or*
- Amoxicillin 2 g IV 6 times daily

4. Adults aged >60 years, or with risk factors in (3) above, in areas with a significant incidence of penicillin resistance in the community

As for (2) but add:
- Ampicillin 2 g IV 6 times daily *or*
- Amoxicillin 2 g IV 6 times daily

5. Patients with a clear history of anaphylaxis to β-lactams

- Chloramphenicol 25 mg/kg IV 4 times daily *plus*
- Vancomycin 15–20 mg/kg IV twice daily
  If over the age of 60 years, add: co-trimoxazole 10–20 mg/kg (of the trimethoprim component) in four divided doses

6. Adjunctive treatment (see text)

- Dexamethasone 10 mg 4 times daily for 2–4 days

*N.B. Antibiotic recommendations depend on local epidemiology of organisms and antibiotic resistance. Local guidance should always be sought.
British Infection Association Guideline in Journal of Infection 2016; 72:405–438.

28

<table>
<tr><td colspan="3">➕ 28.63 Chemotherapy of bacterial meningitis when the cause is known (based on the British Infection Association Guideline 2016)[1]</td></tr>
</table>

Pathogen	Regimen of choice	Alternative agents
Neisseria meningitidis	Cefotaxime 2 g IV 4 times daily or ceftriaxone 2 g IV twice daily for 5–7 days	Benzylpenicillin 2.4 g IV 6 times daily or Chloramphenicol[2,3] 25 mg/kg 4 times daily for 5–7 days
Streptococcus pneumoniae (sensitive to β-lactams, MIC ≤0.06)	Cefotaxime 2 g IV 4 times daily or Ceftriaxone 2 g IV twice daily for 10–14 days	Chloramphenicol[2,3] 25mg/kg 4 times daily for 10–14 days
Strep. pneumoniae (resistant to β-lactams)	As for sensitive strains but add: Vancomycin 15–20 mg/kg IV twice daily or Rifampicin 600 mg IV twice daily for 14 days	Chloramphenicol[3] 25 mg/kg 4 times daily for 14 days
Haemophilus influenzae	Cefotaxime 2 g IV 4 times daily or Ceftriaxone 2 g IV twice daily for 10 days	Moxifloxacin 400 mg daily for 10 days
Listeria monocytogenes	Amoxicillin 2 g IV 6 times daily for 21 days	Co-trimoxazole 10–20 mg/kg (of the trimethoprim component) daily in four divided doses for 21 days
Streptococcus suis	Cefotaxime 2 g IV 4 times daily or Ceftriaxone 2 g IV twice daily for 10–14 days	Chloramphenicol[2,3] 25 mg/kg 4 times daily for 10–14 days

[1]N.B. Antibiotic recommendations depend on local epidemiology of organisms and antibiotic resistance. Local guidance should always be sought. [2]For patients with a history of anaphylaxis to β-lactam antibiotics. *British Infection Association Guideline in Journal of Infection 2016; 72:405–438.* [3]If the patient is recovering reduce the dose of chloramphenicol to 12.5 mg/kg to reduce the risk of dose-related anaemia. *From Erratum to reference in note 2.* (MIC = minimum inhibitory concentration)

Tuberculous meningitis

Tuberculous meningitis is now uncommon in high-income countries except in immunocompromised individuals, although it is still seen in those born in endemic areas and in low- and middle-resource countries. It is seen more frequently as a secondary infection in patients with HIV infection.

Pathophysiology

Tuberculous meningitis most commonly occurs shortly after a primary infection in childhood or as part of miliary tuberculosis. The usual local source of infection is a caseous focus in the meninges or brain substance adjacent to the CSF pathway. The brain is covered by a greenish, gelatinous exudate, especially around the base, and numerous scattered tubercles are found on the meninges.

Clinical features

The clinical features and staging criteria are listed in Box 28.65. Onset is much slower than in other bacterial meningitis – over 2–8 weeks. If untreated, tuberculous meningitis is fatal in a few weeks but complete recovery is usual if treatment is started at stage I (Box 28.65). When treatment is initiated later, the rate of death or serious neurological deficit may be as high as 30%.

<table>
<tr><td colspan="2">ℹ 28.64 Chemoprophylaxis following meningococcal exposure</td></tr>
</table>

Close contacts warranting chemoprophylaxis

- Household contacts (including persons who ate or slept in the same dwelling as the patient during the 7 days prior to disease onset)
- Child-care and nursery-school contacts
- Persons having contact with patient's oral secretions during the 7 days prior to disease onset:
    Kissing
    Sharing of toothbrushes
    Sharing of eating utensils
    Mouth-to-mouth resuscitation
    Unprotected contact during endotracheal intubation
- Aircraft contacts for persons seated next to the patient for > 8 hr

Persons at low risk in whom chemoprophylaxis is not recommended

- Casual contact (e.g. at school or work) without direct exposure to patient's oral secretions
- Indirect contact only (contact with a high-risk contact and not a case)
- Health-care worker without direct exposure to patient's oral secretions

<table>
<tr><td colspan="2">ℹ 28.65 Clinical features and staging of tuberculous meningitis</td></tr>
</table>

Symptoms

- Headache
- Vomiting
- Low-grade fever
- Lassitude
- Depression
- Delirium
- Behaviour changes

Signs

- Meningism (may be absent)
- Oculomotor palsies
- Papilloedema
- Depression of conscious level
- Focal hemisphere signs

Staging of severity

- Stage I (early): non-specific symptoms and signs without alteration of consciousness
- Stage II (intermediate): altered consciousness without coma or delirium *plus* minor focal neurological signs
- Stage III (advanced): stupor or coma, severe neurological deficits, seizures or abnormal movements

Investigations

Lumbar puncture should be performed if the diagnosis is suspected. The CSF is under increased pressure. It is usually clear but, when allowed to stand, a fine clot ('spider web') may form. The fluid contains up to 500×10^6 cells/μL, predominantly lymphocytes, but can contain neutrophils. There is a rise in protein, often marked, and a similarly marked fall in glucose. The tubercle bacillus may be detected in a smear of the centrifuged deposit from the CSF but a negative result does not exclude the diagnosis. The CSF should be cultured but, as this result will not be known for up to 6 weeks, treatment must be started without waiting for confirmation. The WHO recommends use of additional nucleic acid amplification tests (NAATs), specifically Xpert MT/RIF Ultra. This should be used in addition to smear and culture studies, as NAATs are not sensitive enough to exclude tuberculous meningitis when negative. Brain imaging may show hydrocephalus, brisk particularly basal meningeal enhancement on enhanced CT or MRI, and/or uncommonly an intracranial tuberculoma.

Management

As soon as the diagnosis is made or strongly suspected, chemotherapy should be started using one of the regimens that include pyrazinamide, described on page 522. The use of glucocorticoids in addition to antituberculous therapy has been controversial. Recent evidence suggests that it improves mortality, especially if given early, but not focal neurological damage whether associated with HIV infection or not. Surgical ventricular drainage may be needed if obstructive hydrocephalus develops. Skilled nursing is essential during the acute phase of the illness, and adequate hydration and nutrition must be maintained.

Fungal meningitis

Fungal meningitis is uncommon and usually occurs in the immunosuppressed. The yeast *Cryptococcus neoformans* is the commonest and an important cause of meningitis in those immunosuppressed by HIV infection. It does occur in the immunocompetent although non-HIV forms of immunocompromise should be sought. The presentation may be atypical with subacute or chronic meningism, fever, headache and symptoms of raised intracranial pressure occur. The CSF opening pressure is often very raised, with 20–200 cells x10⁶/L mainly lymphocytes, elevated protein and low glucose levels (similar to findings in tuberculous meningitis) (Box 28.6). In some regions the India ink test and cryptococcal PCR are used to detect cryptococci in the CSF. Cryptococcal antigen is present in the CSF and sometimes serum. Treatment is discussed on p. 363. Treatment of raised CSF pressure may be complex and frequent, sometimes daily, lumbar punctures are required.

Other meningitides

In some areas, meningitis may be caused by spirochaetes (leptospirosis, Lyme disease and syphilis; rickettsiae (typhus fever) or protozoa (primary amoebic meningoencephalitis, PAM).

Meningitis can also be due to non-infective pathologies. This is seen in recurrent aseptic meningitis resulting from systemic lupus erythematosus (SLE), Behçet's disease or sarcoidosis, as well as a condition of previously unknown origin known as Mollaret syndrome, in which the recurrent meningitis is associated with epithelioid cells in the spinal fluid ('Mollaret' cells). Recent evidence suggests that this condition may be due to herpes simplex virus type 2 and is therefore infective after all. Meningitis can also be caused by direct invasion of the meninges by neoplastic cells ('malignant meningitis'; see Box 28.59).

Subdural empyema

This is a rare complication of frontal sinusitis, osteomyelitis of the skull vault or middle ear disease. A collection of pus in the subdural space spreads over the surface of the hemisphere, causing underlying cortical oedema or thrombophlebitis. Patients present with severe pain in the face or head and pyrexia, often with a history of preceding paranasal sinus or ear infection. The patient then becomes drowsy, with seizures and focal signs such as a progressive hemiparesis.

The diagnosis rests on a strong clinical suspicion in patients with a local focus of infection. Careful assessment with contrast-enhanced CT or MRI may show a subdural collection with underlying cerebral oedema. Management requires aspiration of pus via a burr hole and appropriate parenteral antibiotics. Any local source of infection must be treated to prevent re-infection.

Spinal epidural abscess

The characteristic clinical features are back pain, often in a nerve root distribution and progressive transverse spinal cord syndrome with paraparesis, sensory impairment and sphincter dysfunction. There may be fever and raised inflammatory markers. Features of the primary focus of infection may be less obvious and thus can be overlooked. The resurgence of resistant staphylococcal infection and injection drug use has contributed to a recent marked rise in incidence.

Once the diagnosis is suspected, an MRI scan of the spine should be carried out (or myelography if MRI is not available). MRI is often negative in early disease, so if it is non-diagnostic and the clinical suspicion remains, it should be repeated after a week or so. Obtaining a bacteriological diagnosis is a high priority, and antibiotics are not usually started until this has been achieved (or at least attempted),

e.g. by blood culture and tissue aspiration or biopsy. If there is spinal cord compression surgical treatment is required (e.g. decompressive laminectomy with abscess drainage). However, in the absence of neurological impairment, treatment with antibiotics alone is often attempted, usually using intravenous antibiotics for at least 6 weeks, guided by clinical and biochemical response.

Parenchymal viral infections

Infection of the substance of the nervous system will produce symptoms of focal dysfunction (deficits and/or seizures) with general signs of infection, depending on the acuteness of the infection and the type of organism.

Viral encephalitis

A range of viruses can cause encephalitis but only a minority of patients report recent systemic viral infection (Box 28.66). The relative importance of specific viruses depends on location and the specific population involved, e.g. immunosuppressed. In high-income countries, the most serious cause of viral encephalitis is herpes simplex, which probably reaches the brain via the olfactory nerves. The development of effective therapy for some forms of encephalitis has increased the importance of clinical diagnosis and virological examination of the CSF.

Pathophysiology

The infection provokes an inflammatory response that involves the cortex, white matter, basal ganglia and brainstem. The distribution of lesions varies with the type of virus. For example, in herpes simplex encephalitis, the temporal lobes are usually primarily affected, whereas cytomegalovirus can involve the areas adjacent to the ventricles (ventriculitis). Inclusion bodies may be present in the neurons and glial cells, and there is an infiltration of polymorphonuclear cells in the perivascular space. There is neuronal degeneration and diffuse glial proliferation, often associated with cerebral oedema.

Clinical features

Viral encephalitis presents with acute onset of headache, fever, focal neurological signs (aphasia and/or hemiplegia, visual field defects) and seizures. Disturbance of consciousness ranging from drowsiness to deep coma supervenes early and may advance dramatically. Meningism occurs in many patients. Additional clues to the causative virus are listed in Box 28.66. Rabies presents a distinct clinical picture and is described below.

Investigations

Imaging by CT scan may show low-density lesions in the temporal lobes but MRI is more sensitive in detecting early abnormalities. Lumbar puncture should be performed once imaging has excluded a mass lesion. The CSF usually contains excess lymphocytes but polymorphonuclear cells may predominate in the early stages. The CSF may be normal in up to 10% of cases. Some viruses, including the West Nile virus, may cause a sustained neutrophilic CSF. The protein content may be elevated but the glucose is normal. The EEG is usually abnormal in the early stages, especially in herpes simplex encephalitis, with characteristic periodic slow-wave activity in the temporal lobes. Virological investigations of the CSF, including PCR, may reveal the causative organism but treatment initiation should not await this.

Management

Optimum treatment for herpes simplex encephalitis (aciclovir 10 mg/kg IV 3 times daily for 2–3 weeks) has reduced mortality from 70% to around 10%. This should be given early to all patients suspected of having viral encephalitis.

Some survivors will have residual epilepsy or cognitive impairment. For details of post-infectious encephalomyelitis, see page 1163. Antiepileptic treatment may be required and raised intracranial pressure may indicate the need for dexamethasone.

28

i	28.66 Causes of viral encephalitis (location dependent)		
Virus	**Locations**		**Comment**
Sporadic encephalitides			
Herpes simplex virus type 1	Commonest cause; especially high resource areas		Treatable, important to consider diagnosis early
Herpes simplex virus type 2	Around 10% of herpes simplex virus infections		Usually meningoencephalitis, may be recurrent
Varicella zoster virus	Increasing globally		Before, with or few days after vesicular rash. More common in immunosuppressed. Post infectious cerebellitis and cerebral vasculitis may occur
Enterovirus 70 and 71	Global, Enterovirus 71, particularly Asia–Pacific region		Haemorrhagic conjunctivitis (Enterovirus 70), hand foot and mouth disease and brainstem encephalitis (Enterovirus 71)
Human immunodeficiency virus	Global		Around seroconversion
Measles and mumps	Global		Measles: post infectious or long-term subacute sclerosing panencephalitis. Mumps: before or after parotitis
Arbo- and zoonotic viruses (spread by ticks, mosquitoes and other vectors)			
West Nile virus	West and Central Asia, Middle East, Africa, Southern Europe and North America		*(Mosquito)* Profound flaccid weakness and rash; parkinsonism, myoclonus
Japanese encephalitis virus	Asia, Western Pacific		*(Pigs and wading birds)* Seizures very common, abnormal behaviour/psychosis, asymmetric flaccid paralysis, abnormal movement/parkinsonian
Dengue viruses	Asia, Pacific, Africa, Americas, Southern Europe		*(Mosquito)* Fever, arthralgia, rash, haemorrhagic manifestations, leukopenia
Chikungunya	Africa, Asia, Europe, Indian and Pacific Ocean islands, Americas		*(Mosquito)* Excruciating joint pain/arthritis, rash
Nipah and Hendra viruses	Asia–Pacific region, Hendra in Australia		*(Bats, human to human, intermediate transmission pigs, horses; Hendra – horse contact)* Nipah – segmental myoclonus, cerebellar signs, areflexia, multiple small (< 5 mm) lesions on MRI
Rabies virus	Latin America, Caribbean, Asia, Africa, Central Asia and Middle East		*(Bats, dogs, cats)* Hyperactivity, painful pharyngeal and inspiratory muscle spasms, autonomic instability, hydrophobia
Other: St Louis virus, eastern, western, Venezuelan equine, La Crosse viruses/ Colorado tick fever virus, Powassan virus	Americas mainly		*(Mosquitos/ticks)*
Zika virus	Africa, South-east Asia, Pacific islands, Americas, Carribbean		*(Mosquitos, human to human)* Pruritic rash, conjunctivitis, arthralgia hands and feet

(MRI = magnetic resonance imaging)

Brainstem encephalitis

This presents with ataxia, dysarthria, diplopia or other cranial nerve palsies. The CSF is lymphocytic, with a normal glucose. The causative agent is presumed to be viral. However, *Listeria monocytogenes* may cause a similar syndrome with meningitis (and often a polymorphonuclear CSF pleocytosis) and requires specific treatment with ampicillin (2 grams 6 times daily; see Box 28.63).

Rabies

Rabies is caused by a rhabdovirus that infects the central nervous tissue and salivary glands of a wide range of mammals. It is usually conveyed by saliva through bites or licks on abrasions or on intact mucous membranes. Humans are most frequently infected from dogs and bats. In Europe, the maintenance host is the fox. The incubation period varies in humans from a minimum of 9 days to many months but is usually between 4 and 8 weeks. Severe bites, especially if on the head or neck, are associated with shorter incubation periods. Human rabies is a rare disease, even in endemic areas. However, because it is usually fatal, major efforts are directed at limiting its spread and preventing its importation into uninfected countries, such as the UK.

Clinical features

At the onset there may be fever, and paraesthesia at the site of the bite. A prodromal period of 1–10 days, during which the patient becomes increasingly anxious, leads to the characteristic 'hydrophobia'. Although the patient is thirsty, attempts at drinking provoke violent contractions of the diaphragm and other inspiratory muscles. Delusions and hallucinations may develop, accompanied by spitting, biting and mania, with lucid intervals in which the patient is markedly anxious. Cranial nerve lesions develop and terminal hyperpyrexia is common. Death ensues, usually within a week of the onset of symptoms.

Investigations

During life, the diagnosis is usually made on clinical grounds but rapid immunofluorescent techniques can detect antigen in corneal impression smears or skin biopsies.

Management

Established disease

Only a few patients with established rabies have survived. All received some post-exposure prophylaxis (see below) and needed intensive care facilities to control cardiac and respiratory failure. Otherwise, only palliative treatment is possible once symptoms have appeared. The patient should be heavily sedated with diazepam, supplemented by chlorpromazine if needed. Nutrition and fluids should be given intravenously or through a gastrostomy.

Pre-exposure prophylaxis

Pre-exposure prophylaxis with rabies vaccine is required by those who handle potentially infected animals professionally, work with rabies virus in laboratories or live at special risk in rabies-endemic areas.

Post-exposure prophylaxis

The wounds should be thoroughly cleaned, preferably with a quaternary ammonium detergent or soap; damaged tissues should be excised and the wound left unsutured. Rabies can usually be prevented if treatment is started within a day or two of biting. Delayed treatment may still be of value. For maximum protection, hyperimmune serum and vaccine are required.

The safest anti-rabies antiserum is human rabies immunoglobulin. The dose is 20 IU/kg body weight; half is infiltrated around the bite and half is given intramuscularly at a different site from the vaccine. Hyperimmune animal serum may be used but hypersensitivity reactions, including anaphylaxis, are common.

The safest vaccine, free of complications, is human diploid cell strain vaccine. Post-exposure treatment is complex and depends on a composite risk based on the risk by country and the category of exposure. Detailed advice may be available locally or on the UK website https://www.gov.uk/government/publications/rabies-post-exposure-prophylaxis-management-guidelines. For example, an unimmunised individual from a high-risk country exposed to direct contact with terrestrial mammal saliva should receive human rabies immunoglobulin and four doses of vaccine on days 0, 3, 7 and 21. If immunocompromised, they should receive five doses of vaccine on days 0, 3, 7, 14 and 30. In contrast, an individual in a low-risk country and no physical contact with terrestrial mammal saliva would not require post-exposure prophylaxis.

Human immunodeficiency virus (HIV) infection

Box 28.67 summarises the neurological manifestations of HIV infection. These are covered in detail in Chapter 14.

Poliomyelitis

Disease is caused by one of three polioviruses, which constitute a subgroup of the enteroviruses. Poliomyelitis has become much less common following the introduction of the Global Polio Eradication initiative. Incidence dropped from more than 350 000 cases in 1988 to 33 in 2018. However, incomplete immunisation still results in small numbers of cases. Transmission usually occurs through faecal–hand–oral contamination with primary replication in the lymphatic tissue of the gastrointestinal and oropharyngeal tracts.

The virus causes a lymphocytic meningitis and infects the grey matter of the spinal cord, brainstem and cortex. There is a particular propensity to damage anterior horn cells, especially in the lumbar segments.

Many patients recover fully after the initial phase of a few days of mild fever and headache. In other individuals, after a week of well-being, there is a recurrence of pyrexia, headache and meningism. Weakness may start later in one muscle group and can progress to widespread paresis. Respiratory failure may supervene if intercostal muscles are paralysed or the medullary motor nuclei are involved. Poliomyelitis virus may be cultured from CSF and stool. Second attacks are very rare but occasionally

i | **28.67 Neurological manifestations of human immunodeficiency virus (HIV) infection and treatment side-effects**

Neurocognitive manifestations

- HIV-associated neurocognitive disorder
- HIV-associated encephalopathy: subcortical dementia (psychomotor slowing and memory loss), depression, movement disorders

Stroke

- Ischaemic stroke (90%): HIV-associated vasculopathy (accelerated atherosclerosis, aneurysm, vasculitis, small vessel disease), cardioembolism (cardiomyopathy, ischaemic heart disease, endocarditis), opportunistic infection (causing meningitis or vasculitis), lymphoma involving blood vessels, coagulopathy
- Cerebral haemorrhage (< 10%): HIV-associated vasculopathy, thrombocytopenia, mycotic aneurysm

Other brain/cranial nerve involvement

- Bell palsy (often around seroconversion)
- Meningitis: aseptic around seroconversion, cryptococcal meningitis, tuberculous meningitis
- Mass lesions: toxoplasmosis, lymphoma, tuberculosis
- Encephalitis: HIV around seroconversion, cytomegalovirus, Epstein–Barr virus, varicella zoster virus (can also result in vasculitis)
- Progressive multifocal leukoencephalopathy
- Seizures
- Immune reconstitution syndrome*

Spinal cord, motor neuron and nerve root

- Motor neuron disease
- Vacuolar myelopathy (late stage)
- Other viral myelopathy (particularly herpes group of viruses)
- Radiculopathy (caused by cytomegalovirus, or tuberculous meningitis)

Peripheral nerve and plexus

- Acute inflammatory demyelinating polyneuropathy (AIDP)
- Chronic inflammatory demyelinating polyneuropathy (CIDP)
- Mononeuritis multiplex (vasculitic)
- Distal symmetric peripheral neuropathy
- Diffuse infiltrative lymphocytosis syndrome
- Brachial plexopathy
- Antiretroviral-associated neuropathy*

Muscle

- HIV-associated myopathy (inflammatory myopathy)
- Antiretroviral-associated myopathy*

*Treatment effect.

patients show late deterioration in muscle bulk and power many years after the initial infection (this is termed the 'post-polio syndrome').

Prevention of poliomyelitis is by immunisation with live Sabin vaccine, a collection of live attenuated polio viruses (OPV – oral poliovirus vaccine) in low- and middle-income regions. The advantages of OPV include cost, ease of administration and transmission of the vaccine virus to unimmunised contacts. In high-income countries where polio is now very rare, the live vaccine has been replaced by the Salk vaccine (IPV), a collection of inactivated polio viruses. Advantages include avoidance of vaccine-associated paralytic poliomyelitis and effective combination with other routine childhood vaccines.

Herpes zoster (shingles)

Herpes zoster is the result of reactivation of the varicella zoster virus that has lain dormant in a nerve root ganglion following chickenpox earlier in life. Reactivation may be spontaneous (as usually occurs in middle-aged or older adults) or due to immunosuppression (as in patients with diabetes, malignant disease or HIV).

Subacute sclerosing panencephalitis

This is a rare, chronic, progressive and eventually fatal complication of measles, presumably a result of an inability of the nervous system to eradicate the virus. It occurs in children and adolescents, usually many years after the primary virus infection. There is generalised neurological deterioration and onset is insidious, with intellectual deterioration, apathy and clumsiness, followed by myoclonic jerks, rigidity and dementia.

The CSF may show a mild lymphocytic pleocytosis and the EEG demonstrates characteristic periodic bursts of triphasic waves. Although there is persistent measles-specific IgG in serum and CSF, antiviral therapy is ineffective and death ensues within a few years.

Progressive multifocal leucoencephalopathy

This was originally described as a rare complication of lymphoma, leukaemia or carcinomatosis but is seen in untreated HIV/AIDS or secondary to immunosuppression, e.g. following organ transplantation or use of disease-modifying drugs for MS, in particular natalizumab. It is an infection of oligodendrocytes and other neuroglial cells by human polyomavirus JC, causing widespread demyelination of the white matter of the cerebral hemispheres. Clinical signs include dementia, hemiparesis and aphasia, which progress rapidly, usually leading to death within weeks or months. Areas of low density in the white matter are seen on CT but MRI is more sensitive, showing diffuse high signal in the cerebral white matter on T2-weighted images, sometimes with contrast enhancement. The only treatment available is restoration of the immune response (by treating HIV/AIDS or reversing immunosuppression) which can lead to the development of an immune reconstitution inflammatory syndrome (PML-IRIS).

Parenchymal bacterial infections

Cerebral abscess

Bacteria may enter the cerebral substance through penetrating injury, by direct spread from paranasal sinuses or the middle ear, or secondary to sepsis. Untreated congenital heart disease is a recognised risk factor. The site of abscess formation and the likely causative organism are both related to the source of infection (Box 28.68). Initial infection leads to local suppuration followed by loculation of pus within a surrounding wall of gliosis, which in a chronic abscess may form a tough capsule. Haematogenous spread may lead to multiple abscesses.

Clinical features

A cerebral abscess may present acutely with fever, headache, meningism and drowsiness, but more commonly presents over days or weeks as a cerebral mass lesion with little or no evidence of infection. Seizures, raised intracranial pressure and focal hemisphere signs occur alone or in combination. Distinction from a cerebral tumour may be impossible on clinical grounds.

Investigations

Lumbar puncture is potentially hazardous in the presence of raised intracranial pressure and CT should always precede it. CT reveals single or multiple low-density areas, which show ring enhancement with contrast and surrounding cerebral oedema (Fig. 28.34). There may be an elevated white blood cell count and ESR in patients with active local infection. The possibility of cerebral toxoplasmosis or tuberculous disease secondary to HIV infection should always be considered. MRI with diffusion weighted imaging may be helpful in distinguishing between cerebral abscess (hyperintense) and tumour (hypointense or variable increase lower than found in abscess).

Management and prognosis

Antimicrobial therapy is indicated once the diagnosis is made. The likely source of infection should guide the choice of antibiotic (see Box 28.68).

i	**28.68 Aetiology and treatment of bacterial cerebral abscess**		
Site of abscess	Source of infection	Likely organisms	Recommended treatment
Frontal lobe	Paranasal sinuses / Teeth	Streptococci / Anaerobes	Cefotaxime 2–3 g IV 4 times daily *plus* Metronidazole 500 mg IV 3 times daily
Temporal lobe	Middle ear	Streptococci Enterobacterales *Pseudomonas* species Anaerobes	Ampicillin 2–3 g IV 3 times daily *plus* Metronidazole 500 mg IV 3 times daily *plus either*
Cerebellum	Sphenoid sinus	*Pseudomonas* species Anaerobes	Ceftazidime 2 g IV 3 times daily *or* Gentamicin* 5 mg/kg IV daily
Any site	Penetrating trauma	Staphylococci *Clostridium* species	Vancomycin 15–20 mg/kg IV 2–3 times daily *plus*
Multiple	Metastatic (bacteraemia or endocarditis) and cryptogenic	Streptococci Anaerobes Staphylococci	Metronidazole 500 mg IV 3 times daily

*Monitor gentamicin levels.
(IV = intravenous)

Surgical drainage by burr-hole aspiration or excision may be necessary, especially where the presence of a capsule may lead to a persistent focus of infection. Epilepsy frequently develops and is often resistant to treatment.

Despite advances in therapy, mortality remains 10%–20% and may partly relate to delay in diagnosis and treatment.

Lyme disease

Infection with *Borrelia burgdorferi* can cause numerous neurological problems, including polyradiculopathy, meningitis, encephalitis and mononeuritis multiplex.

Neurosyphilis

Neurosyphilis may present as an acute or chronic process and may involve the meninges, blood vessels and/or parenchyma of the brain and spinal cord. The decade to 2008 saw a 10-fold increase in the incidence of syphilis. The clinical manifestations are diverse and early diagnosis and treatment are essential.

Clinical features

The clinical and pathological features of the three most common presentations are summarised in Box 28.69. Neurological examination reveals signs indicative of the anatomical localisation of lesions. Delusions of grandeur suggest general paresis of the insane, but more commonly there is simply progressive dementia. Small and irregular pupils that react to convergence but not light, as described by Argyll Robertson (see Box 28.21), may accompany any neurosyphilitic syndrome but most commonly tabes dorsalis.

Investigations

Routine screening for syphilis is warranted in many neurological patients. Treponemal antibodies are positive in the serum in most patients, but

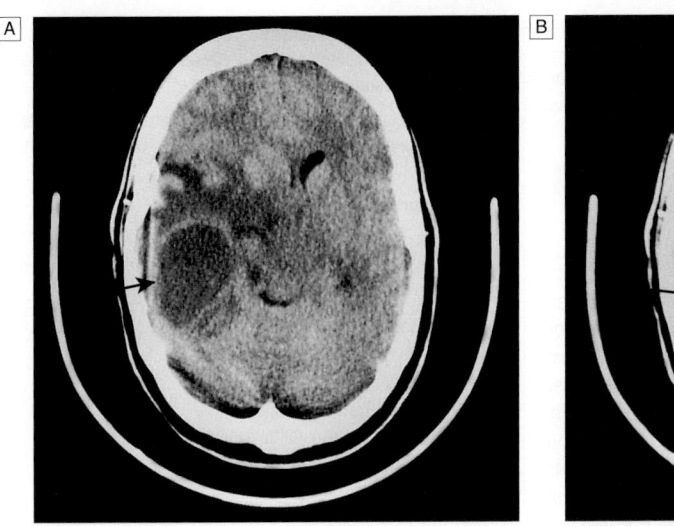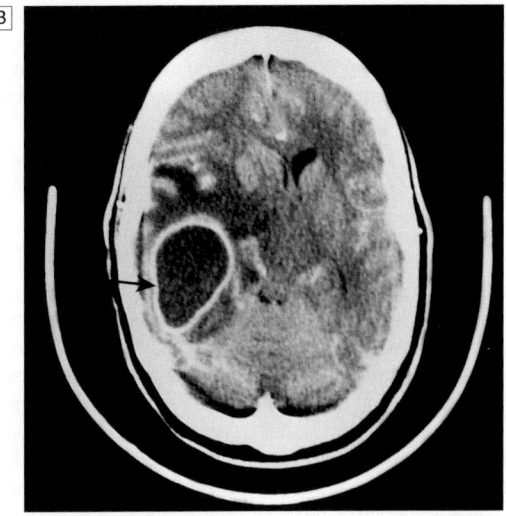

Fig. 28.34 Right temporal cerebral abscess (arrows), with surrounding oedema and midline shift to the left. A Unenhanced computed tomography (CT) image. B Contrast-enhanced CT image.

28.69 Clinical and pathological features of neurosyphilis		
Type and interval from primary infection	Pathology	Clinical features
Meningovascular (5 to 12 years)*	Endarteritis obliterans Meningeal exudate (often basal meningitis) Granuloma (gumma)	Stroke Cranial nerve palsies Seizures/mass lesion
General paralysis of the insane (2–15 years)*	Degeneration in cerebral cortex/ cerebral atrophy Thickened meninges	Dementia Tremor Bilateral upper motor signs Delusions Paranoia
Tabes dorsalis (5–20 years)*	Degeneration of sensory neurons Wasting of dorsal columns Optic atrophy	Lightning pains Sensory ataxia Visual failure Abdominal crises Incontinence Trophic changes
Any of the above		Argyll Robertson pupils (see Box 28.21)

*All forms can occur earlier or later than noted.

CSF examination is essential if neurological involvement is suspected. Active disease is suggested by an elevated cell count, usually lymphocytic, and the protein content may be elevated to 0.5–1.0 g/L. Serological tests in CSF are usually positive but progressive disease can occur with negative CSF serology.

Management

Aqueous crystalline penicillin G intravenously or intramuscular injection of procaine benzylpenicillin (procaine penicillin) and probenecid for 10–14 days is essential in the treatment of neurosyphilis of all types. Further courses of penicillin must be given if symptoms are not relieved, if the condition continues to advance or if the CSF continues to show signs of active disease. The cell count returns to normal within 3 months of completion of treatment, but the elevated protein takes longer to subside and some serological tests may never revert to normal. Evidence of clinical progression at any time is an indication for renewed treatment.

The spinal cord can be involved by other infections, including HTLV1, TB, bilharzia and echinococcus.

Parenchymal parasitic infections

Neurocysticercosis

Neurocysticercosis is the commonest parasitic neurological disease globally. Most infections occur in low-resource regions, but it occurs in high-resource regions in travellers and immigrants. Cysts may be asymptomatic, often for years, or symptomatic, the symptoms depending on the site of the cysts. Seizures are the commonest manifestation. Parenchymal cysts occur in the brain or in the convexity sulci, while extra-parenchymal cysts occur in the ventricles, cisterns and the spinal cord, and present most often with raised intracranial pressure. Investigation and management are discussed on p. 342.

Cerebral malaria

Cerebral malaria should be suspected in anyone presenting with fever, altered awareness or behaviour living in or returning from travel to a malaria endemic area. Drowsiness may progress over a few days, but coma can occur within hours. Level of consciousness may fluctuate and seizures occur, but focal neurological signs are unusual. The eyes frequently diverge with roving eye movements, but cranial nerve involvement and papilloedema are uncommon and suggest other causes, e.g. meningitis. Cerebral malaria is a serious condition with a case fatality rate of 15%–20% and requires rapid diagnosis and treatment (see Box.13.56).

Neuroschistosomiasis

Schistosomiasis is commonest in sub-Saharan Africa and neuroschistosomiasis should be considered in individuals in endemic areas and returning travellers presenting with neurological signs. The brain, but more commonly spine (particularly conus medullaris) and cauda equina can be involved. Spinal cord involvement often results in a rapidly progressive transverse myelitis, leg pain, bladder and bowel involvement. Investigation and management are discussed on p. 338.

28

Parenchymal fungal infections

Fungal infections of brain parenchyma are uncommon but occur particularly in the immunocompromised, in the presence of intraventricular devices and as an extension of sinus infection.

Diseases caused by bacterial toxins

Tetanus

This disease results from infection with *Clostridium tetani*, a commensal in the gut of humans and domestic animals that is found in soil. Infection enters the body through wounds, which may be trivial. It is rare in the UK, occurring mostly in gardeners and farmers, but a recent increase has been seen in injection drug users. By contrast, the disease is common in many countries, where dust contains spores derived from animal and human excreta. Unhygienic practices soon after birth may lead to infection of the umbilical stump or site of circumcision, causing tetanus neonatorum. Tetanus is still one of the major killers of adults, children and neonates in low-income countries, where the mortality rate can be nearly 100% in the newborn and around 40% in others.

In circumstances unfavourable to growth of the organism, spores are formed and these may remain dormant for years in the soil. Spores germinate and bacilli multiply only in the anaerobic conditions that occur in areas of tissue necrosis or if the oxygen tension is lowered by the presence of other organisms, particularly if aerobic. The bacilli remain localised but produce an exotoxin with an affinity for motor nerve endings and motor nerve cells.

The anterior horn cells are affected after the exotoxin has passed into the blood stream and their involvement results in rigidity and convulsions. Symptoms first appear from 2 days to several weeks after injury: the shorter the incubation period, the more severe the attack and the worse the prognosis.

Clinical features

By far the most important early symptom is trismus – spasm of the masseter muscles, which causes difficulty in opening the mouth and in masticating; hence the name 'lockjaw'. Lockjaw in tetanus is painless, unlike the spasm of the masseters due to dental abscess, septic throat or other causes. Conditions that can mimic tetanus include functional neurological disorders and phenothiazine overdosage, or overdose in injection drug users.

In tetanus, the tonic rigidity spreads to involve the muscles of the face, neck and trunk. Contraction of the frontalis and the muscles at the angles of the mouth leads to the so-called 'risus sardonicus'. There is rigidity of the muscles at the neck and trunk of varying degree. The back is usually slightly arched ('opisthotonus') and there is a board-like abdominal wall.

In the more severe cases, violent spasms lasting for a few seconds to 3–4 minutes occur spontaneously, or may be induced by stimuli such as movement or noise. These episodes are painful and exhausting, and suggest a grave outlook, especially if they appear soon after the onset of symptoms. They gradually increase in frequency and severity for about 1 week and the patient may die from exhaustion, asphyxia or aspiration pneumonia. In less severe illness, periods of spasm may not commence until a week or so after the first sign of rigidity, and in very mild infections they may never appear. Autonomic involvement may cause cardiovascular complications, such as hypertension. Rarely, the only manifestation of the disease may be 'local tetanus' – stiffness or spasm of the muscles near the infected wound – and the prognosis is good if treatment is commenced at this stage.

Investigations

The diagnosis is made on clinical grounds. Laboratory testing supports the diagnosis, but treatment should not be delayed while waiting for results. Wound tissue samples or a wound swab may be sent in cooked meat broth for PCR and culture of *C. tetani*. Serum samples should be

28.70 Treatment of tetanus (consult local guidance)

Neutralise absorbed toxin

- Human tetanus antitoxin IM/IV (local guidance varies) or where human tetanus antitoxin is not available (e.g. in the UK), IVIG (human intravenous immunoglobulin) IV*

Prevent further toxin production

- Débride wound
- Give metronidazole 500 mg IV every 6–8 hours ideally, or penicillin G 2–4 million units IV every 4–6 hours for 7–10 days

Control spasms

- Nurse in a quiet room
- Avoid unnecessary stimuli
- Give IV diazepam
- If spasms continue, paralyse patient and ventilate

General measures

- Maintain hydration and nutrition
- Treat secondary infections
- Vaccination following recovery

*For dose, depending on specific IVIG used, see https://assets.publishing.service.gov.uk/government/uploads/system/uploads/attachment_data/file/820628/Tetanus_information_for_health_professionals_2019.pdf

(IM = intramuscular; IV = intravenous)

collected, before immunoglobulin is given, for tetanus toxin and antibodies against tetanus toxoid.

Management

Established disease

Management of established disease should begin as soon as possible, as shown in Box 28.70.

Prevention

Tetanus can be prevented by immunisation and prompt treatment of contaminated wounds by débridement and antibiotics. In patients with a contaminated wound, a 7–10-day course of metronidazole (500 mg intravenously every 6–8 hours) or penicillin G (2–4 million units every 4–6 hours) are recommended. Alternative antibiotics include tetracyclines, macrolides, clindamycin, cephalosporins and chloramphenicol. Tetanus toxoid containing vaccine and human tetanus immunoglobulin use should follow local guidelines, and depend on the level of risk associated with a wound, prior immunisation and time since last tetanus vaccination.

Botulism

Botulism is caused by the neurotoxins of *Clostridium botulinum*, which are extremely potent and cause disease after ingestion of even picogram amounts. Its classical form is an acute onset of bilateral cranial neuropathies associated with symmetric descending weakness.

Anaerobic conditions are necessary for the organism's growth. It may contaminate and thrive in many foodstuffs, where sealing and preserving provide the requisite conditions. Contaminated honey has been implicated in infant botulism, in which the organism colonises the gastrointestinal tract. Wound botulism is a growing problem in injection drug users.

The toxin causes predominantly bulbar and ocular palsies (difficulty in swallowing, blurred or double vision, ptosis), progressing to limb weakness and respiratory paralysis. Criteria for the clinical diagnosis are shown in Box 28.71.

Management includes assisted ventilation and general supportive measures until the toxin eventually dissociates from nerve endings 6–8 weeks following ingestion. A polyvalent antitoxin is available for

28.71 US Centers for Disease Control (CDC) definition of botulism

Three main syndromes

- Infantile
- Food-borne
- Wound infection

Clinical features

- Absence of fever
- Symmetrical neurological deficits
- Patient remains responsive
- Normal or slow heart rate and normal blood pressure
- No sensory deficits with the exception of blurred vision

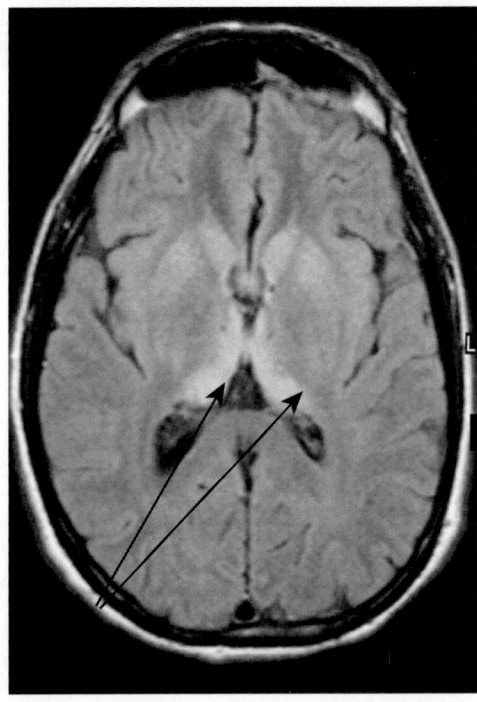

Fig. 28.35 Magnetic resonance imaging in variant Creutzfeldt–Jakob disease. Arrows indicate bilateral pulvinar hyperintensity.

28.72 Prion diseases affecting humans

Disease	Mechanism
Creutzfeldt–Jakob disease	
Sporadic	Unknown: spontaneous PrP^C to PrP^{SC} conversion or somatic mutation
Familial	Genetic: mutations in the *PrP* gene
Variant	Dietary ingestion: infection from bovine spongiform encephalopathy
Gerstmann–Sträussler–Scheinker disease	Genetic: mutations in the *PrP* gene
Fatal familial insomnia	Genetic: mutations in the *PrP* gene
Sporadic fatal insomnia	Genetic: spontaneous PrP^C to PrP^{SC} conversion or somatic mutation
Kuru	Dietary: ingestion of affected human brain

post-exposure prophylaxis and for the treatment of suspected botulism. It specifically neutralises toxin types A, B and E and is not effective against infant botulism (in which active growth of the organism allows continued toxin production).

Prion diseases

Prions are unique amongst infectious agents in that they are devoid of any nucleic acid. They appear to be transmitted by acquisition of a normal mammalian protein (prion protein, PrP^C) that is in an abnormal conformation (PrP^{SC}, containing an excess of beta-sheet protein). The result is accumulation of protein that forms amyloid in the CNS, causing a transmissible spongiform encephalopathy (TSE) across several species.

Human prion diseases (Box 28.72) are characterised by the histopathological triad of cortical spongiform change, neuronal cell loss and gliosis. Associated with these changes there is deposition of amyloid, made up of an altered form of a normally occurring protein, the prion protein. Prion proteins are not inactivated by cooking or conventional sterilisation, and transmission is thought to occur by consumption of infected CNS tissue or by inoculation (e.g. via depth EEG electrodes, corneal grafts, cadaveric dura mater grafts and pooled cadaveric growth hormone preparations). The same diseases can occur in an inherited form, due to mutations in the *PrP* gene.

The apparent transmission of bovine spongiform encephalopathy (BSE) to humans was thought to be responsible for the emergence of a new variant of Creutzfeld–Jakob disease (vCJD) in the UK (see below). This outbreak led to nationwide precautionary measures, such as leuco-depletion of all blood used for transfusion, and the mandatory use of disposable surgical instruments wherever possible for tonsillectomy, appendicectomy and ophthalmological procedures.

Creutzfeldt–Jakob disease

Creutzfeldt–Jakob disease (CJD) is the best-characterised human TSE. Some 10% of cases arise from a mutation in the gene coding for the prion protein. The sporadic form is the most common, occurring in middle-aged to older patients. Clinical features usually involve a rapidly progressive dementia, with myoclonus and a characteristic EEG pattern (repetitive slow-wave complexes), although a number of other features, such as visual disturbance or ataxia, may also be seen. These are particularly common in CJD transmitted by inoculation (e.g. by infected dura mater grafts). Death occurs after a mean of 4–6 months. There is no effective treatment.

Variant Creutzfeldt–Jakob disease

This type of CJD (vCJD) emerged in the late 1990s, affecting a small number of patients in the UK. The causative agent appears to be identical to that causing BSE in cows, and the disease may have been a result of the epidemic of BSE in the UK a decade earlier. Patients affected by vCJD are typically younger than those with sporadic CJD and present with neuropsychiatric changes and sensory symptoms in the limbs, followed by ataxia, dementia and death. Progression is slightly slower than in patients with sporadic CJD (mean time to death is over a year). Characteristic EEG changes are not present, but MRI brain scans show typical high-signal changes in the pulvinar thalami in a high proportion of cases (Fig. 28.35). Brain histology is distinct, with very florid plaques containing the prion proteins. Abnormal prion protein has been identified in tonsil specimens from patients with vCJD, leading to the suggestion that the disease could be transmitted by reticulo-endothelial tissue (like TSEs in animals but unlike sporadic CJD in humans). It was the emergence of this form of the disorder that led to the changes in public health and farming policy in the UK; while the incidence of vCJD has declined dramatically, surveillance and research continue.

28

i 28.73 Common causes of raised intracranial pressure

Mass lesions

- Intracranial haemorrhage (traumatic or spontaneous):
    Extradural haematoma
    Subdural haematoma
    Intracerebral haemorrhage
- Cerebral tumour (particularly posterior fossa lesions or high-grade gliomas: see Box 28.75)
- Infective:
    Cerebral abscess
    Tuberculoma
    Cysticercosis
    Hydatid cyst
- Colloid cyst (in ventricles)

Disturbance of cerebrospinal fluid circulation

- Obstructive (non-communicating) hydrocephalus: obstruction within ventricular system
- Communicating hydrocephalus: site of obstruction outside ventricular system

Obstruction to venous sinuses

- Cerebral venous thrombosis
- Trauma (depressed fractures overlying sinuses)

Diffuse brain oedema or swelling

- Meningo-encephalitis
- Trauma (diffuse head injury, near-drowning)
- Subarachnoid haemorrhage
- Metabolic (e.g. water intoxication)
- Idiopathic intracranial hypertension

i 28.74 Clinical features of intracranial mass lesions

Presentation	Features
Seizures	Focal onset ± generalised spread
Focal symptoms	Progressive loss of function Weakness Numbness Dysphasia Cranial neuropathy
False localising signs	Unilateral/bilateral 6th nerve palsies Contralateral 3rd nerve (usually pupil first)
Raised intracranial pressure (usually aggressive tumours causing vasogenic oedema or obstructive hydrocephalus)	Headache worse on lying/straining Vomiting Diplopia (6th nerve involvement) Papilloedema Bradycardia, raised blood pressure Impaired conscious level
Stroke/TIA-like symptoms	Acute haemorrhage into tumour Paroxysmal 'tumour attacks'
Cognitive/behavioural change	Usually frontal mass lesions
Endocrine abnormalities	Pituitary tumours
Incidental finding	Asymptomatic but identified on imaging (meningiomas commonly)

(TIA = transient ischaemic attack)

Intracranial mass lesions and raised intracranial pressure

Many different types of mass lesion may arise within the intracranial cavity (Box 28.73). In low-income countries tuberculoma and other infections are frequent causes, but in the West intracranial haemorrhage and brain tumours are more common. The clinical features depend on the site of the mass, its nature and its rate of expansion. Symptoms and signs (see Box 28.74) are produced by a number of mechanisms.

Raised intracranial pressure

Raised intracranial pressure (RICP) may be caused by mass lesions, cerebral oedema, obstruction to CSF circulation leading to hydrocephalus, impaired CSF absorption and cerebral venous obstruction (see Box 28.73).

Clinical features

In adults, intracranial pressure is less than 10–15 mmHg. The features of RICP are listed in Box 28.74. The speed of pressure increase influences presentation. If it is slow, compensatory mechanisms may occur, including alteration in the volume of fluid in CSF spaces and venous sinuses, minimising symptoms. Rapid pressure increase (as in aggressive tumours) does not permit these compensatory mechanisms to take place, leading to early symptoms, including sudden death. Papilloedema is not always present, either because the pressure rise has been too rapid or because of anatomical anomalies of the meningeal sheath of the optic nerve.

A false localising sign is one in which the pathology is remote from the site of the expected lesion; in RICP, the 6th cranial nerve (unilateral or bilateral) is most commonly affected but the 3rd, 5th and 7th nerves may also be involved. Sixth nerve palsies are thought to be due either to stretching of the long slender nerve or to compression against the

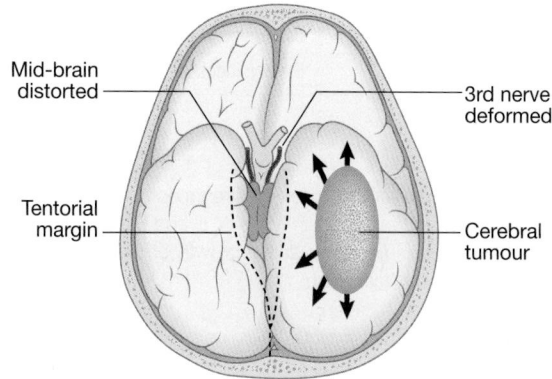

Fig. 28.36 Cerebral tumour displacing medial temporal lobe and causing pressure on the mid-brain and 3rd cranial nerve.

petrous temporal bone ridge. Transtentorial herniation of the uncus may compress the ipsilateral 3rd nerve and usually involves the pupillary fibres first, causing a dilated pupil; however, a false localising contralateral 3rd nerve palsy may also occur, perhaps due to extrinsic compression by the tentorial margin. Vomiting, coma, bradycardia and arterial hypertension are later features of RICP.

The rise in intracranial pressure from a mass lesion may cause displacement of the brain. Downward displacement of the medial temporal lobe (uncus) through the tentorium due to a large hemisphere mass may cause 'temporal coning' (Fig. 28.36). This may stretch the 3rd and/or 6th cranial nerves or cause pressure on the contralateral cerebral peduncle (giving rise to ipsilateral upper motor neuron signs) and is usually accompanied by progressive coma. Downward movement of the cerebellar tonsils through the foramen magnum may compress the medulla – 'tonsillar coning' (Fig. 28.37). This may result in brainstem haemorrhage and/or acute obstruction of the CSF pathways. As coning progresses, coma and death occur unless the condition is rapidly treated.

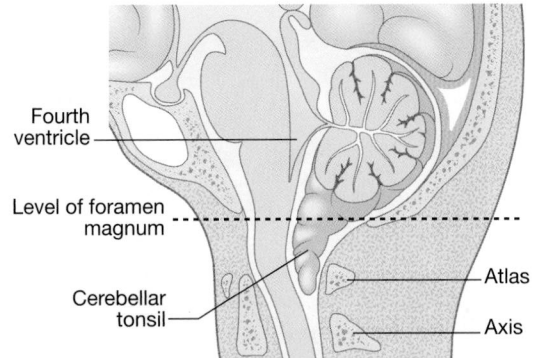

Fourth ventricle

Level of foramen magnum

Cerebellar tonsil

Atlas

Axis

Fig. 28.37 Tonsillar cone. Downward displacement of the cerebellar tonsils below the level of the foramen magnum.

Management

Primary management of RICP should be targeted at relieving the cause (e.g. surgical decompression of mass lesion, glucocorticoids to reduce vasogenic oedema or shunt procedure to relieve hydrocephalus). Supportive treatment includes maintenance of fluid balance, blood pressure control, head elevation and use of diuretics such as mannitol. Intensive care support may be needed.

Brain tumours

Primary brain tumours are a heterogeneous collection of neoplasms arising from the brain tissue or meninges and vary from benign to highly malignant. Primary malignant brain tumours (Box 28.75) are rare, accounting for 1% of all adult tumours but a higher proportion in children. The most common benign brain tumour is a meningioma. Primary brain tumours do not metastasise due to the absence of lymphatic drainage in the brain. There are rare pathological subtypes, however, such as medulloblastoma, which do have a propensity to metastasise; the reasons for this are not clear. Most cerebral tumours are sporadic but may be associated with genetic syndromes such as neurofibromatosis or tuberous sclerosis. Brain tumours are not classified by the usual TNM system but by the World Health Organization (WHO) grading I–IV; this is based on histology (e.g. nuclear pleomorphism, presence of mitoses and presence of necrosis), with grade I the most benign and grade IV the most malignant. Gliomas account for 60% of brain tumours, with the aggressive glioblastoma multiforme (WHO grade IV) the most common glioma, followed by meningiomas (20%) and pituitary tumours (10%). Although the lower-grade gliomas (I and II) may be very indolent, with prognosis measured in terms of many years, these may transform to higher-grade disease at any time, with a resultant sharp decline in life expectancy.

Most malignant brain tumours are due to metastases, with intracranial metastases complicating about 20% of extracranial malignancies. The rate is higher with primaries in the bronchus, breast and gastrointestinal tract (Fig. 28.38). Metastases usually occur in the white matter of the cerebral or cerebellar hemispheres but there are diffuse leptomeningeal types.

Clinical features

The presentation is variable and usually influenced by the rate of growth. High-grade disease (WHO grades III and IV) tends to present with a short (weeks) history of mass effect (headache, nausea secondary to RICP), while more indolent tumours can present with slowly progressive focal neurological deficits, depending on their location (see Box 28.74); generalised or focal seizures are common in either. Headache, if present, is usually accompanied by focal deficits or seizures, and isolated stable headache is almost never due to intracranial tumour.

The size of the primary tumour is of far less prognostic significance than its location within the brain. Tumours within the brainstem will result in early neurological deficits, while those in the frontal region may be quite large before symptoms occur.

i 28.75 Primary brain tumours

Histological type	Common site	Age
Malignant		
Glioma (astrocytoma)	Cerebral hemisphere	Adulthood
	Cerebellum	Childhood/adulthood
	Brainstem	Childhood/young adulthood
Oligodendroglioma	Cerebral hemisphere	Adulthood
Medulloblastoma	Posterior fossa	Childhood
Ependymoma	Posterior fossa	Childhood/adolescence
Cerebral lymphoma	Cerebral hemisphere	Adulthood
Benign		
Meningioma	Cortical dura	Adulthood (often incidental finding)
	Parasagittal	
	Sphenoid ridge	
	Suprasellar	
	Olfactory groove	
Neurofibroma	Acoustic neuroma	Adulthood
Craniopharyngioma	Suprasellar	Childhood/adolescence
Pituitary adenoma	Pituitary fossa	Adulthood
Colloid cyst	Third ventricle	Any age
Pineal tumours	Quadrigeminal cistern	Childhood (teratomas) Young adulthood (germ cell)

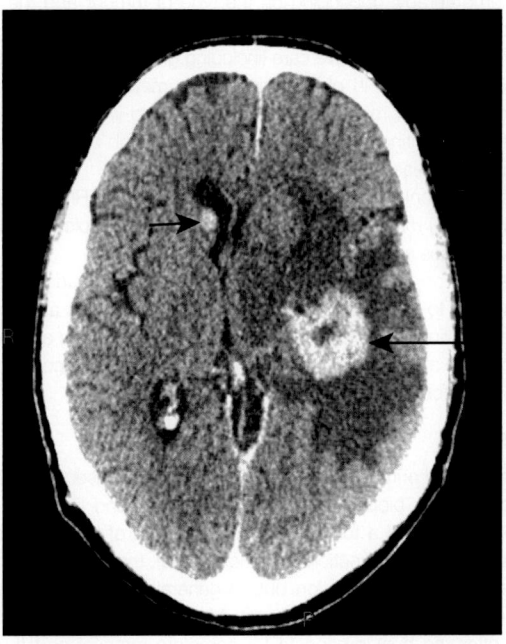

Fig. 28.38 Contrast-enhanced computed tomogram of the head showing a large metastasis within the left hemisphere (long arrow). There is surrounding cerebral oedema, and a smaller metastasis (short arrow) within the wall of the right lateral ventricle. The primary lesion was a lung carcinoma.

Investigations

Diagnosis is by neuroimaging (Figs. 28.39 and 28.40) and pathological grading following biopsy or resection where possible. The more malignant tumours are more likely to demonstrate contrast enhancement on imaging. If the tumour appears metastatic, further investigation to find the primary is required.

28

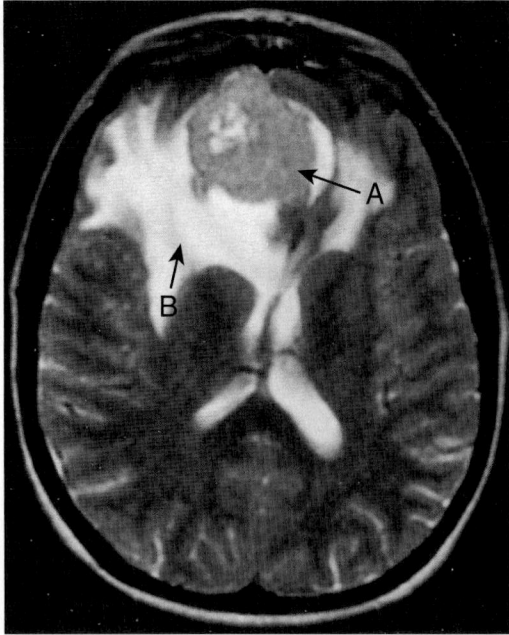

Fig. 28.39 Magnetic resonance image showing a meningioma in the frontal lobe (arrow A) with associated oedema (arrow B).

Management

Brain tumours are treated with a combination of surgery, radiotherapy and chemotherapy, depending on the type of tumour and the patient. Advancing age is the most powerful negative prognostic factor in CNS tumours, so best supportive care (including glucocorticoid therapy) may be most appropriate in older patients with metastases or high-grade disease. Treatment may not always be indicated in low-grade gliomas and watchful waiting may be appropriate, although a more aggressive approach is increasingly favoured.

Dexamethasone given orally (or intravenously where RICP is acutely or severely raised) may reduce the vasogenic oedema typically associated with metastases and high-grade gliomas.

Prolactin- or growth hormone-secreting pituitary adenomas may respond well to treatment with dopamine agonists (such as bromocriptine, cabergoline or quinagolide); in this situation, imaging and hormone levels may be all that is required to establish a formal diagnosis, precluding the need for surgery.

Surgical

The mainstay of primary treatment is surgery, either resection (full or partial debulking) or biopsy, depending on the site and likely radiological diagnosis. Clearly, if a tumour occurs in an area of brain that is highly important for normal function (e.g. motor strip), then biopsy may be the only safe surgical intervention but, in general, maximal safe resection is the optimal surgical management. Meningiomas and acoustic neuromas offer the best prospects for complete removal and thus cure. Some meningiomas can recur, however, particularly those of the sphenoid ridge, when partial excision is often all that is possible. Thereafter, post-operative surveillance may be required, as radiotherapy is effective at preventing further growth of residual tumour. Pituitary adenomas may be removed by a trans-sphenoidal route, avoiding the need for a craniotomy. Unfortunately, gliomas, which account for the majority of brain tumours, cannot be completely excised, since infiltration spreads well beyond the apparent radiological boundaries of the intracranial mass. Recurrence is therefore the rule, even if the mass of the tumour is apparently removed completely; partial excision ('debulking') may be useful in alleviating symptoms caused by RICP, but although there is increasing evidence that the degree of surgical excision may have a positive influence on survival, this has not yet been convincingly demonstrated.

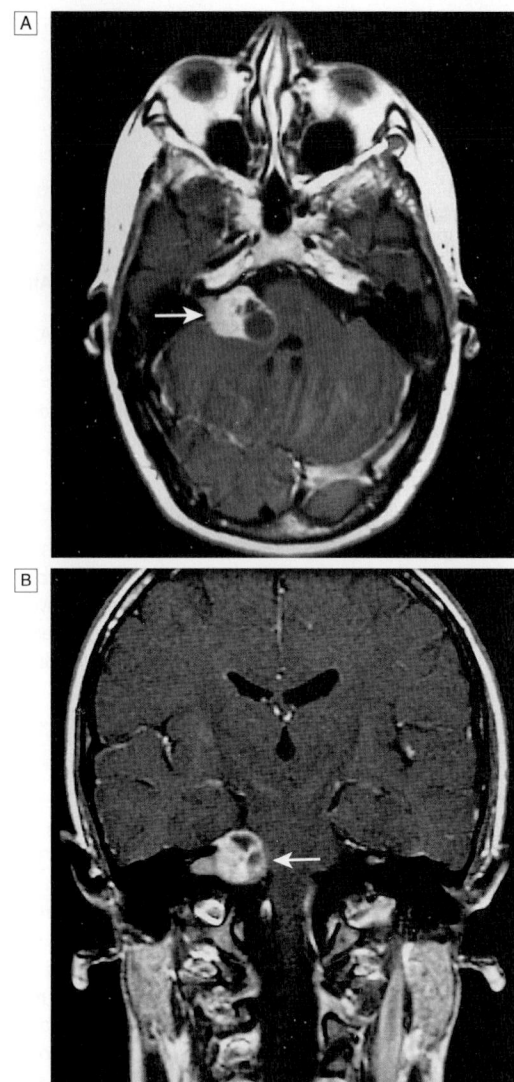

Fig. 28.40 Magnetic resonance image of an acoustic neuroma (arrows) in the posterior fossa compressing the brainstem. [A] Axial image. [B] Coronal image.

Radiotherapy and chemotherapy

In the majority of primary CNS tumours, radiation and chemotherapy are used to control disease and extend survival rather than for cure. Meningioma and pituitary adenoma offer the best chance of life-long remission. The gliomas are incurable; high-grade, WHO grade IV disease still carries a median survival of just over 1 year. In this situation, patient and family should always be involved in decisions regarding treatment. The diagnosis, and often the symptoms, are devastating, and support from palliative care and social work is crucial at an early stage. In WHO grade III disease, prognosis is a little better (2–4 years), and in rarer, more indolent tumours very prolonged survival is possible.

Advances have been made recently in terms of therapeutic outcome. Standard care for WHO grade IV glioblastoma multiforme is now combination radiotherapy with temozolomide chemotherapy; although this improves median survival of the population from only 12 to 14.5 months, up to 25% of patients survive for more than 2 years (compared to approximately 10% with radiotherapy alone). Ten percent will survive more than 5 years with temozolomide (virtually unheard of with radiotherapy alone). Benefits are more likely in well-debulked patients who are younger and fitter. Implantation of chemotherapy gives a small survival benefit.

Understanding of the molecular biology of brain tumours has allowed the use of biomarkers to guide therapy and prognostic discussions.

In patients with methylation of the promoter region of the *MGMT* (methyl guanine methyl transferase) gene (about 30% of the population) within the tumour, 2-year survival is almost 50%. MGMT reduces the cyto-toxicity of temozolomide and this mutation also reduces the enzyme's activity, rendering the tumour more sensitive to chemotherapy. In grade II and III gliomas, the presence of the loss of heterozygosity (LOH) 1p19q chromosomal abnormality confers chemosensitivity and thus improves prognosis. The presence of a rare mutation in the *IDH-1* (isocitrate dehydrogenase) gene confers a more favourable prognosis in patients with glioblastoma.

There is a small group of highly malignant grade IV tumours that can be cured with aggressive therapy. Medulloblastomas have a good chance of long-term remission with maximal surgery followed by irradiation of the whole brain and spine; younger patients may also benefit from concomitant and adjuvant chemotherapy. Older patients do not tolerate this, however.

Once tumours relapse, chemotherapy response rates are low and survival is short in high-grade disease. In the more uncommon low-grade tumours, repeated courses of chemotherapy can result in much more prolonged survival.

In metastatic disease, radiotherapy offers a modest improvement in survival but with costs in terms of quality of life; treatment therefore needs careful discussion with the patient. Benefits may be superior in breast cancer but there is little to separate other pathologies. Occasional chemosensitive cancers, such as small-cell lung cancer, may benefit from systemic chemotherapy but intracerebral metastases represent a late stage of disease and have a short prognosis.

Prognosis

The WHO histological grading system is a powerful predictor of prognosis in primary CNS tumours, though it does not yet take account of individual biomarkers. For each tumour type and grade, advancing age and deteriorating functional status are the next most important negative prognostic features. The overall 5-year survival rate of about 14% in adults masks a wide variation that depends on tumour type.

Acoustic neuroma

This is a benign tumour of Schwann cells of the 8th cranial nerve, which may arise in isolation or as part of neurofibromatosis type 2 (see below). When sporadic, acoustic neuroma occurs after the third decade and is more frequent in females. The tumour commonly arises near the nerve's entry point into the medulla or in the internal auditory meatus, usually on the vestibular division. Acoustic neuromas account for 80%–90% of tumours at the cerebellopontine angle.

Clinical features

Acoustic neuroma typically presents with unilateral progressive hearing loss, sometimes with tinnitus. Vertigo is an unusual symptom, as slow growth allows compensatory brainstem mechanisms to develop. In some cases, progressive enlargement leads to distortion of the brainstem and/or cerebellar peduncle, causing ataxia and/or cerebellar signs in the limbs. Distortion of the fourth ventricle and cerebral aqueduct may cause hydrocephalus (see below), which may be the presenting feature. Facial weakness is unusual at presentation but facial palsy may follow surgical removal of the tumour. The tumour may be identified incidentally on cranial imaging.

Investigations

MRI is the investigation of choice (see Fig. 28.40).

Management

Surgery is the treatment of choice. If the tumour can be completely removed, the prognosis is excellent, although deafness is a common complication of surgery. Stereotactic radiosurgery (radiotherapy) may be appropriate for some lesions.

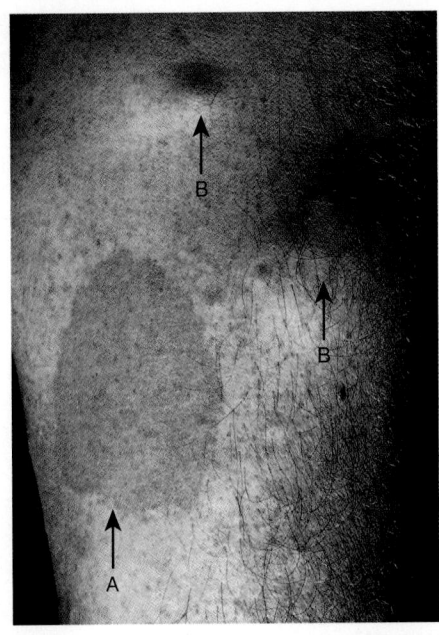

Fig. 28.41 A café au lait spot (arrow A) and subcutaneous nodules (arrows B) on the forearm of a patient with neurofibromatosis type 1.

Neurofibromatosis

Neurofibromatosis encompasses two clinically and genetically separate conditions, with an autosomal dominant pattern of inheritance. The more common neurofibromatosis type 1 (NF1) is caused by mutations in the *NF1* gene on chromosome 17, half of which are new mutations. NF1 is characterised by neurofibromas (benign peripheral nerve sheath tumours) and skin involvement (Fig. 28.41), and may affect numerous systems (Box 28.76). Neurofibromatosis type 2 (NF2) is caused by mutations of the *NF2* gene on chromosome 22 and is characterised by schwannomas (benign peripheral nerve sheath tumours comprising Schwann cells only) with little skin involvement; the clinical manifestations are more restricted to the eye and nervous system (see Box 28.76). Malignant change may occur in NF1 neurofibromas but is rare in NF2 schwannomas. The prevalence of NF1 and NF2 is about 20–50 per 100000 and 1.5 per 100000, respectively.

Von Hippel–Lindau disease

This rare autosomal dominant disease is caused by mutations of the *VHL* tumour suppressor gene on chromosome 3. It promotes development of tumours affecting the kidney, adrenal gland, CNS, eye, inner ear, epididymis and pancreas, which may undergo malignant change. Benign haemangiomas and haemangioblastomas affect about 80% of patients and are mostly cerebellar and retinal.

Paraneoplastic neurological disease

Paraneoplastic neurological syndromes often present before the underlying tumour declares itself and cause considerable disability. They are discussed in full on page 1165.

Hydrocephalus

Hydrocephalus is the excessive accumulation of CSF within the brain, and may be caused either by increased CSF production, by reduced CSF absorption, or by obstruction of the circulation (Fig. 28.42). Symptoms range from none to sudden death, depending on the speed at which and degree to which hydrocephalus develops. The causes are listed in Box 28.77. The terms 'communicating' and 'non-communicating' (also known as obstructive) hydrocephalus refer to blockage either outside or within the ventricular system, respectively (Fig. 28.43).

28

i 28.76 Neurofibromatosis types 1 and 2: clinical features

Neurofibromatosis 1	Neurofibromatosis 2
Skin	
Cutaneous/subcutaneous neurofibromas	Much less commonly affected than in NF1
Angiomas	Café au lait patches (usually < 6)
Café au lait patches (> 6)	Cutaneous schwannomas: plaque lesions
Axillary/groin freckling	Subcutaneous schwannomas
Hypopigmented patches	
Eyes	
Lisch nodules (iris fibromas)	Cataracts
Glaucoma	Retinal hamartoma
Congenital ptosis	Optic nerve meningioma
Nervous system	
Plexiform neurofibromas	Vestibular schwannomas
Malignant peripheral nerve sheath tumours	Cranial nerve schwannomas (not 1 and 2)
Aqueduct stenosis	Spinal schwannomas
Slight tonsillar descent	Peripheral nerve schwannomas
Cognitive impairment	Cranial meningiomas
Epilepsy	Spinal meningiomas
	Spinal/brainstem ependymomas
	Spinal/cranial astrocytoma
Bone	
Scoliosis	
Osteoporosis	
Pseudoarthrosis	
Cardiorespiratory systems	
Pulmonary stenosis	
Hypertension	
Renal artery stenosis	
Compression from neurofibroma causing restrictive lung defect	
Gastrointestinal system	
Gastrointestinal stromal tumour (GIST)	
Duodenal/ampullary neuro-endocrine tumour	

i 28.77 Causes of hydrocephalus

Congenital malformations

- Aqueduct stenosis
- Chiari malformations
- Dandy–Walker syndrome
- Benign intracranial cysts
- Vein of Galen aneurysms
- Congenital central nervous system infections
- Craniofacial anomalies

Acquired causes

- Mass lesions (especially those in the posterior fossa)
- Tumour
- Colloid cyst of third ventricle
- Abscess
- Haematoma
- Absorption blockages due to:
  Inflammation (e.g. meningitis, sarcoidosis)
  Intracranial haemorrhage

Normal pressure hydrocephalus

Normal pressure hydrocephalus (NPH) is a controversial entity, said to involve intermittent rises in CSF pressure, particularly at night. It is described in old age as being associated with a triad of gait apraxia, dementia and urinary incontinence.

Management

Diversion of the CSF by means of a shunt placed between the ventricular system and the peritoneal cavity or right atrium may result in rapid relief of symptoms in obstructive hydrocephalus. The outcome of shunting in NPH is much less predictable and, until a good response can be predicted, the management of individual cases will remain uncertain.

Idiopathic intracranial hypertension

This usually occurs in young women with high BMI. The annual incidence is about 3 per 100 000. RICP occurs in the absence of a structural lesion, hydrocephalus or other identifiable cause. The aetiology is uncertain but there is an association with obesity in females, perhaps inducing a defect of CSF reabsorption by the arachnoid villi. A number of drugs may be associated, including tetracycline, vitamin A and retinoid derivatives.

Clinical features

The usual presentation is with headache, sometimes accompanied by diplopia and visual disturbance (most commonly, transient obscurations of vision associated with changes in posture). Clinical examination reveals papilloedema but little else. False localising cranial nerve palsies (usually of the 6th nerve) may be present. It is important to record visual fields accurately for future monitoring.

Investigations

Brain imaging is required to exclude a structural or other cause (e.g. cerebral venous sinus thrombosis). The ventricles are typically normal in size or small ('slit' ventricles). The diagnosis may be confirmed by lumbar puncture, which shows raised normal CSF constituents at increased pressure (usually > 30 cmH_2O CSF).

Management

Management can be difficult and there is no evidence to support any specific treatment. Weight loss in overweight patients may be helpful if it can be achieved. Acetazolamide or topiramate may help to lower intracranial pressure, the latter perhaps aiding weight loss in some patients. Repeated lumbar puncture is an effective treatment for headache but may be technically difficult in obese individuals and is often poorly tolerated. Patients failing to respond, in whom chronic papilloedema threatens vision, may require optic nerve sheath fenestration or a lumbo-peritoneal shunt.

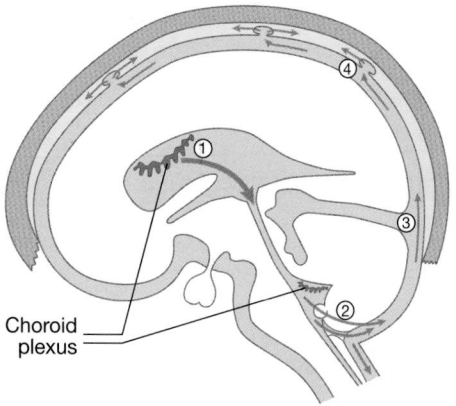

Choroid plexus

Fig. 28.42 The circulation of cerebrospinal fluid (CSF). (1) CSF is synthesised in the choroid plexus of the ventricles and flows from the lateral and third ventricles through the aqueduct to the fourth ventricle. (2) At the foramina of Luschka and Magendie it exits the brain, flowing over the hemispheres (3) and down around the spinal cord and roots in the subarachnoid space. (4) It is then absorbed into the dural venous sinuses via the arachnoid villi.

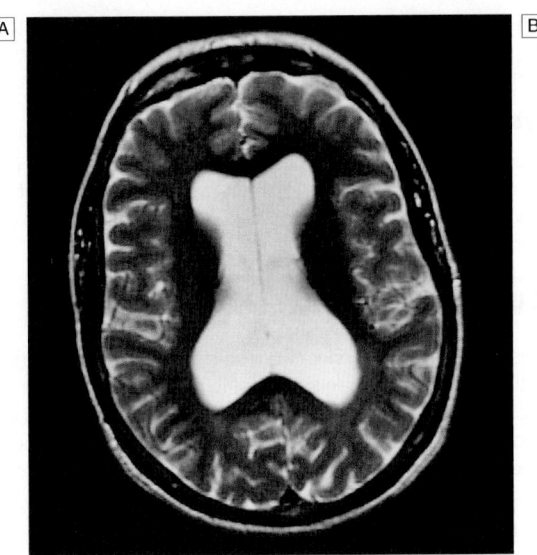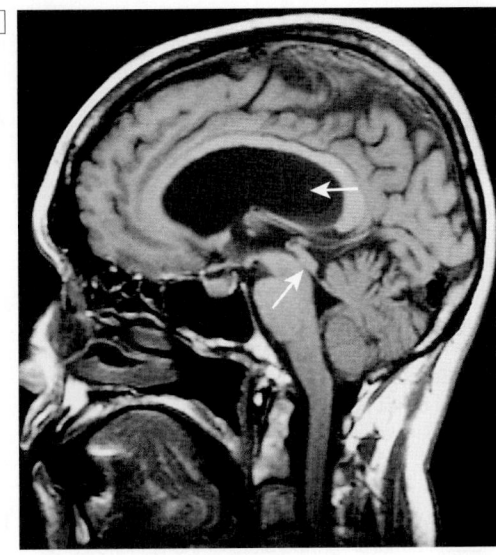

Fig. 28.43 Magnetic resonance image of hydrocephalus due to aqueduct stenosis. [A] Axial T2-weighted image (cerebrospinal fluid appears white): note the dilated lateral ventricles. [B] Sagittal T1-weighted image (cerebrospinal fluid appears black): note the dilated ventricles (top arrow) and narrowed aqueduct (bottom arrow).

Head injury

Diagnosis of head trauma is usually clear either from the history or from signs of external trauma to the head. Brain injury is more likely with skull fracture but can occur without. Individual cranial nerves may be damaged in fractures of the facial bones or skull base. Intracranial effects can be substantial and take several forms: extradural haematoma (collection of blood between the skull and dura); subdural haematoma (collection of blood between the dura and the surface of the brain); intracerebral haematoma; or diffuse axonal injury.

Whatever pathology occurs, the resultant RICP may lead to coning (see Figs. 28.36 and 28.37). Haematomas are identified by CT and management is by surgical drainage, usually via a burr hole. Penetrating skull fractures lead to increased infection risk. Long-term sequelae include headache, cognitive decline and depression, all contributing to significant social, work, personality and family difficulties.

Subdural haematoma may occur spontaneously, particularly in patients on anticoagulants, in old age and with alcohol misuse. There may or may not be a history of trauma. Patients present with subacute impairment of brain function, both globally (obtundation and coma) and focally (hemiparesis, seizures). Headache may not be present. The diagnosis should always be considered in those who present with reduced conscious level.

Beyond the immediate consequences of brain injury, there is increasing suspicion of long-term consequences, including dementia, postulated after either single (moderate or severe) injuries or even after multiple mild injuries, such as in boxers. If substantiated, this would encourage more effort to go into prevention of repeated brain injury in sporting contexts.

Disorders of cerebellar function

Cerebellar dysfunction can manifest as incoordination of limb function, gait ataxia, speech or eye movements. Acute dysfunction may be caused by alcohol or prescription drugs (especially the sodium channel-blocking antiepileptic drugs phenytoin and carbamazepine).

Inflammatory changes in the cerebellum may cause symptoms in the aftermath of some infections (especially herpes zoster) or as a paraneoplastic phenomenon. The hereditary spinocerebellar ataxias are described on page 1169; they manifest as progressive ataxias in middle and old age, often with other neurological features that aid specific diagnosis.

Disorders of the spine and spinal cord

The spinal cord and spinal roots may be affected by intrinsic disease or by disorders of the surrounding meninges and bones. The clinical presentation of these conditions depends on the anatomical level at which the cord or roots are affected, as well as the nature of the pathological process involved. It is important to recognise when the spinal cord is at risk of compression so that urgent action can be taken.

Cervical spondylosis

Cervical spondylosis is the result of osteoarthritis in the cervical spine. It is characterised by degeneration of the intervertebral discs and osteophyte formation. Such 'wear and tear' is extremely common and radiological changes are frequently found in asymptomatic individuals over the age of 50. Spondylosis may be associated with neurological dysfunction. In order of frequency, the C5/6, C6/7 and C4/5 vertebral levels affect C6, C7 and C5 roots, respectively (Fig. 28.44).

Cervical radiculopathy

Acute onset of compression of a nerve root occurs when a disc prolapses laterally. More gradual onset may be due to osteophytic encroachment of the intervertebral foramina.

Clinical features

The patient complains of pain in the neck that may radiate in the distribution of the affected nerve root. The neck is held rigidly and neck movements may exacerbate pain. Paraesthesia and sensory loss may be found in the affected segment and there may be lower motor neuron signs, including weakness, wasting and reflex impairment (Fig. 28.45).

Investigations

Where there is no trauma, imaging should not be carried out for isolated cervical pain. MRI is the investigation of choice in those with radicular symptoms. X-rays offer limited benefit, except in excluding destructive lesions, and electrophysiological studies rarely add to clinical examination with MRI.

Management

Conservative treatment with analgesics and physiotherapy results in resolution of symptoms in the great majority of patients, but a few require surgery in the form of discectomy or radicular decompression.

28

Cervical myelopathy

Dorsomedial herniation of a disc and the development of transverse bony bars or posterior osteophytes may result in pressure on the spinal cord or the anterior spinal artery, which supplies the anterior two-thirds of the cord (see Fig. 28.44).

Clinical features

The onset is usually insidious and painless but acute deterioration may occur after trauma, especially hyperextension injury. Upper motor neuron signs develop in the limbs, with spasticity of the legs usually appearing before the arms are involved. Sensory loss in the upper limbs is common, producing tingling, numbness and proprioception loss in the hands, with progressive clumsiness. Sensory manifestations in the legs are much less common. Neurological deficit usually progresses gradually and disturbance of micturition is a very late feature.

Investigations

MRI (see Fig. 28.44) (or rarely myelography) will direct surgical intervention. The former provides information on the state of the spinal cord at the level of compression.

Management

Surgical procedures, including laminectomy and anterior discectomy, may arrest progression of disability but neurological improvement is not

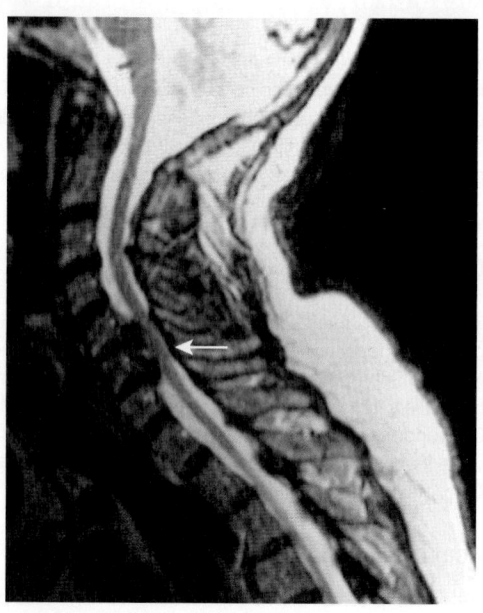

Fig. 28.44 Magnetic resonance image showing cervical cord compression (arrow) in cervical spondylosis.

the rule. The decision as to whether surgery should be undertaken may be difficult. Manual manipulation of the cervical spine is of no proven benefit and may precipitate acute neurological deterioration.

Prognosis

The prognosis of cervical myelopathy is variable. In many patients, the condition stabilises or even improves without intervention. If progression results in sphincter dysfunction or pyramidal signs, surgical decompression should be considered.

Lumbar spondylosis

This term covers degenerative disc disease and osteoarthritic change in the lumbar spine. Pain in the distribution of the lumbar or sacral roots ('sciatica') is almost always due to disc protrusion but can be a feature of other rare but important disorders, including spinal tumour, malignant disease in the pelvis and tuberculosis of the vertebral bodies.

Lumbar disc herniation

While acute lumbar disc herniation is often precipitated by trauma (usually lifting heavy weights while the spine is flexed), genetic factors may also be important. The nucleus pulposus may bulge or rupture through the annulus fibrosus, giving rise to pressure on nerve endings in the spinal ligaments, changes in the vertebral joints or pressure on nerve roots.

Pathophysiology

The altered mechanics of the lumbar spine result in loss of lumbar lordosis and there may be spasm of the paraspinal musculature. Root pressure is suggested by limitation of flexion of the hip on the affected side if the straight leg is raised (Lasègue sign). If the third or fourth lumbar root is involved, Lasègue sign may be negative, but pain in the back may be induced by hyperextension of the hip (femoral nerve stretch test). The roots most frequently affected are S1, L5 and L4; the signs of root pressure at these levels are summarised in Figure 28.46.

Clinical features

The onset may be sudden or gradual. Alternatively, repeated episodes of low back pain may precede sciatica by months or years. Constant aching pain is felt in the lumbar region and may radiate to the buttock, thigh, calf and foot. Pain is exacerbated by coughing or straining but may be relieved by lying flat.

Investigations

MRI is the investigation of choice if available, since soft tissues are well imaged. Plain X-rays of the lumbar spine are of little value in the diagnosis of disc disease, although they may demonstrate conditions affecting the vertebral body. CT can provide helpful images of the disc protrusion and/or narrowing of exit foramina.

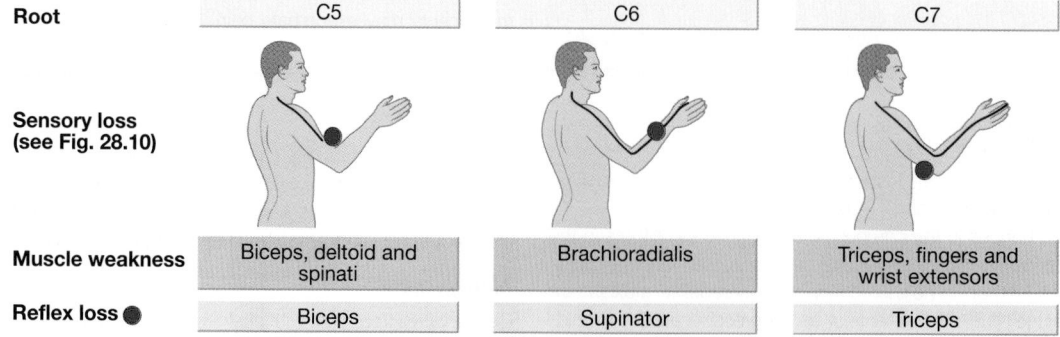

Root	C5	C6	C7
Sensory loss (see Fig. 28.10)			
Muscle weakness	Biceps, deltoid and spinati	Brachioradialis	Triceps, fingers and wrist extensors
Reflex loss ●	Biceps	Supinator	Triceps

Fig. 28.45 Findings in cervical nerve root compression.

Management

Some 90% of patients with sciatica recover following conservative treatment with analgesia and early mobilisation; bed rest does not help recovery. The patient should be instructed in back-strengthening exercises and advised to avoid physical manoeuvres likely to strain the lumbar spine. Injections of local anaesthetic or glucocorticoids may be useful adjunctive treatment if symptoms are due to ligamentous injury or joint dysfunction. Surgery may have to be considered if there is no response to conservative treatment or if progressive neurological deficits develop. Central disc prolapse with bilateral symptoms and signs and disturbance of sphincter function requires urgent surgical decompression.

Lumbar canal stenosis

This occurs with a congenitally narrowed lumbar spinal canal, exacerbated by the degenerative changes that commonly occur with age.

Pathophysiology

The symptoms of spinal stenosis are thought to be due to local vascular compromise secondary to the canal stenosis, rendering the nerve roots ischaemic and intolerant of the increased demand that occurs on exercise.

Clinical features

Patients, who are usually in old age, develop exercise-induced weakness and paraesthesia in the legs ('spinal claudication'). These symptoms progress with continued exertion, often to the point that the patient can no longer walk, but are quickly relieved by a short period of rest. Physical examination at rest shows preservation of peripheral pulses with absent ankle reflexes. Weakness or sensory loss may only be apparent if the patient is examined immediately after exercise.

Investigations

The investigation of first choice is MRI, but contraindications (body habitus, metallic implants) may make CT or myelography necessary.

Management

Lumbar laminectomy may provide relief of symptoms and recovery of normal exercise tolerance.

Spinal cord compression

Spinal cord compression is one of the more common neurological emergencies encountered in clinical practice and the usual causes are listed in Box 28.78. A space-occupying lesion within the spinal canal may damage nerve tissue either directly by pressure or indirectly by interference with blood supply. Oedema from venous obstruction impairs neuronal function, and ischaemia from arterial obstruction may lead to necrosis of the spinal cord. The early stages of damage are reversible but severely damaged neurons do not recover; hence the importance of early diagnosis and treatment.

Clinical features

The onset of symptoms of spinal cord compression is usually slow (over weeks) but can be acute as a result of trauma or metastases (see Figs. 28.44, 28.47 and 28.48), especially if there is associated arterial occlusion. The symptoms are shown in Box 28.79.

Pain and sensory symptoms occur early, while weakness and sphincter dysfunction are usually late manifestations. The signs vary according to the level of the cord compression and the structures involved. There may be tenderness to percussion over the spine if there is vertebral disease and this may be associated with a local kyphosis. Involvement of the roots at the level of the compression may cause dermatomal sensory impairment and corresponding lower motor signs. Interruption of fibres in the spinal cord causes sensory loss and upper motor neuron signs below the level of the lesion, and there is often disturbance of sphincter function. The distribution of these signs varies with the level of the lesion (Box 28.80).

The Brown–Séquard syndrome (see Fig. 28.18E) results if damage is confined to one side of the cord; the findings are explained by the anatomy of the sensory tracts (see Fig. 28.11). With compressive lesions, there is usually a band of pain at the level of the lesion in the distribution of the nerve roots subject to compression.

Investigations

Patients with a history of acute or subacute spinal cord syndrome should be investigated urgently, as listed in Box 28.81. The investigation of choice is MRI (Fig. 28.47), as it can define the extent of compression and associated soft-tissue abnormality (Fig. 28.48). Plain X-rays may show bony destruction and soft-tissue abnormalities. Routine investigations,

✚ 28.78 Causes of spinal cord compression		
Site	Frequency	Causes
Vertebral	80%	Trauma (extradural) Intervertebral disc prolapse Metastatic carcinoma (e.g. breast, prostate, bronchus) Myeloma Tuberculosis
Meninges (intradural, extramedullary)	15%	Tumours (e.g. meningioma, neurofibroma, ependymoma, metastasis, lymphoma, leukaemia) Epidural abscess
Spinal cord (intradural, intramedullary)	5%	Tumours (e.g. glioma, ependymoma, metastasis)

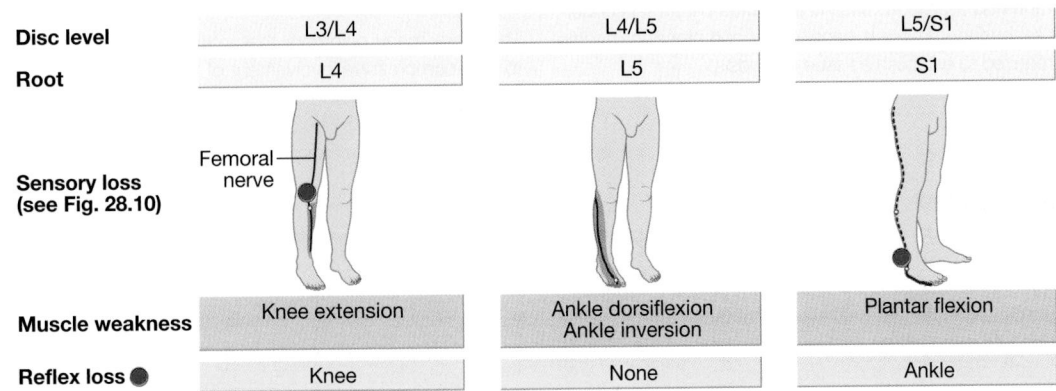

Disc level	L3/L4	L4/L5	L5/S1
Root	L4	L5	S1
Sensory loss (see Fig. 28.10)	Femoral nerve		
Muscle weakness	Knee extension	Ankle dorsiflexion Ankle inversion	Plantar flexion
Reflex loss ●	Knee	None	Ankle

Fig. 28.46 Findings in lumbar nerve root compression.

28

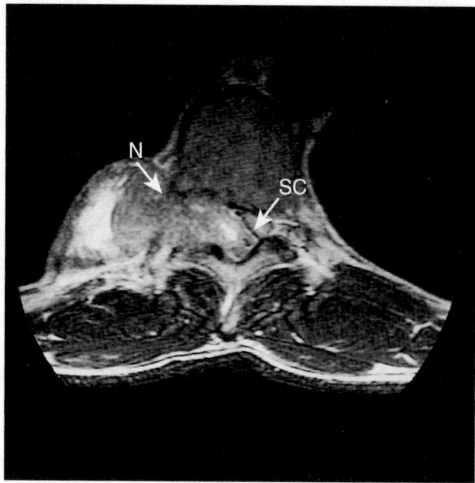

Fig. 28.47 Axial magnetic resonance image of thoracic spine. A neurofibroma (N) is compressing the spinal cord (SC) and emerging in a 'dumbbell' fashion through the vertebral foramen into the paraspinal space.

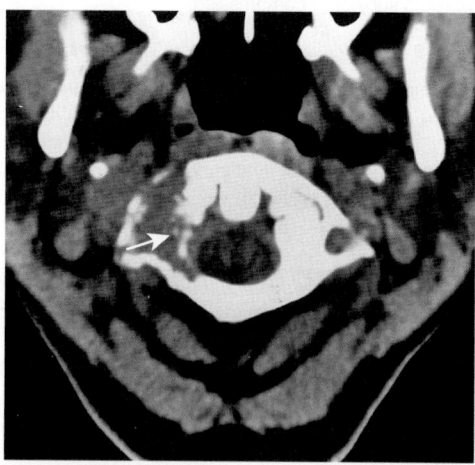

Fig. 28.48 Computed tomographic myelogram of cervical spine at the level of C2 showing bony erosion of vertebra by a metastasis (arrow).

28.79 Symptoms of spinal cord compression

Pain

• Localised over the spine or in a root distribution, which may be aggravated by coughing, sneezing or straining

Sensory

• Paraesthesia, numbness or cold sensations, especially in the lower limbs, which spread proximally, often to a level on the trunk

Motor

• Weakness, heaviness or stiffness of the limbs, most commonly the legs

Sphincters

• Urgency or hesitancy of micturition, leading eventually to urinary retention

28.80 Signs of spinal cord compression

Cervical, above C5

• Upper motor neuron signs and sensory loss in all four limbs
• Diaphragm weakness (phrenic nerve)

Cervical, C5–T1

• Lower motor neuron signs and segmental sensory loss in the arms; upper motor neuron signs in the legs
• Respiratory (intercostal) muscle weakness

Thoracic cord

• Spastic paraplegia with a sensory level on the trunk
• Weakness of legs, sacral loss of sensation and extensor plantar responses

Cauda equina

• Spinal cord ends approximately at the T12/L1 spinal level and spinal lesions below this level can cause lower motor neuron signs only by affecting the cauda equina

28.81 Investigation of acute spinal cord syndrome

• Magnetic resonance imaging of spine or myelography
• Plain X-rays of spine
• Chest X-ray
• Cerebrospinal fluid
• Serum vitamin B12

including chest X-ray, may provide evidence of systemic disease. If myelography is performed, CSF should be taken for analysis; in cases of complete spinal block, this shows a normal cell count with a very elevated protein causing yellow discoloration of the fluid (Froin syndrome). The risk of acute deterioration after myelography in spinal cord compression means that the neurosurgeons should be alerted before it is undertaken. Where a secondary tumour is causing the compression, needle biopsy may be required to establish a tissue diagnosis.

Management

Treatment and prognosis depend on the nature of the underlying lesion. Benign tumours should be surgically excised, and a good functional recovery can be expected unless a marked neurological deficit has developed before diagnosis. Extradural compression due to malignancy is the most common cause of spinal cord compression in developed countries and has a poor prognosis. Useful function can be regained if treatment, such as radiotherapy, is initiated within 24 hours of the onset of severe weakness or sphincter dysfunction; management should involve close cooperation with both oncologists and neurosurgeons (p. 139).

Spinal cord compression due to tuberculosis is common in some areas of the world and may require surgical treatment. This should be followed by appropriate antituberculous chemotherapy for an extended period. Traumatic lesions of the vertebral column require specialised neurosurgical treatment.

Intrinsic diseases of the spinal cord

There are many disorders that interfere with spinal cord function due to non-compressive involvement of the spinal cord itself. A list of these disorders is given in Box 28.82. The symptoms and signs are generally similar to those that would occur with extrinsic compression (see Boxes 28.79 and 28.80), although a suspended sensory loss (see Fig. 28.18F) can occur only with intrinsic disease such as syringomyelia. Urinary symptoms usually occur earlier in the course of an intrinsic cord disorder than with compressive disorders.

Investigation of intrinsic disease starts with imaging to exclude a compressive lesion. MRI provides most information about structural lesions, such as diastematomyelia, syringomyelia (Fig. 28.49) or intrinsic tumours. Non-specific signal change may be seen in the spinal cord in inflammatory (see Fig. 28.28) or infective conditions and metabolic disorders such as vitamin B12 deficiency. Lumbar puncture or blood tests may be required to make a specific diagnosis.

28.82 Intrinsic diseases of the spinal cord

Type of disorder	Condition	Clinical features
Congenital	Diastematomyelia (spina bifida)	Features variably present at birth and deteriorate thereafter LMN features, deformity and sensory loss of legs Impaired sphincter function Hairy patch or pit over low back Incidence reduced by increased maternal intake of folic acid during pregnancy
	Hereditary spastic paraplegia	Onset usually in adult life Autosomal dominant inheritance usual Slowly progressive UMN features affecting legs > arms Little or no sensory loss
Infective/inflammatory	Transverse myelitis due to viruses (HZV), schistosomiasis, HIV, MS, sarcoidosis	Weakness and sensory loss, often with pain, developing over hours to days UMN features below lesion Impaired sphincter function
	Paraneoplastic	May predate tumour diagnosis
Vascular	Anterior spinal artery infarct due to atherosclerosis, aortic dissection, embolus	Abrupt onset Anterior horn cell loss (LMN) at level of lesion UMN features below it Spinothalamic sensory loss below lesion but dorsal column sensation spared
	Spinal AVM/dural fistula	Onset variable (acute to slowly progressive) Variable LMN, UMN, sensory and sphincter disturbance Symptoms and signs often not well localised to site of AVM
Neoplastic	Glioma, ependymoma	Weakness and sensory loss often with pain, developing over months to years UMN features below lesion in cord; additional LMN features in conus Impaired sphincter function
Metabolic	Vitamin B_{12} deficiency (subacute combined degeneration) Copper deficiency Nitrous oxide toxicity	Progressive spastic paraparesis with proprioception loss Absent reflexes due to peripheral neuropathy ± Optic nerve and cerebral involvement Excess dietary zinc Modifies vitamin B_{12} metabolism
Degenerative	Motor neuron disease	Relentlessly progressive LMN and UMN features, associated bulbar weakness No sensory involvement
	Syringomyelia	Gradual onset over months or years, pain in cervical segments Anterior horn cell loss (LMN) at level of lesion, UMN features below it Suspended spinothalamic sensory loss at level of lesion, dorsal columns preserved (see Figs. 28.18F and 28.49)

(AVM = arteriovenous malformation; HIV = human immunodeficiency virus; HZV = herpes zoster virus; LMN = lower motor neuron; MS = multiple sclerosis; UMN = upper motor neuron)

Diseases of peripheral nerves

Disorders of the peripheral nervous system are common and may affect the motor, sensory or autonomic components, either in isolation or in combination. The site of pathology may be nerve root (radiculopathy), nerve plexus (plexopathy) or nerve (neuropathy). Neuropathies may present as mononeuropathy (single nerve affected), multiple mononeuropathies ('mononeuritis multiplex') or a symmetrical polyneuropathy (Box 28.83). Cranial nerves 3–12 share the same tissue characteristics as peripheral nerves elsewhere and are subject to the same range of diseases.

Pathophysiology

Damage may occur to the nerve cell body (axon) or the myelin sheath (Schwann cell), leading to axonal or demyelinating neuropathies. The distinction is important, as only demyelinating neuropathies are usually susceptible to treatment. Making the distinction requires neurophysiology (nerve conduction studies and EMG). Neuropathies can occur in association with many systemic diseases, toxins and drugs (Box 28.84).

Clinical features

Motor nerve involvement produces features of a lower motor neuron lesion. Symptoms and signs of sensory nerve involvement depend on the type of sensory nerve involved; small-fibre neuropathies are often painful. Autonomic involvement may cause postural hypotension, disturbance of sweating, cardiac rhythm and gastrointestinal, bladder and sexual functions; isolated autonomic neuropathies are rare and more commonly complicate other neuropathies.

Investigations

The investigations required reflect the wide spectrum of causes (Box 28.85). Neurophysiological tests are key in discriminating between demyelinating and axonal neuropathies, and in identifying entrapment neuropathies. Most neuropathies are of the chronic axonal type.

Entrapment neuropathy

Focal compression or entrapment is the usual cause of a mononeuropathy. Symptoms and signs of entrapment neuropathy are listed in Box 28.86. Entrapment neuropathies may affect anyone, but diabetes,

28

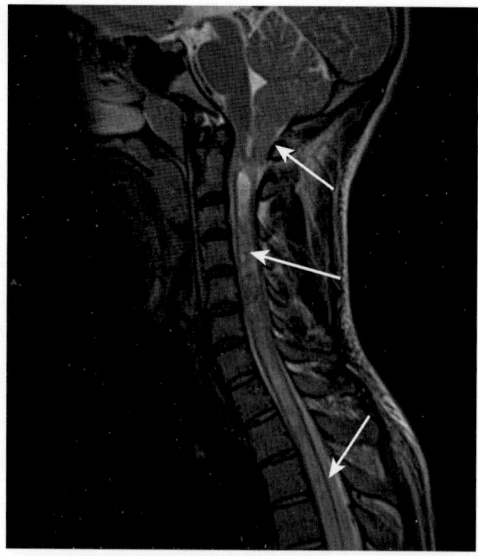

Fig. 28.49 Sagittal magnetic resonance image showing descent of cerebellar tonsils and central syrinx. The MRI shows descent of the cerebellar tonsils (top arrow), with a large central cord syrinx extending down from the cervical cord (middle arrow) to the thoracic cord (bottom arrow).

 28.83 Causes of polyneuropathy

Genetic

- Charcot–Marie–Tooth disease (CMT)
- Hereditary neuropathy with liability to pressure palsies (HNPP)
- Hereditary sensory ± autonomic neuropathies (HSN, HSAN)
- Familial amyloid polyneuropathy
- Hereditary neuralgic amyotrophy

Drugs

- Amiodarone
- Antibiotics (dapsone, isoniazid, metronidazole, ethambutol)
- Antiretrovirals
- Chemotherapy (cisplatin, vincristine, thalidomide)
- Phenytoin

Toxins

- Alcohol
- Nitrous oxide (recreational use)
- Rarely: lead, arsenic, mercury, organophosphates, solvents

Vitamin deficiencies

- Thiamin
- Pyridoxine
- Vitamin B_{12}
- Vitamin E

Infections

- Human immunodeficiency virus
- Leprosy
- Brucellosis

Inflammatory

- Guillain–Barré syndrome
- Chronic inflammatory demyelinating polyradiculoneuropathy
- Vasculitis (polyarteritis nodosa, granulomatosis with polyangiitis (also known as Wegener granulomatosis), rheumatoid arthritis, systemic lupus erythematosus)
- Paraneoplastic (antibody-mediated)

Systemic medical conditions

- Diabetes
- Renal failure
- Sarcoidosis

Malignant disease

- Infiltration

Others

- Paraproteinaemias
- Amyloidosis
- Critical illness polyneuropathy/myopathy

 28.84 Common causes of axonal and demyelinating chronic polyneuropathies

Axonal

- Diabetes mellitus
- Alcohol
- Uraemia
- Cirrhosis
- Amyloid
- Myxoedema
- Acromegaly
- Paraneoplasm
- Drugs and toxins (see Box 28.83)
- Deficiency states (see Box 28.83)
- Hereditary factors
- Infection (see Box 28.83)
- Idiopathic factors

Demyelinating

- Chronic inflammatory demyelinating polyradiculoneuropathy
- Multifocal motor neuropathy
- Paraprotein-associated demyelinating neuropathy
- Charcot–Marie–Tooth disease type I and type X

28.85 Investigation of peripheral neuropathy

Initial tests

- Glucose (fasting)
- Erythrocyte sedimentation rate, C-reactive protein
- Full blood count
- Urea and electrolytes
- Liver function tests
- Serum protein electrophoresis
- Vitamin B_{12}, folate
- ANA, ANCA, ENA
- Chest X-ray
- HIV testing

If initial tests are negative

- Nerve conduction studies
- Vitamins E and A
- Genetic testing (see Box 28.83)
- Lyme serology
- Serum angiotensin-converting enzyme
- Serum amyloid

(ANCA = antineutrophil cytoplasmic antibody; ANA = antineutrophil antibody; ENA = extractable nuclear antigen)

excess alcohol or toxins, or genetic syndromes may be predisposing causes. Unless axonal loss has occurred, entrapment neuropathies will recover, provided the primary cause is removed, either by avoiding the precipitation of activity or by surgical decompression.

Multifocal neuropathy

Multifocal neuropathy (mononeuritis multiplex) is characterised by lesions of multiple nerve roots, peripheral nerves or cranial nerves (Box 28.87). Vasculitis is a common cause, either as part of a systemic disease or isolated to the nerves, or it may arise on a background of a polyneuropathy (e.g. diabetes). Multifocal motor neuropathy (MMN) with conduction block is a rare pure motor neuropathy, typically affecting the arms; it is associated with anti-GM1 antibodies in about 50% and responds to intravenous immunoglobulin.

Polyneuropathy

A polyneuropathy is typically associated with a 'length-dependent' pattern, occurring in the longest peripheral nerves first and affecting the distal lower limbs before the upper limbs. Sensory symptoms and signs develop in an ascending 'glove and stocking' distribution. In inflammatory demyelinating neuropathies, the pathology may be more patchy, affecting the upper rather than lower limbs.

Guillain–Barré syndrome

Guillain–Barré syndrome (GBS) is a heterogeneous group of immune-mediated conditions of acute peripheral nerve inflammation, with an

28.86 Symptoms and signs in common entrapment neuropathies

Nerve	Symptoms	Muscle weakness/ muscle wasting	Area of sensory loss
Median (at wrist) (carpal tunnel syndrome)	Pain and paraesthesia on palmar aspect of hands and fingers, waking patient from sleep. Pain may extend to arm and shoulder	Abductor pollicis brevis	Lateral palm and thumb, index, middle and lateral half fourth finger
Ulnar (at elbow)	Paraesthesia on medial border of hand, wasting and weakness of hand muscles	All small hand muscles, excluding abductor pollicis brevis	Medial palm and little finger, and medial half fourth finger
Radial	Weakness of extension of wrist and fingers, often precipitated by sleeping in abnormal posture, e.g. arm over back of chair	Wrist and finger extensors, supinator	Dorsum of thumb
Common peroneal	Foot drop, trauma to head of fibula	Dorsiflexion and eversion of foot	Nil or dorsum of foot
Lateral cutaneous nerve of the thigh (meralgia paraesthetica)	Tingling and dysaesthesia on lateral border of thigh	Nil	Lateral border of thigh

28.87 Causes of multifocal mononeuropathy

Axonal (defined on nerve conduction studies)

- Vasculitis (systemic or non-systemic)
- Diabetes mellitus
- Sarcoidosis
- Infection (HIV, hepatitis C, Lyme disease, leprosy, diphtheria)

Focal demyelination with/without conduction block

- Multifocal motor neuropathy
- Multiple compression neuropathies (usually in association with underlying disease, such as diabetes or alcoholism)
- Multifocal acquired demyelinating sensory and motor neuropathy (MADSAM)
- Hereditary neuropathy with a predisposition to pressure palsy (autosomal dominant, peripheral myelin protein 22 gene)
- Lymphoma

incidence of 1–2/100 000/year. In Europe and North America, the most common variant is an acute inflammatory demyelinating polyneuropathy (AIDP). Axonal variants, either motor (acute motor axonal neuropathy, AMAN) or sensorimotor, are more common in China and Japan, and account for 10% of GBS in Western countries, often associated with *Campylobacter jejuni*. The hallmark is an acute paralysis evolving over days or weeks, with loss of tendon reflexes. About two-thirds of those with AIDP have a prior history of infection, and an autoimmune response

triggered by the preceding infection is thought to cause peripheral nerve inflammation. A number of GBS variants have been described, associated with specific anti-ganglioside antibodies; the best recognised is Miller Fisher syndrome, which involves anti-GQ1b antibodies.

Clinical features

Distal paraesthesia and pain precede muscle weakness that ascends rapidly from lower to upper limbs and is more marked proximally than distally. Facial and bulbar weakness commonly develops, and respiratory weakness requiring ventilatory support occurs in 20% of cases. Weakness progresses over a maximum of 4 weeks (usually less). Rapid deterioration to respiratory failure can develop within hours. Examination shows diffuse weakness with loss of reflexes. Miller Fisher syndrome presents with internal and external ophthalmoplegia, ataxia and areflexia.

Investigations

The CSF protein is raised, but may be normal in the first 10 days. There is usually no increase in CSF white cell count ($> 50 \times 10^6$ cells/L suggests an alternative diagnosis; though the cell count may be considerably higher in HIV infection). Electrophysiological changes may emerge after a week or so, with conduction block and multifocal motor slowing, sometimes most evident proximally as delayed F waves. Antibodies to the ganglioside GM1 are found in about 25%, usually the motor axonal form. Other causes of an acute neuromuscular paralysis should be considered (e.g. poliomyelitis, botulism, acute intermittent porphyria, diphtheria, spinal cord syndromes or myasthenia), via the history and examination. Nerve roots are an important site of inflammation and contrast uptake is sometimes seen here in contrast-enhanced MRI spinal cord imaging.

Management

Active treatment with plasma exchange or intravenous immunoglobulin therapy shortens the duration of ventilation and improves prognosis. In severe GBS, both intravenous immunoglobulin (IVIg) and plasma exchange started within 2 weeks of onset hasten recovery, with similar rates of adverse effects but IVIg treatment is significantly more likely to be completed than plasma exchange. The choice of treatment often depends on logistical considerations. Overall, 80% of patients recover completely within 3–6 months, 4% die and the remainder suffer residual neurological disability, which can be severe. Adverse prognostic features include older age, rapid deterioration to ventilation and evidence of axonal loss on EMG. Supportive measures to prevent pressure sores and deep venous thrombosis are essential. Regular monitoring of respiratory function (vital capacity) is needed in the acute phase, as respiratory failure may develop with little warning.

Chronic polyneuropathy

The most common axonal and demyelinating causes of polyneuropathy are shown in Box 28.84. A chronic symmetrical axonal polyneuropathy, evolving over months or years, is the most common form of chronic neuropathy. Diabetes mellitus is the most common cause but in about 25%–50% no cause can be found.

Hereditary neuropathy

Charcot–Marie–Tooth disease (CMT) is an umbrella term for the inherited neuropathies. The members of this group of syndromes have different clinical and genetic features. The most common CMT is the autosomal dominantly inherited CMT type 1, usually caused by a duplication in the *PMP-22* gene. Common signs are distal wasting ('inverted champagne bottle' legs), often with pes cavus, and predominantly motor involvement. X-linked and recessively inherited forms of CMT, causing demyelinating or axonal neuropathies, also occur.

28

Chronic demyelinating polyneuropathy

The acquired chronic demyelinating neuropathies include chronic inflammatory demyelinating peripheral neuropathy (CIDP), multifocal motor neuropathy (see above) and paraprotein-associated demyelinating neuropathy. CIDP typically presents with relapsing or progressive motor and sensory changes, evolving over more than 8 weeks (in distinction to the more acute GBS). It is important to recognise, as it usually responds to intravenous immunoglobulin and other immunotherapies such as glucocorticoids or plasma exchange.

Some 10% of patients with acquired demyelinating polyneuropathy have an abnormal serum paraprotein, sometimes associated with a monoclonal gammopathy of uncertain significance (MGUS) or lymphoproliferative malignancy. Those with distal sensory involvement and prominent neuropathic tremor may also demonstrate positive antibodies to myelin-associated glycoprotein (MAG antibodies).

Brachial plexopathy

Trauma usually damages either the upper or the lower parts of the brachial plexus, according to the mechanics of the injury. The clinical features depend on the anatomical site of the damage (Box 28.88). Lower parts of the brachial plexus are vulnerable to infiltration from breast or apical lung tumours (Pancoast tumour) or damage by therapeutic irradiation. The lower plexus may also be compressed by a cervical rib or fibrous band between C7 and the first rib at the thoracic outlet.

Neuralgic amyotrophy (also known as brachial neuritis) presents as an acute brachial plexopathy of probable inflammatory origin. Severe shoulder pain precedes the appearance of a patchy upper brachial plexus lesion, with motor and/or sensory involvement. There is no specific treatment and recovery is often incomplete; it may recur in about 25% and there is a rare autosomal dominant hereditary form. The appearance of vesicles should indicate the alternative diagnosis of motor zoster.

Lumbosacral plexopathy

Lumbosacral plexus lesions may be caused by neoplastic infiltration or compression by retroperitoneal haematomas. A small-vessel vasculopathy can produce a unilateral or bilateral lumbar plexopathy in association with diabetes mellitus ('diabetic amyotrophy') or an idiopathic form in non-diabetic patients. This presents with painful wasting of the quadriceps with weakness of knee extension and an absent knee reflex.

Spinal root lesions

Spinal root lesions (radiculopathy) are described above. Clinical features include muscle weakness and wasting and dermatomal sensory and reflex loss, which reflect the pattern of the roots involved. Pain in the muscles innervated by the affected roots may be prominent.

i	**28.88 Physical signs in brachial plexus lesions**	
Site	Affected muscles	Sensory loss
Upper plexus	Biceps, deltoid, spinati, rhomboids, brachioradialis (triceps, serratus anterior)	Patch over deltoid
Lower plexus	All small hand muscles, claw hand (ulnar wrist flexors)	Ulnar border of hand/forearm
Thoracic outlet syndrome	Small hand muscles, ulnar forearm	Ulnar border of hand/forearm/upper arm

Diseases of the neuromuscular junction

Myasthenia gravis

This is the most common cause of acutely evolving, fatigable weakness and preferentially affects ocular, facial and bulbar muscles.

Pathophysiology

Myasthenia gravis is an autoimmune disease, most commonly (80% of cases) caused by antibodies to acetylcholine receptors in the post-junctional membrane of the neuromuscular junction. The resultant blockage of neuromuscular transmission and complement-mediated inflammatory response reduces the number of acetylcholine receptors and damages the end plate (Fig. 28.50). Other antibodies can produce a similar clinical picture, most notably autoantibodies to muscle-specific kinase (MuSK), which is involved in the regulation and maintenance of acetylcholine receptors.

About 15% of patients (mainly those with late onset) have a thymoma, most of the remainder displaying thymic follicular hyperplasia. Myasthenic patients are more likely to have associated organ-specific autoimmune diseases. Triggers are not always evident but some drugs (e.g. penicillamine) can precipitate an antibody-mediated myasthenic syndrome that may persist after drug withdrawal. Other drugs, especially aminoglycosides and quinolones, may exacerbate the neuromuscular blockade and should be avoided in patients with myasthenia.

Clinical features

Myasthenia gravis usually presents between the ages of 15 and 50 years and there is a female preponderance in younger patients. In older patients, males are more commonly affected. It tends to run a relapsing and remitting course.

The most evident symptom is fatigable muscle weakness; movement is initially strong but rapidly weakens as muscle use continues. Worsening of symptoms towards the end of the day or following exercise is characteristic. There are no sensory signs or signs of involvement of the CNS, although weakness of the oculomotor muscles may mimic a central eye movement disorder. The first symptoms are usually intermittent ptosis or diplopia but weakness of chewing, swallowing, speaking or limb movement also occurs. Resting of the eyelids (looking downwards) may be followed by increased reflex elevation with up-gaze (so-called Cogan's lid twitch sign). Any limb muscle may be affected, most commonly those of the shoulder girdle; the patient is unable to undertake tasks above shoulder level, such as combing the hair, without frequent rests. Respiratory muscles may be involved and respiratory failure is an avoidable cause of death. Aspiration may occur if the cough is ineffectual. Ventilatory support is required where weakness is severe or of abrupt onset. Subtypes of myasthenia gravis include ocular myasthenia, where disease is often confined to eye muscles, and generalised myasthenia, where more widespread muscle involvement is seen which can include bulbar and respiratory muscles. There is often overlap between these subtypes. Congenital (genetic) forms of myasthenia also exist and do not have an autoimmune basis.

Investigations

Serological investigations play an important role in the diagnosis of myasthenia gravis. Acetylcholine receptor antibodies are highly specific, but seronegative cases also exist and further serological testing, e.g. for MuSK antibodies, should be performed if AChR antibodies are negative. Anti-MuSK antibodies are associated with prominent bulbar involvement.

Neurophysiological assessment is important in establishing the diagnosis. Repetitive stimulation during nerve conduction studies may show a characteristic decremental response if the muscle has been clinically affected. Specialised single fibre EMG changes such as 'jitter' may also be seen. All patients should have a thoracic CT or MRI to exclude

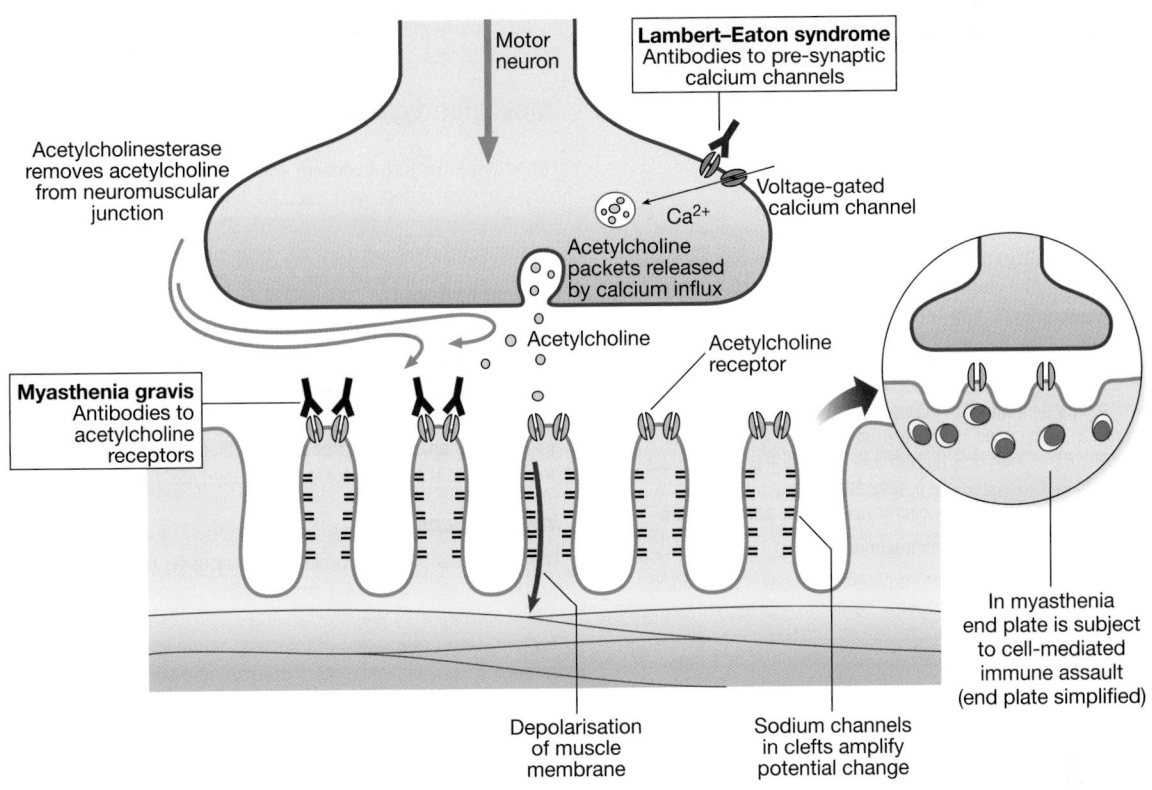

Fig. 28.50 Myasthenia gravis and Lambert–Eaton myasthenic syndrome (LEMS). In myasthenia there are antibodies to the acetylcholine receptors on the post-synaptic membrane, which block conduction across the neuromuscular junction (NMJ). Myasthenic symptoms can be transiently improved by inhibition of acetylcholinesterase (e.g. with Tensilon – edrophonium bromide), which normally removes the acetylcholine. A cell-mediated immune response produces simplification of the post-synaptic membrane, further impairing the 'safety factor' of neuromuscular conduction. In LEMS, antibodies to the pre-synaptic voltage calcium channels impair release of acetylcholine from the motor nerve ending; calcium is required for the acetylcholine-containing vesicle to fuse with the pre-synaptic membrane for release into the NMJ.

thymoma, especially those without anti-acetylcholine receptor antibodies. Screening for associated autoimmune disorders, particularly thyroid disease, is important.

Intravenous injection of the short-acting anticholinesterase edrophonium bromide (the Tensilon test) is less widely used than before and requires specialist involvement in cases where there is diagnostic doubt. Structural imaging (e.g. MRI of brainstem) may be needed to exclude alternative diagnoses that can cause ocular-bulbar weakness.

Management

The goals of treatment are to maximise the activity of acetylcholine at remaining receptors in the neuromuscular junctions and to limit or abolish the immunological attack on motor end plates.

The duration of action of acetylcholine is prolonged by inhibiting acetylcholinesterase. The most commonly used anticholinesterase drug is pyridostigmine. Muscarinic side-effects, including diarrhoea and colic, may be controlled by propantheline.

Myasthenia gravis can cause life-threatening disease, often referred to as 'myasthenic crisis', when bulbar and respiratory failure occurs. Prompt acute immunotherapy, often using intravenous immunoglobulin or plasma exchange is required, together with a longer-term immunosuppressive approach. Supportive respiratory care, and early involvement of intensive care teams, is important during these periods.

Immunological treatment of myasthenia is outlined in Box 28.89. Thymoma should be managed with joint oncology and thoracic surgery input. Prognosis is variable and remissions may occur spontaneously. When myasthenia is entirely ocular, prognosis is excellent and disability slight. Younger seropositive patients with generalised disease may benefit from thymectomy in the absence of thymoma, while older patients are less likely to have a remission despite treatment. Rapid progression of the disease more than 5 years after onset is uncommon.

Some medications, such as aminoglycoside antibiotics, can worsen myasthenia gravis.

Lambert–Eaton myasthenic syndrome

Other rarer conditions can present with muscle weakness due to impaired transmission across the neuromuscular junction. The most common of these is the Lambert–Eaton myasthenic syndrome (LEMS), which can occur as an inflammatory or paraneoplastic phenomenon. Antibodies to pre-synaptic voltage-gated calcium channels (see Fig. 28.50) impair transmitter release. Patients may have autonomic dysfunction (e.g. dry mouth) in addition to muscle weakness but the cardinal clinical sign is absence of tendon reflexes, which return after sustained contraction of the relevant muscle. The condition is associated with underlying malignancy in a high percentage of cases and investigation must be directed towards identifying any neoplasm. Diagnosis is made electrophysiologically on the presence of post-tetanic potentiation of motor response to nerve stimulation at a frequency of 20–50/sec. Treatment is with 3,4-diaminopyridine, or pyridostigmine and immunosuppression.

Diseases of muscle

Muscle disease, either hereditary or acquired, is rare. Most typically, it presents with a proximal symmetrical weakness. Diagnosis is dependent on recognition of clinical clues, such as cardiorespiratory involvement, evolution, family history, exposure to drugs, the presence of contractures, myotonia and other systemic features, and on investigation findings, most importantly EMG and muscle biopsy. Hereditary syndromes include the muscular dystrophies, muscle channelopathies,

28

28.89 Immunological treatment of myasthenia

Acute treatments

Intravenous immunoglobulin

- Lowers production of antibodies and rapidly reduces weakness

Plasma exchange

- Removing antibody from the blood may produce marked improvement; this is usually brief, so is normally reserved for myasthenic crisis or for pre-operative preparation

Long-term treatments

Glucocorticoid treatment

- Improvement can be preceded by marked exacerbation of myasthenic symptoms, so treatment should be initiated cautiously in an environment where deterioration can be managed. In an outpatient setting many neurologists start corticosteroids at a low dose and increase gradually. If urgent high-dose steroids are needed this may require hospital admission
- Usually necessary to continue for months or years, risking adverse effects

Pharmacological immunosuppression treatment

- Azathioprine 2.5 mg/kg daily reduces the necessary dosage of glucocorticoids and may allow withdrawal. Effect on clinical features may be delayed for months
- Mycophenolate mofetil and rituximab are both used, although high-quality evidence is currently lacking

Thymectomy

- Likely to be required for thymoma
- Should be considered in any antibody-positive patient under 45 years with symptoms not confined to extraocular muscles, unless the disease has been established for more than 7 years

metabolic myopathies (including mitochondrial diseases) and congenital myopathies.

Muscular dystrophies

These are inherited disorders with progressive muscle destruction and may be associated with cardiac and/or respiratory involvement and sometimes non-myopathic features (Box 28.90). Myotonic dystrophy is the most common, with a prevalence of about 12/100 000.

Clinical features

The pattern of the clinical features is defined by the specific syndromes. Onset is often in childhood, although some patients, especially those with myotonic dystrophy, may present as adults. Wasting and weakness are usually symmetrical, without fasciculation or sensory loss, and tendon reflexes are usually preserved until a late stage. Weakness is usually proximal, except in myotonic dystrophy type 1, when it is distal.

Investigations

The diagnosis can be confirmed by specific molecular genetic testing, supplemented with EMG and muscle biopsy if necessary. Creatine kinase is markedly elevated in the dystrophinopathies (Duchenne and Becker) but is normal or moderately elevated in the other dystrophies. Screening for an associated cardiac abnormality (cardiomyopathy or dysrhythmia) is important.

Management

There is no specific therapy for most of these conditions but physiotherapy and occupational therapy help patients cope with their

28.90 The muscular dystrophies

Type	Genetics	Age of onset	Muscles affected	Other features
Myotonic dystrophy (DM1)	Autosomal dominant; expanded triplet repeat *DMPK* gene	Any	Face (including ptosis), sternomastoids, distal limb, generalised later	Myotonia, cognitive impairment, cardiac conduction abnormalities, lens opacities, frontal balding, hypogonadism
Proximal myotonic myopathy (PROMM; DM2)	Autosomal dominant; quadruplet repeat expansion in *CNBP* gene	8–50 years	Proximal, especially thigh, sometimes muscle hypertrophy	As for DM1 but cognition not affected Muscle pain
Duchenne	X-linked; deletions in *dystrophin* gene Xp21	<5 years	Proximal and limb girdle	Cardiomyopathy and respiratory failure
Becker	X-linked; deletions in *dystrophin* gene Xp21	Childhood/early adulthood	Proximal and limb girdle	Cardiomyopathy common but respiratory failure uncommon
Limb girdle	Many mutations on different chromosomes	Childhood/early adulthood	Limb girdle	Very variable depending on genetic subtype, some involve cardiac and respiratory systems
Facioscapulohumeral (FSH)	Autosomal dominant; tandem repeat deletion chromosome 4q35	7–30 years	Face and upper limb girdle, distal lower limb weakness	Pain in shoulder girdle common, deafness Cardiorespiratory involvement rare
Oculopharyngeal	Autosomal dominant and recessive; triplet repeat expansion in *PABP2* gene chromosome 14q	30–60 years	Ptosis, external ophthalmoplegia, dysphagia, tongue weakness	Mild lower limb weakness
Emery–Dreifuss	X-linked recessive; mutations in *emerin* gene	4–5 years	Humero-peroneal, proximal limb girdle later	Contractures develop early Cardiac involvement leads to sudden death

disability. Glucocorticoids can be used in Duchenne muscular dystrophy but side-effects should be anticipated and avoided by dose modification. Treatment of associated cardiac failure or arrhythmia (with pacemaker insertion if necessary) may be required; similarly, management of respiratory complications (including nocturnal hypoventilation) can improve quality of life. Improvements in non-invasive ventilation have led to significant improvements in survival for patients with Duchenne muscular dystrophy. Genetic counselling is important.

Inherited metabolic myopathies

There are a large number of rare inherited disorders that interfere with the biochemical pathways that maintain the energy supply (adenosine triphosphate, ATP) to muscles. These are mostly recessively inherited deficiencies in the enzymes necessary for glycogen or fatty acid (β-oxidation) metabolism (Box 28.91). They typically present with muscle weakness and pain.

Mitochondrial disorders

Mitochondrial diseases are discussed on page 47. Mitochondria are present in all tissues and dysfunction causes widespread effects on vision (optic atrophy, retinitis pigmentosa, cataracts), hearing (sensorineural deafness) and the endocrine, cardiovascular, gastrointestinal and renal systems. Any combination of these should raise the suspicion of a mitochondrial disorder, especially if there is evidence of maternal transmission.

Mitochondrial dysfunction can be caused by alterations in either mitochondrial DNA or genes encoding for oxidative processes. Genetic abnormalities or mutations in mitochondrial DNA may affect single individuals and single tissues (most commonly muscle). Thus, patients with exercise intolerance, myalgia and sometimes recurrent myoglobinuria may have isolated pathogenic mutations in genes encoding for oxidation pathways.

Inherited disorders of the oxidative pathways of the respiratory chain in mitochondria cause a group of disorders, either restricted to the muscle or associated with non-myopathic features (Box 28.92). Many of these mitochondrial disorders are inherited via the mitochondrial genome, down the maternal line. Diagnosis is based on clinical appearances, supported by muscle biopsy appearance (usually with 'ragged red' and/or cytochrome oxidase-negative fibres), and specific mutations either on blood or, more reliably, muscle testing. Mutations may be due either to point mutations or to deletions of mitochondrial DNA.

A disorder called Leber hereditary optic neuropathy (LHON) is characterised by acute or subacute loss of vision, most frequently in males, due to bilateral optic atrophy. Three point mutations account for more than 90% of LHON cases.

Channelopathies

Inherited abnormalities of the sodium, calcium and chloride ion channels in striated muscle produce various syndromes of familial periodic paralysis, myotonia and malignant hyperthermia, which may be recognised by their clinical characteristics and potassium abnormalities (Box 28.93). Genetic testing is available.

Acquired myopathies

These include the inflammatory myopathies, or myopathy associated with a range of metabolic and endocrine disorders or drug and toxin exposure (Fig. 28.51).

i	28.91 Inherited disorders of muscle metabolism		
Disease	**Clinical features**	**Diagnosis**	
Carbohydrate (glycogen) metabolism			
Myophosphorylase deficiency (McArdle disease): autosomal recessive	Exercise-induced myalgia, stiffness, weakness (with 'second wind' phenomenon), myoglobinuria	Creatine kinase (CK) elevated Muscle biopsy Enzyme assay	
Acid maltase deficiency (Pompe disease): autosomal recessive	Infantile form: death within 2 years Childhood: death in twenties or thirties Adult: progressive proximal myopathy with respiratory failure	CK elevated Blood lymphocyte analysis for glycogen granules Muscle biopsy Enzyme assay	
Lipid metabolism (β-oxidation)			
Carnitine-palmitoyl transferase (CPT) deficiency	Myalgia *after* exercise, myoglobinuria, weakness	CK normal between attacks Urinary organic acids Enzyme assays Muscle biopsy	

i	28.92 Mitochondrial syndromes	
Syndrome	**Clinical features**	
Myoclonic epilepsy with ragged red fibres (MERRF)	Myoclonic epilepsy, cerebellar ataxia, dementia, sensorineural deafness ± peripheral neuropathy, optic atrophy and multiple lipomas	
Mitochondrial myopathy, encephalopathy, lactic acidosis and stroke-like episodes (MELAS)	Episodic encephalopathy, stroke-like episodes often preceded by migraine-like headache, nausea and vomiting	
Chronic progressive external ophthalmoplegia (CPEO)	Progressive ptosis and external oculomotor palsy, proximal myopathy ± deafness, ataxia and cardiac conduction defects	
Kearns–Sayre syndrome	Like CPEO but early age of onset (< 20 years), heart block, pigmentary retinopathy	
Mitochondrial neurogastrointestinal encephalomyopathy (MNGIE)	Progressive ptosis, external oculomotor palsy, gastrointestinal dysmotility (often pseudo-obstruction), diffuse leucoencephalopathy, thin body habitus, peripheral neuropathy and myopathy	
Neuropathy, ataxia and retinitis pigmentosa (NARP)	Weakness, ataxia and progressive loss of vision, along with dementia, seizures and proximal weakness	

28

i   28.93 Muscle channelopathies

Channel	Muscle disease	Gene and inheritance	Clinical features
Sodium	Paramyotonia congenita	*SCN4A* (17q35) Autosomal dominant	Cold-evoked myotonia with episodic weakness provoked by exercise and cold
	Potassium-aggravated myotonia	*SCN4A*	Pure myotonia without weakness provoked by potassium
	Hyperkalaemic periodic paralysis	*SCN4A*	Brief (mins to hours), frequent episodes of weakness provoked by rest, cold, potassium, fasting, pregnancy, stress
		Autosomal dominant	Less common than hypokalaemic periodic paralysis
	Hypokalaemic periodic paralysis	*SCN4A* Autosomal dominant (one-third new mutations)	Longer (hours to days) episodic weakness triggered by rest, carbohydrate loading, cold

Chloride	Myotonia congenita:
	    Thomsen disease
	    Becker disease
		CLCN1
		Autosomal dominant
		CLCN1
		Autosomal recessive
			Myotonia usually mild, little weakness
			Myotonia often severe, transient weakness

Calcium	Hypokalaemic periodic paralysis Malignant hyperthermia	*CACNA1S* Autosomal dominant *CACNA1S, CACNL2A* Autosomal dominant	Episodic weakness triggered by carbohydrate meal Hyperpyrexia due to excess muscle activity, precipitated by drugs, usually anaesthetic agents; most common cause of death during general anaesthetic
Potassium	Hypokalaemic periodic paralysis with cardiac arrhythmia	*KCNJ2* Autosomal dominant	Similar to hypokalaemic periodic paralysis, associated with cardiac and non-myopathic features (skeletal and facial)
Ryanodine receptor	Malignant hyperthermia Central core and multicore disease	*RYR1* (19q13)*RYR1* Mostly autosomal dominant	As malignant hyperthermia above Present in infancy with mild progressive weakness

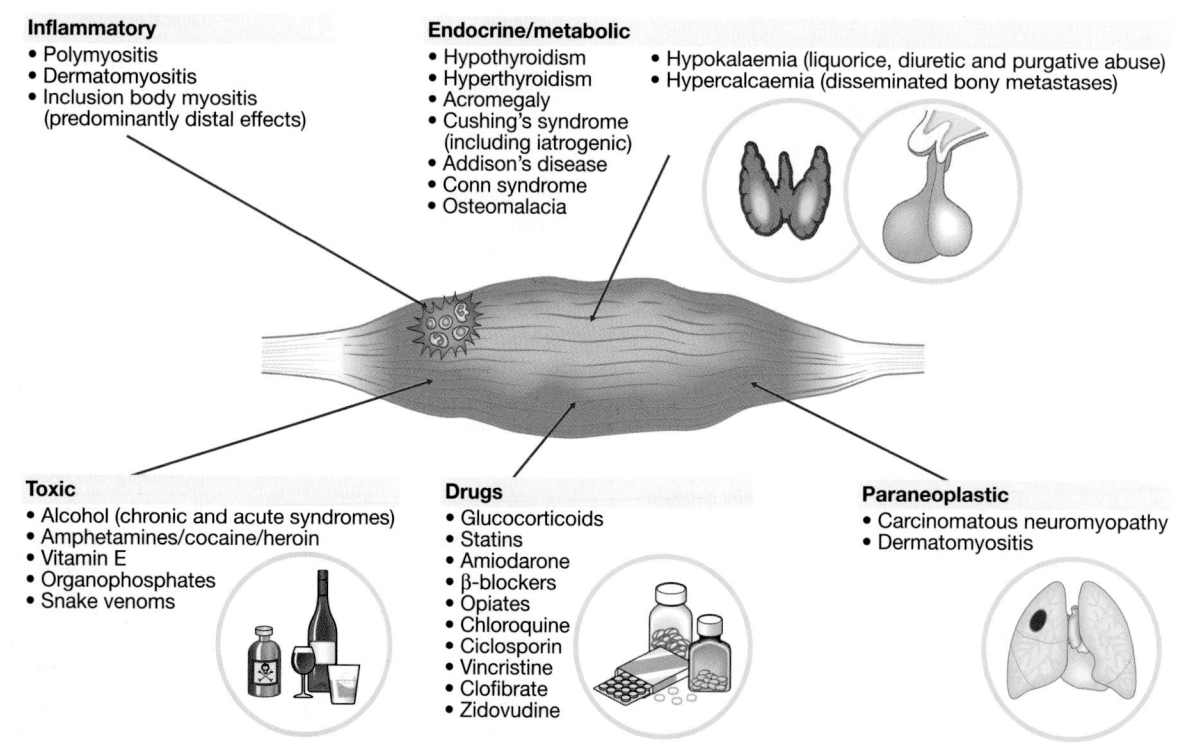

Inflammatory
- Polymyositis
- Dermatomyositis
- Inclusion body myositis (predominantly distal effects)

Endocrine/metabolic
- Hypothyroidism
- Hyperthyroidism
- Acromegaly
- Cushing's syndrome (including iatrogenic)
- Addison's disease
- Conn syndrome
- Osteomalacia

- Hypokalaemia (liquorice, diuretic and purgative abuse)
- Hypercalcaemia (disseminated bony metastases)

Toxic
- Alcohol (chronic and acute syndromes)
- Amphetamines/cocaine/heroin
- Vitamin E
- Organophosphates
- Snake venoms

Drugs
- Glucocorticoids
- Statins
- Amiodarone
- β-blockers
- Opiates
- Chloroquine
- Ciclosporin
- Vincristine
- Clofibrate
- Zidovudine

Paraneoplastic
- Carcinomatous neuromyopathy
- Dermatomyositis

Fig. 28.51 Causes of acquired proximal myopathy.

Further information

Journal articles

Evidence-Based Guideline: Treatment of Convulsive Status Epilepticus in Children and Adults: Report of the Guideline Committee of the American Epilepsy Society. Epilepsy Curr 2016; 16(1):48–61.

Operational classification of seizure types by the International League Against Epilepsy. Epilepsia 2017; 58(4):522–530.

Scolding N, Barnes D, Cader S, et al. Association of British Neurologists: revised (2015) guidelines for prescribing disease-modifying treatments in multiple sclerosis. Pract Neurol 2015;15(4):1–7.

Sussman J, Farrugia ME, Maddison P, et al. Myasthenia gravis: Association of British Neurologists' management guidelines. Pract Neurol 2015;15:199–206.

UK joint specialist societies guideline on the diagnosis and management of acute meningitis and meningococcal sepsis in immunocompetent adults. J Infect 2016; 72:405–438.

Websites

myana.org *American Neurological Association*.

brainandspine.org.uk *Brain and Spine Foundation*

dizziness-and-balance.com/disorders *Diagnosing benign paroxysmal positional vertigo.*

epilepsydiagnosis.org *International League Against Epilepsy: free access to videos of different seizure types and clinical summaries of the epilepsies.*

headinjurysymptoms.org *Symptoms and management of mild and moderate head injury.*

ihs-classification.org/en/ *International Headache Society: full access to 3rd edition of International Classification of Headache Disorders.*

neurosymptoms.org *Advice on managing functional neurological symptoms.*

ninds.nih.gov *National Institute of Neurological Disorders and Stroke.*

sign.ac.uk *Scottish Intercollegiate Guidelines Network: SIGN 107 Diagnosis and management of headache in adults; SIGN 110 Early management of patients with a head injury; SIGN 113 Diagnosis and pharmacological management of Parkinson's disease; SIGN 143 Diagnosis and management of epilepsy in adults; SIGN 155 Pharmacological management of migraine.*

wfneurology.org *World Federation of Neurology.*

28

W Whiteley
R Woodfield

Stroke medicine

Clinical examination in stroke

4 **Higher cerebral function**
Dysphasia or dysarthria
Attention and neglect
Abbreviated mental test

3 **Blood pressure, carotid bruits and cardiac auscultation**

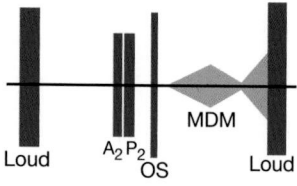

Loud   A₂ P₂ MDM   Loud
A_2 P_2
OS

2 **Pulse**
Rate and rhythm

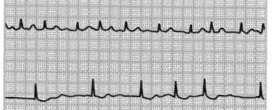

▲ Atrial fibrillation

1 **General appearance**
Conscious level
Gaze deviation
Facial symmetry

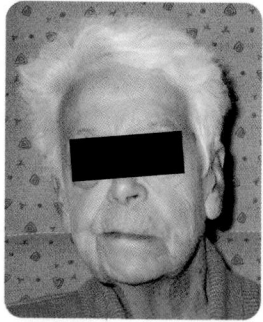

▲ Left upper motor neuron pattern of facial weakness

5 **Cranial nerve function**
Swallow
Horner syndrome
Internuclear opthalmoplegia
Cranial nerve palsy, e.g. 3rd, 6th, 7th or 12th
Visual field loss

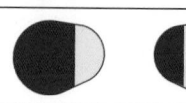

▲ Visual field defect – left homonymous hemianopia

6 **Motor system**
Tone
Strength, including pronator drift
Co-ordination
Tendon reflexes
Plantar reflexes

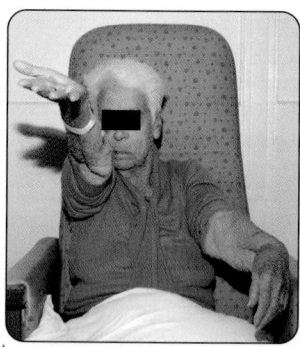

▲ Left pronator drift

7 **Sensory system**
Touch sensation
Cortical sensory function: sensory inattention or neglect
Joint position sense

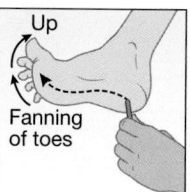

Up
Fanning of toes

▲ Extensor plantar reflex

8 **Gait**
Sitting balance
Standing balance
Ataxic gait pattern
Hemiparetic gait pattern

ℹ️ General examination

Skin

- Xanthelasma
- Rash (e.g. vasculitic, splinter haemorrhages)
- Colour change (limb ischaemia, deep vein thrombosis)
- Pressure sores or early pressure injury

Eyes

- Diabetic retinopathy
- Hypertensive retinopathy
- Cholesterol emboli
- Papilloedema (unexpected in stroke)
- Subhyaloid haemorrhages (after subarachnoid haemorrhage)

Cardiovascular system

- Atrial fibrillation
- Blood pressure (high or low)
- Carotid bruit
- Cardiac murmurs (source of embolism, e.g. endocarditis)
- Peripheral pulses and bruits (generalised arteriopathy)

Respiratory system

- Signs of pulmonary oedema or infection
- Oxygen saturation

Abdomen

- Palpable bladder (urinary retention)
- Organomegaly

Locomotor system

- Injuries sustained during collapse
  (e.g. hip fracture)
- Comorbidities that influence recovery
  (e.g. osteoarthritis)

ℹ️ Rapid clinical assessment of suspected stroke

Exclusion of hypoglycaemia

- Bedside blood glucose testing

Measure blood pressure

- Significant hypertension may require treatment (e.g. in acute intracerebral haemorrhage, or if thrombolysis is being considered)

National Institutes of Health Stroke Scale (NIHSS)

A formalised neurological examination and a measure of stroke severity which can be useful for organising acute stroke assessment, monitoring and communicating stroke severity.

1A Level of consciousness

Alert; keenly responsive	0
Arouses to minor stimulation	+1
Arouses to pain	+2
Abnormal postures or unresponsive	+3

1B Ask month and age

Both questions right	0
One question right or dysarthric or intubated	+1
No questions right or aphasic	+2

1C Ask to 'close eyes' and 'squeeze hands'

Performs both tasks	0
Performs one task	+1
Performs no tasks	+2

2 Horizontal extraocular movements

Normal	0
Partial gaze palsy: can be overcome or corrects	+1
Complete gaze palsy: cannot be overcome	+2

3 Visual fields

No visual loss	0
Partial hemianopia	+1
Complete hemianopia	+2
Bilateral blindness or hemianopia	+3

4 Facial palsy

Normal symmetry	0
Minor paralysis (flat nasolabial fold)	+1
Partial paralysis (lower face only)	+2
Unilateral or bilateral complete paralysis	+3

5A Left arm motor drift (ask patient to hold out arm for 10 seconds while you count aloud)

No drift for 10 seconds	0
Drift, but doesn't hit bed	+1
Drift and hits bed, or some effort against gravity	+2
No effort against gravity	+3
No movement	+4

5B Right arm motor drift (perform and score following instructions for left arm)

6A Left leg motor drift (ask patient to raise leg for 5 seconds while you count aloud)

No drift for 5 seconds	0
Drift, but doesn't hit bed	+1
Drift and hits bed, or some effort against gravity	+2
No effort against gravity	+3
No movement	+4

6B Right leg motor drift (perform and score following instructions for left leg)

7 Limb ataxia (finger–nose–finger and heel–shin testing, all four limbs)

No ataxia or doesn't understand or paralysed	0
Ataxia in one limb	+1
Ataxia in two limbs	+2

8 Sensation

Normal, no sensory loss	0
Mild–moderate sensory loss	+1
Complete sensory loss or unresponsive	+2

9 Language (check comprehension 'lift your arms', 'close your eyes'. Ask the patient to name people or objects, e.g 'nurse', 'pen', 'watch', to check for nominal dysphasia)

Normal, no dysphasia	0
Mild–moderate dysphasia but no major limitation	+1
Severe dysphasia, e.g meaning of speech is unclear	+2
Global aphasia or mute or coma	+3

10 Dysarthria (check articulation, e.g repeat 'tip-top', or 'fifty-fifty')

Normal or intubated and unable to test	0
Mild–moderate, e.g slurring but understandable	+1
Severe, unintelligible or mute	+2

11 Inattention (test sensation and visual fields on both sides simultaneously. The affected side will not be felt or seen)

Inattention to one modality (sense or vision)	+1
Inattention to both modalities or severe neglect (e.g doesn't recognise own hand)	+2

Score (0 to 42): 0 to 5 mild, 5 to 15 moderate, more than 16 severe

Tips: Score what you see, score the first response (not the best response) and don't coach the patient. Check if the patient can sit up or stand without support.
The NIHSS does not measure well the severity of posterior circulation and non-dominant hemisphere stroke syndromes.

29

A stroke is a sudden onset focal cerebral dysfunction due to vascular disease of the brain (Fig. 29.1). Stroke is the third most common cause of disability in the world after ischaemic heart disease and congenital disorders. In Europe, most strokes (about 80%) are caused by cerebral ischaemia and fewer are due to haemorrhage, although there are probably a similar number of deaths due to ischaemic and haemorrhagic stroke worldwide. Subarachnoid haemorrhage (SAH) and cerebral venous thrombosis (CVT) are discussed later in this chapter. Vascular dementia is described on page 1246.

Functional anatomy and physiology

The paired internal carotid and vertebral arteries supply blood to the brain. Each internal carotid artery bifurcates into the anterior and middle cerebral arteries which supply the anterior cerebrum ('anterior circulation'). The vertebral arteries join to form the basilar artery (supplying the brainstem, cerebellum and pons) which bifurcates into the posterior cerebral arteries which supply the posterior cerebrum ('posterior circulation') (Fig. 29.2). The function of each brain area is described on page 1122. Communicating arteries connect the anterior with the posterior and the left with the right circulations. These anastomoses form the circle of Willis that – if complete – maintains cerebral circulation even if one carotid or vertebral artery is blocked. In health, autoregulation maintains a constant cerebral blood flow across a wide range of arterial blood pressures to meet the high cerebral metabolic activity. This autoregulatory mechanism can be disrupted after stroke. The venous system is formed by a collection of sinuses over the surface of the brain which drain into the jugular veins (Fig. 29.3).

Investigations

Brain imaging

Brain imaging helps to determine the cause of stroke symptoms. Non-contrast (unenhanced) computed tomography (CT) scanning is rapid, sensitive for intracranial haemorrhage and can show cerebral ischaemia or other diagnoses, but does use ionising radiation. In patients with a clinical diagnosis of an acute stroke, a CT scan that shows no intracerebral haemorrhage makes an ischaemic stroke the likelier diagnosis.

Magnetic resonance imaging (MRI) is more sensitive than CT for changes of cerebral ischaemia and provides very detailed images of brain anatomy, although it takes longer than CT to perform (Fig. 29.4). MRI uses powerful magnets that can interfere with medical devices (such as pacemakers) or metal implants, and can be claustrophobic for patients. Diffusion-weighted MRI adds sensitivity for cerebral ischaemia compared with other MRI sequences.

Vascular imaging

Imaging of the carotid artery and of intra- and extracranial vessels can influence practice by demonstrating carotid stenosis which guides decisions about carotid endarterectomy, and by showing major vessel occlusion in acute stroke which guides decisions about thrombectomy.

The first-line imaging techniques for vessels supplying the brain can be ultrasound, CT angiography or MR angiography, depending on availability and expertise. Intra-arterial angiography is used less frequently as a primary investigation, although it is often done during neuro-interventional procedures to confirm findings from non-invasive techniques or guide treatment (Fig. 29.5). Vascular imaging can show also major vessel dissection, changes of cerebral vasculitis, intracranial aneurysms or arteriovenous malformations. Transcranial Doppler sonography is used in some centres to identify intracranial stenosis or occlusion.

Blood tests

The choice of blood tests should be guided by the clinical situation. A full blood count, electrolytes and renal function are usually indicated. Blood glucose (usually fasting) can diagnose unrecognised diabetes (or poor diabetes control), lipids (cholesterol fractions and triglycerides) may guide lipid-lowering therapy, and C-reactive protein or erythrocyte sedimentation rate may identify an inflammatory response (for example in giant cell arteritis or endocarditis).

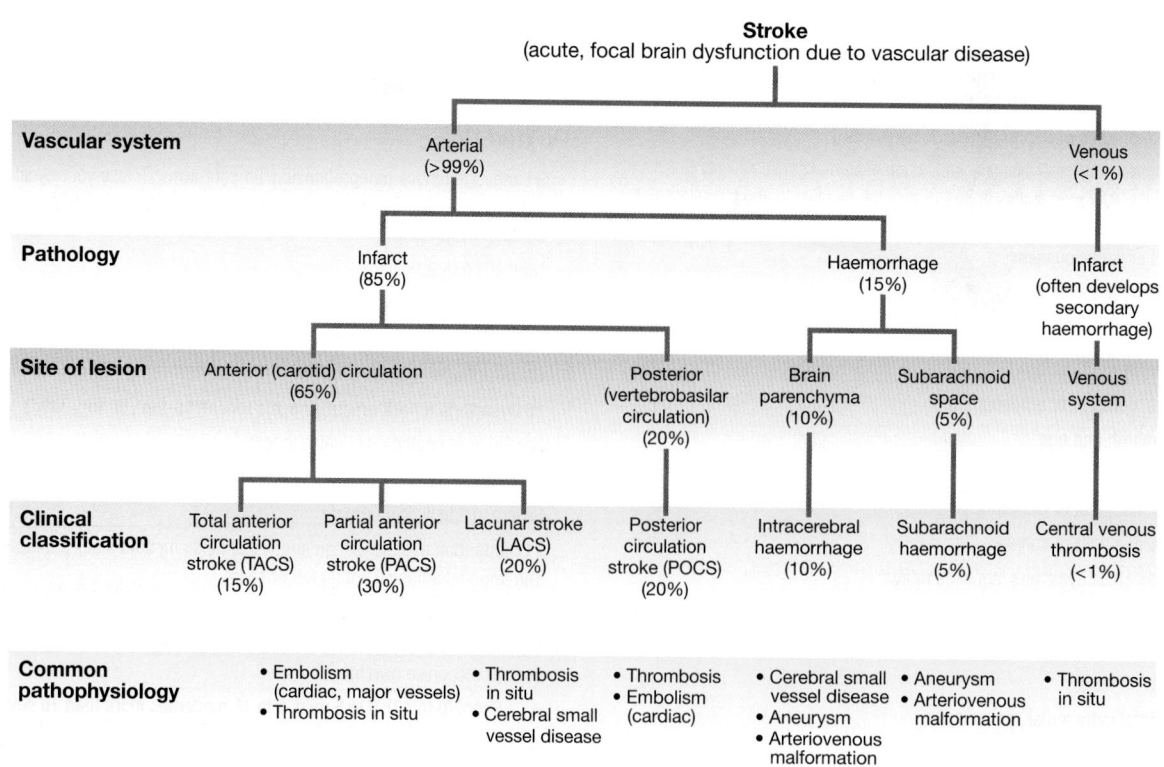

Fig. 29.1 A classification of stroke.

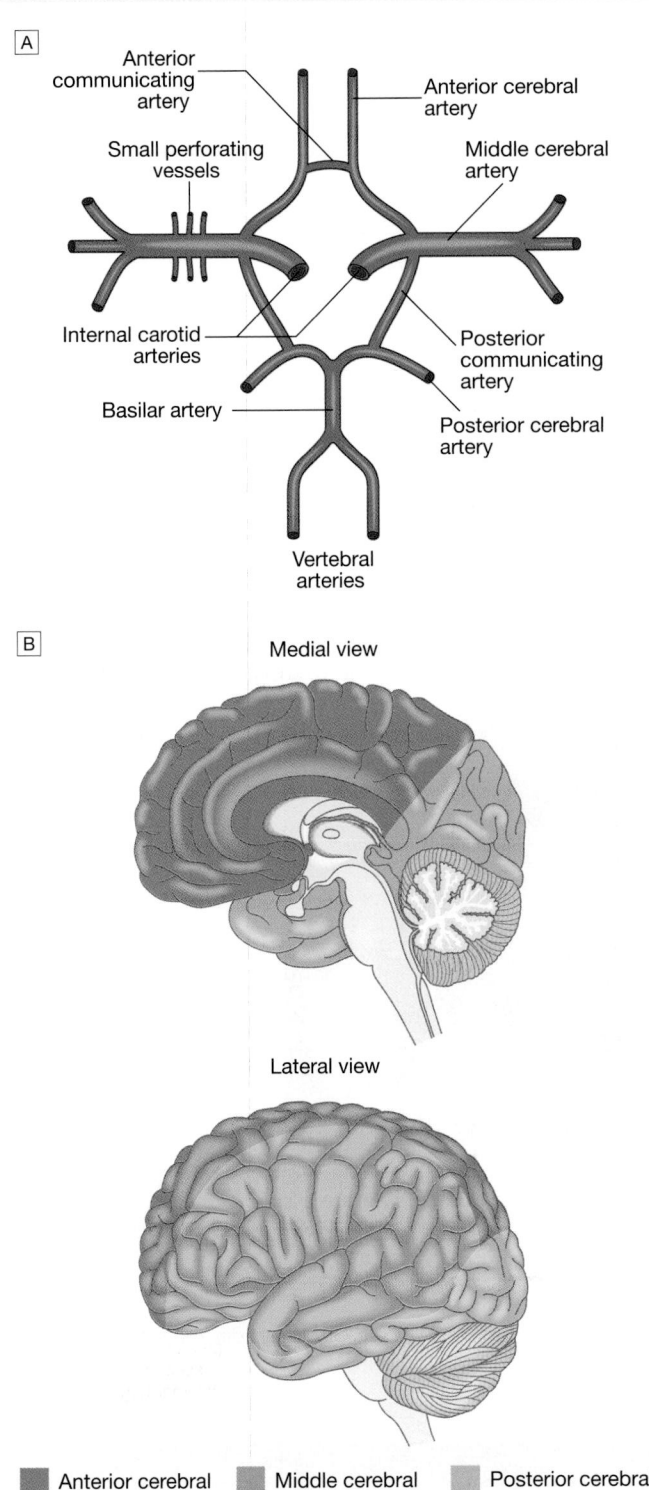

Fig. 29.2 **Arterial circulation of the brain.** [A] Circle of Willis. [B] Anterior, middle and posterior cerebral artery territories. *(B) Adapted from Amin HP, Schindler J. Vascular neuroanatomy. In: Amin H, Schindler J (eds), Vascular Neurology Board Review. Cham: Springer; 2017. https://doi.org/10.1007/978-3-319-39605-7_3.*

Monogenic disorders are a rare cause of stroke, and genetic testing is usually guided by particular clinical or radiological syndromes (e.g. cerebral autosomal dominant arteriopathy with subcortical infarcts and leukoencephalopathy, CADASIL), but needs careful discussion with patients and families so the implications of a genetic diagnosis are understood.

Lumbar puncture

Cerebrospinal fluid can show evidence of subarachnoid haemorrhage, but is not used for most stroke patients.

Cardiac investigations

A 12-lead ECG may show atrial fibrillation (AF), an important stroke risk factor, evidence of prolonged hypertension (left ventricular hypertrophy), or previous myocardial infarction. Prolonged ECG monitoring may reveal short periods of AF ('paroxysmal' AF), which leads to anticoagulation for prevention of future ischaemic stroke. Management can change when an echocardiogram shows a right-to-left shunt (e.g. a patent foramen ovale), endocarditis or a cardiac tumour.

Presenting problems

Most strokes develop suddenly within a matter of minutes or hours, and are one of the differential diagnoses of patients with almost any acute focal neurological presentation.

Weakness

In severe stroke, involvement of large areas of the cortex or smaller areas of the deep white matter in the cerebrum or brainstem leads to a hemiparesis (see Fig. 28.17). Other patterns of weakness include: face only (usually an upper motor neuron pattern affecting the lower face only); face and arm; leg only (anterior cerebral artery involvement); hand only (often a clumsiness); or a quadraparesis (with brainstem stroke).

Speech disturbance

Stroke can lead to a number of speech abnormalities. Cortical strokes (usually dominant frontal or parietal lobe) can cause dysphasia, with difficulties understanding speech (a receptive dysphasia) or difficulties producing grammatically correct speech (an expressive dysphasia). Stroke in the cortex, deep white matter, cerebellum or brainstem can lead to slurred speech (dysarthria). More rarely, isolated difficulties with reading (alexia) or writing (agraphia) occur, but they are more usually associated with other symptoms (see Box 28.2).

Visual deficit

Occlusion of the ophthalmic artery by thrombus leads to sudden blindness in one eye. If the blindness is transient, this is called 'transient monocular blindness' or 'amaurosis fugax'. These symptoms should lead to a similar search for risk factors and cause as stroke symptoms.

Stroke affecting the occipital lobe or optic tracts or radiation leads to a contralateral hemianopia or, in smaller lesions, a partial field defect (see p. 1145).

Visuo-spatial dysfunction

Damage to the non-dominant cortex often results in contralateral visuo-spatial dysfunction, e.g. sensory or visual neglect and apraxia (inability to perform complex tasks despite normal motor, sensory and cerebellar function). Confusion or dysphasia after stroke are sometimes misdiagnosed as delirium.

Ataxia

Stroke causing damage to the cerebellum and its connections can present with an acute ataxia and there may be associated brainstem features such as diplopia and vertigo. The differential diagnosis includes vestibular disorders.

29

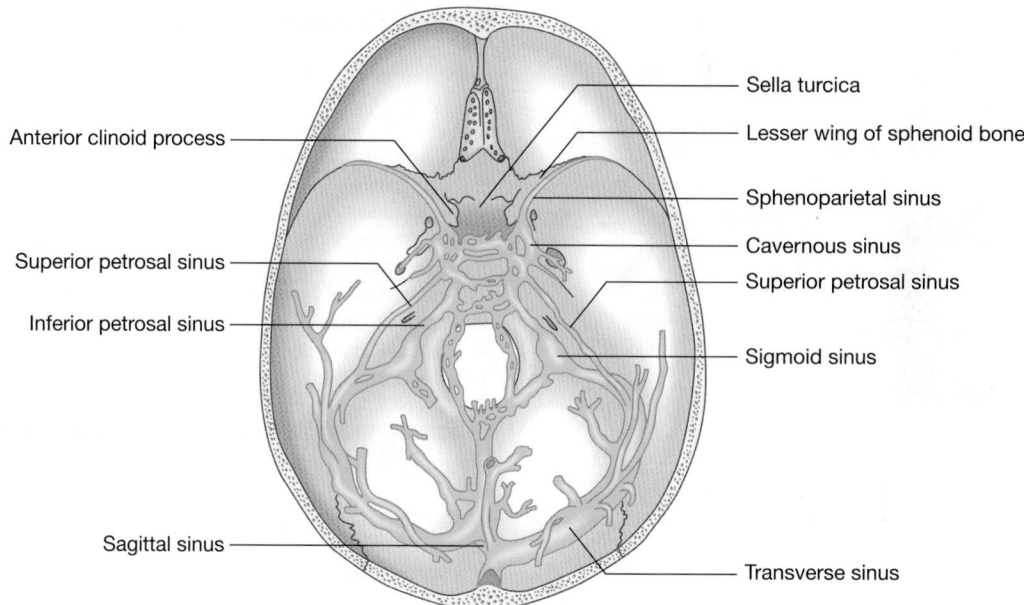

Fig. 29.3 Veins of the brain. *Adapted from Anatomy, imaging and surgery of the intracranial dural venous sinuses. https://doi.org/10.1016/B978-0-323-65377-0.00017-9.*

- Anterior clinoid process
- Superior petrosal sinus
- Inferior petrosal sinus
- Sagittal sinus
- Sella turcica
- Lesser wing of sphenoid bone
- Sphenoparietal sinus
- Cavernous sinus
- Superior petrosal sinus
- Sigmoid sinus
- Transverse sinus

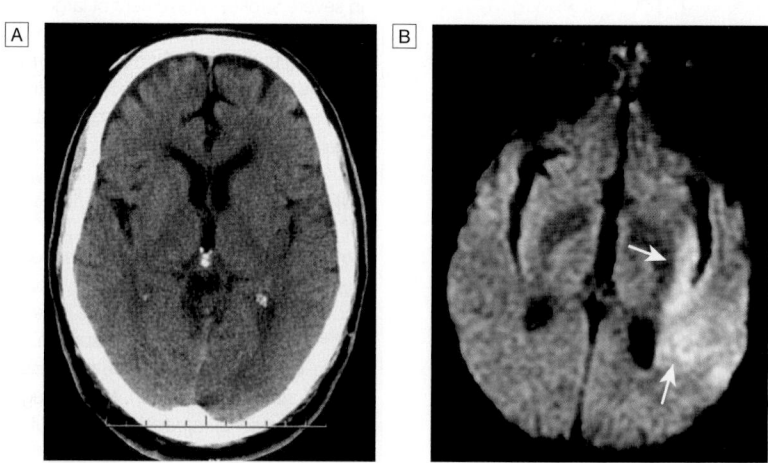

Fig. 29.4 Acute stroke seen on computed tomography (CT) scan with corresponding magnetic resonance imaging (MRI) appearance. [A] CT may show no evidence of early infarction. [B] A corresponding image seen on MRI diffusion weighted imaging (DWI) with changes of infarction in the middle cerebral artery (MCA) territory (arrows). *(A, B) Courtesy of Prof. A. Farrell and Prof. J. Wardlaw.*

Headache

Sudden severe headache is the cardinal symptom of SAH but also occurs in intracerebral haemorrhage. Although headache is common in acute ischaemic stroke, it is rarely a dominant feature.. Headache also occurs in cerebral venous thrombosis and in giant cell arteritis. Migraine is a weak risk factor for stroke, and sometimes a stroke can precipitate a migraine attack.

Seizure

Epileptic seizures are unusual in acute ischaemic stroke. Focal onset seizures can occur during stroke recovery, or during acute intracerebral haemorrhage or acute cerebral venous thrombosis (particularly of the cortical veins).

Coma

If a stroke patient presents with coma, it is usually due to a large intracerebral haemorrhage or brainstem stroke. Cortical ischaemic stroke patients can become comatose if they develop space occupying cerebral oedema, or develop complications of stroke such as pneumonia (see Box 9.31).

Stroke

Stroke is a common medical emergency. In the UK about 150 per 100 000 people have a stroke each year. It is commoner with increasing age, greater poverty and with vascular risk factors (Box. 29.1).

Pathophysiology

Cerebral infarction

Cerebral infarction is usually due to atherothromboembolism. The source of embolism can be the heart, particularly when there is AF, or the rupture of large artery atherosclerosis and subsequent thromboembolism

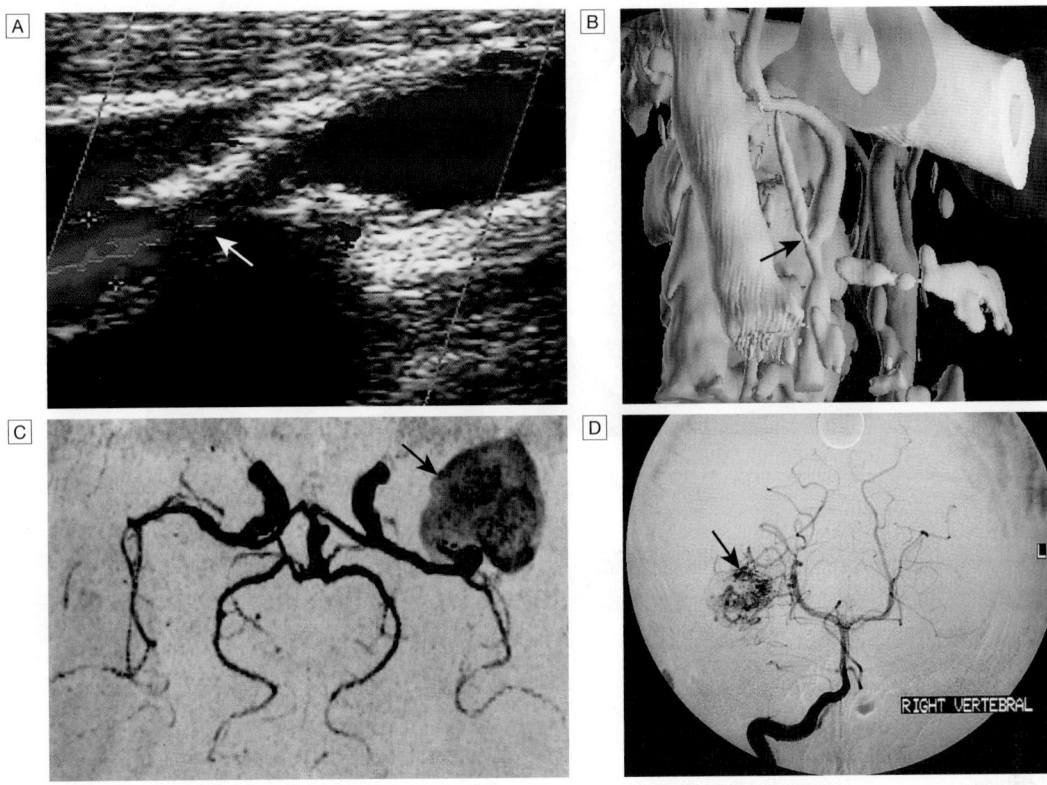

Fig. 29.5 Different techniques for imaging blood vessels. [A] Doppler scan showing 80% stenosis of the internal carotid artery (arrow). [B] Three-dimensional reconstruction of CT angiogram showing stenosis at the carotid bifurcation (arrow). [C] MR angiogram showing giant aneurysm at the middle cerebral artery bifurcation (arrow). [D] Intra-arterial angiography showing arteriovenous malformation (arrow). *(A–D) Courtesy of Dr D. Collie.*

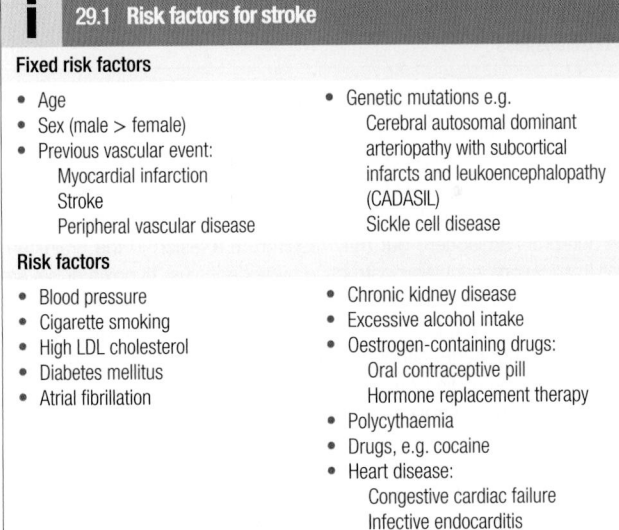

i 29.1 Risk factors for stroke

Fixed risk factors

- Age
- Sex (male > female)
- Previous vascular event:
  Myocardial infarction
  Stroke
  Peripheral vascular disease
- Genetic mutations e.g.
  Cerebral autosomal dominant arteriopathy with subcortical infarcts and leukoencephalopathy (CADASIL)
  Sickle cell disease

Risk factors

- Blood pressure
- Cigarette smoking
- High LDL cholesterol
- Diabetes mellitus
- Atrial fibrillation
- Chronic kidney disease
- Excessive alcohol intake
- Oestrogen-containing drugs:
  Oral contraceptive pill
  Hormone replacement therapy
- Polycythaemia
- Drugs, e.g. cocaine
- Heart disease:
  Congestive cardiac failure
  Infective endocarditis

from carotid arteries, vertebral arteries and aortic arch. Intracranial atheroma can lead to in situ thrombosis. Occlusion of the small perforating lenticulostriate arteries in patients with sporadic or genetic small vessel diseases leads to 'lacunar' infarctions. Spontaneous cervical artery dissection is an important mechanism in younger people. Infarction can also be the result of low arterial flow, for example severe hypotension (sometimes intraoperative), vessel inflammation in children or adults with vasculitis, or failure in energy production in mitochondrial disease.

After the occlusion of a cerebral artery, the supply of oxygen, glucose and other nutrients to tissue falls, and neuronal functions begin to fail. If there are adequate collateral vessels, these may dilate and restore normal blood flow, or maintain a reduced blood flow that keeps tissue alive but not active. Cerebral tissue begins to die if there are inadequate collateral vessels, or the vessel is not re-opened by endogenous thrombolysis, thrombolytic medication or thrombectomy. The process of cell death leads to oedema of dying tissue, which can be life-threatening if it expands to increase intracranial pressure. Although reopening blood vessels is of overall benefit, restoration of blood supply can lead to a secondary injury which is most obvious clinically in haemorrhagic transformation of an infarct, which is not infrequent (~3%) after thrombolytic therapy,

If the patient survives the acute stages of infarction, healing begins with inflammation to clear dying tissue, recovery of some neurons and reorganisation of some cerebral function to other brain areas.

Intracerebral haemorrhage

The commonest cause of intracerebral haemorrhage is the rupture of small blood vessels. Small vessels can be damaged by hypertension, diabetes, amyloid deposition or genetic causes. Rupture of abnormalities of larger vessels such as arteriovenous or cavernous malformations, and sometimes intracranial aneurysms (which usually presents as SAH) can also lead to intracerebral haemorrhage (Fig. 29.6). Haemorrhage leads to harm by direct pressure of the haematoma which can continue to grow after presentation, mass effect from surrounding oedema, and inflammation due to degrading blood products. Haemorrhage recovers with the resorption of blood products, resolution of oedema, healing of neurons and cerebral re-organisation (Box 29.2)

Clinical features

Both acute stroke and transient ischaemic attack (TIA) are characterised by a rapid-onset, focal deficit of brain function. Symptoms can be transient (TIA) or persistent (stroke). The symptoms of a typical stroke progress over minutes, affect an identifiable area of brain and are 'negative' (i.e. loss of function) (Box 29.3). If symptoms progress over hours or days, or

29

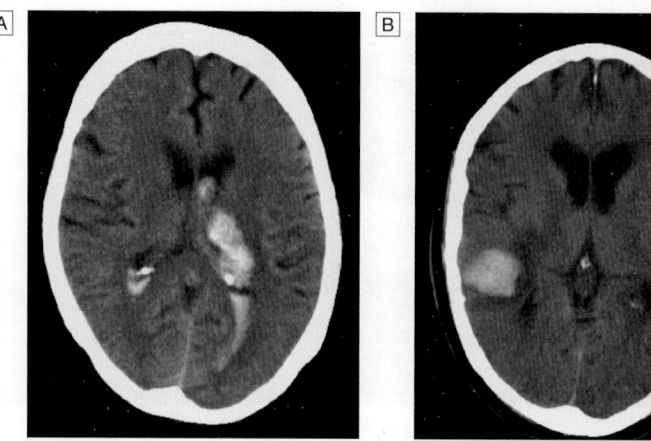

Fig. 29.6 CT scans showing intracerebral haemorrhage. A Basal ganglia haemorrhage with intraventricular extension. B Small cortical haemorrhage. *(A, B) Courtesy of Prof. A. Farrell and Prof. J. Wardlaw.*

29.2 Risk factor and causes of intracerebral haemorrhage

Disease	Risk factors
Small-vessel disease with disruption of vessel wall	Age Hypertension
Amyloid angiopathy	Familial (rare) Age
Impaired blood clotting	Anticoagulant therapy Thrombocytopenia Thrombolytic therapy Intracranial venous thrombosis
Vascular anomaly	Arteriovenous malformation Cavernous haemangioma Aneurysms
Substance misuse	Alcohol Amphetamines Cocaine

29.4 Characteristic features of stroke and non-stroke syndromes ('stroke mimics')

Feature	Stroke	Non-stroke
Symptom onset	Sudden (minutes)	Often slower onset
Symptom progression	Rapidly reaches maximum severity	Often gradual onset
Symptom type	Negative (e.g. weakness)	Positive (e.g. abnormal movements)
Pattern of deficit	Hemispheric pattern	May be non-specific with delirium, memory loss, balance disturbance
Loss of consciousness	Uncommon	More common

29.3 Differential diagnosis of stroke and transient ischaemic attack

- Seizure, particularly focal
- Syncope if history is unclear
- Sepsis presenting with delirium
- Migraine with aura
- Brain tumours
- Functional neurological symptoms
- Neuropathies
- Vertigo due to labyrinthopathy
- Multiple sclerosis
- Subdural haematoma
- Demyelination

if significant 'positive' features are present (e.g. spreading paraesthesiae, abnormal movements), other diagnoses are more likely (Box 29.3). Persistent or transient symptoms that cannot be localised to one brain area, e.g. syncope, amnesia, delirium and dizziness, are more likely to have causes other than TIA or stroke (see Fig. 9.4 and Box 29.4). It is important to remember that anxiety is common in people presenting with stroke or TIA, but also that people with functional neurological disorders can present with acute onset weakness or collapse (see Chapter 28).

The clinical syndrome of an ischaemic stroke depends on the arterial territory involved and the size of the lesion (see Fig. 29.1). These will both have a bearing on management, such as suitability for carotid endarterectomy. The presence of a unilateral motor deficit, a higher cerebral function deficit such as aphasia or neglect, or a visual field defect usually places the lesion in the cerebral hemisphere. Ataxia, diplopia, vertigo or bilateral weakness usually indicates a lesion in the brainstem or cerebellum. Different combinations of these deficits define several ischaemic stroke syndromes (Fig. 29.7), which reflect the site and size of the lesion and may provide clues to the underlying arterial occlusion.

Reduced conscious level usually indicates a large-volume lesion in the cerebral hemisphere but may result from a lesion in the brainstem or complications such as obstructive hydrocephalus, hypoxia or severe systemic infection (usually pneumonia). The combination of severe headache and vomiting at the onset of the focal deficit is suggestive of intracerebral haemorrhage, although headache is also a feature of giant cell arteritis and arterial dissection.

The definitions of strokes and TIA, are:

- *Transient ischaemic attack (TIA):* a transient focal neurological dysfunction caused by brain or retinal ischaemia with no evidence of infarction, where symptoms resolve within 24 hours.
- *Cerebral ischaemic stroke:* acute focal neurological dysfunction caused by focal infarction at single or multiple sites of brain or retina, with evidence of infarction either from neuroimaging or symptom duration longer than 24 hours.
- *Intracerebral haemorrhage:* acute focal neurological disturbance caused by haemorrhage within the brain parenchyma or ventricular system.

Investigations

Investigation of suspected stroke aims to confirm the vascular nature of a lesion, distinguish infarction from haemorrhage and identify the underlying vascular disease and risk factors (Boxes 29.5 and 29.6).

Clinical syndrome	Common symptoms	Common cause	CT scan features
Total anterior circulation syndrome (TACS) 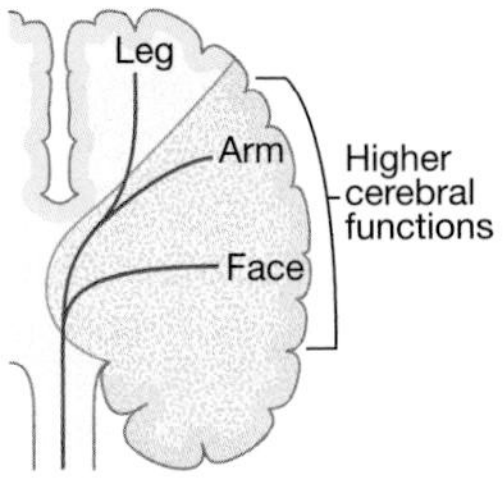 Leg / Arm / Face — Higher cerebral functions	Combination of: Hemiparesis Higher cerebral dysfunction (e.g. aphasia) Hemisensory loss Homonymous hemianopia (damage to optic radiations)	Middle cerebral artery occlusion Embolism from heart or major vessels	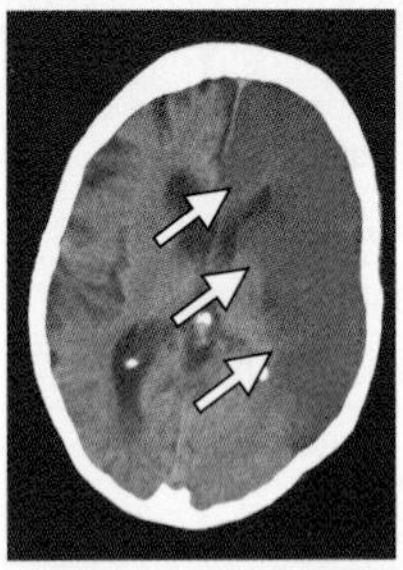
Partial anterior circulation syndrome (PACS) 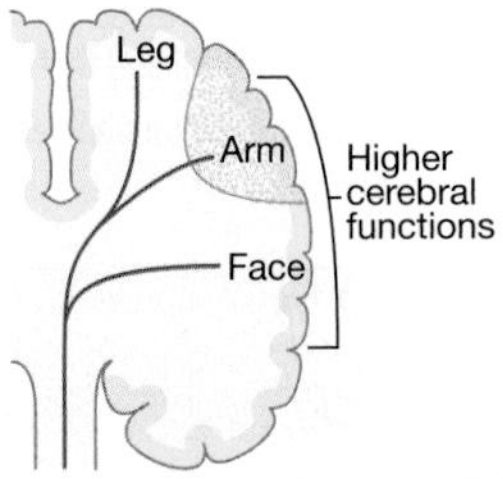 Leg / Arm / Face — Higher cerebral functions	Isolated motor loss (e.g. leg only, arm only, face) Isolated higher cerebral dysfunction (e.g. aphasia, neglect) Mixture of higher cerebral dysfunction and motor loss (e.g. aphasia with right hemiparesis)	Occlusion of a branch of the middle cerebral artery or anterior cerebral artery Embolism from heart or major vessels	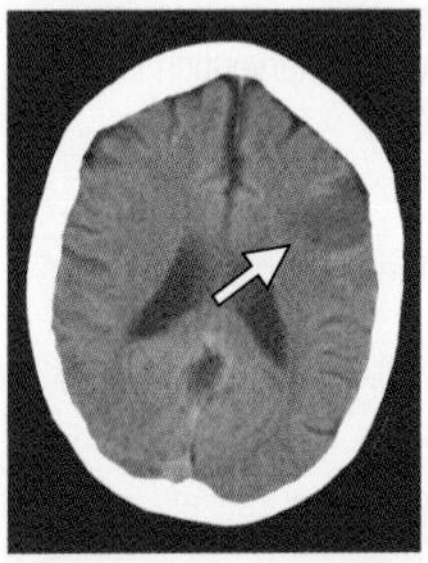
Lacunar syndrome (LACS) 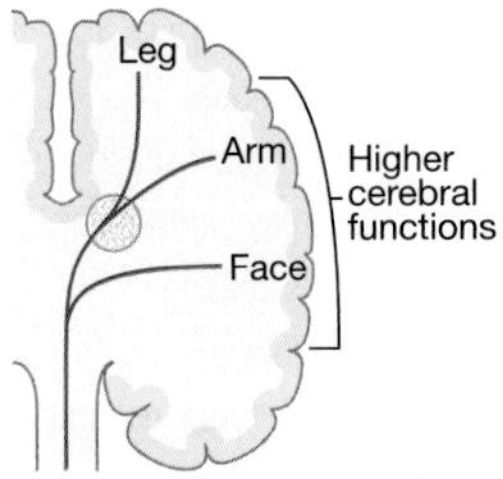 Leg / Arm / Face — Higher cerebral functions	Pure motor stroke – affects two limbs Pure sensory stroke Sensory-motor stroke No higher cerebral dysfunction or hemianopia	Thrombotic occlusion of small perforating arteries Thrombosis in situ	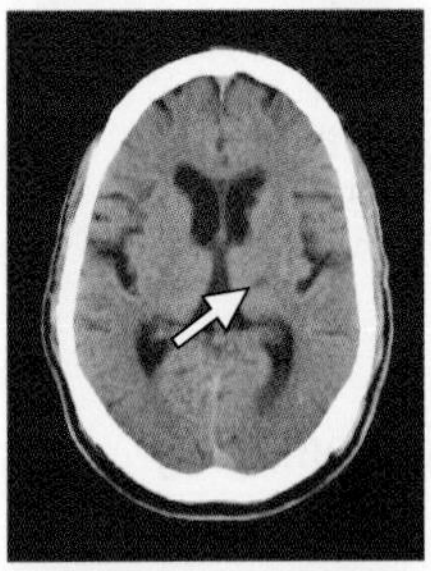
Posterior circulation stroke (POCS) (lateral view) 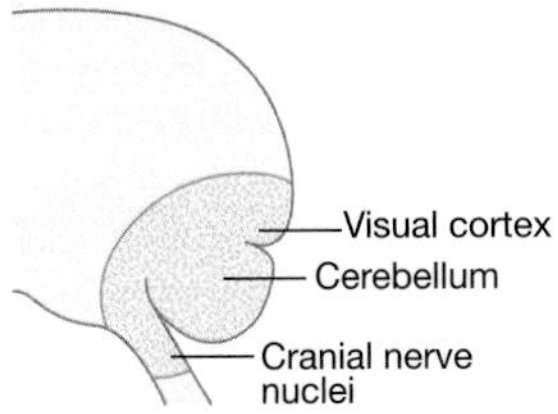 Visual cortex Cerebellum Cranial nerve nuclei	Homonymous hemianopia (damage to visual cortex) Cerebellar syndrome Cranial nerve syndromes	Occlusion in vertebral, basilar or posterior cerebral artery territory Cardiac embolism or thrombosis in situ	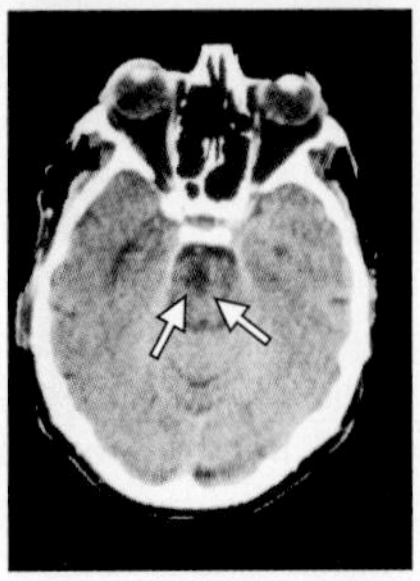

Fig. 29.7 Clinical and radiological features of the stroke syndromes. The top three diagrams show coronal sections of the brain and the bottom one shows a sagittal section. The anatomical locations of cerebral functions are shown with the nerve tracts in green. A motor (or sensory) deficit (shown by the areas shaded red) can occur with damage to the relevant cortex (PACS), nerve tracts (LACS) or both (TACS). The corresponding CT scans show horizontal slices at the level of the lesion, highlighted by the arrows.

Neuroimaging

CT is the most widely available method of imaging the brain. It has reasonable sensitivity for some non-stroke lesions, such as subdural haematomas, subarachnoid haemorrhage and brain tumours, but not others, such as the changes of early multiple sclerosis (see Fig. 29.6). CT has a high sensitivity for acute intracranial haemorrhage (see Fig. 29.6). However, soon after symptom onset, CT changes in cerebral infarction may be absent, or very subtle. Signs of infarction develop over time but small cerebral infarcts may never show up on CT imaging. Immediate brain imaging is a help and sometimes essential (see Box 29.7).

Perfusion of brain tissue can be demonstrated with CT after injection of contrast media (i.e. CT perfusion scanning). After ischaemic stroke, this technique can identify areas of brain with low perfusion that might be reversed with thrombolysis or thrombectomy.

MRI scanning times are longer than CT, but MRI diffusion weighted imaging (DWI) can detect ischaemia earlier than CT. It may not show changes in up to a third of stroke patients (see Fig. 29.4). MRI is more sensitive than CT in detecting strokes affecting the brainstem and cerebellum, and, unlike CT, can reliably distinguish haemorrhagic from ischaemic stroke weeks after the onset. CT and MRI may reveal clues as to the nature of the arterial lesion. For example, there may be a small, deep lacunar infarct indicating small-vessel disease, or a more peripheral infarct suggesting other causes (see Fig. 29.7). The location of an intracerebral haemorrhage might indicate the presence of an underlying vascular malformation, aneurysm or amyloid angiopathy.

A 'positive scan' is not needed to make a diagnosis of acute ischaemic stroke. A typical stroke syndrome with a normal CT (or a CT with no acute changes of stroke) means that an ischaemic stroke is the likeliest diagnosis. This means clinical skills are very important in stroke diagnosis.

29

Vascular imaging

It is important to identify carotid stenosis in patients with recent ischaemic stroke or TIA. The presence or absence of a carotid bruit is not a reliable indicator of the degree of carotid stenosis. Carotid stenosis can be non-invasively identified with duplex ultrasound, magnetic resonance or computed tomography angiography (MRA or CTA) (see Fig. 29.5), or very occasionally with intra-arterial contrast radiography. Although many patients have intracranial, vertebral artery or aortic arch atherosclerosis, at the time of writing there are no evidenced-based interventions for these lesions. In patients with spontaneous intracerebral haemorrhage, imaging (MRA, CTA or CT venogaphy (CTV)) may identify an underlying macrovascular cause, e.g intracranial aneurysm, arteriovenous malformation (AVM), or venous sinus thrombosis (see Fig. 29.5). CTA is an important technique to demonstrate large artery occlusion to identify patients who are suitable for thrombectomy.

Cardiac investigations

Approximately 20% of ischaemic strokes are due to embolism from the heart. The most common cause is atrial fibrillation, but prosthetic heart valves, endocarditis, other valve abnormalities and recent myocardial infarction may also lead to cardioembolism.

Atrial fibrillation can be identified on a 12-lead ECG, or more prolonged ECG recording with devices that can record between a few days and many months. A transthoracic or transoesophageal echocardiogram in selected stroke patients can identify endocarditis, atrial myxoma, intracardiac thrombus or patent foramen ovale (PFO). A PFO is a right-to-left cardiac shunt that is usually asymptomatic but can act as a conduit for thrombi from the venous system.

Blood tests

Blood tests can identify high fasting glucose levels, anaemia, electrolyte disturbances or evidence of an inflammatory response (e.g. in temporal

arteritis or vasculitis). Clotting abnormalities are a rare cause of ischaemic or haemorrhagic stroke, and tests for thrombophilia or haemophilia without other clinical pointers rarely lead to a change in management. However, in selected patients (for example those with both venous and arterial events) tests for inherited thrombophilia or anti-phospholipid antibodies may be helpful. Intracranial haemorrhage is frequently due to prescribed anticoagulants (direct oral anticoagulants or coumarins like warfarin) and monitoring may be important when reversing the effect of these agents.

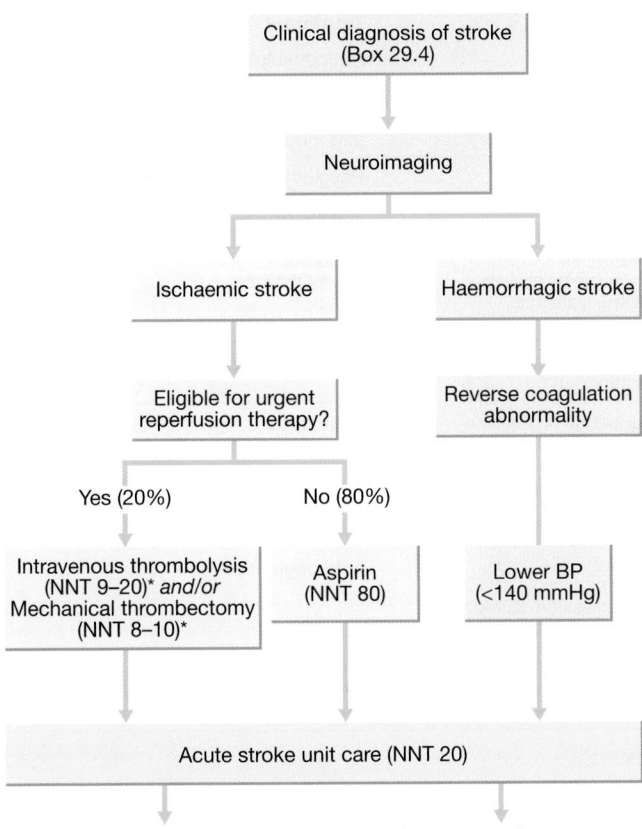

Fig. 29.8 Emergency management of stroke. *Varies with patient selection and delay in treatment. (BP = blood pressure; NNT = number needed to treat to avoid one death or long-term disability)

Management

Management (Fig. 29.8) is aimed at identifying the cause, minimising the volume of brain that is irreversibly damaged, preventing complications (Fig. 29.9), reducing the patient's disability and handicap through rehabilitation, and reducing the risk of recurrent stroke or other vascular events. With TIA there is no major persisting brain damage and disability, so the priority is to reduce the risk of stroke.

Reperfusion (thrombolysis and thrombectomy)

Rapid reperfusion in ischaemic stroke can reduce the extent of brain damage.

Intravenous thrombolysis with recombinant tissue plasminogen activator (alteplase) improves recovery if given within 4.5 hours of symptom onset to carefully selected patients. The main contraindications to thrombolysis are a high bleeding risk (recent haemorrhage, anticoagulant therapy, recent surgery or trauma at a non-compressible site) and delay to treatment: the earlier treatment is given, the greater the benefit (Fig. 29.10).

Intravenous thrombolysis fails to re-perfuse the brain in up to 30% of patients presenting with a large-vessel occlusion. Mechanical clot retrieval (thrombectomy) performed up to 6 hours after onset of symptoms can greatly improve the chances of avoiding disability in these patients (see Fig. 29.8 and Fig. 29.11). Treatment of patients presenting later, or where symptoms onset is unknown (e.g. waking from sleep), is possible if there is evidence of 'salvageable' tissue with brain imaging.

Supportive care

Rapid admission of patients to a specialised stroke unit facilitates coordinated care from a multidisciplinary team and reduces mortality and disability amongst survivors. For every 1000 patients managed in a stroke unit, an extra 50 will avoid death or long-term disability, compared to those managed in non-specialist wards. Rehabilitation should begin at the same time as acute medical management. Dysphagia is common and can be detected by an early bedside test of swallowing. This allows hydration, feeding and medication to be given safely, if necessary by nasogastric tube. In the acute phase, a checklist may be useful (Box 29.8) to ensure that all the factors that might influence outcome have been addressed.

Neurological deficits may worsen during the first few hours or days after their onset. This may be due to further infarction, haemorrhagic transformation of infarction (most commonly after thrombolysis), or the development of oedema with consequent mass effect. It is important to distinguish these patients from those who are deteriorating as a result of complications such as hypoxia, sepsis, epileptic seizures or metabolic abnormalities that may be reversed more easily. Patients with cerebellar haematomas or infarcts with mass effect may develop obstructive hydrocephalus and some will benefit from insertion of a ventricular drain or decompressive surgery. Some patients with large haematomas or infarction with massive oedema in the cerebral hemispheres may benefit from anti-oedema agents, such as mannitol, or artificial ventilation. Surgical decompression with hemicraniectomy to reduce intracranial pressure should be considered in patients where survival with severe disability is acceptable and surgery is possible within 48 hours.

Antiplatelet agents

In the absence of contraindications, aspirin (300 mg daily) should be started immediately after a major ischaemic stroke unless thrombolysis has been given, in which case it should be withheld for at least 24 hours. Aspirin reduces the risk of early ischaemic stroke recurrence and has a small but clinically worthwhile effect on disability (see Fig. 29.8 and Fig. 29.12); it may be given by rectal suppository or by nasogastric tube in dysphagic patients. In minor ischaemic stroke or TIA, two antiplatelet agents (for example clopidogrel and aspirin) for a few weeks reduce the risk of early recurrent stroke.

Considerations specific to use of anticoagulants in old age are given in Box 29.9.

Coagulation abnormalities

In patients with intracerebral haemorrhage, coagulation abnormalities should be reversed as quickly as possible to reduce haematoma expansion. This is a problem in patients taking anticoagulant therapy. There is no evidence that clotting factors are useful in the absence of a clotting defect.

Blood pressure

Early reduction of blood pressure (<180 mmHg) reduces haematoma expansion and may improve the overall outcome in patients with acute intracerebral haemorrhage. Blood pressure lowering in acute ischaemic stroke does not improve later disability, but reduces intracranial haemorrhage after thrombolysis.

However, reducing blood pressure is very important in the longer term to reduce the risk of recurrent stroke.

Management of risk factors

The approaches used are summarised in Fig. 29.12. The average risk of a further stroke is 5%–10% within the first week of an ischaemic stroke or TIA, 15% over the first year (including the early period) and 5% per year thereafter. Patients with ischaemic stroke or TIA should be offered long-term antiplatelet drugs and statins to lower low density lipoprotein cholesterol (LDL-C). For patients in atrial fibrillation, the risk can be reduced substantially with oral anticoagulation with direct oral anticoagulants or warfarin (in selected patients, see Box 29.9). The risk of recurrence after

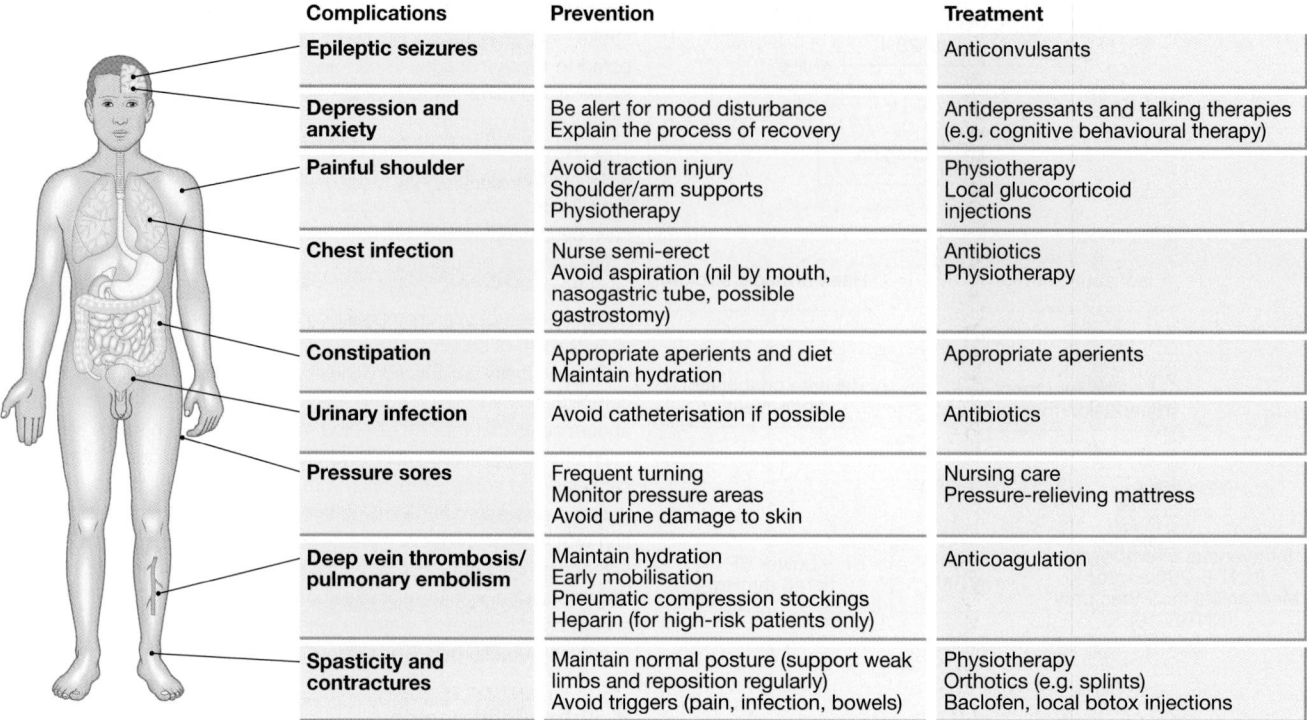

Complications	Prevention	Treatment
Epileptic seizures		Anticonvulsants
Depression and anxiety	Be alert for mood disturbance Explain the process of recovery	Antidepressants and talking therapies (e.g. cognitive behavioural therapy)
Painful shoulder	Avoid traction injury Shoulder/arm supports Physiotherapy	Physiotherapy Local glucocorticoid injections
Chest infection	Nurse semi-erect Avoid aspiration (nil by mouth, nasogastric tube, possible gastrostomy)	Antibiotics Physiotherapy
Constipation	Appropriate aperients and diet Maintain hydration	Appropriate aperients
Urinary infection	Avoid catheterisation if possible	Antibiotics
Pressure sores	Frequent turning Monitor pressure areas Avoid urine damage to skin	Nursing care Pressure-relieving mattress
Deep vein thrombosis/ pulmonary embolism	Maintain hydration Early mobilisation Pneumatic compression stockings Heparin (for high-risk patients only)	Anticoagulation
Spasticity and contractures	Maintain normal posture (support weak limbs and reposition regularly) Avoid triggers (pain, infection, bowels)	Physiotherapy Orthotics (e.g. splints) Baclofen, local botox injections

Fig. 29.9 Complications of acute stroke.

both ischaemic and haemorrhagic strokes can be reduced by blood pressure reduction, even for those with relatively 'normal' blood pressures. Patients should stop smoking. The evidence for change in diet or increasing exercise is weaker, but it is probable these interventions reduce recurrent stroke.

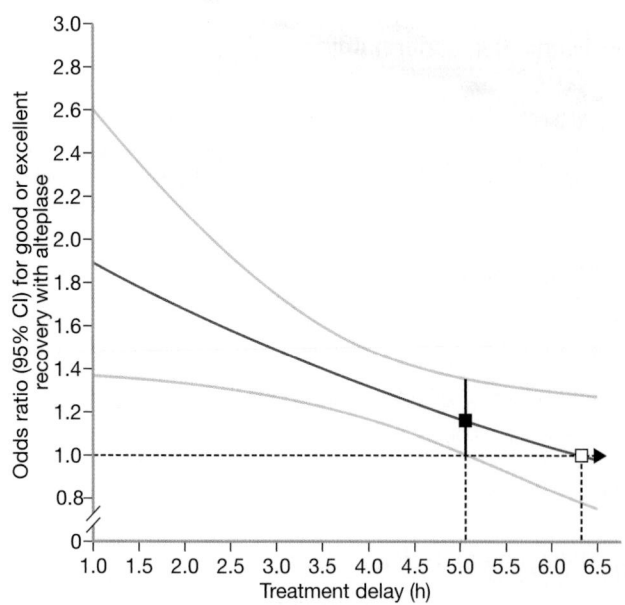

Fig. 29.10 Effect of timing of alteplase treatment on recovery from stroke. The solid blue line shows how the estimated recovery for patients given alteplase (compared with patients given control treatment) falls as the delay to treatment increases. The black box (at 5 hours) shows the point at which treatment with alteplase is no more effective than control (the lower 95% confidence interval for the estimated treatment effect first crosses 1.0 at this point). *From Emberson J et al. The Lancet 2014; 384:1929–1935.*

Carotid endarterectomy and arterial angioplasty

Some patients with a carotid territory ischaemic stroke or TIA have >50% stenosis of the carotid artery on the side of the brain lesion. These patients have a greater than average risk of stroke recurrence. For those without major residual disability, removal of the stenosis by carotid endarterectomy reduces the risk of recurrent stroke although the operation itself carries about a 3%–4% stroke risk, depending on the surgical centre. Surgery is most effective in patients with more severe stenoses (70%–99%) and when it is performed within the first couple of weeks after the TIA or ischaemic stroke. Carotid angioplasty and stenting are technically feasible but have not been shown to be as effective as endarterectomy for the majority of eligible patients. Endarterectomy of asymptomatic carotid stenosis reduces stroke risk. but it has a smaller absolute benefit. Whilst stenting of other arteries (vertebral or intracranial) could reduce stroke incidence, at present there is no evidence to support their use in clinical practice.

Rehabilitation

Stroke survivors are often disabled by reduced mobility or upper limb weakness, impaired communication, cognitive impairment, dyspraxia, poor coordination, or visual impairment. Around a third of patients develop dementia after stroke. A minority have persistent dysphagia and some need long-term enteral feeding with a gastrostomy tube. Other long-term stroke complications include neuropathic pain (particularly common after thalamic stroke), limb spasticity, shoulder pain, epilepsy, incontinence, fatigue and anxiety or depression.

The purpose of rehabilitation is to maximise functional recovery and prevent complications. The speed and degree of recovery varies between individuals. Severe strokes (total anterior circulation syndrome or NIHSS score >15) are more likely to cause severe disability and loss of independent living. Other predictors of poor recovery are older age, pre-existing disability, multi-morbidity and pre-existing cognitive impairment.

The goals set during rehabilitation should be achievable, and reached by discussion between the patient and a multidisciplinary team on a dedicated stroke unit, including doctors, nurses, physiotherapists, speech and language therapists, occupational therapists, psychologists and dieticians. Supportive family and social networks are important.

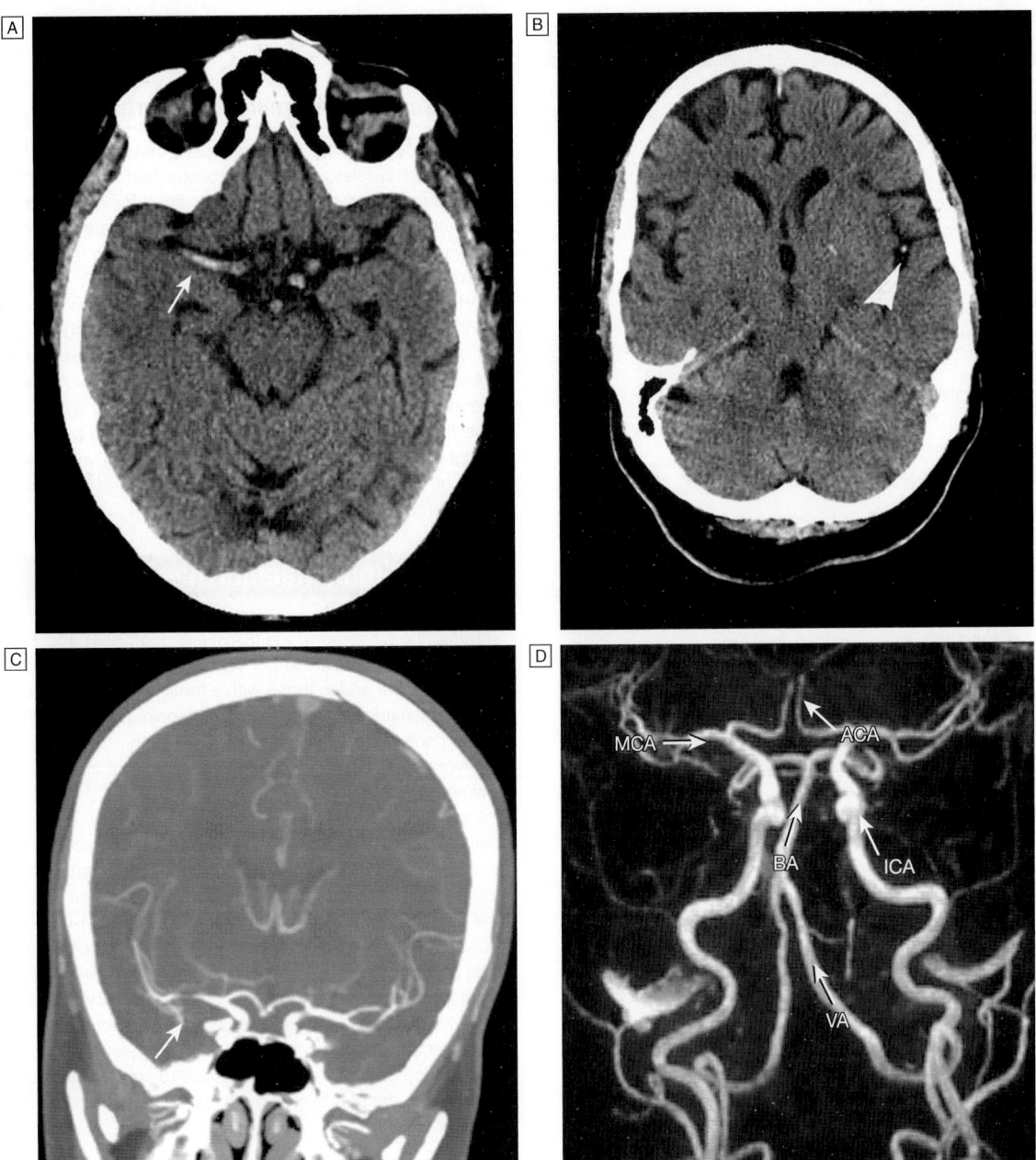

Fig. 29.11 Imaging of major arteries in ischaemic stroke. **A** CT scan showing a proximal hyperdense artery sign (arrow) in the M1 segment of MCA. **B** Non-contrast CT showing a distal hyperdense artery sign in the sylvian fissure (arrowhead). **C** Angiogram of the circle of Willis showing occlusion of the right MCA. **D** Contrast-enhanced MR angiography showing normal circle of Willis in the frontal plane. (ACA = anterior cerebral artery; BA = basilar artery; ICA = internal carotid artery; MCA = middle cerebral artery; VA = vertebral artery). *(A, B) From Li Q, Davis S, Mitchell P, Dowling R, Yan B. PLoS ONE 2014; 9:e96123; (C) from Campbell BCV, Khatri P. The Lancet 2020; 396:10244; (D) from Aminoff MJ, Daroff RB (eds). Encyclopedia of the neurological sciences. New York: Academic Press; 2003.*

There are three main phases of recovery. Early recovery (first few days) is due to resolution of cerebral oedema and cerebral reperfusion. The second phase – 'neuroplasticity' – is when new areas of brain take over from damaged areas of brain. This 'rewiring' can occur for a year or even later after stroke but most happens within the first few months. Intensive rehabilitation should begin as early as possible after the first 24 hours, because very early mobilisation (<24 hr) may be harmful. Repetitive practice of lost skills has been shown to increase neuroplasticity. The third phase is adaptive recovery. In this period the patient may learn new strategies to live with their disability and provision can be made for mobility aids, communication aids, or adaptations to the home. Intense therapy in the longer term may be beneficial to some patients and is an area of active research.

It is important not to underestimate the long-term emotional and financial impacts of stroke. Many stroke survivors face an initial loss of identity, loss of income and relationship strain. It is common for stroke survivors to feel fear, anxiety, frustration, anger, sadness and a sense of grief over physical and mental losses. Stroke survivors hoping to return to education or work need specialist vocational support.

Barriers to effective rehabilitation include physical illness: post-stroke pneumonia or delirium, which can delay rehabilitation sessions; pre-existing cognitive impairment or physical frailty; poor motivation and apathy (common in non-dominant hemisphere strokes); fatigue; depression; or pain. When improvements in lost function slow down the focus of therapy shifts to adaptive recovery. Milestones can be used to discuss rehabilitation goals with patients and their carers and to set out realistic expectations for recovery. Physical milestones include sitting balance (e.g. 1 minute unsupported sit), followed by standing balance (e.g. 1 minute), followed by stepping (e.g. 10 steps on the spot) and then walking (e.g. 10 metres).

29

29.8 How to manage a patient with acute stroke

Airway

- Perform bedside swallowing screen and consider nasogastric tube for feeding if swallowing is unsafe

Breathing

- Check respiratory rate

Circulation

- Check peripheral perfusion, pulse and blood pressure

Hydration

- If signs of dehydration, give fluids parenterally or by nasogastric tube

Nutrition

- Assess nutritional status and provide supplements if needed
- If unable to swallow, consider feeding via nasogastric tube

Medication

- If dysphagic, consider other routes for essential medications

Blood pressure

- Haemorrhagic stroke: consider lowering systolic blood pressure to 130–140 mmHg and maintain this blood pressure for at least 7 days
- Ischaemic stroke: unless there is heart or renal failure, evidence of hypertensive encephalopathy or aortic dissection, do not lower blood pressure abruptly
- Check blood glucose and treat if diabetes is diagnosed
- Avoid hypoglycaemia

Temperature

- If pyrexial, investigate and treat underlying cause
- Control temperature with antipyretics

Pressure areas

- Reduce risk of skin breakdown:
  Treat infection
  Maintain nutrition
  Provide pressure-relieving mattress
  Turn immobile patients regularly

Incontinence

- Check for constipation and urinary retention; treat these appropriately
- Avoid urinary catheterisation unless patient is in acute urinary retention or incontinence is threatening pressure areas

Prevention of deep vein thrombosis

- Consider intermittent pneumatic compression stockings in immobile patients

Mobilisation

- Avoid bed rest after the first 24 hours

Research in technologies to assist stroke rehabilitation is ongoing, including transcranial direct current stimulation and vagal stimulators for motor recovery and mirror therapy for limb pain and visuospatial neglect.

Causes of ischaemic stroke

Large artery atherosclerosis, small vessel disease and cardioembolism from AF are the commonest causes of ischaemic stroke. Carotid or vertebral artery dissection occasionally leads to stroke . The presenting history often includes minor injury and face or neck pain. After confirmation on angiography (MRA or CTA), treatment is with either antiplatelet drugs or anticoagulation, (the latter are more effective). The cause of dissection is unknown in most cases, but collagen disorders, e.g. Ehlers–Danlos syndrome (type 4), are occasionally responsible.

Giant cell arteritis, a vasculitis of large and medium-sized blood vessels, may present with transient monocular blindness, usually with head tenderness, shoulder pain or jaw claudication on chewing. It is important to identify because blindness can be prevented with steroids. Other large artery vasculitis can very rarely present with stroke.

Causes of intracerebral haemorrhage

Most intracerebral haemorrhages result from disease of the small cerebral blood vessels, either due to sporadic small vessel disease or amyloid angiopathy. Anticoagulants, given for AF or metal prosthetic heart valves, increase the risk of intracerebral haemorrhage but almost always to a smaller degree than their reduction in the risk of ischaemic stroke.

Arteriovenous or cavernous malformations ('cavernomas') are more commonly discovered after intracerebral haemorrhage in younger people. To reduce the risk of further haemorrhage, it is possible to treat some of these malformations with surgery or radio-surgery. Arteriovenous malformation can be treated by surgical removal, by ligation of the blood vessels that feed or drain the lesion, or most often by radiological injection of material to occlude the fistula or draining veins. However, treatment of these malformations when they are asymptomatic probably leads to more harm than benefit.

Subarachnoid haemorrhage

Subarachnoid haemorrhage (SAH) (see Fig. 29.1) affects about 6 per 100 000 of the population per year. SAH is more common in women, in older people and in those with a family history, or vascular risk factors (particularly smoking and hypertension). About 30% of patients with an aneurysmal SAH die within a month of their bleed; untreated survivors have a recurrence (or rebleed) rate of about 40% in the first 4 weeks.

Most (85%) SAHs are due to saccular or 'berry' aneurysms at bifurcations of cerebral arteries (see Fig. 29.2), particularly in the circle of Willis. The most common sites are in the anterior communicating artery (30%), posterior communicating artery (25%) and middle cerebral artery (20%). There is an increased risk in first-degree relatives of those with saccular aneurysms, in patients with polycystic kidney disease and congenital connective tissue disorders such as Ehlers–Danlos syndrome. A minority of SAHs are not associated with aneurysms – the clinical syndrome of 'peri-mesencephalic haemorrhage', which have a characteristic appearance on CT and a benign prognosis. Small cortical surface SAH is thought to be due to amyloid angiopathy. Around 5% of SAHs are due to arteriovenous malformations or vertebral artery dissection.

Clinical features

SAH usually presents with a sudden, severe, 'thunderclap' headache, which is usually persistent, often accompanied by vomiting, raised blood pressure and neck stiffness or pain. It can occur spontaneously, on physical exertion, straining or during sex. There may be loss of consciousness so SAH should be considered if a patient is found comatose. About 1 patient in 8 with a sudden severe headache has SAH and, in view of this, all who present in this way require investigation to exclude it (Fig. 29.13).

On examination, the patient may be distressed, in pain, with photophobia. There may be neck stiffness due to subarachnoid blood, but this may take some hours to develop. Focal hemisphere signs, such as hemiparesis or aphasia, may be present at onset if there is an associated intracerebral haematoma. A third nerve palsy may be present due to local pressure from an aneurysm of the posterior communicating artery, and patients presenting with a painful third nerve palsy should be investigated urgently for the presence of an expanding aneurysm. Fundoscopy may reveal a subhyaloid haemorrhage, which represents blood tracking along the subarachnoid space around the optic nerve.

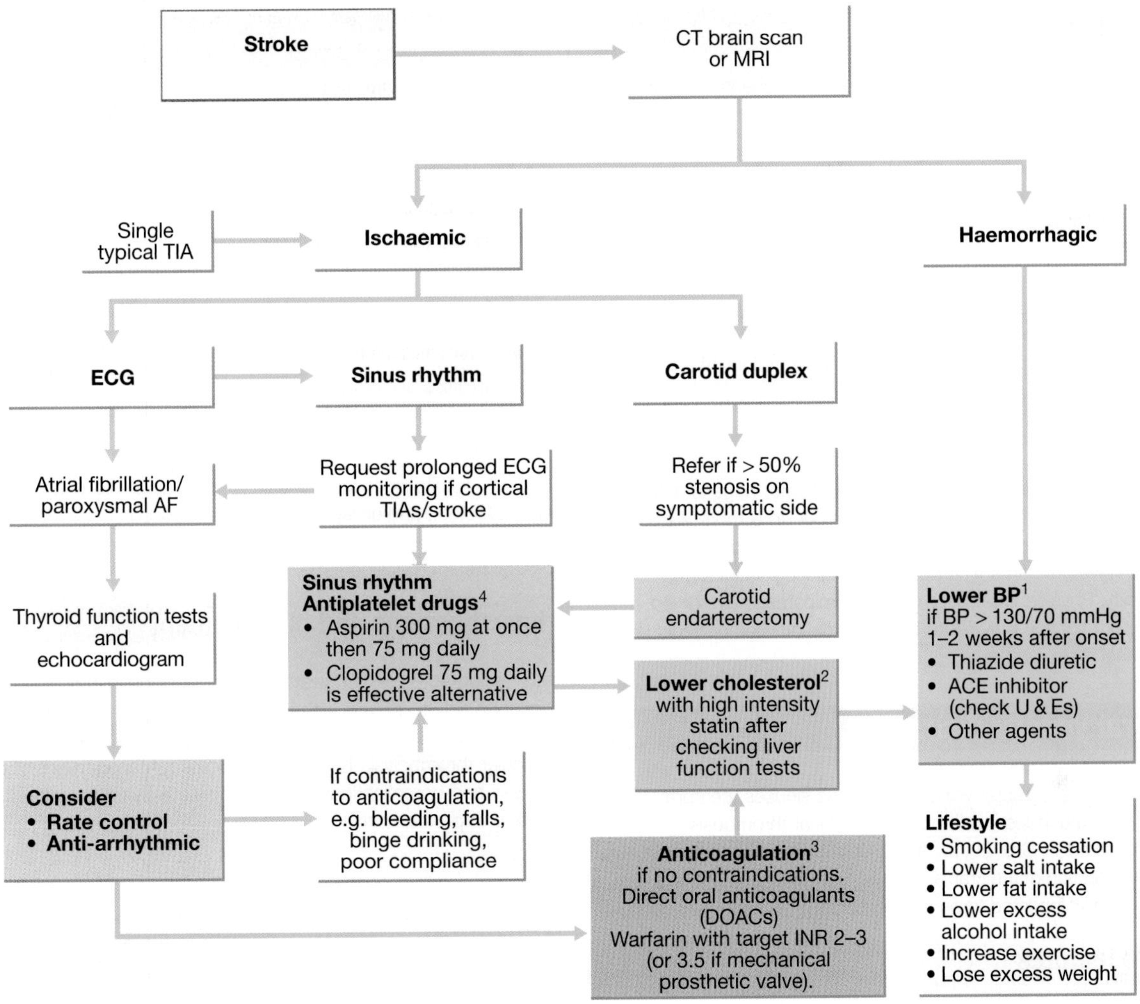

Stroke
CT brain scan or MRI
Single typical TIA
Ischaemic
Haemorrhagic
ECG
Sinus rhythm
Carotid duplex
Atrial fibrillation/ paroxysmal AF
Request prolonged ECG monitoring if cortical TIAs/stroke
Refer if > 50% stenosis on symptomatic side
Thyroid function tests and echocardiogram
Sinus rhythm Antiplatelet drugs4
• Aspirin 300 mg at once then 75 mg daily
• Clopidogrel 75 mg daily is effective alternative
Carotid endarterectomy
Lower cholesterol2 with high intensity statin after checking liver function tests
Lower BP1 if BP > 130/70 mmHg 1–2 weeks after onset
• Thiazide diuretic
• ACE inhibitor (check U & Es)
• Other agents
Consider
• Rate control
• Anti-arrhythmic
If contraindications to anticoagulation, e.g. bleeding, falls, binge drinking, poor compliance
Anticoagulation3 if no contraindications. Direct oral anticoagulants (DOACs) Warfarin with target INR 2–3 (or 3.5 if mechanical prosthetic valve).
Lifestyle
• Smoking cessation
• Lower salt intake
• Lower fat intake
• Lower excess alcohol intake
• Increase exercise
• Lose excess weight

Fig. 29.12 Strategies for secondary prevention of stroke. [1]Lower blood pressure with caution in patients with postural hypotension, renal impairment or severe bilateral carotid stenosis. [2]Other statins can be used as an alternative to simvastatin in patients on warfarin or digoxin. [3]Warfarin and aspirin have been used in combination in patients with prosthetic heart valves. [4]The combination of aspirin and clopidogrel is indicated short term (≤ 21 days) in patients with high-risk TIA (ABCD2 score > 4) or mild stroke (NIHSS <3) and low bleeding risk. Afterwards these patients should continue either aspirin or clopidogrel long term. (ACE = angiotensin-converting enzyme; AF = atrial fibrillation; BP = blood pressure; CT = computed tomography; ECG = electrocardiogram; INR = International Normalised Ratio; MRI = magnetic resonance imaging; TIA = transient ischaemic attack; U&Es = urea and electrolytes)

Emergency CT
Negative (<10% of subarachnoid haemorrhage)
Shows subarachnoid haemorrhage
Blood/xanthochromia
CSF (after 12 hours)
Traumatic lumbar punctures do not cause xanthochromia in that specimen
Refer to neurosurgeons Resuscitate Nimodipine 60 mg
If CT and CSF at 12 hours are negative the patient has not had a subarachnoid haemorrhage

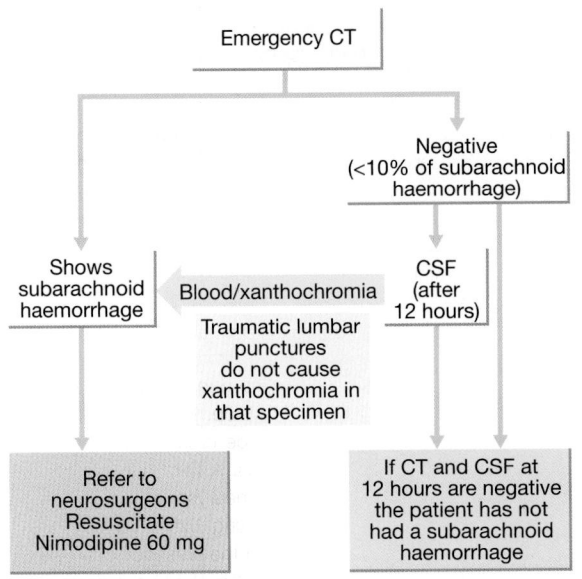

Fig. 29.13 Investigation of subarachnoid haemorrhage. (CSF = cerebrospinal fluid; CT = computed tomography)

29.9 Anticoagulation in old age

- Randomised trials of anticoagulation versus aspirin in older people with atrial fibrillation demonstrate a halving of the risk of stroke from about 4% to about 2% per year. Any increased risk of bleeding is much smaller.
- **AF and increased risk of stroke**: older age and previous stroke increase the risk of stroke in the presence of atrial fibrillation, and bleeding risk with anticoagulation.
- **Falls risk**: older patients are more prone to falls, including head injuries, which may increase bleeding risk.

Investigations

The diagnosis of SAH can usually be made by a timely CT read by an expert radiologist but a negative result does not completely exclude it, since small amounts of blood in the subarachnoid space may not be detected by CT, especially if the presentation is delayed by more than a day (see Fig. 29.13). Lumbar puncture should be performed 12 hours after symptom onset if possible, to allow detection of xanthochromia. If either of these tests is positive, CT or digital subtraction cerebral angiography (see Fig. 29.5) is needed to identify an aneurysm.

Management

Nimodipine is given to prevent delayed cerebral ischaemia in the acute phase. Insertion of platinum coils into an aneurysm (via an endovascular procedure) or surgical clipping of the aneurysm neck reduces the risk of both early and late recurrent SAH. Coiling is associated with fewer perioperative complications and better outcomes than surgical clipping: where feasible, it is now the procedure of first choice. Treatment may also be needed for complications of SAH, which include obstructive hydrocephalus (that may require drainage via a shunt), delayed cerebral ischaemia due to vasospasm (which may be treated with vasodilators), hyponatraemia (best managed by fluid restriction) and systemic complications associated with immobility, such as chest infection and venous thrombosis.

Rehabilitation

The pattern of recovery after subarachnoid haemorrhage is different to ischaemic or haemorrhagic stroke, perhaps due to a more widespread brain injury. Even those who make a good physical recovery from a mild SAH often have problems with headache, thinking, fatigue and change in personality. Physical disabilities due to hemiparesis, arm or leg weakness or incoordination may relate to ischaemic or haemorrhagic lesions following aneurysm rupture.

Cerebral venous disease

Thrombosis of the cerebral veins and venous sinuses (cerebral venous thrombosis) is much less common than arterial thrombosis. The main causes are listed in Box 29.10. It may be idiopathic, associated with pregnancy, infection of the cranial sinuses, severe dehydration, or due to other acquired or inherited thrombophilias.

Clinical features

Cerebral venous sinus thrombosis usually presents with symptoms of raised intracranial pressure, seizures and focal neurological symptoms. The clinical features vary according to the sinus involved (Box 29.11 and see Fig. 29.3). Cortical vein thrombosis presents with focal

---

i 29.10 Causes of cerebral venous thrombosis

Predisposing systemic causes

- Dehydration
- Pregnancy
- Behçet's disease
- Thrombophilia
- Hypotension
- Oral contraceptive use

Local causes

- Paranasal sinusitis
- Meningitis, subdural empyema
- Penetrating head and eye wounds
- Facial skin infection
- Otitis media, mastoiditis
- Skull fracture

---

i 29.11 Clinical features of cerebral venous thrombosis

Cavernous sinus thrombosis

- Proptosis, ptosis, headache, external and internal ophthalmoplegia, papilloedema, reduced sensation in trigeminal first division
- Often bilateral, patient ill and febrile

Superior sagittal sinus thrombosis

- Headache, papilloedema, seizures
- Clinical features may resemble idiopathic intracranial hypertension (p. 1186)
- May involve veins of both hemispheres, causing motor and sensory focal deficits

Transverse sinus thrombosis

- Hemiparesis, seizures, papilloedema
- May spread to jugular foramen and involve cranial nerves 9, 10 and 11

---

cortical deficits such as aphasia and hemiparesis (depending on the area affected), and epilepsy (focal or generalised). Occlusion of the larger veins may present with severe illness, but also with a milder illness of headache and papilloedema.

Investigations and management

MR venography demonstrates a filling defect in the affected vessel. Anticoagulation, initially with heparin followed by warfarin, is beneficial, even in the presence of venous haemorrhage. In selected patients, endovascular thrombolysis has been advocated. Management of underlying causes and complications, such as persistently raised intracranial pressure, is important.

Further information

Websites

eso-stroke.org *European Stroke Organisation guidelines.*
nhs.uk/conditions/stroke/symptoms *NHS website, includes the FAST (face, arms, speech, time) acronym used to raise public awareness of the emergency nature of stroke.*
nice.org.uk/guidance *National Institute for Health and Care Excellence CG180 'Tools and resources' includes a patient decision aid – Atrial fibrillation: medicines to help reduce your risk of a stroke – what are the options?*
stroke.cochrane.org *Systematic reviews of stroke treatments.*
chsselearning.org.uk *STARs – Stroke Training and Awareness Resources.*
mdcalc.com/ *Useful calculators for stroke and other disorders.*
ed.ac.uk/clinical-sciences/edinburgh-imaging/education-teaching/short-courses/training-tools/acute-cerebral-ct-evaluation-stroke-study-access *How to read a CT brain scan in acute stroke.*

JA Olson

30

Medical ophthalmology

The ability to see is an important aspect of everyday life. Although rarely a cause of mortality, visual impairment can have a profoundly negative impact on socioeconomic status.

Globally, although refractive errors and cataract remain the main causes of visual impairment, significant progress has occurred in prevention and treatment. Public health measures have reduced diseases of poor hygiene and unclean water, such as trachoma and onchocerciasis, and greater access to surgery has reduced the burden of untreated cataract and glaucoma. However, conditions associated with longevity, such as age-related macular degeneration, diabetic retinopathy and retinal vein occlusion, are increasing.

Traditionally, ophthalmology relied on other specialties to undertake extraocular investigation and treatment. Medical ophthalmology bypasses that co-dependence, allowing patients with visual disorders to receive overarching care within ophthalmology. As such, it requires a good grounding in medicine and many of its sub-specialties. Medical ophthalmology presents a challenge for a medical textbook as it overlaps with almost all other specialties, but particularly neurology. In this book neuro-ophthalmology is mainly covered in Chapter 28. This chapter concentrates on intraocular inflammation, which was the prime drive to create the specialty, and conditions that require intravitreal injection therapy. It does not therefore represent the totality of the medical ophthalmologist's workload.

Ophthalmological conditions that are usually managed within non-ophthalmological specialties are discussed in the corresponding chapters, although for ease of reference the more common ophthalmic features of non-ophthalmological conditions are listed throughout this chapter (haematological disease in Box 30.1, diabetes and endocrine disease in Box 30.2, cardiovascular disease in Box 30.3, respiratory disease in Box 30.4, rheumatological/musculoskeletal disease in Box 30.5, gastrointestinal disease in Box 30.6 and skin disease in Box 30.7).

Functional anatomy and physiology

Visual pathways, innervation of the eye and the control of eye movement are discussed in Chapter 28.

Orbit

The orbit is the fat-filled cavity in which the eye is suspended. It is shaped like a square pyramid, the perimeter of its base being the orbital rim. The orbital periosteum ('periorbita') is continuous with the periosteal layer of cranial dura mater. The dura and arachnoid form the optic nerve sheath, its subarachnoid space containing cerebrospinal fluid in continuity with the third ventricle.

Eyelid/orbital septum/conjunctiva

In primary gaze, the eyelids just cover the superior and inferior cornea. The eyelids contain the orbital septum and the tarsal plate.

Within the tarsal plates, modified sebaceous (Meibomian) glands produce an oily surfactant to slow tear evaporation.

The conjunctiva, a mucous membrane, lines the posterior surface of the eyelid, adhering only to the tarsal plates and the scleral/corneal junction. The accessory lacrimal glands provide basal tear production; mucus produced by goblet cells stabilises the tear film by lowering surface tension.

Lacrimal gland/lacrimal drainage

The lacrimal gland lies within the periorbita of the anterolateral roof of the orbit. Its secretions (tears) wash away surface irritants and convey emotion. Excess tears drain, via canaliculi in the lids, into the lacrimal sac, nasolacrimal duct and inferior nasal meatus.

i 30.1 Ophthalmic features of haematological disease	
Condition	Ophthalmic findings
Severe anaemia of any cause (retinopathy of anaemia)	Flame haemorrhages Cotton wool spots Roth spots Pre-retinal haemorrhage
Megaloblastic anaemia	Optic neuropathy
Sickle cell anaemia	Conjunctival vasculopathy Peripheral retinal neovascularisation
Thalassaemia	Desferrioxamine-associated pigmentary retinopathy
Leukaemia (leukaemic retinopathy)	Pseudohypopyon Flame haemorrhages Roth spots Retinal oedema Retinal vein occlusion
Lymphoma Non-Hodgkin lymphoma Central nervous system lymphoma	Lacrimal gland infiltration Posterior uveitis (atypical choroiditis)
Myeloproliferative disorders Hyperviscosity Cerebral venous thrombosis	Retinal vein occlusion Papilloedema
Paraproteinaemias Waldenström's macroglobulinaemia Multiple myeloma	Retinal vein engorgement/occlusion
Thrombophilia Cerebral venous thrombosis	Papilloedema

Extraocular muscles

The extraocular muscles (Fig. 30.1) consist of four recti, two obliques and one levator. The recti originate from a circular condensation of periorbita, the annulus of Zinn, which encircles the superior orbital fissure and the optic canal. They extend forwards to insert into the anterior sclera.

The levator palpebrae superioris originates above the optic canal and inserts into the tarsal plate and overlying skin of the upper eyelid. The superior tarsal muscle (Müller's muscle) originates from the inferior aspect of the levator and also inserts into the tarsal plate.

The superior oblique originates superonasal to the recti, and runs along the roof of the orbit, its tendon passing horizontally through the trochlea at the orbital rim to insert into the anterior sclera.

The inferior oblique originates from the floor of the anterior orbit, just posterior to the lacrimal sac. It turns horizontally, passing beneath the inferior rectus, to insert into the inferior anterior sclera.

Eye

The optic vesicle develops from the diencephalon. The eye is therefore contiguous with the brain. This is reflected in the three-layer structure of the eye:

- the sclera/cornea, a fibrous outer layer analogous to the meningeal dura
- the choroid, ciliary body and iris (together known as the uveal tract), a vascular middle layer analogous to the pia-arachnoid
- the retina, an inner layer analogous to white matter.

The major structures of the eye are shown in Figure 30.2.

During embryogenesis, overlying ectoderm sinks into the neuroectoderm of the optic vesicle to form the lens vesicle, thus inducing the optic vesicle to form the two-layered optic cup. The inner and outer layers of the optic cup form the neurosensory retina and the retinal pigment epithelium, respectively. The intervening space is continuous with the third

30.2 Ophthalmic features of diabetes and other endocrine disease

Condition	Ophthalmic findings
Diabetes	Proliferative retinopathy Macular oedema Small pupils (autonomic neuropathy) Cataract (including 'snowflake' cataract)
Thyrotoxicosis (any cause)	Eyelid retraction
Graves' disease (TSH receptor antibody-positive)	Exposure keratopathy Conjunctival and periorbital oedema Restrictive ocular motility Proptosis Optic neuropathy
Parathyroid disease	Band keratopathy Corneal calcium deposition
Phaeochromocytoma	Hypertensive retinopathy Cotton wool spots Flame haemorrhages Optic disc oedema with or without macular oedema
Cushing's syndrome	Posterior subcapsular cataract Diabetic retinopathy Central serous retinopathy
Thyroid carcinoma	Horner syndrome with absent unilateral facial sweating

(TSH = thyroid stimulating hormone)

30.3 Ophthalmic features of cardiovascular disease

Condition	Ophthalmic findings
Arteriosclerosis	Arteriovenous nipping Retinal vein occlusion, caused by arteriovenous nipping Retinal artery macroaneurysm Ischaemic optic neuropathy Pupil-sparing third and/or sixth nerve palsy, caused by infarction of the vasa nervosum
Hypertension	Hypertensive retinopathy Cotton wool spots Flame haemorrhages Optic disc oedema, with or without macular oedema
Infective endocarditis	Flame haemorrhages Roth spots Endophthalmitis, caused by haematogenous spread of infection
Drugs	Vortex keratopathy (corneal epithelial deposits), caused by amiodarone (also seen in Fabry's disease) Bilateral optic neuropathy, caused by amiodarone
Thromboembolic disorders (including thromboembolus from atrial fibrillation)	Retinal artery occlusion, caused by artery-to-artery embolism Homonymous hemianopia, caused by embolic stroke

30.4 Ophthalmic features of respiratory disease

Condition	Ophthalmic findings
Chronic obstructive pulmonary disease	Optic disc oedema (type 2 respiratory failure)
Cystic fibrosis	Diabetic retinopathy
Tuberculosis	Anterior uveitis Choroidal granuloma Serpiginous choroiditis Peripheral retinal arteritis Optic neuropathy, visual loss and disturbance of colour vision (adverse effects of ethambutol and isoniazid)
Sarcoidosis	Anterior uveitis (granulomatosis) Mutton fat keratitic precipitates Iris nodules Choroidal granuloma Panuveitis Multifocal choroiditis Retinal periphlebitis Sicca syndrome, caused by lacrimal gland infiltration Exposure keratopathy, caused by corneal exposure secondary to facial nerve palsy Optic neuropathy, caused by optic disc oedema secondary to meningeal infiltration
Lung cancer	Horner syndrome Cancer-associated retinopathy

Initially, the hyaloid artery supplies the lens and vitreous. In its final form, the vitreous develops from the retina and the hyaloid artery regresses, leaving only the central retinal artery and its branches.

Mesenchyme forms the tarsal plates of the eyelid, the stroma and the endothelium of the cornea, the sclera and the choroid.

Surface ectoderm, as well as forming the lens, forms the epidermis of the eyelid, the conjunctiva, the epithelium of the cornea and the lacrimal gland.

Sclera/cornea

The sclera lends shape to the eye and provides attachment for the ocular musculature. It makes up five-sixths of the eyeball, the other sixth being formed by transparent cornea.

The limbus lies at the junction between the cornea and sclera, and contains stem cells and Schlemm's canal. The stem cells allow continuous regeneration of the corneal epithelium. Schlemm's canal, with its overlying trabecular meshwork, drains aqueous fluid from the anterior chamber into the external veins of the episclera and conjunctiva.

The avascular cornea is nourished by diffusion from the anterior chamber, limbal capillaries and oxygen dissolved in the tear film. The cornea, assisted by the lens and the length of the eye, determines the refractive ability of the eye.

The sclera is pierced posteriorly by the optic nerve at the lamina cribrosa, a sieve-like conduit. Its outer layer, the episclera, consists of loose connective tissue, separating it from Tenon's capsule, the soft-tissue socket of the eye.

Choroid, ciliary body and iris – the uveal tract

Posteriorly, the choroid acts as a conduit for branches of the ophthalmic artery and veins. The choriocapillaris, a network of wide-bore, fenestrated capillaries, abuts the retinal pigment epithelium.

The ciliary body forms the junction between the choroid and the iris and lies just inferior to the limbus. Anteriorly, its ciliary processes produce aqueous (fluid) that circulates through the pupil into the anterior chamber. Posteriorly, it constitutes the pars plana and forms

ventricle of the diencephalon. The cilia on the ependymal cells that line the third ventricle are continuous with the cilia on the neurosensory retinal cells, and the latter form the outer segments of the photoreceptors (rods and cones).

30

i **30.5 Ophthalmic features of rheumatological/musculoskeletal disease**

Rheumatoid arthritis
- Keratoconjunctivitis sicca
- Peripheral ulcerative keratitis ('corneal melt')
- Painless episcleritis
- Scleritis and scleromalacia

Seronegative spondyloarthropathies
- Conjunctivitis (chlamydia-associated sexually acquired reactive arthritis, SARA)
- Anterior uveitis

Connective tissue diseases

Dermatomyositis
- Periorbital oedema with violaceous eyelid rash

Sjögren syndrome
- Dry eyes

Treatment effects
- Bull's eye maculopathy (hydroxychloroquine)
- Viral retinitis (immunosuppression)

Systemic vasculitides

Giant cell arteritis
- Central/branch retinal artery occlusion
- Ischaemic optic neuropathy

Behçet's disease
- Occlusive retinal vasculitis (posterior uveitis)
- Anterior uveitis with hypopyon

Granulomatosis with polyangiitis
- Scleritis with involvement of adjacent cornea (sclerokeratitis)
- Retro-orbital inflammation (see Fig. 26.53)

Polyarteritis nodosa
- Peripheral ulcerative keratitis
- Scleritis
- Retinal arteritis

Others/non-specific
- Necrotising scleritis/sclerokeratitis/peripheral ulcerative keratitis
- Anterior ischaemic optic neuropathy
- Extraocular myositis (painful diplopia)
- Retinal arteritis
- Pupil-sparing 3rd nerve palsy
- 6th nerve palsy
- Proptosis
- Occipital lobe infarction

Diseases of bone

Paget's disease, polyostotic fibrous dysplasia
- Optic neuropathy

Others/non-specific
- Anterior uveitis (adverse effect of bisphosphonates)

i **30.6 Ophthalmic features of gastrointestinal disease**

Malabsorption
- Corneal and conjunctival keratinisation
- Rod photoreceptor loss

Chronic pancreatitis
- Diabetic retinopathy

Inflammatory bowel disease
- Episcleritis
- Non-necrotising scleritis
- Anterior uveitis

Large bowel tumours
- Atypical congenital retinal pigment epithelium hypertrophy (familial adenomatous polyposis)

Inherited liver disease
- Kayser–Fleischer corneal rings, sunflower cataracts (Wilson's disease)
- Diabetic retinopathy (haemochromatosis)

i **30.7 Ophthalmic features of skin disease**

Rosacea
- Posterior blepharitis
- Keratitis

Acne vulgaris
- Dry eye (adverse effect of isotretinoin)
- Papilloedema (adverse effect of tetracycline)

Psoriasis
- Anterior uveitis

Eczema
- Atopic keratoconjunctivitis

Urticaria
- Angioedema

Bullous diseases
- Ocular cicatricial pemphigoid
- Stevens–Johnson syndrome

Alopecia areata
- Eyebrow and eyelash loss

Cutaneous melanoma
- Melanoma-associated retinopathy

Skin tumours
- Eyelid tumours (basal cell carcinoma, squamous cell carcinoma, keratoacanthoma, naevus, melanoma)

Skin infections
- Stye (eyelash folliculitis)
- Acute blepharoconjunctivitis (herpes simplex)
- Chronic conjunctivitis (molluscum contagiosum)

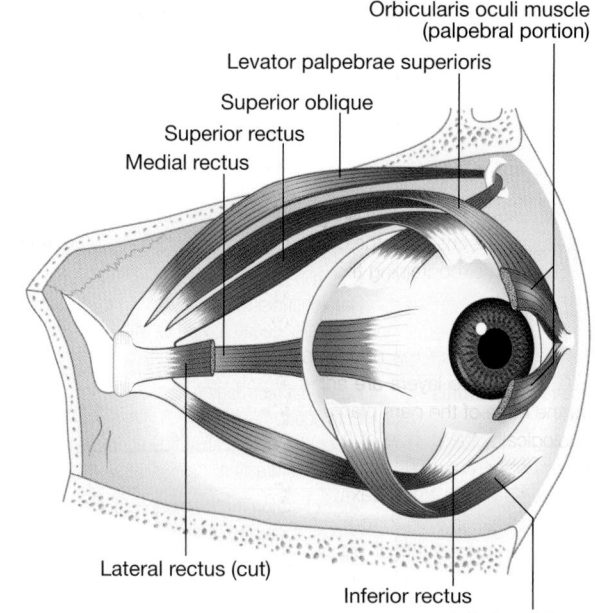

Fig. 30.1 The extraocular musculature (right eye). *Adapted from Batterbury M, Bowling B, Murphy C. Ophthalmology. An illustrated colour text, 3rd edn. Ednburgh: Churchill Livingstone, Elsevier Ltd; 2009.*

the attachments for the suspensory ligaments of the lens. The ciliary muscle encircles the eye within the ciliary body. Contraction of this muscle relaxes the suspensory ligaments of the lens, bringing near objects into focus.

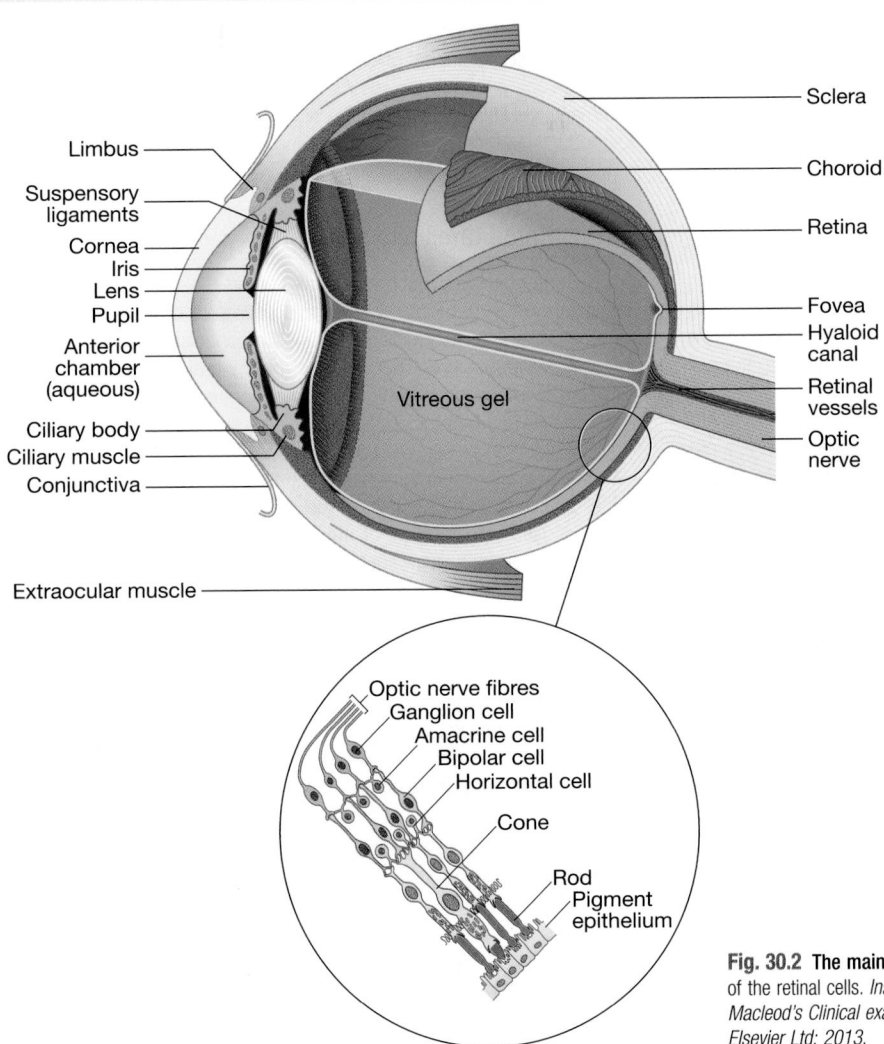

Sclera
Choroid
Retina
Fovea
Hyaloid canal
Retinal vessels
Optic nerve

Limbus
Suspensory ligaments
Cornea
Iris
Lens
Pupil
Anterior chamber (aqueous)
Ciliary body
Ciliary muscle
Conjunctiva

Vitreous gel

Extraocular muscle

Optic nerve fibres
Ganglion cell
Amacrine cell
Bipolar cell
Horizontal cell
Cone
Rod
Pigment epithelium

Fig. 30.2 The main structures of the eye. The inset shows the arrangement of the retinal cells. *Inset adapted from Douglas G, Nicol F, Robertson C (eds). Macleod's Clinical examination, 13th edn. Edinburgh: Churchill Livingstone, Elsevier Ltd; 2013.*

The iris bows gently forwards as it lies against the lens. It is divided into a pupillary zone, containing the circumferential sphincter pupillae muscle, and a ciliary zone, containing the dilator pupillae.

Retina

The retina consists of the neurosensory retina and the retinal pigment epithelium. The two layers are adherent only adjacent to the optic disc and at the edge of the pars plana.

Histologically, the centre of the retina is termed the macula lutea, its yellowish appearance caused by the presence of the xanthophylls (yellow pigments) lutein and zeaxanthin. At the centre of the macula, the neurosensory retina dips to form the fovea.

The single-layered retinal pigment epithelium is highly metabolically active and is essential for the maintenance and survival of the overlying photoreceptors.

The neurosensory retina initiates the visual pathway. Its photoreceptors synapse with radially arranged bipolar neurons, which in turn synapse with circumferentially arranged optic nerve ganglion cells.

'Horizontal' and amacrine cells within the plexiform layers modulate neuronal activity between bipolar cells, photoreceptors and the ganglion cells. At the fovea, a one-to-one relationship between cones, bipolar neurons and ganglion cells leads to the highest acuity. In the peripheral retina, many rods converge on to a bipolar neuron, and many bipolar neurons converge on to a ganglion cell, leading to lower acuity. In effect, the peripheral retina conveys black-and-white sentinel vision, alerting the brain to move the higher-acuity colour vision of the fovea into gaze.

Photoreceptors are specialised neurons that cause neurotransmitters to be released in response to light ('phototransduction'). There are three types of photoreceptors: namely, rods, cones and ganglion cells, the last of which independently respond to blue light, influencing circadian rhythms.

Lens

The lens is a transparent flexible structure suspended between the iris and the vitreous. Its flexibility enables objects over a range of distances to be focused on the retina. It has a capsule, a central nucleus and a peripheral cortex. It continues to grow throughout life, becoming less flexible with age.

Vitreous

The vitreous gel is 99% water and 1% collagen/hyaluronic acid. The outer edge (cortex) of the vitreous condenses to form the anterior and posterior hyaloid membranes. The base of the vitreous strongly adheres to the ora serrata/pars plana and the optic disc rim, where the internal limiting membrane of the retina is thinnest. Lesser degrees of adhesion occur at the parafoveal retina and along the retinal vessels.

Blood supply of the orbit/eye

The main blood supply of the orbit originates from the intracranial internal carotid artery. The ophthalmic artery, the first branch of the internal carotid artery, traverses the subarachnoid space to enter the optic canal

30

within the dural sheath of the optic nerve. On leaving the optic canal, it emerges from the dural sheath to course briefly along, and then over, the optic nerve to reach the medial wall of the orbit.

Several arterial circles are formed. The major arterial circle of the iris is formed within the ciliary body by anterior ciliary arteries anastomosing with the posterior ciliary arteries. The pial branches of the optic nerve and the short ciliary arteries join together, as the circle of Zinn, to supply the intraocular optic nerve.

The infraorbital artery, a branch of the maxillary artery, also contributes to the orbital blood supply, in particular the inferior rectus, the inferior oblique and the lacrimal sac.

The orbit is drained by the superior and inferior ophthalmic veins, which converge to drain through the superior orbital fissure into the cavernous sinus.

Investigation of visual disorders

History is the key to diagnosing visual disorders, with examination and investigations used to confirm or refute the expectations formed by the history.

Perimetry

In the era before modern radiology, manual perimetry was utilised as a non-invasive form of 'neuroimaging'. Nowadays, perimetry is largely automated and its main role lies in the monitoring of glaucoma; it also has a lesser role in assessing neuro-ophthalmic disorders. All methods of perimetry are subjective and rely on patient cooperation and mental agility.

Amsler chart

The Amsler chart (Fig. 30.3) is the simplest method of documenting the visual field, and is easy for both patient and clinician to understand and perform. It can be used for all forms of visual field loss but is best suited to follow up the central scotomata of macular disorders, which are often too subtle for other methods of perimetry.

Tangent/Goldmann kinetic perimetry

Manual perimetry methods, such as tangent screen and Goldmann kinetic perimetry, appeal to the non-specialist, as they produce easily interpretable contoured maps of the visual field.

The tangent screen is a piece of black cloth attached to a wall, in front of which the operator introduces moving targets into the patient's field of

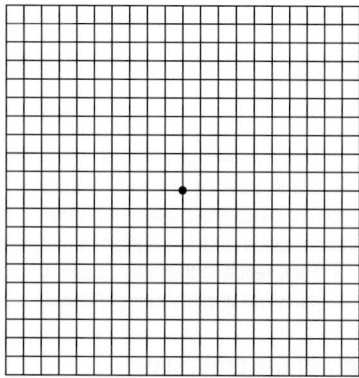

Fig. 30.3 Amsler chart. The Amsler chart is a grid of 0.5 cm squares with a dot in the centre. The subject is asked to fix on the central dot with one eye and any distorted or missing lines are recorded.

view. It retains an important role in the positive identification of functional peripheral field loss (tunnel vision) versus pathological peripheral field loss (funnel vision), although the results are somewhat operator-dependent. Goldmann perimetry is a mechanical improvement on tangent screen perimetry, which utilises targets of varying size and illumination. An automated version is available.

Automated threshold perimetry

Automated visual fields test the threshold of the eye's ability to see at various points within the visual field, forming complex outputs that can be stored digitally. Internal quality assurance mechanisms monitor stability of fixation, false positives due to trigger-happy patients and false negatives due to performance fatigue. Many patients need practice before accurate results are obtained; first-time fields are rarely reliable and often show spurious and misleading findings.

Most automated perimetry assesses only central vision. Few neurological disorders start peripherally, the exception being unilateral loss of peripheral field with disease of the anterior pole of the occipital lobe. However, retinal pathology, such as retinal detachment and retinitis pigmentosa, may be missed if reliance is placed on automated perimetry rather than clinical examination.

Visual field defects on perimetry that affect the whole of the superior or inferior half of the visual field need to be differentiated by confrontation into arcuate visual field defects, which affect central field only, and altitudinal field defects, which affect both central and peripheral vision. Arcuate visual field defects localise a lesion to the optic nerve head, whereas a lesion anywhere along the optic nerve can cause an altitudinal defect.

Imaging

See Figure 30.4.

Photography

Digital photography is utilised to document surface anatomy. Colour images are ideal for lesions affecting the skin and cornea. For the retina, however, red-free imaging brings additional benefits, particularly for discriminating red haemorrhages or abnormal new vessels from the red background of the retina. Wide-field imaging is increasingly replacing the need to examine the fundus clinically.

Optical coherence tomography (OCT)

Optical coherence tomography is the optical equivalent of ultrasound, using light rather than sound waves to create its images. It is invaluable, not least for assessing the integrity of the layers of the retina and detecting macular oedema of any cause.

Autofluorescence

The retinal pigment epithelium contains autofluorescent lipofuscin, which can be excited by blue- and green-coloured light and captured by digital imaging.

Increased autofluorescence occurs when there is abnormal accumulation of lipofuscin, as seen with certain inherited retinal dystrophies; excess retinal pigment epithelium metabolic activity, such as at the edge of evolving atrophic macular degeneration; or drug deposition, such as with hydoxychloroquine.

Fundus angiography

Fluorescein angiography is an invasive technique with risks including local extravasation of dye at the site of intravenous injection and anaphylaxis. Currently, its role is limited to the diagnosis of retinal vasculitis, retinal and choroidal neovascularisation, and capillary occlusion. Non-invasive

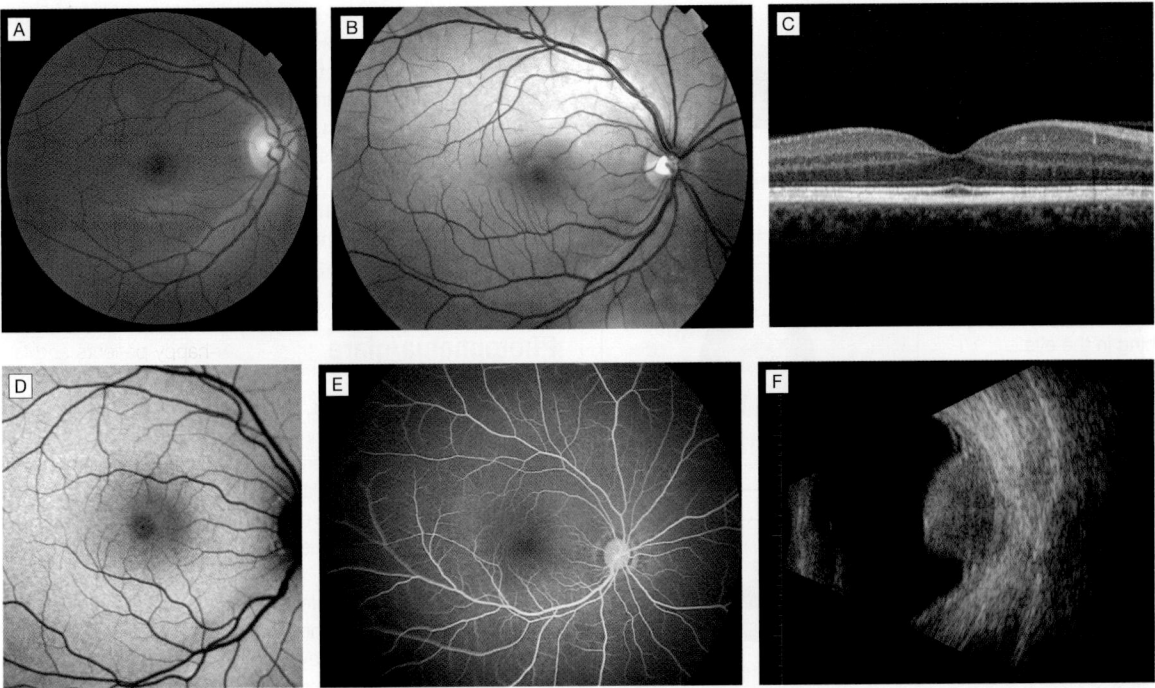

Fig. 30.4 Ocular imaging. A Colour retinal photograph from a healthy subject. B Red-free retinal photograph from a healthy subject. C Optical coherence tomogram of a normal eye, showing the layers of the retina. In this image, the macula shows normal foveal indentation. D Fundus autofluorescence (FAF) of the right eye in a normal subject. Distribution of FAF intensity shows typical background signal with reduced signal at the optic disc (absence of autofluorescent material) and retinal vessels (absorption). Intensity is markedly decreased over the fovea due to the absorption of the blue light by yellow macular pigment. E Fundal fluorescein angiogram of a normal adult retina. F Ocular ultrasound image showing typical biconvex appearance of a choroidal melanoma. *(A, B, C and F) Courtesy of Aberdeen Royal Infirmary. (D) From Schmitz-Valckenberg S, Fleckenstein M, Hendrik PN, et al. Fundus autofluorescence and progression of age-related macular degeneration. Surv Ophthalmol 2009; 54(1):96–117. (E) From Witmer MT, Szilárd K. Wide-field imaging of the retina. Surv Ophthalmol 2013; 58(2):143–154.*

angiography is now possible using optical coherence tomography, but its applicability is limited by small field of view and inability to demonstrate flow or leakage.

Indocyanine angiography directly images the choroidal circulation and is particularly useful in guiding laser treatment for the choroidal polyps of polypoidal choroidal vasculopathy.

Ocular ultrasound

The main role of ultrasound is where the retina is obscured: for instance, by cataract or vitreous haemorrhage. It also has an important role in diagnosing choroidal melanoma, based on its distinctive internal reflectivity.

Visual electrophysiology

Electrophysiology is used to localise disorders to the photoreceptors (electroretinogram), the retinal ganglion cells (pattern electroretinogram) or the optic pathways (visual evoked potential). The site of photoreceptor involvement can be further localised to specific regions of the retina (multifocal electroretinogram) or the macula itself (pattern electroretinogram).

Electrophysiology requires cooperation, correction of refractive errors and the ability to fixate. Voluntary suppression of the electrical responses is possible by simply not focusing on the target. Despite this, it remains the investigation of choice for visual symptoms unexplained by clinical examination.

Presenting problems in ophthalmic disease

Presenting problems that are ophthalmological manifestations of predominantly neurological disease (e.g. ptosis, diplopia, oscillopsia, nystagmus and pupillary abnormalities) are discussed in Chapter 28.

Watery/dry eye

The most common cause of a watery eye is a dry eye triggering reflex lacrimation. Patients with dry eye may complain of a foreign body or gritty sensation in the eye or intermittent visual blurring, triggered by reduced blinking, as occurs when reading or when concentrating on a distant object, such as the television.

Pruritus

Common causes of itch are an acute allergic response to either airborne allergens or direct contact. A significant proportion of people are allergic to topical chloramphenicol, a first-line treatment for many minor ocular ailments.

Pain/headache

The key consideration in deciding whether or not ocular pain and/or headache originates from the eye is whether there is a ciliary flush (red eye) or no ciliary flush (white eye).

Red eye

The presence of a ciliary flush in the region of the limbus is a key finding in intraocular causes of pain. The presence of watering or watery discharge is not a discriminatory feature, and over-reliance on this symptom often results in anterior uveitis being misdiagnosed as viral conjunctivitis. The features that are used to distinguish between different causes of red eye are illustrated in Figure 30.5.

White eye

In the absence of a ciliary flush (see Fig. 30.5), ocular or periorbital pain is most commonly caused by migraine.

30

Normal eye anatomy

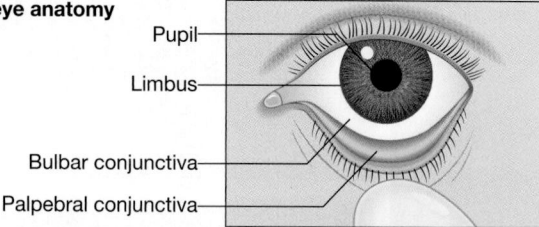

Blepharitis
- Red eyelid margin, symptoms of dry eye, irritation, feeling of something in the eye
- Common in all age groups and may be associated with rosacea or seborrhoeic dermatitis

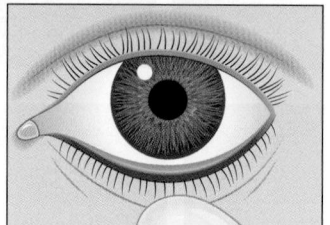

Conjunctivitis
- Maximal redness in palpebral conjunctiva, rest of eye may or may not be red
- The discharge of viral conjunctivitis may be hard to differentiate from reflex lacrimation due to photophobia of any cause

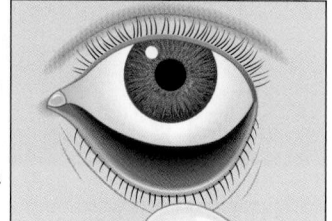

Ciliary flush
- Redness first appears at limbus and then spreads outwards
- Early sign of intraocular inflammation, e.g. anterior uveitis, keratitis or acute angle closure glaucoma

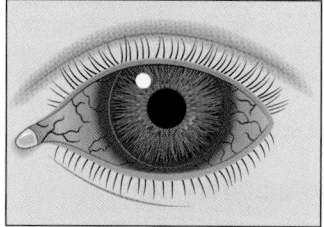

Subconjunctival haemorrhage
- Bright red in colour, note sparing of limbus
- Patient often unconcerned, unless part of severe head injury. Usually spontaneous, triggered by Valsalva manoeuvre

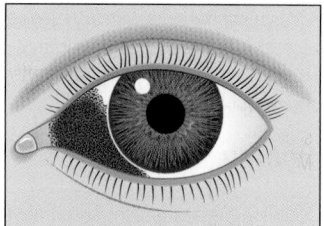

Scleritis
- Usually extensive, often bilateral, true extent often hidden by lids
- Unlike episcleritis, this is always painful, often waking the patient at night

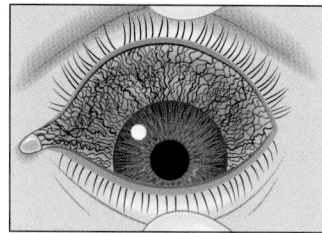

Fig. 30.5 Common causes of red eye.

Pain on eye movement is a cardinal feature of optic neuritis and scleritis. In optic neuritis the eye is white, whereas in scleritis, except for posterior scleritis, it is red.

Posterior scleritis, in which the visible sclera is white, should be diagnosed only in the setting of positive signs such as disc swelling and exudative retinal detachment, or with confirmation by ocular ultrasound. A more common cause of severe ocular/periocular pain, with associated photophobia and lacrimation, is cluster headache, which is often misdiagnosed as scleritis. Just like scleritis, cluster headache responds to oral glucocorticoids, adding to the diagnostic confusion.

Intermittent, subacute angle closure glaucoma can cause headache, but usually accompanying corneal oedema causes haloes (a form of glare with rainbow colours), elicited by looking at lights or blurring of vision.

Giant cell arteritis (see Ch. 26) occasionally presents with sudden painless visual loss in the absence of raised inflammatory markers. Diagnosis can be made by demonstrating absence of choroidal blood flow on fluorescein angiography.

Photophobia/glare

Excessive sensitivity to light, rather than fear of light, usually indicates ciliary muscle spasm due to inflammation in the iris. Common causes are corneal abrasion, acute anterior uveitis and contact lens-related keratitis.

Occasionally, photophobia can be a symptom of congenital retinal dystrophies, especially cone photoreceptor deficiency. Photophobia may also be a feature of meningitis, usually with accompanying neck stiffness and headache (meningism).

Glare is a common early feature of cataract, particularly triggered by oncoming car headlights when driving at night. It is a relatively common indication for surgery. It may also be an issue where there is insufficient melanin in the retinal pigment epithelium, e.g. in atrophic age-related macular degeneration, in ocular albinism or following extensive pan-retinal laser therapy. If surgery is not an option, or while surgery is awaited, the symptom of glare may be reduced by wearing a broad-brimmed hat.

Photopsia

A flickering light sensation is indicative of photoreceptor activity, either through traction, as in the setting of posterior vitreous detachment, or inflammation, as in the setting of autoimmune or paraneoplastic retinopathy. Rarely, photopsia is a symptom of occipital lobe epilepsy, in which case there is usually an accompanying homonymous hemianopia.

Blurred vision

Blurred vision describes the situation in which patients are able to see what they are looking at, but what they are looking at is out of focus. The most common cause of intermittent blurred vision is dry eye; the most common cause of permanent blurred vision is cataract. If blurred vision is worse in the morning and eases as the day progresses, this suggests macular oedema.

Loss of vision

In visual loss, patients are no longer able to see all or part of what they are looking at. This may be manifested as either negative visual phenomena, in which part or all of what is being looked at is missing, or positive visual phenomena, in which the object of regard appears to be hidden by something in the way. In positive phenomena the obstruction is often white or coloured, and may either expand across the visual field or remain in a constant position, sometimes shimmering. The most common cause of transient visual loss is the aura of migraine, which is described in Chapter 28.

Negative visual phenomena are a cardinal feature of ocular, usually retinal, ischaemia, with complete absence of vision (blackness) occupying part or all the visual field. Transient ocular ischaemia is usually embolic in nature but is occasionally seen in giant cell arteritis, where it suggests critical optic nerve ischaemia. Permanent monocular negative visual phenomena usually indicate previous optic nerve or retinal infarction. Tiny negative visual phenomena may also be seen in capillary disorders such as diabetic retinopathy, where patchy macular capillary occlusion may, for instance, cause letters to be missing from words on reading.

The clinical features and causes of visual loss (including neurological causes) are summarised in Box 30.8. Some symptoms associated with visual loss require urgent ophthalmological assessment (Box 30.9).

Distortion of vision

Distortion is a cardinal symptom of disruption of foveal photoreceptor alignment. The most common cause is choroidal neovascularisation. Less commonly, it can be caused by epiretinal membrane formation, where posterior hyaloid surface scarring causes foveal traction.

Usually with distortion, objects are not only misshapen but also smaller (micropsia), due to the photoreceptors being pulled apart. Macropsia, where objects look bigger than normal, is uncommon. It is sometimes seen in the 'Alice in Wonderland' syndrome, a paediatric variant of migraine, where there is altered visual perception of body images.

Eyelid retraction

Eyelid retraction is usually caused by inflammatory thyroid eye disease or thyrotoxicosis (see Ch. 20 and Fig. 20.9).

The first muscle to be affected in thyroid eye disease is the inferior rectus. The enlarged muscle tethers the eye and restricts upgaze. Compensatory increased innervation to the superior rectus and the levator palpebrae superioris, as well as direct inflammation, leads to eyelid retraction.

In thyrotoxicosis, increased sympathetic nervous activity leads to bilateral eyelid retraction. This, however, resolves with beta-blockade and treatment of thyrotoxicosis.

✚ 30.9 Red flag symptoms in visual loss*

Symptom	Possible causes
Sudden onset	Retinal artery occlusion Ischaemic optic neuropathy
Headache	Giant cell arteritis if age >55 years
Eye pain	Angle closure glaucoma Keratitis Scleritis Anterior uveitis
Pain on eye movement	Optic neuritis Scleritis

Distortion	Choroidal neovascular membrane:
	    Age-related macular degeneration
	    Pathological myopia
	    Posterior uveitis
	    Idiopathic
	Macular hole

Worse in the morning	Macular oedema:
	    Diabetic macular oedema
	    Retinal vein occlusion
	    Uveitis

*The presence of any of these symptoms in a patient with visual loss requires emergency referral to an ophthalmologist.

ℹ 30.8 Clinical manifestations of visual field loss

Site of lesion	Common causes	Complaint	Visual field loss	Associated physical signs
Retina/optic disc	Vascular disease (including vasculitis) Glaucoma Inflammation	Partial/complete visual loss depending on site, involving one or both eyes	Altitudinal field defect Arcuate scotoma	Reduced acuity Visual distortion (macula) Abnormal retinal appearance Reduced colour vision Relative afferent pupillary defect (RAPD, Fig. 30.6)
Optic nerve	Optic neuritis Sarcoidosis Tumour Leber's hereditary optic neuropathy	Partial/complete loss of vision in one eye Often painful Central vision particularly affected	Central or paracentral scotoma Monocular blindness	Reduced acuity Reduced colour vision RAPD Optic atrophy (late)
Optic chiasm	Pituitary tumour Craniopharyngioma Sarcoidosis	May be none Rarely, diplopia ('hemifield slide')	Bitemporal hemianopia	Pituitary function abnormalities Reduced acuity Reduced colour vision RAPD Optic atrophy (late)
Optic tract	Tumour Inflammatory disease	Disturbed vision to one side of midline	Incongruous contralateral homonymous hemianopia	
Temporal lobe	Stroke Tumour Inflammatory disease	Disturbed vision to one side of midline	Contralateral homonymous upper quadrantanopia	Memory/language disorders
Parietal lobe	Stroke Tumour Inflammatory disease	Disturbed vision to one side of midline Bumping into things	Contralateral homonymous lower quadrantanopia	Contralateral sensory disturbance Asymmetry of optokinetic nystagmus
Occipital lobe	Stroke Tumour Inflammatory disease	Disturbed vision to one side of midline Difficulty reading Bumping into things	Homonymous hemianopia (may be macula-sparing)	Damage to other structures supplied by posterior cerebral circulation

30

Rarely, bilateral eyelid retraction is a sign of dorsal mid-brain pathology (Collier's sign), where it is accompanied by a supranuclear upgaze palsy and convergence–retraction nystagmus.

Optic disc swelling and papilloedema

Optic disc swelling (Box 30.10) can be a developmental variant of normal (pseudopapilloedema), a manifestation of optic nerve pathology, or a reflection of more widespread nerve-fibre oedema, as with retinal vein occlusion.

Papilloedema is optic disc swelling occurring as a result of raised intracranial pressure. In this situation obstructed axoplasmic flow from retinal ganglion cells results in swollen nerve fibres, which in turn cause capillary and venous congestion, producing papilloedema. The earliest

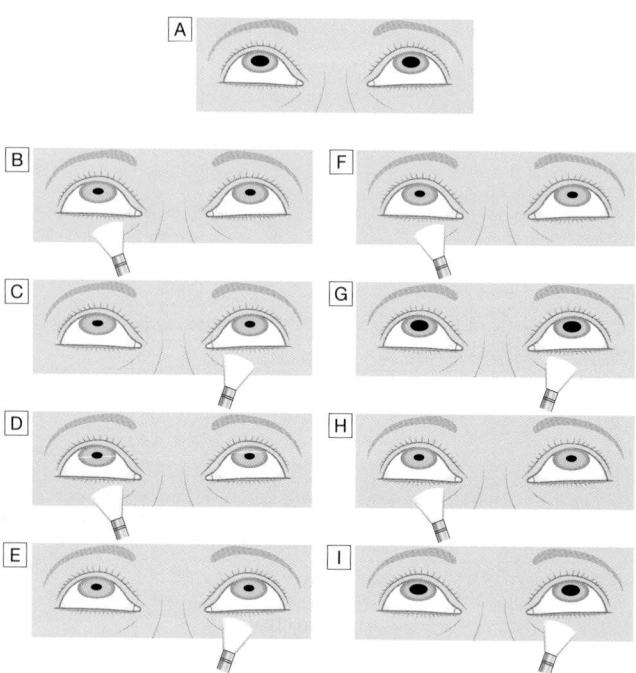

Fig. 30.6 Relative afferent pupillary defect (RAPD). The eyes are examined in upgaze. [A] Pupils in ambient light. [B–E] When a light is swung back and forth to each eye both pupils constrict equally. [F–I] With a left-sided RAPD the constricting effect of shining the light into the left eye is reduced on both sides, so the pupils dilate each time the light swings to the left eye.

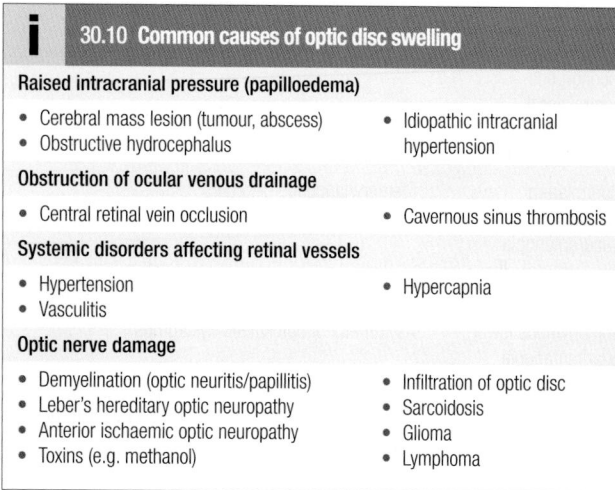

i | **30.10 Common causes of optic disc swelling**

Raised intracranial pressure (papilloedema)

- Cerebral mass lesion (tumour, abscess)
- Obstructive hydrocephalus
- Idiopathic intracranial hypertension

Obstruction of ocular venous drainage

- Central retinal vein occlusion
- Cavernous sinus thrombosis

Systemic disorders affecting retinal vessels

- Hypertension
- Vasculitis
- Hypercapnia

Optic nerve damage

- Demyelination (optic neuritis/papillitis)
- Leber's hereditary optic neuropathy
- Anterior ischaemic optic neuropathy
- Toxins (e.g. methanol)
- Infiltration of optic disc
- Sarcoidosis
- Glioma
- Lymphoma

sign is the cessation of venous pulsation seen at the disc, progression causing the disc margins to become red (hyperaemic). Disc margins become indistinct and haemorrhages may occur in the retina (Fig. 30.7). The absence of papilloedema does not exclude the possibility of raised intracranial pressure.

Normal variations of disc appearance (e.g. optic nerve drusen) may mimic disc swelling.

Proptosis

Proptosis, particularly if bilateral and symmetrical, is often first recognised when it is quite advanced. Accompanying eyelid retraction is a typical feature of thyroid eye disease. By far the most common cause is thyroid eye disease, when proptosis is termed exophthalmos.

Proptosis is a sign of retro-orbital expansion and may be intraconal or extraconal. When expansion is within the cone of extraocular muscles, then movement forwards will be in line with the visual axis. When outside, the eye is additionally displaced to the side.

The primary clinical concern is whether vision is at risk due to optic nerve compression or corneal exposure. In addition, there may be double vision. In thyroid eye disease, diplopia may be absent if the disease is symmetrical. Instead, restricted ocular movements make patients move their head en bloc when looking at objects deviating from the primary position of gaze. To the patient, however, the overarching concern is often the change in appearance.

Optic atrophy

Loss of nerve fibres causes the optic disc to appear pale, as the sclera becomes visible (Fig. 30.8). A pale disc (optic atrophy) follows optic nerve damage; causes include previous optic neuritis or ischaemic damage, long-standing papilloedema, optic nerve compression, trauma and degenerative conditions (e.g. Friedreich's ataxia, see Box 28.55).

Specialist ophthalmological conditions

Ocular inflammation

Inflammation can affect any part of the eye. In structures in direct contact with the environment, particularly the cornea and the conjunctiva, inflammation is most likely to be caused by infection. In other structures, such as the uveal tract and sclera, inflammation is more likely to be caused by autoimmune conditions, although it may also be a manifestation of infection or malignancy. Although the latter conditions may present with indicative ocular signs, their presence is often appreciated only retrospectively, after failure to respond to immunosuppression.

Most non-infective forms of ocular inflammation are idiopathic; all are more common in the presence of other autoimmune conditions. Some may be directly associated but asynchronous in disease activity, such as the anterior uveitis of ankylosing spondylitis. Others are direct manifestations of an overarching, underlying, inflammatory condition such as the keratoscleritis of granulomatosis with polyangiitis (formerly known as Wegener's granulomatosis).

Sjögren syndrome

Sjögren syndrome is the archetypal autoimmune disease and its secondary form is associated with a large number of other autoimmune conditions (see Box 26.64). The cardinal features are inflammation of the lacrimal gland, its conjunctival accessory glands and the parotid gland, leading to hyposecretion of tears and saliva. Involvement of the lacrimal gland alone causes keratoconjunctivitis sicca, a syndrome of dry eyes and corneal and conjunctival irritation. Keratoconjunctivitis sicca, however, can also be caused by reduced function of the lacrimal glands and/or lacrimal ducts from other causes.

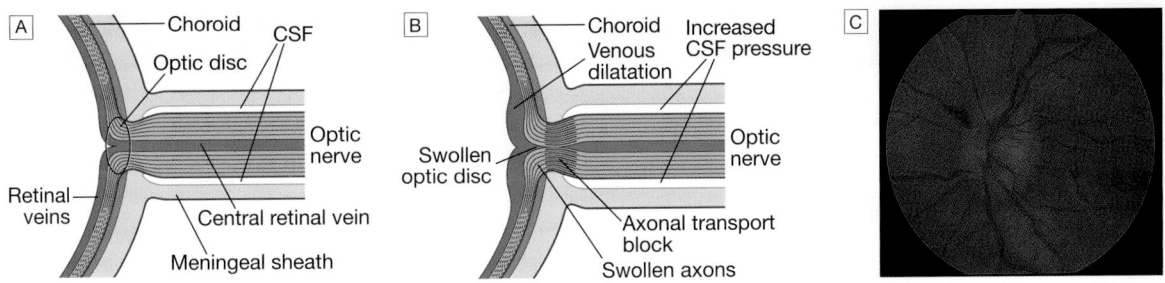

Fig. 30.7 Mechanism of optic disc oedema (papilloedema). [A] Normal. [B] Disc oedema (e.g. due to cerebral tumour). [C] Fundus photograph of the left eye showing optic disc oedema with a small haemorrhage on the nasal side of the disc. (CSF = cerebrospinal fluid) *(C) Courtesy of Dr B. Cullen.*

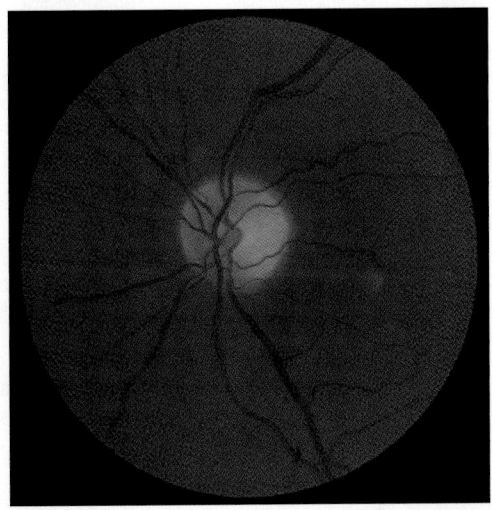

Fig. 30.8 Fundus photograph of the left eye of a patient with familial optic atrophy. Note the marked pallor of the optic disc.

Treatment of the ophthalmological manifestations of Sjögren syndrome is symptomatic, and consists of supplementing tear production with artificial tears (e.g. hypromellose) and reducing tear loss by humidification and avoidance of dry environments. If these measures are insufficient, tear drainage may be reduced with surgical options such as punctal plugs and punctal occlusion.

Peripheral ulcerative keratitis

Peripheral ulcerative keratitis ('corneal melting') is an autoimmune disorder affecting the corneal limbus, where it may be accompanied by adjacent scleritis. It may be directly associated with inflammatory disorders in which immune complexes are formed, particularly rheumatoid arthritis, systemic lupus erythematosus and granulomatosis with polyangiitis. Pain and redness are helpful indicators but may not always be present. Systemic immunosuppression is always required but topical glucocorticoids should be used cautiously due to the risk of aggravating keratolysis (corneal thinning). Secondary infection should be prevented with topical antibiotics and attention should be paid to corneal hydration, through the use of artificial tears and lubricants.

More common causes of peripheral corneal ulceration are blepharitis and acne rosacea, which cause ocular irritation rather than frank pain. Hypersensitivity to staphylococcal exotoxin leads to stromal infiltrate adjacent to, but sparing, the limbus (marginal keratitis). Resolution of this self-limiting condition can be assisted by the use of topical chloramphenicol, with or without topical glucocorticoids. Prevention is through management of the underlying condition, usually with ocular lid hygiene for simple blepharitis and metronidazole gel for rosacea.

Scleritis

Scleritis is usually accompanied by severe pain, worse on eye movement and often waking the patient through the night. Diagnosis of anterior scleritis is usually straightforward, with the eye showing diffuse or nodular erythema (although it may have to be searched for under the eyelids). Posterior uveitis is often accompanied by reduced vision and oedema of the retina, choroid and extraocular muscles.

White patches of necrosis (pallor) within the erythema are an ominous sign, indicative of systemic vasculitis. Non-necrotising scleritis is commonly idiopathic but may be associated with other autoimmune conditions, particularly rheumatoid arthritis and inflammatory bowel disease. It is also common with herpes zoster ophthalmicus, intraocular involvement being indicated by the involvement of the lateral external nose (Hutchison's sign).

Necrotising scleritis requires aggressive immunosuppression; non-necrotising scleritis can occasionally be managed by topical glucocorticoids or non-steroidal anti-inflammatory drugs (NSAIDs) but usually requires oral glucocorticoids.

Some patients with recurrent episodes of scleritis, or in whom inflammation is gradual and prolonged, may develop scleral thinning (scleromalacia), revealing the underlying blue choroid.

Episcleritis

Episcleritis is a benign self-limiting condition of uncertain aetiology, occasionally associated with other inflammatory disorders. Sectoral redness of the episclera is usual, although nodules can form. Often confused with scleritis, although usually less symptomatic, the diagnostic topical application of phenylephrine turns the inflamed episclera white but has no effect on the redness of scleritis. Treatment is with cold artificial tears, although occasionally topical NSAIDs or topical glucocorticoids are required.

Uveitis

Uveitis is an overarching term for inflammation anywhere in the uveal tract, retina or vitreous. It may be classified according to speed of onset, location, specific features, or aetiology (Box 30.11). Syphilis can cause all forms of uveitis. Active tuberculosis may present with an occlusive vasculitis or serpiginous (snake-like) choroiditis emanating from the optic disc. Latent tuberculosis is a particular concern because treatment of the uveitis with biologics may induce active systemic infection. Furthermore, the type of biologic most commonly used for uveitis, anti-tumour necrosis factor therapy (e.g. adalimumab, infliximab), may trigger demyelination.

The most common form of uveitis is anterior uveitis, which is usually idiopathic and may be associated with other autoimmune conditions, particularly HLA-B27-related spondyloarthropathies (Ch. 26); it is rarely caused directly by infection. Acutely, dilating drops are used to prevent the inflamed iris from sticking to the lens (posterior synechiae) and obstructing the outflow of aqueous fluid, while a tapering dose of topical

30

i 30.11 Aetiology of uveitis

Idiopathic

- Anterior uveitis often associated with the HLA-B27 haplotype, even in the absence of other manifestations

Primary ophthalmic conditions

- Trauma, including penetrating injury and ophthalmic surgery
- Fuchs heterochromic cyclitis
- Posner–Schlossman syndrome

Rheumatological

- HLA-B27-associated (seronegative) spondyloarthropathies: ankylosing spondylitis, psoriatic arthritis, reactive arthritis
- Juvenile idiopathic arthritis

Systemic vasculitides

- Behçet's disease
- Polyarteritis nodosa
- Granulomatosis with polyangiitis (Wegener's)

Systemic infections (only the more common causes are listed)

- Brucellosis
- Herpes virus infections (cytomegalovirus, herpes simplex virus, varicella zoster virus)
- Leptospirosis
- Lyme borreliosis
- Syphilis
- Toxoplasmosis
- Tuberculosis
- Whipple's disease

Gastrointestinal conditions

- Inflammatory bowel disease (Crohn's disease, ulcerative colitis)

Malignancy

- Primary central nervous system lymphoma (rare)

Systemic conditions of unknown cause

- Multiple sclerosis
- Sarcoidosis

i 30.12 Common causes of infectious keratitis

Organism	Features/comments	Treatment
Viruses		
Herpes simplex	Characteristic 'dendritic' ulcer is the most common form, often recurrent	Topical/systemic acyclovir (with topical glucocorticoid for stromal keratitis once the epithelium is healed)
Varicella zoster	Herpes zoster ophthalmicus	Systemic aciclovir
Bacteria		
Pseudomonas aeruginosa *Staphylococcus aureus* Coagulase-negative staphylococci *Cutibacterium* (formerly *Propionibacterium*) spp.	Coagulase-negative staphylococci and *Cutibacterium* spp. are members of the skin flora, and must not be dismissed as contaminants	Topical fluoroquinolone with Gram-positive and Gram-negative cover (e.g. ofloxacin) Subsequent treatment depends on sensitivity testing results
Fungi		
Fusarium sp. *Aspergillus* sp. *Candida* sp.	*Fusarium* and *Aspergillus* keratitis are often associated with soil and/ or corneal trauma; may also be contact lens-related *Candida* causes post-keratoplasty keratitis	Options include topical natamycin (if available), amphotericin B, voriconazole and other azoles (e.g. econazole), and systemic fluconazole or voriconazole
Parasites		
Acanthamoeba castellanii (free-living amoeba)	Associated with poor contact lens hygiene	Topical polyhexamethylene biguanide
Onchocerca volvulus (nematode)	See Chapter 13	

glucocorticoids, usually over 4–6 weeks, mitigates the local signs and symptoms of the self-resolving inflammation. Inadequate treatment can lead to pupil block glaucoma and cataract. Posterior complications can also develop, predominantly macular oedema, the main cause of visual impairment in all forms of uveitis.

With intermediate uveitis, inflammation occurs at the pars plana, with most symptoms, predominantly floaters, being a result of inflammation of the vitreous base. Unlike anterior uveitis, pure intermediate uveitis is not associated with iris inflammation; instead, white blood cells are seen predominantly in the anterior vitreous, with a lesser amount overspilling into the anterior chamber. Treatment is challenging. Topical therapy is ineffective, as it does not penetrate beyond the anterior chamber, but symptoms of floaters are not often sufficient to justify systemic immunosuppression. In some cases, vitritis (vitreous inflammation), or more commonly macular oedema, may cause visual impairment. Occasionally, retinal neovascular proliferation may occur, either as an inflammatory response or as a direct result of capillary occlusion. Intermediate uveitis may be associated with demyelination, sarcoidosis and inflammatory bowel disease.

Posterior uveitis tends to present with visual impairment secondary to macular oedema, vitritis or choroiditis. More chronic forms also exist and these tend to present with photopsia, visual field defects or distortion inducing choroidal neovascular membranes.

Infectious conditions

Conjunctivitis

Conjunctivitis is predominantly caused by bacteria or viruses and is usually self-limiting in 7–10 days. Bacterial conjunctivitis is associated with a purulent discharge and viral conjunctivitis with a watery discharge, the latter often being confused with the photophobia and reflex lacrimation of anterior uveitis. Underlying chlamydial infection should always be considered if there is a persistent thick, mucopurulent discharge.

Allergic conjunctivitis is also common, either as a component of hay fever (allergic rhinitis) or as an allergy to chloramphenicol, which is commonly used to treat conjunctivitis.

Rarely, conjunctivitis may be associated with inflammatory systemic mucus membrane disorders, such as ocular mucus membrane (cicatricial) pemphigoid or Stevens–Johnson syndrome. The secondary effects of loss of conjunctival function can be devastating to the cornea. Other causes of conjunctival scarring include trachoma, chemical burns and orbital radiotherapy.

Infectious keratitis/corneal ulceration

Inflammation of the cornea should always raise concern about underlying infection (Box 30.12). Central ulceration is always more serious than peripheral, through involvement of the visual axis. Cultures from corneal scraping or biopsy may be required, although much infectious keratitis is treated empirically on the basis of site, morphology and response to treatment.

Herpes simplex virus type 1 (occasionally type 2) is a common cause of infectious keratitis (Fig. 30.9). All layers of the cornea may be involved: the epithelium in the form of dendritic ulceration; the stroma in the form of white infiltrate and occasionally necrosis; and the endothelium in the form of localised oedema and keratitic precipitates. Loss of corneal sensation is common following herpes simplex keratitis, and occasionally

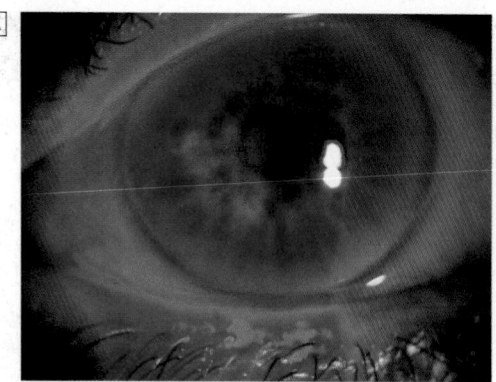 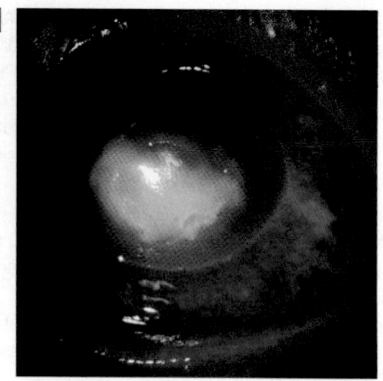

Fig. 30.9 Infective keratitis. [A] Herpes simplex dendritic ulcer stained with fluorescein. [B] Fusarium keratitis. An irregularly edged lesion suggests a fungal cause but is not pathognomonic. *(A) Courtesy of McPherson Optometry, Aberdeen. (B) From Macsai MS, Fontes BM. Rapid diagnosis in ophthalmology: anterior segment. Elsevier Inc.; 2008 (courtesy of the External Eye Disease and Cornea Section, Federal University of São Paulo, Brazil).*

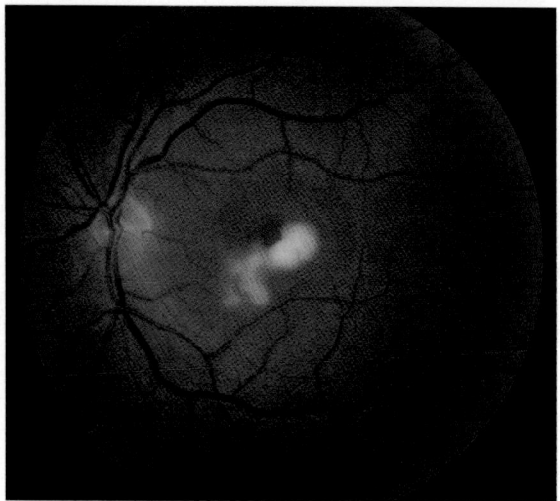

Fig. 30.10 Focal chorioretinitis in clinically suspected endogenous *Candida* **endophthalmitis.** This patient was an injection drug user and improved with empirical oral fluconazole. *From Ryan SJ (ed). Retina, 5th edn. Philadelphia: Saunders, Elsevier Inc.; 2013 (case courtesy of Jeffrey K. Moore, MD).*

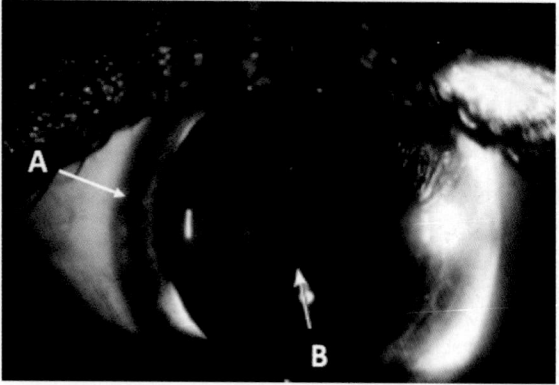

Fig. 30.11 Kayser–Fleischer ring (arrow A) and sunflower cataract (arrow B) in Wilson's disease. *Modified from Kaiser PK, Friedman NJ (eds). Massachusetts Eye and Ear Infirmary Illustrated manual of ophthalmology, 4th edn. Philadelphia: Saunders, Elsevier Inc.; 2014.*

neurotrophic keratopathy may result. Epithelial disease is self-limiting but treatment with topical or oral antivirals reduces the risk of stromal involvement and scarring. Stromal and endothelial disease requires additional topical glucocorticoids, but only once any epithelial defect has healed. Herpes simplex keratitis is analogous to herpes labialis; recurrences are therefore common and, if frequent, may warrant long-term oral antivirals. Corneal grafting may be required but the risk of recurrence remains.

Bacteria also cause infectious keratitis, especially following corneal trauma or contact lens misuse. Other risk factors for microbial keratitis include topical glucocorticoids and pre-existing ocular surface disease. Bacterial keratitis has many causes, some of which do not respond to chloramphenicol, so topical quinolones are used as first-line agents. Rarely, the free-living amoeba *Acanthamoeba castellanii* may be a cause of contact lens-associated keratitis, presenting subacutely and leading to corneal nerve infiltration, keratitis and accompanying scleritis.

Fungal keratitis is the most common cause of infectious keratitis in low income countries, particularly if there has been corneal trauma and contact with soil or plant matter. It is usually caused by *Fusarium*. Fungal keratitis has no particular distinguishing features and delayed diagnosis is common. If it is suspected, cultures should be undertaken and antifungal treatment, which is hampered by poor corneal penetration of antifungals, started promptly. Corneal transplantation is often required.

Endophthalmitis

Endophthalmitis is infection of the anterior and posterior chambers of the eye. It may be exogenous (e.g. from penetrating trauma or following surgery) or, less commonly, endogenous, caused by haematogenous spread of microorganisms within the blood, which gain entry to the eye via the choroid and ciliary body. The causes of endogenous endophthalmitis are therefore the causes of blood-stream infection (Chapter 13) Gram-positive bacteria are most common, followed by Gram-negative bacteria and then fungi, mainly *Candida*.

Clinical presentation is with visual blurring and/or visual loss, which are usually unilateral. Ocular findings range from a few deposits in the retina/choroid (chorioretinitis) to panendophthalmitis, in which there is a severe inflammatory reaction in both the anterior and posterior chambers. A specific appearance of the retina is described for *Candida* endophthalmitis, which characteristically causes creamy-white retinal or chorioretinal lesions (Fig. 30.10). It is vitally important to sample the vitreous, as this may provide the only opportunity to determine the most appropriate therapy.

Treatment is with systemic and/or intravitreal antibiotics or antifungal agents, depending on the cause and severity. Vitrectomy may also be required.

Cataract

Cataract is permanent opacity of the lens (Fig. 30.11). Globally, untreated cataract is the most common cause of visual impairment.

30

The normal lens thickens and opacifies with age, and cataract can be detected in more than half the population over the age of 65 (senile cataract). Many ocular and systemic diseases can predispose to cataract formation, the most common being uveitis and diabetes mellitus. Wilson's disease (hepatolenticular degeneration) causes a characteristic 'sunflower' cataract. Excessive exposure to ultraviolet light, ionising radiation and glucocorticoid therapy are also predisposing factors.

The characteristic symptoms of cataract are progressive loss of vision and glare. If these become serious enough to require treatment, surgical intervention will be required, usually in the form of ultrasonic phacoemulsification with intraocular lens (IOL) implant.

Common ophthalmological findings in older people are shown in Box 30.13. Findings and management issues in adolescence and pregnancy are shown in Boxes 30.14 and 30.15, respectively.

Diabetic eye disease

Diabetic retinopathy

Diabetic retinopathy is one of the most common causes of visual impairment in people of working age in high-income countries. The prevalence of diabetic retinopathy increases with the duration of diabetes. Almost all individuals with type 1 diabetes, and most of those with type 2 diabetes, will have some degree of retinopathy after 20 years. Fortunately, most patients develop only mild forms of retinopathy.

Pathogenesis

The underlying pathogenesis of diabetic retinopathy is local vascular endothelial growth factor production initiated by hyperglycaemia-induced capillary occlusion. This occlusion stimulates increased production of retinal vascular endothelial growth factor, which not only increases capillary permeability, leading to retinal oedema, but also stimulates angiogenesis, leading to new vessel formation.

Clinical features

The initial clinical feature of diabetic retinopathy, capillary occlusion, is visible only on retinal angiography. Capillaries adjacent to the occluded capillary form discrete swellings (microaneurysms), which leak fluid and blood, causing oedema and retinal haemorrhages (Fig. 30.12).

30.14 Medical ophthalmology in adolescence

Inherited conditions

- **Stargardt disease**: autosomal recessive macular dystrophy that commonly presents in adolescence/early adulthood, causing significant bilateral impairment of central vision.

Developmental anomalies

- **Pathological myopia**: due to elongated ocular axial length rather than refractive index of cornea and lens. Increased risk of retinal detachment and choroidal neovascular membrane formation.
- **Optic disc drusen**: come to prominence during adolescence and usually first detected during routine examination. Often mistaken for papilloedema, particularly in the setting of coincidental daily headache.
- **Amblyopia**: occasionally detected after the age of 7 years, particularly in the absence of pre-school screening, when it is unlikely to respond to patching of the other eye.
- **Keratoconus**: presents with increasing astigmatism (distortion of vision due to abnormal corneal topography). Hard contact lenses are the mainstay of therapy. Further progression may be prevented through 'cross-linking' surgery.

Deterioration of existing conditions

- **Diabetic retinopathy**: in type 1 diabetes, retinopathy usually first presents at least 5 years after diagnosis, which often coincides with adolescence. Puberty may accelerate progression. Greatest risk is disengagement with diabetes care, including retinal screening, significantly increasing later presentation with advanced symptomatic retinopathy.
- **Adult manifestations of retinopathy of prematurity**: clinical features depend on the type of treatment used in the neonatal period and include retinal detachment, angle closure glaucoma, severe myopia and cataract.

Sexual activity

- **Chlamydia conjunctivitis**: onset of sexual activity may lead to this ocular condition, which may be associated with reactive arthritis (SARA). Untreated coexistent genital tract infection may cause infertility.

Transition to adult services

- Neurofibromatosis type 1.
- Optic nerve astrocytoma/glioma: often develops in late childhood or early adolescence.

Sports medicine

- **Contact sports**: eye protection is important for all, especially if there is only one functional eye, e.g. with amblyopia.

30.13 Common ophthalmological findings in older people

- **Small pupils that dilate poorly with mydriatics**: common neurodegenerative finding, particularly with diabetes.
- **Spurious findings on automated perimetry**: decreasing manual dexterity and cognitive function often render automated perimetry findings unreliable.
- **Lens opacities**: cataract is ubiquitous but requires treatment only if symptomatic.
- **Drusen**: common from mid-life onwards. Larger (soft) drusen are more likely to herald age-related macular degeneration than smaller (hard) drusen.
- **Glaucoma**: angle closure glaucoma is more common as the increasing size of the lens shallows the anterior chamber. Once it is identified, both eyes are always treated to prevent development/recurrence. Chronic open angle glaucoma is more common in those with a family history or ocular hypertension (isolated raised intraocular pressure).
- **Impaired upgaze**: common. It is differentiated from progressive supranuclear palsy by the doll's head manoeuvre, the full range of vertical movement being retained in progressive supranuclear palsy PSP.
- **Ptosis**: mechanical ptosis is common due to degenerative disinsertion of the levator palpebrae superioris aponeurosis. A high skin crease and preserved ability to elevate help differentiate it from other causes.
- **Late-onset presentation of congenital conditions**: adult pseudovitelliform macular 'degeneration' is an autosomal dominant retinal dystrophy, which causes mild visual impairment. Oculopharyngeal muscular dystrophy is an autosomal dominant condition characterised by later-onset chronic progressive external ophthalmoparesis and swallowing difficulties.

30.15 Visual disorders and pregnancy

- **Ocular inflammation**: pregnancy appears to have a protective effect on many inflammatory disorders, although not systemic lupus erythematosus. Most patients can taper treatment during pregnancy. Mycophenolate mofetil is teratogenic. Glucocorticoids and tacrolimus appear safe. The use of biologics during pregnancy should be based on a balance of risks, and professional guidelines should be consulted.
- **Diabetic retinopathy**: may be accelerated during pregnancy because the placenta is a potent source of angiogenic growth factors. Retinal screening each trimester is recommended.
- **HELLP/pre-eclampsia/eclampsia**: retinal features of accelerated hypertension may be seen, including optic disc oedema, flame haemorrhages and cotton wool spots. Occasionally, exudative retinal detachments occur. Vasogenic oedema (posterior reversible encephalopathy syndrome), affecting the posterior occipital and parietal lobes, may cause cortical visual impairment. All features tend to resolve with delivery or control of blood pressure.

Clinically, microaneurysms appear as isolated red dots, the capillaries being too small to visualise. At the edge of any leaking fluid, lipids precipitate out to form exudate, like the tidemark of the sea.

In turn, capillaries with microaneurysms also occlude, their microaneurysms turning white before disappearing entirely from clinical view.

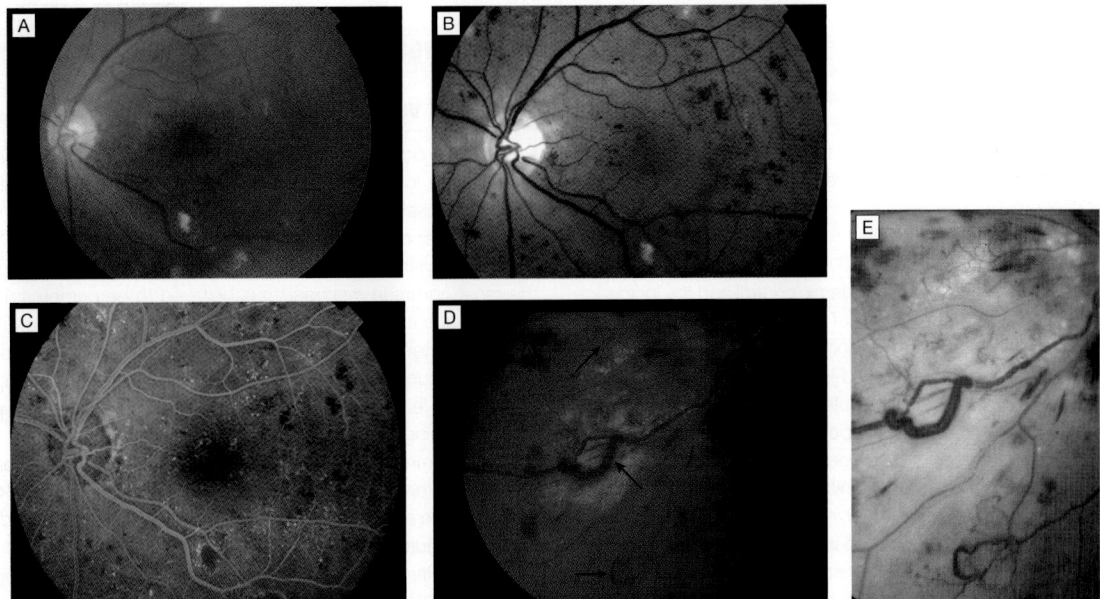

Fig. 30.12 Diabetic retinopathy. [A] Colour photograph of severe background diabetic retinopathy: multiple blot haemorrhages indicative of capillary occlusion; dot haemorrhages indistinguishable from microaneurysms or microaneurysmal bleeds; and cotton wool spots indicative of arteriolar occlusion. [B] Red-free image shows the presence of extensive haemorrhages more clearly; the more haemorrhages, the greater the degree of likely capillary occlusion. [C] Fluorescein angiogram now reveals extensive entrapment of fluorescein within multiple microaneurysms. [D] Colour photograph showing three cardinal consequences of capillary occlusion: intra-retinal microvascular anomalies occurring within an area of capillary occlusion (top arrow); venous reduplication (rare finding), with venous beading, extending from the reduplication towards the optic disc, occurring where capillaries are occluded either side of the vein (middle arrow); and new vessel formation occurring at the border between the diseased and health retina (bottom arrow). [E] Red-free image shows these features, particularly intra-retinal microvascular anomalies, more clearly. Note the relative pallor compared to the right-hand side of the image, which is indicative of widespread capillary occlusion. Absolute pallor never occurs, as it is 'masked' by the highly vascularised choroid lying underneath. *(A–E) Courtesy of Aberdeen Royal Infirmary.*

As more and more capillaries occlude, larger patches of retinal ischaemia form, leading to sufficient vascular endothelial growth factor production to induce the growth of new vessels at the border of diseased and undiseased retina.

Within patches of retinal ischaemia, diseased remnants of partially perfused capillaries form intra-retinal microvascular abnormalities (IRMAs) and retinal veins develop multiple diffuse swellings (venous beading). These signs are best seen on fluorescein angiography.

New vessels and their glial tissue (like a cabbage leaf) grow from retinal veins, through the overlying internal limiting membrane into the vitreous, triggering local inflammation and contracting scars. The vitreous is strongly adherent to the pars plana. It pulls back on the new vessel, triggering further bleeding, growth, inflammation and scarring. If the scarring is sufficient, then tractional retinal detachment and complete blindness may occur.

Other retinal lesions, not unique to capillary occlusion, are also seen in diabetic retinopathy. These include flame haemorrhages and cotton wool spots (soft exudates). Flame haemorrhages are horizontal streaky haemorrhages in the retinal nerve-fibre layer. They are also seen in any severe anaemia, e.g. bacterial endocarditis and leukaemia. Cotton wool spots are also situated in the nerve-fibre layer and are usually most numerous nasal to the optic disc, where the nerve fibres crowd together. They are also seen in accelerated hypertension, after severe hypoglycaemia and occasionally in giant cell arteritis. A cotton wool spot combined with an enclosing flame haemorrhage is termed a Roth spot. Roth spots have traditionally been associated with endocarditis, although they may be seen with any cause of a flame haemorrhage.

Management of proliferative diabetic retinopathy

If untreated, proliferative retinopathy eventually causes severe visual impairment through recurrent vitreous haemorrhage and retinal detachment. Pan-retinal laser photocoagulation therapy is extremely effective at preserving vision, if applied before complications set in.

Historically, laser therapy was used empirically to ablate the retina extensively outside the macula. However, this caused secondary optic atrophy and night blindness (nyctalopia), which interfered with the ability to drive. Modern application of laser is lighter, more tailored to the sites of underlying capillary ischaemia and relatively free of side-effects, only occasionally resulting in loss of the ability to drive. In the UK there is a requirement to inform the driver licensing authority if retinopathy is (or has been) present in both eyes, irrespective of treatment history.

Intravitreal injections of anti-vascular endothelial growth factor (e.g. ranibizumab, aflibercept, bevacizumab) also cause temporary regression of proliferative retinopathy, whereas, after pan-retinal laser therapy, background and proliferative types of retinopathy regress permanently. If both eyes have been treated with laser, patients can be safely discharged to a retinal screening programme.

Management of diabetic macular oedema

Traditionally, oedema seen on slit-lamp biomicroscopy was categorised according to three patterns of leakage elucidated from fluorescein angiogram studies:

- focal leakage from microaneurysms
- diffuse leakage from diseased capillaries
- ischaemia (no leakage) from thrombosis of the perifoveal capillaries.

Laser was applied, either directly on leaking microaneurysms or empirically by placing a grid of burns on the affected macula, to reduce leakage. The main aim was to treat oedema before the fovea was affected, as laser therapy for oedema affecting the fovea was never particularly effective.

However, retinal screening programmes have demonstrated that extrafoveal macular oedema often resolves spontaneously, and the introduction of intravitreal injection therapy, which rescues vision in 50% of those treated regardless of the mechanism of oedema, has led to

30

a paradigm shift in management. Now, rather than laser treatment of asymptomatic oedema that does not involve the centre of the fovea, the emphasis has shifted to treating those who are symptomatic from centre-involving foveal oedema (confirmed on optical coherence tomography) with anti-vascular endothelial growth factor injections. Although this method of treatment is more effective, monthly injections may be required indefinitely.

Prevention

There is a clear relationship between glycaemic control and the incidence of diabetic retinopathy. A combination of good glycaemic and blood pressure control also slows the progression of retinopathy.

When blood glucose is rapidly lowered in patients with type 1 diabetes, however, there can be a transient deterioration of retinopathy, predominantly in the form of cotton wool spot formation, but occasionally triggering new vessel formation. The trigger is believed to be increased systemic insulin growth factor release, which is most likely to occur with sudden correction of eating disorders or reinstitution of insulin therapy in those who miss out injections, often to induce weight loss. This often occurs during hospitalisation for other reasons.

Although, ideally, any improvement in glycaemic control should be gradual, in many circumstances this is hard to achieve, particularly if the patient suddenly decides to comply with treatment, leading to dramatic improvement in glycaemic control.

Screening

Systematic screening for asymptomatic proliferative retinopathy has been shown to be cost-effective. It has led to the introduction of population-based screening programmes in the UK and other countries, where health care is funded centrally. There is little evidence that screening asymptomatic patients for macular oedema is cost-effective, although a by-product of screening is that suspected macular oedema has become the most common reason for referral from retinal screening to ophthalmology.

Although hand-held ophthalmoscopy has been shown to have poor sensitivity compared to examination by slit-lamp biomicroscopy or retinal photography, any form of screening is better than none where resources are scarce. Currently, optical coherence tomography is being added to the screening pathway to reduce false-negative referrals for macular oedema.

Historically, annual screening has been advocated. However, evidence now indicates that patients with repeated normal screens, particularly those with type 2 diabetes, can be safely screened every 2 years.

In pregnancy, the placenta is a source of angiogenic growth factors. For this reason, although the risk of developing significant retinopathy during pregnancy remains low, pregnant women should be screened every trimester until the placenta is delivered.

Other causes of visual loss in people with diabetes

Around 50% of visual loss in people with type 2 diabetes results from causes other than diabetic retinopathy. These include cataract, age-related macular degeneration, retinal vein occlusion, retinal arterial occlusion, non-arteritic ischaemic optic neuropathy and glaucoma. Some of these conditions are to be expected in this group, as they relate to cardiovascular risk factors (e.g. hypertension, hyperlipidaemia and smoking), all of which are prevalent in people with type 2 diabetes.

In diabetes, metabolic changes in the lens (which are not yet fully elaborated) cause premature and/or accelerated cataract formation. A rare type of 'snowflake' cataract occurs in young patients with poorly controlled diabetes. This does not usually affect vision but tends to make fundal examination difficult. The indications for cataract surgery in diabetes are similar to those in the non-diabetic population, but an additional indication in diabetes is when adequate assessment of the fundus and/or retinal laser therapy becomes impossible.

Retinal vascular occlusion

Retinal vein occlusion (thrombosis)

Retinal vein occlusion is an important vascular cause of visual impairment, visual loss resulting from macular oedema or occasionally from neovascularisation, both of which are managed in a similar way to diabetic macular oedema or proliferative diabetic retinopathy.

Although pathogenesis of retinal vein occlusion is not fully understood, the most common mechanism is believed to be compression of a vein by an adjacent arteriosclerotic artery. Retinal vessels are unusual in that, where the arteries and veins cross over each other, they share a common outer layer (tunica adventitia). This means that arteriosclerotic thickening of an artery leads directly to compression of the adjacent vein (arteriovenous nipping).

A less common cause of retinal vein occlusion is inflammation of the retinal vein (periphlebitis), also called retinal vasculitis (unlike systemic vasculitis, the arterial system is not involved). Periphlebitis should be suspected in younger patients and in patients with no obvious risk factors for arteriosclerosis. Diagnosis is made by fluorescein angiography and treatment is with systemic immunosuppression, with or without adjunctive intravitreal therapy.

Retinal vein occlusion is associated with systemic hypertension and may rarely result from hyperviscosity due to a myeloproliferative disorder, multiple myeloma, Waldenström's macroglobulinaemia or leukaemia. Glaucoma is associated with retinal vein occlusion but whether this is a direct cause or merely a comorbidity in older people is not known.

Clinical presentation is with unilateral painless loss of central vision (central retinal vein thrombosis) or an area of peripheral vision (branch retinal vein thrombosis). Fundoscopic features include flame haemorrhages, cotton wool spots, macular oedema and a swollen optic disc (Fig. 30.13).

The management of retinal vein occlusion is twofold: management of the underlying aetiology and management of the consequences of retinal vein occlusion. Where an underlying risk factor for arteriosclerosis is clearly present secondary prevention measures should be commenced. However, the role of secondary prevention of arteriosclerosis in isolated retinal vein occlusion, although common practice by some, remains controversial.

Retinal artery occlusion

Retinal artery occlusion is usually an embolic phenomenon. Common predisposing factors are therefore (predominantly carotid) atherosclerosis, valvular heart disease, arrhythmias and infective endocarditis. The next most common cause is vasculitis, mainly giant cell arteritis.

Fig. 30.13 Central retinal vein occlusion (thrombosis), showing flame haemorrhages, cotton wool spots, macular oedema and a swollen optic disc. *Courtesy of Aberdeen Royal Infirmary.*

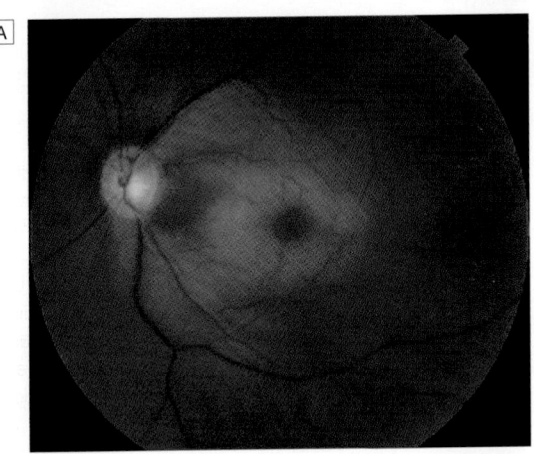

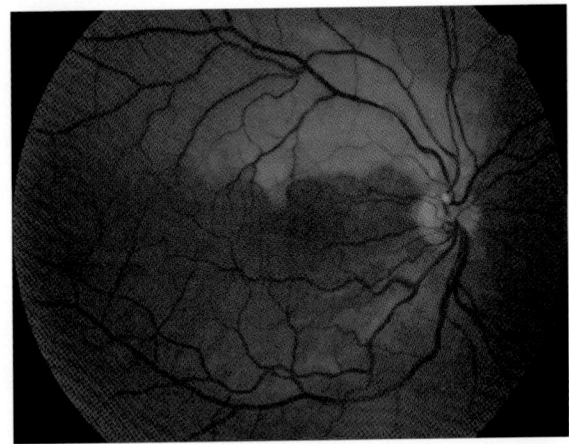

Fig. 30.14 Retinal artery occlusion. A Colour fundus photograph of central retinal artery occlusion, showing a classic cherry-red spot and a superior optic disc haemorrhage. B Superior branch retinal artery occlusion due to an embolus at the disc branch retinal artery occlusion, showing a pale segment of retina. *(A) From Duker JS, Waheed NK, Goldman DR. Handbook of retinal OCT. Philadelphia: Saunders, Elsevier Inc.; 2014. (B) From Bowling B. Kanski's Clinical ophthalmology, 8th edn. Oxford: Elsevier Ltd; 2016.*

Retinal artery occlusion presents with painless unilateral visual loss, the extent and location of which depend on whether there is a central occlusion or a branch occlusion (peripheral occlusions may be asymptomatic). Transient occlusion of the internal carotid or ophthalmic artery causes transient visual loss, or amaurosis fugax. The typical fundoscopic finding in a central occlusion is a transiently pale retina with a 'cherry-red' spot at the macula, the appearance developing over an hour or so after the occlusion (Fig. 30.14). In branch occlusions there is no cherry-red spot and the retinal pallor is regional.

Age-related macular degeneration

Age-related macular degeneration is the most common cause of visual impairment in high income countries. There are two basic forms: atrophic (dry) and neovascular (wet). The underlying mechanism is dysfunction of the retinal pigment epithelium, leading to overlying photoreceptor death. Choroidal neovascularisation, growing under and into the overlying retina, may occur, distorting the anatomy of the photoreceptors and ending in scar formation. Both forms are preceded by deposits under the retinal pigment epithelium ('drusen'), often followed by the development of focal areas of macular hypo- and hyperpigmentation, where diseased retinal pigment epithelial cells have precipitated their pigment (age-related maculopathy).

The atrophic form presents with gradual onset of central visual blurring, accompanied, to a lesser degree, by visual distortion. Large (geographic), central patches of atrophy are seen with areas of adjacent hyperpigmentation. In the neovascular form, sudden onset of central distortion, progressing within weeks, is the predominant symptom. Apart from age, the main risk factor appears to be smoking.

The advent of anti-vascular endothelial growth factor injectors has led to effective therapy for the neovascular form, in many but not all. Unfortunately, treatment is expensive and requires considerable financial and staff resources to treat in timely fashion; delayed treatment can lead to irreversible visual loss. For whichever type, whether treatable or not, visual rehabilitation, through the use of appropriate magnifiers, alteration in lighting and specialised adaptation of everyday living objects, remains important adjunctive therapy.

Further information

Websites

jrcptb.org.uk/specialties/medical-ophthalmology *How to train in medical ophthalmology in the UK.*

ndrs.scot.nhs.uk *Scottish Diabetic Retinopathy Screening Collaborative: aspects of screening for diabetic retinopathy, including rationale, organisation, delivery and an on-line training handbook.*

rcophth.ac.uk *Royal College of Ophthalmologists, London: as part of its role in championing excellence, produces a range of pragmatic surgical and medical guidelines.*

sun.scot.nhs.uk *Scottish Uveitis Network: standards of care, treatment guidelines and information leaflets.*

RM Steel
SM Lawrie

31

Medical psychiatry

Psychiatric disorders have traditionally been considered as 'mental' rather than as 'physical' illnesses. This is because they manifest with disordered functioning in the areas of emotion, perception, thinking and memory, and formerly had no clearly biological basis. However, as biochemical and structural abnormalities of the brain are identified in an increasing number of psychiatric disorders, and psychological and behavioural factors are identified in many medical illnesses, the distinction between mental and physical illness has become questionable.

The World Health Organization (WHO) periodically publishes its International Classification of Disease (ICD), which provides definitions for every recognised clinical condition. The 10th Revision (ICD-10) comprises 22 chapters. The diagnoses listed in Chapter V, 'Mental and behavioural disorders' (Box 31.1), are used by psychiatrists around the world in everyday clinical practice and it is these conditions that provide the focus for this chapter.

Psychiatric disorders are among the most common of all human illnesses. The WHO's Global Burden of Disease study found 'Mental, neurological and substance misuse disorders' to be the leading cause of 'Years Lost to Disability' (YLDs), accounting for almost 20% of global YLDs, with anxiety and mood disorders alone accounting for over 10%. As with most clinical conditions, the prevalence of mental disorders varies with the setting. In the general population, depression, anxiety disorders and adjustment disorders are most common (>10%) and psychosis is rare (<2%); in acute medical wards of general hospitals, organic disorders such as delirium are very common, with prevalence highest among sick, older patients; in specialist general psychiatric services, psychoses are the most common disorders (Box 31.2).

Clinical examination

As in other areas of medicine, the psychiatric assessment comprises a structured clinical history and examination followed by appropriate investigations. However, psychiatric assessment differs from a standard medical assessment in the following ways:

- There is greater emphasis on the history and relatively less reliance on investigations.
- A large part of the clinical examination component is conducted as the history is being taken rather than as a discrete set of procedures afterwards.
- It commonly includes the interviewing of an informant, usually a relative or friend who knows the patient, especially when the illness affects the patient's ability to give an accurate history.

i 31.1 World Health Organization classification of psychiatric disorders (ICD-10)	
Chapter V (F00–F99) **Mental and behavioural disorders**	**Examples**
F00–F09 Organic mental disorders	Dementias Delirium Other mental disorders due to brain damage or disease
F10–F19 Disorders due to psychoactive substances: alcohol, opioids, cannabinoids etc.	Intoxication Harmful use Dependence Withdrawal
F20–F29 Schizophrenia and delusional disorders	Schizophrenia
F30–F39 Mood [affective] disorders	Depression Bipolar disorder
F40–F48 Neurotic, stress-related and somatoform disorders	Phobias Generalised anxiety disorder Obsessive–compulsive disorder Post-traumatic stress disorder Adjustment disorders Somatoform disorders
F50–F59 Behavioural syndromes associated with physiological disturbances	Eating disorders: anorexia and bulimia nervosa Sexual dysfunction
F60–F69 Disorders of adult personality and behaviour	Specific personality disorders Trichotillomania Gender identity disorders
F70–F79 Mental retardation	Mild, moderate, severe or profound
F80–F89 Disorders of psychological development	Autism Asperger syndrome
F90–F98 Behavioural and emotional disorders of childhood	Hyperkinetic disorders Tic disorders

From WHO. International Classification of Diseases and Related Health Problems. 10th Revision (ICD-10). Geneva: World Health Organization.

i 31.2 Prevalence of psychiatric disorders by medical setting

	Medical/surgical			General psychiatric services
	General practice	Outpatients	Inpatients	
Delirium	–	–	+++	–
Alcohol/substance abuse	++	++	+++	+++
Schizophrenia	–	–	–	+++
Bipolar disorder	–	–	–	+++
Depression	++	++	+++	+++
Anxiety disorders	++	++	++	+++
Adjustment disorders	++	++	+++	+
Somatoform disorders	+	+++	++	–
Personality disorders	+	+	+	+++

– 'rare' (<2%); + 'uncommon' (2%–5%); ++ 'common' (5%–10%); +++ 'very common' (>10%)

A full psychiatric history (Box 31.3) incorporating a detailed mental state examination may take an hour or more because of its complexity. A brief mental state examination, usually taking no more than a few minutes (see below), should be part of the assessment of *all* patients, not merely those deemed to have psychiatric illnesses.

The psychiatric interview

The aims of the interview are to:

- establish a therapeutic relationship with the patient
- elicit the symptoms, history and background information (Box 31.3)
- examine the mental state
- provide information, reassurance and advice.

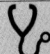

31.3 How to structure a psychiatric interview

Presenting problem

Reason for referral

- Why the patient has been referred and by whom

Presenting complaints

- The patient should be asked to describe the main problems for which help is requested and what they want the doctor to do

History of present illness

- The patient should be asked to describe the course of the illness from when symptoms were first noticed
- The interviewer asks direct questions to determine the nature, duration and severity of symptoms, and any associated factors

Background

Family history

- Description of parents and siblings, and a record of any mental illness in relatives

Personal history

- Birth and early developmental history, major events in childhood, education, occupational history, relationship(s), marriage, children, current social circumstances

Previous medical and psychiatric history

- Previous health, accidents and operations
- Use of alcohol, tobacco and other drugs
- Direct questions may be needed concerning previous psychiatric history since this may not be volunteered: 'Have you ever been treated for depression or nerves?' or 'Have you ever suffered a nervous breakdown?'

Previous personality

- The patterns of behaviour and thinking that characterise a person, including their relationships with other people and reactions to stress (useful information may be obtained from an informant who has known the patient well for many years)

The mental state examination

The mental state examination (MSE) is a systematic examination of the patient's thinking, emotion and behaviour. As with the clinical examination in other areas of medicine, the aim is to elicit objective clinical signs. While many aspects of the patient's mental state may be observed as the history is being taken, specific enquiries about important features should always be made.

General appearance and behaviour

Any abnormalities of alertness or motor behaviour, such as restlessness or retardation, should be noted. The level of consciousness should be determined, especially in the assessment of possible delirium.

Speech

Speed and fluency should be observed, including slow (retarded) speech and word-finding difficulty. 'Pressure of speech' describes rapid speech that is difficult to interrupt.

Mood

This can be judged by facial expression, posture and movements. Patients should also be asked if they feel sad or depressed and if they lack ability to experience pleasure (anhedonia). Are they anxious, worried or tense? Is mood elevated with excess energy and a reduced need for sleep, as in (hypo)mania?

Thoughts

The content of thought can be elicited by asking 'What are your main concerns?' Is thinking negative, guilty or hopeless, suggesting depression? Are there thoughts of self-harm? If so, enquiry should be made about plans. Are patients excessively worried about many things, suggesting anxiety? Do they think that they are especially powerful, important or gifted (grandiose thoughts), suggesting mania?

The form of thinking may also be abnormal. In schizophrenia, patients may display loosened associations between ideas, making it difficult to follow their train of thought. There may also be abnormalities of thought possession, when patients experience the intrusion of alien thoughts into their mind or the broadcasting of their own thoughts to other people.

Abnormal beliefs

A delusion is a false belief, out of keeping with a patient's cultural background, which is held with conviction despite evidence to the contrary.

Abnormal perceptions

Illusions are misperceptions of real stimuli. Hallucinations are sensory perceptions that occur in the absence of external stimuli, such as hearing voices when no one is present.

Cognitive function

Cognitive function has many components: memory, concentration, visuospatial abilities, executive function and so on. In most cases, a brief assessment of orientation (person, place and time – the patient is asked their name, age, date of birth, what building they are in, the current date and day of the week) and attention ('serial 7 s' – the patient is asked to subtract 7 from 100 and then 7 from the answer, and so on) is sufficient to exclude clinically significant cognitive impairment. Where there is reason to suspect cognitive impairment, a standardised screening tool should be used. In delirium, cognitive impairment typically fluctuates over time so may be missed by a single assessment.

The Montreal Cognitive Assessment (MoCA) is a useful screening questionnaire that covers all the main domains of cognitive function (Fig. 31.1). It is designed to be easy to use and is freely available online in many different languages. Another widely used screening test is the Mini-Mental State Examination (MMSE), although this is subject to copyright, unlike the MoCA. The Addenbrooke's Cognitive Examination – 3rd edition (ACE-III) offers a more comprehensive assessment and brief training courses for clinicians wishing to use it. These resources are available online (see 'Further information').

Patients' own understanding of their symptoms

Patients should be asked what they think their symptoms are due to and whether they warrant treatment. The failure of a patient to understand their own symptoms is referred to as 'lack of insight'. Psychotic patients characteristically have lack of insight and fail to accept that they are in need of treatment.

Investigations in medical psychiatry

In many areas of medicine, laboratory or radiological tests play a central role in diagnosis. Such tests are often performed in psychiatry but are typically used to exclude non-psychiatric illness rather than to confirm a psychiatric diagnosis. For example, in a patient presenting with symptoms of anxiety it may be appropriate to check thyroid function to exclude thyrotoxicosis as a cause of their symptoms. Specific investigations are recommended in certain psychiatric conditions such as

31

VISUOSPATIAL / EXECUTIVE

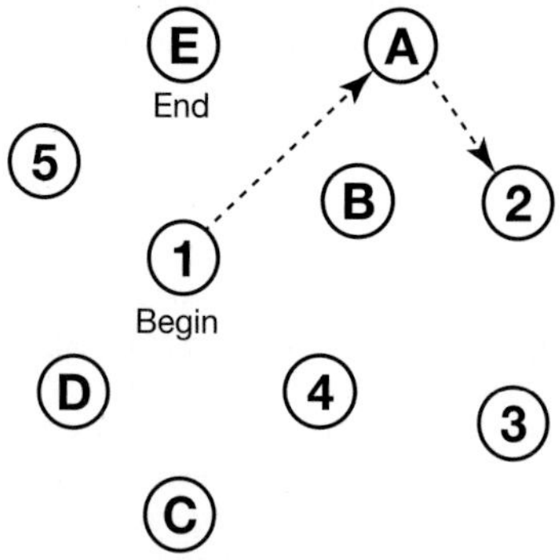

[ ]

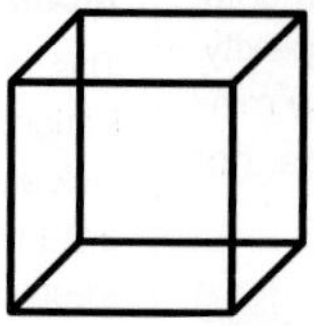

Copy cube

[ ]

Draw CLOCK (Ten past eleven) (3 points)

[ ] Contour [ ] Numbers [ ] Hands

POINTS: ___/5

NAMING

[ ] [ ] [ ]

___/3

MEMORY Read list of words, subject must repeat them. Do 2 trials, even if 1st trial is successful. Do a recall after 5 minutes.

	FACE	VELVET	CHURCH	DAISY	RED
1st trial					
2nd trial					

No points

ATTENTION Read list of digits (1 digit/ sec.)

Subject has to repeat them in the forward order [ ] 2 1 8 5 4

Subject has to repeat them in the backward order [ ] 7 4 2

___/2

Read list of letters. The subject must tap with his hand at each letter A. No points if ≥ 2 errors

[ ] FBACMNAAJKLBAFAKDEAAAJAMOFAAB

___/1

Serial 7 subtraction starting at 100 [ ] 93 [ ] 86 [ ] 79 [ ] 72 [ ] 65

4 or 5 correct subtractions: **3 pts**, 2 or 3 correct: **2 pts**, 1 correct: **1 pt**, 0 correct: **0 pt**

___/3

LANGUAGE Repeat: I only know that John is the one to help today. [ ]

The cat always hid under the couch when dogs were in the room. [ ]

___/2

Fluency / Name maximum number of words in one minute that begin with the letter F [ ] _____ (N ≥ 11 words)

___/1

ABSTRACTION Similarity between e.g. banana – orange = fruit [ ] train – bicycle [ ] watch – ruler

___/2

DELAYED RECALL	Has to recall words	FACE	VELVET	CHURCH	DAISY	RED	Points for UNCUED recall only
	WITH NO CUE	[ ]	[ ]	[ ]	[ ]	[ ]	___/5
Optional	Category cue						
	Multiple choice cue						

ORIENTATION [ ] Date [ ] Month [ ] Year [ ] Day [ ] Place [ ] City ___/6

 www.mocatest.org Normal ≥ 26 / 30 TOTAL ___/30

Add 1 point if ≤ 12 yr edu

Administered by: ________________

Fig. 31.1 Montreal Cognitive Assessment (MoCA). A widely used screening tool for cognitive impairment. © *Z. Nasreddine MD, www.mocatest.org*.

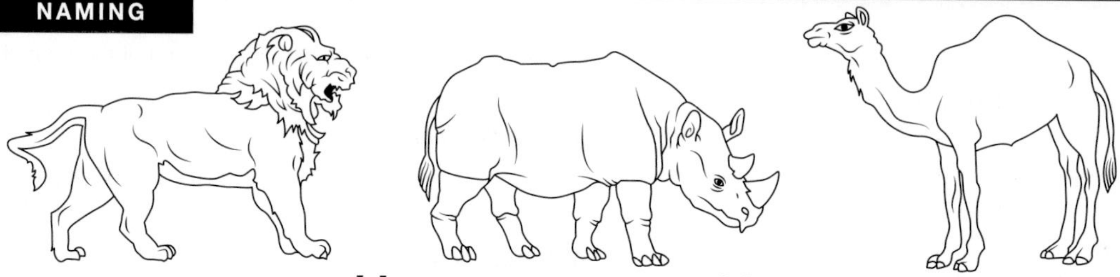

dementia, delirium, substance misuse and eating disorders, as shown in Box 31.4. Further details of each of these disorders are discussed later in the chapter,

Functional anatomy and physiology

Most psychiatric disorders result from a complex interplay between psychological, social, environmental and genetic factors. Each of these factors may play a role in predisposing to, precipitating or perpetuating a disorder (Box 31.5).

Biological factors

Genetic

Genetic factors play a predisposing role in many psychiatric disorders, including schizophrenia and bipolar disorder. However, while some

i | 31.4 Investigations in psychiatry

Presentation	Investigation
Dementia	FBC, ESR
	U&Es, TFTs, LFTs, calcium, cholesterol, CRP
	Glucose (fasting)
	Vitamin B_{12}, folate
	CT brain
	HIV*, VDRL*
	MRI*
	EEG*
	Lumbar puncture*
Substance misuse	
Alcohol	Breath alcohol
	FBC
	U&Es, LFTs, albumin, γGT
	CT brain*
	FibroScan*
Other psychoactive substances	Urine drug screen
	HIV, Hep B, Hep C serology
	ECG*
Psychosis	Urine drug screen
	FBC
	U&Es, TFTs
	HIV*, VDRL*
	CT brain*
Mood disorders	
Depression	FBC
	U&Es, TFTs, LFTs
	Vitamin B_{12}*, folate*, vitamin D*
	EBV serology*
Mania	Urine drug screen
	FBC
	U&Es, TFTs
	CT brain*
Anxiety disorders	FBC
	U&Es, TFTs, calcium
	Urine drug screen*
	γGT*
	Serum/urine metanephrine
Eating disorders	
Anorexia nervosa	FBC
	U&Es, TFTs, LFTs, albumin, cholesterol, amylase
	Calcium, magnesium, phosphate
	Glucose (fasting)
	ECG
	Bone mineral density scan
Bulimia nervosa	FBC
	U&Es
	Calcium, magnesium, phosphate
	Vitamin B_{12}, folate, ferritin
	ECG

*When indicated in specific cases
(CRP = C-reactive protein; CT = computed tomography; ESR = erythrocyte sedimentation rate; EBV = Epstein–Barr virus; ECG = echocardiogram; EEG = electroencephalogram; FBC = full blood count; γGT = gamma-glutamyltransferase; Hep = hepatitis; HIV = human immunodeficiency virus; LFTs = liver function tests; MRI = magnetic resonance imaging; TFTs = thyroid function tests; U&Es = urea and electrolytes; VDRL = Venereal Diseases Research Laboratory)

i | 31.5 Classification of risk factors for psychiatric disorders

Classification	Examples
Predisposing	
Established in utero or in childhood	Genetic and epigenetic factors
	Congenital defects
Increase susceptibility to psychiatric disorder	Disturbed family background
Operate throughout patient's lifetime	Chronic physical illness
Precipitating	
Trigger an episode of illness	Stressful life events
Determine its time of onset	Acute physical illness
	Misuse of alcohol or drugs
Perpetuating	
Delay recovery from illness	Lack of social support
	Chronic physical illness

Brain structure and function

Brain structure is grossly normal in most psychiatric disorders, although abnormalities may be observed in some conditions, such as generalised cerebral atrophy in Alzheimer's disease and enlarged ventricles with a slightly decreased brain size in schizophrenia. Functioning of the brain, however, is commonly altered due to changes in neurotransmitters such as dopamine, noradrenaline (norepinephrine) and 5-hydroxytryptamine (5-HT, serotonin). Functional differences in specific areas of the brain are increasingly being recognised using advanced imaging techniques. For example, positron emission tomography (PET) studies of dopamine ligand binding in schizophrenia have consistently demonstrated increased dopamine synthesis in the striatum, even in untreated patients, while a smaller body of PET evidence points towards reductions in 5-HT transporter binding in the mid-brain and amygdala in depression.

Pattern classification approaches to structural magnetic resonance imaging (MRI) data can accurately predict the development of schizophrenia in at-risk populations, and generalised grey matter loss over time is a poor prognostic guide. Increased anterior cingulate activity in depression is a consistent predictor of good response to both antidepressants and cognitive behaviour therapy. While these and other imaging techniques show potential as diagnostic, prognostic and therapeutic aids, they remain research tools at the present time.

It is also increasingly clear that psychiatric disorders are associated with disruptions in neuronal systems rather than single sites. These can be characterised using diffusion tensor imaging (DTI) of white-matter projection fibres and resting-state/task-based functional MRI (fMRI) studies of inter-regional connectivity. For example, DTI has shown reduced white-matter density in limbic ('emotional') system tracts, such as the fornix and cingulum, in many disorders. Resting-state fMRI studies consistently identify 'default mode', salience and executive control networks of interconnected neuronal populations for certain mental activities. These pathways are implicated in several psychiatric disorders but, as yet, in non-specific ways.

Psychological and behavioural factors

Early environment

Early childhood adversity, such as emotional deprivation or abuse, predisposes to most psychiatric disorders, such as depression, eating disorders and personality disorders in adulthood.

Personality

The relationship between personality and psychiatric disorder can be difficult to assess because the development of psychiatric disorder can impact on a patient's personality. Some personality types predispose the

disorders, such as Huntington's disease, are due to mutations in a single gene, the genetic contribution to most psychiatric disorders is polygenic in nature and mediated by the combined effects of several genetic variants, each with modest effects and modulated by environmental factors.

31.6 Medical psychiatry in old age

- **Organic psychiatric disorders**: especially common, so cognitive function should always be assessed; if impaired, an associated medical condition or adverse drug effect should be suspected.
- **Disturbed behaviour**: delirium is the most common cause.
- **Depression**: common. Just because a person is old and frail does not mean that depression is 'to be expected' and that it should not be treated.
- **Self-harm**: associated with an increased risk of completed suicide.
- **Medically unexplained symptoms**: common and often associated with depressive disorder.
- **Loneliness, poverty and lack of social support**: must be taken into consideration in management decisions.

individual to develop a psychiatric disorder, however; for example, an obsessional ('anankastic') personality increases the risk of obsessive–compulsive disorder. A disordered personality may also perpetuate a psychiatric disorder once it is established, leading to a poorer prognosis.

Behaviour

A person's behaviour may predispose to the development or perpetuation of a disorder. Examples include excess alcohol intake leading to dependence, dieting in anorexia or persistent avoidance of the feared situation in phobia.

Social and environmental factors

Social isolation

The lack of a close, confiding relationship predisposes to some psychiatric disorders, such as depression, and this may be particularly relevant in older adults where social isolation is common (see Box 31.6). As well as predisposing to psychiatric disorders the reduced social support that results from having a psychiatric disorder may also act to perpetuate it.

Stressors

Social and environmental stressors often play an important role in precipitating psychiatric disorder in those who are predisposed, such as trauma in post-traumatic stress disorder, losses (such as bereavement) in depression, and events perceived as threatening (such as potential loss of employment) in anxiety.

Presenting problems in psychiatric illness

Delirium

Delirium is a medical disorder that is common in older adults and in patients in high-dependency and intensive care units. The causes, assessment and management of delirium are described in Chapter 14.

Alcohol misuse

Misuse of alcohol is a major problem worldwide. It presents in a multitude of ways, which are discussed later on in this chapter and summarised in Box 31.23. In many cases, the link to alcohol is obvious; in others, it may not be, since denial and concealment of alcohol intake are common.

Clinical assessment

The patient should be asked to describe a typical week's drinking, quantified in terms of units of alcohol (1 unit contains approximately 8 g alcohol and is the equivalent of half a pint of beer, a single measure of spirits or a small glass of wine). The history from the patient may need corroboration by the general practitioner (GP), earlier medical records and family members.

Investigations

Abnormalities in routine biochemistry and haematology can support the diagnosis of alcohol excess (such as the finding of a raised mean cell volume (MCV) and/or raised γ-glutamyl transferase (GGT)), but such tests are abnormal in only half of problem drinkers; consequently, normal results on these tests do not exclude an alcohol problem. When abnormal, these measures may be helpful in challenging denial and monitoring treatment response. Transient elastography (also known as FibroScan) is an ultrasound-based technique that measures fibrosis and steatosis. It is used in specialist services to complement information derived from tests of MCV and GGT.

Management

The prevention and management of alcohol-related problems are discussed later in this chapter.

Substance misuse

The misuse of drugs of all kinds is also widespread. As well as the general headings listed for alcohol problems in Box 31.23, additional problems may occur in association with substance misuse (Box 31.7). These can be broken down into two broad categories:

- problems linked with the route of administration, such as intravenous injection
- problems arising from pressure applied to doctors to prescribe the misused substances.

Assessment and management are described later in this chapter in the section on substance misuse.

Delusions and hallucinations

Delusions and hallucinations are abnormal beliefs and perceptions that have no rational basis. They are often due to psychiatric illness but can be secondary to substance misuse, physical illness or neurological disorders, such as epilepsy.

Delusions

A delusion is a false belief, out of keeping with a patient's cultural background, which is held with conviction despite evidence to the contrary. It is common to classify delusions on the basis of their content. They may be:

- persecutory – such as a conviction that others are out to harm one
- hypochondriacal – such as an unfounded conviction that one has cancer
- grandiose – such as a belief that one has special powers or status
- nihilistic – such as 'My head is missing', 'I have no body' or 'I am dead'.

31.7 Substance misuse

Complications arising from the route of use

Intravenous
- Local: abscesses, cellulitis, thrombosis
- Systemic: bacterial (endocarditis), viral (hepatitis, human immunodeficiency virus (HIV))

Nasal ingestion
- Erosion of nasal septum, epistaxis

Smoking
- Oral, laryngeal and lung cancer

Inhalation
- Burns, chemical pneumonitis, rashes

Pressure to prescribe misused substance
- Manipulation, deceit and threats
- Factitious description of illness
- Malingering

Hallucinations

Hallucinations are defined as sensory perceptions occurring without external stimuli. They can occur in any sensory modality but most commonly are visual or auditory. Typical examples are hearing voices when no one else is present, or seeing 'visions'. Hallucinations have the quality of ordinary perceptions and are perceived as originating in the external world, not in the patient's own mind (when they are termed 'pseudo-hallucinations'). Those occurring when falling asleep ('hypnagogic') and on waking ('hypnopompic') are a normal phenomenon and not pathological. Hallucinations should be distinguished from illusions, which are misperceptions of real external stimuli (such as mistaking a shrub for a person in poor light).

Clinical assessment

Careful and tactful enquiry is required because agitation, terror or the fear of being thought 'mad' may make patients unable or unwilling to volunteer or describe their abnormal beliefs or perceptions. The nature of hallucinations can be important diagnostically; for example, 'running commentary' voices that discuss the patient are strongly associated with schizophrenia. In general, auditory hallucinations suggest schizophrenia, while hallucinations in other sensory modalities, especially vision but also taste and smell, suggest an organic cause, such as substance misuse, delirium or temporal lobe epilepsy.

Hallucinations and delusions often co-occur. If their content is consistent with coexisting emotional symptoms, they are described as 'mood-congruent'. Thus, patients with severely depressed mood may believe themselves responsible for all the evils in the world, and hear voices saying, 'You are worthless. Go and kill yourself.' In this case, the diagnosis of depressive psychosis is made on the basis of the congruence of different phenomena (mood, delusion and hallucination). Incongruence between hallucinations, delusions and mood suggests schizophrenia.

Investigations

The presence of hallucinations and/or delusions should not automatically trigger a round of expensive investigations; rather, careful clinical assessment of the nature, extent and time course of the patient's symptoms will generate a list of likely diagnoses, and investigations can then be intelligently deployed to differentiate between these. When hallucinations and/or delusions arise in the context of disturbed consciousness and impaired cognition, the diagnosis is usually an organic disorder, most commonly delirium and/or dementia, and should be investigated accordingly.

Management

The management of hallucinations and/or delusions is primarily the management of the underlying condition (such as delirium, schizophrenia, mania or psychotic depression). Certain principles apply, however, whatever the underlying cause.

Hallucinations and delusions can be very real to, and often frightening for, the person who is experiencing them. Patients will often seek reassurance from the doctor. The doctor should acknowledge that these experiences are real *for the patient* while avoiding being drawn into colluding with the patient's false beliefs or perceptions. Statements such as 'Sometimes when we are unwell our brain plays tricks on us' can help to reassure a patient. Where the patient lacks insight, however, a more neutral 'We will have to agree to disagree' may be necessary to avoid conflict.

Antipsychotic medication can reduce psychotic symptoms, such as hallucinations and delusion, and is often used in combination with other sedating medication (such as a benzodiazepine) to alleviate acute distress and reduce behavioural disturbance.

Low mood

It is not uncommon for general hospital patients to report low mood. It is important to differentiate an understandable, self-limiting reaction to adversity (such as physical illness or bad news), which is normal and requires support rather than 'treatment', from a depressive disorder, which is characterised by a more severe and persistent disturbance of mood and requires specific treatment.

Clinical assessment

Depression is a relatively common illness, with a prevalence of approximately 5% in the general population and 10%–20% in medical patients. It is important to note that depression has physical as well as mental symptoms (Box 31.8). The diagnosis of depression in the medically ill, who may have physical symptoms of disease such as weight loss, fatigue, disturbed sleep, reduced appetite and so on that overlap with the physical symptoms of depression, relies on detection of the core psychological symptoms of 'anhedonia' (inability to experience pleasure) and the negative cognitive triad (see Box 31.18).

In some cases, depression may occur as a result of a direct effect of a medical condition or its treatment on the brain, when it is referred to as an 'organic mood disorder' (Box 31.9).

Investigations

When a patient appears to be low in mood, it is good practice to ask them specifically about their mood. Do they *feel* low (nausea, over-sedation, parkinsonism and so on can all cause a patient to *appear* low in mood). If so, how long have they been feeling low? Are they still able to enjoy things? To what do they attribute their low mood? If the low mood is persistent, not adequately explained by circumstances and/or associated with anhedonia, the patient should be investigated for depression. Where a patient's mood is extremely low, the clinician should ask about suicide. Asking about suicide does not increase the risk of it occurring, whereas failure to enquire denies the opportunity to prevent it. The assessment of suicide risk is described in the self-harm section later in this chapter.

31.8 Symptoms of depressive disorders	
Psychological	
• Depressed mood	• Loss of interest
• Reduced self-esteem	• Loss of enjoyment (anhedonia)
• Pessimism	• Suicidal thinking
• Guilt	
Somatic	
• Reduced appetite	• Loss of libido
• Weight change	• Bowel disturbance
• Disturbed sleep	• Motor retardation (slowing of activity)
• Fatigue	

31.9 Organic mood disorders*	
Neurological	**Infections**
• Cerebrovascular disease	• Infectious mononucleosis
• Cerebral tumour	• Herpes simplex
• Multiple sclerosis	• Brucellosis
• Parkinson's disease	• Typhoid
• Huntington's disease	• Toxoplasmosis
• Alzheimer's disease	
• Epilepsy	**Connective tissue disease**
	• Systemic lupus erythematosus
Endocrine	**Drugs**
• Hypothyroidism	• Phenothiazines
• Hyperthyroidism	• Phenylbutazone
• Cushing's syndrome	• Glucocorticoids, oral contraceptives
• Addison's disease	• Interferon
• Hyperparathyroidism	
Malignant disease	

*Diseases that may cause organic affective disorders by direct action on the brain.

31

Management

Where a patient's low mood is an understandable reaction to adversity, the clinical team can support the patient by minimising uncertainty through open and effective clinical communication and by addressing isolation (allowing access to visitors, telephone and so on). More details of the strategies available for management of depression are provided later in this chapter.

Elevated mood

Elevated mood is much less common than depressed mood, and in medical settings is often secondary to drug or alcohol misuse, an organic disorder or medical treatment. Where none of these applies, the patient may be experiencing a manic (or, if less severe, 'hypomanic') episode as part of a bipolar affective disorder. Mania is the converse of depression. It may manifest as infectious joviality, over-activity, lack of sleep and appetite, undue optimism, over-talkativeness, irritability, and recklessness in spending and sexual behaviour. When elated mood is severe, psychotic symptoms are often evident, like delusions of grandeur such as believing erroneously that one is royalty.

Investigations

The first investigation for any medical patient presenting with persistent and inexplicable elevated mood in the absence of a history of bipolar affective disorder is a medication review. Mania is a relatively common side-effect of certain classes of drug, such as glucocorticoids, and is a rare side-effect of many other drugs. Recreational, herbal and over-the-counter preparations should also be considered. Second-line investigations include tests for Cushing's disease, thyrotoxicosis, syphilis and encephalitis.

Management

The management of bipolar disorder and disturbed or aggressive behaviour are discussed in the relevant sections later in this chapter. The management of organic mania involves identifying and addressing the underlying cause.

Anxiety

Anxiety may be transient, persistent, episodic or limited to specific situations. The symptoms of anxiety are both psychological and physical (Box 31.10). The differential diagnosis of anxiety is shown in Box 31.11. Most anxiety is part of a transient adjustment to stressful events: adjustment disorders. Other more persistent forms of anxiety are described in detail on page 1254.

Investigations

Anxiety may occasionally be a manifestation of a medical condition such as thyrotoxicosis (see Box 31.11). Tests to exclude or confirm these conditions should be considered, particularly if anxiety is a new symptom that has arisen in the absence of an obvious stressor.

31.10 Symptoms of anxiety disorder

Psychological

- Apprehension
- Irritability
- Worry
- Poor concentration
- Fear of impending disaster
- Depersonalisation

Somatic

- Palpitations
- Fatigue
- Tremor
- Dizziness
- Sweating
- Diarrhoea
- Frequent desire to pass urine
- Chest pain
- Initial insomnia
- Breathlessness
- Headache

31.11 Differential diagnosis of anxiety

- Normal response to threat
- Adjustment disorder
- Generalised anxiety disorder
- Panic disorder
- Phobic disorder
- Organic (medical) cause:
  - Hyperthyroidism
  - Paroxysmal arrhythmias
  - Phaeochromocytoma
  - Alcohol and benzodiazepine withdrawal
  - Hypoglycaemia
  - Temporal lobe epilepsy

Management

The management of specific anxiety disorders is discussed later in this chapter. Benzodiazepines and related drugs, while extremely effective in the short term, cause tolerance and unpleasant or even dangerous withdrawal syndromes if used for more than a few weeks.

Psychological factors affecting medical conditions

Psychological factors may influence the presentation, management and outcome of medical conditions. Specific factors are shown in Box 31.12. The most common psychiatric diagnoses in the medically ill are anxiety and depressive disorders. Often these appear understandable as adjustments to illness and its treatment; however, if the anxiety and depression are severe and persistent, they may complicate the management of the medical condition and active management is required. Anxiety may present as an increase in somatic symptoms, such as breathlessness, tremor or palpitations, or as the avoidance of medical treatment. It is most common in those facing difficult or painful treatments, deterioration of their illness or death. Depression may manifest as increased physical symptoms, such as pain, fatigue and disability, as well as with depressed mood and loss of interest and pleasure. It is most common in patients who have suffered actual or anticipated losses, such as receiving a terminal diagnosis or undergoing disfiguring surgery.

Treatment is by psychological and/or pharmacological therapies, as described later in this chapter in the section on depression. Care is required when prescribing psychotropic drugs to the medically ill in order to avoid exacerbation of the medical condition and harmful interactions with other prescribed drugs.

Medically unexplained somatic symptoms

Medically unexplained somatic symptoms (MUS) is the term used to describe the situation where patients have symptoms that cannot be explained on the basis of a physical disorder (see Fig. 31.6). They fall into characteristics patterns (Box 31.13), and are very common in patients

31.12 Risk factors for psychological problems associated with medical conditions

- Previous history of depression or anxiety
- Lack of social support
- New diagnosis of a serious medical condition
- Deterioration of, or failure of treatment for, a medical condition
- Unpleasant, disabling or disfiguring treatment
- Change in medical care, such as discharge from hospital
- Impending death

Medical specialty	Somatic syndromes
Gastroenterology	Irritable bowel syndrome, functional dyspepsia
Gynaecology	Pre-menstrual syndrome, chronic pelvic pain
Rheumatology	Fibromyalgia
Cardiology	Atypical or non-cardiac chest pain
Respiratory medicine	Hyperventilation syndrome
Infectious diseases	Chronic (post-viral) fatigue syndrome
Neurology	Tension headache, non-epileptic attacks, functional gait disorder
Dentistry	Temporomandibular joint dysfunction, atypical facial pain
Ear, nose and throat	Globus syndrome
Allergy medicine	Multiple chemical sensitivity

attending general medical outpatient clinics. Almost any symptom can be medically unexplained, including:

- pain (including back, chest, abdominal, pelvic and headache)
- fatigue
- fits, 'funny turns', dizziness and feelings of weakness.

Patients with MUS may receive a medical diagnosis of a so-called 'functional somatic syndrome', such as irritable bowel syndrome (Box 31.13), and may also merit a psychiatric diagnosis on the basis of the same symptoms. The most frequent psychiatric diagnoses associated with MUS are anxiety or depressive disorders. When these are absent, a diagnosis of somatoform disorder may be appropriate. Somatoform disorders are discussed in more detail later in this chapter.

Self-harm

Self-harm (SH) is a common reason for presentation to medical services. The term 'attempted suicide' is potentially misleading, as most of these patients are not trying to kill themselves. Most cases of SH involve overdose, of either prescribed or non-prescribed drugs (Ch. 10). Less common methods include asphyxiation, drowning, hanging, jumping from a height or in front of a moving vehicle, and the use of firearms. Methods that carry a high chance of being fatal are more likely to be associated with serious psychiatric disorder. Self-cutting is common and often repetitive, but rarely leads to contact with medical services.

The incidence of SH varies over time and between countries. In the UK, the lifetime prevalence of suicidal ideation is 15% and that of acts of SH is 4%–5%. SH is more common in women than men, and in young rather than older adults. (In contrast, completed suicide is more common in men and older people; Box 31.14.) There is a higher incidence of SH among lower socioeconomic groups, particularly those living in crowded, socially deprived urban areas. There is also an association with alcohol misuse, child abuse, unemployment and recent relationship problems.

Clinical assessment

The main differential diagnosis is from accidental poisoning and so-called 'recreational' overdose in drug users. It must be remembered that SH is not a diagnosis but a presentation, and may be associated with any psychiatric diagnosis, the most common being adjustment disorder, substance and alcohol misuse, depressive disorder and personality disorder. In many cases, however, no psychiatric diagnosis can be made.

- Psychiatric illness (depressive illness, schizophrenia)
- Older age
- Male sex
- Living alone
- Unemployment
- Recent bereavement, divorce or separation
- Chronic physical ill health
- Drug or alcohol misuse
- Suicide note written
- History of previous attempts (especially if a violent method was used)

Management

A thorough psychiatric and social assessment should be attempted in all cases (Fig. 31.2), although some patients will discharge themselves before this can take place. The need for psychiatric assessment should not delay urgent medical or surgical treatment, though, and may need to be deferred until the patient is well enough for interview. The purpose of the psychiatric assessment is to:

- establish the short-term risk of suicide
- identify potentially treatable problems, whether medical, psychiatric or social.

Topics to be covered when assessing a patient are listed in Box 31.15. The history should include events occurring immediately before and after the act, and especially any evidence of planning. The nature and severity of any current psychiatric symptoms must be assessed, along with the personal and social supports available to the patient outside hospital.

Most SH patients have depressive and anxiety symptoms on a background of chronic social and personal difficulties (often complicated by use of alcohol or other substances), but no psychiatric disorder. They do not usually require psychotropic medication or specialised psychiatric treatment but may benefit from personal support and practical advice from a GP, social worker or community psychiatric nurse. Admission to a psychiatric ward is necessary only for persons who display one or more of the following:

- an acute psychiatric disorder
- high short-term risk of suicide
- need for temporary respite from intolerable circumstances
- requirement for further assessment of their mental state.

Approximately 20% of SH patients make a repeat act during the following year and 1%–2% kill themselves. Factors associated with suicide after an episode of SH are listed in Box 31.14.

Disturbed and aggressive behaviour

Disturbed and aggressive behaviour is common in general hospitals, especially in emergency departments. Most behavioural disturbance arises not from medical or psychiatric illness, but from alcohol intoxication, reaction to the situation and personality characteristics.

Clinical assessment

The key principles of management are, firstly, to establish control of the situation rapidly and thereby ensure the safety of the patient and others; and secondly, to try to determine the cause of the disturbance in order to remedy it. Establishing control requires the presence of an adequate number of trained staff, an appropriate physical environment and sometimes sedation (Fig. 31.3). The assistance of hospital security staff and sometimes the police may be required. In all cases, the staff approach is important; a calm, non-threatening manner expressing understanding of the patient's concerns is often all that is required to defuse potential aggression (Box 31.16).

31

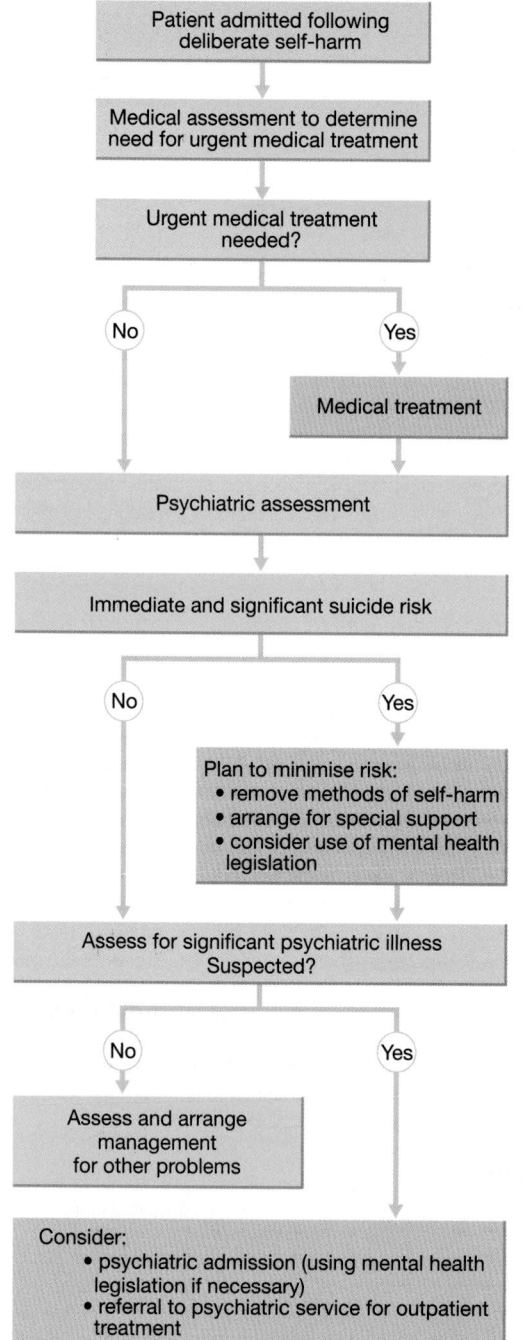

Fig. 31.2 **Assessment of patients admitted following self-harm.**

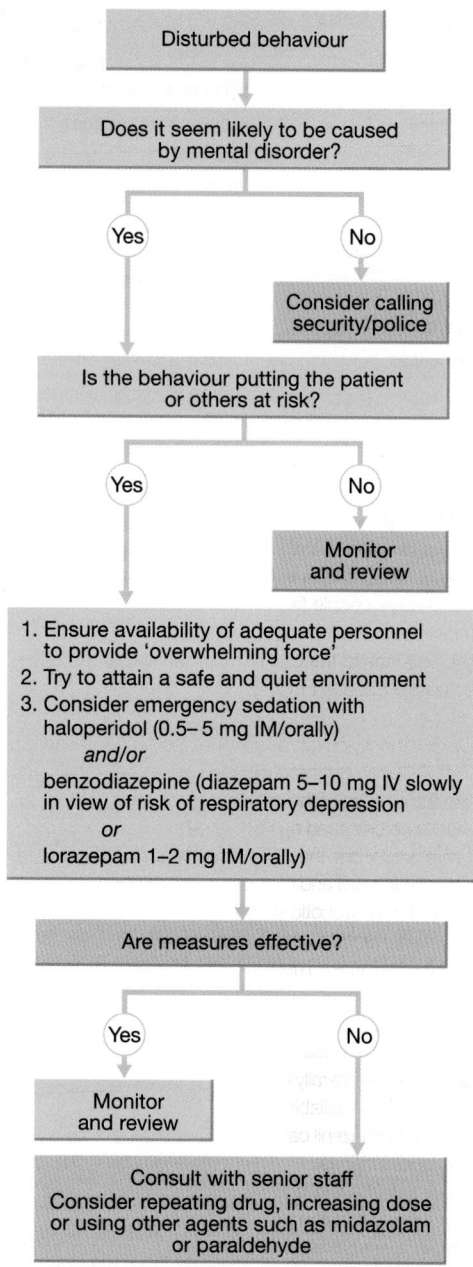

Fig. 31.3 **Acute management of disturbed behaviour.** (IM = intramuscular; IV = intravenous)

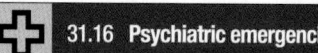

31.15 **Assessment of patients after self-harm**

Current attempt

- Patient's account
- Degree of intent at the time: preparations, plans, precautions against discovery, note
- Method used, particularly whether violent
- Degree of intent now
- Symptoms of psychiatric illness

Background

- Previous attempts and their outcome
- Family and personal history
- Social support
- Previous response to stress
- Extent of drug and alcohol misuse

31.16 **Psychiatric emergencies**

- Intervene as necessary to reduce the risk of harm to the patient and to others
- Adopt a calm, non-threatening approach
- Arrange availability of other staff and parenteral medication
- Consider diagnostic possibilities of drug intoxication, acute psychosis and delirium
- Involve friends and relatives as appropriate

An attempt should be made to try to identify the factors that are contributing to the disturbed behaviour. When the patient is cooperative, these factors are best determined at interview. Other sources of information about the patient include medical and psychiatric records, and discussion with nursing staff, family members and other informants, including the patient's GP. The following information should be sought:

- psychiatric, medical (especially neurological) and criminal history
- current psychiatric and medical treatment

- alcohol and drug misuse
- recent stressors
- the time course and accompaniments of the current episode in terms of mood, belief and behaviour.

Observation of the patient's behaviour may also yield useful clues. Do they appear to be responding to hallucinations? Are they alert or variably drowsy and confused? Are there physical features suggestive of drug or alcohol misuse or withdrawal? Are there new injuries or old scars, especially on the head? Do they smell of alcohol or solvents? Do they bear the marks of drug injection? Are they unwashed and unkempt, suggesting a gradual development of their condition?

Investigations

Depending on the results of clinical assessment, routine biochemistry, haematology and analysis of blood or urine for illicit drugs or alcohol may be required.

Management

Measures such as restraint and sedation may be required in patients with acute behavioural disturbance in order to identify the cause and to protect the patient and other people from harm. While this potentially raises legal issues, in most countries, including the UK, common law confers on doctors the right, and indeed the duty, to intervene against a patient's wishes if this is necessary. Sedation may be required and can be achieved with antipsychotic drugs (such as haloperidol) and/or benzodiazepines (such as lorazepam or diazepam). The choice of drug, dose, route and rate of administration depends on the patient's age, gender and physical health, as well as the likely cause of the disturbed behaviour. The benefits of sedation must always be balanced against the potential risks. When prescribing benzodiazepines, consider the risk of respiratory depression (particularly in patients with lung disease) and encephalopathy (in those with liver disease). When prescribing antipsychotic drugs for acute sedation, consider the risk of acute dystonias (such as 'oculogyric crisis') and acute arrhythmias (in patients with heart disease). Thus for a frail older woman with emphysema and delirium, sedation may be achieved with a low dose (0.5mg) of oral haloperidol, while for a strong young man with an acute psychotic episode, 10mg or more of intravenous diazepam and a similar dose of haloperidol may be required. A parenterally administered anticholinergic agent, such as procyclidine, should be available to treat extrapyramidal effects from haloperidol if they arise. Flumazenil can be used to reverse respiratory depression caused by benzodiazepines.

If the initial assessment suggests that the patient has an acute psychiatric disorder, then admission to a psychiatric facility may be indicated. If a medical cause is more likely, psychiatric transfer is usually inappropriate and the patient should be managed in a medical setting, with whatever nursing and security support is required. Where it is clear that there is no medical or psychiatric illness, the person should be removed from the hospital, to police custody if necessary.

Many countries, such as the UK, also have specific mental health legislation that may be used to detain patients if necessary.

Principles of management

The multifactorial origin of most psychiatric disorders means that there are multiple potential targets for treatment. It is useful to consider management strategies within a bio-psycho-social framework. This can help to address the biological factors that contribute to the illness with medication and other physical treatments such as electroconvulsive therapy, while also considering the potential role for psychological therapies and changes to the patient's social environment.

Pharmacological treatments

These aim to relieve psychiatric disorder by modifying brain function. The main biological treatments are psychotropic drugs. These are widely used for various purposes; a pragmatic classification is set out in Box 31.17. It should be noted that some drugs have applications to more than one condition; for example, antidepressants are also widely used in the treatment of anxiety *and* chronic pain. The specific subgroups of psychotropic drugs are discussed in the sections on the appropriate disorders below.

Electroconvulsive therapy

Electroconvulsive therapy (ECT) entails producing a convulsion by the brief administration of a high-voltage direct-current impulse to the head while the patient is anaesthetised and paralysed by muscle relaxant. If properly administered, it is remarkably safe, has few side-effects and is of proven efficacy for severe depressive illness. There may be headaches and amnesia for events occurring a few hours before ECT (retrograde) and after it (anterograde). Pronounced amnesia can occur but is infrequent and difficult to distinguish from the effects of severe depression.

Other forms of electromagnetic stimulation

Clinical trials of transcranial magnetic stimulation (TMS) and vagal nerve stimulation (VNS) suggest they may have a limited role in patients with depression refractory to conventional treatments.

Surgery

Surgery to the brain (psychosurgery) has a very limited place and then only in the treatment of severe chronic psychiatric illness resistant to other measures. Frontal lobotomies are never done now, and pre-frontal leucotomies are very rare. Operations these days usually target specific sub-regions and tracts of the brain.

i 31.17 Classification of commonly used psychotropic drugs

Action	Main groups	Clinical use
Antipsychotic	Phenothiazines Butyrophenones Second-generation antipsychotics	Schizophrenia Bipolar mania Delirium
Antidepressant	Tricyclics and related drugs Serotonin and noradrenergic re-uptake inhibitors Monoamine oxidase inhibitors Esketamine	Depression/anxiety Obsessive-compulsive disorder Depression/anxiety Adjunctive therapy in treatment of resistant depression
Mood-stabilising	Lithium Sodium valproate Lamotrigine	Treatment and prophylaxis of bipolar disorder Adjunctive therapy in bipolar disorder
Anti-anxiety	Benzodiazepines β-adrenoceptor antagonists	Anxiety/insomnia (short term) Alcohol withdrawal (short term) Anxiety (somatic symptoms)

31

Psychological therapies

These treatments are useful in many psychiatric disorders and also in non-psychiatric conditions. They are based on talking with patients, either individually or in groups. Sometimes discussion is supplemented by 'homework' or tasks to complete between treatment sessions. Psychological treatments take a number of forms based on the duration and frequency of contact, the specific techniques applied and their underlying theory.

General supportive psychotherapy

General psychotherapy should be part of all medical treatment. It involves empathic listening to the patient's account of their symptoms and associated fears and concerns, followed by the sympathetic provision of accurate information that addresses these.

Cognitive therapy

This therapy is based on the observation that some psychiatric disorders are associated with systematic errors in the patient's conscious thinking, such as a tendency to interpret events in a negative way or see them as unduly threatening. A triad of 'cognitive errors' has been described in depression (Box 31.18). Cognitive therapy aims to help patients to identify such cognitive errors and to learn how to challenge them. It is widely used for depression, anxiety, and eating and somatoform disorders, and also increasingly in psychoses.

Behaviour therapy

This is a practically orientated form of treatment, in which patients are assisted in changing unhelpful behaviour, such as helping patients to implement carefully graded exposure to the feared stimulus in phobias.

Cognitive behaviour therapy

Cognitive behaviour therapy (CBT) combines the methods of behaviour therapy and cognitive therapy. It is the most widely available and extensively researched psychological treatment.

Problem-solving therapy

This is a simplified brief form of CBT, which helps patients actively tackle problems in a structured way (Box 31.19). It can be delivered by non-psychiatric doctors and nurses after appropriate training and is commonly used to help patients who self-harm in response to a situational crisis.

i	**31.18** **The negative cognitive triad associated with depression**
Cognitive error	**Example**
Negative view of self	'I am no good'
Negative view of current life experiences	'The world is an awful place'
Negative view of the future	'The future is hopeless'

i	**31.19** **Stages of problem-solving therapy**

- Define and list problems
- Choose one to work on
- List possible solutions
- Evaluate these and choose the best
- Try it out
- Evaluate the result
- Repeat until problems are resolved

Psychodynamic psychotherapy

This treatment, also known as 'interpretive psychotherapy', was pioneered by Freud, Jung and Klein, among others. It is based on the theory that early life experience generates powerful but unconscious motivations. Psychotherapy aims to help the patient to become aware of these unconscious factors on the assumption that, once identified, their negative effects are reduced. The relationship between therapist and patient is used as a therapeutic tool to identify issues in patients' relationships with others, particularly parents, which may be replicated or transferred to their relationship with the therapist. Explicit discussion of this relationship is the basis for the treatment, which traditionally requires frequent sessions over a period of months or even years.

Interpersonal psychotherapy

Interpersonal psychotherapy (IPT) is a specific form of brief psychotherapy that focuses on patients' current interpersonal relationships and is an effective treatment for mild to moderate depression.

Social interventions

Some adverse social factors, such as unemployment, may not be readily amenable to intervention but others, such as access to benefits and poor housing, may be. Patients can be helped to address these problems themselves by being taught problem-solving. Befrienders and day centres can reduce social isolation, benefits advisers can ensure appropriate financial assistance, and medical recommendations can be made to local housing departments to help patients obtain more appropriate accommodation.

Psychiatric disorders

Dementia

Dementia is a clinical syndrome characterised by a loss of previously acquired intellectual function in the absence of impaired arousal. It affects 5% of those over 65 and 20% of those over 85. It is defined as a global impairment of cognitive function and is typically progressive and non-reversible. There are many subtypes (Box 31.20) but Alzheimer's disease and diffuse vascular dementia are the most common. Rarer causes of dementia should be actively sought in younger patients and those with short histories.

Pathogenesis

Dementia may be divided into 'cortical' and 'subcortical' types, depending on the clinical features.

Clinical features

The usual presentation is with a disturbance of personality or memory dysfunction. A careful history is essential and it is important to interview both the patient and a close family member. Simple bedside tests, such as the MoCA, are useful in assessing the nature and severity of the cognitive deficit, although a more intensive neuropsychological assessment may sometimes be required, especially if there is diagnostic uncertainty. It is important to exclude a focal brain lesion. This is done by determining that there is cognitive disturbance in more than one area. Mental state assessment is important to seek evidence of depression, which may coexist with or occasionally cause apparent cognitive impairment. Many of the primary degenerative diseases that cause dementia have characteristic features that may allow a specific diagnosis during life. Creutzfeldt–Jakob disease, for example, is usually quickly progressive (over months) and is associated with myoclonus. The more slowly progressive dementias are more difficult to distinguish during life, but

i 31.20 Subtypes and causes of dementia

Type	Common	Less common	Rare
Vascular	Diffuse small-vessel disease	Amyloid angiopathy Multiple emboli	Cerebral vasculitis Systemic lupus erythematosus
Inherited	Alzheimer's disease	Fronto-temporal dementia Leukodystrophies Huntington's disease Wilson's disease Dystrophia myotonica Lewy body dementia Progressive supranuclear palsy	Mitochondrial encephalopathies Cortico-basal degeneration
Neoplastic	Secondary deposits	Primary cerebral tumour	Paraneoplastic syndrome (limbic encephalitis)
Inflammatory	–	Multiple sclerosis	Sarcoidosis
Traumatic	Chronic subdural haematoma Post-head injury	Punch-drunk syndrome	–
Hydrocephalus		Communicating/non-communicating 'normal pressure' hydrocephalus	–
Toxic/nutritional	Alcohol	Thiamin deficiency Vitamin B_{12} deficiency	Anoxia/carbon monoxide poisoning Heavy metal poisoning
Infective	–	Syphilis Human immunodeficiency virus (HIV)	Post-encephalitis Whipple's disease Subacute sclerosing panencephalitis
Prion diseases	–	Sporadic Creutzfeldt–Jakob disease (CJD)	Variant CJD Kuru Gerstmann–Sträussler–Scheinker disease

fronto-temporal dementia typically presents with signs of temporal or frontal lobe dysfunction, whereas Lewy body dementia may present with visual hallucinations. The course may also help to distinguish types of dementia. Gradual worsening suggests Alzheimer's disease, whereas stepwise deterioration is typical of vascular dementia.

Investigations

The aim is to seek treatable causes and to estimate prognosis. This is done using a standard set of investigations (Box 31.21). Imaging of the brain can exclude potentially treatable structural lesions, such as hydrocephalus, cerebral tumour or chronic subdural haematoma, though the only abnormality usually seen is that of generalised atrophy. An electroencephalogram (EEG) may be helpful if Creutzfeldt–Jakob disease is suspected, as characteristic abnormalities of generalised periodic sharp wave pattern are usually observed. If the initial tests are negative, more invasive investigations, such as lumbar puncture or, very rarely, brain biopsy, may be indicated.

Management

This is mainly directed at addressing treatable causes and providing support for patients and carers. Tackling risk factors may slow deterioration, such as by management of hypertension in vascular dementia, or abstinence and vitamin replacement in toxic/nutritional dementias. Psychotropic drugs may have a role in alleviating symptoms, such as disturbance of sleep, perception or mood, but should be used with care because of an increased mortality in patients who have been treated long-term with these agents. Sedation is not a substitute for good care of patients and carers or, in the later stages, attentive residential nursing care. In the UK, incapacity and mental health legislation may be required to manage patients' financial and domestic affairs, as well as to determine their safe placement. If the diagnosis is Alzheimer-type dementia, cholinesterase inhibitors and memantine may slow progression for a time.

Alzheimer's disease

Alzheimer's disease is the most common form of dementia. It increases in prevalence with age and is rare in people under 45 years.

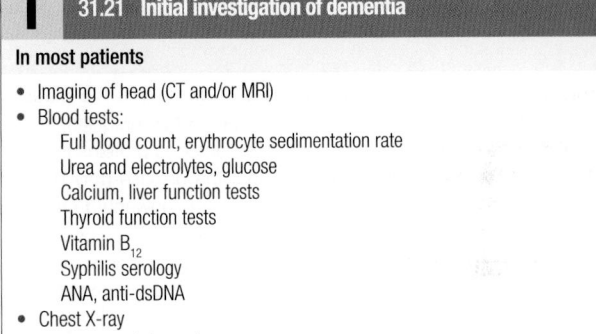

i 31.21 Initial investigation of dementia

In most patients
- Imaging of head (CT and/or MRI)
- Blood tests:
  - Full blood count, erythrocyte sedimentation rate
  - Urea and electrolytes, glucose
  - Calcium, liver function tests
  - Thyroid function tests
  - Vitamin B_{12}
  - Syphilis serology
  - ANA, anti-dsDNA
- Chest X-ray
- Electroencephalography

In selected patients
- Lumbar puncture
- HIV serology
- Brain biopsy

(ANA = antinuclear antibody; anti-dsDNA = anti-double-stranded DNA; CT = computed tomography; HIV = human immunodeficiency virus; MRI = magnetic resonance imaging)

Pathogenesis

Genetic factors play an important role and about 15% of cases are familial. These cases fall into two main groups: early-onset disease with autosomal dominant inheritance and a later-onset group where the inheritance is polygenic. Mutations in several genes have been described but most are rare and/or of small effect. The inheritance of one of the alleles of apolipoprotein ε (apo ε4) is associated with an increased risk of developing the disease (2–4 times higher in heterozygotes and 6–8 times higher in homozygotes). Its presence is, however, neither necessary nor sufficient for the development of the disease and so genetic testing for ApoE4 is not clinically useful. The brain in Alzheimer's disease is macroscopically atrophic, particularly the cerebral cortex and hippocampus. Histologically, the disease is characterised by the presence of senile plaques and neurofibrillary tangles in the cerebral cortex. Histochemical

31

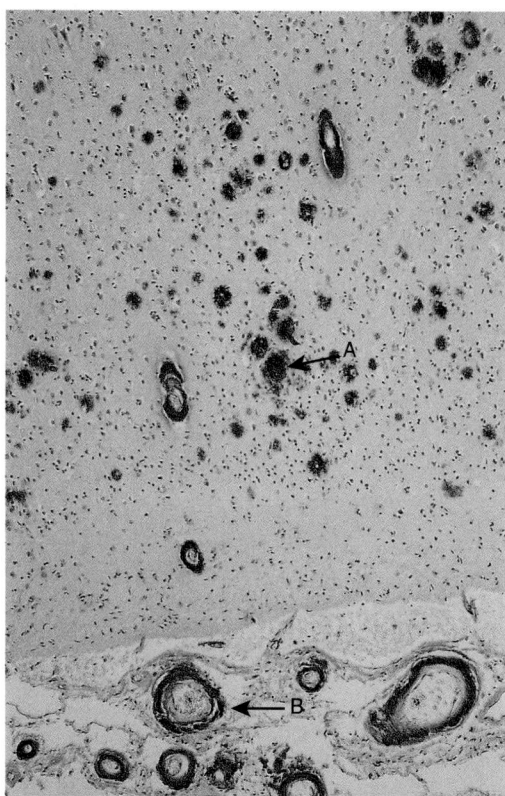

Fig. 31.4 Alzheimer's disease. Section of neocortex stained with polyclonal antibody against βA4 peptide showing amyloid deposits in plaques in brain substance (arrow A) and in blood-vessel walls (arrow B). *Courtesy of Dr J. Xuereb.*

staining demonstrates significant quantities of amyloid in the plaques (Fig. 31.4); these typically stain positive for the protein ubiquitin, which normally is involved in targeting unwanted or damaged proteins for degradation. This has led to the suggestion that the disease may be due to defects in the ability of neuronal cells to degrade unwanted proteins. Many different neurotransmitter abnormalities have also been described. In particular, there is impairment of cholinergic transmission, although abnormalities of noradrenaline (norepinephrine), 5-HT, glutamate and substance P have also been described.

Clinical features

The key clinical feature is impairment of the ability to remember new information. Hence, patients present with gradual impairment of memory, usually in association with disorders of other cortical functions. Short- and long-term memory are both affected but defects in the former are usually more obvious. Later in the course of the disease, typical features include apraxia, visuospatial impairment and aphasia. In the early stages of the disease patients may notice these problems, but as the disease progresses it is common for patients to deny that there is anything wrong (anosognosia). In this situation, patients are often brought to medical attention by their carers. Depression is commonly present. Occasionally, patients become aggressive, and the clinical features can be made acutely worse by intercurrent physical disease.

Patients typically present with subjective memory loss, sometimes getting lost in familiar locations. A history of progressive memory loss and associated functional impairment, corroborated by an informant, is the key to making the diagnosis. Cognitive testing and neuroimaging can be helpful but in themselves are not diagnostic.

Investigations

Investigation is aimed at excluding treatable causes of dementia (see Box 31.20), as histological confirmation of the diagnosis usually occurs only after death.

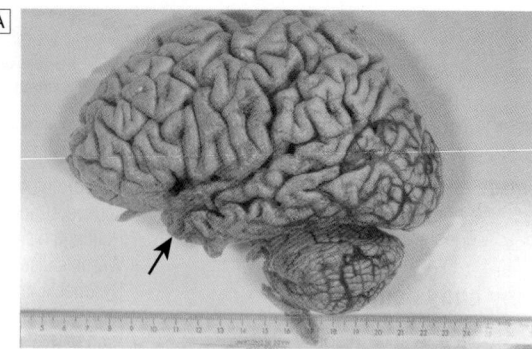

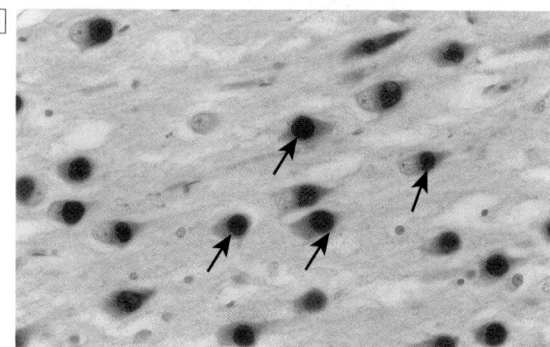

Fig. 31.5 Fronto-temporal dementia. Ⓐ Lateral view of formalin-fixed brain from a patient who died of Pick's disease, showing gyral atrophy of frontal and parietal lobes and a more severe degree of atrophy affecting the anterior half of the temporal lobe (arrow). Ⓑ High power (×200) view of hippocampal pyramidal layer, prepared with monoclonal anti-tau antibody. Many neuronal cell bodies contain sharply circumscribed, spherical cytoplasmic inclusion bodies (Pick bodies, arrows). *(A and B) Courtesy of Dr J. Xuereb.*

Management

Treatment with anticholinesterases, such as donepezil, rivastigmine and galantamine, has been shown to be of some benefit at slowing progression of cognitive impairment in the early stages of the disease while post-synaptic cholinergic receptors are still available. The N-methyl-D-aspartate (NMDA) receptor antagonist memantine slightly enhances learning and memory in early disease and can also be useful in selected patients with more advanced disease. Novel treatments are under development to block amyloid plaque formation directly, by inhibiting the enzyme γ-secretase. Non-pharmacological approaches include the provision of a familiar environment for the patient and support for the carers. Many patients are anxious or depressed, and if this is confirmed, treatment with antidepressant medication may be helpful.

Fronto-temporal dementia

Fronto-temporal dementia encompasses a number of different syndromes characterised by behaviour abnormalities and impairment of language. Symptoms usually occur before the age of 60 and the prevalence has been estimated at 15 per 100 000 in the population aged between 45 and 65 years. The three major clinical subtypes are behavioural-variant fronto-temporal dementia, primary progressive aphasia and semantic dementia. Pick's disease is a common cause of the first two in particular. Genetic factors play an important role and familial cases have been described caused by mutations in several genes, including *MAPT*, which encodes microtubule-associated protein tau, *GRN*, *TPD43*, *FUS*, *VCP* and *C9orf72*. The causal mutations trigger abnormal accumulation of tau and other proteins in brain tissue, which are seen as cytoplasmic inclusion bodies on histological examination (Fig. 31.5). It is of interest that some gene mutations that cause fronto-temporal dementia, such as *VCP*, are also associated with amyotrophic lateral sclerosis, inclusion body myopathy and Paget's disease of bone, suggesting that these disorders share a similar pathogenic basis in which cellular degeneration is caused by accumulation of abnormal proteins. The clinical presentation may be with personality change due to frontal lobe involvement or with language disturbance due to temporal lobe involvement. In contrast to Alzheimer's disease, memory is relatively preserved in the early stages. There is no specific treatment. Disinhibition and compulsive behaviours can be helped by selective serotonin re-uptake inhibitors (SSRIs). Although fronto-temporal dementia shares certain symptoms with Alzheimer's, it cannot be treated with anticholinesterases because cholinergic systems are not affected.

Lewy body dementia

This neurodegenerative disorder is clinically characterised by dementia and signs of Parkinson's disease. It is often inherited and mutations in the α-synuclein and β-synuclein genes have been identified in affected patients. These mutations result in accumulation of abnormal protein aggregates in neurons that contain the protein α-synuclein in association with other proteins, including ubiquitin (see Fig. 28.30). The cognitive state often fluctuates and there is a high incidence of visual hallucinations. Affected individuals are particularly sensitive to the side-effects of anti-Parkinsonian medication and also to antipsychotic drugs. There is no curative treatment but anticholinesterase drugs can be helpful in slowing progression of cognitive impairment.

Alcohol misuse and dependence

Alcohol consumption associated with social, psychological and physical problems constitutes misuse. The criteria for alcohol dependence, a more restricted term, are shown in Box 31.22. Approximately one-quarter of male patients in general hospital medical wards in the UK have a current or previous alcohol problem.

Pathogenesis

Availability of alcohol and social patterns of use appear to be the most important factors. Genetic factors predispose to dependence. The majority of people who misuse alcohol do not have an associated psychiatric disorder, but a few drink heavily in an attempt to relieve anxiety or depression.

Clinical features

The modes of presentation of alcohol misuse and complications are summarised below.

Social problems

Common features include absenteeism from work, unemployment, marital tensions, child abuse, financial difficulties and problems with the law, such as violence and traffic offences.

Low mood

Low mood is common since alcohol has a direct depressant effect and heavy drinking creates numerous social problems. Attempted and completed suicide are associated with alcohol misuse.

Anxiety

People who are anxious may use alcohol as a means of relieving anxiety in the short term and this can develop into dependence. Conversely, alcohol withdrawal increases anxiety.

31.22 Criteria for alcohol dependence
- Narrowing of the drinking repertoire
- Priority of drinking over other activities (salience)
- Tolerance of effects of alcohol
- Repeated withdrawal symptoms
- Relief of withdrawal symptoms by further drinking
- Subjective compulsion to drink
- Reinstatement of drinking behaviour after abstinence

Alcohol withdrawal syndrome

The features are described in Box 31.23. Symptoms usually become maximal about 2–3 days after the last drink and can include seizures. The term 'delirium tremens' is used to describe severe alcohol withdrawal syndrome characterised by both delirium (characteristically, agitation and visual hallucinations) and physiological hyper-arousal (tremor, sweating and tachycardia). It has a significant mortality and morbidity (see Box 31.23).

Hallucinations

Hallucinations (characteristically visual but sometimes in other modalities) are common in delirium tremens. Less common is the phenomenon called 'alcoholic hallucinosis', where a patient with alcohol dependence experiences auditory hallucination in clear consciousness at a time when they are not withdrawing from alcohol.

Wernicke–Korsakoff syndrome

This is a rare but important indirect complication of chronic alcohol misuse. It is an organic brain disorder resulting from damage to the mamillary bodies, dorsomedial nuclei of the thalamus and adjacent areas of periventricular grey matter caused by a deficiency of thiamin (vitamin B_1). The syndrome most commonly results from long-standing heavy drinking and an inadequate diet but can also arise from malabsorption or even protracted vomiting. Wernicke's encephalopathy (nystagmus or ophthalmoplegia with ataxia and delirium) often presents acutely and, without prompt treatment (see below), can progress and become irreversible. Korsakoff syndrome (severe short-term memory deficits and confabulation) can develop chronically or acutely (with Wernicke's).

Alcohol-related brain damage

The term alcohol-related brain damage (ARBD) is often used as a collective description of the many brain pathologies associated with alcohol excess,

31.23 Presentation and consequences of chronic alcohol misuse

Acute intoxication
- Emotional and behavioural disturbance
- Medical problems: hypoglycaemia, ketoacidosis, aspiration of vomit, respiratory depression
- Accidents, injuries sustained in fights

Withdrawal phenomena
- Psychological symptoms: restlessness, anxiety, panic attacks
- Autonomic symptoms: tachycardia, sweating, pupil dilatation, nausea, vomiting
- Delirium: agitation, hallucinations (classically 'Lilliputian'), illusions, delusions
- Seizures

Consequences of harmful use
Medical
- Neurological: peripheral neuropathy, cerebellar degeneration, cerebral haemorrhage, dementia
- Hepatic: fatty change and cirrhosis, liver cancer
- Gastrointestinal: oesophagitis, gastritis, pancreatitis, oesophageal cancer, Mallory–Weiss syndrome, malabsorption, oesophageal varices
- Respiratory: pulmonary tuberculosis, pneumonia
- Skin: spider naevi, palmar erythema, Dupuytren's contractures, telangiectasias
- Cardiac: cardiomyopathy, hypertension
- Musculoskeletal: myopathy, fractures
- Endocrine and metabolic: pseudo-Cushing's syndrome, hypoglycaemia, gout
- Reproductive: hypogonadism, fetal alcohol syndrome, infertility

Psychiatric and cerebral
- Depression
- Alcoholic hallucinosis
- Alcoholic 'blackouts'
- Wernicke's encephalopathy: nystagmus or ophthalmoplegia with ataxia and delirium
- Korsakoff syndrome: short-term memory deficits leading to confabulation

31

which often coexist in the same patient. Acute alcohol intoxication causes ataxia, slurred speech, emotional incontinence and aggression. Very heavy drinkers may experience periods of amnesia for events that occurred during bouts of intoxication, termed 'alcoholic blackouts'. Established alcohol dependence may lead to 'alcoholic dementia', a global cognitive impairment resembling Alzheimer's disease, but which does not progress and may even improve if the patient becomes abstinent. Heavy alcohol use can damage the brain indirectly through Wernicke–Korsakoff syndrome (see above), head injury, hypoglycaemia and encephalopathy.

Effects on other organs

These are protean and virtually any organ can be involved (see Box 31.23). These effects are discussed in detail in other chapters in this book.

Diagnosis

The diagnosis of alcohol excess may emerge while taking the patient's history, but many patients do not tell the truth about their alcohol intake. Alcohol misuse may also present through its effects on one or more aspects of the patient's life, as listed above. Alcohol dependence commonly presents with withdrawal in those admitted to hospital, as they can no longer maintain their high alcohol intake in this setting.

Management

For the person misusing alcohol, provision of clear information from a doctor about the harmful effects of alcohol and safe levels of consumption is often all that is needed. In more serious cases, patients may have to be advised to alter leisure activities or change jobs to help them to reduce their consumption. Psychological treatment is used for people who have recurrent relapses and is usually available at specialised centres. Support to stop drinking is also provided by voluntary organisations, such as Alcoholics Anonymous (AA) in the UK.

Alcohol withdrawal syndromes can be prevented, or treated once established, with long-acting benzodiazepines. Large doses may be required (such as diazepam 20 mg 4 times daily), tailed off over a period of 5–7 days as symptoms subside. Prevention of the Wernicke–Korsakoff syndrome requires the immediate use of high doses of thiamin, which is initially given parenterally in the form of Pabrinex (two vials 3 times daily for 48 hrs, longer if symptoms persist) and then orally (100 mg 3 times daily). There is no treatment for Wernicke–Korsakoff syndrome once it has arisen. The risk of side-effects, such as respiratory depression with benzodiazepines and anaphylaxis with Pabrinex, is small when weighed against the potential benefits of treatment.

Acamprosate (666 mg 3 times daily) may help to maintain abstinence by reducing the craving for alcohol. Disulfiram (200–400 mg daily) can be given as a deterrent to patients who have difficulty resisting the impulse to drink after becoming abstinent. It blocks the metabolism of alcohol, causing acetaldehyde to accumulate. When alcohol is consumed, an unpleasant reaction follows, with headache, flushing and nausea. Disulfiram is always an adjunct to other treatments, especially supportive psychotherapy. Treatment with antidepressants may be required if depression is severe or does not resolve with abstinence. Antipsychotics, such as chlorpromazine (100 mg 3 times daily), are needed for alcoholic hallucinosis. Although such treatment may be successful, there is a high relapse rate.

Prognosis

Between 80% and 90% of patients with established alcohol dependence syndrome who embark on medically supervised detoxification will successfully complete detoxification without encountering significant complications. Sustaining abstinence is more challenging than achieving it, however. Studies indicate that 1 year after successful detoxification, only 20% of patients will remain abstinent. This figure rises to approximately 30% for patients who are engaged with alcohol services, and to over 40% if such specialist support is combined with supervised disulfiram treatment.

Substance misuse disorder

Dependence on and misuse of both illegal and prescribed drugs is a major problem worldwide. Drugs of misuse are described in detail in Chapter 7. They can be grouped as follows.

Sedatives

These commonly give rise to physical dependence, the manifestations of which are tolerance and a withdrawal syndrome. Drugs include benzodiazepines, opiates (including morphine, heroin, methadone and dihydrocodeine) and barbiturates (now rarely prescribed). Overdosage with sedatives can be fatal, primarily as a result of respiratory depression (Ch. 10). Withdrawal from opiates is notoriously unpleasant, and withdrawal from benzodiazepines and barbiturates can cause prolonged anxiety and even hallucinations and/or seizures.

Intravenous opiate users are prone to bacterial infections, hepatitis B, hepatitis C and HIV infection through needle contamination. Accidental overdose is common, mainly because of the varied and uncertain potency of illicit supplies of the drug. The withdrawal syndrome, which can start within 12 hours of last use, presents with intense craving, rhinorrhoea, lacrimation, yawning, perspiration, shivering, piloerection, vomiting, diarrhoea and abdominal cramps. Examination reveals tachycardia, hypertension, mydriasis and facial flushing.

Stimulants

Stimulant drugs include amphetamines and cocaine. They are less dangerous than the sedatives in overdose, although they can cause cardiac and cerebrovascular problems through their pressor effects. Physical dependence syndromes do not arise, but withdrawal causes a rebound lowering in mood and can give rise to an intense craving for further use, especially in any form of drug with a rapid onset and offset of effect, such as crack cocaine. Chronic ingestion can cause a paranoid psychosis similar to schizophrenia. A 'toxic psychosis' (delirium) can occur with high levels of consumption. Unpleasant tactile hallucinations described as 'like ants crawling under the skin' (formication) may be prominent in either acute intoxication or withdrawal.

Hallucinogens

The hallucinogens are a disparate group of drugs that cause prominent sensory disturbances. They include cannabis, ecstasy, lysergic acid diethylamide (LSD), *Psilocybin* (magic mushrooms) and a variety of synthetic cannabinoids (as one of the so-called 'legal highs' or 'novel psychoactive substances'). A toxic confusional state can occur after heavy cannabis consumption. Acute psychotic episodes are well recognised, especially in those with a family or personal history of psychosis, and there is evidence that prolonged heavy use increases the risk of developing schizophrenia. Paranoid psychoses have been reported in association with ecstasy. A chronic psychosis has also been documented after regular LSD use.

Organic solvents

Solvent inhalation (glue sniffing) is popular in some adolescent groups. Solvents produce acute intoxication characterised by euphoria, excitement, dizziness and a floating sensation. Further inhalation leads to loss of consciousness; death can occur from the direct toxic effect of the solvent, or from asphyxiation if the substance is inhaled from a plastic bag.

Pathogenesis

Many of the causal factors for alcohol misuse also apply to substance misuse. The main factors are the psychological and behavioural vulnerabilities described above, cultural pressures, particularly within a peer group, and availability of a drug. In the case of some drugs such as opiates, medical over-prescribing has increased their availability, but there has also been a relative decline in the price of illegal drugs. Most drug users take a range of drugs; this is termed 'polydrug misuse'.

Diagnosis

As with alcohol, the diagnosis either may be apparent from the history and examination, or may be made only once the patient presents with a complication. Drug screening of samples of urine or blood can be valuable in confirming the diagnosis, especially if the patient persists in denial.

Management

The first step is to determine whether patients wish to stop using the drug. If they do not, they can still benefit from advice about how to minimise harm from their habit, such as how to obtain and use clean needles for those who inject. For those who are physically dependent on sedative drugs, substitute prescribing (using methadone, for example, in opiate dependence) may help stabilise their lives sufficiently to allow a gradual reduction in dosage until they reach abstinence. Some specialist units offer inpatient detoxification. The medical management of overdose is discussed in Chapter 10. The drug lofexidine, a centrally acting α-agonist, can be useful in treating the autonomic symptoms of opiate withdrawal, as can clonidine, although this carries a risk of hypotension and is best used by specialists. Long-acting opiate antagonists, such as naltrexone, may also have a place, again in specialist hands, in blocking the euphoriant effects of the opiate, thereby reducing addiction.

In some cases, complete opiate withdrawal is not successful and the patient functions better if maintained on regular doses of oral methadone as an outpatient. This decision to prescribe long-term methadone should be taken only by a specialist, and carried out under long-term supervision at a specialist drug treatment centre.

Substitute prescribing is neither necessary nor possible for the hallucinogens and stimulants, but the principles of management are the same as those that should accompany prescribing for the sedatives. These include identifying problems associated with the drug misuse that may serve to maintain it, and intervening where possible. Intervention may be directed at physical illness, psychiatric comorbidity, social problems or family disharmony.

Relapsing patients and those with complications should be referred to specialist drug misuse services. Support can also be provided by self-help groups and voluntary bodies, such as Narcotics Anonymous (NA) in the UK.

Schizophrenia

Schizophrenia is characterised by delusions, hallucinations and lack of insight. Acute schizophrenia may also present with disturbed behaviour, disordered thinking, or with insidious social withdrawal and other so-called negative symptoms and less obvious delusions and hallucinations. Schizophrenia occurs worldwide in all ethnic groups with a prevalence of about 0.5%. It is more common in men (1.4 to 1). Children of an affected parent have an approximate 10% risk of developing the illness, but this rises to 50% if an identical twin is affected. The usual age of onset is the mid-twenties but can be older, particularly in women.

Pathogenesis

There is a strong genetic contribution, usually involving many susceptibility genes, each of small effect, but 2%–3% of cases can be attributed to increased or decreased copies of genes (so-called 'copy number variations'). Environmental risk factors include a history of obstetric complications at the time of the patient's birth, childhood adversity and urban upbringing. Brain imaging techniques have identified subtle structural abnormalities in groups of people with schizophrenia, including an overall decrease in brain size (by about 3% on average), with a relatively greater reduction in temporal lobe volume (5%–10%). Episodes of acute schizophrenia may be precipitated by social stress and also by cannabis, which increases dopamine turnover. Consequently, schizophrenia is now viewed as a neurodevelopmental disorder, caused by abnormalities of brain development associated with genetic predisposition and early environmental influences, but precipitated by later triggers.

Clinical features

Acute schizophrenia should be suspected in any individual with bizarre behaviour accompanied by delusions and hallucinations that are not due to organic brain disease or substance misuse. The characteristic clinical features are listed in Box 31.24. Hallucinations are typically auditory but can occur in any sensory modality. They commonly involve voices from outside the head that talk to or about the person. Sometimes the voices repeat the person's thoughts. Patients may also describe 'passivity of thought', experienced as disturbances in the normal privacy of thinking, such as the delusional belief that their thoughts are being 'withdrawn' from them and perhaps 'broadcast' to others, and/or that alien thoughts are being 'inserted' into their mind. Other characteristic symptoms are delusions of control: believing that one's emotions, impulses or acts are controlled by others. Another phenomenon is delusional perception, a delusion that arises suddenly alongside a normal perception, such as 'I saw the moon and I immediately knew he was evil.' Other, less common, symptoms may occur, including thought disorder, as manifest by incomprehensible speech, and abnormalities of movement, such as those in which the patient can become immobile or adopt awkward postures for prolonged periods (catatonia).

Diagnosis

The diagnosis is made primarily on clinical grounds but investigations may be required to rule out organic brain disease. The main differential diagnosis of schizophrenia (Box 31.25) includes:

---

i | **31.24 Symptoms of schizophrenia**

First-rank symptoms of acute schizophrenia

- A = Auditory hallucinations – second- or third-person/écho de la pensée
- B = Broadcasting, insertion/withdrawal of thoughts
- C = Controlled feelings, impulses or acts ('passivity' experiences/phenomena)
- D = Delusional perception (a particular experience is bizarrely interpreted)

Symptoms of chronic schizophrenia (negative symptoms)

- Flattened (blunted) affect
- Apathy and loss of drive (avolition)
- Social isolation/withdrawal (autism)
- Poverty of speech (alogia)
- Poor self-care

---

i | **31.25 Differential diagnosis of schizophrenia**

Alternative diagnosis	Distinguishing features
Other functional psychoses	
Delusional disorders	Absence of specific features of schizophrenia
Psychotic depression	Prominent depressive symptoms
Manic episode	Prominent manic symptoms
Schizoaffective disorder	Mood and schizophrenia symptoms both prominent
Puerperal psychosis	Acute onset after childbirth
Organic disorders	
Drug-induced psychosis	Evidence of drug or alcohol misuse
Side-effects of prescribed drugs	Levodopa, methyldopa, glucocorticoids, antimalarial drugs
Temporal lobe epilepsy	Other evidence of seizures
Delirium	Visual hallucinations, impaired consciousness
Dementia	Age, established cognitive impairment
Huntington's disease	Family history, choreiform movements, dementia

31

- *Other functional psychoses*, particularly psychotic depression and mania, in which delusions and hallucinations are congruent with a marked mood disturbance (negative in depression and grandiose in mania). Schizophrenia must also be differentiated from specific delusional disorders that are not associated with the other typical features of schizophrenia.
- *Organic psychoses*, including delirium, in which there is impairment of consciousness and loss of orientation (not found in schizophrenia), typically with visual hallucinations.
- *Drug misuse*, particularly in young people.
- *Auto-immune or infectious encephalitis*.
- *Temporal lobe epilepsy*, with psychotic symptoms, in which olfactory and gustatory hallucinations may occur.

Many of those who experience acute schizophrenia go on to develop a chronic state in which the acute, so-called positive symptoms resolve, or at least do not dominate the clinical picture, leaving so-called negative symptoms that include blunt affect, apathy, social isolation, poverty of speech and poor self-care. Patients with chronic schizophrenia may also manifest positive symptoms, particularly when under stress, and it can be difficult for those who do not know the patient to judge whether or not these are signs of an acute relapse.

Investigations

As in dementia, investigations are focused on excluding a treatable cause, such as a slow-growing brain tumour, temporal lobe epilepsy, neurosyphilis or various autoimmune conditions. These are required only in patients with neurological or other organic symptoms or signs.

Management

First-episode schizophrenia often requires admission to hospital because patients lack the insight that they are ill and are unwilling to accept treatment. In some cases, they may be at risk of harming themselves or others. Subsequent acute relapses and chronic schizophrenia are now usually managed in the community.

Drug treatment

Antipsychotic agents are effective against the positive symptoms of schizophrenia in the majority of cases. They take 2 weeks or so to be maximally effective but have some beneficial effects shortly after administration. Treatment is then ideally continued to prevent relapse. In a patient with a first episode of schizophrenia this will usually be for 1 or 2 years, but in patients with multiple episodes treatment may be required for many years. The benefits of prolonged treatment must be weighed against the adverse effects, which include extrapyramidal side-effects (EPSE) like acute dystonic reactions (which may require treatment with parenteral anticholinergics), akathisia and parkinsonism. For long-term use, antipsychotic agents are often given by slow-release (depot) injections to improve adherence.

A number of antipsychotic agents are available (Box 31.26). These may be divided into first-generation drugs such as chlorpromazine and haloperidol, and second-generation drugs such as olanzapine and clozapine. In general, the newer drugs are less likely to produce unwanted EPSE but tend to cause greater weight gain and metabolic disturbances, such as dyslipidaemia. All work by blocking D_2 dopamine receptors in the brain, with the possible exception of clozapine. Clozapine can be remarkably effective in those who do not respond to other antipsychotics but can cause agranulocytosis in about 1% of patients in the first few months. Prescription therefore requires regular monitoring of white blood cell count, initially on a weekly basis, then fortnightly and monthly thereafter. Clozapine, like all antipsychotics, should not be stopped suddenly because of the likelihood of relapse. Adverse effects of antipsychotic drugs are listed in Box 31.27. Two serious adverse effects deserve special mention.

Neuroleptic malignant syndrome

This is a rare but serious condition characterised by fever, tremor and rigidity, autonomic instability and delirium. Characteristic laboratory

31.26 Antipsychotic drugs

Group	Drug	Usual adult dose[1]
Phenothiazines	Chlorpromazine	400–600 mg daily
Butyrophenones	Haloperidol	8–12 mg daily
Thioxanthenes	Flupentixol decanoate	40 mg fortnightly (depot injection)
Diphenylbutylpiperidines	Pimozide	8–10 mg daily
Substituted benzamides	Sulpiride	800–1200 mg daily
Dibenzodiazepines[2]	Clozapine	300–600 mg daily
Benzisoxazole[2]	Risperidone	4–6 mg daily
Thienobenzodiazepines[2]	Olanzapine	10–15 mg daily
Dibenzothiazepines[2]	Quetiapine	300–600 mg daily

[1]Lower or higher doses may be required in some patients. [2]Second-generation antipsychotics.

31.27 Adverse effects of antipsychotic drugs

Weight gain due to increased appetite

Effects due to dopamine blockade*

- Acute dystonia
- Akathisia (motor restlessness)
- Parkinsonism
- Tardive dyskinesia
- Gynaecomastia
- Galactorrhoea

Effects due to cholinergic blockade

- Dry mouth
- Blurred vision
- Impotence
- Constipation
- Urinary retention

Hypersensitivity reactions

- Blood dyscrasias (neutropenia with clozapine)
- Cholestatic jaundice
- Photosensitive dermatitis

Ocular complications

- Corneal and lens opacities (long-term use)

*Less severe with clozapine, quetiapine and olanzapine, possibly because of strong 5-hydroxytryptamine-blocking effect and relatively weak dopamine blockade.

findings are an elevated creatinine phosphokinase and leucocytosis. Antipsychotic medication must be stopped immediately and supportive therapy provided, often in an intensive care unit. Treatment includes ensuring hydration and reducing hyperthermia. Dantrolene sodium and bromocriptine may be helpful. Mortality is 20% untreated and 5% with treatment.

Cardiac arrhythmias

Antipsychotic medications cause prolongation of the QTc interval, which may be associated with ventricular tachycardia, torsades de pointes and sudden death. If this occurs, treatment should be reviewed, with careful electrocardiographic monitoring and treatment of serious arrhythmias if necessary.

Psychological treatment

Psychological treatment, including general support for the patient and family, is now seen as an essential component of management. CBT may help patients to cope with symptoms. There is evidence that personal and/or family education, when given as part of an integrated treatment package, reduces the rate of relapse.

Social treatment

After an acute episode of schizophrenia has been controlled by drug therapy, social rehabilitation may be required. Recurrent illness is likely to cause disruption to patients' relationships and their ability to manage their accommodation and occupation; consequently, patients with schizophrenia often need help to obtain housing and employment. A graded return to employment and sometimes a period of supported accommodation may be required.

Patients with chronic schizophrenia have particular difficulties and may need long-term, supervised accommodation. This now tends to be in supported accommodation in the community. Patients may also benefit from sheltered employment if they are unable to participate effectively in the labour market. Ongoing contact with a health worker allows monitoring for signs of relapse, sometimes as part of a multidisciplinary team working to agreed plans (the 'care programme approach'). Partly because of a tendency to inactivity, smoking and a poor diet, patients with chronic schizophrenia are at increased risk of cardiovascular disease, diabetes and stroke, and require proactive medical as well as psychiatric care.

Prognosis

About one-third of those who develop an acute schizophrenic episode have a good outcome. One-third develop chronic, incapacitating schizophrenia, and the remainder largely recover after each episode but suffer relapses. Most affected patients cannot work or live independently. Schizophrenia is associated with suicide and up to 10% of patients take their own lives.

Mood disorders

Mood or affective disorders include:

- *unipolar depression*: one or more episodes of low mood and associated symptoms
- *bipolar disorder*: episodes of elevated mood interspersed with episodes of depression
- *dysthymia*: chronic low-grade depressed mood without sufficient other symptoms to count as 'clinically significant' or 'major' depression.

Depression

Major depressive disorder has a prevalence of 5% in the general population and approximately 10%–20% in chronically ill medical outpatients, including older adults (see Box 31.6). It is a major cause of disability and suicide. If comorbid with a medical condition, depression magnifies disability, diminishes adherence to medical treatment and rehabilitation, and may even shorten life expectancy.

Pathogenesis

There is a genetic predisposition to depression, especially when of early onset. The genetic predisposition is mediated by variants in a large number of genes and loci of small effect rather than mutations in single genes. Adversity and abuse early in life also predispose to depression. Depressive episodes are often, but not always, triggered by stressful life events (especially those that involve loss or imposed change), including medical illnesses. Associated biological factors include hypofunction of monoamine neurotransmitter systems, including 5-HT and noradrenaline (norepinephrine), and abnormalities of the hypothalamic–pituitary–adrenal (HPA) axis, which results in elevated cortisol levels that do not suppress with dexamethasone.

Diagnosis

The symptoms are listed in Box 31.8. Depression may be mild, moderate or severe. It may also be recurrent or chronic. It can be both a complication of a medical condition and a cause of MUS (see below), so physical examination is essential; an associated medical condition should always be considered, particularly where there is no past history of depression and no apparent psychological precipitant.

Investigations

Investigations are not usually required unless there are clinical grounds for suspicion of an underlying medical disorder, such as Cushing's syndrome or hypothyroidism.

Management

Pharmacological and psychological treatments both work in depression. In practice, the choice is determined by patient preference and local availability. Severe depression complicated by psychotic symptoms, dehydration or suicide risk may require ECT.

Drug treatment

Antidepressant drugs are effective in moderate and severe depression, whether it is primary or secondary to a medical illness. The most suitable drug for an individual patient will depend on their previous response, likely side-effects, their concurrent illnesses and potential drug interactions. Commonly used antidepressants are shown in Box 31.28.

The different classes of antidepressant have similar efficacy and about three-quarters of patients respond to treatment. Successful treatment requires the patient to take an appropriate dose of an effective drug for an adequate period. For those who do not respond, a proportion will do so if changed to another class of antidepressant. The patient's progress must be monitored and, after recovery, treatment should be continued for at least 6–12 months to reduce the high risk of relapse. The dose should then be tapered off over several weeks to avoid discontinuation symptoms. The Scottish Intercollegiate Guidelines Network (SIGN) and National Institute for Health and Care Excellence (NICE) have published treatment guidelines.

Tricyclic antidepressants

Tricyclic antidepressant (TCA) agents inhibit re-uptake of the amines noradrenaline (norepinephrine) and 5-HT at synaptic clefts. The

i 31.28 Antidepressant drugs		
Group	**Drug**	**Usual adult dose***
Tricyclic antidepressants	Amitriptyline	75–150 mg daily
	Imipramine	75–150 mg daily
	Dosulepin	75–150 mg daily
	Clomipramine	75–150 mg daily
Selective serotonin re-uptake inhibitors (SSRIs)	Citalopram	20–40 mg daily
	Escitalopram	10–20 mg daily
	Fluoxetine	20–60 mg daily
	Sertraline	50–200 mg daily
	Paroxetine	20–50 mg daily
Monoamine oxidase inhibitors	Phenelzine	45–90 mg daily
	Tranylcypromine	20–40 mg daily
	Moclobemide	300–600 mg daily
Noradrenaline (norepinephrine) re-uptake inhibitors and SSRIs	Venlafaxine	75–375 mg daily
	Duloxetine	60–120 mg daily
Noradrenaline and specific serotonergic inhibitor	Mirtazapine	15–45 mg daily
N-methyl D-aspartate antagonists	Esketamine	28 mg initially, then 28–84 mg twice weekly, then weekly, then every 1–2 weeks

*Higher doses may be required in some patients: see guidelines. With the exception of esketamine, which is given intranasally, other drugs are given orally.

31

therapeutic effect is noticeable within a week or two. Adverse effects, such as sedation, anticholinergic effects, postural hypotension, lowering of the seizure threshold and cardiotoxicity, can be troublesome during this period. TCAs may be dangerous in overdose and should be used with caution in people who have coexisting heart disease, glaucoma and prostatism.

Selective serotonin re-uptake inhibitors

Selective serotonin reuptake inhibitors (SSRIs) are less cardiotoxic and less sedative than TCAs, and have fewer anticholinergic effects. They are safer in overdose but can still cause QTc prolongation, headache, nausea, anorexia and sexual dysfunction. They can also interact with other drugs increasing serotonin (5-HT), to produce 'serotonin syndrome'. This is a rare syndrome of neuromuscular hyperactivity, autonomic hyperactivity and agitation, and potentially seizures, hyperthermia, delirium and even death.

Noradrenaline (norepinephrine) re-uptake inhibitors

These agents primarily inhibit noradrenaline uptake at the synaptic cleft but have additional pharmacological effects. Venlafaxine and duloxetine also act as serotonin re-uptake inhibitors, whereas mirtazapine also acts as an antagonist at 5-HT2a, 5-HT2c and 5-HT3 receptors. These drugs have similar efficacy to the agents listed above but a different adverse-effect profile.

Monoamine oxidase inhibitors

Monoamine oxidase inhibitors (MAOIs) increase the availability of neuro-transmitters at synaptic clefts by inhibiting metabolism of noradrenaline (norepinephrine) and 5-HT. They are now rarely prescribed in the UK, since they can cause potentially dangerous interactions with drugs such as amphetamines and certain anaesthetic agents, and with foods rich in tyramine (such as cheese and red wine). This is due to accumulation of amines in the systemic circulation, causing a potentially fatal hypertensive crisis.

Esketamine

Esketamine has recently been licensed for treatment-resistant major depressive disorder. It acts as an antagonist at NMDA receptors and is typically used in patients who have not responded to at least two different treatments

ECT and related treatments

Electroconvulsive therapy (ECT) is a highly effective and relatively safe treatment for severe depression but, whilst valuable in the acute setting, its use as a maintenance treatment presents challenges. Transcranial magnetic stimulation (TMS) and the related vagal nerve stimulation (VNS) have shown promise in clinical trials but are not in widespread clinical use.

Psychological treatment

Both CBT and interpersonal therapy are as effective as antidepressants for mild to moderate depression. Antidepressant drugs are, however, preferred for severe depression. Drug and psychological treatments are more effective in combination.

Prognosis

Over 50% of people who have had one depressive episode and over 90% of people who have had three or more episodes will have another. The risk of suicide in an individual who has had a depressive disorder is 10 times greater than in the general population.

Bipolar disorder

Bipolar disorder is an episodic disturbance with interspersed periods of depressed and elevated mood; the latter is known as hypomania when mild or short-lived, or mania when severe or chronic. The lifetime risk of developing bipolar disorder is approximately 1%–2%. Onset is usually in the twenties, and men and women are equally affected.

Pathogenesis

Bipolar disorder is strongly heritable (approximately 70%). Relatives of patients have an increased incidence of both bipolar and unipolar affective disorder. More than a hundred genetic variants of small effect have been identified by genome-wide association studies. Life events, such as physical illness, sleep deprivation and some medications, such as steroids, may also play a role in triggering episodes.

Diagnosis

The diagnosis is based on clear evidence of episodes of depression and mania. Isolated episodes of hypomania or mania do occur but they are usually preceded or followed by an episode of depression. Psychotic symptoms may occur in both the depressive and the manic phases, with delusions and hallucinations that are usually in keeping with the mood disturbance. This is described as an affective psychosis. Patients who present with symptoms of both bipolar disorder and schizophrenia in equal measure may be given a diagnosis of schizoaffective disorder.

Management

Depression should be treated as described above. If antidepressants are prescribed, however, they should be combined with a mood-stabilising drug (see below) to avoid 'switching' the patients into (hypo)mania. Manic episodes and psychotic symptoms usually respond well to antipsychotic drugs (see Box 31.26).

Prophylaxis to prevent recurrent episodes of depression and mania with mood-stabilising agents is important. The main drugs used are lithium and sodium valproate but lamotrigine, olanzapine, quetiapine and risperidone are increasingly employed. Caution must be exercised when stopping these drugs, as a relapse may follow.

Lithium carbonate is the drug of first choice. It is also used for acute mania, and in combination with a tricyclic as an adjuvant treatment for resistant depression. It has a narrow therapeutic range, so regular blood monitoring is required to maintain a serum level of 0.5–1.0 mmol/L. Toxic effects include nausea, vomiting, a coarse tremor and convulsions. With long-term treatment, weight gain, hypothyroidism, increased calcium and parathyroid hormone (PTH), nephrogenic diabetes insipidus and renal failure can occur. Thyroid and renal function should be checked before treatment is started and regularly thereafter. Lithium may be teratogenic and should not be prescribed during the first trimester of pregnancy.

Anticonvulsants, such as sodium valproate and lamotrigine, and some antipsychotic drugs can all be used as prophylaxis in bipolar disorder, usually as a second-line alternative to lithium. Valproate conveys a high risk of birth defects and should not be used in women of child-bearing age. Olanzapine can cause significant weight gain. (For a list of the adverse effects of antipsychotic drugs see Box 31.27.)

Prognosis

The relapse rate of bipolar disorder is high, although patients may be perfectly well between episodes. After one episode, the annual average risk of relapse is about 10%–15%, which doubles after more than three episodes. There is a substantially increased lifetime risk of suicide of 5%–10%.

Anxiety disorders

These are characterised by the emotion of anxiety, worrisome thoughts, avoidance behaviours and the somatic symptoms of autonomic arousal. Anxiety disorders are divided into three main subtypes: phobic, paroxysmal (panic) and generalised (Box 31.29). The nature and prominence of the somatic symptoms often lead the patient to present initially to medical services. Anxiety may be stress-related and phobic anxiety may follow an unpleasant incident. Many patients with anxiety also have depression.

i	**31.29 Classification of anxiety disorders**		
	Phobic anxiety disorder	Panic disorder	Generalised anxiety disorder
Occurrence	Situational	Paroxysmal	Persistent
Behaviour	Avoidance	Escape	Agitation
Cognitions	Fear of situation	Fear of symptoms	Worry
Symptoms	On exposure	Episodic	Persistent

Clinical features

Phobic anxiety disorder

A phobia is an abnormal or excessive fear of a specific object or situation, which leads to avoidance of it (such as excessive fear of dying in an air crash, leading to avoidance of flying). A general phobia of going out alone or being in crowded places is called 'agoraphobia'. Phobic responses can develop to medical procedures such as venepuncture.

Panic disorder

Panic disorder describes repeated attacks of severe anxiety, which are not restricted to any particular situation or circumstances. Somatic symptoms, such as chest pain, palpitations and paraesthesia in lips and fingers, are common. The symptoms are in part due to involuntary over-breathing (hyperventilation). Patients with panic attacks often fear that they are suffering from a serious illness, such as a heart attack or stroke, and seek emergency medical attention. Panic disorder may coexist with agoraphobia.

Generalised anxiety disorder

This is typically a recurrent or a chronic anxiety state associated with uncontrollable worry. The associated muscle tension often leads to a variety of medical presentations.

Diagnosis

The diagnosis is made on the basis of clinical history and typical symptoms, as described above. Where a diagnosis of panic disorder is suspected, it can be confirmed by asking the patient to hyperventilate deliberately for 1–2 minutes and observing whether the symptoms are reproduced. A finding of respiratory alkalosis on arterial blood gas measurement is indicative of chronic hyperventilation.

Management

Psychological treatment

Explanation and reassurance are essential, especially when patients fear they have a serious medical condition. Specific treatment may be needed. Treatments include relaxation, graded exposure (desensitisation) to feared situations for phobic disorders, and CBT.

Drug treatment

Antidepressants are the drugs of first choice. The therapeutic dose can be higher – and response delayed – for anxiety disorders than for depression and there is some evidence that, within their respective classes, escitalopram (SSRI), duloxetine (SNRI) and clomipramine (TCA) have greatest efficacy against anxiety disorders. Activating side-effects of some antidepressants can lead to a worsening of anxiety symptoms in the first 2 weeks and patients should be warned of this.

Benzodiazepines are useful in the short term but regular long-term use carries a high risk of dependence. Regular prescriptions should therefore be limited to 3 weeks; beyond that, prescriptions should be restricted to occasional use as required, with periodic review to guard against dose escalation. Short-acting benzodiazepines, such as lorazepam, have a rapid onset and provide symptomatic relief for up to 2 hours but have

the greatest potential for dependence. Longer-acting drugs, such as diazepam, can take an hour to take effect when given orally but provide symptomatic relief for up to 12 hours. The GABA analogue pregabalin is an effective alternative but can also lead to tolerance and dependence. A β-blocker, such as propranolol, can help when somatic symptoms are prominent.

Obsessive–compulsive disorder

Obsessive–compulsive disorder (OCD) is characterised by 'obsessions' – thoughts, images or impulses that are recurrent, unwanted and usually anxiety-provoking, but recognised as one's own. In many cases, the obsessions give rise to 'compulsions', which are repeated acts performed to relieve the anxiety. Unlike the anxiety disorders discussed above, which are more common in women, OCD is equally common in men and women.

Clinical features

Common examples include fears of contamination, giving rise to repeated and ritualised hand-washing, and concerns about having forgotten something, giving rise to time-consuming repeated checking. The differential diagnoses include normal checking behaviour and delusional beliefs about thought possession.

Diagnosis

The diagnosis is made on the basis of the typical history, as described above.

Management

Obsessive–compulsive disorder usually responds to some degree to antidepressant drugs (high-dose clomipramine or SSRI; see Box 31.28) and to 'exposure response prevention' – a form of CBT in which patients are encouraged to expose themselves to the feared thought or situation without performing the anxiety-relieving compulsions. Relapses are common, however, and the condition often becomes chronic.

Stress-related disorders

Acute stress reaction

Following a traumatic or life-threatening event, such as an assault or a major accident, some people develop a characteristic pattern of symptoms: an initial state of 'daze' or bewilderment is followed by altered activity (withdrawal or agitation), often with anxiety. The symptoms are transient and usually resolve completely within a few days. The lay media often describes this as 'shock'.

Adjustment disorder

A more common psychological response to a major stressor such as a serious medical diagnosis is a less severe but more prolonged emotional reaction.

Clinical features

The predominant symptom is usually depression and/or anxiety, which is insufficiently persistent or intense to merit a diagnosis of depressive or anxiety disorder. There may also be anger, aggressive behaviour and associated excessive alcohol use. Symptoms develop within a month of the onset of the stress, and their duration and severity reflect the course of the underlying stressor.

'Pathological grief' describes a grief reaction that is abnormally intense or persistent, and such abnormalities are a particular type of adjustment disorder. They manifest as a brief period of emotional numbing, followed by a period of distress lasting several weeks, during which sorrow, tearfulness, sleep disturbance, a sense of futility, anger and 'bargaining' are common. Perceptual distortions may occur, including misinterpreting sounds as the dead person's voice or 'seeing' the dead person.

31

Diagnosis

The diagnosis is made on the basis of the typical history, with a strong presumed relationship between the stressful life event and the onset of symptoms described above.

Management

Ongoing contact with and support from a doctor or another person who can listen, reassure, explain and advise are often all that is needed. Most patients do not require psychotropic medication, although benzodiazepines reduce arousal and they and antidepressants can aid sleep.

Post-traumatic stress disorder

Post-traumatic stress disorder (PTSD) is a delayed and/or protracted response to a stressful event of a life-threatening or catastrophic nature. Examples of such events include natural disasters, terrorist activity, serious accidents and witnessing violent deaths. It may also sometimes occur after distressing medical treatments or admissions to intensive care.

Clinical features

The development of PTSD is usually delayed from a few days to several months between the traumatic event and the onset of symptoms. Typical symptoms are recurrent intrusive memories (flashbacks) of the trauma; sleep disturbance, especially nightmares (usually of the traumatic event) from which the patient awakes in a state of anxiety; symptoms of autonomic arousal (anxiety, palpitations, enhanced startle); emotional numbing; and avoidance of situations that evoke memories of the trauma. Anxiety and depression are often associated and excessive use of alcohol or drugs frequently complicates the clinical picture.

Diagnosis

The diagnosis is made on the basis of the typical clinical features following a traumatic life event.

Management

In the immediate aftermath of a significant trauma, the main aim is to provide support, direct advice and the opportunity for emotional catharsis (routine debriefing may actually be harmful). In established PTSD, structured psychological approaches (CBT, eye movement desensitisation and reprocessing (EMDR) and stress management) are effective. Antidepressant drugs are moderately effective.

Prognosis

Most patients recover within 2–3 years. In a small proportion, the symptoms become chronic.

Somatoform disorders

The essential feature of these disorders is that the somatic symptoms are not explained by a medical condition (medically unexplained symptoms, MUS), nor better diagnosed as part of a depressive or anxiety disorder. The derivation of the term 'somatoform' is 'body-like'. Several syndromes are described within this category; there is considerable overlap between them, both in the underlying causes and in the clinical presentation.

Pathogenesis

The cause of somatoform disorders is incompletely understood but contributory factors include depression and anxiety, the erroneous interpretation of somatic symptoms as evidence of disease, excessive concern with physical illness and a tendency to seek medical care. A family history or previous history of a particular condition may have shaped the patient's beliefs about illness. Doctors may exacerbate the problem, either by dismissing the complaints as non-existent or by over-emphasising and investigating the possibility of disease.

Clinical features

Somatoform disorders can present in several different ways, as described below.

Somatoform autonomic dysfunction

This describes somatic symptoms referable to bodily organs that are largely under the control of the autonomic nervous system. The most common examples involve the cardiovascular system ('cardiac neurosis'), respiratory system ('psychogenic hyperventilation') and gut ('psychogenic vomiting' and 'irritable bowel syndrome'). Antidepressant drugs and CBT may be helpful.

Somatoform pain disorder

This describes severe, persistent pain that cannot be adequately explained by a medical condition. Antidepressant drugs (especially tricyclics and dual action drugs such as duloxetine) are helpful, as are some of the anticonvulsant drugs, particularly carbamazepine, gabapentin and pregabalin. CBT and multidisciplinary pain management teams are also useful.

Chronic fatigue syndrome

Chronic fatigue syndrome (CFS) is characterised by excessive fatigue after minimal physical or mental exertion, poor concentration, dizziness, muscular aches and sleep disturbance. This pattern of symptoms may follow a viral infection such as infectious mononucleosis, influenza or hepatitis. Symptoms overlap with those of depression and anxiety. There is good evidence that many patients improve with carefully graded exercise and with CBT, as long as the benefits of such treatment are carefully explained.

Dissociative conversion disorders

Dissociative conversion disorders are characterised by a loss or distortion of neurological functioning that is not fully explained by organic disease ('functional neurological disorder'). These may be psychological functions such as memory ('dissociative amnesia'), sensory functions such as vision ('dissociative blindness'), or motor functions ('functional gait disorder') (Box 31.30). The cause is unknown but there is an association with recent stress and with adverse childhood experiences, including physical and sexual abuse. Organic disease may precipitate dissociation and provide a model for symptoms. For example, non-epileptic seizures often occur in those with epilepsy. Treatment with CBT may be of benefit.

Somatisation disorder

This is defined as the occurrence of multiple medically unexplained physical symptoms affecting several bodily systems. It is also known as Briquet syndrome after the physician who first described the presentation. Symptoms often start in early adult life but somatisation disorder can arise later, usually following an episode of physical illness. The disorder is much more common in women. Patients may undergo a multitude of negative investigations and unhelpful operations, particularly hysterectomy and cholecystectomy. There is no proven treatment except to try to ensure that unnecessary investigations and surgical procedures are avoided to minimise iatrogenic harm.

Hypochondriacal disorder

Patients with this condition have a strong fear or belief that they have a serious, often fatal, disease (such as cancer), and that fear persists despite appropriate medical reassurance. They are typically highly anxious and seek many medical opinions and investigations in futile but repeated attempts to relieve their fears.

i	**31.30 Common presentations of dissociative (conversion) disorder**
• Gait disturbance	• Non-epileptic seizures
• Loss of function in limbs	• Sensory loss
• Aphonia	• Blindness

Hypochondriacal disorder often resembles OCD, but in a small proportion of cases the conviction that disease is present reaches delusional intensity. The best-known example is that of parasitic infestation ('delusional parasitosis'), which leads patients to consult dermatologists. Treatment with CBT can be helpful. Patients who suffer delusions may benefit from antipsychotic medication. The condition may become chronic.

Body dysmorphic disorder

This is defined as a preoccupation with bodily shape or appearance, with the belief that one is disfigured in some way (previously known as 'dysmorphophobia'). People with this condition may make inappropriate requests for cosmetic surgery. Treatment with CBT or antidepressants may be helpful. The belief in disfigurement may sometimes be delusional, in which case antipsychotic drugs can help.

Management

The management of the various syndromes of medically unexplained complaints described above is based on the general principles outlined in Box 31.31 and discussed in more detail below.

Reassurance

Patients should be asked what they are most worried about. Clearly, it may be unwise to state categorically that the patient does not have any disease, as that is difficult to establish with certainty. However, it can be emphasised that the probability of having a disease is low and that doctors often see patients with physical symptoms but no physical disease. If patients repeatedly ask for reassurance about the same health concern despite reassurance, they may have hypochondriasis.

Explanation

Patients need a positive explanation for their symptoms. It is unhelpful to say that symptoms are psychological or 'all in the mind'. Rather, a term such as 'functional' (meaning that the symptoms represent a reversible disturbance of bodily function) may be more acceptable. When possible, it is useful to describe a plausible physiological mechanism that is linked to psychological factors such as stress and implies that the symptoms are reversible. For example, in irritable bowel syndrome, psychological stress results in increased activation of the autonomic nervous system, which leads to constriction of smooth muscle in the gut wall, which in turn causes pain and bowel disturbance.

Advice

This should focus on how to overcome factors perpetuating the symptoms: for example, by resolving stressful social problems or by practising relaxation. The doctor can offer to review progress, to prescribe (for example) an antidepressant drug and, if appropriate, to refer for physiotherapy or psychological treatments such as CBT. The attitudes of relatives may need to be addressed if they have adopted an over-protective role, unwittingly reinforcing the patient's disability.

Drug treatment

Antidepressant drugs are often helpful, even if the patient is not depressed.

---

i | **31.31 General management principles for medically unexplained symptoms**

- Take a full sympathetic history
- Exclude disease but avoid unnecessary investigation or referral
- Seek specific treatable psychiatric syndromes
- Demonstrate to patients that you believe their complaints
- Establish a collaborative relationship
- Give a positive explanation for the symptoms, including but not over-emphasising psychological factors
- Encourage a return to normal functioning

Psychological treatment

There is evidence for the effectiveness of CBT. Other psychological treatments such as IPT may also have a role.

Rehabilitation

Where there is chronic disability, particularly in dissociative (conversion) disorder, conventional physical rehabilitation may be the best approach.

Shared care

Ongoing planned care is required for patients with chronic intractable symptoms, especially those of somatisation disorder. Review by the same specialist, interspersed with visits to the same GP, is probably the best way to avoid unnecessary multiple re-referral for investigation, to ensure that treatable aspects of the patient's problems, such as depression, are actively managed and to prevent the GP from becoming demoralised.

Eating disorders

There are two well-defined eating disorders, anorexia nervosa (AN) and bulimia nervosa (BN); they share some overlapping features. Ninety per cent of people affected are female. There is a much higher prevalence of abnormal eating behaviour in the population that does not meet diagnostic criteria for AN or BN but may attract a diagnostic label such as 'binge eating disorder'. In developed societies, obesity is arguably a much greater problem but is usually considered to be more a disorder of lifestyle or physiology than a psychiatric disorder.

Anorexia nervosa

The lifetime risk of anorexia nervosa for women living in Europe is approximately 1%–2% (for men it is <0.5%) with a peak age of onset of 15–19 years. Predisposing factors include familiality (both genetic and shared environmental factors appear to play a role) and 'neurotic' personality traits. The illness is often precipitated by weight loss, whether due to non-pathological dieting/increased exercise or physical illness such as gastrointestinal disorders or diabetes mellitus. Many sufferers do not engage with specialist services and it is not uncommon for the first presentation to be with a medical problem (Box 31.32) rather than to psychiatric services.

Clinical features

There is marked weight loss, arising from food avoidance, often in combination with bingeing, purging, excessive exercise and/or the use of

---

 | **31.32 Medical consequences of eating disorders**

Cardiac

- ECG abnormalities: T-wave inversion, ST depression and prolonged QTc interval
- Arrhythmias, including profound sinus bradycardia and ventricular tachycardia

Haematological

- Anaemia, thrombocytopenia and leucopenia

Endocrine

- Pubertal delay or arrest
- Growth retardation and short stature
- Amenorrhoea
- Sick euthyroid state

Metabolic

- Uraemia
- Renal calculi
- Osteoporosis

Gastrointestinal

- Constipation
- Abnormal liver function tests

---

diuretics and laxatives. Body image is profoundly disturbed so that, despite emaciation, patients still feel overweight and are terrified of weight gain. These preoccupations are intense and pervasive, and the false beliefs may be held with a conviction approaching the delusional. Anxiety and depressive symptoms are common accompaniments. Downy hair (lanugo) may develop on the back, forearms and cheeks. Extreme starvation is associated with a wide range of physiological and pathological bodily changes. All organ systems may be affected, although the most serious problems are cardiac and skeletal (see Box 31.32).

Pathogenesis

The underlying cause is unclear but probably includes personality (high neuroticism), genetic (twin studies indicate heritability of 0.3–0.5) and environmental factors, including, in many societies, the social pressure on women to be thin.

Diagnosis

Diagnostic criteria are shown in Box 31.33. Differential diagnosis is from other causes of weight loss, including psychiatric disorders such as depression, and medical conditions such as inflammatory bowel disease, malabsorption, hypopituitarism and cancer, although it is important to remember that AN can coexist with any of these. The diagnosis is based on a pronounced fear of fatness despite being thin, and on the absence of an adequate alternative explanation for weight loss.

Management

The aims of management are to ensure patients' physical well-being while helping them to gain weight by addressing the beliefs and behaviours that maintain the low weight. Treatment is usually given on an outpatient basis. Inpatient treatment should be reserved for those at risk of death from medical complications or from suicide. There is a limited evidence base for CBT-based psychological treatments. Family behaviour therapy has efficacy for adolescent but not adult patients. Psychotropic drugs are of no proven benefit in AN but antidepressant medication may be indicated in those with clear-cut comorbid depressive disorder.

Weight gain is best achieved in a collaborative fashion. Compulsory admission and refeeding (including tube feeding) are very occasionally resorted to when patients are at risk of death and other measures have failed. While this may produce a short-term improvement in weight, it rarely changes long-term prognosis.

Prognosis

Two-thirds of patients with AN no longer meet diagnostic criteria at 5-year follow-up. However, long-term follow-up studies suggest that many sufferers continue to have a relatively low body mass index (BMI), suggesting that the symptoms do not completely resolve. Approximately 20% of patients develop a chronic, intractable disorder. Long-term follow-up studies demonstrate that minimum lifetime BMI is the strongest prognostic indicator (BMI <11.5 is associated with a standardised mortality ratio of 4–5). Other indicators of poor prognosis are comorbid BN and atypical demographics (very early or relatively late onset, male gender). Forty per

cent of additional deaths are due to suicide, the remainder being due to complications of starvation.

Bulimia nervosa

The prevalence of BN is difficult to determine with precision, as only a small proportion of sufferers come to medical attention. It is believed to be more common than AN, with a similar gender ratio. Peak age of onset is slightly later than for AN, typically late adolescence or early adult life.

Clinical features

Patients with BN are usually at or near normal weight (unlike in AN), but display a morbid fear of fatness associated with disordered eating behaviour. They recurrently embark on eating binges, often followed by corrective measures such as self-induced vomiting.

Diagnosis

Diagnostic criteria are shown in Box 31.33. Physical signs of repeated self-induced vomiting include pitted teeth (from gastric acid), calluses on knuckles ('Russell's sign') and parotid gland enlargement. There are many associated physical complications, including the dental and oesophageal consequences of repeated vomiting, as well as electrolyte abnormalities, cardiac arrhythmias and renal problems (see Box 31.32).

Investigations

Self-induced vomiting and/or abuse of laxatives and diuretics can lead to clinically significant electrolyte disturbances, including hypokalaemia leading to cardiac arrhythmias. Hence it is good practice to measure urea and electrolytes and obtain an ECG whenever these behaviours are prominent in any patient and when BN is suspected in any medical inpatient. Repeated vomiting can also give rise to Mallory–Weiss tears and even oesophageal rupture; if symptoms are suggestive of these, an endoscopy should be performed.

Management

Treatment of bulimia with CBT achieves both short-term and long-term improvements. Guided self-help and IPT may also be of value. There is also evidence for benefit from the SSRI fluoxetine, but high doses of up to 60 mg daily may be required for a prolonged period of up to 1 year; this appears to be independent of the antidepressant effect.

Prognosis

Bulimia is not associated with increased mortality but a proportion of sufferers go on to develop anorexia. At 10-year follow-up, approximately 10% are still unwell, 20% have a subclinical degree of bulimia, and the remainder have recovered.

Personality disorders

Personality refers to the set of characteristics and behavioural traits that best describes an individual's patterns of interaction with the world. The intensity of particular traits varies from person to person, although certain ones, such as shyness or irritability, are displayed to some degree by most people. A personality disorder (PD) is diagnosed when an individual's personality causes persistent and severe problems for the person or for others.

Pathogenesis

Some PDs appear to have an inherited aspect (especially schizotypal and paranoid subtypes) but most are more clearly related to adverse childhood experiences.

Clinical features

Personality disorders present in various ways. For example, anxiety may be so pronounced that the individual rarely ventures into any situation where they fear scrutiny. Dissocial traits, such as disregard for the

---

 31.33 Diagnostic criteria for eating disorders

Anorexia nervosa

- Weight loss of at least 15% of total body weight (or body mass index ≤17.5)
- Avoidance of high-calorie foods
- Distortion of body image so that patients regard themselves as fat even when grossly underweight
- Amenorrhoea for at least 3 months

Bulimia nervosa

- Recurrent bouts of binge eating
- Lack of self-control over eating during binges
- Self-induced vomiting, purgation or dieting after binges
- Weight maintained within normal limits

well-being of others and a lack of guilt concerning the adverse effects of one's actions on others, may occur. If pronounced, they may lead to damage to others, to criminal acts or to successful careers, such as in politics. They usually persist throughout life and are not readily treated. While they typically become less extreme with age, they can re-emerge in the context of cognitive decline.

Diagnosis

It is possible to classify PD into several subtypes (such as emotionally unstable, antisocial or dependent), depending on the particular behavioural traits in question. A patient who meets diagnostic criteria for one subtype may also meet criteria for others. As allocation to one particular subtype gives little guidance to management or prognosis, classification is of limited value. Diagnosis requires a longitudinal perspective, with clear evidence that the patient's behavioural traits and patterns of interaction with the world have been present throughout their adult life, have been evident across a range of settings and have caused repeated and persistent problems. It can be difficult to achieve this during a single interview, and most psychiatrists warn against making a diagnosis of personality disorder until the patient has been seen several times and corroborative accounts have been obtained. It is common for PD to accompany other psychiatric conditions, making treatment of the latter more difficult and therefore affecting their prognosis.

Management

Treatment options are limited but there is some evidence that emotionally unstable PD may respond to dialectical behavioural therapy (DBT). Anxious (avoidant) and obsessional (anankastic) PD may benefit from prescription of anxiolytic drugs, while paranoid/schizotypal PD may be improved by treatment with low doses of antipsychotic agents.

The problematic and inflexible patterns of interaction that characterise a PD are often apparent in the patient's interaction with health services and can present a challenge to both the service and the patient. Clear clinical communication supported by robust documentation can help to minimise any potential disruption.

Factitious disorder and malingering

Factitious disorder describes the repeated and deliberate production of the signs or symptoms of disease to obtain medical care.

Pathogenesis

It is difficult to understand what motivates a person to act in this way. Several theories have been proposed but the deception that lies at the heart of the condition makes it difficult to gather accurate data from which to draw reliable conclusions.

Clinical features

The disorder feigned is usually medical but can be a psychiatric illness (for example, false reports of hallucinations or symptoms of depression). An example of a medical factitious disorder is dipping of a thermometer into a hot drink to fake a fever. Factitious disorder is uncommon and is important to distinguish from somatoform disorders. A suggested diagnostic algorithm is shown in Figure 31.6.

Münchausen syndrome

This refers to a severe chronic form of factitious disorder. Patients characteristically travel widely, sometimes visiting several hospitals in one day. Although the condition is rare, such patients are memorable because they present so dramatically. The history can be convincing enough to persuade doctors to undertake investigations or initiate treatment, including exploratory surgery. It may be possible to trace the patient's history and show that they have presented similarly elsewhere, often changing name several times. Some emergency departments hold lists of such patients.

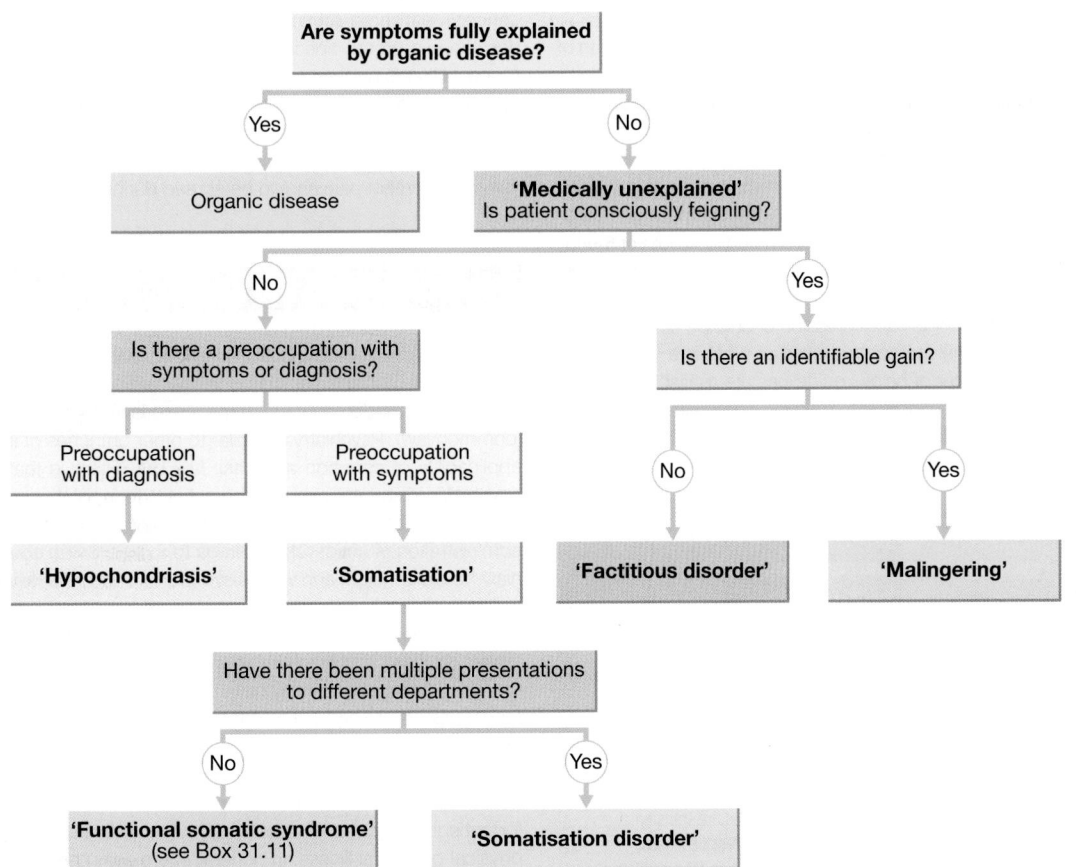

Fig. 31.6 Differential diagnosis of medically unexplained symptoms.

31

Malingering

Malingering is a description of behaviour, not a psychiatric diagnosis. It refers to the deliberate and conscious simulation of signs of disease and disability for an identifiable gain (patients have motives that are clear to them but which they initially conceal from doctors). Examples include the avoidance of burdensome responsibilities (such as work or court appearances) or the pursuit of financial gain (fraudulent claims for benefits or compensation). Malingering can be hard to detect at clinical assessment but is suggested by evasion or inconsistency in the history.

Management

Management is by gentle but firm confrontation with clear evidence of the fabrication of illness, together with an offer of psychological support. Treatment is usually declined but recognition of the condition may help to avoid further iatrogenic harm.

Puerperal psychiatric disorders

There are three important psychiatric presentations following childbirth. When managing these conditions, it is important always to consider both the mother and the baby, and their relationship (Box 31.34).

Post-partum blues

This is characterised by irritability, labile mood and tearfulness. About 80% of women are affected to some degree. Symptoms begin soon after childbirth, typically peak on about the fourth day and then resolve spontaneously within a few weeks. While the aetiology of post-partum blues is not fully understood, it is likely to be related to hormonal or physiological changes associated with childbirth. No treatment is required, other than to reassure the mother and to remain vigilant for development of post-partum depression.

Post-partum depression

This occurs in 10%–15% of women, with onset typically within a month of delivery (although women often suffer for some time before presenting). It can usually be differentiated from post-partum blues by the duration and severity of the symptoms, in particular anhedonia (loss of capacity for pleasure) and negative thoughts. Risk factors include a previous history of depression, a previous history of post-partum depression, antenatal depression and antenatal anxiety. Unlike depression arising at other times, post-partum depression is not more common in lower socioeconomic groups; the prevalence is similar across all social backgrounds. Diagnosis, explanation and reassurance are important. The usual psychological and drug treatments for depression should be considered to minimise the impact on the mother and child at what is a very important time for both. A number of helpful guidelines are available to inform prescribing decisions (see 'Further information'). The potential risks to both mother and child should be considered and, if hospital admission is required, it should ideally be to a mother and baby unit.

31.34 Psychiatric illness and pregnancy

- **Psychiatric disorder and pregnancy**: always consider effects on mother, fetus and child.
- **Bipolar disorder**: women should have pre-conceptual advice because there is a very high risk of relapse following delivery and some mood stabilisers are teratogenic.
- **Psychiatric treatments and pregnancy**: always make an individual assessment of the risks and benefits taking into consideration effects on mother, fetus and child.
- **Post-partum low mood ('blues')**: weeks 1–3; most cases are transient.
- **Persistent low mood and anhedonia**: may indicate depressive illness.
- **Puerperal psychosis**: progresses rapidly and is an indication for psychiatric admission.

Puerperal psychosis

This has its peak onset in the first 2 weeks after childbirth but can arise several weeks later. It is a rare but serious complication affecting approximately 1 in 500 women. There is a strong association with a personal or familial history of bipolar disorder. It usually takes the form of a manic or depressive psychosis but with sudden onset and fluctuation in severity. Delirium is rare with modern obstetric management but should still be considered in the differential diagnosis. Suspiciousness, concealment and impulsivity are common features of puerperal psychosis; hence the risks to both mother and baby are considerable. The clinical priority is to ensure the safety of both mother and baby and so psychiatric admission, ideally to a psychiatric mother and baby unit, is usually necessary. Pharmacological treatment reflects the clinical picture; antipsychotic medication is almost always indicated, augmented by antidepressants if the picture is of psychotic depression and/or by mood stabilisers if the picture is bipolar. Most women recover but the risk of recurrence following subsequent deliveries is 50% and some women will progress to psychotic episodes not associated with childbirth, usually bipolar disorder.

Psychiatric disorders during pregnancy

Pregnancy can affect the course of psychiatric illnesses and of bipolar affective disorder in particular. Mood-stabilising drugs such as lithium and sodium valproate, which are prescribed for prophylaxis in bipolar disorder, are teratogenic and should be avoided. Most guidelines recommend deferring conception until mood-stabilising medication is not required, or replacing the mood stabiliser with an antipsychotic such as chlorpromazine. Furthermore, the immediate post-partum period is associated with a dramatically increased risk of relapse in bipolar disorder: studies report relapse rates of up to 60% in the first 3 months after delivery in the absence of prophylactic medication. When relapse occurs following childbirth, not only are the stakes higher than at other times but also the onset of illness is more rapid, the symptoms more severe and concealment more pronounced. Post-partum relapse of bipolar disorder requires urgent specialist treatment, usually comprising admission to a psychiatric mother and baby unit. Ideally, women with major mental disorders such as bipolar disorder should be offered expert pre-conception advice to help them make informed decisions about medication and other aspects of their psychiatric care. A comprehensive post-partum risk management plan should be agreed during pregnancy.

Psychiatry and the law

Medicine takes place in a legal framework, made up of legislation (statute law) drafted by parliament or other governing bodies, precedent built up from court judgments over time (case law) and established tradition (common law). Psychiatry is similar to other branches of medicine in the applicability of common and case law but differs in that patients with psychiatric disorders can also be subject to legislative requirements to remain in hospital or to undergo treatments they refuse, such as the administration of antipsychotic drugs to a patient with acute schizophrenia who lacks insight and whose symptoms and/or behaviour pose a risk to himself/herself or to others.

The UK has three different Mental Health Acts, covering England and Wales, Scotland and Northern Ireland, and all of these have recently been revised. Other countries may have very different provisions. It is important for practitioners to be familiar with the relevant provisions that apply in their jurisdictions and are likely to arise in the clinical settings in which they work.

All the countries that make up the UK have also introduced Incapacity Acts in recent years, with detailed provisions covering medical treatments for patients incapable of consenting, whether this incapacity arises from physical or mental illness. In general, the guiding principle in British law is that people should be free to make their own decision about any proposed medical treatment, except where their ability to make and/or communicate that decision is demonstrably impaired (by mental illness or physical incapacity). Any restrictions or compulsions applied should be the minimum necessary, they should be applied only for as long as is necessary, and there should be a benefit to the patient that balances the restrictions imposed. There should also be provisions for appeals and oversight.

Further information

Books and journal articles

Hofer H, Pozzi A, Joray M, et al. Safe refeeding management of anorexia nervosa inpatients: an evidence-based protocol. Nutrition 2014;30:524–530.

Mitchell JE, Peterson CB. Anorexia nervosa. N Engl J Med 2020;382:1343–1351.

Steel RM. Factitious disorder (Münchausen's syndrome). J R Coll Phys Edinb 2009;39:343–347.

Taylor D, Meader N, Bird V, et al. Pharmacological interventions for people with depression and chronic physical health problems: systematic review and meta-analyses of safety and efficacy. Br J Psychiatry 2011;198:179–188.

Vos T, Limm SS, Abbafati C, et al. Global burden of 369 diseases and injuries in 204 countries and territories, 1990–2019: a systematic analysis for the Global Burden of Disease Study 2019. Lancet 2020;396:1204–1222.

Websites

neurovascularmedicine.com/ace.pdf *Addenbrooke's Cognitive Examination – ACE -III.*

mind.org.uk *Information on depression.*

mocatest.org *Montreal Cognitive Assessment.*

neurosymptoms.org *A guide to medically unexplained neurological symptoms.*

niaaa.nih.gov/ *Information on alcoholism.*

nice.org.uk *National Institute for Health and Care Excellence: treatment guidelines for depression.*

ocdaction.org.uk *Useful information about obsessive–compulsive disorder.*

rcpsych.ac.uk/info/ *Royal College of Psychiatrists: mental health information.*

sign.ac.uk *Scottish Intercollegiate Guidelines Network: treatment guidelines for depression, including Guideline 127 – Management of perinatal mood disorders.*

who.int/health-topics/mental-health *World Health Organization: mental health and brain disorders.*

www4.parinc.com/ *Mini-Mental State Examination.*

L Mackillop
FEM Neuberger

Maternal medicine

Clinical examination in pregnancy

6 Breasts
Increase in size and vascularity

5 Heart
Ejection systolic murmur may be part of normal pregnancy
Diastolic murmurs are always pathological

4 Face
Conjunctival pallor (physiological anaemia of pregnancy)

▲ Jaundice in acute fatty liver of pregnancy

▲ Melasma

3 Blood pressure
Lower in 2nd and 3rd trimesters

2 Pulse
Pulse rate increased by 10–20 bpm
Bounding pulse

1 Hands

▲ Palmar erythema

7 Respiratory system
Mild breathlessness common
Respiratory rate unchanged

▲ Increased risk of varicella pneumonia

Observation
Plethoric
Mood/affect

8 Abdomen
Scars
Excoriations
Umbilicus eversion
Obstetric examination

▲ Linea nigra

▲ Striae gravidarum

▲ Striae albicans

9 Legs
Varicose veins

▲ Peripheral oedema
Mild oedema in normal pregnancy
Rapid-onset oedema suggests pre-eclampsia

10 Urine dipstick

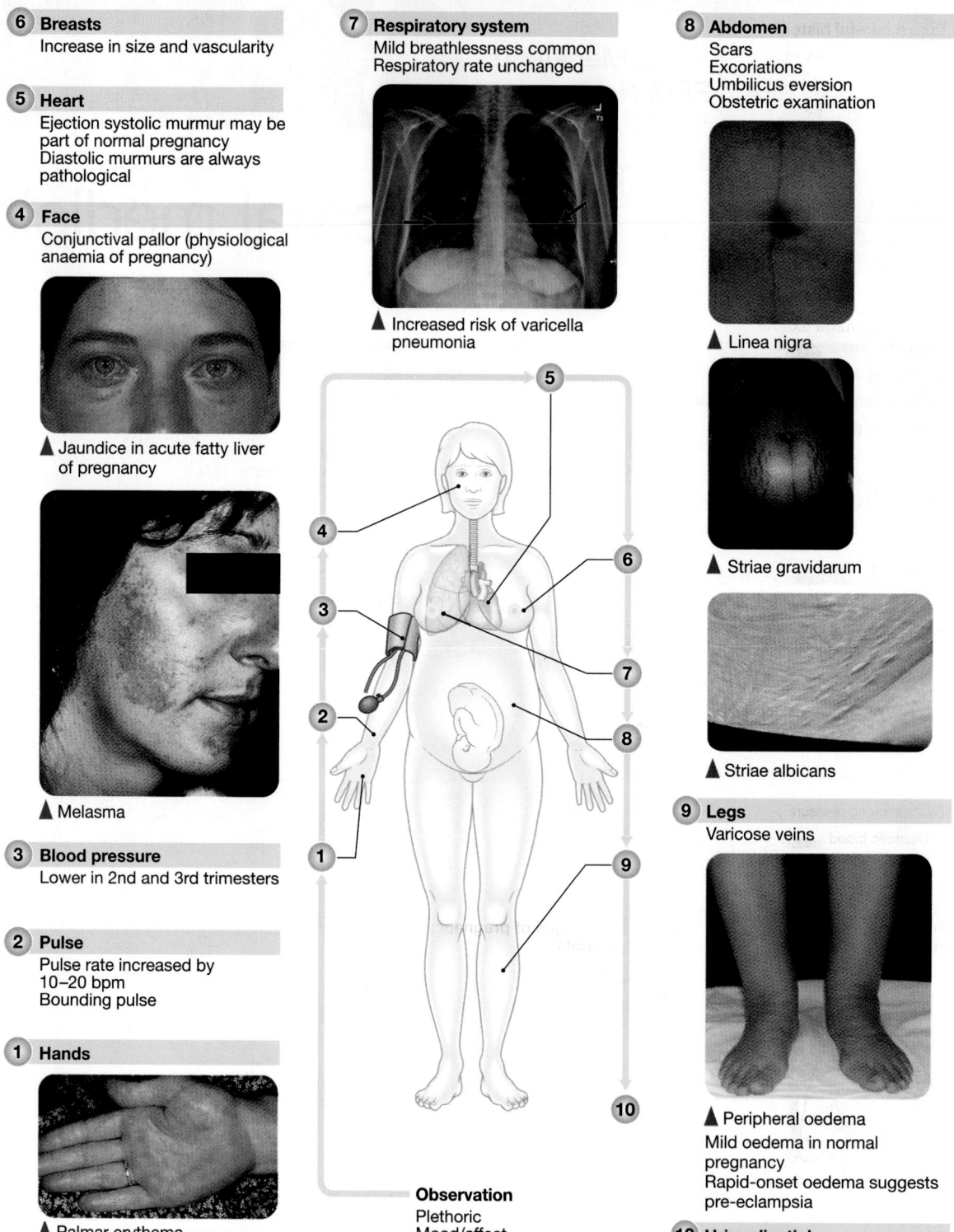

Insets: (Palmar erythema) From Fitzpatrick JE, Morelli JG. Dermatology secrets plus, 5th edn. Philadelphia: Saunders, Elsevier Inc.; 2016; (Melasma) From Lawrence CM, Cox NH. Color atlas and text of physical signs in dermatology. London: Wolfe; 1993; (Jaundice) From Morse SA, Ballard RC, Holmes KK, et al. Atlas of sexually transmitted diseases and AIDS, 4th edn. Philadelphia: Saunders, Elsevier Inc.; 2010; (Varicella pneumonia) From Voore N, Lai R. Varicella pneumonia in an immunocompetent adult. Can Med Assoc J 2012; 184(17):1924; (Linea nigra) From Bolognia JL, Schaffer JV, Duncan KO, et al. Dermatology essentials. Philadelphia: Saunders, Elsevier Inc.; 2014, Courtesy of Jean L. Bolognia;

Clinical evaluation in maternal medicine

Take a careful history

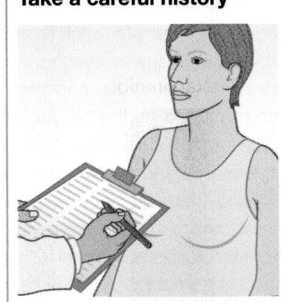

Ask specifically about:
- Cardiac disease
- Renal disease
- Diabetes
- Rheumatic disease
- Inflammatory bowel disease
- Epilepsy

Take a careful drug history

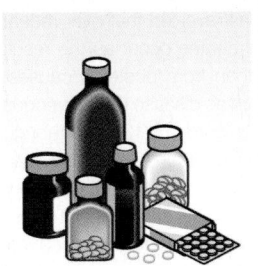

Stop fetotoxic drugs before conception

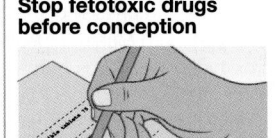

- Methotrexate
- Leflunomide
- Mycophenolate
- Valproate

Perform general examination

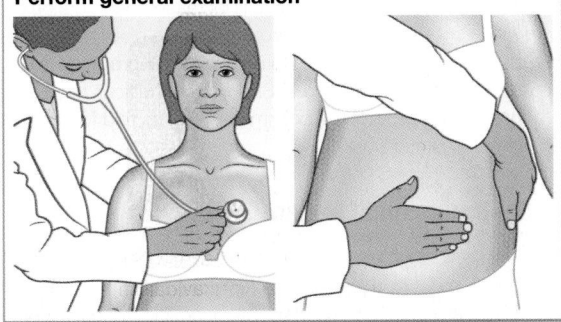

Palmar erythema

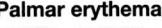
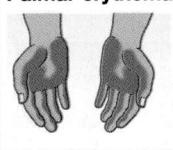

Check for anaemia and jaundice

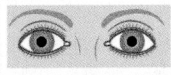

Check for oedema and deep venous thrombosis

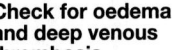
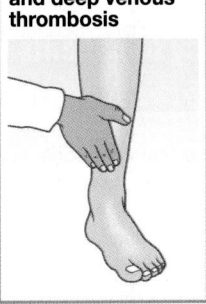

Check blood pressure

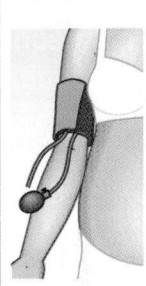

Consider cardiovascular adaptations during pregnancy

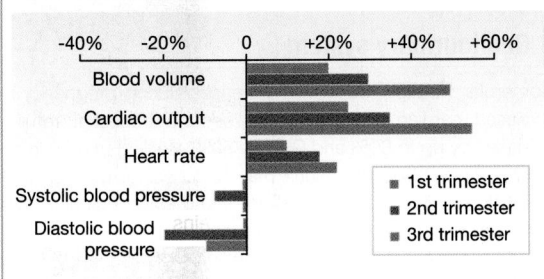

	-40%	-20%	0	+20%	+40%	+60%
Blood volume						
Cardiac output						
Heart rate						
Systolic blood pressure						
Diastolic blood pressure						

- 1st trimester
- 2nd trimester
- 3rd trimester

Perform urinalysis

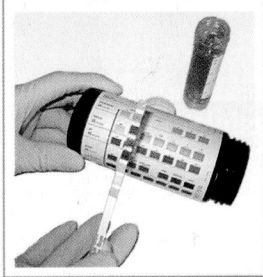

Perform further investigations if appropriate

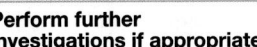
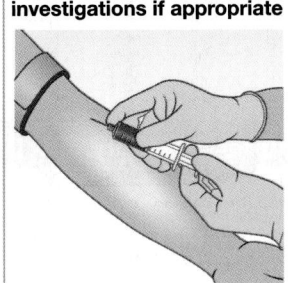

Perform X-ray imaging if indicated

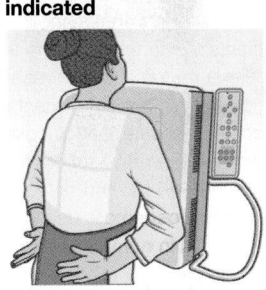

Remember changes of pregnancy when interpreting laboratory results

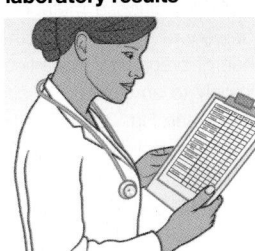

- Anaemia
- Altered thyroid function tests
- Low creatinine/urea
- Low CO_2
- Raised alkaline phosphatase
- Glycosuria

Consider mother and fetus when prescribing

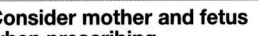
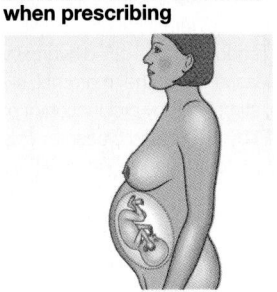

(Striae gravidarum) From Buchanan K, Fletcher HM, Reid M. Prevention of striae gravidarum with cocoa butter cream. Int J Gynecol Obstet 2009; 108(2010):65–68; (Striae albicans) From Cantisano-Zilkha M. Aesthetic oculofacial rejuvenation. Philadelphia: Saunders, Elsevier Inc.; 2010; (Peripheral oedema) From Huang H-W, Wong L-S, Lee C-H. Sarcoidosis with bilateral leg lymphedema as the initial presentation: a review of the literature. Dermatologica Sinica 2016; 34:29–32.

Major physiological changes occur during pregnancy, which impact on several organ systems. These are necessary to support the growing fetus, to prepare for delivery and to support lactation. These changes can adversely affect the activity and progression of many pre-existing medical conditions. Emphasising this fact, information from the UK Confidential Enquiry into Maternal Deaths has revealed that over recent years, approximately two-thirds of maternal deaths occur as the result of pre-existing medical conditions, rather than from obstetric causes. The most common causes of death were cardiac disease (23%), venous thromboembolism (16%) and neurological disorders (13%). Although some diseases can undergo remission during pregnancy, others can worsen, potentially jeopardising the health and well-being of the mother and fetus. In this chapter we review the physiological changes that occur during pregnancy and the impact of pregnancy on the diagnosis, clinical course and management of common medical conditions. In addition, we review the pathogenesis and management of several medical conditions specific to pregnancy.

Planning pregnancy in patients with medical conditions

Patients with pre-existing medical conditions require careful counselling when planning a pregnancy to make them aware of the risks that pregnancy might pose, as well as the changes in symptoms that might be expected to occur during pregnancy. Although each disease is different, as is discussed later in this chapter, the general principles are to ensure that drugs that may be fetotoxic are stopped before pregnancy is attempted; that high-risk patients are kept under close surveillance during their pregnancy; and that new symptoms that emerge during pregnancy are treated seriously and fully investigated where appropriate.

Functional anatomy and physiology

The most important changes that occur in the anatomy and physiology of major organ systems during pregnancy are discussed below.

Bone metabolism

Major changes in bone metabolism take place to meet the demands of the growing fetus. Intestinal calcium absorption increases, due in part to increased production of 1,25-dihydroxyvitamin D (1,25(OH)$_2$D). Calcium is also released from the maternal skeleton due to increased bone resorption, stimulated by production of parathyroid hormone-related protein (PTHrP) by breast and placenta. This results in loss of bone from the maternal skeleton during pregnancy that continues until lactation ceases and then recovers. Serum concentrations of alkaline phosphatase (ALP) can increase by up to fourfold but this is due to release of ALP from the placenta rather than bone.

Cardiovascular system

Heart rate and stroke volume increase during pregnancy; when combined with peripheral vasodilatation and a reduction in systemic blood pressure, this causes a hyperdynamic circulatory state and an increase in cardiac output. Diaphragmatic elevation may affect the electrocardiogram (ECG), causing left axis deviation of up to 15°. Other changes include T-wave inversion in leads III and aVF, ST depression, small Q waves and a sinus tachycardia. Supraventricular and ventricular beats are common. Echocardiography shows a modest increase in the dimensions of the cardiac chambers.

Endocrine system

During early pregnancy there is secretion of human chorionic gonadotrophin (hCG) by trophoblast cells, which act on the corpus luteum in the ovary to stimulate oestradiol and progesterone production (Fig. 32.1). Levels of hCG rise rapidly during early pregnancy to reach a peak around 8 weeks, and then fall before stabilising at a lower level from 20 weeks until term. There is a progressive rise in oestradiol and progesterone levels; initially, these hormones are produced by the corpus luteum but placental production takes over after about 12 weeks. The high levels of gonadal hormones suppress pituitary gonadotrophin production but prolactin levels rise about 10-fold and there is an increase in volume of the anterior pituitary. Serum levels of free T$_4$ increase during the first trimester but, paradoxically, thyroid-stimulating hormone (TSH) levels fall by almost 50%. This is because hCG is homologous to TSH and mimics the effect of TSH on the thyroid, stimulating both T$_3$ and T$_4$ production. The raised levels of T$_3$ and T$_4$ feed back to the pituitary and reduce TSH secretion. Later in pregnancy, there is increased degradation of thyroxine by the placenta and levels of thyroxine-binding globulin (TBG) rise, causing the normal range for free T$_4$ and T$_3$ to fall progressively during the course of pregnancy. Although TSH levels are difficult to interpret early in pregnancy, they provide the best measure of thyroid function after about 16 weeks' gestation.

Gastrointestinal system

The high levels of progesterone during pregnancy lead to relaxation of smooth muscle in the gastrointestinal tract. This causes the lower oesophageal sphincter to relax, predisposing to gastro-oesophageal reflux and reduced gastrointestinal transit; this in turn leads to delayed gastric emptying and constipation.

Genitourinary system

Glomerular filtration rate (GFR) increases during pregnancy due to an increased cardiac output. By the second trimester, renal perfusion increases by up to 80% and GFR by 50%, leading to a fall in serum urea and creatinine. Mild glycosuria may be observed during normal pregnancy due mainly to an increase in filtered load of glucose. The ureters and renal pelvis are slightly dilated, most prominently on the left side, leading to the physiological hydronephrosis of pregnancy.

Glucose metabolism

Maternal glucose metabolism changes during pregnancy to optimise delivery of glucose and other nutrients to the fetus. During the second half of pregnancy in particular, there is maternal insulin resistance due largely to an increase in circulating levels of human placental lactogen (hPL) (see Fig. 32.1). The net effect is to ensure that glucose is preferentially supplied to the fetus rather than the mother. Following delivery of the placenta, there is a rapid decline in hPL and reversal of insulin resistance. During pregnancy, fasting plasma glucose decreases slightly, while post-prandial blood glucose may increase. Glycosuria may occur, even in women who do not have diabetes, due to the increased GFR. Insulin secretion in the fetus is driven by fetal glucose levels, which in turn are dependent on maternal glucose concentrations. Accordingly, in women with diabetes, maternal hyperglycaemia stimulates fetal insulin secretion, which increases fetal growth, resulting in increased birth weight or macrosomia.

Haematological system

Haemoglobin normally falls by about 20% during pregnancy since plasma volume increases more than red cell volume: the so-called physiological anaemia of pregnancy. The reduction in haematocrit lowers

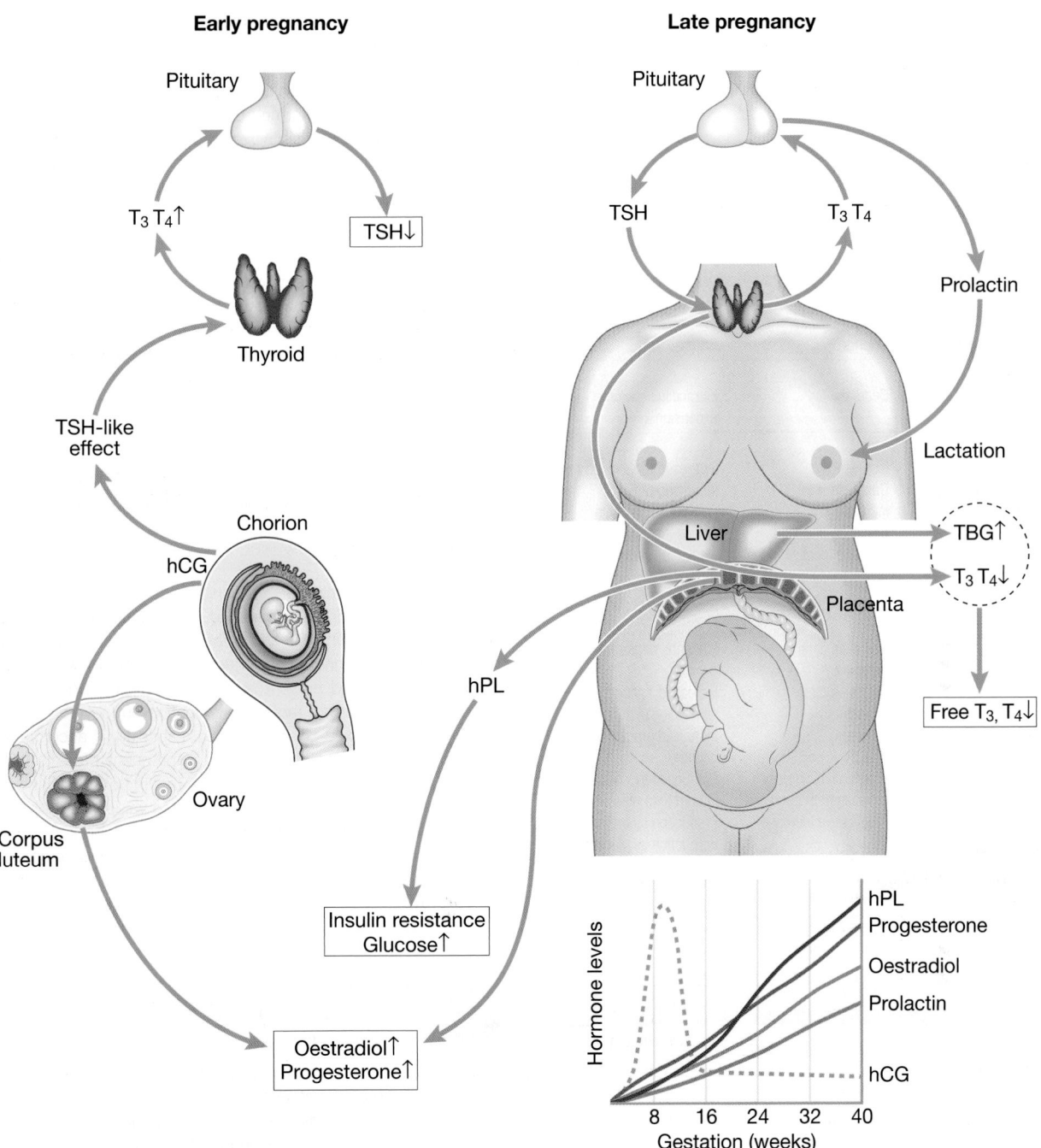

Fig. 32.1 Hormonal changes in pregnancy. In early pregnancy, oestradiol and progesterone are mainly derived from the corpus luteum in response to human chorionic gonadotrophin (hCG), secreted by the trophoblast. The raised levels of hCG also act on the thyroid to stimulate T_3 (triiodothyronine) and T_4 (thyroxine) production, which in turn suppresses thyroid-stimulating hormone (TSH) production by the pituitary. Later in pregnancy, oestradiol and progesterone are derived from the placenta, which also produces human placental lactogen (hPL), impairing glucose tolerance. There is a progressive reduction of free T_3 and T_4 during pregnancy as the result of T_3 and T_4 degradation by the placenta and increased secretion of thyroxine-binding globulin (TBG) by the liver.

blood viscosity but this is offset by an elevation in levels of several clotting factors, resulting in a hypercoagulable state that increases the risk of venous and arterial thrombosis.

Respiratory system

Tidal volume (TV) increases during pregnancy due to an increased vital capacity and reduced residual volume, and by term the increase in TV is about 200 mL. These changes are required to meet the 20% increase in oxygen demand that occurs during pregnancy. The PCO_2 level decreases

but this is offset by an increase in renal excretion of bicarbonate, such that the blood pH remains relatively stable. Respiratory rate is unaffected by pregnancy.

Investigations

The profound changes in physiology and anatomy that occur during pregnancy cause changes in the normal reference ranges for several hormones, electrolytes and other analytes, as summarised in Box 32.1. While many investigations can proceed as normal during pregnancy, invasive procedures should generally be avoided unless the potential benefit clearly outweighs the risk. Investigations that can be performed in pregnancy are shown in Box 32.2.

Imaging

Imaging during pregnancy should be undertaken only when the clinical benefit outweighs the potential risks to mother and fetus. In suspected pulmonary embolus, radionuclide ventilation/perfusion ($\dot{V}/\dot{Q}$) scanning is preferred over computed tomographic pulmonary angiography (CTPA) in women with a normal chest X-ray since ($\dot{V}/\dot{Q}$) scans expose the maternal breast and lungs to less radiation than CTPA. However, if the chest X-ray is abnormal, CTPA should be performed, since it is more likely to yield a definitive diagnosis. The radiation exposure for both investigations is well below the maximum recommended fetal radiation dose in pregnancy (5 rad). Chest X-rays may also be performed safely at any gestation during pregnancy if clinically indicated, since the radiation exposure is very low for the fetus. Magnetic resonance imaging (MRI) is safe in the second and third trimesters and is useful in the assessment of proximal deep vein thrombosis (DVT) and neurological disorders. However, gadolinium-containing contrast agents should be used only if absolutely necessary. If gadolinium contrast agents are used in women who are breastfeeding, the milk should be discarded for 24 hours. Ultrasound imaging is safe during pregnancy and useful in the assessment of patients with DVT or intra-abdominal pathology.

Presenting problems in pregnancy

Breathlessness

The causes of breathlessness during pregnancy are summarised in Box 32.3. Many women experience mild breathlessness as part of normal pregnancy, which is known as physiological breathlessness of pregnancy. It is thought to be progesterone-mediated and is classically of gradual onset and present at rest and on exercise. Physiological breathlessness does not require investigation but severe or persistent breathlessness should be investigated, especially if accompanied by chest pain. The diagnostic approach in pregnant patients with suspected pulmonary embolism differs from that in non-pregnant women. Measurement of D-dimer is not helpful since values normally increase progressively throughout pregnancy. Accordingly, the first-line investigation in suspected pulmonary embolism is a ($\dot{V}/\dot{Q}$) scan in a patient with a normal chest X-ray and CTPA in a patient with an abnormal chest X-ray.

i	32.1 Common laboratory changes during pregnancy		
Laboratory test	**Change**	**Cause**	
Haematology			
Haematocrit	Decrease	Extracellular volume expansion	
Routine biochemistry			
GFR	Increase	Increased renal blood flow	
Urea and creatinine	Decrease	Increased GFR	
Alkaline phosphate	Increase	Release by placenta	
Glucose	Decrease (fasting)	Raised insulin	
	Increase (post-prandial)	Insulin resistance	
Hormones			
T_4	Increase (first trimester)	Stimulation of thyroid by hCG	
	Decrease (later pregnancy)	Placental degradation	
TSH	Decrease (first trimester)	Increased T_4 due to stimulation of thyroid by hCG	
Prolactin	Increase	Increased production by pituitary	
Oestradiol)	Progressive increase	Production by corpus luteum then placenta	
Progesterone)	Increase then decrease		
hCG	Progressive increase	Production by trophoblast	
hPL		Production by placenta	

(GFR = glomerular filtration rate; hCG = human chorionic gonadotrophin; hPL = human placental lactogen; TSH = thyroid-stimulating hormone)

i	32.2 Investigations in pregnancy*		
Investigation	**Use during pregnancy**	**Comment**	
Renal biopsy	Can be performed during pregnancy	< 22 weeks is safest; 23–28 weeks is period of highest risk	
Upper gastrointestinal endoscopy	Safe during pregnancy	Fetal monitoring should be offered pre- and post-procedure	
	Left lateral position is recommended in the second half of pregnancy	Low-dose sedation recommended	
Colonoscopy	Safe during pregnancy	Fetal monitoring should be offered pre- and post-procedure	
		Low-dose sedation recommended	
Flexible sigmoidoscopy	Safe during pregnancy	Fetal monitoring should be offered pre- and post-procedure	
		Low-dose sedation recommended	
Magnetic resonance imaging	Not contraindicated at any gestation		
Computed tomography	Can be performed at any gestation	Radiation exposure to fetus and mother must be considered and addressed in counselling	
Chest X-ray	Safe at any gestation		
Ultrasound	Safe at any gestation		
Echocardiogram	Safe at any gestation		
Ambulatory electrocardiogram	Safe at any gestation		

*For any investigation, the potential benefit must outweigh the risk.

i **32.3 Breathlessness during pregnancy**

Cause	Management
Physiological breathlessness of pregnancy	No treatment required
Asthma	Treatment as in non-pregnant women
Pneumonia	Treatment with antibiotic as in non-pregnant women
Valvular heart disease	Treatment as in non-pregnant women
Heart failure	Treatment as in non-pregnant women
Peripartum cardiomyopathy (PPCM)	Treatment as in non-pregnant women Early delivery if haemodynamic deterioration
Pulmonary embolus	Treatment as in non-pregnant women

i **32.4 Differential diagnosis of severe nausea and vomiting in pregnancy**

Gastrointestinal

- Peptic ulcer disease
- Gastroenteritis
- Appendicitis
- Pancreatitis

Endocrine and metabolic

- Thyrotoxicosis
- Addison's disease
- Hyperparathyroidism
- Diabetic ketoacidosis

Neurological

- Space-occupying lesion
- Migraine

Pregnancy-associated conditions

- Hydatidaform mole
- Acute fatty liver of pregnancy
- Hyperemesis gravidarum

Genitourinary

- Urinary tract infection

Psychological

- Bulimia nervosa

Cardiovascular

- Myocardial infarction

Chest pain

Chest pain does not occur during normal pregnancy but the incidences of acute coronary syndrome (ACS) and aortic dissection are both increased. Accordingly, if a pregnant woman develops acute severe chest pain suggestive of either of these conditions, she should be investigated and treated in the same way as a non-pregnant woman.

Circulatory collapse

The differential diagnosis of circulatory collapse is wide and causes unrelated to pregnancy are discussed in Chapter 9. Obstetric causes include pulmonary embolism, haemorrhage and amniotic fluid embolism (AFE). This usually presents with collapse and profound shock during delivery or immediately afterwards, often accompanied by a severe coagulopathy. It can be difficult to differentiate AFE from other causes of maternal collapse, and the diagnosis is often made on clinical grounds when other causes of collapse have been excluded. Management is supportive, with oxygenation, careful fluid balance and correction of coagulopathies where necessary, ventilatory support and vasopressors.

Another important cause of circulatory collapse is obstetric haemorrhage, which can be divided into ante-partum and post-partum subtypes. Ante-partum haemorrhage is defined as bleeding from the vagina after 24 weeks' gestation. Primary post-partum haemorrhage is defined as occurring in the first 24 hours after delivery, and secondary post-partum haemorrhage after 24 hours. Haemorrhage may be concealed, and physiological changes such as hypotension, tachycardia and tachypnoea may be late signs. Management is supportive with administration of blood, intravenous fluids and oxygen. Patients with post-partum haemorrhage may also benefit from uterotonic agents such as oxytocin. If the bleeding fails to settle, surgical intervention or interventional radiology may be required.

Headache

Migraine and tension headache may occur during pregnancy and should be assessed along the usual lines, as described in Chapter 28. Important causes of headache that are specific to pregnancy are pre-eclampsia, which should be suspected in patients with hypertension, oedema and proteinuria, and cerebral venous thrombosis, which should be suspected when there is a neurological deficit or seizures.

Nausea and vomiting

Nausea and vomiting are common during the first trimester of pregnancy and do not usually require any specific investigation or treatment. Other causes of nausea and vomiting are summarised in Box 32.4. Severe vomiting with significant weight loss and/or electrolyte disturbance suggests hyperemesis gravidarum, which is discussed in more detail later in this chapter.

Oedema

A mild degree of ankle oedema can occur in normal pregnancy but significant oedema raises suspicion of pre-eclampsia and this should be considered in patients who are also hypertensive and those with proteinuria (Fig. 32.2).

Seizures

The causes and management of seizures during pregnancy are summarised in Box 32.5. An important cause is eclampsia, which should be borne in mind in patients with no previous history of seizures and accompanying features such as hypertension, oedema and proteinuria. Seizures can also occur secondary to electrolyte disturbances associated with hyperemesis gravidarum or hypoglycaemia. Other disorders that are more common during pregnancy and can present with seizures include cerebral venous thrombosis and thrombotic thrombocytopenic purpura (TTP).

32

Medical disorders in pregnancy

Many disorders present specific management problems before pregnancy, during pregnancy and in the puerperium; the most important of these are discussed in more detail below.

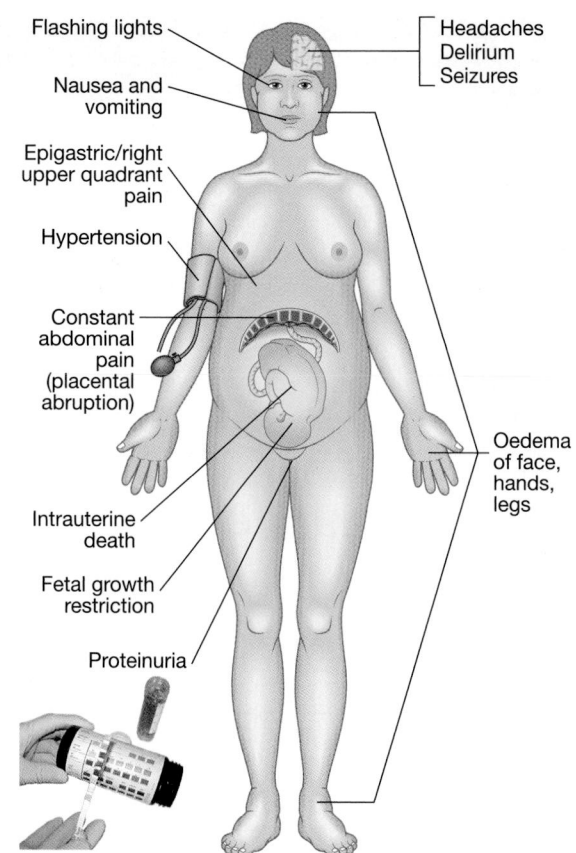

Flashing lights

Nausea and vomiting

Epigastric/right upper quadrant pain

Hypertension

Constant abdominal pain (placental abruption)

Intrauterine death

Fetal growth restriction

Proteinuria

Headaches
Delirium
Seizures

Oedema of face, hands, legs

Fig. 32.2 Symptoms and signs of pre-eclampsia.

32.6 Classification of hypertension during pregnancy

Hypertension	Definition
Hypertension in pregnancy	Blood pressure ≥ 140/90 mmHg on two separate occasions, at least 4 hrs apart
Pre-existing hypertension	Hypertension prior to pregnancy or occurring before 20 weeks' gestation
Gestational hypertension	Hypertension occurring after 20 weeks' gestation without proteinuria or any other features of pre-eclampsia
Pre-eclampsia	Hypertension occurring after 20 weeks' gestation with proteinuria, maternal organ dysfunction or uteroplacental dysfunction
Eclampsia	Generalised seizures in a pregnant woman with pre-eclampsia
White coat hypertension	Hypertension that only occurs in a clinical environment

Adapted from Brown A, Magee L, Kenny L, et al. Hypertensive disorders of pregnancy 2018. International Society for the Study of Hypertension in Pregnancy (ISSHP) classification, diagnosis, and management recommendations for international practice.

32.7 Drug treatment of hypertension during pregnancy

Medication	Dosage
Labetalol	100 mg twice daily to 600 mg four times a day
Nifedipine	5 mg once daily to 10 mg once daily
Amlodipine	10mg B.D. to 40mg B.D.
Methyldopa	250 mg twice daily to 1000 mg three times a day
Doxazosin	0.5 mg twice daily to 8 mg three times a day

32.5 Causes of seizures during pregnancy

Cause	Management
Epilepsy	Similar to that in non-pregnant women Avoid valproate
Eclampsia	Antihypertensives Magnesium sulphate Careful fluid balance
Hypoglycaemia	Glucose
Hyponatraemia	Saline infusion
Alcohol withdrawal	Supportive treatment
Drugs	Supportive treatment
Stroke	As in non-pregnant women
Cerebral venous thrombosis	Low-molecular-weight heparin
Thrombotic thrombocytopenic purpura	Plasma exchange Immunosuppressives

Hypertension

Hypertension is one of the most common medical problems during pregnancy, occurring in about 10%–15% of women. The causes and classification are summarised in Box 32.6.

Pre-existing hypertension

If hypertension is discovered during the first half of pregnancy, it usually indicates that there was pre-existing hypertension. This is most likely to be due to essential hypertension but secondary causes also need to be considered. Hypertension during pregnancy should be managed with vasodilators or methyldopa (Box 32.7), taking care to avoid hypotension. Angiotensin-converting enzyme (ACE) inhibitors should be stopped in hypertensive women who are planning to become pregnant and should be avoided during pregnancy since they have fetotoxic effects. Diuretics should also be avoided unless there is heart failure, as they can reduce circulating volume and cause placental hypoperfusion.

Gestational hypertension

Gestational hypertension usually presents in the second half of pregnancy and most often resolves by 3 months post partum. It should be managed actively with one of the drugs listed in Box 32.7, to reduce the risk of progression to pre-eclampsia.

Pre-eclampsia and eclampsia

Pre-eclampsia is a disorder of vascular endothelial dysfunction that affects about 10% of all pregnancies worldwide. The risk factors for pre-eclampsia are shown in Box 32.8 and the clinical features illustrated in Figure 32.2. Management includes control of blood pressure, administration of magnesium sulphate as prophylaxis against seizures, correction of coagulation abnormalities and monitoring of fluid balance. If pre-eclampsia occurs early in pregnancy, medical management should be initiated with the aim of controlling the condition and maintaining the fetus in utero as long as possible. If these measures are ineffective and eclampsia supervenes (see below), then urgent delivery should be considered, provided the fetus is viable, since this results in an immediate cure.

Eclampsia occurs in about 1% of pregnancies and is associated with significant mortality. It usually presents with seizures on a background of pre-eclampsia but rarely can occur before the onset of hypertension and proteinuria. Treatment is with intravenous magnesium sulphate 4 g intravenously over 15 mins followed by an infusion of 1 g/hr titrated to serum magnesium for 24 hr, and delivery of the fetus as soon as possible. Women with pre-eclampsia are more likely to develop hypertension, chronic kidney disease, and cerebrovascular and ischaemic heart disease in later life.

Respiratory disease

Asthma

Women with asthma should be managed aggressively during pregnancy, since poorly controlled asthma is associated with pre-eclampsia, fetal growth restriction, low birth weight and pre-term birth. The management is very similar to that in non-pregnant individuals. Short-acting and long-acting β-agonists, inhaled and oral glucocorticoids, intravenous magnesium and theophylline can be used freely. Biologic agents such as the monoclonal anti-IgE antibody omalizumab can be given for severe allergic asthma. There is less experience with leukotriene receptor agonists during pregnancy but they can be given if necessary. It is advisable to involve an anaesthetist or intensivist at an early stage in patients with severe exacerbations of asthma since airway management is more difficult in late pregnancy.

Respiratory infection

The most common causes of pneumonia during pregnancy are summarised in Box 32.9. Diagnosis and management are broadly the same as in non-pregnant patients. Prompt treatment of infections is important since mothers with pneumonia are more likely to deliver early and have low-birth-weight infants compared with healthy pregnant women.

Bacterial infections

Antibiotics should be given, depending on the causal organism and sensitivities, along with supplemental oxygen and fluids as required. Penicillins, cephalosporins and macrolides such as erythromycin are all safe during pregnancy but tetracyclines should be avoided because they may be fetotoxic and can cause staining of the teeth in the fetus (see Box 6.20).

Viral infections

Viral pneumonia is more common and often more severe during pregnancy. Varicella zoster pneumonia in particular is associated with a high fetal and maternal mortality rate. It presents with cough, breathlessness and pyrexia, and is usually preceded by a vesicular rash up to 1 week before. Varicella infection can be diagnosed clinically, with laboratory confirmation by culture or polymerase chain reaction (PCR) of fluid from vesicles, or by serology. Varicella pneumonia causes an interstitial

pneumonitis with a characteristic nodular appearance on chest X-ray (p. 1264). Women with confirmed varicella zoster pneumonia should be admitted to hospital for supportive care and treatment with intravenous aciclovir for 7–10 days.

Tuberculosis

Tuberculosis (TB) may occur during pregnancy and in the UK is more common among African and Asian women. Untreated TB is associated with premature delivery and low birth weight. Transmission to the fetus can occur but is unusual. If the diagnosis of TB is confirmed, then antituberculous chemotherapy should be given as normal, since the benefit of treating TB in pregnancy outweighs any potential risks from the medication. A proportion of pregnant women with TB have coexisting human immunodeficiency virus (HIV) infection, which confers a poorer prognosis and also requires treatment with antiretroviral therapy, as described in Chapter 14.

COVID-19

Pregnant women are not disproportionately affected by COVID-19 and should this occur during pregnancy, the same principles of treatment should be followed as for the non-pregnant population.

Gastrointestinal disease

Hyperemesis gravidarum

Hyperemesis gravidarum is a serious condition that affects about 0.5% of pregnant women. It typically presents during the first trimester with severe nausea, vomiting and other clinical features (Box 32.10). It is associated with significant morbidity and mortality, due to malnutrition and electrolyte imbalance. Wernicke's encephalopathy may develop as the result of thiamin deficiency. Recurrence is common in successive pregnancies. The cause is unknown and the diagnosis is one of exclusion, since alternative causes of severe nausea and vomiting need to be ruled out, particularly if the onset of symptoms occurs after the first trimester. Management is with lifestyle advice and support, intravenous fluids, electrolyte replacement and antiemetics. Thiamin and glucocorticoids may be required in the most severe cases.

Inflammatory bowel disease

Women with inflammatory bowel disease (IBD) should be counselled prior to planning a pregnancy. Medications such as azathioprine, sulfasalazine, 5-aminosalicylic acid (5-ASA), glucocorticoids and tumour

32

necrosis factor alpha (TNF-α) inhibitors can be continued as normal during pregnancy during the first and second trimesters but methotrexate must be stopped at least 3 months before conception because of its teratogenic effects. Since poorly controlled IBD is associated with an increased risk of pre-term birth, low birth weight and miscarriage, it is important for the disease to be well controlled before conception. The activity of IBD can increase during pregnancy and ulcerative colitis is more likely to flare than Crohn's disease. Women who experience disease flares should be managed by multidisciplinary teams including medicine and obstetrics, and monitored closely. It is usual to stop TNF-α inhibitors in the third trimester because most drugs in this class are actively transported across the placenta, potentially causing immunosuppression in the neonate. Should TNF-α inhibitors be required in the third trimester, certolizumab pegol is a good choice since it does not cross the placenta in significant amounts. Most women with uncomplicated IBD can have a normal vaginal delivery and do not need a caesarean section, but the need for this should be assessed on an individual basis by obstetric and medical teams.

Diabetes

It is important to institute meticulous glucose control in pregnancy, as maternal diabetes is associated with increased risks of congenital malformations, stillbirth, pre-eclampsia, pre-term delivery, operative delivery, neonatal hypoglycaemia and admission to neonatal intensive care.

Gestational diabetes

Gestational diabetes is defined as diabetes with first onset or recognition during pregnancy. This definition will include a few patients who develop type 1 diabetes during pregnancy, where prompt action and early insulin treatment will be required, and some patients who develop type 2 diabetes, or had unknown pre-existing type 2 diabetes, in whom the diabetes does not remit after pregnancy. However, in most cases, gestational diabetes develops due to an inability to increase insulin secretion adequately to compensate for pregnancy-induced insulin resistance, and most women can expect to return to normal glucose tolerance immediately after pregnancy. Risk factors for gestational diabetes are shown in Box 32.11.

The diagnosis of gestational diabetes is based on maternal blood glucose measurements that are associated with increased fetal growth. An international consensus recommended that glucose values diagnostic of gestational diabetes should be lower than those for non-gestational diabetes (see Box 32.12). Controversy remains about who should be screened, and the screening strategy depends, in part, on the population risk. It is widely accepted that women at high risk for gestational diabetes should have an oral glucose tolerance test at 24–28 weeks, and some guidelines recommend that all high-risk women should be screened by measuring HbA_{1c}, fasting blood glucose or random blood glucose at the first booking visit. It should be noted that measurements of HbA_{1c} cannot reliably be used to diagnose diabetes in early pregnancy and until 3 months post partum, since HbA_{1c} levels fall due to increased red cell turnover.

Management

The aim is to normalise maternal blood glucose concentrations and reduce the risk of excessive fetal growth. The first element of management is dietary modification, in particular by reducing consumption of refined carbohydrate. Women with gestational diabetes should undertake regular pre- and post-prandial self-monitoring of blood glucose, aiming for pre-meal blood glucose levels of < 5.3 mmol/L (96 mg/dL) and a 1-hour post-prandial level of <7.8 mmol/L (142 mg/dL) or a 2-hour post-prandial level of < 6.4 mmol/L (109 mg/dL). If pharmacological treatment is necessary, metformin, glibenclamide or insulin can all be used. Glibenclamide should be used rather than other sulphonylureas because it does not cross the placenta. Other oral therapies or injectable incretin-based therapies should not be given in pregnancy.

32.11 Risk factors for gestational diabetes

- Body mass index > 30 kg/m²
- Previous macrosomic baby weighing ≥ 4.5 kg
- Previous gestational diabetes
- Family history of diabetes (first-degree relative with diabetes)
- Family origin with a high prevalence of diabetes:
  - South Asian (specifically women whose country of family origin is India, Pakistan or Bangladesh)
  - African Caribbean
  - Middle Eastern

32.12 Diagnosis of gestational diabetes

- Fasting plasma glucose of ≥ 5.1 mmol/L (92 mg/dL)
- 1 hour plasma glucose ≥ 10 mmol/L (180 mg/dL) after a 75 g glucose load
- 2 hour plasma glucose ≥ 8.5 mmol/L (153 mg/dL) after a 75 g glucose load

After delivery, maternal glucose usually returns to pre-pregnancy levels. In the UK, it is currently recommended that women with gestational diabetes should have a fasting blood glucose measured at 6 weeks post partum and have HbA_{1c} concentrations measured annually to screen for the development of diabetes. This is because even those whose glucose tolerance returns to normal post partum are at increased risk for developing type 2 diabetes, with a 5-year risk between 15% and 50%, depending on the population. Therefore, all women who have had gestational diabetes should be given diet and lifestyle advice to reduce their risk of developing type 2 diabetes later in life.

Pregnancy in women with established diabetes

Maternal hyperglycaemia early in pregnancy (during the first 6 weeks post conception) can adversely affect fetal development, causing cardiac, renal and skeletal malformations, of which the caudal regression syndrome (abnormal development of the lower part of the spine) is the most characteristic. The risk of fetal abnormalities is about 2% for non-diabetic women and about 4% for women with well-controlled diabetes (HbA_{1c} <53 mmol/mol) but more than 20% for those with poor glycaemic control (HbA_{1c} >97 mmol/mol). Therefore, it is important for women with diabetes to aim to achieve good glycaemic control before becoming pregnant. In addition, high-dose folic acid (5 mg daily, rather than the usual 400 µg) should be initiated before conception to reduce the risk of neural tube defects.

As for gestational diabetes, mothers should attempt to maintain near-normal blood glucose levels while avoiding hypoglycaemia throughout their pregnancy, as this minimises excessive fetal growth and neonatal hypoglycaemia. This is often difficult to achieve, however. Pregnancy is also associated with an increased risk of ketosis, particularly, but not exclusively, in women with type 1 diabetes. Ketoacidosis during pregnancy is dangerous for the mother and is associated with a high rate (10%–35%) of fetal mortality.

Pregnancy is linked with a worsening of diabetic complications, most notably retinopathy and nephropathy, so careful monitoring of eyes and kidneys is required throughout pregnancy. If heavy proteinuria and/or renal dysfunction exist prior to pregnancy, there is a marked increase in the risk of pre-eclampsia, and renal function can deteriorate irreversibly during pregnancy. These risks need to be carefully discussed before a woman with diabetes is considering pregnancy. The outlook for mother and child has been vastly improved over recent years but pregnancy outcomes are still not equivalent to those of non-diabetic mothers. Perinatal mortality rates remain 3–4 times those of the non-diabetic population (at around 30–40 per 1000 pregnancies) and the rate of congenital malformation is increased five- to sixfold.

Endocrine disease

Thyroid disease

Iodine deficiency

Iodine deficiency is a major public health issue in many countries, particularly in South-east Asia, the Western Pacific and Central Africa. Severe iodine deficiency in pregnancy is associated with miscarriage, stillbirth and cretinism, with significant cognitive impairment, gait abnormalities and deafness in the affected child. More moderate iodine deficiency is associated with milder forms of cognitive impairment and affects millions of people. The World Health Organization recommends a daily iodine intake of 250 µg/day for pregnant women. Treatment of iodine deficiency in the first and second trimesters can prevent impaired cognitive development but is less effective if started in the third trimester.

Hypothyroidism

Hypothyroidism occasionally presents during pregnancy, with symptoms such as weight gain, constipation and lethargy, though more commonly, women with hypothyroidism are already diagnosed before they become pregnant. The diagnosis is easily missed since these symptoms are common in normal pregnancy. If suspected, the diagnosis can be confirmed by checking thyroid function tests, which show a raised TSH and low free T_4. The reference range for thyroid function tests is different in pregnancy, and results should be checked using a local gestation-specific reference range.

Women with hypothyroidism should aim for optimal disease control before conceiving, and throughout the pregnancy. Untreated hypothyroidism is associated with miscarriage, pre-eclampsia and anaemia. During pregnancy, women should have their thyroid function checked every trimester, and dose adjustments made depending on the results, and blood tests repeated 4–6 weeks after any alterations. Some women may require an increase in their thyroxine dose during pregnancy to maintain normal TSH levels because there is an increased requirement for thyroxine during pregnancy. TSH should be < 2.5mIU/L for women on treatment prior to pregnancy.

Subclinical hypothyroidism is more common. There is no evidence that treating women with subclinical hypothyroidism and negative thyroid peroxidase (TPO) antibodies is beneficial. For TPO antibody-positive women, there are some data to suggest treating TSH above the upper limit of the reference range but less than 10 mIU/L may be beneficial for pregnancy outcome.

Hyperthyroidism

The coexistence of pregnancy and thyrotoxicosis is unusual, since anovulatory cycles are common in thyrotoxic patients and autoimmune disease tends to remit during pregnancy, due to suppression of the maternal immune response. Thyroid function tests must be interpreted in the knowledge that thyroid-binding globulin, and hence total T_4 and T_3 levels, are increased in pregnancy and that the normal range for TSH is lower (see Box 35.10). Despite this, a fully suppressed TSH is usually indicative of Graves' disease. When thyroid disease during pregnancy is being dealt with, both mother and fetus must be considered, since maternal thyroid hormones, TSH receptor antibodies (TRAb) and antithyroid drugs can all cross the placenta to some degree, exposing the fetus to the risks of thyrotoxicosis, iatrogenic hypothyroidism and goitre. Moreover, poorly controlled thyrotoxicosis can result in fetal tachycardia, intrauterine growth retardation, prematurity, stillbirth and possibly even congenital malformations.

Antithyroid drugs are the treatment of first choice for thyrotoxicosis in pregnancy. Newly diagnosed hyperthyroidism during pregnancy can be treated with β-adrenoceptor antagonists (β-blockers) in the short term, followed by antithyroid drugs. Propylthiouracil (PTU) is the preferred antithyroid drug because treatment with carbimazole during the first trimester has been associated with the occurrence of choanal atresia and aplasia cutis. Hyperthyroid women who become pregnant while taking carbimazole or PTU should be advised to continue their current drug in pregnancy, with close monitoring. Both carbimazole and PTU cross the placenta and are effective in treating thyrotoxicosis in the fetus caused by transplacental passage of TRAb. To avoid fetal hypothyroidism, which can affect brain development and cause goitre, it is important to use the smallest dose of antithyroid drug (typically < 150 mg PTU or 15 mg carbimazole per day) that will maintain maternal free T_4, T_3 and TSH concentrations within their respective reference ranges. Thyroid surgery is sometimes necessary because of poor drug adherence, drug hypersensitivity or failure of medical treatment and is most safely performed during the second trimester. Radioactive iodine is absolutely contraindicated throughout pregnancy, as it invariably induces fetal hypothyroidism. Frequent review of mother and fetus (monitoring heart rate and growth) is important during pregnancy and in the puerperium. Serum TRAb levels can be measured in the third trimester to predict the likelihood of neonatal thyrotoxicosis. PTU is the drug of choice in the breastfeeding mother, as it is excreted in the milk to a much lesser extent than carbimazole. Thyroid function should be monitored periodically in the breastfed child.

Post-partum thyroiditis

Post-partum thyroiditis typically presents 3–4 months after delivery. It is discussed in more detail in Chapter 20.

Pituitary disease

Prolactinoma

Prolactinomas are the most common pituitary tumours in young women. Although fertility is reduced in patients with prolactinoma, pregnancies can occur and if this happens the tumour may enlarge as part of the physiological pituitary enlargement that takes place during normal pregnancy. Macroprolactinomas (≥ 10mm) are at greater risk of enlarging and may cause optic chiasm compression. If women known to have a prolactinoma become pregnant, they should have visual field testing each trimester, followed by pituitary imaging by MRI if enlargement is suspected from changes in visual fields or from symptoms. Measurement of serum prolactin is generally not helpful, since levels increase anyway as part of normal pregnancy. Dopamine receptor agonists such as cabergoline and bromocriptine should normally be stopped during pregnancy, but can be reintroduced if necessary in patients with an enlarging prolactinoma that is threatening the visual fields.

Diabetes insipidus

Women with pre-existing diabetes insipidus may find that their symptoms worsen in pregnancy due to placental production of vasopressinase, a protease that degrades vasopressin (antidiuretic hormone, ADH). Because of this, pregnant women with diabetes insipidus may need higher doses of desmopressin until delivery. The development of symptoms suggestive of diabetes insipidus, such as thirst and polyuria, during pregnancy should raise suspicion of acute fatty liver of pregnancy (AFLP), the syndrome of haemolysis, elevated liver enzymes and low platelets (HELLP) or pre-eclampsia, as all of these conditions are also associated with decreased breakdown of vasopressinase by the liver.

Sheehan syndrome

This is a form of post-partum hypopituitarism caused by infarction of the pituitary, usually associated with hypotension from major post-partum haemorrhage. It can present with failure to establish lactation after birth, amenorrhoea or other features of hypopituitarism. The diagnosis can be confirmed by tests of pituitary function and treated with hormone replacement, as described in Chapter 20.

Parathyroid disease

Primary hyperparathyroidism

Primary hyperparathyroidism (PHPT) is uncommon in women of child-bearing age, but if pregnancy does occur in a patient with pre-existing PHPT, careful monitoring is required. Women with mild disease can be managed conservatively but if serum calcium levels rise above 2.85 mmol/L (11.5 mg/dL), consideration should be given to parathyroidectomy, as fetal mortality is high (up to 40%) in patients with severe hypercalcaemia. If parathyroidectomy is required, it should ideally be performed during the second trimester. Anecdotal evidence suggests that the calcimimetic drug cinacalcet can be used for medical management of PHPT during pregnancy.

Familial hypocalciuric hypercalcaemia

Familial hypocalciuric hypercalcaemia (FHH) is a benign disorder caused by mutations in the calcium-sensing receptor, which is described in Chapter 20. Although FHH poses no risk for pregnant women, the hypercalcaemia can suppress PTH secretion in neonates that do not inherit the FHH mutation, resulting in severe hypocalcaemia. Infants of mothers with FHH should have their serum calcium levels monitored during the first few days of life; if hypocalcaemia is detected, intravenous calcium should be given.

Adrenal disease

Women with known adrenal insufficiency can continue their glucocorticoid and mineralocorticoid replacement during pregnancy as normal. Rarely, adrenal insufficiency can present for the first time during pregnancy. If this occurs, the diagnosis is challenging because total cortisol normally increases during pregnancy, and short Synacthen tests can be falsely normal. Specialist assessment is required. In women with Conn syndrome who become pregnant, amiloride should be substituted for spironolactone to prevent anti-androgenic effects on a male fetus.

Human immunodeficiency virus infection

The course of HIV disease is not altered by pregnancy but treatment with antiretroviral therapy should be given during pregnancy to women who are HIV-positive, as outlined in Chapter 14. In some societies routine HIV testing is recommended at an early stage in pregnancy in all women.

Inflammatory rheumatic disease

Most women with inflammatory rheumatic disorders have successful pregnancies but it is critically important for them to be given pre-conception counselling and to review medication use, optimise disease control and make them aware of the risks that pregnancy might pose to their condition and vice versa.

Rheumatoid arthritis

Women with rheumatoid arthritis should have a medication review; methotrexate, leflunomide, mycophenolate and JAK inhibitors should be stopped and an alternative substituted before conception if necessary (Box 32.13). Rheumatoid arthritis often improves during pregnancy, particularly in those who are negative for rheumatoid factor or anti-cyclic citrullinated peptide antibodies. There is an increased risk of pre-eclampsia, pre-term birth and small babies for women with active disease, emphasising the importance of maintaining disease control during pregnancy. Glucocorticoids, hydrochloroquine, azathioprine and sulfasalazine can all be continued as normal but non-steroidal anti-inflammatory drugs (NSAIDs) should be avoided after 28 weeks (see Box 32.13). Inhibitors of TNF-α are safe during pregnancy and can be continued if necessary to maintain control of the disease. Many TNF-α inhibitors are actively transported across the placenta and this can lead to immunosuppression in the neonate. Accordingly, infants of mothers who have been treated with TNF-α inhibitors during the second and third trimesters should not be given live vaccines and should be monitored closely for any signs of infection, particularly if treatment is continued into the third trimester. An exception is certolizumab pegol, which is a pegylated antibody that is not transported across the placenta but this is used infrequently in IBD. Experience with other biologic therapies such as ustekinumab and vedolizumab during pregnancy is limited, but increasing and clinical experience suggests that these drugs may be used until at least the third trimester. Disease flares are common in the post-partum period, regardless of serology, and this can pose a problem for breastfeeding and care of the infant. Glucocorticoids are a good short-term option to control such flares, pending reintroduction of other disease-modifying antirheumatic drugs (DMARDs) that might have been stopped prior to pregnancy.

Systemic sclerosis

Pregnancy in women with diffuse systemic sclerosis (SSc), those with pulmonary hypertension or renal involvement and those with disease of recent onset (< 4 years) poses risks to mother and fetus. In milder forms of the disease, however, the prognosis is better (Box 32.14). Raynaud's phenomenon

i | 32.13 Safety of antirheumatic drugs during pregnancy and breastfeeding

Drug	Safe during pregnancy	Safe during breastfeeding	Comment
Azathioprine	Yes	Yes	
Ciclosporin	Yes	Yes	Data on breastfeeding limited
Cyclophosphamide	No	No	
Glucocorticoids	Yes	Yes	A good short-term option for disease flares
Hydroxychloroquine	Yes	Yes	
Janus activated kinase	No	No	Stop before planning pregnancy
Leflunomide	No	No	Stop 2 years before planning pregnancy
Methotrexate	No	No	Stop 3 months before planning pregnancy
Mycophenolate	No	No	Stop before planning pregnancy
Non-steroidal anti-inflammatory drugs (NSAIDs)	Yes (< 28 weeks)	Yes	
Sulfasalazine	Yes	Yes	Co-prescribe with folic acid
Tacrolimus	Yes	Yes	
Tumour necrosis factor (TNF) inhibitors	Yes	Yes	Avoid live vaccines in the neonate for 6 months

Adapted from Ateka-Barrutia O, Nelson-Piercy C. Connective tissue disease in pregnancy. Clin Med 2013; 131:580–584.

i	**32.14 Systemic sclerosis (SSc) and pregnancy**	
Subtype	Effect of disease on pregnancy	
Localised SSc	Good prognosis Raynaud's may improve Oesophagitis may worsen	
CREST syndrome	Good prognosis Raynaud's may improve Oesophagitis may worsen	
Diffuse SSc	Increased risk of: Pre-term delivery Pre-eclampsia Fetal growth restriction Low-birth-weight babies Maternal and fetal mortality	

(CREST = calcinosis, Raynaud's phenomenon, oesophageal involvement, sclerodactyly and telangiectasia)

i	**32.15 Differential diagnosis of lupus flare during pregnancy**		
Clinical finding	Lupus flare	Pre-eclampsia	Normal pregnancy
Hypertension	Yes	Yes	No
Proteinuria	Yes	Yes	No
Red cells/casts in urine	Yes	No	No
Liver function tests	Normal	Abnormal	Normal
Anti-double-stranded DNA	Increase	Unchanged	Unchanged
C3 and C4	Low	Elevated or unchanged from baseline	Unchanged

often improves during pregnancy due to vasodilatation but oesophageal symptoms may worsen. Renal crises are no more frequent during pregnancy, but if one occurs, ACE inhibitors should be given. Although these are normally contraindicated in pregnancy, the potential benefit in this situation outweighs the risk to the fetus. Glucocorticoids, which can be given to promote fetal lung maturation in premature babies, should be avoided in women with SSc where possible because they may provoke renal crisis.

Systemic lupus erythematosus

Pregnancy in women with systemic lupus erythematosus (SLE) poses several risks to both mother and fetus, especially if there is renal involvement. There is an increased risk of pre-eclampsia, thrombosis, fetal growth restriction, pre-term delivery, miscarriage and fetal death. There is also a higher risk of lupus flare during the puerperium. Good control of disease is paramount, since women with SLE who conceive when their disease has been quiescent for at least 6 months are less likely to have complications than those who conceive when their disease has recently been active. It can be difficult to assess disease activity during pregnancy because symptoms such as oedema, hair loss, joint pain and fatigue, which occur in active SLE, are also common during normal pregnancies. The features in Box 32.15 can help differentiate between an SLE flare, normal pregnancy and pre-eclampsia.

All women with SLE should be tested for anti-Ro and anti-La antibodies, since they can cross the placenta and cause neonatal complete heart block or cutaneous lupus, respectively. Medications should be reviewed prior to pregnancy, to ensure they are safe, and an alternative substituted if necessary (see Box 32.13). The management of patients with antiphospholipid antibodies (aPL) is described below.

Antiphospholipid syndrome

Primary antiphospholipid syndrome (APS) is associated with an increased risk of adverse pregnancy outcomes, including thrombosis, miscarriage, fetal death and pre-eclampsia. This applies to primary APS and that associated with connective tissue diseases such as SLE. During pregnancy, women with APS should be managed with low-dose aspirin in combination with low-molecular-weight heparin (LMWH).

Bone disease

Osteoporosis can rarely present for the first time during pregnancy. Typically, this is with either hip or back pain in the third trimester or puerperium due to fractured neck of femur or multiple vertebral fractures, respectively. The cause is unknown but it has been speculated that in some cases this may be due to amplification of the bone loss that normally occurs during pregnancy in women who have pre-existing low bone density. In other women, known risk factors for osteoporosis may be identified such as inflammatory disease or corticosteroids. Pregnancy-associated osteoporosis improves even without treatment but patients with severe disease may be left with chronic back pain due to vertebral deformity. Bisphosphonates and other osteoporosis treatments are often given empirically post partum in an attempt to increase bone density but the effects on fracture outcomes are unclear. Another presentation is with a localised form of osteoporosis affecting the femoral head, which presents with hip pain. This is thought to be a manifestation of chronic regional pain syndrome type 1 (CRPS-1). The diagnosis can be confirmed by MRI scan which shows bone marrow oedema at the affected site. Treatment is symptomatic and the condition usually resolves spontaneously post partum.

Cardiac disease

Congenital heart disease

Women who have a history of surgically corrected congenital heart disease generally tolerate pregnancy well, but are more likely to have babies with congenital heart disease and should be offered fetal cardiac scans. Acyanotic heart diseases, such as atrial septal defect, ventricular septal defect and patent ductus arteriosus, all have a good prognosis in pregnancy. Unrepaired cyanotic heart disease has a very poor prognosis in pregnancy, as does pulmonary hypertension, regardless of the underlying cause. Women with mechanical heart valves require anticoagulation throughout pregnancy but their anticoagulation should be planned with consideration of substituting warfarin with LMWH and aspirin during the first trimester to reduce the risk of warfarin embryopathy. If necessary, warfarin can be used during pregnancy, particularly in the second and third trimesters.

Valvular heart disease

The physiological changes of pregnancy may also unmask previously undiagnosed valvular disease. Women with regurgitant lesions, such as mitral regurgitation and aortic regurgitation, tolerate pregnancy better than those with stenotic lesions. Mitral stenosis causes a reduction in blood flow from the left atrium to left ventricle in diastole, which worsens during pregnancy due to the increased heart rate and hypervolaemia. Those with moderate to severe mitral stenosis (valve area < 1.5 cm^2) are at particular risk and may develop arrhythmias, tachycardia and pulmonary oedema. Most patients can be managed medically with β-blockers, LMWH and furosemide as necessary. Surgical intervention is indicated if there is continued haemodynamic compromise despite optimal medical management.

32

Myocardial infarction

Pregnancy increases the risk of myocardial infarction. While atherosclerosis is the main cause in non-pregnant individuals, coronary artery dissection and coronary thrombosis secondary to the hypercoagulable state are more common causes during pregnancy. Management is similar to that of non-pregnant women, except that statins and glycoprotein IIb/IIIa inhibitors such as tirofiban should be avoided where possible. Clopidogrel can be given but should be stopped around the time of delivery to reduce the risk of uterine bleeding and to allow spinal anaesthesia to be used if necessary. There is little evidence regarding ticagrelor, an alternative antiplatelet drug, during pregnancy. Stenting can be performed, but bare-metal stents are preferred because drug-eluting stents require dual antiplatelet therapy that cannot be continued around the time of delivery.

Aortic dissection

Pregnancy is an independent risk factor for aortic dissection and this should be considered when a woman presents with acute severe chest pain during pregnancy. The vast majority of cases in pregnancy are 'type A', involving the ascending aorta (see Fig. 16.71), and require careful control of hypertension, caesarean section to deliver the fetus, and emergency surgery to treat the aneurysm.

Peripartum cardiomyopathy

Peripartum cardiomyopathy (PPCM) presents with heart failure secondary to left ventricular systolic dysfunction towards the end of pregnancy or in the months following delivery. It is a diagnosis of exclusion, made when other causes of heart failure have been ruled out. The cause is unknown but PPCM is more prevalent in women who are older, multiparous, hypertensive and African Caribbean. It is treated by conventional medications for heart failure, including ACE inhibitors if necessary, and delivery of the baby. Many women recover within 3–6 months of diagnosis but the prognosis is variable. There is a significant chance of reduction in cardiac function in subsequent pregnancies.

Dilated cardiomyopathy

Dilated cardiomyopathy carries a poor prognosis if the pre-pregnancy ejection fraction is below 30% or if symptoms are in New York Heart Association grades 3 or 4. Management is as described for PPCM.

Renal disease

Renal tract infection

Pregnancy predisposes women to urinary tract infection. If asymptomatic bacteriuria is discovered during pregnancy it should be treated promptly with antibiotics, to prevent ascending renal tract infection. Pyelonephritis is more common in pregnancy due to the physiological dilatation of the upper renal tract; if it does occur, it can trigger premature labour.

Acute kidney injury

Acute kidney injury (AKI) may occur during pregnancy or in the puerperium due to a variety of causes (Box 32.16). Women with AKI caused by pre-eclampsia are prone to pulmonary oedema. Particularly close attention to fluid balance is very important for these women. Intravenous fluid is rarely indicated for women with pre-eclampsia, and most will undergo a diuresis in the days following the diagnosis and the AKI will resolve. If there is a coexisting condition such as sepsis with associated hypotension, then intravenous fluids may be helpful. It is wise to enlist the assistance of critical care medicine specialists early for such patients.

In the post-partum period, AKI may occur as the result of post-partum haemorrhage or pre-eclampsia, and sometimes these occur in combination. Although pre-eclampsia resolves after delivery, AKI can be at its worst in the first few days post partum, especially when exacerbated by obstetric haemorrhage.

Glomerular disease

Proteinuria caused by glomerular disease is usually exacerbated during pregnancy, and nephrotic syndrome may develop without any alteration in the underlying disease activity in individuals who had only slight

i	32.16 Causes of acute kidney injury in pregnancy	
Mechanism	**Cause**	**Features**
Pre-renal	Hyperemesis gravidarum	Nausea and vomiting
		Dehydration
		Presentation in first trimester
	Post-partum haemorrhage	Vaginal bleeding immediately post partum
	Placental abruption	Abdominal pain or vaginal bleeding in second or third trimester
	Septic abortion	Presentation with hypotension, shock and pyrexia
Renal	Pre-eclampsia	Presentation in second and third trimesters with new-onset hypertension and proteinuria
	Thrombotic thrombocytopenic purpura	Possible antenatal or post-partum presentation with headache, irritability and drowsiness
		Haematology shows thrombocytopenia and microangiopathic haemolytic anaemia
	Acute fatty liver of pregnancy	Presentation with vomiting and abdominal pain in third trimester
		Abnormal liver function tests
		Liver ultrasound can be normal
	Acute interstitial nephritis	Most common cause is use of non-steroidal anti-inflammatory drugs
Post-renal	Acute urinary retention	Usual presentation is in third trimester due to enlarged uterus causing ureteric obstruction; sometimes presents post partum

Adapted from Palma-Reis I, Vais A, Nelson-Piercy C, et al. Renal disease and hypertension in pregnancy. Clin Med 2014; 13:57–62.

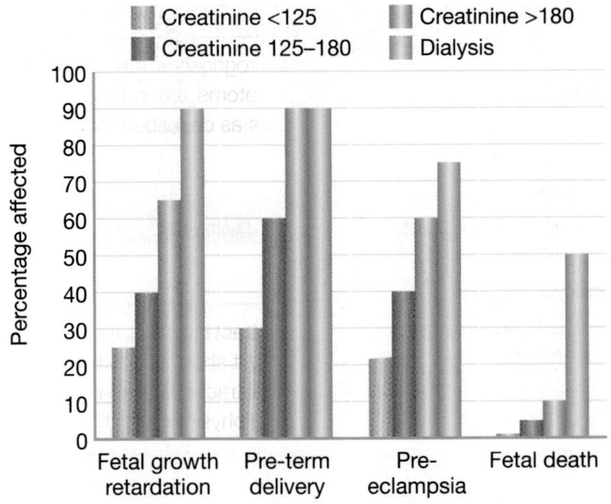

Fig. 32.3 Adverse pregnancy outcomes in chronic kidney disease. (Creatinine is in µmol/L. To convert to mg/dL, multiply by 0.011.) *Data from Williams D, Davison D. Chronic kidney disease in pregnancy. BMJ 2008; 336:211–215.*

i | **32.17 Criteria for diagnosis of acute fatty liver of pregnancy**

- Vomiting
- Abdominal pain
- Polydipsia/polyuria
- Encephalopathy
- Elevated bilirubin (> 14 µmol/L (> 0.82 mg/dL))
- Low glucose (< 4 mmol/L (< 72.4 mg/dL))
- Elevated urate (> 340 µmol/L (> 5.7 mg/dL))
- Leucocytosis (> 11 ×10⁹/L)
- Ascites or bright liver on ultrasound
- Elevated transaminases (alanine/aspartate aminotransferase (ALT/AST) > 42 U/L)
- Elevated ammonia (> 47 µmol/L (> 81.7 mg/dL))
- Renal impairment (creatinine > 150 µmol/L (> 1.7 mg/dL))
- Coagulopathy (prothrombin time > 14 secs or activated partial thromboplastin time > 34 secs)
- Microvascular steatosis on liver biopsy

Acute fatty liver of pregnancy can be diagnosed when ≥ 6 of the above features are present in the absence of another explanation.

Adapted from Ch'ng CL, Morgan M, Hainsworth I, et al. Prospective study of liver dysfunction in pregnancy in Southwest Wales. Gut 2002; 51:876–880.

proteinuria before pregnancy. This further increases the risk of venous thromboembolism, the leading cause of maternal deaths in higher-income countries.

Chronic kidney disease

Women with chronic kidney disease (CKD) are at increased risk of pre-eclampsia, fetal growth restriction, miscarriage, pre-term delivery and fetal death (Fig. 32.3). Pregnancy can also cause acceleration of maternal renal decline. The factors that influence pregnancy outcome for women with CKD are baseline renal function, hypertension, degree of proteinuria and the underlying cause of CKD. Women with CKD should have pre-pregnancy counselling, be closely monitored by a multidisciplinary team throughout pregnancy, and be given low-dose aspirin as prophylaxis against pre-eclampsia.

Renal replacement therapy

Fertility is reduced among women on renal replacement therapy and there is increased risk of adverse pregnancy outcomes. Despite this, many women receiving renal replacement therapy have successful pregnancies. More intensive dialysis is recommended in pregnancy, and particular attention should be paid to addressing issues around blood pressure, fluid balance and anaemia.

Renal transplant recipients

Pregnancy should be delayed for a minimum of 12 months following renal transplantation, to allow the graft to stabilise, on minimum immunosuppressive drugs. The outcome is best for women with a well-functioning graft, with no proteinuria or hypertension. Women with renal transplants can deliver vaginally but in practice there is a higher incidence of caesarean section in this group, due to the higher incidence of pre-term delivery.

Liver disease

Specific causes of liver disease during pregnancy are discussed below.

Acute fatty liver of pregnancy

Acute fatty liver of pregnancy (AFLP) is a rare and serious condition that typically presents in the third trimester with vomiting, abdominal pain, jaundice and other symptoms (Box 32.17). It is more common in first pregnancies and multiple pregnancies, and is associated with male fetuses. Rarely, fulminant liver failure may occur. The diagnosis can usually be made on the basis of the clinical features, abnormal liver function tests (LFTs) and the appearances of fatty liver on ultrasound. A liver biopsy is rarely needed to make the diagnosis but shows microvascular steatosis. Management is with supportive care and by delivery of the fetus. The development of AFLP has been linked in some cases with an inherited deficiency of the enzyme long-chain acyl-CoA dehydrogenase (LCHAD) in the baby.

HELLP syndrome

The syndrome of haemolysis, elevated liver enzymes and low platelets (HELLP) is thought to be part of the spectrum of pre-eclampsia. It usually presents antenatally but can also appear for the first time in the postnatal period. The presenting symptoms can be the same as those of pre-eclampsia but can also include headache, right upper quadrant pain and visual disturbance. HELLP can be complicated by liver haematoma and capsular rupture. Management involves supportive care, control of hypertension, correction of coagulopathy and delivery of the fetus.

Obstetric cholestasis

Obstetric cholestasis is estimated to affect about 1% of pregnancies in women of European descent, although the prevalence is about 1.5% in women of Indian-Asian and Pakistani-Asian descent. The cause is incompletely understood but the condition is thought to be due in part to the cholestatic effect of high oestrogen levels. The typical presentation is in the third trimester with pruritus, particularly affecting the soles and palms. Laboratory testing reveals raised levels of bile acids and abnormal LFTs. The diagnosis can be made on the basis of these clinical features when other causes of liver dysfunction and pruritus have been excluded. Treatment is with ursodeoxycholic acid (UDCA) at a starting dose of 250 mg twice daily, to improve symptoms and liver function. However, this treatment does not reduce the risk of adverse fetal outcomes. Rifampicin may be given as an additional therapy if UDCA is ineffective, and vitamin K should be given if clotting is abnormal. Aqueous cream with menthol can also be effective in soothing pruritus There is an increased risk of fetal mortality with evidence of a particularly high risk when bile acid levels are over 100 µmol/L. Some centres induce labour before 40 weeks in an effort to reduce the risk. The risk of recurrence in future pregnancies is high.

32

Viral hepatitis

The course of hepatitis B is unchanged in pregnancy, but it is important to identify women who have active infection to reduce the risk of vertical transmission to the fetus; this risk is up to 90% in women who are hepatitis B e-antigen-positive. Vaccinations and immunoglobulin should be given to infants of mothers who test positive for hepatitis B, and antiviral agents should be given to the mother after delivery. Vertical transmission rates of hepatitis C are low in the absence of HIV infection and so no action is required for the infant, unless there is co-infection with HIV; in this case, antiviral drugs should be considered. Pregnant women are at greater risk of contracting hepatitis E than the non-pregnant population. It is transferred via the faeco-oral route, and is usually a mild self-limiting illness outside of pregnancy. However, it can cause fulminant hepatic failure in up to 20% of pregnant women.

Neurological disease

Epilepsy

Women with epilepsy should have pre-pregnancy counselling, should be advised to take high-dose folic acid from pre-conception, and should have their their antiepileptic drugs (AEDs) reviewed. Many AEDs are associated with teratogenicity, and the risk increases with dose and use of multiple medications. Sodium valproate in particular is associated with a 40% risk of persistent neurodevelopmental disorders and a 10% risk of physical birth defects, which is considerably higher than for other AEDs. Ideally, sodium valproate should be avoided in women of child-bearing potential and an alternative AED substituted with a better safety profile, such as lamotrigine, levetiracetam or carbamazepine if it is safe to do so. The minimum number of drugs at the lowest effective dose required for control of epilepsy should be given, and women should be reminded of general safety advice, such as showering instead of bathing. Emergency management of seizures in a pregnant woman with epilepsy (without eclampsia) is the same as that in non-pregnant women. While pregnancy does not generally affect the frequency of seizures in women with well-controlled epilepsy, those who enter pregnancy with poorly controlled epilepsy are likely to deteriorate. The plasma levels of some AEDs such as lamotrigine can fall in pregnancy. Seizures are more common at the time of delivery and women should be advised to deliver in a unit staffed with personnel able to manage this.

Idiopathic intracranial hypertension

Idiopathic intracranial hypertension (IIH) may worsen during pregnancy due to weight gain. Treatment with acetazolamide can be continued during pregnancy but should be avoided in the first trimester due to lack of safety data. Therapeutic lumbar puncture can also be helpful. The mode of delivery is not affected by IIH and spinal analgesia can be given as normal.

Migraine

Migraine often improves during pregnancy but if attacks occur they should be managed with simple analgesia and antiemetics. If necessary, prophylaxis can be given with aspirin, β-blockers or tricyclic antidepressants. Safety data on use of triptans during pregnancy are limited but reassuring. Triptans can therefore be used for the treatment of migraine if other therapies are ineffective.

Stroke

Stroke is twice as common in pregnant women as in non-pregnant women of the same age. The risk is highest during the third trimester and puerperium. The management of stroke during pregnancy is similar to that in non-pregnant patients. The risk of cerebral venous thrombosis is greatly increased during pregnancy. The presentation is with headache,

---

i	**32.18 Causes of anaemia in pregnancy**

Microcytic

- Iron deficiency
- Haemoglobinopathies
- Thalassaemia

Normocytic

- Anaemia of chronic disease
- Haemorrhage
- Haemolysis

Macrocytic

- Vitamin B_{12}/folate deficiency
- Liver disease
- Alcohol excess

---

i	**32.19 Causes of thrombocytopenia during pregnancy**

- Gestational thrombocytopenia
- Idiopathic thrombocytopenic purpura
- Systemic lupus erythematosus
- HELLP (haemolysis, elevated liver enzymes and low platelets)
- Haemolytic uraemic syndrome
- Thrombotic thrombocytopenic purpura

---

seizures and neurological deficits such as hemiparesis. If the diagnosis is suspected, neuroimaging should be performed with MRI or CT venography. Management of acute infarct should be as for the non-pregnant patient and include consideration of thrombolysis.

Psychiatric disorders

Mood changes are common during pregnancy but more severe psychiatric disorders, such as depression or psychosis, typically present within 2–4 weeks of delivery (see Box 31.34). These disorders are discussed in more detail in Chapter 31.

Haematological disease

Anaemia

The causes of anaemia during pregnancy are summarised in Box 32.18. Iron deficiency anaemia is most commonly due to a 20% increased demand for iron. In most cases, it responds well to oral iron supplementation, with a rise in haemoglobin of approximately 0.8 g/L per week. If the haemoglobin does not rise following a 4-week trial of iron supplementation, alternative causes of anaemia should be considered. Non-adherence to oral iron is common and intravenous iron should be considered in women with iron deficiency and failure of oral treatment. It is generally not necessary to investigate iron deficiency anaemia during pregnancy unless there is clinical evidence of gastrointestinal blood loss, which should be investigated in the normal way.

Rhesus disease

Women who are negative for the Rhesus antigen should be offered treatment with anti-RhD immunoglobulin around the time of delivery to reduce the risk of haemolytic disease of the newborn. More details are provided in Chapter 25 and Box 25.19.

Thrombocytopenia

The causes of thrombocytopenia during pregnancy are summarised in Box 32.19. The most common cause is gestational thrombocytopenia, which typically occurs towards the end of pregnancy and resolves spontaneously after delivery. It is not associated with adverse pregnancy outcomes and requires no specific intervention. Pregnancy may occur in women with pre-existing idiopathic thrombocytopenic purpura (ITP). This should be managed with glucocorticoids and/or immunoglobulin, with the aim of maintaining the platelet count above 80×10^9/L at the time of delivery, in case spinal anaesthesia or caesarean section is required. Thrombocytopenia may also occur as a component of haemolytic uraemic syndrome (HUS) and thrombotic thrombocytopenic purpura (TTP). Both are characterised by microangiopathic haemolytic anaemia, acute kidney injury and thrombocytopenia, but in TTP neurological symptoms and fever also occur. These conditions are rare but important to recognise since up to one-quarter of cases occur during pregnancy and the post-partum period. TTP is managed with plasma exchange, fresh frozen plasma and sometimes glucocorticoids or rituximab. Platelet transfusion should be avoided.

Venous thromboembolism

The risk of venous thromboembolism (VTE) is 4–5 times higher in pregnancy than in non-pregnant women. Women should receive risk assessments for VTE during their pregnancy, based on individualised risk factors (see Box 32.20). On the basis of their personal level of risk, women will be given general advice such as ensuring adequate hydration and mobility, and those at higher risk will be advised to take daily low-molecular-weight heparin (LMWH) during pregnancy and the post-partum period. It is a safe drug in pregnancy, and does not cross the placenta. Deep venous thrombosis (DVT) is the most common presentation and more commonly affects the left leg in pregnancy. Treatment with LMWH should be started once the clinical suspicion has been raised (unless there is a strong contraindication), and diagnostic imaging sought. Measurement of D-dimer is not useful in pregnancy because levels rise as part of normal pregnancy, and clinical decision rules such as Wells score are not validated for use in pregnancy.

Doppler ultrasound scan is the investigation of choice. If the initial Doppler ultrasound scan is negative, and clinical suspicion low, treatment with LWMH can be stopped. However, if the clinical suspicion remains high, treatment can be stopped, and the scan repeated on day 3 and/or day 7. If proximal DVT is suspected, then an MRI of the abdomen should be considered.

Pulmonary embolism (PE) is a significant cause of death in pregnancy. It usually presents with symptoms such as breathlessness, pleuritic chest pain and haemoptysis, and signs such as tachypnoea, tachycardia, hypoxia and hypotension. Initial investigations should include an ECG, CXR and blood tests, including a troponin. Further details of investigations for possible PE are in the Imaging section earlier in this chapter.

Treatment of VTE in pregnancy is with LMWH at a higher dose than outside of pregnancy, based on the patient's weight. For women with massive PE, systemic or catheter-directed thrombolysis should be considered.

Women with a previous history of VTE who are receiving warfarin or direct oral anticoagulants as prophylaxis should have these stopped prior to conception and LMWH should be substituted. Women on treatment dose LMWH need careful planning around the time of delivery, to balance the need for anticoagulation against bleeding risk from epidural/spinal anaesthetic techniques, and delivery. LMWH and warfarin are both safe in breastfeeding. There is insufficient evidence regarding direct oral anticoagulants in breastfeeding, and they are considered unsafe.

---

i | **32.20 Risk factors for VTE in pregnancy**

Pre-existing risk factors

- Previous VTE
- Thrombophilia (inherited and acquired)
- Medical comorbidities, e.g. cancer, active IBD, active SLE, nephrotic syndrome
- Age > 35
- Obesity
- Smoking
- Gross varicose veins
- Parity ≥3

Obstetric risk factors

- Multiple pregnancy
- Pre-eclampsia
- Prolonged labour > 24 hours
- Mid-cavity of rotational operative delivery
- Stillbirth
- Pre-term birth
- PPH

Transient risk factors

- Surgery while pregnant
- Hyperemesis gravidarum
- Ovarian hyperstimulation syndrome
- Immobility
- Systemic infection
- Long-distance travel

Adapted from RCOG Green-top Guideline 37A: Reducing the risk of venous thromboembolism during pregnancy and the puerperium, April 2015.

Further information

British Society for Rheumatology and British Health Professionals in Rheumatology guideline on prescribing drugs in pregnancy and breastfeeding. BSR/BHPR; September 2016.

British Thoracic Society/Scottish Intercollegiate Guidelines Network. SIGN 158 – British guideline on the management of asthma. Edinburgh: Health Improvement Scotland; 2019. *Useful asthma guidelines.*

Royal College of Obstetricians and Gynaecologists. Thromboembolic disease in pregnancy and the puerperium: acute management. Green-top guideline. London: RCOG; April 2015. *A useful evidence-based guideline on the investigation of pulmonary embolism in pregnancy.*

Websites

npeu.ox.ac.uk/mbrrace-uk *National Perinatal Epidemiology Unit: a very useful resource with detailed and extensive information on causes of maternal deaths, stillbirths and infant deaths in the UK.*

RJ Mann

33

Adolescent and transition medicine

Historically, childhood illnesses were characterised by a series of acute episodes, often infective, on a background of an otherwise healthy patient. Adult medicine traditionally comprised patients with progressive conditions, and increasing pathology with advancing age. A number of factors have led to the recognition that boundaries between adult medicine and paediatric care are not clear-cut, and recent evidence has confirmed that anticipating and carefully planning the transition of children with long-term conditions (LTCs) into adult services improves care and outcomes. About 14% of children in the industrialised world are diagnosed with an LTC and in the majority of patients the disorder will persist into adulthood. Common illnesses include asthma, epilepsy, congenital heart disease, diabetes and childhood cancer (Box 33.1). Similar trends are developing worldwide, with increasing survival rates of children with complex pathology, and increasing prevalence of lifestyle-related conditions such as obesity, hypertension and type 2 diabetes. Specific factors that make transition planning important in young people with LTCs are outlined in Figure 33.1.

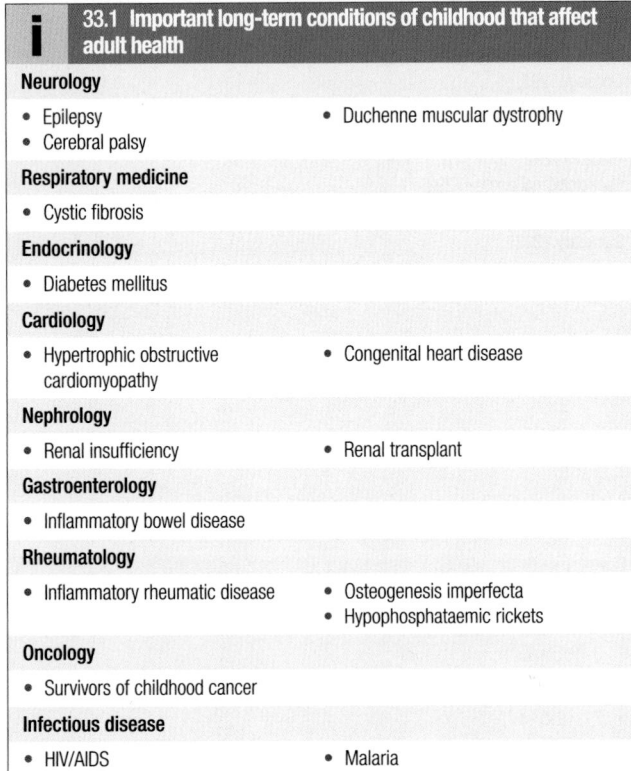

i	33.1 Important long-term conditions of childhood that affect adult health

Neurology
- Epilepsy
- Cerebral palsy
- Duchenne muscular dystrophy

Respiratory medicine
- Cystic fibrosis

Endocrinology
- Diabetes mellitus

Cardiology
- Hypertrophic obstructive cardiomyopathy
- Congenital heart disease

Nephrology
- Renal insufficiency
- Renal transplant

Gastroenterology
- Inflammatory bowel disease

Rheumatology
- Inflammatory rheumatic disease
- Osteogenesis imperfecta
- Hypophosphataemic rickets

Oncology
- Survivors of childhood cancer

Infectious disease
- HIV/AIDS
- Malaria

Planning the process of transition from paediatric to adult health services and improving the assessment of young people as they enter those adult services have been shown to impact positively on long-term health outcomes. There is a need for physicians to gain new skills in the care of young people and adults who have conditions that have arisen in childhood. This includes developing specific skills in the management of adolescents and young adults, managing the process of transition and developing knowledge of relevant medical conditions. The overall approach to transition medicine, as well as important disease-specific issues, will be considered in this chapter.

Transition from paediatric to adult health services

Effectiveness of transition planning

A review of the effectiveness of transition planning has confirmed improved health outcomes when specific interventions to improve coordination between adult and paediatric services are implemented. Most research in this field has been undertaken with young people with diabetes, and many of the outcome measures relate to that condition. The principles of transition planning and the potential benefits are, however, likely to be generalisable to other LTCs that present in childhood. Young people with serious LTCs are among the most complex and high-risk patients to care for in adulthood, and it is important to work closely with them as they move to adult services, to try to improve their long-term outcome.

General principles of transition planning

Paediatric services are organised and delivered in a very different way to adult medical services. They encompass a period of life that spans from infancy to independence, and progress from taking parents' views as paramount to needing to recognise the wishes of the young person. After transition, young people move from medical services that have been family-centred and focused around maximising the child's development, to a service that encourages patient autonomy, in which employment and reproduction are important measures of outcome. At the same time as undergoing transition within medical services, young people are making multiple other transitions in their lives as they move from a dependent to an independent way of living (Fig. 33.2). They often move away from the family home, and parents who formerly held responsibility for patient

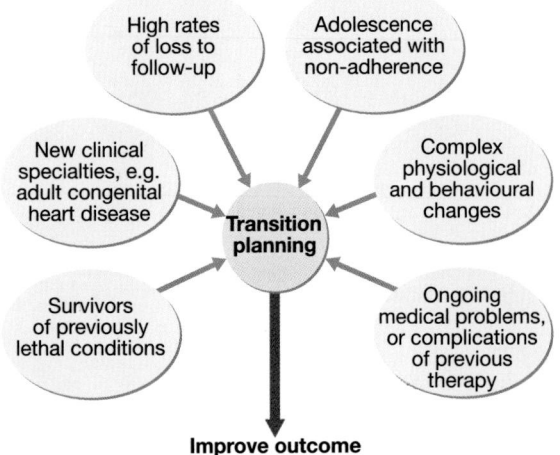

Fig. 33.1 Reasons to consider transition planning.

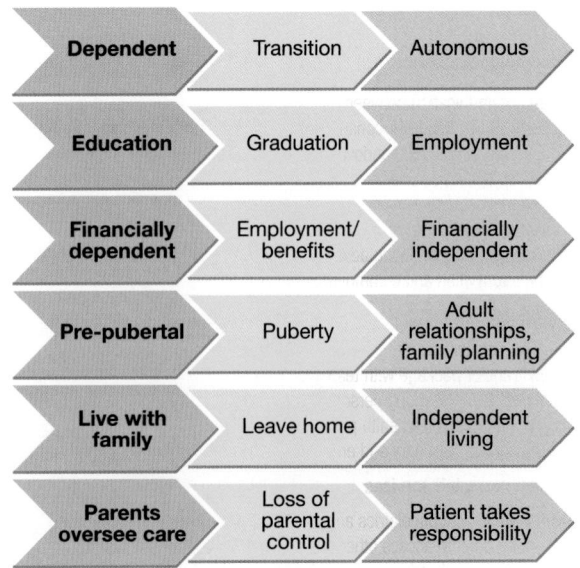

Fig. 33.2 Lifestyle changes during transition to adulthood.

management, coordination of care, communication and consent to treatments will be demoted to an advisory role. Paediatric services are not well placed to meet this change in focus from the patient as a child to the patient as an independent adult, and young people benefit from the move to adult services as long as their specific needs as a young adult are recognised.

Principles of prescribing during transition

Hepatic drug metabolism increases from neonatal levels during childhood, eventually decreasing to adult levels after puberty. Once puberty has been completed, adolescents can be considered, in pharmacokinetic and pharmacodynamic terms, to behave like adults. It is important to remember that many young people have considerably lower body mass and therefore body mass index (BMI) than adults, and care needs to be taken to avoid excessive dosage in physically smaller patients. Medicines are often prescribed on a dose per kilogram basis in children, to ensure that they are not exposed to inappropriately high drug concentrations. In young people who are obese (those in whom actual body weight is >20% of their ideal weight), this can potentially lead to problems if the calculated dose per kilogram exceeds the standard adult dose. Accordingly, the ideal weight for the patient's height rather than actual body weight should be used to calculate drug dosages when prescribing for obese young people. This can be easily done in clinical practice using centile charts to calculate ideal body weight based on the patient's age and height. Whether or not the patient is obese it is important not to exceed the recommended adult dose when prescribing for young people.

A systematic approach to transition planning

Several steps need to be undertaken to develop a successful programme for transition of care. The key components are summarised in Box 33.2.

> **i** **33.2 Core elements in developing a transitional care programme**
>
> **Establishing transition policy**
> - Develop policy, with input from young people
> - Train staff in operation of policy
>
> **Tracking and monitoring**
> - Establish process to identify patients
> - Develop systems to track individual progress
> - Incorporate transition planning into clinical care
>
> **Transition readiness**
> - Identify suitable adult care provider
> - Establish process for introduction to adult team
> - Provide written information about joint first consultation
>
> **Transition planning**
> - Ensure communication between paediatric and adult teams
> - Identify need for handover consultation
> - Prepare written medical handover:
>   - Diagnosis
>   - Current treatment
>   - Previous key issues
> - Send relevant information in advance
> - Provide information and community support
>
> **Transfer to adult services**
> - Arrange first consultation
> - Review transfer package with team
> - Identify concerns of young person
> - Review young person's health priorities
> - Update medical summary and emergency care plans
>
> **Integration into adult services**
> - Communicate with paediatrics and confirm transfer
> - Help young adult to access other adult services
> - Continue individualised care plan tailored to young person
> - Seek feedback from young adult about transition

The first step is to establish a policy in consultation with young people and train staff in the policy. Subsequently, systems need to be developed to identify patients in need of transition and track them as they pass through the programme. Adult health-care providers need to be identified and processes developed for introducing the young person to the adult team. This should be followed by written communication between the paediatric and adult teams, and then a first consultation with the adult team at which the transfer can be reviewed and a care plan developed. There should subsequently be written communication between the adult and paediatric teams to confirm that handover has occurred, followed eventually by integration of the young person's care into the adult service.

A number of organisations have published guidelines to planning transition services. Two of the best known include the 'Ready Steady Go' programme in the UK and the American Academy of Pediatrics' 'Got Transition' (see 'Further information'). Details of the sorts of competencies that a young person might need before making a full transition to adult medical services are outlined in Box 33.3.

When should transition happen?

The optimum timing for transition is not specifically defined; it is a process that evolves over a number of years, during which puberty and then adolescence occur. Transition should generally be initiated at around

> **i** **33.3 Key features in assessing readiness for transition to adult services**
>
> **(K) Knowledge**
> 1. Describes condition, effects and prognosis
> 2. Understands medication purpose and effects
> 3. Understands treatment purposes and effects
> 4. Knows key team members and their roles
>
> **(S) Self-advocacy**
> 1. Can attend part/whole clinic appointment on their own
> 2. Knows how to make appointments/alter appointments
> 3. Has understanding of confidentiality
> 4. Orders repeat prescriptions
> 5. Takes some/complete responsibility for medication/other treatment
> 6. Knows where to get help
>
> **(H) Health and lifestyle**
> 1. Understands importance of diet/exercise/dental care
> 2. Understands impact of smoking/alcohol/substance use
> 3. Understands sexual health issues/pregnancy/sexually transmitted infections
>
> **(A) Activities of daily living**
> 1. Self-care/meal preparation
> 2. Independent travel/mobility
> 3. Trips/overnight stays away from home
> 4. Benefits/financial independence
>
> **(V) Vocational**
> 1. Current and future education/impact of condition on career plans
> 2. School attendance and performance
> 3. Work experience and access to careers advice
> 4. Outside activities and interests
> 5. Disclosure to school/employer
>
> **(P) Psychosocial**
> 1. Self-esteem/self-confidence
> 2. Body/self-image
> 3. Peer relationships/bullying
> 4. Support networks/family/disclosure to friends
> 5. Coping strategies
>
> **(T) Transition**
> 1. Understands concept of transition
> 2. Agrees transition plan
> 3. Attends transition clinic
> 4. Visits adult unit (if appropriate)
> 5. Sees primary care team/other clinical staff independently

33

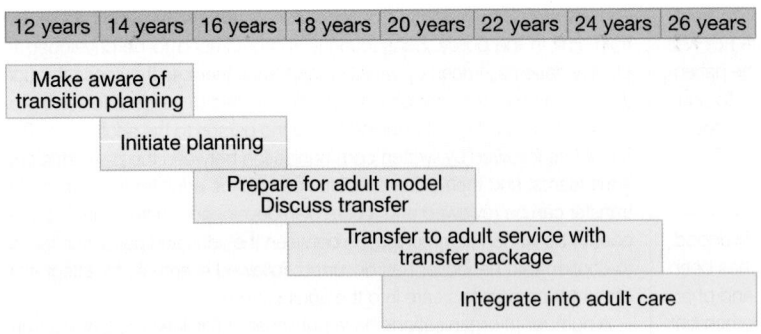

Fig. 33.3 Timing of transition.

12 years of age. Completion time then varies from person to person, also depending on the model of adult services available. Most commonly, full transition occurs between 16 and 18 years of age (Fig. 33.3). This coincides with many other areas where young people are considered to have made the transition to adulthood, such as the completion of formal education.

Functional anatomy and physiology

Puberty and adolescence are developmental stages through which children progress during the second decade of life. During this phase, several physical, biochemical and emotional changes occur. The most important are discussed in more detail below.

Endocrine changes

The hormonal and physical stages of progression through puberty in males and females are summarised in Figure 33.4. Puberty is initiated by pulsatile increases in gonadotrophin-releasing hormone (GnRH) by the hypothalamus, which in turn stimulates pulsatile release of luteinising hormone (LH) and follicle-stimulating hormone (FSH) by the pituitary. In males, the increased production of LH stimulates Leydig cells in the testes to produce testosterone, and FSH acts on Sertoli cells to stimulate sperm production, as described on page 667 and shown in Figure 20.14. The rise in testosterone increases skeletal growth, promotes development of the male genital organs and stimulates growth of pubic, facial and axillary hair. In females, FSH and LH act on the ovary to promote follicle production, ovulation and menstruation, as described on page 667 and shown in Figure 20.15. Other hormonal changes in all adolescents include a rise in adrenal androgens and a rise in growth hormone, which in turn stimulates production of insulin-like growth factors 1 and 2 (IGF-1 and IGF-2). Insulin production also rises by about 30% during puberty. These hormonal changes contribute to the biological, morphological and psychological changes seen during the teenage years. Adolescence (as opposed to puberty) comprises not only the physical changes of puberty, but also the wider emotional and psychological changes of progression into early adulthood. The emotional and psychological changes are associated with physical maturation but also with sociocultural influences. The feelings and behavioural development of normal adolescence are complex but tend to follow fairly predictable patterns.

Physical changes

In girls, there is an increased rate of growth, followed soon after by the development of breasts and pubic hair. Menstruation typically starts after the rate of growth has peaked. In boys, puberty begins with testicular enlargement, followed soon after by a growth spurt and the development of pubic hair. In clinical practice, Tanner staging is used as a method of documenting progression of physical changes that occur during puberty (Fig. 33.5). The average age at onset of puberty in the UK is about 11 years in girls and 12 years in boys, but normal puberty has a very wide range of onset. Factors that are important in predicting age of onset of normal puberty include family history (age of onset is strongly predicted by the parents' pattern of onset) and body mass, with heavier children entering puberty at a younger age. The current trends towards improved nutritional status and increased obesity in particular are driving earlier onset of puberty. Delayed puberty is defined to have occurred when the age at onset is more than 2.5 standard deviations above the national average, which in the UK is about 13 years in girls and 14 years in boys. If puberty is delayed beyond this point, investigations may be needed to determine the underlying cause. Many children who have had long-term health conditions during childhood experience a delayed onset of puberty because chronic ill health slows longitudinal growth and causes functional hypogonadotrophic hypogonadism. Glucocorticoid therapy also contributes to growth retardation in children with chronic inflammatory diseases. An X-ray of the left wrist can be used to assess bone age accurately, and a bone age that is more than 2 years behind the chronological age should prompt consideration of further investigations.

Cognitive and behavioural changes

As young people move from their early teenage years to later adolescence there is a move away from the family towards personal independence. This is often characterised by change from a self-centred focus, associated with a sense of awkwardness and worries about being normal, towards increased self-confidence and an awareness of weaknesses in parents and others in authority. In late adolescence, young people reach a stage of self-reliance, increased emotional stability and improved ability to think ideas through. Finally, young adults begin to develop firm belief systems, autonomy and independence. With time, there is reduced conflict with parents and other figures in authority and full maturity develops.

In terms of cognition, there is a transition from being mostly interested in the present, in short-term outcomes and instant gratification, through to increased concern for the future and a greater focus on one's longer-term role in life. Sexuality and relationships clarify during adolescence, and individuals move from early awkwardness and uncertainty to a firmer sense of their sexual identity, and then development of more serious and longer-term relationships. In terms of morals and values, young people move from a period of risk-taking behaviour and experimentation through to understanding the potential consequences of such behaviour for their future health and well-being. Young adults develop a greater capacity for setting personal goals and an increased focus on self-esteem. Finally, family, social and cultural traditions regain some of their previous importance, and by the time young people emerge from adolescence, they

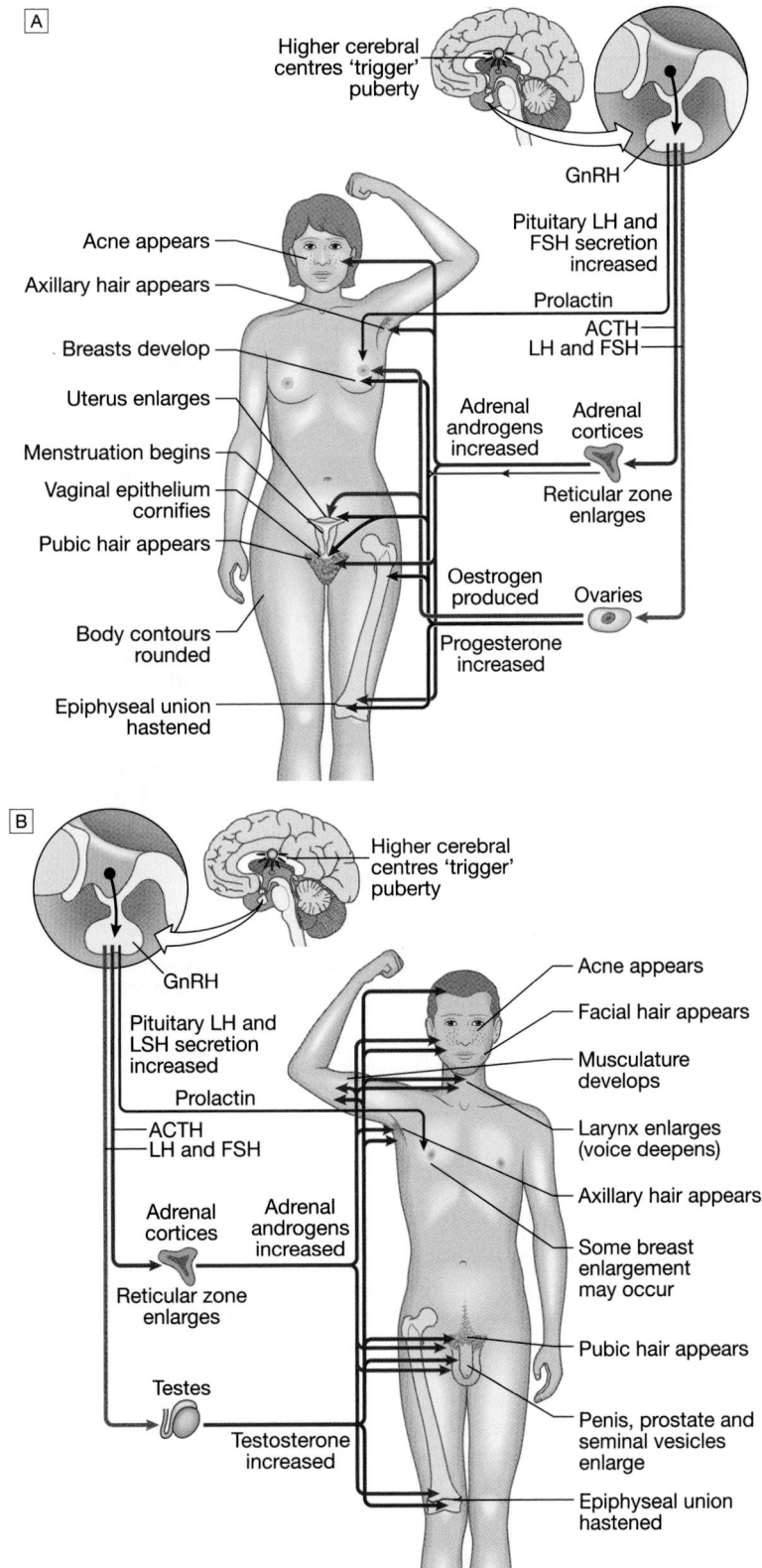

Fig. 33.4 Hormonal events of puberty. [A] In the ovary, FSH acts on granulosa cells to stimulate oestrogen production, whereas LH acts on theca cells to stimulate progesterone production. Androgens are also produced in small amounts by theca cells in response to LH (not shown). [B] In the male, LH acts on interstitial Leydig cells to stimulate testosterone production. FSH with testosterone acts on Sertoli cells to stimulate spermatogenesis. (ACTH = adrenocorticotrophic hormone; FSH = follicle-stimulating hormone; GnRH = gonadotrophin-releasing hormone; LH = luteinising hormone) *From Smith RP. Netter's Obstetrics and gynecology, 2nd edn. Philadelphia: Saunders, Elsevier, Inc.; 2008.*

33

Tanner stage	I	II	III	IV	V
Female					
Breast	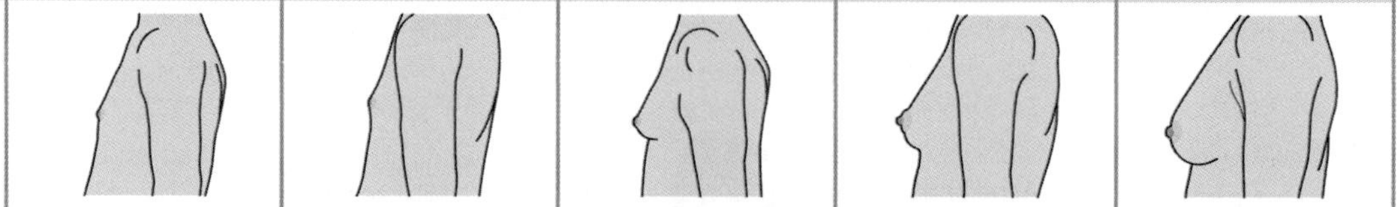 Pre-adolescent	Elevation of breast and papilla as a small mound	Further enlargement of breast and areola with no separation of contours	Projection of areola and papilla to form mound above breast	Mature stage. Projection of papilla with recession of areola to contour of breast
Pubic hair	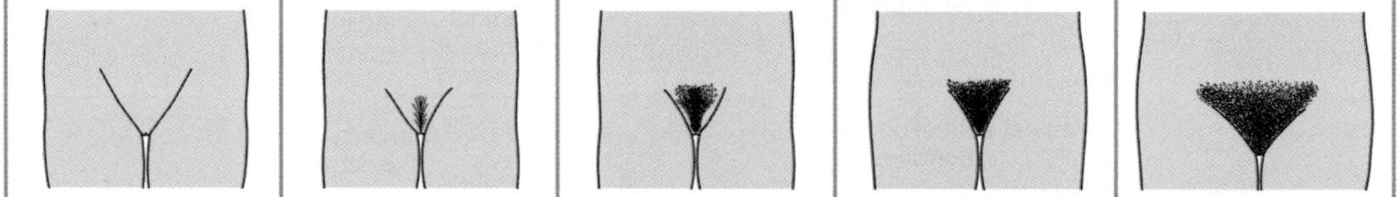 None	Sparse, long and straight	Darker, coarse and curled hair	Darker, coarse and curled hair but covering smaller area than in adult. No spread to medial surface of thighs	Dark, coarse and curled hair extending to inner thighs
Male					
Genitalia	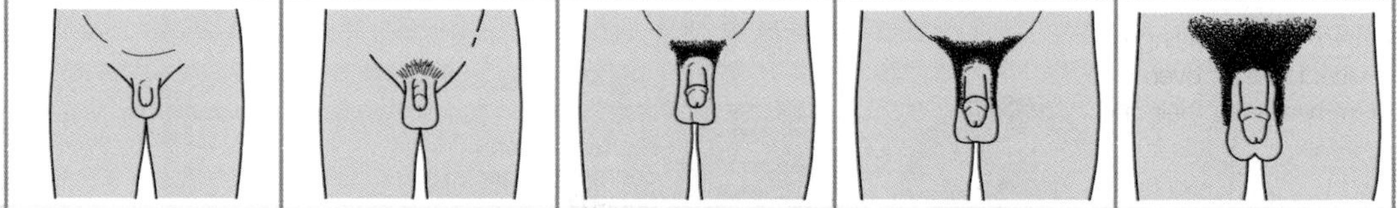 Pre-adolescent	Growth of testes and scrotum. Skin on scrotum reddens and becomes wrinkled	Growth of penis and further growth of testes and scrotum. Skin of scrotum becomes darker and more wrinkled	Further growth in length and width of penis, testes and scrotum	Penis, testes and scrotum of adult size
Pubic hair	None	Sparse, long and straight	Darker, coarse and curled hair	Darker, coarse and curled hair but covering smaller area than in adult	Dark, coarse and curled hair extending toward umbilicus

Fig. 33.5 Tanner staging of puberty.

have usually developed insight and a greater focus on long-term well-being. It is the development of these more mature personality traits that are important for the more active role in health care that is needed for patients to function well within an adult model of medicine. Some young people do vary slightly from these broad patterns but the feelings and behaviours described are, in general, considered normal for each stage of adolescence. Understanding these changes in emotional and psychological behaviour underpins the approaches that are needed to meet the challenges of managing long-term conditions in older adolescents and young adults.

Investigations

Several changes take place during adolescence in terms of skeletal growth, organ development and body composition, which can influence the interpretation of results. Examples include fusion of the epiphyses as puberty progresses, increases in bone mineral content and density as the skeleton grows, and changes in the reference range of certain biochemical tests. Most of these changes occur gradually during puberty and there are rarely abrupt alterations in adult biochemical concentrations. It is important to use age-adjusted biochemical reference ranges until puberty has been completed. Several biochemical changes take place in the composition of body fluids between infancy and puberty.

Some of the key changes in biochemical markers are outlined in Box 33.4. More detail on reference ranges for specific analytes is provided in Box 35.9. The elevation in alkaline phosphatase (ALP) levels during adolescence relates to the bone isoenzyme produced by osteoblasts in the growing skeleton during the growth spurt. Further investigations for raised levels of ALP are not required in adolescence, as long as other liver function tests, including γ-glutamyl transferase (GGT), are normal.

In general, under normal physiological conditions, the reference ranges of most biochemical tests remain fairly constant between puberty and menopause in women and between puberty and middle age in men.

Clinical assessment

The initial patient consultation at transition is of vital importance for establishing a potentially life-long professional relationship with the

i	33.4	Biochemical changes during transition

Analyte	Comment
Alanine aminotransferase (ALT)	Increased during adolescence Activity may continue to rise, at least in men, until middle age
Alkaline phosphatase (ALP)	Activity higher in infancy, decreases during childhood, and rises again with skeletal growth during puberty Peak in females at median 11 years and in males at 13 years Levels decrease rapidly after puberty, particularly in girls; adult levels achieved after epiphyses fused
Insulin-like growth factor 1	Levels 30% higher during adolescence
Serum creatinine	Increases steadily from infancy to puberty parallel to development of skeletal muscle; until puberty, there is little difference in concentration between males and females
Uric acid concentration	Decreases from high levels at birth until 7–10 years of age, then increases, especially in boys, until 16 years

i	33.5	Features in transition assessment

Features of history and/or examination	Reason
History*	
Main/presenting condition and detailed review of clinical course	Understand detail and severity of illness; understand which treatments have been undertaken and which have been successful
Family history: Draw family tree of all first-degree and any relevant/affected second-degree family members	Many long-term conditions arising during childhood have significant genetic and familial factors to be taken into account
Current drug therapy, significant previous therapies	Many drugs have significant long-term implications, levels may need monitoring, may have teratogenic effects to consider
Any surgical or other relevant medical history	Understand which treatments have been undertaken and which have been successful
Pubertal status/age of menarche	Helps assess disease severity plus patterns of growth Informs about patient's reproductive health and family-planning wishes
Social history: In education or in work? Receiving appropriate benefits/support? Financial or other practical concerns? Living with parents/left home?	Assesses wider effects of patient's health on their independent living, as well as their financial and practical circumstances Can be a proxy measure of disease severity and identifies their support mechanisms, which also helps in the assessment of their current needs
Systems enquiry	Any other related/unrelated symptoms or problems
Physical examination	
Height, weight, calculation of body mass index Blood pressure Urinalysis if relevant Assessment of pubertal status General physical examination	Although young people are often accompanied by a parent, examine them separately and use this opportunity to consider asking about private matters, such as partners, sexual activity and drug or alcohol use

*Throughout the first consultation, confidence and competence in decision-making/capacity to consent should be assessed. If there are concerns about capacity, clarify key decision-makers.

patient, as well as identifying key features in the history, examination and assessment of their overall needs. Parents commonly attend a first adult appointment with their son or daughter, and it is usually necessary to allow longer for this initial assessment. Often, the first transition appointment is undertaken jointly with the paediatrician in a specialist transition clinic and this will enable a thorough face-to-face handover of all the key facts.

A detailed transition referral letter should clearly describe the diagnosis, current and previous treatments, and key interventions that have been undertaken while the patient was under the care of paediatric services. It is important to check the main details with the young person and to make sure there are no other factors that they feel are of relevance. There are a few features in the history that merit special attention, particularly at the first consultation, as outlined in Box 33.5. Many young people with an LTC attend their first adult outpatient department consultation with their parents, and it is important either to create a time to ask personal and lifestyle-related questions separately from the main history – that is, privately – or to make sure that these can be confidentially explored in future.

Presenting problems

Adherence

Adherence is defined as 'the extent to which a person's behaviour, in terms of taking medications, following diets or executing lifestyle changes, coincides with medical or health advice'. The term 'adherence' is used in preference to 'compliance' because it focuses on whether a person actively adheres to the regimen rather than passively follows the doctor's orders. It also implies partnership and cooperation between the patient and the care-giver. More recently, clinicians have moved to seeking patients' concordance with management plans. 'Concordance' refers to a consultation process that has an underlying ethos of shared decision-making. It has become clear that current levels of adherence do not deliver the full benefits of medication. Historical paternalistic medical practice does not maximise the chances of patients adopting the changes and treatments they need to improve their outcomes. Reaching a concordant position with patients involves

a range of approaches (such as patient-centredness or shared decision-making) and a number of specific actions (such as exploring anxieties about medication side-effects, individualising regimens to suit the patient's lifestyle, offering a range of treatment options) and has not been evaluated comprehensively.

Adherence to clinic attendance, investigation and treatment often falls significantly in adolescence and during transition to adult services. Measurement of adherence is challenging and reported rates vary according to the method of assessment. Adolescents may also have varying adherence levels within their treatment regimen. An important example is in patients who have undergone organ transplantation, in whom low adherence to immunosuppressive medication is a significant cause of graft rejection and may cause death. Adherence merits careful consideration when caring for adolescents and young adults, and focusing on strategies to improve adherence at this initial stage of patient management can deliver life-long improvements in health outcomes. Young teenagers mainly believe in things that they have directly experienced and do not fully appreciate the unseen consequences of not taking their medications. In time, adolescents learn to

33

develop hypothetical thinking and to analyse more complex information and decision-making. The ability to engage in formal thinking is inconsistent at first, and at times of stress (such as during an illness) adolescents may regress to more simple ways of problem-solving. Despite their maturing skills, they may remain self-centred and feel invincible. Factors that positively and negatively affect adherence are outlined in Box 33.6. Interventions to improve adherence are summarised in Box 33.7.

Recent literature suggests that two-way communication between patients and professionals about medicines leads to improved satisfaction with care, knowledge of the condition and treatment, adherence, health outcomes and fewer medication-related problems. Younger adults and those coming to adult services following transition from paediatric services have very different expectations in terms of the nature of the patient–doctor relationship and are more likely to require a more collaborative approach to development of management plans to maximise their concordance with treatment in the long term.

High-risk behaviour

The high-risk behaviour that can be undertaken by adolescents is well documented and is seen across many cultures. It is important to assess this by history-taking at the time of transition (Box 33.8). Adolescents who have had LTCs during childhood are at greater risk of undertaking harmful behaviour and there is evidence that a poor long-term health outlook is associated with risk-taking behaviour earlier in life.

Globally, the leading causes of death among adolescents are road injury, human immunodeficiency virus (HIV) infection, suicide, lower respiratory infections and interpersonal violence; many of these deaths are linked to risk-taking behaviours such as excess alcohol and drug intake. Quite apart from mortality, there are other significant adverse events linked to risk-taking behaviour in adolescents: excess alcohol ingestion is also associated with non-fatal road traffic accidents, unwanted and unprotected sexual activity, and violence as both perpetrator and victim.

There are a number of theories about the neurodevelopmental changes associated with these behaviour changes. At around 11 years of age, the prefrontal cortex (PFC) and parietal lobes begin a period of pruning of neuronal axons. It is theorised that these changes represent the start of the process of increasing frontal lobe control. A separate process that occurs at the same time predisposes the adolescent to risk-taking behaviour and impulsivity: frontostriatal reward circuits mature relatively early and encourage the adolescent towards adult activities such as alcohol and drug use, and sexual intercourse, which carry potential health risks. At this stage, the PFC has not yet matured to the point where the individual can assess risk adequately. The PFC and its connections are structurally unable to provide sufficient control. It is thought

33.6 Factors affecting adherence

Negative factors

- Older adolescent
- Mental health issues with care-giver
- Family conflicts
- Complex therapy
- Medication with side-effects
- Denial of illness

Positive factors

- Positive family functioning
- Close friends
- Internal locus of control
- Treatment with immediate benefits
- Patient's belief in seriousness of illness and efficacy of treatment
- Physician empathy

33.7 SIMPLE strategies to improve adherence

Simplify regimen

- Use once daily/twice daily regimens if possible
- Match regimen to bedtime and meals
- Use pill box or alarms on phone
- Organise services around patient (combined clinics, flexible timing and appointments)

Impart knowledge

- Share decision-making
- Provide clear instructions:
  Limit to three or four major points
  Use simple, everyday language
  Use written information or pamphlets and verbal education at all encounters
- Supply addresses of quality websites
- Provide advice on how to cope with medication costs

Modify patient beliefs

- Empower patients to self-manage their condition:
  Ask about their needs
  Ask what might help them become and remain adherent
  Ensure they understand the risks of not taking their medication
  Address fears and concerns about taking the medication

Provide communication

- Improve interviewing skills
- Practise active listening

- Provide emotional support – treat the whole patient and not just the disease
- Provide clear, direct and thorough information
- Elicit the patient's input in treatment decisions
- Allow adequate time for patients to ask questions
- Build trust

Leave the bias

- Learn more about low health literacy and how it affects patient outcomes
- Consider care of ethnically and socially diverse patient populations
- Acknowledge biases in medical decision-making (intentional or unintentional)
- Address dissonance of patient–provider race/ethnicity and language
- Take extra time to overcome cultural barriers
- Ask specifically about attitudes, beliefs and cultural norms around medication
- Use culturally and linguistically appropriate targeted patient interventions
- Increase engagement, activation and empowerment
- Tailor education to the patient's level of understanding

Evaluate adherence

- Direct:
  Number of repeat prescriptions
  Biomarkers of response
  Measurement of drug levels
- Indirect:
  Self-reporting: 'When did you last forget your medicine?'; 'How often have you forgotten your medicines this week?'

Excerpted with permission from the American College of Preventive Medicine. Medication Adherence: Improving Health Outcomes Time Tool: A Resource from the American College of Preventive Medicine. 2011. Retrieved from https://ogg.osu.edu/media/documents/agingconnections/MedicationAdherenceTool_syndromes-screenings.pdf.

that this maturational gap in PFC control of the pleasure-seeking brain systems is responsible for the risk-taking lifestyle that characterises the period of adolescence.

A number of studies have investigated personality and other factors that contribute to different risk-taking behaviours during adolescence: essentially, younger adolescents and females tend to rate activities as being more risky, and are therefore less likely to undertake them. Older males and those of lower educational status are higher-risk takers. Specific protective factors include high self-esteem and a strong orientation to an internal locus of control; young people who feel they have less control and influence over themselves and their behaviour are more likely to undertake high-risk activities. Many young people with serious long-term health conditions are disempowered in a number of ways and there is evidence that they are predisposed to be high-risk takers during adolescence. Examples of risk-taking behaviour include not only alcohol and drug intake, but also non-adherence to medicines and other aspects of health care, such as diet in diabetes.

It is not easy to affect behaviour during this period of non-adherence. Isolated educational intervention is not sufficient to improve outcome; for example, there is a wealth of evidence showing that adolescents know about the behaviours needed to prevent transmission of HIV, but many do not adhere to this advice. Long-term health-care providers have an invaluable role in supporting adolescents during this period of their development as adults, as many important health-related and lifestyle habits are established during this period: more than 90% of smokers start smoking in adolescence, and life-long habits around eating and exercise are laid down during the teenage years. Focusing on the needs of the emerging adult for autonomy and using the highest levels of communication and patient engagement significantly improve outcomes for patients with LTCs.

Unplanned pregnancy

In many parts of the world, females commonly undergo their first pregnancy during or just after adolescence. The median age for first pregnancy varies from 19 years in India and parts of Asia, through to 25 years in the United States and around 30 years in Australia and Western Europe. Teenage pregnancy rates are high across the world (Box 33.9). Information from the UK suggests that 1 in 6 pregnancies is unplanned, and 1.5% of women between the ages of 18 and 45 face an unplanned pregnancy each year. It is therefore vital to anticipate and discuss the issues surrounding reproductive health with all young people before and during transition, as well as during early adulthood. Young people with serious LTCs have a number of additional factors to be taken into consideration when discussing reproduction, and these discussions need to take place long before a family is planned. General physicians do not need to be able to undertake complex genetic counselling and investigation, but should be able to provide advice about the recurrence risk of common inherited conditions, as well as that of the more common multifactorial LTCs, many of which have an inherited or genetic component.

Clinical presentations

In almost every clinical setting, there is the potential for a young adult with a serious LTC that has arisen during childhood to present to adult physicians. Medical services can improve the care and outcome for this vulnerable group by planning a systematic approach to transition, as described above, and by focusing the clinical consultation on issues of relevance and importance to each particular patient. The key issues to consider for a number of the most common LTCs of childhood are discussed below.

i	**33.8 History-taking in adolescent patients**

Home life

- Relationships
- Social support
- Household chores

Education

- School
- Exams
- Work experience
- Career
- University
- Financial issues

Activities

- Peers, people that patients can rely on
- Exercise and sport

Driving

- Aged 16 if disabled

Drugs

- Cigarettes and alcohol: how much, how often
- Non-prescription drugs

Diet

- Nutritional content (calcium, vitamin D)
- Weight
- Caffeine (diet drinks)
- Binges/vomiting

Sex

- Concerns
- Periods
- Contraception (in relation to medication)

Sleep

- Amount
- Difficulty getting to sleep
- Frequent waking
- Early waking?

Suicide

- Depression
- Mood
- Disabled adolescent men high risk

From Segal TY. Adolescence: what the cystic fibrosis team needs to know. J R Soc Med 2008; 101(Suppl 1):15–27.

i	**33.9 Adolescent pregnancy rates/1000 women aged 15–19 years (2018)**	
Region		**Pregnancy rate**
World		42
Arab world		46
Caribbean small states		50
Central Europe and the Baltics		19
East Asia and Pacific		21
East Asia and Pacific (excluding high income)		22
Euro area		7
Europe and Central Asia		17
Europe and Central Asia (excluding high income)		25
European Union		9
Fragile and conflict-affected situations		91
Heavily indebted poor countries (HIPC)		100
Latin America and Caribbean		62
Latin America and Caribbean (excluding high income)		63
Least developed countries: UN classification		93
Middle East and North Africa		40
Middle East and North Africa (excluding high income)		44

Data from: https://data.worldbank.org/indicator/SP.ADO.TFRT.

33

Neurological disease

Epilepsy

Epilepsy is a chronic disorder, the hallmark of which is recurrent, unprovoked seizures. Epilepsy that has presented during childhood, as opposed to adulthood, is less often associated with underlying central nervous system malignancy and is well controlled with first-line anticonvulsants in around 80% of cases. Young people who still have epilepsy or are on anticonvulsant therapy as they progress into adulthood are more likely to have underlying structural brain disease, such as cerebral palsy, or have more complex or syndromic epilepsy. In many of them, epilepsy may be associated with learning difficulties or other neurological conditions.

Epilepsy presents several problems during transition. Adherence to medication can be an issue and patients with low adherence to epilepsy medicines have higher mortality, higher hospital admission rates and higher Emergency Department attendances. Conversely, high adherence rates at initiation of epilepsy therapy are associated with improved long-term seizure freedom and higher seizure freedom at 4 years. Epilepsy can also affect employment options for young people, as about 30% of patients still have breakthrough seizures while on treatment. Certain types of employment, such as working within the emergency services or armed forces, or becoming a pilot or driver of a heavy goods vehicle, may therefore not be possible. Driving restrictions may also limit options for some other occupations. Young women with epilepsy should be advised that oral contraceptives are less effective with enzyme-inducing antiepileptic drugs; they should also be made aware of the risk of teratogenicity with many antiepileptic drugs, most notably sodium valproate, which should be avoided in pregnancy if at all possible. Pre-conceptual counselling is desirable for all young girls with epilepsy and pre-conceptual folic acid supplementation is advisable to reduce the risk of neural tube defects.

Alcohol use in moderation does not affect seizure control in the majority of patients, but withdrawal from alcohol in dependent patients is epileptogenic and heavy alcohol use should be discouraged. Information about marijuana and epilepsy risk is lacking, but regular marijuana use and excess drinking are associated with poor adherence to medication regimens and increased seizure risk.

Cerebral palsy

Cerebral palsy comprises a range of non-progressive neurological impairments, present from the time of birth or arising in early childhood. Although the neuropathology is non-progressive, the manifestation of problems can evolve, with progressive motor dysfunction related to increased spasticity and possibly progressive seizure activity.

Patients with severe cerebral palsy present specific problems during transition and early adulthood. They may be paraplegic or quadriplegic and most non-ambulatory individuals have significant intellectual disability. This group of patients will be unable to live independently during adulthood and need ongoing long-term care. Delivering medical care to these individuals poses several problems, including practical issues such as consideration of capacity and consent to treatment. Other comorbidities include gastro-oesophageal reflux (often related to abnormal lower oesophageal function), seizures and feeding difficulties often requiring gastrostomy. These individuals usually require a complex care package involving many members of the multidisciplinary team. There are also risks of abuse and neglect in the care of adults with severe disability and this needs to be borne in mind when considering atypical problems or unusual presentations in this vulnerable patient group. Depending on the severity of the patient's condition, end-of-life care may need to be discussed and planned with the family and other care-givers.

Muscular dystrophy

The muscular dystrophies are a group of diseases that cause progressive weakness and loss of muscle mass. The disorders differ in terms of which muscle groups are affected, the degree of weakness and the rate of disease and symptom progression. All the inherited muscular dystrophies that present during childhood need active management during transition. One of the most important and most severe conditions is Duchenne muscular dystrophy (DMD), which is associated with a progressive decline in mobility, coupled with cardiac dysfunction due to cardiomyopathy, and respiratory failure requiring respiratory support as the disease progresses. Physicians should ensure that the whole family is aware of the wider genetic issues. Female carriers of the DMD gene mutations can suffer muscle fatigue and are at risk of cardiomyopathy, as well as there being obvious risks for their male offspring. On average, patients with DMD survive until their late teens to early twenties, and those with less severe muscular dystrophies, such as Becker dystrophy, survive until their thirties. Although fertility is reduced, young men with these conditions may themselves father children. Male offspring will be unaffected but all female infants of affected males will be carriers.

As the muscular dystrophies progress, a complex package of care involving a multidisciplinary team is necessary; it should include respiratory input to assess the need for ventilatory support, which is a common endpoint for many patients. At the present time, there is no definitive treatment. Glucocorticoids (prednisolone at 0.75 mg/kg/day) have been shown to improve muscle strength and are frequently used, but carry an increased risk of osteoporosis and vertebral fractures. New therapeutic approaches are being developed with the aim of ameliorating disease progression in patients with nonsense mutations. One involves the use of drugs such as ataluren, which promotes binding of transfer RNA (tRNA) molecules at the site of stop codons with a mismatch in one base (near-cognate tRNAs) which results in read-through of the stop codon causing a full-length protein to be produced with an amino acid substitution rather than a truncated non-functional protein. Other potential treatment options for patients with DMD include the use of drugs that are targeted at splice sites to promote exon skipping. Eteplirsen is one such drug which promotes skipping of exon 51 in patients who have a mutation within this exon. Another is golodirsen, which promotes skipping of exon 53 in patients with mutations in this exon. Another approach that is under investigation is to use idebenone, which an antioxidant drug that facilitates electron transport in mitochondria. At the moment, however, the evidence for clinical benefit of all of these drugs remains somewhat limited.

Patients with DMD usually require social and financial support. It is important to consider end-of-life care plans with patients and family members. Involvement from palliative care teams, as well as psychological, spiritual and wider non-medical support, is essential.

Respiratory disease

Cystic fibrosis

Cystic fibrosis (CF) is a single-gene autosomal recessive disorder that affects about 1 in 2000 to 1 in 3000 individuals of European descent (p. 510). Clinical manifestations are caused by defects in an ion transporter termed the cystic fibrosis transmembrane conductor regulator (CFTR) protein. With improved supportive care, the median survival in the UK is now more than 50 years. It is well recognised that young people with life-limiting conditions face particular challenges during transition: individuals often exhibit high-risk behaviour during adolescence, and this was particularly true in the past when long-term survival rates were poor. The rates of non-concordance with medication and with time-consuming physiotherapy and nebuliser regimens are high and adversely affect outcome and survival. Exercise tolerance and employment are likely to be restricted as time progresses, and patients need particular support managing the slow decline in function and well-being that occurs throughout their adult lives.

In terms of fertility and child-bearing potential, the picture is complex and merits detailed discussion with patients. It is not often discussed openly by the paediatrician or during childhood, other than with the parents when the patient is young. The vas deferens is absent in 98% of males with CF and seminal vesicular dysfunction means that ejaculates are low in volume. While boys are infertile, newer reproductive therapies, such as the availability of intracytoplasmic sperm injection, mean that fatherhood is possible. The opportunity for assisted reproduction should be discussed early so that people can make informed choices at an appropriate stage of their lives. Females with CF who have good nutritional status and reasonable health status have normal fertility and genetic counselling should be offered early. Contraception needs to be discussed with women who are not planning a pregnancy, since pulmonary hypertension is an absolute contraindication for the oral contraceptive pill (OCP). Women also need to be advised about the effects of antibiotics on OCP effectiveness. New orally available small-molecule therapies, including lumacaftor and ivacaftor, have recently been licensed; they can partially rectify functional defects in the CTFR and have improved outcome. These drugs are having a positive effect on symptom control and are potentially disease-modifying. The triple drug combination of elexacaftor–tezacaftor–ivacaftor is an important new therapy for individuals who have at least one *F508del* mutation, which includes approximately 85% of people with CF in the United States. Other therapeutic approaches, including gene therapy and mRNA-editing therapies, are also being explored as treatments for CF. Common issues encountered during transition of CF patients are summarised in Box 17.34.

Cardiovascular disease

Congenital heart disease

Congenital heart disease (CHD) is the most common congenital anomaly, affecting about 1% of live births. Among birth defects, CHD is the leading cause of mortality. Maternal illnesses such as rubella and injection of teratogenic agents during pregnancy, along with paternal age, all play roles in pathogenesis. Although some chromosomal anomalies, such as trisomy 13, 18 and 21 and monosomy X (Turner syndrome), are strongly associated with CHD, these account for only 5% of cases. Microdeletion and single-gene mutations can also be important, such as in DiGeorge syndrome (22q11.2 microdeletion). Overall, the most common congenital valvular anomalies are aortic and pulmonary stenosis. The most common structural anomaly is ventricular septal defect.

There is a wide range of severity of CHD but many patients with life-limiting conditions (usually complex structural anomalies such as tetralogy of Fallot or hypoplastic left heart syndrome) survive to adulthood. Genetic counselling of affected individuals is important, as there is a 1%–2% recurrence risk of any cardiac anomaly in offspring. Affected patients should be transitioned to a cardiologist with experience in CHD since this has become a subspecialty in own right. More details are provided on page 465 and in Box 16.103.

Hypertrophic obstructive cardiomyopathy

Hypertrophic obstructive cardiomyopathy (HOCM) is characterised by left ventricular wall hypertrophy, impaired diastolic filling and abnormalities of the mitral valve. These features can cause dynamic obstruction of the left ventricular outflow tract, diastolic dysfunction, myocardial dysfunction and an increased risk of supraventricular and ventricular tachyarrhythmias. HOCM is a genetic disorder caused by mutations affecting the genes that encode cardiac sarcomere proteins and is most frequently transmitted as an autosomal dominant trait. It may present for the first time during adolescence with cardiac arrest or sudden cardiac death. Predictive genetic testing is possible but challenging because of the large number of causal mutations. In clinical practice, careful analysis of the family history can be useful in identifying those at risk of inheriting the disease. If no gene anomaly has been identified within a family, first-degree relatives may need screening by electrocardiography (ECG) and echocardiography. Identification of a genetic anomaly is most helpful in allowing identification of family members who do not need echocardiograms or clinical follow-up. Children of affected parents should be screened every 3 years until puberty, and then annually until 20 years of

age. If there is no evidence of HOCM in early adulthood, it is unlikely that the condition will develop in later life.

Oncology

Around 1 child in 500 will develop cancer by the age of 14 years. Leukaemia is the most common, accounting for about 33% of cases; central nervous system tumours are the next most common, accounting for around 25% of all childhood cancers. Fifty years ago, 75% of children diagnosed with cancer died, but overall survival rates now range from 75% to 80%. Between 60% and 70% of young adults who have survived childhood cancer will develop at least one medical disability, most commonly as a result of their therapy rather than their primary cancer. There is a three- to sixfold increased risk of a second cancer, with an absolute risk of about 10% before 50 years of age. It is therefore important for these individuals to be kept under surveillance during transition and beyond.

Endocrine and reproductive disturbances are the most common late effects, affecting 40%–60% of survivors. Infertility can be an issue in both males and females receiving cytotoxic medications, unless it has been possible to store semen and ovarian tissue in advance of treatment. Other long-term risks include hypopituitarism, growth hormone deficiency and pubertal delay (especially in boys) from brain irradiation. Radiotherapy to the neck can cause hypothyroidism and increases the risk of thyroid cancer. Total-body irradiation offered as conditioning for bone marrow transplantation affects both ovarian and testicular function, and many of the chemotherapeutic agents used have adverse effects on fertility. Chemotherapy-induced ovarian failure is typically associated with high-dose alkylating agents such as cyclophosphamide, and this is an independent risk factor for premature ovarian failure. In recent years, patients have been offered ovarian and testicular tissue retention and fertility issues are being discussed with families during childhood, but often the patients themselves have limited levels of knowledge of the details. Chemotherapy and radiotherapy in childhood significantly reduce ovarian reserves. When combined with the progressive ovarian decline that occurs in all women throughout adulthood there is a significant risk of premature menopause or ovarian failure, with 8% of survivors affected. Young women need to be aware of these risks during their early adulthood to help with family and lifestyle planning; for example, they may wish to plan to have children earlier in their adult life rather than risking ovarian decline.

Cardiomyopathy is another complication of anthracyclines such as doxorubicin and daunorubicin. Serious cardiac complications include arrhythmias, dilated cardiomyopathy from myocardial necrosis, and angina or myocardial infarction arising from vaso-occlusion or vasospasm.

In addition to physical effects, children who have faced life-threatening illness in childhood may experience psychological and family difficulties during adulthood. Cognitive impairment is more common in children who have received chemotherapy or radiotherapy to the brain, and problems can include lower IQ, problems with memory and attention, poor hand–eye coordination and behaviour or personality problems, combined with the well-recognised and physical complications of cancer treatment in childhood.

Increasing recognition of these issues has resulted in active monitoring programmes for survivors of childhood cancer, who are best seen in specialist 'late effects' multidisciplinary clinics, where teams include oncologists, psychologists and specialists from other relevant disciplines.

Renal disease

Chronic kidney disease (CKD) accounts for some of the most complex long-term illnesses in childhood. The most common causes during childhood and adolescence are shown in Box 33.10. The primary pathology can be varied and many conditions have no specific treatment, but the overall approach to management of progressive renal insufficiency is the same. Internationally agreed definitions of CKD staging in children differ

---

i | **33.10 Causes of renal impairment in childhood and adolescence**

- Obstructive uropathy
- Renal hypoplasia/dysplasia
- Reflux nephropathy
- Focal segmental glomerular sclerosis
- Polycystic kidney disease

---

i | **33.11 Staging of chronic kidney disease (CKD) in children over 2 years of age***

Stage	Glomerular filtration rate (GFR) (mL/min/1.73 m²)	Description
1	>90	Normal or high
2	60–89	Mildly decreased
3a	45–59	Mildly to moderately decreased
3b	30–44	Moderately to severely decreased
4	15–29	Severely decreased
5	<15	Kidney failure

*Kidney Disease: Improving Global Outcomes (KDIGO) 2012 classification. Chronic kidney disease is defined either as GFR <60 mL/min/1.73 m² for >3 months, regardless of whether other CKD markers are present, or as GFR <60 mL/min/1.73 m² accompanied by evidence of structural damage or other markers of kidney abnormalities, including proteinuria, albuminuria and pathological abnormalities in histology or imaging. In adults, albumin excretion is also included in CKD staging as the level of albuminuria correlates with outcome. These data are lacking in children and so albuminuria is not used to classify paediatric CKD.

from those in adults and are summarised in Box 33.11. In adults the rate of albumin excretion is included in CKD definitions, as outcome correlates with the level of albuminuria, but in children similar data are lacking and so the staging system is based on glomerular filtration rate alone. The majority of children with CKD stage 3 or higher will ultimately require renal replacement therapy but the timescale for reaching this stage can vary widely. The mainstay of support is to delay progression by treatment of secondary factors that are known to be associated with progressive decline in renal function: namely, hypertension, proteinuria and anaemia.

Organ transplantation

Children requiring renal replacement therapy are the most common recipients of kidney transplants in childhood. Liver and heart transplantation, followed by lung and small bowel transplantation, are well recognised but less commonly undertaken procedures. Non-adherence to immunosuppressive regimens during adolescence is a well-known risk factor for graft failure. The reported incidence of graft failure due to non-adherence is 10%–15% but this is likely to be an under-estimate. Rates of non-adherence are highest among adolescents and young adults. As well as non-adherence to immunosuppression, non-adherence to testing and clinic attendance adversely affects the care and outcome of around 1 in 8 kidney transplant patients. Poor adherence is associated with patients with worse psychological status and family dysfunction; adherence has been shown to improve with education and increased motivational factors, as might be expected. This offers the opportunity to improve graft survival. At present, 50% of cadaveric grafts and around 68% of live donor grafts are still functioning 10 years post transplant. There is no clear difference between children and adults in survival of transplanted kidneys.

Many medications used in transplant medicine and in renal disease can have long-term effects on health. Inhibition of linear growth is seen even with low doses of glucocorticoids, such as prednisolone 0.125 mg/kg/day on a long-term basis. Alternate-day regimens are generally considered preferable in childhood. The height reduction associated with long-term glucocorticoid use in childhood is dose-dependent, and even for children with

---

i | **33.12 Impact of transition planning on outcome in diabetes**

Intervention	Outcome measures
Disease-specific education	Lower HbA$_{1C}$
Generic education/skills training	Fewer acute complications: Hypoglycaemia Admissions with ketoacidosis
Transition coordinator	Lower rate of loss to follow-up
Joint paediatric/adult clinic	Fewer chronic complications: Hypertension Nephropathy Retinopathy
Separate young adult clinic	Improved self-management Improved disease-specific knowledge
Out-of-hours phone support	Improved screening for complications
Enhanced follow-up	Better quality-of-life scores

asthma treated with inhaled glucocorticoids, an average height reduction of 1.2 cm is reported. This is can also be associated with delayed puberty, as well as an increased risk of osteoporosis in adulthood. Post-transplant lymphoproliferative disorders (PTLDs) are a well-recognised and potentially life-threatening complication in solid organ recipients. PTLD is the most common malignancy complicating solid organ transplantation, accounting for 20% of all cancers. They represent a range of lymphoproliferative disorders, from infectious mononucleosis and lymphoid hyperplasia to malignant lymphoma. Most cases of PTLD are associated with Epstein–Barr virus (EBV), leading to uncontrolled B-cell proliferation and tumour formation. Up to 10% of solid organ transplant recipients develop PTLD but the risk is almost four times higher in patients under 20 years of age, as opposed to those aged 20–50. This increased risk relates mainly to the development of EBV infection after transplantation; most adults are already EBV-seropositive at the time of transplantation and therefore at lower risk of this complication. The type of organ transplant that has been undertaken predicts PTLD risk, with the cumulative incidence over 5 years ranging from 1% to 2% in haematopoietic cell transplant and liver transplants, 1%–3% in renal transplants, 2%–6% in heart transplants and 2%–9% in lung transplants to as high as 11%–33% in intestinal or multi-organ transplants. The different rates possibly relate to the varying degrees of immunosuppression required. The incidence of PTLD is highest in the first year after transplantation, when it is associated with the highest levels of immunosuppression.

Diabetes

Adherence and concordance with medication are a particular challenge in adolescents who have developed diabetes during childhood. Studies of adolescents with type 1 diabetes have revealed that 25% were neglecting insulin injections, 81% were not following their diet, and 29% were not measuring their glucose level and were completing a daily diary with fictitious results. Research has also shown that the outcome of diabetes is improved with a formal transition programme (Box 33.12). Good control of diabetes is particularly important during this phase since microvascular disease often emerges around time of transition, although it can occur sooner in patients with early-onset diabetes.

Gastrointestinal disease

Inflammatory bowel disease

The prevalence of inflammatory bowel disease (IBD) in childhood is increasing, and the incidence of Crohn's disease (CD) in particular is rising in both children and adults, probably due to currently undefined environmental factors. Current treatment aims are outlined in Box 33.13. Standard measures

> **i** | **33.13 Treatment strategy in Crohn's disease**
>
> - Induce and maintain clinical remission
> - Optimise nutrition
> - Optimise bone health
> - Optimise growth and pubertal progress
> - Minimise adverse drug effects

include exclusive enteral nutrition for 6–8 weeks using a whole-protein (polymeric) formula, which induces initial remission in 80% of children. This is equivalent to glucocorticoid therapy but offers improved nutritional status and superior mucosal healing. Glucocorticoids can also be used to induce remission, as well as to treat exacerbations, but should be followed up by immunosuppressive therapy with azathioprine or methotrexate. Adolescents and children are more likely than adults to require biologics and around 20% need treatment with tumour necrosis factor alpha (TNF-α) inhibitors such as infliximab or adalimumab. Around 20% of children with CD require surgery within 5 years of diagnosis; limited resections and stricturoplasty are considered best practice to preserve gut length and prevent short bowel syndrome.

Children with ulcerative colitis (UC) are more likely than adults to present with pancolitis (approximately 80% versus 40%–50% in adults). Mild disease should be treated initially with oral 5-ASA preparations such as mesalamine or sulfasalazine. If the response is inadequate, oral glucocorticoids can be used, but caution must be exercised because of the adverse effects on skeletal growth and bone mineral density. Thiopurines such as 6-mercaptopurine or azathioprine are frequently used as steroid-sparing agents, with progression to anti-TNF-α therapy for those who still do not respond. There is less evidence for efficacy of TNF-α inhibitors in adolescents with UC than those with CD; they seem to be effective at inducing an initial response but less useful for maintaining long-term remission, since a significant proportion of patients still require colectomy (20% at 1 year) or long-term glucocorticoids. Ciclosporin is probably more effective than infliximab in adolescents with refractory UC. As with other young people who have long-term conditions, adherence to medication is particularly important to reduce the risk of relapse. In terms of lifestyle advice, smoking is a particular risk since it increases both the rate and severity of relapses. Body image can be a particular challenge for young adults with IBD, and those with colostomies or fistulae, for example, can find this part of their illness particularly difficult. Delayed puberty and short stature are important comorbidities, partly related to medication side-effects and also to the nature of the inflammatory bowel disease itself.

Rheumatology and bone disease

Juvenile idiopathic arthritis

Juvenile idiopathic arthritis (JIA) is the term used to describe a wide variety of inflammatory rheumatic diseases that present during childhood. Oligoarticular juvenile arthritis has a good prognosis and often remits during adulthood, and so transitioning patients to adult rheumatology services may not always be required. The same does not hold true for systemic JIA and polyarticular JIA, which often require long-term immunosuppressive therapy through transition and beyond into adulthood. Smoking is a risk because it increases the activity of inflammatory disease and reduces the effectiveness of biologics. Adherence to and concordance with medication remain a challenge, as in other chronic diseases. Functional limitation secondary to joint damage may limit employment opportunities. Contraceptive advice is important in patients on methotrexate.

Glucocorticoid-induced osteoporosis

Osteoporosis is a complication of long-term glucocorticoid therapy that may be required in patients with inflammatory disease, transplantation and DMD.

There is a paucity of evidence about best practice in glucocorticoid-induced osteoporosis in children and adolescents, but in general the teenage years are a period of considerable bone mineral deposition and offer a chance to enhance bone mineral density significantly. It is important to ensure adequate calcium and vitamin D intake and to supplement if necessary. Therapy with bisphosphonates is often initiated in patients with clinical vertebral fractures although the evidence base for prevention of fractures with treatment in childhood and adolescence is limited.

Osteogenesis imperfecta

Osteogenesis imperfecta (OI) is a genetic disorder most commonly caused by mutations in the type 1 collagen genes which typically presents with multiple low-trauma fractures during infancy and childhood. The incidence of fractures falls substantially in adolescence, probably because of the increase in bone mass which occurs as the result of skeletal growth. However, the incidence of fractures in OI during transition and in young adults is about 10–100 times higher throughout life as compared with the general population. Intravenous bisphosphonates such as pamidronate and zoledronic acid are widely used in the treatment of children with osteogenesis imperfecta (those with long-bone deformities, vertebral compression fractures, and three or more fractures per year, in whom the benefit/risk ratio is thought to be positive), although the evidence base for prevention of fractures is poor and mainly based on observational studies.

There is much debate about whether continuing bisphosphonate therapy into adulthood is beneficial due to concerns about suppression of bone turnover in the long term. Affected individuals and their parents can find this change in treatment strategy confusing and it is important to explain the underlying rationale in order to manage expectations.

Hypophosphataemic rickets

Hypophosphataemic rickets is a rare genetic disorder caused by mutations in genes that regulate phosphate excretion. Adherence to phosphate supplements and, to a lesser extent, vitamin D metabolites represents an important issue in optimising management during childhood and this becomes even more challenging in transitioning patients. The treatment of X-linked hypophosphataemic rickets (XLH) in children has, however, been revolutionised by burosumab, a neutralising antibody to FGF23 given by subcutaneous injection once monthly which corrects the metabolic disorder and has been shown in clinical trials to be significantly more effective in the treatment of XLH than standard care. While skeletal deformity does not progress following closure of the epiphyses, different problems arise in adolescent patients when there is suboptimal control of hypophosphataemia, including painful pseudofractures and arthralgia associated with enthesopathy. The renal phosphate leak tends to improve to an extent during adolescence and early adulthood and the requirement for phosphate is reduced, but many patients still require treatment in adulthood.

Summary

Young people who have suffered long-term conditions during childhood represent a particularly high-risk group of patients as they progress through adolescence to become young and, finally, mature adults. They bring with them specific medical risks and complications related to their previous medical treatment, and knowledge of these is important to identify the long-term complications of the therapies to which they have been exposed. They are a patient group that can display complex and often abnormal illness behaviour. Understanding this and implementing an effective process for transition from paediatric to adult services can reduce the significant risks that these patients face in early adulthood. As they mature and develop more adult intellectual and emotional behaviour patterns, the risks to their health and well-being reduce. Patients in transition can be a particularly challenging group to manage, but investment of time and effort at this stage of their lives can be extremely rewarding and can bring significant improvements in long-term health-related outcomes.

Further information

Books and journal articles

Atreja A, Bellam N, Levy SR. Strategies to enhance patient adherence: Making it simple. Med Gen Med 2005;7:4.

Crowley R, Wolfe I, Lock K, McKee M. Improving the transition between paediatric and adult healthcare: a systematic review. Arch Dis Child 2011;96:548–553.

Nagra A, McGinnity P, Davis N, et al. Implementing transition: Ready Steady Go. Arch Dis Child Educ Pract Ed. 2015;100:313–320.

Segal TY. Adolescence: what the cystic fibrosis team needs to know. J R Soc Med 2008;101(Suppl 1):15–27.

Websites

acpm.org/?Adherence *American College of Preventive Medicine: detailed review of adherence.*

health.org.uk/sites/default/files/QualityImprovementMadeSimple.pdf *Sample clinical tools and measurement resources for quality improvement purposes.*

uhs.nhs.uk *More clinical tools and measurement resources.*

readysteadygo.net *Transition and Patient Empowerment Innovation, Education and Research Network: Ready, Steady, Go programme.*

TJ Quinn

34

Ageing and disease

Assessment of the older adult

7 Cognitive function
Montreal Cognitive Assessment
(see Ch. 31)
Assess for delirium
Assess mood

6 Vision
Visual acuity
Glasses worn/present
Cataract

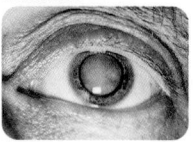

▲ Cataract

5 Hearing
Wax
Hearing aid used

4 Erect and supine blood pressure
Postural hypotension,
see opposite

3 Pulse
Atrial fibrillation

2 Hydration
Skin turgor
Oedema, including sacral
oedema
Mucous membranes

1 Nutrition
Body mass index
(Height calculated from arm
demispan or knee height to
compensate for loss of
vertebral height)
Recent weight loss,
e.g. loose skin folds

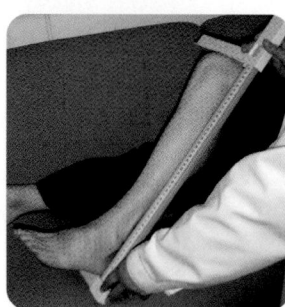

▲ Measurement of knee height
(see Ch. 22)

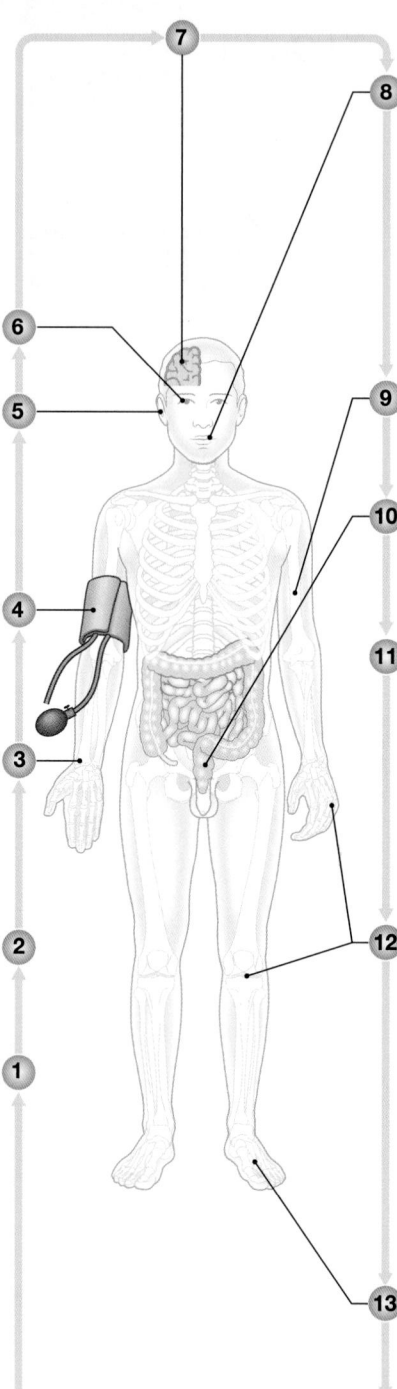

Full systems examination
with particular attention
to the above

8 Oral cavity
Dentition
Swallow assessment

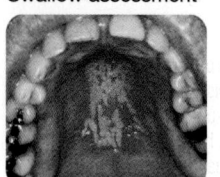

▲ Oral *Candida* and poor
dentition

9 Muscle
Wasting
Strength

10 Bladder and bowel
Faecal impaction
Prostate size/consistency
in men
Palpable bladder

11 Skin
Pressure areas
Pattern of bruising (falls,
non-accidental)

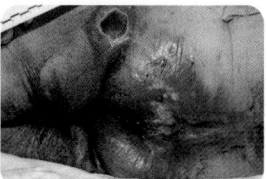

▲ Sacral pressure sore

12 Joints
Deformity
Pain
Swelling
Range of movement

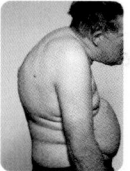

▲ Severe kyphosis

13 Feet
Ulcers
Onychogryphosis
Neuropathy

14 Gait and balance
Get up and go test
(see opposite)
Walking aid used

Insets (kyphosis) From Afzal Mir M. Atlas of clinical diagnosis, 2nd edn. Edinburgh: Saunders, Elsevier Ltd; 2003; (oral candida and poor dentition) From Ibsen O. Oral pathology for the dental hygienist, 7th edn. Philadelphia: Saunders, Elsevier Inc.; 2017; (sacral pressure sore) From Walls R, et al. Rosen's emergency medicine: Concepts and clinical practice, 9th edn. Philadelphia: Elsevier Inc., 2017.

History

Approach

- Find a quiet area free from external distractions
- Ensure the patient can hear
- Slow down the pace
- Carry out a full systematic enquiry

Content

- Establish the person's goals and expectations of treatments
- Medication history, including adherence, recent changes to medications and any non-prescribed drugs or supplements
- Past medical history, even from many years previously
- Establish usual function – change in function is often a sign of illness
- Ask specifically about: mobility, continence, cognition, self-care

Collateral

- Obtain a collateral history from a suitable informant (relative, care-giver or family doctor)
- Ask about care-giver stress

Social assessment

Home circumstances

- Living alone, with another person or in a care home
  Stairs, access to toilet, adequate heating

Activities of daily living (ADL)

- Tasks for which help is needed:
  Basic ADL: bathing, dressing, walking
  Extended ADL: shopping, cooking, housework

Social support

- Informal assistance: relatives, friends, neighbours
- Formal assistance: social care, home help, meals on wheels

Examination – general points

- Thorough and systematic
- Tailored to the patient's stamina and ability to cooperate, may need to be performed in stages
- Includes cognitive function, gait, hearing and vision
- Initial assessment is screening rather than diagnostic; for example, screening visual acuity can be performed using different sizes of print in a newspaper
- Maintains safety; for example, ensure you have appropriate assistance before mobilising an unwell older adult for the first time
- Includes assessment of risk of future events; for example, assessing skin for risk of pressure sores, assessing gait and balance for risk of falls

Cognitive screening

- Sensitively, enquire about level of education and ability in reading and writing.
- Maximise cognitive abilities, ensure glasses are worn, hearing aids turned on.
- Screen for delirium using a validated tool such as 4-A test. If the person struggles with this test then more detailed direct testing may not be possible.
- Use a multidomain cognitive assessment validated for the language of the person being tested (e.g. Montreal Cognitive Assessment, see Ch. 31).
- Complement the cognitive assessment with collateral information, use a structured questionnaire such as the AD8.
- Change in cognition is important; look for results of any previous cognitive tests in medical records.

(4) Assessment for postural hypotension

- Have the person supine and relaxed for at least 5 minutes.
- Measure blood pressure with manual sphygmomanometer.
- Keep the sphygmomanometer cuff on the person's arm.
- Stand the person up rapidly but safely (in some cases lying to sitting measures may be needed).
- Check standing blood pressure immediately and then at 1, 2, 3 minutes.
- Ask about symptoms with each blood pressure check.
- A fall of >20 mmHg systolic or >10 mmHg diastolic defines postural hypotension, but important symptomatic drops may be seen with lesser falls in blood pressure.

(14) Get up and go test

To assess gait and balance, ask the patient to stand up from a sitting position, walk 3 m, turn and go back to the chair. This can be timed and usually takes less than 12 seconds. However, observed performance is more important than precise timing.

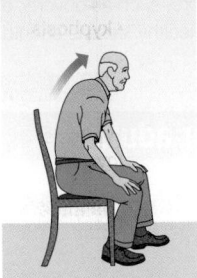 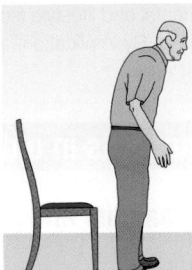 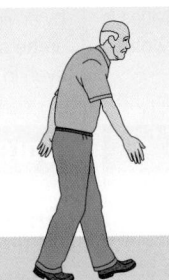 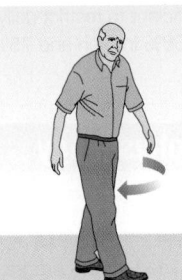 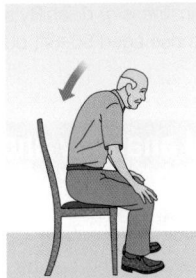

Difficulty rising?   Unsteady on standing?   Unsteady gait?   Unsteady on turning?   Unsteady on sitting down?

Demographic change has meant that older people now represent the core practice of medicine. A knowledge of the effects of ageing and the associated clinical problems is therefore essential for all clinicians. The older population is diverse; a substantial proportion of 90-year-olds enjoy an active healthy life, while some 70-year-olds are severely disabled by chronic disease. The terms 'chronological' and 'biological' ageing have been coined to describe this phenomenon. In the context of medical care, biological age is the more important factor to consider.

Geriatric medicine is concerned particularly with frailty – where physiological capacity is so reduced that even minor illness has serious consequences. Management in frailty differs from that in a robust younger adult in fundamental ways. Disability and multiple comorbidities can complicate both assessment and treatment and acute illness may present with non-specific symptoms. A broad knowledge of medicine is required, as disease in any, and often many, organ systems has to be managed at the same time. Finally, the person's expectations and goals of treatment may differ from younger adults and these should be established as early as possible.

Older people are under-represented in clinical trials. Accordingly, there is often little high-quality evidence on which to base practice. However, some interventions have a compelling evidence base, such as the process of Comprehensive Geriatric Assessment.

Demography

Improvements in health care, lifestyle and public health measures have resulted in prolonged life expectancy across the world. For example, in the UK, the total population has grown by 11% over the past 30 years, but the number of people aged over 65 years has grown by 24%, with the steepest rise in those aged over 80. In contrast, the working age population has remained relatively static. Similarly, the proportion of people aged over 65 in India has increased by 35.5%, which is almost twice the rate of growth of the general population. The rate of population ageing is much faster in developing countries and so there will be less time to adjust to its impact.

Thus, the old-age dependency ratio, which is the ratio of people of working age to people over retirement age, has substantially increased. Since young people support older members of the population both directly and indirectly through taxation and pension contributions, the consequences of this change are far-reaching. It is important to emphasise, however, that many older people also support the younger population, through the care of children and other older people.

Life expectancy gains are seen even in old age (Box 34.1); women aged 80 years can expect to live for a further 10 years. However, rates of disability and chronic illness rise sharply with ageing and have a major impact on health and social services. In the UK, the reported prevalence of a chronic illness or disability sufficient to restrict daily activities is around 25% in those aged 50–64, but 66% in men and 75% in women aged over 85.

Functional anatomy and physiology

Biology of ageing

At a biological level, ageing can be defined as the progressive accumulation of random molecular defects that build up over the life course. Despite multiple repair and maintenance mechanisms, eventually these defects result in functional impairments of tissues and organs.

Genes that contribute to ageing profiles include those involved in regulation of DNA repair, telomere length and insulin signalling. However, genetic factors only account for around 25% of the variance in human lifespan with lifestyle and environmental factors more important determinants.

i	34.1 Mean life expectancy in years, UK and India			
	Males		Females	
	UK	India	UK	India
At birth	79.1	65.1	83.0	67.2
At 60 years	22.8	16.7	25.5	18.9
At 70 years	15.0	10.9	17.1	12.4
At 80 years	8.7	7.5	9.9	8.0

i	34.2 Structural damage contributing to ageing

- *Nuclear chromosomal DNA:* mutations and deletions ultimately lead to aberrant gene function and potential for malignancy.
- *Telomeres:* these structures at the ends of chromosomes shorten with each cell division. When sufficiently eroded, cells stop dividing. This 'biological clock' prevents uncontrolled cell division and cancer. Telomeres are particularly shortened in patients with premature ageing due to progeria.
- *Mitochondrial DNA:* mutations and deletions resulting in reduced cellular energy production and ultimately cell death.
- *Proteins:* glycosylation due to spontaneous reactions between proteins and sugars damages structure and function.

At a cellular level, production of reactive oxygen species is thought to play a major role in ageing. These molecules cause oxidative damage at a number of targets (Box 34.2). The rate at which damage occurs is variable and is influenced by environmental and lifestyle factors. There is evidence in some organisms that this interplay is mediated by insulin signalling pathways and chronic inflammation, so called inflamm-ageing.

Physiological changes of ageing

Physiological features of disease-free, normal ageing have been described (Fig. 34.1). However, ageing is so often associated with concomitant disease that the use of the term 'normal' is debatable. Age-related changes alone are usually not enough to interfere with organ function, but reserve capacity can be significantly reduced with implications for response to an external stressor like disease.

Ageing is characterised by substantial inter-individual variation in function. Thus, each person must be assessed individually, and the same management cannot be applied unthinkingly to all people of a certain age. This heterogeneity in the ageing phenotype is predominantly driven by environmental and lifestyle factors, such as poverty, exercise and cigarette smoking. By implication, a healthy lifestyle should be encouraged even in older age.

Core concepts in older adults

Frailty, disability and multimorbidity

Frailty

Frailty is defined as the inability to withstand minor stresses because of reduced functional reserve in several organ systems. Thus, in frailty even a trivial illness may result in organ failure and death (Fig. 34.2). The term 'frail' has often been used rather vaguely, sometimes to justify a lack of adequate investigation and intervention in older people. Frailty research has substantially increased in the last decades and we now have a better understanding of the meaning and implications of frailty.

There are various complementary approaches to the assessment of frailty (Box 34.3). The cumulative deficit model counts the number of age-related symptoms, signs, diagnoses and test abnormalities. If this count is compared against a pre-defined list of issues, then a frailty index can be calculated. The phenotypic approach is based on a series of common features associated with poor outcomes, such as exhaustion and reduced strength. Finally, the syndromic approach recognises that patients with frailty tend to respond to disease in stereotyped ways. A list of presentations that are markers of underlying frailty was first described by Sir Bernard Isaacs in his text on 'Geriatric Giants'. Formal phenotyping and frailty indexing are mostly used in research settings. In clinical practice, clinicians can often recognise frailty based on initial assessment. Frailty scales, such as that described by Rockwood, offer guidance and illustration to allow the categorisation of clinical frailty into an ordinal scale (Fig. 34.3).

Older people with frailty benefit from a clinical approach that addresses both the acute illness and their underlying loss of reserves. It may be possible to prevent further loss of function through early intervention. For example, a frail woman with myocardial infarction may benefit from cardiovascular secondary prevention medications but may benefit even further from an exercise programme that improves musculoskeletal function, balance and aerobic capacity. Establishing a patient's level of frailty also helps inform decisions regarding further investigation, management and the need for rehabilitation.

Disability

Disability is an umbrella term for describing loss of function that results from complex interactions between health, environmental and personal factors. The WHO International Classification of Functioning, Disability and Health (ICF) provides a framework for understanding this concept at the levels of basic body structure and function, activity limitations (previously called disability) and participation in society (previously called handicap) (Fig. 34.4). Care of the older adult should seek not only to cure or limit disease but also to minimise the resulting disability. Given the multifaceted nature of disability, this often requires a team approach with expertise in differing areas.

Multimorbidity

Multimorbidity describes a state where multiple health conditions coexist in an individual. A related term is comorbidity which describes conditions that exist alongside a disease of interest. There is no consensus on the total number of conditions that should define multimorbidity and with increasing age, accumulation of chronic conditions is almost invariable. Regardless of the definition used, multimorbidity is a driver for future disability, hospitalisation and death. Related to multimorbidity is the concept of polypharmacy, where multiple medications are used to treat each chronic disease individually.

Traditional health-care systems are poorly equipped to manage multimorbidity. When each disease is dealt with by a separate team of specialists, this places a high burden on the patient and can lead to inefficiency,

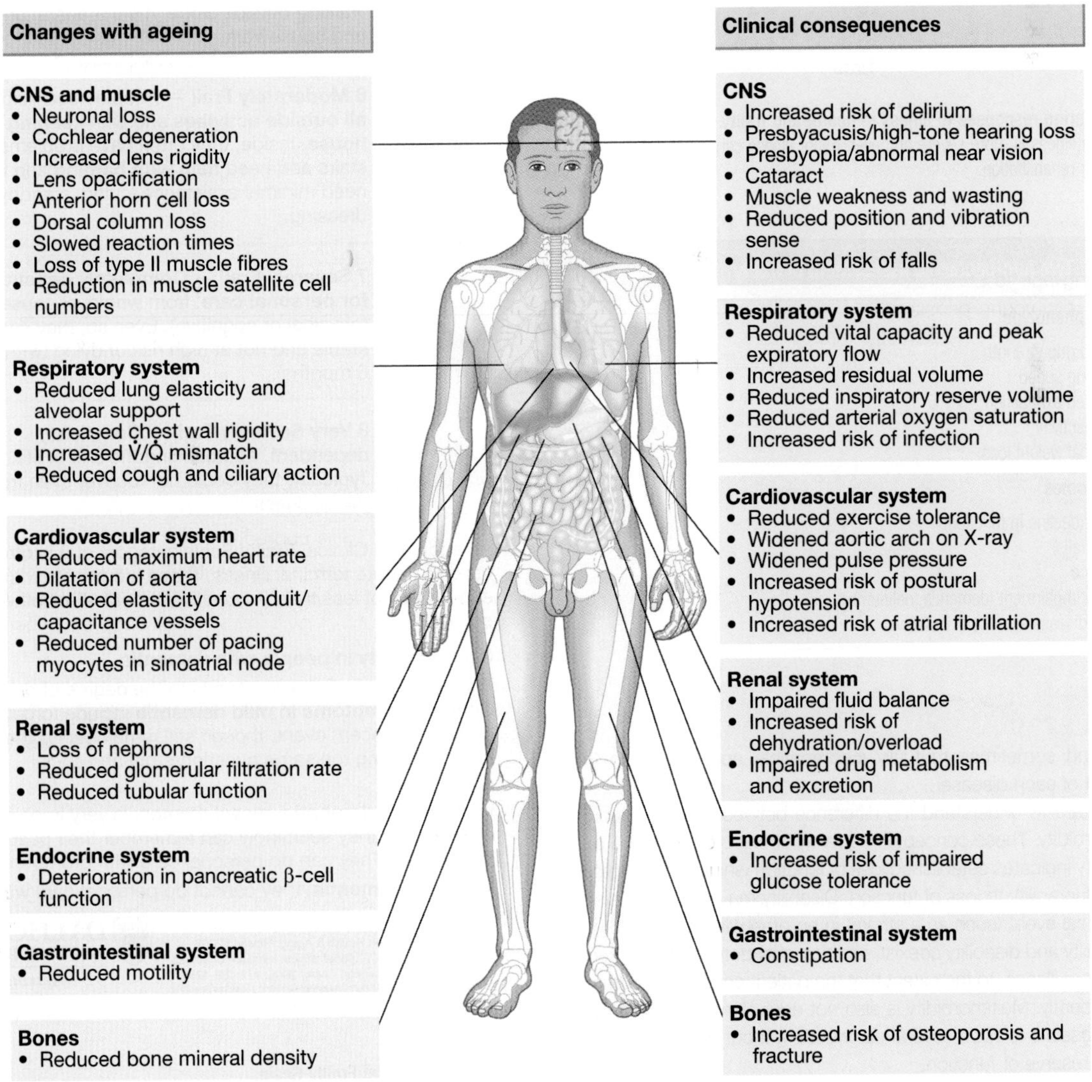

Changes with ageing

CNS and muscle
• Neuronal loss
• Cochlear degeneration
• Increased lens rigidity
• Lens opacification
• Anterior horn cell loss
• Dorsal column loss
• Slowed reaction times
• Loss of type II muscle fibres
• Reduction in muscle satellite cell numbers

Respiratory system
• Reduced lung elasticity and alveolar support
• Increased chest wall rigidity
• Increased V̇/Q̇ mismatch
• Reduced cough and ciliary action

Cardiovascular system
• Reduced maximum heart rate
• Dilatation of aorta
• Reduced elasticity of conduit/capacitance vessels
• Reduced number of pacing myocytes in sinoatrial node

Renal system
• Loss of nephrons
• Reduced glomerular filtration rate
• Reduced tubular function

Endocrine system
• Deterioration in pancreatic β-cell function

Gastrointestinal system
• Reduced motility

Bones
• Reduced bone mineral density

Clinical consequences

CNS
• Increased risk of delirium
• Presbyacusis/high-tone hearing loss
• Presbyopia/abnormal near vision
• Cataract
• Muscle weakness and wasting
• Reduced position and vibration sense
• Increased risk of falls

Respiratory system
• Reduced vital capacity and peak expiratory flow
• Increased residual volume
• Reduced inspiratory reserve volume
• Reduced arterial oxygen saturation
• Increased risk of infection

Cardiovascular system
• Reduced exercise tolerance
• Widened aortic arch on X-ray
• Widened pulse pressure
• Increased risk of postural hypotension
• Increased risk of atrial fibrillation

Renal system
• Impaired fluid balance
• Increased risk of dehydration/overload
• Impaired drug metabolism and excretion

Endocrine system
• Increased risk of impaired glucose tolerance

Gastrointestinal system
• Constipation

Bones
• Increased risk of osteoporosis and fracture

34

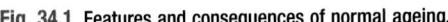

Fig. 34.1 Features and consequences of normal ageing.

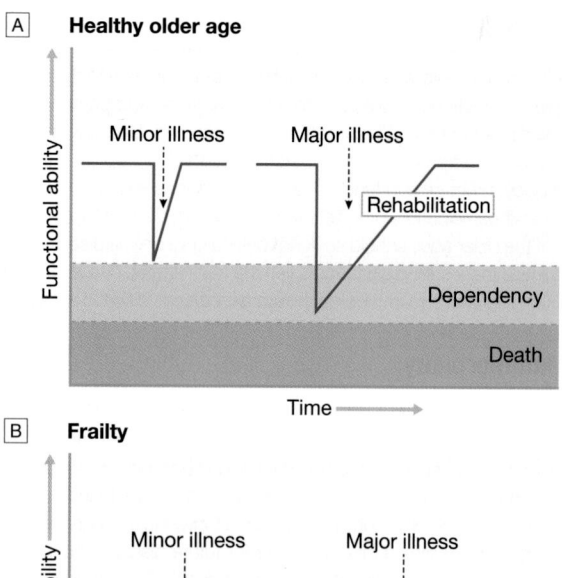

A Healthy older age

B Frailty

Fig. 34.2 **Differing responses to illness in health and frailty.** Note that in frailty the response to illness is more severe and even minor illness can cause functional issues requiring rehabilitation.

i 34.3 Two approaches to assessment of frailty

Fried Frailty phenotype
- Weak hand grip strength
- Slow walking speed
- Self-reported exhaustion
- Physical inactivity
- Unintentional weight loss

Frailty syndromes
- Immobility (decline in function)
- Instability (falls)
- Incontinence
- Intellectual impairment (dementia, delirium)
- Iatrogenic disease and social isolation

replication and sometimes mutually incompatible approaches to the management of each disease.

It is important to understand the difference between frailty, disability and multimorbidity. These concepts frequently coexist, but they are distinct. Disability indicates established loss of function while frailty indicates increased vulnerability to loss of function. Disability may arise from a single pathological event (such as a stroke) in an otherwise robust individual. When frailty and disability coexist, function may deteriorate markedly even with minor illness, to the extent that the patient can no longer manage independently. Multimorbidity is also not equivalent to frailty or disability; it is possible to have several diagnoses without major impact on homeostatic reserve or function.

Clinical Frailty Scale*

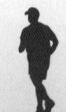 **1 Very Fit** — People who are robust, active, energetic and motivated. These people commonly exercise regularly. They are among the fittest for their age.

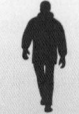 **2 Well** — People who have **no active disease symptoms** but are less fit than category 1. Often, they exercise or are very **active occasionally**, e.g. seasonally.

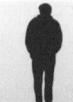 **3 Managing Well** — People whose **medical problems are well controlled**, but are **not regularly active** beyond routine walking.

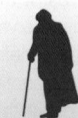 **4 Vulnerable** — While **not dependent** on others for daily help, often **symptoms limit activities**. A common complaint is being "slowed up", and/or being tired during the day.

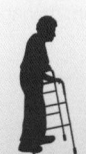 **5 Mildly Frail** — These people often have **more evident slowing**, and need help in **high order IADLs** (finances, transportation, heavy housework, medications). Typically, mild frailty progressively impairs shopping and walking outside alone, meal preparation and housework.

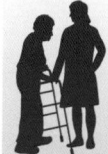 **6 Moderately Frail** — People need help with **all outside activities** and with **keeping house**. Inside, they often have problems with stairs and need **help with bathing** and might need minimal assistance (cuing, standby) with dressing.

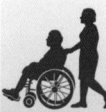 **7 Severely Frail** — **Completely dependent for personal care**, from whatever cause (physical or cognitive). Even so, they seem stable and not at high risk of dying (within 6 months).

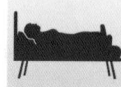 **8 Very Severely Frail** — Completely dependent, approaching the end of life. Typically, they could not recover even from a minor illness.

An additional Clinical Frailty Scale category of 9 is often used to denote terminal illness. These are people with a life expectancy of less than 6 months but not frail by other criteria.

Scoring frailty in people with dementia
The degree of frailty corresponds to the degree of dementia. Common **symptoms in mild dementia** include forgetting the details of a recent event, though still remembering the event itself, repeating the same question/story and social withdrawal.

In **moderate dementia**, recent memory is very impaired, even though they seemingly can remember their past life events well. They can do personal care with prompting.

In **severe dementia**, they cannot do personal care without help.

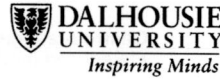 DALHOUSIE UNIVERSITY *Inspiring Minds*

Fig. 34.3 The Clinical Frailty Scale.

Pathology: fracture neck of femur

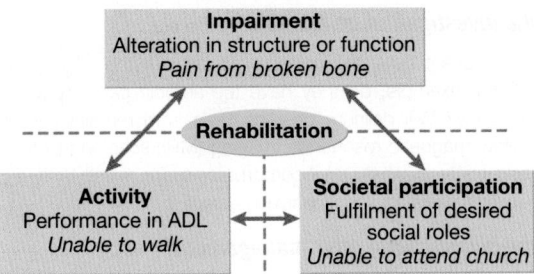

Fig. 34.4 **The WHO international classification of function.** Note that the various levels of function interact, and relationships are potentially bidirectional. For example, while a broken bone (impairment) may directly limit walking (activity), a maladaptive, antalgic gait (activity) may also impair healing (impairment). Pathology may directly and indirectly have an impact at all levels of function. This has implications for treatment and a rehabilitation strategy will need to target all levels of function. (ADL = activities of daily living)

Rehabilitation

Rehabilitation aims to improve the ability of people of all ages to perform activities that are important to them. Rehabilitation is often needed in older adults for two reasons: acute illness can be associated with decline in functional ability and with increasing age comes increasing risk of chronic disabling conditions such as osteoarthritis or stroke.

The rehabilitation process

Rehabilitation is a holistic, problem-solving process focused on improving the patient's physical, psychological and social function. It entails:

- *Assessment*. The nature and extent of the patient's problems can be identified using the WHO ICF (see Fig. 34.4). Doctors tend to focus on health conditions and impairments but patients are often more concerned with daily activity and ability to participate in society. Specific assessment scales, such as the Barthel Index of basic activities of daily living (ADL) (Box 34.4) are useful to quantify function but additional assessment is needed to determine the underlying causes and interventions required.
- *Goal-setting*. Goals should be specific to the patient's problems, should be realistic and agreed between the patient and the rehabilitation team.
- *Intervention*. This includes treatments needed to achieve goals and to maintain health and quality of life. Interventions may include hands-on treatment by therapists using a functional, task-orientated approach, education, training and psychological support. The emphasis on the type of intervention will be individualised, according to the patient's goals and abilities.
- *Re-assessment*. There is ongoing re-evaluation of the patient's function and progress towards the goals by the rehabilitation team, the patient and the care-giver. Interventions may be modified as a result.

Multidisciplinary team working

Effective rehabilitation requires a multidisciplinary team approach; core members of the team are described in Box 34.5. Others may also be involved as needed, such as audiometrists to correct hearing impairment, podiatrists for foot problems and orthoticists where a prosthesis or splinting is required. Good communication and mutual respect are essential. Regular team meetings allow sharing of assessments, agreement on rehabilitation goals and interventions, evaluation of progress and planning for discharge. Rehabilitation is *not* when the doctor orders 'physiotherapy' or 'a home visit' and takes no further role.

34.4 How to assess basic activities of daily living using the Modified Barthel Index*

	Independent	Needs help	Unable to do
Mobility	15	10 5 wheelchair	0
Stairs	10	5	0
Transfers (bed to chair)	15	10 minor help 5 major help	0
Continent bladder	10	5 occasional incontinence	0
Continent bowels	10	5 occasional incontinence	0
Grooming	5	0	0
Toilet use	10	5	0
Feeding	10	5	0
Dressing	10	5	0
Bathing	5	0	0

*The 100-point version is illustrated. If a person is completely unable to perform a task, the score is zero. The total score reflects the degree of dependency.

34.5 Multidisciplinary team (MDT) roles

Team member	Activity assessed and promoted
Physiotherapist	Mobility, balance and upper limb function
Occupational therapist	ADL, home environment and care needs
Dietitian	Nutrition
Speech and language therapist	Communication and swallowing
Social worker	Care needs and discharge planning
Nurse	Self-care, feeding, continence, skin care
Doctor	Diagnosis and management of medical problems

Rehabilitation outcomes

There is evidence that rehabilitation improves functional outcomes and reduces mortality in older people following acute illness like stroke and hip fracture. These benefits accrue from complex multicomponent interventions, but occupational therapy to improve personal ADLs and individualised exercise interventions have been shown to be effective in improving functional outcome in their own right.

Investigation and management

Comprehensive Geriatric Assessment

One of the most powerful tools in the management of older people is Comprehensive Geriatric Assessment (CGA) (Fig. 34.5). The term assessment is in fact a misnomer; CGA is not merely assessment, but a dynamic, iterative process of identifying and managing all factors affecting the health and well-being of an older person. The process should begin as soon as possible following acute illness or functional decline. The outcome should be a coordinated, goal-driven, management plan that not only addresses the acute presenting problems but also seeks to improve the patient's overall health and function.

34

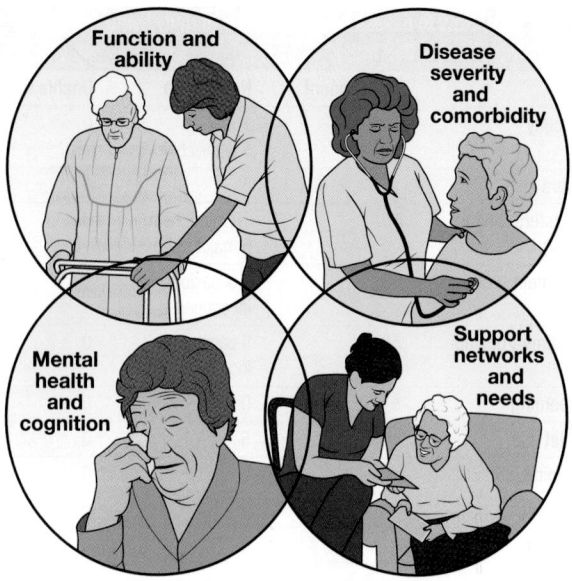

Fig. 34.5 The core elements of Comprehensive Geriatric Assessment.

The CGA approach was pioneered by Dr Marjory Warren in the 1930s. Her comprehensive assessment and rehabilitation of supposedly incurable, bedridden older people revolutionised the approach of the medical profession to frailty and laid the foundations for the modern specialty of geriatric medicine. There is now excellent evidence from systematic reviews that CGA reduces death or deterioration and increases the chances of living independently at home. Current evidence suggests that the process works best when delivered by a dedicated multidisciplinary team on a specialist inpatient unit.

Decisions about investigation and treatment

Accurate diagnosis is important at all ages but management plans in older adults need to be mindful of the implications of frailty, disability and multimorbidity. However, old age alone should not permit denying potentially useful treatments. Change in function should never be dismissed as due to age alone. For example, it would be wrong to supply a wheelchair to a patient struggling to mobilise, when simple tests would have revealed treatable osteoarthritis and angina. So how do clinicians decide when and how far to investigate?

Does the patient want this investigation?

Older people may have strong views about the extent of investigation and the treatment they wish to receive, and these should be sought from the outset. A key issue is to establish what the patient wants from investigation and treatment. Many older people do not desire prolongation of life; rather they aspire to maintain physical function, gain relief from symptoms and preserve the ability to live independently. It can be useful to proactively document the person's wishes, particularly around the interventions that are acceptable to them, so that difficult decisions around ceilings of care do not have to be made in an emergency. There can be situations where a person is unable to sufficiently understand or communicate their circumstances to make informed decisions. Every effort should be made to maximise the patient's ability to participate in decision-making and this may require input from other team members such as speech and language therapy. Family or care-givers may be able to give information on views previously expressed by the patient or on what they believe the patient would have wanted under the current circumstances. However, families should never be made to feel responsible for difficult decisions. Advance directives or 'living wills' allow people to document their views and are used if they no longer are able to make or communicate these decisions. Advance directives and family wishes cannot

authorise a doctor to do anything that, in their professional opinion, is not clinically appropriate.

Will the investigation be feasible?

Does this patient have the capacity to tolerate the proposed investigation? For example, do they have the aerobic capacity to undergo bronchoscopy? Will delirium prevent them from remaining sufficiently still to allow magnetic resonance imaging (MRI) scanning of the brain? Increasing frailty, disability and comorbidity make it less likely a patient will be able to withstand an invasive intervention.

Will the investigation alter management?

Would the patient be fit for, or benefit from, the treatment that would be indicated if investigation proved positive? Again, frailty, disability and comorbidity are more important than age itself in determining this. When a patient with severe heart failure and a previous disabling stroke presents with a suspected cancer on chest X-ray, detailed investigation and staging may not be appropriate if they are not fit for surgery, radical radiotherapy or chemotherapy. On the other hand, if the same patient presented with dysphagia, investigation of the cause would be important, as they might be able to tolerate endoscopic treatment to palliate an obstructing oesophageal lesion and allow resumption of oral diet.

Will management benefit the patient?

It is important to consider whether interventions that might be considered as standard-of-care for younger people are likely to be beneficial in older people living with frailty. For example, while guidelines may recommend tight glycaemic control in diabetes mellitus, such treatment may not accord with the wishes of a patient in a care home who finds regular blood tests distressing, or who is more worried about immediate hypoglycaemia than future vascular complications.

Presenting problems in geriatric medicine

Characteristics of presenting problems in old age

The traditional single-organ, single-disease-based paradigm is rarely helpful in older people. Most presentations are multifactorial, with a social and environmental aspect, and there is rarely a single unifying diagnosis. The diagnostic formulation is more commonly a list of problems, some acute and some chronic. There are certain features of illness presentation that are particular to older patients.

Late presentation

Many people (of all ages) accept ill health as a consequence of ageing and may tolerate symptoms for lengthy periods before seeking medical advice. Comorbidities may also contribute to late presentation. For example, in a patient whose mobility is limited by stroke, angina may only present when coronary artery disease is advanced, as the patient has been unable to exercise sufficiently to cause symptoms at an earlier stage.

Atypical presentation

The classical presentations of diseases are rarely seen in frailty. Infection may present with delirium and no clinical pointers to the organ system affected. Myocardial infarction may present as weakness and fatigue, without chest pain or dyspnoea. The reasons for these atypical presentations are not always easy to establish. Perception of pain is altered, and the pyretic response is blunted in old age. Cognitive impairment may limit the patient's ability to give a history of classical symptoms.

Acute illness and changes in function

A change in functional ability is a common presentation of illness in frailty. Often labels such as 'failure to cope', and 'off feet' are used, but these are *not* diagnoses, and should not prevent a comprehensive assessment for underlying precipitants. It is vital to establish the person's usual level of functioning and the chronicity of any change. Collateral information from a relative or care-giver (by telephone if necessary) can be useful.

Multiple pathology

Presentations in older patients have diverse differential diagnosis, and various contributory problems, both acute and chronic, can coexist. For example, a patient may have recurrent falls because of osteoarthritis of the knees, drug-induced postural hypotension and poor vision from cataracts. All these factors must be addressed to prevent further falls.

Approach to presenting problems in old age

For the sake of clarity, the common presenting problems are described individually but, in reality, older patients often present with several presentations at the same time. Syndromes such as falls, or incontinence represent a final common pathway that is the result of a variety of insults. For most presenting problems in old age the clinician has to search for and treat any acute illness as well as identifying and reversing predisposing risk factors. The initial approach to assessment is often less focused than would be typical in a younger, robust patient (Box 34.6).

Falls and collapse

A commonly used definition describes a fall as an unexpected event in which the person comes to rest on the ground without known loss of consciousness. Around 30% of people over 65 years of age fall each year and this figure rises to more than 40% in those aged over 80.

Important aspects in the assessment of falls include an assessment of the mechanism, risk factors and consequences.

Mechanism

Falls are one of the classic presentations of acute illness in frailty. The reduced reserves in older people's neurological function mean that they are less able to maintain their balance when challenged by an acute illness. The history may give a clear account of an accident, for example a trip on uneven ground. However, a proportion of older people who 'fall' have, in fact, had a syncopal episode. A collateral falls history from a witness is crucial as people who lose consciousness do not always remember having done so. As differentiating syncopal and non-syncopal falls is challenging, all patients who fall should have a 12-lead electrocardiogram and assessment for postural hypotension (see p. 1297).

Risk factors

Risk factors for falls should be considered in the history and examination (Box 34.7). If problems are identified with muscle strength, balance or vision, these should be investigated and treated as needed. Careful assessment of the patient's gait may provide important clues to an underlying diagnosis (Box 34.8).

Management

Older adults who have fallen more than once in the past year and those who are unsteady during a 'get up and go' test (see p. 1297) require further assessment and may benefit from multidisciplinary intervention. Evidence-based interventions to prevent or reduce recurrent falls involve a multifactorial, multidisciplinary approach (Box 34.9). People at low or moderate risk of falls benefit most from balance and strength training delivered by physiotherapists or other suitably trained practitioners. An assessment of the patient's home environment for hazards should be undertaken by an occupational therapist, who may also provide personal alarms so that the person can summon help, should they fall again. A medication review is required, rationalising medications that may be contributing to sedation, syncope or postural hypotension.

Calculation of fracture risk using tools such as FRAX or QFracture should be performed and dual X-ray absorptiometry (DXA) bone density scanning considered in patients with a 10-year risk of major osteoporotic

34.6 Screening investigations for acute illness

- Full blood count
- Urea and electrolytes, liver function tests, calcium and glucose
- Chest X-ray
- Electrocardiogram
- C-reactive protein: useful marker for infection or inflammatory disease
- Procalcitonin: inflammatory marker more specific to bacterial infection
- Lactate: non-specific marker of severe illness
- Urinalysis: although a positive urine dip is not synonymous with urinary tract infection
- Blood cultures if pyrexial

34.7 Risk factors for falls

- Muscle weakness
- History of falls
- Gait or balance abnormality
- Use of a walking aid
- Visual impairment
- Arthritis
- Impaired activities of daily living
- Depression
- Cognitive impairment
- Age over 80 years
- Psychotropic medication

34.8 Abnormal gaits and probable causes

Gait abnormality	Probable cause
Antalgic	Arthropathy
Waddling	Proximal myopathy
Stamping	Sensory neuropathy
Foot drop	Peripheral neuropathy or radiculopathy
Ataxic	Sensory neuropathy or cerebellar disease
Shuffling/festination	Parkinson's disease
Marche à petits pas	Small-vessel cerebrovascular disease
Hemiplegic	Cerebral hemisphere lesion

fracture of more than 10%. If osteoporosis is diagnosed, specific drug therapy may be considered after informing the patient what their absolute risk of a fracture is over the subsequent 5 years with and without treatment. In the frailest patients, such as those in institutional care, calcium and vitamin D_3 supplements have been shown to reduce both falls and fractures.

Dizziness

Dizziness is very common, affecting at least 30% of those aged over 65 years in community surveys. It can be disabling in its own right and is also a risk factor for falls and functional decline.

The management of dizzy spells is complicated by the difficulty that patients have in describing the symptoms. Important questions in the history include establishing timing and whether it is an acute event (suggesting stroke) or a more chronic problem (such as a space-occupying lesion); whether continuous (for example labyrinthitis) or episodic (for example benign positional paroxysmal vertigo) and any provoking or relieving factors (for example the effect of change in posture).

There may be a predominant symptom complex (although more than one of these may be present).

34

i | 34.9 Evidence-based interventions to reduce the risk of falls and fractures

- Exercise (should include components of lower limb strength and balance training):
    Multimodal group exercise and Tai Chi are both effective
- Calcium and vitamin D supplementation:
    Main evidence of effectiveness for patients in institutional care
- Home environment assessment and modification
- Medication review:
    Particularly medications with central actions such as hypnotics but also those with anticholinergic and hypotensive actions
- Cataract surgery:
    Effective if for first cataract
    Other vision interventions ineffective and may increase falls risk
- Anti-slip shoes:
    Effective only in icy conditions
- Cardiac pacemaker for carotid sinus hypersensitivity

i | 34.10 Multicomponent interventions to prevent delirium

Risk factor	Intervention
Bowel and bladder	Assess and treat constipation, avoid urinary catheters
Dehydration	Regular assessment and prompting for fluids and food
Environmental	Orientation and cognitive stimulation activities; limit ward moves
Medications	Medication review and stopping or reducing culprit drugs
Sleep disturbance	Noise reduction (ear plugs), non-pharmacological sleeping aids
Sensory impairment	Screen for visual and hearing impairments, adaptive equipment (large-text, hearing aids)

- *Pre-syncope, light-headedness*, impending faint. Suggestive of reduced cerebral perfusion. While structural cardiac disease (aortic stenosis) and arrhythmia must be considered, autonomic disorders such as postural hypotension are the most common cause. Regardless of cause, antihypertensive medications may exacerbate symptoms and deprescribing may help.
- *Vertigo*, an illusion of movement. Suggestive of (peripheral) labyrinthine or (central) brainstem disease. In older patients this is most commonly due to peripheral causes, but if any brainstem symptoms or signs are present, MRI of the brain is required to exclude a central lesion.
- *Disequilibrium* unsteadiness, off balance, veering to one side. Suggestive of joint or neurological disease.
- *Psychological* anxiety and hyperventilation can be experienced as dizziness, or can complicate dizziness from other causes.

As with many conditions of older age, dizziness is often multifactorial. For example, a patient may have an acute labyrinthitis in the context of small-vessel cerebrovascular disease and peripheral neuropathy. A multifaceted approach is needed and making small improvements in each contributing problem can have a large effect on symptoms and function.

Confusion (dementia and delirium)

Dementia

Dementia is a syndrome characterised by progressive loss of function across multiple cognitive domains (executive function, language, memory etc.). The cognitive deficits should be sufficient to cause problems in everyday activities. Where a person has cognitive impairment but no functional limitation this is often termed mild cognitive impairment. Further details on the assessment and management of dementia are available in Chapter 31.

A common clinical problem is trying to establish whether an older adult presenting with confusion has pre-existing, and potentially undiagnosed cognitive decline, or a more acute change that may suggest a delirium. To complicate the assessment, dementia and delirium commonly coexist. Cognitive screening of the patient can provide useful information and is described in Chapter 31. However, direct assessment of the patient may not always be possible, particularly if the person is medically unwell. Collateral information from someone that knows the person well, often termed an informant, can be useful. Figure 34.6 suggests a short, structured approach to the informant interview to assess for pre-existing cognitive disorders.

Delirium

Delirium is a syndrome characterised by acute cognitive impairment, precipitated by an insult such as illness or surgery. Delirium is common,

affecting around 25% of all hospital inpatients; 50% following hip fracture and 75% in intensive care. Delirium is associated with poor outcomes, including increased length of hospital stay, institutionalisation and mortality. Although traditionally considered a transient phenomenon, longer-lasting effects of delirium are described. In particular, delirium is a powerful risk factor for subsequent dementia and there is considerable overlap between 'persistent delirium' and dementia. The most important risk factors for delirium are frailty, dementia and a previous history of delirium. Other modifiable and non-modifiable risk factors are shown in (Box 34.10).

Presentation

Delirium presents as an acute change (hours to days) in cognition that often fluctuates over time. Collateral information is crucial to assess whether impaired cognition in the context of illness represents an acute change (delirium) or is a more chronic phenomenon (more likely dementia). The defining neuropsychological feature of delirium is a deficit in attention, although this can be accompanied by problems in other cognitive domains. Based on psychomotor patterns, subtypes of delirium are described. Patients with hyperactive delirium are often agitated and restless, whereas hypoactive delirium can present as lethargy and sedation. A mixed picture with periods of hyper- and hypoactivity is common. Hypoactive delirium is more common in frailty and can be easily missed unless specifically looked for.

Clinical assessment

In order to manage delirium effectively, the first step is to make a diagnosis. Screening tools such as the 4AT (Box 34.11) can be used to detect delirium and differentiate it from dementia and these should be applied to all older patients admitted to hospital. Once a diagnosis of delirium has been established, attempts should be made to identify reversible precipitating factors, especially acute illness. An accurate drug and alcohol history is required with a focus on any drugs recently started or stopped. Full physical assessment may be difficult, especially in hyperactive delirium if the person resists examination. Assessment for localising neurological signs and stigmata of head injury are essential as these would suggest the need for neuroimaging.

Management

The best management of delirium is to prevent it happening. The landmark studies of the Hospital Elder Life Program (HELP) demonstrated that a package of non-pharmacological interventions can reduce the incidence of delirium and its severity (see Box 34.10).

Once a diagnosis of delirium is established, the priority is to treat the underlying precipitating factors, recognising that these may be multiple. Life-threatening causes should be assessed for immediately, including sepsis, drug and alcohol intoxication or withdrawal, hypoglycaemia and other metabolic disorders. This should be followed by a systematic

AD8 Dementia Screening Interview

Patient ID#:_____
CS ID#:_____
Date: _____

Remember, "Yes, a change" indicates that there has been a change in the last several years caused by cognitive (thinking and memory) problems	YES, A change	NO, No change	N/A, Don't know
1. Problems with judgement (e.g., problems making decisions, bad financial decisions, problems with thinking)			
2. Less interest in hobbies/activities			
3. Repeats the same thing over and over (questions, stories or statements)			
4. Trouble learning how to use a tool, appliance, or gadget (e.g., VCR, computer, microwave, remote control)			
5. Forgets correct month or year			
6. Trouble handling complicated financial affairs (e.g., balancing chequebook, income taxes, paying bills)			
7. Trouble remembering appointments			
8. **Daily** problems with thinking and/or memory			
TOTAL AD8 SCORE			

Fig. 34.6 Eight-item informant interview to differentiate ageing and dementia (AD8). The AD8 is a screening test for the early cognitive changes that are common to many forms of dementia (Alzheimer's disease, frontotemporal, vascular dementia). The test is best used as part of an interview with an informant, e.g. spouse, care-giver. A score of 2 or more 'Yes' answers suggests that a cognitive syndrome is likely. *From Galvin JE, et al. The AD8: A brief informant interview to detect dementia. Neurology 2005; 65:559–564. Copyright © 2005 Washington University, St Louis, Missouri. All Rights Reserved.*

ℹ 34.11 How to make a diagnosis of delirium: the 4A Test (4AT)

1 Alertness

This includes patients who may be markedly drowsy (e.g. difficult to rouse and/or obviously sleepy during assessment) or agitated/hyperactive. Observe the patient. If asleep, attempt to wake with speech or gentle touch on shoulder. Ask the patient to state their name and address to assist rating:

Normal (fully alert and not agitated, throughout assessment)	0
Mild sleepiness for < 10 secs after waking, then normal	0

2 Four-question abbreviated mental test (AMT4)

Ask the patient their age, date of birth, the place where they are (name of the hospital or building), the current year:

No mistakes	0
1 mistake	1
≥ 2 mistakes/untestable	2

3 Attention

Say to the patient: 'Please tell me the months of the year in backwards order, starting at December.' To assist initial understanding, one prompt of 'What is the month before December?' is permitted:

Achieves ≥ 7 months correctly	0
Starts but scores < 7 months/refuses to start	1
Untestable (cannot start because unwell, drowsy, inattentive)	2

4 Acute change or fluctuating course

Evidence of significant change or fluctuation in: alertness, cognition, other mental function (e.g. paranoia, hallucinations) arising over the last 2 weeks and still evident in last 24 hrs:

No	0
Yes	4

Total 4AT score (maximum possible score 12)

- **≥ 4**: possible delirium ± cognitive impairment
- **1–3**: possible cognitive impairment
- **0**: delirium or severe cognitive impairment unlikely (but delirium still possible if information in 4 incomplete)

---

approach to look for and treat any other potentially reversible precipitants, remembering that in frailty, seemingly trivial factors such as constipation or a urinary catheter may be sufficient to cause or prolong delirium. Interventions that may promote recovery from delirium are similar to those that prevent delirium and include an environment that permits orientation (clocks, windows) and minimises external stimuli. Management also includes prevention of complications by attending to hydration, nutrition and early mobilisation. The role of drug therapy in delirium is controversial and most guidelines recommend non-pharmacological strategies as first line. However, in a patient with psychotic features who is extremely distressed or where safety is at risk, a trial of low-dose antipsychotic medication may be indicated.

Continence

Both urinary and faecal incontinence are common in older age but they are not an inevitable consequence of ageing. These conditions are under-diagnosed and often only come to medical attention when sufficiently severe to cause a social or hygiene problem. Many older adults may not volunteer problems with continence due to embarrassment or wrongly attributing the symptoms as a natural consequence of ageing. Sensitive enquiry into bladder and bowel health should be a routine part of the medical history for this patient group. In the context of frailty, new incontinence can be a sign of acute illness and a sudden change in continence always demands thorough assessment.

Treatment should always begin with lifestyle changes and behavioural approaches (Fig. 34.7). Containment strategies, including catheters and pads, should never be viewed as first-line or definitive management, but may be required as a final resort if the perineal skin is at risk of breakdown or quality of life is affected. True incontinence is not synonymous with 'functional' incontinence, where the problem is an inability to access a toilet in time rather than an issue with the mechanics of excretion.

Bladder health

Urinary incontinence is defined as the involuntary loss of urine. It occurs in all age groups but is especially common in older age and frailty, with up to 80% of care-home residents being incontinent of urine. The initial assessment should seek to identify and address contributory factors and some of these may be easily remedied, for example infection,

34

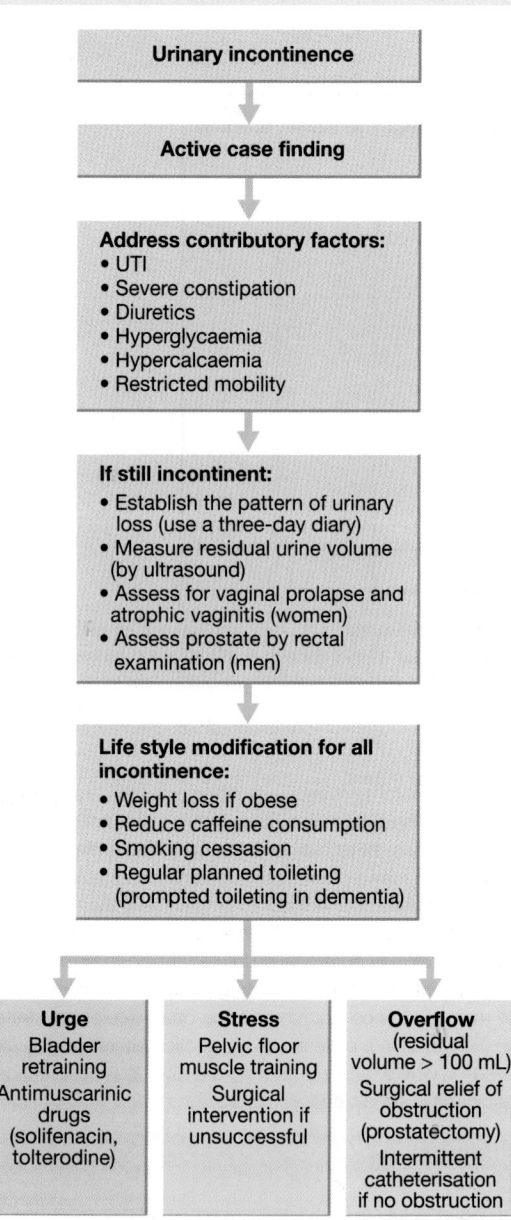

Fig. 34.7 Assessment and management of urinary incontinence in old age. See also Box 18.52. (UTI = urinary tract infection). *Based on European Association of Urology Guidelines 2018.*

constipation, pelvic prolapse. The type of incontinence should be ascertained as this will guide subsequent treatment.

- *Urgency incontinence* is usually due to detrusor over-activity and results in urgency and frequency. Bladder retraining is the first-line intervention, occasionally antimuscarinic medications are needed but these should be used with caution in frailty and cognitive impairment.
- *Stress incontinence* is due to weakness of the pelvic floor muscles, which allows leakage of urine when intra-abdominal pressure rises, such as on coughing. It may be compounded by atrophic vaginitis, associated with oestrogen deficiency in old age, which can be treated with oestrogen pessaries.
- *Overflow incontinence* is demonstrated by a significant post-void residual on bladder scanning. It is most commonly seen in older men with prostatic enlargement, which obstructs bladder outflow.

- *Mixed incontinence* more than one continence issue may be present, most commonly urgency and stress in females and overflow and urgency in males.

Bowel health

Both constipation and faecal incontinence are common in older age and often coexist. Problems with bowel habit are often multifactorial and may result from cognitive factors, local bowel factors and external factors such as immobility. Assessment should include enquiring about diet, medication, previous surgery and lifelong bowel habit. The examination should include an anorectal assessment looking for prolapse, anal tone and faecal loading.

In patients with severe stroke disease or dementia, treatment may be difficult as cortical inhibitory signals are lost. A timed/prompted toileting programme may help.

Infection in the older adult

Infection is one of the commonest reasons for older adults to seek medical attention. All the considerations around disease in older age and frailty that have been discussed in this chapter remain pertinent in relation to infection – non-specific presentations, challenges of comorbidity, competing risks and benefits of interventions. In fact, infection could be considered an exemplar of the need for an adapted management strategy in older age.

Ageing and the immune system

Older adults, particular those living with frailty, face an increased risk and severity of infection. Although absolute numbers of immune cells do not change substantially with age, immune function decreases leading to less efficient responses of both the innate and adaptive immune systems, a phenomenon which is sometimes referred to as immunosenescence. Age-related changes in anatomy and physiology also occur that predispose to infection in certain sites. For example, in the respiratory system, blunting of cough reflex, impaired mucociliary clearance and decreased respiratory muscle strength with subsequent hypoventilation, increase the risk of pulmonary infection. Age-related changes in bladder function and thinning of the skin may partly explain the high prevalence of infection in these sites with older age. Factors that are common in older adults but not part of biological ageing are also important. These include, multiple morbidity, polypharmacy including use of antibiotics and immunosuppressants, and environmental exposures to pathogens.

Assessment

The diagnosis of infection in older age is challenging as symptoms and signs are often atypical and non-specific. Frailty syndromes of delirium and functional decline are common while 'classical' features of the disease such as pyrexia may be absent. Older adults have a lower baseline temperature and blunted or absent fever response to infection. Thus, a core temperature of greater than 38°C is likely to be indicative of important disease. Unfortunately, the temperature response is non-specific in older adults and non-infective causes such as myocardial infarction and deep vein thrombosis need to be considered. The commonest infections seen in older age are respiratory, urinary and skin. However, with frailty, atypical infections and infections in atypical sites are often seen. Thus, the assessment of the unwell older adult always needs to consider infection and physical examination needs to be comprehensive including pressure areas, the oral cavity and intravenous cannulation sites. Consideration of the patient's environment may offer clues to the underlying pathogen. The patient from a care home or who has had a prolonged hospital admission will be at risk from differing causative pathogens to the robust community-dwelling older adult.

Management

Treating infection in the older adult poses further challenges. The pharmacokinetics and pharmacodynamics of antibiotics change with ageing and older adults are at greater risk of adverse drug reactions. Given the

34.12 COVID-19 disease and older adults

Non-specific signs and symptoms

- Fever, breathlessness often absent
- Delirium common and sometimes severe
- Non-pulmonary complications common (thrombosis, gastrointestinal upset)

Variation in outcomes

- Asymptomatic carriage is common, this has implications for infection control
- High morbidity and mortality
- Survivors at risk of functional decline and often require extensive rehabilitation
- Frailty is associated with poor outcomes, but even people with advanced frailty can survive disease
- Frailty assessment can inform management decisions but should not be the only consideration

34.13 Factors leading to polypharmacy in old age

- Multiple pathology
- Poor patient education
- Lack of routine review of all medications
- Patient expectations of prescribing
- Over-use of drug interventions by doctors
- Attendance at multiple specialist clinics
- Poor communication between specialists

34.14 Common adverse drug reactions in old age

Drug class	Adverse reaction
NSAIDs	Gastrointestinal bleeding Renal impairment
Diuretics	Renal impairment, electrolyte disturbance Hypotension, postural hypotension
Warfarin Anticoagulants	Bleeding (any site)
ACE inhibitors	Renal impairment Hypotension, postural hypotension
β-blockers	Bradycardia, heart block Hypotension, postural hypotension
Opiates	Vomiting Urinary retention, constipation
Antidepressants	Hyponatraemia (SSRIs) Hypotension, postural hypotension
Benzodiazepines	Delirium Falls
Anticholinergics	Delirium Urinary retention, constipation

(ACE = angiotensin-converting enzyme; NSAIDs = non-steroidal anti-inflammatory drugs; SSRIs = selective serotonin re-uptake inhibitors)

difficulty of making an initial diagnosis, the use of empirical broad-spectrum antibiotics may seem intuitive, but this approach is strongly discouraged not least due to the risks of *Clostridioides difficile* infection and promoting antibiotic-resistant strains. If the patient is not septic or rapidly deteriorating there should be time for investigations, including relevant cultures, before initiating antibiotic therapy. In liaison with the microbiology laboratory the prescribed therapy can be rationalised as results become available.

The adage 'prevention is better than cure' is particularly relevant in older age. Vaccination programmes for seasonal influenza, pneumococcus and herpes zoster can all reduce incidence, severity or complications from the relevant infections. Health-care associated infection is a particular concern in frailty and all staff working with frail older adults need to be mindful of infection control policies including meticulous hand washing between patient encounters. Without these measures, hospital ward and institutional care settings are at risk of outbreaks of diseases such as norovirus, scabies, methicillin-resistant *Staphylococcus aureus* and more recently COVID-19 (Box 34.12).

Prescribing and deprescribing

The multimorbidity that accompanies ageing often leads to polypharmacy (Box 34.13 and see Box 2.23). This has been defined as the use of four or more drugs, and is associated with adverse outcomes including falls, hospitalisation and increased risk of death. While some of these outcomes are caused by drug–drug interactions and adverse effects, others are due to the underlying problems for which the drugs were prescribed in the first place.

An important component of any older adult assessment is a critical review of medications. This group can be the victim of well-intentioned, but ultimately harmful, prescribing cascades where new medications are introduced to combat effects of other medications and these new medications in turn have adverse effects that result in further prescribing. Of course, for many older people, taking multiple drugs is

entirely appropriate, as such therapy is required to treat multiple diseases. Getting the right balance between over- and undertreatment is a dynamic process and requires frequent, careful exploration of the person's treatment goals.

Adverse drug reactions

The more drugs that are taken, the greater the risk of an adverse drug reaction (ADR) (Box 34.14). ADRs are the cause of around 5% of all hospital admissions but account for up to 20% of admissions in those aged over 65. The risks associated with polypharmacy are compounded by age-related changes in pharmacodynamic and pharmacokinetic factors as described in Chapter 2. Older people are especially sensitive to drugs that can cause postural hypotension or volume depletion and centrally acting drugs can often cause or exacerbate cognitive syndromes. However, the clinical presentations of ADRs are diverse, so for any presenting problem in old age the possibility that the patient's medication is a contributory factor should always be considered. Prescribers must also be mindful of the burden of taking medications at various times, with need for monitoring, lifestyle restrictions and associated expense. It is perhaps not surprising that non-adherence to drug therapy rises with the number of drugs prescribed.

Appropriate prescribing and deprescribing

The key to appropriate prescribing is first to ensure that medications are started only for reasons that accord with the patient's goals and wishes. Thoughtless adherence to specialist guidelines quickly leads to polypharmacy that may be inappropriate. Some medications (such as chronic use of non-steroidal anti-inflammatory medications) are best avoided in older people because of the high risk of ADR. Other medications, such oral bisphosphonates, lack evidence of efficacy in very old people, who may not live for long enough to derive benefit.

Deprescribing is as important as prescribing in older people. Regular review of medications should be undertaken to ensure that medications are still required, to establish that they are still working, to check that they are not causing side-effects, and to ascertain whether the patient is actually taking them. The patient or care-giver should be asked to bring all

i	34.15 Other presenting problems in old age
• Hypothermia	p. 252
• Dizziness and blackouts	p. 184
• Delirium	p. 213
• Infection	pp. 264 and 272
• COVID-19	p. 296
• Fluid balance problems	p. 627
• Prostatic hypertrophy	p. 609
• Heart failure	p. 406
• Atrial fibrillation	p. 414
• Hypertension	p. 449
• Valvular heart disease	p. 460
• Under-nutrition	p. 773
• Diabetes mellitus	p. 718
• Thyroid disease	p. 658
• Anaemia	p. 962
• Painful joints	p. 1000
• Bone disease and fracture	pp. 1002 and 1052
• Stroke	p. 1201
• Dementia	p. 1246

medication for review rather than the doctor relying on previous records. Such reviews should take place regularly, not just at a point of crisis such as after a fall or on hospital admission. Deprescribing of medications that have been taken for years needs to be done in a controlled manner, with dose reduction to ensure that rebound symptoms or withdrawal effects do not occur.

There are tools to assist with rational prescribing choices in older adults. The American Geriatrics Society Beer's criteria is an expert generated list of medications that should be avoided or used with caution in old age. A similar European initiative is STOPP (Screening Tool of Older Person's Prescriptions) and START (Screening Tool to Alert to Right Treatment), which recognises that good prescribing in old age should ensure effective treatments are prioritised as well as discontinuing those medications that may be of limited benefit or potential harm.

Other problems in old age

A vast range of other presenting problems in older people present to many medical specialties. End-of-life care is an important facet of clinical practice in old age and the general principles of this are discussed in Chapter 8. Relevant sections in other chapters are shown in Box 34.15.

Within each chapter, 'In Old Age' boxes highlight the areas in which presentation or management differs from that in younger individuals.

Further information

Websites

americangeriatrics.org *American Geriatrics Society: education, careers vignettes from geriatricians, advocacy and clinical guidelines.*

bgs.org.uk *British Geriatrics Society: useful publications on management of common problems in older people and links to other relevant websites.*

eugms.org *European Union Geriatric Medicine Society: research, position papers and educational resources.*

iagg.info *International Association of Gerontology and Geriatrics: promoting care of older people and the science of gerontology globally; research, policy and educational resources.*

cochrane.org *Cochrane review CD006211 Comprehensive geriatric assessment for older adults admitted to hospital; CD007146 Interventions for preventing falls in older people living in the community.*

profane.co *Prevention of Falls Network Earth: focuses on the prevention of falls and improvement of postural stability in older people.*

shef.ac.uk/FRAX/tool.jsp *Fracture risk calculator: can be used to calculate risk in several populations. Includes option to calculate with or without measurement of hip bone mineral density.*

Qfracture.org *An online calculator to assess risk of osteoporotic fracture (developed and validated for use in the UK).*

geri-em.com/ and gempodcast.com/ *These North American websites contains educational resources, training and blogs on the practice of acute geriatric medicine.*

cgem.ed.ac.uk/research/rheumatological/ORBCalculator/ *ORB calculator. Calculates the absolute benefit of different osteoporosis treatments in preventing fractures.*

SJ Jenks

35

Laboratory reference ranges

Notes on the international system of units (SI units)

Système International (SI) units are a specific subset of the metre–kilogram–second system of units and were agreed on as the everyday currency for commercial and scientific work in 1960, following a series of international conferences organised by the International Bureau of Weights and Measures. SI units have been adopted widely in clinical laboratories but non-SI units are still used in many countries. For that reason, values in both units are given for common measurements throughout this textbook and commonly used non-SI units are shown in this chapter. The SI unit system is, however, recommended.

Examples of basic SI units

Length	metre (m)
Mass	kilogram (kg)
Amount of substance	mole (mol)
Energy	joule (J)
Pressure	pascal (Pa)
Volume	The basic SI unit of volume is the cubic metre (1000 litres). For convenience, however, the litre (L) is used as the unit of volume in laboratory work.

Examples of decimal multiples and submultiples of SI units

Factor	Name	Prefix
10^6	mega-	M
10^3	kilo-	k
10^{-1}	deci-	d
10^{-2}	centi-	c
10^{-3}	milli-	m
10^{-6}	micro-	μ
10^{-9}	nano-	n
10^{-12}	pico-	p
10^{-15}	femto-	f

Exceptions to the use of SI units

By convention, blood pressure is excluded from the SI unit system and is measured in mmHg (millimetres of mercury) rather than pascals.

Mass concentrations such as g/L and μg/L are used in preference to molar concentrations for all protein measurements and for substances that do not have a sufficiently well defined composition.

Some enzymes and hormones are measured by 'bioassay', in which the activity in the sample is compared with the activity (rather than the mass) of a standard sample that is provided from a central source. For these assays, results are given in standardised 'units' (U/L), or 'international units' (IU/L), which depend on the activity in the standard sample and may not be readily converted to mass units.

Laboratory reference ranges in adults

Reference ranges are largely those used in the Departments of Clinical Biochemistry and Haematology, Lothian Health University Hospitals Division, Edinburgh, UK. Values are shown in both SI units and, where appropriate, non-SI units. Many reference ranges vary between laboratories, depending on the assay method used and on other factors; this is especially the case for enzyme assays. Wherever possible an internationally agreed standard reference material is used to calibrate assays and reference ranges and assay nomenclature are standardised between laboratories. The origin of reference ranges and the interpretation of 'abnormal' results are discussed on page 3. No details are given here of the collection requirements, which may be critical to obtaining a meaningful result. Unless otherwise stated, reference ranges shown apply to adults; values in children may be different.

Many analytes can be measured in either serum (the supernatant of clotted blood) or plasma (the supernatant of anticoagulated blood). A specific requirement for one or the other may depend on a kit manufacturer's recommendations. In other instances, the distinction is critical. An example is fibrinogen, where plasma is required, since fibrinogen is largely absent from serum. In contrast, serum is required for electrophoresis to detect paraproteins because fibrinogen migrates as a discrete band in the zone of interest.

i **35.1 Urea and electrolytes in venous blood**

Analysis	Reference range	
	SI units	Non-SI units
Sodium	135–145 mmol/L	135–145 mEq/L
Potassium*	3.6–5.0 mmol/L	3.6–5.0 mEq/L
Chloride	95–107 mmol/L	95–107 mEq/L
Urea	2.5–6.6 mmol/L	15–40 mg/dL
Creatinine		
Male	64–111 μmol/L	0.72–1.26 mg/dL
Female	50–98 μmol/L	0.57–1.11 mg/dL

*Serum values are, on average, 0.3 mmol/L higher than plasma values.

i **35.2 Analytes in arterial blood**

Analysis	Reference range	
	SI units	Non-SI units
Bicarbonate	21–29 mmol/L	21–29 mEq/L
Hydrogen ion	37–45 nmol/L	pH 7.35–7.43
$PaCO_2$	4.5–6.0 kPa	34–45 mmHg
PaO_2	12–15 kPa	90–113 mmHg
Oxygen saturation	>97%	

i 35.3 Hormones in venous blood

Hormone	Reference range	
	SI units	**Non-SI units**
Adrenocorticotrophic hormone (ACTH) (plasma)	1.5–13.9 pmol/L (0700–1000 hrs)	63 ng/L
Aldosterone Supine (at least 30 mins) Erect (at least 1 hr)	 30–440 pmol/L 110–860 pmol/L	 1.09–15.9 ng/dL 3.97–31.0 ng/dL
Cortisol	Dynamic tests are required – see Box 20.51	
Fibroblast growth factor 23 (FGF23)	<100 RU/mL	–
Follicle-stimulating hormone (FSH) Male Female	 1.0–10.0 IU/L 3.0–10.0 IU/L (early follicular) >30 IU/L (post-menopausal)	 – – –
Gastrin (plasma, fasting)	<40 pmol/L	<83 pg/mL
Growth hormone (GH)	Dynamic tests are usually required – see Box 20.54 <0.5 μg/L excludes acromegaly (if insulin-like growth factor 1 (IGF-1) in reference range) >6 μg/L excludes GH deficiency	 <2 mIU/L >18 mIU/L
Insulin	Highly variable and interpretable only in relation to plasma glucose and body habitus	
Luteinising hormone (LH) Male Female	 1.0–9.0 IU/L 2.0–9.0 IU/L (early follicular) >20 IU/L (post-menopausal)	 – – –
17β-Oestradiol Male Female	 <160 pmol/L 75–140 pmol/L (early follicular) <150 pmol/L (post-menopausal)	 <43 pg/mL 20–38 pg/mL <41 pg/mL
Parathyroid hormone (PTH)	1.6–6.9 pmol/L	16–69 pg/mL
Progesterone (in luteal phase in women) Consistent with ovulation Probable ovulatory cycle Anovulatory cycle	 >30 nmol/L 15–30 nmol/L <10 nmol/L	 >9.3 ng/mL 4.7–9.3 ng/mL <3 ng/mL
Prolactin (PRL)	60–500 mIU/L	2.8–23.5 ng/mL
Renin concentration Supine (at least 30 mins) Sitting (at least 15 mins) Erect (at least 1 hr)	 5–40 mIU/L 5–45 mIU/L 16–63 mIU/L	 – – –
Testosterone Male Female	 10–38 nmol/L 0.3–1.9 nmol/L	 290–1090 ng/dL 10–90 ng/dL
Thyroid-stimulating hormone (TSH)	0.2–4.5 mIU/L	–
Thyroxine (free), (free T$_4$)	9–21 pmol/L	0.7–1.63 ng/dL
Triiodothyronine (free), (free T$_3$)	2.6–6.2 pmol/L	0.16–0.4 ng/dL
Vitamin D (25(OH)D) Normal Insufficiency Deficiency	 >50 nmol/L 25–50 nmol/L <25 nmol/L	 >20 ng/mL 10–20 ng/ml <10 ng/mL

Notes

1. A number of hormones are unstable and collection details are critical to obtaining a meaningful result. Refer to local laboratory handbook.
2. Values in the table are only a guideline; hormone levels can often be meaningfully understood only in relation to factors such as gender, age, time of day, pubertal status, stage of the menstrual cycle, pregnancy and menopausal status.
3. Vitamin D levels vary seasonally in many parts of the world, with levels being higher in the summer months in most people due to increased exposure to solar UV-B rays.
4. Reference ranges are usually dependent on the method used for analysis and frequently differ between laboratories. Non-SI units also differ; those shown here are amongst those most widely used. Readers are encouraged to consult their local laboratory for non-SI units for individual analytes and their respective reference ranges.

(RU = relative units. Relative units are used since at the present time there is no agreed international standard for the measurement of FGF-23.)

i 35.4 Other common analytes in venous blood

Analyte	Reference range SI units	Non-SI	Analyte	Reference range SI units	Non-SI units
α_1-antitrypsin	1.1–2.1 g/L	110–210 mg/dL	Glycated haemoglobin (HbA$_{1c}$)	4.0–6.0% 20–42 mmol/mol Hb See Box 21.2 for diagnosis of diabetes mellitus	–
Alanine aminotransferase (ALT)	10–50 U/L	–			
Albumin	35–50 g/L	3.5–5.0 g/dL	Immunoglobulins (Ig)		
Alkaline phosphatase (ALP)	40–125 U/L	–	IgA IgE IgG IgM	0.8–4.5 g/L 0–250 kU/L 6.0–15.0 g/L 0.35–2.90 g/L	– – – –
Amylase	<100 U/L	–			
Aspartate aminotransferase (AST)	10–45 U/L	–	Lactate	0.6–2.4 mmol/L	5.4–21.6 mg/dL
Bile acids (fasting)	<14 µmol/L	–	Lactate dehydrogenase (LDH; total)	125–220 U/L	–
Bilirubin (total)	3–21 µmol/L	0.18–1.23 mg/dL	Lead	<0.5 µmol/L	<10 µg/dL
Caeruloplasmin	0.2–0.47 g/L	20–47 mg/dL	Magnesium	0.75–1.0 mmol/L	1.5–2.0 mEq/L or 1.82–2.43 mg/dL
Calcium (total)	2.1–2.6 mmol/L	4.2–5.2 mEq/L or 8.5–10.5 mg/dL	Osmolality	280–296 mOsmol/kg	–
Carboxyhaemoglobin	0.1–3.0% Levels of up to 8% may be found in heavy smokers	–	Osmolarity	280–296 mOsmol/L	–
			Phosphate (fasting)	0.8–1.4 mmol/L	2.48–4.34 mg/dL
Cholesterol (total)	Ideal level varies according to cardiovascular risk (see p. 637)		Procalcitonin	<0.1 ug/L (indicates absence of bacterial infection) <0.24 (bacterial infection unlikely) 0.25–0.49 (bacterial infection is possible) ≥0.5 (suggestive of the presence of bacterial infection)	–
High-density lipoprotein (HDL)-cholesterol	Ideal level varies according to cardiovascular risk, so reference ranges can be misleading. According to the National Cholesterol Education Programme Adult Treatment Panel III (ATPIII), a low HDL-cholesterol is <1.0 mmol/L (<40 mg/dL)				
Complement					
C3 C4 Total haemolytic complement	0.81–1.57 g/L 0.13–1.39 g/L 0.086–0.410 g/L	– – –	Protein (total)	60–80 g/L	6–8 g/dL
			Triglycerides (fasting)	0.6–1.7 mmol/L	53–150 mg/dL
Copper	10–22 µmol/L	64–140 µg/dL	Troponins	Values consistent with myocardial infarction are crucially dependent on which troponin is measured (I or T) and on the method employed. Interpret in context of clinical presentation. See Box 16.47	
C-reactive protein (CRP)	<5 mg/L Highly sensitive CRP assays also exist that measure lower values and may be useful in estimating cardiovascular risk		Tryptase	0–135 mg/L	–
			Urate		
Creatine kinase (CK; total)*			Male Female	120–420 µmol/L 120–360 µmol/L	2.0–7.0 mg/dL 2.0–6.0 mg/dL
Male Female	55–170 U/L 30–135 U/L	– –	Zinc	10–18 µmol/L	65–118 µg/dL
Creatine kinase MB isoenzyme	<6% of total CK	–			
Ethanol	Not normally detectable				
Marked intoxication Stupor Coma	65–87 mmol/L 87–109 mmol/L >109 mmol/L	300–400 mg/dL 400–500 mg/dL >500 mg/dL			
γ-glutamyl transferase (GGT)	Male 10–55 U/L Female 5–35 U/L	–			
Glucose (fasting)	3.6–5.8 mmol/L See Box 21.2 for definitions of impaired glucose tolerance and diabetes mellitus, and Box 21.14 for definition of hypoglycaemia	65–104 mg/dL			

*CK levels vary according to ethnicity such that people of African and Caribbean origin typically have CK levels 1.5 to 2 times higher than people of European descent.

35.5 Common analytes in urine

Analyte	Reference range	
	SI units	Non-SI units
Albumin	Definitions of albuminuria are given in Box 18.11	
Calcium (normal diet)	Up to 7.5 mmol/24 hrs	Up to 15 mEq/24 hrs or 300 mg/24 hrs
Copper	< 0.6 µmol/24 hrs	< 38 µg/24 hrs
Cortisol	20–180 nmol/24 hrs	7.2–65 µg/24 hrs
Creatinine Male Female	 6.3–23 mmol/24 hrs 4.1–15 mmol/24 hrs	 712–2600 mg/24 hrs 463–1695 mg/24 hrs
5-Hydroxyindole-3-acetic acid (5-HIAA)	10–42 µmol/24 hrs	1.9–8.1 mg/24 hrs
Metadrenalines Normetadrenaline Metadrenaline	 0.4–3.4 µmol/24 hrs 0.3–1.7 µmol/24 hrs	 73–620 µg/24 hrs 59–335 µg/24 hrs
Oxalate	0.04–0.49 mmol/24 hrs	3.6–44 mg/24 hrs
Phosphate	15–50 mmol/24 hrs	465–1548 mg/24 hrs
Potassium*	25–100 mmol/24 hrs	25–100 mEq/24 hrs
Protein	Definitions of proteinuria are given in Box 18.11	Definitions of proteinuria are given in Box 18.11
Sodium*	100–200 mmol/24 hrs	100–200 mEq/24 hrs
Urate	1.2–3.0 mmol/24 hrs	202–504 mg/24 hrs
Urea	170–600 mmol/24 hrs	10.2–36.0 g/24 hrs
Zinc	3–21 µmol/24 hrs	195–1365 µg/24 hrs

*The urinary output of electrolytes such as sodium and potassium is normally a reflection of dietary intake. This can vary widely. The values quoted are appropriate to a 'Western' diet.

35.6 Analytes in cerebrospinal fluid (CSF)

Analysis	Reference range	
	SI units	Non-SI units
Cells	< 5×10⁶ cells/L (all mononuclear)	< 5 cells/mm³
Glucose[1]	2.3–4.5 mmol/L	41–81 mg/dL
IgG index[2]	< 0.65	–
Total protein	0.14–0.45 g/L	0.014–0.045 g/dL

[1]Interpret in relation to plasma glucose. Values in CSF are typically approximately two-thirds of plasma levels. [2]A crude index of increase in IgG attributable to intrathecal synthesis.
(IgG = immunoglobulin G)

35.7 Analytes in faeces

Analyte	Reference range	
	SI units	Non-SI units
Calprotectin	< 50 µg/g	–
Elastase	> 200 µg/g	–

i 35.8 Haematological values

Analysis	Reference range	
	SI units	Non-SI units
Bleeding time (Ivy)	< 8 mins	–
Blood volume		
Male	65–85 mL/kg	–
Female	60–80 mL/kg	–
Coagulation screen		
Prothrombin time (PT)	10.5–13.5 secs	–
Activated partial thromboplastin time (APTT)	26–36 secs	–
D-dimers		
Interpret in relation to clinical presentation	< 500 ng/mL	–
Erythrocyte sedimentation rate (ESR)	Higher values in older patients are not necessarily abnormal	
Adult male	0–10 mm/hr	–
Adult female	3–15 mm/hr	–
Ferritin		
Male (and post-menopausal female)	20–300 µg/L	20–300 ng/mL
Female (pre-menopausal)	15–200 µg/L	15–200 ng/mL
Fibrinogen	1.5–4.0 g/L	0.15–0.4 g/dL
Folate		
Serum	2.8–20 µg/L	2.8–20 ng/mL
Red cell	120–500 µg/L	120–500 ng/mL
Haemoglobin		
Male	130–180 g/L	13–18 g/dL
Female	115–165 g/L	11.5–16.5 g/dL
Haptoglobin	0.4–2.4 g/L	0.04–0.24 g/dL
Iron		
Male	14–32 µmol/L	78–178 µg/dL
Female	10–28 µmol/L	56–157 µg/dL
Leucocytes (adults)	$4.0–11.0 \times 10^9$/L	$4.0–11.0 \times 10^3$/mm^3
Differential white cell count		
Neutrophil granulocytes	$2.0–7.5 \times 10^9$/L	$2.0–7.5 \times 10^3$/mm^3
Lymphocytes	$1.5–4.0 \times 10^9$/L	$1.5–4.0 \times 10^3$/mm^3
Monocytes	$0.2–0.8 \times 10^9$/L	$0.2–0.8 \times 10^3$/mm^3
Eosinophil granulocytes	$0.04–0.4 \times 10^9$/L	$0.04–0.4 \times 10^3$/mm^3
Basophil granulocytes	$0.01–0.1 \times 10^9$/L	$0.01–0.1 \times 10^3$/mm^3
Mean cell haemoglobin (MCH)	27–32 pg	–
Mean cell volume (MCV)	78–98 fL	–
Packed cell volume (PCV) or haematocrit		
Male	0.40–0.54	–
Female	0.37–0.47	–
Platelets	$150–350 \times 10^9$/L	$150–350 \times 10^3$/mm^3
Red cell count		
Male	$4.5–6.5 \times 10^{12}$/L	$4.5–6.5 \times 10^6$/mm^3
Female	$3.8–5.8 \times 10^{12}$/L	$3.8–5.8 \times 10^6$/mm^3
Red cell lifespan		
Mean	120 days	–
Half-life (^{51}Cr)	25–35 days	–
Reticulocytes (adults)	$25–85 \times 10^9$/L	$25–85 \times 10^3$/mm^3
Transferrin	2.0–4.0 g/L	0.2–0.4 g/dL
Transferrin saturation		
Male	25–50%	–
Female	14–50%	–
Vitamin B$_{12}$		
Normal	> 210 ng/L	–
Intermediate	180–200 ng/L	–
Low	< 180 ng/L	–

Laboratory reference ranges in childhood and adolescence

The levels of many analytes in blood vary due to the physiological changes that occur during growth and adolescence. Hospital laboratories may provide reference ranges that are age-adjusted or based on pubertal stage but this is not always the case. It is therefore important for the doctor requesting these tests to understand the impact of age and puberty on interpretation of the results. For example, a creatinine of 70 μmol/L (0.79 mg/dL) is perfectly normal for the majority of adults but may indicate significant renal impairment in a child. Reference ranges for hormone results are described according to the Tanner stages of puberty (see Fig. 33.5).

35.9 Analytes that may be significantly affected by growth and puberty*

Analyte	Age/Pubertal stage	Gender	Reference range	Analyte	Age/Pubertal stage	Gender	Reference range
Alkaline phosphatase (ALP)	<1 year	M, F	80–580 U/L	Luteinising hormone (LH)	Prepubertal	M	<1.0 IU/L (<0.1 μg/L)
	1–16 years	M, F	100–400 U/L		Pubertal stage 2	M	<3.0 IU/L (<0.3 μg/L)
	16–20 years	M	50–250 U/L		Prepubertal and pubertal stage 2	F	<1.0 IU/L (<0.1 μg/L)
		F	40–200 U/L		Pubertal stage 3	M	1.0–4.0 IU/L (0.1–0.4 μg/L)
Creatinine	<1 year	M, F	12–39 μmol/L (0.14–0.44 mg/dL)		Pubertal stages 4–5	M	1.0–5.0 IU/L (0.1–0.6 μg/L)
	1–4 years	M, F	13–42 μmol/L (0.15–0.48 mg/dL)		Pubertal stages 3–5	F	1.0–8.0 IU/L (0.1–0.9 μg/L)
	4–12 years	M, F	20–57 μmol/L (0.23–0.64 mg/dL)	17β-Oestradiol	Prepubertal and pubertal stages 2–3	M	<75 pmol/L (<20 pg/mL)
	12–15 years	M, F	31–67 μmol/L (0.35–0.76 mg/dL)		Prepubertal and pubertal stage 2	F	<100 pmol/L (<27 pg/mL)
	15–18 years	M	39–92 μmol/L (0.44–1.04 mg/dL)		Pubertal stages 4–5	M	<130 pmol/L (<35 pg/mL)
		F	34–72 μmol/L (0.38–0.81 mg/dL)		Pubertal stages 3–5	F	<150 pmol/L (<41 pg/mL)
Follicle-stimulating hormone (FSH)	Prepubertal	M	<3.0 IU/L (<0.6 μg/L)	Testosterone	Prepubertal	M	<0.5 nmol/L (<10 ng/dL)
		F	<3.2 IU/L (<0.64 μg/L)		Pubertal stage 2	F	<0.6 nmol/L (<20 ng/dL)
	Pubertal stage 2	M	<6.6 IU/L (<1.32 μg/L)		Pubertal stage 3	M	<10.6 nmol/L (<310 ng/dL)
		F	<4.1 IU/L (<0.82 μg/L)		Pubertal stage 4	F	<1.4 nmol/L (<40 ng/dL)
	Pubertal stage 3	M	0.7–5.0 IU/L (0.14–1 μg/L)		Pubertal stage 5	M	0.4–30 nmol/L (10–870 ng/dL)
	Pubertal stages 4–5	M	1.5–6.0 IU/L (0.3–1.2 μg/L)		Pubertal stages 3–5	M	5.6–30 nmol/L (160–870 ng/dL)
	Pubertal stages 3–5	F	2.5–13.5 IU/L (0.5–2.7 μg/L)			M	10–30 nmol/L (290–870 ng/dL)
Insulin-like growth factor 1	<7 years	M	15–349 μg/L			F	0.4–1.9 nmol/L (10–50 ng/dL)
		F	17–272 μg/L				
	8–16 years	M	67–510 μg/L				
		F	59–502 μg/L				

*Non-SI equivalents are given in brackets where appropriate.

35

Laboratory reference ranges in pregnancy

The levels of many analytes in blood vary during pregnancy, when many hormonal and metabolic changes occur. The standard adult reference ranges may therefore not be appropriate and it is important for the clinician reviewing the results to be aware of this to enable appropriate interpretation and patient management.

35.10 Analytes that may be significantly affected by pregnancy*

Analyte	Reference range		
	First trimester	Second trimester	Third trimester
Alkaline phosphatase (ALP)	17–88 U/L	25–126 U/L	38–229 U/L
Packed cell volume (PCV) or haematocrit	0.31–0.41	0.30–0.39	0.28–0.40
Haemoglobin	116–139 g/L	97–148 g/L	95–150 g/L
Human chorionic gonadotrophin	4 weeks: 16–156 IU/L 4–9 weeks: 101–233 000 IU/L 9–13 weeks: 20 900–291 000 IU/L	4270–103 000 IU/L	2700–78 300 IU/L
17β-Oestradiol	690–9166 pmol/L (188–2497 pg/mL)	4691–26 401 pmol/L (1278–7192 pg/mL)	12 701–22 528 pmol/L (3460–6137 pg/mL)
Progesterone	25–153 nmol/L (8–48 ng/mL)	Not available	314–1088 nmol/L (99–342 ng/mL)
Prolactin	765–4532 mIU/L (36–213 ng/mL)	2340–7021 mIU/L (110–330 ng/mL)	2914–7914 mIU/L (137–372 ng/mL)
Thyroid-stimulating hormone (TSH)	0.60–3.40 mIU/L	0.37–3.60 mIU/L	0.38–4.04 mIU/L
Thyroxine (free), (free T₄)	10–18 pmol/L 0.77–1.40 ng/dL	9–16 pmol/L 0.70–1.24 ng/dL	8–14 pmol/L 0.62–1.09 ng/dL

*Non-SI equivalents are given in brackets where appropriate.

Further information

Abbassi-Ghanavati M, Greer LG, Cunningham FG. Pregnancy and laboratory studies: a reference table for clinicians. Obstet Gynecol 2009;114:1326–1331.

Neal RC, Ferdinand KC, Ycas J, Miller E. Relationship of ethnic origin, gender and age to blood creatine kinase levels. Am J Med 2009;122:73–78.

Tanner JM, Whitehouse RH. Clinical longitudinal standards for height, weight, height velocity, weight velocity, and stages of puberty. Arch Dis Child 1976;51:170–179.

Woitge HW, Scheidt-Nave C, Kissling C, et al. Seasonal variation of biochemical indexes of bone turnover: results of a population-based study. J Clin Endocrinol Metabol 1998;83:68–75.

Index